THE MERCK VETERINARY MANUAL

Previous Editions

First Edition	1955
Second Edition	1961
Third Edition	1967
Fourth Edition	1973
Fifth Edition	1979
Sixth Edition	1986
Seventh Edition	1991
Eighth Edition	1998

Foreign Language Editions

Croatian/Slovakian—Komora Vetarinarnich Lekarov, Brno

French—Editions d'Apres, Paris

Italian—Cristiano Giraldi Editore, Bologne

Japanese—Gakusosha, Tokyo

Portuguese—Editora Roca, São Paulo

Spanish—Editorial Oceano, Barcelona

THE
MERCK
VETERINARY
MANUAL

Ninth E

THE
MERCK VETERINARY MANUAL

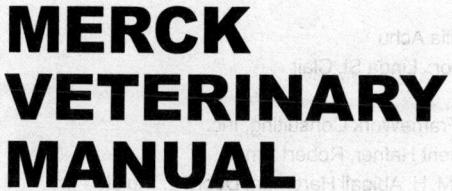

Ninth Edition

Editor: Cynthia M. Kahn, B.A., M.A.
Associate Editor: Scott Line, D.V.M., Ph.D., Dipl. A.C.V.B.

Published by
MERCK & CO., INC.
WHITEHOUSE STATION, N.J., U.S.A.

in educational partnership with
MERIAL LIMITED
A Merck and Aventis Company

2005

Editorial and Production Staff

Editor: Cynthia M. Kahn, B.A., M.A.
Associate Editor: Scott Line, D.V.M., Ph.D., D.A.C.V.B.
Consulting Editor: Susan E. Aiello, B.S., D.V.M., E.L.S.

Project Coordinator: Odilia Achu
Administrative Coordinator: Linda St. Clair
Indexer: Elizabeth Axtell
Designer: Julie Nudler, FrameWork Consulting, Inc.
Technical Assistance: Brent Hafner, Robert Amos
Administrative Support: M. H. Abigail Hardman, Debra L. Triplett

Publisher: Gary Zelko
Advertising and Promotions Supervisor: Pamela J. Barnes-Paul

Dedicated to the Contributors to The Merck Veterinary Manual, *who have made it a leading veterinary reference for 50 years.*

Library of Congress Control Number: 2004111348
ISBN Number: 0-911910-50-6

Printed in the U.S.A.

Composition by Nesbitt Graphics, Inc.
Fort Washington, Pennsylvania

Printed by National Publishing, Inc.
Philadelphia, Pennsylvania

FOREWORD

The publication of the 9th edition of *The Merck Veterinary Manual* is a cause for both celebration and reflection. Celebration is in order because this newest edition is being published on the 50th anniversary of the first edition, which made its debut in 1955. The foreword in that first edition concisely stated the aim of the text: *"The Merck Veterinary Manual* is intended to provide the veterinarian with concise, authoritative, and readily available information on diagnosis and treatment of the diseases of animals kept by man for use or pleasure." This goal still resonates today; it remains the aim of the editors and editorial board to continue to provide clinically useful and up-to-date information as a service to the veterinary profession and its allied disciplines.

This new edition reflects both the remarkable advances in veterinary science and the emergence of new pathogens and new diseases since the publication of the 8th edition of the *Manual*. Every chapter has been carefully reviewed and either revised or rewritten as needed. In addition, more than 30 new chapters or subchapters were added to address emerging diseases (eg, West Nile encephalomyelitis, chronic wasting disease, Lechiguana, Nipah virus infection, and postweaning multisystemic wasting syndrome, to name a few), and to better cover advances in diagnosis and treatment (eg, imaging techniques, pain management, ophthalmic emergencies). Expanded coverage of specialty fields such as cardiology, neurology, ophthalmology, toxicology, and emergency medicine has been undertaken, as well as reorganization and expansion of the section on exotic and laboratory animals to reflect the increasing popularity of exotic pets—and to highlight their potential to transmit zoonotic diseases. The pharmacology section has been strengthened with the addition of chapters on chemical residues and veterinary dosage forms and delivery systems. The table of zoonoses continues to grow; we have added information on clinical manifestations in humans, as veterinarians continue to be at the forefront of control of zoonotic diseases and protection of public health.

To use the *Manual* most effectively, readers are encouraged to become familiar with the Guide for Readers and to use the Table of Contents for each thumb-tabbed section. The extensive Index may be the best first step to locate information on a specific topic. To maintain the handbook style that has been the hallmark of this book, the editors have required concise space limitations of our contributors, and references are not included.

It would be impossible to assemble a book such as this without the efforts of the 470 authors and reviewers who contributed to this edition of the *Manual*. Many are new to this edition and represent contributions from around the globe. Contributors to this edition are from Australia, Belgium, Brazil, Canada, the Czech Republic, Denmark, France, Ireland, Israel, Malaysia, the Netherlands, New Zealand, South Africa, Spain, Sweden, Switzerland, and the United Kingdom, in addition to the United States. Such international collaboration seems appropriate as advances in laboratory and clinical research increasingly come from centers of veterinary excellence throughout the world. The *Manual* is distributed and used worldwide; the previous edition was translated into six languages in addition to English.

Thanks are also due to the many people who have worked tirelessly for the past five years to make this edition—the second to be published in an educational partnership between Merck and Merial—possible. The editorial board reviewed every chapter and provided invaluable suggestions and assistance that shaped the structure of the book. A debt of gratitude is due Susan Aiello, editor of the previous edition, for her guidance and devotion to this endeavor. Management support from Mark Soll and Kevin Schultz at Merial have ensured that this edition could be produced in a timely fashion. Pamela

Barnes-Paul and Gary Zelko of the Merck Publishing Group continue their seamless work in producing, marketing, and distributing this book, and facilitating foreign translations. Last, but certainly not least, my publication team deserves special thanks for their assistance: Odilia Achu, who coordinated virtually every phase of the *Manual*'s development; Linda St. Clair who spent countless dedicated hours in manuscript processing, typing, and coding; and particularly the associate editor of the *Manual*, Scott Line, who edited, revised, and polished every chapter to make it more readable and, hopefully, more useful.

Finally, many of the changes in this and previous editions have come at the suggestion of our readers. We look forward to continued feedback from the users of this edition of the *Manual*.

Cynthia M. Kahn
Editor

GUIDE FOR READERS

■ The Contents shows the title of each section of the *Manual* and the corresponding thumb tab abbreviation.

■ Each section has its own Table of Contents that lists chapter and subchapter titles in that section.

■ Many cross-reference page numbers are found throughout the text to enable the reader to quickly find discussions of related material elsewhere in the book.

■ A number of abbreviations and symbols used routinely throughout the text are listed on p ix and p xi. Other abbreviations used in the text are defined at their first use.

■ Generic (nonproprietary) names of drugs are used in most instances.

■ Running heads on left-hand pages correspond to the chapter title of the text appearing at the top of that page. Running heads on right-hand pages correspond to the chapter title of the text appearing at the bottom of that page. In other words, running heads are used as in a standard dictionary.

■ The Index is the best way to locate specific discussions of a disease, condition, or syndrome for which the name is known.

■ The first half of the *Manual* is arranged into anatomic systems, and specific conditions are located in the system that is primarily affected. Conditions that may affect more than one system are covered in the section Generalized Conditions (GEN). The second half of the *Manual* covers special topics or disciplines.

■ The authors, reviewers, editors, and publisher have made extensive efforts to ensure that treatments, drugs, dosage regimens, and withdrawal times are accurate and conform to the standards accepted at the time of publication. **However, constant changes in information resulting from continuing research and clinical experience, reasonable differences in opinions among authorities, unique aspects of individual clinical situations, and the possibility of human error in preparing such an extensive text require that the reader exercise individual judgment when making a clinical decision and, if necessary, consult and compare information from other sources**. In particular, the reader is advised to check the product information currently provided by the manufacturer of each drug before prescribing or administering it, especially if the drug is unfamiliar or is used infrequently.

OTHER
MERCK HANDBOOKS

The Merck Index
First Edition, 1889

The Merck Manual of Diagnosis and Therapy
First Edition, 1899

The Merck Manual of Geriatrics
First Edition, 1990

The Merck Manual of Medical Information
Home Edition
First Edition, 1997

The Merck Manual of Health and Aging
First Edition, 2004

CONTENTS

CONTENTS

ad lib	as much as desired	**IV**	intravenous(ly)
ALT	alanine aminotransferase	**kcal**	kilocalorie(s)
AST	aspartate aminotransferase	**kg**	kilogram(s)
ATP	adenosine triphosphate	**L**	liter(s)
BID	twice a day	**lb**	pound(s)
bpm	beats per minute	**m**	meter(s)
BUN	blood urea nitrogen	**M**	molar
C	Celsius (Centigrade)	**Mcal**	megacalorie(s)
cal	calorie(s)	**ME**	metabolizable energy
CBC	complete blood count(s)	**mEq**	milliequivalent(s)
cm	centimeter(s)	**mg**	milligram(s)
CNS	central nervous system	**min**	minute(s)
CK	creatine kinase (CPK, cre-	**mL**	milliliter(s)
	atine phosphokinase)	**mm**	millimeter(s)
CSF	cerebrospinal fluid	**mo**	month(s)
cu	cubic	**mol**	mole(s)
dL	deciliter(s)	**mOsm**	milliosmole(s)
DNA	deoxyribonucleic acid	**nm**	nanometer(s)
ECG	electrocardiogram	**MRI**	magnetic resonance imaging
eg	for example	**NRC**	National Research Council
ELISA	enzyme-linked immunosor-	**NSAID**	nonsteroidal anti-
	bent assay		inflammatory drug(s)
EPG	eggs per gram (of feces)	**OIE**	Office International des
et seq	and the following one(s)		Épizooties
EU	European Union	**oz**	ounce(s)
F	Fahrenheit	**p/pp**	page/pages
FDA	Food and Drug Administra-	**PCR**	polymerase chain reaction
	tion	**PCV**	packed cell volume
fL	femtoliter(s)	**pH**	negative logarithm of
ft	foot, feet		hydrogen ion activity
g	gram(s)	**PO**	per os, orally
gal.	gallon(s)	**ppb**	part(s) per billion
GI	gastrointestinal	**ppm**	part(s) per million
GnRH	gonadotropin-releasing	**QID**	four times a day
	hormone	**qs ad**	quantity sufficient to make
H&E	hematoxylin and eosin	**RBC**	red blood cell
Hgb	hemoglobin	**RNA**	riboneucleic acid
hr	hour(s)	**SC**	subcutaneous(ly)
ie	that is	**sec**	second(s)
Ig	immunoglobulin (with class	**SID**	once a day
	following: A, D, E, G, or M)	**SI units**	International System of Units
IM	intramuscular(ly)	**SPF**	specific pathogen free
in.	inch(es)	**sq**	square
IP	intraperitoneal(ly)	**tbsp**	tablespoon(s)
IU	international unit(s)	**TDN**	total digestible nutrients

TID	three times a day	ε	epsilon
tsp	teaspoon(s)	γ	gamma
U	unit(s)	λ	lambda
UK	United Kingdom	μ	micro, mu
USDA	United States Department	κ	kappa
	of Agriculture	σ	sigma
USA	United States of America	°	degree
USSR	Union of Soviet Socialist		
	Republics (former)	/	per
		%	percent
WBC	white blood cell(s)	~	approximately
wk	week(s)	=	equals
wt	weight	>	greater than
yr	year(s)	≥	greater than or equal to
α	alpha	<	less than
β	beta	≤	less than or equal to
σ	delta	±	plus or minus

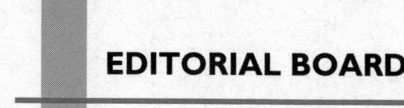

EDITORIAL BOARD

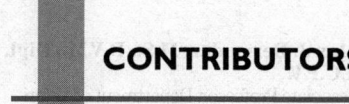

CONTRIBUTORS

Dana G. Allen, D.V.M., M.Sc., Dipl. A.C.V.I.M.
Professor of Internal Medicine, Department of Clinical Studies, Ontario Veterinary College, University of Guelph, Guelph, Ontario, Canada

Diseases of the Stomach and Intestines, Vomiting

Gary C. Althouse, D.V.M., M.S., Ph.D., Dipl. A.C.T.
Associate Professor and Chief, Section of Reproductive Studies, New Bolton Center, University of Pennsylvania, Kennett Square, PA

Management of Reproduction: Pigs

Trevor R. Ames, D.V.M., M.S., Dipl. A.C.V.I.M.
Professor and Chair, Department of Clinical and Population Sciences, College of Veterinary Medicine, University of Minnesota, St. Paul, MN

Respiratory Diseases of Cattle

Christine Andreoni
Senior Manager Immunology, Merial Limited, Lyon, France

Immunopathologic Diseases, Immunopathologic Mechanisms

Max J. Appel, Dr. Med.Vet., Ph.D.
Professor Emeritus, Ithaca, NY

Borreliosis (Lyme Disease)

Donald Armstrong, M.D.
Emeritus Chief, Infectious Disease Service, Memorial Sloan Kettering Cancer Center, NY, Professor of Medicine, Cornell University Medical College, NY

Zoonoses

David A. Ashford, D.V.M., M.P.H., D.Sc.
Associate Director, Region V, U.S. Department of Agriculture, APHIS, International Service, Atlanta, GA

Anthrax

Joerg A. Auer, Dr. Med. Vet., Dipl. A.C.V.S., Dipl. E.C.V.S.
Equine Hospital, Vetsuisse Faculty, University of Zürich, Zürich, Switzerland

Musculoskeletal System, Introduction

Clell V. Bagley, D.V.M.
Extension Veterinarian, Utah State University, Logan, UT

Lameness in Sheep

David G. Baker, D.V.M., M.S., Ph.D., Dipl. A.C.L.A.M.
Director and Professor, Division of Laboratory Animal Medicine, School of Veterinary Medicine, Louisiana State University, Baton Rouge, LA

Eyeworm Disease

Gordon J. Baker, B.V.Sc., Ph.D., M.R.C.V.S., Dipl. A.C.V.S.
Professor, Equine Medicine and Surgery, College of Veterinary Medicine, University of Illinois, Urbana, IL

Dentistry in Large Animals, Diseases of the Esophagus in Large Animals, Diseases of the Mouth in Large Animals, Pharyngeal Paralysis, Pharyngitis

John C. Baker, D.V.M., Ph.D.
Professor and Associate Dean for Research and Graduate Studies, College of Veterinary Medicine, Michigan State University, East Lansing, MI

Respiratory Diseases of Cattle

H. John Barnes, D.V.M., Ph.D., Dipl. A.C.V.P., Dipl. A.C.P.V.
Professor, Poultry Health Management, College of Veterinary Medicine, North Carolina State University, Raleigh, NC

Avian Chlamydiosis, Bloodborne Organisms

Stephen C. Barr, B.V.Sc., M.V.S., Ph.D., Dipl. A.C.V.I.M.
Professor of Medicine, Department of Clinical Sciences, College of Veterinary Medicine, Cornell University, Ithaca, NY
Visceral Leishmaniasis

George M. Barrington, D.V.M., Ph.D., Dipl. A.C.V.I.M.
Assistant Professor, Department of Veterinary Clinical Sciences, College of Veterinary Medicine, Washington State University, Pullman, WA
Metabolic Disorders Introduction, Parturient Paresis in Cows, Transport Tetany in Ruminants

Joseph W. Bartges, D.V.M., Ph.D., Dipl. A.C.V.I.M., Dipl. A.C.V.N.
Professor of Medicine and Nutrition, The Acree Chair of Small Animal Research, Department of Small Animal Clinical Sciences, College of Veterinary Medicine, University of Tennessee, Knoxville, TN
Diagnostic Procedures for the Private Practice Laboratory: Urinalysis

Andrew P. Bathe, M.A., Vet.M.B., Dipl. E.C.V.S., D.E.O., M.R.C.V.S.
Rossdale & Partners, Beaufort Cottage Equine Hospital, Exning, Newmarket, Suffolk, UK
Lameness in Horses: Regional Analgesia

John E. Bauer, D.V.M., Ph.D., Dipl. A.C.V.N.
Professor of Nutrition and Mark L. Morris Professor of Clinical Nutrition, Department of Small Animal Clinical Sciences, College of Veterinary Medicine, Texas A&M University, College Station, TX
Nutrition: Small Animals

Daniela Bedenice, Med.Vet., Dipl. A.C.V.I.M.
Clinical Assistant Professor, Large Animal Clinic, School of Veterinary Medicine, Tufts University, North Grafton, MA
Hypoxic Ischemic Encephalopathy, Septicemia in Foals, Uroperitoneum in Foals

Alex J. Bermudez, M.S., D.V.M., Dipl. A.C.P.V.
Associate Professor, Department of Veterinary Pathobiology, College of Veterinary Medicine, University of Missouri, Columbia, MO
Feeding and Management Practices

Michael Bernstein, D.V.M., Dipl. A.C.V.I.M.
Director, Medical Services, Angell Animal Medical Center, Boston, MA
Hemobartonellosis, Hepatozoonosis and American Canine Hepatozoonosis

J. Dürr Bezuidenhout, D.V.Sc.
Sinoville, South Africa
Sweating Sickness

William G. Bickert, B.S., M.S., Ph.D.
Professor, Biosystems and Agricultural Engineering, Michigan State University, East Lansing, MI
Ventilation

Rob Bildfell, D.V.M., M.Sc., Dipl. A.C.V.P.
Assistant Professor, Department of Biomedical Sciences, College of Veterinary Medicine, Oregon State University, Corvallis, OR
Collection and Submission of Laboratory Samples, Pyrrolizidine Alkaloidosis

William D. Black, M.Sc., D.V.M., Ph.D.
Professor, Department of Biomedical Sciences, Ontario Veterinary College, University of Guelph, Guelph, Ontario, Canada
Bracken Fern Poisoning, Herbicide Poisoning, Insecticide and Acaricide (Organic) Toxicity, Pentachlorophenol Poisoning, Sweet Clover Poisoning

Pat Blackall, B.Sc., Ph.D.
Senior Principal Research Scientist, Animal Research Institute, Yeerongpilly, Australia
Infectious Coryza

Barry R. Blakley, D.V.M., Ph.D.
Professor, Department of Veterinary Biomedical Sciences, Western College of Veterinary Medicine, University of Saskatchewan, Saskatoon, Saskatchewan, Canada
Copper Poisoning, Lead Poisoning, Quercus Poisoning, Sorghum Poisoning

Herman J. Boermans, D.V.M., M.Sc., Ph.D.
Director, Toxicology Program, Associate Professor of Toxicology, Department of Biomedical Sciences, Ontario Veterinary College, University of Guelph, Guelph, Ontario, Canada
Fluoride Poisoning, Mercury Poisoning, Metaldehyde Poisoning, Molybdenum Poisoning

Steven R. Bolin, M.S., D.V.M., Ph.D.
Section Chief, Immunodiagnostics Section, Animal Health Diagnostic Laboratory, Michigan State University, East Lansing, MI
Bovine Viral Diarrhea and Mucosal Disease Complex, Postweaning Multisystemic Wasting Syndrome

Calvin W. Booker, D.V.M., M.Vet.Sc.
Feedlot Health Management Services, Okotoks, Alberta, Canada
Histophilosis

Rosemary J. Booth, B.V.Sc.
Lecturer and Wildlife Veterinarian, School of Animal Studies, University of Queensland, Gatton, Queensland, Australia
Sugar Gliders

Dawn M. Boothe, D.V.M., Ph.D., Dipl. A.C.V.I.M., Dipl. A.C.V.C.P.
Professor, Department of Veterinary Physiology and Pharmacology, College of Veterinary Medicine, Texas A&M University, College Station, TX
Antibacterial Agents, Antifungal Agents, Antiviral Agents and Interferon, Chemotherapeutics Introduction, Pharmacology Introduction

Davin J. Borde, D.V.M., Dipl. A.C.V.I.M. (Cardiology)
Staff Cardiologist, Veterinary Heart Institute, Gainesville, FL
Congenital and Inherited Anomalies of the Cardiovascular System, Heart Disease and Heart Failure

Kenneth R. Boschert, D.V.M., Dipl. A.C.L.A.M.
Associate Director, Division of Comparative Medicine, Washington University, St. Louis, MO
Rodents

Kyle G. Braund, B.V.Sc., M.V.Sc., Ph.D., F.R.C.V.S., Dipl. A.C.V.I.M. (Neurology)
Director, Veterinary Neurological Consulting Services, Dadeville, AL
Congenital and Inherited Anomalies of the Nervous System, Neoplasia of the Nervous System, Paraneoplastic Disorders of the Nervous System

Joseph M. Bricker, Ph.D.
Head, Avian Group, Merial Limited, Athens GA
Erysipelas (Poultry)

Thomas P. Brown, M.S., D.V.M., Ph.D., Dipl. A.C.V.P., Dipl. A.C.P.V.
Professor, Department of Avian Medicine, College of Veterinary Medicine, University of Georgia, Athens, GA
Breast Blisters, Cannibalism, Coronaviral Enteritis of Turkeys, Gout, Myopathies, Poisonings

Scott A. Brown, V.M.D., Ph.D., Dipl. A.C.V.I.M.
Department of Physiology and Pharmacology, College of Veterinary Medicine, University of Georgia, Athens, GA
Noninfectious Diseases of the Urinary System in Small Animals

Cecil F. Brownie, D.V.M., Ph.D., Dipl. A.B.V.T., Dipl. A.B.T., Dipl. A.B.F.E., Dipl. A.B.F.M., F.A.C.F.E.
Professor of Pharmacology/Toxicology, Department of Molecular and Biomedical Sciences, College of Veterinary Medicine, North Carolina State University, Raleigh, NC
Plants Poisonous to Animals

David Bruyette, D.V.M., Dipl. A.C.V.I.M.
Medical Director, VCA West Los Angeles Animal Hospital, Los Angeles, CA
The Adrenal Glands, The Pancreas

Raymond Cahill-Morasco, M.S., D.V.M.
Boston, MA
Zinc Toxicity

Paul P. Calle, V.M.D., Dipl. A.C.Z.M.
Senior Veterinarian, Wildlife Health Sciences, Wildlife Conservation Society, Bronx, NY
Zoo Animals

Clay A. Calvert, D.V.M., Dipl. A.C.V.I.M.
Professor, Department of Small Animal Medicine and Surgery, College of Veterinary Medicine, University of Georgia, Athens, GA

Heartworm Disease

Ranald D. A. Cameron, B.V.Sc., M.V.Sc., Ph.D.
Associate Professor, School of Veterinary Sciences, University of Queensland, Brisbane, Australia

Exudative Epidermitis, Parakeratosis, Pityriasis Rosea in Pigs, Swine Erysipelas

Karen L. Campbell, M.S., D.V.M., Dipl. A.C.V.I.M., Dipl. A.C.V.D.
Professor and Section Head, Specialty Medicine, Department of Veterinary Clinical Medicine, College of Veterinary Medicine, University of Illinois, Urbana, IL

Polycythemia

Sharon Campbell, D.V.M., M.S., Dipl. A.C.V.I.M.
Manager, Pharmacovigilance, Regulatory Affairs, Veterinary Medicine Research and Development, Pfizer Inc., Kalamazoo, MI

Hepatic Disease in Small Animals

Ivan W. Caple, B.V.Sc., Ph.D., M.A.C.V.Sc., M.R.C.V.S.
Dean, Faculty of Veterinary Sciences, Veterinary Clinical Centre, University of Melbourne, Werribee, Victoria, Australia

Disorders of Magnesium Metabolism

Wayne W. Carmichael, Ph.D.
Professor, Aquatic Biology and Toxicology, Department of Biological Sciences, Wright State University, Dayton, OH

Algal Poisoning

Gordon R. Carter, D.V.M., M.S., D.V.Sc.
Professor Emeritus, Virginia-Maryland Regional College of Veterinary Medicine, Virginia Polytechnic Institute and State University, Blacksburg, VA

Hemorrhagic Septicemia, Lechiguana

Christopher K. Cebra, V.M.D., M.A., M.S., Dipl. A.C.V.I.M.
Associate Professor, Large Animal Medicine, College of Veterinary Medicine, Oregon State University, Corvallis, OR

Disorders of Phosphorus Metabolism, Pregnancy Toxemia in Cows

Margaret L. Cebra, V.M.D., M.S., Dipl. A.C.V.I.M.
Philomath, OR

Pasteurellosis of Sheep and Goats

A. Bill Childers Jr., D.V.M., M.S., Dipl. A.C.V.P.M.
Associate Professor, Department of Veterinary Anatomy and Public Health, Texas A&M University, College Station, TX

Meat Inspection

Cheryl L. Chrisman, D.V.M., M.S., Ed.S., Dipl. A.C.V.I.M. (Neurology)
Professor of Veterinary Neurology, College of Veterinary Medicine, University of Florida, Gainesville, FL

Facial Paralysis, Limb Paralysis, Nervous System Introduction

Vern L. Christensen, Ph.D.
Professor, Department of Poultry Science, College of Agriculture and Life Sciences, North Carolina State University, Raleigh, NC

Artificial Insemination (Poultry)

Keith A. Clark, D.V.M., Ph.D.
Retired Director, Zoonosis Control Division, Texas Department of Health, Austin, TX

Snakebite, Spider Bites, Toad Poisoning

Cyril R. Clarke, B.V.Sc., Ph.D., M.S., Dipl. A.C.V.C.P.
Professor and Head, Department of Physiological Sciences, College of Veterinary Medicine, Oklahoma State University, Stillwater, OK

Systemic Pharmacotherapeutics of the Ruminant Digestive System

Michael T. Collins, D.V.M., Ph.D.
Professor of Microbiology, School of Veterinary Medicine, University of Wisconsin-Madison, Madison, WI

Paratuberculosis

Ben H. Colmery III, D.V.M., Dipl. A.V.D.C.
Vet Dentistry, Ann Arbor, MI

Dentistry in Small Animals

Peter D. Constable, B.V.Sc., M.S., Ph.D., Dipl. A.C.V.I.M.
Associate Professor, Department of Veterinary Clinical Medicine, University of Illinois, Urbana, IL

Diseases of the Abomasum, Acute Intestinal Obstructions in Large Animals

George L. Cooper, D.V.M., M.S.
Associate Professor of Clinical Microimmunology and Pathology, School of Veterinary Medicine, University of California, Davis, CA

Gangrenous Dermatitis

Susan M. Cotter, D.V.M., Dipl. A.C.V.I.M. (Internal Medicine and Oncology)
Distinguished Professor, Department of Clinical Sciences, School of Veterinary Medicine, Tufts University, North Grafton, MA

Blood Groups and Blood Transfusions, Hematopoietic System Introduction

Timothy B. Crawford, D.V.M., Ph.D.
Associate Professor, Department of Veterinary Microbiology and Pathology, College of Veterinary Medicine, Washington State University, Pullman, WA

Malignant Catarrhal Fever

Gary L. Cromwell, Ph.D.
Professor, Swine Nutrition, Animal Sciences Department, University of Kentucky, Lexington, KY

Iron Toxicity in Newborn Pigs, Nutrition: Pigs

Benjamin J. Darien, D.V.M., M.S., Dipl. A.C.V.I.M.
Associate Professor of Internal Medicine, School of Veterinary Medicine, University of Wisconsin, Madison, WI

Thrombosis, Embolism, and Aneurysm

Autumn P. Davidson, D.V.M., M.S., Dipl. A.C.V.I.M.
Clinical Professor, Department of Medicine and Epidemiology, School of Veterinary Medicine, University of California, Davis, CA

Management of Reproduction: Small Animals

Harriet J. Davidson, D.V.M., M.S., Dipl. A.C.V.O.
Associate Professor, College of Veterinary Medicine, Kansas State University, Manhattan, KS

Infectious Keratoconjunctivitis

Sherrill Davison, V.M.D., M.S., M.B.A., Dipl. A.C.P.V.
Associate Professor of Avian Medicine and Pathology, School of Veterinary Medicine, University of Pennsylvania, Kennett Square, PA

Salmonelloses (Poultry)

Scott A. Dee, D.V.M., M.S., Ph.D., Dipl. A.C.V.M.
Associate Professor, College of Veterinary Medicine, University of Minnesota, St. Paul, MN

Health-Management Interaction: Pigs, Necrotic Ear Syndrome in Swine, Porcine Cystitis-Pyelonephritis Complex, Porcine Reproductive and Respiratory Syndrome, Pseudorabies, Respiratory Diseases of Pigs

John Deen, D.V.M., M.Sc., Ph.D., Dipl. A.B.V.P.
Associate Professor, College of Veterinary Medicine, University of Minnesota, St. Paul, MN

Gastrointestinal Ulcers in Large Animals: Pigs

Fabio Del Piero, D.V.M., Dipl. A.C.V.P., Ph.D.
Associate Professor of Pathology, Department of Pathobiology and Department of Clinical Studies, School of Veterinary Medicine, New Bolton Center, University of Pennsylvania, Kennett Square, PA

Congenital and Inherited Anomalies of the Reproductive System

Catherine E. Dewey, D.V.M., M.Sc., Ph.D.
Professor, Population Medicine, Ontario Veterinary College, University of Guelph, Guelph, Ontario, Canada
Lameness in Pigs

Joseph A. DiPietro, D.V.M., M.S.
Dean and Professor, College of Veterinary Medicine, University of Florida, Gainesville, FL
Gastrointestinal Parasites of Horses

Thomas J. Divers, D.V.M., Dipl. A.C.V.I.M., Dipl. A.C.V.E.C.C.
Professor of Medicine, College of Veterinary Medicine, Cornell University, Ithaca, NY
Urolithiasis in Ruminants and Horses

John E. Dohms, Ph.D.
Professor, Department of Animal and Food Sciences, University of Delaware, Newark, DE
Botulism (Poultry)

Stanley H. Done, B.A., D.Vet.Med., Ph.D., Dipl. E.C.V.P., F.R.C.V.S., F.R.C.Path.
Veterinary Laboratories Agency-Thirsk, West House, Thirsk, Surrey, UK
Porcine Dermatitis and Nephropathy Syndrome

Patricia M. Dowling, D.V.M., M.S., Dipl. A.C.V.I.M., Dipl. A.C.V.C.P.
Professor of Veterinary Clinical Pharmacology, Veterinary Biomedical Sciences, Western College of Veterinary Medicine, University of Saskatchewan, Saskatoon, Saskatchewan, Canada
Systemic Pharmacotherapeutics of the Monogastric Digestive System, Systemic Pharmacotherapeutics of the Muscular System, Systemic Pharmacotherapeutics of the Respiratory System, Systemic Pharmacotherapeutics of the Urinary System

Michael W. Dryden, D.V.M., M.S., Ph.D.
Professor of Veterinary Parasitology, College of Veterinary Medicine, Kansas State University, Manhattan, KS
Ectoparasiticides Used in Small Animals, Fleas and Flea Allergy Dermatitis

J. P. Dubey, M.V.Sc., Ph.D.
Microbiologist, Animal Parasitic Diseases Laboratory, Animal and Natural Resources Institute, U.S. Department of Agriculture, Beltsville, MD
Neosporosis, Toxoplasmosis

Gregg A. DuPont, D.V.M., Dipl. A.V.D.C., Fellow A.V.D.
Director, Shoreline Veterinary Dental Clinic, Seattle, WA
Diseases of the Mouth in Small Animals

Neil W. Dyer, D.V.M., M.S.
Director, Veterinary Diagnostic Laboratory, North Dakota State University, Fargo, ND
Aspiration Pneumonia, Chlamydial Pneumonia, Hypostatic Pneumonia, Mycotic Pneumonia, Pulmonary Emphysema

Steven Edwards, D.V.M.&S., M.A., M.Sc., Vet.M.B., M.R.C.V.S.
Professor, Veterinary Laboratories Agency, New Haw, Addlestone, Surrey, UK
Classical Swine Fever

Mahmoud El-Begearmi, Ph.D.
Extension Professor of Nutrition and Food Safety, Cooperative Extension, University of Maine, Orono, ME
Nutritional Requirements of Poultry

Ron Erskine, D.V.M., Ph.D.
Professor, Department of Large Animal Clinical Sciences, College of Veterinary Medicine, Michigan State University, East Lansing, MI
Mastitis in Large Animals

Paul Ettestad, D.V.M., M.S.
State Public Health Veterinarian, Office of Epidemiology, New Mexico Department of Health, Santa Fe, NM
Plague

A. K. Eugster, D.V.M., Ph.D.
Executive Director Emeritus, Texas Veterinary Medical Diagnostic Laboratory, College Station, TX
Chlamydial Conjunctivitis, Intestinal Chlamydial Infections, Sporadic Bovine Encephalomyelitis

David L. Evans, B.V.Sc., Ph.D.
Associate Professor, Faculty of Veterinary Science, University of Sydney, New South Wales, Australia
Fatigue and Exercise

Aly M. Fadly, D.V.M., Ph.D., Dipl. A.C.P.V.
Research Leader and Laboratory Director, U.S. Department of Agriculture, Avian Disease Oncology Laboratory, East Lansing, MI
Neoplasms (Poultry)

Timothy M. Fan, D.V.M., Dipl. A.C.V.I.M.
Visiting Assistant Professor (Medical Oncology), Department of Veterinary Clinical Medicine, University of Illinois, Urbana, IL
Canine Malignant Lymphoma

R. Kent Fenton, D.V.M.
Feedlot Health Management Services, Okotoks, Alberta, Canada
Histophilosis

Scott D. Fitzgerald, D.V.M., Ph.D., Dipl. A.C.V.P.
Professor, Department of Pathobiology and Diagnostic Investigation, Diagnostic Center for Population and Animal Health, College of Veterinary Medicine, Michigan State University, East Lansing, MI
Congenital and Inherited Anomalies of the Urinary System

James A. Flanders, D.V.M., Dipl. A.C.V.S.
Associate Professor, Department of Clinical Sciences, College of Veterinary Medicine, Cornell University, Ithaca, NY
Prostatic Diseases in Small Animals

Carol S. Foil, D.V.M., M.S., Dipl. A.C.V.D.
Professor, Department of Veterinary Clinical Sciences, School of Veterinary Medicine, Louisiana State University, Baton Rouge, LA
Congenital and Inherited Anomalies of the Integumentary System, Dermatophytosis (Ringworm)

Jim Foster, B.Sc.
Institute for Animal Health, Edinburgh, UK
Scrapie

James G. Fox, D.V.M., M.S., Dipl. A.C.L.A.M.
Professor and Director, Division of Comparative Medicine, Massachusetts Institute of Technology, Cambridge, MA
Campylobacteriosis

Ruth Francis-Floyd, D.V.M., M.S., Dipl. A.C.Z.M.
Professor, Department of Large Animal Clinical Sciences and Department of Fisheries and Aquatic Sciences, College of Veterinary Medicine, University of Florida, Gainesville, FL
Fish

Don A. Franco, D.V.M., M.P.H., Dipl. A.C.V.P.M.
President, Center for Biosecurity Food Safety and Public Health, Lake Worth, FL
Congenital Erythropoietic Porphyria

Jack M. Gaskin, D.V.M., Ph.D., Dipl. A.C.V.M.
Associate Professor, Department of Pathobiology, College of Veterinary Medicine, University of Florida, Gainesville, FL
Encephalomyocarditis Virus Infection

Clive C. Gay, D.V.M., M.V.Sc., F.A.C.V.Sc.
Professor, Department of Veterinary Clinical Sciences, College of Veterinary Medicine, Washington State University, Pullman, WA
Bloat in Ruminants, Colisepticemia, Intestinal Diseases in Ruminants, Liver Abscesses in Cattle, Health-Management Interaction: Sheep

Kirk N. Gelatt, V.M.D.
Distinguished Professor of Comparative Ophthalmology, Department of Small Animal Clinical Sciences, College of Veterinary Medicine, University of Florida, Gainesville, FL
Neoplasia of the Eye and Associated Structures, Ophthalmic Emergencies, Ophthalmology

Gertruida H. Gerdes, B.V.Sc.
Department of Virology, Onderstepoort
Veterinary Institute, Onderstepoort,
South Africa

Rift Valley Fever, Wesselsbron Disease

Paul Gibbs, B.V.Sc., Ph.D., F.R.C.V.S.
Professor of Virology, Department of
Pathobiology, College of Veterinary Medi-
cine, University of Florida, Gainesville, FL

Pox Diseases

**Robert O. Gilbert, B.V.Sc.,
M.Med.Vet., Dipl. A.C.T., M.R.C.V.S.**
Professor of Theriogenology, Department
of Clinical Sciences, College of Veterinary
Medicine, Cornell University, Ithaca, NY

*Metritis in Large Animals, Retained Fe-
tal Membranes in Large Animals, Systemic Pharmacotherapeutics of the Reproductive System, Ulcerative Posthitis
and Vulvitis, Uterine Prolapse and Eversion, Vaginal and Cervical Prolapse, Vulvitis and Vaginitis*

John R. Glisson, D.V.M., M.A.M., Ph.D.
Professor, Department of Avian Medicine,
University of Georgia, Athens, GA

*Aspergillosis, Flip-over Disease, Fowl
Cholera, Riemerella anatipestifer Infection*

**Eric Gonder, D.V.M., M.S., Ph.D.,
P.A.S., Dipl. A.C.P.V.**
Veterinarian, Goldsboro Milling Company,
Goldsboro, NC

Pendulous Crop

**John-Karl Goodwin, D.V.M., Dipl.
A.C.V.I.M. (Cardiology),** *Deceased*
Director, Veterinary Heart Institute,
Gainesville, FL

*Congenital and Inherited Anomalies of
the Cardiovascular System*

John R. Gorham, D.V.M., Ph.D.
Professor of Veterinary Microbiology and
Pathology, Washington State University,
Pullman, WA

Foxes, Mink

**Richard E. Gough, F.I.M.L.S., C.Biol.,
M.I.Biol.**
Avian Virology, Central Veterinary Labora-
tory, New Haw, Weybridge, Surrey, UK

*Avian Pneumovirus, Goose Parvovirus
Infection*

**Daniel H. Gould, D.V.M., Ph.D., Dipl.
A.C.V.P.**
Department of Microbiology, Immunology
and Pathology, Colorado State University,
Fort Collins, CO

Polioencephalomalacia

**Gregory F. Grauer, D.V.M., M.S., Dipl.
A.C.V.I.M. (Internal Medicine)**
Professor and Head, Department of Clinical
Sciences, College of Veterinary Medicine,
Kansas State University, Manhattan, KS

Ethylene Glycol Toxicity

Deborah S. Greco, D.V.M., Ph.D.
Staff Internist, The Animal Medical Center, New York, NY

The Pituitary Gland

Craig E. Greene, D.V.M., M.S.
Professor, Department of Small Animal
Medicine, College of Veterinary Medicine,
University of Georgia, Athens, GA

*Canine Distemper, Canine Herpesviral
Infection, Infectious Canine Hepatitis,
Rickettsial Diseases*

Paul R. Greenough, F.R.C.V.S.
Professor Emeritus of Veterinary Surgery,
Western College of Veterinary Medicine,
University of Saskatchewan, Saskatoon,
Saskatchewan, Canada

*Lameness in Cattle, Problematic Bovine
Recumbency (Downer Cow)*

Ric R. Grummer, B.S., M.S., Ph.D.
Professor, Department of Dairy Science, University of Wisconsin-Madison, Madison, WI

Fatty Liver Disease of Cattle

**Jorge Guerrero, D.V.M., Ph.D., Dipl.
E.V.P.C.**
Adjunct Professor of Parasitology, Department of Pathobiology, School of Veterinary Medicine, University of Pennsylvania, Philadelphia, PA

Heartworm Disease

P. Timothy Guichon, D.V.M.
Feedlot Health Management Services,
Okotoks, Alberta, Canada

Histophilosis

James S. Guy, D.V.M., Ph.D.
Professor, Department of Population
Health and Pathobiology, College of Veterinary Medicine, North Carolina State University, Raleigh, NC

Viral Encephalitides

Sharon M. Gwaltney-Brant, D.V.M., Ph.D., Dipl. A.B.V.T., Dipl. A.B.T.
Director of Veterinary Toxicology Training, A.S.P.C.A. Animal Poison Control Center, Urbana, IL

Food Hazards, Household Hazards

Carlton L. Gyles, D.V.M., Ph.D.
Professor, Department of Pathobiology,
Ontario Veterinary College, University of
Guelph, Guelph, Ontario, Canada

Clostridial Diseases, Edema Disease, Salmonellosis

Caroline N. Hahn, D.V.M., M.Sc., Ph.D., M.R.C.V.S.
Neuromuscular Disease Laboratory,
Royal (Dick) School of Veterinary Studies,
University of Edinburgh, Midlothian, UK

Dysautonomia

Jean A. Hall, D.V.M., M.S., Ph.D., Dipl. A.C.V.I.M.
Associate Professor, Department of Biomedical Sciences, College of Veterinary
Medicine, Oregon State University, Corvallis, OR

Puerperal Hypocalcemia in Small Animals

Christopher Hamblin, M.I.Biol., C.I.Biol.
Institute for Animal Health, Pirbright Laboratory, Pirbright, Surrey, UK

Ephemeral Fever

Farouk M. Hamdy, D.V.M., M.Sc., Ph.D., M.P.A.
Animal Health Consultant, Silverspring,
MD

African Horse Sickness, Peste des Petits Ruminants, Rinderpest

Robert L. Hamlin, D.V.M., Ph.D., Dipl. A.C.V.I.M.
Stanton Youngberg Professor, College of
Veterinary Medicine, Ohio State University, Columbus, OH

Cardiovascular System Introduction

K. Larry Hammell, D.V.M., M.Sc.
Associate Professor, Department of
Health Management, Atlantic Veterinary
College, University of Prince Edward Island, Charlottetown, Prince Edward Island, Canada

Aquaculture Systems

Harold E. Hammerquist, D.V.M.
Assistant Professor, Department of Environmental and Population Health, Tufts
University, South Woodstock, CT

Parturient Paresis in Sheep and Goats

Larry G. Hansen, Ph.D.
Professor, Department of Veterinary Biosciences, University of Illinois, Urbana, IL

Halogenated Aromatic Poisoning

Russell Reid Hanson, D.V.M., Dipl. A.C.V.S., Dipl. A.C.V.E.C.C.
Associate Professor, Department of Clinical Sciences, College of Veterinary Medicine, Auburn University, Auburn AL

Congenital and Inherited Anomalies of the Musculoskeletal System

Joseph Harari, M.S., D.V.M., Dipl. A.C.V.S.
Veterinary Surgeon, Veterinary Surgical
Specialists, Spokane, WA

Arthropathies and Related Disorders in Small Animals, Lameness in Small Animals, Myopathies in Small Animals, Osteopathies in Small Animals

Joanne Hardy, D.V.M., Ph.D., Dipl. A.C.V.S., Dipl. A.C.V.E.C.C.
Clinical Associate Professor, Large Animal Medicine and Surgery, Texas A&M
University, College Station, TX

Equine Emergency Medicine

Billy M. Hargis, D.V.M., Ph.D., Dipl. A.C.P.V.
Professor, JKS Poultry Health Research Laboratory, Department of Poultry Science, University of Arkansas, Fayetteville, AR

Ascites Syndrome, Round Heart Disease of Turkeys

Kenneth R. Harkin, D.V.M., Dipl. A.C.V.I.M.
Associate Professor, College of Veterinary Medicine, Kansas State University, Manhattan, KS

Leptospirosis

D. L. Hank Harris, D.V.M., Ph.D.
Professor, Department of Animal Science, College of Agriculture, Department of Veterinary Diagnostics and Production Animal Medicine, College of Veterinary Medicine, Iowa State University, Ames, IA

Intestinal Diseases in Pigs

Lynette A. Hart, Ph.D.
Professor, Department of Population Health and Reproduction, Director, UC Center for Animal Alternatives, School of Veterinary Medicine, University of California, Davis, CA

Human-animal Bond

Joe Hauptman, D.V.M., M.S., Dipl. A.C.V.S.
Professor of Surgery, Department of Small Animal Clinical Sciences, College of Veterinary Medicine, Michigan State University, East Lansing, MI

Diaphragmatic Hernia

William W. Hawkins, B.S., D.V.M.
Hawkins Veterinary Service, Dillon, MT

Contagious Ecthyma (Orf), Ulcerative Dermatosis of Sheep

Peter Hellyer, D.V.M., M.S., Dipl. A.C.V.A.
Professor of Anesthesiology, Department of Clinical Sciences, College of Veterinary Medicine & Biomedical Sciences, Colorado State University, Fort Collins, CO

Pain Management

Charles M. Hendrix, D.V.M., Ph.D.
Professor, Department of Pathobiology, College of Veterinary Medicine, Auburn University, Auburn, AL

CNS Diseases Caused by Helminths and Arthropods, Flies

Thomas H. Herdt, D.V.M., M.S., Dipl. A.C.V.N., Dipl. A.C.V.I.M.
Professor and Chairperson, Department of Large Animal Clinical Sciences, Michigan State University, East Lansing, MI

Ketosis in Cattle

Karen Hicks-Alldredge, D.V.M.
Sweetwater Veterinary Hospital, Sweetwater, TX

Ostriches

Robert Higgins, D.V.M., M.Sc., D.Sc., Ph.D.
Professor and Microbiologist, Faculté de Médicine Vétérinaire, Université de Montréal, Saint-Hyacinthe, Quebec, Canada

Streptococcal Infections in Pigs

Dolores E. Hill, Ph.D.
Parasitologist, U.S. Department of Agriculture, Beltsville, MD

Toxoplasmosis

Katrin Hinrichs, D.V.M., Ph.D., Dipl. A.C.T.
Professor, Department of Veterinary Physiology and Pharmacology, College of Veterinary Medicine, Texas A&M University, College Station, TX

Breeding Soundness Examination of the Male, Hormonal Control of Estrus, Embryo Transfer in Farm Animals

J. Christopher Hodgson, B.Sc., Ph.D.
Moredun Research Institute, Edinburgh, Scotland, UK

Watery Mouth Disease in Lambs

Frederic J. Hoerr, D.V.M., Ph.D., Dipl. A.C.V.P., Dipl. A.C.P.V.
Laboratory Director, Veterinary Diagnostic Laboratory, Alabama Department of Agriculture, Auburn, AL

Mycotoxicoses (Poultry)

Charles L. Hofacre, D.V.M., M.A.M., Ph.D., Dipl. A.C.P.V.
Professor, Avian Medicine, College of Veterinary Medicine, University of Georgia, Athens, GA

Necrotic Enteritis

Steven R. Hollingsworth, D.V.M., Dipl. A.C.V.O.
Lecturer, Department of Surgical and Radiological Sciences, School of Veterinary Medicine, University of California, Davis, CA

Equine Recurrent Uveitis

Peter H. Holmes, B.V.M.S., Ph.D., M.R.C.V.S., F.R.S.E.
Professor, University of Glasgow Veterinary School, Glasgow, Scotland, UK

Trypanosomosis

Johnny D. Hoskins, D.V.M., Ph.D.
Small Animal Consultant, Choudrant, LA

Congenital and Inherited Anomalies (Generalized Conditions), Management of the Neonate: Small Animals

Michael J. Huerkamp, D.V.M., Dipl. A.C.L.A.M.
Director, Division of Animal Resources, Emory University, Atlanta, GA

Laboratory Animals, Nonhuman Primates

Michael F. Hutjens, B.S., M.S., Ph.D.
Professor of Animal Sciences and Extension Dairy Specialist, University of Illinois, Urbana, IL

Nutrition: Dairy Cattle

Basil O. Ikede, B.Vet.Med., D.V.M., Ph.D., F.C.V.S.N.
Professor and Chair, Department of Pathology & Microbiology, Atlantic Veterinary College, University of Prince Edward Island, Charlottetown, Prince Edward, Canada

Bovine Petechial Fever

Walter Ingwersen, D.V.M., D.V.Sc., Dipl. A.C.V.I.M.
Specialist, Companion Animals, Boehringer Ingelheim (Canada) Ltd, Vetmedica, Burlington, Ontario, Canada

Congenital and Inherited Anomalies of the Digestive System

Charles J. Issel, D.V.M., Ph.D.
Wright-Market Chair of Equine Infectious Diseases, Gluck Equine Research Center, University of Kentucky, Lexington, KY

Equine Infectious Anemia

Peter G. G. Jackson, M.A., B.V.M.&S., D.V.M.&S., F.R.C.V.S.
Senior Tutor, St. Edmund's College, University of Cambridge, Cambridge, UK

Prolonged Gestation of Cattle and Sheep

Mark W. Jackwood, Ph.D.
Professor, Department of Avian Medicine, College of Veterinary Medicine, University of Georgia, Athens, GA

Bordetellosis (Poultry)

Nemi C. Jain, M.V.Sc., Ph.D.
Professor Emeritus of Clinical Pathology, Department of Veterinary Pathology, Microbiology and Immunology, School of Veterinary Medicine, University of California, Davis, CA

Hemostatic Disorders, Leukocytic Disorders

Eugene D. Janzen, B.A., D.V.M., M.V.S.
Professor, Large Animal Clinical Sciences, Western College of Veterinary Medicine, University of Saskatchewan, Saskatoon, Saskatchewan, Canada

Lightning Strike and Electrocution, Trichomoniasis

Leo B. Jeffcott, M.A., B.Vet.Med., Ph.D., F.R.C.V.S., D.V.Sc., Vet.Dr.
Professor of Veterinary Clinical Studies and Dean of the Veterinary School, University of Cambridge, Cambridge, UK

Lameness in Horses

G. Kee Jim, D.V.M.
Feedlot Health Management Services, Okotoks, Alberta, Canada

Histophilosis

Cheri A. Johnson, D.V.M., M.S., Dipl. A.C.V.I.M. (S.A.I.M.)
Professor and Chief of Staff, Department of Small Animal Clinical Sciences, College of Veterinary Medicine, Michigan State University, East Lansing, MI

Canine Transmissible Venereal Tumor, Reproductive Diseases of the Male Small Animal

Isobel Johnstone, B.Sc.(Honours), Ph.D., B.V.Sc., M.A.C.V.Sc.
Small Animal Clinic, School of Veterinary Science, University of Queensland, Brisbane, Queensland, Australia

Systemic Pharmacotherapeutics of the Nervous System

Wayne K. Jorgensen, Ph.D.
Senior Principal Research Scientist (Parasitology), Department of Primary Industries and Fisheries, Queensland, Australia

Babesiosis

Robert J. Kemppainen, D.V.M., Ph.D.
Professor, Department of Anatomy, Physiology & Pharmacology, College of Veterinary Medicine, Auburn University, Auburn, AL

Endocrine System Introduction

Morag G. Kerr, B.V.M.S., B.Sc., Ph.D., C.Biol., F.I.Biol., M.R.C.V.S.
Director of Science and Laboratories, VetLab Services, Southwater, Horsham, West Sussex, UK

Diagnostic Procedures for the Private Practice Laboratory: Clinical Biochemistry and Hematology

Safdar A. Khan, D.V.M., M.S., Ph.D., Dipl. A.B.V.T.
Director of Toxicology Research, A.S.P.C.A. Animal Poison Control Center, Urbana, IL

Arsenic Poisoning, Salt Toxicity, Selenium Toxicosis, Strychnine Poisoning, Toxicities from Illicit and Abused Drugs, Toxicities from Over-the-counter Drugs, Toxicities from Prescription Drugs

Daniel J. King, D.V.M., Ph.D.
Veterinary Medical Officer, U.S. Department of Agriculture, ARS, Southeast Poultry Research Laboratory, Athens, GA

Newcastle Disease

Rebecca Kirby, D.V.M., Dipl. A.C.V.E.C.C., Dipl. A.C.V.I.M
Chief of Medicine, Animal Emergency Center and Referral Services, Milwaukee, WI

Emergency Medicine Introduction, Evaluation and Initial Treatment of the Emergency Patient, Fluid Therapy, Monitoring Procedures for the Critically Ill Animal, Specific Diagnostics and Therapy

Peter D. Kirkland, B.V.Sc., Ph.D.
Principal Research Scientist, Head, Virology Laboratory, Elizabeth Macarthur Agriculture Institute, Camden, New South Wales, Australia

Akabane Virus Infection

Richard P. Kitching, B.Sc., B.Vet.Med., M.Sc., Ph.D., M.R.C.V.S.
Director, National Centre for Foreign Animal Disease, Winnipeg, Manitoba, Canada

Foot-and-mouth Disease

Thomas R. Klei, Ph.D.
Boyd Professor, Department of Pathobiological Science, School of Veterinary Medicine, Louisiana State University, Baton, Rouge, LA

Helminths of the Skin

Stanley H. Kleven, D.V.M., Ph.D. Dipl. A.C.V.M., Dipl. A.C.P.V.
Regents' Professor, Department of Avian Medicine, College of Veterinary Medicine, University of Georgia, Athens, GA

Mycoplasmosis (Poultry)

Roger J. Klingenberg, D.V.M.
Greeley, CO

Reptiles

Nick J. Knowles, M.Phil.
Institute for Animal Health, Pirbright Laboratory, Pirbright, Surrey, UK

Porcine Enteroviral Encephalomyelitis, Swine Vesicular Disease, Vesicular Exanthema of Swine

Deborah T. Kochevar, D.V.M., Ph.D., Dipl. A.C.V.C.P.
Professor, Department of Veterinary Physiology and Pharmacology, College of Veterinary Medicine, Texas A&M University, College Station, TX

Antineoplastic Agents

Svend E. Kold, Dr. Med.Vet., M.R.C.V.S., R.C.V.S. Specialist in Equine Surgery (Orthopaedics)
Willesley Equine Clinic, North Tetbury, Gloucestershire, UK

Lameness in Horses: Examination, Arthroscopy

Michelle Kopcha, D.V.M., M.S.
Associate Professor, Food Animal Medicine and Surgery, College of Veterinary Medicine, Michigan State University, East Lansing, MI

Respiratory Diseases of Sheep and Goats

Zheko Kounev, D.V.M., Ph.D.
Associate Professor, Avian Health and Food Safety, Animal Disease Diagnostic Laboratory, School of Veterinary Medicine, Purdue University, West Lafayette, IN

Feeding and Management Practices (Poultry)

T. G. Ksiazek, D.V.M., Ph.D.
Chief, Special Pathogens Branch, Division for Viral and Rickettsial Diseases, National Center for Infectious Diseases, Centers for Disease Control and Prevention, Atlanta, GA

Crimean-Congo Hemorrhagic Fever, Nipah Virus Infection

Ned F. Kuehn, D.V.M., M.S., Dipl. A.C.V.I.M. (Internal Medicine)
Chief of Internal Medicine Services, Michigan Veterinary Specialists, Southfield, MI

Respiratory System Introduction, Respiratory Diseases of Small Animals

Mahesh C. Kumar, B.V.Sc. & A.H., M.S., Ph.D., Dipl. A.C.P.V.
Consultant, Poultry Health & Food Safety, St. Cloud, MN

Dissecting Aneurysm

Garrick C. M. Latch, M.Agr.Sc., Ph.D.
Consultant, Palmerston North, New Zealand

Ryegrass Toxicity

Jimmy C. Lattimer, D.V.M., M.S., Dipl. A.C.V.R., Dipl. A.C.V.R.O.
Associate Professor, Veterinary Medicine and Surgery, University of Missouri-Columbia, Columbus, MO

Diagnostic Imaging

D. Bruce Lawhorn, D.V.M., M.S.
Professor and Extension Swine Veterinarian, Department of Large Animal Medicine and Surgery, College of Veterinary Medicine, Texas A&M University, College Station, TX

Potbellied Pigs

Margie D. Lee, D.V.M., Ph.D.
Professor, Department of Avian Medicine, College of Veterinary Medicine, The University of Georgia, Athens, GA.

Avian Campylobacter Infection, Colibacillosis (Poultry)

Steven Leeson, Ph.D.
Professor, Department of Animal and Poultry Science, University of Guelph, Guelph, Ontario, Canada

Fatty Liver Syndrome, Nutritional Deficiencies (Poultry)

Ala E. Lew, B.Sc. (Honours), Ph.D.
Department of Primary Industries and Fisheries, Yeerongpilly, Brisbane, Queensland, Australia

Anaplasmosis

Teresa L. Lightfoot, D.V.M., Dipl. A.B.V.P. (Avian)
Florida Veterinary Specialists, Tampa, FL

Caged Birds

John E. Lloyd, B.S., Ph.D.
Professor of Entomology, University of Wyoming, Laramie, WY

Cattle Grubs, Lice

Jeanne Lofstedt, B.V.Sc., M.S., Dipl. A.C.V.I.M.
Associate Dean of Academic Affairs, Atlantic Veterinary College, University of Prince Edward Island, Charlottetown, Prince Edward Island, Canada

Caprine Arthritis and Encephalitis, Necrobacillosis, Winter Dysentery

Maureen T. Long, D.V.M., Ph.D., Dipl. A.C.V.I.M (Large Animals)
Assistant Professor, Large Animal Clinical Sciences, University of Florida, Gainesville, FL

West Nile Encephalomyelitis

Bertrand J. Losson, D.V.M., Ph.D.
Professor, Department of Parasitology and Parasitic Diseases, Faculty of Veterinary Medicine, University of Liege, Belgium

Mange in Large Animals

Jodie Low Choy, B.V.M.S.
Veterinary Quarantine Facility, Territory Wildlife Park, Palmerston, Australia

Melioidosis

Katharine F. Lunn, B.V.M.S., M.S., Ph.D., M.R.C.V.S., Dipl. A.C.V.I.M.
Research Scientist, Department of Clinical Sciences, Colorado State University, Fort Collins, CO

Fever of Unknown Origin

Robert J. MacKay, B.V.Sc., Ph.D.
Professor, Department of Large Animal Clinical Sciences, University of Florida, Gainesville, FL

Equine Protozoal Myeloencephalitis

Dennis W. Macy, D.V.M., M.S., Dipl. A.C.V.I.M.
Professor of Medicine and Oncology, College of Veterinary Medicine and Biomedical Sciences, Colorado State University, Fort Collins, CO

Feline Infectious Peritonitis and Pleuritis

Charlotte Maddox-Hyttel, D.V.M., Ph.D., D.V.Sc.
Senior Scientist, Section for Parasitology, Danish Institute for Food and Veterinary Research, Copenhagen, Denmark

Gastrointestinal Parasites of Pigs

John E. Madigan, D.V.M., M.S.
Professor, Department of Medicine and Epidemiology, School of Veterinary Medicine, University of California, Davis, CA

Equine Granulocytic Ehrlichiosis, Potomac Horse Fever

John B. Malone, D.V.M., Ph.D.
Professor, Pathobiological Sciences, School of Veterinary Medicine, Louisiana State University, Baton Rouge, LA

Diagnostic Procedures for the Private Laboratory: Parasitology

Richard A. Mansmann, V.M.D., Ph.D.
Clinical Professor, Department of Clinical Sciences, College of Veterinary Medicine, North Carolina State University, Raleigh, NC

Prepurchase Examination of Horses

Steven L. Marks, B.V.Sc., M.S., M.R.C.V.S., Dipl. A.C.V.I.M.
Associate Professor and Head, Small Animal Medicine, Department of Veterinary Clinical Medicine, College of Veterinary Medicine, University of Illinois, Urbana, IL

Canine Nasal Mites, Health-Management Interaction: Small Animals

Guy-Pierre Martineau, D.V.M., Ph.D.
Professor, National Veterinary School of Toulouse, Toulouse, France

Postpartum Dysgalactia Syndrome and Mastitis in Sows

John J. Maurer, B.S., Ph.D.
Associate Professor, Department of Avian Medicine, University of Georgia, Athens, GA

Colibacillosis (Poultry)

Dudley L. McCaw, D.V.M.
Associate Professor, Department of Veterinary Medicine and Surgery, College of Veterinary Medicine, University of Missouri, Columbia, MO

Feline Leukemia Virus and Related Diseases

Diane McClure, D.V.M., Ph.D., Dipl. A.C.L.A.M.
Director, Animal Resource Center, University of California, Santa Barbara, CA

Rabbits

Brian J. McCluskey, D.V.M., Ph.D., Dipl. A.C.V.P.M.
Analytical Epidemiologist, U.S. Department of Agriculture, APHIS, Centers for Epidemiology and Animal Health, Fort Collins, CO

Vesicular Stomatitis

Larry R. McDougald, Ph.D.
Professor of Poultry Parasitology, Department of Poultry Sciences, University of Georgia, Athens, GA

Avian Spirochetosis, Coccidiosis, Fluke Infections, Hexamitiasis, Histomoniasis, Trichomoniasis (Poultry)

C. Wayne McIlwraith, B.V.Sc., Ph.D., D.Sc., F.R.C.V.S., Dipl. A.C.V.S.
Professor of Surgery, Director of Orthopedic Research, Gail Holmes Equine Orthopedic Research Center, Colorado State University, Fort Collins, CO

Arthropathies in Large Animals, Lameness in Horses: Disorders of the Carpus

Quintin A. McKellar, B.V.M.S., Ph.D., D.V.M., Dipl. E.C.V.P.T., C.Biol., F.I.Biol., F.R.Ag.S., M.R.C.V.S., F.R.S.E.
Principal, The Royal Veterinary College, Hatfield, Hertfordshire, UK

Gastrointestinal Parasites of Ruminants

Ross A. McKenzie, B.V.Sc., M.V.Sc., D.V.Sc.
Senior Principal Veterinary Pathologist, Department of Primary Industries, Queensland, Senior Lecturer, University of Queensland, School of Veterinary Science, Brisbane, Queensland, Australia

Plants Poisonous to Animals

Rita McManamon, D.V.M.
Senior Veterinarian, Zoo Atlanta, Atlanta, GA

Nutrition: Exotic and Zoo Animals, Care of Orphaned Native Birds and Mammals

Gavin L. Meerdink, D.V.M., Dipl. A.B.V.T.
Clinical Professor, Veterinary Diagnostic Laboratory, College of Veterinary Medicine, University of Illinois, Urbana, IL

Toxicology Introduction

Mushtaq A. Memon, B.V.Sc., M.S., Ph.D., Dipl. A.C.T.
Theriogenologist, Department of Veterinary Clinical Sciences, Washington State University, Pullman, WA

Reproductive Diseases of the Female Small Animal

Paula I. Menzies, D.V.M., M.P.V.M.
Associate Professor, Ruminant Health Management, Department of Population Medicine, Ontario Veterinary College, University of Guelph, Guelph, Ontario, Canada

Lymphadenitis and Lymphangitis, Pregnancy Toxemia in Ewes

Samia A. (Shawky) Metwally, D.V.M., Ph.D.
Head, Diagnostic Services Section, Foreign Animal Disease Diagnostic Laboratory, U.S. Department of Agriculture, APHIS, Greenport, NY

Nairobi Sheep Disease

G. Meulemans, D.V.M.
Head, Department of Small Stock Diseases, Veterinary and Agrochemical Research Centre, Ukkel, Belgium

Avian Nephritis Viral Infections

Bernard Mignon, D.V.M., Ph.D.
Assistant Professor, Parasitology, Mycology, Université de Liège, Belgium

Mange in Dogs and Cats

Maureen H. Milne, B.V.M.S., M.V.M., D.C.H.P., M.R.C.V.S.
Farm Animal Division, Veterinary Clinical Studies, University of Glasgow, Glasgow, Scotland

Laryngeal Disorders

Dale A. Moore, M.S., D.V.M., M.P.V.M., Ph.D.
Associate Professor, Veterinary Medical Teaching and Research Center, University of California-Davis, Tulare, CA

Besnoitiosis, Sarcocystosis

James N. Moore, D.V.M., Ph.D.
Distinguished Research Professor, Department of Large Animal Medicine, College of Veterinary Medicine, University of Georgia, Athens, GA

Colic in Horses

Lisa E. Moore, D.V.M., Dipl. A.C.V.I.M.
Assistant Professor, Department of Clinical Sciences, College of Veterinary Medicine, Kansas State University, Manhattan, KS

Diseases of the Esophagus in Small Animals

Karen A. Moriello, D.V.M., Dipl. A.C.V.D.
Clinical Associate Professor of Dermatology, School of Veterinary Medicine, University of Wisconsin-Madison, Madison, WI

Acanthosis Nigricans, Cuterebra Infestation in Small Animals, Dermatophilosis, Hygroma, Integumentary System Introduction, Interdigital Furunculosis, Pyoderma

James K. Morrisey, D.V.M., Dipl. A.B.V.P. (Avian Practice)
Department of Clinical Science, College of Veterinary Medicine, Cornell University, Ithaca, NY

Ferrets

W. Ivan Morrison, Ph.D., B.V.M.S.
Professor, Center for Tropical Veterinary Medicine, Royal (Dick) School of Veterinary Studies, University of Edinburgh, Scotland, UK

Theileriases

Karen R. Munana, D.V.M., M.S., Dipl. A.C.V.I.M. (Neurology)
Associate Professor, Department of Clinical Sciences, College of Veterinary Medicine, North Carolina State University, Raleigh, NC

Meningitis and Encephalitis

Lisa A. Murphy, V.M.D.
Veterinary Poison Information Specialist, A.S.P.C.A. Animal Poison Control Center, Urbana, IL

Toxicities from Over-the-counter Drugs

Michael J. Murray, D.V.M., M.S.
Technical Director, Equine, Merial Limited, Duluth, GA

Gastrointestinal Ulcers in Large Animals: Gastric Ulcers in Horses

Sofie Muylle, D.V.M., Ph.D.
Faculty of Veterinary Medicine, Department of Morphology, University of Ghent, Salisburylaan, Merelbeke, Belgium

Dental Development

Syed A. Naqi, B.V.Sc., M.S., Ph.D., Dipl. A.C.V.M.
Professor, Department of Microbiology and Immunology, College of Veterinary Medicine, Cornell University, Ithaca, NY

Infectious Bronchitis (Poultry)

T. Mark Neer, D.V.M., Dipl. A.C.V.I.M. (Internal Medicine)
Professor of Medicine, Department of Clinical Sciences, College of Veterinary Medicine, Louisiana State University, Baton Rouge, LA

Deafness, Demyelinating Disorders, Motion Sickness, Otitis Media and Interna

Peter Nettleton, B.V.M.S., M.Sc., Ph.D., M.R.C.V.S.
Moredun Research Institute, Scotland, United Kingdom

Border Disease

Robin A. J. Nicholas, Ph.D., M.Sc., M.I.Biol.
Department of Bacterial Diseases, Veterinary Laboratories Agency-Weybridge, Addlestone, Surrey, United Kingdom

Contagious Agalactia and Other Mycoplasmal Mastitides of Small Ruminants

Paul Nicoletti, D.V.M., M.S.
Professor, College of Veterinary Medicine, University of Florida, Gainesville, FL

Brucellosis in Large Animals, Brucellosis in Dogs

Jerome C. Nietfeld, D.V.M., Ph.D., Dipl. A.C.V.P.
Associate Professor, Department of Diagnostic Medicine/Pathobiology, College of Veterinary Medicine, Kansas State University, Manhattan, KS

Abortion in Large Animals

Robert A. Norton, B.S., M.S., Ph.D.
Associate Professor, Department of Poultry Science, Auburn University, Auburn, AL

Helminthiasis (Poultry)

Mark J. Novotny, D.V.M., M.S., Ph.D., Dipl. A.C.V.C.P.
Associate Director-Clinical Research Scientist, Scientific Development, Pfizer Global Research & Development, Groton, CT

Systemic Pharmacotherapeutics of the Cardiovascular System

Frederick W. Oehme, D.V.M., Ph.D.
Professor of Toxicology, Pathobiology, Medicine and Physiology, Comparative Toxicology Laboratories, Kansas State University, Manhattan, KS

Rodenticide Poisoning

Garrett R. Oetzel, D.V.M., M.S.
Associate Professor, Food Animal Production Medicine Section, School of Veterinary Medicine, University of Wisconsin-Madison, Madison, WI

Subacute Ruminal Acidosis in Dairy Cattle

Gary D. Osweiler, D.V.M., M.S., Ph.D., Dipl. A.B.V.T.
Professor, Veterinary Diagnostic and Production Animal Medicine, Iowa State University, Ames, IA

Coal-Tar Poisoning, Mycotoxicoses

Raul E. Otalora, D.V.M.
Production Manager, Quail International, Inc., Greensboro, GA

Ulcerative Enteritis (Quail Disease)

Karen L. Overall, M.A., V.M.D., Ph.D., Dipl. A.C.V.B., A.B.S. Certified Applied Animal Behaviorist
Research Associate, Psychiatry Department, Center for Neurobiology & Behavior, University of Pennsylvania, Philadelphia, PA

Behavioral Medicine Introduction, Normal Social Behavior and Behavioral Problems of Domestic Animals

Sheldon Padgett, D.V.M., M.S., Dipl. A.C.V.S.
Metropolitan Veterinary Referral Group, Akron, OH

Dystrophies Associated with Calcium, Phosphorus, and Vitamin D

David J. Paton, M.A., V.M.B., Ph.D.
Pirbright Laboratory, Institute for Animal Health, Pirbright, Surrey, UK

Swine Vesicular Disease, Vesicular Exanthema of Swine

Sharon Patton, M.S., Ph.D.
Professor of Parasitology, Department of Comparative Medicine, College of Veterinary Medicine, University of Tennessee, Knoxville, TN

Amebiasis, Giardiasis

Janusz T. Paweska, D.V.Sc.
Chief Specialist Scientist, Special Pathogens Unit, National Institute for Communicable Diseases, Sandringham, South Africa

Bluetongue

Sarah E. Payne, D.V.M.
Harrington Oncology Program, School of Veterinary Medicine, Tufts University, Grafton, MA

Anemia

Maurice B. Pensaert, D.V.M., M.S., Ph.D.
Emeritus Professor of Animal Virology, Faculty of Veterinary Medicine, Ghent University, Merelbeke, Belgium

Hemagglutinating Encephalomyelitis

Andrew S. Peregrine, B.V.M.S., Ph.D., D.V.M.
Associate Professor, Department of Pathobiology, Ontario Veterinary College, University of Guelph, Guelph, Ontario, Canada

Gastrointestinal Parasites in Small Animals

Tilden Wayne Perry, B.Ed., B.S., M.S., Ph.D.
Emeritus Professor of Animal Nutrition, Purdue University, West Lafayette, IN

Nutrition: Beef Cattle, Nutritional Diseases of Cattle

Donald Peter, D.V.M., M.S., Dipl. A.C.T.
Veterinarian/Owner, Frontier Genetics, Hermiston, OR

Bovine Genital Campylobacteriosis, Equine Coital Exanthema

Mark E. Peterson, D.V.M., Dipl. A.C.V.I.M.
Head, Division of Endocrinology, The Caspary Research Institute and the Bobst Hospital of The Animal Medical Center, New York, NY

The Parathyroid Glands and Disorders of Calcium Metabolism, The Thyroid Gland

James R. Philips, Ph.D.
Associate Professor of Science, Math/Science Division, Babson College, Babson Park, MA

Air Sac Mite, Ectoparasites (Poultry)

F. William Pierson, M.S., D.V.M., Ph.D., Dipl. A.C.P.V.
Associate Professor of Avian Medicine, Center for Molecular Medicine and Infectious Diseases, Virginia-Maryland Regional College of Veterinary Medicine, Virginia Tech, Blacksburg, VA

Hemorrhagic Enteritis and Marble Spleen Disease (Poultry)

Carlos B. J. Pijoan, D.V.M., Dipl. Bact., Ph.D.
Professor, College of Veterinary Medicine, University of Minnesota, Saint Paul, MN

Glässer's Disease

Tom J. Pittman, B.Sc. Agr., D.V.M., P.Ag.
Feedlot Health Management Services, Okotoks, Alberta, Canada

Histophilosis

Karen W. Post, D.V.M., M.S., Dipl. A.C.V.M.
Veterinary Bacteriologist, North Carolina Department of Agriculture and Consumer Services, Rollins Animal Disease Diagnostic Laboratory, Raleigh, NC

Diagnostic Procedures for the Private Practice Laboratory: Clinical Microbiology

D. G. Pugh, D.V.M., M.S., Dipl. A.C.T., Dipl. A.C.V.N.
Fort Dodge Animal Health, Waverly, AL

Nutrition: Goats, Nutrition: Sheep, Nutritional Diseases of Sheep and Goats, Parturient Paresis in Sheep and Goats

Otto M. Radostits, C.M., D.V.M., M.Sc., Dipl. A.C.V.I.M.
Professor Emeritus, Department of Large Animal Clinical Sciences, Western College of Veterinary Medicine, University of Saskatchewan, Saskatoon, Saskatchewan, Canada

Abdominal Fat Necrosis, Biosecurity, Bovine Cystitis and Pyelonephritis, Bovine Leukosis, Coccidiosis, Health-Management Interaction: Cattle, Erysipelas, Grain Overload, Management of Reproduction: Cattle, Peritonitis, Prepurchase Examination of Ruminants and Swine, Ruminal Parakeratosis, Simple Indigestion, Traumatic Reticuloperitonitis, Vagal Indigestion

D. Owen Rae, D.V.M., M.P.V.M.
Associate Professor, College of Veterinary Medicine, University of Florida, Gainesville, FL

Management of Reproduction: Cattle

Sarah L. Ralston, V.M.D., Ph.D., Dipl. A.C.V.N.
Associate Professor, Department of Animal Science, Cook College, Rutgers University, New Brunswick, NJ

Nutrition: Horses

Willie M. Reed, D.V.M., Ph.D., Dipl. A.C.V.P., Dipl. A.C.P.V.
Professor, Chairperson and Director, Diagnostic Center for Population and Animal Health, College of Veterinary Medicine, Michigan State University, East Lansing, MI

Quail Bronchitis, Viral Hepatitis of Turkeys

Philip T. Reeves, B.V.Sc., Ph.D., F.A.C.V.Sc.
Principal Scientist, Residues and Veterinary Medicines, Australian Pesticides and Veterinary Medicines Authority, Canberra, Australia

Drug Action and Pharmacodynamics, Chemical Residues in Food and Fiber, Veterinary Dosage Forms and Delivery Systems

Hugh W. Reid, M.B.E., B.V.M.&S., D.T.V.M., Ph.D., M.R.C.V.S.
TSE Research Co-ordinator, Moredun Research Institute, Edinburgh, Scotland, UK

Louping Ill

Douglas J. Reinemann, Ph.D.
Professor, Biological Systems Engineering, University of Wisconsin-Madison, Madison, WI

Stray Voltage in Animal Housing

Ase Risberg, V.M.D.
Large Animal Internal Medicine, School of Veterinary Medicine, University of Wisconsin-Madison, Madison, WI

Thrombosis, Embolism, and Aneurysm

James F. Roche, Ph.D., D.Sc.
Professor of Animal Husbandry and Production, Faculty of Veterinary Medicine, University College Dublin, Belfield, Dublin, Ireland

Growth Promotants and Production Enhancers

Barton W. Rohrbach, V.M.D., M.P.H., Dipl. A.C.V.P.M. (Epidemiology)
Associate Professor, Department of Large Animal Clinical Sciences, College of Veterinary Medicine, University of Tennessee, Knoxville, TN

Q Fever, Tularemia

A. Gregorio Rosales, D.V.M., M.S., Ph.D.
Vice President of Veterinary Services, Aviagen North America, Huntsville, AL

Disorders of the Reproductive System (Poultry)

Michele R. Rosenbaum, V.M.D., Dipl. A.C.V.D.
Veterinary Specialists of Rochester, Rochester, NY

Tumors of the Ear Canal

John K. Rosenberger, B.S., M.S., Ph.D.
Professor and Department Chairperson, Department of Animal and Food Sciences, College of Agricultural Sciences and Natural Resources, University of Delaware, Newark, DE

Malabsorption Syndrome, Viral Arthritis (Poultry)

Wayne Rosenkrantz, D.V.M., Dipl. A.C.V.D.
Owner-Partner, Animal Dermatology Clinic, Tustin, CA

Eosinophilic Granuloma Complex

Robert C. Rosenthal, D.V.M., M.S., Ph.D., Dipl. A.C.V.I.M., (Small Animals, Oncology), Dipl. A.C.V.R. (Radiation Oncology)
SouthPaws Veterinary Referral Center, Springfield, VA

Mammary Tumors, Neuroendocrine Tissue Tumors

Stanley I. Rubin, D.V.M., M.S., Dipl. A.C.V.I.M.
Director, Veterinary Teaching Hospital, Western College of Veterinary Medicine, University of Saskatchewan, Saskatoon, Saskatchewan, Canada

Digestive System Introduction, Diseases of the Rectum and Anus

Pamela L. Ruegg, D.V.M., M.P.V.M., Dipl. A.B.V.P. (Dairy)
Associate Professor, Department of Dairy Science, University of Wisconsin-Madison, Madison, WI

Udder Diseases

Charles E. Rupprecht, V.M.D., M.S., Ph.D.
Chief, Rabies Section, Centers for Disease Control and Prevention, Atlanta, GA

Rabies

Bonnie R. Rush, D.V.M., M.S., Dipl. A.C.V.I.M.
Professor, Equine Medicine, College of Veterinary Medicine, Kansas State University, Manhattan, KS

Respiratory Diseases of Horses

H. Carolien Rutgers, D.V.M., M.S., Dipl. A.C.V.I.M., Dipl. E.C.V.I.M.-CA, D.S.A.M., M.R.C.V.S.
Senior Lecturer, The Royal Veterinary College, North Mymms, Hertfordshire, UK

Malabsorption Syndromes in Small Animals

Y. M. Saif, D.V.M., Ph.D.
Professor and Head, Food Animal Health Research Program, Ohio Agricultural Research and Development Center, The Ohio State University, Wooster, OH

Infectious Bursal Disease, Rotaviral Infections in Chickens, Turkeys, and Pheasants

Jean E. Sander, D.V.M., M.A.M., Dipl. A.C.P.V.
Associate Dean for Student Affairs, College of Veterinary Medicine, Ohio State University, Columbus, OH

Candidiasis (Poultry), Disposal of Carcasses and Disinfection of Premises, Omphalitis

Sherry L. Sanderson, B.S., D.V.M., Ph.D., Dipl. A.C.V.I.M., Dipl. A.C.V.N.
Assistant Professor, Department of Physiology and Pharmacology, College of Veterinary Medicine, University of Georgia, Athens, GA

Urinary System Introduction

Donald C. Sawyer, D.V.M., Ph.D., Dipl. A.C.V.A., Hon. Dipl. A.B.V.P.
Professor Emeritus, Michigan State University; Manager, Veterinary Product Development and Support, Minrad Inc., Buffalo, NY

Malignant Hyperthermia

K. A. Schat, D.V.M., Ph.D.
Professor, Department of Microbiology and Immunology, College of Veterinary Medicine, Cornell University, Ithaca, NY

Chicken Anemia Virus Infection

Mary M. Schell, D.V.M.
Veterinary Poison Information Specialist, A.S.P.C.A. National Animal Poison Control Center, Urbana, IL

Toxicities from Prescription Drugs

David G. Schmitz, D.V.M., M.S., Dipl. A.C.V.I.M.
Associate Professor of Medicine, Department of Veterinary Large Animal Medicine & Surgery, College of Veterinary Medicine, Texas A&M University, College Station, TX

Cantharadin (Blister Beetle) Poisoning

Norman R. Schneider, D.V.M., M.Sc., Dipl. A.B.V.T.
Veterinary Toxicologist Emeritus, Department of Veterinary and Biomedical Sciences, University of Nebraska-Lincoln, Lincoln, NE

Cyanide Poisoning, Gossypol Poisoning, Nitrate and Nitrite Poisoning, Nonprotein Nitrogen (Urea) Poisoning

Kevin T. Schultz, D.V.M., Ph.D.
Head of Research & Development, Merial Limited, Duluth, GA

Immunopathologic Diseases, Immunopathologic Mechanisms

Oliver C. Schunicht, D.V.M., B.Sc.
Feedlot Health Management Services, Okotoks, Alberta, Canada

Histophilosis

Maya M. Scott, B.S., D.V.M.
Resident, Clinical Pharmacology, Department of Veterinary Physiology and Pharmacology, College of Veterinary Medicine, Texas A&M University, College Station, TX

Antibacterial Agents, Antifungal Agents, Antiviral Agents and Interferon, Chemotherapeutics Introduction, Pharmacology Introduction

Philip R. Scott, D.V.M.&S., M.Phil., D.S.H.P., Cert. C.H.P., F.R.C.V.S., M.I.Biol.
Reader, Easter Bush Veterinary Centre, Roslin, Midlothian, Scotland, UK

Listeriosis

Colin J. Scrivener, B.V.Sc., M.A.C.V.Sc.
Mackinnon Project, Veterinary Clinical Centre, University of Melbourne, Werribee, Victoria, Australia

Management of Reproduction: Sheep

Brad E. Seguin, D.V.M., M.S., Ph.D., Dipl. A.C.T.
Professor, Department of Clinical and Population Sciences, College of Veterinary Medicine, University of Minnesota, St. Paul, MN

Cystic Ovary Disease, Reproductive System Introduction

Susan D. Semrad, V.M.D., Ph.D., Dipl. A.C.V.I.M.
Associate Professor, Department of Medical Sciences, School of Veterinary Medicine, University of Wisconsin-Madison, Madison, WI

Hepatic Disease in Large Animals, Malassimilation Syndromes in Large Animals

Patricia L. Sertich, M.S., V.M.D., Dipl. A. C.T.
Associate Professor-Clinician Educator, School of Veterinary Medicine, New Bolton Center, University of Pennsylvania, Kennett Square, PA

Management of Reproduction: Horses

David M. Sherman, D.V.M., M.S., Dipl. A.C.V.I.M.
Director, Division of Animal Health, Biosecurity and Dairy Services, Massachusetts Department of Agricultural Resources, Boston, MA

Health-Management Interaction: Goats, Lameness in Goats, Management of Reproduction: Goats

Michael Shipstone, B.V.Sc., F.A.C.V.Sc., Dipl. A.C.V.D.
Dermatology for Animals, Stafford Heights, Queensland, Australia

Systemic Pharmacotherapeutics of the Integumentary System

Elizabeth A. Shull, D.V.M., Dipl. A.C.V.I.M. (Neurology), Dipl. A.C.V.B.
Owner, Appalachian Veterinary Specialists, Knoxville, TN

Euthanasia

Bradford B. Smith, D.V.M., Ph.D.
Professor Emeritus, College of Veterinary Medicine, Oregon State University, Corvallis, OR

Llamas and Alpacas

J. Glenn Songer, Ph.D.
Professor, Department of Veterinary Science and Microbiology, University of Arizona, Tucson, AZ

Actinobacillosis, Actinomycosis, Nocardiosis

Sharon J. Spier, D.V.M., Ph.D., Dipl. A.C.V.I.M.
Associate Professor, Department of Veterinary Medicine and Epidemiology, School of Veterinary Medicine, University of California, Davis, CA

Hypocalcemic Tetany in Horses

Richard A. Squires, B.V.Sc., Ph.D., D.V.R., Dipl. A.C.V.I.M., Dipl. E.C.V.I.M., M.R.C.V.S.,
Associate Professor, Institute of Veterinary, Animal, and Biomedical Sciences, Massey University, Palmerston North, New Zealand

Feline Panleukopenia

James H. Steele, D.V.M., M.P.H.
Professor Emeritus, Center for Infectious Diseases, School of Public Health, University of Texas, Houston, TX

Zoonoses

Bryan L. Stegelmeier, D.V.M., Ph.D., Dipl. A.C.V.P.
U.S. Department of Agriculture, Poisonous Plant Research Laboratory, Logan, UT

High-Mountain Disease

Jörg M. Steiner, Dr.Med.Vet., Ph.D., Dipl. A.C.V.I.M., Dipl. E.C.V.I.M.-CA
Clinical Assistant Professor, GI Laboratory, Texas A&M University, College Station, TX

Tests for Pancreatic Disease, The Exocrine Pancreas in Small Animals

David Stiller, M.S., Ph.D.
Research Entomologist, Animal Disease Research Unit, U.S. Department of Agriculture, Agricultural Research Service, Holm Research Center, University of Idaho, Moscow, ID

Ticks

Michael K. Stoskopf, D.V.M., Ph.D., Dipl. A.C.Z.M.
Professor of Wildlife and Aquatic Medicine and of Environmental and Molecular Toxicology, College of Veterinary Medicine, North Carolina State University, Raleigh, NC

Marine Mammals

Bert E. Stromberg, Ph.D.
Professor and Associate Dean, College of Veterinary Medicine, University of Minnesota, St. Paul, MN

Swine Kidney Worm Infection, Trichinellosis

David E. Swayne, D.V.M., M.Sc., Ph.D.
Laboratory Director, U.S. Department of Agriculture, Agricultural Research Service, Southeast Poultry Research Laboratory, Athens, GA

Avian Influenza, Avian Paramyxovirus Infections

Thomas W. Swerczek, D.V.M., Ph.D.
Professor of Veterinary Pathology, Department of Veterinary Science, University of Kentucky, Lexington, KY

Tyzzer's Disease

Joseph Taboada, D.V.M., Dipl. A.C.V.I.M.
Professor of Small Animal Internal Medicine, Office of Student and Academic Affairs, School of Veterinary Medicine, Louisiana State University, Baton Rouge, LA

Fungal Infections

Patricia A. Talcott, M.S., D.V.M., Ph.D., Dipl. A.B.V.T.
Associate Professor, Department of Food Science and Toxicology, Holm Research Center, University of Idaho, Moscow, ID

Photosensitization

Martin G. Taylor, Ph.D., D.Sc.
Professor of Medical Helminthology, Department of Infectious and Tropical Diseases, London School of Hygiene and Tropical Medicine, University of London, London, UK

Schistosomiasis

Mike A. Taylor, B.V.M.S., Ph.D., M.R.C.V.S., Dipl. E.V.P.C., C.Biol., M.I.Biol.
Professor of Veterinary Parasitology, Veterinary Surveillance, Central Science Laboratory, Sand Hutton, York, UK

Ectoparasiticides Used in Large Animals

Stuart M. Taylor, Ph.D., B.V.M.S., M.R.C.V.S., Dipl. E.C.V.P.
VetPar Services, Bangor, UK

Fluke Infections in Ruminants, Lungworm Infection

Charles O. Thoen, D.V.M., Ph.D.
Professor, Veterinary Microbiology and Preventive Medicine, College of Veterinary Medicine, Iowa State University, Ames, IA

Tuberculosis (Poultry), Tuberculosis and Other Mycobacterial Infections

William B. Thomas, D.V.M., M.S., Dipl. A.C.V.I.M. (Neurology)
Associate Professor of Neurology/Neurosurgery, Department of Small Animal Clinical Sciences, University of Tennessee, Knoxville, TN

Diseases of the Peripheral Nerve and Neuromuscular Junction, Diseases of the Spinal Column and Cord

Leland Thompson, B.S., D.V.M.
Bayer Corporation, Shawnee Mission, KS

Anti-inflammatory Agents

Barry H. Thorp, B.V.M.S., Ph.D., M.R.C.V.S.
Aviagen Limited, Midlothian, Scotland, UK

Disorders of the Skeletal System (Poultry)

John F. Timoney, M.V.B., M.S., Ph.D., D.Sc., M.R.C.V.S.
Keeneland Chair of Infectious Diseases, Gluck Equine Research Center, University of Kentucky, Lexington, KY

Glanders

Peter J. Timoney, M.V.B., M.S., Ph.D., F.R.C.V.S.
Chairman and Director, Gluck Equine Research Center, Department of Veterinary Science, University of Kentucky, Lexington, KY

Equine Viral Arteritis, Hendra Virus Infection

Ian Tizard, B.V.M.S., Ph.D.
Richard M. Schubot Professor, Department of Pathobiology, College of Veterinary Medicine, Texas A&M University, College Station, TX

Amyloidosis, Vaccination of Exotic Mammals, Vaccines and Immunotherapy

Susan Tornquist, D.V.M., Ph.D., Dipl. A.C.V.P.
Associate Professor, Department of Biomedical Sciences, College of Veterinary Medicine, Oregon State University, Corvallis, OR

Diagnostic Procedures for the Private Practice Laboratory: Serology

Thomas E. Toth, D.V.M., Ph.D.
Professor of Virology, Center for Molecular Medicine and Infectious Diseases, Virginia-Maryland Regional College of Veterinary Medicine, Blacksburg, VA

Duck Viral Enteritis

Josie L. Traub-Dargatz, D.V.M., M.S., Dipl. A.C.V.I.M.
Professor of Equine Internal Medicine, Department of Clinical Sciences, College of Veterinary Medicine and Biomedical Sciences, Colorado State University, Fort Collins, CO

Intestinal Diseases in Horses and Foals, West Nile Encephalomyelitis

Robert Tremblay, D.V.M., D.V.Sc., Dipl. A.C.V.I.M.
Technical Services Veterinarian, Boehringer Ingelheim (Canada) Ltd, Burlington, Ontario, Canada

Management and Nutrition Introduction

Deoki N. Tripathy, D.V.M., M.S., Ph.D., Dipl. A.C.V.M., Dipl. A.C.P.V.
Professor, Department of Veterinary Pathobiology, College of Veterinary Medicine, University of Illinois, Urbana, IL

Fowlpox, Infectious Laryngotracheitis

Tracy A. Turner, D.V.M., M.S.
Professor, Equine Surgery, College of Veterinary Medicine, University of Minnesota, St. Paul, MN

Lameness in Horses: Imaging Techniques

Wendy E. Vaala, V.M.D., Dipl. A.C.V.I.M.
Clinical Associate, B.W. Furlong and Associates, Oldwick, NJ

Health-Management Interaction: Horses, Management of the Neonate: Large Animals

Stephanie J. Valberg, D.V.M., Ph.D.
Professor, Department of Clinical and Population Sciences, University of Minnesota, St. Paul, MN

Exertional Myopathies in Horses

Louis van der Heide, D.V.M., Ph.D.
Professor Emeritus, Department of Pathobiology, University of Connecticut, Storrs, CT

Avian Encephalomyelitis

John F. Van Vleet, D.V.M., Ph.D.
Professor of Veterinary Pathology, School of Veterinary Medicine, Purdue University, West Lafayette, IN

Myopathies and Myositides in Large Animals

Jozef Vercruysse, D.V.M., Dipl. E.V.P.C.
Professor, Faculty of Veterinary Medicine, University of Ghent, Merelbeke, Belgium

Anthelmintics

Alice Villalobos, B.S., D.V.M.
Animal Oncology Consultation Service, Woodland Hills, Torrance, Hermosa Beach, CA

Tumors of the Skin and Soft Tissues

Pedro Villegas, D.V.M., Ph.D.
Professor, Department of Avian Medicine, College of Veterinary Medicine, University of Georgia, Athens, GA

Egg Drop Syndrome, Inclusion Body Hepatitis/Hydropericardium Syndrome

Stephan W. Vogel, B.V.Sc.
Ridge Animal Hospital, Pretoria, South Africa

Heartwater

Dennis P. Wages, D.V.M., Dipl. A.C.P.V.
Professor, Department of Population Health and Pathobiology, College of Veterinary Medicine, North Carolina State University, Raleigh, NC

Enterococcosis (Poultry), Listeriosis (Poultry), Perirenal Hemorrhage Syndrome of Turkeys, Staphylococcosis (Poultry), Streptococcosis (Poultry)

Cheryl L. Waldner, D.V.M., Ph.D.
Associate Professor, Department of Large Animal Clinical Sciences, Western College of Veterinary Medicine, University of Saskatchewan, Saskatoon, Saskatchewan, Canada

Petroleum Product Poisoning

Michelle Wall, D.V.M., Dipl. A.C.V.I.M.
Oncology Resident, Department of Small Animal Medicine and Surgery, College of Veterinary Medicine, University of Georgia, Athens, GA

Heartworm Disease

Melissa S. Wallace, D.V.M., Dipl. A.C.V.I.M.
Regional Medical Director, VCA Animal Hospitals, Aurora, IL

Infectious Diseases of the Urinary System in Small Animals

David J. Waltisbuhl, B.App.Sc. (Med.Tech.), M.Sc.
Senior Scientist DPI&F Actest, Yeerongpilly Veterinary Laboratory, Yeerongpilly, Queensland, Australia

Cytauxzoonosis, Eperythrozoonosis

Stephen C. Waring, D.V.M., Ph.D.
Assistant Professor, Epidemiology and Environmental Science, Associate Director of Research, Center for Biosecurity and Public Health Preparedness, School of Public Health, University of Texas Health Science Center, Houston, TX

Zoonoses

Yoram Weisman, D.V.M., Ph.D.
Professor, Head Division of Avian Diseases, Kimron Veterinary Institute, Beit-Dagan, Israel

West Nile Virus Infection in Poultry

Nick Whelan, B.Sc., B.V.Sc., M.V.Sc., M.A.C.V.Sc., Dipl. A.C.V.C.P., Dipl. A.C.V.O.
Senior Lecturer in Veterinary Ophthalmology, Institute of Veterinary Animal and Biomedical Sciences, College of Sciences, Massey University, Palmerston North, New Zealand

Systemic Pharmacotherapeutics of the Eye

Brent R. Whitaker, M.S., D.V.M.
Director of Animal Health, National Aquarium in Baltimore, Baltimore, MD

Amphibians

Trevor J. Whitbread, B.Sc., B.V.Sc., M.R.C.V.S., Dipl. E.C.V.P.
Histopathology and Cytology Diagnostic Laboratories, Abbey Veterinary Services, Devon, UK

Diagnostic Procedures for the Private Practice Laboratory: Cytology

Patricia D. White, D.V.M., M.S., Dipl. A.C.V.D.
Atlanta Veterinary Skin & Allergy Clinic, Atlanta, GA

Allergic Inhalant Dermatitis (Atopy), Diseases of the Pinna, Otitis Externa

Stephen D. White, D.V.M., Dipl. A.C.V.D.
Professor, Department of Medicine and Epidemiology, School of Veterinary Medicine, University of California, Davis, CA

Food Allergy, Miscellaneous Systemic Dermatoses, Nasal Dermatoses of Dogs, Saddle Sores, Seborrhea, Urticaria

Susan L. White, D.V.M., M.S., Dipl. A.C.V.I.M.
Professor of Large Animal Internal Medicine, Department of Large Animal Medicine, College of Veterinary Medicine, University of Georgia, Athens, GA

Equine Encephalomyelitis

Mark L. Wickstrom, D.V.M., M.S., Ph.D.
Associate Professor, Department of Veterinary Biomedical Sciences, Western College of Veterinary Medicine, University of Saskatchewan, Saskatoon, Saskatchewan, Canada

Antiseptics and Disinfectants

Brian K. Wildman, D.V.M.
Feedlot Health Management Services, Okotoks, Alberta, Canada

Histophilosis

John W. Wilesmith, B.V.Sc., M.R.CV.S., Dipl. E.C.P.H., Hon. M.F.P.H.M.
Professor, Epidemiology Department, Veterinary Laboratories Agency (Weybridge), New Haw, Addlestone, Surrey, UK

Bovine Spongiform Encephalopathy

Pamela A. Wilkins, D.V.M., M.S., Ph.D., Dipl. A.C.V.I.M., Dipl. A.C.V.E.C.C.
Chief, Section of Emergency/Critical Care and Anesthesia, University of Pennsylvania, New Bolton Center, Kennett Square, PA

Equine Emergency Medicine

Philip J. Wilkinson, M.V.B., Ph.D., M.R.C.V.S.
Disease Security Officer, Institute for Animal Health, Pirbright Laboratory, Pirbright, Surrey, UK

African Swine Fever

Elizabeth S. Williams, B.S., D.V.M., Ph.D., Dipl. D.A.C.V.P.
Professor, Department of Veterinary Sciences, College of Agriculture, University of Wyoming, Laramie, WY

Chronic Wasting Disease

Kevin P. Winkler, D.V.M., Dipl. A.C.V.S.
Carolina Veterinary Specialists, Huntersville, NC

Wound Management

Zerai Woldehiwet, D.V.M., Ph.D., Dipl. Agric., M.R.C.V.S.
Department of Veterinary Pathology, University of Liverpool, Veterinary Teaching Hospital, Neston, Wirral, UK

Tick Pyemia, Tickborne Fever

Peter R. Woolcock, B.Sc., M.Sc., Ph.D.
School of Veterinary Medicine, University of California, Davis, CA; California Animal Health and Food Safety Laboratory System, Fresno, CA

Duck Viral Hepatitis

Patrick J. Wright, B.V.Sc., M.V.Sc., Ph.D.
Department of Veterinary Science, Veterinary Clinical Centre, University of Melbourne, Victoria, Australia

Management of Reproduction: Sheep

Robert Wylie, B.V.Sc., Q.D.A.
Ulladulla Veterinary Hospital, Ulladulla, New South Wales, Australia

Tick Paralysis

CIRCULATORY SYSTEM

THE BLOOD AND LYMPHATICS

HEMATOPOIETIC SYSTEM
INTRODUCTION

Blood supplies cells with water, electrolytes, nutrients, and hormones, and removes waste products. The cellular elements supply oxygen (RBC), protect against foreign organisms and antigens (white cells), and initiate coagulation (platelets). Because of the diversity of the hematopoietic system, its diseases are best discussed from a functional perspective. Function may be classified as either normal responses to abnormal situations (eg, leukocytosis and left shift in response to inflammation) or primary abnormalities of the hematopoietic system (eg, pancytopenia from marrow failure). Furthermore, abnormalities may be quantitative (ie, too many or too few cells) or qualitative (ie, abnormalities in function). (*See also* THE IMMUNE SYSTEM, p 645.)

RED BLOOD CELLS

The function of RBC is to carry oxygen to the tissues at pressures sufficient to permit rapid diffusion of oxygen. This is done by a carrier molecule, hemoglobin (Hgb); a vehicle (RBC) capable of bringing the intact Hgb to the cellular level; and a metabolism geared to protect both the RBC and the Hgb from damage. Interference with synthesis or release of Hgb, production or survival of RBC, or metabolism causes disease.

Hgb is a complex molecule, formed of 4 heme units attached to 4 globins (2 α and 2 β globins). Iron is added in the last step by the ferrochelatase enzyme. Interference with the normal production of heme or globin leads to anemia. Causes include copper or iron deficiency and lead poisoning. Hemoglobinopathies such as thalassemias and sickle cell anemia, important genetic diseases of people, have not been seen in other animals. In these diseases, the production of globins (α or β, or both) does not balance heme production, and the Hgb is not functional. The only known hemoglobinopathy of animals is porphyria. Although described in several species, it is most important as a cause of photosensitivity in cattle (*see* p 794).

Red cell mass, and thus oxygen-carrying capacity, remains constant over time in the healthy animal. Mature RBC have a finite life span; their production and destruction must be carefully balanced, or disease ensues.

Erythropoiesis is regulated by erythropoietin, which increases in the presence of hypoxia and regulates RBC production. In most species, the kidney is both the sensor organ and the major site of erythropoietin production, so chronic renal failure is associated with anemia. Erythropoietin acts on the marrow in concert with other humoral mediators to increase the number of stem cells entering RBC production, to shorten maturation time, and to cause early release of reticulocytes. Other factors that affect erythropoiesis are the supply of nutrients (eg, iron, folate, or vitamin B_{12}) and cell-cell interactions between erythroid precursors, lymphoid cells, and other components of the hematopoietic microenvironment. Factors that may suppress erythropoiesis include chronic debilitating diseases and endocrine disorders (such as hypothyroidism or hyperestrogenism).

Two mechanisms exist for removal of senescent RBC; both conserve the principal constituents of the cell for reuse. Removal of aged RBC normally occurs by phagocytosis by the fixed macrophages of the spleen. As the RBC ages it may change antigenically, acquiring senescent antigens and losing its flexibility due to impaired ATP production. Both of these changes increase the risk that the cell will become trapped in the spleen and be removed by macrophages. After phagocytosis and subsequent disruption of the cell membrane, Hgb is converted to heme and globin. Iron is released from the heme moiety and either stored in the macrophage as ferritin or hemosiderin, or released into the circulation for transport back to the marrow. The remaining heme is converted to bilirubin, which is released by the macrophages into the systemic circulation where it complexes with albumin for transport to the hepatocytes; there, it is conjugated and excreted into the bile. In extravascular hemolytic anemias, RBC have a shortened life span, and the same mechanisms occur at an increased rate.

About 1% of normal aging RBC are hemolyzed in the circulation, and free Hgb is released. This is quickly converted to Hgb dimers that bind to haptoglobin and are transported to the liver, where they are metabolized in the same manner as products from RBC removed by phagocytosis. In intravascular hemolytic anemia, more RBC are destroyed in the circulation (hemoglobinemia) than can be bound to haptoglobin. The excess Hgb and, therefore, iron are excreted in the urine (hemoglobinuria).

The principal metabolic pathway of RBC is glycolysis, and the main energy source in most species is glucose. Glucose enters the RBC by an insulin-independent mechanism, and most is metabolized to produce ATP and reduced nicotinamide adenine dinucleotide (NADH). The energy of ATP is used to maintain RBC membrane pumps so as to preserve shape and flexibility. The reducing potential of the NADH is utilized via the methemoglobin reductase pathway to maintain the iron in Hgb in its reduced form (Fe^{2+}).

The glucose not used in glycolysis is metabolized via a second pathway, the hexose monophosphate (HMP) shunt. No energy is produced via the HMP shunt; its principal effect is to maintain reducing potential in the form of reduced nicotinamide adenine dinucleotide phosphate (NADPH). In conjunction with the glutathione reductase/peroxidase system, NADPH maintains the sulfhydryl groups of globin in their reduced state.

Some disorders are the direct result of abnormal RBC metabolism and interference with glycolysis. Inherited deficiency of pyruvate kinase, a key glycolytic enzyme, causes ATP deficiency, which leads to reduced RBC life span and hemolytic anemia. Excessive oxidant stress may overload the protective HMP shunt or methemoglobin reductase pathways, causing Heinz body hemolysis or methemoglobin formation, respectively. Hemolytic anemias caused by certain drugs, such as phenothiazine in horses or acetaminophen in cats, are examples of this mechanism. (*See also* ANEMIA, p 14.)

A decreased RBC mass (anemia) may be caused by blood loss, hemolysis, or decreased production. In acute blood loss anemia, RBC are lost, but mortality is usually related to loss of circulating volume, rather than to loss of RBC. Iron is the limiting factor in chronic blood loss. Hemolysis may be caused by toxins, infectious agents, congenital abnormalities, or antibodies directed against RBC membrane antigens. Decreased RBC production may result from primary marrow diseases (eg, aplastic anemia, hematopoietic malignancy, or myelofibrosis) or from other causes such as renal failure, drugs, toxins, or antibodies directed against RBC precursors. Malignancy of RBC or their precursors may be acute (eg, erythroleukemia) or chronic (eg, polycythemia vera). Animals with erythroleukemia are anemic despite having a marrow filled with rubriblasts, whereas those with polycythemia vera have erythrocytosis.

WHITE BLOOD CELLS

Phagocytes: The principal function of phagocytes is to defend against invading microorganisms by ingesting and destroying them, thus contributing to cellular inflammatory responses. There are 2 types of phagocytes: mononuclear phagocytes and granulocytes. Mononuclear phagocytes arise primarily from the marrow and are released into the blood as monocytes. They may circulate for hours to a few days before entering the tissues and differentiating to become macrophages. Granulocytes have a segmented nucleus and are classified according to their staining characteristics as neutrophils, eosinophils, or basophils. Neutrophils circulate for only a few hours before travelling to the tissues.

Five distinct stages in the process of phagocytosis have been identified: 1) attraction of phagocytes (chemotaxis) to microorganisms, antigen-antibody complexes, and other mediators of inflammation; 2) attachment to the organism; 3) ingestion; 4) fusion of cell lysosomes with ingested microorganisms and bacterial killing; and 5) digestion. In addition, many phagocytes have other specialized functions. Monocytes form a link to the specific immune system by processing antigen for presentation to lymphocytes and by producing substances like interleukin-1, which initiates fever and lymphocyte activation and stimulates early hematopoietic progenitors.

Eosinophils, while having a role as phagocytes, also have more specific functions that include providing a defense against metazoan parasites and modulating the inflammatory process. They respond chemotactically to histamine, immune complexes, and eosinophil chemotactic factor of anaphylaxis, a substance released by degranulating mast cells. Basophils are not true phagocytes but contain large amounts of histamine as well as other mediators of inflammation. Both eosinophilia and basophilia may be seen in response to systemic allergic reactions and invasion of tissues by parasites.

As with the RBC, the production and circulating numbers of phagocytes are tightly regulated and controlled by various humoral factors, including colony-stimulating factors and interleukins. Unlike the RBC, which remain circulating in the blood, the phagocytes use this compartment as a pathway to the tissues. Consequently, the number of phagocytes in the blood reflects circumstances in the tissues (eg, inflammation) as well as the proliferative function of the bone marrow. The sensitivity with which phagocytes reflect these conditions varies from species to species. Abnormal response, such as neutropenia from marrow failure, infections, drugs, or toxins, is likely to result in secondary bacterial infections. Finally, phagocyte precursors may undergo malignant transformation, which results in acute or chronic myelogenous leukemia.

Lymphocytes: Lymphocytes are responsible for both humoral and cellular immunity. Cells of the 2 branches of the immune system cannot be differentiated morphologically, but they differ in their dynamics of production and circulation. Lymphocyte production in mammals originates in the bone marrow. Some of the lymphocytes destined to be involved in cellular immunity migrate to the thymus and differentiate further under the influence of thymic hormones. These become T cells and are responsible for a variety of helper or cytotoxic immunologic functions. Most circulating lymphocytes are T cells, but T cells are also present in the spleen and lymph nodes. The B cells migrate directly to organs without undergoing modification in the thymus and are responsible for humoral immunity (antibody production).

Thus, lymphoid organs have populations of both B and T lymphocytes. In the lymph nodes, follicular centers are primarily B cells, and parafollicular zones are primarily T cells. In the spleen, most of the lymphocytes of the red pulp are B cells, whereas those of the periarteriolar lymphoid sheaths are T cells. Close association of T cells and B cells within lymphoid organs is essential to immune function.

Lymphocyte function in the cellular immune system features both afferent (receptor) and efferent (effector) components. Long-lived T cells of the peripheral blood are the receptors. In response to antigens to which they have been previously sensitized, they leave the circulation and undergo blast transformation to form activated T cells, which in turn cause other T cells to undergo blast transformation, both locally and systemically. Stimulated T cells produce lymphokines with a wide range of activities, such as attraction and activation of neutrophils, macrophages, and lymphocytes.

The humoral immune system is composed of B cells that produce antibodies of several classes. When sensitized B cells encounter antigen, they divide and differentiate into plasma cells that produce antibody. Therefore, each initially stimulated B cell produces a clone of plasma cells, all producing the same specific antibody.

Antibody molecules (immunoglobulins) fall into several classes, each with its own functional characteristics. For example, IgA is the principal antibody of respiratory and intestinal secretions, IgM is the first antibody produced in response to a newly recognized antigen, IgG is the principal antibody of the circulating blood, and IgE is the principal antibody involved in allergic reactions.

Antibodies perform their function by combining with the specific antigens that stimulated their production. Antigen-antibody complexes may be chemotactic for phagocytes, or they may activate complement, a process that produces both cell lysis and substances chemotactic for neutrophils and macrophages. In this manner, the humoral immune system is related to, and interacts with, the nonspecific immune system.

The humoral immune system also is related to both the nonspecific immune system and the cellular immune system in other ways. Both "helper" (CD4) and "cytotoxic" (CD8) T-cell classes have been described. Helper T cells recognize processed antigen and activate the humoral immune response. Cytotoxic T cells, after sensitization by antigen, are effector cells, especially important in antiviral immunity. Natural killer cells, which are a class of lymphocyte distinct from T cells and B cells, destroy foreign cells (eg, neoplastic cells) even without prior sensitization. Antigen processing by macrophages precedes recognition of an antigen by lymphocytes. These complex processes are involved in routine surveillance against neoplastic cells and recognition of "self."

Lymphocyte response in disease may be appropriate (activation of the immune system) or inappropriate (immune-mediated disease and lymphoproliferative malignancies). (See also THE IMMUNE SYSTEM, p 645.) Immune-mediated disease results from failure of the immune system to recognize host tissues as self. For example, in immune-mediated hemolytic anemia, antibodies are produced against the host's own RBC. Another inappropriate response of the immune system is allergy. In allergic individuals, IgE antibodies to allergens are bound to the surface of basophils and mast cells. When exposure to the allergen occurs, antigen-antibody complexes are formed, and degranulation of the mast cells and basophils releases vasoactive amines. Reaction to this may be mild (as in urticaria or atopy) or life-threatening (as in anaphylaxis).

Lymphocytosis occurs in some species, especially the cat, as a response to epinephrine secretion. Atypical lymphocytes may be seen in the blood in response to antigenic stimulation (eg, vaccination). Persistent lymphocytosis in cattle infected with bovine leukemia virus is a benign polyclonal increase in lymphocyte numbers. Lymphoproliferative malignancies include lymphomas and acute lymphoblastic and chronic lymphocytic leukemias. Lymphopenia may occur most commonly as a response to glucocorticoid secretion.

PLATELETS

Platelets form the initial hemostatic plug whenever hemorrhage occurs. They also are the source of phospholipid, which is needed for the interaction of coagulation factors to form a fibrin clot. Platelets are produced in the bone marrow from megakaryocytes, under the influence of thrombopoietin. Platelet production begins with invagination of the megakaryocyte cell membrane and the formation of cytoplasmic channels and islands. The cytoplasmic islands produce platelets by fragmentation from the megakaryocyte.

Mature circulating platelets are packed with dense granules containing ATP, adenosine diphosphate (ADP), and calcium, as well as serotonin, lysosomes, glycogen, mitochondria, and an intracellular canalicular system. The mitochondria and glycogen are involved in energy production, and the canalicular system serves both as a transport system for granule components and as a source of phospholipid, which is found in high concentration in the membrane lining of the canals.

When vessel walls are damaged, collagen and tissue factor are exposed, and circulating platelets adhere via von Willebrand factor and undergo a change in shape with the accompanying release of ADP. Local platelet aggregation is stimulated by ADP with the ultimate formation of the primary platelet plug. The local accumulation of fibrin and platelets is known as a hemostatic plug. The fibrin clot which then forms is consolidated by the action of platelet contractile proteins.

Platelet disorders are either quantitative (thrombocytopenia or thrombocytosis) or qualitative (thrombocytopathy). Thrombocytopenia is one of the most common bleeding disorders of animals. In general, platelet counts must fall to <30,000/µL before the risk of hemorrhage increases. Consumption, destruction, or sequestration of platelets causes thrombocytopenia associated with increased production by the bone marrow. Consumptive thrombocytopenia occurs with massive hemorrhage or with disseminated intravascular coagulation, secondary to a variety of diseases. Destruction occurs in immune-mediated thrombocytopenia, in which platelets become coated with antiplatelet antibodies and are removed from the circulation by the fixed phagocyte system. Excessive sequestration of platelets by an enlarged spleen (hypersplenism) may occur in conditions such as myeloproliferative diseases. (See also HEMOSTATIC DISORDERS, p 37.)

Decreased production of platelets in the marrow may be caused by drugs, toxins, or by primary marrow disorders such as aplasia, fibrosis, or hematopoietic malignancy. In primary marrow disorders, more than one hematopoietic cell line is often decreased, resulting in pancytopenia.

Thrombocytosis occurs only rarely and is often idiopathic. It may be associated with primary marrow disease such as in megakaryocytic leukemia. Thrombocytosis is often associated with chronic blood loss and iron deficiency because of increased platelet production in the marrow reacting to continued consumption and loss.

Thrombocytopathies comprise a poorly defined group of diseases in which platelet numbers are normal, but their function is impaired. Von Willebrand disease is characterized primarily by a defect in platelet adhesion to the endothelium. The platelets themselves are normal. Other hereditary disorders of platelet function have been described but are relatively rare. Probably the most common platelet function defect is the irreversible inhibition of thromboxane (which is necessary for platelet aggregation) caused by aspirin administration.

ANEMIA

Anemia is defined as an absolute decrease in the red cell mass as measured by RBC count, hemoglobin concentration, and PCV. It can develop from loss, destruction, or lack of production of RBC. Anemia is classified as regenerative or nonregenerative. In a regenerative anemia, the bone marrow responds appropriately to the decreased red cell mass by increasing RBC production and releasing reticulocytes. In a nonregenerative anemia, the bone marrow responds inadequately to the increased need for RBC. Anemias due to hemorrhage or hemolysis are usually regenerative. Anemias that are caused by decreased erythropoietin or an abnormality in the bone marrow are nonregenerative.

Clinical Findings: Clinical signs in anemic animals depend on the degree of anemia, the duration (acute or chronic), and the underlying cause. Acute anemia can result in shock and even death if more than a third of the blood volume is lost rapidly and not replaced. In acute blood loss, the animal usually presents with tachycardia, pale mucous membranes, bounding or weak pulses, and hypotension. The cause of the blood loss may be obvious, eg, trauma. If no evidence of external bleeding is found, a source of internal or occult blood loss must be sought, eg, a ruptured splenic tumor, coagulopathy, GI ulceration or parasites, or other neoplasia. If hemolysis is present, the patient may be icteric. Patients with chronic anemia have had time to adjust, and their clinical presentation is usually more indolent with vague signs of lethargy, weakness, and anorexia. These patients will have similar physical examination findings, pale mucous membranes, tachycardia, and possibly splenomegaly or a new heart murmur, or both.

Diagnosis: A complete history is an important part of the work-up of an anemic animal. Questions might include duration of clinical signs, history of exposure to toxins (eg, rodenticides, heavy metals, toxic plants), drug treatments, vaccinations, travel history, and any prior illnesses.

A CBC, including a platelet and a reticulocyte count, will provide information on the severity of anemia and degree of bone marrow response, and also allow for evaluation of other cell lines. A blood smear should be evaluated for abnormalities in RBC morphology or size and for RBC parasites. The RBC indices (measures of size and hemoglobin concentration) are calculated by automated cell counters calibrated for the species in question. RBC size is expressed by the mean corpuscular volume (MCV) in femtoliters and usually reflects the degree of regeneration. Macrocytosis (an increase in the MCV) usually correlates with a regenerative anemia. Macrocytosis can be a heritable condition in poodles without anemia and may occur in anemic cats infected with feline leukemia virus. Microcytic RBC are the hallmark of iron-deficiency anemia. The hemoglobin concentration of each RBC, measured in g/dL, is defined as the mean corpuscular hemoglobin concentration. Abnormalities in RBC morphology, such as basophilic stippling, can indicate lead intoxication. Heinz body formation indicates oxidant injury to RBC, secondary to toxin exposure (see TABLE 1). Cats are more susceptible to Heinz body formation than other species, and even cats without anemia can have a small number of Heinz bodies.

The reticulocyte count is usually reported as a percent of the RBC mass. This value should be corrected for the degree of anemia in order to evaluate the degree of regeneration. An absolute reticulocyte count (measured by RBC/μL × reticulocyte percentage) of >50,000/μL or >60,000/μL in cats or dogs, respectively, is considered regenerative. In order to correct the percent reticulocytes, this formula can be applied:

$$\text{corrected reticulocyte \%} = (\text{observed reticulocyte \%}) \times \frac{(\text{PCV of the patient})}{(\text{normal PCV for that species})}$$

TABLE I.   Toxic Causes of Anemia

Pathogenic Mechanism	Drugs	Plants, Foods	Toxins, Chemicals	Heavy Metals
Oxidation	Acetaminophen, benzocaine, dapsone, nitrofurans, primaquine, propofol, quinacrine	Fava beans, oak, onions, propylene glycol, red maple	Crude oil, naphthalene	Copper, zinc
Blood loss	Aspirin, naproxen	Bracken fern, sweet clover	Dicoumarol	
Immune-mediated hemolysis	Cephalosporins, levamisole, penicillin, propylthiouracil, sulfonamides		Pirimicarb	
Hemolysis	Fenbendazole, heparin		Indole	Lead, selenium
Decreased marrow production	Amphotericin, azidothymidine, cephalosporins, chloramphenicol, estrogen, fenbendazole, griseofulvin, meclofenamic acid, phenobarbital, phenothiazine, phenylbutazone, propylthiouracil, quinidine, recombinant human erythropoietin, sulfonamides, thiacetarsamide	Bracken fern	Benzene, trichloroethylene	Lead

A corrected reticulocyte percent >1% indicates regeneration in the dog and cat. After acute blood loss or hemolytic crisis, reticulocytosis usually takes 3-4 days to become evident.

A serum chemistry panel and urinalysis evaluate organ function. If GI blood loss is suspected, an examination of the feces for occult blood and parasites can be useful. Radiographs can help identify occult disease, such as a penny (zinc toxicity) in the stomach of a puppy with hemolytic anemia. Bruising or bleeding may be signs of a coagulopathy and indicate the need for a coagulation profile. If hemolytic disease is suspected, blood can be evaluated for autoagglutination and a direct Coombs test might be indicated. A test for autoagglutination can be done by placing a drop of saline on a slide with a fresh drop of the patient's blood; the slide should be gently rotated to mix the drops together, then evaluated grossly and microscopically for macro- and microagglutination. Serology for infectious agents like feline leukemia virus, *Ehrlichia*, equine infectious anemia virus, and *Babesia* may also be helpful in defining the cause of anemia (*see* TABLE 2).

Bone marrow evaluation by aspiration and/or biopsy is indicated in any animal with an unexplained, nonregenerative anemia. If the CBC reveals a decrease in more than one

TABLE 2.   Infectious Causes of Anemia

Infectious Agent	Species Affected	Hemolytic	Marrow Affected
Bacteria			
Clostridium perfringens A	Cattle, sheep	Yes	No
Clostridium haemolyticum	Cattle, sheep	Yes	No
Leptospira interrogans	Cattle, pigs, sheep	Yes	No
Haemobartonella spp	Cattle, cats	±	No
Viruses			
Equine infectious anemia virus	Horses	±	Rarely
Feline leukemia virus	Cats	±	Yes
Feline immunodeficiency virus	Cats	No	Yes
Rickettsia			
Mycoplasma spp	Cattle, goats, llamas, pigs, sheep[*]	Yes (piglets only)	No
Anaplasma spp	Cattle, goats, sheep	Yes	No
Ehrlichia spp	Dogs	Yes	Yes
Protozoa			
Babesia spp	Cattle, cats, dogs, horses, sheep	Yes	No
Theileria spp[†]	Cattle, goats, sheep	±	No
Cytauxzoon spp	Cats	No	Yes
Trypanosoma spp	Cattle, horses, pigs	Yes	No
Sarcocystis cruzi	Cattle	Yes	No

[*]In adults, only clinically relevant in splenectomized or critically ill patients
[†]Pathogenic species of *Theileria* occur in Africa, the Mediterranean, the Middle East, Asia, and Europe. Species found in North America are nonpathogenic.

cell line, possibly indicating a hypoplastic marrow, a biopsy would be indicated along with an aspirate. Biopsies and aspirates are complementary: biopsies are better for evaluating the architecture and degree of cellularity of the marrow, and aspirates allow for better evaluation of cellular morphology. Aspirates also allow for an evaluation of orderly maturation of the red and white blood cell lines, the ratio of red to white blood cell precursors (M:E ratio), and the number of platelet precursors. Iron store can also be evaluated by Prussian blue staining. An M:E ratio of <1 indicates that red cell production is greater than white cell production; with an M:E ratio >1 the opposite is likely. The M:E ratio is always interpreted in light of a recent CBC, because changes in the ratio could also be due to suppression of one cell line compared to the other.

REGENERATIVE ANEMIAS

BLOOD LOSS ANEMIA

Acute blood loss can lead to shock and even death if >30-40% of blood is lost and the hypovolemia that develops is not treated aggressively with IV fluids or compatible blood (see BLOOD TRANSFUSIONS, p 16), or both. Causes of acute loss can be known (eg, trauma, surgery) or occult. Coagulopathies, bleeding tumors, gastric ulceration, and external or internal parasites should be excluded as causes. GI parasites, such as Haemonchus in ruminants and hookworms in dogs, can lead to severe blood loss, especially in young animals. Low-grade, chronic blood loss eventually results in iron deficiency anemia, although some degree of reticulocytosis may persist even after iron stores become depleted. The hallmark of an iron-deficiency anemia is a microcytic, hypochromic anemia. This chronic blood loss can be due to some type of parasitism in young animals (fleas, lice, intestinal parasitism), but in older animals, bleeding from GI ulcers or tumors is more common.

HEMOLYTIC ANEMIA

Hemolytic anemias are typically regenerative and result from lysis of RBC in either the intra- or extravascular space. Intravascular hemolysis results in hemoglobinemia and hemoglobinuria, whereas extravascular hemolysis does not. Both types of hemolysis can result in icterus. In dogs, the most common cause of hemolytic anemia is immune mediated, although toxins, RBC trauma, infections, and RBC membrane defects can also cause hemolysis.

Immune-mediated Hemolytic Anemia: Immune-mediated hemolytic anemia (IMHA, see p 651) can be primary or secondary to neoplasia, infection, drugs, or vaccinations. In IMHA, the body no longer recognizes RBC as self and develops antibodies to circulating RBC, leading to RBC destruction by macrophages and complement. In some cases, antibodies are directed against RBC precursors in the marrow, resulting in pure red cell aplasia and a nonregenerative anemia. Animals with IMHA are usually icteric, sometimes febrile, and may have splenomegaly. Hematologic hallmarks of IMHA are spherocytosis, autoagglutination, and a positive Coombs test.

Animals with IMHA can show mild, indolent signs or be in an acute crisis. It is important to tailor treatment to the animal's signs. Any underlying infections must be treated and unnecessary drug therapy discontinued. Fluid therapy should be started and supplemented with blood transfusions if indicated by the severity of signs. Bovine hemoglobin solutions (Oxyglobin®) may be given if compatible blood is not available. The goal of therapy is to stop the destruction of RBC by treating with immunosuppressive drugs. Prednisone at a dose of 2 mg/kg is usually the first choice for treatment. If the PCV does not stabilize or the patient relapses while receiving prednisone, other immunosuppressive drugs can be added. In the acute hemolytic crisis, drugs like cyclosporine (10 mg/kg, SID initially) or human intravenous immunoglobin (IVIG, 0.5-2 g/kg as a single dose) may have the most benefit. Dogs with adverse effects from prednisone may be gradually tapered off prednisone while being treated with new immunosuppressive drugs. Two such drugs that have been used in conjunction with, or instead of, prednisone are cyclophosphamide (2 mg/kg, once every other day) or azathioprine (2 mg/kg, SID or every other day).

Pulmonary thromboembolism is a risk in dogs with IMHA. The underlying cause is unknown, but the risk may be reduced by supportive care with fluids and transfusions. Fluids are important to maintain renal perfusion and to protect the kidneys from the high concentrations of circulating bilirubin. If thromboemboli are suspected or the risk for forming thromboemboli is high, heparin (100-200 IU/kg, SC, QID) can be used. If the pro-thrombin time and activated partial thromboplastin time are elevated or if signs of dis-seminated intravascular coagulation are present, fresh frozen plasma should be given at a rate of 10 mL/kg, BID until clinical signs or coagulation parameters improve. Mortality rates for IMHA range from 20-75%, depending on the severity of initial clinical signs. Neg-ative prognostic indicators include a rapid drop in PCV, high bilirubin concentration, in-travascular hemolysis, autoagglutination, and thromboembolic complications. Referral to tertiary care facilities may improve survival.

Alloimmune Hemolysis: Neonatal isoerythrolysis (NI) is an immune-mediated hemolytic disease seen in newborn horses, mules, cattle, pigs, cats, and, rarely, in dogs. NI is caused by ingestion of maternal colostrum containing antibodies to one of the neo-nate's blood group antigens. The maternal antibodies develop to specific foreign blood group antigens during previous pregnancies, unmatched transfusions, and from *Babesia* and *Anaplasma* vaccinations in cattle. Cats are unique in that blood type B cats have naturally occurring anti-A antibodies without prior exposure, and their kittens that are type A develop hemolysis after nursing. In horses, the antigens usually involved are A, C, and Q; NI is most commonly seen in Thoroughbreds and mules. Neonates with NI are normal at birth but develop severe hemolytic anemia within 2-3 days and become weak and icteric. Diagnosis is confirmed by screening maternal serum, plasma, or colostrum against the paternal or neonatal RBC. Treatment consists of stopping any colostrum while giving supportive care with transfusions. If necessary, neonates can be transfused with triple-washed maternal RBC. NI can be avoided by withholding maternal colostrum and giving colostrum from a maternal source free of the antibodies. The newborn's RBC can be mixed with maternal serum to look for agglutination before the newborn is al-lowed to receive maternal colostrum.

Microangiopathic Hemolysis: Microangiopathic hemolysis is caused by RBC damage secondary to turbulent flow through abnormal vessels. It can be seen in dogs secondary to severe heartworm infection, vascular tumors (hemangiosarcoma), splenic torsions, and disseminated intravascular coagulation; hemolytic uremic syndrome in calves, equine in-fectious anemia, African swine fever, and chronic classical swine fever are causes in other species. Schistocytes are common in blood smears from these patients. Treatment in-volves correction of the underlying disease process.

Metabolic Causes of Hemolysis: Hypophosphatemia (p 814) causes postparturient hemoglobinuria and hemolysis in cattle, sheep, and goats. It can occur 2-6 wk after par-turition. Hypophosphatemia with secondary hemolysis is seen in dogs and cats second-ary to diabetes mellitus, hepatic lipidosis, and refeeding syndrome. Treatment with ei-ther oral or IV phosphorus is indicated, depending on the degree of hypophosphatemia. Cattle that drink too much water (water intoxication) are at risk of developing hemoly-sis secondary to hypotonic plasma. This is seen in calves 2-10 mo of age and causes respiratory distress and hemoglobinuria. Clinical signs can progress to convulsions and coma. A calf with hemolytic anemia, hyponatremia and hypochloremia, decreased se-rum osmolality, and low urine specific gravity would support the diagnosis of water intoxication. Treatment consists of hypertonic fluids (2.5% saline) and diuretics (eg, mannitol).

Toxins: Toxins and drugs can cause anemia by many mechanisms. Those implicated most frequently in animals and their pathogenic mechanisms are listed in TABLE 1.

Infections: Many infectious agents—bacterial, viral, rickettsial, and protozoal—can cause anemia, by direct damage to RBC, leading to hemolysis, or by direct effects on precursors in the bone marrow (see TABLE 2).

Heritable Diseases: Several heritable RBC disorders cause anemia. Pyruvate kinase (PK) deficiencies are seen in Basenjis, Beagles, West Highland White Terriers, Cairn Terriers, and other breeds, as well as Abyssinian and Somali cats. Phosphofructokinase (PFK) deficiency occurs in English Springer Spaniels. Deficiencies in these enzymes lead to shortened RBC life span and a regenerative anemia. In dogs with PFK deficiency, the hemolytic crises are set off by alkalosis secondary to excessive excitement or exercise. If such situations are minimized, these dogs may have a normal life expectancy. There is no treatment for PK deficiency, and affected dogs will have a shortened life span due to myelofibrosis and osteosclerosis of the bone marrow. Affected cats will have chronic intermittent hemolytic anemia, which is sometimes helped by splenectomy and steroids. Unlike dogs, cats have not been reported to develop osteosclerosis. A hereditary hemoglobinopathy, porphyria (p 804), leads to build up of porphyrins in the body and has been described in cattle, cats, and pigs. It is most prevalent in Holstein cattle and can lead to a hemolytic crisis. Affected calves fail to thrive and are photosensitive. Diagnosis is made by finding increased levels of porphyrins in bone marrow, urine, or plasma. Teeth of affected animals fluoresce under ultraviolet light.

NONREGENERATIVE ANEMIAS

NUTRITIONAL DEFICIENCIES

Nutritional deficiency anemias develop when micronutrients needed for RBC formation are not present in adequate amounts. Anemia develops gradually and may initially be regenerative, but ultimately becomes nonregenerative. Starvation causes anemia by a combination of vitamin and mineral deficiencies as well as a negative energy and protein balance. Deficiencies most likely to cause anemia are: iron, copper, cobalamin (B_{12}), B_6, riboflavin, niacin, vitamin E, and vitamin C (only important in primates and guinea pigs).

Iron deficiency is the most common deficiency seen in dogs and piglets, but occurs less commonly in horses, cats, and ruminants. Iron deficiency is rarely nutritional in origin—it most commonly occurs secondary to blood loss (see BLOOD LOSS ANEMIA, p 11). Young animals have minimal iron stores, and milk contains very little iron. This can be especially important for piglets that grow rapidly and are often raised indoors with no access to iron. Oral iron supplementation is indicated as treatment for iron deficiency; any source of blood loss must be removed.

Copper deficiency can develop in ruminants fed forage grown in copper-deficient soil. Copper is necessary for the metabolism of iron. Copper deficiency may occur secondary to high dietary molybdenum or sulfate in cattle and can develop in pigs fed whey diets. Low blood copper concentrations or low copper concentrations in liver biopsies (more definitive) are diagnostic. Treatment is oral or injectable copper supplementation.

B vitamin deficiencies are rare. Certain drugs (anticonvulsants, drugs that interfere with folate metabolism) have been associated with the development of folate or cobalamin deficiency, leading to a normocytic, normochromic, nonregenerative anemia. Cobalamin malabsorption has been reported in Giant Schnauzers (their enterocytes are unable to absorb cobalamin). These dogs respond to parenteral supplementation with cobalamin. Ruminants also develop a secondary cobalamin deficiency when grazing on cobalt-deficient pasture. Treatment with oral cobalt or parenteral cobalamin is indicated.

ANEMIA OF CHRONIC DISEASE

Anemia of chronic disease can be characterized as mild to moderate, nonregenerative, normochromic, and normocytic. It is the most common form of anemia seen in animals. The anemia can be secondary to chronic inflammation or infection, neoplasia, liver disease, hyper- or hypoadrenocorticism, or hypothyroidism. The anemia is mediated by cytokines produced by inflammatory cells, which lead to decreases in iron availability, RBC survival, and the marrow's ability to regenerate. Treatment of the underlying disease results in resolution of the anemia. The anemia may be reduced by treatment with recombinant human erythropoietin, but the risk of antibody formation to endogenous erythropoietin probably outweighs any potential benefit.

RENAL DISEASE

Chronic renal disease is a common cause of nonregenerative anemia in animals. Erythropoietin is normally produced by the peritubular endothelial cells in the renal cortex. Animals with renal disease produce less erythropoietin, leading to anemia. Recombinant human erythropoietin (44-132 U/kg, 3 times/wk, with most animals starting at 88 U/kg) has been used for treatment. PCV is monitored weekly until the desired improvement is reached (this will vary with the initial degree of anemia), after which the dose is decreased. Animals receiving recombinant human erythropoietin require supplemental iron to support RBC production. (*See also* HEMATINICS, p 1975.)

PRIMARY BONE MARROW DISEASES

Primary bone marrow disease or failure from any cause can lead to nonregenerative anemia and pancytopenia. With diffuse marrow involvement, granulocytes are affected first, followed by platelets and finally RBC.

Aplastic anemia has been reported in dogs, cats, ruminants, horses, and pigs with pancytopenia and a hypoplastic marrow, replaced by fat. Most cases are idiopathic, but known causes include infections (feline leukemia virus, *Ehrlichia*), drug therapy, toxin ingestion, and total body irradiation (*see* TABLE 1 and TABLE 2). Treatment consists of eliminating the underlying cause and providing supportive measures such as broad-spectrum antibiotics, (amoxicillin/clavulanic acid, 20 mg/kg, BID) and transfusions. Recombinant human erythropoietin and granulocyte colony-stimulating factor (5 μg/kg, PO, SID) can be used until the marrow recovers. If the disease is idiopathic or if marrow recovery is unlikely (eg, phenylbutazone toxicity in dogs), bone marrow transplantation is beneficial if a suitable donor is available.

In pure red cell aplasia (PRCA), only the erythroid line is affected. It is characterized by a nonregenerative anemia with severe depletion of red cell precursors in the bone marrow. It has been reported in dogs and cats and may be primary or secondary. Primary cases are most commonly immune mediated and often respond to immunosuppressive therapy. Feline leukemia-positive cats can have PRCA. Recombinant human erythropoietin has been reported to cause PRCA in dogs and horses. Discontinuation of therapy may eventually lead to RBC recovery in some animals.

Primary leukemias are uncommon to rare in domestic species but have been reported in dogs, cats, cattle, goats, sheep, pigs, and horses. Retroviruses are a cause in some cattle, cats, primates, and chickens. Leukemias can develop in myeloid or lymphoid cell lines and are further classified as acute or chronic. Most affected animals have nonregenerative anemia, neutropenia, and thrombocytopenia, with circulating blasts usually present. Acute leukemias, characterized by infiltration of the marrow with blasts, generally respond poorly to chemotherapy. In animals that do respond, remission times are usually short. In acute lymphoblastic leukemia (ALL) in dogs, the response rate to chemotherapy is ~30% with a median survival of 4 mo. Acute myeloblastic leukemias are less common and even less responsive to treatment than ALL. In acute leukemias, the cell lineage is often difficult to identify morphologically, so cytochemical stains or immunologic evaluation of cell surface markers may be necessary for definitive diagnosis. Chronic leukemias, characterized by an overproduction of one hematopoietic cell line, are less likely to cause anemia and more responsive to treatment.

Myelodysplasia (myelodysplastic syndrome, MDS) is considered a preleukemic syndrome characterized by ineffective hematopoiesis, resulting in a nonregenerative anemia or other cytopenias. MDS has been described in dogs, cats, and humans. The disease can be primary or secondary and is commonly seen in cats with feline leukemia. Primary syndromes probably arise from mutations in stem cells. Secondary syndromes are caused by other neoplasia or drug therapy. Some cats and dogs respond to treatment with recombinant human erythropoietin and prednisone. Supportive care with transfusions may be helpful. Survival is variable because MDS can progress to leukemia; many animals are euthanized or die of sepsis, bleeding, or anemia.

Myelofibrosis causes bone marrow failure secondary to replacement of normal marrow elements with fibrous tissue. It has been observed in dogs, cats, humans, and goats. It can be a primary disorder or secondary to malignancies, immune-mediated hemolytic anemia, whole body irradiation, and congenital anemias (eg, pyruvate kinase deficiency). Diagnosis can be made by bone marrow biopsy. Treatment varies with the underlying cause but usually consists of immunosuppressive therapy.

BLOOD GROUPS AND BLOOD TRANSFUSIONS

Blood groups are determined by genetically controlled, polymorphic, antigenic components of the RBC membrane. The allelic products of a particular genetic locus are classified as a blood group system. Some of these systems are highly complex with many alleles defined at a locus; others consist of a single defined antigen. Blood group systems, in general, are independent of each other, and their inheritance conforms to Mendelian dominance. For polymorphic blood group systems, an animal usually inherits 1 allele from each parent and thus expresses no more than 2 blood group antigens of a system. An exception is in cattle, in which multiple alleles or "phenogroups" are inherited. Normally, an individual does not have antibodies against any of the antigens present on its own RBC or against other blood group antigens of that species' systems unless they have been induced by transfusion, pregnancy, or immunization. In some species (human, sheep, cow, pig, horse, cat, and dog), so-called "naturally occurring" isoantibodies, not induced by transfusion or pregnancy, may be present in variable but detectable titers. For example, Group B cats have naturally occurring anti-A antibody. Also, circulating antibodies to animal blood group antigens may be induced by transfusion. With random blood transfusions in dogs, there is a 30-40% chance of sensitization of the recipient, primarily to blood group antigen DEA 1. In horses, transplacental immunization of the mare by an incompatible fetal antigen inherited from the sire may occur. Immunization also may result when some homologous blood products are used as vaccines (eg, anaplasmosis in cattle).

The number of major recognized blood group systems (TABLE 3) varies among domestic species, with cattle being the most complex and cats the simplest. Animal blood groups are typed to aid in the matching of donors and recipients and to identify breeding pairs potentially at risk of causing hemolytic disease in their offspring. Because expression of blood group antigens is genetically controlled and the modes of inheritance are understood,

TABLE 3.	Major Blood Groups of Clinical Interest	
	Species	**Blood Group**
	Canine	DEA 1.1 and 7
	Feline	A, B
	Equine	A, C, Q
	Bovine	B, J
	Ovine	B, R

these systems also have been used to substantiate pedigrees in cattle and horses; however in most cases, DNA testing has replaced blood typing for paternity testing.

Blood Typing

Antisera used to identify blood groups (typing reagents) usually are produced as isoimmune sera. Their in vitro serologic characteristics vary with the species. Many reagents are hemagglutinins; others are hemolytic and require complement to complete the serologic reaction, such as in cattle (because RBC do not readily agglutinate) and horses (because RBC rouleaux are a problem). Other typing reagents, neither hemagglutinating nor hemolytic, combine with RBC antigens in an "incomplete" reaction because they lack additional combining sites to agglutinate other RBC; addition of species-specific antiglobulin is required for agglutination.

Crossmatching

The direct crossmatch procedure, with appropriate controls, is effective for all species. The **major crossmatch** detects antibodies already present in recipient plasma that could cause a hemolytic reaction when donor RBC are transfused; it will not detect the potential for sensitization to develop. Anticoagulant (calcium disodium edetate or citrate) is added to blood samples from donor and recipient; the donor RBC are washed 3 times with 0.9% saline, and a 4% RBC suspension in saline is made from the washed cells. The major crossmatch consists of combining equal volumes (0.1 mL) of the donor RBC suspension and recipient plasma. The control tube contains recipient RBC and recipient plasma. The samples are incubated, centrifuged, and evaluated for hemolysis or agglutination. Hemolysis is evaluated by comparing the color of the supernatant in the test sample with that of the control sample. Each sample is then gently shaken until all cells in the "button" at the bottom of the tube have returned to suspension. Again, the degree of cell clumping of the test sample is compared with that of the control sample. The test is negative or compatible when the plasma is clear and the RBC are readily suspended. A positive or incompatible test can have hemolysis or hemagglutination, or both. All tests judged macroscopically to be negative for hemagglutination should be confirmed microscopically at low power. This is particularly important in horses because their RBC tend to form rouleaux.

The **minor crossmatch** is the reverse of the major crossmatch, ie, recipient cells are combined with donor plasma. The minor crossmatch is important only in species with naturally occurring isoantibodies or if the donor has been previously transfused or, in horses, previously pregnant.

Blood Transfusions

Frequently, the need for blood transfusions is acute, as in acute hemolysis or hemorrhage; transfusions are also appropriate in treatment of acute or chronic anemias. Animals with hemostatic disorders often require repeated transfusions of either whole blood, red cells, plasma, or platelets. Blood transfusions must be given with care because they have the potential for further compromising the recipient. The diversity of blood groups in animals and the lack of commercially available blood-typing reagents make complete typing and matching difficult but should not preclude the clinical use of transfusions. In horses and dogs, the blood group antigens most commonly implicated in transfusion incompatibilities are known; by selecting donor animals that lack these groups, or that match the recipient, the risk of sensitization of the recipient to the most important antigens can be minimized. Previously sensitized recipients can be detected by crossmatching, which will preclude administration of incompatible blood. In the USA, >99% of cats are of blood group A, so the risk of incompatible transfusion is low. However, certain breeds, including Abyssinian, Birman, British Shorthair, Devon Rex, Himalayan, Persian, Scottish Fold, and Somali, have a higher frequency of blood group B. Any incompatible transfusion in cats results in rapid destruction of transfused cells, so typing or crossmatching should be done before any transfusion.

Whole blood frequently is not the ideal product to be administered. If the need is to replace the oxygen-carrying capability of the blood, then packed RBC are more appropriate; if replacement of circulatory volume is needed, crystalloid or colloid solutions may be used to replace volume, with packed RBC added as needed. Platelet numbers rise rapidly after hemorrhage, so replacement is rarely needed. Plasma proteins equilibrate from the interstitial space, so plasma is not needed except in massive hemorrhage (>1 blood volume in 24 hr). Animals that require coagulation factors benefit most from administration of fresh-frozen plasma or cryoprecipitate if the need is specifically for factor VIII, von Willebrand factor, or fibrinogen. Platelet-rich plasma or platelet concentrates may be of value in thrombocytopenia, although immune-mediated thrombocytopenia usually does not respond to administration of platelets because they are removed rapidly by the spleen.

The amount of RBC required to treat anemia is based on the volume necessary to increase the PCV or Hgb concentration to the desired value. All domestic animals have blood volumes of ~7% of their body weight except cats, which have a blood volume of 4% of their body weight. By determining the recipient's blood volume and knowing the animal's PCV, the required replacement RBC volume can be calculated. For example, a 25-kg dog has a total blood volume of ~2,000 mL; with a PCV of 15%, the RBC volume is 300 mL; if the PCV is to be increased to 20%, that equals an RBC volume of 400 mL. Therefore, 100 mL of RBC or 200 mL of whole blood (with PCV of 50%) would be required to increase the recipient's PCV to the desired level. These calculations assume no ongoing losses of RBC through hemorrhage or hemolysis. No more than 25% of a donor animal's blood should be collected at one time.

Collection, storage, and transfusion of blood must be done aseptically. The anticoagulant of choice is citrate phosphate dextrose adenine (CPDA-1). Commercial blood bags containing the appropriate amount of anticoagulant are less damaging to blood cells than are vacuum collection bottles. Heparin should not be used as an anticoagulant because it has a longer half-life in the recipient and causes platelet activation; also, heparinized blood cannot be stored.

Blood collected in CPDA-1 may be safely stored at 4°C for 3 wk. If the blood will not be used immediately, the plasma can be removed and stored frozen for later use as a source of coagulation factors or albumin for acute reversible hypoalbuminemia. Chronic hypoproteinemia is not helped by plasma because the total body deficit of albumin is so large that it could not be improved by the small amount contained in plasma. Plasma must be frozen at -20° to -30°C within 6 hr of collection to assure that levels of factor VIII are adequate and will remain so for 1 yr.

Risks of Transfusion: The most serious risk of transfusion is acute hemolysis. Fortunately, this is rare in domestic animals. Dogs rarely have clinically significant preformed antibodies, so only those that have received repeated transfusions are at risk. The most common hemolytic reaction in dogs that have received multiple transfusions is delayed hemolysis, seen clinically as shortened survival of transfused RBC and a positive Coombs' test. Even crossmatch-compatible RBC given to horses or cattle survive only 2-4 days. Repeated transfusions can cause acute hemolysis. Nonimmune causes of hemolysis include improper collection or separation of blood, freezing or overwarming of RBC, and infusing under pressure through a small needle.

Other complications include sepsis from contaminated blood, hypocalcemia from too much citrate, and hypervolemia (especially in animals with preexisting heart disease or in very small animals). Urticaria, fever, or vomiting are seen occasionally. Transfusions can also spread disease from donor to recipient, such as RBC parasites (eg, *Haemobartonella*, *Anaplasma*, or *Babesia*) and viruses (eg, retroviruses such as feline or bovine leukemia, equine infectious anemia, or other slow viruses). Other diseases, such as those caused by rickettsia or other bacteria, can also be spread if the donor is bacteremic.

Blood Substitutes: Hemoglobin-based Oxygen Carrier Solutions

Because of problems associated with finding compatible donors and disease transmission by transfusion, the search for a red cell substitute has been ongoing for >50 yrs. An ideal substitute would carry and deliver oxygen like red cells, be easy to produce in large quantities, be nonantigenic, and persist in the circulation at least long enough for resuscitation.

One hemoglobin-based oxygen carrier of bovine origin is currently licensed for use in dogs (Oxyglobin®, Biopure Corporation, Cambridge, MA). The hemoglobin is collected aseptically, filtered to removed all red cell stromal elements, and polymerized to allow the product to persist in the circulation for a half-life of ~36 hr. This product has been shown to carry and deliver oxygen efficiently, can be used immediately without need for typing or crossmatching, and has a 3-yr shelf life at room temperature. Because the structure of the hemoglobin molecule is similar between species, bovine hemoglobin is minimally antigenic. Although currently licensed for use only in dogs, it has been used in cats, horses, llamas, birds, and humans. Its colloidal effects are especially useful in resuscitation after trauma with acute blood loss.

In healthy animals, hemoglobin within RBC picks up oxygen from the lungs and deposits it in the tissues via the capillary microcirculation. Only a very small amount of oxygen can be carried dissolved in plasma. In an anemic animal, the hemoglobin within each red cell becomes fully saturated with oxygen, but tissue oxygenation is inadequate simply because fewer red cells are present. In hypotension, hypovolemia, or local tissue ischemia, oxygen delivery may be further impaired because of constriction or decreased perfusion of capillaries. If hemoglobin solution is given, the oxygen content of the plasma improves, and the delivery of oxygen becomes easier because the oxygen is already in contact with endothelium, and has only to diffuse into the tissues. Because the viscosity of the blood is lower after hemoglobin transfusion than it would be after a comparable volume of blood, perfusion of small capillaries is better.

BLOOD PARASITES

ANAPLASMOSIS

Anaplasmosis, formerly known as gall sickness, traditionally refers to a disease of ruminants caused by obligate intraerythrocytic bacteria of the order Rickettsiales, family Anaplasmataceae, genus *Anaplasma*. Cattle, sheep, goats, buffalo, and some wild ruminants can be infected with the erythrocytic *Anaplasma*. Anaplasmosis occurs in tropical and subtropical regions worldwide (~40° N to 32° S), including South and Central America, the USA, southern Europe, Africa, Asia, and Australia.

The *Anaplasma* genus has recently been expanded to include species transferred from the genus *Ehrlichia*, now named *Anaplasma phagocytophilum* (compiled from species previously known as *Ehrlichia phagocytophila, E equi,* and human granulocytic ehrlichiosis agent), *A bovis* (previously *E bovis*), and *A platys* (previously *E platys*), all of which invade blood cells other than erythrocytes of their respective mammalian hosts. Bovine anaplasmosis is of economic significance in the cattle industry.

Etiology: Clinical bovine anaplasmosis is usually caused by *A marginale*. Cattle are also infected with *A centrale*, which generally results in mild disease. *A ovis* may cause mild to severe disease in sheep, deer, and goats.

Transmission and Epidemiology: Anaplasmosis is not contagious. Numerous species of tick vectors (*Boophilus, Dermacentor, Rhipicephalus, Ixodes, Hyalomma,* and *Ornithodoros*) can transmit *Anaplasma* spp. Not all of these are likely significant vectors in the field, and it has been shown that strains of *A marginale* also co-evolve with particular tick strains. *Boophilus* spp are major vectors in Australia and Africa, and *Dermacentor* spp have been incriminated as the main vectors in the USA. After feeding on an infected animal, intrastadial or trans-stadial transmission may occur. Transovarial transmission may also occur, although this is rare, even in the single-host *Boophilus* spp. A replicative cycle occurs in the infected tick. Mechanical transmission via biting dipterans occurs in some regions. Transplacental transmission has been reported and is usually associated with acute infection of the dam in the second or third trimester of gestation. Anaplasmosis may also be spread through the use of contaminated needles or dehorning or other surgical instruments.

There is a strong correlation between age of cattle and severity of disease. Calves are much more resistant to disease (although not infection) than older cattle. This resistance is not due to colostral antibody from immune dams. In endemic areas where cattle first become infected with *A marginale* early in life, losses due to anaplasmosis are minimal. After recovery from the acute phase of infection, cattle remain chronically infected carriers but are generally immune to further clinical disease. However, these chronically infected cattle may relapse to anaplasmosis when immunosuppressed (eg, by corticosteroids), when infected with other pathogens, or after splenectomy. Carriers serve as a reservoir for further transmission. Serious losses occur when mature cattle with no previous exposure are moved into endemic areas or when under endemically unstable situations when transmission rates are insufficient to ensure all cattle are infected before reaching the more susceptible adult age.

Clinical Findings: In animals <1 yr old anaplasmosis is usually subclinical, in yearlings and 2 yr olds it is moderately severe, and in older cattle it is severe and often fatal. Anaplasmosis is characterized by progressive anemia due to extravascular destruction of infected and uninfected erythrocytes. The prepatent period of *A marginale* is directly related to the infective dose and typically ranges from 15-36 days (although it may be as long as 100 days). After the prepatent period, peracute (most severe but rare), acute, or chronic anaplasmosis may follow. Rickettsemia approximately doubles every 24 hr during the exponential growth phase. Generally, 10-30% of erythrocytes are infected at peak rickettsemia, although this figure may be as high as 65%. RBC count, PCV, and hemoglobin values are all severely reduced. Macrocytic anemia with circulating reticulocytes may be present late in the disease.

Animals with peracute infections succumb within a few hours of the onset of clinical signs. Acutely infected animals lose condition rapidly. Milk production falls. Inappetence, loss of coordination, breathlessness when exerted, and a rapid bounding pulse are usually evident in the late stages. The urine may be brown but, in contrast to babesiosis, hemoglobinuria does not occur. A transient febrile response, with the body temperature rarely exceeding 106°F (41°C) occurs at about the time of peak rickettsemia. Mucous membranes appear pale and then yellow. Pregnant cows may abort. Surviving cattle convalesce over several weeks, during which hematologic parameters gradually return to normal.

Bos indicus breeds of cattle appear to possess a greater resistance to *A marginale* infection than *B taurus* breeds, but variation of resistance of individuals within breeds of both species occurs. Difference in virulence between *Anaplasma* strains and the level and duration of the rickettsemia also play a role in the severity of clinical manifestations.

Lesions: Lesions are typical of those occurring in animals with anemia due to erythrophagocytosis. The carcasses of cattle that die from anaplasmosis are generally markedly anemic and jaundiced. Blood is thin and watery. The spleen is characteristically enlarged and soft, with prominent follicles. The liver may be mottled and yellow-orange. The gallbladder is often distended and contains thick brown or green bile. Hepatic and mediastinal lymph nodes appear brown. There are serous effusions in body cavities, pulmonary edema, petechial hemorrhages in the epi- and endocardium, and often evidence of severe GI stasis. Widespread phagocytosis of erythrocytes is evident on microscopic examination of the reticuloendothelial organs. A significant proportion of erythrocytes are usually found to be parasitized after death due to acute infection.

Diagnosis: *A marginale*, together with the hemoprotozoa *Babesia bovis* and *B bigemina*, are the causative agents of tick fever in cattle. These 3 species have similar geographic distributions, except that anaplasmosis occurs in the absence of babesiosis in the USA. Microscopic examination of Giemsa-stained thin and thick blood films is critical to distinguish anaplasmosis from babesiosis (p 20) and other conditions that result in anemia and jaundice, such as leptospirosis (p 525) and theileriosis (p 30). Blood in anticoagulant should also be obtained for hematologic testing. In Giemsa-stained thin blood films, *Anaplasma* spp appear as dense, homogeneously staining blue-purple inclusions 0.3-1.0 μm in diameter. *A marginale* inclusions are usually located toward the margin of the infected erythrocyte, whereas *A centrale* inclusion bodies are located more centrally. *A caudatum* cannot be distinguished from *A marginale* using Giemsa-stained blood films.

Special staining techniques are used to identify this species based on observation of characteristic appendages associated with the bacteria. *A caudatum* has only been reported in North America and could possibly be a morphologic form of *A marginale* and not a separate species. Inclusion bodies contain 1-8 initial bodies 0.3-0.4 μm in diameter, which are the individual rickettsiae.

Chronically infected carriers may be identified with a fair degree of accuracy by serologic testing using msp5 ELISA, complement fixation, or card agglutination tests. DNA-based detection methods are most useful as species and strain differentiation tests.

At necropsy, thin blood films of liver, kidney, spleen, lungs, and peripheral blood should be prepared for microscopic examination.

Treatment: Tetracycline antibiotics and imidocarb are currently used for treatment. Cattle may be sterilized by treatment with these drugs and remain immune to severe anaplasmosis subsequently for at least 8 mo.

Prompt administration of tetracycline drugs (tetracycline, chlortetracycline, oxytetracycline, rolitetracycline, doxycycline, minocycline) in the early stages of acute disease (eg, PCV >15%) usually ensures survival. A commonly used treatment consists of a single IM injection of long-acting oxytetracycline at a dosage of 20 mg/kg. Blood transfusion to partially restore the PCV greatly improves the survival rate of more severely affected cattle. The carrier state may be eliminated by administration of a long-acting oxytetracycline preparation (20 mg/kg, IM, at least 2 injections with a 1-wk interval). Withholding periods for tetracyclines apply in most countries. Injection into the neck muscle rather than the rump is preferred.

Imidocarb is also highly efficacious against *A marginale* as a single injection (as the dihydrochloride salt at 1.5 mg/kg, SC, or as imidocarb dipropionate at 3.0 mg/kg). Elimination of the carrier state requires the use of higher repeated doses of imidocarb (eg, 5 mg/kg, IM or SC, 2 injections of the dihydrochloride salt 2 wk apart). Imidocarb is a suspected carcinogen with long withholding periods and is not approved for use in the USA or Europe.

Prevention: In South Africa, Australia, Israel, and South America, infection with live *A centrale* (originating from South Africa) is used as a vaccine to provide cattle with partial protection against the disease caused by *A marginale*. *A centrale* (single dose) vaccine produces severe reactions in a small proportion of cattle. In the USA, where live vaccines cannot be used, vaccines comprising nonliving *A marginale* purified from infected bovine erythrocytes and adjuvant have been used in the past but may not currently be available. Immunity generated by using multidose killed vaccine protects cattle from severe disease on subsequent infection, but cattle can still be susceptible to challenge with heterologous strains of *A marginale*. Instances of isoerythrolysis in suckling calves have occurred due to prior vaccination of dams with preparations that contained bovine erythrocytic material. Long-lasting immunity against *A marginale* is conferred by preimmunization with live rickettsia, combined with the use of chemotherapy to control severe reactions. The use of attenuated strains of *A marginale* as a live vaccine has been reported, with instances of severe reactions also occurring. *A marginale* grown in tick cell cultures are being investigated as an alternative live vaccine source. Subunit vaccines to control bovine anaplasmosis are also under investigation. In some areas, sustained stringent control or elimination of the arthropod vectors may be a viable control strategy; however, in other areas immunization is recommended.

BABESIOSIS

Babesiosis is caused by intraerythrocytic protozoan parasites of the genus *Babesia*. The disease, which is transmitted by ticks, affects a wide range of domestic and wild animals and occasionally humans. While the major economic impact of babesiosis is on the cattle industry, infections in other domestic animals, including horses, sheep, goats, pigs, and dogs, assume varying degrees of importance throughout the world.

Two important species in cattle—*B bigemina* and *B bovis*—are widespread in tropical and subtropical areas and are the focus of this discussion. However, because there are many common features of the diseases caused by different *Babesia*, much of this information can be applied to other species.

Transmission and Epidemiology: The main vectors of *Babesia bigemina* and *B bovis* are 1-host *Boophilus* spp ticks, in which transmission occurs transovarially. While the parasites can be readily transmitted experimentally by blood inoculation, mechanical transmission by insects or during surgical procedures has no practical significance. Intrauterine infection has also been reported but is rare.

In *Boophilus* spp ticks, the blood stages of the parasite are ingested during engorgement and undergo life cycles in the replete female, eggs, and subsequent parasitic stages. Transmission to the host occurs when larvae (in the case of *B bovis*) or nymphs and adults (in the case of *B bigemina*) feed. The percentage of larvae infected can vary from 0-50% or higher, depending mainly on the level of parasitemia of the host at the time the female ticks engorge. Under field conditions, the rate of tick transmission is generally higher for *B bigemina* than for *B bovis*.

In endemic areas, 2 features are important in determining the risk of clinical disease: 1) calves have a degree of immunity (related both to colostral-derived antibodies and to age) that persists for ~6 mo, and 2) animals that recover from *Babesia* infections are generally immune for life. Thus, at high levels of tick transmission, all newborn calves will become infected with *Babesia* by 6 mo of age, show few if any clinical signs, and subsequently be immune. This situation of endemic stability can be upset by either a natural (eg, climatic) or artificial (eg, acaricide treatment) reduction in tick numbers to levels such that tick transmission of *Babesia* to calves is insufficient to ensure all are infected during this critical early period. Other circumstances that can lead to clinical outbreaks include the introduction of susceptible cattle to endemic areas and the incursion of *Babesia*-infected ticks into previously tick-free areas. Strain variation in immunity has been demonstrated but is probably not of significance in the field.

Clinical Findings and Pathogenesis: The acute disease generally runs a course of ~1 wk. The first sign is fever (frequently 105.8°F [41°C] or higher), which persists throughout, and is accompanied later by inappetence, increased respiratory rate, muscle tremors, anemia, jaundice, and weight loss; hemoglobinemia and hemoglobinuria occur in the final stages. CNS involvement due to adhesion of parasitized erythrocytes in brain capillaries can occcur with *B bovis* infections. Either constipation or diarrhea may be present. Late-term pregnant cows may abort, and bulls may undergo temporary infertility due to transient fever.

With virulent strains of *B bovis*, a hypotensive shock syndrome, combined with generalized nonspecific inflammation, coagulation disturbances, and erythrocytic stasis in capillaries, contribute to the pathogenesis. With most strains of *B bigemina*, the pathogenic effects relate more directly to erythrocyte destruction.

Animals that recover from the acute disease remain infected for a number of years with *B bovis* and for a few months in the case of *B bigemina*. No clinical signs are apparent during this carrier state.

The susceptibility of cattle breeds to *Babesia* infections varies; for example, *Bos indicus* cattle tend to be more resistant to *B bovis* and *B bigemina* infection than are European breeds.

Lesions: Lesions include an enlarged and friable spleen; a swollen liver with an enlarged gallbladder containing thick granular bile; congested, dark-colored kidneys; and generalized anemia and jaundice. The urine is often, but not invariably, red. Other organs, including the brain and heart, may show congestion or petechiae.

Diagnosis: Clinically, babesiosis can be confused with other conditions that cause fever, anemia, hemolysis, jaundice, or red urine. Therefore, confirmation of a diagnosis by microscopic examination of Giemsa-stained blood or organ smears is essential. From the live animal, thick and thin blood smears should be prepared, preferably from capillaries in the ear or tail tip.

Smears of heart muscle, kidney, liver, lung, brain, and from a blood vessel in an extremity (eg, lower leg) should be taken at necropsy.

Microscopically, the species of *Babesia* involved can be determined morphologically, but some expertise is required. *B bovis* is small, with the parasites in paired form at an obtuse angle to each other and measuring ~1-1.5 × 0.5-1.0 mm. *B bigemina* is larger (3-3.5 × 1-1.5 mm), with paired parasites at an acute angle to each other.

A number of serologic tests are available for the detection of carrier animals. The most commonly used are the indirect fluorescent antibody test and ELISA. A procedure that may occasionally be justified to confirm infection in suspected carrier animals is the inoculation of blood (~500 mL) into a fully susceptible animal, preferably a splenecto-mized calf, and subsequent monitoring of the recipient for infection. PCR assays capable of detecting extremely low parasitemias, as occur in carrier animals, and differentiating isolates are available but are not in routine use.

Treatment and Control: A variety of drugs have been used to treat babesiosis in the past, but only diminazene aceturate and imidocarb dipropionate are still in common use. These drugs are not available in all endemic countries, or their use may be restricted. Diminazene is given IM at 3-5 mg/kg. For treatment, imidocarb is given SC at 1.2 mg/kg. At a dosage of 3.0 mg/kg, imidocarb provides protection from babesiosis for ~4 wk and will also eliminate *B bovis* and *B bigemina* from carrier animals. Long-acting tetracy-cline (20 mg/kg) may reduce the severity of babesiosis if treatment begins before or soon after infection.

Supportive treatment is advisable, particularly in valuable animals, and may include the use of anti-inflammatory drugs, antioxidants, and corticosteroids. Blood transfu-sions may be life-saving in very anemic animals.

Vaccination using live, attenuated strains of the parasite has been used successfully in a number of countries, including Argentina, Australia, Brazil, Israel, South Africa, and Uruguay. The vaccine is provided in either a chilled or a frozen form. One vaccination produces adequate immunity for the commercial life of the animal; however, vaccine breakdowns have been reported. Several recombinant antigens have been shown exper-imentally to induce immunity, but commercial vaccines are not available.

While controlling the tick vector can break the transmission cycle, this approach (short of complete eradication) is rarely feasible in the longterm and can lead to instabil-ity in endemic areas.

Zoonotic Risk: A small number of cases of human babesiosis have been reported, but the species involved often has not been identified with certainty. *Babesia divergens*, *B canis*, *B microti*, and an unnamed species (WA-1), have been incriminated. Cases re-ported in splenectomized or otherwise immunocompromised individuals are often fatal.

Numerous cases, varying in severity from inapparent infections to acute illness, have been documented in both splenectomized and nonsplenectomized people in parts of North America. These infections were caused by the rodent parasite *B microti* or an unnamed species (WA-1) whose host appears to be the Bighorn sheep. Human *Babesia* infections are acquired via bites from infected ticks, or through contaminated blood from an infected transfusion donor.

Other Important *Babesia* of Domestic Animals

Cattle: *Babesia divergens* and *B major* are 2 temperate-zone species with features comparable to those of *B bovis* and *B bigemina*, respectively. *B divergens* is a small, pathogenic *Babesia* of considerable importance in the British Isles and northwest Europe, whereas *B major* is a large *Babesia* of lower pathogenicity. *B divergens* is transmitted by *Ixodes ricinus*, and *B major* by *Haemaphysalis punctata*.

Horses: Equine babesiosis is caused by *Theileria* (formerly *Babesia*) *equi* or *B caballi*. *T equi* is a small parasite and is more pathogenic than *B caballi*. *T equi* was reclassified as a *Theileria* (*see* THEILERIASES, p 30) in 1998. Equine babesiosis occurs in Africa, Eu-rope, Asia, South and Central America, and the southern USA. It is transmitted by ticks of the genera *Rhipicephalus*, *Dermacentor*, and *Hyalomma*. Intrauterine infection, par-ticularly with *T equi*, is also relatively common.

Sheep and Goats: The 2 important species of small ruminants are *B ovis* and *B motasi*. Infection is widespread in the Middle East and southern Europe and through tropical and subtropical areas. Ticks of the genera *Rhipicephalus*, *Haemaphysalis*, *Hyalomma*, *Dermacentor*, and *Ixodes* have been incriminated as vectors.

Pigs: *Babesia trautmanni* has been recorded as causing severe disease in pigs. This parasite has been reported from Europe and Africa. Another species, *B perroncitoi*, is of similar pathogenicity but apparently has a limited distribution in the areas mentioned above. The vectors of these *Babesia* have not been clarified, although *Rhipicephalus* spp have been shown to transmit *B trautmanni*.

Dogs and Cats: *Babesia canis* has been reported in dogs from most regions and consists of subspecies *B canis canis*, *B canis vogeli*, and *B canis rossi*. *B canis canis* is transmitted by *Dermacentor reticularis* in Europe, *B canis vogeli* by *Rhipicephalus sanguineus* in tropical and subtropical countries, and *B canis rossi* by *Haemaphysalis leachi* in South Africa. Clinical signs of *B canis* infection vary from a mild, transient illness to acute disease that rapidly results in death. A vaccine based on a *B canis canis* exoantigen is available in Europe but does not protect against the other subspecies. *B gibsoni* is the other important *Babesia* of dogs and is a much smaller parasite. It has a more limited distribution and characteristically causes a chronic disease with progressive, severe anemia as the main sign.

Illness of varying severity due to *B felis* has been reported in domestic cats in Africa and India. An unusual feature is its lack of response to the normal babesiacides. However, primaquine phosphate (0.5 mg/kg, IM, twice with a 24-hr interval) is reported to be effective.

CYTAUXZOONOSIS

Cytauxzoonosis is caused by the *Theileria*-like parasites of the genus *Cytauxzoon* of the family Theileriidae. Currently there is some dispute as to its taxonomic status, but its multiplication by schizogony in mononuclear phagocytes (macrophages) rather than lymphocytes as for *Theileria* spp is a strong argument for its classification in a separate genus.

Etiology and Transmission: *Cytauxzoon* spp infect ungulates in Africa while *C felis* is a natural parasite of wild cats (bobcat [*Lynx rufus*] and the Florida panther [*Felis concolor coryi*]) of North America. *C felis* is transmitted by the Ixodid tick *Dermacentor variabilis*; as a parasite of wild cats its pathogenicity is unknown. Tick transmission to domestic cats results in an acute and almost always fatal disease. Most cases occur in the south and southeast states of the USA and are usually associated with access to wooded areas. However, transmission by blood infection appears to result in disease with variable pathogenicity and often is not fatal. Studies of *C felis* in northwestern Arkansas and northeastern Oklahoma indicate that less virulent strains may be present in these areas. This is evidenced by mild to asymptomatic clinical signs and recovery without treatment for infected cats. *Cytauxzoon* spp in African ungulates are thought to be transmitted by *Rhipicephalus appendiculatus*. Young, stressed, or immunocompromised animals are thought to be at greatest risk.

Clinical Findings and Lesions: Onset of clinical signs for cats infected with *C felis* usually occurs ~10 days after infection by tick transmission. Severe signs are usually evident 6 days later. Cats are febrile, anorectic, weak, depressed, dyspneic, and dehydrated. Temperatures may be as high as 105°F (40.5°C) but usually become subnormal in extremis. Mucous membranes are often icteric.

At necropsy, splenomegaly, hepatomegaly, enlarged lymph nodes, and renal edema are usually observed. The lungs show extensive edema and congestion with petechial hemorrhage on serosal surfaces and throughout the interstitium. There is progressive venous distension, especially the mesenteric and renal veins and the posterior vena cava. Hydropericardium is often seen with petechial hemorrhage of the epicardium.

Diagnosis: Hematology shows a normochromic, normocytic anemia with a declining leukopenia and pronounced lymphopenia. Occasionally, mononuclear phagocytes with schizont-filled cytoplasm are observed in peripheral blood smears. Giemsa-stained peripheral blood smears reveal pleomorphic, intraerythrocytic protozoan parasites that usually appear ~10 days after infection. Parasites may be round, oval, anaplasmoid, bipolar, or rod-shaped. Round forms are 1.0-2.2 μm in diameter, while oval forms are 0.8-1.0 μm × 1.5-2.0 μm. Once the parasitemia is >0.5%, Maltese cross and paired piriforms are seen. Infection with *Cytauxzoon* spp must be differentiated from *Babesia* spp, which may have similar blood forms but do not have a schizont tissue stage, and the chain-forming *Haemobartonella felis*.

The tissue stage of *C felis* is schizonts in the cytoplasm of mononuclear phagocytes that are attached to the endothelium of vessels. These phagocytes (15-250 μm in diameter) can be identified in the interstitium of the spleen, popliteal lymph node, liver, and bone marrow.

Treatment and Control: Attempts to treat this pathogen have met with little success. Parvaquone (20 or 30 mg/kg, IM, SID) and buparvaquone (5 or 10 mg/kg, IM, SID) once parasites were detected were not successful. Treatment with trimethoprim/sulfadiazine (60 mg, SC, BID) with supportive therapy has been unsuccessful (1 cat) while treatment with sodium thiacetarsamide (0.1 mg/kg, IV) for 2-3 days resulted in survival of 1 of 2 cats. More recently, 6 of 7 cats were successfully treated with diminazene aceturate (not approved in the USA) or imidocarb dipropionate (2 mg/kg, IM, 2 injections 3-7 days apart). Exclusion of cats from areas likely to be infested with the tick vector is the best method of control.

EPERYTHROZOONOSIS

A hemolytic, sometimes febrile, disease is caused by rickettsiae of the genus *Eperythrozoon* of the family Rickettsiaceae. Based on phylogenetic similarities, several members of the genus *Eperythrozoon* have recently been transferred to the genus *Mycoplasma*. Cats (*Haemobartonella* [*Eperythrozoon*] *felis*, see HEMOBARTONELLOSIS, p 25), dogs (*E canis*), cattle (*E wenyoni, E tegnodes, E tuomii*), sheep and goats (*E ovis*), and pigs (*E suis*), can be infected. Except for sheep and goats, each *Eperythrozoon* sp is host specific. Members of the genus have a worldwide distribution. Disease is often subclinical with a mild anemia, but stress in animals may result in severe clinical symptoms.

Etiology and Transmission: *Eperythrozoon* spp are transmitted mechanically by arthropods. *H felis* is also transmitted in utero. Transmission may occur via surgical procedures through blood contamination of instruments (eg, Mules operation in sheep, needle contamination during vaccination). Lice are the main method of transmission in pigs, but fleas and mosquitos may also cause transmission in cats, sheep, and goats. Ticks are vectors for dogs (*Rhipicephalus sanguineus*) and cattle.

Clinical Findings and Lesions: Eperythrozoonosis in cattle, dogs, and goats is regarded as an innocuous disease and usually causes only mild anemia. Animals with clinical disease have inappetence, wasting, anemia, malaise, and depression. Body temperature may be elevated but is often normal. Cats with eperythrozoonosis (feline infectious anemia) show pallid mucous membranes and tongue. The spleen can be enlarged and palpable through the abdominal wall. Pigs show fever, staggering or paralysis, paleness of mucous membranes, emaciation, and jaundice. Reproductive failure, weakness in piglets, and ill thrift can be indicative of eperythrozoonosis. Disease in sheep is evident as ill thrift in lambs and weaners; signs are similar to those in pigs.

Hematology shows a macrocytic hemolytic anemia, with anisocytosis, poikilocytosis, and a marked left shift in erythrocyte maturation. The leukocyte count is normal or slightly elevated.

Diagnosis: *Eperythrozoon* spp are usually coccoid (0.5-1.0 μm diameter). In Giemsa-stained peripheral blood smears, they appear attached to the surface of erythrocytes. Occasionally, rod-shaped forms (1-3 μm diameter) can be seen. It is important to differentiate between acute disease, in which the organism is readily identified in peripheral blood smears, and chronic, subclinical disease, in which animals present with a secondary infection and the organism can be difficult to detect in blood smears.

Treatment and Control: In severely affected animals, especially cats, transfusion may be required before treatment can begin. Tetracyclines used at recommended dose rates have proved effective. The use of arsenical-based drugs is no longer permitted in many countries.

Treatment of sheep in flock management practice is not recommended because infected animals develop immunity if supported with good nutrition during the hemolytic crisis, whereas treatment results in a loss of immunity and clinical disease on reinfection. The use of disposable needles and correct sterilization of surgical instruments will minimize accidental transmission. Control of arthropod parasites on pets and pigs is recommended.

Zoonotic Risk: Recent reports from Inner Mongolia, China, suggest that *Eperythrozoon* spp may be zoonotic, with evidence of congenital transmission. The prevalence in humans appeared to be associated with occupation, but there was also seasonal variation. Up to 35.3% of some populations were shown to be infected. The infections were mild except for pregnant women and their children. All of the children of pregnant women were shown to have *Eperythrozoon* spp in their peripheral blood and umbilical cord.

HEMOBARTONELLOSIS
(Feline infectious anemia)

Feline infectious anemia (FIA) is an acute or chronic disease of domestic cats, seen in many parts of the world, caused by a rickettsial agent that multiplies within the vascular system.

Etiology, Transmission, and Pathogenesis: FIA is caused by an epicellular RBC rickettsial parasite, *Haemobartonella felis* (termed *Eperythrozoon felis* in Europe and Australia). Based on genetic similarities, it has recently been proposed to move this organism to the genus *Mycoplasma*. It is gram-negative and nonacid-fast and reproduces by binary fission. In blood smears, *H felis* typically appear as cocci in thick areas of the film and as rings or rods in thin areas. The dimensions vary from 0.2-1 μm in diameter for the coccoid forms and up to 3 μm in length for the rod forms.

The causative organisms are usually found in varying numbers on the surface of the RBC but are occasionally seen free in the plasma. They appear as dark red-violet bodies in thin blood smears stained with Wright-Giemsa stain or as purple to blue organisms attached to RBC when using the May-Grunwald-Giemsa staining procedure; this procedure appears to be superior to other Romanowsky staining techniques. Acridine orange staining and direct immunofluorescence techniques have also been recommended for diagnosis of *H felis*; unfortunately, these techniques require special equipment and training and are not commercially available.

The number of RBC affected varies with the severity of the infection and the stage in the life cycle of the parasite. Blood films should be examined daily for 5-10 days if infection with *H felis* is suspected because organisms are recognized in only 50% of cats in the acute phase of the disease. During the acute phase, numbers of *H felis* organisms increase gradually, then disappear rapidly; clearance of organisms may occur within 2 hrs. In chronically infected cats, organisms appear only sporadically and in small numbers.

FIA can be transmitted experimentally by parenteral or oral transfer of small amounts of infected whole blood into susceptible cats. Intrauterine transmission can also occur, and infections can be transmitted iatrogenically via blood transfusions. However, the natural mode of transmission is believed to be via bloodsucking arthropods (such as fleas) and possibly via bite wounds.

In experimental cases, the incubation period is 1-5 wk, and recovery does not induce immunity to reinfection. Incidence of the naturally occurring disease appears to be higher among 1- to 3-yr-old cats, particularly males. A significant portion of the feline population may carry the infection in a latent form, which becomes exacerbated during debilitating disease or stress. Underlying infection with feline leukemia (p 631) or feline immunodeficiency virus (p 661) should always be investigated in cats with hemobartonellosis.

It is thought that *H felis* may not cause illness in healthy cats, but that it leads to acute disease only when an infected cat is stressed by concurrent illness. Similarly, recovered carrier cats are believed to be prone to relapse with stress.

Immune-mediated mechanisms of RBC injury are also important in the pathogenesis of FIA. Parasitized RBC may be damaged by antibody-complement interactions against *H felis* antigens. In addition, parasite-induced exposure of hidden or altered RBC antigens may lead to RBC destruction; erythrophagocytosis by the reticuloendothelial system appears to be more important than intravascular hemolysis. In experimental infection, the Coombs' test becomes positive 7-14 days after organisms appear in the blood and remains positive throughout the acute phase; the Coombs' test becomes negative during the carrier phase of the disease.

Clinical Findings and Lesions: Any anemic cat may be suspected of having FIA. In acute cases, fever usually reaches 103-106°F (39-41°C); the temperature may drop to subnormal in moribund cats. Experimentally, cats have ≥2 parasitemic episodes before the resulting anemia leads to clinical signs. The severity of clinical signs correlates with the rapidity of onset of anemia. Pallor or jaundice, anorexia, lethargy, depression, weakness, and splenomegaly are common. In chronic or slowly developing cases, there may be normal or subnormal body temperature, weakness, depression, and weight loss or emaciation, but there is less likely to be jaundice and splenomegaly. Dyspnea varies with the degree of anemia. Gross necropsy findings are not pathognomonic; splenomegaly is common, and mesenteric lymph nodes may be enlarged. Hyperplasia of the bone marrow may be seen on histopathologic examination.

Diagnosis: Laboratory confirmation depends on identification of the parasite in the peripheral blood or bone marrow. A series of smears stained with Wright-Giemsa stain over several days may be required for an accurate diagnosis because the erythrocytic bodies exhibit periodicity. Certain artifacts such as Howell-Jolly bodies may be mistaken for blood parasites. The slides should be clean, and the stains should be filtered immediately before use because dirt particles and stain precipitates can mimic the appearance of the organism.

In the southeastern USA, differentiation from feline cytauxzoonosis (p 23) should be made. *Cytauxzoon felis* appears as an intracellular ring, rod, or coccoid-shaped protozoan 0.5-2 μm in diameter within RBC, while *H felis* tends to form chains on the surface of RBC. A PCR test that detects the organism in blood is also available; a positive result confirms active infection.

Expected laboratory abnormalities include a regenerative anemia; typical changes include diffuse basophilic granules in larger erythrocytes, nucleated RBC, polychromasia, anisocytosis, Howell-Jolly bodies, and an increased reticulocyte count. However, if the onset of anemia is rapid, a nonregenerative anemia may be present. RBC counts may fall as low as $1 \times 10^6/\mu L$, and hemoglobin values of ≤7 g/dL may be seen. Mean corpuscular volume may be increased. There may be moderate leukocytosis with monocytosis in acute forms, normal counts in chronic forms, and leukopenia in moribund cases. Erythrophagocytosis and autoagglutination may be present in peripheral blood. Serum biochemical changes often include increased ALT, AST, bilirubin, and total protein levels; moribund cats may be hypoglycemic.

Treatment: Treatment involves both supportive and specific therapies. Without treatment, one-third of acutely ill cats may die. Severely dyspneic cats may require oxygen, and whole blood or packed RBC transfusions may be needed in cats with a PCV of ≤15%, particularly if the anemia is acute. The decision to transfuse should be based on the cat's clinical condition rather than on the PCV.

Tetracycline (20 mg/kg, PO, TID for 21 days) is recommended as a specific antirickettsial agent. Doxycycline (10 mg/kg, PO, SID for 21 days) is also effective. Unfortunately, *H felis* is not completely eliminated by tetracycline therapy, resulting in chronically infected carrier animals. Thiacetarsamide sodium (1 mg/kg, IV, every 48 hr for 2 treatments) has also been recommended for the treatment of hemobartonellosis; however, some reports suggest that this agent is less effective than previously thought. Although chloramphenicol has also shown efficacy against *H felis*, it can cause a significant but reversible erythroid hypoplasia that may interfere with the regenerative response.

The use of glucocorticoids is recommended based on the evidence of immune-mediated RBC injury. Prednisone or prednisolone (2-4 mg/kg, PO, SID) should be used in conjunction with antibiotic therapy, and the dose should be gradually tapered as the PCV increases.

HEPATOZOONOSIS AND AMERICAN CANINE HEPATOZOONOSIS

Etiology, Epidemiology, and Transmission: Hepatozoonosis is a tickborne disease of wild and domestic carnivores caused by the protozoal agent, *Hepatozoon canis*. It is unclear whether or not infections in wild and domestic Felidae are caused by *H canis*, or by another species of *Hepatozoon*. This organism is transmitted by the brown dog tick, *Rhipicephalus sanguineus*, but its mode of transmission is not typical in the classical sense of a tickborne disease; although the tick ingests the organism from the mammalian host during a blood meal, and oocysts develop in the tick, the dog (or cat) actually obtains the disease from an infected tick by ingesting the tick, and not from being bitten by the tick. Unique features of the clinical presentation in North American dogs have suggested that a different strain or species of *Hepatozoon* may be responsible for the disease in North America as compared to other parts of the world; in 1997, this was confirmed. It is now known that the disease in North America is caused by the protozoal agent *H americanum*, which is transmitted by the Gulf Coast tick, *Amblyomma maculatum*, instead of by the brown dog tick. The disease in North America is now referred to as a separate entity, American canine hepatozoonosis.

In much of the world (India, Africa, southeast Asia, the Middle East, southern Europe, and islands in the Pacific and Indian Oceans), most dogs with hepatozoonosis generally have subclinical infections or only mild clinical signs, and immunosuppression caused by concurrent disease or other factors appears to play an important role in the manifestation of significant clinical signs. In the USA, immunosuppression or concurrent disease does not appear necessary to induce the more severe clinical signs typically seen. Most cases in the USA have been diagnosed in Texas (primarily along the Gulf Coast), Oklahoma, and Louisiana, but cases have also been reported as far east as Tennessee, Alabama, Georgia, and Florida. This is an emerging disease that has primarily spread north and east from the Gulf Coast of Texas, where it was originally detected in 1978. The distribution of this parasite parallels the distribution of the Gulf Coast tick. *H americanum* may also be found in Central and South America.

Experimentally, dogs >4-6 mo old are resistant to infection with *H canis*. However, *H americanum* causes severe clinical signs, even in adult dogs. Because disease caused by *H americanum* is much more clinically significant than that caused by *H canis*, the descriptions in the remainder of this chapter refer primarily to American canine hepatozoonosis.

Clinical Findings: The tissue phases of the hepatozoonosis organism induce pyogranulomatous inflammation, which results in clinical signs. These signs, which may be intermittent, include fever, depression, weight loss, poor body condition, muscle atrophy and weakness, mucopurulent ocular discharge, and bloody diarrhea. Surprisingly, many dogs maintain a normal appetite. Severe hyperesthesia or pain over the paraspinal region is a common finding on physical examination; cervical, joint, or generalized pain are also seen. Hyperesthesia manifests as stiffness and reluctance to move, as well as cervical and/or truncal rigidity. Fever, which may fluctuate with the waxing and waning of clinical signs, may range from 102.7-106.0°F (39.3-41.0°C) and is unresponsive to antibiotics. Longterm sequelae include glomerulonephritis and amyloidosis.

Diagnosis: The most consistent laboratory abnormality is a neutrophilic leukocytosis, with counts ranging from 20,000-200,000 cells/μL. This is typically a mature neutrophilia, although a left shift may be present. A mild to moderate normocytic, normochromic, nonregenerative anemia is another common finding. The platelet count is typically normal to elevated. Mildly increased alkaline phosphatase, hypoalbuminemia, and increased CK may also be seen. Although profound hypoglycemia has been reported, this is thought to be an in vitro sampling artifact caused by increased metabolism of glucose due to the high number of leukocytes. On radiographs, periosteal reactions may be seen involving any bone (except the skull), particularly the long bones; these periosteal reactions are most likely related to an inflammatory response to tissue phases of the organism in adjacent muscle.

The definitive diagnosis of hepatozoonosis is made by finding gamonts in neutrophils or monocytes (using Romanowsky-type stains); identifying the typical cysts, meronts, or pyogranulomas in muscle biopsies; or detecting serum antibodies against *H americanum* sporozoites. In some dogs, multiple or sequential muscle biopsies may be necessary to detect the organism. The relatively new serologic method of diagnosis (an ELISA that detects antibodies to *H americanum* sporozoites) appears to be both highly sensitive and specific.

Treatment: Hepatozoonosis is a life-long infection in dogs. No known therapeutic regimen completely clears the body of the organism. In the past, treatment has been frustrating because most dogs showed only temporary improvement, with frequent relapses within 3-6 mo and death within 2 yr of diagnosis. Remission of clinical signs can usually be achieved through combination therapy, referred to as TCP, which includes 3 drugs: trimethoprim-sulfadiazine (15 mg/kg, PO, BID), clindamycin (10 mg/kg, PO, TID), and pyrimethamine (0.25 mg/kg, PO, SID); these drugs should be administered for 14 days. Unfortunately, remission with this therapy has often been short-lived, and dogs frequently relapse within 2-6 mo. However, a relatively new adjunctive treatment using decoquinate (a large animal anticoccidial drug) has been described; decoquinate does not resolve active clinical disease but may prevent clinical relapses; it is given after resolution of clinical signs as an adjunct to TCP therapy. The recommended dose for decoquinate is 10-20 mg/kg, PO, BID continuously for 2 yr. The advent of TCP combination therapy followed by daily decoquinate therapy has resulted in a marked improvement in the prognosis for dogs with hepatozoonosis.

Other treatments include imidocarb dipropionate (5 mg/kg, SC, given once), a combination of imidocarb dipropionate (6 mg/kg, SC, every 14 days) with tetracycline (22 mg/kg, PO, TID for 14 days) or the coccidiostat toltrazuril (5-10 mg/kg, SC or PO, SID for 3-5 days or 5 mg/kg, PO, BID for 4 days). The effect of imidocarb therapy has been inconsistent and may be dependent on the severity of signs and geographic location. Similarly, although excellent initial clinical response to toltrazuril has been reported, relapses occurred, and there was no evidence of clearing of the cyst forms from the muscle tissue.

NSAID may be the best treatment for control of fever and pain, especially during the first few days of TCP therapy. Glucocorticoid administration should be avoided, because although steroids may provide temporary relief, longterm use can exacerbate the disease.

Prevention of access to ticks is the most effective form of control for hepatozoonosis. There is no known zoonotic risk with this disease; whether the lack of reports in humans is due to the minimal risk of ingesting infected ticks or to natural resistance is unknown.

SCHISTOSOMIASIS
(Bilharzia)

Etiology: Schistosomes are thin, elongated flukes, up to 30 mm long, that live in blood vessels of the final host. The female lies in a longitudinal groove of the male. Various water snails act as intermediate hosts. Schistosomes pathogenic to domestic animals belong to the genera *Schistosoma* and *Orientobilharzia* and are widely distributed throughout Africa, the Middle East, Asia, and some countries bordering the

Mediterranean Sea. In many areas, a high percentage of animals are infected and, although many have low burdens and are asymptomatic, severe outbreaks due to heavy infection are reported occasionally. Most species of pathogenic schistosomes are found in the hepatic portal system, and the principal clinical signs are associated with passage of the spined eggs through the tissues to the gut lumen. One species, *S nasale*, is found in the veins of the nasal mucosa of ruminants and horses, where it may cause coryza and dyspnea.

Eggs passed in the feces must be deposited in water if they are to hatch and release the miracidia, which invade suitable water snails and develop through primary and secondary sporocysts to become cercariae. When fully mature, the cercariae leave the snail and swim freely in the water, where they remain viable for several hours. The cercariae invade the final host through the skin and mucous membranes; during penetration, cercariae develop into schistosomula, which are transported via the lymph and blood to their predilection sites. The prepatent period is ~6-9 wk.

In southern and central Africa, *S mattheei* is the predominant species infecting ruminants; in northern and eastern areas, *S bovis* is more common. The latter parasite is also found in certain areas of southern Europe and the Middle East. Other African species infecting ruminants are *S curassoni*, *S margrebowiei*, and *S leiperi*. In Asia, *S spindale*, *S nasale*, *S indicum*, *S incognitum*, and *S japonicum* are widespread in livestock. The latter species is of particular importance because livestock form a reservoir for the disease in humans. Four species of the related genus *Orientobilharzia* also infect livestock in Asia—*O turkestanicum*, *O harinasutai*, *O dattai*, and *O bomfordi*.

Clinical Findings: Hemorrhagic enteritis, anemia, and emaciation, which develop after the onset of egg excretion, are the major clinical signs associated with the intestinal and hepatic forms of schistosomiasis in ruminants. Severely affected animals deteriorate rapidly and usually die within a few months of infection, while those less heavily infected develop chronic disease with growth retardation. Many older cattle in endemic areas of Africa have an effective level of immunity against reinfection. Nasal schistosomiasis is a chronic disease of cattle, horses, and occasionally buffalo. In severe cases, there is a copious mucopurulent discharge, snoring, and dyspnea; milder cases frequently are asymptomatic.

Lesions: In the intestinal and hepatic forms, adult flukes are found in the portal, mesenteric, and intestinal submucosal and subserosal veins. However, the main pathologic effects are associated with the eggs. In the intestinal form, passage of eggs through the gut wall causes the lesions, while in the hepatic form, granulomas form around eggs trapped in the tissues. Other hepatic changes include medial hypertrophy and hyperplasia of the portal veins, development of lymphoid nodules and follicles throughout the organ, and periportal fibrosis in more chronic cases. Extensive granuloma formation also is seen in the intestine. In severe cases, numerous areas of petechiation and diffuse hemorrhage are seen in the mucosa, and large quantities of discolored blood may be found in the intestinal lumen. Frequently, the parasitized blood vessels are dilated and tortuous. Vascular lesions also may be found in the lungs, pancreas, and bladder of heavily infected animals.

In nasal schistosomiasis, adult flukes are found in the blood vessels of the nasal mucosa, but again, the main pathogenic effects are associated with the eggs, which cause abscesses in the mucosa. The abscesses rupture and release eggs and pus into the nasal cavity, which eventually leads to extensive fibrosis. In addition, large granulomatous growths are common on the nasal mucosa and occlude the nasal passages and cause dyspnea.

Diagnosis: Clinical history and signs are insufficient; the characteristic, terminal-spined eggs must be identified in the feces, rectal scrapings, or nasal mucus for confirmation. Eggs of *S bovis* (202 × 58 μm) and *S mattheei* (173 × 53 μm) are spindle-shaped; those of *S spindale* (382 × 70 μm) are more elongated and flattened on one side, and those of *S nasale* (456 × 66 μm) are boomerang-shaped. The oval eggs of *S japonicum* are relatively small (81 × 63 μm), with a rudimentary spine. In chronic cases, it may not be possible to find eggs in the feces or nasal mucus, and the diagnosis must be confirmed at necropsy by finding adult flukes in the blood vessels.

Treatment and Control: Praziquantel (25 mg/kg) is highly effective, although 2 treatments 3-5 wk apart may be required. Control measures are rarely practiced on a large scale, except in China, where infected livestock constitute important reservoirs of human infection. Transmission of the infection can be reduced by large-scale chemotherapy campaigns, by control of the intermediate snail host using molluscicides (eg, niclosamide) or habitat modifications, or by fencing off contaminated bodies of water and providing clean drinking water. These measures not only help reduce the transmission of schistosomiasis but also help control other parasitic trematodes such as *Fasciola gigantica* and *Paramphistomum* spp, which similarly have water snails as intermediate hosts and frequently occur in the same localities as schistosomes. Antischistosome vaccines are under development.

THEILERIASES

Theileriases are a group of tickborne diseases caused by *Theileria* spp. The most important species are *T parva* and *T annulata*, which cause widespread death in cattle in tropical and subtropical areas of the Old World.

Both *Theileria* and *Babesia* are members of the suborder Piroplasmorina. While *Babesia* are primarily parasites of RBC, *Theileria* use, successively, WBC and RBC for completion of their life cycle in mammalian hosts. The infective sporozoite stage of the parasite is transmitted in the saliva of infected ticks as they feed. Sporozoites invade lymphocytes (and also monocytes in the case of *T annulata*) and, within a few days, develop to schizonts. In the most pathogenic species of *Theileria*, development of schizonts causes the host WBC to divide; at each cell division, the parasite also divides. Thus, the parasitized cell population expands and, through migration, becomes disseminated throughout the lymphoid system. Later in the infection, some of the schizonts undergo merogony; the resultant merozoites infect RBC, giving rise to piroplasms. *T parva* piroplasms undergo limited division in RBC, but in other species, notably *T annulata*, *T mutans*, and *T orientalis*, such division represents a second phase of multiplication. Uptake of piroplasm-infected RBC by vector ticks feeding on infected animals is the prelude to a complex cycle of development, culminating in transmission of infection by ticks feeding in their next instar (trans-stadial transmission). There is no transovarial transmission as occurs in *Babesia*. Occurrence of disease is limited to the geographic distribution of the appropriate tick vectors. In some endemic areas, indigenous cattle have a degree of innate resistance. Mortality in such stock is relatively low, but introduced cattle are particularly vulnerable.

East Coast Fever

East Coast fever, an acute disease of cattle, is characterized usually by high fever, swelling of the lymph nodes, dyspnea, and high mortality. Caused by *Theileria parva*, it is a serious problem in east and central Africa.

Etiology and Transmission: *T parva* sporozoites are injected into cattle by infected vector ticks, *Rhipicephalus appendiculatus*, during feeding. Based on clinical and epidemiologic parameters, 3 subtypes of *T parva* are recognized, but these are probably not true subspecies. *T parva parva*, transmitted mainly between cattle, and *T parva lawrencei*, transmitted mainly from buffalo to cattle, are both highly pathogenic and can cause high levels of mortality, whereas *T parva bovis*, transmitted between cattle, is less pathogenic.

Pathogenesis, Clinical Findings, and Diagnosis: An occult phase of 5-10 days follows before infected lymphocytes can be detected in Giemsa-stained smears of cells aspirated from the local draining lymph node. Subsequently, the number of parasitized cells increases rapidly throughout the lymphoid system, and from about day 14 onwards, cells undergoing merogony are observed. This is associated with widespread lymphocytolysis, marked lymphoid depletion, and leukopenia. Piroplasms in RBC infected by the resultant merozoites assume various forms, but typically they are small and rod-shaped or oval.

Clinical signs vary according to the level of challenge and range from inapparent or mild to severe and fatal. Typically, fever occurs 7-10 days after parasites are introduced by feeding ticks, continues throughout the course of infection, and may be >107°F (42°C). Lymph node swelling becomes pronounced and generalized. Lymphoblasts in Giemsa-stained lymph node biopsy smears contain multinuclear schizonts. Anorexia develops and the animal rapidly loses condition; lacrimation and nasal discharge may occur. Terminally, dyspnea is common. Just before death, a sharp fall in body temperature is usual, and pulmonary exudate pours from the nostrils. Death usually occurs 18-24 days after infection. The most striking postmortem lesions are lymph node enlargement and massive pulmonary edema and hyperemia. Hemorrhages are common on the serosal and mucosal surfaces of many organs, sometimes together with obvious areas of necrosis in the lymph nodes and thymus. Anemia is not a major diagnostic sign (as it is in babesiosis) because there is minimal division of the parasites in RBC, and thus no massive destruction of them.

Animals that recover are immune to subsequent challenge with the same strains but may be susceptible to some heterologous strains. Most recovered or immunized animals remain carriers of the infection.

Treatment and Control: Prospects for survival of cattle with clinical East Coast fever or *T annulata* infection were enhanced by the development of the theilericidal compound parvaquone and, subsequently, its derivative buparvaquone. Treatment with these compounds is highly effective when applied in the early stages of clinical disease but is less effective in the advanced stages in which there is extensive destruction of lymphoid and hematopoietic tissues. Immunization of cattle using an infection-and-treatment procedure is practical and is gaining acceptance in some regions. The components for this procedure are a cryopreserved sporozoite stabilate of the appropriate strain(s) of *Theileria* derived from infected ticks and a single dose of long-acting oxytetracycline given simultaneously; although oxytetracline has little therapeutic effect when administered following development of disease, it inhibits development of the parasite when given at the outset of infection. Immunization can also be achieved by administering parvaquone 7-9 days after infection, but this procedure is rarely used because of the requirement to handle the animals on 2 occasions. Cattle should be immunized 3-4 wk before being allowed on infected pasture. Incidence of East Coast fever can be reduced by rigid tick control, but in many areas, this means biweekly acaricidal treatment.

Other Theileriases

Theileria spp in large domestic and wild animals in tick-infested areas of the Old World are almost ubiquitous but, apart from those in cattle, their differentiation into species is unclear. The following species are important.

In cattle, *T annulata* is widely distributed in north Africa, the Mediterranean coastal area, the Middle East, India, the former USSR, and Asia. It causes **tropical or Mediterranean theileriosis** and is transmitted by ticks of the genus *Hyalomma*. *T annulata* can cause mortality of up to 90%, but strains vary in their pathogenicity. Characteristic signs include fever and swollen superficial lymph nodes; cattle rapidly lose condition and hemoglobinuria may occur. The schizonts and piroplasms are morphologically similar to those of *T parva*. Parasitized bovine cells containing the schizont stage can be cultivated in vitro, and attenuated strains produced by serial passage form the basis of vaccines used in several countries, including Israel, Iran, India, and the former USSR.

T orientalis occurs in the Far East and to a lesser extent through Asia and the southern former USSR, where it may cause a disease syndrome in association with *T annulata*. Transmission is by ticks of the genus *Haemaphysalis*. Mildly pathogenic strains of a closely related parasite, *T buffeli*, exist in Europe, Australasia, and North America where *Haemaphysalis* spp are found. The piroplasms are larger than those of *T parva* and *T annulata*, and they multiply principally by intraerythrocytic division. Mortality, particularly in indigenous cattle, is rare, but progressive chronic anemia is common.

T mutans occurs in Africa, where it is transmitted by ticks of the genus *Amblyomma*. Multiplication occurs mainly by intraerythrocytic division. The piroplasms are morphologically indistinguishable from those of *T orientalis* and *T taurotragi* (an African parasite of eland and cattle), but the parasites can be differentiated by serologic tests such as indirect fluorescent antibody. Some strains of *T mutans* are pathogenic as well. In addition, concurrent infection may add to the pathogenicity of *T parva.*

In sheep and goats, 2 species of *Theileria* have been distinguished, largely based on their relative pathogenicity. Mortality can approach 100% with *T lestoquardi* (formerly *T hirci*), which is found in southern Europe, Africa, and throughout Asia. It is transmitted by *Hyalomma anatolicum* ticks in Asia. Schizonts can readily be demonstrated in Giemsa-stained biopsy smears from swollen superficial lymph nodes. Nonpathogenic *Theileria* spp (eg, *T ovis*) are also widely distributed and are mainly transmitted by *R evertsi* ticks in Africa and *Haemaphysalis punctata* ticks in Europe. Piroplasms of these species are polymorphic.

Babesia equi was reclassified as *T equi* in 1998, based on DNA analysis and other biologic data (*see* BABESIOSIS, p 20).

TRYPANOSOMIASIS

Tsetse-transmitted Trypanosomiasis

This group of diseases caused by protozoa of the genus *Trypanosoma* affects all domestic animals. The major species are *T congolense*, *T vivax*, *T brucei brucei*, and *T simiae.*

See TABLE 4 for the animals mainly affected by these tsetse-transmitted trypanosomes and the geographic areas where tsetse-transmitted trypanosomiasis occurs. Cattle, sheep, and goats are infected, in order of importance, by *T congolense*, *T vivax*, and *T brucei brucei*. In pigs, *T simiae* is the most important. In dogs and cats, *T brucei* is probably the most important. It is difficult to assign an order of importance for horses and camels. *T vivax* may occur outside tsetse-infested areas of sub-Saharan Africa.

The trypanosomes that cause tsetse-transmitted trypanosomiasis (sleeping sickness) in humans, *T brucei rhodesiense* and *T brucei gambiense*, closely resemble *T brucei brucei* from animals, and suitable precautions should be taken when working with such isolates. Domestic animals may act as reservoirs of human infections.

Transmission and Epidemiology: Most tsetse transmission is cyclic and begins when blood from a trypanosome-infected animal is ingested by the fly. The trypanosome loses its surface coat, multiplies in the fly, then reacquires a surface coat and becomes infective. *T brucei* spp migrate from the gut to the proventriculus to the pharynx and eventually to the salivary glands; the cycle for *T congolense* stops at the hypopharynx, and the salivary glands are not invaded; the entire cycle for *T vivax* occurs in the proboscis. The animal-infective form in the tsetse salivary gland is referred to as the metacyclic form. The life cycle in the tsetse may be as short as 1 wk with *T vivax* or extend to a few weeks for *T brucei* spp.

TABLE 4. Tsetse-transmitted Animal Trypanosomes

Trypanosoma spp	Animals Mainly Affected	Major Geographic Distribution
T congolense	Cattle, sheep, goats, dogs, pigs, camels, horses, most wild animals	Tsetse region of Africa
T vivax	Cattle, sheep, goats, camels, horses, various wild animals	Africa, Central and South America, West Indies[*]
T brucei brucei	All domestic and various wild animals; most severe in dogs, horses, cats	Tsetse region of Africa
T simiae	Domestic and wild pigs, camels	Tsetse region of Africa

[*]In non-tsetse areas, transmission is by biting flies.

Tsetse flies (genus *Glossina*) are restricted to Africa from about latitude 15°N to 29°S. The 3 main species inhabit relatively distinct environments—*G morsitans* usually is found in savanna country, *G palpalis* prefers areas around rivers and lakes, and *G fusca* lives in high forest areas. All 3 species transmit trypanosomes and all feed on various mammals.

Mechanical transmission can occur through tsetse or other biting flies. In the case of *T vivax*, *Tabanus* spp and other biting flies seem to be the primary mechanical vectors outside the tsetse areas, as in Central and South America. Mechanical transmission requires only that blood containing infectious trypanosomes be transferred from one animal to another.

Pathogenesis: Infected tsetse inoculate metacyclic trypanosomes into the skin of animals, where the trypanosomes grow for a few days and cause localized swellings (chancres). They enter the lymph nodes, then the bloodstream, where they divide rapidly by binary fission. In *T congolense* infection, the organisms attach to endothelial cells and localize in capillaries and small blood vessels. *T brucei* species and *T vivax* invade tissues and cause tissue damage in several organs.

The immune response is vigorous, and immune complexes cause inflammation, which contributes to the signs and lesions of the disease. Antibodies against the surface-coat glycoproteins kill the trypanosomes. However, trypanosomes have multiple genes that code for different surface-coat glycoproteins that are not vulnerable to the immune response; this antigenic variation results in persistence of the organism. The number of antigenic types of glycoprotein that can be made is unknown, but exceeds several hundred. Antigenic variation has prevented development of a vaccine and permits reinfections when animals are exposed to a new antigenic type.

Clinical Findings and Lesions: Severity of disease varies with species and age of the animal infected and the species of trypanosome involved. The incubation period is usually 1-4 wk. The primary clinical signs are intermittent fever, anemia, and weight loss. Cattle usually have a chronic course with high mortality, especially if there is poor nutrition or other stress factors. Ruminants may gradually recover if the number of infected tsetse flies is low; however, stress results in relapse.

Necropsy findings vary and are nonspecific. In acute, fatal cases, extensive petechiation of the serosal membranes, especially in the peritoneal cavity, may occur. Also, the lymph nodes and spleen are usually swollen. In chronic cases, swollen lymph nodes, serous atrophy of fat, and anemia are seen.

Diagnosis: A presumptive diagnosis is based on finding an anemic animal in poor condition in an endemic area. Confirmation depends on demonstrating trypanosomes in stained blood smears or wet mounts. The most sensitive rapid method is to examine a wet mount of the buffy coat area of a PCV tube after centrifugation. Other infections that cause anemia and weight loss, such as babesiosis, anaplasmosis, and theileriosis, should be ruled out by examining a stained blood smear.

Various serologic tests measure antibody to trypanosomes, but their use is more suitable for herd and area screening than for individual diagnosis. Tests for detection of circulating trypanosome species-specific antigens in peripheral blood are becoming available for both individual and herd diagnosis, although their reliability remains unproven.

Treatment and Control: Several drugs can be used for treatment (*see* TABLE 5). Most have a narrow therapeutic index, which makes administration of the correct dose essential. Drug resistance occurs and should be considered in refractory cases.

Control can be exercised at several levels, including eradication of tsetse flies and use of prophylactic drugs. Tsetses can be partially controlled by frequent spraying and dipping of animals, spraying of insecticides on fly-breeding areas, use of insecticide-impregnated screens, bush clearing, and other methods. Animals can be given drugs prophylactically in areas with a high population of trypanosome-infected tsetse. Drug resistance must be carefully monitored by frequent blood examinations for trypanosomes in treated animals.

TABLE 5. Drugs Commonly Used for Trypanosomosis in Domestic Animals

Drug	Animal	*Trypanosoma*	Main Action
Diminazene aceturate	Cattle	*vivax, congolense, brucei*	Curative
Homidium bromide	Cattle	*vivax, congolense, brucei*	Curative, some prophylactic activity
	Equids	*vivax*	
Homidium chloride		As for the bromide salt	
Isometamidium chloride	Cattle	*vivax, congolense*	Curative and prophylactic
Quinapyramine sulfate	Horses, camels, pigs, dogs	*vivax, congolense, brucei, evansi, equiperdum, simiae*	Curative
Quinapyramine dimethylsulfate	Horses, camels, pigs, dogs	*vivax, congolense, brucei, evansi, equiperdum, simiae*	Prophylactic
Suramin	Horses, camels, dogs	*brucei, evansi*	Curative, some prophylactic activity
Melarsomine dichlorhydrate	Camels	*evansi*	Curative

In west Africa, several breeds of cattle have been identified that show innate resistance to trypanosomiasis and play a valuable role in reducing the impact of the disease in this area. However, resistance may be lost due to poor nutrition or heavy tsetse challenge.

Control is ideally achieved by combining methods to reduce the tsetse challenge and by enhancing host resistance with prophylactic drugs.

Surra
(*Trypanosoma evansi* infection)

Surra is separated from the tsetse-transmitted diseases because it is usually transmitted by other biting flies that are found within and outside tsetse fly areas. It occurs in North Africa, the Middle East, Asia, the Far East, and Central and South America. The distribution of *T evansi* in Africa extends into the tsetse areas, where differentiation from *T brucei* is difficult. It is essentially a disease of camels and horses, but all domestic animals are susceptible. The disease can be fatal, particularly in camels, horses, and dogs. *T evansi* in other animals appears to be nonpathogenic, and these animals serve as reservoirs of infection.

Transmission is primarily by biting flies, probably resulting from interrupted feedings. A few wild animals are susceptible to infection and may serve as reservoirs.

Pathogenesis, clinical findings, lesions, diagnosis, and treatment are similar to those of the tsetse-transmitted trypanosomes (*see* above).

Dourine

Dourine is an often chronic venereal disease of horses that is transmitted during coitus and caused by *T equiperdum*. The disease is recognized on the Mediterranean coast of Africa and in the Middle East, southern Africa, and South America; distribution is probably wider.

Signs may develop over weeks or months. Early signs include mucopurulent discharge from the urethra in stallions and from the vagina in mares, followed by gross edema of the genitalia. Later, characteristic plaques 2-10 cm in diameter appear on the skin, and the horse becomes progressively emaciated. Mortality in untreated cases is 50-70%.

Demonstration of trypanosomes from the urethral or vaginal discharges, the plaques on the skin, or peripheral blood is difficult unless the material is centrifuged. Infected horses can be detected with the complement fixation test but only in areas where *T evansi* or *T brucei* are not found because they have common antigens. An ELISA test may become available for diagnosis.

In endemic areas, horses may be treated (TABLE 5). When eradication is required, strict control of breeding and elimination of stray horses has been successful. Alternatively, infected horses may be identified using the complement fixation test; euthanasia is mandatory.

Chagas' Disease
(*Trypanosoma cruzi* infection)

The common transmission cycle of Chagas' disease is between opossums, armadillos, rodents, and wild carnivores, with bugs of the Reduviidae family serving as vectors. Distribution is in Central and South America and localized areas of the southern USA. Chagas' disease is important in South America. Domestic animals may become infected and introduce the trypanosome into human dwellings where the bugs are present; humans then become infected by contamination of eye wounds or by eating food contaminated with insect feces that contain trypanosomes. The trypanosome is pathogenic to humans and occasionally to young dogs and cats; other domestic animals act as reservoir hosts. *T cruzi* should be suspected in endemic areas in dogs that die acutely or have myocarditis.

Nonpathogenic Trypanosomes

Trypanosoma theileri or markedly similar trypanosomes have been detected in cultures of peripheral blood from cattle on every continent. Infection with similar trypanosomes also has been detected in domestic and wild buffalo and various other wild ungulates. In the few areas studied, transmission is by contamination after a cycle of development in species of tabanid flies. Although most parasitemias are subpatent, the trypanosomes may be seen in a blood smear being examined for pathogenic protozoa or in a hemocytometer chamber. Pathogenicity has never been proved experimentally.

T melophagium of sheep also has a worldwide distribution and is transmitted by the sheep ked. *T theodori*, reported in goats, may be a synonym for the same trypanosome.

CANINE MALIGNANT LYMPHOMA

Canine malignant lymphoma is a progressive, fatal disease caused by the malignant clonal expansion of lymphoid cells. Although lymphoid cell neoplastic transformation is not restricted to specific anatomic compartments, lymphoma most commonly arises from organized lymphoid tissues including the bone marrow, thymus, lymph nodes, and spleen. In addition to these primary and secondary lymphoid organs, common extranodal sites include the skin, eye, CNS, testis, and bone. Lymphoma is reported to be the most common hematopoietic neoplasm in dogs, with an incidence reported to approach 0.1% in susceptible, older dogs. Despite the prevalence of malignant lymphoma, its etiology remains poorly characterized. Hypothesized etiologies include retroviral infection, environmental contamination with phenoxyacetic acid herbicides, magnetic field exposure, chromosomal abnormalities, and immune dysfunction.

Clinical Findings: Canine lymphoma is a heterogeneous cancer, with variable clinical signs depending in part on the anatomic region involved and extent of disease.

In dogs, 4 well recognized anatomic forms of lymphoma have been described: multicentric, alimentary, mediastinal, and extranodal (renal, CNS, and cutaneous). Multicentric lymphoma is by far the most common form, accounting for ~80% of all diagnosed cases. An early clinical sign of multicentric lymphoma is the rapid and nonpainful development of generalized lymphadenopathy. In addition to dramatic peripheral lymphadenopathy, malignant lymphocytes may infiltrate internal organs including the spleen, liver, bone marrow, and other extranodal sites. Late in the course of disease, when a significant tumor burden exists, patients may show constitutional signs of illness, including lethargy, weakness, fever, anorexia, and depression.

Alimentary lymphoma accounts for <10% of all canine lymphomas. Dogs with focal intestinal lesions may exhibit clinical signs consistent with partial or complete luminal obstruction (eg, vomiting, abdominal pain). With diffuse involvement of the intestinal tract, dogs with alimentary lymphoma may show significant GI signs, including anorexia, vomiting, diarrhea, and profound weight loss secondary to severe malabsorption and maldigestion.

Mediastinal lymphoma, similar to the alimentary form, comprises only a small fraction of diagnosed cases. It is typically characterized by enlargement of the cranial mediastinal lymph nodes, thymus, or both. Mediastinal lymphoma arising from the thymus is predominantly comprised of malignant T lymphocytes; with advanced disease, clinical signs may include respiratory distress associated with pleural fluid accumulation, direct compression of adjacent lung lobes, or superior vena cava syndrome. In addition to respiratory signs, some dogs with mediastinal lymphoma may exhibit polyuria and polydipsia secondary to the development of hypercalcemia of malignancy, a paraneoplastic syndrome seen in 10-40% of dogs with lymphoma.

The clinical findings associated with extranodal lymphoma (which may involve the skin, lungs, kidneys, eyes, and CNS) can be quite variable and are dictated by the organ infiltrated. Cutaneous lymphoma may appear as solitary, raised, ulcerative nodules or generalized, diffuse, scaly lesions. Clinical signs of lymphoma at other extranodal sites include respiratory distress (lungs), renal failure (kidneys), blindness (eyes), and seizures (CNS).

Lesions: Commonly, all superficial and various internal lymph nodes are 3-10 times normal size (multicentric form). Affected nodes are freely movable, firm, and gray-tan; they bulge on cut surface and have no cortical-medullary demarcation. Frequently, there is hepatosplenomegaly with either diffuse enlargement or multiple, pale nodules of variable size disseminated in the parenchyma. In the alimentary form, any part of the GI tract or mesenteric lymph nodes may be affected. Involvement of the bone marrow, CNS, kidney, heart, tonsils, pancreas, and eyes can be seen but is less common.

Diagnosis: The definitive diagnosis of lymphoma is often uncomplicated and can be obtained by either cytologic or histopathologic evaluation of the affected organ system. In dogs with multicentric lymphoma, fine-needle aspiration of enlarged peripheral lymph nodes usually provides specimens of adequate cellular content and detail to make a definitive diagnosis. Cytologically, lymph node aspirates may identify a monomorphic population of lymphoid cells, either of large (lymphoblastic), intermediate, or small size. Despite the ease of diagnosis, cytology is unable to differentiate or categorize the wide spectrum of lymphomas with regard to morphologic pattern (diffuse versus follicular) and histologic grade (high versus low). Due to these constraints, histopathologic tissue evaluation remains the gold standard for the diagnosis of lymphoma, providing additional morphologic information required for definitive classification.

In rare situations where cytology or histology fails to confirm the diagnosis, new molecular techniques may allow for its identification. The use of PCR allows for the amplification of DNA sequences that confirms the presence of malignant lymphocytes. Although PCR methods are highly sensitive, the methodology should be reserved for cases where conventional cytologic and histologic diagnostic techniques have failed.

Treatment: Treatment of multicentric canine lymphoma with aggressive, multi-agent chemotherapy protocols is often rewarding, with >90% of all dogs achieving some clinical response. The most common chemotherapeutic agents used in combination protocols are vincristine, adriamycin, cyclophosphamide, L-asparaginase, and prednisone. Individual treatment protocols vary with respect to dosage, frequency, and duration of treatment; advantages and disadvantages of each treatment protocol can be found in medical oncology textbooks. With combination chemotherapy, the expected survival time for dogs with B-cell lymphoma is ~9-12 mo. For dogs with T-cell lymphoma, expected survival times are shorter (6 mo). Dogs that fail to respond to traditional combination chemotherapy or that relapse may achieve disease remission, added survival times, or both with the use of various rescue protocols (eg, lomustine, half-body radiation).

Although systemic chemotherapy remains the cornerstone for treating lymphoma, the idea that both induction and maintenance phases of chemotherapy are necessary for achieving durable remission times has recently changed. Short but dose-intense chemotherapy protocols (eg, Madison Wisconsin protocol) without maintenance provide disease-free intervals and survival times equivalent to protocols that include chronic maintenance therapy. Additionally, the use of half-body radiation in replacement of maintenance chemotherapy has demonstrated clinical efficacy and provides another option for maintaining durable remission times without the need for chronic chemotherapy.

Despite the favorable outcomes expected in treating multicentric lymphoma, the successful management of other anatomic forms of lymphoma is often more difficult and less rewarding. Alimentary lymphoma, if focal, can be treated effectively with surgical resection and combination chemotherapy. However, with diffuse involvement of the intestinal tract, low constitutional reserve and severe malabsorption of nutrients and loss of proteins often results in poor clinical responses and short survival times (ie, <3 mo). The use of combination chemotherapy with or without palliative radiation therapy can afford dogs with mediastinal lymphoma considerable improvement in survival times and quality-of-life scores, but the expected median duration of remission is ~6 mo for T-cell lymphoma. Dogs with hypercalcemia of malignancy, often associated with mediastinal lymphoma, are also less likely to achieve prolonged survival times, due to the multi-organ damage associated with chronic elevations in ionized calcium. Lymphoma involving other extranodal sites such as the skin, can be managed with combination therapies including surgery, radiation, and systemic chemotherapy; however, the development of refractory and progressive disease is common.

HEMOSTATIC DISORDERS

Effective hemostasis depends on an adequate number of functional platelets, an adequate concentration and activity of plasma coagulation and fibrinolytic proteins, and a normally responsive blood vasculature. Primary hemostasis is accomplished by interaction of platelets with exposed subendothelial surfaces. Simultaneously, plasma coagulation proteins are activated in a sequential cascade that depends on the phospholipid provided by the activated platelets and calcium ions from plasma to form a stable clot. Circumstances that activate platelets and the coagulation proteins also activate plasma fibrinolytic proteins, which ensure localization of the clot and its timely dissolution.

Bleeding diatheses may be caused by congenital or acquired defects in coagulation proteins, platelets, or the vasculature. Congenital or acquired deficiencies in coagulation proteins usually manifest clinically as delayed deep tissue hemorrhage and hematoma formation, while congenital or acquired defects or deficiencies of platelets usually manifest as superficial petechial and ecchymotic hemorrhages (especially of mucous membranes), epistaxis, melena, or prolonged bleeding at injection and incision sites.

Pathologic thrombosis may occur because of primary or inherited disorders of anticoagulant protein factors or because of secondary or acquired disorders. Often, these conditions are called hypercoagulable states. Anticoagulant proteins identified in animals include antithrombin III and protein C. Systemic diseases that enhance platelet responsiveness to agonists, alter the balance between anticoagulant and procoagulant protein factors, or increase the reactivity of endothelium are more common in animals than are inherited disorders.

Coagulation screening tests can help identify the defective or deficient coagulation protein. However, they have low sensitivity; usually, activity of a coagulation protein must be <30% and sometimes <10% of normal before an abnormality is detected. The prothrombin time (PT) tests the extrinsic and common pathways; the activated partial thromboplastin time (APTT) and the activated coagulation time (ACT) test the intrinsic and common pathways; and the thrombin time (TT) tests the quantity and quality of fibrinogen. Often, specific factors must be quantified to determine which protein is deficient. The APTT differs from the ACT in that the latter relies on platelet phospholipid to support the clotting reaction; therefore, if platelet concentration is <10,000/µL, the ACT may be prolonged. Mucosal bleeding time tests a bleeding defect usually due to a platelet disorder (quantitative or qualitative), but it may also indicate an intrinsic blood vessel problem.

Tests for increased risk or tendency toward thrombosis are not routinely available at commercial laboratories, but they are available through some research laboratories. Measurement of antithrombin III activity requires the least amount of special sample handling and sophisticated laboratory equipment; this test is being offered by increasing numbers of laboratories. Tests for measurement of activities of plasminogen, protein C, α_2-antiplasmin, tissue plasminogen activator, and plasminogen activator inhibitor have been established in some domestic animals. Crude tests, such as fibrin clot lysis tests, often are unreliable and poorly repeatable.

BLEEDING DIATHESES

COAGULATION PROTEIN DISORDERS

Congenital Coagulation Protein Disorders

In a severe deficiency or functional defect of coagulation proteins, clinical signs appear at an early age. Marked reductions in activity of coagulation proteins essential to hemostasis are usually fatal. Animals may be stillborn if there is <1% of normal activity or die shortly after birth owing to massive hemorrhage. Insufficient production of coagulation proteins or limited access to vitamin K by the immature neonatal liver may exacerbate a coagulation defect. If activity of any particular coagulation protein is 5-10% of normal, the neonate may survive, but signs usually appear before 6 mo of age. It is during this time, when numerous routine procedures (eg, vaccination, declawing, tail docking, dewclaw removal, ear cropping, and castration or ovariohysterectomy) are usually done, that a bleeding tendency may become apparent.

Most of the congenital coagulation protein disorders reported in domestic animals are deficiencies or abnormalities of a single factor. Dual or multiple factor defects are rare.

Congenital afibrinogenemia (Factor I deficiency) has been reported in a family of Saanen dairy goats but not in dogs or cats. Hypofibrinogenemia, accompanied by severe bleeding, has been reported in Saint Bernards and Vizslas; the ACT, APTT, PT, and TT were prolonged. Dysfibrinogenemia has been reported in an inbred family of Russian Wolfhounds (Borzois). The ACT, APTT, PT, and TT were prolonged, but fibrinogen was present by quantitative testing. Affected dogs had mild bleeding episodes with epistaxis and lameness, but trauma or surgery resulted in life-threatening bleeding. IV administration of fresh or fresh-frozen plasma or cryoprecipitate is the best treatment to stop the bleeding.

Factor II (prothrombin) disorders are rare. Boxer dogs have been reported to have abnormally functioning prothrombin but normal concentrations; the defect was inherited as an autosomal recessive. A disorder of Factor II has been reported in English Cocker Spaniels; clinical signs in affected puppies (epistaxis and gingival bleeding) decrease with age and adults bruise easily or have dermatitis. In affected puppies, TT is normal, while ACT, APTT, and PT are prolonged. Treatment is by transfusion of fresh whole blood; however, fresh or fresh-frozen plasma are preferable if RBC are not needed.

Factor VII deficiency has been reported in Beagles, English Bulldogs, Alaskan Malamutes, Miniature Schnauzers, Boxers, and mixed-breed dogs. It is inherited in an autosomal pattern with incomplete dominance. Usually, it is not associated with spontaneous clinical bleeding, but affected dogs may have bruising or prolonged bleeding after surgery. Prolonged postpartum hemorrhaging has been reported. Factor VII deficiency is most often diagnosed coincidentally when coagulation screening tests are performed; the PT is prolonged, and other test results are normal.

Factor VIII deficiency (hemophilia A) is the most common inherited bleeding disorder in dogs and cats; it has also been reported in several breeds of horses, including Arabians, Standardbreds, Quarter Horses, and Thoroughbreds. There is an X-linked pattern of inheritance, so usually females are asymptomatic carriers and males are affected. Rarely, in highly inbred families, a carrier female mated with an affected male can produce affected female offspring. In affected puppies, prolonged bleeding is seen from the umbilical vessels after birth, from the gingiva during tooth eruption, and after surgery such as tail docking, dewclaw removal, or ear cropping. Hemarthrosis accompanied by intermittent lameness, spontaneous hematoma formation, and hemorrhagic body cavity effusions also are common clinical findings in dogs with <5% of normal Factor VIII activity. Animals with 5-10% of normal activity often do not bleed spontaneously but exhibit prolonged bleeding after trauma or surgery. Affected cats and, sometimes, small dogs may show prolonged bleeding after surgery or trauma but rarely bleed spontaneously, probably because of their agility and light weight. Affected animals usually have very low concentrations of Factor VIII (<10%) and prolonged ACT and APTT. Von Willebrand's factor (Factor VIII-related antigen) concentrations are normal or greater than normal. Carrier animals have intermediate concentrations of Factor VIII (40-60%), and results of coagulation screening tests are usually normal. Care should be taken in diagnosis if animals are <6 mo old because of possible low production of coagulation factors by an immature liver. Usually, results of coagulation screening tests are normal in carrier animals. Treatment of bleeding diatheses requires repeated transfusions of fresh whole blood, fresh plasma, or fresh-frozen plasma concentrates (6-10 mL/kg) 2-3 times/day until bleeding has been controlled. Plasma is preferable to whole blood because of the possible sensitization of the animal to RBC antigens.

Factor IX deficiency (hemophilia B) is diagnosed less often than Factor VIII deficiency. It has been reported in several breeds of purebred dogs, a mixed-breed dog, Himalayan cats, a family of Siamese-cross cats, and a family of British Shorthaired cats. The defect is X-linked with carrier females and affected males, although affected females can occur in closely inbred families. Clinical presentation is similar to that of animals with Factor VIII deficiency. Animals with extremely low Factor IX activity (<1%) usually die at birth or shortly thereafter. Animals with 5-10% of normal Factor IX activity may spontaneously form hematomas, hemarthroses, hemorrhagic body cavity effusions, or organ hemorrhage. Gingival bleeding during tooth eruption or prolonged bleeding after tail docking or dewclaw removal can occur. Some animals are asymptomatic until trauma or surgery. The ACT and APTT are prolonged. Carrier animals with 40-60% of normal Factor IX activity are usually asymptomatic, and results of coagulation screening tests are normal. Treatment requires transfusion with fresh or fresh-frozen plasma (6-10 mL/kg) every 12 hr until bleeding resolves. Often, internal hemorrhage into the abdomen, thorax, CNS, or between muscle fascial planes occurs and may be undetected until a crisis.

Factor X deficiency has been reported in a single family of American Cocker Spaniels and a mixed-breed dog. In the former, the inheritance pattern was autosomal dominant with variable penetrance. Homozygotes usually die early in life or are stillborn due to massive internal hemorrhage. Heterozygotes have mild to severe bleeding problems. The ACT, APTT, and PT are usually prolonged when animals have <30% normal activity of Factor X. Transfusions with fresh or fresh-frozen plasma are required to control hemorrhage.

Factor XI deficiency has been recognized in Kerry Blue Terriers, a female English Springer Spaniel, a Great Pyrenees dog, Weimaraners, and Holstein cattle. Mild deficiencies usually go undetected. In severe deficiencies with Factor XI at 30-40% or less of normal activity, mild prolonged bleeding may occur after trauma or surgery. Bleeding tendencies usually are not immediate but delayed for 3-4 days. The ACT and APTT are usually prolonged. Transfusion with fresh or fresh-frozen plasma (6-10 mL/kg) is sufficient to stop the bleeding for up to 3 days. Repeat transfusions may be needed. Inheritance is autosomal, but it has not been determined if the gene is dominant or recessive. A single case involving an adult cat with epistaxis and diagnosed with systemic lupus erythematosus was attributed to the presence of a circulating inhibitor against Factor XI.

Factor XII deficiency has been reported in a German Shorthaired Pointer, a Standard Poodle, and a family of Miniature Poodles. Affected animals do not have clinical bleeding problems. The deficiency is usually diagnosed coincidentally when coagulation screening tests are performed. The ACT and APTT are prolonged. People with Factor XII deficiency do not have bleeding problems but are predisposed to thrombosis or infections, which is attributed to the normal role of Factor XII in fibrinolysis and complement activation. Tendencies for thrombosis or infection have not been reported in animals. Factor XII deficiency has been found to coexist with von Willebrand's disease in a dog and with Factor IX deficiency in a cat, but bleeding tendencies were not exacerbated. Factor XII is not present in the plasma of birds, marine mammals, and reptiles, with no untoward effects.

Prekallikrein deficiency has been reported in a Poodle, a family of miniature horses, and a family of Belgian horses. Clinical bleeding problems are not usually apparent. One horse bled excessively after castration. The diagnosis is usually made coincidentally when coagulation screening tests are performed. The ACT and APTT are usually prolonged.

Acquired Coagulation Protein Disorders

Most coagulation proteins are produced primarily in the liver. Therefore, liver disease characterized by necrosis, inflammation, neoplasia, or cirrhosis often is associated with decreased production of coagulation proteins, particularly Factors VII, IX, X, and XI. Because the various coagulation proteins have a relatively short half-life (4 hr to 2 days), mild to marked deficiencies can result secondary to severe hepatopathies. The APTT or PT (or both) are prolonged in 50-66% of dogs with liver disease, meaning that the factor activity is <30% of normal. Coagulation tests are often performed before liver biopsy. Severe hepatic diseases can also lead to disseminated intravascular coagulation. Fibrinogen, an acute phase reactant, and von Willebrand's factor, which is produced extrahepatically, can be increased in liver disease.

Ingestion of anticoagulant rodenticides by dogs and cats causes a coagulopathy owing to the lack of production of functional vitamin K-dependent factors (*see* RODENTICIDE POISONING, p 2508). Inactive precursor coagulation Factors II, VII, IX, and X are still produced by the liver, but γ-carboxylation of the inactive precursors does not occur because the rodenticide inhibits the epoxide-reductase enzyme required for recycling of active vitamin K. There are 2 classes of rodenticides: the coumarin compounds (warfarin, coumafuryl, brodifacoum, and bromadiolone) and the indanedione compounds (diphacinone, pindone, valone, and chlorophacinone). However, the half-life of the coumarins (up to 55 hr) is much shorter than that of the indanedione compounds (15-20 days). Affected animals may have hematoma formation (especially over pressure points) and bruising of superficial and deep tissues. Often, the animals do not bleed within the first 24 hr after ingestion of the toxin. The APTT, PT, and ACT are usually prolonged. Factor VII has the shortest half-life of the vitamin K-dependent coagulation proteins; therefore, the PT is often abnormal before other tests and can be used to monitor response to treatment. Vitamin K_1, 0.25-2.5 mg/kg, PO, for 4-6 days, is recommended for treatment of coumarin toxicity. Doses of vitamin K_1 as high as 5 mg/kg, PO, for 3-6 wk, may be required for treatment of indanedione toxicity; however, these high doses should be administered cautiously because Heinz body anemia has been reported in dogs given 4 mg/kg for 5 days. IV administration of vitamin K_1 is not recommended because anaphylactic reactions can result. Administration of vitamin K_3 is not useful.

Disseminated intravascular coagulation (DIC) is a syndrome characterized by massive activation and consumption of coagulation proteins, fibrinolytic proteins, and platelets. It is not a primary disease, but a disorder secondary to numerous triggering events such as bacterial, viral, rickettsial, protozoal, or parasitic diseases; heat stroke; burns; neoplasia; or severe trauma. In acute, fulminant DIC, the clinical presentation is uncontrolled hemorrhaging and the inability to form a normal clot. Classically, all coagulation screening tests (ACT, APTT, PT, thrombin time) are prolonged, fibrin (or fibrinogen) degradation products are increased, and fibrinogen and platelet concentrations are decreased. Death is caused by extensive microthrombosis or circulatory failure, leading to single or multiple organ failure. If the animal survives the acute DIC event, a chronic form of DIC can exist. Compensatory production of coagulation proteins and platelets by the liver and bone marrow, respectively, can alter the results of coagulation screening tests such that they may be within reference ranges or even shortened, and platelet concentrations may be normal. However, DIC can usually be identified by the presence of at least 3 abnormal coagulation test results. Horses, even in fulminant DIC, most often have hyperfibrinogenemia because their liver can produce much fibrinogen. Treatment should be directed toward correcting the underlying problem. Supportive care is essential. Administration of balanced electrolyte solutions to maintain effective circulating volume is imperative. Administration of heparin is controversial and should be accompanied by administration of plasma to assure adequate antithrombin III activity.

PLATELET DISORDERS

Disorders of platelets can be divided into 4 categories: congenital and acquired thrombocytopenias and congenital and acquired functional disorders.

Congenital Thrombocytopenia

Fetal and neonatal alloimmune thrombocytopenia occur when maternal antibodies are produced against a paternal antigen on fetal platelets. A group of lambs artificially reared and fed bovine colostrum had prolonged bleeding from puncture wounds from ear tag placement, subcutaneous bruising, weakness, and pale mucous membranes. All affected lambs died within 48 hr after birth. Thrombocytopenia was seen in whole blood, and platelets were markedly decreased on blood smears. The presence of antibodies directed against platelets was suspected because the cows from which colostrum was obtained had been used in a previous experiment in which they had been immunized against sheep blood.

Cyclic hematopoiesis in gray Collie dogs (p 51) is characterized by 12-day cycles of cytopenia. All marrow stem cells are affected, but neutrophils are most affected because of their short half-life (usually <24 hr). Mild to severe thrombocytopenia can be seen, and excessive bleeding is a potential complication. This autosomal recessive disorder is fatal; affected dogs usually die from fulminating infections before 6 mo of age. Even dogs that receive intense antibiotic therapy usually die by 3 yr of age with amyloidosis (p 478) secondary to chronic antigenic stimulation from recurrent infections. Treatment with recombinant granulocyte colony-stimulating factor was temporarily successful in alleviating the neutropenic cycles until antibodies were produced against the noncanine proteins.

Acquired Thrombocytopenia

Acquired thrombocytopenias are reported frequently in dogs and cats, less often in horses, and rarely in other species. Numerous causes have been identified, most involving immunologic or direct destruction of platelets.

Ehrlichial diseases, caused by *Ehrlichia platys* and *E canis*, cause mild to severe thrombocytopenia in dogs. *Ehrlichia platys* infection (*see* EHRLICHIOSIS AND RELATED INFECTIONS, p 638) usually is characterized by mild, often cyclic thrombocytopenia in the acute stages of the disease. Chronic infections often have constant mild to moderate thrombocytopenia. Morula (single to multiple, round to oval basophilic inclusions) can sometimes be identified in platelets of infected dogs. The thrombocytopenia is seldom severe enough to result in clinical bleeding tendencies. Ticks are the likely vectors. *E canis* infections (p 638) are characterized by variable alterations in total WBC count,

PCV, and platelet count. In acute infections, there is usually thrombocytopenia and possibly anemia or leukopenia. In chronic infections, there may or may not be thrombocytopenia or anemia; however, there is often leukocytosis and sometimes hyperglobulinemia (monoclonal or polyclonal). Infected dogs may have epistaxis, melena, gingival bleeding, retinal hemorrhage, hematoma formation, and prolonged bleeding after venipuncture or surgery.

Neoplasms like hemangiosarcoma may be associated with consumptive thrombocytopenia. Immunologic and inflammatory mechanisms cause increased platelet consumption and decreased platelet survival. However, bleeding tendencies without thrombocytopenia occasionally exist. Altered platelet function due to an acquired membrane defect has been associated with hyperglobulinemia. Vasculitis also may contribute to the hemostatic disorder. Bovine viral diarrhea virus may cause thrombocytopenia in cattle.

Primary immune-mediated thrombocytopenia (also called idiopathic thrombocytopenia or idiopathic thrombocytopenic purpura) is characterized by immune-mediated destruction of either circulating platelets or, less commonly, marrow megakaryocytes. It has been seen in dogs and horses. Clinical signs include petechiae of the gingivae or skin and ecchymosis, melena, or epistaxis. Platelets are usually <100,000/μL. Low platelet concentration and low mean platelet volume have been noted in the early stages but not in the later stages. Evaluation of megakaryocytes (by bone marrow aspiration) helps determine if circulating platelets or marrow megakaryocytes are targeted by antibody. A test for platelet factor 3 released from damaged platelets has been unreliable or not readily available commercially. A megakaryocyte immunofluorescence assay that detects antibodies on megakaryocytes has been done, but an adequate bone marrow aspiration sample must be obtained. A direct test for the presence of antiplatelet antibodies—an ELISA that detects platelet-bound antibodies—has been reported to have good sensitivity (94%) but is not highly specific for primary immune-mediated thrombocytopenia. A negative test result likely rules out primary immune-mediated thrombocytopenia as the cause of thrombocytopenia; however, a positive test result could indicate either primary immune-mediated thrombocytopenia or secondary immune-mediated thrombocytopenia (eg, thrombocytopenia associated with autoimmune hemolytic anemia, lymphoproliferative diseases, systemic lupus erythematosus). Administration of corticosteroids, starting at a fairly high dose and then tapering (as in the treatment of IMMUNE-MEDIATED HEMOLYTIC ANEMIA, p 11) is recommended. Other treatments reported are administration of danazol and ascorbate. Splenectomy should be reserved as a treatment for animals that have recurrent episodes of thrombocytopenia. Vincristine has been used to enhance the release of platelets from marrow megakaryocytes, but its usefulness to decrease immune destruction of platelets is questionable.

Vaccine-induced thrombocytopenia has been reported in dogs vaccinated repeatedly with modified live adenovirus and paramyxovirus vaccines. The thrombocytopenia occurs 3-10 days after repeat vaccination, is usually transient, and may be sufficiently mild that a bleeding tendency will not be evident unless superimposed on another platelet or coagulation disorder. The thrombocytopenia may develop due to antibody production against viral antigens attached to platelet surfaces or to nonspecific binding of antigen-antibody complexes to platelet surfaces.

Drug-induced thrombocytopenia has been reported in dogs, cats, and horses. One mechanism is marrow suppression of megakaryocytes or generalized marrow stem cell suppression (after administration of estrogen, chloramphenicol, phenylbutazone, diphenylhydantoin, and sulfonamides). Another mechanism is increased platelet destruction and consumption (after administration of sulfisoxazole, aspirin, diphenylhydantoin, acetaminophen, ristocetin, levamisole, methicillin, and penicillin). Drug reactions are idiosyncratic and therefore unpredictable. Platelets usually return to normal shortly after the drug is discontinued. Drug-induced bone marrow suppression may be prolonged.

Congenital Platelet Function Disorders

Congenital disorders of platelet function affect platelet adhesion, aggregation, or secretion. They can be either intrinsic or extrinsic to platelets. Testing of intrinsic platelet function requires careful handling of samples and specialized equipment that is not routinely available in diagnostic laboratories; therefore, the incidence of intrinsic functional defects in platelets is not known accurately. However, if a bleeding disorder (especially mucosal bleeding or superficial petechiation) exists in an animal that has not received any medication and that has normal coagulation screening test results, platelet concentration, and von Willebrand's factor concentration, then an intrinsic platelet defect should be suspected.

Congenital Intrinsic Platelet Function Disorders: Chédiak-Higashi syndrome (p 51) is an autosomal recessive disorder characterized by abnormal granule formation in leukocytes, melanocytes, and platelets. The defect appears to be in microtubule formation; therefore, granules, which are abnormally large but reduced in number, are evident in numerous types of cells. Diluted coat color results from the defect in the melanocytes. Leukocytes may have decreased functional ability to phagocytize and kill organisms (an inconsistent finding in animals), and platelets have decreased aggregation and release reactions. Platelets are almost devoid of dense granules and have markedly decreased storage quantities of adenosine diphosphate and serotonin. Prolonged bleeding in affected blue smoke Persian cats occurs after venipuncture or surgery. The syndrome has been diagnosed in mink, cattle, and beige mice with similar bleeding tendencies.

Canine thrombopathia has been described in Basset Hounds. Affected dogs have epistaxis, petechiation, and gingival bleeding. Results of studies suggest that inheritance is autosomal with variable penetrance. Platelets have abnormal fibrinogen receptor exposure and impaired dense granule release. Basset Hounds with mucosal bleeding and petechiation and normal concentrations of platelets and von Willebrand's factor should be suspected of having thrombopathia. Specific diagnosis of this disorder requires specialized platelet function testing. Results of the clot retraction test are usually normal.

Bovine thrombopathia is an autosomally inherited platelet function defect seen in Simmental cattle. Bleeding can be mild to severe in affected cattle and is exacerbated by trauma or surgery. Platelets have impaired aggregation responses.

Thrombasthenic thrombopathia has been diagnosed in Otterhounds. It is autosomally transmitted. Affected dogs have prolonged bleeding times and form hematomas at sites of venipuncture or injury. Numerous (30-80% of all platelets), bizarre, giant platelets are seen on blood smears. Membrane glycoproteins II and III are reduced. Blood from affected dogs does not have normal clot retraction, and the platelets do not aggregate normally after stimulation with ADP, collagen, or thrombin.

There is no specific treatment for any of the intrinsic platelet function disorders. In instances of severe hemorrhaging, fresh platelet-rich plasma can be administered. Whole blood may be administered if the affected animal is anemic.

Congenital Extrinsic Platelet Function Disorders: Von Willebrand's disease is caused by a defective or deficient von Willebrand's factor (also called Factor VIII-related antigen). It is the most common inherited bleeding disorder in dogs (reported in nearly all breeds and in mixed breeds) and has also been reported in cats, rabbits, and pigs. The disorder is relatively frequent (10-70% prevalence) in several breeds of dogs: Doberman Pinschers, German Shepherds, Golden Retrievers, Miniature Schnauzers, Pembroke Welsh Corgis, Shetland Sheepdogs, Basset Hounds, Scottish Terriers, Standard Poodles, and Standard Manchester Terriers. Two modes of inheritance are known. In the less common autosomal recessive pattern of inheritance, homozygosity is usually fatal, and heterozygosity results in asymptomatic carriers. In the more common inheritance pattern of autosomal dominant with incomplete penetrance, homozygotes and heterozygotes can have variable bleeding tendencies. Affected animals may have gingival bleeding, epistaxis, and hematuria. Some puppies may bleed excessively only after injection, venipuncture, or surgery, such as tail docking, ear cropping, and dewclaw removal. Von Willebrand's factor circulates as a complex with coagulation Factor VIII (also called Factor VIII-coagulant) and mediates platelet adhesion to subendothelial surfaces—the first step in clot formation. Defective or deficient von Willebrand's factor mimics disorders caused by thrombocytopenia or intrinsic platelet defects. Von Willebrand's disease should be suspected in animals with bleeding disorders that have normal results on coagulation screening tests and adequate platelet concentrations. Occasionally, affected animals may have decreased Factor VIII-coagulant and therefore have prolonged APTT and ACT. Quantitative tests of von Willebrand's factor are diagnostic. Drugs known to interfere with normal platelet function should be avoided in animals with suspected disease. Transfusion of fresh whole blood or fresh plasma (6-10 mL/kg) is effective in alleviating a bleeding episode.

Concomitant hemostatic abnormalities may exacerbate von Willebrand's disease. Hypothyroidism (p 461) previously had been thought to be associated with von Willebrand's disease; both conditions are prevalent in many of the same breeds of dogs, eg, Doberman Pinschers and Golden Retrievers. In one study, administration of thyroid supplementation to hypothyroid dogs without deficiency of von Willebrand's factor did not increase von Willebrand's factor activity; in fact, in most of the tested dogs, the activity actually decreased. Therefore, administration of levothyroxine as a treatment of von Willebrand's disease cannot be recommended and may even exacerbate the disease.

Acquired Platelet Function Disorders

Dogs with immune-mediated thrombocytopenia also may have an acquired platelet functional defect. Dogs can have excessive bleeding tendencies without severely decreased platelet concentrations. In dogs with immune-mediated thrombocytopenia, abnormal platelet function in addition to decreased platelet concentration may contribute to their bleeding tendency.

Several diseases have been associated with acquired platelet function disorders. Hyperglobulinemia associated with multiple myeloma induces a platelet membrane defect resulting in impaired hemostatic function. In uremia associated with any form of renal disease, platelet adhesion and aggregation are decreased. Quantitative platelet disorders have been reported in liver disease with or without coagulation protein deficiencies. In 2 studies of cats with thrombocytopenia, 29-50% had infectious diseases, including feline leukemia, feline infectious peritonitis, panleukopenia, or toxoplasmosis. The mechanism of thrombocytopenia has not been identified in many cases. Feline leukemia virus replicates and accumulates in megakaryocytes and platelets; aplasia or hypoplasia of marrow stem cells, immune-destruction of infected platelets, or extravascular sequestration of platelets within lymphoid tissues may contribute to thrombocytopenia in this disease.

Numerous drugs can impair platelet function. Drugs reported to block platelet receptor binding or to change platelet membrane charge or permeability include furosemide, penicillin, carbenicillin, lidocaine, phentolamine, and chlorpromazine. Drugs that inhibit transduction of messages received at the platelet surface include caffeine, theophylline, dipyridamole, and papavarine. Drugs that inhibit execution of platelet responses (aggregation, secretion, or thromboxane production) include aspirin, indomethacin, acetaminophen, phenylbutazone, ticlopidine, pentobarbital, and sulfinpyrazone. Clinical bleeding problems may not be caused by drug-induced impairment of platelet function unless another disorder associated with a hemostatic defect is also present.

VASCULAR DISORDERS

Congenital Vascular Disorders

Cutaneous asthenia (Ehlers-Danlos syndrome, rubber puppy disease) is caused by a defect in the maturation of type I collagen. This causes weak structural support of blood vessels and can result in hematoma formation and easy bruising. The disorder has been reported in dogs, cats, mink, horses, cattle, sheep, and people but is rare in domestic animals. The most striking clinical abnormality is loose, hyperextensible skin that tears easily. No treatment is available.

Acquired Vascular Disorders

Several diseases cause severe, often generalized vasculitis and are characterized by bleeding disorders.

Rocky Mountain spotted fever (p 641) is caused by *Rickettsia rickettsii*, which is transmitted by the ticks *Dermacentor variabilis* and *D andersoni*. The rickettsial organisms invade endothelial cells and cause cellular death with resultant perivascular edema and hemorrhage. Variable degrees of coagulation cascade activation can occur along with thrombocytopenia. Infected dogs may have epistaxis, petechial and ecchymotic hemorrhages, hematuria, melena, or retinal hemorrhages. In severely affected dogs, disseminated intravascular coagulation may occur.

Canine herpesvirus generally affects puppies 7-21 days old. Generalized necrotizing vasculitis is accompanied by perivascular hemorrhage. The disease is usually rapidly fatal, and most puppies die within 24 hr after showing signs.

PATHOLOGIC THROMBOSIS

Primary or Inherited Anticoagulant Disorders

Human infants with congenital deficiencies in anticoagulant proteins often die shortly after birth or in infancy owing to massive thrombosis. Congenital deficiency of any anticoagulant protein has not been recognized in domestic animals. If such a condition exists, it is probably incompatible with life.

Secondary or Acquired Anticoagulant Disorders

Certain diseases in animals have been associated with increased risk of thrombosis. Cats with cardiomyopathy, more commonly the dilated form but also the hypertrophic and restrictive forms, can form large thromboemboli in the aorta or brachial artery. Thrombosis has been seen in dogs with protein-losing nephropathies, hyperadrenocorticism, chronic hypothyroidism accompanied by atherosclerosis, and rare instances of autoimmune hemolytic anemia. Thrombi and thromboemboli have been seen in horses with systemic inflammatory diseases (such as colic, laminitis, or equine ehrlichial colitis) and in instances of prolonged jugular catheter placement and infusion of drugs that irritate the vasculature.

In protein-losing nephropathies (eg, glomerulopathies, nephrotic syndrome, renal amyloidosis), a deficiency of antithrombin III has been well documented. Antithrombin III has a molecular weight of 57,000 kilodaltons (kD), which is similar in size to albumin (60,000 kD); therefore, glomerular lesions sufficient to result in albumin loss also result in loss of antithrombin III. Other abnormalities identified in renal disease include increased responsiveness of platelets to agonists, increased procoagulant activities, and decreased antiplasmin activity. At present, the etiology of thrombosis is thought to be multifactorial.

Hypercholesterolemia has been associated with increased risk of thromboembolism. It is hypothesized that endothelial and platelet membrane phospholipid concentrations are altered, which leads to damaged vasculature and increased platelet responsiveness to agonists, respectively. Increased production of thromboxane via the cyclooxygenase pathway in platelets has been seen. Diseases characterized by hypercholesterolemia include hyperadrenocorticism, diabetes mellitus, nephrotic syndrome, hypothyroidism, and pancreatitis. All have been associated with increased risk of thrombus formation, often pulmonary thrombosis.

Cats with cardiomyopathy have increased risk of thromboembolism. Endomyocardial lesions and turbulent blood flow through the heart chambers and valves secondary to altered myocardial functioning are thought to initiate thrombus formation. Specific deficiencies of anticoagulant or fibrinolytic proteins have not been seen. Interestingly, antithrombin III is markedly increased but does not provide protective benefits. Cats with cardiac disease secondary to hyperthyroidism are often administered drugs (eg, propranolol, atenolol, or diltiazem) that abate clinical signs of cardiac dysfunction. These drugs appear to protect against increased risk of thrombosis by altering platelet responsiveness to agonists.

Horses with colic associated with endotoxemia have decreased plasminogen activity and protein C antigen concentration. These horses have increased mortality and risk for thrombus formation. Laminitis is thought to be the end result of several diverse systemic disorders. Microthrombi in the vasculature of the hoof lamina have been identified in the early stages of laminitis. One theory is that endotoxin has direct effects on the vasculature and activates contact factors in the coagulation cascade. Ischemia of the lamina secondary to edema, vascular compression, and possible blood shunting at the level of the coronet also damage endothelium. When circulation is reestablished, reperfusion injury results, and the exposed subendothelial collagen promotes thrombosis.

The most appropriate treatment of an animal with thrombi or thromboemboli is diagnosis and management of the underlying disease process, along with good supportive care. Maintenance of adequate tissue perfusion is critical. Dissolution of clots and prevention of clot recurrence by administration of anticoagulants (eg, heparin and coumarin) has had mixed success. Heparin facilitates the action of antithrombin III, but to be effective, adequate antithrombin III must be present. In dogs with protein-losing nephropathies or in horses with endotoxemia, plasma transfusion may be necessary before heparin therapy is effective. Coumarin has been most useful for control or prevention, rather than for treatment. Fibrinolytic compounds have been administered to animals to enhance dissolution of clots. Tissue plasminogen activator has more fibrin specificity than does streptokinase or urokinase and, therefore, provides more localized fibrinolytic effects (although not totally). The main deterrent to use of tissue plasminogen activator is its high cost. Streptokinase is more available and less expensive, but the therapeutic dose is difficult to determine. Many animals have naturally occurring antibodies to streptokinase as a result of previous streptococcal infections. Administration of streptokinase must be sufficient to neutralize all antibodies but not produce a systemic fibrinolytic state with resultant bleeding diathesis.

LEUKOCYTIC DISORDERS

LEUKOCYTOSIS AND LEUKOPENIA

Leukocytes, or white blood cells (WBC), in mammalian blood include segmented neutrophils, band neutrophils, lymphocytes, monocytes, eosinophils, and basophils. These cells vary in their site of production, their duration of peripheral circulation and recirculation, and the stimuli that affect their release into and migration out of the vascular bed. Differential counts also vary among species.

Leukocytosis is an increase in the total number of circulating WBC; **leukopenia** is a decrease. Changes in WBC counts and morphologic appearance of various leukocytes are evaluated by comparison with reference ranges for each species. Differential WBC counts may be reported either as total (absolute) cell numbers per volume of blood (μL) or in relative percentages of the total. Valid interpretations can be made only by considering the absolute numbers. *See* TABLE 6, p 2584, for reference values for total WBC and differential WBC counts in absolute numbers and in percentages for common domestic species. In neonates the total WBC count is more variable and often higher than in adults. Age-related reference values should be used to evaluate hemograms in young animals, especially species in which lymphocytes are more numerous (and neutrophils less) than in adults. This may interfere with the identification of lymphopenia. Generally, differential WBC patterns of adults are reached at about the age of sexual maturity.

Differential WBC counts are performed by identifying and classifying the first 100 or 200 intact WBC encountered in the monolayer of a blood smear. The absolute number of each WBC type is then determined by multiplying the percentage of a particular WBC in the differential count by the total WBC count. Smears from buffy coat preparations are sometimes used to concentrate cells for differential counts in cases of marked leukopenia, to find circulating neoplastic cells, to identify intracellular infectious agents, or to perform fluorescent antibody testing.

Increases in any of the various cell types are indicated by the suffix "philia" or "cytosis" (eg, neutrophilia, lymphocytosis, etc); decreases are indicated by the suffix "penia" or "cytopenia" (eg, neutropenia, lymphopenia, etc). An increase in immature nonsegmented neutrophils above species reference values is called a **left shift**, which may be regenerative or degenerative. A regenerative left shift occurs when a leukocytosis is due to a neutrophilia and the absolute number of nonsegmented neutrophils does not exceed the absolute number of segmented neutrophils. A degenerative left shift occurs when nonsegmented neutrophil numbers exceed segmented neutrophil numbers. Occasionally, marked peripheral leukocytosis is difficult to differentiate from granulocytic leukemia due to the magnitude of both the left shift and increase in WBC. When the total WBC count exceeds 30,000/μL in horses and cows, and 75,000/μL in dogs and cats, with a neutrophilia and left shift due to inflammation, these reactions may be termed a **leukemoid response**.

Although nucleated red blood cells (nRBC) are counted as WBC by most counting techniques, they should not be included in the WBC differential count. The total nucleated cell count must be corrected to give an accurate WBC count if >5 nRBC/100 cells are encountered during the WBC differential count. The total WBC count must be corrected for nRBC by the following formula:

$$\frac{100}{100 + (\text{nRBC per 100 WBC})} \times \text{total WBC count} = \text{corrected WBC count}$$

Within blood vessels, WBC occur in 2 subpopulations—the central and the marginal pools. In most species, the ratio of neutrophils in the central pool to neutrophils in the marginal pool is 1:1; however, in cats it is 1:3. WBC in venipuncture samples represent the central pool because venipuncture fails to collect the WBC of the marginal pool along the endothelial surfaces. WBC in the circulating pool can be increased by the following mechanisms: epinephrine can redistribute neutrophils from the marginal pool to the circulating pool, and corticosteroids can prevent neutrophils from adhering to the endothelial surface.

Granulocytes

Granulocytes consist of neutrophils, eosinophils, and basophils, which are produced in the bone marrow from a common progenitor cell, the myeloblast. The proliferative (mitotic) pool consists of myeloblasts, promyelocytes, and myelocytes, which are ~20% of the marrow myeloid cells. The storage (maturation) pool, comprising 80% of the marrow myeloid cells, consists of metamyelocytes, band neutrophils, and segmented neutrophils that are functionally mature. During maturation, promyelocytes first form primary granules (lysosomes) that later become inapparent. During the myelocyte stage, granulocytes form specific granules that have characteristic staining affinity, eg, basophilic for basophils, eosinophilic for eosinophils, and neutral for neutrophils. These cytoplasmic granules protect the body against microbial and parasitic infections or, if not modulated, may result in tissue damage.

Neutrophils: In peripheral blood, neutrophils normally are mature (segmented). Neutrophils from bone marrow enter the peripheral bloodstream, remain for a half-life of ~6 hr, and adhere to the endothelium; when needed, they enter tissues to function primarily in phagocytosis and enzymatic killing of bacteria. They do not return to the vascular bed. The maintenance of normal numbers of neutrophils in the peripheral blood depends on regular replacement from the bone marrow. Small numbers of young (band) neutrophils may normally be found in the peripheral blood of some species such as pigs and dogs (and rarely in horses and cattle).

Morphologic changes in neutrophil cytoplasm, including toxic granulation, diffuse cytoplasmic basophilia, cytoplasmic vacuolation, and Döhle bodies, may occur during systemic bacterial infections or severe inflammation and are referred to as toxic changes. Although all circulating WBC are exposed to the same systemic diseases, only neutrophils are evaluated for toxic changes. Toxic change is graded subjectively as mild, moderate, or marked, based on the number of affected neutrophils and the severity of toxic change. Clinical significance is reflected by the type of toxic change and its severity. Toxic granulation is identified by the presence of pink to purple intracytoplasmic granules within neutrophils; these granules represent primary granules of the neutrophil that have retained their staining affinity. Diffuse cytoplasmic basophilia and cytoplasmic vacuolation frequently occur together. The cytoplasmic basophilia is due to persistent ribosomes, and the cytoplasmic vacuolation possibly due to autodigestion of the cell. Döhle bodies appear as pale blue, intracytoplasmic inclusions within neutrophils. Even when present in high numbers, Döhle bodies alone usually indicate a mild toxic change. They also may occur in clinically healthy cats. Bacterial toxins induce the most severe toxic changes. Severe toxic change is indicated when toxic granulation, diffuse cytoplasmic basophilia, or cytoplasmic vacuolation are present in a moderate to high number of the peripheral blood neutrophils. The presence of many severely toxic neutrophils indicates a guarded to poor prognosis. An autosomal recessive condition in Birman cats results in fine intracytoplasmic eosinophilic granules within neutrophils that may be mistaken for toxic granulation; these cats have normal neutrophil function. Metachromatic intracytoplasmic granules may occur in WBC in metabolic storage diseases.

The magnitude of **neutrophilia** induced by inflammation is a function of the size of the bone marrow storage pool of granulocytes, hyperplasia of the marrow, and rate of WBC migration into the tissues. The storage pool is quite large in dogs and far smaller in cattle; dogs can sometimes have a reactive WBC count of $>100 \times 10^3/\mu L$, while counts of $>30 \times 10^3/\mu L$ are uncommon in cattle. Neutrophilia, often the cause of leukocytosis, generally characterizes bacterial infections and conditions associated with extensive tissue necrosis, including burns, trauma, extensive surgery, and neoplasia. Extreme leukocytosis ($>100,000/\mu L$) may be associated with neoplasms that produce colony-stimulating factors, *Hepatozoon canis* infections, leukemias, and closed cavity infections. In pyometra and abscesses, the wall of the cavity inhibits the migration of neutrophils into the site of infection but does not impair the release of leukocyte chemotactic substances. The net effect is a high peripheral neutrophil count, which often includes an increased number of band neutrophils (regenerative left shift).

Neutropenia may occur due to margination of neutrophils (pseudoneutropenia), excessive tissue demand or destruction of neutrophils, or reduced or ineffective granulopoiesis. Neutropenia may occur with overwhelming bacterial infections, especially gram-negative septicemia or endotoxemia, in all species. Immune-mediated destruction of neutrophils occurs in animals, and assays have been developed to detect antineutrophil antibodies in horses. Idiosyncratic drug reactions may result in neutropenia or sometimes pancytopenia, eg, sulfonamides, penicillins, cephalosporins, phenylbutazone in dogs, and chloramphenicol in cats. Feline leukemia virus has also been associated with neutropenia.

Eosinophils: Eosinophils contain enzymes that modulate products of mast cells or basophils released in response to IgE stimulation. For example, histamine released by basophils or mast cells is modulated by histaminase in eosinophils. The cytoplasmic granules of eosinophils contain proteins that are involved in parasite killing. **Eosinophilia** is induced by substances that promote allergic responses and hypersensitivity (eg, histamine and allied substances) and by IgE. Eosinophils increase in response to parasitic infections, especially those that involve tissue migration, due to the contact of parasite chitin with host tissues. Eosinophilia occurs in ~50% of dogs with dirofilariasis. The severity of eosinophilia produced by fleas depends on both host sensitivity and severity of the infestation. Eosinophilia also may occur with inflammation of the GI, urogenital, or respiratory tracts, or of the skin. **Hypereosinophilic syndrome** has been reported in cats; diagnosis requires the presence of >1,500 eosinophils/μL for 6 mo, tissue infiltration and organ dysfunction due to eosinophils, and lack of a recognized etiology. Less commonly, peripheral eosinophilia may be associated with neoplasia. Localized eosinophilic tissue lesions do not necessarily produce a peripheral eosinophilia, eg, the eosinophilic granuloma dermatopathies and oral lesions of cats. Usual WBC differential count techniques are not sufficiently sensitive to reliably detect eosinopenia in a single blood count. The absence of eosinophils in repeated hemograms indicates **eosinopenia**, which is most commonly reported with corticosteroid-induced (stress) leukograms.

Basophils: Basophils are rare in all common domestic animals. Basophil granules contain histamine, heparin, and sulfated mucopolysaccharides. Although basophils and mast cells have similar functions and enzymatic contents, basophils do not become mast cells and there is no proof of a common precursor cell. Among species, normal peripheral blood basophil numbers vary inversely with the number of tissue mast cells. For example, in dogs, mast cells are numerous in the tissues, and basophils are rare in blood. A peripheral basophilia is uncommon; however, it does occur in some animals with heartworm disease (and other causes of systemic antigenemia) or pathologic lipemias (eg, liver disease, nephrotic syndrome, and hereditary hyperlipoproteinemias). A basopenia is difficult to document and has no diagnostic significance.

Lymphocytes

Lymphocytes originate from a marrow stem cell and mature in lymph nodes, spleen, and associated peripheral lymphoid tissues. Mature lymphocytes consist of 2 subpopulations, B cells and T cells. **B cells** (B for bone marrow or bursa equivalent) are the precursors of plasma cells and produce antibodies for humoral immunity. **T cells** (T for thymus) engage in cellular immunity (eg, histocompatibility and delayed-type hypersensitivity). A lymphocyte in tissue may return to the vascular bed and recirculate. Some lymphocytes are long-lived compared with other WBC and may survive weeks to years.

A peripheral **lymphocytosis** has many possible causes, including a physiologic (epinephrine) lymphocytosis, immune stimulation, and lymphocytic leukemia. Immune (antigenic) stimulation is associated with chronic inflammation and characterized by the presence of reactive (immunologically stimulated) lymphocytes. These lymphocytes have a more basophilic and slightly more abundant cytoplasm due to increased protein synthesis. Reactive lymphocytes may occur in any disease that causes moderate to marked systemic immunostimulation. Lymphocyte counts of up to 17,000/μL, with some cells containing intracytoplasmic azurophilic granules, have been reported in dogs infected with *Ehrlichia canis*. Persistent lymphocytosis in cattle is a B-cell hyperplasia, with lymphocyte counts ranging from 7,000-15,000/μL.

Lymphopenia is a common leukogram abnormality. It is most commonly associated with endogenous (stress) or exogenous corticosteroids and is the result of redistribution or lysis of lymphocytes. Lymphopenia also occurs due to other causes, such as extravasation of lymph (eg, lymphangiectasia, chylous effusion), impaired lymphopoiesis, some viral infections, and hereditary immunodeficiency diseases (eg, combined immunodeficiency disease of Arabian foals).

Monocytes

Monocytes are formed in the bone marrow and mature from monoblasts to promonocytes to monocytes. Monocytes enter the peripheral blood for ~24-36 hr and exit into tissues and become fixed tissue macrophages (eg, Kupffer's cells) or migrating macrophages at sites of inflammation. Monocytes and **macrophages** can perform pinocytosis and phagocytosis and form multinucleated giant cells in the tissue, particularly in response to foreign bodies. Monocytes and macrophages are a major source of colony-stimulating factors and cytokines that regulate inflammatory responses, and they function as antigen-processing cells. **Monocytosis** may be associated with chronic inflammation (particularly mycotic and other granulomatous infections), endocarditis, bacteremia, or corticosteroid or stress responses (especially in dogs). **Monocytopenia** is occasionally seen but usually has no diagnostic significance.

THE LEUKOGRAM

Physiologic Leukocytosis: Leukocytosis may occur as a result of exercise or excitement; this response is mediated by increased epinephrine. Epinephrine centralizes the marginal pool; thus, the effect of excitement may double the total WBC count within minutes. In addition, splenic contraction releases WBC and RBC into the peripheral circulation. The leukocytosis is usually due to a mature neutrophilia without a left shift. A lymphocytosis also may be present, especially in young horses or cats.

Corticosteroid-induced or Stress Leukogram: Treatment with exogenous corticosteroids or endogenous release results in a typical leukogram with lymphopenia as a consistent feature and invariably accompanied by neutrophilia. The net effect on the total WBC count is a function of the species and its normal differential WBC count. In dogs, in which neutrophils are the predominant circulating WBC, corticosteroids produce leukocytosis. In cattle, in which lymphocytes predominate, the WBC count is variable depending on the degree of neutrophilia and lymphopenia. There usually is a reversal of the neutrophil to lymphocyte ratio. Stress leukograms have a characteristic WBC differential count consisting of a mature neutrophilia, lymphopenia, and eosinopenia. Neutrophilia is due to decreased adherence to the vascular endothelium, which prolongs circulating time and shifts the marginating cells to the circulating pool, and increased marrow release of neutrophils. Lymphopenia is due to redistribution or lysis of lymphocytes. Monocyte numbers are variable; however, a monocytosis often occurs in steroid or stress reactions in dogs and horses.

Other Leukogram Alterations: Although the specific features of leukocytosis and leukopenia vary with species, there are some generalities. Radiation and radiomimetic drugs (eg, many antineoplastic drugs) produce leukopenia. Lymphocytes are extremely sensitive to radiation, but mature granulocytes—unlike their precursors in the bone marrow—are not particularly radiosensitive. Pancytopenias, which include leukopenias, may result from drug toxicities (eg, estrogen toxicity in dogs, bracken fern toxicity in cattle), nutritional deficiencies, stem-cell alterations (possibly immune-mediated), and space-occupying lesions of bone marrow (myelophthisis). Generally, viral infections, particularly acute infections not associated with extensive tissue necrosis, produce leukopenia as neutropenia and may have mild lymphocytosis or lymphopenia. In viral infections of longer duration (2-3 wk) with secondary bacterial complications, the total WBC count may be increased or within normal limits due to concurrent neutrophilia and lymphopenia. Ehrlichiosis in dogs is associated with thrombocytopenia, but persistent leukopenia may be seen, especially in chronic cases.

Species-specific Leukograms: In **dogs**, the normal neutrophil to lymphocyte ratio is ~3.5:1. A variety of infectious and noninfectious diseases can induce changes in the leukogram. Inflammation, corticosteroid (stress) reactions, and physiologic (epinephrine) responses are common causes of leukocytosis. A leukocytosis is typically present at parturition in the bitch. Cyclic hematopoiesis of gray Collies (*see* below) produces peripheral neutropenia at 11- to 14-day intervals. Severe panleukopenia with total WBC counts <1 × 10^3/µL often characterizes parvovirus infection, while in coronavirus infection and in infectious hepatitis, neutropenia may be more moderate. In the later stages of canine distemper with secondary bacterial infection, the total WBC count may be normal with neutrophilia, lymphopenia, and sometimes increased band neutrophils and toxic changes.

In **cats**, the neutrophilic response can be strong, although less marked than in dogs. Feline infectious peritonitis generally does not produce a leukopenia but more commonly a neutrophilia and lymphopenia. Feline leukemia virus has a variable effect on peripheral blood cells. In the absence of leukemia or lymphoma (*see* below), it may produce a panleukopenia with marked neutropenia, toxic changes, and mild lymphopenia sometimes with atypical cells that may resemble the leukogram induced by feline panleukopenia virus.

In **horses**, the normal neutrophil to lymphocyte ratio is ~1.1:1. The magnitude of neutrophilic response is much less than in dogs or cats. The highest absolute lymphocyte values are normally present in yearlings. In horses, corticosteroids induce neutrophilia, lymphopenia, eosinopenia, and frequently monocytosis. In equine viral arteritis, an initial leukopenia during the febrile episode is followed by lymphopenia and mild neutrophilia. Leukopenia occurs in equine herpesvirus infection, influenza, and sometimes in the early febrile phase of equine infectious anemia. In equine ehrlichiosis, there may be leukopenia, sometimes accompanied by thrombocytopenia, anemia, or both.

In **cattle** and most ruminants, the normal neutrophil to lymphocyte ratio is ~0.5:1, and the neutrophilic response is weaker than in any other common domestic species. Leukopenia occurs early in bacterial infections in ruminants and persists longer than in other species due to their low bone marrow neutrophil reserve (storage) pool and lymphopenia secondary to endogenous corticosteroid release. A degenerative left shift frequently develops in ruminants with acute inflammatory disease; however, it does not carry the same poor prognosis as in other species unless the WBC count fails to increase in 2-3 days. Cattle with septic infections, including septic mastitis or peritonitis, characteristically have leukopenia, lymphopenia, and neutropenia the first few days. A return to normal of absolute lymphocyte and neutrophil numbers or neutrophilia are good prognostic signs. Persistent leukopenia or toxic changes in the neutrophils indicates an unfavorable prognosis.

In **pigs**, the normal neutrophil to lymphocyte ratio is 0.7:1. Neutrophilic responses may be marked, possibly even more so than in dogs. The stress of venipuncture may result in a doubling of the circulating neutrophil count in 30 min, which persists for 8 hr; this may impair studies that require frequent serial blood sampling. During parturition, sows manifest neutrophilia, lymphopenia, and eosinopenia. Leukopenia is marked ($<10 \times 10^3/\mu L$) in classical swine fever and African swine fever.

LEUKEMIA AND LYMPHOMA

Leukemia and lymphoma with a circulating leukemia should be considered as differential diagnoses in leukocytosis. In some instances of lymphoma without leukemia, necrosis within the tumor induces neutrophilia. Rarely, a diffuse lymphomatous or leukemic infiltration of the bone marrow (myelophthisis) results in leukopenia, generally in association with anemia and thrombocytopenia. Leukemia is defined as malignant neoplastic disease of the WBC or RBC precursors, with neoplastic cells in the peripheral blood and bone marrow. Leukemia is generally recognized by identifying moderate to high numbers of blast cells within the peripheral blood and/or bone marrow. Classifying blast cells (eg, lymphoblasts, rubriblasts, myeloblasts) may be difficult by routine light microscopy, and special stains for cell enzymes (eg, peroxidase) or monoclonal antibodies to lineage-specific antigens may be needed to correctly identify the cell line involved. Leukemia and leukocytosis may resemble one another; sometimes the distinction is difficult. Extreme leukocytosis (leukemoid response) may be confused with leukemia, in particular with chronic myelogenous leukemia, in which a persistent strong leukocytosis exists without the presence of blast cells characteristic of most leukemias.

INHERITED LEUKOCYTIC DISORDERS

Chédiak-Higashi Syndrome: This syndrome, inherited as an autosomal recessive, is characterized by leukocyte dysfunction secondary to abnormal lysosomes. It has been described in humans, mink, foxes, Persian cats, Hereford and Brangus cattle, mice, and killer whales. There is an increased susceptibility to bacterial infections due to impaired WBC function, an increased tendency to bleed due to platelet granule defects, and partial oculocutaneous albinism due to abnormal melanin distribution. The beige mouse and the Aleutian mink exemplify the pigment dilution seen in the syndrome. Abnormal giant granules appear to develop after fusion of lysosomes in neutrophils, eosinophils, renal tubular cells, epithelial cells, and Kupffer's cells of humans, mink, cats, and cattle. In mice, only the WBC appear affected. Pink to magenta staining characteristics of the granules are similar in all species. Diagnosis is based on pigment dilution, presence of giant granules, and increased susceptibility to infections.

Cyclic Hematopoiesis in Gray Collie Dogs: This syndrome, also called Gray Collie syndrome and canine cyclic neutropenia, is an inherited, autosomal recessive immunodeficiency characterized by a profound cyclic neutropenia, overwhelming recurrent bacterial infections, bleeding, and coat color dilution. The molecular basis is thought to be a cyclic bone-marrow maturation defect at the level of the pluripotential hematopoietic stem cells. Arrest of neutrophil maturation occurs at regular cycles of 11- to 14-day intervals; the peripheral neutropenia lasts 3-4 days and is followed by a neutrophilia. All other hematopoietic cells, including lymphocytes, are also cyclic with the same interval but occur at different times compared with the neutropenic phase. Hematopoietic growth factors (eg, erythropoietin) and other hormones (eg, cortisol) also have a cyclic pattern.

Affected puppies often die at birth or during the first week and rarely live >1 yr. Surviving dogs may be stunted and weak and develop serious recurrent bacterial infections during periods of neutropenia, which are characterized by fever, septicemia, pneumonia, and gastroenteritis. They also develop amyloidosis (p 478) in many tissues, including kidney and liver, resulting in renal disease and coagulopathies. All affected dogs have a diluted coat color, known as a pleiotropic effect, with phenotypically black hairs diluted to charcoal-gray and phenotypically brown or sable hairs diluted to silver-gray. Diagnosis is based on clinical signs and repeated complete blood counts over a 2-wk period.

Bone marrow transplantation at an early age eliminates the cyclic hematopoiesis and effects a clinical cure. In one study, administration of human recombinant granulocyte colony-stimulating factors temporarily eliminated the cyclic hematopoiesis until the dogs were assumed to have produced neutralizing antibodies.

Pelger-Huët Anomaly: This condition of humans, cats, rabbits, and dogs, characterized by failure of granulocytes to lobulate from the band form to the segmented form, appears to be inherited as an autosomal dominant trait. The cells, particularly neutrophils, are hyposegmented and the chromatin is condensed; the CBC shows an apparent left shift with a normal WBC count. This anomaly is usually an incidental laboratory finding; WBC function is normal, and heterozygotes do not exhibit clinical signs. The homozygous state, described in rabbits and one kitten, is lethal and associated with skeletal deformities and increased susceptibility to infection. Pseudo-Pelger-Huët anomaly refers to acquired hyposegmentation of granulocytes secondary to chronic infection, viral disease, drug therapy, and neoplasia; it has been reported in rats, dogs, and cattle.

Bovine Leukocyte Adhesion Deficiency: In this lethal, autosomal recessive disorder seen in Holstein cattle, the leukocytes lack or partially lack the glycoproteins (integrins) that are essential for normal leukocyte adherence and emigration. Recurrent bacterial infections, persistent neutrophilia (often >100,000/μL), lymphocytosis, and death (usually between 2 wk and 8 mo of age) are characteristic. Calves often are stunted and have recurrent pneumonia, ulcerative stomatitis, enteritis, and periodontitis. On examination of tissues, there are few neutrophils, except within vessel lumens, because they persist in the circulation and are unable to enter the tissues. Testing is available to detect carriers. Leukocyte adhesion molecule deficiency has also been described in Irish Setters (p 658).

LYMPHADENITIS AND LYMPHANGITIS

CASEOUS LYMPHADENITIS OF SHEEP AND GOATS

Caseous abscessation of lymph nodes and internal organs caused by *Corynebacterium pseudotuberculosis* occurs worldwide and is widely distributed throughout North America. It is an important endemic infection in regions with large sheep and goat populations. Economic losses result mostly from condemnation and trim of infected carcasses and devaluation of hides. Caseous lymphadenitis is also a cause of ill-thrift and sudden death in animals with internal abscesses. However, producers often report that the major impact in the flock is from disagreeable aesthetics, which may result in loss of breeding stock sales as well as early culling. Although principally an infection of sheep and goats, sporadic disease also occurs in horses and cattle (*see* below), camelids, water buffalo, wild ruminants, primates, pigs, and fowl. It rarely causes regional lymphadenitis in humans.

Etiology and Pathogenesis: The small gram-positive rod is a facultative intracellular parasite that is found on fomites and in soil and manure contaminated with purulent exudate. Two biotypes have been identified based on the ability of the bacteria to reduce nitrate: a nitrate-negative group that infects sheep and goats, and a nitrate-positive group that infects horses. Isolates from cattle are a heterogeneous group. All strains produce an antigenically similar exotoxin with enzymatic activity (phospholipase D) that appears to be leukotoxic and that can damage endothelial cells and promote spread from the initial site of infection to regional lymph nodes and visceral organs. The chemical composition of its cell wall (high lipid content) enables the organism to resist being killed by phagocytes and to maintain chronic infection despite a good immune response.

Infection occurs after *C pseudotuberculosis* penetrates through unbroken or abraded skin or through mucous membranes. Most infections occur through wounds contaminated with purulent exudate from ruptured external and pulmonary abscesses. Contaminated dipping vats and shearing, handling, and feeding equipment are responsible for spread of the organism, along with confinement housing at high stocking densities. The pus contains large numbers of bacteria that can survive for months in hay, shavings, and soil. The disease is most often introduced into a flock by entry of an apparently healthy carrier from an infected flock, by contact on shared pastures, or via contaminated fomites such as shearing equipment.

Clinical Findings: Caseous lymphadenitis is a chronic, recurring disease. A slowly enlarging, localized, and nonpainful abscess may develop either at the point of entry into the skin or in the regional lymph node (superficial or external form), from which it may spread via the blood or lymphatic system and cause abscessation of internal lymph nodes or organs (visceral or internal form). Initial infection may cause no clinical signs or may be accompanied by high fever, anorexia, anemia, and cellulitis at the infection site. Superficial abscesses enlarge and may rupture and discharge infectious pus. In sheep on range, most superficial abscesses develop in the prescapular and prefemoral region, with transmission probably occurring when the flock is gathered for group treatments such as shearing. In housed goats and sheep, superficial abscesses develop mainly in the head and neck region, likely due to transmission by contaminated feed, feeders, and other fomites. Animals with superficial abscesses show no obvious ill effects unless the location of the abscess interferes with functions such as swallowing or breathing. Abscessation may recur at the same site. Internal abscesses should be considered as a potential diagnosis for "thin ewe syndrome," in which an adult small ruminant loses condition in the face of adequate nutrition. The visceral form is usually more extensive in sheep than in goats, mostly involving abscesses of the pulmonary parenchyma and mediastinal lymph nodes. Other less common manifestations include caseous bronchopneumonia, arthritis, abortion, CNS abscessation often occurring in the pituitary gland, abscessation of a vertebral body causing paresis or paralysis, scrotal abscessation, and rarely, mastitis. Scrotal (inguinal) abscesses can cause temporary infertility in rams. The incidence of abscesses steadily increases with age; clinical disease is more prevalent in adults, and up to 40% of animals in a flock can have superficial abscesses.

Lesions: The typical gross lesion is a discrete abscess distended by thick and often dry, greenish yellow or white, purulent exudate. In sheep, the abscess often has the classically described laminated "onion-ring" appearance in cross section, with concentric fibrous layers separated by inspissated caseous exudate. In goats, the exudate is usually soft and pasty.

Diagnosis: The diagnosis can usually be based on clinical signs and flock history. For definitive diagnosis, an aspirate of an intact abscess should be submitted for bacteriologic examination; *C pseudotuberculosis* can easily be isolated, although it may be recovered in mixed culture with other pyogenic organisms. Suppurative lymphadenitis and abscesses can also be caused by various other pyogenic organisms, such as *Arcanobacter (Actinomyces) pyogenes*, *Staphylococcus aureus*, *Pasteurella multocida*, and occasionally anaerobes such as *Fusobacterium necrophorum*. Scrotal abscesses may be confused with orchitis due to *A pyogenes* or with epididymitis due to *Histophilus* sp, *Brucella ovis*, or other pyogenic organisms. The differential diagnosis for emaciated animals also should include ovine progressive pneumonia (maedi, visna), caprine arthritis and encephalitis, paratuberculosis (Johne's disease), dental disease, and parasitism.

Serologic testing is available commercially. Most tests detect antibodies to the phospholipase D exotoxin. A positive test should be interpreted as exposure to the exotoxin and may indicate active infection. Infected animals may have a false-negative result, likely because the infection is well walled off in abscesses, or if they are severely debilitated. Colostral titers usually disappear by 3-6 mo of age, so serologic testing of lambs or kids <6 mo old should be interpreted with caution. Vaccinated animals will test positive and should not be included in a serologic program. Goats tend to have higher titers than sheep.

Treatment and Control: Although the organism is susceptible to penicillin, treatment with antibiotics is usually not attempted because the formation of abscesses limits their penetration and effectiveness. Therefore, prophylactic and therapeutic treatment will not eliminate *C pseudotuberculosis* from infected flocks or individuals. Abscesses frequently recur after draining or attempted surgical excision. The practice of injecting abscesses with formalin should be discouraged as this practice is painful to the animal and may leave a residue of a carcinogenic compound in a food-producing animal.

Prevention is based on reducing transmission of the organism from infected to susceptible animals. Emaciated animals and those with recurring abscesses should be culled. When animals are too valuable to cull, those with developing abscesses should be isolated, and the abscesses lanced and flushed with an iodine solution. Any lancing of abscesses should be done so that the purulent material can be collected and environmental contamination prevented. Young animals should be raised in isolation from older, infected animals. Older animals and those with abscesses should be shorn last, and equipment should be disinfected whenever it is contaminated with draining exudate. Skin wounds from shearing or fighting should be treated topically with iodine and sutured if necessary.

Commercial vaccines, currently only licensed for use in sheep, reduce the incidence and prevalence of caseous lymphadenitis within a flock, but they neither prevent all new infections nor cure animals already infected. Currently, all contain phospholipase D toxoid, and some also contain killed whole bacterial cells. Usually, *Clostridium tetani* and *C perfringens* type D, along with other clostridial antigens, are included in the vaccine. Vaccination should start in young stock after colostral immunity has waned (~3 mo of age). Colostral immunity can be improved by administering a booster to pregnant ewes and does 1 mo prior to lambing/kidding. A primary series (2 injections, 4 wk apart) is required in young stock or previously unvaccinated adults; repeat vaccination at least annually will help reduce the prevalence of disease. Vaccination will not cure existing infections, so it is important to ensure that animals are well vaccinated prior to exposure. Evidence suggests that increasing the frequency of vaccination to every 4-6 mo may be of benefit in flocks where exposure is high (eg, confinement housed for at least part of the year). These vaccines should be used with caution in potentially infected goats, as adverse reactions are sometimes reported.

An effective control program must involve vaccinating, culling, and reducing exposure to potentially contaminated fomites, such as shearing blades, dipping fluids, feeders, and feed. Eradication is difficult and requires strict biosecurity and vaccination protocols and rigorous culling of all infected animals. Once the disease is at a low prevalence, vaccination should be stopped and all seropositive, nonvaccinated animals culled. Prevention of disease entry into a clean flock is based on serologic screening and isolation of incoming animals. Seropostive unvaccinated animals should not be accepted into the flock.

If management allows, removal of young stock at birth and rearing separately from the infected flock has been shown to be an effective means of eradication. The infected flock is then culled as quickly as economics allow. Prevention of caseous lymphadenitis in an uninfected flock involves shearing biosecurity and purchase only of uninfected replacement stock. Producers should purchase their own shearing equipment and not share it with other flocks. Shearers should arrive at the flock wearing clean footwear and clothing. Wool bags, shearing boards, moccasins, hands, clothing, and all parts of clippers can be a source of bacteria. If there is a break in biosecurity, disease usually shows up 1-3 mo after exposure, or longer if the initial abscesses are internal or are missed.

CORYNEBACTERIUM PSEUDOTUBERCULOSIS INFECTION OF HORSES AND CATTLE

(Pigeon breast, Pigeon fever, False strangles, Dry land distemper)

In horses, *C pseudotuberculosis* causes **ulcerative lymphangitis** (an infection of the lower limbs), chronic abscesses in the pectoral region, and contagious acne. It is one of the most common and economically important infectious diseases of horses in California and is increasing in prevalence in other dry, western states of the USA. In cattle, the bacteria causes ventral lymphadenitis, abscesses, and ulcerative dermatitis. Sporadic outbreaks have occurred in cattle in the western USA. Large, ulcerative skin lesions and lymphangitis may occur in 2-5% of cows. Location on the animal is variable. Healing often occurs without treatment or with limited topical treatment. Abortion and mastitis may also occur. Rarely, visceral involvement has been reported.

Pathogenesis and Clinical Findings: The onset of ulcerative lymphangitis in horses is slow and usually manifests by painful inflammation, nodules, and ulcers, especially in the region of the fetlock; occasionally, the edematous swelling can extend up the entire limb. The exudate is odorless, thick, greenish white, and blood tinged. Usually, only one leg is involved. Lesions and swelling progress slowly, and the condition can become chronic with relapses.

In the southwestern USA, *C pseudotuberculosis* infection in horses is seasonal, with a peak incidence in late summer and fall. Infection results in abscessation of the lower pectoral region or ventral abdominal wall with secondary dissemination to internal organs. Clinical signs include diffuse or localized swellings, ventral pitting edema, ventral midline dermatitis, lameness, draining abscesses or tracts, fever, weight loss, and depression. Leukocytosis and neutrophilia may be present. A marked or prolonged fever indicates untoward sequelae—chronic discharge, multiple or internal abscessation, or systemic infection with abortion. Abscesses can be large, up to 20 cm in diameter before rupturing, and take months to resolve. Weight loss, colic, or ataxia may be signs of internal abscesses. Dermatitis lesions are painful and mildly pruritic with alopecia, exudation, crusting, and ulceration.

The bacteria probably enter via skin wounds including IM injections, arthropod vectors such as *Habronema* spp larva and stable flies, and contact with fomites such as contaminated tack and grooming equipment. Unhygienic and wet conditions predispose animals to infection, particularly of the lower legs and ventral region. However, the disease also occurs under excellent management conditions.

Diagnosis: Isolation of *C pseudotuberculosis* from lesions is necessary for confirmation. In all forms of lymphangitis in horses, samples for culture include aspirates of abscesses, swabs of purulent exudate beneath crusts associated with folliculitis, and punch biopsies. Differential diagnoses include pyoderma, abscesses, lymphangitis from other bacteria (eg, *Staphylococcus aureus, Rhodococcus equi, Streptococcus* spp, or *Dermatophilus* spp), dermatophytosis, sporotrichosis, equine cryptococcosis, North American blastomycosis, and onchocerciasis.

Treatment: Lymphangitis and early abscess swellings are treated with hot packs, poultices, or hydrotherapy. Abscesses are lanced and flushed with iodine solution. Large abscesses require surgery. Skin lesions and grossly contaminated limbs are scrubbed daily with an iodophor shampoo. Penicillin or trimethoprim-sulfa combinations have been given; however, antimicrobial treatment may prolong the disease by delaying abscess maturation. Phenylbutazone relieves pain and swelling. General supportive and nursing care is indicated. If treatment is successful, the swelling gradually recedes over days or weeks. Severe or untreated cases often become chronic, and fibrosis and induration of the leg occurs. An experimental bacterin-toxoid was not effective in field trials.

STREPTOCOCCAL LYMPHADENITIS OF PIGS
(Jowl abscess, Cervical abscess)

Streptococcal lymphadenitis is a contagious disease characterized by abscessation of the cervical, mandibular, and cephalic lymph nodes. Affected pigs are generally thrifty and grow well. The disease can lead to condemnation of affected heads and increased processing time required for cleanup of the abattoir when an abscess is accidentally incised.

The host for the causative agent, *Streptococcus porcinus* (formerly *Streptococcus* Group E), is the pig, although pyogenic infections from this organism have been reported in humans. These reports include genitourinary infection in reproductive age females as well as infection secondary to wound contamination. There appear to be 2 serotypes—type 1 occurs more often in piglets and type 2 in adults. The bacteria also produces 2 exotoxins: EF and hemolysin. The organism has been recovered in several areas of the world, but the disease has been economically important only in the USA, where incidence has declined considerably since the mid 1960s.

Transmission, Epidemiology, and Pathogenesis: Streptococcal lymphadenitis is endemic; once it occurs on a farm, successive groups of pigs develop abscesses during the growing and finishing period. Pigs may become infected by ingesting *S porcinus* from draining abscesses; however, recovered carrier pigs are the most common and important source of infection. Recovered pigs harbor *S porcinus* in their tonsils and readily transmit the organisms via nose-to-nose contact and by contamination of water and feed. Pigs are resistant to infection for the first 3-4 wk of life.

Scattered miliary abscesses develop in mandibular, parotid, or retropharyngeal lymph nodes within 7 days after infection. By ~21 days, abscesses measuring 5-8 cm in diameter are common; these destroy the internal structure of affected nodes and may involve adjacent tissue. Incidence may be >50% in a given lot of market hogs and sometimes approaches 100%. Developing abscesses may reach the skin, rupture, and drain in 7-10 wk. The drained lesions heal by granulation, leaving a dense, fibrous, subcutaneous tract that resolves after several weeks. Deep-seated abscesses may remain undetected until slaughter; they tend not to drain into the pharynx.

Clinical Findings, Lesions, and Diagnosis: Generally, abscesses are the only sign seen by the producer. Abscesses are most common in the mandibular and retropharyngeal lymph nodes and rare in other nodes. Occasionally the disease may cause meningitis, polyarthritis, or septicemia. Although pigs experimentally exposed to *S porcinus* develop transient fever, leukocytosis, depression, and anorexia; these signs are rarely noticed with natural infection. Diagnosis is by culture and isolation of *S porcinus* from abscess exudate. Infection also can be detected serologically by an agglutination test.

Treatment and Control: In affected herds, piglets should be weaned at 21 days and reared in an environment free of older pigs. Oral administration of broad-spectrum antibiotics (tetracyclines at 50 g/ton of feed) is effective prophylactically; tetracycline fed at 200-400 g/ton of feed has reduced the number of abscesses. However, treatment after infection is established is not effective in eliminating the bacteria. An oral avirulent vaccine has been successfully used and appears to give much better protection than a bacterin.

POLYCYTHEMIA

Polycythemia is a relative or absolute increase in the number of circulating RBC resulting in an increased PCV, RBC count, and hemoglobin concentration.

Relative Polycythemia: A loss of plasma volume will result in an apparent increase in RBC numbers. Relative polycythemia can be caused by any mechanism that results in hemoconcentration, such as dehydration from vomiting or diarrhea, or in a fluid shift from the intravascular to the extravascular space due to increased vascular permeability. **Transient polycythemia** is a type of relative polycythemia that occurs when excitement or fear causes splenic contraction, resulting in the release of large numbers of RBC into the circulation. Transient polycythemia is characterized by an elevated PCV with normal plasma protein concentrations. In both relative and transient polycythemia, the PCV is increased but the total RBC mass is normal. Relative polycythemia is diagnosed by finding an increased PCV and plasma protein concentration. There are breed differences in normal reference ranges of PCV. For example, Greyhounds normally have a PCV of ≥60%. Treatment consists of rehydrating the animal and treating the underlying cause.

Absolute Polycythemia: A real increase in RBC numbers results from increased production. Definitive diagnosis requires direct RBC mass determination, which usually is not clinically available. Clinical diagnosis is based on a persistently increased PCV, without concurrent splenic contraction or dehydration (the latter based on lack of response to fluids). Clinical signs include red mucous membranes, often normal hydration status, bleeding tendencies, polyuria and polydipsia, seizures or behavioral changes, ataxia, weakness, amaurosis, tortuous retinal vessels and hemorrhages, and retinal detachments and blindness.

Absolute polycythemia may be primary or secondary. Primary polycythemia, or **polycythemia rubra vera**, is a myeloproliferative disease of unknown cause. It has been reported in dogs, cats, and cattle. RBC production is dramatically increased, and serum erythropoietin levels are low or low normal. In secondary polycythemia, RBC production increases in response to increased erythropoietin levels. This may be seen in cases of chronic renal hypoxia from severe pulmonary disease, congestive heart failure, or right-to-left blood shunting (such as with tetralogy of Fallot, transposition of great vessels, and reversed shunting patent ductus arteriosis). Excess production of erythropoietin by the kidney has been seen with renal carcinoma, renal cyst, hydronephrosis, and pyelonephritis. Hyperadrenocorticism (p 435) commonly causes an increase in the PCV (rarely >55-60%); the exact mechanism is unknown.

Diagnosis: A baseline CBC, chemistry panel, and urinalysis may be helpful in distinguishing relative from absolute polycythemia (high PCV and plasma protein levels suggest relative polycythemia). An elevated absolute reticulocyte count (>49,000/μL) in an animal with an elevated PCV documents the presence of increased erythropoietic activity and an absolute polycythemia. A bone marrow biopsy is not useful in distinguishing primary from secondary polycythemia.

Increased serum erythropoietin (EPO) levels are diagnostic for secondary polycythemia; however, this test lacks sensitivity as up to half of animals with secondary polycythemia will have EPO levels within normal reference ranges. Assessment of systemic hypoxia is important in differentiating primary from secondary absolute polycythemia. Blood gas pO_2 values <90 mm Hg or pulse oximetry oxygen saturation values <80% suggest hypoxemia as the cause of secondary absolute polycythemia. Radiographs are normal in primary polycythemia but show changes if cardiac or pulmonary disease is present. Echocardiography is necessary to evaluate the heart, and abdominal ultrasonography is used to assess the kidneys and adrenal glands. An IV pyelogram should be done to further assess the renal architecture.

Treatment: Treatment initially consists of reduction in RBC mass and concurrent hyperviscosity using phlebotomy (5 mL/kg repeated daily until PCV is reduced <55%) and replacement of blood volume with isotonic fluids. In secondary polycythemia, the underlying disease process must be addressed; phlebotomy may be contraindicated in animals with hypoxemia. In primary polycythemia, periodic phlebotomies may be required, with or without the administration of hydroxyurea (30 mg/kg, PO, SID until PCV is below 55% and then titrated) or chlorambucil (0.2 mg/kg, PO, SID until PCV is <55% and then titrated).

CARDIOVASCULAR SYSTEM INTRODUCTION

The cardiovascular system comprises the heart, the veins, and the arteries. The atrioventricular and semilunar valves keep blood flowing in one direction through the heart, and valves in large veins keep blood flowing in one direction through them as well. The rate and force of contraction of the heart and the degree of constriction or dilatation of blood vessels are determined by the autonomic nervous system and hormones produced either at the heart and blood vessels (ie, paracrine or autocrine) or at a distance from the heart and blood vessels (ie, endocrine).

Slightly >10% of all domestic animals examined by a veterinarian have some form of cardiovascular disease. Unlike diseases of many other organ systems, cardiovascular diseases generally do not resolve but almost always become more limiting and may lead to death. In addition, cardiovascular diseases may be more difficult to detect and quantify because the heart cannot be seen and is protected so well by the rib cage. Therefore, evaluation of the heart depends on heart sounds and murmurs, pressure pulses and the apex beat, the electrocardiogram, and radiology and echocardiology.

Heart Rate and the Electrocardiogram: The heart beats because of a wave of depolarization that originates in the sinoatrial (SA) node at the juncture of the cranial vena cava and the right atrium. At rest, the SA node discharges ~15 times/min in the horse, >200 times/min in the cat, and 60-160 times/min in the dog. In general, the larger the species, the slower the rate of SA node discharge and the slower the heart rate.

The rate of SA node discharge increases, often to nearly 300 bpm, when norepinephrine is released from the sympathetic nerves and binds to the β_1-adrenoreceptors on the SA node. This cardioacceleration may be blocked by β-adrenergic blocking agents (eg, propranolol, atenolol, metoprolol, esmolol, sotalol). The rate of SA node discharge decreases when acetylcholine released by the parasympathetic (vagus) nerves binds to the cholinergic receptors on the SA node. This vagally mediated cardiodeceleration may be blocked by a parasympatholytic (vagolytic) compound (eg, atropine, glycopyrrolate). When the SA node discharges and the wave of depolarization traverses the atria, the P wave of the ECG is produced, and the atria contract, ejecting a small volume of blood into the respective ventricles.

In quiet, healthy dogs, the heart rate is usually irregular. It increases during inspiration and decreases during expiration. This is termed **respiratory sinus arrhythmia** (RSA) and results from decreased vagal activity during inspiration and increased vagal activity during expiration. Therefore, vagolytic compounds, as well as excitement, pain, or fever, usually abolish or diminish RSA. Heart rate variability synchronized with respirations is a good indicator of health. This variability leaves during excitement or during heart diseases that may reduce the quality or duration of life. It is rare to find an animal that has heart disease with a RSA in which the heart disease is the cause of symptoms (eg, exercise incapacity, dyspnea).

Heart rate is also inversely related to systemic arterial blood pressure. When blood pressure increases, heart rate decreases; when blood pressure decreases, heart rate increases. This relationship is known as the **Marey reflex** and occurs by the following mechanisms. When high-pressure arterial baroreceptors in the aortic and carotid sinuses detect the fall in blood pressure, they send increased afferent volleys to the medulla oblongata, which decreases vagal efferents to the SA node and causes the heart rate to increase. When blood pressure increases, heart rate slows due to increased vagal efferents to the SA node. In heart failure, the baroreceptors (laden with Na^+/K^+-ATPase) "believe" that blood pressure is too low and initiate compensatory mechanisms (eg, arterial and arteriolar constriction, venous constriction, increase in heart rate) designed to increase blood pressure. Unfortunately, these mechanisms injure the heart.

Once the wave of depolarization reaches the atrioventricular (AV) node in the right atrium, it travels slowly through the AV node, giving the atria time to contract and to eject the small volume of blood into the ventricles. The depolarization then travels rapidly to the subendocardium of the ventricles and to the ventricular septum. From these points, it travels slowly through the ventricular myocardium, producing the QRS complex of the ECG as the ventricles contract. Under rare conditions, there may be depolarization without contraction; this is called electromechanical dissociation.

The interval on an ECG between the onset of the P wave and the onset of the QRS complex is termed the PQ or PR interval. It is a measure of the time between when the atria and ventricles were stimulated and contracted, and is termed the AV conduction time. Whatever speeds or slows the rate of discharge of the SA node also speeds or slows conduction through the AV node. Thus, when heart rate is fast, the PR is short; when heart rate is slow, the PR is long.

The T wave of the ECG represents repolarization of the ventricles. It is affected by electrolyte imbalance, myocardial injury, or ventricular enlargement. Repolarization of the atria is often lost in the QRS complex or appears as a "hammock" between the P wave and QRS complex.

Force of Ventricular Contraction: The force with which the ventricles contract is determined by 3 factors: 1) the end-diastolic volume or preload, which is the volume of blood within the ventricles just before they begin to contract; 2) myocardial contractility or the inotropic state, which is the rate of cycling of the microscopic contractile units of the myocardium; and 3) the afterload, which is the hindrance to ejection of blood from the ventricle into and through the arterial tree. The afterload is measured as the peak tension the myocardium must generate to eject blood.

The preload is determined by the difference in end-diastolic pressure between the ventricle and the pleural space, divided by the stiffness of the ventricular myocardium. The end-diastolic pressure of the ventricle is determined by the ratio of blood volume and the capacity of the systemic veins to store the blood. The venous capacity depends on the degree of constriction or relaxation of the venous vascular smooth muscle. In general, the state of venous smooth muscle is under the same control as arterial smooth muscle. The preload is regulated predominantly by low-pressure volume receptors in the heart and large veins. When these receptors are stimulated by an increase in blood volume or by distention of the structures the receptors occupy, the body responds by making more urine and by dilating the veins—an attempt to decrease blood volume and lower the pressures in the veins responsible for venous distention. Stretching of receptors in the atria and in the ventricles causes them to release atrionatriuretic proteins (ANP), brain ANP from the ventricles and ANP from the atria. These proteins, also called atrippewtin, are natriuretic, relax smooth muscle, and in general oppose vasopressin and angiotensin-II.

Myocardial contractility is determined by the rate of liberation of energy from ATP, which is determined, in part, by the amount of norepinephrine binding to β_1-adrenergic receptors in the myocardium. One of the most important factors in heart failure is the down-regulation (decreased number) of β_1-receptors.

The afterload is determined by the relative stiffness of the arteries and by the degree of constriction or dilatation of the arterioles, both of which are determined by the degree of constriction or relaxation of the arterial and arteriolar vascular smooth muscle. The tone of vascular smooth muscle depends on many factors, some of which constrict the muscle (eg, α-1, angiotensin II, vasopressin, endothelin) and some of which relax the muscle (eg, β-2, atriopeptin, bradykinin, adenosine, nitric oxide). Afterload and peak tension are also determined by the preload and thickness of the ventricular wall just before ejecting. In fact, peak tension is equal to the preload times the diastolic arterial blood pressure, all divided by the end-diastolic wall thickness of the ventricle. Afterload is often increased in heart failure, and therapy must be directed at decreasing it.

Oxygen and the Myocardium: Oxygen is essential for the production of energy that permits all body functions (eg, muscle contraction and relaxation, gland secretion, nerve conduction). The amount of oxygen available for production of this energy is termed the **tissue oxygen content**. The myocardial oxygen content is a balance between how much oxygen is delivered to the heart minus how much oxygen is consumed by the heart.

The amount of oxygen delivered to the heart depends on how well the lungs function, how much hemoglobin (Hgb) is present to carry the oxygen, and how much blood carrying the Hgb flows through the heart muscle via the coronary arteries. If the lungs are functioning well and there is sufficient Hgb, coronary blood flow will determine how much oxygen is delivered to the myocardium. Coronary blood flow is determined by the difference in pressure between the aorta (normally 100 mm Hg), from which all coronary blood originates, and the right atrium (normally 5 mm Hg), into which most coronary blood empties. Because coronary blood flows mainly during diastole when the heart is resting, and because the duration of diastole is inversely related to heart rate, then it follows that the lower the heart rate, the longer the period of diastole, and the greater the coronary blood flow. Optimal oxygen is delivered to the myocardium when the lungs function well, there is adequate functional Hgb, blood pressure is high, right atrial pressure is low, and heart rate is low.

The amount of oxygen consumed by the heart is termed **myocardial oxygen consumption**. It is determined, principally, by heart rate, myocardial contractility, and afterload. Myocardial oxygen consumption is higher when each of the determinants is higher, and lower when each of the determinants is lower. Both heart rate and myocardial contractility are increased by β_1-adrenergic stimulation (or by norepinephrine) and are decreased by an increase in parasympathetic stimulation; therefore, autonomic activity also influences myocardial oxygen consumption. Because afterload, or peak tension, is equal to the preload times the diastolic arterial blood pressure, all divided by end-diastolic wall thickness of the ventricle, any factor that increases preload and diastolic systemic arterial blood pressure, or that decreases left ventricular end-diastolic wall thickness, will increase myocardial oxygen consumption.

The importance of heart rate on oxygen balance cannot be overemphasized. An increasing heart rate increases myocardial oxygen consumption and decreases the duration of ventricular diastole when coronary blood flow delivering oxygen occurs; thus increasing heart rate may result in oxygen debt and impaired cardiac performance.

Oxygen is responsible for the production of the vast majority of ATP, and it is the energy transformed from ATP that fuels both contraction and relaxation of the myocardium. Cessation of the cycling and relaxation is permitted by the energy from ATP driving calcium ions from the microscopic units of contraction (troponin) into the saccules (sarcoplasmic reticulum) from which the calcium is unavailable to sustain contraction.

In heart failure, inappropriate handling of calcium may be the most important factor that leads to both reduced force of contraction and reduced rate of relaxation (ie, reduced systolic as well as diastolic function).

Hindrance to the Blood Flow: The hindrance to blood flow, termed **cardiac output**, is the same from left and right ventricles. It flows through the systemic arterial or pulmonary arterial trees and is critical to satisfactory function of the heart and consequent perfusion of organs with adequate quantities of blood and the oxygen it contains. Most (>90%) of the hindrance to blood flow is from the degree of constriction or dilatation of the arterioles, termed the **vascular resistance**; however, some interference is from the stiffness of the portion of the great arteries closest to the ventricles, termed the **impedance**. The ventricles eject a stroke volume into the proximal portion of the great arteries, which expand to accommodate the stroke volume; when the ventricles are relaxed, the distended great arteries constrict and keep blood moving through the arterioles into the capillaries and veins. The semilunar valves close and prevent the stroke volume from returning to the ventricle that ejected it.

One of the most important features of heart failure that leads to morbidity is increased resistance of arterial, arteriolar, and venous smooth muscle because of increased angiotensin II, vasopressin, and endothelin. These increases are due to (incorrect) compensatory feedback from the high-pressure baroreceptors to the medulla indicating that blood pressure is too low, even when it is not. If the left ventricle is unable to eject a normal stroke volume or cardiac output, it is reasonable that the ventricular function might be improved by decreasing both vascular resistance and impedance—which is precisely why drugs that relax vascular smooth muscle are useful (eg, angiotensin-converting enzyme [ACE] inhibitors).

ABNORMALITIES OF THE CARDIOVASCULAR SYSTEM

The following mechanisms can result in abnormalities of the cardiovascular system: 1) the cardiac valves fail to close or open properly (valvular disease); 2) the heart muscle pumps too feebly or relaxes inadequately (myocardial disease); 3) the heart beats too slowly, too rapidly, or too irregularly (arrhythmia); 4) the systemic vessels offer too great an interference to blood flow (vascular disease); 5) there may be holes between chambers of the left side and right side of the heart (cardiac shunts); 6) there is too little or too much blood compared with the ability of the blood vessels to store that blood; and 7) there is parasitism of the cardiovascular system (eg, heartworm disease). The diseases of greatest importance, due to their prevalence, are mitral regurgitation in dogs, hypertrophic cardiomyopathy in cats, dilated cardiomyopathy in dogs, arrhythmic cardiomyopathy in Boxers, and heartworm disease.

Valvular Disease: Inadequate closure of valves leads to regurgitation, which occurs most commonly as **mitral regurgitation**, often as mitral and **tricuspid regurgitation**, and least commonly as **aortic regurgitation**. Regurgitation through the mitral and/or tricuspid valves constitutes >75% of all heart disease in dogs. As blood regurgitates through either set of AV valves, it often does so at a velocity great enough to produce turbulence, and a typical systolic murmur is heard between the first and second heart sounds. The valve orifices may be assessed by color Doppler echocardiography; regurgitant blood produces a clear, colored signal. When blood regurgitates through the mitral or tricuspid valves, excess blood accumulates in the heart chamber and vessels into which the regurgitation occurs. Thus with mitral regurgitation, it is common to see enlargement of the left atrium, pulmonary veins, and left ventricle. The degree of left atrial enlargement as documented by either radiography or echocardiography may be predictive of disease severity. Mitral or tricuspid regurgitation is most common in small-breed dogs and old horses that have valve leaflets thickened and gnarled by infiltration with glycosaminoglycans. Mitral regurgitation occurs more often in Cavalier King Charles Spaniels, and at a younger age, than in any other breed.

Aortic regurgitation occurs most often in large-breed dogs and in older horses after developing infections of the aortic valves. The left ventricle is often massively enlarged because blood enters it, normally, from the left atrium and by regurgitation from the aorta. The murmur produced by blood regurgitating from the aorta into the left ventricle is always a diastolic murmur, heard immediately after the second heart sound. In horses, the murmur of aortic regurgitation is often a very loud humming sound. Pulmonary regurgitation is of little or no clinical significance. Regurgitant flow through the aortic or pulmonic valves may be quantified by color Doppler echocardiography.

Inadequate opening of valves is termed stenosis. **Pulmonic and aortic stenosis** are equally prevalent; **mitral stenosis** is rare. However, **subaortic stenosis**, produced by a fibrous band of tissue just beneath the aortic valves, is prevalent in certain breeds (eg, Golden Retrievers, Boxers, Newfoundlands, German Shepherds). If a valve opens inadequately, either less blood flows through the valve, or a greater pressure must be generated to keep the normal volume of blood flowing through it. The ventricle responsible for pumping blood through the stenotic valve frequently enlarges proportionally to the degree of tightness of the stenosis. The systolic murmurs produced by pulmonic or aortic stenosis are relatively brief and rough and are heard between the first and second heart sound; they are much shorter in duration than the systolic murmur of mitral regurgitation and are transmitted more craniad and dorsad on the thoracic wall. The severity of stenosis can be predicted by the intensity of the murmur. In general, the louder the murmur, the greater the stenosis. Pulmonic stenosis is most common in small-breed dogs; aortic stenosis develops most commonly because of a partially constricting band of fibrous tissue beneath the aortic valve in large-breed dogs. The velocity of blood flowing through a stenosis correlates with the severity of the stenosis and can be measured with great accuracy by Doppler echocardiography.

Myocardial Disease: Impaired force of contraction is termed **reduced systolic function**, which occurs most commonly in dilated cardiomyopathy (in large-breed dogs and in cats receiving too little taurine) and in long-standing mitral regurgitation (most often in small-breed dogs with endocardiosis). When this occurs, the cardiac muscle is said to be in a negative inotropic state, or it has reduced contractility. This is usually termed **idiopathic dilated cardiomyopathy**, because the origin is unknown.

Impaired ventricular relaxation is termed **reduced diastolic function**, which occurs most commonly when the cardiac muscle suffers oxygen debt and the consequent lack of energy to fuel relaxation. Ventricular muscles also relax poorly in hypertrophic cardiomyopathy (ie, when the muscle is too thick), or with pericardial disease when either the thickened pericardium or fluid contained within the pericardial sac interfere with relaxation. Hypertrophic cardiomyopathy is most common in cats. Probably >85% of cats with heart disease have hypertrophic cardiomyopathy. A smaller number of cats will have so-called restrictive cardiomyopathy, in which the heart fills poorly because the walls are stiffer than normal. Pericardial disease is most common in older, large-breed dogs with tumors bleeding into the pericardial sac.

Arrhythmias: A heart beating too fast, too slowly, or too irregularly to sustain an acceptable cardiac output is termed arrhythmia. The most common arrhythmias are atrial fibrillation (seen commonly in horses and in large-breed dogs with an enlarged left atrium), ventricular premature depolarizations (seen most commonly in Boxers and Doberman Pinschers), sick sinus syndrome (seen mainly in aged Miniature Schnauzers), and third-degree AV block. In **atrial fibrillation**, depolarization of the atria is not coordinated, stimulation of the AV node is frequent but random, and the heart rate is rapid and irregular. **Ventricular premature depolarizations** (also called ventricular premature beats or complexes) arise from irritated regions of the ventricles. Such irritations commonly result from chronic stretch of the fibers, as well as from oxygen debt or drug effects. A single premature beat causes no trouble, but premature beats may evolve into short or long bursts that lead to hemodynamic impairment and syncope, or even to a complicated ventricular spasm (ventricular fibrillation) leading to sudden death. This occurs commonly in Boxers afflicted with a disease termed Boxer cardiomyopathy. With either **sick sinus syndrome** (ie, transient arrest of discharge of the SA node) or **complete heart block** (in which no atrial depolarization enters the ventricles), the ventricular rate is exceptionally slow and may lead to hemodynamic impairment and syncope.

Vascular Disease: Interference to blood flow through arterioles often leads to hypertension, which is most common in aging animals with impaired renal function. It is thought that the kidneys produce excessive renin in response to inadequate blood flow, and that this excessive renin catalyzes the angiotensin system, resulting in excessive angiotensin II—a potent activator of vascular smooth muscle.

Cardiac Shunts: Abnormal communications between chambers of the left and right side of the heart are termed intracardiac shunts. These take the form of (in decreasing prevalence) **patent ductus arteriosus** (between the aorta and pulmonary trunk), **ventricular septal defect** (between the left and right ventricles), or **atrial septal defect** (between the left and right atria). Because blood crosses these defects almost always from chambers of the left side of the heart to those of the right side, these defects are termed left-to-right shunts. They result in overcirculation of the lungs and dilatation of the cardiac chambers required to pump or to carry the shunted blood. Chronic dilatation ultimately leads to myocardial failure.

Tetralogy of Fallot (p 73) is a complex congenital anomaly that consists of a hypoplastic pulmonary trunk, an aorta that overrides the interventricular septum (therefore arising from both ventricles), right ventricular hypertrophy, and a ventricular septal defect. Poorly oxygenated blood enters the systemic circulation and produces a bluish tinge (cyanosis) to the mucous membranes and increased numbers of erythrocytes. Tetralogy of Fallot is the most common form of a right-to-left shunt.

Heartworm Disease: Heartworm disease (p 100) is another important heart disease seen predominantly in dogs but also in cats living in regions with high mosquito populations. In heartworm disease, adult heartworms in the pulmonary vessels impede flow through the lungs, and blood dams up in the right side of the heart and systemic veins. The disease progresses at a varying rate in dogs, but usually lasts <2 yr in cats. Both species may die from pulmonary hypertension arising from partial obstruction to the flow of blood through the diseased pulmonary vessels.

Common Endpoints of Heart Disease

Signs associated with any of the above diseases are due either to inadequate organ perfusion (eg, exercise intolerance, weakness, syncope) or to blood damming up in organs in which the venous effluent is emptied inadequately (eg, pulmonary edema, ascites, pitting edema, effusions). An animal showing signs due to relative inadequacy of the cardiovascular system to deliver enough blood to sustain normal function is said to be in heart failure. An animal showing signs caused by blood damming up in poorly drained organs is said to be in congestive heart failure (CHF). When inadequate amounts of oxygen are present in systemic arterial blood and there is too much unoxygenated Hgb, the mucous membranes appear cyanotic, and often there is an increased concentration of erythrocytes.

Animals with heart disease may deteriorate gradually, due most often to pulmonary failure, or they may die suddenly, due to nearly instant circulatory arrest. Pulmonary failure occurs because the lung becomes too stiff to ventilate; the stiffness arises initially from congestion of blood vessels and then from pulmonary edema. The sudden circulatory arrest results either from cessation of discharge of the SA node or from ventricular fibrillation, in which depolarization of the ventricles is not coordinated, and no unified contraction occurs.

Heart Failure, Congestive Heart Failure, and the Failing Heart

The failing heart is described as one with reduced myocardial contractility, which can be determined by a reduced force of contraction from any given preload. More objectively, a failing heart can be described as one with a reduced rate of liberation of energy from the breakdown of ATP, or with a reduced velocity of fiber shortening when the heart contracts during the imaginary situation of contracting against no load. It is difficult to directly measure myocardial contractility and to identify a failing heart. Almost any animal with heart disease leading to chamber enlargement or increased wall thickness has a failing heart, but they are usually compensated and do not manifest symptoms; therefore, they are not in heart failure or CHF. This includes probably 95% of the 11% of dogs and cats with heart disease.

Heart failure and CHF (p 76) are clinical syndromes in which an animal manifests signs referable to a complex interaction between a failing heart and the blood vessels. In heart failure, cardiac output is insufficient to perfuse organs with enough oxygenated blood for the organs to function properly either at rest (termed functional class IV heart failure), during mild exertion (class III), during moderate exercise (class II), or during extreme exercise (class I). In CHF, blood dams up in organs—usually the lungs but occasionally in the systemic organs—and causes the congested organs to function abnormally, become edematous, or both. The functional classification of heart failure is expressed when, during graded exercise, the animal shows signs (eg, dyspnea, cough, collapse) due to the heart disease.

DIAGNOSIS OF CARDIOVASCULAR DISEASE

The following procedures are important in the diagnosis of cardiovascular disease: history and signalment, physical examination (eg, inspection, auscultation, palpation), radiography, electrocardiography, and echocardiography. Clear images must be obtained for radiography, electrocardiography, and echocardiography, or accurate, valid interpretation will not be possible. Most cardiovascular diseases (eg, mitral regurgitation, dilated cardiomyopathy) can be diagnosed by physical examination and radiography. Electrocardiography is specific for diagnosis of rhythm disturbances (eg, atrial fibrillation, sick sinus syndrome). Echocardiography is excellent for confirming tentative diagnoses, for characterizing the form of cardiomyopathy in cats, for detecting cardiac tumors, or for detecting pericardial disease. Heartworm disease is diagnosed best by detecting antigens of or antibodies to mature, female heartworms that circulate in the blood.

Many heart diseases have specific breed prevalences. Any old, male Cocker Spaniel with a cough, labored breathing, and exercise intolerance, or any Cavalier King Charles Spaniel most likely has mitral regurgitation; however, chronic obstructive pulmonary disease with fibrosis may produce nearly identical signs. Any middle-aged, depressed, coughing, exercise-intolerant Doberman Pinscher with a rapid, irregular heart rate likely has dilated cardiomyopathy. Any middle- to old-aged female Miniature Schnauzer with fainting likely has sick sinus syndrome. Any Boxer who faints intermittently is likely to have arrhythmic cardiomyopathy. A middle-aged cat with labored breathing and reluctance to lie down probably has hypertrophic cardiomyopathy; however, cancer and infection may produce nearly identical signs. An old cat is likely to have hyperthyroidism. A young Wirehaired Fox Terrier with cyanosis and exercise intolerance probably has tetralogy of Fallot.

Heart disease should be considered if any of the following are identified on physical examination: 1) the heart rate is rapid, slow, or irregular (and not due to respiratory sinus arrhythmia); 2) respiratory sinus arrhythmia is absent even when the animal is at rest (also occurs due to pain, fever, or excitement); 3) more than 2 heart sounds are heard (eg, producing a "gallop" rhythm) in any animal but a horse (most common in cats with cardiomyopathy); 4) a loud murmur is heard, or a thrill—the palpable manifestation of a loud murmur—is felt; 5) heart sounds are muffled in the absence of obesity (may indicate pericardial effusion); 6) arterial pulsations are rapid, feeble, or irregular with more heart beats than arterial pulsations (a pulse deficit); 7) the animal faints or has reduced exercise tolerance in the absence of skeletal muscle disease or obesity; 8) the mucous membranes are acutely cyanotic in the absence of primary pulmonary disease (however, long-standing cyanosis in dogs not acutely ill is more likely to be due to primary pulmonary disease).

Echocardiography is more effective than radiography—which is more effective than electrocardiography—for detecting enlargement of chambers of the heart and great vessels. In general, the degree of chamber enlargement parallels disease severity. The degree of engorgement of pulmonary veins detected radiographically, or the degree of impairment of left ventricular wall motion or thinning of the left ventricular free wall, may predict the severity of heart failure. Unfortunately, the correlation between hemodynamic or echocardiographic measurements and either signs or likelihood of death is not always good. There appears to be a better correlation between increase in heart, respiratory rates, and exercise incapacity to severity of heart disease.

Diagnosis of specific cardiovascular diseases are discussed in their respective chapters.

PRINCIPLES OF THERAPY

See also SYSTEMIC PHARMACOTHERAPEUTICS OF THE CARDIOVASCULAR SYSTEM, p 1966.

Although therapy is disease-specific, there are some general goals of therapy for heart disease: 1) Chronic stretch on myocardial fibers should be minimized, because chronic stretch injures and irritates fibers, causes them to consume excess quantities of oxygen, and leads to their death and replacement by fibrous connective tissue (remodeling). 2) Edema fluid should be removed because it makes the lungs wet, heavy, and stiff, and causes ventilation-perfusion inequalities and fatigues muscles of ventilation. 3) The circulation should be improved, and the amount of regurgitation (most often mitral regurgitation) decreased. Improved circulation enhances blood flow to important organs, and reducing mitral regurgitation decreases stretch on the left atrium and pulmonary veins, pulmonary capillary pressure, and edema formation. 4) Heart rate and rhythm should be regulated. A heart beating too slowly fails to eject enough blood, while a heart beating too rapidly does not have time to fill adequately and consumes too much oxygen at a time when there is too little coronary blood flow. A heart beating too irregularly may deteriorate into ventricular fibrillation and sudden death. 5) Oxygenation of the blood should be improved. Inadequate oxygenation leads to inadequate energy to fuel both contraction and relaxation of the myocardium. Inadequate oxygenation of the myocardium may also lead to arrhythmia. 6) β_1-adrenergic receptors should be up-regulated; down-regulation of β_1-adrenergic receptors interferes with the ability to fight diseases of other organ systems. 7) The likelihood of thromboembolism should be minimized. Cats with hypertrophic cardiomyopathy may shed emboli from the enlarged left atrium, which may block major arterial branches and lead to ischemia and death. 8) Mature heartworms and microfilariae should be killed. Mature heartworms may initiate severe changes in the pulmonary arteries that ultimately impede blood flow through the lungs.

The ultimate goals of therapy for cardiovascular disease are achieved when the animal can be classified as functional Class I, the respiratory and heart rates are not increased at rest, and there is a respiratory sinus arrhythmia.

Common Therapeutic Agents

Furosemide is a loop diuretic that decreases resorption of provisional urine at the loop of Henle. It is also a venodilator when used IV. It is the most important and effective means for removing edema fluid from animals with heart failure, and frequently is life saving over the short run. However, there are no clinical trials demonstrating that furosemide prolongs life, and in humans it has been shown to shorten life, probably by activating the renin-angiotensin-aldosterone axis, and possibly by producing hypokalemia. Diuresis with furosemide may be augmented by using thiazide diuretics (eg, hydrochlorthiazide). Thiazides suppress resorption at the distal renal tubules. When using a loop diuretic and a diuretic that works at the distal tubules, the ability of the kidneys to conserve water is reduced dramatically and dehydration may develop. This may be signaled by worsening azotemia.

Spironolactone is a potassium-sparing diuretic that blocks aldosterone. Like thiazides, it exerts its diuretic effect principally at the distal convoluted tubule. It also minimizes remodeling of both blood vessels and the heart, and like ACE inhibitors and β-blockers, has been shown to decrease symptoms and to prolong the lives of humans with heart failure. Amiloride and triamterine are also potassium-sparing diuretics.

Digitalis glycosides exert their effects by inhibiting membrane Na^+/K^+-ATPase. This increases intracellular sodium, which activates the sodium-calcium pump that increases intracellular calcium. Digoxin increases the force of myocardial contraction, slows the heart rate, and improves baroreceptor function. The abnormality of baroreceptor function in heart failure stems from excessive activation of the Na^+/K^+-ATPase by aldosterone.

Enalapril (USA, Europe, Canada), benazepril (Canada and Europe), and ramipril (Europe) are ACE inhibitors approved for use in heart failure in dogs. They are all equally effective at blocking the conversion of angiotensin I to angiotensin II. They reduce afterload, thereby improving cardiac output and reducing mitral regurgitation. They minimize remodeling of both blood vessels and myocardium, improve baroreceptor function, and act as venodilators. There is debate over when and for which diseases ACE inhibitors should be used. Some maintain that they should only be used when heart failure is present; others believe they should be instituted at the first signs of cardiomegaly.

Theophylline, a methylxanthine inhibitor of phosphodiesterase, both bronchodilates and strengthens muscles of ventilation. This improves ventilation but also acts as a mild diuretic and positive inotrope. Amrinone and milrinone, analogs of theophylline that deactivate other forms of phosphodiesterase, are potent IV inodilators. That is, they are both positive inotropes and vasodilators. Piomendan, which increases intracellular calcium, is also an inodilator that is approved for use in dogs in Europe.

Both procainamide and quinidine, class IA antiarrhythmics used formerly to manage ventricular arrhythmias, have been superceded by the β-blocker sotalol and the class IB antiarrhythmic mexiletine. They are used most often for ventricular arrhythmias that are not life threatening. Lidocaine, a class IB antiarrhythmic, is used only IV for emergency ventricular arrhythmias. Mexiletine is an oral compound similar to lidocaine.

Atenolol, propranolol, and metoprolol are oral β-blockers, and esmolol is an IV β-blocker, that slow the heart rate, suppress arrhythmias, and up-regulate adrenergic receptors. Carvedilol is a β- and α-adrenergic blocker that scavenges oxygen free radicals. This compound—like ACE inhibitors and spironolactone—has been shown to both prolong life and decrease symptoms in humans with heart failure.

Diltiazem is a calcium-channel blocker that is useful for slowing ventricular rate in animals with atrial fibrillation. It is also used to decrease myocardial stiffness in cats with hypertrophic cardiomyopathy. Verapamil is also a calcium-channel blocker, but it reduces myocardial contractility more than diltiazem. Amiodarone is an excellent antiarrhythmic compound useful for managing all forms of arrhythmias, but there is relatively little clinical experience with it. Contrary to experience in humans, it appears to be safe and effective in animals.

Atropine and glycopyrrolate block the effects of the vagus nerve on the SA node. Because the vagus nerve slows discharge of the SA node and heart rate, these compounds speed heart rate and may be useful when the heart beats too slowly. Nitroglycerine is a venodilator that is usually applied in a paste form to the skin inside the earflap or thigh. By dilating peripheral veins, blood pools in those veins, and left ventricular preload and pulmonary edema are decreased. Aspirin and coumadin are anticoagulants that may prevent thromboembolism in cats with cardiomyopathy. Taurine and l-carnitine are amino acids useful in preventing dilated cardiomyopathy in cats and in a limited number of dogs, respectively. Malarsomine is used to kill mature heartworms; ivermectin, milbemycin, and selamectin are used to kill microfilariae.

Only ACE inhibitors have been proved safe and effective to treat dogs with heart failure or arrhythmias. Furosemide and digoxin are approved, but without data proving either safety or efficacy. Use of other agents to manage heart failure or rhythm disturbances is based on anecdotal evidence or unblinded, uncontrolled reports.

CONGENITAL AND INHERITED ANOMALIES OF THE CARDIOVASCULAR SYSTEM

Congenital anomalies of the cardiovascular system are defects that are present at birth and can occur as a result of genetic, environmental, infectious, toxicologic, pharmaceutical, nutritional, or other factors, or a combination of factors. For several defects, an inherited basis is suspected based on breed predilections and breeding studies. Congenital heart defects are significant not only for the effects they produce but also for their potential to be transmitted to offspring through breeding and thus affect an entire breeding population. In addition to the congenital heart defects, many other cardiovascular disorders have been shown, or are suspected, to have a genetic basis. Diseases such as hypertrophic cardiomyopathy, dilated cardiomyopathy, and degenerative valvular disease of small breeds of dogs may have a significant heritable component.

In one large study of congenital heart disease in dogs, a prevalence of 0.68% was noted; common defects included patent ductus arteriosus (PDA, 28%), pulmonic stenosis (20%), subaortic stenosis (14%), persistent right aortic arch (8%), and ventricular septal defect (7%). Less common congenital cardiac defects (occurring in <5% of cases) include tetralogy of Fallot, atrial septal defect, persistent left cranial vena cava, mitral dysplasia, tricuspid dysplasia, and cor triatriatum dexter. More recent studies have demonstrated an increase in the prevalence of subaortic stenosis, which now exceeds pulmonic stenosis as the second most common congenital cardiac defect in dogs. Due to regional differences, however, the most common congenital canine cardiac defects in the USA vary from those reported in the UK and may likely differ from those in Europe and other regions.

In cats, the prevalence of congenital heart disease has been estimated to be 0.2-1% and includes atrioventricular septal defects (including ventricular septal defect, atrial septal defect, and endocardial cushion defects), atrioventricular valve dysplasia, endocardial fibroelastosis, PDA, aortic stenosis, and tetralogy of Fallot. The most common defects in other species are as follows: cattle—ventricular septal defect, ectopic heart, and ventricular hypoplasia; sheep—ventricular septal defect; pigs—tricuspid valve dysplasia, atrial septal defect, and subaortic stenosis; and horses—ventricular septal defect, PDA, tetralogy of Fallot, and tricuspid atresia. Arabian horses have a relatively higher incidence of congenital defects than other breeds; a variety of defects have been reported for this breed.

Detection, Diagnosis, and Clinical Significance: The early detection of a congenital heart defect is critical for several reasons. Certain defects are surgically correctable, and treatment should be performed before the onset of congestive heart failure (CHF) or irreversible cardiac damage; recently purchased animals may be returned to avoid economic loss; pets with congenital heart defects are likely to die prematurely causing emotional distress; and animals purchased for performance have limited potential and will likely be unsatisfactory. Early detection also prevents incorporation of genetic defects into breeding lines.

The evaluation of most animals with a congenital cardiac defect usually consists of a physical examination, electrocardiography, radiography, and echocardiography. This allows for a definitive diagnosis and an assessment of the severity of the defect. The use of Doppler echocardiography has supplanted the use of invasive cardiac catheterization studies in the evaluation of most cardiac defects. Once the diagnosis has been made and severity determined, treatment options can be developed and a prognosis given.

The clinical significance of congenital heart disease depends on the particular defect and its severity. Mildly affected animals may exhibit no ill effects and live a normal life span. Defects causing significant circulatory derangement will likely cause neonatal death. Such defects, many incompatible with life, also cause fetal death and reduced litter size. Medical or surgical management is most likely to benefit animals with congenital cardiac defects of moderate severity. Left-to-right shunting PDA is one notable exception; surgical correction is indicated in most affected animals as long as no concurrent diseases or abnormalities that would pose a risk to anesthesia or surgery are noted.

Pathophysiology: Congenital heart defects produce signs of cardiac failure through a variety of pathophysiologic mechanisms. Defects such as pulmonic stenosis and subaortic stenosis cause ventricular outflow obstruction and may result in right- and left-sided failure, respectively. PDA and septal defects are examples of abnormal communications between the system and pulmonary circulatory systems and, in most cases, result in left-to-right shunting of blood. The recirculation of blood through the pulmonary circulation and into the left-sided chambers often precipitates signs of left-sided CHF (eg, pulmonary edema, cough, fatigue). Larger defects typically result in a greater degree of volume overcirculation to the left-sided chambers. PDA is a possible exception, with very large defects sometimes contributing to pulmonary hypertension and right-to-left shunting (see below), also called a reversed PDA. Animals with right-to-left shunting defects (tetralogy of Fallot, reversed PDA) may develop right heart failure but more often have clinical signs associated with polycythemia (p 56), which develops subsequent to renal perfusion with deoxygenated blood. This results in an increase in erythropoietin production by the kidneys and consequent polycythemia.

Innocent Murmurs: It is imperative to appreciate that the presence of a heart murmur in a young animal is not pathognomonic for a congenital heart defect. Many young animals will have a low-grade systolic murmur that is the result of mild turbulence and is not associated with a congenital heart defect. These murmurs usually disappear by 6 mo of age in dogs and cats. Innocent murmurs are heard in the absence of any other demonstrable evidence of cardiovascular disease. High-grade systolic murmurs (grade IV/VI or greater) and diastolic murmurs are indicative of cardiac disease and should prompt further investigation.

ANOMALIES OF DERIVATIVES OF THE AORTIC ARCHES

Embryonic aortic arches give rise to the carotid arteries (third pair of arches), the arch of the aorta (left fourth arch), and the pulmonary arteries and ductus arteriosus (sixth pair of arches). The other aortic arches regress, although the first aortic arches also become part of the maxillary arteries. Congenital defects may arise if development or dissolution of the aortic arches is disrupted.

Patent Ductus Arteriosus

In fetal life, oxygenated blood within the main pulmonary artery is shunted into the descending aorta through the ductus arteriosus, bypassing the nonfunctional lungs. At birth, several factors mediate closure of the ductus, which effects separation of the systemic and pulmonary circulatory systems. Inflation of the lungs allows the pulmonary circulation to function as a low-pressure system, and closure of the ductus prevents shunting of blood from the high-pressure systemic circulatory system into the pulmonary artery.

Pathophysiology: Persistence or patency of the ductus with an otherwise normal systemic and pulmonary circulatory system results in significant shunting of blood from left to right, ie, systemic to pulmonary. Because the systemic vascular resistance is always higher than that of the pulmonary circulation, shunting is continuous. The result is volume overload of the pulmonary arteries and veins, left atrium, and left ventricle. Left atrial and left ventricular dilatation may result in cardiac arrhythmias. Chronic volume overload and dilatation of the left-sided cardiac chambers usually result in signs of left-sided CHF. Therefore, most untreated cases develop refractory CHF. Animals with a small ductus may reach adulthood without signs of heart failure but are at an increased risk of infective endocarditis. In some animals with a large PDA, increased pulmonary blood flow may induce pulmonary vasoconstriction and development of pulmonary hypertension, which has several important implications: shunting through the ductus slows and reverses, which causes disappearance of the murmur and occurrence of caudal cyanosis (differential cyanosis); the right ventricle becomes dilated and hypertrophied as a result of pulmonary hypertension; and perfusion of the kidneys with deoxygenated blood causes excessive release of erythropoietin and subsequent polycythemia. Thus, if the ductus shunts right to left, clinical signs of polycythemia will predominate.

Clinical Findings and Treatment: In animals with a PDA that shunts from left to right, a prominent, continuous, machinery-like murmur is present. The murmur is usually loudest at the time of the second heart sound, heard best over the aortic valve area, and is often associated with a precordial thrill. The diastolic component is softer and heard best over the pulmonic valve area, occasionally best at the axillary area (in some cases, the ductus remains open for several days after birth; therefore, a continuous murmur may be detected during examination of the neonate). Occasionally the diastolic component may be inaudible in late diastole. Femoral pulses are typically bounding. Most young animals do not demonstrate clinical signs. Those with a large shunt and older animals often have signs of left-sided CHF. Electrocardiography frequently demonstrates tall R waves in lead II, indicative of left ventricular enlargement. A spectrum of cardiac arrhythmias may also be seen, including both atrial and ventricular premature complexes. Radiographic abnormalities depend on the size of the ductus and, in left to right shunting PDA, may demonstrate left atrial and left ventricular enlargement, prominent pulmonary vessels, aortic and pulmonic aneurysmal dilatations, and variable degrees of pulmonary edema. Echocardiography is valuable in ruling out concurrent congenital cardiac defects as well as documenting presence of the PDA. Continuous turbulence in the main pulmonary artery is characteristic of a left to right shunting PDA. Left ventricular and left atrial dilatation are typically noted, and mild mitral regurgitation may be present.

Surgical ligation of the ductus in patients with left to right shunting PDA is usually curative and is almost always indicated. If present, CHF should be medically managed (with diuretics, vasodilators, etc) before anesthesia and surgery are performed. Interventional closure is an alternative to surgical ligation. This can be accomplished by transcatheter occlusion through placement of a device (eg, Gianturco helical coils, Gianturco-Grifka vascular occlusion device) in the PDA that results in clot formation or physical occlusion of the ductus.

In animals with a PDA that shunts from right to left, there is usually a history of lethargy, exercise intolerance, and collapse. Careful examination may reveal differential cyanosis. The second heart sound may be split, and there may be a soft diastolic murmur of pulmonic insufficiency. A continuous murmur is not present, and femoral pulses are not bounding. The finding of polycythemia in a young animal with the above clinical signs should prompt further diagnostic evaluation of the heart. Electrocardiography demonstrates severe right ventricular enlargement and occasional arrhythmias. In reversed

PDA, right ventricular enlargement and aneurysmal dilatation of the descending aorta can be noted. Echocardiography is indicated in these cases and will demonstrate right ventricular dilatation and hypertrophy. The right ventricular outflow tract is enlarged. Contrast echocardiography can be used to confirm the diagnosis. After the injection of agitated saline into a peripheral vein, microbubbles will be seen within the abdominal aorta but not within the heart. Ligation of the ductus is contraindicated because this results in an increase in pulmonary hypertension (by causing an increase in flow through the already high and fixed pulmonary vascular resistance) and typically death. Therapy in theses cases involves control of polycythemia through periodic phlebotomies. Long-term prognosis is poor.

Persistent Right Aortic Arch

In this vascular ring anomaly, the right aortic arch persists, which causes obstruction of the esophagus at the level of the heart base. The esophagus is encircled by the persistent arch on the right, by the ligamentum arteriosum to the left and dorsally, and by the base of the heart ventrally.

Persistent right aortic arch (PRAA) has been reported in cattle, horses, cats, and dogs (German Shepherds and Irish Setters in particular).

Other vascular ring anomalies have been reported and result in findings similar to PRAA. These congenital defects do not cause clinical signs referable to the cardiovascular system—signs of regurgitation and aspiration pneumonia predominate.

OUTFLOW TRACT OBSTRUCTIONS

This group of congenital cardiac defects includes aortic stenosis, pulmonic stenosis, and coarctation of the aorta. All involve obstruction to either right or left ventricular outflow.

Aortic Stenosis

Left ventricular emptying may be obstructed at 3 locations: 1) subvalvular, also called subaortic, consisting of a fibrous ridge of tissue within the left ventricular outflow tract; 2) valvular; and 3) supravalvular or obstruction distal to the aortic valve. The most common form in dogs is subaortic stenosis. Breed predilections have been identified for Boxers, Golden Retrievers, Rottweilers, German Shepherds, and Newfoundlands.

Pathophysiology: Aortic stenosis induces left ventricular hypertrophy, the degree of which depends on the severity of the stenosis. In severe cases, left ventricular output may be decreased, especially during exercise. The major ramification of left ventricular hypertrophy is the creation of areas of myocardium with poor perfusion. Myocardial ischemia is a major factor in the development of serious life-threatening ventricular arrhythmias.

Clinical Findings and Treatment: Clinical signs do not consistently parallel the severity of stenosis. There may be a history of syncope and exercise intolerance. Animals with no history of illness may die suddenly and the defect is first detected at necropsy. An ejection-type systolic murmur heard best at the aortic valve area is present. The intensity of the murmur correlates fairly well with the degree of stenosis and may increase as animals mature, reflecting progressive stenosis. Puppies without detectable murmurs should not be considered free of disease until they reach 6 mo of age because the murmur may be very soft in the first months of life. In moderate to severe cases, femoral pulse strength is diminished. Electrocardiography may show left ventricular enlargement (tall R waves in lead II) and ventricular premature complexes that may increase in frequency with exercise. Holter monitoring should be used in syncopal animals or in patients with severe disease to define the presence of any arrhythmias, assess arrhythmia severity, and assist in determining the risk of sudden death. A recheck Holter monitor may be considered following initiation of antiarrhythmic therapy to assess efficacy. Radiographically, there is variable left ventricular enlargement and poststenotic dilatation of the aorta. Doppler echocardiography is recommended to confirm the diagnosis and rule out other cardiac abnormalities. The degree of left ventricular hypertrophy and peak systolic flow velocity through the defect can help determine stenosis severity.

Treatment options include medical management of arrhythmias to reduce the incidence of clinical signs of exercise intolerance or syncope, balloon valvuloplasty (typically not very effective), and surgical resection (high morbidity and mortality, high cost, and lack of significant gradient reduction). The use of β-blockers such as atenolol has been advocated to control ventricular arrhythmias in patients with subaortic stenosis and to presumably reduce the chance of sudden death. Mildly affected animals commonly require no treatment and the prognosis can be fair to good in very mildly affected patients. Affected animals should not be used for breeding.

Pulmonic Stenosis

Pulmonic stenosis is common in dogs and infrequent in cats. It results in obstruction to right ventricular outflow due, in most cases, to dysplasia of the pulmonic valve cusps. The stenosis can also occur in the infundibulum, the subvalvular region, or in the supravalvular area.

Pathophysiology: The right ventricle must generate increased pressure during systole to overcome the stenosis, which in moderate to severe cases can lead to dramatic right ventricular hypertrophy and dilatation. As the right ventricle hypertrophies, ventricular compliance diminishes, leading to increased right atrial pressure and venous congestion. The increased flow velocity deforms the wall of the main pulmonary artery, resulting in a poststenotic dilatation. In severe cases, right-sided congestive failure may be noted. Supravalvular pulmonic stenosis is uncommon and may be most often observed in Giant Schnauzers. Concurrent tricuspid valve dysplasia is sometimes noted in animals with pulmonic stenosis. Anomalous coronary artery development has been documented in some affected animals with pulmonic stenosis such as Boxers and English Bulldogs. Typically, the left main coronary artery originates from a single right coronary artery and encircles the right ventricular outflow tract.

Clinical Findings and Treatment: Affected animals may have a history of failure to thrive and exercise intolerance. Right-sided CHF may be present and is characterized by ascites or peripheral edema. A prominent ejection-type systolic murmur is present and heard best at the pulmonic valve area. A corresponding precordial thrill is usually present. Jugular distention and pulsations may also be present. Electrocardiography will demonstrate evidence of right ventricular enlargement in many cases. Radiographic abnormalities include right ventricular enlargement, an aneurysmal dilatation of the main pulmonary artery, and diminished pulmonary perfusion. Echocardiography is indicated in these cases and may demonstrate right ventricular dilatation and hypertrophy, interventricular septal flattening, and thickened and relatively immobile pulmonic valve cusps. In a few cases, supravalvular or discrete subvalvular stenosis can be noted. Pulmonic insufficiency can sometimes be noted in dogs with pulmonic stenosis. Doppler evaluation is valuable in determining the severity of the stenosis. Based on severity (reported as the pressure gradient across the valve), the need for intervention can be assessed. Animals with moderate or severe pulmonic stenosis can benefit from balloon valvuloplasty or surgical intervention (valvulotomy, patch grafting, partial valvulectomy, or conduits). The choice of surgical procedure depends to some degree on the presence and degree of subvalvular muscular hypertrophy. Palliative therapy with oral medications such as diuretics and vasodilators should be initiated if right-sided CHF is present. The prognosis is typically poor if atrial fibrillation or right-sided CHF is present. If atrial fibrillation is noted, use of a digitalis glycoside may be warranted.

Coarctation of the Aorta

This rare condition of dogs and cats involves narrowing of the aorta distal to the subclavian artery, typically in the area of the ductus arteriosus. Other uncommon congenital abnormalities of the aorta include tubular hypoplasia of the ascending aorta and aortic interruption. Surgical correction has been reported.

SEPTAL DEFECTS

Atrial Septal Defects

A communication between the atria may be the result of a patent foramen ovale or a true atrial septal defect. During fetal life, the foramen ovale, a flapped oval opening of the interatrial septum, allows shunting of blood from the right atrium to the left atrium, in order to bypass the nonfunctional lungs. This flapped oval opening develops between 2 septa: the septum primum and septum secundum, both of which make up the interatrial septum. At birth, the drop in right atrial pressure causes the foramen ovale to close and shunting to cease. Increased right atrial pressure may reopen the foramen ovale where the septa have not sealed and allow shunting to resume. This does not represent a true atrial septal defect because the septa have formed normally. A true atrial septal defect is a consistent opening of the interatrial septum, which allows blood to shunt from the atrium with the greater pressure. Septum secundum defects occur high in the interatrial septum, near the foramen ovale, and are the most common type. Septum primum defects are located lower in the interatrial septum, near the atrioventricular junction.

Pathophysiology: In most cases, blood shunts from the left atrium to the right atrium, causing a volume overload of the right-sided chambers. The magnitude of shunting depends on the size of the defect and the pressure gradient across the defect. Excessive blood flow through the right-sided chambers results in their dilation and hypertrophy. Pulmonary vasoconstriction may occur as a consequence of excessive pulmonary blood flow and may precipitate right-sided CHF. In situations in which right atrial pressure increases (eg, pulmonic stenosis) shunting from right to left across a patent foramen ovale or atrial septal defect may occur and cause cyanosis and, potentially, polycythemia.

Clinical Findings and Treatment: Signs of right heart failure (eg, ascites, edema, cyanosis) may be present. An ejection-type systolic murmur is usually present over the pulmonic valve area, reflecting increased blood flow through the pulmonic valve. Blood flow through the defect itself does not produce a murmur. Prolonged ejection time of the right ventricle may result in a split second heart sound. Electrocardiography may reveal evidence of right ventricular or right atrial enlargement (right axis shift, deep S waves, tall P waves). Right bundle branch block and arrhythmias can also be noted. Radiographically, there are variable degrees of right ventricular enlargement and prominence to the pulmonary vessels indicating pulmonary overcirculation. Echocardiography is indicated in these animals and demonstrates varying degrees of right atrial and right ventricular dilatation as well as identifying the defect as a loss of echogenicity at the interatrial septum. The normal loss of echogenicity of the fossa ovale should not be interpreted as an atrial septal defect. Doppler evaluation confirms shunting through the defect and increased ejection velocities across the pulmonic valve. Surgical correction may be attempted but is associated with high expense and mortality. Animals with septum secundum defects can tolerate the defects well and many of these defects are noted as an incidental finding in older animals. Larger defects, such as noted with septum primum defects or endocardial cushion defects, are more likely to cause right-sided CHF; pulmonary hypertension can also occur as a result of pulmonary overcirculation. The prognosis is guarded to poor in these cases.

Ventricular Septal Defects

Ventricular septal defects are most commonly located in the perimembranous portion of the septum, high in the ventricular septum immediately beneath the right and noncoronary aortic valve cusps on the left and just below the cranioseptal tricuspid valve commissure on the right. They vary in size and hemodynamic significance. Defects of the muscular septum may also occur. Ventricular septal defects may occur with other congenital cardiac anomalies. This defect is heritable in miniature swine.

Pathophysiology: Shunting of blood from the left ventricle into the right ventricle and right ventricular outflow tract occurs in most animals due to the higher pressures of the left ventricle. The magnitude of the shunt depends on the size of the defect and the pressure gradient between the ventricles. Blood shunted into the right ventricle is recirculated through the pulmonary vessels and left cardiac chambers, which causes dilatation of these structures. The right ventricle may dilate as well, especially in animals with large nonresistive ventricular septal defects or defects lower in the ventricular septum (which occur rarely). Small defects (highly resistive ventricular septal defects) limit the volume of shunted blood and minimize hemodynamic effects, whereas large defects usually result in severe circulatory derangements and clinical signs. Significant shunting through the pulmonary arteries can induce vasoconstriction of these vessels. As resistance rises, the shunt may reverse (ie, resistance to right ventricular outflow exceeds resistance to left ventricular outflow resulting in right-to-left shunting of blood), resulting in cyanosis and polycythemia. The shunting of blood from right to left through a septal defect as a consequence of pulmonary hypertension is referred to as Eisenmenger's complex.

Clinical Findings and Treatment: Clinical findings depend on the severity of the defect and the shunt direction. A small defect usually causes minimal or no signs. Larger defects may result in acute left-sided CHF. Cattle are prone to developing signs of right-sided failure. The development of Eisenmenger's complex is indicated by cyanosis, fatigue, and exercise intolerance. Most affected animals have a loud systolic murmur that radiates widely with an accompanying left-sided thrill. This murmur is absent or faint when a very large defect is present or when shunting is right to left. On occasion, aortic valvular insufficiency develops secondarily because a subaortic defect may disrupt aortic valve apposition. In these cases, a concurrent diastolic murmur is present, and the combination systolic/diastolic murmur (to-and-fro murmur) may be mistaken as that of a PDA. Chronic turbulence in the area of the defect can erode the endothelium and predispose affected animals to infective endocarditis. Thoracic radiographs can demonstrate generalized cardiomegaly with overcirculation of the pulmonary vessels. The defect can usually be visualized by echocardiography, although small defects may be missed. Doppler echocardiography or contrast studies will confirm the presence of a shunt. Therapy depends on the use of the animal, severity of clinical signs, and direction of the shunt. Animals with small ventricular septal defects do not typically require therapy and the prognosis is good. Animals with a moderate to severe ventricular septal defect more commonly develop clinical signs and treatment should be considered. Surgical closure of the defect; pulmonary artery banding to increase right ventricular outflow tract resistance and thus decrease left-to-right shunting; or use of therapy to reduce systemic vascular resistance (eg, a vasodilator such as hydralazine) may be considered in the treatment of animals with a large ventricular septal defect and left-to-right shunting. With right-to-left shunting, surgical closure of the defect is generally contraindicated. Phlebotomy to relieve the effects of polycythemia or use of hydroxyurea may be considered to relieve clinical signs; however, the prognosis is poor to guarded. Animals diagnosed with a ventricular septal defect should not be bred; the defect has been demonstrated to be heritable in at least 1 breed (English Springer Spaniels).

PERITONEOPERICARDIAL DIAPHRAGMATIC HERNIA (PPDH)

Peritoneopericardial diaphragmatic hernia is the most common congenital pericardial disease in dogs and cats. It results from abnormal development of the dorsolateral septum transversum or from failure of the lateral pleuroperitoneal folds and the ventromedial pars sternalis to unite. The result is herniation of abdominal viscera into the pericardial sac. Liver is most commonly herniated, followed by small intestine, spleen, and stomach. Clinical signs are highly variable, with many patients remaining asymptomatic and the defect being discovered on a necropsy examination. Thoracic radiographs can demonstrate small intestinal loops or liver crossing the diaphragm into the pericardial sac. A contrast radiographic examination using oral barium may also identify small intestinal loops or stomach in the pericardial sac. The diagnosis can be made by the findings of abdominal viscera in the pericardial sac on echocardiography as well. Patients with vomiting, signs of hepatic encephalopathy, or other adverse conditions resulting from PPDH should have a surgical reduction of the hernia.

TETRALOGY OF FALLOT

Tetralogy of Fallot is the most common defect that produces cyanosis. It results from a combination of pulmonic stenosis, a typically high and large ventricular septal defect, right ventricular hypertrophy, and varying degrees of dextropositioning of the aorta. A single conotruncal malformation (cranially displaced formation of the upper portion of the interventricular septum) is believed to result in narrowing of the right ventricular outflow tract (pulmonic stenosis), overriding of the aorta, and the ventricular septal defect. The right ventricular hypertrophy is simply a consequence of these abnormalities. The pulmonic stenosis may be valvular, infundibular, or both. Breeds predisposed to tetralogy of Fallot include Keeshonds, English Bulldogs, Miniature Poodles, Miniature Schnauzers, and Wirehaired Fox Terriers. The trait is inherited in Keeshonds and presumably in other breeds. This defect has been recognized in other breeds of dogs and in cats.

Pathophysiology: The hemodynamic consequences of tetralogy of Fallot depend primarily on the severity of the pulmonic stenosis, on the size of the ventricular septal defect (which is typically large and nonresistive), and on systemic vascular resistance. The direction and magnitude of the shunt through the septal defect depends in large part on the relative resistances to flow between the pulmonic circulation (obstructed by the pulmonic stenosis) and the systemic circulation. Consequences include reduced pulmonary blood flow (resulting in fatigue, shortness of breath) and generalized cyanosis (resulting in polycythemia, weakness) caused by the mixing of deoxygenated blood from the right side circulation with oxygenated blood from the left ventricle in aortic flow. Due to shunting of venous blood into the aorta and consequent hypoxia, the kidneys release erythropoietin, resulting in polycythemia (p 56). The increased blood viscosity associated with polycythemia can have significant hemodynamic effects, such as sludging of blood and poor capillary perfusion. Animals with severe polycythemia often have a history of seizures.

Clinical Findings and Treatment: Typical historical features include stunted growth, exercise intolerance, cyanosis, collapse, and seizures. A precordial thrill may be felt in the area of the pulmonic valve, and in most cases, a murmur of pulmonic stenosis is present. The intensity of the murmur is attenuated when severe polycythemia is present, and in some affected animals, a cardiac murmur is not present. Electrocardiographically, a pattern of right ventricular enlargement is usually seen (deep S waves in left chest leads, right axis shift) and arrhythmias are infrequent. Radiographs demonstrate variable right heart enlargement and undersized pulmonary vessels, often including the main pulmonary artery. Echocardiography confirms the diagnosis. Overriding (rightward displacement) of the aortic root, right ventricular hypertrophy, and a ventricular septal defect are evident. The left-sided chambers may be small as a result of decreased pulmonary venous return. Routine contrast echocardiography demonstrates shunting from right to left at the level of the ventricular septal defect. Flow through the defect can also be detected by Doppler echocardiography.

β-adrenergic blockade has been used to reduce the dynamic component of right ventricular outflow obstruction and to attenuate β-adrenergic-mediated decreases in systemic vascular resistance. Increases in systemic vascular resistance lower the magnitude of shunting. Polycythemia should be controlled by periodic phlebotomy when the PCV exceeds 65%. The prognosis is guarded, but animals with mild to moderate shunting may reach adulthood.

Treatment options include surgical and medical management. Corrective surgery has been reported in dogs but is rarely performed. Palliative surgical techniques to relieve clinical signs associated with tetralogy of Fallot are also rarely performed and include techniques to produce systemic to pulmonary anastomoses. These procedures may reduce signs of pulmonary hypoperfusion and systemic hypoxia. In some cases, reducing pulmonic stenosis is palliative. Surgical valvuloplasty or balloon valvuloplasty of the pulmonic stenosis are also options.

MITRAL VALVE DYSPLASIA

Congenital malformation of the mitral valve complex (mitral valve dysplasia) is a common congenital cardiac defect in cats. Canine breeds predisposed are Bull Terriers, German Shepherds, and Great Danes. Mitral valve dysplasia results in mitral insufficiency and systolic regurgitation of blood into the left atrium. Any component of the mitral valve complex (valve leaflets, chordae tendineae, papillary muscles) may be malformed, and often more than one component is defective.

Pathophysiology: Malformation of the mitral valve complex results in significant valvular insufficiency. Chronic mitral regurgitation leads to volume overload of the left heart, which results in dilatation of the left ventricle and atrium. When mitral regurgitation is severe, cardiac output decreases, which results in signs of cardiac failure. Severe mitral regurgitation can also result in pulmonary venous congestion and left-sided CHF. Dilatation of the left-sided chambers predisposes affected animals to arrhythmias. In some cases, malformation of the mitral valve complex causes a degree of valvular stenosis as well as insufficiency (see MITRAL STENOSIS, below).

Clinical Findings and Treatment: Clinical signs correlate with the severity of the defect. Affected animals usually display signs of left-sided CHF. A holosystolic murmur of mitral regurgitation is prominent at the left cardiac apex. A diastolic heart sound (gallop rhythm) is present in some cases. Affected animals may have a precordial thrill over the left cardiac apex. Electrocardiography may demonstrate atrial arrhythmias (atrial premature complexes, atrial fibrillation), especially in severely affected animals. There may also be evidence of both left atrial (widened P waves) and left ventricular enlargement. Thoracic radiographs may demonstrate severe left atrial enlargement. Left ventricular enlargement and pulmonary venous congestion can also be noted. Echocardiography demonstrates malformation of the mitral valve complex (fused chordae tendineae and thickened, immobile valve leaflets, abnormal appearance to the papillary muscles) and left atrial and ventricular dilatation. Doppler echocardiography demonstrates severe mitral regurgitation. If present, mitral stenosis can be identified (see below).

Prognosis for animals with clinical signs and severe disease is poor. Mildly affected animals may remain free of clinical signs for several years. For therapy of progressive left-sided CHF, see MANAGEMENT OF HEART FAILURE, p 85.

MITRAL STENOSIS

Mitral valve stenosis is a narrowing of the mitral valve orifice caused by abnormalities of the mitral valve, resulting in obstruction to left ventricular inflow. This congenital abnormality is rare in dogs and cats and can occur together with other congenital defects such as subaortic stenosis, mitral valve dysplasia, and pulmonic stenosis.

Pathophysiology: The disease results in increased resistance to left atrial outflow, creating a pressure gradient between the left atrium and left ventricle. This leads to left atrial enlargement and increases in pulmonary venous and capillary wedge pressures. Pulmonary edema can develop as a consequence, and syncope occurs in some cases.

Clinical Findings and Treatment: Mitral stenosis by itself can result in a diastolic heart murmur that is typically low-grade (I-II/VI). If concurrent mitral valve dysplasia is present, a murmur with maximum intensity at the left cardiac apex may be heard. Radiographs demonstrate varying degrees of left atrial enlargement and pulmonary edema in animals with left-sided CHF. Electrocardiography may demonstrate widened P waves (indicating left atrial enlargement) and supraventricular arrhythmias. Echocardiography provides a definitive diagnosis. Doming of the mitral valve leaflets toward the left ventricle during diastole, left atrial enlargement, and thickening of the mitral valve leaflets can be noted. Doppler echocardiography demonstrates turbulent diastolic flow across the mitral valve, beginning at the mitral valve and extending into the left ventricle. A pressure gradient is documented between the left atrium and left ventricle in early diastole.

Medical management of animals with mitral valve stenosis involves use of diuretics and dietary sodium restriction. Excessive diuresis should be avoided as this can reduce cardiac output severely. Surgical or interventional therapy may include closed commisurotomy (disruption of the stenosis without the use of bypass), open commisurotomy, mitral valve replacement, or balloon valvuloplasty (reported in an animal with tricuspid valve stenosis). These are rarely performed in dogs and cats and involve considerable risk and expense.

TRICUSPID DYSPLASIA

Congenital malformation of the tricuspid valve complex is seen occasionally in dogs and cats. Breeds predisposed are Labrador Retrievers and German Shepherds. Tricuspid dysplasia results in tricuspid insufficiency and systolic regurgitation of blood into the right atrium. Rarely, tricuspid valve stenosis can be noted. Chordae tendineae are commonly shortened or absent, and tricuspid valve leaflets may be thickened or adhered to the ventricular or intraventricular septal wall. Other concurrent congenital anomalies such as mitral valve dysplasia, septal defects, subaortic stenosis, or pulmonic stenosis may be present. In Ebstein's anomaly, a variant of tricuspid dysplasia, the tricuspid valve is displaced toward the cardiac apex.

Pathophysiology: Malformation of the tricuspid valve results in significant valvular insufficiency. Chronic tricuspid regurgitation leads to volume overload of the right heart, dilating the right ventricle and atrium. Pulmonary blood flow may be decreased, resulting in fatigue and tachypnea. As the pressure in the right atrium increases, venous return is impaired, causing ascites.

Clinical Findings and Treatment: Clinical signs correlate with the severity of the defect. Affected animals usually display signs of right-sided CHF. A harsh holosystolic murmur of tricuspid regurgitation is prominent at the right cardiac apex. Atrial arrhythmias, especially paroxysmal atrial tachycardia, are common and may cause death. Electrocardiography and radiography typically demonstrate right ventricular and right atrial enlargement. The caudal vena cava may be significantly enlarged. Echocardiography demonstrates malformation of the tricuspid valve and usually severe right atrial and ventricular dilatation. Doppler echocardiography demonstrates severe tricuspid regurgitation.

Prognosis for animals with clinical signs is guarded. Periodic abdominocentesis may be needed to control peritoneal effusions. Diuretics, vasodilators, and digoxin may also be indicated.

ECTOPIC HEART

Ectopic heart is a condition in which the heart is located outside the thoracic cavity, usually in the ventral cervical area. It occurs most commonly in cattle. Displacement through a defective sternum or through ribs usually results in neonatal death, although longterm survival is possible with other types of displacement.

MISCELLANEOUS CONGENITAL CARDIAC ABNORMALITIES

Anomalous pulmonary venous connection is a congenital abnormality in which varying numbers of pulmonary veins (from one to all) attach to the right atrium or a systemic vein. **Endocardial cushion defects** (atrioventricular [AV] canal defects, persistent AV ostium, AV septal defects) involve abnormalities of endocardial cushion development and can produce septum primum defects, AV valve abnormalities, and ventricular septal defects. **Cor triatriatum sinister and dexter** result from a fibrous membrane dividing the left or right atrium, respectively. Cor triatriatum sinister has been reported in cats and cor triatriatum dexter in dogs. The affected atrium is divided into 2 chambers. There are commonly one or more perforations in the separating membrane, allowing communication between the 2 portions of the atrium. Successful balloon valvuloplasty for this disease has been reported. **Dextrocardia**, positioning of the heart in the right hemithorax, can occur as a congenital cardiac defect and by itself is typically benign. It can also occur in combination with **situs inversus** (an abnormal orientation of the organs of the body). The combination of these defects is typically noted in animals with other concurrent abnormalities such as sinusitis, bronchitis, and bronchiectasis. In addition to these defects, several others are reported, including double outlet right ventricle (all of one great artery and the majority of another great artery originate from the right ventricle), interruption of the aortic arch, persistent left cranial vena cava, pulmonary atresia, and transposition of the great arteries.

HEART DISEASE AND HEART FAILURE

Heart disease is defined as any abnormality of the heart and encompasses a wide range of abnormalities including congenital abnormalities (*see* CONGENITAL AND INHERITED ANOMALIES, p 66), as well as anatomic and physiologic disorders of varying etiologies. It can be classified by various methods, including whether the disease was present at birth or not (eg, congenital or acquired), etiology (eg, infectious, degenerative), duration (eg, chronic or acute), clinical status (eg, left heart failure, right heart failure, or biventricular failure), or by anatomic malformation (eg, ventricular septal defect).

Heart failure is any cardiac abnormality that results in failure of the heart to pump blood at a rate that is in accordance with the requirements of metabolizing tissue. It is a clinical syndrome in which congestion or edema, decreased peripheral perfusion, and/or systemic hypotension arise as the final consequence of severe heart disease. Heart disease can be present without ever leading to heart failure. Heart failure, however, can only occur if heart disease is present because it is a consequence of heart disease.

DIAGNOSIS

The diagnosis of heart disease typically involves evaluating the signalment, history, and physical examination findings, as well as results of diagnostic tests such as radiography, electrocardiography, and echocardiography. Occasionally, more specialized tests such as cardiac catheterization or nuclear studies are necessary.

History and Signalment

For patients with suspected heart disease, the signalment (age, breed, sex) helps provide a differential diagnosis list. The signalment influences not only the heart diseases listed, but also their relative importance (eg, endocarditis is rare in cats, but is more common in cows, horses, and dogs).

Animals presenting with heart disease may have a history of exercise intolerance, weakness, dyspnea, tachypnea, abdominal distention (secondary to ascites), syncope (fainting), cyanosis, or anorexia and weight loss. More rarely, peripheral or ventral edema, jaundice, or hemoptysis may be noted. There is also some species variation in presenting complaints. Cats rarely demonstrate cough with heart disease and more commonly present with a history of dyspnea (which may be subtle and go unnoticed by the owner) and anorexia. Dogs with congestive heart failure (CHF), in contrast, commonly demonstrate cough and dyspnea as a presenting complaint.

Physical Examination

A complete physical examination should be performed on any animal being evaluated for heart disease. In addition to auscultation of the thorax, palpation should be performed to assess for the presence of thrills (low frequency vibrations that can be palpated with the fingertips) and alterations in intensity or location of the impulse beat. Concurrent auscultation and palpation of pulses should also be performed. Mucous membrane color and refill time, as well as assessment for jugular pulsation and excessive distention, is recommended. Limbs should be examined for the presence of edema, and the abdomen should be assessed for the presence of ascites.

Heart Sounds and Murmurs: Heart sounds are generated by the rapid acceleration and deceleration of blood and secondary vibrations in the cardiohemic system. Four heart sounds can potentially by ausculted. The first heart sound (S_1) is associated with closure of the atrioventricular (AV) valves, and the second heart sound (S_2) is associated with closure of the semilunar (aortic and pulmonic) valves. The third heart sound (S_3) occurs in early diastole and is a result of rapid ventricular filling, and the fourth heart sound (S_4) is associated with atrial systole. In horses, all 4 sounds can be audible. In cattle, typically only S_1 and S_2 are audible, although S_3 or S_4 can sometimes be heard. IV fluid administration in cattle can result in accentuation of the third and/or fourth heart sounds. In dogs, cats, and ferrets, S_1 and S_2 are normally the only heart sounds audible. Less is known about goats, sheep, and pigs; however, only the first and second heart sounds are believed to be audible in these species.

Gallop Heart Sounds: A gallop heart sound is the presence of the first and second heart sounds accompanied by an interceding sound that is either an accentuated third or fourth heart sound, or both. These are classified as **protodiastolic** (S_3), **presystolic** (S_4), or **summation gallop heart sounds** (fusion of S_3 and S_4). The most common gallop heart sound noted in dogs is a result of an accentuated third heart sound and typically occurs secondary to myocardial disease such as dilated cardiomyopathy or degenerative valve disease. An S_4 gallop heart sound (presystolic) can be audible in cats with cardiomyopathy. Because the heart rate commonly exceeds 160-180 bpm in cats, gallop heart sounds are typically summation gallop heart sounds. A **systolic click** is a short, sharp, often transient sound that can occur during mid- to late systole. These clicks are uncommon in dogs and probably in other domestic species and are most commonly noted in dogs with early myxomatous degeneration of the mitral valve. They usually are single but may be multiple or may disappear completely in some cycles.

Splitting of S_1 or S_2: This may occur in the absence of other cardiac abnormalities. The first heart sound is due to passive closure of the mitral and tricuspid valves. S_1 may be markedly split when the contraction of the 2 ventricles is asynchronous, as in bundle-branch block, cardiac pacing, and certain ectopic ventricular beats, resulting in differential closure of the AV valves. Splitting of S_1 can also occur in normal healthy, large-breed dogs. S_2 may be split during inspiration in dogs (especially large-breed dogs) and typically results from an increase in negative intrathoracic pressure during inspiration, increased right ventricular filling, and consequent delayed closure of the pulmonic valve relative to the aortic valve. Splitting of S_2 is a normal finding in horses during either inspiration or expiration. The second heart sound is produced by passive closure of the aortic and pulmonic valves. Abnormal splitting of S_2 is associated with pulmonary hypertension, as in pulmonary emphysema of horses and heartworm infestation of dogs. Other causes in dogs (and possibly other species) include atrial septal defect, pulmonic stenosis, right or left bundle-branch block, and certain ventricular ectopic beats. Delayed closure of the aortic valve (such as with subaortic stenosis, left bundle branch block, certain ectopic ventricular beats, or systemic hypertension) can result in paradoxical splitting of S_2 (the pulmonic valve closes prior to the aortic valve).

Synchronous Diaphragmatic Flutter: The diaphragm may contract synchronously with the heart to produce loud thumping noises on auscultation and usually visible contraction in the flank area. The syndrome results from stimulation of the phrenic nerve by atrial depolarization and occurs primarily when there is a marked electrolyte or acid-base imbalance, particularly with hypocalcemia. It is most common in horses and dogs and occurs frequently in eclampsia. It is seen most commonly in dogs in association with electrolyte disturbances induced by GI disease.

Murmurs: Heart murmurs are audible vibrations emanating from the heart or major blood vessels and generally are the result of turbulent blood flow or vibrations of cardiac structures such as part of a valve leaflet or chordal structure. Murmurs are typically defined relative to timing, intensity, and location, but can also be characterized by frequency (pitch), quality (eg, musical), and configuration (eg, crescendo-decrescendo). A **systolic murmur** occurs during systole and is typically either ejection (crescendo-decrescendo) or regurgitant (holosystolic, plateau). Ejection systolic murmurs demonstrate the greatest intensity during mid-systole and appear diamond-shaped on phonocardiography. They can be produced by stenotic lesions at the semilunar valves (eg, pulmonic stenosis or subaortic stenosis). Regurgitant systolic murmurs demonstrate a constant intensity throughout systole and can be caused by mitral or tricuspid regurgitation (eg, myxomatous degeneration of the mitral valve). **Diastolic murmurs** are typically decrescendo (decreasing in intensity through diastole) and a result of aortic or pulmonic insufficiency (such as that caused by aortic valve infective endocarditis). **Continuous murmurs** are most commonly a result of patent ductus arteriosus (a congenital cardiac defect) and occur throughout systole and diastole. Continuous murmurs vary in intensity over time, typically being most intense at the end of ventricular ejection and decreasing in intensity through diastole. A **to-and-fro murmur** occurs in patients that demonstrate both a systolic murmur and a diastolic murmur and can occur in patients with a ventricular septal defect and aortic valve insufficiency or in a patient with subaortic stenosis and aortic insufficiency.

In horses, early systolic and diastolic murmurs can be noted in the absence of heart disease or anemia. The point of maximum intensity is typically located over the left heart base. A short, high-pitched, squeaking, early diastolic cardiac murmur is sometimes seen in healthy young horses. Occasionally, systolic murmurs are noted in some cats secondary to an increase in right midventricular flow velocity without significant structural heart disease. Innocent cardiac murmurs are also commonly noted in immature cats and dogs (<6 mo of age) as a result of increased stroke volume.

Heart murmurs are classified as follows: Grade I—the lowest intensity murmur that can be heard, typically detected only while auscultation is performed in a quiet room; Grade II—a faint murmur, easily audible, and restricted to a localized area; Grade III—a murmur immediately audible when auscultation begins; Grade IV—a loud murmur immediately heard at the beginning of auscultation but not accompanied by a thrill; Grade V—a very loud murmur with a palpable thrill, the loudest murmur that is still inaudible when the stethoscope is just removed from the chest wall; or Grade VI—an extremely loud murmur that can be heard when the stethoscope is just removed from the chest wall.

Arrhythmias: Arrhythmias are abnormalities of the rate, regularity, or site of cardiac impulse formation and are noted during auscultation. Other terms such as dysrhythmia and ectopic rhythm are also used to describe arrhythmias. The presence of a cardiac arrhythmia does not necessarily indicate the presence of heart disease; many cardiac arrhythmias are clinically insignificant and require no specific therapy. Some arrhythmias, however, may cause severe clinical signs such as syncope or lead to sudden death. Numerous systemic disorders may be associated with abnormal cardiac rhythms. (For discussion of specific arrhythmias, *see* p 79.)

Pulses: A pulse is the rhythmic expansion of an artery that can be digitally palpated (or visualized) during physical examination. Physiologically, the pulse pressure is the difference between systemic systolic and diastolic pressures. In dogs and cats, pulses are typically palpated at the femoral artery. Jugular venous pulsation can be noted in normal animals. These pulses typically do not extend beyond a third of the distance up the neck of an animal in a standing position. **Pulse deficits** are absent pulses despite auscultation of a heart beat and are thus detected during simultaneous auscultation and pulse palpation. These occur as a result of ectopic ventricular contractions (arrhythmias) that occur so prematurely (rapidly) that the ventricles are unable to fill sufficiently to result in ejection of blood. **Bounding pulses** (an increase in pulse pressure) can be noted in patients with aortic insufficiency or patent ductus arteriosus. **Weak pulses** (a reduction in pulse pressure) can be noted in patients with heart failure or subaortic stenosis. Dogs with severe subaortic stenosis may demonstrate a pulse pressure that slowly increases during ventricular systole and reaches a peak pressure late in systole called **pulsus parvus et tardus**. **Pulsus paradoxus** is a decrease in pulse pressure during inspiration and an increase in pulse pressure during expiration. This is a normal occurrence in animals, but, it is usually too subtle to observe on physical examination. Patients with pericardial effusion and cardiac tamponade, however, demonstrate an exaggeration of this finding. **Pulsus alternans** is an alternating strong and weak pulse while the patient is in sinus rhythm; it can be noted (albeit rarely) in patients with myocardial failure or tachyarrhythmias. **Pulsus bigeminus** is an alternating strong and weak pulse caused by an arrhythmia such as ventricular bigeminy. The weaker pulse (during the ventricular premature contraction) typically follows a shorter time interval than the stronger pulse.

Respiratory Sounds: Pulmonary edema may develop as a result of CHF. On physical examination, this may manifest as respiratory crackles and wheezes. Dyspnea or tachypnea may also be noted in these patients. A decrease in air movement is commonly present during thoracic auscultation in patients that have developed pleural effusion as a result of heart disease. However, respiratory diseases or pleural effusion secondary to other underlying disease can also result in these clinical signs.

Ascites: Abdominal swelling may occur as a result of gas, soft tissue, or fluid accumulation. Patients with heart disease and right-sided heart failure (such as caused by heartworm disease or tricuspid valve dysplasia) can develop ascites.

Radiography

Thoracic radiographs frequently provide valuable information in the assessment of patients suspected of having heart disease. Finding generalized cardiomegaly or enlargement of specific cardiac chambers makes the presence of heart disease more likely and may also provide clues as to the specific disease present. Pulmonary edema is a common finding in patients with CHF; pleural effusion may also be noted. Resolution of these abnormalities on recheck thoracic radiographs can be used as one indication of therapy efficacy. Animals with CHF may also demonstrate distention of the pulmonary vasculature. Although thoracic radiographs are useful in evaluation of patients with heart disease, they have certain limitations. The presence of pulmonary edema does not definitively confirm a cardiogenic origin or rule out another origin such as pulmonary disease, and assessment of overall cardiac size as well as specific chamber enlargement is typically far less accurate compared to echocardiography.

Electrocardiography

Electrocardiography is the recording of cardiac electrical activity from the body surface. It can be used not only to identify cardiac arrhythmias and conduction disturbances, but also chamber enlargement.

Waveform Abnormalities: Chamber enlargement can be indicated by waveform abnormalities. In lead II in dogs and cats, **wide P waves** are suggestive of left atrial enlargement, **tall P waves** of right atrial enlargement, **tall R waves** of left ventricular enlargement, and **deep S waves** of right ventricular enlargement. Wide QRS complexes can occur in patients with ventricular enlargement; however, they can also be due to conduction disturbances (*see* below). While the ECG may suggest chamber enlargement, thoracic radiographs and echocardiography are more sensitive.

Sinus Rhythm: The sinus node initiates each cardiac contraction in a normal animal, sets the normal rate and rhythm, and is called the pacemaker of the heart. **Normal sinus rhythm** is a rhythm that is regular and originates at the sinus node. **Sinus bradycardia** is a regular sinus rhythm that is slower than expected. Clearly, expected heart rate will vary by species or by situation (eg, exercise, anesthetized, resting). Sinus bradycardia may be noted in patients that are overdosed with anesthesia or agents that can result in elevated vagal tone or reduction of sympathetic tone (eg, xylazine, digoxin), hypothermic patients, hypothyroid patients, patients with sick sinus syndrome, or in patients with elevated vagal tone secondary to systemic disease such as respiratory, neurologic, ocular, GI, or urinary tract disease. Treatment for sinus bradycardia is typically not needed unless clinical signs associated with the bradycardia, such as weakness or collapse, are noted. In dogs and cats, atropine (0.04 mg/kg, IV, IM, or SC) may be considered for treatment of bradycardia. The initiating cause should also be corrected.

Sinus tachycardia is the finding of a regular sinus rhythm at an excessive rate. Causes include stress (resulting in high sympathetic drive), hyperthyroidism, fever, hypovolemia, cardiac tamponade, heart failure, or administration of agents that can increase the rate of sinus node discharge (eg, catecholamines). Treatment involves resolving the underlying cause. **Sinus arrhythmia** occurs as a result of irregular discharge of the sinus node. The site of impulse formation remains the sinus node; however, the frequency of the discharge varies. Sinus arrhythmia is a normal finding in dogs and horses; it is abnormal in cats. Heart rate usually increases with inspiration and decreases with expiration. The rhythm is irregular, with >10% variation in the RR interval. The variation in heart rhythm is associated with variation in the intensity of vagal tone. It is abolished by reduced vagal tone or increased heart rate resulting from excitement, exercise, or administration of atropine. It may be associated with a wandering pacemaker (P waves vary in shape) within the sinoatrial (SA) node and a varying PR interval. **Sinoatrial block** occurs when the impulse from the SA node fails to be conducted through the surrounding tissue to the atria and ventricles. Thus, no P waves or QRS complexes are noted on the ECG. In second-degree SA block (which is most common), some of the SA impulses fail to conduct, resulting in a pause that is an exact integer multiple of the normal PP interval.

Sinus arrest is the failure of the SA node to discharge for a short period of time, resulting in a pause between complexes on the ECG (typically accepted as a pause exceeding twice the normal RR interval). **Atrial standstill (sinoventricular rhythm)** occurs as a result of the atria being unable to depolarize. There are no P waves present on the ECG and no atrial fibrillation. The heart rate is typically 40-60 bpm in dogs affected by this condition, depending on the precise etiology. Causes include hyperkalemia (where the atrial myocardium is poisoned), myocarditis, and specific forms of cardiomyopathy where the atrial myocardium is replaced by fibrous tissue. Treatment for hyperkalemia-induced atrial standstill requires treatment of the underlying hyperkalemia. **Sick sinus syndrome** involves the sinus node; however, other portions of the specialized conduction tissue of the myocardium, including the AV node, can be affected. This disease is commonly noted in geriatric dogs such as Miniature Schnauzers and can result in periods of bradycardia caused by sinus arrest or sinoatrial block, tachycardia, or conduction disturbances such as second degree AV block (see below). Initial treatment usually involves sympathomimetics to increase heart rate (eg, extended-release theophylline, 10 mg/kg, PO, BID; or terbutaline, 0.14 mg/kg, PO, BID-TID in dogs). In patients that do not respond to oral therapy, pacemaker implantation may be warranted.

Conduction Disturbances: Atrioventricular (AV) block refers to alteration of impulse conduction from the atria to the ventricles. In **first-degree AV block** (prolonged conduction), the conduction time is increased and is recognized on an ECG as an increased PR interval. In **second-degree AV block** (intermittent conduction), occasional impulses fail to be conducted through the AV junction, and atrial contraction is not followed by ventricular contraction. The block may occur at regular intervals or at random. During the block, there is no S_1 or S_2 and no arterial pulse. In horses, the sound associated with atrial contraction (S_4) is commonly heard, and the occurrence of S_4 not followed by other heart sounds is diagnostic for second- or third-degree heart block. S_4 may also be audible in dogs with second-degree AV block. In all species, an atrial jugular wave may be seen during the block. When the PR intervals preceding the dropped beat progressively lengthen, the condition is known as the Wenckebach or Mobitz type I second-degree AV block. If the PR intervals do not change, the condition is known as a Mobitz type II second-degree AV block.

In **third-degree AV block** or **complete heart block**, none of the impulses are conducted from the atria to the ventricles. The ventricular rhythm is established from an ectopic nodal or ventricular pacemaker that discharges at a slower rate than the SA node, and the atria and ventricles beat independently of each other. The heart and pulse rates are regular, but there is a pronounced bradycardia that is relatively unresponsive to factors that usually increase heart rate (eg, exercise or excitement). The difference in timing between atrial and ventricular contractions results in variation in ventricular filling and consequent variation in intensity of S_1 and arterial pulse pressure. Periodically, the atria contract when the ventricle is in systole, which results in large pulsations in the jugular vein (cannon A waves). In some animals, the faster atrial contractions can be detected with a stethoscope.

The significance of the AV block varies by species. Both first- and second-degree AV block may be present without outward evidence of cardiac disease. First-degree AV block may result from excessive vagal tone and generally is not considered significant in dogs or horses unless other evidence of heart disease is present. In all species, second-degree AV block may be indicative of heart disease. However, in horses, it is more commonly the result of high vagal tone. It is detected at resting heart rates of <40 bpm and, as in SA block, may be induced or abolished by situations that decrease vagal tone. Complete AV block is always abnormal in dogs and cats.

AV block may be caused by fibrosis, neoplasia, other injuries to the AV node, hypoxia, agents that increase vagal tone, or electrolyte abnormalities. Treatment is aimed primarily at correcting the underlying cause. It is frequently associated with syncope, especially during exercise or excitement. Oral therapy, such as extended-release theophylline (10 mg/kg, PO, BID) or terbutaline (0.14 mg/kg, PO, BID-TID in dogs), may be useful in animals with second-degree AV block that are symptomatic (syncope, weakness). Complete heart block is usually associated with irreversible lesions; pharmaceuticals are typically ineffective at resolving the conduction disturbance, and cardiac pacemaker implantation is warranted.

Arrhythmias: Arrhythmias can be divided into bradyarrhythmias, in which the heart rate is excessively slow, and tachyarrhythmias, in which the heart rate is excessively rapid. The former includes sinus bradycardia, sinus arrest, SA block, AV block, and atrial standstill (*see* above). Tachyarrhythmias can be divided into supraventricular and ventricular based on their site of origin. **Supraventricular premature depolarizations** are premature depolarizations that originate from a site outside the sinus node and above the ventricles. They are also called atrial or nodal premature complexes/depolarizations/beats. Possible sites for ectopic depolarizations include the atrial myocardium and junction (proximal AV node, AV node, and bundle of His). Electrocardiographically, supraventricular premature depolarizations include a QRS complex that appears normal but occurs prematurely. A P wave of variable morphology may be noted preceding the supraventricular premature depolarization or may be hidden in the preceding sinus complex. Supraventricular premature depolarizations are most commonly a result of chronic mitral regurgitation in dogs, but may be caused by any heart disease that can result in atrial enlargement, as well as other underlying causes such as myocarditis, sick sinus syndrome, stress, or other causes for increased sympathetic drive. **Supraventricular tachycardia** is a series of supraventricular premature depolarizations occurring consecutively. **Accessory pathways** are congenital abnormalities that allow an electrical connection between the atria and ventricles outside the normal connection (AV node/bundle of His). These pathways or bypass tracts have been recognized in dogs and cats and can result in supraventricular tachyarrhythmias. Treatment may involve radiofrequency catheter ablation of the bypass tract; oral medications such as diltiazem and digoxin (not the drug of choice) have also been tried.

Atrial flutter is a rare arrhythmia that, if present, typically precedes the development of atrial fibrillation. It is in essence a rapid supraventricular tachycardia where P waves commonly appear as a "saw-toothed" baseline. The atrial rate of discharge is so rapid (usually >400 bpm) that only intermittent impulses are conducted because of intermittent AV nodal refractoriness. The ventricular rate may be regular and rapid or irregular and rapid.

Atrial fibrillation is an irregular rhythm that is typically rapid and caused by disorganized depolarization of the atria. Stimulation of the AV node occurs frequently but in a random fashion, resulting in a rapid and irregular rhythm. The irregularity results in variation in the diastolic filling period between contractions and, consequently, variation in intensity of the heart sounds and amplitude of the arterial pulses. With exceptionally short diastolic periods, there is insufficient filling of the ventricles to produce an arterial pulse after ventricular contraction. At rapid heart rates, this produces a pulse rate that is considerably lower than the heart rate (pulse deficit). Electrocardiography demonstrates an absence of P waves, the presence of rapid F waves, and an absolute irregularity in the RR intervals. In dogs and cats, atrial fibrillation with high heart rates usually indicates severe cardiovascular disease. Causes include any heart disease resulting in atrial enlargement (eg, cardiomyopathy, degenerative valve disease), myocarditis, or noncardiac disease such as neoplasia or (less commonly) gastric dilation and volvulus syndrome in dogs. In ruminants, atrial fibrillation is sometimes paroxysmal in association with GI tract disorders, but it also may occur as a sequela for cor pulmonale or with cardiac disease. In horses, atrial fibrillation may occur in conjunction with other cardiac disease such as mitral insufficiency. It also can occur in the apparent absence of serious underlying cardiac disease and, in horses with high vagal tone, may occur with a bradycardia. There is significant irregularity of heart rhythm and variation in heart sound intensity and pulse amplitude but no pulse deficits in these patients. When the resting rate is 26-48 bpm, there may be few signs of cardiac disability except with heavy exercise. The heart rate increases in response to moderate exercise. At very slow rates, several seconds may elapse between some contractions, and syncope may occur. Atrial fibrillation occurs more commonly in draft and other large horses. It occurs in racehorses in association with poor racing performance and may be paroxysmal. Atrial fibrillation with a low, resting heart rate is not incompatible with long life, but affected horses should not be used for riding. Conversion to a sinus rhythm with quinidine at a dosage of 22 mg/kg, PO, every 2 hr is sometimes attempted in horses and is often followed by a return to successful performance in racing animals. The chance for success is greatest when conversion is attempted shortly after the initial onset.

Ventricular premature depolarizations arise from a site within the ventricular myocardium. On an ECG, the complex appears wide and bizarre and is premature relative to the preceding sinus complex. There is no associated P wave. Causes include primary myocardial disease, electrolyte imbalance, acute toxicities, noncardiac disease such as neoplasia (eg, splenic hemangiosarcoma in dogs), gastric distention (such as seen with gastric dilation and volvulus syndrome in dogs), or trauma. **Ventricular tachycardia** is the presence of 3 or more ventricular premature depolarizations consecutively. **Ventricular fibrillation** is a result of microreentrant circuits within the ventricular myocardium resulting in the absence of effective ventricular contractions and is thus a terminal rhythm. An **idioventricular rhythm** is the presence of only ventricular escape complexes on an ECG and is also typically a terminal rhythm. **Accelerated idioventricular rhythm** is a slow form of ventricular tachycardia where the ventricular tachycardia rate is less than ~120 bpm in dogs. This is considered a benign arrhythmia in most animals. While the underlying cause should be sought and treated as necessary, the arrhythmia itself typically results in no clinical signs and requires no specific therapy.

Echocardiography

Echocardiography is the use of ultrasound to evaluate the heart and proximal great vessels. Echocardiography complements other diagnostic procedures by quantifying the dynamic events of the cardiac cycle. Cardiac chamber and wall dimensions can be determined; the anatomy and motion of valves can be visualized; and pressure gradients, blood flow volumes, and several indices of cardiac function can be calculated. Echocardiography can also identify changes in myocardial tissue texture indicative of ischemia and fibrosis and delineate masses, valvular vegetations, pericardial effusion, and many other features previously verifiable only at necropsy. There are 3 main types of echocardiography: two-dimensional, M-mode, and Doppler. **Two-dimensional echocardiography** provides a wedge-shaped, two-dimensional image of the heart in real-time motion. Several standard long-axis and short-axis views obtained from standard imaging windows on the thorax have been developed for dogs, cats, horses, and cows. **M-mode echocardiography** is produced by a one-dimensional beam of ultrasound that penetrates the heart, providing an "ice-pick view." The tissue interfaces that are encountered by the beam are then plotted on a screen. This mode of evaluation is typically used to measure chamber dimensions, wall thickness, valve motion, and great vessel dimensions. **Doppler echocardiography** employs the principle of changing frequency of the ultrasonic beam after it contacts a moving RBC to measure flow velocity and thus identify turbulent or high-velocity flow. This can locate cardiac murmurs.

Cardiac Catheterization

Cardiac catheterization involves the placement of specialized catheters into the heart and surrounding great vessels. Indications include diagnostic evaluation, eg, when other diagnostic tests are insufficient to identify specific cardiac abnormalities or are unable to identify the severity of a lesion, presurgical evaluation, therapeutic intervention, and in clinical research. Diagnostic and presurgical cardiac catheterization, however, have largely been replaced by echocardiography.

HEART FAILURE

Heart failure is not a specific disease or diagnosis, but a syndrome in which severe systolic and/or diastolic dysfunction results in decompensation of the cardiovascular system. There are limited and specific mechanisms by which heart disease can result in decompensation of the cardiovascular system. As a result, there are limited and specific clinical signs that can develop as a result of heart failure. Heart failure can be divided into 4 functional classifications: systolic myocardial failure, impedance to cardiac inflow, pressure overload, and volume overload.

Systolic Myocardial Failure: Systolic myocardial failure is a general reduction in the ability of the myocardium to contract. This can be identified on echocardiography as an increase in end-systolic diameter and end-diastolic diameter, as well as a reduction in the percentage change in volume following ventricular contraction and reduced wall motion during ventricular contraction. If the reduction in contractility is significant, normal cardiac output cannot be maintained. **Primary systolic myocardial failure** is an idiopathic condition resulting in myocardial failure and is called dilated cardiomyopathy (p 91). **Secondary myocardial failure** is myocardial failure resulting from some insult such as neoplasia, heat stroke, electric shock, trauma, infectious disease (bacterial, viral, fungal, protozoal), nutritional deficiency (eg, taurine deficiency), drugs (eg, doxorubicin), or toxins.

Impedance to Cardiac Inflow: Heart failure resulting from impedance to cardiac inflow may result in a decrease to ventricular volume and, as a result, a decrease in cardiac output. This may result from external compression of the heart (eg, pericardial effusion, constrictive pericarditis), diastolic dysfunction resulting in a stiff ventricle and reduced ventricular filling (eg, hypertrophic cardiomyopathy, restrictive cardiomyopathy), or anatomic abnormalities resulting in impedance to ventricular filling (eg, atrial tumor, mitral and tricuspid valve stenosis).

Pressure Overload: Heart failure caused by pressure overload occurs as a result of chronic increases in systolic wall stress. This may result from impedance to cardiac outflow (eg, subaortic stenosis, pulmonic stenosis) or increased vascular resistance (eg, systemic or pulmonary hypertension). The response of the myocardium to these conditions is **concentric hypertrophy** (ie, increased wall thickness of the affected chamber). Pressure overload to the adult right ventricle can result in dilation of the chamber as well as increased wall thickness, however.

Volume Overload: Volume overload heart failure occurs secondary to any disease that results in an increase in ventricular volume. Grossly, the ventricular chamber increases in diameter with a relatively normal wall thickness (**eccentric hypertrophy**). This still represents ventricular hypertrophy because the overall mass of the ventricle is increased. Sarcomeres, however, increase in series (end-on-end) as compared to in parallel (as with concentric hypertrophy). Typically, the process begins with a volume overload to the ventricle (such as volume overload to the left ventricle caused by a left-to-right shunting patent ductus arteriosus), resulting in a compensatory increase in left ventricular chamber diameter/eccentric hypertrophy. Myocardial contractility typically remains normal, but may be reduced (such as when myocardial failure develops). The increase in ventricular volume means that the same degree of ventricular contraction produces an increased cardiac output. Though this can temporarily normalize cardiac output, eventually compensatory mechanisms are overwhelmed and signs of congestive heart failure (CHF) develop. Diseases that result in volume overload myocardial failure include valvular insufficiencies (eg, degenerative valve disease of the AV valves), left-to-right shunts (eg, patent ductus arteriosus, ventricular septal defect), or high-output states (such as those caused by hyperthyroidism or anemia).

Compensatory Mechanisms

The cardiovascular system maintains normal systemic arterial pressure, blood flow to metabolizing tissue, and capillary (systemic and pulmonary) pressures. In heart disease, the body uses compensatory mechanisms to attempt to normalize these functions. In a patient with dilated cardiomyopathy, for example, cardiac output is compromised by reduced cardiac contractility. This leads to reduced systemic arterial blood pressure (due to decreased stroke volume). The body acutely compensates by increasing sympathetic drive to peripheral arterioles, thereby producing peripheral vasoconstriction. Elevation of sympathetic drive also increases myocardial contractility (via β_1-receptor activation) and heart rate. These responses result in normalization of cardiac output and systemic blood pressure. Eventually, however, chronic elevation of sympathetic drive damages the myocardium (and other organs) and β-receptor down-regulation occurs. This returns myocardial contractility to its previously reduced state.

The return to reduced cardiac output results in a decrease in sodium delivery to the juxtaglomerular apparatus of the kidneys, which, along with chronic elevation of sympathetic drive, results in increased renin release, activation of the renin-angiotensin-aldosterone system (RAAS), and conversion of angiotensinogen (produced in the liver) to angiotensin I. Angiotensin I is then converted to angiotensin II by angiotensin-converting enzyme (ACE). This increases sodium and water retention via a direct effect on the renal tubules as well as secondarily via an increase in aldosterone secretion. Other effects of angiotensin II include vasoconstriction, myocardial hypertrophy, increased thirst, norepinephrine release, constriction of efferent renal arterioles, increased antidiuretic hormone release, increased oxygen free radical production, and increased endothelin release. Ultimately, the activation of the RAAS results in increased blood volume and increased cardiac output and is another mechanism by which the body attempts to normalize cardiovascular function. This occurs at the expense of diastolic pressure, which has now increased because of increased end-diastolic blood volume. Blood volume can increase as much as 30% in patients with severe CHF. Eventually, progressive myocardial failure and chronic activation of the RAAS result in pulmonary edema. The cardiovascular system has compromised capillary pressure (pulmonary edema results from an elevation in pulmonary capillary pressures) while maintaining blood flow and systemic arterial pressure. With continued myocardial failure, the latter functions become further compromised with progressive signs of CHF (see below).

Clinical Manifestations

Clinical signs associated with heart failure are typically distinct, depending on the etiology of the heart failure, as well as the chamber affected. Some species variation also occurs.

Left-sided Congestive Heart Failure: With left-sided CHF, clinical signs are associated with an increase in pulmonary venous and capillary hydrostatic pressure (ie, a backup of pressure in the vessels delivering blood to the left ventricle). Pulmonary edema and congestion (cough, dyspnea) are the most common signs. Cats less commonly demonstrate cough; however, dyspnea, tachypnea, anorexia, or exercise intolerance may be noted. In cats, as in humans, increased pulmonary venous pressure can lead to pleural effusion. This phenomenon is less common in dogs. Many dogs with left-sided CHF, especially secondary to degenerative valve disease, demonstrate syncope resulting from activation of the ventricular mechanoreceptors with a consequent surge in vagal tone and withdrawal of sympathetic tone resulting in bradycardia, hypotension, and collapse.

Right-sided Congestive Heart Failure: Right-sided CHF results in an increase in pressure in the vessels delivering blood to the right ventricle—the systemic veins and systemic capillaries. This can result in ascites, pleural effusion, and/or peripheral edema.

Biventricular Failure: This can arise when both the right and left ventricles are dysfunctional, such as in patients with myocardial failure resulting from dilated cardiomyopathy or toxin exposure. Clinical signs attributable to both forms of CHF can be noted, although commonly signs of one will predominate.

Management

Therapy for heart failure is directed primarily at reducing signs of congestion (pulmonary edema, ascites, pleural effusion). The goals of therapeutic management include improving myocardial performance, controlling arrhythmias, reducing deleterious effects of angiotensin II (such as adverse myocardial remodeling and increased peripheral vascular resistance), improving cardiac output, and reducing preload. The specific agents used to achieve these goals vary depending on the etiology and severity of the heart failure, species, and other factors. *See also* SYSTEMIC PHARMACOTHERAPEUTICS OF THE CARDIOVASCULAR SYSTEM, p 1966.

Diuretics: Diuretics are the mainstay therapy in the management of animals with pulmonary edema, pleural effusion, or ascites. Of the several types available, the loop diuretics (eg, furosemide, bumetanide) are most commonly used. **Loop diuretics** inhibit the $Na^+/K^+/2Cl^-$ transporter on the loop of Henle. This results in a decrease in resorption of these ions (ie, increased excretion); water is excreted in concert with them. The dose and frequency of furosemide depends on the severity of pulmonary congestion or ascites, as well as on the degree of respiratory distress. In severe, life-threatening cases, furosemide should be administered IV at relatively high dosages (ie, 4-8 mg/kg). When given IV, the onset of action of furosemide is 5 min; effects peak at 30 min and wane at 2 hr. Once animals with CHF have been stabilized, furosemide is usually continued orally at maintenance dosages of 0.5-1.0 mg/kg, SID-BID. In chronic cases, furosemide should be administered at the lowest dose that will control pulmonary edema and its attendant clinical signs, including cough and respiratory distress. Side effects of furosemide may include volume depletion and prerenal azotemia, hypokalemia, and metabolic alkalosis (via renal loss of hydrogen). Cats appear to be more prone to the adverse effects of furosemide therapy than are dogs.

Thiazide diuretics (eg, hydrochlorthiazide, chlorthiazide) are sometimes added to the therapeutic regimen of CHF patients refractory to furosemide. The combined use of a thiazide and loop diuretic increases the likelihood of adverse effects such as azotemia and hypokalemia. Potassium-sparing diuretics (eg, spironolactone, triamterene, amiloride), specifically spironolactone, have recently been reported to improve survival time and reduce morbidity in humans with CHF already being treated with standard therapy. They inhibit the actions of aldosterone or block sodium entry into the distal tubules and collecting ducts. When used in combination with loop diuretics, potassium loss is frequently reduced.

Diuretic resistance refers to development of refractoriness to diuretic therapy (typically furosemide). There are many causes, including decreased delivery of the drug to the nephron, activation of the RAAS (which counteracts the effects of diuresis), and hypertrophy of the distal convoluted tubular cells with consequent increases in ion transport in this region of the nephron. GI edema secondary to right-sided CHF may decrease absorption of orally administered diuretics and contribute to diuretic resistance. A recent study, however, found no alteration in the pharmacokinetics of furosemide in humans with severe heart failure. Addition of another diuretic, such as a thiazide, to loop diuretic therapy results in increased delivery of the loop diuretic to the nephron. Administering a loop diuretic IV is another option. Finally, concurrent administration of an ACE inhibitor and aldosterone inhibitor can result in inhibition of the RAAS, thereby reducing the counteractive effects of aldosterone and angiotensin II.

Positive Inotropes: These agents increase myocardial contractility and are used primarily in patients with dilated cardiomyopathy or advanced degenerative valve disease with myocardial failure. The **digitalis glycosides** (digoxin, digitoxin) are the most commonly used positive inotropic agents and cause a modest increase in cardiac contractility. They also increase parasympathetic nerve activity to the sinus node, AV node, and atria. This reduces heart rate and is especially useful in the setting of atrial fibrillation with a rapid ventricular response rate or other supraventricular arrhythmias in dogs and cats. Digitalis glycosides also alter baroreceptor function, resulting in a decrease in plasma catecholamine concentration, sympathetic nerve activity, and renin activity. Mild diuretic effects are also noted. Digoxin is the most commonly used digitalis glycoside. When administered orally in dogs, 4-5 days of treatment are required to achieve stable blood levels; therefore, oral digitalization is ineffective in acute myocardial failure. The dosage of digoxin in dogs is 0.005-0.010 mg/kg, PO, BID. For large-breed dogs, dosing digoxin at 0.22 mg/m^2 is recommended to reduce the frequency of side effects. (*See* TABLE 9, p 2589, for weight to body surface area [in m^2] conversion.) In horses, the dosage of digoxin is 11 µg/kg, PO, BID and in cattle the dosage is 5.5 µg/kg, PO, BID. Rapid digitalization commonly results in toxicity and is not recommended. Digoxin should be used with caution in animals with renal insufficiency. In these animals, digitoxin is the preferred digitalis glycoside because blood levels are typically unaffected by azotemia (digitoxin is excreted by the liver). Digitoxin is not recommended in cats because of an excessively long half-life. If digoxin is used in patients with renal insufficiency, the starting dosage is lowered to prevent signs of toxicity. The starting dosage of digoxin is also lowered in patients with ascites (20% reduction with moderate ascites, 30% reduction for severe ascites), or obese patients (because the drug is poorly lipid soluble and does not distribute well to ascitic fluid). Dosage may also require adjustment in patients concurrently administered drugs that can affect hepatic microsomal enzymes such as barbiturates, tetracycline, and phenylbutazone.

Side effects of digitalis glycosides are common and include depression, anorexia, vomiting, diarrhea, and cardiac arrhythmias and conduction disturbances. Serious toxicity can usually be avoided by following these guidelines: 1) Renal function should be determined before beginning digitalis therapy; if renal insufficiency is present, the dosage should be decreased or digitoxin used. 2) The animal's diet should not be changed dramatically when starting digitalis; dietary changes may interfere with appetite, which is monitored as an indicator of toxicity. 3) Client communication is essential—owners should be instructed to call if any signs of toxicity develop. The drug should be temporarily discontinued (usually for 1-2 days) or the dose reduced when side effects are first noted to prevent more serious side effects from occurring. A serum digoxin or digitoxin level after 1-2 wk of therapy helps to ensure that the drug is being dosed appropriately. A serum sample should be obtained 8 hr after the last dose has been administered. For most laboratories, the normal digoxin range is 1.0-2.5 ng/mL. Electrolyte abnormalities, particularly hypokalemia, may increase the risk of toxicity.

Another class of positive inotropes is the **sympathomimetic amines** (dobutamine, dopamine). These drugs stimulate β_1-adrenergic receptors, resulting in increased heart rate, conduction velocity, and contractility. Dobutamine is used more commonly. Its positive inotropic effects on normal myocardium are ~3 times greater than those of the digitalis glycosides. Dobutamine must be administered as a constant rate infusion, preferably by an infusion pump. Because of its rapid onset of action, it is effective in the acute management of patients in CHF secondary to myocardial failure (eg, in dogs with dilated cardiomyopathy and CHF or with degenerative valve disease and concurrent myocardial failure). Dobutamine is diluted with 5% dextrose and administered at a rate of 5-15 µg/kg/min in dogs. Electrocardiographic monitoring during infusion is critical, as dobutamine can cause cardiac arrhythmias. If arrhythmias worsen during the infusion, the rate of administration should be decreased or the infusion stopped. Dobutamine also increases conduction of the AV node; therefore, if atrial fibrillation is present, the ventricular response may increase excessively. For this reason, it is recommended that dogs with atrial fibrillation be adequately digitalized before receiving a dobutamine infusion.

Although plasma dobutamine levels decrease rapidly 3 min after the infusion, beneficial effects often persist for weeks.

Angiotensin-converting Enzyme (ACE) Inhibitors: ACE inhibitors competitively inhibit ACE, reducing the formation of angiotensin II and attenuating its adverse effects (peripheral vasoconstriction, adverse myocardial remodeling and hypertrophy, increased aldosterone levels, etc). In addition, ACE inhibitors are vasodilators. They have become an important tool in the treatment of mild to severe CHF in dogs. By reducing excessive systemic vascular resistance, ACE inhibitors may improve cardiac output and reduce the regurgitant fraction when mitral insufficiency is present.

Clinical benefits are considered moderately good in dogs with CHF treated with ACE inhibitors. A few placebo-controlled trials in dogs with CHF demonstrated that the addition of enalapril to conventional therapy resulted in an improvement in heart failure scores and a decrease in heart rate, frequency of cough, and degree of pulmonary edema. The beneficial effects varied between patients, however, and many patients demonstrated only mild clinical response. There have been no survival studies on clinically ill animals that indicate prolongation of life. Clinical improvement is frequently more dramatic than hemodynamic or echocardiographic improvement.

Side effects are uncommon and include anorexia, vomiting, and azotemia. Hypotension is rare and typically occurs when aggressive therapy is begun in a volume-depleted animal. Cough is not a common side effect. Clinically, the most significant concern is the development of azotemia secondary to reduced renal perfusion. Although the risk is low, it is recommended that renal function be determined before starting therapy. It is also advisable to decrease the dosage of the diuretic by ~25% and to evaluate BUN and creatinine 5-7 days after starting an ACE inhibitor. If azotemia develops or worsens, the dosage of the diuretic should be decreased. If the azotemia persists, enalapril should be discontinued or the dosage further reduced. Renal function should be monitored periodically. Enalapril should be initiated in dogs at a dosage of 0.5 mg/kg, PO, SID. If the response to treatment is inadequate, the dosage may be increased to 0.5 mg/kg, PO, BID. Enalapril is approved in the USA for use in dogs. Other oral ACE inhibitors used (but not approved) include captopril (0.5-1.0 mg/kg, TID), benazepril (0.25 mg/kg, SID), and lisinopril (0.5 mg/kg, SID). Unlike enalapril and captopril, benazepril is excreted by the liver and may be useful in animals with heart failure and renal insufficiency.

Vasodilators: Although enalapril and captopril are most commonly used, other vasodilators are available. **Hydralazine** is a potent arteriolar vasodilator that directly dilates arterioles, presumably by increasing vasodilatory prostaglandins (PGI_2). Hydralazine decreases pulmonary capillary wedge pressure, reduces regurgitant flow, increases forward aortic flow and venous oxygen tension, and reduces systemic vascular resistance by 40% (captopril reduces systemic vascular resistance by 25%). Hypotension and tachycardia are common side effects, and it is recommended that animals be hospitalized and carefully monitored (eg, blood pressure, electrocardiography) when instituting therapy. Because of the potential for serious side effects of hydralazine, as well as the safety and efficacy of ACE inhibitors, hydralazine is now typically reserved for patients that are refractory to ACE inhibitors. The initial dosage is 0.5 mg/kg, PO, BID in dogs receiving an ACE inhibitor (use cautiously in this setting), or 1 mg/kg in dogs not receiving an ACE inhibitor. The dosage is slowly titrated up to 3 mg/kg depending on therapeutic response. The effective dose is then administered BID. Blood pressure monitoring during titration is very important. If hypotension occurs, hydralazine should be discontinued for 24 hr and then resumed at one-half the previous dosage. Persistent tachycardia should also prompt a reduction in the dosage; occasionally, digoxin or β-adrenergic blocker are required to control heart rate. In a significant proportion of cases, the drug must be discontinued because of adverse effects such as vomiting or diarrhea.

Nitroglycerin is a venodilator that is sometimes used in patients with acute pulmonary edema. By increasing venous capacitance, preload is decreased and blood volume is essentially shifted from the central to the peripheral vascular compartments. This results in a decrease in end-diastolic ventricular pressure and a reduction in edema. Nitroglycerin can be applied to the skin (it is transcutaneously absorbed), so administration is not stressful to the animal. The dose of 2% nitroglycerin ointment is 0.3-0.6 cm/kg applied BID-TID in dogs, and 0.3-0.6 cm/kg applied every 4-6 hr in cats. Efficacy has not been documented in these species, however. The person applying the ointment should wear gloves, and care should be taken to avoid contact with the ointment once it has been applied. The previous dose should be removed before applying subsequent doses. Side effects are infrequent, but excessive use may result in hypotension, lethargy, and vomiting. Tolerance has been documented in humans and may occur in animals with chronic use. Nitroglycerin-free periods should therefore be planned every day or two.

Nitroprusside can also be used in acute CHF because it causes rapid vasodilation. It has been demonstrated to be effective in combination with dobutamine in the treatment of dogs with severe heart failure secondary to dilated cardiomyopathy. Unlike nitroglycerin, nitroprusside is a balanced vasodilator, causing dilation of both arterioles and veins. The result is a decrease in both systemic vascular resistance and preload and an increase in cardiac output. Because the half-life is very short, nitroprusside must be administered as a constant rate infusion. In addition, its potential to cause systemic hypotension warrants careful blood pressure monitoring during the infusion. Rebound vasoconstriction exceeding vasoconstriction prior to therapy may occur. Nitroprusside is commonly administered in conjunction with an infusion of dobutamine, which further increases cardiac output and mitigates the hypotensive effects of nitroprusside. The initial infusion rate of nitroprusside should be 1 μg/kg/min, with increases in increments of 1 μg/kg/min every 5 min until the mean arterial pressure is ~70 mm Hg. It is uncommon to exceed 5-7 μg/kg/min; infusions >10 μg/kg/min are not typically needed, nor do they provide any added benefit. If systemic hypotension occurs, infusion should immediately be stopped. Due to the short half-life, blood pressure will increase once infusion has stopped, and it can be restarted at a lower rate. Infusions should not be administered for excessive periods of time (>16 hr), in order to avoid cyanide toxicity.

β-Adrenergic Blockers: Many studies have demonstrated increased cardiac output and exercise tolerance and decreased morbidity in human patients with CHF and dilated cardiomyopathy, as well as in experimental dogs with CHF administered a β-adrenergic blocking drug (eg, atenolol, propranolol, carvedilol). The cause of this benefit has not been completely identified; however, up-regulation of β receptors, or protection of the myocardium from excessive catecholamine levels have been postulated as possible reasons. The adverse effects of β-blockers when used in patients with dilated cardiomyopathy or myocardial failure of other etiology are significant and primarily involve negative inotropic effects that can result in worsening CHF. When β-blockers such as carvedilol are used in the treatment of CHF, very low dosages are initially used (1.5625 mg, PO, SID-BID in large breed dogs such as Doberman Pinschers with dilated cardiomyopathy) and very slowly titrated up to a dosage of ~12.5-25 mg, BID. Carvedilol is a nonselective β-blocker that also has other benefits such as oxygen free radical scavenging as well as some α-blocking capacity resulting in vasodilation.

Calcium Channel Blockers: Calcium channel blockers such as diltiazem are used in the treatment of heart failure secondary to hypertrophic cardiomyopathy. Diltiazem reduces myocardial contractility (mild), reduces heart rate, and improves diastolic function in cats with hypertrophic cardiomyopathy. It is also used in conjunction with digoxin in dogs with atrial fibrillation and a very rapid ventricular response rate. The dosage in cats is 7.5 mg, PO, TID and in dogs 1 mg/kg, PO, BID-TID. Long-acting versions of diltiazem are also available.

Supplementation: A taurine-responsive cardiomyopathy has been noted in cats and some breeds of dogs (Cocker Spaniels, Golden Retrievers, and other breeds). Deficiency can be documented by obtaining whole blood or plasma concentrations of taurine. Dogs are treated with taurine 500-1,000 mg, PO, BID. The dosage in cats is 250 mg, PO, BID. L-carnitine plays a pivotal role in fatty acid metabolism and myocardial energy production.

Deficiency of L-carnitine has been documented in a family of Boxers and in some Doberman Pinschers with dilated cardiomyopathy; supplementation resulted in an improvement in cardiac contractility and a significant increase in survival time compared with dogs that were not carnitine deficient. The incidence of L-carnitine deficiency in the general population of dogs with dilated cardiomyopathy has not been determined but is likely to be low. The dosage is 110 mg/kg, PO, BID. The cost of this compound, along with the fact that an endomyocardial biopsy is required to document deficiency has limited its use. Supplementation with coenzyme Q_{10} increased cardiac contractility and cardiac output in humans with dilated cardiomyopathy who received conventional therapy, although studies have for the most part been poorly controlled. Coenzyme Q_{10} is essential in myocardial energy production. The efficacy of coenzyme Q_{10} in dogs has not been clearly proven.

Low-sodium Diets: Along with diuretics and ACE inhibitors (which reduce total body sodium content and blood volume), a severely sodium-restricted diet is recommended in patients with severe CHF refractory to conventional therapy. In patients with mild to moderate CHF, severe sodium restriction is not needed; however, diets high in sodium should be avoided. Prescription diets tailored for these differing levels of sodium restriction are readily available, and recipes for home-made diets are also available. A list of sodium-free snacks is also helpful for owners. In large animals, access to salt blocks should be prevented. Salt should not be restricted in patients with heart disease that demonstrate no evidence of CHF, because this can result in early activation of the RAAS.

Oxygen Therapy: Patients with severe left-sided CHF and pulmonary edema can become hypoxic, in part as a result of the increased diffusion distance for alveolar oxygen to enter the blood in the pulmonary capillaries. By administering oxygen to these patients, diffusion into the blood is facilitated. The percent inspired oxygen is generally increased to 40-50% (room air is 21%). In patients with severe CHF, 100% oxygen may be needed in the acute treatment phase. Oxygen can be administered via an oxygen cage, tight-fitting mask, or nasal cannula. Stress should be minimized during oxygen administration.

Thoracentesis: CHF patients demonstrating significant pleural effusion can benefit from thoracentesis. Besides the rapid clinical response that can be achieved, there are no significant adverse effects such as can be seen with IV diuretic administration in a patient with concurrent azotemia. Thoracentesis may be necessary as an emergency procedure without the benefit of thoracic radiographs in severely compromised patients when pleural effusion is suspected.

Abdominocentesis: In dogs and cats with severe right-sided CHF, ascites can be severe enough to result in dyspnea and considerable discomfort. Abdominocentesis is a safe and effective means of treating this fluid accumulation and can be performed on a regular basis (every 2-4 wk if needed) as long as the patient is cooperative.

Ancillary Therapy: **Bronchodilator therapy** (eg, theophylline, aminophylline) is generally reserved for patients with chronic airway disease. Alhough these agents also have mild diuretic and positive inotropic effects, they act primarily as bronchodilators and are not typically used to treat CHF. The exception to this is dogs demonstrating syncope secondary to a transient cardiac arrhythmia associated with heart disease such as degenerative valve disease. Sympathomimetic therapy with theophylline (10 mg/kg, PO, BID-TID) can reduce episodes of syncope.

    Cough suppressants are generally contraindicated in the treatment of CHF, because masking clinical signs of cough can worsen the underlying pulmonary edema. If, however, a patient diagnosed with severe heart disease is coughing, and cardiac enlargement on thoracic radiographs demonstrates no pulmonary edema, the clinical signs may result from mainstem bronchial compression by left atrial enlargement. A cough suppressant may be helpful in this setting.

SPECIFIC DISEASES

Degenerative Valve Disease

(Endocardiosis, Chronic valvular disease, Chronic valvular fibrosis)

This acquired disease is characterized by nodular thickening of the cardiac valve leaflets, most severely at their free margins. The most commonly affected valves are the mitral or tricuspid valve leaflets. The etiology is unknown; however, in Cavalier King Charles Spaniels (which are prone to this disease), it is believed to be an inherited trait possibly resulting in a collagen abnormality. Degenerative valve disease is the most common cardiac disease in dogs and accounts for ~75% of cardiovascular disease in this species. Approximately 60% of affected dogs have myxomatous degeneration of the mitral valve, 30% have lesions in both the tricuspid and mitral valves, and 10% have only tricuspid valve disease. In dogs, the disease is age- and breed-related, with older, small-breed dogs demonstrating a higher incidence. There is also a slight predisposition among male dogs. Large animals are also affected by this disease (most commonly affecting the mitral valve leaflets), however it is uncommon in cats. In horses, degenerative valve disease often affects the aortic valve and consists of valvular nodules or fibrous bands at the free borders of the valve. This condition is most common in middle-aged and older horses. In many horses, unlike dogs, clinical signs are uncommon because significant left ventricular volume overload and dilation do not occur.

Insufficiency of the AV valve results in turbulent, systolic (ie, during ventricular contraction) flow at the affected valve. This regurgitation of blood into the atrium results in an increase in pressure within the atrium. If the mitral valve is affected, the elevated left atrial pressures eventually result in elevated pulmonary capillary pressures and, ultimately, pulmonary edema. If the tricuspid valve is affected, elevated systemic venous pressures arise and ascites may develop. The constant, high-velocity, regurgitant jet of blood at the affected mitral valve physically damages the endocardium of the left atrium, resulting grossly in jet lesions and, in severe cases, may result in left atrial rupture. The decrease in the amount of blood ejected by the left ventricle (cardiac output) results in an activation of compensatory mechanisms such as the RAAS (p 84). The body responds to decreases in cardiac output by increasing sympathetic tone and activating angiotensin-converting enzyme (ACE). On a chronic basis, these compensatory mechanisms become deleterious rather than beneficial. Chronically increased sympathetic tone causes sustained tachycardia, which increases the oxygen demand of the heart and predisposes to arrhythmias. ACE activation results in the formation of angiotensin II, which causes sustained arteriolar constriction and increased aldosterone. Vasoconstriction increases cardiac afterload, hampering ventricular ejection of blood. Aldosterone release results in sodium and water retention and predisposes to pulmonary edema.

In dogs there are no clinical signs in the early stages of the disease, although a systolic murmur of low intensity (grade I-II/VI) can be heard with maximum intensity at the left apex. As the disease progresses, exercise intolerance, increased respiratory rate and effort, and cough develop. Syncope may also occur secondary to either compromised cardiac output or, more likely, a transient cardiac arrhythmia. Sudden death is rare, but may occur secondary to left atrial rupture caused by severe and chronic mitral regurgitation. With continued progression, the murmur intensity generally increases (up to a grade VI/VI systolic murmur); however, the intensity does not always coincide with disease severity. Physical examination findings in patients that have developed left-sided CHF include respiratory crackles and wheezes and dyspnea. If tricuspid valve degeneration is significant, signs of right-sided CHF may be noted (eg, ascites, jugular pulses).

A CBC, serum chemistry profile, and urinalysis are usually within normal limits. Left atrial enlargement is the characteristic finding on thoracic radiographs of a patient with myxomatous degeneration of the mitral valve. Other changes include enlargement of the left ventricle and pulmonary veins. As heart failure develops, increased interstitial density to the pulmonary parenchyma occurs and ultimately air bronchograms (indicative of an alveolar pattern and severe pulmonary edema) appear. Echocardiography demonstrates a thickened, enlarged, and irregular valvular leaflet of normal echogenicity. Chordae tendineae may be ruptured, and the AV leaflets may prolapse into the atrium during ventricular contraction. Ventricular enlargement is common. In most cases, contractility is normal initially, but left ventricular fractional shortening is increased due to off-loading of some of the left ventricular ejection into the low resistance left atrium rather than the high resistance aorta. A decrease in contractility suggest the presence of myocardial failure. Electrocardiographically, asymptomatic patients with early degenerative valve disease demonstrate a normal sinus arrhythmia or normal sinus rhythm. As the disease progresses, and especially when CHF develops, left atrial enlargement promotes the occurrence of atrial arrhythmias such as atrial premature complexes and atrial fibrillation. Cardiac hypoxia may result in ventricular arrhythmias. There may be evidence of left atrial enlargement (P-mitrale or widened P waves) and left ventricular enlargement (tall and widened R waves) when the mitral valve is involved.

A recent, large study in asymptomatic Cavalier King Charles Spaniels with degenerative valve disease demonstrated no reduction in time to onset of CHF with use of ACE inhibitors. Thus, treatment in small breed dogs should be reserved for symptomatic animals or those demonstrating cardiogenic pulmonary edema on thoracic radiographs. Treatment for early signs of CHF includes ACE inhibitors to reduce adverse neurohormonal effects caused by activation of the RAAS, and to reduce mitral regurgitation and signs of pulmonary edema. Control of pulmonary edema is also accomplished by use of diuretics (furosemide is the drug of choice). Abnormal arrhythmias such as atrial fibrillation or other severe supraventricular arrhythmias, if present, should either be resolved or rate controlled with use of digitalis glycosides and, if needed, calcium channel blockers or β-blockers to improve cardiac output and reduce signs of CHF. Another indication for digitalis glycosides is the presence of myocardial failure. Optimal therapy should be planned for each stage of disease. In acute and severe CHF, oxygen and nitroglycerin ointment, along with aggressive parenteral furosemide and other medication previously mentioned, would be warranted. Affected dogs can live for years with appropriate therapy.

Valvular Blood Cysts or Hematomas

These benign valvular lesions are present in up to 75% of calves <3 wk of age. They are most commonly located on the AV valves.

Cardiomyopathies

Cardiomyopathy is defined as any disease involving primarily and predominantly the heart muscle. The cardiomyopathies of animals are idiopathic diseases that are not the result of any systemic or primary cardiac disease. In animals (primarily dogs and cats), they have been classified as dilated cardiomyopathy, hypertrophic cardiomyopathy, and restrictive or unclassified cardiomyopathy. If a disease process has been identified as the cause of myocardial dysfunction, these are more correctly identified as secondary myocardial diseases or a descriptive term precedes the term cardiomyopathy (eg, taurine-responsive cardiomyopathy).

Dilated Cardiomyopathy: This acquired disease is characterized by the progressive loss of cardiac contractility of unknown cause. Several forms of secondary dilated cardiomyopathy exist (eg, taurine deficiency in cats, doxorubicin- or parvovirus-induced). Dilated cardiomyopathy has a protracted subclinical phase in dogs, with clinical signs evident for a relatively short period of time. During the subclinical phase, compensatory mechanisms maintain normal hemodynamics. As cardiac contractile function is progressively lost, cardiac output decreases. Increased blood volume and pressure within the chambers causes them to dilate, most dramatically evident in the left atrium and left ventricle. The increased activation of the sympathetic nervous system and the RAAS, after an initial benefit, cause deleterious effects (*see* p 84). Excessive stimulation of the myocardium by the sympathetic nervous system may stimulate ventricular arrhythmias and myocyte death, while excessive activation of the RAAS causes excessive vasoconstriction and retention of sodium and water. Signs of CHF are then inevitable.

Dilated cardiomyopathy is one of the most prevalent acquired heart diseases of dogs, only surpassed by degenerative valve disease and, in some parts of the world, heartworm disease as a major cardiovascular cause of morbidity and mortality. It most commonly affects large-breed dogs and far less commonly small-breed dogs (with a few exceptions such as American Cocker Spaniels, Springer Spaniels, and English Cocker Spaniels). Doberman Pinschers, Boxers, Great Danes, German Shepherds, Irish Wolfhounds, Scottish Deerhounds, Newfoundland Retrievers, Saint Bernards, and Labrador Retrievers, among other large-breed dogs, are particularly at risk. The disease is typically seen in middle-aged dogs; males are affected more than females. The incidence in cats has decreased dramatically since the discovery in 1985 that taurine deficiency was responsible for most cases (taurine-responsive cardiomyopathy). Since then, taurine levels have been increased to acceptable levels in all commercial cat foods. Most cases today are not taurine responsive and reflect primary (or idiopathic) disease.

There is breed variation in the presenting history and clinical signs. Up to 35% of Boxers demonstrate episodes of weakness or collapse as the presenting clinical sign and most demonstrate no myocardial failure at the time of presentation. The syncope typically results from severe ventricular arrhythmias. In those Boxers that do not succumb to sudden death, signs of left-sided CHF (eg, cough, dyspnea) eventually develop as a result of myocardial failure. Doberman Pinschers typically develop concurrent and progressive ventricular arrhythmias along with progressive systolic dysfunction. As with Boxers, collapse and sudden death occur (in up to 20% of Doberman Pinschers), and signs of left-sided CHF eventually develop. Most Doberman Pinschers demonstrate evidence of myocardial failure at the time syncopal episodes are noted, in contrast to Boxers. In other breeds, such as Great Danes and Newfoundlands, sudden death and collapse are far less likely. Signs of right-sided CHF predominate, including weakness, exercise intolerance, pleural effusion, and ascites. Ascites was noted in 35% of Newfoundlands with dilated cardiomyopathy in one study. Cats with dilated cardiomyopathy typically present with severe signs of pleural effusion and dyspnea, and clinical signs are usually rapidly progressive and refractory to therapy.

A low-grade systolic murmur, best heard at the left cardiac apex, is usually present. A third heart sound or gallop heart sound is also frequently present, especially in cats. Femoral pulses may be weak, and an arrhythmia with associated pulse deficits may be noted. The arrhythmia is most commonly a result of ventricular ectopy, but supraventricular arrhythmias such as atrial fibrillation or atrial premature complexes can also be noted, especially in giant breeds. Ascites, dyspnea, or cough may also be noted depending on the type of heart failure that develops.

Blood work may demonstrate elevation of BUN, creatinine, and alkaline phosphatase, as well as a mild reduction in sodium. Thoracic radiographs typically demonstrate mild to marked generalized cardiomegaly. If heart failure is present, pulmonary edema is evident and the pulmonary veins are enlarged. Echocardiography is the ideal test to definitively diagnose dilated cardiomyopathy. There is a dramatic loss of cardiac contractility (evidenced by a reduced left ventricular fractional shortening) and an increase in left ventricular end-systolic diameter. Cardiac chambers, especially the left atrium and left ventricle, are dilated. Mitral or tricuspid insufficiency typically develops as progressive cardiac dilation results in separation of the valve leaflets. Abnormal ECG findings may include ventricular premature complexes and ventricular tachycardia (especially in Doberman Pinschers and Boxers), atrial fibrillation, and atrial premature complexes (especially giant breeds). There may be electrocardiographic evidence of left atrial enlargement (P mitrale or widened P waves) and left ventricular enlargement (tall and wide R waves). Conduction disturbances, such as left bundle-branch block, are uncommon but could indicate severe disease. The occurrence of ventricular premature contractions on a routine ECG in a presumed healthy Doberman Pinscher or Boxer is highly suggestive of cardiomyopathy.

The objectives of therapy are to control the congestive state (eg, with diuretics), improve contractility (eg, with digoxin or dobutamine), and reduce adverse effects of angiotensin II and other neurohormonal changes (eg, with ACE inhibitors). Taurine-responsive myocardial failure occurs in some breeds, particularly American Cocker

Spaniels, Golden Retrievers, and Dalmatians, and in anecdotal reports, Welsh Corgis, Tibetan Terriers, and other breeds. In many of these breeds, taurine deficiency can be diagnosed by low plasma or whole blood levels. Response to taurine supplementation (which may take 2-4 wk) can be dramatic, many times obviating the need for other cardiac medications. Carnitine-responsive cardiomyopathy has been reported in Boxers and Doberman Pinschers. Dogs deficient in L-carnitine cannot be identified without an endomyocardial biopsy, however, and supplementation with L-carnitine may be cost prohibitive. Taurine is less expensive. Coenzyme Q_{10} supplementation has resulted in significant improvements in humans with dilated cardiomyopathy in some small studies. The recommended dose is 30 mg, PO, TID. Administration of fish oil may reduce the severity of cardiac cachexia in patients with dilated cardiomyopathy.

CHF, which may be severe, should be treated as discussed under HEART FAILURE, p 85. As pulmonary edema resolves, furosemide can be administered orally, with oxygen and nitroglycerin continued until clinical signs are controlled. Digoxin and an ACE inhibitor (eg, enalapril, benazepril) should be started. Antiarrhythmic therapy is frequently indicated, especially for Doberman Pinschers and Boxers with severe ventricular arrhythmias. Holter monitoring is the ideal method for evaluating both the severity of arrhythmias and therapy efficacy. In Boxers with severe ventricular arrhythmias without evidence of systolic dysfunction, sotalol (2 mg/kg, PO, BID) may be considered. Mexiletine (4-8 mg/kg, PO, BID-TID), can be added to sotalol if arrhythmia control is inadequate. Mexiletine is also useful in patients with ventricular arrhythmias and concurrent heart failure, as negative inotropy is less than with β-blocker therapy. β-Blockers are very effective at controlling ventricular arrhythmias; however, they must be used with extreme caution because the negative inotropic effects of most β-blockers (eg, atenolol) can predispose dilated cardiomyopathy patients to worsening CHF.

The prognosis is grave for cats with dilated cardiomyopathy (not taurine responsive), with a median survival time of 2 wk. Cats that are taurine responsive also have a high risk of death. However, patients that can be kept alive long enough for taurine to become effective (2-3 wk) have an excellent prognosis. Dogs that are taurine or carnitine responsive also have a fair to good prognosis once signs of CHF abate. The prognosis is poor in most Doberman Pinschers; ~25% die within 2 wk of presenting in heart failure, and 65% die within 8 wk. The prognosis in other breeds is better but remains guarded; 75% die within 6 mo of diagnosis. As expected, dogs with severe heart failure, particularly left-sided CHF, have a worse prognosis than those with milder signs or signs of right-sided CHF at presentation.

Hypertrophic Cardiomyopathy: Hypertrophic cardiomyopathy is characterized by primary concentric left ventricular hypertrophy resulting from an inherent myocardial disorder rather than pressure overload (such as caused by aortic stenosis), hormonal stimulation (such as hyperthyroidism or acromegaly), or other noncardiac disease. With severe disease, significant left ventricular hypertrophy develops; this results in a decrease in size of the left ventricular chamber, and consequently decreased left ventricular end-systolic diameter, sometimes to zero, as well as decreased left ventricular end-diastolic diameter and volume, resulting in reduced stroke volume and activation of the RAAS. Although contractility is not significantly impaired, the hypertrophied ventricular walls lose compliance and resist filling during diastole. Elevation of left ventricular end-diastolic pressure results in increased pressure within the left atrium, causing it to dilate; the pressure is then transmitted to the pulmonary veins, causing pulmonary edema and sometimes pleural effusion. Severe left atrial enlargement can develop, leading to left atrial thrombi and the potential for systemic thromboembolism. Mitral regurgitation also leads to left atrial dilation. This can develop secondary to an anterior displacement of the anterior mitral valve leaflet during ventricular systole, a phenomenon termed systolic anterior motion of the mitral valve. Gross pathology may include increased cardiac weight, left ventricular concentric hypertrophy, papillary muscle hypertrophy, left atrial enlargement, asymmetric septal hypertrophy, and a reduction in left ventricular chamber volume.

Hypertrophic cardiomyopathy is the most common primary heart disease diagnosed in cats but is rare in dogs. It is familial in certain breeds of cats such as Maine Coon cats and American Shorthairs. The disease occurs in cats from 3 mo to 17 yr of age, although most patients are middle aged; male cats are predisposed. The etiology is believed to be genetic mutations resulting in abnormalities of the sarcomeric proteins. Although not proved in cats, it has been documented in humans with this disease.

Affected patients may be asymptomatic or may have signs of acute dyspnea, collapse, or hindlimb paresis/paralysis. Cough is uncommon in cats with heart failure. Physical examination frequently demonstrates abnormal heart sounds, including soft to prominent systolic cardiac murmurs and gallop heart sounds. Increased respiratory sounds may suggest pulmonary edema, and decreased respiratory sounds may indicate pleural effusion. Pulses may be normal, weak, or absent if distal aortic thromboembolism has developed. Distal aortic embolization commonly leads to rear limb paresis or paralysis. Radiographically, there may be pronounced left atrial enlargement and variable left ventricular enlargement. The cardiac silhouette often appears relatively normal even in the presence of moderate left ventricular hypertrophy. Echocardiography allows confirmation of the diagnosis and assessment of additional therapy needed (eg, anticoagulants are most beneficial in cats with severe left atrial enlargement). Systolic anterior motion of the mitral valve, concentric left ventricular hypertrophy, or variable hypertrophy of other portions of the left ventricle such as papillary muscle hypertrophy or asymmetric septal hypertrophy can be noted. ECG abnormalities may include atrial premature complexes, ventricular premature complexes, and ventricular tachycardia. With severe atrial enlargement, atrial fibrillation may develop. Conduction disturbances such as left anterior fascicular block may also be noted.

Treatment is directed at controlling signs of CHF, improving diastolic function, and reducing the incidence of systemic thromboembolism. Furosemide administration, oxygen, and nitroglycerin administration should be considered when acute CHF is present. Diltiazem (7.5 mg, PO, TID), a calcium-channel blocker, improves diastolic function and may also reduce wall thickness and edema formation. Use of β-blockers such as atenolol (6.25-12.5 mg, PO, SID-BID) or propranolol may also be considered. Humans with hypertrophic cardiomyopathy have shown improvement in angina, dyspnea, and exercise intolerance when given β-blockers. If calcium channel blockers are ineffective, switching to β-blockers may be considered. ACE inhibitors may be considered in some cats (enalapril, 0.25-0.5 mg/kg, PO, SID), especially where CHF has developed and activation of the RAAS is a concern. Either aspirin (80 mg, PO, every third day) or warfarin (0.2-0.5 mg, PO, SID) may reduce the incidence of further thrombus formation in cats with thromboembolism or a propensity to develop thrombi (such as a large left atrium on echocardiographic examination). Efficacy has not been well documented, however. Prognosis is highly variable, with many mildly affected patients having a good longterm prognosis. Patients in CHF have a poorer prognosis, with a median survival time of 3 mo. Up to 20% of CHF patients survive for prolonged periods, however.

Restrictive/Unclassified Cardiomyopathy: **Restrictive cardiomyopathy** is characterized by restrictive filling and reduced diastolic volume of either or both ventricles without significant ventricular hypertrophy or abnormalities of systolic function. The disease is seen in cats. Definitive documentation typically requires cardiac catheterization or specific abnormalities to Doppler mitral valve flow patterns that are not readily notable in cats. Although echocardiography can be variable, left atrial enlargement (usually severe) without significant left ventricular hypertrophy is common. Left atrial thrombi may be evident. Systolic function is usually preserved, but abnormalities of the mitral valve apparatus and papillary muscles may be noted. Doppler evaluation may demonstrate mitral regurgitation. Clinical signs and treatment are similar to those for hypertrophic cardiomyopathy (*see* above); however, prognosis seems to be worse, especially in patients with CHF. **Unclassified cardiomyopathy** includes patients with obvious abnormalities to the myocardium on echocardiography that do not clearly fit into any other category. It is also a disease of cats. The causes of restrictive cardiomyopathy and unclassified cardiomyopathy are unknown.

Myocarditis

Myocarditis is a focal or diffuse inflammation of the myocardium with myocyte degeneration or necrosis causing an adjacent inflammatory infiltrate. There are numerous causes, including several viruses and bacteria. Canine parvovirus (p 319), encephalomyocarditis virus (p 574), and equine infectious anemia virus (p 559) tend to cause myocarditis. Myocardial degeneration occurs in lambs, calves, and foals with white muscle disease and in pigs with mulberry heart disease or hepatosis dietetica. *Streptococcus* spp are the most common cause of bacterial myocarditis in horses. *Salmonella, Clostridium*, equine influenza, *Borrelia burgdorferi*, and strongylosis are other recognized causes. Mineral deficiencies (eg, iron, selenium, copper) can also result in myocardial degeneration. Deficiencies of vitamin E or selenium may cause myocardial necrosis. Cardiac toxins include ionophore antibiotics such as monensin and salinomycin, cantharidin (blister beetle toxicosis, p 2351), *Cryptostegia grandiflora* (rubber vine), and *Eupatorium rugosum* (white snakeroot). These diseases cause typical signs of CHF. In horses, signs of right-sided heart failure are common and include ascites, venous congestion, and jugular pulsations. A murmur of mitral or tricuspid regurgitation is usually audible as well as an irregular rhythm. Atrial fibrillation is common, and ventricular or atrial premature complexes may also be seen. Echocardiography reveals chamber dilatation and poor contractility with essentially normal valves. Neutrophilic leukocytosis and hyperfibrinogenemia are common. Cardiac isoenzymes (CK and lactate dehydrogenase) are often increased.

Treatment should be aimed at improving cardiac contractility, relieving congestion, and reducing vasoconstriction. Digoxin and dobutamine are used most commonly to improve contractility. Furosemide is indicated to control signs of pulmonary edema. Corticosteroids are often used when cardiac isoenzymes are increased and a viral infection is deemed unlikely.

Chagas' Myocarditis: *Trypanosoma cruzi*, a protozoan, causes Chagas' disease (p 35). Acutely, ECG abnormalities such as first-, second- or third-degree AV block, right bundle branch block, sinus tachycardia, and depressed R wave amplitude are noted. There are usually no echocardiographic abnormalities during the acute phase; however, sudden death is a concern. An asymptomatic latent phase then develops for 27-120 days in dogs, followed by a chronic stage demonstrating systolic dysfunction indistinguishable from dilated cardiomyopathy. Treatment for the chronic phase is as for dilated cardiomyopathy, but is typically ineffective at controlling signs of progressive myocardial failure.

Lyme Myocarditis: Lyme disease (p 485) is caused by the spirochete *Borrelia burgdorferi*; infection with this organism rarely results in myocardial disease. Patients developing myocardial disease secondary to Lyme infection may have ECG abnormalities such as ventricular arrhythmias or conduction disturbances such as first-, second- or transient third-degree AV block. Myocardial failure similar to dilated cardiomyopathy can also develop. In patients with complete AV block, cardiac pacemaker implantation may be warranted.

Other Causes of Myocardial Failure

In addition to the diseases listed below, histophilosis in cattle (p 606) can result in myocardial infarcts and abscesses.

Atrial Standstill: A form of cardiomyopathy resulting in destruction of the atrial myocardium (and occasionally affecting the ventricular myocardium) has been reported in dogs, especially English Springer Spaniels. Other affected breeds include Old English Sheepdogs, Shi-Tzus, German Shorthaired Pointers, and mixed-breed dogs. The disease has also been reported in some cats with concurrent dilated cardiomyopathy. Initially, atrial myocardial destruction leading to sinoatrial standstill and an AV nodal escape rhythm is noted. Eventually, myocardial failure ensues. Clinical signs are similar to patients with dilated cardiomyopathy, with right or left heart failure being noted.

Treatment is typically unrewarding and is similar to other myocardial failure patients. Pacemaker implantation may improve heart rate and cardiac output.

Doxorubicin-induced Myocardial Failure: Doxorubicin is a common chemotherapeutic agent that causes well-recognized cardiotoxicity. Cardiotoxicity tends to be dose dependent, but some patients show toxicity at far lower dosages than others. Abnormalities include isolated ventricular premature complexes (which develop in 80% of dogs administered 80 mg/m^2/day for 2 days or 25 mg/m^2/wk for 4-11 wk) and periods of ventricular tachycardia. Myocardial failure may also develop and has been documented in 100% of dogs experimentally administered 25 mg/m^2/wk for 20 wk. Sudden death and heart failure were noted in 65% of dogs after administration of ~17 wk of therapy. The cardiotoxic effects are irreversible.

Endocardial Fibroelastosis: This disease of unknown etiology is characterized by focal thickening of the left atrial, left ventricular, and mitral valve endocardium. It is a rare cause of myocardial failure in young dogs and cats. Affected animals are usually <6 mo of age and present with clinical signs of left-sided heart failure. Breeds reported include Labrador Retrievers, Great Danes, English Bulldogs, Springer Spaniels, Boxers, Pit Bulls, and Siamese and Burmese cats (in which the disease is believed to be inherited). Echocardiography demonstrates dilation of the left ventricular and atrial chambers, decreased left ventricular fractional shortening, and increased left ventricular endsystolic diameter and may demonstrate diffuse endocardial thickening. Clinical signs, treatment, and prognosis are similar to dilated cardiomyopathy.

Arrhythmogenic Right Ventricular Cardiomyopathy: This rare cause of myocardial failure in dogs and cats is restricted primarily to the right heart; however, some left ventricular involvement may be noted. It is characterized by a fibrofatty infiltrate of the right ventricular myocardium that results in progressive myocardial failure. Dyspnea, tachypnea, and nonspecific clinical signs such as anorexia and lethargy are reported in affected cats. Syncope secondary to arrhythmias may be noted. ECG abnormalities may include supraventricular tachycardias, ventricular arrhythmias, and conduction disturbances. Echocardiography reveals severe right ventricular and right atrial dilation. Treatment is similar to dilated cardiomyopathy.

Duchenne's Cardiomyopathy: This inherited, X-linked neuromuscular disorder has been reported in dogs, particularly Golden Retrievers. A similar disease called X-linked muscular dystrophy has been reported in Irish Terriers, Samoyeds, and Rottweilers. These diseases may result in myocardial as well as neuromuscular disease. ECG abnormalities include deep and narrow Q waves, shortened PR intervals, sinus arrest, and ventricular arrhythmias. Echocardiography may demonstrate hyperechoic lesions affecting primarily the left ventricular and papillary muscle myocardium. This usually develops by 6-7 mo of age, with the lesions decreasing in size over the next 2 yr. The lesions result from calcification and fibrosis. In patients that survive, myocardial failure may develop.

Infective Endocarditis

Infection of the endocardium typically involves one of the cardiac valves, although mural endocarditis may occur. It is believed that endothelial damage must be present for infective endocarditis to develop. When the endothelium is partially eroded and underlying collagen exposed, platelets adhere and produce a thrombus. Bloodborne bacteria may become enmeshed in this thrombic lattice, resulting in a localized infection that causes a progressive destruction of the valve and results in valvular insufficiency. In dogs, horses, and cats, the aortic and mitral valves are most commonly affected. The tricuspid valve is rarely affected, and pulmonic valve infective endocarditis is exceedingly rare. In contrast, the tricuspid valve is the most commonly affected in cattle. Infective endocarditis is rare in cats, and there are no breed predilections. In dogs, middle-aged, large-breed dogs are predisposed; <10% of dogs diagnosed with infective endocarditis weigh <15 kg. Most affected dogs are >4 yr of age, and males are more commonly affected than females.

Bacteria released from the infected aortic or mitral valves enter the circulation and can colonize other organs; therefore, infective endocarditis can produce a wide spectrum of clinical signs, including primary cardiovascular effects or signs related to the nervous system, GI tract, urogenital system, or joints. A chronic, intermittent fever is usually present. Shifting leg lameness may be reported, and weight loss and lethargy are present in almost all cases. If a right-sided valve is affected (tricuspid, pulmonic), ascites and jugular pulsations may be present. Mastitis and decreased milk production can be noted in affected cattle. Hematuria and pyuria may also be noted. A cardiac murmur is present in most cases; the exact type depends on the valve involved. When the aortic valve is affected, a low-grade diastolic murmur is present, with maximum intensity over the left cardiac base. A systolic murmur caused by increased stroke volume may also be noted. In this instance, arterial pulses are bounding due to diastolic run-off and increased stroke volume. Mitral valve endocarditis results in a murmur similar to that caused by degenerative valve disease—a low- to high-grade systolic murmur (intensity dependent on the degree of mitral insufficiency) heard best over the left cardiac apex.

Bacteria most often isolated from affected small animals include *Streptococcus*, *Staphylococcus*, and *Klebsiella* spp, and *Escherichia coli*. Other bacterial species and fungi may be involved. In humans, 60-80% of patients with infective endocarditis had a predisposing cardiac lesion that facilitated bacterial attachment. In dogs, however, infection appears to develop commonly in patients with no evidence of valve abnormalities. *Streptococcus* and *Actinobacillus* spp are the most common isolates in horses, and *Arcanobacterium (Actinomyces) pyogenes* is most commonly cultured from cattle. A CBC often shows a neutrophilic leukocytosis. Active infection may be associated with the presence of band neutrophils, and chronic infection with a monocytosis (90% of cases in one series). Anemia of chronic disease is frequently present. Serum analysis abnormalities reflect organ involvement secondary to infective emboli and may include increases in liver enzymes, BUN, and creatinine. In patients that develop immune complex glomerulonephritis, significant urinary protein loss and hypoalbuminemia may develop. Blood cultures with sensitivity should be obtained in affected animals. It is preferable to draw 2 or 3 blood samples, each 1-2 hr apart, in a 24-hr period. A strict aseptic technique is required. Radiography demonstrates cardiac chamber enlargement, depending on the location and degree of insufficiency of the involved valve. If the aortic or mitral valve is affected, there will be left atrial and left ventricular dilatation. Evidence of left-sided failure may be seen as an increase in interstitial density or, in severe CHF, an alveolar pattern in the pulmonary parenchyma. If the tricuspid or pulmonic valve is affected, right-sided chamber enlargement is expected. Echocardiography is the diagnostic test of choice, as blood cultures are positive in only 50-90% of dogs. The affected valve is easily detected—the involved area is hyperechoic (bright) and thickened. Doppler echocardiography will confirm insufficiency of the valve, and chamber enlargement on the side of the affected valve is expected when significant insufficiency is present. Electrocardiography may demonstrate atrial and ventricular premature complexes. Infrequently, other arrhythmias such as atrial fibrillation or conduction disturbances are found. The height of the R waves may be increased (suggestive of left ventricular enlargement) and the width of the P wave increased (suggestive of left atrial enlargement).

Therapy is directed at controlling clinical signs of CHF, resolving any significant arrhythmias, sterilizing the lesion, and eliminating the spread of infection. The heart failure may be extreme and intractable if the aortic valve is significantly involved; the prognosis is grave in these cases. The prognosis is much more favorable when infection is mild and limited to one of the AV valves. Controlling heart failure requires the use of diuretics such as furosemide, ACE inhibitors, and, where myocardial failure or supraventricular arrhythmias are present, digoxin. Initially, parenteral antibiotics are indicated for 1-2 wk (which may be cost prohibitive), followed by oral antibiotics for 6-8 wk. Initial broad-spectrum bactericidal antibiotics (ampicillin and gentamicin or cephalothin and gentamicin) should be used and changed, if needed, based on sensitivity studies. Renal function should be monitored with gentamicin therapy. Fluoroquinolones such as enrofloxacin may be considered as an alternative to aminoglycosides if renal failure occurs. The prognosis is poor in most dogs. Those that respond to therapy will likely require longterm cardiac medications (eg, diuretics, vasodilators, digoxin) and frequent reevaluations. In large animals, rifampin (5 mg/kg, PO, BID), together with another broad-spectrum antibiotic, has been demonstrated to improve short-term outlook. Aspirin (100 mg/kg, SID in ruminants and 17 mg/kg every other day in horses) or heparin (30 U/kg, SC, BID in ruminants and horses) may prevent further thrombus and vegetative growth in large animals.

Considering the poor clinical course, prevention is vital. When animals with predisposing cardiac disease (eg, subaortic stenosis, patent ductus arteriosus, ventricular septal defect, cyanotic congenital heart disease) are to be subjected to procedures with a potential to cause bacteremia (eg, dental scaling, tooth extractions), prophylactic use of a broad-spectrum antibiotic, although controversial, may be considered.

Pericardial Disease

When fluid accumulates in the pericardial sac, the pressure within the sac increases and progressively compresses the chambers of the heart. Because the right ventricular and right atrial diastolic pressures are less than those of the left chambers, the rising intrapericardial pressure first equilibrates with right-sided diastolic pressures, a condition termed **cardiac tamponade**. Compression of the right-sided chambers has 2 major consequences: venous return is significantly decreased, causing jugular venous distention and ascites, and blood flow to the lungs is significantly decreased, causing hypoxia and tachypnea.

Pericardial effusion is uncommon compared with other acquired cardiovascular diseases and occurs in both small and large animals. There are no breed predilections in cats. Golden Retrievers, Great Danes, and Great Pyrenees are among the most commonly affected breeds of dogs. Overall, most cases involve middle-aged, predominantly male, large- and giant-breed dogs. **Cardiac neoplasia** is the most common cause of pericardial effusion in dogs; right atrial tumors are the most frequently seen cardiac neoplasm (usually hemangiosarcoma), followed by heart base tumors (most commonly chemodectoma or ectopic thyroid carcinoma). In cats, the most common cardiac neoplasia is lymphoma. Less common causes of pericardial effusion in dogs and cats are infections (eg, feline infectious peritonitis), trauma, chamber rupture, and secondary to CHF. Cattle most often develop pericardial effusion secondary to **traumatic reticulopericarditis** (p 186) or cardiac neoplasia (lymphoma). Lymphoma in cattle can also result in valvular insufficiencies. In horses, **septic pericarditis** and idiopathic pericarditis are most commonly reported.

The severity of clinical signs depends on the rate of pericardial fluid accumulation. Clinical signs include exercise intolerance, anorexia, listlessness, and abdominal swelling (caused by ascites). In horses, there is often a history of respiratory tract infection, fever, anorexia, and depression. Physical examination findings include lethargy, jugular venous distention, muffled heart sounds, and occasionally pericardial friction rubs. Ascites is consistently present in affected dogs, in which pericardial effusion rapidly develops. With slow development of pericardial fluid, the pericardial sac is able to stretch and clinical signs of right-sided CHF may not develop until severe pericardial effusion is present.

CBC, serum chemistry profile, and urinalysis results are usually normal. Mild anemia, neutrophilic leukocytosis, hyperfibrinogenemia, and hyperproteinemia may occur in horses with septic pericarditis and effusion. In horses with suspected septic pericarditis, a culture and sensitivity of the fluid should be performed. In septic pericarditis, there will be a large number of neutrophils with some being degenerate. Protein content of the fluid will be high, and bacteria may be seen. Cytologic features of idiopathic pericardial effusion in horses are variable, with neutrophils, eosinophils, and macrophages present in variable numbers. Cytologic evaluation of the pericardial fluid is usually not helpful in providing a definitive cause for the pericardial effusion in dogs.

Radiographs show an increase in the size of the cardiac silhouette, which takes on a rounded appearance. If the cause is a cardiac tumor, especially a heart base tumor, the cardiac silhouette may appear eccentrically enlarged. The caudal vena cava may be dilated if cardiac tamponade is present. Pleural effusion may also be present if cardiac neoplasia is the cause of the pericardial effusion. The ECG in most cases shows normal sinus rhythm to sinus tachycardia. Occasional atrial premature and ventricular complexes may occur, especially if neoplasia is the cause. The height of the R waves is often decreased (<1 mV in dogs), and there may be a pattern of alternating variation in R wave amplitude, referred to as **electrical alternans**. This results from the swinging motion of the heart within the fluid-filled pericardial sac. Echocardiography is the most sensitive and specific test for the detection of pericardial effusion. A tumor can be visualized in many cases of neoplastic effusion. When cardiac tamponade is present, the walls of the right atrium and right ventricle appear to collapse and flutter. The left-sided chambers are often decreased in size secondary to decreased venous return from the lungs.

Animals with cardiac tamponade require urgent treatment. Medical therapy is typically ineffective at rapidly reducing pericardial effusion. Diuretics are generally contraindicated because they decrease blood volume and cause further collapse of the cardiac chambers. Pericardiocentesis, which is most commonly performed with mild sedation in dogs, should be performed. This is done by placement of a catheter through the chest wall on the right side, just above the costochondral junction at the fourth to fifth intercostal space. Echocardiography can guide catheter placement at the point where the pericardial sac is closest to the thoracic wall and most distended with fluid. A syringe or extension set with stopcock and syringe (preferred) is attached to the catheter. The system must be closed to air at all times once penetration of the chest wall occurs to avoid creating a pneumothorax. The catheter is passed directly toward the heart while intermittently aspirating. When the pericardial sac is entered, fluid (usually serosanguineous) flows freely into the syringe. The catheter should be carefully advanced over the needle into the pericardial sac. If arrhythmias develop, withdrawing the needle slightly usually suffices. Antiarrhythmic therapy is rarely needed. As much fluid as possible should be removed from the sac and a sample submitted for analysis. When performing pericardiocentesis in horses, the left fifth intercostal space should be used in order to avoid the atria, coronary arteries, and right ventricle. Pericardial lavage, with or without antibiotics, is often performed in horses following pericardiocentesis. Pericardiocentesis is relatively easy to perform and serious complications are rare. However, confirming the presence of pericardial effusion by echocardiography is advisable before performing pericardiocentesis.

Broad-spectrum antibiotics and parenteral fluids may be given immediately before and after pericardiocentesis. Corticosteroids have not been shown to be beneficial in benign pericardial effusion in dogs, although they have been used with success in horses. Most tumors that cause neoplastic effusion do not respond to chemotherapy.

When idiopathic pericarditis is suspected (ie, no mass visible by echocardiography), the owner should be instructed to carefully monitor the animal for any signs of recurrence. Should this occur, a repeat pericardiocentesis is indicated and a subtotal pericardectomy is recommended. Heart base tumors are usually benign in dogs, and if pericardial effusion secondary to a heart base tumor is diagnosed, subtotal pericardectomy should be considered. Many dogs survive symptom-free up to 2 yr following successful subtotal pericardectomy.

Systemic and Pulmonary Hypertension

Systemic hypertension is an increase in systemic blood pressure. There are 2 major types of systemic hypertension. Essential hypertension, which is idiopathic (primary) hypertension, is rare in dogs and cats, but common in humans. Secondary hypertension results from a specific underlying disease. In dogs, the most common cause of hypertension is renal disease; in cats, the most common causes are renal disease and hyperthyroidism. Hyperadrenocorticism, diabetes mellitus, and pheochromocytoma are other causes of hypertension in dogs.

The diagnosis of systemic hypertension is made by measurement of blood pressure. The most accurate assessment method is direct measurement via arterial puncture, which is impractical in most instances. The next most accurate method is indirect measurement using a Doppler probe to assess blood flow in an artery (typically the superficial palmar arterial branch of the radial artery) distal to pressure cuff placement (typically on the forelimb). Cuff width should be 30% of the circumference of the forelimb in cats, and 40% of the forelimb circumference in dogs. The hair just proximal to the palmar metacarpal pad is shaved for application of the Doppler probe in order to allow more accurate results. The hindlimb can also be used, in which case the superficial plantar arterial branch of the caudal tibial artery is assessed. The disadvantage of Doppler blood pressure measurement is that only systolic blood pressure is reliably measured. Although indirect blood pressure measurement is less accurate than direct assessment, it can detect trends in blood pressure. Normal values vary with patient stress; values higher than expected for a normal patient often are caused by the stress of hospitalization (white coat syndrome). With certain exceptions, systolic pressures >180 mm Hg are likely to be truly elevated in a patient that appears calm, and values >200 mm Hg should be strongly considered evidence of systemic hypertension.

Patients with severe hypertension may demonstrate no clinical signs. Retinal lesions (eg, retinal hemorrhage, retinal detachments, arterial tortuosity, focal or diffuse retinal edema) were found in 80% of hypertensive cats in one study. Blood work may demonstrate abnormalities consistent with the cause of hypertension (eg, elevated T_4 levels in hyperthyroid cats, elevated BUN and creatinine in patients with renal failure). Treatment should be initiated in patients with consistently measurable and severe hypertension, or in patients with consistently measurable hypertension and documentation of an underlying cause such as renal failure. Treatments in cats include amlodipine (0.625-1.25 mg, PO, SID), enalapril (0.5 mg/kg, PO, SID-BID), diltiazem (0.5-1.5 mg/kg, PO, TID), β-blockers such as atenolol (6.25-12.5 mg/PO, SID-BID), or diuretics such as furosemide (0.5-1 mg/kg, PO, SID-BID). In dogs, treatments that may be effective include enalapril (0.5 mg/kg, PO, SID-BID), atenolol (0.2-1 mg/kg, PO, SID-BID), furosemide (2-4 mg/kg, PO, SID-BID), or amlodipine (0.05-0.2 mg/kg, PO, SID).

Pulmonary hypertension is elevation of blood pressure in the pulmonary circulation. Possible etiologies include increased blood viscosity (eg, polycythemia), increased pulmonary blood flow (eg, ventricular septal defect, patent ductus arteriosus, or atrial septal defect), and decreased overall cross-sectional area of the pulmonary vascular bed (such as caused by pulmonary arterial wall hypertrophy with heartworm disease, stenosis of pulmonary artery branches, pulmonary thromboembolism, or pulmonary vasoconstriction). Primary pulmonary hypertension is rare in dogs. In cattle, the most common cause is hypoxia-induced pulmonary vasoconstriction caused by dwelling at high altitude (see HIGH-MOUNTAIN DISEASE p 107). Chronic ingestion of locoweed (Oxytropis and Astragalus spp), or chronic pulmonary disease caused by bronchopneumonia or lungworm infestation can also result in cor pulmonale (brisket disease). In horses, pulmonary hypertension may occur secondary to left-sided CHF. Clinical signs are typically those of right-sided CHF (ascites, exercise intolerance, collapse); physical examination findings may include evidence of ascites and jugular distention and pulsation. In cattle, subcutaneous edema of the brisket, ventral thorax, and submandibular area is common. Definitive diagnosis requires direct measurement of pulmonary arterial pressures (rarely performed), or estimation of pulmonary pressures by Doppler echocardiography. Echocardiography may demonstrate septal flattening, right ventricular dilation and/or concentric hypertrophy, and right atrial enlargement. Treatment is typically unrewarding and the prognosis is poor. The best chance for a successful outcome is when the underlying disease can be identified and treated.

HEARTWORM DISEASE

(Dirofilariasis)

Heartworm (HW) infection is caused by a filarial organism, Dirofilaria immitis. At least 70 species of mosquitos can serve as intermediate hosts; Aedes, Anopheles, and Culex are the most common genera acting as vectors. Patent infections are possible in numerous wild and companion animal species. Wild animal reservoirs include wolves, coyotes, foxes, California gray seals, sea lions, and raccoons. In companion animals, HW infection is seen primarily in dogs and less commonly in cats and ferrets. HW disease has been reported in most countries with temperate, semitropical, or tropical climates, including the USA, Canada, and southern Europe. In companion animals, infection risk is greatest in dogs and cats housed outdoors. Although any dog, indoor or outdoor, is capable of being infected, most infections are diagnosed in medium- to large-sized, 3- to 8-yr-old dogs.

Infected mosquitos are capable of transmitting HW infections to humans, but there are no reports of such infections becoming patent. Maturation of the infective larvae may progress to the point where they reach the lungs, become encapsulated, and die. The dead larvae precipitate granulomatous reactions called "coin lesions," which are medically significant because radiographically they appear similar to metastatic lung cancer.

HW infection rates in other companion animals such as ferrets and cats tend to parallel those in dogs in the same geographic region, but usually at a lower prevalence. No age predilection has been reported in ferrets or cats, but male cats have been reported to be more susceptible than females. Indoor and outdoor ferrets and cats can be infected. Other infections in cats, such as those caused by the feline leukemia virus or feline immunodeficiency virus, are not predisposing factors.

Life Cycle: Mosquito vector species acquire the first stage larvae (microfilariae) while feeding on an infected host. Development of microfilariae to the second larval stage (L_2) and to the infective third stage (L_3) occurs within the mosquito in ~1-4 wk, depending on environmental temperatures. This development phase requires the shortest time when the ambient temperature is >86°F (30°C). When mature, the infective larvae migrate to the labium of the mosquito. As the mosquito feeds, the infective larvae erupt through the tip of the labium with a small amount of hemolymph onto the host's skin. The larvae migrate into the bite wound, beginning the mammalian portion of their life cycle. A typical *Aedes* mosquito is only capable of surviving the developmental phase of small numbers of HW larvae, usually <10 larvae per mosquito.

In canids and other susceptible hosts, infective larvae (L_3) molt into a fourth stage (L_4) in 2-3 days. After remaining in the subcutaneous tissue for close to 2 mo, they molt into young adults (L_5) that migrate through host tissue, arriving in the pulmonary arteries ~50 days later. Adult worms (males ~15 cm in length, females ~25 cm) develop primarily in the pulmonary arteries of the caudal lung lobes over the next 2-3 mo. They reside primarily in the pulmonary arteries but can move into the right ventricle when the worm burden is high. Microfilariae are produced by gravid females ~6-7 mo postinfection.

Microfilariae are usually detectable in infected canids not receiving macrolide prophylaxis. However, 25% to >50% of infected canids may not have circulating microfilariae. Thus, the number of circulating microfilariae does not necessarily correlate strongly to adult female HW burden. Adults typically live 3-5 yr, while microfilariae may survive for 1-2 yr while awaiting a mosquito intermediate host.

Most dogs are highly susceptible to HW infection, and the majority of infective larvae (L_3) develop into adults. Ferrets are susceptible hosts, and cats are somewhat resistant. A lower percentage of exposed cats develop adult infections and the burden is often only 1-3 worms. Further evidence of relative resistance in cats is the short survival time of many L_5 in the pulmonary arteries; adult worms probably survive no longer than 2 yr. Aberrant migration into different organs, including the CNS, has been described in cats.

Pathogenesis: The severity of cardiopulmonary pathology in dogs is determined by worm numbers, host immune response, duration of infection, and host activity level. Live adult HW cause direct mechanical irritation of the intima and pulmonary arterial walls, leading to perivascular cuffing with inflammatory cells, including infiltration of high numbers of eosinophils. Live worms seem to have an immunosuppressive effect; however the presence of dead worms leads to immune reactions and subsequent lung pathology in areas of the lung not directly associated with the dead HW. Longterm infections, due to all of the factors noted (ie, direct irritation, worm death, and immune response) result in chronic lesions and subsequent scarring. Active dogs tend to develop more pathology than inactive dogs for any given worm burden. Frequent exertion increases pulmonary arterial pathology and may precipitate overt clinical signs, including congestive heart failure (CHF). High worm burdens are most often the result of infections acquired from numerous mosquito exposures. High exposures in young, naive dogs in temperate climates can result in severe infections, causing a vena caval syndrome the following year. In general, due to the worm size and smaller dimensions of the pulmonary vasculature, small dogs do not tolerate infections and treatment as well as large dogs.

HW-associated inflammatory mediators that induce immune responses in the lungs and kidneys (immune complex glomerulonephritis) cause vasoconstriction and possibly bronchoconstriction. Leakage of plasma and inflammatory mediators from small vessels and capillaries causes parenchymal lung inflammation and edema. Pulmonary arterial constriction causes increased flow velocity, especially with exertion, and resultant shear stresses further damage the endothelium. The process of endothelial damage, vasoconstriction, increased flow velocity, and local ischemia is a vicious cycle. Inflammation with ischemia can result in irreversible interstitial fibrosis.

Pulmonary arterial pathology in cats and ferrets is similar to that in dogs, although the small arteries develop more severe muscular hypertrophy. Arterial thrombosis is caused by both blood clots and worms lodged within narrow lumen arterioles. In cats, parenchymal changes associated with dead HW differ from those observed in dogs and ferrets. Rather than type I cellular edema and damage as found in dogs, cats experience type II cellular hyperplasia, which causes a significant barrier to oxygenation. Most significantly, due to restricted pulmonary vascular capacity and subsequent pathology, both ferrets and cats are more likely to die as a result of HW infection.

Clinical Findings: In dogs, infection should be identified by serologic testing prior to the onset of clinical signs; however, it should be kept in mind that HW antigenemia and microfilaremia do not appear until ~5 and 6.5 mo postinfection, respectively. When dogs are not administered a preventative and are not appropriately tested, clinical signs such as coughing, exercise intolerance, unthriftiness, dyspnea, cyanosis, hemoptysis, syncope, epistaxis, and ascites (right-sided CHF) are likely to develop. The frequency and severity of clinical signs correlate to lung pathology and level of patient activity. Signs are often not observed in sedentary dogs, even though the worm burden may be relatively high. Infected dogs experiencing a dramatic increase in activity, such as during hunting seasons, may develop overt clinical signs. Canine HW disease can be classified by physical examination, thoracic radiographs, urinalysis, and PCV. Class I is asymptomatic to mild HW disease, with no clinical or radiographic signs and no laboratory abnormalities. Subjective signs such as loss of condition, decreased exercise tolerance, or occasional cough might be seen. Class II is moderate HW disease, characterized by an occasional cough and mild-to-moderate exercise intolerance. A slight loss of condition, increased lung sounds, and mild to moderate radiographic changes, such as right ventricular enlargement, are present. Laboratory results may show anemia and proteinuria. Class III is severe disease variably characterized by anemia, weight loss, exercise intolerance, tachypnea at rest, severe or persistent coughing, dyspnea, hemoptysis, syncope, and ascites. Severely abnormal radiographs may show right ventricular hypertrophy, enlargement of the main pulmonary artery, and diffuse pulmonary densities. Laboratory results indicate marked anemia, thrombocytopenia, and proteinuria. Electrocardiographic evidence of right ventricular hypertrophy is often present. Class IV, also known as the caval syndrome, is characterized by sudden onset with collapse, hemoglobinuria, and respiratory distress. If surgery is not immediately instituted, this syndrome is usually fatal.

Infected cats may be asymptomatic or exhibit intermittent coughing, dyspnea, vomiting, lethargy, anorexia, or weight loss. The symptoms often resemble those of feline asthma. In general, signs are most prevalent during periods when worms die, including when young adult worms arrive in the lungs. Antigen tests in cats are negative during the early eosinophilic pneumonitis syndrome, although antibody tests may be positive. Subsequently, clinical signs often resolve and may not reappear for months. Cats harboring mature worms may exhibit intermittent vomiting, lethargy, coughing, or episodic dyspnea. HW death can lead to acute respiratory distress and shock, which may be fatal and appears to be the consequence of pulmonary thrombosis.

Diagnosis: The antigen detection test is the preferred diagnostic method for asymptomatic dogs or when seeking verification of a suspected HW infection. This is the most sensitive diagnostic method available to veterinary practitioners. Even in areas where the prevalence of HW infection is high, ~20% of infected dogs may not be microfilaremic. Also, monthly macrolide prophylaxis induces embryo stasis in female dirofilariae.

Available antigen detection tests are very sensitive and specific. To determine when testing might become useful, it is advisable to add a predetection period to the approximate date on which infection may have been possible. A reasonable interval is 7 mo. There is generally no need to test a dog for antigen or microfilariae prior to ~7 mo of age. The level of antigenemia is directly related to the number of mature female worms present. At least 90% of dogs harboring ≥3 adult females will test positive. In general, strong-quick positive reactions correlate with relatively high worm burdens. For low-burden suspects, commercial laboratory-based microwell titer tests are the most sensitive.

In dogs, echocardiography is relatively unimportant as a diagnostic tool. Worms observed in the right heart and vena cava are associated with high-burden infection with or without caval syndrome. Severe, chronic pulmonary hypertension causes right ventricular hypertrophy, septal flattening, underloading of the left heart, and high-velocity tricuspid and pulmonic regurgitation. The ECG of infected dogs is usually normal. Right ventricular hypertrophy patterns are seen when there is severe, chronic pulmonary hypertension and are associated with overt or impending right-sided CHF (ascites). Heart rhythm disturbances are usually absent or mild, but atrial fibrillation is an occasional complication in dogs with Class III disease.

The diagnosis of HW disease in cats is based on historical and physical findings, index of suspicion, thoracic radiographs, echocardiography, and serology. Cats may develop a positive antigen test 8 mo post L_3 inoculation. However, antigen tests are considered too unreliable as the initial screening test for cats because unisex infections are common in cats, light infections may occur with insufficient numbers of mature females to be detectable, and some cats may become ill and be tested before a detectable antigenemia develops at ~5.5-8 mo postinfection. Antiheartworm antibodies, produced by 90% of infected cats, may first appear 2-3 mo post L_3 infection and are usually present by 5 mo. However, antibodies can persist for several months following worm death. Also, antibodies induced by larvae can persist after macrolide prophylaxis has been instituted and has killed the preadults. Thus, a positive antibody test is only an indication of exposure to the parasite and not necessarily of infection. In conjunction with other provocative findings, antibody seropositivity may be useful in making a clinical diagnosis of feline heartworm disease. False-positive results from cross-reactivity have not been observed. A negative antibody test indicates ≥90% probability of the absence of infection. Microfilariae are rarely detected by Knott's or filter tests (<10%).

In cats, worms can usually be imaged on echocardiography. Parallel hyperechoic lines, which are an image from the heartworm cuticle, may be seen in the right heart and pulmonary arteries. High worm burdens may be associated with worms in the right heart. Echocardiography is more important in cats than dogs because of the increased difficulty of diagnosis and the high sensitivity of the test in experienced hands.

In addition to special diagnostic tests in both cats and dogs, a CBC, chemistry profile, urinalysis, and particularly thoracic radiographs are indicated. Laboratory data are often normal. Eosinophilia and basophilia are common and together suggest occult dirofilariasis or allergic lung disease. Eosinophilia surges as the L_5 arrive in the pulmonary arteries. Subsequently, eosinophil counts vary but are usually high in dogs with immune-mediated occult infections, especially if eosinophilic pneumonitis develops (<10% of total infections).

Hyperglobulinemia may be present in dogs and cats due to antigenic stimulation. Hypoalbuminemia in dogs is associated with severe immune-complex glomerulonephritis or right-sided CHF. Serum ALT and alkaline phosphatase are occasionally increased, but do not correlate well with abnormal liver function, efficacy of adulticide treatment, or risk of drug toxicity. Urinalysis may reveal proteinuria that can be semiquantitated by a urine protein:creatinine ratio. Occasionally, severe glomerulonephritis or amyloidosis can lead to hypoalbuminemia and nephrotic syndrome. Dogs with hypoalbuminemia secondary to glomerular disease also lose antithrombin III and are at risk for thromboembolic disease. Hemoglobinuria is associated with Class III disease when RBC are lysed in the pulmonary circulation by fibrin deposition. Heparin therapy (75-100 U/kg, SC, TID) is indicated. Hemoglobinuria is also a classic sign of the vena caval syndrome.

In dogs, thoracic radiography provides the most information on disease severity and is a good screening tool for dogs with clinical signs compatible with dirofilariasis. Class III infections are characterized by a large main pulmonary artery segment and dilated, tortuous caudal lobar pulmonary arteries. If the latter are ≥1.5 times the diameter of the 9th rib at their point of superimposition, then severe pathology is present. Right ventricular enlargement may also be seen. Fluffy, ill-defined parenchymal infiltrates of variable extent often surround the caudal lobar arteries, usually worst in the right caudal lobe, in advanced disease. The infiltrate may improve with cage confinement with or without anti-inflammatory dosages of a corticosteroid.

In cats, cardiac changes are less common. The caudal lobar arteries normally appear relatively large, but are larger still with heartworm infection. Patchy parenchymal infiltrates may also be present in cats with respiratory signs. The main pulmonary artery segment usually is not visible due to its relatively midline location.

Treatment in Dogs: The extent of the preadulticide evaluation will vary depending on the clinical status of the patient and the likelihood of coexisting diseases that may affect the outcome of treatment. Clinical laboratory data should be collected selectively to complement information obtained from a thorough history, physical examination, antigen test, and usually thoracic radiography.

The most important variables influencing the probability of postadulticide thromboembolic complications and the outcome of treatment are the extent of concurrent pulmonary vascular disease and the severity of infection. Assessment of cardiopulmonary status is indispensable for evaluating a patient's prognosis. Postadulticide pulmonary thromboembolic complications are most likely to occur in heavily infected dogs already exhibiting clinical and radiographic signs of severe pulmonary arterial vascular obstruction, especially if CHF is present.

The only available heartworm adulticide is melarsomine dihydrochloride, which is effective against mature (adult) and immature heartworms of both genders. For Class I and II patients, melarsomine is given at 2.5 mg/kg, deep IM in the epaxial (lumbar) musculature in the L3-L5 region using a 22 g needle (1 in. long for dogs <10 kg or 1.5 in. for dogs >10 kg). Pressure is applied during delivery and for 1 min after the needle is withdrawn to prevent SC leakage. The procedure is repeated on the opposite side 24 hr later. Approximately one-third of dogs will exhibit local pain, swelling, soreness with movement, or sterile abscessation at the injection site. Local fibrosis is uncommon.

Dogs with high worm burdens are at risk of severe pulmonary thromboembolism from several days to 6 wk postadulticide. Dogs with Class III infection receive the alternate (split-dose) regimen of 1 injection, followed in 1 mo by 2 injections 24 hr apart. Administration of a single initial dose results in a graded (~50%) worm kill and reduced pulmonary complications. By initially killing few worms and completing the treatment in 2 stages, the cumulative impact of worm emboli on severely diseased pulmonary arteries and lungs can be reduced. This 3-injection protocol is becoming the treatment of choice of many veterinarians regardless of stage of disease, due to its increased safety and efficacy.

Other treatment protocols recommend the administration of prophylactic doses of ivermectin for 1-6 mo prior to administration of melarsomine, if the clinical presentation does not demand immediate intervention. The rationale for this approach is to greatly reduce or eliminate circulating microfilariae and migrating *D immitis* larvae, stunt immature HW, and reduce female worm mass by destroying the reproductive system. This results in reduced antigenic mass, which in turns reduces the risk of pulmonary thromboembolism.

Following melarsomine injection, exercise must be severely restricted for 4-6 wk to minimize thromboembolic lung complications. A low cardiac output should be maintained in order to reduce thrombosis and endothelial damage and facilitate lung repair. Adverse effects of melarsomine are otherwise limited to local inflammation, brief low-grade fever, and salivation. Hepatic and renal toxicity are seldom seen.

Class III patients should be stabilized prior to melarsomine administration. Stabilizing treatment variably includes cage confinement, oxygen, corticosteroids, and heparin (75-100 U/kg, SC, TID) for 1 wk prior to the alternate melarsomine treatment protocol.

Patients with right-sided CHF should be treated with furosemide (1-2 mg/kg, BID), a low-dose angiotensin-converting enzyme (ACE) inhibitor such as enalapril (0.25 mg/kg, BID, possibly increased to 0.5 mg/kg, BID after 1 wk pending renal function test results), and a restricted sodium diet. Digoxin, digitoxin, and arteriolar dilators, such as hydralazine and amlodipine, should not be administered. Digoxin is not effective for cor pulmonale; arteriolar dilators, and occasionally even ACE inhibitors, are likely to cause systemic hypotension.

Postadulticide thromboembolic complications can occur 2-30 days following treatment, with signs most likely 14-21 days after treatment. Clinical signs are coughing, hemoptysis, dyspnea, tachypnea, lethargy, anorexia, and fever. Laboratory findings may include an inflammatory leukogram, thrombocytopenia, and prolonged activated clotting time or prothrombin time. A postinjection increase in serum CK may be noted. Local or disseminated intravascular coagulopathy may occur when platelet counts are <100,000/ μL. Treatment for severe thromboembolism should include oxygen, cage confinement, a corticosteroid at an anti-inflammatory dosage (eg, prednisone at 1.0 mg/kg, PO, SID), and low-dose heparin (75-100 U/kg, SC, TID) for several days to 1 wk. Most dogs respond within 24 hr. Severe lung injury is likely if, after 24 hr of oxygen therapy, no improvement is noted and partial pressures of oxygen remain <70 mm Hg.

Both the standard melarsomine protocol and the alternate regimen kill all or most worms in ~75% of dogs. Antigen testing is performed 6 mo after the first 2 doses of the standard protocol or 4-6 mo after the third dose of the alternate protocol. A positive test result should be followed by retreatment (2 injections, 24 hr apart) if the antigen test is strongly positive, if the patient is still symptomatic, and if the patient is an athlete or a working dog. Mild infection, a weakly positive antigen test, absence of clinical signs, advanced age, and a sedentary dog are factors that may negate the need for a repeat melarsomine treatment. Maintaining dogs on ivermectin/pyrantel pamoate to slowly kill residual worms over the following 20 mo is an alternative in nonperforming dogs with a post-melarsomine weakly positive antigen test result.

Ivermectin/pyrantel pamoate administered monthly for ~2 yr beginning at 5-7 mo post-L_3 inoculation eradicates most adult worms. Further, during this time period, some older worms are also killed. However, the use of ivermectin/pyrantel pamoate is seldom a substitute for melarsomine treatment because the slow kill may allow pulmonary pathology to progress in the interim.

In caval syndrome cases (class IV), surgical removal of worms from the right atrium and orifice of the tricuspid valve is necessary to save the life of the dog. This may be accomplished by using local anesthesia and either a rigid or flexible alligator forceps, or an intravascular retrieval snare, introduced preferentially via the right external jugular vein. With fluoroscopic guidance, if available, the instrument should continue to be passed until worms can no longer be retrieved. Immediately following a successful operation, the clinical signs should lessen or disappear. Fluid therapy may be necessary in critically ill, hypovolemic dogs to restore hemodynamic and renal function. Within a few weeks following recovery from surgery, adulticide chemotherapy is recommended to eliminate any remaining worms, particularly if many are still visible echocardiographically.

Microfilaricide Treatment: At specific preventive dosages, the macrolide preventative drugs are effective microfilaricides, although not approved by the FDA for this purpose. Adverse reactions may occur in dogs with high microfilarial counts (>40,000/μL), depending on the type of macrolide given. However, the microfilarial count is usually lower, and mild adverse reactions occur in ~10% of dogs. Most adverse reactions are limited to brief salivation and defecation, occurring within hours and lasting up to several hours. Dogs, especially small dogs (<10 kg), with high microfilarial counts (>40,000/μL) may develop tachycardia, tachypnea, pale mucous membranes, lethargy, retching, diarrhea, and even shock. Treatment includes IV balanced electrolyte solution and a soluble corticosteroid. Recovery is usually rapid when treatment is administered quickly. Microfilarial counts are not routinely performed, and thus severe reactions are seldom expected. Treatment specifically targeting circulating microfilariae may be started as early as 3-4 wk following adulticide administration. More commonly, microfilariae are eventually eliminated, even from non-adulticide-treated dogs, after several months of treatment with prophylactic doses of the macrocyclic lactones. No drugs are currently approved as microfilaricides by the FDA. However, licensed veterinarians are permitted extra-label use of certain drugs if a valid veterinarian-client-patient relationship exists. The use of monthly administered HW chemoprophylactics as microfilaricides is governed by this regulation. The macrocyclic lactones are the safest and most effective microfilaricidal drugs available. Livestock preparations of these drugs should not be used to achieve higher doses for the purpose of obtaining more rapid results. The macrolide of choice for killing microfilariae quickly is milbemycin (0.5 mg/kg, PO, 1 dose). Performance of a microfilariae test is recommended at the time the antigen test is performed (6 mo after the adulticide treatment).

Developing Larvae: Ivermectin/pyrantel pamoate, administered monthly for 1 yr to dogs with larvae that are no more than 4 mo post-L_3 inoculation, prevents the development of infection. Continuous monthly administration of prophylactic doses of ivermectin, alone or in combination with pyrantel pamoate, is also highly effective against late precardiac larvae and young (<7 mo postinfection) quasi-adult HW. Comparable capability of the other macrocyclic lactones has not been reported. This extended protection is important in dogs of unknown medical history that may have acquired HW infections because of lack of preventive drug administration or lack of compliance.

Treatment in Cats: There is currently no satisfactory treatment approach to heartworm infections in cats. Infection often is lethal, and a safe and effective melarsomine protocol has not yet been developed. Thus, all cats in canine HW-endemic regions should receive drug prophylaxis. The adult heartworm lifespan in cats is probably ≤2 yr, so spontaneous recovery is possible. Cats may remain asymptomatic, experience episodic vomiting and/or episodic dyspnea (resembling asthma), may die suddenly from pulmonary thromboembolism, or rarely, develop CHF. With each worm death, pulmonary complications occur. There does not appear to be an association between the presence, absence, or severity of clinical signs and the likelihood of acute complications.

Many cats are managed conservatively with restricted activity and corticosteroid therapy, such as prednisolone (1.0-2.0 mg/kg, PO, every 24-48 hr). Steroids reduce the severity of vomiting and respiratory signs. The hope is that episodes of pulmonary complications will not prove fatal as the worms die. Barring superinfection, 25-50% of cats may survive with this approach. Serial antibody testing (at 6-mo intervals) can be used to monitor status.

Surgical retrieval of worms from the right atrium, right ventricle, and vena cavae via jugular venotomy can be attempted in patients with high worm burdens detected by echocardiography. An endoscopic basket or horsehair brush can be advanced via the right jugular vein under fluoroscopy.

Prevention: Heartworm infection is completely preventable with macrolide prophylaxis. Preventive therapy in dogs is recommended beginning at 6-8 wk of age. No testing is necessary at this age. When started at ~1 yr of age, an antigen test is recommended. Before starting a prophylactic regime, all mature dogs that may have been infected >7 mo earlier should be antigen tested and, in appropriate instances, tested for presence of microfilariae. The determination of HW status before starting chemoprophylaxis will avoid unnecessary delay in detecting subclinical infections, and potential confusion concerning effectiveness of the preventive program, if a pre-existing infection becomes evident after beginning chemoprophylaxis. Year-round prevention is advised, but in northern climates, chemoprophylaxis is often initiated in the spring and continued through November. Year-round macrolide administration will arrest the development of larval stages

(L_3 and L_4) that might have occurred prior to preventative initiation or when monthly doses were missed.

The macrolide preventives ivermectin, milbemycin oxime, moxidectin, and selamectin are safe and effective as prescribed for all breeds. Ivermectin/pyrantel pamoate (hookworms and roundworms) and milbemycin (hookworms, roundworms, and whipworms) also provide control of intestinal nematodes. Milbemycin, however, kills microfilariae (L_1) quickly and shock can occur in the face of high microfilarial concentrations. Thus, milbemycin is not administered as a preventive in dogs with microfilariae. Selamectin is administered topically at a monthly dosage of ~6 mg/kg and also kills adult fleas and prevents flea eggs from hatching for 1 mo. It also is indicated for the treatment and control of *Otodectes cynotis* in dogs and cats, sarcoptic mange, *Dermacentor variabilis* infestations in dogs, *Ancylostoma tubaeforme*, and *Toxocara cati* in cats.

Annual antigen testing is recommended because overall owner compliance with macrolide prophylaxis is only ~50%. The injectable form of moxidectin is effective for at least 6 mo following 1 injection but use in microfilaremic dogs is not advised. At the time of publication, this formulation was not available in the USA because of concerns regarding toxicity in dogs. With macrolide administration for 6 mo and longer, microfilariae production by female worms ceases and antigen testing is required for detection of infection.

Heartworm prevention is recommended for all cats in endemic regions, regardless of housing status, because of the potential severe consequences. Ivermectin for cats is safe and effective at 25 µg/kg, PO, once monthly. At this dose, the formulation is also effective against *Ancylostoma tubaeforme* and *A braziliense*. Preventive treatment should be initiated in all adult cats, in kittens 6 wk of age, and continued lifelong. Annual antigen and antibody testing is of limited value in cats receiving prophylaxis.

HIGH-MOUNTAIN DISEASE

(Brisket disease, Pulmonary hypertensive heart disease)

High-mountain disease or brisket disease is noninfectious, congestive heart failure (CHF) of cattle. It is primarily caused by pulmonary hypertension associated with high altitudes. The disease affects cattle in mountainous ranges of the world and is seen most commonly at elevations above 2,000 m (~6,500 ft) in the western USA, western Canada, and South America. Rarely, similar lesions have been described in severely stressed and parasitized sheep and deer. Etiologically similar hypoxia-related heart failure has also been described in chickens in the Andes mountains and humans living at extreme elevations. The incidence in cattle on high mountain pastures averages ~2% with variations from 0.5-5%. Though closely associated with altitude, other genetic, physiologic, environmental, and toxic factors play important roles in disease development and progression. Newly introduced cattle tend to be more susceptible than native cattle. Clinical signs and lesions generally take about 2 mo to become obvious. In those areas in North America where cattle spend summer and fall grazing at high altitudes and return to lower elevations later in the fall, the disease is usually manifest in late summer. In areas where cattle live year round at high altitudes, the disease incidence is greatest in winter or early spring. This may be due to the stress of winter weather and late pregnancy. It affects all sexes, ages, and breeds, but not necessarily equally. It is more common, for instance, in steers <1 yr old.

Etiology: Although many factors may contribute to the incidence of high-mountain disease, the pathogenesis seems directly related to the chronic hypoxia, hypocapnia, and respiratory alkalosis of a high-altitude environment. These changes collectively result in pulmonary vasoconstriction, pulmonary hypertension, and ultimately CHF. There is marked interindividual and interspecies variability in hypoxia-induced increases in pulmonary vascular resistance. Strong responses are seen in cattle, horses, and pigs, while humans, dogs, guinea pigs, and llamas are weak responders. These findings and the high incidence of disease in cattle indicate that they are uniquely susceptible.

The role of genetics in high-mountain disease is supported by high familial incidence with marked variation in susceptibility between animals and between species. While the cause or genes involved have not been identified, it may be related to altered chemoreceptor activity and myocardial metabolism. Previous damage, such as that caused by bronchopneumonia, interstitial pneumonia, emphysema, pulmonary fibrosis, anemia, or a ruptured diaphragm, all increase dyspnea, pulmonary vascular resistance, and pulmonary hypertension.

Although various range plants, both browse and nonbrowse-types, have been associated with increased incidence of high-mountain disease, only locoweed has been experimentally shown to induce the disease. When consumed by cattle at high elevation, locoweeds (certain *Oxytropis* and *Astragalus* spp that contain swainsonine), markedly increase the prevalence and severity of CHF. The condition develops relatively more quickly (eg, within 1-2 wk) and the incidence may be as high as 100%. Swainsonine, the locoweed toxin, is excreted in milk, and nursing calves may also develop CHF. Locoweed-poisoned cows often abort and many develop severe hydrops amnii. Poisoned animals have the signs and lesions of both high-mountain disease and locoweed poisoning. Locoweed poisoning probably directly contributes to increased pulmonary vascular resistance and hypertension; immunohistochemistry and electron microscopy studies have shown that poisoning causes severe swelling and cytoplasmic vacuolation of pulmonary intravascular macrophages and endothelial cells. The myocardium also is compromised by locoweed as there is extensive vacuolation of the myocardial interstitial cells. The toxin also inhibits enzymes that have key roles in glycoprotein synthesis, packaging, and excretion. This results in altered glycosylation of key endocrine and paracrine hormones and their receptors. All of these changes probably contribute to the inappropriate pulmonary vascular resistance that appears to be the initiating factor in the pathogenesis of high-mountain disease.

Clinical Findings: The clinical changes of CHF of high-mountain disease usually develop slowly over several weeks. Periods of severe cold or other environmental stress appear to precipitate the onset of signs. Affected animals initially appear depressed and reluctant to move. As the syndrome progresses, subacute edema develops in the brisket region and extends cranially to the intermandibular space and caudally to the ventral abdominal wall. Marked distention and pulsation of the jugular vein are usually prominent, and profuse, fluid diarrhea may develop. Respiration is labored, and animals may appear cyanotic. As the disease progresses, affected cattle become more reluctant to move and may become recumbent. With forced exertion, severely affected animals may collapse and die.

Lesions: Generalized edema is especially severe in the ventral subcutis, skeletal musculature, perirenal tissues, mesentery, and wall of the GI tract. Ascites, hydrothorax, and hydropericardium are consistent findings. The liver lesions, due to chronic passive congestion, vary from an early "nutmeg" appearance to severe lobular and vascular fibrosis. The lungs may have varying degrees of atelectasis, interstitial emphysema, edema, and pneumonia. The heart has marked right ventricular hypertrophy and dilatation; the cardiac apex is displaced to the left, making the enlarged heart appear round. Pulmonary arterial thrombosis is frequent. Microscopically, there is hypertrophy of the media of small arteries and arterioles in the lungs. This disease must be differentiated from other diseases that cause CHF in cattle, eg, traumatic pericarditis, chronic pneumonia, congenital anomalies, and primary myocardial lesions.

Treatment and Control: Affected animals should be moved with minimal restraint, stress, and excitement to a lower altitude. General supportive therapy, including diuretics, may be beneficial. At high altitudes, use of oxygen may be considered for valuable animals. Because the disease may recur, affected animals should not be returned to high altitudes and, because an inherited susceptibility is likely, they should not be retained for breeding. Although it has been suggested that measurement of pulmonary arterial pressure of new sires may allow selection of resistant animals, this has not been proven. Extensive studies in humans exposed to high altitudes have shown that baseline Doppler studies of pulmonary pressures and circulation have little predictive value of tolerance to altitudes.

Because locoweed poisoning has been directly linked to the development of CHF in cattle, care should be taken to minimize the exposure of susceptible animals by ensuring that animals have a good selection of forage. Poisoned animals should be moved to pastures free of locoweed before severe and irreversible damage occurs.

THROMBOSIS, EMBOLISM, AND ANEURYSM

A **thrombus** is an aggregation of blood factors that may form when the blood flow in the arteries or veins is impeded. It frequently causes vascular obstruction at its site of origin. The thrombus can be classified based on its location and the syndrome it produces (eg, venous thrombosis in large animals associated with prolonged venous catheterization, pulmonary arterial thrombosis associated with heartworm disease in dogs). All or part of a thrombus may break off and be carried through the bloodstream as an **embolus** that lodges distally at a point of narrowing. Embolization can also occur when foreign material (eg, bacteria, air, fat, catheter piece) is carried into the bloodstream. Thrombi and emboli can be septic or nonseptic. Poor injection or catheterization techniques and inferior catheter material can all result in vascular thrombosis. However, life-threatening vascular thrombosis is more commonly encountered in patients with underlying disease states that result in coagulopathies, such as systemic inflammation, or endotoxemia. The underlying mechanism shared by all disease processes that potentiate thrombus formation is endothelial cell injury with concomitant platelet and coagulation factor activation. If left untreated or uncontrolled, these hypercoagulable conditions can result in hemorrhagic diathesis and/or disseminated intravascular coagulation (DIC), a life-threatening disorder of hemostasis with deposition of microthrombi with concurrent hemorrhage.

Thrombus formation can occur in both large and small arteries and veins. Horses and cattle are more likely to develop thrombi affecting the postcapillary circulation, while in dogs and cats arterial thrombi are more clinically important. Nonseptic arterial thrombosis and downstream embolization generally result in ischemia of affected tissues. In addition, septic emboli can result in bacterial dissemination and localized infection. Primary arterial occlusive events affecting the heart or CNS are uncommon in animals. Systemic hypercoagulation with thrombus formation can result in primary coronary or cerebrovascular arterial occlusion, or emboli can lodge in the vasculature of the CNS or myocardium. The underlying pathophysiologic mechanisms of arterial occlusive events affecting these organ systems in animals differ from those in humans, where atherosclerotic lesions commonly lead to thrombus formation and arterial occlusion. Atherosclerotic lesions as seen in humans are not well described in animals. Thrombosis of limb arteries causing lameness and gangrene has been reported in adult horses and foals. Similar to the pathogenesis of arterial occlusion within the CNS and myocardium, thrombosis of limb arteries occurs secondary to hypercoagulation and systemic inflammation (eg, septicemia in foals).

An **aneurysm** is a vascular dilation caused by weakening of the tunica media of blood vessels. The weakness might be primary or caused by degenerative or inflammatory changes progressing from an intimal lesion. False aneurysms are caused by damage to all 3 layers of the arterial wall and result in extravascular accumulation of blood. Disruption of the endothelium associated with a true aneurysm can cause formation of a thrombus with subsequent embolization; thus, aneurysms, thrombi, and emboli may be recognized simultaneously.

Clinical Findings and Diagnosis: Acute onset of dyspnea is often associated with pulmonary thrombosis, and some patients may develop hemoptysis. Septic cardiac thrombi are associated with endocarditis; nonseptic cardiac thrombi are associated with myocardial disease. Infarction or embolization within the genitourinary system can present with hematuria, abdominal pain, and splinting. Embolization to the viscera may have similar signs, although small animals may vomit or become incontinent.

In **cattle**, thrombosis of the caudal vena cava occurs in association with hepatic abscessation and erosion of the abscess into the vein. Embolic pneumonia with secondary pulmonary abscessation, thromboembolism, and pulmonary arterial aneurysms are common sequelae. Affected animals may present with coughing, tachypnea, dyspnea, and abnormal lung sounds. Aneurysms in pulmonary arteries that contain septic emboli may rupture and cause intrapulmonary hemorrhage, or pulmonary abscesses may erode into bronchi and result in hemorrhage into the airways. The sequelae to these disorders may include epistaxis, hemoptysis, and death. Clinical pathologic data usually support a diagnosis of vena caval syndrome, but are not specific. Elevated fibrinogen, anemia, and in cases with an active abscess process, elevated liver enzymes may be seen. Ultrasonographic examination may confirm liver abscessation. Pulmonary arterial thromboembolism and embolic pneumonia are also frequent complications of right heart endocarditis in cattle, but aneurysms rarely develop. Intermittent fever and anorexia due to bacteremia at times of embolic showering are often present, and the animal typically has a history of a chronic active infection (eg, foot abscess, reticular abscess). Most cases of right heart endocarditis in cattle are bacterial and are commonly associated with a cardiac murmur, with a point of maximal intensity over the tricuspid valve. Echocardiography and blood cultures are useful in identifying right heart vegetative lesions and diagnosing showering of bacterial emboli, respectively. Thrombosis of the cranial vena cava in cattle produces bilateral jugular engorgement (usually without a jugular pulse); edema of the head, submandibular area, and brisket; and pronounced oral mucosal hyperemia. Significant lingual, pharyngeal, or laryngeal edema may develop and result in dysphagia and dyspnea. Upper respiratory edema may become life-threatening and necessitate tracheostomy.

In **horses**, cranial vena cava thrombosis may result from embolization of a jugular thrombus or extension of a right atrial endocarditis lesion. Jugular vein thrombosis in horses is often associated with phlebitis following catheterization or paravenous injection and will cause swelling, heat, and pain of the affected area with palpable thickening of the jugular vein. Bilateral jugular vein thrombosis can cause edema and swelling of the head and neck due to passive congestion. Ultrasonographic examination of the affected vein can determine the extent of the thrombus and degree of occlusion. A septic thrombus should be suspected if cavitary lesions are present within accompanying soft tissue inflammation; a nonseptic thrombus is usually of more homogenous echogenicity. Doppler ultrasound is a more sophisticated method to determine blood flow and vessel patency. If a catheter-associated thrombophlebitis is suspected, blood culture and catheter-tip culture can be performed. Horses with colitis and other GI disorders are at increased risk for developing jugular thrombosis; ruminants are much less prone to jugular thrombosis than horses.

Migrating *Strongylus vulgaris* larvae (p 267) can cause arteritis with development of thrombi and verminous aneurysms in the aorta, cranial mesenteric, or iliac artery. In some horses, emboli develop and partially or completely occlude terminal branches of the mesenteric arteries. Affected intestinal segments show changes ranging from passive congestion to hemorrhagic infarction. Clinical signs are those of colic, constipation, or diarrhea. The colic usually is recurrent, and attacks may be severe and prolonged. The recent introductions of newer anthelmintics and improved therapeutic regimens have resulted in verminous arteritis becoming an uncommon disorder.

Thrombosis with or without aneurysm of the terminal aorta and proximal iliac arteries produces a characteristic syndrome in horses. Although associated with parasitism, other causes are probable but have not yet been elucidated. Affected horses appear normal at rest; however, graded exercise results in an increasing severity of weakness of the hindlimbs with unilateral or bilateral lameness, muscle tremor, and sweating. Severely affected animals may show signs of exercise intolerance, weakness, and atypical lameness that resolves after a short rest. Subnormal temperature of the affected limbs may be detectable, along with decreased or absent arterial pulsations and delayed and diminished venous filling. Rectal palpation may show variation in pulse amplitude of the internal or external iliac arteries (or both) and asymmetric vasculature. In severe cases, the hind-quarter muscles atrophy, and lameness may become evident with only mild exercise. Complete embolic or thrombotic occlusion of the distal aorta may produce acute bilateral hindlimb paralysis and recumbency in horses. Affected animals are anxious, appear painful, and rapidly go into shock. The hindlimbs are cold, and rectal palpation reveals an absence of pulsation in either iliac artery. Transrectal ultrasound can be helpful in determining bloodflow in the aorta and iliac arteries.

In **dogs**, and less commonly in **cats**, heartworm disease may lead to pulmonary arterial thrombosis; pulmonary embolism is a major secondary effect. Pulmonary thromboemboli most commonly produce dyspnea and tachypnea, and abnormal lung sounds sometimes can be heard during thoracic auscultation. Affected animals are often reportedly normal until sudden onset of respiratory distress. Secondary pulmonary hypertension may cause a split second heart sound. Chest radiographs may be normal or show changes such as an enlarged main pulmonary artery and right heart, underperfusion of the affected region, pleural effusion, or pulmonary hemorrhage or infarction. Blood-gas determinations most often show hypoxemia with low or normal partial pressure of CO_2. Ventilation/perfusion scanning with radionuclide-labeled albumin and gases or pulmonary angiography can confirm the diagnosis. Ancillary tests are essential for the diagnosis of underlying diseases. In both cats and dogs, bacterial endocarditis can lead to pulmonary thromboembolism and embolic pneumonia. In dogs, other diseases associated with pulmonary thromboembolism include ones that result in systemic or metabolic disorders (eg, diabetes mellitus, glomerulonephropathy, hyperadrenocorticism, immune-mediated hemolytic anemia, neoplasia, renal amyloidosis).

In **cats**, aortic thromboembolism is a frequent complication of cardiomyopathy (p 91). Hypertrophic and dilated cardiomyopathy create abnormal circulatory patterns, which predispose to intracavitary thrombus formation. Thrombi may be located in the left atrium, ventricle, or both. Thrombi that dislodge form emboli that may obstruct aortic branches, most commonly at the aortic trifurcation. Such "saddle clots" obstruct the internal and external iliac arteries and the median sacral artery. Clinical signs include paralysis and pain of the extremities, (lack of a palpable femoral pulse, cold distal limbs), and signs related to congestive heart failure. Incomplete occlusion of the aortic bifurcation may cause mild neurologic deficits in both hindlimbs or unilateral paresis. Emboli may also lodge more proximally in the aorta or in other systemic vascular beds. Experimentally, aortic ligation does not reproduce the clinical signs of aortic thromboembolism, while artificial production of a thrombus does, suggesting that factors elaborated by emboli may inhibit collateral circulation. These may include serotonin and thromboxane A_2, both of which are released by activated platelets, causing vasoconstriction and platelet aggregation that likely contribute to development of clinical signs through inhibition of collateral circulation. Inflammation and necrosis of hepatic and skeletal muscle may also occur, leading to elevation of serum CK, AST, and ALT. Echocardiography is the imaging modality of choice to assess cardiac structure and function. Angiocardiography may be used to assess collateral circulation and confirm the diagnosis. However, because it requires general anesthesia, it is often unsafe in cats with cardiomyopathy.

Aneurysms cause no clinical signs unless hemorrhage occurs or an associated thrombus develops. Except for dissecting aneurysm in turkeys (p 2197), aortic or sinus of Valsalva rupture in horses with sudden death, hemorrhage associated with guttural pouch mycosis in horses (p 1222), or pulmonary arterial aneurysm in cattle, spontaneous aneurysmal hemorrhage is rare and clinical signs usually relate to thrombosis. An aneurysm of the abdominal aorta and its branches in large animals may be palpated rectally as a fixed firm swelling with a rough, irregular surface that pulsates with the heart beat. Fremitus may be present. In excess thrombus formation, the pulse may be delayed distally and have a slow rate of rise in pressure, or it may be absent. Other helpful diagnostic modalities include ultrasonography and angiography.

Treatment: Treatment of embolic pneumonia caused by endocarditis includes longterm antibiotics (several weeks) and in some cases intermittent administration of antipyretic and anti-inflammatory drugs. Antibiotic choice should be based on culture and sensitivity results obtained from blood cultures, transtracheal wash, or both. The prognosis for recovery is guarded at best, and the performance of recovered horses and cattle is often decreased.

Treatment of venous thrombosis is usually limited to supportive care, including hydrotherapy of accessible veins, anti-inflammatory agents, and systemic antimicrobials to control secondary sepsis. Surgical removal of thrombosed jugular veins has been performed successfully in horses, but unless both veins are severely affected, inflammation will resolve with medical treatment and formation of collaterals will usually result in sufficient venous circulation. Thrombosis of the cranial or caudal vena cava generally does not respond to therapy and the prognosis is poor.

Measures to minimize trauma to, and bacterial contamination of, veins remain the best means to prevent thrombosis. Extreme care should be taken when placing catheters or giving IV injections to patients at risk for hypercoagulation disorders. The effectiveness of antiplatelet aggregation with aspirin (100 mg/kg, SID), anticoagulant therapy with unfractionated heparin (40-80 IU/kg, SC, BID-TID), and use of low-molecular-weight heparin to facilitate thrombolysis is questionable, but will help prevent formation of additional clots.

In horses, aneurysms due to *Strongylus vulgaris* rarely rupture; the chief concern is thromboembolism of intestinal vasculature with subsequent colic. Generally, the arterial wall is sufficiently involved that thrombus removal is impractical, as another would likely form. Antibacterial treatment and anthelmintics to kill the migrating larvae are of considerable value. The most rational approach to cranial mesenteric and aortic-iliac thrombosis in horses is prevention and control of strongylosis (p 267).

Surgical removal of aortic emboli may be attempted in cats; however, it is difficult and often unrewarding. Most authorities recommend medical therapy only, including analgesics, anticoagulants, careful use of IV fluids (sufficient to maintain hydration and blood pressure but not exacerbate congestive heart failure), and specific therapy for underlying heart disease. Streptokinase (90,000 IU/cat, IV over 20 min followed by 45,000 IU as a continuous infusion for 2-24 hr) can be given to lyse thrombi, but will increase the risk of bleeding. Recombinant tissue-type plasminogen activator (tPA) promotes fibrinolysis by binding to fibrin within thrombi and converting entrapped plasminogen to plasmin. In a study of cats with spontaneous thromboembolism given tPA (0.25-1 mg/kg/hr, IV, up to a total dose of 1-10 mg/kg), 43% survived the therapy and walked within 48 hr of administration. However, 50% of the cats died from reperfusion syndrome, heart failure, or from no obvious cause, suggesting that this therapy should be reserved for cats with serious disease.

Acepromazine (0.2-0.4 mg/kg, SC, TID) and hydralazine (0.5-0.8 mg/kg, PO, TID) have been given to improve vasodilation and collateral circulation, although the benefits are not clear. They may also cause hypotensive side effects or non-uniform arterial dilation. Unfractionated heparin (220 IU/kg, IV initially, followed by maintenance doses of 66 IU/kg, SC, QID) traditionally has been used to prevent further clot formation. Its use for this indication remains controversial, because its efficacy has never been established. Low-molecular-weight heparin may potentially have greater efficacy and safety, but dosages vary widely and are still being investigated. The dosages of both unfractionated and low-molecular-weight heparin should be adjusted to prolong activated partial thromboplastin time to 1.5-2 times pretreatment values. The primary complication is bleeding. Warfarin (0.25-0.5 mg/cat, SID) has been used both to prevent further clot formation after thromboembolism has occurred and prophylactically in cats with cardiomyopathy. The initial oral dosage is adjusted to prolong the prothrombin time to twice the normal reference range. Joint treatment with warfarin and heparin should only be considered for indoor cats that can be monitored frequently, because of the possiblity of serious bleeding; such therapy may have no effect on established thrombi.

Aspirin (25 mg/kg, PO, every 48-72 hr or $^1/_4$ of a 5-grain tablet) is the most widely used preventive therapy for feline thromboembolism. It preserves collateral circulation by inhibiting formation of thromboxane A_2 and irreversibly inhibits platelet aggregation.

However, evidence that aspirin prevents first time or recurrent thromboembolism is lacking.

Many cats with aortic thromboembolism die despite treatment or fail to regain hind-limb function. Some cats that survive the initial cardiovascular crisis recover the ability to walk after several weeks, but residual deficits, including muscle contracture and peripheral neuropathy, are common. The longterm prognosis often depends on the severity of underlying heart disease.

Treatment recommendations for pulmonary thromboembolism in dogs are the same as for aortic thromboemboli in cats.

■ ■ ■

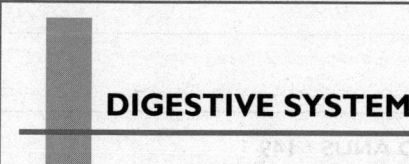

DIGESTIVE SYSTEM

INTESTINAL DISEASES IN PIGS   244

GASTROINTESTINAL PARASITES OF RUMINANTS   254

MALASSIMILATION SYNDROMES 301

ABDOMINAL FAT NECROSIS 306

SMALL ANIMALS

DISEASES OF THE MOUTH 307

DISEASES OF THE ESOPHAGUS   315

DISEASES OF THE STOMACH AND INTESTINES   319

DIGESTIVE SYSTEM
INTRODUCTION

The digestive tract includes the oral cavity and associated organs (lips, teeth, tongue, and salivary glands), the esophagus, the forestomachs (reticulum, rumen, omasum) of ruminants and the true stomach in all species, the small intestine, the liver, the exocrine pancreas, the large intestine, and the rectum and anus. Gut-associated lymphoid tissue (tonsils, Peyer's patches, diffuse lymphoid tissue) is distributed along the GI tract. The peritoneum covers the abdominal viscera and is involved in many GI diseases. Fundamental efforts to manage GI disorders should always be directed toward localizing disease to a particular segment and determining a cause. A rational therapeutic plan can then be formulated.

Function: The primary functions of the GI tract include prehension of feed and water; mastication, ensalivation, and swallowing of feed; digestion of feed and absorption of nutrients; maintenance of fluid and electrolyte balance; and evacuation of waste products. There are 4 primary functions—digestion, absorption, motility, and evacuation—and, correspondingly, 4 primary modes of dysfunction.

Normal GI tract motility involves peristalsis, muscle activity that moves ingesta from the esophagus to the rectum; segmentation movements, which churn and mix the ingesta; and segmental resistance and sphincter tone, which retard aboral progression of gut contents. In ruminants, these movements are of major importance in normal forestomach function.

Pathophysiology: Abnormal motor function usually manifests as decreased motility. Segmental resistance is usually reduced, and transit rate increases. Motility depends on stimulation via the sympathetic and parasympathetic nervous systems (and thus on the activity of the central and peripheral parts of these systems) and on the GI musculature and its intrinsic nerve plexuses. Debility, accompanied by weakness of the musculature, acute peritonitis, and hypokalemia, produces atony of the gut wall (paralytic ileus). The intestines distend with fluid and gas, and fecal output is reduced. In addition, chronic stasis of the small intestine may predispose to abnormal proliferation of microflora. Such bacterial overgrowth may cause malabsorption by injuring mucosal cells, by competing for nutrients, and by deconjugating bile salts and hydroxylating fatty acids.

Vomiting (p 389) is a neural reflex act that results in ejection of food and fluid from the stomach through the oral cavity. It is always associated with antecedent events such as premonition, nausea, salivation, or shivering, and is accompanied by repeated contractions of the abdominal muscles.

Regurgitation is characterized by passive, retrograde reflux of previously swallowed material from the esophagus, stomach, or rumen. In diseases of the esophagus, swallowed material may fail to reach the stomach.

One of the major consequences of subnormal motility is distention with fluid and gas. Much of the accumulated fluid is saliva and gastric and intestinal juices secreted during normal digestion. Distention causes pain and reflex spasm of adjoining gut segments. It also stimulates further secretion of fluid into the lumen of the gut, which exacerbates the condition. When the distention exceeds a critical point, the ability of the musculature of the wall to respond diminishes, the initial pain disappears, and paralytic ileus develops in which all GI muscle tone is lost.

Dehydration, acid-base and electrolyte imbalance, and circulatory failure are major consequences of GI distention. Accumulation of gut fluids stimulates additional secretion of fluids and electrolytes in the anterior segments of the intestine, which can worsen the abnormalities and lead to shock.

Abdominal pain associated with GI disease usually is caused by stretching of the intestinal wall. Contraction of the gut causes pain by direct and reflex distention of neighboring segments. Spasm, an exaggerated segmenting contraction of one section of intestine, results in distention of the immediately anterior segment when a peristaltic wave arrives. Other factors that may cause abdominal pain include edema and failure of local blood supply, eg, in local embolism or twisting of the mesentery.

Specific diseases cause diarrhea by varied and characteristic mechanisms, the recognition of which is useful in understanding, diagnosing, and managing GI diseases. The major mechanisms of diarrhea are increased permeability, hypersecretion, and osmosis. Disorders of motility are often secondary. In healthy animals, water and electrolytes continuously transfer across the intestinal mucosa. Secretions (from blood to gut) and absorptions (from gut to blood) occur simultaneously. In clinically normal animals, absorption exceeds secretion, ie, there is net absorption. Inflammation in the intestines can be accompanied by an increase in "pore size" in the mucosa, permitting increased flow through the membrane ("leak") down the pressure gradient from blood to the intestinal lumen. If the amount exuded exceeds the absorptive capacity of the intestines, diarrhea results. The size of the material that leaks through the mucosa varies, depending on the magnitude of the increase in pore size. Large increases in pore size permit exudation of plasma protein, resulting in protein-losing enteropathies (eg, lymphangiectasia in dogs, paratuberculosis in cattle, nematode infections). Greater increases in pore size result in the loss of RBC, producing hemorrhagic diarrhea (eg, hemorrhagic gastroenteritis, parvovirus infection, severe hookworm infection).

Hypersecretion is a net intestinal loss of fluid and electrolytes that is independent of changes in permeability, absorptive capacity, or exogenously generated osmotic gradients. Enterotoxic colibacillosis is an example of diarrheal disease due to intestinal hypersecretion; enterotoxigenic *Escherichia coli* produce enterotoxin that stimulates the crypt epithelium to secrete fluid beyond the absorptive capacity of the intestines. The villi, along with their digestive and absorptive capabilities, remain intact. The fluid secreted is isotonic, alkaline, and free of exudates. The intact villi are beneficial because a fluid (administered PO) that contains glucose, amino acids, and sodium is absorbed, even in the face of hypersecretion.

Osmotic diarrhea is seen when inadequate absorption results in a collection of solutes in the gut lumen, which cause water to be retained by their osmotic activity. It develops in any condition that results in nutrient malabsorption or maldigestion.

Malabsorption (see p 301 and p 339) is failure of digestion and absorption due to some defect in the villous digestive and absorptive cells, which are mature cells that cover the villi. Several epitheliotropic viruses directly infect and destroy the villous absorptive epithelial cells or their precursors, eg, coronavirus, transmissible gastroenteritis virus of piglets, and rotavirus of calves. Feline panleukopenia virus and canine parvovirus destroys the crypt epithelium, which results in failure of renewal of villous absorptive cells and collapse of the villi; regeneration is a longer process after parvoviral infection than after viral infections of villous tip epithelium (eg, coronavirus, rotavirus). Intestinal malabsorption also may be caused by any defect that impairs absorptive capacity, such as diffuse inflammatory disorders (eg, lymphocytic-plasmacytic enteritis, eosinophilic enteritis) or neoplasia (eg, lymphosarcoma).

Other examples of malabsorption include defects of pancreatic secretion that result in maldigestion. Rarely, because of failure to digest lactose (which, in large amounts, has a hyperosmotic effect), neonatal farm animals or pups may have diarrhea while they are being fed milk. Reduced secretion of digestive enzymes at the surface of villous tip cells is characteristic of epitheliotropic viral infections recognized in farm animals.

The ability of the GI tract to digest food depends on its motor and secretory functions and, in herbivores, on the activity of the microflora of the forestomachs of ruminants, or of the cecum and colon of horses and pigs. The flora of ruminants can digest cellulose; ferment carbohydrates to volatile fatty acids; and convert nitrogenous substances to ammonia, amino acids, and protein. In certain circumstances, the activity of the flora can be suppressed to the point that digestion becomes abnormal or ceases. Incorrect diet, prolonged starvation or inappetence, and hyperacidity (as occurs in engorgement on grain) all impair microbial digestion. The bacteria, yeasts, and protozoa also may be adversely affected by the oral administration of drugs that are antimicrobial or that drastically alter the pH of rumen contents.

Clinical Findings of GI Disease: These include excessive salivation, diarrhea, constipation or scant feces, vomiting, regurgitation, GI tract hemorrhage, abdominal pain and distention, tenesmus, shock and dehydration, and suboptimal performance. The location and nature of the lesions that cause malfunction often can be determined by recognition and analysis of the clinical findings. In addition, abnormalities of prehension, mastication, and swallowing usually are associated with diseases of the oral mucosa, the teeth, the mandible or other bony structures of the head, or the esophagus. Vomiting is most common in single-stomached animals and usually is due to gastroenteritis or nonalimentary disease (eg, uremia, pyometra, endocrine disease). Regurgitation may signify disease of the oropharynx or esophagus and is not accompanied by the premonitory signs seen with vomiting.

Large-volume, fluid diarrhea usually is associated with hypersecretion (eg, in enterotoxigenic colibacillosis in newborn calves) or with malabsorptive (osmotic) effects. Blood and fibrinous casts in the feces indicate a hemorrhagic, fibrinonecrotic enteritis of the small or large intestine, eg, bovine viral diarrhea, coccidiosis, salmonellosis, or swine dysentery. Black, tarry feces (melena) indicate hemorrhage in the stomach or upper part of the small intestine. Tenesmus of GI origin usually is associated with inflammatory disease of the rectum and anus.

Small amounts of soft feces may indicate a partial obstruction of the intestines. Abdominal distention can result from accumulation of gas, fluid, or ingesta, usually due to hypomotility (functional obstruction, adynamic paralytic ileus) or to a physical obstruction (eg, foreign body or intussusception). Distention may, of course, result from something as direct as overeating. A "ping" heard during auscultation and percussion of the abdomen indicates a gas-filled viscus. A sudden onset of severe abdominal distention in the adult ruminant usually is due to ruminal tympany. Ballottement and succussion may reveal fluid-splashing sounds when the rumen or bowel is filled with fluid. Varying degrees of dehydration and acid-base and electrolyte imbalance, which may lead to shock, are seen when large quantities of fluid are lost (eg, in diarrhea or sequestered in intestinal obstruction) or in gastric or abomasal volvulus.

Abdominal pain is due to stretching or inflammation of the serosal surfaces of abdominal viscera or the peritoneum; it may be acute or subacute, and its manifestation varies among species. In horses, acute abdominal pain is common (*see* COLIC, p 202). Subacute pain is more common in cattle and is characterized by reluctance to move and by grunting with each respiration or deep palpation of the abdomen. Abdominal pain in dogs and cats may be acute or subacute and is characterized by whining, meowing, and abnormal postures (eg, outstretched forelimbs, the sternum on the floor, and the hindlimbs raised).

Examination of the GI Tract: A complete, accurate history and routine clinical examination can often determine the diagnosis. In outbreaks of GI tract disease in farm animals, the history and epidemiologic findings are of prime importance. If the history and epidemiologic and clinical findings are consistent with GI disease, the lesion should be localized within the system, and the type of lesion and its cause determined.

The abnormality may be localized to the large or small intestine by history, physical examination, and fecal characteristics (TABLE 1). The distinction is important because it narrows the differential diagnoses and determines the direction of further investigation.

The clinical and laboratory techniques and their applications include the following: 1) visual inspection of the oral cavity, and of the contour of the abdomen for distention or contraction; 2) palpation through the abdominal wall or per rectum to evaluate shape, size, and position of abdominal viscera; 3) abdominal percussion to detect "pings," which suggest gas-filled viscera; 4) auscultation to determine the intensity, frequency, and duration of GI movements, as well as fluid-splashing sounds associated with fluid-filled stomachs and intestines and fluid-rushing sounds associated with diarrheal disease; 5) succussion to reveal fluid-splashing sounds; 6) ballottement to evaluate density and size of abdominal organs by their movement away from and back to the abdominal wall; and 7) gross examination of feces to assess bulk, consistency, color, and presence of mucus, blood, or undigested food particles.

Microscopic studies include examination for parasites. Cytology of a rectal or colonic mucosal smear stained with new methylene blue or Wright's stain for fecal leukocytes is useful to detect inflammatory bowel disease. The following may be useful (or necessary): 1) bacterial culture and virus isolation; 2) endoscopy to visualize the mucosal surface of the esophagus, stomach, duodenum, colon, and rectum; 3) abdominocentesis to collect fluid from distended viscera or from the peritoneal cavity for examination; 4) radiography (contrast) to diagnose obstructive disease; 5) abdominal ultrasonography to detect abdominal masses, intussusceptions, and mesenteric lymphadenopathy in small animals, and to investigate abdominal disorders in horses and cows; 6) biopsy (endoscopic, laparoscopic, surgical) to obtain samples for microscopic examination (samples of intestines

TABLE 1. Differentiation of Small-intestinal from Large-intestinal Diarrhea

Clinical Sign	Small Intestine	Large Intestine
Frequency of defecation	Normal or slightly increased	Very frequent
Fecal volume	Large quantity; bulky or watery	Small quantities often
Urgency	Absent	Usually present
Tenesmus	Absent	Usually present
Mucus in feces	Usually absent	Frequent
Blood in feces	Dark black (melena)	Red (fresh)
Weight loss	May be present	Rare

and liver are useful in diagnosing chronic enteritis and liver disease); and 7) tests for digestion and absorption to estimate and differentiate malabsorption and maldigestion. Common absorption tests include the measurement of the serum concentrations of cobalamin (vitamin B_{12}) and folate. In addition, in small animals, an elevated serum folate concentration in conjunction with a depressed cobalamin is consistent with small intestinal bacterial overgrowth. Pancreatic function can be evaluated by the determination of serum trypsin-like immunoreactivity; laparotomy and biopsy may be indicated in cases in which the diagnosis is not clear or in which surgical correction may be required.

INFECTIOUS DISEASES

The GI tract is subject to infection by many pathogens, which are a major cause of economic loss due to illness, suboptimal performance, and death (see TABLE 2). These infections spread by direct contact or the fecal-oral route. Many of the pathogens are part of the normal intestinal flora, and disease develops only after a stressful event, eg, salmonellosis in horses after transportation, extended anesthesia, or surgery. The intestinal flora becomes established within a few hours after birth, which emphasizes the importance of the early ingestion of colostrum to provide protection against septicemia and intestinal infection.

Definitive etiologic diagnosis of infectious disease of the GI tract depends on demonstrating the pathogen in the tract or in the feces of the affected animal. In herd epidemics, such as an outbreak of acute undifferentiated diarrhea in newborn calves or piglets, the best opportunity to establish a diagnosis is in the earliest stage of the disease by selecting untreated animals and submitting them for necropsy and detailed microbiologic examination of the intestinal flora. When selective necropsy is not an option, a series of carefully collected daily fecal samples should be submitted to a diagnostic laboratory with a request for special culture techniques, depending on the infectious disease that is suspected. ELISA have been developed to demonstrate the presence of viral antigen within the feces, which can provide a definitive diagnosis (eg, canine parvovirus).

Overview of Gastrointestinal Parasitism

The GI tract may be inhabited by many species of parasites. Their cycles may be direct, in which eggs and larvae are passed in the feces and stadial development occurs to the infective stage, which is then ingested by the final host. Alternatively, the immature stages may be ingested by an intermediate host (usually an invertebrate) in which further development occurs, and infection is acquired when the intermediate host or free-living stage shed by that host is ingested by the final host. Sometimes, there is no development in the intermediate host, in which case it is known as a transport or paratenic host, depending on whether the larvae are encapsulated or in the tissues. Clinical parasitism depends on the number and pathogenicity of the parasites, which depend on the biotic potential of the parasites or, when appropriate, their intermediate host and the climate and management practices. In the host, resistance, age, nutrition, and concomitant disease also influence the course of parasitic infection. The economic importance of subclinical parasitism in farm animals is also determined by the above factors, and it is well established that lightly parasitized animals that show no clinical evidence of disease perform less efficiently in the feedlot, dairy, or finishing house.

Feed conversion in light to moderate parasitism is adversely affected and is primarily due to reduced appetite and poor use of absorbed protein and energy. Carcass quality and size also are reduced, which further reduce financial returns. Endoparasites of companion animals can cause severe disease or unthriftiness and are aesthetically undesirable. Furthermore, some of these parasites also infect humans.

Because parasitism is easily confused with other debilitating conditions, diagnosis depends heavily on the seasonal character of parasitic infection; previous farm history; and examination of feces for evidence of oocysts, worm eggs, or larvae. Increased serum pepsinogen levels can support the diagnosis of some abomasal infections, as can increased serum liver enzymes for liver fluke infection. ELISA are being used, and other serologic (including monoclonal antibody) techniques are under development; serodiagnosis

TABLE 2.   Common Pathogens of the Gastrointestinal Tract

	Cattle, Sheep, and Goats	Pigs
Viruses	Bovine viral diarrhea, rotavirus, coronavirus, rinderpest, malignant catarrhal fever, bluetongue, foot-and-mouth disease	Transmissible gastroenteritis, rotavirus, coronavirus, foot-and-mouth disease, vesicular stomatitis, vesicular exanthema
Rickettsiae		
Bacteria	Enterotoxigenic *E coli*, *Salmonella* spp, *Mycobacterium paratuberculosis*, *Fusobacterium necrophorum*, *Clostridium perfringens* (types B, C, and D), *Actinobacillus lignieresii*, *Yersinia enterocolitica*, *Campylobacter jejuni*	Enterotoxigenic *E coli*, *Salmonella* spp, *Serpulina hyodysenteriae*, *Clostridium perfringens* types B and C
Protozoa	*Eimeria* spp, *Cryptosporidium* spp	*Eimeria* spp, *Isospora suis*
Fungi	*Candida* spp (cattle)	*Candida* spp
Algae	*Prototheca* spp	*Prototheca* spp
Parasites (helminths)	*See* GASTROINTESTINAL PARASITES OF RUMINANTS, p 254.	*See* GASTROINTESTINAL PARASITES OF PIGS, p 270.

will likely be used more frequently as the specificity of the tests improves. These tests should be particularly useful in companion animals harboring parasites incriminated in zoonoses.

Advances in epidemiology (particularly regarding factors affecting seasonal development of the free-living stages and their survival), coupled with the discovery of highly efficient broad-spectrum anthelmintics, have made successful treatment and control of GI parasites both possible and practical. Response to therapy is usually rapid, and single treatments usually suffice unless reinfection occurs or the lesions are particularly severe. Preventive control in large animals is generally achieved by integrating grassland management with the use of anthelmintics. Improved methods of administering anthelmintics (eg, the pour-on method or sustained or pulsed-release devices) have also helped. Strategies to prevent parasitism and related production losses are part of any modern herd-health, flock, or stud program. Similar preventive programs are equally important in controlling parasitism in pet animals. Control by vaccination is limited to lungworms; vaccine for cattle is available in several European countries, and vaccine for sheep is available in parts of eastern Europe and in the Middle East.

For estimating parasite load, *see* p 1362.

Treatment of Infectious Diseases

Antimicrobial agents are used for the treatment of bacterial diseases, and anthelmintics for parasitic diseases. There is no specific therapy for treatment of viral diseases.

◀ **TABLE 2.** *(continued)*

Horses	Dogs and Cats
Rotavirus, vesicular stomatitis	Canine parvovirus, canine coronavirus, feline panleukopenia virus, feline enteric coronavirus, canine and feline rotaviruses, canine and feline astroviruses
Ehrlichia risticii (Potomac horse fever [equine monocytic ehrlichiosis])	*Neorickettsia helminthoeca* (salmon poisoning in dogs)
Enterotoxigenic *E coli, Salmonella* spp, *Rhodococcus equi, Actinobacillus equuli, Clostridium perfringens* types B and C	*Salmonella* spp, *Yersinia enterocolitica, Campylobacter jejuni, Bacillus piliformis, Clostridium* spp, *Mycobacterium* spp, *Shigella* spp
Eimeria spp	*Isospora* spp, *Sarcocystis* spp, *Besnoitia* spp, *Hammondia* sp, *Toxoplasma* sp, *Giardia* sp, *Trichomonas* spp, *Entamoeba histolytica, Balantidium coli, Cryptosporidium* spp
Aspergillus fumigatus	*Histoplasma capsulatum, Aspergillus* spp, *Candida albicans,* phycomycetes
Prototheca spp	*Prototheca* spp
See GASTROINTESTINAL PARASITES OF HORSES, p 265.	*See* GASTROINTESTINAL PARASITES OF SMALL ANIMALS, p 352.

Antimicrobials are commonly given PO daily for several days until recovery is apparent, but there is little objective evidence for efficacy. There is evidence that overdosage or prolonged oral treatment may be detrimental (eg, bacterial overgrowth, villous atrophy). Parenteral administration of antimicrobials is indicated when septicemia is apparent or may occur. The choice of antimicrobial agent depends on the suspected disease, previous results, and cost. In herd epidemics, antimicrobials may be added to the feed or water supplies at therapeutic levels for several days, followed by preventive levels for an extended period, depending on the infection pressure in the population. The feed and water supplies of in-contact animals also may be medicated in an attempt to prevent new cases from developing. (*See also* SYSTEMIC PHARMACOTHERAPEUTICS OF THE DIGESTIVE SYSTEM, p 1979.)

Control of Infectious Diseases

Effective control of the common infectious diseases of the GI tract depends on practicing good sanitation and hygiene, developing and maintaining nonspecific resistance in the animal, and in certain cases, providing specific immunity by vaccinating the pregnant dam or susceptible animal.

Effective sanitation and hygiene is achieved primarily by providing adequate space for animals and by regular cleaning of pens and efficient removal of manure from the immediate environment. Development and maintenance of nonspecific resistance depends on the genetic selection of animals that have a reasonable degree of inherent resistance and on the provision of adequate nutrition and housing, which minimizes stress and allows the animals to grow and behave normally. The development of infected but clinically normal animals, which can shed pathogens for weeks or months, is a major problem with some infectious diseases of the GI tract, eg, salmonellosis. Ideally, these carrier animals should be identified by microbiologic means and isolated from the rest of the herd until free of the infection or culled.

Certain diseases (eg, enterotoxigenic colibacillosis in calves and piglets) can be controlled by vaccination of the pregnant dam several weeks before parturition. This method depends on achieving a protective level of antibodies in the colostrum. There are exceptions but, in most cases, systemic immunity provides little protection against the infectious enteritides; effective immunity against GI disease depends on stimulation of local intestinal immunity after the neonatal period. During the neonatal period, protection can be provided through the local action of maternally derived antibodies. For example, secretory IgA progressively increases in sow's milk from the time of farrowing until weaning, which provides the piglet with daily protection during the nursing period.

NONINFECTIOUS DISEASES

The major causes of noninfectious disease of the GI tract include dietary overload or indigestible feeds, chemical or physical agents, obstruction of the stomach and intestines caused by the ingestion of foreign bodies or by any physical displacement or injury to the GI tract that interferes with the flow of ingesta, enzyme deficiencies, abnormalities of the mucosa that interfere with normal function (eg, gastric ulcers, inflammatory bowel disease, villous atrophy, neoplasms), and congenital defects. GI manifestations such as vomiting and diarrhea may occur secondary to systemic or metabolic diseases such as uremia, liver disease, and hypoadrenocorticism. Equine colic (p 202) is a special case because of the prevalence of intestinal lesions due to parasitism, which predispose to subacute and acute dysfunction. The causes are uncertain in several diseases, including abomasal ulcers in cattle, gastric ulcers in pigs and foals, gastric torsion in dogs, and acute intestinal obstruction and displacement of the abomasum in cattle. In noninfectious diseases of the GI tract, usually only a single animal is affected at one time; exceptions are diseases associated with excessive feed intake or poisons, in which herd outbreaks are common.

PRINCIPLES OF THERAPY

See also SYSTEMIC PHARMACOTHERAPEUTICS OF THE MONOGASTRIC AND RUMINANT DIGESTIVE SYSTEMS, p 1979 and p 1993.

Although eliminating the cause of the disease is the primary objective, the major part of treatment is supportive and symptomatic, aimed at relieving pain, correcting abnormalities, and allowing healing to occur.

Elimination of the primary cause may involve antimicrobials, coccidiostats, antifungal agents, anthelmintics, antidotes for poisons, or surgical correction of displacements.

Correction of excessive or depressed motility appears rational, but often the nature and degree of abnormal motility are uncertain; in addition, available drugs may not give consistent results. There is little clinical evidence to recommend the routine use of anticholinergic or opiate drugs to slow intestinal transit. Slowing intestinal transit may be counterproductive to the defense mechanism of diarrhea, which acts to evacuate harmful organisms and their toxins. In general, anticholinergic drugs probably are justified only for short-term symptomatic relief of pain and tenesmus associated with inflammatory diseases of the colon and rectum. In some disorders of gastric or colonic motility, prokinetic drugs (eg, metoclopramide, erythromycin) may be useful.

Replacement of fluid and electrolytes is necessary when dehydration and electrolyte and acid-base imbalance occur as in diarrhea, persistent vomiting, intestinal obstruction, or torsion of the stomach(s), in which large amounts of fluid and electrolytes are sequestered.

Relief of distention medically by stomach tube (as in bloat in ruminants) or surgically (as in acute intestinal obstruction, or in torsion of the abomasum in ruminants or of the stomach in monogastric animals) may be required. The GI tract may become distended with gas, fluid, or ingesta at any level due to physical or functional obstruction.

Relief of abdominal pain by administration of analgesics should be done when the pain is reflexly affecting other body systems (eg, cardiovascular collapse) or when it is causing the animal to injure itself because of rolling, kicking, or throwing itself. Animals treated with analgesics must be monitored regularly to ensure that the relief of pain does not provide a false sense of security; the lesion may be progressively worsening while the animal is under the influence of the analgesic.

Reconstitution of ruminal flora should be done in situations in which the ruminal flora may be seriously depleted (eg, in prolonged anorexia or acute indigestion). Transfaunation (p 1994) involves oral administration of ruminal juice from a normal animal that contains rumen bacteria and protozoa and volatile fatty acids.

CONGENITAL AND INHERITED ANOMALIES OF THE DIGESTIVE SYSTEM

MOUTH

Cleft Palate or Cleft Lip (Harelip) Complex: This is due to a disturbance of the processes that form the jaw and face during embryonic development. Cleft of the lower lip is rare and usually occurs on the midline. Clefts of the upper lip, usually at the junction of the premaxilla and maxilla, may be unilateral or bilateral, complete or incomplete, and often are associated with clefts of the alveolar process and palate. The defect may also involve the palate alone, affecting the hard or soft components of the palate, or both. Developmental anomalies affecting other organ systems are seen in ~8% of dogs and cats with cleft palate or lips. Similarly, in large animals, cleft palate or lip is commonly seen with other defects, such as arthrogryposis, which is inherited in a simple autosomal recessive manner in Charolais cattle. In Texel sheep, a syndrome of bilateral cleavage of the lip with accompanying defects of the maxilla has been reported to have an autosomal recessive mode of inheritance. In small animals, incidence is higher in Beagles, Cocker Spaniels, Dachshunds, German Shepherds, Labrador Retrievers, Schnauzers, Shetland Sheepdogs, and Siamese cats. Brachycephalic breeds can have up to a 30% risk factor. In large animals, cleft palate/lip complex has been reported in cattle, sheep, goats, and horses. The primary etiology is hereditary, although maternal nutritional deficiencies, drug or chemical exposure, mechanical interferences with the fetus, and some viral infections during pregnancy have also been implicated. Ingestion of toxic agents may also play a role; eg, ingestion of lupines (*Lupinus sericeus* and *L caudatus*) during the second and third months of gestation in cattle can potentially result in "crooked calf disease," of which cleft abnormalities may be a component.

Initial signs reflect the extent of the malformation but may include difficulty suckling, dysphagia, and evidence of milk dripping from the nostrils when the newborn attempts to nurse. Respiratory infection due to aspiration of food is common and a grave consequence with a poor prognosis. Examination of the oral cavity generally readily reveals the defect, except in foals having only a cleft of the soft palate that may be difficult to see.

Initial management requires intensive nursing care, including hand or tube feeding to ensure daily nutritional and caloric requirements are met, as well as the occasional need for appropriate antimicrobial therapy to treat secondary infections of the rhinarium or lower respiratory tract. Surgical correction is effective only if the defect is small and is usually done at ~6-8 wk of age in small animals, before their general health is compromised. Various surgical techniques, ranging from simple closure to sliding grafts or prosthetic implants, are used, depending on the severity and location of the defect. More severely affected animals may require multiple surgeries for successful correction. Historically, surgical correction has been associated with a high failure rate; however, newer techniques, such as the bilateral mucosal overlapping pedicle flap repair for soft palate defects, are improving success rates in dogs. Surgical repair should be attempted only after ethical questions have been addressed, and the affected animal should be surgically sterilized or removed from breeding stock to prevent reproducing the anomaly in future offspring.

Occlusal Anomalies: **Brachygnathia** (overshot, short lower jaw, or parrot mouth in horses) is manifest when the mandible is shorter than the maxilla. It can be found, with varying severity and incidence, in all species of animals. In cattle, it is inherited as a polygenetic factor and can be associated with other anomalies such as impacted molar teeth and osteopetrosis (p 849) in Angus calves and Simmental cattle, or with chromosomal aberrations such as trisomy, which is lethal. In small animals, mild forms may be of no clinical significance; however, more severe forms may result in trauma to the hard palate or the restriction of normal mandibular growth secondary to erupting adult mandibular canine teeth. Diagnosis is through careful oral examination. Treatment varies from none to various orthodontic or endodontic procedures, depending on severity. In small animals, the mandibular canine teeth are often removed or shortened, with concurrent pulpotomy or root canal. A range of occlusal defects in sheep, from brachygnathia to mandibular aplasia and agnathia, is reportedly inherited as a simple autosomal recessive. **Craniofacial dysplasia** of Limousin cattle is characterized by a convex profile of the nose, short lower jaw, deficient ossification of frontal sutures, exophthalmos, and a large tongue; it is thought to be due to homozygosity of a simple autosomal recessive gene.

Prognathia (undershot, or monkey or sow mouth in horses) is found when the mandible is longer than the maxilla. It is identified on oral examination by finding the mandibular incisors in contact with or rostral to the maxillary incisors. In brachycephalic dogs and Persian cats, it is considered a normal breed characteristic. Despite being seen to varying degrees, it rarely requires any specific treatment. If a foal is badly affected, suckling may be impossible; treatment, if feasible, consists of rasping or shearing the offending points and projections. In ruminants, it is often seen, to minor degrees, at birth, and it corrects spontaneously as the animal grows. More severe anomalies can impair the ability to graze and masticate and, therefore, have more serious repercussions.

In Angus calves, a facial defect characterized by a broad, short face is accompanied by degenerative joint disease and has a complex genetic transmission.

Tongue Anomalies: **Ankyloglossia** or **microglossia** refers to incomplete or abnormal development of the tongue. It is often referred to as "**bird tongue**" in dogs and may be a component of the fading puppy syndrome. Affected puppies have difficulty nursing and do poorly. Oral examination reveals missing or underdeveloped lateral and rostral thin portions of the tongue that result in prehensile and motility disturbances. It is generally lethal. **Macroglossia**, or large tongue, is seen in belted Galloway cattle but resolves with age and is rarely clinically significant.

Epitheliogenesis imperfecta, or "smooth tongue," is a condition of incomplete development of the lingual filiform papillae that is transmitted as an autosomal recessive trait in Holstein, Friesian, and Brown Swiss cattle. It results in excessive salivation and an unthrifty condition.

Tight-lip Syndrome of Chinese Shar-Peis: Some Shar-Peis have a small or absent lower anterior lip vestibule. The lower lip covers the lower teeth and folds over the lower incisor teeth toward the tongue. Contact between the palatal surface of the upper incisors and the lower lip worsens the lip position and may contribute to the lingual displacement of the lower incisor teeth. Surgical correction requires creating a vestibule through a horizontal release incision, dissecting free the mucosa, then suturing a free mucosal graft over the exposed connective tissue to prevent healing of the cut margins to each other that would result in a relapse.

TEETH

Abnormal Number: In most species, a reduction in the number of teeth (termed **anodontia**) is rare, although in dogs, molars and premolars may fail to develop or erupt. Supernumerary teeth occasionally are found in the incisor or molar regions of horses; in dogs, they are usually unilateral and most often in the upper jaw. In dogs, although rare, improper germination of the permanent dental arcade may lead to splitting of the tooth bud to form 2 teeth. The result may be crowding and subsequent rotation of the teeth, which necessitates extraction to prevent or correct occlusal abnormalities. In horses, supernumerary teeth are either removed or periodically rasped, especially if they interfere with mastication or are irritated by a bit.

Irregularities of Shedding: In premolar teeth of ruminants, the root of the temporary tooth may be absorbed, but the crown may persist as a covering or "cap" to the erupting permanent tooth. These caps are readily removed with forceps if they have not separated spontaneously. Delayed shedding of deciduous teeth in dogs is common and secondary to the failure of the periodontal ligament to detach from the deciduous tooth, with the permanent canine teeth erupting rostrally. This may cause permanent tooth displacement, which can occur within 2-3 wk, and result in malocclusion or food entrapment and subsequent periodontal disease. Therefore, retained deciduous teeth should be removed as soon as possible, taking care not to damage the underlying permanent tooth bud.

Abnormalities in Position, Shape, and Direction: In horses, this may affect the incisors and result in long-axis rotation or overlapping of adjacent teeth. In brachycephalic dogs, the upper third premolar and occasionally other premolar or molar teeth may rotate. Usually, this is of no clinical significance but may require extraction of some involved teeth if crowding or occlusal abnormalities occur. Abnormalities in shape, including dens in dente, are reported in various species and breeds. Clinical significance is variable and based on severity, with most being incidental findings.

Enamel Lesions: Hypoplasia or disruption in enamel formation can occur in both large and small animals. Common causes are pyrexia, trauma, malnutrition, toxicosis (eg, fluorosis in cattle), and infections (eg, distemper virus in dogs). Lesions vary, depending on the severity and duration of the insult, from pitted enamel to the absence of enamel with incomplete tooth development. Affected teeth are prone to plaque and tartar accumulation and subsequent bacterial penetration and formation of caries. In small animals, resin restoration has been used to cover defects, although diligent dental hygiene and home care is critical in reducing the incidence of complications. Enamel may also develop discoloration. In small animals, administration of tetracyclines to pregnant females or to puppies <6 mo old may result in a permanent brownish yellow discoloration of the teeth. In ruminants, the enamel of some teeth may demonstrate flecks of varying color. The condition is thought to have a genetic etiology but generally is of no clinical significance; however, some believe affected teeth may be prone to more rapid wearing.

CYSTS AND SINUSES OF THE HEAD AND NECK

These imperfections in fetal development are important in their differentiation from infections such as abscessation. **Thyroglossal duct cyst** is the result of postnatal persistence of the early embryonic thyroglossal duct. This rare cyst is always single and found in the middle of the neck, usually at the level of the hyoid bone and larynx. It is smoothly rounded with a well-defined border, anchored to the hyoid bone and deep tissues. Unless infection is superimposed, it is seldom attached to the skin. It is not tender and contains fluid.

A **branchial (or lateral cervical) cyst** develops from branchial apparatus malformation, usually of the second branchial cleft. Unilateral or bilateral branchial cysts occupy a lateral position in the upper neck and are usually only slightly mobile. Their size varies considerably, and an individual cyst may change size periodically as its contents escape through a small opening into the throat or through a small cutaneous fistula (branchial or lateral cervical fistula).

Dentigerous cysts are of epithelial origin and arise from abnormal tooth development. They often contain tooth fragments and usually involve the maxilla and mandible to varying degrees. These cysts can be found in young (<3 yr) horses or ruminants (primarily sheep). In young horses, they may be difficult to differentiate from cystic sinuses (osteitis fibrosa cystica), which also typically result in facial or mandibular distortion.

Surgical removal of the cyst(s) is required, with definitive diagnosis based on subsequent histopathologic examination.

ESOPHAGUS

Clinically significant esophageal disorders generally manifest themselves as swallowing dysfunction and regurgitation, especially evident with the introduction of solid food. These disorders, found predominantly in small animals, can be classified as congenital megaesophagus, vascular ring entrapment anomalies, and achalasia. **Congenital megaesophagus** is thought to result from developmental anomalies in esophageal neuromuscular innervation. Incidence is increased in Chinese Shar-Peis, Fox Terriers, German Shepherds, Great Danes, Irish Setters, Labrador Retrievers, Miniature Schnauzers, Newfoundlands, and Siamese cats. In Fox Terriers, it is an autosomal recessive trait, whereas in Miniature Schnauzers, it is an autosomal dominant. Megaesophagus may also be a component of a more diffuse congenital neuropathy. A laryngeal paralysis-polyneuropathy complex that often includes megaesophagus has been reported in young Dalmatians. Also, dog breeds with a defined risk factor for hypothyroidism and hypoadrenocorticism may have a concurrent polyneuropathy that may manifest as megaesophagus. It may also be identified as a paraneoplastic syndrome in young dogs with thymoma (p 1060). **Vascular ring entrapment anomalies** most commonly result from persistence of the right fourth aortic arch during embryonic development, which results in esophageal entrapment at the heart base by the right fourth aortic arch, left atrium, pulmonic artery, and the ligamentum arteriosum. This obstructs food passage and results in food retention and subsequent esophageal dilation anterior to the anomaly. Boston Terriers, German Shepherds, and Irish Setters have higher breed incidences. **Cricopharyngeal achalasia** is a failure, or asynchrony, of the cricopharyngeus muscle to relax during swallowing, thereby preventing the normal passage of a food bolus from the caudal pharynx to the cranial esophagus. It has been mainly identified in toy breeds and rarely in cats. **Lower esophageal sphincter achalasia** is now considered to be a component of a more generalized esophageal motor disturbance (ie, megaesophagus) and no longer a distinct entity.

Identification of an esophageal disorder is generally based on characteristic clinical signs (eg, regurgitation) and contrast radiography or fluoroscopy of the swallowing reflex. Diagnosis of the specific underlying etiology may require further testing, such as endoscopy, endocrine function testing, and elimination of myasthenia gravis. Treatment is directed at the primary etiology. Some mildly affected dogs improve over time; those that do not have a poor longterm prognosis. Aspiration pneumonia is a frequent and often lethal complication. Frequent, elevated feedings of small quantities of a highly digestible diet the consistency of gruel may be helpful. Owner compliance is essential for successful management. Surgical correction of vascular ring anomalies, generally through transection of the ligamentum arteriosum (either during thoracotomy or via thoracoscopy), is effective if done early; otherwise, esophageal damage secondary to esophageal dilation from food retention may result in a permanent disorder of esophageal motility.

Esophageal diverticula may involve the cervical esophagus just cranial to the thoracic inlet or be epiphrenic (just cranial to the diaphragm). Clinical signs depend on severity and are seen in only 10-15% of cases but may include impaction, esophagitis, and rarely rupture or tracheoesophageal fistula formation. Treatment (if necessary) is via surgical removal. Periodic esophageal diverticulization just cranial to the thoracic inlet may be a normal breed variation in English Bulldogs.

HERNIAS

Hernias involving the abdomen are seen when abdominal contents protrude through a natural or abnormal opening in the body wall. They may be congenital or acquired. In acquired hernias, there is usually a history of trauma. Congenital hernias may involve the diaphragm or the abdominal wall. Hernias involving the diaphragm are of 3 main types: **peritoneopericardial**, in which abdominal contents are found extending into the pericardial sac; **pleuroperitoneal**, in which abdominal contents are found within the pleural cavity; and **hiatal**, in which the abdominal esophagus, gastroesophageal junction, and/or portions of the stomach protrude through the esophageal hiatus of the diaphragm into the thoracic cavity. Clinical signs vary from asymptomatic to severe and depend on the amount of herniated tissue and its effect on the organ it is displacing. Hiatal hernias may be "sliding" and result in clinical signs of reflux esophagitis (anorexia, salivation, and/or vomition) that may be intermittent. Diagnosis is through radiology; contrast studies are often needed for confirmation. Fluoroscopy or endoscopy is useful in the diagnosis of sliding hiatal hernias. Correction of the aforementioned hernias is best accomplished through surgery. In the case of hiatal hernias, medical therapy, including the use of systemic antacid preparations and dietary modification, may control signs if mild.

Hernias involving the abdominal wall include umbilical, inguinal, and scrotal. **Umbilical hernias** are secondary to failure of the normal closure of the umbilical ring and result in protrusion of abdominal contents into the overlying subcutis. Size varies depending on the extent of the umbilical defect and the amount of abdominal contents contained within it. The etiology in both large and small animals is likely to have a genetic component; however, excess traction on an oversized fetus or cutting the umbilical cord too close to the abdominal wall are other possible causes. Diagnosis is usually straightforward, especially if the hernia is manually reducible. If irreducible, the hernia must be differentiated from an umbilical abscess, which is common in large animals. Umbilical hernia and umbilical abscess often are seen together, especially in cattle and swine. Exploratory puncture, such as via fine-needle biopsy with cytopathology, may be required for confirmation. Correction is surgical. In small animals, if the hernia is small, surgical correction is often done at the same time as sterilization procedures. In calves, some success has been achieved by applying a binder of broad adhesive bandage (10 cm width) for 3-4 wk. The owner should be advised that the weakness may be heritable.

Inguinal hernias in male pigs are common, and they usually extend into the scrotum. Suspending the piglet by the forelegs and gently shaking, which generally causes even a small hernial bulge to become visible can confirm the diagnosis. In female pigs, this defect is invariably accompanied by arrested genital development; such animals are sterile, and surgery is indicated only when the size of the defect is a threat to the growth of the pig to market weight. Inguinal hernias in male foals often resolve spontaneously during the first year of life. For this reason, early corrective surgery is not indicated unless the hernia is strangulated or of such magnitude that it interferes with gait. Strangulated inguinal hernia in stallions is fairly frequent and is characterized by signs of constant and severe abdominal pain. It is readily recognized by rectal palpation and may be reduced, under general anesthesia, by rectal manipulation. If this fails, immediate surgery is necessary. Inguinal hernias in cattle are rare although sometimes seen in males. Surgical correction to preserve the breeding potential of the bull, when done, is not always successful.

STOMACH

Besides hiatal hernia (*see* above) the most common abnormality involving the stomach with a suspect heritable etiology is **pyloric stenosis**. Pyloric stenosis or hypertrophy results from muscular thickening of the pyloric sphincter, which obstructs pyloric outflow. Affected breeds include brachycephalic and smaller breeds, especially Boxers and Boston Terriers, as well as Siamese cats. Clinical signs reflect delayed gastric emptying and usually manifest as vomiting of food several hours after a meal. Treatment is through dietary modification and motility modifiers, such as metoclopramide or cisapride. In more severely affected cases, pyloromyotomy may be beneficial.

SMALL AND LARGE INTESTINE

Maldigestion or malabsorption disorders usually manifest as chronic, persistent GI signs including vomition, weight loss, small- and/or large-intestinal diarrhea, or a combination of the above. There are many potential etiologies, both heritable and acquired, and most are associated with inflammatory bowel disease (IBD). Congenital conditions may have specific breed predilections. Soft-coated Wheaten Terriers have a high incidence of concurrent **protein-losing enteropathy and nephropathy**. Both IBD and food allergies are considered to be a component of this syndrome. The demonstration of elevated fecal α_1-protease inhibitor concentrations can help confirm abnormal protein loss through the intestinal tract, although final diagnosis is based on intestinal and renal histopathology. Despite hypoallergenic diet trials and immunosuppressive therapy directed at IBD and glomerulonephritis, prognosis is poor. Irish Setters are reported to have a familial tendency for a **gluten-sensitive enteropathy**, with clinical signs beginning as early as 6 mo of age. The wheat sensitivity is both confirmed and treated through the use of gluten-free diets. Basenjis are prone to an **immunoproliferative enteropathy** of unknown mode of inheritance; severe lymphocytic-plasmacytic enteritis is a component, and the condition may progress to lymphoma. Diagnosis is based on histopathologic examination of GI biopsies, usually obtained through endoscopy. Treatment trials with immunosuppressive drugs and hypoallergenic diets are usually unsuccessful unless aggressively initiated in the early stages of the disease. **Lymphangiectasia** is a malformation of the intestinal lymphatic system that results in a protein-losing enteropathy that may be congenital or acquired. The impaired lymphatic drainage results in dilated lacteals and lymphatics of the intestinal wall. It is diagnosed through the exclusion of other protein-losing diseases and confirmed by histopathology of the small-intestinal wall. Most affected animals respond to a combination of dietary manipulation and anti-inflammatory doses of glucocorticoids. Diets should contain minimal fat with an ample amount of high-quality protein and may be supplemented with medium-chain triglycerides. Additional therapeutics include rutin, a drug that is also effective for chylothorax and lymphedema. Some animals do not respond and succumb to severe protein and caloric malnutrition. **Exocrine pancreatic insufficiency** (EPI) has a higher incidence in German Shepherds and is due to pancreatic acinar atrophy; it is an acquired disease (secondary to pancreatitis) in cats. The lack of pancreatic enzymes results in an osmotic diarrhea, in which steatorrhea is a prominent feature. Affected animals either fail to gain weight or, if EPI is acquired later in life, show a dramatic weight loss. Diagnosis is through the measurement of serum trypsin-like immunoreactivity; marked reductions after a fast are diagnostic. More recent tests include canine pancreatic lipase immunoreactivity. Treatment involves the exogenous replacement of pancreatic enzymes and the use of highly digestible diets.

Ileocolonic agangliosis has been reported in white foals produced by matings of Overo horses to each other. Although the foals appear normal at birth, they soon develop colic and die on the second day. The affected horses are white and have blue irises. Diagnosis can be confirmed by the lack of ganglia in the colon. Congenital defects of the rectum and anus generally result from arrested embryonic development.

Inherited atresias of the small- and large-intestinal tracts are relatively common in large animals. **Atresia coli** has been reported in Percheron horses and involves the ascending colon at the pelvic flexure. In Swedish Highland cattle, **atresia ilei** has been recorded, and atresia of the small intestine is seen in lambs. These conditions are invariably fatal. **Anal atresia** has been reported in sheep, pigs, and cattle; it results when the dorsal membrane separating the rectum and anus fails to rupture. Clinical signs are apparent at birth and include tenesmus, abdominal pain and distention, retention of feces, and the absence of an anal opening. Surgical removal of the membrane is indicated.

Segmental aplasia (rectal agenesis) is seen when the rectum terminates in a blind pouch before reaching the anus. Surgical correction is difficult because the location of the terminal section varies, and iatrogenic damage to nerves in the area may occur. **Colonic and rectal duplications** are rare, and affected animals generally show signs of large-bowel disease. Diagnosis is by contrast colonography. Correction is via surgical removal of the duplication, although some cases have multiple concurrent abdominal developmental anomalies that preclude complete surgical correction.

Rectourethral fistula has been reported in English Bulldogs and is seen clinically as simultaneous urination from both the urogenital and anal orifices along with a history of chronic urinary tract infections. Diagnosis is via voiding contrast urethrography or retrograde contrast colonography. Surgical correction is curative. **Rectovaginal fistula** is a fistulous tract that connects the vagina and rectum and usually is seen in conjunction with imperforate anus. Passage of feces through the vulva or signs of colonic obstruction are suggestive. Diagnosis may be confirmed by barium enema, which outlines the extension of the defect into the vagina. Identification of the fistula, surgical correction, and reestablishment of the normal anatomic structures are imperative. Prognosis is usually guarded. Complications are common and include fecal and urinary incontinence.

Urinary and fecal incontinence is often seen in Manx cats as a sequela of heritable spina bifida.

LIVER

The most common congenital liver anomaly is **portosystemic shunt** (PSS). (*See* PORTOSYSTEMIC SHUNTS, p 374, for a complete discussion.) Breeds with a reported increased incidence include Yorkshire Terriers, Miniature Schnauzers, and Himalayan and Persian cats. PSS results in portal blood bypassing the liver and gaining direct access to the systemic vascular system. Shunts may be single and intrahepatic (most often secondary to a patent fetal ductus venosus), single and extrahepatic (with various possible vascular routes between the portal and postcava or azygous vein), or multiple and secondary to intrahepatic arterioportal fistulas. Clinical signs generally manifest as metabolic neurologic disturbances (hepatic encephalopathy) and are usually seen in young animals after a high-protein meal. In the later stages, ascites may develop secondary to portal hypertension. Other concurrent clinical findings may include renomegaly and cystic urate calculi. Definitive diagnosis is via positive-contrast portography, which can identify shunt location and whether the shunt is single or multiple. This procedure also allows assessment of feasibility for surgical correction. Multiple shunts have a poor prognosis because they are often secondary to an underlying, progressive hepatic parenchymal disease (eg, cirrhosis).

Hepatoportal microvascular dysplasia is an intrahepatic circulatory disorder that results in the shunting of portal blood to the systemic circulation. The syndrome is well defined in Cairn Terriers and Yorkshire Terriers, although it has also been reported in Maltese, Dachshunds, Toy and Miniature Poodles, Bichon Frise, Pekingese, Shih Tzus, and Lhasa Apsos. It is generally asymptomatic, with its predominant clinical significance being its differentiation from PSS, as bile acid testing is abnormal in both; this can be done only through the exclusion of a definable macroscopic shunting vessel(s). Dogs that progress to clinical disease are treated medically as described for PSS; with no definable macroscopic shunting vessel, surgery is not a therapeutic option.

Copper-associated hepatopathy is a metabolic derangement of hepatic copper storage resulting in progressive hepatocellular copper accumulation and the subsequent development of chronic hepatitis and hepatic cirrhosis. This condition is well defined in Bedlington Terriers, in which 3 clinical variations are described: acute hepatic necrosis in young (<6-yr-old) dogs; chronic progressive hepatic failure in older dogs; and asymptomatic but affected (carrier) dogs. Elevated copper levels have also been identified in the familial hepatic disease of West Highland White Terriers, Skye Terriers, and Doberman Pinschers, although a causal relationship, as demonstrated in the Bedlington, has not been defined. There are apparent geographic breed variations, with hepatic copper levels worse in Bedlington and West Highland White Terriers of North American descent. Treatment involves the use of copper chelators, low copper diets, and other supportive measures directed at animals with clinical hepatic disease.

Additional hepatic developmental anomalies include **hepatic cysts**, which are generally asymptomatic and of clinical significance only in that they must be differentiated from hepatic abscesses. Finding a hepatic cyst should also prompt the evaluation of renal architecture (especially in cats) as it may coexist with polycystic renal disease.

DENTAL DEVELOPMENT

The morphology of mammalian teeth correlates closely with the animal's alimentation. This explains the large variety in dental morphology between different species of animals. All domestic animals, however, have a diphyodont dentition. The dental formulas are listed in TABLE 3. In an anatomic tooth identification system, permanent teeth are designated as incisor (I), canine (C), premolar (P), and molar (M); deciduous teeth are

TABLE 3. Dental Formulas

	Deciduous	Permanent
Horse	$2(Di_3^3 Dc_0^0 Dp_3^3) = 24$	$2(I_3^3 C_1^1 P_3^3 M_3^3) = 36(-44)^{*\dagger}$
Cow[‡] Sheep Goat	$2(Di_3^0 Dc_1^0 Dp_3^3) = 20$	$2(I_3^0 C_1^0 P_3^3 M_3^3) = 32$
Pig	$2(Di_3^3 Dc_1^1 Dp_3^3) = 28$	$2(I_3^3 C_1^1 P_4^4 M_3^3) = 44$
Dog	$2(Di_3^3 Dc_1^1 Dp_3^3) = 28$	$2(I_3^3 C_1^1 P_4^4 M_3^2) = 42$
Cat	$2(Di_3^3 Dc_1^1 Dp_2^3) = 26$	$2(I_3^3 C_1^1 P_2^3 M_1^1) = 30$

[*]The canine teeth are usually regressed or absent in mares.
[†]Small premolars 1 (wolf teeth) are often present, especially in the upper jaw.
[‡]The canine tooth of domestic ruminants has commonly been counted as a fourth incisor.

designated as Di, Dc, and Dp. Another system that can be used for labeling teeth is the modified Triadan system, which assigns a three-digit number to a specific tooth. The animal's head is divided into 4 quadrants, with the upper right quadrant labeled "1" and the remaining quadrants numbered in a counterclockwise direction. Numbers 1-4 are used to identify the quadrant for permanent teeth, and 5-8 are used for the temporary dentition. The second and third digits identify the specific tooth number; eg, in horses, the left lower second premolar is tooth "306" and the last molar on the right mandible is "411."

Estimation of Age by Examination of the Teeth

In horses, which have a hypsodont dentition, age can be estimated by the eruption times and general appearance of the (lower incisor) teeth. In other species with brachydont incisors, such as cattle and dogs, age determination is less accurate and is mostly based on dental eruption times.

Horses: The most appropriate teeth for estimating age in horses are the (lower) incisors. It must be emphasized, however, that dental appearances are subject to individual and breed variations and differences in environmental conditions. The deciduous incisors are smaller than the permanent teeth, and the surfaces of their crowns are whiter and have several small longitudinal ridges and grooves. Eruption times are listed in TABLE 4. Permanent incisors are larger and more rectangular in shape. Their crown surfaces are largely covered with cement and have a yellowish appearance. The upper incisors have 2 distinct longitudinal grooves on their labial surface, while the lower incisors have only 1.

Equine incisor teeth develop certain wear-related macroscopic features that are traditionally used for estimating age. The dental star consists of yellowish brown secondary dentin that fills up the pulp cavity and appears at the occlusal surface as the tooth wears. Its shape and position, as well as the appearance of the "white spot" in its center, are related to age. The shape, size, and time of disappearance of both the infundibula or "cups" (funnel-like infoldings in the occlusal surface) and the "marks" (enamel infundibular bottoms) are additional but more variable indicators of age. Progressive dental wear causes an alteration of tooth shape. The occlusal surfaces of recently erupted incisors are elliptical, but with age they subsequently become trapezoid, round, and then triangular, with the apex toward the lingual side. Additionally, the arch formed by the incisors of the opposing jaws as they meet changes as the teeth advance from their alveoli and undergo attrition. In young horses, the upper and lower incisors are positioned in a straight line. With increasing age, the angle between upper and lower incisors becomes more acute.

The curvature of the dental arch formed by the lower incisive tables is also age related. In young horses this arch is semicircular, whereas in older individuals it forms a straight line. The Galvayne's groove and the "7-year hook," which have traditionally been used as age indicators, are variable, inconsistent, and thus of little value for age determination in horses. The more useful signs are arranged chronologically in the following list:

Birth to 5 yr: *See* TABLE 4.
5 yr: I 3 is erupting. Dental star in I 1.
6 yr: Dental star in I 2. Cup gone from I 1.
7 yr: Dental star in I 3.
8 yr: I 1 is trapezoid, with white spot in dental star.
9 yr: I 2 is trapezoid, with white spot in dental star.
10 yr: Cup gone from I 2. Mark on I 1 is oval-triangular.
11 yr: White spot in dental star on I 3. I 1 and I 2 have lingual apex. I 3 is triangular with labial apex.
12 yr: Cups gone from all lower incisors.
14 yr: Marks on I 1 and I 2 are small and round.
18 yr: Marks disappear from I 1.
20 yr: Marks are gone from I 2 and I 3.

Cattle: Eruption times of the permanent incisors are primarily used to estimate age up to 5 yr and are listed in TABLE 4. Signs of wear are much less reliable than eruption because wear is largely determined by nutrition, and macroscopic age-related dental features are scarce (dental stars) or absent (cups and marks).

TABLE 4. Eruption of the Teeth[*]

	Horse	Cow	Sheep and Goat	Pig	Dog	Cat
Di 1	0-1 wk	Before birth	0-1 wk	3-4 wk	4-5 wk	2-3 wk
Di 2	4-6 wk	Before birth	1-2 wk	2-3 mo	4-5 wk	3-4 wk
Di 3	6-9 mo	0-1 wk	2-3 wk	Before birth	3-4 wk	3-4 wk
I 1	$2^1/_2$ yr	2 yr	1-$1^1/_2$ yr	12-15 mo	4 mo	4-7 mo
I 2	$3^1/_2$ yr	$2^1/_2$ yr	$1^1/_2$-2 yr	16-20 mo	$4^1/_2$ mo	4-7 mo
I 3	$4^1/_2$ yr	$3^1/_2$ yr	2-$2^1/_2$ yr	8-10 mo	5 mo	4-7 mo
Dc	Does not erupt	0-2 wk	3-4 wk	Before birth	3-4 wk	3-4 wk
C	4-5 yr	$3^1/_2$-4 yr	3-4 yr	6-10 mo	5-6 mo	4-7 mo
Dp 2	0-2 wk	0-3 wk	0-4 wk	4-6 wk	4-6 wk	5-6 wk (upper only)
Dp 3	0-2 wk	0-3 wk	0-4 wk	$1^1/_2$ mo	4-6 wk	5-6 wk
Dp 4	0-2 wk	0-3 wk	0-4 wk	1-5 wk	4-6 wk	5-6 wk
P 1	5-6 mo (wolf tooth)	—	—	5 mo	4-5 mo	—
P 2	$2^1/_2$ yr	2-$2^1/_2$ yr	$1^1/_2$-2 yr	12-15 mo	5-6 mo	4-7 mo (upper only)
P 3	3 yr	2-$2^1/_2$ yr	$1^1/_2$-2 yr	12-15 mo	5-6 mo	4-7 mo
P 4	4 yr	$2^1/_2$-3 yr	$1^1/_2$-2 yr	12-15 mo	5-6 mo	4-7 mo
M 1	9-12 mo	5-6 mo	3-5 mo	4-6 mo	4-5 mo	4-7 mo
M 2	2 yr	1-$1^1/_2$ yr	9-12 mo	8-12 mo	5-6 mo	—
M 3	4 yr	2-$2^1/_2$ yr	$1^1/_2$-2 yr	18-20 mo	6-7 mo	—

[*]Average data, subject to considerable variation

Birth to 5 yr: *See* TABLE 4.
5 yr: All incisors in wear. Occlusal surface of I 1 beginning to level.
6-7 yr: I 1 is leveled and neck is visible.
8 yr: I 2 is leveled and neck is visible.
9 yr: I 3 is leveled and neck is visible. C may be leveled.
10 yr: C is leveled and neck is visible.

As cattle continue to age, the teeth wear shorter and more neck becomes visible; they loosen in the sockets and eventually drop out.

Dogs: The following data were found reliable in ~90% of large dogs. There is more variation in small dogs (especially toy breeds) and in dogs with undershot or overshot jaws. Even, or level, bites usually result in excessive wear.

1½ yr: Cusps worn off lower I 1.
1½-2½ yr: Cusps worn off lower I 2.
3½ yr: Cusps worn off upper I 1.
4½ yr: Cusps worn off upper I 2.
5 yr: Cusps of lower I 3 slightly worn. Occlusal surface of lower I 1 and I 2 rectangular. Slight wear of canines.
6 yr: Cusps worn off lower I 3. Canines worn blunt. Lower canine shows impression of upper I 3.
7 yr: Occlusal surface of lower I 1 elliptical with the long axis sagittal.
8 yr: Occlusal surface of lower I 1 inclined forward.
10 yr: Lower I 2 and upper I 1 have elliptical occlusal surfaces.
12 yr: Incisors begin to fall out (unless care has been taken to maintain healthy gingival and periodontal tissues).

DENTISTRY

LARGE ANIMALS

Most large animals are herbivores, and efficient dental function is the key to food intake and to the maintenance of normal body condition. The teeth of herbivores have evolved to accommodate the results of dental attrition caused by almost continuous grazing or rumination.

The forces of wear have been matched by the development of the hypsodont (high crown) tooth with the continuous eruption of the reserve crown. The dental arcades (6 cheek teeth in horses) have regular serrations that expose sharp enamel edges that shred and crush cellulose material. At the same time, the brittle nature of the enamel of the tooth is protected by the surrounding dentin and peripheral cementum.

Of the common domestic large animals, horses generally require the most dental work. In the swine industry, removal or amputation of deciduous canine teeth in piglets and tusk amputation in breeding boars may be part of routine management. In new world camelids (llamas, etc), blunting the fighting teeth (ie, the upper single incisor and canine and the lower canine teeth) is done to reduce the danger and consequences of fighting. (*See also* LLAMAS AND ALPACAS, p 1521, for additional dental care.) Exotic species may also have various dental conditions, eg, impacted tusks in young elephants or maxillary dental periostitis and actinomycosis in wallabies and kangaroos.

Signs of Dental Disease: Dental disease (eg, broken teeth, irregular dental arcades) is a common underlying cause of unthriftiness, loss of condition, or poor breeding or nursing performance. The classic signs of dental disease in horses include difficulty or slowness in feeding and a reluctance to drink cold water. During the chewing process, the horse may stop for a few moments and then start again. Sometimes, the head is held to one side as if the horse were in pain. Occasionally, the horse may quid, ie, it may pick up its food, form it into a bolus but drop the bolus from the mouth after it has been partially chewed. Occasionally, the semi-chewed mass of feed may become packed between the teeth and the cheek. To avoid using a painful tooth or a sore mouth, the horse may bolt its food and subsequently suffer indigestion or colic. Uncrushed, unmasticated grain may be noticed in the feces. Other signs of dental disease in horses include excessive salivation and blood-tinged mucus in the mouth, accompanied by the fetid breath of dental decay. There may be a lack of desire to eat hard grain accompanied by loss of body condition or poor coat condition. Extensive dental decay and accompanying periostitis and root abscessation may lead to empyema of the paranasal sinuses and intermittent unilateral nasal discharge. There may be facial or mandibular swelling and development of mandibular fistulas from apical infections of the lower cheek teeth.

Horses may be reluctant to take the bit, shake their head when being ridden, or resist training techniques due to irregularly worn cheek teeth and sharp edges on the maxillary cheek teeth and accompanying buccal mucosa laceration. The presence of "wolf" teeth in horses may or may not be associated with resistance to the bit.

Dental Examination: In most cases, history, age, and clinical signs are correlated. A thorough physical examination should always be performed, followed by a detailed and thorough oral and dental examination. In most large animals, including horses, this is greatly facilitated by the use of sedation and an oral speculum; certain animals may require general anesthesia. A thorough oral examination can be facilitated if the mouth is washed out with warm water and if the examiner wears a headlight or an assistant holds a flashlight.

Routine Dental Prophylaxis and Extractions: Routine dental prophylaxis is important in the health care of horses. Enamel edges should be removed twice yearly during the establishment of the permanent dentition and thereafter as frequently as needed, depending on the management of the horse. Horses that graze on free range or grass usually require a yearly dental prophylaxis; horses that are stall confined and are essentially fed hay and grain require at least twice yearly oral examinations and dental prophylaxis.

The objective of dental prophylaxis is to remove the enamel edges of teeth and thereby maintain the normal occlusal surface; by so doing, development of irregularities of wear on the dental arcades is inhibited. Dental prophylaxis can usually be done with simple restraint, a twitch, or the use of sedatives and analgesics. Power equipment is now being used more frequently to grind, balance, and realign the biting surfaces of the incisor and cheek teeth; it should be used carefully to avoid thermal and pressure trauma to dentin and pulp. This means using low-speed grinders with short contact times and light pressure.

Major dental procedures (eg, extractions) usually require general anesthesia. Radiographic evaluation and protection of the airway from debris are necessary in most cases. Some decayed teeth can be extracted per os using compound molar separators, extraction forceps, and cutters. However, in many cases, surgical exposure and tooth repulsion is preferred. Tooth preservation by root end resection and endodontic therapy has demonstrated that extraction is not required in all cases of dental decay in horses.

Congenital and Developmental Anomalies

In horses, the most common oral congenital deformity is parrot mouth, in which the maxilla is relatively longer than the mandible. In equids and cattle, many anomalies of dental development may result from exposure to teratogenic toxins. However, underlying genetic factors should always be considered.

Dental irregularities accompany systemic fluorosis in both cattle and sheep. In the milder forms of fluorosis, only the dentition may be involved. In extreme fluorosis (eg, 40 ppm in the diet for several years), other skeletal abnormalities may be seen (phalanx fracture). (*See also* FLUORIDE POISONING, p 2359.)

Supernumerary teeth (polyodontia) are seen occasionally. In both horses and cattle, double rows of incisor teeth or extra cheek teeth may be seen. Treatment is determined on a case-by-case basis and may require extraction of the extra teeth.

See also CONGENITAL AND INHERITED ANOMALIES OF THE DIGESTIVE SYSTEM, p 131.

Abnormal Tooth Eruption

Abnormal eruption of permanent teeth is commonly a sequela of mandibular or maxillary trauma, eg, symphyseal fractures in cattle and horses in which the developing tooth bud of the permanent tooth is damaged by the fracture itself or by the repair process. In horses, delayed eruption or impaction of cheek teeth is a common cause of apical osteitis and subsequent dental decay. This particularly affects the third cheek tooth (premolar 4 [108, 208, 308, and 408 in the Triadan numbering system]) in both the upper and lower arcades and is a sequela of mild dental overcrowding. Medial displacement of the third cheek tooth is another form of abnormal eruption due to overcrowding.

Irregular Wear

Except for pigs, most large animals have an intermandibular space that is narrower than the intermaxillary space; ie, they are anisognathic. In horses, this, together with limited natural movement of the mandible, results in the development of enamel points on the buccal edges of the upper arcades and on the lingual edges of the lower arcades. In cattle and sheep, because the temporomandibular joint affords greater lateral movement of the mandible, such irregularities do not develop as frequently. Extreme forms of disease, however, are seen in all species and may be influenced by other skeletal deformities of the face or accompanying infections (eg, *Actinomyces* sp). Gross shear mouth may result with exaggerated obliquity of the molar tables. It may be seen in older horses, and treatment is usually unsatisfactory. Dental care should be supplemented by special diets.

Enamel points are best treated by regular dental prophylaxis in horses (ie, floating). This should be done twice annually while the permanent dentition is developing; at the same time, retained caps should be removed if they cause oral ulceration or discomfort.

Wave mouth and **step mouth** are irregularities caused by uneven wear of the teeth and are the result of local pain. In time, secondary gum and socket disease (ie, periodontitis) develop. Such conditions are best prevented by regular, routine dental prophylaxis. Once dental irregularities are severe, results of dental procedures are usually incomplete, although occlusal surfaces may be realigned, and dental care needs to be supplemented by special dietary regimens.

Periodontal Disease

In all animals, a degree of inflammatory change occurs during the eruption of both the deciduous and permanent teeth. However, if malocclusion occurs, severe periodontal disease is inevitable. In horses, this is a common sequela of oral trauma, dental fractures, impactions, and most importantly, irregular wear.

In sheep, periodontal disease of the mandibular rostral teeth (incisors) is often referred to as broken mouth. Sometimes, the viability of grazing sheep is affected dramatically. The productive life of many farm-fed sheep is often 2 yr longer than that of range-fed animals. Little can be done to alter the progress of this disease, although dental prophylaxis and restoration of occlusal regularity of the incisor teeth has been recommended. This can be done by the use of a dental grinder or a fine-bladed tooth rod.

Dental Decay

Infection may be introduced into the pulp chamber of the teeth by various routes, eg, after amputation of teeth. In horses, hypoplasia of the cementum in the enamel lakes of the upper cheek teeth may predispose to caries of cementum and subsequent pulpitis and apical osteitis. Depending on the site of the decayed tooth, there may be accompanying signs of maxillary sinusitis, local cellulitis, periostitis, alveolar periodontitis, and fistula formation. The pathologic features of dental decay are nonspecific. Consequently, the etiology of the apical infection in a draining mandibular dental fistula in a llama or horse may be obscure. Many animals are not examined until the infection is advanced, and tooth fractures may well be secondary rather than primary. It has been suggested that, in some species (eg, the horse), the initiating feature of the establishment of apical osteitis and pulpitis is abnormal eruption and dental impaction. The etiology of apical osteitis in new world camelids and cattle may be similarly influenced.

When dental decay is advanced, extraction of the affected tooth is recommended. In horses, this is usually achieved by surgical exposure of the decayed tooth and then repulsion into the mouth. Recent experience has shown that, with careful technique, sedation, and nerve blocks, the use of general anesthesia may be avoided. The socket should be cleaned carefully to remove all fragments of diseased bone and tooth. Dental acrylics, dental waxes, and wound packs should be used to ensure that the socket can heal properly by protecting it from food material. After dental extractions, the adjacent teeth gradually move to close the gap in the dental arcade. However, this process is never complete, and the occluding arcade will form a "ramp" or hook opposite the missing teeth (both rostral and caudal). Such irregularities in horses can be corrected by grinding and realigning the arcades every 6 mo.

Because of such complications, surgical techniques that preserve the teeth should be considered, at least for horses. Root-end resection after surgical exposure with careful hemostasis is followed by pulp removal and obturation and sterilization of the pulp chamber. The endodontic system is then filled with gutta percha and eugenol, and the root end is sealed after undercutting. Amalgam seals should be carefully placed to ensure complete closure of the root end. The age of the animal and the specifics of local disease should be considered before contemplating root-end resection in horses.

SMALL ANIMALS

Periodontal Disease

Bacterial infection of the tissue surrounding the teeth causes inflammation of the gingivae, periodontal ligament, cementum, and alveolar bone. An early form of periodontal disease, gingivitis, progresses to periodontitis if left untreated. Ultimately, teeth are lost due to the loss of their supporting tissues. This is the major reason for tooth loss in dogs.

Etiology and Pathogenesis: Periodontal disease is caused by gross accumulation of many different bacteria (bacterial plaque) at the gingival margin due in part to a lack of proper oral hygiene. Over time, the flora changes from nonmotile, gram-positive, coccoid, aerobic bacteria to more motile, gram-negative, rod-shaped, anaerobic bacteria. Important flora include *Porphyromonas gingivalis, Bacteroides asaccharolyticus, Fusobacterium nucleatum, Actinomyces viscosus,* and *A odontolyticus* as well as many others. Other contributing factors in disease development may include host response, species and breed, genetics, age, and diet.

As the level of subgingival bacteria increases to 10-20 times normal, gingivitis develops. The accumulation of bacterial metabolic products increases epithelial permeability in crevicular epithelial desmosomes and allows antigens to contact connective tissue. Metabolic products of bacterial metabolism include hydrogen sulfide, ammonia, endotoxin, hyaluronidase, chondroitin sulfatase, mucopeptides, lipoteichoic acids, acetate, butyrate, isovalerate, and propionate. These bacterial products and host defense mechanisms cause tissue necrosis. Polymorphonuclear leukocytes (PMN) migrate through the sulcular epithelium and form a barrier between the subgingival bacteria and the gingiva. With overwhelming bacterial challenge, PMN die in increasing numbers and release breakdown products. The immune system produces lymphokines that participate in tissue destruction, which follows the path of the local vascular supply. Accelerated tissue destruction and inappropriate repair cause loss of periodontal support. Two forms of disease are recognized: gingivitis and periodontitis.

In **gingivitis**, inflammation of the marginal gingival tissues is induced by bacterial plaque and does not affect the periodontal ligament or alveolar bone. There is a change from coral-pink to red or purple, swelling of the gingival margin, and a serous or purulent exudate in the sulcus. The gingivae tend to bleed on contact. Fetid breath is common. Gingivitis is reversible with proper tooth cleaning but, if untreated, may lead to periodontitis. A form of juvenile-onset gingivitis is seen in some cats at 6-8 mo of age; these cats often have gingival hyperemia and halitosis.

In **periodontitis**, the destructive inflammatory process of the periodontium is induced and driven by bacterial plaque that destroy the gingiva, periodontal ligament, alveolar bone, and root cementum. It usually is seen after years of development of plaque, calculus, and gingivitis. There is apical migration of the epithelial attachment and resorption of supporting alveolar bone. It is irreversible and results in permanent loss of tooth support. Affected teeth may show increased mobility, concurrent gingivitis, and subgingival calculus.

Periodontitis is characterized by increased pocket depth, attachment loss, gingival recession, furcation exposure, and horizontal vs vertical patterns of bone loss. Small-breed dogs usually experience more problems than large-breed dogs. Dogs on a hard diet develop fewer problems due to the mechanical cleaning effect on the teeth as the food is chewed. Caudal teeth are affected more often than rostral teeth. The maxilla is affected more severely than the mandible, and buccal surfaces have more disease than lingual surfaces. Gingivitis often becomes evident at ~2 yr of age but resolves if treated. Periodontitis usually begins at 4-6 yr of age and, if untreated, progresses to tooth loss.

Treatment: Gingivitis usually can be treated by thorough cleaning of the teeth, including below the gingival margin (subgingival scaling). If gingivitis does not resolve, further examinations should be performed for the presence of subgingival plaque and calculus, which should be removed in subsequent cleanings. When cleanings are completed, a barrier sealant can be applied to prevent bacterial recolonization and improve healing. Refractory cases should be evaluated for immunocompetence, cellular defects (eg, diminished neutrophil chemotaxis), and systemic disease (eg, diabetes mellitus). Gingivitis reestablishes if the teeth are not kept clean and free of bacteria. Therefore, at-home oral hygiene methods (eg, brushing, plaque prevention gel) and regular cleanings to prevent gingivitis and its progression to periodontitis should be encouraged.

Periodontitis needs to be treated with thorough cleaning above and below the gum line. In areas of increased subgingival depth (>6 mm), surgical means should be used to gain access to the root surface for cleaning, preserving all attached gingiva. Teeth can generally be salvaged until they have lost 75% of their bone support from one or more roots. This can be evaluated by radiography of the jaws, which should be performed if periodontal disease is advanced. Infrabony defects (defects below the crest of the alveolar bone) require flap surgery. Defects on the palatal surface of maxillary canine teeth, which are infrabony in character and invade or approximate the nasal cavity, should be treated with infrabony grafting procedures before a decision is made to extract the tooth. Improper extraction of such teeth frequently results in oronasal fistulas, which require surgical repair; however, the use of proper extraction technique can help avoid this complication. Advanced surgical therapies include guided tissue regeneration using osteoinductive and osteoconductive materials with or without epithelial barriers.

Animals with periodontitis should be maintained postoperatively on oral hygiene methods at home, including mechanical control (daily toothbrushing), dietary changes (providing diets designed to control plaque and calculus), plaque prevention gel, and chemoprophylaxis (such as rinsing with chlorhexidine [10 mL of a 0.2% solution, BID]). Frequent (every 3 mo to 1 yr) prophylactic cleanings should be encouraged to avoid relapse and prevent further bone loss. Dogs with concurrent stomatitis benefit from doxycycline (2.5 mg/kg for 30-60 days).

Prevention: Prevention or reduction of plaque deposition can be achieved with barrier sealants and plaque prevention gels, which use inert polymer sealants to prevent plaque formation on teeth in dogs and cats. The polymer forms a physical (electrostatic) bond to the enamel surface of the teeth, creating a hydrophobic barrier. This barrier effectively repels bacteria-laden saliva from the tooth surface, preventing colonization by oral bacteria and plaque formation.

Mechanical control, in the form of toothbrushing and diets designed to remove tartar and calculus from teeth, can be used proactively to prevent periodontal disease. Consistent use of such products, along with regular dental examinations, are required. The basic principle is that active periodontal disease will not develop around a clean tooth.

Endodontic Disease

Pulpal Hyperemia: The pulp may become acutely inflamed due to trauma or extension of lesions adjacent to the pulp (eg, caries and resorption). Because the pulp is totally confined in dentin, inflammatory swelling may result in pressure necrosis if the insult is prolonged. Severity of the reaction appears to be directly proportional to the extent of injury. Therefore, small injuries that produce transient hyperemia of the pulp may resolve, and a healthy pulp may be reestablished.

Pulpitis: Inflammation of the pulp with pressure necrosis and abscessation may be reversible or irreversible. In general, the abscess cavity is initially sterile unless the tooth has been opened to the oral environment by trauma, resorption, or caries. Teeth with pulpitis often are acutely painful, and the animal resents manipulation or percussion of the tooth. As the pulp dies and gas pressure increases in the pulp cavity, blood is forced into the dentinal tubules and the teeth often change to a reddish brown or dark gray color. Treatment is endodontic therapy and restoration of the tooth structure; as an alternative, teeth that are not vital to the occlusion or function of the dentition may be extracted.

Periapical Lesions: A periapical abscess is a cavitational lesion at the end of the root due to pulpal disease. These areas generally can be seen on radiographs as radiolucent circular areas around the end of the root. This inflammatory response starts as a granuloma that may persist for many months to years but most always evolves into an acute abscess. Such granulomas are rarely palpated over the bony prominence of root ends. When the granulomas become acute they may extend by pressure drainage into adjacent bone and soft-tissue areas and exit extraorally into the soft-tissue space between the jaws, beneath the eye, or into the buccal vestibule by fistula formation. Treatment is endodontic therapy (root canal) on the associated tooth, and the abscess and associated fistula usually resolve within a few weeks. When endodontic therapy cannot be done, the tooth should be extracted.

Gingival Fibroma and Epulides

For a more detailed discussion of oral tumors, *see* DISEASES OF THE MOUTH IN SMALL ANIMALS, p 307.

This benign overgrowth of the epithelial and connective tissue of the gums usually originates near the gingival margin. The tissue is relatively insensitive and tough and has the density of fibrous connective tissue. The growths usually have a broad base of attachment, are the color of the normal gum or more pale, and may grow large enough to completely cover the surfaces of several teeth. Predisposition may exist among brachycephalic breeds, in which the condition is termed **familial gingival hypertrophy**.

Gingival fibroma is most common in older dogs and is usually asymptomatic. Hair, food, and debris may collect between the growth and the teeth and cause irritation and halitosis.

Gingivectomy by electrosurgical techniques is the most satisfactory treatment. Pain control is achieved by maxillary and/or mandibular nerve blocks, butorphenol or morphine injections, and/or fentanyl transdermal patches. After surgery, the mouth should be rinsed daily with 1:1,000 benzalkonium chloride solution or 0.2% chlorhexidine until clinically healed (~2 wk). (*See also* p 312.)

Epulides are benign tumors of the gum that arise from the periodontium. They are the most common benign oral tumors in dogs. This tumor usually is localized to a single tooth. Biopsy is essential for proper diagnosis, treatment, and prognosis.

Feline Odontoclastic Resorptive Lesions
("Neck" lesions, Cervical line erosions)

Feline odontoclastic resorptive lesions (FORL) are the most frequently seen dental lesions in domestic cats. On examination, loss of dental tissue on the crown or at the neck of teeth is evident, often associated with bright red gingival inflammation. The crown may be completely resorbed, and the retained root covered by gingiva. Clinical signs associated with FORL include pain on contact, anorexia, drooling, and general malaise.

The etiology and pathogenesis of FORL has not yet been determined. The lesions are not thought to be infectious; however, abscesses may develop secondarily. Histologically, the lesion is characterized by increased odontoclastic (resorptive) activity. Resorptive lesions are classified according to their severity: Class I, enamel only; Class II, enamel and dentin; Class III, pulp exposure; Class IV, extensive structural damage; and Class V, crown is resorbed but roots are retained. Internal and external root resorption, which can be documented radiographically, often accompany the lesions.

Most teeth affected with FORL should be extracted. Restorative techniques (eg, glass ionomer, dental composite) yield, at best, fair success rates (0-30%), except on very early lesions.

Feline Gingivitis/Stomatitis Syndrome

The oral cavity of the domestic cat may react intensely to disease and result in painful, severe inflammation of the oral cavity. Clinical signs may include oral pain, drooling, halitosis, and anorexia. On examination, inflammation of the gingiva, oral mucosa, palate, caudal fauca, and pharynx may be seen. Soft-tissue biopsy reveals heavy infiltration of plasma cells and lymphocytes. Histologically, plasmacytic-lymphocytic stomatitis signals that one or more severe diseases may be present, and they must be diagnosed accurately to ensure successful treatment. Laboratory data in severe cases usually reveals a polyclonal gammopathy (hypergammaglobulinema) that resolves with treatment.

Initial treatment includes controlling or eliminating the cause and aggressive dental prophylaxis with mandatory home care. Unfortunately, many cats have advanced disease and are far too painful to allow home care. Medical management has been attempted with various drugs. Methylprednisolone acetate (20 mg/cat, every 3-4 wk as needed) has been successful in some reports but is associated with adverse effects, including development of diabetes. The surgical treatment of choice is full-mouth extractions (including any root tips or fragments), although fortunately, the canine teeth can usually be salvaged. (*See also* ULCEROPROLIFERATIVE FAUCITIS/STOMATITIS, p 308.)

Developmental Abnormalities

Malocclusion: Proper growth and development of the oral cavity depends on a series of events that must occur in proper sequence or longterm complications will occur. Preventing major problems with early intervention is in the animal's best interest. Developmental defects can be divided into 3 staging periods. Each stage has its own set of problems, thus requiring close inspection by the veterinarian. Stage 1 is from 0-16 wk of age, Stage 2 is from 16 wk to 7 mo of age, and Stage 3 is from 7 mo to $1\frac{1}{2}$ yr of age. Many developmental abnormalities have a genetic component.

Stage 1: Both kittens and puppies are born with "overshot" maxillas (brachygnathia), which allow the neonate to nurse. As the animal grows and the transition from the mother's milk to solid food occurs, the mandible goes through a growth spurt, nearly catching up to its relative adult percentage of jaw length. If this spurt does not occur and the deciduous dentition erupts, the mandibular canines will most likely be distal to behind the maxillary canines. This creates a malocclusion that can prevent the mandible from developing to its proper length. If this occlusal pattern is noticed in a puppy or kitten, the best therapy is to remove the mandibular canine teeth (cautiously so as not to damage the permanent tooth bud). If the mandibular incisors are excessive in length and occluded behind the dental papilla, they should be extracted using the same care. As a result, the mandible will have the opportunity to reach its genetic potential, thus averting problems with the permanent dentition. If the animal is genetically predetermined to have a significant overbite, this therapy will not affect the outcome.

Another defect seen in Stage 1 is an "underbite" (prognathia), which occurs when the mandible grows faster than usual and becomes too long for the maxilla. This condition becomes evident as early as 8 wk of age. The maxillary incisors occlude inside the mandibular incisors, and the mandibular canines occlude up to or even medial to the maxillary lateral incisors. The treatment of choice is to carefully extract the maxillary central and middle incisors. As a rule, the maxillary lateral incisors are preserved, especially if they are acting as a deterrent to growth of the mandible. Early intervention provides the most favorable outcome.

Other congenital and developmental problems that may require intervention include polydontia (extra teeth should be extracted only if they are causing problems) or gross displacement of a deciduous tooth (the tooth should be extracted if it is causing mechanical interference). Asymmetry of maxilla or mandibular growth is dealt with by extracting the teeth on the underdeveloped side. Although the prognosis for correction is poor, extraction affords the animal every opportunity for "self-correction."

Stage 2: The hallmark of problems in this stage is the retention of deciduous teeth. The normal shedding process begins around 14 wk of age with the loss of the maxillary central incisors. For the next 3 mo, the deciduous teeth are replaced with permanent teeth, plus additional permanent teeth that complete the animal's dentition. If the deciduous teeth are not lost at the time of eruption of the counterpart permanent teeth, occlusal defects in the dentition may result. The treatment of choice is to extract the deciduous tooth as soon as retention becomes evident. Only in rare circumstances will removing a deciduous tooth be an error.

Other developmental defects noted in this stage include lingualversion of the mandibular canine teeth, rostralversion of the maxillary canines, and brachygnathism. When the canine teeth have finished erupting, a window of opportunity exists for simple orthodontic correction of lingual displacement of the mandibular canine teeth with a maxillary bite plate. Because the oral skeletal system is developing at a rapid rate at 6-7 mo of age, orthodontic appliances can be left in an animal's mouth only for 2-3 wk at a time. Thus, any therapy must be accomplished in this short period. Rostralversion of the maxillary canines typically is seen in Shetland Sheepdogs, although it has been reported in many other small breeds as well as in cats. If orthodontic correction is to be attempted it is best to wait as long as possible for the animal to finish growing. The distal dentition does not mature until at least 10 mo of age—the minimum age for orthodontic therapy to begin. If attempted, button brackets and masial chains are the materials of choice. If minimal, brachygnathism can be dealt with using temporary maxillary bite plates. If the brachygnathism is severe (mandibular canine occluding on the palatal side of the maxillary canine), other options such as crown reduction of the mandibular canines or extraction of the maxillary canines should be considered.

Stage 3: Anterior crossbites (incisors in reverse scissors), posterior crossbites (carnassial teeth in reverse position), crowding, tooth rotation, and the final expressions of prognathia and brachygnathia become evident during this final stage of developmental occlusal defects. Anterior crossbites can be dealt with if the remaining dentition is within normal limits (most anterior crossbites are a result of prognathism), using maxillary expansion screw splints or other accepted orthodontic treatments. Posterior crossbites are best dealt with by extracting the maxillary fourth premolar. If orthodontic treatment is attempted, a very cooperative animal and owner are mandatory. Crowding of teeth (large teeth, small space) is resolved by extracting the offending teeth. Likewise, teeth that are rotated >45° (often found in brachycephalic breeds) are removed. If there is any doubt as to which teeth to removed, remember to "establish normal anatomy" and few errors will be made.

Enamel Hypoplasia and Hypocalcification: During the development of enamel (both deciduous and permanent teeth), fevers and deposition of chemicals within the tooth may cause permanent damage. The canine distemper virus is especially damaging in that it attacks the ameleoblasts (enamel-producing cells) and causes a systemic fever. This results in generalized full-thickness loss of enamel, or enamel hypoplasia. Other febrile diseases may result in generalized partial enamel malformation that is not full thickness and is considered enamel hypocalcification. Severe malnutrition in young animals may result in enamel defects. Enamel defects in isolated teeth are most likely the result of trauma or localized infections. Often, the apical abscesses formed in fractured deciduous teeth affect the enamel of the subsequent permanent teeth. Enamel hypoplasia may also be inherited, most notably in Siberian Huskies.

Treatment of enamel hypoplasia includes composite bonding, topical fluoride treatment, and frequent dental prophylaxis. Treatment of enamel hypocalcification includes aggressive polishing of the remaining enamel and possibly composite bonding.

Maxillofacial Trauma

Fractured teeth should be inspected for damage to the pulp. If fractures extend into the pulp, endodontic therapy is required, or extraction must be performed. Restorative techniques (crowns, bonding, and composite restorations) can repair defects in tooth structure over endodontically treated teeth or teeth with manageable defects limited to the hard structure. The periodontal health of affected teeth should also be determined and addressed.

Primary intention closure, when possible, should be used to repair soft-tissue trauma. Results are often good if repaired within a few hours. Use of tension-free closure reduces the risk of failure. Thick tissue that has become avascular due to trauma should be removed.

Bone fractures require stabilization. Acrylic splints, arch bars, interdental wiring, and cerclage wires can be used. In addition, composite bonding reinforced with dental fabrics or enamel retention pins (or both) have the advantage of sparing tooth roots. As long as occlusion is maintained, healing is rapid and most material can be removed in 6-8 wk. Esophageal feeding tubes may be helpful if the animal has difficulty eating during the healing process.

Dental Caries

Dental decay is uncommon in dogs, possibly because of differences in oral flora, diets largely free of readily fermentable carbohydrates, and the slightly alkaline pH of canine saliva. In dogs, decay usually is seen as pits on the occlusal surfaces or on the necks of the molar teeth. Dental caries rarely are seen in cats.

PHARYNGEAL PARALYSIS

Pharyngeal paralysis may be the result of a central or peripheral nervous disorder, or of severe local disease that may cause collapse, obstruction, or malfunction of the pharynx. Of the CNS disorders, rabies (p 1067) is the most important of the viral encephalomyelitides although perhaps not the most frequent. CNS intoxication, lead poisoning, cranial trauma, intracranial abscessation, and tumor formation may also dramatically affect pharyngeal function in many species.

Pharyngeal paralysis of peripheral etiopathogenesis can be the result of pharyngeal trauma or of disease or dysfunction of the pharyngeal adnexa, such as the auditory tube diverticula (guttural pouches) in horses. In many of these cases, the effect on pharyngeal function may not be total paralysis. One-sided lesions (eg, guttural pouch disease) may result in partial pharyngeal malfunction, and the horse may well be able to swallow, although subsequent complications may occur.

Clinical Findings and Lesions: In general, pharyngeal paralysis results in profound dysphagia and the oral and nasal return of food and saliva. In most species, pharyngeal collapse occurs; in horses, this may result in respiratory obstruction. Affected animals are at risk of inhalation pneumonia, dehydration, and circulatory and respiratory collapse. Affected animals have a fever, cough, retch, and choke. Pharyngeal paralysis may result in death.

In many cases, emergency treatment to provide an airway (eg, tracheostomy) may be essential before any clinical diagnostic techniques can be performed.

Diagnosis: The history and clinical signs are usually enough to indicate pharyngeal malfunction and may indicate total pharyngeal paralysis. Use of clinical pathology and hematology to evaluate hemoconcentration, electrolyte depletion, etc, aid in monitoring and evaluating therapeutic regimens. Serology, radiology, ultrasonography, computed tomography, and MRI, as well as endoscopic examination may all be valuable aids to determine whether the underlying etiology is central or peripheral. The use of advanced imaging technologies has particular value in evaluating CNS causes of pharyngeal paralysis in small animals. The possibility of rabies must be kept in mind, especially for any necropsy procedures.

Treatment: In general, treatment is symptomatic, ie, anti-inflammatory drugs, antibiotics to control the complications of inhalation pneumonia, local therapy (including draining the pharyngeal abscesses), and the provision of alternative routes of nutrition. In small animals, intubation and, in large animals, rumenotomy and/or esophagotomy and esophageal feeding may be essential. In many cases, the prognosis is poor, and the welfare of the animal should be considered in management of this condition.

DISEASES OF THE RECTUM AND ANUS

ANAL SAC DISEASE

Anal sac disease is the most common disease entity of the anal region in dogs. Small breeds are predisposed; large or giant breeds are rarely affected. In cats, the most common form of anal sac disease is impaction.

Etiology and Pathogenesis: Anal sacs may become impacted, infected, abscessed, or neoplastic. Failure of the sacs to express during defecation, poor muscle tone in obese dogs, and generalized seborrhea (which produces glandular hypersecretion) lead to retention of sac contents. Such retention may predispose to bacterial overgrowth, infection, and inflammation.

Clinical Findings and Lesions: Signs are related to pain and discomfort associated with sitting. Scooting, licking, biting at the anal area, and painful defecation with tenesmus may be noted. Induration, abscesses, and fistulous tracts are common. In impaction, hard masses are palpable in the area of the sacs; the sacs are packed with a thick, pasty, brown secretion, which can be expressed as a thin ribbon only with a large amount of pressure. When the sacs are infected or abscessed, severe pain and often discoloration of the area are present. Fistulous tracts lead from abscessed sacs and rupture through the skin; these must be differentiated from perianal fistulas. Anal sac neoplasms are usually nonpainful and are associated with perineal edema, erythema, induration, or fistula formation. Apocrine gland adenocarcinomas of the anal sac are typically seen in older female dogs. These dogs are presented for signs secondary to hypercalcemia, such as polyuria and polydipsia, or for problems related to the perineal mass.

Diagnosis of impaction, infection, or abscessation is confirmed by digital rectal examination, at which time the sacs can be expressed. Microscopic examination of the contents from infected sacs reveals large numbers of polymorphonuclear leukocytes and bacteria. A tumor should be suspected (anal sac apocrine adenocarcinoma) in anal sacs that are firm, enlarged, and nonexpressible even with irrigation. In these cases, the diagnosis should be confirmed by biopsy. Regional and systemic metastasis should be evaluated, and serum calcium measured.

Treatment: Impacted anal sacs should be gently manually expressed. A softening or ceruminolytic agent or saline can be infused into the sac if the contents are too dry to express effectively. Infected sacs should be cleaned with antiseptic, followed by local and systemic antibiotic therapy. Hot compresses, applied every 8-12 hr for 15-20 min each, are beneficial for abscesses. Repeated weekly flushings combined with infusion of a steroid-antibiotic ointment may be needed. Adding supplemental fiber to the diet may increase fecal bulk, facilitating anal sac compression and emptying. If medical treatment is ineffective, or if neoplasia is present, surgical excision of the sac is indicated. The closed technique for excision is preferred and has the lowest complication rate. However, fecal incontinence, which is a common complication of anal sac surgery, may result from damage to the caudal rectal branch of the pudendal nerve and may be complete if damage is bilateral. Chronic fistula formation may be seen when sac removal is incomplete or when the sac ruptures. Scar formation in the external anal sphincter may result from surgical trauma and result in tenesmus. (*See also* APOCRINE GLAND TUMORS OF ANAL SAC ORIGIN, p 772.)

PERIANAL FISTULA

Perianal fistula is characterized by chronic, purulent, malodorous, ulcerating, sinus tracts in the perianal tissues. It is most common in German Shepherds and is also seen in Setters and Retrievers. Dogs >7 yr old are at higher risk.

Etiology and Pathogenesis: The cause is unknown, although many theories have been proposed. Contamination of the hair follicles and glands of the anal area by fecal material and anal sac secretions may result in necrosis, ulceration, and chronic inflammation of the perianal skin and tissues. Affected animals may be predisposed to generalized skin problems. Hypothyroidism, an immunologic defect, or an immune-mediated component may contribute to susceptibility. The likelihood of contamination is greater in dogs with a broad-based tail; deep anal folds may cause feces to be retained within rectal glands and play a major role. The draining tracts are lined with chronic inflammatory tissue and often extend to the lumen of the rectum and anus. Infection may spread to deeper structures involving the external anal sphincter and, therefore, should be treated promptly.

Clinical Findings: In dogs, signs include attitude change, tenesmus, dyschezia, anorexia, lethargy, diarrhea, and attempts to bite and lick the anal area. Signs in cats are similar to those in dogs but may include matting of fur and sitting in the litter box.

Treatment: Until recently, management of perianal fistulae was frustrating for both veterinarians and pet owners. Surgical therapy traditionally included anal sacculectomy, in addition to destroying the diseased tissues. Surgical techniques included excision, debridement, fulguration, and cryosurgery. Amputation of the tail at its base was once advocated alone or adjunctively with other therapy. Surgery is now only recommended for fistulae resistant to medical therapy. Sequelae of surgery include fecal incontinence, rectal stricture, and recurrence.

Cyclosporine has been demonstrated to be an effective treatment; it is usually administered for 16 wk and for an additional 4 wk after all fistulae appear to be healed. Concurrent administration of ketoconazole allows the dosage and cost of cyclosporine therapy to be reduced. Prompt treatment with cyclosporine combined with ketoconazole is recommended early in the course of the disease to reduce the likelihood of recurrence. Other aspects of medical management include the use of stool softeners to reduce dyschezia. Perianal cleansing and antibiotics may reduce inflammation.

PERIANAL TUMORS

See HEPATOID GLAND TUMORS, p 773, and APOCRINE GLAND TUMORS OF ANAL SAC ORIGIN, p 772.

PERINEAL HERNIA

Perineal hernia is a lateral protrusion of a peritoneally lined hernial sac between the levator ani and either the external anal sphincter muscle or the coccygeus muscle. Incidence in intact 6- to 8-yr-old male dogs is disproportionately high, and Welsh Corgis, Boston Terriers, Boxers, Collies, Kelpies and Kelpie crosses, Dachshunds and Dachshund crosses, Old English Sheepdogs, and Pekingese are at higher risk.

Etiology and Pathogenesis: Many factors are involved, including breed predisposition, hormonal imbalance, prostatic disease, chronic constipation, and weakness of the pelvic diaphragm due to chronic straining. The higher incidence among sexually intact males is evidence that hormonal influences probably play a primary role. Prostatic hypertrophy attributed to sex-hormone imbalance has been strongly implicated. Both estrogens and androgens have been cited as causative agents.

Clinical Findings and Diagnosis: Common signs include constipation and obstipation, tenesmus, and dyschezia. Stranguria and urinary obstruction may develop secondary to retroflexion of the bladder and prostate. Visceral strangulation may be seen. A perineal swelling ventrolateral to the anus is evident. Herniation may be bilateral, but two-thirds are unilateral and >80% of these are on the right side.

The mass is soft and fluctuant and may be reduced digitally. A firm, painful swelling may be compatible with retropulsion of the bladder and prostate. Determination of contents is often made by rectal examination and perineal centesis (to determine if urine is present). Over 90% of perineal hernias contain a rectal deviation, which is a sacculation of the rectum into the hernial sac, where the layers of the rectal wall remain intact.

Treatment: Perineal hernia is rarely an emergency, except when the bladder has strangulated and the animal is unable to urinate. If catheterization cannot be done, the urine should be removed by cystocentesis and an attempt made to reduce the hernia. An indwelling urinary catheter may be necessary to ensure urethral patency and prevent recurrence of obstruction.

Surgical correction is always indicated, and concurrent castration to reduce recurrence is recommended. The prognosis is guarded because of the high incidence of recurrence (10-46%) and postoperative complications such as infection, rectocutaneous fistula, anal sac fistula, ischiatic and pudendal nerve entrapment, and rectal prolapse.

RECTAL AND ANORECTAL STRICTURES

Strictures are a narrowing of the lumen due to cicatricial tissue. Injury may result from foreign bodies or trauma (eg, bite wounds, accidents) or as a complication of inflammatory disease.

Neoplasia, enlarged prostate, and scar tissue after perianal fistula or anal sac abscess may all predispose to extraluminal constriction. In small animals, anorectal stricture is more common than rectal strictures, but neither is frequent. Strictures are more common in German Shepherds, Beagles, and Poodles.

Rectal stricture in cattle may result from trauma, neoplasia, or fat necrosis impinging on or within the lumen, or from defects associated with rectal and vaginal strictures. Rectal strictures in pigs are seen secondary to enterocolitis, after repair of rectal prolapse, and as a sequela of ulcerative proctitis induced by salmonellae. Treatment is surgical.

RECTAL NEOPLASMS

Malignant rectal neoplasms are usually adenocarcinomas in dogs and lymphosarcomas in cats. Adenocarcinomas are slow growing and infiltrative. Local or systemic metastasis may develop before tenesmus, dyschezia, hematochezia, or diarrhea is seen. Surgery is the treatment of choice for adenocarcinomas, but it may be unrewarding because metastasis has usually occurred before the diagnosis. Cats with rectal lymphosarcoma are treated medically with antineoplastic drugs.

RECTAL POLYPS

Rectal adenomatous polyps are an infrequent, usually benign disease, primarily of small animals. The larger the polyp, the greater the potential for malignancy. Signs include tenesmus, hematochezia, and diarrhea. The polyp is usually palpable per rectum and bleeds easily with surface ulceration. Periodically, the polyp may prolapse through the anal orifice. Surgical excision is usually followed by rapid clinical recovery and lengthy survival time. New polyps may develop after surgery. A biopsy should always be submitted for histopathologic diagnosis.

RECTAL PROLAPSE

In rectal prolapse, one or more layers of the rectum protrude through the anus due to persistent tenesmus associated with intestinal, anorectal, or urogenital disease. Prolapse may be classified as incomplete, in which only the rectal mucosa is everted, or complete, in which all rectal layers are protruded.

Etiology: Rectal prolapse is common in young animals in association with severe diarrhea and tenesmus. Causal factors include severe enteritis, endoparasitism, disorders of the rectum (eg, foreign bodies, lacerations, diverticula, or sacculation), neoplasia of the rectum or distal colon, urolithiasis, urethral obstruction, cystitis, dystocia, colitis, and prostatic disease. Perineal hernia, or other interruption of normal innervation of the external anal sphincter, may also produce prolapse.

Animals of any age, breed, or sex may be affected. Rectal prolapse is probably the most common GI problem in pigs due to diarrhea or weakness of the rectal support tissue within the pelvis. In cattle, it may be associated with coccidiosis, rabies, or vaginal or uterine prolapse; occasionally, excessive "riding" and associated traumatic injury may be causative in young bulls. It is common in sheep with short tail docking and especially in feedlot lambs, in which high-concentrate rations may be causative. The use of estrogens as growth promotants, or accidental exposure to estrogenic fungal toxins, may also predispose large animals to rectal prolapse.

Clinical Findings, Lesions, and Diagnosis: An elongated, cylindrical mass protruding through the anal orifice is usually diagnostic. However, it must be differentiated from prolapsed ileocolic intussusception by passing a probe, blunt instrument, or finger between the prolapsed mass and the inner rectal wall. In rectal prolapse, the instrument cannot be inserted due to the presence of a fornix.

Ulceration, inflammation, and congestion of the rectal mucosa is common. Early, there is a short, nonulcerated, inflamed segment; later, the mucosal surface darkens and may become congested and necrotic.

Treatment: In all animals, identifying and eliminating the cause of prolapse is of primary importance.

In **small animals**, treatment includes prompt replacement of viable prolapsed tissue to its proper anatomic location, or amputation if the segment is necrotic. Small or incomplete prolapses can be manually reduced under anesthesia by using a finger or bougie. Warm saline lavage and lubrication with a water-soluble gel should be applied to the prolapsed tissue prior to reduction. Alternatively, hypertonic sugar solution (50% dextrose or 70% mannitol) applied topically may be used to relieve edematous mucosa. The placement of a loose, anal purse-string suture for 5-7 days is indicated. Straining may be prevented by applying a topical anesthetic (1% dibucaine ointment) or by administering a narcotic epidural injection before or after reduction or correction. Postoperatively, a moistened diet and a fecal softener (eg, dioctyl sodium sulfosuccinate) are recommended. Diarrhea after surgery may require treatment.

When questionable viability of tissue prohibits manual reduction, rectal resection and anastomosis are required. When rectal tissue is viable but not amenable to manual reduction, celiotomy followed by colopexy is indicated to prevent recurrence. As in medical management, epidural anesthesia may be used to reduce straining.

In **large animals**, caudal epidural anesthesia is suggested to reduce straining, facilitate repositioning of the prolapse, and permit surgical manipulations. Reduction and retention with a purse-string suture is recommended. The suture should be loose enough to leave a one-finger opening into the rectum in pigs and sheep, and slightly larger in cattle and horses. Rectal prolapse in mares, if neglected, can lead to prolapse of the small colon. The blood supply to the small colon is easily disrupted. Replacement of a rectal prolapse with prolapse of the small colon followed by purse-string suture of the anus has a poor prognosis. More aggressive treatment of the prolapse is dictated by the condition of the rectum. In general, the prolapse may be salvaged by conservative measures, unless obvious deep necrosis or trauma to the tissue exists, or the everted tissue is firm, indurated, and cannot be reduced. Under these circumstances, submucosal resection or amputation should be considered. Amputation of the rectum should be reserved for severe cases. Complete amputation has a higher incidence of rectal stricture formation, especially in swine. A prolapse ring, syringe case, or plastic tubing may be used as an alternative to surgical amputation in pigs and sheep. Postoperatively, the animal should receive antibiotics. Fecal softeners may be used in horses. Usually, it is not economically feasible to repair rectal prolapses in lambs ready for market.

RECTAL TEARS

A separation, rent, or tear in the rectal or anal mucosa is seen as a result of a laceration inflicted within the lumen. Foreign bodies (eg, sharp bones, needles, and other rough material) have been implicated. Bite wounds and, in large animals, trauma from rectal palpation are common causes. The tear may involve only the superficial layers of the rectum (partial tear) or penetrate all layers (complete tear).

Clinical Findings and Diagnosis: Constipation and reluctance to defecate are usually attributed to pain. Diagnosis is based on tenesmus and hemorrhage, perineal discoloration, and inspection of the rectum and anus; fresh blood found on a glove or on feces after rectal examination is good evidence of a rectal tear. Edema may be present when the injury has persisted. The integrity of the external anal sphincter should be evaluated carefully.

Treatment: In all species, treatment should be initiated immediately. The anorectal area should be cleaned thoroughly and systemic broad-spectrum antibiotics administered. IV fluids and flunixin meglumine may be given to prevent or treat septic and endotoxic shock. In small animals, lacerations should be debrided and may be sutured through the anal orifice, via laparotomy, or through a combination of both depending on the location and degree of the tear. Antibiotics and fecal softeners should be administered postoperatively.

In cattle and horses, accidental perforation during rectal examination necessitates immediate treatment to reduce the risk of peritonitis and death. Exploration throughout the abdomen should be slow, deliberate, and smooth. The temptation to use the fingertips excessively or to push the arm through a region of resistance must be avoided. Rectal tears in horses have been classified according to the tissue layers penetrated. Grade I tears involve the mucosa or submucosa. Grade II tears involve rupture of the muscular layers only. Grade III tears involve mucosa, submucosa, and muscular layers, including tears that extend into the mesorectum. Grade IV tears involve perforation of all layers of the rectum and extension into the peritoneal cavity.

Grade I tears may be treated conservatively with broad-spectrum antibiotics and IV fluids. Flunixin meglumine may be given to prevent or treat endotoxic shock. Mineral oil is given via stomach tube to soften feces, and the diet should consist of pasture grasses or alfalfa. Grade II and III tears require immediate and more extensive surgery. Grade IV tears carry a grave prognosis; they should be repaired only if small and if treatment is instituted before the peritoneal cavity is grossly contaminated.

CAMPYLOBACTERIOSIS

Gastrointestinal campylobacteriosis, caused by *Campylobacter jejuni* or *C coli*, is associated with diarrhea in various animal hosts, including dogs, cats, calves, sheep, ferrets, mink, several species of laboratory animals, zoo animals, and humans. In humans, it is a leading cause of diarrhea. *C jejuni* and *C coli* are also recovered from feces of asymptomatic carriers. (*See also* BOVINE GENITAL CAMPYLOBACTERIOSIS, p 1108). Animals, including dogs and cats (especially those recently purchased from shelters), and wild animals maintained in captivity can serve as sources of human infection. The agents also are isolated frequently from the feces of chickens, turkeys, pigs, and other species. The organism commonly contaminates poultry meat, which serves as one of the major vehicles of spread of *C jejuni* to humans.

The disease is found worldwide; its prevalence appears to be increasing as proper culture techniques for *C jejuni* and *C coli* are refined and updated. Clinical manifestations may be more severe in younger animals. In studies using monoclonal and polyclonal antibodies, *Campylobacter* spp (including *C jejuni*) have been associated with proliferative ileitis in hamsters and proliferative colitis in ferrets. A cause and effect relationship has not been proved experimentally, however. Proliferative bowel disease in these animals is now known to be caused by *Lawsonia intracellularis*.

Etiology: *Campylobacter* is a gram-negative, microaerophilic, slender, curved, motile bacterium with a polar flagellum. *C jejuni* is routinely associated with diarrheal disease; however, *C coli*, distinguished from *C jejuni* on the basis of hippurate hydrolysis, is occasionally isolated from diarrheic animals and is routinely recovered from asymptomatic pigs. Other intestinal, catalase-negative campylobacters, *C upsaliensis* and *C helveticus*, have been isolated from diarrheic dogs and cats as well as asymptomatic dogs and cats. *Campylobacter* was once associated with swine dysentery (p 252), but this is now recognized as being caused by *Treponema hyodysenteriae*. Most believe that *Campylobacter* spp do not produce porcine proliferative enteritis (p 250), even though a new organism, *C hyoilei*, isolated from swine in Australia, has been associated with porcine proliferative enteritis. Its role in this disease, however, is not clearly established. *C mucosalis* and *C hyointestinalis* have also been isolated from swine but are not considered enteric pathogens.

Because of slow growth and microaerobic requirements, standard culture methods require selective media that incorporate various antibiotics to suppress competing fecal microflora. *C jejuni* and *C coli* grow well at 42°C in an atmosphere of 5-10% carbon dioxide and an equal amount of oxygen. Cultures are incubated 48-72 hr; colonies are round, raised, translucent, and sometimes mucoid. The organism can be identified by a series of biochemical tests readily available in any diagnostic laboratory. Recently, PCR assays have been used to identify *Campylobacter* spp. Identification is important to distinguish campylobacters from the growing number of novel enterohepatic helicobacters being isolated from a variety of animals.

Transmission and Epidemiology: As with most intestinal pathogens, fecal-oral spread and food- or waterborne transmission appear to be the principal avenues of infection. One suspected source of infection for pets, as well as mink and ferrets raised for commercial purposes, is ingestion of undercooked poultry and other raw meat products. Asymptomatic carriers can shed the organism in their feces for prolonged periods and contaminate food, water, milk, and fresh processed meats (including pork, beef, and poultry products). The organism can survive in vitro at 41°F (5°C) for 2 mo and can survive in feces, milk, water, and urine. Wild birds also may be important sources of water contamination. Unpasteurized milk has been cited as a principal source of infection in several human outbreaks. Strain identification to study the epizootiology of *C jejuni* and *C coli*, in addition to Penner serotyping, is now done using molecular techniques such as restriction fragment length polymorphism and ribotyping.

Clinical Findings: The diarrhea appears to be most severe in young animals. Typical signs in dogs include mucus-laden, watery, and/or bile-streaked diarrhea (with or without blood) that lasts 3-7 days; reduced appetite; and occasional vomiting. Fever and leukocytosis may also be present. In certain cases, intermittent diarrhea may persist >2 wk; in some, it may be present for months. Gnotobiotic puppies inoculated with *C jejuni* developed malaise, loose feces, and tenesmus within 3 days of inoculation.

In calves, signs vary from mild to moderate. The diarrhea is thick and mucoid with occasionally visible blood flecks; body temperature may be normal. Diarrhea with mucus and blood also has been observed in primates, ferrets, mink, and cats. Organisms with ultrastructure similar to that of *Campylobacter* spp have been seen in hyperplastic ileal epithelial mucosa of hamsters with proliferative ileitis; *C jejuni* has been isolated from these lesions but has failed to reproduce the syndrome. Organisms with *Campylobacter*-like morphology also have been associated with proliferative colitis in ferrets and with hyperplastic intestinal lesions in guinea pigs and rats. *Campylobacter*-like organisms have been described in young rabbits with acute typhlitis. It is now known that these organisms are *Lawsonia intracellularis*, an organism closely related to *Desulfovibrio* spp.

Lesions: In 3-day-old chickens infected with *C jejuni*, the organisms were detected within epithelial cells and mononuclear cells of the lamina propria; the jejunum and ileum were the most severely affected. Congested and edematous colons were found in dogs 43 hr after inoculation; microscopically, epithelial height, brush border, and numbers of goblet cells in the colon and cecum were all reduced. Hyperplastic epithelial glands resulted in a thickened mucosa. Histologic changes in calves primarily involve the jejunum but also can involve the ileum and colon. The lesions vary from mild changes to severe hemorrhagic enteritis. The mesenteric lymph nodes are edematous. Experimentally, some strains of *C jejuni* produce a hepatitis in mice, and the organism has been isolated from inflamed livers of dogs. A cytotoxin, referred to as cytolethal distending toxin, has been identified in *C jejuni*; however, its role in production of intestinal disease is not known. In vitro, the cytotoxin causes distention of cell lines and cell cycle arrest in the G_2M1 phase of the cell cycle.

Diagnosis: The standard method for diagnosis is microaerobic culture of feces at 42°C; a special medium is commercially available. Diagnosis is also possible by using darkfield or phase-contrast microscopy, by which fresh fecal samples are examined for the characteristic darting motility of *C jejuni*. This method is especially useful during the acute stage of diarrhea when large numbers of organisms are more likely to be shed in the feces. Various techniques can detect serum antibodies to various antigens of *Campylobacter* spp. Heat-stable or heat-labile antigen schemes are used routinely to serotype various strains. Serial serum samples to demonstrate rising antibody titers are helpful in diagnosis. Intestinal viruses and other intestinal bacterial pathogens must be ruled out as primary or copathogens in animals with *Campylobacter*-associated diarrhea.

Treatment and Control: Isolation of *C jejuni* or *C coli* from diarrheic feces is not, in itself, an indication for antibiotic therapy. Because *C jejuni* and *C coli* are not routinely cited as potential intestinal pathogens in animals (except for diarrhea in young cats and dogs and in several species of primates), efficacy of antibiotic therapy has been reported infrequently. In certain cases in which animals are severely affected or are a zoonotic threat, antibiotic treatment may be indicated. In general, *C jejuni* and *C coli* isolates from animals are similar to isolates obtained from human populations. Erythromycin, the drug of choice for *Campylobacter* diarrhea in humans, is also effective in other animals, although erythromycin-resistant strains of *Campylobacter* spp have been recovered from swine. Gentamicin, furazolidone, and doxycycline also can be used. Ampicillin is relatively inactive against most strains of *Campylobacter*, and most strains are also resistant to penicillin. Tetracycline and kanamycin resistance in certain *C jejuni* strains is reported to be plasmid-mediated and transmissible within *C jejuni* serotypes. Efficacy of sulfadimethoxine and sulfa combinations is variable. Before therapy is instituted, isolation and sensitivity tests should be done. Some animals continue to shed the organism despite antibiotic therapy. Quinolone antibiotics may be useful in eliminating *C jejuni* and *C coli* in asymptomatic carriers, but drug resistance may develop.

INTESTINAL CHLAMYDIAL INFECTIONS

Chlamydiae have been isolated from fecal samples of clinically normal cattle, goats, sheep, and pigs in many parts of the world. Animals with clinically inapparent intestinal infections may shed chlamydiae in the feces for months and possibly years. Accordingly, the GI tract serves as an important reservoir and source for the transmission of these organisms. Chlamydiae, which may cause abortions (p 1098) and pneumonia (p 1177), can readily be isolated from feces of normal sheep and cattle. They have also been recovered from intestinal samples of animals affected with polyarthritis (p 865), encephalomyelitis (p 1073), and conjunctivitis (p 406). Most fecal isolates from ruminants belong to the species *Chlamydia pecorum* but some isolates belong to *Chlamydophila (Chlamydia) psittaci*. The intestinal infection plays an important role as an initiating event in the pathogenesis of several chlamydia-induced diseases. The intestinal infectious phase also plays an important role in avian chlamydiosis (p 2216).

While most of the intestinal chlamydial infections are clinically quiescent, a primary chlamydia-induced enteritis has been seen under field conditions in newborn calves. Such infections may also lead to a change in the number of *Escherichia coli* in the GI tract, with abnormally high numbers in the abomasum and upper small intestine. Signs are more severe in colostrum-deprived calves or in those with only a partial transfer of colostral immunity. Affected newborn calves may have a transient watery to mucoid diarrhea with slight fever and nasal discharge. Many veterinary diagnostic laboratories do not routinely check diarrheic feces for chlamydiae; therefore, such an examination must be requested specifically. Treatments of choice are high doses of tetracyclines, administered parenterally or orally, or both.

SALMONELLOSIS

Salmonellosis is caused by many species of salmonellae and characterized clinically by one or more of 3 major syndromes—septicemia, acute enteritis, and chronic enteritis. The disease is seen worldwide and in all animals. The incidence has increased with the intensification of livestock production. Young calves, piglets, lambs, and foals usually develop the septicemic form (*see* DIARRHEA IN NEONATAL RUMINANTS, p 228, and DIARRHEAL DISEASES OF FOALS, p 241). Adult cattle, sheep, and horses commonly develop acute enteritis, and chronic enteritis may develop in growing pigs and occasionally in cattle (*see also* the chapters on intestinal diseases in each of the major domestic species, p 220 et seq). Pregnant animals may abort. The clinically normal carrier animal is a serious problem in all host species. Salmonellosis is seen infrequently in dogs and cats and is characterized by acute diarrhea with or without septicemia. The incidence of human salmonellosis has increased in recent years, and animals have been incriminated as the principal reservoir. Transmission to humans occurs via contaminated drinking water, milk, meat, and foods such as cake mixes that use contaminated ingredients; poultry and eggs (p 2262) are particularly important sources of infection.

Etiology, Epidemiology, and Pathogenesis:　While many other *Salmonella* spp may cause disease, the more common ones in each species are as follows: **Cattle**—*Salmonella* serovar *typhimurium*, *Salmonella* serovar *dublin*, and *Salmonella* serovar *newport*; **Sheep and goats**—*S typhimurium*, *S dublin*, *Salmonella* serovar *anatum*, and *Salmonella* serovar *montevideo*; **Pigs**—*S typhimurium* and *Salmonella* serovar *choleraesuis*; **Horses**—*S typhimurium*, *S anatum*, *S newport*, *Salmonella* serovar *enteritidis*, and *Salmonella* serovar IIIa $18:z_4z_{23}$. Although their resulting clinical patterns are not distinct, different species of salmonellae tend to differ in their epidemiology. Plasmid profile and drug-resistance patterns are sometimes useful markers for epidemiologic studies. Feces of infected animals can contaminate feed and water, milk, fresh and processed meats from abattoirs, plant and animal products used as fertilizers or feedstuffs, pasture and rangeland, and many inert materials. The organisms may survive for months in wet, warm areas such as in feeder pig barns or in water dugouts but survive <1 wk in composted cattle manure. Rodents and wild birds also are sources of infection. Pelleting of feeds reduces the level of contamination by salmonellae. The prevalence of infection varies among species and countries and is much higher than the incidence of clinical disease, which is commonly precipitated by stressful situations such as sudden deprivation of feed, transportation, drought, crowding, parturition, and the administration of some drugs. Salmonellosis is common in hospitalized horses that have been subjected to prolonged surgical procedures. Use of oral antimicrobial agents is sometimes a risk factor for the disease.

The usual route of infection is oral and, after infection, the organism multiplies in the intestine and causes enteritis. Greater susceptibility of the young may be due to high gastric pH, absence of a stable intestinal flora, and limited immunity. Penetration of bacteria into the lamina propria likely contributes to gut damage and diarrhea. The inflammatory response is marked, and salmonellae are engulfed by phagocytic cells; however, the bacteria can survive and multiply in these cells. Septicemia may follow with subsequent localization in brain and meninges, pregnant uterus, distal aspects of the limbs, and tips of the ears and tails, which can result, respectively, in meningoencephalitis, abortion, osteitis, and dry gangrene of the feet, tail, or ears. The organism also frequently localizes in the gallbladder and mesenteric lymph nodes, and survivors intermittently shed the organism in the feces.

Calves rarely become carriers but virtually all adults do for variable periods—up to 10 wk in sheep and cattle and up to 14 mo in horses. Adult cattle infected with *S dublin* excrete the organism for years. Infection may persist in lymph nodes or tonsils, with no salmonellae in the feces. Latent carriers may begin shedding the organism or even develop clinical disease under stress. A passive carrier acquires infection from the environment but is not invaded, so that if removed from the environment, it ceases to be a carrier.

Cattle and Sheep: In calves and lambs, the disease is usually endemic on a particular farm, with sporadic explosive outbreaks. Subclinical infection with occasional herd outbreaks may be seen in adult cattle. Stressors that precipitate clinical disease include deprivation of feed and water, minimal levels of nutrition, long transport times, calving, and mixing and crowding in feedlots.

Pigs: Outbreaks of septicemic salmonellosis in pigs are rare and usually can be traced to a purchased, infected pig. Purchase of feeder pigs from salmonellae-free herds and use of the "all-in/all-out" policy in finishing units minimize exposure.

Horses: Many horses may be carriers. In adults, most cases develop after the stress of surgery or transport, especially when horses are moved through sales yards, deprived of feed and water, and then overfed at their destination. Mares may be inapparent shedders and, despite several negative cultures before foaling, may shed the bacteria at parturition and infect the newborn foal. Salmonellosis in horses hospitalized for other causes is a major problem for equine clinics and stud farms. In these circumstances, carriers are constantly reintroduced, the environment is persistently contaminated, and a large population of vulnerable horses is at risk. Septicemic salmonellosis is also common in foals; it may be endemic on a given premises or there may be outbreaks. (*See* also INTESTINAL DISEASES IN HORSES AND FOALS, p 233.)

Dogs and Cats: Many dogs and cats are asymptomatic carriers of salmonellae. Clinical disease is uncommon, but when it is seen, it is often associated with hospitalization, another infection or debilitating condition in adults, or exposure to large numbers of the bacteria in puppies and kittens.

Clinical Findings: **Septicemia** is the usual syndrome in newborn calves, lambs, foals, and piglets, and outbreaks may occur in pigs up to 6 mo old. Illness is acute, depression is marked, fever (105-107°F [40.5-41.5°C]) is usual, and death occurs in 24-48 hr. In pigs, a dark red to purple discoloration of the skin is common, especially of the ears and ventral abdomen. Nervous signs may be seen in calves and pigs; these animals may also suffer from pneumonia. Mortality may reach 100%.

Acute enteritis is the common form in adults as well as in calves that are usually ≥1 wk old. Initially, there is fever (105-107°F [40.5-41.5°C]), followed by severe watery diarrhea, sometimes dysentery, and often tenesmus. In a herd outbreak, several hours may lapse before the onset of diarrhea, at which time the fever may disappear. The feces, which vary considerably, may have a putrid odor and contain mucus, fibrinous casts, shreds of mucous membrane, and in some cases, large blood clots. Rectal examination causes severe discomfort, tenesmus, and commonly dysentery. Milk production often declines precipitously in dairy cows. Abdominal pain is common and severe in horses. Affected horses may be severely dehydrated and may die within 24 hr of the onset of diarrhea; mortality may reach 100%. A marked leukopenia and neutropenia are characteristic of the acute disease in horses. In dogs and cats, clinical disease takes the form of acute diarrhea with septicemia and is seen occasionally in puppies and kittens or in adults stressed by concurrent disease. Pneumonia may be evident. Abortion is likely to occur in pregnant bitches or queens. Conjunctivitis is sometimes seen in affected cats.

Subacute enteritis may develop in adult horses and sheep on farms where the disease is endemic. The signs include mild fever (103-104°F [39-40°C]), soft feces, inappetence, and some dehydration. There may be a high incidence of abortion in cows and ewes, some deaths in ewes after abortion, and a high mortality rate due to enteritis in lambs younger than a few weeks of age. In cattle, the first signs may be fever and abortion, followed several days later by diarrhea.

Chronic enteritis is a common form in pigs and adult cattle. There is persistent diarrhea, severe emaciation, intermittent fever, and poor response to treatment. The feces are scant and may be normal or contain mucus, casts, or blood. In growing pigs, rectal stricture may be a sequela if the terminal part of the rectum is involved. Affected pigs are anorectic and lose weight; the abdomen becomes grossly distended. The stricture is obvious on digital palpation and necropsy.

A number of *Salmonella* spp are found in foxes, especially kits, and produce a peracute enteritis. Fur-bearing and zoo carnivores may be affected. Contaminated feed is often the source of infection. Several rodents (eg, guinea pigs, hamsters, rats, and mice) and rabbits are susceptible. Rodents commonly act as a source of infection on farms where the disease is endemic. Pet turtles were once a common source of infection in humans that has been virtually eliminated by the curtailment of commercial trafficking in turtles.

Diagnosis: This depends on the clinical signs and on the laboratory examination of feces, tissues from affected animals, feed (including all mineral supplements used), water supplies, and feces from wild rodents and birds that may inhabit the premises. The clinical syndromes usually are characteristic but must be differentiated from several similar diseases in each species as follows: **Cattle**—diarrhea due to enterotoxigenic *Escherichia coli*, dysentery due to verotoxigenic *E coli*, coccidiosis, cryptosporidiosis, the alimentary tract form of infectious bovine rhinotracheitis, bovine viral diarrhea, hemorrhagic enteritis due to *Clostridium perfringens* types B and C, arsenic poisoning, secondary copper deficiency (molybdenosis), winter dysentery, paratuberculosis, ostertagiasis, and dietetic diarrhea; **Sheep**—enteric colibacillosis, septicemia due to *Haemophilus* sp or pasteurellae, and coccidiosis; **Pigs**—enteric colibacillosis of newborn pigs and weanlings, swine dysentery, campylobacteriosis, and the septicemias of growing pigs (which include erysipelas, classical swine fever, and pasteurellosis); **Horses**—septicemia (due to *E coli*, *Actinobacillus equuli*, or streptococci) and colitis-X.

The lesions are those of a septicemia or a necrotizing fibrinous enteritis, or both. Lesions are most severe in the lower ileum and the large intestine and vary from shortening of villi with loss of the epithelium to complete loss of intestinal architecture. There is a neutrophilic reaction in the lamina propria, and thrombi may be seen in blood vessels in this region. Hemorrhage and fibrin strands are usually seen. Culture techniques that involve suppression of fecal *E coli* are usually necessary, and several daily fecal cultures may be necessary to isolate the organism. Blood cultures in septicemic animals may be rewarding but are costly. Serologic testing is difficult to interpret.

Treatment: Early treatment is essential for septicemic salmonellosis, but there is controversy regarding the use of antimicrobial agents for intestinal salmonellosis. Oral antibiotics may deleteriously alter the intestinal microflora, interfere with competitive antagonism, and prolong shedding of the organism. There is also concern that antibiotic-resistant strains of salmonellae selected by oral antibiotics may subsequently infect humans.

Broad-spectrum antibiotics are used parenterally to treat the septicemia. Initial antimicrobial therapy should be based on knowledge of the drug resistance pattern found in the area. Nosocomial infections often involve highly drug-resistant organisms. Trimethoprim-sulfonamide combinations are often effective. Alternatives are ampicillin, fluoroquinolones, or third-generation cephalosporins. Treatment should be continued daily for up to 6 days. Oral medication should be given in drinking water because affected animals are thirsty due to dehydration, and their appetite is generally poor. Fluid therapy to correct acid-base imbalance and dehydration is necessary. Calves, adult cattle, and horses need large quantities of fluids. Antibiotics such as ampicillin or cephalosporins lead to lysis of the bacteria with release of endotoxin. NSAID may be used to reduce the effects of endotoxemia. Horses with acute intestinal salmonellosis are severely acidotic and hyponatremic and may need to be treated initially with 5% sodium bicarbonate, IV, at 5-8 L/450 kg body wt. This is followed by balanced electrolytes containing potassium to correct the hypokalemia that may follow correction of the acidosis. In horses, flunixin meglumine is recommended for its antiendotoxic properties. Corticosteroids are not recommended because of their immunosuppressive effects and their potential to exacerbate laminitis. IV administration of plasma with a high titer of *Salmonella* lipopolysaccharide core antibodies may be beneficial in horses. Plasma with serotype-specific antibodies is even more beneficial. Septicemic salmonellosis in pigs usually responds favorably if treated early. However, the intestinal form is difficult to treat effectively in all species. Although clinical cure may be achieved, bacteriologic cure is difficult, particularly in adult animals, because the organisms become established in the biliary system and are intermittently shed into the intestinal lumen, which causes chronic relapsing enteritis and contamination of the environment.

Control and Prevention: These are major problems because of carrier animals and contaminated feedstuffs. Drain swabs or milk filters may be cultured to monitor the salmonellae status of a herd. The principles of control include prevention of introduction and limitation of spread within a herd.

Prevention of Introduction: Every effort must be made to prevent introduction of a carrier; animals should be purchased directly only from farms known to be free of the disease and should be isolated for ≥1 wk while their health status is monitored. Ensuring that feed supplies are free of salmonellae depends on the integrity of the source.

Limitation of Spread Within a Herd: In an outbreak, the following procedures should be implemented: 1) Carrier animals should be identified and either culled or isolated and treated vigorously. Treated animals must be rechecked several times before there can be confidence that they are not carriers. 2) The prophylactic use of antibiotics in feed or water supplies may be considered (but the hazards have been mentioned above). 3) Movement of animals around the farm should be restricted to limit infection to the smallest group. Random mixing of animals should be avoided. 4) Feed and water supplies must be protected from fecal contamination. 5) Contaminated buildings must be vigorously cleaned and disinfected. 6) Contaminated material must be disposed of carefully. 7) All persons should be aware of the hazards of working with infected animals and the importance of personal hygiene. 8) Use of a vaccine should be considered, particularly in an outbreak involving pregnant cattle in which a vaccine has been shown to confer some protection in adults and calves. Commercial killed bacterins or autogenous bacterins may be used. Live attenuated vaccines show considerable promise, but they are not available commercially. 9) Stresses should be minimized. 10) Fetal membranes of mares should be placed in a plastic bag until the mare eliminates them, and the foal should be fed colostrum before contact with the mare.

Salmonella **Vaccines:** Salmonellae are intracellular parasites, and a live vaccine is therefore expected to be necessary for optimal immune protection against disease. Several studies with live attenuated *Salmonella* vaccines in pigs, cattle, and chickens have shown them to be effective in stimulating a strong cell-mediated immune response and protecting animals against disease. A live attenuated *S choleraesuis* vaccine that has been licensed for use in swine appears to be effective in reducing colonization of tissues and protecting pigs from disease following challenge with virulent organisms. This vaccine has also been reported to reduce the prevalence of *Salmonella* infections in pigs under field conditions. This vaccine also protected calves against experimental challenge with *S Dublin* following intranasal or subcutaneous administration of the vaccine. The administration of the *S choleraesuis* vaccine to pregnant dairy cows reduced the frequency of shedding of serogroup C1 salmonellae during the peripartum period. Live *S enteritidis* has been effective in significantly reducing the infection of laying hens challenged with *S enteritidis*. The commercial vaccines available for use in cattle are bacterins and appear to induce a modest level of protection. When given to pregnant cows, they induce antibodies in colostrum, which provide an important measure of protection to calves, which are most susceptible in the first week of life.

Salmonellosis in Veterinary Teaching Hospitals: The risk of equine salmonellosis epidemics is particularly high in veterinary teaching hospitals. A high case load, the presence of animals with severe illnesses, and the stresses of transportation contribute to this risk. The serotype most commonly implicated is *S typhimurium* but other serotypes that have been identified include *Salmonella* serovar *heidelberg*, *Salmonella* serovar *krefeld*, *Salmonella* serovar *infantis*, and *S anatum*. They are frequently resistant to multiple drugs. Contamination of the hospital environment often begins with the introduction of the organisms by a carrier animal. Animals in the hospital (which are often highly susceptible) readily develop diarrhea and contribute to further contamination of the hospital. Infection rates as high as 18% have been reported. Nosocomial infection can be identified by development of salmonellosis ≥3 days after hospitalization and by isolation of hospital-associated *Salmonella* from cases. The identification of hospital-associated *Salmonella* involves determination of serotype, drug resistance patterns, and possibly other strain markers such as pulsed field gel electrophoresis patterns, ribotype, and plasmid profiles. Many hospitals have developed protocols designed to minimize the occurrence of these epidemics, including isolating horses with diarrhea, controlling animal traffic patterns, routinely disinfecting the hospital with an agent of known effectiveness, controlling rodents, using footbaths, limiting access to the hospital area, regularly monitoring drains and other areas of the hospital for salmonellae, routinely repeatedly monitoring horses admitted to the hospital to determine whether they are shedding *Salmonella*, wearing barrier clothing when attending animals at high risk, and educating personnel. Renovations to the hospital may be required to facilitate thorough cleaning. Closing the hospital for a period of time is often necessary to thoroughly clean and disinfect the premises and to break the cycle of transmission. Outbreaks of salmonellosis have been reported among dogs in veterinary teaching hospitals, but these occurrences are uncommon; antibacterial therapy is a predisposing factor.

TYZZER'S DISEASE

Tyzzer's disease is an acute bacterial infection of a wide range of animals (*see also* p 1579 and p 1626) that is seen worldwide. Sporadic fatal infection of foals is common, and acute fatal epidemics occur in laboratory animals. The disease is rare in dogs, cats, and calves. It primarily affects young, stressed animals; however, some species appear resistant unless stressed or immunosuppressed, while others are susceptible without immunosuppression. Immunosuppressive drugs and some antibacterials, especially sulfonamides, predispose animals to the disease.

Etiology and Pathogenesis: The cause is *Clostridium piliforme* (previously *Bacillus piliformis*), a motile, filamentous, gram-negative, sporeforming, obligate, intracellular bacterium. It does not grow in cell-free media but can be cultured in the yolk sac of chick embryos or tissue culture cells. The vegetative phase is very labile; spores may survive in soiled bedding at room temperature for 1 yr and can also survive at ~133°F (60°C) for 1 hr.

The pathogenesis is poorly understood. Infection most likely results from oral exposure. Possible sources include infective spores from the environment, contact with carrier animals, and in foals, ingestion of horse feces. The primary site of infection is the lower intestinal tract with subsequent dissemination via the blood or lymphatics. The bacterium has an affinity for the intestine (epithelial and smooth muscle cells), hepatocytes, and cardiac myocytes. Stress factors such as capture, overcrowding, shipping, and poor sanitation appear to be predisposing. Sulfonamide administration predisposes rabbits to the disease. Mortality is highest at weaning age except in foals, in which the disease is seen between 1 and 6 wk of age, with most cases between 1 and 2 wk. In some species, the disease has been identified concurrently with other diseases, eg, feline infectious peritonitis in cats, distemper and mycotic pneumonia in dogs, and cryptosporidial and coronaviral enteritis in calves.

The disease most often affects well-nourished animals during periods of stress. Under laboratory conditions, stress is created by immunosuppressive drugs or other factors that can be easily identified. With many experiments, stress may be involved as part of the protocol, and when the disease develops, it is devastating.

Clinical Findings: After experimental infection, the incubation period in foals is 3-7 days; under natural conditions, the period is unknown. Most foals are found in a coma or dead. Clinical signs, if seen, are of short duration (a few hours to 2 days). Signs are variable, but may include depression, anorexia, pyrexia, jaundice, diarrhea, and recumbency. Terminally, there are convulsions and coma. Signs vary slightly between species. Laboratory animals may show depression, ruffled coat, and varying degrees of watery diarrhea; at the start of an outbreak, they often are found dead.

Clinicopathologic tests are of little value in laboratory animals because they die so rapidly. In foals, the serum enzymes sorbitol dehydrogenase, AST, alkaline phosphatase, lactate dehydrogenase, and γ-glutamyltransferase are increased. There is also hyperbilirubinemia, leukopenia, hemoconcentration, and terminally profound hypoglycemia.

Lesions: Characteristic lesions are seen in the liver, myocardium, and intestinal tract. In the liver, white, gray, or yellowish foci of necrosis, 2 mm in diameter, are few to disseminated. The hepatic necrosis is most marked and disseminated in foals in which the multiple necrotic foci with slightly depressed hemorrhagic centers appear to infect almost every hepatic lobule. In addition, there is marked hepatomegaly, and the hepatic lymph nodes are hyperplastic. In rabbits, severe lesions develop in the intestines and heart. The terminal ileum, cecum, and proximal colon are diffusely reddened. Diffuse ("paint-brush") hemorrhage is frequently seen on the serosa of the cecum. Patchy areas of mucosal necrosis are present in the cecum and colon, together with marked edema of the wall of the cecum. Mesenteric lymph nodes may be enlarged and edematous. White streaks in the myocardium may be present, especially near the apex. Intestinal and heart lesions are generally milder or absent in other animals.

Microscopically, randomly distributed and coalescing foci of necrosis in the liver are associated with scant to moderate infiltration of neutrophils and macrophages. The causative bacteria are found in a crisscross pattern in viable hepatocytes at the periphery of the necrotic foci. In the cecum and colon of rabbits, patchy areas of necrosis extend as deep as the muscularis externa with associated mucosal and submucosal infiltrates of neutrophils. Organisms may be found in the epithelium, muscularis mucosa, and muscularis externa of the affected intestine. When cardiac lesions are present, they consist of foci of fiber fragmentation, vacuolation, loss of cross-striations, and minimal inflammatory cell infiltration.

Diagnosis: Definitive diagnosis is based on demonstration of organisms in tissue sections with special stains. The organism stains poorly with H&E and Gram's stains. With Giemsa stain, the bacillus stains well in the liver and intestinal epithelium and in smears of infected organs but poorly in smooth muscles and cardiac muscle cells. The Warthin-Starry or Levaditi silver stains are preferable to other stains because the bacillus stains well in the cytoplasm of all infected cells.

Treatment and Control: Little is known about the effectiveness of antibiotics for treatment; some antibiotics are known to aggravate the disease. *C piliforme* is sensitive to tetracycline and partially sensitive to streptomycin, erythromycin, penicillin, and chlortetracycline; it is resistant to sulfonamides and chloramphenicol. In foals, the disease seems to be nearly 100% fatal, although it is likely that some foals survive. A definitive clinical diagnosis is not possible due to the lack of a definitive diagnostic test. Once the disease is present on a farm, it may be seen sporadically year after year. Animals suspected of being infected may be treated IV initially with 50% dextrose, followed by 10% dextrose (slowly), other fluid therapy, and antibiotics. Most foals respond dramatically to the dextrose therapy but relapse into a coma and die in a few hours. Rarely, an occasional foal appears to survive the disease after prolonged treatment with dextrose given slowly IV with antibiotics.

Because the disease in foals is sporadic and not highly contagious, specific preventive measures are usually not indicated. Reducing factors that cause stress and immunosuppression lessens the incidence. When the disease is seen in a colony, treatment is not recommended because it prolongs the disease and possibly produces carrier animals. It is best to destroy all animals in the colony and attempt to restock with disease-free animals.

AMEBIASIS

(Amebiosis)

Amebiasis is an acute or chronic colitis, characterized by persistent diarrhea or dysentery, that is prevalent in tropical and subtropical areas worldwide. Its prevalence has declined in the USA over the past several decades, but the disease is still important in many tropical areas, particularly in times of disasters. It is common in people and nonhuman primates, sometimes seen in dogs and cats, and rare in other mammals. Several species of amebae are found in mammals, but the only known pathogen is *Entamoeba histolytica*. Humans are the natural host for this species and the usual source of infection for domestic animals. Mammals become infected by ingesting food or water contaminated with feces containing infective cysts. *E dispar* is a noninvasive, nonpathogenic amoeba that is molecularly distinct but morphologically indistinguishable from the pathogenic species *E histolytica*. *E invadens* of reptiles is also morphologically identical to *E histolytica*, but it is not transmissible to mammals.

Clinical Findings: *E histolytica* is a pathogen with variable virulence. It lives in the lumen of the large intestine and cecum and may produce no obvious clinical signs or invade the intestinal mucosa and produce mild to severe, ulcerative, hemorrhagic colitis. In acute disease, fulminating dysentery may develop, which may be fatal, progress to chronicity, or resolve spontaneously. Chronic cases may show weight loss, anorexia, tenesmus, and chronic diarrhea or dysentery, which may be continuous or intermittent. In addition to the colon and cecum, amebae may invade perianal skin, genitalia, liver, brain, lungs, kidneys, and other organs. Signs may resemble those of other colonic diseases (eg, trichuriasis, balantidiasis). Invasive amebiasis is exacerbated by immunosuppression.

Diagnosis: Definitive diagnosis depends on finding *E histolytica* trophozoites or cysts in feces. Trophozoites are best seen in direct saline smears or in stained sections of affected colonic tissue. These parasites are difficult to find because many animals with extraintestinal amebiasis have no concurrent intestinal infection. Colonoscopy with scraping or biopsy of ulcerations is more effective than fecal examination in diagnosing amebic colitis. In intestinal infections, repeated examinations may be necessary because parasites may be passed periodically in the feces. Trophozoites range in size from 10-60 μm but usually are >20 μm in diameter, have a single vesicular nucleus, (usually with a central karyosome), are motile, and may contain ingested RBC. Feces should be examined promptly because the trophozoites die quickly once outside the body. Fecal leukocytes may be mistaken for amebae, so fixed and stained fecal smears (iodine, trichrome, iron, hematoxylin, or periodic acid-Schiff reaction) may be necessary for identification. Cysts range from 10-20 μm in diameter; the usual size is 12-15 μm. Mature cysts have 4 nuclei, while immature cysts may have 1 or 2. In primates, the cysts may be recovered and identified on zinc sulfate flotations or in fixed and stained preparations (iodine, trichrome, or iron hematoxylin); however, *E histolytica* cysts are seldom if ever excreted by dogs or cats. An ELISA-based antigen test, available for diagnosis in humans, may also aid diagnosis in other mammals. Immunostaining may also be useful.

Treatment: Scant information on treatment in animals is available. Metronidazole (10-25 mg/kg, PO, BID for 1 wk) or furazolidone (2-4 mg/kg, PO, TID for 1 wk) has been suggested. Dogs may continue to shed trophozoites after therapy.

COCCIDIOSIS

Coccidiosis is a usually acute invasion and destruction of intestinal mucosa by protozoa of the genera *Eimeria* or *Isospora*. Infection is characterized by diarrhea, fever, inappetence, weight loss, emaciation, and sometimes death. Coccidiosis is a serious disease in cattle, sheep, goats, pigs, poultry (p 2201), and also rabbits, in which the liver as well as the intestine can be affected (p 1583). In dogs, cats, and horses, it is less often diagnosed but can result in clinical illness. Other genera, of both hosts and protozoa, can be involved (*see* CRYPTOSPORIDIOSIS, p 168, SARCOCYSTOSIS, p 974, and TOXOPLASMOSIS, p 547).

Etiology and Epidemiology: *Eimeria* and *Isospora* typically require only one host in which to complete their life cycles. Some species of *Isospora* have facultative intermediate (paratenic or transfer) hosts. A new genus name, *Cystoisospora*, has been proposed but has not gained wide acceptance. Coccidia are host-specific, and there is no cross-immunity between species of coccidia.

Coccidiosis is seen universally, most commonly in animals housed or confined in small areas contaminated with oocysts. Coccidia are opportunistic pathogens; if pathogenic, their virulence may be influenced by various stressors. Therefore, clinical coccidiosis is most prevalent under conditions of poor nutrition, poor sanitation, or overcrowding, or after the stresses of weaning, shipping, sudden changes of feed, or severe weather.

In general, for most species of farm animals, the infection rate is high and rate of clinical disease is low (5-10%), although up to 80% of animals in a high-risk group may show signs. Most animals acquire *Eimeria* or *Isospora* infections of varying severity when between 1 mo and 1 yr old. Older animals usually are resistant to clinical disease but may have sporadic inapparent infections. Such clinically healthy, mature animals usually can be sources of infection to young, susceptible animals.

Pathogenesis: Infection results from ingestion of infective oocysts. Oocysts enter the environment in the feces of an infected host, but oocysts of *Eimeria* and *Isospora* are unsporulated and therefore not infective. Under favorable conditions of oxygen, humidity, and temperature, oocysts sporulate and become infective in several days. During sporulation, the amorphous protoplasm develops into small bodies (sporozoites) within secondary cysts (sporocysts) in the oocyst. In *Eimeria* spp, the sporulated oocyst has 4 sporocysts, each containing 2 sporozoites; in *Isospora* spp, the sporulated oocyst has 2 sporocysts, each containing 4 sporozoites.

When the sporulated oocyst is ingested by a susceptible animal, the sporozoites escape from the oocyst, invade the intestinal mucosa or epithelial cells in other locations, and develop intracellularly into multinucleate schizonts (also called meronts). Each nucleus develops into an infective body called a merozoite; merozoites enter new cells and repeat the process. After a variable number of asexual generations, merozoites develop into either macrogametocytes (females) or microgametocytes (males). These produce a single macrogamete or a number of microgametes in a host cell. After being fertilized by a microgamete, the macrogamete develops into an oocyst. The oocysts have resistant walls and are discharged unsporulated in the feces. Oocysts do not survive well at temperatures below −30°C or above 40°C; within this range, they may survive up to 1 yr or more.

Of the numerous species of *Eimeria* or *Isospora* that can infect a particular host, not all are pathogenic. Concurrent infections with 2 or more species, some of which may not normally be considered pathogenic, also influence clinical disease. Within pathogenic species, strains may vary in virulence.

Clinical Findings: Clinical signs of coccidiosis are due to destruction of the intestinal epithelium and, frequently, the underlying connective tissue of the mucosa. This may be accompanied by hemorrhage into the lumen of the intestine, catarrhal inflammation, and diarrhea. Signs may include discharge of blood or tissue, tenesmus, and dehydration. Serum protein and electrolyte levels may be appreciably altered, but changes in Hgb or PCV are seen only in severely affected animals.

Diagnosis: Oocysts can be identified in feces by salt or sugar flotation methods. Finding appreciable numbers of oocysts of pathogenic species in the feces is diagnostic, but because diarrhea may precede the heavy output of oocysts by 1-2 days and may continue after the oocyst discharge has returned to low levels, it is not always possible to find oocysts in a single fecal sample; multiple examinations may be required. The number of oocysts present in feces is influenced by the genetically determined reproductive potential of the species, the number of infective oocysts ingested, stage of the infection, age and immune status of the animal, prior exposure, consistency of the fecal sample, and method of examination. Therefore, the results of fecal examinations must be related to clinical signs and intestinal lesions (gross and microscopic). Furthermore, the species must be determined to be pathogenic in that host. The finding of numerous oocysts of a nonpathogenic species concurrent with diarrhea does not constitute a diagnosis of clinical coccidiosis.

Treatment: The life cycles of *Eimeria* and *Isospora* are self-limiting and end spontaneously within a few weeks unless reinfection occurs. Prompt medication may slow or inhibit development of stages resulting from reinfection and, thus, can shorten the length of illness, reduce discharge of oocysts, alleviate hemorrhage and diarrhea, and lessen the likelihood of secondary infections and death. Sick animals should be isolated and treated individually whenever possible to ensure delivery of therapeutic drug levels and to prevent exposure of other animals. Sulfonamides may be used. Sulfaquinoxaline has been reported to give excellent clinical results in beef and dairy calves, sheep, dogs, and cats. Because the soluble sulfonamides may be given PO or parenterally, they are more effective than intestinal sulfonamides. Amprolium has been reported to be effective during outbreaks in calves, sheep, and goats. In outbreaks in feedlots or on lush pastures, preventive treatment of healthy exposed animals as a safeguard against additional morbidity should be considered.

Prevention: Prevention is based on limiting the intake of sporulated oocysts by young animals so that an infection is established to induce immunity but not clinical signs. Good feeding practices and good management, including sanitation, contribute to this goal. Neonates should receive colostrum. Young susceptible animals should be kept in clean and dry quarters. Feeding and watering devices should be clean and protected from fecal contamination. Stresses (eg, weaning, sudden changes in feed, and shipping) should be minimized.

Preventive administration of coccidiostats is recommended when animals under various management regimens can be predictably expected to develop coccidiosis. In virtually all cases, *Eimeria* spp are implicated. Decoquinate, amprolium, and ionophorous antibiotics are effective in cattle. Continuous low-level feeding of amprolium, decoquinate, lasalocid, or monensin during the first month of feedlot confinement has been reported to have preventive value. Both amprolium and ionophorous antibiotics have been reported to be effective in goat kids, as have sulfas and amprolium in pigs.

Coccidiosis of Cattle

E zuernii, *E bovis*, and *E auburnensis* are the species most often associated with clinical disease in cattle. Experimentally, other species have been shown to be mildly or moderately pathogenic. Coccidiosis is commonly a disease of young cattle (1-2 mo to 1 yr) and usually is sporadic during the wet seasons of the year. "Summer coccidiosis" and "winter coccidiosis" in range cattle probably result from severe weather stress and crowding around a limited water source, which concentrates the hosts and parasites within a restricted area. Although particularly severe epidemics have been reported in feedlot cattle during extremely cold weather, cattle confined to feedlots are susceptible to coccidiosis throughout the year. Outbreaks usually occur within the first month of confinement. The incubation period is 17-21 days.

The most typical syndrome is chronic or subclinical disease in groups of growing animals. Calves may appear unthrifty and have fecal-stained perineal areas. In light infections, cattle appear healthy and oocysts are present in normally formed feces, but feed efficiency is reduced. The most characteristic sign of clinical coccidiosis is watery feces, with little or no blood, and the animal shows only slight discomfort for a few days. Severe infections are rare. Severely affected cattle develop thin, bloody diarrhea that may continue for >1 wk, or thin feces with streaks or clots of blood, shreds of epithelium, and mucus. They may develop a fever; become anorectic, depressed, and dehydrated; and lose weight. Tenesmus is common. During the acute period, some cattle die; others die later from secondary complications (eg, pneumonia). Cattle that survive severe illness can lose significant weight that is not quickly regained or can remain permanently stunted. Calves with concurrent infections (eg, coronavirus) may be more severely affected than calves with coccidia infections alone. In addition, management factors, such as weather, housing, feeding practices, and how animals are grouped, are important in determining the expression of clinical coccidiosis in cattle.

The pathogenic coccidia of cattle can damage the mucosa of the lower small intestine, cecum, and colon. The first-generation schizonts of *E bovis* appear as white macroscopic bodies in the villi of the small intestine.

Nervous signs (eg, muscular tremors, hyperesthesia, clonic-tonic convulsions with ventroflexion of the head and neck, nystagmus) and a high mortality rate (80-90%) are seen in calves with acute clinical coccidiosis. Outbreaks of this "nervous form" have occurred in which 30-50% of all susceptible calves are affected. It has been seen most commonly during, or following, severely cold weather in midwinter in Canada and the northern USA. Affected calves may die <24 hr after the onset of dysentery and nervous signs, or they may live for several days, commonly in a laterally recumbent position with a mild degree of opisthotonos. In spite of intensive supportive therapy, the mortality rate is high. Nervous signs have not been reported in experimental clinical coccidiosis in calves, which suggests that the nervous signs may be unrelated to the dysentery or, indeed, even to coccidiosis.

Diagnosis is by finding oocysts on fecal flotation or direct smear or by the McMaster's technique. Differential diagnoses include salmonellosis, bovine virus diarrhea, malnutrition, toxins, or other intestinal parasites.

Coccidiosis is a self-limiting disease, and spontaneous recovery without specific treatment is common when the multiplication stage of the coccidia has passed. The chemotherapeutic agents in common use for clinical coccidiosis are unlikely to have any effect on the late stages of the coccidia. Most of the coccidiostats have a depressant effect on the early, first-stage schizonts and are used for control.

Drugs that can be used for therapy of clinically affected animals include amprolium (10 mg/kg/day for 5 days) and sulfaquinoxaline (6 mg/lb/day for 3-5 days). Sulfaquinoxaline is particularly useful for feedlot cattle that develop bloody diarrhea after arrival. For prevention, amprolium (5 mg/kg/day for 21 days), decoquinate (22.7 mg/45 kg/day for 28 days) and lasalocid (1 mg/kg/day to a maximum of 360 mg/head/day), or monensin (100-360 mg/head/day) can be used. The major benefits of the coccidiostats are through improved feed efficiency and rate of gain.

In an outbreak, the clinically affected animals should be isolated and given supportive oral and parenteral fluid therapy as necessary. The population density of the affected pens should be reduced. All feed and water supplies should be high enough off the ground to avoid fecal contamination. Mass medication of the feed and water supplies may be indicated in an attempt to prevent new cases and to minimize the effects of an epidemic. Cattle with coccidiosis and nervous signs should be brought indoors, kept well-bedded and warm, and given fluid therapy orally and parenterally. However, the case fatality rate is high despite intensive supportive therapy. Parenteral sulfonamide therapy may be indicated to control the development of secondary bacterial enteritis or pneumonia, which may develop in calves with coccidiosis during very cold weather. Corticosteroids are contraindicated.

Coccidiosis has been difficult to control reliably. Overcrowding of animals should be avoided while they develop an immunity to the coccidial species in the environment. Calving grounds should be well drained and kept as dry as possible. All measures that minimize fecal contamination of hair coats and fleece should be practiced regularly. Feed and water troughs should be high enough to avoid heavy fecal contamination. Control of coccidiosis in feeder calves brought into a crowded feedlot depends on management of population density, or use of chemotherapeutics, to control the numbers of oocysts ingested by the animals while effective immunity develops.

Coccidiostats are used for the control of naturally occurring coccidiosis. The ideal coccidiostat suppresses the full development of the life cycle of the coccidia, allows immunity to develop, and does not interfere with production performance. Sulfonamides in the feed at 25-35 mg/kg for ≥15 days are effective for the control of coccidiosis in calves. Monensin is an effective coccidiostat and growth promotant in calves. Withdrawal of monensin may be followed by development of fatal coccidiosis in some animals, presumably because the drug suppressed the development of immunity. Postweaning coccidiosis in beef calves has been controlled using monensin administered via intraluminal continuous release devices. Lasalocid is related to monensin and is also an effective coccidiostat for ruminants. Mixing lasalocid in the milk replacer of calves beginning at 2-4 days of age is an effective method of controlling coccidiosis. Lasalocid is also effective as a coccidiostat when fed free-choice in salt at a level of 0.75% of the total salt mixture. A level of 1 mg/kg is the most effective and rapid, and is recommended when outbreaks of coccidiosis are imminent. Decoquinate in the feed at 0.5-1.0 mg/kg suppressed oocyst production in experimentally induced coccidiosis of calves. It is most effective in preventing coccidial infections when fed continuously in dry feed at 0.5 mg/kg. Monensin, lasalocid, and decoquinate at the manufacturer's recommended levels are equally effective. Toltrazuril administered at 20 mg/kg as a single dose, 10 days after animals are turned out to pasture, almost completely prevents coccidiosis.

Control of infection should include changes in management factors that contribute to the development of clinical disease. Inadequate housing and ventilation should be corrected, feeding practices adopted that avoid fecal contamination of feed, calves grouped by size, and an "all-in/all-out" method of calf movement from pen to pen adopted.

Coccidiosis of Sheep

Infection with *Eimeria* is one of the most economically important diseases of sheep. Historically, some *Eimeria* spp were thought to be infectious and transmissible between sheep and goats, but the parasites are now considered host-specific. The names of some species of goat coccidia are still erroneously applied to species of similar appearance found in sheep. *E ahsata* and *E ovinoidalis (ninakohlyakimovae)* are pathogens of lambs, usually 1-6 mo old; *E ovina* appears to be somewhat less pathogenic. Older sheep serve as sources of infection for the young. All other *Eimeria* of sheep are essentially nonpathogenic, even when large numbers of oocysts are present in feces.

Signs include diarrhea (sometimes containing blood or mucus), dehydration, fever, inappetence, weight loss, anemia, wool breaking, and death. The ileum, cecum, and upper colon are usually most affected and may be thickened, edematous, and inflamed; sometimes, there is mucosal hemorrhage. Thick, white, opaque patches containing large numbers of *E ovina* oocysts may develop in the small intestine. Because oocysts are prevalent in feces of sheep of all ages, coccidiosis cannot be diagnosed based solely on finding oocysts. Peak oocyst counts of >100,000/g of feces have been reported in 8- to 12-wk-old lambs that appeared healthy. However, diarrhea with oocyst counts of a pathogenic species of >20,000/g is characteristic of coccidiosis in sheep. Immune complex glomerulonephritis has also been attributed to coccidiosis. Fly strike and secondary bacterial enteric infections may accompany coccidiosis.

Lambs 1-6 mo old in lambing pens, intensive grazing areas, and feedlots are at greatest risk as a result of shipping, ration change, crowding stress, severe weather, and contamination of the environment with oocysts from ewes or other lambs. Because occurrence of coccidiosis under these management systems often becomes so predictable, coccidiostats should be administered prophylactically for 28 consecutive days beginning a few days after lambs are introduced into the environment. A concentrated ration containing monensin at 15 g/tonne can be fed to ewes from 4 wk before lambing until weaning, and to lambs from 4-20 wk of age. The toxic level of monensin for lambs is 4 mg/kg.

Lasalocid (15-70 mg/head/day, depending on body wt) may be effective. A combination of monensin and lasalocid at 22 and 100 mg/kg of diet, respectively, is an effective prophylactic against naturally occurring coccidiosis in early weaned lambs under feedlot conditions. Treatment of affected sheep once coccidiosis has been diagnosed is not effective, but severity can be reduced if treatment is begun early. A single treatment of toltrazuril (20 mg/kg) can significantly reduce the oocyst output in naturally infected lambs for ~3 wk after administration. Sulfaquinoxaline in drinking water at 0.015% concentration for 3-5 days may be used for treatment of affected lambs. In groups of lambs at pasture, the frequent rotation of pastures for parasite control will also help control coccidial infection. However, when lambs are exposed to infection early in life as a result of infection from the ewe and a contaminated lambing ground, a solid immunity usually develops and only when the stocking density is extremely high will a problem develop.

Coccidiosis of Goats

Numerous species of *Eimeria* are found in goats in North America. The *Eimeria* spp are host-specific and are not transmitted from sheep to goats.

E arloingi, *E christenseni*, and *E ovinoidalis* are highly pathogenic in kids. Clinical signs include diarrhea with or without mucus or blood, dehydration, emaciation, weakness, anorexia, and death. Some goats are actually constipated and die acutely without diarrhea. Usually, stages and lesions are confined to the small intestine, which may appear congested, hemorrhagic, or ulcerated, and have scattered pale, yellow to white macroscopic plaques in the mucosa. Histologically, villous epithelium is sloughed, and inflammatory cells are seen in the lamina propria and submucosa. In addition, there have been several reports of hepatobiliary coccidiosis with liver failure in dairy goats. Diagnosis of intestinal coccidiosis is based on finding oocysts of the pathogenic species in diarrheal feces, usually at tens of thousands to millions per gram of feces. It is not unusual to find oocyst counts as high as 70,000 in kids without overt disease, but weight gain may be affected.

Angora and dairy goats, raised under different management practices, may have similar patterns of exposure of kids. Just after parturition, nursery pens and surrounding areas may be heavily contaminated with oocysts from does. Resistance to infection is decreased just after shipping, changing rations, introducing new animals, or mixing young with older animals. Coccidiostats can be administered to a herd immediately after diagnosis or as a preventive in predictable situations such as those mentioned above.

Diagnosis and treatment are similar to those for cattle and sheep. Sulfadimidine at 55 g/tonne is also effective for the control of coccidiosis in goats. In nonlactating goats, adding monensin to the feed at 18 g/tonne is preventive.

Coccidiosis of Pigs

Eight species of *Eimeria* and 1 of *Isospora* infect pigs in the USA. Piglets 5-15 days old are characteristically infected with only *I suis*, which produces enteritis and diarrhea. These agents must be differentiated from viruses, bacteria, and helminths that also cause scours in neonatal pigs.

I suis is prevalent in neonatal pigs. Infection is characterized by a watery or greasy diarrhea, usually yellowish to white and foul smelling. Piglets may appear weak, dehydrated, and undersized; weight gains are depressed, and sometimes piglets die. A contributing factor to mortality is that piglets become covered with diarrheic feces and stay damp. Oocysts are usually shed in the feces and can be identified by their size, shape, and sporulation characteristics; however, in peracute infections, diagnosis must be based on finding stages of the parasite in impression smears or histologic sections of the small intestine because pigs can die before oocysts are formed. In severely affected piglets, histologic lesions confined to the jejunum and ileum are characterized by villous atrophy, blunting of villi, focal ulceration, and fibrinonecrotic enteritis with parasite stages in epithelial cells. Preventive control by feeding anticoccidials to sows from 2 wk before farrowing through lactation or to neonatal pigs from birth to weaning has been reported; however, effectiveness of the latter has not been confirmed. Although the sow is a logical source of infection for piglets, this has not been well documented. Thorough removal of feces and disinfection of farrowing facilities between litters greatly decreases infection. Piglets that recover from infection are highly resistant to reinfection.

Although less commonly associated with clinical coccidiosis, *E debliecki, E neodebliecki, E scabra,* and *E spinosa* have been found in pigs ~1-3 mo old with diarrhea. Illness may last 7-10 days, with pigs remaining unthrifty.

Treatment may include sulfamethazine in drinking water. The control of coccidiosis in newborn piglets infected with *I suis* has been unreliable. The use of coccidiostats in the feed of the sow for several days or a few weeks prior to, and following, farrowing has been recommended and used in the field, but the results are variable. Amprolium and monensin are ineffective for the prevention of experimental coccidiosis in piglets. A control program designed to decrease the number of oocysts has been recommended and consists of proper cleaning, disinfection, and steam cleaning of the farrowing housing. Amprolium (25% feed grade) at the rate of 10 kg/tonne of sows' feed started 1 wk before farrowing and continued until the piglets are 3 wk of age has been recommended, but the results are unsatisfactory. A single oral dose of 1.0 mL of toltrazuril given to piglets 3-6 days old reduced the occurrence of coccidiosis from 71% to 22%, and the number of days that oocysts were excreted in the feces was reduced from 4.9 to 2.5.

Coccidiosis of Cats and Dogs

Many species of coccidia infect the intestinal tract of cats and dogs. All species appear to be host-specific. Cats have species of *Isospora, Besnoitia, Toxoplasma, Hammondia,* and *Sarcocystis.* Dogs have species of *Isospora, Hammondia,* and *Sarcocystis.* Neither dogs nor cats have *Eimeria.*

Hammondia has an obligatory 2-host life cycle with cats or dogs as final hosts and rodents or ruminants as intermediate hosts. *Hammondia* oocysts are indistinguishable from those of *Toxoplasma* and *Besnoitia* but are nonpathogenic in either host. *See also* BESNOITIOSIS, p 484, SARCOCYSTOSIS, p 974, and TOXOPLASMOSIS, p 547.

The most common coccidia of cats and dogs are *Isospora.* Some *Isospora* spp of cats and dogs can facultatively infect other mammals and produce in various organs an encysted form that is infective for the cat or dog. Two species infect cats: *I felis* and *I rivolta;* both can be identified easily by oocyst size and shape. Almost every cat eventually becomes infected with *I felis.* Four species infect dogs: *I canis, I ohioensis, I burrowsi,* and *I neorivolta.* In dogs, only *I canis* can be identified by the oocyst structure; the other 3 *Isospora* overlap in dimensions and can be differentiated only by endogenous developmental characteristics.

Clinical coccidiosis, although not common, has been reported in kittens and puppies. In kittens, it is seen primarily during weaning stress. The most common clinical signs in severe cases are diarrhea (sometimes bloody), weight loss, and dehydration. Usually, coccidiosis is associated with other infectious agents, immunosuppression, or stress.

Treatment may be unnecessary in cats because they usually spontaneously eliminate the infection. In clinically affected cats, trimethoprim-sulfa (30-60 mg/kg/day for 6 days) can be used.

In kennel conditions when the need for prophylaxis might be predicted, amprolium is said to be effective, although it is not approved for use in dogs. In severe cases, in addition to supportive fluid therapy, sulfonamides such as sulfadimethoxine (50 mg/kg the first day and 25 mg/kg/day for 2-3 wk thereafter) can be used. Sanitation is important, especially in catteries and kennels, or where large numbers of animals are housed. Feces should be removed frequently. Fecal contamination of feed and water should be prevented. Runs, cages, and utensils should be disinfected daily. Raw meat should not be fed. Insect control should be established.

CRYPTOSPORIDIOSIS

Cryptosporidiosis is recognized worldwide, primarily in neonatal calves but also in lambs, kids, foals, and piglets. It is considered a cause of varying degrees of naturally occurring diarrhea in neonatal farm animals. The parasites commonly act in concert with other enteropathogens to produce intestinal injury and diarrhea.

Etiology and Epidemiology: *Cryptosporidium parvum* infection is common in young ruminants and is found in many species of mammals, including humans. Infection is common in calves. Cryptosporidia have been detected in 70% of 1- to 3-wk-old dairy calves. Infection can be detected as early as 5 days of age, with the greatest proportion of calves excreting organisms between days 9 and 14. Many reports associate infection in calves with diarrhea occurring at 5-15 days of age. *C parvum* is also a common enteric infection in young lambs and goats. Diarrhea can result from a monoinfection, but more commonly is associated with mixed infections. Infection can be associated with severe outbreaks of diarrhea, with high case fatality rates in lambs 4-10 days of age and in goat kids 5-21 days of age. Cryptosporidial infection in pigs is seen over a wider age range than in ruminants and has been observed in pigs from 1 wk of age through market age. The majority of infections are asymptomatic, and the organism does not appear to be an important enteric pathogen in pigs, although it may contribute to postweaning malabsorptive diarrhea. Cryptosporidial infection in foals appears less prevalent and is seen at a later age than in ruminants, with excretion rates peaking at 5-8 wk of age. Infection is not usually detected in yearlings or adults. Most studies indicate that cryptosporidiosis is not a common disease in foals; infections in immunocompetent foals are usually subclinical. Persistent clinical infections are seen in Arabian foals with inherited combined immunodeficiency. Cryptosporidiosis is also recorded in young deer and can be a cause of diarrhea in artificially reared orphans.

Transmission: The source of infection is oocysts that are fully sporulated and infective when excreted in the feces. Large numbers are excreted during the patent period, resulting in heavy environmental contamination. Transmission may occur directly from calf to calf, indirectly via fomite or human transmission, from contamination in the environment, or by fecal contamination of the feed or water supply. A periparturient rise in the excretion of oocysts may occur in ewes. *C parvum* is not host-specific, and infection from other species (eg, rodents, farm cats) via contamination of feed is also possible.

Oocysts are resistant to most disinfectants and can survive for several months in cool and moist conditions. Oocyst infectivity can be destroyed by ammonia, formalin, freeze-drying, and exposure to temperatures <32°F (0°C) or >149°F (65°C). Ammonium hydroxide, hydrogen peroxide, chlorine dioxide, 10% formol saline, and 5% ammonia are effective in destroying oocyst infectivity. Infectivity in calf feces is reduced after 1-4 days of drying.

Concurrent infections with other enteric pathogens, especially rotavirus and coronavirus, are common, and epidemiologic studies suggest that diarrhea is more severe in mixed infections. Immunocompromised animals are more susceptible to clinical disease than immunocompetent animals, but the relationship between disease and failure of passive transfer of colostral immunoglobulins is not clear. Age-related resistance, unrelated to prior exposure, is observed in lambs but not calves. Infection results in the production of parasite-specific antibody, but both cell-mediated and humoral antibody are important in protection, as well as local antibody in the gut of the neonate.

Case fatality rates in cryptosporidiosis are generally low unless complicated by other factors (eg, concurrent infections, energy deficits from inadequate intake of colostrum and milk, chilling from adverse weather conditions).

Pathogenesis: The life cycle of *Cryptosporidium* consists of 6 major developmental events. Following ingestion of the oocyst there is excystation (release of infective sporozoites), merogony (asexual multiplication), gametogony (gamete formation), fertilization, oocyst wall formation, and sporogony (sporozoite formation). Oocysts of *Cryptosporidium* spp can sporulate within host cells and are infective when passed in the feces. Infection persists until the host's immune response eliminates the parasite. In natural and experimentally produced cases in calves, cryptosporidia are most numerous in the lower part of the small intestine and less common in the cecum and colon. Prepatent periods are 2-7 days in calves and 2-5 days in lambs. Oocysts are usually passed in the feces of calves for 3-12 days.

Clinical Findings: Calves usually have a mild to moderate diarrhea that persists for several days regardless of treatment. The age at onset is later, and the duration of diarrhea tends to be a few days longer than are seen in the diarrheas caused by rotavirus, coronavirus, or enterotoxigenic *Escherichia coli*. Feces are yellow or pale, watery, and contain mucus. The persistent diarrhea may result in marked weight loss and emaciation. In most cases, the diarrhea is self-limiting after several days. Varying degrees of apathy, anorexia, and dehydration are present. Only rarely do severe dehydration, weakness, and collapse occur, in contrast to other causes of acute diarrhea in neonatal calves. Case fatality rates can be high in herds with cryptosporidiosis when the calf feeder withholds milk and feeds only electrolyte solutions during the episode of diarrhea. The persistent nature of the diarrhea leads to a marked energy deficit in these circumstances, and the calves die of inanition at 3-4 wk of age.

Lesions: Calves with persistent diarrhea have villous atrophy in the small intestine. Histologically, large numbers of the parasite are embedded in the microvilli of the absorptive enterocytes. In low-grade infections, only a few parasites are present, with no apparent histologic changes in the intestine. The villi are shorter than normal, with crypt hyperplasia and a mixed inflammatory cell infiltrate.

Diagnosis: Diagnosis is based on detection of oocysts by examination of fecal smears with Ziehl-Neelson stains, by fecal flotation, or by immunologically assisted methods. It has been suggested that if the diarrhea is caused by cryptosporidia, there should be 10^5-10^7 oocysts/mL of feces. The oocysts are small (5-6 mm in diameter) and relatively nonrefractile. They are difficult to detect by normal light microscopy but are readily detected by phase-contrast microscopy.

Treatment: There are no currently licensed therapeutics available in the USA for *C parvum* infection in food animals. Anecdotal reports of success with extra-label use of various compounds have not been replicated in controlled trials. Experimental treatments have for the most part been toxic or ineffective. Halofuginone is reported to markedly reduce oocyst output in experimentally infected lambs and naturally and experimentally infected calves; therapy was also reported to prevent diarrhea. Paromomycin sulfate (100 mg/kg, PO, SID for 11 days from the second day of age) proved successful in preventing natural disease in a controlled clinical field trial in goat kids.

Affected calves should be supported with fluids and electrolytes, both orally and parenterally, as necessary until recovery occurs. Cows' whole milk should be given in small quantities several times daily (to the full level of requirement) to optimize digestion and to minimize weight loss. Several days of intensive care and feeding may be required before recovery is apparent. Parenteral nutrition may be considered for valuable calves.

Control: The disease is difficult to control. Reducing the number of oocysts ingested may reduce the severity of infection and allow immunity to develop. Calves should be born in a clean environment, and adequate amounts of colostrum should be fed at an early age. Calves should be kept separate without calf-to-calf contact for at least the first 2 wk of life, with strict hygiene at feeding. Diarrheic calves should be isolated from healthy calves during the course of the diarrhea and for several days after recovery. Great care must be taken to avoid mechanical transmission of infection. Calf-rearing houses should be vacated and cleaned out on a regular basis; an "all-in/all-out" management system, with thorough cleaning and several weeks of drying between batches of calves, should be used. Rats, mice, and flies should be controlled when possible, and rodents and pets should not have access to calf grain and milk feed storage areas.

Hyperimmune bovine colostrum can reduce the severity of diarrhea and the period of oocyst excretion in experimentally infected calves. Protection is not related to circulating levels of specific antibody but requires a high titer of *C parvum* antibody in the gut lumen for prolonged periods. Vaccination with lyophilized *C parvum* given orally shortly after birth gave partial protection to calves challenged experimentally at 1 wk of age. It was not effective in protecting against natural challenge in a field trial, presumably because natural infection occurred too early to allow development of immunity. In the same trial, lactic acid-producing probiotics had no protective effect.

Zoonotic Risk: Infections in domestic animals may be a reservoir for infection of susceptible humans. *Cryptosporidium* is considered to be a relatively common nonviral cause of self-limiting diarrhea in immunocompetent persons, particularly children. Immunocompromised persons, clinical disease may be severe. The infection is transmitted predominantly from person to person, but direct infection from animals and waterborne infection from contamination of surface water and drinking water by domestic or wild animal feces can also be important. Animal handlers on a calf farm can be at high risk of diarrhea due to cryptosporidiosis transmitted from infected calves. Immunocompromised people should be restricted from access to young animals and possibly from access to farms.

GIARDIASIS

(Giardosis, Lambliasis, Lambliosis)

Giardiasis is a chronic, intestinal protozoal infection that is seen worldwide in most domestic and wild mammals, many birds, and people. Infection is common in dogs and cats, occasional in ruminants, and rare in horses and pigs. The number of different species and the zoonotic potential of *Giardia* spp are controversial. There is circumstantial evidence that *Giardia* spp that infect domestic animals can infect people. It appears that some *Giardia* spp isolates are infective to a variety of mammals, while others are more species specific. Wild animals may also be reservoirs. *Giardia* spp have been reported to be found in 1-39% of fecal samples from pet and shelter dogs and cats, with a higher rate of infection in younger animals.

Etiology and Transmission: Flagellate protozoa (trophozoites) of the genus *Giardia* inhabit the mucosal surfaces of the small intestine, where they attach to the brush border, absorb nutrients, and multiply by binary fission. Trophozoites encyst in the small or large intestine and pass in the feces. The cyst is the infective stage, and transmission occurs by the fecal-oral route. Cyst shedding may be continuous over several days and weeks but is often intermittent. Although occasionally passed in the feces, trophozoites are not infective. Incubation and prepatent periods are generally 5-14 days. Cysts can survive in the environment, but trophozoites cannot. Overcrowding and high humidity favor survival of cysts and transmission. Earlier classifications have assigned different species names to the *Giardia* of various hosts; it is generally agreed that all species infecting mammals (except some rodents) are structurally similar.

Clinical Findings and Lesions: *Giardia* infections in dogs and cats may be inapparent or may produce weight loss and chronic diarrhea or steatorrhea, which can be continual or intermittent, particularly in puppies and kittens. Clinical disease is also reported in calves. Feces usually are soft, poorly formed, pale, malodorous, contain mucus, and appear fatty. Watery diarrhea is unusual in uncomplicated cases, and blood is not present in feces; typical small-bowel diarrhea is more common. Occasionally vomiting occurs. Giardiasis must be differentiated from other causes of nutrient malassimilation (eg, exocrine pancreatic insufficiency [p 349], intestinal malabsorption [p 339]). Clinical laboratory findings usually are normal. Pathogenesis of *Giardia* spp infections is poorly understood. Gross intestinal lesions are seldom evident, although microscopic lesions, consisting of villous atrophy and cuboidal enterocytes, may be present. Laboratory studies have demonstrated malabsorption of nutrients, decreased quantities of intestinal disaccharides, increased enterocyte turnover, lymphocytic infiltration, and villous atrophy.

Diagnosis: The motile, piriform trophozoites (10-20 × 7-10 μm) are occasionally seen in saline smears of loose or watery feces. They should not be confused with trichomonads, which have a single rather than double nucleus, an undulating membrane, and no concave ventral surface. The oval cysts (9-15 × 7-10 μm) are best detected in feces concentrated by the zinc sulfate (specific gravity 1.18) flotation technique. Sodium chloride, sucrose, or sodium nitrate flotation media are too hypertonic and severely distort the cysts. Staining cysts with iodine aids identification. Because *Giardia* cysts are excreted intermittently, several fecal examinations should be performed if giardiasis is suspected; eg, 3 samples collected and examined over 3-5 days. About 70% of infected dogs can be identified with a single zinc sulfate flotation; 93% can be identified with 2. In dogs, duodenal aspiration for trophozoite detection is useful; however, in cats, *Giardia* spp are more prevalent in the mid to lower small intestine. An ELISA that detects *Giardia* antigen in the feces of dogs and cats is available, but field data on sensitivity and specificity are lacking.

Treatment: No drugs are approved for treating giardiasis in animals. Fenbendazole (50 mg/kg/day) effectively removes *Giardia* cysts from the feces of dogs; no side effects are reported, and it is safe for pregnant and lactating animals. This dosage is approved for controlling and removing *Toxocara canis*, *Trichuris vulpis*, and *Ancylostoma caninum* in dogs. Recently, a combination product of praziquantel, pyrantel pamoate, and febantel decreased cyst excretion in infected dogs. Fenbendazole is not approved in cats, but may reduce clinical signs and cyst shedding at 50 mg/kg/day, PO, for 3-5 days. Albendazole is effective at 25 mg/kg, PO, BID for 2 days in dogs and for 5 days in cats, but should not be used in these animals because it has led to bone marrow suppression and is not approved for use in these species. *Giardia*-infected calves may be treated with albendazole or fenbendazole. Oral fenbendazole may also be an option in large animals and some birds. Metronidazole (25 mg/kg, PO, BID for 5-7 days) is ~65% effective in eliminating *Giardia* spp from infected dogs but may be associated with acute development of anorexia and vomiting, which may occasionally progress to pronounced generalized ataxia and vertical positional nystagmus. Metronidazole may be administered to cats at 10-25 mg/kg, PO, BID for 5 days. Furazolidone at 4 mg/kg, PO, BID for 7 days, is also effective in cats and small dogs, although diarrhea and vomiting are possible side effects; it is also suspected of teratogenicity. A killed vaccine, available for dogs and cats, reportedly reduces clinical signs and the number and duration of cysts shed into the environment.

Control: *Giardia* cysts are immediately infective when passed in the feces and survive in the environment. Cysts are a source of infection and reinfection for animals, particularly those in crowded conditions (eg, kennels and catteries). Prompt removal of feces from cages, runs, and yards limits environmental contamination. Cysts are inactivated by most quaternary ammonium compounds, household bleach (1:32 or 1:16 dilution), steam, and boiling water.

To increase the efficacy of disinfectants, solutions should be left for 5-20 min before being rinsed off kennel or run surfaces. Disinfection of grass yards or runs is impossible. These areas should be considered contaminated for at least a month after infected dogs last had access. Cysts are susceptible to desiccation, and areas should be allowed to dry thoroughly after cleaning. Cysts contaminating the hair of dogs and cats may be a source of reinfection. Shampooing and rinsing the animals well can help remove cysts from hair. The killed vaccines that are available for dogs and cats aid in disease prevention by decreasing or preventing cyst shedding.

DISEASES OF THE MOUTH IN LARGE ANIMALS

Lip Lacerations: Wounds of the lips and cheeks are most common in horses. They may be caused by a fall, a kick, or the use of inappropriate bits or restraint devices or, more commonly, from the horse having its lips and sometimes mandible caught as it "plays" in its stall. Lip lacerations may be accompanied by mandibular or incisive bone and dental fractures and avulsions in some cases (eg, if the horse panics). Because of the vascularity of the region, healing is usually rapid. However, once the wound has penetrated into the mouth, careful management is needed to avoid formation of a fistula. First-stage healing is best achieved by the construction of intraoral mucosal flaps to achieve an oral seal. Subsequent skin or mucosal grafts may be necessary to correct large defects or fistulae.

Glossoplegia (Paralysis of the Tongue): This may be seen in newborns as a result of the placement of obstetric snares. Such neonates need to be managed carefully to ensure that they are able to eat; ingestion of colostrum is particularly important. Fluid therapy (IV) and anti-inflammatory treatments are required. If the condition persists for >10 days after birth, the likelihood of regaining normal function is slight. Inflammatory diseases and trauma may also result in transient glossoplegia. Glossoplegia of central origin may accompany or follow such conditions as strangles, upper respiratory infections, meningitis, botulism, encephalomyelitis, leukoencephalomalacia, or cerebral abscessation in horses.

In cattle, glossoplegia may accompany severe actinobacillosis (p 476). There may be complete paralysis of the tongue accompanied by necrosis of the tip. Such conditions are occasionally seen in outbreaks in feedlot cattle and may follow an initiating viral stomatitis.

Neoplasia: Neoplasia of the mouth and lips other than viral papillomas are uncommon in younger animals. In gray horses, melanomas may develop and infiltrate the commissures of the mouth and cause hard, thickened, tumorous plaques that may not be detected until well advanced. Treatment of oral and lip melanomas in the horse is unrewarding, although prolonged cimetidine therapy may be palliative. Both verrucose and fibrous forms of equine sarcoid around the mouth should be treated as early as possible to maintain lip function. (*See also* TUMORS OF THE SKIN AND SOFT TISSUES, p 764.)

Slaframine Toxicosis: The causes are ingestion of forages, particularly clovers, infected with the fungus *Rhizoctonia leguminicola*, which produces the toxic alkaloid slaframine. The only clinical signs that may be diagnostic are profuse salivation; no lesions have been described within the mouth. Usually, there is complete recovery. Differential diagnoses in large animals, particularly in ruminants, include bluetongue, vesicular stomatitis, vesicular exanthema, and foot-and-mouth disease. Removal of infected forages results in rapid recovery.

Stomatitis: Inflammation of the mouth is a clinical sign of many diseases in large animals. Oral trauma or contact with chemical irritants (eg, horses that lick at their legs after having been blistered) may result in transient stomatitis. Traumatic injury from the ingestion of the awns of barley, foxtail, porcupine grass, and spear grass, as well as feeding on plants infested with hairy caterpillars, also will result in severe stomatitis in horses and cattle.

Frothy salivation and reluctance to eat or resistance to oral examination are the clinical signs of acute active stomatitis. The animal should be sedated, and the mouth examined carefully with a speculum. Any ulcers should be curetted to expose embedded foreign material, eg, grass awns, etc. If the etiology is ingestion of foreign material, changing the quality and quantity of the hay may effect recovery. Differential diagnoses include actinobacillosis, foot-and-mouth disease, malignant catarrhal fever, and bovine viral diarrhea. Epidemic diseases such as bluetongue in ruminants, swine vesicular disease, and vesicular stomatitis in horses must be differentiated from other forms of acute noninfectious or contagious stomatitis.

Papillar Stomatitis: Viral papillomas are found around the lips and mouths of all young animals, particularly in cattle from 1 mo to 2 yr old. In some instances, the rate of occurrence may be 100%. The lesions are characteristic and usually resolve spontaneously. However, in some cases, the lesions may coalesce to form cosmetically unacceptable masses around the muzzles of young horses, and owners may request therapy. Application of cryogenetics (liquid nitrogen), use of autologous vaccines, or combinations of such therapies may be effective.

DISEASES OF THE ESOPHAGUS IN LARGE ANIMALS

ESOPHAGEAL OBSTRUCTION (CHOKE)

Esophageal obstruction or choke, in which the esophagus is obstructed by food masses or foreign objects, is by far the most common esophageal disease in large animals. Horses most frequently obstruct on greedily eaten dried grains or hay. Cattle more usually obstruct on a single solid object, eg, apples, beets, potatoes, turnips, corn stalks, or ears of corn.

Clinical Findings: In **horses**, the classic clinical findings associated with esophageal obstruction are overflow of esophageal food and regurgitation of that food through the nostrils. Nasal discharge of saliva and food material, which usually also spills from the pharynx into the airway, induces coughing. The horse is anxious and may stretch and arch its neck but may still attempt to continue to either eat or drink.

In **cattle**, acute and complete esophageal obstruction is an emergency because it prohibits the eructation of ruminal gases, and free-gas bloat develops. This in turn may result in asphyxia as the expanding rumen puts pressure on the diaphragm and reduces return of blood to the heart. The cow may be bloated and in distress or recumbent, or there may be protrusion of the tongue, extension of the head, and grinding of the teeth with excess salivation.

Diagnosis: The clinical signs are extremely suggestive. Objects lodged in the cervical esophagus may be located via palpation. Endoscopic evaluation and the inability to pass a stomach or nasogastric tube in horses or cattle can also confirm the diagnosis. Each case should be carefully evaluated independently because, in many instances, the complications of esophageal disease (eg, aspiration pneumonia) may prohibit or limit the effectiveness of treatment. In such cases, thoracic radiography, hematology, and biochemical serum analyses are indicated.

Treatment: In **horses**, many cases of obstruction caused by greedily eaten grain or hay may resolve spontaneously. The horse should be held off feed and water, and mild sedation and smooth muscle relaxants may be effective. (Compounds such as acepromazine have some effect in these cases, even though the esophagus has striated muscle, ie, special visceral muscle.) Oxytocin may be useful to facilitate relaxation and esophageal movement. Horses should be monitored because spontaneous resolution may take from a few hours to several days. However, the longer the horse is obstructed, the greater the danger of pressure necrosis or esophagitis and complications of aspiration pneumonia. If the obstruction does not resolve spontaneously and the horse resists attempts at passage of a nasogastric tube and subsequent irrigation, then irrigation of the esophagus under general anesthesia is recommended. A nasogastric tube should be placed before general anesthesia is induced; a cuffed endotracheal tube must be used to protect the airway. Repeated pumping and siphoning of warm water usually loosens the impacted food material. Oral food should be introduced gradually. The horse should receive parenteral antibiotics and analgesics, and the esophagus should be examined endoscopically to monitor the healing of mucosal ulcers.

In **cattle**, esophageal obstruction accompanied by ruminal tympany is an emergency, and if clinical signs of distress indicate, the bloat (p 181) must be relieved by trocarization through the left sublumbar fossa. Once the tympany has been relieved, then solid objects (eg, potatoes) may often be massaged free or spontaneously dislodge as their outer surfaces are softened by saliva. Caution should be used if any attempt is made to push an offending object down the esophagus using a probang; esophageal rupture and fatal septic mediastinitis may result.

In both horses and cattle, elective esophagotomy may be used in some cases to relieve cervical choke.

Complications of Esophageal Obstruction

In both horses and cattle, inhalation pneumonia and resultant fulminating septic pleural pneumonia may be complications of esophageal obstruction. Longterm obstruction may be associated with pressure necrosis of the esophageal mucosa due to prolonged contact with the foreign body. A 360° mucosal slough may result in development of a postobstruction esophageal stricture. When large animals gulp food material and become obstructed, the etiology may be esophageal spasm; therefore, if the animal's respiratory system is healthy, conservative management should be practiced in most cases before any attempts to irrigate, siphon, or use a probang to loosen the object.

Intrathoracic esophageal rupture is a fatal event. Cervical esophageal rupture can be managed in horses by local drainage, wound hygiene, and nasogastric feeding. If secondary healing does not occur, delayed surgical repair may be effective.

Esophageal Obstruction Secondary to Extraesophageal Disease

Cervical and prethoracic trauma may result in scar formation that may lead to constriction of the esophagus. Such cases may be diagnosed from a history of recurrent choke or recurrent obstruction. The use of radiography and contrast material may delineate the site of the obstruction within the esophagus. If the lesion is extrathoracic, it may be explored and relieved surgically.

ESOPHAGEAL STRICTURES

Idiopathic esophageal strictures are seen in foals. Initial diagnosis based on clinical signs may be difficult in that horses may be presented because they are thought to have either cleft palates or pharyngeal cysts. The diagnosis is confirmed by endoscopic evaluation of the esophagus. Treatment is based on either dilation (bougienage) or surgical relief of the lesion. Critical cases should be referred to advanced surgical centers, and esophagomyotomy or esophageal resection and anastomosis may be attempted.

ESOPHAGEAL NEOPLASIA

In ruminants, bovine viral papillomas (ie, warts) occasionally develop in the cranial esophagus and pharynx and, in the presence of other agents, may result in development of esophageal carcinoma. In some areas of the world (eg, Scotland and South America), such disease may follow ingestion of natural bracken fern toxins. There is also a causal relationship between such bracken fern tumors and bladder cancers in cattle. (*See also* BRACKEN FERN POISONING, p 2349.)

GASTROINTESTINAL ULCERS IN LARGE ANIMALS

Gastric ulcers are important in adult horses, foals, and pigs. Abomasal ulcers (p 196) in mature cattle and calves appear to be increasing in importance.

GASTRIC ULCERS IN HORSES

Mild gastric ulcers are seen in ~50% of foals. In most cases, these ulcers heal without treatment or clinical signs. The prevalence of clinical signs from ulcers in foals is not known. In adult horses, ~30% have mild gastric erosions, and the prevalence and severity of ulcers increase as the intensity of work increases—90% of race horses have gastric lesions, and in 50% the lesions are moderate to severe. Prevalence also varies by location of ulcers within the stomach and tends to be highest in the nonglandular squamous mucosa. Within the glandular mucosa, prevalence differs between the mucosa of the corpus (<10%) and that of the antrum and pylorus (>50%).

Duodenal ulceration in foals has been considered part of the ulcer syndrome and hence a peptic (acid-induced) disorder. Duodenitis appears, instead, to be an enteritis syndrome. Duodenal ulceration, perforation, and stricture can occur, and it is not known whether these problems develop solely as a result of enteritis (duodenitis) or whether peptic factors have a role.

Etiology: Causes of gastric ulcers vary and can differ for nonglandular squamous mucosa and glandular mucosa. Horses' stomachs secrete hydrochloric acid continuously and gastric acidity of a horse or foal is very high between periods of eating or nursing Ulcers in the squamous mucosa result from increased exposure to hydrochloric acid which can be secondary to prolonged periods of not eating or nursing, intensive exercise, or delayed gastric emptying. The effects of different feeds on gastric acidity and ulcerogenesis have not been thoroughly studied, although one report indicated that alfalfa hay was associated with reduced ulcer severity in research horses. The causes of most ulcers in the glandular mucosa of the stomach are not known. Excessive doses of NSAID are known to induce ulceration, but most horses with ulcers in this part of the stomach have had no recent exposure to NSAID. Recent research suggests that horses may be infected with a species of *Helicobacter*, but a role for this organism in equine gastric ulcers has not been shown.

Clinical Findings: Most foals with gastric ulcers do not exhibit clinical signs. Clinical signs become apparent when the ulceration is widespread or severe. The classic clinical signs for gastric ulcers in foals include diarrhea, bruxism, poor nursing, dorsal recumbency, and ptyalism. None of these signs is specific for gastric ulcers. In fact, ptyalism is a sign of esophagitis, which in most foals is secondary to gastric outflow obstruction and gastroesophageal reflux. Other causes, including esophageal obstruction and *Candida* infection, should be considered. Importantly, when a foal exhibits clinical signs, the ulcers are severe and should be diagnosed and treated immediately. Sudden gastric perforation without prior signs occurs sporadically in foals. Adult horses with ulcers display nonspecific signs that can include abdominal discomfort (colic), poor appetite, mild weight loss, poor body condition, and attitude changes.

Complications related to gastric ulcers are most frequent and severe in foals and include perforation, delayed gastric emptying, gastroesophageal reflux and esophagitis and megaesophagus secondary to chronic gastroesophageal reflux. Ulcers in the proximal duodenum or at the pylorus can cause fibrosis and stricture. The latter complication is seen in both foals and adult horses. In rare cases, severe gastric ulceration causes fibrosis and contracture of the stomach.

Diagnosis: Neither clinical signs nor laboratory tests are specific for gastric ulcers and an abnormality in a laboratory test does not preclude the possibility that another disorder may be present. Gastric ulcers can develop secondary to problems in many organ systems. Endoscopy is the only reliable method of diagnosis.

Treatment. Suppression of gastric acidity is the primary treatment objective. This can be accomplished with over-the-counter antacids, with the histamine type-2 receptor antagonists (cimetidine and ranitidine), and with the proton pump inhibitor omeprazole. Of these, omeprazole is the most effective, and antacids are the least effective. Ranitidine (6.6 mg/kg, PO) is effective in healing and preventing gastric ulcers, but recent evidence suggests that cimetidine is not effective. Omeprazole is the only medication approved by the FDA for treatment of gastric ulcers in horses. It is effective for treatment and prevention of ulcers in race horses and other types of horses. Sucralfate binds to the gastric glandular mucosa and may promote healing there, although no efficacy data is available to support its use in horses.

GASTRIC ULCERS IN PIGS

Ulcers affect the pars esophagea in pigs and cause sporadic cases of acute gastric hemorrhage resulting in death or slow growth due to chronic ulceration.

Etiology: The specific causes are unknown. Ulcers are seen in pigs of all ages but are most common in growing pigs (100-200 lb [45-90 kg]) fed pelleted feed or finely ground rations, and also in pigs fed large quantities of skimmed milk or whey. It is thought that promotants of hyperacidity may contribute to ulcer development. A combination of finely ground feeds, transportation, hot weather, deprivation of feed and water, and mixing with unfamiliar pigs results in a significant increase in the incidence of gastric ulcers in rapidly growing pigs. Variability in daily feed intake secondary to a systemic illness, particularly pneumonias, also result in an increased incidence of ulcers. This condition is particularly significant in pigs gathered for slaughter at abattoirs, especially those transported long distances.

Clinical Findings: In the peracute form, the pig dies quickly; it is found dead with paleness as the only sign. In the acute form, hemorrhage results in anorexia, weakness, anemia, and black, tarry feces; death can occur in hours or days. In the chronic form, unthriftiness, anemia, and black, tarry feces are characteristic; the pig may survive for several weeks. Pigs with the subclinical form may not reach maturity at the expected time; in these pigs, the ulcer usually heals and a scar remains. In some herds, up to 90% of pigs may be affected; in other herds, the incidence is sporadic. In findings at abattoirs, the incidence of ulcers may be quite high in pigs that have grown normally, although the lesion may have developed in some during transport. Clinical disease apparently develops only after hemorrhage of the ulcer.

Lesions: The typical terminal lesion is found in the gastric mucosa near the esophageal opening in a rectangular area of white, glistening, nonglandular, squamous epithelium. It is common to find a crater ≥2.5-5 cm in diameter encompassing the entrance of the esophagus. The crater appears as a cream or gray, punched-out area and may contain blood clots or debris. In acute hemorrhage, the stomach and upper small intestine contain dark blood. Earlier lesions are characterized by hyperkeratosis and parakeratosis of the squamous epithelium in the area of the esophageal opening into the stomach. Later, the proliferative lesion erodes to form the ulcer. The healed ulcer appears as a stellate scar.

Diagnosis and Treatment: Appearance in a pen of 1 or 2 listless, anorectic pigs that show weight loss, anemia, dark feces, and sometimes dyspnea is suggestive of gastric ulceration, as is the sudden death of an apparently healthy pig. No economically feasible treatments are currently available. Palliative care—removing the affected pig from the pen and feeding a coarse and fibrous diet—can be attempted. Early marketing of affected pigs should be considered. Controlling chronic respiratory disease is important. Feeding meal rather than pellets with a recommended particle size ≥600-700 μm in diameter is of value but may have a negative effect on feed conversion. Strategic use of such diets during stages of production that are at higher risk is useful.

DISEASES OF THE RUMINANT FORESTOMACH

SIMPLE INDIGESTION
(Mild dietary indigestion)

Simple indigestion is a minor disturbance in ruminant GI function that is seen in cattle and rarely in sheep. It is usually related to a change in the quality or quantity of the diet.

Etiology: Almost any dietary factor that can alter the ruminal environment can cause simple indigestion. The disease is common in hand-fed dairy and beef cattle because of variability in the quality and quantity of their feed. Dairy cattle may suddenly eat excessive quantities of highly palatable feeds such as corn or grass silage; beef cattle may eat excessive quantities of relatively indigestible, poor-quality roughage during winter. During drought, cattle and sheep may be forced to eat large quantities of poor-quality straw, bedding, or scrub. Simple indigestion can result from suddenly changing the feed, using spoiled or frozen feeds, introducing urea to a ration, turning cattle onto a lush cereal grain pasture, or introducing feedlot cattle to a high-level grain ration. It can also result from ingestion of placentas by postparturient cows.

Simple indigestion, which is primarily ruminal atony, may follow a sudden change in the pH of the ruminal contents caused by excessive fermentation or putrefaction of ingested feed. The simple accumulation of excessive quantities of relatively indigestible feed may physically impair rumen function for 24-48 hr.

Clinical Findings: The signs depend on the type of animal affected and cause of the disorder. Silage overfeeding causes anorexia and a moderate drop in production in dairy cattle. The rumen is usually full, firm, and doughy; primary contractions are absent, but secondary contractions may be present. Temperature, pulse, and respiration are normal. The feces are normal to firm in consistency but reduced in amount. Recovery usually is spontaneous within 24-48 hr.

Simple indigestion due to excessive feeding of grain results in anorexia and ruminal stasis. The rumen is not necessarily full and may contain excessive fluid. The feces are usually soft and foul smelling. The affected animal is bright and alert and usually begins to eat within 24 hr. A more severe upset from the same cause is described as grain overload (*see* p 178).

Diagnosis: This is based largely on elimination of other possibilities and a history of a change in the nature or amount of the diet. The systemic reaction and painful responses to deep palpation of the xiphoid in traumatic reticuloperitonitis are not seen. The history and the absence of ketonuria help eliminate ketosis from consideration. The possibility of displaced abomasum usually can be eliminated by auscultation.

Vagal indigestion and abomasal torsions become more readily detectable as they progress because they have a longer course, but initial differentiation may be difficult. Grain overload is distinguishable by its greater severity and the pronounced fall in the pH of the rumen contents. Phytobezoars cause partial or complete anorexia and scant feces; on rectal examination, distended loops of intestine and the firm phytobezoar masses are palpable.

Treatment: Treatment is aimed at correcting the suspected dietary factors. Spontaneous recovery is usual. Administration of 20-40 L of warm water or saline via a stomach tube, followed by vigorous kneading of the rumen, may help restore rumen function. Magnesium hydroxide PO seems to be useful when excessive amounts of high-energy feeds have been ingested. If too much urea (*see* p 2426) or protein has been ingested, acetic acid or vinegar may be administered PO. If the activity of the ruminal microbes is reduced, administration of 4-8 L of ruminal fluid from a healthy cow will help. (*See* RUMINAL FLUID TRANSFER, p 1994.)

GRAIN OVERLOAD
(Lactic acidosis, Carbohydrate engorgement, Rumen impaction)

Grain overload is an acute disease of ruminants that is characterized by indigestion, rumen stasis, dehydration, acidosis, toxemia, incoordination, collapse, and frequently death.

Etiology and Pathogenesis: The disease is most common in cattle that accidentally gain access to large quantities of readily digestible carbohydrates, particularly grain. It also is common in feedlot cattle when they are introduced to heavy grain diets too quickly. Wheat, barley, and corn are the most readily digestible and oats less digestible. Less common causes include engorgement with apples, grapes, bread, batter's dough, sugar beets, mangels, or sour wet brewer's grain that was incompletely fermented in the brewery. The amount of a feed required to produce acute illness depends on the kind of grain, previous experience of the animal with that grain, the nutritional status and condition of the animal, and the nature of the microflora. Cattle accustomed to heavy grain diets may consume 30-45 lb (15-20 kg) of grain and develop only moderate illness, while others may become acutely ill and die after eating 20 lb (10 kg) of grain.

Ingestion of toxic amounts of highly fermentable carbohydrates is followed within 2-6 hr by a change in the microbial population in the rumen. The number of gram-positive bacteria (*Streptococcus bovis*) increases markedly, which results in the production of large quantities of lactic acid. The rumen pH falls to ≤5, which destroys protozoa, cellulolytic organisms, and lactate-utilizing organisms, and impairs rumen motility. The low pH allows the lactobacilli to utilize the carbohydrate and to produce excessive quantities of lactic acid. The superimposition of lactic acid and its salt, lactate, on the existing solutes in the rumen liquid causes osmotic pressure to rise substantially, which results in the movement of excessive quantities of fluid into the rumen, causing dehydration.

The lactic acid causes a chemical rumenitis, and its absorption results in lactic acidosis. In addition to acidosis and dehydration, the pathophysiologic consequences are hemoconcentration, cardiovascular collapse, renal failure, muscular weakness, shock, and death. Animals that survive may develop mycotic rumenitis in several days, hepatic necrobacillosis several weeks or months later, or chronic laminitis, as well as evidence of ruminal scars at slaughter.

Clinical Findings: Carbohydrate engorgement results in conditions ranging from simple indigestion (p 177) to a rapidly fatal acidosis. The interval between overeating and onset of signs is shorter with ground feed than with whole grain, and severity increases with the amount eaten. A few hours after engorgement, the only detectable abnormality may be an enlarged rumen and possibly some abdominal pain (manifest by belly kicking). In the mild form, the rumen movements are reduced but not entirely absent, the cattle are anorectic but bright and alert, and diarrhea is common. The animals usually begin eating again 3-4 days later without any specific treatment.

Within 24-48 hr of the onset of severe overload, some animals will be recumbent, some will be staggering, and others will be standing quietly; all will be completely off feed. Immediately after consuming large quantities of dry grain, cattle may engorge themselves on water, but once ill they usually do not drink at all.

Body temperature is usually below normal, 98-101°F (36.5-38.5°C); however, in animals exposed to the sun in hot weather, it may be increased to 106°F (41°C). Respirations tend to be shallow and rapid, up to 60-90/min. The heart rate usually is increased in accordance with severity of the acidosis; prognosis is poor for cattle with rates of 120-140/min. Diarrhea is common and usually profuse. The feces are soft to liquid, yellow or tan, and have an obvious sweet-sour odor. The feces frequently contain undigested kernels of the feed that has induced the overload. In mild cases, dehydration equals 4-6% body wt; in severe cases, up to 10-12%.

In severe overload, the primary contractions of the rumen are completely absent, although the gurgling sounds of gas rising through the large quantity of fluid are usually audible on auscultation. Ballottement and auscultation of the left flank may elicit fluid-splashing sounds in the rumen. The contents of the rumen, as palpated through the left paralumbar fossa, may feel firm and doughy in cattle that were previously on a roughage diet and have consumed a large amount of grain. In cattle that have become ill on smaller amounts of grain, the rumen will feel not necessarily full, but rather resilient because of the excessive fluid. Severely affected animals stagger and may bump into objects; their palpebral reflex is sluggish or absent, and the pupillary light reflex is usually present but slower than normal. They commonly lie quietly, often with the head turned into the flank, and their response to any stimulus is much decreased so that they resemble cases of parturient paresis (p 806).

Acute laminitis may be present and is most common in those animals that are not severely affected; chronic laminitis may develop weeks or months later. Anuria is a common finding in acute cases, and diuresis after fluid therapy is a good prognostic sign.

Death may occur in 24-72 hr, and rapid development of acute signs, particularly recumbency, indicates an urgent need for radical treatment. A reduction in heart rate, rise in temperature, return of ruminal movement, and passage of large amounts of soft feces are more favorable signs. However, some animals appear to improve temporarily but become severely ill again 3-4 days later, probably because of severe fungal rumenitis; death from acute diffuse peritonitis usually follows in 2-3 days. In pregnant cattle that survive the severe form of the disease, abortion may occur 10-14 days later.

Diagnosis: The diagnosis is usually obvious if the history is available. It may be confirmed by the clinical findings, a low ruminal pH (<5), and examining the microflora of the rumen for the presence of live protozoa. When only one animal is involved and there is no history of engorgement, the diagnosis is less obvious, but the clinical signs—a static rumen with gurgling fluid sounds, diarrhea, ataxia, and a normal temperature—are characteristic.

Although parturient paresis (p 806) may resemble rumen overload, diarrhea and dehydration are not typical, the intensity of heart sounds is reduced, and the response to calcium injection is usually dramatic. Peracute coliform mastitis and acute diffuse peritonitis may also resemble overload, but usually a careful examination will reveal the cause of the toxemia.

To avoid an increase in pH on exposure to air, rumen fluid obtained by stomach tube or paracentesis should be checked promptly. Normally, the pH in cattle on roughage is 6-7; in those on a grain diet, 5.5-6. Values below those ranges are strongly suggestive of overload, and a pH <5 indicates severe acidosis. Wide-range (2-11) pH indicator paper is suitable for field use. Ruminal fluid may be examined microscopically; 5-7 protozoa are normally seen under low power. In acidosis, the protozoa are virtually absent. A Gram's stain of the fluid will reveal a change from predominantly gram-negative bacteria (normal) to predominantly gram-positive bacteria in acidosis.

Increased blood lactate and inorganic phosphate levels, mild hypocalcemia, and reduced urinary pH are also seen, but it is seldom necessary to check such values to make a firm diagnosis. The diagnostic problem is to properly assess which animals require vigorous therapy (or slaughter), which require supportive therapy, which have only a mild indigestion that will correct itself if water and grain intake are restricted and hay and exercise are provided, and which need nothing beyond their routine care and ration. In an outbreak of overload involving several animals, it is necessary to identify those animals that need the most intensive therapy and those that will recover with minimal medical therapy.

If the cattle are found while still eating, it is possible that some of the group will fall into each category, and close monitoring is necessary to minimize losses. Cattle found while engorging or shortly thereafter should be allowed no more concentrate or water, but plenty of good hay for up to 24 hr, and forced to exercise periodically. Cattle that appear normal at the end of the first day are probably in good health, although if even one is ill, all should be monitored closely for 48 hr. Most of those that have eaten enough concentrate to be affected seriously show signs within 6-8 hr.

Treatment: For all cattle suspected of having eaten large quantities of concentrate, it is important to restrict water intake for the first 18-24 hr. If overload is serious, slaughter for salvage should be considered; in feeders nearing the end of their feeding period, it may well be the most economical choice. Mortality is high in severely affected animals unless vigorous therapeutic measures are initiated early. In such animals, removal of rumen contents and replacement with ingesta taken from healthy animals is necessary. In animals that are still standing, rumen lavage may be accomplished with a large stomach tube if sufficient water is available. A large-bore tube (2.5 cm inside diameter, 3 m long) should be used, and enough water added to distend the left paralumbar fossa; gravity flow is then allowed to empty out what it will. Repeating this 15-20 times achieves the same results (and requires about as much time) as using rumenotomy to empty and wash out the rumen with a siphon.

Emptying the rumen should be followed by rumen inoculation (p 1994) and, if not accomplished before signs of severe toxicosis are evident, by rigorous fluid therapy to correct the acidosis and dehydration and to restore renal function. Initially, over a period of ~30 min, 5% sodium bicarbonate solution should be given IV (5 L/450 kg). During the next 6-12 hr, a balanced electrolyte solution, or a 1.3% solution of sodium bicarbonate in saline, may be given IV, up to as much as 60 L/450 kg body wt. Urination should resume during this period. Usually, it is unnecessary and even undesirable to also administer antacids PO (or intraruminally).

In less severe cases, emptying the rumen is unnecessary. In these, magnesium hydroxide (500 g/450 kg body wt) should be added to warm water, pumped into the rumen, and mixed therein via kneading the flank. This may be all that is necessary if the rumen pH is >5, and the animal is still standing and reasonably alert several hours after the engorgement. A heart rate of 70-85 bpm, weak ruminal contractions, normal body temperature, and especially willingness to eat are additional reassurances that this therapy will suffice. If any question remains, additional fluids should be given. During the convalescent period, which may last 2-4 days, good-quality hay and no grain should be given, and the grain then reintroduced gradually. If good appetite returns within 3 days, the prognosis is good. However, if treatment was not started early enough to prevent acidification of the ruminal contents, and mycotic infection of the rumen wall ensues, relapse is likely within 3-5 days, and the prognosis is grave.

Prevention: Accidental access to concentrates for which the cattle have developed an appetite, in quantities to which they are unaccustomed, should be avoided. Feedlot cattle should be introduced gradually to concentrate rations over a period of ~3 wk, beginning with a mixture of ≤50% concentrate in the milled feed containing roughage.

SUBACUTE RUMINAL ACIDOSIS
(Chronic ruminal acidosis, Subclinical ruminal acidosis)

Ruminant animals are adapted to digest and metabolize predominantly forage diets; however, growth rates and milk production are increased substantially when they consume high-grain diets. One consequence of feeding excessive amounts of rapidly fermentable carbohydrates in conjunction with inadequate fiber to ruminants is subacute ruminal acidosis, characterized by periods of low ruminal pH, depressed feed intake, and subsequent health problems. Chronic disease conditions secondary to subacute ruminal acidosis can negate the production gains accomplished by high grain feeding. Dairy cattle, feedlot cattle, and feedlot sheep are all at high risk for developing this condition. Although dairy cattle are typically fed diets that are higher in forage and fiber compared with feedlot animals, this advantage is offset by their much higher dry-matter intakes.

Field observations suggest that periparturient cows are at risk of subacute ruminal acidosis because of the time required for the rumen microflora and papillae to adapt to increased intakes of concentrates immediately before parturition and during early lactation when feed intake increases rapidly to meet the energy needs of high-producing dairy cows. The adaptation of the ruminal microflora and papillae from a system appropriate for forage to a system capable of utilizing high-energy lactation rations requires a gradual change over a period of 3-5 wk.

Etiology: Ruminal pH drops below ~5.5 (the normal physiologic nadir) when ruminants consume excessive amounts of rapidly fermentable carbohydrates. Any additional intake puts the ruminant at risk of subacute ruminal acidosis because it results in the fermentation of carbohydrates into volatile fatty acids (VFA). Ruminal pH typically drops 0.5-1.0 pH units after the major meal of the day.

The ability of the rumen to rapidly absorb organic acids contributes greatly to the stability of ruminal pH. It is rarely difficult for peripheral tissues to utilize VFA already absorbed from the rumen; however, absorption of these VFA from the rumen can be an important bottleneck.

VFA from the rumen are absorbed passively across the rumen wall. This passive absorption is enhanced by finger-like papillae, which project away from the rumen wall. Ruminal papillae increase in length when cattle are fed higher-grain diets; this presumably increases ruminal surface area and absorptive capacity, which protects the animal from acid accumulation in the rumen. If the absorptive capacity of these cells is impaired (eg, chronic rumenitis with fibrosis), it becomes much more difficult for the animal to maintain a stable ruminal pH following a meal.

Intake depression is the ruminant's last resort for regulating ruminal pH. Depressed dry-matter intake becomes especially evident if ruminal pH falls to <~5.5. Intake depression may be mediated by pH receptors and/or osmolality receptors in the rumen. Inflammation of the ruminal epithelium (rumenitis) could cause pain and contribute to intake depression during subacute ruminal acidosis.

Unfortunately, lactate production at low ruminal pH can offset gains from VFA absorption. As pH drops, lactate-synthesizing bacteria such as *Streptococcus bovis* begin to ferment glucose to lactate instead of VFA. This is a dangerous situation, since lactate has a much lower pK_a than VFA (3.9 vs 4.8) and lactate is 5.2 times less dissociated than VFA at pH 5.0. As a result, lactate stays in the rumen longer and contributes to the downward spiral in ruminal pH.

Additional adaptive responses are invoked if lactate production begins. Lactate-utilizing bacteria, such as *Megasphaera elsdenii* and *Selenomonas ruminantium*, begin to proliferate. These beneficial bacteria convert lactate to other VFA, which are then easily protonated and absorbed. However, the turnover time of lactate utilizers is much slower than that of lactate synthesizers. Thus, this mechanism may not be invoked quickly enough to fully stabilize ruminal pH. Periods of very high ruminal pH, as during feed deprivation, may inhibit populations of lactate utilizers (which are sensitive to higher ruminal pH) and leave them more susceptible to severe ruminal acidosis.

Besides disrupting microbial balance, feed deprivation causes cattle to overeat when feed is reintroduced. This creates a double effect in lowering ruminal pH. Cycles of feed deprivation and refeeding are critical risk factors for subacute ruminal acidosis.

Low ruminal pH during subacute ruminal acidosis also reduces the number of species of bacteria in the rumen, although the metabolic activity of the bacteria that remain is very high. Protozoa populations are limited as ruminal pH approaches 5.0. When fewer species of bacteria and protozoa are present, the ruminal microflora are less stable and less able to maintain normal ruminal pH during periods of sudden dietary change. Thus, pre-existing subacute ruminal acidosis increases the risk of acute ruminal acidosis in the event of accidental ingestion of excessive amounts of grain.

Pathogenesis: Ruminal epithelial cells are not protected by mucus, so they are vulnerable to chemical damage by acids. Low ruminal pH leads to rumenitis, erosion, and ulceration of the ruminal epithelium. Once the ruminal epithelium is inflamed, bacteria may colonize the papillae and leak into the portal circulation. These bacteria may cause liver abscesses, which may eventually lead to peritonitis around the site of the abscess. If the ruminal bacteria clear the liver (or if bacteria from liver infections are released into circulation), they may colonize the lungs, heart valves, kidneys, or joints. The resulting pneumonia, endocarditis, pyelonephritis, and arthritis are often difficult to diagnose antemortem. Postmortem evaluation of these conditions in animals that are slaughtered, culled, or that died on the farm can be very beneficial.

Caudal vena cava syndrome can cause hemoptysis and peracute deaths due to massive pulmonary hemorrhage in affected cows. In these cases, septic emboli from liver abscesses can lead to lung infections, which ultimately invade pulmonary vessels and cause them to rupture.

Subacute ruminal acidosis has also been associated with laminitis and subsequent hoof overgrowth, sole abscesses, and sole ulcers. The severity of laminitis depends on the duration and frequency of metabolic insult. These foot problems generally do not appear until weeks or months after the initiating event. The mechanism by which subacute ruminal acidosis increases the risk of laminitis has not been fully characterized.

Clinical Findings: The major clinical manifestation is reduced or cyclic feed intake, or both. Other associated signs include decreased efficiency of milk production, reduced fat test, poor body condition score despite adequate energy intake, unexplained diarrhea, and episodes of laminitis. High rates of culling or unexplained deaths may be noted in the herd. Sporadic nosebleeds due to caudal vena cava syndrome may also be observed. The clinical signs are delayed and insidious. Actual episodes of low ruminal pH are not identified; in fact, by the time an animal is observed to be off-feed, its ruminal pH has probably been restored to normal. Diarrhea may follow periods of low ruminal pH; however, this finding is subtle and difficult to evaluate.

Diagnosis: Subacute ruminal acidosis is diagnosed on a group rather than individual basis. Measurement of pH in the ruminal fluid of a representative portion of apparently healthy animals in a group has been used to assist in making the diagnosis of subacute ruminal acidosis in dairy herds. Animal selection should be from high-risk groups, eg, in the first 60 days of lactation. Ruminal fluid is collected by rumenocentesis or stomach tube and can be measured in the field using wide-range pH (2-12) indicator paper, although a pH meter yields more accurate results. Twelve or more animals are typically sampled at ~2-4 hr after a grain feeding (in component-fed herds) or 6-10 hr after the first daily total mixed ration feeding. If >25% of the animals tested have a ruminal pH <5.5, then the group is considered to be at high risk of subacute ruminal acidosis. This type of diagnostic tool should be used in conjunction with other factors such as ration evaluation, evaluation of management practices, and identification of health problems on a herd basis.

Milk fat depression is a poor and insensitive indicator of subacute ruminal acidosis in dairy herds. Cows and herds with severe subacute ruminal acidosis may have normal milk fat tests. Thus, it is vitally important not to exclude the diagnosis in a dairy herd that has a normal milk-fat test.

Treatment: Because subacute ruminal acidosis is not detected at the time of depressed ruminal pH, there is no specific treatment for it. Secondary conditions may be treated as needed.

Prevention: The key to prevention is reducing the amount of readily fermentable carbohydrate consumed at each meal. This requires both good diet formulation (proper balance of fiber and nonfiber carbohydrates) and excellent feed bunk management. Animals consuming well-formulated diets remain at high risk for this condition if they tend to eat large meals because of excessive competition for bunk space or following periods of feed deprivation.

Field recommendations for feeding component-fed concentrates to dairy cattle during the first 3 wk of lactation are usually excessive. Feeding excessive quantities of concentrate and insufficient forage results in a fiber-deficient ration likely to cause subacute ruminal acidosis. The same situation may be seen during the last few days before parturition if the ration is fed in separate components; as dry-matter intake drops before calving, dry cows preferentially consume concentrate over fiber and develop acidosis.

Subacute ruminal acidosis may also be caused by errors in delivery of the rations or by formulation of rations that contain excessive amounts of rapidly fermentable carbohydrates or a deficiency of fiber. Recommendations for the fiber content of dairy rations are available in the National Research Council report, *Nutrient Requirements of Dairy Cattle* (*see* NUTRITION: DAIRY CATTLE, p 1828). Dry-matter content errors in total mixed rations are commonly related to a lack of adjustment for changes in moisture content of forages.

Including long-fiber particles in the diet reduces the risk of subacute ruminal acidosis by encouraging saliva production during chewing and by increasing rumination after feeding. However, long-fiber particles should not be easily sorted away from the rest of the diet; this could delay their consumption until later in the day or cause them to be refused completely.

Ruminant diets should also be formulated to provide adequate buffering. This can be accomplished by feedstuff selection and/or by the addition of dietary buffers such as sodium bicarbonate or potassium carbonate. Dietary anion-cation difference is used to quantify the buffering capacity of a diet.

Supplementing the diet with direct-fed microbials that enhance lactate utilizers in the rumen may reduce the risk of subacute ruminal acidosis. Yeasts, propionobacteria, lactobacilli, and enterococci have been used for this purpose. Ionophore (eg, monensin sodium) supplementation may also reduce the risk by selectively inhibiting ruminal lactate producers; however, ionophores are not currently approved for use in lactating dairy cows in North America.

BLOAT
(Ruminal tympany)

Bloat is an overdistention of the rumenoreticulum with the gases of fermentation, either in the form of a persistent foam mixed with the ruminal contents—called primary or frothy bloat, or in the form of free gas separated from the ingesta—called secondary or free-gas bloat. It is predominantly a disorder of cattle but may also be seen in sheep. The susceptibility of individual cattle to bloat varies and is genetically determined.

Etiology and Pathogenesis: In **primary ruminal tympany**, or **frothy bloat**, the cause is entrapment of the normal gases of fermentation in a stable foam. Coalescence of the small gas bubbles is inhibited, and intraruminal pressure increases because eructation cannot occur. Several factors, both animal and plant, influence the formation of a stable foam. Soluble leaf proteins, saponins, and hemicelluloses are believed to be the primary foaming agents and to form a monomolecular layer around gas rumen bubbles that has its greatest stability at about pH 6.0. Salivary mucin is antifoaming, but saliva production is reduced with succulent forages. Bloat-producing pastures are more rapidly digested and may release a greater amount of small chloroplast particles that trap gas bubbles and prevent their coalescence. The immediate effect of feeding is probably to supply nutrients for a burst of microbial fermentation. However, the major factor that determines if bloat will occur is the nature of the ruminal contents. Protein content and rates of digestion and ruminal passage reflect the forage's potential for causing bloat. Over a 24-hr period, the bloat-causing forage and unknown animal factors combine to maintain an increased concentration of small feed particles and enhance the susceptibility to bloat. Bloat is most common in animals grazing legume or legume-dominant pastures, particularly alfalfa, ladino, and red and white clovers, but also is seen with grazing of young green cereal crops, rape, kale, turnips, and legume vegetable crops. Legume forages such as alfalfa and clover have a higher percentage of protein and are digested more quickly. Other legumes, such as sainfoin, crown vetch, milk vetch, and birdsfoot trefoil, are high in protein but do not cause bloat, probably because they contain condensed tannins, which precipitate protein and are digested more slowly than alfalfa or clover. Leguminous bloat is most common when cattle are placed on lush pastures, particularly those dominated by rapidly growing leguminous plants in the vegetative and early bud stages, but can also be seen when high-quality hay is fed.

Frothy bloat also is seen in feedlot cattle, and less commonly in dairy cattle, on high-grain diets. The cause of the foam in feedlot bloat is uncertain but is thought to be either the production of insoluble slime by certain species of rumen bacteria in cattle fed high-carbohydrate diets or the entrapment of the gases of fermentation by the fine particle size of ground feed. Fine particulate matter, such as in finely ground grain, can markedly affect foam stability as can a low roughage intake. Feedlot bloat is most common in cattle that have been on a grain diet for 1-2 mo. This timing may be due to the increase in the level of grain feeding or to the time it takes for the slime-producing rumen bacteria to proliferate to large enough numbers.

In **secondary ruminal tympany**, or **free-gas bloat**, physical obstruction of eructation is caused by esophageal obstruction due to a foreign body (eg, potatoes, apples, turnips, kiwifruit), stenosis, or pressure from enlargement outside the esophagus (as from lymphadenopathy). Interference with esophageal groove function in vagal indigestion and diaphragmatic hernia may cause chronic ruminal tympany. This also occurs in tetanus. Tumors and other lesions of the esophageal groove or the reticular wall are less common causes of obstructive bloat. There also may be interference with the nerve pathways involved in the eructation reflex. Lesions of the wall of the reticulum (which contains tension receptors and receptors that discriminate between gas, foam, and liquid) may interrupt the normal reflex that is essential for escape of gas from the rumen.

Ruminal tympany also can be secondary to the acute onset of ruminal atony that occurs in anaphylaxis and in grain overload; this causes a reduction in rumen pH and possibly an esophagitis and rumenitis that can interfere with eructation. Ruminal tympany also develops with hypocalcemia. Chronic ruminal tympany is relatively frequent in calves up to 6 mo old without apparent cause; this form usually resolves spontaneously.

Unusual postures, particularly lateral recumbency, are commonly associated with secondary tympany. Ruminants may die of bloat if they become accidentally cast in dorsal recumbency or other restrictive positions in handling facilities, crowded transportation vehicles, or irrigation ditches.

Clinical Findings: Bloat is a common cause of sudden death. Cattle not observed closely, such as pastured and feedlot cattle and dry dairy cattle, usually are found dead.

In lactating dairy cattle, which are observed regularly, bloat commonly begins within 1 hr after being turned onto a bloat-producing pasture. Bloat may develop on the first day after being placed on the pasture but more commonly develops on the second or third day.

In primary pasture bloat, the rumen becomes obviously distended suddenly, and the left flank may be so distended that the contour of the paralumbar fossa protrudes above the vertebral column; the entire abdomen is enlarged. As the bloat progresses, the skin over the left flank becomes progressively more taut and, in severe cases, cannot be "tented." Dyspnea and grunting are marked and are accompanied by mouth breathing, protrusion of the tongue, extension of the head, and frequent urination. Occasionally, vomiting occurs. Rumen motility does not decrease until bloat is severe. If the tympany continues to worsen, the animal will collapse and die. Death may occur within 1 hr after grazing began but is more common ~3-4 hr after onset of clinical signs. In a group of affected cattle, there are usually several with clinical bloat and some with mild to moderate abdominal distention. Death rates as high as 20% are recorded in cattle grazing bloat-prone pasture, and in pastoral areas, the annual mortality rate from bloat in dairy cows may approach 1%. There is also economic loss from depressed milk production in nonfatal cases and from suboptimal use of bloat-prone pastures. Bloat can be a significant cause of mortality in feedlot cattle.

In secondary bloat, the excess gas is usually free on top of the solid and fluid ruminal contents, although frothy bloat may be seen in vagal indigestion when there is increased ruminal activity. Secondary bloat is seen sporadically. There is tympanic resonance over the dorsal abdomen left of the midline. Free gas produces a higher pitched ping on percussion than frothy bloat. The distension of the rumen can be detected on rectal examination. In free-gas bloat, the passage of a stomach tube or trocarization releases large quantities of gas and alleviates distention.

Lesions: Necropsy findings are characteristic. Congestion and hemorrhage of the lymph nodes of the head and neck, epicardium, and upper respiratory tract are marked. The lungs are compressed, and intrabronchial hemorrhage may be present. The cervical esophagus is congested and hemorrhagic, but the thoracic portion of the esophagus is pale and blanched—the demarcation known as the "bloat line" of the esophagus. The rumen is distended, but the contents usually are much less frothy than before death. The liver is pale due to expulsion of blood from the organ.

Diagnosis: Usually, the clinical diagnosis of frothy bloat is obvious. The causes of secondary bloat must be ascertained by clinical examination to determine the cause of the failure of eructation.

Treatment: In life-threatening cases, an emergency rumenotomy may be necessary; it is accompanied by an explosive release of ruminal contents and, thus, marked relief for the cow. Recovery is usually uneventful with only occasional minor complications.

A trocar and cannula may be used for emergency relief, although the standard-sized instrument is not large enough to allow the viscous, stable foam in peracute cases to escape quickly enough. A larger bore instrument (2.5 cm in diameter) is necessary, but an incision through the skin must be made before it can be inserted through the muscle layers and into the rumen. If the cannula fails to reduce the bloat and the animal's life is threatened, an emergency rumenotomy should be performed. If the cannula provides some relief, an antifoaming agent can be administered through the cannula, which can remain in place until the animal has returned to normal, usually within several hours.

When the animal's life is not immediately threatened, passing a stomach tube of the largest bore possible is recommended. A few attempts should be made to clear the tube by blowing and moving it back and forth in an attempt to find large pockets of rumen gas that can be released. In frothy bloat, it may be impossible to reduce the pressure with the tube, and an antifoaming agent should be administered while the tube is in place. If the bloat is not relieved quickly by the antifoaming agent, the animal must be observed carefully for the next hour to determine if the treatment has been successful or if an alternative therapy is necessary.

A variety of antifoaming agents are effective, including vegetable oils (eg, peanut, corn, soybean) and mineral oils (paraffins), at doses of 250-500 mL. Dioctyl sodium sulfosuccinate (docusate), a surfactant, is commonly incorporated into one of the above oils and sold as a proprietary antibloat remedy, which is effective if administered early. Poloxalene (25-50 g, PO) is effective in treating legume bloat but not feedlot bloat. Placement of a rumen fistula provides short-term relief for cases of free-gas bloat associated with external obstruction of the esophagus.

Control and Prevention: Prevention of **pasture bloat** can be difficult. Management practices that have been used to reduce the risk of bloat include feeding hay before turning cattle on pasture, maintaining grass dominance in the sward, or using strip grazing to restrict intake, with movement of animals to a new strip in the afternoon, not the early morning. For hay to be effective, it must be at least one-third of the diet. Feeding hay or strip grazing may be reliable when the pasture is only moderately dangerous, but these methods are less reliable when the pasture is in the prebloom stage and the bloat potential is high. Mature pastures are less likely to cause bloat than immature or rapidly growing pastures.

The only satisfactory method available to prevent pasture bloating is continual administration of an antifoaming agent during the risk period. This is widely practiced in grassland countries such as Australia and New Zealand. The most reliable method is drenching twice daily (eg, at milking times) with an antifoaming agent. Spraying the agent onto the bloatprone pasture is equally effective, provided that the animals have access only to treated pasture. This method is ideal for strip grazing but not when grazing is uncontrolled. The antifoaming agent can be added to the feed or water or incorporated into feed blocks, but success with this method depends on adequate individual intake. The agent can be "painted" on the flanks of the animals, from which it is licked during the day, but animals that do not lick will be unprotected.

Available antifoaming agents include oils and fats and synthetic nonionic surfactants. Oils and fats are given at 60-120 mL/head/day; doses up to 240 mL are indicated during most dangerous periods. Poloxalene, a synthetic polymer, is a highly effective nonionic surfactant that can be given at 10-20 g/head/day and up to 40 g/head/day in high-risk situations. It is safe and economical to use and is administered daily through the susceptible period by adding to water, feed grain mixtures, or molasses. Alcohol ethoxylate detergents are equally effective and are more palatable than poloxalene. Ionophores are effective in preventing bloat, and a sustained-release capsule that is administered into the rumen and releases 300 mg of monensin daily for a 100-day period protects against pasture bloat and improves milk production on bloat-prone pastures.

The ultimate aim in control is development of a pasture that permits high production, while keeping incidence of bloat low. The use of pastures of clover and grasses in equal amounts comes closest to achieving this goal. Bloat potential varies between cultivars of alfalfa, and low-risk LIRD (low initial rate of digestion) cultivars are available commercially. The addition of legumes with high condensed tannins to the pasture seeding mix (10% sainfoin) can reduce the risk of bloat where there is strip grazing, as can the feeding of sainfoin pellets.

To prevent **feedlot bloat**, rations should contain ≥10-15% cut or chopped roughage mixed into the complete feed. Preferably, the roughage should be a cereal, grain straw, grass hay, or equivalent. Grains should be rolled or cracked, not finely ground. Pelleted rations made from finely ground grain should be avoided. The addition of tallow (3-5% of the total ration) may be successful occasionally, but it was not effective in controlled trials. The nonionic surfactants, such as poloxalene, have been ineffective in preventing feedlot bloat, but the ionophore lasalocid is effective in control.

TRAUMATIC RETICULOPERITONITIS
(Hardware disease, Traumatic gastritis)

Traumatic reticuloperitonitis develops as a consequence of perforation of the reticulum. It is important in differential diagnosis of other diseases marked by stasis of the GI tract because it causes similar signs. It is most common in mature dairy cattle, occasionally seen in beef cattle, and rarely reported in other ruminants.

Cattle commonly ingest foreign objects because they do not discriminate against metal materials in feed and do not completely masticate feed before swallowing. The disease is common when greenchop, silage, and hay are made from fields that contain old rusting fences or baling wire, or when pastures are on areas or sites where buildings have recently been constructed, burned, or torn down. The grain ration may also be a source due to accidental addition of metal.

Etiology: Swallowed metallic objects, such as nails or pieces of wire, fall directly into the reticulum or pass into the rumen and are subsequently carried over the ruminoreticular fold into the cranioventral part of the reticulum by ruminal contractions. The reticulo-omasal orifice is elevated above the floor, which tends to retain heavy objects in the reticulum, and the honeycomb-like reticular mucosa traps sharp objects. Contractions of the reticulum promote penetration of the wall by the foreign object. Compression of the ruminoreticulum by the uterus in late pregnancy, straining during parturition, and mounting during estrus increase the likelihood of an initial penetration of the reticulum and may also disrupt adhesions caused by an earlier penetration.

Perforation of the wall of the reticulum allows leakage of ingesta and bacteria, which contaminates the peritoneal cavity. The resulting peritonitis is generally localized and frequently results in adhesions. Less commonly, a more severe peritonitis develops. Diffuse peritonitis is rare. The object can penetrate the diaphragm and enter the thoracic cavity (causing pleuritis and sometimes pneumonitis) and the pericardial sac (causing pericarditis, sometimes followed by myocarditis, endocarditis, and septicemia). Occasionally, the liver or spleen may be pierced and become infected.

Clinical Findings: The initial attack is characterized by sudden onset of ruminoreticular atony and a sharp fall in milk production. Fecal output is decreased. The rectal temperature is often mildly increased. The heart rate is normal or slightly increased, and respiration is usually shallow and rapid. Initially, the cow exhibits an arched back; an anxious expression; a reluctance to move; and an uneasy, careful gait. Forced sudden movements as well as defecating, urinating, lying down, getting up, and stepping over barriers may be accompanied by groaning. A grunt may be elicited by applying pressure to the xiphoid or by elevating this area firmly and then pinching the withers, which causes extension of the thorax and lower abdomen. The grunt can be detected by placing a stethoscope over the trachea and applying pressure or pinching the withers at the end of an inspiration. Tremor of the triceps and abduction of the elbow may be seen.

In chronic cases, feed intake and fecal output are reduced, and milk production remains low. Signs of cranial abdominal pain become less apparent, and the rectal temperature usually returns to normal as the acute inflammation subsides and peritoneal contamination is walled off. Some cattle develop chronic vagal indigestion, possibly due to the adhesions that form after foreign body perforation, particularly those on the ventromedial reticulum.

Cows with pleuritis or pericarditis due to foreign body perforation usually are depressed, tachycardic (>90 bpm), and pyrexic (104°F [40°C]). Pleuritis is manifest by fast, shallow respiration; muffled lung sounds; and possibly pleuritic friction rubs. Thoracentesis may yield several liters of fluid. Traumatic pericarditis usually is characterized by muffled heart sounds, possibly with pericardial friction rubs, and occasionally by gas and fluid splashing sounds on auscultation. This has been described as a washing machine murmur. Jugular vein distention with a pronounced jugular pulse is present early in the course, and congestive heart failure with marked submandibular and brisket edema is a frequent sequela. Prognosis is grave with these complications. Penetration through the myocardium usually results in extensive hemorrhage into the pericardial sac and sudden death.

Diagnosis: This can be based on history (when available) and clinical findings if the cow is examined when signs initially appear. Without an accurate history and when the condition has been present for several days or longer, diagnosis is more difficult. Other causes of peritonitis, particularly perforated abomasal ulcers, can be difficult to distinguish from traumatic reticuloperitonitis. Differential diagnoses should include conditions that can produce variable or nonspecific GI signs, eg, indigestion, lymphosarcoma, or intestinal obstruction. Abomasal displacement or volvulus should be ruled out by simultaneous auscultation and percussion. Pleuritis or pericarditis of nontraumatic origin produces signs similar to those associated with foreign body perforation.

Although not always necessary, laboratory tests may be helpful. In many cases, there is a neutrophilia with a left shift. Fibrinogen and, in chronic cases, total plasma protein concentrations may be high. The acid-base status and serum electrolyte levels are typically normal because abomasal and small-intestinal absorption can remain normal. However, marked hypokalemic, hypochloremic metabolic alkalosis can be seen, presumably because adynamic ileus from peritonitis can affect abomasal and GI motility and resorption of abomasal secretions. The metabolic alkalosis can be created or exacerbated by treatment with alkalinizing agents such as magnesium hydroxide used as a laxative. Peritoneal fluid analysis can be helpful in determining if peritonitis is present. However, the nucleated cell count and the protein level return to normal as the contamination is walled off.

Radiographs may detect metallic material in the reticulum. To determine whether the reticulum has been perforated, the foreign body must be visible beyond the border of the reticulum or be positioned off the floor of the reticulum. Depression in the cranioventral aspect of the reticulum or identification of an abscess (by gas accumulation outside a viscus), soft-tissue masses, or a fluid line in the cranial abdomen are also reliable radiographic findings. Portable radiographic units cannot penetrate the reticular area of standing adult cattle, and the cow may need to be transported to where there is equipment with sufficient power. The area can be radiographed using portable equipment if the systemic condition does not preclude placing the cow in dorsal recumbency. A perforating foreign body will remain in the ventral aspect of the reticulum and be surrounded by gas.

Electronic metal detectors can identify metal in the reticulum but do not distinguish between perforating and nonperforating foreign bodies.

Ultrasonography of the heart and thorax is useful in the diagnosis of pleuritis and pericarditis.

Treatment: Treatment of the typical case seen early in its course may be surgical or medical. Either approach improves the chances of recovery from ~60% in untreated cases to 80-90%. Surgery involves rumenotomy with manual removal of the object or objects; if an abscess is adhered to the reticulum, it should be aspirated (to confirm that it is an abscess) and then drained into the reticulum. Antibiotics should be administered perioperatively. Medical treatment involves administration of antibacterials to control the peritonitis and a magnet to prevent recurrence. Because of the mixed bacterial flora in the lesion, a broad-spectrum antimicrobial agent such as oxytetracycline (6.6-11 mg/kg) should be used. Penicillin (22,000 IU/kg, IM, BID) is used widely and is effective in many cases despite its limited spectrum. Affected cows should be confined for 1-2 wk; placing them on an inclined plane (elevated in front) may limit further penetration of the foreign object. Supportive therapy, such as oral or occasionally IV fluids and SC calcium borogluconate, should be administered as needed. Rumen inoculation is beneficial in some cases with prolonged ruminal stasis and loss of normal flora.

More advanced cases, those with obvious secondary complications, or those that do not respond to initial medical or surgical therapy should be evaluated from an economic perspective; if the cow is of limited value, slaughter should be considered if the carcass is likely to pass inspection.

Prevention: Preventive measures include avoiding the use of baling wire, passing feed over magnets to remove metallic objects, keeping cattle away from sites of new construction, and completely removing old buildings and fences. Additionally, bar magnets may be administered PO, preferably after fasting for 18-24 hr. Usually, the magnet remains in the reticulum and holds any ferromagnetic objects on its surface. There is good evidence that giving magnets to all herd replacement heifers and bulls at ~1 yr of age minimizes incidence of traumatic reticuloperitonitis.

VAGAL INDIGESTION
(Chronic indigestion)

Vagal indigestion is characterized by gradual development of rumenoreticular and abdominal distention thought to be the result of lesions affecting the vagus nerve. However, vagal nerve involvement is not present in all cases. The most common cause is traumatic reticuloperitonitis (see p 186). Vagal indigestion is seen in cattle and has been reported in sheep.

Etiology and Pathogenesis: Various diseases can cause vagal indigestion due to injury, inflammation, or pressure on the vagal nerve. However, conditions resulting in mechanical obstruction of the cardia or reticulo-omasal orifice (eg, papillomas or ingested placenta) also have been included in the syndrome if ruminoreticular distention is present and the condition is subacute to chronic.

There are 4 types of vagal indigestion based on the site of the functional obstruction. Type I is failure of eructation or free-gas bloat, Type II is a failure of omasal transport, type III is abomasal impaction, and type IV is partial obstruction of the forestomach.

Type I vagal indigestion, or failure of eructation, results in free-gas bloat. It is most commonly due to inflammatory lesions in the vicinity of the vagus nerve, such as localized peritonitis, adhesions (usually after an episode of traumatic reticuloperitonitis), or chronic pneumonia. Less common causes include pharyngeal trauma, which affects a more proximal part of the vagus nerve, and esophageal compression by abscesses or neoplasia, such as lymphosarcoma. Free-gas bloat can also be seen with esophageal obstruction by intraluminal foreign bodies or masses. However, this typically is an acute condition, which does not fit the definition of vagal indigestion.

Type II vagal indigestion, or failure of omasal transport, develops as a result of any condition that prevents ingesta from passing through the omasal canal into the abomasum. Adhesions and abscesses (reticular or single liver abscesses) are the most common causes. They are usually on the right or medial wall of the reticulum near the route of the vagus nerve. Reticular abscesses and adhesions are almost invariably the result of traumatic reticuloperitonitis. Mechanical obstruction of the omasal canal by ingested material (eg, placenta) or masses (eg, lymphosarcoma, squamous cell carcinoma, granulomas, or papillomas) can also cause chronic ruminoreticular distention due to failure of omasal transport.

Type III vagal indigestion is abomasal impaction, which tends to develop due to feeding of dry, course roughage, such as straw, in a chopped or ground form with restricted access to water and usually during extremely cold temperatures (see DIETARY ABOMASAL IMPACTION, p 198). Secondary impactions are seen after an episode of traumatic reticuloperitonitis or as a sequela of right abomasal displacement or abomasal volvulus or, less commonly, of obstruction of the pylorus (eg, by placenta or trichobezoars). Vagal indigestion can develop in cattle after abomasal volvulus without abomasal impaction. These cases would presumably fall into the category of failure of omasal transport (type II) with damage to the vagal nerve found more cranial in its course.

Type IV vagal indigestion, or partial forestomach obstruction, is poorly defined. It typically develops in cattle during gestation. It may be related to the enlarging uterus shifting the abomasum to a more cranial position, which inhibits normal motility.

Clinical Findings: The clinical signs vary to some extent with the location of the obstruction. In all cases, there is a gradual development (over days to weeks) of ruminoreticular and abdominal distention. Distention of the dorsal and ventral sacs of the rumen result in an "L-shaped" rumen on rectal examination. Left dorsal and left and right ventral distention of the abdomen causes a "papple" (pear plus apple) shape.

Cattle with vagal indigestion have a diminished appetite, which typically improves temporarily if distention is relieved. Milk production gradually decreases, fecal output is reduced and often contains long hay particles, and the rumen develops a "splashy" fluid consistency. The feces are characteristically very scant and sticky. The strength of rumen contractions is decreased; however, rumen motility is often increased (3-4 contractions/min). It is commonly possible to see movements of the left abdominal wall that mirror the movements of the hyperactive rumen. However, rumen contraction sounds are not audible because the contents have become frothy due to the prolonged contractions and failure of the rumen to empty.

Temperature and respiratory rate are usually normal; however, these can be increased depending on the cause. Bradycardia is present in 25-40% of cases. Because bradycardia is uncommonly associated with other conditions, vagal indigestion should be considered in the differential diagnosis in any case in which bradycardia is present. Tachycardia develops as the disease progresses. Over time, the animal develops a rough hair coat, loses condition, and becomes weak (in some cases to the point of recumbency) and dehydrated.

On rectal palpation, the rumen is distended with gas or froth that occupies the entire left abdomen, pushing the left kidney to the right of the midline. The ventral sac of the rumen is enlarged and palpable to the right of the midline (the characteristic "L-shaped" rumen). Palpation of the lower half of the right side of the abdomen below the costochondral junction may detect an impacted abomasum that feels doughy. Hematologic findings vary. The PCV can be increased because of dehydration or decreased because of bone marrow depression (anemia of chronic disease). The WBC may be normal, increased, or decreased. If an inflammatory condition such as peritonitis is present, the neutrophil to lymphocyte ratio is typically reversed, and a neutrophilia may be present. Lymphocytosis can be seen with vagal indigestion due to lymphosarcoma. Leukopenia may be present with diffuse peritonitis. Increased serum globulin and total protein can be seen with abscesses.

Metabolic status is normal, or metabolic alkalosis may be present. The chloride level varies with the site of the obstruction. Low chloride indicates reflux of chloride from the abomasum into the rumen and obstruction at the level of the abomasum. The chloride levels of the rumen fluid may be increased. Metabolic alkalosis is typically present if serum chloride is decreased. The chloride is usually normal if the lesion is cranial to the abomasum. Potassium is usually low due to decreased potassium intake in the feed. Calcium is often moderately decreased because of ongoing milk production; however, it can be low enough to cause recumbency. BUN and creatinine increase with dehydration due to prerenal azotemia.

Diagnosis: Diagnosis is based on the presence of subacute to chronic ruminoreticular and abdominal distention. Because vagal indigestion is by definition a subacute to chronic disease, this diagnosis should not be made in cattle that have not been sick for at least several days, which rules out acute rumen tympanites and acute frothy bloat. Other causes of abdominal distention, such as ascites and uterine enlargement, are included in the differential diagnosis and can almost invariably be ruled out by rectal palpation due to the absence of ruminoreticular distention. Occasional cases of longstanding obstruction of the cecum or small intestine can cause severe ruminoreticular and abdominal distention; however, palpable cecal or small-intestinal distention is also palpable rectally. In addition, the rumen is distended but not L-shaped, and a characteristic ping is present in the case of cecocolic volvulus.

Diagnosing the specific cause of vagal indigestion is more difficult but is important because of differences in treatment and prognosis. Physical examination, rectal examination, CBC, blood acid-base determination, and serum chemistry values are often useful. Peritoneal fluid analysis can support the diagnosis of peritonitis if total protein or nucleated cells are increased. Radiographs of the reticulum should be taken to identify a radiopaque linear foreign body (eg, wire) or reticular abscess. Definitive diagnosis often requires exploratory surgery (left paralumbar fossa laparotomy and rumenotomy).

Treatment and Prognosis: If the value of the animal justifies treatment, surgery is almost always needed to identify the underlying cause. Medical management alone is ineffective. A left paralumbar fossa laparotomy and rumenotomy provides the opportunity for definitive treatment in some cases. Emptying the rumen at the time of surgery may help restore normal rumen motility. Stimulation of low-threshold tension receptors in the reticulum occurs under normal circumstances and causes reflex reticuloruminal contractions. However, severe distention causes stimulation of high-threshold receptors that have the opposite effect and inhibit contractions.

Supportive or symptomatic therapy should be provided in all cases, which typically involves correcting dehydration as well as calcium and electrolyte deficits, commonly with oral fluids and electrolytes. Severely dehydrated animals and those with longstanding disease require IV fluids. Fresh water and normal feed should be available. Transfaunation at surgery and/or via stomach tube may help reestablish normal rumen flora in cattle with chronic anorexia. Antibiotics should be given if the underlying cause is infectious or if a rumen fistula is created. Choice of antibiotic should be based on culture results if possible.

Treatment of type I vagal indigestion (failure of eructation) also typically involves creating a rumen fistula to allow free gas to escape. If surgery is not economically feasible and the underlying cause of vagal indigestion has been identified and treated, a rumen trocar can be placed temporarily. Such trocars are commercially available and must be secure and self-retaining to prevent potentially fatal leakage of rumen contents into the peritoneal cavity. The trocar should not be removed for at least 2 wk to allow firm adhesions to form between the rumen and body wall.

The prognosis for animals with type I vagal indigestion is usually favorable. After creation of a rumen fistula, the signs of vagal indigestion resolve in nearly all cases. However, animals with chronic respiratory disease or pharyngeal trauma may not recover from the underlying condition. Leakage of ingesta from fistulas can cause off-flavored milk. Peritonitis can develop from leakage around the fistula or as a sequela of rumenotomy; however, this should not happen with good surgical technique.

Type II vagal indigestion (failure of omasal transport) rarely responds to supportive or symptomatic therapy without surgical intervention. Left paralumbar fossa laparotomy and rumenotomy can be used to identify adhesions in the vicinity of the reticulum, reticular or hepatic abscesses, or obstruction of the omasal canal. Removal of foreign bodies, wires, and some masses at surgery affords an excellent prognosis. A diagnosis of lymphosarcoma at surgery warrants a grave prognosis. Reticular abscesses identified at surgery should be cautiously drained into the reticulum, and antibiotics given for 10-14 days. Reportedly, 83% of cattle with reticular abscesses respond favorably to treatment. Identification of adhesions in the vicinity of the reticulum warrants a fair to good prognosis with surgery, antibiotic therapy, and appropriate supportive treatment. Hepatic abscesses must be drained by a second surgery. Large-bore cannulas placed through the body wall, through the adhesions, and into the abscess will drain the pus. However, recurrence is more of a problem with hepatic abscesses than with reticular abscesses.

Animals with type III vagal indigestion (abomasal impaction) diagnosed without surgery usually do not receive further treatment because of the poor prognosis, particularly if there is a history of traumatic reticuloperitonitis or abomasal volvulus. If the diagnosis is made at surgery or if the abomasal impaction is thought to be dietary, dioctyl sodium sulfosuccinate or magnesium sulfate can be infused directly into the abomasum via the reticulo-omasal orifice after emptying the rumen. A nasogastric tube can be passed into the abomasum at surgery and left in place for continued treatment. If possible, impacted material should be removed manually through the reticulo-omasal orifice. Other lesions, such as abscesses, should be identified and drained. Abomasotomy and removal of abomasal contents, using a right paracostal approach with the cow in left lateral recumbency, can be performed as a last resort. However, recurrence of the impaction is common. Pyloric obstruction in cattle is rare and is most often due to a foreign body obstructing the lumen. Pyloromyotomy is almost never effective in resolving abomasal impactions.

Type III vagal indigestion has a poor prognosis regardless of the cause or the treatment. However, some cattle with primary abomasal impactions will respond to therapy, although severely affected animals will not (*see* DIETARY ABOMASAL IMPACTION, p 198). Cattle with secondary impactions due to traumatic reticuloperitonitis or as a sequela of right abomasal displacement or abomasal volvulus seldom recover. Animals with foreign bodies (eg, trichobezoars) obstructing the pylorus have a good prognosis if the obstruction is removed.

Therapeutic abortion has been recommended for treatment of cattle with type IV vagal indigestion (partial forestomach obstruction), and some cows have improved with this treatment; however, because type IV vagal indigestion is a poorly defined condition, the prognosis is always guarded. A more specific prognosis is based on response to therapy and identification of a specific lesion at exploratory celiotomy and rumenotomy.

Prevention: The most common cause of vagal indigestion is traumatic reticuloperitonitis, which causes adhesions and abscesses that interfere with vagal nerve function. Therefore, prevention of traumatic reticuloperitonitis is important. Good management practices will prevent some cases of vagal indigestion resulting from chronic pneumonia. Early diagnosis of right-sided abomasal displacements and abomasal volvulus, and surgical correction the day the diagnosis is made, may prevent some cases. Prompt removal of the placenta from the cow's enclosure after parturition will keep it from obstructing the cardia, reticulo-omasal orifice, or pylorus.

RUMINAL DRINKERS
(Ruminal drinking)

Ruminal drinkers refers to calves that develop chronic indigestion because milk is deposited into the rumen as a result of failure of the reticular groove reflex during drinking.

The disease is most common in bucket-fed calves, especially veal calves 2-8 wk old. Calves that "gulp" rather than sip milk are at greatest risk. The milk retained in the rumen ferments and produces acetic acid, butyric acid, and lactate; the pH in the rumen falls; and dyskeratosis of the ruminal mucosa develops. Secondary changes include villous atrophy in the small intestine and reduced disaccharidase activity of the brush border. Affected calves show inappetence, ventral abdominal distention, and poor growth. They pass sticky, clay-like feces that may adhere to the tail, perineum, and hindlegs. Chronically affected calves are small for their age and have a poor prognosis. Fluid-splashing sounds, audible on auscultation over the left flank while the calf is drinking, are diagnostic. Rancid-smelling fermented material can be obtained by stomach tube from the rumen. A ruminal pH of <6 leads to systemic acid-base disturbance.

Treatment consists of removing the fermented material and flushing the rumen with saline. With subsequent feedings, an attempt is made to induce reticular groove closure by inducing vigorous sucking activity with the fingers before feeding milk. Calves that relapse should be fed by nipple-bottle or weaned. A rubber nipple floating on the surface of bucket-fed milk may prevent the syndrome. Failure of the reticular groove reflex and putrefactive rumenitis also is seen in calves <2 wk old and can be an important cause of sporadic cases of diarrhea in this age group.

RUMINAL PARAKERATOSIS

Ruminal parakeratosis is a disease of cattle and sheep characterized by hardening and enlargement of the papillae of the rumen. It is most common in animals fed a high-concentrate ration during the finishing period. It also is seen in cattle fed rations of heat-treated alfalfa pellets. It does not appear to be related to the feeding of antibiotics or protein concentrates. Incidence in a group may be as high as 40%. The lesions are thought to be caused by the lowered pH and the increased concentration of volatile fatty acids (VFA) in the rumen juice (*see also* SIMPLE INDIGESTION, p 177). The lesions usually do not develop in cattle fed unprocessed whole grain (on which animals gain weight as readily), which may be related to the higher pH and higher concentration of acetic acid compared with the longer chain VFA in the rumen juice.

Many of the papillae are enlarged and hardened, and several may adhere together to form bundles. The papillae of the anterior ventral sac are commonly affected. In cattle, the roof of the dorsal sac may show multiple foci (each 2-3 cm^2) of parakeratosis. In sheep, abnormal papillae may be visible and palpable through the wall of the intact rumen. Affected papillae contain excessive layers of keratinized epithelial cells, particles of food, and bacteria. The rumens of affected cattle are difficult to clean in the preparation of tripe. The abnormal epithelium, by interfering with absorption, may reduce efficiency of feed utilization and rate of gain, although there is little evidence to support this theory.

Ruminal parakeratosis may be prevented by finishing animals on rations that contain unground ingredients in the proportion of 1 part roughage to 3 parts concentrate. The necessity and economics of prevention are not well defined.

DISEASES OF THE ABOMASUM

Abomasal disorders include left displaced abomasum (LDA), right displaced abomasum (RDA), abomasal volvulus, ulcers, and impaction. Displacement or volvulus is seen most commonly in dairy cows, but can also be seen in dairy bulls and calves. Except for abomasal volvulus, abomasal displacement is rare in beef cattle and essentially undiagnosed in small ruminants. Ulcers are seen in dairy and beef cattle and in calves and lambs; they are rarely diagnosed in small ruminants. Impactions can be primary, which is most frequent in beef cattle, or secondary, which develop most often in dairy cows as a form of vagal indigestion. Impactions may have a hereditary basis in some black-faced sheep.

LEFT OR RIGHT DISPLACED ABOMASUM AND ABOMASAL VOLVULUS

Because the abomasum is suspended loosely by the greater and lesser omenta, it can be moved from its normal position on the right ventral part of the abdomen to the left or right side (LDA, RDA), or it can rotate on its mesenteric axis while displaced to the right (abomasal volvulus). It can shift from its normal position to left displacement or to right displacement over a relatively short period. Abomasal volvulus can develop rapidly or slowly from an uncorrected RDA.

Etiology: Although LDA, RDA, and abomosal volvulus (previously referred to as RTA for right torsion of the abomasum) are often considered separately, there is evidence of a common underlying etiology; they may be different manifestations of the same or a similar disease process.

The etiology is multifactorial, although abomasal hypomotility and gas production contribute to development of displacement or volvulus. Important contributing factors include abomasal hypomotility associated with hypocalcemia and concurrent diseases (mastitis, metritis) associated with endotoxemia and decreased rumen fill, periparturient changes in the position of intra-abdominal organs, and genetic predisposition, particularly in deep-bodied cows. Hypomotility is also related to ingestion of high-concentrate, low-roughage diets, which reduce abomasal motility through a poorly defined mechanism that may involve increased concentrations of volatile fatty acids. In addition, high-concentrate diets result in a linear increase in gas production (mostly carbon dioxide, methane, and nitrogen). Finally, subclinical and clinical ketosis increase the risk of abomasal displacement through an unknown mechanism that may be associated with decreased rumen fill.

About 80% of displacements are seen within 1 mo of parturition; however, they can be seen at any time. LDA is much more common than RDA (30:1); cases of volvulus are also more common than RDA (10 LDA to 1 volvulus). Abomasal volvulus is preceded by RDA.

Pathogenesis: In LDA, as a result of abomasal hypomotility and gas production, the partially gas-distended abomasum becomes displaced upward along the left abdominal wall lateral to the rumen. It is primarily the fundus and greater curvature of the abomasum that become displaced, which in turn causes displacement of the pylorus and duodenum.

The omasum, reticulum, and liver are also rotated to varying degrees. The abomasal obstruction is partial, and although the segment contains some gas and fluid, a certain amount can still escape, and the distention rarely becomes severe. Because there is no interference with blood supply, the effects of displacement are entirely due to interference with digestion and passage of ingesta, which lead to decreased appetite and dehydration. A mild metabolic alkalosis with hypochloremia and hypokalemia are common. The hypochloremic metabolic alkalosis is due to abomasal hypomotility, continued secretion of hydrochloric acid into the abomasum, and the partial abomasal outflow obstruction, with sequestration of chloride in the abomasum and reflux into the rumen. Hypokalemia is due to decreased intake of feeds high in potassium, sequestration of potassium in the abomasum, and dehydration. Secondary ketosis is common and may be complicated by development of fatty liver disease (p 824).

In RDA, hypomotility, gas production, and displacement of the partially gas-filled abomasum occur as in LDA. Mild hypokalemic, hypochloremic, metabolic alkalosis develops as well. After this dilatation phase, rotation of the abomasum on its mesenteric axis leads to volvulus and local circulatory impairment and ischemia (hemorrhagic strangulating obstruction). The volvulus is usually in a counterclockwise direction when viewed from the rear and the right side of the animal. The omasum is displaced medially and can be involved in the volvulus with occlusion of its blood supply (called an omasalabomasal volvulus). The liver and reticulum usually are displaced also. In rare cases, the reticulum can be involved (called a reticular-omasal-abomasal volvulus). A large quantity of fluid accumulates in the abomasum; chloride is sequestered there as well. Hypochloremic, hypokalemic metabolic alkalosis develops. The blood supply to the abomasum, and often the omasum and proximal duodenum, is compromised, eventually resulting in ischemic necrosis of the abomasum as well as dehydration and circulatory failure. As this progresses, a metabolic acidosis is superimposed on the metabolic alkalosis.

Clinical Findings: The typical history of displacement includes anorexia (most commonly a lack of appetite for grain with a decreased or normal appetite for roughage) and decreased milk production (usually significant but not as dramatic as with traumatic reticuloperitonitis or other causes of peritonitis). In abomasal volvulus, anorexia is complete, milk production is more markedly and progressively reduced, and clinical deterioration is rapid. In abomasal displacement, temperature, heart rate, and respiratory rate are usually normal. The caudal part of the rib cage on the side of the displacement may appear "sprung." Hydration appears subjectively normal with displacements except in some chronic cases. Rumen motility may be normal but often is reduced in frequency and strength of contraction. Feces are usually reduced in quantity and more fluid than normal.

The most important diagnostic physical finding is a ping on simultaneous auscultation and percussion of the abdomen, which should be performed in the area marked by a line from the tuber coxae to the point of the elbow, and from the elbow toward the stifle. The ping characteristic of an LDA is most commonly located in an area between ribs 9 and 13 in the middle to upper third of the abdomen; however, the ping can be more ventral or more caudal, or both. Pings associated with a rumen gas cap are usually more dorsal, less resonant, and extend more caudally through the paralumbar fossa. Rectal examination can confirm a gas-filled rumen or an extremely empty rumen that correlates with the rumen ping in these cases. Pings associated with pneumoperitoneum typically are less resonant, present on both sides of the abdomen, and inconsistent in location on repeated evaluation. Frequently, secondary ketosis develops and ketones are present in the urine or milk. Ketosis that develops in association with abomasal displacement responds only transiently to treatment and recurs (as compared with primary ketosis, which develops early in lactation in high-producing cows and responds to therapy permanently if instituted early). *See also* KETOSIS, p 830.

The ping associated with RDA also is most commonly located in the area between ribs 10 and 13. Differentiation between various causes of a right-sided ping is difficult in some cases. A small ping underlying ribs 12 or 13 and extending as far forward as rib 10 is common in cows with functional ileus from a number of causes. It is most often associated with gas in the ascending colon and resolves with correction of the underlying condition. Cecal dilatation and rotation are characterized by a right-sided ping. The ping extends through the dorsal paralumbar fossa in cecal dilatation and usually is located more caudally (well into the paralumbar fossa) in cecal rotation compared with the ping of RDA. Palpation per rectum is helpful in differentiating an RDA from cecal dilatation or rotation. Other right-sided pings are produced by pneumoperitoneum or gas in the rectum, descending colon, duodenum, or uterus.

Spontaneous fluid splashing or gas tinkling sounds may be heard on auscultation of the area of the ping or on simultaneous ballottement and auscultation of the abdomen (succussion). The characteristic rectal examination findings with LDA include a medially displaced rumen and left kidney. The abomasum is rarely palpable in LDA and only occasionally in RDA.

The clinical signs associated with abomasal volvulus are more severe than with simple displacements because of the vascular compromise. However, an early abomasal volvulus can be difficult to distinguish from an RDA except by the presence of a right-sided ping cranial to rib 10 (indicating medial displacement of the liver by the abomasal volvulus) and the anatomic position identified at surgery. In contrast to cases of displacement, an animal with abomasal volvulus has tachycardia proportional to the severity of the condition. The area of the ping is usually larger (extending as far forward as rib 8), and the amount of succussible fluid is greater. The animal is more depressed, and signs of weakness, toxemia, and dehydration develop as the disease progresses. The caudal extent of the abomasum is usually palpable per rectum. Without therapy, the animal often becomes recumbent within 48-72 hr after developing volvulus. Death occurs from shock and dehydration and is sudden if the ischemic abomasum ruptures.

Diagnosis: For displacement or volvulus, diagnosis is based on the presence of the characteristic ping on simultaneous auscultation and percussion and excluding other causes of left- or right-sided pings. Recent parturition, partial anorexia, and decreased milk production suggest displacement. A ketosis that is only temporarily responsive to treatment is consistent with abomasal displacement, which may be intermittent. The typical signs on physical examination (in addition to the ping), rectal examination, and laboratory evaluation also support the diagnosis. Melena or signs of peritonitis (eg, fever, tachycardia, localized abdominal pain, pneumoperitoneum) with an LDA may indicate a bleeding or perforated abomasal ulcer, respectively.

Treatment: Open (surgical) and closed (percutaneous) techniques can be used to correct displacements. Rolling a cow through a 70° arc after casting her on her right side corrects most LDA; however, recurrence is very likely. LDA can be corrected surgically using right flank pyloric omentopexy, right paramedian abomasopexy, left paralumbar abomasopexy, or combined left flank and right paramedian laparoscopy. Blind suture techniques (toggle-pin fixation or the "big needle" [blind-stitch] method), performed in the right paramedian area, are percutaneous methods for correction of LDA; however, the exact location of the suture is not known. Potentially fatal complications following blind suture techniques can develop, although the reported success is similar to that of surgical correction. With toggle-pin fixation, the pH can be checked to confirm that the pin is in the abomasum, which reduces the likelihood of attaching rumen, small intestine, or omentum to the body wall rather than the abomasum. RDA and abomasal volvulus are corrected surgically (using right paralumbar fossa omentopexy or right paramedian abomasopexy) when economically feasible. The right paramedian abomasopexy should be used only for correcting RDA and abomasal volvulus in cattle that are unable to stand.

Ancillary treatment of animals with displacements include treating any concurrent disease (eg, metritis, mastitis, ketosis). Calcium borogluconate SC or calcium gels PO help restore normal abomasal motility in many cases. In simple displacement, fluid and electrolyte abnormalities correct spontaneously with access to water and a salt block. Providing electrolyte water (60 g sodium chloride and 30 g potassium chloride in 19 L of water) via stomach tube is helpful in cases of longer duration. Animals with significant dehydration and metabolic derangement require IV therapy, which is typically administered as hypertonic saline (7.2% NaCl, 5 mL/kg, IV over 5 min). Occasionally, animals with abomasal displacement or volvulus have atrial fibrillation, thought to be of metabolic origin. Correction of the displacement or volvulus almost always results in correction of the atrial fibrillation within 1 wk. Aggressive treatment of ketosis plays an important role in the successful treatment of abomasal displacement, as most of the cattle that die following surgical correction of LDA and RDA do so from the metabolic consequences of prolonged anorexia.

The prognosis after correction of simple LDA or RDA is good, with survival rates of 95%. Abomasal volvulus has a variable and less favorable prognosis (average survival rate of 70%); a high heart rate, moderate to severe dehydration, a longer period of illness, a large quantity of fluid in the abomasum, and the presence of omasal-abomasal or reticulo-omasal-abomasal volvulus are associated with a poor prognosis.

Prevention: The incidence of displacements can be decreased by ensuring a rapid increase in rumen volume following calving, feeding a total mixed ration rather than feeding grain twice daily ("slug feeding"), avoiding rapid dietary changes, maintaining adequate roughage in the diet, avoiding postparturient hypocalcemia, and minimizing and promptly treating concurrent disease and ketosis.

ABOMASAL ULCERS

Abomasal ulcers affect mature cattle and calves and have several different manifestations.

Etiology and Pathogenesis: Except for lymphosarcoma of the abomasum and the erosions of the abomasal mucosa that develop in viral diseases such as bovine viral diarrhea, rinderpest, and bovine malignant catarrhal fever, the causes of abomasal ulceration are not well understood. Many different causes have been suggested. Although abomasal ulcers can be seen any time during lactation, they are common in high-producing, mature dairy cows within the first 6 wk after parturition. The most likely cause is prolonged inappetence, which results in sustained periods of low abomasal pH.

Abomasal ulcers may also arise in association with lymphosarcoma, abomasal disorders (displacement or volvulus), or increased intraluminal pressure causing ischemia of abomasal mucosa; they may also appear to be unrelated to other disease.

Abomasal ulcers are very common in milk-fed calves after they have consumed milk or milk replacer for 4-12 wk. Most of these are subclinical and nonhemorrhagic. Occasionally, milk-fed calves <2 wk old are affected by acute, hemorrhagic abomasal ulcers that may perforate and cause rapid death. Well-nourished suckling beef calves, 2-4 mo old, may be affected by acute abomasal ulcers. Abomasal trichobezoars are common in these calves, but do not appear to increase the risk of ulcer formation.

Clinical Findings: The syndrome varies, depending on whether ulceration is complicated by hemorrhage or perforation and by the severity of such hemorrhage or peritonitis.

A system of classification is based on the depth of penetration or the degree of hemorrhage or peritonitis caused by the ulcer: Type I is an erosion or ulcer without hemorrhage, Type II is hemorrhagic, Type III is perforated with acute localized peritonitis, and Type IV is perforated with acute diffuse peritonitis. There may be only a single ulcer or many acute and chronic ulcers.

Cattle with bleeding abomasal ulcers may be asymptomatic except for intermittent occult blood in the feces, or they can die acutely from massive hemorrhage. Common clinical signs include mild abdominal pain, bruxism, sudden onset of anorexia, tachycardia (90-100 bpm), and fecal occult blood or melena that may be intermittent. Signs of blood loss are seen with major hemorrhage and may include tachycardia (100-140 bpm), pale mucous membranes, weak pulse, cool extremities, shallow breaths, tachypnea, and melena. More severe signs include acute rumen stasis, generalized abdominal pain with a reluctance to move and an audible grunt or groan with each breath, weakness, and dehydration. Melena may not be present in peracute cases because it takes at least 8 hr for abomasal blood to be detected in the feces. As the condition progresses, body temperature drops, and the animal becomes recumbent and dies within 6-8 hr.

In general, bleeding ulcers do not perforate, and perforating ulcers do not bleed into the GI tract sufficiently to produce melena. However, hemorrhage and perforation are seen together occasionally, usually in cases that are chronic or associated with abomasal displacement.

Calves with abomasal ulceration and hairballs may have a distended gas- and fluid-filled abomasum that is palpable behind the right costal arch. Deep palpation may reveal abdominal pain associated with local peritonitis due to a perforated ulcer. In calves, perforating ulcers are more common than bleeding ulcers.

Lesions: Ulceration is most common in the fundic region in adult cattle and in the pyloric antrum in milk-fed calves. The single or multiple ulcers measure from a few millimeters to 5 cm in diameter. The affected artery is usually visible after ingesta and necrotic tissue are removed from a bleeding ulcerated area. Most cases of perforation are walled off by the omentum, which forms a cavity 12-15 cm in diameter that contains degenerated blood and necrotic debris. Material from this cavity may infiltrate widely through the omental fat. Adhesions may form between the ulcer and surrounding organs or the abdominal wall.

Diagnosis: In cases with only slight bleeding and mild clinical signs, diagnosis is difficult and may require repeated fecal evaluations for occult blood. Other conditions that can cause partial anorexia and decreased milk production should be excluded by physical examination and laboratory tests, including abdominocentesis. In cases with melena, the diagnosis can be based on physical examination alone. The PCV can help to determine the degree of hemorrhage. An occult blood test of the feces can confirm melena. Other conditions that result in blood in the feces should be eliminated. Blood from portions of the GI tract distal to the abomasum reacts on fecal occult blood tests; it is usually bright red if from the large intestine or raspberry-colored if from the small intestine. Animals with abomasal lymphosarcoma can have a bleeding syndrome similar to that associated with abomasal ulcers but do not respond to therapy. Occasionally, oral, pharyngeal, and laryngeal lesions bleed, and the swallowed blood appears in the feces. Similarly, pulmonary abscesses that form as a sequela of rumenitis by embolization to the lungs and liver can erode blood vessels and result in hemoptysis; if the blood is swallowed, this can also result in melena. Fecal occult blood may also be due to abomasal volvulus or to bloodsucking helminths.

Diagnosis of perforating abomasal ulcers is based on physical examination and excluding other causes of peritonitis. Abomasal ulceration with perforation and local peritonitis may be indistinguishable from chronic traumatic reticuloperitonitis. A magnet in the reticulum (confirmed by use of a compass) or an accurate history of having given the cow a magnet before the onset of signs decreases the likelihood of traumatic reticuloperitonitis. Reticular radiographs may confirm or exclude the presence of radiopaque foreign bodies in the reticulum. In some cases, there is a neutrophilia, possibly with a left shift. Evaluation of peritoneal fluid will confirm peritonitis if total protein and nucleated cell count are increased. Intracellular bacteria or degenerate neutrophils are rarely seen because, in most cases, the infection is rapidly walled off. The diagnosis of diffuse peritonitis due to perforation is based on physical examination and excluding other causes. Rupture of a distended viscus, such as can occur with abomasal volvulus or cecal rotation, produces similar signs. Regardless of the cause of diffuse peritonitis, the prognosis is grave because of overwhelming infection and cardiovascular deterioration. There is neutrophilia with a marked left shift and hemoconcentration. Abdominal fluid is usually readily obtainable in large quantities, and the protein level is increased; the nucleated cell count may be increased, or it may be normal due to dilution or utilization.

Treatment: Most cases of abomasal ulcers are undiagnosed and therefore untreated. Occasionally, a presumptive diagnosis is made and medical treatment instituted. The most important treatment is to get the animal to eat, as food is an excellent buffer and continual flow of forestomach contents (pH 6.0-7.0) into the abomasum helps increase abomasal pH. Broad-spectrum antibiotic therapy (given for ≥5 days or until the rectal temperature is normal for 48 hr) is indicated for perforating ulcers. Antacids are effective in increasing abomasal pH in milk-fed calves when administered at 4- to 6-hr intervals in a manner that induces esophageal groove closure; however, their efficacy is extremely questionable in adult ruminants because of ruminal dilution. H_2-receptor antagonists are effective in increasing abomasal pH in milk-fed calves; however, the oral doses required for cimetidine (100 mg/kg, TID) and ranitidine (50 mg/kg, TID) are high. Because NSAID can contribute to ulceration, their use is contraindicated. The prognosis for localized peritonitis associated with perforating abomasal ulcers is good with medical therapy and dietary alteration. Recovery generally takes 1-2 wk, and animals that are fully recovered for 1-2 wk generally do not experience recurrence. Surgery is indicated for perforating abomasal ulcers only when the abomasum is displaced; however, significant abdominal contamination can occur in the process of breaking down adhesions and resecting or oversewing the ulcer. Animals in which the ulcerated area is resected or oversewn usually recover.

Animals with diffuse peritonitis after perforation of an abomasal ulcer rarely respond to therapy, and the prognosis is grave. Treatment consists of rapid and continued IV fluid therapy (based on the current metabolic status) and IV broad-spectrum antibiotics. The few animals that recover from diffuse peritonitis usually have massive abdominal adhesions.

For bleeding ulcers, blood transfusions and fluid therapy may be necessary in addition to dietary management, stall confinement, and oral antacids. If hemorrhage is acute, the PCV may not reflect the severity because equilibration between intravascular and extravascular fluid after blood loss takes at least 4 hr. Generally, a blood transfusion is required whenever weakness and lethargy are present; a decision regarding transfusion should be based on clinical signs rather than PCV. Cross-matching is not usually necessary; a single transfusion of 4-6 L of blood is required. Some cattle require more than one transfusion over the course of several days. Complete recovery usually takes 1-2 wk. The prognosis is good if weakness and lethargy have not developed before treatment is started.

Prevention: Animals should be encouraged to keep eating to avoid prolonged periods of inappetence and low abomasal pH.

DIETARY ABOMASAL IMPACTION

Impaction of the abomasum develops in pregnant beef cows during cold winter months when cattle have decreased water intake and are fed poor-quality roughage. It also has been seen in feedlot cattle fed a variety of mixed rations containing chopped or ground roughage (straw, hay) and cereal grains and in late-pregnancy dairy cows on similar feeds.

Etiology: The cause is unknown but considered to be consumption of excess roughage that is low in both digestible protein and energy. Impaction with sand can occur if cattle are fed hay or silage on sandy soils, or root crops that are sandy or dirty. Outbreaks may affect up to 15% of all pregnant cattle on individual farms when the ambient temperature drops to -14°F (-26°C) or lower for several days.

Pathogenesis: The pathogenesis is unknown but is related to diet. Once the abomasum becomes impacted, subacute obstruction of the upper GI tract develops. Ions of hydrogen and chloride are continually secreted into the abomasum in spite of the impaction, and atony and alkalosis with hypochloremia result. Varying degrees of dehydration develop because fluids are not moving beyond the abomasum into the duodenum for absorption. Sequestration of potassium ions in the abomasum results in hypokalemia. Dehydration, alkalosis, electrolyte imbalance, and progressive starvation are seen. Impaction of the abomasum may be severe enough to cause irreversible abomasal atony.

Clinical Findings and Lesions: Complete anorexia, scant feces, moderate distention of the abdomen, weight loss, and weakness are usually the initial signs. Body temperature is usually normal but may be subnormal during cold weather. A mucoid nasal discharge tends to collect at the external nares and on the muzzle; the muzzle is usually dry and cracked due to the failure of the animal to lick its nostrils and to the effects of dehydration. The heart rate may be increased, and mild dehydration is common.

Most often, the rumen is static and distended with dry contents, but it may contain excess fluid if the cow has been fed finely ground feed. The pH of the ruminal fluid is usually normal (6.5-7). Protozoal activity in the rumen ranges from normal to a marked reduction in numbers and activity (assessed microscopically under low power). The impacted abomasum is usually in the right lower quadrant on the floor of the abdomen. Deep palpation and strong percussion of the right flank may indicate the presence of a large, firm mass (impacted abomasum) and elicit a grunt (as is common in acute traumatic reticuloperitonitis), probably because of distention of the abomasum and stretching of its serosa.

Severely affected cattle die 3-6 days after the onset of signs. The abomasum ruptures in some cases, and death from acute, diffuse peritonitis and shock occurs precipitously in a few hours. In sand impaction, there is considerable weight loss, chronic diarrhea with sand in the feces, weakness, recumbency, and death in a few weeks.

Metabolic alkalosis, hypochloremia, hypokalemia, and hemoconcentration are common, as are total and differential WBC counts within the normal range. At necropsy, the abomasum is commonly enlarged (up to 8 times normal size) and impacted with dry rumen-like contents. The omasum may be similarly enlarged and impacted. The rumen is grossly enlarged and filled with dry contents or fluid. The GI tract beyond the pylorus is characteristically empty and has a dry appearance. Varying degrees of dehydration and emaciation are also present. If the abomasum has ruptured, lesions of acute diffuse peritonitis are present.

Diagnosis: Clinical diagnosis is based on the nutritional history, clinical evidence of impaction, and laboratory results. The disease must be differentiated from secondary abomasal impaction as a form of vagal indigestion.

Impaction of the abomasum as a complication of traumatic reticuloperitonitis usually is seen in late pregnancy, and commonly only in one animal. A mild fever may or may not be present, and there may be a grunt on deep palpation of the xiphoid. The rumen is enlarged and may be hypermotile (early) or atonic (late). In many cases, it is impossible to distinguish between the 2 causes of impacted abomasum, and a right flank laparotomy may be necessary to explore the abdomen for peritoneal lesions.

Treatment: The challenge is to recognize the cases that will respond to treatment and those that will not, ie, to determine those that should be slaughtered immediately for salvage. Cows that are weak, have a severely impacted abomasum, and have a marked tachycardia (100-120 bpm) are poor treatment risks. In cows that are treated, the metabolic alkalosis, hypochloremia, hypokalemia, and dehydration should be corrected. Lubricants and cathartics can be used in an attempt to move the impacted material, or the abomasum should be emptied surgically. Balanced electrolyte solutions are infused IV continuously for up to 72 hr at a daily rate of 80-120 mL/kg. Some cows respond well to this therapy and begin ruminating and passing feces in 48 hr.

Mineral oil can be administered at 4L/day for 3 days. Alternatively, dioctyl sodium sulfosuccinate (DSS) can be given by stomach tube at 120-180 mL of a 25% solution for a 1,000-lb (450-kg) animal mixed with ~20 L of warm water and repeated daily for 3-5 days. This dose rate will kill rumen protozoa. Mineral oil and DSS should not be administered simultaneously because DSS may potentiate the absorption of mineral oil. A beneficial response cannot be expected in <24 hr; in cattle that respond, improvement is usually seen by the end of day 3 after treatment begins.

Surgery may be considered, but results are often unsuccessful, probably because of abomasal atony, which appears to worsen after surgery. An alternative may be a rumenotomy to empty the rumen and infuse mineral oil directly into the abomasum through the reticulo-omasal orifice in an attempt to soften and promote the evacuation of the abomasal contents. Cattle with secondary impactions that develop as a sequela of traumatic reticuloperitonitis or abomasal volvulus usually show signs of vagal indigestion, and abomasal impaction may be diagnosed at the time of exploratory surgery.

The induction of parturition using dexamethasone (20 mg, IM) may be indicated in affected cattle within 2 wk of term and in which the response to treatment for a few days has been unsuccessful. Parturition may assist recovery because of a reduction in intra-abdominal volume. For sand impaction, affected cattle should be moved off the sandy soil and fed good hay and a grass mixture containing molasses and minerals. Severely affected cattle should be treated with mineral oil (4 L/day for 3 days).

Prevention and Control: Prevention is possible by providing the necessary nutrient requirements for wintering pregnant beef cattle. When low-quality roughage is used, it should be analyzed for crude protein and digestible energy. Based on the analysis, grain is usually added to the ration to meet energy and protein requirements.

The nutrient requirements of beef cattle (p 1811) are guidelines for use under average conditions; higher nutrient levels than those indicated may be necessary, particularly during periods of severe cold stress. Adequate fresh drinking water should be supplied at all times; the practice of forcing wintering cows to obtain their water requirements by eating snow while on low-quality roughage is hazardous.

ACUTE INTESTINAL OBSTRUCTIONS IN LARGE ANIMALS

Intestinal obstructions are seen in all large animal species but are most common in horses. Cattle are the most commonly affected ruminants; diagnosis in sheep and goats is rare. Other than inguinal hernias, obstructions are infrequently recognized in pigs. In general, obstructions are mechanical or functional, and can be seen in any part of the intestinal tract. They can interrupt the flow of ingesta, and vascular integrity may or may not be compromised (strangulating or simple obstruction, respectively).

Etiology and Pathogenesis: The inciting cause of an intestinal obstruction often is not determined. Functional obstructions are associated with altered intestinal motility, often due to dietary or management factors, parasite infection, enteritis, or peritonitis. Mechanical obstructions (physical blockage of ingesta) occur due to abnormalities in the bowel lumen, in the wall, or outside the tract. Congenital obstructions (atresia jejuni, coli, recti, and ani in calves, atresia ani in lambs and pigs) result in the lack of passage of feces since birth.

In horses, transient functional obstructions are common, as are feed impactions, which usually involve the pelvic flexure. Parasite infection or migration, dental abnormalities, and dietary or management factors are often implicated. Impactions and other luminal obstructions can result from coarse feeds, reduced water intake, enteroliths, or ingested foreign material. Sites of impaction other than the pelvic flexure are the small colon, transverse colon, right dorsal colon, cecum, and ileum. Other causes of intestinal obstruction in horses are volvulus (twist on the mesenteric axis), torsion (twist along the long axis of the bowel), displacement of the ascending (large) colon, and volvulus of part or all of the small intestine. Altered motility and possibly strenuous exercise and rolling may be initiating causes. Broodmares may be predisposed to volvulus, torsion, or displacement of the ascending colon during gestation and shortly after parturition. Obstruction occurs either due to incarceration of the intestine (usually small) by herniation through the inguinal canal, diaphragm, mesenteric defects, umbilicus, or epiploic foramen; or because of fibrous bands (adhesions, mesodiverticular bands, or stalks of pedunculated lipomas). Standardbred stallions and colts develop inguinal and scrotal hernias more commonly than other breeds. Diaphragmatic hernias and mesenteric defects may be congenital or traumatically induced. Adhesions in horses are most often the sequela of parasite migration or abdominal surgery; however, most adhesions are clinically silent. Pedunculated lipomas are common in older horses. Ileocecal, cecocecal, cecocolic, and small-intestinal intussusceptions also are seen. Lymphosarcoma and other abdominal neoplasms as well as abdominal abscesses can cause intestinal obstruction.

In cattle, specific causes include intussusception; volvulus of the jejunoileal flange of the small intestine; volvulus at the root of the mesentery; cecocolic volvulus; and atresia coli, recti, and ani. Intussusceptions are thought to be the result of irregular peristaltic movements related to enteritis, intestinal parasitism, dietary disorders, and mural masses. Altered intestinal motility may also cause intestinal volvulus. Obstructions of the small intestine can develop due to a variety of fibrous bands (eg, adhesions, parovarian bands, falciform ligament, spermatic cord retraction into the abdomen after surgical castration), mural thickening (eg, intestinal adenocarcinoma), extramural masses (eg, lymphosarcoma, fat necrosis, abdominal abscesses), herniation (inguinal or umbilical), or hemorrhagic jejunitis (which results in luminal blood clots and obstruction). Adhesions and abdominal abscesses can form subsequent to peritonitis, intraperitoneal injections, or previous abdominal surgery. Decreased motility caused by accumulation of volatile fatty acids, possibly related to high-concentrate rations or an abrupt increase in the concentrate:forage ratio, have been suggested as causes of cecocolic volvulus in cattle. They also are associated with advanced pregnancy and ileus from concurrent disease. Atresia coli develops most commonly in Holstein calves secondary to in utero ischemia of the developing spiral colon.

Clinical Findings and Diagnosis: Intestinal obstruction in horses generally manifests as abdominal pain (*see* COLIC, p 202). In cattle, signs of abdominal pain include treading, stretching, and kicking at the abdomen, and less commonly rolling and bellowing. These signs are generally more subtle than in horses and are usually referable to small-intestinal distention, tension on the intestinal mesentery (by the weight of distended bowel), or vascular impairment. Signs of pain are relatively consistent but often transient with intussusceptions and are seen in some cases of cecocolic volvulus. Cattle with volvulus of the small intestine at the root of the mesentery are severely affected.

Usually, cattle with intestinal obstruction are anorectic and pass few or no feces, and milk production in lactating cows drops suddenly. The feces that are passed may be covered with mucus, or mixed or coated with blood. Thick, raspberry-colored blood mixed with scant feces is characteristic of small-intestinal bleeding, particularly that associated with intussusception. Blood from the colon or rectum is generally brighter red. Melena is typical of abomasal bleeding. Calves with atresia coli are normal at birth but have progressive abdominal distention and decreased appetite over the first few days of life. (*See also* CONGENITAL AND INHERITED ANOMALIES OF THE DIGESTIVE SYSTEM, p 131.)

Abdominal distention, usually with a ping on simultaneous auscultation and percussion, in the upper right caudal abdominal quadrant occurs with cecocolic volvulus. Cecal dilatation does not produce abdominal distention, but a ping is generally present in the caudal dorsal paralumbar fossa. In cecocolic volvulus, one or more large distended loops of large intestine are present. Rumen motility is usually present, and metabolic and cardiovascular derangement tend to be mild except in cecocolic volvulus of long duration.

Abdominal distention in the lower right abdominal quadrant is sometimes seen with small-intestinal distention. Distended loops of bowel may be palpable on rectal examination, and fluid may be heard on simultaneous ballottement and auscultation of the right side of the abdomen. Small areas of tympanic resonance may be heard on simultaneous auscultation and percussion. Intussusceptions and fibrous bands that cause small-intestinal obstruction can be palpated rectally in some cases.

Profound changes in cardiovascular parameters, such as tachycardia, abnormal color of the mucous membranes, prolonged capillary refill time, and dehydration, are most commonly associated with hemorrhagic strangulating obstructions such as volvulus of the jejunal-ileal flange of the small intestine. Volvulus of the jejunal-ileal flange and volvulus at the root of the mesentery are characterized by acute onset and rapid cardiovascular deterioration. This is in contrast with cecocolic volvulus or intussusception, which can continue for several days.

Metabolic derangements range from hypokalemic, hypochloremic metabolic alkalosis in longstanding small-intestinal and duodenal obstructions to severe metabolic acidosis with hemorrhagic strangulating obstructions. Usually, there are no metabolic derangements in mild functional obstructions and early (simple) mechanical obstructions, particularly if a relatively distal part of the intestinal tract is involved. Hypocalcemia can develop, presumably due to decreased calcium absorption from the duodenum.

Peritoneal fluid changes reflect the degree of peritonitis and may aid in the diagnosis in both cattle and horses, although results are more variable in cattle. Hemorrhagic strangulating obstructions are characterized by an increase in RBC, with subsequent increases in total protein and nucleated cell counts due to extravasation through the bowel wall. Neutrophils become degenerative, and intracellular gram-positive and gram-negative bacteria are seen as the integrity of the bowel wall is lost. Plant material in the peritoneal cavity is indicative of bowel rupture or inadvertent enterocentesis. Simple obstructions with severe dilatation of the bowel can be associated with increases in total protein and, less commonly, nucleated cell counts. Peritoneal fluid analysis is normal with most simple mechanical and functional obstructions. When neoplasms are present, neoplastic cells are sometimes identified in peritoneal fluid.

Treatment: For treatment of obstruction in horses, *see* COLIC, p 202. Treatment of functional obstructions in cattle is generally symptomatic and supportive after identifying and eliminating the inciting cause (eg, excessive grain intake) and allowing time for normal intestinal motility to return. If present, dehydration and electrolyte imbalances should be corrected by appropriate fluid therapy (PO or IV). Lactating cows often benefit from calcium gels administered orally or calcium borogluconate administered SC, and secondary ketosis should be treated if present. Occasionally, surgical decompression is required in cases of functional obstruction.

Mechanical obstructions almost always require surgery. Antibiotic therapy should be started preoperatively; supportive therapy, such as fluids, electrolytes, and calcium, should be administered if needed. The prognosis with most functional obstructions is good with appropriate supportive therapy, particularly if the inciting cause is identified and eliminated.

Horses that require exploratory celiotomy to correct an intestinal obstruction have an overall longterm survival rate of 50%. The survival rate is lower for horses with hemorrhagic strangulating obstructions than for horses with simple obstructions, but early surgical intervention can improve the prognosis.

In cattle, 70-80% of those with cecocolic volvulus survive, although 10% of cases recur. For cows with small-intestinal obstruction amenable to resection and anastomosis, 30-40% survive and lead a productive life. For cows with volvulus of the jejunal-ileal flange of the small intestine or at the root of the mesentery, ~50% survive if surgical correction is performed within a few hours of onset. Only 30% of calves with atresia coli survive to adulthood. Surgical correction is not recommended in Holstein calves because the condition is probably inherited in this breed, although vascular damage secondary to amniotic vesicle palpation in the first 6 wk of embryonic development can also lead to intestinal ischemia and atresia in calves.

Prevention: Prevention of all, or even most, cases of intestinal distention is not possible. However, abrupt changes in feeding and management, inadequate water intake, parasite infection, dental abnormalities, and access to coarse feeds and foreign material should be avoided or corrected.

COLIC IN HORSES

In its strictest definition, the term "colic" means abdominal pain. Over the years, it has become a broad term for a variety of conditions that cause the horse to exhibit clinical signs of abdominal pain. Consequently, it is used to refer to conditions of widely varying etiologies and severity. To understand these etiologies, make a diagnosis, and initiate appropriate treatments, veterinarians must first appreciate the clinically relevant aspects of equine GI anatomy, the physiologic processes involved in movement of ingesta and fluid along the GI tract, and the extreme sensitivity of the horse to the deleterious effects of bacterial endotoxin that normally exists within the lumen of the intestine.

GI Anatomy: The horse is a monogastric animal, with a relatively small stomach (capacity 8-10 L) that is located on the left side of the abdomen beneath the rib cage. The junction of the distal esophagus and the cardia is a functional 1-way valve, permitting gas and fluid to move into the stomach but not out. Consequently, conditions that impede the normal aboral movement of gas and fluid through the small intestine may result in severe dilation and rupture of the stomach. Because of its position, the stomach is difficult to visualize with radiography or ultrasonography in large adult horses. The smaller size of the foal, however, permits assessment of gastric emptying by contrast radiography.

The small intestine comprises the duodenum, jejunum, and ileum, with the latter joining the cecum at a distinct ileocecal junction. The duodenum is positioned primarily dorsally on the horse's right side, where it is suspended from the dorsal body wall by a small mesentery of 3-5 cm. Consequently, the duodenum is not involved in small-intestinal displacements involving the mesentery (volvulus). At the base of the cecum in the right paralumbar fossa region, the duodenum turns toward the midline. It is at this point that the duodenum, if distended with gas or fluid (eg, in horses with proximal enteritis), can be felt on rectal examination.

As the small intestine reaches the dorsal midline, it becomes the jejunum. The characteristic long mesentery allows loops of the jejunum to rest on the contents of the ventral portion of the abdomen. The jejunum is ~65 ft (19.5 m) long; its length, coupled with its long mesentery, allow it to be involved in small intestinal volvulus and incarcerations. At the end of the jejunum, the wall of the intestine becomes more muscular, the lumen is narrowed, and an additional mesenteric attachment becomes apparent. The last 18 in. (45 cm) of the small intestine, the ileum, joins the cecum at its dorsal medial aspect. This junction is identified by the attachment of the ileocecal fold from the ileum to the dorsal band of the cecum. This ileocecal fold is used as a landmark to locate the ileum at surgery.

From the ileum, the ingesta enters the cecum, a large, blind-ended fermentation vat that is situated primarily on the horse's right side, extending from the region of the paralumbar fossa to the xiphoid cartilage on ventral midline. The cecum is 4-5 ft (1.2-1.5 m) long and can hold 27-30 L of feed and fluid. Under the influence of the cecal musculature, the ingesta in the cecum is massaged, mixed with microorganisms capable of digesting cellulose, and eventually passed through the cecocolic opening into the right ventral colon. The attachment of the cecum to the dorsal body wall is wide, thus minimizing the likelihood that the cecum can become displaced or twisted on its own.

The right ventral colon is divided into sacculations that help mix and retain plant fibers until they are digested. It is located on the ventral aspect of the abdomen from the flank region to the rib cage. The ventral colon then turns toward the left, becoming the sternal flexure and then the left ventral colon. The left ventral colon, which also is large and sacculated, passes caudally to the left flank area. Near the pelvic region, the diameter of the colon decreases markedly, and the colon folds back on itself. This region, which is called the pelvic flexure, is the initial portion of the unsacculated left dorsal colon. Presumably due to the abrupt decrease in diameter, the junction between the left ventral colon and pelvic flexure is the most common location for impactions.

The diameter of the dorsal colon is maximal either at its diaphragmatic flexure or at the right dorsal colon. There are no sacculations in either the left or right portion of the dorsal colon. The right dorsal colon is closely attached to the right ventral colon by a short intercolic fold and to the body wall by a tough common mesenteric attachment with the base of the cecum. In contrast, neither the left ventral nor the left dorsal colons are attached directly to the body wall, allowing these portions of the colon to become displaced or twisted.

Ingesta moves from the large right dorsal colon into the short transverse colon, which has a diameter of ~10 cm and is fixed firmly to the most dorsal aspect of the abdominal cavity by a strong, short, fibrous mesentery. The transverse colon is located cranial to the cranial mesenteric artery. Finally, the ingesta enters the sacculated descending colon, which is 10-12 ft (3-3.6 m) long.

Blood Supply to the GI Tract: The celiac and cranial mesenteric arteries (branches of the abdominal aorta) supply blood to the GI tract. The celiac artery supplies arterial blood to the stomach, pancreas, liver, spleen, and the first portion of the duodenum. The cranial mesenteric artery supplies arterial blood to the remaining portion of the duodenum; to all of the jejunum, ileum, cecum, large colon, and transverse colon; and to the first portion of the descending colon. Because the large colon is attached to the body wall only in the region near the cranial mesenteric artery, the blood supplying all portions of the colon must traverse the entire length of the colon. The pelvic flexure receives its blood supply from 2 branches of the cranial mesenteric artery; one branch supplies the right dorsal and left dorsal colons before reaching the pelvic flexure, and the other branch supplies the right and left ventral colons before reaching the pelvic flexure. Thus, volvulus of the large colon near the junction of the colon and cecum may impede the flow of blood to the entire left colon.

The major branches of the cranial mesenteric artery can be damaged by the migrating forms of *Strongylus vulgaris* (*see* p 267).

Natural Openings in the Abdomen: There are several natural openings or spaces within the abdominal cavity that can be important in conditions causing colic. The inguinal canal provides an opening through which intestine might pass and become trapped. Although inguinal hernias are common in young foals, they rarely cause clinical problems; the situation is considerably different in stallions. Similarly, if the ventral abdominal wall fails to form properly around the umbilicus, an opening remains and the potential exists for intestinal problems to develop secondary to an umbilical hernia. The epiploic foramen, a natural opening between the portal vein, the caudal vena cava, and the caudate lobe of the liver, can be the site of intestinal incarcerations. Finally, there is a natural space between the dorsal aspect of the spleen and the left kidney. This space is bounded by the renosplenic ligament, a strong band of tissue that connects the dorsomedial aspect of the spleen with the fibrous capsule of the left kidney. This ligament provides a "shelf" over which large colon can be displaced.

Colonic Motility Patterns: Normograde peristalsis in the left ventral colon moves ingesta toward the left dorsal colon, and the muscles in the wall of the left dorsal colon contract to move the ingesta toward the diaphragmatic flexure. There is evidence, however, that the muscles in the left ventral colon contract in a retrograde fashion, from the pelvic flexure region toward the sternal flexure. Furthermore, these contractions originate from a pacemaker region in the pelvic flexure. It has been hypothesized that this pacemaker senses either the size or the consistency of the feed particles in the ingesta and then initiates the appropriate motility pattern. If the ingesta has been digested sufficiently, it is moved in a normograde direction; if additional digestion is necessary, the ingesta is moved in a retrograde direction to retain it in the ventral colon. This theory has been proposed to account for the common clinical occurrence of obstruction at or near the pelvic flexure.

Clinical Findings: Numerous clinical signs are associated with colic. The most common include pawing repeatedly with a front foot, looking back at the flank region, curling the upper lip and arching the neck, repeatedly raising a rear leg or kicking at the abdomen, lying down, rolling from side to side, sweating, stretching out as if to urinate, straining to defecate, distention of the abdomen, loss of appetite, depression, and decreased number of bowel movements. It is uncommon for a horse with colic to exhibit all of these signs. Although they are reliable indicators of abdominal pain, the particular signs do not indicate which portion of the GI tract is involved or whether surgery will be needed.

Diagnosis: A diagnosis can be made and appropriate treatment begun only after thoroughly examining the horse, considering the history of any previous problems or treatments, determining which part of the intestinal tract is involved, and identifying the cause of the particular episode of colic. In most instances, colic develops for one of 4 reasons: 1) The wall of the intestine is stretched excessively by either gas, fluid, or ingesta. This stimulates the stretch-sensitive nerve endings located within the intestinal wall, and pain impulses are transmitted to the brain. 2) Pain develops due to excessive tension on the mesentery. 3) Ischemia develops, most often as a result of incarceration or severe twisting of the intestine. 4) Inflammation develops and may involve either the entire intestinal wall (enteritis) or the covering of the intestine (peritonitis). Under such circumstances, proinflammatory mediators in the wall of the intestine decrease the threshold for painful stimuli.

The list of possible conditions that cause colic is long, and it is reasonable first to determine the most likely type of disease and begin appropriate treatments and then to make a more specific diagnosis, if possible. The general types of disease that cause colic include excessive gas in the intestinal lumen (flatulent colic), simple obstruction of the intestinal lumen, obstruction of both the intestinal lumen and the blood supply to the intestine (strangulating obstruction), interruption of the blood supply to the intestine alone (nonstrangulating infarction), inflammation of the intestine (enteritis), inflammation of the lining of the abdominal cavity (peritonitis), erosion of the intestinal lining (ulceration), and "unexplained colic." In general, horses with strangulating obstructions and complete obstructions require emergency abdominal surgery, whereas horses with the other types of disease can be treated medically.

The history of the present colic episode and previous episodes, if any, must be ascertained to determine if the horse has had repeated or similar problems, or if this episode is an isolated event. The duration of the episode, the rate of deterioration of cardiovascular status, the severity of pain, whether feces have been passed, and the response to treatment are important information. It is also critical to determine the horse's deworming history (schedule, treatment dates, drugs used), when the teeth were floated last, if any changes in feed or water supply or amount have occurred, and whether the horse was at rest or exercising when the colic episode started.

The physical examination should include assessment of the cardiopulmonary and GI systems. The oral mucous membranes should be evaluated for color, moistness, and capillary refill time. The mucous membranes may become cyanotic or pale in acute cardiovascular compromise and eventually hyperemic or muddy as peripheral vasodilation develops later in shock. The capillary refill time (normal ~1.5 sec) may be shortened early but usually becomes prolonged as vascular stasis (venous pooling) develops. The membranes become dry as the horse becomes dehydrated. The heart rate increases due to pain, hemoconcentration, and hypotension; therefore, higher heart rates have been associated with more severe intestinal problems (strangulating obstruction). However, not all conditions requiring surgery are accompanied by a high heart rate.

An important aspect of the physical examination is passing a nasogastric tube. Because horses can neither regurgitate nor vomit, adynamic ileus, obstructions involving the small intestine, or distention of the stomach with gas or fluid may result in gastric rupture. Passing a stomach tube may, therefore, save the horse's life and assist in diagnosis of these conditions. If fluid reflux occurs, the volume and color of the fluid should be noted.

The abdomen and thorax should be auscultated, and the abdomen percussed. The abdomen should be auscultated over several areas (cecum on the right, small intestine high on the left, colon lower on the left). Intestinal sounds associated with episodes of pain may indicate an intraluminal obstruction (eg, impaction, enterolith). Gas sounds may indicate ileus or distention of a viscus. Fluid sounds may indicate impending diarrhea associated with colitis. A complete lack of sounds is usually associated with adynamic ileus or ischemia. Percussion will assist in identifying a grossly distended segment of intestine (cecum on right, colon on left) that may need to be trocarized. The respiratory rate may be increased due to fever, pain, acidosis, or an underlying respiratory problem. Diaphragmatic hernia is also a possible cause of colic.

The most definitive part of the examination is the rectal examination. The veterinarian should develop a consistent method of palpating for the following: aorta, cranial mesenteric artery, cecal base and ventral cecal band, duodenum, bladder, peritoneal surface, inguinal rings in stallions and geldings or the ovaries and uterus in mares, pelvic flexure, spleen, and left kidney. The intestine should be palpated for size, consistency of contents (gas, fluid, or impacted ingesta), distention, edematous walls, and pain on palpation.

A sample of peritoneal fluid (obtained via paracentesis performed aseptically on midline) often reflects the degree of intestinal damage. The color, cell count and differential, and total protein concentration should be evaluated. Normal peritoneal fluid is clear to yellow, contains <5,000 WBC/μL, most of which are mononuclear cells, and <2.5 g of protein/dL.

The age of the horse is important because a number of age-related conditions cause colic. The more common of these include the following: in foals—atresia coli, meconium retention, uroperitoneum, and gastroduodenal ulcers; in yearlings—ascarid impaction; in the young—small-intestinal intussusception, nonstrangulating infarction, and foreign body obstruction; in the middle-aged—cecal impaction, enteroliths, and large-colon volvulus; and in the aged—pedunculated lipoma and mesocolic rupture.

Ultrasonographic evaluation of the abdomen may help clinicians differentiate between diseases that can be treated medically and those that require surgery. The technique also can be applied transrectally to clarify findings noted on rectal palpation. In foals, echoes from the large colon and small intestine are commonly identified from the ventral abdominal wall, whereas only large colon echoes are usually seen in adult horses. The large colon can be identified by its sacculated appearance. The duodenum can be identified in the tenth intercostal space and traced around the caudal aspect of the right kidney. The jejunum is rarely identified during transabdominal ultrasonographic examination of normal adult horses, whereas the thick-walled ileum can be identified by transrectal examination.

The most common abnormalities identified by ultrasonography include inguinal hernia, renosplenic entrapment of the large colon, sand colic, intussusception, enterocolitis, right dorsal colitis, and peritonitis. Stallions with inguinal hernia have incarcerated intestine on the affected side; it is possible to identify the intestine, and to obtain information concerning the thickness of its wall and presence or lack of peristalsis can be obtained. In horses with renosplenic entrapment of the large colon, the tail of the spleen or the left kidney cannot be imaged, or the gas-filled large colon is present in the caudodorsal aspect of the abdomen in the region of the renosplenic space. Horses with sand colic have granular hyperechoic echoes originating from the affected portion of the colon. The characteristic finding in horses with intussusception is the "bull's eye" appearance of the affected portion of the small intestine. Very often the intestine proximal to the intussusception is distended and the strangulated portion is thickened. Horses with enterocolitis frequently have evidence of hyperperistalsis, thickened areas of the bowel wall, and fluid distention of the intestine. In contrast, horses with right dorsal colitis commonly have marked thickening of the wall of the right dorsal colon. In horses with peritonitis, the peritoneal fluid may be anechoic or there may be evidence of flocculent material and fibrin between serosal surfaces of the viscera.

Treatment: Horses with colic may need either medical or surgical treatments. Almost all require some form of medical treatment, but only those with certain mechanical obstructions of the intestine need surgery. The type of medical treatment is determined by the cause of colic and the severity of the disease. In some instances, the horse may be treated medically first and the response evaluated; this is particularly appropriate if the horse is mildly painful and the cardiovascular system is functioning normally. Ultrasonography can be used to evaluate the effectiveness of nonsurgical treatment. If necessary, surgery can be used for a diagnosis as well as a treatment.

If evidence of intestinal obstruction with dry ingesta is found on rectal examination, a primary aim of treatment is to hydrate and evacuate the intestinal contents. If the horse is severely painful and has clinical signs indicating loss of fluid from the bloodstream (high heart rate, prolonged capillary refill time, and discoloration of the mucous membranes), the initial aims of treatment are to relieve pain, restore tissue perfusion, and correct any abnormalities in the composition of the blood and body fluids (*see* TABLE 5). If damage to the intestinal wall (as a result of either severe inflammation or a displacement or strangulating obstruction) is suspected, steps should be taken to prevent or counteract the ill effects of bacterial endotoxin that leaves the intestine and enters the bloodstream. Finally, if there is evidence that the colic episode is caused by parasites, one aim of treatment is to eliminate the parasites.

Pain Relief: In most cases of colic, pain is mild, and analgesia is all that is needed. In these instances, the cause of colic is presumed to be spasm of intestinal muscle or excessive gas in a portion of the intestine. If, however, the pain is due to an intestinal twist or displacement, some of the stronger analgesics may mask the clinical signs that

TABLE 5. General Concepts Regarding Fluid Needs in Dehydrated Horses*

Determining Factor	Formula Used	Amount for a 500 kg Horse
Fluid deficit	% dehydration × body weight (kg)	4-10% × 500 = 20-50 L
Maintenance	50 mL/kg/24 hr	50 × 500 = 25 L/24 hr
Fluid losses	Estimate reflux or diarrhea volume	
Rate of administration	50% in 1-2 hr; 50% throughout rest of day	20-35 L in first 1-2 hr; remainder distributed over next 23 hr

*Adapted, with permission, from Zimmel D.N., Management of pain and dehydration in horses with colic. In *Current Therapy in Equine Medicine*, 5, 2003, Robinson N.E., (ed.), Elsevier.

would be useful in making a diagnosis. For these reasons, a thorough physical examination should be completed before any medications are given. However, because horses with severe colic or pain may hurt themselves and become dangerous to people nearby, analgesics often must be given first. Additionally, many horses with less severe problems may need pain relief until the other treatments have time to be effective. An analgesic that has the fewest side effects and causes the least alteration in the horse's attitude should be selected.

Medications used commonly for abdominal pain are NSAID that reduce the production of prostaglandins. When these drugs are used as recommended, their toxic effects on the kidneys and GI tract occur infrequently. Clinical experience suggests that flunixin meglumine may mask the early signs of conditions that require surgery and, therefore, must be used carefully in horses with colic.

The most commonly used sedative for colic is xylazine, an α_2-agonist. Within a few minutes after administration, the horse stands quietly and is less responsive to pain. Unfortunately, the effects of xylazine are short-lived, and it inhibits the intestinal muscles; it also decreases cardiac output and thus reduces blood flow to the tissues. Detomidine, a more potent α_2-agonist that is much longer-acting, is used successfully under similar circumstances.

Of the narcotic analgesics, butorphanol is used most often in horses with colic. Butorphanol has few adverse effects on the GI tract or heart. However, when given in large doses, narcotics can cause excitement, and the horse may become unstable. Butorphanol is frequently combined with an α_2-agonist to produce a more prolonged period of analgesia.

Although pain relief usually is provided by analgesics, there are other important ways to reduce the degree of pain. For example, passing a nasogastric tube (also an important part of the diagnostic workup) may remove any fluid that has accumulated in the stomach because of an obstruction of the small intestine. The removal of this fluid not only relieves pain from gastric distention but also prevents rupture of the stomach.

Fluid Therapy: Many horses with colic benefit from fluid therapy to prevent dehydration and maintain blood supply to the kidneys and other vital organs. The fluids may be given either through the nasogastric tube or IV, depending on the particular intestinal problem (*see* TABLE 5). Horses with strangulating obstruction or enteritis must be given fluids IV because absorption of fluids from the diseased intestine is reduced and fluid may be secreted into the lumen of the intestine. The latter mechanism causes a buildup of fluid in the intestine, which must be removed from the stomach through a nasogastric tube. This abnormal movement of body fluids into the intestine contributes to the development of circulatory shock, which is often the ultimate cause of death.

Most of the fluid is reabsorbed from the ingesta in the cecum and colons. In fact, ~95% of the fluid that normally enters the lumen of the large intestine is returned to the bloodstream. Therefore, horses with intestinal obstructions near the pelvic flexure usually require relatively small amounts of IV fluids, whereas horses with small-intestinal obstructions need extremely large amounts.

The volume and type of fluid to be given are determined by the severity and cause of the problem. Laboratory tests to determine the degree of hemoconcentration and whether concentrations of electrolytes are abnormal are critical for accurate treatment of a horse with severe colic. The balance of body fluids can be reestablished by administering IV fluids formulated to replenish the deficient electrolyte(s). In most instances, however, fluid therapy must be started before laboratory results are available, particularly when the horse is showing clinical signs of circulatory shock.

When IV fluids are needed but the clinical signs are mild to moderate, the horse is usually given 8-10 L of a sterile replacement fluid that contains electrolytes in concentrations that normally exist in the blood. This volume is administered over 1-2 hr, and the horse is reevaluated to determine if additional fluids are needed. Horses in circulatory shock require much larger volumes of IV fluids, given as rapidly as possible; up to 20 L in 1 hr may be needed to reestablish tissue perfusion. In severe cases, hypertonic saline (7% NaCl) may be given to rapidly increase plasma volume. Depending on the cause of colic, IV fluids may be needed for several days until intestinal function has returned, electrolyte concentrations are balanced, and the horse can maintain its fluid needs by drinking. Under such circumstances, the daily IV fluid requirements may range from 30 to 100 L.

Fluids are sometimes given through the nasogastric tube as part of the treatment of impactions of the colon. Many clinicians believe that the same result can be accomplished by giving large volumes of fluids IV. If the horse will not drink voluntarily and there is no obstruction in the small intestine, hydration may be maintained by administering fluids through the tube. Fluids or medications should not be given through the nasogastric tube if fluid reflux is being removed from the stomach, as this indicates either the stomach or the small intestine is not emptying properly.

Protection Against Bacterial Endotoxin: Endotoxin, a part of the outer coating of enteric gram-negative bacteria, is released when the bacteria die or multiply rapidly. Normally, endotoxin is restricted to the intestinal lumen, but if the intestinal mucosal lining is damaged due to ischemia, endotoxin moves into the peritoneal cavity or the bloodstream. It then interacts with mononuclear phagocytes and triggers an inflammatory response that can include fever, depression, hypotension, coagulation abnormalities, and eventually death. Minimizing the inflammatory responses to endotoxemia is a vital part of colic therapy.

Prostaglandins are involved in causing many of endotoxin's early ill effects. Flunixin meglumine reduces the cellular production of prostaglandins and can help prevent some of their effects. Because flunixin can help prevent some of the early effects of endotoxemia at dosages less than the recommended dosage (1.1 mg/kg), smaller dosages (0.25 mg/kg) can be administered without masking clinical signs associated with conditions that require surgery.

There is considerable controversy regarding the efficacy of plasma or serum that contains antibodies designed to neutralize endotoxin. These antibodies are directed against the components of endotoxins that are consistent among different gram-negative bacteria. The results of clinical studies using such antibodies have been conflicting, with evidence of protection being seen in some studies and no positive effects identified in others. Because endotoxin itself stimulates the generation of a wide array of inflammatory substances that ultimately produce the pathophysiologic effects, neutralizing antibodies should be used as early in the course of the disease as possible.

As an alternative approach, polymyxin B has been used to prevent endotoxin from interacting with the horse's inflammatory cells. Polymyxin B has well documented nephrotoxicity; however, concentrations of polymyxin B that bind endotoxin are far less than those that cause toxic effects. Polymyxin B has been evaluated in several recent experimental studies of endotoxemia and currently is being used in clinical cases at 1,000-5,000 U/kg, BID-TID. This form of therapy should be initiated as early as possible in the clinical course of the disease. In addition, fluid replacement therapy should be maintained in hypovolemic animals, and serum creatinine concentration should be closely monitored. This latter concern is especially relevant to azotemic neonatal foals, as they appear to be more susceptible to the nephrotoxic side effects of polymyxin B.

Intestinal Lubricants and Laxatives: A common cause of colic in horses is simple obstruction of the large intestine by dried ingesta, sometimes mixed with sand. These impactions of the large intestine generally develop near the pelvic flexure or in the right dorsal colon but may involve any portion of the large colon, descending colon, or cecum. In most instances, lubricants or fecal-softening agents given through a nasogastric tube soften the impacted ingesta, allowing it to be passed. This form of therapy can be aided by the simultaneous administration of IV fluids. Keeping the horse muzzled is advised to prevent further impaction of feed material while the obstruction is softening.

Mineral oil is the most commonly used medication in the treatment of a large colon impaction. It coats the inside of the intestine and aids the normal movement of ingesta along the GI tract. It is administered through a nasogastric tube, up to 4 L, SID-BID, until the impaction is resolved. Although mineral oil is safe, it is not highly effective in treating severe impactions or sand impactions because it may simply pass by the obstruction without softening it.

Dioctyl sodium sulfosuccinate (DSS) is a soap-like compound that acts by drawing water into the dry ingesta. It is more effective than mineral oil in softening impactions; however, it may interfere with the normal fluid absorptive functions of the colon and can be toxic. Thus, DSS can be given safely only in small quantities 2 times 48 hr apart.

A safe and useful compound for treating impactions, especially those containing sand, is psyllium hydrophilic mucilloid. When mixed with water, it forms a gelatinous mass that carries ingesta along the GI tract. Although usually given through a nasogastric tube to horses with impactions, psyllium also may be used as a preventive by mixing the dry powder into the feed. Horses that live in a sandy environment or that persistently develop impactions may be given psyllium powder, 400 g/500 kg, SID in their feed for 7 days. This treatment is repeated 2-3 times each year in an effort to prevent the development of sand impactions.

Strong laxatives that stimulate intestinal contractions are not commonly used to treat impactions and, in fact, may worsen the problem. Occasionally, horses with extremely hard impactions are treated with magnesium sulfate, which draws body fluids into the GI tract. Side effects include dehydration and an increased risk of diarrhea.

Fluid therapy, whether the fluids are administered through a nasogastric tube or IV, is an important and effective part of treating horses with colonic or cecal impactions. If an impaction does not start to break down within 3-5 days, surgery may be necessary to evacuate the intestine and aid in restoring normal motility.

Larvicidal Deworming: The normal migratory routes of the larvae of large bloodworms, particularly *Strongylus vulgaris*, have been implicated in many cases of colic. In response to the migratory and maturation processes of the larvae in the cranial mesenteric artery, the wall of the artery becomes thickened and forms loose plaques of inflammatory tissue. It has been hypothesized that these plaques activate coagulation, resulting in thromboembolism. The blood supply to the intestine may be reduced, resulting in altered intestinal motility, a change in the absorption of nutrients from the intestine, or death of the intestine. Thus, thromboembolism has been presumed to be a cause of recurrent episodes of colic and weight loss.

Modern deworming medications, such as ivermectin and moxidectin, have activity against migrating *S vulgaris* larvae. Fenbendazole kills migrating strongyles if given at twice the recommended dosage daily for 5 days or at 10 times the recommended dosage daily for 3 days. As a result of common use of these anthelmintics, chronic intermittent colic once thought to be caused by thromboembolism or parasite larval migration has largely been eliminated from equine practice.

There is considerable evidence that damage caused by cyathostomes causes colic, diarrhea, and loss of condition, particularly in young horses. These signs are seen on a seasonal basis and are synchronous with the emergence of large numbers of encysted larvae into the lumen of the large colon. In temperate areas of the Northern hemisphere, the larvae encyst during the winter months and emerge in the late winter and spring causing ulceration, edema, and inflammation of the mucosa of the large colon. This may result in diarrhea, protein loss, weight loss, and mild intermittent colic and fever. Horses with cyathostomiasis require treatment with larvacidal dosages of anthelmintics such as ivermectin, moxidectin, and fenbendazole. Some horses require analgesics, supportive care, and proper nutritional support.

See also GASTROINTESTINAL PARASITES OF HORSES, p 265, for a detailed discussion of treatment for large and small strongyles.

Surgery: Surgery usually is necessary if there is a mechanical obstruction to the normal flow of ingesta that cannot be corrected medically or if the obstruction also interferes with the intestinal blood supply. The latter conditions cause death of the horse unless surgery is performed quickly. Occasionally, surgery is indicated as an exploratory diagnostic procedure for horses with chronic colic that have not responded to routine medical therapy.

Under most circumstances, horses exhibiting signs of severe abdominal pain nonresponsive to analgesic therapy require emergency abdominal surgery. Generally, the lumen of the intestine is completely obstructed, such as is caused by strangulating obstruction or severe displacement. Similarly, horses with an abnormally distended intestine on rectal examination and peritoneal fluid with an increased total protein concentration and number of RBC probably have a strangulating lesion that requires surgical correction. These classic findings that characterize horses requiring emergency surgery often are the exception rather than the rule. Some horses with mild or moderate pain may also require surgery, and a judgment must be based on a thorough physical examination and other methods of evaluation. Some of the more commonly used indications for surgery in horses with colic include uncontrollable pain; >4 L of fluid reflux from the stomach; no borborygmi on auscultation; peritoneal fluid with increased protein, erythrocytes, and toxic neutrophils; and a tightly distended intestine, displaced colon, or enterolith or foreign body identified on rectal examination.

Performing surgery (if indicated) early is critical to success and improves the prognosis for survival. Therefore, it is more important to decide if the horse should be referred to a clinic where surgery could be performed if needed, rather than trying to determine if emergency surgery is definitively required. It is generally prudent to refer the following types of cases: 1) a horse that responds initially to an analgesic but requires additional analgesic therapy a few hours later, 2) a horse that continues to exhibit signs of pain despite administration of analgesics, 3) a horse that remains painful but has normal peritoneal fluid, 4) a horse with distended small intestine on rectal examination but lacking fluid reflux, or 5) a horse with large quantities of fluid removed from the stomach but no distended small intestine palpable on rectal examination.

When surgery is required, in most instances, the horse is anesthetized and positioned on its back, and the surgical incision is made on the ventral midline. Once the peritoneal cavity is entered, portions of the intestine should be examined to determine the definitive cause of the colic. Correction may involve repositioning a displaced portion of intestine, removing an obstruction, or resecting devitalized intestine. When devitalized segments of intestine must be removed or an enterotomy performed, postoperative care may include antibiotics, IV fluids, polymyxin B, antibodies directed against endotoxin, and NSAID to combat endotoxemia. When a displaced segment of intestine is simply returned to its normal location, the postoperative care is much less intense. Each horse must be handled individually, and its treatment needs are based on its response to surgery and the development of complications.

Prognosis: A large retrospective study in the USA documented an overall survival rate of 60% for horses with colic, and a survival rate of 50% for those horses undergoing abdominal surgery, including those euthanized on the surgery table for inoperable conditions. Survival rates for horses with strangulating obstruction and inflammatory diseases were only 24% and 42%, respectively. In contrast, horses with an undefined cause for the colic episode had a survival rate of 94%. When the segment of the GI tract was considered, the survival rates for conditions affecting the small intestine and stomach were poorer than for those affecting the large colon. In addition, conditions that interfered with both the passage of ingesta and the intestinal blood supply dramatically decreased the chances of survival. The results of more recent studies are far more promising, with survival rates for horses undergoing emergency abdominal surgery often >80%. Furthermore, there have been reports documenting survival rates of 70% for horses requiring resection of strangulated small intestine or correction of large colon volvulus. In earlier retrospective studies, these conditions were associated with survival rates ≤30%. Although data on longterm survival (ie, the horse returning to its intended use) are more difficult to obtain, recent findings indicate that most horses that die or are euthanized because of serious problems do so within 3 mo after surgery.

Values obtained from several variables are often combined to predict survival in horses with colic. Prognostic indicators include pain assessment, intestinal distention, mucous membrane color, and cardiovascular system function. Survival rates are highest for horses with mild abdominal pain and are lowest for horses with severe pain. Horses with palpable intestinal distention have lower survival rates than horses lacking evidence of intestinal distention, and survival rates are even lower if no intestinal sounds are audible on auscultation of the abdomen. Red mucous membranes are frequently associated with bacterial endotoxemia, which decreases the survival rate. Cardiovascular system function reflects the degree of shock and, therefore, correlates with the prognosis for survival. For instance, horses with low systolic blood pressure or a high heart rate have a decreased chance of survival.

Of the laboratory analyses used to predict survival, blood lactate concentration and the anion gap are used most often. Measurement of blood lactate has been used as an indicator of tissue perfusion, with increasing concentrations of lactic acid corresponding with poor tissue perfusion. Similarly, the anion gap (the calculated difference between the measured cations and the measured anions) reflects the generation of organic anions, most notably lactic acid, due to reduced tissue perfusion. The concentration of protein in the peritoneal fluid also has been used to predict survival, with higher concentrations associated with a poorer prognosis.

DISEASES ASSOCIATED WITH COLIC BY ANATOMIC LOCATION

Stomach

Gastric Dilatation and Gastric Rupture: The most common cause of gastric dilatation in horses is excessive gas or intestinal obstruction. Gastric dilatation may be associated with overeating fermentable feedstuffs such as grains, lush grass, and beet pulp. Presumably the large increase in production of volatile fatty acids inhibits gastric emptying. If untreated, gastric dilatation associated with overeating can rapidly lead to gastric rupture. If intestinal obstruction is the cause, the obstruction most often involves the small intestine. The fluid from the obstructed small intestine accumulates in the lumen of the stomach, causing dilatation of the stomach and retrieval of gastric reflux on passage of the nasogastric tube. Gastric dilatation also may develop in some horses with certain colonic displacements, most notably right dorsal displacement of the colon around the cecum (see p 215). It is presumed that the displaced colon obstructs duodenal outflow. Gastric dilatation with fluid also is a characteristic of proximal enteritis-jejunitis.

Rupture of the stomach is a fatal complication of gastric dilatation. The stomach generally tears along its greater curvature. About two-thirds of all gastric ruptures occur secondary to mechanical obstruction, ileus, and trauma; the remaining cases are due to overload or to idiopathic causes.

Clinical signs associated with gastric dilatation include severe abdominal pain, tachycardia, and retching. The mucous membranes may be pale. Classically, these acute signs are replaced by relief, depression, and toxemia after the stomach has ruptured. The prognosis for survival may be excellent in most cases of gastric dilatation, but gastric rupture is fatal.

Gastric Impaction: Impaction of the stomach is an uncommon cause of colic. Although it may be associated with ingestion of certain feedstuffs (beet pulp, pelleted feeds, persimmon seeds, straw, barley), contributing factors (diseased teeth, inadequate intake of water, and rapid eating) should also be considered. Because the incidence of this condition is low, it is difficult to determine which factors may be most important. The most striking clinical sign associated with gastric impaction is severe abdominal pain. Due to the lack of other characteristic findings, the diagnosis most often is made at surgery, and the decision for surgery is based on unrelenting pain.

Treatment usually involves intragastric administration of saline or water through a needle passed into the mass. After the fluid has been injected into the mass, the stomach then is massaged and the obstruction is broken down. If a nasogastric tube is in place at the time of surgery, water may be pumped into the stomach and the mass massaged. Gavage is continued after surgery with the hopes of removing some of the impacted material. The prognosis is favorable if the decision to perform exploratory surgery is made early, and the impaction can be broken down manually at surgery.

Small Intestine

Clinical signs of colic may arise due to obstruction, inflammation, or strangulating obstruction of the small intestine. The prognosis for conditions affecting the small intestine is often guarded. Hence, rapid diagnosis and appropriate treatment are critical.

Ileal Impaction: The most common condition producing simple obstruction of the lumen of the small intestine is ileal impaction. It is most common in the southeastern USA, Germany, and The Netherlands. Although high-fiber hays may be important in the pathogenesis, a cause and effect relationship has not been proved. The results of recent clinical studies in the UK indicate that infection with the intestinal tapeworm *Anoplocephala perfoliata* and ileal impaction are strongly associated. In a similar study performed in the USA, 2 risk factors for ileal impaction were identified—the lack of administration of pyrantel pamoate, an anthelmintic with some efficacy against *A perfoliata*, within 3 mo and the feeding of Coastal Bermuda hay. Further, it has been suggested that the impaction develops secondary to spastic contractions of the ileal musculature against ingesta.

Clinical signs include the onset of mild to severe abdominal pain, followed by reduced intestinal sounds, gastric reflux, and tachycardia. Although early rectal examination may permit identification of the impaction in the ileum low in the right caudal abdominal quadrant, subsequent distention of the jejunum may make this identification difficult or impossible. The most common differential diagnosis is proximal jejunitis, and distinguishing the 2 conditions can often be difficult. Because the horse's condition initially may remain stable and the degree of abdominal pain may be mild, many horses with this condition are not referred for intensive care or surgery for >18 hr. The protein concentration of the peritoneal fluid may increase if the impaction has persisted for this long.

Treatment most often requires surgery, although it has also been reported that the condition responds to treatment with fluids and mineral oil, if identified early. If surgery is indicated, the impacted mass may be mixed with saline or carboxymethylcellulose and massaged into the cecum, or an enterotomy may be performed in the distal jejunum and the ingesta removed through the incision. Ileus may develop after surgery. Depending on the degree of damage to the serosal surface of the small intestine at the time of surgery, complications may develop several weeks after surgery due to intra-abdominal adhesions (*see* below).

Adhesions: Intra-abdominal adhesions generally affect the small intestine and usually cause obstruction of the intestinal lumen, although they may cause strangulating obstruction. These adhesions develop in response to peritoneal injury and, most often, are the result of previous small-intestinal surgery, chronic small-intestinal distention, peritonitis, or larval parasite migration. The tissue response to ischemia, traumatic tissue handling, foreign material, hemorrhage, or dehydration results in the formation of fibrinous (and subsequently fibrous) adhesions. Clinical signs are seen if the adhesion causes kinking, compression, or stricture of the intestine.

Adhesions should be considered if the horse has had prior abdominal surgery and a more recent history of recurrent abdominal pain. Clinical signs associated with intra-abdominal adhesions range from mild, recurrent colic to severe unrelenting pain. Most commonly, intra-abdominal adhesions cause clinical signs within 90 days of the initial surgery if they are going to be a significant problem for the horse.

Surgical treatment involves transection of the adhesion, resection of the affected intestine, and anastomosis to achieve normal flow of ingesta. Therapeutic agents purported to reduce the subsequent formation of additional adhesions then are used. These include the systemic administration of antimicrobials, NSAID, and instillation of sterile carboxymethylcellulose into the abdomen at the time of closure. The owner should be informed that adhesions are likely to recur and that the longterm prognosis for horses with extensive adhesions is poor.

Ascarid Impaction: Young horses, particularly those on farms with inadequate parasite control programs, may develop ascarid impactions of the small intestine. These impactions are seen after administration of an anthelmintic with high efficacy against *Parascaris equorum*. The anthelmintics most commonly associated with this condition are ivermectin, piperazine, and organophosphates. These drugs paralyze the ascarids, resulting in accumulation of masses of the worms in the small-intestinal lumen. It has been suggested that disruption of the surface of the ascarid releases antigenic fluids that inhibit intestinal muscular activity, thereby increasing the likelihood of intestinal obstruction.

Clinical signs range from mild to severe abdominal pain, evidence of toxemia, and gastric reflux that may contain ascarids. Ascarid impaction should be suspected if the affected horse is a weanling or yearling, in poor condition, and has a recent history of deworming. Medical treatment with fluids and intestinal lubricants may be successful in some cases. Other horses may require surgical intervention and removal of the ascarids through multiple enterotomies. The prognosis is guarded if surgery has to be performed. The owner should be advised that other young horses on the premises should be treated with anthelmintics that have lower efficacy against ascarids, such as fenbendazole. These initial treatments can then be followed with more efficacious compounds.

Proximal Enteritis-jejunitis: This poorly understood disease affects the proximal portion of the small intestine and has various names including proximal enteritis-jejunitis, anterior enteritis, and duodenitis-jejunitis. The condition initially was recognized in the southeastern USA but has been reported to occur in the northeastern USA, England, and on the European continent. The cause is unknown. The affected intestine contains lesions varying from hyperemia to necrosis and infiltration of the submucosa with inflammatory cells. Often, there is edema and hemorrhage in the various layers of the intestinal wall.

Varying degrees of abdominal pain, ranging from mild to severe, are characteristic. When the prevalence of the condition peaked in the 1980s, it was characterized by voluminous amounts of gastric reflux, progression from pain to depression, and moderate to severe distention of the small intestine on rectal examination. In addition, the distended duodenum often was palpated as it coursed around the base of the cecum. The peritoneal fluid often contained an increased concentration of protein (>3 g/dL) with a normal number of WBC, but this finding did not consistently distinguish the condition from other causes of small-intestinal disease. Based on anecdotal reports, the prevalence and clinical severity of the condition have decreased in the past decade, at least in regions of the country where the condition characteristically had a more severe course and was accompanied by a high incidence of laminitis.

Treatment may be either medical or surgical. Medical treatment includes continued gastric decompression until the gastric reflux abates, IV fluids, and analgesics, as required. Many clinicians administer penicillin and low doses of flunixin meglumine; some also administer neostigmine, lidocaine, or metoclopramide to stimulate small-intestinal motility. Some surgeons, particularly in the UK, believe exploratory laparotomy and intestinal decompression result in a more rapid recovery. The survival rate associated with proximal enteritis-jejunitis is reported to be 44%.

The feet should receive particular attention because acute laminitis has been reported as a common complication; the prevalence of acute laminitis in horses with proximal enteritis-jejunitis has been reported to be ~25%.

Intussusception: Most intussusceptions that develop in horses are jejuno-jejunal, ileal-ileal, or ileocecal. The length of intestine that has become invaginated (the intussusceptum) into the more distal segment of intestine (the intussuscipiens) may range from a few centimeters to as much as a meter. Although the precise cause of most intussusceptions remains speculative, alterations in peristalsis due to enteritis, surgical trauma, parasite damage, anthelmintics, and *Anaplocephala perfoliata* infection have been suggested. Horses <3 yr old are affected most commonly.

Abdominal pain may be either acute due to complete obstruction of the intestinal lumen or chronic due to partial occlusion of the lumen. If the occlusion of the intestinal lumen is complete, the horse is acutely painful and has gastric reflux, and distended loops of small intestine are palpable per rectum. It may be possible to palpate the turgid intussusception, especially if the ileum is involved. Because the strangulated intussusceptum is contained within the intussuscipiens, the WBC count in the peritoneal fluid may not reflect the degree of intestinal damage.

Treatment requires surgery to reduce the intussusception, if possible, followed by resection and anastomosis. Due to the edema and hemorrhage in the wall of the affected intestine, it may be difficult to assess the viability of the bowel. Additionally, the damage to the intussusceptum may result in the development of adhesions. If the jejunum is involved, a jejuno-jejunal anastomosis must be performed. If the intussusception involves only the ileum, the affected intestine must be resected and a jejuno-cecal anastomosis performed. If the ileum has invaginated into the cecum, the terminal portion of the ileum should be transected close to the cecum and a jejuno-cecal anastomosis performed. The prognosis for survival is good if surgery is performed before the intussusception has become irreducible. The prognosis is fair to poor in the latter case due to the development of peritonitis, ileus, adhesions, and abscess formation.

Volvulus: A small-intestinal volvulus is seen when the intestine rotates on its mesenteric axis >180°. As the degree of the rotation increases, the vascular supply to the intestine is lost. Presumably because of its attachment to the cecum, the distal aspect of the volvulus is the ileum in most cases.

Horses with small-intestinal volvulus are acutely painful, and have an increased heart rate, a prolonged capillary refill time, and gastric reflux. Due to the loss of fluid into the intestine and stomach, these horses are dehydrated and have increased PCV and plasma protein concentrations. The horse's status may deteriorate rapidly due to hypovolemia and endotoxemia. Rectal examination generally reveals turgid distended loops of small intestine, and the peritoneal fluid contains increased numbers of WBC and protein.

Treatment involves surgical correction of the volvulus via a ventral midline celiotomy. If the intestine is nonviable, it must be resected and an anastomosis performed. The prognosis for survival depends on the duration of illness and amount of intestine that must be resected. Prognosis is good with early detection and surgery. Horses with a longer period of illness preoperatively, or postoperative ileus and peritonitis, are at increased risk for adhesion formation. It has been suggested that euthanasia is warranted if >50% of the length of the small intestine must be removed. However, results of an experimental study in ponies indicated that removal of 70% of the small intestine did not result in malabsorption provided the ponies were fed several (8) small pelleted meals each day.

Pedunculated Lipomas: Colic due to pedunculated lipomas is seen in horses >10 yr old. Pedunculated lipomas are suspended from the mesentery by a stalk or pedicle, which wraps around a segment of intestine, occluding the lumen of the intestine and interfering with its blood supply. The lipoma frequently forms a knot with the pedicle.

Clinical signs range from depression to severe abdominal pain, gastric reflux, and rapid deterioration in metabolic status. Distended loops of small intestine are palpable on rectal examination; the lipoma can also be felt per rectum in selected cases. The peritoneal fluid contains an increased number of WBC and RBC and an increased protein content.

Treatment requires transection of the pedicle and, if necessary, resection of the devitalized intestine. The prognosis depends on the time between onset of clinical signs and surgery. If surgery is performed early, the prognosis is good; however, if surgery is not performed until signs of cardiovascular deterioration are present, the prognosis for survival is fair to poor.

Internal Incarceration: The most common sites for internal incarcerations are mesenteric rents and the epiploic foramen. **Mesenteric rents** are defects in the small-intestinal mesentery. Problems develop when a segment of small intestine passes through the mesenteric defect, and the intestine becomes incarcerated. Because the intestine distends with fluid and blood, volvulus of the affected segment frequently occurs. Mesenteric rents are seen in horses of all ages.

The **epiploic foramen** is a natural opening bounded by the caudate lobe of the liver, the portal vein, and the caudal vena cava. The distal jejunum and ileum are the most common portions of the intestine that become incarcerated through the epiploic foramen. Although generally the intestine passes from right to left to enter the omental bursa, it may pass in the opposite direction pushing the omentum ahead of it. Although it has been reported that horses >7 yr old are affected most frequently, the results of recent studies indicate that the condition often develops in horses <7 yr old.

Clinical signs may be vague and similar to those of horses with proximal enteritis or pedunculated lipomas. The diagnosis may have to be made at surgery. Furthermore, in some cases, because of the position of the affected intestine within the omental bursa, the peritoneal fluid available for analysis may be normal.

Treatment of horses with either mesenteric rents or epiploic foramen entrapments is surgical. The affected segment of intestine must be exteriorized, its viability evaluated, and, if necessary, a resection and anastomosis performed. The prognosis for survival depends on the time between onset and surgery. If surgery is performed early in the course of the disease, the prognosis is good. However, because the clinical signs may be vague, the decision to perform surgery may be delayed, worsening the prognosis.

Inguinal Hernia: Inguinal hernias generally develop in stallions after breeding a mare, trauma, or a hard workout. Hernias appear to be most common in Tennessee Walking Horses, American Saddlebreds, and Standardbreds. In most cases, the hernia results in acute colic. The intestine descends through the vaginal ring in most cases and lies next to the testis and epididymis. Physical examination reveals a swollen testis that is firm and cool to the touch. If the hernia has occurred within hours, the intestine may be palpated in the inguinal canal. In this situation, an attempt may be made to reduce the hernia by pulling down on the testis to tighten the boundaries of the inguinal canal and then forcing the intestine up toward the vaginal ring. Once the incarcerated intestine, which frequently includes the ileum, has become edematous, it is not possible to reduce the hernia manually. Rectal examination will reveal distended loops of small intestine, with one of the loops tracing to the vaginal ring on the affected side. There will be gastric reflux, and the horse's condition will deteriorate rapidly. Peritoneal fluid generally reflects the degree of ischemia.

Surgery involves a ventral midline celiotomy and inguinal approach to reduce the hernia. Often, the testicle on the affected side must be removed, and the affected intestine resected. The prognosis for survival seems to be breed-dependent, with Standardbred horses having a good prognosis and Tennessee Walking Horses having a fair to poor prognosis. Presumably, this reflects the fact that many Tennessee Walking Horse stallions with inguinal hernias show little evidence of pain.

Cecum and Large Intestine

Impaction: The most common sites of impaction are the pelvic flexure region of the left colon, the junction of the right dorsal colon with the transverse colon, and the base and body of the cecum. The pelvic flexure and transverse colon regions are anatomically predisposed to obstruction because of the dramatic changes in size. The underlying reason for impaction of the cecum is unknown, although it has been speculated that cecal muscular activity is abnormal in affected horses. Other predisposing factors include feed that is too coarse, diseased or poorly managed teeth, and insufficient water intake. In one clinical study, Morgan, Arabian, and Appaloosa breeds were over-represented among horses with cecal impaction, and it has been proposed that the condition may develop secondary to infection with the tapeworm *Anoplocephala perfoliata*. Impactions also may develop secondary to other intestinal diseases and may be associated with prolonged hospitalization. Consequently, the fecal output of horses being treated for other abnormalities should be assessed on a routine basis. This is especially important in horses receiving NSAID on a daily basis.

Horses with simple impactions of the cecum or large colon exhibit mild intermittent signs of colic, and there is minimal evidence of systemic deterioration unless the impaction has a prolonged course. Generally, the heart rate is only slightly increased. Intestinal sounds are usually heard on auscultation of the abdomen and may be associated with the onset of pain as the affected portion of the intestine contracts against the obstruction. Diagnosis is made on rectal examination. Although the most common site of obstruction is considered to be the pelvic flexure region of the large colon, the impacted ingesta actually fills much or all of the left ventral colon. The impacted mass may be felt extending cranially in the abdomen, and the affected segment of bowel identified by palpating the longitudinal bands on the surface of the ventral colon. Impaction of the cecum is relatively easy to identify because the mass is situated in the right paralumbar region. The cecum can be definitively identified by palpating the taut ventral cecal band and the fat and blood vessels overlying the medial cecal band. Peritoneal fluid analysis may be normal, or the total protein concentration may be increased as the course becomes more prolonged.

Cecal impactions tend to be a primary cause of colic in horses >8 yr old. Alternatively, impactions may be seen in horses hospitalized for other reasons and are often associated with abrupt rupture of the cecum in these cases. Consequently, there is some controversy regarding the best method of treatment. Because medical therapy in some clinical studies has been unsuccessful in 50% of the cases, surgical removal of the impacting mass followed by an ileocolostomy has been strongly recommended. Other veterinarians report good results with aggressive medical therapy, particularly if abdominal pain associated with the cecal impaction was the primary reason the horse required veterinary attention.

Medical treatment of horses with cecal or large-colon impaction involves the administration of analgesics as necessary, large volumes of balanced IV fluids, and intragastric administration of either mineral oil or dioctyl sodium sulfosuccinate and water. Feed should be restricted until the impaction is relieved. Many veterinarians consider aggressive fluid therapy to be the mainstay of treatment. Balanced electrolyte solutions are administered to induce movement of fluid from the plasma into the lumen of the intestine. This form of treatment may require administration of >50 L of fluid/day to a 450-kg horse until the impaction is resolved. Recently, interest has increased in using enteral fluid therapy to treat horses with impactions, primarily because enteral fluid therapy is significantly less expensive than IV fluid therapy. The clinical results with enteral fluid therapy have been rewarding, and the results of experimental work in healthy horses have shown that enteral fluid therapy is more effective than IV fluid therapy in promoting hydration of colonic contents.

If the large-colon impaction fails to resolve with medical management, surgery can be performed. Generally, the impaction is approached via a ventral midline celiotomy, with the affected portion of the colon gently exteriorized and positioned on a sterile colon tray. An enterotomy then is made in the pelvic flexure and the contents of the colon removed.

Surgery for treatment of cecal impactions requires general anesthesia, a ventral midline celiotomy, isolation of the cecum from the celiotomy site, and removal of the contents of the cecum via an enterotomy. Because impactions have recurred after simple evacuation, the cecum is bypassed with an ileocolostomy.

The prognosis associated with impactions involving the large colon is excellent, with a survival rate of >95%. In contrast, the survival rate associated with cecal impactions remains 50-55%, which may reflect the poor prognosis associated with cecal impactions that develop in hospitalized horses.

In some geographic areas, the offending material may be sand, especially if there is an insufficient amount of pasture grass and the horses are fed on the ground. The sand accumulates in the right dorsal colon and transverse colon. Intermittent signs of abdominal pain may occur due to the weight of the sand in the intestine. More severe signs of pain occur when the impaction occludes the lumen of the transverse colon. Under such circumstances, the colon proximal to the obstruction distends with gas, and the horse may become extremely painful. It may not be possible to distinguish this condition from an intestinal displacement or volvulus. Sand also may be identified in the feces by mixing fecal material with water in a plastic rectal examination sleeve.

Treatment of sand impaction may be either medical or surgical. Medical treatment generally involves intragastric administration of psyllium (400 g/500 kg body wt, daily for 7 days) to purge the sand from the lumen. The psyllium flakes are added to 7.5 L of warm water and rapidly pumped into the stomach. These treatments are accompanied by analgesics as needed and IV fluids to promote movement of fluid into the intestinal lumen.

Surgery via a ventral midline celiotomy is necessary if the sand completely obstructs the lumen of the transverse colon. The left colon is exteriorized on a sterile colon tray, and the sand is removed via an enterotomy. The prognosis is usually good. Problems sometimes develop during surgery if the colon was damaged due to the extensive weight of the sand or while the sand is being removed from the intestine. *See also* p 240.

Enterolithiasis: Enteroliths are concretions composed of magnesium ammonium phosphate crystals around a nidus (eg, wire, stone, nail). Enteroliths may be seen singly or in groups and are commonly found in horses in certain parts of the USA, including California, the southwest, Indiana, and Florida. Enterolithiasis commonly affects Arabian horses, but the fact that these horses are extremely popular in the aforementioned areas confounds the question regarding breed association. Most horses with enteroliths are ~10 yr old; enterolithiasis rarely is seen in horses <4 yr old. Although not all factors that contribute to the formation of enteroliths have been identified, the results of recent clinical studies indicate that large colon contents from horses with enteroliths have higher mineral (magnesium, calcium, and phosphorus) concentrations and pH than contents from horses with colic not due to enteroliths. A common factor associated with enterolithiasis is the consumption of alfalfa hay, which results in a higher pH and increased concentrations of calcium, magnesium, and sulfur in the large colon.

Many horses with enterolithiasis have a history of recurring colic, presumably indicating that the enterolith(s) had caused partial or temporary obstruction of the colonic lumen. If the enterolith becomes lodged at the origin of the transverse colon, the colon proximal to the obstruction distends with gas and the pain is severe. Distention of the abdomen may be marked. Heart and respiratory rates are increased, and the mucous membranes may be pale or pink. Generally, colonic and cecal distention is evident on rectal examination, but the mass rarely is palpable because the transverse colon is cranial to the cranial mesenteric artery. Analysis of the peritoneal fluid is usually within normal limits unless ischemia of the colonic wall has developed over the enterolith. In areas where the problem is endemic, radiography may be used to identify the enteroliths.

Treatment involves surgery via a ventral midline celiotomy to decompress the colon and cecum and then to remove the stone(s). The left portion of the large colon is exteriorized and positioned on a sterile colon tray, the ingesta removed via an enterotomy, and then the enterolith(s) removed. If the stone has a flat side or a polyhedral shape, the rest of the large and small colons must be thoroughly checked for other stones. The prognosis is excellent, with practices in endemic areas reporting survival rates of 95%.

Left Dorsal Displacement: Left dorsal displacement of the colon is seen when either the pelvic flexure or the entire left colon becomes displaced over the renosplenic ligament. Because the renosplenic ligament is not attached to the most dorsal aspect of the spleen, a natural cleft exists between the spleen and left kidney. Although all ages and sexes of horses are affected equally, results of a clinical study indicate that the displacement is common in young horses.

Because left dorsal displacement results in simple obstruction of the colon at the point where it hangs across the ligament, the condition usually is associated with moderate abdominal pain or a prolonged course of intermittent painful episodes. The mucous membranes remain normal, and the heart rate is increased only slightly. The diagnosis usually is made on rectal examination (palpating the pelvic flexure over the ligament, palpating the bands of the left ventral colon running dorsocranially to the left kidney, and detecting that the spleen is displaced toward the middle of the abdomen). The condition also may be identified using ultrasonography. A paracentesis may yield blood if the spleen is displaced toward the midline.

Four forms of treatment have been used: 1) withholding feed to determine whether evacuation of the intestinal contents will allow the colon to return to its normal position, 2) rolling the horse to dislodge the colon from the ligament, 3) administering phenylephrine and/or jogging the horse to cause splenic contraction and correction of the displacement, or 4) performing surgery to return the colon to its correct position. The rolling procedure involves short-term anesthesia (generally xylazine or detomidine and ketamine), elevation of the horse's hindlimbs, and rolling the horse 360°. Surgery is performed via a ventral midline celiotomy. The advantage of surgery is that the viability of the colon can be assessed. Overall, the prognosis is good, with most studies reporting survival rates >80%.

Right Dorsal Displacement: The left colons move laterally around the base of the cecum to lie between the cecum and the right body wall. With the most common form of this displacement, the pelvic flexure ends up positioned near the diaphragm. In many instances, the displacement may be complicated by twisting of the colon near the base of the cecum. Although there may be some interference with venous drainage from the affected colon, usually the arterial supply remains intact.

Most horses with right dorsal displacements exhibit moderate degrees of pain, and there is slow development of systemic deterioration. In some cases, however, the pain may be severe. Rectal examination may reveal the taenia of the colon running transversely across the pelvic inlet. It may not be possible to palpate the ventral cecal band on rectal examination. Some horses with this condition have gastric reflux, presumably due to occlusion of the lumen of the duodenum.

Some horses with this condition appear to be stable and may show intermittent signs consistent with mild abdominal pain. Treatment may be conservative, involving attention to fluid needs and administration of mild analgesics. For painful horses, however, surgery must be performed to locate the pelvic flexure, to exteriorize and decompress the left portion of the colon, if possible, and then to relocate the colon to its normal position by rotating it around the cecal base. The twisting of the colon must be identified and corrected. The prognosis for survival is good, provided that the colonic wall is not damaged during surgery.

Right Dorsal Colitis: Right dorsal colitis has been recognized with increasing regularity in the past decade, particularly in, but not limited to, horses receiving excessive amounts of NSAID. Because the condition has been identified in horses receiving recommended doses of these drugs, it appears that some horses are particularly sensitive to their toxic effects. The drug most commonly associated with right dorsal colitis is phenylbutazone, but this may reflect the common and often chronic use of this drug. The most common lesions reported in horses with right dorsal colitis are ulceration and thickening and/or fibrosis of the wall of the right dorsal colon.

Horses commonly present with abdominal pain, anorexia, and lethargy. In many cases, the signs are consistent with severe abdominal pain, fever, endotoxemia, and diarrhea. Horses with the more chronic form of the disease present with intermittent abdominal pain, weight loss, lethargy, and anorexia. In most cases, hypoproteinemia is a common finding on hematology, and may account for ventral edema in some horses with the chronic form of the disease. The diagnosis is usually based on the history, clinical signs, and hematologic findings. In some cases, ultrasonographic evaluation of the colon via the twelfth to fifteenth intercostal spaces may provide evidence of marked thickening of the colonic wall.

Treatment of affected horses includes discontinuation of NSAID, rest, and a change in diet to a complete pelleted feed that contains ≥30% dietary fiber. Some clinicians recommend the feeding of many small meals daily, many recommend the inclusion of psyllium to promote mucosal healing, and some administer sucralfate or metronidazole. Horses with uncontrollable pain may require surgery to resect or bypass the affected portion of the right dorsal colon. The prognosis for horses with right dorsal colitis is guarded.

Volvulus of the Large Colon: Although the term "torsion" has been used for years to indicate that the colon has twisted on itself, the involvement of the mesentery between the ventral and dorsal colons indicates that the condition is a volvulus. When viewed from the most common site of the volvulus (the junction between the right ventral colon and the cecum), the volvulus most often occurs in a clockwise direction; the cecum may or may not be involved. If the volvulus is <270°, there may be obstruction of the bowel lumen without ischemia. If the volvulus is >360°, there is strangulating obstruction of the entire left colon.

The onset of colic is sudden, and the degree of pain may be mild to moderate if the volvulus results only in obstruction of the intestinal lumen. When the twist is more extensive, the pain is severe and the horse may fail to respond to analgesics. The colon is extremely enlarged, and the mesentery between the dorsal and ventral colons is edematous on rectal examination. The heart rate is rapid, the horse's condition deteriorates rapidly, and there is poor peripheral perfusion. Distention of the abdomen usually is marked. Generally, results of peritoneal fluid analysis and the degree of colonic involvement are poorly correlated.

Although the cause of colonic volvulus remains unknown, it is presumed to be associated with a disproportionate amount of gas in the colon. On broodmare farms, the condition frequently is associated with recent (within 90 days) or impending parturition, a grass diet, or highly fermentable feeds. The presence of a foal at the mare's side (recent history of parturition) is an additional risk factor.

Treatment of colonic volvulus requires surgery to correct the volvulus and remove affected bowel, if necessary. Although the technique for removal of 90% of the colon has been perfected in healthy horses, extreme difficulty can be encountered if the colon is edematous. Because the recurrence rate has been estimated to be as high as 20% in some clinical studies, colopexy procedures have been devised to reduce the recurrence of the condition in broodmares. Although the results of a study involving several university hospitals reported a 27% survival rate, survival rates >85% are common for practices situated near broodmare farms.

Impaction and Foreign Body Obstruction of the Descending Colon: Abnormalities involving the descending (small) colon are infrequent, accounting for <5% of conditions characterized by colic in one study. The more common causes include meconium retention, impaction, and foreign body obstruction. Meconium retention is seen in newborn male foals within the first 24 hr of life. Affected foals swish their tails from side to side, strain to defecate, and roll. The diagnosis is made by careful digital examination. Treatment involves gentle administration of a warm, soapy water enema. The prognosis is excellent.

Impaction of the descending colon is seen in ponies, miniature horses, and adult horses with limited access to drinking water or with other causes of intestinal stasis. Most recently, the condition has been associated with salmonellosis, although a cause and effect relationship has not been proved. Pain may be severe if the obstruction is complete. In such cases, tympany of the colon occurs secondarily, and ileus results. The diagnosis is made in adult horses by palpating the obstructing mass in the ventral portion of the abdomen on rectal examination. Foreign body obstruction of the descending colon must be considered if the horse is <3 yr old; the offending material may be rubber fencing, nylon fibers from halters or lead shanks, hay net, or feed sacks. Horses with impactions may be treated medically with analgesics, IV fluids, and gentle enemas. Often, however, surgery is required to evacuate the colon due to severity of pain and gas distention. The prognosis associated with impaction of the descending colon is fair unless it is complicated by severe colitis after the obstruction has been removed. The prognosis is good.

INTESTINAL DISEASES IN RUMINANTS

INTESTINAL DISEASES IN CATTLE

Determination of the cause of intestinal disease in cattle is based on clinical, epidemiologic, and laboratory findings. Nonspecific therapy includes replacement of fluid and electrolytes. An overview is given below; specific therapy and prevention are detailed under the individual disease headings. Intestinal diseases of neonates are discussed separately, although some of the causes also affect older animals.

Bovine Viral Diarrhea and Mucosal Disease Complex

Bovine viral diarrhea (BVD) is most common in young cattle (6-24 mo old) and generally is accompanied by typical mucosal lesions; it must be distinguished from other viral diseases that produce diarrhea and mucosal lesions. These include malignant catarrhal fever (p 609), which usually is a sporadic disease in more mature cattle, and rinderpest (p 619), which can be seen in outbreak form but is exotic in most countries.

Bovine viral diarrhea virus (BVDV), the causal agent of BVD and mucosal disease complex, is classified in the genus Pestivirus in the family Flaviviridae. Although cattle are the primary host for BVDV, several reports suggest most even-toed ungulates are also susceptible. Isolates of BVDV are separated into noncytopathic and cytopathic biotypes based on cytopathic effects observed in infected cell cultures. Noncytopathic BVDV are the predominant viral biotype in nature. Cytopathic BVDV are relatively rare and arise in cattle that are persistently infected with noncytopathic BVDV. The switch in viral biotype is triggered by mutations that often involve recombination of noncytopathic viral RNA with itself, with heterologous viral RNA, or with host cell RNA. Based on viral RNA sequence, there are at least 2 viral genotypes of BVDV that can be further divided into subgenotypes. The viral genotypes are termed BVDV type 1 and BVDV type 2, and both cytopathic and noncytopathic BVDV are represented in each viral genotype. Although the viral genotypes are antigenically related, serologic assays can separate BVDV type 1 from BVDV type 2.

Etiology and Epidemiology: Serologic surveys indicate that BVDV is distributed worldwide. The prevalence of antiviral antibody in cattle varies among countries and may vary between geographic regions within a country. Prevalence of antiviral antibody may be >90% if vaccination is practiced commonly in a geographic region. Although cattle of all ages are susceptible, most cases of overt clinical disease are seen in cattle that are between 6 mo and 2 yr of age.

Cattle that are persistently infected with noncytopathic BVDV serve as a natural reservoir for virus. Persistent infection develops when noncytopathic BVDV is transmitted transplacentally during the first 4 mo of fetal development. The calf is born infected with virus, remains infected for life, and usually is immunotolerant to the resident noncytopathic virus. Transplacental infection that occurs later in gestation results in abortion, congenital malformations, or birth of normal calves that have antibody against BVDV. The prevalence of persistent infection varies among countries and between regions within a country. In some areas, the prevalence of persistent infection in calves may be as high as 1-2% of cattle <1 yr of age. On a given farm, persistently infected cattle are often found in cohorts of animals that are approximately the same age. Persistently infected cattle can shed large amounts of BVDV in their secretions and excretions and readily transmit virus to susceptible herdmates. Clinical disease and reproductive failure often are seen after healthy cattle come in contact with a persistently infected animal.

Biting insects, fomites, semen, biologic products, and possibly wild ruminants also can spread BVDV.

Clinical Findings and Lesions: Disease induced by BVDV varies in severity, duration, and organ systems involved. Acute disease results from infection of susceptible cattle with either noncytopathic or cytopathic BVDV. Acute BVD, also termed transient BVD, often is an inapparent to mild disease of high morbidity and low mortality. Biphasic fever (~104°F [40°C]), depression, decreased milk production, transient inappetence, rapid respiration, excessive nasal secretion, excessive lacrimation, and diarrhea are typical signs of acute BVD. Clinical signs of disease usually are seen 6-12 days after infection and last 1-3 days. Transient leukopenia may be seen with onset of signs of disease. Recovery is rapid and coincides with production of viral neutralizing antibody. Gross lesions seldom are seen in cases of mild disease. Lymphoid tissue is a primary target for replication of BVDV, which may lead to immunosuppression and enhanced severity of intercurrent infections.

Some isolates of BVDV induce clinically severe disease that manifests as high fever (~107°F [41-42°C]), oral ulcerations, eruptive lesions of the coronary band and interdigital cleft, diarrhea, dehydration, leukopenia, and thrombocytopenia. In thrombocytopenic cattle, petechial hemorrhages may be seen in the conjunctiva, sclera, nictitating membrane of the eyes; and on mucosal surfaces of the mouth and vulva. Prolonged bleeding from injection sites also occurs. Swollen lymph nodes, erosions and ulcerations of the GI tract, petechial and ecchymotic hemorrhages on the serosal surfaces of the viscera, and extensive lymphoid depletion are associated with severe forms of acute BVD. The duration of overt disease may be 3-7 days. High morbidity with moderate mortality is common. Severity of acute BVD is related to the virulence of the viral strain infecting the animal and does not depend on viral biotype or genotype.

In pregnant cattle, BVDV may cross the placental barrier and infect the fetus. The consequences of fetal infection usually are seen several weeks to months after infection of the dam and depend on the stage of fetal development and on the strain of BVDV. Infection of the dam near the time of fertilization may result in reduced conception rates. Infection during the first 4 mo of fetal development may lead to embryonic resorption, abortion, growth retardation, or persistent infection. Congenital malformations of the eye and CNS result from fetal infections that occur between months 4-6 of development. Fetal mummification, premature birth, stillbirth, and birth of weak calves also are seen after fetal infection.

Persistent infection is an important sequela of fetal infection with noncytopathic BVDV. Persistently infected calves may appear healthy and normal in size, or they may show stunted growth and be prone to respiratory or enteric ailments. They often have a short lifespan, and death before 2 yr of age is common. Persistently infected cows give birth to persistently infected calves, but most calves sired by a persistently infected bull will not be infected with virus in utero. Lesions attributable to BVDV often are not seen in persistently infected cattle at necropsy. Antibody against BVD seldom is detected in persistently infected cattle in the absence of vaccination or superinfection with an antigenically heterologous BVDV. Persistently infected cattle exposed to BVDV that is antigenically different from their resident noncytopathic virus can produce antiviral antibody. Therefore, screening for persistent infection using the viral neutralization test to identify animals that lack antiviral antibody may not detect some persistently infected cattle.

Mucosal disease is a highly fatal form of BVD that may be acute or chronic and is seen infrequently in persistently infected cattle. Mucosal disease is induced when persistently infected cattle become superinfected with cytopathic BVDV. The origin of the cytopathic BVDV is usually internal, resulting from a mutation of the resident persistent, noncytopathic BVDV. In those cases, the cytopathic virus is antigenically similar to the resident noncytopathic virus. External origins for cytopathic BVDV include other cattle and modified live virus vaccines. Cattle that develop mucosal disease due to exposure to a cytopathic virus of external origin often produce antiviral antibody. Prevalence of persistent infection usually is low, and many persistently infected cattle do not develop mucosal disease, regardless of exposure. Acute mucosal disease is characterized by fever, leukopenia, dysenteric diarrhea, inappetence, dehydration, erosive lesions of the nares and mouth, and death within a few days of onset. At necropsy, erosions and ulcerations may be found throughout the GI tract. The mucosa over Peyer's patches may be hemorrhagic and necrotic. Extensive necrosis of lymphoid tissues, especially gut-associated lymphoid tissue, is seen on microscopic examination.

Clinical signs of chronic mucosal disease may last several weeks to months and are less severe than those of acute mucosal disease. Intermittent diarrhea and gradual wasting are common. Coronitis and eruptive lesions on the skin of the interdigital cleft cause lameness in some cattle. Lesions found at necropsy are less pronounced than, but similar to, those seen in acute mucosal disease. Often, the only gross lesions seen are focal ulcerations in the mucosa of the cecum, proximal colon, or rectum, and the mucosa over, Peyer's patches of the small intestine may appear sunken.

Diagnosis: BVD is diagnosed tentatively from disease history, clinical signs, and gross and microscopic lesions. Diagnostic laboratory support is required when clinical signs and gross lesions are minimal. Laboratory support also is required in some outbreaks of mucosal disease or clinically severe acute BVD because either disease may appear similar to rinderpest (p 619) or malignant catarrhal fever (p 609).

Laboratory tests for BVDV include virus isolation and assays that detect antibody in serum or detect viral RNA or viral antigen in clinical specimens and tissues. Because antibody against BVDV is prevalent in most cattle populations, a single serologic test is seldom sufficient for diagnosis. A >4-fold increase in antibody titer in paired serum samples obtained 2 more weeks apart is necessary to verify recent infection. Isolation of BVDV from blood, nasal swab specimens, or tissues confirms active infection. Identification of persistent infection requires detection of virus in clinical specimens obtained at least 3 wk apart. At necropsy, tissues of choice for viral isolation include spleen, lymph node, and ulcerated segments of the GI tract.

Alternatives to viral isolation include antigen-capture ELISA from blood or serum, immunohistochemistry to detect viral protein in frozen or fixed tissues, PCR to detect viral RNA in clinical specimens, and PCR or in situ hybridization to detect viral RNA in fresh or fixed tissues. Differentiation of viral genotypes usually is done by PCR or PCR followed by nucleic acid sequencing. Monoclonal antibody binding assays and nucleic acid hybridization assays also differentiate viral genotypes.

Treatment and Control: Treatment of BVD is limited primarily to supportive therapy. Control is based on sound management practices that include use of biosecurity measures, elimination of persistently infected cattle, and vaccination. Replacement cattle should be tested for persistent infection before entry into the herd. Quarantine or physical separation of replacement cattle from the resident herd for 2-4 wk should be considered, and vaccination of replacement cattle for BVD should be done before commingling with the resident herd. Embryo donors and recipients also should be tested for persistent infection. If vaccination of embryo donors or recipients is warranted, it should be done at least 1 estrous cycle before embryo transfer is performed. Because BVDV is shed into semen, breeding bulls should be tested for persistent infection before use. Artificial insemination should be done only with semen obtained from bulls free of persistent infection.

Screening cattle herds for persistent infection is done by virus isolation from serum or buffy coat cells, antigen-capture ELISA from serum or buffy coat, or antigen detection in skin biopsies. Several strategies, based on herd size, type of herd being screened, financial limitations of the herd owner, and testing ability of the diagnostic laboratory being used, are available to screen herds for persistent infection. When identified, persistently infected cattle should be sold for slaughter as soon as possible.

Inactivated and modified live virus vaccines are available. They contain a variety of strains of BVDV representing both viral biotypes and viral genotypes 1 and 2. Antigenic diversity among BVDV may affect the efficacy of a given vaccine if the vaccine virus or viruses differ significantly from the challenge virus. Proper and safe immunization of cattle with either inactivated or modified live virus vaccines requires adherence to the manufacturer's instructions. Because BVDV is fetotropic and may be immunosuppressive, use of modified live virus vaccines is not recommended in cattle that are pregnant or showing signs of disease. Inactivated viral vaccines may be used in pregnant cattle. Protection conferred by inactivated vaccines may be of short duration, and frequent vaccination may be necessary to prevent disease or reproductive failure. Colostral antibody confers partial to complete protection against disease in most calves for 3-6 mo after birth. Vaccination of neonatal cattle that have acquired colostral antibody may not stimulate a protective immune response, and revaccination at 5-9 mo of age may be necessary.

Winter Dysentery

Winter dysentery is an acute, highly contagious GI disorder that affects housed adult dairy cattle, primarily during winter. Clinical features include explosive diarrhea (sometimes accompanied by dysentery), a profound drop in milk production, variable anorexia and depression, and mild respiratory signs such as coughing. The disease has a high morbidity but low mortality, and spontaneous recovery within a few days is typical.

Etiology: The precise etiology of winter dysentery is unclear. In recent years, a bovine coronavirus (BCV), closely related to the virus that causes diarrhea in neonatal calves, has been implicated as the etiologic agent. Evidence for BCV as the cause of winter dysentery includes the following: 1) clinical signs and pathologic findings are consistent with disease induced by BCV, 2) seroconversion to BCV has been demonstrated in affected cattle, 3) the virus is frequently isolated from diarrheic feces of cattle exhibiting clinical signs of winter dysentery, and 4) the disease has been reproduced by briefly exposing BCV seronegative, lactating cows to a calf experimentally infected with feces from cows with winter dysentery. Despite this evidence, it has not been possible to consistently reproduce winter dysentery through oral inoculation of adult cattle with BCV. Concurrent risk factors, such as changes in diet, cold temperatures, and presence of other microorganisms, may be required before BCV will cause clinical disease in adult cattle. Agents previously suggested as causes of winter dysentery include *Campylobacter jejuni*, bovine parvovirus, enteroviruses, infectious bovine rhinotracheitis virus, and bovine viral diarrhea virus.

Transmission, Epidemiology, and Pathogenesis: BCV is transmitted via the fecal-oral route through ingestion of feed or water contaminated with feces from clinical cases or clinically normal carrier animals. Viral particles present in respiratory secretions of affected animals may further enhance transmission. Transmission of disease is promoted by close confinement. Winter dysentery is highly contagious and easily introduced to barns by visitors, carrier animals, and fomites. Winter dysentery is common in northern climates where animals are housed indoors for extended periods during the winter months. It is seen frequently in the northern USA, Canada, the UK, Europe, Australia, New Zealand, Israel, and Japan. Coronaviruses survive best at low temperatures and at low ultraviolet light intensities, which can lead to a buildup of virus in the environment during the colder months. Adult lactating cows that have recently calved are most severely affected, but the disease can affect younger or older animals and males. Mortality rates associated with winter dysentery are generally low (1-2%), but morbidity in affected herds is high, with 20-50% of the animals in a herd exhibiting clinical signs within a few days and close to 100% of animals in the herd exhibiting signs within a week. Some degree of immunity to winter dysentery appears to develop because recurrences, if seen in the same herd, are noted at 1- to 5-yr intervals.

Inflammatory mediators that cause hypersecretion in the small intestine and colon are thought to contribute to the voluminous diarrhea seen in cattle with winter dysentery. In addition, destruction of epithelial cells in the colonic crypts results in transudation of extracellular fluid and blood, explaining the hemorrhagic nature of the diarrhea in some cases.

Clinical Findings: The clinical syndrome is characterized by an acute onset of fluid diarrhea and a profound decrease in milk production (25-95% production loss). Feces are liquid and homogenous with little odor, dark green to black, and rarely contain blood or mucus. A sweet, musty, unpleasant odor is reported in barns with large numbers of affected cattle. Nasolacrimal discharge or cough may accompany or precede the diarrhea. Other signs include mild colic, dehydration, depression, a brief period of anorexia, and some decrease in body condition. Occasionally, animals exhibit more severe signs such as passage of feces with variable amounts of blood, severe dehydration, and weakness. Fatalities are rare. Diarrhea in individual animals has a short course, and feces return to normal in 2-3 days in most animals. Disease in the herd typically subsides in 1-2 wk, but milk production may take weeks to months to return to normal.

Lesions: The small intestine may be dilated and flaccid. Lesions are primarily seen in the large intestine and consist of cecal and colonic mucosal hyperemia, linear streaks or pinpoint-sized hemorrhages mostly along the colonic mucosal ridges, and blood in the lumen of the large intestine. Histologic findings may include widespread degeneration and necrosis of colonic glandular epithelium.

Diagnosis: A diagnosis can be confirmed by demonstrating coronaviral particles in fecal samples via ELISA or electron microscopy. Seroconversion to coronavirus in acute and convalescent serum samples, taken 8 wk apart, also aids in confirming a diagnosis of winter dysentery.

Differential diagnoses for acute diarrhea in adult cattle include bovine viral diarrhea (BVD), coccidiosis, and enteric salmonellosis. These diseases can be ruled out by absence of mucosal lesions (BVD), negative fecal cultures (*Salmonella* spp), and negative fecal flotation (coccidiosis), as well as by the characteristic clinical presentation of winter dysentery (rapid onset of diarrheal disease of short duration in a herd with high morbidity but low mortality).

Treatment and Control: Most affected cattle recover spontaneously. Fresh water, palatable feed, and free-choice salt should be available at all times. The use of astringents, protectants, and adsorbents is controversial. IV fluid therapy or blood transfusions may be required in severely affected cattle.

There is no vaccine for winter dysentery. Isolation of newly introduced cattle for 2 wk and isolation of any adult cow with diarrhea is advised to decrease the likelihood of disease introduction into a herd. In an outbreak, access to the premises should be restricted, and all persons in contact with affected cattle should ensure that their footwear and clothing are clean before leaving an affected farm.

Other Intestinal Diseases of Cattle

Infection with *Salmonella* spp (p 156) can produce diarrhea in animals of all ages, especially those that are stressed, closely stocked, or exposed to a heavily contaminated feed or water supply. In older animals, the disease is manifest by dysentery and toxemia, and mortality can be significant.

Rotavirus and coronavirus occasionally cause outbreaks of diarrhea in suckling calves 2-3 mo old. The feces are voluminous and may contain mucus. Toxemia is not evident and mortality is negligible, but growth is decreased. *See also* DIARRHEA IN NEONATAL RUMINANTS, p 228.

Necrotic enteritis of unknown etiology is seen in beef cattle 5-12 wk old, commonly affecting several calves within the herd. There is sudden onset of fever, depression, and profuse diarrhea. The feces are initially dark green, contain blood, and frequently stain the perineum. Circular erosions may be present in the oral mucosa. A proportion of calves recover after a clinical course of 3-5 days. The clinical course is longer in fatal cases; animals have scant mucohemorrhagic feces that are passed with tenesmus and develop a severe nonregenerative leukopenia. A secondary fibrinous bronchopneumonia may develop. Mortality is high despite intensive antibiotic treatment. At necropsy, there is ulcerative necrosis of the terminal small intestine and the large intestine.

Coccidiosis (p 163) usually is seen in cattle <1 yr old, especially in situations of heavy stocking density and overgrazing. It is characterized by dysentery and tenesmus and may be accompanied by nervous signs. Intestinal helminthiasis, particularly ostertagiasis (p 258), is seen in cattle of the same age group. Type I ostertagiasis is seen in cattle on pasture, but Type II ostertagiasis may be seen in housed animals.

Explosive outbreaks of diarrhea in mature cattle are associated most commonly with winter dysentery (p 223) but also with salmonellosis when there is heavy contamination of feed or water.

Chronic diarrhea with unthriftiness and wasting, seen as a sporadic disease, most commonly is associated with paratuberculosis (p 612) but also may be caused by chronic salmonellosis and chronic BVD infections. Diarrhea with wasting also may be seen in cattle with congestive heart failure, uremia, or chronic peritonitis. Persistent diarrhea with unthriftiness, and occasionally wasting in yearling and mature cattle, can be associated with a secondary copper deficiency due to excess molybdenum in the pastures. Diarrhea may also accompany selenium-responsive ill-thrift syndromes in growing cattle.

Individual cases or outbreaks of diarrhea may be associated with dietary indiscretions. Diarrhea may follow cases of simple indigestion and is common in rumen overload (p 178). It also follows ingestion of toxic amounts of chemicals (eg, arsenic, copper, zinc, and molybdenum) or certain poisonous plants and mycotoxicoses; dipyridyl and organophosphate poisoning can also cause diarrhea.

Cattle may also harbor organisms such as *Escherichia coli* O157:H7, *Yersinia enterocolitica*, and *Campylobacter jejuni* in the intestine; although these are rarely associated with clinical disease in cows, fecal contamination of milk may lead to outbreaks of gastroenteritis in people who consume unpasteurized milk or cheese products. Retail meat products can also be infected if there has been fecal contamination of the carcass at slaughter.

Intestinal adenocarcinoma, commonly seen in association with bovine enzootic hematuria, is believed to result from the interaction of a carcinogen (ptaquiloside) in bracken fern (*Pteridium* spp, p 2349) and papilloma virus.

Jejunal hemorrhage syndrome has emerged as an important disease in dairy cattle in North America in recent years and is believed by some to be caused by toxins of *Clostridium perfringens* type A. It is manifest by sudden onset of abdominal pain, shock, sternal recumbency, rapid death, and a segmental hemorrhagic enteritis in the upper small intestine.

Intestinal obstructions are seen sporadically (*see also* p 200). Cecal dilatation and volvulus are seen predominantly in adult cattle in the postparturient period. Intussusception occurring at the distal jejunum or proximal ileum is the most common cause of complete obstruction in both adult cattle and calves. Ileocecocolic, cecocolic, and colonic intussusceptions are seen less frequently in calves and not at all in adult cattle due to the greater strength of the ileocecal ligament and the presence of mesenteric fat, which stabilize this region of the bowel in older cattle. Intestinal volvulus and volvulus around the mesenteric root are seen sporadically at all ages. Rarely, intestinal obstruction is caused by incarceration and entrapment of the small intestine by persistent urachal or umbilical remnants, by obstruction of the small intestine or descending colon by phytobezoars and enteroliths, or by compression from fat necrosis or lipoma. Intestinal obstruction can also be caused by congenital disease (p 131), most commonly by atresia coli (which is seen both sporadically and in clusters on a farm and may be caused by rectal palpation of the amniotic vesicle at 35 and 41 days of pregnancy) but also by atresia ani (which may be accompanied by urogenital defects and defects of the tail).

INTESTINAL DISEASES IN SHEEP AND GOATS

The causes and circumstances of diarrhea in neonatal lambs and kids are similar to those in newborn calves. Intensive lambing practices and shed-lambing increase the potential for disease and buildup of infectious agents and can be associated with serious outbreaks of diarrhea. The serotypes of enteropathogenic *Escherichia coli* that cause secretory diarrhea in calves also do so in lambs, and the approach to diagnosis, treatment, and control is similar. Similarly, rotavirus, coronavirus, and cryptosporidia (p 168) also cause outbreaks of diarrhea in lambs. *See also* DIARRHEA IN NEONATAL RUMINANTS, p 228. Lamb dysentery caused by *Clostridium perfringens* type B (p 493) is a distinct intestinal disease of lambs in the first week of life. It is seen principally in hill breeds of sheep in the UK and is characterized by sudden death or diarrhea, dysentery, and toxemia. In the USA, *C perfringens* type C causes a similar syndrome. Watery mouth or rattle belly (*see* below), a disease of uncertain etiology associated with low concentrations of circulating immunoglobulins, is seen predominantly in the UK. It also affects young lambs but is manifest by GI stasis. Coccidiosis (p 163) and GI helminthiasis (p 262), except for haemonchosis, are important causes of diarrhea in older nursing and weaned sheep. Terminal ileitis and villous atrophy, both of unknown etiology, are often present in the intestine of lambs culled because of poor growth.

GI helminthiasis is the most common cause of diarrhea in pastured sheep. Coccidiosis develops in association with overstocking or intensive indoor housing and poor sanitation. Salmonellosis (p 156) can cause diarrhea in all ages; the circumstances in young lambs are similar to those in calves. It also can cause outbreaks of diarrhea late in pregnancy and is frequently accompanied by abortion. Salmonellosis is more common when sheep or goats are congregated intensively or stressed, particularly by shipping. *Yersinia pseudotuberculosis* and *Y enterocolitica* have both been associated with enterocolitis and diarrhea in young sheep at pasture that are debilitated from factors such as starvation and cold weather. Diarrhea may be present in bluetongue in sheep (p 590) and is accompanied by typical mucosal lesions. In goats, diarrhea is often prominent in enterotoxemia associated with *C perfringens* type D (p 493). This is not a feature of the clinical disease in sheep but may be present in flockmates of affected sheep. In feedlot sheep, diarrhea most commonly is associated with grain overload, salmonellosis, or coccidiosis.

Other intestinal diseases of adult sheep may manifest with diarrhea. Infection with *C perfringens* type C (struck, p 493) manifests with abdominal pain, tenesmus, and rapid death. Intestinal obstruction due to intestinal accidents occur sporadically but are usually not seen clinically. Sheep with paratuberculosis (p 612) usually show progressive emaciation without diarrhea. Progressive emaciation also is the primary sign in adult sheep with intestinal adenocarcinoma, which can be prevalent in certain areas, associated with ingestion of bracken fern (*see* p 2349).

WATERY MOUTH DISEASE IN LAMBS
(Slavery mouth, Slavers, Rattle belly)

Throughout the UK, watery mouth disease accounts for ~25% of all lamb deaths in indoor intensive lambing systems. It is not seen in extensively managed flocks. The disease develops quickly and affects predominantly lambs 12-72 hr old that have had inadequate or delayed access to colostrum. Morbidity in a flock can be as high as 30% and, if untreated, most affected lambs die. A similar syndrome has been reported in lambs in Spain and goat kids in France and Canada.

Etiology and Pathogenesis: Newborn lambs deprived of adequate colostrum because of sibling competition, weakness, poor mothering, or inadequate maternal supply are at greatest risk. The disease develops after ingestion of gram-negative bacteria, particularly *Escherichia coli*, from contaminated fleece or bedding. The strains of *E coli* involved do not possess the K99 antigen and are normally regarded as nonenteropathogenic and nonenterotoxigenic.

The unique digestive physiology of the newborn lamb and absence of gut or systemic antibodies allow ingested bacteria to survive and translocate from the gut to the bloodstream. The resultant bacteremia is initially tolerated by the lamb; however, bacteremias $>10^4$ colony-forming units/mL are associated with the release of free endotoxin, and endotoxic shock rapidly develops.

The newborn lamb is particularly vulnerable to disease resulting from ingestion of environmental bacteria for the following reasons. First, it is immunocompromised because it lacks circulating antibodies. Second, neutral conditions in the abomasum may allow viable bacteria to pass to the small intestine. Third, rapid multiplication of bacteria within the gut is enhanced by the normal depression in gut motility that occurs during the first 48 hr of life. Fourth, *E coli* are able to attach to receptors present on the intestinal epithelium and be absorbed into the systemic circulation. Intensive indoor lambing systems increase the degree of environmental bacterial contamination and, thus, the incidence of disease.

Watery mouth disease is more common in twins and triplets than in single lambs, particularly when born to ewes in poor body condition. Although male lambs are considered more prone to watery mouth disease than female lambs, controlled experiments have found no significant link between sex and susceptibility to disease; however, the stress caused by early castration may reduce the intake of colostrum by male lambs at a critical time and lead to a higher incidence of disease.

Clinical Findings: Affected lambs are dull, stop feeding and, classically, have long strings of saliva drooling from the mouth. Less obvious cases may have a wet muzzle; others may show no external signs of excess salivation, but the mouth may be cold to the touch and contain frothy saliva. Lacrimation may also be seen. As the disease progresses, lambs become hypothermic, gut motility is depressed or absent, and the abomasum may become distended and give the deceptive appearance of a well-fed lamb. If these lambs are lifted and shaken gently, accumulated liquid in the gas-filled stomach may make the noise associated with the alternative name of "rattle belly." Scours may be seen but is not a common finding.

Lesions: Necropsy may reveal an inflamed GI tract distended with fluid and gas, retained meconium, pale kidneys and muscle, a dehydrated carcass, and mesenteric lymph nodes that are enlarged and reactive.

Diagnosis: Diagnosis requires clinical examination in the early stages of disease before the secondary effects of starvation, toxemia, and abdominal tympany supervene. Biochemical and hematologic changes and necropsy findings in affected lambs are consistent with endotoxemia and the clinical diagnosis of endotoxic shock. Terminally, lambs develop leukopenia, severe hypoglycemia, lactic acidemia, and metabolic acidosis. Differential diagnoses include joint ill or navel ill, hypothermia, primary starvation, and infectious enteritis.

Treatment: There is no specific treatment. Affected lambs may be saved by providing parenteral antibiotics daily and a minimum of 50 mL of an electrolyte and 10% glucose solution containing a water-soluble, oral antibiotic preparation (neomycin and/or streptomycin) fed by stomach tube TID. If the lamb is not sucking, the volume of each feeding should be increased to 100-200 mL. Oral purgatives or enemas may help overcome gut stasis and expel the infecting bacteria. Treatment should be continued until the signs resolve and the lamb is sucking again. Boosting body temperature by external warming may also be required. However, such care is time-consuming and expensive and carries no guarantee of success.

Prevention: Prevention is the best option. Good management practices are important. Yards, pens, ewes, and equipment should be kept as clean as possible throughout lambing to help control the buildup of *E coli* and keep the incidence of disease low. Ewes should be well nourished to ensure a plentiful supply of colostrum, of which lambs should ingest a minimum of 50 mL/kg within 6 hr of birth. It may be necessary to supplement the lamb's colostrum intake with stored colostrum (ewe, cow, or goat) or commercial colostrum substitute. Lambs should not be castrated with rubber rings in the first 24 hr because this depresses colostrum intake. Lambs that obtain colostrum late or in small quantities remain at risk.

In controlled experiments, a single dose of oral antibiotic given within 2 hr of birth to colostrum-deprived lambs delivered into a contaminated indoor environment was as effective as ewe colostrum in preventing neonatal disease and death in all lambs up to 3 days old, despite the absence of maternal antibodies. Thus, antibiotic treatment can provide simple, quick, and inexpensive protection against watery mouth disease and is an attractive option for the busy sheep farmer. However, it is important that such treatment be targeted to lambs in the high-risk categories specified above because indiscriminate dosing may encourage antibiotic resistance. Additionally, all colostrum-deprived lambs born indoors become bacteremic within 4-8 hr of birth, indicating that antibiotic treatment should be timed to avoid the possibility of lysing bloodborne bacteria and precipitating endotoxic shock.

DIARRHEA IN NEONATAL RUMINANTS
(Scours)

Diarrhea is common in newborn calves, lambs, and kids. The acute disease is characterized by progressive dehydration and death, sometimes in as few as 12 hr. In the subacute form, diarrhea may persist for several days and result in malnutrition and emaciation. This discussion emphasizes the disease in calves, but the principles of pathophysiology and treatment apply to lambs and kids as well.

Etiology: Several enteropathogens are associated with neonatal diarrhea. Their relative prevalence varies geographically, but the most prevalent infections in most areas are *Escherichia coli*, rotavirus, coronavirus, and *Cryptosporidium parvum*. Cases of neonatal diarrhea are commonly associated with more than one of these agents, and the cause of most outbreaks is multifactorial. Determining the particular agents associated with an outbreak of diarrhea can be important because specific therapy is available for some. Also, some agents have zoonotic risk. Diarrhea is also present in septicemic colibacillosis.

Bacteria: *E coli* is the most important bacterial cause of diarrhea in calves; at least 2 distinct types of diarrheal disease are produced by different strains of this organism. One type is associated with enterotoxigenic *E coli*, which has 2 virulence factors associated with the production of diarrhea. Fimbrial antigens enable them to attach to and colonize the villi of the small intestine. Strains in calves most commonly possess K99 (F5) or F41 fimbrial antigens, or both. These antigens are the focus of immunologic protection. Enterotoxigenic *E coli* also elaborate a thermostable, nonantigenic enterotoxin (Sta) that influences intestinal ion and fluid secretion to produce a noninflammatory secretory diarrhea. Diarrhea in calves and lambs also has been associated with enteropathogenic *E coli* that adhere to the intestine to produce an attaching and effacing lesion, with dissolution of the brush border and loss of microvillous structure at the site of attachment, a decrease in enzyme activity, and changes in ion transport in the intestine. These enteropathogens are also called "attaching and effacing *E coli*." Some produce verotoxin, which may be associated with a more severe hemorrhagic diarrhea. The infection most frequently is in the cecum and colon, but the distal small intestine can also be affected. The damage in severe infections can result in edema and mucosal erosions and ulceration, leading to hemorrhage into the intestinal lumen.

Salmonella spp, especially *S typhimurium* and *S Dublin*, but occasionally other serovars, cause diarrhea in calves 2-12 wk old. Salmonellae produce enterotoxins but are also invasive and produce inflammatory change within the intestine. In calves, infection commonly progresses to a bacteremia. *See also* SALMONELLOSIS, p 156.

Clostridium perfringens types A, B, C, and E produce a variety of necrotizing toxins and cause a rapidly fatal hemorrhagic enteritis in calves. The disease in calves is rare and usually sporadic. Infection with type B or C is a common cause of enteritis and dysentery in lambs (*see also* p 493). *Campylobacter jejuni* and *Yersinia enterocolitica* may be present in the feces of calves and lambs with diarrhea but also may be found in the feces of healthy animals.

Viruses: Rotavirus is the most common viral cause of diarrhea in calves and lambs. Groups A and B rotavirus are involved, but group A is most prevalent and clinically important and contains several serotypes of differing virulence. Rotavirus replicates in the mature absorptive and enzyme-producing enterocytes on the villi of the small intestine, leading to rupture and sloughing of the enterocytes with release of virus to infect adjacent cells. Rotavirus does not infect the immature cells of the crypts. With virulent strains of rotavirus, the loss of enterocytes exceeds the ability of the intestinal crypts to replace them; hence, villous height is reduced, with a consequent decrease in intestinal absorptive surface area and intestinal digestive enzyme activity.

Coronavirus is also commonly associated with diarrhea in calves. It replicates in the epithelium of the upper respiratory tract and in the enterocytes of the intestine, where it produces similar lesions to rotavirus but also infects the epithelial cells of the large intestine to produce atrophy of the colonic ridges.

Other viruses, including Breda virus, a calicilike virus, astrovirus, and parvovirus, have been demonstrated in the feces of calves with diarrhea and can produce diarrhea in calves experimentally. However, these agents can also be demonstrated in the feces of healthy calves. The importance of these agents in the syndrome of neonatal diarrhea has yet to be determined. The viruses of bovine virus diarrhea and infectious bovine rhinotracheitis are reported to cause calf diarrhea, but this is not a common manifestation of these infections.

Protozoa: *C parvum* (p 168) is a common cause of diarrhea in calves and lambs. The parasite does not invade but adheres to the apical surface of enterocytes in the distal small intestine and the colon. This results in loss of microvilli, decreased mucosal enzyme activity with villous blunting and fusion (leading to a reduced villous surface absorptive area), and inflammatory changes in the submucosa. Mammalian cryptosporidia lack host specificity. *Giardia duodenalis* is a common asymptomatic infection in the intestine of young calves and lambs. It has been demonstrated in the feces of poorly growing calves that have a chronic mucoid diarrhea, but there is little evidence for a causative association of this organism with diarrhea in calves or lambs.

Other Causes: Calves that are fed large amounts of milk or inappropriately formulated milk replacers produce a large volume of feces with a greater than normal fluid content but do not have a fluid diarrhea with weight loss. Similarly, calves sucking highproducing beef cows grazing lush pasture may have loose feces. Milk replacers with poor quality, heat-denatured proteins or with excessive amounts of soybean or fish protein or carbohydrates of nonmilk origin have a higher risk of producing diarrhea.

There is some evidence that the oral administration of chloramphenicol, neomycin, or tetracycline to young calves for 3-5 days can result in villous change with resultant malabsorption and mild diarrhea. Prolonged and high-dose antibiotic treatment of calves can lead to diarrhea associated with bacterial superinfection of the intestine. Colisepticemia (p 600) and ruminal drinking (p 192) can also be accompanied by diarrhea.

Epidemiology and Transmission: Enteropathogens associated with diarrhea are commonly found in the feces of healthy calves; whether intestinal infection leads to diarrhea depends on a number of determinants, including differences in virulence of different strains of a pathogen and the presence of more than one pathogen. The resistance of the calf is of major importance and is largely determined by successful passive transfer of colostral immunoglobulins. Colostrum-deprived calves are highly susceptible to infection with enteropathogens and develop severe and often fatal disease. The progression of infection, the severity of lesions produced, and the severity of the diarrhea can be modulated by immunoglobulins received via colostrum. Immunoglobulins act directly on pathogens in the intestinal lumen during the period of colostrum ingestion as well as after, because significant amounts of circulating immunoglobulins are re-secreted into the intestine, especially when the concentration of circulating immunoglobulin is high. The lack of specific antibodies in dams that have not been exposed to specific pathogens, and the use of specific vaccines, further modulate this influence. Stress caused by a poor environment, inadequate protection from the weather, or an insufficient or inappropriate diet also increases the risk for disease. With all of the enteropathogens, healthy adult cattle may be carriers and periodically excrete the organism in feces. Excretion may increase with the stress of parturition and be more frequent in primiparous cows. This can lead to contaminated calving areas and infection of the udder and perineum of the dam. Other sources of infection include the feces of healthy calves and the feces of diarrheic calves, which contain large numbers of organisms early in the course of infection. A few scouring calves can result in severe contamination of the calf-rearing area. Transmission is by fecal-oral contact, fecal aerosol, and, in the case of coronavirus, also by respiratory aerosol.

Pathogenesis: Diarrhea in neonatal ruminants is usually associated with disease of the small intestine and can be caused by either hypersecretion or malabsorption. Hypersecretory diarrhea develops when an abnormal amount of fluid is secreted into the gut, exceeding the resorptive capacity of the mucosa. In malabsorptive diarrhea, the capacity of the mucosa to absorb fluid and nutrients is impaired to the extent that it cannot keep up with the normal influx of ingested and secreted fluids. This is usually the result of villous atrophy, in which the loss of mature enterocytes at the tips of the villi results both in a decrease in villous height (with a consequent decrease in the surface area for absorption) and in loss of the brush border digestive enzymes. The extent and distribution of villous atrophy varies with different pathogens and can explain variation in the severity of clinical disease. Malabsorptive diarrhea may be aggravated by the colonic fermentation of nutrients that normally would have been absorbed in the small intestine. Fermentation products, especially lactic acid, appear to draw water into the colon osmotically, which contributes to the severity of diarrhea. Inflammation contributes to the pathophysiology of diarrhea in most intestinal infections, and mediators of inflammation can affect ion flux within the intestine. Inflammation also leads to vascular and lymphatic damage and to structural damage of the crypt-villus unit. Most infectious forms of diarrhea have hypersecretory, inflammatory, and malabsorptive components, although one usually predominates. These lead to a net loss of water, sodium, potassium, and bicarbonate; if severe, the calf develops hypovolemia, hyponatremia, acidosis, and prerenal azotemia.

Enterotoxigenic *E coli* produce the enterotoxin Sta, which stimulates marked hypersecretion by activating guanylate cyclase and by inducing a net secretion of sodium and chlorine. The membrane-bound sodium-glucose cotransport system remains functional. Salmonellae also elaborate enterotoxins. Inflammation, leading to necrosis of the enterocyte, submucosal inflammatory infiltration, and villous atrophy, is also a major component of the pathophysiology of diarrhea produced by salmonellae, as well as of diarrhea produced by enteropathogenic *E coli* and by toxigenic *Clostridium perfringens*. Infections with verotoxin-producing enteropathogenic *E coli* result in accumulation of fluid within the large intestine and extensive damage to the large intestinal mucosa, with edema, hemorrhage, and erosion and ulceration of the mucosa, which results in blood and mucus in the lumen.

Viruses usually produce a malabsorptive diarrhea by destroying the absorptive cells of the mucosa, thus shortening the intestinal villi. The mechanism by which cryptosporidia produce diarrhea is not completely understood, but it appears to have both malabsorptive and inflammatory components.

Inappropriately formulated milk replacers produce diarrhea by 2 mechanisms, both associated with malabsorption. Vegetable (especially soybean) products are commonly used as protein sources in the manufacture of milk replacers. Depending on the degree of refinement, these products may contain carbohydrates that are indigestible in young calves. Such carbohydrates are not absorbed in the small intestine and may contribute to diarrhea via colonic fermentation. In addition, most calves <3 wk old appear to have an allergic reaction to soy proteins that results in villous atrophy, leading to diarrhea that is probably malabsorptive.

Clinical Findings: The major signs are diarrhea, dehydration, profound weakness, and death within one to several days of onset.

Diarrhea due to enterotoxigenic (K99-bearing) *E coli* is seen in calves <3-5 days old, rarely later. However, the age of susceptibility may be extended in the presence of other pathogens. Onset is sudden. Profuse amounts of liquid feces are passed, and the calves rapidly become depressed and recumbent. Calves may lose over 12% of body weight in fluid, and hypovolemic shock and death may occur in 12-24 hr. Body temperature may be increased but is commonly normal or subnormal. If fluid and electrolyte therapy is administered early, response is usually good. Disease produced by attaching and effacing *E coli* is seen predominantly in calves from 4 days to 2 mo old and may manifest with diarrhea or primarily as dysentery with blood and mucus in the feces. The clinical course is short. Diarrhea due to *Salmonella* spp usually is not seen in calves <14 days old. It is characterized by feces that are foul smelling and contain blood, fibrin, and copious amounts of mucus. Septicemia, with high fever and depression progressing to prostration and coma, is the salient manifestation of salmonellosis in calves and, although diarrhea is present, death is usually from septicemic rather than from hypovolemic shock. Calves with salmonellosis usually lose weight rapidly and often die in spite of vigorous therapy. Hemorrhagic enterotoxemia due to *C perfringens* type B or C is characterized by acute onset of depression, weakness, bloody diarrhea, abdominal pain, and death within a few hours. It usually develops in vigorous calves that are just a few days old that have large appetites and a ready source of milk. Calves affected with *C perfringens* usually die before treatment can be instituted.

Diarrhea due to rotavirus, coronavirus, and other viruses usually is seen in calves 5-15 days old but can affect calves to several months of age. Affected calves are only moderately depressed and often continue to suck or drink milk. The feces are voluminous, soft to liquid, and often contain large amounts of mucus. Diarrhea commonly persists for three to several days, with some cases of coronaviral diarrhea becoming chronic. Cases of viral diarrhea that are uncomplicated by other pathogens commonly respond within a few days to fluid and electrolyte therapy and adequate nutritional support.

Cryptosporidiosis (p 168) is seen in calves 5-35 days old but most commonly in the second week of life. It is characterized by persistent diarrhea that does not respond to therapy. Diarrhea due solely to *Cryptosporidium* spp is often mild and self-limiting, although the severity may be related to the general strength of the calf and to the intensity of challenge with the organism. Combination infections with cryptosporidia, rotavirus, and coronavirus are common and result in persistent diarrhea often characterized by emaciation and death. Death from hypoglycemia also occurs as a sequela of cryptosporidiosis in calves 3-4 wk of age that have recovered from diarrhea but are still emaciated. Death often occurs during a bout of cold weather and is more likely to occur on farms where there is a policy of reducing the amount of milk fed to calves during periods of diarrhea.

Dietary diarrheas are seen in calves <3 wk old and are characterized by voluminous feces of pasty to gelatinous consistency. Initially, the calves are bright and alert and have good appetites. Eventually, however, they become weak and emaciated if the diet is not corrected. Infectious forms of diarrhea are often complicated by poor-quality diets or insufficient nutritional intake.

Diagnosis: Usually, it is difficult to make a definite etiologic diagnosis based solely on clinical findings. However, the history, age of the animal(s) affected, and clinical signs may permit a presumptive diagnosis. Fecal samples can be submitted for isolation and characterization of the common enteropathogens. Samples should be taken from several untreated calves in the early stages of diarrhea. Special techniques are necessary for the demonstration of viruses, cryptosporidia, and K99-bearing *E coli*. The interpretation of fecal microbiology can be difficult because of mixed infections and because enteropathogens are commonly present in the feces of healthy calves. The best diagnostic information is usually obtained by submitting untreated, acutely affected animals for necropsy. This allows examination of intestinal mucosa for evidence of diagnostic lesions and for the presence of enteropathogens such as cryptosporidia. It may be the only way that disease such as that associated with attaching and effacing strains of *E coli* can be diagnosed. The diagnostic value of a necropsy diminishes quickly with time after death; important lesions can disappear within minutes due to autolysis. Complete laboratory examination can be expensive, and it has also been argued that there is little value in expending large amounts of money on diagnosis unless there are specific control procedures that can be implemented based on the information gained. In all cases, information on total milk or milk replacer consumption should be obtained. When milk replacer is being fed, the composition of the diet should be evaluated. Nonspecific immunity should be assessed by determining immunoglobulin and vitamin A concentrations in serum.

Treatment: Many of the factors involved in disease resistance are nonspecific; thus, important preventive measures can be taken and therapy can be initiated before an etiologic diagnosis has been established. Treatment includes fluid and electrolyte replacement, alterations of the diet, antimicrobial and immunoglobulin therapy, and use of antidiarrheal drugs and adsorbents. Fluid and electrolyte therapy is most important and should be instituted as soon as possible regardless of whether clinical evidence of dehydration has developed (clinical signs of dehydration are not apparent until the calf has lost at least 6% of its body weight in fluid). Calves that are still able to stand and that are willing and able to suck can often be treated with oral electrolytes alone. Fluids for oral rehydration should promote the cotransport of sodium with glucose and amino acids and should contain sodium, glucose, glycine or alanine, potassium, and either bicarbonate or citrate or acetate as a bicarbonate precursor. Several commercial preparations are available. These can be administered by nipple bottle or, if necessary, by stomach tube. The solutions should be used liberally until the animal is rehydrated.

Whether or not milk should be fed during the rehydration period is controversial. Feeding milk may increase fecal volume, but it provides energy to the calf and may promote gut healing. Calves have large energy requirements and little reserve. Electrolyte solutions do not meet calf energy requirements, and milk should not be withheld for >24-36 hr.

Calves that are recumbent and weak and show evidence of water loss ≥8% of their body weight require IV fluid and electrolyte therapy. These calves are usually acidotic, and the fluid and base deficits can be corrected initially by administering an isotonic (13 g/L) solution of sodium bicarbonate, ideally at 100 mL/kg over 4-6 hr. Because the calves are frequently hypoglycemic, addition of 25-50 g of dextrose to the bicarbonate solution is often beneficial. The bicarbonate solution should be followed by continuous IV fluid therapy with a physiologically balanced electrolyte solution administered at 5-8 mL/kg/hr for the next 20 hr; higher rates may be necessary depending on the severity of diarrhea. Oral electrolyte solutions should probably be used concurrently with IV therapy.

The use of antimicrobials is not supported by most clinical trials and not indicated in diarrhea induced by viruses or protozoa. Antibiotics may be of value in treating diarrhea associated with enterotoxigenic or attaching and effacing *E coli*. The route of administration should be oral, and the choice based on sensitivity testing. When septicemic disease, due to inadequate transfer of colostral immunoglobulins, is suspected as a complication, parenterally administered antibiotics are also indicated. Salmonellosis should be treated with parenteral antimicrobials. Several drugs, such as flunixin meglumine, indomethacin, loperamide, diphenoxate, and bismuth subsalicylate, have antisecretory and anti-inflammatory activity and are used in treatment, but there are no clinical trials of their efficacy in calves. Intestinal gels and adsorbents, such as kaolin and pectin, are in general use, but their only established effect is to increase fecal consistency; they do not reduce the loss of water and ions.

Prevention and Control: Because of the complex nature of diarrhea in neonates, it is unrealistic to expect total prevention—economical control is the major objective. The incidence of clinical disease and the case fatality rate depend on the balance between the levels of exposure to infectious agents and the resistance in the calf. Differences in herd size; availability of facilities, land, and labor; and general management objectives make it impossible to recommend specific management procedures that are applicable to all situations. However, 3 broad principles apply in all herds: 1) the degree of exposure of neonates should be reduced by isolating diseased animals or by moving calving and calf rearing to a separate area, and by practicing good general hygiene; 2) nonspecific resistance should be maximized by providing good nutrition to the dam and neonate and assuring that newborn calves consume ≥5% of their body wt of high-quality colostrum, preferably within 2 hr and certainly within 6 hr of birth, followed by equivalent amounts at 12-hr intervals for the next 48 hr; and 3) the specific resistance of the newborn should be increased by vaccinating the dam or the newborn. A significant portion of both naturally sucking dairy calves and calves handfed colostrum do not acquire adequate amounts of immunoglobulin because of delayed sucking or feeding, ingestion of an inadequate volume of colostrum, or ingestion of colostrum of inferior immunoglobulin concentration. When time constraints on labor preclude an ensured intake of colostrum by nipple-bottle feeding, administration of 3.8 L of colostrum by esophageal feeder within the first 2 hr of life can be the best colostrum feeding policy. (*See also* DISEASE-MANAGEMENT INTERACTION: CATTLE, p 1707, and MANAGEMENT OF REPRODUCTION: CATTLE, p 1747.)

Immunization of calves against colibacillosis by vaccination of pregnant dams can control enterotoxigenic colibacillosis. The pregnant dam is vaccinated 6 and 2 wk before parturition to stimulate antibodies to strains of enterotoxigenic *E coli*; these antibodies are then passed on to the newborn through the colostrum (provided the calf ingests it). A single booster is given in subsequent years. Monoclonal K99 *E coli* antibody is commercially available for oral administration to calves immediately after birth. It is an effective substitute for the K99-specific antibody in the colostrum of vaccinated cows, although calves that receive this product should also receive colostrum for its nonspecific protection.

Vaccination of pregnant cows with rotavirus and coronavirus vaccines increase the amount of specific antibody in colostrum and milk, but the concentration of antibodies in milk may be insufficient to provide local antibody in the intestinal lumen during the period of peak prevalence of infection which, in calves, is 5-15 days of age. Controlled trials of commercial vaccines have shown variable results. The addition of small amounts of immune colostrum to milk fed during the period of susceptibility can provide some protection against disease.

Zoonotic Risk: Several of the agents that produce diarrhea in calves can also produce diarrheal disease in humans. *Cryptosporidium parvum* and *Salmonella* serovar *typhimurium* can produce serious disease, particularly in immunocompromised individuals. These organisms are commonly present as subclinical infections in the gut of calves and lambs; immunocompromised people should avoid contact with young ruminants and possibly all farm animals. Cattle, including calves, are one of the reservoirs for the verotoxic *E coli* serotype O157:H7 that is associated with human hemorrhagic colitis and the hemolytic uremic syndrome. Infection in humans is usually acquired by consumption of contaminated food, but the infective dose is low, and the possibility of infection by direct contact exists. Other verotoxic *E coli* associated with human disease can also be isolated from the feces of healthy cattle.

INTESTINAL DISEASES IN HORSES AND FOALS

Intestinal disease in horses and foals is suggested by diarrhea, weight loss, hypoproteinemia, and abdominal pain. (*See also* COLIC, p 202.)

DIARRHEAL DISEASE

A definitive etiology can be determined in <50% of cases. Yet, treatment of most horses and foals with diarrhea is similar and thus allows therapeutic management despite the lack of a definitive diagnosis.

Diarrhea in adult horses can be acute or chronic. Infectious agents that have been cited as potential causes of acute diarrhea in adult horses include *Salmonella enteritica* of various serovars, *Neorickettsia (Ehrlichia) risticii*, *Clostridium difficile*, *C perfringens*, *Aeromonas hydrophila*, and cyathastomiasis. Other differential diagnoses for acute diarrhea in horses include ingestion of a toxicant(s), antimicrobial-induced colitis, toxicity due to NSAID, and sand enterocolopathy. An acute, fatal diarrheal disease of unknown etiology is known as colitis-X. Diarrhea that persists >1 mo is considered chronic and is often a diagnostic challenge. Chronic diarrhea can be caused by inflammatory or neoplastic conditions involving the intestine or by disruption of the normal physiologic process in the bowel. Differential diagnoses include sand enterocolopathy and infiltrative lesions, such as those associated with inflammatory bowel disease. The body's response to certain components of feed may play a role in chronic diarrhea of horses due to bowel inflammation, but has not frequently been established as an etiology.

Noninflammatory conditions of the colon can also result in diarrhea. These include altered fermentation in the large colon, which is potentially the result of altered intestinal flora or milieu secondary to antimicrobial treatment, alteration in diet, or unknown etiologies. Nonintestinal causes of chronic diarrhea include congestive heart failure and chronic liver disease. The diagnostic approach to these cases is aimed at differentiation of infiltrative diseases of the intestine from physiologic causes of diarrhea.

Because of the large volume of the colon and cecum of horses, massive fluid losses can occur in a short time. Thus, diarrhea in adult horses can be an explosive event with morbidity and mortality exceeding that associated with diarrheal diseases in other animals and humans.

SALMONELLOSIS

Salmonellosis is one of the most commonly diagnosed infectious causes of diarrhea in adult horses. Clinical manifestations range from no abnormal clinical signs (subclinical carrier) to acute, severe diarrhea and even death. The disease most commonly is seen sporadically but may become an epidemic depending on the virulence of the organism, level of exposure, and host factors. Infection can occur via contamination of the environment, feed, or water or by contact with animals actively shedding the bacteria. Stress appears to play an important role in the pathogenesis—a history of surgery, transportation, or change in feed; concurrent disease, particularly GI disorders (colic); or treatment with broad-spectrum antimicrobial drugs often precedes the diarrhea. Salmonellae are subdivided into serogroups and then further into types or serovars based on testing with specific antisera. Serovars are named after the clinical condition, host, or geographic region from which the organism was first identified. For example, *Salmonella typhimurium* is now referred to as *Salmonella enteritica* serovar *typhimurium* or *S typhimurium*. In the USA, the types of *Salmonella* isolated from samples of ill equids are reported annually by the National Veterinary Services Laboratory in Ames, IA. Although the list may vary slightly from year to year, certain types are consistently in the top 10. *Salmonella* of the serogroup B (which includes *S typhimurium* and *S agona*) are consistently in the top 10 isolates from horses with clinical disease. Serogroup C, which is further divided into serogroup C_1 (includes *S infantis*, *S braenderup*, *S montevideo*, *S thompson*, *S ohio*, *S oranienburg*) and serogroup C_2 (includes serovars *S javiana*, *S newport*, *S hadar*, *S muenchen*), appears to be on the increase as a cause of disease in horses. The other serogroup often identified in clinical disease of horses is serogroup E (includes *S krefeld*, *S muenster*, *S anatum*). Knowledge of the type of *Salmonella* may aid in development of a prognosis. Some types (eg, *S typhimurium*) appear to be more pathogenic than others. Knowing the serovar and antibiogram can aid in tracking or monitoring the type or serovar of salmonellae affecting any given group or population of horses (eg, in tracking nosocomial spread within a veterinary hospital).

Clinical Findings: Three forms have been recognized in adult horses. One is the subclinical carrier, which may or may not be actively shedding the organism but has the potential of transmitting the bacteria to susceptible animals either by direct contact or by contamination of the environment, water, or feed sources. Multiple fecal cultures may be necessary to identify carriers because the organism is shed in the feces intermittently and in small numbers. If stressed, the carrier may develop clinical disease. Based on one 1998 study, the national prevalence of fecal shedding of *Salmonella* spp by horses in the USA is estimated to be 0.8%, and ~1.8% of horse operations had 1 or more horses shedding *Salmonella* spp in their feces. The percent of horses that chronically shed may be higher. The most common serovars identified among the general population of horses were *S muenchen* and *S newport* (both serogroup C_2).

The second form of the disease is characterized by a mild clinical course, with signs of depression, fever, anorexia, and soft but not watery feces. Affected horses may have an absolute neutropenia. Clinical disease may last 4-5 days and usually is self-limiting, and *Salmonella* spp can be isolated from the feces. Recovered horses may continue to excrete the organism in their feces for days to months; therefore, isolation of the shedding horse and thorough cleaning and subsequent disinfection of the contaminated area are recommended.

The third form is characterized by an acute onset of severe depression, anorexia, profound neutropenia, and frequently abdominal pain. Diarrhea develops in 6-24 hr; feces are fluid and foul smelling. Affected horses dehydrate rapidly, and metabolic acidosis and electrolyte losses occur as the horse deteriorates. The severe form of salmonellosis often results in a protein-losing enterocolopathy. Plasma protein levels may become dangerously low after a few days of diarrhea. Occasionally, these horses become bacteremic. If untreated, this form of salmonellosis is often fatal.

Diagnosis: Diagnosis is based on clinical signs, severe neutropenia, and isolation of salmonellae from feces, blood, or tissues. Submission of 1-2 g of feces for culture has been more successful in identifying salmonellae than has culturing fecal swabs. It is important to collect and submit feces based on the recommendations of the laboratory that will be performing the culture. Working with a diagnostic laboratory that uses enrichment techniques along with agars specifically selected to optimize recovery of *Salmonella* spp is advisable. Because salmonellae cannot be consistently cultured from feces, multiple samples (generally 3-5) should be collected daily from each horse. Culturing of rectal mucosal biopsies increases the probability of isolating the organism; however, the technique is not without risk to the horse. Fecal samples that must be mailed should be placed in transport media suitable for enteric pathogens at the time of collection. A PCR test is available and, depending on the primers used, appears to be more sensitive than routine bacterial culture for detection of salmonellae. However, the biologic significance of a positive PCR test has yet to be determined.

Treatment: Treatment of the severe form of salmonellosis is based on IV fluid and electrolyte replacement and efforts to control the host's responses initiated by endotoxemia. A polyionic isotonic fluid with bicarbonate precursors is used for volume replacement. Because of active secretion of fluid and electrolytes into the lumen of the intestine, IV fluid volumes of 40-80 L/day may be necessary. Electrolyte and acid-base deficiencies are common and are corrected by use of oral and/or IV fluids supplemented with electrolytes. It is difficult to predict the electrolyte status of affected horses. Deficits should be determined by serum biochemical analysis; supplementation with sodium chloride, potassium chloride, and occasionally sodium bicarbonate may be indicated.

Antimicrobial treatment in adult horses with salmonellosis is controversial and does not appear to alter the course of the colitis or to decrease shedding of salmonellae; however, it may reduce the likelihood of septicemia. Selection of an antimicrobial is not easy and should be based on the sensitivity of the organism isolated. Resistance patterns vary among *Salmonella* isolates and can change over the course of an outbreak. There is potential nephrotoxicosis from aminoglycoside antibiotics in volume-depleted horses; therefore, the hydration status of the horse should be taken into consideration when selecting an antimicrobial. The ideal antibiotic should also be lipid soluble.

The use of GI protectants (eg, biosponge, bismuth subsalicylate, activated charcoal) may be beneficial. These substances may bind bacterial toxins. NSAID, such as flunixin meglumine, help counteract the effect of endotoxin, control pain, and possibly help prevent laminitis. The dosage of NSAID used has been quite variable. Serious side effects, such as gastric and colonic ulceration and renal nephrotoxicosis, can result from NSAID treatment, so the minimum effective dosage should be used. Equine plasma can be administered to correct hypoproteinemia and to supply coagulation factors and, depending on the source of the plasma, specific antibodies to endotoxin. Colloidal plasma substitutes such as hetastarch may be necessary to maintain oncotic pressure in horses with substantial protein loss into the GI tract. These colloidal plasma substitutes may be less expensive and better tolerated than equine plasma in some horses. Often, equine plasma and colloidal plasma substitutes are both used in horses with hypoproteinemia due to colitis.

Low-dose polymyxin B (3,000 units/kg, BID) has also been advocated to bind circulating endotoxin. In controlled trials, polymyxin B ameliorated some of the known effects of endotoxemia in horses. Antimicrobial doses of polymyxin B are substantially higher than the dose used to bind endotoxin and may be nephrotoxic. The nephrotoxicity of polymyxin in horses that are dehydrated or have pre-existing renal compromise is unknown, but should be considered.

Prevention: Prevention of salmonellosis is difficult because the organism is present in the environment as well as in the feces of some healthy animals. Certainly, in a hospital environment where horses are stressed by transport, may be off feed, and are often receiving antimicrobial treatment, aggressive identification and strict isolation of salmonellae-infected horses is indicated. Biosecurity practices to minimize cross contamination between hospitalized horses are also advisable.

Owners should be made aware of the zoonotic risk of *Salmonella* spp infection. People working with infected animals should practice strict hygiene.

POTOMAC HORSE FEVER
(Equine monocytic ehrlichiosis, Ditch fever, Shasta River crud, Equine ehrlichial colitis)

Potomac horse fever (PHF) is an acute enterocolitis syndrome producing mild colic, fever, and diarrhea in horses of all ages, as well as abortion in pregnant mares. The causative agent, formerly known as *Ehrlichia risticii*, has recently been renamed *Neorickettsia risticii* because of its lesser genetic relationships to other *Ehrlichia* groups. The infection of enterocytes of the small and large intestine results in acute colitis, which is one of the principal clinical signs of PHF. The disease is seen in spring, summer, and early fall and is associated with pastures bordering creeks or rivers. Recently, the epidemiology of PHF has been shown to involve a trematode vector. Sporadic disease caused by *N risticii* has been reported in dogs and cats; cattle appear to be resistant to infection. PHF has been reported in many areas of the USA and Canada using an indirect fluorescent antibody test as evidence of exposure; however, recent studies indicate a high rate of false-positive titers with this test, and the true geographic range of distribution is not known. Isolation or detection of the causative agent from clinical cases of PHF using conventional cell culture or PCR assay has been reported only from California, Illinois, Indiana, Kentucky, Maryland, Michigan, New York, New Jersey, Ohio, Oregon, Pennsylvania, Texas, and Virginia.

Etiology and Pathogenesis: *N risticii* is a gram-negative obligate intracellular bacterium with a trophism for monocytes. Initial morphologic studies of this organism isolated from cell culture, as well as the serologic responses of *N risticii*, caused this bacterium to be assigned to the genus *Ehrlichia*. Recent DNA analyses have revealed *N risticii* is most closely related to *N helminthoeca*, the agent of salmon poisoning in dogs, and *Ehrlichia sennetsu*, a disease of humans in Japan. The organism is not visible in monocytes in blood films from clinical cases in contrast to *Ehrlichia (Anaplasma) equi*, which is readily identifiable in granulocytes of infected horses.

Recently *N risticii* has been identified in freshwater snails and isolated from trematodes released from the snails. *N risticii* DNA was detected in 13 species of immature and adult caddisflies (Trichoptera), mayflies (Ephemeroptera), damselflies (Odonata, Zygoptera), dragonflies (Odonata, Anisoptera), and stoneflies (Plecoptera). Transmission studies using *N risticii*-infected caddisflies have reproduced the clinical disease. One route of exposure is believed to be inadvertent ingestion of aquatic insects that carry *N risticii* in the metacercarial stage of a trematode. The incubation period is ~10-18 days. The causative organism is present in the feces of experimentally infected horses, but the biologic significance of this is unknown. Clinically ill horses are not contagious and can be housed with susceptible horses. Future studies are needed to determine the exact role of the vector and helminth hosts in the complex maintenance cycle of *N risticii*.

Clinical Findings and Lesions: The clinical features of PHF are typified initially by mild depression and anorexia, followed by a fever ranging from 102-107°F (38.9-41.7°C). At this stage, intestinal sounds can be decreased. Within 24-48 hr, a moderate to severe diarrhea, with feces ranging in consistency from that usually seen in cows to watery, develops in ~60% of affected horses. The onset of diarrhea is often accompanied by mild abdominal discomfort. Some horses develop severe toxemia and dehydration. Laminitis can supervene as a severe complication of PHF in up to 40% of affected horses. Hematologic findings vary in the early stage of PHF from leukopenia (characterized by neutropenia and lymphopenia) to a normal hemogram, despite evidence of systemic toxicity. A common finding in cases of PHF is a marked leukocytosis, which is normally observed within a few days of onset. PHF may present with all or any combination of these clinical signs.

Several months following clinical disease in pregnant mares, abortion due to fetal infection with *N risticii* may occur. Experimentally, pregnant mares infected at 100-160 days of gestation abort at 190-250 days of gestation. The abortion is accompanied by placentitis and retained placenta. Fetal lesions include colitis, periportal hepatitis, and lymphoid hyperplasia of mesenteric lymph nodes and spleen. Necropsy findings in nonpregnant horses with enterocolitis are nonspecific and reveal diffuse inflammation, mainly in the large intestines.

Diagnosis: A provisional diagnosis of PHF often is based on the presence of typical clinical signs and the seasonal and geographic occurrence of the disease. A definitive diagnosis of PHF should be based on isolation or detection of *N risticii* from the blood or feces of infected horses. Serologic testing is of limited value as a diagnostic tool, although many infected horses have high antibody titers at the time of infection. Because of the high prevalence of false-positive titers, interpretation of the indirect fluorescent antibody test in individual horses is difficult. Isolation of the agent in cell culture, although possible, is time-consuming and not routinely available in many diagnostic laboratories. A recently developed real-time PCR assay allows the detection of *N risticii* DNA within 2 hr, making this a much more feasible test for routine diagnostic examination. To enhance the chances of detection of *N risticii*, the assay should be performed on a blood as well as a fecal sample, as the presence of the organism in blood and feces may not necessarily coincide.

Treatment: PHF can be treated successfully with oxytetracycline (6.6 mg/kg, IV, BID), if given early in the clinical course of the disease. A response to treatment is usually seen within 12 hr. This is associated with a drop in rectal temperature, followed by an improvement in demeanor, appetite, and borborygmal sounds. If therapy is begun early, clinical signs frequently resolve by the third day of treatment. Generally, antimicrobial therapy is for no more than 5 days. In animals exhibiting signs of enterocolitis, fluids and NSAID should be administered. Laminitis, if it develops, is usually severe and often refractory to treatment.

Prevention: Several inactivated, whole-cell vaccines based on the same strain of *N risticii* are commercially available. Although vaccination has been reported to protect 78% of experimentally infected ponies, it has been marginally protective in the field. Vaccine failure has been attributed to antigenic and genomic heterogeneity among the >14 different strains of *N risticii* isolates from naturally occurring cases. Furthermore, vaccine failure may also be due to lack of antibody protection at the site of exposure, because the natural route of transmission has been determined to be oral ingestion of the agent. Reduction of snail numbers in rivers and ditches may be attempted to lessen sources of infection. No zoonotic risk is known.

CLOSTRIDIA-ASSOCIATED ENTEROCOLITIS

Clostridium spp have been incriminated as a cause of enterocolitis in horses and foals and appear to be part of a complex disease process. The role of *Clostridium* spp in equine enterocolitis has been debated. The sporadic occurrence of the disease, the variety of clostridial species involved, and the difficulty in experimental reproduction of the disease suggest a poorly defined multifactorial syndrome. (*See also* p 493.)

Clostridium spp that have been associated with equine enterocolitis include *C perfringens* (types A, B, C, and D), *C sordellii*, *C difficile*, and *C cadaveris*. Alteration of the normal intestinal milieu appears to be necessary for this disease to develop. The clinical enterocolitis syndrome due to clostridial infection has been best characterized in foals but appears to occur in adult horses as well. Possibly, certain factors may predispose horses to overgrowth of *C perfringens*, resulting in disease. Approximately one third of healthy broodmares and >90% of foals in the general population shed *C perfringens* in their feces. The most common type identified is type A, with type C being very rarely identified in the feces or environment of normal broodmares and their foals. A recently discovered toxin, which can be produced by any of the types of *C perfringens*, is called β2 toxin due to the clinical signs it induced in experimental challenge models, ie, pathology similar to that induced by β1 toxin. The role that *C perfringens* with the β2 gene plays in enterocolitis in horses or foals is yet to be fully defined.

Antimicrobial use, food deprivation, and other stressors have been suggested to predispose horses to the overgrowth of either or both *C perfringens* and *C difficile*, leading to GI disease. In one report, mares whose foals were being treated with erythromycin developed fatal enterocolitis associated with *C difficile*.

Clinical Findings: Clinical signs include sudden death, diarrhea with or without blood, colic, reduced feed intake, and lethargy. These clinical signs are also consistent with other causes of enterocolitis. Foals affected at <3 days old with *C perfringens*-associated enterocolitis often have bloody diarrhea and colic. *C perfringens* type C infection in neonatal foals has consistently been associated with severe GI disease. Several foals on a particular farm may be affected, but the disease is typically sporadic. The role of *C perfringens* type A in enterocolitis in neonatal foals is less clear; it has been reported that >90% of foals at 3 days of age shed this organism in their feces and that *C perfringens* type A is likely one of the first bacteria to colonize the intestinal tract of newborn foals, irrespective of hygiene protocols. *C difficile* has been associated with enterocolitis in newborn foals as well as in adult horses. It has been identified as a nosocomial infection in humans, and this may also be seen in horses.

The mortality rate associated with *C perfringens* enterocolitis, especially type C, is high, even with intensive medical treatment.

Diagnosis: Diagnosis is based on clinical signs, microbiologic identification of the bacteria in feces and tissues if available, gross necropsy, and histopathology. Microbiology should include isolation of the organism and ideally identification of toxins in the fecal or intestinal contents or tissues. Fecal material should be submitted using a method that will maintain the sample in an anaerobic environment. Isolation of clostridial organisms requires anaerobic conditions and, depending on the organism, special growth media. Communicating to the laboratory that clostridial enterocolitis is a differential diagnosis is critical as many veterinary laboratories do not routinely culture fecal samples anaerobically unless specifically requested to do so. *C difficile* is particularly difficult to culture if the sample is shipped to the laboratory overnight vs delivered directly to the laboratory for culture. Diagnosis of clostridial enterocolitis is often made at necropsy and is based primarily on identification of intestinal necrosis associated with large gram-positive rods in intestinal smears. Tissue and fecal specimens must be taken immediately after death to avoid degradation of toxins or an overgrowth of clostridial organisms. A PCR test, available at selected laboratories, allows differentiation of *C perfringens* types A, B, C, D, and E, as well as identification of the gene coding for the β2 toxin. The only commercially available test kit for the detection of toxins of *C perfringens* detects only the enterotoxin, not α, β, ε, or ι toxins.

Treatment: Treatment is similar to that for other causes of equine enterocolitis but often is unrewarding in neonatal foals infected with *C perfringens* type C. Treatment includes IV fluids and NSAID. In neonatal foals, treatment to prevent gastric ulceration may be indicated. Broad-spectrum systemic antibiotics are indicated if the horse is suspected of being septic or is severely leukopenic. Oral metronidazole has been used with some success to treat foals with suspected clostridial enterocolitis; however, the most appropriate dose and potential side effects of this drug in foals have not been fully determined. An injectable form of metronidazole has been used in some foals with colic that cannot be treated orally. The pharmacokinetics and appropriate dose of the injectable form in foals are unknown. Specific antitoxin for *C perfringens* type C and D has also been used in foals; however, it is not approved for this use. The benefit of type C and D antitoxin in disease associated with type A or β2 toxin is unknown, but based on production methods, the α and β2 toxins are unlikely to be present in high levels in this toxoid. A product with *Saccharomyces boulardii* has been advocated for the potential it may have in adhering to the toxin binding sites in the intestine, but its efficacy and safety in neonatal foals have not been determined.

Foals with colic associated with ingestion of milk often require IV fluids and parenteral nutritional support. Continuous infusion of fluids is optimal but labor intensive and requires separation of the foal and mare. Intensive treatment may be required for several days, ie, until the enterocolitis resolves.

Prevention: No proven efficacious biologic products are available to immunize horses or foals against clostridial enterocolitis. When the disease is a problem in multiple foals on a farm, preventive measures have been implemented, but the efficacy and safety of these interventions have yet to be critically evaluated. These measures included administering oral probiotics to foals soon after birth, vaccinating pregnant mares twice at 2- to 4-wk intervals at least 1 mo before foaling with *C perfringens* type C and D toxoid (bacterin products and those with oil adjuvants should be avoided), using *C perfringens* type C and D antitoxin prophylactically, PO, in newborn foals, administering antimicrobials (eg, metronidazole) prophylactically to foals for the first 3-5 days of life, minimizing the amount of lactation by the mare in the first week after foaling through dietary management, and keeping the foaling area and mare as clean as possible during the perinatal period. The *C perfringens* type C and D toxoid and antitoxin are not approved for use in horses; however, these products have been used by some owners because of the high mortality rate in foals with clostridial enterocolitis on problem farms. Adverse reactions to the *C perfringens* type C and D toxoid have been reported in broodmares.

COLITIS-X

This peracute, fatal disease of horses is characterized by sudden onset of profuse, watery diarrhea and development of hypovolemic shock. Many affected horses have a history of stress. The cause of colitis-X is unknown, although multiple causes have been proposed, including peracute salmonellosis, clostridial enterocolitis, and endotoxemia.

Clinically, there may be a short febrile period, but body temperature soon returns to normal or subnormal. Tachypnea, tachycardia, and marked depression are present. An explosive diarrhea develops, followed by extreme dehydration. Hypovolemic and endotoxic shock are manifest by poor capillary refill time, purplish mucous membranes, and cold extremities. Death may occur within 3 hr of onset of clinical signs. In less acute cases, death occurs within 24-48 hr. The mortality rate approaches 100%. At necropsy, edema and hemorrhage in the wall of the large colon and cecum are pronounced, and the intestinal contents are fluid and often blood-stained.

Typically, the PCV is >65% even shortly after the onset of clinical signs. The leukogram ranges from normal to neutropenia with a degenerative left shift. Metabolic acidosis and electrolyte disorders are also present.

Disease onset is often closely associated with stress, eg, surgery or transport. Signs are similar to those of other diarrheal diseases, including peracute salmonellosis, toxemia caused by *Clostridium* spp, Potomac horse fever, experimental endotoxic shock, and anaphylaxis. A similar condition may be seen after administration of tetracycline or lincomycin to horses. Colitis-X is the term reserved for those cases in which no definitive diagnosis can be made and the horse dies.

Treatment for colitis-X usually is not effective but would be similar to that for salmonellosis (*see* p 156). Large volumes of IV fluids are needed to counter the severe dehydration, and electrolyte replacement is often necessary. Flunixin meglumine may help block the effects of toxemia.

PARASITISM

Both large and small strongyles have been incriminated as a cause of chronic diarrhea in horses and foals. The condition associated with small strongyles in horses is termed cyathomostomiasis and has been reported to result in recurrent colic, diarrhea, and weight loss. (*See* GASTROINTESTINAL PARASITES OF HORSES, p 265.)

Giardiasis (p 171) has been reported in a limited number of cases as a cause of intermittent diarrhea in horses. Cryptosporidia (p 168) have been identified in the feces of both healthy and diarrheic foals. There is evidence that *Cryptosporidium* spp can cause diarrhea and even death in immunocompetent foals; they have been described as a cause of outbreaks of foal diarrhea on some farms.

SAND ENTEROCOLOPATHY

Consumption of large amounts of sand, which then accumulates in the large intestine, can produce diarrhea, weight loss, or colic. Sand is ingested when the horse or foal is kept on sandy pasture or is fed hay or grain in a sandy area (paddock, stall, or pasture). Some horses or foals preferentially eat dirt and sand if it is in their environment. A diagnosis is based on history of a sandy environment, the presence of sand in the feces, "sand sounds" on auscultation of the ventral abdomen, and (if available) abdominal radiographs that reveal the presence of sand in the large colon. Treatment involves use of a hemicellulose product (psyllium seed hull) administered via nasogastric tube or added to the grain daily. Diarrhea generally resolves within 2-3 days of initiation of treatment. Generally, 3-4 wk of treatment is necessary to remove all the sand and may need to be repeated if the horse or foal is not removed from the source of sand. Preventive psyllium treatment (daily for 1 wk each month) has been used where sand enterocolitis is common. There are several psyllium products on the market; many horses prefer the pelleted over the powdered form. (*See also* p 215.)

RECURRENT DIARRHEA

Some horses develop semiformed feces when first introduced to lush pastures, alfalfa hay, or a temporarily stressful situation (eg, trailer ride, racing, showing, visit to a veterinary hospital). This change in fecal consistency is not of medical significance as long as the horse is healthy in all other regards, but owners may be concerned. It is important that horses with diarrhea have a physical examination and appropriate laboratory tests to rule out infectious causes and to determine whether treatment is required. Usually, the fecal consistency returns to normal when the horse adapts to its new diet or the stressful situation resolves.

INFILTRATIVE COLONIC DISEASE

Any process that causes a thickening of the wall of the large colon may interfere with absorption of fluid and result in chronic diarrhea, weight loss, and sometimes hypoproteinemia. Thickening may be due to neoplasia, inflammatory cells (such as lymphocytes, plasma cells, macrophages, or eosinophils), or scar formation from previous acute colitis. Rectal palpation may help detect bowel thickening and mesenteric lymphadenopathy. Abdominal fluid cytology may reveal neoplastic cells. Ultrasonography can be used to determine the degree of thickening of the bowel wall (if the affected area of bowel can be imaged) and may reveal masses in the liver or spleen or on the peritoneal surfaces; a percutaneous biopsy could provide a histopathologic diagnosis of neoplasia or inflammatory cell infiltrate. A biopsy of the rectal mucosa may be beneficial in diagnosis of inflammatory bowel disease but is not without risk to the horse. A surgically obtained colonic biopsy is more reliable for diagnosis of inflammatory bowel disease (p 243) but is more expensive and involves risks of general anesthesia and poor postoperative healing.

Treatment of abdominal neoplasia or inflammatory bowel disease is generally unrewarding and seldom undertaken. However, improvement of clinical signs and laboratory parameters with high-dose dexamethasone (0.1 mg/kg, SID) treatment has been reported in 3 horses with clinical signs of alimentary tract lymphoma of T-cell origin. In 2 horses, the high-dose dexamethasone was followed by a lower dosage (0.01-0.95 mg/kg, SID) once clinical improvement occurred. Favorable responses persisted for >9 mo. The third horse had to be maintained on the higher dose of dexamethasone throughout treatment, as signs recurred whenever the dose was lowered. Clinical signs recurred despite high doses of dexamethasone, and after 2 mo of treatment the horse was euthanized. The mechanism of action of the steroid is speculated to be control of inflammation associated with the condition, as opposed to glucocorticoid-induced apoptosis.

MISCELLANEOUS CAUSES OF DIARRHEA

Other causes of diarrhea or semiformed to watery feces in horses include grain overload, thromboembolic disease of the colon, peritonitis, antibiotic treatment, renal failure, numerous toxicoses (eg, blister beetles [cantharidin], salt poisoning, slaframine, amitraz, propylene glycol, phosphorus, selenium, nicotine, reserpine, arsenic, mercury, monensin, organophosphates, oleander, Japanese yew, castor bean, avocado, thorn apple, potatoes, heath, algae, acorn or oak, *Hypericum*, corn cockle, mycotoxicoses, and horse tail [scouring rush]), hyperlipidosis, and resolving impaction of the large intestine.

DIARRHEAL DISEASE IN FOALS

Foal Heat Diarrhea: From 4 to 14 days after birth, foals often develop a mild, self-limiting diarrhea. During this time, the dam is usually undergoing her first estrous cycle, hence the name "foal heat diarrhea." Although the cause is unknown, it may be associated with alterations in the foal's intestinal microbial flora or alteration in diet as the foal begins to eat small amounts of hay and grain.

The foal remains active and alert and has a normal appetite. Vital signs remain normal. Feces are semiformed to watery and not malodorous. Monitoring is important to ensure the foal's condition does not deteriorate. Specific treatment is usually not necessary, but application of a protectant to the skin around the perineum helps prevent scalding of the buttocks.

Bacterial Diarrhea in Foals: Bacterial enterocolitis in neonatal foals can be a component of neonatal septicemia. Organisms that may be involved in diarrhea in neonatal foals include *Salmonella* spp, *Escherichia coli*, *Klebsiella* spp, and *Clostridium* spp. Intensive antimicrobial treatment, correction of fluid loss and electrolyte abnormalities, and nursing care are needed. Foals should be evaluated to determine if adequate passive transfer of colostral antibodies has occurred; if not, a plasma transfusion is indicated. (*See also* SEPTICEMIA IN FOALS, p 567.) Markedly hypoproteinemic foals will benefit from plasma transfusion and/or the administration of a plasma substitute such as hetastarch for the improvement of oncotic pressure. IV fluid treatment without correction of the severe hypoproteinemia may induce pulmonary or peripheral edema.

An acute, fulminant, hemorrhagic diarrhea syndrome with high mortality in young foals <3 days old has been associated with *Clostridium perfringens* type C infection (p 237). Enterocolitis has also been associated with *C perfringens* type A with or without b2 toxin gene. The significance of this association is less clear than with type C, as type A has been identified in the feces of >90% of healthy neonatal foals in a farm-based study. It is possible that the number of bacteria and the phase of growth predispose to disease from type A. Infections may be sporadic or be seen as outbreaks in multiple foals on a farm. Severe lethargy and rapid deterioration of cardiovascular status is followed by death in 24-48 hr in most cases. Intraluminal hemorrhage and extensive mucosal necrosis of the small intestine and, in some cases, the colon are found on necropsy.

Other bacteria that have been associated with diarrhea in foals are *Bacteroides fragilis*, *Clostridium difficile*, *Aeromonas hydrophila*, and *Rhodococcus (Corynebacterium) equi*. The first 3 are seen in foals <2 wk old, and infected foals require intensive supportive care. Although *R equi* primarily causes respiratory disease (p 1209), both acute and chronic enteritis can be seen; diarrhea is seen in foals 1-4 mo old. The diagnosis is more straightforward if pneumonia is also present. When cultured from tracheal wash fluid, *R equi* is considered a pathogen; however, a positive fecal culture is not as helpful because *R equi* can be found in the feces of healthy foals. Erythromycin combined with rifampin is the treatment of choice for *R equi* infection in foals.

Enteric infection with *Lawsonia intracellularis* has been associated with outbreaks of diarrhea, rapid weight loss, colic, subcutaneous edema, and protein-losing enteropathy in weanling foals on breeding farms in Canada and the USA. Several foals on affected farms died of the disease prior to identification of the cause. Marked hypoproteinemia was noted along with increased creatine kinase, anemia, hyponatremia, and leukocytosis in some foals. A diagnosis was made at necropsy when the characteristic intracellular bacteria were seen in silver-stained tissues. *L intracellularis* can be confirmed using PCR analysis and immunohistochemistry on tissues collected at necropsy. Serology can be used to detect antibodies to *L intracellularis*, but discrimination of infected from exposed foals is uncertain. Thus, PCR and special stains of tissues acquired at necropsy remain the only definitive methods of diagnosis. Treatment with oxytetracycline (6.6 mg/kg, IV, BID for 3-5 days), followed by doxycycline (10 mg/kg, BID for 14 days) has been successful. Because it is difficult to make an antemortem diagnosis, some clinicians initiate treatment for *L intracellularis* in foals when other causes of diarrhea have been ruled out and there is serologic evidence of exposure to this agent. Response to treatment is considered confirmation of the diagnosis.

Viral Diarrhea in Foals: Viruses appear to cause diarrhea in foals but not in adult horses. Rotavirus is the main cause of viral diarrhea in foals; however, other viruses (eg, coronavirus) have been implicated. Diarrhea induced by rotavirus is characterized by depression, anorexia, and profuse, watery, malodorous feces. It is usually seen in foals <2 mo old; younger foals typically have more severe clinical signs. The diarrhea usually lasts 4-7 days, although it can persist for weeks.

Rotavirus destroys the enterocytes on the tip of the villi in the small intestine, which results in malabsorption. Lactase becomes deficient, so lactose passing into the large intestine induces an osmotic diarrhea. Diagnosis is made by identification of virus in the feces; several test methods are available. Requesting that the laboratory test specifically for rotavirus, collecting feces early in the course of disease, and sampling several foals improve the chances of viral detection.

Treatment is generally supportive. Certain farm management practices and disinfection techniques have effectively limited the spread of rotavirus during outbreaks. Sick foals are highly contagious and should be isolated in the stall in the barn in which the foal originally became ill or moved to a designated isolation facility. Personnel should wear disposable gloves and cleanable boots and wash their hands with soap before and after handling diarrheic foals. Foot dips containing phenolic disinfectants outside the stalls of sick foals should also be used. Specific stall-cleaning equipment should be designated only for cleaning the stalls of diarrheic foals. Once the stall has been vacated, it should be cleaned of particulate material, washed with detergent, and then disinfected with phenolic compounds that meet EPA standards. Bleach, chlorhexidine, and quaternary compounds do not appear to be effective disinfectants for rotavirus. Fecal material of sick foals removed from stalls should not be spread on pastures that are used for horses and foals, and care should be taken to avoid fecal contamination of alleyways. All stall-cleaning equipment should be disinfected. Stalls with dirt floors are difficult to adequately clean and disinfect. Removal of the top layers of dirt may be required.

Arriving horses and foals, including those returning from veterinary hospitals, should be isolated for ≥7 days before being introduced to the resident population. A vaccine for pregnant mares to induce colostral antibodies directed at reducing the risk of rotavirus infection in their foals is available.

Miscellaneous Causes of Diarrhea in Foals: Nutritional diarrhea can result from overfeeding (eg, when a foal is reunited with the mare after a period of separation) and improper nutrition (eg, orphan foals being fed calf milk replacer or sucrose). Lactose intolerance in foals is rare and can be determined by lactose tolerance challenge tests. Diarrhea can also develop when foals consume indigestible substances such as roughage, sand, dirt, and rocks. Diarrhea in foals has been reported to be associated with infection by *Strongyloides westeri*, *Parascaris equorum*, and *Cryptosporidium* spp. (*See* GASTROINTESTINAL PARASITES OF HORSES, p 265.)

WEIGHT LOSS AND HYPOPROTEINEMIA

The causes for weight loss in horses are numerous and can involve many body systems. This discussion is confined to diseases of the GI tract. Protein loss may or may not be associated with weight loss. The disorders commonly associated with either of these signs are neoplasia, inflammatory bowel disease, and toxicosis from treatment with NSAID.

GASTROINTESTINAL NEOPLASIA

Squamous cell carcinoma of the stomach and the alimentary form of lymphosarcoma are the most common forms of neoplasia involving the GI tract in horses. Chronic weight loss may be the primary clinical sign. Chronic diarrhea and hypoalbuminemia may develop when lymphosarcoma has infiltrated the wall of the intestine.

Because the incidence of GI neoplasia is low, other causes of weight loss should be investigated first. Diagnosis is usually made by exclusion of other causes of weight loss and by histopathologic examination of the tissue collected during exploratory surgery or at necropsy. Squamous cell carcinoma of the stomach can be diagnosed by gastroscopy. An endoscope 2-3 m long is necessary to examine the gastric mucosa of adult horses. In horses with lymphosarcoma, enlarged mesenteric lymph nodes or thickened bowel may be detected by rectal palpation or by ultrasonographic examination. Occasionally, neoplastic cells are identified by cytologic examination of abdominal fluid. Ultrasonography may reveal masses in the liver or spleen as well as facilitate percutaneous biopsy of the masses. An exploratory laparotomy with biopsy of intestinal or other masses can provide a definitive diagnosis.

Treatment of GI neoplasia in horses is generally not attempted, and the prognosis is grave. There have been a few reports of surgical removal of the affected segment of bowel.

INFLAMMATORY BOWEL DISEASE
(Granulomatous enteritis, Chronic eosinophilic gastroenteritis, Plasmacytic-lymphocytic enteritis)

This disease is characterized by infiltration of the small and large intestine and regional lymph nodes with inflammatory cells, including lymphocytes, plasma cells, macrophages, and eosinophils. The inflammatory condition may be limited to only a short segment of the bowel or be more diffuse. Malabsorption and a protein-losing enterocolopathy result. Diarrhea may or may not be a clinical feature. Inflammatory bowel disease should be considered in the differential diagnosis of horses with weight loss, recurrent colic, or hypoproteinemia as well as in some horses with generalized skin disease.

Diagnosis is based on clinical signs, the presence of thickened bowel or enlarged mesenteric lymph nodes on rectal palpation, low serum protein concentration, and intestinal or rectal biopsy. Failure to absorb oral glucose or D-xylose verifies malabsorption from the small intestine. The pathophysiology is not understood. An altered immune response to a common intestinal factor (eg, feed, parasites, bacteria) has been suggested.

Various medical treatments have been tried with limited success. Corticosteroids, dietary alterations, metronidazole, and the antimetabolite azathioprine have been used. Supportive nutritional care should involve frequent feeding of good-quality, high-energy feeds. The prognosis is grave. If only a limited and accessible section of the bowel is affected, surgical removal may be successful.

NONSTEROIDAL ANTI-INFLAMMATORY DRUG TOXICOSIS

Phenylbutazone administered at high doses or for prolonged periods can cause a protein-losing enterocolopathy in horses. Clinical signs include oral ulceration, anorexia, lethargy, weight loss, diarrhea, colic, and ventral edema. Toxicosis can develop from oral or parenteral administration of NSAID. Hypoproteinemia is seen due to loss of protein into the intestinal lumen, which can occur without visible ulceration. Gastric and colonic ulceration are potential sequelae of phenylbutazone toxicosis. Scarring of the right dorsal colon with subsequent recurrent colic and hypoproteinemia is also a sequela. Renal papillary necrosis may be seen. Administration of flunixin meglumine at high doses or for prolonged periods can result in a similar toxicosis.

A tentative diagnosis can be made based on the history of NSAID administration, clinical signs, and presence of hypoproteinemia. Gastric ulceration can be confirmed by gastroscopy but requires an endoscope 2-3 m long.

Treatment includes discontinuing use of phenylbutazone or any other NSAID. Reducing production of gastric acid with cimetidine, ranitidine, or omeprazole may be beneficial; sucralfate may be indicated as well. Surgery may be required if scarring of the bowel has resulted in partial obstruction of the intestine.

SMALL-INTESTINAL FIBROSIS

Extensive fibrosis of the submucosa of the small intestine has been associated with weight loss and recurrent colic in adult horses on pasture in northern Colorado. All affected horses died or were euthanized due to their deteriorating condition. The cause is unknown.

INTESTINAL DISEASES IN PIGS

Pigs of all ages are susceptible to intestinal diseases, and diarrhea is the sign common to nearly all such disorders. Transmission of infectious agents that cause enteropathies is by the fecal-oral route. At least 12 different etiologic agents, including bacteria, viruses, and parasites, can cause primary intestinal disease. Diarrhea in a herd may be due to a single agent, but concurrent infections are common. Because some diseases are age-dependent, differential diagnosis is best considered by age group (TABLE 6).

TABLE 6.   Age Distribution of Diarrheal Diseases in Pigs

	Age Group		
	Nursing	Weaning	Growing-finishing or Breeding
Bacterial Diseases			
Clostridium difficile	+++	+	+
C perfringens type C enteritis	++	–	–
Enteric colibacillosis	+++	+++	–
Intestinal spirochetosis	–	++	+++
Porcine proliferative enteritis	–	++	+++
Salmonella enteritis	+	++	+++
Swine dysentery	+	+	+++
Parasitism			
Cryptosporidium sp	+	+	–
Isospora suis	+++	+	–
Strongyloides ransomi	+	+	+
Trichuris suis	–	–	++
Viral Diseases			
Porcine epidemic diarrhea	+	++	+++
Rotaviral enteritis	+++	+++	+
Transmissible gastroenteritis	+++	+++	++

– Rare or does not occur
+ Uncommon
++ Common
+++ Very common

CLOSTRIDIUM DIFFICILE DISEASE

C difficile is an important emerging pathogen that causes diarrhea primarily in neonatal swine. The agent was first recognized as a cause of antibiotic-associated diarrhea in humans. It most commonly causes disease in piglets 1-7 days old and in other domestic and laboratory animals.

Etiology and Pathogenesis: *C difficile* is an anaerobic, gram-positive, sporeforming rod that is more oxygen-sensitive than *C perfringens*. The organism can be demonstrated in the intestine by direct Gram's stain of smears. Survival of *C difficile* in the environment and shedding by carrier sows is believed to be important in transmission. *C difficile* produces "large clostridial toxins" A and B, which are thought to be involved in lesion production. Toxin A is an enterotoxin that causes fluid secretion into the gut lumen, and toxin B is a cytotoxin.

Clinical Findings: Affected piglets may have dyspnea, abdominal distention, and scrotal edema. Diarrhea may not be present in all pigs affected.
Lesions: Ascites, hydrothorax, and edema of the ascending colon have been reported. Urates are commonly present in the kidneys. Pasty to watery colonic contents may be observed. Microscopically, the colon is primarily affected with multifocal exudation of mucus and fibrin plus submucosal edema.

Diagnosis: Gross lesions are not pathognomonic, and diagnosis must be confirmed by culture or demonstration of either toxin A or B and histopathology. *C difficile* can be cultured on selective medium containing cefoxitin, cycloserine, taurocholate, and fructose under anaerobic conditions. The genes of toxins A and B are identified readily by PCR. The toxins can also be detected directly in suspensions of intestinal contents by commercially available enzyme immunoassays.

Treatment and Control: Based on minimum inhibitory concentration determinations, it has been suggested that erythromycin, tetracycline, and tylosin may be useful for treatment of suckling piglets, and tiamulin and virginiamycin may be helpful in reducing levels of the organism in adult swine. No controlled studies on the effect of antibiotics on clinical disease have been reported.

CLOSTRIDIUM PERFRINGENS TYPE C ENTERITIS

Infection of the small intestine by type C strains of *C perfringens* causes a highly fatal, necrohemorrhagic enteritis. It most commonly affects piglets 1-5 days old but may be seen in pigs up to 3 wk old (and in other species, *see also* p 493).

Etiology and Pathogenesis: The organism penetrates between the absorptive cells of the upper jejunum and elaborates β toxin, a potent, heat-labile, trypsin-sensitive exotoxin that causes necrosis of all structural components of the villi. Necrotizing inflammation usually extends to the mucosal crypts. The infection may continue caudally and involve the ileum, but it rarely affects the colon. Necrosis of the mucosa is accompanied by blood loss into the intestinal wall and lumen.

Clinical Findings: Sudden onset of hemorrhagic diarrhea followed by collapse and death is characteristic in piglets 1-3 days old. In less acute cases, brownish liquid feces develop at 3-5 days. Infrequently, pigs develop a persistent, pasty, gray diarrhea and become progressively emaciated. In peracute cases, the perineal region is blood stained.
Lesions: The small intestines are dark red, hemorrhagic, and filled with hemorrhagic liquid. Less acute cases at 3-5 days may have gas bubbles in the wall of the jejunum and necrosis of the mucosa of the jejunum and ileum. More chronic cases have a thickened small intestine that is lined by a pale yellow or gray necrotic membrane tightly adhered to the submucosa.

Diagnosis: Necropsy is usually sufficient to establish the diagnosis in the peracute hemorrhagic form and in the acute form with jejunal emphysema. A rapid presumptive diagnosis can be made by demonstrating large rod-shaped bacteria in gram-stained mucosal impression smears. Histologic demonstration of villous necrosis with mucosal colonization by numerous large gram-positive rods is adequate for confirmation. Subacute and chronic forms of the disease in pigs 6-14 days old are easily confused at necropsy with *Isospora suis* enteritis, but diagnosis is usually possible by histologic examination of the jejunum and ileum or by observing clostridia in mucosal smears stained with Gram's or Giemsa stain. Isolates of *C perfringens* may be genotyped for the presence of genes that code for β toxin.

Treatment and Control: Treatment of pigs with clinical signs is of little benefit because lesions usually are irreversible at the onset of diarrhea. In an acute outbreak, prophylactic administration of type C antitoxin or antibiotic (or both) parenterally or PO is protective if given to piglets within 2 hr of birth. The disease tends to recur on infected premises. Vaccination of gestating sows at 6 and 3 wk before parturition with type C bacterin-toxoid confers some passive lactogenic immunity to subsequent litters, provided piglets consume colostrum soon after birth. Once immunized with 2 doses of bacterin-toxoid, sows should receive one dose ~3 wk before each subsequent farrowing.

EDEMA DISEASE
(Escherichia coli enterotoxemia)

Edema disease is an acute, highly fatal, neurologic disorder that usually is seen 5 days to 2 wk after weaning and may be accompanied by diarrhea. (*See* p 573.)

ENTERIC COLIBACILLOSIS

Enteric colibacillosis is a common disease of nursing and weanling pigs caused by colonization of the small intestine by enterotoxigenic strains of *Escherichia coli.*

Etiology and Pathogenesis: Certain strains of *E coli* possess fimbria or pili that allow them to adhere to or colonize the absorptive epithelial cells of the jejunum and ileum. The common antigenic types of pili associated with pathogenicity are K88, K99, 987P, and F41. Pathogenic strains produce enterotoxins that cause fluid and electrolytes to be secreted into the intestinal lumen, which results in diarrhea, dehydration, and acidosis. Infection in neonates is commonly caused by K88 and 987P strains, whereas postweaning colibacillosis is nearly always due to the K88 strain.

Clinical Findings: Profuse watery diarrhea with rapid dehydration, acidosis, and death is common. Rarely, pigs may collapse and die before diarrhea begins.

Lesions: Dehydration and distention of the small intestine with yellowish, slightly mucoid fluid is characteristic. The colon contains similar fluid. The fundic portion of the gastric mucosa is often reddened. Pigs dying suddenly may have patchy cutaneous erythema. Histologically, the villi are usually of normal length and have many small bacterial rods adhered to the absorptive enterocytes.

Diagnosis: Confirmation is based on histologic observation of villous colonization; demonstration of K88, K99, 987P, or F41 pilus antigens in intestinal scrapings by immunofluorescence or other immunologic procedures; and isolation of the organism from the small intestine. Because *E coli* is a common secondary agent, the possibility of involvement of other agents such as viruses or coccidia should be considered.

Treatment and Control: Therapy includes prompt treatment with antibacterials and restoration of fluid and electrolyte balance. Bacterial antibiotic sensitivity testing is helpful to identify effective medication. Prevention includes reducing predisposing factors, such as dampness and chilling; improving sanitation, such as by replacing solid or slatted concrete flooring with wire-mesh flooring; and vaccinating gestating sows with pilus-specific vaccines. Pigs lacking receptors for K88 have been shown to be resistant to disease caused by enterotoxin-positive K88-positive *E coli.*

HEMORRHAGIC BOWEL SYNDROME
(Mesenteric torsion of the small intestine)

Hemorrhagic bowel syndrome affects rapidly growing swine 4-6 mo of age. Pigs die suddenly without evidence of diarrhea, but the small intestine is thin walled on necropsy and filled with either clotted or unclotted blood. The large intestine usually contains tarry fecal material but no lesions suggestive of swine dysentery, salmonellosis, proliferative enteritis, or intestinal spirochetosis. The condition can be prevented by the administration of either bacitracin or chlortetracycline in the feed. When performing a necropsy, the mesenteric root should be palpated prior to opening the abdomen. A peracute form of proliferative enteritis may have similar clinical and gross lesions; however, histology and culture of the intestine will discern the presence or absence of epithelial proliferation and *Lawsonia intracellularis*.

The cause in most cases is believed due to intestinal volvulus. Predisposing factors may include vigorous exercise, handling, fighting, piling, or irregular feeding. Long-loined pigs may be more likely to develop mesenteric torsion than shorter pigs. Rotation of the entire intestine, including the posterior part of the duodenum and the anterior part of the rectum, around the root of the mesentery obstructs venous outflow of blood, which causes blood to pool and stagnate in the intestine and soon results in infarction. Rotation may be only partial and difficult to demonstrate at necropsy, which makes diagnosis more challenging.

INTESTINAL SALMONELLOSIS

Enteropathogenic salmonellae cause inflammation and necrosis of the small and large intestines, resulting in diarrhea that may be accompanied by generalized sepsis. All ages are susceptible, but the disease is most common in weaned and growing-finishing pigs.

Etiology and Pathogenesis: *Salmonella choleraesuis kuzendorf (S choleraesuis)* is one of the most common salmonella species affecting pigs. It sometimes produces necrotizing enterocolitis but far more common is a septicemic disease characterized by hepatitis, pneumonia, and cerebral vasculitis. *S typhisuis* infection of the intestine results in necrotizing, nonsuppurative inflammation of the mucosa and submucosa of the ileum, cecum, and colon; frequently, the mucosa is ulcerative. Usually, there is extension to regional lymph nodes and, occasionally, generalized septicemia. Sources of infection for *S choleraesuis* and *S typhisuis* are primarily asymptomatic carrier pigs but also may include rodents and contaminated feed and premises. (*See also* SALMONELLOSIS, p 156.)

Numerous other serotypes of salmonellae are seen in pigs, some of which have been associated with human foodborne illness. Common serotypes seen in pigs are *S typhimurium, S Heidelberg, S Worthington*, and *S infantis*. These serotypes may cause mild to moderate diarrhea in swine and may be resistant to multiple drugs.

Clinical Findings: Nursing pigs may develop diarrhea but usually succumb to generalized septicemia. Weaning or growing-finishing pigs are febrile and have liquid feces that may be yellow and contain shreds of necrotic debris.

Lesions: Pigs infected with *S choleraesuis* have an inflamed, slightly thickened ileum and colon, usually with necrotic debris on the mucosal surface. Mesenteric lymph nodes are enlarged, edematous, and sometimes red. Mucosal ulceration may or may not be evident. A small amount of hemorrhage may be seen in acute cases. Occasionally, rectal strictures (p 151) may develop. Other enteropathogenic salmonellae, except for *S typhisuis*, produce lesions similar to but less severe than those of *S choleraesuis*. Lesions of *S typhisuis* enteritis are distinctive, typically yellow, round (button) ulcers in the colon, cecum, and less commonly the ileum.

Diagnosis: Culture of feces or intestinal mucosa in a selective medium may yield the organism. However, salmonellae often are isolated (and more reliably) from enlarged mesenteric lymph nodes by direct streaking on selective medium such as brilliant green agar or by inoculation of enrichment media. Histologic examination of affected intestine and liver to differentiate salmonellosis from proliferative enteritis and swine dysentery is a valuable adjunct procedure.

Treatment and Control: Live avirulent vaccines administered either intranasally or via the water are very efficacious for the prevention of disease caused by *S choleraesuis*. Avirulent vaccines may also be effective in reducing levels of salmonellae in the tissues of swine at slaughter. Parenteral administration of antibacterials to acutely ill pigs and medication of the affected group via water or feed may decrease the severity of the outbreak. Neomycin and lincomycin-spectinomycin are the most often used water medications. Carbodox in the feed is often used as a preventive. Susceptibility testing of the isolated organism is useful in selecting an appropriate antibacterial. Thorough cleaning and disinfection of contaminated facilities and elimination of the source of the organism decrease the likelihood of repeated epidemics.

INTESTINAL SPIROCHETOSIS

Intestinal spirochetosis is a disease of the large intestine seen in the absence of *Brachyspira hyodysenteriae*. (*See* SWINE DYSENTERY, p 252.) This disease syndrome is being recognized more frequently worldwide.

Etiology and Pathogenesis: The primary cause of intestinal spirochetosis is *B pilosicoli*. There have been reports of other *Brachyspira* being associated with the condition, but recent molecular characterizations indicate that *B innocens*, *B murdochi*, and *B intermedia* are likely nonpathogens. *B pilosicoli* is emerging as a significant pathogen of humans, especially in indigenous populations, homosexuals, and immunosuppressed patients. The organism is transmitted orally and survives extremely well in the environment. *B pilosicoli* has been isolated from a wide variety of animals including waterbirds, rodents, and dogs. It has been shown to cause diarrheal disease in pigs, chickens, and humans by experimental inoculation and in natural occurrence. The pathogenesis is not well studied, but apparently the end-on attachment of the spirochete to the mucosal surface interferes with the absorptive capacity of the colon, resulting in diarrhea.

Clinical Findings: Pigs initially have sticky feces on the perineum. The feces will appear as wet cement, and a mild diarrhea may result. Affected pigs may be inappetent and grow slowly.

Lesions: The lesions in the large intestine are milder than those caused by *B hyodysenteriae* in swine dysentery. The volume of the large intestine may be increased and distended with thickening of the mucosa. In some pigs, a mucohemorrhagic colitis develops in association with enlarged mesenteric lymph nodes. Microscopically, spirochetes may be seen attached end-on to the mucosal surface and give the appearance of a false brush border. The mucosal surface has focal erosions with mild catarrhal exudate. Colonic crypts are often dilated containing numerous spirochetes.

Diagnosis: Important differential diagnoses include salmonellosis, proliferative enteritis, swine dysentery, and whipworm infection. *B pilosicoli* can be isolated on selective agar containing spectinomycin under anaerobic conditions. Biochemical tests and preferably PCR should be performed on *Brachyspira* isolates to confirm species identification.

Treatment and Control: Treatment and prevention of intestinal spirochetosis is similar to that of swine dysentery. Drugs such as tiamulin, lincomycin, and carbadox are effective. It is unknown if the agent can be eradicated without total depopulation as in swine dysentery, but due to the reservoir hosts and environmental survival it is doubtful.

PARASITISM

See also p 270 and p 163.

Ascaris suum is the most common intestinal nematode of pigs. Adults in the intestine reduce feed efficiency, and heavy infections cause emaciation. Larval migration incites inflammation in the liver and lungs.

Cryptosporidium sp is a coccidium that attaches to the mucosal epithelium of the intestine of pigs ≥10 days old. It causes villous atrophy in the lower small intestine. Malabsorption and diarrhea may result.

Eimeria spp are common in pigs, but overt disease is seldom seen. Heavy infections may cause significant enterocolitis in young growing pigs.

Hyostrongylus rubidus is the common stomach worm found in pasture-raised pigs. It usually causes little harm.

Isospora suis is a common and important cause of coccidiosis in pigs 6 days to 3 wk old. Infection causes necrosis and villous atrophy of the ileum and jejunum. Secondary bacterial infection of the injured intestinal mucosa is common. Mortality often is 20-25%, and many pigs are stunted. Diagnosis can be based on identification of immature coccidial forms in the intestinal mucosa by direct mucosal smear stained with Giemsa stain or by histologic examination of the affected intestine. Successful prevention most commonly depends on thorough cleaning of farrowing facilities to minimize the number of oocysts. After cleaning, thorough disinfection with 50% bleach has been useful. Coccidiostats are sometimes fed to sows 2 wk before farrowing or administered PO to pigs from birth to 3 wk of age.

Adult nodular worms of *Oesophagostomum* spp in the large intestine cause little harm, but heavy infection by larvae encysted in the intestinal wall may lead to emaciation.

Strongyloides ransomi (intestinal threadworm) larvae can be transmitted via colostrum or acquired from contaminated skin of the dam. Heavily infected piglets develop severe diarrhea when 10-14 days old, with high mortality. Diagnosis is based on direct microscopical observation of mucosal scrapings.

Trichuris suis (whipworms) penetrate the mucosa of the cecum and colon and cause multifocal inflammation. Heavy infections cause diarrhea and emaciation. The feces are hemorrhagic; therefore, heavy whipworm infections may be confused clinically with swine dysentery or proliferative enteritis. Diagnosis is based on direct observation of whipworms in the large intestine or on fecal flotation.

PORCINE EPIDEMIC DIARRHEA

This coronaviral diarrhea (not yet recognized in the western hemisphere) affects pigs of all ages and clinically resembles transmissible gastroenteritis (TGE, p 253) in several respects.

Etiology and Epidemiology: The porcine epidemic diarrhea (PED) virus is not related to any other member of the Coronaviridae. Pigs are the only known host. Antibodies to the virus have not been found in wild pigs or in other animal species. Infections have been seen in most European countries and in China. Large epidemics occurred in Europe in 1969; no antibodies have been found in sera collected before 1969. Since then, the virus has become widespread and endemic in several European countries, and acute outbreaks have become rare. On large breeding farms, the virus persists in consecutive litters of pigs after weaning and after they lose their immunity from antibody in the milk. On these farms, the virus may be associated with weaning diarrhea. In Belgium, the virus is most frequently associated with diarrhea in feeder pigs, which develops shortly after they are gathered from different breeding farms and assembled in large fattening units. The virus was demonstrated in fecal material in 80% of these groups. Epidemiologic data from other countries are scarce. Spread of the virus mainly occurs directly through infected pigs and indirectly through virus-contaminated fomites and via transport trucks.

Pathogenesis: The pathogenesis and immune mechanisms are similar to those reported for TGE. Oral infection results in viral replication in the epithelial cells of the small intestinal villi. Cells on colonic villi also become infected. No other tissue tropisms have been shown. Virus is excreted in the feces.

Clinical Findings: Diarrhea is the only direct virus-induced clinical sign observed. An acute outbreak on a susceptible breeding farm resembles a TGE outbreak and is characterized by watery diarrhea in pigs of all ages. However, as compared with TGE, the incubation period is longer (3-4 days), not all the litters of suckling pigs may become sick, and mortality in neonatal pigs is lower (average 50%). Also, the disease within the farm spreads more slowly. In all outbreaks, signs are most consistently seen in feeders, finishers, and adults, which appear to be most susceptible because outbreaks often start in these age groups. Older pigs are more lethargic and depressed with PED than with TGE. Sick pigs appear to have colic.

Acute outbreaks in susceptible finishing pigs are characterized by watery diarrhea, but a markedly increased number of acute deaths may be seen, particularly in pigs infected toward the end of the finishing period and in stress-sensitive breeds. Death may even occur during the incubation period.

Lesions: Macroscopic lesions are confined to the small intestine with villous shortening as the main characteristic. These lesions closely resemble those seen with TGE. No lesions have been described in the colon. A consistent finding is acute necrosis of back muscle.

Diagnosis: Clinical differentiation from TGE is difficult. TGE in its typical epidemic form causes a rapidly spreading diarrhea in animals of all ages with high mortality in neonates. With PED, the diarrhea spreads at a slower rate, and although diarrhea is seen in most of the litters, some litters may remain healthy even in the absence of immunity. Morbidity is 100% in older pigs, and they are severely sick. Acute deaths in adults and finishing pigs due to muscle necrosis and occurring during an outbreak of diarrhea are typical of PED and are not seen with any other infectious diarrhea.

Laboratory diagnosis in neonates is made by direct immunofluorescence on cryostat sections of small intestine or colon. ELISA to detect viral antigens in feces or intestinal contents is more useful for older pigs. Antibodies can be detected in paired serum samples through ELISA-blocking.

Control: No specific treatment is available. Measures taken during an outbreak are of a general nature. Pigs with diarrhea should have free access to water, and finishing pigs should have feed withheld for 1-2 days.

On breeding farms, in the face of an outbreak, spread of virus to the farrowing house can be prevented temporarily by sanitary measures and, if performed together with a deliberate infection of pregnant sows, losses in neonates may be lowered. No vaccine is available.

PORCINE PROLIFERATIVE ENTERITIS
(Porcine intestinal adenomatosis, Proliferative hemorrhagic enteropathy, Ileitis)

Porcine proliferative enteritis is a common diarrheal disease of growing-finishing and young breeding pigs characterized by hyperplasia and inflammation of the ileum and colon. It often is mild and self-limiting but sometimes causes persistent diarrhea, severe necrotic enteritis, or hemorrhagic enteritis with high mortality.

Etiology and Pathogenesis: The etiology is an intracellular gram-negative small rod-shaped bacterium called *Lawsonia intracellularis*. The organism has been cultivated only in cell cultures, and attempts to propagate it in cell-free medium have failed. Koch's postulates have been fulfilled by inoculation of pure cultures of *L intracellularis* into conventionally reared pigs; typical lesions of the disease were produced, and *L intracellularis* was reisolated from the lesions. Inoculation of *L intracellularis* into gnotobiotic pigs does not cause the disease; therefore, other factors in the conventionally reared pig may contribute to development of lesions.

Clinical Findings: The more common, nonhemorrhagic form of the disease often affects 40- to 80-lb (18- to 36-kg) pigs and is characterized by sudden onset of diarrhea. The feces are watery to pasty, brownish, or faintly blood stained. After ~2 days, pigs may pass yellow fibrinonecrotic casts that have formed in the ileum. Most affected pigs recover spontaneously, but a significant number develop chronic necrotic enteritis with progressive emaciation. The hemorrhagic form is characterized by cutaneous pallor, weakness, and passage of hemorrhagic or black, tarry feces. Pregnant gilts may abort.

Lesions: Lesions may be seen anywhere in the lower half of the small intestine, cecum, or colon but are most frequent and obvious in the ileum. The wall of the intestine is thickened, and the mesentery may be edematous. The mesenteric lymph nodes are enlarged. The intestinal mucosa appears thickened and rugose, may be covered with a brownish or yellow fibrinonecrotic membrane, and sometimes has petechial hemorrhages. Yellow necrotic casts may be found in the ileum or passing through the colon. Diffuse, complete mucosal necrosis in chronic cases causes the intestine to be rigid, resembling a garden hose. Proliferative mucosal lesions often are in the colon but are detected only by careful inspection at necropsy. In the profusely hemorrhagic form, there are red or black, tarry feces in the colon and clotted blood in the ileum.

Diagnosis: Confirmation is based on histologic observation of characteristic proliferation and inflammation of mucosal crypts. *L intracellularis* (comma-shaped, resembling *Campylobacter*) can usually be demonstrated by silver stains. A PCR test has been developed and is useful for confirmation of the presence of *L intracellularis* in lesions. Bacterial culture of intestine and lymph nodes to exclude *Salmonella* infection, together with histologic examination and culture of cecum and colon to exclude swine dysentery, are essential additional procedures. The colon also should be examined for whipworms. *L intracellularis* is present in most swine herds, so demonstration of the organism in feces by PCR or the presence of antibody in clinically normal pigs is of little diagnostic value.

Treatment and Control: Various antibacterials administered parenterally to acutely affected pigs and by feed or water to the remainder of the group help reduce severity of the enteritis and prevent development of chronic, irreversible, necrotic enteritis. Porcine proliferative enteritis is one of the first diseases to be seen in new herds established by surgical derivation. A live avirulent vaccine administered via the water is highly efficacious. It should be administered to gilts and boars during acclimatization prior to introduction into a herd.

RECTAL STRICTURES

In growing pigs, rectal strictures are sequelae of severely traumatized rectal prolapses (p 151) or of infections that interfere with rectal blood supply. The former cause sporadic cases; the latter may be epidemic. One cause is *Salmonella typhimurium* infection (p 247), which produces an ulcerative proctitis that heals in such a manner that normal function is not restored. The stricture is reportedly the result of fibrosis of the rectal tissue due to persistent ischemia caused by infection in an area of limited blood supply.

Clinical Findings: Several bloated pigs in varying stages of emaciation are generally observed in a group of growing pigs. Other clinical signs, including prior outbreaks of severe debilitating diarrhea, are common but not always reported. An index finger rarely can be passed into the rectum without considerable resistance.

Lesions: At necropsy the colon is grossly distended, and the intestine is filled with gas and green feces. The predominant lesion is a narrowed rectal canal, due to annular fibrotic ulcers or rectal strictures found 2-5 cm cranial to the anus.

Diagnosis: An epidemic of rectal strictures without prior rectal prolapses is indicative of *S typhimurium* infection. Culture of feces and regional lymph nodes usually yields *S typhimurium*. However, it is not possible to determine whether the lesion or the infection occurred first.

Treatment and Control: Early diagnosis and treatment of diarrhea is imperative for control. Good housing, management, and sanitation, with "all-in/all-out" movement of pigs is the best method to prevent further outbreaks. Surgery is not thought to be economically feasible.

ROTAVIRAL ENTERITIS

Rotaviral enteritis is a common disease of the small intestine of pigs. All ages are susceptible, but significant diarrheal disease usually is seen in nursing or postweaning pigs.

Etiology and Pathogenesis: The causal rotavirus infects and destroys villous enterocytes throughout the small intestine, but lesions are most severe in the middle third of the intestine. Loss of villous epithelium results in partial villous atrophy, malabsorption, and osmotic diarrhea. Multiple antigenic types of rotavirus affect pigs. They are easily spread by direct contact. Healthy carrier sows may be fecal shedders during the periparturient period, thereby exposing their litters to infection.

Clinical Findings: If neonatal pigs do not receive protective levels of maternal antibody, they are likely to develop profuse watery diarrhea in 12-48 hr. More commonly, the infection is endemic in a herd, and sows have varying levels of antibody in the colostrum and milk, which provide varying degrees of passive protection to nursing pigs. Diarrhea often begins in pigs 5 days to 3 wk old, or immediately after weaning. The feces of nursing pigs often are yellow or gray and pasty in the early stages and progress to gray and pasty after ~2 days. Diarrhea persists for 2-5 days. Diarrheic pigs become gaunt and rough-haired, but mortality usually is low. Weaned pigs have watery feces that contain poorly digested feed. Weaners become inappetent and noncompetitive, which results in emaciation, stunting, and probably predisposition to pneumonia and other diseases.

Lesions: The small intestine appears thin walled, and the cecum and colon contain liquid feces.

Diagnosis: Laboratory procedures are required. Confirmation is based on histologic demonstration of villous atrophy in the jejunum, electron microscopic demonstration of virions in the intestinal contents, and immunodiagnostic procedures to demonstrate viral antigen in the intestinal mucosa or feces. Differential diagnoses include endemic transmissible gastroenteritis, *Isospora suis* enteritis, and enteric colibacillosis.

Treatment and Control: There is no specific treatment. Minimizing heat loss and providing adequate water to maintain hydration are helpful. Vaccination of sows may be useful. Concurrent infection by enterotoxigenic *Escherichia coli* is common; therefore, antibiotic therapy may reduce mortality. Providing diarrheic weaned pigs with a warm, dry, draft-free environment and frequent limited feedings help prevent starvation, secondary diseases, and permanent stunting.

STREPTOCOCCUS DISPAR ENTERITIS

This diarrheal disease of nursing piglets usually 5-10 days old has been associated with colonization of the small intestine with *S dispar*. Diagnosis may be aided by observation of gram-positive cocci adhered to the villous epithelial cells. Antibacterials such as penicillin should be useful in treatment.

SWINE DYSENTERY
(Bloody scours)

Swine dysentery is a common, mucohemorrhagic diarrheal disease of pigs that affects the large intestine.

Etiology and Pathogenesis: The essential causal agent is *Brachyspira (Serpulina) hyodysenteriae*, an anaerobic spirochete that produces a hemolysin, although other organisms may contribute to the severity of lesions. It proliferates in the large intestine and causes degeneration and inflammation of the superficial mucosa, hypersecretion of mucus by mucosal epithelium, and multifocal bleeding points on the mucosal surface. The organism does not penetrate beyond the intestinal mucosa. Decreased ability of the mucosa to reabsorb endogenous secretions from the unaffected small intestine results in diarrhea.

Clinical Findings: The first signs are partial anorexia, passage of soft feces, and possibly fever. The course is variable. Some pigs die peracutely. More commonly, a mucoid diarrhea with flecks of blood and mucus develops and progresses to a watery mucohemorrhagic diarrhea. After several days, the feces are brown and contain flecks of fibrin and debris. Diarrheic pigs are dehydrated, profoundly weak, gaunt, and emaciated.

Lesions: The diffuse lesions are confined to the cecum, spiral colon, and rectum. The affected mucosa is covered with a layer of transparent or gray mucus, often with suspended flecks of blood in early stages; a mixture of blood, fibrin, and necrotic debris in more advanced cases; and a yellow, necrotic debris late in the course.

Diagnosis: Clinical signs and necropsy findings are usually sufficient for a presumptive diagnosis. Confirmation is based on demonstration of typical histologic lesions in the large intestine and isolation of *B hyodysenteriae* by anaerobic culture. *B hyodysenteriae* must be differentiated in culture from other anaerobic spirochetes. Biochemical tests and preferably PCR should be used on *Brachyspira* isolates to confirm species identification. Concurrent diseases are not uncommon. Differential diagnoses include intestinal spirochetosis, proliferative enteritis, salmonellosis, and heavy whipworm infections.

Treatment and Control: Therapeutic use of antibacterials is effective if started early. Water medication is preferred at first. Because drug-resistant strains are prevalent, it is essential to choose a drug to which the organism is sensitive. Bacitracin, carbadox, lincomycin, tylosin, tiamulin, and virginiamycin are commonly used. The disease may be eradicated from infected premises without total depopulation by a persistent and carefully planned program that includes treatment of carrier pigs with bactericidal drugs and thorough cleaning and disinfection of vacated facilities. Mice are an important reservoir of infection for *B hyodysenteriae*, and any eradication attempt must include elimination/reduction of the mouse population on the farm. In addition, *B hyodysenteriae* will survive >60 days in pig waste at refrigerator temperatures.

TRANSMISSIBLE GASTROENTERITIS

Transmissible gastroenteritis (TGE) is a common viral disease of the small intestine that causes vomiting and profuse diarrhea in pigs of all ages.

Etiology and Pathogenesis: The causal coronavirus infects and destroys villous epithelial cells of the jejunum and ileum, which results in severe villous atrophy, malabsorption, osmotic diarrhea, and dehydration. The incubation period is ~18 hr. The infection spreads rapidly by aerosol or contact exposure. Severe epidemics are more common during winter due to survival of the virus in colder temperatures.

Clinical Findings: In nonimmune herds, vomiting often is the initial sign, followed by profuse watery diarrhea, dehydration, and excessive thirst. Feces of nursing pigs often contain curds of undigested milk. Mortality is nearly 100% in piglets <1 wk old, whereas pigs >1 mo old seldom die. Gestating sows occasionally abort, and lactating sows often exhibit vomiting, diarrhea, and agalactia. Diarrhea in surviving nursing piglets continues for ~5 days, but older pigs may be diarrheic for a shorter period.

In large herds with endemic TGE, clinical signs are variable, depending on the level of immunity and magnitude of exposure. Immunity from antibody in the sow's milk usually is sufficient to protect pigs until they are 4-5 days old. As the antibody level in milk decreases, infection and mild disease may occur. Depending on the level of immunity and exposure, diarrhea may be mild in some litters but severe in others. If passive protection is sufficient to protect pigs throughout the nursing period, diarrhea often develops during the first few days after weaning.

Lesions: Piglets dying of TGE are severely dehydrated, and the skin is soiled with liquid feces. The stomach usually contains milk curd but may be empty. The small intestine is thin walled, and the entire intestine contains greenish or yellow watery fluid and clumps of undigested milk. Older pigs have few remarkable lesions except that the colon contains liquid rather than formed feces. Villous atrophy can be observed by examining the mucosa of the small intestine with a hand lens.

Diagnosis: Clinical signs in the epidemic form of TGE usually justify a presumptive diagnosis. In the mild endemic form, laboratory procedures are required. Histologic and immunofluorescent examinations of the small intestine to demonstrate typical lesions and the presence of TGE viral antigen provide confirmatory evidence. In some outbreaks, hemagluttinating encephalomyelitis (p 577) may cause similar signs.

Treatment and Control: There is no specific treatment. Increasing farrowing room temperature to minimize body heat loss and providing electrolyte solutions to combat dehydration are helpful. Administration of swine immunoglobulins has been reported to be beneficial. Weaning older nursing pigs that are consuming creep feed may reduce mortality.

Protective immunity depends on presence of antibody in the small intestine. Passive protection of piglets is provided by continual nursing of immune sows. Active, protective immunity develops after infection of the intestinal mucosa with virulent TGE virus. Active infection of the intestine with virulent virus provides protective immunity for 6-18 mo due to a secretory IgA response. Vaccination of naturally immune sows boosts immunity sufficiently to protect neonates and is particularly useful in endemically infected herds. Vaccination of swine in herds free of TGE may not be economically beneficial because vaccines do not induce complete immunity.

Planned infection of pregnant sows at least 2-4 wk before farrowing in herds known to be infected with virulent virus usually provides adequate immunity. This may be accomplished by mixing ground, TGE-virus-infected intestine and feces in the gestation ration. Because of the obvious hazards associated with this procedure, it should be undertaken only if a later epidemic in the farrowing house seems inevitable. The infectious material should be used only in the same herd from which it was collected, and the tissues should be as free as possible from other pathogens of pigs. TGE virus can be eliminated from herds without total depopulation by maximizing immunity with planned infection of the sow herd; an "all-in/all-out" management of farrowing, nursery, and grower rooms; and good sanitation.

Because TGE virus is easily spread during an epidemic by persons, animals, and fomites, special care should be taken to prevent spread to unexposed groups of pigs and to neighboring herds.

OTHER INTESTINAL VIRUSES OF PIGS

Other viruses have been isolated from the intestines of pigs but appear not to be associated with economically significant disease. These include adenovirus and enterovirus. Porcine circoviruses may be isolated from the intestine and are associated with postweaning multisystemic wasting syndrome (p 583).

GASTROINTESTINAL PARASITES OF RUMINANTS

Clinical Findings and Diagnosis: The clinical signs associated with GI parasitisms are shared by many diseases and conditions; however, presumptive diagnosis based on signs, grazing history, and season is often justified. Infection usually can be confirmed by demonstrating nematode eggs or tapeworm segments on fecal examination. However, in clinical evaluation of fecal examinations, 2 points should be remembered: an egg per gram of feces (EPG) count is not always an accurate indication of the number of adult worms present, and specific identification of eggs is impractical except in specialized laboratories. EPG counts can be negative or deceptively low in the presence of large numbers of immature worms; even when many adult parasites are present, the count can be low if egg production has been suppressed by immune reaction or previous anthelmintic treatment. Variations in the egg-producing capability of different worms (significantly lower for *Trichostrongylus*, *Ostertagia*, and *Nematodirus* than for *Haemonchus*) also may distort the true picture. The ova of *Nematodirus*, *Bunostomum*, *Strongyloides*, and *Trichuris* are distinctive, but reliable differentiation of the more common species of ruminant nematode ova is difficult. Fecal cultures can produce distinctive third-stage larvae if differentiation is important premortem.

The advent of safe and effective broad-spectrum anthelmintics has largely reduced the need for differentiating the genera and species of these parasites. In areas where *Ostertagia* spp predominate, the analysis of sera for increased plasma pepsinogen levels is a useful diagnostic aid. Generally, tyrosine levels >3 IU reflecting pepsinogen activity are associated with clinical signs. Problems of interpretation may arise in immune animals under challenge, in which there are no clinical signs but the pepsinogen levels may be increased because of a hypersensitivity-type reaction in the abomasal mucosa. Where *Haemonchus* spp predominate, a PCV estimate provides a quick guide to the degree of anemia. In some countries, serologic diagnosis (ELISA) of important species such as *Ostertagia* and *Cooperia* infections in cattle is used. As yet, there is insufficient information on the correlation between serologic titers and parasite load.

In many management situations, high levels of infection can be expected, particularly after favorable temperatures and rainfall conditions in certain seasons. "Diagnostic drenching" is recommended when eggs are few or absent, yet history and signs suggest infections. A clinical response to a broad-spectrum anthelmintic permits a retrospective diagnosis, but the animals should be placed on "clean" pastures after treatment to avoid reinfection.

Necropsy is the most direct method to identify and quantitate GI parasitisms. Routine postmortem examinations can provide valuable parasitologic data about the status of the rest of the herd or flock.

On necropsy, *Haemonchus*, *Bunostomum*, *Oesophagostomum*, *Trichuris*, and *Chabertia* adults (or advanced immature worms) can be seen easily. *Ostertagia*, *Trichostrongylus*, *Cooperia*, and *Nematodirus* are difficult to see except by their movement in fluid digesta, and clinically important infections are easily overlooked with these genera. The total contents and all washings should be combined to a known volume, and a worm count done to evaluate the severity of the infection. Measured samples of GI contents and scrapings of the mucosa should be examined microscopically under low power. These smaller nematodes can be stained (5 min) with a strong iodine solution. After the background digesta and tissue are decolorized with 5% sodium thiosulfate, small nematodes are easily seen. The significance of the numbers of worms present varies according to species of worms and host species. For example, only 100 *Haemonchus* are of clinical significance in lambs, whereas 5,000-10,000 *Ostertagia* are probably required to be clinically significant. If the animals have been diarrheic for a few days, worms may have been shed, and the type and severity of gross lesions may also be of considerable diagnostic value.

Multiple causes should be considered in evaluating clinical, laboratory, and necropsy findings. Mixed parasite infections are the rule.

Diagnosis of ostertagiasis in cattle during the period of larval inhibition presents technical problems, particularly for the feedlot industry in the USA. Fecal egg counts and plasma pepsinogen analysis do not provide useful information. Predisposing factors for inhibition of larvae include age and geographic source of cattle, time of year or season of arrival, previous grazing history and management, weather conditions prevailing during the last grazing period, and prevalence of *Ostertagia ostertagi* in the source region.

Information on such factors usually is not available for feedlot cattle. If cattle have arrived after spring grazing in the south of the USA or fall grazing in the north, they could have heavy burdens of inhibited larvae. Lighter calves from areas where prevalence of parasites is high may also have such a problem. It is becoming more widely accepted that a significant cause of clinical disease or feed efficiency problems in feedlot cattle is parasitism, possibly ostertagiasis. When cattle are received from a suspect area and at a suspect time of year, it may be advisable to treat the new arrivals promptly with an anthelmintic effective against inhibited larvae.

Treatment: Effective worm control cannot always be achieved by drugs alone; however, anthelmintics play an important role. (*See also* p 2124.) They may be used to reduce pasture contamination, particularly at times when seeding of the pasture with parasite eggs is a prerequisite for the development of an infective challenge necessary to cause clinical parasitism. Coordination with other methods of control, such as alternate grazing of different host species, integrated rotational grazing of different age groups within a single host species (including creep grazing), and alternation of grazing and cropping, are other management techniques that can provide safe pasture and give economic advantage when combined with anthelmintic treatment.

The "ideal" anthelmintic should be safe, highly effective against adults and immature stages (including hypobiotic larvae) of the important worms, available in convenient formulations, economical, and compatible with other commonly used compounds. Several drugs satisfy all or most of these requirements. Thiabendazole was the forerunner of the modern anthelmintics and set a new standard in efficacy and safety. Despite ineffectiveness against hypobiotic *Ostertagia* larvae in cattle and 1 or 2 other worm species, it is still widely used. After thiabendazole and mebendazole, other benzimidazoles (such as fenbendazole, oxfendazole, and albendazole) and the probenzimidazoles (thiophanate, febantel, and netobimin) were developed; these compounds are effective against most of the major GI parasites of ruminants and have varying levels of activity against hypobiotic larvae. Levamisole, morantel, and pyrantel also are highly effective, safe, wide-spectrum anthelmintics but have little activity against hypobiotic larvae in cattle. Avermectins and milbemycins are highly effective against adults and larval stages, including hypobiotic larvae of all the common GI nematodes of ruminants, and some of the important ectoparasites. Avermectins and milbemycins may persist in some ruminant species for some time after single subcutaneous or topical administration and may confer protection against reinfection during this period. Moxidectin is also persistent following oral administration. Some narrow-spectrum anthelmintics, such as the salicylanilides, closantel, and rafoxanide, have excellent activity against *Haemonchus contortus* in sheep and also remain in the host for a long time, which confers considerable prophylactic activity after administration.

Routes of administration other than drenching or injection (eg, incorporating into feed, drinking water, and mineral or energy blocks) are used to reduce labor costs and may be useful under drylot conditions or when grazing animals are being given supplemental feed. Another advantage of these "in-feed" routes is that continuous low-level administration of a drug can be achieved and pasture contamination reduced during periods that are optimal for free-living development of the parasites. Disadvantages include erratic consumption of anthelmintic, tissue residues (requiring observance of recommended withdrawal periods), and possible encouragement of drug resistance by continuous exposure. Another labor-saving route of administration is the "pour-on" topical treatment, used for some of the organophosphates (eg, trichlorfon), levamisole, and avermectins. A number of bolus preparations (eg, morantel, levamisole, ivermectin, or benzimidazoles) release drug in a sustained fashion or in pulses at intervals approximately equal to the prepatent periods of the most important GI parasites. The boluses used in cattle have been designed to give entire season pasture control in temperate areas if administered at turn-out to set-stocked herds. Boluses are also available that provide treatment and subsequent prophylaxis of animals already exposed to contaminated pasture and harboring parasites. Boluses in sheep may be used to reduce the periparturient rise in fecal egg output and thus the pasture contamination responsible for disease in their offspring later in the grazing season.

Niclosamide, morantel, praziquantel, and the newer benzimidazoles (albendazole, fenbendazole, and oxfendazole) are effective against tapeworms (*Moniezia* spp) in cattle and sheep. Treatment of *Thysanosoma actinioides* has presented problems, but niclosamide has been reported to be effective at 250 mg/kg. Additionally, bithionol (200 mg/kg) has been used.

When treating clinically affected animals, the following should be considered: 1) providing adequate nutrition, 2) treating all animals in the group, as a preventive measure and to reduce further pasture contamination, and 3) moving stock to "clean" pastures to minimize reinfection. The definition of safe pastures varies in different climates and depends on local knowledge of the seasonal mortality of infective larvae. Some authorities have suggested treating only the most severely affected animals in a flock or herd. This can be achieved by assessing the severity of anemia by observation of the color of the sclera of the eye for haemonchosis in sheep, or the severity of diarrhea or by quantitative fecal egg counts for parasitic gastroenteritis in sheep or cattle. The rationale for this strategy is based on the knowledge that a very large proportion of the parasite egg output (and thus pasture contamination) is associated with a relatively small proportion of the host animal population. Treatment of only these animals significantly reduces pasture contamination and reduces the overall selection pressure exerted by the use of an anthelmintic. Concerns also exist with respect to treatment and movement of stock to clean pasture. If any parasites with resistance genes survive the treatment, then the "clean pasture" will become seeded with a wholly resistant population.

Finally, development of drug resistance by populations of *Haemonchus contortus*, *Trichostrongylus* spp, and *Ostertagia* spp in sheep and goats to benzimidazoles, levamisole, and avermectins/milbemycins has been demonstrated. While such resistance is currently a problem only in certain areas, it should be considered when response to therapy is suboptimal and other factors can be excluded, eg, improper dosage, rapid reinfection, poor nutrition, or some disease state other than parasitism. Drug resistance in parasites of cattle has been demonstrated; overuse and otherwise indiscriminate treatment should be avoided.

General Control Measures: "Control" generally implies the suppression of parasite burdens in the host below that level at which economic loss occurs. To do this effectively requires a comprehensive knowledge of the epidemiologic and ecologic factors that govern pasture larval populations and the role of host immunity to infection.

The goals of control are as follows: 1) prevent heavy exposure in susceptible hosts (recovery from heavy infection is always slow), 2) reduce overall levels of pasture contamination, 3) minimize the effects of parasite burdens, and 4) encourage the development of immunity in the animals (less important in fattening animals than in those that are to be kept for breeding purposes).

Strategic use of anthelmintics is designed to reduce worm burdens and, thereby, the contamination of pastures. Timing of administration is based on knowledge of the seasonal changes in infection and the regional epidemiology of the various helminthoses. Prompt recognition of circumstances likely to favor development of parasitic disease, eg, weather, grazing behavior, and loss of weight and condition, is essential.

For example, in the UK, where the pattern of disease caused by *Nematodirus battus* infection in sheep is clearly defined, strategic treatments with 2 or 3 doses of anthelmintic at 2- to 3-wk intervals, beginning just before the disease characteristically appears, are recommended. Similarly, in the northern USA, Canada, or western Europe, pasture levels of *Ostertagia* and other parasites increase substantially after mid July, ie, the general pattern of infectivity is minimal in spring but increases rapidly to peak levels in late summer and early fall. Current practices in these areas indicate the effectiveness of 2 or more anthelmintic treatments (usually at intervals of 3-5 wk) given when cattle first go to grass in spring. Single treatments with subsequent transfer of animals to safe pasture and treatment associated with delayed spring turn-out also have been effective.

In other countries of either cool or warm temperate climate, similar controls may be used if the seasonal pattern of the disease is known, but in most regions a tactical use of anthelmintics is used, eg, during warm, moist conditions.

Cattle—Special Considerations: Worm problems are seen most frequently in young beef cattle from time of weaning and several months thereafter, and in segregated groups of dairy calves during the first season at grass. Immunity to GI nematodes is acquired slowly; 2 grazing seasons may be required before a significant level is attained. In endemic areas, cows may continue to harbor low burdens, which may be the cause of suboptimal production. GI parasitism in young stock may be controlled by use of broad-spectrum anthelmintics in conjunction with pasture management to limit reinfection; the latter includes a move to "clean" pastures (eg, grass conservation areas or silage or hay aftermath) or alternate grazing with other host species, or integrated rotational grazing in which susceptible calves are followed by immune adults. Alternate grazing with other host species may be ineffective in areas where parasite species (eg, *Nematodirus*) infect both hosts; simple pasture rotation is not effective because the bovine fecal mass can protect larvae from adverse environmental conditions for several months, possibly causing reinfection in rotating calves at a later date.

In beef herds, anthelmintic treatment at weaning is of value, particularly if the young cattle are to be retained, eg, as replacement heifer stock or as steers to be fed. Cattle finished on grass should receive treatment at weaning and at intervals during the next 12 mo and, if possible, should be moved to safe pastures.

When cattle cannot be moved readily to other pastures, strategic treatments may be given to limit contamination of pastures and rapid reinfection. Alternatively, rumen boluses may be used in countries where they are approved. In warm temperate regions of the world, such as Australia and New Zealand, the southern USA, and the large cattle-raising regions of southern Brazil, Uruguay, and Argentina, young cattle may be given 2 or more treatments from late summer and into fall for prevention of large increases in pasture contamination and infection during winter and spring. Two or three strategic treatments, administered with a short interval, from the time of weaning in such regions could be just as effective as spring treatments in cool temperate regions. However, survival of infective larvae on pasture from the time of fall weaning in warm temperate regions is most often persistent, and longer intervals between treatments (eg, at weaning, during winter, and in late spring) may be more applicable. In many areas, anthelmintics are simply given at regular intervals after weaning. Intervals between treatments must necessarily vary according to the local epidemiology and the prophylaxis conferred by the persistence of the anthelmintic. When Type II ostertagiasis is a problem, treatment with an anthelmintic effective against hypobiotic larvae is recommended before the expected time of outbreak.

Sheep—Special Considerations: A special strategic treatment is required in most regions to counter the postparturient relaxation of immunity (periparturient rise, etc) seen in ewes. The precise timing of such treatment varies between regions and for different species of parasites, but in general, treatment within the month before and again within the month after parturition appears desirable and may confer a production benefit on the ewe. Unfortunately, the periparturient rise may last for up to 8 wk in some flocks and 2 treatments with most anthelmintics are not effective in reducing pasture contamination sufficiently to ensure "safe" grazing for offspring later in the season. Bolus preparations containing albendazole or ivermectin are available in some countries and are more effective for this purpose. Furthermore, moxidectin has sufficient persistence in sheep to confer an epidemiologic benefit of treatment for the most important parasitic species. A treatment 2 wk before breeding, as part of a "flushing" program, is another strategic application of anthelmintics. Supportive management after treatment includes movement of sheep from contaminated pastures to cattle pastures, grass conservation areas, root crops, or pasture not grazed by sheep for several months. The latter period varies according to the seasonal pattern of larval mortality in different countries and may be as long as 1 yr in some temperate countries.

Sheep are more consistently susceptible to the adverse effects of worms than other livestock, and clinical disease is more common. Immunity to the parasites is acquired slowly and is generally incomplete. Frequent treatments may be required, particularly during the first year of life.

GASTROINTESTINAL PARASITES OF CATTLE

Haemonchus, Ostertagia, and Trichostrongylus spp

The common stomach worms of cattle are *Haemonchus placei* (barber's pole worm, large stomach worm, wire worm), *Ostertagia ostertagi* (medium or brown stomach worm), and *Trichostrongylus axei* (small stomach worm, p 269). In some tropical countries, *Mecistocirrus digitatus*, a large worm up to 40 mm long, is present. *Haemonchus placei* is primarily a parasite in tropical regions, whereas *O ostertagi* and, to a lesser extent, *T axei* are found in more temperate climates. Adult male *Haemonchus* are up to 18 mm long, females up to 30 mm. *Ostertagia* adults are 6-9 mm long, and *Trichostrongylus*, ~5 mm.

The preparasitic life cycles of the 3 groups are generally similar. Larvae hatch shortly after the eggs are passed in the feces and reach the infective stage in ~2 wk under optimal temperatures (~75°F [24°C]). Development to the infective stage is delayed during cold weather. In areas with narrow diurnal temperature variations, those months with a mean maximum temperature of 65°F (18°C) and with rainfall >2 in. (5 cm) are favorable for development of the free-living stages of *H placei*, but where wide fluctuations occur, a mean minimum temperature of 50°F (10°C) may effectively limit development. The preparasitic forms of *O ostertagi* and *T axei* develop and survive better in cooler conditions, and their upper limits for survival are lower than those for *H placei*. If the temperature is unfavorable or drought conditions exist, infective larvae may remain dormant in the feces for weeks until conditions become favorable again, after which large numbers of infective larvae emerge.

The prepatent period of *O ostertagi* is normally 18-25 days. Ingested larvae enter the lumen of the abomasal glands and molt by the fourth day; they remain there during the prepatent period, growing and undergoing a final molt before emerging to the lumen of the abomasum as young adults. Larvae in gastric glands cause cellular hyperplasia and result in nodules, which may be discrete or confluent. Severe epithelial cytolysis may be seen when the larvae emerge. At this time, the parietal cells are replaced by undifferentiated, rapidly dividing cells. As a consequence, in heavy infections, the pH in the abomasum rises from 2 to >6. A protein-losing gastropathy results and, together with anorexia and impaired protein digestion, leads to hypoproteinemia and weight loss. Diarrhea is persistent. In **Type I ostertagiasis**, which results from recent infection, most worms present are adults and the response to anthelmintic treatment is good. Type I disease is seen primarily in calves 7-15 mo old. It is most common from time of weaning and ensuing months in warm temperate regions, and in young cattle during summer and early fall in cool temperate regions.

In **Type II ostertagiasis**, large numbers of larvae, which had become dormant or inhibited in development at the early fourth larval stage, emerge from the glands. This is seen primarily in cattle 12-20 mo old. In warm temperate regions, inhibition-prone larvae are acquired in spring, and disease may result when large numbers of larvae resume development to the adult stage in late summer or fall. In cold temperate regions, inhibition-prone larvae are acquired during late autumn and mature during late winter or early spring.

Larval inhibition (hypobiosis) in *O ostertagi* and other nematodes is thought to be analogous to diapause in insects. It has been interpreted as a survival mechanism in which the preparasitic stages on pasture avoid the adverse conditions of winter in cool regions and of hot and dry (or hot and alternately wet and dry) conditions of many warm regions. The factors that cause inhibition are not completely known, but experimental cold conditioning of infective larvae was found to be important in a cool temperate region. In warm regions of both northern and southern hemispheres, conditioning of preparasitic stages to inhibition develops principally during spring before the hot and dry conditions of summer. Factors involved in maturation are even less well defined but may include effects of parturition, nutrition, concurrent infection, host immune response, or simply lapse of time.

H placei also may become dormant over winter; they then resume development in the spring and infect the pastures with eggs at a time suitable for their development. Both the larval and adult stages are pathogenic due to their blood-sucking ability. *T axei* causes gastritis with superficial erosion of the mucosa, hyperemia, and diarrhea. Protein loss from the damaged mucosa and anorexia cause hypoproteinemia and weight loss. Hypobiosis does not occur to the same degree.

Clinical Findings: Young animals are more often affected, but adults not previously exposed to infection frequently show signs and succumb. *Ostertagia* and *Trichostrongylus* infections are characterized by profuse, watery diarrhea that usually is persistent. In haemonchosis and *Mecistocirrus* infection, there may be little or no diarrhea but possibly intermittent periods of constipation. Anemia of variable degree is a characteristic sign of both these infections.

Concurrent with the diarrhea of *O ostertagi* and *T axei* infections, and the anemia of heavy *Haemonchus* infection, there is often hypoproteinemia and edema (rare in *O ostertagi* infections), particularly under the lower jaw (**bottle jaw**) and sometimes along the ventral abdomen. Heavy infections can result in death before clinical signs appear. Other variable signs include progressive weight loss, weakness, rough coat, and anorexia.

Lesions: Worms can readily be seen and identified in the abomasum, and small petechiae may be seen where the worms have been feeding. The most characteristic lesions of *Ostertagia* infection are small, umbilicated nodules 1-2 mm in diameter throughout the abomasum. These may be discrete, but in heavy infections they tend to coalesce and give rise to a "cobblestone" or "morocco leather" appearance. Nodules are most marked in the fundic region but may cover the entire abomasal mucosa. The pH may rise to 6-7. Pepsinogen may be poorly converted to pepsin and may leak across damaged epithelium; high levels can be found in the plasma. There is also evidence that adult *Ostertagia* can cause direct hypersecretion of pepsinogen. The increased abomasal pH may also stimulate production of gastrin and thus hypergastrinemia. Edema is often marked and, in severe cases, may extend over the abomasum and into the small intestine and omentum.

In *T axei* infections, the mucosa of the abomasum may show congestion and superficial erosions, which are sometimes covered with a fibrinonecrotic exudate.

Diagnosis, Treatment, and Control: *See* p 254 et seq.

Cooperia spp

Several species of *Cooperia* occur in the small intestine of cattle; *C punctata, C oncophora,* and *C pectinata* are the most common. The red, coiled adults are 5-8 mm long, and the male has a large bursa. They may be difficult to observe grossly. Their life cycle is essentially the same as that of other trichostrongylids. These worms apparently do not suck blood. Most of them are found in the first 10-20 ft (3-6 m) of the small intestine. The prepatent period is 12-15 days.

The eggs usually can be differentiated from those of the common GI nematodes by their practically parallel sides, but a larval culture of the feces is necessary to definitively diagnose *Cooperia* infection in the living animal. In heavy infections with *C punctata* and *C pectinata*, there is profuse diarrhea, anorexia, and emaciation, but no anemia; the upper small intestine shows marked congestion of the mucosa with small hemorrhages. The mucosa may show a fine lace-like superficial necrosis. *C oncophora* produces a milder disease but can be responsible for weight loss and poor productivity. It is usually necessary to make scrapings of the mucosa to demonstrate *Cooperia* spp, which must be differentiated from *Trichostrongylus* spp, *Strongyloides papillosus,* and immature *Nematodirus* spp.

For diagnosis, treatment, and control, *see* p 254 et seq.

Bunostomum sp

The adult male *Bunostomum phlebotomum* is ~15 mm long, and the female ~25 mm. Hookworms have well-developed buccal capsules into which the mucosa is drawn; cutting plates at the anterior edge of the buccal capsule are used to abrade the mucosa during feeding. The prepatent period is ~2 mo. Infection is by ingestion or skin penetration; the latter is more common.

Larval penetration of the lower limbs may cause uneasiness and stamping, particularly in stabled cattle. Adult worms cause anemia and rapid weight loss. Diarrhea and constipation may alternate. Hypoproteinemic edema may be present, but bottle jaw is rarely as severe as in haemonchosis. During the patent period, a diagnosis may be made by demonstrating the characteristic eggs in the feces.

On necropsy, the mucosa may appear congested and swollen, with numerous small hemorrhagic points where the worms were attached. The worms are readily seen in the first few feet of the small intestine, and the contents are often blood-stained. As few as 2,000 worms may cause death in calves. Local lesions, edema, and scab formation may result from penetration of larvae into the skin of resistant calves.

For diagnosis, treatment, and control, *see* p 254 et seq.

Strongyloides sp

The intestinal threadworm, *Strongyloides papillosus,* has an unusual life cycle. Only females are in the parasitic phase of the cycle. They are 3.5-6 mm long and are embedded in the mucosa of the upper small intestine. Small, embryonated eggs are passed in the feces, hatch rapidly, and may develop directly into infective larvae or free-living adults. The offspring of these free-living adults may develop into another generation of infective larvae or free-living adults. The host is infected by penetration of the skin or by ingestion; infective larvae can be transmitted in colostrum as in other species of the genus. The prepatent period is ~10 days.

Infections are most common in young calves, particularly dairy stock. Although signs are rare, they may include intermittent diarrhea, loss of appetite and weight, and sometimes blood and mucus in the feces. Large numbers of worms in the intestine produce catarrhal enteritis with petechiae and ecchymoses, especially in the duodenum and jejunum.

For diagnosis, treatment, and control, see p 254 et seq.

Nematodirus spp

Nematodirus helvetianus is generally recognized as the most common species in cattle, although several other species, eg, *N spathiger* and *N battus*, can also infect cattle. The adult males of *N helvetianus* are ~12 mm long, and the females 18-25 mm. The eggs develop slowly; the infective third stage is reached within the egg in 2-4 wk and may remain within the egg for several months. Eggs may accumulate on pastures and hatch in large numbers after rain to produce heavy infections over a short period. The eggs are highly resistant, and those passed by calves in one season may remain viable and infect calves the next season. After ingestion of infective larvae, the adult stage is reached in ~3 wk. Worms are most numerous 10-20 ft (3-6 m) from the pylorus.

Signs, which include diarrhea and anorexia, usually develop during the third week of infection before the worms are sexually mature; clinical infections may be seen in dairy calves from 6 wk onward. Diagnosis is difficult during the prepatent period, but during the patent period diagnosis is easily made on the basis of the characteristic eggs. Relatively small numbers of eggs are produced. Immunity to reinfection develops rapidly. Necropsy may show only a thickened, edematous mucosa.

For diagnosis, treatment, and control, see p 254 et seq.

Toxocara sp

The ascarid *Toxocara vitulorum* is a stout, whitish worm (males 20-25 cm, females 25-30 cm) found in the small intestine of calves <6 mo old; older calves are resistant. Larvae hatching from ingested eggs pass to the tissues and, in pregnant cows, are mobilized late in pregnancy and passed via the milk to calves. Eggs appear in the feces of calves from 3 wk of age and are easily recognized by their thick, pitted shells. In some parts of the world, the infection is considered serious, particularly in buffalo calves.

For diagnosis, treatment, and control, see p 254 et seq.

Oesophagostomum sp

Adults of *Oesophagostomum radiatum* (nodular worm) are 12-15 mm long, and the head is bent dorsally. Because the eggs are very similar to those of *Haemonchus placei*, they are often grouped together on routine fecal examination. The life cycle is direct. The larvae penetrate primarily into the wall of the lower 10-20 ft (3-6 m) of the small intestine but also into the cecum and colon, where they remain for 5-10 days and then return to the lumen as fourth-stage larvae. The prepatent period in susceptible animals is ~6 wk. However, in subsequent reinfections, larvae become arrested for some time, and many never return to the lumen (host encystment).

Young animals suffer from the effects of adult worms, whereas in older animals, the effect of the nodules is more important. Infection causes anorexia; severe, constant, dark, persistent, fetid diarrhea; weight loss; and death. In older, resistant animals, the nodules surrounding the larvae become caseated and calcified, thus decreasing the motility of the intestine. Stenosis or intussusception occasionally occurs. Nodules can be palpated per rectum, and the worms and nodules can be seen readily at necropsy.

For diagnosis, treatment, and control, see p 254 et seq.

Chabertia sp

Adults of the large-mouth bowel worm, *Chabertia ovina*, are ~12 mm long and bent ventrally at the anterior end. There is a typical direct life cycle. The larvae penetrate the mucosa of the small intestine shortly after ingestion and later emerge and pass to the colon. The prepatent period is ~7 wk. Larvae and adults may cause small hemorrhages with edema in the colon and passage of feces coated with mucus. Clinical chabertiasis is seldom, if ever, seen in cattle.

For diagnosis, treatment, and control, *see* p 254 et seq.

Trichuris spp

Trichuris spp infections are common in young calves and yearlings, but numbers of worms are seldom large. The eggs are resistant, and infections are likely to persist on problem premises. Clinical signs are unlikely, but in occasional heavy infections, dark feces, anemia, and anorexia may be seen.

For diagnosis, treatment, and control, *see* p 254 et seq.

Tapeworms

The anoplocephalid tapeworms *Moniezia expansa* and *M benedeni* are found in young cattle. The worms of this group are characterized by the absence of a rostellum and hooks, and the segments usually are wider than they are long. The eggs are triangular or rectangular and are ingested by free-living oribatid mites, which live in the soil and grass. After 6-16 wk, infective cysticercoids are present in the mites. Infection occurs by ingestion of the mites; the prepatent period is ~5 wk. *Moniezia* are commonly considered nonpathogenic in calves, but intestinal stasis has been reported.

For diagnosis, treatment, and control, *see* p 254 et seq.

GASTROINTESTINAL PARASITES OF SHEEP AND GOATS

Many species of nematodes and cestodes cause parasitic gastritis and enteritis in sheep and goats. The most important of these are *Haemonchus contortus, Ostertagia circumcincta, Trichostrongylus axei*, intestinal species of *Trichostrongylus, Nematodirus* spp, *Bunostomum trigonocephalum*, and *Oesophagostomum columbianum*. *Cooperia curticei, Strongyloides papillosus, Trichuris ovis*, and *Chabertia ovina* also may be pathogenic in sheep; these and related species are discussed under GI parasites of cattle (p 258).

Haemonchus, Ostertagia, and Trichostrongylus spp

The principal stomach worms of sheep and goats are *Haemonchus contortus, Ostertagia circumcincta, O trifurcata, Trichostrongylus axei* (p 258), and in some tropical regions, *Mecistocirrus digitatus*. Cross-transmission of *Haemonchus* between sheep and cattle can occur but not as readily as transmission between homologous species. Sheep are more susceptible to the cattle species than cattle are to the sheep species. For descriptions and life cycles, *see* GASTROINTESTINAL PARASITES OF CATTLE, p 258.

Haemonchus is most common in tropical or subtropical areas or in those areas with summer rainfall, while *Ostertagia* and *T axei* are more common in winter rainfall areas. The latter species is predominant in temperate zones.

Haemonchosis in sheep may be classified as hyperacute, acute, or chronic. In the hyperacute disease, death may occur within 1 wk of heavy infection without significant signs. The acute disease is characterized by severe anemia accompanied by generalized edema; anemia is also characteristic of the chronic infection, often of low worm burdens, and is accompanied by progressive weight loss. Diarrhea is not a sign of haemonchosis; the lesions are those associated with anemia. The abomasum is edematous and, in the chronic phase, the pH increases, which causes gastric dysfunction. Mature sheep may develop heavy, even fatal infections, particularly during lactation.

The lesions, pathogenesis, and signs of *Ostertagia* and *T axei* infections are similar to those found in cattle. Even subclinical infection depresses appetite, impairs gastric digestion, and reduces use of metabolizable energy and protein. *Ostertagia* is the principal genus involved in the periparturient rise in fecal egg counts in sheep, and heavy infections may cause diarrhea and depress milk production in ewes. This output of eggs serves as the main source of contamination for the lambs. The same type of inhibited development (hypobiosis) seen in cattle has been seen with both *Ostertagia* and *Haemonchus* in sheep.

For diagnosis, treatment, and control, *see* p 254 et seq.

Intestinal Trichostrongylosis

The life cycle of intestinal *Trichostrongylus* (*T colubriformis*, *T vitrinus*, *T rugatus*) is direct. The developing larvae burrow superficially in the crypts of the mucosa and develop to egg-laying adults in 18-21 days.

Anorexia, persistent diarrhea, and weight loss are the main signs. Villous atrophy results in impaired digestion and malabsorption; protein loss occurs across the damaged mucosa. There are no diagnostic lesions; a total worm count should be done to evaluate the condition.

For diagnosis, treatment, and control, *see* p 254 et seq.

Bunostomum and *Gaigeria* spp

Adult *Bunostomum trigonocephalum* (hookworm) are found in the jejunum. The life cycle and clinical findings are essentially the same as for the cattle hookworm (p 260). As few as 100 worms may cause clinical signs. *Gaigeria pachyscelis* is found in Africa and Asia and resembles *Bunostomum* in size and form (2-3 cm). Larvae of *G pachyscelis* infect the host only by skin penetration. *G pachyscelis* is a voracious bloodsucker and probably the most pathogenic hookworm.

For diagnosis, treatment, and control, *see* p 254 et seq.

Nematodirus spp

The species of *Nematodirus* found in the small intestine of sheep are similar in morphology and life cycle to *N helvetianus* (p 261). Clinical infections are of considerable importance in the UK, New Zealand, and Australia, where death losses of 20% of the lambs in affected flocks have been reported. The parasites are endemic in some parts of the Rocky Mountain states of the USA, where they occasionally cause clinical disease in lambs.

In areas where clinical infections are common, the disease often has a characteristic seasonal pattern. Many of the eggs passed by affected lambs lie dormant through the remainder of the grazing season and the winter, with large numbers of larvae appearing during the early grazing period of the following year. Thus, the lambs of one season contaminate the pastures for the next season's lambs, but the life cycle can be broken if the same area is not used for lambing each year. Most clinical infections are seen in lambs 6-12 wk old.

N battus is seen in the UK and other parts of Europe and also in North America. Eggs hatch after a period of chill and then a rise in ambient temperature to a day/night mean of 10°C. This occurs in late spring in temperate areas. The hatching requirements mean that there is generally one annual generation of *N battus*, although in the UK, outbreaks in the autumn have been reported. Disease may be associated with developing larval stages and may be seen within 2 wk of challenge. Other *Nematodirus* spp often are found in low-rainfall regions (eg, the Karroo in South Africa and inland Australia) where other parasites are rarely seen.

Nematodirosis is characterized by sudden onset, "loss of bloom," unthriftiness, profuse diarrhea, and marked dehydration, with death as early as 2-3 days after an outbreak begins. Nematodirosis is commonly confined to lambs or weaner sheep, but in low-rainfall country where outbreaks are sporadic, older sheep may have heavy infections. The lesions usually consist of dehydration and a mild catarrhal enteritis, but acute inflammation of the entire small intestine may develop. Counts of ≥10,000 worms, together with characteristic signs and history, are indicative of clinical infections. Affected lambs may pass large numbers of eggs, which can be identified easily; however, because the onset of disease may precede the maturation of the female worms, this is not a constant finding.

For diagnosis, treatment, and control, *see* p 254 et seq.

Oesophagostomum sp

The nodular worm of sheep, *Oesophagostomum columbianum*, has a similar morphology and life cycle to the nodular worm of cattle (p 261).

Diarrhea usually develops during the second week of infection. The feces may contain excess mucus as well as streaks of blood. As the diarrhea progresses, sheep become emaciated and weak. These signs often subside near the end of the prepatent period, but the continuing presence of numerous adult worms may result in a chronic infection in which signs may not develop for several months. The sheep become weak, lose weight despite a good appetite, and show intermittent diarrhea and constipation.

As immunity develops, nodules form around the larvae; they may become caseated and calcified. Nodule formation usually is more pronounced in sheep than in cattle. Affected sheep walk with a stilted gait and often have a humped back. Stenosis and intussusception may develop in severe cases. Diagnosis is difficult during the prepatent period, at which time it must be based largely on clinical signs.

For diagnosis, treatment, and control, *see* p 254 et seq.

Chabertia sp

Adult worms cause severe damage to the mucosa of the colon with resulting congestion, ulceration, and small hemorrhages. Infected sheep are unthrifty; the feces are soft, contain much mucus, and may be streaked with blood. Immunity develops quickly, and outbreaks are seen only under conditions of severe stress.

For diagnosis, treatment, and control, *see* p 254 et seq.

Strongyloides sp

Heavy infections with adult worms cause a disease resembling trichostrongylosis. Infection is usually by skin penetration but can also occur via the milk. Damage to the skin between the claws, produced by skin-penetrating larvae, resembles the early stages of foot rot and may aid penetration of the causal agents of foot rot. Most infections are transitory and inconsequential.

For diagnosis, treatment, and control, *see* p 254 et seq.

Trichuris spp

Heavy infections with whipworms are not common but may be seen in very young lambs or during drought conditions when sheep are fed grain on the ground. The eggs are very resistant. Congestion and edema of the cecal mucosa, accompanied by diarrhea and unthriftiness, are seen.

For diagnosis, treatment, and control, *see* p 254 et seq.

Tapeworms

The pathogenicity of *Moniezia expansa* in sheep has long been debated. Many earlier observations, which associated this infection with diarrhea, emaciation, and weight loss, did not accurately differentiate between tapeworm infections and infection with certain small nematodes (eg, *Trichostrongylus colubriformis*). Tapeworms are relatively nonpathogenic, but heavy infections can result in mild unthriftiness and GI disturbances. Diagnosis may be made by finding yellowish to pearl-white, bell-shaped proglottids in the feces or protruding from the anus or by demonstrating the characteristic eggs on fecal examination. The life cycle involves an oribatid mite that lives in the mat of pastures. The prepatent period is 6-7 wk. Lambs develop resistance quickly, and infections are unusual after ~4-5 mo of age.

Thysanosoma actinioides, the "fringed tapeworm," inhabits the small intestine, the bile ducts, and the pancreatic ducts. It is commonly found in sheep from the Rocky Mountain areas of the USA. Although it has not been associated with clinical disease, it is of economic importance because livers are condemned when tapeworms are found in the bile duct.

For diagnosis, treatment, and control, *see* p 254 et seq.

GASTROINTESTINAL PARASITES OF HORSES

GASTEROPHILUS SPP

Horse bots, which are found in the stomach, are the larvae of botflies, *Gasterophilus* spp. Three major species are distributed worldwide, and a number of minor species are found in parts of Europe, Africa, and Asia. The adult flies are not parasitic and cannot feed; they exist long enough to mate and lay eggs and die as soon as the nutrients remaining from the larval stage are used, usually in ~2 wk. The 3 important species can be differentiated in any stage of their development. The eggs of *G intestinalis* (the common bot) are glued to the hairs of almost any part of the body but especially the forelimbs and shoulders. The larvae hatch in ~1 wk when stimulated, usually by the animals' licking. The eggs of *G haemorrhoidalis* (the nose or lip bot) are attached to the hairs of the lips. The larvae emerge in 2-3 days without stimulation and crawl into the mouth. *G nasalis* (the throat bot) deposits eggs on the hairs of the submaxillary region. They hatch in ~1 wk without stimulation.

The larvae of all 3 species apparently stay embedded in the tongue or the mucosa of the mouth for ~1 mo, after which they pass to the stomach where they attach themselves to the cardiac or pyloric portions and, in the case of *G nasalis*, to the mucosa of the first part of the small intestine. After development for ~8-10 mo, they pass out in the feces and pupate in the soil for 3-5 wk, after which the adult emerges. The main pathogenic effect is caused by larvae, which attach by oral hooks to the lining of the stomach. This induces erosions and ulcerations at the site of attachment and a hyperplastic reaction around it. However, oral stages may cause sinus tracts in which mucopurulent discharges form, especially along the lingual border of the upper, more posterior cheek teeth.

Clinical Findings and Diagnosis: Bots cause a mild gastritis, but large numbers may be present with no clinical signs. The first instars migrating in the mouth can cause stomatitis and may produce pain on eating. The adult flies may annoy horses when they lay their eggs. Specific diagnosis of *Gasterophilus* infection is difficult and can be made by demonstrating larvae as they pass in the feces. In the USA, the presence of gastric infections during the winter months is often assumed. History of the individual horses, knowledge of the local seasonal cycle of the fly, and observation of the yellow to cream-white bot eggs (1-2 mm) on the horse's hairs are all helpful.

Treatment: In temperate areas, it is assumed that most animals are infected by the end of summer. Ivermectin is effective against oral and gastric stages of bots and, when used as part of a routine parasite control program, provides effective bot control throughout the season. Moxidectin is effective against gastric stages. Current recommendations for control include minimally 2 treatments annually, one ~1 mo after the first bot egg is seen on hair coats and one at the end of the botfly season. In some locations where the botfly season is long, additional treatments may be necessary. Although there is no satisfactory method for protecting exposed horses from attack by the adult flies, bot control programs, when applied on a regional basis to all horses, markedly reduce fly numbers and larval infections.

HABRONEMA SPP

The stomach worms *Habronema muscae*, *H microstoma*, and *Draschia megastoma* are widely distributed. The adults are 6-25 mm in size. *Draschia* are found in tumor-like swellings in the stomach wall. The other species are free on the mucosa. The eggs or larvae are ingested by larvae of house or stable flies, which serve as intermediate hosts. Horses are infected by ingesting flies that contain infective larvae or by free larvae that emerge from flies as they feed around the lips. (*See also* CUTANEOUS HABRONEMIASIS, p 735.)

A catarrhal gastritis may result from heavy infections with adult worms. *Draschia* produces the most severe lesions—tumor-like enlargements up to 10 cm in diameter. These are filled with necrotic material and a large number of worms and are covered by intact epithelium, except for a small opening through which the eggs pass. Rarely, these nodules rupture and cause fatal peritonitis. Larvae of *Habronema* spp and *Draschia* have been found in the lungs of foals associated with *Rhodococcus equi* abscesses (p 1209). Clinical signs usually are absent except when granulomas associated with *Draschia* infection lead to mechanical obstruction or rupture.

Antemortem diagnosis is difficult because the thin-shelled eggs or larvae are easily missed in fecal examinations. Worms and eggs may be found by gastric lavage. Most anthelmintics have not been tested against *Habronema* spp or *Draschia* sp, although ivermectin is effective against their cutaneous larvae and against adults of *H muscae*. Moxidectin is effective against adult *H muscae*.

OXYURIS SP

Adult pinworms, *Oxyuris equi*, are more common in horses <18 mo old and are found primarily in the terminal portion of the large intestine. The females are 7.5-15 cm long; males are smaller and fewer in number. The gravid females pass toward the rectum to lay their eggs, "cementing" them to the perineum around the anus. Masses of eggs and cement around the anus appear as a white to yellow, crusty mass. The eggs, which are flattened on one side, become embryonated in a few hours and are infective in 4-5 days.

Adult pinworms are of little significance in the intestine but cause perineal irritation after egg laying. Rubbing of the tail and anal regions, with resulting broken hairs and bare patches around the tail and buttocks, is characteristic and suggests the presence of pinworms. Fecal examination may or may not reveal a pinworm infection. Samples collected around the perineal region may contain dried female worms or eggs. Application of cellophane tape to the skin of the perineum or scraping the area with a tongue depressor may recover ova for microscopic examination but is likely to result in a large number of false-negative tests.

Most of the broad-spectrum drugs recommended for treatment of strongyles (*see* p 267 and p 267) are effective against pinworms.

PARASCARIS SP

Adult *Parascaris equorum* are stout, whitish worms, up to 30 cm long, with 3 prominent lips. The life cycle is similar to that of *Ascaris suum* (the roundworm of pigs, p 270), with a prepatent period of 10-12 wk. Large numbers of infective eggs can remain viable for years in contaminated soil. Adult animals usually harbor very few worms. The principal sources of infection for young foals are pastures, paddocks, or stalls contaminated with eggs from foals of the previous year.

In heavy infections, the migrating larvae may produce respiratory signs ("summer colds"). In heavy intestinal infections, foals show unthriftiness, loss of energy, and occasionally colic. Intestinal obstruction and perforation have been reported. Intestinal stages compete for absorption of essential amino acids. Diagnosis is based on demonstration of eggs in the feces. If disease due to prepatent infection is suspected, diagnosis may be confirmed by administration of an anthelmintic, after which large numbers of immature worms may be seen in the feces.

On farms where the infection is common, most foals become infected soon after birth. As a result, most of the worms are maturing when the foals are ~4-5 mo old. Treatment should be started when foals are ~8 wk old and repeated at 6- to 8-wk intervals until they are yearlings. All broad-spectrum equine anthelmintics are effective against the adult and immature worms in the small intestine and, therefore, ascarids are readily controlled by routine anthelmintic administration. In cases in which verminous pneumonia due to *Parascaris* migration has developed, therapeutic benefit may be achieved by treatment with ivermectin or fenbendazole (the latter at 10 mg/kg/day for 5 consecutive days) concurrent with appropriate antimicrobial therapy. *Parascaris* infection can be effectively prevented by daily administration of pyrantel tartrate once foals are eating grain regularly.

LARGE STRONGYLES

The large strongyles of horses are also known as blood worms, palisade worms, sclerostomes, or red worms. The 3 major species are *Strongylus vulgaris* (up to 25 mm), *S edentatus* (up to 40 mm), and *S equinus* (up to 50 mm). (*See also Triodontophorus* spp, p 267.) Under favorable conditions, the larvae develop to the infective stage within 1-2 wk after the eggs are passed. Infection is by ingestion of infective larvae, which exsheath in the intestine and migrate extensively before developing to maturity in the large intestine. The prepatent period is 6-11 mo. The larvae of *S vulgaris* migrate extensively in the cranial mesenteric artery and its branches, where they may cause parasitic thrombosis and arteritis. Larvae of the other 2 species may be found in various parts of the body, including the liver, perirenal tissues, retroperitoneal tissues, and pancreas. These species do not produce lesions in the mesenteric arteries. Mixed infections of large and small strongyles are the rule.

Clinical Findings: Adult large strongyles have large buccal capsules and are active blood feeders; they ingest mucosal plugs as they move about in the intestine. The associated blood loss may lead to anemia. Weakness, emaciation, and diarrhea are also common. *S vulgaris* is important because of the damage it does to the cranial mesenteric artery and its branches. As a result of the interference with the flow of blood to the intestine and thromboembolism, any of several conditions may follow, including colic; gangrenous enteritis; or intestinal stasis, torsion or intussusception, and possibly rupture. Cerebrospinal nematodiasis (p 1036) can cause a variety of lesions and signs depending on the part of the CNS affected.

Diagnosis and Treatment: Diagnosis of mixed strongyle infection is based on demonstration of eggs in the feces. Specific diagnosis can be made by identifying the infective larvae after fecal culture. When colic due to verminous arteritis is suspected, a painful enlargement at the root of the mesentery may be palpable per rectum. Serologic diagnosis based on a rise in β-globulins has been recommended but is not specific for *S vulgaris*. Parasitic arterial lesions have been demonstrated using arteriography.

Colic due to arterial lesions has been successfully controlled by anthelmintic treatments. Ivermectin and moxidectin at standard dosages are effective against the larval stages (L_4 and L_5) of *S vulgaris*; fenbendazole and oxfendazole, at dosages higher than that for adult parasites, are also effective against larval infections. Daily administration of pyrantel tartrate is effective in preventing the establishment of arterial stages of *S vulgaris*. A number of anthelmintics, including the benzimidazoles, pyrantel, and ivermectin, are active against adult large strongyles.

Parasite control programs are designed to minimize the level of pasture contamination and thereby reduce the risks associated with migrating larvae. Routine anthelmintic treatments do this by preventing fecal excretion of strongyle eggs (*see also* SMALL STRONGYLES, below).

SMALL STRONGYLES

Over 40 species of small strongyles in several genera have been found in the cecum and colon of domestic equids, each with its own site of preference. They belong to the subfamily Cyathostominae of the family Strongylidae and ~10 species are particularly prevalent. Most are appreciably smaller than the "large strongyles," but *Triodontophorus* spp (sometimes classified as nonmigratory large strongyles) are almost as long as *Strongylus vulgaris*.

Unlike the large strongyles, small strongyles do not migrate extraintestinally, as early development is confined to the wall of the intestine. Third-stage larvae may progress to the fourth stage without interruption, or they may undergo hypobiosis and resume development after prolonged periods of dormancy. When these worms emerge from the gut wall, they feed superficially on the mucosa and may rupture capillaries but are less pathogenic than the large strongyles, as their buccal cavities are much smaller. An exception is *T tenuicollis*, which can produce severe ulcers in the wall of the colon. Generally, however, the resulting erosions of the mucosa are slight and hard to visualize. Consequently, it is common to recover thousands of adult worms from apparently healthy horses that have received limited anthelmintic treatment. In heavier infections, however, disruption may be extensive enough to disturb digestive and absorptive function, resulting in loss of condition and even a catarrhal enteritis of the large intestine.

Larval Cyathostomiasis: An acute syndrome of sudden weight loss, often with severe diarrhea, is seen in temperate areas in late winter and spring, particularly in young ponies and horses (<5 yr old). This is associated with the mass emergence of previously hypobiotic larvae from the intestinal wall and, although of relatively low incidence, is nevertheless of concern as response to treatment is variable, and prognosis must be guarded even with intensive therapy. It is seen more frequently in Europe than in the USA, where it has been reported in New York and Tennessee.

Horses with larval cyathostomiasis generally have a neutrophilia and hypoalbuminemia. Hyperglobulinemia, particularly involving the β-globulin fraction described as characteristic in some reports, has been a less consistent finding. Eosinophilia is not a consistent finding. Often, strongyle eggs are not seen on fecal examination. However, gross observation of fourth- or fifth-stage larvae, which are often bright red, in the feces is helpful in making a diagnosis. Biopsy of large intestine via laparotomy also may assist in diagnosis; rectal biopsy is less reliable. Gross pathologic findings include typhlitis or colitis with mucosal hyperemia, hemorrhage, congestion, ulceration, or necrosis; in protracted cases, there may be only mucosal thickening. At necropsy, cyathostome larvae can be seen as small, gray dots (1-2 mm) in the mucosa, giving it a gritty sensation on palpation. Transillumination of the mucosa from the serosal surface may aid in visualizing the larvae.

Treatment: Adult cyathostomes are easily removed from the gut lumen by a wide range of anthelmintics, provided that the worm population is susceptible to the chosen drug. Benzimidazole-resistant strains of small strongyles are common in some regions, and pyrantel resistance has been demonstrated in some locations. Drug efficacy and the presence of anthelmintic resistance may be determined by comparing the worm egg count at the time of treatment and 10-14 days later. An effective drug should reduce the egg count to 0 or to very low levels. If resistance is present, a different anthelmintic class must be used because side resistance occurs within chemical groups.

Small-strongyle larvae in the intestinal mucosa are much more difficult to effectively remove with anthelmintics. Ivermectin has been used with mixed results; lack of efficacy has been reported at and above label dosages. Treatment with large dosages of fenbendazole (10 mg/kg for 5 consecutive days) or with moxidectin has been reported as effective and can be used during the winter to reduce the risk of larval cyathostomiasis. Horses already suffering from this disease may not respond to treatment if submucosal inflammation is too severe. Consequently, treatment must be augmented by corticosteroids and other appropriate supportive therapy.

Prevention: Routine or interval treatments are traditional and are intended to minimize the level of pasture contamination, thereby reducing the risks associated with the accumulation of mucosal larvae and adult worms. Alternatively, infection may be prevented by daily administration of pyrantel tartrate. The interval between routine treatments depends on the duration a particular drug keeps the feces free of eggs and varies from 4-13 wk. The frequency of treatment is also influenced by the value of the horses and the perceived level of risk, which varies with access to pasture, stocking density, and management practices. Control measures should be designed to minimize the risk of resistance developing in the worm population. Fewer treatments may be effective if given strategically according to local epidemiologic and climatic considerations. Removal of feces from paddocks and pastures aids in control and may also reduce the number of anthelmintic treatments required.

Generally in parasite control programs, all horses on a farm should be treated, and those commingled on the same pasture or paddock should be treated at the same time. Boarded horses or horses returning after having been off the premises for an extended time should be quarantined and dewormed before being admitted to the herd. In administering the anthelmintic, all horses should receive the proper dose, as determined by an accurate estimation of body weight. Rotating different classes of anthelmintics in a fast rotation scheme (eg, every few months) or a slow rotation scheme (annually) is widely practiced to prevent development of resistant parasite strains, but there is little evidence to support the utility of this procedure. Whatever program is used, fecal samples should be examined periodically to monitor the effectiveness of the program. Treatment can be restricted to those horses in a group with positive egg counts, if this information is available.

STRONGYLOIDES SP

Strongyloides westeri is found in the small intestine in foals. Adult horses rarely harbor patent infections, but mares often have larval stages within their tissues that are activated by parturition to move into the mammary tissue and, subsequently, are transmitted to foals in the milk. However, the relationship of *S westeri* infection with diarrhea in foals from 10 days of age has not been clearly established. The life cycle of the worm in horses is not known to differ significantly from that of *Strongyloides* in pigs (p 272). Diagnosis can be made based on observation of eggs somewhat more oval and about one-third the length of strongyle eggs that contain larvae. Ivermectin and oxibendazole are effective in removing *S westeri*. Transmission of larvae to foals in mare's milk may be prevented by routine treatment of mares with ivermectin within 24 hr postpartum.

TAPEWORMS

Three species of tapeworms are found in horses: *Anoplocephala magna*, *A perfoliata*, and *Paranoplocephala mamillana*. They are 8-25 cm long (the first usually being the longest, and the last the shortest). *A magna* and *P mamillana* usually are in the small intestine but may also be in the stomach; *A perfoliata* is found mostly in the cecum but may also be in the small intestine. The life cycle is similar to that of *Moniezia* spp in ruminants (p 262) and involves free-living oribatid mites as intermediate hosts. Diagnosis is by demonstration of the characteristic eggs in the feces, but because the discharge of proglottids is sporadic, a single fecal examination may not be diagnostic. In light infections, no signs of disease are present; in heavy infections, GI disturbances may be seen. Unthriftiness and anemia have been reported. Ulceration of the mucosa is quite common in the area of attachment of *A perfoliata* and has been suggested as one cause of intussusception. Intestinal perforation, peritonitis, and subsequent colic have been associated with *Anoplocephala* infections. Colic from disturbances of the ileocecal area is more likely in horses with tapeworm infections than in those not infected. Colic due to tapeworm infections often recurs. The site of attachment of tapeworms frequently becomes secondarily infected or abscessed. *Anoplocephala* spp can be effectively treated with pyrantel salts; normal dosages (6.6 mg/kg) of pyrantel pamoate are 87% effective, while double the normal dosage is >93% effective. Daily administration of pyrantel tartrate (2.65 mg/kg) removes *Anoplocephala* spp. Praziquantel (0.75-1.0 mg/kg) is 89-100% effective in the removal of *A perfoliata*. Praziquantel (at 1 mg/kg) appears to be effective in removing *P mamillana*, pyrantel salts are not.

On facilities where tapeworms are prevalent, clinical signs of tapeworm infections can be prevented by pyrantel salts, either routinely administered daily during the grazing season, or administered at the standard dosage or double the standard dosage within an interval deworming program. Treatment of horses according to the latter program with pyrantel pamoate immediately before turn out and at the end of the grazing season is likely to be most beneficial.

TRICHOSTRONGYLUS SP

The small stomach worm (hairworm) of horses, *Trichostrongylus axei*, is also found in ruminants (p 258) and, consequently, is generally a clinical problem only in horses commingled or rotated on pasture with ruminants. Adult *T axei* are slender and measure up to 8 mm long. Details of the life cycle in Equidae have not been carefully studied, but it is known that the larvae penetrate the mucosa. These worms produce a chronic catarrhal gastritis, which may result in weight loss. The lesions comprise nodular areas of thickened mucosa surrounded by a zone of congestion and covered with a variable amount of mucus. The lesions may be rather small and irregularly circumscribed, or they may coalesce and involve most or all of the glandular portion of the stomach, and erosions and ulcerations may be seen.

Definitive diagnosis based on fecal examination is difficult because the eggs are similar to strongyle eggs. The feces can be cultured and, in ~7 days, the infective larvae identified. Some of the benzimidazoles and ivermectin are effective against *T axei*.

GASTROINTESTINAL PARASITES OF PIGS

See also COCCIDIOSIS OF PIGS, p 167.

In pigs, GI helminths are ever present; their main effects are loss of appetite, reduction in daily gain, poor feed utilization, and potentiation of other pathogens. Only rarely do they cause death. A periparturient relaxation of immunity occurs in sows from 2 wk before parturition to 6 wk after; if they harbor a strongyle infection, the fecal egg count may increase markedly. At weaning, fecal egg output may drop abruptly and many worms, particularly *Oesophagostomum*, are eliminated. This phenomenon is less constant in pigs than in sheep but has considerable epidemiologic importance because the environment of the young is contaminated.

Apart from good basic hygiene in pig houses, which should be emphasized, control of GI helminths is based on anthelmintic treatments and preventive measures, such as removing the pigs from contact with intermediate hosts. To reduce the risk of development of resistance, anthelmintic use should be preceded by helminth surveillance of a representative number of animals, and should be initiated only on demonstration of parasite eggs in the feces of the examined age groups. In-feed products include benzimidazoles, ivermectin, levamisole, and dichlorvos. A simple anthelmintic program is to treat sows and gilts ~10 days before breeding and again before farrowing, weaners and feeders before entering clean pens, and boars at 6-mo intervals. Alternatively, an injection of ivermectin, also effective against lice and mange mites, may be given in a similar program. A different approach is to treat all pigs in the herd on the same day and to repeat every 3-6 mo or less, with the dosing interval being determined by fecal egg counts. Notwithstanding, a good management system incorporates practices aimed at preventing infections and does not use anthelmintic treatment as the sole method of controlling parasites.

ASCARIS SP

Adults of the large roundworm, *Ascaris suum*, are found principally in the small intestine but may migrate into the stomach or bile ducts. They are ~30 cm long, whitish, and quite thick. Large numbers of eggs are produced (as many as 250,000/day); they can develop to the infective stage (containing the L_3 larva) in 2-3 wk in warm conditions. The eggs are resistant to chemical agents, but conditions with low humidity, heat, or direct sunlight may reduce their survival significantly. When the eggs are ingested, the larvae hatch in the intestine, penetrate the large intestinal wall, and enter the portal circulation. After a period in the liver, they are carried by the circulation to the lungs, where they pass through the capillaries into the alveolar spaces. About 9-10 days after ingestion, the larvae pass up the bronchial tree to return to the GI tract. On arrival in the small intestine the majority of the larvae are expelled; remaining larvae develop into mature adult worms. The first eggs are passed $1^1/_2$-$2^1/_2$ mo after infection.

Clinical Findings: Adult worms may significantly reduce the growth rate of young pigs; if sufficiently numerous, they may cause mechanical obstruction of the intestine, or migrate into and occlude the bile ducts, producing icterus. Migration of larvae through the liver causes hemorrhage and fibrosis that appears as "white spots" under the capsule and leads to condemnation of the liver at slaughter. In heavy infections, the larvae can cause pulmonary edema and consolidation as well as exacerbate swine influenza and endemic pneumonia. Affected pigs show abdominal breathing, commonly referred to as "thumps." In addition to the respiratory signs, marked unthriftiness and weight loss are seen. Permanent stunting may result in pigs up to 4-5 mo old. The infection generally induces the development of resistance to reinfection.

Diagnosis: During the patent period, diagnosis can be made by demonstrating the typical eggs (golden brown, thick pitted outer wall, 50-70 × 40-60 μm) in the feces. However, many young pigs show signs (especially respiratory) during the prepatent period. A presumptive diagnosis can be made based on history and signs and confirmed by demonstrating immature worms on necropsy. In acute cases in which no worms are found in the intestine, it may be possible to recover larvae from affected lung tissue.

Treatment: Supportive therapy, including treatment for secondary bacterial invaders, may be necessary during the respiratory phase of infection. Many drugs have been used to remove adult ascarids. Piperazine preparations have low toxicity and are moderately priced. The benzimidazoles and probenzimidazoles, dichlorvos, ivermectin, levamisole, and pyrantel are effective and have a broader spectrum of activity than piperazine. Hygromycin is active against ascarids when administered as a low-level additive to the feed. Less information is available concerning the control of migratory stages; pyrantel and fenbendazole show activity.

MACRACANTHORHYNCHUS SP

Adult *Macracanthorhynchus hirudinaceus* (thorny-headed worm) are usually seen in the small intestine. They are 10 cm (males) to ~35 cm (females) long, 3-9 mm thick, and slightly pink with a transversely wrinkled outer covering. The anterior end bears a spiny, retractable proboscis or rostellum used for firm attachment to the intestinal wall. The eggs (dark brown, embryonated, with 3 embryonic envelopes, 90-110 × 50-65 μm) are ingested by the grubs of various beetles that serve as intermediate hosts. Pigs become infected by ingesting either grubs or adult beetles. The prepatent period is 2-3 mo and the female lays ~260,000 eggs/day for several months.

Signs are not specific; antemortem diagnosis is difficult because the ova do not float reliably in salt solutions and thus should be looked for in the sediment. The site of attachment may have a necrotic center surrounded by a zone of inflammation. These lesions usually can be seen through the serosa. The rostellum may perforate the intestinal wall and cause peritonitis and death.

Levamisole and ivermectin are effective for treatment. Control depends on avoiding use of contaminated hog lots or pastures or by regular removal of feces when pigs are kept in sties or small runs.

OESOPHAGOSTOMUM SPP

Oesophagostomum spp are prevalent worldwide; *O dentatum* is the most common species, while *O quadrispinulatum* appears to be more pathogenic. The adults are found in the lumen of the large intestine; they are 8-12 mm long, slender, and white or gray. The life cycle is direct. Infection results from ingestion of larvae, which penetrate the mucosa of the large intestine within a few hours after ingestion and return to the lumen in 6-20 days. The prepatent period is 17-35 days. Sows may have a periparturient rise in worm egg output, which is an important source of infection for piglets. Most infections are asymptomatic, but heavily infected pigs may show anorexia, emaciation, and GI disturbances. The serosa shows small nodules, their size reflecting species and previous exposure. In severe cases, the intestinal wall may be thickened and necrotic. Infection induces only moderate immunity, hence prevalence of nodular worms tends to be higher in the older age groups (sows, boars). In patent infections, typical strongyle eggs (66-80 × 38-47 μm) are found in feces, often in large numbers. These can be differentiated from those of *Hyostrongylus* by larval culture (*Oesophagostomum* larvae are shorter, thicker, and move more slowly). At necropsy, the worms and lesions are readily seen The benzimidazoles, levamisole, piperazines, dichlorvos, pyrantel tartrate, and ivermec tin are effective. A diet composed of highly degradable carbohydrates may suppor worm control by creating unfavorable conditions, which decrease worm establishmen and fecundity.

STOMACH WORMS

Three types of stomach worms are seen in pigs: a thin worm, *Hyostrongylus rubidu:* (the red stomach worm), and 2 thick stomach worms, *Ascarops strongylina* and *Physo cephalus sexalatus. H rubidus* is ~6 mm long and slender and has a direct life cycle. The thick stomach worms are ~10-20 mm long and much stouter and have coprophagous beetles as intermediate hosts.

Clinical Findings: These worms are more common in grazing pigs. When present in large numbers or when the host's condition is reduced by poor nutrition or other factors they may cause variable appetite, anemia, diarrhea, or weight loss. *Hyostrongylus* sp characteristically is found under a heavy catarrhal or mucous exudate and may produce mucosal lesions similar to those of *Ostertagia* spp in ruminants, except that hemor rhages are more common. Retarded development of larval stages in the mucosa is analo gous to that of *Ostertagia*. In sows, inhibited larvae may resume development near par turition and may cause severe gastritis and, in addition, contaminate the environment o' the young pigs. Egg excretion per female *Hyostrongylus* worm is generally low com pared with that of other nematode genera.

Diagnosis: Clinical signs other than unthriftiness are not obvious. Fecal examinations may show the distinctive ova of *Physocephalus* and *Ascarops*—small ($35\text{-}40 \times 17\text{-}20$ mm) thick-shelled eggs containing an active larva. *Hyostrongylus* ova resemble those of other strongyle worms (*Oesophagostomum, Globocephalus*), and fecal cultures are required to obtain infective larvae for differential diagnosis.

At necropsy, adult worms, especially *Physocephalus* and *Ascarops*, are readily seen Mucosal scrapings for microscopic examination are essential for detection of immature *Hyostrongylus.*

Treatment: The newer benzimidazoles, probenzimidazoles, and ivermectin are highly effective against adult and immature stages (including hypobiotic larvae) of *Hyo strongylus*. Ivermectin has activity against adult *Ascarops.*

STRONGYLOIDES SP

The life cycle of *Strongyloides ransomi* (intestinal threadworm) is apparently simi lar to that of *S papillosus* of cattle (p 260). Transmission of *S ransomi* larvae in the co lostrum is the most common route of infection in neonatal pigs and explains the serious nature of the infection. The adult worms (only females in the parasitic cycle) burrow into the wall of the small intestine. The prepatent period is 4-9 days, depending on the mode of infection. In light and moderate infections, the pigs usually show no signs. In heavy infections, diarrhea, anemia, and emaciation may be seen, and death may result. Infection induces strong immunity, hence older pigs are usually not clinically affected.

Demonstration of the characteristic small, thin-shelled, embryonated eggs ($20\text{-}35 \times 40\text{-}55$ μm) in the feces, or of the adults in scrapings from the intestinal mucosa is diag nostic. *Strongyloides* ova must be differentiated from the larger *Metastrongylus* (swine lungworm) ova ($33\text{-}42 \times 51\text{-}63$ μm), which also are embryonated in fresh feces. At necropsy, immature worms may be recovered from minced tissues placed in a Baermann isolation apparatus.

The benzimidazoles and levamisole are effective against intestinal infections. If ad ministered in the feed for several days before and after parturition, they reduce infections in suckling piglets. Ivermectin is effective against adults and, if given to the sow 1-2 wk before farrowing, controls transmission to the piglets. A high level of hygiene in the pig sty is necessary to diminish free-living larvae and thus decrease the infection risk.

TRICHURIS SP

Trichuris suis is 5-8 cm long and whip-shaped; the anterior slender portion embeds in the wall of the large intestine, especially the cecum, with the thickened posterior third lying free in the lumen. Infection is by ingestion of embryonated ova. Heavy infections may cause inflammatory lesions in the cecum and adjacent large intestine and be accompanied by (bloody) diarrhea and unthriftiness. Infection is most often seen in young animals; resistance is both acquired and age-related. The double-operculated yellowish eggs (50-68 × 21-31 μm) are diagnostic, with egg excretion commencing ~6 wk after infection. However, trichurids are sporadic egg layers, thus little significance can be given to numbers of eggs per gram of feces. Dichlorvos, levamisole, some benzimidazoles, and ivermectin are effective against the adult worms. The eggs are comparable to *Ascaris* eggs—they are highly resistant and may remain infective for up to 11 yr; hence, control relies on thorough cleaning of the affected area and moving the animals to clean plots.

FLUKE INFECTIONS IN RUMINANTS

Fasciola hepatica, the most important trematode of domestic ruminants, is the most common cause of liver fluke disease in temperate areas of the world. In the USA, it is endemic along the Gulf Coast, the West Coast, the Rocky Mountain region, and other areas. It is present in eastern Canada, British Columbia, and South America, and is of particular economic importance in the British Isles, western and eastern Europe, Australia, and New Zealand. *F gigantica* is economically important in Africa and Asia and is also found in Hawaii. *F magna* has been reported in at least 21 states (USA) and in Europe. In North America, *Dicrocoelium dendriticum* is confined mainly to New York, New Jersey, Massachusetts, and the Atlantic provinces of Canada. It is also widespread in some areas in Europe and Asia. *Eurytrema* spp, the pancreatic flukes, parasitize sheep, pigs, and cattle in Brazil and parts of Asia. Several species of paramphistomes or rumen flukes are found throughout much of the world.

FASCIOLA HEPATICA
(Common liver fluke)

Etiology: *F hepatica* (30 × 2-12 mm and leaf-shaped) is distributed worldwide and has a broad host range. Economically important infections are seen in cattle and sheep in 3 forms: chronic, which is rarely fatal in cattle but often fatal in sheep; subacute or acute, which is primarily in sheep and often fatal; and in conjunction with "black disease" (INFECTIOUS NECROTIC HEPATITIS, p 288), which is most common in sheep and usually fatal.

Eggs passed in the feces develop into miracidia in ~2-4 wk, depending on temperature, and hatch in water. Miracidia infect lymnaeid snails, in which development and multiplication occur through the stages of sporocysts, rediae (sometimes daughter rediae), and cercariae. After ~2 mo (or longer if temperatures are low), cercariae emerge from snails and encyst on aquatic vegetation. Snails may extend the period by hibernating during the winter. Encysted cercariae (metacercariae) may remain viable for many months unless they become desiccated.

After ingestion by the host, usually with herbage, young flukes are released in the duodenum, penetrate the intestinal wall, and enter the peritoneal cavity. The young flukes penetrate the liver capsule and wander in the parenchyma for several weeks, growing and destroying tissue. They usually enter the bile ducts 6-8 wk after ingestion, mature, and begin to produce eggs. The prepatent period is usually 2-3 mo, depending on the fluke burden. Adult flukes may live in the bile ducts of sheep for years; most are shed from cattle within 5-6 mo. Prenatal infections have been reported in cattle.

Clinical Findings: Fasciolosis ranges in severity from a devastating disease in sheep to an asymptomatic infection in cattle. The course usually is determined by the number of metacercariae ingested over a short period. In sheep, acute fasciolosis occurs seasonally and is manifest by a distended, painful abdomen; anemia; and sudden death. Deaths can occur within 6 wk of infection. The acute syndrome must be differentiated from "black disease." In subacute disease, survival is longer (7-10 wk), even in cases with significant hepatic damage, but deaths occur due to hemorrhage and anemia. Chronic fasciolosis is seen in all seasons; signs include anemia, unthriftiness, submandibular edema, and reduced milk secretion, but even heavily infected cattle may show no clinical signs. Heavy chronic infection is fatal in sheep.

Sheep do not appear to develop resistance to infection, and chronic liver damage is cumulative over several years. In cattle, there is evidence of reduced susceptibility after fibrosis of liver tissues and calcification of bile ducts.

Lesions: Immature, wandering flukes destroy liver tissue and cause hemorrhage. In acute fasciolosis, damage is extensive; the liver is enlarged and friable with fibrinous deposits on the capsule. Migratory tracts can be seen, and the surface has an uneven appearance. In chronic cases, cirrhosis develops. Mature flukes damage the bile ducts, which become enlarged, or even cystic, and have thickened, fibrosed walls. In cattle, the duct walls become greatly thickened and often calcified. Flukes may be found in aberrant sites, eg, lungs. Mixed infections with *Fasciola magna* can be seen in cattle.

Tissue destruction by wandering flukes may create a microenvironment favorable to activation of clostridial spores.

Diagnosis: The oval, operculated, golden brown eggs, 130-150 × 65-90 μm, must be distinguished from those of paramphistomes (rumen flukes), which are larger and clear. Eggs of *F hepatica* cannot be demonstrated in feces during acute fasciolosis. In subacute or chronic disease in cattle, the number varies from day to day, and repeated fecal examination may be required. Diagnosis can be aided by an ELISA (commercially available in Europe) that enables diagnosis ~2-3 wk after infection and well before the prepatent period. Plasma concentrations of γ-glutamyltransferase, which are increased with bile duct damage, are also helpful during the late maturation period when flukes are in the bile ducts. At necropsy, the nature of the liver damage is diagnostic. Adult flukes are readily seen in the bile ducts, and immature stages may be squeezed or teased from the cut surface.

Control: Control measures for *F hepatica* ideally should involve removal of flukes in affected animals, reduction of the intermediate host snail population, and prevention of livestock access to snail-infested pasture. In practice, only the first of these is used in most cases. While molluscicides can be used to reduce lymnaeid snail populations, those that are available all have drawbacks that restrict their use. Copper sulfate, if applied before the snail population multiplies each year, is effective but toxic to sheep, which must be kept off treated pasture for 6 wk after application. Prevention of livestock access to snail-infested pasture is frequently impractical because of the size of the areas involved and the consequent expense of erecting adequate fencing.

Several drugs are available to treat infected ruminants, including triclabendazole, clorsulon (cattle and sheep only), albendazole, netobimin, closantel, rafoxanide, and oxyclozanide. Not all are approved in all countries (eg, only clorsulon and albendazole are approved in the USA), and most have long withdrawal periods before slaughter if used in meat-producing animals and before milk from treated livestock can be used for human consumption. The timing of treatment is also important so that the pharmacokinetics of the drug used will result in the optimal removal of flukes—each flukicide has varying efficacy against different ages of fluke. Traditionally, some treatments are determined by local epidemiologic factors and additional treatments by unusually suitable conditions for parasite multiplication. For example, in the Gulf Coast states of the USA, cattle should be treated before the fall rainy season and again in the late spring. In northwestern USA and in northern Europe, cattle should be treated at the end of the pasture season and, if not housed, again in late January or February. In European countries with large susceptible sheep populations, computerized prediction systems are used to determine the likely prevalence of *F hepatica* infections. In areas where heavy infections are expected, sheep may require treatment in September or October, January or February, and again in April or May to reduce both the chances of acute or chronic infections and the output of fluke eggs for development of future disease.

FASCIOLA GIGANTICA
(Giant liver fluke)

Fasciola gigantica is similar in shape to *F hepatica* but is larger (75 mm), with less clearly defined shoulders. It is found in warmer climates (Asia, Africa) in cattle and buffalo, in which it is responsible for chronic fasciolosis, and in sheep, in which the disease is frequently acute and fatal. The life cycle is similar to that of *F hepatica* except for species of snail intermediate hosts. The pathology of infection, diagnostic procedures, and control measures are similar to those for *F hepatica* (*see* above).

FASCIOLOIDES MAGNA
(Large American liver fluke, Giant liver fluke)

Fascioloides magna is up to 100 mm long, thick, and oval; it is distinguished from *Fasciola* spp by the lack of an anterior projecting cone. It is found in domestic and wild ruminants; deer are the normal hosts. The life cycle resembles that of *Fasciola* spp.

The life cycle is not completed in cattle. In this host, pathogenicity is low, and losses are confined primarily to liver condemnations. In sheep and goats, a few parasites can cause death due to extensive fluke migration in the liver parenchyma. In deer, there is little tissue reaction, and the parasites are enclosed in thin, fibrous cysts that communicate with bile ducts. In cattle, *Fascioloides magna* causes severe tissue reaction, resulting in thick-walled encapsulations that do not communicate with bile ducts. In sheep, encapsulations do not develop, and the parasites migrate in the liver and other organs, causing tremendous damage. Histologically, infected livers of cattle, sheep, and deer show black, tortuous tracts formed by migrations of young flukes.

While the eggs of *Fascioloides magna* resemble those of *Fasciola hepatica*, this is of limited use; eggs usually are not passed in cattle and sheep. Recovery of the parasites at necropsy as well as differentiation of *Fasciola hepatica* and *Fasciola gigantica* is necessary for definite diagnosis. When domestic ruminants and deer share the same grazing, the presence of disease due to *Fascioloides magna* should be kept in mind. Mixed infections with *Fasciola hepatica* are seen in cattle.

Oxyclozanide has been reported to be effective against *Fascioloides magna* in white-tailed deer, and rafoxanide has been used successfully against natural infections in cattle. Albendazole (7.5 mg/kg), clorsulon (15 mg/kg), and closantel (15 mg/kg) have shown efficacy against this fluke in sheep. Currently no products are approved for use against this fluke in the USA. Deer are required for completion of the life cycle; if they can be excluded from the areas grazed by cattle and sheep, control may be effected. Control of the intermediate host (lymnaeid snails) may be possible once it has been identified in a region and the nature of its habitat examined.

DICROCOELIUM DENDRITICUM
(Lancet fluke, Lesser liver fluke)

Dicrocoelium dendriticum is slender and 6-10 mm long. It is widely distributed in many countries and infects a wide range of final hosts, including domestic ruminants. Another species, *D hospes*, is common in Africa.

The first intermediate host is a terrestrial snail (*Cionella lubrica*, in the USA), from which cercariae emerge and are aggregated in a mass of sticky mucus (slimeball). The cercariae are ingested by the second intermediate host, which is an ant (*Formica fusca*, in the USA), and encyst in the abdominal cavity. One or two metacercariae in the subesophageal ganglion of the ant cause abnormal behavior in which the ants attach themselves to the herbage, which in turn increases the probability of ingestion by the final host. The young flukes do not migrate through the liver tissue but reach the bile ducts from the intestine and begin laying eggs ~10-12 wk after infection.

There appears to be no immunity, and heavy infections may accumulate (up to 50,000 flukes in a mature sheep). Cirrhosis develops, and the bile ducts may be thickened and distended. Economic loss is due primarily to condemnation of livers. Clinical signs are not obvious but may be seen in massive infections. The eggs contain a miracidium and are very small (40×25 µm), lopsided, and yellowish brown.

The complex life cycle makes control of intermediate hosts almost impossible, because widespread chemical use has damaging ecologic effects on other similar organisms. Effective anthelmintic treatments in cattle are albendazole at 15 mg/kg in a single dose or 2 doses of 7.5 mg/kg on successive days, or netobimin at 20 mg/kg.

EURYTREMA SPP
(Pancreatic fluke)

These flukes have a thick body and are 8-16 mm long and 6 mm wide. They are parasites of the pancreatic ducts and occasionally of the bile ducts of sheep, pigs, and cattle in Brazil and Asia. Three species, *Eurytrema pancreaticum*, *E coelomaticum*, and *E ovis* are recognized. The first intermediate hosts are terrestrial snails (*Bradybaena* spp), and the cercariae encyst in grasshoppers (*Conocephalus* spp), which are the second intermediate host. After the animal ingests a grasshopper, the immature flukes are released and migrate to the pancreatic duct, where they mature and produce eggs in ~11-14 wk.

There are no obvious clinical signs. *Dicrocoelium*-like eggs can be demonstrated in feces. Light infections cause proliferative inflammation of the pancreatic duct, which may become enlarged and occluded. In heavy infections, fibrotic, necrotic, and degenerative lesions develop. Losses are reported due to condemned pancreas, but the pathogenesis suggests an additional loss of production.

As with *Dicrocoelium*, the control of intermediate hosts may not be practical. Treatment with praziquantel (20 mg/kg, for 2 days) or albendazole (7.5 mg/kg for sheep, 10 mg/kg for cattle) have been reported to be effective.

PARAMPHISTOMES
(Amphistomes, Rumen flukes, Conical flukes)

There are numerous species of paramphistomes (*Paramphistomum*, *Calicophoron*, *Cotylophoron*) in ruminants worldwide. The adult parasites are pear-shaped, pink or red, up to 15 mm long, and attach to the lining of the rumen. Immature forms are found in the duodenum and are 1-3 mm long.

Eggs are passed in the feces, and miracidiae hatch in the water and infect planorbid or bulinid snails. Development in the snail is similar to that in the life cycle of *Fasciola hepatica*, with the snail shedding cercariae that encyst on the herbage. In the ruminant host, the young flukes excyst and remain in the small intestine for 3-5 wk before migrating forward through the reticulum to the rumen. Eggs are produced 7-14 wk after infection.

Adult flukes do not cause overt disease, and large numbers may be encountered. The immature flukes attach to the duodenal and, at times, the ileal mucosa by means of a large posterior sucker and cause severe enteritis, possibly necrosis, and hemorrhage. Affected animals exhibit anorexia, polydipsia, unthriftiness, and severe diarrhea. Extensive mortality may occur, especially in young cattle and sheep. Older animals can develop resistance to reinfection but may continue to harbor numerous adult flukes.

The large, clear, operculated eggs are readily recognized, but in acute paramphistomosis there may be no eggs in the feces. Known occurrence in the area and examination of the fluid feces may reveal immature flukes, many of which are passed in these cases. Diagnosis is commonly made at necropsy.

Control measures to reduce the host snail population are as for control of fasciolosis (p 273). Treatments with reported success (efficacies >90%) are resorantel, oxyclozanide, and the combination of bithional and levamisole.

HEPATIC DISEASE IN LARGE ANIMALS

Hepatic disease is common in large animals, especially horses. Increases in serum hepatic enzymes and total bile acid concentration may indicate hepatic dysfunction, insult, disease, or failure. Diseases that frequently result in hepatic failure in horses include Theiler's disease, Tyzzer's disease, pyrrolizidine alkaloid toxicosis, hepatic lipidosis, suppurative cholangitis, cholelithiasis, chronic active hepatitis, and ferrous fumarate toxicosis. Obstructive biliary disease associated with intestinal displacement, aflatoxicosis, leukoencephalomalacia, pancreatic disease, duodenal ulcerations, kleingrass or alsike clover poisoning, portal caval shunts, hepatic abscess, hepatic neoplasia, and perinatal herpesvirus 1 infections sporadically result in hepatic failure. Less frequently, hepatic failure is associated with endotoxemia, steroid administration, inhalant anesthesia, systemic granulomatous disease, drug-induced amyloidosis, or parasite damage. In ruminants, hepatobiliary disease is associated with hepatic lipidosis, hepatic abscesses, endotoxemia, pyrrolizidine alkaloid and other plant toxicities, certain clostridial diseases, liver flukes, mycotoxicosis, and mineral toxicity (copper, iron, zinc) or deficiency (cobalt). Vitamin E or selenium deficiency (hepatosis dietetica), aflatoxicosis, ascarid migration, bacterial hepatitis, and ingestion of toxic substances (eg, coal tar, cyanamide, blue-green algae, plants, gossypol) are associated with hepatic injury in swine. Although the exact incidence of hepatic disease in camelids (llamas, alpacas) is unknown, it appears to be common in North America. Hepatic lipidosis (secondary more often than primary) is reportedly the most common liver disease in llamas and alpacas, but bacterial (*Salmonella* sp, *Escherichia coli, Listeria* sp, *Clostridium* sp) cholangiohepatitis, adenoviral hepatitis and pneumonia, fungal hepatitis (coccidioidomycosis), toxic hepatopathy (copper), halothane-induced hepatic necrosis, hepatic neoplasia (lymphosarcoma, hemangiosarcoma, adenoma), and liver fluke infestation have been reported.

The liver can respond to insult in only a limited number of ways. Fat droplets in the liver may be an early and often reversible change. Biliary hyperplasia is also reversible if the insult is removed early. Necrosis of hepatocytes indicates more recent damage. The dead cells are removed by an inflammatory process and replaced with either new hepatocytes or fibrosis. Unless the dysfunction is acute and hepatocellular regeneration is evident, prognosis for animals with liver failure is usually unfavorable. Early hepatic fibrosis may be reversible with prompt recognition and intervention. Chronic disease with extensive loss of hepatic parenchyma and fibrosis warrants a poor prognosis.

Clinical Findings: Clinical signs of hepatic disease may not be evident until >60-80% of the liver parenchyma is nonfunctional or when hepatic dysfunction is secondary to disease in another organ system. Signs of hepatic encephalopathy and liver failure commonly present acutely whether the hepatic disease process is acute or chronic. The clinical signs and severity of hepatic pathology reflect the degree of compromise of one or more of the liver's vital functions, including blood glucose regulation; fat metabolism; production of clotting factors, albumin, fibrinogen, nonessential amino acids, and plasma proteins; bile formation and excretion; bilirubin and cholesterol metabolism; conversion of ammonia to urea; polypeptide and steroid hormone metabolism; synthesis of 25-hydroxycholecalciferol; and metabolism and/or detoxification of many drugs and toxins.

Icterus, weight loss, or abnormal behavior are common in horses with liver disease and hepatic failure. Photosensitization, and less commonly inspiratory stridor, diarrhea, or constipation, are present. Affected cattle usually show inappetence, decreased milk production, and weight loss. Tenesmus and ascites are seen in cattle but are not commonly noted in affected horses. Weight loss is a common clinical sign in chronic liver disease and may be the only sign associated with liver abscesses. Icterus is common in acute liver failure in horses but is variably present in chronic liver failure or in ruminants. Fasting hyperbilirubinemia is a more common cause of icterus in horses and is not associated with hepatic disease. Occasionally, persistent hyperbilirubinemia (primarily indirect or unconjugated bilirubin) may be seen in healthy horses without evidence of hemolysis or hepatic disease. In ruminants, icterus is more commonly due to hemolysis and primarily involves increases in indirect bilirubin. Hyperbilirubinemia caused by obstructive biliary conditions is rare in goats.

Hepatic encephalopathy is associated with behavioral changes in horses, ruminants, and swine. The severity of hepatic encephalopathy often reflects the degree of hepatic failure but does not differentiate between acute or chronic liver failure. Signs of hepatic encephalopathy range from nonspecific depression and lethargy to head pressing, circling, aimless walking, dysphagia, ataxia, dysmetria, persistent yawning, increased friendliness, aggressiveness, vicious behavior, stupor, seizures, or coma. Pharyngeal or laryngeal collapse with loud, stertorous inspiratory noises and dyspnea occurs in some cases of hepatic failure, especially in ponies. The pathogenesis of hepatic encephalopathy is unknown, but proposed theories include ammonia as a neurotoxin, alterations in monoamine neurotransmission (serotonin, tryptophan) or catecholamine neurotransmitters, imbalance between aromatic and short branch chain amino acids resulting in increased inhibitory neurotransmitters (γ-aminobutyric acid, L-glutamate), neuroinhibition due to increased cerebral levels of endogenous benzodiazepine-like substances, increased permeability of the blood-brain barrier, and impaired CNS energy metabolism. Although the signs can be dramatic, hepatic encephalopathy is potentially reversible if the underlying hepatic disease is resolved.

Photosensitization, which can be seen with acute or chronic liver failure, must be differentiated from primary photosensitization (p 794). Hepatogenous photosensitization develops when compromised hepatic function results in phylloerythrin, a photodynamic metabolite of chlorophyll, entering the skin. Phylloerythrin in the skin reacts with ultraviolet light and releases energy, causing inflammation and skin damage. Signs of photosensitization are varied but include uneasiness, pain, pruritus, mild to severe dermatitis with erythema, extensive subcutaneous edema, skin ulceration, sloughing of skin and ophthalmia with lacrimation, photophobia, and corneal cloudiness. Dermatitis and edema are particularly evident on nonpigmented, light-colored or hairless areas of the body and areas exposed to sun. Mucocutaneous junctions and patches of white hair are the most common sites of photosensitization in cattle. Occasionally, the underside of the tongue may be affected. Blindness, pyoderma, loss of condition, and occasionally death are possible sequelae. Pruritus may result from photosensitization or from deposition of bile salts in the skin secondary to alterations in hepatic excretion.

Diarrhea or constipation may be seen in animals with hepatic disease. Diarrhea is more commonly seen in cattle than in horses with chronic liver disease or in animals with chronic fascioliasis and hepatotoxic plant poisonings. Ponies and horses with hyperlipemia and hepatic failure may develop diarrhea, laminitis, and ventral edema. Some animals with liver disease have alternating diarrhea and constipation. Horses with liver failure and hepatic encephalopathy frequently develop colonic impaction due to decreased water intake. Constipation is characteristic of *Lantana* poisoning in goats and other ruminants.

Recurrent colic, intermittent fever, icterus, weight loss, and hepatic encephalopathy may be seen in horses with choleliths that obstruct the common bile duct. Infectious or inflammatory hepatic disease or failure of the liver to prevent endotoxin from gaining access to the systemic circulation may also result in intermittent fever and colic. Abdominal pain, due to pressure on the liver capsule from parenchymal swelling, often is seen in animals with acute diffuse hepatitis or trauma to the capsule itself. Affected animals stand with an arched back, are reluctant to move, or show signs of colic. In ruminants, pain may be localized to the liver by palpation over the anterior ventrolateral aspect of the abdomen or the last few ribs on the right side. Tenesmus followed by rectal prolapse is seen in some ruminants with liver disease. It may be associated with diarrhea, hepatic encephalopathy, or edema of the bowel from portal hypertension.

Hypoalbuminemia is not as frequently associated with liver disease in horses as previously thought. Due to the long half-life (19 days) and liver reserve for albumin production, hypoalbuminemia is usually a very late event in the disease process. Serum total protein concentrations may be normal or elevated due to an increase in β-globulins in horses with liver disease. Hypoalbuminemia and hypoproteinemia most commonly develop in chronic liver disease, and they are common findings in llamas with liver disease.

Generalized ascites or dependent edema may result. Ascites is related to portal hypertension caused by venous blockage and increased hydrostatic pressure and to protein leakage into the peritoneal cavity. The abdominal fluid present with liver disease usually is a modified transudate. Hypoalbuminemia can aggravate the ascites, but if it is seen alone, it more likely will cause intermandibular, brisket, or ventral edema. Ascites is difficult to appreciate in horses and adult cattle unless it is extensive. Ascites is a common finding in calves with liver cirrhosis.

Anemia may be seen in animals with liver dysfunction due to parasitic diseases, chronic copper toxicity, some plant poisonings, or chronic inflammatory disease. Anemia in acute fascioliasis results from severe hemorrhage into the peritoneal cavity as the larvae penetrate the liver capsule. Trauma and feeding activity of adult flukes within the bile ducts cause anemia and hypoproteinemia in animals with chronic fascioliasis. Chronic inflammatory disease (eg, hepatic abscesses, neoplasia) may cause anemia without accompanying hypoproteinemia.

Clinical signs of severe or terminal hepatic failure include coagulopathies and hemorrhage due to decreased production of clotting factors by the liver and possibly increased utilization in septic or inflammatory processes. A prolonged prothrombin time is usually seen first because factor VII has the shortest plasma half-life. Horses may develop a terminal hemolytic crisis caused by increased RBC fragility. This has not been reported in ruminants.

Fecal color rarely changes in adult herbivores with liver disease. In young ruminants and monogastric animals, cholestasis may result in lighter color feces being passed due to loss of stercobilin, a metabolite of bilirubin.

Liver disease should always be considered when nonspecific clinical signs, such as depression, weight loss, intermittent fever, and recurrent colic, are present without an apparent cause. Differentiation between acute and chronic hepatitis or failure based on the duration of clinical signs before presentation may be misleading because the disease process is often advanced before clinical signs are evident. Early vague signs of depression and decreased appetite may be overlooked. Liver biopsy to determine the type of pathology, degree of hepatic fibrosis present, and the regenerative capabilities of the liver parenchyma is necessary for developing a treatment plan and giving an accurate prognosis.

Laboratory Analyses: Laboratory tests often detect liver disease before hepatic failure occurs. Routine biochemical tests such as serum enzyme concentrations are sensitive indicators of liver disease, but they do not assess hepatic function. Dynamic biochemical tests that assess hepatic clearance provide quantitative information regarding hepatic function. Tests of hepatic function are useful diagnostic and prognostic tools and provide a guide for the modification of drug-dosing regimens.

Serum Enzyme Concentrations: Serum concentrations of liver-specific enzymes are generally higher in acute liver disease than in chronic liver disease. They may be within normal limits in the later stages of subacute or chronic hepatic disease. Careful interpretation of laboratory values in conjunction with clinical findings is essential.

Sequential measurements of serum γ-glutamyl transpeptidase or transferase (GGT), sorbitol dehydrogenase (SDH; also called iditol dehydrogenase, IDH), aspartate amino transferase (AST), bilirubin, and bile acids are commonly used to assess hepatic dysfunction and disease in large animals. Serum GGT, bilirubin and total bile acid concentrations, and sulfobromophthalein (BSP®) clearance are not sensitive indicators of liver disease in young calves. Although GGT is primarily associated with microsomal membranes in the biliary epithelium, it is also present in the canalicular surfaces of the hepatocytes, pancreas, kidneys, and udder. Due to urinary and milk excretion of GGT and rarity of pancreatitis in large animals, increased serum GGT concentrations most commonly indicate bile duct or liver disease. Some consider GGT to be the single test of highest sensitivity for liver disease in adult large animals. Increase of GGT is most pronounced with obstructive biliary disease. In acute hepatic disease in horses, GGT may continue to increase for 7-14 days despite clinical improvement and return toward normal of other laboratory tests. Reportedly, serum GGT concentrations become elevated within a few days of liver damage and remain elevated until the terminal phase. Chronic hepatic fibrosis is the only liver disease in which an abnormal increase in GGT might not be seen. Neonatal foals and young horses, especially those in training, may show a nonspecific increase in GGT that is not associated with liver disease or other increases in liver enzymes or serum bile acid concentration. GGT is of little value in diagnosing liver disease in neonatal calves or lambs because it is present in colostrum and milk. GGT activity may also be increased with colonic displacement or administration of drugs (eg, corticosteroids, rifampin, benzimidazole, anthelmintics). Some liver-derived enzymes are higher in young calves (GGT, alkaline phosphatase [AP], glutamate dehydrogenase, lactate dehydrogenase) and foals (AP, GGT, SDH, AST) because they are transiently elevated or come from sources other than the liver. Serum levels of hepatic enzymes also vary in goats with age, breed, and sex. Reference ranges must be appropriate for the species and age group being evaluated.

SDH, arginase, ornithine carbamoyltransferase (OCT), AST, isoenzyme 5 lactate dehydrogenase (LDH-5), glutamate dehydrogenase (GLDH), and AP are also used to assess hepatic dysfunction and disease. Arginase, SDH, and OCT are liver-specific enzymes in horses, most ruminants, and swine. SDH is most predictive for active hepatocellular disease, with marked increases in enzyme activity following hepatocellular damage. Mild increases in SDH can also occur with obstructive GI lesions, endotoxemia, anoxia from shock, acute anemia, hyperthermia, and anesthesia. Because of their short half-lives, SDH and LDH-5 are useful in assessing acute, ongoing liver disease. Both enzymes usually return to near-normal values 4 days after liver insult, and neither is usually increased in chronic liver disease. Arginase and GLDH are considered specific for acute liver disease because both have high tissue concentrations in the liver and short half-lives in the blood. AST is highly sensitive for liver disease but lacks specificity because high concentrations come from both liver and skeletal muscle. Other AST sources include cardiac muscle, erythrocytes, intestinal cells, and the kidneys. When CK is simultaneously measured to rule out muscle disease and the serum is not hemolyzed, increases in AST and LDH-5 are caused by hepatocellular disease. AST may remain increased 10-14 days or more after an acute, transient insult to the liver. AST values are often normal in chronic hepatic disease. SDH and AST may be markedly increased with intrahepatic cholestasis and mildly increased with extrahepatic cholestasis. Increases in AP and GGT are associated with irritation or destruction of biliary epithelium and biliary obstruction. AP comes from the placenta, bone, macrophages, intestinal epithelium, and liver. AP is increased in very young calves and foals, probably because of the placental or bone source. In young calves, AP levels up to 1,000 IU/L at birth and 500 IU/L at several weeks of age are considered normal. AP levels from 152-2,835 IU/L are reported in foals (<12 hr old), and AP activity may remain elevated compared with adult levels for 1-2 mo. In calves (<6 wk old), none of the common tests (bilirubin, GGT, GLDH, AP, LDH, AST, or alanine transaminase) for liver damage or function are clinically useful for detection of hepatic disease when used alone. AST and GLDH are the most sensitive of the enzymes for hepatic injury, but AST also increases with muscle damage. AST levels in foals may be elevated compared with values of adults for many months. This elevation is also likely related to muscle development. Transient and mild increases in SDH activity may be noted in some foals <2 mo old.

Serum Total Bile Acid Concentration: Serum concentration of bile acids is highly specific for liver dysfunction but does not define the type of insult or disease present. Serum bile acid concentrations increase with hepatocellular damage, cholestasis, or shunts from the portal system to the vena cava. Elevations are highest with biliary obstruction and portosystemic shunts. Serum bile acid concentrations rise early in liver disease and often remain elevated through the later stages. Concentrations of serum bile acids >20 μmol/L have a high sensitivity and positive predictive value for determining liver disease in **horses** but not in ruminants. Serum total bile acid concentration in most normal horses is <10 μmol/L. Total bile acid concentration remains increased in horses with chronic liver disease. In horses, there is no diurnal variation, no postprandial rise, and no significant hour-to-hour variation in bile acid concentrations. Prolonged, but not short-term (<14 hr), fasting may cause increased serum bile acid concentrations in horses.

Interpretation of total bile acid concentrations is difficult in foals <1 wk old. In **dairy cattle**, serum bile acid measurement is of little value in recognizing fatty liver or liver disease or failure due to significant hour-to-hour variations. In recently freshened cows, serum total bile acid concentrations are significantly higher than in cows in mid-lactation or in 6-mo-old heifers. Total bile acid concentration may be the best single test for hepatic disease in young **calves**. In calves, concentrations >35 μmol/L may indicate liver disease, bile obstruction, or a portosystemic shunt. Reported reference intervals for serum concentration of bile acids are 1.1-22.9 μmol/L for **llamas** >1 yr old and 1.8-49.8 μmol/L for llamas <1 yr old. Feeding and sampling time of day revealed a variation in bile acid concentrations in individual llamas, but values remained within the reference interval.

Serum Bile Pigments: Evaluation of serum bilirubin (direct and indirect) concentration is useful for determining hepatic dysfunction in horses and ruminants. Increases in bilirubin result from hemolysis, hepatocellular disease, cholestasis, or physiologic causes. Anorexia in horses causes a physiologic increase in total serum bilirubin to usually <6-8 mg/dL and rarely as high as 10.5-12 mg/dL. The indirect bilirubin increases 2- to 3-fold, while the direct bilirubin remains within the reference range. In foals, indirect more than direct bilirubin may be increased with prematurity, neonatal isoerythrolysis, septicemia, or a portocaval shunt. Enteritis, umbilical infection, intestinal obstruction, and certain drugs (corticosteroids, heparin, halothane) may also cause hyperbilirubinemia. Icterus and hyperbilirubinemia in neonatal calves and foals may result from a normal physiologic condition involving breakdown of fetal erythrocytes and from inefficiency in bilirubin excretion. In normal calves <72 hr old, total bilirubin may be as high as 1.5 mg/dL and up to 0.8 mg/dL in 1-wk-old calves. Direct bilirubin is usually <0.3 mg/dL in young calves. In healthy foals (<2 days old), total bilirubin concentrations may range from 0.9-4.5 mg/dL, with the majority being due to unconjugated bilirubin (0.8-3.8 mg/dL). Bilirubin concentrations in foals should be within adult reference ranges by the time they are 2 wk of age. Normal values for total bilirubin in goats are 0-0.1 mg/dL.

Horses with hepatic disease and failure most often have significant increases in both indirect and direct bilirubin. With liver damage in horses or ruminants, most of the retained bilirubin is indirect (unconjugated), and the direct-to-total ratio usually is <0.3. Increases in indirect bilirubin fraction in horses are most likely to occur with acute hepatocellular disease. However, an increase in direct bilirubin is a more sensitive indicator of hepatocellular disease. Hepatocellular disease should be considered when the direct bilirubin fraction is >25% of the total bilirubin value. In biliary obstruction, total bilirubin concentrations are increased, with the percentage of direct bilirubin often being >25-30%. With bile blockage or intrahepatic cholestasis, the direct-to-total ratio may be >0.3 in horses or 0.5 in cows. In chronic liver disease, bilirubin concentrations are often within normal limits. Adult cattle and calves may have severe liver disease without any increase in serum bilirubin. In cattle, goats, and sheep, circulating bilirubin levels increase only modestly with severe, generalized hepatic disease. The most dramatic increases in serum or plasma bilirubin are due to hemolytic crises rather than to liver dysfunction.

Urobilinogen: Urobilinogen may be detected by dipstick analysis in normal horses. Increased levels of urobilinogen in urine without hemolysis are suggestive of a hepatic dysfunction, portosystemic shunting, or increased production by intestinal bacteria. Urobilinogen in the urine indicates the presence of a patent bile duct. Absence of urobilinogen may indicate complete biliary blockage, liver disease, or failure to excrete bilirubin into the intestine, reduce it by intestinal bacteria, or absorb it from the ileum. The correlation between urobilinogen and hepatocellular disease in animals is poor. Urobilinogen is unstable in the urine; thus, analysis must be done within 1-2 hr, or the amount will be decreased or undetectable.

Serum and Plasma Proteins: Serum albumin and protein concentrations are variable in horses and cattle with hepatic disease. Hypoproteinemia is not common in horses with acute liver disease. Serum albumin is most likely to be reduced in chronic liver disease due to decreased functional hepatic parenchyma. In one study of 84 horses, 13% were hypoalbuminemic. Albumin concentrations were below minimum reference values in 18% of horses with chronic liver disease and 6% with acute liver disease. Globulin concentrations were elevated in 64% of the horses. Hyperproteinemia due to hyperglobulinemia (polyclonal gammopathy or increase in β-globulins) may develop in horses with severe acute or chronic liver disease. Total plasma protein concentration is often normal, but the albumin to globulin ratio may be decreased.

Plasma fibrinogen concentration may not be a sensitive test in horses with hepatic insufficiency. Low fibrinogen concentrations may result from parenchymal insufficiency or disseminated intravascular coagulopathy. A high fibrinogen concentration is associated with an inflammatory response in horses with cholangiohepatitis.

Prothrombin Time: Abnormalities in prothrombin time (PT) are often the first detected because factor VII, a liver-synthesized vitamin K-dependent factor, has the shortest half-life. Serum PT may be rapidly prolonged with hepatic failure and is one of the first function tests to return to normal with recovery from acute hepatic disease. A normal PT determination, however, does not rule out coagulopathy due to vitamin K deficiency. Prolonged activated partial thromboplastin time (APTT) or other indications of coagulopathy may be noted in animals with severe hepatic disease. As a number of factors may influence measurement of PT or APTT values in horses, the ratio of clotting time of the animal with suspected hepatic disease to that of a normal horse's value should be >1.3 for the test to be interpreted as abnormal.

Urea, Glucose, and Ammonia: Serum concentration of urea may be decreased in both acute and chronic liver failure. Hypoglycemia is uncommon in adult horses and ruminants with hepatic dysfunction but is more likely in chronic liver disease. Plasma triglyceride concentrations are markedly increased in ponies, miniature horses, donkeys, and adult horses with hepatic lipidosis. Alterations in triglycerides, very-low-density lipoproteins, and esterified cholesterol levels are more common in ruminants than in horses with hepatic insufficiency. Neonatal foals have higher blood cholesterol and trigylceride concentrations than adult horses. Plasma ammonia levels may be increased with hepatic insufficiency but do not correlate well with severity of hepatic encephalopathy except during portocaval shunts. Increased levels of blood ammonia and signs of hepatic encephalopathy without hepatic failure are reported in Morgan weanlings with hyperornithinemia, hyperammonemia, and normocitrullinuria syndrome and in adult horses with primary or idiopathic hyperammonemia. Ingestion of urea or ammonium salts may cause increases of blood ammonia and encephalopathy in horses and cattle.

Dye Excretion and Clearance Tests: Sulfobromophthalein (BSP®) or indocyanine green dyes can be used to assess hepatobiliary transport. The BSP half-life is prolonged when >50% of hepatic function is lost. The normal clearance half-life of BSP is <3.7 min in horses, 2.13 ± 0.19 min in goats, and ≤4.0 min in sheep. BSP clearance is longer in calves (5-15 min) than in adult cattle (≤5 min). Although dye excretion tests are usually prolonged with hepatic dysfunction, they may still be within the normal range. Hyperbilirubinemia, decreased hepatic blood flow, and significant cholestasis may falsely prolong and hypoalbuminemia may falsely shorten BSP clearance. BSP clearance in goats is most often prolonged with generalized hepatic lipidosis secondary to pregnancy toxemia. Determination of BSP clearance time, rather than half-life, reportedly is more useful in detection of liver disease. BSP clearance time in healthy fed and 3-day fasted horses is 10 mL/min/kg and 6 mL/min/kg, respectively. These tests, however, are of limited use in clinical practice due to the lack of commercially available pharmaceutical-grade BSP. Expense, procedural limitations, and equipment requirements for quantitation of indocyanine green clearance have limited its use as a diagnostic test.

Scintigraphy: Biliary patency and hepatocyte function, structure, and blood flow may be evaluated by hepatobiliary scintigraphy. Radionucleotide liver scans and biliary scans can detect alterations in blood flow or hepatic masses and biliary obstruction (atresia, cholangitis, cholelithiasis), respectively. Scintigraphy has been used in pigs, foals, and lambs to differentiate biliary obstruction from other causes of hyperbilirubinemia.

Ultrasonography: Ultrasonography can be used to evaluate liver size, appearance (shape, texture), and location in horses and ruminants for diagnosis of hepatomegaly, hepatolithiasis, biliary dilatation, cholelithiasis, or focal lesions. Tumors, cysts, abscesses, and granulomas may be observed. Diffuse diseases are harder to detect than focal processes because the former cause less distortion of normal hepatic architecture.

Diagnosis of diffuse liver disease should be substantiated by biopsy and histopathology. Ultrasound can be used to guide collection of liver biopsy specimens and to perform cholecystocentesis and aspiration of abscesses, masses, or bile samples (fluke eggs, bile acids, culture). It is also an accurate, noninvasive means for monitoring the progression or resolution of disease. In horses, the liver should be imaged from both the right and left sides of the animal.

Liver Biopsy: Percutaneous liver biopsy is the definitive means of diagnosing hepatic disease. Histologic evaluation of the liver provides valuable information regarding etiology and severity of the disease process. Most cases of liver disease are diffuse so the sample will be representative of the disease. Samples can be obtained blindly, but ultrasonographic guidance decreases the risk of complications (peritonitis due to bile leakage or intestinal puncture, hemorrhage, or pneumothorax). Liver biopsies can also be obtained during laparoscopy, which offers the additional advantage of being able to visualize the surface of the liver and other abdominal organs for evidence of disease.

Samples should be placed in media for bacterial culture and sensitivity and in formalin for histologic evaluation. Coagulation profiles (prothrombin time, partial thromboplastin time, fibrinogen, fibrin degradation products, and optional platelet count) may be performed before liver biopsy to reduce the risk of hemorrhage. Liver biopsy may not be advised in an animal with clinical or clinicopathologic evidence of a coagulopathy or a hepatic abscess because hemorrhage or contamination of the peritoneal cavity may result.

Radiography: Contrast abdominal radiography in foals is beneficial in diagnosing gastroduodenal obstructions and secondary cholangiohepatitis. Portosystemic shunts in foals or young calves can be identified with mesenteric portovenography by injecting radiopaque contrast solution into a jejunal mesenteric vein followed by fluoroscopy or sequential survey radiographs to monitor the hepatic blood flow.

Treatment and Management: Initial treatment of animals with signs of hepatic disease or insufficiency is often supportive and started before the underlying cause and extent of hepatic damage is known. History, clinical signs, and laboratory data may give some clue as to the nature of the hepatic disease process, but liver biopsy is usually required to make a definitive diagnosis and to determine the degree of hepatic injury. Specific therapies for hepatic disease depend on etiology, presence of liver failure, chronicity, degree of hepatic fibrosis or biliary obstruction, and species affected. Increases in hepatic enzymes without hepatic disease may not require specific therapy for the liver but rather for the primary disease.

Therapy is most successful when intervention is early, hepatic fibrosis is minimal, and there is evidence of regeneration in the liver. Horses with severe or bridging fibrosis respond poorly due to inadequate potential for liver regeneration. The goals for treatment of large animals with hepatic disease or insufficiency are to control hepatic encephalopathy, to treat the underlying disease process, to provide supportive care to allow time for liver regeneration, and most importantly, to prevent injury to the animal and persons working with the animal. Animals with hepatic encephalopathy often show aggressive and unpredictable behavior that can result in injury to self or handlers.

Hepatic Encephalopathy: Horses with hepatic encephalopathy may be aggressive or demonstrate repetitive behaviors that make restraint difficult. To ensure safety of the animal and handlers, sedation is required. Because most sedatives and tranquilizers are metabolized by the liver, their elimination half-life may be prolonged in animals with hepatic failure; therefore, dosages should be minimized. A reduced drug dose is initially given to assess its effect. Xylazine or detomidine given in small doses to effect can be used to control horses exhibiting abnormal behavior. Diazepam should be avoided in animals with hepatic encephalopathy because it may enhance the effect of γ-aminobutyric acid on inhibitory neurons and worsen neurologic signs. Acepromazine should also be avoided because it may lower the seizure threshold.

Dehydration, acid-base and electrolyte imbalances, and hypoglycemia should be corrected with appropriate IV fluids. Initially, a balanced polyionic solution (preferably without lactate) is administered for rehydration. Potassium (10-40 mEq/L, depending on infusion rate) supplement is added if the animal is hypokalemic or hypophagic. If IV infusion is not possible in ruminants, rehydration may be attempted by oral administration of fluids if rumen motility is normal. Some horses with hepatic disease have polycythemia, making evaluation of hydration status by PCV difficult. Severe acidosis may be present. Because rapid correction of the acidosis may exacerbate neurologic signs, acidosis should be corrected gradually by IV administration of fluids with a high concentration of electrolytes. If this fails or if blood pH is <7.1 (bicarbonate <14 mEq/L), bicarbonate should be administered cautiously. Supplemental vitamins are optional. Adequate fresh water should be available if the animal can swallow normally.

Factors that may contribute to the hepatic encephalopathy should be eliminated. Glucose as a 5-10% solution is given to correct hypoglycemia if present. A continuous IV infusion of glucose (5% at 2 mL/kg/hr or 10% at 1 mL/kg/hr) should be given even to animals that are not hypoglycemic. The rate should be adjusted so that the adult animal is not receiving >50 g of glucose (1 L of 5%) per hour. Induction of moderate to severe hyperglycemia, rapid changes in glucose level, and glucosuria should be avoided. IV glucose is best used in combination with a balanced electrolyte solution.

Therapies directed toward decreasing either ammonia production in or absorption from the bowel include administration of mineral oil, neomycin, lactulose, and metronidazole. Administration of mineral oil decreases absorption and facilitates removal of ammonia. Passing a nasogastric tube in an animal with hepatic encephalopathy must be done cautiously because nasal bleeding may be difficult to control due to decreased clotting factors. In addition, blood swallowed may exacerbate the neurologic signs. Oral administration of neomycin (20-30 mg/kg, QID for 1 day; 5.0 mg/kg, TID for 2 days; or 10-100 mg/kg, QID) is used to decrease ammonia-producing bacteria in the intestine. Lactulose (0.2 mL/kg, BID; 0.3 mL/kg, PO, QID; or 90-120 mL/450 kg, TID-QID) is metabolized to organic acids by bacteria in the ileum and colon. Reduction in colonic pH reportedly fosters an increased bacterial assimilation of ammonia, decreased ammonia production, ammonia trapping in the bowel, intestinal microflora changes, and osmotic catharsis. Metronidazole (10-15 mg/kg, PO, TID-QID) decreases ammonia-producing organisms in horses but should not be used in food animals. If the animal can swallow, oral drugs can be mixed with Karo syrup or molasses and given via dose syringe to avoid trauma and risk of passing a nasogastric tube. Neomycin, lactulose, and metronidazole may all potentially induce mild to severe diarrhea (salmonellosis) due to disruption of GI flora. Use of the drugs in combination is more likely to induce diarrhea than any one of the drugs given alone.

Until the nature of the underlying hepatic disease is known, treatment with broad-spectrum antimicrobials is warranted if infectious hepatitis is suspected. A trimethoprim-sulfa combination is a good empiric choice because of its activity against gram-negative bacteria and its high concentration in bile. Penicillin in combination with an aminoglycoside has a broad spectrum of action and may be of benefit if a *Streptococcus* sp or an anaerobic or gram-negative coliform is suspected. First- and second-generation cephalosporins have been used in foals and in other species. Metronidazole (15 mg/kg, PO, TID-QID) may be administered when anaerobic infection is suspected in horses. Specific antimicrobial therapy based on culture and sensitivity of a liver biopsy is ideal.

Pain may be controlled with low doses of NSAID (eg, flunixin meglumine, 0.5 mg/kg, IV or IM, BID-TID). In foals, butorphanol (0.07 mg/kg, IM) may be preferred. Vitamin K_1 (40-50 mg/450 kg, SC) and plasma transfusions (1-2 L/100 kg) may be given when coagulopathies develop.

Dietary Management: Dietary management is essential for management of animals with hepatic encephalopathy or acute or chronic hepatopathy. Affected animals should be fed carefully because dysphagia may be a problem. The diet should be fed frequently in relatively small amounts. It should meet dietary energy needs with readily digestible carbohydrates, provide adequate but not excessive protein, have a high ratio of branched-chain amino acids to aromatic amino acids, and be high in starch to decrease need for hepatic glucose synthesis. Fat and salt should not be added to the diet. Feeds used successfully in horses include grass or oat hay, corn, and sorghum. Small amounts of molasses may be added to make the diet more palatable and to add energy.

Large amounts of molasses may make the feed less palatable and can induce diarrhea. Linseed meal and soybean meal have an excellent branched-chain to aromatic amino acid ratio and may be used as a protein supplement in small quantities. Beet pulp may be substituted for oat or grass hay. Beet pulp should be soaked first to allow full expansion before being fed. Choke may be a problem in some animals eating beet pulp. The feeding of alfalfa hay, alfalfa-containing feeds, or other legume hays to horses with hepatic disease is controversial. Although alfalfa hay has a better branched-chain to aromatic amino acid ratio than grass hay, it may have too high a protein content. Feeding grass hay is preferred for animals with hyperammonemia or signs of hepatic encephalopathy. A mixed grass/alfalfa hay can be fed to horses without central neurologic signs if weight loss is a problem and the added protein is tolerated. Grazing grass pastures is allowable as long as signs of hepatic encephalopathy are controlled and exposure to sunlight is avoided. Other feeds high in branched-chain amino acids include sorghum, bran, or milo. Parenteral or enteral supplement with branched-chain amino acids helps restore the normal ratio of branched-chain to aromatic amino acids. Supplement of vitamins A, D, and B_1 and folic acid, possibly with vitamins C and E, might be indicated. Vitamin K_1 may be indicated in animals with a coagulopathy. Large amounts of fat should not be fed to meet energy requirements; feeding an excess of it may lead to fatty liver.

Transfaunation (p 1994) with rumen fluid from a healthy cow may help re-establish normal ruminal flora and enhance the appetite of affected cattle. Animals that will not eat voluntarily must be force fed. A gruel may be given by nasogastric tube in horses and swine or by orogastric tube or rumen fistula in ruminants. In ruminants, forced feeding of alfalfa-meal (15% protein) and dried brewer's grain or beet pulp with potassium chloride and normal rumen fluid has been recommended. Alfalfa hay and alfalfa-containing feeds may be better tolerated by cattle than by horses with hepatic disease. IV polyionic fluids with 5% dextrose, potassium chloride, and B vitamins may also be needed in animals that are not consuming adequate amounts.

ACUTE HEPATITIS

Infectious, toxic, and undefined etiologies may cause acute hepatitis. Clinical signs may appear suddenly with horses appearing lethargic, anorectic, and icteric. Photosensitization, diarrhea, and clotting abnormalities also may be seen. Neurologic signs resulting from hypoglycemia and hepatic encephalopathy can be most severe in animals with acute fulminant liver disease. Signs of endotoxemia may be present, depending on the underlying etiology and the ability of the Kupffer's cells to remove endotoxin from the systemic circulation. Increases in serum SDH and AST activities indicate acute hepatocellular injury. GGT is increased with cholestasis secondary to hepatocyte swelling. Cholestasis results in hyperbilirubinemia, with the direct (conjugated) fraction ranging from 15-35% of total in horses. Increased serum total bile acid concentration, decreased glucose and BUN concentrations, and prolonged BSP® clearance and coagulation times become evident as hepatic function progressively worsens. Anorexia can lead to hypokalemia. The CBC is variable because it may reflect an inflammatory response with a neutrophilia or an endotoxemia with a neutropenia, increased band neutrophils, and toxic changes.

Idiopathic Acute Hepatic Disease

(Theiler's disease, Serum hepatitis, Postvaccinal hepatitis, Acute hepatic necrosis, Acute hepatic atrophy)

Idiopathic acute hepatic disease (IAHD) is the most common cause of acute hepatitis in horses.

Etiology and Epidemiology: About 20% of horses with IAHD show clinical signs of hepatic failure 4-10 wk after receiving an equine origin biologic, such as tetanus antitoxin (TAT). In some cases, the affected horse may not have received TAT but may have been in contact with another horse that received TAT. Others affected have no prior history of exposure to such a product. Subclinical IAHD can also develop after administration of TAT.

Most commonly, only one horse on the premises is affected, although outbreaks may occur or other horses on the farm may have evidence of liver disease (increased enzyme levels) without clinical signs. Occurrence of the disease in groups of adult horses during the late summer or early fall (August to November) suggests an infectious (viral) or vector-spread etiology, although supporting evidence is lacking. The seasonal occurrence could reflect the fact that many foaling mares receive TAT in the spring of the year along with their newborn foals. Lactating mares that receive TAT at foaling seem to be more susceptible. A Type III (immune-complex mediated) hypersensitivity reaction also has been proposed.

Clinical Findings: Onset of clinical signs is acute. Acute mortality may be 50-60% with overall mortality as high as 88% in affected horses. Horses with IAHD typically present with anorexia, hepatic encephalopathy, and icterus. The CNS signs are variable, ranging from lethargy to aggression or maniacal behavior, central blindness, and ataxia. Photosensitivity and discolored urine due to high bilirubin concentrations may be seen. Fever is present in ~50% of cases. Weight loss (uncommon), ventral edema with jugular pulses, and acute respiratory distress have been seen in some horses with IAHD. These findings suggest there may be a subclinical phase before development of overt hepatic failure. Most cases are sporadic, but epidemics with several horses involved have been reported. Recognition of IAHD in one horse indicates horses on the same premises should be carefully observed for clinical or serum biochemical signs of hepatic disease.

Serum levels of GGT, AST, and SDH are increased. GGT is frequently further increased during the first few days of illness, despite clinical improvement and eventual recovery in an affected horse. Horses with AST values >4,000 IU/L have a poor prognosis. AST decreases within 3-5 days in horses that improve, and SDH decreases even more rapidly. Total serum bilirubin concentration is generally higher in horses with IAHD than in horses with anorexia. Hyperbilirubinemia is common, with the unconjugated form being >70% of the total. Moderate to severe acidosis, hypokalemia, polycythemia, increased plasma aromatic amino acids, and hyperammonemia may also be present. Serum total bile acid concentration will also be increased.

Lesions: At necropsy, icterus and varying degrees of ascites are present. The liver is usually small to normal in size but may be enlarged (peracute cases), with a mottled and bile-stained surface. Histologically, there is marked centrilobular-to-midzonal hepatocellular necrosis, mild to moderate mononuclear infiltrate and a few neutrophils, and moderate bile duct proliferation.

Diagnosis: This is based on history, abrupt onset on clinical signs and laboratory alterations suggestive of hepatic insufficiency. In some cases, the liver is shrunken and difficult to visualize with ultrasonographic examination. A definitive diagnosis can be made only by liver biopsy. Differential diagnoses include acute pyrrolizidine toxicosis, hepatotoxins, acute infectious hepatitis, acute mycotoxicosis, cerebral disease, and hemolytic disease.

Treatment and Prognosis: Supportive therapy and treatment of the hepatic encephalopathy are often successful. Stressful situations, such as moving the animal or weaning the mare's foal, may exacerbate the clinical signs of hepatic encephalopathy and should be avoided. Sedation should be used only to control behavior that could lead to injury of the animal and to allow therapeutic procedures.

Recovery depends on the degree of hepatocellular necrosis. Affected horses that remain stable for 3-5 days and that continue to eat often recover. Decreases in the SDH and prothrombin time along with improvement in appetite are the best positive predictive indicators of recovery. Horses with rapid progression of clinical signs and uncontrollable encephalopathy have a poor prognosis. For affected horses that do recover, the longterm prognosis is excellent.

Prevention: Use of TAT is not without risk. Routine administration of TAT to parturient mares is strongly discouraged. Use of TAT should be restricted to situations necessitating tetanus prophylaxis and in which a history of active tetanus toxoid immunization is absent or unknown.

Acute Hepatic Necrosis in Cattle

Epidemiology and Pathogenesis: Acute hepatic disease and failure in cattle most commonly results from a toxic insult. Hepatocellular necrosis with clinical and laboratory evidence of hepatic failure may develop in cattle after mastitis or metritis with clinical signs of endotoxemia. Endotoxin induces hepatocellular necrosis through both direct or indirect effects on the liver. Endotoxin can cause Kupffer's cells to release lysosomal enzymes, prostaglandins, and collagenase that damage hepatocytes, or it may interact directly with the hepatocytes, causing lysosomal damage, decreased mitochondrial function, and necrosis. Endotoxin-related hepatocellular necrosis may be due in part to decreased hepatic blood flow and liver hypoxia.

Clinical Findings and Lesions: Clinical signs include weight loss, anorexia, and cessation of milk production. Photosensitization and mild icterus are variable. Serum SDH, GGT, and AST concentrations are mildly to severely increased. Fatty liver or ketosis is not characteristic. The liver may be normal in size or mildly enlarged. Histologically, there is marked hydropic change with varying degrees of hepatic necrosis.

Diagnosis: Diagnosis is based on a history of hepatic-related signs developing concurrently or after a primary disease and endotoxemia. Increases in hepatic and biliary enzymes and absence of ketosis support the diagnosis. Definitive diagnosis is based on liver biopsy and by excluding other infectious, toxic, and inflammatory causes of hepatic dysfunction. Differential diagnoses include other causes of subacute or chronic liver disease (eg, hepatotoxins, hepatic lipidosis, primary photosensitivity) and conditions causing weight loss and hypophagia.

Treatment: Nutritional and fluid support is often successful in affected cows with acute hepatic necrosis after transient insults. Forced feeding of alfalfa meal (15% protein) and dried brewers' grain or beet pulp with potassium chloride and normal rumen fluid is recommended. IV polyionic fluids with 5% dextrose, potassium chloride, and B vitamins may also be needed. Control of endotoxemia and treatment of the primary disease condition are essential.

INFECTIOUS HEPATITIS AND HEPATIC ABSCESSES

Tyzzer's Disease

Tyzzer's disease, due to *Clostridium piliforme*, causes an acute necrotizing hepatitis, myocarditis, and colitis in foals 8-42 days old. (*See* p 160 for clinical findings, diagnosis, and treatment). Tyzzer's disease has been reported in 2 calves—a 1-wk-old Jersey bull calf with enteritis and multifocal necrotizing hepatitis and a second calf with concurrent cryptosporidiosis and coronaviral enteritis. In the latter animal, *C piliforme* was identified in hepatocytes and epithelium and smooth muscle cells of the ileum and cecum. Clinical signs included hypophagia, generalized weakness, dullness, and decreased fecal passage.

Cholangiohepatitis

Cholangiohepatitis is a severe inflammation of the bile passages and adjacent liver, which sporadically causes hepatic failure in horses and ruminants. It is occasionally associated with cholelithiasis in horses.

Etiology: Bacteremia due to an organism (eg, *Salmonella*) eliminated in the bile, an ascending infection of the biliary tract after intestinal disturbance, or ileus are thought to be related to the development of cholangiohepatitis. In foals, duodenal ulceration and duodenitis may result in bile stasis, hepatic duct obstruction, and cholangiohepatitis. Parasite migration through the liver may predispose to cholangiohepatis in some animals. Gram-negative organisms, including *Salmonella* sp, *Escherichia coli*, *Pseudomonas* sp, and *Actinobacillus equuli* are frequently isolated from the liver. *Clostridium* sp, *Pasteurella* sp, and *Streptococcus* sp are less frequently recovered.

Clinical Findings: Depending on the severity of infection and virulence of the organism, clinical signs may be acute with severe toxemia, subacute, or chronic. Most typically, cholangiohepatitis is a subacute or chronic disease process with affected animals showing signs of weight loss, anorexia, intermittent or persistent fever, or colic. Icterus, photosensitivity, and signs of hepatic encephalopathy are variable. SDH, AST, GGT, bilirubin, and total bile acid concentrations are usually increased. Peripheral WBC counts are variable, depending on the degree of inflammation and endotoxemia present. Acute, suppurative cholangiohepatitis may occasionally result in severe septicemia and death.

Lesions: In acute cases, the liver is swollen, soft, and pale. Suppurative foci may be visible beneath the capsule or on cut surface. Lesions in other systems may reflect septicemia and jaundice. Microscopically in acute cases, neutrophils are present in the portal triads and degenerate parenchyma. Purulent exudate is evident in the ducts. In subacute or chronic cholangiohepatitis, the inflammation is more proliferative and bile duct proliferation more pronounced. Areas of atrophy, regenerative hyperplasia, and periportal fibrosis may be evident.

Diagnosis: Liver biopsy should be performed to confirm the diagnosis and to obtain a liver sample for aerobic and anaerobic culture and sensitivity. Differential diagnoses include other causes of acute to chronic hepatic disease, weight loss, colic, or sepsis. If neurologic signs are present, cerebral diseases must be considered. Because cholangiohepatitis is frequently associated with cholelithiasis in horses, the presence of one or more calculi must be ruled out.

Treatment: Treatment based on culture and sensitivity results from liver tissue often gives favorable results. Therapy should be continued for 4-6 wk or longer. Liver enzyme (GGT) levels and biopsies should be repeated to monitor response to therapy. If no organism is cultured, broad-spectrum antimicrobial therapy against gram-negative, gram-positive, and anaerobic organisms should be administered. A combination of penicillin with either a trimethoprim-sulfa or an aminoglycoside or enrofloxacin may be used. Ampicillin or a cephalosporin can be used instead of penicillin. Metronidazole can be used in horses to treat anaerobic bacteria. Prognosis is good if fibrosis is not severe.

Equine Rhinopneumonitis

Equine rhinopneumonitis due to equine herpesvirus 1 is a sporadic cause of interstitial pneumonia, hepatic disease, and often death in newborn foals. *See* p 1211 for clinical findings, diagnosis, and treatment.

Infectious Necrotic Hepatitis
(Black disease)

Infectious necrotic hepatitis, caused by *Clostridium novyi* type B, affects primarily sheep but also cattle, horses, and pigs. *See* p 489 for clinical findings, lesions, and control.

Bacillary Hemoglobinuria

Clostridium haemolyticum is the anaerobic organism that causes bacillary hemoglobinuria in cattle, other ruminants, and rarely horses. *See* p 487 for clinical findings, diagnosis, and control.

Hepatic Abscesses

The primary etiologic agent of liver abscesses in cattle is *Fusobacterium necrophorum.* In goats, most abscesses are due to *Corynebacterium pseudotuberculosis. Arcanobacterium (Actinomyces) pyogenes* and *Escherichia coli* are also common. Organisms less frequently isolated include *Proteus* sp, *Mannheimia (Pasteurella) haemolytica, Staphylococcus epidermidis, S aureus, Rhodococcus equi, Erysipelothrix rhusiopathiae,* and the yeast *Candida krusei.* In horses, hepatic abscesses often contain *Streptococcus, (S equi equi, S equi zooepidemicus), C pseudotuberculosis,* or enterobacteria after ascending cholangiohepatitis or intestinal disease. In pigs, hepatic abscesses develop after migration of ascarids into the bile ducts.

The liver is particularly susceptible to abscess formation because it receives blood from the hepatic artery, the portal system, and the umbilical vein in the fetus and the newborn. Hepatic abscesses are most prevalent in ruminants and uncommon in horses. Abscesses are associated with bacteremia, septic portal vein thrombosis, parasite migration, or extension from intestinal disease. In neonates and young animals, abscesses may develop secondary to ascarid migration, bacterial septicemia, or ascending infection of the umbilical vein. In horses and cattle, signs may be similar to those seen with other abdominal abscesses and include intermittent colic, intermittent fever, and weight loss. Often, liver abscesses are subclinical in cattle.

HEPATOTOXINS

Hepatotoxins manifest their toxicity by one or more mechanisms: periacinal (centrilobular) necrosis, midzonal necrosis, periportal necrosis, cholestasis, biliary hyperplasia, fatty or hydropic change near necrotic zones, or venous occlusion. Fatal hepatic insufficiency may result if the initial injury is acute and severe. More commonly, the hepatic damage from toxins is subacute or chronic. In chronic processes, the longterm result may be cirrhosis. Many hepatotoxins, especially those in plants, exert toxic effects on multiple organs, particularly kidneys, lungs, and the GI tract.

Definitive diagnosis may be difficult. Careful history, inspection of the environment, laboratory evaluations, liver biopsy, or necropsy may be needed to determine the offending agent. With acute plant toxicities, evidence of hepatotoxic plants may be seen in the stomach contents or rumen.

Specific antidotes for hepatotoxins are limited. Removal of the animals from the source is essential to decrease additional exposure. Administration of laxatives (eg, mineral oil, magnesium sulfate) or absorbants (eg, activated charcoal or mineral oil) or rumenotomy may decrease absorption of toxic elements in acute poisonings. These may not be helpful in chronic intoxications (ie, pyrrolizidine alkaloid toxicity), in which the toxic agent has been ingested over weeks to months before signs of toxicity are evident. Supportive care includes correction of electrolyte, metabolic, and glucose disorders via fluid therapy and dietary management. Hepatic encephalopathy must be controlled. Sunlight should be avoided if photosensitization is present. Antimicrobials may be considered to prevent secondary pyoderma. Prognosis is guarded and depends on the particular hepatotoxin.

Chemical and Drug-related Causes of Toxic Hepatopathy

For COAL-TAR POISONING, see p 2352.

Iron Toxicosis: Newborn foals are exceptionally sensitive to iron because of the high serum iron levels, increased ability to absorb iron, and oversaturation of transferrin at birth. In adult horses, injectable iron increases body iron concentration more substantially than most oral supplements. Iron toxicosis has been reported in calves and young bulls injected with a ferric ammonium citrate alone or in combination with ferrous gluconate.

Foals given iron at birth, especially before nursing colostrum, develop clinical signs of hepatic encephalopathy in 2-5 days. Concentrations of serum bilirubin (both conjugated and unconjugated) and blood ammonia are high, and prothrombin time is prolonged. Alterations in serum hepatic enzymes are more variable. In foals, acute iron toxicity is commonly fatal; in adult horses, although less commonly a problem, it causes enteric irritation and cardiovascular collapse with sudden death. Signs of more chronic hepatic failure, including weight loss, icterus, and depression, may be seen with repeated oral administration of iron. Possible sources of excess iron include inappropriate supplementation, forages high in iron, injectable iron, and leaching of iron into water or feed. Calves with iron toxicosis have trembling, vocalizing, bruxism, colic, and convulsions.

Hepatic lesions are variable. Most livers are friable and are swollen or shrunken. The liver is pale tan or mottled red-brown in color. Hemorrhages may be present in the stomach, intestines, and bladder.

Diagnosis is based on the history of iron supplementation, clinical signs, and necropsy lesions. Serum and liver iron concentrations may be normal or increased. Normal iron concentrations in serum and liver tissue in horses are 66-204 µg/dL and 100-300 ppm, respectively. Because serum iron concentration correlates poorly with total iron stores, serum ferritin levels are better used as an estimate of total iron.

Treatment is generally supportive with fluids and nutritional supplementation. Chelation therapy with deferoxamine is unlikely to be successful in either acute iron toxicosis or chronic hemochromatosis. Repeated phlebotomy has been attempted for hemochromatosis. The prognosis is poor.

Copper Toxicosis: Acute copper toxicosis with severe hepatic necrosis and death may be seen in cattle 1-4 days after injection of copper salt. Copper toxicosis is seen in sheep and young calves after excess dietary intake of copper and in young goat kids fed calf milk replacer containing copper. The primary condition associated with copper toxicosis is hemolytic anemia and liver damage. (*See also* p 2353.)

Miscellaneous Chemicals and Drugs Associated with Hepatotoxicity: Exposure to carbon tetrachloride, chlorinated hydrocarbons, hexachlorethane, carbon disulfide, arsenic, monensin, pentachlorophenols, phenol, paraquat, halothane (goat, llama), isoflurane, phenobarbital, tannic acid, copper disodium edetate, and high doses of ivermectin may cause centrilobular necrosis and hepatic failure. Phosphorus causes primarily periportal changes. Active hepatitis to cirrhosis may be seen after use of isoniazid, nitrofuran, halothane, aspirin, or dantrolene in large animals. Erythromycin, rifampin, anabolic steroids, phenothiazine tranquilizers, some diuretics, quinidine sulfate, and diazepam have been associated with cholestasis and icterus.

Mycotoxicoses

Aflatoxins and fumonisins can cause hepatic injury and failure in ruminants, swine, and horses. *Fusarium* toxicosis is the most common mycotoxicosis causing liver failure in horses, while aflatoxins only sporadically cause hepatic failure in this species. (*See* MYCOTOXICOSES, p 2408.)

Blue-green Algae Intoxication

Acute hepatotoxicosis may be seen after ingestion of hepatotoxic cyanobacteria. (*See* ALGAL POISONING, p 2344.)

Hepatotoxic Plants

Pyrrolizidine Alkaloid Toxicity: Pyrrolizidine alkaloid toxicity most commonly is a chronic, progressive hepatopathy, but acute intoxication can occur. (*See* PYRROLIZIDINE ALKALOIDOSIS, p 2506.)

Kleingrass Toxicosis: Kleingrass (*Panicum coloratum*) can produce toxicosis in horses and ruminants. Kleingrass toxicosis is a problem in the southwestern USA from late spring to early fall. Young growing plants are most hazardous due to their high sapogenin content, believed to be the toxic principle. A similar syndrome is seen in horses in the eastern USA grazing pasture or fed hay containing high concentrations of fall *Panicum*.

Clinical signs include icterus, photosensitivity, intermittent colic and fever, weight loss, and hepatic encephalopathy. Photosensitivity may develop around the coronary band and cause lameness. Lesions include hepatic and portal fibrosis and biliary hyperplasia. GGT, bilirubin, and blood ammonia levels are increased. Sheep with photosensitivity caused by kleingrass ingestion commonly have a crystalline material in the bile ducts, canaliculi, and macrophages.

Presumptive diagnosis of plant-induced hepatopathy is based on history of exposure to plants and multiple affected animals on a farm or in an area. Affected animals should be removed from the kleingrass source, fed good-quality hay, and protected from sunlight. Local treatment of the photodermatitis with antimicrobial or softening creams may be needed in severe cases.

Alsike Clover Toxicosis: Alsike clover (*Trifolium hybridium*) causes 2 syndromes in horses in the USA and Canada—photosensitivity (trifobiasis) and Alsike clover poisoning ("big liver disease"). Alsike clover grows well on heavy clay soil, and an increased incidence of toxicity is reported during wet seasons. The disease is seen mostly when the blossom of the plant is eaten and the predominant forage being fed is the Alsike clover. The toxic principle is an unidentified phototoxin. Photosensitivity has been reported in horses, sheep, cattle, and pigs.

Alsike photosensitivity is also known as "dew poisoning" because it is seen mostly when pastures of clover are wet and horses' skins are moist. It is characterized by reddened skin after exposure to sun, followed by dry necrosis of the skin or edema and serous discharge. The muzzle, tongue, and feet are frequently affected. If the stomatitis is severe, anorexia and weight loss develop.

Alsike clover poisoning may be fatal with progressive loss of condition and signs of hepatic failure and neurologic disturbances. Colic, diarrhea, and other signs of GI disturbances have been noted. Affected hoses may be markedly depressed or excited. Prolonged exposure is usually required before signs of hepatic insufficiency are evident. Serum chemistry alterations include increased GGT and AST activities, and hyperbilirubinemia, with direct bilirubin frequently being ≥25% of the total.

Presumptive diagnosis of plant-induced hepatopathy is based on history of exposure to plants and multiple animals on a farm or in an area affected. Horses in which photosensitivity is the primary finding may recover quickly after being removed to Alsike-free pasture. Those with severe stomatitis or dermatitis require supportive care and local treatment of the stomatitis until they heal.

Mycotoxic Lupinosis: Mycotoxic lupinosis is a worldwide disease of sheep and cattle that consume lupines containing a hepatic mycotoxin produced by the fungus *Phomopsis leptostromiformis*. *See* p 2420 for clinical findings, diagnosis, and control.

Xanthium (Cocklebur) Toxicosis: Cockleburs, including *Xanthium strumarium*, may be found throughout the world. Poisoning is most frequent after ingestion of the palatable 2-leaf seedling stage or ground seeds. The burs are highly toxic but rarely eaten. The mature plant is less toxic and generally unpalatable. The toxic principle is carboxyatractyloside, which directly affects the liver.

Within hours of toxin ingestion, swine, cattle, and horses develop signs of depression, nausea, weakness, ataxia, and subnormal temperature. Spasms of the cervical muscles, vomiting, dyspnea, and convulsions may occur. Death may occur within hours of the onset of signs. Animals that survive initial acute poisoning frequently develop chronic liver disease.

Affected animals require intensive supportive care. Mineral oil or activated charcoal may be given orally to delay absorption of the toxic principle. Physostigmine (5-30 mg, IM) has also been recommended.

Miscellaneous Plant Hepatotoxicosis: Hepatotoxins are found in numerous plants, including *Nolina texana*, *Agave lecheguilla*, *Phyllanthus abnormis*, and *Lantana camara*. (*See* RANGE PLANTS OF TEMPERATE NORTH AMERICA, p 2433.)

CHOLELITHIASIS, CHOLEDOCHOLITHIASIS, AND HEPATOLITHIASIS

Etiology and Epidemiology: Cholelithiasis in horses may cause biliary obstruction and concurrent liver disease or may be an incidental finding at necropsy. It most commonly affects middle-aged (6-15 yr old) horses with no sex or breed predilection. Solitary or multiple calculi may be present in the common bile duct (choledocholithiasis), intrahepatic bile ducts (hepatolithiasis), or bile duct or gallbladder in ruminants (cholelithiasis). The cause of cholelith formation in horses is not known. Ascending biliary tract (cholangiohepatitis), intestinal bacterial infection resulting in bile stasis, and a change in bile composition or cholesterol concentration have been proposed. Choleliths also may form around a foreign body or parasites may occlude the common bile duct. Cholelithiasis and hepatolithiasis reportedly are not recognized as a clinical problem in sheep and goats.

Clinical Findings: Clinical signs commonly seen in horses with choleliths or cholangiohepatitis include weight loss, abdominal pain, icterus, depression, and intermittent fever. Signs of hepatic failure, including encephalopathy, photosensitivity, and coagulopathy, occur less frequently. Clinical signs are often intermittent. Complete obstruction of the common bile duct often is accompanied by persistent abdominal pain. Laboratory abnormalities include hyperbilirubinemia with increased direct (conjugated) bilirubin, a marked increase in serum GGT activity, and increased serum total bile acid concentration. SDH and AST activities are increased but to a lesser degree. Serum urea nitrogen, glucose, and potassium concentration may be decreased. Metabolic tests indicate reduced hepatic function. Activated partial thromboplastin time and one-stage prothrombin time may be prolonged. Leukocytosis, anemia of chronic disease, hyperproteinemia, hyperglobulinemia, and hyperfibrinogenemia are often present due to inflammation. Histologic changes include periportal and intralobular fibrosis, moderate bile duct dilatation and proliferation, and cholestasis. Culture of the liver may reveal a bacterial infection.

Lesions: At necropsy, the liver may be enlarged or shrunken. The liver is red to green-brown and firmer than normal. Hepatic ducts and the common bile duct are dilated and may contain one or more calculi.

Diagnosis: Cholelithiasis should be considered in horses with a history of fever, icterus, abdominal pain, and signs of hepatic failure. A marked increase in serum GGT with hyperbilirubinemia (direct bilirubin >25%) is supportive. Ultrasonographic examination may reveal hepatomegaly with increased echogenicity of the liver, thickened distended bile ducts, and hyperechoic regions suggestive of choleliths. Choleliths in horses are most often visualized in the most cranioventral portion of the right lobe of the liver, especially in the sixth to eighth intercostal spaces. Choleliths may be hyperechoic, casting an acoustic shadow, or sonolucent. Stones may be seen as discrete calculi or less discrete sludge deposits within the biliary tract. The thickened distended bile ducts may appear as dilated channels adjacent to portal veins. Because of the large lung field of horses, choleliths may be missed on ultrasound examination.

Treatment: Although biliary obstruction in horses is often fatal, choledocholithotripsy and choledocholithotomy have been performed successfully. Prognosis in cases requiring choledocholithotomy depends on the severity of concurrent cholangiohepatitis and on the size of the horse. The procedure is difficult because of limited exposure and poor visibility of the common hepatic duct. Complications include bile contamination, bile peritonitis, dehiscence, bile duct stricture, cholelith reformation, and enteritis (eg, stress-induced, salmonellosis). The prognosis is better if the obstruction is corrected by choledocholithotripsy. When small calculi or less discrete sludge deposits are present, resolution may be attempted medically by "flushing" the bile duct(s) through IV administration of large volumes of polyionic fluids. In addition, dissolution of bilirubinate stones, which are common in horses, may be facilitated by concurrent administration of IV dimethyl sulfoxide (<20% solution at 0.5-1.0 mg/kg). Dimethyl sulfoxide should be used cautiously or avoided in horses with coagulopathies or signs of hemolysis. Antiinflammatory agents are administered to reduce inflammation and provide analgesia. As cholangitis is often present, longterm broad-spectrum antimicrobial therapy is indicated. Antimicrobial choice is best guided by culture and sensitivity of the bacteria from a liver biopsy, bile duct aspirate, or from the cholelith. Supportive care is provided to manage any degree of accompanying hepatic insufficiency.

CHRONIC ACTIVE HEPATITIS

Chronic active hepatitis describes any progressive inflammatory process within the liver. It is a histopathologic diagnosis in which there is evidence of sustained, aggressive, chronic liver disease. The histologic diagnosis is often cholangiohepatitis because the inflammatory response is mainly in the periportal areas.

Etiology: The exact etiology is not known. Infectious, immune-mediated, or toxic processes are thought to be involved. The early stages are associated with inflammation of the bile ducts and portal areas of the liver. Extension of bacterial infection through the bile duct or portal venous drainage may be responsible for the lesions in animals with suppurative cholangiohepatitis. When lymphocytes and plasma cells predominate in the cellular infiltrate, an immune-mediated process is more likely. Many causes of acute hepatic failure can progress to chronic active hepatitis.

Clinical Findings: The predominant clinical signs are weight loss, anorexia, depression, and lethargy. Icterus, behavioral changes, diarrhea, photosensitization, and hemorrhage are variably present. Fever may be persistent or intermittent, depending on the degree of cholangiohepatitis and fibrosis present. Dermatitis of the coronary band with regional sloughing of skin may develop. Recent or concurrent abdominal disease is often reported. Duration of clinical signs is variable, extending over days to months. Neurologic signs may seem to appear abruptly even though there is histologic evidence of chronic disease. GGT and AP are moderately increased, as are SDH and glutamate dehydrogenase, which indicates ongoing hepatocyte damage. In cases with marked hepatic fibrosis, enzyme activity may be normal, and BUN and albumin concentrations may be decreased. Serum total protein is either increased or normal. Globulins are usually increased. Serum total bile acid concentration is increased, and BSP® clearance prolonged. Cholestasis may cause hyperbilirubinemia with >25% of total bilirubin being direct. With diminishing hepatic function, serum glucose and coagulation factors decrease, and one-stage prothrombin time and activated partial thromboplastin time become prolonged. Blood ammonia levels may be elevated. There may be a neutrophilia or neutropenia with a left shift if endotoxemia develops. Anorexia can lead to hypokalemia. Ultrasonography generally reveals increased echogenicity in the liver indicative of hepatic fibrosis. The liver may be smaller than normal.

Lesions: Grossly, the liver is firm, pale brown to green in color, and often small. Irregular markings may be seen on the cut surface. Histologic lesions are predominantly in the periportal areas. Inflammatory cell infiltration may consist primarily of mononuclear cells, neutrophils with bacteria (often coliforms), or lymphocytes and plasma cells. The character of the infiltrate may indicate the nature of the primary disease process. Biliary hyperplasia may be marked if there is cholangiohepatitis. Variable degrees of necrosis and fibrosis are present.

Diagnosis: Histologic examination of a liver biopsy is needed for a definitive diagnosis. The tissue should also be cultured, although in most cases significant isolates are not identified.

Treatment: Supportive care should be provided, including fluid therapy with potassium chloride, glucose, and vitamin supplementation; dietary management (a low-protein, high branched-chain amino acid, high-carbohydrate diet); and prevention of exposure to the sun if photodermatitis is present.

Corticosteroid therapy has been used successfully in horses with a lymphocytic-plasmacytic infiltrate on liver biopsy. Different therapeutic regimens using prednisolone and dexamethasone have been recommended. The risk of inducing laminitis or abortion in pregnant animals with corticosteroids must be discussed with the owner before initiating therapy. Alternatively, an antifibrotic agent, colchicine (0.03 mg/kg/day, PO) has been recommended, but its efficacy in hepatic failure and safety in pregnant animals is unproved. Possible adverse reactions to colchicine in horses include laminitis and diarrhea. Malaise, vomiting, diarrhea, abdominal pain, myopathy, alopecia, and bone marrow suppression have been reported in humans and other species. In cases complicated with septic cholangiohepatitis, broad-spectrum antimicrobials are indicated. Ideally, antimicrobial therapy should be based on bacterial culture and sensitivity from the biopsy specimen.

Prognosis: The prognosis is generally guarded to poor and is best based on liver biopsy and response to therapy. The prognosis is fair to good in animals with less severe lesions, especially those with a lymphocytic-plasmacytic cellular infiltrate that responds well to corticosteroid therapy. Prognosis is poor in horses with hepatic failure, widespread fibrosis, and loss of normal hepatic parenchyma.

HYPERLIPEMIA AND HEPATIC LIPIDOSIS IN HORSES, DONKEYS, AND CAMELIDS

Epidemiology and Pathogenesis: Poor feed quality or decrease in feed intake, particularly during a period of high-energy requirement (eg, pregnancy, systemic disease), may result in hyperlipemia syndrome. Hyperlipemia is seen most commonly in ponies, miniature horses, and donkeys, and less frequently in standard-size adult horses. Pathogenesis of hyperlipemia is complex, with a negative energy balance triggering excessive mobilization of fatty acids from adipose tissue leading to increased hepatic triglyceride synthesis and secretion of very low density lipoproteins, concomitant hypertriglyceridemia, and fatty infiltration of the liver. The biochemical etiology of hyperlipemia is overproduction of triglyceride, rather than failure of triglyceride catabolism.

Onset of disease is associated with stress, decreased feed intake, fat mobilization and deposition in the liver, and overproduction of triglycerides, which may be precipitated by insulin resistance. In ponies, hyperlipemia is usually a primary disease process associated with obesity, pregnancy, lactation, stress, or transportation. Hyperlipemia may develop secondary to any systemic disease that results in anorexia and a negative energy balance. Secondary hyperlipemia is more common than primary hyperlipemia in miniature breeds. Hyperlipemia secondary to a systemic disease can be seen in horses of any age and in any condition. Female, stressed, and obese donkeys are at highest risk of developing hyperlipemia regardless of pregnancy status. Hyperlipemia is most commonly seen in the winter and spring.

Clinical Findings: Signs are nonspecific, variable, and may not relate to loss of liver function. They include lethargy, weakness, inappetence, decreased water intake, and diarrhea. Often, there is a history of prolonged anorexia, rapid weight loss, and previous obesity. Emaciation, ventral edema, colic, and trembling may be seen. Serum biochemical values and coagulation testing in miniature horses and ponies with hyperlipemia indicate that impairment of hepatic function is common. Affected animals have grossly opalescent blood and lipemic plasma. The blood concentrations of all lipids are increased, especially triglycerides, nonesterified fatty acids, and very-low-density lipoproteins. Donkeys have higher plasma triglyceride concentrations than do other equids. Hypoglycemia is a common finding in ponies but not in miniature horses with hyperlipemia. Total bile acid concentration and BSP® clearance are often normal, but BSP clearance may be prolonged in some animals. Activated partial thromboplastin time and one-stage prothrombin time may be prolonged. AST and SDH may be normal or increased. Increased creatinine, isosthenuria, and metabolic acidosis may develop secondary to renal disease. BUN and creatinine values are variable. Anorexia can lead to hypokalemia. Animals may become neutropenic with increased band neutrophils. Concurrent pancreatitis has been reported.

Prolonged increase in serum triglyceride concentrations is associated with lipid accumulation in the liver, kidneys, myocardium, and skeletal muscles, impairing function of these organs. The liver and kidneys become friable, and death may result from acute hepatic rupture.

Alpacas and llamas may develop hyperlipemia and ketonuria in late stages of gestation or secondary to disease states. Nonspecific clinical signs include lethargy, anorexia, and recumbency. Hypertriglyceridemia, hypercholesterolemia, increased SDH activity, metabolic acidosis, azotemia, and ketonuria may be seen. Secondary renal failure may develop. Camelids appear to be similar to both horses (hyperlipidemia) and cattle (ketosis) in their response to severe energy imbalance in late gestation. Hepatic lipidosis is the most common liver disease found in llamas and alpacas. Camelids of various ages and energy requirements are susceptible, and the pathogenesis is multifactorial. Common clinical findings include anorexia, weight loss, high concentrations of bile acids, high activities of GGT and AST, and hypoproteinemia. Some animals have high nonesterified fatty acids and β-hydroxybutyrate concentrations.

Lesions: The liver and kidneys are often pale, swollen, and friable with a greasy texture. Microscopically, there is variable fat deposition within the hepatocytes and epithelium of the bile ducts. The hepatic sinusoids may appear compressed and anemic with severe fatty infiltration. Gross and microscopic lesions of the primary disease process in ponies and horses may predominate.

Diagnosis: Clinical diagnosis is often based on the signalment, history, clinical signs, and gross observation of a white to yellow discoloration of the plasma. Plasma or serum triglyceride levels >500 mg/dL confirm the diagnosis. Cholesterol may also be increased, indicating an increase in lipoprotein. Laboratory evidence of hepatic dysfunction is supportive.

Treatment: Correction of the underlying disease, IV fluids, and nutritional support are the most essential factors in treatment of hyperlipemia. Nutritional support reverses the negative energy balance, increases serum glucose concentrations, promotes endogenous insulin release, and inhibits mobilization of peripheral adipose tissue. Polyionic electrolyte solution containing supplemental dextrose (50 g/hr/450 kg) and potassium (20-40 mEq of potassium chloride/L) should be given IV to hypoglycemic, hypokalemic animals. Glucose administration may cause refractory hyperglycemia in animals with insulin resistance. Glucose levels, renal function, urine output, and serum electrolyte concentrations should be monitored closely. IV fluids must be administered cautiously in camelids with hepatic lipidosis as many are already hypoproteinemic. Intermittent bolus administration of IV fluids rather than continuous infusion may be more effective for maintaining hydration without exacerbating existing hypoproteinemia.

Voluntary enteral nutrition is preferred if the affected animal will consume adequate quantities of nutritionally valuable feeds; however, most will not. Frequent feedings of a high-carbohydrate, low-fat diet are preferred. In animals with inadequate oral intake, supplemental tube feeding is necessary. Commercially available high-calorie enteral formulations provide adequate short-term nutritional support. Recipes for home-prepared, liquid tube-feeding diets for horses are also available. Small frequent feedings are required to meet caloric needs without overloading the GI tract. Animals should be observed after each feeding for signs of abdominal discomfort. Body weight, total fluid intake, and fecal consistency should be monitored daily. In animals that survive, hyperlipemia usually resolves in 5-10 days, but enteral feeding should be continued until voluntary feed intake is adequate. Enteral nutritional supplementation and treatment of the primary disease is often successful in reversing hyperlipemia in miniature horses and donkeys but not in ponies.

For horses that are totally anorectic, parenteral nutrition may be used. The lipid portion of the solution is omitted. Blood glucose concentration should be monitored twice daily to ensure that euglycemia is maintained and that substantial hyperglycemia (≥180 mg/dL) is avoided.

In camelids, partial parenteral nutrition with enteral supplementation can be used to maintain adequate energy intake and minimize further fat mobilization. Because of the distinct metabolism of camelids, parenteral nutrition products must contain higher amounts of amino acids (relative to nonprotein calories) than traditional formulations used in other species. Glucose concentrations must be carefully monitored, as these animals do not assimilate exogenous glucose well.

Exogenous insulin administration is recommended for treatment of iatrogenic hyperglycemia and hyperlipemia. Insulin decreases mobilization of peripheral adipose tissue by stimulating lipoprotein lipase activity and by inhibiting adipocyte hormone-sensitive lipase activity. The appropriate dose of insulin to be used in horses has not been well established. When insulin is used, response to therapy must be closely monitored and the dose adjusted accordingly. Insulin administration may fail to lower serum triglyceride or glucose concentrations in hyperlipemic animals when an insulin-resistant state is present. Insulin treatment is not well documented in camelids but was reportedly effective in the treatment of llamas with hepatic lipidosis.

Heparin is used in treatment of hyperlipemia because it promotes peripheral utilization of triglycerides and enhances lipogenesis via stimulation of lipoprotein lipase activity. Heparin may be given IV or SC with recommended dosages of 40-100 IU/kg, BID. Use of heparin is questionable in affected animals with increased hepatic production of triglycerides and without impaired peripheral removal of triglycerides. Heparin administration may potentiate bleeding complications and is contraindicated in animals with coagulopathies from liver dysfunction.

Nutritional supplementation to prevent hyperlipemia is indicated in miniature horses and donkeys, ponies, and horses with systemic disease associated with hypophagia and high metabolic demands.

Prognosis: Clinical biochemical parameters are not useful prognostic indicators of survival in ponies with hyperlipemia. Death from hyperlipemia is rare in miniature breeds. In most instances, survival depends on the ability to successfully treat the primary disease. Prognosis is often poor in ponies, standard-size horses, and camelids.

FATTY LIVER DISEASE AND HEPATIC LIPIDOSIS IN CATTLE AND SMALL RUMINANTS

Fatty liver disease is a complex metabolic disease seen primarily in dairy cattle (p 824). In goats, hepatic lipidosis has been associated with cobalt deficiency. Histologic lesions are consistent with those characteristic of ovine white liver disease in sheep.

HEPATIC NEOPLASIA

Primary hepatic tumors are uncommon in horses and ruminants. They include hepatocellular carcinoma, cholangiocarcinoma, and rarely lymphoma, hepatoblastoma, and mixed hamartoma. Cholangiocarcinoma is the most common and is primarily found in middle-aged or older horses. Hepatic carcinomas arise from hepatocytes, bile ducts, or metastasis. Hepatocellular carcinomas generally are found in yearlings to young adult horses and have also been reported in llamas and goats. Adenomas or adenocarcinomas of the liver have been reported in cattle. Hepatic fibrosarcoma and bile duct carcinoma with metastasis to the lungs have been reported in goats. Erythrocytosis, large areas of extramedullary hemopoiesis, and metastasis to the thoracic cavity have been reported in horses with hepatoblastoma.

Lymphosarcoma is the most common neoplasia of the hematopoietic system in horses. As many as 37% of horses with lymphosarcoma have neoplastic involvement of the spleen, and 41% have neoplastic involvement of the liver. Metastasis of lymphosarcoma of the liver has been reported in cattle, llamas, and goats.

The predominant clinical findings with hepatic carcinoma are lethargy and weight loss. A progressively enlarging abdomen, erythrocytosis, persistent hypoglycemia, icterus, and hepatic failure may also be seen. Cholangiocarcinoma causes pronounced weight loss before the onset of hepatic failure. Liver hepatocellular and biliary enzymes may be increased with hepatic carcinoma or cholangiocarcinoma. Serum GGT activity in affected horses is usually very high. Hepatocellular carcinomas are characteristically uniform in appearance on ultrasonographic examination.

Clinical manifestations of lymphosarcoma in horses are variable. Early in the disease, nonspecific signs such as weight loss, anorexia, and lethargy are seen. Lymphoma occasionally may diffusely infiltrate the liver and produce signs of hepatic failure, jaundice, and severe depression. Laboratory findings include hypoglycemia, mild to moderate increases in liver enzymes, hyperbilirubinemia, and abnormally low levels of IgM. Ultrasonographic examination helps to detect splenic and hepatic neoplasia. In ruminants, signs produced by growth in other organs (lymph nodes, abomasum, heart, uterus, spinal cord) are often most predominant.

The presence and character of the hepatic neoplasia can be confirmed by liver biopsy and microscopic examination of the tissue. Atypical lymphocytes or lymphoblasts may be seen in peritoneal fluids and peripheral blood of some affected animals. Increased serum α-fetoprotein concentration may support, but is not pathognomonic for, hepatoblastoma, as levels may also be elevated with hepatocellular carcinoma.

MISCELLANEOUS LIVER DISEASES

Hepatic Failure in Foals

Hepatic failure in neonatal foals may follow septicemia (especially *Actinobacillus equuli*), endotoxemia, *Leptospira pomona* infection, perinatal asphyxia, biliary atresia, hepatic duct obstruction secondary to gastroduodenal obstruction, and iron toxicity. Gastric ulcers and duodenitis in foals can cause strictures of the duodenum and subsequent cholangiohepatitis due to bile stasis. Neonatal isoerythrolysis and hemolysis may cause hypoxic and cholestatic hepatic disease. Administration of total parenteral nutrition may cause cholestasis and concurrent hepatic disease.

Biliary Atresia

Biliary atresia (extrahepatic) has been reported in 2 foals and in a neonatal lamb. Affected foals presented for anorexia, depression, lethargy, poor growth, colic, polydipsia, polyuria, pyrexia, and icterus at 1 mo of age. Markedly increased serum GGT and bilirubin with mildly increased SDH supported biliary obstruction. Diagnosis of biliary atresia was confirmed at necropsy.

Hemochromatosis

Hemochromatosis is an iron storage disease in which hemosiderin is deposited in the parenchymal cells, causing damage and dysfunction of the liver and other tissues. The disease is either primary (idiopathic) or secondary. It is reported in humans, Mynah birds, Salers cattle, and horses.

Etiology: In Salers cattle, the condition appears to be a homozygous recessive condition with inappropriate intestinal absorption of iron, excessive hepatic storage, and eventual loss of hepatic function. In horses, there is no evidence of a familial tendency or of excessive iron being consumed in the diet. Rather, it appears there is cirrhosis of the liver with secondary iron overload. In both horses and cattle, increased iron is deposited in the liver.

Clinical Findings and Lesions: In horses, primary clinical signs are weight loss, lethargy, and intermittent anorexia. In cattle, signs include decreased weight gain, poor body condition, dull hair coat, and diarrhea. In both species, liver enzymes, including GGT, AP, AST, and SDH are increased. Serum total bile acid concentrations are increased in horses, and serum iron, total iron binding capacity (TIBC), and percent saturation of the TIBC are usually normal. In some cases, serum iron and ferritin may be increased but TIBC is not saturated. In cattle, total serum iron, TIBC, and saturation of transferrin are increased. Iron content of the liver tissue is greatly increased in both horses (normal 100-300 ppm) and cattle (normal 84-100 ppm). Hepatomegaly and hemosiderin accumulation in the liver, lymph nodes, pancreas, spleen, thyroid, kidney, brain, and glandular tissue are typically present.

Diagnosis: Diagnosis is based on history, clinical signs, and laboratory findings. Finding abundant hemosiderin in the hepatocytes on histopathologic examination of a liver biopsy supports the diagnosis. High iron levels in liver tissue in animals with no history of excess iron intake helps confirm the diagnosis. Differential diagnoses include iron toxicosis from exogenous sources and diseases causing chronic weight loss and hepatic dysfunction or disease.

Treatment: Phlebotomies to remove blood and reduce the iron stores have been used in treatment of people with hemochromatosis. Similar treatment in horses and cattle has been unsuccessful. Deferoxamine is also used in people to induce a negative ion balance and reduce the rate at which iron accumulates. The effect in cattle and horses has not been evaluated.

Right Hepatic Lobe Atrophy in Horses

The right lobe of the liver is the largest lobe in young horses but frequently atrophies in older animals and becomes fibrous. Right hepatic lobe atrophy was previously considered an incidental postmortem finding, but some consider it to be a pathologic condition.

Right hepatic lobe atrophy has been proposed to result from chronic compression of this portion of the liver by the right dorsal colon and base of the cecum. Feeding horses high-concentrate, low-fiber diets may contribute to atony of the right dorsal colon with resultant distention; this compresses the right hepatic lobe against the visceral surface of the diaphragm. Although there is no morphologic evidence of direct vascular impairment to the right hepatic lobe, vascular compromise may result secondary to compression. With chronicity, the portal circulation to the right lobe is impaired, resulting in hepatic anoxia, deprivation of nutrients, and gradual atrophy of the right lobe of the liver.

No evidence of biliary tract disease has been noted. Colic may be seen. Some horses may have signs not related to the GI tract.

Hepatic Lobe Torsion

Hepatic lobe torsion can cause colic in horses. Liver enzymes and fibrinogen are increased, but abdominal fluid analysis is variable in affected animals. Bacteria, including *Clostridium* sp, may be found in the necrotic portion of liver. Exploratory celiotomy may be required for diagnosis.

Hepatic Amyloidosis

Amyloidosis refers to disease characterized by the extracellular deposition of amyloid, a proteinaceous fibril substance, in the tissue. Deposition of amyloid within an organ distorts normal tissue architecture and possibly function. In horses, the liver and spleen are the most common organs affected by systemic amyloidosis. Reactive or secondary systemic amyloidosis with deposition of amyloid A (AA) fibrils in the liver has been associated with severe parasitism and chronic infection or inflammation in horses.

Congenital Hepatic Fibrosis

Retrospective study of the records from the University of Berne, Institute of Animal Pathology, identified 30 Swiss Freiberger foals with pathologic lesions compatible with congenital hepatic fibrosis. Affected foals were 1-12 mo old (average 3.7 mo). The majority showed signs and had clinicopathologic changes reflecting severe liver damage. Pedigree analysis traced the disease back to one stallion. Results suggest that congenital hepatic fibrosis in Swiss Freiberger horses is a recessively inherited autosomal genetic defect. A similar condition has been reported in a calf.

HYPERAMMONEMIA AND HYPERBILIRUBINEMIA SYNDROMES WITH LITTLE OR NO EVIDENCE OF LIVER DISEASE

Primary Hyperammonemia of Adult Horses

In this syndrome of hyperammonemia, blindness and severe neurologic signs are seen in adult horses. The etiology is unknown, but a primary intestinal problem with overgrowth of urease-producing bacteria within the intestine is suspected.

The syndrome is nearly always associated with enteric disease, diarrhea, or colic. Diarrhea and, in some cases, protein-losing enteropathy may persist for several days. In most cases, diarrhea or colic precedes the neurologic signs by 24-48 hr. Laboratory abnormalities include increased blood ammonia levels (200-400 μm/L), severe metabolic acidosis, low plasma bicarbonate ($\leq$12 mEq/L) concentration, and profound hyperglycemia (250-400 mg/dL). Serum concentrations of liver enzymes, total bile acids, and bilirubin are normal.

In most horses, neurologic signs resolve within 2-3 days with supportive treatment (IV fluids, potassium chloride, glucose, sodium bicarbonate) and administration of drugs to reduce ammonia absorption (lactulose, neomycin).

Portosystemic Shunts

Portosystemic shunts are seen in foals and calves. Hyperammonemia and neurologic signs result from liver dysfunction with little laboratory or microscopic evidence of liver disease.

Clinical Findings and Lesions: Clinical signs are first seen when affected foals are ~2 mo of age and start to ingest larger amounts of grain and forage. Neurologic signs include staggering, wandering, blindness, circling, and seizures. Poor growth and intermittent neurologic signs (ataxia, weakness, depression, bruxism, tenesmus) have been reported in 2- to 3-mo-old calves. Serum levels of hepatic enzymes are often normal. Blood ammonia and total bile acid concentration are increased, and BSP® clearance is prolonged.

The liver is often small with a smooth surface and normal in color and texture. Microscopically, the hepatocytes are small. Portal veins in the triads may be small or absent. Hepatic arteries are often prominent and multiple.

Diagnosis: A portosystemic shunt should be suspected in foals or calves exhibiting repeated episodes of cerebral signs without obvious reasons. Signs may be most pronounced and associated with feedings. Catheterizing the mesenteric vein and performing a portogram or nuclear scintigraphy can confirm and locate the shunt. In some cases, the shunt may be seen on ultrasonographic examination of the liver.

Treatment: Surgical repair may be attempted in animals in which the site of the shunt can be identified, but the prognosis is guarded. Clinical signs in some foals may be controlled by restricting protein intake and by careful dietary management. Neomycin or lactulose are given orally to decrease ammonia production within the bowel. Supportive care with polyionic fluids, potassium, and dextrose may be needed to help decrease neurologic signs.

Hyperammonemia of Morgan Weanlings

A syndrome of ill thrift and hyperammonemia with variable hepatic involvement are seen in Morgan foals. Affected foals have been related, but the cause of the syndrome is undetermined. Clinical signs are usually first seen around weaning time. Liver enzymes and blood ammonia levels are increased. Bilirubin level is often normal.

HYPERBILIRUBINEMIA SYNDROMES

Gilbert's Syndrome

Gilbert's syndrome is a congenital hyperbilirubinemia seen in humans, inherited as an autosomal dominant trait, and Southdown sheep. It is an unconjugated hyperbilirubinemia in the presence of normal erythrocyte life span. A defect in carrier proteins or conjugating enzyme is suspected. Affected Southdown sheep have increased conjugated and unconjugated plasma bilirubin levels. Hepatic bilirubin clearance is defective, and affected sheep cannot excrete BSP® into the bile. Icterus is variable. Histopathologic lesions are absent except for pigment in the hepatocytes.

Dubin-Johnson Syndrome

Dubin-Johnson syndrome sporadically is seen in humans and Corriedale sheep. It is a failure of conjugated bilirubin to enter the bile canaliculi. Excretion of bilirubin and other conjugated organic anions may be impaired. Affected sheep may be icteric or hyperbilirubinemic. Serum conjugated and unconjugated bilirubin concentrations are increased, and BSP clearance and bile acid excretion may be delayed in affected Corriedale sheep. Histologically, the hepatocytes contain a black melanin-like pigment.

LIVER ABSCESSES IN CATTLE

Liver abscesses are seen in all ages and breeds of cattle wherever cattle are raised. They are most common in feedlot and dairy cattle fed rations that predispose to rumenitis. Cattle with liver abscesses have reduced production efficiency. Affected livers are condemned at slaughter, and adhesions to surrounding organs or the diaphragm may necessitate carcass trimming. Liver abscess can also lead to disease syndromes associated with posterior vena caval thrombosis.

Etiology and Pathogenesis: *Fusobacterium necrophorum*, a gram-negative, obligate anaerobic bacterium, and a component of normal rumen microflora, is the primary etiologic agent. Infection in the liver usually originates from a necrobacillary rumenitis. Two biovars have been implicated. Biovar A (*F necrophorum necrophorum*), the more virulent, is the predominant biovar in the rumen microflora and is isolated, usually in pure culture, from most cases of liver abscessation. Biovar B (*F necrophorum funduliforme*) is commonly isolated from microabscesses in the rumen wall but is less commonly isolated from liver abscesses, in which it is always found in mixed culture with biovar A or other bacterial species. *Arcanobacterium (Actinomyces) pyogenes*, streptococci, staphylococci, and *Bacteroides* spp are most frequently recovered from mixed cultures.

Rumenitis is usually the result of rapid intraruminal fermentation of dietary carbohydrate with subsequent production of lactic acid and increased acidity of the ruminal fluid. Rations with high levels of carbohydrate are the principal cause in both dairy and feedlot cattle, but the texture of the feed and method of feeding can be modifying factors. The incidence of rumenitis in feedlot cattle is significantly higher when they are transferred directly from a roughage ration to a finishing ration, and when there is poor feed bunk management. *F necrophorum*, alone or with other bacteria, colonizes through the area of superficial necrosis produced by the acid rumen contents. Leukotoxin may facilitate resistance to phagocytosis. Bacterial emboli from the lesions invade the hepatic portal venous system and are transported to the liver, where they can establish infectious foci of necrobacillosis that eventually develop into abscesses.

Other sources of infection in liver abscesses include foreign body penetration from the reticulum, direct extension of infection from omphalophlebitis in neonatal calves, and bacteremic diseases.

Clinical Findings, Lesions, and Diagnosis: Cattle with liver abscesses seldom exhibit clinical signs. Detailed clinical examination may show periodic fever, inappetence, and evidence of pain when pressure is applied to the xiphisternum and posterior rib cage on the right side. Grunting and other signs of pain may occur with movement or when the animal lies down. Clinical signs of omphalophlebitis are always present when there is liver abscessation resulting from extension of omphalophlebitis. Acute-phase proteins are increased early in the course of the disease, and serum sialic acid concentrations have been used for antemortem diagnosis. When there are several abscesses, or a large abscess, leukocytosis with neutrophilia and increased fibrinogen levels develop. Ultrasonography is an aid to diagnosis but abscesses in the left side of the liver may not be visualized. Feedlot cattle with abscessed livers have reduced feed efficiency, and those with severely abscessed livers gain 5-15% less per day than cattle without abscesses. Most liver abscesses are occult lesions that regress to a sterile scar. Untoward sequelae include peritonitis after abscess rupture into the peritoneal cavity, and sudden death from an anaphylactic or toxic reaction when there is rupture of an abscess into hepatic blood vessels. Rupture into hepatic veins can also lead to thrombophlebitis of the posterior vena cava with thromboembolic disease, endocarditis, pulmonary thromboembolism, multiple pulmonary abscesses, and chronic suppurative pneumonia. Aneurysms of the pulmonary artery consequent to pulmonary thromboembolism may rupture into airways to result in hemoptysis, epistaxis, and death. Caudal vena caval thrombosis may also lead to portal hypertension with a resulting syndrome of hepatomegaly, ascites, and diarrhea.

The ruminal lesions are characterized by a marked inflammatory reaction and necrosis. Occasionally, abscesses are found in the deeper layers of the rumen wall. Hepatic necrobacillosis lesions of <6 days duration are pale yellow and spherical with irregular outlines; they are characterized by coagulation necrosis of the hepatocytes with a surrounding intense zone of hyperemia and inflammation. Older abscesses have a core that is progressively encapsulated by fibrous connective tissue. Abscesses are usually 4-6 cm in diameter. Affected livers usually have 3-10 abscesses but may have up to 100.

Liver condemnation rates as high as 40% were recorded in a large survey of cattle slaughtered in the USA. Culture is seldom done to confirm the diagnosis. Occasionally, liver abscesses due to *F necrophorum* must be distinguished from those resulting from traumatic reticuloperitonitis (p 186).

Treatment and Control: Tylosin phosphate fed at 10 g/ton of feed significantly reduces the number of liver abscesses and increases feed efficiency and weight gain but has little, if any, effect on prevalence of ruminal lesions. Virginiamycin fed at 16 g/ton of feed or chlortetracycline fed continuously at 70 mg/head/day during the finishing period is also used. Leukotoxoid vaccines reduce abscess incidence and severity.

The primary control is by controlling ruminal acidosis through the method of feeding, diet composition, diligent feed bunk management, and the use of buffers in the diet.

Fewer ruminal lesions develop when the ratio of concentrate to roughage is decreased and when the transition period from a roughage to a finishing ration is lengthened. Increased roughage in the ration and multiple daily feedings increase the time of mastication and saliva flow; this increases buffer to the rumen and provides a continuous and uniform fermentation that reduces intraruminal acidity, which in turn lowers the number of ruminal lesions and, indirectly, the number of liver abscesses.

MALASSIMILATION SYNDROMES IN LARGE ANIMALS

Malassimilation is a defect in the ability of the GI tract to incorporate nutrients into the body either due to malabsorption or maldigestion. Malabsorption is the failure of passage of nutrients from the lumen of the bowel into the bloodstream, while maldigestion is the failure of intraluminal degradation of dietary constituents due to a defect in pancreatic exocrine function, bile acid content, or brush border enzymes. Maldigestion alone is an infrequent cause of malassimilation in large animals. Maldigestion syndromes are uncommon in horses compared with other domestic species. Diseases of malabsorption are much more common in horses than are diseases of maldigestion. The equine pancreas normally secretes only low concentrations of digestive enzymes and probably plays a small role in nutrient digestion. Some disease processes involve both maldigestion and malabsorption, such as is seen in young animals with lactase deficiency.

Etiology and Pathogenesis: Many diseases, by altering the normal absorptive mechanisms of the small intestine, induce a malabsorption syndrome. In horses, these include the following: 1) inflammatory or infiltrative disorders—diffuse lymphosarcoma of the small intestine (alimentary lymphoma); enteritis due to eosinophilic, lymphocytic-plasmacytic, or monocytic infiltrate; granulomatous enteritis; intestinal ischemia and damage due to migration of *Strongylus vulgaris* larvae, small strongyles, or *Strongyloides westeri* (foals) infection; cryptosporidia; postinfarction inflammation; amyloid A-associated gastroenteropathy; multiple abscessation in the bowel; tuberculosis; histoplasmosis; intestinal *Rhodococcus equi* infection; invasive enterocolitis (*Salmonella* spp); 2) biochemical or genetic abnormalities—congenital or acquired lactase deficiency (lactose intolerance), dietary-induced enteropathy, monosaccharide transport defect, pancreatic exocrine insufficiencies; 3) diseases causing inadequate absorptive area—villous damage or atrophy due to viral infection (rotavirus, coronavirus), cryptosporidia, intestinal resection; 4) cardiovascular disorders—congestive heart failure, intestinal ischemia; 5) lymphatic obstruction—lymphosarcoma, mesenteric lymphadenopathy, intestinal lymphangiectasia, abscessation, thoracic duct obstruction; and 6) miscellaneous—drug-induced, heavy metal toxicity, zinc deficiency.

Malabsorption syndromes in cattle are poorly documented but likely are seen most frequently in calves with diarrhea. Diseases that cause malabsorption syndromes in ruminants and swine include viruses (rotavirus, coronavirus), cryptosporidia, local or generalized ischemia, protein malnutrition, small-intestinal resection (short-bowel syndrome), congestive heart failure, lymphatic obstruction, parasitism (trichostrongylosis of sheep and cattle), tuberculosis, and Johne's disease in ruminants. Oral antibiotics may alter absorptive epithelial cells and cause an imbalance in GI tract flora. Treatment with high doses of ampicillin, neomycin, or tetracycline significantly decreases and delays glucose absorption during oral glucose tolerance tests in calves.

Maldigestion syndromes are uncommon and poorly understood in large animals. They may be due to alterations in gastric function or activity of rumen microflora, abnormal bacterial proliferation in the small intestine, or a decrease or lack of small-intestinal brush border enzyme (lactase deficiency). Less likely causes include drug-induced alteration in secretion or excretion of bile salts (induced by drugs or by hepatic or intestinal disease), or deficiency or inactivation of pancreatic lipase. Changes in bile salt concentration may not impair digestion in the adult herbivore but may exacerbate diarrheal states in milk-fed neonates. Surgical resection or bypass of the distal small intestine may facilitate bacterial overgrowth with associated bile salt abnormalities.

Lactose is a disaccharide composed of glucose and galactose. The small-intestinal brush border enzymes of foals and calves include lactase, which catalyzes the degradation of lactose into its component monosaccharides that are then absorbed. Primary lactase deficiency is inherited as an autosomal recessive trait in humans, but its occurrence and the mode of inheritance in large animals is poorly documented. Acquired or secondary lactase deficiency is more common. It is seen in foals and calves as a result of intestinal mucosal changes induced by viral, protozoal, and bacterial enteritis. Sloughing of the small-intestinal epithelial cells, loss of villous tips, and loss of some or all of the crypt cells result in some degree of lactase deficiency due to loss of lactase-secreting epithelial cells. Morphologic changes may include partial villous atrophy, crypt hyperplasia, and infiltration of the lamina propria. Osmotic diarrhea results in lactose-deficient foals and calves due to presence of osmotically active particles (lactose) and retention of water and electrolytes in the small intestine.

Malabsorption is commonly seen in animals with GI disease. It may arise from structural or functional disorders of the small intestine or be multifactorial. Often, malabsorption is seen concurrently with enteric protein loss. Either may cause loss of nutrients in the feces and weight loss. Malabsorption is not synonymous with diarrhea in any species, although diarrhea may be a feature. Function of the large intestine may be secondarily altered due to changes in the small intestine. Transient diarrhea may result as abnormal quantities of bile acids, fatty acids, and carbohydrates enter the large bowel in ileal effluent. These substances can directly or indirectly enhance secretion or decrease absorption rates.

Malabsorption of nutrients may result from insufficient absorptive surface area, an intrinsic defect in the mucosal or submucosal morphology of the intestinal wall, or lymphatic obstruction. Rotavirus infection in younger animals may cause destruction of intestinal villous epithelial cells, which results in maldigestion due to decreased activity of brush border disaccharidase enzymes and in malabsorption due to decreased absorptive surface area. Coronavirus and cryptosporidia may have similar effects. Decreased absorptive surface area can also result from small-intestinal resection (short-bowel syndrome) or from villous atrophy due to granulomatous enteritis. Local infiltrative or inflammatory disease, edema, or lymphatic obstruction (granulomatous enteritis, lymphosarcoma) secondary to local or systemic causes may interfere with the ability of the intestinal wall to absorb nutrients. Inefficient absorption also may develop due to increased mucosal permeability caused by cellular damage. Metabolic abnormalities may alter the epithelial cells and decrease the available energy for active transport and maintenance of the carrier proteins or brush border enzymes. Congenital deficiencies of enzymes that are normally present on the microvilli are not well recognized in domestic animals. However, neonates and ruminants have low levels of maltase, and ruminants lack sucrase. In most species, lactase levels decline with age.

Clinical Findings: Clinical signs are variable, depending on the underlying disease condition and the presence or absence of concurrent protein-losing enteropathy. A negative energy balance, weight loss, and possibly low serum protein concentrations characterize malassimilation syndromes. Chronic weight loss or reduced growth rate is the predominant clinical sign. Frequently, enteric protein loss may coexist with and prove more debilitating than malabsorption.

Appetite of affected animals may be normal, increased, or decreased. Polyphagia may be seen due to failure of assimilated nutrients to stimulate satiety centers. More commonly with small-intestinal malabsorption, hypophagia or anorexia is present because the primary disease process causes loss of appetite. Feces are frequently normal in consistency and volume. Diarrhea may be present but is not a consistent feature. Small-intestinal disease may be extensive before diarrhea develops because the colon can compensate and absorb the increased fluid load. In adult horses and ruminants, diarrhea indicates large-intestinal disease.

Clinical signs may also include poor condition, muscle wasting, exercise intolerance, normal or lethargic attitude, and variable thirst. Vital signs are usually normal until late in the disease. Pyrexia may be seen with inflammatory and neoplastic conditions. Abnormal pain may result from bowel inflammation, mesenteric or mural abscesses, adhesions, or partial obstruction. Ascites, dependent edema, and weakness may develop later in the disease process, especially if enteric protein loss is present. Skin and ocular lesions, vasculitis, arthritis, hepatitis, and renal disease may indicate immunologic reactions, particularly with inflammatory bowel disease. Skin lesions seen with malabsorption-related dermatosis include a thin hair coat, patchy alopecia, and focal areas of scaling and crusting that are often symmetrically distributed.

Foals and calves with lactose intolerance commonly have diarrhea, poor growth rate, and an unthrifty appearance. Some may experience flatulence, mild abdominal discomfort, or bloating after intake of milk. In young animals with acquired lactase deficiency, clinical signs (diarrhea, dehydration, weight loss) and clinicopathologic alterations (acidosis, hypoglycemia, electrolyte abnormalities) may be indistinguishable from those of the primary enteropathy. The animal's condition may improve quickly, and diarrhea may resolve when milk is withdrawn or replaced with enzymatically treated milk.

Pancreatic exocrine insufficiencies are an uncommon cause of maldigestion in horses. Affected ponies and draft horses were reported to have progressive weight loss and intermittent colic. The 2 ponies had clinicopathologic evidence of diabetes mellitus.

Lesions: The carcass is thin to emaciated, depending on the duration and severity of the malassimilation disease. Specific lesions depend on the primary underlying disease process. Overt signs of malabsorption do not always correlate with gross and histopathologic changes, emphasizing the importance of functional disorders.

Diagnosis: Small-intestinal malabsorption cannot be determined by clinical examination or by routine laboratory data. More common causes of weight loss must be excluded before a diagnosis of a malassimilation syndrome can be made. Determination of the primary underlying disease process is also necessary to establish an appropriate treatment regimen and prognosis.

A complete history should focus on duration of condition, precipitating factors, nutritional history, deworming and routine health care program, previous or concurrent diseases, as well as the number, age, and proximity of other affected animals. A thorough physical examination is performed to correlate physical findings with clinical signs and history. Rectal palpation is performed to determine the presence of intra-abdominal masses, enlarged lymph nodes, adhesions, abnormal positioning or thickening of bowel segments, or abnormalities in the cranial mesenteric artery. The kidneys, bladder, and related structures should also be evaluated.

A CBC, fibrinogen, and serum chemistry panel aid in determining the animal's general health status; presence of inflammation or an infectious process; involvement of body systems; and metabolic, electrolyte, and serum protein status. Urinalysis; abdominocentesis; and fecal examination for parasite ova, larvae, protozoa, and occult blood should also be performed. Plasma protein electrophoresis; fecal pH, culture, and leukocyte count; and immunologic studies may be indicated. Intracolonic fermentation of malabsorbed carbohydrates will often reduce the fecal pH in foals and calves. Protein-losing enteropathy can be diagnosed presumptively by excluding other causes of protein loss, such as renal disease or loss into a third space (peritoneum, pleural space), and by excluding the possibility of decreased albumin production (eg, as in liver disease). Contrast radiography of the bowel may be feasible in foals and small ponies. Ultrasonography may be used to help assess bowel thickness, presence of intra-abdominal masses, and vascular abnormalities in the cranial mesenteric artery in larger animals.

When malassimilation is suspected, a carbohydrate absorption test may be performed to assess small-intestinal function. For absorption tests to be diagnostic, the intestinal disorder either must be diffuse or must affect the delivery to and transit through the small intestine. An abnormal or flattened absorption curve is suggestive of small-intestinal dysfunction. Gastroscopy to eliminate the presence of lesions in the stomach (granulomas, tumor, ulcers) and duodenum or retention of ingesta should be done before absorption tests are performed.

Although absorption tests may indicate malassimilation is present, an etiologic diagnosis requires a biopsy of intestinal mucosa and possibly lymph node. A few cases can be diagnosed by rectal biopsy, which may reveal focal or diffuse inflammatory infiltration. Culture of the biopsy and fecal examination for leukocytes and epithelial cells may confirm the presence of salmonellae or other invasive organisms. In many cases, exploratory celiotomy is required to obtain the intestinal or lymph node biopsy. Surgery may not be advisable in a debilitated animal because wound healing is poor, and dehiscence is a potential problem. If undertaken, intestinal and lymph node biopsies should be obtained for culture, histopathology, enzymology, and immunology. Because of the risk and cost of obtaining appropriate tissue samples, malassimilation syndrome is often presumptively diagnosed with the aid of absorption tests.

Clinically applicable absorption tests include the D-glucose and D-xylose absorption tests. These tests may be useful in assessing small-intestinal function in preruminant calves, foals, and horses. Oral carbohydrate tolerance studies are not useful in ruminants because the sugar is degraded in the rumen. The D-glucose absorption test has the advantages of being easy and inexpensive, and methods to determine blood glucose concentrations are available in most clinical laboratories. The main disadvantage is that results are influenced by cellular uptake and metabolism of glucose, as well as by intestinal absorption. The D-xylose absorption test more directly measures intestinal absorptive capacity and is not influenced by endogenous factors and intestinal enzymatic activity. However, D-xylose is expensive, and availability of both xylose and laboratories that can perform plasma xylose determinations are limited.

Glucose or galactose may inhibit the absorption of D-xylose; therefore, fasting is necessary before the test is performed. The protocols of both tests require prolonged fasting, which may be deleterious to sick young foals and calves. The results of both tests are also affected by gastric emptying rate, small-intestinal transit time, and the animal's diet and length of fasting period before testing. The shape of the D-xylose absorption curve is influenced by renal clearance, hypoxia, anemia, systemic bacterial infections, and IgG concentrations in foals. Age of the animal being evaluated also affects absorption and digestion of glucose, lactose, and xylose. Therefore, the control animals must be within a few days of age of the affected animal if reference ranges are not available for its age group.

A delayed peak in the absorption curve of both D-glucose and D-xylose tests may result from delayed gastric emptying resulting from hypertonicity of the glucose or xylose mixture, excitement, pain, or retained gastric contents, or from changes in GI transit time and motility or partial obstruction. A flat absorption curve may be seen in a horse with normal absorptive capacity due to a transient decrease in intestinal blood flow or to bacteria in the lumen of the small intestine that metabolize the test sugar. Xylose rapidly equilibrates with many body fluids (in ascites), which lowers the blood level of xylose and may give a flat curve. Indications for an oral D-xylose absorption test in foals or calves include persistent diarrhea not attributable to infectious agents, poor growth despite normal intake, and other signs of maldigestion (repeated episodes of gas colic, bloating, ileus).

D-Xylose Absorption Test: This test measures absorptive capacity of the small-intestinal mucosa because functional enterocytes actively transport xylose across the mucosa and into the bloodstream. Subnormal absorption supports a diagnosis of malabsorption. Age and diet also affect xylose absorption in normal horses. Foals <3 mo old have a higher peak concentration of xylose after administration than adults. Adult horses maintained on a high-roughage, low-energy diet have a higher peak concentration of xylose after administration than those fed a high-energy diet. Food deprivation can alter D-xylose absorption in horses without overt GI tract disease. This effect must be considered when interpreting results in horses that are anorectic regardless of cause.

D-Xylose (0.5-1 g/kg in a 10% solution) is administered via nasogastric tube to a horse that has been fasted overnight (18-24 hr). Heparinized venous blood samples are collected 30 min before xylose administration and at 30-min intervals afterward for up to 2.5-4 hr. Expected peak values (20-25 mg/dL) vary between reports and laboratories. The curve, however, should be bell-shaped with a definable peak plasma xylose concentration 1-2 hr after administration. Peak absolute plasma values should be at least ≥15 mg/dL above baseline values in normal horses.

D-Glucose Absorption Test: Glucose absorption curves are steeper in pasture-fed horses than in those fed a higher energy ration. Lower peak values are seen in horses on a high-concentrate ration. The length of the pretest fast influences the absorption curve. Prolonged fasting may delay or decrease peak glucose concentration, thus giving a false-positive result. In two studies, >90% of adult horses with evidence of "total" glucose malabsorption had severe infiltrative lesions of the small intestine. The majority of horses (18/25) classified with "partial" glucose malabsorption also had obvious pathologic abnormalities of the small intestine.

Performance of the D-glucose absorption test is similar to that of the D-xylose absorption test except samples are collected into sodium fluoride tubes. Reportedly, in the normal horse, blood glucose concentrations are expected to rise by 15-20% or double the resting baseline value at 120 min after administration. One of the major disadvantages to the oral glucose absorption test is that using the conventional protocol, sampling is over a 6-hr period. One reported modified protocol requires only 2 test samples at 0 and 120 min after administration. This modification reportedly did not affect the reliability of the test result.

Oral Lactose Tolerance Test: Diagnosis of acquired lactase deficiency is usually presumptive based on history, clinical signs, and confirmation of presence of associated pathogens. Definitive diagnosis can be made with an oral lactose tolerance test. Lactose is hydrolyzed within the brush border of the small-intestinal enterocytes by lactase to constituent D-glucose and galactose before it is absorbed. Oral lactose tolerance testing is directed specifically at assessing whether lactase activity is present or not. Adult horses (>3 yr old) are lactose intolerant, and the test is unsuitable for ruminants. The oral lactose tolerance test is of value in evaluating young foals and preruminant calves with diarrhea or poor growth. Lactose intolerance has been documented in foals and calves. An oral lactose tolerance test does not distinguish maldigestion from malabsorption and requires fasting for several hours. Feeding enzymatically treated milk to animals suspected of being lactose intolerant may be tried before subjecting animals to the lengthy fast (18 hr) required before this test is performed. Before performing an oral lactose intolerance test, grain and hay should be withheld from the dam and foal for 18 hr. The foal should be muzzled for ≥4 hr before administering 20% lactose (1 g/kg via nasogastric tube); the muzzle should be kept in place for the duration of the test. Blood glucose levels are measured before dosing and at 30, 60, and 90 min (120 min is optional). The glucose level should peak within 60-90 min of lactose administration and should be ≥35 mg/dL higher than baseline in healthy foals.

Lack of an appropriate rise in blood glucose after lactose administration could be due to maldigestion or malabsorption. Therefore, if the lactose tolerance test is abnormal, a D-glucose or D-xylose absorption test should be performed to determine whether malabsorption or maldigestion alone is the problem. Casein hypersensitivity is distinguished from lactose intolerance by assessing the animal's response to enzymatically treated and untreated milk. Definitive confirmation of lactase deficiency is through direct measurement of mucosal lactase activity in the intestinal tissue. However, this is rarely undertaken in the clinical setting because a surgical biopsy of the mucosa is required.

Treatment: The etiology of the primary underlying disease process must be determined before specific therapy can be initiated. Specific therapy for most causes of malassimilation is not available, except for lesions due to parasite damage. Larvacidal dewormings with ivermectin or high-dose benzimidazoles may be corrective. Anti-inflammatory agents (eg, NSAID, corticosteroids) may also be beneficial in decreasing the inflammatory response within the affected bowel.

Malabsorption and chronic weight loss in horses may follow viral enteritis. Sloughing of the villous tips with loss of intestinal epithelial cells results in insufficient intestinal absorptive surface for adequate uptake of nutrients from the gut. Supportive care and facilitation of nutrient absorption from the hindgut must be encouraged until the intestinal epithelium recovers and new villous cells are produced. Maturation and healing of the intestinal absorptive surfaces may take weeks to months in severe cases.

Calves and foals with acquired lactase deficiency after diarrheal disease often respond well to supportive care (correction of acid-base, electrolyte, and glucose abnormalities) and feeding of enzymatically treated milk until the small-intestinal mucosa has regenerated.

Foals and calves that can tolerate it should be fed small amounts of high-quality roughage or grain to help meet their energy needs. Young foals and calves may benefit from intestinal rest (withdrawal of milk feeding) while the intestinal mucosa heals. These animals need alternate sources of energy and nutrients such as short-term feeding (≤24 hr) of glucose-containing electrolyte solutions or, in more severe cases, partial or total parenteral nutrition. Dietary change to a soy-based, non-lactose-containing milk replacer and early weaning are advised for animals with nonresponsive lactose intolerance.

Treatment of granulomatous enteritis has been attempted but is often unsuccessful. Anti-inflammatory agents (eg, corticosteroids) can be useful; sulfasalazine and isoniazid have also been recommended. The usefulness of dimethyl sulfoxide in the treatment of intestinal amyloidosis is unknown. Animals with anaerobic or aerobic bacterial overgrowth as a problem may respond to antimicrobial administration. Adequate penetration of antimicrobials into inflammatory bowel lesions (*Rhodococcus equi* in foals and Johne's in ruminants) is doubtful.

Horses with malabsorption due to a disease process or after small-bowel resection must be fed a diet that optimizes digestion of feeds in the large intestine. The diet should provide easily absorbed protein, carbohydrates, fat, and water-soluble vitamins and maintain mineral balance. Increased concentrate-to-forage ratios decrease digestion of feeds in the large intestine and should be avoided. Horses benefit from a fiber-based diet. To enhance digestion in the large intestine, easily fermentable roughages (eg, alfalfa) should be fed. High-quality fiber, metabolized in the cecum and colon to volatile fatty acids, may partially compensate for small-intestinal losses. In young animals, the diet may be supplemented with milk protein if lactase deficiency is not present. Fat may be added to the diet to enhance caloric intake. Calcium, magnesium, phosphate, zinc, copper, and iron may need to be supplemented because they are absorbed in the horse only in the small intestine. Water-soluble (especially vitamin B_{12}) and fat-soluble vitamins should be supplemented parenterally as needed. Oversupplementation, which could lead to toxicity, should be avoided.

Horses that will not eat may have to be force-fed with a gruel via nasogastric tube. The horse should be fed small, frequent meals to take advantage of the limited remaining absorptive ability of the small intestine without overloading it. Preruminant calves that are repeatedly tube-fed may develop ruminal acidosis due to deposition of feed material into the rumen rather than the abomasum. IV feeding, using partial or total parenteral nutrition, may be necessary for animals that refuse to eat or for those that cannot tolerate force-feeding. However, parenteral nutrition is difficult to continue on a longterm basis.

Prognosis: Efforts should be made to determine an etiologic diagnosis once malassimilation has been confirmed so that an accurate prognosis can be given and appropriate therapy prescribed. Most conditions causing malassimilation in adult large animals warrant a poor prognosis, and treatment is commonly unsuccessful. However, parasitic infestation of the bowel or its blood supply can respond to anthelmintic therapy. Occasionally, a non-neoplastic infiltration of the bowel may respond to corticosteroids, but the response may be transient in some cases. Calves and foals with lactase deficiency usually respond well to supportive care and dietary management.

ABDOMINAL FAT NECROSIS

(Lipomatosis)

Hard masses of necrotic fat are relatively common in the peritoneal cavity of adult cattle, especially the Channel Island breeds. The disease has also been seen in some species of deer maintained on pastures consisting primarily of tall fescue. The masses are commonly mistaken for a developing fetus because they feel like "floating corks" similar to cotyledons; they may result in episodes of intestinal obstruction characterized by moderate abdominal pain and the passage of small amounts of feces. The lipomatous masses are located in the small omentum, large omentum, and mesentery in cattle and more diffusely in sheep and goats. The composition of the fatty deposits is identical to that of fat of normal cows, and there is no suggestion that the disease is neoplastic.

Fat necrosis may also be seen in cattle ≥2 yr old after prolonged grazing of tall fescue infected with *Acremonium coenophialum* (*see also* FESCUE POISONING, p 2418). The condition is seen throughout the USA where tall fescue is used as the primary pasture plant. Over 90% of such pastures are infected. Hard masses of necrotic fat form in the omentum, mesentery, and perirenal fat and may cause clinical disease when they compress the intestine, obstruct the birth canal, or compress ureters. Rectal examination is useful in diagnosis and in determining prevalence in a herd. Removal of cattle from endophyte-infected pastures or dilution of intake by supplying legume or other grass pasture promotes slow reduction in the size of masses. In affected deer herds, 90% of the females may be involved. Clinical signs include anorexia, depression, and uremia associated with large masses of necrotic abdominal fat constricting the ureters, causing hydroureter and hydronephrosis.

A second form, less well defined, appears to be related to pancreatic problems. Although not associated with a clinical syndrome, the lesions (discrete or confluent masses of necrotic adipose tissue) may be found throughout the abdomen and are not a rare finding at necropsy.

A third form, a focal necrosis of abdominal and retroperitoneal fat, is seen most often in sheep but also in pigs, horses, and other species.

DISEASES OF THE MOUTH IN SMALL ANIMALS

For a discussion of developmental diseases of the mouth, *see* p 131. For EOSINOPHILIC GRANULOMA COMPLEX, *see* p 790.

The primary and most important function of the mouth is to obtain and introduce food into the digestive tract. Some of its additional functions include communication and social interaction, grooming, protection, and heat regulation (particularly in canines). The oral cavity shares many of the characteristics of the entire alimentary tract, including maintaining a large bacterial flora in the normal healthy state that lives primarily in biofilm communities. Unlike other areas of the body, the mouth also contains nonvital surfaces (enamel of teeth) that have neither local immune system defenses nor the ability to regenerate their surface through sloughing cells. The gingiva and mucosa have excellent vascular circulation, and the tightly adherent gingiva protect the underlying bone from trauma, thermal injury, and bacterial invasion.

Food prehension requires a complex interaction of the muscles of mastication, the teeth, the tongue, and the pharyngeal muscles. When any of these functions become compromised through disease or trauma, malnutrition and dehydration may result.

A complete oral examination should be included in physical examinations because oral diseases are most effectively treated with early diagnosis. Otherwise, many will remain hidden in the mouth, progressing to an advanced stage.

ORAL INFLAMMATORY AND ULCERATIVE DISEASE

Inflammation of the oral tissues may be either primary or secondary. Inflammation in the oral cavity may affect the gingiva (gingivitis), periodontium (periodontitis), oral mucosa (stomatitis), tongue (glossitis), glossopalatine arches (faucitis), palate (palatitis), or pharynx (pharyngitis). The nature and severity of the lesions vary greatly depending on the etiology and duration of the disease.

Periodontal disease, including gingivitis and periodontitis, is the most common oral problem in small animals. Gingivitis is a normal gingival inflammatory response to the presence of bacterial plaque on the adjacent tooth surface. Periodontitis (loss of periodontal ligament attachment) develops from a combination of bacterial periodontal pathogens and the immune response of susceptible individuals that together destroy the bone and tissues that support the tooth. (*See also* PERIODONTAL DISEASE, p 143.)

Periapical infection caused by endodontic disease and periodontal abscess can both cause a parulis, or gum boil, that manifests as a circular raised area of inflamed granulation tissue on the gingiva, with a central draining fistula. The tract can be followed to the primary periodontal or periapical lesion, and the etiology resolved (*see also* ENDODONTIC DISEASE, p 144).

Other causes for oral inflammatory conditions include immunopathy (eg, autoimmune, immune deficiency), chemical agents, infectious disease, trauma, metabolic disease, developmental anomalies or conformational anatomy that predisposes to irritation or inflammation, burns, radiation therapy, or neoplasia. Infectious agents that have been associated with gingivitis, glossitis, stomatitis, faucitis, and oral ulcerations are feline herpesvirus, feline calicivirus, feline leukemia virus, feline immunodeficiency virus, canine distemper virus, *Leptospira canicola*, and *L icterohaemorrhagiae*. Traumatic stomatitis may be seen after oral exposure to plant material (embedded plant awns) or fiberglass insulation. *Dieffenbachia* spp may cause oral inflammation and ulcers if chewed. Thallium is the major heavy metal responsible for oral lesions; incidence of this toxicity is low. Uremia can cause stomatitis and oral ulcers. Recurrent oral ulcerations are seen in gray Collies with cyclic hematopoiesis (p 51).

Signs vary widely with the cause and extent of inflammation. Anorexia may be seen, especially in cats. Halitosis and drooling are common with stomatitis, glossitis, and faucitis, and saliva may be blood tinged. The animal may paw at its mouth and resent any attempt to examine the oral cavity because of pain. Regional lymph nodes may be enlarged.

Ulceroproliferative Faucitis/Stomatitis
(Plasma cell stomatitis, Lymphocytic-plasmacytic stomatitis)

Cats with ulceroproliferative faucitis/stomatitis (UPFS) present with progressively worsening gingivitis and stomatitis. More significantly, the glossopalatine arches (fauces) have readily apparent lesions that are often very severely ulcerated, friable, inflamed, and proliferative. When a severe oral inflammation extends to involve this area in the back of the mouth that connects the upper and lower molar regions, UPFS should be suspected. The cause is unproved, but is suspected to result from an inappropriate inflammatory response in affected individuals to an unidentified antigen on the tooth surfaces, including the root surfaces and periodontal ligament.

The most immediate sign is severe pain on opening the mouth. Cats vocalize and jump when they yawn or open their mouth to prehend food. Halitosis, ptyalism, and dysphagia may be seen. Cats often show an "approach-avoidance" behavior as they approach their food in hunger, then hiss and run off in anticipation of discomfort. If the condition is severe and of long duration, weight loss may be evident. The disease is slowly progressive, and if soft, palatable foods are being fed, it may be fairly severe before signs are recognized. Submandibular lymphadenopathy is sometimes present. Frequently, because of pain, the oral cavity cannot be visualized adequately without sedation or anesthesia.

Diagnosis: A complete history, oral examination, and evaluation for systemic disease (eg, renal failure) is the minimum database that should be obtained. Oral biopsy for histopathology and immunodiagnostic testing, virus isolation (eg, calicivirus), and retroviral testing may also be needed to determine a prognosis; affected cats generally require surgery. Histopathologic evaluation is required to exclude oral neoplasia or other specific oral disorders. Most biopsy samples collected from chronic inflammatory or ulcerated lesions reveal a predominance of lymphocytes and plasma cells, which indicate the chronic inflammatory nature of the lesion without elucidating the primary etiology.

Treatment: Extraction of all the premolars and molars and removal of the associated periodontal ligaments by alveolar curettage is the only treatment that has provided some improvement and aided in overall longterm control. If any teeth are missing, dental radiographs are required to check for retained roots, which must be removed. Antibiotics (eg, amoxicillin-clavulanate, clindamycin, metronidazole) should be administered if primary or secondary bacterial infections are present. Culturing the lesions and performing susceptibility tests are rarely indicated even in chronic or recurrent infections. Symptomatic treatment for stomatitis includes dietary changes, antibiotics, and topical antiseptics (eg, 0.1% chlorhexidine solution or gel). Animals that are unable or unwilling to eat and drink should be given parenteral or subcutaneous fluids to prevent dehydration. Placement of a nasoesophageal, pharyngostomy, or gastrostomy tube should be considered in debilitated animals that do not respond to therapy. Frequent feedings of palatable liquids and, later, semisolid foods encourage eating.

Many other treatments for UPFS have been reported, including maintaining good oral hygiene, treating periodontal disease, regular dental prophylaxis, gold salts, azathioprine, hypoallergenic diets, CO_2 laser, cryotherapy, electrofulguration, and radiosurgery. None of these provide longstanding resolution. Glucocorticoid administration usually results in significant and immediate clinical improvement due to modulation of the excessive inflammatory response, but is not recommended. Repeated injections (methylprednisolone) or oral maintenance therapy (prednisone) are frequently required, as the treatment becomes progressively less effective and eventually completely ineffective. In addition, animals treated with glucocorticoids have a poorer prognosis once the teeth are extracted. Extraction of all premolars and molars or full-mouth extractions generally result in significant improvement or complete resolution of the inflammation if performed early in the course of the disease and before multiple glucocorticoid treatments. (See also FELINE GINGIVITIS/STOMATITIS SYNDROME, p 146.)

Chronic Ulcerative Stomatitis

Characteristics of chronic ulcerative stomatitis (also called chronic ulcerative paradental syndrome or CUPS) include severe gingival inflammation, multiple sites of gingival recession and dehiscence, and large areas of ulcerated labial mucosa adjacent to the surfaces of large teeth. The problem commonly affects Greyhounds, but it has also been seen in Maltese, Miniature Schnauzers, Labrador Retrievers, and other breeds. The characteristic feature is the contact ulcer that develops where the lip mucosa contacts the tooth surface, most commonly on the inner surface of the upper lip adjacent to the upper canine teeth. These lesions have also been termed "kissing ulcers" because they are found where the lips "kiss" the teeth. The underlying pathology is an immunopathy that results in an excessive local inflammatory response to the antigens in dental plaque.

Stringent plaque control through professional cleaning and excellent home oral hygiene may resolve the problem. Supplemental antibacterial measures, eg, topical chlorhexidine rinses or gels, also help. In severe cases, topical anti-inflammatory preparations to modulate the inflammatory response may provide comfort. Discomfort caused by the ulcers complicates efforts to brush the teeth and give oral medications. In the worst cases, in which discomfort is severe and the owners are unable or unwilling to brush the teeth, extraction of the adjacent teeth may be necessary to remove the contact surfaces on which plaque accumulates. Although this may aid in control of the lesions, it is not curative, as plaque grows on all mucosal surfaces in the mouth. In many cases with complete extractions, animals continue to develop lesions due to hyperimmune response to the plaque.

Lip Fold Dermatitis and Cheilitis

Lip fold dermatitis is a chronic moist dermatitis seen in breeds that have pendulous upper lips and lower lateral lip folds (eg, spaniels, English Bulldogs, Saint Bernards) that accumulate saliva. These lesions may be exacerbated when poor oral hygiene results in high salivary bacterial counts. The lower lip folds can become very malodorous, inflamed, uncomfortable, and swollen.

Lip wounds, resulting from fights or chewing on sharp objects, are common and vary widely in severity. Thorns, grass awns, plant burrs, and fishhooks may embed in the lips and cause marked irritation or severe wounds. Irritants such as plastic or plant material may produce inflammation of the lips. Lip infections may develop secondary to wounds or foreign bodies or may be associated with inflammation of adjacent areas. Direct extension of severe periodontal disease or stomatitis can produce cheilitis. Licking areas of bacterial dermatitis or infected wounds may spread the infection to the lips and lip folds. Inflammation of the lips also can be associated with parasitic infections, autoimmune skin diseases, and neoplasia.

Clinical Findings and Diagnosis: Inflammation of the lips and lip folds can be acute or chronic. Animals with cheilitis may paw, scratch, or rub at their mouth or lip; have a foul odor on the breath; and occasionally salivate excessively or be anorectic. With chronic infection of the lip margins or folds, the hair in these areas is discolored, moist, and matted with a thick, yellowish or brown, malodorous discharge overlying hyperemic and sometimes ulcerated skin.

Cheilitis due to extension of infection from the mouth or another area of the body usually is detected easily because of the primary lesion.

Treatment: Medical management of lip fold dermatitis includes clipping the hair, cleaning the folds 1-2 times/day with benzoyl peroxide or a mild skin cleanser, and keeping the area dry. Topical diaper rash cream applied daily may be helpful. Surgical correction of deep lip folds is a more longlasting remedy.

Cheilitis that is unrelated to lip folds usually resolves with minimal cleansing, appropriate antibiotics if a bacterial infection is present, and specific treatment of primary etiologies (eg, autoimmune skin disease). Wounds of the lips should be cleaned and sutured if necessary. Treatment of periodontal disease or stomatitis is necessary to prevent recurrence.

Infectious cheilitis that has spread from a lesion elsewhere usually improves with treatment of the primary lesion, but local treatment also is necessary. With severe infection, hair should be clipped from the lesion and the area gently cleaned and dried. Antibiotics are indicated if the infection is severe or systemic.

Mycotic Stomatitis

Mycotic stomatitis, caused by overgrowth of *Candida albicans*, is an uncommon cause of stomatitis in dogs and cats. It is characterized by the appearance of creamy white plaques on the tongue or mucous membranes. It is usually thought to be associated with other oral diseases, longterm antibiotic therapy, or immunosuppression. The underlying tissue is frequently red and ulcerated. There may be smaller plaques surrounding a larger main plaque. The periphery of the lesion is usually reddened. The lesions may coalesce as the disease progresses, and similar lesions may be seen in the oral pharynx and at other mucocutaneous junctions. Diagnosis may be confirmed by culture of the organism from the lesion and by histologic evidence of tissue invasion. Histologic diagnosis may be confirmatory in the absence of a positive culture.

Any existing underlying local or systemic diseases affecting the oral cavity should be treated. Ketoconazole or a related benzimidazole should be administered until the lesions resolve, after which antibiotic therapy should be discontinued. An adequate level of nutrition should be maintained. The prognosis is guarded if predisposing diseases cannot be adequately treated or controlled.

Acute Necrotizing Ulcerative Gingivitis (ANUG)
(Necrotizing ulcerative gingivostomatitis, Ulceromembranous stomatitis, Necrotizing ulcerative stomatitis, Vincent's stomatitis, Trenchmouth)

This relatively uncommon disease of dogs is characterized by severe gingivitis, ulceration, and necrosis of the oral mucosa. *Fusobacterium* spp and spirochete organisms (*Borrelia vincenti*), normal inhabitants of the mouth, have been suggested to cause this disease after some predisposing factor increases their levels or decreases the local resistance of the oral mucosa. The role, if any, of these organisms in causing disease is unknown. More recently, it has been found in humans that *Bacteroides melanogenicus intermedius* may play a more important role. Other potential factors are stress, excess glucocorticoid administration in susceptible dogs, and poor nutrition.

The disease appears first as reddening and swelling of the gingival margins and interdental papillae, which are painful, bleed easily, and may progress to gingival recession. Extension to other areas of the oral mucosa is common, resulting in ulcerated, necrotic mucous membranes and exposed bone in severe cases. Halitosis is severe, and the animal may be anorectic due to pain. Ptyalism may be present, and the saliva may be blood tinged. Differential diagnoses include severe periodontal disease, autoimmune skin disease, uremia, neoplasia, and other systemic disease associated with oral lesions.

Diagnosis is made by exclusion of other etiologies.

Treatment of periodontal disease, debridement of lesions, oral hygiene, antibiotics (amoxicillin-clavulanate, ampicillin, clindamycin, metronidazole, tetracyclines), and oral antiseptics (0.1% chlorhexidine solution or gel) are indicated.

Glossitis

Glossitis, an acute or chronic inflammation of the tongue, may be due to infectious (calicivirus, herpesvirus, rhinotracheitis virus, leptospirosis), physical (irritation from excess calculus and periodontal disease, foreign bodies that penetrate or become lodged under the tongue, traumatic wounds), or chemical agents; metabolic disease (uremia, hypoparathyoidism, protein-losing hepatopathy); or other causes such as electrical burns and insect stings. Foreign body glossitis is especially a problem in longhaired dogs that attempt to remove plant burrs from their coats.

Drooling and a reluctance to eat are common signs, but the cause may go undiscovered unless the mouth is carefully examined. Periodontitis may result in reddening, swelling, and occasionally ulceration of the edge of the tongue. A thread, string, or other linear foreign body may get caught under the tongue. There may be no inflammation of the dorsal surface of the tongue, but the ventral surface is painful, shows acute or chronic irritation, and frequently is lacerated by the foreign body. Porcupine quills, plant material, and other foreign materials may become embedded so deeply that they are not palpable. Insect stings cause an acute swelling of the tongue.

In chronic cases of ulcerative glossitis, a thick, brown, foul-smelling discharge (occasionally with bleeding) may be present. Frequently, the animal is reluctant to allow oral examination.

Fissured, or plicated, tongue (lingua dissecta) describes a textural variation of the dorsum of the tongue with a deep central groove. The fissure deepens with age and is therefore felt to be acquired from some extrinsic factor. However it may also represent a developmental anomaly. The groove often becomes deeply filled with hairs that act as a local irritant causing inflammation and discomfort.

For any glossitis, foreign bodies and hairs should be removed, and broken or diseased teeth removed or treated. Bacterial infectious glossitis should be treated with an appropriate systemic antibiotic. Debridement and 0.12% chlorhexidine mouthwashes are beneficial in some cases. Lingual curettage may be required if foreign material is embedded in the tongue. A soft diet and parenteral fluids may be necessary. If the animal is debilitated and unable to eat well for a prolonged period, a nasoesophageal, pharyngostomy, or gastrostomy tube to allow for nutritional support should be considered. Acute glossitis due to insect stings may require emergency treatment.

If the glossitis is secondary to another condition, the primary disease should be treated. The tongue tissues heal rapidly after irritation and infection have been eliminated.

SOFT TISSUE TRAUMA

Cheek-biting

A proliferative, verrucous lesion along the bite-plane of the cheek may result from self-trauma when the tissue becomes entrapped between the teeth during chewing. This is similar to morsicato buccarum and morsicato labiorum in humans. It can also affect the sublingual tissues in dogs and cats, similar to morsicato linguarum. Surgical removal of the excess tissue prevents further trauma.

Mouth Burns

Thermal, chemical, or electrical burns involving the mouth are not uncommon. The animal should be evaluated and treated for systemic involvement, which may be life-threatening in some cases. The tongue, lips, buccal mucosa, and palate are frequently involved with electrical burns. The injuries may be mild, with only temporary discomfort, or may be very destructive with loss of tissue, scar formation, and subsequent deformity or tissue deficits. Chewing on an electrical cord is most frequently a problem in puppies. These animals often have a linear scar across the dorsum of the tongue, outlining the path of the electrical cord. One or both lip commisures may have a scar or wound, and the adjacent carnassial teeth may be discolored and eventually require endodontic treatment.

The owner may have observed the incident, thus providing a history. The animal hesitates to eat or drink, drools, and resents handling of its mouth or face. If tissue destruction is marked, ulcerative or gangrenous stomatitis may develop, with secondary bacterial infections. If contact with a corrosive chemical is seen and the chemical is alkaline, the mouth may be flushed with mild solutions of vinegar or citrus juice; if the chemical is acidic, a solution of sodium bicarbonate may be used. Copious flushing of the mouth with water may help remove some of the chemical substances. More commonly, the animal is seen too long after the exposure for neutralization to be effective.

Animals showing a reddened oral mucosa without tissue defects require no specific treatment other than a soft or liquid diet until the lesion has healed. If tissue damage is extensive, treatment includes lavage with dilute chlorhexidine solution and conservative tissue debridement. The risk of secondary infection should be minimized with systemic antibiotic therapy for several days.

VIRAL WARTS AND PAPILLOMAS

Viral warts (verruca vulgaris) are benign growths caused by a virus (*see also* p 774). The oral mucosa and commissures of the lip are most frequently involved, but the masses (single or, more frequently, multiple) can involve the palate and oropharynx. Viral warts are most common in young dogs and often appear suddenly, with rapid growth and spread. Signs are seen when the growths interfere with prehension, mastication, or swallowing. Occasionally, if the growths are numerous, the dog may bite them when chewing, causing them to bleed and become infected. They may regress spontaneously within a few weeks, and removal is generally not necessary. If necessary, debulking of the exophytic lesion can be accomplished with electro- or radiosurgery, or by sharp resection. Surgical removal of one or more of the warts may initiate regression. The use of commercial or autogenous wart vaccines is usually disappointing. The self-limiting character of the disease makes evaluation of any treatment difficult.

Papillomas (p 774) are benign exophytic proliferations of squamous epithelium. They are clinically indistinguishable from virus-induced warts. Unlike viral warts, papillomas are generally slow growing and solitary. They most commonly remain benign, and surgical removal is curative.

ORAL TUMORS

Epulides

Epulides are firm masses involving the gingival tissue and are the most common benign oral tumors in dogs (*see also* p 145). Cats less commonly have benign oral tumors. These tumors may be seen in dogs of any age but generally are found in those >6 yr old. The 3 histologic types of epulides were previously classified as fibromatous epulis, ossifying epulis, and acanthomatous epulis. This classification was based on their clinical appearance and behavior. Fibromatous and ossifying epulides are now considered to be peripheral odontogenic fibromas. The ossifying form is a fibromatous mass that has developed centers of ossification. They are generally solitary, although multiple lesions may be present. The tumors are noninvasive, but may become quite extensive. They arise from the periodontal ligament of the subjacent tooth, and complete surgical removal must include tissues up to and including the periodontal ligament. This often necessitates en bloc removal of the affected tooth or teeth. Complete excision is curative.

Acanthomatous epulis is now called canine peripheral ameloblastoma or canine acanthomatous ameloblastoma. These routinely aggressively invade local tissues including bone. They generally do not metastasize, but due to their locally aggressive nature surgical excision must include a full 1-cm margin of clinically normal tissue (again including bone) to prevent recurrence. Radiation treatment may minimize disfigurement when treating large tumors. Adequate surgical removal is curative.

Due to the varied behavior of gingival growths, they should always be biopsied before surgery.

Malignant Oral Tumors

Tumors of the mouth and pharynx are common and likely to be malignant. In dogs, the 3 most common are malignant melanoma, squamous cell carcinoma, and fibrosarcoma. The gingiva is affected most frequently. The incidence of malignant oral tumors is higher in dogs >8 yr old.

Squamous cell carcinomas are by far the most common malignant oral neoplasms in cats; they commonly involve the gingiva and tongue and are locally highly invasive. Fibrosarcomas are the next most common; in cats, they are locally invasive and have a poor prognosis.

Clinical Findings: Signs vary depending on the location and extent of the neoplasm. Halitosis, reluctance to eat, and hypersalivation are common. If the oropharynx is involved, dysphagia may be present. The tumors frequently ulcerate and bleed. The face may become swollen as the tumor enlarges and invades surrounding tissue. Regional lymph nodes often become swollen before oral and pharyngeal tumors are seen.

Diagnosis: A cytologic diagnosis from impression smears of a fine-needle aspirate is possible in some cases. Biopsy is usually required for definitive diagnosis. Malignant melanomas are variable in appearance, pigmented or nonpigmented, and should be considered in the diagnosis of any oral tumor. Squamous cell carcinomas commonly involve the gingiva or tonsils, and lymphosarcoma should be a differential diagnosis for an enlarged tonsil. Regional lymph nodes and the lungs should be evaluated for metastases.

Treatment: Malignant melanomas are highly invasive and metastasize readily; consequently, the prognosis is guarded to poor. Surgical resection can extend survival and may be curative, particularly with masses in the rostral areas of the mouth. However, local recurrence is common. Nontonsillar squamous cell carcinomas are locally invasive with a low rate of metastasis, and the prognosis is good with aggressive surgical resection or radiation therapy, or both. Tonsillar squamous cell carcinomas are aggressive and have a poor prognosis. Fibrosarcomas have a guarded prognosis because of their locally aggressive nature. Recurrence of tumor growth after resection is common.

In cats, squamous cell carcinoma has a poor prognosis, and longterm survival is seen only if diagnosed and treated early. Local tumor removal often requires mandibulectomy.

SALIVARY DISORDERS

Ptyalism

Ptyalism, or sialosis, describes hypersecretion of saliva that is characterized clinically by drooling. Pseudoptyalism is seen when there is a normal quantity of saliva but an increase in drooling secondary to conformational abnormalities or swallowing disorders. Both are discussed together as ptyalism.

Ptyalism may result from the following: 1) drugs, eg, organophosphates or poisons; 2) local irritation or inflammation associated with stomatitis, glossitis (especially in cats), oral foreign bodies, neoplasms, injuries, or other mucosal defects; 3) infectious diseases (eg, rabies), the nervous form of distemper, or other convulsive disorders; 4) motion sickness, fear, nervousness, or excitement; 5) reluctance to swallow from irritation of the esophagus or from stimulation of GI receptors in gastritis or enteritis;

6) sublingual lesions (eg, linear foreign body, tumor); 7) tonsillitis; 8) administration of medicine (particularly in cats); 9) conformational defects; 10) metabolic disorders (eg, hepatic encephalopathy [especially in cats]) or uremia; 11) abscess or other inflammatory blockage or condition of the salivary gland.

The possibility of rabies should be eliminated before oral examination. The underlying cause, local or systemic, should be determined and treated. Acute moist dermatitis of the lips and face may develop if the skin is not kept as dry as possible. Cleansing with a dilute chlorhexidine solution or benzoyl peroxide may be helpful.

Salivary Mucocele

In a salivary mucocele (or sialocele), mucoid saliva accumulates in the subcutaneous tissue after damage to the salivary duct or gland. This is the most common salivary gland disorder of dogs. While any of the salivary glands may be affected, the sublingual and mandibular glands are involved most commonly. Usually, the saliva collects at the intermandibular or cranial cervical area (cervical mucocele). It may also collect in the sublingual tissues on the floor of the mouth (ranula). A less common site is in the pharyngeal wall.

The cause may be traumatic or inflammatory blockage or rupture of the duct of the sublingual, mandibular, parotid, or zygomatic salivary gland. Usually, the cause is not determined, but a developmental predisposition in dogs has been suggested.

Signs depend on the site of saliva accumulation. In the acute phase of saliva accumulation, the inflammatory response results in the area being swollen and painful. Frequently, this stage is not seen by the owner, and the first noticed sign may be a nonpainful, slowly enlarging, fluctuant mass, frequently in the cervical region. A ranula may not be seen until it is traumatized and bleeds. A pharyngeal mucocele may obstruct the airways and result in moderate to severe respiratory distress.

A mucocele is detectable as a soft, fluctuant, painless mass that must be differentiated from abscesses, tumors, and other retention cysts of the neck. Pain or fever may be present if the mucocele becomes infected. A salivary mucocele usually can be diagnosed by palpation and aspiration of the characteristic golden or blood-tinged, viscous saliva. Usually, careful palpation with the animal in dorsal recumbency can determine the affected side; if not, sialography may be helpful.

Surgery is recommended to remove the damaged salivary gland and duct. Cervical mucoceles can be managed with periodic drainage if surgery is not an option. Drainage, marsupialization, or gland removal has been recommended for treatment of ranulas. Complete gland and duct removal is recommended for pharyngeal mucoceles to avoid future life-threatening airway obstruction.

Salivary Fistula

Salivary fistulas, which are rare, may result from trauma to the mandibular, zygomatic, or sublingual salivary glands. Wounds of the parotid gland are more likely to develop a fistula. Parotid duct injury may be the result of a traumatic wound (eg, bite wound), abscess drainage, or prior surgery in the area with iatrogenic rupture. The constant flow of saliva prevents healing, and a fistula develops.

History of injury in the gland area, location of the fistula, and nature of the discharge are characteristic. A salivary fistula must be differentiated from a draining sinus (due to a penetrating foreign body or endodontic disease of a mandibular tooth) in the neck or from sinuses arising from congenital defects. Surgical ligation of the duct usually results in resolution, but excision of the associated gland may also be necessary.

Salivary Gland Tumors

Salivary gland tumors are rare in dogs and cats, although cats are affected twice as frequently as dogs. Most are seen in dogs and cats >10 yr old. There is no breed or sex predilection, although Poodles and Spaniel breeds may be predisposed. Most salivary gland tumors are malignant, with carcinomas and adenocarcinomas the most common. Local infiltration and metastasis to regional lymph nodes and lungs are common, as is local recurrence after surgical excision. Radiotherapy, with or without surgery, offers the best prognosis.

Sialadenitis

Sialadenitis, or inflammation of the salivary gland, is rarely a clinical problem in dogs and cats. However, it is frequently an incidental finding on histopathology at necropsy.

The cause may be trauma, commonly from penetrating wounds such as bites, or systemic infection affecting the salivary gland or surrounding tissue. Sialadenitis as a component of systemic disease has been reported with rabies, distemper, and the paramyxovirus that causes mumps in people.

Signs include fever, depression, and painful, swollen salivary glands. Rupture of an abscessed gland discharges pus into the surrounding tissue or the mouth. Rupture through the skin may cause a salivary fistula to form. Swelling of the parotid gland is most prominent below the ear, swelling of the mandibular gland at the angle of the jaw, and swelling of the zygomatic gland just caudal to the eye. Zygomatic gland involvement may result in retrobulbar swelling, divergent strabismus of the affected eye, exophthalmos, excess tearing, and reluctance to open the mouth or eat. Abscesses of the zygomatic and parotid glands are acutely painful; the animal may hold its head rigidly and resent any manipulation involving the head or neck.

Radiographs and laboratory tests are usually not helpful, although evaluation of fluid in an abscess can lead to a diagnosis. Histopathology of salivary gland tissue can reveal acute or chronic inflammatory changes or necrosis.

Mild sialadenitis requires no treatment, and recovery is usually rapid and complete. A developed abscess should be drained through the overlying skin or, if involving the zygomatic gland, behind the last upper molar on the affected side. Systemic antibiotics should be administered.

Lack of resolution or recurrence necessitates cytology of aspirated material, biopsy, or surgical removal of the affected gland.

Xerostomia

Xerostomia, or aptyalism, is a decreased secretion of saliva, characterized by a dry mouth. It can cause significant discomfort and difficulty with eating. It is uncommon in dogs and cats, but is very common in humans that have undergone orthoradiation treatment for tumors of the head and neck and have had collateral radiation injury to the salivary glands. As radiation treatment is used more commonly in veterinary medicine, this condition may become more frequent in animals. Decreased salivary secretion may also result from use of certain drugs (eg, atropine), extreme dehydration, pyrexia, or anesthesia. It is seen in some dogs with keratoconjunctivitis sicca and may be immune-mediated. Occasionally, it is due to disease of the salivary gland. Determination and treatment of the underlying cause is of primary importance. Physiologically balanced mouthwashes relieve the discomfort that results from xerostomia. Fluids may be administered to correct dehydration, if present. Immunosuppressive therapy is indicated if immune-mediated disease is suspected.

DISEASES OF THE ESOPHAGUS IN SMALL ANIMALS

CRICOPHARYNGEAL ACHALASIA

Cricopharyngeal achalasia is characterized by inadequate relaxation of the cricopharyngeal muscle, which leads to a relative inability to swallow food or liquids. It is seen primarily as a congenital defect, but is occasionally seen in adult dogs. Repeated attempts to swallow are followed by gagging and regurgitation. Aspiration pneumonia is a common complication. The cause is generally unknown, but may be associated with acquired neuromuscular disorders in adult animals. An accurate diagnosis requires fluoroscopic evaluation of swallowing after oral administration of contrast material alone and mixed with food. Abnormal function (lack of relaxation) of the cricopharyngeal muscle results in retention of barium in the posterior pharynx.

Treatment consists of cricopharyngeal myotomy, which usually results in normal swallowing immediately after surgery. The success rate of surgery approaches 70%. Dogs with acquired neuromuscular disorders are less likely to respond to surgery, but may respond to treatment of the underlying disease. Aspiration pneumonia should be treated aggressively if present.

DILATATION OF THE ESOPHAGUS
(Megaesophagus)

Megaesophagus may be due to a congenital defect or may be an adult-onset, acquired disorder. Congenital defects that may result in megaesophagus include vascular ring anomalies, esophageal diverticula, and an idiopathic form. (*See also* CONGENITAL AND IN-HERITED ANOMALIES, p 134.) Adult-onset megaesophagus may be primary (idiopathic) or secondary to systemic disease. Secondary megaesophagus may be due to myasthenia gravis, systemic lupus erythematosus, polymyositis, hypoadrenocorticism, heavy metal (lead) toxicity, dysautonomia, CNS disorders including neoplasia, and possibly hypothyroidism. Esophageal dilatation may also develop cranial to an esophageal lesion such as an esophageal stricture, foreign body, neoplasia, or extraesophageal compression.

The cardinal sign is regurgitation. A puppy with congenital megaesophagus characteristically begins to regurgitate at weaning when it starts to eat solid food. Affected pups are generally unthrifty and smaller than their littermates. Pressure applied to the abdomen may cause ballooning of the esophagus at the thoracic inlet. Aspiration pneumonia is a complication with associated signs of cough, fever, and sometimes nasal discharge. Adult animals that develop megaesophagus also start to regurgitate and ultimately lose weight. Respiratory signs may predominate, with little or no apparent regurgitation. Thoracic radiographs reveal air, fluid, or food in a dilated esophagus. The esophagus is usually uniformly dilated. A large ventral deviation may be present cranial to the heart. Megaesophagus secondary to a stricture, foreign body, neoplasia, or vascular ring anomaly is visualized as a dilatation of the esophagus cranial to the defect only. Strictures, foreign bodies, or vascular ring anomalies can be excluded with an esophagram and/or esophagoscopy.

In adult dogs, associated diseases (eg, myasthenia gravis) should be excluded or, if found, treated. Surgery is indicated for a vascular ring anomaly. Surgery may not successfully resolve the clinical signs in longstanding cases with severe esophageal dilatation cranial to the anomaly. Medical management is indicated for congenital or acquired idiopathic megaesophagus. Congenital megaesophagus may resolve as the animal ages, usually by 6 mo of age. The consistency of the diet that best prevents regurgitation varies from dog to dog; a soft gruel works for some, while dry food works for others. Another possibility is canned food formed into a meatball shape. Frequent, small meals work best for most dogs. Feeding from an elevated position with the forelimbs higher than the hindlimbs and holding that position for at least 10-15 min after eating allows gravity to assist food passage into the stomach. Neither surgery nor medications help esophageal function. Most animals succumb to a bout of aspiration pneumonia or, ultimately, fibrosis of the lungs secondary to recurrent pneumonia.

ESOPHAGEAL STRICTURES
(Esophageal stenosis)

Esophageal stricture is a pathologic narrowing of the lumen that may develop after trauma (eg, foreign body, caustic substance, certain drugs such as doxycycline), esophagitis, gastroesophageal reflux, or tumor invasion. Most strictures develop in the thoracic portion of the esophagus. Esophageal tumors are rare, but esophageal sarcomas may be associated with *Spirocerca lupi* infection (p 352), requiring consideration in areas where this parasite is prevalent.

Clinical signs are similar to those associated with foreign bodies and include regurgitation, ptyalism, dysphagia, and pain. An esophagram under fluoroscopy is the preferred tool for diagnosis, as it allows visualization of the number, length, location, and severity of strictures. Esophagoscopy can also be diagnostic but does not allow visualization beyond the stricture unless esophageal balloon dilation is also performed.

Treatment with balloon catheter dilation has been the most successful. Bougienage is another, less available, technique but is thought to cause more damage to the esophagus. Surgical resection of a single stricture is another option; however, it is also less successful. These treatments are likely to induce some degree of esophagitis, which must be treated to decrease the chance of stricture reformation. The use of corticosteroids, either systemically or intralesionally, to help prevent stricture reformation is controversial, and no data exist regarding the success of this adjunct therapy for esophageal strictures in dogs and cats.

ESOPHAGITIS

Inflammation of the esophagus is usually caused by foreign bodies, gastroesophageal reflux, and occasionally certain drugs (eg, doxycycline). Gastroesophageal reflux is usually associated with anesthesia, drugs that decrease lower esophageal sphincter tone (eg, atropine, acepromazine), and acute or chronic vomiting. Other causes of esophagitis include ingestion of an irritating or caustic substance, neoplasia, and *Spirocerca lupi* infection (p 352). Feeding tubes that traverse the gastroesophageal junction may also result in gastroesophageal reflux. Calicivirus in cats may also cause esophagitis.

Regurgitation is the classic sign of esophagitis; others include ptyalism, repeated swallowing attempts, pain, depression, anorexia, dysphagia, and extension of the head and neck. Mild esophagitis may have no associated clinical signs.

Endoscopy is the diagnostic tool of choice. It allows visualization of any associated problems (eg, foreign body) and direct assessment of esophageal damage. Plain radiographs are of little or no benefit in the diagnosis of esophagitis. An esophagram under fluoroscopy demonstrates any associated esophageal motility defects secondary to the esophagitis and may demonstrate esophageal wall defects if severe.

Mild esophagitis may require no treatment. If clinical signs are present, medical therapy should be instituted. Esophagitis secondary to gastroesophageal reflux is treated by decreasing gastric acidity, increasing lower esophageal sphincter tone, increasing the rate of gastric emptying, and providing pain control. In most cases, H_2-receptor antagonists (eg, ranitidine, famotidine) are sufficient to decrease gastric acid production; however, in severe cases of esophagitis a proton pump inhibitor (eg, omeprazole) is preferred. Cisapride and metoclopramide increase lower esophageal tone and the rate of gastric emptying. Cisapride is more potent than metoclopramide. A sucralfate slurry may also be administered orally for esophageal cytoprotection. Soft food, low in fat and fiber, should be fed in small, frequent meals. Systemic analgesics may be used for pain relief.

If esophagitis is severe, a gastrostomy tube may be used to completely rest the esophagus. The administration of corticosteroids to prevent esophageal stricture formation is controversial, but may be tried for 2-3 wk. Broad-spectrum antibiotics are also usually used with moderate to severe esophagitis in an attempt to prevent bacterial invasion and infection.

ESOPHAGEAL FOREIGN BODIES

Esophageal foreign bodies are more common in dogs than cats. Bones are the most common foreign body, but needles, fishhooks, wood, and rawhide pieces may also become lodged in the esophagus. Objects usually lodge in the areas of the esophagus with the least distensibility, eg, the thoracic inlet, bases of the heart, or the caudal esophagus just cranial to the diaphragm. Occasionally, an object may lodge in other locations such as the upper esophageal sphincter.

Ptyalism, gagging, dysphagia, regurgitation, and repeated attempts to swallow are signs of an esophageal foreign body. Often, the owner may see the animal eat the foreign body. The signs depend on the location of the foreign body and the degree and duration of obstruction. A partial obstruction may allow fluids but not food to pass. With a chronic obstruction, anorexia, weight loss, and lethargy are common.

Perforation of the cervical esophagus may result in local abscessation or subcutaneous emphysema; perforation of the thoracic esophagus may result in pleuritis, mediastinitis, pyothorax, pneumothorax, or bronchoesophageal fistula formation. Esophagitis, mucosal laceration, esophageal stricture, and esophageal diverticulum formation are potential complications. Esophageal stricture formation is the most common complication associated with an esophageal foreign body. Aspiration pneumonia may also be seen secondary to the regurgitation.

Many esophageal foreign bodies are radiopaque and can be seen on plain radiographs. A contrast esophagram or esophagoscopy is often required to identify radiolucent foreign bodies. If a perforation is suspected, an iodinated contrast medium should be used instead of barium suspensions. Esophagoscopy permits evaluation of both the foreign body and the esophageal wall and often allows therapeutic intervention.

Once diagnosed, esophageal foreign bodies should be removed immediately. Most often, a foreign body can be removed per os with a flexible endoscope and forceps. A rigid endoscope can also be used if a flexible scope is not available, but care must be taken when manipulating the scope in the esophagus to prevent lacerations or perforations. If the foreign body is smooth, a Foley catheter can be inserted distal to the foreign body, inflated, then removed orally bringing the foreign body with it. A large endotracheal tube can be placed over the endoscope to remove sharp foreign bodies such as fish hooks, which can be drawn up into the endotracheal tube and removed without damaging the esophagus on the way out. If a foreign body cannot be removed per os, it may be pushed into the stomach where it can either be digested (eg, bones), passed, or removed via a gastrotomy. Surgery is indicated if a perforation has occurred or the foreign body cannot be removed via endoscopy. If surgery is required, the prognosis is poor due to poor wound healing ability of the esophagus and the potential for stricture formation. Esophagitis, if present, should be treated as above.

ESOPHAGEAL DIVERTICULA

Diverticula are pouch-like dilatations of the esophageal wall and may be congenital or acquired. They are rare in dogs and cats. Acquired diverticula are of 2 types: pulsion or traction. **Pulsion diverticula** are caused by increased intraluminal pressure or deep esophageal inflammation, which can lead to mucosal herniation. Predisposing diseases include esophagitis, esophageal stricture, foreign bodies, vascular ring anomalies, megaesophagus, and hiatal hernia. This type of diverticulum consists of esophageal epithelium and connective tissue. **Traction diverticula** result from inflammation in the chest cavity in close proximity to the esophagus. Fibrous tissue is produced, which then contracts, pulling the esophageal wall outwards. This diverticulum consists of all 4 layers of the esophagus.

Small diverticula may be subclinical. Large diverticula allow food to become trapped in the pouch leading to postprandial dyspnea, regurgitation, and anorexia. Survey radiographs may show the diverticulum if it is full of ingesta or air, but contrast radiographs are best to demonstrate the pouch. Endoscopy will also allow visualization and can identify ulceration and scarring.

Small diverticula may be treated with a bland, soft diet fed with the animal in an upright position. Large diverticula require surgical excision and reconstruction of the esophageal wall. The prognosis after surgery is fair to good.

BRONCHOESOPHAGEAL FISTULA

Bronchoesophageal fistulas are rarely seen in dogs and cats. They most commonly develop secondary to foreign body penetration of the esophagus. Fistulas may develop between the esophagus and any part of the respiratory tree. A congenital form has been described, and Cairn Terriers may be predisposed. The most common clinical sign is coughing after eating or drinking. Regurgitation may also be seen, and anorexia, fever, and lethargy may be related to pneumonia.

Survey radiographs may reveal a radiopaque foreign body and pneumonia. Contrast esophograms will show the communication between the esophagus and airways. Use of a small amount of barium is recommended—iodinated contrast agents are hyperosmolar and can cause pulmonary edema.

Surgical correction consisting of a lung lobectomy and repair of the defect in the esophagus is required. The prognosis after surgery is good.

DISEASES OF THE STOMACH AND INTESTINES IN SMALL ANIMALS

CANINE PARVOVIRUS

Etiology and Pathophysiology: The origin of the canine parvovirus has not been established. The virus is very stable in the environment, able to withstand wide pH ranges and high temperatures. It is resistant to a number of common disinfectants and may survive for several months in contaminated areas. Rottweilers, American Pit Bull Terriers, Doberman Pinschers, and German Shepherds are at increased risk of disease. Toy Poodles and Cocker Spaniels appear at decreased risk for developing the enteric disease. Mortality associated with canine parvovirus infection is variably reported to be 16-48%.

The virus is transmitted by direct contact with infected dogs. Indirect transmission, eg, from fecal-contaminated fomites, is also an important source of infection. The virus is shed in the feces of infected dogs for up to 3 wk after infection. Recovered dogs may serve as carriers and shed the virus periodically.

After ingestion, the virus replicates in lymphoid tissue of the oropharynx; from there, it spreads to the bloodstream. It attacks rapidly dividing cells throughout the body, especially those in the bone marrow, lymphopoietic tissue, and the crypt epithelium of the jejunum and ileum. Early lymphatic infection is accompanied by lymphopenia and precedes intestinal infection and GI signs. Replication in the bone marrow and lymphopoietic tissue causes neutropenia and lymphopenia, respectively. By 3 days after infection, rapidly dividing intestinal crypt cells are infected. Viral shedding in the feces begins 3-4 days after infection and peaks when clinical signs appear. Viral shedding decreases rapidly and may no longer be detected 10-14 days after initial infection. Replication of the virus in the crypt epithelium of the gut causes collapse of intestinal villi, epithelial necrosis, and hemorrhagic diarrhea. Normal enteric bacteria, eg, *Clostridium perfringens* and *Escherichia coli* enter the denuded mucosa and may gain entry to the bloodstream, resulting in bacteremia.

Clinical Findings: Infected dogs are often asymptomatic. Clinical disease may be triggered by stress (eg, boarding), and clinical signs may be exacerbated by concurrent infection with opportunistic enteric pathogens (eg, *Salmonella*, *C perfringens*, *E coli*, *Campylobacter*, coronavirus, and various parasites). The dose of virus required to cause clinical disease may also be a factor. Prolonged contact with a dog shedding high levels of virus increases the likelihood of disease. The incubation period is 3-8 days. Viral shedding may begin on day 3, before the onset of clinical signs.

Initially, 2 common clinical forms of the disease were recognized—myocarditis and gastroenteritis. Myocarditis was seen in young pups, especially in the early neonatal period. Infection led to myocardial necrosis with either acute cardiopulmonary failure (causing pulmonary edema, cyanosis, and collapse) or scarring of the myocardium and progressive cardiac insufficiency. However, myocarditis is no longer seen because effective immunization of bitches protects pups during this early period of life.

Gastroenteritis is most common in pups 6-20 wk old, ie, the period when maternal antibody protection falls and vaccination has not yet adequately protected the pup against infection. Most affected dogs (~85%) are <1 yr old. In dogs >6 mo old, intact males are more likely to develop enteritis than intact females, reflecting the tendency of male dogs to roam. Dogs with the enteric form suffer from an acute onset of lethargy, anorexia, fever, vomiting, and diarrhea. The feces are loose and may contain mucus or blood. The severity of clinical signs varies. Most dogs recover within a few days with appropriate supportive care; others can die within hours of the onset of clinical signs. A common complication is pulmonary edema or alveolitis.

Other clinical problems that have been associated with canine parvovirus include birth defects and infertility; however, supportive evidence is lacking.

Diagnosis: Diagnosis is based on an appropriate history and clinical signs and confirmed by a positive fecal ELISA or hemagglutination test. The ELISA may be positive on the first day of clinical signs and for 3-4 more days. The ELISA may be false negative if run too early in the disease course; it should be repeated if the history and clinical signs support the likely presence of the virus. Leukopenia or lymphopenia is seen in most infected dogs during the course of illness. Neutropenia is suggestive of the disease. Hypoalbuminemia, hyponatremia, hypokalemia, and hypochloremia may be seen. Serum ALT levels are increased in some dogs. Diagnosis may also be confirmed by a 4-fold increase in serum IgG titer over 7-14 days, detection of serum IgM antibody to parvovirus in dogs that have not been vaccinated within the last 3-4 wk, or the detection of parvovirus particles in the feces using immunofluorescence, immunoperoxidase staining, or electron microscopy.

Treatment: There is no specific therapy to eliminate the virus. Most dogs recover with appropriate supportive care directed to restoration of fluid balance. Oral electrolyte solutions may be used in mildly dehydrated dogs without a history of vomiting. More severely affected dogs should receive IV fluid therapy (lactated Ringer's and 5% dextrose with additional potassium chloride [10-20 mEq/L]) to counter dehydration and maintain fluid balance. Monitoring of electrolyte changes is advisable. Most dogs that survive the first 2-3 days of disease recover. Persistent vomiting can be controlled with metoclopramide, 0.2-0.5 mg/kg, PO or SC, QID, or 1-2 mg/kg/day, slow IV).

Routine use of antibiotics is discouraged. More severe cases (eg, dogs with severe blood loss, fever, or loss of intestinal integrity) are predisposed to bacteremia and septicemia. In these cases, a combination of either ampicillin or a first- or second-generation cephalosporin, plus an aminoglycoside or enrofloxacin, provide broad-spectrum coverage.

Food and water should be withheld until vomiting has subsided. After this, small amounts of a bland diet (eg, cottage cheese and rice or a commercially available prescription diet) should be offered frequently. A small volume of warm, salted meat broth should be given concurrently. If GI signs recur after feeding, the dog should be fasted for an additional 12-24 hr before feeding again. If food can be tolerated, the bland diet is continued for 7-14 days, after which the dog's regular diet can be gradually reintroduced.

Prevention and Control: Contaminated areas should be thoroughly cleaned. Household bleach (1:30 dilution) or commercial products labeled for use against parvovirus are potent inactivators of the virus. The same solutions may be used as footbaths to disinfect footwear. Disinfection of hands, clothing, and food and water bowls is recommended. Pups should be kept isolated from adult dogs returning from shows or field trials.

Vaccination is critical in the control of the disease. Variants of the virus have appeared since the disease was first recognized, but current vaccines protect dogs against all strains of the virus. Vaccines containing live attenuated canine parvovirus generally induce more effective immunity than inactivated virus vaccines. The high-titer canine parvovirus vaccines now available effectively protect puppies against viral challenge, even during the period when maternal antibody titers remain high enough to interfere with active immunization but have declined enough to predispose pups to infection. Vaccination of pups should begin at 5-8 wk of age, preferably with a high antigen-density vaccine. The last vaccination should be given at 16-20 wk of age, and annual vaccination thereafter is recommended.

COLITIS

The colon helps maintain fluid and electrolyte balance and absorb nutrients; it also temporarily stores feces and provides an environment for microorganisms. Pathology of the colon impairs these functions, and diarrhea ensues. It has been estimated that about one-third of dogs with a history of chronic diarrhea have colitis. The mean age of dogs with idiopathic large-bowel diarrhea is 6 yr. Colitis has been classified into 4 forms: eosinophilic, plasmacytic-lymphocytic, histiocytic, and granulomatous. Hypereosinophilic syndrome of cats is a variant of eosinophilic enteritis with eosinophilic involvement not only of the bowel but also of the liver, spleen, mesenteric lymph nodes, kidney, adrenal glands, and heart.

Etiology and Pathophysiology: Inflammation of the colon may be acute or chronic. In most cases, the inciting factors are unknown. Bacterial (eg, *Salmonella* spp, *Clostridium* spp, and *Campylobacter* spp), parasitic, fungal, traumatic, uremic, and allergic causes have been postulated. Inflammation may be the result of a defect in mucosal immunoregulation. After initial mucosal injury, submucosal lymphocytes and macrophages become exposed to luminal antigens and subsequently initiate an inflammatory process. An exaggerated reaction to dietary or bacterial factors within the lumen of the bowel, genetic predisposition, psychologic pathology affecting the neurologic or vascular supply to the colon, or sequelae of previous infectious or parasitic disease have also been implicated.

Rectal cytology samples are often normal. In acute colitis, there is mucosal infiltration with neutrophils and epithelial disruption and ulceration. Chronic colitis is most often characterized by mucosal infiltration of plasma cells and lymphocytes, fibrosis, and sometimes ulceration. Goblet cells are stimulated to secrete excessive quantities of mucus. Absorption of water and electrolytes is impaired, and motility is reduced. Inflammation disrupts intracellular tight junctions and reduces the transmucosal electrical potential difference interrupting the ability of the colon to absorb sodium. Cytokines may stimulate colonic secretion. Normal segmentation is inhibited, giant migrating muscular contractions proceed down the length of the colon, and luminal contents are rapidly expulsed. The inflamed bowel is more sensitive to stretch, and contents entering the colon stimulate strong giant migrating muscular contractions, an urge to defecate, and abdominal discomfort.

Fructo-oligosaccharides (FOS) enhance colonic microflora and assist the prevention and treatment of colonic disease. These complex carbohydrates are not digested in the small intestine. They are fermented by specific colonic bacteria that use them as an energy source. FOS promote the growth of beneficial bacteria and inhibit growth of potentially harmful bacteria. They are responsible for the production of short-chain fatty acids (SCFA).

SCFA (acetate, propionate, butyrate) are an important energy source essential for maintenance of normal mucosal health. They also serve as a substrate for cellular lipid synthesis and are the primary cations in the colonic lumen, participating in sodium and water fluxes. The acidic environment they favor reduces the ionization of long-chain fatty acids and bile acids (both of which are colonic irritants), increases the concentration of ammonium ions that are unable to cross the cell membrane and are excreted in the feces, and reduces the sporulation and overgrowth of pathogenic bacteria. SCFA help maintain intestinal motility and ameliorate intestinal inflammation. Alteration of fatty acids leads to mucosal atrophy and injury.

Clinical Findings: Animals with inflammation of the colon have a history of tenesmus and frequent passage of mucus-laden feces, sometimes with frank blood. Feces are often of a small volume and a more liquid consistency. Weight loss is uncommon, and vomiting is seen in ~30% of cases.

Diagnosis: The initial approach should include a complete history and physical examination, including rectal palpation and evaluation of feces. Fecal smears for *Giardia* and fungal elements, fecal flotation for parasite identification, and culture for bacteria is suggested in cases of chronic colitis. Complete evaluation of the colon includes endoscopy and biopsy. A normal mucosal biopsy or one with evidence of a hyperplastic mucosa in conjunction with clinical signs supportive of large-intestinal diarrhea is compatible with irritable bowel syndrome. Peripheral eosinophilia is invariably present in cats with hypereosinophilic syndrome.

Treatment and Control: If possible, the inciting cause should be identified and eliminated. Food should be withheld for an initial 24-48 hr in animals with acute colitis in an effort to "rest" the bowel. The addition of soluble fiber to a highly digestible commercial diet results in a very good to excellent clinical response in most dogs with chronic idiopathic large-bowel diarrhea; over time, the fiber dose can be reduced or eliminated in some dogs and a standard dog food substituted without causing a return of the diarrhea. When feeding is begun, the protein source used should be one to which the animal has not previously been exposed, ie, a "novel protein." In one study, clinical signs associated with lymphocytic-plasmacytic colitis resolved in all dogs within ~2 wk after feeding of a low-residue, digestible, hypoallergenic diet (1 part low-fat cottage cheese and 2 parts boiled white rice). Thereafter, most dogs were maintained without recurrence of clinical signs on commercially available prescription diets they had not been previously fed. Currently, there are a number of commercially available diets that contain rice with mutton or lamb, venison, or rabbit. If feeding a high fiber or novel protein diet is not beneficial, a commercial low residue diet may be tried, especially a low residue diet that contains FOS. Cats with lymphocytic-plasmacytic colitis may respond to dietary management alone (eg, lamb and rice, horsemeat, or a commercially available diet). In another study, cats were initially treated with dietary fiber, or dietary fiber and pharmacologic intervention (prednisone, tylosin, or sulfasalazine). Most cats were eventually maintained on high-fiber diets or a highly digestible diet.

Supplementation of the diet with fiber (1-6 tsp psyllium hydrophilic mucilloid or 1-4 tbsp of coarse wheat bran per feeding) improves diarrhea in many animals. Dietary fiber reduces free fecal water, prolongs luminal transit time (increasing the opportunity to absorb water), absorbs toxins, increases fecal bulk and stretches the colonic smooth muscle, and improves contractility. However, the addition of fiber alone rarely results in complete resolution of clinical signs of large-intestinal diarrhea in dogs, and beneficial effects may take as long as 6 wk to become evident.

Clinical signs resolve more rapidly when concurrent anti-inflammatory medication is added to the change in diet. Those drugs most commonly used in the management of colitis include sulfasalazine, prednisone or prednisolone, and azathioprine. Sulfasalazine (dogs: 12.5 mg/kg, QID for 14 days, then 12.5 mg/kg, BID for 28 days; cats: 10-20 mg/kg/day for 14 days) is the drug most often used to treat lymphocytic-plasmacytic colitis, the most common form of idiopathic colitis. Longterm use is discouraged because it predisposes to keratoconjunctivitis sicca. Prednisone is reportedly not as effective as sulfasalazine in the management of lymphocytic-plasmacytic colitis but may be considered. In some cases, prednisone is used in conjunction with sulfasalazine in cases unresponsive to more conventional therapy. Azathioprine (1 mg/kg, SID for 2 wk), alone or in combination with prednisone, has been used to control clinical signs associated with lymphocytic-plasmacytic colitis. Azathioprine may be considered in cases poorly responsive to prednisone or to prednisone with sulfasalazine. Eosinophilic colitis generally responds to prednisone (2-4 mg/kg/day for 2 wk and then tapered over 6-10 wk). Histiocytic colitis of Boxers is treated with a combination of controlled diet, sulfasalazine, and prednisone.

Some animals require additional short-term use of motility modifiers until inflammation is brought under control. Loperamide (0.1-0.2 mg/kg, BID-QID) stimulates segmental activity and slows passage of fecal contents. Loperamide also decreases colonic secretion, enhances salt and water absorption, and increases anal sphincter tone.

Most cases of lymphocytic-plasmacytic idiopathic colitis respond to appropriate dietary and medical changes. Stricture formation and extensive fibrosis warrant a more guarded prognosis. Eosinophilic colitis in dogs responds favorably to controlled diets and glucocorticoid therapy. In cats, the prognosis is more guarded, and more aggressive treatment with immunosuppressive agents is required. The prognosis for cats with hypereosinophilic syndrome is guarded to poor; generally, high doses of prednisone (3 mg/kg, BID) are required for maintenance. Histiocytic colitis of Boxers carries a grave prognosis unless treatment is started early in the course of the disease. The immunoproliferative enteropathy of Basenjis also carries a poor prognosis; most dogs die within 2 yr of diagnosis, although some have been reported to live as long as 5 yr. Similarly, the prognosis for the diarrheal syndrome reported in Lundehunds is also poor.

CONSTIPATION AND OBSTIPATION

Constipation is a common clinical problem in small animals. In most instances, the problem is easily rectified; however, in more debilitated animals, accompanying clinical signs can be severe. As feces remain in the colon longer, they become drier, harder, and more difficult to pass. Obstipation is intractable constipation, in which the animal is unable to successfully defecate.

Etiology and Pathophysiology: Chronic constipation may be due to intraluminal, extraluminal, or intrinsic (ie, neuromuscular) factors. Intraluminal obstruction is most common and is due to the inability to pass poorly digestible, often firm matter (eg, hair, bones, litter) mixed with fecal material. The lack of water intake or the reluctance to defecate on a regular basis due to environmental (stress) or behavioral (dirty litter box) situations or to painful anorectal disease predisposes to the formation of hard, dry feces. Intraluminal tumors may also impede the passage of feces. Extraluminal obstruction may be caused by compression of the colon or rectum by a narrowed pelvic inlet following inappropriate healing of pelvic fractures or by compression of the colon or rectum by enlarged sublumbar lymph nodes or prostate gland. Colonic stricture due to trauma or neoplasia should also be considered. Finally, some animals (usually cats) with chronic constipation or obstipation may have megacolon, likely caused by a lesion of the neuromuscular bed of the colon. The etiology of megacolon often remains undiagnosed. Other diseases that affect neuromuscular control of the colon and rectum include hypothyroidism, dysautonomia, and lesions of the spinal cord or pelvic nerves. Hypokalemia and hypercalcemia also adversely affect muscular control. Some drugs (eg, opioids, diuretics, antihistamines, anticholinergic agents, sucralfate, aluminum hydroxide, potassium bromide, and calcium channel-blocking agents) promote constipation via differing mechanisms.

Peristaltic waves are responsible for the aboral movement of fecal material in the colon. Giant migrating waves that occur intermittently throughout the day move this matter farther and more rapidly. These waves constitute the "gastrocolic reflex" and are common after ingestion of a meal. A reduction or loss of this wave activity may contribute to constipation. Similarly, an increase in segmentation wave activity may predispose to constipation. However, diet is the most important local factor affecting colonic function.

Clinical Findings: The classic clinical signs are tenesmus and the passage of firm, dry feces. If the passage of feces is hindered by an enlarged prostate or sublumbar lymph nodes, the feces may appear thin or "ribbon-like" in appearance. Abdominal palpation and rectal examination can confirm the presence of large volumes of retained fecal matter. Passed feces are often putrid. Some animals are quite ill and also have lethargy, depression, anorexia, vomiting, and abdominal discomfort.

Diagnosis: A history of dietary indiscretion and physical evidence of retained feces confirms the diagnosis. Abdominal palpation and rectal examination, including evaluation of the prostate and sublumbar lymph nodes, should be performed. Plain abdominal radiographs may help establish the inciting factor(s) of fecal retention and give some indication of what the feces contain (eg, bones). A barium enema or colonoscopy may facilitate demonstration of obstructive lesions or predisposing causes of chronic constipation.

A CBC, biochemical profile including a serum T_4 level, urinalysis, and detailed neurologic examination should be completed in cases of chronic or recurring constipation.

Treatment and Control: Affected animals should be adequately hydrated. Mild constipation can often be treated by dietary adjustment consisting of avoidance of dietary indiscretion, ready access to water and high-fiber diets, and the use of suppository laxatives. Continued or longterm use of laxatives should be discouraged unless absolutely necessary to deter constipation.

In more severe cases, retained feces must be evacuated using enemas or manual extraction while under general anesthesia. Complete removal of all feces may require 2-3 attempts over as many days. Concurrent fluid and electrolyte abnormalities should also be corrected.

Laxatives are classified as bulk-forming, lubricant, emollient, osmotic, or stimulant types. Most act on fluid transport mechanisms and colonic motor stimulation. They should be avoided in the presence of dehydration. High-fiber bulk-forming laxatives are added to the diet. These products absorb water, soften feces, add bulk, stretch the colonic smooth muscle, and improve contractility. Supplementation of the diet with fiber (eg, 1-6 tsp per feeding of psyllium hydrophilic mucilloid, or 1-4 tbsp of coarse wheat bran) is adequate. For longterm control of constipation, commercial high-fiber diets should be fed. Mineral oil (5-25 mL, PO, BID) and petrolatum products are lubricants and are given to affected animals between meals. Mineral oil should be flavored to avoid accidental inhalation of this otherwise tasteless product. Docusate sodium (cats: 50-mg capsule, SID; dogs: 50-mg capsule, 1-4/day) and docusate calcium (cats: 50-mg capsule, 1-2/day; dogs: 50-mg capsule, 2-3/day) are emollient laxatives. These mild laxatives soften feces by promoting water absorption. Osmotic laxatives (eg, lactulose, 0.5 mL/kg, PO, BID-TID) osmotically retain water in the bowel to soften fecal material. Lactulose, a nonabsorbable disaccharide, is also useful in management of hepatic encephalopathy because it decreases luminal pH, reduces the bacterial production of ammonia, and favors the formation of ammonium ions that are poorly absorbed. Stimulant laxative products (eg, bisacodyl [cats and small dogs: 5 mg; medium-sized dogs: 10 mg; large dogs: 15-20 mg]) increase the propulsive activity of the bowel. They are contraindicated in the presence of bowel obstruction.

Enema solutions are frequently used to moisten and soften feces making them easier to pass. Warm isotonic saline or tap water (5-10 mL/kg) with or without a mild soap (without hexachlorophene) to act as an irritant is practical and effective. Docusate sodium (cats and small dogs: 5-10 mL; medium-sized dogs: 10-20 mL; large dogs: 20-30 mL) is another option. Sodium phosphate enemas are sometimes used to relieve constipation in dogs but should not be used if dehydration, cardiac disease, nausea, or vomiting are present. They are also contraindicated in small dogs and cats and in animals with renal dysfunction. Clinical signs of toxicity are seen within 1 hr of use and include depression, ataxia, tetany, seizures, vomiting, hemorrhagic diarrhea, tachycardia, pallor, and stupor. Associated biochemical abnormalities may include hyperphosphatemia, hypernatremia, hypocalcemia, hyperglycemia, hyperosmolality, and metabolic acidosis with a high anion gap (increased lactic acid). Death has been reported with the use of these agents in cats. Mineral oil (5-20 mL) can be directly instilled into the rectum to help facilitate passage of hard feces.

To prevent recurrence, animals are encouraged to eat high-fiber diets, ready access to water should be maintained, and frequent opportunities to defecate allowed.

Chronic constipation that has been unresponsive to medical management may respond to subtotal or total colectomy. Cases that present with simple intraluminal obstruction due to dietary indiscretion respond well to bowel evacuation and prevention of this habit in the future. Cats with megacolon that do not respond to medical management alone respond well to subtotal colectomy.

FELINE ENTERIC CORONAVIRUS

Feline enteric coronavirus is an enveloped single-stranded RNA virus that is highly contagious among cats in close contact. Although the feline enteric coronavirus is antigenically similar to the virus of feline infectious peritonitis (FIP, p 628), the pathogenesis of each differs. The enteric form of infection is limited to the GI tract. Death from the enteric form of disease is uncommon.

Etiology and Pathophysiology: The virus is shed in the feces of seropositive cats. Close contact between cats is required for effective transmission, although the possibility of transmission via fomites also exists. The close antigenic relationship of the enteric form of the virus and that causing clinical signs of FIP has led to speculation that FIP virus may be a mutated form of enteric coronavirus. Cross-protection is not induced by either virus to the other, and recent evidence refutes the supposition that preexisting infection with the enteric form of disease accelerates or enhances the severity of disease associated with FIP.

Feline coronavirus infects the apical columnar epithelium of intestinal villi of the duodenum, jejunum, and ileum, and causes the tips of villi to slough, fuse with adjacent villi, and atrophy.

Clinical Findings: In catteries, the virus may be a cause of inapparent to mildly severe enteritis in kittens 6-12 wk old. Recently weaned kittens may exhibit fever, vomiting, and diarrhea that may last 2-5 days. More severely affected kittens may also be anorectic for 1-3 days. Adult cats often have subclinical infection. Transient neutropenia may appear with the onset of diarrhea in more severely affected kittens.

Diagnosis: Most FIP infections result in seroconversion without progression to the fatal form of the disease. Positive coronavirus antibody titers are seen in ~10-40% of cats in the general cat population and in 80-90% of cats in catteries, but only 8% develop FIP. Serologic tests (serum ELISA and immunofluorescent antibody) do not differentiate the enteric form of the virus from that causing clinical signs associated with FIP. Furthermore, these tests do not differentiate between past exposure to the virus or an actively infected cat. Titers >1:3,200 are suggestive of FIP, as opposed to the enteric form of disease. Titers between 1:100 and 1:3,200 may be found in cats with effusive or noneffusive disease and in cats with the enteric form. Some commercial vaccines containing bovine serum components may induce antibody production that may react with antigenically similar bovine serum components in cell cultures used to propagate target FIP viruses for immunochemical tests, thus causing a false-positive test in recently vaccinated (<4 mo previously) cats. Consequently, antibody testing is only useful as a screening tool to detect the presence or absence of virus in a household, to recognize potential carriers or shedders when introducing new cats into an antibody-negative population, and as an aid in the clinical diagnosis of FIP.

Cytologic evaluation of effusions from cats with the wet form of FIP have a high protein content and a variable cell count consisting of neutrophils, macrophages, and lymphocytes. The neutrophils are nondegenerate and do not show signs of toxicity, and the lymphocytes are morphologically normal.

Treatment and Control: The virus is ubiquitous in cats, and many cats that recover from the infection remain carriers. Enteric coronavirus infection can be prevented only by minimizing exposure to infected cats and their feces. Cats with the enteric disease do not progress to develop clinical signs of FIP. Most cats develop an effective immune response on exposure and recover from infection. However, once clinical signs of disease develop in cats with FIP, the disease is invariably fatal. Management consists only of supportive therapy, ie, fluids when indicated. Vaccination with the temperature-sensitive intranasal vaccine for FIP may protect against challenge with virulent enteric coronavirus.

GASTRIC DILATATION-VOLVULUS
(Bloat)

Gastric dilatation-volvulus (GDV) is a life-threatening emergency. Successful management depends on prompt diagnosis and appropriate medical and surgical treatment.

Etiology and Pathophysiology: GDV tends to primarily affect large, deep-chested dogs. Stress may precipitate an acute episode of GDV. There is no apparent sex or age predisposition, but incidence increases with age, being most common in dogs 7-10 yr old. A familial tendency has been reported but not substantiated. Doberman Pinschers, German Shepherds, Standard Poodles, Great Danes, Saint Bernards, Irish Setters, and Gordon Setters are affected most commonly. An association between GDV and inflammatory bowel disease has been suggested, but the relationship is unclear.

Dilatation likely precedes volvulus. Dilatation develops secondary to the accumulation of gas or fluid (or both) within the stomach, the outflow from which is obstructed. Obstruction may be caused by neoplasia, pyloric stenosis, foreign body, or compression of the duodenum against the body wall by the expanding stomach. Prolonged gastric emptying, chronic dilatation secondary to pyloric dysfunction, and hypotonic gastric and pyloric musculature associated with the ingestion of large meals at protracted intervals have been incriminated in the pathogenesis of GDV. However, there is a lack of evidence for gastric emptying disorders in dogs that develop GDV. Distention of the stomach by gas may be associated with aerophagia, diffusion from the bloodstream, release of carbon dioxide after the reaction of hydrochloric acid and bicarbonate, or bacterial fermentation.

Viewed from a caudal to cranial direction, the stomach rotates 90-360° in a clockwise fashion about the distal esophagus. The pylorus is displaced to the left of the midline, the duodenum becomes entrapped between the distal esophagus and the stomach, and the spleen may vary in position from left posterodorsal to right anterodorsal (depending on the extent of volvulus). If the volvulus is >180°, the distal esophagus becomes occluded.

Clinical Findings: Clinical signs may include an acute onset of restlessness, apparent discomfort, abdominal pain, repeated unproductive retching, excessive salivation, and abdominal distention. Progression to volvulus predisposes to hypovolemic shock. Abnormalities on physical examination include tachypnea or dyspnea, rapid and weak arterial pulses, pale mucous membranes, and prolonged capillary refill time indicative of hypovolemic shock. An irregular heart rate and associated pulse deficits indicate cardiac arrhythmias. Decrease in venous return, cardiac output, and arterial blood pressure, as well as hypovolemic shock, are caused by compression of the caudal vena cava; sequestration of blood in dilated splanchnic, renal, and posterior muscular capillary beds; loss of fluid into the obstructed stomach; and a lack of water intake. Endotoxemia, hypoxemia, metabolic acidosis, and hypotension predispose to disseminated intravascular coagulation.

Diagnosis: A history of ingestion of a large meal followed by exercise and repeated attempts to vomit is common. Dogs not in a state of shock may appear anxious. Hypersalivation and abdominal distention with gas are noted on physical examination.

Abdominal radiographs taken in right lateral recumbency are preferred for the diagnosis of volvulus. The gas-filled pylorus is located dorsal and slightly cranial to the gas-filled gastric fundus. A compartmentalization line between the pylorus and fundus that represents folding of the pyloric antral wall back onto the fundic wall is frequently seen.

Systemic hypotension predisposes to prerenal azotemia with increases in serum urea and creatinine concentrations. Serum phosphorus increases similarly. After decompression and the "wash out" of sequestered blood, serum levels of ALT and AST increase. CK levels also increase due to striated muscle damage, and serum potassium levels increase subsequent to cell membrane injury.

Treatment and Control: The principal goals of initial treatment are to stabilize the animal and decompress the stomach.

Initial management for shock should include the administration of IV fluids (eg, 0.45% saline in 2.5% dextrose or balanced electrolyte solutions) at an initial rate of 90 mL/kg over the first hour. The rate is adjusted thereafter based on clinical response and the need to maintain adequate blood pressure and cardiac output. The rate of administration can be reduced as much as 40% if pentastarch, hetastarch, or dextran 70 (20 mL/kg over 15-30 min) is administered. Dogs in severe shock may benefit from the use of 5% or 7.5% hypertonic saline (4 mL/kg over 5-10 min), followed by isotonic fluids as indicated above, until clinical signs of shock have dissipated. Glucocorticoids (hydrocortisone sodium succinate, 10 mg/kg, IV bolus, followed by dexamethasone, 2-4 mg/kg, every 6 hr) may be used as part of the regimen for shock, but efficacy remains controversial. Because endotoxemia may complicate the disease process, antibiotics (eg, ampicillin at 22 mg/kg, QID, and continued for 2-3 days after surgery) are often given.

Metabolic acidosis frequently accompanies GDV. Adequate fluid therapy and gastric decompression generally correct this problem. Electrolyte abnormalities should be addressed if present.

Gastric decompression should be accomplished as soon as possible. Initially, an attempt should be made to pass a well-lubricated orogastric (stomach) tube. The distance from the incisors to the xiphoid or costal arch should be measured and marked by a piece of tape on the stomach tube. This distance indicates the maximum length of tube that can be safely passed; marking this length decreases the likelihood of passing the stomach tube through a devitalized stomach wall. The dog is positioned in sternal or lateral recumbency. A 2-in. roll of tape or an oral speculum is placed in the dog's mouth, and the muzzle taped closed around it. The tube can then be readily passed through the center of the roll of tape or the speculum. Some resistance is usually felt as the tube passes through the esophageal-gastric juncture. If resistance is met, the tube should be gently rotated while attempting to advance it. Undue force may tear the esophagus. Successful passage of a tube does not rule out concurrent gastric volvulus. Once the tube enters the stomach, gastric gas readily escapes. Excess fluid and ingesta are removed via gravity and suction. After the stomach has been decompressed, it should be lavaged with warm water or saline to remove any remaining debris.

If a tube cannot be readily passed into the stomach, excess gas may be relieved by inserting a large-bore (16-18 gauge) "over the needle" catheter into the stomach percutaneously. An area (10 cm × 10 cm) on the right abdominal wall caudal to the last rib and ventral to the transverse vertebral process should be shaved and prepared in an aseptic fashion. Before the needle is inserted, the area should be percussed to avoid accidental puncture of an overlying spleen. Gastric decompression generally facilitates the passage of a stomach tube and lavage of the stomach.

If sedation is required, oxymorphone hydrochloride (0.05-0.10 mg/kg, 3 mg maximum) or, alternatively, butorphanol (0.2-0.4 mg/kg, IM or SC) may be used.

Temporary gastrotomy may be useful to decompress the stomach and evacuate its contents while avoiding the need for general anesthesia. This procedure is useful in dogs too critical for immediate general anesthesia and can be used to delay exploratory laparotomy until the animal is stabilized. An area caudal to the right costal arch should be shaved and prepared as indicated above. Local anesthesia is provided by the injection of 2% lidocaine hydrochloride administered in an inverted "L" block pattern. A 5-cm skin incision is made ~2 cm caudal and parallel to the costal arch. Abdominal muscles are separated, and the stomach is exposed. A stay suture is used to anchor the stomach to each end of the skin incision. The skin is sutured to the stomach in a continuous pattern. The stomach thus exposed can be decompressed, its contents evacuated, and the body lavaged. A potential disadvantage of this procedure is that an exploratory laparotomy, including inspection of the stomach and restoring it to its customary position, is delayed. Immediate inspection of the stomach permits evaluation of the extent of injury and the possible need for resection. Gastric wall necrosis, rupture, peritonitis, and sepsis are the most common causes of death in these dogs. Delayed exploratory laparotomy may also predispose to cardiac arrhythmias, which develop in ~40-50% of dogs with GDV.

The goals of surgical management are to assess the integrity of the stomach and spleen, to reposition the stomach to its normal location, and to fix the stomach to the abdominal body wall in an attempt to decrease the likelihood of recurrence of volvulus. A midline celiotomy provides access to the stomach and visualization of the spleen and adjacent abdominal structures. Most often, the stomach and pylorus have shifted to the left (clockwise when viewed caudally to cranially), and the gastric fundus has shifted from its normal position in the left dorsal abdomen to the right ventral sector of the abdomen. Splenic congestion generally resolves after the stomach has been repositioned. Gastric wall resection or splenectomy is reserved for cases in which tissue viability has been compromised.

Several surgical techniques have been used to prevent recurrence of volvulus, and recurrence rates are similar (5-11%) for all. Techniques include simple incisional gastropexy, tube gastrotomy, and circumcostal gastropexy. A recent prospective study indicated that the median survival times for dogs that underwent gastropexy was 547 days compared with 188 days for those that did not. The value of pyloromyotomy and pyloroplasty in an effort to promote gastric emptying has not been substantiated. Medical management alone results in a 75% recurrence rate within a 12-mo period.

Food should be withheld for 24-48 hr after surgery. If vomiting continues, metoclopramide (0.2-0.5 mg/kg, SC, or 1-2 mg/kg/day, constant rate IV infusion) can be administered.

Of dogs that die of GDV, 24% do so within the first 7 days after surgery. Many dogs develop ventricular arrhythmias, the cause of which may include myocardial ischemia, autonomic imbalance, acid-base and electrolyte imbalance, catecholamine release, and the release of myocardial depressant factor. Arrhythmias that warrant medical therapy include those that significantly impair cardiac output, multifocal premature ventricular contractions, a ventricular rate persistently >140 bpm, and the "R on T wave" pattern (a phenomenon that predisposes to ventricular fibrillation). If predisposing factors have been addressed and persistent ventricular arrhythmias warrant therapy, 2% lidocaine hydrochloride without epinephrine (2-4 mg/kg, slowly IV) is given and repeated twice during a 30-min period if necessary. Continuous IV infusion (30-80 μg/kg/min) may be indicated to control arrhythmias. Cardiac arrhythmias associated with GDV are often difficult to control. If the arrhythmia is poorly responsive to this therapy, procainamide (6-10 mg/kg, IV over 15 min) should be given. Life-threatening arrhythmias may respond to 20% magnesium sulfate (0.15-0.3 mEq/kg, or 12.5-35 mg/kg, IV over 15-60 min).

Dogs with a tendency to develop dilatation and volvulus should be fed smaller meals more frequently over the course of the day. Excessive exercise should be avoided to decrease the likelihood of volvulus, and consumption of large volumes of water after exercise should be avoided to limit gastric distention.

GASTRITIS

Gastritis may be acute or chronic. Several different histologic forms of gastritis have been identified. Most are likely secondary to the ingestion of various substances that cause injury to the gastric mucosa. Continued mucosal damage may initiate an immune-mediated reaction. Other factors, including allergic reactions, immune mechanisms, and hormonal factors, may play a part in the etiology of chronic gastritis.

Acute gastritis is usually caused by dietary indiscretion leading to damage of the gastric mucosa. Chronic gastritis is caused by a variety of diseases, including chronic superficial gastritis, chronic atrophic gastritis, chronic hypertrophic gastritis, and eosinophilic gastritis. **Chronic superficial gastritis** is characterized histologically by infiltration of the superficial mucosa and lamina propria with lymphocytes, plasma cells, and fibrosis. Caustic agents, including aspirin, may cause these lesions. Dietary factors may also be responsible. **Chronic atrophic gastritis** is characterized by a thin mucosa, a variable inflammatory cell infiltrate, and a reduction in the size and depth of gastric glands. The number of chief and parietal cells is decreased, and that of mucus-secreting cells increased. Chronic atrophic gastritis may represent the sequela of long-standing chronic superficial gastritis or immune-mediated disease directed against the gastric mucosa and parietal cells. It is reported more often in the Norwegian Lundehund breed. **Chronic hypertrophic gastritis** is identified by a diffuse or focal thickening of the gastric mucosa and large rugal folds that result from hypertrophy and hyperplasia of mucosal glands. Gastric outflow obstruction (p 330) may follow. Inflammatory infiltrate invariably accompanies these changes, and ulceration may be seen as a result of chronic mucosal inflammation. Trophic factors, eg, histamine and gastrin, may also initiate abnormalities. For example, increased histamine production from dogs with mast cell tumors, and excessive gastrin levels in dogs with renal dysfunction, predispose to hypertrophic gastritis. The disease is more common in Basenjis, Lhasa Apsos, Shih Tzus, Maltese, Miniature Poodles, and other small-breed dogs. Males are predisposed, and older dogs are most often affected. **Eosinophilic gastritis** is uncommon. It is characterized by diffuse eosinophilic infiltration and granulation of the gastric wall. Eosinophilia in a vomiting animal is strongly suggestive of eosinophilic gastritis or eosinophilic gastroenteritis. The etiology is unknown but is suspected to be secondary to exposure to dietary allergens or as a consequence of an immune response to other antigens, eg, migrating parasites.

Vomiting (p 389) is the characteristic clinical sign of gastritis. In cases of acute gastritis, the vomitus may contain evidence of whatever substances the pet ingested (eg, grass). Bile, froth, frank blood, or digested blood that appears like "coffee grounds" may also be present. Occasionally, abdominal pain is signaled by the animal displaying a "praying" position (hindquarters raised and chest and forelegs held close to floor), a position that apparently gives some sense of relief. Polydipsia is often followed by immediate vomiting in dogs with acute gastritis. Acute or sporadic vomiting is generally not associated with other abnormalities. Diarrhea from concurrent intestinal involvement may also be noted.

Chronic vomiting may be associated with weakness, lethargy, weight loss, dehydration, and electrolyte imbalance and acid-base disorders.

For diagnosis, treatment, and control, see VOMITING, p 389. In addition to the treatments discussed under vomiting, therapy for chronic atrophic gastritis includes the use of corticosteroids, azathioprine, and H_2-blocking agents. Similarly, H_2-blocking agents are indicated in the management of chronic hypertrophic gastritis. Clinical disease associated with focal or discoid areas of hypertrophy respond well to simple surgical resection. Therapy for eosinophilic gastritis includes elimination of its cause, eg, parasites or dietary hypersensitivity, and the use of corticosteroids and commercial or homemade hypoallergenic diets.

Prognosis depends on the nature of the disease and the ability to eradicate or control it. Acute gastritis responds well to fasting and avoiding further dietary indiscretion. The prognosis for chronic gastritis is variable, depending somewhat on the owner's ongoing cooperation in dietary trials and continued therapy with H_2-blocking agents. Response to treatment is better and seen more often in chronic superficial gastritis than in chronic atrophic gastritis. Dogs with focal hypertrophic lesions respond well to surgical resection. Hypertrophic gastritis associated with hypergastrinemia and hyperchlorhydria have a guarded prognosis and tend to require continued medical therapy. Dogs with eosinophilic gastritis respond to dietary and corticosteroid therapy but often require continued longterm management. Azathioprine has been used in more intractable cases.

GASTROINTESTINAL NEOPLASIA

Neoplasia of the GI system is uncommon and represents <1% of all cancers in small animals. GI cancer most commonly develops in the rectum and colon of dogs and in the small intestine of cats. Older animals are predisposed, and adenocarcinoma and lymphosarcoma are seen more frequently in male dogs. Colorectal tumors are more prevalent in Boxers, German Shepherds, Poodles, Great Danes, and spaniels.

Etiology and Pathophysiology: No specific cause(s) has been identified for most GI tumor types, although alimentary lymphoma in cats is believed to be caused by the feline leukemia virus (FeLV), even in FeLV-negative cats. It has been suggested that the severe form of inflammatory bowel disease in cats may transform into lymphosarcoma, although to date no substantive evidence exists. Intestinal neoplasms tend to be malignant in small animals (88% of nonlymphoid tumors in dogs and all nonlymphoid tumors in cats).

Clinical Findings: Clinical signs vary depending on the location and extent of the tumor and associated paraneoplastic consequences, eg, hypercalcemia (p 444). Vomiting sometimes with blood, diarrhea also with blood, weight loss, constipation, tenesmus, abdominal pain, ascites, and peritonitis associated with rupture of affected bowel have been reported. Affected animals may also have clinical signs of anemia.

Adenomas are extremely rare in dogs and cats. In dogs, adenomas most often involve the rectum but have also been found in the stomach and colon. These tumors tend to form polyps that may range in size from 0.5-3 cm. Adenomatous polyps may progress to carcinoma in dogs. Affected dogs may have clinical signs of GI obstruction or bleeding.

Adenocarcinoma is the most common GI tumor type in dogs, in which the stomach, colon, and rectum are most frequently involved. In cats, the small intestine is most often affected. Gastric adenocarcinomas of the stomach tend to affect the pylorus and may ulcerate or invade the muscularis, which gives the stomach a "leather bottle-like" appearance. Metastasis to mesenteric lymph nodes is common, and adhesions and peritoneal implantation occur.

Leiomyomas and leiomyosarcomas appear as firm, white, lobulated masses throughout the GI tract, most commonly in the cecum and jejunum. Gastric leiomyomas appear as round, smooth, mucosal-covered masses, most often located along the lesser curvature near the cardia. They may be ulcerated. Leiomyosarcomas are locally invasive and slow to metastasize. Dogs with leiomyosarcoma tend to be aged (~12 yr). Biopsy is required to differentiate the benign from the malignant forms of the disease.

Lymphosarcomas may arise anywhere throughout the GI tract but are more often seen in the stomach of dogs and in the ileum of cats. Lymphoma was thought to be the most common tumor involving the GI tract in cats, but more recent reports indicate that adenocarcinoma may be the most common malignant neoplasm of the large intestine in cats. Lymphoma tends to affect older cats, most of which are FeLV-negative. These tumors tend to have a large, swollen, ellipsoid appearance and may invade all layers of the gut. Ulceration and metastasis to local mesenteric lymph nodes are common.

Mast cell tumors are found in cats and are located in the muscularis of the small intestine. They are also reported in the large intestine of cats. These tumors appear pale, firm, and diffusely swollen. A primary mast cell tumor of the ileocecal area has been reported in a dog.

Diagnosis: Diagnosis is based on an appropriate history and physical examination and confirmed by histologic evaluation. A mass may be detected on abdominal palpation and confirmed by plain and contrast radiographs or by abdominal ultrasound. Rectal examination may reveal evidence of a palpable mass lesion or bleeding. Biopsy samples may be taken at the time of a laparotomy or endoscopically. If samples are taken during endoscopy, it is important to take several samples from different areas and to take deep biopsies of suspect areas in an attempt to establish the diagnosis and to determine its extent. Deep-seated tumors, eg, leiomyomas and leiomyosarcomas, may not be detected by endoscopic biopsy because generally only the mucosa and superficial submucosa are sampled. In another study, 30% of canine rectal lesions were incorrectly diagnosed by endoscopic biopsy because samples were insufficient.

A CBC, biochemical profile, and urinalysis should be completed to determine the extent of concurrent illness. Other than anemia or hypoproteinemia, these tests are often normal. Pulmonary metastasis is rarely documented on thoracic radiographs.

Treatment: Surgical resection is the preferred treatment. Margins of 4-8 cm should be included in the resected area. Biopsies of suspect lesions in other areas should also be taken to determine the extent of metastatic disease.

Prognosis depends on tumor type and the ability to remove all of it. The prognosis for longterm survival of dogs is poor with leiomyosarcoma but excellent with leiomyomas. Recurrence after surgical resection is uncommon. Metastasis develops in up to 74% of dogs with gastric adenocarcinoma; efficacy of chemotherapy is unknown, and clinical signs have recurred from 3 days to 10 mo after surgery. The longterm prognosis is poor.

Local canine lymphoma responds better to chemotherapy than the diffuse form of disease. Local resection of feline intestinal lymphosarcoma has occasionally been curative. Cats with alimentary lymphoma treated with L-asparaginase, vincristine, cyclophosphamide, methotrexate, and prednisone had a mean survival time of 25.3 wk. In the same study, cats that received prednisone alone had a mean survival time of 7.3 wk. Cats with alimentary lymphoma are reported poorly responsive to treatment with vincristine, cyclophosphamide, and prednisone (median survival 50 days), but a few affected cats may have long survival times.

High-dose radiotherapy may be considered for select cases of rectal adenocarcinoma. The affected section of rectum is prolapsed with stay sutures, and doses of radiation are directly applied to the tumor and immediate area. Cats with colonic adenocarcinoma should undergo subtotal colectomy; adding doxorubicin may increase survival times.

GASTROINTESTINAL OBSTRUCTION

Gastric outflow obstruction can result from neoplasia, foreign bodies, polyps, ulcers, and gastric mucosal hypertrophy. Pyloric stenosis secondary to chronic hypertrophic gastropathy is the most common cause of gastric outflow obstruction. It is seen as a congenital lesion and is most often reported in brachycephalic breeds; it also is seen as an acquired lesion in older dogs. In dogs, there is a history of chronic intermittent vomiting and gastric distention. The etiology of pyloric stenosis is unknown, but it may be hormonally (eg, gastrin) or neurologically mediated. Positive-contrast abdominal radiographs show the obstructed stomach. Primary gastric neoplasia is uncommon. It tends to affect middle-aged to older dogs. Benign tumors include polyps and leiomyomas. Adenocarcinoma is the most common malignant form of tumor in dogs; metastasis is common, and the prognosis is poor. Therapy for gastric outflow obstruction is generally surgical. Response of chronic hypertrophic pyloric gastropathy to surgery is good to excellent.

Intestinal obstruction may be partial or complete and may be caused by foreign bodies, intussusception, gastric dilatation-volvulus, incarceration, and neoplasia. Strangulated obstructions impede blood flow to the affected intestine; simple obstructions do not. Linear foreign bodies (eg, string, pantyhose, fabric, or plastic materials) may become fixated at one end (eg, base of tongue or pylorus) or elsewhere in the GI tract. If a string becomes fixed and there is sufficient length to trail into the intestines, normal intestinal movement tends to cause a sawing or cutting motion of the string on the gut, predisposing to intestinal perforation and peritonitis. Obstruction secondary to neoplastic infiltration of the intestine is uncommon.

Pathophysiology: Intussusception tends to develop when one segment of the intestine is hypermotile. It may also be seen with mass lesions (eg, tumors, granulomas, or scars) that become fixed and tend to get thrust into an adjacent lumen of intestine. The area involved most commonly is the ileocecocolic junction, where the smaller segment of ileum may slide into the larger lumen of the colon.

Gastroesophageal (GEI) and pylorogastric intussusceptions are more acute and severe. The prognosis for GEI is poor, with a 95% mortality rate. Clinically, vomiting and regurgitation are seen most often. With intestinal intussusceptions, vomiting, diarrhea, hematochezia or melena, anorexia, and weight loss are common clinical findings. A palpable mass is present in 50-70% of cases and is most often palpated in the cranial abdomen. Contrast radiographs or abdominal ultrasound are most useful in confirming a diagnosis. The recurrence rate for intussusception is estimated at 3-25%, and usually a different site is affected.

Distention with gas and fluid develops proximal to the obstruction. Strangulation or incarceration of bowel is seen with entrapment of intestinal loops in hernias or mesentery. Venous return is impaired although arterial supply remains intact, leading to venous congestion, anoxia, and necrosis. Loss of blood into the intestinal lumen and peritoneal cavity and the subsequent emigration of bacteria and toxins from the devitalized tissue ensues. The most common toxin-producing bacteria are *Escherichia coli* and clostridia.

Grossly, wall edema and hemorrhage and mucosal sloughing are apparent within 1-3 hr. After 4 hr, the affected segment of intestine is turgid, and whole blood collects within the lumen. At 8-12 hr, the affected gut appears black, distended, and elongated. Gross necrosis is evident by 20 hr.

Clinical Findings: Clinical signs of small-intestinal obstruction may include lethargy, anorexia, vomiting, diarrhea, abdominal pain, abdominal distention, fever or subnormal body temperature, dehydration, and shock. Gaseous bowel distention develops within the initial 12-35 hr after obstruction and is followed by the loss of fluid into the intestinal lumen. Without treatment, death due to hypovolemia ensues within 3-4 days.

Upper or duodenal obstruction tends to present as frequent vomiting. In general, the closer the obstruction to the pylorus, the more severe the vomiting. Obstruction of the lower small intestine (eg, distal jejunum and ileum) is infrequently associated with vomiting. Lethargy, anorexia, weight loss, and ultimate starvation in untreated dogs lead to death within 3 wk or longer.

Intussusception may result in luminal obstruction, mucosal congestion, or infarction, depending on the length of the intussusception and the size of the intestinal loops involved. Clinical signs vary and may include vomiting, abdominal pain, and scant bloody diarrhea. In more chronic cases of intussusception, diarrhea with or without blood is seen. Intussusception is more common in young dogs (< 6-8 mo old).

In intestinal incarceration, a history of abdominal pain that rapidly progresses to hypovolemia and shock is typical. Incarceration of the affected intestine leads to bacterial proliferation within the stagnant bowel loop and to devitalization of tissue predisposing to hypovolemia and septic shock. It most commonly is seen secondary to hernia formation associated with abdominal trauma.

Diagnosis: A careful history including information about the animal's eating habits is important. Many animals with a history of dietary indiscretion continue that practice even after having experienced discomfort in the past. Access to string or sewing needles or missing objects (eg, toys) may be important historical facts. Examination of the oral cavity and, in cats, the base of the tongue is vital. Linear foreign bodies most often lodge at the base of the tongue in cats and at the level of the pylorus in dogs. Careful abdominal palpation examining for evidence of pain (ruptured bowel, peritonitis), organomegaly, thickened bowel loops (intussusception), and tympany (dilatation-volvulus), and a rectal examination for evidence of dietary indiscretion or blood (suggestive of strangulation) are important components of the physical examination. Intussusception can be difficult to identify on abdominal palpation because the affected segments of intestine are not always turgid. Bowel loops that are incarcerated often become distended and painful.

Plain abdominal radiographs may demonstrate the presence of foreign objects, masses, obstruction, or abdominal fluid. Radiographic signs of intestinal obstruction include accumulation of fluid, gas, or ingesta proximal to the obstruction and delayed intestinal transit time. Abdominal radiographs are often diagnostic for gastric dilatation-volvulus (p 325). Gastric distention with gas and a "shelf" of tissue causing compartmentalization is diagnostic of gastric dilatation-volvulus. Linear foreign bodies cause a pleating or bunching up of the affected intestines. The jejunum often becomes gathered in the cranial to midventral abdomen. The presence of small, eccentrically located luminal gas bubbles (3 or more) that appear tapered at one or both ends has a high correlation with linear foreign objects in cats. Gathering of the small intestine to the right side of the abdomen on the ventrodorsal abdominal view is also a common radiographic indication of linear foreign bodies in cats. The presence of free abdominal gas on survey radiographs is associated with high mortality rates. Barium contrast radiographs are best for demonstration of ileocolic intussusception. Plain radiographs are often unrewarding. Incarceration of intestine causes dilation of the affected loops, which can be seen on plain radiographs. Abdominal ultrasound is useful for diagnosing intestinal intussusception. Transverse sonographic images of intestinal intussusception often show a "target-like" appearance.

Barium-impregnated polyethylene spheres are capsules containing radiopaque plastic spheres. They are being used for the diagnosis of GI obstruction and motility disorders in dogs and cats.

Flexible endoscopic examination is useful in the identification of foreign objects, mass lesions, and ileocolic intussusception.

In animals that are systemically ill, a CBC, biochemical profile including electrolytes, and a urinalysis should be completed before therapy is initiated. Strangulation of gut causes a leukocytosis with a left shift early in the course of disease or leukopenia later and a low PCV. Initially, fluid lost into the intestinal lumen is isotonic. With time, there is an increased secretion of sodium, potassium, and albumin into the intestine. The additional loss of bicarbonate-rich secretions contributes to metabolic acidosis. Hypoproteinemia, with or without iron deficiency anemia due to GI blood loss, is common in chronic intussusception.

If abdominal fluid is detected on physical examination, abdominal radiographs, or ultrasonography, it should be aspirated and characterized as a transudate, exudate, chyle, blood, or urine. Pink to dark red peritoneal fluid may be seen with strangulation of the gut. Perforation of gut or peritonitis increases the likelihood of death.

If an obstructive lesion is documented and it cannot be resolved via endoscopy (eg, removal of a foreign object), the animal should be stabilized and an exploratory laparotomy performed. Similarly, animals with acute abdominal signs of unknown etiology, and those that continue to deteriorate clinically, should also have an exploratory laparotomy.

Treatment: Animals that are systemically ill benefit from IV fluid therapy (eg, lactated Ringer's or normal saline). Restoring vascular volume is vital to improve tissue perfusion. There is no difference in survival for animals undergoing small- versus large-intestinal surgery. The overall mortality rate for intestinal surgery is reported to be 12%. Large-intestinal surgery tends to be associated with longer surgery and recovery times. Animals requiring both resection and anastomosis and enterotomy are less likely to survive. Those with concurrent peritonitis reportedly have a mortality rate of up to 31%. Animals requiring more than one procedure tend to have higher mortality rates. Surgery and multiple enterotomies are necessary in most cats for the removal of linear foreign objects, yet many recover well. Peritonitis and death associated with linear foreign objects is much more common in dogs than in cats.

GASTROINTESTINAL ULCERS IN SMALL ANIMALS

The awareness of GI ulcers as a cause of GI disease has markedly increased with the advent of endoscopy in veterinary medicine, but the incidence of GI ulcers in small animals remains to be established.

Etiology and Pathophysiology: GI ulcers result from a breakdown of the normal gastric mucosal barrier and are aggravated by an increase in hydrochloric acid or pepsin production. The gastric mucosal barrier consists of a thick mucous layer and the mucosal cells that make up the epithelial membrane. Mucus has only a weak neutralizing and buffering capacity. The epithelial cells constitute the most important anatomic barrier to acid. A healthy gastric mucosal barrier is supported by adequate mucosal blood flow, a thick mucous layer, bicarbonate secretion, epithelial cell turnover, and an electrical potential difference. Prostaglandins maintain integrity of gastric mucosa by inhibiting gastric acid secretion, enhancing gastric bicarbonate production, preserving mucosal blood flow, stimulating epithelial cell turnover, and promoting the secretion of gastric mucus with an increased protein content. Injury to the mucosal barrier results in "back diffusion" of luminal acid into the mucosa, which initiates a series of events that result in cellular damage. The small amount of acid that normally diffuses into the mucosa is rapidly cleared by mucosal blood flow. Mucosal blood flow also serves to deliver oxygen and nutrients to the epithelium. Damage to the mucosal barrier increases mucosal permeability and the amount of acid diffusing back into the mucosa. Mast cells in the submucosa and lamina propria degranulate on contact with acid, releasing histamine. Histamine stimulates parietal cell secretion of hydrochloric acid and promotes cellular injury. The back diffusion of hydrochloric acid is the principal factor eliciting mucosal erosion and ulceration. Conditions predisposing to increased acid production or mucosal damage facilitate ulcer production. Acid also damages local blood vessels and nerves.

Potential causes of GI ulceration include the following: 1) drugs—NSAID (including aspirin, phenylbutazone, ibuprofen, indomethacin, carprofen, flunixin meglumine, naproxen, and piroxicam) and corticosteroids; 2) neoplasia—lymphosarcoma, adenocarcinoma, gastrinoma (Zollinger-Ellison syndrome), and mastocytosis; 3) systemic disease—renal or hepatic disease, hypovolemic shock, hypoadrenocorticism, sepsis, spinal injury, and pancreatitis; 4) other causes—*Helicobacter* spp, pyloric outlet obstruction, inflammatory bowel disease, chronic gastritis.

Aspirin, an NSAID, directly injures gastric epithelial cells and impairs prostaglandin E production. Standard formulations of buffered aspirin do not provide sufficient buffering to neutralize gastric acid or prevent mucosal injury. In people, enteric-coated aspirin causes less gastric irritation but absorption is less consistent. Corticosteroids potentiate the effects of mucosal damage by decreasing cell turnover and mucus production and by stimulating gastrin and hence acid production.

Gastrinoma and mastocytosis cause ulcer formation by increasing acid production.

Renal failure results in the retention of uremic toxins and gastrin that damage the gastric mucosa and blood vessels of the gastric wall and result in increased acid production.

The exact mechanism(s) by which liver failure favors ulcer production is unknown but may include reduced mucosal blood flow, increased serum levels of gastrin and histamine, and contribution to a loss of the normal mucosal barrier.

Hypotension, hypovolemic shock, and sepsis impair normal gastric microcirculation leading to ischemia and cell death. Spinal cord lesions may affect autonomic nervous control of blood vessels to the gut causing vasodilation, vascular stasis, and ischemia. Dogs with spinal cord lesions undergoing surgery and receiving corticosteroids are prone to hemorrhagic gastroenteritis (p 336) and perforating gastric ulcers. Stress may precipitate sympathetic-mediated vasoconstriction and increase the production of endogenous corticosteroids, vasoactive catecholamines, and serotonin, which contribute to mucosal injury. Reflux of bile acids and pancreatic enzymes damage mucosal cells by directly damaging the mucosal barrier. Reflux may be due to a number of factors, including disorders of pyloric function.

Clinical Findings: Animals with gastric ulceration may be asymptomatic or have a history that includes vomiting, sometimes with frank or digested blood, and abdominal discomfort that may appear less severe after a meal. Melena and pale mucous membranes supportive of anemia may be apparent. Clinical signs may be indicative of the causative factor of the ulcer, eg, clinical signs related to renal failure.

Diagnosis: The diagnostic approach to animals with a history of vomiting, abdominal discomfort, anorexia, or weight loss of unknown etiology should begin with a CBC, biochemical profile, trypsin-like immunoreactivity analysis, urinalysis, and fecal parasite evaluation. When indicated, abdominal ultrasonography should be performed or radiographs taken. In cases in which the etiology remains obscure or in those with apparent GI pathology, gastroduodenoscopy and biopsy should be completed.

Treatment and Control: The primary goal of ulcer management is to determine and eliminate or control the cause of the ulceration and provide supportive care. Medication directed at the ulcer itself reduces gastric acidity, prevents further destruction of GI mucosa, and promotes ulcer healing. In general, antiulcerative therapy should be continued for 6-8 wk.

Gastric acid production is stimulated by histamine (most potent), gastrin, and acetylcholine. H_2-blocking agents reversibly bind H_2-receptors and impede endogenous histamine occupation of the receptor. H_2-blocking agents include cimetidine, ranitidine, and famotidine. Cimetidine (10 mg/kg, PO, IM, or IV, TID) inhibits gastric acid secretion for 3-4 hr and requires dosing 3-4 times daily. Although no drug is more efficacious than another in promoting ulcer healing, ranitidine (dogs: 2 mg/kg, PO or IV, TID; cats: 2.5 mg/kg, IV, BID, or 3.5 mg/kg, PO, BID) is 4-10 times more potent than cimetidine, and famotidine (0.5-1 mg/kg, PO or IV, SID-BID) is 20-40 times more potent. Nizatidine (dogs and cats: 2.5-5 mg/kg/day, PO) is an H_2-blocking agent similar to cimetidine but up to 10 times more potent. It is primarily used as a prokinetic agent.

Omeprazole (0.7 mg/kg, PO, SID) inhibits the hydrogen-potassium ATPase responsible for hydrogen ion production in the parietal cell. It is 2-10 times more potent than cimetidine in decreasing intragastric acidity. In a study in dogs, SID administration of omeprazole was as effective as cimetidine given TID in lessening aspirin-induced gastritis.

Cytoprotective agents include antacids and sucralfate. Antacids are as effective as other antiulcerative agents but require more frequent dosing (eg, aluminum hydroxide in dogs is given at $1/2$-1 tablet, QID, and in cats at $1/4$ tablet, QID). One antacid tablet containing aluminum hydroxide given QID is as effective as higher doses of liquid antacids and cimetidine in promoting ulcer healing. Sucralfate (dogs: 0.5-1 g, PO, BID-TID; cats: 0.25 g, PO, BID-TID) forms a complex with proteinaceous exudates that adheres to the ulcer, providing a protective barrier to the penetration of acid. It also stimulates prostaglandin production, increases mucus production and mucosal turnover, inactivates pepsin, and absorbs bile acids. Sucralfate is as effective as H_2-receptor antagonists in promoting healing of ulcers in people.

Misoprostol (dogs: 2-5 µg/kg, PO, TID) is a synthetic prostaglandin E_1 analog. It decreases gastric acid secretion; increases bicarbonate and mucus secretion, epithelial cell turnover, and mucosal blood flow; and has a cytoprotective effect. It is reportedly effective in the prevention of NSAID-induced GI ulceration, whereas cimetidine and sucralfate have a therapeutic effect only if NSAID are discontinued. In spite of its efficacy, misoprostol has not been reported to decrease the frequency of GI pain associated with NSAID use. It is as effective as other antiulcerative drugs in treating GI ulcers in cases other than those associated with NSAID use, but in these cases, it offers no clear advantage over these other drugs. Misoprostol mitigates NSAID-induced gastroduodenal injury.

Although partial protection is provided, gastritis may still develop and contribute to vomiting. The drug does not prevent GI hemorrhage in dogs treated with methylprednisolone and is not effective in the healing or prevention of gastric mucosal lesions in dogs with acute degenerative disk disease treated with corticosteroids. Neither does omeprazole, cimetidine, or sucralfate. Dietary management should include the use of bland diets (eg, cottage cheese and rice or chicken and rice).

Ideally, ulcer healing should be monitored with gastroduodenoscopy. Failure of ulcers to respond to appropriate medical management necessitates biopsy of the stomach and small bowel. Several biopsies should be taken because obvious lesions may not be apparent or may be located sporadically throughout the gut.

The prognosis for animals with peptic ulcers and benign gastric neoplasia is good. Prognosis is poor for those with ulcers associated with renal or hepatic failure and for animals with gastric carcinoma and gastrinoma.

HELICOBACTER INFECTION

Helicobacter pylori has been associated with gastritis, peptic ulcer, and gastric adenocarcinoma in people. The mode of transmission of the disease is not clear, and reservoir hosts have not been clearly identified. Although the prevalence of gastric *Helicobacter* spp in dogs and cats is high, *H pylori* has not been found in dogs and is rarely identified in cats. Isolation of the bacteria from domestic cats raises the possibility that the organism may be a zoonotic pathogen, although the risk is minimal. Fecal-oral transmission is suggested, but gastric *Helicobacter* organisms have not been isolated from the feces of dogs or cats.

Etiology and Pathophysiology: The causative organism is a spiral-shaped, gramnegative, microaerophilic bacteria. Several different species of *Helicobacter* have been isolated from the stomachs of dogs, cats, ferrets, cheetahs, and nonhuman primates. Spiralshaped bacteria are most commonly detected in the gastric fundus but can be isolated from all parts of the stomach and, to a lesser extent, from the duodenum and lower GI tract. The organism resides in the glandular lumina, intracellular canaliculi of parietal cells, and mucous layer of the stomach, where it is protected from the acidic gastric environment.

In people, gastritis caused by *H pylori* is characterized by inflammation consisting of both a polymorphonuclear and a mononuclear infiltrate. The clinical significance of the organism in dogs and cats is unclear. In most infected animals, the presence of these bacteria have been associated with inflammatory changes (increased intraepithelial neutrophils, lymphocytes, mucosal edema, and infiltration of the lamina propria with lymphocytes, plasma cells, and eosinophils, as well as prominent lymphoid nodules) that support an associated pathology.

Clinical Findings: Clinical signs of disease have been produced by experimental inoculation of *Helicobacter* organisms in germ-free dogs and pathogen-free kittens. In the natural setting, fecal-oral or oral-oral transmission is suspected. Spiral organisms were found in several Persian cats with clinical signs of chronic gastroenteritis. Intermittent vomiting in dogs, sometimes containing bile, has been linked to this organism. Most evidence to date suggests that the organism causes a mild subclinical gastritis. Whether presence of the organism predisposes the animal to food allergy, inflammatory bowel disease, ulceration, or neoplasia remains to be seen.

Diagnosis: The rapid urease test, touch cytology, and histopathology are highly accurate, invasive tests for gastric *Helicobacter*-like organisms in dogs and cats. A history of persistent vomiting should prompt gastroscopy and biopsy. A presumptive diagnosis can be made based on the fact that *Helicobacter* organisms produce large quantities of urease. Biopsy samples are incubated in a urea broth. A change in color of the broth, signaling a change in pH associated with the production of ammonia from urea, constitutes a positive test. Gastric mucosal scrapings can be examined under darkfield microscopy for evidence of motile helical organisms. Histologic examination may reveal the presence of *Helicobacter*-like organisms on the gastric mucosa or in the mucous layer. Culture and

PCR are required to identify the organism to the species level. Definitive diagnosis requires culture and isolation of the specific species of organism. *H heilmannii*, the most common spiral organism in dogs and cats, cannot be cultured on artificial media; *H felis* can be cultured but is difficult to isolate. Urea breath and blood tests or serology are noninvasive tests that can be used to diagnosis *Helicobacter* spp.

Treatment: Although specific recommendations for dogs and cats are lacking, *H felis* can be transiently eliminated with a 4-wk course of bismuth (17-20 mg/kg, PO, BID) or a 10-day course of metronidazole (dogs: 15-20 mg/kg, PO, BID; cats: 12.5 mg/kg, PO, BID). A 10-day course of amoxicillin (20 mg/kg, PO, BID) reduces bacterial numbers. An uncontrolled clinical trial in dogs and cats with gastritis and *Helicobacter* infection showed a beneficial response in 90% of patients following treatment with metronidazole, amoxicillin, and famotidine (0.5 mg/kg, PO, SID-BID). Most therapeutic studies in dogs and cats have not demonstrated longterm eradication of the organism; whether this is due to reinfection or recrudescence is unknown. Patients that do not respond to this regimen are treated with immunosuppressive agents (eg, prednisone) for inflammatory bowel disease.

HEMORRHAGIC GASTROENTERITIS

Hemorrhagic gastroenteritis (HGE) is characterized by an acute onset of bloody diarrhea in formerly healthy dogs. Young, toy, and miniature breeds of dogs appear predisposed. Mortality is high in untreated dogs.

Etiology and Pathophysiology: The etiology is unknown. An abnormal response to bacteria, bacterial endotoxins, or diet may be involved, but evidence is lacking. *Clostridium perfringens* has been cultured from some dogs with HGE, although its significance is unknown. *Escherichia coli* has also been identified from some dogs with the disease, but no toxigenic strains have been isolated. There is no sex predilection, and dogs of any age may be affected. King Charles Spaniels, Shetland Sheepdogs, Pekingese, Yorkshire Terriers, Poodles, and Schnauzers may be more frequently affected than other breeds. Hyperactivity and stress are possible contributing factors.

Although no definitive cause has been found, a marked increase in vascular and mucosal permeability is likely. RBC, plasma, and fluid leak into the bowel lumen. Inflammation and necrosis are rarely seen. The increase in bowel permeability may represent a type I hypersensitivity reaction. Inciting factors may include food allergens, bacterial products, or intestinal parasites. Splenic contraction and the loss of fluid into the bowel contributes to the increased PCV and the maintenance of a low or normal serum total protein.

Clinical Findings: The disease is often seen in dogs 2-4 yr old and is characterized by an acute onset of vomiting and bloody diarrhea, anorexia, and depression. Dogs are not clinically dehydrated, but unless fluid support is initiated, hypovolemic shock may develop. The disease is not contagious and may be seen without obvious changes in diet, environment, or daily routine; the history is unremarkable.

Diagnosis: Diagnosis is based on the clinical sign of acute, bloody diarrhea accompanied by an increased PCV, which is often >60%. Findings on physical examination and biochemical profile tend to be normal. Other causes of GI bleeding that should be considered include parvovirus, coronavirus, *Campylobacter* spp, *Salmonella* spp, *Clostridium* spp, *Escherichia coli*, and leptospirosis, as well as whipworms, hookworms, coccidiosis, and giardiasis. Coagulopathies (including warfarin toxicity and thrombocytopenia), GI neoplasia, ulceration, colitis, and hypoadrenocorticism are other potential causes of GI bleeding.

Treatment: Most dogs respond to supportive treatment, including fluid therapy (eg, lactated Ringer's) and antibiotics (eg, ampicillin at 20 mg/kg, IV, TID and gentamicin at 2.2 mg/kg, SC, TID). Potassium chloride should be added to the IV fluids. Less severely affected dogs may be treated with amoxicillin, trimethoprim-sulfa, fluoroquinolone, or cephalosporin antibiotics. Food and water should be withheld for 2-3 days. When vomiting has ceased, food can be gradually reintroduced. Because of the possibility that food sensitivity may be an inciting factor, the protein source chosen should be one not previously fed to the dog, eg, cottage cheese, lamb, or tofu, mixed with rice. This diet is fed for 1-2 wk, after which the dog's regular diet can be gradually reintroduced.

Serious complications are uncommon but may include disseminated intravascular coagulation. Most dogs recover. Fewer than 10% of treated dogs die, and 10-15% have repeated occurrences.

INFLAMMATORY BOWEL DISEASE

Idiopathic inflammatory bowel disease (IBD) constitutes a group of GI diseases characterized by persistent clinical signs and by histologic evidence of inflammatory cell infiltrate of unknown etiology. The various forms of IBD are classified by anatomic location and the predominant cell type involved. Included in this group are lymphocytic-plasmacytic enteritis of cats (the most common form of IBD in cats), chronic lymphocytic-plasmacytic colitis of dogs, eosinophilic gastroenteritis and colitis, granulomas, histiocytic colitis, granulomatous enteritis (rare) and colitis, transmural granulomatous enterocolitis, suppurative colitis, and the diarrheal syndromes of the Basenji and Lundehund. German Shepherds may be predisposed to lymphocytic-plasmacytic enteritis.

Etiology and Pathophysiology: The etiology of IBD is unknown. Suspected factors include defective immunoregulation of gut-associated lymphoid tissue (GALT); permeability defects; genetic, ischemic, biochemical, and psychosomatic disorders; infectious and parasitic agents; dietary allergens; and adverse drug reactions. Defective immunoregulation of GALT results in exposure and adverse reaction to antigens that normally would not evoke such a response. Although dietary allergy is an unlikely cause of IBD (except in eosinophilic gastroenteritis), it may contribute to increased mucosal permeability and food sensitivity.

Current evidence supports the likely involvement of hypersensitivity reactions to antigens (eg, food, bacteria, mucus, epithelial cells) in the intestinal lumen or mucosa. More than one type of hypersensitivity reaction is involved in IBD. For example, type I hypersensitivity is involved in eosinophilic gastroenteritis, whereas type IV hypersensitivity is likely involved in granulomatous enteritis. The hypersensitivity reaction incites the involvement of inflammatory cells that results in mucosal inflammation. Inflammation impairs the mucosal barrier, facilitating increased intestinal permeability to additional antigens. Persistent inflammation results in fibrosis.

Clinical Findings: There is no apparent age, sex, or breed predisposition associated with IBD. However, it may be more common in German Shepherds, Yorkshire Terriers, Cocker Spaniels, and purebred cats. The mean age reported for the development of clinical disease is 6.3 yr in dogs and 6.9 yr in cats, but IBD has been documented in dogs <2 yr old. Clinical signs are often chronic and sometimes cyclic or intermittent. Vomiting, diarrhea, changes in appetite, and weight loss may be seen. In a retrospective study of cats with lymphocytic-plasmacytic enterocolitis, weight loss, intermittent vomiting progressing to more frequent vomiting on a daily basis, diarrhea, and anorexia were seen most often. Vomiting, melena, and cranial abdominal pain are often seen with gastroduodenal ulceration and erosion. When erosion or ulceration does occur, it is seen most often in the areas that do not produce acid (ie, the fundus, antrum, and pylorus). The duodenum has also been implicated as a frequent site for this problem. Clinical signs of large-intestinal diarrhea, including anorexia and watery diarrhea, are not uncommon.

An association between gastric dilatation-volvulus (p 325) and IBD in dogs has also been postulated. In this case, inflammation of the bowel may cause alterations in gastric motility and emptying and in GI transit time, thus predisposing to dilatation-volvulus.

An association between inflammatory hepatic disease, pancreatitis, and IBD has been reported in cats, although an etiology for this triad of diseases has not been established. However, cats with cholangiohepatitis should also be evaluated for IBD and pancreatitis. Although as yet unproved, it has been suggested that severe IBD in cats may progress to lymphosarcoma.

Diagnosis: Thickened intestinal loops may be palpated in >50% of cats with lymphocytic-plasmacytic enterocolitis; 50% of affected cats are thin or cachectic in appearance. Diagnosis requires intestinal mucosal biopsy.

There are no consistent abnormalities on CBC, biochemical evaluations, or radiographs. Erythrocytosis associated with fluid loss from vomiting and diarrhea and a stress leukogram may be seen. Thrombocytopenia has been observed in dogs with IBD. It may resolve in some dogs with successful management of the disease. The degree of thrombocytopenia does not correlate with the severity of the intestinal lesions, nor does it lead to clinical evidence of bleeding. Histologic infiltrates with eosinophils may be found in some dogs and cats with absolute eosinophilia. Nonresponsive anemia, if present, likely reflects anemia of chronic or inflammatory disease.

Hypoproteinemia due to reduced dietary intake and malabsorption or increased loss via the GI tract, may be seen. Increases in serum amylase as a consequence of inflammation of the bowel is also reported. Hypokalemia secondary to anorexia, potassium loss from vomiting and diarrhea, and low serum levels of folate and cobalamin are also documented. Additionally, mild increases in serum levels of liver enzymes can be expected. Hypocholesterolemia was reported to be the most common biochemical abnormality noted in one study of cats with the disease and was attributed to malabsorption.

Radiographic changes may include gas or fluid distention of the stomach and increased total diameter of small-intestinal loops. Contrast films may show diffuse or focal mucosal irregularities suggestive of infiltrative disease. Abdominal ultrasound may reveal thickened intestinal walls.

Gross mucosal lesions seen endoscopically may be evident in ~50% of cases and may include erythema, friability, enhanced granularity, erosion, and ulceration. In one report, 28% of cats had endoscopic evidence of disease of the stomach and 50% of the duodenum. In many cases, the endoscopic appearance is normal. Even in the absence of gross changes, biopsy samples should always be taken. Small populations of lymphocytes, plasma cells, macrophages, eosinophils, and neutrophils are normal components of intestinal mucosal tissue. Increased numbers of plasma cells, lymphocytes, eosinophils, and neutrophils in the lamina propria are seen in IBD. However, these morphologic features may also be seen with other causes of GI disease (eg, *Giardia*, *Campylobacter*, *Salmonella*, lymphangiectasia, and lymphosarcoma). The interpretation of histologic specimens of intestinal tissues from dogs and cats appears to vary substantially among pathologists. A histologic diagnosis of intestinal pathology may be made in a clinically normal dog, normal intestinal mucosa may be reported from dogs dying of intestinal disease, and tissue samples from clinically normal dogs have been described as having neoplastic infiltrates. Biopsy must always be considered in relation to clinical signs, and the animal treated accordingly.

Treatment and Control: The goals of therapy are to reduce diarrhea, promote weight gain, and decrease intestinal inflammation. If a cause can be identified (eg, dietary, parasitic, bacterial overgrowth, drug reaction, etc), it should be eliminated. Dietary manipulation by itself may be effective in some cases (eg, in chronic colitis); in other cases, it can enhance the efficacy of concurrent medical therapy allowing for the drug dosage to be reduced or for drug therapy to be discontinued once clinical signs are in remission. Corticosteroids, azathioprine, sulfasalazine, tylosin, and metronidazole are among the drugs most often used in the management of IBD.

Dietary modification generally involves feeding a hypoallergenic or elimination diet, ie, feeding a source of protein that the animal has not been previously exposed to such as homemade diets of lamb and rice or venison and rice or commercial diets. This diet should be the sole source of food for a minimum of 4-6 wk, and no treats of any kind should be fed. Novel protein diets alone are effective in controlling clinical signs in cats with IBD, but not in cats with food sensitivity or food allergy. Dogs with large-intestinal diarrhea may benefit from diets high in insoluble fiber content. Supplementation of dietary fiber alone is rarely effective in cases with severe inflammatory cell infiltrate.

Corticosteroids may be useful for small- as well as large-intestinal disease. Initial dosages recommended are 2.2 mg/kg/day for prednisone or prednisolone and 0.22 mg/kg/day for dexamethasone. Budesonide (dogs: 2 mg/dog/day, PO; cats: 1 mg/cat/day, PO) has a high topical glucocorticoid activity and a substantial first-pass elimination. The drug is rapidly inactivated in the liver, resulting in lower systemic bioavailablility and reduced effects on the hypothalamic-pituitary-adrenal axis, making iatrogenic hyperadrenocorticism less common. In cats with mild to moderate IBD or relapse of clinical signs, and in those in which administration of oral medication is difficult, methylprednisolone at a dose of 20 mg, SC or IM, every 2 wk for 2-3 doses, then every 2-4 wk, may be effective as the sole treatment or as an adjunct to prednisone and metronidazole. Dosages should be gradually reduced every 7-10 days to the lowest possible dose required to control clinical signs and, if possible, discontinued altogether. Animals in which this is not possible should be closely monitored for adverse effects associated with longterm or high-dose corticosteroid therapy. Prednisone alone or in combination with another drug is effective in controlling clinical signs in most cats with lymphocytic-plasmacytic enterocolitis. When combination therapy is indicated in cats, prednisone is often combined with metronidazole.

Azathioprine is commonly used in the management of IBD in dogs and cats. However, because of the potential adverse effects (eg, hepatotoxicity, myelosuppression, pancreatitis), it should be used only in cases refractory to dietary manipulation and corticosteroid therapy. Recommended dosages of azathioprine are 2.2 mg/kg, PO, SID, for dogs, and 0.3 mg/kg, every other day, PO, for cats. Cats are especially prone to bone marrow toxicity, and the dosage is decreased accordingly. Clinical signs typically improve in 3-5 wk. A CBC should be completed at 2-wk intervals to monitor for evidence of myelosuppression.

Sulfasalazine is used in the management of colitis in dogs. In the colon, this drug is split to release 5-aminosalicylic acid, which exerts its anti-inflammatory activity in the mucosa. The principal adverse effects noted in dogs are keratoconjunctivitis sicca and vasculitis. A dosage of 3-4.5 mg/kg, BID-TID for 7-10 days, is recommended in cats. Other newer aminosalicylic drugs without some of the adverse effects of sulfasalazine are available, eg, olsalazine (10-20 mg/kg, PO, TID in dogs) and mesalamine (10 mg/kg, PO, TID in dogs).

Metronidazole (10-20 mg/kg, PO, BID-TID) is also commonly used for the treatment of IBD in dogs and cats. Management for gastric ulcer or erosion may include misoprostol, omeprazole, cimetidine or ranitidine, or sucralfate. Cyclosporine has been recommended in people with severe, unresponsive IBD.

Ursodeoxycholic acid (10-15 mg/kg/day, PO), an agent used to treat chronic inflammatory cholestatic liver disease, primary biliary cirrhosis, chronic persistent hepatitis, cirrhosis, and biliary atresia, promotes biliary flow, has anti-inflammatory properties and may also have a role in reducing inflammation associated with IBD in cats.

The prognosis for feline IBD is good for adequate control but poor for cure. It has been reported that 79% of cats with IBD treated with a combination of diet and prednisone had a positive clinical response. A more guarded prognosis is reported in cases with severe histologic lesions, mucosal fibrosis, eosinophilic enteritis, or hypereosinophilic syndrome. Relapses occur and are most often precipitated by dietary indiscretion.

MALABSORPTION SYNDROMES

Malabsorption implies defective absorption of a dietary constituent resulting from interference with its digestion or absorption. Interference with food digestion in small animals is typically due to exocrine pancreatic insufficiency (EPI), whereas most cases of absorption failure are caused by small intestinal disease.

The primary functions of the small intestine include mixing and propulsion of luminal contents, absorption of water and ions, digestion and absorption of nutrients, and secretion of hormones. Digestion and absorption of nutrients occur in 3 sequential phases: intraluminal digestion, mucosal digestion and absorption, and delivery of nutrients to the circulation. Many GI diseases cause chronic malabsorption by interfering with these processes. Malabsorptive syndromes in dogs have been studied in more detail; however, basic diagnostic and therapeutic principles are relevant to other species.

Physiology: The normal digestive processes convert dietary nutrients into forms that can cross the brush border of intestinal absorptive epithelial cells, or enterocytes. The majority of digestive enzymes are secreted by the pancreas; EPI is thus a major cause of malabsorption. Some terminal digestion prior to absorption can be performed by brush border enzymes.

Main dietary carbohydrates are starch, glycogen, sucrose, and lactose. Starch and glycogen are first hydrolyzed by pancreatic amylase to the oligosaccharides maltose, maltotriose, and α-limit dextrins. Oligosaccharides and ingested disaccharides (sucrose, lactose) are further hydrolyzed to monosaccharides by enzymes located on the brush border of the intestinal epithelial cell. Brush border lactase declines after weaning, especially in cats, and animals may become lactose-intolerant. The final products of mucosal hydrolysis (glucose, galactose, and fructose) are actively transported into the enterocyte by a protein-carrier-mediated process. Once in the cell, monosaccharides diffuse down a concentration gradient through the lamina propria and into the portal venous circulation.

Protein digestion and absorption follow a similar pattern. Proteolytic enzymes from the stomach and pancreas degrade protein into a mixture of short-chain oligopeptides, dipeptides, and amino acids. Oligopeptides are further hydrolyzed by brush-border peptidases to dipeptides and amino acids that cross the brush-border membrane on specific carrier proteins.

Fat-soluble molecules do not need specific carriers to cross the phospholipid barrier of the brush border. However, intraluminal degradation of large lipids is essential. Fat in the duodenum stimulates release of cholecystokinin, which, in turn, stimulates secretion of pancreatic lipase. After solubilization by bile salt micelles, triglycerides are digested by pancreatic lipase to monoglycerides and free fatty acids. At the cell membrane, the monoglycerides and free fatty acids disaggregate from the micelle and are passively absorbed into the cell. Released bile acids remain within the lumen and are ultimately reabsorbed by the ileum. Once inside the cell, the monoglycerides and free fatty acids are re-esterified to triglycerides and incorporated into chylomicrons, which subsequently enter the central lacteals of the villus and are delivered to the venous circulation via the thoracic duct. However, medium-chain triglycerides can be absorbed directly into the portal blood, thus providing an alternative route for fat uptake in case of lymphatic obstruction.

Etiology and Pathophysiology: Malabsorption is a consequence of interference with mechanisms responsible for either the degradation or absorption of dietary constituents (TABLE 7).

Diseases that disrupt the synthesis or secretion of digestive pancreatic enzymes cause maldigestion with subsequent malabsorption. An important cause is EPI (p 349), which occurs if there is a loss of ~85-90% of exocrine pancreatic mass. EPI is characterized by severe maldigestion-malabsorption of starch, protein, and most notably, fat. In dogs, EPI is most commonly due to acinar atrophy; chronic pancreatitis is less common, and pancreatic hypoplasia is a rare cause. EPI in dogs is often complicated by small-intestinal bacterial overgrowth (SIBO), which further disrupts nutrient digestion and absorption. EPI is relatively uncommon in cats and is mostly due to chronic pancreatitis.

Intraluminal effects of bacteria in SIBO can also have important consequences. Bacterial deconjugation of bile salts interferes with micelle formation, which results in malabsorption of lipid. Deconjugated bile salts and hydroxy fatty acids exacerbate diarrhea by stimulation of colonic secretion. The causes of SIBO can include defective gastric acid secretion, interference with normal motility or mechanical obstruction of the intestine, interference with the function of the ileocecal valve, and local immunodeficiency; often, the cause is unknown. SIBO may also develop secondary to diffuse small-intestinal disease. It is not clear whether SIBO is seen in domestic species other than dogs; recent evidence suggests it is not a clinical problem in cats, which normally harbor relatively large numbers of anaerobes in the small intestine.

TABLE 7. Mechanisms of Malabsorption

Location	Disease	Mechanism
Luminal	Exocrine pancreatic insufficiency	Lack of pancreatic enzymes (maldigestion)
	Small intestinal bacterial overgrowth	Bile salt deconjugation, fatty acid hydroxylation, competition for cobalamin and nutrients
Mucosal	Inflammatory bowel disease, infectious enteropathies, dietary sensitivities, neoplastic infiltration, small intestinal bacterial overgrowth	Mucosal inflammation, brush border defects, disturbed enterocyte function (reduction of surface area)
	Villous atrophy	Reduction in surface area
	Brush border enzyme deficiencies	Lactase deficiency, diffuse small-intestinal disease
Postmucosal	Lymphangiectasia	Lymphatic obstruction
	Vasculitis, portal hypertension	Impaired absorption

Fat malabsorption may also be seen with a deficiency of intraluminal bile salts due to cholestatic liver disease, biliary obstruction, or ileal disease, resulting in defective absorption of conjugated bile salts.

Small-intestinal disease can cause malabsorption by reduction of the number or function of individual enterocytes. Diffuse diseases of the mucosa can result in reduced activities of brush border enzymes, decreased carrier-protein function, decreased mucosal absorptive surface area, and interference with final transport of nutrients into the circulation. Weight loss may be due to compromised nutrient intake. In addition, malabsorbed nutrients exert strong intraluminal osmotic effects that diminish intestinal and colonic absorption of water and electrolytes, resulting in diarrhea. This may be exacerbated if mucosal damage is accompanied by intestinal inflammation, which can cause secretory and permeability diarrhea.

Potential causes of mucosal damage include inflammatory bowel disease, enteric pathogens (eg, enteric viruses, pathogenic bacteria, giardiasis, histoplasmosis), dietary sensitivity, SIBO, and intestinal neoplasia (lymphosarcoma). Histologic changes such as villous atrophy and infiltration with inflammatory cells indicate intestinal disease but do not identify the underlying cause. For example, lymphocytic-plasmacytic enteritis may be a common response of the intestinal mucosa to more than one provocative agent, particularly microbial and dietary antigens. Definite associations with parasites and pathogenic bacteria, SIBO, and dietary sensitivity have been demonstrated in dogs, but often the underlying cause cannot be identified.

Mucosal damage may also be seen without obvious histologic changes. This is typified by infection with enteropathogenic *Escherichia coli* (which specifically cause ultrastructural damage to microvilli in an attaching-effacing lesion) and sometimes also by SIBO in the proximal small intestine (which in dogs can cause biochemical damage to the intestinal brush border interfering with enterocyte function).

The main brush border enzyme deficiency reported is a relative lactase deficiency in adult dogs and cats. Acquired brush border defects also may be seen in the course of generalized intestinal disease.

Postmucosal obstruction may be seen with lymphatic obstruction (especially lymphangiectasia) and vascular compromise (portal hypertension, vasculitis). Intestinal lymphangiectasia causes severe fat malabsorption as well as intestinal protein loss.

Usually there is malabsorption of a number of ingredients with consequent diarrhea; malabsorption of a single ingredient without GI signs is rare (eg, selective cobalamin malabsorption in Giant Schnauzers). Furthermore, the large absorptive capacity of the colon may prevent overt diarrhea despite significant malabsorption (with or without weight loss).

Clinical Findings: The clinical signs of malabsorption are mainly the result of lack of nutrient uptake and losses in the feces. The duration, severity, and primary cause determine the severity of signs, which typically include chronic diarrhea, weight loss, and altered appetite (anorexia or polyphagia). The absence of diarrhea does not exclude the possibility of severe GI disease. Weight loss may be substantial despite a ravenous appetite, sometimes characterized by coprophagia. Typically, animals with malabsorption are systemically well unless there is severe inflammation or neoplasia. Nonspecific signs may include dehydration, anemia, and ascites or edema in cases of hypoproteinemia. Thickened bowel loops or enlarged mesenteric lymph nodes may be palpable, especially in cats.

Diagnosis: Chronic diarrhea and weight loss are nonspecific signs common to a variety of systemic and metabolic diseases, as well as malabsorption. A thorough diagnostic approach in dogs and cats with signs suggestive of malabsorption is therefore needed to help exclude association with possible underlying systemic or metabolic disease. A precise diagnosis is also important for determining treatment and prognosis.

The history is particularly important because it may suggest specific dietary intolerance, indiscretion, or sensitivity. Weight loss may indicate malabsorption or protein-losing enteropathy but may also be due to anorexia, vomiting, or extra-GI disease. Small- and large-intestinal diarrhea may be distinguished by a number of features (TABLE 1, p 126). This distinction is more helpful in dogs than in cats, which rarely have exclusively large-intestinal disease. Suspected large-intestinal disease in dogs may be further evaluated by visualizing and taking a biopsy of the mucosa via endoscopic examination. However, if signs of large-intestinal disease are accompanied by weight loss or large volumes of feces, then the small intestine is probably also diseased.

A thorough physical examination should be performed. Abdominal palpation is essential to identify abnormalities, and rectal examination is required even when no lower-intestinal disease is suspected to provide a stool sample and possibly reveal previously unreported melena. In cats, the thyroid should be palpated carefully and serum T_4 assayed, as signs of hyperthyroidism can closely mimic those of malabsorption.

Initial evaluation should include a CBC, biochemical profile, urinalysis, fecal examination, abdominal ultrasonography and, when indicated, radiography. Hematologic correlates of intestinal diseases include anemia of chronic blood loss (microcytic, hypochromic) or chronic inflammation (normocytic, normochromic); neutrophilia and/or monocytosis associated with inflammatory bowel diseases, infectious enteropathies, or neoplasia; eosinophilia associated with parasitism, eosinophilic enteritis, or hypoadrenocorticism; and lymphopenia that may be associated with intestinal lymphangiectasia in dogs.

Biochemical tests and urinalysis help to exclude systemic diseases that cause chronic diarrhea, most notably hypoadrenocorticism, renal failure, and liver disease. Hypoproteinemia frequently is secondary to a protein-losing enteropathy; in most cases, serum albumin and globulin are both low, but a low albumin alone does not rule it out. Inflammatory bowel disease and neoplasia may be associated with hyperglobulinemia as well as hypoalbuminemia. Liver enzymes (ALT, AST) may be elevated as a consequence of increased intestinal permeability allowing more antigens to reach the liver; in such cases, a bile acid stimulation test as well as ultrasonography should be performed to exclude primary liver disease. Hypocholesterolemia may develop with fat malabsorption and is notable in lymphangiectasia. Urinalysis is important to exclude renal causes of hypoalbuminemia and/or renal disease. However, sometimes both may be seen together (eg, the familial protein-losing enteropathy and nephropathy of Soft-coated Wheaten Terriers). In cats, serologic tests for feline leukemia virus and feline immunodeficiency virus should be performed, not only because both may be associated with secondary chronic diarrhea but also because they are important prognostic factors. Feline infectious peritonitis and toxoplasmosis have also been described occasionally as causes of chronic diarrhea in cats. Suspected hyperthyroidism can be excluded by measuring serum T_4 levels.

Feces should be examined for parasites (especially *Giardia*) and potentially pathogenic bacteria (including *Salmonella* and *Campylobacter*). Pathogenic *Escherichia coli* are emerging as a potentially important problem in dogs, but sophisticated molecular techniques to identify genes encoding pathogenicity determinants are required for diagnosis. *Giardia* can be detected using serial fecal flotations or with a commercially available ELISA; the latter is easier to perform but less reliable. The presence of fat, undigested muscle fibers, or starch may provide indirect evidence for malabsorption but these are unreliable. Detection of excessive leukocytes on fecal cytology may indicate chronic inflammatory bowel disease or presence of enteric pathogens such as *Salmonella* or *Campylobacter*. Cytology of colonic scrapings may reveal *Histoplasma* organisms.

Abdominal radiography is more useful when vomiting is present or palpable abnormalities are detected. Ultrasonography is an important part of the investigation of most small-intestinal diseases. It can be used to measure intestinal wall thickness, layering, and luminal diameter, and to detect other intestinal lesions (masses, intussusception), mesenteric lymphadenopathy (in neoplasia and inflammatory bowel disease), and abnormalities in other organs.

Once obvious dietary, systemic, parasitic, and infectious causes of chronic small-intestinal diarrhea have been eliminated, the next step is differentiation of EPI from intestinal malabsorption while that; the diagnosis of EPI is relatively straightforward, while that of small-intestinal disease is more complicated. Numerous tests of exocrine pancreatic function have been recommended for dogs and cats with suspected EPI, but except for fecal proteolytic activity, they are too inaccurate or impractical to be recommended. Instead, assay of serum trypsin-like immunoreactivity (TLI), which is a highly sensitive and specific test for the diagnosis of EPI in dogs, is used. This assay measures trypsinogen that normally leaks from the pancreas into the blood, thereby providing an indirect assessment of functional pancreatic tissue. In dogs with EPI, functional exocrine tissue is severely depleted and serum TLI concentrations are extremely low, clearly distinguishing EPI from other causes of malabsorption. This test requires a fasted serum sample in dogs but not in cats. In cats, measurement of fecal proteolytic activity was formerly the most reliable widely available test of EPI, but a species-specific feline TLI test has recently been developed and validated.

Diagnosis of small-intestinal disease is difficult due to limitations of routine screening procedures, the need for biopsy, and frequently the absence of diagnostic histologic changes.

Assay of serum folate and cobalamin (vitamin B_{12}) concentrations can be a helpful initial test in the assessment of small-intestinal disease. Folate is absorbed primarily by the proximal small intestine (jejunum), whereas cobalamin is absorbed by the distal small intestine (ileum). As a result, serum folate concentrations can be decreased in proximal small-intestinal diseases, serum cobalamin concentrations can be decreased in distal diseases, and both can be decreased in severe diffuse enteropathies. In addition, SIBO (also called antibiotic-responsive diarrhea) may be suspected by finding increased serum folate or decreased serum cobalamin concentrations, reflecting the ability of many enteric bacteria to synthesize folate (which is subsequently absorbed in the proximal intestine) and to bind cobalamin (which is then unavailable for uptake in the ileum). These tests have a moderate specificity for the detection of SIBO but a low sensitivity, emphasizing that normal serum folate and cobalamin concentrations do not exclude the possibility of small-intestinal disease. Other factors such as the severity, extent, and duration of a mucosal abnormality; the type and numbers of organisms present in SIBO; vitamin supplementation; and dietary intake also influence these concentrations. In addition, EPI can affect serum folate and cobalamin concentrations. The validity of serum folate and cobalamin assays for the investigation of small-intestinal disease in cats is less clear, but low serum cobalamin concentrations may be found with both small-intestinal disease and feline EPI. Measurement of serum folate appears to be of little value in cats, because most cats normally have high serum folate concentrations.

A further indirect approach to the detection of small-intestinal disease is the assessment of intestinal function and permeability by the oral administration of test substances that are subsequently measured in blood or urine samples. Intestinal function has typically been assessed by the xylose absorption test. However, this is an insensitive test; results are frequently normal in dogs with small-intestinal disease, and the test does not appear to work well in cats. As an alternative approach in humans, D-xylose has been given with 3-O-methyl-D-glucose to provide a differential absorption test that exploits the contrasting effect of impaired intestinal absorption on these 2 markers. This appears to be an effective approach in dogs, but the sugar analyses are technically demanding and likely to be available only in specialized laboratories.

Assessment of intestinal permeability provides information about the physical integrity rather than the functional capacity of the mucosa. This new and extremely sensitive approach to the detection of small-intestinal damage involves measurement of urinary or blood concentrations of orally administered probes that cross the intestinal mucosa by unmediated permeation through 2 possible pathways. An intercellular aqueous pathway is represented by a few relatively large "pores." Damage to the mucosa can open these intercellular pathways and result in enhanced permeability to larger probes such as ^{51}Cr-EDTA, cellobiose, and lactulose. A second transcellular pathway is thought to consist of a greater number of small "pores," which act as aqueous channels in enterocytes. These pores are permeable to smaller probe molecules such as mannitol and rhamnose and are reduced in a number of diseases that decrease intestinal surface area. Calculation of the ratio of the urinary excretion of a mixture of 2 probes of different sizes, such as lactulose and rhamnose, has been used successfully not only for the diagnosis of small-intestinal disease in dogs but also to monitor response to treatment (eg, to document dietary sensitivity or SIBO). Unfortunately, this approach does not appear to be useful in cats because intestinal permeability in healthy cats is so high.

IV administration of ^{51}Cr-labeled albumin, or ^{51}Cr, involves a different principle and has been used successfully to document protein-losing enteropathy in dogs. Measurement of 3-day fecal excretion of this radioactive marker provides an estimation of albumin and hence protein loss into the intestinal lumen. This test is preferred for diagnosis of intestinal protein loss, but its use is limited to large institutions due to the use of radioactive markers. An alternative approach is the measurement of α-1 protease inhibitor in the feces. This plasma protein is lost into the intestinal lumen together with albumin, but unlike albumin it is excreted in the feces essentially intact. A species-specific canine assay has recently been developed, but further studies are needed to assess its usefulness in the management of protein-losing enteropathy.

Hydrogen breath testing after oral administration of individual sugars has been used extensively in humans to assess bacterial colonization of the small intestine and carbohydrate malabsorption. This test works on the principle that intestinal bacteria ferment intraluminal carbohydrate and produce hydrogen gas, some of which is absorbed into the blood and excreted by the lungs. Increased breath hydrogen concentrations after oral carbohydrate may therefore reflect either bacterial colonization in the proximal small intestine, where carbohydrate concentration is relatively high, or malabsorption of carbohydrate, which then reaches the flora normally present in the distal small intestine and large intestine. This is a promising, simple procedure to detect SIBO in dogs and to assess transit time in cats, but it is likely to be available only at specialist centers.

A new method that can be used to diagnose SIBO in dogs is measurement of serum unconjugated bile acids. Many of the bacterial species that overgrow have the ability to deconjugate bile acids, which then readily diffuse across the mucosa and can be found in the blood. The test is technically difficult, but studies suggest it may be useful.

Definitive diagnosis of chronic small-intestinal disease typically includes histologic examination of intestinal biopsies taken by endoscopy or at laparotomy. Endoscopy is noninvasive and allows visualization of the mucosa and targeted biopsy sampling. However, endoscopic mucosal biopsies may not always give an adequate representation of deeper disease and are limited to the part of the duodenum that can be visualized. Surgery is the preferred option when there is a concern about deeper and extraintestinal disease or a focal lesion. If a laparotomy is performed, multiple thin, longitudinal biopsy samples should be collected from at least the duodenum, jejunum, and ileum; mesenteric lymph nodes should be biopsied and other organs examined.

Histologic examination of intestinal biopsy specimens can identify morphologic changes in inflammatory bowel diseases, including lymphocytic-plasmacytic enteritis and eosinophilic enteritis, intestinal lymphangiectasia, villous atrophy, and intestinal neoplasia. The description of morphologic abnormalities can provide a baseline to evaluate response to treatment, although indirect assessments such as intestinal permeability are clearly more practical than sequential intestinal biopsies. Morphologic abnormalities also provide some indication of prognosis because the more severe enteropathies tend to be more difficult to manage. However, there may be minimal or no obvious abnormalities in certain disorders despite considerable interference with intestinal function. Furthermore, histologic descriptions alone provide little information on possible etiology or underlying mechanisms of damage, which would clearly assist effective management.

Bacteriologic culture of duodenal juice obtained endoscopically or at laparotomy is needed for a definitive diagnosis of SIBO. The exact cut-off point when small-intestinal bacterial numbers are considered excessive is still a matter of debate. An association between >10^5 total or >10^4 obligate anaerobic colony-forming units (CFU)/mL, clinical disease, and mucosal damage has been established in dogs. However, higher numbers may be found in apparently clinically healthy dogs, depending on circumstances including environment, diet, scavenging, and coprophagia. The most frequent isolates typically include enterococci and *E coli* in dogs with aerobic overgrowth and *Clostridium* in dogs with anaerobic overgrowth. High numbers of anaerobic bacteria are most likely to be pathogenic.

Treatment: Treatment of malabsorption involves dietary therapy, management of complications, and treatment of the primary cause (if identified). Management of EPI in dogs is relatively straightforward (*see* p 349). It should include feeding a low-fiber diet that contains moderate levels of fat or highly digestible fat, very digestible carbohydrate, and high-quality protein. Specific treatment involves lifelong supplementation of each meal with pancreatic extract. Powdered extracts (2 tsp/20 kg body wt) are preferable to tablets, capsules, and enteric-coated preparations. Fresh or frozen pancreas can be used as an alternative (100 g/meal for an adult German Shepherd). If response to pancreatic replacement therapy is poor, SIBO may be suspected, and the animal treated with oral antibiotics for ≥1 mo (*see* below). H_2-receptor blockers, such as cimetidine at 5-10 mg/kg or ranitidine at 2 mg/kg, may be given 20 min before a meal to inhibit acid secretion and to minimize degradation of enzymes in the pancreatic extract, but their efficacy is questionable. Oral multivitamin supplementation should be considered as supportive therapy, but cobalamin (500 mg/mo) should be given parenterally. Dietary requirements of cats with EPI can generally be met by conventional commercial diets, but pancreatic replacement therapy is still needed, as well as parenteral cobalamin supplementation in cats with low serum cobalamin levels.

Effective treatment of **small-intestinal disease** depends on the nature of the disorder, but therapy may be empirical when a specific diagnosis cannot be made. In dogs with SIBO, a low-fat diet may help by minimizing secretory diarrhea due to bacterial metabolism of fatty acids and bile salts. Oral broad-spectrum antibiotic therapy with oxytetracycline (10-20 mg/kg, TID for 28 days) has been successful. Metronidazole (10-20 mg/kg, BID) and tylosin (20 mg/kg, TID) are effective alternatives. Repeated or longterm treatment may be necessary in dogs with idiopathic SIBO. Vitamin supplementation may be helpful, particularly cobalamin by injection (eg, 500 mg/mo for 6 mo) for dogs with cobalamin deficiency. Secondary SIBO usually resolves with appropriate management of the underlying disease, but idiopathic SIBO can be difficult to control, especially in German Shepherds, which are predisposed to developing the condition.

Dietary modification is an important aspect of the management of small intestinal disease in both dogs and cats. Diets generally contain moderate levels of limited protein sources and highly digestible carbohydrates (to reduce protein antigenicity, reduce osmolar effects, and improve nutrient availability), and low to moderate levels of fat (to reduce steatorrhea and decrease secretogogues). In addition, they are lactose and gluten free, may be fiber-restricted, and may contain increased levels of antioxidants, prebiotics (fructo-oligosaccharides), or omega-3 fatty acids. These additives are thought to modulate the inflammatory response and increase the health of the bacterial gut flora. Treatment with an exclusion diet consisting of a single novel protein source should be used as trial therapy when dietary sensitivity is suspected. In addition, intestinal inflammation is sometimes a manifestation of dietary sensitivity, and an exclusion food trial is also indicated in mild cases of inflammatory bowel disease. Boiled white rice and potato are suitable carbohydrate sources, while lamb or chicken are often used as a protein source, depending on the dietary history. Cottage cheese, horsemeat, rabbit, venison, or fish may be acceptable alternatives. Commercial exclusion diets may be generally less suitable than home-cooked diets for diagnosing food hypersensitivity in dogs, although not necessarily in cats; however, they are preferred for maintenance to reduce dietary imbalances. Protein hydrolysate diets may be most effective in eliminating dietary sensitivity. The exclusion diet generally does not need to be fed for >3 wk. Oral prednisolone (0.5 mg/kg, BID for 2-4 wk, followed by a reducing dose) may be useful in some animals with dietary sensitivity if the initial response to the exclusion diet is disappointing.

Treatment of **idiopathic intestinal disease** in dogs should initially attempt to eliminate or control an underlying antigenic stimulus that may be playing a primary or secondary role in the damage. This is particularly important if there is evidence of intestinal inflammation. Treatment should first involve the use of an exclusion or protein hydrolysate diet for suspected dietary sensitivity as described above. The diet should comprise digestible carbohydrate, (preferably rice, which is most digestible) and high-quality protein. Restriction of fat content may also be valuable and can minimize the secretory diarrhea that is a consequence of bacterial metabolism of fatty acids and bile salts. Oral prednisolone (0.5 mg/kg, BID for 1 mo, followed by a reducing dose) is indicated in cases of intestinal disease with an obvious inflammatory component, such as lymphocytic-plasmacytic enteritis and eosinophilic enteritis. Higher dosages (1-2 mg/kg, BID) may be indicated in more severe cases. In rare severe cases, it may be necessary to use azathioprine (2-2.5 mg/kg, SID).

Cats with **inflammatory bowel disease** have a higher incidence of dietary sensitivity than dogs, emphasizing the importance of a dietary trial with an exclusion diet. If this fails, treatment may be needed with oral prednisolone at a dosage of 1-2 mg/kg, daily for 2-4 wk, gradually decreasing until clinical signs resolve. Severe cases often require higher dosages and longterm therapy. Cats that do not respond may be given adjunct metronidazole (10 mg/kg, BID). The beneficial effect of metronidazole might be due to an inhibition of cell-mediated immune responses as well as to its anaerobic antibacterial activity. If remission is not maintained on this combination, other immunosuppressive drugs such as chlorambucil or azathioprine can be attempted, although the latter has many side effects in cats.

For treatment of cases of **idiopathic villous atrophy**, prednisolone, antibiotics, and an exclusion diet can be considered. In **lymphangiectasia**, a severely fat-restricted, calorie-dense, highly digestible diet is essential. Supplementation with fat-soluble vitamins is advised, and additional medium-chain triglycerides have been recommended as an easily absorbable fat source that bypasses the lymphatics, although their efficacy has recently been questioned. Prednisone therapy may be beneficial for its anti-inflammatory and immunosuppressive effects, especially if there are associated lymphangitis and lipogranulomas. The response to treatment is variable; clinical signs may sometimes abate for months or even years, but the longterm prognosis is grave. **Giardiasis** can be treated with metronidazole or fenbendazole, and **histoplasmosis** with itraconazole (cats) or ketoconazole (dogs), with or without amphotericin B. In cases of **lymphosarcoma**, treatment involves an appropriate chemotherapy regimen.

THE EXOCRINE PANCREAS

The pancreas has both endocrine and exocrine functions. The exocrine pancreas is made up of pancreatic acinar cells and a duct system that opens into the proximal duodenum. Pancreatic acinar cells synthesize and secrete digestive enzymes, which are essential for the digestion of complex dietary components such as proteins, triglycerides, and complex carbohydrates. The exocrine pancreas also secretes large amounts of bicarbonate, which buffers gastric acid.

PANCREATITIS

Pancreatitis is the most common exocrine pancreatic disease in both dogs and cats. It can be acute or chronic, depending on whether or not the disease has led to permanent changes of the pancreatic parenchyma. Both acute and chronic pancreatitis can be severe and associated with pancreatic necrosis and systemic complications. Thus a distinction between the two is clinically of little significance.

Etiology and Pathogenesis: Most cases of pancreatitis in dogs and cats are idiopathic. However, dietary indiscretion is believed to be a common risk factor in dogs. Severe trauma or surgery can also lead to pancreatitis. However, anesthesia-induced hypotension may be more important in inducing pancreatitis than trauma from handling of the pancreas. Infectious diseases have been implicated, but the evidence for a cause and effect relationship is weak, except for *Toxoplasma gondii* and *Amphimerus pseudofelineus* in cats. Many drugs have been implicated in causing pancreatitis in humans but very few have been confirmed in dogs and cats. In general, most drugs should be viewed as potential causes of pancreatitis; anticholinesterases, calcium, L-asparaginase, estrogen, salicylates, azathioprine, thiazide diuretics, and vinca alkaloids are probably the most likely. Corticosteroids were long considered to be a risk factor for pancreatitis but have recently been removed from the list of drugs that may induce pancreatitis in humans. Similarly, there is no credible evidence that corticosteroids are a risk factor for pancreatitis in dogs or cats.

Many different insults may ultimately lead to pancreatitis through a common mechanism. Secretion of pancreatic juice decreases during the initial stages of pancreatitis. This is followed by localization of both zymogen granules and lysosomes, leading to activation of trypsinogen. Trypsinogen in turn activates more trypsinogen and also other zymogens. Prematurely activated digestive enzymes lead to local damage of the exocrine pancreas with pancreatic edema, bleeding, inflammation, necrosis, and peripancreatic fat necrosis. The inflammatory process also leads to recruitment of WBC and cytokine production. The activated enzymes, and more importantly, the cytokines circulate in the bloodstream and lead to distant complications such as generalized inflammation, disseminated intravascular coagulation, disseminated lipodystrophy, pancreatic encephalopathy, hypotension, renal failure, pulmonary failure, or even multiorgan failure.

Clinical Findings: Anorexia (91%), vomiting (90%), weakness (79%), abdominal pain (58%), dehydration (46%), and diarrhea (33%) are the most common clinical signs reported in dogs with severe pancreatitis. Clinical signs in cats with severe pancreatitis are even less specific with lethargy (100%), anorexia (97%), dehydration (92%), hypothermia (68%), vomiting (35%), and abdominal pain (25%) most commonly reported. The low rate of abdominal pain reported is remarkable given that >90% of human patients with pancreatitis report abdominal pain.

Diagnosis: A history of dietary indiscretion combined with vomiting and abdominal pain may suggest pancreatitis in dogs, but most cats present with nonspecific histories and clinical signs. Findings on CBC and serum biochemistry profiles may suggest an inflammatory disease process but are nonspecific. In dogs, thrombocytopenia and neutrophilia with a left shift are common. Azotemia and elevations in liver enzymes and bilirubin are common, nonspecific findings in both dogs and cats. Abdominal radiographs may show decreased detail in the proximal abdominal cavity and displacement of abdominal organs, but these findings are also nonspecific and a diagnosis based on radiographic findings alone is not reliable. Abdominal ultrasound, if stringent criteria are applied, is highly specific for pancreatitis, but pancreatic enlargement and fluid accumulation around the pancreas alone are not sufficient for diagnosis. A combination of pancreatic enlargement, fluid accumulation around the pancreas, changes in echogenicity (decreased echogenicity in cases of pancreatic necrosis, increased echogenicity in cases of fibrosis), and/or a pancreatic mass effect are highly specific for pancreatitis. Unfortunately, the sensitivity of abdominal ultrasound is highly operator-dependent, with sensitivities as high as 35% in cats and 65% in dogs in the most experienced hands.

Several diagnostic markers for pancreatitis have been evaluated in dogs and cats. Serum lipase and amylase activities have limited clinical usefulness in dogs and no usefulness in cats. In dogs with suspected pancreatitis, serum amylase and lipase can be used as a diagnostic indicator until a more definitive diagnostic test (eg, abdominal ultrasonography or serum pancreatic lipase immunoreactivity [PLI] concentration) can be performed. Serum trypsin-like immunoreactivity (TLI) concentration is also of limited clinical usefulness for the diagnosis of pancreatitis in dogs. Although highly specific for exocrine pancreatic function, it has a sensitivity of only 30-60%, depending on the study. In both dogs and cats, serum PLI concentration is highly specific for exocrine pancreatic function and is also the most sensitive currently available diagnostic test for pancreatitis (sensitivity >80%). The canine and feline PLI assays are currently performed only by the GI Laboratory at Texas A&M University.

Abdominal exploratory laparotomy can also be used to definitively diagnose pancreatitis. However, even if the presence of pancreatitis seems obvious (eg, pancreatic congestion can easily be misdiagnosed as pancreatitis on gross examination), a biopsy specimen should be collected, as the definitive diagnosis of pancreatitis requires the identification of an inflammatory infiltrate. It is difficult to exclude pancreatitis during abdominal exploratory laparotomy. In many cases, pancreatitis is localized to one lobe of the pancreas and may be missed when a single biopsy is being collected. Also, patients with severe pancreatitis are often poor anesthetic risks, and exploratory laparotomy may not be justified.

Treatment: The mainstay of therapy is supportive care with fluid therapy, vigorous monitoring, and early intervention to prevent systemic complications. In those few cases in which the etiology is known, specific therapy against the inciting cause may be initiated. Antibiotics are of questionable value. Resting the exocrine pancreas by giving the patient nothing per os (NPO) for 3-4 days is still recommended in most cases, although the validity of this approach has been questioned. Patients that vomit may be held NPO. However, patients held NPO should be given alternative nutritional support. This is especially important in cats that are at risk for secondary hepatic lipidosis. Total parenteral nutrition and jejunostomy tubes have both been suggested. However, these are often not feasible in a general practice setting; nasogastric and gastric tubes may be viable alternatives in patients that are not vomiting incessantly. Abdominal pain should be assumed to be present and treated until contrary evidence is available. Traditionally, meperidine and butorphanol have been used, but many opioids, such as fentanyl or morphine are also useful. Intra-abdominal lidocaine has also been used. Plasma appears to be helpful in severe cases of canine pancreatitis. It should be given daily until improvement is significant or until adverse effects are identified. Many other treatments have been investigated in dogs, cats, and humans, but unfortunately none has been shown to be useful.

Prognosis: The prognosis in mild cases is good, but prognosis in severe cases of pancreatitis is poor in both dogs and cats. About 50% of human patients with severe pancreatitis die, and the mortality rate appears to be similar in dogs and cats. A challenge in both human and veterinary medicine is the identification of severe cases early during the disease process and the prevention of complications.

Mild Chronic Pancreatitis

Many dogs—and particularly cats—have mild forms of chronic pancreatitis. Once pancreatitis has been diagnosed, risk factors for pancreatitis can be excluded from the history. Also, hypercalcemia and hypertriglyceridemia can be excluded by clinical pathology. Cats with mild chronic pancreatitis should be evaluated for concurrent chronic small-intestinal disease. This is most easily accomplished by measuring serum cobalamin and folate concentrations.

Patients should be switched to a low-fat diet and low-fat treats. Pancreatic enzyme supplementation can be tried in cases in which abdominal pain is present or for animals with consistently poor appetites, which may be the only indicator of abdominal pain. Finally, patients with mild, chronic pancreatitis should be monitored for potential complications, such as exocrine pancreatic insufficiency.

EXOCRINE PANCREATIC INSUFFICIENCY

Exocrine pancreatic insufficiency (EPI) is a syndrome caused by insufficient synthesis and secretion of digestive enzymes by the exocrine portion of the pancreas. It is much more common in dogs than cats.

Etiology and Pathogenesis: Pancreatic acinar atrophy is the most common cause of EPI in dogs, while chronic pancreatitis is the most common cause in cats. Less common causes of EPI in dogs and cats are pancreatic or extrapancreatic masses that lead to obstruction of the pancreatic duct. The exocrine pancreas has a remarkable functional reserve, 90% of which must be lost before clinical signs of EPI develop. Pancreatic acinar enzymes play an integral role in the assimilation of all major dietary components, and a lack of pancreatic digestive enzymes leads to maldigestion and malabsorption (*see also* MALABSORPTION SYNDROMES, p 339). The nutrients remaining in the intestinal lumen lead to loose, voluminous stools and steatorrhea. The lack of nutrients also causes weight loss and may lead to vitamin deficiencies. In animals with EPI caused by chronic pancreatitis, destruction of pancreatic tissue may not be limited to the acinar cells, and concurrent diabetes mellitus may develop.

Clinical Findings: EPI due to pancreatic acinar atrophy is most frequent in young adult German Shepherds. Dogs and cats with EPI due to other causes are usually middle-aged to older and can be of any breed. Clinical signs most commonly reported are polyphagia, weight loss, and diarrhea. Vomiting and anorexia are observed in some animals with EPI and may be a sign of concurrent conditions. The feces are most commonly pale, loose, and voluminous and may be malodorous. In rare cases watery diarrhea may be seen. The high fat content of the feces can lead to a greasy appearance of the hair coat, especially in the perianal and tail region of cats.

Diagnosis: A serum trypsin-like immunoreactivity (TLI) concentration of ≤2.5 µg/L (dogs) or ≤8.0 µg/L (cats) is diagnostic for EPI. A few German Shepherds with subclinical EPI had severely decreased serum TLI concentrations, a lack of exocrine pancreatic tissue at abdominal exploratory, but no or only intermittent clinical signs of EPI. Recently, a new assay for measurement of fecal elastase in dogs has been developed and validated. Unfortunately, some healthy dogs or dogs with chronic small-intestinal disease may have a decreased fecal elastase concentration, making this test less reliable than serum TLI concentration.

Treatment: Most dogs and cats with EPI can be successfully treated by dietary supplementation with pancreatic enzymes. Powder is more effective than tablets, capsules, and especially enteric-coated products. Initially, 2 tsp/20 kg body wt should be given with each meal for dogs and 1 tsp/cat with each meal for cats. Oral bleeding has been reported in 3 of 25 dogs with EPI treated with pancreatic enzyme supplements; the bleeding stopped in all 3 dogs after a dose reduction. Moistening the food and pancreatic powder mix may also decrease the frequency of this side effect. When clinical signs have resolved, the amount of pancreatic enzymes given can be gradually decreased to the lowest effective dose, which may vary from animal to animal, and from batch to batch of the pancreatic supplement. Fresh pancreas may be a viable alternative to the use of powder; 1-3 oz (30-90 g) of raw chopped pancreas can replace 1 tsp of pancreatic extract. Because of a slight risk of transmission of Aujeszky's disease from raw porcine pancreas, only raw bovine pancreas should be used. Raw pancreas can be kept frozen for several months without loss of enzymatic activity. Preincubation of the food with pancreatic enzymes or supplementation with bile salts is not necessary. Concurrent antacid therapy has little effect on overall digestive ability and is unnecessary in almost all EPI patients.

Even though pancreatic enzyme supplementation decreases the clinical signs in almost all animals, nutrient absorption, especially of fats, is not normalized. Feeding low-fat diets to accommodate impaired fat digestion has been suggested, but this may further decrease fat assimilation and lead to deficiencies of fat-soluble vitamins and/or essential fatty acids. Some types of dietary fiber interfere with pancreatic enzyme activity, and a diet low in insoluble or nonfermentable fiber should be fed.

Enzyme supplementation alone may not lead to complete resolution of clinical signs; cobalamin deficiency should be considered as a possible cause. Cobalamin absorption depends on adequate synthesis and secretion of intrinsic factor. In cats, ~99% of intrinsic factor is secreted by the exocrine pancreas, and most cats with EPI are cobalamin deficient. In contrast, in dogs, ~90% of intrinsic factor is secreted by the exocrine pancreas, and cobalamin deficiency is seen in slightly <50% of dogs with EPI. Thus, serum cobalamin and folate concentrations should be routinely evaluated in small animals with suspected EPI. Dogs and cats with cobalamin deficiency, suggested by a severely decreased serum cobalamin concentration, should be treated with cobalamin parenterally. Other hypovitaminoses have been reported. For example, vitamin K deficiency leading to a coagulopathy has been reported in some cats with EPI. Some animals may not respond to enzyme supplementation and cobalamin therapy and likely have concurrent small-intestinal disease. Dogs with EPI commonly have concurrent small-intestinal bacterial overgrowth and may need antibiotic therapy, while cats with EPI often have concurrent inflammatory bowel disease.

Prognosis: EPI results from an irreversible loss of pancreatic acinar tissue in most cases, and recovery is rare. However, with appropriate management and monitoring, these animals usually gain weight quickly, pass normal stools, and can live a normal life for a normal life span.

PANCREATIC NEOPLASMS

Neoplasias of the exocrine pancreas can be primary or secondary and can be classified as benign or malignant. Pancreatic adenomas are benign tumors that are usually singular and can be differentiated from pancreatic nodular hyperplasia by the presence of a capsule. Pancreatic adenocarcinoma is the most common neoplastic condition of the exocrine pancreas in dogs and cats. Epidemiologic studies based on necropsy findings suggest that pancreatic adenocarcinoma is common in both dogs and cats. However, pancreatic adenocarcinoma is rarely diagnosed clinically in either species. A few cases of pancreatic sarcomas, ie, spindle cell sarcoma and lymphosarcoma, have also been reported.

Pathogenesis: Benign neoplasms can lead to transposition of organs of the cranial abdominal cavity. However, these changes are subclinical in most cases, and the diagnosis is often made as an incidental finding during necropsy. In rare cases, the neoplastic growth can obstruct the pancreatic duct and cause secondary atrophy of the remaining exocrine pancreas, leading to EPI. Adenocarcinomas may lead to tumor necrosis, if the tumor outgrows its blood supply. Tumor necrosis causes local inflammation, which can lead to clinical signs of pancreatitis. Malignant neoplasms may also spread to neighboring or distant organs.

Clinical Findings: The presentation of dogs and cats with exocrine pancreatic neoplasia is nonspecific, and many cases remain subclinical until late in the disease. Some animals show clinical signs suggestive of pancreatitis. Obstructive jaundice may be seen if bile duct obstruction develops. Clinical signs related to metastatic lesions have also been reported in some cases of pancreatic adenocarcinoma and may present as lameness, bone pain, or dyspnea. Recently, paraneoplastic alopecia has been reported in cats with pancreatic adenocarcinoma.

Diagnosis: Several nonspecific findings, such as neutrophilia, anemia, hypokalemia, bilirubinemia, azotemia, hyperglycemia, and elevated hepatic enzymes, have been reported in dogs and cats with pancreatic adenocarcinoma. However, results of routine blood tests may be unremarkable. Elevated serum lipase and amylase activities have not been commonly reported in either dogs or cats with pancreatic adenocarcinoma, but some dogs with pancreatic adenocarcinoma have extremely high serum lipase activities, reaching as high as 25 times the upper limit of the reference range.

Radiographic findings are also nonspecific in most cases. Abnormal findings include decreased contrast in the cranial abdomen suggesting peritoneal effusion, transposition of the spleen caudally, and shadowing in the pyloric region. In some cases, abdominal radiographs suggest a cranial abdominal mass. Abdominal ultrasound generally shows a soft-tissue mass near the pancreas, but in many if not most cases, continuation of the mass with pancreatic tissue cannot be demonstrated conclusively. Neoplastic lesions of neighboring organs also may be falsely presumed to be pancreatic. Finally, animals with severe pancreatitis may show an ultrasonographic mass effect in the area of the pancreas that must not be confused with a pancreatic adenocarcinoma. If peritoneal effusion is present, a sample should be aspirated and evaluated cytologically. However, in most cases neoplastic cells do not readily exfoliate into the peritoneal effusion, and no neoplastic cells are identified on cytology. Fine needle aspiration or transcutaneous biopsy under ultrasonographic guidance can be attempted when suspicious masses are identified. Ultrasonographic-guided biopsy of the pancreatic mass has been reported infrequently but will allow a definitive diagnosis in up to 50% of cases. In many cases, the diagnosis is made at exploratory laparotomy or necropsy.

Treatment and Prognosis: Pancreatic adenomas are benign and theoretically do not require therapy unless they cause clinical signs. However, because the final diagnosis of pancreatic adenocarcinoma is often made at exploratory laparotomy, a partial pancreatectomy should be performed even in cases of suspected pancreatic adenoma. The prognosis in these cases is excellent. Pancreatic adenocarcinomas often present at a late stage of disease. Metastatic disease at the time of diagnosis is common in both dogs and cats. Common sites for metastasis are the liver, abdominal and thoracic lymph nodes, mesentery, intestines, and lungs, but other metastatic sites have also been reported. In those few cases when gross metastatic lesions are not identified at the time of diagnosis, surgical resection of the tumor may be attempted, but clean surgical margins can almost never be achieved and owners should be forewarned. Both chemotherapy and radiation therapy have shown little success in human or veterinary patients with pancreatic adenocarcinomas. Thus, the prognosis for dogs and cats with pancreatic adenocarcinoma is grave.

PANCREATIC ABSCESSES

A pancreatic abscess is a collection of pus, usually in proximity to the pancreas, containing little or no pancreatic necrosis. Pancreatic abscesses are considered a complication of pancreatitis. A bacterial infection may or may not be present, but almost all cases reported in small animals have been sterile. Clinical signs are nonspecific and may include vomiting, depression, abdominal pain, anorexia, fever, diarrhea, and dehydration. In some animals, abdominal palpation reveals a mass in the cranial abdomen. Common clinicopathologic findings are neutrophilia with a left shift, elevated serum amylase and lipase activities, elevated hepatic enzyme activities, and hyperbilirubinemia. Surgical drainage and aggressive antimicrobial therapy are the treatments of choice in human patients with a pancreatic abscess. Dogs and cats may also respond favorably to surgical drainage. However, in one report only slightly >50% of animals survived the immediate postsurgical period. Thus, given the mixed results and risks, difficulties, and expenses associated with anesthesia, surgery, and postoperative care, surgery may not be warranted unless there is clear evidence of an enlarging mass and/or sepsis in a medically managed animal.

PANCREATIC PSEUDOCYST

A pancreatic pseudocyst is a collection of sterile pancreatic fluid enclosed by a wall of fibrous or granulation tissue; these structures are also considered a complication of pancreatitis. Recently, several cases of pancreatic pseudocysts in dogs and cats have been described. Clinical signs are usually nonspecific and mimic those of pancreatitis. Vomiting is the most consistent clinical sign reported in both dogs and cats. In some cases, a mass can be palpated in the cranial abdomen. On abdominal ultrasonography, a cystic structure in close proximity to the pancreas can be identified. Aspiration of the pseudocyst is relatively safe and should be attempted for diagnostic and therapeutic purposes. Fluid from a pancreatic pseudocyst should have few cells and should not contain any evidence of inflammation. Pancreatic pseudocysts can be treated medically or surgically. Medical management involves ultrasonographic-guided percutaneous aspiration and close monitoring of the size of the pseudocyst. Surgery may be indicated in animals with persistent clinical signs or when the pseudocyst fails to regress over time.

GASTROINTESTINAL PARASITES OF SMALL ANIMALS

SPIROCERCA LUPI
(Esophageal worm)

Adult *Spirocerca lupi* are bright red worms, 40 mm (male) to 70 mm (female) long, generally located within nodules in the esophageal, gastric, or aortic walls. Infections are seen in southern areas of the USA as well as in most tropical regions worldwide. Dogs are infected by eating an intermediate host (usually dung beetle) or a transport host (eg, chickens, reptiles, or rodents). The larvae migrate via the wall of the thoracic aorta, where they usually remain for ~3 mo. Eggs are passed in feces ~5-6 mo after infection.

Clinical Findings: Most dogs with *S lupi* infection show no clinical signs. When the esophageal lesion is very large (usually when it has become neoplastic), the dog has difficulty swallowing and may vomit repeatedly after trying to eat. Such dogs salivate profusely and eventually become emaciated. In addition, dogs may develop spondylitis or enlargement of the extremities characteristic of hypertrophic osteopathy. These clinical signs are suggestive of spirocercosis in regions where the parasite is prevalent. Occasionally, a dog dies suddenly as the result of massive hemorrhage into the thorax after rupture of the aorta damaged by the developing worms.

Lesions: The characteristic lesions are aneurysm of the thoracic aorta, reactive granulomas of variable size around the worms in the esophagus, and deformative ossifying spondylitis of the posterior thoracic vertebrae. Esophageal sarcoma, often with metastases, is sometimes associated (apparently causally) with *S lupi* infection, particularly in hound breeds. Dogs with *Spirocerca*-related sarcoma often develop hypertrophic osteopathy (p 973).

Diagnosis: Diagnosis can be made by demonstrating the characteristic small (11-15 × 30-37 μm), elongated eggs (by $NaNO_3$ [specific gravity 1.36] flotation) that contain larvae in the feces. However, eggs are sporadically voided in feces and can be difficult to find. Gastroscopy occasionally reveals a nodule or an adult worm. A presumptive diagnosis can be made by radiographic examination when it reveals dense masses in the esophagus; a positive-contrast barium study may help define the lesion.

Most infections are not diagnosed until necropsy. The granulomas vary greatly in size and location in the esophagus but usually are so characteristic as to be diagnostic, even if the worms are no longer present. Worms and granulomas may be present in the lungs, trachea, mediastinum, stomach wall, or other abnormal locations. Healed aneurysms of the aorta persist for the life of the dog and are diagnostic of previous infection. When sarcomas are associated with the infection, the esophageal lesion usually is larger and often contains cartilage or bone; metastases frequently are present in the lungs, lymph nodes, heart, liver, or kidneys.

Treatment and Control: In endemic areas, dogs should be prevented from eating dung beetles, frogs, mice, lizards, etc, and not fed raw chicken scraps. Treatment is often not practical. However, efficacy has been demonstrated with disophenol (10 mg/kg, SC, 2 doses 1 wk apart) and doramectin (0.2 mg/kg, SC, 3 doses at 2-wk intervals; 0.4 mg/kg, SC, 6 doses at 2-wk intervals; 0.8 mg/kg, SC, 2 doses 1 wk apart; additional treatments may be required), although these treatments are not approved. Surgical removal usually is unsuccessful because of the large areas of the esophagus involved.

PHYSALOPTERA SPP
(Stomach worm)

Several species of these stomach nematodes of dogs and cats are seen throughout the world. They are usually firmly attached to the gastric or duodenal mucosa. The males are ~30 mm and the females ~40 mm long. The eggs are oval, 32×55 µm, thick-shelled, and larvated.

Encysted infective larvae of *Physaloptera* spp have been found in several species of insects, including beetles, cockroaches, and crickets. Mice and frogs may be paratenic hosts. After the dog or cat ingests the intermediate or paratenic host, development of larvae to adults is direct. These parasites may cause gastritis or duodenitis, which can result in vomiting, anorexia, and dark feces. Bleeding, ulcerated areas remain on the gastric mucosa when the parasites move to other locations; in heavy infections, anemia and weight loss may develop. Gastroscopy is the most efficient means of diagnosis, and immature worms are often found in the vomitus of puppies or kittens. The eggs are difficult to find in feces because they do not readily float. In cats, pyrantel pamoate (5 mg/kg, PO, 2 doses 2-3 wk apart; 20 mg/kg, PO, once) and ivermectin (0.2 mg/kg, SC, once) can be used for *Physaloptera* infections. In dogs, fenbendazole (50 mg/kg, PO, SID for 3 days), pyrantel pamoate (5 mg/kg, PO, once; 15 mg/kg, PO, 2 doses 2-3 wk apart; 20 mg/kg, PO, once), and ivermectin (0.2 mg/kg, PO, once) can be used. None of these medications is approved for treatment of *Physaloptera* in either dogs or cats.

OLLULANUS SP

Ollulanus tricuspis is a small worm, ≤1 mm long, that infects several animal species and occasionally induces a mild erosive or catarrhal gastritis in cats. Vomiting minutes to a few hours after eating is a common sign. The females are viviparous, so massive infections can build up endogenously. Transmission is via vomitus. Diagnosis is by microscopic demonstration of worms in the vomitus. The use of a Baermann apparatus enables the separation of the worms from ingesta, after which they are easier to observe. Therapeutic efficacy in cats has been demonstrated with fenbendazole (20-50 mg/kg, PO, SID for 3 days) and levamisole (5 mg/kg, SC, once), although these are not approved treatments.

STRONGYLOIDES SP

Strongyloides stercoralis is a small, slender nematode that when fully mature is located at the base of the villi in the anterior half of the small intestine of dogs and cats. The worms are almost transparent and all but impossible to see grossly at necropsy. Usually, infections are associated with warm, wet, crowded, unsanitary housing. The species found most often in dogs is identical to that found in people.

The parasitic worms are all females. The eggs embryonate rapidly, and most larvae hatch before being passed in the feces. Under appropriate conditions of warmth and moisture, extracorporeal development is rapid. The third larval stage may be reached in little more than a day. Some of these larvae develop into infective filariform larvae; others develop into free-living worms that mate and produce progeny similar to that of the parasitic female. The filariform larvae penetrate the skin but also may infect a host via the oral cavity. Transmammary transmission is possible. Progeny may be shed in the feces 7-10 days after infection. Autoinfection caused by larvae that developed to the infective stage within the GI tract can result in infections in which dogs shed larvae for lengthy periods.

Clinical Findings: The presence of clinical signs indicates that a heavy infection has been building up for some weeks. A blood-streaked, mucoid diarrhea, usually seen in young animals during hot humid weather, is characteristic. Emaciation is often prominent, and reduced growth rate may be one of the first signs. Appetite usually is good, and the dog is normally active in the earlier stages of the disease. In the absence of concurrent secondary infections, there is little or no fever. Usually in advanced stages, there is shallow, rapid breathing and pyrexia, and the prognosis is grave. Autoinfection may be induced by the use of corticosteroids or other factors that affect immunocompetence. There may be larvae in tissues, and these dogs are more likely to die. At necropsy, there can be evidence of verminous pneumonia with large areas of consolidation in the lungs as well as marked enteritis with hemorrhage, mucosal exfoliation, and much secretion of mucus.

Diagnosis: Larvae are identified by direct microscopic evaluation of a small quantity of feces. Usually, the Baermann technique is used to separate larvae from fecal material. It is important to use fresh fecal material obtained from the infected dog so that the larvae can be easily differentiated from hookworm larvae or free-living soil nematodes. Adult female worms can be identified by scraping the mucosa of the small intestine. They are only ~2 mm long, but the presence of eggs in the uterus easily differentiates them from larvae of other nematodes.

Treatment and Control: Poor sanitation and mixing of susceptible with infected dogs can lead to a rapid buildup of the infection in all dogs in a kennel or pen. Dogs with diarrhea should be promptly isolated from dogs that appear healthy. Direct sunlight, increased soil or surface temperatures, and desiccation are deleterious to all free larval stages. Thorough washing of wooden and impervious surfaces with steam or concentrated salt or lime solutions, followed by rinsing with hot water, effectively destroys the parasite. Because the disease in humans can be serious, caution should be exercised in handling infected dogs. The disease in people (as in dogs) is much more likely to be severe if the person is immunosuppressed.

Infections in dogs can be treated with ivermectin (0.2 mg/kg, SC or PO, once, with a second dose required in some animals; 0.8 mg/kg, PO, once) or thiabendazole (100-150 mg/kg, PO, SID for 3 days, repeated weekly until larvae are not detected in feces—toxicity may be observed with this regimen). In cats, fenbendazole (50 mg/kg, PO, SID for 3 days) can be used. These are not approved regimens in either cats or dogs. In all animals, feces should be examined regularly for at least 6 mo after treatment to confirm efficacy.

ROUNDWORMS
(Ascariasis)

The large roundworms (ascaridoid nematodes) of dogs and cats are common, especially in puppies and kittens. Of the 3 species *Toxocara canis, Toxascaris leonina,* and *Toxocara cati,* the most important is *T canis,* not only because its larvae may migrate in people (as do larvae of *T cati*), but also because fatal infections may be seen in young pups. *T leonina* is seen in adult dogs and in cats. These species also infect wild carnivores, especially those in zoos or other captive settings.

In puppies, the usual mode of infection with *T canis* is transplacental transfer. If pups <3 mo old ingest embryonated eggs, the hatched larvae penetrate the intestinal mucosa, reach the lungs via the liver and bloodstream, are coughed up, swallowed, and mature to egg-producing adults in the small intestine. However, when embryonated infective eggs of *T canis* are swallowed by older dogs, the larvae hatch, penetrate the intestinal mucosa, and migrate to the liver, lungs, muscles, connective tissue, kidneys, and many other tissues, where development is arrested. In pregnant bitches, these dormant larvae mobilize and migrate into the developing fetus; they can be found in the intestine of the puppies as early as 1 wk after birth. Some larvae migrate to the mammary gland, so that pups may also be infected via the milk. During this perinatal period, the immunity of the bitch to ascarid infection is partially suppressed, and substantial numbers of eggs may be passed in feces. Development of these patent infections appears to be associated with maturation of arrested larvae in the bitch, which migrate to the intestine via the lungs, and to ingestion and maturation of larvae that are passed in the feces of puppies.

Larvae of ascaridoid nematodes may migrate into the tissues of many animals and thus provide an alternative source of infection, particularly for cats and wild carnivores. Such migration also occurs if larvated eggs are swallowed by people. Most human infections are asymptomatic, but fever, persistent eosinophilia, and hepatomegaly (sometimes with pulmonary involvement) may occur, resulting in a condition known as **visceral larva migrans**. Rarely, a larva may settle in the retina and impair vision, resulting in a condition known as **ocular larva migrans**.

The life cycles of *T cati* and *T leonina* are similar except that, in the former, no prenatal infection is seen, while in the latter, migration is restricted to the intestinal wall so that neither prenatal nor transmammary transmission occurs.

Clinical Findings and Lesions: The first indication of infection in young animals is lack of growth and loss of condition. Infected animals have a dull coat and often are "potbellied." Worms may be vomited and are often voided in the feces. In the early stages, migrating larvae may cause an eosinophilic pneumonia, which can be associated with coughing. Diarrhea with mucus may be evident.

In puppies with severe infections, verminous pneumonia, ascites, fatty liver, and mucoid enteritis are common. Cortical kidney granulomas containing larvae are frequent in young dogs.

Diagnosis: Infection in dogs and cats is diagnosed by detection of eggs in feces. Distinguishing the spherical, pitted-shelled eggs of *Toxocara* spp from the oval, smooth-shelled eggs of *Toxascaris leonina*, is important because of the public health significance of the former.

Treatment and Control: In dogs, compounds licensed for treatment of roundworm infections include dichlorvos, diethylcarbamazine, fenbendazole, flubendazole, mebendazole, milbemycin, nitroscanate, piperazine, and pyrantel (TABLE 8). In Europe, selamectin is approved to treat *T canis* infections with a single dose, while in Canada approved treatment requires 2 doses 1 mo apart. The following drug combinations can also be used: praziquantel/pyrantel/febantel, pyrantel/febantel, and pyrantel/oxantel. Preventive programs for heartworm infection using milbemycin oxime, milbemycin/lufenuron, pyrantel/ivermectin, selamectin, or oxibendazole/diethylcarbamazine also control intestinal ascarid infections. However, selamectin is approved for this indication in only some countries.

Drugs licensed for treatment of ascarid infections in cats include dichlorvos, diethylcarbamazine, fenbendazole, flubendazole, mebendazole, piperazine, pyrantel, selamectin, and the combination formulation praziquantel/pyrantel (TABLE 8). Heartworm-preventive programs that use milbemycin or selamectin also control ascarid infections in cats.

Environmentally resistant larvated eggs on the ground and somatic larvae in the bitch are the main reservoirs of infection. Perinatal transmission of infection can be greatly reduced by treating bitches with 1) daily doses of fenbendazole (50 mg/kg, PO) from day 40 of gestation to day 14 after whelping, 2) ivermectin (0.3 mg/kg, SC) on days 0, 30, and 60 of gestation, and 10 days after whelping, 3) ivermectin (0.5 mg/kg) on days 38, 41, 44, and 47 of gestation, and 4) ivermectin (1.0 mg/kg) on days 20 and 42 of gestation. Otherwise, to minimize egg output, pups should be treated as early as possible; ideally, treatment should be given 2 wk after birth and repeated at 2- to 3-wk intervals to 3 mo of age. Nursing bitches should be treated at the same times. Because the eggs adhere to many surfaces and become mixed in soil and dust, strict hygiene should be observed by people, particularly children, exposed to potentially contaminated animals or areas.

TABLE 8. Drugs with Approved Activity Against Intestinal Helminths of Dogs and Cats

Drug/Drug Combination	Dog	Cat
Dichlorophene	200 mg/kg, PO (UK) 220 mg/kg, PO (USA)	200 mg/kg, PO (UK)
Dichlorvos	27-33 mg/kg, PO for adults (extra-label) 11 mg/kg, PO for all ages (USA)	11 mg/kg, PO (USA)
Diethylcarbamazine citrate	55-110 mg/kg, PO; repeat 10-20 days later (USA, CAN)	55-110 mg/kg, PO; repeat 10-20 days later (CAN)
Diethylcarbamazine citrate + oxibendazole (daily HW)	6.6 mg/kg + 5 mg/kg, respectively, PO (USA)	
Epsiprantel	5.5 mg/kg, PO (USA, CAN)	2.75 mg/kg, PO (USA, CAN)
Fenbendazole	50 mg/kg, PO, SID for 3 days (USA, CAN, UK) 100 mg/kg, PO for adults (UK)	50 mg/kg, PO, SID for 3 days (UK) 100 mg/kg, PO for adults (UK)
Flubendazole	22 mg/kg, PO, SID for 2 days for roundworms and hookworms; SID for 3 days for *Trichuris vulpis* and *Taenia pisiformis* (UK)	22 mg/kg, PO, SID for 2 days for roundworms and hookworms; SID for 3 days for *Taenia taeniaeformis* (UK)
Ivermectin (monthly HW)		0.024 mg/kg (USA, CAN)
Ivermectin + pyrantel (monthly HW)	0.006 mg/kg + 5 mg/kg, respectively, PO (USA, CAN)	
Mebendazole	50-200 mg total, PO, BID for 2-5 days; depends on age and weight (UK)	50-200 mg total, PO, BID for 2-5 days; depends on age and weight (UK)
Milbemycin oxime (monthly HW + therapy)	0.5 mg/kg, PO (USA, CAN, UK)	2.0 mg/kg, PO (USA, CAN)
Milbemycin oxime + lufenuron (monthly HW)	0.5 mg/kg + 10 mg/kg, respectively, PO (USA, CAN, UK)	
Moxidectin	0.17 mg/kg, SC; 6-mo HW injectable (USA, CAN)	
Nitroscanate	50 mg/kg, PO (CAN, UK)	
Piperazine	55-62 mg/kg, PO for roundworms, re-treat 10 days after first treatment (USA, CAN); 80-100 mg piperazine hydrate/kg, PO for roundworms (UK); 120-240 mg piperazine hydrate/kg, PO for hookworms (UK)	55-62 mg/kg, PO for roundworms, re-treat 10 days after first treatment (USA, CAN); 80-100 mg piperazine hydrate/kg, PO for roundworms (UK); 120-240 mg piperazine hydrate/kg, PO for hookworms (UK)

TABLE 8. (continued)

Drug/Drug Combination	Dog	Cat
Praziquantel	Follow label dose PO, SC, IM (USA, CAN) 5 mg/kg, PO (UK) 5.68 mg/kg, SC, IM (UK)	Follow label dose PO, SC, IM (USA, CAN) 5 mg/kg, PO (UK) 5.68 mg/kg, SC, IM (UK) Follow label dose for topical formulation (UK)
Praziquantel + pyrantel		Follow label dose, PO (USA, CAN, UK)
Praziquantel + pyrantel + febantel	Follow label dose, PO (USA, CAN, UK)	
Pyrantel	5 mg/kg, PO for dogs >2.3 kg (USA) 10 mg/kg, PO for dogs <2.3 kg (USA) 5 mg/kg, PO for all weights (USA, CAN, UK)	20 mg/kg, PO; repeat 7-10 days later (CAN) 5-10 mg/kg, PO; repeat 2 wk later (extra-label)
Pyrantel + febantel	14.4 mg/kg + 15 mg/kg, respectively, PO (UK)	
Pyrantel + oxantel	5 mg/kg + 20 mg/kg, respectively, PO (CAN)	
Selamectin (monthly HW + therapy)	6 mg/kg, topical (CAN, UK)	6 mg/kg, topical (USA, CAN, UK)

*See text for specific approvals; (USA) = approved in the USA; (UK) = approved in the UK; (CAN) = approved in Canada; HW = heartworm prevention.

HOOKWORMS

Ancylostoma caninum is the principal cause of canine hookworm disease in most tropical and subtropical areas of the world. *A tubaeforme* of cats has a similar but more sparse distribution. *A braziliense* of dogs and cats is sparsely distributed from Florida to North Carolina in the USA. *Uncinaria stenocephala* is the principal canine hookworm in cooler regions; it is the canine hookworm in Canada and the northern fringe of the USA, where it is primarily a fox parasite. *U stenocephala* also is seen in cats. *A caninum* males are ~12 mm long, females, 15 mm; the other species are somewhat smaller. The infective larvae of canine hookworms, particularly those of *A braziliense*, may penetrate and wander under the skin of people and cause either **cutaneous larva migrans** or eosinophilic enteritis.

The elongate (>65 μm), thin-walled, hookworm eggs in the early cleavage stages (2-8 cells) are first passed in the feces 15-20 days after infection; they complete embryonation and hatch in 24-72 hr on warm, moist soil. Transmission may result from ingestion of infective larvae from the environment or, in the case of *A caninum*, via the colostrum or milk of infected bitches. Infections with either *A caninum* or *A braziliense* can also result from larval invasion through the skin, but this route is of little significance for *U stenocephala*. Skin penetration in young pups is followed by migration of the larvae through the blood to the lungs, where they are coughed up and swallowed to mature in the small intestine. However, in animals >3 mo old, *A caninum* larvae, after migration through the lungs, are arrested in the somatic tissues. Arrested development may also occur in the mucosa of the small intestine. These arrested larvae are activated after removal of adult worms from the intestine or during pregnancy when they accumulate in the mammary glands.

Clinical Findings: An acute normocytic, normochromic anemia followed by hypo chromic, microcytic anemia in young puppies is the characteristic, and often fatal, clinical manifestation of *A caninum* infection. Surviving puppies develop some immunity and show lesser clinical signs. Nevertheless, debilitated and malnourished animals may con tinue to be unthrifty and suffer from chronic anemia. Mature, well-nourished dogs may harbor a few worms without showing signs; they are of primary concern as the direct or indirect source of infection for pups. Diarrhea with dark, tarry feces accompanies severe infections. Anemia, anorexia, emaciation, and weakness develop in chronic disease.

Lesions: Anemia results directly from the bloodsucking and the bleeding ulcer ations that result when *A caninum* shift feeding sites. The amount of blood loss due to a single worm in 24 hr has been estimated to be up to 0.1 mL. There is no interference with erythropoiesis in uncomplicated hookworm disease. The liver and other organs may ap pear ischemic with some fatty infiltration of the liver. Neither *A braziliense* nor *U steno cephala* is an avid blood feeder, and anemia rarely develops. However, hypoproteinemia is characteristic, and serum seepage around the site of attachment in the intestine may reduce blood protein by >10%. Hemorrhagic enteritis with a swollen intestinal mucosa that shows red, small ulcers and attached worms is usually seen in acute, fatal cases.

Dermatitis due to larval invasion of the skin may be seen with any of the hookworms but has been seen most frequently in the interdigital spaces with *U stenocephala*. Pneu monia and lung consolidation may result from overwhelming infections in pups.

Diagnosis: The characteristic thin-shelled, oval eggs are easily seen on flotation of fresh feces from infected dogs. Acute anemia and death from infections acquired via milk may be seen in young pups before eggs are passed in their feces, ie, as early as 1-2 wk of age.

Treatment and Control: Bitches should be free of hookworms before breeding and kept out of contaminated areas during pregnancy. Bitches should whelp and the pups suckle in sanitary quarters. Concrete runways that can be washed at least twice a week in warm weather are best. Sunlit clay or sandy runways can be decontaminated with sodium borate (1 kg/2 m^2).

In dogs, the following drugs and drug combinations are approved for treatment of *A caninum* and *U stenocephala* infections: dichlorvos, fenbendazole, flubendazole, me bendazole, nitroscanate, piperazine, pyrantel, pyrantel/febantel, pyrantel/oxantel, and praziquantel/pyrantel/febantel. Milbemycin is also licensed for treatment of *A caninum* infections (TABLE 8). When anemia is severe, chemotherapy may have to be supported by blood transfusion or supplemental iron, and followed by a high-protein diet until the Hgb level is normal. Heartworm prevention with milbemycin, milbemycin/lufenuron, and di ethylcarbamazine/oxibendazole also controls *A caninum*, while pyrantel/ivermectin controls *A caninum*, *A braziliense*, and *U stenocephala*. Finally, the injectable formula tion of moxidectin for heartworm prevention in dogs also has significant efficacy against infection with *A caninum* and *U stenocephala* for at least 3 mo.

In cats, drugs approved for treatment of *A tubaeforme* include dichlorvos, flubendazole, mebendazole, milbemycin, piperazine, pyrantel, pyrantel/praziquantel, and selamectin (TABLE 8). Dichlorvos, flubendazole, mebendazole, and piperazine are also approved for treatment of *U stenocephala* infections. Heartworm prevention with ivermectin, milbemy cin, and selamectin controls *A tubaeforme*, while ivermectin also controls *A braziliense*.

When neonatal pups die due to hookworm infection, subsequent litters from the bitch should be treated weekly for *A caninum* for ~12 wk beginning at 2 wk of age. In addition, fenbendazole (50 mg/kg, PO) given daily to pregnant bitches from day 40 of preg nancy to day 14 after whelping greatly reduces transmammary transmission to the pups. Likewise, treatment of the bitch with ivermectin (0.5 mg/kg) on 2 occasions (4-9 days before whelping and 10 days later) has the same effect.

WHIPWORMS
(Trichuriasis)

Adult *Trichuris vulpis* are 40-70 mm long and consist of a long, slender anterior por tion and a thick posterior third. They commonly inhabit the cecum of dogs where they are firmly attached to the wall, with their anterior end embedded in the mucosa. Thick-shelled eggs with bipolar plugs are passed in the feces and become infective in 2-4 wk in a warm, moist environment. Although eggs may remain viable in a suitable environment for up to 5 yr, they are susceptible to desiccation. The life cycle is direct. After infective eggs are ingested, the larvae develop in the jejunal wall, and the adults mature in the cecum in ~11 wk. They may remain for up to 16 mo.

No signs are seen in light infections, but as the worm burden increases and the in-flammatory (and occasionally hemorrhagic) reaction in the cecum becomes more pro-nounced, weight loss and diarrhea become evident. Fresh blood may be seen in the feces of heavily infected dogs, and anemia occasionally follows.

Trichuris infections rarely are seen in cats in North America but may occasionally be associated with clinical signs similar to those described for dogs.

Treatment and Control: The eggs are susceptible to desiccation; therefore, by main-taining cleanliness and eliminating moist areas, the risk of infection in dogs can be reduced considerably, although *T vulpis* infections can be difficult to control. For anthelmintic treatment of dogs, licensed compounds include fenbendazole, flubendazole, mebendazole, milbemycin, and the combination formulations praziquantel/pyrantel/febantel, pyrantel/febantel, and pyrantel/oxantel (TABLE 8). Treatment should be repeated 3 times at monthly intervals because of the long prepatent period. Finally, milbemycin oxime, milbemycin/lufenuron, and diethylcarbamazine/oxibendazole, when administered for heartworm pre-vention, are also approved for control of *T vulpis* infections.

Effective therapy has yet to be described for *Trichuris* infections in cats. If required, treatment should be attempted on an experimental basis using a compound with li-censed activity against *T vulpis*.

ACANTHOCEPHALANS
(Thorny-headed worms)

Oncicola sp

Oncicola canis are rarely found in the small intestine of dogs and cats in the western hemisphere. They are white and ~12 mm long, and their thorny heads are embedded in the mucosa. The females lay brown, thick-shelled, embryonated, wide oval eggs (45 × 65 μm). The life cycle is not completely known, but it is thought to include an arthropod interme-diate host and paratenic hosts such as turkeys or armadillos. Most infections cause no clinical signs.

Macracanthorhynchus sp

Macracanthorhynchus ingens, naturally a parasite of raccoons, is occasionally found in dogs. The usual observation is of a large (8-12 cm), white, wrinkled worm passed in the feces. No clinical signs have been definitively associated with the infection. The life cycle requires a millipede as an intermediate host, but other animals may serve as paratenic hosts. The eggs look similar to those of *Oncicola canis* but are larger (~50 × 100 μm). Diagnosis of patent infections is unlikely because experimentally in-duced infections did not persist after 1-12 days of patency. No treatment is necessary.

TAPEWORMS
(Cestodes)

Most urban dogs and cats eat prepared foods and have restricted access to natural prey. Such animals may acquire *Dipylidium caninum* (the double-pored dog tape-worm) from fleas. Cats with access to infected house (or outdoor) mice and rats also can acquire *Taenia taeniaeformis*. Suburban, rural, and hunting dogs have more access to various small mammals, in addition to raw meat and offal from domestic and wild ungu-lates. A number of cestodes can be expected in such dogs (*see* TABLE 9). On sheep ranges

TABLE 9. Cestodes of Dogs and Cats in North America ▶

Cestode	Definitive Host	Intermediate Host and Organs Invaded*
Dipylidium caninum	Dog, cat, coyote, wolf, fox, other animals	Fleas and more rarely lice; free in body cavity
Taenia taeniaeformis	Cat, dog, lynx, wolf, other animals	Various rats, mice, other rodents; in large cysts in liver
Taenia pisiformis	Dog, cat, fox, wolf, coyote, lynx, other animals	Rabbits and hares, rarely squirrels and other rodents; in pelvic or peritoneal cavity attached to viscera
Taenia hydatigena	Dog, wolf, coyote, lynx, rarely cat	Domestic and wild cloven-hoofed animals, rarely hares and rodents; in liver and abdominal cavity
Spirometra mansonoides	Cat, dog, raccoon, bobcat	Copepods, frogs, rodents, snakes, connective tissue
Diphyllobothrium spp	Human, dog, cat, other fish-eating animals	Encysted in various organs, or free in body cavity of various fish

TABLE 9. *(continued)*

Diagnostic Features of Adult Worm	Comments	Approved Treatment[†]
Strobila 15-70 cm long and up to 3 mm in maximum width, 30-150 rostellar hooks of rose-thorn shape in 3 or 4 circles; large hooks 12-15 μm, smallest 5-6 μm long. Segments shaped like cucumber seeds with pore near middle of each lateral margin.	Probably most common tapeworm of dogs, less common in cats; cosmopolitan. Occasionally infects humans, particularly infants.	Dogs and cats: dichlorophene, epsiprantel, praziquantel Dogs only: nitroscanate, praziquantel/pyrantel/ febantel Cats only: praziquantel/ pyrantel
Strobila 15-60 cm long, 5-6 mm in maximum width, 26-52 rostellar hooks in double row; large hooks 380-420 μm, small hooks 250-270 μm long. No neck. Sacculate lateral branches of uterus difficult to count.	Common cestode of cats, rare in dogs; cosmopolitan	Cats: epsiprantel, flubendazole, praziquantel, praziquantel/pyrantel, dichlorophene, fenbendazole, mebendazole
Strobila 60 cm to 2 m long, 5 mm in maximum width, ~34-48 rostellar hooks in double row; large hooks 225-290 μm, small hooks 132-177 μm long. Each side of gravid uterus has 5-10 lateral branches.	Particularly common in suburban, farm, and hunting dogs that eat rabbits and rabbit viscera.	Dogs: epsiprantel, fenbendazole, flubendazole, praziquantel, praziquantel/ pyrantel/febantel, nitroscanate, dichlorophene, fenbendazole, mebendazole
Strobila to 5 m long and 7 mm in maximum width; ~26-44 rostellar hooks in double row; large hooks 170-220 μm, small hooks 110-160 μm long. Each side of gravid uterus 5-10 lateral branches.	In farm dogs, more rarely hunting dogs; cosmopolitan	Dogs: praziquantel, nitroscanate, dichlorophene, fenbendazole, mebendazole
Strobila 0.5 m long, 8 mm in maximum width. Scolex with 2 grooves and no hooks. Genital pores ventral midline of segment.	Eastern and Gulf Coast, North America	*See* text for extra-label treatment
Strobila to 10 m long, 20 mm in maximum width but usually smaller. Scolex with 2 grooves (bothria) and no hooks. Genital pores ventral midline of segment	Canada, Alaska and various other states of the USA, Siberia, and other areas	*See* text for extra-label treatment

(continued)

TABLE 9.   Cestodes of Dogs and Cats in North America (continued) ▶

Cestode	Definitive Host	Intermediate Host and Organs Invaded[*]
Echinococcus granulosus	Dog, wolf, coyote, possibly fox, and several other wild carnivores	Sheep, goats, cattle, pigs, horses, deer, moose, some rodents, occasionally humans and other animals; commonly in liver and lungs, occasionally in other organs and tissues
Echinococcus multilocularis	Arctic, red, and gray foxes; coyote, cat, dog	Microtine rodents, occasionally in humans; in the liver
Mesocestoides spp	Many wild canids, felids, mustelids; other animals, including dog and cat	Complete life cycle unknown; arthropod intermediate hosts suspected; juvenile tetrathyridia in abdominal cavity and elsewhere of various mammals, birds, and reptiles; tetrathyridia from body cavity of dogs may enter intestine through intestinal wall.
Taenia multiceps	Dog, coyote, fox, wolf	Sheep, goats, and other domestic or wild ruminants, rarely humans; usually in brain and spinal cord
Taenia serialis	Dog, coyote, fox, wolf	Rabbit, hare, squirrel, rarely humans; in subcutaneous connective tissue or retroperitoneally

◀ **TABLE 9.** (continued)

Diagnostic Features of Adult Worm	Comments	Approved Treatment[†]
Strobila 2-6 mm long with 3-5 segments; 28-50 (usually 30-36) rostellar hooks in double row; large hooks 27-40 μm, small hooks 21-25 μm.	Foci among North American range sheep and dogs associating with them are known; sylvatic moose-wolf cycle where these animals are found; probably cosmopolitan	Dogs: praziquantel, mebendazole, praziquantel/pyrantel/febantel
Strobila 1.2-2.7 mm long with 2-4 segments; along with above species smallest tapeworm in dogs; 26-36 rostellar hooks in double row; large hooks 23-29 μm, small hooks 19-26 μm.	Eastern Europe, former USSR, Alaska and midwestern USA, and Canada; thus far, significant cycle in cats and dogs in North America not recognized	Dogs: praziquantel, mebendazole, praziquantel/pyrantel/febantel Cats: praziquantel, mebendazole
Strobila 10 cm long and 2-5 mm wide. Scolex with 4 suckers but no rostellum or hooks. Genital pore ventral in midline of worm. Gravid segments with paruterine organ.	Reported in dogs and cats in midwest and west; in wild animals elsewhere in USA and Canada; probably cosmopolitan	Dogs: praziquantel
Strobila 40-100 cm long and up to 5 mm wide. Scolex with 4 suckers and 22-32 hooks in double row; large hooks 150-170 μm, small hooks 90-130 μm. Vagina with reflexed curve near lateral excretory canal; 9-26 lateral branches on gravid uterus.	Rare in domestic carnivores in western North America; more common in wild animals; probably cosmopolitan	Dogs: dichlorophene, fenbendazole, mebendazole, nitroscanate
Strobila 20-72 cm long and 3-5 mm wide; 26-32 hooks in double row; large hooks 110-175 μm, small hooks 68-120 μm. Vagina with reflexed curve near lateral excretory canal; 20-25 lateral branches on gravid uterus.	Primarily in wild canids; considered by some authorities as not distinct from *T multiceps*	Same as for *T multiceps*

(continued)

TABLE 9. Cestodes of Dogs and Cats in North America (*continued*) ▶

Cestode	Definitive Host	Intermediate Host and Organs Invaded[*]
Taenia crassiceps	Dog, coyote, fox, wolf	Various rodents, perhaps other animals, a few records in humans; subcutaneous and in body cavities
Taenia krabbei	Dog, coyote, wolf, bobcat	Moose, deer, reindeer; in striated muscle
Taenia ovis	Dog, cat (rarely)	Sheep and goat; in musculature, rarely elsewhere

[*]In all cases in which the life cycle is known, cats and dogs become infected by eating animals (or parts) that contain the infective metacestode. These intermediate hosts become infected by ingesting tapeworm eggs (except in *Mesocestoides* spp, *Spirometra*, and *Diphyllobothrium* spp, which have an extra stage in the life cycle), which are passed in the feces of the definitive host.

and wherever wild ungulates and wild canids are common, dogs may acquire *Echinococcus granulosus* (the hydatid tapeworm). Sylvatic *E multilocularis* (the alveolar hydatid tapeworm), previously known only from arctic North America, has been found in midwestern and western USA and Canada but, thus far, infections in cats or dogs are rare. *Spirometra mansonoides* is an uncommon (but not rare) parasite of cats and occasionally of dogs along the eastern and Gulf Coast areas of North America.

Association with infected dogs may result in human infection with metacestodes of *E granulosus*, *E multilocularis*, *Taenia multiceps*, *T serialis*, or *T crassiceps* in various tissues (by ingestion of eggs passed in dog feces), or adult *D caninum* in the intestine (by ingestion of infected fleas). The presence of metacestodes in livestock may limit commercial use of such carcasses or offal meats. Thus, cestodes of dogs and cats may be of both economic and public health importance (*see* TABLE 10).

Adult cestodes in the intestine of dogs and cats rarely cause serious disease, and clinical signs, if present, may depend on the degree of infection, age, condition, and breed of host. Clinical signs vary from unthriftiness, malaise, irritability, capricious appetite, and shaggy coat to colic and mild diarrhea; rarely, intussusception of the intestine, emaciation, and seizures are seen.

Diagnosis is based on finding proglottids or eggs in the feces. The eggs of *Taenia* spp and *Echinococcus* spp cannot be differentiated by microscopic examination. Direct

◀ TABLE 9. (continued)		
Diagnostic Features of Adult Worm	Comments	Approved Treatment[†]
Strobila 70-170 mm long and 1-2 mm wide. Scolex with 30-36 hooks in double row; large hooks 158-187 μm, small hooks 119-141 μm. Uterus has 16-21 lateral branches, sometimes becoming diffuse.	Reported from Canada and northern USA, including Alaska	Same as for *T multiceps*
Strobila ~20 cm long and up to 9 mm wide. Scolex small with 26-36 hooks in double row; large hooks 146-195 μm, small hooks 85-141 μm. Gravid uterus has 18-24 straight and narrow lateral branches.	Reported from Canada and northern USA, including Alaska; considered by some a subspecies of *T ovis*	Same as for *T multiceps*
Strobila 45-110 cm long and up to 4-8.5 mm wide. Scolex with 32-38 hooks in double row; large hooks 160-202 μm. Gravid uterus has 20-25 lateral branches. Vagina crosses ovary on poral side of segment.	Occasionally from farm dogs in western North America; cosmopolitan	For dogs: praziquantel (5 mg/kg, once PO or SC; extra-label); otherwise same as for *T multiceps*

[†]See TABLE 8 for drug dosages.

microscopic examination of fecal samples or fecal flotation may reveal the eggs of *Spirometra mansonoides*, which are sometimes mistaken for trematode eggs, although they are larger and possess an operculum that is often difficult to see.

Control of tapeworms of dogs and cats requires therapy and prevention. Animals that roam freely usually become reinfected by ingestion of metacestodes in carrion or prey animals. *Dipylidium caninum* is different because it can cycle through fleas that may be associated with confined infected animals. An accurate diagnosis is necessary for effective advice on preventing reinfection.

Effective treatment should remove the attached scolices from the small intestine of infected animals. (*See* TABLE 9 for specific approved treatments.) For dogs, it should be noted that dichlorophene, fenbendazole, mebendazole, and nitroscanate are approved for treatment of *Taenia* spp, and that mebendazole is approved for treatment of *Echinococcus* spp. Likewise, for cats, dichlorophene, fenbendazole, and mebendazole are approved for treatment of *Taenia* spp, and mebendazole and praziquantel are approved for treatment of *Echinococcus* spp.

Praziquantel at 7.5 mg/kg, PO, for 2 consecutive days is effective against *Diphyllobothrium* sp in dogs. Furthermore, a single dose of 35 mg/kg, PO, eliminates *D latum* from infected cats.

Infections with *S mansonoides* in dogs can be treated with praziquantel at 7.5 mg/kg, PO, for 2 consecutive days. *Spirometra* sp infections in cats can be treated with a single dose of praziquantel at 30 mg/kg, SC, IM, or PO.

TABLE 10. Cestodes of Public Health Importance* ▶

Cestode	Host of Adult Worm	Name or Metacestode Intermediate
Taenia saginata	Humans only	Cysticercus "beef measles"
Taenia solium	Humans only	Cysticercus "pork measles"
Diphyllobothrium spp	Humans, dogs, cats, and other fish-eating mammals and birds	Procercoid in copepod, plerocercoid in fish
Echinococcus granulosus	Dogs, wolves, foxes, and several other wild carnivores	Hydatid cyst
Echinococcus multilocularis	Canids and domestic cats	Multilocular or alveolar "cyst" or hydatid

*Human infections with the metacestodes of *Taenia crassiceps, T multiceps, T serialis, Mesocestoides* spp, and other cestodes occur rarely. Children may become infected with adult *Dipylidium caninum*, which appears to have no medical significance but important aesthetic aspects.

FLUKES

Intestinal Flukes

Nanophyetus (Troglotrema) salmincola, the "salmon poisoning" fluke, is a small (0.5 × 0.3 mm), oval fluke found in the small intestine of dogs, cats, and many wild carnivores in the northwestern USA, southwestern Canada, and Siberia. The eggs, which pass in the feces of infected hosts, are light brown, 55 × 45 μm, and indistinctly operculated with a small knob at one pole. The life cycle includes an extended period (3 mo) of embryonation. The first intermediate hosts are snails found in endemic locations (eg, *Oxytrema silicula* in the USA). The cercariae from these snails penetrate the skin of young salmonid fishes and encyst as metacercariae in their muscles and organs. Dogs and other animals become infected by eating raw or improperly prepared infected fish.

Because these flukes embed deeply between the villi of the intestine, infection with a large number may cause enteritis. Most infections, however, are complicated through development of the salmon poisoning complex caused by rickettsial organisms, which the fluke transmits (*see* p 642). Praziquantel (6.7-38.7 mg/kg, SC or IM, once) and fenbendazole (50 mg/kg, PO, SID for 10-14 days) are both effective treatments for dogs.

Alaria alata, A canis, and other *Alaria* spp are small (0.5-1.5 mm) flukes usually found in the small intestine of dogs, cats, foxes, and mink in the western hemisphere, as well as in Europe, Australia, and Japan. The anterior part of the body is flat, and the posterior part is conical. The eggs are oval, light brown, and fairly large (120 × 65 μm). The life cycle includes freshwater snails (eg, *Helisoma* spp) as first intermediate hosts. Cercariae emerge from the snails, penetrate tadpoles, and develop into mesocercariae. Frogs, snakes, and mice then acquire infection by eating tadpoles; the mesocercariae transfer to their tissues and remain as this life-cycle stage. Dogs and other definitive hosts become infected by feeding on these animals. The young flukes migrate through various organs of the definitive host, including the diaphragm and lungs, before reaching the small intestine. Although the flukes are generally considered to be nonpathogenic, large numbers may cause pulmonary hemorrhages during migration or enteritis when they mature in the small intestine. These flukes may infect humans. Infections can be treated with praziquantel using the approved cestocidal dosage (*see* TABLE 9).

TABLE 10. *(continued)*

Measurements of Metacestode	Principal Intermediate Hosts	Site of Metacestode
9 × 5 mm	Cattle	Skeletal and cardiac muscle
6-10 × 5-10 mm	Pigs, dogs (humans may be both definitive and intermediate hosts)	Skeletal and cardiac muscle, occasionally nervous system
2-25 × 2.5 mm	Copepod, then fish	Mesenteric tissues, testes, ovary, muscles
Diameter 50-100 mm, sometimes ≥150 mm	Sheep, cattle, pigs, horses, moose, deer; rarely dogs, cats, humans	Commonly in liver and lungs, occasionally in other organs and tissues
Variable, penetrates like neoplastic tissue	Field mice, voles, lemmings, sometimes domestic mammals and humans	Various organs and tissues

Other species of flukes, usually not pathogenic, have been found occasionally in the intestine of dogs, cats, and other carnivores; these include *Heterophyes heterophyes* in some north African and Asian countries; *Metagonimus yokogawai* in Asia; *Cryptocotyle lingua* in the USA, Canada, Japan, Siberia, and Europe; and *Apophallus donicum* in North America and eastern Europe. Their life cycles include snails as first intermediate hosts and fish as second intermediate hosts, in which metacercariae become encysted.

Heterobilharzia americana is found in the mesenteric veins of dogs and wild animals in southeastern USA. The eggs pass through the tissues of the intestine to the lumen and then are voided with the feces. From the snail intermediate host, the cercariae escape into water and penetrate the skin of dogs and other definitive hosts, migrate to the liver, mature, and move to the mesenteric vessels. Granulomas form around the eggs in the wall of the intestine, the liver, and other parts of the body. Enteritis and wasting may develop in heavy infections. "Water dermatitis" is sometimes seen when cercariae penetrate the skin. The eggs do not readily float and, if placed in water, hatch within minutes; therefore, a sedimentation method using 0.85% saline is useful in separating eggs from ingesta. In infected dogs, eggs are passed intermittently, so on a given day they may not be found in feces. Fenbendazole at 40 mg/kg, PO, SID for 10 days, is an effective treatment. Praziquantel at the approved dosage also appears to be effective.

Hepatic Flukes

Flukes in the bile ducts and gallbladder cause mild to severe fibrosis. Many species of distome trematodes have been reported from the liver of dogs and cats in most parts of the world. Mild infections may pass unnoticed; however, in severe infection, dogs may develop progressive weakness, ending in complete exhaustion, coma, and death. The following are some of the most commonly encountered trematodes.

Opisthorchis felineus (tenuicollis) is parasitic in the bile duct, pancreatic duct, and small intestine of dogs and cats in eastern Europe and parts of Asia. *O viverrini* is seen in dogs as well as in domestic and wild cats in southeast Asia. They are small (9 × 2 mm) and elongate. Their life cycle includes certain snails (*Bithynia* sp) and cyprinid fishes as intermediate hosts. A related species, *Clonorchis sinensis*, the Oriental liver fluke of humans, also has been found in the bile ducts and pancreatic ducts of dogs, cats, and other animals. It is larger than *Opisthorchis* spp. The operculated eggs of these parasites may be identified in the feces of infected animals.

Longterm presence of these flukes in the bile duct causes adenomatous thickening and fibrosis of the duct wall. Carcinomas in the liver or pancreas have been seen in chronic and severe cases. Treatment of *Opisthorchis* spp infections in dogs may be attempted with fenbendazole (200 mg/kg, PO, SID for 3 days) or praziquantel (100 mg/kg, PO, once).

Platynosomum concinnum (fastosum) is a small fluke (6 × 2 mm) found in the bile and pancreatic ducts of Felidae in southeastern USA, Puerto Rico and other Caribbean Islands, South America, some of the Pacific islands, and parts of Africa. Its life cycle includes the snail *Sublima octona* as intermediate host and certain lizards as paratenic hosts. Cats acquire the parasite by feeding on infected lizards. In mild cases, vague chronic signs of unthriftiness may be seen. Severe infections, however, may cause the "lizard poisoning" syndrome, which is characterized by anorexia, persistent vomiting, diarrhea, and jaundice, leading to death. Treatment with praziquantel (20 mg/kg, once) and nitroscanate (100 mg/kg, once, PO) has been successful, although they are not approved for this use.

Metorchis albidus and *M conjunctus* are 2 minute flukes (5 × 1.5 mm) that have been found in the bile ducts and gallbladder of dogs, cats, and other carnivores in North America, Europe, and the former USSR. They seldom cause any recognizable clinical signs. Their eggs are small (27 × 15 μm), and the life cycle includes certain freshwater snails and cyprinid fish as intermediate hosts.

Eurytrema procyonis is a small fluke (2.1 × 1.0 mm) that commonly is seen in the pancreatic duct of raccoons in the eastern USA, and has occasionally been found in the pancreatic duct, bile duct, and gallbladder of domestic cats. Infection may be associated with weight loss and intermittent vomiting. The eggs are medium sized (49 × 33 μm), and the life cycle involves a land snail and a second intermediate host that is thought to be an arthropod. Treatment may be attempted with fenbendazole (30 mg/kg, PO, SID for 6 days), although it is not approved for this use.

HEPATIC DISEASE IN SMALL ANIMALS

The liver performs numerous functions that include but are not limited to lipid, carbohydrate, and protein metabolism; storage and metabolism of vitamins; storage of minerals, glycogen, and triglycerides; extramedullary hematopoiesis; and coagulation homeostasis. The liver also has immunologic activity, contributes to digestion by producing bile acids, and is essential for detoxification of many endogenous and exogenous compounds. The liver has a large storage capacity and functional reserve and is capable of regeneration. These properties are somewhat protective against permanent damage. However, the liver is also predisposed to secondary injury because of its ability to metabolize, detoxify, and store various compounds.

Clinical Findings and Pathophysiology: Clinical signs can vary and include anorexia, vomiting, gastric ulceration, diarrhea, hepatic encephalopathy, fever, coagulation abnormalities, jaundice, ascites, polyuria and polydipsia, hepatomegaly or microhepatia, and weight loss. Understanding the pathophysiology of specific clinical signs facilitates appropriate treatment.

Hepatic encephalopathy is seen in a number of liver diseases. Clinical signs suggestive of hepatic encephalopathy include circling, head pressing, aimless wandering, weakness, ataxia, blindness, ptyalism, aggression, dementia, seizures, and coma. Although the pathophysiology is not completely understood, a synergistic effect between the failure of the liver to clear several neurotoxins (ammonia, mercaptins, and short-chain fatty acids) and an imbalance in plasma amino acids (γ-aminobutyric acid [GABA], aromatic amino acids) along with an increased sensitivity of the brain to these changes are considered to be the major contributing factors.

Currently ammonia is considered the primary neurotoxin contributing to the clinical signs of hepatic encephalopathy. Colonic bacteria metabolize proteins and urea into un-ionized **ammonia**, which is readily absorbed into the portal circulation. In animals with normal liver function, most of the ammonia is removed by hepatocytes and converted into amino acids or urea. However, with liver failure or in the case of portosystemic shunts, in which the portal blood bypasses the liver, blood ammonia levels remain high because of inadequate detoxification. Blood ammonia levels can also be increased during GI bleeding, azotemia, alkalosis, hypokalemia, and anorexia. Elevated ammonia levels have an inhibitory effect on the CNS.

GABA is an endogenously produced neuroinhibitor. Levels of GABA in the CNS are increased in hepatic disease by 2 means. Ammonia is a substrate for GABA; therefore, increased ammonia levels result in increased GABA levels in the CNS. Also, GABA-like compounds are produced by intestinal bacteria, and clearance is decreased in hepatic dysfunction, resulting in increased CNS uptake. GABA receptors are complexed with receptors for diazepam and barbiturates. An increase in the number or affinity of GABA receptors may explain why the use of these drugs can exacerbate signs of hepatic encephalopathy in animals with liver dysfunction.

Clinical signs have also been attributed to an imbalance of the ratio of branched-chain amino acids to aromatic amino acids. In liver dysfunction, the ratio of branched-chain amino acids to aromatic amino acids is decreased because of increased utilization of branched-chain amino acids by myocytes and decreased hepatic clearance of aromatic amino acids. Increased CNS uptake of aromatic amino acids is favored due to the imbalance.

Mercaptans are produced by intestinal bacteria as a result of metabolism of sulfur-containing amino acids (methionine). Mercaptan levels increase with decreased liver clearance. Elevated levels of ammonia and short-chain fatty acids compete with mercaptans for metabolism by the liver. The neurotoxic effects of mercaptans are thought to work synergistically with elevations of ammonia levels to contribute to hepatic encephalopathy.

Short-chain fatty acids have a barbiturate-like effect on the brain. Decreased liver catabolism results in increased blood levels, which have both a direct effect on the CNS and an indirect effect by interfering with hepatic metabolism of ammonia and mercaptans.

Ascites in patients with liver disease is secondary to a combination of portal hypertension and an imbalance in sodium and water homeostasis. Portal hypertension can be hepatic, due to intrahepatic obstruction; posthepatic, due to obstruction of the portal veins or increased portal blood volume; or prehepatic, due to obstruction or kinking of the caudal vena cava or secondary to right heart failure. Causes of hepatic portal hypertension include inflammation, fibrosis, necrosis, regenerative nodules, arteriovenous fistulas, or neoplastic masses. Imbalance in sodium and water homeostasis can either precede or result from portal hypertension. Ascites can be exacerbated by hypoalbuminemia. Cytologic evaluation of the ascitic fluid seen with hepatic failure is usually consistent with a modified transudate.

GI bleeding can be seen in animals with liver disease due to ulceration or coagulation abnormalities. The cause of ulceration is multifactorial. Hypoalbuminemia can lead to decreased turnover of gastric mucosal cells. The integrity of the gastric mucosal layer can also be affected negatively by portal hypertension and increased levels of histamine, both of which can cause mucosal edema. Increased bile acids within the GI lumen can both decrease the effectiveness of the mucosal barrier and increase lumen pH.

Laboratory Analyses: Either regenerative or nonregenerative anemia can be seen in liver disease, depending on the underlying cause. Conversely, severe or acute anemia can inhibit liver function because of hypoxia. Leukocytosis can be seen with inflammatory diseases; leukopenia with sepsis. In general, changes in WBC counts are nonspecific. Platelet number and function can be decreased, and coagulation times prolonged. Coagulation abnormalities can be seen due to decreased production or activation of coagulation factors that are produced by the liver (Factors V, VII, IX, X, XI, XII, fibrinogen, prothrombin, antithrombin III, plasminogen, α_2-macroglobulin, and α_1-antitrypsin).

Decreased GI absorption of vitamin K because of decreased bile production can also lead to coagulopathies.

Liver enzyme activity is often an indicator of liver dysfunction, although levels may be normal in certain situations, eg, end-stage liver disease. ALT and AST are cytosolic enzymes. Changes in cell permeability, hepatocellular degeneration or necrosis, and inflammation can cause release of ALT and AST from hepatocytes and subsequent increase of serum values. AST is a less reliable indicator of liver disease because it is not liver specific (AST is also present in heart, skeletal muscle, kidney, and brain); AST levels within hepatocytes are much lower than ALT levels and may return to normal before ALT as disease resolves. However, in dogs with hepatic metastases, AST may be a more sensitive indicator of disease than ALT or alkaline phosphatase (AP). ALT levels rise rapidly after hepatobiliary necrosis or inflammation. Extrahepatic biliary obstruction results in a more gradual increase in ALT. Drugs that induce microsomal enzymes, including anticonvulsants and prednisone, may cause an increase in ALT in dogs, although levels usually are lower than those associated with disease. Decrease in ALT levels with acute disease is usually a good prognostic indicator. However, in chronic disease, a decrease in ALT may be due to recovery or to a severe decrease in hepatocyte population, as seen with end-stage disease.

AP is a membrane-bound enzyme found in a number of different tissues. In dogs, significant increases in AP activity can be attributed to bone isoenzyme (young animals, panosteitis, bone tumors, and secondary renal hyperparathyroidism), corticosteroid isoenzyme (excessive corticosteroids, either exogenous or endogenous), or liver isoenzymes. With acute hepatocellular necrosis, AP values lag behind an increase in ALT values; they are usually mildly to moderately increased and can return to normal in 2-3 wk. Highest values are noted with cholestatic disease, extrahepatic bile duct obstruction, hepatic neoplasia, and enzyme induction. Increased AP levels can also be caused by hepatic inflammation and systemic infection or inflammation and have been reported as a possible paraneoplastic syndrome seen with mammary adenocarcinoma. Minor increases in AP activity can be seen in numerous diseases, including hypothyroidism, hyperthyroidism, diabetes mellitus, pancreatitis, anoxia, hyperthermia, thromboembolism, hypotension, septicemia, and endotoxemia. Anticonvulsants, glucocorticoids, thiacetarsamides, and ketoconazole can also cause an increase in AP.

AP increases in cats are liver-specific and tend to be less severe than in dogs. In cats, AP is primarily derived from the liver and has a significantly shorter half-life than in dogs, and there is no corticosteroid isoenzyme. Therefore, mild increases of AP in cats are significant indicators of liver disease. (Placental enzymes may cause slight increases late in pregnancy.) AP in cats is rarely affected by anticonvulsants or glucocorticoids but can be increased in diabetes mellitus, hyperthyroidism, and pancreatitis. Highest levels are seen in hepatic lipidosis. Increase of AP precedes increase of bilirubin in both dogs and cats with cholestasis.

The liver is the primary contributor to serum γ-glutamyl transferase (GGT), which increases with intrahepatic and extrahepatic cholestasis and pancreatitis. The kidney and pancreas also have high tissue levels of GGT but do not contribute to serum values. In dogs, GGT activity can be stimulated by glucocorticoids and anticonvulsants. In cats, GGT is increased to a greater degree than AP in cirrhosis, bile duct obstruction, and intrahepatic cholestasis. Little to no increase in GGT levels is seen with acute hepatic necrosis. GGT levels are lower than AP levels in cats with hepatic lipidosis.

Albumin levels during hepatic disease can be decreased due to decreased synthesis or increased volume of distribution (ascites). Decreased albumin level is usually an indicator of severe or chronic liver disease. Glomerular disease or protein-losing enteropathy must be excluded as a cause for hypoalbuminemia. Serum globulins that are synthesized in the liver (α- and β-globulins) can be decreased in chronic liver disease. However, immunoglobulin (γ-globulin) levels are usually increased in liver disease due to inflammation or immune stimulation.

Serum bilirubin levels >2.5-3.0 mg/dL result in clinical icterus. Bilirubin levels can be increased due to prehepatic causes (such as hemolysis) or to intrahepatic or extrahepatic cholestasis. Extrahepatic cholestasis usually results in higher levels of hyperbilirubinemia than intrahepatic causes. AP values increase before serum bilirubin values with intrahepatic cholestasis. In dogs, bilirubinuria can be detected before bilirubinemia because the renal threshold for bilirubin is very low. Cats have a much higher renal threshold, and bilirubinemia is detected before bilirubinuria. Common causes of hyperbilirubinemia in cats include idiopathic hepatic lipidosis, feline infectious peritonitis, toxoplasmosis, cholangiohepatitis, pancreatitis, lymphosarcoma, and myeloproliferative disease. Icteric cats with anemia should always be tested for hemobartonellosis.

Biliprotein, a form of bilirubin that is tightly bound to albumin, is not excreted in the urine and remains in the circulation for a prolonged time. When a significant amount of biliprotein is present, animals can be icteric without bilirubinuria and can remain icteric for several weeks to months after the cholestatic disease has resolved.

BUN can be decreased in animals with liver disease because of decreased conversion of ammonia to urea. Anorexia or a low-protein diet can also cause lower BUN values. Increased BUN may be seen in hepatic disease if the animal is dehydrated (prerenal azotemia).

Hypoglycemia can be seen with hepatic disease because the liver is essential for glucose metabolism. Hypoglycemia is also reported with portosystemic shunts, as a paraneoplastic syndrome in animals with hepatic neoplasia, and in animals with liver disease associated with sepsis.

Cholesterol values may be normal; increased due to decreased excretion and increased production with cholestasis; or decreased due to decreased synthesis, malabsorption, or increased bile acid synthesis. Hypercholesterolemia is seen in cats with cholestasis. Hypocholesterolemia can be seen in portosystemic shunts or end-stage liver disease.

Bile acid levels are used to evaluate liver function. Measurement of serum bile acids after fasting and postprandially reflect the degree of hepatocyte uptake, biliary secretion, and portal circulation—the 3 components of the enterohepatic pathway. Fasting levels >20 μmol/L in dogs and >15 μmol/L in cats, and postprandial levels of >25 μmol/L in dogs and >20 μmol/L in cats, indicate liver dysfunction. Postprandial bile acids may be more sensitive in determining liver dysfunction than fasting samples. Because icterus is an indicator of defective bile metabolism, measurement of serum bile acids is not necessary in icteric animals. When serum bile acid values are increased, a liver biopsy is recommended to determine the specific cause of dysfunction. Bile acids may be increased in certain nonhepatic diseases, including inflammatory bowel disease, hyperadrenocorticism, and pancreatitis.

Two other methods of evaluating liver function are a fasting blood ammonia level and an ammonia tolerance test. If fasting blood ammonia levels are within normal limits, but liver disease is suspected, then an ammonia tolerance test can be conducted. Ammonium chloride is given at 100 mg/kg in a 5% solution orally or at 2 mL/kg of a 5% solution rectally (30 min after a cleansing enema). Rectal administration may be preferable because oral administration often induces vomiting. Blood ammonia is measured 20 and 40 min after administration. An ammonia tolerance test should be done with caution when hepatic encephalopathy is suspected because it can exacerbate clinical signs in these animals. Because ammonia is not affected by cholestasis, it can help differentiate between biliary and hepatic disease. Difficult sample handling limits use of this test in private practice.

Radiography is useful in determining liver size, irregular liver borders, choleliths, and diseases of the gallbladder that involve gas-producing bacteria. Ultrasonography can help to determine common bile duct obstruction and other biliary disease, differentiate between diffuse and focal lesions, and identify portosystemic shunts. Ultrasonographic-guided fine-needle aspirates or biopsy are relatively noninvasive procedures to obtain diagnostic liver specimens. In some situations, a wedge biopsy may be preferred to assure that the sample provides an accurate diagnosis. A complete coagulation profile should be done before attempting to collect any biopsy samples. Biopsy samples should be submitted for aerobic and anaerobic bacterial culture, cytology and histopathology, and, when appropriate, copper or toxicologic analysis. Nuclear scintigraphy is a valuable tool for identifying portosystemic shunts and other vascular anomalies.

Treatment and Management: Early and appropriate therapy is critical for animals with acute and fulminate hepatic failure. Specific treatment should be administered if an underlying cause is identified. Attention to electrolyte and acid-base balance and proper nutrition provides the best environment for regeneration. In cases of chronic or end-stage liver disease, and in cases of acute liver disease when no underlying cause has been identified, supportive treatment is directed at slowing progression of disease and minimizing complications.

Hepatic Encephalopathy: Treatment of acute hepatic encephalopathy is aimed at providing supportive therapy and rapidly reducing the neurotoxins being produced by the colon. Affected animals are usually comatose or semicomatose. Benzodiazepines and other sedatives should not be administered. Food should be withheld until the animal's neurologic status improves. Fluids (2.5% dextrose and 0.45% saline with potassium chloride and vitamin B complex added) should be administered to correct dehydration and electrolyte and acid-base imbalances. Lactated Ringer's solution should be avoided. Cleansing enemas of warm soapy water, followed by retention enemas of either lactulose (3 parts lactulose to 7 parts water at 20 mL/kg), 10% povidone-iodine solution (20 mL/kg), or neomycin (22 mg/kg) should be given every 6 hr until the animal is stable. Retention enemas should be maintained for 15-20 min; retention can be facilitated by use of a Foley catheter. Lactulose is a nonabsorbable disaccharide that interacts with bacterial flora and decreases encephalopathic toxin production. The sugars are not absorbed but are fermented in the colon to organic acids; this lowers colonic pH and traps ammonia in the ionized form, which prevents absorption. Disaccharides also provide an alternate substrate for bacterial metabolism and, therefore, decrease the amount of ammonia produced. In addition, disaccharides are osmotic cathartics and decrease noxious substances and ammonia-producing bacteria by purging. Neomycin and povidone-iodine directly alter the colonic bacterial population, decreasing the population of ammonia-producing bacteria.

Once the animal has been stabilized, treatment is aimed at preventing recurrence. Protein-restricted diets should be fed. If needed, oral lactulose (0.1-0.5 mL/kg, PO, BID-TID) along with antibiotic therapy, either neomycin (22 mg/kg, PO, BID) or metronidazole (7.5 mg/kg, PO, BID) are recommended. Antibiotic therapy works synergistically with lactulose.

The clinical signs can be exacerbated by GI bleeding, infection, glucocorticoid use (resulting in increased catabolism of tissue protein), neoplasia, fever, azotemia or dehydration (due to increased blood urea concentration), constipation (causing increased generation of colonic neurotoxins), metabolic alkalosis (favoring both production of ammonia by the kidneys and uptake of urea by the blood-brain barrier), and use of diazepam and barbiturates (synergetic neuroinhibitors). Use of H_2-receptor antagonists and sucralfate, control of fever and infection, proper hydration, and minimal (if any) use of antiseizure medication can help alleviate these complications.

Ascites: The first step in control of ascites is dietary sodium restriction. However, sodium-restricted diets alone are often not sufficient, and diuretics are recommended. Diuretic therapy should be directed at slowly reducing ascites without causing dehydration, metabolic alkalosis, and hypokalemia. Spironolactone (1-3 mg/kg, PO, BID) is recommended initially; if spironolactone is not effective, furosemide (1-2 mg/kg, PO, BID) can be added. If ascites is causing respiratory compromise, then abdominocentesis is recommended to temporarily reduce fluid buildup. Periodic abdominocentesis is also recommended if ascites is refractory to treatment. Possible complications when removing large volumes of fluid by abdominocentesis include hypotension and hypoalbuminemia. Therefore, as little fluid as possible should be removed to keep the animal comfortable.

Coagulation Abnormalities: In cases of acute hepatic failure, bleeding disorders are usually associated with disseminated intravascular coagulation (DIC). Treatment for DIC with anemia requires fresh whole blood transfusion, which is preferred over packed RBC for presence of clotting factors. (Fresh whole blood is also preferred over stored blood in animals with hepatobiliary disease because ammonia tends to build up during storage.) Alternatively, if anemia is not present, fresh frozen plasma transfusion can be used. Regardless of whether fresh whole blood or plasma is used, the unit should be incubated with heparin (100 U/kg) for 30 min. Additional heparin therapy is recommended at 50 U/kg, SC, TID for 24 hr, then 25 U/kg, SC, TID for 24 hr, then 10 U/kg, TID until the coagulation profile is within normal limits.

In chronic liver disease, coagulopathies are generally due to decreased production and/or absorption of coagulation factors. Vitamin K deficiency can be prevented by administration of vitamin K_1 at 0.5 mg/kg, SC or IM, BID for 3 days. In cholestasis or severe hepatic disease, chronic therapy with parenteral vitamin K_1 (0.5 mg, every 7-20 days, SC or IM) is indicated.

Bacterial Infections and Sepsis: Animals with acute hepatic failure and chronic hepatobiliary disease are predisposed to bacterial infections. In acute hepatic failure, septicemia may be masked as fever; hypoglycemia and leukocytosis might be mistaken for manifestation of the hepatic disease and not associated with sepsis. Ampicillin and cephalosporins are active against both gram-positive and anaerobic organisms, enrofloxacin and gentamicin against gram-negative bacteria. In chronic disease, the infection is more likely to be intrahepatic, and both aerobic and anaerobic cultures should be performed. Empiric use of antibiotics should include drugs specifically active against GI flora and avoid drugs that are extensively metabolized by the liver. Appropriate choices pending culture and sensitivity include ampicillin (22 mg/kg, PO or IV, TID-QID), metronidazole (7.5 mg/kg, PO, BID), cephalexin (22 mg/kg, PO or IV, TID), enrofloxacin (2.5-5 mg/kg, PO, IM, or IV, BID) and amikacin (5 mg/kg, SC, IM, or IV, BID-TID). Combination antibiotic therapy may be necessary to adequately cover the spectrum of bacteria associated with infection.

Nutrition: Adequate calorie intake, with the bulk of energy supplied by carbohydrates (20-40% of the diet) in the form of complex carbohydrates such as rice and pasta, is recommended for most animals with liver disease. (Exceptions include cats with hepatic lipidosis and animals with hepatocutaneous syndrome.) A higher soluble fiber diet may be beneficial because fermentation of fiber in the colon, through various mechanisms, decreases ammonia production and absorption and reduces incidence of hepatic encephalopathy. Because it is difficult to maintain adequate caloric requirements with high-fiber diets, they should not be used in debilitated animals.

Fat restriction is not a major consideration in animals with hepatobiliary disease unless decreased bile acid production prevents dietary fat absorption and results in steatorrhea. If malabsorption of dietary fat is a factor, medium-chain triglycerides may be used as a source of fats.

Protein restriction is recommended only for animals with hepatic disease that are at risk of having clinical signs of hepatic encephalopathy. Protein levels should be sufficient to prevent tissue catabolism and maintain albumin levels without leading to hepatic encephalopathy by ammonia production. The amount of protein may not be as important as the type of protein. Vegetable and dairy protein sources such as soy, peanuts, and cheese are better sources than meat proteins.

Zinc may have antifibrotic and hepatoprotective properties by preventing the absorption of copper from the gut. Supplementation of zinc may be beneficial in dogs, although some dogs may not tolerate zinc because it is a gastric irritant.

Hypokalemia and decreased levels of B vitamins are common complications with liver disease, especially in cats, and supplementation is recommended. Vitamin C deficiency has been reported in dogs with hepatobiliary disease, and supplementation may be beneficial. Parenteral use of vitamin K is recommended in animals with bleeding tendencies.

If animals are anorectic, tube feeding should be considered. Nasogastric tubes are inexpensive, easily placed, and can provide a short-term solution to feeding anorectic animals. Esophagostomy tubes are also inexpensive, but require more expertise to place and esophageal and respiratory problems may develop with longterm use. Percutaneous gastrostomy tubes can be placed with or without an endoscope and should be used in animals that need longterm nutritional support. Gastrostomy tubes should remain in place for a minimum of 7 days to prevent complications at the gastrostomy site.

Choleretic Agents: In cases in which there is evidence of intrahepatic cholestasis but not biliary obstruction, choleretic agents may be helpful. Ursodeoxycholic acid (10-15 mg/kg, PO, SID) stimulates flow of bile and may also have hepatoprotective and immunomodulating effects.

Anti-inflammatory Drugs: Use of these drugs in treatment of chronic hepatobiliary disease is controversial. However, corticosteroids or azathioprine may be indicated if there is no evidence of infection, if an immune-mediated disease is associated with chronic hepatobiliary disease, or to decrease inflammation, which can contribute to ongoing necrosis and fibrosis. Corticosteroid therapy (eg, prednisone, 1-2 mg/kg, PO, divided BID, and reduced to 0.5 mg/kg, every other day) has been effective in Doberman Pinschers with chronic hepatobiliary disease and in cats with chronic cholangiohepatitis. Other cases of chronic hepatobiliary disease may benefit from anti-inflammatory therapy only if there is evidence of an underlying immune-mediated disease or active inflammatory disease without evidence of sepsis.

Detrimental effects of glucocorticoids in chronic hepatobiliary disease include sodium and water retention (which can either exacerbate or promote ascites formation), catabolic effects (which can promote hepatic encephalopathy), GI ulceration, pancreatitis, predisposition to secondary infections, glucose intolerance, and iatrogenic hyperadrenocorticism.

Azathioprine (2 mg/kg, PO, SID decreased to every 48 hr) has been recommended for use in chronic hepatobiliary disease either with or without glucocorticoids. Adverse effects of azathioprine include bone marrow suppression, pancreatitis, and GI toxicity. Azathioprine is not recommended in cats.

Limiting Fibrosis: Hepatic fibrosis can eventually lead to cirrhosis. However, fibrosis is potentially reversible. Colchicine is both antifibrotic and anti-inflammatory. The dosage is 0.03 mg/kg, PO, SID. Adverse effects of colchicine include nausea, vomiting, and hemorrhagic diarrhea. Colchicine is available in formulations with and without probenecid. Formulations without probenecid should be used because probenecid can cause nausea and vomiting.

Zinc may also be useful in decreasing fibrosis. The recommended dosage is 1-2.2 mg/kg, PO, BID, 1 hr before meals. Zinc levels should be monitored every 2 wk, and plasma levels should be maintained at 200-300 µg/dL. Zinc therapy should be discontinued if levels are >1,000 µg/dL because of potential toxicity.

PORTOSYSTEMIC SHUNTS

The most common circulatory anomaly of the liver in both dogs and cats is the portosystemic shunt (PSS). A PSS is a connection between the portal vessels and systemic circulation that diverts blood flow, in varying degrees, from the liver. Decreased blood flow results in liver atrophy and subsequent dysfunction, decreasing liver metabolism of neurotoxins. Clinical signs of hepatic encephalopathy are frequently noted and can be most severe postprandially, especially after a high-protein meal.

Congenital PSS are seen primarily in purebred dogs, including Miniature Schnauzers, Yorkshire Terriers, Cairn Terriers, Maltese, Scottish Terriers, Pugs, Irish Wolfhounds, Golden Retrievers, Labrador Retrievers, German Shepherds, and Poodles. In cats, congenital PSS are seen more frequently in mixed breeds, but Himalayans and Persians are affected more commonly than other purebreds. Cats and small-breed dogs usually have extrahepatic shunts, whereas large-breed dogs have intrahepatic shunts. Extrahepatic shunts arise from the portal vein, left gastric vein, or splenic vein and connect to the caudal vena cava (most common), the azygous vein, or other systemic vessels. Congenital intrahepatic shunts usually are due to failure of the fetal ductus venosus to close at birth.

Clinical Findings and Diagnosis: Animals with congenital PSS are often smaller than littermates, show failure to thrive, and can have other congenital abnormalities (eg, cryptorchidism in dogs and cats, heart murmurs in cats). Male cats may be more prone to congenital shunts than females. Clinical signs are usually seen by 6 mo of age in cats and between 6 mo and 1 yr of age in dogs. If clinical signs are mild, diagnosis may be not be made until the animal is several years old. Hepatic encephalopathy is the most common clinical sign. Other clinical signs include vomiting, diarrhea, pica, nausea, and anorexia. Polyuria and polydipsia are common in dogs but not in cats. Hematuria, pollakiuria, stranguria, or urethral obstruction due to ammonia biurate urolithiasis have been reported. Hypersalivation is a common clinical sign in cats; blindness and excessive vocalization have also been reported.

Abnormalities in laboratory data include a microcytic, nonregenerative anemia, poikilocytosis, target cells, hypoproteinemia, hypoalbuminemia, hypoglycemia (especially toy-breed dogs), low BUN, hypocholesterolemia, normal to mildly increased enzymes (ALT, AST, and AP), normal bilirubin, hyposthenuria or isothenuria, and ammonia urate crystals in the urine. Cats can have a microcytosis without anemia, decreased creatinine and BUN levels, and increased ALT and AP. After a prolonged fast, both the fasting bile acid and resting ammonia values may be normal, but postprandial bile acids and ammonia tolerance test will be abnormal.

Microhepatica and renomegaly are usually noted on abdominal radiographs. Ultrasonography is a useful noninvasive tool for identifying the shunt, determining if the shunt is intrahepatic or extrahepatic, and identifying radiolucent uroliths in the kidneys or bladder. Contrast portography is a more invasive method to identify the shunt but is the best way to evaluate portal vessel anatomy. Rectal portal scintigraphy is noninvasive but is not widely available and cannot differentiate between intrahepatic and extrahepatic shunts or determine location of the shunt. Liver biopsy is indicated in shunt repair or if multiple shunts are noted to determine the primary underlying disease.

Treatment: The treatment of choice for single congenital PSS is surgical attenuation or ligation. Whether ligation is total or partial depends on portal pressures (should be <20 cm H_2O). If only partial ligation can be achieved at the time of the first surgery, then additional surgery may be indicated if clinical signs do not resolve. The most common postsurgical complication is acute portal hypertension, which manifests as accumulation of abdominal effusion, bloody diarrhea, abdominal pain, ileus, endotoxic shock, and cardiovascular collapse. If this develops, immediate medical treatment for shock and removal of the ligature is necessary. Postsurgical seizures have been reported. Acquired shunts can develop after surgery if the portal vein is unable to dilate and compensate for the increased portal hypertension induced by surgical ligation.

Acute portal hypertension can be prevented if an ameroid constrictor band is used to attenuate a single extrahepatic shunt. The band is impregnated with cellulose that absorbs abdominal fluid; as the cellulose swells, the shunt is slowly ligated over an extended period of time.

In cases in which either surgery is not possible or clinical signs are minor, medical management can be used. Although medical management can lessen clinical signs initially, signs eventually worsen because liver atrophy in congenital PSS is progressive.

Overall, the prognosis is good if complete correction can be achieved before 1 yr of age in dogs with single extrahepatic congenital PSS. The prognosis is less favorable with partial correction, multiple shunts, and intrahepatic shunts. Poor prognosis after 2 yr of age is attributed to progressive liver atrophy. Overall prognosis postsurgically for cats with congenital shunts is not as favorable as for dogs. Cats appear to be more likely to develop multiple shunts after ligation. Delay in diagnosis and treatment may partially explain the difference.

Acquired PSS are caused by portal hypertension. Acquired shunts are usually seen in older animals, more frequently in dogs than in cats, and are usually multiple. Acquired shunts develop to prevent fatal portal hypertension, which develops as a result of chronic, severe, diffuse intrahepatic disease (eg, chronic hepatitis, cirrhosis, and hepatic fibrosis). The vessels involved are connections between the splenic and mesenteric veins through the renal veins, gonadal veins, or the venous sinuses within the spinal cord to the caudal vena cava. These vessels are fetal vasculature that open as a compensatory mechanism to shunt blood to the lower pressure systemic circulation as a response to portal hypertension. During acquired PSS, these vessels become tortuous. Possible causes of portal hypertension in younger dogs include hepatic arteriovenous fistulas hepatoportal vascular hypoplasia veno-occlusive disease in Cocker Spaniels, or porta vascular atresia.

Clinical signs include polydipsia, vomiting, and diarrhea. Ascites is a common findin in acquired portosystemic shunts but is rarely seen in congenital shunts unless hypoalbu minemia is severe (<.15 g/dL). Laboratory abnormalities consistent with the primar underlying hepatic disease can be seen, including microcytosis, hyperbilirubinemia decreased BUN, and increased AP and ALT. Ligation of multiple acquired PSS is contra indicated because this is a compensatory response, and correction can lead to acute porta hypertension. However, banding of the caudal vena cava can increase pressure within th vena cava to be slightly above portal pressure and reduce the signs of hepatic encephalop athy. Medical treatment of the underlying disease along with banding of the caudal ven. cava can result in a favorable prognosis for some animals with acquired PSS.

Other Vascular Anomalies

Hepatic arteriovenous fistulas, hepatic venous outflow obstruction, and hepatopor tal microvascular dysplasia are other vascular anomalies. An arteriovenous fistula is a connection between the high-pressure hepatic artery and the low-pressure portal vein It causes a retrograde flow of blood into the portal vessels, which results in portal hy pertension, ascites, and acquired PSS. The right medial lobe is most often affected. Con genital hepatic arteriovenous fistulas are more common in dogs and cats than acquire arteriovenous fistulas, which are rare. Clinical signs are seen in young animals, are usu ally acute in onset, and are consistent with portal hypertension. On abdominal ausculta tion, a murmur, representing the anomalous flow of blood through the fistula, can be heard over the affected liver lobe. Laboratory abnormalities are similar to those seen with PSS. The presence of ascites is one distinguishing sign between the 2 diseases Abdominal ultrasonography can identify the fistula and may detect multiple acquire PSS; portal angiography and scintigraphy are also diagnostic tools. Exploratory laporat omy locates the fistula, which grossly appears as thin-walled, tortuous, pulsating distor tions of the liver lobe. Lobectomy is recommended if one lobe is involved. Liver func tion may not return to normal if acquired PSS have formed. Banding of the caudal ven: cava may be effective in controlling clinical signs but not in restoring function to nor mal. Longterm medical management is usually necessary to prevent hepatic encephal opathy and other clinical signs. Prognosis is guarded, but some animals do well afte surgery.

Outflow obstruction of hepatic venous flow can be caused by heart disease that leads to passive congestion of the caudal vena cava (eg, right heart failure, pericardial disease congenital defects, and cardiac tumors), obstruction of the caudal vena cava (eg, post caval syndrome associated with heartworm disease, kinking of the caudal vena cava thrombosis or neoplasia of the caudal vena cava, diaphragmatic hernia that compresses the caudal vena cava), or obstruction of the efferent hepatic venous system (eg, liver lobe torsion, compression of hepatic mass, idiopathic postsinusoidal venous obstructio and veno-occlusive disease of Cocker Spaniels). Clinical signs include hepatomegaly ascites, multiple acquired PSS, and signs suggestive of underlying disease. Laboratory abnormalities include modified transudate ascitic fluid, normal bile acids, hypoproteine mia, mild increases in liver enzymes, hypercholesterolemia, hyperglycemia, and mild hy perbilirubinemia. Thoracic and abdominal radiographs help to define cardiac vs other disease. Cardiac ultrasonography can differentiate between pericardial disease, cardiac tumors, congenital disease, or intrathoracic masses compressing the caudal vena cava Additional diagnostics include abdominal ultrasonography, cardiac catheterization, an giography, venous pressure measurements, or exploratory surgery. Treatment and prog nosis depend on the underlying disease.

Hepatoportal microvascular dysplasia is often seen in animals predisposed to con genital PSS, including mixed-breed cats and small-breed dogs (particularly Yorkshire Terriers and Cairn Terriers). Affected animals may be asymptomatic or show clinical signs, which include anorexia, vomiting, diarrhea, hepatic encephalopathy, and dysuria due to ammonia biurate crystals. Asymptomatic animals may not be able to tolerate drugs that are metabolized by the liver, but otherwise do not seem to be affected by the condition. Dogs that show clinical signs can experience progressive disease with worsening signs and develop portal hypertension and ascites over time. Laboratory data are usually within normal limits, fasting bile acids are usually mildly increased, and postprandial bile acids may be markedly increased. The hepatic mass appears normal on radiographs. There is no identifiable shunt on ultrasonography; however, portal vasculature appears decreased. Rectal portal scintigraphy is within normal limits. There is no evidence of portal shunting with portograms. Histopathologic changes are similar to those seen with PSS.

Asymptomatic dogs require no therapy, except for special considerations when prescribing drugs for other conditions. Prognosis for asymptomatic dogs is excellent. Treatment for symptomatic dogs includes a diet that is rich in carbohydrates and a nonmeat protein source, and use of lactulose and neomycin or metronidazole as needed to control clinical signs of hepatic encephalopathy. Symptomatic dogs that respond well to therapy have a good prognosis. Dogs with hepatic encephalopathy that is difficult to control with medical treatment have a poor prognosis.

HEPATOTOXINS

Many drugs have been associated with hepatic dysfunction. These include anticonvulsants (especially primidone, phenytoin, and phenobarbital), glucocorticoids, thiacetarsamide, mebendazole, oxibendazole-diethylcarbamazine, NSAID, trimethoprim-sulfadiazine, tetracyclines, griseofulvin, ketoconazole, itraconazole, halothane, methoxyflurane, acetaminophen, methimazole, glipizide, and diazepam in cats. Griseofulvin-associated hyperbilirubinemia and increased ALT in cats are thought to be idiosyncratic, and clinical signs are usually mild and reversible. Mebendazole has also been associated with idiosyncratic reactions; however, the acute hepatic necrosis and hepatitis that is seen with toxicity is usually fatal. Glipizide and tetracyclines cause an increase in ALT and AP, but clinical signs do not usually develop. Thiacetarsamide and acetaminophen in cats have relatively small margins of safety.

Effects on liver pathology vary with different drugs. Increases in AP and, to a lesser extent, ALT are seen as soon as 2 days following glucocorticoid administration in dogs. A similar glucocorticoid-induced increase in liver enzymes is not seen in cats. Vacuolar hepatopathy (steroid hepatopathy) is a benign reversible change seen with high-dose, longterm glucocorticoid use. Thiacetarsamide usually causes increased ALT values but can also cause jaundice, which is an indication to discontinue therapy; changes are reversible. Longterm oxibendazole-diethylcarbamazine use can lead to increased ALT and AP, hyperbilirubinemia, and subsequent periportal hepatitis and fibrosis. Clinical signs resolve after discontinuation. Acetaminophen causes hepatic necrosis at dosages higher than therapeutic ranges in dogs (acute toxicity at >100 mg/kg, chronic use at 42 mg/kg, QID for 6 wk). Methemoglobinemia is also seen. Toxicity in cats is seen acutely at a much lower dosage (56 mg/kg). Methemoglobinemia is the primary toxic effect; hepatic necrosis is not seen frequently. Trimethoprim-sulfonamide can cause reversible cholangiostatic hepatopathy or acute and subacute massive hepatic necrosis, sometimes after only a few doses. Hepatic necrosis is seen as an idiosyncratic reaction that can be fatal in dogs receiving the recommended dose. NSAID are associated with an idiosyncratic acute hepatocellular necrosis. Diazepam administered orally to cats can cause an idiosyncratic fatal acute massive hepatic necrosis and failure. Methimazole can cause hepatocellular degeneration and necrosis, which is reversible after discontinuation of the drug.

Specific nondrug chemicals that are toxic to the liver include aflatoxins, amanita mushrooms, and blue-green algae. All are rare but cause acute hepatic necrosis that can be life-threatening. Other chemicals reported to be hepatotoxic include heavy metals, certain herbicides, fungicides, insecticides, and rodenticides.

Important steps to minimize absorption of ingested toxins or overdose of oral drugs include inducing vomiting and decreasing absorption. Vomiting can be induced 30 min to 2 hr after ingestion by administering hydrogen peroxide (5 mL, PO, every 15 min) or syrup of ipecac (1-2 mL/kg). Activated charcoal (2 g/kg, repeated every 6-8 hr) should be administered to reduce absorption only if the animal is conscious and not vomiting. Gastric lavage is also important to prevent absorption in unconscious animals. Treatment for acetaminophen toxicity consists of N-acetylcysteine (140 mg/kg, PO or IV, initial dose, followed by 70 mg/kg, PO or IV, QID for 48 hr), ascorbic acid (30 mg/kg, PO, QID for 48 hr), and cimetidine (5-10 mg/kg, PO or IV, TID for 48 hr). If there is no specific treatment for a hepatotoxin, supportive therapy should be provided.

INFECTIOUS DISEASES OF THE LIVER

Viral Diseases

Viral diseases associated with liver dysfunction include infectious canine hepatitis, feline infectious peritonitis, canine acidophil hepatitis, and canine herpesvirus.

Infectious canine hepatitis is caused by canine adenovirus 1 (CAV-1). In addition to acute hepatic necrosis, chronic hepatitis and hepatic fibrosis can also be noted. *See* p 637 for clinical findings, diagnosis, treatment, and control.

Feline infectious peritonitis virus is a coronavirus that causes a diffuse pyogranulomatous inflammation and vasculitis. Icterus, abdominal effusion, vomiting, diarrhea, and fever are common clinical signs. *See* p 628 for clinical findings, diagnosis, treatment, and control.

Canine acidophil hepatitis and **canine herpesvirus** are uncommon. Canine acidophil hepatitis is caused by an unidentified virus that, apparently, is unrelated to CAV-1. It has been reported in Great Britain. Clinical disease varies from acute hepatitis that is severe and fatal to chronic hepatitis and eventually cirrhosis. Intermittent fevers and spikes in ALT levels are noted in chronic disease. Prognosis is poor, and treatment consists of supportive care. Canine herpesvirus affects neonatal puppies, causing hepatic necrosis as well as other systemic changes, and is fatal.

Leptospirosis

Leptospira interrogans, especially serotype *icterohemorrhagiae* and, to a lesser extent, chronic infections with *grippotyphosa* are associated with liver disease. Diagnosis depends on positive serologic testing and identification of the organism using Warthin-Starry stains in biopsy specimens. Treatment includes supportive care and specific antibiotic therapy. Penicillin drugs are drugs of choice for the acute phase, eg, ampicillin (22 mg/kg, IV, QID) or amoxicillin (22 mg/kg, PO, BID). Aminoglycosides or doxycycline (5 mg/kg, PO, BID for 4 wk) are recommended to treat the carrier phase. Special precautions are recommended when handling animals suspected of or having leptospirosis (and their urine specimens) because of the zoonotic potential. (*See also* p 525.)

Tyzzer's Disease

Tyzzer's disease (p 160) is a rare but fatal condition caused by *Bacillus piliformis*. Clinical signs are acute in onset and rapidly progress to death within 24-48 hr. Special stains are needed to identify the organism, which will not grow in routine bacterial culture media. There is no effective treatment.

Extrahepatic Bacterial Infections

Icterus associated with overwhelming extrahepatic bacterial infections is thought to be due to structural and functional changes in the liver induced by endotoxins. Other possible mechanisms include bacteria invading the liver or damage to the liver caused by fever, hypoxia, and malnutrition. Bilirubin, AP, and serum bile acids are increased. Specific antibiotic therapy to control the bacterial infection and supportive care usually result in a favorable prognosis.

Mycotic Infections

The most common mycotic infections associated with liver dysfunction are coccidioidomycosis (p 513) and histoplasmosis (p 516). Clinical signs include ascites, jaundice, and hepatomegaly, in addition to signs associated with other systems involved. Because liver involvement in histoplasmosis is seen with the disseminated form of the disease, aggressive chemotherapy (including a combination of either itraconazole or ketoconazole and amphotericin B) is recommended. Depending on the level of debilitation, prognosis is often poor. Coccidioidomycosis can be treated successfully with longterm (6-12 mo) ketoconazole or itraconazole. However, relapses have been reported.

Toxoplasmosis

Toxoplasmosis (p 547) can cause acute hepatic failure due to hepatic necrosis. *Toxoplasma gondii* is more commonly seen in cats positive for feline immunodeficiency virus. Icterus, abdominal effusion, fever, lethargy, vomiting, and diarrhea are seen in addition to clinical signs consistent with CNS or ocular involvement. Liver disease associated with toxoplasmosis in dogs is most often seen in young dogs; a high percentage are also infected with canine distemper virus, and the disease is acute in onset and rapidly fatal. Diagnosis can be difficult, but a positive IgM titer is indicative of clinical disease. Clindamycin (12.5 mg/kg, PO or IM, BID for 3 wk) is the drug of choice. Prognosis depends on the degree of debilitation.

FELINE IDIOPATHIC HEPATIC LIPIDOSIS

Feline idiopathic hepatic lipidosis is the most common cause of feline hepatopathy. The etiology is undetermined but is associated with a period of anorexia (few days to several weeks), especially in obese cats. Factors that may trigger anorexia include a change of diet to initiate weight loss or other stressful events (eg, moving, boarding, death of other pets or owners). Secondary hepatic lipidosis is associated with either a primary metabolic (eg, diabetes mellitus) or GI disease (eg, inflammatory bowel disease, gastric foreign bodies, pancreatitis, or cholangiohepatitis) that can cause anorexia. Regardless of the inciting cause, the end result is excessive accumulation of triglycerides (fat) within the liver, which leads to severe intrahepatic cholestasis and hepatic failure.

Clinical Findings: Clinical signs are variable but can include dramatic weight loss (30-40% of body weight, experimentally) due to anorexia, vomiting, lethargy, and diarrhea. Signs of hepatic encephalopathy are unusual, as are bleeding tendencies, but can be noted in advanced disease. Icterus or pale mucous membranes, ptyalism, hepatomegaly, and decreased body condition with retention of abdominal fat are commonly seen. Laboratory abnormalities include a nonregenerative anemia with poikilocytosis, stress leukogram, hyperbilirubinemia and bilirubinuria, mild to moderate increases in AST and ALT and marked increase in AP; GGT values are usually normal or mildly elevated. Hypoalbuminemia, prolonged coagulation profile, and hyperammonemia have been reported in advanced disease. If the cat is not icteric, bile acids can be evaluated. Postprandial values may be difficult to obtain if the cat cannot be force-fed. However, in most cases, fasting bile acids will be abnormal, precluding the need for the postprandial sample. Peritoneal effusion may be seen on radiographs. On ultrasonographic evaluation, the liver often appears diffusely hyperechoic when compared with the falciform ligament. If pancreatitis is also present, abdominal effusion and pancreatic changes can be identified with ultrasonography. Histopathology or cytology reveals vacuolated hepatocytes and cholestasis; lipid is identified within the vacuoles using Sudan black or oil Red O stain.

Treatment: Treatment is primarily supportive, unless an underlying cause can be found. Fluid therapy, with a polyionic, isotonic solution supplemented with potassium and thiamine, is recommended to correct dehydration. Potassium phosphate should be added if the cat is hypophosphatemic. Administration of dextrose fluids can exacerbate signs of hepatic lipidosis by stimulating hepatic fat synthesis and should be avoided unless the cat is hypoglycemic. Feeding as soon as possible is essential. Occasionally, appetite stimulants (eg, diazepam or cyproheptidine) may be helpful. However, diazepam can cause fulminant hepatic necrosis and should be used with caution. Usually, placement of a nasoesophageal, pharyngostomy, esophagostomy, or gastrotomy tube is necessary. A nasoesophageal tube can be used initially until the cat is stable and can withstand anesthesia to have a longterm feeding tube placed. A high-protein, calorie-dense, balanced diet is recommended unless the cat shows signs of hepatic encephalopathy, in which case a low-protein diet should be used. Supplementation with taurine, carnitine, and/or arginine (250 mg of each, BID) can be considered. Initially, feedings are small and given frequently. On the first day, one-third to one-half of the cat's ideal caloric intake is fed; the amount fed is gradually increased over the next 3-4 days until the total ideal caloric requirement is fed in 3-4 feedings. Vomiting associated with tube feeding can be controlled with metoclopramide. Another complication associated with tube feeding is hypophosphatemia, which can lead to hemolytic anemia; therefore, phosphorus levels should be routinely evaluated. Gastritis can be controlled with H_2-blockers (eg, famotidine or ranitidine) and carafate. If clinical signs of hepatic encephalopathy are present, lactulose and metronidazole are also recommended. If pancreatitis is concurrent, total parenteral nutrition may be necessary to prevent pancreatic secretions. Prognosis is good if the diagnosis is made early, treatment is begun, and the underlying disease, if any, can be treated. Concurrent pancreatitis is a poor prognostic indicator. Monitoring AP of obese cats on a weight-reducing diet may be effective in diagnosing preclinical hepatic lipidosis and preventing clinical signs from developing. Early dietary support for obese cats that become anorectic because of other underlying disease is also recommended to prevent hepatic illness.

CHOLANGITIS AND CHOLANGIOHEPATITIS
(Inflammatory liver disease)

Inflammatory liver disease is the second most common hepatopathy reported in cats but is rare in dogs. Classification for inflammatory liver disease in cats includes cholangiohepatitis (acute and chronic) and lymphocytic portal hepatitis.

Cholangiohepatitis is defined as inflammation of the biliary tract that extends into the hepatic parenchyma. Concurrent inflammatory bowel disease and pancreatitis have been reported in cats with cholangiohepatitis.

Acute Cholangiohepatitis

Acute cholangiohepatitis is often associated with bacterial, fungal, or protozoal infections, or less frequently, liver fluke infection. It is suspected that the bacteria originate from the gut and ascend via the bile duct due to some predisposing condition, such as biliary stasis, choleliths, chronic pancreatitis, inflammatory bowel disease, or anatomic abnormalities of the gallbladder. Clinical signs are usually of short duration and include fever, hepatomegaly, abdominal pain, icterus, lethargy, vomiting, anorexia, and weight loss. Laboratory abnormalities include neutrophilia with left shift; nonregenerative anemia; hyperbilirubinemia; moderate to marked increases in ALT, AST, and GGT; and a mild increase in AP. Serum bile acids are usually increased, especially postprandial values. Histopathologic changes include neutrophilic inflammatory infiltrates in the hepatic parenchyma and bile ducts, periportal necrosis, bile duct hyperplasia, and fibrosis. Cholestasis and inspissation of bile can cause extrahepatic biliary obstruction and predispose to cholelith formation. Biopsy samples should be cultured for both aerobic and anaerobic bacteria. Commonly isolated bacteria include *Escherichia coli*, *Streptococcus*, *Clostridium*, *Bacteroides*, and *Actinomyces*. Cultures may be negative due to prior antibiotic administration or failure to culture for anaerobic bacteria. Treatment consists of fluid therapy to correct dehydration and longterm (3-6 mo) antibiotics as determined by culture and sensitivity. Ampicillin (20-40 mg/kg, TID), metronidazole (10-25 mg/kg, SID), and chloramphenicol (50 mg/kg, SID) are recommended while cultures are pending, because of the spectrum of activity provided and because the active forms of these antibiotics are excreted in the bile. Combination antibiotic therapy may be more effective, especially if multiple species of bacteria are present. If extrahepatic biliary obstruction is not present, ursodeoxycholic acid (10-15 mg/kg, SID) can be used as a choleretic. If biliary obstruction is present, a cholecystojejunostomy should be performed.

Chronic Cholangiohepatitis

Chronic cholangiohepatitis may be a chronic form of acute cholangiohepatitis; an immune-mediated disease, or secondary to infectious agents including feline infectious peritonitis, feline leukemia, toxoplasmosis, or liver fluke infections. Incidence may be higher in Persian cats. Ascites and icterus are the most frequently reported clinical signs, and lymphadenopathy may be present. Other clinical signs are similar to those seen with acute cholangiohepatitis, although fever may not be as common. If the disease has progressed to cirrhosis, then clinical signs of hepatic encephalopathy may also be seen. Laboratory abnormalities are similar to those reported for acute cholangiohepatitis; however, in advanced disease, hypergammaglobulinemia, hypoalbuminemia, low BUN, and coagulopathies due to vitamin K deficiency can be seen. Histopathologic changes include portal and biliary infiltration with lymphocytes and neutrophils; marked bile duct proliferation, degeneration, and fibrosis; and periportal necrosis and fibrosis. Progression to cirrhosis or end-stage liver disease is possible.

Supportive fluid therapy, antibiotics, and ursodeoxycholic acid can be used, with recommendations similar to those for acute cholangiohepatitis (see above). In addition, treatment with prednisone (2.2-6.6 mg/kg, PO, SID initially, then tapered to 2-4 mg/kg every 48 hr) is recommended because of the suspected immune-mediated component. Prognosis is variable. Some cats respond well to initial therapy, others relapse repeatedly, and some do not respond and succumb to the disease.

Biliary Cirrhosis

Biliary cirrhosis refers to portal fibrosis and biliary hyperplasia that develop after longterm inflammation; it is thought to be the sequela of chronic cholangiohepatitis. Biliary cirrhosis is uncommon, possibly because animals succumb before this condition develops. Clinical signs include icterus, anorexia, hepatomegaly, cachexia, and ascites. Liver enzymes may be normal. Hypoalbuminemia, hyperglobulinemia, hyperbilirubinemia, and coagulopathies are common laboratory abnormalities. The liver is large on radiographs and appears nodular on ultrasonographic evaluation. Biopsies are needed for a definitive diagnosis. Often, coagulation defects necessitate a whole blood transfusion before a biopsy can be taken. Treatment is symptomatic. Higher-protein diets are recommended to correct hypoalbuminemia unless hepatic encephalopathy is present. Angiotensin-converting-enzyme inhibitors (eg, enalapril) or loop diuretics (eg, furosemide) and low-salt diets are indicated to control ascites. However, the effectiveness of enalapril may be minimized because hepatic matabolism provides the active metabolite. Loop diuretics may cause electrolyte abnormalities and lead to anorexia, so animals should be monitored closely. Spironolactone can be used with furosemide to control ascites. Corticosteroids are contraindicated. Ursodeoxycholic acid may slow progression of cirrhosis. Prognosis is poor.

Lymphocytic Portal Hepatitis

Lymphocytic portal hepatitis is an inflammatory disease of the liver that does not appear to be related to cholangiohepatitis. An immune-mediated etiology has been suggested, but the definitive cause is unknown. Incidence is increased in hyperthyroid cats, although a direct association has not been proved. Clinical signs include anorexia, weight loss, and less frequently vomiting, diarrhea, lethargy, and fever. Hepatomegaly is noted in ~50% of cats. Increased poikilocytosis, AP, and ALT and normal to mildly increased bilirubin are common laboratory abnormalities. Bile acids are increased. Histopathologic changes include periportal lymphocytic plasmacytic infiltration, portal fibrosis, and bile duct proliferation. Combination antibiotic and immunosuppressive corticosteroid therapy has been tried with variable results. Nonsteroidal immunosuppressive drugs may be more effective.

CANINE CHOLANGIOHEPATITIS

Cholangiohepatitis in dogs is rare and is associated with ascending biliary tract infections (Salmonella, Campylobacter jejuni), choleliths, coccidiosis, and surgery of the biliary tract. Clinical signs include anorexia, vomiting, diarrhea, lethargy, polyuria, polydipsia, fever, and abdominal pain. Laboratory abnormalities are typical for cholestasis and include hyperbilirubinemia, and elevated AP and GGT. Histopathologic changes include a suppurative or mononuclear infiltrate; samples should be submitted for aerobic and anaerobic culture and sensitivity. Antibiotics and treatment for specific underlying diseases are recommended.

CANINE CHRONIC HEPATITIS

Chronic hepatitis is more common in dogs than in cats. Several breeds are predisposed, including Bedlington Terriers, Cocker Spaniels, Doberman Pinschers, Skye Terriers, Standard Poodles, and West Highland White Terriers. Although there is an identifiable etiology for some categories of chronic hepatitis, in most cases the cause is unknown. Copper accumulation is found in a number of cases of chronic hepatitis. Other associated conditions are infectious canine hepatitis, acidophil hepatitis, leptospirosis, and drug toxicities. Terminology that reflects specific etiology or breed predilection, such as drug-induced chronic hepatitis, infectious chronic hepatitis, copper-associated chronic hepatitis of Bedlington Terriers, etc, is preferred. The term idiopathic chronic hepatitis is used when etiology cannot be determined. Histopathologic changes are similar in all cases of chronic hepatitis, regardless of the underlying cause, and include lymphocytic-plasmacytic inflammation, piecemeal necrosis, and in severe cases, bridging necrosis.

Chronic Hepatitis of Bedlington Terriers

Chronic hepatitis of Bedlington Terriers is a result of chronic progressive copper accumulation within the hepatocytes due to an abnormal binding protein. The defect in copper metabolism is attributed to an autosomal recessive trait. Failure to excrete copper through the biliary system can cause minimal damage initially but can progress to chronic hepatitis or cirrhosis. Increased copper accumulation is first detected in young animals when ~1 yr old. Copper levels progressively increase until ~6 yr of age and then decline. Normal hepatic copper levels are <400 μg/g. Affected dogs may have hepatic copper levels as high as 12,000 μg/g at 1 yr of age. Liver damage is usually seen when copper levels are >2,000 μg/g. Excessive copper levels cause oxidative injury to hepatocyte mitochondria.

There are 3 distinct clinical presentations. The first is acute hepatic necrosis and is seen in Bedlington Terriers <6 yr old. Clinical signs include hepatomegaly, vomiting, depression, anorexia, icterus, copper-associated hemolytic anemia, and hemoglobinuria. Copper-associated hemolytic anemia is seen if there is a rapid release of copper from necrotic hepatocytes. Death may occur within 48-72 hr of onset of clinical signs. If the dog survives, recurrent bouts can be noted and may be induced by stressful situations. The second clinical presentation is chronic hepatitis. Clinical signs include chronic weight loss, hepatic encephalopathy, ascites, and icterus. The third presentation is seen in young, clinically healthy dogs that have increased liver enzymes and hepatic copper levels on liver biopsy. The condition may progress to acute hepatic necrosis or chronic hepatitis, or the dog may remain asymptomatic.

Screening for affected dogs includes monitoring liver enzymes and serum bile acids and performing a liver biopsy of dogs >1 yr old for quantitative copper analysis. Radioisotope studies may identify asymptomatic dogs. Hepatic copper levels should be measured in dogs selected for breeding at 5-7 mo and again at 14-15 mo. Recessive carriers can be eliminated from the gene pool because the copper levels are increased at 5-7 mo, but are decreased at 14-15 mo. In other affected dogs, hepatic copper levels are decreased at both 5-7 mo and 14-15 mo.

Treatment to control or decrease hepatic copper levels includes copper chelators (either D-penicillamine or trientine hydrochloride) and vitamin C to enhance urinary excretion of copper, zinc acetate or zinc sulfate to prevent intestinal absorption of copper, and feeding a low-copper diet. Choleretic effects of ursodeoxycholic acid may also be beneficial, and antioxidant effects of vitamin E (400-600 IU, SID) may decrease oxidative damage to hepatocytes. D-penicillamine (10-15 mg/kg, PO, BID, 30 min before meals) decreases hepatic copper levels slowly; a significant decrease in copper levels may take >1 yr. Trientine (10-15 mg/kg, PO, BID) is used if D-penicillamine is not tolerated. Lifelong use of chelator therapy is needed because copper levels decline slowly, and copper will reaccumulate if therapy is discontinued. Zinc acetate or sulfate (100-200 mg, PO, BID, 1 hr before meals for 3-6 mo, then 50 mg, PO, BID) can be used in combination with copper chelators. Zinc acetate alone may decrease copper levels in young dogs that are asymptomatic. Foods high in copper, including red meat, liver, shellfish, and fish, should be avoided. Chicken, dairy products, and rice have a low copper content. Therapy is lifelong. Prognosis is guarded if the dog is showing clinical signs. Early screening and treatment are recommended.

Chronic Hepatitis of West Highland White Terriers

West Highland White Terriers also have a copper-associated chronic hepatitis. The disease in West Highland White Terriers differs from that in Bedlington Terriers (p 382) in the following ways: 1) mode of inheritance has not been determined, 2) maximum copper accumulation is seen by 6 mo of age and then may decline, 3) overall hepatic copper concentrations are lower than those in Bedlington Terriers, and 4) hemolytic anemia has not been reported.

Focal hepatitis is seen in early disease, and dogs are usually asymptomatic. Jaundice, ascites, anorexia, diarrhea, and vomiting are commonly reported. Increases in liver enzymes, bilirubin, and serum bile acids are noted in advanced disease. Histopathologic changes include multifocal hepatitis, necrosis, and cirrhosis. Therapy includes use of copper chelators and zinc acetate as described above (p 382). Therapy is not warranted in dogs >2 yr of age that have hepatic copper levels <2,000 μg/g.

Idiopathic Chronic Hepatitis

Idiopathic chronic hepatitis is defined as chronic periportal hepatitis with no identifiable cause. Most affected animals are 5-6 yr old. Any breed can be affected, with males and females equally affected. Clinical signs include those typical for chronic liver disease and include anorexia, vomiting, diarrhea, weight loss, jaundice, polyuria and polydipsia, ascites, depression, and weakness. Common laboratory abnormalities include marked increases in ALT, moderate to marked increases of AP, bilirubinuria and hyperbilirubinemia, increased serum bile acids, and an abnormal ammonia tolerance test. Hypoalbuminemia, hyperglobulinemia, nonregenerative anemia, and abnormal coagulation profile are also reported. Radiographs may demonstrate a small liver, and nodular lesions may be detected on ultrasonographic studies. Definitive diagnosis is by liver biopsy. Histopathologic findings include lymphocytic-plasmacytic inflammation, piecemeal necrosis advancing to bridging necrosis, and in advanced cases, cirrhosis. Biopsy specimens should be submitted for both aerobic and anaerobic cultures.

Supportive care and use of specific therapy as indicated (eg, antibiotics if bacterial cultures are positive), along with choleretics, antifibrotic agents, and low-protein diets may be effective. Ursodeoxycholic acid is used if significant cholestasis is noted without biliary obstruction. The use of colchicine as an antifibrotic agent may be limited by side effects that include nausea, vomiting, and hemorrhagic diarrhea. Use of immunosuppressive drugs is controversial but recommended if there is no evidence of infectious disease, if there is strong evidence of immune-mediated disease, or if active disease is evident on biopsy. Prednisolone can be given at 1-2 mg/kg, divided BID until clinical remission, after which the dosage is slowly reduced. Complete remission is difficult to evaluate clinically and may require a followup biopsy. Prognosis depends on the amount of damage sustained by the liver and the degree of fibrosis but can be favorable if damage is mild to moderate and if initial therapy is effective.

Chronic Hepatitis of Doberman Pinschers

Chronic hepatitis and cirrhosis of Doberman Pinschers is an idiopathic disease. Copper levels are increased in affected dogs, but this may be due to increased retention as a result of decreased biliary excretion and not to a primary disorder of copper excretion. However, hepatitis and increased hepatic copper levels without cholestasis have been reported in some cases, suggesting that copper accumulation may be an inciting factor.

Increased copper levels may also be a breed variation because normal Doberman Pinschers have exceptionally high hepatic copper levels.

The disease primarily affects middle-aged females, although age can vary. Clinical signs include anorexia, weight loss, vomiting, diarrhea, ascites, jaundice, polyuria, and polydipsia; bleeding abnormalities and hepatic encephalopathy are indicators of advanced disease. Laboratory abnormalities include increased levels of liver enzymes, bilirubin, blood ammonia, and serum bile acids, as well as hypoalbuminemia. Coagulation disorders may be secondary to hepatic failure or concurrent von Willebrand's disease. Radiography and ultrasonography show microhepatica, ascites, and splenomegaly. Ultrasonography may identify nodular lesions in the liver.

Treatment consists of symptomatic and supportive care and immunosuppressive therapy. Prednisone at 1.1 mg/kg, PO, BID, is used initially, and azathioprine at 2.2 mg/kg, PO, SID, may be added. Use of ursodeoxycholic acid may be beneficial. Copper chelators may also be effective in reducing copper levels, but their use is controversial because the exact role of copper in this disease is poorly understood. Prognosis is usually poor because the disease is often advanced before it is detected.

There is a subclinical stage of Doberman hepatitis. Affected dogs are clinically normal but have elevated ALT values and evidence of hepatitis on liver biopsy. Treatment with anti-inflammatory doses of prednisone is thought to be beneficial.

Chronic Hepatitis of Skye Terriers and Cocker Spaniels

Chronic hepatitis in Skye Terriers and Cocker Spaniels is associated with increased hepatic copper concentrations. However, increased copper levels are attributed to cholestasis and decreased biliary excretion of copper and not to a primary copper retention disorder. Young male Cocker Spaniels (American and English) appear to be most affected. Ascites is the most common physical abnormality; other clinical signs include depression, icterus, dehydration, and melena. The most common laboratory abnormalities are mild anemia; mature neutrophilia; low BUN; hypoalbuminemia; bilirubinuria; bilirubinemia; and elevated AP, blood ammonia, and serum bile acids. Treatment is supportive and symptomatic, including prednisone, D-penicillamine, ursodeoxycholic acid, and dietary management. Prognosis is poor due to the extent of liver damage at the time of diagnosis.

Hepatitis can affect Skye Terriers at any age. Dogs can be asymptomatic or in end-stage liver failure. Three separate stages of liver disease have been described and vary from mild inflammation with no evidence of cirrhosis or copper accumulation to advanced macronodular cirrhosis, cholestasis, and marked copper accumulation.

Lobular Dissecting Hepatitis

Lobular dissecting hepatitis is an idiopathic disease reported primarily in young to middle-aged Standard Poodles. Ascites is the most common clinical sign. Laboratory abnormalities include hypoalbuminemia and increased serum bile acids; AP values may be normal or slightly increased. Multiple portosystemic shunts may develop secondary to advanced hepatic failure and portal hypertension. The disease can progress to cirrhosis. Copper levels are not consistently increased. Supportive treatment is recommended.

METABOLIC DISEASES AFFECTING THE LIVER

Endocrine Diseases

Diabetes mellitus, hyperadrenocorticism, and hyperthyroidism can cause changes in the liver.

Hepatic lipidosis develops secondary to diabetes mellitus because of increased lipid metabolism and mobilization. Hepatomegaly and increased liver enzymes are noted. Dogs with diabetes mellitus rarely have liver dysfunction although AP and, to a lesser degree, ALT may be increased. Cats have increased ALT, hyperbilirubinemia, and normal or mildly increased AP. Liver function tests may be abnormal. Hepatic lipidosis may or may not resolve with insulin replacement. Diabetic animals are also at increased risk for pancreatitis, extrahepatic bacterial infections, or hepatocutaneous syndrome.

In dogs with hyperadrenocorticism, changes in the liver are similar to those seen in glucocorticoid toxicity and resolve with appropriate treatment of hyperadrenocorticism.

In cats with hyperthyroidism, increased AP and ALT and possibly hyperbilirubinemia are seen. Liver function is usually normal. Possible causes for the changes noted in the liver include toxic effects of excessive thyroid hormone, malnutrition, or if cardiac thyroid toxicosis is present, hypoxia due to congestive heart failure. Liver enzymes return to normal with treatment; however, treatment with methimazole can lead to liver toxicity.

Hepatocutaneous Syndrome
(Superficial necrolytic dermatitis, Metabolic epidermal necrosis, Necrolytic migratory erythema)

Hepatocutaneous syndrome is rare, chronic, progressive, and usually fatal. Although usually associated with a hepatopathy, this syndrome can also be seen in animals with pancreatic or neuroendocrine tumors. Diabetes mellitus is a common concurrent disease. Bilaterally symmetric crusting and ulcerative lesions on the footpads, mucocutaneous junctions, ears, periorbital region, and pressure points are typical dermatologic changes. Anorexia, weight loss, and lethargy are also reported. Marked increase in AP, moderate increases in ALT and AST, hyperglycemia, decreased plasma amino acids, hypoalbuminemia, increased bile acids, and normocytic, normochormic anemia are usually reported. Hyperglucagonemia is not a consistent finding, as it is in people with a similar condition. Liver size varies radiographically. Multiple hypoechoic nodules surrounded by hyperechoic strands are seen diffusely scattered throughout the liver on ultrasonography, and this "starry sky" pattern is thought to be pathognomonic. Possible reasons for skin lesions associated with liver disease include hypoaminoacidemia resulting in a reduction in epidermal cell turnover or abnormal zinc metabolism. Histopathologic changes include vacuolization of hepatocytes, liver parenchymal collapse, and nodular regeneration. Recommended treatments include appropriate antifungal and antibiotic therapy for skin infections, zinc and vitamin supplementation, high-protein diets (eg, egg yolks or amino acid supplements), control of diabetes mellitus with insulin therapy, and topical cleansing of skin lesions. Treatment has little effect on the course of the disease. Corticosteroids are contraindicated. Prognosis is guarded to poor.

HEPATIC CYSTS AND NODULAR HYPERPLASIA

Hepatic cysts (cytoadenomas) can be acquired (usually single nodules) or congenital (usually multiple). They are found in both dogs and cats. Congenital polycystic disease of the liver has been reported in Cairn Terriers, West Highland White Terriers, and Persian cats and may be seen with polycystic kidneys. In cats, hepatic cysts are usually incidental findings at necropsy. Occasionally, the cysts can become large and cause abdominal distention and other clinical signs such as lethargy, vomiting, and polydipsia. Masses that are palpable on physical examination are usually nonpainful. Ascites can be present, and the ascitic fluid is usually a modified transudate. Laboratory data are usually normal. Lesions can be identified with radiographs or ultrasonography. Definitive diagnosis is by biopsy. Surgical removal is usually curative.

Nodular hyperplasia is a benign, age-related change in dogs that does not usually cause clinical disease but is often accompanied by mild to moderate increases in ALT and AP; serum bile acids are normal. Lesions on ultrasonography vary in size and appear as hypoechoic or hyperechoic areas. Because ultrasonographic findings of nodular hyperplasia cannot be differentiated from those of hepatocellular carcinoma, a biopsy may be necessary for differentiation. A wedge biopsy is preferred over a needle biopsy. Hepatocytes are enlarged (hyperplastic) and contain either lipid or glycogen or undergo hydropic degeneration; fibrosis is not seen. Iron concentration is increased in hepatic macrophages. Nodular hyperplasia rarely affects liver function.

HEPATIC NEOPLASIA

Primary hepatic neoplasms are less common than metastatic neoplasms of the liver and are either carcinomas, sarcomas, or of hemolymphatic origin. Metastatic neoplasia of the liver can originate from several organs.

Primary tumors are seen in older animals (>10 yr) and can be either malignant or benign. They include hepatocellular adenomas and carcinomas, biliary adenomas and carcinomas, and hemangiosarcomas. Leiomyosarcomas are also reported, although infrequently. Bile duct adenomas and adenocarcinomas are the most common intrahepatic neoplasias in cats. Hepatocellular carcinomas are the most common primary liver tumor in male dogs; biliary carcinomas are more frequently reported in female dogs. Primary malignant tumors can be seen as a single mass in one liver lobe with or without smaller masses in other lobes (massive), as discrete nodules located in multiple lobes (nodular), or as infiltrative disease throughout the liver without the presence of discrete nodules (diffuse). A solitary mass is the most common in dogs; cats tend to have multiple lobe involvement. Hepatic carcinoids are rare tumors that metastasize readily and are referred to as APUDomas (amine precursor uptake and decarboxylase tumors). Metastatic disease from primary liver tumors is common and can involve the lymph nodes, peritoneum, and lungs.

Lymphoma is the most common hemolymphatic tumor found in the liver in both dogs and cats. Lymphosarcoma of the liver is often seen with lymphosarcoma of the intestines and stomach. Other myeloproliferative diseases such as leukemia, multiple myleoma, and mast cell tumor are reported.

The most common **metastatic tumors** in dogs include pancreatic carcinoma, mammary carcinoma, pheochromocytoma, intestinal carcinoma, thyroid carcinoma, fibrosarcoma, osteosarcoma, and transitional cell carcinoma. Metastatic tumors of the liver are less common in cats, but the most common ones include pancreatic, intestinal, and renal cell carcinomas. Metastatic tumors are usually multifocal.

Clinical signs can be nonspecific or specific and include polyuria and polydipsia, vomiting, weight loss, jaundice, bleeding dyscrasias, hepatic encephalopathy, and ascites. Seizures may develop because of hepatic encephalopathy, hypoglycemia due to a paraneoplastic process, or metastatic lesions in the brain. Cats are usually anorectic and lethargic; ascites is seldom seen. Hepatomegaly or a cranial abdominal mass may be found on abdominal palpation. Animals may be pale (due to hemorrhage or anemia of chronic disease) or icteric.

Laboratory data is similar to that seen in other diseases of the liver. Animals with lymphoma or myeloproliferative disease may have circulating blast cells. Eosinophilia can be seen with mast cell tumors. Liver enzymes are generally increased more frequently with primary tumors than with metastatic disease. AP and ALT are often increased in dogs; ALT and AST are increased in cats. Hyperbilirubinemia and increased AST are seen more frequently in canine metastatic disease than with primary tumors. Radiographic findings are variable. Ultrasonographic findings can confirm single lobe involvement, multiple nodular changes, or diffuse disease. Biopsy is needed for a definitive diagnosis. If one liver lobe is involved, surgical removal is recommended. If hemangiosarcoma, lymphoma, or mastocytosis is diagnosed, appropriate chemotherapy may be effective. The prognosis is poor for primary hepatic tumors that involve multiple lobes, as there is no effective therapy.

MISCELLANEOUS LIVER DISEASES

Glycogen Storage Disease

Of the 3 glycogen storage diseases reported in dogs, types I and III directly affect the liver. In general, glycogen storage diseases are caused by a deficiency of certain enzymes and result in failure of glycogen to be released from the cell. Therefore, glycogen accumulates within the liver and other organs and is unavailable for conversion to glucose. Type Ia glycogen storage disease results from a deficiency in glucose-6-phosphatase and has been reported in toy-breed dogs. Type III is caused by a deficiency in amylo-1,6-glucosidase and has been reported in German Shepherds. Clinical signs for both include hepatomegaly, retarded growth, and weakness and depression due to hypoglycemia.

Enzyme analysis of fresh frozen samples of liver, muscle, or skin is needed for diagnosis. Treatment is symptomatic and includes frequent small meals of high-carbohydrate food. Prognosis is poor, and most dogs succumb to these diseases at a young age.

Hepatic Amyloidosis

Amyloidosis is a familial disease of Abyssinian, Siamese, and oriental cats and Chinese Shar-Peis. Shar-Peis are more likely to have episodic fever and swollen hocks, with or without renal failure, but the liver may also be affected in these dogs. Although affected Abyssinian cats usually present with clinical signs of renal failure, occasionally clinical signs may be consistent with liver disease. Oriental and Siamese cats with amyloidosis generally have hepatic disease. Other conditions associated with hepatic amyloidosis include hypervitaminosis A (cats) and coccidioidomycosis (dogs). Although some affected animals may be asymptomatic, typical clinical signs include anorexia, polydipsia, and polyuria, vomiting, icterus, and hepatomegaly. Affected animals may present in an acute state of collapse with pale mucous membranes due to rupture of the liver and subsequent hemorrhage. Diagnosis is made by identifying amyloid deposits in liver biopsy samples using Congo red stain; amyloid has a birefringent apple-green appearance. Colchicine and dimethyl sulfoxide have been used to slow progression of the disease, with limited success. Amyloidosis is progressive and the prognosis is poor, especially if the diagnosis is made late in the disease. (*See also* AMYLOIDOSIS, p 478.)

Idiopathic Hepatic Fibrosis

Hepatic fibrosis in young dogs that is not associated with any underlying inflammatory conditions is referred to as idiopathic hepatic fibrosis. Affected dogs are usually <2 yr of age, but older dogs have been diagnosed with this disease. Three different categories have been described, based on the location of fibrosis. Excessive fibrosis around the centrilobular veins is referred to as central perivenous fibrosis, and German Shepherds appear to be predisposed. When fibrosis is intralobular, surrounding the hepatocytes, the condition is termed diffuse pericellular fibrosis. Again, German Shepherds are affected more commonly than other breeds. Periportal fibrosis is characterized as fibrosis in the portal areas. There appears to be no breed predisposition to periportal fibrosis.

Clinical signs are similar for all 3 forms and include ascites and hepatic encephalopathy due to portal hypertension and portosystemic shunting. Jaundice is uncommon, but may be present in dogs with diffuse pericellular fibrosis. Other signs include weight loss, vomiting, and diarrhea. Microcytic anemia, elevated AP and ALT, hypoalbuminemia, and markedly increased postprandial bile acids are common laboratory findings. Microhepatica is noted on radiographs, and portosystemic shunts can be identified by ultrasonography. Symptomatic treatment for management of hepatic encephalopathy and ascites is recommended. The effect of antifibrotic therapy has not been thoroughly evaluated. Prognosis is guarded.

DISEASES OF THE GALLBLADDER AND EXTRABILIARY SYSTEM

Icterus is often the presenting sign of diseases of the gallbladder and extrahepatic biliary system. Ascites may be present if bile is leaking into the abdomen, causing bile peritonitis. Higher bilirubin levels in the abdominal effusion than in the serum can confirm leakage of bile into the abdomen or bile duct rupture. Icterus may not be the presenting sign in malignancies of the gallbladder.

Obstructive Diseases of the Extrahepatic Biliary System

Obstructive diseases of the extrahepatic biliary system are most often associated with pancreatic disease (*see* p 347). Pancreatic edema, inflammation, or fibrosis due to pancreatitis can cause compression of the common bile duct. Diagnosis is based on laboratory data (increased AP, bilirubinuria with or without bilirubinemia) and on radiographic and ultrasonographic evidence of pancreatic disease. Medical management of pancreatitis is often the only treatment necessary to relieve biliary obstruction. If this is not successful, then either temporary compression of the gallbladder with a catheter or cholecystoduodenostomy may be necessary. Choleliths rarely cause obstruction, but when this does occur, cholecystectomy is preferred over choledochectomy (incision of the common bile duct, which can lead to stricture postsurgically). Neoplasia of the pancreas, bile ducts, liver, intestines, and lymph nodes can also cause obstructive disease. Biopsy is needed to confirm the diagnosis. Cholecystojejunostomy may be palliative, but a cure can rarely be achieved. Other than for lymphoma, chemotherapy is generally not effective.

Cholecystitis

Cholecystitis is usually caused by bacterial infections that either are intestinal in origin and ascend up the common bile duct or are from hematogenous spread. The infection can remain within the gallbladder, resulting in either necrotizing or emphysematous cholecystitis. With necrotizing cholecystitis, the wall of the gallbladder is damaged, and bile leaks into the abdomen causing a severe septic peritonitis, which can be lethal. If the bile that leaks is inspissated, then peritonitis will be local. Anorexia, abdominal pain, icterus, fever, and vomiting are common clinical signs. The animal may present in a state of shock due to bile peritonitis. Radiographic evidence of gas in the area of the gallbladder is consistent with emphysematous cholecystitis. Ultrasonography can assist with the diagnosis. Stabilizing the animal, cholecystectomy, appropriate antibiotic therapy, and management for peritonitis (p 537) are necessary for treatment. Prognosis is poor, unless diagnosis and treatment are early in the disease.

Cholecystitis can also spread to the surrounding bile ducts and liver parenchyma, resulting in bacterial cholangitis and cholangiohepatitis. *Escherichia coli* is the most frequently isolated bacteria. Icterus, vomiting, and anorexia are the most common clinical signs. Bilirubin and liver enzymes are frequently increased. Diagnosis can be confirmed by biopsy for both aerobic and anaerobic cultures and for histopathology. Prognosis is favorable if appropriate antibiotic therapy is initiated early.

Choleliths

Choleliths rarely cause disease. When it does occur, disease is usually seen in older, female, small-breed dogs. In cats, choleliths are generally associated with cholangitis and cholangiohepatitis. Clinical signs include vomiting, icterus, abdominal pain, and fever. Unlike gallstones in humans, which primarily contain cholesterol, choleliths in dogs and cats contain bilirubin pigments. Treatment consists of removal of the stones by cholecystotomy or cholecystoduodenostomy or jejunostomy and appropriate antibiotic therapy.

Extrahepatic Infection and Sepsis

Extrahepatic infection and sepsis can cause cholestasis and hyperbilirubinemia. Increases in serum bilirubin levels are often moderate to marked, while those of AP levels are only mild to moderate. Appropriate treatment of the underlying septic condition returns bile flow to normal.

Parasitic Infection

The liver fluke *Platynosomum concinnum* is an uncommon cause of biliary tract disease in cats. Affected cats are found in Florida, the Caribbean, and Hawaii. The life cycle of the fluke includes lizards and toads as intermediate hosts, which are then eaten by cats. The flukes can exist in the biliary system without causing signs, or they can cause obstruction and severe hepatic dysfunction. Clinical signs depend on the severity of the worm burden. Vomiting, diarrhea, icterus, and hepatomegaly are signs of biliary obstruction. Changes in the biliary system range from cholecystitis to cholangiohepatitis and fibrosis in animals with chronic heavy infections. Flukes can migrate into the pancreas and cause pancreatic atrophy. Eosinophilia and increased ALT, AP, and bilirubin are seen. Finding ova in a fecal specimen is diagnostic, but ova will not be seen if the biliary tract is completely obstructed. Praziquantel (20 mg/kg, SC, SID for 3 days, or 20 mg/kg, PO, every 12 wk) is recommended for treatment. Treatment results are variable. Prognosis is favorable for mild forms of the disease. Other rare parasites of the biliary tract include *Amphimerus pseudofelineus*, *Metorchis conjunctus*, and *Eurytrema procyonis*.

Rupture of the Gallbladder

Rupture of the gallbladder is most often seen with cholelithiasis, necrotizing cholecystitis, or blunt trauma. Rupture of the extrahepatic biliary system can be associated with blunt trauma, cholelith obstruction, neoplasia, or parasites. Trauma may rupture the cystic duct, hepatic ducts, or, most commonly, the common bile duct. Regardless of the cause, the end result is bile peritonitis. Diagnostic peritoneal lavage may be useful in early diagnosis. If diagnosis is delayed, necrosis, bacterial peritonitis, and adhesions can develop, which increases the difficulty of repair and management and worsens the prognosis. Surgical intervention consists of bile duct ligation, cholecystectomy, or cholecystojejunostomy as indicated.

VOMITING

Vomiting is the forceful ejection of the contents of the stomach and proximal small intestine. It is a vigorously active motion signaled by hypersalivation, retching, and forceful contractions of the abdominal muscles and the diaphragm. Vomiting must be differentiated from regurgitation, which is a passive motion facilitated by gravity and body position of the animal. With regurgitation, the expelled food and fluid tends to be undigested, has a neutral pH depending on the composition of the diet, and may have a cylindrical shape reflecting the shape of the esophagus. Dyspnea or cough is more often associated with regurgitation, which indicates a lesion of the oral cavity, pharynx, or esophagus.

Etiology, Pathophysiology, and Clinical Findings: Vomiting represents a coordinated effort of the GI, musculoskeletal, and nervous systems to expel food, fluid, or debris from the GI tract. It is initiated by direct stimulation of the vomiting center in the brain stem or indirectly via the chemoreceptor trigger zone (CTZ) or abdominal afferent nerves. Stimulation of receptors in the semicircular canals of the vestibular system, or inflammation within the CNS and increases in intracranial pressure, can also promote vomiting. The CTZ responds to substances in the blood, eg, drugs, ketones, or uremic or bacterial toxins. Most of the receptors involved in the vomiting reflex are found in the abdominal viscera, especially in the duodenum. Abdominal afferent neural stimulation may arise from GI tract inflammation; stretching or distention of the bowel; or irritation or inflammation of the liver, pancreas, kidneys, spleen, genitourinary tract, or peritoneum. Motor efferent innervation of the vomiting reflex is mediated from the spinal and phrenic nerves, which innervate muscles of the abdominal wall and diaphragm.

Vomiting can be due to primary GI disease, renal or hepatic failure, electrolyte abnormalities (eg, hypoadrenocorticism), pancreatitis, or CNS disorders (including toxin ingestion).

Anxiety, depression, hypersalivation, and repeated swallowing accompanied by relaxation of the gastroesophageal sphincter are followed by retching. The proximal small intestine and gastric antrum contract, propelling their contents into the body of the stomach where movement is inhibited. The gastroesophageal sphincter moves into the thoracic cavity, rendering it incompetent and facilitating gastroesophageal reflux. Esophageal and pharyngoesophageal sphincter motility is repressed, and the nasopharynx closes to prevent nasal regurgitation. Forceful contractions of the abdominal muscles and diaphragm against a closed glottis and increases in intra-abdominal pressure force expulsion of food, fluid, or debris.

Diagnosis: The diagnostic approach to vomiting varies depending on whether the vomiting is acute or chronic. Acute or even sporadic vomiting is generally not associated with other abnormalities. Chronic vomiting may be associated with weakness, lethargy, weight loss, dehydration, electrolyte imbalance, and acid-base disorders.

When vomiting has been of a short duration, ie, <3-4 days, and without associated adverse clinical signs, the diagnostic approach may be limited to a detailed history (including questions related to possible ingestion of garbage or toxins), a physical examination (including abdominal palpation), examination of the oropharynx, and a rectal examination (checking for evidence of dietary indiscretion). If nothing of significance is found, symptomatic therapy may be administered.

Chronic vomiting, vomiting that occurs more often than once or twice daily, and vomiting accompanied by hematemesis, abdominal pain, depression, dehydration, weakness, fever, or other adverse clinical signs should be approached more vigorously. In addition to a detailed history and physical examination, an initial database should include a CBC, biochemical profile (including serum electrolytes), urinalysis, and abdominal radiographs (and abdominal ultrasonography if available). A more detailed database will be dictated by any identified abnormalities. In many cases, endoscopic evaluation and biopsy of the stomach and small intestine is the only test that can determine the nature of the disease.

Treatment and Control: Control of vomiting should be directed to identifying the inciting cause and (if possible) eliminating it and to controlling accompanying secondary changes.

Symptomatic therapy for acute vomiting includes fasting and withholding water for 24 hr to rest the GI tract. (Water can be provided in the form of ice.) Animals predisposed to hypovolemia, eg, animals with concurrent renal insufficiency or cardiac disease, should receive parenteral fluid therapy. If the vomiting has stopped after 24 hr, the animal may be offered small amounts of water initially. If no further vomiting occurs, small amounts of a commercial low-fat diet can be fed 4-6 times the first day or so, after which the animal can be fed its standard diet.

Therapy for chronic vomiting is also directed to elimination of the primary cause and, in addition, to correction of dehydration, electrolyte imbalances, and acid-base disorders. The vomiting reflex should be suppressed. (Specific treatment regimens are detailed under respective disease headings.) If untreated, persistent vomiting may result in prerenal azotemia. Vomiting associated with GI obstruction (p 330) commonly results in hypokalemia, hypochloremia, metabolic alkalosis, and paradoxical aciduria due to losses of secretions rich in potassium, chloride, and hydrogen. However, continued vomiting, lack of water intake, insensible water losses, and catabolism of body energy stores contribute to dehydration, poor tissue perfusion, hypoxia, and lactic acidosis. In the absence of gastric obstruction, the loss of bicarbonate from duodenal secretions may predispose to metabolic acidosis. It is therefore difficult to accurately predict the acid-base status of a vomiting animal, especially when the cause or duration of vomiting is unknown.

Antiemetic therapy is indicated in animals with intractable vomiting, dehydration, and weakness. (*See also* p 1981.) Commonly used antiemetics include antispasmodic medication, agents that depress the CTZ, drugs that suppress the emetic center, drugs that have peripheral activity, and the newer serotonin-antagonist agents. Drugs that act directly on the emetic center are very effective but tend to be less effective in the control of vomiting associated with severe GI disease. Drugs that act on the emetic center as well as the CTZ are more efficacious.

Antispasmodic agents (eg, scopolamine, 0.03 mg/kg, SC or IM, QID) inhibit cholinergic activity from visceral receptors. Consequently, they may inhibit vomiting associated with excessive contraction of GI smooth muscle. These drugs are rarely effective in small animals.

Drugs that depress the CTZ are used primarily to control motion sickness in people and may be useful to prevent nausea caused by drugs. They include dimenhydrinate (8 mg/kg, PO, TID) and trimethobenzamide (3 mg/kg, BID-TID). Trimethobenzamide is not as consistently effective as the phenothiazine antiemetic agents.

Diphenhydramine (2-4 mg/kg, PO, TID), an antihistamine, works by blocking H_1 receptors in the vestibular apparatus and, to a lesser extent, the CTZ. It may be useful in management of motion sickness.

Drugs acting directly on the emetic center include the phenothiazine tranquilizers such as prochlorperazine (0.3 mg/kg, TID, PO; 0.1 mg/kg, IM, QID; or 0.1-0.5 mg/kg, SC, TID) and chlorpromazine (0.5 mg/kg, PO, QID; 0.5 mg/kg, IM, TID; or 1 mg/kg, rectally, TID). Phenothiazine agents also inhibit activity of the CTZ and have weak anticholinergic effects. The antiemetic effects are seen at dosages lower than those required to cause tranquilization.

Dopaminergic antagonists such as metoclopramide (0.2-0.5 mg/kg, PO or SC, QID, or 1-2 mg/kg/day, slow IV or 1.3 µg/kg/min) and domperidone (0.05-0.1 mg/kg, PO, SID-BID) act at the level of the CTZ and peripheral receptors and are useful in the management of vomiting associated with toxins in the blood. Ondansetron (0.5-1 mg/kg, PO, SID-BID, or 30 min before chemotherapy, PO) is a potent antiemetic agent. It is a selective serotonin-receptor antagonist with both central and peripheral activity. It should be considered in cases unresponsive to other antiemetic agents. Dolasetron (0.6-1.0 mg/kg, IV, PO) is a serotonin type III antagonist used to reduce nausea and vomiting secondary to anesthesia, chemotherapy, enteritis, and renal and hepatic disease. To date, no side effects have been reported in pets.

■ ■ ■

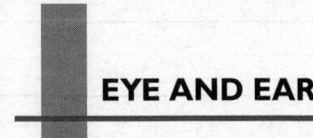

EYE AND EAR

OPHTHALMOLOGY

PHYSICAL EXAMINATION OF THE EYE

The initial examination of the eye should assess symmetry, conformation, and gross lesions; the eye should be viewed from 2-3 ft (≤1 m) away, in good light, and with minimal restraint of the head. The anterior ocular segment and pupillary light reflexes are examined in detail with a strong light and under magnification in a darkened room. Baseline tests like the Schirmer tear test, fluorescein staining, and tonometry (intraocular pressure measurement), may be followed by ancillary tests such as taking corneal and conjunctival cytology and cultures, everting the eyelids for examination, and flushing the nasolacrimal duct to evaluate the external parts of the eye, including the anterior segment. Diseases of the vitreous and ocular fundus are evaluated by direct and indirect ophthalmoscopy (usually performed after inducing mydriasis) and vision testing (menace reflex, obstacle course, etc).

Schirmer tear tests and cultures should be performed before topical anesthetic is instilled. Fluorescein staining and eversion of the eyelids need not require topical anesthesia, but tonometry, examination of the bulbar surface of the nictitating membrane, conjunctival and corneal cytology, gonioscopy, and lavage of the nasolacrimal duct usually do. To avoid false positives, samples for corneal and conjunctival cytology that will be analyzed by fluorescent antibody procedures should be collected before topical fluorescein staining.

Special examinations such as slit-lamp biomicroscopy, ultrasonography, fluorescein angiography, and electroretinography may require sedation or local, regional, or general anesthesia.

EYELIDS

Conformational Abnormalities

Entropion is an inversion of all or part of the lid margins that may involve one or both eyelids and the canthi. It is the most frequent inherited eyelid defect in many canine and ovine breeds, and may also follow cicatrix formation, and severe blepharospasm due to ocular or periocular pain. Inversion of the cilia (or eyelashes) or facial hairs causes further discomfort, conjunctival and corneal irritation, and if protracted, corneal scarring, pigmentation, and possibly ulceration. Early spastic entropion may be reversed if the inciting cause is removed, or if pain is alleviated by everting the lid hairs away from the eye with mattress sutures in the lid, by subcutaneous injections (eg, of procaine penicillin) into the lid adjacent to the entropion, or by palpebral nerve blocks. Established entropion may require surgical correction.

Ectropion is a slack, everted lid margin, usually with a large palpebral fissure. It is a common bilateral conformational abnormality in a number of dog breeds, including the Bloodhound, Bull Mastiff, Great Dane, Newfoundland, St. Bernard, and several Spaniel breeds. Contracting scars in the lid or facial nerve paralysis may produce unilateral ectropion in any species. Conjunctival exposure to environmental irritants and secondary bacterial infection can result in chronic or recurrent conjunctivitis. Topical antibiotic-corticosteroid preparations may temporarily control intermittent infections, but surgical lid-shortening procedures are often indicated. Mild cases can be controlled by repeated, periodic lavage with mild decongestant solutions.

Lagophthalmos is an inability to fully close the lids and protect the cornea from drying and trauma. It may result from extremely shallow orbits (in brachycephalic breeds), exophthalmia due to a space-occupying orbital lesion, or facial nerve paralysis. Corneal scarring, pigmentation, and ulceration usually result. Unless the cause can be corrected, the therapy is frequent topical lubrication and surgical shortening or closure of the canthi either temporarily or permanently. Excessive nasal skin folds and facial hair may aggravate the damage caused by lagophthalmos.

Abnormalities of the cilia include extra (distichia) or misdirected eyelashes on the lid margin. Epiphora, corneal vascularization, and corneal ulceration and scarring may result. In many instances, anomalous cilia are very fine and result in neither clinical signs nor damage. However, ectopic cilia protruding through the dorsal palpebral conjunctiva can cause profound pain. If the corneal or conjunctival damage is caused by the extra cilia, excision or cryothermy of the cilia follicles is indicated. Anomalies of the cilia are common in some dog breeds and probably inherited.

Inflammation

Blepharitis (inflammation of the eyelids) can result from extension of a generalized dermatitis, conjunctivitis or local glandular infections, or irritants such as plant oils or solar exposure. The lids can be the original site of involvement for agents that progress to a generalized dermatitis. Dermatophytes, *Demodex canis*, and bacteria such as staphylococci often are involved. The mucocutaneous junction of the skin and conjunctiva can be the site of lesions of immune-mediated diseases such as pemphigus. Skin scrapings, cultures, and biopsies may be required for an accurate diagnosis. Localized glandular infections may be acute or chronic (stye and chalazion).

In generalized blepharitis, systemic therapy often is indicated in addition to topical treatment. Supportive therapy of hot packing and frequent cleansing is indicated in acute cases. Nonophthalmic preparations can be used to treat the eyelids, but caution in application is indicated to avoid corneal and conjunctival contact and possible irritation.

NASOLACRIMAL AND LACRIMAL APPARATUS

Hypertrophy and prolapse of the gland of the nictitating membrane (**cherry eye**) is common in young dogs and certain breeds (eg, American Cocker Spaniel and English Bulldog). In the acute stage, the red glandular mass swells and protrudes over the leading margin of the nictitans, and there is a mucopurulent discharge. Although the swelling may recede for short periods, it eventually often remains prolapsed. Because it is a major tear gland, it should be preserved if possible; the gland should be replaced and anchored with sutures to the orbital rim or periorbital fascia, or covered with adjacent mucosa (envelope or pocket techniques). Partial excision should be avoided. Complete excision may predispose to keratoconjunctivitis sicca (*see* below) in 30-40% of dogs in later life. Surgical or medical resolution of cherry eye still predisposes ~20% of these dogs to keratoconjunctivitis sicca.

Dacryocystitis (inflammation of the lacrimal sac) usually is caused by obstruction of the nasolacrimal sac and proximal nasolacrimal duct by inflammatory debris, foreign bodies, or masses pressing on the duct. It results in epiphora, secondary conjunctivitis refractory to treatment, and occasionally a draining fistula in the medial lower eyelid. Irrigation of the nasolacrimal duct reveals an obstruction of the duct, reflux of mucopurulent discharge from the lacrimal puncta, or both. Radiographs of the skull after injection of contrast material into the duct (dacryocystorhinography) may be necessary to establish the site, cause, and prognosis of chronic obstructions. Therapy consists of maintaining patency of the duct and instilling topical antibiotic solutions. Tubing (polyethylene or silicone) or 2-0 monofilament nylon suture temporarily catheterized in the duct may be necessary to maintain patency. When the nasolacrimal apparatus has been irreversibly damaged, a new drainage pathway can be constructed surgically (conjunctivorhinostomy or conjunctivoralostomy) to empty tears into the nasal cavity, sinus, or mouth.

Imperforate lacrimal puncta are an infrequent cause of epiphora in young dogs. In foals, atresia of the nasal (distal) end of the nasolacrimal duct is a common cause of epiphora and chronic conjunctivitis. In calves, multiple openings of the nasolacrimal duct may empty tears onto the lower eyelid and medial canthus, causing chronic dermatitis. Therapy in dogs and foals consists of surgically opening the blocked orifice and maintaining patency by catherization during healing.

Keratoconjunctivitis sicca (KCS) is due to an aqueous tear deficiency and usually results in persistent, mucopurulent conjunctivitis and corneal ulceration and scarring. KCS occurs in dogs, cats, and horses. In dogs, it is often associated with an autoimmune dacryoadenitis of both the lacrimal and nictitans glands. Distemper, systemic sulfonamide therapy, heredity, and trauma are less frequent causes of KCS in dogs. KCS occurs infrequently in cats and has been associated with chronic feline herpesvirus-1 infections. In horses, KCS may follow head trauma. Topical therapy consists of artificial tear solutions, ointments, and, if there is no corneal ulceration, antibiotic-corticosteroid combinations. Lacrimogenics such as topical cyclosporin A (0.2-2%, BID) may increase tear production in ~80% of dogs with Schirmer tear test values of 2 mm wetting/min or higher. Ophthalmic pilocarpine mixed in food may be useful for neurogenic KCS (a 20-30 lb [10-15 kg] dog should be started on 2-4 drops of 2% pilocarpine, BID). Mucolytic agents (eg, 10% acetylcysteine) lyse excess mucus and restore the spreading ability of other topical agents. In chronic KCS refractory to medical therapy, parotid duct transplantation is indicated.

CONJUNCTIVA

Subconjunctival hemorrhage may arise from trauma or blood dyscrasias and certain infectious diseases. It does not require therapy, but close inspection is warranted to determine if more important intraocular alterations have occurred. If definite evidence or history of trauma is not present, then systemic examination is indicated to determine the cause of the spontaneous hemorrhage.

Chemosis, or **conjunctival edema**, occurs to some degree with all cases of conjunctivitis, but the most dramatic examples are seen with trauma, hypoproteinemia, allergic reactions, and insect bites. The latter are treated with topical corticosteroids and usually resolve rapidly. Specific therapy for the etiologic agent is indicated.

Conjunctivitis is common in all domestic species. The etiologic agent(s) vary from infectious to environmental irritants. The signs are hyperemia, chemosis, ocular discharge, follicular hyperplasia, and mild ocular discomfort. The appearance of the conjunctiva usually is not sufficiently distinctive to suggest the etiologic agent, and specific diagnosis depends on history, physical examination, conjunctival scrapings and culture, Schirmer tear test, and occasionally biopsy. Unilateral conjunctivitis may result from a foreign body, dacryocystitis, or keratoconjunctivitis sicca (*see* above). In cats, herpesvirus-1 (FHV-1), *Mycoplasma*, or *Chlamydophila (Chlamydia) psittaci* may produce conjunctivitis that begins in one eye and becomes bilateral after ~1 wk. Specific diagnosis is made most rapidly by demonstrating the inclusions or the agent in conjunctival scrapings. Bilateral conjunctivitis is common in viral infections in all species. Herpesviruses produce conjunctivitis in cats, cattle, horses, and pigs. Purulent discharge indicates a bacterial component, but this may be opportunistic due to debilitation of the mucous membrane. Environmental irritants and allergens are common causes of conjunctivitis in all species. If a mucopurulent exudate is present, topical antibiotic therapy is indicated but may not be curative if other predisposing factors are involved. Mechanical factors such as foreign bodies, environmental irritants, parasites, and eyelid conformational defects should be removed or corrected. Topical tetracycline is indicated for chlamydial and mycoplasmal infections; topical antiviral preparations (eg, 1% idoxuridine, 3% adenine arabinoside, or 1% trifluorothymidine) are indicated for herpesvirus infections when both the cornea and conjunctiva are involved. Oral supplementation in cats with 250-500 mg L-lysine daily may reduce the severity and frequency of recurrence of FHV-1 conjunctivitis and keratitis.

CORNEA

Superficial keratitis is common in all species and is characterized by corneal vascularization and opacification, which may be due to edema, cellular infiltrates, pigmentation, or fibroplasia. If ulceration is present, pain—manifest by epiphora and blepharospasm—is an outstanding sign. Unilateral keratitis frequently is traumatic in origin. Mechanical factors, such as lid conformational defects and foreign bodies, should always be eliminated as possible causes because improvement will not occur until they are resolved. Ulcerative keratitis may be complicated by secondary invasion by bacteria and, in horses, by saprophytic fungi. Bilateral superficial keratitis may be immune-mediated or associated with a lack of tears, eyelid conformational defects, or infectious agents.

Pannus or Uberreiter's disease is a specific, bilateral, progressive, proliferative, chronic, superficial keratitis that begins laterally at the limbus and eventually extends from all quadrants to cover the cornea. It is common in German Shepherds, Belgian Tervurens, Border Collies, Greyhounds, Siberian Huskies, and Australian Shepherds. Specific therapy consists of topical antibiotics, antiviral or antimycotic agents when appropriate, removal of any mechanical irritants, tear replacement when deficient, and corticosteroids or cyclosporin A (or both) when immune-mediated. The latter may need to be continued indefinitely and the frequency varied depending on the response.

Interstitial keratitis is a deep involvement of the corneal stroma that is present with all chronic and many acute cases of anterior uveitis. The corneal vascularization is less branching, finer, and deeper than in superficial keratitis; if the endothelium has been disrupted, corneal edema is often marked. Systemic diseases, such as infectious canine hepatitis, malignant catarrhal fever, systemic mycoses, and septicemias that localize in the eye, can cause bilateral or unilateral interstitial keratitis. Therapy is directed at the anterior uveitis, the systemic infection, or both. A specific, nonulcerative, peripheral, stromal keratitis and persistent anterior uveitis (keratouveitis) occurs in horses; prognosis and response to treatment are poor.

Ulcerative keratitis may be superficial, deep, deep with descemetocele, or perforating. Pain, corneal irregularity, edema, and eventually vascularization are signs of ulceration. A dense, white infiltrate at the ulcer margin indicates strong leukotaxis and bacterial involvement. To detect small ulcers, topical fluorescein may be required. In dogs and horses, most ulcers are mechanical in origin; in cattle, sheep, goats and reindeer, infectious agents and mechanical causes are important; in cats and horses, herpesvirus infection is a frequent cause. All ulcers have the potential for secondary bacterial contamination or endogenous proteinase "melting" of the stroma. Therapy for superficial ulcers is usually medical and consists of topical broad-spectrum antibiotic(s), correction of any mechanical factors, and topical atropine for iridocycloplegia and reduction of ocular pain. Adverse effects of atropine-induced reduced tear production in all species and colic in horses must be considered.

Syndromes of very slow-healing and recurrent superficial ulcers occur in dogs, cats, and horses; in dogs, they may be due to basement membrane disease causing faulty attachment of the corneal epithelium, while in cats and horses, herpesvirus should be suspected. Initial therapy is ulcer debridement followed by topical antibiotics and atropine. For refractory cases in dogs, multiple punctures or cross-hatching (grid and punctate keratotomies) of affected corneas with a 22-gauge needle stimulates most indolent ulcers to heal within 7-10 days. Early reports suggest these keratotomies in cats may predispose to corneal sequestration, and should be employed with great care. Nictitating membrane flaps (or soft contact lenses or collagen shields) act as a pressure bandage and often are therapeutic for shallow ulcers. Medical treatment of deep ulcers is similar to that of superficial ulcers, but many deep ulcers also require conjunctival grafts to strengthen the cornea.

Corneal sequestration and keratitis appear to be unique to the cat. There is a painful, central to paracentral, brown to black opacity composed of necrotic stroma, vascularization, and surrounding inflammation. Treatment consists of superficial keratectomy and, with deeper lesions, conjunctival grafts.

Corneal stromal abscesses in horses may be sequelae of healing corneal ulcers or defects and the trapping of bacteria or fungal organisms (or both) within the stroma after re-epithelialization. A variable, white to yellow, stromal infiltrate is surrounded by an intense stromal keratitis and vascularization, and a variable but sometimes intense anterior uveitis. Treatment consists of intensive topical and occasional systemic antibiotics (and if indicated, antifungals), iridocycloplegics, nonsteroidal anti-inflammatory drugs, and often surgical removal of the abscess with conjunctival and tectonic corneal graft.

Corneal degeneration and dystrophies occur in dogs, cats, and horses. Corneal degenerations are often unilateral and usually secondary to ocular or systemic diseases. The corneal dystrophies are bilateral, appear inherited or breed-predisposed in dogs, and often consist of triglyceride, cholesterol, and calcium deposits within the corneal stroma. Treatment is not usually necessary.

ANTERIOR UVEA

Persistent pupillary membranes are remnants of the normal prenatal vascular network that fills the pupillary region. Persistence of pigmented strands across the pupil from one area of the iris to another, or to the lens or cornea, is not uncommon in dogs and occurs occasionally in other species. In Basenjis, the condition is inherited.

Atrophy of the iris is common in older dogs and may involve the pupillary margin or the stroma. Atrophy of the pupillary margin creates a scalloped border and a weakening of the sphincter muscle, which is manifest as a dilated pupil(s) or by sluggish pupillary light reflexes. Stromal atrophy results in dramatic holes in the iris, and often, displacement of the pupil. Neither form of atrophy appears to affect vision. Animals lacking a functional iridal sphincter may show increased sensitivity to bright light.

Iridic cysts are seen in dogs, cats, and horses. In dogs, they usually are free-floating, pigmented spheres in the aqueous humor within the pupil and anterior and posterior chambers. Although innocuous in most breeds of dogs, anterior uveal cysts (iris and ciliary body) in Golden Retrievers are associated with chronic uveitis, glaucoma, and cataract formation. In cats, the cysts frequently are attached at the pupillary margin. In horses, they are present in the stroma of the iris and more frequently involve blue irides. Therapy is rarely necessary, but aspiration or laser-induced deflation can be performed. Transillumination will usually demonstrate their cystic nature and differentiate them from neoplasms. Enlarged and cystic dorsal corpora nigra may impair vision and mimic iridic melanomas in horses. Surgical excision or aspiration may be indicated.

Anterior uveitis or **iridocyclitis**, when acute, is manifest by miosis, increased protein and cells in the anterior chamber, low intraocular pressure, bulbar conjunctival hyperemia, iridal swelling, photophobia, and blepharospasm. Secondary glaucoma, cataract, and corneal opacification may be complications. Concurrent posterior uveitis or choroiditis is frequent. Causes of anterior uveitis can be separated into exogenous and endogenous. Penetrating and nonpenetrating trauma and, rarely, intraocular neoplasms or intraocular helminths are causes of unilateral uveitis. Common causes of bilateral uveitis include immune-mediated diseases and infectious diseases such as infectious canine hepatitis, feline infectious peritonitis, feline leukemia, feline immunodeficiency, toxoplasmosis, systemic mycoses, canine brucellosis, leptospirosis, malignant catarrhal fever, infectious bovine rhinotracheitis, equine viral arteritis, classical swine fever, canine ehrlichiosis, and neonatal bacterial infections (joint, navel, and gut) of calves and foals. Recurrent uveitis that is at least in part immune-mediated affects horses (periodic ophthalmia or moon blindness) and dogs (panuveitis with dermal depigmentation or uveodermal syndrome). A thorough history, examination of the cornea for injuries, physical examination, serum serology, and centesis of the aqueous for culture, serology, and cytology aid in diagnosis.

Nonspecific therapy consists of topical mydriatics to maintain pupillary dilation and movement, topical corticosteroids (if nonbacterial), a darkened environment, and prostaglandin inhibitors (such as aspirin, flunixin meglumine, or phenylbutazone). If bacterial in origin, topical, systemic, and perhaps intraocular antibiotics are indicated. Treatment of immune-mediated processes may require systemic or subconjunctival as well as topical corticosteroids and oral azathioprine.

GLAUCOMA

The glaucomas represent a group of diseases characterized by increased intraocular pressure with resultant retinal and optic disk destruction. Low-tension glaucoma, characterized in humans by normal levels of intraocular pressure and progressive optic disk damage, has not been documented in domestic animals. In dogs, the glaucomas occur in ~1.7% of the canine population in North America. The frequency of bilateral breed-predisposed glaucomas in purebred dogs is the highest of any animal species, except humans (0.9%). In cats, the glaucomas are predominately secondary to anterior uveitis and neoplasms; however, primary open-angle glaucoma occurs. In horses, the glaucomas appear underdiagnosed because applanation tonometry is not routinely done; they appear most frequently in older animals, Appaloosas, and with concurrent anterior uveitis. In cattle, the glaucomas have been associated with congenital iridocorneal anomalies and anterior uveitis.

Diagnostic procedures essential to manage the glaucomas include tonometry, ophthalmoscopy (direct and indirect), and gonioscopy (visualization of the iridocorneal angle and anterior ciliary cleft). Newer techniques, such as pattern electroretinograms and visual evoked potentials, estimate damage to the retinal ganglion cells and their axons, and appear to be sensitive indicators of glaucoma-related destruction of these cells. In small animals, both Schiotz indentation and applanation tonometers are used to estimate intraocular pressure; in horses and cattle, only applanation-type tonometers can be used. Intraocular pressure is reasonably consistent in most species (see TABLE 1) and diurnal variations have been documented in the dog, cat, and rabbit. Ophthalmoscopy permits detection of the intraocular pressure-related damage to the retina and optic disk. Gonioscopy is the basis for classification of all glaucomas; it detects iridocorneal outflow changes as the glaucoma progresses and helps determine the most appropriate medical and surgical treatments. Ultrasound biomicroscopy permits further examination of the anterior chamber angle and the entire ciliary cleft.

Clinical signs are traditionally divided into acute and chronic; in reality, most cases of acute glaucoma are superimposed on chronic glaucoma rather than occurring as singular events. Most dogs with early to moderate chronic glaucoma are not taken to the veterinarian because the early clinical signs—sluggish to slightly dilated pupils, mild bulbar conjunctival venous congestion, and early enlargement of the eye (buphthalmia or megaloglobus)—are so subtle. To detect early glaucoma, tonometry should be routinely performed on high-risk breeds of dogs as part of the general physical examination. The clinical signs of acute and often markedly increased levels of intraocular pressure are a dilated, fixed, or sluggish pupil; bulbar conjunctival venous congestion; corneal edema; and a firm globe. With prolonged increases of intraocular pressure, secondary enlargement of the globe, lens displacement, and breaks in Descemet's membrane of the cornea result. Pain usually is manifest by behavioral changes and occasional periorbital pain rather than by blepharospasm.

Classification of the glaucomas assists in the optimal plan for clinical management and preservation of vision. The choice of medical or surgical treatment, or most frequently a combination of both, is based on the progressive iridocorneal angle closure that occurs in most of the canine glaucomas. For open-angle glaucoma in dogs, short- and

TABLE 1.   Intraocular Pressure (IOP) by Applanation Tonometry

Species	Tonometer	IOP (mm Hg) Mean ± SD[*]
Dog	MacKay-Marg	15.7 ± 4.2
		18.8 ± 5.5
	Tono-Pen™	16.7 ± 4.0
		19.2 ± 5.9
Cat	Tono-Pen	19.7 ± 5.6
Rabbit	Pneumatonograph	19.5 ± 1.8
		17.9 ± 2.1
Horse	Tono-Pen	29.6 ± 6.2
		23.3 ± 6.9
Cow	Tono-Pen	26.9 ± 6.7
Llama/alpacas	Tono-Pen	16.6 ± 3.6
Monkey (ketamine)	Tono-Pen	13.6 ± 3.7
Alligator	Tono-Pen	23.7 ± 2.1
Ferret	Tono-Pen	22.8 ± 5.5
Rat	Tono-Pen	17.3 ± 5.3
Hawks	Tono-Pen	20.6 ± 3.4
Owl	Tono-Pen	10.8 ± 3.6

[*]Duplicate figures represent different reports for that species.

longterm management is by treatment with miotics, topical and systemic carbonic anhydrase inhibitors, prostaglandins, osmotics, and β-blocking adrenergics. These same treatments are used for initial control of narrow and closed-angle glaucoma, but short- and longterm management often requires surgery, eg, filtering procedures, anterior chamber shunts, cyclocryotherapy, or laser transcleral cyclophotocoagulation. Short- and longterm management of end-stage glaucoma with buphthalmia and blindness in dogs also requires surgery, eg, intrascleral prosthesis, enucleation, cyclocryothermy, or intravitreal gentamycin (10-25 mg) combined with 1 mg dexamethasone. Surgical procedures in dogs have traditionally provided only short-term resolution because the filtering fistulas eventually scar over and fail. More recently, anterior chamber shunts, with and without valves, offer improved results. Antifibrotic drugs, such as mitomycin C and 5-fluorouracil, may delay or prevent scarring of the alternate aqueous outflow channels and prolong their function.

LENS
Cataracts are an opacity of the lens or its capsule and should be differentiated from the minor lens imperfections in young dogs and the normal increase in nuclear density (nuclear sclerosis) that occurs in older animals. Cataracts usually are classified by their age of onset (congenital, juvenile, senile), anatomic location, cause, degree of opacification (incipient, immature, mature, hypermature), and shape. Most cataracts can be detected by dilating the pupil and examining the pupillary region against the retroillumination of the tapetal fundus. Slit lamp biomicroscopy permits optimal direct examination of the lens. Cataracts (often inherited) are more common in dogs than in other species (see TABLE 2). Other etiologies include diabetes mellitus, malnutrition, radiation,

TABLE 2. Inherited Cataracts in Domestic Animals

Breed	Age of Onset	Initial Localization	Mode of Inheritance
Dogs			
Afghan Hound	6-12 mo	Equatorial/posterior cortex	Autosomal recessive
American Cocker Spaniel	≥6 mo	Posterior/anterior cortex	Autosomal recessive polygenetic
Bichon Frise	>2 yr	Posterior/anterior cortex	Autosomal recessive
Boston Terrier	Congenital, late onset	Posterior sutures/cortex	Autosomal recessive
Chesapeake Bay Retriever	≥1 yr	Nuclear/cortex	Incomplete dominant
German Shepherd	≥8 wk	Posterior sutures/cortex	Incomplete dominant
Golden Retriever	≥6 mo	Posterior subcapsular (triangular)	Incomplete dominant
Labrador Retriever	≥6 mo	Posterior subcapsular (triangular)	Incomplete dominant
Miniature Schnauzer	Congenital	Nuclear/posterior cortex	Autosomal recessive
	≥6 mo	Posterior cortex	Autosomal recessive
Norwegian Buhund	≥1 yr	Nuclear/cortex	Autosomal dominant
Old English Sheepdog	Congenital	Nuclear/cortex	Autosomal recessive
Rottweiler	≥10 mo	Posterior polar/complete	Unknown
Siberian Husky	≥6 mo	Posterior subcapsular/posterior sutures	Autosomal recessive
Staffordshire Bull Terrier	≥6 mo	Posterior sutures/cortex	Autosomal recessive
Standard Poodle	≥1 yr	Equatorial cortex	Autosomal recessive
Welsh Springer Spaniel	Congenital	Nuclear/posterior cortex	Autosomal recessive
West Highland White Terrier	Congenital	Posterior sutures	Autosomal recessive
Horses			
Belgian	Congenital	Nuclear/cortex	Autosomal dominant
Morgan	Congenital	Nuclear	Autosomal dominant

(continued)

TABLE 2. Inherited Cataracts in Domestic Animals (*continued*)

Breed	Age of Onset	Initial Localization	Mode of Inheritance
Cattle			
Holstein-Freisian	Congenital	Nuclear/cortex	Autosomal recessive
Jersey	Congenital	Nuclear	Autosomal recessive
Sheep			
New Zealand Romney	Congenital	Anterior/posterior cortex	Autosomal dominant

inflammation, and trauma. In cats and horses, most cataracts are secondary to anterior uveal inflammation. Sight may be regained in young dogs, cats, and horses when cataracts undergo sufficient spontaneous resorption; congenital nuclear cataracts in young animals may reduce in size with growth of the lens to permit restoration of vision as the animal matures. Animals with immature and incomplete cataracts may benefit from topical ophthalmic atropine 2-3 times/wk, which allows vision around a central cataract. In general, the only definitive therapy for cataracts is surgical removal of the lens. In dogs, cataract extraction, often by phacoemulsification, yields best results when performed before cataract maturation is complete and lens-induced uveitis, due to leakage of lens material, is established. Lens-induced uveitis is intensified by cataract surgery and contributes substantially to postoperative complications. In animals in which cataract surgery is not performed, continued clinical monitoring is important. The secondary lens-induced anterior uveitis often requires longterm corticosteroid therapy and occasional mydriasis. Secondary glaucoma and phthisis bulbus formation are possible complications.

Lens displacement (subluxation, anterior or posterior luxation) occurs in all species but is common as a primary inherited defect in several terrier breeds. Complete displacement into the anterior chamber produces acute signs and frequently is accompanied by glaucoma and corneal edema. Treatment is surgical removal. Posterior displacement into the vitreous cavity is asymptomatic or associated with ocular inflammation or glaucoma. Subluxated lenses are recognized by an aphakic crescent and trembling of the iris (iridodonesis) and lens (phacodonesis). The decision to remove subluxated lenses is based on the severity of ocular disease that can be attributed to the lens displacement. Lens displacements also can be produced by trauma, enlargement of the globe with glaucoma, and degenerative zonular changes with hypermature cataracts. Procedures to remove the lens for lens displacement are associated with higher levels of postoperative complications of glaucoma and retinal detachment.

OCULAR FUNDUS

Diseases of the ocular fundus (retina, choroid, optic disk) may be primary or may be manifestations of systemic diseases. Inherited abnormalities may be congenital or appear later, and are important in the pathogenesis of retinopathies in dogs and cats. Trauma, metabolic disturbances, systemic infections, neoplasms, blood dyscrasias, hypertension, and nutritional deficiencies are possible underlying causes for retinopathies in all species.

Inherited Retinopathies

Collie eye anomaly is a congenital, recessively inherited, ocular defect with variable expression in rough- and smooth-coated Collies. It also occurs in Shetland Sheepdogs, Border Collies, Australian Shepherds, and Lancashire Heelers. The basic lesion is an area of choroidal or chorioretinal hypoplasia that on ophthalmoscopy appears as a focal, variable-sized, pale area lateral to the optic disk. More severely affected dogs (10-20%) can have additional colobomatous lesions of the optic papilla or peripapillary region, and occasional retinal detachments. Intraocular hemorrhage may occur. Vision is not appreciably affected unless retinal detachment is present.

Retinal dysplasia is a congenital, focal, geographic, or generalized maldevelopment of the retina that may arise from trauma, genetic defect, or intrauterine damage, such as viral infections. Most forms of retinal dysplasia in dogs are inherited. Maternal viral infections, especially during early fetal development, can result in multiple ocular anomalies with retinal dysplasia in kittens (panleukopenia), lambs (bluetongue disease), puppies (herpesvirus), and calves (bovine viral diarrhea). Breeds of dogs with focal, geographic, and generalized retinal dysplasia thought to be inherited as an autosomal recessive trait include American Cocker Spaniels, Beagles, Labrador Retrievers, Rottweilers, and Yorkshire Terriers. Focal areas of retinal maldevelopment may be asymptomatic or interfere with central vision. Generalized retinal dysplasia with retinal detachment, visual impairment, or blindness is inherited in English Springer Spaniels, Bedlington Terriers, Sealyham Terriers, Labrador Retrievers, Doberman Pinschers, and Australian Shepherds. Other ocular anomalies, including microphthalmia and congenital cataracts, often accompany the generalized forms. In Labrador Retrievers and Samoyeds, retinal dysplasia may be associated with skeletal dysplasia (shortening) of the forelegs.

Progressive retinal atrophy (PRA) is a group of degenerative retinopathies consisting of inherited photoreceptor dysplasia and degenerations that have a similar clinical appearance. The photoreceptor dysplasias inherited as autosomal recessive traits in which clinical signs develop in the first year occur in Irish Setters, Collies, Norwegian Elkhounds, Miniature Schnauzers, and Belgian Sheepdogs. The photoreceptor degenerations inherited as autosomal recessive traits in which clinical signs develop at 3-5 yr occur in Miniature and Toy Poodles, English and American Cocker Spaniels, Labrador Retrievers, Tibetan Terriers, Miniature Longhaired Dachshunds, Akitas, and Samoyeds. In Siberian Huskies, PRA is inherited as an X-linked trait, while in Bull Mastiffs, PRA is inherited as an autosomal dominant. Many other breeds of dogs are also suspected of having inherited PRA. In Abyssinian cats, PRA occurs as both photoreceptor dysplasia and degeneration. Night blindness is noted early and progresses to total blindness over months to years. Ophthalmoscopic lesions are a bilateral symmetric increase in reflectivity of the tapetal fundus, decreased pigmentation of the nontapetal fundus, attenuation and a decrease in the number of retinal vessels, and eventual atrophy of the optic papilla. Electroretinography is often used to investigate and diagnose the condition. Cortical cataracts are common late in the course of PRA in many breeds and may mask the underlying retinopathy. No effective therapy is available. Blood and buccal mucosa-based DNA marker and specific gene tests have been developed to detect carrier and affected dogs before clinical signs develop in many breeds.

Retinal pigment epithelial dystrophy (central progressive retinal atrophy) occurs in Labrador Retrievers, smooth and rough Collies, Border Collies, Shetland Sheepdogs, and Briards. The condition is inherited in Labrador Retrievers as a dominant trait with variable penetrance. Early ophthalmoscopic findings (often before clinical signs are apparent) are small foci of irregular pigmentation in the tapetal fundus, which eventually coalesce and fade as reflectivity of the tapetal fundus increases. The pigmented nontapetal fundus becomes mottled, the retinal vasculature gradually decreases, and the optic disk atrophies. Progressive visual impairment occurs gradually over several years. Cataract formation occurs late in the disease. There is no treatment. Recent studies suggest vitamin E disorders may also be important in the pathogenesis of this disease complex.

Chorioretinitis

Chorioretinitis frequently is a manifestation of systemic infectious disease; it is important as both a convenient diagnostic clue and a prognosticator of visual function.

Unless the lesions are generalized or involve the optic nerve, they often are "silent." Scars may be differentiated from active lesions by the haze and ill-defined borders of the latter. Routine ophthalmoscopic examinations of all animals with systemic diseases often permit rapid diagnosis of many specific diseases. Chorioretinitis may be present with canine distemper, systemic mycoses, protothecosis, toxoplasmosis, tuberculosis, bacterial septicemias, feline infectious peritonitis, thromboembolic meningoencephalitis, malignant catarrhal fever, classical swine fever, leptospirosis in horses, and onchocerciasis. Therapy is directed at the systemic disease.

Retinal Detachments

Retinal detachments occur in most species. In dogs, retinal detachment or separation of the neurosensory retina from the retinal pigment epithelium is associated with congenital retinal disorders (retinal dysplasia and Collie eye anomaly), chorioretinitis, trauma, intraocular surgery, and posterior segment neoplasia. In cats, retinal detachments occur with chorioretinitis associated with feline infectious peritonitis, feline viral leukemia, and systemic hypertension. In horses, the most frequent causes are trauma, intraocular surgery, and recurrent uveitis.

Retinal detachments are divided clinically into nonrhegmatogenous (serous, exudative, hemorrhagic, secondary to vitreal syneresis) and rhegmatogenous (with retinal breaks [hole or tear]). Clinical signs include mydriasis, aniscoria, vision impairment, and intraocular hemorrhage. Diagnosis is by ophthalmoscopy and, in eyes with an opaque cornea or lens, ocular ultrasonography.

Nonrhegmatogenous retinal detachments are usually treated medically with therapy directed at the primary disease. Retinal reattachment occurs with resolution of the subretinal exudates and hemorrhage. Variable retinal degeneration may follow in the detached areas. Rhegmatogenous retinal detachments with retinal breaks generally require surgical correction.

OPTIC NERVE

Optic nerve hypoplasia may be inherited in Miniature Poodles; in kittens and calves, it may result from in utero infections with panleukopenia and bovine viral diarrhea, respectively. In calves, the cause may be maternal avitaminosis A. The condition may be unilateral or bilateral, and it can occur with or without other ocular anomalies. Bilateral involvement is manifest as blindness in the neonate; unilateral involvement is often an incidental finding later in life or becomes manifest if the other eye acquires a blinding disease.

Papilledema is infrequent in animals and often associated with orbital masses. Increased intracranial pressure does not usually result in papilledema in animals, except in calves with avitaminosis A. The optic disk appears raised above the surface of the adjacent retina, and venous congestion is present. Vision and the light pupillary reflexes are not usually affected unless optic atrophy develops.

Optic atrophy may occur after glaucoma, trauma, advanced retinal degeneration, prolonged ocular hypotension, or inflammation. The optic disc appears depressed and smaller than normal; it is often pigmented, with marked reduction in the optic nerve and retinal vasculature. Both direct pupillary reflex and vision are absent. There is no treatment.

ORBIT

The signs of **orbital cellulitis** are acute pain on opening the mouth, eyelid swelling, unilateral prolapse of the nictitating membrane, forward displacement of the globe, and conjunctivitis. Keratitis may develop from lagophthalmos. The condition is seen predominantly in large and hunting breeds of dogs and is rare in other species. Foreign bodies (eg, migrating grass awns) and zygomatic sialadenitis are additional causes. Orbital hemorrhage and neoplasia may mimic inflammation except there is usually no pain on opening the mouth. In acute cases, systemic broad-spectrum antibiotics are usually curative, but if swelling behind the last molar is present, drainage of this area is indicated. Warm compresses and topical lubricants to protect the cornea are also indicated. Relapses may occur, and radiographs and ultrasonography of the adjacent teeth, sinuses, and nasal cavity are recommended.

PROLAPSE OF THE EYE

Acute prolapse or proptosis of the eye occurs as a result of trauma. It is common in dogs and infrequent in cats. Prognosis depends on the extent of the trauma, the breed of dog, depth of the orbit, duration of the proptosis, resting pupil size, condition of the exposure keratitis, and other periocular damage. In cats, proptosis usually results from severe trauma to the head; often, other facial bones are fractured. The globe should be replaced as soon as possible if the animal's physical condition will permit induction of general anesthesia. The lateral canthus is usually incised, increasing the palpebral fissure, to permit replacement of the swollen orbital tissues and the globe. The upper and lower eyelids are apposed temporarily by several partial-thickness eyelid sutures to protect the damaged eye and prevent recurrence. Treatment consists of systemic antibiotics and occasionally corticosteroids, combined with topical antibiotics and mydriatics. Although the prognosis for retention of vision is guarded, the globe is usually saved. Return of vision occurs in ~50% of dogs and is infrequent in cats.

OPHTHALMIC MANIFESTATIONS OF SYSTEMIC DISEASES

Ophthalmic manifestations of systemic diseases are not uncommon with inherited, infectious, degenerative, and neoplastic disorders in animals. In dogs, ophthalmic diseases, such as retinal dysplasia, microphthalmia, and cataracts have been associated with dwarfism, albinism, and merling. Infectious diseases often involve the uveal tract and present as iridocyclitis, choroiditis, and panuveitis. They may be caused by viruses (distemper, infectious hepatitis), rickettsial diseases (ehrlichiosis and Rocky Mountain spotted fever), bacteria (*Brucella canis* and *Borrelia burgdorferi*), fungi (*Blastomyces, Coccidioides, Histoplasma, Cryptococcus,* and *Aspergillus*), protozoa (*Toxoplasma, Neospora, Leishmania,* and *Hepatozoon*), algae (*Prototheca*), or parasites (*Dirofilaria, Toxocara,* and *Diptera* spp). Metabolic diseases associated with eye diseases in the dog include diabetes mellitus (cataract formation), hypocalcemia (cataracts), hyperadrenocorticism (corneal disease, cataracts, and lipemia retinalis), and hypothyroidism (keratoconjunctivitis sicca, intraocular hemorrhages from elevated systemic blood pressure, and lipemia retinalis [hyperlipidemia]). Blood and vascular disorders may present as intraocular hemorrhage, retinal detachment, secondary glaucoma, and papilledema. Metastatic neoplasms, such as lymphosarcoma, most often affect the uvea, presenting as persistent uveitis, overt intraocular masses, intraocular hemorrhage, secondary glaucoma, or retinal detachment.

In cats, systemic diseases frequently affect the ophthalmic system. Eyelid inflammations are often associated with systemic *Demodex, Notoedres cati* (scabies), ringworm, and immune-mediated skin diseases. The pathogens that commonly cause infectious diseases of cats, ie, feline herpesvirus-1, *Chlamydia,* and *Mycoplasma* frequently present as acute and recurrent conjunctivitis. Feline herpesvirus-1 is also associated with ulcerative and stromal keratitis, proliferative keratoconjunctivitis, corneal sequestrum, corneal symblepharon, and keratoconjunctivitis sicca. Feline infectious peritonitis, toxoplasmosis, feline immunodeficiency, and feline leukemia virus often present as anterior and posterior uveitis, chronic uveitis, retinal detachment, and secondary glaucoma. Acute vision loss with intraocular hemorrhage and retinal detachment in older cats may be secondary to systemic hypertension and is often associated with chronic renal failure or hyperthyroidism. Resolution of intraocular hemorrhages, repair of the retinal detachment, and possible restoration of vision depends on the successful lowering of blood pressure to normal levels, often using the oral calcium channel blocker, amlodipine, 0.625 mg/day.

In horses, systemic infectious diseases, such as adenovirus in immunodeficient Arabian foals, equine influenza, strangles (*Streptococcus equi*), *Rhodococcus equi* infection, leptospirosis, Lyme disease (*Borrelia burgdorferi*), and salmonellosis, may present as conjunctivitis, anterior uveitis, or posterior uveitis. Ophthalmic onchocerciasis can be markedly reduced by the frequent administration of ivermectin, but can present with anterior and posterior uveitis, peripapillary chorioretinitis, keratitis, keratoconjunctivitis, or lateral conjunctival vitiligo. Habronemiasis presents with inflammatory conjunctival masses of the periocular area (especially the medial canthus) associated with the aberrant migration of larvae of *Habronema muscae*, *H microstoma*, and *Draschia megastoma*. Therapy is usually systemic ivermectin.

In cattle, microphthalmia, cataracts, retinal dysplasia, and retinal detachments are associated with hydrocephalus and in utero infection of calves with bovine viral diarrhea. The same ophthalmic defects occur in lambs affected in utero with bluetongue virus. Vitamin A deficiency in piglets causes microphthalmia, and in calves blindness and optic nerve hypoplasia. Vitamin A deficiency in adult or growing cattle results in night blindness, mydriasis, and eventually total blindness. Ophthalmoscopic abnormalities include papilledema, retinal degeneration, and optic nerve atrophy. Vitamin A supplementation may restore vision in animals with night blindness only. Lymphosarcoma in cattle may present as bilateral progressive exophthalmia. Many infectious diseases, such as rhinotracheitis, malignant catarrhal fever, thromboembolic meningoencephalitis, and neonatal septicemia, may present with conjunctivitis or anterior or posterior uveitis. Intoxications such as male fern poisoning (*Dryopteris filix*), bracken fern poisoning (*Pteridium aquilinum*) in sheep, coumarin poisoning (sweet clover poisoning) in cattle, and phenothiazine toxicity in cattle present with clinical signs of blindness from retinal degeneration, intraocular hemorrhage, or corneal edema. (*See also* TOXICOLOGY, p 2337.)

CHLAMYDIAL CONJUNCTIVITIS

Etiology and Epidemiology: Different strains of *Chlamydophila* (*Chlamydia*) *psittaci* and *Chlamydia pecorum* cause significant eye infection in cats, lambs, goats, and guinea pigs. These infections are occasionally transmitted to humans. (*See also* INTESTINAL CHLAMYDIAL INFECTIONS, p 155.) Trachoma and inclusion conjunctivitis in humans are caused by *C trachomatis*.

The disease in cats is also known as feline pneumonitis, which is largely a misnomer because chlamydiae rarely cause pneumonia in cats. The infection usually involves the eye and mucosa of the upper respiratory tract (rhinitis, sinusitis, pharyngitis). Serologic surveys indicate that 2-12% of cats, depending on age and geographic location, have complement-fixing chlamydial antibodies.

Chlamydial keratoconjunctivitis in lambs and goats can have significant economic impact, particularly in confinement flocks, in which up to 90% can become affected. Concurrently, lambs often have chlamydial polyarthritis (p 865). Also, chlamydial abortions (p 1103) have been seen in a goat herd affected simultaneously with chlamydial keratoconjunctivitis. Chlamydial keratoconjunctivitis has been reported in dogs, cattle, horses, and pigs and can be produced experimentally in these species.

Conjunctival chlamydial infections, sometimes asymptomatic, are common in guinea pig herds (*see* p 1631). Conjunctivitis is usually seen in 4- to 8-wk-old animals. Genital infections cause salpingitis and cystitis in female guinea pigs, and urethritis in males.

Clinical Findings: Signs in cats range from serous to mucopurulent conjunctivitis and rhinitis. Early signs are unilateral, reddened, slightly swollen conjunctivae. The incubation period after exposure to an infected cat is 3-10 days. Bilateral conjunctivitis develops after a few days, and the conjunctivae become hyperemic and chemotic, with prominent follicles on the inside of the third eyelid in more severe cases. The signs are most severe 9-13 days after onset and then subside over 2-3 wk. Some cats develop, with or without secondary bacterial or mycoplasmal infections, vascular keratitis, pannus, and corneal scarring. In some cats, clinical signs can last for weeks despite treatment, and recurrence is not uncommon.

Similar eye lesions occur in sheep and goats. Secondary infections in lambs and goats are also common and, if untreated, can lead to severe complications.

Lesions: Inflammatory reactions in the conjunctivae are prominent, and various cells such as neutrophils, lymphocytes, plasma cells, and macrophages infiltrate early in the disease. These cells, together with conjunctival epithelial cells containing chlamydial inclusions, are found in smears made from conjunctival scrapings. Ulcerative keratitis with resultant penetration of the anterior chamber can also be found in severely affected cats or those with secondary infections.

Diagnosis: Diagnosis can be confirmed by demonstration of chlamydial inclusions in exfoliative cytologic preparations or by isolation of the chlamydial organism. Scrapings are prepared by lightly but firmly moving a spatula or sharp teaspoon over the conjunctiva and smearing the scraped material onto a glass slide; the preparation is air-dried and stained. The elementary bodies appear basophilic or purple if stained with Giemsa, and reddish if stained with Gimenez. Scrapings may also be submitted for isolation of chlamydiae in chicken embryos or cell cultures or for PCR testing. A serologic diagnosis is difficult and requires paired samples taken during the acute and convalescent phases of the disease to compare antibody levels; occasionally, false seronegative results occur.

Chlamydial conjunctivitis in cats should be differentiated from herpesvirus and calicivirus infections, and in lambs and goats from mycoplasmal and other bacterial infections (eg, "pinkeye").

Prevention and Treatment: Vaccines are available for chlamydiosis in cats but not for other species. The feline chlamydial vaccine does not completely protect the cat but significantly reduces severity and infection rates.

All *C psittaci* isolates are susceptible to tetracyclines. In cats, ophthalmic ointments that contain tetracycline may be the only therapy necessary. However, in severe or recurring cases, oral or parenteral treatment with tetracyclines is advisable. Cats that are pregnant or have kidney disease should be treated with erythromycin.

Systemic rather than ophthalmic treatment with oxytetracycline (20 mg/kg/day) or tylosin starting early in the course of the disease is advisable in lambs and goats. Daily feeding of 150-200 mg of chlortetracycline to affected lambs in feedlots also reduces the incidence of conjunctivitis and polyarthritis.

To reduce recurrence, treatment in cats, lambs, and goats should be continued for 7-10 days after clinical signs disappear.

EQUINE RECURRENT UVEITIS

(Periodic ophthalmia, Moon blindness, Equine uveitis)

Equine recurrent uveitis is one of the most common ocular diseases in horses, classically characterized by episodes of active inflammation followed by varying periods of quiescence. During the so-called quiescent periods, low-grade, subclinical inflammation may continue in at least some individuals. Regardless of the specific course, the inflammatory events eventually lead to secondary changes. It is these adverse secondary complications that make this syndrome the most common cause of blindness in horses worldwide.

Etiology and Pathogenesis: Equine recurrent uveitis is an immune-mediated disease with many potential initiating causes. The common denominator is damage to the uveal tract, which may be initiated by trauma (both penetrating and blunt) or systemic disease. Specific conditions or agents implicated in the pathogenesis include leptospirosis, brucellosis, strangles (*Streptococcus equi* infection), onchocerciasis, equine influenza, tooth root abscess, and hoof abscess. The most widely investigated of these are the *Leptospira* spp, in particular *L interrogans* serovar *pomona*, although other serogroups have been implicated. As active uveitis often does not occur for months, or even years, after the systemic disease, the exact relationship between leptospirosis and equine recurrent uveitis remains obscure. Although onchocerciasis is less common due to the routine use of ivermectin, equine recurrent uveitis is thought to be stimulated by dead or dying microfilaria that have aberrantly migrated to the eye. Therefore, active episodes of uveitis can be seen following normal worming.

Even though the immunologic basis for the recurrent nature of uveitis has been extensively studied, detailed understanding of the factors involved remains elusive. Sequestration of organisms, antigen, or antibody-antigen complexes within the anterior uvea has been advanced as an explanation for the chronicity of the ocular inflammation long after the initiating cause has resolved. Additionally, T lymphocytes have been found to be the predominant inflammatory cell type in clinical cases; their presence suggests a cytokine-driven, immune-mediated inflammatory response. The mechanisms by which this response is activated (or deactivated) remain unknown.

Clinical Findings and Lesions: The clinical signs associated with equine recurrent uveitis include both acute signs of active inflammation and chronic secondary side effects. Damage to the uveal tract leads to the release of inflammatory mediators such as leukotrienes, prostaglandins, and histamines, which in turn causes increased permeability of anterior uveal vessels, breakdown of the blood-aqueous barrier, iris sphincter spasm, and ciliary body muscle spasm. The compromise of the blood-aqueous barrier allows for leakage of protein, fibrin, and cells into the aqueous. These responses account for the classic signs of acute uveitis: blepharospasm, epiphora, episcleral injection, corneal edema, aqueous flare, fibrin clots in the anterior chamber, and miosis. Often, the anterior segment signs restrict the visibility of the posterior segment. If visible, posterior segment signs of an acute episode may include an inflammatory cell infiltrate involving the retina and/or choroid, focal or diffuse retinal separation, retinal hemorrhage, and a hazy appearance to the vitreous secondary to infiltration by inflammatory or red blood cells. One or both eyes may be affected. When bilateral, it is not unusual for one eye to be more severely inflamed.

Corneal scarring, iridal fibrosis, blunting of the corpora nigra, posterior synechia, glaucoma, cataracts, and pigment clumping of the nontapetal fundus (retinal degeneration) are all signs consistent with chronic equine recurrent uveitis. The importance of careful fundoscopy as a part of prepurchase or soundness examinations cannot be overstated. Horses with chronic uveitis can have few or no anterior segment signs but may manifest equine recurrent uveitis by retinal degeneration. Such horses usually have normal or near-normal pupillary light responses and may not exhibit overt signs of visual compromise until late in the disease course. However, any horse with significant retinal degeneration must be suspected of having equine recurrent uveitis and therefore also regarded as a likely candidate for future vision compromise.

Diagnosis: While the diagnosis is based on the presence of characteristic clinical signs, an attempt should be made to identify the underlying cause. Because an acute episode of uveitis can be the first sign of systemic disease, a thorough physical examination should always be performed in addition to the ophthalmic examination. A CBC and serum chemistry panel are often included as part of the minimum database. Specific tests may aid in finding an underlying cause of the initial episode of uveitis. Serologic testing for *Leptospira* spp is frequently advocated, although a recent study did not find a correlation between serology for *Leptospira* spp and leptospiral antibodies or organisms in the aqueous humor of horses with equine recurrent uveitis. Serologic testing for *Brucella* may be done, but the marked reduction of brucellosis from cattle has probably lessened its role as a causative agent. Conjunctival biopsies from the lateral aspect of the bulbar conjunctiva may be examined for *Onchocerca* microfilaria, but results must be interpreted with caution as horses without equine recurrent uveitis may also exhibit these microfilaria. Paracentesis of either the anterior chamber or the vitreous cavity offers the possibility of identifying a causative agent; however, the procedure may cause severe intraocular damage, especially if attempted in a conscious patient.

Treatment, Prevention, and Control: Therapy is initiated as soon as possible once signs of the acute phase are recognized. If a specific underlying cause can be identified, it should be addressed as part of the initial treatment protocol. In addition to dealing with the causative agent, or in instances where no specific cause is found, aggressive therapy with both topical and systemic anti-inflammatory medications is started to minimize the damage associated with intraocular inflammation. Both steroidal and nonsteroidal topical medications are commonly used. Prednisolone acetate (steroid, 1% suspension), dexamethasone (steroid, 0.1% suspension or ointment), flurbiprofen (nonsteroidal, 0.03% solution), and diclofenac (nonsteroidal, 0.1% solution) have all been successfully used. When selecting a topically applied steroid, either prednisolone or dexamethasone are preferred to hydrocortisone, which penetrates the cornea poorly and is not sufficiently potent to be an effective medication for anterior uveitis. Frequency of application depends on severity of the inflammation, but administration 4-6 times a day is common. As the signs resolve, the frequency can be slowly reduced. It is recommended that therapy be continued for 1 mo after the signs of acute inflammation have resolved. Topical atropine (1% solution or ointment) benefits patients with acute anterior uveitis by paralyzing the iris sphincter and ciliary body musculature. These effects reduce the likelihood of posterior synechia formation and markedly decrease the pain associated with ciliary body muscle spasm. Atropine is applied topically BID-TID until the pupil is widely dilated. The frequency can then be reduced to SID or once every other day as needed to maintain mydriasis. Although such a dosage schedule is well tolerated in most horses, gut motility should be monitored, as topically applied atropine can potentially lead to ileus.

Flunixin meglumine administered systemically, and particularly when given IV, may be the single most effective treatment of acute anterior uveitis in horses. The usual initial IV dose is 1.1 mg/kg, administered at the time of diagnosis. This is followed by a 5- to 7-day course at a dosage of 0.25-1.1 mg/kg, BID, PO. Because of the potential for GI and renal problems with the longterm use of flunixin meglumine, it is common to switch to oral phenylbutazone (2-4 mg/kg, SID-BID) after the initial treatment period. Alternatively, some horses respond better to aspirin (25 mg/kg, SID-BID, PO) after flunixin meglumine. Systemic steroids, specifically prednisolone (100-300 mg/day) and dexamethasone (5-10 mg/day) have also been successfully used to treat acute uveitis episodes, but their longterm use has been associated with laminitis. As the severity of the clinical signs lessens, the dosage and frequency of oral anti-inflammatory medications can be tapered over the 2- to 3-mo treatment period. If frequent topical medication is not feasible, subconjunctival injections of triamcinolone (10-40 mg), methylprednisolone acetate (10-40 mg), or betamethasone (5-15 mg) can supply therapeutic intraocular anti-inflammatory levels. However, these should be used with caution as they cannot be easily removed once injected and can have devastating consequences should an infectious component be present or a corneal ulcer develop. Except in instances when bacterial infection is present, systemic antibiotics are not indicated.

Historically, horses with frequent recurrences or chronic, low-grade uveitis were managed medically with daily (or every other day) doses of oral phenylbutazone or aspirin. Although most horses tolerate this regimen well, these medications can have adverse GI and hematologic side effects and the need for daily administration can lead to adherence problems. In addition, these regimens frequently do not eliminate recurrence. Recently, in an attempt to address the problems of medical management alone, 2 surgical procedures have been developed. **Core vitrectomy** removes virtually all of the vitreous through an incision ~1 cm posterior to the dorsolateral aspect of the limbus. The vitreous is then replaced with either saline or balanced salt solution. The theorized benefit of this procedure is that T lymphocytes and/or organisms in the vitreous significantly contribute to the chronic inflammation of equine recurrent uveitis. By removing these elements, the frequency and severity of the inflammatory events can be minimized. Although the core vitrectomy procedure has been successful in achieving this goal, postoperative formation of cataracts has led to significant vision compromise in ~50% of patients. An alternative procedure has recently been introduced—**suprachoroidal cyclosporine implant**. In this procedure, a cyclosporine A disk ~5 mm in diameter is implanted under a scleral flap created ~8 mm posterior to the dorsolateral aspect of the limbus. Although this procedure is still regarded as experimental, early results have been encouraging.

Good husbandry practices such as effective fly control, frequent bedding changes, routine worming and vaccinations, minimizing contact with cattle or wildlife, draining stagnant ponds or restricting access to swampy pastures, and maximizing nutrition have all been advocated as means to reduce the effects of equine recurrent uveitis. While such measures provide overall benefits for individual horses, the extent to which they impact the clinical course of equine recurrent uveitis is debatable.

EYEWORM DISEASE

(Thelaziasis)

EYEWORMS OF LARGE ANIMALS

Etiology and Epidemiology: Eyeworms (*Thelazia* spp) are common parasites of horses and cattle in many countries, including several areas of North America. Horses are infected primarily by *T lacrymalis*; cattle mainly by *T gulosa*, *T skrjabini*, and *T rhodesii*. The latter is the most common and harmful to cattle in many countries, but it has been conspicuously absent in recent reports on cattle from North America. *Thelazia* spp are also found in pigs, sheep, goats, deer, water buffalo, dromedaries, hares, dogs and cats (*see* below), birds, and humans.

The face fly, *Musca autumnalis*, is the vector of *T lacrymalis*, *T gulosa*, and *T skrjabini* in North America. Feeding habits of this fly include a preference for ocular secretions, which is ideal for transmission. The life cycle of *Thelazia* is as follows: female worms are ovoviviparous and discharge larvae into the ocular secretions; the larvae are ingested by the fly and become infective in 2-4 wk. Infective third-stage larvae emerge from the labellae of infected flies and are mechanically deposited in the host's eye by the fly during feeding. Development of sexually mature worms takes 1-4 wk in cattle, depending on worm species, and 10-11 wk for *T lacrymalis* in horses. Infections may be found year-round, but clinical disease outbreaks, particularly in cattle, usually are associated with the warm season activities of the flies. *Thelazia* sp larvae may overwinter in face flies. Infection rates generally tend to increase with advancing host age, although some studies report maximum levels in hosts 2-3 yr of age.

Pathogenesis: The lacrimal gland and its ducts are common sites for *Thelazia lacrymalis* and *T gulosa*; the glands of the nictitating membrane and the nasolacrimal ducts, less so. *T skrjabini* is normally found within the lacrimal ducts of the nictitating membrane. Superficial locations on the cornea, in the conjunctival sac, and under the eyelids and nictitating membrane are more typical for *T rhodesii*, but *T lacrymalis*, *T skrjabini*, and *T gulosa* may be found in these sites too. Worms may also be found on the periorbital hair or skin during anesthesia or following migration after death of the host. Localized irritation and inflammation is likely due to the serrated cuticle of the worms, especially for *T rhodesii*. Invasion of the lacrimal gland and excretory ducts may cause inflammation and necrotic exudation. Inflammation of the lacrimal ducts and sac has also been reported in horses. Mild to severe conjunctivitis and blepharitis are common. Also, keratitis, including opacity, ulceration, perforation, and permanent fibrosis, may develop in severe cases, particularly with *T rhodesii* infections in cattle.

Clinical Findings and Diagnosis: Asymptomatic infections in both horses and cattle appear to be typical of thelaziasis in North America. Infection may be encountered incidentally during surgery, and reports have indicated a surprisingly high prevalence when a specific search is made at necropsy. However, *Thelazia* infections in cattle in North America may not always be innocuous. They may produce mild conjunctivitis, excessive lacrimation, localized edema, corneal clouding, and occasionally, subconjunctival cysts. In Europe and Asia, thelaziasis is commonly associated with severe clinical manifestations, including conjunctivitis, photophobia, and keratitis. Characteristically, there is chronic conjunctivitis with lymphoid hyperplasia and a seromucoid exudate.

A clinically feasible technique for reliable detection of adult eyeworms is lacking. Gross inspection of the eyes may reveal the worms and is generally recommended for *T rhodesii*, commonly found in the conjunctival sac. However, *T gulosa* and *T skrjabini* in cattle, and *T lacrymalis* in horses tend to be more invasive and are less apt to be seen. Topical anesthetics allow for tissue manipulation and so are helpful for detection and recovery of worms. Microscopic examination of lacrimal fluids for embryonated eggs or larvae may be attempted.

Clinical signs may be helpful in differential diagnosis. Thelaziasis tends to cause a chronic conjunctivitis. In cattle, infectious keratoconjunctivitis (p 412) is an acute, rapidly spreading infection of the cornea. In horses, infective larvae of the stomach worms *Draschia* and *Habronema* sp may also produce ophthalmic lesions. These tend to occur near the medial canthus of the eyelid and are raised, ulcerative granulomas, often containing characteristic yellow, plaque-like "sulfur granules" 1-2 mm in diameter. Likewise, microfilariae of *Onchocerca* sp invade the eye and may result in ophthalmic manifestations. Small (<1 mm), raised, white nodules in the pigmented conjunctiva adjacent to the temporal limbus are pathognomonic of *Onchocerca* infection. Depigmentation of the bulbar conjunctiva in this area also frequently occurs. Other lesions of onchocerciasis involve the cornea and include edema and punctate or streaking opacities of the stroma, superficial erosions, and a wedge-shaped sclerosing keratitis emanating from the temporal limbus. Intraocular structures also may be affected by microfilariae of *Onchocerca* sp (p 736).

Treatment and Control: Mechanical removal with forceps after instillation of a local anesthetic is useful for *Thelazia rhodesii* in cattle. This also may be feasible for the more invasive *T gulosa* or *T skrjabini* in cattle or *T lacrymalis* in horses. Irrigation of the eyes with 50-75 mL aqueous solution of 0.5% iodine and 0.75% potassium iodide has been recommended for *T gulosa* and *T skrjabini*. This also may be effective for *T lacrymalis* in horses. Topical application of 0.03% echothiophate iodide or 0.025% isoflurophate (both organophosphates) has been successful for *T lacrymalis* in horses. Concurrent use of an antibiotic-steroid ointment for the inflammation and secondary invaders is recommended. These topical agents should also be useful for *T gulosa* and *T skrjabini* in cattle. Certain systemic anthelmintics have exhibited activity against eyeworms. In cattle, levamisole at 5 mg/kg, SC, and ivermectin and doramectin, both at 0.2 mg/kg, SC or IM, have shown activity against *Thelazia* spp. Pour-on formulations of ivermectin or doramectin, delivered to achieve a dosage of 0.5 mg/kg, have also proven highly effective. Doramectin has been approved in the USA for the treatment of adult eyeworms in cattle. For *T lacrymalis* in horses, single doses of the commonly used anthelmintics, including ivermectin, administered via stomach tube at 0.2 mg/kg, have had limited, if any, effect on eyeworms. In contrast, the multidose regimen of fenbendazole (10 mg/kg, SID for 5 days) is efficacious against *T lacrymalis*.

Fly control measures, directed especially against the face fly, aid in the control of thelaziasis in both cattle and horses. Cattle on dry, open pastures have fewer face flies than those on pastures where shade and water are present.

EYEWORMS OF SMALL ANIMALS

Thelazia californiensis and *T callipaeda* are found in dogs, cats, and other animals, including humans, in the western USA and Asia, respectively. They are whitish, 7-19 mm long, and move in a rapid serpentine motion across the eye. Up to 100 eyeworms may be seen in the conjunctival sac, tear ducts, and on the conjunctiva under the nictitating membrane and eyelids. Filth flies (*Musca* spp, *Fannia* spp) serve as intermediate hosts and deposit infective larvae on the eye while feeding on ocular secretions.

Clinical signs include excessive lacrimation, conjunctivitis, corneal opacity and ulceration, and rarely, blindness. After local anesthesia, diagnosis and treatment are readily accomplished by observing and removing the parasites with forceps. Some have reported the successful elimination of *Thelazia* spp infections from dogs with SC injection of ivermectin at 0.2 mg/kg. Ocular solutions (2% levamisole) or ointments (1% levamisole or 4% morantel) also may be effective.

INFECTIOUS KERATOCONJUNCTIVITIS

(Pinkeye, Infectious ophthalmia)

Infectious keratoconjunctivitis of cattle, sheep, and goats is characterized by blepharospasm, conjunctivitis, lacrimation, and varying degrees of corneal opacity and ulceration.

In cattle, *Moraxella bovis* with multiple serovars is the most commonly recognized cause of infectious keratoconjunctivitis. Most other ocular infections of cattle are characterized by conjunctivitis and minimal or absent keratitis. The primary differential diagnosis is infectious bovine rhinotracheitis (IBR), which causes severe conjunctivitis and edema of the cornea near the corneoscleral junction, but corneal ulceration is uncommon. Other organisms that may cause conjunctivitis of cattle, either alone or in conjunction with *M bovis*, include *Mycoplasma* spp and *Neisseria* spp. Infection with IBR or other microbes may increase the severity of infection with *M bovis*.

In sheep, infection with *Chlamydophila (Chlamydia) pecorum* is most common. Nonchlamydophilal infections may be caused by rickettsia-like organisms (*Colesiota conjunctivae*), *Mycoplasma* spp, and aerobic bacteria, notably *Neisseria ovis*. In goats, mycoplasmal infections are most common, although aerobic bacteria also have been isolated. Although much of the syndrome in young goats is caused by *Mycoplasma agalactiae* (*see* CONTAGIOUS AGALACTIA, p 1114), it may be caused by other mycoplasmal species, notably *M conjunctivae*.

Clinical Findings: The disease usually is acute and tends to spread rapidly. One or both eyes may be affected. In cattle, dry, dusty environmental conditions; shipping stress; bright sunlight; and irritants such as pollens, grasses, and flies tend to predispose to or exacerbate the disease. Flies also serve as vectors. In all species, young animals are affected most frequently, but animals of any age are susceptible. The initial signs are photophobia, blepharospasm, and epiphora; later, the ocular discharge may become mucopurulent. Conjunctivitis, with or without varying degrees of keratitis, is always present. In sheep and goats, concurrent polyarthritis may be present. In goats, mammary gland and uterine infection may also occur simultaneously with keratoconjunctivitis. Appetite may be depressed due to ocular discomfort or visual disturbance that results in inability to locate food. The clinical course varies from a few days to several weeks unless complicated by other diseases.

Lesions: Lesions vary in severity. In cattle, 1 or more small ulcers occur near the center of the cornea (but occasionally near the limbus), often preceded by cloudiness of the central cornea. Initially, the cornea around the lesion is clear, but within a few hours a faint haze appears that subsequently becomes denser. Lesions may regress in the early stages or may continue to progress. After 48-72 hr in severe cases, the entire cornea may be opaque, blinding the animal in that eye. Blood vessels may invade the cornea from the limbus and move toward the ulcer at ~1 mm/day. Corneal opacity may result from edema (hazy white to blue corneas), which is a part of the inflammatory process, or leukocyte infiltration (milky white to yellow corneas), which indicates severe infection. Continued active ulceration may cause corneal rupture. In sheep and goats, disease rarely advances beyond a mild corneal opacity, with the accompanying ulcer and conjunctivitis. Relapse may occur at any stage of recovery, but late lesions are not as severe as initial lesions.

Diagnosis: In all species, presumptive diagnosis is based on ocular signs and concurrent systemic disease. It is important to distinguish that the lesions are not due to foreign bodies or parasites (*see* EYEWORMS OF LARGE ANIMALS, p 410). In IBR, upper respiratory signs and conjunctivitis predominate, while keratitis accompanied by ulceration is rare. In bovine malignant catarrhal fever, respiratory signs are prominent with primary uveitis and associated keratitis. Microbial culture may be beneficial in confirming the causative organisms. *Chlamydophila* and *Mycoplasma* spp require special media; the diagnostic laboratory should be consulted prior to sample collection. Cytologic evaluation of stained slides prepared from conjunctival scrapings of sheep and goats may reveal *Chlamydophila* or *Mycoplasma* organisms. However, the intracytoplasmic inclusion bodies can be difficult to recognize. PCR analysis can be used to detect *Chlamydophila* and *Mycoplasma* spp.

Prevention and Treatment: Good management practices are of paramount importance in reducing or preventing spread of infection in cattle, sheep, and goats. Separation of infected animals is beneficial when possible. Temporary isolation and preventive treatment of animals newly introduced to the herd may be helpful, because some of these animals may be asymptomatic carriers. Ultraviolet radiation from sunlight may enhance disease (particularly in cattle); therefore, affected animals should be provided with shade. Dust bags or insecticide tags can be used to reduce the number of face flies (*Musca autumnalis*), an important vector for *M bovis*. *M bovis* bacterins are available and can be administered before the beginning of fly season. The efficacy of these bacterins is controversial. Although they are unlikely to prevent *M bovis* infections, immunization may reduce the severity and duration of infection in affected animals. IBR infection may predispose cattle to infection with *M bovis*; thus, vaccination of herds against IBR may reduce outbreaks of *M bovis*. However, cattle should not be vaccinated during an outbreak with *M bovis*.

M bovis is susceptible to a variety of antibiotics. Because antibiotic susceptibility may vary in different geographic locations, bacterial culture and susceptibility testing is advised. Ampicillin, penicillin, gentamicin, and kanamycin can be injected subconjunctivally; best results are obtained with injection into the bulbar conjunctiva. Oxytetracycline is generally considered the drug of choice for systemic therapy because it is concentrated in corneal tissue. It cannot, however, be injected in the subconjunctiva because it will cause conjunctival necrosis. Two injections (20 mg/kg, IM) of a long-acting oxytetracycline formulation (200 mg/mL) at 72-hr intervals is the treatment of choice. Sulfonamides (eg, sulfadiazine and sulfamethazine) may also be effective when administered systemically because most of them pass readily into the tear film. Florfenicol (20 mg/kg, IM, 2 doses or 40 mg/kg, SC, 1 dose) and tilmicosin (10 mg/kg, IM, 1 dose) may also be used systemically. Systemic therapy can be augmented with topical applications of antibiotic, subconjunctival injection, or both. Topical applications of ophthalmic preparations should be applied at least TID to be effective, and thus are often not cost-effective or practical. Effective antibiotics for topical ophthalmic use include triple antibiotic, gentamicin, and a combination oxytetracycline/polymyxin B ointment. A third-eyelid flap or partial tarsorrhaphy, which will shade the cornea from sunlight, together with subconjunctival injection, may help severely affected animals. A temporary eye patch glued to the hair surrounding the eye is an inexpensive and easily applied treatment. The eye patch provides shade and prevents exposure to flies, decreasing spread of the organism.

For sheep and goats, in which chlamydophilal and mycoplasmal infections are most likely, respectively, topical tetracycline, oxytetracycline/polymyxin B, or erythromycin ointments are the treatments of choice. These preparations are all effective against *Chlamydophila* or *Mycoplasma* and should be applied 3-4 times daily. If topical therapy is not practical, an injection of long-acting oxytetracycline (10-20 mg/kg, IM) or the addition of oxytetracycline to the feed (80 mg/animal/day) may be beneficial.

Animals with substantial uveitis secondary to keratoconjunctivitis that is particularly painful may benefit from topical ophthalmic application of 1% atropine ointment 1-3 times daily. This will prevent painful ciliary body spasms and reduce the likelihood of posterior synechia formation that occurs with miosis. Because of mydriasis caused by atropine, treated animals should be provided with shade. Systemic NSAID may be used to provide relief from the secondary uveitis.

NEOPLASIA OF THE EYE AND ASSOCIATED STRUCTURES

The different tissues of the eye and associated structures can develop primary neoplasms or can be the site of metastatic neoplasms. Ophthalmic neoplasms vary in frequency and importance in different species, and are a significant group of diseases in veterinary ophthalmology.

Cattle

The most frequent ophthalmic neoplasms in cattle are the squamous cell carcinoma complex and the orbital infiltration associated with lymphosarcoma (p 593). The latter, with extensive invasion of the orbital structures, results in progressive exophthalmia, reduced ocular mobility, exposure keratitis, and corneal ulcerations that can lead to perforation.

Ocular squamous cell carcinoma (cancer eye) is the most common neoplasm of cattle. It results in significant economic loss due to condemnation at slaughter and a shortened productive life. It occurs more frequently in the *Bos taurus* than the *Bos indicus* breeds, and is seen most often in Herefords, less often in Simmentals and Holstein-Friesians, and rarely in other breeds. The peak age of incidence is 8 yr; actual incidence varies from 0.8% to 5.0% among herds. The etiology is multifactorial with heritability, sunlight, nutrition, eyelid pigmentation, and perhaps viral involvement playing roles. The medial and lateral limbal regions (corneoscleral junction) are affected most frequently, but the eyelids, conjunctivae, and nictitating membrane may be affected. Bilateral involvement varies but can be as high as 35%. Eyelid and conjunctival pigmentation are highly inheritable and can reduce the frequency of lid squamous cell carcinomas, but have less effect on the development of tumors of the conjunctiva and nictitating membrane. The cancerous or precancerous lesions are bilateral or multiple in the same eye in ~28% of cases. Ultraviolet radiation and a high plane of nutrition are contributing influences. The viruses of infectious bovine rhinotracheitis and papilloma have been isolated from the neoplasms, but their significance is unknown.

The lesions usually begin as benign, smooth, white plaques on the conjunctival surfaces; they may progress to a papilloma and then a squamous cell carcinoma, or go directly to the malignant stage. The lid lesions usually begin as either an ulcerative or a hyperkeratotic lesion (cutaneous horn). While in this benign stage, ~30% may spontaneously regress. The tumor may become quite large without invading the globe, but invasion into the eye and orbit and metastasis to parotid and submandibular lymph nodes occur in late stages of the disease. Diagnosis usually is made by the typical clinical appearance but can be confirmed rapidly by cytologic examination of impression smears. The intraocular tumor invasion must be differentiated from severely disorganized eyes after trauma or infectious keratoconjunctivitis (p 412).

Squamous cell carcinomas may respond to excision, cryotherapy, hyperthermia, radiation therapy, and immunotherapy, or a combination of these therapies. Surgical excision is indicated for small lesions or for debulking the larger lesions before cryotherapy or hyperthermia. Superficial keratectomy can be used to excise the limbal plaques, papillomas, and squamous cell carcinomas. Both cryotherapy and hyperthermia have yielded excellent short-term results, but recurrence at the same or a different site is ~25%.

For advanced lesions confined to the globe, enucleation is recommended. When adjacent tissues are affected, removal of the globe and all orbital contents (exenteration) should be performed. Immunotherapy is still experimental, and the resulting tumor regression may be temporary. Radiation therapy is not practical in the field but may be an option for valuable animals.

Owners of problem herds should be advised of the heritability factor, and affected animals and their offspring culled to decrease the incidence of tumors.

Horses

In horses, tumors of the skin, eye, and genital system are the most frequent, and ~80% of eye neoplasms are malignant. Neoplasms of the eyelids and conjunctivae are the most frequent ophthalmic tumors in horses; most are either squamous cell carcinoma or sarcoid. Orbital neoplasms are rare and are usually local extensions of eyelid, conjunctiva, or sinus tumors or systemic neoplasms, including lymphosarcoma. Intraocular neoplasms, usually malignant melanomas, are rare.

Squamous cell carcinoma occurs most frequently in horses 8-10 yr old and may occur more frequently in those with lightly- or non-pigmented eyelids. The Appaloosa and draft breeds are affected most frequently. Ultraviolet radiation may be important, because the incidence in North America is higher in southern and western areas and in areas of increased altitude or mean solar radiation. The eyelids, conjunctivae, nictitating membrane, and limbal regions can be affected with ulcerative or proliferative masses. Bilateral involvement occurs infrequently (~15%). Squamous cell carcinoma of the nictitans is more likely to invade the orbit than are those from other sites. Treatment of ophthalmic squamous cell carcinoma in horses is similar to that in cattle, although presentation for treatment is usually earlier, and greater emphasis is placed on cosmetic appearance after therapy. Repeated intratumoral injections of cisplatin (mean dosage 0.97 mg/cm^3 of tumor tissue) often cause successful tumor regression.

The equine sarcoid generally affects young horses (average 3.8 yr old) and represents ~40% of all neoplasms in horses. Because sarcoids are locally destructive and have a high recurrence rate after surgery, effective treatment when the periocular tissues are involved presents cosmetic and functional problems. Sarcoids are grouped into occult, verrucose, nodular, fibroblastic, mixed, and malignant types. They appear initially as subcutaneous masses in the eyelids or canthi; they usually enlarge rapidly and may invade the skin, appearing as red, fleshy masses. Treatment by surgery, hyperthermia, cryotherapy, chemotherapy, radiation, or a combination of these therapies. After attempts to surgically remove the sarcoid, recurrence may be rapid and precede the wound healing. Immunotherapy using BCG (bacille Calmette-Guérin) as a potentiator of the cellular immune system is often successful (~70%). After surgically debulking large sarcoids, the BCG preparation (7.5 mg purified cell-wall extract suspended in 10 mL saline solution) is injected directly into the remaining mass (2 mL/site). Injections should be repeated at 2- to 4-wk intervals until the mass disappears. Systemic corticosteroids and antiprostaglandins before and after treatment may decrease the likelihood of systemic anaphylactic reactions. Gamma radiation therapy using platinum-sheathed iridium^{192} is highly successful (~95%) but less convenient and usually requires a total average dose of 7,000-9,000 rads.

Dogs

Eyelid neoplasms are the most frequent group of ophthalmic neoplasms in dogs. Adenoma and adenocarcinoma of the meibomian gland are the most common lid neoplasms (~60%); local disfigurement and irritation necessitate local excision, which is usually successful. Sebaceous adenocarcinomas are locally invasive and histologically malignant but are not known to metastasize. Lid melanomas, exhibited as spreading pigmented masses on the eyelid margins, should be widely excised. Other frequent eyelid neoplasms include histiocytoma, mastocytoma, and papilloma.

Orbital neoplasms in dogs produce exophthalmia, conjunctival and eyelid swelling, strabismus, and exposure keratitis. The globe cannot be retropulsed. Usually, there is no pain. Because ~90% of the neoplasms are malignant and ~75% arise within the orbit, the prognosis for longterm survival is often poor. The neoplasm type should be determined histologically, and the extent of the mass determined by physical examination, skull radiographs (including special contrast procedures, computed tomography, and MRI), and ultrasonography before treatment by surgical excision or radiation. Excision of the orbital mass with the globe and all orbital tissues (including adjacent bone) may decrease the possibility of recurrence.

Corneal and limbal neoplasms are uncommon in dogs and can be confused with nodular fasciitis and proliferative keratoconjunctivitis in Collies. Limbal or epibulbar malignant melanomas are focal, usually superficial, pigmented masses that extend both onto the cornea and caudally toward the globe's equator. After close intraocular examination, including gonioscopy and B-scan ultrasonography, to detect possible penetration of the sclera, partial- to full-thickness surgical excision with scleral grafts, cryotherapy, or laser photocoagulation is usually successful. If intraocular extension occurs, enucleation is performed.

Malignant melanomas are the most common uveal neoplasm, are usually pigmented, and most frequently involve the iris and ciliary body. Clinical signs of anterior uveal melanomas may include an obvious mass, persistent iridocyclitis, hyphema, glaucoma, and pain. Ciliary body adenoma and adenocarcinoma are the most frequent epithelial neoplasms of the anterior uvea. Signs may include hyphema, glaucoma, and usually a nonpigmented mass behind the iris and in the pupil. Neoplasms of neuroectodermal origin are rare. Treatment is usually enucleation. Recent studies in iridal melanomas, especially in Labrador Retrievers, suggest noninvasive diode laser photocoagulation may be effective and can be repeated if necessary. Secondary uveal adenocarcinomas are relatively infrequent and originate from a number of distant sites. Other neoplasms such as the transmissible venereal tumor and hemangiosarcoma may metastasize to the anterior uvea. Lymphosarcoma frequently involves the anterior uvea and other ocular structures, and may present as bilateral disease. Systemic therapy with topical and/or systemic anti-inflammatory treatment for intraocular lymphoma may be attempted using one of several available lymphoma protocols (eg, Madison, WI or Animal Medical Center: combination of cyclophosphamide, prednisolone, vincristine, and/or doxorubicin), but dogs with intraocular lymphoma have shorter survival times.

Cats

Ophthalmic neoplasms are less frequent in cats than in dogs. About 2% of feline patients present with neoplasia, and of these, 2% are affected with ophthalmic tumors. Eyelid and conjunctival tumors are the most frequent primary ophthalmic neoplasms. These neoplasms are usually malignant and more difficult to treat in cats than in dogs. Squamous cell carcinomas, which are more common in white cats with nonpigmented eyelid margins, can involve the eyelids, conjunctivae, and the nictitating membrane; they are pink, roughened, irregular masses or thickened ulcerations. Other less frequent neoplasms include adenocarcinomas, fibrosarcomas, neurofibrosarcomas, and basal cell carcinomas. Treatment varies with the tumor type, location, and size and includes surgical excision, radiation therapy, and cryotherapy.

The most common primary intraocular neoplasm in cats is diffuse iridal melanoma, which presents as progressive hyperpigmentation of the iris with an expanding irregular surface. Pupillary abnormalities, secondary glaucoma due to iridocorneal angle obstruction, and buphthalmia occur late in the disease. Enucleation is recommended because the masses are fast-growing and metastasis is frequent in advanced cases.

Post-traumatic intraocular sarcoma occurs in older cats with a history of chronic uveitis and previous intraocular damage. Clinical signs are either glaucoma, phthisis bulbi, or chronic uveitis. Intraocular cartilage and osteoid production is common. Early enucleation is recommended.

Feline lymphosarcoma-leukemia complex (FeLLC) is the most common secondary ocular neoplasm. Cats with ocular FeLLC have clinical signs ranging from isolated ocular lesions, affecting one or both eyes, to severe systemic illness. Corneal abnormalities may include keratitis, edema, neovascularization, corneal infiltrates, and hemorrhages within the stroma. Ulcerative keratitis may result. Masses can be found in the orbit, globe, conjunctivae, and eyelids. Pupillary abnormalities include mydriasis, anisocoria, spastic pupil syndrome, 'D' or reverse 'D' pupil shape, and lack of light-induced pupillary reflexes. Anterior uveitis is the most common clinical finding in FeLLC. Other findings include ocular hypotension, changes in iridal pigmentation, keratic precipitates, hyphema, anterior and posterior synechiae, miosis, and aqueous flare. Posterior segment changes include retinal hemorrhages, tortuous dilated vessels, perivascular cuffing, and detachment and degeneration of the retina. Few therapy studies of cats with ophthalmic lymphoma exist, but cats with lymphoma and feline leukemia virus infection have lower overall survival times.

DEAFNESS

Acquired deafness may result from occlusion of the external ear canal as occurs in chronic otitis externa, or it may be secondary to destruction of the middle or inner ear. Other causes include trauma to the petrous temporal bone, loud noises (eg, gunfire), demyelinating conditions, ototoxic drugs (eg, aminoglycoside antibiotics [gentamicin, kanamycin, neomycin, streptomycin] or salicylates), neoplasms involving the ear or brain stem, and degeneration of the cochlea in aged dogs. Unilateral deafness or partial hearing loss, or both, is possible in some of these instances. Cochlear degeneration in aged dogs is the most common cause of acquired deafness.

Congenital deafness can be inherited or result from damage (toxic or viral) to the developing fetus. An autosomal gene in cats causes white fur, blue eyes, and deafness; it is dominant with complete expression for white fur and incomplete expression for blue eyes and deafness. Deafness in this instance is due to cochleosaccular degenerative changes that are expressed in the first week of life. Merle and white coat colors are associated with congenital deafness in dogs and other animals. Dog breeds commonly affected include the Dalmatian, Australian Heeler, Catahoula, English Setter, Australian Shepherd, Boston Terrier, Old English Sheepdog, Great Dane, West Highland White Terrier, and Boxer. The list of affected breeds (now >48) continues to expand and may change due to breed popularity and elimination of the defect through selective breeding. For example, Cocker Spaniels were known to have hereditary deafness, but the trait is no longer common in the breed.

Diagnosis requires careful observation of the animal's response to sound. It is helpful to consider the owner's description of behavior and to ask appropriate questions. The response to visual, tactile, and olfactory stimuli must be differentiated from the response to sound. In young animals or in animals kept in groups, deafness may be difficult to detect, because the suspect individual will follow the response of others in the group. If the animal is observed as an individual after an age when responses to auditory stimuli are predictable (~3-4 wk for dogs and cats), then the deafness may be detected. The primary sign of deafness is failure to respond to an auditory stimulus, eg, failure of noise to awaken a sleeping dog or failure to alert to the source of a sound. Other signs include unusual behavior such as excessive barking, unusual voice, hyperactivity, confusion when given vocal commands, and lack of reflex-alerting and attention movements of the pinnae. An animal that has gradually become deaf, as in old age, may become unresponsive to the surroundings and refuse to answer the owner's call. These signs should be differentiated from cognitive dysfunction (*see also* OTHER CANINE BEHAVIORAL PROBLEMS, p 1320). Unilateral deafness is difficult to detect, except by astute observation or by electrodiagnostic procedures. Otoscopic examination of the external ear, radiography of the tympanic bullae, and neurologic examination may reveal the cause, especially in cases of acquired deafness. In congenital deafness, these procedures usually reveal normal anatomic structures, but the animal shows no evidence of hearing, except in cases of unilateral deafness. Brain stem auditory evoked responses (BAER, an electrodiagnostic test) are used to determine the presence and level of an auditory defect from either or both ears. This test is useful in assessing hearing in puppies of breeds prone to congenital deafness. Impedance audiometry can evaluate the integrity of the middle ear and the conduction system.

Deafness due to occlusion of the external ear canal usually responds to appropriate surgical or medical treatment. This deafness is consistent with conduction deafness based on BAER testing and is usually not a complete deafness. Deafness due to bacterial infections of the middle and inner ear may respond to appropriate antibiotic treatment, which should be based on culture and sensitivity results. Recovery from deafness due to persistent intense noise, trauma, or viral infections may be complete, partial, or nil. Recovery from deafness caused by ototoxic drugs is rare. Hereditary deafness may be eliminated from a breed by removal of identifiable carriers from the breeding program. The mode of inheritance of the deafness trait may be determined by study of pedigrees or by test mating. More recently, the BAER test has been used to identify both unilaterally and bilaterally affected dogs, which can then be eliminated from the breeding program.

DISEASES OF THE PINNA

A variety of dermatologic conditions affect the pinna. Most conditions cause lesions elsewhere as well. Rarely, a disease affects the pinna alone, or the pinna is the initial site affected. As with all dermatologic conditions, a diagnosis is best made with the results of a thorough history, a complete physical and dermatologic examination, and with careful selection and evaluation of specific diagnostic tests.

Insects and parasites commonly cause **pinnal dermatitis** either through direct damage from the bite of the parasite or as a result of hypersensitivity. Ticks can cause irritation at the site of attachment and may be found on the pinna or in the ear canal. The spinous ear tick (*Otobius megnini*), found in the southwestern USA, south and central Americas, southern Africa, and India, is a soft-shelled tick whose larval and nymphal forms parasitize the external ear canal of horses, cattle, sheep, goats, deer, rabbits, cats, and dogs. Clinical signs include head shaking, head rubbing, or drooped pinnae. Both the animal and the environment should be treated. Pyrethrin/pyrethroid products are effective.

Fly strike is a worldwide problem caused by the stable fly, *Stomoxys calcitrans*, and typically affects dogs and horses. The fly bite causes small papules and wheals with central hemorrhagic crusts that itch. Lesions are found on the tips or on the folded surface of the pinnae of dogs with flopped ears. However, in horses this fly can cause a hypersensitivity reaction or severe dermatitis resulting in lesions on the dorsal and/or ventral trunk and face in addition to the pinna. Treatment includes fly repellents, controlling the fly population with environmental clean up (manure, etc), and insecticides.

Equine aural plaques (papillary acanthoma, ear papillomas) are caused by a papillomavirus. Black flies (*Simulium* spp) are likely the mechanical vector. These flies are active at dawn and dusk, when they attack the head, ears, and ventral abdomen of horses. Clinically, the lesions are characterized by depigmented, hyperkeratotic, coalescing papules and plaques localized to the concave aspect of the pinna. Often both pinnae are affected. Similar lesions may be present around the anus and external genitalia. Lesions are usually asymptomatic, but in some cases the direct effect of the fly bite causes dermatitis and discomfort. Histologically, the lesions are characterized by mildy papillated epidermal hyperplasia and marked hyperkeratosis. Increased size of keratohyalin granules, poikilocytosis, and hypomelanosis may also be present in the epidermis. Intranuclear viral particles have been seen in electron microscopic studies. Treatment includes frequent applications of fly repellent and stabling the horse during the fly's feeding times. Lesions typically do not regress.

An allergic reaction to mosquito bites can cause an **ulcerative and crusted dermatitis** of the pinnae, nose, and rarely the footpads and eyelids of cats. Lesions progress from papules to crusted ulcers that coalesce to affect extensive areas. Pruritus is variable and lymphadenopathy may occur. Histologically, the lesions are characterized by severe superficial and deep perivascular to interstitial eosinophilic dermatitis, often associated with folliculitis and furunculosis. The differential diagnoses include pemphigus foliaceus, other causes of eosinophilic dermatitis (food allergy, atopy, idiopathic), *Notoedres cati*, and dermatophytosis. Treatment includes keeping the animal inside and using a pyrethrin repellent when exposure to mosquitos is anticipated. Systemic glucocorticoids may be necessary in severe cases.

Sarcoptiform mite infestation (*Sarcoptes scabiei, Notoedres cati*) is common in pigs, dogs, and cats throughout the world. In the USA, sarcoptic mange is rare in horses, cattle, and sheep and is considered a reportable disease. Papular eruptions progress to scaling, crusting, and excoriations of the ear margins and other parts of the body. Pruritus is severe. Transmission is by direct contact with infected animals. Diagnosis is based on clinical signs, history of exposure, and discovery of mites on multiple skin scrapings. Negative scrapings do not rule out the diagnosis, however, as the mite is often difficult to find. If the diagnosis is suspected, treatment should be instituted. Treatment options include lime sulfur dips (safe in all species) every 5 days for 3-5 treatments, insecticidal dips such as amitraz (in dogs only) 2-3 treatments 2 wk apart, and ivermectin at 200-300 µg/kg, PO or SC, every 1-2 wk for 2-4 treatments. Ivermectin is widely used to treat sarcoptic mange in dogs, and has been used to treat notoedric mange in cats, but is not approved by the FDA for this indication. Therefore, every caution should be taken and clients specifically informed of inherent risks with this drug. It should not be used in Collies, Shetland Sheepdogs, Australian Shepherds, and Old English Sheepdogs. Oral milbemycin oxime has been reported to be effective in the treatment of canine sarcoptic mange but is not FDA approved for this purpose. The recommended treatment protocol is 2 mg/kg once weekly for 4 treatments. Because mites can survive off the host for a variable amount of time, all bedding, brushes, tack, and fomites should be treated as well.

Nonburrowing psoroptic mites cause a pruritic otitis externa in horses. Horses may present with head shaking and a drooping ear. Diagnosis is confirmed by finding the mites on skin scraping or in otic exudate, but mites may be difficult to find in the ear canal. Psoroptic mange is a reportable disease in some regions. Ivermectin at 200 µg/kg, PO, every 2 wk for 2 treatments has been shown to be effective.

Several **ear margin dermatoses** characterized by alopecia have been described in dogs. Periodic pinnal alopecia in Miniature Poodles is characterized by progressive bilateral alopecia of the convex surfaces of the ear. The hair loss is acute in onset and progresses over several months, but hair may spontaneously regrow. There are no other clinical signs. Treatment is unnecessary.

Pinnal alopecia has been reported in Dachshunds, Chihuahuas, Italian Greyhounds, and Whippets and is thought to have a hereditary predisposition. The age of onset is ≤1 yr of age. Lesions start as thinning of the hair coat, and complete pinnal alopecia may occur by 8-9 yr of age. Other commonly affected areas are the ventral neck and thorax and the caudal medial thighs. The hair loss is asymptomatic. Differential diagnoses for this condition are endocrinopathies (eg, hypothyroidism, hyperadrenocorticism, sex hormone imbalance). Histologically, the skin is normal and hair follicles are diminished in size but normal in appearance. No effective treatment has been reported, but pentoxifylline (10 mg/kg, BID-TID), melatonin (3 mg for small breeds and 6 mg for large breeds, BID-TID), and topical minoxidil have anecdotally been described as helpful.

Ear margin seborrhea or ear margin dermatosis is common in Dachshunds, although other breeds with pendulous pinnae may be affected. Lesions usually affect the apex of the pinnae on both sides but can progress to involve the whole ear margin. The cause is unknown. Lesions appear as waxy gray to yellow scale adherent to the base of hair shafts. Plugs of hair can be easily epilated leaving behind a shiny surface to the skin. In severe cases the ear margins are edematous, and fissured. Histologic findings include severe hyperkeratosis and follicular keratosis with dilated follicles filled with keratin debris. Differential diagnoses include sarcoptic mange, pinnal alopecia, proliferative thrombovascular necrosis, dermatophytosis, and frostbite. Dermatophytosis in particular can cause a scaling pinnal dermatitis in dogs, cats, and horses but the ear margin is not typically involved and other areas of the body are generally affected as well. Treatment includes antiseborrheic shampoos (eg, sulfur, salicylic acid, benzoyl peroxide), keratolytic products, dioctyl sodium sulfosuccinate (DSS), and systemic medications that may help normalize the abnormal keratinization process (vitamin A and synthetic retinoids; essential fatty acids). Topical or oral glucocorticoids and pentoxifylline (10 mg/kg, BID-TID) may be beneficial when severe inflammation and fissures develop.

Several immune-mediated diseases such as pemphigus foliaceus, pemphigus erythematosus, drug eruption, toxic epidermal necrolysis, and immune vasculitis may affect the pinna and the ear canal. (*See also* AUTOIMMUNE SKIN DISORDERS, p 653.) Other areas of the body are typically affected and may include footpads, mucous membranes, mucocutaneous junctions, nails and nail beds, and the tip of the tail. Immune-mediated diseases are confirmed with biopsy of primary lesions (papules, vesicles, pustules, erythematous margins of secondary lesions) with histologic evaluation by a dermatopathologist.

Acquired **folded ear tips** in cats are most often associated with longterm glucocorticoid therapy (eg, daily eye or otic preparations). It may also be caused by solar radiation damage. Ear folding may not be reversible.

Feline solar dermatitis or actinic dermatitis is seen most commonly in white cats or cats with white pinnae that have been chronically exposed to sun. Lesions first appear as erythema and scaling on the sparsely-haired tips of the ears. Crusting, exudation, and ulceration may develop as the actinic keratosis undergoes transformation into a squamous cell carcinoma. During early stages of the disease, treatment consists of limiting exposure to ultraviolet light through confinement indoors between the hours of 10 am and 4 pm, and the use of topical sunscreens. Squamous cell carcinoma of the pinnae is treated with surgical excision followed by radiation therapy.

Auricular hematomas are small to large fluid-filled swellings that develop on the concave surface of the pinnae in dogs, cats, and pigs. The pathogenesis for the development of the lesions is unknown, but head shaking or ear scratching due to pruritus is always involved. In dogs, the condition is seen with atopy and food allergy in which the ear canals are the primary sites of allergic inflammation and pruritus. In pigs, sarcoptic mange, pediculosis, and meal in the ears (from overhead feeders) have been implicated as a cause of head-shaking that has led to auricular hematomas. Bites from other pigs also may be at fault (*see* NECROTIC EAR SYNDROME, below). Treatment is surgical to allow drainage. After draining and flushing, several mattress sutures can be placed to eliminate the pocket. The addition of a drain made out of a teat tube, piece of soft urinary catheter, or IV catheter increases the success rate of the surgery. Drainage and glucocorticoid instillation are successful in ~50% of cases. Drainage is best obtained with a butterfly connection or an IV catheter. Glucocorticoids are instilled to fill the cavity without causing skin distention. A short course of a low anti-inflammatory dose of oral glucocorticoids is commonly added to this treatment.

Proliferative vascular necrosis of the pinnae is rare in dogs. There are no known breed, sex, or age predilections and the etiology is also unknown. Lesions, which consist of scaly, thickened, hyperpigmented skin surrounding a necrotic ulcer, begin at the apex of the ear and spread along the concave surface. Eventually, necrosis may deform the margin of the pinna.

Auricular chondritis has been reported rarely in cats and in 1 dog. Clinical signs include pain, swelling, erythema, and deformation of the pinnae. Both ears are typically affected. Lesions consist of lymphoplasmacytic infiltrates, basophilia, and necrosis of cartilage. Treatment may not be required if the condition is nonpainful. Systemic glucocorticoids have been reported to be ineffective, but dapsone (1 mg/kg, SID) has induced remission in some cases.

Frostbite may occur in animals poorly adapted to cold climates and is more likely in wet or windy conditions. It typically affects body regions that are poorly insulated, including the tips of the ears. The skin may be pale or erythematous, edematous, and painful. In severe cases, necrosis and sloughing of the tips may follow. Treatment consists of rapid, gentle warming and supportive care. Amputation of affected regions may be required but should be delayed until the extent of viable tissue is determined.

Canine juvenile cellulitis is an uncommon disorder of puppies and is characterized by granulomatous, sterile pustules of the face, pinnae, and submandibular lymph nodes. It occurs in puppies 3 wk to 4 mo of age and rarely in older animals. Golden Retrievers, Gordon Setters, and Dachshunds appear to be at greater risk than other breeds. A pustular otitis externa is common, along with edematous, thickened pinnae. The diagnosis can be confirmed by biopsy, which shows a pyogranulomatous inflammatory infiltrate with no microorganisms, and by negative bacteriologic culture. Early treatment is recommended to avoid scarring. Prednisone or prednisolone (2 mg/kg, PO, divided BID) should be tapered slowly over 4-6 wk or until the disease is inactive. Antibiotics may be needed to treat secondary bacterial infection.

Necrotic Ear Syndrome in Swine
(Ear necrosis, Necrotic auricular dermatitis)

Pigs with necrotic ear syndrome have unilateral or bilateral necrosis of the pinnae, are unthrifty, and commonly develop septic arthritis or die from secondary bacterial septicemia. The condition occurs sporadically in weaned and growing pigs under all management systems.

Etiology, Transmission, and Pathogenesis: The causes have not been determined conclusively. Circumstantial evidence strongly suggests that the disease is due to trauma (fighting) and subsequent bacterial invasion of the damaged tissue. Another potential factor that may contribute to the problem is inadequate dietary lysine levels in the feed.

Histologic and microbiologic findings suggest that the aggressive erosive lesion is due to secondary bacterial infection. In the early phases of the disease, large numbers of *Staphylococcus hyicus* and low to moderate numbers of β-hemolytic streptococci are found in the surface exudate; later, during the ulcerative and necrotic stage, large numbers of the streptococci are found deep in the lesion. It is hypothesized that *S hyicus* colonizes the traumatized tissue, which prepares the way for the highly invasive streptococci that induce the changes that lead to ulceration and necrosis. Efforts to reproduce the disease by experimental inoculation of the 2 organisms have been unsuccessful.

Clinical Findings, Lesions, and Diagnosis: The nature and extent of clinical signs depend on the severity of the local lesion and development of secondary bacterial septicemia. Thus, a spectrum of signs, including unthriftiness, inappetence, fever, septic arthritis, collapse, and death, may be seen.

Mild lesions consist of superficial scratches covered with thin, dry, brown crusts. Mild edema or erythema may be present near the scratches. In more severe cases, thick, brown, moist scabs cover deep ulcers. In the most severe cases, there is extensive necrosis. The lesions evolve from mild, superficial dermatitis to severe, deep inflammation with exudation, ulceration, thrombosis, and necrosis. In mild cases, resolution occurs with no loss of ear tissue; in severe cases, the margins, tips, or even the entire pinna may be lost.

Diagnosis is made on the appearance of the affected ears.

Control: Tincture of iodine, applied topically BID for 1 wk, has reduced the incidence and severity of the disease. Antibacterial drugs administered in the feed are effective in some herds but not in others. Lack of effectiveness could be due to drug resistance. In cases of antibacterial ineffectiveness, specimens should be collected aseptically from the deep aspect of the ulcerative lesions for culture and sensitivity testing. Traumatizing events should be minimized. Management practices (ventilation, location and functioning of waterers, pen design, group size, mixing) and proper levels of dietary lysine should be checked and corrected if deficiencies are detected. (*See also* HEALTH-MANAGEMENT INTERACTION: PIGS, p 1740.)

OTITIS EXTERNA

Otitis externa is an acute or chronic inflammation of the epithelium of the external ear canal. It may develop anywhere from the tympanic membrane to the pinna. It is variably characterized by erythema, edema, increased sebum or exudate, and desquamation of the epithelium. The ear canal may be painful or pruritic depending on the cause or duration of the condition. It is the most common disease of the ear canal in dogs and cats, is occasionally seen in rabbits (in which it is usually due to the mite *Psoroptes cuniculi*), and is uncommon in large animals. Internal and external factors may directly induce inflammation and pruritus in the ear canal. Identifying these factors is key to successful management.

Etiology: The causes of otitis externa have been grouped into 3 areas. Primary factors are disease conditions that directly cause the otitis. Predisposing factors are conditions that place an individual at risk for developing otitis. Perpetuating factors tend to prevent the resolution of the otitis once it develops. Often all 3 factors are involved, but each category must be identified and addressed separately. In this way a more accurate prognosis can be provided, a specific and safe therapeutic plan formulated, and the best possible outcome from treatment assured.

Primary factors include parasites (*Otodectes, Psoroptes, Sarcoptes, Demodex* spp), foreign bodies (grass awn, concreted wax, medications), tumors (cerumin gland adenoma, inflammatory polyps), hypersensitivity (atopy, food sensitivity, contact dermatitis), disorders of keratinization, hypothyroidism, autoimmune diseases, juvenile cellulitis, and irritants (cleaners, plucking fur, etc).

Predisposing factors are often congenital or environmental and include conformation (pinnal carriage, narrow ear canal, excessive hair or ceruminous glands), maceration of the ear canal from overtreatment or swimmer's ear, and systemic disease. Small changes in the otic microclimate may alter the delicate balance of normal secretions and microflora and result in opportunistic infections. Any disease that affects normal responses to pathogens can predispose the ear canal to opportunistic infections.

Perpetuating factors include bacteria, yeasts, otitis media, and progressive pathologic changes. Once the environment of the ear canal has been altered by a combination of primary and predisposing factors, opportunistic infections and pathologic changes occur, which prevent resolution of the disease. Chronic pathologic changes in the ears may also reflect a generalized systemic or skin disease. Unless all the causes are identified and treated, recurrence may be expected.

Clinical Findings and Diagnosis: Signalment and a thorough dermatologic history provide information suggestive of primary problems (eg, genetic, hypersensitivity, keratinization disorders). A thorough physical and dermatologic examination provide diagnostic clues related to hormonal, endocrine, and immune disorders that also affect the ear. Skin scrapings, cytologic evaluation of exudate, a Wood's lamp examination, and dermatophyte culture should be done in every case.

The pinnae and periauricular regions should be inspected for evidence of self-trauma, erythema, and primary and secondary skin lesions. Pinnal deformities, hyperplastic tissue in the canal, and head-shaking suggest chronic otic discomfort.

For animals with unilateral signs, the unaffected ear should be examined first to prevent iatrogenic contamination of the unaffected ear with organisms (eg, *Pseudomonas aeruginosa* or *Proteus mirabilis*) that may be present in the diseased ear. The unaffected ear may, in fact, be diseased, requiring an adjustment of the differential diagnosis list to include causes of bilateral otitis.

Sedation or anesthesia may be needed for a thorough otoscopic examination. This is especially true if the ear is painful, if the canal is obstructed with exudate or proliferative inflammatory tissue, or if the animal is uncooperative. An otoscopic examination will allow identification of deep otic foreign bodies, impacted debris, low-grade infections with *Otodectes cynotis*, and ruptured or abnormal tympanic membranes.

During an otoscopic examination, the ear canal should be inspected for changes in diameter, pathologic changes in the skin, quantity and type of exudate, parasites, foreign bodies, neoplasms, and changes in the tympanic membrane. The tympanic membrane should be examined for evidence of disease or rupture. However, in many cases of otitis externa, the tympanic membrane cannot be visualized at all until the exudate is gently flushed from the canal.

Cytologic evaluation of exudate or cerumen taken from the horizontal ear canal may provide immediate diagnostic information. Exudate obtained with a cotton-tipped applicator can be rolled onto a glass slide, heat fixed, stained with a 3-step quick stain or modified Wright's stain, and examined under a microscope. Smears should be examined first under low-power magnification and then under high-power (preferably using immersion oil) for numbers and morphology of bacteria, yeasts, and WBC; evidence of phagocytosis of microorganisms; fungal hyphae; and acantholytic or neoplastic cells.

The external ear canals of most dogs and cats harbor small numbers of commensal gram-positive cocci. These organisms may become pathogenic if the microenvironment is changed to encourage overgrowth of these organisms. A stained smear can quickly determine if microbial overgrowth is present. Coccal organisms are usually staphylococci or streptococci. Rod-shaped organisms are usually *Pseudomonas aeruginosa* or *Proteus mirabilis*; their appearance in large numbers indicates that a bacterial culture with antibiotic sensitivity should be performed because of their known resistance to many antimicrobial agents. The presence of many neutrophils phagocytizing bacteria confirms the pathogenic nature of the organisms.

The yeast *Malassezia pachydermatis* is found in low numbers in the ear canals of many normal dogs and cats. Because yeasts colonize the surface of the ear canal, they are most easily found adhered to clumps of exfoliated squamous epithelial cells. *M pachydermatis* is identified readily on microscopic examination and its numbers easily assessed. No more than 2-3 organisms per high-power field should be present on any aggregate of cells from a normal animal. When unidentified yeasts or hyphal organisms are seen in significant numbers in cytologic smears, the species should be identified through culture. Concurrent bacterial infections, especially with gram-positive cocci, are common.

A dark exudate in the canal usually signals the presence of either *Malassezia* spp or a parasite, but may also be seen with a bacterial or mixed infection. In addition to stained cytology, otic exudate should be examined for eggs, larvae, or adults of the ear mite *Otodectes cynotis* in dogs and cats, and *Psoroptes cuniculi* in rabbits and goats. Smears are made by combining cerumen and otic discharge with a small quantity of mineral oil on a glass slide. A coverglass should be used, and the smear examined under low-power magnification. Rarely, refractory ceruminous otitis externa may be associated with localized proliferation of *Demodex* sp in the external ear canals of dogs and cats and may be the only area on the body affected.

Microbial cultures are taken before otoscopy is completed and before any cleaning takes place. Samples for culture should be taken with a sterile culturette from the horizontal canal (the region where most infections arise) or from the middle ear in cases of tympanic rupture. A bacterial culture and antibiotic sensitivity and an antibiotic mean inhibitory concentration (MIC) should be done.

Histopathologic changes associated with chronic otitis externa are often nonspecific. Histopathologic evidence of a hypersensitivity response may support a recommendation for intradermal allergy testing or for a hypoallergenic diet trial. Additionally, biopsies from animals with chronic, obstructive, unilateral otitis externa may reveal whether neoplastic changes are present.

Radiography of the osseous bullae is indicated when proliferative tissues prevent adequate visualization of the tympanic membrane, when otitis media is suspected as a cause of relapsing bacterial otitis externa, and when neurologic signs accompany otitis externa. Fluid densities and proliferative or lytic osseous changes provide evidence of middle ear involvement. Unfortunately, radiographs are normal in many otitis media cases. Computed tomography or MRI, if available, should be performed for cases of severe, chronic otitis.

Treatment: Underlying primary, predisposing, and perpetuating causes should be identified and corrected. The periauricular area should be clipped of fur, and hair removed from the ear canal to improve ventilation, facilitate cleaning and drying of the canals, and to increase adherence to treatment recommendations.

Topical medications are inactivated by exudates, and excessive cerumen may prevent medications from reaching the epithelium. The ears should be gently cleaned and should be dry before treatment is started. In animals with painful ears, proper cleaning requires general anesthesia. The ears may be flushed with an antibacterial cleansing solution (chlorhexidine or povidone iodine) or with a ceruminolytic solution such as carbamide peroxide or dioctyl sodium sulfosuccinate (DSS). There are many appropriate products available for use if the otitis is limited to the external canal. Thorough rinsing with warmed saline to remove the cleaning agent must always follow after all debris has been removed. If the tympanic membrane is ruptured, detergents and DSS are contraindicated; milder cleansers (eg, saline, saline plus povidone iodine, Tris EDTA) should be used to flush the ear.

Medical therapy should be specific and simple. Contributing causes should be treated specifically and aggressively. In treatment of acute bacterial otitis externa, antibacterial agents in combination with corticosteroids may be used to reduce exudation, pain, and swelling, and decrease glandular secretions. The least potent corticosteroid that will reduce the inflammation should be used. Animals with recurring bacterial otitis externa and a history of infection with *Otodectes cynotis* should be treated with a topical product that contains antibacterial and antiparasitic agents to ensure that undetected low-grade parasitic infections are eliminated. Parasites may also affect extra-auricular sites. A general topical or systemic parasiticide will be most effective in suspected or confirmed recurring cases.

Topical therapy should be based on the character of the disease. Properly applied, the ideal medication coats the epithelium of the external ear canal as a thin film. Nonocclusive solutions or lotions should be used for acute or chronic exudative otitis externa and proliferative conditions. Occlusive oil-based ointments should be reserved for dry, scaly lesions within the ear canals. Changes in the skin of the ear canals during treatment may indicate a need for a different vehicle or base.

Irritating medications should be avoided. They cause swelling of the lining of the ear canal and an increase in glandular secretions, which predispose to opportunistic infections. Substances that are usually not irritating in normal ear canals may cause irritation in an ear that is already inflamed. This is particularly true of propylene glycol. Powders, such as those used after plucking hair from the canal, can form irritating concretions within the ear canal and should not be used.

Systemic therapy should be incorporated into the treatment regimen in most cases of chronic otitis and in any case in which otitis media is suspected. In cases of severe atopy or idiopathic seborrhea, systemic corticosteroids may be necessary to control the inflammation. Failure to use systemic antimicrobial therapy is an important perpetuating cause of chronic ear disease in dogs. Systemic antibiotics should be used when neutrophils or rod-type bacteria are found on cytology, in cases of therapeutic failure with topical antimicrobial agents, in chronic recurring ear infections, and in all cases of otitis media.

Duration of treatment will vary depending on the individual case but should continue until the infection is resolved. Animals with bacterial and yeast infections should be physically examined and cytologies evaluated weekly to every other week until there is no evidence of infection. For most acute cases, this takes 2-4 wk. Chronic cases may take months to resolve, and in some instances, a therapeutic regimen must be continued indefinitely. Animals with *Otodectes cynotis* or *Psoroptes cuniculi* should receive appropriate parasiticide treatment in the ears and on the whole body for at least 2-4 wk. *Otobius megnini* infestations are best treated by manual removal of the ticks, followed by an acaricide/corticosteroid otic preparation.

Pseudomonas otitis (caused by *Pseudomonas aeruginosa*) has emerged as one of the most frustrating and difficult perpetuating causes of otitis because of the development of resistance to most common antibiotics. It is often chronic in course (>2 mo) and associated with marked suppurative exudation, severe epithelial ulceration, pain, and edema of the canal. Successful treatment of chronic *Pseudomonas* otitis is multifaceted and should include the following steps: 1) identify the primary cause of the otitis and manage it, 2) remove the exudate and dry the canal, 3) identify and treat concurrent otitis media, 4) select an appropriate antibiotic from the results of culture and MIC on the organism and use it at an effective dose for an appropriate duration, and 5) treat both topically and systemically until the infection resolves (weeks to months).

The best treatment of chronic otitis is prevention. In addition to identifying the cause of acute otitis, topical and/or systemic medications should be chosen based on cytology or culture; they should have a narrow spectrum and be specific for the current condition. Aminoglycosides and fluoroquinolone antibiotics should not be used unless absolutely required for successful treatment. Polymyxin B and fluoroquinolone antibiotics have shown the best success in controlling infections in cases in which resistance has been identified through culture. However, resistance is developing to fluoroquinolones.

Maintenance Care: Owners should be shown how to properly clean the ears. The frequency of cleaning usually decreases over time from daily to once or twice weekly as a preventive maintenance procedure. The ear canals should be kept dry and well ventilated. Using topical astringents in dogs that swim frequently and preventing water from entering the ear canals during bathing should minimize maceration of the ear canal. Chronic maceration impairs the barrier function of the skin, which predisposes to opportunistic infection. Preventive otic astringents may decrease the frequency of bacterial or mycotic infections in moist ear canals. Clipping hair from the inside of the pinna and around the external auditory meatus, and plucking it from hirsute ear canals, improves ventilation and decreases humidity in the ears. However, hair should not routinely be removed from the ear canal if it is not causing a problem, because doing so can induce an acute inflammatory reaction.

OTITIS MEDIA AND INTERNA

Otitis media, inflammation of the middle ear structures, is usually due to extension of infection from the external ear canal or to penetration of the tympanic membrane by a foreign object. It is seen in all species but is most common in dogs, cats, and rabbits. Extension of infection through the auditory tube occurs in dogs, cats, and pigs. Hematogenous spread of infection to these areas is possible but rare. Otitis media may lead to otitis interna and inflammation of the inner ear structures. This can in turn lead to loss of equilibrium and deafness.

Clinical Findings and Diagnosis: The signs of otitis media and otitis externa (p 421) may be similar. Head shaking, rubbing the affected ear on the floor, and rotating the head toward the affected side are often noted. The ear is usually painful, with a discharge and inflammatory changes in the ear canal. Because the facial and sympathetic nerves course through the middle ear, facial nerve paralysis or Horner's syndrome (miosis, ptosis, enophthalmos, and protrusion of the nictitans), or both, may be present on the same side as the otitis media. If there is concurrent otitis interna, head tilt toward the affected side will be more pronounced. Additionally, the animal with otitis interna may circle and fall toward the affected side and will have generalized incoordination that may be severe enough to cause difficulty in rising and ambulating. Nystagmus may also be seen with otitis interna and is characterized as a spontaneous, horizontal to rotary type, with the fast phase away from the affected side and head tilt. Rarely, infection may ascend the vestibulocochlear and facial nerves to the brain stem and result in meningitis, a brain-stem abscess, and death.

Otitis media should be suspected in cases of severe purulent otitis externa; chronic, recurrent otitis externa; or whenever the tympanic membrane has been penetrated by a foreign object or has ruptured secondary to chronic otitis. The diagnosis can be confirmed by bulging, discoloration, or rupture of the tympanic membrane. Fluid in the tympanic cavity or sclerotic changes of the osseous tympanic bullae may be detected radiographically, although computerized tomography is the imaging modality of choice for this region. Cytologic examination (Gram's stain and Wright's stain) and culture of the exudate may be beneficial, along with sensitivity testing of any microbial isolates.

Otitis interna should be strongly suspected if peripheral vestibular signs are present. Otoscopic examination and radiographs of the tympanic bulla may confirm the presence of concurrent otitis media.

Treatment and Prognosis: Because of the possibility of hearing loss and damage to the vestibular apparatus, longterm (3-6 wk) systemic antibacterial therapy should be instituted as soon as the diagnosis is made. Chloramphenicol, cephalosporins, trimethoprim-sulfa combinations, or fluoroquinolones should be used until the results of bacterial sensitivity tests are known. If the eardrum is ruptured, the tympanic cavity should be carefully cleaned with visualization through an otoscope and the use of long alligator forceps, flushes of warm saline, and low vacuum suction. Small perforations of the eardrum usually heal in 2-3 wk. Any associated otitis externa should be treated concurrently. Additionally, anti-inflammatory doses of glucocorticoids (0.5 mg/kg/day) during the first 5-7 days of treatment may decrease inflammatory changes in the vestibulocochlear, facial, or sympathetic nerves.

In animals with otitis media and interna in which the external ear is clean and normal, but the tympanum is bulging or discolored, it may be advantageous to perforate the tympanum (perform a myringotomy) to permit culture of the fluid, to relieve the pressure (and thus the pain) within the middle ear, and to permit removal of the inflammatory exudate; however, perforation of the tympanum could result in permanent diminished hearing loss. Systemic antibiotic therapy based on sensitivity testing should be continued for 3-4 wk and possibly up to 6 wk if otitis interna exists. In chronic otitis media, if radiographic changes are consistent with osteomyelitis or fluid in the tympanic bulla, a bulla osteotomy is usually necessary to allow for drainage and adequate resolution of the infection.

Otitis media with an intact tympanum usually responds well to systemic antibiotic therapy; however, if chronic otitis externa exists and the tympanum is ruptured, the chances of successful treatment are reduced. If facial and sympathetic nerve deficits develop, they may persist even after the infection has been cleared. Otitis interna usually responds well to longterm antibiotic therapy, but some neurologic deficits (eg, incoordination, head tilt, deafness) may persist for life. Animals recovering from otitis interna should be given adequate time to adapt to any persistent neurologic deficiencies.

TUMORS OF THE EAR CANAL

Ear canal tumors may develop from any of the structures lining or supporting the ear canal, including the squamous epithelium, the ceruminous or sebaceous glands, or the mesenchymal tissues. Tumors arising from the external ear canal and pinna are more common than tumors originating from the middle or inner ear. Ear canal tumors are more common in cats than in dogs. These tumors are relatively uncommon compared with cutaneous tumors elsewhere on the body.

Although the precise cause of ear canal tumors is unknown, several theories have been postulated. Chronic inflammation of the ear canal may lead to tissue hyperplasia, followed by dysplasia, and finally neoplasia. Inspissated apocrine secretions from hyperplastic ceruminous glands during otitis externa episodes may stimulate carcinogenesis in the ear canal. Feline nasal-pharyngeal polyps may be congenital or due to viral (calicivirus) or bacterial respiratory infections.

Cocker Spaniels have an increased incidence of benign and malignant ear canal tumors when compared with other breeds. Middle-aged to older dogs and cats are predisposed to benign and malignant ear canal tumors, while young cats (3 mo-5 yr) are more likely to develop nasopharyngeal polyps. Clinical signs of ear canal tumors include usually unilateral chronic otic discharge (ceruminous, purulent, or hemorrhagic) and necrotic odor, head shaking and ear scratching, swelling or draining abscesses in the parotid region below the affected ear, deafness, and vestibular signs if there is middle or inner ear involvement, including head tilt, ataxia, nystagmus, and Horner's syndrome. In any case of medically refractory unilateral otitis, a neoplasm of the ear canal should be suspected.

Ear canal tumors are more likely to be malignant than benign in both dogs and cats, although cats have a higher incidence of malignant tumors. The most common pinnal neoplasms in dogs are sebaceous gland tumors, histiocytomas, and mast cell tumors. In cats, common pinnal neoplasms include squamous cell carcinoma, basal cell tumors, hemangiosarcomas, and melanocytic tumors. The most common external ear canal tumors reported in dogs are ceruminous gland adenomas and ceruminous gland adenocarcinomas. Other tumors reported in the external ear canal of dogs include inflammatory polyps, papillomas, sebaceous gland adenomas, histiocytomas, plasmacytomas, melanomas, fibromas, squamous cell carcinomas, and hemangiosarcomas. The most common external ear canal masses reported in cats are nasopharyngeal polyps, squamous cell carcinomas, and ceruminous gland adenocarcinomas. Lymphoma, fibrosarcoma, and squamous cell carcinoma are rarely seen in the middle or inner ear of dogs and cats. (*See also* TUMORS OF THE SKIN AND SOFT TISSUES, p 764.)

Ceruminous Gland Tumors
(Ceruminous gland adenoma, Adenocarcinoma)

Benign or malignant neoplasms that develop from the modified apocrine or cerumen glands in the external ear canal are most common in cats but also occur in dogs, usually in middle-aged or older animals. Although rare, ceruminous gland adenocarcinomas are more common than adenomas in both dogs and cats. Cats have a higher percentage of adenocarcinomas than dogs. Animals with a history of chronic hyperplastic otitis are predisposed to the development of ceruminous gland tumors, and Cocker Spaniels are particularly over-represented. These neoplasms appear as firm, dome-shaped, pink-white, often pedunculated nodules or plaques that may be ulcerated. Because many tumors completely obstruct the ear canal, they are often associated with secondary otitis externa or media with purulent to hemorrhagic discharge. Vestibular signs may be present if there is middle ear involvement. Ceruminous gland adenocarcinomas are locally invasive and may metastasize to regional lymph nodes and to the parotid salivary gland. Distant metastasis to the lungs is rare.

Diagnosis of ceruminous gland tumors is by deep otoscopic examination under sedation or general anesthesia, with flushing and suction removal of purulent discharge as needed to visualize the deep vertical and horizontal canals. Use of a videographic otoscope greatly facilitates this procedure. Computed tomography or MRI may be very useful in assessing the tympanic bulla more completely and in determining the extent of tumor invasion, especially in malignant tumors. Definitive diagnosis is made by histopathology after surgical removal of the mass.

Surgical removal of benign ear canal tumors may be accomplished via lateral ear canal resection in most cases, unless there is involvement of the tympanic bulla. Laser surgery has also been used. Total ear canal ablation with bulla osteotomy is the only recommended surgery for removal of malignant ear canal tumors. Lateral ear canal resection is associated with a 75% recurrence rate. Median survival time of animals with malignant ear canal tumors has been reported to be >58 mo in dogs and >11.7 mo in cats. Dogs with extensive tumor involvement had a less favorable prognosis. Cats with invasive tumors, squamous cell carcinoma, or neurologic signs at the time of diagnosis had a poorer prognosis. Radiation therapy can be used to treat incompletely excised ceruminous gland adenocarcinomas in dogs and cats, with a 56% 1-yr survival rate reported.

Feline Nasopharyngeal Polyps

Nasopharyngeal polyps are uncommon, benign, smooth, pink-red, fleshy, pedunculated, inflammatory growths of fibrous connective tissue that are found in the external ear canals of young cats. They may arise from the mucosal lining of the tympanic bulla, the pharyngeal mucosa, or the auditory tube. These polyps may be congenital or due to viral (calicivirus) or bacterial infection. Bacterial otitis externa or media due to obstruction of the ear canal or tympanic bulla may be present.

Diagnosis involves sedation and deep otoscopic examination of the vertical and horizontal ear canals. Purulent discharge may need to be gently suctioned from the ear canal to visualize the polyp. Use of a videographic otoscope greatly enhances the ability to evaluate the deep horizontal canal for polyps. Polyps originating from the eustachian tube may be seen by gently retracting the soft palate rostrally. Computed tomography or MRI may be helpful if a mass is suspected in the tympanic bulla that cannot be seen otoscopically. Definitive diagnosis is made via histopathology.

Surgical removal is curative as long as the entire polyp and stalk are removed. This often involves performing a bulla osteotomy, as the base of the polyp is often in the tympanic bulla. Incomplete removal of the base of the polyp leads to rapid regrowth and return of clinical signs.

■ ■ ■

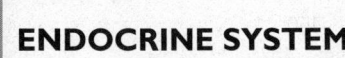

ENDOCRINE SYSTEM

ENDOCRINE SYSTEM INTRODUCTION

The endocrine system encompasses a group of tissues that release hormones into circulation for travel to distant targets. An endocrine tissue is typically a ductless gland (eg, pituitary, thyroid) that releases its hormones into capillaries permeating the tissue. These glands are richly supplied with blood. It is, however, increasingly clear that non-typical endocrine tissues also contribute important hormones to circulation, eg, secretion of atrial natriuretic peptide from the heart, erythropoietin from the kidney, insulin-like growth factor from the liver, and leptin from fat. New hormones continue to be discovered. Some act only on a single tissue, while others have effects on virtually all cells of the body. The effects of hormones on their targets are varied—from enhancement of nutrient uptake to altering cell division and differentiation, among many others.

GENERAL CHEMICAL STRUCTURE AND FUNCTION

There are 3 main chemical categories of hormones: protein/polypeptides, steroids, and those made from modified amino acids.

Protein/polypeptide Hormones: Examples of protein/polypeptide hormones include adrenocorticotropin (ACTH) from the pituitary, insulin from the pancreas, and parathyroid hormone (PTH). These hormones range in size from 3 amino acids (thyrotropin-releasing hormone) to considerably larger proteins with subunit structure (eg, luteinizing hormone). They are produced in their endocrine tissue of origin by transcription/translation of the gene coding for the hormone and synthesized initially as larger products (prepro- or pre-forms) that undergo processing to authentic hormone inside the cell prior to secretion. Embedded in the gene coding for protein structure are amino acid sequences (signal peptides) that communicate to the cell that these molecules are destined for the regulated secretory pathway. Other post-translational modifications may occur during processing including folding, glycosylation, disulfide bond formation, and subunit assembly. The folded and processed hormone is then stored in secretory granules or vesicles in preparation for release by the exocytotic process. Release of hormone is triggered by unique signals; eg, secretion of PTH is stimulated by a decline in the concentration of ionic or free calcium present in the extracellular fluid bathing the parathyroid chief cells. In most cases, cells producing protein/polypeptide hormones store significant amounts of these substances intracellularly; therefore, they can respond quickly when increased amounts are needed in circulation. Generally, protein/polypeptide hormones have relatively short half-lives in blood (minutes) and do not travel in blood-bound carrier proteins (exceptions exist, eg, insulin-like growth factor 1 is highly protein bound).

Protein/polypeptide hormones act on their target cells by binding to receptors located on the cell surface. These receptors are proteins and glycoproteins embedded in the cell membrane that traverse the membrane at least once so that the receptor is exposed to both the extracellular and intracellular environments. There are several classes or types of cell surface hormone receptors that translate the hormonal message to the cell interior by different means. Some are the G-protein (guanosine) coupled type, with 7 transmembrane spanning domains. After hormone binding, these receptors activate a G-protein that is also located in the membrane. One or more of the G-protein subunits affects other downstream molecules (known as effectors) such as enzymes (eg, adenylate cyclase or phospholipase C) or ion channels. Activation may result in production of a second messenger, such as cyclic AMP, that can then bind to protein kinase A causing its activation and subsequent phosphorylation of other proteins. Thus, signal transduction is a cascading and often amplifying series of events triggered when a hormone binds to its receptor. The ultimate effects in target cells are multiple and include such things as triggering secretion, increasing uptake of a molecule, or activating mitosis.

Cell surface receptors are dynamic; their numbers and/or activity change with physiologic conditions. In some cases, such as exposure to excessive amounts of hormone, receptor down-regulation can occur. Down-regulation and a decline in target tissue responsiveness may be due to internalization of receptors following ligand binding or to desensitization whereby the receptor is chemically modified and becomes less active. Conversely, a lack of hormonal exposure can lead to an increase in receptor numbers on target cells (up-regulation). Diseases have been linked to mutations in hormone receptors, which can result in inactivation or constitutive or nonhormonal activation of the pathway. In some instances, a single amino acid substitution is responsible.

Steroid Hormones: Steroid hormones are derivatives of cholesterol and include products of the adrenal cortex, ovaries, and testes as well as the related molecule, vitamin D. Unlike protein/polypeptide hormones, steroid hormones are not stored in large amounts. When needed they are rapidly synthesized from cholesterol by a series of enzymatic reactions. Most of the cholesterol needed for rapid steroid hormone synthesis is stored intracellularly in the tissue of origin. In response to appropriate signals, the precursor is moved to organelles (mitochondria and smooth endoplasmic reticulum), where a series of enzymes (eg, isomerases, dehydrogenases) rapidly convert the molecule to the appropriate steroid hormone. The identity of the final steroidal product is thus dictated by the set of enzymes expressed in that tissue.

Steroid hormones are hydrophobic and pass through cell membranes easily. In the blood, they are bound to a great extent to carrier proteins. Albumin binds many steroids fairly loosely; in addition, specific binding globulins exist for many steroid hormones. The majority of the steroid hormone in circulation is bound to carrier proteins, and a small fraction circulates free or unbound. This latter fraction is thought to be available for target cell entry, ie, the biologically active portion. A rapid equilibrium exists between protein-bound and unbound steroid in extracellular fluid. Possible roles for steroid hormone binding proteins include aiding in tissue delivery of steroids by providing an even distribution to all cells within a target tissue, buffering against large fluctuations in free hormone, and prolonging the half-life of steroids in blood. Relative to protein/polypeptide hormones, steroids usually have longer half-lives, often in the range of many minutes to hours.

Steroid hormones act on target cells via receptors located in the cell interior. These receptors are generally found in the nucleus, although some appear to reside, when unoccupied, in the cytoplasm. There are several classes of steroid receptors—those for glucocorticoids, mineralocorticoids, progestins, etc. Steroid receptors comprise a family of related proteins that also show homology to receptors for the thyroid hormones and vitamin D. The receptor has regions or domains that carry out specific tasks: one for recognition and binding of the steroid, another for binding to a specific region on chromosomal DNA, and a third for helping regulate the transcriptional complex. Steroid hormones enter targets by diffusing through the cell membrane and then binding to the receptor, causing a conformational change in the new complex. This, in turn, leads to release of associated proteins (eg, heat shock proteins) and movement to the nucleus (if necessary), followed by binding of the complex to regions of DNA located near specific steroid-regulated genes. The result is an alteration in the rate of transcription of specific genes, either increasing or decreasing their expression. Thus, steroid hormones primarily function by affecting the production rates of specific messenger RNA and proteins in targets. Steroid action is relatively slow in onset (hours) but may be long lasting because of the duration of production and half-lives of the messenger RNA and proteins induced in target cells. Some evidence exists to support the idea of "nongenomic" actions of steroids, with many of these effects occurring rapidly following steroid hormone exposure.

Steroids in the blood are eliminated by metabolism in the liver. Reduced forms are produced and subsequently conjugated to glucuronic acid and sulfate. These metabolites are freely soluble in blood and are eliminated from the body by renal excretion and elimination through the GI tract. Small amounts of free steroid hormone are also directly excreted by the kidneys.

Modified Amino Acid Hormones: This class of hormones is made by chemical modification of amino acids, mainly tyrosine. They include thyroid hormones and the catecholamines epinephrine and norepinephrine. Thyroxine (T_4) and triiodothyronine (T_3) are stored in the thyroid as a part of thyroglobulin; secretion of these hormones involves thyroidal cell uptake and breakdown of this large molecule liberating T_4 and T_3. Thyroid hormones act on targets much like steroids; they are relatively water insoluble, transported by carrier proteins in blood, and act on targets via intracellular receptors. Catecholamines are manufactured by hydroxylation, decarboxylation, and methylation of tyrosine and are secreted into the blood from the adrenal medulla. They have exceedingly short half-lives (<5 min), are not protein bound, and act on targets via cell surface receptors (α- and β-adrenergic receptors).

MEASUREMENT OF HORMONES

Because hormones circulate in low quantities in blood, accurate measurement of these substances requires sensitive assays, usually in the form of a competitive immunoassay. The original method (still widely used) is radioimmunoassay employing an antibody directed against the hormone and a radio-labeled form of the hormone. The labeled hormone competes with unlabeled hormone for antibody-binding sites. A standard curve containing known amounts of hormone is used for comparison to calculate the concentration of hormone in patient samples. The use of radioactive tags permits detection of low concentrations of hormone, which typically circulate in the pico- (10^{-12}) or nanomolar (10^{-9}) range. In recent years, nonradioactive tags, "sandwich-type" assays, and ELISA methods have been developed for hormone measurement.

Accurate measurement in veterinary species presents some challenges, because normal concentrations of a given hormone can vary significantly between species. For example, normal total T_4 concentrations in dogs and cats are approximately 4 times lower than those in humans. Concern about cross-reactivity is important; protein/polypeptide hormones vary in amino acid composition and in other structural ways (eg, patterns of glycosylation) across species. As a consequence, antibodies made against a particular hormone may not recognize that material from another species. Finally, while steroid hormones are structurally identical across species (cortisol in a dog is identical to the human form), substances present in the serum of a given species can sometimes interfere in an assay, leading to inaccurate results. Overall, it is important that a laboratory providing measurement of a particular hormone in a species demonstrate that the assay is valid in that species and that the laboratory has established normal ranges.

REGULATION OF ENDOCRINE SYSTEMS

Secretion of hormones is regulated by a system of sensing elements possessing the means to detect need for both increased and decreased secretion. The particular sensing network, feedback elements, and network of control responses are unique for each hormone. Hormonal pathways maintain homeostasis, and adjustments in secretion usually result in changes that will help maintain the status quo. In addition, secretion and activity of a particular hormone may be adjusted upward or downward in response to challenges such as chronic stress, disease, or alteration in nutritional status. The concept of negative feedback and its relationship to control of hormonal pathways is important in understanding pathway regulation and evaluation of endocrine function tests. For example, insulin is released in response to an increase in glucose concentration bathing the β-cells in the pancreatic islets of Langerhans. One of insulin's actions is to lower glucose concentrations in extracellular fluid by enhancing its uptake in target tissues. This decline in glucose leads to reductions in insulin secretion. In patients suspected of having an insulin-secreting tumor, the finding of a low blood glucose concentration (hypoglycemia) together with an elevated insulin concentration demonstrates inappropriate feedback, characteristic of such a tumor. In another example, patients showing elevated blood calcium concentrations should have low levels of PTH in circulation. Measurement of high PTH levels in such patients indicates a malfunction at the level of the parathyroid, most often associated with parathyroid adenoma.

Secretory patterns of hormones vary tremendously. The thyroid hormones tend to have less variability than the steroid hormones and show only moderate daily or weekly variation. In contrast, blood levels of the adrenal steroid cortisol show much more fluctuation with occasional bursts of secretion followed by periods of low activity (low blood levels) occurring throughout the day.

PATHOGENESIS OF ENDOCRINE DISEASE

Endocrine diseases can arise from many possible causes. Hormones can be over- or underproduced, receptors can malfunction, and normal pathways for hormone removal may be disrupted. Clinical signs consistent with malfunction in an endocrine tissue may develop because of a problem originating in the source of the hormone itself or may be due to disruption in another location that is secondarily affecting hormone secretion or action.

In veterinary medicine, the most common types of endocrine disease are hormonal overproduction associated with either a tumor or hyperplastic tissue manufacturing excessive amounts of hormone, and hormonal deficiency due to destruction of the endocrine tissue source. Common diseases associated with hormonal overproduction are hyperthyroidism in cats and hyperadrenocorticism (Cushing's disease) in dogs. Often the abnormal endocrine tissue not only overproduces hormone, it also fails to respond normally to feedback signals, contributing to inappropriate release of hormone. Hormonal overproduction from an endocrine tissue can also result from stimulation arising from a secondary source; eg, renal disease can result in parathyroid hyperplasia and oversecretion of PTH. Hyperphosphatemia occurs as a consequence of some types of renal disease. This leads to decreased formation of the active form of vitamin D, 1,25-dihydroxycholecalciferol (calcitriol). In turn, low calcitriol concentrations contribute to low calcium levels in extracellular fluid, which act as a stimulus for PTH secretion. Nonendocrine tissues can produce and secrete hormones in sufficient amounts to cause clinical signs; eg, certain tumors (apocrine gland tumors of the anal sac in dogs, lymphoma) can manufacture PTH-related protein that can mimic PTH action, resulting in hypercalcemia.

Syndromes associated with deficient or absent hormone secretion also have multiple causes. Endocrine tissue destruction secondary to cell-mediated autoimmune attack is often believed to be the cause. Examples of endocrine hypofunction resulting from primary tissue loss include canine hypothyroidism, type 1 diabetes mellitus, primary hypoparathyroidism, and primary hypoadrenocorticism. In early stages of tissue loss, compensatory mechanisms involving feedback pathways stimulate activity (hormone production) from the remaining tissue. For example, in primary hypoadrenocorticism (Addison's disease), secretion of pituitary ACTH increases as the adrenal cortex disappears. The increased trophic support results in full activation of the remaining tissue and often provides sufficient hormone secretion to delay signs of deficiency until tissue loss simply eliminates the hormonal source. Disorders resulting in clinical signs of endocrine hypoactivity may also occur due to disruption in tissues distant from the hormone source. Secondary hypothyroidism results from pituitary thyroid-stimulating hormone insufficiency that reduces the stimulus needed at the thyroid for T_4 and T_3 production and secretion. Patients receiving glucocorticoid therapy may experience atrophy of the cortisol-producing zones in the adrenal cortex. The exogenous steroid initiates negative feedback on the pituitary gland, suppressing ACTH secretion and leading to adrenal cortical atrophy. Another potential cause for endocrine hypofunction relates to tissue loss secondary to compressive and/or destructive growth of nonfunctional tumors.

Endocrine disease and related maladies also result from alterations in tissue responsiveness to hormones. An important example is type 2 or non-insulin-dependent diabetes mellitus, in which relative insensitivity to insulin is observed, often associated with obesity. Nephrogenic diabetes insipidus is due to renal insensitivity to the actions of vasopressin (antidiuretic hormone). The renal insensitivity to vasopressin in this syndrome may relate to congenital abnormalities in the vasopressin receptor but more often is secondary to other diseases (eg, pyometra, hyperadrenocorticism) or abnormalities in ion concentrations (eg, hypokalemia, hypercalcemia).

PRINCIPLES OF THERAPY

Endocrine diseases involving hyperactivity may be treated surgically (tumor removal), by radiotherapy (eg, ^{131}I for hyperthyroidism), or medically (eg, methimazole as an antithyroid drug). Syndromes of hormone deficiency are often successfully managed by simply replacing the missing hormone(s), such as insulin treatment of diabetes mellitus or thyroid hormone replacement therapy in hypothyroidism. Replacement therapy for deficiencies related to protein/polypeptide hormones can present a challenge. Often the species-specific version of the hormone is not available, the drug may need to be injected several times per day, and the possibility of antibody formation and anaphylaxis must be considered. Steroid and thyroid hormones can usually be administered orally. Some protein/polypeptide hormones or analogs are effective when given by routes other than injection (eg, the antidiuretic hormone analog desmopressin acetate is effective when administered by a variety of routes).

Hormonal replacement therapy should be monitored by assessment of clinical response and other suitable measures such as therapeutic blood monitoring (eg, post-pill measurement of T_4 concentrations, measurement of sodium and potassium in serum in patients with primary hypoadrenocorticism). Replacement therapy is often required for a time following surgical removal of an endocrine tumor. However, remaining normal tissue that was atrophied as a consequence of the disease often recovers activity in a fairly short period of time, obviating need for lifelong replacement therapy. Animals show significant variation in drug bioavailability; thus, a proper dosing schedule should be tailored to each patient.

Glucocorticoids are commonly used therapeutic drugs, particularly because of their anti-inflammatory and anti-allergic activity. Proper use requires an understanding of the side effects, including the potential appearance of signs of hyperadrenocorticism resulting from longterm therapy or from use of potent derivatives. Such adverse effects can be minimized by use of orally administered glucocorticoids given on alternate days.

THE ADRENAL GLANDS

The adrenal glands of mammals are located near the cranial pole of the kidneys. They consist of 2 distinct parts, the outer cortex and inner medulla, that differ in morphology, function, and origin.

ADRENAL CORTEX

The adrenal cortex is subdivided into 3 layers or zones, although the demarcation between zones often is indistinct. The zona glomerulosa (multiformis), the outer zone, is responsible for the secretion of mineralocorticoid hormones. The zona fasciculata, the middle zone, comprises ~70% of the cortex and is composed of cells that contain abundant cytoplasmic lipid and the glucocorticoid hormones. The zona reticularis, the inner zone, is responsible for the secretion of sex steroids.

Mineralocorticoids, of which the most potent naturally occurring one is aldosterone, are adrenal steroids that have their principal effects on ion transport by epithelial cells, resulting in a loss of potassium and retention of sodium. Sweat glands and the electrolyte "pumps" in epithelial cells of the renal tubule respond similarly. In the distal convoluted tubule of the mammalian nephron, a cation-exchange mechanism resorbs sodium from the glomerular filtrate and secretes potassium into the lumen. These reactions are accelerated by mineralocorticoids and proceed more slowly in their absence. A lack of secretion of mineralocorticoids (Addison's disease) may result in a lethal retention of potassium and loss of sodium.

Cortisol and lesser amounts of corticosterone are the most important glucocorticoid hormones secreted by the adrenal gland in many species. In general, the actions of glucocorticoids on carbohydrate, protein, and lipid metabolism result in sparing of glucose and a tendency to hyperglycemia and increased glucose production. In addition, they decrease lipogenesis and increase lipolysis in adipose tissue, which results in release of glycerol and free fatty acids.

Glucocorticoids also suppress inflammatory and immunologic responses, thereby attenuating associated tissue destruction and fibroplasia. However, high levels of glucocorticoids reduce resistance to bacteria, viruses, and fungi, which favors the spread of infection. Glucocorticoids may impair the immunologic response at any stage from the initial interaction and processing of antigens by cells of the reticuloendothelial system, through the induction and proliferation of immunocompetent lymphocytes and subsequent antibody production. Inhibition of a number of lymphocyte functions forms part of the basis for immunosuppression.

Glucocorticoids can have a profound negative effect on wound healing. High therapeutic levels of adrenal corticosteroids or the syndrome of hyperadrenocorticism may cause wound dehiscence after surgery. The inhibition of fibroblast proliferation and collagen synthesis leads to a decrease in scar tissue formation.

Progesterone, estrogens, and androgens are adrenal sex hormones. Excess secretion may be associated with a neoplasm of the zona reticularis. The manifestation of virilism, precocious sexual development, or feminization depends on which steroid is secreted in excess, sex of the individual, and age of onset.

HYPERADRENOCORTICISM
(Cushing's disease)

Hyperadrenocorticism may be the most frequent endocrinopathy in adult to aged dogs but is infrequent in other domestic animals. The clinical signs and lesions result primarily from chronic excess of cortisol. Increased cortisol levels in dogs may result from one of several mechanisms. The most common is an adenoma or hyperplasia of the adrenocorticotropic hormone (ACTH)-containing cells of the pituitary gland (pars distalis or pars intermedia), which results in bilateral adrenal cortical hypertrophy and hyperplasia. This form of the disease is referred to as pituitary-dependent hyperadrenocorticism (Cushing's disease) and occurs in ~90% of cases. Functional adrenal tumors, a far less frequent cause of hyperadrenocorticism in dogs, may secrete cortisol or sex steroids resulting in a variety of clinical signs. Many of the signs and lesions of naturally occurring hyperadrenocorticism can be induced by longterm, daily administration of large doses of corticosteroids. Dogs develop a spectrum of clinical signs and laboratory abnormalities as a result of the combined gluconeogenic, lipolytic, protein catabolic, and anti-inflammatory effects of the glucocorticoid hormones on many organ systems. The disease is insidious and slowly progressive. (See THE PITUITARY GLAND, p 451, for discussion of the clinical signs, laboratory abnormalities, diagnosis, and treatment of hyperadrenocorticism.)

HYPOADRENOCORTICISM
(Addison's disease)

A deficiency in adrenocortical hormones is seen most commonly in young to middle-aged dogs and occasionally in horses. The disease may be familial in Standard Poodles, Bearded Collies, and Portuguese Water Dogs. The cause of primary adrenocortical failure usually is not known, although most cases probably result from an autoimmune process. Other causes include destruction of the adrenal gland by granulomatous disease, metastatic tumor, hemorrhage, infarction, or overdose of mitotane (o,p'-DDD).

Clinical Findings: Many of the functional disturbances of chronic adrenal insufficiency are not highly specific; they include recurrent episodes of gastroenteritis, a slowly progressive loss of body condition, and failure to respond appropriately to stress. Although hypoadrenocorticism occurs in dogs of any breed, sex, or age, idiopathic adrenocortical insufficiency is most common in young female adult dogs. This may be related to its suspected immune-mediated pathogenesis.

A reduction in secretion of aldosterone, the principal mineralocorticoid, results in marked alterations of serum levels of potassium, sodium, and chloride. Potassium excretion by the kidneys is reduced and results in a progressive rise in serum potassium levels. Hyponatremia and hypochloremia result from renal tubular loss. Severe hyperkalemia may result in bradycardia and an irregular heart rate with alterations in the ECG. Some dogs develop a pronounced bradycardia (heart rate ≤50 bpm) that predisposes to weakness or circulatory collapse after minimal exertion.

Although the development of clinical signs is often inapparent, acute circulatory collapse and evidence of renal failure frequently occur. A progressive decrease in blood volume contributes to hypotension, weakness, and microcardia. Increased excretion of water by the kidneys, due to decreased reabsorption of sodium and chloride, results in progressive dehydration and hemoconcentration. Emesis, diarrhea, and anorexia are common and contribute to the animal's deterioration. Weight loss is frequently severe. Similar clinical signs are seen in cats with hypoadrenocorticism.

Decreased production of glucocorticoids results in several characteristic functional disturbances. Decreased gluconeogenesis and increased sensitivity to insulin contribute to the development of moderate hypoglycemia. In some dogs, hyperpigmentation of the skin occurs due to the lack of negative feedback on the pituitary gland and increased ACTH release. Atypical Addison's disease has been reported in dogs and is associated with hypocortisolemia with normal electrolytes. Clinical signs are similar to those seen in dogs with both glucocorticoid and mineralocorticoid insufficiency.

Lesions: The most common lesion in dogs is bilateral idiopathic adrenocortical atrophy, in which all layers of the cortex are markedly reduced in thickness. The adrenal cortex is reduced to one-tenth or less of its normal thickness and consists primarily of the adrenal capsule. The adrenal medulla is relatively more prominent and, with the capsule, makes up the bulk of the remaining adrenal glands.

All 3 zones of the adrenal cortex are involved, including the zona glomerulosa which is not under ACTH control; however, no obvious pituitary lesions have been seen in dogs with idiopathic adrenal cortical atrophy.

A destructive pituitary lesion that decreases ACTH secretion is characterized by severe atrophy of the inner 2 cortical zones of the adrenal gland; the zona glomerulosa remains intact.

Diagnosis: A presumptive diagnosis is based on the history and supportive (although not specific) laboratory abnormalities, including hyponatremia, hyperkalemia, a sodium:potassium ratio of <25:1, azotemia, mild acidosis, and a normocytic, normochromic anemia. Severe GI blood loss has also been reported. Occasionally, mild hypoglycemia is present. The hyperkalemia results in ECG changes: an elevation (spiking) of the T wave, a flattening or absence of the P wave, a prolonged PR interval, and a widening of the QRS complex. Ventricular fibrillation or asystole may occur with potassium levels >11 mEq/L.

Differential diagnoses include primary GI disease (especially whipworm infection), renal failure, acute pancreatitis, and toxin ingestion. For definitive diagnosis, evaluation of adrenal function is required. After obtaining a baseline blood sample, ACTH (gel or synthetic) is administered IM and a second blood sample obtained 1-2 hr later. Affected dogs have low baseline cortisol levels, and there is little response to ACTH administration in classic and atypical cases. This test can be completed in most animals before replacement hormone therapy is started.

Treatment: An adrenal crisis is an acute medical emergency. An IV catheter should be inserted and a 0.9% saline infusion begun. If the dog is hypoglycemic, the saline can include 5% dextrose. The hypovolemia is corrected rapidly by administering 0.9% saline (60-70 mL/kg over the first 1-2 hr). Urine output should be assessed to determine whether the dog is anuric. Fluids should be continued, at a rate appropriate to match ongoing losses, until the clinical signs and laboratory abnormalities have resolved.

Prednisolone sodium succinate (22-30 mg/kg) or dexamethasone sodium phosphate (2.2-4.4 mg/kg) may be used in the initial management of shock. Dexamethasone will not interfere with cortisol measurements during the ACTH stimulation test. Prednisolone or prednisone should be given at 1 mg/kg, BID, for the first few days of therapy and then at 0.25-0.5 mg/kg/day. Mineralocorticoid replacement therapy (see below) is also begun to help with electrolyte imbalances and hypovolemia. Electrolytes, renal function, and glucose should be monitored regularly to assess response to therapy.

In cases of severe, nonresponsive hyperkalemia, 10% glucose (4.4-11 mL/kg) in 0.9% saline can be given over 30-60 min to increase potassium movement into the cells. Regular insulin (0.28-1.1 U/kg) administered IM will enhance glucose and potassium uptake, but 10% glucose (20 mL per unit of insulin) should be administered IV concurrently to avoid hypoglycemia.

For longterm maintenance therapy, the mineralocorticoid fludrocortisone acetate is administered PO at 10-30 µg/kg/day. Serum electrolytes should be monitored weekly until the proper dose is determined. Alternatively, desoxycorticosterone pivalate may be administered at 2.2 mg/kg, IM or SC, every 25-28 days. Electrolytes should be measured at 3 and 4 wk after the first few injections to determine the duration of action. Sodium may be added to the diet (1-5 g/day) if hyponatremia persists despite normal serum potassium concentration. Some dogs also require daily oral glucocorticoid therapy to adequately control clinical signs. Replacement doses of prednisone (0.2-0.4 mg/kg/day) are required in ~50% of dogs. Additional glucocorticoid supplementation may be required (2-10 times maintenance) during times of illness or stress. Dogs with atypical Addison's disease only require replacement doses of prednisone, although it is recommended that electrolytes be monitored every 3 mo for the first year after diagnosis. Dogs with chronic hypoadrenocorticism should be reexamined every 3-6 mo.

Treatment of horses with hypoadrenocorticism is similar—aggressive replacement of fluids, steroids, and glucose if needed in an adrenal crisis. Supportive therapy and rest are indicated in cases of chronic Addison's disease.

ADRENAL MEDULLA

The adrenal medulla, although apparently not essential to life, plays an important role in response to stress or hypoglycemia. It secretes epinephrine and norepinephrine, which increase cardiac output, blood pressure, and blood glucose, and decrease GI activity.

Pheochromocytomas may develop in domestic animals, most often in cattle and dogs. These secrete epinephrine, norepinephrine, or both. Clinical signs are often absent, and tumors may be incidental findings during the workup for other conditions or at necropsy. In some dogs, clinical signs may include polyuria, polydipsia, tachycardia, restlessness, abdominal distention, and collapse. Due to the lack of routine availability of validated assays for catecholamines in dogs and cats, the diagnosis is often made on the basis of clinical signs and ultrasound. Treatment involves surgery (if feasible) and management of hypertension. Other adrenal tumors, such as neuroblastomas and ganglioneuromas, may arise in the chromaffin cells of the sympathetic nervous system.

THE PANCREAS

The endocrine function of the pancreas is performed by small groups of cells, the islets of Langerhans, that are completely surrounded by acinar (exocrine) cells that produce digestive enzymes. The endocrine and exocrine portions of the pancreas are closely related during development, and evidence suggests that islet, acinar, and ductal cells arise from a common multipotential precursor cell.

Pancreatic islets contain α, β, and δ cells, each of which synthesize a unique polypeptide hormone. β cells account for 60-70% of the islet-cell population and secrete insulin, α cells secrete glucagon, and δ cells secrete somatostatin.

The pancreatic islets function as discrete microendocrine organs. They are distributed throughout the pancreas with a characteristic pattern of cellular interrelationships to assure an appropriate balance of hormones. Afferent vessels and nerves enter the islet in the peripheral tricellular region. The close anatomic relationship of α, β, and δ cells in this heterogeneous cortical region allow it to function as a local glucose sensor, permitting a coordinated output of insulin and glucagon in response to fluctuations in blood glucose. Specialized tight junctions between membranes of adjacent endocrine cells tend to partition the intercellular space and may permit somatostatin to exert a direct local (paracrine) inhibitory effect on glucagon and insulin release.

Insulin is formed initially as a single polypeptide chain of 81-86 amino acid residues. This prohormone (proinsulin) contains the A and B chains of the insulin molecule, plus a connecting peptide. Proinsulin is converted enzymatically to insulin before storage in membrane-limited secretory granules.

The major physiologic stimulus for the release of insulin from β cells is an increase in the concentration of glucose in the extracellular fluid. Specific glucoreceptors that bind with glucose exist on the plasma membrane of β cells. An appropriate level of extracellular calcium is required for insulin secretion. In certain hypocalcemic disorders (eg, parturient hypocalcemia in cows), insulin secretion may be inhibited due to the low extracellular fluid calcium concentration, resulting in hyperglycemia. Other sugars (fructose, mannose, ribose), amino acids (leucine, arginine), hormones (glucagon, secretin), drugs (sulfonylurea, theophylline), short-chain fatty acids, and ketone bodies may also stimulate insulin secretion under certain conditions. Pancreatic β cells are able to respond to a specific physiologic stimulus with release of stored hormone in a modulated fashion, rather than releasing all of the stored hormone at once.

Insulin affects, either directly or indirectly, the function of every organ in the body. Tissues that are especially responsive to insulin include skeletal and cardiac muscle, adipose tissue, fibroblasts, liver, WBC, mammary glands, cartilage, bone, skin, aorta, pituitary gland, and peripheral nerves. The main function of insulin is to stimulate anabolic reactions involving carbohydrates, fats, proteins, and nucleic acids. Liver, adipose cells, and muscle are 3 principal target sites for insulin. Insulin catalyzes the formation of macromolecules used in cell structure and energy stores, and it regulates many cell functions. In general, insulin increases the transfer of glucose and certain other monosaccharides, some amino acids and fatty acids, and potassium and magnesium ions across the plasma membrane of target cells. It also decreases the rate of lipolysis, proteolysis, ketogenesis, and gluconeogenesis.

Glucagon is secreted in response to a reduction in blood glucose. It promotes mobilization of stores of energy-yielding nutrients by increasing glycogenolysis, gluconeogenesis, and lipolysis. At physiologic concentrations, glucagon increases both hepatic glycogenolysis and gluconeogenesis, thereby increasing blood glucose.

Insulin and glucagon act in concert to maintain the concentration of glucose in extracellular fluids within relatively narrow limits. A glucose sensor in the pancreatic islets controls the relative amounts of insulin and glucagon secreted. Glucagon controls glucose release from the liver into the extracellular space, and insulin controls glucose transport from the extracellular space into insulin-sensitive tissues such as fat, muscle, and liver.

DIABETES MELLITUS

Diabetes mellitus is a chronic disorder of carbohydrate metabolism due to relative or absolute insulin deficiency. Most cases of spontaneous diabetes occur in middle-aged dogs and cats. In dogs, females are affected twice as often as males, and incidence appears to be increased in certain small breeds such as Miniature Poodles, Dachshunds, Schnauzers, Cairn Terriers, and Beagles, but any breed can be affected. In one study, male cats were more commonly affected than females; no breed predilection is seen in cats.

Etiology and Pathogenesis: The pathogenic mechanisms responsible for decreased insulin production and secretion are multiple, but usually they are related to destruction of islet cells, secondary to either immune destruction or severe pancreatitis (dogs) or amyloidosis (cats). Chronic relapsing pancreatitis with progressive loss of both exocrine and endocrine cells and their replacement by fibrous connective tissue results in diabetes mellitus. The pancreas becomes firm and multinodular and often contains scattered areas of hemorrhage and necrosis. Later in the course of disease, a thin, fibrous band of tissue near the duodenum and stomach may be all that remains of the pancreas. Selective infiltration of islets with amyloid, glycogen, and collagen with destruction of islet cells are less frequent causes of diabetes mellitus in dogs than in cats. In other cases, the numbers of β cells are decreased, and the cells become vacuolated; in chronic cases, the islets are difficult to find. Insulin resistance and secondary diabetes mellitus are also seen in many dogs with hyperadrenocorticism, and chronic administration of glucocorticoids or progestins can predispose to diabetes mellitus. In dogs, but not cats, progesterone leads to release of growth hormone, resulting in hyperglycemia and insulin resistance. Obesity also predisposes to insulin resistance in both dogs and cats.

Complete expression of the complex metabolic disturbances in diabetes mellitus appears to be the result of a bihormonal abnormality. Although a relative or absolute deficiency of insulin action in response to a rising extracellular glucose concentration has long been recognized as the major hormonal abnormality, the importance of an absolute or relative increase of glucagon secretion has been appreciated more recently. Hyperglucagonemia in diabetes may be the result of increased secretion of pancreatic glucagon, enteroglucagon, or both. Increased glucagon appears to contribute to development of severe hyperglycemia by mobilizing hepatic stores of glucose and to development of ketoacidosis by increasing the oxidation of fatty acids in the liver.

Cats with diabetes mellitus usually have specific degenerative lesions localized selectively in the islets of Langerhans, whereas the remainder of the pancreas appears to be normal. The selective deposition of amyloid in islets, with degenerative changes in β cells, is the most common pancreatic lesion in many cats with diabetes. The amyloid appears to arise from islet-associated polypeptide (IAPP), which is secreted together with insulin from the β cells. Cats seem unable to process IAPP normally, which leads to excessive accumulation and conversion into amyloid. As cats age, a greater percentage of their islets contain amyloid. Cats with diabetes have a greater percentage of their islets affected with larger amounts of amyloid than age-matched cats without diabetes. The amyloid or IAPP (or both) lead to both physical disruption of the β cell and insulin resistance, resulting in diabetes.

Infection with certain viruses in humans may cause selective islet damage or pancreatitis and has been suggested to be responsible for certain cases of rapidly developing diabetes mellitus. This has yet to be documented in dogs or cats. The selective degeneration and necrosis of β cells is accompanied by infiltration of the islets by lymphocytes and macrophages. Stress, obesity, and administration of corticosteroids or progestogens may increase the severity of clinical signs.

Clinical Findings: The onset of diabetes is often insidious, and the clinical course chronic. Common signs in dogs include polydipsia, polyuria, polyphagia with weight loss, bilateral cataracts, and weakness. The disturbances in water metabolism develop primarily due to an osmotic diuresis. The renal threshold for glucose is ~180 mg/dL in dogs and ~240 mg/dL in cats.

Diabetic animals have decreased resistance to bacterial and fungal infections and often develop chronic or recurrent infections such as cystitis, prostatitis, bronchopneumonia, and dermatitis. This increased susceptibility to infection may be related in part to impaired chemotactic, phagocytic, and antimicrobial activity associated with decreased neutrophil function. Radiographic evidence of emphysematous cystitis (rare) is suggestive of diabetes mellitus because of infections with glucose-fermenting organisms such as *Proteus* sp, *Aerobacter aerogenes*, and *Escherichia coli*, which result in gas formation in the wall and lumen of the bladder. Emphysema also may develop in the wall of the gallbladder in diabetic dogs.

Hepatomegaly due to lipid accumulation is common in diabetic dogs and cats. The fatty liver results from increased fat mobilization from adipose tissue. Individual liver cells are greatly enlarged by the accumulation of multiple droplets of neutral lipid. In cats, hepatic lipidosis may occur in conjunction with diabetes mellitus.

Cataracts develop frequently in dogs (not cats) with poorly controlled diabetes mellitus. The lenticular opacities appear initially along the suture lines of lens fibers and are stellate ("asteroid") in shape. Cataract formation in dogs is related to the unique sorbitol pathway by which glucose is metabolized in the lens, which leads to edema of the lens and disruption of normal light transmission. Other extrapancreatic lesions associated with diabetes mellitus in humans, such as nephropathy, retinopathy, and micro- and macrovascular angiopathy, are rare in dogs and cats.

Diagnosis: A diagnosis of diabetes mellitus is based on persistent fasting hyperglycemia and glycosuria. The normal fasting value for blood glucose in dogs and cats is 75-120 mg/dL. In cats, stress-induced hyperglycemia is a frequent problem, and multiple blood and urine samples may be required to confirm the diagnosis. Measurement of serum glycosylated hemoglobin or fructosamine (or both) can assist in differentiating between stress-induced hyperglycemia and diabetes mellitus. In all cases, a search should be made for drugs or diseases that predispose to diabetes.

Treatment: Longterm success depends on the understanding and cooperation of the owner. Treatment involves a combination of weight reduction, diet, insulin, and possibly oral hypoglycemics. Intact females should be neutered. In cats, recent evidence has supported the use of high protein, low carbohydrate diets (canned kitten foods). In dogs, diets that are high in fiber and complex carbohydrates are preferred. Diet and weight reduction alone will not control the disease, so initial therapy with insulin is required. Most dogs require 2 doses of insulin a day. In general NPH or lente is the initial insulin of choice at a dose of 0.5 U/kg BID. With twice daily injections, 2 meals of equal calories are given at the time of insulin administration. Diets high in simple sugars (semimoist foods) should be avoided. Clinical signs and serial blood glucose determinations are used to monitor therapy after initial stabilization at home for 5-7 days. In cats, high protein diets along with insulin therapy or oral hypoglycemics are initiated and the pet re-evaluated in 5-7 days. NPH, lente, or PZI insulin is preferred in cats. Initial starting doses range from 1-3 units BID.

The use of oral hypoglycemic agents (glipizide) has been evaluated in diabetic cats. Glipizide is a sulfonylurea that stimulates the release of insulin from functional β cells. Glipizide should not be used in thin or ketonuric cats when absolute insulin deficiency is likely and exogenous insulin administration is required. Glipizide is administered at an initial dose of 2.5 mg, BID, PO, in conjunction with dietary management. Clinical response is seen at 3-4 wk. Short-term success is seen in 50% of treated cats with longterm success rates (>1 yr) of ~15%. Alternatively, glimepiride (another sulfonylurea) may be administered to cats at 2 mg once a day. Acarbose, an oral α-glucosidase inhibitor, has also been used in cats at a dosage of 12.5-25 mg, BID-TID, in conjunction with diet and/or insulin to control hyperglycemia.

Ketoacidosis is a serious complication of diabetes mellitus and should be regarded as a medical emergency. Therapy includes correcting dehydration by administration of IV fluids, such as 0.9% NaCl or lactated Ringer's solution; reducing hyperglycemia and ketosis by administration of crystalline zinc (regular) insulin; maintaining serum electrolyte levels, especially potassium, through supplemental administration of appropriate electrolyte solutions; and identifying and treating underlying and complicating diseases, such as acute pancreatitis or infections.

Numerous insulin regimens have been used in treatment of ketoacidotic diabetes mellitus. In the intermittent insulin regimen, regular insulin at 0.2 U/kg IM is the initial dose, followed by hourly administration of 0.1 U/kg. Once the serum glucose is <250 mg/dL, the insulin is administered SC at 0.25-0.5 U/kg, every 4-6 hr, with careful monitoring of the serum glucose at 1- to 2-hr intervals. During aggressive treatment with insulin, blood glucose levels may fall rapidly, and the addition of 2.5-5% dextrose to the IV fluids may be required.

When insulin therapy has been instituted, the blood glucose should be checked frequently until an adequate maintenance dose has been determined. Once the animal is on maintenance therapy and its condition is stable, it should be reassessed every 4-6 mo.

FUNCTIONAL ISLET CELL TUMORS

The most frequent pancreatic islet tumor is an islet cell carcinoma derived from insulin-secreting β cells. These neoplasms frequently are hormonally active and secrete excessive amounts of insulin, which causes hypoglycemia. Endocrine pancreatic tissue appears to be derived from multipotential ductal epithelial cells, which differentiate into one of the several cell types present within the islets. Gastrin, somatostatin, pancreatic polypeptide, and vasoactive intestinal peptide may also be produced in excess in islet cell tumors. β-cell neoplasms of the pancreatic islets (insulinomas) are seen most frequently in dogs 5-12 yr old. They have also been less frequently reported in cats and in older cattle.

Clinical Findings: The clinical signs seen with insulinomas result from excessive insulin secretion, which leads to an increased rate of transfer of glucose from the extracellular fluid to body tissues, and thus to severe hypoglycemia. The clinical signs are a reflection of the hypoglycemia and are not specific for hyperinsulinism associated with β-cell neoplasms. Initial signs include posterior weakness, fatigue after exercise, generalized muscular twitching and weakness, ataxia, mental confusion, and changes of temperament. Dogs are easily agitated, and there are intermittent periods of excitability and restlessness. Periodic seizures may occur, and episodes of collapse resembling syncope have also been reported.

Clinical signs are characteristically episodic and occur initially at widely spaced intervals but become more frequent and prolonged as the disease progresses. Hypoglycemic attacks may be precipitated by physical exercise (increased use of glucose) or fasting (decreased availability of glucose), as well as by ingestion of food (stimulation of insulin release). Administration of glucose rapidly alleviates the signs.

The predominance of clinical signs relating to the CNS demonstrates the primary dependence of the brain on the metabolism of glucose for energy. When the brain is not supplied with glucose, cerebral oxidation decreases and manifestations of anoxia appear. Because clinical signs are compatible with primary disease of the CNS, functional islet cell tumors may be misdiagnosed as idiopathic epilepsy, brain tumors, or other organic neurologic disease. Repeated episodes of prolonged and severe hypoglycemia may result in irreversible neuronal degeneration throughout the brain. Permanent neurologic disability probably accounts for the terminal coma, unresponsiveness to glucose, and eventual death of some dogs.

Lesions: Insulinomas usually appear as single, yellow to dark red, spherical, small (1-3 cm) nodules visible from the serosal surface. They occur singly or occasionally as multiple nodules in the same or different lobes of the pancreas. They are of similar consistency to or slightly firmer than the surrounding pancreatic parenchyma. A thin layer of fibrous connective tissue separates the neoplasm from the adjacent parenchyma. Insulinomas frequently metastasize to regional lymph nodes or the liver (or both) before diagnosis. True benign adenomas of islet cells are rare.

Diagnosis: A blood glucose determination should be done on all older dogs with a history of periodic weakness, collapse, or seizures. Fasting hypoglycemia (≤60 mg/dL) in a middle-aged to older dog is strong support for an insulinoma. Serum insulin concentrations taken at the time of hypoglycemia are normal to increased in animals with an insulinoma. Differential diagnoses for hypoglycemia include hypoadrenocorticism, hepatic failure, large extrapancreatic neoplasms, sepsis, polycythemia, insulin overdosage, and laboratory error.

Treatment: Although insulinomas are usually solitary in dogs, the entire pancreas should be examined carefully for multiple tumors. Complete excision of the tumor ameliorates the hypoglycemia and associated neurologic signs, unless there have been irreversible changes in the CNS. If there are nonvisible metastases, hypoglycemia may persist after surgery. Even though the potential for malignancy of insulinomas is high, many dogs live >1 yr with acceptable quality of life if all visible tumors are debulked at surgery. Dogs with inoperable tumors may be managed fairly well with multiple feedings/day and glucocorticoid administration (0.5-1 mg/kg/day). Diazoxide (20-80 mg/kg/day, TID) may also alleviate clinical signs in some dogs, though problems with availability have limited its use. The chemotherapeutic agent, streptozotocin, has recently been investigated for the treatment of islet cell tumors in dogs and may be considered following surgical resection.

GASTRIN-SECRETING ISLET CELL TUMORS

Gastrinomas of the pancreas have been reported in humans, dogs, and a cat. Hypersecretion of gastrin in humans results in the Zollinger-Ellison syndrome, consisting of hypersecretion of gastric acid and recurrent peptic ulceration in the GI tract. The tumors, derived from ectopic amine precursor uptake decarboxylase (APUD) cells in the pancreas, produce an excess of the hormone gastrin, which normally is secreted by cells of the antral and duodenal mucosa.

Clinical Findings: These tumors are rare; they occur less frequently than the insulin-secreting β-cell neoplasms. The few documented cases have had anorexia, hematemesis, intermittent diarrhea (usually with dark blood present), progressive weight loss, and dehydration. The prominent functional disturbances appear to result from multiple ulcerations of the GI mucosa that develop from gastrin hypersecretion.

Lesions: Animals studied with the Zollinger-Ellison syndrome have had single or multiple tumors of varying size in the pancreas. The tumors were firm on palpation due to an increase of fibrous connective tissue in the stroma, and all had evidence of metastasis before diagnosis.

Diagnosis: Serum gastrin levels have been evaluated in a limited number of dogs with gastrinomas. Gastrin levels in a dog with a Zollinger-Ellison-like syndrome varied from 155-2780 pg/mL, whereas the mean serum gastrin in clinically normal (control) dogs was 70.9 pg/mL. Recurrent gastric or duodenal ulcers in dogs with no identified cause warrants exploratory surgery and careful inspection of the pancreas.

Treatment: Excision of the gastrin-secreting mass in the pancreas can be attempted. However, all such tumors that have been studied in dogs have had evidence of local invasion into adjacent parenchyma and had metastasized to regional lymph nodes and liver. The dogs had either single or multiple ulcerations in the gastric or duodenal mucosa associated with free blood in the lumen. Medical management with H_2-receptor antagonists (famotidine or ranitidine) or the proton-pump inhibitor omeprazole may temporarily alleviate clinical signs in animals with inoperable disease.

THE PARATHYROID GLANDS AND DISORDERS OF CALCIUM METABOLISM

The physiology and disorders of calcium and phosphate metabolism, the function of vitamin D (which acts more like a hormone than a vitamin), and the formation of bone are all tied together in a common system along with 2 other regulatory hormones—parathyroid hormone (PTH) and calcitonin. Therefore, PTH, calcitonin, and vitamin D will be discussed in this chapter together with the associated disorders of calcium homeostasis.

Because aberrant calcium and phosphorus metabolism is reflected in the skeletal system, specific syndromes are presented in that section. (*See also* DYSTROPHIES ASSOCIATED WITH CALCIUM, PHOSPHORUS, AND VITAMIN D, p 852.)

CALCIUM-REGULATING HORMONES

The concentration of calcium in the blood of mammals is ~10 mg/dL, with some variation due to species (eg, up to 13 mg/dL is normal in horses and rabbits), age, dietary intake, and analytic method. The blood calcium is composed of protein-bound and diffusible fractions. Diffusible calcium consists of calcium complexed to anions, such as phosphate and citrate, plus biologically active free (ionic) calcium.

The calcium ion is an essential structural component of the skeleton and plays a key role in muscle contraction, blood coagulation, enzyme activity, neural excitability, secondary messengers, hormone release, and membrane permeability. Precise control of calcium ion in extracellular fluids is vital to health. Three major hormones (PTH, vitamin D, and calcitonin) interact to maintain a constant concentration of calcium, despite variations in intake and excretion. Other hormones, such as adrenal corticosteroids, estrogens, thyroxine, somatotropin, and glucagon, may also contribute to the maintenance of calcium homeostasis.

Parathyroid Hormone: PTH is synthesized and stored in the chief cells of the parathyroid glands. Synthesis is regulated by a feedback mechanism involving the level of blood calcium (and, to a lesser degree, magnesium). In addition, biological amines, peptides, steroids, and several classes of drugs can influence PTH secretion.

The primary function of PTH is to control calcium concentration in the extracellular fluid, which it does by affecting the rate of transfer of calcium into and out of bone, resorption in the kidneys, and absorption from the GI tract. The effect on the kidneys is the most rapid, causing reabsorption of calcium and excretion of phosphorus. The major initial effect on bone is to mobilize calcium from the bone to the extracellular fluid; later, bone formation may be enhanced. PTH does not directly affect calcium absorption from the gut. Its effect is mediated indirectly by regulation of synthesis of the active metabolite of vitamin D.

Vitamin D: The second major hormone involved in the regulation of calcium metabolism and skeletal remodeling is vitamin D, which includes cholecalciferol (vitamin D_3) of animal origin, as well as ergocalciferol (vitamin D_2) of plant origin. Vitamin D has long been considered an essential dietary ingredient, but in several species, including sheep, cattle, horses, pigs, and humans, vitamin D can be formed in the skin from a cholesterol metabolite (7-dehydrocholesterol) after exposure to ultraviolet light. In contrast, dogs and cats are not able to synthesize vitamin D_3 adequately in the skin and are mainly dependent on dietary intake.

Vitamin D must be metabolically activated before it can function physiologically. The biologic actions of vitamin D depend on hydroxylation in the liver and kidney to form the biologically active 1,25-dihydroxyvitamin D (calcitriol). This conversion in the kidneys is the rate-limiting step in vitamin D metabolism, and it is partly responsible for the delay between vitamin D administration and expression of its biologic effects. PTH and conditions that stimulate its secretion, as well as hypophosphatemia, increase the formation of the active vitamin D metabolite. High circulating phosphorus concentrations have the opposite effect. Under certain conditions, prolactin, estradiol, placental lactogen, and possibly somatotropin have a similar enhancing effect. Increased secretion of these hormones, either alone or in combination, appears to be important in the efficient adaptation to the major calcium demands of pregnancy, lactation, and growth.

Calcitonin: Calcitonin is a 32-amino acid polypeptide hormone secreted by the parafollicular cells (C-cells) of the thyroid gland in mammals and by ultimobranchial tissue in avian and other nonmammalian species. The concentration of calcium ion in extracellular fluids is the principal stimulus for the secretion of calcitonin by C-cells. In hypercalcemia, the rate of secretion of calcitonin is increased greatly by rapid discharge of stored hormone from C-cells into interfollicular capillaries. Hyperplasia of C-cells occurs in response to longterm hypercalcemia. When blood calcium is lowered, the stimulus for calcitonin secretion is diminished. The storage of large amounts of preformed hormone in C-cells and rapid release in response to a moderate rise in circulating calcium probably reflect the physiologic role of calcitonin as an "emergency" hormone to protect against development of hypercalcemia.

Calcitonin exerts its effects by interacting with target cells, primarily in bone and kidney. The actions of PTH and calcitonin are antagonistic on bone resorption but synergistic on decreasing the renal tubular reabsorption of phosphorus. The hypocalcemic effects of calcitonin are primarily the result of decreased entry of calcium from the skeleton into plasma, resulting from a temporary inhibition of PTH-stimulated bone resorption. The hypophosphatemia develops from a direct action of calcitonin, which increases the rate of movement of phosphorus out of plasma into soft tissue and bone and inhibits the bone resorption stimulated by PTH and other factors. Although many effects have been attributed to calcitonin at pharmacologic doses, their physiologic relevance is suspect. Physiologically, calcitonin has at best a minor role in regulating blood concentrations of calcium. Neither chronically high (eg, as in animals with medullary thyroid cancer) nor chronically low (eg, as in animals after surgical removal of the thyroid gland) circulating calcitonin concentrations result in any alterations in the serum calcium concentration.

HYPERCALCEMIA IN DOGS AND CATS

The development of clinical signs from hypercalcemia depends on the magnitude of the calcium elevation, how quickly it develops, and its duration. Serum total calcium concentrations of ≤15 mg/dL may not be associated with systemic signs, but serum concentrations of >18 mg/dL are often associated with severe, life-threatening signs. Polydipsia and polyuria are the most common signs of hypercalcemia and result from an impaired ability to concentrate urine and a direct stimulation of the thirst center. Anorexia, vomiting, and constipation can also develop as a result of decreased excitability of GI smooth muscle. Decreased neuromuscular excitability may lead to signs of generalized weakness, depression, muscle twitching, and seizures.

In dogs, hypercalcemia is most commonly associated with malignancy, hypoadrenocorticism (Addison's disease), and renal disease. Less common causes of hypercalcemia in dogs include primary hyperparathyroidism, vitamin D toxicosis, granulomatous disease, and miscellaneous conditions. In cats, renal failure, neoplasia, and a recently recognized syndrome of idiopathic hypercalcemia are the most common causes of hypercalcemia.

Hypercalcemia of Malignancy

Malignancy is the most common cause of persistent hypercalcemia in dogs and is a common cause in cats. In hypercalcemia of malignancy, the hypercalcemia primarily results from increased osteoclastic bone resorption, but increased renal tubular resorption and increased intestinal absorption may also play a role. Factors that may be produced by tumors and result in humoral hypercalcemia of malignancy include PTH, PTH-related protein, transforming growth factor, 1,25-dihydroxyvitamin D, prostaglandin E_2, osteoclast-activating factor, and other cytokines (interleukin-1, interleukin-2, and γ-interferon). Although many tumors have been associated with hypercalcemia in humans, in dogs malignancy-associated hypercalcemia has been most commonly linked to lymphoma, adenocarcinoma of the apocrine glands of the anal sac, and multiple myeloma. Other tumors (thymoma, squamous cell carcinoma, nasal carcinoma, hemangiosarcoma, and undifferentiated adenocarcinoma) have also been associated with hypercalcemia in dogs. In cats, humoral hypercalcemia of malignancy occurs less frequently than in dogs but has been reported with squamous cell carcinoma, multiple myeloma, and lymphoproliferative diseases.

Lymphoma (Lymphosarcoma):
The most common tumor associated with hypercalcemia in dogs, lymphoma is also one of the tumors associated with hypercalcemia in cats. The pathogenesis of the hypercalcemia may involve 2 general mechanisms. One is local elaboration of an osteolytic factor that induces resorption of bone and mobilization of calcium when the bone marrow is infiltrated by tumors cells. The other, probably more important, is humoral hypercalcemia in which neoplastic cells produce a humoral factor that acts at a distance from the tumor. As evidence for secretion of a humoral

substance by tumor cells, increased bone resorption, phosphaturia, and urinary excretion of cyclic adenosine monophosphate (cAMP) have been documented in dogs with lymphoma. Serum concentrations of both PTH and 1,25-dihydroxyvitamin D are generally low in these dogs, but a peptide related to PTH (PTH-related peptide) has been detected in dogs with lymphoma (TABLE 1).

Of dogs with lymphoma, 10-40% have concurrent hypercalcemia, and a large number of these cases also have the mediastinal form of lymphoma. Although detectable lymphadenopathy is usually present, hypercalcemia may be the first abnormality noted. A thorough physical examination, together with thoracic chest and abdominal radiographs, abdominal ultrasonography, multiple lymph node aspirates or biopsies, and multiple bone marrow aspirates may be necessary to make the diagnosis. Treatment with glucocorticoids (eg, prednisone) will lower the serum calcium concentrations; however, steroids are lympholytic and will make identification of lymphoma difficult. Although

TABLE 1. Characteristic Laboratory Abnormalities of Common Causes of Hypercalcemia

Diagnosis	Total Calcium	Ionized Calcium	Intact PTH	1,25-OH₂ Vitamin D	Phosphorus	PTH-related Protein
Primary hyperthyroidism	High	High	Normal to high	Low to normal	Normal to low	Negative
Malignant hypercalcemia	High	High	Low to low-normal	Low to normal	Normal to low	Positive (sometimes)
Hypoadrenocorticism (Addison's disease)	Low, normal, or high	Normal	Normal	Normal	Normal to high	Negative
Chronic renal failure	Low, normal, or high	Normal to low	Normal to high	Low to normal	High	Negative
Hypervitaminosis D (calcitriol or calcitriol analog)	High	High	Low to low-normal	Low to normal	Normal to high	Negative
Hypervitaminosis D (D₂ or D₃ toxicity)	High	High	Low to low-normal	High	Normal to high	Negative
Granulomatous disease	High	High	Low to low-normal	Low to normal	Normal to high	Negative
Idiopathic hypercalcemia of cats	High	High	Normal	Normal	Normal	Negative

remission rates in dogs with lymphoma and hypercalcemia are not statistically different from those without hypercalcemia, survival times are considerably less, indicating that hypercalcemic lymphomas have a poorer prognosis. (*See also* CANINE MALIGNANT LYMPHOMA, p 35, and FELINE LEUKEMIA VIRUS AND RELATED DISEASES, p 631.)

Adenocarcinoma of the Apocrine Glands of the Anal Sac: This tumor usually occurs in older female dogs, with hypercalcemia developing in ~90% of cases. Humoral mechanisms are most likely responsible for the hypercalcemia as a PTH-like protein has been identified from tumor tissue in dogs. This tumor is usually malignant and has metastasized to regional lymph nodes by the time of diagnosis. Surgical resection is associated with reduction of serum calcium. Failure to remove all of the tumor or recurrence of the tumor usually results in recurrence of hypercalcemia. Despite surgical excision, radiation, and various chemotherapy protocols, the tumor usually recurs within a few months, and prognosis is poor.

Multiple Myeloma: This malignancy in dogs and cats has been associated with hypercalcemia in 10-15% of cases. The pathogenesis of the hypercalcemia is most likely multifactorial. Myeloma cells are known to produce osteoclast-activating factor in humans, which may partially account for the hypercalcemia. The presence of extensive bony lysis may also contribute to the increased serum calcium. Although serum protein concentration is usually increased in multiple myeloma, increased protein binding of calcium rarely accounts for the hypercalcemia. Treatment of multiple myeloma with chemotherapy has been associated with longterm survival, but the presence of associated hypercalcemia, light chain proteinuria, and extensive bony lesions is associated with a shorter survival time.

Hypercalcemia Associated with Hypoadrenocorticism

Mild hypercalcemia (≤15 mg/dL) has been reported in up to 30% of dogs with hypoadrenocorticism (Addison's disease). Multiple factors may result in the hypercalcemia, including increased calcium citrate (complexed calcium), hemoconcentration (relative increase), increased renal resorption of calcium, and increased affinity of serum proteins for calcium. Although total serum calcium concentrations may be increased, the ionized fraction usually is normal. The hypercalcemia resolves quickly with successful treatment for hypoadrenocorticism.

Renal Failure

In cats, chronic renal failure (usually associated with chronic interstitial nephritis) appears to be the most common cause of hypercalcemia. The pathogenesis of the hypercalcemia is not known, but the ionized calcium concentrations remain normal. In dogs, renal failure caused by familial renal disease is more often associated with hypercalcemia than are other forms of chronic renal failure. Hypercalcemia may also be present in acute renal failure during the polyuric phase, but this is rare.

Primary Hyperparathyroidism

Primary hyperparathyroidism results from excessive secretion of PTH by one or more abnormal (usually neoplastic) parathyroid glands. It is relatively rare in dogs and cats. Persistent hypercalcemia is characteristic.

Etiology: Solitary adenoma of the external or internal parathyroid gland is the most common cause of primary hyperparathyroidism, whereas parathyroid carcinoma has been infrequently reported. Hyperplasia of 1 or all 4 parathyroid glands has been described but is very rare.

Clinical Findings: Polydipsia, polyuria, anorexia, lethargy, and depression are the most common signs, but many animals with milder degrees of hypercalcemia may be asymptomatic. Constipation, weakness, shivering, twitching, vomiting, stiff gait, and facial swelling are less often reported.

Diagnosis: Hypercalcemia, normal to low serum phosphorus, and low urine specific gravity are the most consistent findings. Azotemia commonly develops as a consequence of moderate to severe hypercalcemia. In hypercalcemic animals that still have relatively normal renal function (normal serum creatinine and urea nitrogen concentrations), determination of serum PTH is helpful in diagnosis. The finding of high-normal to high serum PTH concentrations in hypercalcemic animals with normal renal function is consistent with primary hyperparathyroidism, whereas the finding of low PTH concentrations is consistent with hypercalcemia of malignancy. Exploratory surgery of the cervical region is a diagnostic alternative if no other cause of hypercalcemia can be determined.

Treatment: Treatment for primary hyperparathyroidism is most often surgical excision of the parathyroid adenoma or carcinoma. A less commonly used treatment is ethanol injection of the parathyroid tumor, which results in necrosis and destruction of the adenoma or carcinoma. The ethanol must be injected carefully with use of ultrasound guidance to avoid any leakage or damage to adjacent soft tissues, otherwise serious complications (eg, vocal cord paralysis) may result. Attempts to lower the serum calcium concentration with IV fluids (saline) and furosemide before surgery may be beneficial (*see* PRINCIPLES OF TREATMENT OF HYPERCALCEMIA, below).

Other Causes of Hypercalcemia

Hypervitaminosis D: Vitamin D toxicity refers to the effects of excessive intake of bioactive metabolites of vitamin D. Toxicity caused by ergocalciferol (vitamin D_2) or cholecalciferol (vitamin D_3) can occur from excessive dietary supplementation (most common in young growing dogs) for treatment of primary hypoparathyroidism. Both of these forms of vitamin D have a slow onset of action and prolonged duration, making correct dosing difficult. Treatment is directed at discontinuing the supplement or decreasing the dose of vitamin D. Toxicity caused by calcitriol (1,25-dihydroxyvitamin D), the most active form of vitamin D, most commonly occurs following treatment of primary hypoparathyroidism. Calcitriol is also the active ingredient in some rodenticides, but these products are no longer widely available, at least in the USA.

In dogs, a newly emerging cause of vitamin D toxicity is ingestion of the calcitriol analog, calcipotriene (also called tacalcitol), which is a topical preparation used to treat psoriasis in people. Calcipotriene toxicity in dogs can result in severe metastatic calcification in the GI tract, kidney, and other tissues; the condition is commonly fatal.

Granulomatous Disease: Hypercalcemia associated with granulomatous disease arises from an alteration of endogenous vitamin D metabolism. Macrophages activated in response to granulomatous inflammation can develop the capability to convert vitamin D precursors to the active form of vitamin D (ie, calcitriol) in an unregulated manner. A similar alteration of vitamin D metabolism in humans may explain hypercalcemia in non-Hodgkin's lymphoma, Hodgkin's lymphoma, and lymphomatoid granulomatosis.

In companion animals, hypercalcemia related to granulomatous disease has been reported in disseminated histoplasmosis, blastomycosis, coccidiomycosis, tuberculosis, and schistosomiasis. Animals with hypercalcemia related to granulomatous disease are expected to have high serum concentrations of ionized calcium and low values for PTH. Serum calcium concentrations return to normal with treatment (ie, antifungal drugs and surgical removal).

Idiopathic Hypercalcemia of Cats: In recent years, a hypercalcemic syndrome in cats has emerged. Affected cats range in age from 2-13 yr, with no gender predilection. Clinical signs are nonspecific and may include vomiting, weight loss, anorexia, lethargy, and evidence of lower urinary tract disease. Crystalluria or calcium oxalate urolithiasis is often an underlying cause of the urinary tract signs. Many affected cats have received urine-acidifying diets.

The most consistent laboratory abnormality is hypercalcemia (high total and ionized calcium concentration), usually accompanied by normal serum phosphorus and normal renal function. In cats with idiopathic hypercalcemia, diagnostic evaluation does not identify malignancy, primary hyperparathyroidism, or vitamin D excess.

Treatment options include dietary modification, glucocorticoids, or both. A high-fiber diet is thought to be beneficial because the fiber content may decrease availability of dietary calcium for absorption. If dietary modification is unsuccessful, some cats respond to treatment with prednisone, administered at an initial dose of 5 mg BID and increased to 10 mg BID, if needed. If a response occurs, the prednisone dose can be tapered to the minimum daily dosage required to maintain normocalcemia.

Houseplants: Certain house plants (eg, *Cestrum diurnum* [the day-blooming jessamine], *Solanum malacoxylon, Triestum flavescens*) may contain a substance similar to vitamin D that may cause hypercalcemia when ingested.

Osteolytic Lesions: Hypercalcemia resulting from tumor invasion or metastasis to bone develops very rarely in animals. Primary bone tumors (eg, osteosarcoma) and neoplastic cells within the bone marrow (eg, multiple myeloma) may occasionally produce hypercalcemia. The mechanisms whereby bony neoplasia may produce hypercalcemia include mechanical destruction by the infiltrating cells (as occurs with metastatic tumors and osteosarcoma) and local production of osteoclast-activating factor (as occurs with multiple myeloma). Bacterial and mycotic osteomyelitis can also occasionally produce hypercalcemia. The hypercalcemia may result from direct bone lysis or may be mediated by bone-resorbing factors (eg, prostaglandins, osteoclast-activating factor).

Principles of Treatment of Hypercalcemia

The definitive treatment of hypercalcemia is treating or removing the underlying cause. Unfortunately, the etiology may not be apparent, and supportive measures must be taken to decrease the serum calcium concentration.

Fluid Therapy: Volume expansion with 0.9% saline, ~100-125 mL/kg/day, IV, decreases hemoconcentration and increases renal calcium loss by improving glomerular filtration rate and sodium excretion, which results in less calcium reabsorption.

Diuretics: Loop diuretics such as furosemide (2-4 mg/kg, every 8-12 hr) increase calcium excretion by the kidneys; however, higher doses may be needed. If dehydration is present, fluid therapy should be instituted first because volume contraction and further hemoconcentration may worsen the hypercalcemia. Thiazide diuretics are contraindicated in hypercalcemia because these agents decrease calcium excretion by the kidneys and worsen the hypercalcemia.

Sodium Bicarbonate: Bicarbonate given as an IV bolus (1 mEq/kg) or as a continuous infusion has been shown to decrease serum total calcium concentrations. Although the magnitude of calcium reduction is mild, alkalosis also favors the shift of ionized calcium to protein-bound calcium. Sodium bicarbonate therapy is more beneficial when combined with other treatments.

Glucocorticoids: Administration of glucocorticoids (eg, prednisone, 1-2 mg/kg, BID) decreases bone resorption of calcium and intestinal calcium absorption and increases renal calcium excretion, leading to a substantial decrease in serum calcium concentration in animals with hypercalcemia secondary to lymphoma, myeloma, hypervitaminosis D, and hypoadrenocorticism.

Miscellaneous Agents: Calcitonin has been reported as an antidote to cholecalciferol toxicity, but the decrease in serum calcium may be short (hours), requiring multiple treatments. Diphosphonates inhibit osteoclastic bone resorption, but their use in veterinary medicine has been limited. Mithramycin is a potent inhibitor of osteoclastic bone resorption; however, this drug has been associated with many adverse effects, such as thrombocytopenia, hepatic necrosis, renal necrosis, and hypocalcemia.

HYPOCALCEMIA IN DOGS AND CATS

Hypocalcemia causes the major clinical manifestations of hypoparathyroidism by increasing the excitability of both the central and peripheral nervous systems. Peripheral neuromuscular signs classically include muscle tremors, twitches, and tetany. Generalized convulsions, resembling those of an idiopathic seizure disorder, are the predominant CNS manifestation of hypoparathyroidism.

Hypoparathyroidism

Hypoparathyroidism is a metabolic disorder characterized by hypocalcemia and hyperphosphatemia and either transient or permanent PTH insufficiency. The spontaneous disorder is uncommon in dogs and rarely reported in cats. Iatrogenic injury or removal of the parathyroid glands during thyroidectomy for treatment of hyperthyroidism is the most common cause in cats. Postoperative hypoparathyroidism secondary to parathyroidectomy for parathyroid tumor may occur due to atrophy of the remaining glands in either dogs or cats.

Diagnosis: Diagnosis is based on history, clinical signs, laboratory evidence of hypocalcemia and hyperphosphatemia, and exclusion of other causes of hypocalcemia (eg, hypoproteinemia, malabsorption, pancreatitis, renal failure). If idiopathic hypoparathyroidism is suspected, it should be confirmed by histologic examination of the parathyroid glands and documentation of parathyroid atrophy or destruction. Because the parathyroid glands are not grossly evident in animals with hypoparathyroidism, a unilateral thyroidectomy should be performed to ensure that adequate parathyroid tissue is available for examination. Determination of serum PTH concentrations might be helpful in the diagnosis of idiopathic hypoparathyroidism and may thereby eliminate the need for cervical exploratory surgery and histologic verification.

Treatment: Treatment is directed at restoring the serum calcium concentration to the low end of the normal range. This should include use of calcium supplements and vitamin D for either iatrogenic or idiopathic forms of hypoparathyroidism. If hypocalcemic tetany or seizures are present, calcium should be administered IV immediately. For maintenance of normocalcemia, oral calcium should be administered together with a vitamin D preparation.

The major complication associated with treatment of hypoparathyroidism is hypercalcemia, which develops as a consequence of overtreatment with calcium and vitamin D. If this occurs, calcium and vitamin D therapy should be temporarily discontinued; saline and furosemide should be administered if hypercalcemia is severe (*see* PRINCIPLES OF TREATMENT OF HYPERCALCEMIA, above). With idiopathic hypoparathyroidism, long-term management with vitamin D (with or without calcium supplementation) is necessary. In contrast, with iatrogenic hypoparathyroidism, spontaneous recovery of parathyroid function or accommodation of calcium-regulating mechanisms to the absence of PTH may occur weeks to months after surgery.

Other Causes of Hypocalcemia

Renal Disease: Chronic renal failure is probably the most frequently encountered cause of hypocalcemia. Azotemia and hyperphosphatemia result from decreased glomerular filtration rates. Mechanisms of hypocalcemia include decreased renal tubular calcium resorption, hyperphosphatemia, decreased formation of 1,25-dihydroxyvitamin D, hypoalbuminemia, and chelation of calcium with oxalate. Parathyroid gland hyperplasia occurs to maintain serum calcium in normal ranges. High PTH concentrations result in increased bone resorption. The hypocalcemia associated with renal failure, however, is rarely clinically significant (ie, muscle tremors, twitches, tetany, or convulsions do not develop). In addition, most animals with chronic renal failure have normal serum calcium concentrations. Treatment should be directed at lowering the serum phosphate concentrations by dietary restriction of phosphorus and intestinal phosphate binders. (*See also* RENAL DYSFUNCTION, p 1267.)

Hypoproteinemia: Animals with hypoalbuminemia may be hypocalcemic because of a decrease in the protein-bound fraction of calcium, but the ionized calcium fraction may remain normal. Clinical signs of hypocalcemia do not usually develop. The magnitude of hypocalcemia is usually mild.

Pancreatitis: Hypocalcemia, when it occurs in animals with pancreatitis (p 347), is usually mild and subclinical. The exact mechanism is unknown, but a commonly accepted theory is that calcium is precipitated in the form of insoluble soaps through saponification of peripancreatic fatty acids formed subsequent to release of the pancreatic enzyme lipase. More recent work suggests that hypocalcemia may result from a shift of calcium into soft tissues, especially muscle.

Puerperal Tetany: Puerperal tetany (eclampsia, p 809) is an acute, life-threatening disease caused by an extreme fall in circulating calcium concentrations in the lactating bitch or queen. Severe hypocalcemia associated with eclampsia develops during the nursing period (several days to several weeks postpartum). The pathophysiology remains poorly understood but appears to result from an imbalance between the rate of inflow (eg, bone resorption, GI absorption) and outflow (eg, mammary gland) from the extracellular calcium pool. Treatment consists of slow IV administration of calcium (*see* PRINCIPLES OF TREATMENT OF HYPOCALCEMIA, below) and weaning of the litter, if possible.

Phosphate Enema Toxicity: Hypertonic sodium phosphate (eg, Fleet®) enemas may result in severe biochemical abnormalities, especially when administered to dehydrated cats with colonic atony and mucosal disruption. Hypernatremia and hyperphosphatemia result from the colonic absorption of sodium and phosphate from the enema solution, as well as transfer of intravascular water to the colonic lumen (because of the hypertonic enema). Hyperphosphatemia leads to precipitation of serum calcium with resultant hypocalcemia. Clinical signs of phosphate enema toxicosis, which result from these electrolyte and fluid alterations, include shock and neuromuscular irritability. Treatment consists of IV volume expansion with an electrolyte-poor solution (eg, 5% dextrose in water), as well as treatment of hypocalcemia (*see* below).

Chelating Agents: EDTA (ethylenediaminetetraacetic acid), citrated blood, and oxalic acid (a metabolite of the ethylene glycol in antifreeze) all complex calcium and can cause hypocalcemia. Animals with ethylene glycol intoxication (p 2357) also demonstrate severe metabolic acidosis, azotemia, and hyperphosphatemia from the oliguric renal failure, which results from calcium oxalate crystal precipitation in the renal tubules.

Principles of Treatment of Hypocalcemia

The definitive treatment for hypocalcemia is to eliminate the underlying cause. Supportive measures, including the following, to restore normocalcemia can be administered pending the diagnosis.

Parenteral Calcium: Hypocalcemic tetany or convulsions are indications for the immediate IV administration of 10% calcium gluconate (1.0-1.5 mL/kg), which should be slowly infused over a 10-min period. Close monitoring is mandatory; if bradycardia or shortening of the QT interval occurs, the IV infusion should be slowed or temporarily discontinued.

Once the life-threatening signs of hypocalcemia have been controlled, calcium can be added to the IV fluids and administered as a slow continuous infusion (eg, 10% calcium gluconate, 2.5 mL/kg every 6-8 hr). The rate of calcium administration should be adjusted as necessary to maintain a normal serum calcium concentration, and the infusion should be continued for as long as necessary to prevent recurrence of hypocalcemia. Although this continuous calcium infusion will maintain normocalcemia, its effects are short-lived; hypocalcemia will recur within hours of stopping the infusion unless other treatment is given.

Oral Calcium: Oral calcium supplementation may be beneficial in some conditions (eg, hypoparathyroidism, puerperal tetany). The daily requirements are 1-4 g for dogs and 0.5-1 g for cats. The daily dose of calcium should be based on the amount of elemental calcium in the product, rather than on the weight of the calcium salt.

Vitamin D: In some conditions, vitamin D supplementation is necessary to increase calcium absorption from the intestines. There are 3 main preparations of vitamin D available, including vitamin D_2 (ergocalciferol), dihydrotachysterol, and 1,25-dihydroxyvitamin D (calcitriol). The dosage and duration of response of these drugs depends on the form used. For vitamin D_2, the initial required dosages are generally 4,000-6,000 IU/kg/day, whereas the final dosages required to maintain normocalcemia range from 1,000-2,000 IU/kg, once daily to once weekly. For dihydrotachysterol, initial loading dosages of 0.02-0.03 mg/kg/day are usually administered, with maintenance dosages of 0.01-0.02 mg/kg given every 24-48 hr. For 1,25-dihydroxyvitamin D, a daily dosage of 0.025-0.06 μg/kg (25-60 ng/kg/day) is generally required. Because the available capsule sizes (250 and 500 ng) are not well formulated for the small body size of most dogs and cats, and these capsules cannot be readily divided, it may be desirable to contact a pharmacist who can reformulate these products to a size that is appropriate for the individual pet. With all vitamin D preparations and dosage regimens, the development of iatrogenic hypercalcemia is a common complication of treatment.

THE PITUITARY GLAND

The pituitary gland (hypophysis) is composed of the adenohypophysis (anterior lobe) and the neurohypophysis (posterior lobe).

Adenohypophysis: The adenohypophysis, which surrounds the pars nervosa of the neurohypophyseal system to varying degrees in different species, consists of the pars distalis, the pars tuberalis, and the pars intermedia. The pars distalis is the largest part and contains multiple populations of endocrine cells. The pars tuberalis functions primarily as a scaffold for the capillary network of the hypophyseal portal system. The pars intermedia forms the junction between the pars distalis and pars nervosa. It contains 2 populations of cells in dogs, one of which synthesizes adrenocorticotropic hormone (ACTH).

A specific population of endocrine cells in the pars distalis (and in the pars intermedia for ACTH in dogs) synthesizes and secretes each of the pituitary trophic hormones. Pituitary cells have a secretory cycle and enter an actively synthesizing phase in response to increased demand for a particular hormone. Secretory cells in the adenohypophysis are often subdivided into chromophils (acidophils, basophils) and chromophobes based on interaction of the secretory granules with pH-dependent histochemical stains.

Acidophils are further subdivided into somatotrophs that secrete growth hormone (GH, somatotropin) and lactotrophs that secrete prolactin. Basophils include gonadotrophs that secrete both luteinizing hormone (LH) and follicle-stimulating hormone (FSH), and thyrotrophs that secrete thyrotropic hormone (thyroid-stimulating hormone [TSH]). Chromophobes include the endocrine cells involved in the synthesis of ACTH and melanocyte-stimulating hormone (MSH), nonsecretory follicular cells, and undifferentiated stem cells.

Endocrine cells in the adenohypophysis are under the control of corresponding hypothalamic-releasing hormones. These releasing hormones are conveyed by the hypophyseal portal system to specific cells in the adenohypophysis, where they stimulate the rapid release of preformed trophic hormones.

Separate hypothalamic-releasing hormones regulate the rate of secretion of each trophic hormone from the adenohypophysis. For most pituitary trophic hormones, negative feedback control is accomplished by a feedback loop involving the blood concentration of the hormone produced by the target endocrine gland (eg, thyroid gland, adrenal cortex, ovary, and testis). Hormones such as prolactin, GH, and MSH have more complex feedback mechanisms. For example, prolactin affects primarily the mammary gland, and GH has its principal effect on the liver—both nonendocrine tissues. The negative feedback in such cases includes metabolites and other messengers (eg, insulin-like growth factor I produced by the liver). In the case of GH, there is an inhibitory (somatostatin) as well as stimulatory (GH-releasing hormone) hypothalamic regulator.

Neurohypophysis: The neurohypophysis (pars nervosa, posterior lobe) has 3 anatomic subdivisions. Secretion granules that contain the neurohypophyseal hormones, ie, antidiuretic hormone (ADH, vasopressin) and oxytocin, are synthesized in the hypothalamus but are released into the bloodstream in the pars nervosa. The infundibular stalk joins the pars nervosa to the overlying hypothalamus.

ADH, an octapeptide synthesized in the hypothalamus, is packaged into membrane-limited granules with a corresponding binding protein (neurophysin) and transported to the pars nervosa, where it is released into the circulation. ADH binds to specific receptors in the distal part of the nephron and collecting duct of the kidney; it increases the renal tubular reabsorption of water from the glomerular filtrate.

The output of ADH is directly related to the degree of hydration of the body. Hydration of the body inhibits release of ADH, while dehydration or injection of hypertonic electrolyte solutions favors release of ADH, which in turn causes increased water resorption from the glomerular filtrate, resulting in dilution and decreased osmolarity of body fluids. Barbiturates, ether, chloroform, morphine, acetylcholine, nicotine, and pain increase ADH release, which leads to less urine formation. Ethanol inhibits ADH release, which leads to diuresis.

The pressor effect of ADH is less prominent than the antidiuretic effect. At a dosage several hundred times larger than the antidiuretic dosage, ADH has a pronounced pressor effect, which may also lead to coronary constriction. The contractile mechanism of the capillaries, as well as GI and uterine muscle, is stimulated, and a prolonged increase in blood pressure follows.

Oxytocin has specific effects on the smooth muscle of the uterus and the myoepithelial cells of the mammary gland. It has no established physiologic function in the male, although an effect on sperm transport has been suggested.

HYPERADRENOCORTICISM
(Cushing's disease)

Functional tumors in the pituitary gland, derived from corticotroph (ACTH-secreting) cells in either the pars distalis or the pars intermedia, result in a clinical syndrome of cortisol excess. This disease is common in dogs but not other species. Miniature Poodles, Dachshunds, Boxers, Boston Terriers, and Beagles are at increased risk of the disease. In ~85% of affected dogs, the hyperadrenocorticism is pituitary dependent (PDH), while ~15% have functional adrenal tumors. Differentiation of PDH from adrenal tumors is necessary for appropriate treatment.

Clinical Findings: Hyperadrenocorticism is a disease of middle-aged to older dogs (7-12 yr). A sex predilection for females is seen in some dogs with hyperadrenocorticism secondary to adrenal tumors. The most common clinical signs are polydipsia (PD), polyuria (PU), polyphagia, heat intolerance, lethargy, abdominal enlargement or "potbelly," panting, obesity, muscle weakness, and recurrent urinary tract infections. Dermatologic manifestations are numerous and often include truncal alopecia, thin skin, phlebectasias, comedones, bruising, cutaneous hyperpigmentation, calcinosis cutis, pyoderma, dermal atrophy, secondary demodicosis, and seborrhea. Cutaneous mineralization (calcinosis cutis) is a characteristic although infrequent finding in dogs. Although mineral deposition may occur anywhere in the skin, the dorsal midline, ventral abdomen, and inguinal region are affected most frequently. Numerous mineral crystals are deposited along collagen and elastin fibers in the dermis and outer subcutis and may protrude through the atrophic and thinned epidermis. In less severe cases, the epidermis remains intact and appears irregularly elevated by the firm, opaque, white deposits of mineral. A narrow rim of hyperemia and foreign-body granulomatous inflammation often surrounds the areas of mineralization. The mineral deposits occur despite normal blood calcium and phosphorus levels probably because of the gluconeogenic and protein catabolic actions of cortisol. Mineralization may also occur in other tissues of the body, most frequently the airways and blood vessels.

Uncommon clinical manifestations include hypertension, pulmonary thromboembolism, testicular atrophy, polyneuropathy and myopathy, congestive heart failure, prostatomegaly in male castrated dogs, clitoral hypertrophy, bronchial calcification, behavioral changes, corneal ulceration (nonhealing), blindness, neuralgic disease, pseudomyotonia, cranial cruciate rupture (small dogs), and perianal adenoma in female or castrated male dogs.

Adenomas of the adrenal cortex are seen most frequently in old dogs and sporadically in horses, cattle, and sheep. They usually occur as well-demarcated, single nodules in one adrenal gland but may be bilateral. Larger cortical adenomas are yellow to red, distort the external contour of the affected gland, and are partially or completely encapsulated. Adjacent cortical parenchyma is compressed, and the tumor may extend into the medulla.

Carcinomas of the adrenal cortex occur with equal frequency to adenomas and have been reported most often in adult to older cattle and dogs, with no apparent breed or sex predilection. Adrenal carcinomas are larger then adenomas and more likely to be bilateral.

In dogs, they are composed of a variegated, yellow-red, friable tissue that incorporates the affected adrenal gland. They often are fixed in location because of extensive invasion of surrounding tissues (posterior vena cava, kidney, and aorta) and may result in a large tumor thrombus. In cattle, carcinomas may attain considerable size ($\geq$10 cm in diameter), have multiple areas of mineralization or ossification, and usually completely obliterate the affected adrenal.

Some carcinomas and adenomas of the adrenal cortex in dogs are functional and secrete excess cortisol, sex steroids, or both. They may compress adjacent organs, invade the aorta or posterior vena cava (which leads to intra-abdominal hemorrhage), and metastasize to distant sites (eg, liver, kidneys, mesenteric lymph nodes, and lungs). Functional cortisol-secreting cortical adenomas and carcinomas are associated with profound atrophy of the contralateral cortex because of inhibition of pituitary ACTH secretion due to increased blood cortisol levels. The adrenal medulla appears expanded and is more conspicuous because of the lack of cortical parenchyma.

Laboratory Abnormalities: In dogs, serum chemistry abnormalities associated with hypercortisolemia include increased serum alkaline phosphatase and ALT, hypercholesterolemia, hyperglycemia, and decreased BUN. The hemogram is often characterized by evidence of regeneration (erythrocytosis, nucleated red blood cells) and a classic "stress leukogram" (mature neutrophilia, lymphopenia, and eosinopenia). Basophilia is occasionally seen.

Many dogs have evidence of urinary tract infection without pyuria (positive culture), bacteriuria, and proteinuria resulting from glomerulosclerosis. Thyroid status is often affected, as evidenced by decreased basal thyroxine (T_4) and triiodothyronine (T_3), caused by euthyroid sick syndrome and by an attenuated response to TSH stimulation due to the effect of cortisol and overcrowding on pituitary thyrotrophs. Overt diabetes mellitus may result from the insulin antagonism caused by hypercortisolemia in ~10-25% of dogs with hyperadrenocorticism and in an even higher percentage of cats. In addition, hyperadrenocorticism can be a cause of insulin resistance and poor glycemic control in diabetic dogs. A consistent finding is the excretion of large amounts of dilute urine with a low specific gravity ($\leq$1.015).

Diagnosis: Diagnosis can be challenging; it should be based on clinical signs and laboratory abnormalities and confirmed via an appropriate screening test for hyperadrenocorticism. If results of screening tests are inconclusive or if laboratory abnormalities associated with hyperadrenocorticism are noted in a dog without clinical signs, the dog should be retested 3-6 mo later.

The low-dose dexamethasone suppression (LDDS) test is the screening test of choice for hyperadrenocorticism in dogs. It is sensitive; only 5% of dogs with hyperadrenocorticism exhibit suppressed cortisol concentrations at 8 hr. In addition, 30% of dogs with PDH exhibit suppression at 3 or 4 hr followed by "escape" of suppression at 8 hr—this pattern is diagnostic for PDH. The major disadvantage of the LDDS test is the lack of specificity in dogs with nonadrenal illness (diabetes mellitus, chronic renal disease, liver disease); these dogs should be treated for the nonadrenal illness and stabilized before the LDDS test is performed.

The ACTH stimulation test is used to diagnose a variety of adrenopathic disorders, including endogenous or iatrogenic hyperadrenocorticism and spontaneous hypoadrenocorticism. As a screening test for the diagnosis of naturally occurring hyperadrenocorticism, the ACTH stimulation test has a diagnostic sensitivity of ~85-90% and a higher specificity than the LDDS test.

The urine cortisol/creatinine ratio (UCCR) is a rapid and easy screening test; however, it is very sensitive and can be associated with false-positive results. Therefore, a normal UCCR can only effectively rule out the diagnosis of hyperadrenocorticism, whereas an increased UCCR requires an LDDS or ACTH stimulation test to confirm the diagnosis. Collection of the first urine sample in the morning may be a better reflection of cortisol production over time than random urine samples obtained throughout the day when the time since the last urination may have been only a few hours.

Measurement of ciALP as a screening test appears to lack both sensitivity and specificity. An increased ciALP is suggestive but not diagnostic.

Pituitary- Versus Adrenal-Dependent Disease: Once the diagnosis of hyper-adrenocorticism has been confirmed, differentiation of pituitary- versus adrenal-dependent disease may be necessary. Although most dogs with hyperadrenocorticism have PDH, in atypical cases (eg, the anorectic dog with hyperadrenocorticism), a differentiation test is appropriate. In particular, differentiation of PDH (often macroadenomas) from adrenal tumors is often necessary in large breeds of dogs.

Measurement of endogenous plasma ACTH concentrations is the most reliable method of differentiating between PDH and adrenal tumors. Dogs with adrenal tumors have low to undetectable ACTH concentrations; in contrast, dogs with PDH have normal to increased ACTH concentrations. The high-dose dexamethasone suppression (HDDS) test works on the principle that ACTH secretion has already been suppressed maximally in dogs with functioning adrenal tumors; therefore, administration of dexamethasone, no matter how high the dose, will not suppress serum cortisol concentrations. In dogs with PDH, however, high doses of dexamethasone are able to suppress ACTH and hence cortisol secretion. One caveat is that in dogs with pituitary macroadenomas (15-50% of dogs with PDH) cortisol concentrations do not suppress on the HDDS test.

Diagnostic imaging of the pituitary or adrenal glands can be accomplished via abdominal radiography, ultrasonography, computed tomography (CT), or MRI. Abdominal radiographs should be performed in all dogs that do not suppress on an HDDS; in ~30-50% of dogs with adrenal tumors, a mineralized mass in the area of the adrenal glands can be seen. Abdominal ultrasonography is a more sensitive method of identifying adrenal tumors. In addition, liver metastasis or invasion into the vena cava may be demonstrated in dogs with adrenal carcinomas. CT and/or MRI of the abdomen or brain in dogs that do not suppress on the HDDS may show unilateral adrenal enlargement, pituitary macroadenoma, or pituitary microadenoma.

Treatment: Dogs with PDH may be treated using the adrenolytic agent mitotane (o,p′-DDD), beginning with an induction dose of 25-50 mg/kg/day for 7-10 days. Dogs should be monitored for signs of hypoadrenocorticism, such as anorexia, vomiting, and diarrhea; if such signs occur, mitotane therapy should be discontinued and glucocorticoids administered. Water consumption or appetite may be measured to provide an endpoint for therapy; water consumption should decrease to <60 mL/kg/day (dogs). After 7-10 days of therapy with mitotane or a reduction in water consumption, an ACTH response test should be performed to determine if cortisol suppression is adequate. The pre- and post-ACTH cortisols should both be in the normal range. To maintain suppression of cortisol secretion, mitotane is administered at a dosage of 50 mg/kg/wk. Dogs on longterm treatment with mitotane should have an examination and ACTH response test every 3-4 mo. Gradually increasing doses of the drug are often required to maintain adequate clinical remission.

Side effects of mitotane at the recommended dose include GI irritation (vomiting and anorexia), CNS disturbances (ataxia, weakness, seizures), mild hypoglycemia, and a moderate increase in serum alkaline phosphatase. If signs such as depression or ataxia develop, they can usually be alleviated by dividing the daily dose into 2 equal parts administered at 8- to 12-hr intervals. Persistence of CNS signs after mitotane is discontinued suggests an expanding pituitary macroadenoma.

Ketoconazole, which affects steroid biosynthesis, is an alternative therapy for hyperadrenocorticism in dogs. It is given at 5 mg/kg, BID, PO, initially for 7 days. If no problems (such as anorexia or icterus) are noted, the dosage is increased to 10 mg/kg, BID. After 14 days, an ACTH response test is performed. If cortisol secretion is not adequately suppressed, the dosage may be increased to 15 mg/kg, BID. The disadvantages of ketoconazole are its cost, twice daily administration indefinitely, and a failure rate of 20-25%.

L-deprenyl (selegiline hydrochloride) is approved by the FDA for the management of PDH in dogs. In initial studies it was effective in 70-80% of cases of PDH with mild to moderate clinical signs, although other investigators have found it to be less effective. Its use is associated with few side effects. Its mechanism of action is through inhibition of monoamine oxidase, resulting in increased concentrations of dopamine with subsequent inhibition of endogenous ACTH. The initial dosage is 1 mg/kg, SID, and dogs are monitored based on clinical response. If no response is seen after 2 wk, the dosage can be increased to 2 mg/kg, SID. Because L-deprenyl does not cause hypoadrenocorticism, routine endocrine evaluations are not warranted.

Recent reports have demonstrated the efficacy of the adrenal enzyme inhibitor trilostane in the treatment of PDH in dogs. As is the case with ketoconazole, trilostane must be administered daily and results in glucocorticoid insufficiency without effects on aldosterone concentrations.

Surgical removal of unilateral adrenal adenomas or adenocarcinomas may be indicated in some cases; however, surgical and anesthetic complications (eg, hypotension) may develop secondary to hypoadrenocorticism, which occurs immediately after surgical removal of the tumor. Medical treatment of adrenal tumors is difficult because they tend to be resistant to the effects of mitotane. Finally, if the dog is showing neurologic signs (eg, anorexia, stupor, or seizures) and a large pituitary tumor (macroadenoma) is identified, radiation therapy of the pituitary gland is indicated. However, radiation therapy is expensive and time-consuming (3 wk). Results of radiation therapy in dogs show that this is an effective method of treatment with low morbidity; however, it may take several months for the signs of PDH to subside. These dogs do well in the longterm, however, because the primary disease process (pituitary tumor) has been addressed.

NONFUNCTIONAL PITUITARY TUMORS

These tumors are uncommon in most species. Chromophobe adenomas appear to be endocrinologically inactive, but they may cause compression atrophy of adjacent portions of the pituitary gland and extend into the overlying brain. Clinical disturbances occur because of either a lack of secretion of pituitary trophic hormones and diminished target organ function (eg, adrenal cortex), or dysfunction of the CNS. Affected animals often are depressed, incoordinated, and weak and may collapse with exercise. (*See also* ADULT-ONSET PANHYPOPITUITARISM, p 456.)

Endocrinologically inactive pituitary adenomas often attain considerable size before they cause obvious signs (or death). The proliferating tumor cells incorporate the remaining structures of the adenohypophysis and infundibular stalk. The entire hypothalamus may become compressed and replaced by the tumor.

HIRSUTISM ASSOCIATED WITH ADENOMAS OF THE PARS INTERMEDIA
(Hypertrichosis)

Hirsutism develops in older horses, more often in mares, and usually is associated with a pituitary adenoma derived from cells of the pars intermedia. Such adenomas often severely compress the overlying hypothalamus. The hypothalamus is the primary center for homeostatic regulation of body temperature, appetite, and cyclic shedding of hair.

Clinical Findings and Lesions: Signs are polyuria, polydipsia, ravenous appetite, weakness, somnolence, intermittent hyperpyrexia, and generalized hyperhidrosis. Hirsutism often becomes evident because of failure of the cyclic seasonal shedding of hair. The hair over most of the trunk and extremities is long (up to 4-5 in. [10-12 cm]), abnormally thick, wavy, and often matted.

Horses with larger tumors may have hyperglycemia (insulin-resistant) and glycosuria, probably because of a down-regulation of insulin receptors on target cells induced by the chronic overeating and hyperinsulinemia.

These are the most common pituitary tumors in horses. They are yellow to white, multinodular, and incorporate the pars nervosa. Plasma cortisol and immunoreactive adrenocorticotropin levels are modestly increased; the cortisol levels lack the normal diurnal rhythm and are not suppressed by either high or low doses of dexamethasone.

Diagnosis: Hyperglycemia and some insulin insensitivity are highly suggestive of pituitary adenoma in horses. Other nonspecific findings include an absolute or relative neutrophilia, eosinopenia, and lymphopenia; lipemia; hypercholesterolemia; and a mild, normochromic, normocytic anemia. Liver enzymes may be increased. Electrolytes are usually normal. Urinalysis is normal except for occasional glycosuria and a low to normal specific gravity.

Definitive diagnosis is based on response to tests that suppress the pituitary-adrenal axis or measurement of endogenous ACTH. Baseline cortisol is in the high-normal to modestly increased range. Dexamethasone (40 μg/kg, IM) often will not suppress cortisol levels to at least 30% of baseline or to <1 μg/dL, as it does in normal horses 6 hr after administration.

Differential diagnoses include syndromes resulting in chronic debilitation, eg, poor management and nutrition, parasitism, and chronic systemic diseases. The polyuria and polydipsia (PU/PD) must be differentiated from that due to chronic renal disease or diabetes insipidus. The hyperglycemia, glycosuria, and PU/PD must be differentiated from that due to primary diabetes mellitus. Pheochromocytomas (p 467) may cause hyperhidrosis, hyperglycemia, and tachypnea, although they usually are nonfunctional and only found incidentally at necropsy.

Treatment: Few horses have been treated successfully, but daily cyproheptadine (0.13-0.26 mg/kg, PO) may be beneficial. PU/PD should decrease within 1-2 mo if the therapy is successful. After 3 mo, alternate-day therapy can be tried. Pergolide, a dopaminergic agonist, also has been used successfully in a few horses at a daily dosage of 4-11 μg/kg, PO. The vasoconstrictive action of the drug could potentially result in side effects, although they have not been reported.

ADULT-ONSET PANHYPOPITUITARISM

Endocrinologically inactive, nonfunctional pituitary tumors develop most commonly in adult to aged animals; there is no apparent breed predisposition. The most common cause is a chromophobe adenoma arising in the pars distalis. Other infrequent causes include extensive inflammatory destruction of pituitary tissue, ischemic necrosis of the pituitary due to infarction from invasion of tumor cells, parasitic or septic emboli, diffuse necrosis associated with toxemia, invasion by neoplasms arising in adjacent structures (eg, meninges, sphenoid bone, nasal cavity, etc), and widespread hemorrhage and subsequent scarring after traumatic injury. Dogs and cats with nonfunctional adenomas develop clinical disturbances related to a lack of secretion of pituitary trophic hormones and diminished target organ function or to dysfunction of the CNS.

Clinical Findings: Affected animals often are depressed and incoordinated and collapse with exercise. Occasionally, they exhibit a change in attitude, become unresponsive to people, and develop a tendency to hide at the slightest provocation. In chronic cases, there may be evidence of blindness with dilated and fixed pupils due to compression and disruption of optic nerves by dorsal extension of the pituitary tumor. Affected dogs often show a progressive weight loss with muscle atrophy due to loss of the protein anabolic effect of growth hormone. Compression of the cells that secrete gonadotropic hormones or the corresponding releasing hormone from the hypothalamus results in atrophy of the gonads. Disturbances of water balance result from interference with the synthesis of antidiuretic hormone or its release into capillaries of the pars nervosa. The posterior lobe, infundibular stalk, and hypothalamus are compressed or disrupted by neoplastic cells.

Animals with panhypopituitarism appear dehydrated, despite increased water consumption. Dogs and cats with large nonfunctional pituitary tumors usually excrete large volumes of dilute urine with a low specific gravity (≤1.007) and may break housetraining. Clinical signs are not highly specific and can be confused with other CNS disorders (eg, brain tumors or encephalitis) or chronic renal disease.

Hypopituitarism caused by pituitary tumors should be included in the differential diagnosis of diseases characterized by incoordination, depression, polyuria, blindness, and sudden behavioral changes in adult or aged animals. Because the blindness is central in origin, ophthalmoscopic examination usually fails to reveal significant lesions. There is no effect on body stature associated with compression of the pars distalis and probable interference of growth hormone secretion because these tumors usually arise in dogs that have already completed their growth. Parakeets with chromophobe adenomas often develop exophthalmos due to extension of neoplastic cells along the optic nerve.

Lesions: Endocrinologically inactive pituitary adenomas usually reach considerable size before they cause obvious signs or death. The proliferating tumor cells incorporate the remaining structures of the adenohypophysis and infundibular stalk. The entire hypothalamus may be compressed and replaced by tumor.

Thyroid glands in dogs and cats with large pituitary adenomas often are smaller than normal, although to a much lesser degree than the adrenal cortex. The adrenal glands are small and consist primarily of medullary tissue surrounded by a narrow zone of cortex. Seminiferous tubules are small and show little evidence of active spermatogenesis.

Skin atrophy and loss of muscle mass may be related to a lack of protein anabolic effects of growth hormone in an adult dog or cat. Interference with the secretion of pituitary trophic hormones often results in gonadal atrophy resulting in either decreased libido or anestrus.

JUVENILE-ONSET PANHYPOPITUITARISM
(Pituitary dwarfism)

Pituitary dwarfism occurs most frequently in German Shepherds, but has been reported in other breeds such as the Spitz, Miniature Pinscher, and Karelian Bear Dog. It is inherited as a simple autosomal recessive trait.

Pituitary dwarfism is usually associated with a failure of the oropharyngeal ectoderm of the cranial pharyngeal duct (Rathke's pouch) to differentiate into trophic-hormone-secreting cells of the pars distalis. Consequently, the adenohypophysis is not completely developed. The second most common cause is craniopharyngioma, a benign tumor derived from the oropharyngeal ectoderm of Rathke's pouch. Compared with other types of pituitary neoplasms, these tumors tend to develop in younger dogs. Craniopharyngiomas cause subnormal secretion of growth hormone, which results in dwarfism.

Clinical Findings: Dwarf pups are indistinguishable from normal littermates up to 2 mo of age. Subsequently, the slower growth rate compared with littermates, retention of puppy coat, and lack of primary guard hairs gradually become evident. German Shepherds with pituitary dwarfism appear coyote- or fox-like owing to their small size and soft, woolly coat. Bilaterally symmetric alopecia develops gradually and often becomes complete except for the head and tufts of hair on the legs. Permanent dentition is delayed or completely absent. Closure of the epiphyses is delayed as long as 4 yr depending on the severity of the hormonal insufficiency and is caused by deficiencies of both thyroid-stimulating hormone and growth hormone. The testes and penis are small, calcification of the os penis is delayed or incomplete, and the penile sheath is flaccid. The ovarian cortex is hypoplastic, and estrus is irregular or absent. Lifespan is shortened because of the resulting secondary endocrine dysfunction, such as hypothyroidism and hypoadrenocorticism. Puppies with panhypopituitarism often have a shrill bark.

Lesions: Pituitary cysts fill with mucus and eventually occupy the entire pituitary area, resulting in severe compression of the pars nervosa and infundibular stalk. Craniopharyngiomas are large, solid, cystic areas that extend into the overlying hypothalamus. They may also grow along the ventral aspect of the brain, where incorporation of several cranial nerves results in specific nerve function deficits.

Diagnosis: Levels of thyroxine, triiodothyronine, and cortisol are reduced or in the low-normal range. In those animals with an equivocal change in basal hormone level, the responses to challenge by exogenous thyrotropin or adrenocorticotropin are subnormal, owing to the hypoplasia or atrophy of the thyroid gland and adrenal cortex. Other useful diagnostic aids include comparison of height with that of littermates, evidence of delayed epiphyseal closure or dysgenesis on skeletal radiographs, and skin biopsy. Cutaneous lesions include hyperkeratosis, follicular keratosis, hyperpigmentation, adnexal atrophy, loss of elastin fibers, and a loose network of collagen fibers in the dermis. Hair shafts are absent, and hair follicles are primarily in the telogen stage of the growth cycle.

The activity of somatomedin C (insulin-like growth factor 1) is low in dwarf dogs. Intermediate somatomedin C activity is present in phenotypically normal ancestors suspected to be heterozygous carriers. Assays for somatomedin C provide an indirect measurement of circulating growth hormone activity in dogs with suspected pituitary dwarfism. Basal levels of circulating canine growth hormone are reported to be detectable but low (normal range: 1.75 ± 0.17 mg/mL) in pituitary dwarfs and fail to increase after a provocative test for secretion via clonidine injection (30 µg/kg, IV) as they do in normal dogs. Insulin hypersensitivity has been demonstrated in pituitary dwarf dogs, probably due to a change in insulin receptor numbers or affinity of binding in response to the low level of growth hormone.

DIABETES INSIPIDUS

Central diabetes insipidus is caused by reduced secretion of antidiuretic hormone (ADH). When target cells in the kidney lack the biochemical machinery necessary to respond to the secretion of normal or increased circulating levels of ADH, nephrogenic diabetes insipidus results. It occurs infrequently in dogs, cats, and laboratory rats, and rarely in other animals.

Etiology: The hypophyseal form develops as a result of compression and destruction of the pars nervosa, infundibular stalk, or supraoptic nucleus in the hypothalamus. The lesions responsible for the disruption of ADH synthesis or secretion in hypophyseal diabetes insipidus include large pituitary neoplasms (endocrinologically active or inactive), a dorsally expanding cyst or inflammatory granuloma, and traumatic injury to the skull with hemorrhage and glial proliferation in the neurohypophyseal system.

Clinical Findings: Affected animals excrete large volumes of hypotonic urine and drink equally large amounts of water. Urine osmolality is decreased below normal plasma osmolality (~300 mOsm/kg) in both hypophyseal and nephrogenic forms, even if the animal is deprived of water. The increase of urine osmolality above that of plasma in response to exogenous ADH in the hypophyseal form, but not in the nephrogenic form, is useful in the clinical differentiation of the 2 forms of the disease.

Lesions: The posterior lobe, infundibular stalk, and hypothalamus are compressed or disrupted by neoplastic cells. This interrupts the nonmyelinated axons that transport ADH from its site of production (hypothalamus) to its site of release (pars nervosa).

Diagnosis: This is based on chronic polyuria that does not respond to dehydration and is not due to primary renal disease. To evaluate the ability to concentrate urine, a water deprivation test should be done if the animal is not dehydrated and does not have renal disease. The bladder is emptied, and water and food are withheld (usually 3-8 hr) to provide a maximum stimulus for ADH secretion. The animal should be monitored carefully to prevent a loss of >5% body wt and severe dehydration. Urine and plasma osmolality should be determined; however, because these tests are not readily available to most practitioners, urine specific gravity is frequently used instead. At the end of the test, urine specific gravity is >1.025 in those animals with only a partial ADH deficiency or with antagonism to ADH action caused by hypercortisolism. There is little change in specific gravity in those animals with a complete lack of ADH activity, whether due to a primary loss of ADH or to unresponsiveness of the kidneys.

An ADH response test should follow to differentiate among conditions that may result in large volumes of urine that is chronically low in specific gravity but otherwise normal. These include nephrogenic diabetes insipidus (an inability of the kidneys to respond to ADH), psychogenic diabetes insipidus (a polydipsia in response to some psychological disturbance but a normal response to ADH), and hypercortisolism (which results in a partial deficiency of ADH activity due to the antagonistic effect of cortisol on ADH activity in the kidneys). This test also can be used to evaluate animals in which a water deprivation test could not be performed. Urine specific gravity is determined at the start of the test; desmopressin acetate is administered (2-4 drops in the conjunctival sac); the bladder is emptied at 2 hr; and urine specific gravity is measured 4, 8, 12, 18, and 24 hr after ADH administration. Specific gravity peaks at >1.026 in animals with a primary ADH deficiency, is significantly increased above the level induced with water deprivation in those with a partial deficiency in ADH activity, and shows little change in those with nephrogenic diabetes insipidus.

If osmolality is measured, the ratio of urine to plasma osmolality after water deprivation is >3 in normal animals, 1.8-3 in those with moderate ADH deficiency, and <1.8 in those with severe deficiency. The ratio of urine osmolality after ADH administration as compared with water deprivation is >2 in animals with primary ADH deficiency, between 1.1 and 2 in those with inhibitors to ADH action, and <1.1 in those unresponsive to ADH.

As an alternative to the water deprivation test, or in cases in which this test fails to establish a definitive diagnosis, a closely monitored therapeutic trial with desmopressin (see below) can be performed. Again, all other causes of polyuria and polydipsia should initially be ruled out, limiting the differential diagnosis to central diabetes insipidus, nephrogenic diabetes insipidus, and psychogenic polydipsia. For cats, the owner should measure the animal's 24-hr water intake 2-3 days before the therapeutic trial with desmopressin, allowing free-choice water intake. The intranasal preparation of desmopressin is administered in the conjunctival sac (1-4 drops, BID) for 3-5 days. A dramatic reduction in water intake (>50%) during the first treatment day would strongly suggest an ADH deficiency and a diagnosis of central diabetes insipidus or partial nephrogenic diabetes insipidus.

Diabetes insipidus also needs to be distinguished from other diseases with polyuria. The most common are diabetes mellitus with glycosuria and high urine specific gravity, and chronic nephritis with a urine specific gravity that is usually low and shows evidence of renal failure (protein, casts, etc).

Treatment: Polyuria may be controlled using desmopressin acetate, a synthetic analog of ADH. The initial dose is 2 drops applied to the nasal mucosae or conjunctivae; this is gradually increased until the minimal effective dose is determined. Maximal effect usually occurs in 2-6 hr and lasts for 10-12 hr. Water should not be restricted. Treatment should be continued SID or BID for the life of the animal.

FELINE ACROMEGALY

Acromegaly, or hypersomatotropism, results from chronic, excessive secretion of growth hormone in the adult animal. Acromegaly in cats is caused by a growth-hormone-secreting tumor of the anterior pituitary. In cats, these tumors grow slowly and may be present for a long time before clinical signs appear.

Clinical Findings: Feline acromegaly occurs in older (8-14 yr) cats and appears to be more common in males. Clinical signs of uncontrolled diabetes mellitus are often the first sign of acromegaly in cats; therefore, polydipsia, polyuria, and polyphagia are the most common presenting signs. Net weight gain of lean body mass in cats with uncontrolled diabetes mellitus is a key sign of acromegaly. Organomegaly including renomegaly, hepatomegaly, and enlargement of endocrine organs is also seen. Some cats show the classic enlargement of extremities, body size, jaw, tongue, and forehead that is characteristic of acromegaly in people. Some of the most striking manifestations occur in the musculoskeletal system and include an increase in muscle mass and growth of the acral segments of the body including the paws, chin, and skull. Cardiovascular abnormalities such as cardiomegaly (radiographic and echocardiographic), systolic murmurs, and congestive heart failure develop late in the disease course. Azotemia also develops late in the course of the disease in ~50% of acromegalic cats. Neurologic signs of acromegaly in humans, such as peripheral neuropathies (paresthesias, carpal tunnel syndrome, sensory and motor defects) and parasellar manifestations (headache and visual field defects), are not generally detected in acromegalic cats.

Impaired glucose tolerance and insulin resistance resulting in diabetes mellitus are seen in all cats with acromegaly. Measurement of endogenous insulin reveals dramatically increased serum insulin concentrations. Despite severe insulin resistance and hyperglycemia, ketosis is rare. Feline acromegaly should be suspected in any diabetic cat that has severe insulin resistance (insulin requirement >20 U/cat/day). Hypercholesterolemia and mild increases in liver enzymes are attributed to the diabetic state. Hyperphosphatemia without azotemia is also a common clinicopathologic finding. Urinalysis is unremarkable except for persistent proteinuria.

Lesions: Gross necropsy findings in acromegalic cats may include a large expansile pituitary mass, hypertrophic cardiomyopathy with marked left ventricular and septal hypertrophy (early) or dilated cardiomyopathy (late), hepatomegaly, renomegaly, degenerative joint disease, lumbar vertebral spondylosis, moderate enlargement of the parathyroid glands, adrenocortical hyperplasia, and diffuse enlargement of the pancreas with multifocal nodular hyperplasia. Histopathologic examination of the endocrine glands reveals acidophil adenoma of the pituitary; adenomatous hyperplasia of the thyroid gland; and nodular hyperplasia of the adrenal cortices, parathyroid glands, and pancreas.

Diagnosis: A definitive diagnosis requires measurement of increased plasma growth hormone or insulin-like growth factor 1 (IGF-1) concentrations in suspected cases. Unfortunately, feline growth hormone assays are no longer available. Serum IGF-1 concentrations are often dramatically increased in acromegalic cats (as in affected people). Currently, the most definitive diagnostic test is computed tomography of the pituitary region. Results of computed tomography, coupled with the exclusion of other disorders that cause insulin resistance (hyperthyroidism, hyperadrenocorticism) and clinical signs and laboratory abnormalities, support a diagnosis of acromegaly.

Treatment and Prognosis: Medical therapy in people includes the use of dopamine agonists, such as bromocriptine, and somatostatin analogs (octreotide). Treatment with octreotide has been unsuccessful in acromegalic cats. The lack of efficacy of the long-acting somatostatin analogs may result from species-specific tissue binding. Radiation therapy probably offers the greatest chance for success with low rates of morbidity and mortality. The disadvantages include the slow rate of tumor shrinkage (>3 yr) and the occurrence of hypopituitarism, cranial and optic nerve damage, and radiation injury to the hypothalamus.

The short-term prognosis in cats with untreated acromegaly is fair to good. Insulin resistance is generally controlled satisfactorily by using large doses of insulin divided into several daily doses. Mild cardiac disease can be managed with diuretics and vasodilators. The longterm prognosis is relatively poor, however, and most cats die of congestive heart failure, chronic renal failure, or signs of an expanding pituitary mass. The longterm prognosis may improve with early diagnosis and treatment.

THE THYROID GLAND

All vertebrates have a thyroid gland. In mammals, it is usually bilobed and located just caudal to the larynx, adjacent to the lateral surface of the trachea. The 2 lobes may be connected by a fibrous isthmus (eg, ruminants, horses), or a connecting isthmus may be indistinct (eg, dogs, cats). The gland is extremely vascular. In birds, it is found within the thoracic cavity; both lobes are located near the syrinx, adjacent to the carotid artery near the origin of the vertebral artery.

Ectopic or accessory thyroid tissue is relatively common in most species, especially dogs and cats. It may be located anywhere from the larynx to the diaphragm and may be responsible for maintaining normal thyroid function after surgical thyroidectomy. In addition, ectopic thyroid tissue occasionally is the site of hyperplasia or neoplasia.

Physiology: Thyroid hormones are the only iodinated organic compounds in the body. Thyroxine (T_4) is the main secretory product of the normal thyroid gland. However, the gland also secretes 3,5,3'-triiodothyronine (T_3), reverse T_3, and other deiodinated metabolites. T_3 is ~3-5 times more potent than T_4, while reverse T_3 is thyromimetically inactive.

Although all T_4 is secreted by the thyroid, a considerable amount of T_3 is derived from T_4; therefore, T_4 has been called a prohormone. Its activation to the more potent T_3 is a step regulated individually by peripheral tissues.

Thyroid hormone secretion is regulated primarily via negative-feedback control through the coordinated response of the hypothalamic-pituitary-thyroid axis: thyrotropin-releasing hormone (TRH) binds to the thyrotroph cell in the pituitary and stimulates secretion of thyrotropin (thyroid-stimulating hormone, TSH), which binds to the follicular cell membrane and stimulates thyroid hormone synthesis and secretion.

Thyroid hormones are water-insoluble lipophilic compounds that are bound to plasma proteins (thyroxine-binding protein, thyroxine-binding prealbumin [transthyretin], and albumin). The major function of the thyroid-hormone-binding proteins is probably to provide a hormone reservoir in the plasma and to "buffer" hormone delivery into tissue. In the healthy euthyroid animal, 0.1% of total serum T_4 is free (not bound to thyroid-hormone-binding proteins), whereas ~1% of circulating T_3 is free. Current evidence suggests that the fractions of circulating free T_4 and free T_3 determine the amount of hormone that is available for uptake by tissues.

Action of Thyroid Hormones: Thyroid hormones act on many different cellular processes; however, no single reaction or metabolic event can be equated with their action. Although both T_4 and T_3 have intrinsic metabolic activity, T_3 is 3-5 times more potent in binding to the nuclear receptors and similarly more potent in stimulating oxygen consumption.

Effects of thyroid hormones generally are divided into 2 categories: those that manifest within minutes to hours after hormone receptor binding and do not require protein synthesis, and those that manifest later (usually >6 hr) and require synthesis of new proteins. About half the increase in oxygen consumption produced by thyroid hormones is related to activation of the plasma-membrane-bound Na^+/K^+ATPase; thyroid hormones also stimulate mitochondrial oxygen consumption. These changes are linked directly to the calorigenic effect of thyroid hormones. More chronic effects invariably are related to the cellular actions that require interaction with nuclear T_3 receptors, followed by an increase in protein synthesis crucial to physiologic processes such as growth, differentiation, proliferation, and maturation.

Thyroid hormones, in physiologic quantities, are anabolic. In conjunction with growth hormone and insulin, protein synthesis is stimulated and nitrogen excretion is reduced. However, in excess (hyperthyroidism), they can be catabolic, with increased gluconeogenesis, protein breakdown, and nitrogen wasting.

HYPOTHYROIDISM

In hypothyroidism, impaired production and secretion of the thyroid hormones result in a decreased metabolic rate. This disorder is most common in dogs but also develops rarely in other species, including cats, horses, and other large domestic animals.

Etiology: Although dysfunction anywhere in the hypothalamic-pituitary-thyroid axis may result in thyroid hormone deficiency, >95% of clinical cases of hypothyroidism in dogs appear to result from destruction of the thyroid gland itself (primary hypothyroidism). The 2 most common causes of adult-onset primary hypothyroidism in dogs include lymphocytic thyroiditis and idiopathic atrophy of the thyroid gland. Lymphocytic thyroiditis, probably immune-mediated, is characterized histologically by a diffuse infiltration of the gland by lymphocytes, plasma cells, and macrophages, and results in progressive destruction of follicles and secondary fibrosis. Idiopathic atrophy of the thyroid gland is characterized histologically by loss of thyroid parenchyma and replacement by adipose tissue. (*See also* AUTOIMMUNE THYROIDITIS, p 656.)

In dogs, the most common cause of secondary hypothyroidism is destruction of pituitary thyrotrophs by an expanding, space-occupying tumor. Because of the nonselective nature of the resulting compressive atrophy and replacement of pituitary tissue by such large tumors, deficiencies of other (one or more) pituitary hormones also usually occur.

Other rare forms of hypothyroidism in dogs include neoplastic destruction of thyroid tissue and congenital (or juvenile-onset) hypothyroidism. Congenital primary hypothyroidism may result from one of various forms of thyroid dysgenesis (eg, athyreosis, thyroid hypoplasia) or from dyshormonogenesis (usually an inherited inability to organify iodide). Congenital secondary hypothyroidism (associated with clinical signs of disproportionate dwarfism, lethargy, gait abnormalities, and constipation) has been documented in a family of Giant Schnauzers. Congenital secondary hypothyroidism also has been reported in German Shepherds with pituitary dwarfism associated with a cystic

Rathke's pouch. However, the degree of TSH deficiency in these dogs is variable, and clinical signs are usually caused primarily by deficiency of growth hormone (rather than thyroid hormone).

In cats, iatrogenic hypothyroidism is the most common form. Hypothyroidism develops in these cats after treatment for hyperthyroidism with radioiodine, surgical thyroidectomy, or use of an antithyroid drug. Although naturally occurring hypothyroidism is an extremely rare disorder in adult cats, congenital or juvenile-onset hypothyroidism does also occur. Recognized causes of congenital hypothyroidism in the cat include intrathyroidal defects in thyroid hormone biosynthesis (dyshormonogenesis), an inability of the thyroid gland to respond to TSH, and thyroid dysgenesis. All reported cats with hypothyroidism have had the primary (thyroidal) disorder. Secondary (pituitary) or tertiary (hypothalamic) hypothyroidism have not been described in either the juvenile or adult cat.

In foals, congenital hypothyroidism may develop when pregnant mares graze plants that contain goitrogens, or are fed diets either deficient in or containing excessive amounts of iodine. Most commonly, congenital hypothyroidism develops in association with a specific syndrome of neonatal foals characterized by thyroid gland hyperplasia together with multiple congenital musculoskeletal anomalies. This syndrome, reported most commonly in western Canada, has been referred to as either thyroid hyperplasia and musculoskeletal deformities syndrome, or congenital hypothyroidism and dysmaturity syndrome and may be related to feeding a high nitrate diet to pregnant mares (see CONGENITAL HYPOTHYROIDISM AND DYSMATURITY SYNDROME OF FOALS, p 466). In adult horses, hypothyroidism appears to be very rare but, as in other species, is commonly misdiagnosed.

Clinical Findings: Although onset is variable, hypothyroidism is most common in dogs 4-10 yr old. It usually affects mid- to large-size breeds and is rare in toy and miniature breeds. Breeds reported to be predisposed include the Golden Retriever, Doberman Pinscher, Irish Setter, Miniature Schnauzer, Dachshund, Cocker Spaniel, and Airedale Terrier. There does not appear to be a sex predilection, but spayed females appear to have a higher risk of developing hypothyroidism than intact females.

A deficiency of thyroid hormone affects the function of all organ systems; as a result, clinical signs are diffuse, variable, often nonspecific, and rarely pathognomonic. While the disorder should be highly suspect, overdiagnosis should be avoided, because many diseases, especially those of the skin, can easily be misdiagnosed as hypothyroidism.

Many of the clinical signs associated with canine hypothyroidism are directly related to slowing of cellular metabolism, which results in development of mental dullness, lethargy, intolerance of exercise, and weight gain without a corresponding increase in appetite. Mild to marked obesity develops in some dogs. Difficulty maintaining body temperature may lead to frank hypothermia; the classic hypothyroid dog is a heat-seeker. Alterations in the skin and coat are common. Dryness, excessive shedding, and retarded regrowth of hair are usually the earliest dermatologic changes. Nonpruritic hair thinning or alopecia (usually bilaterally symmetric) that may involve the ventral and lateral trunk, the caudal surfaces of the thighs, dorsum of the tail, ventral neck, and the dorsum of the nose occurs in about two-thirds of dogs with hypothyroidism. Alopecia, sometimes associated with hyperpigmentation, often starts over points of wear. Occasionally, secondary pyoderma (which may produce pruritus) is observed.

In moderate to severe cases, thickening of the skin occurs secondary to accumulation of glycosaminoglycans (mostly hyaluronic acid) in the dermis. In such cases, myxedema is most common on the forehead and face, resulting in a puffy appearance and thickened skin folds above the eyes. This puffiness, together with slight drooping of the upper eyelid, gives some dogs a "tragic" facial expression. These changes also have been described in the GI tract, heart, and skeletal muscles.

In intact dogs, hypothyroidism may cause various reproductive disturbances: in females, failure to cycle (anestrus) or sporadic cycling, infertility, abortion, or poor litter survival; and in males, lack of libido, testicular atrophy, hypospermia, or infertility.

Myxedema coma, a rare syndrome, is the extreme expression of severe hypothyroidism. The course can develop rapidly; lethargy progresses to stupor and then coma. The common signs of hypothyroidism (eg, hair loss) are usually present, but other signs, such as hypoventilation, hypotension, bradycardia, and profound hypothermia, are usually seen as well.

During the fetal period and in the first few months of postnatal life, thyroid hormones are crucial for growth and development of the skeleton and CNS. Therefore, in addition to the well-recognized signs of adult-onset hypothyroidism, disproportionate dwarfism and impaired mental development (cretinism) are prominent signs of congenital and juvenile-onset hypothyroidism. In primary congenital hypothyroidism, enlargement of the thyroid gland (goiter) also may be detected, depending on the cause of the hypothyroidism. Radiographic signs of epiphyseal dysgenesis (underdeveloped epiphyses throughout the long bones), shortened vertebral bodies, and delayed epiphyseal closure are common.

In dogs with congenital hypopituitarism (pituitary dwarfism, p 457), there may be variable degrees of thyroidal, adrenocortical, and gonadal deficiency, but clinical signs are primarily related to growth hormone deficiency. Signs include proportionate dwarfism (rather than the disproportionate form of dwarfism characteristic of congenital hypothyroidism), loss of primary guard hairs with retention of the puppy coat, hyperpigmentation of the skin, and bilaterally symmetric alopecia of the trunk.

In adult cats, clinical signs associated with hypothyroidism usually include lethargy, dullness, nonpruritic seborrhea sicca, hypothermia, and occasionally bradycardia. Obesity may develop, especially in cats with iatrogenic hypothyroidism, but it is not a consistent sign. Bilaterally symmetric alopecia, with the exception of pinnal involvement, does not appear to develop, but focal areas of alopecia over the craniolateral carpi, caudal hocks, and dorsal and lateral tailbase have occasionally been observed. In young cats with congenital or juvenile-onset hypothyroidism, the clinical signs include disproportionate dwarfism, severe lethargy, mental dullness, constipation, and bradycardia.

Diagnosis: In dogs, hypothyroidism is probably one of the most overdiagnosed diseases. Many diseases and conditions can mimic hypothyroidism, and some of the clinical signs, even in dogs with normal thyroid function, can improve following administration of exogenous thyroid hormone. In addition, a variety of nonthyroidal factors (eg, nonthyroid illness and prior administration of certain drugs) can lead to low serum thyroid hormone measurements in euthyroid dogs, cats, and other species. Definitive diagnosis of canine hypothyroidism requires careful attention to clinical signs, routine laboratory testing, and demonstration of low serum concentrations of total or free thyroid hormones that are unresponsive to TSH administration.

There are well-recognized clinicopathologic abnormalities associated with hypothyroidism, the severity of which usually correlates with the severity and chronicity of the hypothyroid state. These alterations are nonspecific and may be associated with many other diseases in dogs. Their presence, however, adds supportive evidence for a diagnosis of hypothyroidism in a dog with appropriate clinical signs. The classic hematologic finding associated with hypothyroidism is a normocytic, normochromic, nonregenerative anemia. The classic serum biochemical abnormality is hypercholesterolemia, which occurs in ~80% of dogs with hypothyroidism. The value of serum cholesterol determination as a screening test for hypothyroidism cannot be overemphasized, as cholesterol concentrations represent a sensitive but inexpensive biochemical marker for this disease in dogs. Other clinicopathologic abnormalities may include high serum concentrations of triglycerides, alkaline phosphatase, and creatine kinase.

Because T_3 is the most potent thyroid hormone at the cellular level, it would seem logical to measure its concentration for diagnostic purposes. However, serum T_3 concentrations may be low, normal, or (occasionally) high in dogs with documented hypothyroidism. The diagnostic value of a serum T_3 determination is particularly weak during early thyroid failure because the "failing" thyroid tends to increase the relative synthesis and secretion of T_3 versus T_4. In the hypothyroid dog in which values for serum T_3 are high, anti-T_3 antibodies, which produce spurious results in most T_3 radioimmunoassays, should be suspected.

The determination of basal serum total T_4 concentration by radioimmunoassay techniques may provide important information to rule out a diagnosis of hypothyroidism.

Because T_4 is produced only by the thyroid gland, hypothyroid animals can, in most cases, be distinguished based on a low resting serum total T_4 concentration. However, many nonthyroidal illnesses and administration of various drugs including glucocorticoids, sulfonamides, anticonvulsants (eg, phenobarbital), NSAID, and radiocontrast agents may "falsely" lower serum T_4 concentrations in dogs. Even when historical and physical findings do not suggest other factors that would lower serum T_4, the diagnosis of hypothyroidism is best confirmed by measuring free T_4 concentration (by dialysis), which is affected to a much lesser degree by nonthyroidal illness or drug therapy than is the total T_4 concentration.

Free T_4 is the fraction of circulating thyroxine that is not bound to plasma proteins (normally 0.1% of total T_4). Because the free concentration of T_4 reflects the hormone available for entry into cells, free T_4 determinations provide a more consistent assessment of thyroid status at the tissue level than measurement of total T_4. Furthermore, free T_4 is not as likely as total T_4 to be affected by nonthyroidal illness or drug therapy. Determination of free T_4 is most accurately performed by methods that include a dialysis step (eg, equilibrium dialysis). The finding of a low free T_4 concentration is consistent with the diagnosis of hypothyroidism, as concentrations usually remain within the reference range in animals with nonthyroidal illness.

Determination of serum TSH concentrations by use of a valid species-specific TSH assay can be a useful adjunctive test for hypothyroidism in dogs and horses. Animals with primary hypothyroidism (by far the most common type) would be expected to have low serum T_4 and/or free T_4 concentrations with high endogenous TSH concentrations. Unfortunately, serum TSH concentrations remain within the reference range in 20-40% of dogs with confirmed hypothyroidism. Although a few dogs with normal serum TSH concentrations have secondary hypothyroidism, pituitary TSH deficiency is extremely rare, and most dogs with normal TSH concentrations (ie, a false-negative result) have primary hypothyroidism. In contrast, falsely high serum TSH concentrations (ie, a false-positive result) are occasionally found in euthyroid dogs with nonthyroidal illness. Thus, serum TSH determinations should never be evaluated alone, but always in conjunction with the dog's history, routine laboratory abnormalities, and total or free T_4 concentrations.

Circulating antithyroglobulin antibodies can be detected in up to half of dogs with hypothyroidism and are believed to reflect a state of autoimmune thyroiditis. Measurement of these antibodies in breeding studs and bitches has been proposed as a method to identify dogs with autoimmune thyroid disease. Serum thyroglobulin autoantibody determinations may be a useful adjunctive diagnostic aid for hypothyroidism but should not be used alone. Identification of these autoantibodies support the diagnosis if the dog has clinical signs and other laboratory data consistent with the disorder.

Although extremely rare in dogs, circulating thyroid hormone autoantibodies (anti-T_3 or anti-T_4 antibodies) are occasionally detected and also are believed to reflect a state of autoimmune thyroiditis. These antibodies, which can be formed against either T_3 or T_4 (or both), produce a spurious increase in the apparent T_3 or T_4 concentrations, into the hyperthyroid range in most dogs. Of all the thyroid hormones, only measurement of free T_4 (by dialysis) is not affected by autoantibodies directed at T_4 or T_3 because the serum autoantibodies are removed in the dialysis step. Therefore, if hypothyroidism is suspected in a dog with circulating thyroid hormone autoantibodies, serum free T_4 concentration should be determined to help confirm the diagnosis.

Treatment: Thyroxine (T_4) is the thyroid hormone replacement compound of choice in dogs. With few exceptions, replacement therapy is necessary for the remainder of the dog's life; careful initial diagnosis and tailoring of treatment is essential. The reported replacement dosages for T_4 in dogs range from a total dose of 0.01-0.02 mg/lb (0.02-0.04 mg/kg), daily, given once or divided BID.

The most important indicator of the success of therapy is clinical improvement. Reversal of changes in coat and body weight should be assessed only after 1-2 mo of therapy. When clinical improvement is marginal or signs of thyrotoxicosis are seen, the clinical observations can be supported by therapeutic monitoring of serum thyroid hormone concentrations ("post-pill testing"). With once-daily administration of T_4, the peak serum concentration of T_4 generally should be slightly high to high-normal 4-8 hr after dosing and should be low-normal to normal 24 hr after dosing. Animals on BID administration probably can be checked at any time, but peak concentrations can be expected at the middle of the dosing interval (4-8 hr) and the nadir just before the next dose. When the dose is stabilized, serum T_4 (with or without T_3) concentrations should be checked 1-2 times per year.

If clinical signs of hypothyroidism remain despite the use of reasonable doses of thyroid hormone, the following must be considered: 1) the dose or frequency of administration is improper; 2) the owner is not complying with instructions or is not successfully administering the product; 3) the animal is not absorbing the product well, or is metabolizing and/or excreting it too rapidly; 4) the product is outdated; or 5) the diagnosis is incorrect.

NON-NEOPLASTIC ENLARGEMENT OF THE THYROID GLAND
(Goiter)

Non-neoplastic and noninflammatory enlargements of the thyroid gland develop in all domestic mammals as well as birds. The major causes of goiter include iodine deficiency, goitrogenic substances, dietary iodine excess, and inherited enzyme defects in the biosynthesis of thyroid hormones. Many animals with goiter appear to remain euthyroid, but clinical signs of hypothyroidism may develop in some, especially in newborns.

Iodine Deficiency: Thyroid hyperplasia due to iodine deficiency was common in many goitrogenic areas throughout the world before the widespread supplementation of iodized salt to animal diets. Although outbreaks of iodine-deficient goiter are now sporadic and fewer animals are affected, iodine deficiency is still responsible for most goiters seen in large domestic animals.

Insufficient iodine reduces the ability of the thyroid to make thyroid hormone. With reduced circulating thyroid hormone levels, the pituitary secretes more TSH, which acts as a stimulus for hyperplasia of the thyroid gland and goiter. The hyperplastic gland may, and usually does, compensate for the reduced availability of iodine; therefore, goiter is in no way synonymous with hypothyroidism. However, animals born to females on iodine-deficient diets are more likely to develop severe thyroid enlargement and have clinical signs of hypothyroidism.

Goiter caused by iodine deficiency is most common in newborn pigs, lambs, calves, and foals in iodine-deficient areas. The thyroid lobes of the young animal usually are at least twice normal size, soft, and dark red. In severe cases, there is an accompanying lack of hair (especially in pigs) or wool (lambs). The neck is usually grossly enlarged, and the skin and other tissue may be thickened, flabby, and edematous. In mildly affected animals, treatment with iodized salt (containing >0.007% iodine) may resolve the goiter and associated clinical signs, but many die before or soon after birth. Prophylaxis is more effective than treatment. The use of stabilized iodized salt is recommended in all areas known or suspected to be iodine deficient.

Iodine Toxicity: Foals of dams fed excess iodine may develop extreme thyroid enlargement and die before birth or shortly thereafter. Clinical signs include general weakness, long hair, and marked limb abnormalities.

Goitrogenic Substances: Certain plants may produce goiter when ingested in sufficient amounts, especially in the absence of adequate iodine intake. Soybeans are most notable, but cabbage, rape, kale, and turnips all contain less potent goitrogens. Cooking or heating (and the usual processing of soybean meal) destroys the goitrogenic substance in these plants. All of the goitrogenic substances act by interfering with production of thyroid hormone. As with iodine deficiency, the pituitary responds to the reduced circulating thyroid hormone levels by increasing its secretion of TSH, which results in thyroid gland enlargement. In adult animals the disease is usually not significant, but severe thyroid enlargement and hypothyroidism may develop in newborns.

Congenital Hypothyroidism and Dysmaturity Syndrome of Foals: This syndrome of neonatal foals first recognized in the early 1980s is characterized by hyperplasia of the thyroid gland and multiple congenital musculoskeletal anomalies. It is most common in western Canada. Foals with this syndrome are born weak or dead with hyperplasia of the thyroid gland, flexural deformities of the forelimbs, ruptured tendons of the common digital extensor muscles, mandibular prognathia, and immature carpal and tarsal bones. The underlying etiology is unknown but may be the result of diets that contain high levels of nitrate (eg, greenfeed).

Familial Dyshormonogenetic Goiter: This has been reported in sheep, cattle, goats, and pigs, and appears to be inherited as an autosomal recessive trait. Essentially, it is a genetic enzyme defect in the biosynthesis of thyroid hormones. As with iodine deficiency, reduced thyroid hormone production leads to secretion of increased levels of TSH and subsequent goiter. Clinical signs may include subnormal growth rate, absence of normal wool development or a sparse coat, myxedematous swelling of subcutaneous tissues, and weakness. Many affected animals die shortly after birth or are very sensitive to adverse environmental conditions.

HYPERTHYROIDISM

Excessive secretion of the thyroid hormones, T_4 and T_3, results in signs that reflect an increased metabolic rate and produces clinical hyperthyroidism. It is most common in middle-aged to old cats but also develops rarely in dogs.

Functional thyroid adenoma (adenomatous hyperplasia) is the most common cause of feline hyperthyroidism; in ~70% of cases, both thyroid lobes are enlarged. Thyroid carcinoma, the primary cause of hyperthyroidism in dogs, is rare in cats (1-2% of hyperthyroidism cases).

Clinical Findings and Diagnosis: The most common signs include weight loss, increased appetite, hyperexcitability, polydipsia, polyuria, and palpable enlargement of the thyroid gland. GI signs are also common and may include vomiting, diarrhea, and increased fecal volume. Cardiovascular signs include tachycardia, systolic murmurs, dyspnea, cardiomegaly, and congestive heart failure. Rarely, hyperthyroid cats will exhibit apathetic signs (eg, anorexia, lethargy, and depression); weight loss remains a common sign in these cats.

High basal serum total thyroid hormone concentration is the hallmark of hyperthyroidism and confirms the diagnosis. Although serum total T_4 concentrations are high in most cats with hyperthyroidism, ~5-10% of cats have normal T_4 values. Most cats with normal serum T_4 values have either mild or early hyperthyroidism or hyperthyroidism with concurrent nonthyroidal illness, which has caused suppression of a high total T_4 concentration to within reference range limits. In these cats, a high free T_4 concentration along with consistent history and physical examination findings is diagnostic of hyperthyroidism.

Treatment: Cats with hyperthyroidism can be treated by radioiodine therapy, thyroidectomy, or chronic administration of an antithyroid drug. Radioactive iodine provides a simple, effective, and safe treatment and is considered the treatment of choice. The radioiodine is concentrated within the thyroid tumor, where it selectively irradiates and destroys hyperfunctioning thyroid tissue.

Surgical thyroidectomy is also an effective treatment for hyperthyroidism in cats. With unilateral thyroid tumors, hemithyroidectomy corrects the hyperthyroid state, and thyroxine supplementation usually is not necessary. For bilateral thyroid tumors, complete thyroidectomy is indicated, but parathyroid function must be preserved to avoid postoperative hypocalcemia. Thyroxine supplementation should be started 1-2 days after complete thyroidectomy. If iatrogenic hypoparathyroidism develops, treatment with vitamin D and calcium is also indicated.

Treatment with methimazole, an antithyroid drug, controls hyperthyroidism by blocking thyroid hormone synthesis. Propylthiouracil, another antithyroid drug, is not recommended for use in cats because of the high incidence of serious side effects (especially hemolytic anemia and thrombocytopenia). The recommended initial daily dose of methimazole is 10-15 mg in 2 or 3 divided doses. The dose is adjusted to maintain circulating thyroid hormone concentrations within the normal range and is given daily. Adverse effects, the more serious of which are agranulocytosis and thrombocytopenia, develop in <5% of treated cats. If this occurs, methimazole should be discontinued and supportive therapy instituted; these adverse reactions should resolve within 2 wk. To maintain normal levels of thyroid hormone and to monitor for adverse reactions during the first 3 mo of treatment (when the most serious side effects associated with methimazole therapy develop), complete blood counts and serum thyroid hormone determinations should be repeated at 2- to 4-wk intervals, and the drug dose adjusted as necessary. Subsequently, serum T_4 concentrations should be measured at 3- to 6-mo intervals to monitor dosage requirements and response to treatment.

NEUROENDOCRINE TISSUE TUMORS

Neuroendocrine tissues derived from the embryonic neural crest are widely dispersed throughout the body. In mammals, they are in the center of the adrenal gland and are concerned with the synthesis and secretion of the catecholamine hormones (epinephrine and norepinephrine). C-cells in the mammalian thyroid gland also are derived from the neural crest and, during early embryonic development, are incorporated into the last (ultimobranchial) pharyngeal pouch, which subsequently fuses with each thyroid lobe. C-cells are involved in the biosynthesis of calcitonin, a hormone involved in the regulation of calcium homeostasis and skeletal turnover.

Tumors develop occasionally from neuroendocrine cells in the adrenal medulla, thyroid, and aortic and carotid bodies. They are clinically significant due to physical disruption of adjacent normal tissues by the enlarging mass and possibly to autonomous secretion of excess hormone.

ADRENAL MEDULLA

Adrenal Medullary Hyperplasia: Diffuse or nodular adrenal medullary hyperplasia appears to precede the development of pheochromocytoma in bulls with C-cell tumors of the thyroid gland. This diffuse proliferation of chromaffin cells is nonencapsulated but compresses the surrounding adrenal cortex. In bulls with prominent diffuse medullary hyperplasia, there are often a few small foci of intense nodular proliferation of medullary cells.

Pheochromocytomas: These tumors of chromaffin cells are almost always located in the adrenal glands. They are the most common tumors in the adrenal medulla of animals; they develop most often in cattle, laboratory rats, and dogs, and are infrequent in other domestic animals. In bulls and rats, pheochromocytomas develop concurrently with calcitonin-secreting C-cell tumors of the thyroid gland, possibly as a neoplastic transformation of multiple types of endocrine cells of neuroectodermal origin in the same individual. Malignant pheochromocytoma designates a medullary tumor that invades through the adrenal capsule into adjacent structures (eg, posterior vena cava) or metastasizes to distant sites (eg, liver, regional lymph nodes, or lungs), or both. Functional pheochromocytomas are reported infrequently in animals; however, several dogs and horses with pheochromocytomas have had tachycardia, edema, and cardiac hypertrophy attributed to excess catecholamine secretion. It appears that horses may have a syndrome similar to the multiple endocrine neoplasia noted in humans with concurrent adrenal and thyroid disease.

Although size varies considerably, pheochromocytomas may be large (≥10 cm in diameter) and incorporate most of the affected adrenal. A small remnant of the adrenal gland often can be found at one pole. Smaller tumors are well encapsulated by a thin, compressed rim of adrenal cortex. Large pheochromocytomas are multilobular and variegated, and they may exert pressure on and invade adjacent tissues, particularly the vena cava and aorta. In dogs, ~50% of pheochromocytomas metastasize to the liver, regional lymph nodes, spleen, and lungs.

THYROID C-CELL TUMORS

Tumors derived from C-cells (parafollicular, ultimobranchial cells) of the thyroid gland are most common in adult to aged bulls and horses and in certain strains of laboratory rats. A high percentage of aged bulls has been reported to develop C-cell tumors (≥30%) or hyperplasia of C-cells and ultimobranchial derivatives (≥15-20%). These have not been seen in cows fed similar diets. The incidence in bulls increases with advancing age and is often associated with development of increased vertebral density. Multiple endocrine tumors, especially bilateral pheochromocytomas and occasionally pituitary adenomas, are detected coincidentally in bulls with C-cell tumors. A high frequency of thyroid C-cell tumors and pheochromocytomas has been reported in a family of Guernsey bulls, which suggests an autosomal dominant pattern of inheritance. A diffuse or nodular hyperplasia of secretory cells in the adrenal medulla often precedes the development of pheochromocytoma.

Adenomas: C-cell adenomas appear in one or both thyroid lobes as discrete, single or multiple, gray to tan nodules. Adenomas are smaller (~1-3 cm in diameter) than carcinomas and are separated from the thyroid parenchyma by a thin, fibrous connective tissue capsule. The adjacent thyroid is compressed but not invaded by the tumor. In horses, C-cell adenomas may result in a palpable enlargement in the anterior cervical region. Larger C-cell adenomas incorporate most of the thyroid lobe, but a rim of dark brown-red thyroid often is present on one side.

Carcinomas: Thyroid C-cell carcinomas cause extensive multinodular enlargements of one or both thyroid lobes and may incorporate the entire thyroid gland. Multiple metastases in anterior cervical lymph nodes usually are large and have areas of necrosis and hemorrhage. Pulmonary metastases are infrequent and appear as discrete tan nodules throughout all lobes of the lung.

The chronic stimulation of C-cells by longterm dietary intake of excess calcium may be related to the high incidence of these tumors in bulls; adult bulls frequently were fed diets with 3.5-6 times the amount of calcium normally recommended for maintenance, and incidence of the tumors declined significantly when calcium intake was reduced.

Syndromes associated with abnormalities in the secretion of calcitonin are recognized much less frequently than disorders involving parathyroid hormone (PTH). Hypersecretion of calcitonin has been reported in people, bulls, and laboratory rats with medullary (ultimobranchial) thyroid neoplasms derived from C-cells. Osteosclerotic changes have been reported in bulls with this syndrome, but the relationship of longterm excess calcitonin secretion to the pathogenesis of the skeletal lesions and their occurrence in other species is unclear.

In dogs, the histologic grading of thyroid carcinoma has been important in prognosis, although histologic type has not. Of greater importance is the volume of tumor and its relationship to the potential for metastasis; also, the more deeply fixed the tumor is to underlying structures, the less likely surgical resection will be complete. Surgery is the primary therapy, but some form of adjuvant therapy is reasonable because of the potential for metastatic spread and residual nonresectable tissue. A combination of radiotherapy and chemotherapy would be ideal in theory, and there is increasing interest in such combined therapy. For the rather rare functional thyroid carcinoma in dogs, treatment with ^{131}I would be a reasonable choice, but institutions where such therapy can be done are few and the technical problems (disposal of all urine and feces in accordance with proper radiation safety guidelines) are great.

CHEMORECEPTOR ORGANS

Chemoreceptor organs are sensitive barometers of changes in the carbon dioxide and oxygen content and pH of the blood and aid in the regulation of respiration and circulation. Although chemoreceptor tissue appears to be widely distributed in the body, tumors develop principally in the aortic (more frequent in animals) and carotid bodies (more frequent in humans). These tumors are found primarily in dogs and rarely in cats and cattle. Brachycephalic breeds of dogs, such as the Boxer and Boston Terrier, are predisposed to tumors of the aortic and carotid bodies.

Aortic body tumors appear most frequently as single masses or as multiple nodules within the pericardial sac near the base of the heart. They vary considerably in size (0.5-12.5 cm), with carcinomas generally larger than adenomas. Solitary, small adenomas either are attached to the adventitia of the pulmonary artery and ascending aorta, or are embedded in the adipose connective tissue between these major vascular trunks. Larger adenomas may indent the atria or displace the trachea, are multilobular, and partially surround the major arterial trunks at the base of the heart.

In dogs, malignant aortic body tumors occur less frequently than adenomas. Carcinomas may infiltrate the wall of the pulmonary artery to form papillary projections into the lumen or invade through the wall into the lumen of the atria. Although tumor cells often invade blood vessels, metastases to the lungs and liver are infrequent in dogs with aortic body carcinomas. Nonetheless, the local and physiologic effects are important, including those of adenomas.

Aortic body tumors in animals are not functional (ie, they do not secrete excess hormone into the circulation) but, as space-occupying lesions, may result in various functional disturbances. These include manifestations of cardiac decompensation due to pressure on the atria or vena cava (or both) associated with larger aortic body adenomas and carcinomas. Aortic body tumors tend to be more benign than carotid body tumors. They grow slowly by expansion and exert pressure on the vena cava and atria. Aortic body carcinomas may invade locally into the atria, pericardium, and adjacent large, thin-walled vessels.

Carotid body tumors arise near the bifurcation of the common carotid artery, usually as a unilateral slow-growing mass. Adenomas are usually 1-4 cm in diameter. The bifurcation of the carotid artery is incorporated in the mass, and tumor cells are firmly adherent to the tunica adventitia. Complete excision or biopsy often is difficult due to the high degree of vascularity and intimate relationship with major arterial trunks in the neck.

Malignant carotid body tumors are larger and more coarsely multinodular then adenomas. Although carcinomas appear to be encapsulated, tumor cells invade the capsule and penetrate into the walls of adjacent vessels and lymphatics. The external jugular vein and several cranial nerves may be incorporated by the neoplasm. Metastases of carotid body tumors occur in ~30% of cases and have been found in the lung, bronchial and mediastinal lymph nodes, liver, pancreas, and kidneys. Multicentric neoplastic transformation of chemoreceptor tissue occurs frequently in brachycephalic breeds of dogs.

The histologic characteristics of chemoreceptor tumors ("chemodectomas") are essentially similar whether derived from the carotid or aortic body.

Although the etiology of carotid and aortic body tumors is unknown, it has been suggested that a genetic predisposition aggravated by chronic hypoxia may account for the higher risk in certain brachycephalic breeds. Carotid bodies of several mammalian species, including dogs, have undergone hyperplasia when subjected to chronic hypoxia by living in a high-altitude environment.

■ ■ ■

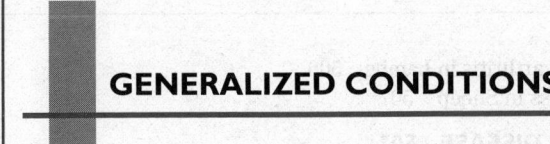

GENERALIZED CONDITIONS

ACTINOBACILLOSIS

Actinobacillosis, caused by gram-negative coccobacilli in the genus *Actinobacillus*, may present in several different forms, depending on the specific agent and the host. Soft-tissue infections are common, and lymph node involvement is frequently a step in systemic spread; adjacent bony tissue may also be affected.

A pleuropneumoniae (*Haemophilus pleuropneumoniae, H parahaemolyticus*) causes contagious pleuropneumonia in pigs (p 1227). Disease ranges from acute, severe pleuropneumonia to subacute or chronic infection with pleuritis and pulmonary abscessation. Immune complexes formed as a result of host response may damage endothelial cells, resulting in vasculitis and thrombosis, with edema, necrosis, infarction, and hemorrhage. Infection is usually restricted to pigs <5 mo of age. *A pleuropneumoniae* may be normal mucosal flora in pigs, cattle, and sheep. Vaccines are available, and treatment usually involves use of penicillins, tetracycline, erythromycin, spectinomycin, or cephalosporins.

The natural host of *A equuli* is the horse; infections are seen in both foals and adult horses. Two subspecies, *equuli* and *haemolyticus*, have been described recently. Disease in foals may manifest as diarrhea, followed by meningitis, pneumonia, purulent nephritis, or septic polyarthritis (sleepy foal disease or joint-ill). Infection may be acquired through a contaminated umbilicus, or by inhalation or ingestion. The incidence of foal infection is reduced with greater attention to sanitation in the birthing environment and when maternal antibodies in colostrum have the desired antibacterial effect. Abortions, septicemia, nephritis, and endocarditis may result from *A equuli* infection in adult horses. Infection may be treated with chloramphenicol, gentamicin, sulfonamides, ampicillin, or third-generation cephalosporins, depending on the nature of the infection and the ability to achieve therapeutic concentrations at the site of infection.

A arthritidis is a newly described species, previously classified as Bisgaard taxon 9, which has been isolated from horses with arthritis and septicemia.

A lignieresii causes tumorous abscesses of the tongue, usually referred to as wooden tongue. It is seen primarily in cattle but also in sheep, horses, pigs, and dogs. It is a rare cause of disease in chickens. The organism may also cause pyogranulomatous lesions in soft tissues associated with the head, neck, limbs, and occasionally the lungs, pleura, udder, and subcutaneous tissue. The organism is part of the normal mucosal flora of the upper GI tract and causes disease when it gains access to adjacent soft tissue via penetrating wounds. It causes localized infections and can spread via the lymphatics to other tissues. Pus from the abscesses may contain microcolonies surrounded by clublike spicules of calcium phosphate, giving the appearance of sulfur granules <1 mm diameter. This form of actinobacillosis is found worldwide, but is sporadic and thus difficult to prevent. Surgical debridement may be useful in treatment; potassium iodide can be administered PO (although not to food-producing animals), and systemic antibacterial agents, such as tetracycline, erythromycin, or tilmicosin, may be effective.

A suis is part of the normal flora of the oral cavity of pigs. It causes septicemia in young pigs and arthritis, pneumonia, and pericarditis in older pigs. It may also cause septicemia, arthritis, pneumonia, and purulent nephritis in neonatal and postnatal foals. Disease follows a break in the integrity of the oral mucosa or may be associated with immunosuppression. The organism is typically susceptible to tetracycline, sulfonamides, and cephalosporins.

A actinomycetemcomitans is a common agent of human periodontal disease, and a rare cause of human endocarditis and ram epididymitis. It is found naturally on mucous membranes. *A capsulatus* is occasionally associated with septic arthritis in rabbits. "*A seminis*" has been associated with epididymitis in rams and with purulent polyarthritis in lambs.

Actinobacillus (Pasteurella) ureae has caused upper respiratory tract infections in humans and abortions in pigs.

A actinoides has been associated with suppurative pneumonia in calves and seminal vesiculitis in bulls, but is not a valid species.

Three new *Actinobacillus* species, *A minor*, *A porcinus*, and *A indolicus*, are members of the normal flora of the porcine upper respiratory tract. Their possible role in disease remains undefined.

ACTINOMYCOSIS

Actinomyces spp are normal flora of the oral and nasopharyngeal mucous membranes. Members of the genus *Actinomyces* are gram-positive, non-acid-fast rods, many of which are filamentous or branching. Branches are <1 μm in diameter, as opposed to fungal filaments, which are >1 μm in diameter. Several species are associated with diseases in animals.

A bovis is the etiologic agent of lumpy jaw in cattle. It has also been isolated from nodular abscesses in the lungs of cattle and from infrequent infections in sheep, pigs, dogs, and other mammals, including chronic fistulous withers and chronic poll evil in horses. Lumpy jaw is a chronic, progressive, indurated, granulomatous, suppurative abscess that most frequently involves the mandible, the maxillae, or other bony tissues in the head. Disease is seen when *A bovis* is introduced to underlying soft tissue, via penetrating wounds of the oral mucosa from wire or coarse hay or sticks. Involvement of adjacent bone frequently results in facial distortion, loose teeth (making chewing difficult), and dyspnea from swelling into the nasal cavity. Diagnosis can be based on clinical signs alone, but demonstration of gram-positive rods in yellowish "sulfur granules" from aspirated purulent material, as well as bacteriologic culture and histopathology, are confirmatory. The organism appears as long filaments, rods, and cocci in exudate from active lesions. Treatment is rarely successful in chronic cases in which bone is extensively involved, due to poor penetration of antibacterial agents into the site of infection. In less advanced cases, penicillin may be effective. Systemic treatment with potassium iodide has been used successfully in the past, but is no longer recommended due to food safety issues.

A hordeovulneris causes localized abscesses and systemic infections, such as pleuritis, peritonitis, visceral abscesses, and septic arthritis in dogs. A common predisposing factor is the presence of tissue-migrating foxtail grass (*Hordeum* spp) particles. History and clinical signs may contribute to the diagnosis, but demonstration of the causative agent by Gram's stain and bacteriologic culture is necessary for confirmation of etiology. Treatment includes surgical debridement and drainage and longterm treatment with penicillin or clindamycin.

A israelii is primarily associated with chronic granulomatous infections in humans, but has also been isolated rarely from pyogranulomatous lesions in pigs and cattle. Treatment involves surgical debridement and administration of penicillin. Clindamycin is also effective in porcine infections.

A naeslundii has been isolated from suppurative infections in several animal species, the most common being aborted porcine fetuses.

A (Corynebacterium) pyogenes has now been reclassified as *Arcanobacterium pyogenes*. It is associated with infections in many organ systems in multiple species of domestic animals; it is perhaps most common in cattle, but is found in goats, sheep, pigs, and others. Conditions include acute and chronic suppurative mastitis, suppurative pneumonia (usually as a sequela of acute bovine respiratory disease caused by *Mannheimia haemolytica* or *Pasteurella multocida*), septicemia, vegetative endocarditis, endometritis, septic arthritis, wound infections including umbilical infections, seminal vesiculitis (bulls and boars), and summer mastitis. Liver abscesses in feedlot cattle often involve *A pyogenes*, alone or in combination with *Fusobacterium necrophorum*. Diagnosis is accomplished easily by bacteriologic culture and identification of the organism. Surgical debridement and drainage may be useful in treatment, and antimicrobials such as penicillin may be useful as well. Tylosin is commonly used as a preventive in feedlot rations.

A suis causes pyogranulomatous porcine mastitis, characterized by small abscesses containing viscid, yellow pus surrounded by a wide zone of dense connective tissue. Yellow "sulfur granules" may be scattered throughout the pus, as in *A bovis* in cattle. Chronic, deep-seated abscesses may fistulate. Sows may also develop ventral subcutaneous granulomatous lesions, and occasional pyogranulomatous infections develop in lungs, spleen, kidneys, and other organs. Diagnosis is based on clinical signs and on isolation and identification of the etiologic agent. Treatment is rarely successful, primarily due to the inability of an antibacterial agent to penetrate the infected tissue. Infected tissue is often surgically removed to salvage sows for slaughter.

A viscosus causes chronic pneumonia, pyothorax, and localized subcutaneous abscesses in dogs. Thoracic lesions are pyogranulomas, whereas cutaneous lesions are granulomatous abscesses, often with fistulous tracts. Lesions generally develop after a traumatic injury such as a bite wound. Diagnosis may be based on history and clinical signs, including the presence of soft, grayish white granules in the pus or exudate, and isolation and identification of *A viscosus*. Treatment of pyothorax with penicillin or clindamycin may be successful if begun early in the clinical course. A successful outcome is more likely with cutaneous infections, which should also be treated with the same antimicrobials.

AMYLOIDOSIS

Amyloidoses are protein misfolding diseases. When new proteins are made, they normally fold automatically into their correct configuration. Sometimes, however, mistakes are made and incorrectly folded protein gets deposited in tissues. This misfolded protein consisting of very stable β-sheets is called amyloid. Amyloid may be deposited in a localized fashion or may be widely distributed throughout the body. It causes damage by displacement of normal cells. If critical organs such as the kidneys, liver, or heart are involved, the disease may be fatal. Amyloidosis can affect all domestic mammals, and minor, asymptomatic deposition of amyloid is common in aged animals.

Many different proteins can misfold, and amyloidosis can be classified on the basis of these fibril proteins. The most common form of amyloid is generated by misfolding of the acute-phase protein, serum amyloid A. Its misfolded product, AA amyloid, develops as a sequela of chronic inflammatory diseases, chronic bacterial infections, and malignant tumors. It is a common cause of death in horses aggressively immunized for antiserum production. AA amyloid is commonly deposited in parenchymal organs and may not cause clinical signs. The spleen is commonly affected. If the kidneys are involved, the presence of amyloid in glomeruli may lead to proteinuria, eventually resulting in renal failure.

A second common form of amyloid, AL amyloid, is generated by misfolding of immunoglobulin light chains. Its deposition results from the overproduction of monoclonal light chains in animals with multiple myeloma. It tends to be deposited in mesenchymal tissues, especially nervous tissues and joints.

At least 20 other proteins have been shown to misfold and become deposited in the tissues as amyloid. Thus, there are many recognized forms of hereditary amyloidoses, such as those described in Abyssinian cats and Shar-Pei dogs. Some amyloid is formed in all aged animals (senile systemic amyloidosis); eg, in aged dogs, amyloid is commonly deposited in the media of meningeal and cortical arteries. Localized deposits of amyloid are not uncommon, and it is believed that they result from the local production of fibril precursors. Tumor-like amyloid nodules and subcutaneous amyloid have been reported in horses.

Some forms of amyloid are transmissible. The most important of these are the transmissible spongiform encephalopathies, such as bovine spongiform encephalopathy (p 991) and scrapie (p 1071). These are caused by misfolded prion proteins. Indeed, there is evidence that AA amyloid is somewhat transmissible; experimental administration of small amounts of amyloid protein to an animal has been shown to accelerate its development.

Because of its diffuse distribution and insidious onset, amyloidosis is difficult to diagnose clinically. However, amyloidosis should be suspected if renal or hepatic failure develops in animals with chronic infections or inflammation. There is no specific therapy that can prevent the development of amyloidosis or promote the resorption of fibrils. Animals with conditions such as chronic abscesses or multiple myeloma should be treated to reduce the availability of fibril precursor protein. Amyloidosis is readily recognized at necropsy and in histologic sections by its affinity for Congo red dye.

ANTHRAX

(Splenic fever, Siberian ulcer, Charbon, Milzbrand)

Anthrax is a zoonotic disease caused by the sporeforming bacterium *Bacillus anthracis*. Anthrax is most common in wild and domestic herbivores (eg, cattle, sheep, goats, camels, antelopes) but can also be seen in humans exposed to tissue from infected animals, contaminated animal products or directly to *B anthracis* spores under certain conditions. Depending on the route of infection, host factors, and potentially strain-specific factors, anthrax can have several different clinical presentations. In herbivores, anthrax commonly presents as an acute septicemia with a high fatality rate, often accompanied by hemorrhagic lymphadenitis; in dogs, humans, horses, and pigs, it is usually less acute. *B anthracis* spores can remain infective in soil for many years. During this time, they are a potential source of infection for grazing livestock, but generally do not represent a direct infection risk for humans. Grazing animals may become infected when they ingest sufficient quantities of these spores from the soil. In addition to direct transmission, biting flies may mechanically transmit *B anthracis* spores from one animal to another. The relative importance of this mode of transmission during epizootics or epidemics has yet to be quantified but is frequently suspected. Feed contaminated with bone or other meal from infected animals can serve as a source of infection for livestock, as can hay that is heavily contaminated with infected soil. Raw or poorly cooked contaminated meat is a source of infection for carnivores and omnivores; anthrax resulting from contaminated meat consumption has been reported in pigs, dogs, cats, mink, wild carnivores, and humans.

Epidemiology: Underdiagnosis and unreliable reporting make it difficult to estimate the true incidence of anthrax worldwide. However, anthrax has been reported from nearly every continent and is most common in agricultural regions with neutral or alkaline, calcareous soils. In these regions, anthrax periodically emerges as epizootics among susceptible domestic and wild animals. These epizootics are usually associated with drought, flooding, or soil disturbance, and many years may pass between outbreaks. During interepidemic periods, sporadic cases may help maintain soil contamination.

Human cases may follow contact with contaminated animals or animal products. The risk of human disease in these settings is comparatively small in developed countries, partly because humans are relatively resistant to infection and less likely to be exposed to virulent spores. However, in Africa each affected cow can result in up to 10 human cases for a variety of cultural, economic, and epidemiologic reasons. In cases of natural transmission, humans exhibit primarily cutaneous disease (>95% of all cases). GI anthrax (including pharyngeal anthrax) may be seen among human populations following consumption of contaminated raw or undercooked meat. Under certain artificial conditions (eg, laboratories, animal hair processing facilities, exposure to weaponized spore products), humans may develop a highly fatal form of disease known as inhalational anthrax or woolsorter's disease. Inhalational anthrax is an acute hemorrhagic lymphadenitis of the mediastinal lymph nodes, often accompanied by hemorrhagic pleural effusions, severe septicemia, meningitis, and a high mortality rate. Inhalational anthrax among humans has not been reported following exposure to contaminated soil or infected animals.

In the USA, anthrax has been reported among domestic and wild animals nearly every year since records have been available. The precise incidence of anthrax among animals in the USA is unknown. Over the past hundred years, animal infections have occurred in nearly all states, with highest frequency from the Midwest and West. Presently, anthrax is enzootic in west Texas and northwest Minnesota; sporadic in south Texas, Nevada, eastern North and South Dakota; and only occasionally seen elsewhere. The annual incidence of human anthrax in the USA has declined from ~130 cases annually in the beginning of the last century to 1 case in 2002.

In addition to causing naturally occurring anthrax, *B anthracis* has been manufactured as a biologic warfare agent. *B anthracis* was used successfully as a weapon of terrorism in 2001, killing 5 people and causing disease in 22. Probably due to the method of delivery (via mail), no known animal disease resulted from this attack. Historically, *B anthracis* was selected for production as a weapon because of its respiratory route of infection, the high mortality of inhalational anthrax, and the greater stability of *B anthracis* spores compared with other potential biologic warfare agents. Weaponized spores represent a threat to both human and animal populations. The World Health Organization has estimated that 50 kg of *B anthracis* released upwind of a population center of 500,000 could result in 95,000 deaths and 125,000 hospitalizations. The effect on animal populations has not been estimated, but because livestock are more susceptible to *B anthracis* infection than primates, the outcome of an attack with *B anthracis* spores against livestock would result in higher and earlier mortality and morbidity rates than among a human population. Thus, livestock could serve as sentinels for a bioterrorism event.

Pathogenesis: *B anthracis* spores have a high affinity for macrophages. After wound inoculation, ingestion, or inhalation, spores infect macrophages, germinate, and proliferate. In cutaneous and GI infection, proliferation can occur at the site of infection and the lymph nodes draining the site of infection. Lethal toxin and edema toxin are produced by *B anthracis* and respectively cause local necrosis and extensive edema, which is a frequent characteristic of the disease. As the bacteria multiply in the lymph nodes, toxemia progresses and bacteremia may ensue. With the increase in toxin production, the potential for disseminated tissue destruction and organ failure increases. After vegetative bacilli are discharged from an animal following death (by carcass bloating, scavengers, or postmortem examination), the oxygen content of air induces sporulation. Spores are relatively resistant to extremes of temperature, chemical disinfection, and dessication. Necropsy is discouraged because of the potential for vegetative cells to be exposed to air, resulting in large numbers of spores being produced. Because of the rapid pH change following death and decomposition, vegetative cells in an unopened carcass quickly die without sporulating.

Clinical Findings: Typically, the incubation period is 3-7 days (range 1-14 days). The clinical course ranges from peracute to chronic. The peracute form (common in cattle and sheep) is characterized by sudden onset and a rapidly fatal course. Staggering, dyspnea, trembling, collapse, a few convulsive movements, and death may occur in cattle, sheep, or goats with only a brief evidence of illness.

In acute anthrax of cattle and sheep, there is an abrupt fever and a period of excitement followed by depression, stupor, respiratory or cardiac distress, staggering, convulsions, and death. Often, the course of disease is so rapid that illness is not observed and animals are found dead. The body temperature may reach 107°F (41.5°C), rumination ceases, milk production is materially reduced, and pregnant animals may abort. There may be bloody discharges from the natural body openings. Some (chronic?) infections are characterized by localized, subcutaneous, edematous swelling that can be quite extensive. Areas most frequently involved are the ventral neck, thorax, and shoulders.

The disease in horses may be acute. Signs may include fever, chills, severe colic, anorexia, depression, weakness, bloody diarrhea, and swellings of the neck, sternum, lower abdomen, and external genitalia. Death usually occurs within 2-3 days of onset.

Although relatively resistant, pigs may develop an acute septicemia following ingestion of B anthracis, characterized by sudden death, oropharyngitis, or more usually a mild chronic form. Oropharyngeal anthrax is characterized by rapidly progressive swelling of the throat, which may cause death by suffocation. In the chronic form, pigs show systemic signs of illness and gradually recover with treatment. Some later show evidence of anthrax infection in the cervical lymph nodes and tonsils when slaughtered (as apparently healthy animals). Intestinal involvement is seldom recognized and has nonspecific clinical characteristics of anorexia, vomiting, diarrhea (sometimes bloody), or constipation.

In dogs, cats, and wild carnivores, the disease resembles that seen in pigs. In wild herbivorous animals, the expected course of illness and lesions varies by species but resembles, for the most part, anthrax in cattle.

Lesions: Rigor mortis is frequently absent or incomplete. Dark blood may ooze from the mouth, nostrils, and anus with marked bloating and rapid body decomposition. If the carcass is inadvertently opened, septicemic lesions are seen. The blood is dark and thickened and fails to clot readily. Hemorrhages of various sizes are common on the serosal surfaces of the abdomen and thorax as well as on the epicardium and endocardium. Edematous, red-tinged effusions commonly are present under the serosa of various organs, between skeletal muscle groups, and in the subcutis. Hemorrhages frequently occur along the GI tract mucosa, and ulcers, particularly over Peyer's patches, may be present. An enlarged, dark red or black, soft, semifluid spleen is common. The liver, kidneys, and lymph nodes usually are congested and enlarged. Meningitis may be found if the skull is opened.

In pigs with chronic anthrax, the lesions usually are restricted to the tonsils, cervical lymph nodes, and surrounding tissues. The lymphatic tissues of the area are enlarged and are a mottled salmon to brick-red color on cut surface. Diphtheritic membranes or ulcers may be present over the surface of the tonsils. The area around involved lymphatic tissues generally is gelatinous and edematous. A chronic intestinal form involving the mesenteric lymph nodes is also recognized.

Diagnosis: A diagnosis based on clinical signs alone is difficult. Confirmatory laboratory examination should be attempted if anthrax is suspected. Because the vegetative cell is not robust and will not survive 3 days in transit, the optimal sample is a cotton swab dipped in the blood and allowed to dry. This results in sporulation and the death of other bacteria and contaminants. Because pigs with localized disease are rarely bacteremic, a small piece of affected lymphatic tissue that has been collected aseptically should be submitted. Before submission, the receiving reference laboratory should be contacted regarding appropriate specimen labelling, handling, and shipping procedures.

Specific diagnostic tests include bacterial culture, PCR tests, and fluorescent antibody stains to demonstrate the agent in blood films or tissues. Western blot and ELISA tests for antibody detection are available in some reference laboratories. Lacking other tests, fixed blood smears stained with Loeffler's or MacFadean stains can be used and the capsule visualized; however, it can result in some 20% false positives.

In livestock, anthrax must be differentiated from other conditions that cause sudden death. In cattle and sheep, clostridial infections, bloat, and lightning strike may be confused with anthrax. Also, acute leptospirosis, bacillary hemoglobinuria, anaplasmosis, and acute poisonings by bracken fern, sweet clover, and lead must be considered in cattle. In horses, acute infectious anemia, purpura, colic, lead poisoning, lightning strike, and sunstroke may resemble anthrax. In pigs, acute classical swine fever, African swine fever, and pharyngeal malignant edema are diagnostic considerations. In dogs, acute systemic infections and pharyngeal swellings due to other causes must be considered.

Treatment, Control, and Prevention: Anthrax is controlled through vaccination programs, rapid detection and reporting, quarantine, treatment of asymptomatic animals (postexposure prophylaxis), and burning or burial of suspect and confirmed cases. In livestock, anthrax can be controlled largely by annual vaccination of all grazing animals in the endemic area and by implementation of control measures during epizootics. The nonencapsulated Sterne-strain vaccine is used almost universally for livestock immunization. Vaccination should be done 2-4 wk before the season when outbreaks may be expected. Because this is a live vaccine, antibiotics should not be administered within 1 wk of vaccination. Before vaccination of dairy cattle during an outbreak, all of the procedures required by local laws should be reviewed and followed. Human anthrax vaccines currently licensed and used in the USA and Europe are based on filtrates of artificially cultivated *B anthracis*.

Early treatment and vigorous implementation of a preventive program are essential to reducing losses among livestock. Livestock at risk should be immediately treated with a long-acting antibiotic to stop all potential incubating infections. This is followed by vaccination ~7-10 days after antibiotic treatment. Any animals becoming sick after initial treatment and/or vaccination should be retreated immediately and revaccinated a month later. Simultaneous use of antibiotics and vaccine is inappropriate, as the Sterne vaccine is live. Animals should be moved to another pasture away from where the bodies had lain and any possible soil contamination. Suspected contaminated feed should be immediately removed. Domestic livestock respond well to penicillin if treated in the early stages of the disease. Oxytetracycline given daily in divided doses also is effective. Other antibacterials, including amoxicillin, chloramphenicol, ciprofloxacin, doxycycline, erythromycin, gentamicin, streptomycin, and sulfonamides also can be used, but their effectiveness in comparison with penicillin and the tetracyclines has not been evaluated under field conditions.

In addition to therapy and immunization, specific control procedures are necessary to contain the disease and prevent its spread. These include the following: 1) notification of the appropriate regulatory officials; 2) rigid enforcement of quarantine (after vaccination, 2 wk before movement off the farm, 6 wk if going to slaughter); 3) prompt disposal of dead animals, manure, bedding, or other contaminated material by cremation (preferable) or deep burial; 4) isolation of sick animals and removal of well animals from the contaminated areas; 5) cleaning and disinfection of stables, pens, milking barns, and equipment used on livestock; 6) use of insect repellents; 7) control of scavengers that feed on animals dead from the disease; and 8) observation of general sanitary procedures by people who handle diseased animals, both for their own safety and to prevent spread of the disease. Contaminated soils are very difficult to completely decontaminate, but formaldehyde will be successful if the level is not excessive. The process generally requires removal of soil.

Human infection is controlled through reducing infection in livestock, veterinary supervision of animal production and slaughter to reduce human contact with potentially infected livestock or animal products, and in some settings either pre- or postexposure prophylaxis. Trade restrictions of hides and wool from countries known to have anthrax reduce the risk to the public. In countries where anthrax is common and vaccination coverage in livestock is low, humans should avoid contact with livestock and animal products that were not inspected before and after slaughter. In general, consumption of meat from animals that have exhibited sudden death, meat obtained via emergency slaughter, and meat of uncertain origin should be avoided. Routine vaccination against anthrax is indicated for individuals engaged in work involving large quantities or concentrations of *B anthracis* cultures or activities with a high potential for aerosol production. Laboratory workers using standard Biosafety Level 2 practices in the routine processing of clinical samples are not at increased risk of exposure to *B anthracis* spores.

The risk for workers who come into contact with imported animal hides, furs, bone meal, wool, animal hair, or bristles has been reduced by improvements in industry standards and import restrictions. Routine pre-exposure vaccination is recommended for people in this group only when these standards and restrictions are insufficient to prevent exposure to anthrax spores. Routine vaccination of veterinarians in the USA is not recommended due to the low incidence of animal cases. However, vaccination may be indicated for veterinarians and other high-risk persons handling potentially infected animals in areas where there is a high incidence of anthrax cases.

The US Centers for Disease Control and Prevention (CDC) has recommended that those at risk of repeated exposure to *B anthracis* spores in response to a bioterrorism attack should be vaccinated. Those groups include some emergency first responders, federal responders, and laboratory workers. Because recommendations regarding preexposure vaccination should be based on some sense of a calculable risk assessment, and because the target population for a bioterrorist release of *B anthracis* and the risk of exposure cannot be predetermined, vaccination in anticipation of a terrorist attack is not recommended for other populations.

For humans, post-exposure prophylaxis against *B anthracis* is recommended following an aerosol exposure to *B anthracis* spores. Such exposure may occur following a laboratory accident or a terrorist incident. Prophylaxis may consist of antibiotic therapy alone or the combination of antibiotic therapy and vaccination, if vaccine is available, as most human vaccines are not live. Though there is no approved regimen, the CDC has suggested that antibiotics may be discontinued after 3 doses of vaccine have been administered according to the standard schedule (0, 2, and 4 wk). Because of availability and ease of dosing, doxycycline or ciprofloxacin may be chosen initially for antibiotic chemoprophylaxis until the susceptibility of the infecting organism is determined. Penicillin and doxycycline are approved by the FDA for the treatment of human anthrax, and have traditionally been considered the drugs of choice. Both ciprofloxacin and ofloxacin have demonstrated in vitro activity against *B anthracis*. Although naturally occurring *B anthracis* resistance to penicillin is infrequent, it is reported; resistance to other antibiotics has been noted. Antibiotics are effective against the germinated form of *B anthracis*, but are not effective against the spore form of the organism. Spores may survive in the mediastinal lymph nodes in the lung for months without germination in nonhuman primates. There are currently no approved vaccination regimens for postexposure prophylaxis following *B anthracis* exposures. Although postexposure chemoprophylaxis using antibiotics alone has been shown to be effective in animal models, the definitive length of treatment remains unclear. Antibiotic chemoprophylaxis may be switched to penicillin VK or amoxicillin in children or pregnant women once antibiotic susceptibilities are known and the organism is found to be susceptible to penicillin. The safety and efficacy of anthrax vaccine in children or pregnant women has not been studied; therefore, a recommendation for the use of vaccine in these groups cannot be made. Although the shortened vaccine regimen has been shown to be effective when used in a postexposure regimen that includes antibiotics, the duration of protection from vaccination is not known. The existing evidence suggests that vaccine protection is adequate for 12 mo. If subsequent exposures occur, additional vaccinations may be required.

There is little published science to guide the postexposure prophylaxis recommendations following cutaneous or GI exposures of humans to *B anthracis*. However, based on the slow progression of disease, low fatality rate, and ease of antibiotic treatment of cutaneous anthrax, and the general low risk of cutaneous disease following natural exposure, postexposure prophylaxis is not recommended following direct cutaneous exposure to contaminated animals or animal products. However, immediate washing of the exposed areas is advised. Those exposed should be advised of the signs of cutaneous anthrax (ie, an inflamed but painless area with or without circumferential small vesicles, enlargement of the regional lymph nodes) and should seek medical assistance if illness develops. Because of the high fatality rate and rapid progression of GI anthrax, serious consideration should be given to initiating postexposure antibiotic prophylaxis for those who consume contaminated undercooked or raw meat. There is no current indication for vaccination following either cutaneous exposure or ingestion, because there is no evidence of longterm survival of *B anthracis* spores in these forms of anthrax.

BESNOITIOSIS

Besnoitiosis is a protozoan disease of the skin, subcutis, blood vessels, mucous membranes, and other tissues.

Etiology and Transmission: The causal agent of the cutaneous disease is *Besnoitia besnoiti* in cattle and *B bennetti* in horses and burros. *B jellisoni* and *B wallacei* have been described from rodents; *B tarandi* from reindeer or caribou; *B darlingi* from lizards, opossums, and snakes; and *B sauriana* from lizards. Viscerotropic strains of *B besnoiti* have been isolated from African antelope; an unidentified *Besnoitia* sp has been found in goats in Iran, New Zealand, and Kenya. Wildlife in Australia and blue duiker, impala, and blue wildebeest in Africa have been affected. *B besnoiti* has been reported from southern Europe, Africa, Asia, and South America, but it has not been reported in cattle in North America. *B bennetti* has been reported from Africa, southern France, Mexico, and in 2 imported burros in the USA.

These *Toxoplasma*-like organisms multiply in endothelial, histiocytic, and other cells and produce characteristic large, thick-walled cysts filled with bradyzoites.

Experimental cyclic transmission with intestinal sexual stages in a definitive host—the cat—has been reported for *B besnoiti, B wallacei,* and *B darlingi.* Transmission of *B besnoiti* from cattle to cats has not been substantiated by subsequent studies. Biting flies (eg, tsetse) or ticks may transmit *B besnoiti* mechanically from chronically infected cattle; some *Besnoitia* spp can be transmitted artificially to suitable hosts by needle inoculation of tissues that contain cysts. Contamination of water or feed by infected cat feces are other possible routes of transmission. Individual isolates appear to be fairly specific for intermediate hosts.

Clinical Findings: Infected cattle often show no clinical signs other than a few cysts in the scleral conjunctiva. Illness begins with fever followed by warm, painful swellings ventrally (anasarca). Swollen lymph nodes, diarrhea, inappetence, photophobia, rhinitis, and orchitis also are seen. Anasarca gives way to sclerodermatitis. The skin becomes hard, thick, and wrinkled and develops cracks that allow secondary bacterial infection and myiasis to develop; movement is painful. There is loss of hair and epidermis. In addition to the skin lesions, there may be focal, disseminated myositis, keratitis, periostitis, endostitis, lymphadenitis, pneumonia, periorchitis, orchitis, epididymitis, arteritis, and perineuritis. Severely affected animals become emaciated.

A diagnostic finding is the appearance of cysts in the scleral conjunctiva and nasal mucosa. Diagnosis can also be made by finding crescent-shaped bradyzoites in skin scrapings, biopsy, or conjunctival scrapings.

Although mortality is low, convalescence is slow in severe cases. Severely affected bulls can become permanently sterile. Affected animals remain carriers for life.

The disease in goats is similar to that in cattle. In horses, the clinical signs are similar but tend to be less severe or invasive.

Prevention and Treatment: *B besnoiti* infections are economically important to cattle owners in endemic areas because of mortality (although usually <10%), sterility (which may be temporary or permanent), loss of condition and lower market value, and damage to the hide.

In some countries, cattle are immunized with a live, tissue-culture-adapted vaccine. Affected animals should be isolated and treated symptomatically. Reduction of biting insects and ticks also may reduce transmission. In limited studies of *B besnoiti* in rabbits, both antimony and sulfanilamide complex prevented cyst development. Oxytetracycline also may have some therapeutic value if given early in the course of the disease.

BORRELIOSIS

(Lyme disease)

Borreliosis is a tickborne, bacterial disease of domestic animals and humans. Areas of greatest incidence in the USA include the Atlantic seaboard, upper midwest, and Pacific coast. Borreliosis also is seen in Europe, Asia, Australia, and elsewhere. The importance of borreliosis as a zoonotic disease is increasing; although the incidence of disease in a geographic area is similar in animals and humans, animals, especially dogs, are at significantly higher risk.

Etiology and Transmission: In the USA, proven tick vectors of *Borrelia burgdorferi*, the causative agent of borreliosis, are *Ixodes pacificus* on the west coast and *I scapularis* elsewhere. The *Ixodes* tick vectors are 3-host ticks that hatch from eggs as uninfected larvae. Both larvae and nymphs may acquire infections by feeding on infected reservoir hosts and, after molting, can transmit infection to their host. Small mammals, especially rodents, play a major role as reservoir hosts, although experimental findings have shown that dogs can also serve as a reservoir. Risk of transmission is highest during periods when the nymphs (spring) and adults (spring and fall) are actively seeking hosts.

Clinical Findings and Diagnosis: Numerous clinical syndromes have been seen in domestic animals, including limb and joint disease and neurologic, cardiac, and renal abnormalities. In dogs, lameness, fever, anorexia, lethargy, and lymphadenopathy with or without swollen, painful joints constitute the most common clinical syndrome. Renal, cardiac, and neurologic forms of the disease are characterized by clinical and laboratory abnormalities in the affected systems. Renal borreliosis is the second most common canine syndrome and is generally fatal. It is characterized by uremia, hyperphosphatemia, and severe protein-losing nephropathy, often accompanied by peripheral edema. Conduction abnormality with bradycardia is typical of the rare cardiac form. Facial paralysis and seizure disorders have been reported in the neurologic form.

Diagnosis is based on history, clinical signs, elimination of other diagnoses, laboratory data, epidemiologic considerations, and response to antibiotic therapy. Clinical signs are appropriate for the affected organ system, while autoimmune panels, CBC, blood chemistry, radiographs, and other laboratory data are generally normal, except for results pertaining directly to the affected system (eg, uremia in renal disease, heart block on ECG in cardiac disease, and soft-tissue swelling in limb and joint disease).

Serologic testing for antibodies to *B burgdorferi* is an adjunct to clinical diagnosis. Presence of antibodies detected by ELISA, immunofluorescent antibody (IFA), or protein immunoelectrophoresis (Western blot) assays indicates exposure. However, long incubation periods, persistence of antibodies for months to years, and the disassociation of the antibody response from the clinical stage of disease make diagnosis by blood testing alone impossible. Recent studies of Western blot data indicate that the immune response to tickborne spirochetes is notably deficient in production of antibodies against the outer surface proteins A and B (Osp A and Osp B) of *B burgdorferi*. This is significant because antibodies directed against these, as well as other *Borrelia* proteins, are protective against infection and disease in several animal models. High ELISA and IFA titers in borreliosis may be attributed to rapid sequestration of spirochetes in fibroblasts and endothelial cells and to production of antigen by these spirochetes. Persistence of antibodies after therapy and similarity of Western blot profiles in all stages of disease and convalescence further demonstrate the limitations of serology in diagnosis. More recently, a membrane ELISA bench test has been introduced. It measures antibody to the C-6 *B burgdorferi* protein. The test is convenient and eliminates antibody responses to Lyme vaccines. However, 10% false-positive reactions were recently reported in field samples.

Isolation or detection by PCR of *B burgdorferi* from joints, periarticular tissue, blood, or other sources may also be helpful in diagnosis. Interpretation of culture results must include consideration of incubation period, the possibility of asymptomatic infection, and the technical difficulty of culturing these organisms.

Treatment and Control: Antibiotic therapy is indicated in all cases. Antimicrobials in the penicillin and tetracycline groups are effective, and rapid response is seen in limb and joint disease in most cases, although incomplete or transient resolution of signs is seen in a significant number of affected animals. Clinical and research data indicate that infection in animals, including humans, may persist in spite of antibiotic therapy. In dogs, standard antibiotic doses and treatment for 2 wk have been evaluated and demonstrated to be as effective as higher doses and longer durations. Symptomatic therapy directed toward the affected organ system and clinicopathologic abnormalities is also important, especially in renal, cardiac, and neurologic disease. In limb and joint disease, the use of NSAID concurrent with antibiotic therapy may lead to confusion over the source of clinical improvement and make diagnosis based on therapeutic response difficult. Corticosteroid treatment causes a clinical relapse in persistently infected dogs.

Tick avoidance plays a role in disease control. While highly effective products (permethrin spray, amitraz collar, and fipronil spot-on) are available for use on dogs, lack of owner compliance in application is often a barrier to effective, longterm tick avoidance. Furthermore, tick control products are evaluated by the EPA (USA) for their efficacy against the vectors (ticks), not for their ability to prevent disease transmission. Killed, whole-cell bacterins for the prevention of borreliosis in dogs have been in use since June 1990. Immunized dogs have strong antibody titers to Osp A and Osp B and produce antibodies that kill *B burgdorferi* in vitro. In one field efficacy study, dogs vaccinated with a commercially available bacterin before tick exposure had the highest degree of protection against disease. Analysis of postvaccination Western blots indicated that these dogs lacked the response to antigens typically seen in natural infections. In 1996, a canine vaccine containing only Osp A was introduced in the USA. While it was once believed that Osp A was the first *B burgdorferi* protein to which the immune system of the infected dog was exposed, it has been demonstrated that when a tick attaches to a warm-blooded animal, the *B burgdorferi* in that tick stop producing Osp A and begin producing a new protein, Osp C. However, antibodies to Osp A block transmission of *B burgdorferi* from the midgut of infected, engorging ticks and prevent infection. Development of vaccines that contain multiple *B burgdorferi* antigens is being pursued.

Strategically, in endemic areas, young dogs should be vaccinated before natural exposure to ticks to attain the highest percentages of protection. Prevaccination infection, long incubation, and persistence of infection after antibiotic therapy, rather than vaccine failure, may lead to disease in immunized dogs. In newly emerging areas of canine borreliosis, vaccination programs should be started before large numbers of dogs are exposed to infected ticks. Two doses of either type of vaccine are administered SC to dogs ≥9 wk old at 3-wk intervals, and annual revaccination is recommended.

CLOSTRIDIAL DISEASES

Clostridia are relatively large, anaerobic, sporeforming, rod-shaped organisms. The spores are oval, sometimes spherical, and are central, subterminal, or terminal in position. The vegetative forms of clostridia in tissue fluids of infected animals occur singly, in pairs, or rarely in chains. Differentiation of the various pathogenic and related species is based on cultural characteristics, spore shape and position, biochemical reactions, and the antigenic specificity of toxins or surface antigens. The natural habitats of the organisms are the soil and intestinal tract of animals, including humans. Pathogenic strains may be acquired by susceptible animals either by wound contamination or by ingestion. Diseases thus produced are a constant threat to successful livestock production in many parts of the world.

Clostridial diseases can be divided into 2 categories: 1) those in which the organisms actively invade and reproduce in the tissues of the host, with the production of toxins that enhance the spread of infection and are responsible for death (sometimes referred to as the gas-gangrene group); and 2) those characterized by toxemia resulting from the absorption of toxins produced by organisms within the digestive system (the enterotoxemias), in devitalized tissue (tetanus), or in food or carrion outside the body (botulism). If treatment for diseases in the first category is attempted, large doses of antibiotic are indicated to establish effective levels in the center of necrotic tissue where clostridia are found.

BACILLARY HEMOGLOBINURIA
(Red water disease)

Bacillary hemoglobinuria is an acute, infectious, toxemic disease caused by *Clostridium haemolyticum* (*C novyi* type D). It affects primarily cattle but has also been found in sheep and rarely in dogs. It occurs in the western part of the USA, along the Gulf of Mexico, in Venezuela, Chile, Great Britain, the middle East, and other parts of the world.

Etiology: *C haemolyticum* is a soilborne organism that may be found naturally in the GI tract of cattle. It can survive for long periods in contaminated soil or in bones from carcasses of infected animals. After ingestion, latent spores ultimately become lodged in the liver. The incubation period is extremely variable, and the onset depends on the presence of a locus of anaerobiosis in the liver. Such a nidus for germination is most often caused by fluke infection, much less often by high nitrate content of the diet, accidental liver puncture, liver biopsy, or any other cause of localized necrosis. When conditions for anaerobiosis are favorable, the spores germinate, and the resulting vegetative cells multiply and produce β toxin (phospholipase C), which causes intravascular hemolysis and its sequelae, including hemolytic anemia and hemoglobinuria.

Clinical Findings: Cattle may be found dead without premonitory signs. Usually, there is a sudden onset of severe depression, fever, abdominal pain, dyspnea, dysentery, and hemoglobinuria. Anemia and jaundice are present in varying degrees. Edema of the brisket may occur. Hgb and RBC levels are quite low. The duration of clinical signs varies from ~12 hr in pregnant cows to ~3-4 days in other cattle. The mortality in untreated animals is ~95%. Some cattle suffer from subclinical attacks of the disease and thereafter act as immune carriers.

Lesions: Dehydration, anemia, and sometimes subcutaneous edema are present. There is bloody fluid in the abdominal and thoracic cavities. The lungs are not grossly affected, and the trachea contains bloody froth with hemorrhages in the mucosa. The small intestine and occasionally the large intestine are hemorrhagic; their contents often contain free or clotted blood. An anemic infarct in the liver is virtually pathognomonic; it is slightly elevated, lighter in color than the surrounding tissue, and outlined by a bluish red zone of congestion. The kidneys are dark, friable, and usually studded with petechiae. The bladder contains purplish red urine. After death, rigor mortis sets in more rapidly than usual.

Diagnosis: The general clinical picture usually permits a diagnosis. The most striking sign is the typical port-wine-colored urine, which foams freely when voided or on agitation. The presence of the typical liver infarct is sufficient for a presumptive diagnosis. The normal size and consistency of the spleen serve to exclude anthrax and anaplasmosis. Bracken fern poisoning and leptospirosis also should be considered. Diagnosis can be confirmed by isolating *C haemolyticum* from the liver infarct, but the organism is difficult to culture. Rapid and accurate diagnosis can be made by demonstrating the organism in the liver tissue by a fluorescent antibody or immunohistochemical test or by demonstrating the toxin in the fluid in the peritoneal cavity or in a saline extract of the infarct.

Control: Early treatment with penicillin or broad-spectrum antibiotics is essential. Whole blood transfusions and fluid therapy also are helpful. *C haemolyticum* bacterin prepared from whole cultures confers immunity for ~6 mo. In areas where the disease is seasonal, one preseasonal dose is usually adequate; where the disease occurs throughout the year, semiannual vaccination is necessary. Cattle that are in contact with animals from areas where this disease is endemic should be vaccinated, as the latter may be carriers.

BIG HEAD

Big head is an acute, infectious disease, caused by *Clostridium novyi, C sordellii*, or rarely *C chauvoei*, characterized by a nongaseous, nonhemorrhagic, edematous swelling of the head, face, and neck of young rams. This infection is initiated in young rams by their continual butting of one another. The bruised and battered subcutaneous tissues provide conditions suitable for growth of pathogenic clostridia, and the breaks in the skin offer an opportunity for their entrance. Treatment is with broad-spectrum antibiotics or penicillin.

BLACKLEG

Blackleg is an acute, febrile disease of cattle and sheep caused by *Clostridium chauvoei (feseri)* characterized by emphysematous swelling, usually in the heavy muscles. It is found worldwide.

Etiology: *C chauvoei* is found naturally in the intestinal tract of animals. It probably can remain viable in the soil for many years, although it does not actively grow there. Contaminated pasture appears to be a source of organisms. Outbreaks of blackleg have occurred in cattle on farms in which recent excavations have occurred, which suggests that disturbance of soil may activate latent spores. The organisms probably are ingested, pass through the wall of the GI tract, and after gaining access to the bloodstream, are deposited in muscle and other tissues.

In cattle, blackleg infection is endogenous, in contrast to malignant edema (p 489). Lesions develop without any history of wounds, although bruising or excessive exercise may precipitate some cases. Commonly, the animals that contract blackleg are of the beef breeds, in excellent health, gaining weight, and usually the best animals of their group. Outbreaks occur in which a few new cases are found each day for several days. Most cases are seen in cattle from 6-24 mo old, but thrifty calves as young as 6 wk and cattle as old as 10-12 yr may be affected. The disease usually occurs in summer and fall and is uncommon during the winter. In sheep, the disease is not restricted to the young, and most cases follow some form of injury such as shearing cuts, docking, crutching, or castration. Endogenous blackleg in sheep is uncommon in the USA; it is much more common in New Zealand where blackleg is seen more frequently in sheep than in cattle.

Clinical Findings and Lesions: Usually, onset is sudden, and a few cattle may be found dead without premonitory signs. Acute lameness and marked depression are common. Initially, there is a fever but, by the time clinical signs are obvious, body temperature may be normal or subnormal. Characteristic edematous and crepitant swellings develop in the hip, shoulder, chest, back, neck, or elsewhere. At first, the swelling is small, hot, and painful. As the disease rapidly progresses, the swelling enlarges, there is crepitation on palpation, and the skin becomes cold and insensitive as the blood supply to the area diminishes. General signs include prostration and tremors. Death occurs in 12-48 hr. In some cattle, the lesions are restricted to the myocardium and the diaphragm, with no reliable antemortem evidence of the localized lesion.

Diagnosis: A rapidly fatal, febrile disease in well-nourished young cattle, particularly of the beef breeds, with crepitant swellings of the heavy muscles suggests blackleg. The affected muscle is dark red to black and dry and spongy; it has a sweetish odor and is infiltrated with small bubbles but with little edema. The lesions may be in any muscle, even in the tongue or diaphragm. In sheep, because the lesions of the spontaneously occurring type are often small and deep, they may be overlooked. Occasionally, the tissue changes caused by *C septicum, C novyi, C sordellii*, and *C perfringens* may resemble those of blackleg. At times, both *C septicum* and *C chauvoei* may be isolated from blackleg lesions, particularly when the carcass is examined ≥24 hr after death, which allows time for postmortem invasion of the tissues by *C septicum*. Field diagnoses are confirmed by laboratory demonstration of *C chauvoei* in affected muscle. The samples of muscle should be taken as soon after death as possible. The fluorescent antibody test for *C chauvoei* is rapid and reliable.

Control: A bacterin containing *C chauvoei* and *C septicum* is safe and reliable for both cattle and sheep. Calves should be vaccinated twice, 2 wk apart, at 2-6 mo of age; in high-risk areas, revaccination may be necessary at 1 yr and every 5 yr thereafter. When outbreaks are encountered, all susceptible cattle should be vaccinated and treated prophylactically with penicillin to prevent new cases, which may develop for up to 10 days, at which the bacterin provides protection. In some areas, multicomponent clostridial vaccines are warranted. Treatment of clinical cases with parenteral and multiple local injections of penicillin may be attempted but is frequently unsuccessful.

INFECTIOUS NECROTIC HEPATITIS
(*Clostridium novyi [oedematiens]* infection, Black disease)

Infectious necrotic hepatitis is an infectious disease of sheep that is sometimes seen in cattle and is rare in pigs and horses.

Etiology and Pathogenesis: The etiologic agent, *Clostridium novyi* type B, is soilborne and frequently present in the intestines of herbivores; it may be present on skin surfaces and is a potential source of wound infections. Fecal contamination of pasture by carrier animals is the most important source of infection. The organism multiplies in areas of liver necrosis caused by migration of liver flukes and produces a powerful necrotizing toxin. The disease is worldwide in distribution, wherever sheep and liver flukes are both found.

C novyi has been suspected but not yet confirmed as a cause of sudden death in cattle and pigs fed high-level grain diets, and in which preexisting lesions of the liver were not detectable. The lethal and necrotizing toxins (primarily α toxin) damage hepatic parenchyma, thereby permitting the bacteria to multiply and produce a lethal amount of toxin.

Clinical Findings: Usually, death is sudden with no well-defined signs. Affected animals tend to lag behind the flock, assume sternal recumbency, and die within a few hours. Most cases occur in the summer and early fall when liver fluke infection is at its peak. The disease is most prevalent in 1- to 4-yr-old sheep and is limited to animals infected with liver flukes. Differentiation from acute fascioliasis may be difficult, but peracute deaths of animals that show typical lesions on necropsy should arouse suspicion of infectious necrotic hepatitis.

Lesions: The most characteristic lesions are the grayish yellow, necrotic foci in the liver that often follow the migratory tracks of the young flukes. Other common findings are an enlarged pericardial sac filled with straw-colored fluid, and excess fluid in the peritoneal and thoracic cavities. Usually, there is extensive rupture of the capillaries in the subcutaneous tissue, which causes the adjacent skin to turn black (hence the common name, black disease).

Control: The incidence may be lowered by reducing the numbers of snails, usually *Lymnaea* spp, that act as intermediate hosts for the liver flukes or by otherwise reducing the fluke infection of sheep. However, these procedures are not always practical, and active immunization with *C novyi* toxoid is more effective. Longterm immunity is produced by one vaccination. After this, only new introductions to the flock (lambs and sheep brought in from other areas) need to be vaccinated. This is best done before the late summer.

MALIGNANT EDEMA
Malignant edema is an acute, generally fatal toxemia of cattle, horses, sheep, goats, and pigs usually caused by *Clostridium septicum*, often accompanied by other clostridial species. Other clostridia implicated in wound infections include *C chauvoei*, *C perfringens*, *C novyi*, and *C sordellii*. The disease occurs worldwide. A similar infection in humans is not uncommon.

Etiology: *C septicum* is found in soil and intestinal contents of animals (including humans) throughout the world. Infection ordinarily occurs through contamination of wounds containing devitalized tissue, soil, or some other tissue-debilitant. Wounds caused by accident, castration, docking, insanitary vaccination, and parturition may become infected.

Clinical Findings: General signs, such as anorexia, intoxication, and high fever, as well as local lesions, develop within a few hours to a few days after predisposing injury. The local lesions are soft swellings that pit on pressure and extend rapidly because of the formation of large quantities of exudate that infiltrates the subcutaneous and intramuscular connective tissue of the affected areas. The muscle in such areas is dark brown to black. Accumulations of gas are uncommon. Severe edema of the head of rams develops after infection of wounds inflicted by fighting. Malignant edema associated with lacerations of the vulva at parturition is characterized by marked edema of the vulva, severe toxemia, and death in 24-48 hr.

Diagnosis: Similarity to blackleg (p 488) is marked, and differentiation made on necropsy is unreliable; laboratory confirmation is the only certain procedure. Horses and pigs are susceptible to malignant edema but not to blackleg. (*C septicum* also causes **braxy** in sheep, a highly fatal infection characterized by toxemia and inflammation of the abomasal wall. This disease seems to be confined mostly to European sheep fed on "frosted" pasture.)

Diagnosis can be confirmed rapidly on the basis of fluorescent-antibody staining of *C septicum* from a tissue smear. However, *C septicum* is an extremely active postmortem invader from the intestine, and its presence in a specimen taken from an animal that has been dead for ≥24 hr is not significant.

Control: Bacterins are used for immunization. *C septicum* usually is combined with *C chauvoei* in a blackleg/malignant edema vaccine and is available in multicomponent vaccines. In endemic areas, animals should be vaccinated before they are castrated, dehorned, or docked. Calves should be vaccinated at ~2 mo of age. Two doses 2-3 wk apart generally give protection. In high-risk areas, annual vaccination is indicated, as is revaccination after severe trauma.

Treatment with high doses of penicillin or broad-spectrum antibiotics is indicated early in the disease. Although injection of penicillin directly into the periphery of the lesion may minimize spread of the lesion, usually the affected tissues still slough.

BOTULISM
(Lamziekte)

Botulism is a rapidly fatal motor paralysis caused by ingestion of the toxin of *Clostridium botulinum*. The organism proliferates in decomposing animal tissue and sometimes in plant material.

Etiology: Botulism is an intoxication, not an infection, and results from ingestion of toxin in food. There are 7 types of *C botulinum*, differentiated on the antigenic specificity of the toxins: A, B, C_1, D, E, F, and G. Types A, B, and E are most important in botulism in people; C_1 in most animal species, notably wild ducks, pheasants, chickens, mink, cattle, and horses; and D in cattle. Only 2 outbreaks, both in humans, are known to have been caused by type F. Type G, which was isolated from soil in Argentina, is not known to have been involved in any outbreak of botulism either in humans or other animals. The usual source of the toxin is decaying carcasses or vegetable materials such as decaying grass, hay, grain, or spoiled silage. Toxins of all types have the same pharmacologic action. Like tetanus toxin, botulinum toxin is a zinc-binding metalloprotease that cleaves specific proteins in synaptic vesicles.

The incidence of botulism in animals is not known with accuracy, but it is relatively low in cattle and horses, probably more frequent in chickens, and high in wild waterfowl. Probably 10,000-50,000 birds are lost in most years, with losses reaching 1 million or more during the great outbreaks in the western USA. Most affected birds are ducks, although loons, mergansers, geese, and gulls also are susceptible. (*See also* BOTULISM IN POULTRY, p 2286.) Dogs, cats, and pigs are comparatively resistant to all types of botulinum toxin when administered orally.

Most botulism in cattle occurs in South Africa, where a combination of extensive agriculture, phosphorus deficiency in soil, and *C botulinum* type D in animals creates conditions ideal for the disease. The phosphorus-deficient cattle chew any bones with accompanying bits of flesh that they find on the range; if these came from an animal that had been carrying type D strains of *C botulinum*, intoxication is likely to result. A gram or so of dried flesh from such a carcass may contain enough toxin to kill a mature cow. Any animal eating such material also ingests spores, which germinate in the intestine and, after death of the host, invade the musculature, which in turn becomes toxic for other cattle. Type C strains also cause botulism in cattle in a similar fashion. This type of botulism in cattle is rare in the USA, although a few cases have been reported from Texas under the name of **loin disease**, and a few cases have occurred in Montana. Hay or silage contaminated with toxin-containing carcasses of birds or mammals and poultry litter fed to cattle have also been sources of type C or type D toxin for cattle. Botulism in sheep has been encountered in Australia, associated not with phosphorus deficiency as in cattle, but with protein and carbohydrate deficiency, which results in sheep eating carcasses of rabbits and other small animals found on the range. Botulism in horses often results from forage contaminated with type C or D toxin.

Toxicoinfectious botulism is the name given the disease in which *C botulinum* grows in tissues of a living animal and produces toxins there. The toxins are liberated from the lesions and cause typical botulism. This has been suggested as a means of producing the **shaker foal syndrome**. Gastric ulcers, foci of necrosis in the liver, abscesses in the navel and lungs, wounds of the skin and muscle, and necrotic lesions of the GI tract are predisposing sites for development of toxicoinfectious botulism. This disease of foals and adult horses appears to resemble "wound botulism" in humans. Type B toxin is often implicated in botulism in horses and foals in the eastern USA.

Botulism in mink usually is caused by type C strains that have produced toxin in chopped raw meat or fish. Type A and E strains are occasionally involved. Botulism has not been reported in cats but occurs sporadically in dogs. Type C toxin is usually responsible, but there have been reports in which type D was incriminated.

Clinical Findings and Lesions: The signs of botulism are caused by muscle paralysis and include progressive motor paralysis, disturbed vision, difficulty in chewing and swallowing, and generalized progressive weakness. Death is usually due to respiratory or cardiac paralysis. The toxin prevents release of acetylcholine at motor endplates. Passage of impulses down the motor nerves and contractility of muscles are not greatly hindered; only the passage of impulses from nerves to motor endplates is affected. No characteristic lesions develop, and pathologic changes may be ascribed to the general paralytic action of toxin, particularly in the muscles of the respiratory system, rather than to the specific effect of toxin on any particular organ.

Epidemics have occurred in dairy herds in which up to 65% of adult cows developed clinical botulism and died 6-72 hr after the onset of recumbency. Major clinical findings included drooling, inability to urinate, dysphagia, and sternal recumbency that progressed to lateral recumbency just before death. Skin sensation is usually normal, and withdrawal reflexes of the limbs are weak. Initially, clinical signs resemble second-stage milk fever (p 806), but the cows do not respond to calcium therapy.

In the shaker foal syndrome, foals are usually <4 wk old. They may be found dead without premonitory signs; most often, they exhibit signs of progressive symmetric motor paralysis. Stilted gait, muscular tremors, and the inability to stand for >4-5 min are salient features. Other clinical signs include dysphagia, constipation, mydriasis, and frequent urination. As the disease progresses, dyspnea with extension of the head and neck, tachycardia, and respiratory arrest occur. Death occurs most often 24-72 hr after the onset of clinical signs. The most consistent necropsy findings are pulmonary edema and congestion and excessive pericardial fluid, which contains free-floating strands of fibrin.

Diagnosis: Although sporadic cases of botulism often are suspected because of the characteristic motor paralysis, it is sometimes difficult to establish the diagnosis by demonstrating the toxin in animal tissues or sera or in the suspect feed. Commonly, the diagnosis is made by eliminating other causes of motor paralysis. Filtrates of the stomach and intestinal contents should be tested for toxicity in mice, but a negative answer is unreliable. Primary supportive evidence is provided by feeding suspect material to susceptible animals. In peracute cases, the toxin may be detectable in the blood by mouse inoculation tests but usually is not detectable in the average field case in farm animals. Use of ELISA methodology for detection of the toxin makes it feasible to test large numbers of samples, increasing the chances of diagnosis confirmation. In toxicoinfectious botulism, the organism may be cultured from tissues of affected animals.

Control: Any dietary deficiencies should be corrected and carcasses disposed of, if possible. Decaying grass or spoiled silage should be removed from the diet. Immunization of cattle with types C and D toxoid has proved successful in South Africa and Australia. Toxoid is also effective in immunizing mink and has been used in pheasants.

Botulinum antitoxin has been used for treatment with varying degrees of success, depending on the type of toxin involved and the species of host. Treatment of ducks and mink with type C antitoxin is often successful; however, such treatment is rarely used in cattle. Treatment with guanidine hydrochloride, 11 mg/kg body wt, has been reported to overcome some of the paralysis caused by the toxin; however, its use has not been extensive enough to determine its value.

CLOSTRIDIA-ASSOCIATED ENTEROCOLITIS IN HORSES

Clostridium difficile and *C perfringens* have been implicated in this acute, sporadic disease of horses characterized by diarrhea and colic. Because of uncertainty about the etiology, the condition has also been referred to as idiopathic colitis, but there is now good evidence that these organisms are responsible for enterocolitis in horses. *See also* p 237.

Etiology: *C difficile* is found only infrequently and *C perfringens* is found in low concentrations in the feces of normal horses. Both organisms may be present in soil or the environment and be ingested by horses. The factors that trigger disease are not well known, but it is presumed that some alteration in the normal flora permits excessive multiplication of the bacteria, which produce toxins capable of causing intestinal damage and systemic effects.

Predisposing factors that have been suggested include change in diet and antibiotic therapy. Other host factors that may determine whether disease develops include age, immunity, and presence or absence of intestinal receptors for the clostridial toxins. *C difficile* produces protein toxin A or B or both in the intestine. Toxin A is an enterotoxin that causes hypersecretion of fluid into the intestinal lumen and also causes tissue damage. Toxin B is a potent cytotoxin that induces inflammation and necrosis. Recent antibiotic therapy is a common feature of the history of horses with *C difficile*-induced diarrhea. Certain antibiotics, notably erythromycin, β-lactam antibiotics, and trimethoprim/ sulfonamide, are more likely than others to be associated with *C difficile* colitis. Mares with foals that are being treated with erythromycin appear to be at high risk. Elimination of roughage from the diet prior to surgery is also reported to predispose to *C difficile* colitis.

C perfringens type A is believed to cause diarrhea by elaboration of an enterotoxin (CPE), which is released during sporulation and stimulates intestinal epithelial cells to secrete excess fluid into the lumen. A novel necrotizing toxin, called β2, produced by some strains of *C perfringens*, has recently been strongly associated with colitis in horses.

Clinical Findings: Foals and adult horses may be affected. Typically there are signs of abdominal pain and diarrhea with or without blood. There may be abdominal distention, especially in cases of *C difficile*-induced diarrhea. Dehydration, toxemia, and shock may develop, and the mortality rate is variable. One or several animals on a farm may be affected.

Lesions: The characteristic lesion is a necrotizing enterocolitis. There is severe loss of colonic and cecal mucosal epithelial cells, hemorrhagic colitis and typhlitis, and thrombosis in capillaries of the intestinal mucosa.

Diagnosis: Clinical features of the disease are similar to those of acute salmonellosis (p 156), Potomac horse fever (p 236), or monocytic ehrlichiosis. The identification of *C perfringens* as the cause of diarrhea in horses depends on demonstration of the presence of enterotoxin or the gene for CPE in the feces or intestinal fluid and the absence of other likely etiologic agents. Most *C perfringens* found in the intestine of horses lack the gene for CPE. Demonstration of large numbers of bacterial spores or a high concentration of *C perfringens* in the feces are also aids to a diagnosis. The diagnosis of *C difficile* diarrhea is suggested by a history of recent treatment with antibiotics and is confirmed by demonstration of the presence of *C difficile* toxin A and/or B in a freshly passed or frozen fecal sample submitted to a laboratory. Toxin may be rapidly detected by an enzyme immunoassay, or the toxin gene may be identified by PCR.

Control: Steps may be taken to reduce the opportunity for *C difficile* infections in horses. The use of antibiotics may be unavoidable in veterinary hospitals, but selection of antibiotics such as metronidazole and chloramphenicol for oral administration to high-risk horses is recommended. The sources of *C difficile* spores may be attacked by surface disinfection with a sporicidal disinfectant, and the spread may be reduced by hand washing and by isolation of infectious horses and foals. There are no control measures available for prevention of *C perfringens*-induced diarrhea. Oral metronidazole is recommended for treatment of either of these clostridial infections.

CLOSTRIDIUM DIFFICILE IN SWINE

Clostridium difficile has emerged in recent years as an important cause of diarrhea in neonatal swine. In some studies, it has been identified as the second most frequent cause of diarrhea in 1- to 7-day-old pigs. *C difficile* has been discussed in association with disease in horses (*see* above), and critical virulence factor has been identified as toxins A and B. Mesocolonic edema is a characteristic feature of the disease seen in almost all affected pigs, but this lesion is not pathognomonic. Diagnosis of the disease depends on detection of toxins as described for the disease in horses.

ENTEROTOXEMIAS

(Clostridium perfringens infection)

Clostridium perfringens is widely distributed in the soil and the GI tract of animals and is characterized by its ability to produce potent exotoxins, some of which are responsible for specific enterotoxemias. Five types (A, B, C, D, and E) have been identified, but type E is of questionable significance in disease.

Enterotoxemia Caused by Clostridium perfringens Type A

Type A strains of *C perfringens* are commonly found as part of the normal intestinal microflora of animals and lack some of the powerful toxins produced by strains of other types. Nonetheless, they produce the lethal and necrotizing α toxin and are incriminated in necrotic enteritis in poultry (p 2210) and dogs, in colitis in horses, and in diarrhea in pigs. *C perfringens* type A is clearly implicated in a rarely occurring hemorrhagic diarrhea in dogs. The disease is characterized by a necrotic enteritis in which there is massive destruction of the villi and coagulation necrosis of the small intestine. These organisms are also associated with chronic intermittent diarrhea in dogs but have not been confirmed as the causal agent. Typically, large numbers of large, gram-positive rods are visible in fecal smears, and large numbers of *C perfringens* type A are recovered on anaerobic culture of feces. Other known enteric pathogens are usually absent. Untyped *C perfringens* has also been shown to proliferate in the intestines of dogs with parvoviral enteritis, but its contribution to disease is not clear. Production of enterotoxin by type A strains of *C perfringens* can induce diarrhea in humans, but this has not been demonstrated in dogs. Type A strains from pigs with diarrhea have produced enterotoxin in vitro, and anti-enterotoxin antibodies in sows indicate that enterotoxin is produced in vivo in pigs. Enterotoxin has also been demonstrated in the feces of pigs with diarrhea but not in feces of healthy pigs. However, recent studies have shown that *C perfringens* isolated from pigs with diarrhea are typically nonenterotoxigenic but produce the cytotoxic β2 toxin, which has been suggested to play a role in disease. Experimental disease has been produced in pigs challenged orally with *C perfringens* type A.

Enterotoxemia Caused by *Clostridium perfringens* Types B and C

Infection with *Clostridium perfringens* types B and C causes severe enteritis, dysentery, toxemia, and high mortality in young lambs, calves, pigs, and foals. Types B and C both produce the highly necrotizing and lethal β toxin that is responsible for severe intestinal damage. This toxin is sensitive to proteolytic enzymes, and disease is associated with inhibition of proteolysis in the intestine. Sow colostrum, which contains a trypsin inhibitor, has been suggested as a factor in the susceptibility of young piglets. Type C also causes enterotoxemia in adult cattle, sheep, and goats. The diseases are listed below, categorized as to cause and host. *C perfringens* also has been associated with hemorrhagic enteritis in dogs. (*See also* INTESTINAL DISEASES IN HORSES, p 233.)

Lamb dysentery: type B in lambs up to 3 wk of age. **Calf enterotoxemia**: types B and C in well-fed calves up to 1 mo. **Pig enterotoxemia**: type C in piglets during the first few days of life. **Foal enterotoxemia**: type B in foals in the first week of life. **Struck**: type C in adult sheep. **Goat enterotoxemia**: type C in adult goats.

Clinical Findings: Lamb dysentery is an acute disease of lambs <3 wk old. Many may die before signs are seen, but some newborn lambs stop nursing, become listless, and remain recumbent. A fetid, blood-tinged diarrhea is common, and death usually occurs within a few days.

In calves, there is acute diarrhea, dysentery, abdominal pain, convulsions, and opisthotonos. Death may occur in a few hours, but less severe cases survive for a few days, and recovery over a period of several days is possible. Pigs become acutely ill within a few days of birth and there is diarrhea, dysentery, reddening of the anus, and a high fatality rate; most affected piglets die within 12 hr. In foals, there is acute dysentery, toxemia, and rapid death. Struck in adult sheep is characterized by death without premonitory signs.

Lesions: Hemorrhagic enteritis with ulceration of the mucosa is the major lesion in all species. Grossly, the affected portion of the intestine is deep blue-purple and appears at first glance to be an infarction associated with mesenteric torsion. Smears of intestinal contents can be examined for large numbers of gram-positive, rod-shaped bacteria, and filtrates made for detection of toxin and subsequent identification by neutralization with specific antiserum.

Control: Treatment is usually ineffective because of the severity of the disease, but if available, specific hyperimmune serum is indicated, and oral administration of antibiotics may be helpful. The disease is best controlled by vaccination of the pregnant dam during the last third of pregnancy: initially, 2 vaccinations 1 mo apart, and annually thereafter. When outbreaks occur in newborn animals from unvaccinated dams, antiserum should be administered immediately after birth.

Type D Enterotoxemia
(Pulpy kidney disease, Overeating disease)

This classic enterotoxemia of sheep is seen less frequently in goats and rarely in cattle. It is worldwide in distribution and may be seen in animals of any age. It is most common in lambs that are either <2 wk old or weaned in feedlots and on a high-carbohydrate diet or, less often, on lush green pastures. The disease has been suspected in well-nourished beef calves nursing high-producing cows grazing lush pasture and in sudden death syndrome in feedlot cattle; however, supportive laboratory evidence in the latter is lacking.

Etiology: The causative agent is *C perfringens* type D. However, predisposing factors also are essential; the most common of these is the ingestion of excessive amounts of feed or milk in the very young and of grain in feedlot lambs. In young lambs, the disease usually is restricted to the single lambs, because a ewe with twins seldom gives enough milk to allow enterotoxemia to develop. In the feedlot, the disease usually is seen in lambs switched rapidly to high-grain diets. As the starch intake increases, it provides a suitable medium for growth of the causative bacteria, which produce ε toxin. A major effect of the toxin is to cause vascular damage, particularly of capillaries in the brain. Many sheep carry strains of *C perfringens* type D as part of the normal microflora of the intestine and serve as the source of organisms to infect the newborn. Most such carriers have nonvaccinal antitoxin titers.

Clinical Findings: Usually, sudden deaths in the best-conditioned lambs are the first indication of enterotoxemia. In some cases, excitement, incoordination, and convulsions occur before death. Opisthotonos, circling, and pushing the head against fixed objects are common signs of CNS involvement; frequently, hyperglycemia or glycosuria is seen. Diarrhea may or may not develop. Occasionally, adult sheep are affected; they show weakness, incoordination, and convulsions and die within 24 hr. In goats, the course of disease ranges from peracute to chronic, with signs that vary from sudden death to watery diarrhea with or without blood. Acutely affected calves not found dead show mania, convulsions, blindness, and death in a few hours. Subacutely affected calves are stuporous for a few days and may recover. In goats, diarrhea and nervous signs are seen, and death occurs in several weeks. Type D enterotoxemia occasionally is seen in young horses that have overeaten.

Lesions: Necropsy may reveal only a few hyperemic areas on the intestine and a fluid-filled pericardial sac. This is particularly the case in young lambs. In older animals, hemorrhagic areas on the myocardium may be found as well as petechiae and ecchymoses of the abdominal muscles and serosa of the intestine. Bilateral pulmonary edema and congestion frequently occur but usually not in young lambs. The rumen and abomasum contain an abundance of feed, and undigested feed often is found in the ileum. Edema and malacia can be detected microscopically in the basal ganglia and cerebellum of lambs. Rapid postmortem autolysis of the kidneys has led to the popular name, pulpy kidney disease; however, pulpy kidneys are by no means always found in affected young lambs and are seldom found in affected goats or cattle. Hemorrhagic or necrotic enterocolitis may be seen in goats.

Diagnosis: A presumptive diagnosis of enterotoxemia is based on sudden, convulsive deaths in lambs on carbohydrate-rich feed. Smears of intestinal contents reveal many short, thick gram-positive rods. Confirmation requires demonstration of ε toxin in the small-intestinal fluid. Fluid, not ingesta, should be collected in a sterile vial within a few hours after death and sent under refrigeration to a laboratory for toxin identification. Chloroform, added at 1 drop for each 10 mL of intestinal fluid, will stabilize any toxin present. Although immunologic tests have been developed to replace the traditional mouse assay for detection of toxin, they are less sensitive than the mouse assay. A PCR protocol for detection of the gene for ε toxin is effective in identifying isolates as either type B or D.

Control: The method of control depends on the age of the lambs, the frequency with which the disease appears on a particular property, and the method of husbandry. If the disease is seen consistently in young lambs on a property, ewe immunization probably is the most satisfactory method of control. Breeding ewes should be given 2 injections of type D toxoid their first year, and 1 injection 4-6 wk before lambing and each year thereafter.

Enterotoxemia in feedlot lambs can be controlled by reducing the amount of concentrate in the diet. However, this may not be economical, in which case, immunization of all lambs with toxoid when they first enter the feedlot probably will reduce losses to an acceptable level. Two injections, 2 wk apart, will protect lambs through the feeding period. When alum-precipitated toxoids or bacterins are used, the injection should be given at such a site that the cold abscesses, which commonly develop at the site of injection, can be removed easily during normal dressing and not blemish the carcass.

TETANUS

Tetanus toxemia is caused by a specific neurotoxin produced by *Clostridium tetani* in necrotic tissue. Almost all mammals are susceptible to this disease, although dogs are relatively resistant, and cats seem much more resistant than any other domestic or laboratory mammal. Birds are quite resistant; the lethal dose for pigeons and chickens is 10,000-300,000 times greater (on a body wt basis) than that for horses. Horses are the most sensitive of all species, with the possible exception of humans. Although tetanus is worldwide in distribution, there are some areas, such as the northern Rocky Mountain section of the USA, where the organism is rarely found in the soil and where tetanus is almost unknown. In general, the occurrence of *C tetani* in the soil and the incidence of tetanus in humans and horses is higher in the warmer parts of the various continents.

Etiology and Pathogenesis: *C tetani*, an anaerobe with terminal, spherical spores, is found in soil and intestinal tracts. In most cases, it is introduced into the tissues through wounds, particularly deep puncture wounds, that provide a suitable anaerobic environment. In lambs, however, and sometimes in other species, it often follows docking or castration. Sometimes, the point of entry cannot be found because the wound itself may be minor or healed.

The spores of *C tetani* are unable to grow in normal tissue or even in wounds if the tissue remains at the oxidation-reduction potential of the circulating blood. Suitable conditions for multiplication occur when a small amount of soil or a foreign object causes tissue necrosis. The bacteria remain localized in the necrotic tissue at the original site of infection and multiply. As bacterial cells undergo autolysis, the potent neurotoxin is released. The neurotoxin is a zinc-binding protease that cleaves synaptobrevin, a vesicle-associated membrane protein. Usually, toxin is absorbed by the motor nerves in the area and passes up the nerve tract to the spinal cord, where it causes ascending tetanus. The toxin causes spasmodic, tonic contractions of the voluntary muscles by interfering with the release of neurotransmitters from presynaptic nerve endings. If more toxin is released at the site of the infection than the surrounding nerves can take up, the excess is carried off by the lymph to the bloodstream and thus to the CNS, where it causes descending tetanus. Even minor stimulation of the affected animal may trigger the characteristic muscular spasms. The spasms may be so severe as to cause bone fractures. Spasms affecting the larynx, diaphragm, and intercostal muscles lead to respiratory failure. Involvement of the autonomic nervous system results in cardiac arrhythmias, tachycardia, and hypertension.

Clinical Findings: The incubation period varies from one to several weeks but usually averages 10-14 days. Localized stiffness, often involving the masseter muscles and muscles of the neck, the hindlimbs, and the region of the infected wound, is seen first; general stiffness becomes pronounced ~1 day later, and tonic spasms and hyperesthesia become evident. Because of their high resistance to tetanus toxin, dogs and cats often have a long incubation period and frequently develop localized tetanus; however, generalized tetanus does develop in these species.

The reflexes increase in intensity, and the animal is easily excited into more violent, general spasms by sudden movement or noise. Spasms of head muscles cause difficulty in prehension and mastication of food, hence the common name, **lockjaw**. In horses, the ears are erect, the tail stiff and extended, the anterior nares dilated, and the third eyelid prolapsed. Walking, turning, and backing are difficult. Spasms of the neck and back muscles cause extension of the head and neck, while stiffness of the leg muscles causes the animal to assume a "sawhorse" stance. Sweating is common. General spasms disturb circulation and respiration, which results in increased heart rate, rapid breathing, and congestion of mucous membranes. Sheep, goats, and pigs often fall to the ground and exhibit opisthotonos when startled. Consciousness is not affected. In dogs and cats, localized tetanus often presents as stiffness and rigidity in a limb with a wound. The stiffness progresses to involve the opposing limb and may advance anteriorly. The appearance in generalized tetanus is similar to that described for horses except that the partially open mouth with the lips drawn back (as seen in humans) is usually evident.

Usually, the temperature remains slightly above normal, but it may rise to 108-110°F (42-43°C) toward the end of a fatal attack. In mild attacks, the pulse and temperature remain nearly normal. Mortality averages ~80%. In animals that recover, there is a convalescent period of 2-6 wk; protective immunity usually does not develop after recovery.

Diagnosis: The clinical signs and history of recent trauma are usually adequate for a diagnosis of tetanus. It may be possible to confirm the diagnosis by demonstrating the presence of tetanus toxin in serum from the affected animal. In cases in which the wound is apparent, demonstration of the bacterium in gram-stained smears and by anaerobic culture may be attempted.

Control: Active immunization can be accomplished with tetanus toxoid. If a dangerous wound occurs after immunization, another injection of toxoid to increase the circulating antibody should be given. If the animal has not been immunized previously, it should be treated with 1,500-3,000 IU or more of tetanus antitoxin, which usually provides passive protection for up to 2 wk. Toxoid should be given simultaneously with the antitoxin and repeated in 30 days. Yearly booster injections of toxoid are advisable. Mares should be vaccinated during the last 6 wk of pregnancy and the foals vaccinated at 5-8 wk of age. In high-risk areas, foals may be given tetanus antitoxin immediately after birth and every 2-3 wk until they are 3 mo old, at which time they can be given toxoid. The decision to vaccinate lambs or calves depends on the prevalence of the disease in the area.

All surgical procedures should be conducted with the best possible techniques. After surgery, animals should be turned out on clean ground, preferably grass pastures. Only the oxidizing disinfectants such as iodine or chlorine dependably kill the spores.

When administered in the early stages of the disease, curariform agents, tranquilizers, or barbiturate sedatives, in conjunction with 300,000 IU of tetanus antitoxin BID, have been effective in the treatment of horses. Good results have been obtained in horses by injecting 50,000 IU of tetanus antitoxin directly into the subarachnoid space through the cisterna magna. Such therapy should be supported by draining and cleaning the wounds and administering penicillin or broad-spectrum antibiotics. Good nursing is invaluable during the acute period of spasms. The horse should be placed in a quiet, darkened box stall with feeding and watering devices high enough to allow use without lowering the head. Slings may be useful for horses having difficulty standing or rising. The same approach as described for horses is used in treatment of dogs and cats, except that caution must be exercised in the IV administration of antitoxin because the equine antitoxin may induce anaphylaxis. A combination of chlorpromazine and phenobarbital may be used to reduce hyperesthetic reactions and convulsions.

CLOSTRIDIAL VACCINES

Vaccination is frequently practiced for protection of animals against clostridial diseases. A wide variety of vaccines is available, singly or in combinations that consist of bacterins, toxoids, or mixtures of bacterins and toxoids. Tetanus toxoid is commonly used as a single vaccine in horses but is often used in combination in sheep, goats, and cattle. In sheep and goats, a common combination is tetanus toxoid plus *Clostridium perfringens* types C and D. In cattle, a combination frequently used in feedlots is a "4-way" vaccine that consists of killed cultures of *C chauvoei*, *C septicum*, *C novyi*, and *C sordellii* to protect against blackleg and malignant edema. A more complex clostridial vaccine that contains *C perfringens* types C and D in addition to the components of the 4-way vaccine may be used to protect cattle against enterotoxemias as well. The addition of *C haemolyticum* extends the protection to include infectious necrotic hepatitis. The clostridial vaccines often cause tissue reactions and swelling and should therefore be administered to cattle in the neck and by the SC rather than the IM route.

CONGENITAL AND INHERITED ANOMALIES

A variety of structural and functional defects have been described in animals; these defects are usually classified by the body system primarily affected. Defective neonates are adapted survivors from a disruptive event during embryonic or fetal development. Defective development may also be expressed as embryonic loss, fetal death, mummification, abortion, stillbirth, or a nonviable neonate. (*See also* discussions of CONGENITAL AND IN-HERITED ANOMALIES in various body systems, located via the index.)

Susceptibility to injurious environmental or genetic agents varies with the stage of development and species and decreases with fetal age. The zygote is resistant to teratogens but susceptible to genetic mutations and chromosomal aberrations. The embryo is highly susceptible to teratogens, but susceptibility decreases with age as the critical developmental periods of various organs or organ systems are passed. The fetus becomes increasingly resistant to teratogens except for later-differentiating structures such as the cerebellum, palate, and urogenital system.

The frequency of individual defects varies with the species, breed, geographic location, season, and other environmental factors. The incidence is estimated as 0.2-3.5% of all births of calves, lambs, foals, and dogs. Cats have the lowest incidence of congenital defects.

Commonly reported congenital and inherited defects by species include the following: in cattle—arthrogryposis, cleft palate, internal hydrocephalus, syndactyly, umbilical hernia, schistosomus reflexus; in horses—contracted tendons, hydrocephalus, cryptorchidism, patellar luxation, cataracts, pervious urachus; in sheep—agnathia, brachygnathia, entropion, cleft palate, cryptorchidism, atresia ani, hypospadias, limb defects; in pigs—atresia ani, arthrogryposis, cleft palate, cryptorchidism, hydrocephalus, myoclonia congenita; in dogs—neurologic defects, eye defects, cardiac defects, skeletal muscle defects, cryptorchidism, hip and elbow dysplasia; and in cats—cerebellar hypoplasia, eye and eyelid defects, cardiac defects, cleft palate, cryptorchidism, polydactyly, diaphragmatic and umbilical hernias.

Most congenital defects have no clearly established cause; others are caused by genetic or environmental factors or interaction between these factors (*see* TABLE 1).

Genetic Factors

Inherited defects resulting from mutant genes or chromosomal abnormalities are seen in families in typical intergenerational and intragenerational patterns of inheritance such as the common simple autosomal recessive, eg, syndactyly in cattle, patellar luxation in foals, agnathia in sheep, and diaphragmatic hernia in cats. Other inheritance patterns are dominant (eg, polydactyly in foals and cats, polycystic kidneys in Persian cats), overdominant, incomplete dominant, polygenic (eg, hip dysplasia in dogs, and dermoids, umbilical hernia, and polydactyly in cattle), and sex-linked.

Lysosomal storage diseases in domestic animals are increasingly reported; most are inherited as autosomal recessive traits. α-Mannosidosis of Angus cattle (also reported in Galloway and Murray Grey breeds) is the most extensively studied storage disease of domestic animals. β-Mannosidosis is described in Salers cattle and Anglo-Nubian goats.

Citrullinemia (argininosuccinate synthase deficiency) has been reported in Holstein cattle, dogs, and humans. It is characterized in neonatal calves by rapid onset of CNS disease and death within 5 days of birth. Maple syrup urine disease in Herefords and polled Shorthorns is also characterized by rapid onset of severe neurologic disease in neonates within 24 hr of birth and death within 5 days.

Deficiency of uridine monophosphate synthase in Holsteins is characterized by early fetal death at 30-60 days of gestation. Protoporphyria (ferrochelatase deficiency) in Limousin cattle is an extreme form of photosensitization that is evident almost from birth.

Chromosomal abnormalities are divided into 2 basic categories, numerical and structural. Some are self-limiting and result in sterility, abnormal growth, increased embryonic mortality, or reduced litter size, eg, calico cats, polyploidy in puppies, and aneuploidy in Miniature Schnauzers resulting in male pseudohermaphroditism. Viruses, certain drugs, and radiation are common causes of chromosome damage.

The complex interaction between genetic and environmental factors is becoming better understood, eg, in spastic paresis, kyphoscoliosis, and torticollis in cattle.

Environmental Factors

Teratogenic factors include toxic plants, viruses, drugs, trace elements, nutritional deficiencies, and physical agents such as irradiation, hyperthermia, uterine positioning, and pressure during rectal examination. They may be difficult to identify, often follow seasonal patterns and stress, and may be linked to maternal disease. They do not follow a familial pattern as do genetic causes.

Toxic Plants: *See also* PLANTS POISONOUS TO ANIMALS, p 2432. Crooked calf disease, characterized by joint contractures, torticollis, scoliosis or kyphosis, cleft palate, and combinations of these defects is seen in calves of in cows fed *Lupinus laxiflorus, L caudatus, L sericeus,* or *L nootkatensis* between days 40 and 70 of gestation. The quinolizidine alkaloid anagyrine is the teratogen. Ingestion of *L formosus* causes similar skeletal defects and cleft palate in cattle and goats; the teratogen is the alkaloid piperidine. Fetal development is at greatest risk when lupines are grazed early in plant growth or during seed formation. *Conium maculatum* (poison hemlock) causes contracture-type defects and occasionally cleft palate in calves, goats, sheep, and pigs. It may be a contributing factor in contracted tendons in foals. Both the plant and seed are toxic and teratogenic. Other plants suspected of causing similar defects in calves include *Senecio, Cycadales, Blighia, Papaveraceae, Colchicum, Vinca* spp, and *Indigofera spicata* and related plants. Ingestion of *Nicotiana tabacum* produces skeletal defects in pigs similar to those induced in cattle and pigs by *Lupinus* and *Conium. Nicotiana glauca* also induces contracture-type defects and cleft palate in cattle, sheep, and goats. Sudan grass (*Sorghum vulgare*) is incriminated as a cause of arthrogryposis in horses, and *S sudanese* may cause arthrogryposis in calves.

Epidemics of giantism with cyclopian defects occurred in bands of sheep in south-central and southwestern Idaho while grazing *Veratrum californicum* (skunk cabbage) on certain alpine ranges in early pregnancy.

Locoweed poisoning by plants of the genera *Oxytropis* and *Astragalus* in all types of range livestock (most commonly cattle, sheep, and horses) resulted in various clinical signs such as emaciation, visual impairment, neurologic signs, habituation, abortion, and congenital defects. Locoweed produces musculoskeletal defects in calves and lambs, and hypoplastic testicles and enlarged seminal vesicles in rams. Swainsonia and locoweed poisoning in growing cattle have similarities to genetic mannosidosis in Angus cattle because the alkaloid indolizidine-1,2,8-triol is a potent and specific inhibitor of the hydrolytic enzyme α-mannosidase.

Viruses: Certain prenatal viral infections are teratogenic in cattle, sheep, goats, pigs, dogs, and cats but have not been incriminated in defects in horses. Akabane virus (*see* below) causes abortion, premature birth, and arthrogryposis and hydranencephaly in cattle, sheep, and goats. Cache Valley virus causes similar defects in sheep.

Bovine viral diarrhea virus may cause cerebellar dysplasia, brachygnathia, alopecia, ocular defects, internal hydrocephalus, dysmyelination, and impaired immunocompetence. Fetal bluetongue virus infection may cause hydranencephaly, porencephaly, and arthrogryposis in sheep, and abortion, stillbirths, arthrogryposis, campylognathia, prognathia, hydranencephaly, and "dummy calf" syndrome in cattle. Other orbiviruses such as epizootic hemorrhagic disease and Chuzan viruses may cause abortion, congenital defects, and neonatal losses similar to bluetongue virus.

Wesselsbron disease virus (p 624) in South Africa is reported to cause primarily neurologic defects such as arthrogryposis, hydranencephaly, porencephaly, and cerebellar hypoplasia in ruminant fetuses.

Border disease ("hairy shaker" or "fuzzy" lambs, p 503) virus infection is manifest by embryonic and fetal death and various congenital defects involving the nervous, skeletal, integumentary, endocrine, and immune systems. Defects include arthrogryposis, brachygnathia, hypomyelination (particularly of the spinal cord), depressed immune responsiveness, and birth of small, weak lambs with poor growth and viability. The defective myelinogenesis is partially reversible if the lamb survives.

Classical swine fever virus (p 570), a togavirus, is teratogenic in piglets and causes congenital tremors, demyelination, internal hydrocephalus, arthrogryposis, and cerebellar hypoplasia. Japanese B encephalitis virus infection may result in hydrocephalus, cerebellar hypoplasia, and spinal hypomyelinogenesis in piglets.

TABLE I. Congenital Disorders with a Known Molecular Basis

Species	Disorder
Cat	Gangliosidosis, GM$_2$ Hyperlipoproteinemia
	α-Mannosidosis
	Mucopolysaccharidosis I, VI, VII
	Muscular dystrophy, Duchenne and Becker types
Dog	C3 deficiency
	Coat color, extension
	α-Fucosidosis
	Glycogen storage disease I, VII
	Hemophilia B
	Krabbe disease
	Leukocyte adhesion deficiency
	Mucopolysaccharidosis I, VII
	Muscular dystrophy, Duchenne and Becker types
	Myotonia
	Narcolepsy
	Nephritis, X-linked
	Pyruvate kinase deficiency of RBC
	Retinal pigment epithelial dystrophy
	Rod-cone dysplasia-1, -3
	Severe combined immunodeficiency disease, X-linked
	Tremor, X-linked
	von Willebrand's disease III
Cattle	Chédiak-Higashi syndrome
	Chronic interstitial nephritis with diffuse zonal fibrosis
	Citrullinemia
	Coat color, extension
	Coat color, roan
	Deficiency of uridine monophosphate synthetase
	Ehlers-Danlos syndrome
	Glycogen storage disease II, V
	Goiter, familial
	Leukocyte adhesion deficiency
	α-Mannosidosis
	β-Mannosidosis
	Maple syrup urine disease
	Muscular hypertrophy
	Protoporphyria
	Sex reversal: XY female
	Spherocytosis
Goat	Goiter, familial
	β-Mannosidosis
	Mucopolysaccharidosis III
	Reduced casein concentration
Pig	Coat color, dominant white
	Hypercholesterolemia
	Malignant hyperthermia
	Meat quality
Sheep	Ceroid lipofuscinosis
	Chondrodysplasia
	Coat color, extension
	Glycogen storage disease V

TABLE I. *(continued)*

Species	Disorder
Horse	Coat color, extension
	Megacolon
	Periodic paralysis II
	Severe combined immunodeficiency disease, autosomal
	Sex reversal: XY female
Bird	Dwarfism, sex-linked in chicken
	Feather color, albinism in chicken
	Feathering, Z-linked in chicken
	Henny feathering in chicken
	Hypotrophic axonopathy in quail
	Nanomelia in chicken
	Resistance to avian sarcoma and leukosis viruses, subgroup b in chicken
	Riboflavinuria in chicken
	Ribosomal DNA deficiency in chicken
Rabbit	Adrenal hyperplasia
	C8 deficiency
	Tremor, X-linked

Natural and experimental infection of pregnant cats with feline panleukopenia virus (p 635) causes cerebellar hypoplasia in neonatal kittens. Infection of pregnant ferrets in utero with feline panleukopenia virus also resulted in cerebellar hypoplasia.

Nutritional Factors: Deficiency of one or more nutrients during pregnancy may result in congenital defects in the newborn. Severe deficiencies may interrupt pregnancy or result in weak or nonviable young. Iodine deficiency is endemic in certain areas and may cause goiter or cretinism in all species. Congenital musculoskeletal abnormalities such as forelimb contracture and ruptured common digital extensor tendon have been reported in foals with hypothyroidism. Copper deficiency causes enzootic ataxia in lambs; manganese deficiency causes limb deformities in calves. Vitamin D deficiency may cause neonatal rickets, and vitamin A deficiency may cause eye defects or harelip. Experimentally, teratogenic effects have been induced by deficiencies of choline, riboflavin, pantothenic acid, cobalamin, and folic acid, and by hypervitaminosis A.

Physical Agents: Atresia of the gut, particularly the colon, may result from external pressure on the amnion during rectal palpation between days 35 and 40 of gestation. Torticollis, scoliosis, and frequently one or more defective limbs in foals have been associated with intrauterine fetal positioning, especially in caudal and transverse presentation. Pervious urachus in foals is reported to be associated with twisting of the umbilical cord.

AKABANE VIRUS INFECTION

Akabane is an insect-transmitted virus that causes congenital abnormalities of the CNS in ruminants. Disease due to Akabane virus has been recognized in Australia, Israel, Japan, and Korea; antibodies to it have been found in a number of countries in southeast Asia, the Middle East, and Africa. The disease affects fetuses of cattle, sheep, and goats. Asymptomatic infection has been demonstrated serologically in horses, buffalo, and deer (but not in humans or pigs) in endemic areas.

Etiology, Epidemiology, and Transmission: The causal agent, Akabane virus, is a member of the Simbu serogroup of the family Bunyaviridae. It is spread by biting midges (*Culicoides* spp) in Australia, Japan, and Kenya.

Akabane virus is common in many tropical and subtropical areas between ~35°N and 35°S. In these endemic areas, herbivores are bitten by the vectors, become infected at an early age, and develop a longlasting immunity by the time of breeding; thus, congenital abnormalities are seldom seen. However, under favorable environmental conditions such as an extended humid summer, the vector (and hence the virus) may spread beyond its usual range into new areas, and outbreaks of congenital infection may be expected. These outbreaks usually occur at the northern or southern limits of the vector distribution or in areas of higher altitude. Similarly, pregnant ruminants from virus- and vector-free areas moved to virus-infected areas are at risk.

The incidence of Akabane virus-induced disease is influenced by the time of gestation at which infection occurs and also by the strain of virus. Infections in the last 3 mo of pregnancy result in a relatively low incidence of disease (5-10% of calves are affected). The peak incidence is seen after infection in the third and fourth months, when up to 40% of calves may be born with defects. Some strains of Akabane virus produce a very low incidence of abnormalities (<20%), even at the most susceptible stages of gestation, whereas the most severe can cause disease in up to 80% of infected animals.

In sheep and goats, disease is observed but the distinct sequential manifestation of different abnormalities seen in cattle does not occur due to the shorter period of gestation and the shorter period of susceptibility. Most abnormalities develop following infection between 28-56 days of gestation. Few, if any, abnormalities are observed after infection at other times. However, it is not known whether infection in large or small ruminants very early in gestation results in a lethal infection, with abortion of the fetus.

Clinical Findings and Lesions: The clinical signs and pathology depend on the species of animal and time of infection. In a herd of cattle with an extended or year-round calving period, the full range of abnormalities may be seen. The most severe defects are seen after susceptible cows have been infected between ~80-150 days of gestation; however, calves can be affected at most times after the first 2 mo of gestation. Calves infected late in pregnancy may be born alive but unable to stand and may have a flaccid paralysis of the limbs, or may be incoordinated and on necropsy show a disseminated encephalomyelitis. Those infected earlier (120-180 days of gestation) have rigid fixation of limbs, usually in flexion (arthrogryposis), and sometimes also torticollis, kyphosis, and scoliosis with associated neurogenic muscle atrophy due to loss of spinal motor neurons. These abnormalities usually cause dystocia, and can result in severe obstetric complications, sometimes resulting in infertility and even death of cows. The first calves born with arthrogryposis are less severely affected than those born during the next 4-6 wk. Initially only 1-2 joints may be affected on a single limb, but later cases can have severe fixation of multiple joints on several or all limbs. Calves infected at 80-120 days of gestation are usually born alive and, if able to stand, walk poorly and are depressed and blind. These calves have varying degrees of cavitation of cerebral hemispheres, ranging from porencephaly to severe hydranencephaly. The latter is common, especially among those infected in the earlier stages of pregnancy. Some calves may be affected with both arthrogryposis and hydranencephaly.

Calves with severe hydranencephaly may be aborted in midgestation. A useful differential diagnostic feature is the virtual absence of either gross or histologic lesions in the cerebellum, distinguishing Akabane virus infection from other teratogenic viruses such as bovine viral diarrhea virus (BVDV).

In small ruminants, the lesions of arthrogryposis and hydranencephaly are often seen concurrently and are common in the same animals. In lambs and kids, a range of other defects may occur, including pulmonary hypoplasia and hypoplasia of the spinal cord. Most Akabane-infected lambs or kids are stillborn or die soon after birth. Abortions are also seen.

Akabane virus-induced congenital abnormalities (especially arthrogryposis and hydranencephaly) have been suspected in horses, but laboratory confirmation has been inconclusive.

Diagnosis: A presumptive diagnosis can be made on the gross CNS lesions, but the disease must be differentiated from other infectious and genetic conditions. Infection can be confirmed by testing sera or body fluids (eg, pericardial or pleural fluid) from unsuckled, affected offspring and their dams for serum neutralizing antibodies against Akabane virus. While the detection of antibody does not confirm Akabane as an etiologic agent, its absence is definitive for exclusion.

Other vectorborne viruses (and also nonvectorborne viruses such as BVDV) can cause congenital defects identical to those of Akabane virus. Aino virus, a relative of Akabane, is found in Australia, Japan, and several other countries where Akabane virus is found and has been an infrequent cause of disease in cattle. In Japan, Chuzan virus, a reovirus, is transmitted by *Culicoides oxystoma* and causes congenital infection in calves similar to Akabane virus. In the USA, Cache Valley virus, another vectorborne bunyavirus unrelated to Akabane virus, has been associated with congenital defects in sheep and perhaps cattle in some states.

Treatment and Control: There is no specific treatment for affected animals. Measures should be directed at the prevention of infection of susceptible animals with Akabane virus during pregnancy. Introduction of stock from nonendemic to endemic areas should be done well before first breeding. Effective vaccines are available in Japan.

BORDER DISEASE
(Hairy shaker disease)

Border disease (Britain) or hairy shaker disease (Australia and New Zealand) is a congenital disorder of lambs characterized by low birth weight and viability, poor conformation, tremor, and an excessively hairy birth coat in normally smooth-coated breeds. Kids may also be affected, and a similar condition occasionally occurs in calves. The disease has been recognized in most sheep-rearing areas of the world, including the western USA.

Etiology, Pathogenesis, and Epidemiology: Border disease is caused by infection of the fetus in early pregnancy with a pestivirus (Flaviviridae) closely related to the viruses of classical swine fever (hog cholera, p 570) and bovine viral diarrhea/mucosal disease (p 220). Surviving lambs are persistently viremic, and the virus is present in their excretions and secretions, including semen. Ruminants and possibly also pigs can be readily infected by contact with these persistent excretors or with acutely infected sheep. Acute infections in immunocompetent animals usually are transient and subclinical and result in immunity to challenge with homologous but not heterologous strains of virus.

Virus acquired in early pregnancy by previously unexposed animals crosses the placenta and invades the fetus. Placentitis occurs 10-30 days after infection and may cause fetal death with expulsion, resorption, or mummification. Abortion may occur at any stage of pregnancy and may pass unnoticed because there is little maternal malaise.

In sustained pregnancies, the virus becomes widely distributed in fetal tissues, but pathologic changes are most obvious in the skin, skeleton, and CNS. Affected lambs may be born 2-3 days early, and many die before or at weaning. In survivors, the clinical signs gradually regress, but such animals remain infected and excrete virus for the remainder of their lives, exposing their progeny and flockmates. Death from a syndrome similar to bovine mucosal disease may occur in these "recovered" hairy-shaker sheep at any time.

In flocks in the first season of a new infection, up to 50% or more of lambs born may be affected with border disease. Thereafter, prevalence declines, although the disease may become endemic when "recovered" lambs are retained for breeding. The virus is most commonly introduced into susceptible flocks by the addition of persistently infected sheep. However, it is not uncommon for sheep to acquire infection from persistently infected cattle. For practical purposes, it should be assumed that sheep and cattle are equally susceptible to all strains of border disease virus and bovine viral diarrhea virus, even though at least 3 antigenic groups of pestiviruses have been identified in ruminants.

Clinical Findings: Affected flocks probably are recognized first at lambing time by an increase in the number of barren ewes and in the birth of undersized lambs with excessively hairy and sometimes excessively pigmented fleece. Some lambs exhibit involuntary muscular tremors, particularly of the trunk and hindlegs. The tremors are reduced at rest and exacerbated by purposeful movement. In others, skeletal defects such as dropped pasterns and mandibular brachygnathia may predominate. Affected lambs have a poor survival rate. In survivors, nervous signs gradually disappear within 3-4 mo. Even in the absence of typical hairy-shaker lambs, outbreaks of low fertility in ewes and poor viability and ill-thrift in lambs are becoming associated more often with border disease virus infection.

Lesions: In severe cases, cavitation of the cerebrum may be seen at necropsy. Otherwise, the characteristic lesions are microscopic and involve the white matter of the CNS. There is a deficiency of myelin and an increase in interfascicular glial cells, in which myelin-like lipid droplets may accumulate. These changes are most obvious in the newborn and gradually resolve.

Diagnosis: Clinical findings usually allow a diagnosis, although abnormal hairiness of the birth coat may not be apparent in rough-coated breeds of sheep. The diagnosis can be confirmed by histologic demonstration of the pathognomonic lesions in the CNS with immunocytochemical staining of the virus. In typical hairy-shaker lambs, the virus may be demonstrated readily in blood and tissues. Precolostral blood is ideal because colostral antibody can mask virus for up to 2 mo. Virus can be isolated from serum or buffy coat cells in cell cultures, but a viral antigen detection ELISA using heparinized or EDTA blood is available. Reverse transcriptase-PCR can also be used for detecting viral RNA in clinical specimens and for typing ruminant pestiviruses.

Other causes of ovine abortion (eg, *Chlamydia, Salmonella, Campylobacter, Rickettsia* spp, and *Toxoplasma gondii*) should be considered in the differential diagnosis. In live-born lambs, border disease must be differentiated from swayback (enzootic ataxia), bacterial meningoencephalitis, focal symmetric encephalomalacia, and "daft lamb" disease.

Control: There is no effective treatment. Serology should be done on the dams of affected lambs. Most should have high levels of antibody and be immune to further challenge with the same strain of virus in subsequent pregnancies. Those that do not have antibody titers should be screened for virus to identify any that are persistently infected. Recovered lambs should not be retained for breeding but can be mixed with replacement stock well before breeding season to maximize opportunities for the latter to become infected and develop immunity before subsequent matings. There is no effective vaccine. Bovine viral diarrhea vaccines for cattle cannot be recommended for use in sheep because border disease viruses most commonly isolated from sheep are antigenically distinct from bovine viral diarrhea viruses most common in cattle.

ERYSIPELAS

Erysipelothrix rhusiopathiae (insidiosa) is distributed worldwide and can live in water, soil, decaying organic matter, slime on the bodies of fish, and in carcasses, even after processing. The bacterium has a variable survival time in soil, but not usually >35 days; however, carrier pigs (or other hosts) may cause recontamination. It causes swine erysipelas in its various forms; nonsuppurative arthritis in lambs and less frequently in calves and kids; postdipping lameness in sheep; uncommonly, joint-ill in goats (p 896); and acute septicemia in turkeys, ducks, and occasionally geese and other birds (*see* p 2225). In humans, the infection is usually localized and is termed erysipeloid. (It should not be confused with erysipelas in humans, a superficial cellulitis caused by group A β-hemolytic streptococci.)

In acute disease, *E rhusiopathiae* usually appears as a slender, gram-positive rod, ~1-2 μm long. In chronic lesions and old cultures, it often appears as a mixture of rods and filaments up to 20 μm long. It is resistant to certain commonly used antiseptics, such as formaldehyde, phenol, hydrogen peroxide, and alcohol, but is readily destroyed by caustic soda and hypochlorites. It is very sensitive to penicillin and ceftiofur but less so to the tetracyclines. The many strains vary markedly in pathogenicity.

SWINE ERYSIPELAS

Erysipelas is an infectious disease caused by *Erysipelothrix rhusiopathiae* seen mainly in growing pigs and characterized clinically by sudden death, fever, arthritis, and skin lesions. The disease may be acute, subacute, or chronic. Although acute septicemic swine erysipelas can result in a high mortality rate, the greatest economic loss probably occurs from the chronic, nonfatal forms of the disease.

Etiology: *E rhusiopathiae* is a gram-positive bacillus. Colonies on agar media are grayish translucent and nonhemolytic with smooth or rough morphology. At least 28 different serovars exist. Serovars 1 and 2 and strains forming smooth colonies are most commonly isolated from pigs with the septicemic form of the disease. *E rhusiopathiae* can survive for several months in animal tissue, eg, frozen or chilled meat, cured and smoked ham, and dry blood. It can survive in swine feces for up to 6 mo at temperatures below 54°F (12°C).

On farms where the organism is endemic, pigs are exposed naturally to *E rhusiopathiae* when they are young; their maternal antibodies provide a degree of active immunity without visible disease. The organism is excreted by infected pigs in feces and/or oronasal secretions and survives for short periods in most soils. Recovered pigs and those chronically infected may be carriers of the organism, possibly for life. The mode of entry is by ingestion and through skin abrasions. Following ingestion, the organism most likely enters the body via the tonsils or lymphoid tissue of the GI tract.

Clinical Findings: The acute, subacute, and chronic forms of swine erysipelas may occur in sequence or separately. Pigs with the acute septicemic form may die suddenly without previous signs. This occurs most frequently in finishing pigs (100-200 lb [45-90 kg]). Acutely infected pigs are febrile (104-108°F [40-42°C]), walk stiffly on their toes, lie on their sternums separately rather than piling in groups, and are reluctant to move. They squeal plaintively when handled and may shift weight from foot to foot when standing. Anorexia and thirst are common. Skin discoloration may vary from widespread erythema and purplish discoloration of the ears, snout, and abdomen, to diamond-shaped skin lesions almost anywhere on the body, but particularly the lateral and dorsal parts. The lesions may occur as pink or light-purple areas of varying size that become raised and firm to the touch within 2-3 days of illness. They may disappear or progress to a more chronic type of lesion such as diamond-skin disease. If untreated, necrosis and separation of large areas of skin can occur, but more commonly, the tips of the ears and tail may become necrotic and slough.

Clinical disease is usually sporadic, and affects individuals or small groups, but sometimes larger outbreaks occur. Mortality is 0-100%, and death may occur up to 6 days after the first signs of illness. Acutely affected pregnant sows may abort, probably due to the fever, and suckling sows may show agalactia. Untreated pigs may develop the chronic form, usually characterized by chronic arthritis, vegetative valvular endocarditis, or both; such lesions may also be seen in pigs with no previous signs of septicemia. Valvular endocarditis is most common in mature or young adult pigs and is frequently manifest by death, usually from embolism or cardiac insufficiency. Chronic arthritis, the most common form of chronic infection, produces mild to severe lameness; the affected joints may be difficult to detect but tend to become hot and painful to touch and later visibly enlarged and firm, resulting in lameness. Dark purple, necrotic skin lesions that commonly slough may be seen. Mortality in chronic cases is low, but growth rate is retarded.

Lesions: In acute infection, in addition to skin lesions, lymph nodes are usually enlarged and congested, the spleen is swollen, and the lungs are edematous and congested. Petechiae may be found in the kidneys, heart, and occasionally elsewhere.

In chronic erysipelas, valvular endocarditis is seen as proliferative, granular growths on the heart valves, and embolisms and infarctions may develop. Arthritis may involve joints of one or more legs or the intervertebral articulations; the joint enlargement is proliferative but nonsuppurative, and tags of granulation tissue form in the articular cavity. In chronic cases, there may be proliferation and erosion of the articular cartilage; this may be followed by fibrosis and ankylosis of the joint.

Diagnosis: Acute erysipelas is difficult to diagnose in individual pigs showing only fever, poor appetite, and listlessness; however, in outbreaks involving several animals, the presence of skin lesions and lameness is likely to be seen in at least some cases and would support a clinical diagnosis. Erysipelas responds extremely well to penicillin—a marked improvement within 24 hr also supports the diagnosis. The typical diamond-shaped skin lesions are diagnostic. Arthritis and endocarditis are difficult to diagnose in live animals because other agents can cause similar syndromes (*see* LAMENESS IN PIGS, p 932). Serology can prove unreliable, although a rising titer in an agglutination test (with controls) is helpful, as is the complement fixation test. An ELISA has been developed and is considered reliable for chronic infections on a herd basis.

At necropsy, demonstration of the organism in stained smears or cultures confirms the diagnosis, although in chronic arthritis cases, organisms may not be cultured. *E rhusiopathiae* can be isolated readily on blood agar plates from spleen, kidney, and long bones of acutely sick pigs (and from the tonsils and other lymph nodes of many apparently healthy ones).

Treatment: Penicillin is the drug of choice for the treatment of acutely affected pigs, and it has been used concurrently with antiserum. Penicillin should be given daily for 2-3 days; alternatively, a long-acting form may be used. Improvement is usually seen in 24 hr. Treatment of chronic infection is usually ineffective or not cost effective, and such pigs should be culled. If acute cases develop suddenly in an unvaccinated herd, antiserum, if available, may be administered to in-contact pigs. It may be more cost effective to use a long-acting form of penicillin or tetracyclines before implementing a vaccine program.

Prevention: Prevention is best achieved by regular vaccination using killed bacterins or, in some countries, attenuated vaccines prepared by serial passage or strains of low virulence for pigs. The formalin-killed, aluminum-hydroxide-adsorbed bacterin confers an immunity that, in most instances, protects growing pigs from acute disease until they reach market age. An oral vaccine of low virulence is also used. Young breeding stock, including boars, should be vaccinated twice at intervals of 3-5 wk at selection or before entering the herd, and then revaccinated every 6 mo or after each litter. Piglets born to vaccinated sows will be protected for 10-12 wk. Further protection will require vaccination at 12 wk. A booster vaccination 3-5 wk later is recommended. Vaccination of heavily pregnant sows is not advisable.

Vaccination raises the level of immunity but does not provide complete protection. Acute cases may develop after stress, and protection may not be provided against the arthritic or cardiac forms of the disease. Antigenic variation exists between bacterial strains, so a vaccine may not be equally effective against all wild strains.

Good sanitation, efficient disposal of feces, and regular disinfection of pens is also important in the prevention of erysipelas.

NONSUPPURATIVE POLYARTHRITIS IN LAMBS

This is an acute or, more commonly, chronic arthritis of one or more of the joints, usually of the limbs in lambs. Calves and kids are sometimes affected.

Etiology: The infective agent, *Erysipelothrix rhusiopathiae*, usually enters the body through wounds in young lambs, sometimes through the navel but more commonly after docking and castration. After a transient septicemia, the organism localizes in joints, without leaving evidence of infection at the site of entry. Poor condition of the lambs at the time of surgery, or adverse weather afterward, may predispose to a high infection rate.

Clinical Findings and Lesions: In the acute form, the characteristic lesion is a nonsuppurative arthritis manifest by heat and pain but only slight swelling of the joint tissues. The joints most commonly involved are the hock, stifle, elbow, and knee. Affected lambs are reluctant to move, and growth is often severely depressed, but complete recovery may occur in 2-3 wk. In ~10-15% of cases, however, the infection persists, and chronic arthritis with permanent enlargement of the joint develops. Mortality is usually low, but some lambs die from acute septicemia or complications arising from recumbency.

In outbreaks after docking and castration, the incubation period is remarkably constant; the first cases appear 9-19 days after the procedure, and practically all subsequent cases develop within 5 days. The incidence may reach 50%, but in most outbreaks it is <10%.

In the chronic form, signs usually are not seen until lambs are 2-6 mo of age. Typically, several joints are affected, causing the lambs to have a stiff gait.

Diagnosis: In outbreaks after docking and castration, a presumptive diagnosis can be made from the history and clinical signs. In sporadic cases, isolation and identification of the organism from affected joints should be attempted. The disease must be distinguished from polyarthritis due to other bacteria (eg, streptococcal joint-ill), white muscle disease, and other causes of lameness.

Prevention and Treatment: Adopting strict antiseptic techniques and maintaining hygienic conditions for docking and castration are recommended but cannot be relied on for prevention. The so-called "bloodless" methods of performing both procedures may reduce the chances of wound contamination, but outbreaks are known to follow all of the common methods. Vaccination should be considered where the disease is a recurring problem. Penicillin given early in acute disease is the best therapy but is of no value in the chronic form.

POSTDIPPING LAMENESS IN SHEEP

This cellulitis and laminitis arises from an extension of a focal cutaneous infection caused by the penetration of *Erysipelothrix rhusiopathiae* through small skin abrasions in the region of the hoof. Postdipping lameness, which normally occurs in outbreaks, has been described in most sheep-raising countries.

Etiology: With time and repeated use, dipping solutions or suspensions of insecticidal agents, which have little or no bacteriostatic activity, become heavily charged with various species of bacteria. *E rhusiopathiae* is a common contaminant, and its presence in the vat, sometimes in enormous numbers, leads to infection of skin wounds during dipping. Small skin abrasions in the region of the hoof and fetlock joint are a common portal of entry. Lesions extending from these leg wounds to the laminae of the hoof cause the acute postdipping lameness. Outbreaks may also occur when sheep must walk through muddy areas heavily contaminated with the organism.

Clinical Findings: Two to 4 days after dipping, a variable number (up to 90%) of sheep in the flock may be lame in one or more legs. Affected legs appear normal except for the hoof and pastern regions, which are hot and painful. Later, there is a variable degree of hair loss, sometimes extending as far as the carpus or tarsus. Most sheep recover spontaneously in 2-4 wk with nothing more serious than a slight loss of body weight. In some outbreaks, however, mortality may reach 5% and, particularly in young sheep, much body condition may be lost. Acute and chronic arthritis are rare sequelae.

Prevention and Treatment: The addition of copper sulfate to the dip (0.04%) should provide effective control, although dips heavily contaminated with organic matter are best discarded. Penicillin is the antibiotic of choice, and early treatment should speed recovery.

FOOT-AND-MOUTH DISEASE

Foot-and-mouth disease (FMD) is a highly infectious viral disease of cattle, pigs, sheep, goats, buffalo, and artiodactyl wildlife species. It is characterized by fever and vesicles in the mouth and on the muzzle, teats, and feet. In a susceptible population, morbidity approaches 100%. The disease is rarely fatal except in young animals. All species of deer and antelope, elephant, and giraffe are susceptible to FMD, but Old World camels are resistant to natural infection. South American camelids such as alpacas and llamas, although susceptible, are probably of no epidemiologic significance. Rats, mice, and guinea pigs can be infected experimentally.

FMD is endemic in the Middle East, Iran, the southern countries of the former Soviet Union, India, and southeast Asia. Sporadic outbreaks occurred in South Korea in 2000 and 2002, Japan in 2000, and in peninsular Malaysia. FMD is restricted to Luzon island in the Philippines. Australasia and Indonesia are free of FMD, as are Central and North America. In South America, Chile, southern Argentina, Guyana, Surinam, and the region of Colombia bordering Panama are free; large outbreaks of FMD in Uruguay and central Argentina during 2001 were brought under control, and these areas together with Paraguay and large parts of Brazil are now considered free areas in which vaccination is still used. Most of sub-Saharan Africa has endemic FMD, and also Egypt, Ethiopia, and Eritrea; FMD has returned to Zimbabwe associated with economic and social changes, and sporadic outbreaks have also occurred in the previously FMD-free zones of South Africa, Namibia and Botswana. In Europe, an outbreak in Greece on the border with Turkey in 2000 was quickly eliminated, but in 2001, FMD was introduced into the UK, from where it spread to the Republic of Ireland, the Netherlands, and France. The strain causing the outbreak was the same as that found throughout Asia, and was eventually brought under control in the UK following the slaughter of >4 million animals, without the use of vaccination. Vaccination was used in the Netherlands, and all vaccinated animals were subsequently slaughtered. Europe is currently free of FMD.

Etiology: FMD is caused by an aphthovirus of the family Picornaviridae. There are 7 immunologically distinct serotypes: A, O, C, Asia 1, and SAT (Southern African Territories) 1, 2, and 3. Within each serotype, there are a large number of strains that exhibit a spectrum of antigenic characteristics; therefore, more than one vaccine strain for each serotype, particularly O and A, is required to cover the antigenic diversity. Strains are characterized by their genomic relationships and their antigenic similarities with established vaccine strains. (Previous classification into subtypes became untenable as the number of subtypes rapidly increased.)

The virus is quickly inactivated outside the pH range of 6.0-9.0 and by desiccation and temperatures > 56°C, although residual virus may survive a considerable time when associated with animal protein (for instance, a proportion of FMD virus in infected milk will survive pasteurization at 72°C for 15 sec). FMD virus is resistant to lipid solvents such as ether and chloroform. Because of the sensitivity of the virus to acid and alkaline pH, sodium hydroxide, sodium carbonate, and citric or acetic acid are effective disinfectants.

Transmission, Epidemiology, and Pathogenesis: Transmission of FMD is generally by contact between susceptible and infected animals. Infected animals have a large amount of aerosolized virus in their exhaled air, which can infect other animals via the respiratory or oral routes. All excretions and secretions from the infected animal contain virus, and virus may be present in milk and semen for up to 4 days before clinical signs appear. Aerosolized FMD virus can spread a considerable distance as a plume, depending on weather conditions, particularly when the relative humidity is >60% and when the topography of the surface over which it is dispersing does not cause turbulence. FMD has been transmitted to calves via infected milk, and milk tankers carrying infected milk have been implicated in the spread of disease between farms. Fodder can become contaminated after contact with infected animals and iatrogenic spread of FMD has been reported. Although horses, dogs, and cats are not affected by FMD, they can act as mechanical vectors, as can humans. Also, avian species are not susceptible to infection, but they can carry virus on their feet and feathers and will excrete virus after ingesting infected material. Therefore, birds may carry the virus, although their role in dissemination is unclear. A typical scenario for the introduction of FMD into a previously clear area is for pigs to be fed imported food derived from an infected animal (as meat, offal, or milk); virus then spreads by aerosol from the infected pigs to cattle, which are the most likely species to be infected by the respiratory route because of their large respiratory volume. FMD virus can survive in dry fecal material for 14 days in summer, in slurry up to 6 mo in winter, in urine for 39 days, and on the soil between 3 (summer) and 28 (winter) days.

Ruminants that have recovered from infection and vaccinated ruminants that have contact with live FMD virus can serve as foci of infection and carry the virus in the pharyngeal region for up to 3.5 years in cattle, 9 mo in sheep, and ≥5 years in African buffalo. Experimentally, it has not been possible to show transmission from a carrier bovid to an in-contact susceptible animal, but there is evidence that under field conditions these carrier animals initiate new outbreaks of disease. FMD virus can be recovered from carrier animals by culturing a sample of pharyngeal mucus and superficial cells (collected using a probang cup) on susceptible tissue culture, such as primary bovine thyroid cells. However, the technique is probably only 50% reliable in identifying a carrier using a single sample because the quantity of virus found in the pharynx varies on different occasions.

The primary site of infection and replication is usually the mucosa of the pharynx, although the virus can enter through skin abrasions or the GI tract. Virus is distributed through the lymphatic system to sites of replication in the epithelium of the mouth, muzzle, feet, and teats, and also to areas of damaged skin (eg, the knees and hocks of pigs kept on concrete). Vesicles develop at these sites and rupture, usually within 48 hr. The viremia persists for ~3 days.

Clinical Findings: The incubation period for FMD is 2-14 days, depending on the infecting dose, susceptibility of the host, and strain of virus—in pigs, it may be as short as 18 hr with some strains of FMD virus. The clinical signs are more severe in cattle and intensively reared pigs than in sheep and goats, and FMD has frequently been ignored or misdiagnosed in small ruminants. In cattle and pigs, after the incubation period, anorexia and fever of up to 106°F (41°C) may develop. Cattle salivate and stamp their feet as vesicles develop on the tongue, dental pad, gums, lips, and on the coronary band and interdigital cleft of the feet. Vesicles may also appear on the teats and udder, particularly of lactating cows and sows, and on areas of skin subject to pressure and trauma, such as the legs of pigs. Young calves, lambs, kids, and piglets may die before showing any vesicles because of virus-induced damage to the developing cells of the myocardium. Milk yield drops dramatically in milking animals, and all animals show a loss in condition and growth rate that may persist after recovery. Sheep and goats may develop only a few vesicles on the coronary band and in the mouth. Vesicles in the mouth, even when severe, usually heal within 7 days, although recovery of the tongue papillae takes longer. Lesions on the mammary gland and feet frequently develop secondary infections, resulting in mastitis, underrunning of the sole, and chronic lameness. In pigs, the complete horn of the toe may be lost. Cattle and deer may also lose one or both horns of the foot, and deer may shed their antlers.

Diagnosis: In cattle and pigs, the clinical signs of FMD are indistinguishable from those of vesicular stomatitis (p 555), and in pigs from those of swine vesicular disease (p 588) and vesicular exanthema (p 590). Samples of vesicular epithelium or vesicular fluid should be sent in phosphate-buffered saline (pH 7.4) to the national laboratory responsible for the diagnosis of FMD, or otherwise to the OIE/FAO World Reference Laboratory for FMD, Pirbright, UK, by previous arrangement. Samples must be kept as close as possible to pH 7.4 to prevent destruction of the FMD virus and antigen. They should be securely packed in double leak-proof containers that comply with national and, when appropriate, international regulations for the shipment of pathologic and hazardous material. Samples are prepared as a 10% suspension, inoculated onto susceptible tissue culture, and directly typed by ELISA. Isolated FMD virus is characterized by antigenic comparison with existing FMD vaccine strains, and the nucleotide sequence of a segment of the 1D gene is determined for comparison with other strains of the same serotype to identify a possible origin of the outbreak. ELISA are available to show serologic evidence of vaccination against FMD or recovery from infection: either the liquid phase blocking ELISA, or the more recently introduced solid phase competition ELISA, which is equally sensitive but more specific. Tests for antibodies to the nonstructural proteins (NSP) of FMD virus can be used to distinguish an animal that has been infected from one that has been vaccinated, as only infected animals will have supported live replicating FMD virus, which express the NSP as part of their replication cycle. Virus in FMD vaccine is dead, and consequently there is no expression of NSP; therefore, no antibodies are formed in the host to these proteins. However, there may be sufficient NSP contamination in some vaccines to cause an antibody response, particularly to the 3D protein, in some animals that have received multiple vaccinations. Conversely, vaccinated animals that have had contact with live virus and become carriers of live FMD virus may fail to produce antibody to NSP, as the immunity provided by the vaccination suppresses viral replication. Rapid diagnostic kits are becoming available for on-farm diagnosis, but they will require stringent validation. PCR is also becoming more frequently used for rapid diagnosis; although difficult to fully validate, this test is likely to be more widely used in the future.

Treatment and Control: The occurrence of FMD in countries previously free of the disease can have a major effect on local and international trading arrangements. Many countries free of FMD have a policy of slaughter of all affected and in-contact susceptible animals and strict restrictions on movement of animals and vehicles around infected premises. After slaughter, the carcasses are either burned or buried on or close to the premises, and the buildings are thoroughly washed and disinfected with mild acid or alkali and by fumigation. Tracing is done to identify the source of the outbreak and premises to which FMD virus could have already been transmitted by infected animals or animal products, by contaminated vehicles or people, or aerosol. In areas or countries free of FMD in which this is not possible, control is by movement restriction, quarantine of affected premises, and vaccination around (and possibly within) the affected premises. This has the disadvantage that many carrier animals may remain after the outbreak, and quarantine may not be sufficiently long to prevent their subsequent movement. In countries in which FMD is endemic, protection, particularly of high-yielding dairy cattle, is by a combination of vaccination and prevention of FMD virus entering the dairy premises. This can be difficult if prevalence of FMD in the unvaccinated population is high and climatic conditions are suitable for aerosol transmission. FMD vaccine is a killed preparation and, at best, affords good protection against challenge for 4-6 mo. However, the antigenic diversity of virus strains within each of the serotypes is an additional complication, so it is necessary to ensure that vaccines contain strains antigenically similar to the potential outbreak strains. Otherwise, the duration of immunity provided by vaccines containing dissimilar strains may be very short. FMD vaccines for pigs require an oil adjuvant, whereas those for ruminants may contain an oil or aluminum hydroxide/saponin adjuvant. There are currently no recommended alternatives to vaccine antigens derived from whole virus grown in tissue culture and then chemically inactivated.

FUNGAL INFECTIONS

(Mycoses)

Systemic mycoses are infections with fungal agents that exist in the environment and disseminate in the host from a single portal of entry. The soil reservoir is the primary source of most infections, which can be acquired by inhalation, ingestion, or traumatic introduction of fungal elements. (*See also* DERMATOPHILOSIS, p 690.)

Pathogenic fungi establish infection in apparently normal hosts, and such diseases as histoplasmosis, coccidioidomycosis, blastomycosis, and cryptococcosis are regarded as primary systemic mycoses. Opportunistic fungi usually require a host that is debilitated or immunosuppressed (eg, by such stresses as captivity, metabolic acidosis, malnutrition, viral infections, or neoplasia) to establish infection. Prolonged administration of antimicrobials or immunosuppressive agents appears to increase the likelihood of infection by the opportunistic fungi that cause diseases such as aspergillosis and candidiasis, which may be focal or systemic.

Clinical findings and gross lesions are not definitively diagnostic of systemic mycoses; microscopic identification, culture of the organism, or PCR are required. Identification of the fungus and the tissue reaction via microscopic examination of exudates and biopsy material is adequate for diagnosis of histoplasmosis, cryptococcosis, blastomycosis, coccidioidomycosis, and rhinosporidiosis. Other diseases, such as candidiasis, aspergillosis, zygomycosis, phaeohyphomycosis, hyalohyphomycosis, and oomycosis (pythiosis and lagenidiosis), require more than microscopic evaluation for a definitive diagnosis. Some of these fungi are also common contaminants of cultures; thus, tissue invasion and reaction must be demonstrated for the culture isolation to be considered significant. Serology may be useful for diagnosis (and prognosis) of some mycotic diseases such as cryptococcosis, coccidioidomycosis, pythiosis, and lagenidiosis. For others, such as histoplasmosis and blastomycosis, its use is questionable.

For treatment, *see* discussions of specific systemic mycoses (below) and SYSTEMIC PHARMACOTHERAPEUTICS OF THE INTEGUMENTARY SYSTEM, p 2001.

ASPERGILLOSIS

Aspergillosis is caused by several *Aspergillus* spp, especially *A fumigatus* and *A terreus*. It is found worldwide and in almost all domestic animals and birds as well as in many wild species. It is primarily a respiratory infection that may become generalized; however, tissue predilection varies among species. The most common forms are pulmonary infections in poultry and other birds, mycotic abortion in cattle, guttural pouch mycosis in horses, and infections of the nasal and paranasal tissues, intervertebral sites, and kidneys of dogs. Pulmonary and intestinal forms have been described in domestic cats.

Clinical Findings and Lesions: In **birds**, aspergillosis (p 2296) is primarily bronchopulmonary, with dyspnea, gasping, and polypnea accompanied by somnolence, anorexia, and emaciation. Mycotic tracheitis has also been described. Torticollis and disturbances of equilibrium are seen when infection disseminates to the brain. Yellow nodules of varying size and consistency or plaque lesions are found in the respiratory passages, lungs, air sacs, or membranes of body cavities. Fur-like growth of fungus may be found on the thickened walls of air sacs. Other species with bronchopulmonary aspergillosis may have nodular lesions in the lungs, or an acute pneumonia accompanied by serosanguineous fluid in the pleural cavity and a fibrinous pleuritis.

In **ruminants**, aspergillosis may be asymptomatic, appear in a bronchopulmonary form, cause mastitis, or cause placentitis and abortion. Mycotic pneumonia may be rapidly fatal. Signs include pyrexia; rapid, shallow, stertorous respiration; nasal discharge; and a moist cough. The lungs are firm, heavy, and mottled and do not collapse. In subacute to chronic mycotic pneumonia, the lungs contain multiple discrete granulomas, and the disease grossly resembles tuberculosis (p 549).

In the absence of pneumonia, infected cows generally have no signs except for abortion; a dead fetus is aborted at 6-9 mo gestation, and the fetal membranes are retained. Lesions are found in the uterus, fetal membranes, and often the fetal skin. In the uterus, the intercaruncular areas are grossly thickened, leathery, dark red to tan, and contain elevated or eroded foci covered by a yellow-gray adherent pseudomembrane. Maternal caruncles are dark red to brown, and the adherent fetal cotyledons are markedly thickened. Cutaneous lesions in aborted fetuses consist of soft, red to gray, elevated, discrete foci that resemble ringworm.

In **horses**, epistaxis and dysphagia are common complications of gutturomycosis (*see also* p 1222). The infected guttural pouch is characterized by a necrotizing inflammation and is thickened, hemorrhagic, and covered by a friable pseudomembrane. Mycotic rhinitis characterized by dyspnea and nasal discharge has also been described. Aspergillosis can be a rapidly fatal disease associated with diffuse pulmonary invasion. In these cases, acute enteritis is often a predisposing factor. The colitis is thought to result in a profound neutropenia that decreases the immunocompetence of the host, followed by the invasion of *Aspergillus* from disrupted intestinal mucosa. Locomotor and visual disturbances, including blindness, may occur when the infection spreads to the brain and optic nerve.

In **dogs**, aspergillosis is typically localized to the nasal cavity or paranasal sinuses and is usually caused by infection with *A fumigatus*. Nasal aspergillosis is seen mainly in dolichocephalic breeds; it begins in the posterior region of the ventral maxilloturbinate with signs of lethargy, nasal pain, ulceration of the nares, sneezing, unilateral or bilateral sanguinopurulent nasal discharge, frontal sinus osteomyelitis, and epistaxis. Gross lesions vary considerably with site of infection, but the mucosa of the nasal and paranasal sinuses may be covered by a layer of gray-black necrotic material and fungal growth. The mucosa and the underlying bone may be necrotic with loss of bone definition on radiographs.

Disseminated disease in dogs is seen most often in German Shepherds and usually involves *A terreus* and *A deflectus*. The clinical signs of disseminated aspergillosis may include lethargy, lameness, anorexia, weight loss, pyrexia, hematuria, urinary incontinence, generalized lymphadenopathy, and neurologic deficits. Lesions are frequently found in the kidneys, spleen, and vertebrae. Discospondylitis is common.

Diagnosis: Radiographs in dogs with nasal aspergillosis may show generalized radiolucence of the nasal chambers secondary to turbinate tissue destruction. Frontal sinus osteomyelitis is seen in up to 80% of dogs. Visualization of fungal plaques by rhinoscopy together with serologic and either mycologic or radiographic evidence of disease is often how a diagnosis is made. A diagnosis based on culture results alone is not appropriate because aspergilli are ubiquitous and can be isolated from the nasal cavities of healthy dogs. Positive culture results should be supported by demonstration of narrow, hyaline, septate, branching hyphae within lesions or by serologic tests. The agar-gel double-diffusion test for serum antibody is a reliable technique for diagnosis; improved sensitivity may be possible with techniques such as ELISA. Immunofluorescent procedures can be used to identify hyphae in tissue sections.

Treatment: In dogs, topical treatment is considered the treatment of choice for nasal and paranasal aspergillosis. Several surgical techniques and drug regimens have been used with varying success. Clotrimazole is generally considered the first-line treatment. It can be administered through indwelling tubes trephined into the frontal sinuses or via the nares as a single infusion. If infusion is via the nares, Foley catheters are used to instill 0.5 g in each side of the nasal cavity. The infused solution is left in place for 1 hr, during which the dog's position is changed periodically to maximize penetration. There is an ~80% success rate using local infusions in this manner. Enilconazole, 10 mg/kg, instilled BID for 7-14 days, via tubes implanted surgically into the frontal sinuses, has also been used with a similar success rate. Drugs given systemically have included ketoconazole, itraconazole, and fluconazole. Ketoconazole (5-10 mg/kg, BID for 6-8 wk) is not as effective as fluconazole (2.5-10 mg/kg, divided BID) and itraconazole (5-10 mg/kg, SID).

In horses, surgical exposure and curettage have been used to treat gutturomycosis. Topical natamycin and oral potassium iodide have been reported effective in cases of *Aspergillus* infection. Recently, itraconazole, 3 mg/kg, BID given for 84-120 days, was reported effective in equine *Aspergillus* rhinitis.

Bovine mastitis has been treated successfully with combined intra-arterial and intra-mammary injection with miconazole.

CANDIDIASIS

Candidiasis is a localized mucocutaneous disease, which is distributed worldwide in a variety of animals, caused by species of the yeast-like fungus, *Candida*, most commonly *C albicans*. *C albicans* is a normal inhabitant of the nasopharynx, GI tract, and external genitalia of many species of animals and is opportunistic in causing disease. Factors associated with candidal infections are disruption of mucosal integrity; indwelling, intravenous, or urinary catheters; administration of antibiotics; and immunosuppressive drugs or diseases. The organism most frequently infects birds (p 2201), in which it involves the oral mucosa, esophagus, and crop. Superficial infections limited to the mucous membranes of the intestinal tract have been described in pigs and foals.

Systemic candidiasis has also been described in cattle, calves, sheep, and foals secondary to prolonged antibiotic or corticosteroid therapy. In cats, candidiasis is rare but has been associated with oral and upper respiratory disease, pyothorax, ocular lesions, intestinal disease, and urocystitis. Infections are rare in dogs and horses. However, *Candida* spp have been considered a cause of arthritis in horses and mastitis and abortion in cattle.

Clinical Findings and Lesions: Signs are variable and nonspecific and may be associated more with the primary or predisposing conditions than with the candidiasis itself. Calves with forestomach candidiasis have watery diarrhea, anorexia, and dehydration, with gradual progression to prostration and death. Affected chicks are listless and have reduced feed intake and growth rate. Porcine candidiasis affects the oral, esophageal, and gastric mucosa, with diarrhea and emaciation the most consistent signs.

Gross lesions of the skin and mucosae are generally single or multiple, raised, circular, white masses covered with scabs. The organism can penetrate keratinized epithelium and cause marked keratinous thickening of the mucosae of the tongue, esophagus, and rumen. In birds, the crop and esophageal lesions are white, circular ulcers with raised surface scabs that produce thickening of the mucosa; an easily removed pseudomembrane is common.

Diagnosis: Fungal organisms are numerous in proliferating epithelial tissue, and diagnosis can be made by examination of scrapings or biopsy specimens from mucocutaneous lesions. *C albicans* are ovoid, budding yeast cells (2-4 μm in diameter) with thin walls, or they occur in chains that produce pseudohyphae when the blastospores remain attached after budding division. Filamentous, regular, true hyphae also may be visible. The fungal cells generally are limited to epithelial tissue and rarely extend deeper.

Treatment: Nystatin ointment or topical application of amphotericin B or 1% iodine solution may be useful in the treatment of oral or cutaneous candidiasis. Amphotericin B, 500 g in 1 L of 5% dextrose, was administered IV, every 48 hr for 24 days and then every 72 hr for 15 days, to successfully resolve arthritis induced by *C fumata* in a horse. Fluconazole, 5 mg/kg, PO, SID for 4-6 wk, was also used to successfully treat disseminated candidiasis in foals. Itraconazole and amphotericin B lipid complex are considered the treatments of choice in dogs, but few cases have been treated.

COCCIDIOIDOMYCOSIS

Coccidioidomycosis is a dustborne, noncontagious infection caused by the dimorphic fungus *Coccidioides immitis*. Infections are limited to arid and semiarid regions of the southwestern USA and to similar areas of Mexico and Central and South America. While many species of animals, including humans, are susceptible, only dogs are affected significantly. Placental infection leading to abortion and osteomyelitis have been described in horses. Ruminants and pigs may have subclinical infections with lesions restricted to foci in the lungs and to thoracic lymph nodes. Inhalation of fungal spores is the only established mode of infection, and spores may be carried on dust particles. Epidemics may occur when rainy periods are followed by drought, resulting in dust storms. Most bovine infections are contracted in dusty feedlots.

Clinical Findings and Lesions: The disease varies from inapparent (cattle, sheep, pigs, dogs, cats) to progressive, disseminated, and fatal (dogs, nonhuman primates, cats, and humans). Coccidioidomycosis is primarily a chronic respiratory disease, but canine infections disseminate to many tissues, especially eyes and bone. Clinical signs can vary greatly, depending on organ involvement and severity of infection. Dogs with disseminated disease may have chronic cough, anorexia, cachexia, lameness, enlarged joints, fever, and intermittent diarrhea. Dissemination to the skin with draining ulceration may occur, but primary infection through the skin is rare. Cats infected with *C immitis* most often present with dermatologic problems (draining skin lesions, subcutaneous granulomatous masses, abscesses), fever, inappetence, and weight loss. Less common clinical signs in cats include respiratory (dypsnea), musculoskeletal (lameness), neurologic, and ophthalmologic abnormalities.

Gross lesions may be limited to the lungs, mediastinum, and thoracic lymph nodes, or may be disseminated to various organs. Lesions are discrete, variable-sized nodules with a firm, gray-white cut surface, and resemble those of tuberculosis (p 549). The nodules are pyogranulomas composed of epithelioid and giant cells, and the center of some foci may contain purulent exudate and fungal organisms. Some lesions may have mineralized foci.

Diagnosis: In endemic areas, coccidioidomycosis should be considered in dogs with chronic bronchopulmonary disease and when pulmonary nodules and enlarged lymph nodes are found on thoracic radiographs. The lesions are pyogranulomas that contain *C immitis* free in the exudate and in epithelioid and multinucleate giant cells. The organisms vary in size and appear as relatively large (20-80 μm, up to 200 μm) spherules with a double-contoured wall. The mature spherules (sporangia) contain endospores (sporangiospores) 2-5 μm in diameter. Diagnosis is established by demonstrating the spherules in tissues. Serum can also be tested by agar gel immunodiffusion for detection of precipitin and complement-fixing antibodies. A presumptive diagnosis can be made when serology is positive in an animal with consistent clinical signs. Attempts to culture the fungus should be restricted to those laboratories equipped to handle such dangerously infective cultures.

Treatment: Disease is often self-limiting, but if chronic respiratory signs or multisystemic disease are present, longterm antifungal therapy is needed; with disseminated infection, treatment of at least 6-12 mo is typical. Ketoconazole (10-30 mg/kg/day) or itraconazole (10 mg/kg/day) is commonly used to treat dogs with coccidioidomycosis. Amphotericin B may be indicated in animals that either do not improve or are unable to tolerate the azole antifungals. Fluconazole may also be effective. The use of longterm fluconazole (2-3 mg/kg/day) resulted in a 55% success rate in monkeys with coccidioidomycosis. Coccidioidomycotic osteomyelitis in a horse has been successfully treated with itraconazole, 2.6 mg/kg, BID for 6 mo.

CRYPTOCOCCOSIS

Cryptococcosis is a systemic fungal disease that may affect the respiratory tract (especially the nasal cavity), CNS, eyes, and skin (particularly of the face and neck of cats). The causal fungus, *Cryptococcus neoformans*, exists in the environment and in tissues in a yeast form. Infection occurs worldwide. The fungus is found in soil and fowl manure, especially in pigeon droppings. Transmission is by inhalation of spores or contamination of wounds. In avian droppings, it may occur in a noncapsulated form as small as 1 μm, which can be inhaled into the deeper portions of the lungs. Cryptococcosis is most common in cats but also is seen in dogs, cattle, horses, sheep, goats, birds, and wild animals. In humans, many cases are associated with a defective cell-mediated immune response.

Clinical Findings and Lesions: Bovine cryptococcosis has been associated only with cases of mastitis, and many cows in a herd may be infected. Affected cows have anorexia, decreased milk flow, swelling and firmness of affected quarters, and enlarged supramammary lymph nodes. The milk becomes viscid, mucoid, and gray-white, or it may be watery with flakes. The disease in horses almost invariably is a respiratory ailment with obstructive growths in the nasal cavities.

In cats, upper respiratory signs secondary to nasal cavity infection are most common and include sneezing; mucopurulent, serous, or hemorrhagic unilateral or bilateral chronic nasal discharge; polyp-like mass(es) in the nostril; and/or a firm, subcutaneous swelling over the bridge of the nose. Cutaneous lesions are also common and are characterized by papules and nodules that are fluctuant to firm. Larger lesions tend to ulcerate, leaving a raw surface with a serous exudate. Neurologic signs associated with cryptococcosis of the CNS may include depression, changes in temperament, seizures, circling, paresis, and blindness. Ocular abnormalities may also develop, including dilated unresponsive pupils and blindness due to exudative retinal detachment, granulomatous chorioretinitis, panophthalmitis, and optic neuritis.

In contrast to cats, dogs often have disseminated disease, with CNS or ocular involvement. Clinical signs are often related to meningoencephalitis, optic neuritis, and granulomatous chorioretinitis. Lesions in the nasal cavity of many dogs have been reported, but they are usually not the primary finding or reason for presentation. About 50% of dogs have lesions in the respiratory tract, usually the lungs, and most have granulomas present in multiple systems. Structures often involved in order of decreasing frequency are kidneys, lymph nodes, spleen, liver, thyroid, adrenals, pancreas, bone, GI tract, muscle, myocardium, prostate, heart valves, and tonsils.

Lesions associated with cryptococcosis vary from a gelatinous mass, consisting of numerous organisms with minimal inflammation, to granuloma formation. The lesion is usually composed of aggregates of encapsulated organisms within a connective tissue reticulum. The cellular response is primarily macrophages and giant cells with a few plasma cells and lymphocytes. Epithelioid giant cells and areas of caseous necrosis are less common than with the other systemic mycoses.

Diagnosis: The most rapid method of diagnosis is cytologic evaluation of nasal exudate, skin exudate, CSF, or samples obtained by paracentesis of the aqueous or vitreous chambers of the eye or by impression smears of nasal or cutaneous masses. Gram's stain is most useful; the organism retains the crystal violet while the capsule stains lightly red with safranin. India ink is also used to visualize the organism, which appears unstained and silhouetted against a black background. It is not as definitive as Gram's stain unless budding is seen, because lymphocytes, fat droplets, and aggregated India ink particles may be confused with the organism. Wright's stain has been used most often in diagnosing canine and feline cases, but this stain can cause the organism to shrink and the capsule to become distorted. New methylene blue and periodic acid-Schiff (PAS) stains are considered to be better than Wright's stain for this reason. Because of the rapidity of cytologic evaluation, impression smears or potassium hydroxide preparations should always be made of suspected cryptococcal lesions. If no organisms are seen, a biopsy of the lesion can be taken, with part of the sample used for culture and the rest processed for routine histology. The organism can be stained with H&E, but the capsule does not stain. The organism is more easily visualized with PAS and Gomori's methenamine silver stains, but the capsule does not stain with these either. The best stain for *Cryptococcus* is Mayer's mucicarmine because of its ability to stain the capsule. Immunofluorescent staining can also be used. The large capsule and thin cell wall of *Cryptococcus* differentiate it from *Blastomyces*. *Cryptococcus*, by its budding and lack of endospores, can be distinguished from *Coccidioides immitis*.

Detection of cryptococcal capsular antigen in serum, urine, or CSF is a useful, rapid method of diagnosis in those suspected cases in which the organism is not identified. A latex agglutination test is commercially available in kit form. The antigen titer can also be used to help determine response to therapy.

The organism can be cultured from exudate, CSF, urine, joint fluid, and tissue samples fairly easily if a large enough sample volume is available. Sabouraud's agar with antibiotics is used if bacterial contamination is likely.

Treatment: Fluconazole (2-10 mg/kg/day) or itraconazole (10 mg/kg/day) are considered the treatments of choice. Amphotericin B can be given SC, (0.5-0.8 mg/kg diluted in 0.45% saline containing 2.5% dextrose; 400 mL for cats, 500 mL for dogs <20 kg, 1,000 mL for dogs >20 kg) 2-3 times per week. Amphotericin B lipid complex can also be used (1-2 mg/kg for cats or 2-3 mg/kg for dogs) given 3 times a week for 12-15 treatments. Flucytosine can be used alone; however, drug resistance may develop, so combination therapy with amphotericin is recommended.

EPIZOOTIC LYMPHANGITIS

Epizootic lymphangitis is a chronic granulomatous disease of the skin, lymph vessels, and lymph nodes of the limbs and neck of Equidae caused by the dimorphic fungus *Histoplasma farciminosum*. The disease is seen in Asian and Mediterranean areas but is unknown in the USA. The fungus forms mycelia in nature and yeast forms in tissues and has a saprophytic phase in soil. Infection probably is acquired by wound infection or transmission by bloodsucking insects.

Clinical Findings and Lesions: Clinically, the disease is characterized by freely movable cutaneous nodules, which originate from infected superficial lymph vessels and nodes and tend to ulcerate and undergo alternating periods of discharge and closure. Affected lymph nodes are enlarged and hard. The skin covering the nodules may become thick, indurated, and fused to the underlying tissues. Lesions also may be present in the lungs, conjunctiva, cornea, nasal mucosa, and other organs. The nodules are pyogranulomas with a thick, fibrous capsule and contain thick, creamy exudate and the causative organisms.

Diagnosis: The clinical features are highly suggestive. Diagnosis can be confirmed by microscopic examination of exudates and biopsy specimens. The yeast forms of the organisms distend the cytoplasm of macrophages and appear in H&E sections as globose or oval bodies (3-4 μm) with a central basophilic body surrounded by an unstained zone. The organism closely resembles *H capsulatum*.

Treatment: No completely satisfactory treatment is known. Surgical excision of lesions combined with antifungal drugs (amphotericin B) could be used.

GEOTRICHOSIS

Geotrichosis is a rare mycosis due to infection with *Geotrichum candidum*, a ubiquitous saprophytic fungus of soil, decaying organic matter, and contaminated food. *G candidum* is part of the normal flora of the mouth and intestinal tract in humans. The organism has caused systemic disease in dogs, abortion and mastitis in cattle, and caseous nodules in the lymph nodes of pigs. It has been isolated from feces of dogs, ocelots, and apes with enteritis; cutaneous lesions in snakes and flamingos; and the respiratory system of horses, penguins, chickens, and humans.

Clinical Findings and Lesions: Clinical signs vary with organ involvement and may be nonspecific. In dogs with disseminated geotrichosis, clinical signs may include coughing elicited by tracheal palpation, fever, anorexia, polydipsia, progressive dypsnea, vomiting, and icterus. Radiographic findings include nodular densities with confluence in some regions of the lungs. Disseminated disease progresses rapidly. Lesions, found in various organs, appear as multiple, yellow-gray, firm, fleshy nodules, which microscopically are well-defined granulomas.

Diagnosis: Definitive diagnosis is based on cultural and microscopic characteristics. Fungal elements may be abundant, both free and in macrophages and multinucleated giant cells, as ovoid yeast-like cells (3-7 μm in diameter) and as short, jointed chains of round yeast cells forming pseudohyphae. In histologic sections of tissues stained with H&E, *G candidum* resembles *Candida albicans* and *Histoplasma capsulatum*.

Treatment: Nystatin given as an oral suspension was effective in treatment of gorillas with watery diarrhea associated with isolation of *G candidum* from fecal wet mounts. The use of antifungal drugs for treating disseminated geotrichosis in animals has not been reported.

HISTOPLASMOSIS

Histoplasmosis is a chronic, noncontagious, disseminated, granulomatous disease of humans and other animals caused by the dimorphic fungus *Histoplasma capsulatum*. The organism is commonly found in soil that contains bird and bat manure. It produces mycelial growth in the soil and in culture at room temperature and grows in a yeast form in tissues and in cultures at 37°C.

Histoplasmosis is found worldwide. Endemic areas in the USA include the Mississippi and Ohio River valleys. Infection has been described in many animal species, but disease is uncommon to rare in all but dogs and cats. Infection is commonly via aerosol contamination of the respiratory tract, and the lungs and thoracic lymph nodes are the sites of primary infection, although the GI tract may be a primary site of infection, especially in dogs. The organisms enter the bloodstream from a primary focus and become disseminated throughout the body; they may localize in bone marrow or the eyes where they produce chorioretinitis or endophthalmitis.

Clinical Findings and Lesions: The signs vary and are nonspecific, reflecting the various organ involvement. Many dogs have a protracted course of weight loss to emaciation, chronic cough, persistent diarrhea, fever, anemia, hepatomegaly, splenomegaly, lymphadenopathy, and nasopharyngeal and GI ulceration. Obstructive respiratory difficulty due to tracheobronchial lymphadenopathy also has been found in dogs. Dissemination may involve the skin, in which weeping, ulcerated, nodular lesions develop. Polyarthropathy, chorioretinitis, and retinal detachment have also been reported in a dog with disseminated histoplasmosis. Acute histoplasmosis may be fatal after 2-5 wk. In cats, disseminated infection is common. Clinical signs may be nonspecific but often include respiratory difficulty, fever, depression, anorexia, and weight loss. Lymphadenopathy, hepatomegaly, ocular disease (conjunctivitis, granulomatous chorioretinitis, retinal detachment, optic neuritis), lameness, and cutaneous nodules or ulcers may also be seen.

Gross lesions include enlargement of the liver, spleen, and mesenteric lymph nodes; ascites; yellow-white, variable-sized nodules in the lungs; and enlargement of bronchial lymph nodes. The enlarged liver may have multiple, scattered, irregular-shaped, pale yellow foci of granulomatous inflammation. Pale foci may be present in the myocardium, and the small intestine may have thickened, gray walls and ulceration of the mucosa.

Diagnosis: Histoplasmosis and other fungal infections should be considered when the clinical signs include respiratory distress, diarrhea, enlarged bronchial lymph nodes, and pulmonary nodules. *Histoplasma* organisms are usually numerous in affected tissues, and a definitive diagnosis can often be made by fine-needle aspiration and exfoliative cytology. Tissue biopsy may be required if cytology is not diagnostic. *Histoplasma* organisms are difficult to detect with routine H&E stain but stain well with PAS, Gomori's methenamine silver, and Gridley's fungal stains. Yeast forms in macrophages and giant cells are round to ovoid (1-4 μm) structures with a thin cell wall and a thin, clear zone between the cell wall and cellular cytoplasm. *H capsulatum* can also be cultured from tissue specimens, fine-needle aspirates, and body fluids.

Treatment: Itraconazole (10 mg/kg/day) is the treatment of choice for disseminated histoplasmosis in dogs and cats. Ketoconazole, 10-15 mg/kg, BID for 4-6 mo, may be effective in early or mild cases of histoplasmosis in dogs. For severe cases, concurrent treatment with amphotericin B or amphotericin B lipid complex is suggested.

HYALOHYPHOMYCOSIS

Hyalohyphomycosis is infection caused by nonpigmented fungi (other than the genera *Aspergillus* or *Penicillium* or the class Zygomycetes) that in tissue form hyphal elements with hyaline or clear walls. Examples of genera causing hyalohyphomycosis in humans and other animals include *Acremonium, Fusarium, Geotrichum, Paecilomyces, Pseudallescheria,* and *Scedosporium.* Hyalohyphomycosis occurs much less frequently than phaeohyphomycosis.

Clinical Findings: Lesions range from local cutaneous, subcutaneous, corneal, or nasal mucosal disease to disseminated disease involving the lungs and multiple other organ systems.

Diagnosis: The several causative fungi cannot be identified by their histologic features in tissues; culture isolation and/or PCR are required.

Treatment: Surgical removal with or without topical antifungal therapy is the treatment of choice for local disease. Disseminated disease typically carries a grave prognosis. Treatment with newer azole antifungals and/or amphotericin B lipid complex may be attempted.

MYCETOMAS

Mycetomas are granulomatous nodules of the subcutaneous tissues that contain tissue grains or granules. Within the grains are dense colonies of the organism. When such lesions are caused by fungi, they are known as eumycotic mycetomas. The causal agents of eumycotic mycetomas include a variety of saprophytic geophilic fungi. Eumycotic mycetomas caused by pigmented fungi such as *Curvularia* spp and *Madurella* spp are called black- or dark-grain mycetomas. White-grained mycetomas are caused by unpigmented fungi such as *Acremonium* spp and *Scedosporium apiospermum* (the asexual state of *Pseudallescheria boydii*).

Clinical Findings and Lesions: Most eumycotic mycetomas are confined to the subcutaneous tissue, but white-grain mycetomas may be extensions of abdominal cavity disease. Peritonitis or abdominal masses are typically seen in white-grain mycetomas. Black-grain mycetomas are usually characterized by relatively poorly circumscribed cutaneous nodules on the extremities or face. The lesions may ulcerate or form fistulas. When the feet or limbs are involved, the infection may extend to the underlying bone.

The fungal mycelia proliferate in the lesions and organize into aggregates known as granules or grains. In these granules, the mycelium is compact and frequently bizarre and distorted in form. Chlamydospores are frequent, especially at the periphery, and the mycelium may or may not be embedded in an amorphous cement-like substance. Histologically, the granules are frequently surrounded by eosinophilic deposits. Granules may be of various colors and sizes, depending on the species of fungus involved.

Diagnosis: A presumptive diagnosis can be made if there are grains within the exudate of draining tracts. For cytology, the grains should be examined for the presence of fungal elements. If no tissue grains are found in the exudate, a biopsy of the lesion should be taken for histopathologic examination. Cultures should be performed to confirm cytologic findings and to identify the causative agent. Either tissue grains or biopsy specimens should be cultured.

Treatment: The prognosis for abdominal mycetomas is guarded because tissue involvement is usually extensive. Cutaneous mycetomas, while not life-threatening, are often difficult to resolve. Radical surgical excision, including limb amputation, may be effective for some cases of cutaneous mycetomas. Effectiveness of antifungal chemotherapy has been reported in only a few cases. In one report, fluconazole, 50 mg/day for 6 wk, was used to successfully treat a dog with intra-abdominal maduromycosis. In another report, longterm treatment with itraconazole, 5-10 mg/kg/day, failed to resolve a disseminated *Acremonium* infection in a dog.

NORTH AMERICAN BLASTOMYCOSIS

North American blastomycosis, caused by the dimorphic fungus *Blastomyces dermatitidis*, is characterized by pyogranulomatous lesions in various tissues. It is most common in humans, dogs, and cats but has also been described in such widely divergent species as horses, ferrets, deer, wolves, African lions, bottlenosed dolphins, and sea lions. It appears not to be a disease of cattle, sheep, or pigs. Blastomycosis is generally limited to North America, and most cases have occurred in the Mississippi, Missouri, Tennessee, and Ohio River basins and along the Great Lakes and the St. Lawrence Seaway. Even within these river basins, the organism is found in geographically restricted areas. Beaver dams and other habitats where soil is moist, acidic, and rich in decaying vegetation may serve as the ecologic niche for the organism, but it is often difficult to find in the environment. The organism has also been recovered from pigeon and bat feces. Rain, dew, or fog may play a critical role in liberating the infective conidia, which then are aerosolized and inhaled. When respiratory defenses are overwhelmed or immunosuppressed, disseminated disease occurs via hematogenous spread from the lungs. Cutaneous lesions may result from a primary entry through the skin or, more commonly, by dissemination from a pulmonary focus. Needle-stick injuries to veterinary personnel following aspiration of cutaneous lesions from infected animals have resulted in primary cutaneous infection. Ocular lesions tend to develop first in the posterior segment, resulting in granulomatous chorioretinitis and retinal detachment. Anterior segment involvement often follows, resulting in anterior uveitis and panophthalmitis.

Clinical Findings and Lesions: The signs vary with organ involvement and are not specific. Weight loss may be accompanied by coughing, anorexia, lymphadenopathy, dyspnea, ocular disease, lameness, skin lesions, and fever. Dry, harsh lung sounds from lung lesions are extremely common in dogs with blastomycosis. Signs of pulmonary involvement are seen in up to 85% of affected dogs. Severe pulmonary involvement results in hypoxemia, which indicates a poor prognosis. Lymph node involvement is seen in about half of affected dogs, which is about the same proportion of dogs that have cutaneous involvement. Skin lesions may include proliferative granulomas and subcutaneous abscesses that ulcerate and drain a serosanguineous discharge. The skin lesions are often very small and multifocal in dogs, but large abscesses are occasionally seen, especially in cats. The planum nasale, face, and nail beds are most often involved. Signs of ocular blastomycosis are seen in 30-50% of affected dogs and include blindness, uveitis, glaucoma, and retinal detachment. Lameness associated with fungal osteomyelitis or severe paronychia occurs in about one quarter of affected dogs. CNS signs are uncommon, occurring in <5% of dogs, but they may be more common in cats. The pattern of systemic involvement is similar in cats, but cats are affected far less commonly than dogs. Hematuria, nocturia, and dysuria with tenesmus may be seen with urogenital blastomycosis.

Gross lesions consist of few to numerous, variable-sized, irregular, firm, gray to yellow areas of pulmonary consolidation and nodules in the lungs and thoracic lymph nodes. Dissemination may result in nodular lesions in various organs but especially the skin, eyes, and bone. Cutaneous lesions are single or multiple papules, or chronic, draining, nodular pyogranulomas.

Diagnosis: Blastomycosis should be considered in dogs with draining cutaneous nodules and signs of respiratory disease. In cats, respiratory tract involvement is seen most frequently, followed by involvement of the CNS, regional lymph nodes, skin, eyes, and GI and urinary tracts. Radiographic findings in the lungs include noncalcified nodules or consolidation, and enlargement of the bronchial and mediastinal lymph nodes. The predominant patterns on thoracic radiographs are those of diffuse nodular interstitial and peribronchial densities. Commonly, the bronchial lymph nodes are greatly enlarged and appear in radiographs as dense masses. Diagnosis can be made from biopsy tissue or aspirated specimens taken from cutaneous lesions or other involved organs by the presence of thick-walled yeast that often have daughter cells budding from a broad base. These round to ovoid, pale pink (H&E) blastospores measure 8-25 μm and have a refractile, double-contoured wall. They may be empty or contain basophilic nuclear material and have single broad-based buds. An antibody response, detected by agar gel immunodiffusion, usually occurs, but this response is neither sensitive nor specific when attempting to make a definitive diagnosis.

Treatment: Itraconazole (5 mg/kg/day) is the treatment of choice for dogs and cats with blastomycosis. A minimum of 2 mo of treatment is necessary, and the drug should be continued until active disease is not apparent. Clinical cure can be expected in ~70% of dogs, with recurrence in ~20% of treated dogs months to years after treatment. Most dogs will again respond to retreatment with itraconazole. In fulminating cases of blastomycosis, especially those with evidence of hypoxemia, combination therapy with amphotericin B and itraconazole is recommended. Short courses of anti-inflammatory doses of glucocorticoids have been advocated during the first few days of treatment by some, but steroid use is controversial and may actually worsen the prognosis. The prognosis is best for dogs without lung disease or with only mild lung disease, is more guarded for dogs with moderate to severe lung disease, and is poorest for dogs with CNS involvement.

OOMYCOSIS
(Pythiosis, Lagenidiosis)

Oomycosis is caused by pathogens in the class Oomycetes. These organisms are not true fungi but are aquatic pathogens in the kingdom Stramenopila. They are more closely related to algae than fungi but cause disease that closely resembles zygomycosis (p 524).

Organisms of significance in veterinary medicine include various species of *Saprolegnia* and *Achyla* (eg, *S diclina*), which are the common agents of cutaneous disease in fishes; *Pythium insidiosum*, the cause of a cutaneous and subcutaneous mycosis in horses (bursatti, swamp cancer, leeches), a cutaneous, subcutaneous, and GI disease in dogs, and a cutaneous and paranasal disease of cats; and *Lagenidium* spp, the cause of cutaneous and systemic lesions and large vessel aneurysms in dogs. Pythiosis is a common disease of domestic animals in some tropical and subtropical areas of the world. In dogs, pythiosis is most often encountered in Southeast Asia, eastern coastal Australia, South America, and in the USA, especially along the Gulf coast. In the USA, the disease most often is seen in fall and winter months.

Clinical Findings and Lesions: In horses, lesions are large, roughly circular, granulomatous, ulcerated, fistulated nodules, or subcutaneous swellings with yellow-gray necrotic masses or cores. The lesions are most common on the legs (especially the lower limbs), abdomen, chest, and genitalia. Distribution of lesions is attributable to the aquatic nature of the organism. The lesions are pruritic, discharge a mucosanguineous exudate, and often are self-traumatized. The granulomas contain firm, yellowish coralliform masses of necrotic tissue known as "kunkers," which may be removed intact. Kunkers are foci of coagulative necrosis in vessels that have become sequestered from the surrounding tissue; they contain broad, branching aseptate hyphae and are 1-10 μm in diameter. Bone involvement may be a feature of chronic pythiosis. Enteric pythiosis in horses is characterized by fibrosing and stenotic GI lesions containing intralesional foci of caseous material and fungal hyphae.

Specimens removed at surgery or necropsy consist of fibrous tissue with irregularly spaced, firm, focal areas of necrosis that vary in size and color. Microscopically, alterations vary from foci of acute exudative inflammation with numerous eosinophils to a granulomatous reaction with sequestered areas of necrosis and a framework of hyphae that are thick-walled, branching, and slightly irregular in width.

GI and cutaneous forms of pythiosis are seen and are characterized by severe granulomatous and eosinophilic inflammation. *P insidiosum* infection is seen most often in the GI tract of young adult dogs, especially Labrador Retrievers. The stomach, proximal small intestine, and ileocolic junction are affected most commonly, but any part of the intestine, esophagus, and colon can be diseased. Clinical signs include vomiting, weight loss, and anorexia. The weight loss can be severe, but affected dogs usually do not appear systemically ill until late in the disease. The lesions are typically characterized by severe transmural thickening of the gastric or intestinal wall, with mesenteric lymphadenopathy in which the lymph nodes are embedded in a large, firm granulomatous mass involving the surrounding mesentery. Bowel ischemia, infarction, or acute hemoabdomen may develop due to extension of disease into mesenteric vessels. Enteric pyogranulomas typically consist of necrotic foci infiltrated and surrounded by neutrophils, eosinophils, epithelioid macrophages, plasma cells, and multinucleated giant cells. Etiologic agents may not be apparent on sections stained with H&E. Sections stained with Gomori's methenamine silver show branching, rarely septate hyphae.

Cutaneous pythiosis is typified by nonhealing wounds, invasive masses, and ulcerated nodules with draining tracts. The extremities, tail head, ventral neck, or perineum are affected most commonly. Pythiosis in cats is rare and typified by either cutaneous or nasopharyngeal lesions.

Lagenidiosis is a recently described oomycotic infection of dogs characterized by multifocal cutaneous lesions and regional lymphadenopathy. In contrast to the clinical course of cutaneous pythiosis, dogs with lagenidiosis often have involvement at distant sites. Hematogenous spread is likely as the infection causes a vasculitis. Lymph nodes, lungs, and especially great vessels may be affected. Great vessel aneurysms may acutely rupture, resulting in sudden death.

Diagnosis: In horses, lesions of pythiosis are similar to those of zygomycosis (p 524) and may be confused with cutaneous habronemiasis (p 735), excessive granulation tissue, and certain equine neoplasms. In pythiosis, the necrotic cores are distinct from the surrounding tissue, and a seropurulent discharge from the sinus tracts is prominent. The lesions contain irregular, branching (at right angles), rarely septate hyphae, 4-8 μm in diameter.

In dogs, diagnosis can be made by isolation of *P insidiosum* from infected tissues. Culture identification or PCR have been used. An ELISA for detection of anti-*P insidiosum* antibodies is available and appears to be both sensitive and specific. The histologic features of lagenidiosis are similar to those of pythiosis and zygomycosis. However, *Lagenidium* hyphae are usually much larger and visible on H&E-stained tissues. Serology can be used for presumptive diagnosis, but definitive diagnosis of lagenidiosis is best made by culture and PCR.

Treatment: In dogs with GI pythiosis, the prognosis is poor. Complete surgical excision is the treatment of choice, but the disease is often too extensive at the time of diagnosis to allow complete resection. Medical therapy for pythiosis should include itraconazole (10 mg/kg/day) and terbinafine (5-10 mg/kg/day). Treatment with amphotericin B lipid complex can also be attempted. Approximately 20% of dogs will respond to longterm therapy. Medical therapy for lagenidiosis has not been described. In horses, the prognosis is guarded, and timely recognition and treatment are essential for successful management. Factors that influence the prognosis include size and site of lesion and duration of infection. Small lesions of short duration that have not invaded critical structures usually respond best to treatment. Surgical excision, immunotherapy, or a combination of both may be effective. Immunotherapy consists of a series of intradermal or SC injections of killed, sonicated, whole-cell hyphal antigens or precipitated soluble antigens of the causative fungus. Subcutaneous abscesses at the sites of injection, osteitis, or deep-seated laminitis may be a complication of such therapy. Surgical removal plus systemic or local administration of amphotericin B may be a satisfactory treatment if the disease is localized.

PAECILOMYCOSIS

Systemic (mainly pulmonary) mycoses caused by *Paecilomyces* spp have been described in humans and various other animals, especially those with lowered body temperatures. Infection in captive reptiles and amphibians is probably fairly common; other hosts include dogs, horses, cats (nasal granuloma), and goats (mastitis). More significant causal fungi are *P lilacinus* and *P variotii*. The fungi, usually considered nonpathogenic, are widely distributed in soil and decaying organic matter. Infection usually has been secondary to debilitation, immunosuppression, and/or alteration of normal microbial flora by prolonged administration of antibiotics.

Clinical Findings and Lesions: Signs vary and are not specific but may reflect tissue or organ involvement. Involved organs are enlarged and contain raised, gray-white nodules. Granulomatous lesions (multiple, pale foci) that contain septate pseudohyphae (2-3 μm in diameter), oval conidia, and spherical to oval, thin-walled spores (3-6 μm) are found in many tissues (eg, lungs) in disseminated cases and are closely associated with small and medium-sized arterioles.

Diagnosis: The gross lesions can be confused with those of other systemic mycoses. However, the septate hyphae, conidia, and spores of this fungus differ from common pathogenic fungi such as *Aspergillus* spp and those of mucormycosis. Diagnosis can be made by cultural isolation of the fungus from multiple specimens of lesions. With most species, growth may be absent or restricted at 37°C but good at 5-30°C.

Treatment: No treatment regimens have been described. *Paecilomyces* spp vary greatly in sensitivity to antifungal agents; *P lilacinus* appears highly resistant to amphotericin B and flucytosine but sensitive to ketoconazole, while *P variotii* is sensitive to the first 2 drugs.

PENICILLIOSIS

Infections with *Penicillium* spp are rare in domestic animals. However, the fungus has been isolated from a case of feline dermatosis; from orbital cellulitis and sinusitis with pneumonia in another cat; from invasive destructive disease of nasal tissues in dogs; from invasive lesions in the lungs, air sacs, liver, and other tissues in captive toucanets (*P griseofulvum*); and from systemic disease in bamboo rats (*P marneffei*) in southeast Asia. *Penicillium* spp are widely distributed in nature and are found in soils, grains, and various foods and feeds.

Clinical Findings and Lesions: Dogs with nasal penicilliosis have chronic sneezing and an acute to chronic nasal discharge that varies from intermittent hemorrhagic to intermittent or continuous mucoid or mucopurulent. Radiographic findings include areas of turbinate destruction with increased radiolucency. Grossly, the nasal mucosa has foci of necrosis and ulceration; microscopically, fungal hyphae may form a thick mat over an intact mucosa adjacent to these foci.

Diagnosis: Diagnosis is based on fungal culture, character of the lesions and presence of fungal hyphae, and a positive agar-gel double-diffusion test. Cultural isolation of a *Penicillium* sp must be accompanied by demonstration of tissue invasion by the fungus for confirmation. In tissues, *P marneffei* closely resemble the yeast phase of *Histoplasma capsulatum*.

Treatment: Surgical turbinectomy with curettage has been combined with flushing of the nasal cavity with 1% tincture of iodine or povidone-iodine (10:1) and oral thiabendazole. Fluconazole, 2.5-5.0 mg/kg/day for 2 mo, has been used to successfully treat some dogs with nasal penicilliosis.

PHAEOHYPHOMYCOSIS

Phaeohyphomycosis is a broad clinicopathologic designation that refers to chronic cutaneous, subcutaneous, or mucosal infection caused by one of several genera and species of pigmented fungi of the family Dematiaceae. Several fungal genera have been reported to affect humans and other animals including *Alternaria, Bipolaris, Cladophialophora (Xylohypha, Cladosporium), Curvularia, Exophiala, Fonsecaea, Moniliella, Phialophora, Ramichloridium,* and *Scolecobasidium*. Fungi in this category are saprophytic, widely distributed organisms found in soil, water, and decaying vegetable matter. Infection may result from fungal implantation into tissue at the site of an injury.

Clinical Findings and Lesions: Phaeohyphomycosis has been described in cows, cats, horses, and dogs. The most common clinical presentations include ulcerated cutaneous nodules, upper respiratory signs, and nasal/paranasal masses. Slowly enlarging, subcutaneous or submucosal masses are found about the head, nasal mucosa, limbs, and chest. The nodules may ulcerate and have draining fistulous tracts. These pyogranulomas contain pigmented, septate hyphae with irregular enlargements and thin-walled, budding yeast-like forms.

Diagnosis: Phaeohyphomycosis can be diagnosed by microscopic examination of exudate and biopsy specimens, which reveals pigmented or hyaline filamentous hyphae (2-6 μm in diameter), with terminal and intercalated vesicles (6-12 μm), and spores. The several causative fungi cannot be identified by their histologic features in tissues; cultural isolation and/or PCR are required. The differential diagnosis should include neoplasia, other granulomas, and epidermoid cysts.

Treatment: In most cases, the infection is confined to the skin and subcutaneous tissues. In a favorable location, cure can be effected by wide excision of the lesion. Chemotherapy with amphotericin B or itraconazole may be considered in cases when surgery is not possible.

RHINOSPORIDIOSIS

Rhinosporidiosis is a chronic, nonfatal, pyogranulomatous infection, primarily of the nasal mucosa and occasionally of the skin of horses, cattle, dogs, cats, and aquatic birds, caused by the fungus *Rhinosporidium seeberi*. Uncommon in North America, it is seen most often in India, Africa, and South America. The organism has not been cultured, and its natural habitat is unknown. Trauma may predispose to infection, which is not considered transmissible.

Clinical Findings and Lesions: Infection of the nasal mucosa is characterized by polypoid growths that may be soft, pink, friable, lobulated with roughened surfaces, and large enough to occlude the nasal passages. The cutaneous lesions may be single or multiple, sessile or pedunculated. The nasal polyps and cutaneous lesions have a granulomatous, fibromyxoid inflammatory component and contain the fungal organism.

Diagnosis: Rhinosporidiosis may be confused with other granulomatous lesions of the nasal mucosa and skin, including aspergillosis, entomophthoromycosis, "nasal granuloma," and cryptococcosis. Microscopic demonstration of spherules (sporangia) of *R seeberi* in biopsy specimens confirms the diagnosis. The spherules may be numerous, vary in size (up to 300 μm), have thick walls that stain periodic acid-schiff positive, and contain endospores 4-19 μm in diameter. Developing stages of varying size without spores are distributed throughout the lesion.

Treatment: Surgical excision of the lesions is considered standard, but recurrence is common.

SPOROTRICHOSIS

Sporotrichosis is a sporadic chronic granulomatous disease of humans and various domestic and laboratory animals caused by *Sporothrix schenckii*. The organism is dimorphic and forms mycelia on vegetation and in Sabouraud's dextrose agar at 25-30°C but is yeast-like in tissue and media at 37°C. It is ubiquitous in soil, vegetation, and timber; is distributed worldwide; and in the USA is most commonly found in coastal regions and river valleys. Infection usually results from direct inoculation of the organism into skin wounds via contact with plants or soil or penetrating foreign bodies. Disseminated disease caused by inhalation of spores is rare. Sporotrichosis has been reported in dogs, cats, horses, cows, camels, dolphins, goats, mules, birds, pigs, rats, armadillos, and humans. Zoonotic infections can occur. The cat may be the species with the greatest zoonotic potential, and transmission from cat to human has been reported without evidence of trauma. In contrast, transmission from other infected species appears to require inoculation of previously traumatized skin. The large number of organisms shed from the wound and in the feces of infected cats is believed to be responsible for the increased zoonotic potential of feline sporotrichosis.

Clinical Findings and Lesions: Sporotrichosis may be grouped into 3 forms—lymphocutaneous, cutaneous, and disseminated. The lymphocutaneous form is the most common. Small, firm dermal to subcutaneous nodules, 1-3 cm in diameter, develop at the site of inoculation. As infection ascends along the lymphatic vessels, cording and new nodules develop. Lesions ulcerate and discharge a serohemorrhagic exudate. Although systemic illness is not seen initially, chronic illness may result in fever, listlessness, and depression. The cutaneous form remains localized to the site of inoculation, although lesions may be multicentric. Disseminated sporotrichosis is rare but potentially fatal and may develop with neglect of cutaneous and lymphocutaneous forms. Infection develops via hematogenous or tissue spread from the initial site of inoculation to the bone, lungs, liver, spleen, testes, GI tract, or CNS. In humans, the incidence of systemic sporotrichosis appears to be rising, primarily due to infection of immunocompromised people.

Diagnosis: Diagnosis can be made by cultural (samples obtained from unopened lesions) or microscopic examination of the exudate or biopsy specimens. In tissues and exudate, the organism is present as few to numerous, cigar-shaped, single cells within macrophages. The fungal cells are pleomorphic and small (2-10 × 1-3 μm); buds may be present and give the appearance of a ping-pong paddle. A fluorescent antibody technique has been used to identify the yeast-like cells in tissues. In species other than cats, *Sporothrix* organisms are often sparse in exudate and infected tissue so that diagnosis usually requires culturing the organism. In cultures, a true mycelium is produced, with fine, branching, septate hyphae bearing pear-shaped conidia on slender conidiophores.

Treatment: Few treatments have been critically evaluated, but itraconazole (10 mg/kg/day) is considered the treatment of choice. Treatment is continued 3-4 wk beyond apparent clinical cure. Alternatively, a saturated solution of potassium iodide, administered PO, has been used with some success; therapy is continued 30 days beyond apparent clinical cure. During treatment, the animal should be monitored for signs of iodide toxicity—anorexia, vomiting, depression, muscle twitching, hypothermia, cardiomyopathy, cardiovascular collapse, and death. Cats are especially sensitive to iodides and the development of iodism.

Zoonotic Risk: Sporotrichosis should be considered a zoonosis because cases of animal-to-human transmission are well documented. Strict hygiene must be observed when handling animals with suspected or diagnosed sporotrichosis. People who are in contact with infected animals should be informed of the contagious nature of the disease when therapeutic options are discussed.

ZYGOMYCOSIS
(Basidiobolomycosis, Conidiobolomycosis, Entomophthoromycosis)

Zygomycosis is used to describe infection with fungi in the class Zygomycetes and 2 genera in the order Entomophthorales, *Basidiobolus* and *Conidiobolus*. True zygomycete infections are rare, but conidiobolomycosis and basidiobolomycosis are more common and cause pyogranulomatous lesions that are grossly and histologically similar to those caused by pythiosis and lagenidiosis. This is primarily an infection of the nasal mucosa and subcutaneous tissue of horses and rarely other animals (llamas, sheep) by *Conidiobolus coronatus*, *C incongruus*, *C lamprauges*, or *B ranarum*. These ubiquitous fungi are present in soil and decaying vegetation and, in the case of basidioboli, the GI tracts of amphibians, reptiles, and macropods. *C coronatus* affects almost exclusively the mucosa of the nose and mouth. *Basidiobolus* infects the lateral aspects of the head, neck, and body. *C coronatus* is also an important insect pathogen.

Clinical Findings and Lesions: Ulcerative pyogranulomas of the mucous membrane of the nostril or mouth, or nodular growths of the nasal mucosa and the lips caused by *C coronatus* may cause mechanical blockage, resulting in dyspnea and nasal discharge. Lesions caused by *B ranarum* are large, usually single, circular, ulcerative, pruritic nodules of the skin of the upper body. Fistulous tracts discharge a serosanguineous fluid from the lesions, which frequently are traumatized. Extension to regional lymph nodes results in swelling of the nodes and development of yellow necrotic foci. Lesions may contain a creamy, yellow central core of necrotic tissue. Disseminated basidiobolomycosis is rare but has been described in dogs and a mandrill.

In excised tissues or necropsy specimens, a thickened fibrotic dermis has scattered, red or creamy white areas. The lesions, which contain hyphal forms, a heavy infiltrate of eosinophils, and sequestered areas of necrosis, have histologic features of infectious granulomas.

Diagnosis: Clinically, zygomycosis may be confused with cutaneous habronemiasis (p 735) and oomycosis (p 519) but can be differentiated by microscopic examination of tissues. In H&E sections, the fungus appears as holes and elongated channels, and many hyphae have an eosinophilic cuff; in sections stained for fungi, the organism consists of large, branching, sometimes septate, 4-20 μm hyphae. Cultural examination is required to identify the causative fungus.

Treatment: Surgical excision or immunotherapy, or both, have been successful. The immunotherapy consists of intradermal injections of 0.02-0.1 mL particulate fungal material. Localized mycotic disease has been treated with amphotericin B given systemically or locally, or both. Ideally, treatment includes early surgical removal of the lesion, followed by administration of amphotericin B.

LEPTOSPIROSIS

Leptospirosis is a worldwide zoonotic disease of domestic animals and wildlife. It is caused by a spirochete bacteria classified under the *Leptospira*, of which there are ~17 species. The taxonomy of the genus is confusing, with a number of species, including *interrogans* (sensu stricto), *kirschneri*, and *santarosai*. Serovars, as defined by agglutination cross-absorption, are the primary grouping below the species designation. This can add even greater confusion, as some serovars are grouped under more than one species. The term *Leptospira interrogans* (sensu lato) is used to describe the broad group of pathogenic leptospires associated with animal hosts.

The same disease processes are seen in all animals, although some species are more resisistant to acute infections. Infections may be asymptomatic or cause various signs, including fever, icterus, hemoglobinuria, renal failure, infertility, abortion, and death. After acute infection, leptospires frequently localize in the kidneys or reproductive organs and are shed in the urine, sometimes in large numbers for months or years, especially with host-adapted serovars. Because the organisms survive in surface waters, such as swamps, streams, and rivers, for extended periods, the disease is often waterborne. The organism survives well in mud and moist, alkaline soil, such as river banks; floods frequently result in an increase of disease outbreaks.

Infection is commonly acquired by contact of skin or mucous membranes with urine and, to a lesser extent, by intake of urine-contaminated feed or water. Ingestion of infected animals and venereal transmission can also be routes of infection. Infections can be readily established via the conjunctiva, vaginal mucosa, or skin abrasions. Development of disease depends on multiple factors, including the initial inoculum. Leptospires spread rapidly via the lymphatics to the blooodstream and then to all tissues. In the immunologically naive animal, initial replication occurs in the lungs, followed by the liver and spleen, and then multiple organs. If the animal mounts an immune response and survives, leptospires will be cleared from most organs and the bloodstream. However, infection persists in sites hidden from the immune system, such as the proximal renal tubules, brain, anterior chamber of the eyes, and genital tract. Persistence in the kidneys results in a carrier state; the animal may shed leptospires in the urine for ≥1 yr. If shedder animals are introduced into a herd previously free of the disease, leptospires are rapidly disseminated. Clinical signs may be severe, mild, or inapparent. Abortions and stillbirths may occur, most frequently during the middle or last third of gestation. Abortions may be followed by retention of fetal membranes, and fertility may be impaired. Disease outbreaks in small herds are often self-limiting. However, control of enzootic infections in large herds generally requires immunization, chemotherapy, fencing the herd from surface waters, and limiting contact with rodents and other wildlife carriers.

Of >200 antigenically distinct pathogenic leptospiral serovars, only a small number have been isolated from domestic animals in the USA, although others have been isolated from wildlife. Cross-immunity between serovars is minimal, and infections with 2 and 3 serovars have been reported. The microscopic agglutination test (MAT) is the most commonly used serologic test for diagnosis. It measures both IgM and IgG antibodies; IgM antibodies usually appear 6-12 days after infection, and IgG after 2-3 wk. MAT titers rise rapidly, then generally decline over several months to moderate levels that may persist for weeks to years. A single seropositive test is of limited diagnostic significance because it can be the result of a recent vaccination, passive immunity in calves, or a current or past infection. Diagnosis can be confirmed by a rising titer in paired serum samples if the first is taken during the acute stage and the second after 7-10 days, or by a single high titer (>1:800) in an animal with clinical disease consistent with leptospirosis. A delayed rise in convalescent titers may occur, depending on the initiation of therapy, but titers should peak by 4 wk in all cases. Some carrier or shedder animals in which the infection has localized do not have diagnostic titers.

Vaccination with bacterins can stimulate a low titer to the MAT, although titers up to 1:3,200 have been reported following vaccination. Titers decline in several weeks; however, protective immunity may last up to 12 mo, especially in cattle. An ELISA to measure

IgM and IgG is helpful in distinguishing titers due to natural infections from those due to vaccination. The ELISA IgM should be positive prior to the MAT, which may aid in early diagnosis; however, the ELISA is not widely available.

Demonstration of leptospires in urine or tissues is helpful in diagnosis. Older techniques, such as darkfield microscopy of urine and Warthin-Starry silver staining of tissues, are not sensitive or specific. Newer tests include fluorescent antibody techniques and PCR.

Definitive confirmation of leptospirosis is made by isolation of the organism from urine or tissue of infected animals. However, because leptospires are not easily cultured, isolation is not usually performed in clinical cases.

Humans are susceptible to all pathogenic serovars found in domestic animals, and transmission from wildlife generally occurs after contact with tissues of infected animals or surface waters contaminated by urine from infected animals. Because of these origins, the disease in humans often is occupationally or recreationally related. In people, as in other animals, the disease varies from subclinical to severe and can be fatal when renal or hepatic failure occurs. The most common signs are fever, headaches, rash, ocular pain, myalgia, and malaise. The flu-like symptoms often have a peracute onset, distinguishing leptospirosis from other diseases with similar symptoms. Laboratory techniques are necessary for a definitive diagnosis. Animal owners should be informed of the potential zoonotic risk of leptospirosis.

LEPTOSPIROSIS IN CATTLE
(Redwater of calves)

In the USA, disease in cattle is primarily due to the *Leptospira* serovars *hardjo*, *pomona*, and *grippotyphosa*. However, serovars *canicola*, *bratislava*, *autumnalis*, and *icterohaemorrhagiae*, among others, also have been isolated. Cattle are the reservoir host for serovar *hardjo*, type *hardjobovis*.

Clinical Findings: Acute leptospirosis can be severe in calves. Serovar *pomona* results in the most severe disease, however other serovars can cause similar disease. Calves may have fever, anorexia, dyspnea from pulmonary congestion, icterus, hemoglobinuria, and hemolytic anemia. Body temperature may rise suddenly to 105-106°F (40.5-41°C). Hemoglobinuria rarely lasts longer than 48-72 hr. The anemia begins to improve by 4-5 days and returns to normal 7-10 days later. Serovar *hardjo* being a host-adapted strain, does not typically result in the acute syndrome. Morbidity and mortality are higher in calves than in adult cattle.

In older cattle, signs vary greatly and diagnosis is more difficult. Enzootic infections of naive cattle with serovar *hardjo*, which usually result in abnormal milk, are more obvious in dairy than in beef cattle. Signs usually are restricted to a sudden drop in milk production; a hemolytic crisis does not occur. The milk is thick, yellow, and blood-tinged, with thick clots and a high somatic cell count; milk production can drop 10-75%, depending on the infecting strain. The udder is typically soft and flabby, which is unique for leptospirosis. Milk production can return to normal in 10-14 days even in the absence of treatment; however, cows with a severe drop in production may not recover to full production during that lactation cycle.

The chronic forms of leptospirosis manifest as abortion and stillbirths, and occur with infections of serovars *pomona* and *hardjo*. Abortion generally occurs 6-12 wk after initial infection and is more common during the third trimester. Stillbirths and birth of premature or weak infected calves also occur. An abortion storm in a breeding herd is often the first indication of leptospirosis infection, because the mild initial signs often pass unnoticed. In endemically infected herds, abortions occur mostly in younger animals and are sporadic. Calves reared by previously infected cows are protected by colostral antibodies for up to 6 mo. The calves generally have an antibody titer similar to that of their dams. Infertility may also be a problem in endemically infected herds, possibly as a consequence of localization of infection in the uterus and oviducts.

Lesions: In the acute form, anemia, icterus, hemoglobinuria, and submucosal hemorrhages are prominent. The kidneys are swollen and dark, with multifocal petechial and ecchymotic hemorrhages, and later develop pale foci of interstitial cell infiltrates. The liver may be swollen, pale, and friable, with minute areas of focal necrosis. Petechiae in other organs are seen in fulminating cases; however, in the more prevalent serovar *hardjo* infections, the lesions are primarily restricted to the kidneys.

Diagnosis: Serology with paired serum samples, direct culture in special media, or fluorescent antibody techniques on tissues are used to confirm clinical and postmortem findings. In herd evaluation, sera should be obtained from various age groups. Isolation of the causative agent constitutes the most definitive diagnostic method, but because leptospires are difficult to culture, it is not commonly performed. Elimination of brucellosis, campylobacteriosis, and trichomoniasis as the cause of an abortion outbreak is suggestive of leptospirosis. MAT titers may peak before abortion because the acute infection occurred several weeks previously. Abortion due to serovar *hardjo* infections may occur with low or negative serologic titers.

Treatment: Tetracycline and oxytetracycline have been reported to be successful if given early in acute cases. Erythromycin, enrofloxacin, tiamulin, and tylosin are also effective in acute cases. Oxytetracycline, amoxicillin, and enrofloxacin may be useful to treat chronic infections. Blood transfusions may be indicated if anemia approaches a critical level. Treatment has limited effect on the course of disease once uremia has developed.

Management of infected herds merits special consideration. When leptospirosis is diagnosed in pregnant beef cows during the early epizootic phase, further abortions can be prevented by prompt vaccination of the entire herd and simultaneous treatment of all animals with appropriate antibiotics. Antibiotics reduce the number of leptospires in the kidneys and other tissues, at least during treatment, and provide a measure of protection until immunity is induced by vaccination. In dairy herds, generally only the sick animals should be treated with antibiotics because the loss of market milk after treatment must be considered.

Prevention: Annual vaccinations, confinement rearing, and chemoprophylaxis are used for control. Annual vaccination should be used in closed herds, whereas semiannual vaccination should be considered for open herds. Bacterins may confer protection against abortions and death and reduce renal infections, although some infections do occur. Management methods to reduce transmission include rat control, fencing cattle from potentially contaminated streams and ponds, separating cattle from pigs and wildlife, selecting replacement stock from herds that are seronegative for leptospirosis, and chemoprophylaxis and vaccination of replacement stock. Serology may fail to identify carrier animals, however, as many will have titers <1:100.

LEPTOSPIROSIS IN DOGS

Dogs are considered the reservoir host for serovar *canicola*. Based on studies that focused on urban populations of dogs, serovars *canicola* and *icterohemorrhagiae* were considered the most prevalent serovars infecting dogs. Studies that have included more rural and suburban populations of dogs document the predominance of serovars of *grippotyphosa* and *pomona* as causative agents of canine leptospirosis. Other serovars, particularly *bratislava*, have also been implicated. A variety of factors, such as increased exposure to raccoons and opossums in suburban and rural areas, communities encroaching on wildlife habitats, and poor farming practices, may explain the rise of previously low-prevalence serovars. Rodents continue to play an important role as reservoirs in urban settings.

Clinical Findings: There is no age or gender predilection, although German Shepherds may be at increased risk compared with other breeds. The incubation period is 4-12 days but may be as short as 2 days. Acute renal failure occurs in 80-90% of dogs that develop clinically significant disease. Early findings are nonspecific and include fever, depression, lethargy, anorexia, arthralgia or myalgia, and oculonasal discharge. This may progress within a few days to a uremic crisis characterized by vomiting, dehydration, lumbar pain from renomegaly and nephritis, and tongue-tip ulceration and necrosis. Icterus and bilirubinuria, suggestive of cholestasis and/or hepatic necrosis, develop in ~20% of these cases and may be present without renal failure. In dogs that develop milder forms of renal failure, polyuria and polydipsia may be the primary sign. Other syndromes reported in dogs include intussusception, pulmonary hemorrhage, uveitis, pneumonitis, chronic hepatitis, and reproductive failure.

The most common hematologic abnormality is a mild to moderate neutrophilic leukocytosis without a left shift, although a normal WBC count may be seen. A mild anemia is seen in 25-35% of cases, often as a result of subclinical hemolysis. Thrombocytopenia occurs in only 10-20% of dogs but is rarely severe enough to be a source of bleeding. Vasculitis is typically the cause of hemorrhage associated with leptospirosis. Azotemia is the most common finding on a serum biochemistry profile. When liver values are abnormal, elevations in serum alkaline phosphatase are typically more pronounced than elevations in ALT and AST. Serum bilirubin is elevated in ~20% of cases. Isosthenuria or hyposthenuria is typically present on the urinalysis, and hematuria, proteinuria, and granular casts are identified in ~30% of cases. Pyuria is less frequently seen, and glycosuria may be identified on occasion as a result of renal tubular damage.

Lesions: Gross findings can include petechial or ecchymotic hemorrhages on any organ, pleural, or peritoneal surface; hepatomegaly; and renomegaly. The liver is often friable with an accentuated lobular pattern and may have a yellowish brown discoloration. The kidneys may have white foci on the subcapsular surface. Microscopic findings in the liver may include hepatocytic necrosis, nonsuppurative hepatitis, and intrahepatic bile statis, while swollen tubular epithelial cells, tubular necrosis, and a mixed inflammatory reaction may be seen in the kidneys. Chronic hepatitis and chronic interstitial nephritis are described in less severe cases.

Diagnosis: Serology is the most useful and frequently used diagnostic test for dogs. Acute and convalescent titers may be necessary to confirm a diagnosis. Other diagnostic tests, such as darkfield microscopy, fluorescent antibody, PCR, culture, and histopathology are less frequently used antemortem. Demonstration of leptospires in tissues with silver staining or fluorescent antibody testing are preferred postmortem.

Treatment: Renal failure and liver disease are treated with fluid therapy and other supportive measures to maintain normal fluid, electrolyte, and acid-base balance. Antibiotic therapy consists of sodium penicillin G, ampicillin, or doxycycline to eliminate leptospiremia, followed by doxycycline to eliminate the renal carrier phase. The fluoroquinolone antibiotics such as enrofloxacin also appear to be leptospirocidal. Doxycycline is preferred over tetracycline, particularly in azotemic patients. First-generation cephalosporins are not effective at any stage of the disease. Previously described regimens of IM procaine penicillin G and dihydrostreptomycin should not be used.

Prevention: Commercial bacterins for dogs are available for serovars *canicola*, *icterohaemorrhagiae*, *grippotyphosa*, and *pomona*. There does not appear to be good cross-immunity between serovars, and vaccinated dogs may still be susceptible to infections with other serovars. Vaccination is recommended at yearly intervals but may be needed more frequently in enzootic areas. Dogs that have recently been exposed to leptospirosis may be treated prophylactically with oral amoxicillin or doxycycline for 7-10 days to prevent infection.

LEPTOSPIROSIS IN HORSES

Leptospirosis in horses is most commonly associated with uveitis or abortions. The disease is typically seen as a self-limiting mild fever with anorexia, although in severe forms hemolysis and vasculitis can result in petechial hemorrhages on mucosal surfaces, hemoglobinuria, anemia, icterus, conjunctival suffusion, depression, and weakness. Renal failure has been documented in foals. Recurrent uveitis (moon blindness) develops anytime from 2-8 mo following the initial infection (p 407). Leptospirosis appears to be a significant cause of recurrent uveitis in horses, accounting for up to 67% of the cases. Serovar *pomona* and an unidentified serovar have been isolated from the aqueous humor of horses with uveitis. It is not clear whether the uveitis is due to intraocular infection or is immune-mediated. Leptospirosis is responsible for 3-4% of all equine abortions annually, although flooding and other environmental catastrophes may result in abortion outbreaks. In the USA, serovar *pomona* type kennewicki appears to be the most significant cause of abortion. The prevalence of leptospirosis in horses is unknown, but serologic evidence indicates a higher incidence than is apparent clinically. In the USA, seroconversion to serovar *bratislava* is reported in up to 40% of horses in large population studies; horses may be a reservoir host for serovar *bratislava*.

Measures for control and treatment are similar to those for cattle and pigs, but specific bacterins have not been developed for horses. Uveitis is treated symptomatically to reduce inflammation and prevent synechiae.

LEPTOSPIROSIS IN PIGS

Although *pomona* was the serovar most commonly found in pigs, recent serologic surveys indicate *bratislava* is the most widespread. Infection usually is from contact with the urine of other pigs or wildlife. Other *Leptospira* serovars reported in pigs include *pomona, grippotyphosa, tarassovi, muenchen,* and *canicola.* Serovars *bratislava, tarassovi,* and *pomona* are host-adapted to swine and can be shed for long periods. Rodents play a significant role in disease maintenance within confinement operations and other swine facilities.

Abortions occurring 2-4 wk before term are the most common manifestation of leptospirosis in pigs. Piglets produced at term may be dead or weak and may die soon after birth. Differential diagnoses include brucellosis, parvovirus, and SMEDI (stillbirth, mummification, embryonic death, and infertility). Suboptimal fertility may be a consequence in sows infected with serovar *bratislava* at the time of breeding or in early gestation. Venereal transmission from carrier boars and sows may play a role in maintenance of the disease. Acute leptospirosis, as described in calves, has been described in piglets but is rare. Treatment and control are similar to those described for cattle.

LEPTOSPIROSIS IN SHEEP

Prevalence of leptospirosis in sheep is lower than in cattle, possibly due to less intensive husbandry methods and the tendency of sheep to avoid contact with surface water. In the USA, *pomona, grippotyphosa, hardjo,* and *bratislava* have been the most common *Leptospira* serovars isolated from sheep. Clinical features, diagnosis, and management of the disease are essentially as described above for mature cattle and calves.

LIGHTNING STROKE AND ELECTROCUTION

Injury or death of an animal due to high-voltage electrical currents may be the result of lightning, fallen transmission wires, faulty electrical circuits, or chewing on an electrical cord. Lightning strike is seasonal and tends to be geographically restricted. Investigation of possible electrocution should always proceed with caution because the electrification resulting from broken transmission wires, for example, may still be present. Once it is evident that the site is safe, the investigation should include the location of the dead animals, examination of all affected animals, and necropsy of those that died.

Certain types of trees, especially hardwoods such as oaks and those that are tall and have spreading root systems just beneath the ground surface, tend to be struck by lightning more often than others. Electrification of such roots charges a wide surface area, particularly when the ground is already damp; passage of charged roots beneath a shallow pool of water causes it to become electrified. A tile drain may spread an electric charge throughout its course. Fallen or sagging transmission wires also may electrify a pool of water, fence, or building, and an animal may also directly contact such wires. Differences exist in conductivity of soil; loam, sand, clay, marble, and chalk are good conductors (in decreasing order), while rocky soil is not.

Accidental electrocution of farm animals in a barn or adjacent confinement pen usually occurs as a result of faulty wiring. Electrification of a water or milk line stanchion, or a metal creep or guard rail can result in widespread distribution of an electric current throughout the stable (*see also* STRAY VOLTAGE IN ANIMAL HOUSING, p 1697) that may result in signs of water deprivation or feed refusal.

Death from electric shock usually results from cardiac or respiratory arrest. Passage of current through the heart usually produces ventricular fibrillation, and involvement of the CNS may affect the respiratory or other vital centers.

Clinical Findings: Varying degrees of electric shock may occur. In most instances of lightning strike, death is instantaneous and the animal falls without a struggle. Occasionally, the animal becomes unconscious but may recover in a few minutes to several hours; residual nervous signs (eg, depression, paraplegia, cutaneous hyperesthesia) may persist for days or weeks or be permanent. Singe marks on or damage to the carcass, damage to the immediate environment, or both, occur in ~90% of cases of lightning stroke but are less likely to be found if the animal is electrocuted by standing on electrified earth. Singe marks tend to be linear and are more commonly found on the medial sides of the legs, although rarely much of the body may be affected. Beneath the singe marks, capillary congestion is common; the arboreal pattern characteristic of lightning strike can be visualized best from the dermal side of the skin by subcutaneous extravasations of blood. Singe marks are rarely found on recovered animals. Smaller animals such as pigs that contact electrified water bowls or creeps may be killed instantly or be thrown some distance by the strength of the shock. Electrocuted pigs are often recumbent and have sustained spinal, pelvic, or limb fractures, resulting from severe muscular contractions.

Diagnosis: The diagnosis is almost always made on circumstantial evidence, ie, location of the cadaver(s) and the absence of any disease processes when examined by necropsy. The presence of dead animals under a tree, hanging through or near a wire fence, or clustered around a light pole is strong evidence of lightning strike even in the absence of physical evidence like recent burning of tree bark or splitting of poles or boards in a fence.

Rigor mortis develops and passes quickly. Postmortem distention of the rumen occurs rapidly and must be differentiated from antemortem ruminal tympany (*see* BLOAT, p 183); in both conditions, the blood tends to clot slowly or not at all. The mucosae of the upper respiratory tract, including the turbinates and sinuses, are congested and hemorrhagic; linear tracheal hemorrhages are common, and large blood clots are occasionally found in the trachea, but the lungs are not compressed as in bloat. All other viscera are congested, and petechiae and ecchymoses may be found in many organs. Due to postmortem ruminal distention, the poorly clotted blood is passively moved to the periphery of the body, resulting in postmortem extravasation of blood in muscles and superficial lymph nodes of the head, neck, and thoracic limbs, and to a lesser extent in the hindquarters. Probably the best indication of instantaneous death is the presence of hay or other feed in the animal's mouth; supportive evidence includes the presence of normal ingesta (especially in the rumen), lack of frothy ingesta (frothy bloat), and presence of normal feces in the lower tract and occasionally on the ground behind the animal. Few conditions affecting livestock will cause such peracute death clustered in a small area.

Farm animals often are insured against lightning strike, and the insurance claims agent or the veterinarian requested to sign an insurance form should closely observe the situation that initiated the claim. The investigator should ascertain that the animal actually died in the high-risk location rather than having been moved after death. This could be done to merely clean up or to deliberately confuse the investigation. A well-documented description of where the animal(s) died and the results of a necropsy examination are acceptable to support an insurance claim of lightning strike.

Treatment: Those animals that survive may require supportive and symptomatic therapy. Euthanasia is indicated for those animals recumbent with fractures or severe muscle injuries.

LISTERIOSIS

(Listerellosis, Circling disease)

Listeriosis is a sporadic bacterial infection that affects a wide range of animals, including humans and birds. It is seen worldwide, more frequently in temperate and colder climates. There is a high incidence of intestinal carriers. Encephalitis or meningoencephalitis in adult ruminants is the most frequently recognized form.

Etiology and Epidemiology: *Listeria monocytogenes* is a small, motile, gram-positive, nonsporeforming, extremely resistant, diphtheroid coccobacillus that grows under a wide temperature range, 39-111°F (4-44°C). Its ability to grow at 4°C is an important diagnostic aid (the "cold enrichment" method) for isolation of the organism from brain tissue but not from placental or fetal tissues. Primary isolation is enhanced under microaerophilic conditions. It is a ubiquitous saprophyte that lives in a plant-soil environment and has been isolated from ~42 species of domestic and wild mammals and 22 species of birds, as well as fish, crustaceans, insects, sewage, water, silage and other feedstuffs, milk, cheese, meconium, feces, and soil.

The natural reservoirs of *L monocytogenes* appear to be soil and mammalian GI tracts, both of which contaminate vegetation. Grazing animals ingest the organism and further contaminate vegetation and soil. Animal-to-animal transmission occurs via the fecal-oral route.

Listeriosis is primarily a winter-spring disease of feedlot or housed ruminants. The less acidic pH of spoiled silage enhances multiplication of *L monocytogenes*. Outbreaks may occur ≥10 days after feeding poor-quality silage. Removal or change of silage in the ration often stops the spread of listeriosis; feeding the same silage months later may result in new cases.

Pathogenesis: *Listeria* organisms that are ingested or inhaled tend to cause septicemia, abortion, and latent infection. Those that gain entry to tissues have a predilection to localize in the intestinal wall, medulla oblongata, and placenta or to cause encephalitis via minute wounds in buccal mucosa.

The various manifestations of infection occur in all susceptible species and are associated with characteristic clinical syndromes: abortion and perinatal mortality in all species, encephalitis or meningoencephalitis in adult ruminants, septicemia in neonatal ruminants and monogastric animals, and septicemia with myocardial or hepatic necrosis (or both) in poultry (*see* p 2240).

Listeric encephalitis affects sheep, cattle, goats, and occasionally pigs. It is essentially a localized infection of the brain stem that develops when *L monocytogenes* ascends the trigeminal nerve. Clinical signs vary according to the function of damaged neurons but often are unilateral and include depression, trigeminal and facial nerve paralysis, and less commonly, circling.

Septicemic or visceral listeriosis is most common in monogastric animals, including pigs, dogs, cats, domestic and wild rabbits, and many other small mammals. These animals may play a role in transmission of *L monocytogenes*. This form is also found in young ruminants before the rumen is functional. Though rare, septicemia has been reported in older domestic ruminants and deer. The septicemic form affects organs other than the brain, the principal lesion being focal hepatic necrosis.

The uterus of all domestic animals, especially ruminants, is susceptible to infection with *L monocytogenes* at all stages of pregnancy, which can result in placentitis, metritis, fetal infection and death, abortion, stillbirths, neonatal deaths, and possibly viable carriers. The metritis has little or no effect on subsequent reproduction; however, *Listeria* may be shed for ≥1 mo via the vagina and milk.

Infections acquired via ingestion tend to localize in the intestinal wall and result in inapparent infection and prolonged fecal excretion. It has been postulated that contaminated silage results in numerous latent infections, often approaching 100% of the exposed herd or flock, but clinical listeriosis in only a few animals.

Clinical Findings: Encephalitis is the most readily recognized form of listeriosis in ruminants. It affects all ages and both sexes, sometimes as an epidemic in feedlot cattle or sheep. The course in sheep and goats is rapid, and death may occur 24-48 hr after onset of signs; however, the recovery rate can be up to 30% with prompt, aggressive therapy. In cattle, the course is less acute, and the recovery rate approaches 50%. Lesions are localized in the brain stem, and the signs indicate dysfunction of the third to seventh cranial nerves.

Initially, affected animals are anorectic, depressed, and disoriented. They may propel themselves into corners, lean against stationary objects, or circle toward the affected side. Facial paralysis with a drooping ear, deviated muzzle, flaccid lip, and lowered eyelid often develops on the affected side, as well as lack of a menace response and profuse, almost continuous, salivation; food material often becomes impacted in the cheek due to paralysis of the masticatory muscles. Terminally affected animals fall and, unable to rise, lie on the same side; involuntary running movements are common.

Listeric encephalitis may recur on the same premises in successive years. The number of animals clinically involved in an outbreak usually is <2% but in exceptional circumstances may reach 10-30% in a flock of sheep.

Listeric abortion usually occurs in the last trimester without premonitory signs. Fetuses usually die in utero, but stillbirths and neonatal deaths occur. The abortion rate varies and has been up to 20% in sheep flocks. Fatal septicemia of the dam secondary to metritis is rare. Encephalitis and abortion usually do not occur simultaneously in the same herd or flock. However, the clinical pattern in sheep in the UK has been changing; abortions, encephalitis, and diarrhea are increasing, and outbreaks of abortions and encephalitis occur together in the same flock.

Listeriosis is relatively uncommon in pigs, with septicemia occurring in those <1 mo old and encephalitis in older pigs; it has a rapid, fatal course of 3-4 days.

Lesions: In listeric encephalitis, there are few gross lesions except for some congestion of meninges. Microscopic lesions are confined primarily to the pons, medulla oblongata, and anterior spinal cord.

In septicemic listeriosis, small necrotic foci may be found in any organ, especially the liver. In calves that die when <3wk old, in addition to focal hepatic necrosis, there is frequently marked hemorrhagic gastroenteritis.

In aborted fetuses, there is slight to marked autolysis, clear to blood-tinged fluid in the serous cavities, and numerous small necrotic foci in the liver, especially in the right half. Necrotic foci may be found in other viscera such as lung and spleen. Shallow erosions, 1-3 mm, may be present in abomasal mucosa. Autolytic changes may mask these lesions. Gram-stained smears of abomasal contents reveal numerous gram-positive, pleomorphic coccobacilli.

Diagnosis: Samples of lumbosacral CSF can be collected under local anesthesia. In cases of listeriosis, the CSF has an increased protein concentration (0.6-2.0 g/L [normal 0.3 g/L]) and a mild pleocytosis composed of large mononuclear cells.

Listeriosis is confirmed only by isolation and identification of *L monocytogenes*. Specimens of choice are brain from animals with CNS involvement and aborted placenta and fetus. If primary isolation attempts fail, ground brain tissue should be held at 39°F (4°C) for several weeks and recultured weekly. Occasionally, *L monocytogenes* has been isolated from spinal fluid, nasal discharge, urine, feces, and milk of clinically ill ruminants. Serology is not used routinely for diagnosis because many healthy animals have high *Listeria* titers. Immunofluorescence is effective for rapidly identifying *L monocytogenes* in smears from animals dead or aborted from listeriosis and from milk, meat, and other sources.

Listeriosis can be differentiated from pregnancy toxemia in ewes (p 828) or ketosis in cattle (p 830) by careful clinical examination, CSF changes, and 3-OH butyrate concentrations well below 3.0 mmol/L. Furthermore, facial and ear paralysis are absent in pregnancy toxemia or ketosis. In cattle, the unilateral signs of trigeminal and facial paralysis (often subtle) help differentiate listeriosis from bovine spongiform encephalopathy (p 991), thromboembolic encephalitis (p 606), polioencephalomalacia (p 1061), sporadic bovine encephalomyelitis (p 1073), and lead poisoning (p 2404). Rabies (p 1067) must always be considered in the differential diagnosis of listeriosis. Animals with brain abscesses and coenurosis (p 1035) present with circling, contralateral blindness, and proprioceptive deficits, but no cranial nerve deficits.

Treatment and Control: *L monocytogenes* is susceptible to penicillin (the drug of choice), ceftiofur, erythromycin, and trimethoprim/sulfonamide. High doses are required because of the difficulty in achieving minimum bactericidal concentrations in the brain. Recovery depends on early, aggressive antibiotic treatment. If signs of encephalitis are severe, death usually occurs despite treatment.

Penicillin G should be given at 44,000 U/kg body wt, IM, daily for 1-2 wk; the first injection should be accompanied by the same dose given IV. Supportive therapy, including fluids and electrolytes, is required for animals having difficulty eating and drinking.

Results with vaccines have been equivocal, which together with the sporadic nature of the disease, lead to questions about the cost-benefit of vaccination. In an outbreak, affected animals should be segregated. If silage is being fed, use of the particular silage should be discontinued on a trial basis. Spoiled silage should be avoided. Corn ensiled before being too mature and grass silage containing additives are likely to have a more acid pH, which discourages multiplication of *L monocytogenes*.

Zoonotic Risk: Whether animals serve as a reservoir of infection for humans may be questioned, because *Listeria* organisms have been isolated from feces of a significant number of apparently healthy people as well as other animals. However, despite this and the apparently low invasiveness of *L monocytogenes*, all suspected material should be handled with caution. Aborted fetuses and necropsy of septicemic animals present the greatest hazard. In cases with encephalitis, *L monocytogenes* is usually confined to the brain and presents little risk of transmission unless the brain is removed. People have developed fatal meningitis, septicemia, and papular exanthema on the arms after handling aborted material. Pregnant animals (including women) should be protected from infection because of danger to the fetus, with possible abortion, stillbirth, and infection of neonates. While human listeriosis is rare (upper estimate of 12 cases per million population per yr), mortality can reach 50%. Most cases involve elderly patients, pregnant women, or immunocompromised people.

L monocytogenes can be isolated from milk of mastitic, aborting, and apparently healthy cows. Excretion in milk is usually intermittent but may persist for many months. Infected milk is a hazard because the organism may survive certain forms of pasteurization. *Listeria* also have been isolated from milk of sheep, goats, and women.

MELIOIDOSIS

Melioidosis is a bacterial infection of humans and animals. It is often associated with suppurative or caseous lesions, comprising a mixed purulent and granulomatous response that can occupy any body organ.

Etiology and Epidemiology: The etiologic agent is *Burkholderia pseudomallei* (*Bacillus pseudomallei, Bacterium whitmori, Pfeifferella pseudomallei, Malleomyces pseudomallei, Pseudomonas pseudomallei*), an oval, motile, gram-negative, facultative anaerobic bacillus with bipolar staining. The organism is ubiquitous throughout southeast Asia, northern Australia, and the South Pacific. Its distribution is predominantly tropical and subtropical with "hyperendemicity" in the top end of the Northern Territory of Australia and northeast Thailand. The true boundaries of its endemicity are ambiguous due to movement of the organism and its ability to travel to and exist in temperate regions (southwest Australia and France), where it may cause sporadic disease and outbreaks. *B pseudomallei* has been introduced to new environments with the export of animals, and shipments of contaminated soil and water could potentially produce the same results. Reports of possible autochthonous melioidosis have also come from India, Pacific islands, Central and South America, the Caribbean, Africa, and the Middle East.

B pseudomallei is a widespread saprophyte and has been isolated from various soil types and surface water of varying depths. Melioidosis outbreaks have coincided with heavy rainfall and flooding associated with high humidity or temperature. Major excavations and disturbances in plumbing resulting in contamination of water supplies have also resulted in outbreaks.

Melioidosis has been diagnosed in sheep, goats, pigs, cattle, horses, deer, camels, an alpaca, dogs, cats, dolphins, wallabies, a tree kangaroo, koala, primates, birds, tropical fish, reptiles, and humans. Laboratory animals affected by melioidosis include hamsters, guinea pigs, rabbits, mice, and rats. Host susceptibility and disease manifestations vary between species. The introduction of naive livestock to endemic regions may predispose them to disease, as seen with sheep, goats, pigs, and camelids. Other species (eg, dogs and cats) may succumb to infection due to immunocompromising conditions.

Transmission: Infection is thought to be opportunistic and primarily a result of transmission from the environment rather than from animal to animal. The most common routes of infection are via percutaneous inoculation, contamination of wounds, ingestion of soil or contaminated carcasses, or inhalation. Transplacental infection resulting in abortion has been reported in goats. Sexual transmission and other means of host-to-host transmission are possible but not documented. Laboratory-acquired infection and iatrogenic infection via contaminated antiseptics, injections, or other hospital or surgical equipment have been reported.

Pathogenesis: The virulence of *B pseudomallei* appears to vary among isolates, but these virulence factors are not well understood. Molecular-typed clonal outbreaks have produced a range of different clinical presentations, which indicate that host factors and infecting dose may be just as important in determining the severity of disease. *B pseudomallei* is a facultative intracellular pathogen that can remain dormant for many years before emerging as an active infection.

Clinical Findings and Lesions: Signs can vary widely within a species, depending on the site of infection, and range from acute to chronic. Subclinical infection is common. Infection may be associated with single or multiple suppurative or caseous nodules/abscesses, which can be located in any organ tissue with variable effects. Disease most likely due to percutaneous inoculation often develops at distant sites without evidence of active infection at the inoculation site. The organs most commonly affected include the lungs, spleen, liver, and associated lymph nodes. Goats often develop mastitis, and aortic aneurysms are common findings. The respiratory system is involved preferentially in sheep. CNS disease has been seen in cattle, horses, sheep, and goats. Pigs often have asymptomatic lesions on the spleen that are incidental findings at slaughter. Lameness due to septic arthritis and osteomyelitis can occur. Fatalities often occur in association with acute fulminating infections or when vital organs are affected.

Diagnosis: The clinical signs of melioidosis are not diagnostic due to the protean nature of the disease. For a definitive diagnosis, isolation and identification of the organism are required. The organism can be isolated from lesions and discharges. It is readily cultured on routine diagnostic media and has a characteristic colony form and odor (especially in Ashdown's media). Gram-stained smears of exudate or pus can sometimes identify bipolar "safety-pin"-shaped gram-negative rods. Serologic tests such as complement fixation and indirect hemagglutination are effective herd surveillance tools. More recently, DNA probes and PCR tests have been developed.

Treatment and Prevention: Treatment can be expensive, prolonged, and often unsuccessful, with the risk of recrudescence once treatment is discontinued. The possibility of underlying immunosuppressive conditions should be investigated in less susceptible species. Treatment regimens using guidelines for human melioidosis include initial intensive therapy using the newer β-lactams (ceftazidime and the carbepenems), possibly in combination with cotrimoxazole for up to 2 mo. This should be followed by subsequent eradication therapy for a minimum of 3 mo with high-dose cotrimoxazole or conventional combination therapy using chloramphenicol, cotrimoxazole, and doxycycline or amoxicillin/

clavulanate. Preventive measures are more practical and economical in intensive farming environments and involve raising the animals off the soil and providing clean drinking water via chlorination and filtration. Minimization of environmental contamination by diseased animals is also an important control measure. Although there is no effective vaccine, promising vaccine candidates are currently being researched and developed.

Zoonotic Risk: Melioidosis has zoonotic potential, although this remains unsubstantiated. Mastitis in goats is a common manifestation, and *B pseudomallei* has been isolated from milk, resulting in the requirement for pasteurization of commercial goats' milk in the tropics. Infected animal carcasses are condemned at the abattoir.

NEOSPOROSIS

Neosporosis has been recognized in dogs, cattle, sheep, goats, deer, horses, and experimentally rodents, pigs, monkeys, and cats. It is a major cause of abortion in dairy cattle.

Etiology and Transmission: *Neospora caninum* is an obligate intracellular protozoan parasite that has been confused previously with *Toxoplasma gondii*. The dog is the definitive host. Infection can be acquired by ingesting food and water contaminated with oocysts excreted in feces of dogs, by ingesting infected tissues, or transplacentally. Vertical transmission is a major route of transmission in cattle and dogs. Tachyzoites are 5-7 × 1-5 μm, depending on the stage of division. They divide by endodyogeny. Tachyzoites are found in myocytes, neural cells, dermal cells, macrophages, and other cells. Tissue cysts up to 100 μm in diameter are found in neural cells; the cyst wall is amorphous and up to 4 μm thick. Cysts have no septa and enclose slender bradyzoites (7 × 1.5 μm). Oocysts are ~10-12 μm in diameter.

Clinical Findings and Lesions: In **dogs**, both pups and older dogs are affected. Not all littermates are affected. Most severe infections are in young pups, which typically develop an ascending paralysis of the limbs, particularly the hindlimbs. The paralysis is often progressive and results in rigid contracture of the muscles of affected limbs. In some dogs, only neural signs are seen. The syndrome of polyradiculoneuromyositis appears typical of neosporosis. Ulcerative dermatitis, hepatitis, pneumonia, and encephalitis may also occur.

In **dairy cattle**, *N caninum* is a major cause of abortion in many countries. Calves may be aborted; stillborn; born underweight, weak, or paralyzed; or they may become paralyzed within 4 wk of birth. Nonsuppurative encephalitis is the main lesion in aborted fetal tissues. Abortion can occur throughout gestation, and some cows may abort again; dams of these calves are clinically normal.

Diagnosis: An immunoperoxidase test using specific antibodies can identify *N caninum* in tissue sections or biopsy specimens. An indirect fluorescent antibody test and several ELISA can be used to detect antibodies.

Treatment and Control: Drugs used to treat toxoplasmosis (sulfadiazine, daraprim, clindamycin) show some success in treating neosporosis. Dogs should not be allowed to defecate in cattle feed. There is no proven vaccine.

NOCARDIOSIS

The nocardioform actinomycetes comprise a suprageneric group of bacteria that cause a chronic, noncontagious disease (nocardiosis) in humans and domestic animals. Nocardiae are gram-positive, strictly aerobic, nonmotile, pleomorphic, and nonsporeforming; organisms in this genus may take the form of rods, cocci, or diphtheroids, and they sometimes produce branching filaments and aerial hyphae. Most reduce nitrate, produce catalase, and oxidize sugars. Some are partially acid-fast.

Epidemiology and Pathogenesis: Nocardiae are found commonly in soil, decaying vegetation, compost, and other environmental sources. They enter the body through contamination of wounds or by inhalation. Species in this genus include *N amarae*, *N brevicatena*, *N carnea*, *N pinensis*, *N seriolae*, *N transvalensis*, *N vaccini*, *N brasiliensis*, and *N otitidiscaviarum (N caviae)*; *N asteroides*, the type species, together with *N farcinica*, and *N nova*, constitute the *N asteroides* complex. *N asteroides* is found frequently in temperate regions, while *N brasiliensis* is more common in tropical and subtropical areas.

Cell wall mycolic acids, including trehalose 6,6'-dimycolate, contribute to virulence of nocardiae, perhaps by inhibiting phagosome-lysosome fusion; membrane-bound catalase and superoxide dismutase probably mediate resistance to killing by neutrophils. Filamentous forms prominent in log phase are more virulent than the coccoid forms of stationary phase. A mouse-toxic secreted product of *N otitidis caviarum* may be involved in pathogenesis. Resistance to nocardiosis is likely primarily cell-mediated.

Clinical Findings: Anorexia, fever, lethargy, and weight loss are common nonspecific signs associated with all infection sites. The first clinical sign of *N asteroides* infection is the appearance of an indurated nodule or pustule, which ruptures and suppurates. Discrete lesions may become joined by sinuses, with frequent development of chronic, progressive disease. Infection of the bovine mammary gland causes the mammary tissue to become enlarged and firm, often with draining tracts. Milk from infected glands contains a viscid exudate, with discrete blood clots and microcolonies of *N asteroides*. The organism can disseminate from the mammary gland to other organs, where it causes suppurative granulomatous lesions. Canine and feline infections are often localized, with subcutaneous lesions, mycetomas, and lymphadenitis. Nocardial stomatitis manifests as gingivitis and ulceration of the oral cavity, with severe halitosis. Canine thoracic nocardiosis often involves suppurative pleuritis or peritonitis; abscessation of heart, liver, kidneys, and brain are common. Occasionally, young dogs experience a disseminated form that begins in the lower respiratory tract following inhalation of the organism. Skin infection and lymph node abscessation are common presentations in horses, with respiratory or disseminated disease in the immunosuppressed. Nocardial abortion may occur in horses and pigs, and respiratory infection of monkeys is common in research colonies.

N brasiliensis has been isolated from suppurative wounds in various animal species on rare occasions. *N brasiliensis* is isolated from horses with pneumonia and pleuritis. *N otitidiscaviarum* was named for its occurrence in guinea pig ear infections, but it is perhaps more important as a cause of bovine mastitis and pneumonia and disseminated infections in other animals. *N farcinica* is associated with bovine farcy, and its importance has increased in recent years. *N salmonicida* and *N seriolae* cause granulomatous lesions in salmonid fish and other fresh and saltwater fish, respectively.

Nocardioform actinomycetes from placentitis and abortion in horses in some areas of the USA have been placed in the genus *Crossiella*, eg, *C equi*.

Diagnosis: Presumptive diagnosis can be based on pathology and the presence of gram-positive, acid-fast, branching, beaded filaments in smears of affected tissues. Specimens should be plated on blood or Sabouraud's agar, incubated at 25°C and at 37°C for 4-5 days. The resulting cultures have the odor of wet dirt. Microscopic morphology is best determined by observation of undisturbed colonies in slide cultures on tap water agar or corn meal agar without dextrose, incubated at 25°C for 2-3 wk. Finely filamentous subsurface hyphae are dichotomously branched at right angles. The presence of aerial hyphae differentiates nocardiae from related genera. Colonies adhere to the surface of blood or chocolate agar, with the leading edge embedded in the agar. Nocardiae may be hemolytic, but *N asteroides* is usually nonhemolytic. Aerial hyphae of *N otitidiscaviarum* are sparse and off-white; colonies are usually pale tan, but may vary from cream-colored, to gray, peach, or purplish. *N salmonicida* substrate mycelium is extensively branched and fragments into rod- to coccoid-shaped elements. Identification of species is based on phenotypic properties, including decomposition of casein, xanthine, hypoxanthine, and tyrosine.

Treatment: β-Lactam antimicrobial agents are not therapeutically effective for any nocardial infection, due to antimicrobial resistance. Udder infusions of novobiocin, combined with nitrofurazone, for 3-5 days has been successful for treatment of bovine nocardial mastitis. Nonmastitic forms can be treated with sulfamethoxazole-trimethoprim, sulfonamides, novobiocin, ampicillin, or tetracyclines. Therapy must often be continued for >3 mo. The prognosis is guarded, due to the long treatment time and the likelihood of relapse.

PERITONITIS

Inflammation of the peritoneum may be acute or chronic, local or diffuse, and most commonly is secondary to contamination of the peritoneal cavity. It is often accompanied by abdominal pain, fever, toxemia, and reduced fecal output.

Etiology: Primary peritonitis is infrequent. It may be caused by infectious agents such as feline infectious peritonitis virus (p 628), *Nocardia* spp, or *Mycobacterium* spp. Access to the peritoneal cavity is generally by the hematogenous route. Progression of primary peritonitis tends to be chronic (days to weeks).

Secondary peritonitis is often acute and results in rapid, progressive, systemic illness. It is most commonly associated with GI perforation or dehiscence of abdominal wound closure, or with perforation of other infected viscera (eg, prostatic or hepatic abscess, pyometra). Penetrating abdominal injuries may lacerate viscera or inoculate the peritoneal cavity with foreign material and microorganisms. Peritonitis may also occur secondary to chemical irritants (eg, bile, urine) and to other disease processes that allow transmural migration of bacteria (eg, neoplasia, visceral ischemia). Peritonitis from chemical irritation or foreign bodies (eg, sponge) may be septic or nonseptic. Septic peritonitis may remain localized if the omentum or mesentery contains the septic process, which sometimes results in formation of an abdominal abscess.

In large animals, peritonitis is most commonly seen in cattle, less often in horses, and rarely in pigs, sheep, and goats. As well, it is a serious and often fatal condition in small animals, with mortality suggested to be as high as 68%.

In large animals, peritonitis most commonly results from injury to the serosal surface of the GI tract, which allows intestinal contents to leak into the peritoneal cavity. Other causes include traumatic perforations of the abdominal wall or reproductive tract and introduction of pathogens or irritants via injection or surgery (TABLE 2).

Microorganisms associated with septic peritonitis reflect the source of contamination. A mixed bacterial population is seen in GI perforation (coliforms, anaerobes), whereas perforation of nongastrointestinal viscera (eg, gallbladder, uterus, prostate) may be associated with aerobic organisms including *Escherichia coli*, *Staphylococcus*, *Proteus* spp, and less commonly, *Klebsiella*, *Enterobacter*, *Pseudomonas*, and *Corynebacterium*. In horses, *Streptococcus equi* and *Rhodococcus equi* may be associated with peritonitis.

Pathogenesis: Toxemia and septicemia, shock, hemorrhage, abdominal pain, paralytic ileus, fluid accumulation, and adhesions all contribute to the clinical signs and progression of peritonitis. Toxins produced by bacteria and tissue breakdown are readily absorbed through the peritoneum. Bacterial or chemical irritants increase serosal capillary permeability resulting in leakage of plasma proteins, solutes, and water into the peritoneal cavity. Exudation of protein-rich fluid can result in hypoproteinemia and bacterial

TABLE 2.   Common Causes of Peritonitis in Livestock

Species	Cause
All species	Traumatic perforation of abdominal wall; faulty surgical asepsis; leakage of infarcted GI wall; spread from subperitoneal sites in spleen, liver, umbilical vessels
Cattle	Traumatic reticuloperitonitis; abomasal ulcer perforation; abomasal volvulus; rumenitis secondary to carbohydrate indigestion; cesarean section; intestinal, rectal, uterine, or vaginal rupture; deposition of semen into peritoneal cavity; injection of sterile hypertonic or nonsterile solutions
Goats	Serositis caused by *Mycoplasma* spp
Horses	Infectious, chemical, or parasitic injury; cecal, colonic, gastric, or rectal rupture
Pigs	Secondary to Glässer's disease; ileal perforation
Sheep	*Esophagostomum* spp intestinal abscess rupture; serositis caused by *Mycoplasma* spp

proliferation. Endotoxins absorbed from the peritoneal cavity have systemic effects leading to hypotension, shock, and systemic inflammatory response syndrome (SIRS) and disseminated intravascular coagulation (DIC). Endotoxins, myocardial depressant factor, acid-base, and electrolyte disturbances directly affect the cardiac function, leading to reduced cardiac output. The combined effect of large fluid losses into the peritoneal cavity and vasodilatory effects of absorbed toxins can produce profound hypotension and hypovolemia. Rupture of the GI tract, with spillage of large volumes of intestinal contents, leads to acute peritonitis. Death due to endotoxic shock may occur suddenly with limited clinical signs or lesions. Shock and hemorrhage associated with rupture of the gut or uterus often lead to death in animals with infection of the GI or reproductive tracts; however, shock and hemorrhage may be minor following uterine rupture in cows. Peritonitis may not develop if the uterine contents are not contaminated, but it may follow if the uterus is not repaired or healed within a few days. Paralytic ileus is a frequent result of acute peritonitis and may also follow intestinal obstruction or surgery, leading to functional obstruction and increased mortality rate if it persists. Large volumes of inflammatory exudates may be secreted into the peritoneal cavity during peritonitis and may lead to impaired respiration by impinging on the diaphragm. Peritoneal trauma leads to secretion of fibrinogen and formation of fibrinous adhesions. Such adhesions help localize the inflammation but may cause mechanical or functional obstruction of the GI tract.

Clinical Findings: Signs are nonspecific and vary depending on the type of peritonitis (primary or secondary). Abdominal pain may be generalized and severe, so that the animal guards the abdomen, walks with a stiff gait, or is recumbent. Cattle may have a shuffling, cautious gait, with a rigid, arched back; grunting when walking or when passing urine or feces is common. Deep, firm palpation of the abdominal wall results in an easily recognized pain response in cattle. Pain responses in all species are most evident in the early stages of the disease. Fever is common but may be suppressed by prostaglandin inhibitors. Fever (103.5-106°F [39.7-41.1°C]) is a common clinical finding in dogs with peritonitis, while cats may be hypothermic with peritonitis and concomitant shock. Abdominal distention, which may be inapparent, usually is due to accumulation of peritoneal exudate and may be accompanied by hemorrhage, septicemia, toxemia, paralytic ileus, shock, and adhesions. Fluid transudation sequesters electrolytes and protein in the abdominal cavity and atonic gut, and venous stasis leads to hypotension, acid-base disturbances, and circulatory collapse. Toxemia and bacteremia contribute to shock.

Icterus may be present in generalized biliary peritonitis. Animals with secondary peritonitis may also exhibit signs of the primary illness.

In small animals, anorexia and depression are often accompanied by vomiting, and feces may not be passed. Dehydration, hypovolemia, and sepsis may result in hypothermia and death due to loss of extravascular fluid volume. In large animals, complete anorexia may be seen in acute, diffuse peritonitis, while decreased appetite may occur in less severe and chronic cases.

In horses, clinical signs include severe colic, ileus, distended intestines on rectal examination, gastric reflux, and occasionally diarrhea. Intestinal stasis leads to reduced peristaltic sounds but sounds of paralytic ileus may be audible and should be differentiated from normal gut sounds. The horse is restless and may lie down and roll intermittently. Tachycardia, weak pulses, poor peripheral perfusion, and fever are common. Septic peritonitis is frequently fatal, despite intensive treatment.

In cattle, rumination ceases and milk production drops. In chronic cases, ruminal contractions may be present but reduced in intensity. Abdominal percussion may detect ruminal tympany. Fever (103°F [39.5°C]) is typical during the first 24-36 hr in cattle with acute, local peritonitis. High fever (up to 106°F [41.5°C]) suggests acute, diffuse peritonitis.

Fecal output in large animals is reduced, although there may be an increased frequency of defecation in the early stages of peritonitis that gives the impression of increased production. Feces may be completely absent for as long as 3 days, even in animals that recover. Rectal palpation may reveal tacky, dry mucosa and fibrinous adhesions between intestinal loops.

Peracute, diffuse peritonitis is associated with extreme weakness, depression, and circulatory failure (tachycardia with a weak pulse). Body temperature is often subnormal (99-100°F [37-37.5°C]). Abdominal pain is not evident. In cases of cecal rupture during foaling, mares suddenly stop straining, and progress toward parturition stops. Shock develops, followed by death in 4-5 hr.

Chronic peritonitis is associated with development of fibrous adhesions. Cattle may have chronic indigestion and toxemia, with periods of acute, severe illness caused by partial intestinal obstruction. Liters of turbid, infected peritoneal fluid may be produced but may be difficult to distinguish from ruminal contents on physical examination. Weight loss, intermittent pain, and diminished gut sounds may be observed in horses with chronic peritonitis.

Diagnosis: Diagnosis can be difficult because the clinical signs are nonspecific.The most reliable indicators of peritonitis include abnormal feces (in large animals, amount and composition), intestinal stasis, abdominal pain (diffuse or focal), fibrinous or fibrous abdominal adhesions, abnormal peritoneal fluid with an increased WBC count, and a normal or low peripheral WBC count with a degenerative left shift. Peritonitis is rarely diagnosed antemortem in pigs, sheep, or goats.

In dogs with septic effusion, peritoneal glucose concentration is often lower than blood glucose concentration. A blood-to-fluid glucose difference of >20 mg/dL has been found to be 100% sensitive and specific for diagnosis of septic peritonitis. In addition, a blood-to-fluid lactate difference of <2.0 mmol/L is equally sensitive and specific. In cats, blood-to-fluid glucose difference was 86% sensitive and 100% specific for septic peritonitis.

Abdominal radiographs may reveal GI obstruction (bowel dilatation, free abdominal air), ascites, or radiodense foreign material. Loss of serosal detail (a "ground glass" appearance) is indicative of abdominal fluid. Ultrasonography is a valuable adjunct test to evaluate size, shape, and contents of other viscera (eg, gallbladder, prostate gland) suspected to be the source of peritonitis. Rectal palpation in large animals is a useful means of evaluating the intestines. Abdominal paracentesis should be used in large and small animals to obtain fluid for cytologic examination and culture (TABLE 3, TABLE 4). Diagnostic peritoneal lavage is used when small amounts of fluid cannot be obtained by paracentesis. Cytologic examination of abdominal fluid may reveal septic or nonseptic suppurative inflammation with one or more bacterial infections. Neutrophils are degenerative in the presence of sepsis.

TABLE 3.	Characteristics of Adult Bovine and Equine Peritoneal Fluid ▶				
Classification of Fluid	Physical Appearance	Total Protein (g/dL)	Specific Gravity	Total RBC (× 10^6/μL)	Total WBC (× 10^6/μL)
Cattle					
Normal	Amber, crystal clear; 1-5 mL per sample	0.1-3.1; does not clot	1.005-1.015	Few from capillary puncture during sampling	0.3-5.3
Moderate inflammation	Amber to pink, slightly turbid	2.8-7.3; may clot	1.016-1.025	0.1-0.2	2.7-40.7
Severe inflammation	Serosanguineous, turbid, viscous; 10-20 mL per sample	3.1-5.8; often clots	1.026-1.040	0.3-0.5	2.0-31.1
Horses[*]					
Normal	Pale yellow; crystal clear	0.5-1.5; does not clot	1.000-1.015	None	0.5-5.0
Suspected inflammation	Slightly cloudy, yellow	1.6-2.5; usually does not clot	1.016-1.020	0.05-0.1	5.0-15.0
Moderate inflammation	Yellow-pink, turbid, viscous	2.6-4.0; may clot	1.021-1.025	0.1-0.2	15.0-60.0
Severe inflammation	Pink to serosanguineous; turbid, thick viscous	4.1-7.0; commonly clot	>1.025	0.3-0.6	>60.0

[*]Normal peritoneal fluid in foals from 13-134 days of age has total cell count of 60-1,420 × 10^6/μL with rare eosinophils, rare cytophagia, and variable percentages of neutrophils and mononuclear cells. In foals, peritoneal fluid cell counts >1,500 × 10^6/μL are considered elevated.

Adapted, with permission, from Radostits OM et al, *Veterinary Medicine*, 9th ed., Elsevier, 2000.

The presence of intra- or extracellular bacteria confirms septic peritonitis. A number of serum biochemical abnormalities may accompany peritonitis. Anemia is commonly associated with any inflammatory disease process in dogs and cats. Hypoglycemia may develop but is not reliably present. Cats <6 mo of age appear more likely to present with a low blood glucose concentration (likely due to decreased glycogen and body fat reserves). Hypoalbuminemia and hyperbilirubinemia are frequently present in dogs and cats. Many septic dogs show cholestasis histopathologically, but this has not been found in septic cats. In contrast to reported findings in other species, cats rarely have an associated increase in serum alkaline phosphatase. Additional causes of icterus in septic animals might include hemolysis (immune-mediated, toxic, or secondary to electrolyte derangements), with or without a decreased capacity for hepatic hemoglobin metabolism.

◀ **TABLE 3.** *(continued)*

Differential WBC Count	Bacteria	Particulate Matter (Plant Fiber)	Interpretation
Cattle			
Polymorphonuclear and mononuclear cells, ratio 1:1	None	None	Increased amounts in late gestation and congestive heart failure
Nontoxic neutrophils, 50-90%; macrophages may predominate in chronic peritonitis	None	None	Early stages of strangulation, destruction of intestine; traumatic reticuloperitonitis; ruptured bladder; chronic peritonitis
Segmented neutrophils, 70-90%; presence of (toxic) degenerate neutrophils containing bacteria	Usually present	May be present	Advanced stages of strangulation obstruction; acute diffuse peritonitis; perforation of abomasal ulcer; rupture of uterus, stomachs, or intestine
*Horses**			
Polymorphonuclear and mononuclear cells, ratio 1:1	None	None	Increased in late gestation and congestive heart failure
Segmented neutrophils 50-60%; mesothelial cells	None	None	Modified transudate
Segmented neutrophils 70-80%; few toxic neutrophils	May be present	None	Early stages of strangulation, obstruction, uterine torsion, colonic torsion
Segmented neutrophils 70-90%; toxic or degenerate neutrophils containing bacteria	Commonly present	May be present	Infarction of intestine, perforation or rupture of viscus

Total and differential WBC counts are helpful in establishing a diagnosis and determining severity of peritonitis. Acute, diffuse peritonitis with toxemia is usually accompanied by leukopenia, neutropenia, and a marked increase in immature neutrophils (degenerative left shift). In less severe acute peritonitis, leukocytosis may occur as a result of increased neutrophil production. Acute, localized peritonitis may reveal a normal WBC count with a regenerative left shift. The total WBC count in chronic peritonitis may be normal, with an occasional increase in lymphocytes and monocytes.

Treatment: Initial treatment must be directed toward stabilizing the metabolic consequences of peritonitis (electrolytes, acid-base, coagulation abnormalities) as well as determining the nidus of inflammation/infection and correcting or excising it. Replacement fluids, electrolytes, plasma, or whole blood may be necessary to maintain cardiac output. Broad-spectrum antimicrobial therapy should be initiated, usually by a parenteral route, once appropriate samples have been collected for cytologic evaluation and culture and sensitivity. Aminoglycoside or quinoline antibiotics are effective against gram-negative organisms, and penicillins or cephalosporins are effective against gram-positive organisms. The antimicrobial selected may be changed after sensitivity testing has been

TABLE 4. Peritoneal Fluid Characteristics and Classification in Dogs and Cats

Effusion Type	Color/ Turbidity	Total Protein (g/dL)	Specific Gravity	WBC (#/μL)	Predominant Cell Type(s)
Transudate	Colorless/ clear	<2.5	<1.017	<1,000	Mesothelium, mononuclear phagocytes
Modified transudate	Light yellow to medium yellow/clear	>2.5	1.017-1.025	>1,000	Mononuclear
Exudate	Medium yellow to tan/ cloudy	>3.0	>1.025	>5,000	Neutrophils (nonseptic: nondegenerate; septic: degenerate)

performed. There are no published clinical reports of the effectiveness of antimicrobials for treating peritonitis in cattle and horses. Cattle are typically treated with broad-spectrum antimicrobials; the specific choice depends on ease of use and drug withdrawal times. Antimicrobials used for peritonitis in horses include gentamicin (2.2-3.3 mg/kg, IV, BID-TID), penicillin (22,000 IU/kg, IV or IM, BID-QID), and metronidazole (15-25 mg/kg, PO).

In small animals, antimicrobial choice is often empirical initially. Multiple isolates are likely, including gram-negative, gram-positive, aerobic, and anaerobic organisms. For combination therapy, enrofloxacin or aminoglycosides (for gram-negative organisms) may be combined with penicillins, first-generation cephalosporins, or clindamycin (for gram-positive anaerobic organisms). Second- or third-generation cephalosporins or imipenum are good candidates for single-agent therapy. Appropriate antibiotics should be started once septic peritonitis is confirmed and fluid samples are obtained for culture and sensitivity.

Once the animal is stabilized, surgery is done to explore the abdomen and to repair any defects (eg, a ruptured viscus). This is followed by thorough peritoneal lavage with an isothermic, isotonic, balanced electrolyte solution. There is no proven clinical benefit in adding an antimicrobial to the lavage solution. Solutions containing antiseptics (eg, povidone-iodine) may induce chemical peritonitis and likewise have no proven clinical benefit. Abdominal drains to allow postoperative lavage and open peritoneal drainage (small animals) are sometimes used to treat severe peritonitis. Survival in dogs and cats managed with closed versus open drainage is very similar. The decision to manage a small animal patient with open peritoneal drainage is often based on experience level and severity of the case. Maintaining patency of drains can be difficult, especially in cattle. In animals treated by open peritoneal drainage, serum protein and electrolyte levels should be monitored periodically, because both are lost with drainage of exudate. Parenteral antimicrobials are continued postoperatively based on either empiric choice or culture and sensitivity data if available. Nutritional support should be anticipated, as many animals with peritonitis will not eat postoperatively. Enteral nutrition helps maintain the health of the intestinal mucosa; however, vomiting or anorexia may force the consideration of alternatives. Feeding tube placement in small animals (esophagostomy, gastrostomy, or jejunostomy tubes) at the time of surgical closure is easily performed. In certain patients, parenteral nutrition (total or partial) may be viewed as a way to provide a portion of the nutritional requirements while enteral nutrition is being initiated. Hyperalimentation, or alimentation by feeding-tube gastrostomy and catheter jejunostomy may be needed in anorectic animals.

In animals with toxemia and shock, IV fluids and electrolytes are crucial elements of treatment, especially during the first 24-72 hr following surgery in horses. Flunixin meglumine (0.25-1.1 mg/kg, IV, BID-TID) is recommended for treatment of shock, although efficacy is unknown.

PLAGUE

Plague, caused by *Yersinia pestis*, is an acute and sometimes fatal bacterial zoonosis that is transmitted primarily by the fleas of rats and other rodents. Enzootic foci of sylvatic plague exist in the western USA and throughout the world, including Eurasia, Africa, and North and South America. In addition to rodents, other mammalian species that have been naturally infected with *Y pestis* include lagomorphs, felids, canids, mustelids, and some ungulates. Domestic cats and dogs have also developed plague from oral mucous membrane exposure to infected rodent tissues, typically when they are allowed to roam and hunt in enzootic areas. Birds and other nonmammalian vertebrates appear to be resistant to plague. On average, 10 human plague cases are reported each year in the USA; the majority are from New Mexico, California, Colorado, and Arizona. Most human cases result from the bite of an infected flea, although direct contact with infected wild rabbits, rodents, and occasionally other wildlife and exposure to infected domestic cats are also risk factors.

Etiology: *Y pestis* is a gram-negative, nonmotile, coccobacillus belonging to the Enterobacteriacae family. It exhibits a bipolar staining, "safety pin" appearance when stained with Wright, Giemsa, or Wayson stains. *Y pestis* grows slowly even at optimal temperatures (28°C) and can require ≥48 hr to produce colonies. Several types of media can be used to grow *Y pestis* including blood agar, nutrient broth, and unenriched agar. Colonies are small (1-2 mm), gray, nonmucoid, and have a characteristic "hammered copper" appearance. Different virulence factors are expressed by the organism at different temperatures and environments, allowing the organism to survive in flea vectors and then be transmitted to and multiply in mammalian hosts. The organism does not survive for long at high temperatures or in dry environments.

Epidemiology and Transmission: *Y pestis* is maintained in the environment in a natural cycle between susceptible rodent species and their associated fleas. Commonly affected rodent species include ground squirrels (*Spermophilus* spp) and wood rats (*Neotoma* spp). Cats and dogs are usually exposed to *Y pestis* by mucous membrane contact with secretions or tissues of an infected rodent or rabbit or by the bite of an infected flea. Humans are usually exposed by an infected flea bite but are sometimes exposed due to contact with infected animals or via respiratory droplet transmission from pneumonic cases. Risk factors for cats acquiring plague include hunting and eating rodents and rabbits, visiting an enzootic plague area, finding dead rodents around the yard or areas that the animal frequents, and exposure to infected fleas. Plague epizootics cause nearly 100% mortality in affected wild rodent and rabbit populations. Once their host has died, *Y pestis*-infected rodent and rabbit fleas will seek other hosts, including cats and dogs, and potentially be transported into homes. Rodent and rabbit flea species are different from dog and cat fleas (*Ctenocephalides* spp), although most veterinarians and pet owners will not be able to visually distinguish flea species. Dog and cat fleas are rare in most plague-enzootic areas of the western USA; therefore, fleas on pets in these areas may be more likely to be fleas from wildlife, including rodents or rabbits.

Pathogenesis: Fleas become infected with *Y pestis* when feeding on a bacteremic mammal. The bacteria multiply and block the flea's digestive tract, preventing it from digesting the blood meal. Such fleas will regurgitate plague bacteria, inoculating the host on which they are attempting to feed with *Y pestis*. In mammalian hosts, plague presents clinically in 1 of 3 forms: bubonic, septicemic, or pneumonic. After inoculation into the skin by a flea bite or into mucous membranes by contact with infectious secretions or tissues, the bacteria travels via lymphatic vessels to regional lymph nodes. These infected lymph nodes are called buboes, the typical lesion of bubonic plague.

Secondary septicemic plague can develop when the organism spreads from the affected lymph nodes via the bloodstream, but can also occur without prior lymphadenopathy (primary septicemic plague), affecting numerous organs including the spleen, liver, heart, and lungs. Pneumonic plague can develop from inadequately treated septicemic plague (secondary pneumonic plague) or from infectious respiratory droplets (primary pneumonic plague), typically from a coughing pneumonic plague patient.

Clinical Findings and Lesions: The clinical presentation of plague in cats is most commonly bubonic plague. The incubation period ranges from 1-4 days. Cats with bubonic plague typically present with fever, anorexia, lethargy, and an enlarged lymph node that may be abscessed and draining. Oral and lingual ulcers, skin abscesses, ocular discharge, diarrhea, vomiting, and cellulitis have also been documented. Such cats typically develop lymphadenitis in a single lymph node or single nodal cluster; symmetrically affected lymph nodes are very unusual. The affected lymph nodes show necrosuppurative inflammation, edema, and hemorrhages, and contain numerous *Y pestis* organisms. In experimentally infected cats, fever was as high as 106°F (41°C), peaking ~3 days after exposure; mortality was as high as 60% in untreated cats. Ten of 16 (62.5%) cats exposed orally developed enlarged lymph nodes in the medial retropharyngeal, submandibular, sublingual, and tonsillar regions, palpable 4-6 days after exposure. *Y pestis* was isolated from the throats of 15 of these cats. In 6 subcutaneously exposed cats (mimicking a flea bite), none had palpably enlarged lymph nodes in the head or neck region, but 4 had subcutaneous abscesses at the inoculation site. A retrospective review of 119 naturally infected cats found that 53% of cats had bubonic plague; of those, 75% had submandibular lymphadenopathy.

Cats with primary septicemic plague have no obvious lymphadenopathy but present with fever, lethargy, and anorexia. Septic signs may also include diarrhea, vomiting, tachycardia, weak pulse, prolonged capillary refill time, disseminated intravascular coagulopathy, and respiratory distress. Primary pneumonic plague has not been documented in cats. Cats with secondary pneumonic plague may present with all the signs of septicemic plague along with a cough and other abnormal lung sounds. Characteristic necropsy findings can include livers that are pale with light-colored necrotic nodules, enlarged spleens with necrotic nodules, and lungs with diffuse interstitial pneumonia, focal congestion, hemorrhages, and necrotic foci.

Dogs infected with plague are less likely to develop clinical illness than cats. Symptomatic plague infection has been documented in 3 naturally infected dogs; clinical signs included fever, lethargy, submandibular lymphadenopathy, a purulent intermandibular lesion, oral cavity lesions, and cough.

Cattle, horses, sheep, and pigs are not known to develop symptomatic illness from plague, while clinical illness has been documented in goats, camels, mule deer, pronghorn antelope, nonhuman primates, and 1 llama. Infected mountain lions and bobcats have shown clinical signs and mortality similar to those of domestic cats.

Diagnosis: Plague must be differentiated from other bacterial infections including tularemia (p 553), abscesses due to wounds (cat fight bites), and staphylococcal and streptococcal infections. During acute illness, preferred antemortem samples for culture include whole blood, lymph node aspirates, swabs from draining lesions, and oral/pharyngeal swabs of cats with oral lesions or pneumonia. Diagnostic samples should be taken before antibiotics are administered. *Y pestis* cultures can take 48 hr for visible growth to develop. An air-dried glass slide smear of a bubo aspirate can be used for a fluorescent antibody test that detects the F1 antigen on *Y pestis* cells. This test can be performed in a matter of hours in an experienced laboratory and is both sensitive and specific.

Postmortem specimens should include samples of liver, spleen, and lung (for pneumonic cases) and affected lymph nodes. Serologic antibody tests can be confirmatory but require acute and convalescent samples taken 2-3 wk apart, demonstrating a 4-fold rise in antibody titer. Single acute sera are often negative or can be problematic in an enzootic area where animals may retain antibody titers from previous exposures.

Treatment: Due to the rapid progression of this disease, treatment for suspected plague (and infection control practices) should be started before a definitive diagnosis is obtained. Streptomycin has been considered the drug of choice in human cases but is difficult to obtain and rarely used today. Gentamicin is currently used to treat most human plague cases and should be the drug of choice in veterinary medicine for seriously ill patients.

Doxycycline is appropriate for treatment of less complicated cases. Tetracycline and chloramphenicol are also options. Penicillins are not effective in treating plague. In treatment studies with experimentally infected mice, the fluoroquinolones performed as well as streptomycin. However, no veterinary clinical trials have been performed and fluoroquinolones are not recommended for treating plague at this time.

The duration of infectivity in treated cats is not definitively known, but cats are thought to be noninfectious after 72 hr of appropriate antibiotic therapy with indications of clinical improvement. During this infectious period, cats should remain hospitalized, especially if there are signs of pneumonia. Human cases have occurred in cat owners trying to give oral medications at home, exposing them to contact with the oral cavity and associated infectious secretions.

Prevention and Zoonotic Risk: Along with treatment and diagnostic considerations, protection of people and other animals and initiation of public health interventions are critical when an animal is suspected to have plague. Animals with signs suggestive of plague should be placed in isolation, and infection control measures implemented for the protection of staff and other animal patients without waiting for a definitive diagnosis. The use of gloves, surgical masks, eye protection (if splashes or sprays are anticipated), patient isolation, and standard hygiene and disinfection procedures for protection from potentially contaminated respiratory droplets, body fluids, and secretions from the patient are essential. Of the 23 patients who developed cat-associated plague in the USA between 1977 and 1998, 6 were veterinary staff; the rest were cat owners or others handling a sick cat. After pneumonia has been ruled out or once there is evidence of clinical improvement after 72 hr of appropriate therapy, isolation procedures may be relaxed, but standard disinfection and hygiene procedures should continue. Local or state public health officials should be notified promptly when plague is suspected to aid in conducting appropriate diagnostic tests, initiating an environmental investigation, and assessing the need for fever watch or prophylactic antibiotics in potentially exposed people. To decrease the risk of pets and humans being exposed to plague, pet owners in enzootic areas should keep their pets from roaming and hunting, limit their contact with rodent or rabbit carcasses, and use appropriate flea control.

Q FEVER

Q fever is a zoonotic bacterial infection associated primarily with parturient ruminants, although domestic animals such as cats and a variety of wild animals have also been associated with human infections. Q fever occurs more frequently in persons with occupational contact with high-risk species. Q fever has a highly variable clinical presentation in humans, ranging from a self-limiting influenza-like illness to pneumonia, hepatitis, and endocarditis. It is highly infectious, and a single organism can reportedly cause infection via the aerosol route in humans. Q fever is considered a potential agent of bioterrorism due to its high rate of infectivity, stability in the environment, and potential for aerosol dispersion.

Etiology, Epidemiology, and Transmission: Q fever is caused by the gram-negative coccobacillus *Coxiella burnetii*. Although classically considered a rickettsial agent, recent phylogenetic analyses suggest that *C burnetii* is more closely related to *Legionella* and *Francisella* than to the genus *Rickettsia*. It resides and reproduces in phagolysosomes of host monocytes and macrophages. Two forms exist—the large cell variant is a vegetative form found in infected cells, and the small cell variant is the extracellular infectious form that is shed in milk, urine, and feces and found in high concentration (10^9 ID_{50}/g) in placental tissue and amniotic fluid. The small cell variant is resistant to heat, drying, and many common disinfectants and remains viable for weeks to months in the environment. Once a domestic ruminant is infected, *C burnetii* can localize in mammary glands, supramammary lymph nodes, placenta, and uterus, from which it may be shed in subsequent parturitions and lactations.

The epidemiology of *C burnetii* is complex because there are 2 major patterns of transmission: in one, the organism circulates between wild animals and their ectoparasites, mainly ticks; the other occurs in domestic ruminants, independent of the wild animal cycle. Ixodid and argasid ticks can act as reservoirs of the organism. Distribution is worldwide (except New Zealand) and the host range includes various wild and domestic mammals, arthropods, and birds. The disease is enzootic in most areas where cattle, sheep, and goats are kept. In the USA, seroprevalence studies have shown antibodies to *C burnetii* in 41.6% of sheep, 16.5% of goats, and 3.4% of cattle.

The greatest risk of transmission occurs at parturition by inhalation, ingestion, or direct contact with birth fluids or placenta. The organism is also shed in milk, urine, and feces. High-temperature pasteurization effectively kills the organism. Ticks may transmit the disease among domestic ruminants, but are not thought to play an epidemiologically important role in transmission of disease to humans.

Clinical Findings and Diagnosis: Infection in ruminants is usually subclinical but can cause anorexia and late abortion. Reports have implicated *C burnetii* as a cause of infertility and sporadic abortion with a necrotizing placentitis in ruminants. Experimental infection in cats causes transient fever, dullness, and anorexia lasting several days.

In domestic ruminants, gross lesions are nonspecific, and differential diagnosis should include infectious and noninfectious agents that cause abortion. Immunofluorescence test on paired sera taken ≥2 wk apart can be used to detect recent infection; however, shedding of *C burnetii* may occur in the absence of a measurable serum antibody titer. Culture, immunohistochemical, and PCR tests may be used to identify the organism in tissues.

Treatment and Control: Q fever in humans is a notifiable disease in the USA, primarily because of its status as a possible bioterrorism agent; reporting is not usually required for animals unless associated with human infection. Vaccines for people and animals have been developed but are not commercially available in the USA. Vaccination has prevented infection when administered to uninfected calves and has improved fertility and reduced shedding in previously infected animals.

For treatment of ruminants, oral tetracycline at the therapeutic dose may be given for 2-4 wk. In known infected herds, segregating pregnant animals indoors, burning or burying reproductive offal, or administering tetracycline (8 mg/kg/day) prophylactically in the water supply prior to parturition may reduce spread of the organism.

Zoonotic Risk: The majority of outbreaks in people have associated with wind dispersion of desiccated reproductive products, contaminated with *C burnetii*, from sites where sheep, goats, or cattle are kept. Farmers and veterinarians are at risk while assisting birthing. Slaughterhouse workers are at risk from contact with infected carcasses, hair, and wool. Transmission may also occur by consumption of unpasteurized milk. Handling of infected tissue poses a threat to laboratory personnel. Q fever has been seen in personnel and human patients in medical institutions where latently infected sheep were used for research. Medical facilities using pregnant ruminants in research should screen animals for antibodies to *C burnetii* prior to use. In addition, workers should use adequate personal protective equipment to protect against small droplet and aerosol exposure during high-risk medical procedures.

SWEATING SICKNESS

Sweating sickness is an acute, febrile, tickborne toxicosis characterized mainly by a profuse, moist eczema and hyperemia of the skin and visible mucous membranes. It is essentially a disease of young calves, although adults are also susceptible. Sheep, pigs, goats, and a dog have been infected experimentally. It occurs in eastern, central, and southern Africa, and probably in Sri Lanka and southern India.

Etiology: The cause is an epitheliotropic toxin produced by females of certain strains of *Hyalomma truncatum*. The toxin develops in the tick, not in the vertebrate host. The potential to produce toxin is retained by ticks for up to 20 generations, and possibly longer. Attempted experimental transmissions between affected and normal animals by contact or inoculations of blood have been unsuccessful.

Graded periods of infestation of a susceptible host by "infected" ticks have different effects on the host. A very short period has no effect; the animal remains susceptible. A period just long enough to produce a reaction may confer immunity, but if the exposure is >5 days, severe clinical signs and death may result. Recovery confers a durable immunity, which may last ≥4 yr. Other closely related forms of *H truncatum* toxicoses have been described.

Clinical Findings: After an incubation period of 4-11 days, signs appear suddenly and include hyperthermia, anorexia, listlessness, watering of the eyes and nose, hyperemia of the visible mucous membranes, salivation, necrosis of the oral mucosa, and hyperesthesia. Later, the eyelids stick together. The skin feels hot, and a moist dermatitis soon develops, starting from the base of the ears, the axillae, groin, and perineum, and extending over the entire body. The hair becomes matted, and beads of moisture may be seen on it. The skin becomes extremely sensitive and emits a sour odor. Later, the hair and epidermis can be readily pulled off, exposing red, raw wounds. The tips of the ears and the tail may slough. Eventually, the skin becomes hard and cracked and predisposed to secondary infection or screwworm infestation. Affected animals are sensitive to handling, show pain when moving, and seek shade.

Often, the course is rapid, and death may occur within a few days. In less acute cases, the course is more protracted and recovery may occur. Mortality in affected calves is 30-70% under natural conditions. Morbidity in endemic areas is ~10%. The severity of infection is influenced by the number of ticks as well as by the length of time they remain on the host.

Lesions: Emaciation, dehydration, diphtheroid stomatitis, pharyngitis, laryngitis, esophagitis, vaginitis or posthitis, edema and hyperemia of the lungs, atrophy of the spleen, and congestion of the liver, kidneys, and meninges are found in addition to the skin lesions.

Diagnosis: For diagnosis, it is essential to determine the presence of the vector. Typically, there is a generalized hyperemia with subsequent desquamation of the superficial layers of the mucous membranes of the upper respiratory, GI, and external genital tracts, and profuse moist dermatitis followed by superficial desquamation of the skin.

Prevention and Treatment: Control of tick infestation is the only effective preventive measure. Removal of ticks, symptomatic treatment, and good nursing care are indicated. Non-nephrotoxic antibiotics and anti-inflammatory agents are useful to combat secondary infection. Immune serum can be used to good effect as a specific treatment.

TOXOPLASMOSIS

Toxoplasma gondii is a protozoan parasite that infects humans and other warm-blooded animals, including birds. It has been found worldwide from Alaska to Australia.

Etiology and Pathogenesis: Felids are the only definitive hosts of *T gondii*; both wild and domestic cats therefore serve as the main reservoir of infection. There are 3 infectious stages of *T gondii*; tachyzoites (rapidly multiplying form), bradyzoites (tissue cyst form), and sporozoites (in oocysts).

T gondii is transmitted by consumption of infectious oocysts in cat feces, consumption of tissue cysts in infected meat, and by transplacental transfer of tachyzoites from mother to fetus. *T gondii* initiates enteroepithelial replication in unexposed cats after ingestion of uncooked meat containing tissue cysts. Bradyzoites are released from tissue cysts by digestion in the stomach and small intestine, invade intestinal epithelium, and undergo sexual replication, culminating in the release of oocysts (10 μm diameter) in the feces. Oocysts are first seen in the feces at 3 days after infection and may be released for up to 20 days. Oocysts sporulate (become infectious) outside the cat within 1-5 days, depending on aeration and temperature, and remain viable in the environment for several months. Cats generally develop immunity to *T gondii* after the initial infection and therefore shed oocysts only once in their lifetime.

Following consumption of uncooked meat containing tissue cysts (carnivores) or feed or drink contaminated with cat feces containing oocysts (all warm-blooded animals), *T gondii* initiates extraintestinal replication. Bradyzoites and sporozoites, respectively, are released and infect intestinal epithelium. After several rounds of epithelial replication, tachyzoites emerge and disseminate via the bloodstream and lymph. Tachyzoites infect tissues throughout the body and replicate intracellularly until the cells burst, causing tissue necrosis. Tachyzoites measure $4\text{-}6 \times 2\text{-}4$ μm in diameter and stain with Giemsa. Young and immunocompromised animals may succumb to generalized toxoplasmosis at this stage. Older animals mount a powerful cell-mediated immune response to the tachyzoites (mediated by cytokines) and control infection, driving the tachyzoites into the tissue cyst or bradyzoite stage. Tissue cysts are usually seen in neurons but also occur in other tissues. Individual cysts are microscopic, up to 70 μm in diameter, and may enclose hundreds of bradyzoites in a thin, resilient cyst wall. Tissue cysts in the host remain viable for many years, and possibly for the life of the host.

Clinical Findings: The tachyzoite is the stage responsible for tissue damage; therefore, clinical signs depend on the number of tachyzoites released, the ability of the host immune system to limit tachyzoite spread, and the organs damaged by the tachyzoites. Because adult immunocompetent animals control tachyzoite spread efficiently, toxoplasmosis is usually a subclinical illness. However, in young animals, particularly puppies, kittens, and piglets, tachyzoites spread systemically and cause interstitial pneumonia, myocarditis, hepatic necrosis, meningoencephalomyelitis, chorioretinitis, lymphadenopathy, and myositis. The corresponding clinical signs include fever, diarrhea, cough, dyspnea, icterus, seizures, and death. *T gondii* is also an important cause of abortion and stillbirth in sheep and goats and sometimes in pigs. After infection of a pregnant ewe, tachyzoites spread via the bloodstream to placental cotyledons, causing necrosis. Tachyzoites may also spread to the fetus, causing necrosis in multiple organs. Finally, immunocompromised adult animals (eg, cats infected with feline immunodeficiency virus) are extremely susceptible to developing acute generalized toxoplasmosis.

Diagnosis: Diagnosis is made by biologic, serologic, or histologic methods, or by some combination of the above. Clinical signs of toxoplasmosis are nonspecific and are not sufficiently characteristic for a definite diagnosis. Antemortem diagnosis may be accomplished by indirect hemagglutination assay, indirect fluorescent antibody assay, latex agglutination test, or ELISA. IgM antibodies appear sooner after infection than IgG antibodies but generally do not persist past 3 mo after infection. Increased IgM titers (>1:256) are consistent with recent infection. In contrast, IgG antibodies appear by the fourth week after infection and may remain increased for years during subclinical infection. To be useful, IgG titers must be measured in paired sera from the acute and convalescent stages (3-4 wk apart) and must show at least a 4-fold increase in titer. Additionally, CSF and aqueous humor may be analyzed for the presence of tachyzoites or anti-*T gondii* antibodies. Postmortem, tachyzoites may be seen in tissue impression smears. Additionally, microscopic examination of tissue sections may reveal the presence of tachyzoites or bradyzoites. *T gondii* is morphologically similar to other protozoan parasites and must be differentiated from *Sarcocystis* spp (in cattle), *S neurona* (in horses), and *Neospora caninum* (in dogs).

Treatment: For animals other than humans, treatment is seldom warranted. Sulfadiazine (15-25 mg/kg) and pyrimethamine (0.44 mg/kg) act synergistically and are widely used for treatment of toxoplasmosis. While these drugs are beneficial if given in the acute stage of the disease when there is active multiplication of the parasite, they will not usually eradicate infection. These drugs are believed to have little effect on the bradyzoite stage. Certain other drugs, including diaminodiphenylsulfone, atovaquone, and spiramycin are also used to treat toxoplasmosis in difficult cases. Clindamycin is the treatment of choice for dogs and cats, at 10-40 mg/kg and 25-50 mg/kg respectively, for 14-21 days.

Prevention and Zoonotic Risk: *T gondii* is an important zoonotic agent. In some areas of the world, up to 60% of the human population have serum IgG titers to *T gondii* and are likely to be persistently infected. Toxoplasmosis is a major concern for people with immune system dysfunction (eg, people infected with human immunodeficiency virus). In these individuals, toxoplasmosis usually presents as meningoencephalitis and results from the emergence of *T gondii* from tissue cysts located in the brain as immunity wanes rather than from primary *T gondii* infection. Toxoplasmosis is also a major concern for pregnant women because tachyzoites can migrate transplacentally and cause birth defects in human fetuses. Infection of women with *T gondii* may occur after ingestion of undercooked meat or accidental ingestion of oocysts from cat feces. To prevent infection, the hands of people handling meat should be washed thoroughly with soap and water after contact, as should all cutting boards, sink tops, knives, and other materials. The stages of *T gondii* in meat are killed by contact with soap and water. *T gondii* organisms in meat can also be killed by exposure to extreme cold or heat. Tissue cysts in meat are killed by heating the meat throughout to 67°C or by cooling to -13°C. *Toxoplasma* in tissue cysts are also killed by exposure to 0.5 kilorads of gamma irradiation. Meat of any animal should be cooked to 67°C before consumption, and tasting meat while cooking or while seasoning should be avoided. Pregnant women should avoid contact with cat litter, soil, and raw meat. Pet cats should be fed only dry, canned, or cooked food. The cat litter box should be emptied daily, preferably not by a pregnant woman. Gloves should be worn while gardening. Vegetables should be washed thoroughly before eating because they may have been contaminated with cat feces.

At present there is no vaccine to prevent toxoplasmosis in humans.

TUBERCULOSIS AND OTHER MYCOBACTERIAL INFECTIONS

Tuberculosis (TB) is an infectious, granulomatous disease caused by acid-fast bacilli of the genus *Mycobacterium*. Although commonly defined as a chronic, debilitating disease, TB occasionally assumes an acute, rapidly progressive course. The disease affects practically all species of vertebrates, and before control measures were adopted, was a major disease of humans and domestic animals. Bovine TB is still a significant zoonosis in many parts of the world. Signs and lesions are generally similar in the various species.

Etiology: Three main types of tubercle bacilli are recognized: human, bovine, and avian, respectively, *M tuberculosis*, *M bovis*, and *M avium* complex (*M avium-intracellulare-scrofulaceum*). The 3 types differ in cultural characteristics and pathogenicity. The 2 mammalian types are more closely related to each other than to the avian type. More than 30 serovars of *M avium* complex are recognized; however, only serovars 1, 2, and 3 are pathogenic for birds. Mycobacteria may survive on pasture for 2 mo or more.

All 3 types may produce infection in host species other than their own. *M tuberculosis* is most specific; it rarely produces progressive disease in animals other than people and nonhuman primates and occasionally in dogs, pigs, and birds. *M bovis* can cause progressive disease in most warm-blooded vertebrates, including humans. *M avium avium* is the only species of consequence in birds, but it has a wide host range and is also pathogenic for pigs, cattle, sheep, deer, mink, dogs, cats, and some cold-blooded animals. Mycobacteria other than tubercle bacilli (p 553) are infrequently isolated from exotic and domestic animals.

Pathogenesis: Inhalation of infected droplets expelled from the lungs is the usual route of infection, although ingestion, particularly via contaminated milk, also occurs. Intrauterine and coital methods of infection are recognized less commonly. Inhaled bacilli are phagocytosed by alveolar macrophages that may either clear the infection or allow the mycobacteria to proliferate. In the latter instance, a primary focus may form, mediated by cytokines associated with a hypersensitivity reaction that consists of dead and degenerate macrophages surrounded by epithelioid cells, granulocytes, lymphocytes, and later, giant cells. The purulent to caseous, necrotic center may calcify, and the lesion may become surrounded by granulation tissue and a fibrous capsule to form the classic "tubercle." The primary focus plus similar lesions formed in the regional lymph node is known as the "primary complex." In alimentary forms of disease, the primary focus may be found in the pharynx or mesenteric lymph nodes or, less commonly, in the tonsils or intestines. The cellular composition of and presence of acid-fast bacilli in tuberculous lesions differ between and within host species.

The primary complex seldom heals in animals and may progress slowly or rapidly. Dissemination through vascular and lymphatic channels may be generalized and rapidly fatal, as in acute miliary TB. Nodular lesions may form in many organs, including the pleura, peritoneum, liver, kidney, skeleton, mammary glands, reproductive tract, and CNS. A prolonged, chronic course may also ensue, with lesions usually having a more localized pattern of distribution.

Clinical Findings: The clinical signs reflect the extent and location of lesions plus the underlying toxemia. Generalized signs include progressive emaciation, lethargy, weakness, anorexia, and a low-grade, fluctuating fever. The bronchopneumonia of the respiratory form of the disease causes a chronic, intermittent, moist cough with later signs of dyspnea and tachypnea. The destructive lesions of the granulomatous bronchopneumonia may be detected on auscultation and percussion. Superficial lymph node enlargement may be a useful diagnostic sign when present. Affected deeper lymph nodes cannot always be palpated, but they may cause obstruction of the airways, pharynx, and gut, leading to dyspnea and ruminal tympany.

In pigs, lesions caused by *M avium avium* are most often seen in lymph nodes associated with the GI tract, although generalized disease does not occur.

Diagnosis: The single most important diagnostic test for TB is the intradermal tuberculin test. Diagnosis on clinical signs alone is very difficult, even in advanced cases. Radiography is useful in nonhuman primates and small animals. Microscopic examination of sputum and other discharges is sometimes used. Necropsy findings of the classic "tuberculous" granulomas are often very suggestive of the disease. Confirmation of diagnosis is by isolation and identification of the organism, with culture usually taking 4-8 wk, or by PCR, which requires only a few days.

The delayed-type hypersensitivity response of the host, responsible for much of the pathology of TB, is fundamental to the tuberculin skin test that is widely used for diagnosis in large animals. The single intradermal (SID) test involves inoculation of mycobacterial antigen prepared from a filtrate of cultures of either *M bovis* or *M tuberculosis*. Purified protein derivative (PPD) preparations of the mycobacteria improve specificity. In a reactor, the antigen stimulates a local infiltrate of inflammatory cells and causes skin swelling that can be detected by palpation and measured by calipers. The reaction is read at 48-72 hr for maximum sensitivity and at 96 hr for maximum specificity. Test sites used vary in sensitivity and between countries and include the neck region, anal or caudal fold at the tail base, and vulval lip. One disadvantage of the *M bovis* SID test is its poor specificity, with cross-reactions occurring in animals infected with *M avium*, *M tuberculosis*, *M paratuberculosis*, and even *Nocardia* spp.

In areas with a high incidence of either avian TB, atypical mycobacteriosis, or paratuberculosis, the comparative test can be used, with biologically balanced *M bovis* and *M avium* PPD tuberculins inoculated simultaneously but at separate sites in the neck. The agent causing sensitization provokes the greater skin reaction. Other diagnostic tests used for TB include the thermal test, which may detect a pyrexic peak (104°F [>40°C]) at 6-8 hr after SC inoculation with tuberculin. The Stormont test uses an intradermal inoculation of PPD followed by a second inoculum at the same site 7 days later. The test is read for swelling 24 hr later. (*See also* p 1536.)

False-negative results may occur in animals with poor immunity such as those in the early stages of infection, anergic cases in advanced disease, or old animals. Cattle that have recently calved may also have false negative results. Current research is focused on the identification of antigens such as secretory proteins of *M bovis* for use in improved diagnostic tests. Serologic tests such as ELISA appear to be of limited diagnostic use, consistent with the lesser role of antibody compared with the cellular immune response in TB. In vitro cellular assays have been developed (ie, interferon-γ assay) using blood lymphocytes stimulated with *M bovis* antigen and show promise as an alternative to the widely used SID test; however, they have not come into widespread use.

Control: The main reservoirs of infection are humans and cattle. However, other animals have been found to be reservoirs in some countries, including badgers and red deer (England, Ireland); opossums and ferrets (New Zealand); mule deer, white-tailed deer, elk, and bison (North America); buffalo (South Africa); and water buffalo (Australia). Kudu, llamas, and domestic and feral pigs have also been found to be infected with *M bovis*. The prevalence of disease in such reservoirs influences the incidence of disease in other species.

The 3 principal approaches to the control of TB are test and slaughter, test and segregation, and chemotherapy. The test and slaughter policy is the only one assured of eradicating TB and relies on the slaughter of reactors to the tuberculin test. In an affected herd, testing every 3 mo is recommended to rid the herd of individuals that can disseminate infection. Routine hygienic measures aimed at cleaning and disinfecting contaminated food, water troughs, etc, are also useful. Test and slaughter has been used widely in the UK, USA, Canada, New Zealand, and Australia. In most European countries, where test and slaughter would have been impractical, varying forms of test and segregation have been used, with test and slaughter used only in the final stages of eradication.

Treatment of cases of TB in elephants and nonhuman primates has been attempted using drugs that have had success in humans, eg, isoniazid, ethambutol, and rifampin. Efficacy is limited, and there are overriding arguments against therapy, based on the removal of infected animals, zoonotic risks, and the danger of encouraging drug resistance. Treatment is illegal in some countries. The BCG (bacille Calmette-Guérin) vaccine, sometimes used to control TB in humans, has proved to provide little protection in most animal species, and inoculation often provokes a severe local granulomatous reaction.

Cattle

Most of the general discussion above applies to bovine TB. The introduction of milk pasteurization was a major step in the fight against human TB and continues to be an important control procedure in many countries.

Sheep and Goats

Lesions caused by *M bovis* in the lungs and lymph nodes of sheep and goats are similar to those seen in cattle, and the organism may sometimes disseminate to other organs. Sheep and goats are quite resistant to *M tuberculosis* and *M avium* infection. The SID test is commonly used for diagnosis.

Deer and Elk

Tuberculosis due to *M bovis* is an important problem in most species of farmed and wild cervids. Deer appear to be unusually susceptible to mycobacterial infections, and *M avium* infections may produce similar lesions. *M tuberculosis* infection seems to be uncommon. Tuberculous lesions may be confined to isolated lymph nodes, or they may be found extensively in lymph nodes and organs after a rapid, fulminating disease course. Abscessation in deer should always raise suspicions of TB. Diagnosis may be assisted by the tuberculin skin test, blood lymphocyte stimulation test, serology, or a combination of these. Infection should be confirmed by an organism-based test.

Horses

Horses are relatively resistant to TB caused by all 3 bacillus species. When TB does develop, tuberculous, noncalcified lesions are often found in the liver, mesenteric lymph nodes, lungs, and other sites. Tuberculin test results are rather erratic.

Elephants

Tuberculosis due to *M tuberculosis* has been reported in captive elephants. Lesions most often involve the lung and associated lymph nodes. Nonspecific responses are observed on immunologic tests; therefore, diagnosis should be made on an organism-based test of trunk washes. Multidrug regimens have been developed that eliminate shedding of tubercle bacilli in discharges and minimize development of drug-resistant strains.

Pigs

Pigs are susceptible to all 3 types of tubercle bacilli. *M avium avium* is most frequently isolated; serologic identification of isolates is useful in epidemiologic investigations. Granulomatous lesions are most often found in the cervical, submandibular, and mesenteric lymph nodes, but lesions may also be found elsewhere. Typically, enlarged nodes contain small, white or yellow, caseous foci, usually without any evidence of mineralization. Pigs with disease due to *M tuberculosis* may have similar regionalized lesions. Pigs are particularly susceptible to *M bovis*, which is usually acquired from shared grazing or ingestion of dairy products. This can cause a rapidly progressive, disseminated disease with caseation and liquefaction of lesions. The SID test conducted on the dorsal surface of the ear is useful for diagnosis.

Dogs

Dogs may be infected with *M tuberculosis*, *M bovis*, and occasionally with *M avium* or *M fortuitum*, commonly from a human or bovine source. Tuberculous lesions are usually found in the lungs, liver, kidney, pleura, and peritoneum; they have a gray appearance, usually with a noncalcified, necrotic center. Lesions are often exudative and can produce a large quantity of straw-colored fluid in the thorax. False-negative tuberculin tests are common in dogs. Radiographs and a thorough history are useful in diagnosis. Affected dogs should be euthanized because of public health concerns.

Cats

Cats are resistant to infection with *M tuberculosis* but are susceptible to *M bovis* and *M avium* complex or *M microti* bacilli. Some unclassified bacillus forms have also been isolated. Contaminated milk causing GI tract lesions, typically in the mesenteric lymph nodes, is the most common circumstance, and historically this was responsible for a very high percentage of tuberculous cats in Europe. Rapid, hematogenous dissemination to other organs, including the lungs and regional lymph nodes, can occur. Infected skin or deeper wounds sometimes give rise to tuberculous sinuses. Lesions have a central area of necrosis, usually without calcification. The tuberculin skin test is considered unreliable in cats. Diagnosis may be assisted by radiography or culture of the organism. Affected cats should be euthanized because of public health concerns.

Nonhuman Primates

In monkeys and large apes, *M bovis*, *M tuberculosis*, and *M avium* can cause severe disease of the lungs and other organs. Epidemics in primate colonies may be caused by contact with infected human caregivers. Transmission is usually by aerosol with respiratory infection, but the oral route is also possible. Bacilli may also be shed in the urine. The tuberculin PPD skin test developed for animals is superior to the human preparations for diagnosis.

Captive Exotic Hoofed Animals

Numerous species are susceptible to *M bovis* infection. Tuberculous lesions vary in consistency from purulent to caseous and often involve the lungs and regional lymph nodes, with liver, spleen, and serosal surfaces as other potential sites. Tuberculin skin tests may be useful for diagnosis.

MYCOBACTERIAL INFECTIONS OTHER THAN TUBERCULOSIS

Mycobacteria found in soil and water have been isolated from tissues of animals. *Mycobacterium fortuitum*, a rapidly growing organism that is highly resistant to penicillin G, streptomycin, ampicillin, sulfamethoxazole, and chloramphenicol, has been associated with mastitis in cows, pulmonary infections in dogs, lymph node lesions in pigs and certain exotic animals, and cutaneous lesions in cats and dogs. Drug susceptibility tests indicate the organism is inhibited by capreomycin and by ethionamide. *M chelonei*, another rapidly growing mycobacterium similar to *M fortuitum* in biochemical reactions, has been isolated from contaminated wounds and injection abscesses. These organisms must be distinguished from *M phlei*, *M smegmatis*, and *M vaccae*, which are rarely if ever pathogenic.

Fish and other cold-blooded animals can be infected with *M avium intracellulare* or with *M marinum*, which have been recognized as human pathogens. A photochromogenic organism, *M kansasii*, has been isolated from pigs, cattle, and nonhuman primates. These organisms can be differentiated on biochemical and seroagglutination tests.

M avium paratuberculosis, the cause of Johne's disease, has been isolated from domestic and wild ruminants (*see also* PARATUBERCULOSIS, p 612). It is a slowly progressive diarrheal disease resulting in weight loss and emaciation. Lesions are most often observed in the ileocecal valve and associated lymph nodes. Diagnosis should be based on an organism-based test. No treatment is available.

M scrofulaceum, a scotochromogen, has been isolated from lymph node lesions in pigs, cattle, and certain nonhuman primates. *M xenopi*, a slowly growing scotochromogen, has been isolated from pigs, seafowl, and amphibians. These organisms should be differentiated from *M gordonae* and *M flavescens* and from other slowly growing scotochromogenic mycobacteria that are common contaminants of water.

Numerous nonpathogenic, nonphotochromogenic mycobacteria that closely resemble potential pathogens can be isolated from water and soil: *M nonchromogenicum*, *M gastri*, *M triviale*, and *M terrae*, which closely resemble strains of the *M avium* complex, may be differentiated by in vitro laboratory examinations.

Although opportunistic mycobacteria usually fail to produce progressive disease, they may be important in inducing transient tuberculin skin sensitivity in animals. The application of comparative skin tests, using biologically balanced PPD tuberculins prepared from culture filtrates of *M bovis* and *M avium*, provides useful information on the possible cause of tuberculin skin sensitivity. Tuberculins prepared for veterinary use, containing ~5,000 tuberculin units per test dose, should be used for skin tests in domestic, wild, and exotic animals.

M lepraemurium, a nonphotochromogenic, slow-growing, acid-fast bacillus, causes a disease in cats and rats similar in some respects to leprosy in humans. It can be grown on media containing cytochrome C and α-ketoglutarate. *M leprae*, the cause of leprosy in humans, has been found in spontaneously occurring disease in armadillos. This organism has not been grown on artificial culture medium.

TULAREMIA

Tularemia is a bacterial septicemia that affects >250 species of wild and domestic mammals, birds, reptiles, fish, and people.

Etiology: The causative bacterium, *Francisella tularensis*, is a nonsporulating, gram-negative coccobacillus that is antigenically related to *Brucella* spp. It is a facultative intracellular parasite that is killed rapidly by heat and proper disinfection but survives for weeks or months in a moist environment. It is fastidious in growth but can be cultured readily. There are 2 types of organisms based on their biochemistry and virulence. Type A has been found predominantly in North America and is more virulent; in people, the mortality rate may be 5-7% if untreated. Type B is less virulent and is most commonly isolated from aquatic animals and water-associated infections in North America and Eurasia. Both types have been isolated from arthropod vectors.

Epidemiology and Transmission: In domestic animals, sheep are the primary host, but clinical infection has been reported in dogs, pigs, and horses. Cats are at increased risk due to predatory behavior and appear to have an increased susceptibility, while cattle appear to be resistant. Little is known of the true incidence and spectrum of clinical disease in domestic animals. Important wild animal hosts include cottontail and jackrabbits, beaver, muskrat, meadow voles, and sheep in North America, and other voles, field mice, and lemmings in Europe and Asia.

Natural foci of infection exist in North America and Eurasia, where the organism circulates between arthropod vectors and various mammals, birds, reptiles, and fish. Although found in every state except Hawaii, tularemia is most often reported in the southcentral and western USA (eg, Missouri, Oklahoma, South Dakota, and Montana).

Tularemia is a classic zoonosis, capable of being transmitted by aerosol, direct contact, ingestion, or arthropods. Inhalation of aerosolized organisms (as in the laboratory or as an airborne agent in an act of bioterrorism) can produce a pneumonic form. Direct contact with, or ingestion of, infected carcasses of wild animals (eg, cottontail rabbit) can produce the ulceroglandular, oculoglandular, oropharyngeal (local lesion with regional lymphadenitis), or typhoidal form. Immersion in or ingestion of contaminated water can result in infection in aquatic animals. Ticks can maintain infection trans-stadially and transovarially, which makes them an efficient reservoir as well as a vector. Recognized vectors in the USA include *Dermacentor andersoni* (the wood tick), *Amblyomma americanum* (the lone star tick), *Dermacentor variabilis* (the dog tick), and *Chrysops discalis* (the deer fly).

The most common source of infection for people and herbivores is the bite of an infected tick, but persons who dress, prepare, or eat improperly cooked wild game are also at increased risk. Dogs, cats, and other carnivores may acquire infection from ingestion of an infected carcass. A few case reports have implicated cats as a source of infection in people.

Clinical Findings: The incubation period is 1-10 days. In sheep and most mammals, the disease is characterized by sudden onset of high fever, lethargy, anorexia, stiffness, reduced mobility, or other signs associated with septicemic disease. Pulse and respiratory rates are increased. Coughing, diarrhea, and pollakiuria may develop. Prostration and death may occur in a few hours or days. Sporadic cases are best recognized by signs of septicemia. Outbreaks in untreated lambs may have up to 15% mortality. Subclinical cases may be common.

Lesions: The most consistent lesions are miliary, white to off-white foci of necrosis in the liver and sometimes in the spleen and lymph nodes. Enlargement of the liver, spleen, and lymph nodes is common. Organisms can be readily isolated from necropsy specimens by use of special media. Risk of infection during necropsy or to laboratory personnel is significant; special procedures and facilities are essential.

Diagnosis: Tularemia must be differentiated from other septicemic diseases (especially plague) or acute pneumonia. When large numbers of sheep show typical signs during periods of heavy tick infestation, tularemia or tick paralysis (p 1073) should be suspected. Tularemia should be considered in cats with signs of acute lymphadenopathy, malaise, oral ulcers, and history of recent ingestion of wild prey.

Diagnosis of acute infection is confirmed by culture and identification of the bacterium, direct or indirect fluorescent antibody test, or a 4-fold increase in antibody titer between acute and convalescent serum specimens. A single titer of ≥1:80 by the tube agglutination test is presumptive evidence of prior infection. When tularemia is suspected, laboratory personnel should be alerted to reduce the risk of laboratory-acquired infection.

Treatment and Control: Streptomycin, gentamicin, chloramphenicol, and tetracyclines are effective at recommended dose levels; however, tetracycline and chloramphenicol have been associated with relapses in people. Early treatment should prevent death loss. Control is difficult and is limited to reducing tick infestation and to rapid diagnosis and treatment. Prolonged treatment may be necessary because many organisms are intracellular. Use of a vaccine previously available for people at high risk of infection (eg, laboratory personnel) is currently under review. Recovery confers long-lasting immunity.

VESICULAR STOMATITIS

Vesicular stomatitis is a viral disease caused by 2 distinct serotypes of vesicular stomatitis virus—New Jersey and Indiana. Vesiculation, ulceration, and erosion of the oral and nasal mucosa and epithelial surface of the tongue, coronary bands, and teats are typically observed in clinical cases, along with crusting lesions of the muzzle, ventral abdomen, and sheath. Clinical disease has been observed in cattle, horses, and pigs and very rarely in sheep, goats, and llamas. Serologic evidence of exposure has been found in many species including cervids, nonhuman primates, rodents, birds, dogs, antelope, and bats. The viruses are zoonotic and may cause influenza-like disease in people working in close contact with the virus (eg, laboratory exposure, direct contact with lesions in infected animals).

Etiology: The viruses are members of the family Rhabdoviridae and genus Vesiculovirus. Vesicular stomatitis viruses are the prototypes of the Vesiculovirus genus. They are bullet shaped and generally 180 nm long and 75 nm wide. The genomic structure is a single strand of negative sense RNA composed of 5 genes (N, P, M, G, and L, representing the nucleocapsid protein, phosphoprotein, matrix protein, glycoprotein, and the large protein, respectively). Although there are many members of the Vesiculovirus genus, the New Jersey and Indiana serotypes are of particular interest in the Western hemisphere. These 2 viruses are similar in size and morphology but generate distinct neutralizing antibodies in infected animals. They have both been isolated in recent outbreaks in the USA.

Epidemiology and Transmission: Vesicular stomatitis is seen sporadically in the USA. Outbreaks historically occurred in all regions of the country but since the 1980s have been limited to southwestern states. Vesicular stomatitis viruses are endemic in South America, Central America, and parts of Mexico but have not been seen naturally outside the Western hemisphere. The virus can be transmitted through direct contact with infected animals with clinical disease (those with lesions) or by blood-feeding insects. In the southwestern USA, black flies (Simulidae) are the most likely biologic insect vector. In endemic areas, sand flies (*Lutzomyia*) are proven biologic vectors. Other insects may act as mechanical vectors. The prevalence of clinical cases in a herd is generally low (10-20%), but seroprevalence within the herd may approach 100%. No reservoir or amplifying host of vesicular stomatitis viruses has been identified.

Clinical Findings: The incubation period is 2-8 days and is typically followed by a fever. Ptyalism is often the first sign of disease. Vesicles in the oral cavity are rarely observed in naturally occurring cases due to rupture soon after formation; therefore, ulcers are the most common lesion observed during primary examination. Ulcers and erosions of the oral mucosa, sloughing of the epithelium of the tongue, and lesions at the mucocutaneous junctions of the lips are commonly seen in both cattle and horses. Ulcers and erosions on the teats are not uncommon in cattle and may result in secondary cases of mastitis in dairy cows. Coronitis with erosions at the coronary band are observed in cattle, horses, and pigs with subsequent development of lameness. Crusting lesions of the muzzle, ventral abdomen, sheath, and udder of horses are typical during outbreaks in the southwestern USA. Loss of appetite due to oral lesions and lameness due to foot lesions are normally of short duration, as the disease is generally self-limiting with complete resolution within 10-14 days. Virus neutralizing antibodies to either serotype persist, potentially for ≥5 yr, but reinfection can occur following a second exposure.

Diagnosis: In most areas, including the USA, vesicular stomatitis is a reportable disease. Samples for diagnostic purposes are generally taken by regulatory veterinarians and are tested by government laboratories. Diagnosis is based on the presence of typical clinical signs and either antibody detection through serologic tests, viral detection through isolation, and/or detection of viral genetic material by molecular techniques. Samples for viral isolation may include vesicular fluid, epithelial tags from lesions, or swabs of lesions. Vesicular stomatitis viruses are easily propagated in cell culture. Three commonly used serologic tests are competitive ELISA, virus neutralization, and complement fixation. PCR may also be used to identify the virus. Of primary concern in diagnosis is differentiation of vesicular stomatitis from clinically indistinguishable but much more devastating viral diseases including foot-and-mouth disease, swine vesicular disease, and vesicular exanthema of swine. Horses are not susceptible to foot-and-mouth disease.

Treatment, Control, and Prevention: No specific treatment is available or warranted. Cachexia can be avoided by providing softened feeds. Cleansing lesions with mild antiseptics may help avoid secondary bacterial infections. Management factors suggested to reduce risk of exposure to the virus include limiting time on pasture, providing shelters or barns during insect feeding times, and implementing other procedures that reduce animal contact with insects including application of insecticides. When affected animals are identified, they should be isolated, and movement of other animals from the affected premises restricted. Vesicular stomatitis is a reportable disease in most areas, including the USA, so animal health officials must be notified when it is suspected. Commercially produced vaccines are not available in the USA, but vaccines are available in some Latin American countries.

AFRICAN HORSE SICKNESS

African horse sickness (AHS) is an acute or subacute, insectborne, viral disease of Equidae that is endemic to Africa. It is characterized by clinical signs and lesions associated with respiratory and circulatory impairment.

Etiology and Epidemiology: AHS is caused by an orbivirus, 55-70 nm in diameter, of the family Reoviridae. There are 9 immunologically distinct types. Extracts of mouse brain infected with AHS virus hemagglutinate horse RBC. The virus is inactivated at a pH of <6 or ≥12, or by formalin, β-propiolactone, acetylethyleneimine derivatives, or radiation.

Appearance of AHS is preceded by seasons of heavy rain that alternate with hot and dry climatic conditions. Outbreaks in central and east Africa have extended to Egypt, the Middle East, and southern Arabia. In 1950-1960, a major epidemic extended from India to the Near Eastern countries; an estimated 300,000 Equidae were destroyed. A second epidemic in 1966 occurred in northeast Africa and southern Spain. In 1987, the disease entered Spain via imported zebra from Namibia. These 2 outbreaks in Spain were controlled, but another occurred in 1988, and sporadic cases occurred through early 1989. Recent AHS outbreaks (through 2001) have been reported only in Botswana and Namibia. In Botswana there were fewer cases in 2000 than in 1999. The disease was reported in horses and donkeys in the western regions. In 2001, 11 outbreaks were reported in Botswana. Two outbreaks were reported in Namibia in 2000, and 7 outbreaks in 2001. In a survey in Egypt, antibodies to AHS virus were detected in sheep, goats, camels, buffalo, and dogs.

Transmission: *Culicoides* spp are the principal vectors of transmission. AHS is seen during warm, rainy, seasons, which favor propagation of the vectors, and disappears after frost. The virus was isolated from blood of clinically healthy street dogs, the dog tick *Rhipicephalus sanguineus sanguineus*, and the camel tick *Hyalomma dromedarii* during winter in the Aswan region of southern Egypt where the disease is endemic. AHS has been experimentally transmitted by infected mosquitos. Limited studies in Egypt using dogs that had recovered from experimental infection revealed that 3 successive daily attacks by groups of *Culex pipiens* activated latent AHS virus and initiated viremia and fever. It has been suggested that the virus may overwinter in dogs with persistent infection. However, the full role of arthropods in transmission of the disease is unclear.

Clinical Findings and Lesions: Mortality depends on virulence of the viral strain and susceptibility of the host. It may reach 90% in epidemics. The acute respiratory form is characterized by an incubation period of 3-5 days, interlobular edema, and hydropericardium; death occurs in ~1 wk. A fever of 40-40.5°C (104-105°F) for 1-2 days is followed by dyspnea, spasmodic coughing, and dilated nostrils; the animal stands with its legs apart and head extended. The conjunctiva is congested and the supraorbital fossa may be swollen. Recovery is rare, and the animal dies of anoxia. At necropsy, pulmonary edema is especially visible in the intralobular spaces. The lungs are distended and heavy, and frothy fluid may be found in the trachea, bronchi, and bronchioles. There may be pleural effusion. Thoracic lymph nodes may be edematous, and the gastric fundus may be congested. Petechiae are found in the pericardium, and there is an increase in pericardial fluid; however, cardiac lesions usually are not outstanding. The abdominal viscera may be congested. A frothy exudate may ooze from the nostrils. The pulmonary form is the usual form in dogs.

The cardiac form is subacute with an incubation period of 1-2 wk. A fever of <1 wk is followed by swelling of the supraorbital fossa, which is pathognomonic. Swelling usually extends to the eyelids, facial tissues, neck, thorax, brisket, and shoulders. Death usually occurs within 1 wk and may be preceded by colic. The mortality rate is ~50%. Petechiae and ecchymoses on the epicardium and endocardium are prominent. The lungs are usually flaccid or slightly edematous. There are yellow, gelatinous infiltrations of the subcutaneous and intramuscular tissues, especially along the jugular veins and ligamentum nuchae. Other lesions include hydropericardium, myocarditis, hemorrhagic gastritis, and petechiae on the ventral surface of the tongue and peritoneum. A mixed pulmonary and cardiac form is usually found in outbreaks, with signs and lesions of one type predominating.

Diagnosis: In endemic areas, clinical signs and lesions may lead to a provisional diagnosis. However, laboratory confirmation is essential for definitive diagnosis and determination of the serotype; the latter is important for control measures. Blood specimens should be obtained at the peak of fever, preserved in OCG solution (50% glycerol, 0.5% potassium oxalate, 0.5% phenol), and transported (at 4°C) to the laboratory. Spleen samples collected from freshly dead animals should be preserved in 10% buffered glycerin. For virus isolation, infant mice or cell cultures are used. Infected mice may develop nervous and paralytic signs and should be observed for 3 wk. To obtain a high-titered antigen from mouse brains for the complement fixation test, 2 or 3 passages may be necessary. Brains from paralyzed mice only are harvested for antigen preparation. The complement fixation test is useful for disease diagnosis; virus neutralization and/or hemagglutination-inhibition tests are used for serotyping.

Prevention and Control: Surviving Equidae develop solid immunity to the homologous serotype but remain susceptible to other serotypes. There are vaccines for all 9 serotypes. These are either cell-culture adapted or mouse-brain attenuated and provide long-lasting protection. Inactivated vaccines are available; 2 doses are required to provide adequate immunity. These vaccines induce local reaction at the site of inoculation and a short protection period.

When the disease first appears in an area, affected horses should be eliminated immediately, and noninfected Equidae should be vaccinated with polyvalent vaccine and rested for 2 wk. When the virus isolate has been typed, animals that received polyvalent vaccine should be revaccinated with the homologous vaccine. Vector control is also initiated by using insecticides and repellents. Vaccinated horses should be kept in insect-proof housing because vaccine failure may occur. Aircraft flying from endemic areas to countries free of the disease should be sprayed with insecticides on arrival. In the USA, equids from African countries are quarantined for 2 mo and then tested for the virus. Presence of antibodies does not interfere with importation of Equidae into countries free of the disease.

EQUINE GRANULOCYTIC EHRLICHIOSIS

Equine granulocytic ehrlichiosis is an infectious, noncontagious, seasonal disease, seen chiefly in the USA in northern California but also recognized in several other states; it also occurs in Europe and South America. (*See also* POTOMAC HORSE FEVER, p 236.)

Etiology, Epidemiology, and Transmission: The causal rikettsial agent was initially termed *Ehrlichia equi*, but based on DNA sequence relationships, the organism is now referred to as *Anaplasma phagocytophila*. The organism has a wide host range; naturally occurring infections have been seen in horses, burros, dogs, llamas, and rodents. A rickettsia closely resembling *A phagocytophila*, the human granulocytic ehrlichiosis (HGE) agent, has recently been implicated in cases of human illness in the upper midwestern and northeastern states in the USA.

A phagocytophila frequently infects horses in the foothills of northern California. Other states in which clinical infection has been confirmed include Connecticut, Illinois, Arkansas, Washington, Pennsylvania, Colorado, Minnesota, and Florida. It has also been confirmed in British Columbia, Sweden, Great Britain, and South America.

A phagocytophila resembles the etiologic agents of tickborne fever, bovine petechial fever, and the HGE agent based on morphology, cell tropism, and 16S rRNA gene sequence data. It is present in cytoplasmic vacuoles of neutrophils and occasionally eosinophils during the acute phase. Blood smears stained with Giemsa or Wright-Leishman stains reveal one or more loose aggregates (morulae or inclusion bodies, 1.5-5 μm in diameter) of blue-gray to dark blue coccoid, coccobacillary, or pleomorphic organisms within the cytoplasm of neutrophils.

The infection can be transmitted experimentally to susceptible horses by whole blood from infected horses or from people with HGE. The incubation period is 1-2 wk. *Ixodes pacificus* (the western black-legged tick) can transmit *A phagocytophila* to horses.

The zoonotic risk is unknown at this time. Although horses and people appear to be infected with strains of the same agent, it is believed that human exposure occurs through tick bites, and not by direct transmission from horses to people.

Clinical Findings: Severity of signs varies with age of the animal and duration of the illness. Signs may be mild. Horses <1 yr old may have a fever only; horses 1-3 yr old develop fever, depression, mild limb edema, and ataxia. Adults exhibit the characteristic signs of fever, partial anorexia, depression, reluctance to move, limb edema, petechiation, and icterus. The fever, which is highest during the first 1-3 days of infection at 103-104°F (39.5-40°C), persists at 102-104°F (39-40°C) for 6-12 days. Signs become more severe over several days. Rarely, myocardial vasculitis may cause transient ventricular arrhythmias. Any concurrent infection (eg, a leg wound or respiratory infection) can be exacerbated. Cytoplasmic inclusion bodies are few during the first 48 hr and increase to 30-40% of circulating neutrophils at days 3-5 of infection. The disease is seasonal in California, occurring in the late fall, winter, and spring.

Lesions: Gross petechiation, ecchymoses, and edema develop in the subcutis and fascia. Vasculitis is regional, with the subcutis and fascia of the legs predominantly affected.

Diagnosis: Demonstration of the characteristic cytoplasmic inclusion bodies in a standard blood smear is diagnostic. PCR can detect *A phagocytophila* DNA in unclotted blood or buffy coat smears. An indirect fluorescent antibody test can detect rising antibody titers to *A phagocytophila*. Differential diagnoses include viral encephalitis, primary liver disease, equine infectious anemia, purpura hemorrhagica, and viral arteritis.

Treatment and Control: Oxytetracycline is extremely effective against *A phagocytophila*, and tetracycline, 7 mg/kg, IV, SID for 8 days, has eliminated the infection. Penicillin, chloramphenicol, and streptomycin have no inhibitory effect. Horses with severe ataxia and edema may benefit from short-term corticosteroid treatment (dexamethasone, 20 mg, SID for 2-3 days). Recovered horses are solidly immune for ≥2 yr and are not carriers. Tick control measures are mandatory for control of disease. There is no vaccine.

EQUINE INFECTIOUS ANEMIA

Equine infectious anemia (EIA) affects Equidae and is caused by an equid-specific lentivirus in the retrovirus family, equine infectious anemia virus (EIAV). Although the majority of persistent infections appear to have minimal clinical consequences, EIA may be seen in epizootic form with high morbidity and mortality. Infection can be accurately diagnosed with laboratory tests. Because there are no effective and safe vaccines, many countries have established control programs based on serologic testing.

Transmission and Pathogenesis: EIA is a bloodborne infection; virus can be found free in the plasma or cell-associated. Infection with EIAV appears to persist for life and, in nature, blood-feeding insects initiate most infections by mechanical transfer of infective blood between horses in close proximity. Tabanids, horseflies, and deer flies appear to be the most efficient vectors because the pain of their bite initiates host defensive behavior that interrupts feeding and results in additional host-seeking behavior. As EIAV has not been shown to multiply in insects, infected equids appear to be the only reservoir of the virus. Iatrogenic transmission has a high epizootic potential that can be avoided by standard precautions, eg, disposal or decontamination of needles and equipment between horses.

Clinical Findings: Exposed equids generally support viral replication for days to weeks before antibodies to EIAV can be detected. The incubation period ranges from 10 to ≥45 days, usually lasting 21-42 days after natural transmission. Peak viremia often occurs during a febrile episode before the horse becomes test-positive. These acute signs often go unrecognized in horses on pasture and may be accompanied by a mild reduction in platelet counts and transient inappetence. Often, infection is noted only after routine surveillance testing for EIA or when the horse develops recurring clinical bouts of fever accompanied by marked platelet reductions, petechial hemorrhages, anemia, depression, weight loss, cachexia, and dependent edema (hallmarks of the chronic form of EIA). EIAV infection can therefore present as an inapparent infection or as an acute or chronic disease. The clinical manifestations are determined in part by the viral strain and dose, and the genetic makeup and status of the immune system of the equid. For example, strains of EIAV adapted by rapid serial passage in horses can kill horses within 14 days of infection but may have no clinical effect on donkeys. Likewise, strains that produce no or mild clinical disease in adults have killed immunologically immature fetuses or immunodeficent foals. Frequently, EIAV enters a herd and is transmitted silently until the chronic form of the disease is noted. By that time, a high percentage of the herd can be infected.

    Lesions: In acute cases, the spleen and splenic lymph nodes are enlarged. In chronic cases, necropsy reveals emaciation, pale mucous membranes, subcutaneous dependent edema, splenomegaly, and enlarged abdominal lymph nodes.

    Microscopically, there is proliferation of reticuloendothelial cells in many organs, and periportal and perisinusoidal collections of round cells in the liver with accumulations of hemosiderin in Kupffer's cells. Perivascular lymphoid accumulations may be seen in other organs also. In some horses, there is proliferative glomerulitis with glomerular deposition of immunoglobulins (IgG) and complement.

Diagnosis: Clinical diagnosis should be confirmed by serology. The agar gel immunodiffusion (AGID, Coggins) test is internationally accepted; antigen sources include cell culture-propagated virus and recombinant proteins. ELISA tests for detection of antibody against EIAV antigens are accepted in many countries and aid in the practical diagnosis of EIAV infection. The ELISA tests can be done in minutes (compared with 1-2 days for AGID test results) and used under field conditions. In all cases, positive ELISA tests should be confirmed by AGID before regulatory actions are taken because of the higher rate of false positive results. When combined, ELISA and AGID testing affords the highest level of sensitivity and specificity.

Treatment and Control: No specific treatment or vaccine is available. As EIAV-infected equids present the only known source of infection, antibody-positive animals should be kept at a safe distance (~200 m) from other equids. The only recognized exception to this rule is the progeny of test-positive mares, which may possess maternal antibodies to EIAV. In the majority of cases, passive antibody against EIAV wanes to negative on AGID tests by 6-8 mo of age.

The risk associated with maintaining EIAV-infected breeding stock varies. Field studies have indicated excellent success in raising test-negative foals from inapparent carriers of EIAV. The risks of infection in utero increase dramatically if clinical signs of EIA are seen in the mare prior to parturition. Unfortunately, it is not possible to accurately determine the risk posed by any EIAV-infected equid. As EIAV persists in each infected equid for life, most regulatory agencies assume all EIAV-positive equids pose the same high risk.

EQUINE VIRAL ARTERITIS

(Epizootic cellulitis-pinkeye, Equine typhoid, Rotlaufseuche)

Equine viral arteritis (EVA) is an acute, contagious, viral disease of equids caused by equine arteritis virus. It is characterized by fever, depression, dependent edema (especially of the limbs, scrotum, and prepuce in the stallion), conjunctivitis, nasal discharge, abortion, and infrequently, death in young foals.

Etiology and Pathogenesis: Equine arteritis virus is a small, enveloped RNA virus and the prototype virus of the genus Arterivirus, family Arteriviridae, order Nidovirales. While only one serotype of the virus has been identified—the prototype Bucyrus strain—there is ample evidence of genomic and antigenic variation among temporally and geographically disparate isolates. Furthermore, strains of the virus vary in their ability to produce disease, including abortion, with some causing only a mild to moderate fever.

After aerosol exposure, the virus multiplies in the bronchial and alveolar macrophages and, within 48 hr of infection, can be found in the regional lymph nodes. This is followed by a leukocyte-associated viremia, during which the virus becomes widely disseminated in various tissues and fluids throughout the body. The virus localizes in the vascular endothelium of the smaller blood vessels, especially the arterioles, and in the epithelium of certain tissues, particularly the adrenals, seminiferous tubules, thyroid, and liver. Characteristic vascular lesions include endothelial swelling and degeneration, neutrophil infiltration, and necrosis of the tunica media of affected vessels. The vascular lesions give rise to edema and hemorrhage in many tissues and organs.

The pathogenesis of abortion caused by equine arteritis virus is still open to speculation. It may result from myometritis in the pregnant mare, leading to impairment of placental circulation and eventually death of the fetus.

Except for certain stallions, infectious virus is no longer detectable in most tissues or body fluids beyond day 28 after infection. A variable percentage of stallions can remain infected for extended periods. The virus is localized primarily in certain accessory sex glands (especially the ampulla of the vas deferens) in the carrier stallion.

Epidemiology and Transmission: The natural and experimental host range of equine arteritis virus appears to be restricted to equids. Based on the findings of serologic surveys and reported outbreaks of EVA, the virus is present in horse populations in many countries throughout the world; Japan and Iceland are notable exceptions. However, outbreaks of EVA are uncommon and usually associated with the movement of horses or shipment of semen. While the virus is known to infect many breeds of horses, the prevalence of infection varies widely, usually being highest in Standardbreds and Warmbloods. There is little evidence of infection in populations of wild equids.

The epidemiology of EVA involves virus-, host-, and environment-related factors, including variability in pathogenicity among naturally occurring strains of the virus, routes of transmission, existence of the carrier state in the stallion, and the nature of acquired immunity to infection. Outbreaks of EVA are usually linked to the movement of animals or the shipment of semen. Viral transmission can be widespread at racetracks or on breeding farms; such occurrences are not always associated with the appearance of clinical illness characteristic of EVA. In fact, the vast majority of cases of natural infection with the virus are asymptomatic.

Transmission of EAV infection can occur by respiratory, venereal, congenital, or indirect means. Aerosol transmission is the principal mode of spread by horses acutely infected with the virus. It is primarily responsible for dissemination of infection among horses at racetracks, shows, sales, veterinary clinics, and on breeding farms. The virus can also be transmitted venereally by the acutely infected mare and by the acutely or chronically infected (carrier) stallion. Mares can be infected by the venereal route either following natural service or artificial insemination with infective semen. The virus can also be transmitted indirectly through the use of virus-contaminated fomites (eg, shanks, twitches, head collars, and breeding shed equipment) and on the hands or clothing of animal handlers.

Unlike mares, geldings, or sexually immature colts, carrier stallions are viral reservoirs and are primarily responsible for persistence of the virus in different horse populations throughout the world. The virus is shed constantly in the semen. Such animals transmit infection to >85% of susceptible mares to which they are bred. While the duration of the carrier state varies between individuals, the virus may persist in some clinically healthy stallions for years. Such stallions do not suffer any apparent decrease in fertility. Spontaneous resolution of the carrier state has been observed in a variable percentage of persistently infected stallions.

Clinical Findings: Exposure to equine arteritis virus may result in clinical or inapparent infection, depending on the virus strain involved, viral dose, age, and physical condition of the animal(s), and various environmental factors. Studies have shown that most cases of natural infection are subclinical. The onset of clinical signs is preceded by an incubation period of 3-14 days, which varies mainly with the route of exposure. Signs vary widely in range and severity between outbreaks of EVA and among affected individuals in the same outbreak. Typically, any combination of the following may be seen: fever of 2-9 days duration, leukopenia, depression, anorexia, limb edema (especially of the hindlimbs), and edema of the prepuce and scrotum. Less consistent signs include conjunctivitis, lacrimation and photophobia, periorbital or supraorbital edema, rhinitis and nasal discharge, edema of the ventral body wall (including the mammary glands of mares), an urticarial-type skin reaction that is frequently localized to the sides of the neck or head (although it can sometimes be generalized), stiffness of gait, dyspnea, diarrhea, icterus, and ataxia.

Abortion may occur late in the acute phase or early in the convalescent phase of the disease. It may also supervene in subclinically infected mares. Mares may abort any time from 3 mo to over 10 mo of gestation. In natural outbreaks, abortion rates can vary from <10% to as high as 50%. Abortion does not result from a mare being bred to a carrier stallion or inseminated with infective semen. Mares that abort are already pregnant at time of exposure, which principally occurs by the respiratory route from an acutely infected in-contact animal. Mares infected late in gestation may not abort, but give birth to a congenitally infected foal.

Stallions affected with EVA may undergo a period of short-term subfertility. This is believed to result from increased intratesticular temperature caused by the high fever and severe scrotal edema that can be experienced by acutely infected stallions.

Clinical signs are more severe in young, old, and debilitated animals. Mortality is rare in natural outbreaks; it has been reported infrequently in young foals from a few days to several months of age that succumb from a fulminating pneumonia or pneumoenteritis.

Lesions: The gross and microscopic lesions reflect the extensive and considerable vascular damage caused by the virus. The most prominent gross findings include edema, congestion, and hemorrhages, especially in the subcutis of the limbs and abdomen; excess peritoneal, pleural, and pericardial fluid; and edema and hemorrhage of the intra-abdominal and thoracic lymph nodes and of the small and large intestine, especially the cecum and colon. Pulmonary edema, emphysema and interstitial pneumonia, enteritis, and infarcts in the spleen have been described in fatal cases of the disease in foals.

Aborted fetuses are usually partly autolyzed, and gross lesions, if present, may be limited to an excess of fluid in body cavities and a variable degree of interlobular pulmonary edema. The characteristic vascular lesions and immune-mediated changes seen in mature animals are not always a significant feature in fetuses infected with the virus.

The characteristic microscopic lesion is a vasculitis, involving primarily small arteries but also small veins. Histologically, the changes can range from vascular and perivascular edema, with occasional lymphocytic infiltration and endothelial cell hypertrophy in mild cases, to fibrinoid necrosis of the tunica media, extensive lymphocytic infiltration, necrosis and loss of endothelium, and thrombus formation in severe cases. Microscopic lesions are not a constant feature in abortions. Vasculitis, if present, has been observed in placenta, brain, liver, spleen, and lungs of the fetus. Fatal cases of infection in young foals are characterized by interlobular edema, congestion and mononuclear cell infiltration in the lungs, lymphoid depletion and hemorrhage in lymphoreticular tissues, and when there is an associated enteritis, focal hemorrhages and necrosis of the mucosa of the small intestine.

Diagnosis: Because of the clinical similarity of EVA to other respiratory and certain nonrespiratory diseases of horses, a clinical diagnosis cannot be made without corroborative virologic, serologic, or histopathological findings. Equine influenza; infection with equine herpesvirus 1 and 4, equine rhinitis A and B viruses, or equine adenoviruses; and streptococcal infections, with particular reference to purpura hemorrhagica, are among the more common diseases that clinically resemble EVA. The latter must also be differentiated from sporadic cases of equine infectious anemia and toxicosis caused by hoary alyssum (*Berteroa incana*). Among the exotic equine diseases that clinically mimic EVA are Getah virus infection and African horse sickness (p 556).

Abortion caused by equine arteritis virus can be differentiated from abortion caused by equine herpesvirus 1 (and rarely 4) in that the mare seldom displays any premonitory signs in herpesviral abortion. Furthermore, fetuses aborted due to herpesvirus infection are invariably fresh at expulsion and often have characteristic gross and microscopic lesions. In contrast, fetuses aborted due to equine arteritis virus are usually partly autolyzed and frequently devoid of any diagnostic lesions.

Appropriate specimens for confirmation of a diagnosis include nasopharyngeal and conjunctival swabs and unclotted blood samples (preferably citrated or EDTA samples) for virus isolation or detection by PCR. These should be obtained as early as possible following the onset of clinical signs. Acute and convalescent sera taken 3-4 wk apart should also be collected for serologic examination using the microneutralization or a validated ELISA test. Placental and fetal fluids, together with placenta, lung, lymphoreticular, and other fetal tissues, can be productive sources of virus from suspect cases of equine arteritis virus abortion. The carrier state can be readily confirmed in seropositive stallions by demonstration of the virus in semen that includes the sperm-rich fraction of the ejaculate either by virus isolation or PCR. When death has occurred and infection with equine arteritis virus is suspected, specimens of body cavity fluids, lung, and reticuloendothelial tissues, especially the lymph nodes associated with the GI and respiratory tracts, should be taken for virus isolation or PCR. These tissues should also be submitted for histopathologic and immunohistochemical examination for the characteristic vascular lesions. It is advisable to consult with a qualified laboratory before collecting specimens for virologic or serologic testing.

Swabs for attempted virus isolation should be transferred to a suitable viral transport medium and shipped (together with any fluids or tissues collected for either virus isolation or PCR) refrigerated or frozen in an insulated container via an overnight delivery service. Unclotted blood samples must be transported refrigerated but not frozen.

Treatment, Prevention, and Control: There is no known specific antiviral treatment for EVA. Because virtually all acutely affected horses recover completely, symptomatic treatment (eg, antipyretic, anti-inflammatory, and diuretic agents) is indicated only in severe cases, especially in stallions in which prolonged fever and extensive scrotal edema can result in short-term subfertility. Good nursing care and rest with a gradual return to normal activity are desirable. As yet, there is no proven therapeutic means of successfully eliminating the carrier state in stallions.

EVA is a preventable disease that can be controlled by sound management practices and selective use of a commercial, modified live virus vaccine. While the vaccine is both safe and immunogenic for stallions and nonpregnant mares, it is not recommended for use in pregnant mares, especially in the last 2 mo of gestation, or in foals <6 wk old, unless there is a high risk of exposure to natural infection.

Most prevention and control programs are focused on preventing or curtailing dissemination of equine arteritis virus in breeding populations, to minimize the risk of virus-related abortion or death in young foals and establishment of the carrier state in stallions. Such programs are based on good breeding management practices, identification of any carrier stallions, and immunization of the noncarrier breeding stallion population. Carrier stallions should be managed separately to avoid the risk of inadvertent viral spread to previously uninfected or unvaccinated horses on the premises. They should be bred only to naturally seropositive mares or mares adequately immunized against EVA. The natural reservoir of the virus may be reduced by vaccinating all colts against the disease at 6-12 mo of age, while they are still prepubertal and before there is any significant likelihood of natural exposure to infection.

Infective fresh-cooled or frozen semen also constitutes an important source of infection. Semen used for artificial insemination, especially if imported, should be tested for virus. Provided that precautions equivalent to those recommended when breeding a mare to a carrier stallion are observed, infective semen can be used with minimal risk of spread of the virus to other horses on the premises.

GLANDERS

(Farcy)

Glanders is a contagious, acute or chronic, usually fatal disease of Equidae caused by *Burkholderia (Pseudomonas) mallei* and characterized by serial development of ulcerating nodules that are most commonly found in the upper respiratory tract, lungs, and skin. Humans, Felidae, and other species are susceptible, and infections are usually fatal. Glanders is one of the oldest diseases known and once was prevalent worldwide. It has now been eradicated or effectively controlled in many countries, including the USA. In recent years, the disease has been reported in Iraq, Turkey, Pakistan, India, Mongolia, China, Brazil, and the United Arab Emirates.

Etiology: *Burkholderia mallei* is present in nasal exudates and ulcerated skin of infected animals, and the disease is commonly contracted by ingesting food or water contaminated by the nasal discharge of carrier animals. The organism is susceptible to heat, light, and disinfectants; it may survive in a contaminated area for >1 yr. Humid, wet conditions favor survival of the organism. A polysaccharide capsule is an important virulence factor and enhances survival in the environment.

Clinical Findings: After an incubation period of ~2 wk, affected animals usually have septicemia and high fever (up to 106°F [41°C]) and, subsequently, a thick, mucopurulent nasal discharge and respiratory signs. Death occurs within a few days. The chronic disease is common in horses and is seen as a debilitating condition with nodular or ulcerative cutaneous and nasal lesions. Infected animals may live for years and disseminate the organism. The prognosis is unfavorable. Recovered animals may not develop immunity.

Nasal, pulmonary, and cutaneous forms of glanders are recognized, and an animal may be affected by more than one form at a time. In the **nasal form,** nodules develop in the mucosa of the nasal septum and lower parts of the turbinates. The nodules degenerate into deep ulcers with raised irregular borders. Characteristic star-shaped cicatrices remain after the ulcers heal. In the early stage, the submaxillary lymph nodes are enlarged and edematous, and later become adherent to the skin or deeper tissues.

In the **pulmonary form,** small tubercle-like nodules, which have caseous or calcified centers surrounded by inflammatory zones, are found in the lungs. If the disease process is extensive, consolidation of the lung tissue and pneumonia may be present. The nodules tend to break down and may discharge their contents into the bronchioles, resulting in extension of the infection to the upper respiratory tract.

In the **cutaneous form** ("farcy"), nodules appear along the course of the lymph vessels, particularly of the extremities. These nodules degenerate and form ulcers that discharge a highly infectious, sticky pus. The liver and spleen also may show typical nodular lesions.

Diagnosis: The typical nodules, ulcers, scar formation, and debilitated condition may provide sufficient evidence for a clinical diagnosis. However, because these signs usually do not develop until the disease is well advanced, specific diagnostic tests should be used as early as possible. The mallein test is the procedure of choice. Complement fixation is also accurate, although occasionally a false-positive result occurs. An ELISA has been shown to be more sensitive than complement fixation but has not been widely used. Culture of exudate from lesions reveals the presence of the causative organism. PCR based on 16S and 23S rRNA gene sequences may be used for specific identification.

Prevention and Treatment: There is no vaccine. Prevention and control depend on early detection and elimination of affected animals, as well as complete quarantine and rigorous disinfection of the area involved. Treatment is given only in endemic areas. Doxycycline, ceftrazidime, gentamicin, streptomycin, and combinations of sulfazine or sulfamonomethoxine with trimethoprim were found to be efficient in the prevention and treatment of experimental glanders.

HENDRA VIRUS INFECTION

(Equine morbillivirus pneumonia, Acute equine respiratory syndrome)

Equine morbillivirus pneumonia is an acute viral respiratory infection of horses caused by Hendra virus. Characteristic clinical signs include fever, anorexia, depression, increased respiratory and heart rates, respiratory distress, and death in a high percentage of affected animals. Facial edema, frothy nasal discharge, cyanotic/jaundiced mucous membranes and mild neurologic signs have been less frequently observed in field and/or experimental cases of the disease.

Etiology and Pathogenesis: Hendra virus is a large, pleomorphic enveloped RNA virus, and the prototype virus of the genus *Henipavirus*. Although initially considered to be more closely related to members of the genus *Morbillivirus* than to other genera in the family Paramyxoviridae, studies have shown only low-level sequence homology with respiroviruses, morbilliviruses, and rubuloviruses and negligible immunologic cross-reactivity with other paramyxoviruses, reacting very weakly by immunofluorescence and protein immunoblot analysis with antiserum to rinderpest virus. Hendra virus is antigenically related to Nipah virus (p 578), with which it shares ~90% amino acid homology. Both viruses have been classified in a new genus, *Henipavirus*, in the subfamily Paramyxovirinae, family Paramyxoviridae. Hendra and Nipah viruses vary with regard to the species they infect and mode(s) and ease with which each can be transmitted.

Interstitial pneumonia of variable severity is the principal finding in natural or experimental cases of infection in horses exposed by the respiratory or parenteral routes. Hendra virus, unlike morbilliviruses such as measles and distemper, has a specific tropism for vascular tissues, regardless of route of challenge. In early infection, the vascular lesions range from edema and hemorrhage of vessel walls, fibrinoid degeneration with pyknotic nuclei in endothelial and tunica media cells, to the presence of numerous giant cells in the endothelium and sometimes the tunica media of affected vessels (both venules and arterioles). As the disease progresses, there is destruction of alveolar walls, with the appearance of alveolar and intravascular macrophages. There is evidence that virus becomes more widely distributed in various tissues throughout the body, presumably as a result of a leukocyte-associated viremia. The virus has been demonstrated in the vascular endothelium of subarachnoid and cerebral vessels and also affects the vasculature of the renal glomerulus and pelvis, lamina propria of the stomach, spleen, various lymph nodes and myocardium. In addition to its vascular tropism, Hendra virus can also be neurotropic, causing neuronal necrosis and focal gliosis.

Epidemiology and Transmission: Naturally occurring disease caused by Hendra virus has been reported only in horses and humans. Experimentally, disease has been produced in cats and guinea pigs, but not in mice, rats, rabbits, chickens, or dogs. The clinical response and pathologic findings in cats are very similar to those observed in horses. Serologic surveys have revealed a high prevalence of neutralizing antibodies to Hendra virus in wild-caught flying foxes or fruit bats (*Pteropus* spp) in Australia and Papua New Guinea. Fruit bats experience subclinical infection and are considered the natural reservoir of the virus. Natural outbreaks of disease have been infrequent and reported only in Australia. The geographic distribution of the virus appears to be limited to Australia and Papua New Guinea. Hendra virus appears to be minimally contagious. Under field conditions, transmission between infected and noninfected horses occurs infrequently. Experimentally, attempted aerosol transmission from virus-infected horses to in-contact horses or cats was unsuccessful. Nonetheless, the possibility of respiratory transmission cannot be completely ruled out. The frothy nasal discharge commonly observed in naturally affected horses, which represents virus-rich exudate from the lungs, could potentially provide a source of virus for aerosol transmission. Although absent in the nasal cavities, trachea, conjunctival sacs, mouth, and feces, Hendra virus has been found in the urine of experimentally infected horses and cats. This route of infection may have been responsible for transmission of the virus from cat to horse in one experimental study. Based on available field and laboratory data, infection of humans or animals appears to require direct contact with virus-infective secretions (lung exudates), excretions (urine), or tissues.

Available epidemiologic, serologic, and virologic evidence implicates pteropid bats as the natural reservoir of Hendra virus. There is field and experimental proof of vertical transmission, with isolates recovered from the uterine fluid and fetal tissues of a grey-headed flying fox (*Pteropus poliocephalus*) and a black flying fox (*P alecto*). The infrequent occurrence and sporadic nature of outbreaks suggest that exposure of horses to Hendra virus is a chance event. While horses may have been infected through contact with food or water contaminated with material from infected pteropid bats (secretions, excreta, or tissues from mothers or fetuses), the mechanism of spread remains to be determined.

Clinical Findings: Natural or experimental exposure to Hendra virus results in a high rate of clinical infection. The incubation period in field cases of the disease is usually 8-14 days, but ranges from 5-10 days in experimentally infected horses. Clinical signs include fever (up to 106°F [41°C]), anorexia, lethargy, elevation in respiratory and heart rates, respiratory distress, pneumonia, and frothy clear to blood-tinged nasal discharge, which has been observed only in natural cases of the disease. Additional clinical signs seen in some affected horses include cyanotic or jaundiced mucous membranes, dependent edema (intermandibular space, cheeks, infraorbital fossae, limbs, prepuce), and neurologic signs (ataxia, muscle fasciculation, head pressing). Case fatality may be >60-70% in cases of natural or experimentally acquired infection, with terminal cases dying in extremis. The course of the disease is short; death may occur within 1-3 days. Clinical recovery occurs occasionally.

Lesions: The principal gross lesions are severe edema and congestion of the lungs and marked dilatation of the subpleural lymphatics. The airways are filled with thick froth, which is often blood-tinged. Additional lesions seen in some affected horses include increased pleural and pericardial fluids, congestion of lymph nodes, hemorrhages in various organs, and slight jaundice.

Microscopically, the primary lesions are those of an acute interstitial pneumonia. Severe vascular damage, with serofibrinous alveolar edema, hemorrhage, thrombosis of capillaries, necrosis of alveolar walls, and alveolar macrophages are evident in the lungs. Widespread fibrinoid degeneration of small blood vessels is seen in many organs, including the lungs, heart, kidneys, spleen, lymph nodes, meninges, alimentary tract, skeletal muscle, and bladder.

The presence of large endothelial syncytial cells is characteristic of infection. Although most prominent in pulmonary capillaries and arterioles, these cells are also observed in other organs (lymph nodes, spleen, heart, stomach, kidneys, and brain). Antigen specific for Hendra virus can be demonstrated in the vascular lesions and along alveolar walls by immunohistochemical staining. Intracytoplasmic viral inclusion bodies can be seen in infected endothelial cells by electron but not light microscopy. Lesions of nonsuppurative meningitis or meningoencephalitis, including perivascular cuffing, neuronal degeneration, and focal gliosis, have been observed in some infected horses.

Diagnosis: Hendra virus infection should be considered in horses that die after a short febrile illness with prominent necropsy findings of severe interstitial pneumonia with marked distention of the subpleural lymphatics. Confirmation of the diagnosis is based on laboratory examination of appropriate specimens for the detection of Hendra virus, viral antigen, viral nucleic acid, or specific antibodies. Specimens of lung, kidney, spleen, liver, lymph nodes, and brain should be submitted for viral isolation or detection by PCR. The virus can be isolated in a range of cell lines; Vero cells are the cell line of choice. Viral cytopathic effect, which develops after ~3 days, is characterized by syncytia formation in infected cells. Serologic confirmation of infection is based on testing acute and convalescent sera collected 3-4 wk apart, either in a neutralization or a validated ELISA. A comprehensive range of tissues should be collected from suspect fatal cases of the disease for histopathologic examination. Presence of the characteristic vascular lesions is highly suggestive of the infection; specificity of the lesions can be confirmed by immunochemical labeling with Hendra virus reference antiserum.

African horse sickness can clinically mimic Hendra virus infection, and should be considered in the differential diagnosis. Other causes of sudden death that must be ruled out include anthrax, botulism, certain bacterial infections (eg, pasteurellosis, equine influenza, peracute equine herpesvirus 1 infection), and plant or chemical poisoning.

Treatment, Prevention, and Control: There is no specific antiviral treatment and no vaccine for the disease caused by Hendra virus.

In view of the limited transmissibility under conditions of natural exposure to the virus and the sporadic and infrequent nature of outbreaks of the disease, there is little justification for implementation of a specific control program. The few outbreaks that have occurred in Australia have been dealt with by slaughtering all known infected horses and by imposing movement restrictions within a defined area around affected premises. Contact between horses and bat urine or uterine fluids should be avoided, when feasible.

Zoonotic Risk: Hendra virus is transmissible to humans. The infection has been fatal in a high percentage of the cases recorded so far, either from a fulminant interstitial pneumonia or from a nonsuppurative encephalitis. Direct contact with infectious respiratory secretions, urine, or tissues appears to be necessary for viral transmission. Special precautions should be taken when conducting a clinical examination or necropsy on a horse suspected of having the disease.

SEPTICEMIA IN FOALS

Septicemia is a systemic disease involving the presence and persistence of bacteria or their toxins in the blood. The condition implies an extensive, whole body insult from a single or multiple sources of infection.

Etiology and Pathogenesis: The predominant bacteria involved in neonatal foal septicemia are the gram-negative organisms *Escherichia coli, Klebsiella* spp, *Enterobacter* spp, *Actinobacillus* spp, and *Pseudomonas* spp. About 50% of infections also involve gram-positive bacteria, with *Streptococcus* spp being the most common isolates. Anaerobic pathogens are involved in 30% of cases. The routes of entry for these bacteria include the placenta, umbilicus, lungs, and GI tract.

Clinical signs of septicemia and septic shock mainly result from the release of endotoxins related to gram-positive infections. Endotoxins stimulate macrophages to release an array of cytokines (eg, IL-6, IL-1, TNF-α) and activate pro-inflammatory enzymes (eg, phospholipase A_2). Together, these factors lead to signs of inflammation such as fever, vasodilation, hypoglycemia, myocardial depression, procoagulant activity, and eventually disseminated intravascular coagulation (DIC). Bacterial infection accounts for nearly one third of all foal mortality. Septicemia is the second most common problem of equine neonates, second only to failure of passive transfer of maternal antibodies.

Certain immunologic and management factors predispose foals to septicemia. Although foals can respond immunologically in utero to bacterial or viral infections, their ability to do so is less than that of adults. The major risk factor for septicemia in foals is failure to receive an adequate quality and quantity of colostral antibodies. Other factors that influence disease incidence include unsanitary environmental conditions, gestational age of the foal (prematurity), health and condition of the dam, difficulty of parturition, and the presence of new pathogens in the environment against which the mare has no antibodies.

Clinical Findings: Clinical signs largely depend on the stage of the animal's illness and the primary body systems involved. Frequently affected organ systems include the umbilical remnants, CNS, respiratory, cardiovascular, musculoskeletal, renal, ophthalmic, hepatobiliary, and GI organs. Foals in the early stages of sepsis display some degree of depression and lethargy and may lie down more than usual. The mare's udder is often distended with milk, indicating that the foal is not nursing with normal frequency.

In the advanced stage of illness (septic shock), foals are severely depressed, recumbent, dehydrated, and tachycardic. The mucous membranes are muddy, and hypotension, which manifests clinically as cold extremities, thready pulse, and poor capillary refill time, is evident. Foals may be hyper- or hypothermic. In septicemia, bacteria spread hematogenously to various organs, such as the lungs, intestines, eyes, CNS, bones, and joints. The foal may show evidence of single or multiple organ dysfunction. Sepsis can manifest as respiratory distress, pneumonia, diarrhea, uveitis, meningitis, osteomyelitis, or septic arthritis.

Diagnosis: A good perinatal history and physical examination can provide clues in the diagnosis. Depending on the specific organ systems involved, an umbilical, abdominal, and synovial ultrasound examination; arterial blood gas analysis; arthrocentesis; cerebrospinal centesis; and chest, abdominal, and distal limb radiographs may be indicated. Advanced diagnostic imaging techniques (eg, computed tomography of the distal limbs) may further serve as a prognostic aid.

Septic foals are often neutropenic with a high ratio of band to segmented neutrophils. The neutrophils may exhibit toxic changes, which are highly suggestive of sepsis. Foals <24 hr old are often hypoglycemic. Fibrinogen levels >600 mg/dL in a foal <24 hr old is indicative of an in utero infection. Other chemistry abnormalities that may be evident include azotemia due to inadequate renal perfusion and increased bilirubin secondary to endotoxin damage to the liver. A high anion gap (>20 mEq/L), hypoxemia, hypercapnia, and a mixed respiratory and metabolic acidosis may be found on arterial blood gas analysis.

Because of the high correlation between failure of passive transfer of antibodies and septicemia, serum IgG levels should be measured in any questionably sick equine neonate. IgG levels <200 mg/dL indicate complete failure of passive transfer of maternal antibodies. IgG levels >800 mg/dL are optimal.

A definitive diagnosis of neonatal sepsis is based on clinical signs, laboratory data, and evidence of failure of passive antibody transfer. These data can be combined to determine the animal's sepsis score, which helps synthesize laboratory results into a coherent whole. A positive blood culture also correlates to sepsis, but a negative culture does not rule out the possibility of infection. Differential diagnoses include hypoxic ischemic encephalopathy (p 1039), hypoglycemia, hypothermia, neonatal isoerythrolysis (p 12), white muscle disease (p 948), prematurity, neonatal pneumonia, and uroperitoneum (p 1262).

Treatment: Foals suspected of being septic should be placed on broad-spectrum antibiotics active against both gram-positive and gram-negative organisms. Penicillin (22,000 IU/kg, IV, QID) in combination with amikacin sulfate (20-25 mg/kg, IV, SID) provides good initial coverage until culture results are available. Metronidazole (10-15 mg/kg, PO or IV, TID) may be necessary if an anaerobic infection (eg, *Clostridium*) is suspected. A third-generation cephalosporin (eg, ceftiofur, 4.4-6 mg/kg, IV, BID-QID) may be used as a broad-spectrum agent in patients with compromised renal function.

In all cases of neonatal sepsis, immunologic support, in the form of IV plasma transfusions (1-2 L), to raise the IgG levels to >800 mg/dL is important. Effective IV fluid therapy is needed to combat endotoxic shock. Foals may require 100 mL/kg/day of maintenance therapy using polyionic isotonic crystalloid fluids (eg, lactated Ringer's solution) after fluids have been administered for shock. Because many foals are hypoglycemic, dextrose should be added to make a 2.5-5% dextrose solution. Isotonic bicarbonate solution may be given to help correct moderate to severe metabolic acidosis, but can worsen respiratory acidosis. In these cases, mechanical ventilation should be used to decrease $PaCO_2$ before giving bicarbonate.

Treatment with hyperimmune antiendotoxin serum should be considered in patients with endotoxemia. Antiprostaglandin drugs counteract several of the clinical and hemodynamic changes associated with endotoxemia and septic shock. Low doses of flunixin meglumine (0.25 mg/kg, IV, TID) may help reduce signs of endotoxemia. Additionally, administration of low doses of polymyxin B (6,000 IU/kg, diluted in 300-500 mL of saline, slow IV) is an investigational treatment used to neutralize systemic endotoxin.

Because sepsis creates a catabolic state in the foal, nutritional support is important. If the foal is not nursing adequately, it should be fed mare's milk or a milk substitute at 15-25% of its body weight over each 24-hr period. An indwelling nasogastric tube should be placed in foals with a decreased suckle reflex. Parenteral nutrition may also be helpful to provide adequate nutrients. Administration of gastric protectants (eg, ranitidine, cimetidine, omeprazole) has been proposed as an adjunct therapy in sick neonates.

System-specific therapy includes lavaging septic joints with sterile fluids and providing nasal oxygen (2-10 L/min) or ventilation for foals with septic pneumonia. Corneal ulceration may be treated with low doses of topical atropine (although it may cause ileus), NSAID, and broad-spectrum topical antimicrobials. Entropion generally requires mattress sutures of the lower eyelid. Surgical removal of infected umbilical remnants may be indicated.

Recovery from neonatal sepsis depends on the severity and manifestation of the infection. Current survival rates are 50-65% in referral centers. A minimum of 1-4 wk of intensive care should be expected. Early recognition and intensive treatment of neonatal sepsis improves the outcome. If the foal survives the initial problems, it has the potential of becoming a healthy and useful adult.

AFRICAN SWINE FEVER

African swine fever (ASF) is a highly contagious hemorrhagic disease of pigs that produces a wide range of clinical signs and lesions that closely resemble those of classical swine fever (p 570). It is an economically important disease that is enzootic in many African countries and the Mediterranean island, Sardinia.

Etiology and Epidemiology: ASF virus is a large, enveloped DNA virus that replicates primarily in cells of the mononuclear phagocytic system. It is currently classified as the only member of a family called African swine fever-like viruses (Asfarviridae). The prolonged period during which ASF has been an enzootic disease in Africa has led to the selection of viruses of varying virulence. No distinct antigenic types have been identified, but distinct genotypes have been differentiated by restriction enzyme analysis of the genomes of viruses obtained from different geographic areas over a long period of time. The virus is highly resistant to a wide pH range and to a freeze/thaw cycle and can remain infectious for many months at room temperature or when stored at 4°C. Virus in body fluids and serum is inactivated in 30 min at 60°C, but virus in unprocessed pig meat, in which it can remain viable for several weeks, can be inactivated only by heating to 70°C for 30 min. Although ASF virus can be adapted to grow in cells from different species, it does not replicate readily in any species other than swine.

The disease is limited to all breeds and types of domestic pigs and European wild boar. All age groups are equally susceptible. In Africa, the virus produces inapparent infection in 2 species of wild swine—wart hog (*Phacochoerus aethiopicus*) and bush pig (*Potamochoerus porcus*)—and in the soft tick *Ornithodoros moubata*. When the disease was endemic in southern Spain and Portugal, a different species of soft tick, *Ornithodoros erraticus*, became infected with the virus. Several other *Ornithodoros* spp that are not usually associated with pigs or wild swine have been infected experimentally.

ASF has been reported in a large number of countries in Africa, south of the Sahara, either as an enzootic disease or as sporadic epidemics in domestic pigs. The first spread of the disease outside Africa was into Europe in 1957; this was almost certainly successfully eradicated. The second introduction in 1960 resulted in ASF becoming enzootic in Spain and Portugal and, subsequently (1978), in Sardinia. During the 1970s, it spread to the Caribbean and South America and serious, but limited, outbreaks in Europe occurred in Belgium (1985) and the Netherlands (1986). Rigorous eradication programs ended with the successful eradication of the disease from both Portugal (1993) and Spain (1995).

Transmission and Pathogenesis: ASF virus is maintained in Africa by a natural cycle of transmission between wart hogs and the soft tick vector *O moubata*, which inhabits wart hog burrows and from which it is unlikely ever to be eliminated. The spread of virus from the wildlife reservoirs to domestic pigs can be either by the bite of an infected soft tick or by ingestion of wart hog tissues. Virulent viruses produce acute disease, and all body fluids and tissues contain large amounts of infectious virus from the onset of clinical disease until death. Pigs infected with less virulent isolates can transmit virus to susceptible pigs up to 1 mo after infection; blood is infectious up to 6 wk, and transmission can occur if blood is shed. Pigs usually become infected via the oronasal route by direct contact with infected pigs or by ingestion of waste food containing unprocessed pig meat or pig meat products. The primary route of infection is the upper respiratory tract, and virus replicates in the tonsil and lymph nodes draining the head and neck; generalized infection rapidly follows via the bloodstream. High concentrations of virus are then present in all tissues. The factors that produce the hemorrhagic lesions are not defined, but the severe disruptions to the blood clotting mechanism play a major role. Virus is excreted mainly from the upper respiratory tract and is also present in secretions and excretions containing blood.

Pigs that survive infection with the less virulent isolates are probably persistently infected for life and have circulating antibody, although they do not excrete virus or transmit virus to their offspring in utero. Their role in the epidemiology of the disease is not known, but they are resistant to disease when challenged with related virus genotypes. This challenge virus may replicate and be transmitted, either directly or indirectly, to other pigs.

The main factor in the persistence of the disease in domestic pigs in Africa is the presence of large numbers of free-ranging village pigs and, in some areas, soft tick vectors in pig pens.

Clinical Findings and Lesions: Peracute, acute, subacute, and chronic forms occur, and mortality rates vary from 0 to 100%, depending on the virulence of the virus with which pigs are infected. Acute disease is characterized by a short incubation period of

5-7 days, followed by high fever (up to 42°C) and death in 7-10 days. The least variable clinical signs are loss of appetite, depression, and recumbency; other signs include hyperemia of the skin of the ears, abdomen, and legs; respiratory distress; vomiting; bleeding from the nose or rectum; and sometimes diarrhea. Abortion is sometimes the first event seen in an outbreak. The severity and distribution of the lesions also vary according to virulence of the virus. Hemorrhages occur predominantly in lymph nodes, kidneys (almost invariably as petechiae), and heart; hemorrhages in other organs are variable in incidence and distribution. Some isolates produce an enlarged and friable spleen; straw-colored or blood-stained fluid in pleural, pericardial, and peritoneal cavities; or edema and congestion of the lungs. Some viruses of low virulence have been isolated in Europe and produce nonspecific clinical signs and lesions. Chronic disease is characterized by emaciation, swollen joints, and respiratory problems. This form of the disease is rarely seen in outbreaks.

Diagnosis: ASF cannot be differentiated from classical swine fever (hog cholera) by either clinical or postmortem examination. Samples of blood, serum, spleen, tonsil, and gastrohepatic lymph nodes from suspected cases should be submitted to the laboratory for confirmation. Virus can be isolated by inoculation of primary cultures of pig monocytes, in which it produces hemadsorption of pig red cells to the surface of infected cells. Classical swine fever virus does not replicate in these cells. There are nonhemadsorbing viral isolates, some of which produce virulent disease. These isolates produce only a cytopathic effect in pig leukocytes. Confirmation of ASF in these cases has to be performed by either PCR or an antigen-detection ELISA. Viral antigen can be detected in infected tissue smears or sections by staining with labelled antibodies (several enzyme-labelled tests are available, eg, immunofluorescence), and viral DNA by PCR or hybridization of nucleic acid probes to tissue sections. The most appropriate tests for detecting antibody in serum or tissue fluids are the ELISA, indirect immunofluorescence, and counterimmunoelectrophoresis; a number of other useful tests are available.

Other differential diagnoses include hemorrhagic bacterial infections and certain types of poisons.

Control: There is no treatment, and all attempts to develop a vaccine have been unsuccessful. Pigs that recover from infection with less virulent viral isolates are resistant to challenge with viruses of a different genotype in the absence of neutralizing antibody. Prevention therefore depends on ensuring that neither infected live pigs nor pig meat products are introduced into areas free of ASF. All successful eradication programs have involved the rapid diagnosis, slaughter, and disposal of all animals on infected premises. Sanitary measures must also be applied and include control of movement and treatment of waste food. Subsequently, a serologic survey of all pig farms within a specific control zone must be done to ensure that all infected pigs have been identified.

CLASSICAL SWINE FEVER

(Hog cholera, Swine fever)

Classical swine fever is a contagious febrile disease of pigs. It was first described in the early 19th century in the USA. Later, a condition in Europe termed swine fever was recognized to be the same disease. Both names continue in use, although in Europe it is now called classical swine fever to distinguish it from African swine fever (p 568), which is clinically indistinguishable but caused by an unrelated virus.

Classical swine fever has the potential to cause devastating epidemics, particularly in countries that are free of the disease and do not practice vaccination, so that their total pig population is susceptible. For example, an outbreak in the Netherlands in 1997-98 involved 429 herds; >12 million pigs were killed either to control the spread of disease or for associated welfare reasons. Awareness and vigilance are essential so that outbreaks are detected early and control measures are instituted rapidly to prevent further spread.

Etiology and Epidemiology: Classical swine fever is caused by a small, enveloped RNA virus in the pestivirus group of the family Flaviviridae. Classical swine fever virus is antigenically related to the other pestiviruses, namely bovine viral diarrhea (BVD) virus of cattle (p 220) and border disease virus of sheep (p 503). The latter 2 are widespread in ruminant populations and can occasionally infect pigs; therefore, laboratory tests using monoclonal antibody reagents or genetic sequence recognition methods must be done to differentiate classical swine fever from ruminant pestiviruses.

Classical swine fever virus infects only pigs and wild boar, although experimental infections can be induced in other species. It will grow in porcine cell cultures, notably the PK15 cell line, but does not generally cause a visible cytopathic effect in culture so that immunolabeling methods are essential to detect viral growth. The virus has only one serotype, although some minor antigenic variability between strains can be shown. Strain typing for epidemiologic mapping purposes can be done by genetic sequencing of the virus combined with phylogenetic analysis.

The virus is moderately fragile and does not persist in the environment or spread long distances by the airborne route. It can survive for prolonged periods in a moist, protein-rich medium such as meat, other tissues, and body fluids, particularly if kept cold or frozen. Virus survival times of several years in frozen pig meat, or months in chilled or cured meat, have been reported.

Classical swine fever is distributed worldwide. It is endemic in much of Latin America, some Caribbean islands, and pig-producing countries of Asia. It has not been reported in mainland Africa. Australia, New Zealand, Canada, and the USA are free of classical swine fever, as is most of western and central Europe, although sporadic outbreaks have occurred in a number of European countries during the past decade.

The main source of infection is the pig—either live animals or uncooked pig products. In endemic areas, the major concern is spread of disease by movement of infected pigs, which can be a cause of remote outbreaks where there is large-scale transport of pigs for finishing. In parts of Europe, the wild boar population may harbor the virus, although the significance of wild boar as a reservoir for domestic pigs remains controversial.

Another major risk is accidental introduction of the virus through imported pig meat and meat products that readily find their way into the porcine food chain through the feeding of waste food. The virus is readily inactivated by cooking, which emphasizes the importance of enforcing regulations on heat treatment of swill. Many countries have completely banned swill feeding.

Mechanical transmission on vehicles and equipment, as well as by personnel (notably veterinarians) travelling between pig farms, are also significant means of spread within an infected area.

If sows are infected with low to moderately virulent strains of virus during pregnancy and then recover, there is a high risk that their offspring may be carriers. Not all such carriers will show clinical signs of disease. Therefore, it is particularly important to investigate herds that have a high level of unexplained reproductive failure, congenital tremor, or other congenital abnormalities.

Clinical Findings and Lesions: The disease has acute and chronic forms, and virulence varies from severe, with high mortality, to mild or even subclinical. Low virulence strains are a special diagnostic problem; the only expression may be poor reproductive performance and the birth of piglets with neurologic defects (eg, congenital tremor, p 996).

The severe acute form is characterized by fever, inappetence, and depression. The incubation period is typically 2-6 days, with death at 10-20 days after infection. Fever (>41°C) persists until the terminal stage of disease, when body temperature may become subnormal. Constipation is common, followed by diarrhea. The principal lesion is a generalized vasculitis, seen in live pigs as hemorrhages and cyanosis in the skin, notably of the extremities. There may also be a generalized erythema. Vasculitis in the CNS may produce incoordination or even convulsions. At necropsy, the principal findings are widespread petechial and ecchymotic hemorrhages, especially in lymph nodes, kidneys, spleen, bladder, and larynx. Infarction may be seen, notably in the spleen. Most pigs show a nonsuppurative encephalitis with vascular cuffing.

In chronic disease, pigs often survive >30 days. After an initial acute febrile phase, pigs may show apparent recovery but then relapse, with anorexia, depression, fever, and progressive loss of condition. Histologically, there is atrophy of the thymus and lymphoid depletion. Button ulcers may develop in the intestine, particularly near the ileocecal junction.

Diagnosis: Differential diagnoses include other febrile hemorrhagic diseases of pigs such as African swine fever, bacterial septicemias (eg, salmonellosis, erysipelas, etc), anticoagulant poisoning (coumarin derivatives), and hemolytic disease of the newborn. Hemorrhagic lesions must be distinguished from those that are seen in porcine dermatitis and nephropathy syndrome (p 579) and postweaning multisystemic wasting syndrome (p 583), which have become widespread in many pig-producing countries. With low virulence strains of classical swine fever virus, a variety of other cases of low reproductive performance and congenital tremors should be considered, including pseudorabies, parvovirus, BVD, border disease, and noninfectious causes.

Virologic tests are essential to confirm a diagnosis. Advice on sample submission should be sought from the laboratory. Suitable tissues are tonsil, maxillary or submandibular lymph nodes, mesenteric lymph nodes, spleen, ileum, and kidney. Whole blood with EDTA as anticoagulant can be used for virus isolation from a live acute case, or for antigen or nucleic acid detection. Clotted blood samples are taken when serologic tests for antibody are required. Serology is unlikely to be of use for acute disease but may be the method of choice for testing sows that have given birth to congenitally affected litters.

Antigen detection can be performed using direct immunofluorescence on frozen tissue sections, particularly of tonsil. Reading the sections requires highly skilled and experienced personnel. Its main advantage is a rapid result. Antigen detection can also be done using ELISA, which can be useful for large-scale screening of pigs for viremia in infected areas, eg, as a premovement check.

For virus isolation, cell cultures are inoculated with tissue suspensions and tested daily by immunofluorescence for the presence of virus. Final results may not be available for 4-7 days.

Virus characterization using virus-specific monoclonal antibodies is performed as a differential diagnostic test for BVD and border disease. Positive results of antigen detection or virus isolation tests should not be confirmed until virus characterization is done.

Nucleic acid detection is performed via reverse transcriptase-PCR to detect classical swine fever virus in clinical samples. With the use of suitable primers, it can differentiate the virus from BVD and border disease. Standardized methods have been described that permit scale-up to screen large numbers of blood samples, giving rapid results while retaining high sensitivity. This is particularly useful for screening herds during an outbreak.

The most widely used serologic tests are virus neutralization and ELISA. Because the virus is noncytopathogenic in culture, the neutralization test requires an additional immunolabeling stage (using fluorescent or enzyme labels). The ELISA is more suited to large-scale serology, ie, for surveillance. Blocking ELISA can distinguish classical swine fever from BVD antibodies by use of appropriate monoclonal antibody reagents, although confirmatory testing is advised in cases of doubt. ELISA methods have been developed that can detect antibodies to a specific viral protein that is absent from so-called "marker vaccines." Although potentially useful for identifying pigs infected with wild-type virus among a population vaccinated with the gene-deleted vaccine, the technique has not as yet found much acceptance for field use, and the ELISA for the deleted protein has rather low sensitivity.

Control: No treatment should be attempted. Classical swine fever is on the OIE List A. Reporting the disease to authorities is compulsory in many countries. Confirmed cases and in-contact animals should be slaughtered, and measures taken to protect other pigs. This may involve herd slaughter combined with area restrictions on pig movements, or vaccination, depending on local disease control regulations.

Live attenuated vaccines are widely used in endemically infected areas; these are either derivatives of the lapinized "C" strain or strains adapted from cell cultures. They are effective at controlling clinical disease but allow the virus to continue circulating subclinically; therefore, vaccination is inappropriate in countries or regions with an eradication policy. Recently, genetic manipulation has resulted in the production of marker vaccines that do not express one of the viral glycoproteins. Because naturally infected pigs develop antibodies to this protein, the combination of marker vaccine and specific diagnostic test (*see* above) enables the theoretical differentiation of vaccinated from infected pigs. Although the vaccines have been granted marketing authorizations in Europe, their use in the field has not yet been permitted by disease control authorities. Such an approach may be adopted in the event of a major outbreak.

EDEMA DISEASE

(*Escherichia coli* enterotoxemia)

Edema disease is a peracute toxemia caused by specific pathotypes of *Escherichia coli* that affects primarily healthy, rapidly growing nursery pigs. Other names for edema disease include "gut edema" or "bowel edema," due to the prominent edema of the submucosa of the stomach and mesocolon.

Etiology and Pathogenesis: Edema disease is caused by hemolytic *E coli* that produce F18 pili and Shiga toxin 2e (also known as verotoxin 2e). The F18 pili have 2 antigenic variants, F18ab and F18ac, with F18ab being characteristic of edema disease strains and F18ac being associated primarily with enterotoxigenic *E coli*. The Shiga toxin-producing *E coli* implicated in edema disease most commonly belong to 4 specific serotypes: O138:K81:NM, O139:K12:H1, O141:K85a,b:H4, and O141:K85ac:H4.

Pigs become infected initially by contaminated environment or the sow. Spread of infection among penmates is facilitated by the large numbers of pathogenic *E coli* that are shed by colonized pigs. Some strains of *E coli* that cause edema disease also carry genes for enterotoxins and can cause diarrhea as well as edema disease. Ingestion of edema disease strains of *E coli* is followed by colonization of the intestine in pigs in which intestinal epithelial cells carry receptors for the F18 pili. Expression of the receptors is age-related, so younger pigs are less susceptible to colonization than older pigs. Furthermore, some pigs carry a specific mutation in a gene required for expression of the receptors and are thereby resistant to infection. Resistance/susceptibility is determined by a single locus with a dominant susceptibility allele and a recessive resistant allele; it is possible to select resistant pigs, which can be identified by a simple PCR test that identifies presence or absence of the specific mutation.

High-protein diets have increased the susceptibility of pigs to the disease. Factors associated with weaning, including the stresses of mixing pigs, changes in diet, and the loss of milk antibodies from the intestine, appear to be important elements in enhancing the susceptibility of weaned pigs to the disease.

Shiga toxin 2e produced in the intestine of colonized pigs is responsible for the major clinical signs and pathology that are observed. This cytotoxin inhibits protein synthesis, leading to cell death. The toxin is absorbed from the intestine and targets vascular endothelium in specific sites believed to have high concentrations of the toxin receptor globotetraosyl ceramide. These sites include the submucosa of the stomach, the colonic mesentery, the subcutaneous tissues of the forehead and eyelids, the larynx, and the brain. Damage to vascular endothelium results in edema, hemorrhage, intravascular coagulation, and microthrombosis.

Clinical Findings and Lesions: Clinical signs range from peracute death with no signs of illness to CNS involvement with ataxia, paralysis, and recumbency. Edema disease usually occurs 1-2 wk after weaning and typically involves the healthiest animals in a group. The disease is seen occasionally in nursing pigs or in adult pigs. The average morbidity is 30-40%, and the mortality among affected pigs is often as high as 90%. Periocular edema, swelling of the forehead and submandibular regions, dyspnea, and anorexia are common. Edema disease is primarily a disease of the vasculature, and gross lesions consist of subcutaneous edema and edema in the submucosa of the stomach, particularly in the glandular cardiac region. The edema fluid is usually gelatinous and may extend into the mesocolon. The edema may be accompanied by hemorrhage. Fibrin strands may be found in the peritoneal cavity, and serous fluid may be found in both the pleural and peritoneal cavities. Microscopically, a degenerative angiopathy affecting arteries and arterioles and necrosis of the smooth muscle cells in the tunica media are present. Lesions of focal encephalomalacia in the brain stem are characteristic and thought to result from vascular damage, leading to edema and ischemia.

Diagnosis: The clinical history of peracute death in healthy, well-conditioned, recently weaned pigs, along with visual observation of periocular edema and extensive edema of the stomach and mesocolon, are helpful in diagnosis. There may be a characteristic squeal due to edema of the larynx. Diarrhea may precede the signs of edema disease if the *E coli* responsible also possesses genes for enterotoxins. Characteristically, the stomach is full of dry feed. Diagnosis is easily made in an outbreak in which the full range of clinical signs and pathologic features are likely to occur. It is more difficult when only a few animals are affected or when the disease occurs in an atypical age group. Isolation and characterization of the *E coli* are needed for a definitive diagnosis. Culture of the small intestine and colon typically yields a heavy growth of hemolytic *E coli*, but in some cases the organism may no longer be present in the intestine at the time of death. Demonstration that the hemolytic *E coli* isolated is an edema disease strain may be done by PCR amplification of the genes for the F18 pili and Shiga toxin 2e. Serotyping of the isolate is useful for tracking the persistence of a particular type of the organism on a farm. However, the F18 pili are not readily expressed in vitro and they may not be detected on organisms that are cultured routinely.

Treatment and Control: Because the onset of disease is often sudden and the course rapid, treatment is often ineffective. Oral medication via the drinking water may be used to protect clinically unaffected pigs in a herd in which cases of the disease have been detected. Antibiotic sensitivity should be determined on the isolate from an affected pig; medication should be changed if the initial choice was ineffective. Control is also difficult. Several experimental approaches have been shown to be effective, but none are economical to date. These methods include feeding a high fiber and low protein diet, reducing the amount of feed given to weaned pigs, vaccination by a systemic route with a Shiga toxin 2e toxoid, oral vaccination with an F18+ nontoxigenic *E coli*, passive systemic immunization with antitoxin, and passive oral immunization with anti-F18 antibodies.

ENCEPHALOMYOCARDITIS VIRUS INFECTION

Encephalomyocarditis (EMC) is a specific viral infection of swine and exotic mammals that is caused by members of the genus Cardiovirus in the family Picornaviridae. It has been recognized in many parts of the world, and molecular studies have revealed a genetic homogeneity of viral isolates from some geographic areas but not others.

Swine may die acutely at any age due to associated myocardial failure or may be affected with near-term abortions, fetal mummification, and apparent reproductive failure. A variety of exotic mammals have been fatally afflicted with EMC in zoologic parks in the USA, Australia, and other parts of the world, and have included African elephants, rhinoceroses, hippopotamuses, sloths, llamas, various antelope species, and many types of nonhuman primates (chimpanzees, orangutans, baboons, cynomologous monkeys, lemurs, etc). An episode of lion deaths at a zoo in the USA was associated with the feeding of the carcass of an African elephant that had died of EMC, and a spontaneous outbreak of fatal EMC was reported in free-ranging African elephants at Kruger National Park in South Africa in 1995.

Serologic studies have revealed that subclinical infections are common in EMC outbreaks. Humans appear to be resistant to fatal infections with EMC viruses; although EMC antibodies are frequently detected, no deaths have been confirmed.

Epidemiology: Cardioviruses are small, nonenveloped viruses that are almost always associated with rodents, and disease in other mammalian species has often been attributed to spillover from populations of mice and rats. These, and presumably other rodent species, shed the viruses in feces and urine, which may contaminate food and water supplies of large mammals. Ingestion of rodents dead or dying of EMC may be another means of infection. Pigs shed virus in nasal secretions and feces during the first 3 days of experimental infection. During this short period, the virus may be transmitted to other pigs by contact. Cardioviruses are resistant to adverse environmental influences and may remain infective for weeks to months under favorable conditions.

Clinical Findings and Lesions: The disease is named for its predilection for the CNS and cardiovascular systems of experimental mice, and both encephalotropic and cardiotropic strains have been defined. In swine and zoologic species, however, acute and subacute deaths are almost always attributed to the destructive effects of the virus on the myocardium, with resultant cardiac insufficiency, pulmonary edema, and frothy transudation in the respiratory tract. Affected animals often appear to have asphyxiated in their own respiratory fluids. Other clinical signs may include fever, anorexia, listlessness, trembling, staggering, dyspnea, and paralysis. Mortality approaching 100% has been described in suckling swine but becomes successively lower in older age groups. Strains of EMC viruses that target the pancreas and are diabetogenic in experimental mice have been recovered, but the significance of this finding for other mammals has not been established.

EMC viruses are known to cross the placenta in swine and have been recovered from conceptuses in cases of reproductive failure due to near-term abortions (107-111 days of gestation), stillbirths, and mummifications. Reproductive problems often persist in affected herds for 2-3 mo and may affect sows of all parities.

Diagnosis: Because the pale necrotic heart muscle lesions that may be observed in fatal EMC infections also are seen in septic infarction or vitamin E/selenium deficiency, a definitive diagnosis requires virus recovery and identification. Myocardial tissue and spleen collected from acutely dead animals or abortuses are the specimens of choice for virus isolation. Because EMC viruses are very stable, they may be recovered from frozen tissues.

Serologic diagnosis via virus neutralization, hemagglutination-inhibition, or ELISA is possible if acute and convalescent sera are collected, but the frequency of subclinical EMC infections makes single serum determinations of little value in aborting sows. Detection of antibody against EMC viruses in stillborn or large mummified fetuses is significant for fetal infection, however, because maternal immunoglobulins are not transferred across the placenta in swine.

Treatment and Control: There is no specific treatment for EMC, but mortality may be minimized by avoiding stress or excitement in animals at risk. EMC viruses appear to cycle in rodents and are most likely to affect swine and zoo animals when rodent populations are high. Rodent control is thus important for minimizing exposure of susceptible species. Prompt and proper disposal of animals that have died of the disease is also recommended. EMC viruses are inactivated by the judicious use of many disinfectants labeled for livestock use.

Killed vaccines for the prevention of myocarditis in weaned swine are available. Pigs are inoculated IM at ≥4 wk of age, revaccinated 2-3 wk later, and semiannually thereafter. These vaccines have been used extra-label in susceptible exotic animal species in zoos and amusement parks where EMC has been problematic.

GLÄSSER'S DISEASE

(Porcine polyserositis, Infectious polyarthritis)

Haemophilus parasuis is a commensal organism of the upper respiratory tract of swine that cause severe systemic disease characterized by fibrinous polyserositis, arthritis, and meningitis. Disease caused by *H parasuis* has a sudden onset, short course, and high morbidity and mortality. Young animals (6-8 wk) are primarily affected, although sporadic disease can be observed in adults (eg, introduction of a naive adult to a normal herd). Survivors can develop severe fibrosis in the abdominal and thoracic cavities, which can result in reduced growth rate and carcass condemnation at slaughter. Glässer's disease is seen worldwide, and its incidence appears to have increased since the introduction of porcine reproductive and respiratory syndrome (p 581).

Etiology: The causal agent, *H parasuis*, is a gram-negative coccobacillus that requires V factor (NAD) supplementation for growth. Fifteen serovars of *H parasuis* have been reported, but a high percentage of the evaluated isolates are nontypable. The factors involved in systemic invasion by *H parasuis* are still unknown.

Clinical Findings: Clinical signs are observed mainly in pigs 6-8 wk old, although the age of affected animals may vary, depending on the level of acquired maternal immunity. Acute disease has a short course and may result in sudden death without the presence of characteristic gross lesions. Clinical signs include high fever (41.5°C), severe coughing, abdominal breathing, swollen joints, and CNS signs such as lateral decubitus, paddling, and trembling. These signs may be seen jointly or independently. Chronically affected animals may have a reduced growth rate as a result of severe fibrosis in the thoracic and peritoneal cavities.

Lesions: Systemic infection is characterized by the development of fibrinous polyserositis, arthritis, and meningitis. The fibrinous exudate can be observed on the pleura, pericardium, peritoneum, synovia, and meninges and is usually accompanied by an increased amount of fluid. Fibrinous pleuritis may be accompanied by anteroventral pneumonia, which is characterized by consolidation of the lung as a result of infiltration of inflammatory cells and severe congestion. Hyperacute cases have increased fluid in the thoracic and abdominal cavities, without the presence of fibrin. Lack of characteristic gross lesions is also common in swine showing CNS signs. Chronically affected animals usually have severe fibrosis of the pericardium and pleura, which may or may not extend to the peritoneal cavity.

Diagnosis: Diagnosis is based on the observation of characteristic clinical signs and lesions, in association with isolation of *H parasuis* from affected swine. Only samples from systemic sites such as pleura, pericardium, peritoneum, joints, and brain should be submitted for bacterial isolation. Isolation of *H parasuis* from the upper respiratory tract has no relevance in the diagnosis of systemic infection. *H parasuis* is a fastidious organism that can disappear quickly following death of affected animals. Samples collected from clinically affected animals that were euthanized increase the chances of isolation. *H parasuis* is initially isolated using sheep blood agar with V factor supplementation, which can be provided by a nurse streak of *Staphylococcus aureus*. Growth is characterized by the presence of translucent small colonies near the *Staphylococcus* streak (satellitism). Differential diagnoses include *Actinobacillus pleuropneumonia* and Vitamin E deficiency.

Treatment and Control: *H parasuis* is one of the few gram-negative organisms that can be successfully treated with synthetic penicillin. Other antimicrobials that have been used include ceftiofur and sulfonamides. Individual treatments are given parenterally. Preventive treatments can be given via water or feed medication. Either commercial or autogenous vaccines can be used to control *H parasuis* infection. The broad range of potentially pathogenic serovars has impaired the development of a universal vaccine for *H parasuis*. Homologous protection between isolates from the same serovar group is satisfactory, while heterologous protection is restricted to a few serovars.

HEMAGGLUTINATING ENCEPHALOMYELITIS

(Vomiting and wasting disease, Coronaviral encephalomyelitis)

This viral disease of young pigs characterized by vomiting, constipation, and anorexia results either in rapid death or chronic emaciation. Motor disorders due to acute encephalomyelitis (hemagglutinating encephalomyelitis) also may be seen during some outbreaks.

Etiology, Epidemiology, and Pathogenesis: The causal coronavirus, hemagglutinating encephalomyelitis virus, is of a single antigenic type, and it grows in several types of porcine cell cultures, in which it causes syncytia. It agglutinates RBC of several animal species. Pigs are the only natural host. The virus is spread via aerosol.

Infection appears to be widespread in North America, western Europe, and Australia. It usually remains subclinical. The virus is endemic in most breeding herds, and a herd immunity exists. Immune sows transfer maternal antibodies to their piglets, which are protected until they have developed an age resistance; thus, clinical outbreaks are rare. However, if the virus enters a susceptible herd with neonatal piglets, morbidity and mortality may be high.

The virus first replicates in the nasal mucosa, tonsils, lungs, and to a very limited extent, in the small intestine. From these sites of entry, the virus invades defined nuclei of the medulla oblongata via the peripheral nervous system and subsequently spreads to the entire brain stem, and possibly to the cerebrum and cerebellum. Vomiting is thought to be caused by viral replication in the vagal sensory ganglion. Wasting is due to vomiting and delayed emptying of the stomach, which is the result of virus-induced lesions in the intramural plexus. Infection of cerebral and cerebellar neurons may rarely cause motor disorders.

Clinical Findings: Both clinical syndromes, the vomiting and wasting disease (VWD) and the encephalitic forms, are confined almost exclusively to pigs <4 wk old. The VWD form has an incubation period of 4-7 days. Repeated retching and vomiting are seen. Pigs start suckling but soon stop, withdraw from the sow, and vomit the milk they have ingested. They dip their mouths into water bowls but drink little, possibly indicative of pharyngeal paralysis. The persistent vomiting results in a rapid decline of condition. Neonatal pigs become dehydrated, cyanotic, and comatose, and die. Older pigs continue to vomit, although less frequently than in the early stage of the disease. They lose appetite and become emaciated. A large distention of the cranial abdomen can develop. This "wasting" state may persist for 1-6 wk until the pigs die of starvation. Mortality approaches 100% within the litter, and survivors remain permanently stunted.

The encephalomyelitic form also starts with vomiting, usually 4-7 days after birth. Vomiting continues intermittently for 1-2 days, but it is rarely severe and does not result in dehydration. After 1-3 days, generalized muscle tremors and hyperesthesia are seen. The pigs tend to walk backward, often ending in a dog-sitting position. They soon become weak, are unable to rise, and paddle their limbs. Blindness, opisthotonos, and nystagmus also occur. After a few days, they become dyspneic, comatose, and die.

From onset to disappearance, an outbreak on a farm lasts 2-3 wk. Disappearance of disease coincides with the development of immunity in sows in late pregnancy, which subsequently protects piglets via maternal antibodies.

Lesions: Cachexia and abdominal distention are seen in chronically affected pigs. Their stomachs are dilated and filled with gas. Microscopically, perivascular cuffing, gliosis, and neuronal degeneration are found in the medulla in 70-100% of pigs with nervous signs, and in 20-60% of pigs with VWD. Neuritis of peripheral sensory ganglia, particularly the trigeminal ganglia, is seen regularly. Degeneration of the ganglia of the stomach wall and perivascular cuffing are found in 15-85% of pigs with VWD. The lesions are most pronounced in the pyloric gland area.

Diagnosis: A laboratory diagnosis can be made routinely by virus isolation from the brain stem if the pigs are euthanized within 2 days after clinical signs appear. It is difficult to isolate the virus from pigs that have been affected for >2 days.

A significant rise in antibody titer can be demonstrated in paired serum samples. The acute serum sample must be collected immediately after the start of disease, because pigs may already have built up a low antibody titer when the first signs appear.

Differential diagnoses include pseudorabies (p 1065) and porcine enteroviral encephalomyelitis (p 1064). Respiratory signs in older pigs and abortions in sows are part of a pseudorabies outbreak. In porcine enteroviral encephalomyelitis, older pigs are usually involved.

Control: There is no treatment. Once signs are evident, the disease runs its course. Spontaneous recoveries are rare. Piglets born from nonimmune sows during an outbreak can be protected by injecting, at birth, either hyperimmune serum or serum from sows randomly selected at slaughter. However, the time lapse between diagnosis and cessation of the disease is usually too short for this procedure to be effective. Maintaining the virus on the farm (thus retaining naturally induced immunity in the sows) avoids outbreaks in piglets.

NIPAH VIRUS INFECTION

(Porcine respiratory and neurologic syndrome, Barking pig syndrome)

Nipah virus disease is a newly discovered disease of swine and humans associated with infection with a new paramyxovirus given the name Nipah virus. This disease emerged in Malaysia in 1998 and 1999. It was linked to severe encephalitis among humans occupationally exposed to infected pigs in Malaysia and Singapore. The disease was eradicated from the national commercial swine population by control efforts. Fruit bats of the genus *Pteropus* appear to be reservoirs of the virus.

Etiology and Epidemiology: The etiologic agent, Nipah virus (genus Henipavirus, family Paramyxoviridae), is an enveloped negative-sense, single-stranded RNA virus. The virus is closely related to Hendra virus (p 564), the only other member of the genus. The human outbreak in Malaysia and Singapore followed contact with infected swine and resulted in encephalitis and ~40% case mortality. The virus is assumed to have been introduced into the swine population from 1 of the 2 species of *Pteropus* found with Nipah virus antibodies during investigation of the outbreak. The geographic range of *Pteropus* includes all of southeast and south Asia, and several species have been found with antibodies, suggesting that the virus or closely related viruses occur in other areas within the range of this genus of bats. In Malaysia, genetic analysis of virus from human and swine clinical materials strongly supported a single introduction of the virus with spread through the commercial swine population. There was evidence of infection among several other species of domestic animals including dogs, cats, and horses.

Transmission and Pathogenesis: Infection in pigs is assumed to have been a transfer from the reservoir bat species to pigs. Once the virus was introduced into an intensive swine husbandry setting, infection of animals within premises was rapid, and serologic tests suggested that nearly all pigs on an infected premise were infected. Transmission between premises was thought to be by poor biosecurity procedures and movement of infected animals. Experimental infection of swine with Nipah virus in a high biosecurity facility in Geelong supported that transmission between swine in close contact occurred readily.

Clinical Findings: Because of the danger of human infection and the emergency setting, clinical observations were not detailed in the field during the epidemic. Most pigs developed a febrile respiratory disease with a severe cough that led to the local names for the disease, "barking pig syndrome" and "one-mile cough." Encephalitis was also noted, particularly in the sows and boars in affected facilities. The proportion of animals with each form of the disease is uncertain, although the respiratory form predominated. Overall mortality within affected facilities was also not well documented but it probably was not >5% among all age groups.

Diagnosis: Laboratory diagnosis can be made by isolation of the virus, identification of the RNA by use of reverse transcriptase-PCR, detection of antigens in tissues by immunohistochemical staining with specific antibodies, or serologic tests such as indirect ELISA and virus neutralization tests. The virus is considered biosafety level 4 in the USA and Australia, and stringent laboratory containment at limited laboratories is a special consideration.

Treatment: Treatment of affected swine was not attempted during the Malaysian emergency. Humans required intensive care with ventilation support to manage the encephalitis; no specific treatment is available. Ribavirin was administered to some patients and results of one study suggested that it may reduce mortality, but subsequent studies in laboratory animals suggest that it is ineffective.

Control and Prevention: Control of the epidemic/epizootic in Malaysia was dependent on the initiation of strict quarantine procedures and the slaughter of all swine from affected facilities. Adherence to appropriate biosecurity and quarantine procedures within facilities, as with other contagious diseases, is of paramount importance in preventing spread of the infection. An active surveillance and slaughter program successfully eliminated the virus from the national commercial swine population and it has remained free of infection. Presence of the virus in reservoir species of bats in a wide geographic range emphasizes the importance of good disease surveillance and biosecurity practices to promote early detection and confine the disease to initial premises should reintroduction occur.

Zoonotic Risk: Transmission of the virus from infected pigs to humans was largely in an occupational setting, and a study of risk factors associated with human infection suggests that close contact with live infected swine is the means of infection of nearly all human Nipah virus infections.

PORCINE DERMATITIS AND NEPHROPATHY SYNDROME

Porcine dermatitis and nephropathy syndrome (PDNS) was first described in Chile in 1976 under the name proliferative glomerulonephritis in young pigs. Since then the sporadic form of this disease has been widely reported from all pig-producing areas around the world. It has become prevalent since the occurrence of postweaning multisystemic wasting syndrome (PMWS, p 583), although its link with porcine circovirus type 2 (PCV2), considered the causal agent of PMWS, has not been definitively proved. PDNS is characterized by vasculitis in many organs, particularly the skin and kidneys, with resulting clinical signs. The pathologic changes of PDNS suggest an immune complex disorder, with severe renal lesions causing azotemia that results in the death of affected pigs, usually in the growing and finishing areas. The incidence of PDNS is generally low (<1%), but during the late 1990s, an epizootic version of PDNS, which was clinically and macroscopically very similar to classical swine fever (p 574) or African swine fever (p 568), was reported in the UK.

Epidemiology and Pathogenesis: PDNS occurs in all types of swine production systems with different health status and management procedures. Disease presentation tends to be sporadic with incidence <1%; however, incidence of up to 10-20% or even higher (epizootic presentation) has been described. Most reports suggest that PDNS appears without any changed management, husbandry, or dietary practices. Many other diseases, clinical signs, and gross lesions appear to coincide with occurrence of PDNS, including PMWS, porcine reproductive and respiratory syndrome (PRRS), conjunctivitis, gastric ulcers, and a variety of respiratory, digestive, and systemic bacterial infections.

Microscopic lesions of PDNS strongly suggest an immune complex-mediated disease. Immunoreactants such as IgM, IgA, and occasionally IgG, and complement factors C3 and C1q, have been detected within renal glomeruli and affected vessel walls. However, the responsible antigen(s) involved in the immune complex-mediated disorder is currently unknown, and several etiologic possibilities have been postulated. PCV2, PRRS virus, and *Pasteurella multocida* are the most studied, but the definitive role of any of these antigens in the disease pathogenesis has not been determined. More recently, PCV2 has been further indirectly linked to PDNS because the affected pigs have extremely high levels of PCV2 antibodies.

Clinical Findings: The disease usually has an acute onset in a single pig or in a group of pigs. Multiple or coalescing skin lesions occur in ~90% of cases. Cutaneous manifestations, however, may vary and may be confused with classical and African swine fever, swine erysipelas, septicemic salmonellosis, infection with *Actinobacillus suis*, porcine stress syndrome, transit erythema (urine-soaked floors, chemical burns, etc), and other bacterial septicemias.

Affected pigs typically weigh 25-70 kg. Morbidity is usually <1% but may be 0.05-30%; case mortality is usually 80-90%. Often there is a short clinical illness (a few hours to 3 days), with some sudden deaths. Pigs with skin conditions usually die despite treatment. Many pigs are pyrexic (up to 41.5°C) with anorexia and listlessness; some are depressed, prostrate, or unwilling to stand or move. Many pigs have edema of the lower limbs and ventral body surfaces. A few pigs with skin lesions survive, with resolution of the lesions (as scars) over 2-3 wk. Some pigs show very mild effects, which may range from a vague malaise to more obvious illness with reduced feed intake and weight loss; those pigs with milder clinical signs usually have no or only slight kidney lesions.

   Lesions: The skin lesions are the most striking feature but are not always present. They may be multifocal, flat, discrete lesions (1 cm or less) with an irregular margin, but are more commonly seen as larger, coalescing lesions on any part of the body. Lesions are usually worse on the hindlimbs, perineum, ventral abdomen, and flanks. Erythema may be intense, giving a rosette appearance on close inspection. Occasionally the skin lesions turn purple or black, signalling the onset of dermal necrosis. In some animals, blackened skin across the rear and perineum develops and may even ulcerate; these pigs always die.

In addition to skin lesions, gross necropsy findings include enlarged kidneys with petechial hemorrhages in the cortices, enlarged and congested lymph nodes, excess fluid in body cavities, serosal surface and subcutaneous hemorrhages, and serosanguineous fluid in joint cavities. Other lesions, such as cranial lung lobe pneumonia, hyperkeratosis and ulceration of the stomach, and pericarditis, are considered features of concurrent diseases or conditions.

Histopathologic findings are essentially those of a systemic necrotizing vasculitis with hemorrhage, edema, and fibrinoid necrosis, affecting medium- and small-sized arteries of many tissues (virtually all vascularized tissues may be affected). Kidney lesions vary from a marked, acute, fibrinous glomerulitis with hyaline casts in the tubules and some degree of interstitial nephritis (acute cases) to glomerular sclerosis, nonsuppurative interstitial inflammation, and fibrosis in pigs that survive the acute phase and develop chronic lesions.

Diagnosis: Definitive diagnosis is based on histopathologic findings. There are 2 major criteria for diagnosis: the presence of compatible gross lesions in skin and kidney, and the presence of systemic necrotizing vasculitis and fibrinous glomerulitis. Serum analyses may help differentiate PDNS from other diseases such as classical and African swine fever; in PDNS, urea (normal 8.2-24.6 mg/dL) and creatinine (normal 69.6-207.7 mmol/dL) are markedly increased. Serum globulins (mainly γ-globulins) also increase, and proteinuria is pronounced in all cases. There are no etiologic diagnostic laboratory tests, as no definitive agent has yet been determined.

Treatment and Prevention: No treatment has proved successful. Rapid hospitalization and supportive care may enable a few affected pigs to survive. Only those epizootic

PDNS cases with moderate to high morbidity and mortality rates may be of importance in terms of economic losses. Treatment using a wide range of antimicrobial agents has been unsuccessful. Some field experiences have suggested that the use of anti-inflammatory drugs and multivitamin supplements to control PDNS and PMWS, together with the minimization of stress factors, may be of benefit.

Because the pathogenesis of PDNS is not known, no preventive recommendations have been indicated to be of value in control.

PORCINE REPRODUCTIVE AND RESPIRATORY SYNDROME

Porcine reproductive and respiratory syndrome (PRRS) was first reported in the USA in 1987. Since then, outbreaks of PRRS and successful isolation of the virus have been confirmed throughout North America and Europe.

Etiology and Epidemiology: The etiologic agent is a virus in the group Arteriviridae. The virus is enveloped and ranges in size from 45 to 80 mm. Inactivation is possible after treatment with ether or chloroform; however, the virus is very stable under freezing conditions, retaining its infectivity for 4 mo at -70°C. As the temperature rises, infectivity is reduced (15-20 min at 56°C).

Following infection of a naive herd, exposure of all members of the breeding population is inconsistent, leading to the development of naive, exposed, and persistently infected subpopulations of sows. This situation is exacerbated over time through the addition of improperly acclimated replacement gilts and leads to shedding of the virus from carrier animals to those that have not been previously exposed.

The primary vector for transmission of the virus is the infected pig. Contact transmission has been demonstrated experimentally, and the spread of virus from infected seedstock originating from a single source has been described. Introduction of infected seedstock can lead to the introduction and coexistence of genetically diverse isolates of PRRS virus on the same farm. Controlled studies have indicated that infected swine may be longterm carriers, with adults able to shed PRRS virus for up to 86 days after infection, while weaned pigs may harbor virus for 157 days. Experimentally infected boars can shed virus in the semen up to 93 days after infection.

Aerosol transmission of the virus has been considered to be a potential route of transmission, particularly under conditions of high humidity, low temperatures, and low wind speeds; however, this has been difficult to consistently reproduce under controlled field conditions and in the laboratory. PRRS virus can also be transmitted by fomites, such as contaminated needles, boots, coveralls, transport vehicles, and shipping containers. Farm personnel are not a risk, unless hands are contaminated with blood from viremic pigs. Finally, transmission via certain species of insects (mosquitos [Aedes vexans] and house flies [Musca domestica]) has been reported. The role of migratory waterfowl has not been determined. While biologic transmission of PRRS virus has been documented in immature Mallard ducks, results have not been reproducible experimentally using adult Mallards, nor have infected pigs been able to transmit virus to adult Mallards housed under field conditions.

Clinical Findings: PRRS appears to have 2 distinct clinical phases: reproductive failure and postweaning respiratory diseases. The reproductive phase of the disease includes increases in the number of stillborn piglets, mummified fetuses, premature farrowings, and weak-born pigs. Stillbirths and mummies may increase up to 25-35%, and abortions can be >10%. Anorexia and agalactia are evident in lactating sows and result in increased (30-50%) preweaning mortality. Suckling piglets develop a characteristic thumping respiratory pattern, and histopathologic examination of lung tissue reveals a severe, necrotizing, interstitial pneumonia. PRRS is capable of crossing the placenta in the third and possibly second trimester of gestation. Piglets may also be born viremic and transmit the virus for 112 days after infection. Performance after weaning is also affected. Infection with PRRS virus results in destruction of mature alveolar macrophages, which has led to the hypothesis that infection results in the suppression of the immune system; however, controlled studies indicate that the virus may actually enhance specific parameters of the immune response.

Outbreaks of the reproductive form of PRRS have been reported to last 1-4 mo, depending on the facilities and initial health status of the pigs. In contrast, the postweaning pneumonic phase can become chronic, reducing daily gain by 85% and increasing mortality to 10-25%. Numerous other pathogens are commonly isolated along with PRRS virus from affected nursery or finishing pigs. Other bacteria such as *Streptococcus suis*, *Escherichia coli*, *Salmonella choleraesuis*, *Haemophilus parasuis*, and *Mycoplasma hyopneumoniae* have been reported, as well as viruses such as porcine respiratory coronavirus and swine influenza virus. Finally, differences in the clinical response to PRRS virus may also be due to strain variation. Studies have demonstrated the ability of different isolates to induce varying degrees of interstitial pneumonia in CD/CD (cesarean-derived/colostrum-deprived) piglets after intranasal inoculation.

Diagnosis: The most commonly used tests are the ELISA or the indirect fluorescent antibody test. These tests measure IgG antibodies to PRRS virus. They cannot measure the level of immunity in an animal or predict whether the animal is a carrier. Titers are detected within 7-10 days after infection and can persist for up to 144 days. High titers may indicate recent exposure, and viral shedding may be occurring within the sampled population. Tests for PRRS virus include PCR, virus isolation, and immunohistochemistry. Recently, nucleic acid sequencing of the open reading frame 5 region of the virus has become commercially available, and has proved to be an excellent tool for epidemiologic investigations in the field to confirm similarity between isolates recovered from different sites.

Treatment and Control: Currently, there are no effective treatment programs for acute PRRS. Attempts to reduce fever using NSAID (aspirin) or appetite stimulants (B vitamins) appear to have minimal benefit. The use of antibiotics or autogenous bacterins to reduce the effects of opportunistic bacterial pathogens have also been reported; however, results have been mixed.

Prevention of infection appears to be the primary means of control. Understanding the PRRS status of replacement gilts and boars, as well as proper isolation and acclimatization of incoming stock are critical measures to prevent viral introduction. Pigs should be retested on arrival at the isolation facility and 45-60 days later, before entry to the herd. Elimination of existing infection by multisite production and segregated early weaning has also been described. While these strategies have had some success, the longterm risks of reinfection appear high. Prevention of viral spread by nursery depopulation has been described. This is successful when virus transmission is not occurring in the sow herd (usually 12-18 mo after initial outbreak), but the nurseries and growing/finishing pigs are still infected. All nursery pigs are removed from the farm to be finished elsewhere. The nurseries are then aggressively washed and disinfected and left empty for 7-14 days, after which they can be used normally. The technique has successfully eliminated PRRS virus from several herds, in which pigs have remained seronegative (for >1 yr) to market age, and production in the nurseries has improved, both in growth rate and mortality.

Commercial vaccines, both modified live and killed, have been licensed and have been effective in controlling outbreaks and preventing economic losses.

Recently, eradication of PRRS has been demonstrated to be possible on an individual farm basis. Methods such as whole herd depopulation-repopulation, test and removal, and herd closure have been documented as effective methods for eliminating PRRS virus from endemically infected herds. Unfortunately, a number of eradication efforts have failed due to the introduction of new isolates through unidentifiable routes.

POSTWEANING MULTISYSTEMIC WASTING SYNDROME

Postweaning multisystemic wasting syndrome (PMWS) of swine was identified in western Canada in 1991; however, retrospective studies from several countries indicate PMWS was present in the previous decade. PMWS is distributed worldwide and most swine-producing countries report variable prevalence of the disease. The primary manifestations are poor growth rate, ill thrift, and/or wasting. PMWS often occurs after weaning in pigs 4-14 wk old. The disease can also be seen in older pigs, particularly finishing pigs that weigh 45-70 kg. Morbidity is typically 5-20% among cohorts in the nursery or finishing stages. Mortality in swine that show signs of PMWS often is >50%. In addition to death loss, PMWS in finishing pigs may prevent, or substantially delay, affected pigs from reaching market weight, which can result in economic loss for the producer.

Etiology and Pathogenesis: PMWS is a multifactorial disease in which porcine circovirus type 2 (PCV2) is the necessary infectious agent. Circoviruses are small (17-22 nm in diameter), nonenveloped viruses that contain a single strand of circular DNA. There are 2 genotypes of porcine circovirus; only PCV2 has been shown to induce PMWS. Serologic cross-reaction occurs between PCV1 and PCV2, but antigenic differences between the viral genotypes allow separation of viruses using some serologic assays. Serologic surveys show that PCV2 is widespread in swine. Some reports have suggested that animals other than swine may be infected with PCV2 or PCV-like viruses. However, results of serologic studies for antibody against PCV in cattle and other livestock have been contradictory, and experimental induction of disease using PCV1 or PCV2 in species of livestock other than swine has not been successful.

Initially, PMWS was identified in high health herds that were free of most common swine pathogens but were infected with PCV2. Results from retrospective serologic studies indicate that PCV2 infected swine decades before PMWS was identified. Comparison of DNA from numerous recent isolates has shown high nucleic acid sequence homology exists among PCV2 and has not revealed a genetic determinant for virulence. Under field conditions, swine that show signs of PMWS usually are infected with multiple agents, but PCV2 is present consistently. Porcine parvovirus, porcine reproductive and respiratory syndrome virus, *Actinobacillus*, *Pasteurella*, *Staphylococcus*, and *Streptococcus* are common pathogens frequently isolated from pigs that show signs of PMWS.

The frequent finding of mixed infection in nursery pigs with PMWS may be attributable to waning protection from colostral antibody, making the pig more susceptible to simultaneous infection with PCV2 and multiple other pathogens. Affected pigs are probably immunosuppressed. Pigs that show signs of PMWS have reduced populations of $CD8^+$ and IgM^+ lymphocytes in circulation. Microscopically, affected pigs show generalized lymphocyte depletion in lymphoid tissue. Substantial amounts of viral antigen and DNA are found in the cytoplasm of macrophages, dendritic cells, and other antigen presenting cells.

Severe disease has been reproduced in pigs co-infected with PCV2 and other viruses or immunostimulant noninfectious products; however, the mechanism of this synergy is not known. Because PCV2 replication depends on cellular enzymes expressed during the S phase of the cell cycle, it has been hypothesized that previous activation of those cells supporting viral replication (not yet fully known) may promote replication of PCV2. Enhanced viral replication might lead to extensive loss of lymphoid cells and promote onset of PMWS. However, under field conditions, stimulation of the immune system of piglets with adjuvants, or with commercially available vaccines, appears to favor induction of PMWS after infection with PCV2.

Epidemiology and Transmission: Transmission may be by direct contact with infected pigs, and although not clearly demonstrated, by semen, contact with contaminated fomites, exposure to contaminated feeds or biologic products, multiple use of hypodermic needles, or by biting insects. The virus is found in blood, saliva, feces, urine, and semen of infected swine. PCV2 is known to persist in swine for several months under either experimental or field conditions. Convalescent swine may carry virus for extended periods and be important in disease transmission. PCV2 is fairly resistant to commonly used disinfectants and to irradiation, probably allowing it to accumulate in an environment and be infective for new groups of susceptible pigs if rigorous sanitary measures are not followed.

Longitudinal serologic studies show that the decline of colostral antibody titer in pigs is associated with onset of PMWS in nursery or finishing pigs. Transplacental infection with PCV2 has been documented. Transplacentally infected cohorts entering a nursery from a farrowing facility are a potential source of virus for other pigs in the nursery. Similarly, convalescent pigs or those subclinically infected with PCV2 in the nursery may carry virus and serve as a source of infection for cohorts in the finishing building.

Clinical Findings: Wasting, ill thrift, and dyspnea are the clinical signs seen most frequently in outbreaks of PMWS. Pallor, anemia, jaundice, diarrhea, and palpable lymphadenopathy also are seen is some affected pigs. A low-grade fever (104-106°F [40-41°C]) of several days' duration may be seen in affected pigs. Overcrowding, poor air quality, insufficient air exchange, and commingled age groups seems to exacerbate PMWS. Usually, only a few pigs in a group show signs of PMWS. The onset of disease may be acute, leading to death within a few days in some pigs. Other pigs show a more chronic disease and fail to gain weight or thrive.

Abortion, congenital tremors in neonatal pigs, and porcine dermatitis and nephropathy syndrome have been associated with PCV2 and may occur independently of PMWS (however, the link between PCV2 and some of these conditions remains controversial).

Lesions: Gross and microscopic lesions of PMWS vary among affected pigs. Lymph nodes may be substantially enlarged, pale on cut surface, and show lymphocytic depletion and/or granulomatous inflammation on microscopic examination. Epithelioid macrophages and multinucleated giant cells are the main inflammatory cells. Variably sized, basophilic, intracytoplasmic inclusion bodies may be found in the histiocytic cells. Similar lesions are seen in the tonsils, spleen, thymus and Peyer's patches of the intestine.

Lesions in the lung are common; their severity is influenced by duration of disease and presence of concurrent infections. Gross lung lesions may include failure to collapse, firmness, diffuse pulmonary edema, mottling, and consolidation.

Microscopic lesions vary from mild, multifocal lymphohistiocytic interstitial pneumonia to granulomatous bronchointerstitial pneumonia with bronchiolitis and bronchiolar fibrosis.

Grossly, the liver may appear icteric and/or atrophic in a low proportion of PMWS-affected pigs. Interlobular connective tissue may be prominent. Microscopic lesions range from single cell necrosis (apoptosis) with mild lymphocytic infiltration of portal zones to extensive lymphohistiocytic periportal hepatitis with diffuse necrosis of hepatocytes. The kidneys may be enlarged and show scattered to diffuse white foci on the cortical surface. Microscopic lesions include interstitial lymphohistiocytic infiltration, nonsuppurative vasculitis, tubular atrophy, and in some cases extensive tubular necrosis. Other lesions seen in pigs with PMWS include gastric ulceration and occasional multifocal lymphohistiocytic myocarditis. Lesions in the kidneys and heart are more prominent in pigs that are chronically affected with PMWS.

Diagnosis: PMWS is diagnosed on the basis of clinical signs of wasting or ill thrift, presence of gross and microscopic lesions that are consistent with the disease, and presence of viral antigen or DNA in the microscopic lymphoid lesions. Differential diagnoses include salmonellosis, chronic respiratory disease, porcine reproductive and respiratory syndrome, swine dysentery, and porcine proliferative enteritis. Because PCV2 is ubiquitous and may infect swine for an extended period, isolation of virus or detection of antiviral antibody in serum is not sufficient to establish a diagnosis of PMWS. Similarly, detection of viral DNA in tissues or clinical specimens by PCR does not establish a diagnosis.

Antibody against PCV2 may be detected by ELISA, indirect fluorescent antibody, or immunoperoxidase staining of infected cell cultures. Several porcine cell lines support replication of PCV2. Viral isolation can be done using serum, bronchiolar lavage fluid, or tissue homogenates of lymphoid tissue, kidney, liver, or lung. Viral DNA can also be detected using PCR in most tissues or in serum from affected pigs. Visualization of viral DNA or antigen in lesions is usually done using in situ hybridization or immunohistochemistry, respectively. Several tissue samples from multiple pigs may be required for detection of virus in cases of chronic disease.

Treatment and Control: There is no treatment for PMWS. Antibiotic therapy to control other infectious agents does not appear to affect the course once clinical signs appear. However, use of antibiotics may help prevent additional cases through control of intercurrent infections. Control of PMWS is possible through use of biosecurity and sanitary measures such as isolation of affected pigs and disinfection of pens after their use. Decreasing stressors (eg, high stocking density, inadequate ventilation, inadequate temperature control) is important. Other prevention and control measures that have been used on young pigs prior to the anticipated time of onset of PMWS include injection of vitamins, IP injection of serum harvested from finishing pigs, and vaccination against common pathogens.

STREPTOCOCCAL INFECTIONS IN PIGS

Streptococcal and enterococcal bacteria are found in tonsils, intestines, or feces of clinically healthy pigs. *Streptococcus intestinalis, S hyointestinalis, S alactolyticus, S bovis, Enterococcus faecalis, E faecium, E durans, E hirae,* and *E cecorum* are part of the intestinal microflora. *S suis, S porcinus,* and *S dysgalactiae* are potential pathogens.

STREPTOCOCCUS SUIS INFECTION

S suis is a bacterium of increasing importance in the swine industry. Most of the serotypes have been found in clinically healthy pigs, but a limited number of serotypes are more often associated with clinical infections such as meningitis, septicemia, endocarditis, arthritis, or pneumonia.

Etiology and Pathogenesis: *S suis* is an α-hemolytic streptococci related to Lancefield group D. A total of 35 serotypes have been described, along with subtypes defined as different genotypes within these serotypes. *S suis* isolated from diseased pigs generally belong to serotypes 1-8. A higher prevalence of serotypes 9-34 is noted in nasal and vaginal swabs in tissues taken from diseased pigs. Even when the carrier rate is near 100%, the disease incidence varies and is usually <5%. Although most weaned piglets carry *S suis* strains, few carry strains capable of inducing disease after weaning.

S suis is found in the upper respiratory tract, particularly the tonsils and nasal cavities, and the genital and alimentary tracts of pigs. Clinical infections are seen mainly in weaners or growing pigs and less frequently in suckling piglets. *S suis* has been isolated from a wide range of animal species, eg, cattle, sheep, goats, horses, and birds, as well as humans. Its presence in the environment is transitory.

Most studies on virulence factors have been done with serotype 2 strains. Serotype 2 virulent and avirulent strains exist, but characterization of virulence factors is incomplete. Capsular polysaccharide is so far the only proven virulence factor. Virulence-related proteins (MRP and EF), suilysin, and adhesins are potential virulence factors.

Epidemiology and Transmission: *S suis* is present in all parts of the world where the swine industry is important. Serotype 2 is responsible for the majority of the infections in diseased pigs in most countries. Isolates belonging to serotypes other than 2 have been associated with serious disease and cases of bronchopneumonia in Europe and North America, serotype 3 was associated with severe pneumonia in Argentina, serotype 9 was implicated in cases of systemic disease in several countries, and serotype 14 was associated with clinicopathologic findings similar to those associated with serotype 2 in the UK.

Most clinically healthy pigs are carriers of multiple serotypes of *S suis*. During parturition piglets become colonized with *S suis* from vaginal secretions or while suckling. Colonized piglets carry *S suis* into the nursery. Transmission between herds occurs usually by the movement of healthy carrier pigs. Their introduction into a noninfected herd usually results in the subsequent onset of disease in weaners and/or growing pigs. However, some infected herds that show no illness may develop clinical disease in the presence of other predisposing factors, eg, porcine reproductive and respiratory syndrome virus. *S suis* can also be transmitted via fomites and flies. The importance of other animal species or birds as reservoirs or vectors of the infection is unknown.

Clinical Findings: The earliest sign is usually fever, which may occur initially without other obvious signs. It is accompanied by a detectable bacteremia or pronounced septicemia that may persist for several days if untreated. During this period, there is usually a fluctuating fever and variable degrees of inappetence, depression, and shifting lameness. In peracute cases, pigs may be found dead with no premonitory signs. Meningitis is the most striking feature and the one on which a presumptive diagnosis is usually based. Early nervous signs include incoordination and adoption of unusual stances, which soon progress to inability to stand, paddling, opisthotonos, convulsions, and nystagmus. Endocarditis is also a frequent finding in older piglets—affected pigs may die suddenly or show various levels of dyspnea, cyanosis, and wasting. Septicemia, arthritis, and pneumonia are less common signs. Rhinitis, abortions, and vaginitis may also occur.

Lesions: Lesions are mainly seen in weaners and growing pigs and are associated with meningitis, arthritis, serositis, and endocarditis. Lesions may include fibrinopurulent exudates in the brain, swollen joints, fibrinous serositis, and cardiac valvular vegetations. Less frequently, lesions of septicemia are seen. *S suis* can also cause lesions of pneumonia, but generally these are considered to be secondary to other diseases. Lesions of septicemia, meningitis, or polyarthritis can be seen in suckling piglets.

Diagnosis: Presumptive diagnosis is generally based on clinical signs, age of animals, and gross lesions. Isolation and serotyping of the infectious agent and evaluation of microscopic lesions in affected tissues confirms the diagnosis. Serology is not routinely available. Genetic characterization is done in some laboratories and is particularly useful for epidemiologic studies.

Differential diagnoses include polyserositis caused by *Haemophilus parasuis* or *Mycoplasma hyorhinis*; meningitis caused by *H parasuis*; endocarditis caused by *Erysipelothrix rhusiopathiae*; septicemia caused by *H parasuis, Actinobacillus suis, Escherichia coli, E rhusiopathiae,* or *Salmonella choleraesuis*; and polyarthritis caused by other streptococci, staphylococci, *E coli,* or *A suis.*

Treatment, Control, and Prevention: Prompt recognition of the early clinical signs of streptococcal meningitis, followed by immediate parenteral treatment of affected pigs with an appropriate antibiotic, is currently the best method to maximize pig survival. The early stages of meningitis may be difficult to detect, so groups of pigs should be checked 2-3 times daily. The sensitivity rate to amoxicillin and ampicillin is ~90%. A high degree of resistance among *S suis* isolates to some antibacterial agents such as tetracycline, clindamycin, erythromycin, kanamycin, neomycin, and streptomycin has been reported. Susceptibility to trimethoprim-sulfamethoxazole is variable. Adjunctive therapy with an anti-inflammatory agent is recommended for treatment of *S suis* meningitis in pigs.

Along with sanitary measures, antimicrobial preventive medication may be used. Penicillins should be orally administered through drinking water to reduce the interference in absorption due to feed. Amoxicillin has advantages over natural penicillins for mass medication—its body clearance is lower than that of penicillin V, and higher serum concentrations are obtained.

Most vaccines used to protect against *S suis* infections have been commercial or autogenous bacterins and results have been inconsistent. In general, because *S suis* is a very early colonizer, it is felt that it cannot be eliminated by medicated early weaning.

Zoonotic Risk: Human cases are not frequent but are serious. Over 200 cases have been reported worldwide. Meningitis is the most common manifestation, followed by septicemia and endocarditis. Because hospital laboratories are not familiar with *S suis*, human disease is possibly underdiagnosed. The majority of human cases have been attributed to *S suis* serotype 2. In nearly all reported cases, patients had close contact with pigs, eg, were farmers, butchers, abattoir workers, or veterinarians, or handled pork products. The most frequent transmission route is through skin abrasions or cuts.

STREPTOCOCCUS DYSGALACTIAE INFECTION

S dysgalactiae dysgalactiae includes α- and nonhemolytic streptococci of Lancefield group C found in animals; β-hemolytic streptococci belonging to groups C, G, or L are classified as *S dysgalactiae equisimilis*. In swine, the *S dysgalactiae* group C and L serovars are β-hemolytic. The former are commonly found in nasal and throat secretions, tonsils, and vaginal and preputial secretions. They are the most important β-hemolytic streptococci involved in lesions in pigs. Vaginal secretions and milk from postparturient sows are the most likely sources of infection in piglets. Streptococci enter the bloodstream via skin wounds, the navel, and tonsils. A bacteremia or septicemia occurs, and the organisms then settle in one or more tissues, giving rise to arthritis, endocarditis, or meningitis. *S dysgalactiae* is not recognized as a zoonotic pathogen.

Clinical Findings and Lesions: Infection is usually first seen in pigs 1-3 wk old. Joint swelling and lameness are the most obvious and persistent clinical signs. Elevated temperatures, lassitude, roughened hair coat, and inappetence may also be noted. Early lesions consist of periarticular edema; swollen, hyperemic synovial membranes; and turbid synovial fluid. Necrosis of articular cartilage may be seen 15-30 days after onset and may become more severe. Fibrosis and multiple focal abscessation of periarticular tissues and hypertrophy of synovial villi also occur. Endocarditis occurs but is difficult to diagnose premortem. Lesions consist of yellow or white vegetations of different sizes, often covering the entire surface of the affected valve.

Diagnosis: Diagnosis of streptococcal septicemia, arthritis, or endocarditis is best accomplished by necropsy and bacteriologic examination of representative affected pigs. Only small numbers of organisms or no organisms may be isolated from affected joints, especially when inflammation is advanced.

Treatment and Prevention: β-hemolytic streptococci are sensitive to β-lactam antibiotics. Long-acting antibacterial agents may be beneficial, and treatment should be given before inflammation is well advanced. There are no recent reports about vaccination against these streptococci. Autogenous bacterins have been used, and there are reports of a reduction in incidence of arthritis when sows were vaccinated before farrowing.

Effective preventive measures should be undertaken. Adequate intake of colostrum may ensure that piglets receive protective antibodies. Traumatic injuries to the feet and legs should be minimized by reducing the abrasiveness of the floor surface in the nursing area.

STREPTOCOCCUS PORCINUS INFECTION

S porcinus was proposed in 1984 as a species that includes streptococci of Lancefield groups E (formerly *S infrequens*), P, U, and V. This bacterium can be isolated from tonsils, pharynx, and nasal cavities of clinically healthy pigs.

S porcinus group E was associated, particularly in the USA, with a contagious clinical entity in growing pigs known as streptococcal lymphadenitis, jowl abscesses, or cervical abscesses. The importance of this disease has considerably declined, and it is not recognized as an important economic entity in other countries where the bacterium only represents a few percent of the microorganisms isolated from abscesses in swine. Transmission is possible by contact or ingestion of food or water contaminated by abscess discharge or infected feces. Organisms enter the host through the mucosa of the pharyngeal or tonsillar surfaces and are carried to the lymph nodes, primarily of the head and neck region, where abscesses are formed. *S porcinus* is also occasionally found in the vaginal mucus of sows and the semen and prepuce of boars. It is generally considered to be a secondary invader.

S porcinus groups P, U, and V have been isolated from pig lungs, genital organs, or brains. Members of groups P and V were associated with abortions in pigs, and group P was involved in a case of tracheitis.

S porcinus is sensitive to penicillins. Nonetheless, antibiotic treatment is not usually successful in treating swine with abscesses or in eliminating carriers. Resistance to tetracycline has been reported. Vaccination is possible but has not been widely used, as cervical abscesses are not widespread.

There is no evidence that *S porcinus* has zoonotic potential.

SWINE VESICULAR DISEASE

Swine vesicular disease (SVD) is typically a transient disease of pigs in which vesicular lesions appear on the feet and snout and in the mouth. It does not cause severe production losses, and recent outbreaks of infection have been mainly subclinical. However, infection is of major economic importance because it must be differentiated from foot-and-mouth disease, eradication is costly, and embargoes on export of pigs and pork products are often imposed on nations not free of SVD.

Although infection in laboratory workers has occurred, and the virus may be present in sheep or cattle, pigs are said to be the only natural host. The disease was first identified in Italy in 1966 and subsequently in Hong Kong, Japan, Taiwan, and 16 countries in Europe. Although SVD virus was eradicated from Japan in the mid-1970s and most European countries by the mid-1980s, it has remained endemic in Italy and caused sporadic outbreaks of disease in other European countries during the 1990s and in Portugal in 2003 and 2004.

Etiology: The causal agent is an enterovirus of the family Picornaviridae. It belongs to the species human enterovirus B and is thought to have evolved from the human pathogen coxsackievirus B5, with which it shares a close antigenic and genetic relationship. There is only 1 serotype of SVD virus, although isolates may be differentiated by antigenic or genetic typing and may differ in virulence. SVD virus is transmitted by direct or indirect contact or by feeding infected pork or pork products. Infection can give rise to viremia and generalized vesicles that contain large amounts of virus.

Clinical Findings and Lesions: The primary signs are fresh or healing vesicular lesions on the feet, especially the coronary band, and in other areas such as the mouth, lips, or snout. The lesions may be mild or inapparent, especially when pigs are kept on soft bedding. The lesions are similar to those of foot-and-mouth disease (p 507), vesicular exanthema of swine (p 590), and vesicular stomatitis (p 555); however, affected pigs do not lose condition, and the lesions heal rapidly. Nervous signs have been described but are rarely seen in the field.

Diagnosis: Diagnosis is confirmed by laboratory tests on epithelial samples, feces, or serum. Virus detection is by antigen-detection ELISA, virus isolation, or reverse transcriptase-PCR. Serology is by antibody-detection ELISA or virus neutralization test.

Control: Countries free of the disease can remain so by controlling the import of pigs and pork products or by ensuring that pork products are treated (heat or otherwise) to kill the virus. Any suspected outbreak should be reported to the proper authorities. If disease does appear, control measures include thorough cooking (according to regulations) of all garbage fed to pigs and control of pig movement. Extensive serosurveillance is necessary to detect subclinically infected herds. The virus remains infective for long periods; thus, disinfection of premises, trucks, and equipment must be thorough. The most effective disinfectants are strong alkalis, although hypochlorites or acid-containing iodophors can be used when organic material is not present.

TRICHINELLOSIS

(Trichinosis)

Trichinellosis is a parasitic disease of public health importance caused by the nematode *Trichinella spiralis*. Human infections are established by consumption of insufficiently cooked infected meat, usually pork or bear, although other species have been implicated. Natural infections occur in wild carnivores; trichinellosis has also been found in horses, rats, beavers, opossums, walruses, whales, and meat-eating birds. Most mammals are susceptible.

Etiology and Epidemiology: *Trichinella* spp are considered to be a complex of 5 species, with 8 genotypes (T1 to T8) that have been identified by DNA analysis. There are few distinct morphologic differences, and species identification is based on characteristics such as reproductive isolation, infectivity to certain hosts, and resistance to freezing. *T spiralis* (T1) is the most common species affecting humans and domestic animals in most temperate regions; it has high infectivity for pigs and rodents and low resistance to freezing. The other species include *T nativa* (T2)—found in arctic carnivores, with low infectivity for rats and pigs and resistance to freezing; *T nelsoni* (T7)—found primarily in wild carnivores in the southern hemisphere, including Africa, with low infectivity for rats and pigs and relatively low virulence; *T pseudospiralis* (T4)—lacks the cyst in muscle and is primarily a parasite of birds; and *T britovi* (T3)—recently described in southern Europe and similar to *T nelsoni* in biologic characteristics.

Infection occurs by ingestion of larvae encysted in muscle. The cyst wall is digested in the stomach, and the liberated larvae penetrate into the duodenal and jejunal mucosa. Within ~4 days, the larvae develop into sexually mature adults. After mating, the females (3-4 mm) penetrate deeper into the mucosa and discharge living larvae (up to 1,500) over 4-16 wk. After reproduction, the adult worms die and usually are digested. The young larvae (0.1 mm) migrate into the lymphatics, are carried via the portal system to the peripheral circulation, and reach striated muscle where they penetrate individual muscle cells. They grow rapidly (to 1 mm) and begin to coil within the cell, usually 1 per cell. Capsule formation begins ~15 days after infection and is completed by 4-8 wk, at which time the larvae are infective. The cell degenerates as the larva grows, and then calcification occurs (at different rates in various hosts). Larvae may remain viable in the cysts for years, and their development continues only if ingested by another suitable host. The diaphragm, tongue, masseter, and intercostal muscles are among those most heavily involved in pigs.

If larvae pass through the intestine and are eliminated in the feces before maturation, they are infective to other animals.

Clinical Findings and Diagnosis: Most infections in domestic and wild animals go undiagnosed. In humans, heavy infections may produce serious illness with 3 clinical phases (intestinal, muscle invasion, and convalescent) and occasionally death.

Although antemortem diagnosis in animals other than humans is rare, trichinellosis may be suspected if there is a history of eating rodents or raw, infected meat. Microscopic examination of a muscle biopsy sample (usually tongue) may confirm but not necessarily rule out trichinellosis. ELISA is a reliable test to detect anti-*Trichinella* antibodies. Seroconversion may not occur for weeks after infection, although as little as 0.01 larvae per gram of meat can be detected.

Control: Treatment is generally impractical in animals. The objective is to prevent ingestion by any animal, including humans, of viable *Trichinella* cysts in muscle (trichinae). In pigs, this may be accomplished with good management, including controlling rodents, cooking garbage (fed to the pigs) for 30 min at 212°F (100°C), and preventing cannibalism (ie, tail biting) and access to wildlife carcasses.

Inspection of meat for viable trichinae at the time of slaughter (by trichinoscopic or digestion methods) is effective in preventing human infection in many countries. In North America, the assumption is that pork may be infected; therefore, those products that appear as "ready to eat" must be processed by adequate heating, freezing, or curing to kill trichinae before marketing. Other pork should be cooked to assure that all tissue is heated to an internal temperature of ≥137°F (58°C). Freezing pork at an appropriate temperature for an appropriate time is also effective (5°F [-15°C] for 20 days, -9.4°F [-23°C] for 10 days, or -22°F [-30°C] for 6 days). Freezing cannot be relied on to kill trichinae in meat other than pork.

VESICULAR EXANTHEMA OF SWINE

(San Miguel sea lion virus disease)

Vesicular exanthema of swine (VES) is an acute, highly infectious disease characterized by fever and formation of blisters on the snout, oral mucosa, soles of the feet, the coronary band, and between the toes.

Since 1972, a virus indistinguishable from VES virus (VESV), designated as San Miguel seal lion virus (SMSV), has been isolated from throat and rectal swabs from premature and 4-mo-old California sea lion pups, dead and weanling northern fur seal pups, and nursing northern elephant seal pups. It has also been isolated from vesicular lesions on marine mammals, commercial seal meat produced in Alaska, and perch-like fish collected from tidal pools off the southern California coast. SMSV isolated from both fish and marine mammals is capable of producing VES in pigs. In addition, caliciviruses isolated from throat and rectal swabs from dairy calves cause clinical vesicular exanthema in exposed pigs. One calicivirus serotype, SMSV-5, has been recovered from vesicular lesions on the palms and soles of a researcher working with the virus.

VESV, SMSV, and related viruses are members of the genus Vesivirus in the family Caliciviridae. Many immunologically distinct serotypes have been demonstrated (13 types of VESV from pigs and 16 types of SMSV from marine sources). Additionally, a number of serotypes have been named after the host species from which they were isolated: bovine, primate, cetacean, walrus, skunk, mink, and reptile caliciviruses. In some cases, serotypes initially isolated in terrestrial animals (eg, reptile calicivirus) have subsequently been found in marine mammals. All of these viruses (except for SMSV-8, SMSV-12, and mink calicivirus) form a single species, vesicular exanthema of swine virus.

In pigs, the clinical disease is indistinguishable from foot-and-mouth disease (p 507), vesicular stomatitis (p 555), and swine vesicular disease (p 588). Originally confined to California, the disease became widespread in the USA during the 1950s, but a vigorous campaign to eradicate the disease was successful. In 1959, the USA was declared free of VES, and the disease was designated a foreign animal disease; it has never been reported as a natural infection of pigs in any other part of the world.

Presumptive diagnosis in pigs is based on fever and the presence of typical vesicles, which break within 24-48 hr to form erosions. Diagnosis can be confirmed by complement-fixation tests, ELISA, and electron microscopy on epithelial tissue, or after passage in swine tissue cultures. Serum neutralization tests and immunoelectron microscopy are also used. Various reverse transcriptase-PCR have been developed for the identification of vesiviruses, but none have been evaluated for diagnostic use.

Suspected cases of vesicular exanthema should be reported immediately to the proper authorities. Garbage and fish should be cooked before being fed to pigs.

BLUETONGUE

Bluetongue is an infectious, noncontagious arthropodborne viral disease primarily of domestic and wild ruminants. Infection with bluetongue virus is common worldwide but is usually subclinical or mild in most infected ruminants. Bluetongue is almost exclusively a disease of sheep, particularly the fine-wool and mutton breeds, although white-tailed deer (*Odocoileus virginianus*), and pronghorn (*Antilocapra americana*) and desert bighorn sheep (*Ovis canadensis*) may develop severe clinical disease in North America.

Etiology and Transmission: Bluetongue virus is the type-species of the genus Orbivirus in the family Reoviridae. There are 24 serotypes worldwide, although not all serotypes exist in any one geographic area, eg, only 5 serotypes (2, 10, 11, 13, and 17) have been reported in the USA. Distribution throughout the world parallels the spatial and temporal distribution of vector species of *Culicoides* biting midges, which are the only significant natural transmitters of the virus. Of more than 1,400 *Culicoides* species worldwide, fewer than 20 are actual or possible vectors of bluetongue virus. Continued cycling of the virus among competent *Culicoides* vectors and susceptible ruminants is critical to viral ecology. In the USA, the principal biologic vector is *C variipennis sonorensis*, which limits distribution of the virus to southern and western regions. In Australia the principal vector is *C brevitarsis*, while in Africa, Europe, and the Middle East it is *C imicola*. In each geographic region, secondary vector species may attain local importance. Vectors become infected with bluetongue virus by imbibing blood from infected vertebrates; transovarial transmission has not been reported. High affinity of the virus to blood cells, especially the sequestering of viral particles in invaginations of RBC membranes, contributes to prolonged viremia in the presence of neutralizing antibody. The extended viremia in cattle (up to 9 wk), and the host preference of most vector species of *Culicoides* for cattle, provides a mechanism for year-round transmission in domestic ruminants. Mechanical transmission by other bloodsucking insects is of minor significance. Bluetongue virus is not contagious, and concentrations in secretions and excretions are minimal, making oral or aerosol transmission unlikely. However, semen from viremic bulls can serve as a source of infection for cows through natural service or artificial insemination. Embryo transfer is regarded as safe, provided that donors are not viremic and an appropriate washing procedure for embryos is used. Accidental infection has been reported in dogs in the USA following administration of a modified live virus vaccine that was contaminated with the virus. Serologic evidence of infection with bluetongue virus has been found in large carnivores in Africa, perhaps as a result of ingesting virus-infected viscera.

Clinical Findings: The course of the disease in sheep can vary from peracute to chronic, with a mortality rate of 2-30%. Peracute cases die within 7-9 days of infection, mostly as a result of severe pulmonary edema leading to dyspnea, frothing from the nostrils, and death by asphyxiation. In chronic cases, sheep may die 3-5 wk after infection, mainly as a result of bacterial complications, especially pasteurellosis, and exhaustion. Mild cases usually recover rapidly and completely. The major production losses include deaths, unthriftiness during prolonged convalescence, wool breaks, and possibly reproductive loss. In sheep, bluetongue virus causes vascular endothelial damage, resulting in changes to capillary permeability and subsequent intravascular coagulation. This results in edema, congestion, hemorrhage, inflammation, and necrosis. The clinical signs in sheep are typical. After an incubation period of 4-6 days, a fever of 105-107.5°F (40.5-42°C) develops. The animals are listless and reluctant to move. Clinical signs in young lambs are more apparent, and the mortality rate is higher (up to 30%). About 2 days after onset of fever, additional clinical signs such as edema of lips, nose, face, submandibular area, eyelids, and sometimes ears; congestion of mouth, nose, nasal cavity, conjunctiva, and coronary bands; and lameness and depression may be seen. A serous nasal discharge is common, later becoming mucopurulent. The congestion of nose and nasal cavity produces a "sore muzzle" effect, the term used to describe the disease in sheep in the USA. Sheep eat less because of oral soreness and will hold food in their mouths to soften before chewing. They may champ to produce a frothy oral discharge at the corners of the lips. On close examination, small hemorrhages can be seen on the mucous membranes of the nose and mouth. Ulceration develops where the teeth come in contact with lips and tongue, especially in areas of most friction. Some affected sheep have severe swelling of the tongue, which may become cyanotic ('blue tongue") and even protrude from the mouth. Animals walk with difficulty as a result of inflammation of the hoof coronets. A purple-red color is easily seen as a band at the junction of the skin and the hoof. Later in the course of disease, lameness or torticollis is due to skeletal muscle damage. In most affected animals, abnormal wool growth resulting from dermatitis may be observed.

The pathogenesis of bluetongue in cattle seems to differ from that in sheep and is based on immediate IgE hypersensitivity reactions. Clinical signs in cattle are rare but may be similar to those seen in sheep. They are usually limited to fever, increased respiratory rate, lacrimation, salivation, stiffness, oral vesicles and ulcers, hyperesthesia, and a vesicular and ulcerative dermatitis. Susceptible cattle and sheep infected during pregnancy may abort or deliver malformed calves or lambs. The malformations include hydranencephaly or porencephaly, which results in ataxia and blindness at birth. White-tailed deer and pronghorn antelope develop severe hemorrhagic disease leading to sudden death. Pregnant dogs abort or give birth to stillborn pups and then die in 3-7 days.

Diagnosis and Lesions: The typical clinical signs of bluetongue enable a presumptive diagnosis, especially in areas where the disease is endemic. Suspicion is confirmed by the presence of petechiae, ecchymoses, or hemorrhages in the wall of the base of the pulmonary artery and focal necrosis of the papillary muscle of the left ventricle. These highly characteristic lesions are usually obvious in severe clinical infections but may be barely visible in mild or convalescent cases. These lesions are often described as pathognomonic for bluetongue, but they have also been observed occasionally in other ovine diseases such as heartwater, pulpy kidney disease, and Rift Valley fever. Hemorrhages and necrosis are usually found where mechanical abrasion damages fragile capillaries, such as on the buccal surface of the cheek opposite the molar teeth and the mucosa of the esophageal groove and omasal folds. Other autopsy findings include subcutaneous and intermuscular edema, skeletal myonecrosis, myocardial and intestinal hemorrhages, hydrothorax, hydropericardium, pericarditis, and pneumonia. In many areas of the world, bluetongue in sheep, and especially in other ruminants, is subclinical and, therefore, laboratory confirmation based on virus isolation in embryonated chicken eggs, susceptible sheep, or cell cultures, or the identification of viral RNA by PCR is necessary. The identity of isolates may be confirmed by the group-specific antigen-capture ELISA, immunofluorescence, immunoperoxidase, serotype-specific virus neutralization tests, or hybridization with complementary gene sequences of group- or serotype-specific genes. For virus isolation, blood (10-20 mL) is collected as early as possible from febrile animals into an anticoagulant such as heparin, sodium citrate, or EDTA and transported at 4°C to the laboratory. For longterm storage where refrigeration is not possible, blood is collected in oxalate-phenol-glycerin (OPG). Blood to be frozen should be collected in buffered lactose peptone and stored at or below -70°C. Blood collected at later times during the viremic period should not be frozen, as lysing of the RBC or thawing releases the cell-associated virus, which may then be neutralized by early humoral antibody. The virus does not remain stable for long at -20°C. In fatal cases, specimens of spleen, lymph nodes, or red bone marrow are collected and transported to the laboratory at 4°C as soon as possible after death. A serologic response in ruminants can be detected 7-14 days after infection and is generally lifelong. Current recommended serologic techniques for the detection of bluetongue virus antibody include agar gel immunodiffusion and competitive ELISA. The latter is the test of choice and does not detect cross-reacting antibody to other orbiviruses, especially anti-EHDV (epizootic hemorrhagic disease virus) antibody. Various forms of virus neutralization test, including plaque reduction, plaque inhibition, and microtiter neutralization can be used to detect type-specific antibody.

Prevention and Control: Prophylactic immunization of sheep remains the most effective and practical control measure against bluetongue in endemic regions. Three polyvalent vaccines, each comprising 5 different bluetongue virus serotypes attenuated by serial passage in embryonated hens' eggs followed by growth and plaque selection in cell culture, are widely used in southern Africa and elsewhere, should epizootics of bluetongue occur. A monovalent modified live virus vaccine propagated in cell culture is available for use in sheep in the USA. Live-attenuated vaccines should not be used during *Culicoides* vector seasons because they may transmit the vaccine virus(es) from vaccinated to nonvaccinated animals, eg, other ruminant species. This may result in reassortment of genetic material and give rise to new viral strains. Abortion or malformation, particularly of the CNS, of fetuses may follow vaccination of ewes and cows with attenuated live vaccines during the first half and the first trimester of pregnancy, respectively. Passive immunity in lambs usually lasts 4-6 mo. The control of bluetongue is different in areas where the disease is not endemic. During an outbreak, when one or a limited number of serotypes may be involved, vaccination strategy depends on the serotype(s) that are causing infection. Use of vaccine strains other than the one(s) causing infection affords little or no protection. The vector status, potential risk from vaccine virus reassortment with wild-type viral strains, virus spread by the vectors to other susceptible ruminants, and reversion to virulence of vaccine virus strains or even the production of new serotypes also should be considered. Although a number of noninfectious vaccines are in development, they are not yet commercially available. Control of vectors by using insecticides or protection from vectors by moving animals into barns during the evening hours lowers the number of *Culicoides* bites and subsequently the risk of exposure to bluetongue virus infection.

BOVINE LEUKOSIS

(Bovine lymphosarcoma, Leukemia, Malignant lymphoma)

Enzootic bovine leukosis is a viral disease of adult cattle characterized by neoplasia of lymphocytes and lymph nodes. The prevalence of infection in a herd may be high, but only a few animals develop fatal lymphosarcoma. Infection is spread by contact with contaminated blood from an infected animal. Sporadic bovine leukosis consists of juvenile, thymic, and cutaneous lymphosarcomas. These may resemble enzootic bovine leukosis, but affected animals are seronegative for bovine leukemia virus (BLV).

Outbreaks of lymphosarcoma in sheep have been observed with clinical, epidemiologic, hematologic, and necropsy findings similar to those of enzootic bovine leukosis. Infection of other species with BLV has not been demonstrated. Epidemic occurrences of lymphosarcoma have been observed in pigs. Cases in horses are sporadic.

Etiology, Transmission, and Epidemiology: Enzootic bovine leukosis is caused by BLV, an exogenous C-type oncovirus in the family Retroviridae. Infection occurs by iatrogenic transfer of infected lymphocytes and is followed by a permanent antibody response and, less frequently, development of persistent lymphocytosis or lymphosarcoma. This form is rarely seen in animals <2 yr of age and is most common in the 4- to 8-yr age group. Sporadic bovine leukosis occurs in 3 forms: 1) juvenile in calves <6 mo old, characterized by multiple lymph node enlargement; 2) thymic in cattle <2 yr old, characterized by a swelling in the neck causing bloat and edema; and 3) cutaneous in cattle 1-3 yr old, characterized by the development of nodes and plaques in the skin. There is no evidence that these forms of sporadic bovine leukosis are caused by an infectious agent.

Prevalence rates within cattle herds in the USA range from 0-100%. The disease does not spread rapidly, but in infected herds the number of seropositive animals may be 80%. Dairy cattle are more commonly infected than beef cattle and have a higher incidence of lymphosarcoma. In severely affected dairy herds, the annual mortality rate may be as high as 5%. All breeds of cattle are susceptible to BLV infection. Infection occurs rarely in animals <2 yr of age and increases in incidence with increasing age. Lymphosarcoma is one of the 3 main causes of condemnation at slaughter.

Horizontal transmission is the usual method of spread. Close physical contact and exchange of contaminated biologic materials are required. The virus is present mostly in lymphocytes and can be found in the blood, milk, and tumors. Susceptible cattle usually become infected by exposure to infected lymphocytes. Natural transmission occurs mostly in cattle >1.5 yr old, usually during the summer months between in-contact animals and possibly by insect or bat transmission of infected lymphocytes in whole blood. An increased risk of infection in dairy cattle during the periparturient period suggests that vaginal secretions, exudates and placentas from cows, and contaminated calving instruments may serve as sources of infected blood cells.

Transmission can occur via contaminated surgical instruments, eg, dehorning gouges, ear tattooing pliers, and hypodermic needles. Transmission can also occur during blood transfusions, tuberculin testing, and administration of vaccines containing blood. Transmission via infective milk is possible by the passage of infected lymphocytes through intestinal mucosal epithelium during the first few hours of life. However, infection via this route is rare, possibly because of the presence of maternal antibodies in the milk. Congenital infection is seen in 4-8% of calves born from BLV-positive cows, presumably as a result of transplacental exposure to the virus during gestation.

Infection is not synonymous with clinical disease. Lymphosarcoma, the terminal stage of BLV infection involving the clonal transformation of infected B cells, occurs in <5% of BLV-infected cattle.

Outbreaks of leukosis typically follow the introduction of BLV-infected animals in farms or areas previously free of the virus. The level of calf management in dairy herds is also a major risk factor. Any environmental factor or management practice that allows newborn calves access to infective blood, such as prolonged close contact of cow and calf immediately after parturition, use of colostrum or milk from seropositive cows, use of contaminated equipment or needles, and large fly populations in calf barns, will increase infection rates in calves.

Pathogenesis: Exposure of cattle to BLV leads to 4 possible outcomes: 1) failure of the animal to become infected, probably due to genetic resistance, 2) establishment of a permanent infection and the development of detectable antibody levels (latent carriers), 3) establishment of a permanent infection and a persistent benign lymphocytosis, or 4) development of malignant lymphosarcoma, with or without persistent lymphocytosis. Whether the animal becomes infected or develops any of the other forms of the disease depends on its genetic constitution and immune status and on the infective dose of virus.

Clinical Findings: Enzootic bovine leukosis is characterized by multiple cases of adult, multicentric lymphosarcoma within a herd, with tumors developing rapidly in many sites and thus variable clinical signs. The usual incubation period is 4-5 yr. Persistent lymphocytosis without clinical signs occurs earlier, but rarely before 2 yr of age. Many cows remain in the preclinical stage for years, often for their complete productive lifetime, without any apparent reduction in performance.

In 5-10% of clinical cases the course is peracute; often affected animals die suddenly without prior evidence of illness. Involvement of the adrenal glands, rupture of an abomasal ulcer, or an affected spleen followed by acute internal hemorrhage are known causes. In most clinical cases, the course is subacute (up to 7 days) to chronic (several months) and initiated by an unexplainable loss of body condition, anorexia, pallor, and muscular weakness. Production may drop abruptly in dairy cows. The heart rate is not increased unless the myocardium is involved, and the temperature is normal unless tumor growth is rapid and extensive, when it rises to 103-104°F (39.5-40°C). Once signs of clinical illness and tumor development are detectable, the course is rapid and death occurs in 2-3 wk.

The superficial lymph nodes enlarge in 75-90% of cases, and this is often an early clinical finding. It is usually accompanied by small (1 cm diameter) subcutaneous lesions, often on the flanks and perineum. However, peripheral lesions may be completely absent in many cases with advanced visceral involvement. Enlargement of visceral lymph nodes is common, but this is usually subclinical unless they compress other organs such as intestine or nerves. They may be palpable on rectal examination, and special attention should be give to the deep inguinal and iliac nodes. In advanced cases, extensive spread to the peritoneum and pelvic viscera occurs, and the tumor masses are easily palpable. The enlargement may be confined to the pelvic nodes or to one or more subcutaneous nodes. Involvement of the nodes of the head is sometimes observed, often with exophthalmos. The affected nodes are smooth and resilient; in dairy cows, they are easily seen and may be marked by local edema. Occasionally, the entire body surface is covered with subcutaneous masses 5-11 cm in diameter.

In addition to the lymph nodes, tissues most commonly affected include the abomasum, heart, spleen, kidneys, uterus, spinal meninges, and retrobulbar lymphatic tissue. Heart sounds are commonly muffled, and other cardiac abnormalities may be obvious. Neural lymphomatosis may lead to the gradual onset of posterior paralysis over several weeks.

The calf, thymic, and cutaneous forms are designated sporadic bovine leukosis. Clinical signs of calf lymphosarcoma include gradual weight loss, sudden generalized lymph node enlargement, depression, and weakness. Fever, tachycardia, and posterior paresis are less frequent signs. Death occurs in 2-8 wk. Signs of pressure on internal organs, including bloat and congestive heart failure, may occur.

Bone and bone marrow necrosis, with associated unthriftiness and inactivity, posterior ataxia, superficial lymph node enlargement, lameness, and respiratory distress have been recorded.

Thymic lymphosarcoma is a common finding in animals 1-2 yr of age and is characterized by massive thymic enlargement in the brisket area and lesions in bone marrow and regional lymph nodes. Jugular vein engorgement and marked brisket edema extending to the submandibular region are common. Moderate bloat due to inability to eructate because of esophageal compression may occur. The thymic mass is usually not palpable. This form is more common in beef than in dairy cattle. An atypical lymphosarcoma in a mature cow negative for BLV and similar to the thymic form has been reported.

The cutaneous form is most common in cattle 1-3 yr of age. It is rare and manifest by cutaneous plaques (1-5 cm diameter) appearing on the neck, back, croup, and thighs. Spontaneous regression may occur. Relapse may occur in 1-2 yr with reappearance of cutaneous lesions and involvement of internal organs as in the enzootic form of the disease.

Lesions: Firm, white tumors may be found in any organ, although 2 patterns of distribution are apparent. In newborn and young animals, the common sites are the kidneys, thymus, liver, spleen, and peripheral and internal lymph nodes. In adults, the heart, abomasum, and spinal cord are often involved. In the heart, the tumor masses invade particularly the right atrium, although they may be found throughout the myocardium and extend to the pericardium. The abomasal wall may show gross, uneven thickening with tumor material in the submucosa, particularly in the pyloric region. Similar lesions are common in the intestinal wall. Deep ulcerations in the affected area are not uncommon. Involvement of the nervous system usually includes thickening of the peripheral nerves coming from the last lumbar or first sacral cord segment, or more rarely, in a cranial cervical site. This may be associated with one or more circumscribed thickenings in the spinal meninges. Affected lymph nodes may be enlarged and composed of both normal and neoplastic tissue.

Lymphosarcoma may appear as discrete nodular masses or a diffuse tissue infiltrate. The latter pattern results in an enlarged, pale organ and can be easily misinterpreted as a degenerative change rather than neoplasia. Histologically, the tumor masses are composed of densely packed, monomorphic lymphocytic cells.

Diagnosis: Because of the wide range of clinical findings, a definitive diagnosis is often difficult. Enlargement of peripheral lymph nodes without fever or lymphangitis is unusual in other diseases, except for tuberculosis, which can be differentiated by the tuberculin test. Diagnosis of the viral infection is made by serology or virology, persistent lymphocytosis is identified by hematology, and neoplastic tumors are identified by histologic examination of biopsies.

Agar gel immunodiffusion (AGID) is a good screening test for identifying infected animals or herds. It has an estimated specificity of 99.8% and sensitivity of 98.5%. This test is recognized by most governments as the official standard for testing imported animals. Radioimmunoassay is useful for the detection of BLV antibodies in cattle exposed ≤2 wk, in milk samples, and in serum samples from periparturient dams. Serum ELISA is more sensitive than other serologic tests and may also be used on milk. The ELISA may be used for pooled serum samples and allows detection of antibodies in herds with a prevalence of <1%. The bulk tank milk ELISA is useful for identification of herds that are negative for BLV infection. Herds identified as positive by the ELISA require further testing at the individual or herd level to definitively establish their BLV status.

In a control and eradication program, early detection of infected calves is difficult because colostral antibodies to BLV cannot be differentiated from antibodies resulting from natural infection. Calves that have ingested colostrum from seropositive cows usually have maternal antibodies; PCR is necessary to distinguish between infected and virus-free calves in such cases.

PCR is a sensitive and specific assay for direct diagnosis of BLV infection in peripheral blood lymphocytes. The test can identify proviral DNA of BLV in the lymphocytes of neonates born to infected cows, differentiate uninfected newborn calves with colostral antibodies from BLV-infected calves, and detect the presence of the virus in the presence of antibodies.

Enzootic bovine leukosis cannot be distinguished from sporadic bovine leukosis on histopathologic examination. ELISA is recommended to differentiate between enzootic and sporadic bovine leukosis because it is rapid, reliable, and sensitive. In cases in which no blood or other fluids are obtained, PCR is the most useful method for direct detection of BLV.

Treatment and Control: There is no treatment, but the disease can be eradicated from a herd or country or controlled at a low level. Significant costs are associated with control and eradication programs. Denmark established a national program for control of the disease in 1959, Sweden introduced a control program in 1990 with the aim of complete eradication of BLV from the Swedish cattle population, and Britain introduced a national testing program in 1992. Voluntary eradication programs using the AGID test have been effective in other member countries of the European Community in the last 20 yr in reducing the prevalence of infection and disease. These programs have been successful in part because of the low prevalence of infection, and because the economic losses from culling seropositive cows has not been large.

In Canada and the USA, it is economically cost prohibitive to cull and slaughter all seropositive cattle because of the high prevalence of infection. Thus, all control and eradication programs in these countries are herd-based and strictly voluntary. The efficiency of such programs depends on the accuracy of the test used to identify the infected animals and repetition of the test at an appropriate interval. The recommended procedure is: 1) identify infected animals using the AGID test, 2) cull and slaughter seropositive animals immediately, 3) retest the herd 30-60 days later, and 4) use PCR to test young calves and as a complementary test for clarifying doubtful test results in herds with a low prevalence of infection. Testing is repeated until the herd tests negative. Testing is then repeated every 6 mo and the herd declared free when there have been no positive reactors for 2 yr. Future introductions into the herd are managed most safely by artificial insemination, fertilized ovum transfer, or importation of animals that have been tested and are seronegative on 2 tests, done 30 and 60 days prior to arrival.

In herds with a high prevalence of infection, in which the test and slaughter method of eradication is not economically viable, various methods of testing and segregation may be used to control infection. Seropositive cows cannot be exported to many countries.

Prevention: Several management techniques can be used to prevent infection in calves. Feeding newborn calves colostrum and milk from seronegative cows has been widely accepted as effective in preventing infection. The use of colostrum and milk from seronegative cows permits early serologic detection of infected calves. However, feeding colostrum from seropositive cows can provide significant protection from infection during the first 3 mo of life. The replacement of whole milk feeding with high-quality milk replacer may also be considered. Bloody milk should not be fed to calves.

Transmission to newborn calves can also be reduced by avoiding exposure to maternal blood at the time of parturition, housing calves in individual hutches with individual feeders and waterers, and implementing management techniques that avoid iatrogenic transmission. When handling a group of calves, the youngest ones should be handled first and the older and sick calves last. Equipment that could act as fomites in transferring blood should be disinfected with chlorhexidine between calves.

Dehorning calves by electrocautery before 2 mo of age can reduce the prevalence of infection compared with gouge dehorning, which allows the transfer of infected blood between calves. Handling facilities that become contaminated with blood should be cleaned between calves. Single disposable needles should be used for vaccination, treatments, and blood collection. Transmission can be reduced by segregation of seropositive and seronegative cows. Use of individual sleeves for rectal palpation may also be considered.

Infection in a herd can be prevented by ensuring that all imports into the herd have tested seronegative at least 30 days prior to arrival. Control of biting insect vectors is desirable. Blood transfusions and vaccines containing blood, such as those used for babesiosis and anaplasmosis are particularly potent means of spreading the disease, and donors must be carefully screened. Embryo transfer from valuable, pedigreed seropositive cows may aid in reducing prenatal infection. Insemination is not a method of transmission.

BOVINE PETECHIAL FEVER

(Ondiri disease)

Bovine petechial fever is a rickettsiosis of cattle characterized by hemorrhages and edema. Occurrence has been confirmed only in Kenyan highlands at altitudes >5,000 ft (1,500 m), although it is considered likely to occur in neighboring countries with similar topography. The importance of bovine petechial fever lies in its threat to dairy development in the highlands of eastern Africa.

Etiology and Epidemiology: The disease is caused by *Ehrlichia ondiri*, an intracellular rickettsia that resides in cytoplasmic vacuoles of circulating leukocytes. The organism can multiply after experimental infection in cattle, sheep, goats, bushbuck, impala, Thomson's gazelles, and wildebeest, and hence, probably in most domestic and wild ruminants. *E ondiri* is believed to be endemic in wild ruminants, particularly bushbuck, and it sporadically overspills into domestic cattle grazing forest edges or scrubs.

The disease is restricted to scrub or forest edge areas that have heavy shade, a thick layer, and high relative humidity. It occurs sporadically throughout the year in imported breeds of cattle. It is not known how the disease is transmitted. As in other rickettsial infections, an arthropod vector is suspected, but extensive attempts to incriminate ticks, biting insects, and mites have failed. Bushbuck (*Tragelaphus scriptus*) and other wild ruminants may serve as amplifying and reservoir hosts.

Pathogenesis: The route of infection is not known, but *E ondiri* can be seen in circulating granulocytes (neutrophils and eosinophils) and monocytes while cattle are ill, and in the spleen at necropsy. Electron microscopic studies have shown that *E ondiri* can also infect endothelial and Kupffer cells, and it may be free in capillary lumens in the heart. It is believed that *E ondiri* initially multiplies in the spleen, with subsequent spread to other areas. Damage to the vascular endothelium would explain the hemorrhages and edema, as in many other rickettsial infections.

Clinical Findings: The disease is characterized by a high fluctuating fever, apathy, lowered milk yield, and widespread petechiation of mucous membranes. After an incubation period of 4-14 days, animals develop a high fever; 2-3 days later, most animals appear dull, and petechiae appear on mucous membranes, particularly the lower surface of the tongue and the vaginal mucosa. These hemorrhages enlarge over several days and then regress as the animal begins to recover. Marked conjunctival edema and hemorrhage ("poached egg eye") are characteristic in some severe cases. The conjunctival sacs are swollen and everted around a tense and protruding eyeball, and there may be blood in the aqueous humor. Pregnant cows may abort, most likely from the high fever. Other clinical signs are absent. The case mortality rate in untreated cases can be as high as 50% in imported animals or in animals newly introduced to the area. Latent infections develop after recovery in some animals, especially in indigenous stock. Immunity lasts for several years.

Lesions: Typically, eosinopenia and lymphopenia are marked, followed by an equally pronounced neutropenia. Anemia is characteristically a sequela, and organisms can be demonstrated in Giemsa-stained smears of blood or spleen. At necropsy, widespread hemorrhages and edema are accompanied by lymphoid hyperplasia. The edema is characterized by gelatinous fluid in the intermuscular connective tissue, lymph nodes, and abomasum. No characteristic histologic abnormalities have been described.

Diagnosis: In areas where the disease is endemic, a history of movement to forest edge areas, coupled with clinical signs and postmortem lesions, allows for a presumptive diagnosis. Definitive diagnosis requires demonstration of the causal organism in Giemsa-stained smears of blood or spleen or by electron microscopy. *E ondiri* stains blue with Giemsa and can be seen as small bodies (0.4 μm), larger bodies (1-2 μm), groups of small and large bodies, and groups or morulae of small bodies. They are seen in cytoplasmic vacuoles and are most commonly seen in neutrophils. Tissue suspensions (spleen) can also be inoculated into susceptible cattle or sheep. Blood smears from the recipient animal should be made daily for up to 10 days, by which time *E ondiri* should be detectable in neutrophils. The disease is difficult to differentiate from other hemorrhagic diseases of cattle such as Rift Valley fever, acute trypanosomosis (hemorrhagic *Trypanosoma vivax*), acute theileriosis, heartwater, hemorrhagic septicemia, and bracken fern poisoning.

Treatment and Control: Dithiosemicarbazone and tetracyclines have been used successfully to treat early experimental cases. The former is said to be more effective. In endemic areas, the disease can be prevented by avoiding areas associated with previous cases. However, this may not always be practical.

CAPRINE ARTHRITIS AND ENCEPHALITIS

Caprine arthritis and encephalitis (CAE) virus infection is manifested clinically as polyarthritis in adult goats and less commonly as progressive paresis (leukoencephalomyelitis) in kids. Subclinical or clinical interstitial pneumonia, indurative mastitis ("hard udder"), and chronic wasting have also been attributed to infection with this virus. Most CAE virus infections, however, are subclinical. Infection with the CAE virus decreases the lifetime productivity of dairy goats and is a barrier to exportation of goats from North America.

CAE virus infection is widespread among dairy goats in most industrialized countries but rare among indigenous goat breeds of developing countries unless they have been in contact with imported goats. In countries such as Canada, Norway, Switzerland, France, and the USA, seroprevalence of CAE virus is >65%.

Etiology, Epidemiology, and Pathogenesis: The CAE virus is an enveloped, single-stranded RNA lentivirus in the family Retroviridae. There are several genetically distinct isolates of the virus that differ in virulence.

Under natural conditions, CAE virus appears to be host-specific, but experimental infection of sheep with this virus is possible. Prolonged commingling of naive sheep with infected goats usually does not result in infection or seroconversion, but lambs allowed to suckle infected goats seroconvert and develop persistent CAE virus infections. Experimental inoculation of CAE virus into the joints of lambs produces arthritis, seroconversion, and virus-positive joints.

CAE virus infection is widespread in dairy goat breeds but uncommon in meat- and fiber-producing goats. This has been attributed to genetics, management practices such as feeding colostrum and milk from a single dam to multiple kids, and industrialized farming practices (eg, frequent introductions of new animals into a herd). Prevalence of infection increases with age but is not influenced by sex. Most goats are infected at an early age, remain virus positive for life, and develop disease months to years later.

The chief mode of spread of CAE is through ingestion of virus-infected goat colostrum or milk by kids. The feeding of pooled colostrum or milk to kids is a particularly risky practice, because a few infected does will spread the virus to a large number of kids. Horizontal transmission also contributes to disease spread within herds and may occur through direct contact, exposure to fomites at feed bunks and waterers, ingestion of contaminated milk in milking parlors, or serial use of needles or equipment contaminated with blood. Unlikely methods of transmission, as indicated by experimental studies, include in utero transmission to the fetus, infection of the kid during parturition, and infection through breeding or embryo transfer.

The pathogenesis of CAE is not fully understood. Virus-infected macrophages in colostrum and milk are absorbed intact through the gut mucosa. Infection is subsequently spread throughout the body via infected mononuclear cells. Periodic virus replication and macrophage maturation induces the characteristic lymphoproliferative lesions in target tissues such as the lungs, synovium, choroid plexus, and udder. Persistence of the CAE virus in the host is facilitated by its ability to become sequestered as provirus in host cells. Infection induces a strong humoral and cell-mediated immune response, but neither is protective.

Clinical Findings: Arthritis is the syndrome exhibited by adult goats infected with CAE virus. Clinical signs include joint capsule distention and varying degrees of lameness. The carpal joints are most frequently involved. The onset of arthritis may be sudden or insidious, but the clinical course is always progressive. Affected goats lose condition and usually have poor hair coats. Encephalomyelitis is generally seen in kids 2-4 mo old but has been described in older kids and adult goats. Affected kids initially exhibit lameness, ataxia, and hindlimb placing deficits. Hypertonia and hyperreflexia are also common. Over time, signs progress to paraparesis or tetraparesis and paralysis. Depression, head tilt, circling, opisthotonos, torticollis, and paddling have also been described. The interstitial pneumonia component of CAE virus infection rarely produces clinical signs in kids. However, in adult goats with serologic evidence of CAE virus infection, chronic interstitial pneumonia that leads to progressive dyspnea has been documented. The "hard udder" syndrome attributed to CAE virus infection is characterized by a firm, swollen mammary gland and agalactia at the time of parturition. Milk quality is usually unaffected. Although the mammary gland may soften and produce close to normal amounts of milk, production remains low in many goats suffering from indurative mastitis.

Lesions: Pathologic lesions of CAE virus infection are generally described as lymphoproliferative with degenerative mononuclear cell infiltration. Lesions in joints are characterized by thickening of the joint capsule and marked proliferation of synovial villi. In chronic cases, soft-tissue calcification involving joint capsules, tendon sheaths, and bursae is not uncommon. Severe cartilaginous destruction, rupture of ligaments and tendons, and periarticular osteophyte formation have also been described in advanced cases. Microscopic features of articular lesions include synovial cell hyperplasia, subsynovial mononuclear cell infiltration, villous hypertrophy, synovial edema, and synovial necrosis. Gross lesions associated with the neurologic form of CAE include asymmetric, brownish pink, swollen areas, most commonly in the cervical and lumbosacral spinal cord segments. Histopathologically, these lesions are characterized by multifocal, mononuclear cell inflammatory infiltrates and varying degrees of demyelination. On gross examination, lungs of affected goats are firm and gray-pink with multiple, small, white foci, and do not collapse. The bronchial lymph nodes are invariably enlarged. Histologic findings include chronic interstitial pneumonia with mononuclear cell infiltration in alveolar septae and in perivascular and peribronchial regions. In does with udder induration, mononuclear infiltration of periductular stroma obliterates normal mammary tissue.

Diagnosis: A presumptive diagnosis can be based on clinical signs and history. Traumatic arthritis, and infectious arthritis caused by *Mycoplasma* spp, are differential diagnoses for arthritis induced by CAE virus. Differential diagnoses for the progressive paresis and paralysis exhibited by young kids should include enzootic ataxia, spinal cord abscess, cerebrospinal nematodiasis, spinal cord trauma, and congenital anomalies of the spinal cord and vertebral column. If neurologic examination indicates brain involvement, polioencephalomalacia, listeriosis, and rabies should be considered as possible causes. The pulmonary form of caseous lymphadenitis may have a similar clinical presentation to the pulmonary form of CAE in adult goats.

Serologic tests available for diagnosis are the agar gel immunodiffusion (AGID) and ELISA. In general, the ELISA is more sensitive than the AGID, but the latter test is more widely available in North America. A positive test result in an adult goat implies infection but does not confirm that the clinical signs are caused by CAE virus. Kids infected at birth develop a measurable antibody response 4-10 wk after infection. However, positive test results in kids <90 days old usually reflect colostral antibody transfer. Negative test results do not reliably rule out CAE virus infection, because the time for postinfection seroconversion is variable and occasional goats have a very low titer that may not be detectable. Low antibody titers are common in late pregnancy. Because of the limitations of serologic testing, definitive diagnosis of clinical CAE requires demonstration of characteristic lesions in biopsy specimens or at necropsy. Virus isolation should be performed to further substantiate the diagnosis.

Treatment and Control: There are no specific treatments for any of the clinical syndromes associated with CAE virus infection. However, supportive treatments may benefit individual goats. The condition of goats with the arthritic form of CAE may be improved with regular foot trimming, use of additional bedding, and administration of NSAID such as phenylbutazone or aspirin. Goats with encephalomyelitis can be maintained for weeks with good nursing care. Antimicrobial therapy is indicated to treat secondary bacterial infections that may complicate the interstitial pneumonia or indurative mastitis components of CAE virus infection. Providing high-quality, readily digestible feed to goats positive for CAE virus may delay the onset of the wasting syndrome. In commercial herds, one or more of the following have been recommended for control of CAE: 1) permanent isolation of kids beginning at birth; 2) feeding of heat-treated colostrum (56°C for 60 min) and pasteurized milk; 3) frequent serologic testing of the herd (semiannually), with identification and segregation of seronegative and seropositive goats; and 4) eventual culling of seropositive goats. If the control program includes segregation of herds into seropositive and seronegative groups, shared equipment should be disinfected using phenolic or quaternary ammonium compounds.

COLISEPTICEMIA

(Septicemic colibacillosis, Septicemic disease)

Septicemia caused by *Escherichia coli* is a common disease of calves, and to a lesser extent lambs, <1 wk old. It may present with signs of acute septicemia or as a chronic bacteremia with localization.

Etiology and Epidemiology: The disease is caused by specific serotypes of *E coli* that possess virulence factors enabling them to cross mucosal surfaces and produce bacteremia and septicemia. However, the main determinant of the disease is deficiency of circulating immunoglobulins as the result of a failure in passive transfer of colostral immunoglobulin; septicemic disease due to invasion by *E coli* occurs only in immunoglobulin-deficient calves.

Colisepticemia is seen during the first week of life, most commonly at 2-5 days of age. Chronic disease with localization can be seen up to 2 wk of age. The disease is usually sporadic and is more common in dairy than beef calves.

Transmission and Pathogenesis: Invasion occurs primarily through the nasal and oropharyngeal mucosa but can also occur across the intestine or via the umbilicus and umbilical veins. There is a period of subclinical bacteremia that, with virulent strains, is followed by rapid development of septicemia and death from endotoxemic shock. A more prolonged course, with localization of infection, polyarthritis, meningitis, and less commonly uveitis and nephritis, is seen with less virulent strains. Chronic disease also develops in calves that have acquired marginal levels of circulating immunoglobulin. The organism is excreted in nasal and oral secretions, urine, and feces; excretion begins during the preclinical bacteremic stage. Initial infection can be acquired from a contaminated environment. In groups of calves, transmission is by direct nose-to-nose contact, urinary and respiratory aerosols, or as the result of navel-sucking or fecal-oral contact.

Clinical Findings and Diagnosis: In the acute disease, the clinical course is short (3-8 hr), and signs are related to the development of septic shock. Pyrexia is not prominent, and the rectal temperature may be subnormal. Listlessness and an early loss of interest in sucking are followed by depression, poor response to external stimuli, collapse, recumbency, and coma. Tachycardia, a poor pulse pressure, and a prolonged capillary refill time are seen. The feces are loose and mucoid, but severe diarrhea is not seen in uncomplicated cases. Mortality approaches 100%. With a more prolonged clinical course, the infection may localize. Polyarthritis and meningitis are common; tremor, hyperesthesia, opisthotonos, and convulsions are seen occasionally, but stupor and coma are more common.

A moderate but significant leukocytosis and neutrophilia are seen early, but leukopenia is marked in the terminal stages. The joint fluid contains increased inflammatory cells and protein, and the CSF shows pleocytosis and an increased protein concentration; organisms may be evident on microscopic examination. Less commonly, other bacteria, including other Enterobacteriaceae, *Streptococcus* spp, and *Pasteurella* spp, produce septicemic disease in young calves. These organisms are more common in sporadic cases than as causes of outbreaks. They produce similar clinical disease, but they can be differentiated by culture. As with colisepticemia, the primary determinant of these infections is a failure of passive transfer of immunoglobulins.

The diagnosis is based on history and clinical findings, demonstration of a severe deficiency of circulating IgG, and ultimately, demonstration of the organism in the blood or tissues. Zinc sulfate or total protein estimation can be used for rapid estimation of IgG (p 1811).

Treatment: Treatment requires aggressive use of antibiotics. Because there is no time for sensitivity testing, the initial choice should be a bactericidal drug that has a high probability of efficacy against gram-negative organisms. Antibacterial therapy should be coupled with aggressive fluid, drug, and other therapy for endotoxic shock. Mortality is high despite aggressive treatment.

Control and Prevention: Calves that acquire adequate concentrations of immunoglobulin from colostrum are resistant to colisepticemia. Therefore, prevention depends primarily on management practices that ensure an adequate and early intake of colostrum. The adequacy of the farm's practice of feeding colostrum should be monitored, and corrective strategies applied as required. In dairy herds, natural sucking does not guarantee adequate concentrations of circulating immunoglobulins, and calves should be fed 2-4 L of first-milking colostrum, using a nipple bottle or an esophageal feeder, within 2 hr of birth, followed by a second feeding at 12 hr. The circulating concentration of immunoglobulin required to protect against colisepticemia is low; however, high concentrations of circulating immunoglobulins are desirable because they decrease susceptibility to other neonatal infectious diseases.

When natural colostrum is not available for a newborn calf, commercial colostrum substitutes containing 25 g IgG will provide sufficient immunoglobulin for protection against colisepticemia if fed early in the absorptive period. Plasma containing at least 4 g and preferably 8 g IgG, administered parenterally, will provide some protection for older calves that have not been fed colostrum and are unable to absorb immunoglobulins from the intestine. Small-volume hyperimmune serum is of benefit only when it contains antibody specific to the particular serotype associated with an outbreak. The risk of early infection should be minimized by hygiene in the calving area and disinfection of the navel at birth. To minimize transmission, calves reared indoors should be in separate pens (without contact) or reared in calf hutches.

CRIMEAN-CONGO HEMORRHAGIC FEVER

Crimean-Congo hemorrhagic fever (CCHF) is a severe hemorrhagic viral disease of humans acquired from infected ticks, tissues of infected wild or domestic animals, and from human patients with the disease.

Etiology and Epidemiology: The etiologic agent, CCHF virus (genus Nairovirus, family Bunyaviridae) is an enveloped negative-sense, single-stranded RNA virus. The virus has been reported in a wide area from South Africa through southern Europe, Eurasia, and into parts of western China. The virus is principally associated with ticks of the genus *Hyalomma*, although it has also been isolated from other genera of ixodid ticks. The global distribution of the virus roughly approximates that of *Hyalomma* spp ticks. Recent analyses of the genome of the virus suggest that there is significant genetic diversity somewhat correlated with geographic origin of the virus. However, anomalies to this pattern suggest that dispersal of host ticks by migratory wildlife such as birds or the movement of livestock by humans may act to perturb the "normal" geographic distribution of CCHF virus subpopulations.

Transmission and Pathogenesis: The virus replicates in the host tick as it passes from larval through adult stages (trans-stadial transmission) and can also be transmitted from one generation to the next (transovarial transmission). Thus, the tick not only is a vector but also can be a reservoir of the virus via vertical transmission. Vertebrates ranging from small rodents, lagomorphs, and birds have all been incriminated as sources of infection of immature stages of the tick, while most *Hyalomma* spp ticks are multihost and use larger vertebrates as the host for the adult stage of their life cycle.

Clinical Findings and Diagnosis: In experimental inoculations, sheep and cattle become infected but develop only transient and mild increases of body temperature with little evidence of clinical disease. Viremia levels and duration are relatively low and short, and antibodies are detectable shortly after cessation of viremia. Some tests (principally IgG ELISA) can detect antibodies for the remainder of the life of the animal, while other tests, such as complement fixation and indirect fluorescent antibody, can detect antibodies for shorter periods after infection. Antibody prevalence in adult livestock species in endemic regions can be >50%.

Treatment: The antiviral drug ribavirin has been used in treatment of human disease in South Africa, although placebo-controlled trials have not been completed. Lack of significant clinical disease in livestock warrants no treatment considerations.

Control and Prevention: Control strategies for human infection include the avoidance of tick bites through use of repellents and appropriate protection when slaughtering or grooming animals. Medical personnel should use appropriate barrier nursing techniques and universal precautions when handling suspect patients.

EPHEMERAL FEVER

(Three-day sickness)

Ephemeral fever is an insect-transmitted, noncontagious, viral disease of cattle and water buffalo that is seen in Africa, the Middle East, Australasia (excluding Papua New Guinea and New Zealand), and Asia south of the former USSR. Inapparent infections can develop in cape buffalo, hartebeest, waterbuck, wildebeest, deer, and possibly goats.

Etiology and Epidemiology: Ephemeral fever virus is classified as a Rhabdovirus (single-stranded, negative sense RNA). It is best isolated from infected cattle by inoculation of mosquito (*Aedes albopictus*) cell cultures with defibrinated blood, followed by transfer to baby hamster kidney (BHK-21) or monkey kidney (Vero) cell cultures after 15 days. Suckling mice may also be used for primary isolation by intracerebral inoculation. Both BHK-21 and Vero cell lines can be used to grow the virus and to conduct serologic tests.

The virus can be transmitted from infected to susceptible cattle by IV inoculation; as little as 0.005 mL of blood collected during the febrile stage is infective. Although the virus has been recovered from several *Culicoides* species and from Anopheline and Culicine mosquito species collected in the field, the identity of the major vectors has not been proved. Transmission by contact or fomites does not occur, and the virus does not appear to persist in recovered cattle. Most recovered cattle have a lifelong immunity.

The prevalence, geographic range, and severity of the disease vary from year to year, and epidemics occur periodically. During epidemics, onset is rapid; many animals are affected within days or 2-3 wk. Ephemeral fever is most prevalent in the wet season in the tropics and in summer to early autumn in the subtropics or temperate regions (when conditions favor multiplication of biting insects); it disappears abruptly in winter. Morbidity may be as high as 80%; overall mortality is usually 1-2%, although it can be higher in lactating cows, bulls in good condition, and fat steers (10-30%).

Clinical Findings: Signs, which occur suddenly and vary in severity, include biphasic to polyphasic fever, shivering, inappetence, lacrimation, serous nasal discharge, drooling, dyspnea, atony of forestomachs, depression, stiffness and lameness, and a sudden decrease in milk yield. Affected cattle may become recumbent and paralyzed for 8 hr to >1 wk. After recovery, milk production often fails to return to normal levels until the next lactation. Abortion, with total loss of the season's lactation, occurs in ~5% of cows pregnant for 8-9 mo. The virus does not appear to cross the placenta or affect the fertility of the cow. Bulls, heavy cattle, and high-lactating dairy cows are the most severely affected, but spontaneous recovery usually occurs within a few days. More insidious losses may result from decreased muscle mass and lowered fertility in bulls.

Lesions: Ephemeral fever is an inflammatory disease. The most common lesions include polyserositis affecting joint, tendon, pleural, and peritoneal surfaces; cellulitis; and focal necrosis of skeletal muscles. Generalized edema of lymph nodes and lungs and atelectasis may also be present.

Diagnosis: Diagnosis is based almost entirely on clinical signs in an epidemic. All clinical cases have a neutrophilia with the presence of many immature forms, although this is not pathognomonic.

Laboratory confirmation is by serology, rarely by virus isolation. Whole blood should be collected from sick and apparently healthy cattle in affected herds. Samples must be sufficient to provide 2 air-dried blood smears, 5 mL in anticoagulant (not EDTA), and 20 mL for serum.

Isolated viruses are identified by neutralization tests using specific ephemeral fever virus antisera and by ELISA using specific monoclonal antibodies. The neutralization test and the blocking ELISA are recommended for antibody detection and give similar results. A 4-fold rise in antibody titer between paired sera collected 2-3 wk apart confirms infection.

Treatment and Control: Complete rest is the most effective treatment, and recovering animals should not be stressed or worked because relapse is likely. Anti-inflammatory drugs given early and in repeated doses for 2-3 days are effective. Oral dosing should be avoided unless the swallowing reflex is functional. Signs of hypocalcemia are treated as for milk fever (p 806). Antibiotic treatment to control secondary infection and rehydration with isotonic fluids may be warranted.

Attenuated virus vaccines appear to be effective but should be used only in endemic areas. Inactivated virus vaccines have not produced longterm protection against experimental challenge with virulent virus and cannot guarantee lasting immunity, but they may boost immunity produced by live virus vaccine. The efficacy of vector control remains uncertain because the insect vectors have not been fully identified.

HEARTWATER

(Cowdriosis)

Heartwater is an infectious, noncontagious, rickettsial disease of ruminants in areas infested by ticks of the genus *Amblyomma*. These include regions of Africa south of the Sahara and the islands of the Comores, Zanzibar, Madagascar, Sao Tomé, Réunion, and Mauritius. Heartwater and its vector are also endemic on the islands of Guadeloupe and Antigua. Possible spread to the American mainland threatens the livestock industry of regions from northern South America to Central America and the southern USA. Many ruminants, including some antelope species, are susceptible. Some animals may become subclinically infected and act as reservoirs. Indigenous African cattle breeds (*Bos indicus*) appear more resistant than *B taurus* breeds.

Etiology and Transmission: The causative organism is an obligate intracellular parasite, previously known as *Cowdria ruminantium*. Molecular evidence led to reclassification of several organisms in the order Rickettsiales, and it is now classified as *Ehrlichia ruminantium*. Under natural conditions, *E ruminantium* is transmitted by *Amblyomma* ticks. These 3-host ticks become infected during either larval or nymphal stages and transmit the infection during one of the subsequent stages (trans-stadial transmission). The progeny of an infected female tick are most probably not infective (ie, there is no epidemiologically significant transovarial transmission). Therefore, the infection rate in tick populations tends to be low. Intrastadial transmission by male ticks may also occur, as well as some degree of vertical transmission from cow to calf (eg, via colostrum), in areas where the disease is endemic.

E ruminantium can be propagated experimentally by serial passage, either by inoculating infective blood into, or by feeding infected nymphal or adult stages of a vector tick on susceptible animals. The organism can also be propagated in tissue culture, most reliably in endothelial cells, but also in primary neutrophil cultures and macrophages. At room temperature, infective material loses its infectivity within a few hours, but the organisms, together with suitable cryoprotectants, may be viably preserved in liquid nitrogen for years.

Immunity to heartwater appears to be chiefly, if not exclusively, cell mediated. There is no, or only partial, cross-protection between different strains (stocks) of *E ruminantium*. Most of these stocks are infective for, but cannot be serially passaged in, mice; however, a few are pathogenic to mice infected by the IV route. One of these, the Kümm stock, can even be passaged by the intraperitoneal route. Molecular analysis recently established that the traditional Kümm stock actually was made up of organisms of 2 distinct genotypes.

Clinical Findings, Pathogenesis, and Lesions: The signs are dramatic in the peracute and acute forms. In peracute cases, animals develop fever, followed rapidly by hyperesthesia, lacrimation, and convulsions. In the acute form, animals show anorexia and nervous signs such as depression, a high-stepping stiff gait, exaggerated blinking of eyes, and chewing movements. Both forms terminate in prostration and convulsions. Diarrhea is occasionally seen. In subacute cases, the signs are less marked, and CNS involvement is inconsistent.

E ruminantium seems to initially reproduce in macrophages and then invades and multiplies in the vascular endothelium. During the febrile stage, and for a short while thereafter, the blood is infective to susceptible animals if subinoculated. Signs and lesions are associated with functional injury to the vascular endothelium, resulting in increased vascular permeability. The concomitant fluid effusion into tissues and body cavities precipitates a fall in arterial pressure and general circulatory failure. The lesions in peracute and acute cases are hydrothorax, hydropericardium, edema and congestion of the lungs and brain, splenomegaly, petechiae and ecchymoses on the mucosal and serosal surfaces, and occasionally hemorrhage into the GI tract, particularly the abomasum.

Diagnosis: Clinical cases must be differentiated from a wide range of infectious and noninfectious diseases, especially plant poisonings, that manifest with CNS signs. In acute clinical cases in endemic areas, clinical signs alone may suggest the etiology, but demonstration of colonies of organisms in the cytoplasm of capillary endothelial cells is necessary for definitive diagnosis. Traditionally, this is done with "squash" smears of cerebral or cerebellar gray matter, stained with Romanowsky-type stains, of which low concentration Giemsa affords the best color differentiation. Organisms in autolyzed material lose their stainability, and diagnosis then becomes difficult. For the "brain squash smear," a piece of gray matter (~3 × 3 mm) is macerated between 2 glass slides; the softened material is then spread like a blood smear. A slight lifting of the spreader slide about every 5-10 mm creates several thick ridges across the slide, from which capillaries are arranged straight and parallel in the thin sections of the smear for easier examination. The endothelial cells of all capillaries on a smear should be carefully scrutinized for the presence of the dark purple rickettsial colonies of *E ruminantium*. Using an immunoperoxidase staining method, a definitive diagnosis can be made on any formalinized tissue samples, even from autolyzed carcasses. The contrasting color makes the search much faster, although the substructure of the rickettsial colonies should be identified before the diagnosis is confirmed. Due to the nature of the test, false-positive reactions may arise with some closely related organisms. *Chlamydophila pecorum* on brian squash smears may be confused with *E ruminantium*, but histopathology or the immunoperoxidase technique allow differentiation. Serodiagnosis of animals previously exposed to the disease, ie, recovered from subclinical or clinical infection, still poses problems. Several tests are currently in use, including several indirect fluorescent antibody and ELISA tests. All serologic tests, including an ELISA that uses recombinant antigen, are plagued by cross reaction with sera from animals infected with one of several *Ehrlichia* or *Anaplasma* organisms (false positive) and the fact that immune cattle on repeated exposure may become seronegative (false negative). Several DNA probes, available at research institutions, can be used together with PCR technology. A combination of a pCS20 probe and probes to 16S rRNA of several of the stocks are routinely used to examine samples from animals when permits for importation into nonendemic areas are required.

Treatment and Control: There is as yet no widely effective and safe vaccine available to immunize against *E ruminantium*. Control of tick infestation is a useful preventive measure in some instances but may be difficult and expensive to maintain in others. Excessive reduction of tick numbers, however, interferes with the maintenance of adequate immunity through regular field challenge in endemic areas and may result in heavy losses. For immunization, the "infection and treatment method" is still in use in southern Africa—infected sheep blood, containing fully virulent organisms, is used for infection, followed by monitoring of rectal temperature and antibiotic therapy after fever develops. In certain conditions, the controlled infection is followed by preventive "block treatment" without temperature recording (cattle on day 14 [susceptible *Bos taurus* breeds] or day 16 [resistant *B indicus* breeds], and small stock on day 11). In South Africa, a doxycycline implant is available for SC deposition behind the ear at the time of infection. Young calves (<6-8 wk old) and lambs and kids (<1 wk old) are fairly resistant and may recover spontaneously from natural or induced infections. If immunized at that early age, block treatment can be avoided. Oxytetracycline at 10 mg/kg or doxycycline at 2 mg/kg usually effect a cure, if administered early in the course of the disease. In sheep, goats, and susceptible cattle breeds, a higher dosage (10-20 mg/kg) of oxytetracycline may be required, particularly if treatment begins late during the febrile reaction or after other clinical signs appear. In such cases, the first treatment should preferably be given IV. A second and third treatment may be necessary before the fever abates, or a second injection IM with a long-acting tetracycline formulation may be given. In the USA, the appropriate withdrawal times for milk and meat after treatment with doxycycline or short- or long-acting oxytetracyclines must be observed. Corticosteroids have been used as supportive therapy (prednisolone, 1 mg/kg), although there is debate as to their effectiveness and appropriateness of their use in an active infectious disease. Inactivated, attenuated and recombinant vaccines are currently being developed but are at an experimental stage.

HISTOPHILOSIS

(Thrombotic meningoencephalitis)

Histophilosis is a common disease in North American, primarily Canadian, cattle feedlots. It also is seen sporadically in individual beef and dairy cattle worldwide. *Histophilus somni* (formerly *Haemophilus somnus*) can cause an acute, often fatal, septicemic disease that can involve the respiratory, cardiovascular, musculoskeletal, or nervous systems, either singly or together. The reproductive system is often affected but usually without clinical signs and without other systemic involvement.

Etiology and Transmission: *H somni* is a gram-negative, nonmotile, nonsporeforming, nonencapsulated, pleomorphic coccobacillus that requires an enriched medium and a microaerophilic atmosphere for culture. Hemolysis on blood agar occurs within 48 hr due to an exotoxin produced by most disease-causing isolates. Pathogenic and nonpathogenic strains have been differentiated. The virulence of the organism may vary by region and age group.

H somni is considered a commensal of bovine mucous membranes. Pathogenic and nonpathogenic strains of *H somni* are found in the sheath and prepuce of males, the vagina of females, and in the nasal passages of both sexes. Nasal and urogenital secretions are believed to be sources of the organism. The organism may colonize the respiratory tract, presumably after inhalation, and gain access to the bloodstream via that route. Colonization of the male and female reproductive tracts may involve venereal spread.

Epidemiology: All feedlot cattle are at risk of histophilosis for the duration of the feeding period. However, recently weaned calves are at higher risk of infection and death from histophilosis than are previously weaned older calves, yearlings, or mature animals. The risk of infection with *H somni* is highest early in the feeding period with high-risk calves in the feedlot establishing peak titers to *H somni* at ~21-23 days on feed. Although calves are generally exposed to *H somni* earlier in the feeding period, the average days on feed at death of calves that die of histophilosis is 30-60 days. Sudden death due to peracute septicemia, especially, may occur throughout the feeding period. Sporadic reproductive disease manifestations, including sporadic abortion and mastitis, are seen in individual beef and dairy cattle.

Pathogenesis: Septicemia is likely required for most forms of histophilosis. Strains of *H somni* that cause disease adhere to the endothelium of vessels, resulting in contraction, exposure of collagen, platelet adhesion, and thrombus formation. The primary lesion likely involves a thrombus, rather than a thromboembolism as once thought. Strains may adhere to endothelium in vessels of the pleura, myocardium, pericardium, synovium, or a variety of other tissues (eg, brain, larynx). Interruption of the blood supply in those areas results in destruction of tissue and the development of clinical signs associated with the organ system involved. The susceptibility of individual animals and variations in the preference of strains of the organism for vessels in different tissues may be important in the development of the different forms of the disease, but the mechanisms involved are incompletely understood. Reproductive problems may not necessarily be preceded by bacteremia, but the pathogenesis in those situations is poorly defined.

Clinical Findings: Sudden death is often the first indication of *H somni* infection in a feedlot animal. A profound depression is often the most noticeable clinical sign of histophilosis. Fever is also a common finding; however, animals diagnosed with undifferentiated fever may be suffering from *Mannheimia* pneumonia, histophilosis, or both. Other findings are determined by the system(s) involved and may include rapid respiration, stiffness, muscle weakness, ataxia, paralysis, and opisthotonos. Specifically, animals affected with the fibrinous pleuritic form of the disease may exhibit extreme dyspnea; animals with myocarditis may exhibit sudden collapse and death on exertion (eg, being moved through a handling facility); and animals with the nervous form are predominantly depressed with occasional signs of hyperesthesia (eg, convulsions) prior to death.

Animals found dead and confirmed with *H somni* infection often have a history of having been treated for undifferentiated fever or depression in the previous 14 days.

Lesions: Feedlot cattle that die of peracute or acute disease may exhibit postmortem lesions including fibrinous pleuritis, a myocardial infarct or abscess in the papillary muscle of the left ventricle, fibrinous pericarditis, fibrinopurulent bronchopneumonia, polyarthritis, and a fibrinous or abscessed laryngitis. Less common gross postmortem lesions include polyserositis, visible fibrin in the stifle joint fluid, and a fibrinopurulent meningitis with cloudy CSF. Lesions of the reproductive tract may include suppurative vaginitis, cervicitis, and endometritis.

Diagnosis: A definitive diagnosis is based on sampling and examination of affected tissues collected during a postmortem or clinical examination. Isolation of the organism from CSF, brain, blood, urine, joint fluid, or other sterile, internal organs or fluids confirms the diagnosis. Because *H somni* is a commensal of the mucous membranes of cattle, the bacterium should be isolated in predominant or pure culture from the respiratory or urogenital tract to be considered a significant etiologic agent. Characteristic histologic lesions include severe vasculitis, vascular thrombosis, infarction, necrosis, and heavy infiltrations of neutrophils in all tissues where localization of the bacteria occurs. Treatment often interferes with recovery of the organism; as a result, the diagnosis may need to be confirmed with immunohistochemical staining techniques.

Treatment and Prevention: A major hindrance to successful antimicrobial treatment of individual histophilosis cases is the difficulty in identifying affected animals early in the course of disease due to its often rapidly fatal nature. Antimicrobial treatment is most effective in the early stages of disease. Prophylactic administration of injectable oxytetracycline on arrival at the feedlot (or within a few days of arrival) has not significantly affected mortality due to histophilosis. However, a commercially available, oral formulation of chlortetracycline and sulfamethazine fed for the first 56 days of the feeding period has significantly reduced overall mortality due to histophilosis. *H somni* is susceptible in vitro to a wide range of antimicrobials including florfenicol, tilmicosin, tetracyclines, trimethoprim-sulfadoxine, fluoroquinolones and ceftiofur. Florfenicol (20 mg/kg, IM, repeated in 48 hr, or 40 mg/kg, SC, once) may be the antimicrobial of choice if *H somni* is a major cause of mortality in feedlot calves.

Bacterins containing different strains of the organism have been used to immunize cattle against *H somni*. The humoral response generated by different commercial vaccines has been described, but the ability of current vaccines to protect cattle from *H somni*-associated morbidity and mortality is not completely understood.

HEMORRHAGIC SEPTICEMIA

Hemorrhagic septicemia (HS) is an acute pasteurellosis, caused by particular serotypes of *Pasteurella multocida* and manifested by an acute and highly fatal septicemia principally in cattle and water buffaloes; the latter are thought to be more susceptible. HS is seen infrequently in swine and even less commonly in sheep and goats. It has been reported in bison, camels, elephants, horses, and donkeys, and there is evidence of its occurrence in yak. An acute pasteurellosis indistinguishable from HS is seen infrequently in deer, elk, and probably other feral ruminants. Laboratory rabbits and mice are highly susceptible to experimental infection.

HS is a major disease of cattle and water buffalo in Asia, Africa, and some countries of southern Europe and the Middle East. Although it may be seen at any time of year, the worst epidemics occur during the rainy season. It is most common in the river valleys and deltas of southeast Asia among buffaloes used in rice cultivation. The only true outbreaks in North America have occurred in bison in Yellowstone National Park. Occurrence in Central and South America has not been confirmed.

The HS serotypes of *P multocida* have not been recovered from human infections. However, because many serotypes of *P multocida* have the potential to infect humans, appropriate precautions should be taken.

Etiology: Epidemic HS is caused by 1 of 2 serotypes of *P multocida*, designated B:2 and E:2. Serotype E:2 has been recovered only in Africa; B:2 causes the disease elsewhere and also has been recovered from cases in Egypt and the Sudan. Serotypes closely related antigenically to serotype B:2 have been implicated in limited outbreaks of a disease indistinguishable from HS in deer and elk. *P multocida* is an extracellular parasite, and immunity is primarily humoral.

Transmission, Epidemiology, and Pathogenesis: Animals are infected by direct or indirect contact. The source of infective bacteria is thought to be the nasopharynx of bovine or buffalo carriers. As many as 5% of cattle and water buffaloes may be carriers in endemic regions.

It is hypothesized that animals become susceptible as a result of various stresses, eg, the inanition seen in cattle and water buffalo at the beginning of the rainy season. Natural infection is acquired by ingestion or inhalation. The initial site of proliferation is thought to be the tonsillar region. In susceptible animals, a septicemia develops rapidly, and death due to endotoxemia ensues within 8-24 hr after the first signs develop. Exotoxins have not been demonstrated.

The mortality rate is high when the agent is introduced to virgin or nonendemic regions. Losses vary widely in endemic areas. The heaviest losses occur during the monsoon rains in southeast Asia, and it is thought that the organisms, which can survive for hours and probably days in the moist soil and water, are transmitted widely at this time.

Clinical Findings: Most cases are acute or peracute, resulting in death within 8-24 hr after onset. Because the course is so short, clinical signs may easily be overlooked. Animals first evince dullness, then reluctance to move, fever, salivation, and serous nasal discharge. Edematous swelling is frequently seen, beginning in the throat region and spreading to the parotid region, neck, and brisket. Mucous membranes are congested. There is respiratory distress, and usually the animal goes down and dies within hours. Occasional cases linger for several days. Recovery is rare. There appears to be no chronic form.

Lesions: The most obvious changes in affected animals are the edema, widely distributed hemorrhages, and general hyperemia. In most cases, there is an edematous swelling of the head, neck, and brisket region. Incision of the swellings reveals a clear or straw-colored serous fluid. The edema is also found in the musculature, and the subserous petechial hemorrhages, which are found throughout the animal, are particularly characteristic. Blood-tinged fluid is often found in the pericardial sac and in the thoracic and abdominal cavities. Petechial hemorrhages are particularly prominent in the pharyngeal and cervical lymph nodes. Gastroenteritis is seen only occasionally and, unlike in pneumonic pasteurellosis, pneumonia usually is not extensive.

Diagnosis: Some characteristic epidemiologic and clinical features aid in the recognition of HS. Of particular significance is a history of earlier outbreaks and a recent failure to vaccinate. Sporadic cases are more difficult to diagnose clinically. The season of the year, rapid course, and high herd incidence, with fever and edematous swellings indicate typical HS. Characteristic necropsy lesions support the clinical diagnosis. Although typical outbreaks are not difficult to recognize clinically, particularly in endemic regions, acute salmonellosis, anthrax, pneumonic pasteurellosis, and rinderpest should be considered.

A presumptive diagnosis is based on the isolation of *P multocida* from the blood and vital organs of an animal with typical signs. Definitive diagnosis depends on identifying the serotype as B:2 (or closely related serotypes) or E:2. Other serotypes cause various infections in cattle and buffalo but not typical HS. The passive mouse protection test using specific B:2 and E:2 immune rabbit sera is used in Asia and Africa to identify these serotypes. More precise tests, such as indirect hemagglutination, coagglutination, and counterimmunoelectrophoresis and immunodiffusion tests, are available in some laboratories.

If there is postmortem decomposition, the causative agent may be obscured by overgrowth of extraneous bacteria. In such cases, the subcutaneous inoculation of mice or rabbits with small amounts of blood and tissue suspensions facilitates the recovery of the pasteurellae in pure or nearly pure culture.

Serologic tests are of no value in diagnosis. However, the indirect hemagglutination procedure and passive mouse protection test are of value in determining the immune status of animals.

Treatment and Prevention: Various sulfonamides, tetracyclines, penicillin, and chloramphenicol (where its use is permitted) are effective if administered early. Because of the rapid course of the disease and the frequent difficulty of access to animals, antimicrobial therapy often is not practicable. Although multiple antibiotic resistance has been reported for some strains of *P multocida*, it has not been described for the HS serotypes.

The principal means of prevention is by vaccination. Three kinds of vaccine are widely used: plain bacterin, alum-type precipitated bacterin, and oil-adjuvant bacterin. The most effective bacterin is the oil-adjuvant—one dose provides protection for 9-12 mo; it should be administered annually. The alum-precipitated-type bacterin is given at 6-mo intervals. Maternal antibody interferes with vaccine efficacy in calves. The oil-adjuvant vaccine has not been popular because of difficulty in syringing and occasional adverse tissue reactions. A live intranasal vaccine prepared from a B:3,4 serotype of deer origin is being used with reported success in southeast Asia.

MALIGNANT CATARRHAL FEVER

(Malignant head catarrh, Snotsiekte, Catarrhal fever, Gangrenous coryza)

Malignant catarrhal fever (MCF) is an infectious systemic disease that presents as a variable complex of lesions affecting mainly ruminants and rarely swine. It is principally a disease of domestic cattle, water buffalo, Bali cattle (banteng), American bison, and deer. In addition to these farmed animals, MCF has been described in a variety of captive ruminants in mixed zoologic collections. In some species, such as bison and some deer, MCF is acute and highly lethal, capable of affecting large numbers of animals. With occasional exceptions, the disease in cattle normally is seen sporadically and affects single animals. MCF is typically fatal; however, there are outbreaks in which several animals are affected, with evidence of recovery and mild or inapparent infections in some cases. It also occasionally presents as chronic alopecia and weight loss. Its distribution is essentially worldwide, mirroring that of the principal carriers, domestic sheep and wildebeest. MCF has long been a major problem in farmed deer operations, and in recent years has emerged as a severe threat to the commercial bison industry.

Etiology: MCF results from infection by one of several members of a group of closely related ruminant gammaherpesviruses of the Rhadinovirus genus. While the MCF group of ruminant rhadinoviruses currently comprises about 10 known members, only a few are known to be pathogenic under natural conditions. The principal carriers and their viruses are sheep (ovine herpesvirus-2), wildebeest (alcelaphine herpesvirus-1), and goats (caprine herpesvirus-2). Another strain of unidentified origin has caused MCF in white-tailed deer. Virtually all clinical cases are caused by the sheep or wildebeest viruses.

The viruses are maintained within the sheep and wildebeest populations in similar but not identical patterns. Lambs are infected usually at 1-2 mo of age by aerosol transmission from other individuals within the flock and begin to actively shed virus at ~6 mo of age. Shedding decreases at ~10 mo, with adults shedding at a much lower rate than adolescents. Wildebeest calves, in contrast, are infected in the perinatal period by horizontal and occasional intrauterine transmission, and actively shed virus until 3-4 mo of age. Transmission is by transfer of virus-laden nasal secretions by direct contact or poorly defined airborne routes. In Africa, most wildebeest-associated MCF is seen around the time of calving; however, sheep-associated MCF (SA-MCF) does not follow the same pattern. Ewes do not shed virus in placental tissues or secretions and do not experience more frequent shedding episodes around lambing time. The only rational and established factors contributing to seasonality of SA-MCF are climatic influences on virus survival and the age-related shedding patterns in lambs. The epidemiology of the caprine MCF virus appears similar to that of sheep.

The severity of SA-MCF outbreaks depends on factors such as the total numbers, population density, and species of susceptible hosts involved; the closeness of contact; and the amount of shed virus available for transmission. Cases usually are seen sporadically in European breeds of cattle (*Bos taurus*), as they are a relatively resistant species. By contrast, Bali cattle, bison, and some but not all cervid species (eg, white-tailed deer, Pere David's deer) are highly susceptible. As agricultural systems involving bison and deer production have developed, MCF has become more troublesome. It is a leading cause of infectious disease losses on New Zealand deer farms. In bison exposed to large numbers of adolescent sheep, losses can be devastating. About 800 head died in one outbreak in the USA in 2003.

Among animals that survive, infection is lifelong; some susceptible species may be latently infected. Recrudescence of latent infections is common and must be considered for cases with no known history of contact with carriers.

MCF is transmitted only between carriers and clinically susceptible animals. Affected animals do not transmit MCF to their cohorts.

Clinical Findings: Acute MCF cases caused by ovine herpesvirus-2 and alcelaphine herpesvirus-1 are similar clinically and pathologically. Disease course may range from peracute to chronic. Cases in deer are often peracute with sudden death. Deer that survive for a few days and bison usually develop hemorrhagic diarrhea, bloody urine, and corneal opacity before expiring. High fever (106°-107°F [41-41.5°C]) and depression are common. Other signs that may be present include catarrhal inflammation; erosions and mucopurulent exudation affecting the upper respiratory, ocular, and oral mucosa; swollen lymph nodes; lameness; and CNS signs (depression, trembling, hyporesponsiveness, stupor, aggressiveness, convulsions). Historically, MCF has been described as having several "forms"—mild, peracute, head and eye, intestinal, etc. There is little basis for this division and it is of little utility. Variation in organ system involvement sometimes can be seen in the same outbreak, and is at least partially related to survival time after disease onset. On average, the time to death in European cattle breeds is somewhat longer than in deer, bison, water buffalo, and Bali cattle. In cattle, swollen lymph nodes and severe eye lesions (panophthalmitis, hypopyon, corneal erosions) are more frequent, and hemorrhagic enteritis and cystitis less frequent, than in deer and bison. Skin lesions (erythema, exudation, cracking, crust formation) are common in animals that do not succumb quickly. Up to 25% of cattle experience chronic disease, and sometimes the disease waxes and wanes. Most eventually die, but ~5% clinically recover. Hematologic parameters are not rewarding.

In a few outbreaks, the goat MCF virus (caprine herpesvirus-2) induced disease in white-tailed and Sika deer. These cases were subacute to chronic, with weight loss, dermal inflammation, and alopecia as the primary signs. Whether this strain of virus causes disease in species other than deer is not known.

Lesions: The disease is systemic, and lesions may be found in any organ, although severity and frequency varies greatly. The principal lesions are inflammation and necrosis of respiratory, alimentary, or urinary mucosal epithelium; subepithelial lymphoid infiltration; generalized lymphoid proliferation and necrosis; and widespread vasculitis. Mucosal ulcerations and hemorrhage are common. Hemorrhages any be present in many parenchymatous organs, particularly lymph nodes. A classic but not pathognomonic histologic lesion is fibrinoid necrosis of small muscular arteries, but vessels of all types may be inflamed, including those in the brain. Prominent white nodules representing intramural and perivascular proliferation may be apparent, particularly in the kidney.

Diagnosis: Diagnosis of MCF is based on clinical signs, gross and histologic lesions, and laboratory confirmation. Primary differential diagnoses include bovine viral diarrhea/

mucosal disease, rinderpest, infectious bovine rhinotracheitis, and East Coast fever (theileriosis). When CNS involvement is prominent, MCF can resemble rabies and the tickborne encephalitides. A history of contact with a carrier species (sheep, goats, or wildebeest) can be helpful, although recrudescent cases can be seen without such a history. Reliable and specific laboratory assays for antibody and for viral DNA are available. The test of choice for clinical diagnosis is PCR to detect viral DNA. Preferred tissues for testing are anticoagulated blood, kidney, intestinal wall, lymph node, and brain.

Serology is used for surveying normal animals and is indicative only of infection—latent infection among susceptible animals may render serology alone inconclusive evidence of current disease. Several seroassays are available, including viral neutralization, immunoperoxidase, immunofluorescence, and ELISA. The polyclonal assays are hampered by cross-reactivity. The monoclonal-based competitive ELISA is currently the most specific and detects antibody against all of the known MCF group viruses. Only PCR can discriminate between the different viruses.

Treatment and Control: The prognosis is grave. No treatment has been found to provide any consistent benefit. Stress reduction of subclinical or mildly affected animals is indicated. No vaccine is available. Sheep can be produced that are free of virus by early weaning and isolation. The only other effective control strategy is separation of carriers from susceptible species. When large numbers of potent shedders are present, such as in lamb feedlots, considerable distances are necessary to protect highly susceptible species such as bison.

NAIROBI SHEEP DISEASE

Nairobi sheep disease is a tickborne viral disease of sheep and goats characterized by fever and hemorrhagic gastroenteritis, abortion, and high mortality. It has been reported in Kenya, Uganda, Tanzania, Somalia, Ethiopia, Botswana, Mozambique, and Republic of Congo. Although humans are susceptible, human infections are rare. It is a reportable disease in the USA and is on List B of the OIE.

Etiology and Transmission: The causal nairovirus, family Bunyaviridae, is possibly the most pathogenic virus known for sheep and goats. It is identical to or closely related to Ganjam virus, a tickborne infection of sheep, goats, and humans in India; and is serologically related to Dugbe virus, another tickborne infection in cattle, and to Crimean-Congo hemorrhagic fever virus (p 602). It is transmitted transovarially and trans-stadially by the brown ear tick, *Rhipicephalus appendiculatus*, in which it can survive for up to 800 days. Other *Rhipicephalus* spp and *Amblyomma variegatum* ticks also may transmit the disease. The virus is shed in urine and feces, but the disease is not spread by contact.

Clinical Findings: A prodromal fever lasting 1-3 days follows an incubation period of 4-5 days. Sometimes, the fever is diphasic. Illness is manifest by depression; anorexia; mucopurulent, blood-stained, nasal discharge; and fetid dysentery that causes painful straining. Pregnant animals frequently abort. Death may occur in the early febrile viremic phase or follow ~2 days after remission of the fever. Experimental infection has shown that indigenous Persian fat-tailed and European breeds of sheep are equally susceptible; however, mortality rate in the field is as high as 70-90% for indigenous breeds of sheep and 30% for exotic and cross breeds. The disease in goats is usually less severe, although 80% mortality has been reported.

Lesions: The main lesions are enlarged and edematous lymph nodes and hemorrhages in the GI (particularly the abomasum), respiratory, and female genital tracts; gallbladder; spleen; and heart. Petechial and ecchymotic hemorrhages in the mucosa of the cecum and colon frequently appear as longitudinal striations and are sometimes the only lesion evident. Subserosal hemorrhages may be seen in the cecum, colon, gallbladder, and kidney.

Conjunctivitis with dried crusts around the nostrils is often noted. Common histopathologic lesions are hyperplasia of lymphoid tissues, myocardial degeneration, nephrosis, and necrosis of the gallbladder.

Diagnosis: The occurrence of a disease in sheep or goats with high mortality accompanied by a tick infestation is suggestive, especially if it follows movements into endemic areas or changes in tick populations that have been induced by heavy and prolonged rainfall. Confirmation of suggestive signs and lesions requires detection of virus or viral antigen and antibodies. The preferred specimens are plasma from febrile animals, mesenteric lymph nodes, spleen, and serum. Mouse inoculation and cell cultures can be used for primary isolation of virus. Agar gel immunodiffusion, complement fixation, and ELISA can be valuable for detection of antigen in the infected tissues or tissue culture. Antibodies in infected or recovered animals can be detected by immunodiffusion, complement fixation, indirect fluorescent antibody tests, hemagglutination, and ELISA.

Differential diagnoses should include rinderpest, peste des petits ruminants, Rift Valley fever, heartwater, and salmonellosis.

Treatment and Control: No specific antiviral agent is available for treatment. Unaffected animals in the flock may be treated with acaricides (eg, pyrethroids in a grease, cypermethrin "pour on" products, various dip preparations). Longterm tick control is not cost effective in endemic areas.

In endemic areas, clinical signs are not seen unless susceptible animals are introduced. Such animals should be vaccinated, as should those exposed when the range of the tick vector extends. Two types of experimental vaccines have been developed—a modified live virus vaccine attenuated in mouse brain and an inactivated oil adjuvant vaccine. A single dose of the modified live vaccine produces rapid immunity; however, revaccination is necessary to maintain full protection. Two doses of the inactivated vaccine are required to elicit good protection. Neither of these vaccines is produced commercially.

PARATUBERCULOSIS

(Johne's disease)

Paratuberculosis is a chronic, contagious granulomatous enteritis characterized in cattle by persistent diarrhea, progressive weight loss, debilitation, and eventually death. It is considered a List B disease by the OIE. The etiologic agent, *Mycobacterium paratuberculosis*, is believed capable of infecting and causing disease in all other ruminants (eg, sheep, goats, llamas, deer) and in captive and free-ranging wildlife. The infection has also been recognized in omnivores and carnivores such as wild rabbits, foxes, weasels, as well as nonhuman primates. Distribution is worldwide. National control programs include those established in Australia, Norway, Iceland, Japan, The Netherlands, and the USA. The highest published prevalence is in dairy cattle with 20-50% of herds infected in many of the major dairy-producing countries. Limited information is available about the prevalence in other species. The disease is of economic importance for the goat industry in Spain and the sheep industry in Australia.

Etiology and Pathogenesis: *M paratuberculosis* is excreted in large numbers in feces of infected animals and in lower numbers in their colostrum and milk. It is resistant to environmental factors and can survive on pasture for >1 yr; survival in water is longer than in soil. The infection is usually acquired through the fecal-oral route; the dose needed to infect an animal is not known. Introduction of the disease into a noninfected herd is usually through herd expansion or replacement purchases; the infection is introduced via subclinically infected carriers.

Infection is acquired early in life—often soon after birth—but clinical signs rarely develop in cattle <2 yr old because progression to clinical disease occurs slowly. Resistance to infection increases with age, and cattle exposed as adults are much less likely to become infected. Infection is acquired by ingestion of the organism when nursing on contaminated teats; consumption of milk, solid feed, or water contaminated by the organism; or licking and grooming behavior in a contaminated environment. In the later, bacteremic stages of infection, intrauterine infections can be seen. After ingestion, and uptake in the Peyer's patches of the lower small intestine, this intracellular pathogen infects macrophages in the GI tract and in associated lymph nodes. It is possible that some animals may eliminate infection through a cell-mediated immune response that encourages microbiocidal activity in macrophages, but the frequency with which this occurs is unknown. In most cases, the organisms multiply and eventually provoke a chronic granulomatous enteritis that interferes with nutrient uptake and processing, leading to the cachexia typical of advanced infection. This may take months to years to develop and is usually paralleled by a decline in cell-mediated immunity, a rise in serum antibody, and bacteremia with dissemination of the infection beyond the GI tract. Fecal shedding begins before clinical signs are apparent, and animals in this "silent" stage of infection are important sources of transmission.

Clinical Findings: The disease in cattle is characterized by weight loss and diarrhea in the late phases of infection, but infected animals can appear healthy for months to years. In cattle, diarrhea may be constant or intermittent; in sheep, goats, and other ruminants, diarrhea may not be seen. It typically does not contain blood, mucus, or epithelial debris and is passed without tenesmus. Over weeks or months, the diarrhea becomes more severe, further weight loss occurs, coat color may fade, and ventral and intermandibular edema may develop due to a protein-losing enteropathy. This leads to low concentrations of total protein and albumin in plasma, although gamma globulin levels are normal. In dairy cattle and goats, milk yield may drop or fail to reach expected levels. Animals are alert, and temperature and appetite are usually normal, although thirst may be increased. The disease is progressive and ultimately terminates in emaciation and death. In infected herds, the mortality rate may be low for a number of years, but up to 50% of animals may be infected subclinically with associated production losses. The disease in sheep and goats is similar, but diarrhea is not a common feature and advanced cases may shed wool easily. In cervids (deer and elk), the course of the disease may be more rapid.

 Lesions: A diverse array of pathology may be seen in infected animals, ranging from a complete lack of gross lesions to a thickened and corrugated intestine with enlarged and edematous neighboring lymph nodes. Often, there is no correlation between clinical signs and the severity of lesions. Carcasses may be emaciated with loss of pericardial and perirenal fat in the more advanced, cachectic cases. Intestinal lesions can be mild, but typically the distal small-intestinal wall is diffusely thickened with a nonulcerated mucosa thrown into prominent transverse folds. Lesions may extend proximally and distally to the jejunum and colon. Serosal lymphangitis and enlargement of mesenteric and other regional lymph nodes are usually apparent. Histologically, there is a diffuse granulomatous enteritis characterized by the progressive accumulation of epithelioid macrophages and giant cells in the mucosa and submucosa of the gut. Sparse to myriad acid-fast organisms may be seen within the macrophages. Often, there is no correlation between clinical signs and the severity of lesions. Sheep, goats, and deer sometimes develop foci of caseation with calcification in the intestinal wall and lymph nodes.

Diagnosis: There are many commercially available tests for paratuberculosis, each with their own advantages, disadvantages, and appropriate application. The assays focus on detecting the organism in feces or tissue (culture, PCR), on finding evidence of cellular immune response to infection (skin testing, gamma interferon), or on detecting antibody to *M paratuberculosis* antigens (ELISA, agar gel immunodiffusion). Use of different tests in combination can increase diagnostic sensitivity. Given the biology of the infection and the need to manage it on a herd basis, diagnostic information should be gathered for a group of animals rather than for an individual case. An animal showing clinical signs of disease is more likely to provide diagnostic evidence of the infection (shedding, antibody production) than an animal at the preclinical stage of infection. Necropsy with culture and histopathology on multiple tissues is the gold standard for definitive diagnosis. Ziehl-Neelsen stains of tissue samples for acid-fast bacteria usually reveal abundant mycobacteria in lesions; however, in some cases, a careful search may still not reveal their presence. Acid-fast staining of an impression smear made from the ileum of a cow with typical pathology is a quick, low-cost (albeit insensitive) method to arrive at a preliminary diagnosis. Biopsy of full-thickness sections of ileum and regional lymph nodes for culture and histopathology may provide a definitive diagnosis; however, this approach is usually restricted to particularly valuable animals. *M paratuberculosis* has been isolated from a wide variety of tissue sites, but the mesenteric and ileocecal lymph nodes, ileum, and liver are most frequently recommended for diagnostic sampling.

Serologic tests are rapid, low-cost methods for antemortem confirmation of a clinical diagnosis; sensitivity is >85% in clinically affected animals. They are also useful tools for detection of infection in clinically normal cattle in the later stages of infection that are shedding large numbers of *M paratuberculosis*; sensitivity is ~45%. Of the serologic tests, those based on ELISA technology offer the highest sensitivity and specificity and are best used to determine the infection prevalence in a herd. Quantitative use of ELISA to identify animals for selective culling or isolation in herds may be a cost-effective strategy for disease control; higher ELISA values are associated with higher probabilities of infection and higher rates of fecal shedding. Fecal culture is more sensitive and more specific than serology, but the organism grows very slowly (2-4 mo) and the assay is more costly than serology. Pooling of fecal samples (eg, 5 samples per pool) can establish a herd's infection status at a lower cost, despite some reduction in test sensitivity. Proficiency at isolation of this pathogen varies significantly among laboratories. Use of a laboratory that has passed a proficiency test is recommended. Most strains infecting sheep will not grow on solid media but may be isolated using liquid culture media systems. Genetic probes for an element specific for *M paratuberculosis* DNA, such as IS900, can be used in conjunction with culture or directly on fecal samples. Some laboratories report that the PCR can be almost as sensitive and specific as fecal culture and is much more rapid; others do not find this to be true. Cost is its primary disadvantage. The performance of the PCR, as with other assays validated for use in cattle, may be different when used with samples from other species.

Tests of cell-mediated immunity, such as the intradermal Johnin test, lymphocyte transformation test, and γ–interferon, are used more on a research basis and may be negative in advanced clinical cases. The genome of *M paratuberculosis* has recently been described and may provide the basis for new diagnostic approaches.

Tests that have fallen out of favor due to reports of low sensitivity and/or specificity are microscopic examination of Ziehl-Neelsen-stained fecal samples and the IV Johnin test. The complement fixation (CF) test also reportedly is less accurate than other serologic tests. The CF test is still required by many countries for importation of animals, although many of the reagents used in the CF test are made to different specifications in different countries, resulting in a lack of standardization.

Control: No satisfactory treatment is known. Control requires good sanitation and management practices aimed at limiting the exposure of young animals to the organism. Calves, kids, or lambs should be birthed in areas free of manure, removed from the dam immediately after birth in the case of dairy cattle, bottle-fed colostrum that has been pasteurized or obtained from dams that test negative and then reared segregated as much as possible from adults and their manure until >1 yr old. Use of milk replacer is recommended instead of waste milk unless the milk has been pasteurized. A routine testing program for adults can help focus efforts in controlling the disease. Herds with confirmed cases should be tested to determine the infection prevalence. Animals testing positive, particularly those that are heavy shedders or have strong-positive ELISA results, should be sent to slaughter as soon as economically feasible. Retesting at least annually should be continued until herd tests indicate a low (<5%) infection prevalence. Because intrauterine infection can occur, in the more aggressive control programs, calves from dams that have or develop signs of the disease should be culled. Herd replacements should be obtained from herds believed to be free of the disease, and the replacements themselves should be tested prior to introduction to the new herd. More general procedures to minimize fecal contamination on the farm can also help, eg, elevating food and water troughs, providing piped water in preference to ponds, and harrowing frequently to disperse feces on pasture. Herd owners should be advised that paratuberculosis control takes at least 5 yr.

The formulation of *M paratuberculosis* vaccines vary by manufacture and, in many countries, their use is subject to approval by regulatory agencies and may be restricted to heavily infected herds. Vaccination of calves <1 mo of age can be effective in reducing disease incidence but does not prevent shedding or new cases of infection in the herd. Vaccination thus does not eliminate the need for good management and sanitation. In the goat industry in Spain, vaccination has increased productive herd life, and its use is being studied in sheep in Australia. Cattle inoculated with inactivated whole-cell, mineral-oil vaccine develop granulomas, one to several inches in diameter, at the site of inoculation (brisket) and may react positively on subsequent tuberculin tests. Accidental self-inoculation can result in severe acute reactions with sloughing and chronic synovitis and tendinitis.

Zoonotic Risk: There are conflicting data on the involvement of the causative organism in Crohn's disease, a chronic enteritis in humans of unknown etiology. However, *M paratuberculosis* has a broad host range, including nonhuman primates and, in rare cases, immunosuppressed humans. Animals with paratuberculosis thus should be considered as zoonotic risks until the situation is clarified.

PASTEURELLOSIS OF SHEEP AND GOATS

Pasteurella and *Mannheimia* organisms are nonmotile, nonsporeforming, aerobic, fermentative, gram-negative coccobacilli. They are distributed worldwide, and diseases caused by them are common in sheep and goats of all ages. *Mannheimia (Pasteurella) haemolytica* and *Pasteurella trehalosi* (formerly *P haemolytica* biotype T) are the species most often associated with disease. These organisms are the primary agents involved in respiratory disease, septicemia, arthritis, meningitis, and mastitis and may also be important secondary invaders in respiratory diseases of ruminants. There are 12 serotypes of *M haemolytica* and 4 of *P trehalosi* currently recognized on the basis of capsular antigens. *M haemolytica* is most commonly associated with pneumonic pasteurellosis (p 1232), while *P trehalosi* mainly causes septicemia and systemic pasteurellosis (*see* below) in young, weaned sheep. The virulence of *M haemolytica* and *P trehalosi* is mediated by the action of several factors (including endotoxin, leukotoxin, and capsular polysaccharide) that afford the bacteria advantages over host immunity and are important in the pathogenesis of disease. Pneumonic pasteurellosis can also be caused primarily or secondarily by *P multocida* in sheep and goats, and outbreaks worldwide lead to high mortality and great economic loss. *M haemolytica*, *P trehalosi*, and *P multocida* are common commensal organisms of the tonsils and nasopharynx of healthy sheep and goats. Transition from infection to disease appears to be facilitated by various stressors, including concurrent infections; changes in climate, pasture, or feed; and other management factors.

SYSTEMIC PASTEURELLOSIS

The systemic form of pasteurellosis is caused by *P trehalosi* and develops when the organism moves from the tonsils to the lungs and passes into the blood. This results in septicemia or localization of the infection in one or more tissues such as the joints, udder, meninges, or lungs. Systemic pasteurellosis is more common in sheep than goats. It most commonly is seen in young, weaned sheep (~6 mo old) during the late fall and winter after transport or a sudden feed change, but it can be seen in sheep of any age throughout the year. Sheep with septicemia often die quickly without premonitory signs. In some animals, pyrexia, dullness or coma, recumbency, dyspnea, and a frothy discharge from the mouth may be noted before death. Sheep or goats in which the infection becomes localized may survive long enough to demonstrate signs specific to the affected organ(s), but most do poorly in spite of treatment. Diagnosis is often based on clinical findings of sudden death, isolation of *P trehalosi* from a range of tissues, and gross and histopathologic findings. Lesions include subcutaneous hemorrhage; epithelial necrosis of the tongue, pharynx, esophagus, or occasionally the abomasum and intestine; enlargement of tonsils and retropharyngeal lymph nodes; and peracute, multifocal, embolic, necrotizing lesions in the lung and liver associated with bacteria of a consistent morphology. Treatment is frequently unrewarding due to diffuse infection or damage to organs but consists of antibiotics, fluid support, and anti-inflammatory agents. Gradual changes of feed and minimizing transport and other stressors may help decrease the incidence. Preventive vaccination may be beneficial.

PESTE DES PETITS RUMINANTS

Peste des petits ruminants (PPR) is an acute or subacute viral disease of goats and sheep characterized by fever, necrotic stomatitis, gastroenteritis, and pneumonia. It is also known as pseudorinderpest of small ruminants, pest of small ruminants, pest of sheep and goats, Kata, stomatitis-pneumoenteritis syndrome, contagious pustular stomatitis, and pneumoenteritis complex. It was first reported in the Ivory Coast in 1942 and subsequently in Senegal, Ghana, Togo, Benin, and Nigeria. Sheep are less susceptible than goats; cattle are only subclinically infected. Humans are not at risk.

Etiology and Epidemiology: The causal virus, a morbillivirus of the family Paramyxoviridae, has a particular affinity for lymphoid tissues and epithelial tissue of the GI and respiratory tracts, where it produces characteristic lesions.

PPR is present in west and central Africa and the Middle East. Generally, outbreaks that affect only a few animals are not reported; epidemics occur when the population of susceptible animals increases. Such an epidemic may eliminate the goats or sheep in an area. Because of strengthening surveillance and disease monitoring, as well as the establishment of good reporting systems in Africa and Asia as part of the global strategy to eradicate rinderpest, the prevalence of PPR has been better recognized, and reporting to OIE on PPR has increased.

Transmission: Transmission is by close contact, and confinement seems to favor outbreaks. Secretions and excretions of sick animals are the sources of infection. As in rinderpest, in PPR it is generally accepted that there is no carrier state; however, subclinical cases of PPR may spread the infection during the incubation phase. White-tailed deer are fully susceptible; these and other wild ruminants may play a role in the epidemiology of the disease. Pigs with experimentally induced subclinical infections do not transmit the disease to susceptible pigs or goats; therefore, pigs may have no role in PPR epidemiology. Although cattle are susceptible to infection, they usually do not exhibit clinical signs or transmit the disease.

Clinical Findings: The acute form of PPR is accompanied by a sudden rise in body temperature to 104-106°F (40-41.3°C). Affected animals appear ill and restless and have a dull coat, dry muzzle, congested mucous membranes, and depressed appetite. Early, the nasal discharge is serous; later, it becomes mucopurulent and gives a putrid odor to the breath. The incubation period is usually 4-5 days. Small areas of necrosis may be observed on the mucous membrane on the floor of the nasal cavity. The conjunctiva is frequently congested, and the medial canthus may exhibit a small degree of crusting. Some affected animals develop a profuse catarrhal conjunctivitis with matting of the eyelids. Necrotic stomatitis affects the lower lip and gum and the gumline of the incisor teeth; in more severe cases, it may involve the dental pad, palate, cheeks and their papillae, and the tongue. Diarrhea may be profuse and is accompanied by dehydration and emaciation; hypothermia and death follow, usually after 5-10 days. Bronchopneumonia, characterized by coughing, may develop at late stages of the disease. Pregnant animals may abort. Morbidity and mortality rates are higher in young animals than in adults. Latent infections may be activated and complicate the clinical picture.

Lesions: Emaciation, conjunctivitis, and stomatitis are seen; necrotic lesions are observed inside the lower lip and on the adjacent gum, the cheeks near the commissures, and on the ventral surface of the tongue. In severe cases, the lesions may extend to the hard palate and pharynx. The erosions are shallow, with a red, raw base and later become pinkish white; they are bounded by normal epithelium that provides a sharply demarcated margin. The rumen, reticulum, and omasum are rarely involved. The abomasum exhibits regularly outlined erosions that have red, raw floors and ooze blood.

Severe lesions are less common in the small intestines than in the mouth, abomasum, or large intestines. Streaks of hemorrhages, and less frequently erosions, may be present in the first portion of the duodenum and terminal ileum. Peyer's patches are severely affected; entire patches of lymphoid tissue may be sloughed. The large intestine is usually more severely affected, with lesions developing around the ileocecal valve and at the cecocolic junction and rectum. The latter exhibits streaks of congestion along the folds of the mucosa resulting in the characteristic "zebra-striped" appearance.

Petechiae may appear in the turbinates, larynx, and trachea. Patches of bronchopneumonia may be present.

Diagnosis: A presumptive diagnosis is based on clinical, pathologic, and epidemiologic findings and may be confirmed by viral isolation and identification. The specimens required are unclotted blood, lymph nodes, tonsils, spleen, and whole lung. Detection of viral antigens by complement fixation or agar-gel precipitin tests does not differentiate the disease from rinderpest. Detection of virus-neutralizing antibodies with a rising titer in surviving animals is diagnostic. PPR must be differentiated from other acute GI infections (eg rinderpest), respiratory infections (eg, contagious caprine pleuropneumonia), and such other diseases as contagious ecthyma, heartwater, coccidiosis, and mineral poisoning.

Control: State and federal authorities should be notified when PPR is suspected. Eradication is recommended when the disease appears in previously PPR-free countries; rinderpest eradication methods are useful. There is no specific treatment; however, treatment for bacterial and parasitic complications decreases mortality in affected flocks or herds. An attenuated vaccine has been prepared in embryonic caprine kidney cell culture; it affords protection from natural disease for ~1 yr. Rinderpest cell culture vaccine also has been used successfully for immunization against PPR.

RIFT VALLEY FEVER

Rift Valley fever (RVF) is a peracute or acute zoonotic disease of domestic ruminants in Africa and, recently, the Arabian Peninsula. Signs of the disease tend to be nonspecific, rendering it difficult to recognize individual cases. During epidemics, the occurrence of numerous abortions and deaths among young animals, together with an influenza-like disease in humans, tends to be characteristic.

Etiology and Epidemiology: RVF virus belongs to the genus Phlebovirus, and is a typical Bunyavirus. It has a 3-segmented, single-stranded, negative-sense RNA genome with a molecular weight of $4\text{-}6 \times 10^6$, and each of the segments, L (large), M (medium), and S (small), is contained in a separate nucleocapsid within the virion. No significant antigenic differences have been demonstrated between RVF isolates from many countries, but differences in pathogenicity are seen. The disease is endemic in tropical regions of mainly eastern and southern Africa, although an epidemic was reported in 2000 in Saudi Arabia and Yemen. Cyclic epidemics have occurred at 5- to 20-yr intervals in drier areas. The cycles are normally associated with periods of abnormally heavy rainfall. In the periods between epidemics, the virus is believed to be dormant in eggs of the mosquito *Aedes mcintoshi (linneatopennis)* in the dry soil of grassland depressions (dambos). Although transovarial transmission is believed to be the most important interepidemic survival strategy of the virus, inapparent cycling of disease may occur at forest edge habitats. RVF may spread by windborne mosquitos or introduction of viremic animals. With adequate rainfall, the infected maintenance mosquitos develop and infect ruminants, which amplify the virus. The virus is spread epidemically by many species of mosquitos or mechanically by other insects characteristic of different regions. The incidence of RVF peaks in late summer. After the first frost, both the disease and vectors may disappear. In warmer climates where insect vectors are present continuously, seasonality is usually not seen.

Humans are also readily infected through aerosols from infected animals when humidity is high, or by exposure to infected animal tissues, aborted fetuses, mosquito bites, and laboratory procedures, and have the potential to introduce the disease (via mosquitos) to animals in uninfected areas.

Clinical Findings: The incubation period is 12-36 hr in lambs. A biphasic fever of up to 106°F (41°C) may develop. Affected animals are listless and reluctant to move or feed and may show signs of abdominal pain. Lambs usually die within 2 days. Older animals may die acutely or develop an inapparent infection. Sick animals may regurgitate and develop a bad-smelling diarrhea and icterus, which is common in cattle. Sometimes, abortion may be the only sign of infection. In pregnant ewes, the mortality and abortion rates vary from 5 to almost 100% in different outbreaks and on different farms. The rates in cattle are usually <10%.

Lesions: The hepatic lesions are similar in all species and vary mainly with the age of the infected individual. The most severe lesions seen in aborted fetuses and newborn lambs are moderately to greatly enlarged, soft, friable livers with irregular congested patches. Numerous grayish white necrotic foci are invariably present but may not be clearly visible. Hemorrhage and edema of the wall of the gallbladder and mucosa of the abomasum are common. Intestinal contents are dark chocolate-brown. In all animals, the spleen and peripheral lymph nodes are enlarged and edematous and may have petechiae. In humans, RVF is usually inapparent or associated with moderate to severe, nonfatal influenza-like illness. A minority may develop severe disease with ocular lesions, encephalitis, and severe hepatic lesions with hemorrhages.

Diagnosis: RVF should be suspected when abnormally heavy rains are followed by the widespread occurrence of abortions and mortality among newborn animals characterized by necrotic hepatitis, and when hemorrhages and influenza-like disease are seen in people handling animals or their products. Histopathologically, the liver lesions in lambs are pathognomonic. The virus can readily be isolated from tissues of aborted fetuses and the blood of infected animals. The viral titer in these tissues is often high enough to use organ suspensions as antigen for a rapid diagnosis in neutralization, complement fixation, ELISA, agar gel diffusion tests, or staining of organ impression smears; however, these tests should be supplemented by isolation in suckling mice or hamsters injected intracerebrally or in cell cultures such as baby hamster kidney (BHK21), monkey kidney (Vero), CER and mosquito cells, or primary kidney and testis cell cultures of lambs. Detection of viral nucleic acid by PCR is possible, and 2 reverse transcriptase-PCR tests have been described.

All conventional serologic tests can be used to detect antibody against RVF virus and are helpful in epidemiologic studies. In some areas, however, serologic surveys may be complicated by cross-reactions between RVF virus and other phleboviruses. An IgM ELISA can demonstrate recent infection using a single serum sample.

Control and Prevention: Control of vectors, movement of stock to higher altitudes, and confinement of stock in insect-proof stables are usually not practical, instituted too late, and of little value. Immunization remains the only effective way to protect livestock. The mouse neuro-adapted Smithburn strain of RVF virus can readily be produced in large quantities, is inexpensive, and induces a durable immunity 6-7 days after inoculation. It should normally not be used for the protection of pregnant animals because it may cause abortion, congenital defects, and hydrops amnii of the ewe; however, its use in pregnant ewes may be contemplated during an outbreak when its adverse effects may be outweighed by the dangers of a natural infection. Although not proved, it is theoretically possible for the attenuated virus to revert to full virulence. A small-plaque variant and a mutagen-induced strain have been investigated as potential vaccine strains but have not been accepted as replacements for the Smithburn strain. Outbreaks of RVF cannot be predicted and are usually of sudden onset. Therefore, routinely immunizing lambs on a regular basis at 6 mo of age, which should afford lifelong protection, is advisable. The offspring of susceptible ewes can be immunized at any age. It is not advisable to use live, attenuated vaccines in nonendemic countries; subunit DNA vaccines are being developed and will offer a better alternative.

Pregnant ewes and cattle should preferably be vaccinated with a formalin-inactivated vaccine. Revaccination after 3 mo is advisable to induce an immunity that will last ~1 yr and to confer colostral immunity to the offspring.

Zoonotic Risk: People involved in the livestock industry should be made aware of the potential dangers of exposure to RVF-infected animals and tissues.

RINDERPEST

(Cattle plague)

Rinderpest is a disease of cloven-hoofed animals characterized by fever, necrotic stomatitis, gastroenteritis, lymphoid necrosis, and high mortality. In epidemic form, it is the most lethal plague known in cattle. All species of the order artiodactyla are variably susceptible to rinderpest. Susceptibility is high in African buffalo, giraffes, wild Suidae, Tragelaphinae, and breeds of cattle such as Ankole, Channel Islands, and Japanese Black; moderate in wildebeest and East African zebus; and mild in gazelles and small domestic ruminants. Rinderpest is subclinical in European pigs and hippopotami. It is endemic in many countries of Asia and Africa. Historically, rinderpest virus has been widely distributed throughout Europe and Africa but has never established itself in North America, Central America, the Caribbean Islands, South America, Australia, or New Zealand. Rinderpest is included in OIE List A.

Etiology and Pathogenesis: The infectious agent is a morbillivirus, closely related to the viruses causing peste des petits ruminants (p 616), canine distemper (p 625), and measles. Strains of rinderpest virus may vary markedly in host range and virulence. Sera from recovered or vaccinated cattle cross-react with all strains in neutralization tests, but minor antigenic differences have been demonstrated. The virus is fragile and becomes rapidly inactivated by heat and light, but remains viable for long periods in chilled or frozen tissues.

Rinderpest virus is present in small amounts of nasal secretions 1-2 days before fever; levels are high in secretions and excretions during the first week of clinical disease and decrease rapidly as animals develop specific antibodies and begin to recover. Transmission requires direct or close indirect contact; infection is via the nasopharynx. There is no carrier state; the virus maintains itself by continual transmission among susceptible animals. In endemic areas, young cattle become infected after maternal immunity disappears and before vaccine immunity begins, with possible auxiliary cycles in sheep, goats, and wild ungulates. In epidemic areas, the virus infects most susceptible animals and tends to limit itself unless the population is large enough to support endemicity.

Following primary growth in lymph nodes associated with the nasopharynx, the virus proliferates throughout the lymphoid tissue and spreads via the blood to the mucosa of the GI and upper respiratory tracts. Tissue damage is caused by viral cytopathology. Viral antigens induce a potent immune response that controls the infection and allows recovery if tissue damage is not too severe.

Clinical Findings: An incubation period of 3-15 days is followed by fever, anorexia, and depression; oculonasal discharge develops 1-2 days later. Within 2-3 days, pinpoint necrotic lesions, which rapidly enlarge to form cheesy plaques, appear on the gums, buccal mucosa, and tongue. The hard and soft palates are often affected. The oculonasal discharge becomes mucopurulent, and the muzzle appears dry and cracked. Diarrhea, the final clinical sign, may be watery and contain blood, mucus, and mucous membranes. Animals show severe abdominal pain, thirst, and dyspnea and may die from dehydration. Convalescence is prolonged and may be complicated by concurrent infections due to immunosuppression. In endemic areas, morbidity is low and clinical signs are often mild; in epidemic areas, morbidity is often 100% and mortality is up to 90%.

Lesions: Gross pathologic changes are evident throughout the GI and upper respiratory tracts, either as areas of necrosis and erosion, or congestion and hemorrhage, the latter creating classic "zebra-striping" in the rectum. Lymph nodes may be enlarged and edematous, with white necrotic foci in the Peyer's patches. Histologic examination reveals lymphoid and epithelial necrosis with viral-induced syncytia and intracytoplasmic inclusions.

Diagnosis: Clinical and pathologic findings may be sufficient for diagnosis in endemic areas and after initial laboratory confirmation of an outbreak. In areas where rinderpest is uncommon or absent, laboratory tests must be used to differentiate it from bovine viral diarrhea in particular, as well as East Coast fever, foot-and-mouth disease, infectious bovine rhinotracheitis, and malignant catarrhal fever. Viral isolation and detection of specific viral antigens in affected tissues are standard tests, and demonstration of rising antibody titers is useful. Simple, rapid tests for antigen detection (immunodiffusion, counterimmunoelectrophoresis, and competitive ELISA) are valuable in the field.

Specimens for the laboratory must be collected from several animals during the early stages of clinical disease, preferably before the onset of diarrhea. Whole blood, lymphoid tissue, spleen, and gut lesions should be collected aseptically and transported swiftly at 4°C or on ice.

Control: Treatment usually is not attempted, but nursing care with supportive fluid and antibiotic therapy (for secondary bacterial infections) may aid recovery of valuable animals. Active immunity is usually lifelong; maternal immunity lasts 6-11 mo. Control in endemic areas is by immunization of all cattle and domestic buffalo >1 yr old with attenuated cell culture vaccine. In these areas, outbreaks are controlled by quarantine and "ring vaccination" and sometimes by slaughtering. In epidemic areas, the disease is best eliminated by imposing quarantine and slaughtering affected and exposed animals. Control of animal movement is paramount because most outbreaks are due to introduction of infected cattle. Countries that are free of the disease and that border endemic areas must be extremely vigilant or vaccinate as a precaution.

In the last 15 yr, the prevalence of rinderpest has been declining. The Food and Agriculture Organization (FAO) of the United Nations, with the leading veterinary officials of rinderpest-affected countries and international experts on rinderpest, has developed a strategy for the worldwide eradication of rinderpest. The OIE has promoted this goal by encouraging disease reporting, sharing information, and developing international animal sanitary standards. Article 2.1.4.4 of the OIE International Animal Health Code requires that, for a country to declare itself or a zone free of rinderpest, it should fulfill certain conditions, including disease absence for at least 2 yr in the presence of disease surveillance and monitoring, a reporting system, a preventive program, and cessation of vaccination. Many countries have now achieved that status; others have made progress in rinderpest eradication and have declared provisional free zones.

TICKBORNE FEVER

(Pasture fever)

Tickborne fever (TBF) is a febrile disease of domestic and free-living ruminants in the temperate regions of Europe. TBF is prevalent in sheep and cattle in the UK, Ireland, Norway, Finland, The Netherlands, Austria, and Spain. It is transmitted by the hard tick *Ixodes ricinus*. A similar disease transmitted by other ticks has been described in India and South Africa. The main hosts are sheep and cattle, but goats and deer are also susceptible.

Etiology: The causative agent is now classified as a member of the order Rickettsiales, family Anaplasmataceae, as *Anaplasma (Ehrlichia) phagocytophilum*, which includes the granulocytic ehrlichiae *A phagocytophilum*, *Ehrlichia equi*, and the agent of human granulocytic ehrlichiosis.

The organism infects eosinophils, neutrophils, and monocytes, in that order. Cytoplasmic inclusions are visible as grayish blue bodies in Giemsa-stained blood smears and may contain one or more rickettsial particles of variable size and shape. The varied morphologic types in the cytoplasmic inclusions do not represent stages of development, as in chlamydiae, but rather are rickettsial colonies within cytoplasmic vacuoles.

The disease is transmitted by the tick *I ricinus*. Adult ticks infected as larvae or nymphs can transmit the disease as can nymphs infected as larvae, but infections do not appear to pass from the adult female to the larva via the egg. The rickettsiae can survive in infected ticks for long periods and, because *I ricinus* can survive unfed for >1 yr awaiting a new host, ticks infected in their previous instar can still be infective after long periods of hibernation. The ready transmission of infection by injecting infected blood suggests that the organism could be transmitted mechanically by biting insects. In addition, if the organisms reported to cause a similar disease in ruminants in India and South Africa are indeed *A phagocytophilum*, it is most likely that ticks other than *I ricinus* are involved.

Clinical Findings: After infestation with infected ticks, the incubation period may be 5-14 days, but after injection with infected blood, the incubation period is 2-6 days. In sheep, the main clinical sign is a sudden fever (105-108°F [40.5-42.0°C]) for 4-10 days. Other signs are either absent or mild, but the animals generally appear dull and may lose weight. Respiratory and pulse rates are usually increased, and a cough often develops.

In cattle, the disease is known as pasture fever in many parts of Europe, including Finland, Norway, Austria, Spain, and Switzerland. The disease occurs as an annual minor epidemic when dairy heifers and cows are turned out to pasture in the spring and early summer. Within days, the cows are dull and depressed, with a marked loss of appetite and milk yield. Affected cows usually suffer from respiratory distress and coughing. Clinical signs are more obvious and last longer in newly purchased animals than in home-bred animals. Often, veterinary advice is sought after an abrupt fall in milk yield.

Abortions affect susceptible ewes and cows newly introduced onto tick-infested pastures during the last stages of gestation, with abortions occurring 2-8 days after the onset of fever. Except for aborting ewes, death due to TBF is rare. The quality of the semen of infected rams and bulls may be greatly reduced. Variations in severity of the clinical effects may be related to differences between strains of *A phagocytophilum* or in host susceptibility.

Perhaps the most significant effect of TBF infection is its serious impairment of humoral and cellular defense mechanisms, which results in increased susceptibility to secondary infections such as tick pyemia, pneumonic pasteurellosis, louping ill, and listeriosis.

Lesions: TBF is characterized by transient but distinct hematologic changes. A modest neutrophilia develops 2-4 days after natural or experimental infection and is followed by a severe leukopenia due to lymphocytopenia and neutropenia. The lymphocytopenia lasts for 4-6 days, while the neutropenia develops more progressively and becomes more marked ~10 days after infection. Studies with monoclonal antibodies that recognize surface markers for lymphocyte subsets have shown that both T and B lymphocytes are reduced. The number of circulating eosinophils is also depressed for up to 2 wk. After the febrile period has subsided, the number of monocytes may increase. At the peak of reaction, >90% of circulating neutrophils and eosinophils may be infected. The monocytes are predominantly infected during the later stages of bacteremia, while the granulocytes are usually infected throughout the period of bacteremia. The number of circulating thrombocytes is also reported to be depressed during the febrile period, and the occasional hemorrhagic syndromes associated with TBF are probably related to the reduction in circulating thrombocytes.

Diagnosis: In sheep, the onset of high fever in tick-infested areas during the spring and summer in association with hematologic changes and the presence of inclusions within granulocytes is diagnostic. The clinical disease usually is seen only in young lambs born in tick-infested areas or in older animals newly introduced to such areas. Blood smears should indicate the association of TBF and cases of tick pyemias and abortions, particularly when abortions occur after pregnant animals are moved from tick-free to tick-infested pastures. TBF could be established retrospectively as a cause of abortions by demonstrating a rise in antibody titers by indirect immunofluorescence.

In affected dairy cattle, the main clinical signs are abortions and a sudden drop in milk yield. The other clinical sign commonly associated with TBF in cattle is respiratory illness after a herd is introduced to tick-infested pastures. TBF must also be considered when abortions and stillbirths, particularly in heifers, occur soon after their introduction to tick-infested pastures. Therefore, in areas where TBF is enzootic, blood smears must be examined for the presence of organisms in all cases of abortion in sheep and cattle and when milk yield is suddenly reduced soon after the animals have returned to pasture.

Treatment and Control: The short-acting oxytetracyclines are regarded as the most effective treatment because other antibiotics such as penicillin, streptomycin, and ampicillin do not prevent relapses. Sulfamethazine has also proved useful. If dairy cattle are treated with oxytetracyclines within a few days of infection, the pyrexia is reduced quickly and milk yield restored.

There are 3 important aspects of control: vector control, chemotherapy, and immunity. Effective control can be achieved by eliminating or markedly reducing contact with the tick vector either by grazing sheep and cattle on tick-free pastures in lowland areas or by use of acaricides. In sheep practice, this commonly involves keeping ewes and lambs in a fenced, relatively tick-free pasture until the lamb is ~6 wk old. The lamb also benefits from improved nutrition of the ewe. Dipping lambs within 1-2 wk of birth is not commonly practiced because of difficulties of gathering the lambs on widely dispersed hill farms, the risks of mismothering, and the relatively short duration of protection provided by acaricides, possibly because of the short fleece and rapid growth rate of lambs. However, dipping twice with a 2- to 3-wk interval or use of pour-on preparations or smears applied before lambs are moved from lambing fields to hill pastures are reported to be effective in controlling ticks. Pregnant animals should not be moved from tick-free to tick-infested pastures.

In enzootic areas, treatment with long-acting tetracyclines may be used as a prophylactic measure against TBF. When susceptible animals, particularly pregnant ewes and cows and newborn lambs, are to be moved from tick-free to tick-infested areas, it may be necessary to combine dipping with prophylactic use of long-acting tetracyclines. Such treatment of lambs in the first 2-3 wk of life can be protective for up to 3 wk and helps reduce secondary infections such as tick pyemia, pasteurellosis, and colibacillosis. It may also improve growth rate.

Several aspects of immunity remain controversial, but it is generally accepted that sheep and cattle are immune to challenge after recovery from 1 or 2 bouts of clinical disease caused by TBF. The immunity may last for several months but wanes rapidly if the animals are removed from tick-infested areas. Secondary infections are usually milder as residual immunity persists. There is a variable degree of cross-protection among strains of *A phagocytophilum*. No effective vaccines are available to protect ruminants from clinical TBF. However, if susceptible animals are being brought into tick-infested pastures, it may be sensible to deliberately infect them before introduction and treat them with oxytetracyclines before or immediately after the onset of fever. This allows multiplication of the organism and therefore stimulation of immune responses without uncontrolled clinical disease; a minimum duration of bacteremia may be required for protective immunity to develop. Because not all strains of *A phagocytophilum* are cross-protective, strains specific to the area must be used.

TICK PYEMIA

Tick pyemia affects lambs 2-12 wk old and is characterized by debility, crippling lameness, and paralysis. Pyemic abscesses are common in joints but may be found in virtually any organ. The disease causes significant economic loss through debilitation and death of lambs. The disease is enzootic in many regions of the UK and Ireland where the tick *Ixodes ricinus* is common, and it is likely to be present in other parts of Europe where the same tick is found.

Etiology: *Staphylococcus aureus* is regarded as the main cause of the pyemic abscesses because it has been isolated consistently from superficial and deep-seated lesions and it is rare to find other bacteria. The bacteria are believed to gain entry into the bloodstream either by direct inoculation during tick feeding, from local superficial wounds, or through the infected umbilicus. However, there is clinical and experimental evidence that *I ricinus* does not simply act as a vector directly injecting staphylococci into the bloodstream. The main role of *I ricinus* is as a vector of the rickettsial agent *Anaplasma (Ehrlichia) phagocytophilum*, which causes tickborne fever (TBF, p 620), which in turn creates factors favorable to development of pyemia. Lambs affected with TBF have severe leukopenia, and their peripheral blood neutrophils are less capable of phagocytizing and killing *S aureus*. Experimental studies have shown that lambs with TBF were more susceptible to experimental infections with *S aureus* during the period of neutropenia and that up to 30% of lambs with TBF may develop staphylococcal infections.

The epidemiology of the disease is closely related to the biology of *I ricinus*. The disease is limited to areas populated by *I ricinus* and to seasons of the year climatically favoring high tick population and activity.

Clinical Findings: Abscesses form in various parts of the body, mainly in the joints, tendon sheaths, and muscles, resulting in lameness—hence the common use of the term "crippled lambs." In some outbreaks, >30% of lambs may be affected; they are usually dull and lame and often suffer from loss of body condition. Internal abscesses without joint lesions may result in no clinical signs other than the loss of condition, but when lesions are present in the CNS, there may be ataxia, paraplegia, or other nervous signs. The crippling disease lasts for days or weeks, but the disease may also appear as an acute septicemia. On occasion, there may be sudden deaths resulting from multiple internal abscesses without other visible signs. Up to 50% of affected lambs may die, and the survivors recover slowly.

Lesions: Apart from the joints and other superficial structures, abscesses are commonly found in the liver, lungs, and kidneys. They may also be present in the meninges of the spinal cord and in the pericardium and myocardium. The diaphragm, thymus, and adrenal glands are less commonly affected. Ticks are often found attached to an inflamed area.

Diagnosis: History and clinical signs are valuable indicators. The restriction of the disease to tick-infested areas, its occurrence during seasons of tick activity, and the demonstration of *A phagocytophilum* in blood smears of affected lambs or other sheep in the flock are diagnostic features. Isolation of *S aureus* from lesions and the absence of other bacteria will help to confirm tick pyemia. The loss of condition and ill-thrift without lameness may be difficult to recognize as tick pyemia, and the acute condition can be confused with other septicemic diseases. Tick pyemia may also resemble other suppurative infections of the newborn, including navel ill and joint ill due to infections by other bacteria such as streptococci and *Arcanobacterium (Actinomyces) pyogenes*.

Treatment and Control: Treatment of clinical cases of tick pyemia with penicillin or tetracycline can be effective, provided the lesions are not too advanced.

Control of tick infestation is the most effective prevention. This can be achieved either by restricting lambs and ewes to low-ground, tick-free pastures for the first few weeks of life or by dipping ewes before lambing and administering acaricides as dips or smears on lambs. In young lambs, pour-on preparations of cypermethrin or smears applied before lambs are moved from lambing fields to hill pastures are reported to be effective in controlling ticks.

Administration of long-acting oxytetracycline at the time of risk can help prevent both TBF and tick pyemia during the first weeks of life. A single injection at double the standard dose at 3 wk of age can significantly reduce mortality and morbidity in young hill lambs on tick-infested pasture and improve weight gains and condition in the remainder. Prophylactic treatment with a long-acting antibiotic may prevent development of TBF for up to 3 wk, without pyrexia and immunosuppression, so that the incidence of tick pyemia and other infections such as pasteurellosis and colibacillosis are reduced. Although treatment with oxytetracycline may inhibit the development of immunity to TBF, if the lambs eventually develop TBF, they are several weeks older and apparently less susceptible to tick pyemia. Deliberate exposure of lambs to TBF by injections, followed by treatment with oxytetracycline, could provide some immunity to TBF before the lambs enter tick-infested areas; however, strains specific to the area must be used because some strains of *A phagocytophilum* have no cross-immunity.

WESSELSBRON DISEASE

Wesselsbron disease is an acute, arthropodborne flavivirus infection of sheep, cattle, and goats. Infection is common but clinical disease is infrequent. Mortality in newborn animals may reach 27% in lambs and 18% in goat kids. Infection in adults is usually subclinical, but disease may be severe in the presence of pre-existing liver pathology. Occasional abortion in ewes, together with congenital malformation of the CNS with arthrogryposis of the ovine fetus and hydrops amnii in ewes, is also seen. In humans, it causes a nonfatal influenza-like disease.

Etiology and Epidemiology: The virus, with properties typical of a hemagglutinating flavivirus, has not been well characterized. It has been isolated from vertebrates and arthropods from several African countries, and serologic surveys provide evidence of its occurrence in others. From the distribution of aedine mosquitos associated with Wesselsbron disease, it can be surmised that the incidence is greater than is generally realized. The high prevalence of antibodies in warmer and moister areas suggests that domestic herbivores may play a significant role in maintenance of the virus, and activity appears to occur year round. In drier areas, however, disease outbreaks are irregular and tend to occur in conjunction with Rift Valley fever (p 617) when abnormally heavy rains favor floodwater-breeding mosquitos.

Clinical Findings: After an incubation period of 1-3 days in newborn lambs, nonspecific signs of illness, including fever, anorexia, listlessness, weakness, and increased respiration, become evident. Wesselsbron disease and Rift Valley fever share many clinical and pathologic features. However, Wesselsbron disease is usually mild, producing much lower mortality and abortion and less destructive liver lesions. The virus appears to be more neurotropic than that of Rift Valley fever because severe fetal teratology of the CNS is seen after experimental infection.

Lesions: In newborn and young animals, a moderate to severe icterus and hepatomegaly are seen; the liver is yellowish to orange brown. Petechiae and ecchymoses are commonly found in the mucosa of the abomasum, the contents of which are chocolate-brown in color. Histopathology reveals mild to extensive necrosis of the parenchyma and individual or small, scattered groups of necrotic hepatocytes. Lesions in adult animals are usually much milder.

Diagnosis: The clinical signs and epidemiology, together with a relative high mortality in lambs, are an indication of the disease. The virus can be isolated from almost all organs of lambs that have died during the clinical stage of the disease. Intracerebral inoculation of newborn mice is the best method of isolation. The virus can be distinguished from that of Rift Valley fever by intraperitoneal inoculation of weaned mice; Wesselsbron disease virus will not kill such mice whereas Rift Valley fever virus will. Confirmation of the viral identity can be accomplished by virus neutralization.

Serodiagnosis has been based on hemagglutination-inhibition, complement fixation, and virus neutralization. Flavivirus cross-reactivity is marked in hemagglutination-inhibition tests. Nevertheless, homologous Wesselsbron titers greatly exceed heterologous flavivirus titers.

Control: Production of an attenuated vaccine was discontinued shortly before 2000. Incidence of disease is low in sheep, and injudicious use of the vaccine in pregnant ewes resulted in severe economic losses in the past due to abortion and fetal malformations. Attempts to control mosquito vectors are of little value as a preventive measure.

CANINE DISTEMPER

(Hardpad disease)

Canine distemper is a highly contagious, systemic, viral disease of dogs seen worldwide. Clinically, it is characterized by a diphasic fever, leukopenia, GI and respiratory catarrh, and frequently pneumonic and neurologic complications. The disease is seen in Canidae (dogs, foxes, wolves), Mustelidae (eg, ferret, mink, skunk), most Procyonidae (eg, raccoon, coatimundi), and some Viveridae (binturong).

Etiology and Pathogenesis: Canine distemper is caused by a paramyxovirus closely related to the viruses of measles and rinderpest. The enveloped virus is sensitive to lipid solvents and most disinfectants and is relatively unstable outside the host. The main route of infection is via aerosol droplet secretions from infected animals. Some infected dogs may shed virus for several months.

Virus initially replicates in the lymphatic tissue of the respiratory tract. A cell-associated viremia results in infection of all lymphatic tissues, which is followed by infection of respiratory, GI, and urogenital epithelium, as well as the CNS and optic nerves. Disease follows virus replication in these tissues. The degree of viremia and extent of spread of virus to various tissues is moderated by the level of specific humoral immunity in the host during the viremic period.

Clinical Findings: A transient fever usually occurs 3-6 days after infection, and there may be a leukopenia (especially lymphopenia) at this time; these signs may go unnoticed or be accompanied by anorexia. The fever subsides for several days before a second fever occurs, which lasts <1 wk. This may be accompanied by serous nasal discharge, mucopurulent ocular discharge, and anorexia. GI and respiratory signs may follow and are usually complicated by secondary bacterial infections. An acute encephalomyelitis may occur in association with or following the systemic disease, or in the absence of systemic manifestations. Hyperkeratosis of the footpads ("hardpad" disease) and epithelium of the nasal plane may be seen. Neurologic signs are frequently seen in those dogs with hyperkeratosis. CNS signs include the following: 1) localized involuntary twitching of a muscle or group of muscles (myoclonus, chorea, flexor spasm, hyperkinesia), such as in the leg or facial muscles; 2) paresis or paralysis, often most noticeable in the hindlimbs as ataxia, followed by tetraparesis and tetraparalysis; and 3) convulsions characterized by salivation and often chewing movements of the jaw ("chewing-gum fits"). The seizures become more frequent and severe, and the dog may fall on its side and paddle its legs; involuntary urination and defecation (grand mal seizure, epileptiform convulsion) often occur. A dog may exhibit any or all of these neurologic signs in addition to others in the course of the disease. Infection may be mild and inapparent or lead to severe disease manifest by most of the above signs. The course of the systemic disease may be as short as 10 days, but the onset of neurologic signs may be delayed for several weeks or months.

Chronic distemper encephalitis (old dog encephalitis, [ODE]), a condition often marked by ataxia, compulsive movements such as head pressing or continual pacing, and incoordinated hypermetria, may be seen in adult dogs without a history of signs related to systemic canine distemper. The development of neurologic signs is often more progressive. Although canine distemper antigen has been detected in the brain of some dogs with ODE by fluorescent antibody staining, dogs with ODE are not infectious and replication-competent virus has not been isolated. Genetic methods may be needed to document infection. The disease is caused by an inflammatory reaction associated with persistent canine distemper virus infection in the CNS.

Lesions: Thymic atrophy is a consistent postmortem finding in infected young puppies. Hyperkeratosis of the nose and footpads is often found in dogs with neurologic manifestations. Depending on the degree of secondary bacterial infection, bronchopneumonia, enteritis, and skin pustules may also be present. Histologically, canine distemper virus produces necrosis of lymphatic tissues, interstitial pneumonia, and cytoplasmic and intranuclear inclusion bodies in respiratory, urinary, and GI epithelium. Lesions found in the brain of dogs with neurologic complications include neuronal degeneration, gliosis, demyelination, perivascular cuffing, nonsuppurative leptomeningitis, and intranuclear inclusion bodies predominately within glial cells.

Diagnosis: Distemper should be considered in the diagnosis of any febrile condition in puppies with multisystemic manifestations. While the typical clinical case is not difficult to diagnose, the characteristic signs sometimes fail to appear until late in the disease. The clinical picture may be modified by concurrent toxoplasmosis, neosporosis, coccidiosis, parasitoses, and numerous viral and bacterial infections. Distemper is sometimes confused with other systemic infections such as leptospirosis, infectious canine hepatitis, or Rocky Mountain spotted fever. Intoxicants such as lead or organophosphates can cause simultaneous GI or neurologic sequelae. A febrile catarrhal illness with neurologic sequelae justifies a clinical diagnosis of distemper. At necropsy, diagnosis is usually confirmed by histologic lesions or immunofluorescent assay for viral antigen in tissues, or both. In dogs with multisystemic signs, conjunctival, tracheal, vaginal, or other epithelium, or the buffy coat of the blood can be examined by immunofluorescent assay. These samples are usually negative when the dog is showing only neurologic manifestations or when circulating antibody is present (or both). The diagnosis can then be made by serologic demonstration of virus-specific IgM or an increased ratio of CSF to serum virus-specific IgG.

Treatment: Treatments are directed at limiting secondary bacterial invasion, supporting fluid balance, and controlling nervous manifestations. Antibiotics, balanced electrolyte solutions, parenteral nutrition, dietary supplements, antipyretics, nasal preparations, analgesics, and anticonvulsants are used. No single treatment is specific or uniformly successful. Dogs may recover completely from systemic manifestations, but good nursing care is essential. Despite intensive care, some dogs do not make a satisfactory recovery. Unfortunately, treatment for acute neurologic manifestations of distemper is unsuccessful. If the neurologic signs are progressive or severe, the owner should be appropriately advised. Dogs with some of the more chronic progressive or vaccine-induced forms of neurologic disease may respond to immunosuppressive therapy with anti-inflammatory or greater dosages of glucocorticoids.

Prevention: Successful immunization of pups with canine distemper modified live virus (MLV) vaccines depends on the lack of interference by maternal antibody. To overcome this barrier, pups are vaccinated with MLV vaccine when 6 wk old and at 2- to 4-wk intervals until 16 wk old. Measles virus induces immunity to canine distemper virus in the presence of relatively greater levels of maternal distemper antibody. An MLV measles vaccine and a combination of MLV measles and MLV canine distemper vaccine are available. Measles vaccines must be administered IM. Pups 6-7 wk old should receive the measles or combination vaccine and at least 2 more doses of MLV distemper vaccine when 12-16 wk old. Many varieties of attenuated distemper vaccine are available and should be used according to manufacturers' directions. MLV vaccines can produce postvaccinal illness in some immunosuppressed dogs. A recombinant canarypox vector vaccine expressing distemper virus proteins is available. Annual revaccination has been suggested because of the breaks in neurologic distemper that can occur in stressed, diseased, or immunosuppressed dogs. Longer than yearly intervals of administration have been suggested with MLV vaccines; however, this should be tempered with the prevalence of the disease and other potential risk factors.

CANINE HERPESVIRAL INFECTION

Canine herpesvirus is a severe, often fatal, viral infection of puppies worldwide. It also may be associated with upper respiratory infection or a vesicular vaginitis or posthitis in adult dogs. Only canids (dogs, wolves, coyotes) are known to be susceptible.

Etiology: The disease is caused by an enveloped DNA canine herpesvirus (CHV) that is sensitive to lipid solvents and most disinfectants. CHV is relatively unstable outside the host.

Transmission usually occurs by contact between susceptible puppies and the infected oral, nasal, or vaginal secretions of their dam or oral or nasal secretions of dogs allowed to commingle with puppies during the first 3 wk of life. In utero transmission may occur.

Infection of newborn susceptible puppies results in replication of CHV in the surface cells of the nasal mucosa, pharynx, and tonsils. If the pups become hypothermic, viremia and invasion of visceral organs occur.

Clinical Findings: Deaths due to CHV infection usually occur in puppies 1-3 wk old, occasionally in puppies up to 1 mo old, and rarely in pups as old as 6 mo. Typically, onset is sudden, and death occurs after an illness of ≤24 hr. Older dogs exposed to or experimentally inoculated with CHV may develop a mild rhinitis or a vesicular vaginitis or posthitis. In utero infections may be associated with abortions, stillbirths, and infertility.

Lesions: The characteristic gross lesions consist of disseminated focal necrosis and hemorrhages. The most pronounced lesions are seen in the lungs, cortical portion of the kidneys, adrenal glands, liver, and GI tract. All lymph nodes are enlarged and hyperemic, and the spleen is swollen. Lesions may also be found in the CNS. The basic histologic lesion is necrosis with hemorrhage in the adjacent parenchyma. Most often there is no inflammatory reaction. Single, small, basophilic, intranuclear inclusion bodies are most common in areas of necrosis in the lung, liver, and kidneys; occasionally, they are seen as faintly acidophilic bodies located within the nuclear space.

Diagnosis: CHV infection may be confused with infectious canine hepatitis (p 637), but it is not accompanied by the thickened, edematous gallbladder often associated with the latter. The focal areas of necrosis and hemorrhage, especially those that occur in the kidneys, distinguish it from hepatitis and neosporosis (p 535). CHV causes serious disease only in very young puppies. The rapid death and characteristic lesions distinguish it from canine distemper (p 625). The virus can be isolated from fresh lung, liver, kidney, and spleen by cell culture techniques. The tissues should be submitted to the laboratory refrigerated but not frozen.

Control: No vaccine is available. Infected bitches develop antibodies, and litters subsequent to the first infected litter receive maternal antibodies in the colostrum. Puppies that receive maternal antibodies may be infected with the virus, but disease does not result.

Removing puppies from affected bitches by cesarean section and rearing them in isolation has prevented deaths under experimental conditions. However, infections have been noted even in puppies delivered by cesarean section. Deaths may be reduced when infected puppies are reared in incubators at increased temperatures (95°F [35°C], 50% relative humidity) and given adequate fluids and supportive therapy. The prognosis of puppies that survive neonatal infections of CHV is guarded because damage to lymphoid organs, brain, kidneys, and liver may be irreparable.

FELINE INFECTIOUS PERITONITIS AND PLEURITIS

(Feline coronaviral vasculitis)

Feline infectious peritonitis (FIP), caused by a feline coronavirus, is seen worldwide. Although a large number of cats may be infected with the feline coronavirus, only a few develop clinical FIP. The disease is progressive and may manifest clinically as a continuum between the effusive (serositis or wet) and noneffusive (granulomatous or dry) forms. A distinct clinical form of noneffusive FIP affecting only the eyes or brain (or both) may be seen. Mortality, even with therapy, approaches 100%. Although primarily a disease of domestic cats, FIP has been recognized in exotic Felidae, including the large and small wild cats. Among larger cats, FIP is seen in lions, leopards, jaguars, mountain lions, and especially cheetahs. Smaller cats susceptible to FIP include the sand cat, lynx, caracal, and pallas cat.

Etiology: Field strains of feline coronavirus vary in their ability to induce FIP. Some isolates cause FIP (feline infectious peritonitis virus [FIPV]); others cause more localized GI disease (feline enteric coronavirus, p 324). Mutations from feline enteric coronavirus to FIPV occur. The exact relationship between low virulence FIPV strains and feline enteric coronavirus, which is relatively nonpathogenic, is not clear. FIPV is antigenically related to and serologically cross-reacts (by current ELISA and immunofluorescent antibody tests) with a subgroup of mammalian coronaviruses, including transmissible gastroenteritis virus of swine, human coronavirus 229-E, canine coronavirus, and feline enteric coronavirus. FIPV and canine coronavirus are very closely related antigenically and may have crossed between hosts. Strains of FIPV may differ considerably in antigenicity.

Feline coronaviruses are fairly stable in the environment and, once dry, can survive for 4-6 wk. They are enveloped viruses and are destroyed by most household disinfectants, particularly household bleach at a 1:32 dilution.

Transmission, Epidemiology, and Pathogenesis: Most FIPV infections probably result from ingestion of the virus; however, aerosol transmission is also possible. Close contact with an infected cat or its excreta, most likely feces and saliva, is required for virus transmission. Because cats shed viral particles in feces, litter box exposure and mutual grooming are important sources of infection. Cats living in multiple cat households are at greater risk of contracting feline coronavirus and developing FIP because of sharing multiple strains of the virus and stress-associated immunosuppression. Transplacental transmission is suggested by the occasional observation of FIP in stillborn kittens, but the frequency with which this occurs is unknown. In the past, up to 50% of cats with FIP were co-infected with feline leukemia virus (FeLV); FeLV potently suppresses cell-mediated immunity, which is required for resistance to FIP. Currently, the co-infection rate is only 5%, due to FeLV testing and vaccination.

Cats of all ages and either sex can develop the disease, but incidence is highest in cats 6-24 mo old, decreased in cats 5-13 yr old, and increased in those 14-15 yr old. Kittens raised in infected colonies may contract the virus from their mothers or asymptomatic carriers when their maternal immunity wanes at 5-10 wk of age. These kittens typically may develop FIP weeks or months after they are placed in new homes. The prevalence of clinical FIP is <1% of cat-containing households, even though 20-35% of cats are infected with coronavirus. Losses are often sporadic and unpredictable, and morbidity and mortality may be greatly increased, sometimes up to 35% or more in some breeding catteries and households with multiple cats. Generally, the morbidity rate in cattery-bred kittens is ≤10%. The prevalence of FIPV infection in the general cat population is difficult to determine because current serologic tests for detecting FIPV antibodies cannot discriminate between FIPV and other feline coronaviruses that do not produce disease and that may be more prevalent.

After ingestion of virus or aerosol exposure, FIPV initially replicates in tonsil or intestinal epithelium and then is transported via macrophages and monocytes to primary target organs such as liver, spleen, and visceral lymph nodes. The development of FIP, and the particular clinical form of disease (ie, effusive or noneffusive) depends on the intrinsic immune responses of the cat. Cats with a strong humoral immunity and a weak or absent cell-mediated immune response against FIPV develop a persistent viremia and effusive FIP. The effusive disease results from widespread formation and deposition of immune complexes in blood vessels and from complement activation leading to vasculitis, vessel damage, and leakage of serum and protein into body cavities. Cats with partial cell-mediated immune responses along with humoral immunity develop the more chronic noneffusive FIP, which is characterized by immune-mediated (delayed hypersensitivity-like), granulomatous, frequently perivascular lesions in abdominal viscera, lungs, eyes, and brain. Cats with strong cell-mediated immune responses with or without humoral responses can either completely recover or become persistently infected asymptomatic carriers. The latter may infect contact cats and may themselves later develop FIP, usually after periods of stress or co-infection with FeLV. Some asymptomatic, seropositive carrier cats subsequently may become seronegative and stop excreting virus.

Clinical Findings: The acute or primary infection often is asymptomatic, but in some cases, fever of unknown origin, conjunctivitis, and other upper respiratory signs and diarrhea may occur. This stage may last several days or weeks or longer before signs of effusive or noneffusive FIP develop. Cats with effusive FIP are often presented after the owner notices progressive distention of the abdomen due to ascites. About one-third of cats with effusive FIP have pleural involvement and dyspnea, often accompanied by chronic fluctuating fever (102-106°F [39-41°C]) lasting 2-5 wk, anorexia, weight loss, and depression.

Cats with noneffusive FIP may have a history of vague illness, including chronic fever, malaise, weight loss, and occasionally major organ failure (renal, hepatic). Overt ocular and CNS signs may occur simultaneously or independently. About 50% of all cats with noneffusive FIP have signs related to intra-abdominal involvement (kidney, liver, spleen, pancreas, lymph nodes); ~60% of cases exhibit either CNS or ocular signs, or both; and ~15% present with ocular signs only. Only 10-15% of noneffusive cases have lesions of the pleural cavity. Many cats have elements of both the effusive and noneffusive forms of FIP.

Ocular disease may manifest as a bilateral anterior uveitis with iritis or iridocyclitis, hyphema, aqueous flare, hypopyon, or keratic precipitates in the anterior chamber. Posterior chamber involvement may include chorioretinitis with subretinal fluid exudation or hemorrhage and secondary bullous or linear retinal detachment. Fundic lesions may include perivascular cuffing, engorgement of retinal veins, and retinal hemorrhage.

Involvement of the CNS in the noneffusive form may cause focal or diffuse lesions in the brain or spinal cord; ~40% of these cases have CNS signs occurring either alone (25%) or in combination with other organ involvement. Clinical signs are variable and may reflect primary spinal cord, cranial, or cerebellar disease. The most common neurologic signs, in order of decreasing frequency, are posterior incoordination and paresis progressing to generalized ataxia, dorsal hyperesthesia, convulsions, personality changes, and hyperesthesia.

Lesions: In classic effusive FIP, there is diffuse peritonitis or pleuritis (or both) characterized grossly by variable amounts of viscous abdominal or thoracic fluid, deposition of gray-white exudate, and disseminated necrotic plaques (0.5-3.0 mm) on the visceral and parietal peritoneum or pleura. Fibrinous adhesions, particularly between the liver and diaphragm and between loops of bowel, can develop in protracted cases; occasionally, the omentum may be contracted into the anterior abdomen as a thickened mass of fibrinous adhesions. Histologically, lesions are characterized by perivascular necrosis and fibrinonecrotizing or pyogranulomatous inflammation; FIPV particles are seen within macrophages at the periphery of lesions.

Gross lesions in noneffusive FIP consist of multiple, gray-white, raised nodules (0.5-2 cm or larger) in kidneys, visceral lymph nodes, liver, intestines, lungs, eyes, and brain. A single, obstructive, granulomatous intestinal mass is seen in some cases. Histologically, the lesions are perivascular granulomas or pyogranulomas with systemic vasculitis or thrombovasculitis. Ocular lesions may affect either anterior or posterior chambers causing anterior uveitis and iridocyclitis or chorioretinitis, retinitis, retinal hemorrhage and detachment, and optic neuritis. Lesions in the CNS affect the brain and spinal cord and can cause either focal granulomatous masses or more diffuse fibrinonecrotizing or pyogranulomatous meningitis and ependymitis. Occasionally, CSF flow is obstructed by inflammatory exudate, and obstructive hydrocephalus develops.

Diagnosis: Presumptive diagnosis of FIP is based on history, clinical signs, and results of laboratory tests. Diagnosis of effusive FIP is based largely on analysis of the characteristic exudate. The fluid typically is sterile, viscous or ropey, and yellow to tan; it may contain fibrin strands, has a high specific gravity (1.017-1.047) and high protein content (5-12 g/dL), and is composed of variable amounts of mixed inflammatory cells (1,600-25,000/μL). Mixtures of neutrophils, lymphocytes, macrophages, and fewer mesothelial cells in a granular, eosinophilic, proteinaceous background are seen on Wright's-stained smears. Protein determinations and electrophoresis of the exudate may be useful in diagnosis. Exudates with total protein >3.5 g/dL (of which >50% is gamma globulin) and cytology consistent with FIP have a positive predictive value of >90%. In addition, the albumin:globulin ratio of the effusion is usually <0.8; a ratio <0.45 is usually predictive of effusive FIP. Documentation of a coronavirus infection by either a positive titer or coronavirus RNA by reverse-transcriptase PCR support a diagnosis of effusive FIP.

About 50% of cats with effusive FIP (and up to 70% of cats with noneffusive FIP) have an increased total plasma protein (>7.8 g/dL), often with hyperglobulinemia (>4.6 g/dL) and a hypergammaglobulinemia. Serum protein electrophoresis may show increases in α_2-globulins and polyclonal (occasionally monoclonal) increases in gamma globulin. Hematologic changes in both effusive and noneffusive FIP, although variable, most consistently show a neutrophilic leukocytosis (>19,000 cells/μL) and a relative lymphopenia (>1,500 cells/μL). Forty to 50% of cats develop a progressive normochromic, normocytic anemia (PCV <24%) that may be severe and nonregenerative if FIP is accompanied by FeLV or infection with *Haemobartonella felis*. Serologic tests (ELISA, immunofluorescent antibody) that detect antibodies against coronaviral proteins are not specific for FIPV and also detect antibodies against feline enteric coronavirus. The coronavirus titer in cats with FIP is usually increased (1:100 to 1:3,200); some cats with clinical FIP have negative or very low titers. PCR does not differentiate between feline coronaviruses and may be interpreted the same as a positive antibody titer.

Noneffusive FIP is a greater diagnostic challenge. Serum protein abnormalities in debilitated cats with nonresponsive fever, weight loss, multisystemic signs (including ocular and CNS signs), and increased coronavirus titers are suggestive of noneffusive FIP. Blood changes in the noneffusive form must be viewed collectively. Cats that have clinical signs of FIP, lymphopenia, and hyperglobulinemia of >5.1 g/dL have an almost 90% probability of having FIP. In cats that do not meet all 3 criteria, there is a 99% probability that FIP is not the diagnosis. A thorough ophthalmic examination is indicated because nearly 40% of noneffusive cases have ocular lesions. Other ancillary laboratory tests may be helpful; clinical chemistries may indicate organ dysfunction in liver, kidney, or pancreas. In cases of neurologic disease with diffuse meningeal involvement, CSF analysis may show increased protein content (90-2,000 mg/dL) and increased numbers of cells (90-9,250 cells/μL), predominantly neutrophils. The most definitive antemortem diagnostic technique is laparotomy and organ punch biopsy of lesions with subsequent demonstration of typical histopathologic changes.

FIP should be considered in the differential diagnosis of any condition that causes peritoneal or thoracic fluid accumulation and in any chronic wasting disease of cats. Effusive FIP with peritoneal involvement should be differentiated from ascites due to congestive heart failure or hypoproteinemia (renal and liver disease, glomerulonephritis, malabsorption, parasitism), neoplasia, bacterial peritonitis, pansteatitis, toxoplasmosis, tuberculosis, pregnancy, and trauma. Differential diagnoses of effusive FIP with pleural effusion include cardiac insufficiency, neoplasia (lymphoma), pyothorax, chylothorax, cryptococcosis, lung lobe torsion, diaphragmatic hernia, and trauma (hemothorax). Differential diagnosis of noneffusive FIP includes neoplasia and other systemic infectious diseases such as toxoplasmosis, nocardiosis, actinomycosis, tuberculosis, and deep mycotic disease (cryptococcosis, coccidioidomycosis, histoplasmosis, blastomycosis).

Treatment: There is no known treatment that can cure FIP once clinical signs arise. Although spontaneous remission in treated cats has been reported, it is uncommon. The mortality rate of clinical FIP is 95%. Cats with the effusive form progress rapidly, usually within 2 mo. The noneffusive form usually is associated with a more prolonged clinical course, with many cats living several months to a year. Treatment with anti-inflammatory and immunosuppressive drugs, along with supportive care, can make the cat more comfortable; in some cats (probably ≤10%), therapy may extend survival time by several months. Treatment is best advised in cats that are in good physical condition, are still eating, have no neurologic signs, and that do not have concurrent FeLV-induced malignancy or bone marrow suppression.

Treatment is directed toward controlling the immune-mediated vasculitis and reducing viral load. The most effective treatments are combinations of prednisolone (4 mg/kg or 50-100 mg/m^2, PO, SID) and cyclophosphamide (2-4 mg/kg, PO, SID for 4 consecutive days of each week). Alternatively, the cyclophosphamide can be given at 50 mg/m^2, PO, every 48 hr or 200-300 mg/m^2, every 2-3 wk. Other cytotoxic agents may be substituted for the cyclophosphamide, such as chlorambucil at 10 mg/m^2, PO, every 2-3 wk. Because this cytotoxic therapy may suppress bone marrow cells, the hemogram should be monitored weekly and the cat observed carefully for signs of sepsis. Supportive therapy for FIP is important and includes broad-spectrum antibiotics, adequate nutrition and fluid intake, and high doses of ascorbic acid (125-250 mg, BID). The use of low doses of aspirin (10 mg/kg every 48-72 hr) may be useful as an anti-inflammatory and possibly antithrombotic agent when used along with the steroids and cytotoxic agents. Treatment directed toward controlling the virus includes systemic interferon-α (10,000 U/kg, SC, SID or 1.3 million U/m^2, SC, 3 times/wk).

Prevention and Control: An intranasal, modified live virus vaccine to help prevent FIP is available. It protects 60-90% of the cats vaccinated as determined by experimental challenge several weeks after vaccination. The protection afforded by the vaccine appears to be related to secretory IgA, which neutralizes the virus before entry. The duration of significant protection is unknown but is thought to be limited. Its use has not been associated with causing FIP or accelerated disease either in the general cat population or in catteries with endemic FIP, and it has shown efficacy in preventing FIP losses in large cat shelters with endemic FIP when given to uninfected cats. Because FIP in the general cat population is relatively rare, vaccination of individual pet cats that live mostly or entirely indoors appears to be unwarranted.

Vaccination alone cannot be relied on to control endemic FIP within a cat facility. Other measures to reduce exposure include frequent removal of feces (the primary source of coronavirus), early weaning, isolation of cats that test positive for coronavirus antibodies, isolation and testing of cats after shows, proper sanitation and cleaning using virucidal disinfectants, and immunization against other feline viruses. These should be combined in an overall preventive health program. Increasing the number of litter boxes to at least 1 litter box per 2 cats and reducing crowding stress will reduce FIP losses. A control program based on the presence of serum antibodies to coronaviruses is not warranted. No healthy cat should be euthanized on the basis of a positive coronavirus serum antibody test. The risk of developing FIP following FIPV infection has been shown to have a strong genetic influence. Thus, prevention programs in catteries should include pedigree analysis of disease incidence so that only FIP-resistant breeding stock are used.

FELINE LEUKEMIA VIRUS AND RELATED DISEASES

(Feline lymphoma and leukemia, Lymphosarcoma)

Despite the widespread use of vaccines, feline leukemia virus (FeLV) remains one of the most important causes of morbidity and mortality in cats. It causes a variety of malignancies, but persistent infection can also cause severe immunosuppression and profound anemia. The virus is present worldwide. In nature, FeLV infects domestic cats and a few other Felidae. In the laboratory, cells from a much wider range of species can be infected by some strains of the virus.

Etiology and Epidemiology: FeLV is a retrovirus in the family Oncovirinae. Other oncoviruses include feline sarcoma virus, mouse leukemia viruses, and 2 human T-lymphotropic viruses. Although oncogenesis is one of their more dramatic effects, oncoviruses cause many other diseases, including degenerative, proliferative, and immunologic disorders.

There are 3 main FeLV subgroups of clinical importance. Subgroup A viruses are found in all naturally infected cats. FeLV-A, the original, archetypical form of the virus, is efficiently transmitted among cats. FeLV-A viruses tend to be less pathogenic than viruses of the other subgroups, but some strains cause severe immunosuppression. Almost all naturally infected cats are originally infected by FeLV-A. Within the infected cat, FeLV-A is sometimes altered to produce FeLV-B and FeLV-C viruses. FeLV-B is found in ~50% of naturally infected cats, along with FeLV-A. FeLV-A and FeLV-B together are more frequently associated with neoplastic diseases than is FeLV-A alone. FeLV-C viruses are isolated from only 1% of naturally infected cats, along with FeLV-A and sometimes both FeLV-A and FeLV-B. The presence of FeLV-C in an infected cat is strongly associated with the development of erythroid hypoplasia and consequent severe anemia. Viruses of all 3 subgroups are detected (but cannot be distinguished) by commonly used FeLV diagnostic test kits.

The incidence of FeLV infection is directly related to the population density of cats. Infection rates are highest in catteries and multicat households, especially when cats have access to the outdoors. In the USA, 1-2% of healthy stray urban cats are persistently viremic. Not surprisingly, much higher percentages of sick, "at risk" cats are found to be infected.

Persistently infected, healthy cats are the major reservoir of FeLV. Carriers excrete large quantities of virus in saliva. Lesser amounts of virus are excreted in tears, urine, and feces. Oronasal contact with infectious saliva or urine is the most likely mode of transmission. Nose-to-nose contact, mutual grooming, and shared litter trays and food dishes facilitate transmission. Bite wounds from infected cats are an efficient mode of transmission but occur relatively infrequently in cats kept indoors 100% of the time. Bites may be a more important mode of transmission in indoor-outdoor cats.

Age resistance is significant. Young kittens are much more susceptible than adults. The virus may be transmitted vertically (in utero or by milk) or horizontally (by secretions and excretions). Because FeLV is a fragile, enveloped virus and because of age resistance, horizontal transmission between adults usually requires prolonged, intimate contact. In addition, the dose required for oronasal transmission of the virus is relatively high.

Pathogenesis: After oronasal inoculation, the virus first replicates in oropharyngeal lymphoid tissue. From there, virus is carried in blood mononuclear cells to spleen, lymph nodes, epithelial cells of the intestine and bladder, salivary glands, and bone marrow. Virus later appears in secretions and excretions of these tissues and in peripheral blood leukocytes and platelets. Viremia is usually evident 2-4 wk after infection. The acute stage of FeLV infection (2-6 wk after infection) is rarely detected. It is typically characterized by mild fever, malaise, lymphadenopathy, and blood cytopenias.

In ~70% of adult cats, viremia and virus shedding are transient, lasting only 1-16 wk. A few cats continue to shed virus in secretions for several weeks to months after they cease to be viremic. Virus may persist in bone marrow for a longer period, but even this latent, or sequestered, infection usually disappears within 6 mo. Some FeLV-exposed cats (~30%) do not mount an adequate immune response and go on to become persistently (ie, permanently) viremic. Persistently viremic cats develop fatal diseases after a variable time period.

Disorders Caused by FeLV: FeLV-related disorders are numerous and include immunosuppression, neoplasia, anemia, immune-mediated diseases, reproductive problems, and enteritis.

The **immunosuppression** caused by FeLV is similar to that caused by feline immunodeficiency virus (p 661). There is an increased susceptibility to bacterial, fungal, protozoal, and other viral infections. Numbers of neutrophils and lymphocytes in the peripheral blood of affected cats may be reduced, and those cells that are present may be dysfunctional. Many FeLV-positive cats have low blood concentrations of complement; this contributes to FeLV-associated immunodeficiency and oncogenicity because complement is vital for some forms of antibody-mediated tumor cell lysis. Much of the immunodeficiency caused by FeLV is thought to be due to the high degree of viral antigenemia.

Lymphoid or myeloid tumors (eg, lymphoma, lymphoid leukemia, erythremic myelosis) develop in up to 30% of cats persistently infected with FeLV. Although FeLV-negative (ie, nonviremic) cats also develop these tumors, they may still be induced by FeLV, as many negative cats with lymphoma have viral sequences that can be detected by immunohistochemistry and PCR. Such cats may have been previously infected with FeLV despite negative test results for the virus. The transient presence of FeLV could have triggered lymphoma. However, the persistence of FeLV antigen increases the risk of lymphoma by as much as 60-fold compared with an FeLV-negative cat. Lymphoma is the most frequently diagnosed malignancy of cats. Most American cats with mediastinal, multicentric, or spinal forms of lymphoma are FeLV-positive. However, in some parts of the world, these forms of lymphoma are becoming much less common, and the proportion occurring in FeLV-positive cats is decreasing. This may be related to effective control of FeLV. Renal and GI forms of lymphoma are more likely to be found in FeLV-negative cats.

Leukemia is a neoplastic proliferation of hematopoietic cells originating in the bone marrow. The cell lines that become neoplastic are neutrophils, basophils, eosinophils, monocytes, lymphocytes, megakaryocytes, and erythrocytes. In cats, the leukemias are strongly associated with FeLV infection and sometimes (but not always) associated with neoplastic cells circulating in the blood. Lymphoid leukemias are further divided as acute and chronic. Acute lymphocytic leukemia is characterized by lymphoblasts circulating in the blood. In chronic lymphocytic leukemia, there is an increased number of circulating lymphocytes that have normal morphology.

The **anemia** caused by FeLV is usually nonregenerative and normochromic. There is frequently an idiosyncratic macrocytosis. About 10% of FeLV-related anemias are hemolytic and regenerative. This form of anemia may be associated with hemobartonellosis or immune-mediated hemolysis, or both.

Immune complexes formed in the presence of moderate antigen excess can cause systemic vasculitis, glomerulonephritis, polyarthritis, and a variety of other immune disorders. In FeLV-infected cats, immune complexes form under conditions of antigen excess, because FeLV antigens are abundant and anti-FeLV IgG antibodies are sparse. These conditions are ideal for the development of immune-mediated disease.

Reproductive problems are common; 68-73% of infertile queens have been reported to be FeLV-positive, and 60% of queens that abort are FeLV-positive (although abortion is a relatively uncommon cause of feline infertility). Fetal death, resorption, and placental involution may occur in the middle trimester of pregnancy, presumably as a result of in utero infection of fetuses by virus transported across the placenta in maternal leukocytes. Occasionally, infected queens give birth to live, viremic kittens. Latently infected (ie, nonviremic) queens may pass virus on to their kittens in milk.

Enteritis, resembling feline panleukopenia both clinically and histopathologically, may develop. Clinical signs include anorexia, depression, vomiting, and diarrhea (which may be bloody). Because of the concurrent immunosuppression associated with FeLV infection, septicemia may develop. Evidence suggests that FeLV and feline panleukopenia virus may act synergistically to produce this syndrome.

Other disorders may also develop. FeLV occasionally causes a neuropathy leading to anisocoria, urinary incontinence, or hindlimb paralysis. Certain FeLV-induced lymphomas can produce identical clinical signs. If antineoplastic therapy is planned, it is important to distinguish neoplasia from neuropathy. FeLV can also cause quasineoplastic disorders such as multiple cartilaginous exostoses (osteochondromatosis).

Diagnosis: Two types of tests are readily available for clinical use. The immunofluorescence assay (IFA) tests for the presence of FeLV structural antigens (eg, p27 or other core antigens) in the cytoplasm of cells suspected to be FeLV-infected. In clinical practice, peripheral blood smears are usually used for the IFA, but cytologic preparations of bone marrow or other tissues can also be used. The IFA is considered to be the most reliable but requires submission to a commercial laboratory, so results are delayed. IFA-positive cats are considered to be persistently viremic and have a poor longterm prognosis.

The more convenient ELISA can be performed in the veterinary clinic and tests for the presence of soluble FeLV p27. FeLV antigen may be present in the absence of intact, infectious viral particles because excess FeLV antigens are released from infected cells free of viral particles. The ELISA detects antigenemia rather than viremia. Several different test kits are available; most have sensitivities and specificities of 98%. Accuracy can be improved by running both the IFA and ELISA on the same cat.

Diagnosis of FeLV-induced neoplasia is similar to that of other tumors. Cytologic examination of fine-needle aspirates of masses, lymph nodes, body cavity fluids (eg, pleural effusion), and affected organs may reveal malignant lymphocytes. Bone marrow examination may reveal leukemic involvement, even when the peripheral blood appears normal. Biopsy and histopathologic examination of abnormal tissues is often necessary for diagnostic confirmation.

Treatment: Ideally, an FeLV-infected cat would be identified early and treated to eradicate the retroviral infection before FeLV-related diseases had time to develop. Unfortunately, eradication of retroviral infections at any stage of disease is extremely difficult. Most infected cats are persistently viremic by the time infection is diagnosed.

Many treatments have been administered in an attempt to reverse viremia or decrease clinical signs associated with FeLV infection. Anecdotal reports of antiviral agents and immunotherapeutic agents reversing viremia, improving clinical signs, and prolonging survival are abundant. Controlled studies using naturally infected cats have been unable to substantiate a benefit from these therapies.

FeLV-positive cats can live without major diseases for several years. Stress and sources of secondary infection should be avoided. The cat should remain indoors 100% of the time to reduce the risk of exposure to infectious agents and to prevent transmission of the virus to other cats. Routine prophylactic care for FeLV-infected cats is more important than for uninfected cats. Routine vaccinations should be administered based on the risk to the cat, with rabies vaccinations given to comply with local laws. FeLV vaccinations should not be administered, as there is no evidence to suggest a benefit. Physical examinations focusing on external parasites, skin infections, dental disease, lymph node size, and body weight should be performed every 6 mo. Administration of an anthelmintic at these visits is recommended. All infected cats should be neutered. Owners should be advised to watch for signs of FeLV-related disease, particularly secondary infections. Therapy for such infections or other illnesses should be more aggressive and of longer duration, as the immunocompromised condition renders the cat less able to fight diseases naturally.

Lymphoma Treatment: Feline lymphoma can be treated with cytotoxic drugs. These drugs may cause significant toxicities if not dosed and administered properly. (*See also* ANTINEOPLASTIC AGENTS, p 2138.) Most cytotoxic drugs are also carcinogens and must be handled properly. Before undertaking treatment with these drugs, veterinarians should familiarize themselves with proper dosing and administration, appropriate monitoring of the patient, toxicities and complications, and safe handling to prevent exposure of veterinary personnel and owners to the agents and their metabolites. Treated properly, most cats do not experience significant toxicities and enjoy a good quality of life.

About 50% of cats with lymphoma that are treated will obtain a complete remission (ie, no clinical evidence of disease). FeLV-negative cats that attain a complete remission live an average of 9 mo, and FeLV-positive cats have an average survival of 6 mo. Cats not treated or those not responding to treatment survive ~6 wk.

Many protocols for treatment of feline lymphoma have been published; most use similar drugs with differing schedules of administration. One widely used protocol consists of an intensive induction phase (vincristine 0.75 mg/m^2, IV, weekly for 4 wk, cyclophosphamide 300 mg/m^2, PO every 3 wk on the same day as vincristine, and prednisone 10 mg/cat, PO, SID throughout the protocol), followed by a less intensive maintenance phase (vincristine and cyclophosphamide given every 3 wk on the same day, prednisone continued daily). Treatment is continued for 1 yr or until relapse. With this protocol, 79% of cats attained remission and average survival was 150 days. Changing the maintenance protocol to doxorubicin 25 mg/m^2, IV, every 3 wk, provided an average remission of 281 days. When relapse occurs, the drug regimen can be changed and a second remission achieved; however, second remissions seldom last as long as the first.

Acute lymphocytic leukemia is treated with the same protocol as lymphoma, but only ~25% of cats obtain remission. For those that obtain remission, the average length is 7 mo. Chronic lymphocytic leukemia is best treated with chlorambucil (2 mg/cat, PO) and prednisone (40 mg/m^2, PO), given every other day on alternating days. Leukemias other than lymphocytic are rarely treated because the cats are extremely ill and very few respond to therapy.

Prevention and Control: Testing should be mandatory in the following situations: 1) all kittens at their first veterinary visit, so the owners can be counseled regarding a cat that tests positive (as is routinely done for congenital abnormalities), 2) all cats prior to entering a household with existing uninfected cats, 3) all cats in an existing household prior to admission of a new, uninfected cat, and 4) all cats prior to their first FeLV vaccination.

FeLV vaccines are intended to protect cats against FeLV infection or, at least, to prevent persistent viremia. Types of vaccines include killed whole virus, subunit, and genetically engineered. Vaccines may vary in protective effect, and manufacturers' claims and independent comparative studies should be carefully noted. Vaccines are indicated only for uninfected cats; there is no benefit in vaccinating an FeLV-positive cat. The cat's risk, of exposure to FeLV-positive cats should be assessed, and vaccines used only for those cats at risk. Although the risk of tumor development is low, FeLV vaccines have been associated with the development of sarcomas at the vaccination site. Uninfected cats in a household with infected cats should be vaccinated; however, other means of protecting uninfected cats (eg, physical separation) should also be used. Constant exposure to FeLV-infected cats is likely to result in viral transmission regardless of vaccination status.

Zoonotic Risk: Some strains of FeLV can be grown in human tissue cultures. This has led to concerns of possible transmission to humans. Several studies have addressed this concern; none have shown any evidence that any zoonotic risk exists.

FELINE PANLEUKOPENIA

(Feline infectious enteritis, Feline distemper)

Panleukopenia is a highly contagious, sometimes fatal, viral disease of cats that is seen worldwide. Kittens are affected most severely. The causative parvovirus is very resistant; it can persist for months in the environment unless potent disinfectants are used to inactivate it. Panleukopenia is now seen infrequently by veterinarians, presumably as a consequence of the widespread vaccine use. However, infection rates remain high in unvaccinated cat populations, and the disease occasionally is seen in vaccinated, pedigreed kittens that have been exposed to a high virus challenge.

Etiology, Transmission, and Pathogenesis: Feline panleukopenia virus (FPV) is closely related to mink enteritis virus and the type 2 canine parvoviruses (CPV-2, CPV-2a, CPV-2b). FPV can cause disease in all Felids and some members of related families (eg, raccoon, mink, and coatimundi), but it does not harm Canids. Conversely, CPV-2a and CPV-2b have recently been shown to cause a panleukopenia-like illness in domestic cats and large Felids. In a study of German and American cats with a clinical diagnosis of panleukopenia, CPV-2a or CPV-2b, rather than FPV, was isolated from ~10% of cases. In a Vietnamese study, 80% of parvoviruses isolated from healthy cats were canine rather than feline.

Virus particles are abundant in all secretions and excretions during the acute phase of illness and can be shed in the feces of survivors for up to 6 wk after recovery. Parvoviruses are extremely resistant to inactivation; they can survive >1 yr in a suitable environment and can be transported long distances via fomites (eg, shoes, clothing). However, parvoviruses are destroyed by exposure to a 6% solution of household bleach (aqueous sodium hypochlorite) for 10 min at room temperature. Peroxygen disinfectants are also highly effective.

Cats are infected oronasally by exposure to infected animals, their secretions, or fomites. Most free-roaming cats are exposed to the virus during their first year of life. Those that develop subclinical infection or survive acute illness mount a robust, long-lasting, protective immune response.

FPV infects and destroys actively dividing cells in bone marrow, lymphoid tissues, intestinal epithelium, and—in very young animals—cerebellum and retina. In pregnant queens, the virus may spread transplacentally to cause embryonic resorption, fetal mummification, abortion, or stillbirth. Alternatively, infection of kittens in the perinatal period may destroy the germinal epithelium of the cerebellum, leading to cerebellar hypoplasia, incoordination, and tremor. FPV-induced cerebellar ataxia has become a relatively rare diagnosis, because most queens passively transfer sufficient antibodies to their kittens to protect them during the period of susceptibility.

Clinical Findings: Most infections are subclinical, as evidenced by the high seroprevalence of anti-FPV antibodies among unvaccinated, healthy cats. Those that become ill are usually <1 yr old. Peracute cases may die suddenly with little or no warning (fading kittens). Acute cases show fever (104-107°F [40-41.7°C]), depression, and anorexia after an incubation period of 2-7 days. Vomiting usually develops 1-2 days after the onset of fever; it is typically bilious and unrelated to eating. Diarrhea may begin a little later but is not always present. Extreme dehydration develops rapidly. Affected cats may sit for hours at their water bowl, although they may not drink much. Terminal cases are hypothermic and may develop septic shock and disseminated intravascular coagulation.

Physical examination typically reveals profound depression, dehydration, and sometimes abdominal pain. Abdominal palpation—which can induce vomiting—may reveal thickened intestinal loops and enlarged mesenteric lymph nodes. In cases of cerebellar hypoplasia, ataxia and tremors with normal mentation are seen. Retinal lesions, if present, appear as discrete gray foci.

The duration of this self-limiting illness is seldom >5-7 days. Mortality is highest in young kittens <5 mo of age.

Lesions: There are typically few gross lesions, although dehydration is usually marked. Bowel loops are usually dilated and may have thickened, hyperemic walls. There may be petechiae or ecchymoses on the intestinal serosal surfaces. Perinatally infected kittens may have a noticeably small cerebellum. Histologically, the intestinal crypts are usually dilated and contain debris consisting of sloughed necrotic epithelial cells. Blunting and fusion of villi may be present. Eosinophilic intranuclear inclusion bodies are only occasionally seen in formalin-fixed specimens.

Diagnosis: A presumptive diagnosis is usually based on compatible clinical signs and the presence of panleukopenia (nadir 50-3,000 WBC/μL). Neutropenia is a more consistent finding than lymphopenia. Total WBC counts <2,000 cells/μL are associated with a poor prognosis. During recovery from infection, there is typically a rebound neutrophilia with a marked left shift. Diagnosis can be confirmed by showing the presence of FPV antigen in feces. Some of the in-office immunochromatographic test kits for detection of fecal CPV antigen can also detect FPV antigen during the acute phase of infection.

Differential diagnoses include other causes of profound depression, leukopenia, and GI signs. Salmonellosis and infections with feline leukemia virus (FeLV) and feline immunodeficiency virus should be considered. Concurrent infection with FeLV and FPV can cause a panleukopenia-like syndrome in adult cats.

Treatment and Prevention: Successful treatment of acute cases requires vigorous fluid therapy and supportive nursing care in the isolation unit. Electrolyte disturbances (eg, hypokalemia), hypoglycemia, hypoproteinemia, anemia, and opportunistic secondary infections often develop in severely affected cats. Anticipation of these possibilities, close monitoring, and prompt intervention are likely to improve outcome. IV fluid replacement and maintenance with a balanced isotonic crystalloid solution (eg, lactated Ringer's solution with calculated potassium supplementation) is the foundation of therapy. B vitamins should be added to the infusion, together with 5% glucose if hypoglycemia is suspected or proved. In addition to crystalloid infusion, transfusion of fresh-frozen plasma helps support plasma oncotic pressure and provides clotting factors to severely ill, hypoproteinemic kittens. Whole blood is preferable for severely anemic patients. Parenteral, broad-spectrum antibiotic therapy is indicated; however, nephrotoxic drugs (eg, gentamicin, amikacin) should be avoided until dehydration has been corrected. Antiemetic therapy (eg, metoclopramide) may provide some relief and allow earlier enteral feeding of soft, easily digested food. Parenteral nutrition is indicated for severely affected cases.

Excellent inactivated and modified live virus vaccines that provide solid, longlasting immunity are available for prevention of FPV infection. Live vaccines should not be given to cats that are pregnant, immunosuppressed, or sick, or to kittens <4 wk old. Most vaccine manufacturers recommend that kittens should receive 2 or 3 modified live vaccine doses, 3 wk apart. The first vaccination is usually given at 6-9 wk of age. The last dose of the initial vaccination series should not be administered before the kitten is 12-14 wk old, to ensure that interfering maternal antibodies do not inactivate the modified live virus. Exposure to virus should be avoided until 1 wk after the vaccination series has been completed. Most manufacturers recommend annual booster revaccination, although other authorities recommend triennial boosters.

INFECTIOUS CANINE HEPATITIS

Infectious canine hepatitis (ICH) is a worldwide, contagious disease of dogs with signs that vary from a slight fever and congestion of the mucous membranes to severe depression, marked leukopenia, and prolonged bleeding time. It also is seen in foxes, wolves, coyotes, and bears; other carnivores may become infected without developing clinical illness. In recent years, the disease has become uncommon in areas where routine immunization is used.

Etiology and Pathogenesis: ICH is caused by a nonenveloped DNA virus, canine adenovirus 1 (CAV-1), which is antigenically related only to CAV-2 (one of the causes of infectious canine tracheobronchitis, p 1247). CAV-1 is resistant to lipid solvents and survives outside the host for weeks or months, but a 1-3% solution of sodium hypochlorite (household bleach) is an effective disinfectant.

Ingestion of urine, feces, or saliva of infected dogs is the main route of infection. Recovered dogs shed virus in their urine for ≥6 mo. Initial infection occurs in the tonsillar crypts and Peyer's patches, followed by viremia and infection of endothelial cells in many tissues. Liver, kidneys, spleen, and lungs are the main target organs. Chronic kidney lesions and corneal clouding ("blue eye") result from immune-complex reactions after recovery from acute or subclinical disease.

Clinical Findings: Signs vary from a slight fever to death. The mortality rate is highest in very young dogs. The incubation period is 4-9 days. The first sign is a fever of >104°F (40°C), which lasts 1-6 days and is usually biphasic. If the fever is of short duration, leukopenia may be the only other sign, but if it persists for >1 day, acute illness develops. Tachycardia out of proportion to the fever may occur. On the day after the initial temperature rise, leukopenia develops and persists throughout the febrile period. The degree of leukopenia varies and seems to be correlated with the severity of illness.

Signs are apathy, anorexia, thirst, conjunctivitis, serous discharge from the eyes and nose, and occasionally abdominal pain and vomiting. Intense hyperemia or petechiae of the oral mucosa, as well as enlarged tonsils, may be seen. There may be subcutaneous edema of the head, neck, and trunk.

Clotting time is directly correlated with the severity of illness. It may be difficult to control hemorrhage, which is manifest by bleeding around deciduous teeth and by spontaneous hematomas, because of underlying disseminated intravascular coagulation. Respiratory signs usually are not seen in dogs with ICH; however, CAV-1 has been recovered from dogs with signs of infectious tracheobronchitis and from dogs with respiratory signs induced by exposure to the nebulated virus. Although CNS involvement is unusual, severely infected dogs may develop convulsions from forebrain damage; brain stem hemorrhages, resulting in paresis, are common. Foxes more consistently have CNS signs and intermittent convulsions during the course of illness, and paralysis may involve one or more limbs or the entire body.

On recovery, dogs eat well but regain weight slowly. Bilateral corneal opacity develops 7-10 days after the acute signs disappear in ~25% of recovered dogs and usually disappears spontaneously. In mild cases, transient corneal opacity may be the only sign of disease.

Chronic hepatitis may develop in dogs having low levels of passive antibody when exposed. Simultaneous infection with CAV-1 and distemper virus is sometimes seen.

Lesions: Endothelial damage results in "paint brush" hemorrhages on the gastric serosa, lymph nodes, thymus, pancreas, and subcutaneous tissues. Hepatic cell necrosis produces a variegated color change in the liver, which may be normal in size or swollen. The gallbladder wall may be edematous and thickened; edema of the thymus may be found. Grayish white foci may be seen in the kidney cortex.

Diagnosis: Usually, the abrupt onset and bleeding suggest ICH. Clinical evidence is not always sufficient to differentiate ICH from distemper (p 625), although the gross changes in the liver and gallbladder are more conclusive. Diagnosis is confirmed by virus isolation, immunofluorescence, or characteristic intranuclear inclusion bodies in the liver.

Treatment: Blood transfusions may be necessary in severely ill dogs. In addition, 5% dextrose in isotonic saline should be given, preferably IV. In dogs with prolonged clotting time, SC administration of fluids may be dangerous. A broad-spectrum antibiotic should be given. Because tetracyclines may cause discoloration of the teeth during tooth development, they should not be used in puppies before their permanent teeth erupt. Although the transient corneal opacity (that may be seen during the course of ICH or be associated with vaccination with attenuated CAV-1 vaccines) usually requires no treatment, atropine ophthalmic ointment may alleviate the painful ciliary spasm that is sometimes associated with it. Dogs with corneal clouding should be protected against bright light. Systemic corticosteroids are generally contraindicated for treatment of corneal opacity associated with ICH.

Prevention: Modified-live virus vaccines are available and are often combined with other vaccines. Vaccination against ICH is recommended at the time of canine distemper vaccinations. Attenuated CAV-1 vaccines have produced transient unilateral or bilateral opacities of the cornea, and the virus may be shed in urine. CAV-2 attenuated live virus strains, which provide cross protection against CAV-1, are preferentially used because they have very little tendency to produce corneal opacities or uveitis, and the virus is not shed in urine. Annual revaccination against ICH is often practiced. Maternal antibody from immune bitches interferes with active immunization in puppies until they are 9-12 wk old.

RICKETTSIAL DISEASES

EHRLICHIOSIS AND RELATED INFECTIONS

In the past, a number of obligate intracellular organisms that infect eukaryotic cells were classified in the genus *Ehrlichia* on morphologic and ecologic grounds and were grouped according to the cell type they inhabit. With newer genetic analyses, these agents have been reclassified into the genera of *Ehrlichia*, *Anaplasma*, and *Neorickettsia*. Although no longer technically correct, usage of the term ehrlichiosis persists when describing infection caused by these agents.

Etiology: Classical canine monocytic ehrlichiosis is caused by *Ehrlichia canis*, which infects the mononuclear cells of dogs; canine monocytic ehrlichiosis may also be caused by *E chaffeensis*, the etiologic agent of human monocytic ehrlichiosis. A monocytic ehrlichiosis has been identified in cats in Africa, France, and the USA; however, the exact species has not been determined. *E ewingi* is a granulocytic species that has been isolated from dogs and humans in the southern, western, and midwestern USA. Human granulocytic ehrlichiosis, caused by *Anaplasma phagocytophilum* is seen in the northern midwestern, northeastern, and western coastal regions of the USA and in Europe and Asia. The host range of infection and illness for various strains within this genogroup also includes horses and ruminants; dogs and cats may occasionally be infected. *Anaplasma (Ehrlichia) platys* is the cause of infectious cyclic thrombocytopenia of dogs. The following discussion of ehrlichiosis primarily describes infection in dogs caused by *E canis*.

Epidemiology: *E canis* and *A platys* are enzootic in many parts of the USA and worldwide. These agents are transmitted by the brown dog tick, *Rhipicephalus sanguineus*. *Rhipicephalus* ticks become infected with *E canis* after feeding on infected dogs, and ticks transmit infection to other dogs during blood meals taken in successive life stages. Blood transfusions, or other means by which infected WBC can be transferred, may also transmit the pathogens. Other *Ehrlichia* and *Anaplasma* species have sylvan cycles in the environment involving various other tick species and wildlife reservoir hosts. In the USA, *E chaffeensis* and *E ewingii* are transmitted by *Amblyomma americanum*, the lone star tick. *Anaplasma phagocytophilum* is transmitted by *Ixodes* species of ticks; in the northeastern USA, infection is transmitted by *I scapularis*, the black-legged tick, whereas infection in western states is primarily associated with *I pacificus*, the Western black-legged tick. People, dogs, cats, and other domestic animals are incidental hosts of these pathogens.

Clinical Findings: In *E canis* infections, signs arise from the involvement of the hemic and lymphoreticular systems and commonly progress from acute to chronic, depending on the strain of organism and immune status of the host. In acute cases, there is reticuloendothelial hyperplasia, fever, generalized lymphadenopathy, splenomegaly, and thrombocytopenia. Variable signs of anorexia, depression, loss of stamina, stiffness and reluctance to walk, edema of the limbs or scrotum, and coughing or dyspnea may occur. Most acute cases are seen in the warmer months, coincident with the greatest activity of the tick vector.

During the acute phase of *E canis* infection in dogs, the hemogram is usually normal but may reflect a mild normocytic, normochromic anemia; leukopenia; or mild leukocytosis. Thrombocytopenia is common, but petechiae may not be evident, and platelet decreases may be mild in some animals. Vasculitis and immune-mediated mechanisms induce a thrombocytopenia and hemorrhagic tendencies. Lymph node aspiration reveals hyperplasia. Death is rare during this phase; spontaneous recovery may occur, the dog may remain asymptomatic, or chronic disease may ensue.

Chronic ehrlichiosis caused by *E canis* may develop in any breed, but certain breeds, eg, German Shepherds, may be predisposed. Seasonality is not a specific hallmark of chronic infection, as appearance of chronic signs may be variably delayed following acute infection. In chronic cases, the bone marrow becomes hypoplastic, and lymphocytes and plasmacytes infiltrate various organs. Clinical findings vary based on the predominant organs affected, and may include marked splenomegaly, glomerulonephritis, renal failure, interstitial pneumonitis, anterior uveitis, and meningitis with associated cerebellar ataxia, depression, paresis, and hyperesthesia. Severe weight loss is a prominent finding.

The hemogram is usually markedly abnormal in chronic cases. Frequently, severe thrombocytopenia may cause epistaxis, hematuria, melena, and petechiae and ecchymoses of the skin. Variably severe pancytopenia (mature leukopenia, nonregenerative anemia, thrombocytopenia, or any combination thereof) may occur. Aspiration cytology reveals reactive lymph nodes and, usually, marked plasmacytosis. Frequently, polyclonal, or occasionally monoclonal, hypergammaglobulinemia occurs.

Dogs infected with *A platys* generally show minimal to no signs of infection despite the presence of the organism in platelets. The primary finding is cyclic thrombocytopenia, recurring at 10-day intervals. Generally, the cyclic nature diminishes, and the thrombocytopenia becomes mild and slowly resolves. Other ehrlichial infections not caused by *E canis* appear clinically similar to acute *E canis* infection, but the clinical course is usually more self-limiting. Shifting leg lameness and fever of unknown origin may be present. Thrombocytopenia and mild leukopenia or leukocytosis may occur during the acute course of infection, which is clinically more discrete. Chronic disease, as seen with *E canis* infection, is not typically seen in other ehrlichial infections.

Lesions: During the acute or self-limiting phase of *E canis* infections, lesions generally are nonspecific, but splenomegaly is common. Histologically, there is lymphoreticular hyperplasia, and lymphocytic and plasmacytic perivascular cuffing. In chronic cases, these lesions may be accompanied by widespread hemorrhage and increased mononuclear cell infiltration in perivascular regions of many organs.

Diagnosis: Because thrombocytopenia is a relatively consistent finding of infection with *Ehrlichia* and *Anaplasma* species, a platelet count is an important screening test. Clinical diagnosis may be confirmed by demonstrating the organisms within WBC, seen in intracytoplasmic inclusion bodies called morulae. This method of diagnosis lacks sensitivity, as low numbers of organisms make demonstration difficult. More commonly, a diagnosis is made by a combination of clinical signs, positive indirect serum fluorescent antibody titer, and response to treatment. The antibody response may be delayed up to 28 days; thus, serologic testing may not be a reliable diagnostic tool early in the course of the disease, and testing of paired sera and demonstration of increased antibody titers is recommended to confirm infection. Serologic cross-reactivity is strong between *E canis*, *E chaffeensis*, and *E ewingi*; minimal cross-reactivity to *Anaplasma phagocytophilum* is also seen. These reactions should be considered in appropriate geographic areas. In some areas, ~50% of dogs infected with *E canis* also have a titer to *A platys*, which likely reflects co-infection; cross-reactivity between these agents is not observed.

PCR has been used to detect and identify specific *Ehrlichia* species in infected people and animals. Samples appropriate for PCR include blood, tissue aspirates, or biopsy specimens of reticuloendothelial organs such as lymph nodes, spleen, liver, or bone marrow. PCR can also be used to detect the effectiveness of treatment in clearing infection. PCR is not routinely available through commercial laboratories, although some veterinary schools and research institutions may offer it.

During the acute stage, differential diagnoses include other causes of fever and lymphadenomegaly (eg, Rocky Mountain spotted fever, brucellosis, blastomycosis, endocarditis), immune-mediated diseases (eg, systemic lupus erythematosus), and lymphosarcoma. During the chronic stage of *E canis* infection, differential diagnoses include estrogen toxicity, myelophthisis, immune-mediated pancytopenia, and other multisystemic diseases associated with specific organ dysfunction (eg, glomerulonephritis).

Treatment: The drug of choice for all forms of infection caused by these organisms is doxycycline because of its superior intracellular penetration. The recommended dosage is 5-10 mg/kg, PO or IV, SID for 10-21 days. Tetracycline (22 mg/kg, PO, TID) can also be used for ≥2 wk in acute cases and 1-2 mo in chronic cases. Two doses of imidocarb dipropionate (5-7 mg/kg, IM), 2 wk apart, are variably effective against both ehrlichiosis and some strains of babesiosis. In acute cases receiving appropriate antibiotic therapy, body temperature is expected to return to normal within 24-48 hr after treatment. In chronic cases, the hematologic abnormalities may persist for 3-6 mo, although clinical response to treatment often occurs much sooner. Supportive therapy may be necessary to combat wasting and specific organ dysfunction; platelet or whole-blood transfusions may be required if hemorrhage is extensive. Concurrent broad-spectrum antibiotics may be needed if the dog has severe leukopenia. The *E canis* antibody titer should be measured again within 6 mo of illness to confirm a low or seronegative status indicative of successful therapy. Serum titers that persist at lower but positive levels should be rechecked in another 6 mo to ensure that they are not increasing.

Prevention: Prevention is enhanced by controlling ticks and using seronegative screened blood donors. Prophylactic administration of tetracycline at a lower dose

(6.6 mg/kg, PO, SID) is effective in preventing *E canis* infection in kennels where disease is endemic. Treatment must be extended for many months through at least one tick season if the endemic cycle is to be successfully eliminated.

ROCKY MOUNTAIN SPOTTED FEVER
(*Rickettsia rickettsii* infection, Tick fever)

Etiology: Rocky Mountain spotted fever (RMSF) is a disease of humans and dogs that is caused by *Rickettsia rickettsii*. *R rickettsii* and closely related members of the spotted fever group of rickettsiae are considered endemic throughout much of North, South, and Central America. These pathogens are transmitted primarily through the bites of infected ticks. Because of their susceptibility, dogs are an excellent sentinel of *R rickettsii* infection in humans. Clusters of disease are frequently reported in defined geographic areas, and temporally associated infections may be seen in both dogs and their owners.

Epidemiology: In the USA, *Dermacentor variabilis* (the American dog tick) and *D andersoni* (the Rocky Mountain wood tick) are considered the primary vectors for *R rickettsii*. The pathogen is acquired by larval and nymph stages of ticks while feeding on infected vertebrate hosts, and is also passed from female ticks to progeny through transovarial transmission. An estimated 1-3% of *Dermacentor* spp of ticks carry *R rickettsii*, even in areas considered highly endemic.

Seroprevalence in dogs from endemic areas ranges from 4.3 to 63.4%, but these values do not accurately reflect infection rates due to the detection of cross-reacting antibodies to other spotted fever group rickettsiae. Because rickettsemia may be present during the acute stages, blood and tissue specimens should be handled with care. RMSF transmission through blood transfusion has been documented in a single human case, and should be considered when selecting canine blood donors. Direct transmission from dogs to humans has not been reported, although human infection may occur following contact of abraded skin or conjunctiva with tick hemolymph or excreta during removal of engorged ticks from pets.

Clinical Findings: Dogs are highly susceptible to clinical infection with *R rickettsii*; in contrast, RMSF infection is rarely diagnosed in cats. Early signs in dogs may include fever (up to 105°F [40.5°C]), anorexia, lymphadenopathy, polyarthritis, coughing or dyspnea, abdominal pain, vomiting and diarrhea, and edema of the face or extremities. Petechial hemorrhages of the conjunctiva and oral mucosa may be observed in severe cases. Focal retinal hemorrhage may be observed during the early course of disease. Neurologic manifestations such as altered mental states, vestibular dysfunction, and paraspinal hyperesthesia may occur.

Thrombocytopenia is common. Leukopenia develops during the early stages of infection and, in untreated cases, is followed by progressive leukocytosis. Serum biochemical abnormalities may include hypoproteinemia, hypoalbuminemia, azotemia, hyponatremia, hypocalcemia, and increased liver enzyme activities. Case fatality rates of ~1-10% are expected.

Lesions: Vascular endothelial damage is due to direct cytopathic effects of the rickettsiae. Severity of the necrotizing vasculitis can be directly correlated to the infective dose. Vascular endothelial damage and thrombocytopenia contribute to development of petechiae and ecchymoses. Necrosis of the extremities (acryl gangrene) or disseminated intravascular coagulation can develop in severely affected dogs.

Diagnosis: Indirect fluorescent antibody titer is preferred for serologic testing. However, because of the high incidence of cross-reacting antibodies to a variety of nonpathogenic spotted fever group rickettsiae, as well as longterm persistence of antibodies following acute RMSF infection, demonstration of a 4-fold rise in titer should be documented in conjunction with a compatible clinical syndrome. Differential diagnoses include other causes of fever of unknown origin. The therapeutic response is usually dramatic, as it is in other canine rickettsial diseases. Animals with neurologic dysfunction may have residual deficits. Immunity appears to be lifelong after natural infection; therefore, recurrent episodes should not be attributed to RMSF.

Treatment: Antibiotic treatment should be administered based on clinical suspicion, without waiting for results of serologic tests, because delayed administration of anitbiotics may result in higher rates of severe or fatal outcome. Doxycycline should be administered at a dosage of 5-10 mg/kg, PO or IV, SID for 10-21 days. Tetracycline at 22 mg/kg, PO, TID for 2 wk, is also effective. Supportive care for dehydration and hemorrhagic diathesis may be necessary. Due to alterations in vascular integrity, conservative rates of fluid administration are advised. Precautions should be taken for the safe removal and control of ticks.

SALMON POISONING DISEASE AND ELOKOMIN FLUKE FEVER
(*Neorickettsia* spp infection)

Salmon poisoning disease (SPD) is an acute, infectious disease of canids, in which the infective agent is transmitted through the various stages of a fluke in a snail-fish-dog life cycle. The name of the disease is misleading because no toxin is involved. Elokomin fluke fever (EFF) is an acute infectious disease of canids, ferrets, bears, and raccoons that resembles SPD but has a wider host range.

Etiology: SPD is caused by *Neorickettsia helminthoeca* and is sometimes complicated by a second agent, *N elokominica*, which causes EFF. The vector of both agents is a small fluke, *Nanophyetus salmincola*. Dogs and other animals become infected by ingesting trout, salmon, or Pacific giant salamanders that contain encysted metacercariae of the rickettsia-infected fluke. In the dog's intestine, the larval flukes excyst, embed in the duodenal mucosa, and introduce the rickettsiae. The fluke infection itself produces little or no clinical disease.

Epidemiology: The life cycle is maintained by the passage of infected fluke ova in the feces of the host. Miracidia develop from these ova and infect the snail *Oxytrema plicifer* to form rediae. Rediae develop into cercariae that are released from the snail, penetrate the salmon or trout, and develop into infective, encysted metacercariae. The cycle is completed when a dog eats the fish and becomes infected with the rickettsiae. Transmission by cage-to-cage contact, rectal thermometers, or aerosols is rare.

There are no age, sex, or breed predilections; however, the disease prevalence is higher when the availability of fish is greater. Infected fish are found in the Pacific Ocean from San Francisco to the coast of Alaska, but SPD is more prevalent from northern California to Puget Sound. It is also seen inland along the rivers of fish migration. Apparently, the snail is the geographically limiting factor.

Clinical Findings: In SPD, signs appear suddenly, usually 5-7 days after eating infected fish, but may be delayed as long as 33 days, and persist for 7-10 days before culminating in death in up to 90% of untreated animals. Body temperature peaks at 104-107.6°F (40-42°C) 1-2 days later, then gradually declines for 4-8 days and returns to normal. Frequently, animals are hypothermic before death. Fever is accompanied by depression and complete anorexia in virtually all cases. Persistent vomiting usually occurs by day 4 or 5. Diarrhea develops by day 5-7; it often contains blood and may be severe. Dehydration and extreme weight loss occur. When severe, the GI signs are clinically indistinguishable from those of canine parvoviral infection. Generalized lymphadenopathy develops in ~60% of cases. Nasal or conjunctival exudate may be present and mimic signs of distemper. Neutrophilia is common, but a marked, absolute leukopenia with a degenerative left shift may occur. Thrombocytopenia is reported in 94% of the cases. Serum chemistry values are normal.

Clinically, EFF is a milder infection than SPD. Severe GI signs are less commonly seen in EFF infections, and lymphadenopathy may be a more pronounced finding. Case fatality rates with EFF are lower, occurring in ~10% of untreated cases.

Lesions: Infection appears to chiefly affect the lymphoid tissues and intestines. There is enlargement of the GI lymph follicles, lymph nodes, tonsils, thymus, and to some extent, the spleen, with microscopic necrosis, hemorrhage, and hyperplasia. A variable but often severe hemorrhagic enteritis, which seems to arise from damaged lymph follicles, is seen throughout the intestine with SPD, but is less commonly observed with EFF.

Microscopic foci of necrosis also appear apart from the follicles. Flukes embedded in the duodenum account for little tissue damage. Nonsuppurative meningitis or meningoencephalitis has been identified in some dogs.

Diagnosis: Fluke ova are found on fecal examination in ~92% of cases, which supports the diagnosis. The ova are oval, yellowish brown, rough-surfaced, and ~87-97 × 35-55 μm, with an indistinct operculum and a small, blunt point on the opposite end. During the first day or two, few ova may be passed. Intracellular organisms have been demonstrated via lymph node aspiration in ~70% of the cases. Other causes of fever of unknown origin, generalized lymphadenopathy, vomiting, and diarrhea are differential diagnoses. When diarrhea and exudative conjunctivitis occur, distemper should be considered.

Prevention and Treatment: Currently, the only means of prevention is to prevent the ingestion of uncooked salmon, trout, steelhead, and similar freshwater fish. In animals that recover, a profound humoral immune response persists, but there is no cross-resistance between *N helminthoeca* and *N elokominica*. Various sulfonamides given PO or parenterally are effective, as are chlortetracycline, oxytetracycline, and chloramphenicol. Animals usually succumb because of dehydration, electrolyte and acid-base imbalances, and anemia. Therefore, general supportive therapy to maintain hydration and acid-base balance, while meeting nutritional requirements and controlling diarrhea, is often essential. Judicious use of whole blood transfusions may be helpful.

VISCERAL LEISHMANIASIS

Visceral leishmaniasis is a chronic, severe, protozoal disease of humans, dogs, and certain rodents characterized by cutaneous or mucocutaneous lesions, lymphadenopathy, weight loss, anemia, lameness, renal failure, and occasionally epistaxis or ocular lesions.

Infection in dogs is prevalent in Central and South America, the Middle East, Asia, and in the Mediterranean region. The disease is endemic in Foxhounds in North America. Isolated cases are diagnosed around the world in animals that have visited endemic areas. Cats and other domestic animals are rarely infected and usually only develop cutaneous ulcers, without showing signs of visceral disease.

Canine leishmaniasis is a zoonosis, and dogs act as a reservoir of the parasite for humans where there is a competent vector.

Etiology, Transmission, and Pathogenesis: *Leishmania infantum* and *L donovani* are the causative agents in the Mediterranean area and Middle East, whereas *L chagasi*, *L braziliensis*, and *L mexicana* are the major species in Central and South America. The parasites are transmitted as flagellated forms (promastigotes) by the bite of several species of phlebotomine sandflies, which are found worldwide. The flies do not fly long distances and complete their life cycles in an area with a diameter of <1 km. The females take blood only from vertebrates and move at dawn and dusk in search of food. Once inoculated in the skin of the mammalian host, the promastigotes are engulfed by macrophages, in which they transform to amastigotes, an aflagellated form. Inside the macrophages, the amastigotes divide and spread to different organs, especially the bone marrow, lymph nodes, skin, spleen, liver, and kidneys. At least 2 different pathogenic mechanisms are responsible for the signs and lesions of the disease—the production of granulomatous inflammatory reactions and the formation of circulating immune complexes that deposit in the renal glomeruli, blood vessels, and joints.

Clinical Findings: The incubation period is quite variable, ranging from 3 mo to several years. The clinical features vary widely; main clinical presentations are skin lesions, loss of weight or poor appetite, local or generalized lymphadenopathy, ocular lesions, renal failure, epistaxis, lameness, and anemia. Occasionally, some dogs have chronic diarrhea or liver failure. The most common cutaneous lesions are alopecia with severe dry desquamation, usually beginning on the head and extending to the rest of the body. Other animals develop chronic ulceration, located particularly on the head and limbs. The signs invariably show a slow, progressive evolution.

The results of blood and urine tests also vary greatly. Most animals have a polyclonal hyperproteinemia. Nonregenerative anemia is present in 50% of dogs. Some animals show leukopenia, whereas others have leukocytosis. In animals with renal lesions, it is also usual to find increased plasma urea and creatinine, proteinuria, and hematuria.

Diagnosis: The most reliable diagnostic test for canine leishmaniasis is direct observation of the parasite in bone marrow or lymph node smears. The amastigotes appear as oval basophilic bodies (4 μm) in the cytoplasm of macrophages. However, it is sometimes impossible to detect the parasite in infected animals, especially in lymph node smears. Serologic methods are useful in diagnosis; indirect immunofluorescence and ELISA are widely used. The results of a serologic test should be interpreted in conjunction with the clinical picture. Although these tests are reliable, a few infected dogs remain seronegative, and there are also seropositive dogs that never develop the disease.

Treatment and Control: For treatment, the drugs of choice are the pentavalent antimony derivatives, particularly N-methylglucamine antimoniate (80-100 mg/kg/day, IM or SC [not approved for use in dogs in the USA]) and sodium stibogluconate (75 mg/kg, SC, BID [available only from the CDC in the USA]). During the first month, the dog is treated with either drug and allopurinol (20 mg/kg, PO, SID; during the next 5 mo, the dog is treated with only allopurinol, which is less expensive and less toxic. Amphotericin B given IV (0.5-0.8 mg/kg, diluted in 10-60 mL of 5% dextrose given over 45 sec every 48 hr for a total cumulative dose of 8-15 mg/kg is reached) or SC 2-3 times/wk (0.5-0.8 mg/kg added to 500 mL of 0.45% saline and 2.5% dextrose for a total cumulative dosage of 8-26 mg/kg) has also been effective. Relapses after treatment are common with either protocol. In endemic areas, rapid treatment of infected dogs, control of stray and homeless dogs, and action against the insect vectors are recommended methods of control. Treatment of dogs in nonendemic areas is questionable and probably unwise if a competent vector is present. At present, there is no effective vaccine against canine leishmaniasis.

IMMUNE SYSTEM

IMMUNOPATHOLOGIC MECHANISMS

The primary role of the immune system is the discrimination of self and non-self. The fundamental purpose of recognition of non-self is to protect against invading microorganisms, chemical agents, or other foreign substances. To eliminate non-self agents, the immune system has developed a variety of mechanisms, including inactivation of biologic agents, lysis of foreign cells, agglutination or precipitation of molecules or cells, or phagocytosis of foreign materials. Generating the right class of immune response is under the control of dendritic cells (DC). DC can be considered immunologic sensors—they are scattered throughout the body, sense environmental stimuli, and convey this information to naïve lymphocytes to tune the relevant immune response. For example, in response to intracellular microbes such as viruses or certain bacteria, DC secrete interleukin-12 (IL_{12}), inducing T-helper cells (T_H) to differentiate into T_H1. T_H1 cells promote cell-mediated immunity through production of γ-interferon (IFNγ) and IL_2. In contrast, extracellular pathogens such as helminths lead DC to secrete IL_4 and to trigger the naïve T_H cells toward T_H2 differentiation. T_H2 cells promote antibody production through the secretion of IL_4, IL_5, IL_{10}, and IL_{13}, which increase IgE production, eosinophils and mast cells. The protective immune response against a non-self agent is a complex program including the nature of the stimuli, DC subsets, T_H subsets, and polarized cytokine profiles.

However, under certain circumstances, these normally protective responses can result in significant tissue damage; these immunopathologic mechanisms are called immune-mediated diseases. There are 4 general classical classifications of these diseases, which are mediated either through antibodies (Types I, II, and III) or by cells (Type IV). Many theories exist to explain immune-mediated diseases including external environmental factors, genetic predisposition, and hormonal influences. Recently immune-mediated diseases have been categorized in light of T_H1 and T_H2 polarization. T_H1 cells are associated with autoimmune diseases (Type II) and T_H2 cells with allergic diseases, immune complex disorders, and delayed-type hypersensitivity (Types I, III, and IV).

Corticosteroids, with or without other immunosuppressive drugs, are currently the mainstay of immune-mediated disease treatment. The primary challenge in this area is to find specific agents that precisely correct the dysregulation of T_H1/T_H2 homeostasis.

TYPE I REACTIONS
(Anaphylaxis)

Anaphylaxis is an acute systemic manifestation of the interaction of an antigen (allergen) binding to IgE antibodies, which are bound to mast cells and basophils. This binding of antigens to cell-bound IgE antibodies triggers the release of chemical substances from the mast cells and basophils. The major biologically active mediators produced by mast cells and basophils include histamine, leukotrienes, eosinophilic chemotactic factor, platelet activating factor, kinins, serotonins, and proteolytic enzymes. These chemicals directly affect both the vascular system, causing vasodilation and increased vascular permeability, and smooth muscles, causing contraction. Additionally, they result in the migration of eosinophils to the triggering site. The severity of the reaction depends on the type of antigen, the amount of IgE antibodies produced, and the amount of antigen and route of exposure. Agents that can cause anaphylactic and allergic reactions are numerous and include the venom of stinging and biting insects, vaccines, drugs of any kind, foods, and blood products.

Clinical signs can be localized or generalized and include restlessness and excitement, pruritis around the head or site of exposure, facial edema, salivation, lacrimation, vomiting, abdominal pain, diarrhea, dyspnea, cyanosis, shock, incoordination, collapse, convulsions, and death. Dogs differ from other domestic animals in that the major organ affected by anaphylactic shock is the liver, rather than the lungs. Signs in dogs are associated with constriction of hepatic veins, which results in portal hypertension and visceral pooling of blood. Therefore, GI signs rather than respiratory signs are more apt to be seen in dogs. Supportive therapy, in addition to treating respiratory distress, consists of the administration of epinephrine (both locally and systemically as needed), IV fluids for the treatment of shock, antihistamines (systemically for severe acute anaphylaxis or orally as a means to control chronic signs of allergy or milder allergic signs), and corticosteroids if needed.

TYPE II REACTIONS
(Antibody-mediated cytotoxic reactions)

Type II reactions occur when an antibody binds to an antigen present on the surface of the cell. This antibody-antigen complex then can activate the complement pathway, resulting in cell lysis or, through an antibody-mediated or complement-fragment-mediated receptor binding of a phagocytic cell, an antibody-mediated cytotoxicity. It is unclear what triggers this antibody-mediated cytotoxicity but, as with all immune-mediated pathologic events, the combination of external factors and an infectious process in a genetically predisposed animal can lead to the development of immunopathologic disorders. It has been hypothesized that acute viral infections can lead to changes in immune regulatory pathways that result in an overreaction of the immune system or to conversion of the protective immune response into a pathologic process. Also, cross-reactive antibodies can develop during an infectious process. These cross-reactive antibodies directed toward an infectious agent will bind to normal tissue and result in antibody-mediated cytotoxicity. For example, in streptococcal infection in horses a cross-reaction between streptococcal antigen and vascular basement membranes can occur, leading to an immunopathologic disease. Lastly, certain pathogens such as *Babesia* or *Haemobartonella* may parasitize tissues, causing an immune response that destroys those tissues as part of the protective mechanism.

Clinical signs of a Type II hypersensitivity are variable and depend on the organ in which the reaction is occurring. They can include fever, cutaneous signs, polyarthritis, pain or joint swelling, and CNS signs. Glomerular nephritis is recognized by proteinuria or acute renal failure. Hematologic abnormalities such as hemolytic anemia, thrombocytopenia, neutropenia, or lymphopenia may be seen. Vague signs such as vomiting, diarrhea, or abdominal pain may also be seen. The diagnosis is primarily made by elimination of more obvious causes for the signs mentioned above and by histopathologic and immunohistopathologic analysis of organ biopsies. Supportive treatment consists of elimination of the offending infectious agent (if determined) and anti-inflammatory or immunosuppressive drug therapy.

TYPE III REACTIONS
(Immune complex disease)

Type III reactions occur when antigen-antibody complexes are deposited along the endothelium. These complexes stimulate, both directly and via the complement pathway, a neutrophilic inflammatory response and vascular damage. The result is a multisystemic vasculitis. The most commonly affected sites include the joints, skin, kidneys, lungs, and brain.

The prerequisite for the development of such disease is continued presence of soluble antigen and continuous production of antibody. When there is slightly more antigen than antibody, the soluble complexes become deposited along endothelial cells. The reason for their deposition is not entirely clear; however, it is presumed that large complexes are removed by phagocytosis and very small complexes can easily pass through the cellular membrane, whereas complexes of intermediate size become trapped on the basement membrane of endothelial cells. These deposited immune complexes then activate the complement cascade. Complement fragments cleaved from precursor molecules in this cascade incite inflammatory cells and are also directly vasoactive. The end result is a vasculitis. There are a number of reasons for the continuous presence of antigen, including chronic persistent infections (due to viruses, bacteria, fungi, protozoa, or parasites) and certain neoplastic conditions, particularly lymphoreticular neoplasms. Drug administration can result in an animal mounting an antibody response to the drug. Chronic antigen exposure is possible with repository medications or if the drug is continually administered. Lastly, some animals respond to self antigens, which represent a source of chronic antigen. In many cases, the origin of the antigen cannot be determined and, therefore, the cause of the disease is unidentifiable.

Clinical signs are variable but include fever, cutaneous signs (such as erythema multiforme), and polyarthritis (demonstrated by the presence of a shifting-leg lameness or painful, swollen joints). Other signs include ataxia, behavior change, proteinuria, isosthenuria, polydipsia, polyuria, or vague signs such as vomiting, diarrhea, or abdominal pain. Diagnosis is based on the elimination of more common causes of clinical signs. Supporting evidence to confirm the diagnosis includes establishing a temporal relationship if a drug is suspected as the cause, identifying chronic infections or malignancies, and performing various laboratory tests (such as a Coombs' test or an antinuclear antibody test) as well as histopathology and immunohistochemistry analyses to identify immune-mediated vasculitides or nephritis. Therapy should include supportive treatment associated with the affected organ and removal of the causative agent or treatment of the underlying disorder (eg, appropriate antibiotic therapy for bacterial infections, surgical drainage of abscesses or infected tissue, therapy for heartworm disease, the withdrawal of drugs, etc). Immunosuppression and anti-inflammatory therapy may be needed to stop the continued formation of immune complexes and to lessen some of the inflammation associated with deposition of immune complexes.

TYPE IV REACTIONS
(Cell-mediated immune reactions)

Cell-mediated immune reactions occur when T_H cells respond to foreign antigen or small molecules bound to cell tissue to form a complete antigen. T cells elaborate a variety of cytokines. IL_1 and other cytokines attract mononuclear phagocytes to the site of antigen. The infiltration of mononuclear cells and the elaboration of a variety of substances from these cells result in the pathologic processes of cell-mediated immune reactions. The antigens usually responsible for the development of Type IV reactions include intercellular bacteria or parasites, some viruses, chemicals, and (in certain situations) cell antigen. This type of reaction can occur in any organ and, therefore, the clinical signs will vary. The diagnosis is based on ruling out other causes for organ-specific diseases and by a classic histologic description of delayed-type hypersensitivity reaction in tissue. The goals of treatment are to provide supportive therapy based on the organ-specific disease process, to identify (if possible) and eliminate the source of antigen that is responsible for the reaction, and to provide anti-inflammatory or immunosuppressive therapy if needed.

IMMUNOPATHOLOGIC DISEASES

Specific disease entities with an immune basis have been best characterized in companion and laboratory animal species. The clinical manifestations and treatment usually are similar among species, except for the relative frequencies of these various disorders.

DISEASES INVOLVING ANAPHYLACTIC REACTIONS
(Type I reactions, Atopic disease)

Type I reactions are either systemic or localized. If the animal has been previously exposed to an allergen (antigen) and produces IgE antibodies, then injection of the sensitizing antigens directly into the bloodstream can result in anaphylactic shock or more focal reactions (eg, hives, urticaria, facial-conjunctival edema). If the sensitizing allergen enters through the mucous membranes or the skin, more localized reactions usually occur.

Systemic Anaphylaxis
(Generalized anaphylactic reactions)

Anaphylactic shock occurs in sensitized animals after parenteral injection of vaccines or drugs, ingestion of foods, or insect bites. Clinical signs occur within seconds to minutes after exposure to the allergen. This latent period is the time required for the allergen to bind to sensitized mast cells and for vasoactive mediators to be released. In people and most domestic animals, lungs are the primary target organ and the portal-mesenteric vasculature is secondary; this is reversed in dogs. Mast cell degranulation in the pulmonary vasculature causes constriction of bronchial airways or pulmonary veins and pooling of blood in the pulmonary vascular bed, which results in severe respiratory distress. Mast cell degranulation in the portosystemic vasculature causes venous dilatation and pooling of blood in the intestines and liver, with resultant shock, agitation, colic, nausea, vomiting and diarrhea, hypersalivation, dyspnea, cyanosis, and in severe cases, death.

Anaphylactic shock is treated with an IV injection of epinephrine to counteract bronchial constriction and portal-mesenteric vasodilation. Ancillary support of blood pressure and respiration may be necessary. Because of the peracute onset of signs, antihistamines are of little therapeutic benefit. Antihistamines are more effective in treating urticarial reactions and facial-conjunctival edema, but even in those cases, antihistamines are more effective when used to prevent attacks in animals with a known allergic predisposition.

Urticarial reactions (hives or angioedematous plaques) of the skin and subcutaneous tissue and acute edema of the lips, conjunctiva, and skin of the face (facial-conjunctival angioedema) are less severe manifestations of a systemic allergic reaction. Hives are the least severe reaction and are seldom associated with other clinical abnormalities. Facial-conjunctival edema is more severe and can be associated with mild to moderately severe systemic anaphylaxis. These reactions usually follow administration of vaccines or drugs, ingestion of certain foods, or insect bites. Urticarial reactions and facial-conjunctival edema occur in most species and usually resolve spontaneously within 24 hr. Not all urticarial reactions are mediated by IgE antibody. (*See also* URTICARIA, p 689.)

Milk allergy occurs occasionally in cows and less frequently in mares. This can happen when intramammary pressure increases enough that normally sequestered milk components, notably casein, gain access to the circulation; these "foreign" proteins induce a Type I hypersensitivity. The reaction can be localized or systemic. Recovery usually is prompt once the gland is emptied.

Localized Anaphylactic Reactions

Allergic rhinitis is manifest by serous nasal discharge and sneezing. It is less common in other animals than in people. Often, it is seasonal, correlating with pollen exposure. Nonseasonal rhinitis may be associated with exposure to ubiquitous allergens, such as molds, danders, bedding, and feeds. Recurrent airway obstruction in horses (p 1213) may be a sequela of low-grade respiratory allergies. Summer snuffles is a seasonal allergic rhinitis occurring commonly in Guernsey or Jersey cattle placed on certain types of flowering pastures in late summer and early autumn. Allergic rhinitis can be diagnosed tentatively by the following: 1) identification of eosinophils in the nasal exudate, 2) demonstration of a favorable response to antihistamines, 3) disappearance of signs when the offending allergen is removed, or 4) occasionally, its seasonal nature. Unlike in people, skin testing is not an accurate means to diagnose nasal allergies in animals.

Chronic allergic bronchitis has been best characterized in dogs. A dry, harsh, hacking cough that is easily precipitated by exertion or by pressure on the trachea is a characteristic clinical sign. The disease may be seasonal or occur year-round. Usually, it is not associated with other signs of illness. The bronchial exudate is rich in eosinophils and free of bacteria. Chest radiographs are normal, and there may or may not be a low-grade peripheral eosinophilia. The condition is treated with bronchial dilators and expectorants (aminophylline and potassium iodide or guaifenesin), which aid in the removal of thick, tenacious mucus. Glucocorticoids dramatically alleviate clinical signs, especially when their use can be limited to certain seasons or to low-dose, alternate-day therapy. Avoidance of the offending allergen(s) usually is not possible because only rarely is it identifiable.

Allergic bronchiolitis is most common in cats. It is manifest by a low-grade cough, wheezing, some dyspnea, and increased peribronchiolar density on radiographs, and it may be mistaken for other conditions (allergic asthma or lungworm disease). Early in the course of the disease, clinical signs can be modified by antihistamine therapy, but if the disease increases in severity, moderate to high dosages of corticosteroids may be necessary. The offending allergen usually is not identified.

Pulmonary infiltration with eosinophilia (PIE syndrome) occurs most frequently in dogs but has been recognized in all species. It is associated with diffuse inflammatory infiltrates in the lungs and a pronounced peripheral eosinophilia; frequently, the serum globulins are increased. Unlike in allergic bronchitis, affected animals are often dyspneic or tire easily with exercise. Diffuse bronchial exudate contains numerous eosinophils. The specific offending allergen usually is not identified. Glucocorticoids are the treatment of choice. A PIE-like syndrome is also associated with resident or migratory parasitic infections of the lungs in young animals.

Allergic asthma is less common in other animals than in humans. Among animals, it is most frequent in cats, in which the signs are similar to those in humans. It occurs more frequently in summer and after going outdoors; individual attacks can be transient and mild, or protracted and severe (status asthmaticus). Mild attacks may manifest as wheezing and coughing; in severe attacks, there may be expiratory dyspnea, hyperinflation of the lungs, aerophagia, cyanosis, and frantic attempts to obtain air.

Intestinal allergies (food allergies) are principally seen in dogs and cats, particularly kittens. (*See also* p 688 and p 1927.) Allergic gastritis is manifest by vomiting, which occurs 1 to >12 times weekly, within 1-2 hr of eating. The vomitus may be tinged with bile. In cats, vomiting may be the sole sign; dogs may also have loose feces intermittently. Cats and dogs with allergic gastritis are usually healthy except for vomiting, although there can be loss of weight and coat condition in severe cases. Allergic enteritis is associated with a mild inflammation of the small intestine but with little or no eosinophilia. Feces usually are normal in volume and frequency, but consistency varies from semiformed to watery. They may be extremely odorous, especially in cats. Affected animals may be excessively thin despite good appetite. Skin lesions and poor coat are commonly associated with food allergies in cats but less commonly in dogs. The allergy often follows bouts of viral, bacterial, or protozoal enteritis (a phenomenon known as allergic breakthrough). Food allergy may be a cause of diarrhea in newly weaned piglets, although the supporting evidence is not clear; the diarrhea is usually treated as an infection rather than an allergy. Eosinophilic enteritis, the most severe form of allergic intestinal disease, manifests by moderate to severe inflammation of the intestines and a pronounced eosinophilia. Diarrhea, weight loss, and poor coat condition are usually evident. The prevalence of allergic colitis is greater in cats than in dogs, although in general it is not common. In dogs, it is often associated with frequent defecation and soft, mucusladen and sometimes bloody feces; in cats, it most frequently manifests by more normal feces coated or spotted with fresh blood.

Spike tests and allergen-specific IgE levels should not be used as a first approach to diagnosing food allergies. Both diagnosis and treatment of intestinal allergies is by a strictly controlled diet. Dogs should be fed low-protein feeds that contain as few ingredients as possible. A basic diet of rice, cottage cheese (or tofu), and mutton, supplemented with vitamins and minerals, is a good starting diet. When the signs (usually diarrhea) have disappeared, additional foods can be introduced one at a time. Commercial prescription diets are also available. Low doses of glucocorticoids given daily or every other day also can provide excellent relief for dogs that are not helped by dietary changes. Allergic enteritis in cats is treated by feeding exclusively meat protein. Ground, cooked turkey and lamb are good hypoallergenic foods for cats. If the cat is not also allergic to these foods, feces, weight, coat quality, and skin lesions improve dramatically within 1-2 wk. Once a response occurs, new foods are introduced one at a time at intervals of ≥2 wk. Kittens with food allergies often grow out of them, while older animals may need hypoallergenic diets for life.

Atopic dermatitis is a pruritic, chronic skin disorder that occurs in many species but has been studied mostly in dogs. Animals with atopic dermatitis have a genetic predisposition that leads to excessive production of reaginic (IgE) antibodies. It has been estimated that ~10% of all dogs suffer from atopy, with a breed predisposition in terriers, Dalmatians, and retrievers. Atopic dermatitis of dogs often is due to inhaled allergens, eg, house dust mites, pollens, molds, and danders, but the predominant infiltration of T_H2 cells into skin lesions indicates that a Type IV reaction could be associated with the disease progression. The skin is the target tissue in dogs. Atopic dogs often chew at their feet and axillae. Excessive sweating is especially noticeable in hairless areas. The skin lesions are greatly increased in severity by licking, scratching, flea infestation, and secondary bacterial or yeast infection. Atopic skin lesions in cats are either miliary (small scabs) and widespread, or larger and more localized. Localized lesions are often pruritic.

In cats, food allergens probably are a more common cause of skin lesions than are inhaled allergens. Sweet itch (p 717) is a seasonal allergic dermatitis of horses associated with certain insect bites, especially night-feeding *Culicoides*. Intensely pruritic lesions appear along the dorsum from the ears to tail head and perianal area. Similar allergic skin reactions to insect bites can be seen about the ears and face of cats and dogs.

Treatment consists of identifying the offending allergens by intradermal skin testing combined with antigen-specific IgE assay and eliminating (or avoiding) them whenever possible. The "wheal and flare" reaction seen when the offending allergen is injected into the dermis is a focal manifestation of the allergic state. Hyposensitization consists of an extended series of injections of the offending allergen until improvement is noted; it is effective in ~60% of dogs with atopic dermatitis. If hyposensitization fails, or is not used, alternate-day glucocorticoid therapy is beneficial. Antihistamines are less effective in stopping the clinical manifestation of the disease. However, many animals improve significantly with antihistamine therapy and, therefore, antihistamines should be tried either before or with corticosteroid therapy. Cyclosporine A can be used locally instead of methylprednisolone in cases of severe disease.

DISEASES INVOLVING CYTOTOXIC ANTIBODIES
(Type II reactions)

Autoimmune Hemolytic Anemia and Thrombocytopenia

These are the most common Type II reactions. Antibody and complement attach to RBC either directly or indirectly via an absorbed antigen and mediate RBC destruction, resulting in a severe, life-threatening anemia. Concurrent thrombocytopenia is found in 60% of cases. Type II reactions can be associated with systemic lupus erythematosus (SLE [more common in dogs]) or with lymphoreticular malignancies (more common in horses and cats). Drugs, vaccines, or infections also can precipitate attacks of hemolytic anemia or thrombocytopenia in most species. More often than not, the triggering cause is unknown. However, as more information becomes available about rickettsia, these intracellular pathogens may be found responsible for many of the idiopathic immune-mediated disorders.

Autoimmune hemolytic anemia (AIHA) has 4 basic forms: peracute, acute or subacute, chronic, and pure red cell aplasia. Most forms are treatable, and relapses are uncommon. (*See also* p 11.)

Peracute AIHA is seen mainly in middle-aged, larger breeds of dogs. Affected dogs are acutely depressed and within 24-48 hr have a fulminant decrease in PCV with bilirubinemia, variable icterus, and sometimes hemoglobinuria. Initially, the anemia is nonresponsive, but it becomes responsive within 3-5 days. Thrombocytopenia and thrombotic phenomena may be accompanying features. The Coombs' test is often negative, and spherocytes may or may not be present, but in-tube or slide agglutination of RBC is marked. The autoagglutination is not dispersed by saline dilution, hence the term hemolytic anemia with in-saline agglutinins. The serum usually contains autoantibodies that cause agglutination of most donor RBC (including heterospecies). The prognosis of peracute AIHA is poor even with prompt and vigorous therapy. The most effective therapy involves immediate use of high dosages of glucocorticoids plus cyclophosphamide. Incompatible blood transfusions should be avoided if possible, because they will provide more foreign material to provoke the failing immune system. If incompatible blood must be used, the animal should first be heparinized and maintained on heparin for the first 10 days. Even without transfusion, heparinization may be beneficial for the first 2 wk or more. Bovine hemoglobin blood substitute and human immunoglobulin can be used to support the patient until immunosuppressive treatment reduces the destruction of RBC.

Acute AIHA is the most common form of the disease, with a breed predilection in Cocker Spaniels. Initial signs are pallor, fatigue, and less commonly, icterus. Hepatosplenomegaly is a prominent sign. The WBC count often is increased due to bone marrow hyperplasia. Autoagglutination of RBC is uncommon, and the Coombs' test is generally positive. These animals usually respond well to glucocorticoid therapy. If a favorable response is not seen within 7-10 days, cytotoxic drugs (cyclophosphamide or azathioprine) should be added to the regimen.

Chronic AIHA differs from the acute form in that the PCV falls to a constant level and remains there for weeks or months. The bone marrow is either normal or hyperresponsive, and the Coombs' test is often negative. Chronic AIHA is relatively more common in cats than in dogs. Usually, the anemia is responsive early in the course of disease but responds minimally or not at all by the time it becomes severe. Initial treatment is with glucocorticoids; if there is no response within 2 wk, cytotoxic drugs are added to the regimen.

Pure red cell aplasia (p 14) is a variant of the above disorders and is most common in dogs. It occurs in 2 forms, one in postweanling to adolescent puppies and the other in adults. Unlike AIHA, the bone marrow shows a selective depression of erythroid elements; granulocytes and platelets are unaffected. Therefore, the peripheral anemia is unresponsive. The immune attack apparently is directed at RBC precursors, and the Coombs' test is usually negative. However, there is often some difficulty in identifying compatible donors. Treatment is usually as for chronic AIHA.

Autoimmune thrombocytopenia is common, especially in dogs. It occurs more often in females than males. The most frequent clinical signs are hemorrhages of the skin and mucous membranes. Melena, epistaxis, and hematuria may be accompanying features and can cause profound anemia. Hemolytic anemia and thrombocytopenia sometimes occur together. Autoimmune thrombocytopenia usually is diagnosed on the basis of low peripheral platelet counts despite a pronounced megakaryocytosis in the marrow. Occasionally, megakaryocytes may be selectively absent from the marrow—a condition analogous to pure red cell aplasia. Tests for antiplatelet antibodies are difficult to conduct and may be positive in ≤70% of cases. The diagnosis is usually made on clinical appearance and response to therapy, rather than on antiplatelet antibody tests. (*See also* p 41.)

Animals with autoimmune thrombocytopenia that show only petechial and ecchymotic hemorrhages, with no significant blood loss and megakaryocytes in the marrow, are usually treated initially with glucocorticoids alone. The clinical signs should abate and the platelet count begin to rise after 5-7 days. If the platelet count has not increased significantly by days 7-10, either cyclophosphamide, azathioprine, or vincristine can be added to the glucocorticoid regimen. In animals with megakaryocytes in the marrow and severe blood loss, a more rapid response to therapy is desirable. Such animals are treated with a single injection of vincristine combined with daily glucocorticoids; a favorable response usually occurs after 3-5 days. If the blood loss is life-threatening, platelet-rich whole blood should be administered. If the platelet count has risen by day 7, remission is maintained on glucocorticoids alone. If there is no response after 7 days, a second dose of vincristine is given. If the platelet count is still low after 2 wk, vincristine is discontinued and either cyclophosphamide or azathioprine is added. Animals with thrombocytopenia and no megakaryocytes respond much more slowly to glucocorticoids, or to glucocorticoids and vincristine. Preferred treatment for these animals is with prednisolone and cyclophosphamide, and a response should not be expected much earlier than 1-2 wk after beginning therapy. Therapy can be discontinued in most animals with autoimmune thrombocytopenia 1-3 mo after the platelet count returns to normal. Some animals have more or less persistent thrombocytopenia despite drug therapy, or they can be maintained in remission only with chronic high-dose treatment. The alternatives are to allow the animal to live with the thrombocytopenia if signs are minimal or to use long-term combination drug therapy with glucocorticoids and either vincristine, azathioprine, or cyclophosphamide. Splenectomy may be helpful; it is seldom curative by itself but may allow use of lower and safer dosages of immunosuppressive drugs.

Cold agglutinin (hemolytic) disease is an AIHA that has been recognized most often in dogs and horses. It is often idiopathic but can be secondary to a chronic infection, other autoimmune diseases, or a neoplastic process. The IgM autoantibodies can be agglutinating or nonagglutinating. Complete agglutination is not seen at body temperature but rather at some lower temperature, thus it is more frequent in colder climates and seasons. Initial signs may be of a hemolytic disease; in the agglutinating type, there also may be microcapillary stasis with subsequent acrocyanosis and necrosis of the nose, tips of the ears and tail, digits, scrotum, and prepuce. Diagnosis is based on a reversible autoagglutination that occurs only at a cool temperature. The direct Coombs' reaction is usually negative for IgG, frequently positive for C3, and usually positive for IgM if the reaction is performed in the cold. Mortality is high. In the absence of precipitating disorders, eg, infection or neoplasia, the disease is best controlled with high doses of glucocorticoids used in combination with cyclophosphamide. Cyclophosphamide is withdrawn when the anemia disappears and cold agglutinins are no longer detected.

Autoimmune Skin Disorders

In these immunologic skin disorders, antibodies are directed against intracellular cement substances at the basal cell layer, which results in separation of the epidermal cells (acantholysis).

Pemphigus foliaceus is more common in dogs than in cats and horses but is still an uncommon disease. It is characterized clinically by erosions, ulcerations, and thick encrustations of the skin and mucocutaneous junctions. The absence of lesions in the mouth, and the widespread thick, crusty nature of the skin lesions, tend to differentiate pemphigus foliaceus from pemphigus vulgaris. Autoantibodies are present in the skin and react with intracellular cement substance. These autoantibodies cause a separation of the cornified from uncornified cell layers. High doses of glucocorticoids are used initially, but low-dose, alternate-day therapy is used once the disease is under control. More potent immunosuppressive drugs such as cyclophosphamide or azathioprine are used with glucocorticoids in cases unresponsive to steroids. Gold salts, in conjunction with low doses of glucocorticoids, are sometimes helpful in maintaining remission in animals in which steroids alone are ineffective. Animals that respond poorly to initial therapy, or require high dosages of drugs to control lesions, have a poor longterm prognosis.

Pemphigus vulgaris is rarer than pemphigus foliaceus. It is characterized by bullous lesions along the mucocutaneous junctions of the mouth, anus, prepuce, and vulva, and in the oral cavity. Other areas of the skin are only mildly involved. Because the epidermis of animals is relatively thin (compared with human skin), the bullae rupture rapidly and form erosions; consequently, characteristic bullae are seldom seen. The bullae occur as a result of suprabasilar acantholysis. Secondary bacterial infection often complicates the lesions, and if untreated, the disorder is often fatal. It is treated with high doses of glucocorticoids alone or in combination with other drugs such as cyclophosphamide, azathioprine, or gold salts. The disease is difficult to maintain in remission, and the longterm prognosis is fair to poor.

Bullous pemphigoid has been recognized in dogs, most often in Collies and Doberman Pinschers. Lesions are often widespread but tend to be concentrated in the groin. The involved skin resembles a severe scald. Bullae also may be seen; they are subepidermal and may be full of eosinophils. Autoantibodies to the basal lamina proteins are seen in immunohistopathologic sections. The treatment of choice is prednisolone and azathioprine used in combination; remission is frequent, but continuous drug therapy at relatively high dosages may be required to keep the disease under control. The longterm prognosis is poor.

Myasthenia Gravis

The acquired form of myasthenia gravis occurs in dogs and rarely in goats and cats. Affected animals produce autoantibodies to acetylcholine receptors, which bind to the receptor and reduce acetylcholine. The clinical manifestations mimic those produced by curare. Extreme generalized muscle weakness, accentuated by mild exercise, is common. Megaesophagus is a frequent primary or accompanying complaint in dogs. Thymomas are often associated with myasthenia gravis in humans, but this is uncommon in other animals. Administration of a short-acting anticholinesterase (edrophonium chloride) produces a dramatic increase in muscle strength. Treatment is with a long-acting anticholinesterase. Chronic immunosuppressive drug therapy for this disease is logical and should be investigated. Autoantibodies to the acetylcholine receptors can be detected in the serum of affected animals by an indirect immunohistopathologic analysis using normal muscle as a substrate.

DISEASES INVOLVING IMMUNE COMPLEXES
(Type III reactions)

Immune complex disorders are among the most common of the immunologic diseases. They may be idiopathic or of secondary origin. The site of deposition of the immune complexes determines the nature of the disease.

Glomerulonephritis (p 1272) is caused by deposition of antigen-antibody complexes in the subendothelial or subepithelial surface of the glomerular basement membrane. Secondary glomerulonephritis occurs as a side effect of chronic infectious, neoplastic, or immunologic disorders. Animals with idiopathic glomerulonephritis (>50% of cases) usually have signs of renal disease, whereas secondary glomerulonephritis is often a relatively minor part of a more serious disease.

Hypersensitivity pneumonitis is caused by deposition of immune complexes in the alveoli; it is most common in large animals that are exposed to antigenic dusts. The most potent antigens of this type are those contained in the spores of thermophilic actinomycetes from moldy hay. Inhalation of these spores causes farmer's lung disease in humans and a similar condition in cattle (p 1200). Hypersensitivity pneumonitis is characterized by the onset of respiratory distress 4-6 hr after exposure to moldy hay. The most effective treatment is removal of the source of the antigen; otherwise, corticosteroid therapy may help.

Systemic lupus erythematosus (SLE) occurs in dogs, is rare in cats, and has been reported in large animals. It has 2 immunologic features: immune complex disease and a heightened antibody responsiveness with a tendency to produce autoantibodies. Therefore, it is a combination of Type II and III diseases. Antibodies to nucleic acid are the diagnostic hallmark of SLE, but in some individuals, antibodies to RBC, platelets, lymphocytes, clotting factors, immunoglobulin (rheumatoid factors), and thyroglobulin also may be present. These autoantibodies, in particular those to nucleic acids, are not always pathogenic by themselves. Rather, they should be considered markers of the disease. Although combinations of autoantibodies and self-antigens may contribute to the total pool of immune complexes, they are not the sole source of immune complexes. Usually, either the immune complex or the autoantibody aspect of the disease predominates in a given animal. Immune complex deposition around small blood vessels leads to synovitis, dermal reactions, oral erosions and ulcers, myositis, neuritis, meningitis, arteritis, myelopathy, glomerulonephritis, and pleuritis. Glomerulonephritis is one of the major life-threatening complications of SLE in cats but not in dogs. Psychosis, a major sign of SLE in people, is also seen in animals with SLE. Autoimmune hemolytic anemia or thrombocytopenia, or both, are the most common autoantibody manifestations of SLE in animals.

SLE is characterized by the presence of antinuclear antibodies (ANA), and tests for these or the associated LE cells may help in diagnosis. However, some healthy animals may have ANA, and not all animals with SLE have detectable ANA in their blood. Diagnosis of SLE should be based on the entire clinical syndrome—not just on the presence or absence of ANA.

SLE usually can be treated with glucocorticoids. Initially, they are used in high daily doses, and when remission occurs, alternate-day, low-dose therapy is used. Drug treatment should be continued for ≥2-3 mo after all clinical signs have disappeared. Cyclophosphamide or azathioprine, or both, are used in combination with glucocorticoids in animals with SLE that is difficult to control with glucocorticoids alone.

Vasculitis mediated by immune complexes occurs in animals, especially dogs and horses. Lesions are most prevalent in the dermis of the distal limbs and mucous membranes of the mouth, particularly the palate and tongue (dogs) and lips (horses). Involvement of the nose, ears, eyelids, cornea, and anus is less common. Early lesions are seen as reddened areas that rapidly form shallow erosions. A scab quickly forms over dermal erosions. Edema of the limbs is common in horses and a less frequent but equally striking sign in dogs. Vasculitis is a feature of SLE in some animals but most often is idiopathic. Drug-induced vasculitis has been well recognized in dogs. The vasculitis is detected on histopathologic and immunohistopathologic examination of superficial and deep biopsies taken from the margins of lesions.

Vasculitis is treated by withdrawal of offending drugs (if implicated in the cause) or by immunosuppressive drug therapy. Glucocorticoids used alone or in combination with other agents such as azathioprine or cyclophosphamide are usually used to treat non-drug-induced cases. (*See also* PERIARTERITIS NODOSA, below.)

Purpura hemorrhagica of horses is a form of nonthrombocytopenic purpura (p 41) that often is a sequela of an earlier *Streptococcus equi* respiratory infection; it is mediated by immune complexes of antibody and streptococcal antigen in vascular basement membranes.

Anterior uveitis (p 398) often involves immune-complex-mediated reactions; it frequently occurs in the recovery stage of infectious canine hepatitis (p 637) due to the reaction of serum antibodies with uveal endothelial cells that contain canine adenovirus 1. Similarly, equine recurrent uveitis (p 407) or anterior uveitis of horses may be associated with immunologic reactions to *Leptospira* or *Onchocerca* spp. Uveitis caused by *Toxoplasma* and feline infectious peritonitis virus infections of cats also has an immunologic basis.

Canine rheumatoid arthritis manifests initially as a shifting lameness with soft-tissue swelling around involved joints. Within weeks or months, the disease localizes in individual joints, and characteristic radiographic changes develop. The earliest radiographic changes consist of soft-tissue swelling and a loss of trabecular bone density in the area of the joint. Lucent, cyst-like areas frequently are seen in the subchondral bone. The prominent lesion is a progressive erosion of cartilage and subchondral bone in the area of synovial attachments, which results in loss of articular cartilage and collapse of the joint space. Angular deformities often occur, and luxation of the joint is a frequent sequela. Deformities are most frequent in the carpal, tarsal, and phalangeal joints, and less frequent in the elbow and stifle. Synovial fluid changes indicate a sterile, inflammatory synovitis, with increased total cell count and a high proportion of neutrophils in the synovial fluid cell population. The condition is believed to be due to deposition of immune complexes in the synovia.

A rheumatoid arthritis also has been recognized in cats. It tends to occur in older male cats and frequently is associated with feline leukemia virus infection. The development of disease in cats is much more insidious than in dogs.

Plasmacytic-lymphocytic synovitis, possibly a variant of rheumatoid arthritis, occurs in medium and large breeds of dogs. Although multiple joints often are involved, the disease has a predisposition for the stifles. The most common clinical sign is hindlimb lameness and anterior drawer motion of the stifles. Lymphocytes and polymorphonuclear neutrophils predominate in the synovial fluid, although in some cases the fluid is essentially normal. Gross inspection of the joint reveals a yellowish proliferation of the synovial membrane and stretching or rupture of the cruciate ligaments.

Canine rheumatoid arthritis and plasmacytic-lymphocytic synovitis respond poorly to systemic glucocorticoids alone. Cyclophosphamide and azathioprine frequently are used with glucocorticoids to treat these disorders; NSAID (eg, aspirin, carprofen, etodolac, meloxicam) may help bring relief.

Idiopathic polyarthritis is most common in large dogs, particularly German Shepherds, Doberman Pinschers, retrievers, spaniels, and pointers. In toy breeds, it is most frequent in Toy Poodles, Yorkshire Terriers, and Chihuahuas, or mixes of these breeds. There is no evidence of a primary chronic infectious disease process or systemic lupus erythematosus; joint disease is often the sole manifestation. Diagnosis is based on the history of cyclic antibiotic-unresponsive fever, malaise, and anorexia, with stiffness or lameness. Bony changes are not seen on radiographs until the disease is well established. Even then, radiographic changes are mild and can mimic degenerative joint disease. Synovial fluid is inflammatory in nature but sterile. The disease may be controlled with daily high-dose glucocorticoids followed by low-dose, alternate-day therapy. Treatment usually can be discontinued after 3-5 mo. Dogs that do not respond well to such therapy (>50%) are treated with more potent immunosuppressive drugs such as azathioprine or cyclophosphamide in addition to glucocorticoids. Gold salts may be helpful in augmenting glucocorticoid therapy in some animals.

Periarteritis nodosa (polyarteritis nodosa, necrotizing polyarteritis) is a rare, idiopathic disease of domestic animals that usually occurs as a secondary immunologic manifestation caused by deposition of immune complexes and inflammation in walls of small and medium-sized arteries. Among farm animals, it is most common in pigs, usually associated with erysipelas and streptococcal infections, and is attributed to a hypertensive arterial reaction to these bacteria or to their vaccines. It has been reported in cats, although it is often mistaken for the noneffusive form of feline infectious peritonitis.

Immune-mediated meningitis is believed to occur in dogs. The condition also has been called periarteritis nodosa, although its relationship to the human syndrome is uncertain. A steroid-responsive meningitis has been seen in adolescent or young adult Beagles, Boxers, German Shorthaired Pointers, and Akitas, but is very rare in other pure and mixed breeds. The clinical signs in Beagles, Boxers, and German Shorthaired Pointers consist of cyclic bouts of fever, severe neck pain and rigidity, reluctance to move, and depression. Each attack lasts 5-10 days, with intervening periods of complete or partial normalcy lasting ≥1 wk. During attacks, protein and neutrophils in the CSF are increased. The lesion is an arteritis, primarily of the meningeal vessels, but occasionally of other organs as well. The disease is often self-limiting over several months; attacks become milder and less frequent. Glucocorticoid therapy reduces the severity of attacks. In some animals, the disease becomes chronic and only partially amenable to therapy.

A more severe form of this meningitis has been reported in a litter of young Bernese Mountain Dogs. The disease in this litter was somewhat cyclical, but the resolution in intervening periods was less than in the disorder of Beagles, German Shorthaired Pointers, and Boxers. CSF abnormalities resembled those of the disease in other breeds. The condition was less self-limiting and required longterm, high-dose glucocorticoid therapy to keep the animals comfortable.

A syndrome of meningitis, often associated with polyarthritis, is seen in Akitas as young as 12 wk old. The dogs show severe (but somewhat cyclical) bouts of fever, depression, cervical pain and rigidity, and generalized stiffness. Affected dogs grow at a slower rate and often appear unthrifty. The condition responds poorly to glucocorticoid and combination immunosuppressive therapy, and most dogs are euthanized as young adults. In older Akitas, a milder and more drug-responsive form of the disease is seen, which may be associated with pemphigus foliaceus, uveitis, and plasmacytic-lymphocytic thyroiditis.

DISEASES INVOLVING CELL-MEDIATED IMMUNITY
(Type IV reactions)

Granulomatous reactions to microorganisms such as mycobacteria, *Coccidioides*, *Blastomyces*, and *Histoplasma* spp, and possibly feline infectious peritonitis virus, may be due to chronic cell-mediated immune reactions. Although cell-mediated immunity effectively controls these types of infection in most individuals, for poorly understood reasons, these same mechanisms are only partially effective in others. A granulomatous reaction occurs, characterized by a fibrous stroma and an infiltration of macrophages, giant cells, and lymphocytes

Lymphocytic choriomeningitis is a viral infection of mice (p 1653) in which CNS damage is due to the destruction of virus-infected cells by thymus-derived lymphocytes. **Old-dog encephalitis** (p 625) also may result from cell-mediated immune mechanisms directed against cells persistently infected with canine distemper virus. The initiating canine distemper virus infection is usually clinically inapparent and may precede the encephalitis by years.

Contact hypersensitivity results from chemicals reacting with dermal proteins, which modify self-proteins. These modified proteins are antigenic, and the host's cell-mediated immune response against these chemically altered dermal proteins damages the skin, eg, poison oak and poison ivy reactions in humans. This reaction has been described in both dogs and horses and usually occurs as a result of contact with sensitizing chemicals incorporated in plastic food dishes, plastic collars, and drugs placed on the skin.

Autoimmune thyroiditis has been recognized in dogs and is characterized by destruction of the thyroid gland by an autoimmune process that has both humoral (Type II)

and cell-mediated (Type IV) components. The disease is particularly prevalent in Doberman Pinschers, Beagles, Golden Retrievers, and Akitas. Hypothyroidism (p 461) may be the sole manifestation of the disease or may be a clinical or subclinical component of a broader autoimmune disorder such as systemic lupus erythematosus, idiopathic polyarthritis, immune-mediated meningitis (periarteritis nodosa), panendocrinopathy, and rheumatoid arthritis.

Autoimmune adrenalitis has been reported in dogs. The adrenal glands are slowly destroyed by a plasmacytic-lymphocytic infiltrate. When sufficient glandular tissue is destroyed, the dogs develop Addison's syndrome (adrenocortical insufficiency, p 436). The condition is sometimes associated with a similar immune attack against other endocrine glands, in particular the thyroid.

Keratitis sicca occurs in dogs, with a genetic predisposition in Cocker Spaniels. It can occur in either a primary form or secondary to chronic use of sulfonamides. It is associated with an immune-mediated destruction of the lacrimal glands and is somewhat analogous to Sjögren's syndrome of humans, which is caused by disease of the salivary glands and a lack of saliva. Of affected dogs, ≥50% respond favorably to eyedrops that contain cyclosporine, which selectively inhibits disorders mediated by T lymphocytes.

IMMUNE-DEFICIENCY DISEASES

Tests used to diagnose immune-deficiency diseases are listed in TABLE 1, p 658.

Deficiencies in Phagocytosis

Phagocytosis is an essential feature of the immune system. Phagocytes are found underlying the mucous membranes and skin and in the bloodstream, spleen, lymph nodes, meninges, synovial membrane, bone marrow, and around blood vessels throughout the body. Phagocytes are either in the tissue (histiocytes, synovial macrophages, Kupffer cells, etc) or in the blood (polymorphonuclear leukocytes, monocytes). Phagocytes have immunoglobulin and complement receptors on their surfaces that assist in the engulfment (opsonization) of foreign material coated with specific antibody (opsonins) or complement, or both. Phagocytosis involves chemotaxis of the phagocyte to foreign, noxious, or damaged material; adherence of the material to the plasma membrane of the phagocyte; incorporation of the material into a pinocytotic vesicle; formation of a phagosome; and activation of the respiratory burst and lysosomal enzymes in the phagosome.

Deficiencies in phagocytosis can involve acquired or congenital defects in any of these steps, or can be due to the available number of phagocytes. They often manifest as an increased susceptibility to bacterial infections of the skin, respiratory system, and GI tract. These infections respond poorly to antibiotics. Acquired phagocytic deficiencies include disorders that lead to profound and chronic depressions of WBC. Feline leukemia virus infection, feline panleukopenia virus infection, feline immunodeficiency virus infection, tropical canine pancytopenia, idiopathic granulocytopenias, drug-induced granulocytopenias (anticancer drugs, estrogens, anticonvulsants, sulfonamides, etc), and myeloproliferative disorders are a few conditions in which secondary infections can develop as life-threatening complications.

A cyclic decrease of all cellular elements, most notably neutrophils, occurs in the peripheral blood and lowers the resistance to infection of gray Collies and Collie crosses. (*See* CYCLIC HEMATOPOIESIS IN GRAY COLLIE DOGS, p 51.)

Congenital abnormalities that lead to impaired phagocytosis are well documented in humans. Deficiencies of opsonins, complement factors, chemotactic abilities, myeloperoxidase, and lysosomal enzyme activation have been recognized in humans but not in other animals. Chronic granulomatous disease has been recognized as an X-linked defect in some Irish Setters (canine granulocytopathy syndrome). Some lines of Weimaraners develop bacterial septicemias (usually manifested by bone and joint infections) as puppies. The underlying cause for this phenomenon is unknown; some of the affected dogs have lower than normal levels of IgM and IgG, and preliminary research indicates that WBC have a bactericidal defect.

TABLE 1. Laboratory Tests for Immune-deficiency Diseases in Dogs ▶

Disease	Leukocyte Count (Hematology Counter)	Globulin Profile (Electrophoresis)	IgM, IgA, IgG Level (Radial Immunodiffusion)
Phagocytosis deficiency	Neutropenia		Deficit
Leukocyte adhesion deficiency	Leukocytosis		
Hypogammaglobulinemia		Possible gammopathy	Deficit
Transient hypogammaglobulinemia			Deficit
Complement deficiency			
Thymic aplasia			
Combined immunodeficiency	Lymphopenia		Deficit
Viral-induced immunodeficiency	Lymphopenia, followed by leukocytosis		Deficit

Leukocyte Adhesion Deficiency

Leukocyte adhesion deficiency (canine granulocytopathy syndrome) is a primary immunodeficiency disorder inherited as an autosomal recessive trait. It has been described in humans, Irish Setters, and Holstein cows. This deficiency is the result of a deficient expression of leukocyte surface glycoproteins. Clinically, it is characterized by recurrent, severe bacterial infections; impaired pus formation; and delayed wound healing. Infected animals usually have severe pyrexia, anorexia, and weight loss; response to antibiotic therapy is usually poor. Extreme, persistent leukocytosis may occur (>100,000 WBC/μL) and consists predominantly of mature neutrophils.

Deficiencies in Immunoglobulins

These may be acquired or congenital. Acquired deficiencies occur in neonates that do not receive adequate maternal antibodies (failure of passive transfer) or in older animals due to conditions that decrease active immunoglobulin synthesis. Failure of passive transfer of immunoglobulin occurs occasionally in all species that have colostrum as the major source of maternal antibodies. It is commonly associated with clinical problems in calves, lambs, and foals. Failure of passive transfer can occur when the young animal fails to nurse properly during the first several days of life or when the dam's colostrum contains low levels of specific antibodies. Theoretically, problems with the intestinal absorption of immunoglobulin in the milk also can occur. Immunoglobulin levels <400 mg/dL in a postnursing serum sample indicate a failure of passive transfer in foals. Removing calves from their dams too soon is a frequent problem in dairy herds and is a leading cause of failure of passive transfer in dairy calves. Newborn animals that do not obtain adequate maternal antibodies often succumb to fatal bacterial or viral infections of the GI and respiratory tracts.

Idiopathic (essential) hypogammaglobulinemia has not been described in animals other than humans, but undoubtedly it occurs. It is associated with excessive regulatory cell activity that depresses antigen-stimulated immunoglobulin synthesis to B lymphocytes.

◀ **TABLE I.** *(continued)*

Complement Level (Coombs' Test, Radial Immunodiffusion)	Cell Immunophenotyping (Flow Cytometry)	Antibody Response to Vaccination (ELISA)
	Normal	Normal
Deficit		
	Low CD3, elevated CD4/CD8 ratio	
	Low CD3 and CD79a, normal or decreased CD4/CD8 ratio	

Hypogammaglobulinemia of clinical significance can be associated with any disorder that interferes with immunoglobulin synthesis. Tumors, such as plasma cell myelomas or lymphosarcomas that occasionally secrete large amounts of monoclonal antibody, can be associated with profound deficiencies of normal beneficial antibodies. This may be because the tumor cells are competing for necessary substrate substances with normal immunoglobulin-producing cells, or because thymus-derived regulatory lymphocytes in the blood nonselectively inhibit the abnormal immunoglobulin production. Animals with tumors that produce monoclonal antibodies can have severe secondary infections. Some viral infections, eg, canine distemper and canine parvovirus, may damage the lymphoreticular system so severely that normal antibody production is virtually stopped.

Congenital hypogammaglobulinemia (common variable immunodeficiency) has been recognized either by itself or in combination with deficiencies in cell-mediated immunity (combined immunodeficiency, *see* below). Deficiencies in IgG subclass synthesis have been seen in some breeds of cattle; IgM deficiency has been described in horses; and IgA deficiencies have been described in Beagles, German Shepherds, and Shar-Peis. Cattle with IgG subclass deficiency are usually asymptomatic. Older foals with IgM deficiencies develop respiratory infections. Dogs with IgA deficiency, like their human counterparts, suffer mainly from chronic skin infections, chronic respiratory infections, and possibly allergies. The IgA deficiency of Beagles appears to be due to a defect in the secretion of IgA, because IgA-positive cells are present in normal numbers. Some German Shepherds seem to have lower IgA levels than other breeds and a higher incidence of GI allergies. IgA deficiency in Shar-Peis is highly variable; some have negligible serum and secretory levels, and some have normal serum levels and low or negligible secretory levels. Like the German Shepherds, affected Shar-Peis have more problems than expected with allergies. Patients with common variable immunodeficiency have a higher than usual incidence of autoimmune disorders and autoantibodies (eg, autoimmune hemolytic anemia, thrombocytopenia, systemic lupus erythematosis). Longterm treatment with broad-spectrum antibiotics is required and IV human γ-globulin is usually needed.

Transient hypogammaglobulinemia has been recognized most frequently in foals and puppies. It may be more common in Spitz-type puppies than in other breeds. It is congenital and manifest by a delay in development of active immunity associated with a maturational defect of both T_H function and the B cell response to foreign antigens. Puppies with this condition develop recurrent respiratory infections at 1-6 mo of age but recover and are essentially normal by 8 mo of age. Affected foals frequently develop clinical signs of hypogammaglobulinemia (usually respiratory infections) at ~6 mo of age when their maternal antibody reaches a very low level. After another 3-5 mo, they begin to produce immunoglobulin. Appropriate antibiotic treatment is often sufficient.

Deficiencies in Cell-mediated Immunity

Pure deficiencies in cell-mediated immunity are rare in humans and have not yet been described in other animals. In general, deficiencies in cell-mediated immune responses are associated with **thymic aplasia**, an absent or very small thymus. This is seen in some inbred lines of dogs and cattle; these animals were deficient in cell-mediated immune functions, such as lymphocyte blastogenesis, as well as having pituitary dysfunction.

Combined Immunodeficiency Disease

An autosomal recessive type of this disease has been identified in Arabian foals and Basset Hounds. Sporadic cases of combined immunodeficiency, probably heritable, have also been seen in Toy Poodle, Rottweiler, and mixed-breed puppies. Affected dogs are frequently asymptomatic during the first several months of life but become progressively more susceptible to microbial infections as maternal antibody wanes. Puppies with combined immunodeficiency disease generally are normal until 6-12 wk old. The most common cause of death from this condition is canine distemper as a consequence of routine immunization with modified live virus distemper vaccine. Arabian foals with the disorder frequently succumb to adenovirus pneumonia or other infections when ~2 mo old. The foals are persistently lymphopenic. Precolostral serum samples have no detectable IgM antibody. Immunoglobulin levels are normal after nursing but progressively decrease after that time compared with levels in normal foals. At necropsy, the thymus gland is difficult to identify and is architecturally abnormal. Lymphoid elements are markedly depleted in the lymph nodes, Peyer's patches, and spleen.

Complement Deficiencies

A congenital deficiency of C3 has been described in an inbred line of Brittany Spaniels. These dogs developed recurrent bacterial infections, especially skin diseases and pneumonias. Although complement is necessary for opsonization and neutrophil chemotaxis, bacterial infections do not always develop in people or laboratory animals with these deficiencies. This is mainly because the existence of 2 pathways provides a way of activating the system even if one pathway is blocked.

Congenital deficiency in the C1 inhibitor has been recognized in humans and occurs rarely in dogs. Affected animals suffer from recurrent bouts of facial edema. Diagnosis is based on a blood test showing <30% of the normal C3 level. There is no specific treatment for complement deficiencies. Vaccination and antibiotics are used to prevent and treat infection.

Selective Immunodeficiencies

Rottweiler puppies have a breed predilection for severe and often fatal canine parvovirus infections (p 319). Their resistance to other diseases is essentially normal, and the basis of this selective immunodeficiency is unknown.

Persian cats have a predilection toward severe, and sometimes protracted, dermatophyte infections (p 704). In some Persian cats, the fungal infections invade the dermis and cause granulomatous disease (mycetomas).

Mink with the Aleutian coat color mutation are susceptible to chronic parvovirus infection and develop a disorder called Aleutian disease (p 1545). Other strains of mink are susceptible to infection with this virus but do not develop clinical disease.

Focal and systemic aspergillosis (p 2296), and mycoses due to related fungi, affect certain types of dogs. Long-nosed breeds, in particular German Shepherds and shepherd-crosses, are prone to develop focal aspergillosis in the nasal passages. Systemic aspergillosis is seen almost exclusively in German Shepherds, and more commonly in western Australia than elsewhere. It is characterized by fungal pyelonephritis, osteomyelitis, and discospondylitis. The organism can be isolated readily from blood and urine.

Viral-induced Immunodeficiencies

These have been caused by a number of agents in animals. Canine distemper virus causes a profound combined immunodeficiency in affected puppies. The infection is associated with a progressive decline in levels of antibody globulin and increased susceptibility to agents normally contained by cellular immunity, eg, *Toxoplasma, Nocardia*.

Parvoviral infection in both dogs and cats causes a profound and transient depression in the number of neutrophils and in lymphocyte responsiveness. This has led to an increased incidence of fungal infections (aspergillosis, mucormycosis, candidiasis) in the immediate post-recovery period. A severe immunodeficiency syndrome induced by parvovirus has also been seen in mice.

Retroviral-induced immunodeficiency has received increased scrutiny since the appearance of acquired immunodeficiency syndrome (AIDS) in humans. Feline leukemia virus (FeLV) infection is associated with acquired immunodeficiency and increased incidence of secondary and opportunistic infections. Acquired immunodeficiency in FeLV infection is multifactorial and broad in nature. Infected cats can have deficiencies of neutrophils, decreased synthesis of antibodies (especially to bacterial antigens), decreased cellular immunity, and variable levels of complement. Immune responses to FeLV infection also appear to inhibit ongoing feline infectious peritonitis (FIP) virus immunity specifically, which leads to reactivation of quiescent FIP.

Simian type D retrovirus (types 1-5 and Mason-Pfizer monkey virus) infection of macaques has a similar pathogenesis to that of FeLV infection of cats but can induce even more severe immunodeficiency. Each serotype tends to be found in specific species of macaques in the wild and within defined geographic areas. Type D retrovirus infection of macaques can cause severe disease in adolescent animals from zoos and in primate centers with large breeding groups. Although the infection rate in the wild may be high, these viruses cause a less severe syndrome in wild than in captive populations. Affected macaques either die within several months with fever, lymphadenopathy, and opportunistic infections of the CNS, respiratory tract, and intestines; become lifelong asymptomatic carriers; or recover fully. A progressive retroperitoneal fibrosis is a feature with some serotypes. Healthy monkeys can be antibody positive and have virus in their blood and saliva (asymptomatic carriers) or can be antibody positive without isolatable virus (immune). Animals with clinical signs are always viremic but may or may not have serum antibodies, depending on disease severity.

Simian immunodeficiency virus (SIV) is a lentivirus with considerable genetic homology to human immunodeficiency virus (HIV). Many strains of SIV exist in nature. The common hosts are African primates such as African green monkeys, sooty mangabeys, mandrills, baboons, and other guenons. Transmission between infected and noninfected monkeys is probably by bites and in utero exposure. SIV is not present in native populations of Asian primates. It rarely causes disease in the host African species. If infected animals are under heavy stress, as in captivity, some may develop AIDS-like disease. SIV, especially of sooty mangabey origin, causes severe disease in macaques (rhesus, stump-tail, pig-tail, bonnet, etc). Most affected macaques have come from zoos and primate centers where contact is allowed between African and Asian species, and tissues and body fluids are often exchanged between animals for research purposes. The immunosuppression associated with SIV can last for weeks or years. Encephalitis (usually asymptomatic except for wasting) and lymphomas are frequent sequelae of SIV infection in macaques. Infected animals, whether healthy or diseased, carry the infection for life. Monkeys that are infected with SIV usually make serum antibodies that are detectable by a number of procedures. Because the infection is lifelong, the presence of serum antibodies to SIV indicates the presence of virus in the body.

Feline immunodeficiency virus (FIV, originally feline T-lymphotropic lentivirus) is a related lentivirus that has been identified in domestic cats and cheetahs. The infection is endemic in cats throughout the world. Virus is shed mainly in the saliva, and the principal mode of transmission is through bites. Free-roaming (feral and pet), male, and aged cats are at the greatest risk of infection. FIV infection is uncommon in closed purebred catteries. After infection, there is a transient period of fever, lymphadenopathy, and neutropenia. Most cats recover from this stage and appear normal for months or years before immunodeficiency occurs. The percentage of infected cats that enter the terminal phase of the illness is unknown. Cats with acquired immunodeficiency induced by FIV develop chronic secondary and opportunistic infections of the respiratory, GI (including mouth), and urinary tracts, as well as the skin. FIV-infected cats have a higher than expected incidence of FeLV-negative lymphomas, usually of the B-cell type, and myeloproliferative disorders (neoplasias and dysplasias). Of affected cats, ~5% have neurologic signs referable to cerebral cortex disease (behavioral abnormalities, psychomotor disturbances, dementia, convulsions). Cats remain infected for life; the presence of serum antibodies is directly correlated with the ability to isolate virus from blood cells and saliva.

Bovine immunodeficiency-like virus is a lentivirus that was originally isolated from bovine leukemia virus (BLV)-negative cattle with persistent lymphocytosis and hemolymphadenopathy. It also has been isolated from cattle with BLV-negative lymphosarcomas. The overall incidence in cattle appears to be ~1% although in some herds it may be ≥15%. Preliminary evidence indicates that the virus is not a cause of immunodeficiency in cattle. Some infected cattle can be detected by serologic tests for viral antibodies. Virus isolation from blood appears to be the most accurate way to detect infected animals.

TUMORS OF THE IMMUNE SYSTEM

Studies of the immunologic response to tumors conducted in the past 15 years have changed the definition of cancer, which is now perceived as a chronic immune disease. In response to genotoxic stress, carcinogens, or viruses, the targeted cells induce expression of stress proteins and tumor-associated antigens. These mark the abnormal cells for the immune system, which eliminates them through cell-mediated cytoxicity. In cancer patients, tumor cells escape from the immune attack by relying on both immunoparalysis and tumor cell modification. The demonstration that even bulky, invasive tumors can undergo complete remission under appropriate stimulation (eg, IL_2) has shown that it is indeed possible to treat cancer successfully by immune manipulation.

Cancer is the number one cause of death in dogs; 45% of dogs ≥10 yr old die of cancer. Lymphoma is one of the most prevalent tumors in dogs and cats. Boxers, Basset Hounds, and Rottweilers are predisposed to developing lymphomas. The normal immune response requires a burst of rapid proliferation of lymphocytes. On occasion however, this proliferation may be uncontrolled, and lymphoid neoplasms result. Because lymphocytes are present in all organs, tumor development can occur in any organ. Lymphomas can be multicentric, mediastinal, gastrointestinal, renal, nervous, or leukemic. Less commonly, they occur in the eyes, skin, or nose. To determine the stage of the disease, CBC, serum chemistry profiles, abdominal ultrasound, abdominal radiographs, and bone marrow analyses are useful. Immunofluorescent staining can be performed in dogs and cats to characterize lymphomas. They may be either T cell or B cell in origin.

Most cases of canine lymphosarcoma, Marek's disease, calf leukosis, and feline leukemia are of T-cell origin, as are thymomas. Thymomas, which are relatively uncommon in domestic animals, generally cause loss of condition and respiratory distress. They are commonly confirmed by radiography. In humans, thymomas may be associated with signs of myasthenia gravis. While this association has been reported in dogs, it is uncommon. Many T-cell lymphomas are associated with a simultaneous immunosuppression manifest by a predisposition to recurrent infections.

Adult bovine and ovine leukosis, alimentary feline leukemia, and avian leukosis are usually of B-cell origin. Under some circumstances, neoplastic B cells may develop into plasma cells. Plasma-cell tumors are known as myelomas. Because neoplastic plasma cells can secrete immunoglobulins, they give rise to gammopathies.

Combination chemotherapy (eg, vincristine, L-asparaginase, cyclophosphamide, doxorubicin, prednisone) is recommended for lymphoma treatment. Side effects include vomiting, diarrhea, lack of appetite, and fever. Hair loss is not observed in dogs and cats.

Lymphomas are rarely cured, but remission of up to 1 yr is common after combination chemotherapy.

GAMMOPATHIES

Gammopathies are conditions in which serum immunoglobulin levels are greatly increased. Using electrophonetic patterns, they can be classified either as polyclonal (increases in all major immunoglobulin classes) or monoclonal (increases in a single homogeneous immunoglobulin).

Polyclonal gammopathies in animals are seen in chronic pyodermas; chronic viral, bacterial, or fungal infections; granulomatous diseases; abscessation; chronic parasitic infections; chronic rickettsial diseases, such as tropical canine pancytopenia; chronic immunologic diseases, such as systemic lupus erythematosus, rheumatoid arthritis, and myositis; or with neoplasia. They also may be idiopathic. In some animals, the gammopathy may appear initially to be monoclonal because of a predominance of 1 immunoglobulin class (usually IgG). Examples of this phenomenon have been seen in cats with noneffusive feline infectious peritonitis and in dogs with chronic tropical canine pancytopenia.

Monoclonal gammopathies are characterized by the presence of a homogeneous serum immunoglobulin protein. Uninvolved immunoglobulin classes are usually depressed. Monoclonal gammopathies are either benign (ie, associated with no underlying disease), or potentially associated with immunoglobulin-secreting tumors. In humans, benign gammopathies may become malignant at a later date; in other animals, they are rare and are not associated with a demonstrable tumor or clinical illness.

Tumors that secrete monoclonal antibodies originate either from plasma cells (myeloma) or lymphoblasts (lymphosarcoma). Plasma-cell myelomas can secrete intact proteins of any immunoglobulin class or immunoglobulin subunits (light chains or heavy chains). Myeloma proteins in dogs are commonly IgG or IgA types and less commonly IgM. Myelomas of the IgA type are particularly common in Doberman Pinschers. Monoclonal immunoglobulin produced by lymphosarcoma are often of the IgM class, regardless of species. Myeloma proteins in cats and horses usually are IgG and, uncommonly, IgM, IgG (T) (horses), or IgA.

Clinical signs depend on the location and severity of the primary neoplasm and on the amount and type of immunoglobulin secreted. Plasma-cell myelomas frequently develop in marrow cavities of flat bones of the skull, ribs, and pelvis, and in the vertebrae. Pathologic fractures of diseased bone can lead to CNS or spinal disorders or to pain and lameness. Lymphosarcomas frequently involve parenchymatous organs; therefore, clinical signs are more diverse.

Clinically evident illness can result from the presence of the monoclonal protein itself. Amyloidosis (p 478) can be due to increased immunoglobulin catabolism. Hyperviscosity syndrome appears in 20% of dogs with monoclonal gammopathy, especially with IgM or IgA monoclonal proteins, and can occur if the protein levels in blood are high. In this syndrome, plasma viscosity can be many times normal, which leads to profound vascular disturbances, thrombosis, and bleeding diathesis. Depression, blindness, and neurologic manifestations can be due to hemorrhage in the nervous system and retina. Some IgM monoclonal proteins act as cryoglobulins and aggregate in vitro and in vivo when the plasma is cooled. Animals with cryoglobulinemia often develop gangrenous sloughs of the ear tips, eyelids, digits, and tip of the tail, especially during cold weather. (*See also* **cold hemolytic disease** under AUTOIMMUNE HEMOLYTIC ANEMIA AND THROMBOCYTOEENIA, p 651.) Myelomas that produce autoantibodies to various tissues have been identified in humans, but not in other animals. Finally, animals with monoclonal gammopathies may have greatly depressed levels of normal immunoglobulins and, therefore, may develop serious secondary infections.

Immunoglobulin-secreting tumors usually are treated with glucocorticoids and alkylating drugs. The prognosis for remission after therapy is much better in dogs than cats. Even in dogs, however, the longterm prognosis is poor and relapse is common after 6-12 mo. Plasmapheresis may be needed to lower serum viscosity in animals with clinical signs of hyperviscosity syndrome. Antibiotics and globulin injections may help prevent secondary infections.

■ ■ ■

INTEGUMENTARY SYSTEM

NEOPLASTIC SKIN DISEASES

TUMORS OF THE SKIN AND SOFT TISSUES   764

INTEGUMENTARY SYSTEM INTRODUCTION

The skin is the largest organ of the body and, depending on the species and age, may represent 12-24% of an animal's body weight. The skin has many functions, including serving as an enclosing barrier and providing environmental protection, regulating temperature, producing pigment avitamin D, sensory perception, etc. Anatomically, the skin consists of the following structures: epidermis, basement membrane zone, dermis, appendageal system, and subcutaneous muscles and fat.

Epidermis: The epidermis is composed of multiple layers of cells consisting of keratinocytes, melanocytes, Langerhans cells, and Merkel cells.

Keratinocytes function to produce a protective barrier. They are produced from columnar basal cells attached to a basement membrane. The rate of cell mitosis and subsequent keratinization are controlled by a variety of factors, including nutrition, hormones, tissue factors, immune cells in the skin, and genetics. Evidence is mounting that the dermis may also exert significant control over the growth of the epidermis. It has been hypothesized that photoperiod and reproduction cycles may affect the epidermis in animals. Glucocorticoids decrease mitotic activity; disease and inflammation also alter normal epidermal growth and keratinization. As keratinocytes migrate upward, they undergo a complex process of programmed cell death or keratinization. The goal of this process is to produce a compact layer of dead cells called the stratum corneum, which functions as an impermeable barrier to the loss of fluids, electrolytes, minerals, nutrients, and water, while preventing the penetration of infectious or noxious agents into the skin. The structural arrangement of keratin and the lipid content of the skin are critical to this function. The vitamin D precursor, 7-dehydrocholesterol, is formed in the epidermis. The epidermis is thickest in large animals. The stratum corneum is continuously shed or desquamated.

Melanocytes are located in the basal cell layer, outer root sheath, and ducts of sebaceous and sweat glands. They are responsible for the production of skin and hair pigment (melanin). Production of pigment is under hormonal and genetic control.

Langerhans cells are mononuclear dendritic cells that are intimately involved in regulating the immune system of the skin. They are damaged by excessive UV light exposure and glucocorticoids. Antigenic and allergenic material is processed by these cells and transported to local and nodal T cells to induce hypersensitivity reactions. Epidermal proteins may also conjugate with exogenous haptens, rendering them antigenic.

Merkel cells are specialized sensory cells associated with skin sensory organs, eg, whiskers and tylotrich pads.

Basement Membrane Zone: This area services as a site for attachment of basal epidermal cells and as a protective barrier between the epidermis and dermis. A variety of skin diseases, including several autoimmune conditions, can cause damage to this zone. Vesicles are an example of a damaged basement membrane zone.

Dermis: The dermis is a mesenchymal structure that supports, nourishes, and to some degree, regulates the epidermis and appendages. The dermis consists of ground substance, dermal collagen fibers, and cells (fibroblasts, melanocytes, mast cells, and occasionally eosinophils, neutrophils, lymphocytes, histiocytes, and plasma cells). Blood vessels responsible for thermoregulation, nerve plexuses associated with cutaneous sensation, and both myelinated and unmyelinated nerves are present in the dermis. Motor nerves are primarily adrenergic and innervate blood vessels and arrector pili muscles. Except in horses, apocrine glands do not appear to be innervated. Sensory nerves are distributed in the dermis, hair follicles, and specialized tactile structures. The skin responds to the sensations of touch, pain, itch, heat, and cold.

Appendageal System: These structures grow out of (and are continuous with) the epidermis and consist of hair follicles, sebaceous and sweat glands, and specialized structures (eg, claw, hoof). The hair follicles of horses and cattle are simple, ie, the follicles have one hair emerging from each pore. The hair follicles of dogs, cats, sheep, and goats are compound, ie, the follicles have a central hair surrounded by 3-15 smaller hairs all exiting from a common pore. Animals with compound hair follicles are born with simple hair follicles that develop into compound hair follicles.

The growth of hair is controlled by a number of factors, including nutrition, hormones, and photoperiod. The growing stage of the hair is referred to as anagen, and the resting stage (mature hair) is referred to as telogen. The transitional stage between anagen and telogen is catagen. Animals normally shed their hair coat in response to changes in temperature and photoperiod; most animals undergo a shed in the early spring and early fall. The size, shape, and length of hair is controlled by genetic factors but may be influenced by disease, exogenous drugs, nutritional deficiencies, and environment. Hormones have a significant effect on hair growth. Thyroxine initiates hair growth, and glucocorticoids inhibit hair growth. The primary functions of the hair coat are to provide a mechanical barrier, to protect the host from actinic damage, and to provide thermoregulation. In most species, trapping dead air space between secondary hairs conserves heat. This requires that the hairs be dry and waterproof; the cold-weather coat of many animals is often longer and finer to facilitate heat conservation. The hair coat can also help cool the skin. The warm-weather coat of animals, particularly large animals, consists of shorter thicker hairs and fewer secondary hairs. This anatomic change allows air to move easily through the coat, which facilitates cooling. The hair coat also helps conceal or camouflage the animal.

Sebaceous glands are simple or branched alveolar, holocrine glands that secrete sebum into the hair follicles and onto the epidermal surface. They are present in large numbers near the mucocutaneous junction, interdigital spaces, dorsal neck area, rump, chin, and tail area; in some species, they are part of the scent-marking system. For example, in cats sebaceous glands are present on the face, dorsum, and tail in high concentration; cats mark territories by rubbing their face on objects and depositing a layer of sebum laced with feline facial pheromones. Sebum is a complex lipid material containing cholesterol, cholesterol esters, triglycerides, diester waxes, and fatty acids. Sebum is important for keeping the skin soft and pliable and for maintaining proper hydration. Sebum gives the hair coat sheen and has antimicrobial properties.

Sweat glands (epitrichial [formerly apocrine] and atrichial [formerly eccrine]) are part of the thermoregulatory system. The evaporation of sweat from the skin is the primary cooling mechanism of the body for horses and primates and, to a lesser degree, pigs, sheep, and goats. There is some clinical evidence to suggest that limited sweating occurs in dogs and cats, and that it may have a minor role in cooling of the body. Dogs and cats thermoregulate primarily via panting, drooling, and spreading saliva on their coats (cats). However, cats will sweat through their paws especially when excited; this is most commonly seen as wet paw prints on surfaces, eg, examination tables.

Subcutaneous Muscles and Fat: The "twitch muscle" (panniculus carnosus) is the major subcutaneous muscle. The subcutaneous fat (panniculus adiposus) serves many functions, including insulation; reservoir for fluids, electrolytes, and energy; and shock absorber.

DERMATITIS

Inflammation of the skin can be produced by numerous agents, including external irritants, burns, allergens, trauma, and infection (bacterial, viral, parasitic, or fungal). It can be associated with concurrent internal or systemic disease; hereditary factors also may be involved. Allergies form an important group of etiologic factors, especially in small animals.

The skin's response to insult is generically called dermatitis and manifests as any combination of pruritus, scaling, erythema, thickening or lichenification of the skin, hyperpigmentation, oily seborrhea, odor, and hair loss. The usual progression of a skin disease involves an underlying trigger (disease syndrome) that causes primary lesions such as papules, pustules, and vesicles. Pruritus is a common clinical sign in many diseases, and in those that are not inherently pruritic, is often present because of secondary infections or as a result of the production of inflammatory mediators. As the inflammatory changes progress, crusting and scaling develop. If the process involves the deeper dermis, exudation, pain, and sloughing of the skin may occur. Secondary bacterial and yeast infections commonly develop as a result of skin inflammation. As dermatitis becomes chronic, acute signs of inflammation (eg, erythema) subside and primary lesions become obscured by signs of chronic inflammation (thickening of the skin, hyperpigmentation, scaling, seborrhea). Often the skin becomes drier; if pruritus is not a component of the underlying trigger, it will often develop at this stage. Resolution of dermatitis requires identification of the underlying cause and treatment of secondary infections or other complications.

DERMATOLOGIC PROBLEMS

Dermatitis is a nonspecific term usually used until the dermatologic history, clinical signs, and physical examination can more precisely define the problem. Dermatologic problems describe a major category of clinical findings that can be caused by a number of skin diseases; many skin diseases look alike and are differentiated by working through diagnostic flow charts and a process of elimination. The most common dermatologic problems include pruritus, alopecia, crusting and scaling, otitis, nonhealing wounds, nodules and tumors, and ulcerative disorders. In some species, for example cats, there may be well-recognized subcategories of dermatologic problems (eg, head and neck pruritus, symmetric alopecia, eosinophilic exudation/dermatitis, etc). Identification of the patient's dermatologic problem is the key to making a diagnosis. A flow chart can be used as a guide for the diagnostic approach. Defining the major dermatologic problem will help create a patient-specific differential diagnosis list and aid selection of appropriate diagnostic tests. It is important to note that the patient's dermatologic problem may or may not be the client's chief complaint. It is important to be sensitive to clients' perceptions of problems or complaints, especially if odor or aesthetics are involved, and to be sure to address them (eg, bathing to minimize odor while the key problem is being evaluated).

DIAGNOSIS OF SKIN DISEASES

Definitive diagnosis of the causes of various skin diseases requires a detailed history, physical examination, and appropriate diagnostic tests. Many skin diseases look alike, and a definitive diagnosis is made over time by ruling in or out possible causes, by evaluating responses to therapy, and/or by process of elimination.

History

A careful dermatologic history is critical to interpreting the physical examination findings and to choosing appropriate diagnostic tests. A complete general history should be obtained, including information about prior illnesses; vaccinations, husbandry (housing, feeding practices, etc), changes in attitude and food consumption; elimination practices; exposure to other animals; and travel within the past 6-12 mo. This should be followed by a detailed dermatologic history. Use of a preprinted history form can be very useful for chronic or complicated cases. A good history is important because many skin diseases that look similar are differentiated based on interpreting clinical signs and historical patterns.

The following information should be obtained: 1) the primary complaint; 2) the length of time the problem has been present; 3) the age at which the skin disease started (distinct age predilections are seen in many diseases, eg, demodicosis and dermatophytosis in pediatric animals and signs of atopy in animals 1-3 yr old); 4) the breed (breed predilections include a predisposition of Cocker Spaniels to primary disorders of keratinization, and of terriers to atopy); 5) the presence and severity of pruritus (including licking, rubbing, scratching, or chewing behaviors—owners often do not realize licking may be a sign of pruritus); 6) how the disease started and its progression (diseases that begin with pruritus may lead to self-trauma and subsequent development of secondary skin lesions [alopecia, seborrhea] or infections [bacterial or yeast pyoderma]); 7) the type of lesions the owner saw develop; 8) evidence of seasonality (suggesting fleas, allergic skin disease, or weather-related diseases); 9) area on the body the problem was first noticed (ie, regional patterns seen in atopy [typically the face and feet], cheyletiellosis [primarily dorsal], scabies [primarily ventral], and endocrine hair loss [usually involves the trunk and spares the head and legs]); 10) any previous treatments and the responses to such (ie, antibiotic-responsive skin diseases suggest a bacterial etiology; pruritus that responds to small doses of glucocorticoids, antihistamines, or essential fatty acids suggests allergic dermatitis); and 11) frequency of bathing and when the last bath was given (recent bathing may obscure or change important clinical lesions, excessive bathing and wetting of the skin can predispose to skin disease); 12) presence of fleas, ticks, or mites; 13) other contact animals (ie, evidence of contagion, which suggests fleas, scabies, cheyletiella, or dermatophytosis); and 14) the environment of the animal (housing changes can influence the development of certain skin diseases, eg, contact dermatitis, contagious diseases).

Physical Examination

A complete physical examination should always be performed. Many skin diseases are manifestations of systemic diseases, eg, hypothyroidism, systemic lupus erythematosus. (See also MISCELLANEOUS SYSTEMIC DERMATOSES, p 792.) A good dermatologic examination requires very close inspection of the entire hair coat and skin under strong lighting; flashlights may be necessary to examine the skin of large animals. It is important to examine the ventrum of the animal, where many primary lesions and cutaneous parasites are found.

Clinical lesions are described in a variety of ways. Gross lesions can be described as focal, multifocal, or diffuse in distribution, followed by a description of the affected region (eg, mucocutaneous, truncal). On closer inspection, lesions may be further described as primary or secondary. Primary lesions include macules or patches (nonelevated areas of discoloration); papules or plaques (elevated lesions, the latter coalescing); pustules, vesicles, or bullae (fluid-filled lesions); wheals (flat-topped, steep-walled, solid elevations of the skin arising from histamine release); or nodules or tumors (large solid elevations of the skin). Secondary lesions include epidermal collarettes (late stage of a pustule), scars, excoriation (areas of self-trauma), erosions or ulcers (loss of the epidermis), fissures, lichenification (increased thickening and hyperpigmentation of the skin), and calluses. Some lesions may be either primary or secondary, depending on the etiology of the disease. These include alopecia, scale, crusts, follicular casts (plugging of hair follicles with visible keratin), comedos (blackheads), and pigmentary changes.

Laboratory Procedures for Skin Diseases

Skin Scrapings: Skin scrapings are part of the basic database for all skin diseases. There are 2 types of skin scrapings, superficial and deep. Superficial scrapings do not cause capillary bleeding and provide information from the surface of the epidermis. Deep skin scrapings collect material from within the hair follicle; capillary bleeding indicates that the sampling was deep enough. Skin scrapings are used primarily to determine the presence or absence of mites. Skin scrapings are best performed using a skin-scraping spatula, which is a thin metal weighing spatula commonly found in pharmacy or chemical supply catalogs. These spatulas are reusable and will not injure patients.

Combing of the Hair Coat: This technique, commonly referred to as "flea combing," is useful for collecting large amounts of skin debris and for trapping cutaneous parasites. Combings are particularly useful for finding fleas, ticks, lice, and some mites. A clean scrub brush or curry comb can be used to collect material into a flat container (eg, pie plate) in large animals.

Examination of Hairs: Microscopic examination of hair shafts can be used to look for evidence of self-trauma, dermatophyte infections (requires clearing agents and special staining), dysplastic hairs, and sometimes genetic diseases of the hair coat.

Cytology: Cutaneous and auricular cytology is helpful in identifying bacterial, fungal, and possibly neoplastic skin diseases. At least 4-6 impression smears should be made; several slides should be saved for examination by a reference laboratory if necessary. When performing impression smears of the skin, the glass slide should be placed directly over the site to be sampled. An index finger or thumb should be placed directly over the slide and very firm pressure exerted. Adequate sampling will produce a "thumb print" from the surface. At least one slide should be heat fixed with a match or lighter prior to staining. In most cases, Diff-Quick stain is adequate. In pruritic patients, material should be scraped from beneath nail beds and smeared onto glass slides for heat fixing, staining, and cytologic examination. Specimens should be examined under 4×, 10×, and oil immersion magnification.

Fungal Cultures: Dermatophyte infections are best identified with a fungal culture on either dermatophyte test medium or on plain Sabouraud's agar. Plates that are easily inoculated are preferred; glass screw-topped jars are difficult to inoculate and obtain samples from and are best avoided. Cats are best sampled using a new toothbrush aggressively combed over the affected lesions. Dogs can be sampled with either a toothbrush or via a hair plucking technique. In large animals, hairs should be gently wiped with alcohol before collecting to minimize contaminant growth. Intermediate and deep fungal organisms are best cultured by a reference laboratory using a skin biopsy specimen (6-8 mm in size).

Bacterial Cultures: Intact pustules can be cultured by rupturing the pustule with a sterile needle and swabbing the lesion with a sterile culture swab. Lesions should not be scrubbed before sampling. Deep pyodermas are best cultured from a skin biopsy (6-8 mm).

The reference laboratory should be informed as to what pathogens are suspected as this may affect how the exudate is cultured. Systemic and topical agents should be withheld for at least 72 hr prior to sampling.

Biopsy: Skin biopsies are indicated in any case that appears severe, unusual, or does not respond to appropriate therapy. Lesions should not be scrubbed before biopsy because surface pathology is important in the diagnosis of many skin diseases. Several samples from a variety of lesions should be submitted for examination. It is important to try to sample primary lesions; otherwise, the report is often not very helpful in making a diagnosis or narrowing a list of differential diagnoses. Biopsy specimens require examination by a pathologist familiar with skin diseases of animals. Direct immunofluorescence is not necessary to diagnose autoimmune skin diseases; routine histopathology is the test of choice.

Routine Blood and Urine Tests: In most dermatologic cases, these tests do not help to make a definitive diagnosis. If systemic signs of an illness are present, then a CBC, serum chemistry panel, and urinalysis may be helpful in identifying the etiology. In dogs with recurrent infections, these tests may identify an underlying subclinical disease.

Intradermal Skin Testing: This test is not necessarily required to make a diagnosis of atopy. A positive intradermal skin test reaction indicates past exposure to a particular allergen. Inhalant allergies are best diagnosed based on a compatible history, physical examination findings, and judicious use of intradermal skin testing or in vitro testing for allergies. Intradermal skin testing is recommended for animals in which immunotherapy is indicated due to the severity or duration of allergic signs. The potential drug interactions that can interfere with testing should be considered before intradermal skin testing is performed.

In Vitro Diagnostic Tests: In vitro diagnostic tests (ELISA or RAST tests) are an alternative to intradermal skin testing. Although in vitro tests are considered less reliable because of the large number of false positive reactions, most complications in interpretation are the result of poor patient selection.

COMMON DERMATOLOGIC PROBLEMS

The 2 most common dermatologic problems are alopecia and pruritus.

ALOPECIA
(Hair loss)

Alopecia is the partial or complete lack of hairs in areas where they are normally present. If a patient is presented for the problem of hair loss and the animal is pruritic, the problem of pruritus should be investigated first (*see* PRURITUS, p 676).

Etiology: There are many causes of alopecia; any disease that can affect hair follicles can cause hair loss. There are 2 broad etiologic categories of alopecia—congenital or hereditary and acquired. Acquired alopecia is further divided into 2 categories: inflammatory and noninflammatory.

Congenital or hereditary alopecia (p 679) has been described in cows, horses, dogs, cats, and pigs. Hairless breeds of mice, rats, cats, and dogs have been bred and developed for personal and research interests. Congenital alopecia may or may not be hereditary; it is caused by a lack of development of hair follicles and is apparent at or shortly after birth. Animals with tardive alopecias are born with normal coats, and focal or generalized hair loss occurs when the animal sheds its juvenile coat or when it becomes a young adult. Examples of this include pattern baldness of Dachshunds, color dilution alopecia (most commonly seen in Doberman Pinschers), and certain types of follicular dysplasias.

Acquired alopecia encompasses all other causes of hair loss. In this type of alopecia, the animal is born with a normal hair coat, has or had normal hair follicles at one time, and is or was capable of producing structurally normal hairs. Acquired alopecia may be noninflammatory, as is seen in endocrine alopecia or some types of immune-mediated alopecia, or inflammatory. Inflammatory acquired alopecia is the most common cause of alopecia. Acquired alopecia develops because a disease destroys the hair follicle or shaft, interferes with the growth of hair or wool, or causes the animal discomfort (eg, pain, pruritus) leading to self-trauma and loss of hair.

Diseases that can directly cause destruction or damage to the hair shaft or follicle include bacterial skin diseases, dermatophytosis, demodicosis, severe inflammatory diseases of the dermis (eg, juvenile cellulitis, deep pyoderma), traumatic episodes (eg, burns, radiation), and (rarely) poisonings caused by mercury, thallium, and iodine. These diseases tend to be inflammatory.

Diseases that can directly inhibit or slow hair follicle growth include nutritional deficiencies (particularly protein deficiencies), hypothyroidism, hyperadrenocorticism, and excessive estrogen production or administration (hyperestrogenism, Sertoli cell tumors, estrogen injections for mismating). Temporary alopecia in horses, sheep, and dogs can occur during pregnancy, lactation, or several weeks after a severe illness or fever. These types of alopecia tend to be noninflammatory unless a secondary infection of the skin develops.

Pruritus or pain is a common cause of acquired inflammatory alopecia in animals. Diseases that commonly cause pruritus or pain include infectious skin diseases (eg, bacterial pyoderma and dermatophytosis), ectoparasites, allergic skin diseases (eg, atopy, food allergy, contact, insect hypersensitivity), and less commonly neoplastic skin diseases. Friction may cause local hair loss, eg, poorly fitted halters or collars. Rarely, excessive grooming may be the cause of hair loss in some animals, particularly cats.

Feline endocrine alopecia is no longer recognized as a bona fide syndrome; the new name is feline acquired symmetric alopecia. To date, there is no documented evidence of an endocrine disease in these cats, and the symmetric alopecia seen is a clinical sign of an underlying disease, most commonly a pruritic disease.

Clinical Findings and Lesions: The clinical signs of hair loss may be obvious or subtle, depending on the disease. Congenital or hereditary hair loss is commonly symmetric and not accompanied by many inflammatory changes; in some cases, the areas of hair loss are localized to one region (eg, ear flaps) or to well-demarcated areas.

The clinical signs of acquired hair loss are varied and often influenced by the underlying cause(s); the pattern of hair loss may be focal, multifocal, symmetric, or generalized. Inflammatory changes such as hyperpigmentation, lichenification, erythema, scaling, excessive shedding, and pruritus are common. Some causes of acquired alopecia may predispose the animal to the development of secondary skin diseases, such as a bacterial pyoderma or seborrhea. Pruritus is variable, depending on the primary cause. In endocrine alopecias, the hair loss usually develops in a symmetric pattern, often in wear areas first; pruritus is uncommon unless there is a secondary infection. Contrary to previous thought, hair loss is not generally an early clinical sign of an endocrine alopecia.

Many owners seek veterinary assistance because of perceived excessive shedding. Shedding may be abnormal (excessive) if it results in obvious loss of the hair coat and areas of alopecia. A common cause of abnormal shedding is bacterial pyoderma. If, however, the shedding is not accompanied by development of patchy or symmetric hair loss, it is likely that it is just a stage in the natural replacement of the hair coat. Owners frequently do not recognize that the development and growth of a new hair is accompanied by the expulsion or shedding of the old hair.

Diagnosis: An accurate diagnosis of the cause of alopecia requires a careful history and physical examination. Key points in the history include recognition of breed predispositions for congenital or hereditary alopecias; the duration and progression of lesions; and the presence or absence of pruritus, evidence of contagion, or nondermatologic problems, eg, polyuria and polydipsia. On physical examination, the distribution of lesions should be noted (focal, multifocal, symmetric, generalized), and the hairs examined to determine if they are being shed from the hair follicle or broken off—the latter suggesting pruritus. Signs of secondary skin infections or ectoparasites should be noted, and a careful nondermatologic examination should be performed.

Initial diagnostic tests include skin scrapings for ectoparasites (particularly *Demodex* mites); combing of the hair coat for fleas, mites, and lice; impression smears of the skin for evidence of bacterial or yeast infections; fungal cultures for identification of dermatophytosis; and examination of plucked hairs, looking at both the shaft and the ends for evidence of dermatophytosis or that the hairs were chewed off. In many cases of bacterial pyoderma, impression smears of the skin do not show neutrophils and/or cocci, but rather large numbers of shed keratinocytes. Neutrophils and cocci are seen if pustules or recently ruptured pustules are sampled.

If these tests do not identify or suggest an underlying cause, a skin biopsy may be indicated to evaluate hair follicle structures, numbers, and anagen/telogen ratios and to look for evidence of bacterial, fungal, or parasitic skin infections. In addition, skin biopsies are often needed to confirm congenital or tardive causes of hair loss and to identify inflammatory or neoplastic causes of hair loss. Skin biopsies from normal and abnormal sites should be submitted for evaluation. CBC, serum chemistry panels, and urinalyses are generally only helpful when an endocrinopathy is suspected. Specific endocrine function tests can be performed based on findings of routine laboratory work or clinical signs.

Treatment: Successful therapy depends on the underlying cause and specific diagnosis.

PRURITUS
(Itching)

Pruritus is defined as an unpleasant sensation within the skin that provokes the desire to scratch.

Pathophysiology: Pruritus may be well or poorly localized. It may manifest as a sharp or diffuse, burning sensation. Although the skin is richly innervated, there are no known specialized pruritus receptors. The sensation of itch is transmitted via a specialized set of afferent fibers. Myelinated fibers that conduct sensations at 10-20 m/sec carry the well-localized pricking itch sensation. In contrast, the sensation of burning itch is transmitted via nonmyelinated fibers that conduct sensations at 2 m/sec. Both of these fibers enter the dorsal root of the spinal cord, ascend through the dorsal column, and cross into the lateral spinothalamic tract. From there they go to the thalamus and on to the sensory cortex.

The mediators of pruritus are controversial and may vary depending on the species. These putative mediators include histamines (released from mast cell degranulation), proteolytic enzymes (proteases), and leukotrienes. Proteases are released by fungi, bacteria, and mast cell degranulation, and during antigen-antibody reactions. Leukotrienes, prostaglandins, and thromboxane A_2, which are broken down from arachidonic acid, are pro-inflammatory. Essential fatty acids, particularly γ-linolenic acid, have been used to counter the inflammation mediated by leukotrienes and thromboxane A_2. The sensation of pruritus may be affected by a variety of factors including boredom, competing sensations, and anxiety. Stress may potentiate pruritus via the release of opioid peptides.

Etiology: Pruritus is a clinical sign and not a diagnosis or specific disease. In general, the most common causes of pruritus are parasites, infections, allergic skin diseases, and miscellaneous causes (eg, cutaneous neoplasia). Many diseases that are nonpruritic (eg, endocrinopathies) become pruritic when the patient develops secondary bacterial or yeast infections.

Diagnosis: A thorough dermatologic history and physical examination should be performed. Parasitic causes of pruritus, including *Demodex*, fleas and ticks, contagious mites, and lice, should be ruled out, as they are most common. Skin scrapings can rule in or out various mite infestations including *Demodex*. However, some mite infestations (eg, *Sarcoptes, Cheyletiella, Psoroptes, Chorioptes*) might be missed on skin scrapings. If a mite infestation is suspected, a response to therapy trial should be undertaken. The most commonly used drug in these cases is ivermectin. Fleas can be ruled in or out on the basis of a history of flea control, response to flea control, or finding evidence of flea infestation via a flea combing. Flea control practices will also rule out louse infestations.

The next most important group of pruritic diseases to rule out is infectious causes of skin disease. These include bacterial infections (primarily staphylococcal infections,

Malassezia overgrowth, and dermatophytosis). A fungal culture should be performed in any cat presented for pruritus. It is also highly recommended in dogs that are newly acquired, any animal with a possible history of exposure and/or compatible clinical signs, or when there is a history of humans with skin disease. Concurrent bacterial and yeast infections are increasingly recognized as a common cause of pruritus in dogs, cats, and large animals. Infectious causes of pruritus commonly induce clinical signs of hair loss, scaling, scales piercing hairs, odor, and/or greasy seborrhea. Marked pedal pruritus and facial rubbing are common in animals with concurrent yeast and bacterial infections. Before pursuing allergies as a cause of pruritus or performing skin biopsies or other more expensive and/or invasive diagnostic testing, a concurrent bacterial and yeast infection should be ruled out. A 21-30 day concurrent course of an antibiotic effective against *Staphylococcus* spp (eg, cephalexin 30 mg/kg, PO, BID) and a systemic antifungal (eg, ketoconazole or itraconazole 5-10 mg/kg, PO, SID) should be prescribed. If the pruritus resolves, then existing pruritus was due to a microbial infection. It is possible that the initial trigger is long gone or seasonal. However, if the animal's pruritus is unchanged or only somewhat better, the most likely underlying cause is allergic (assuming parasitic causes have been ruled out). The most common causes of allergic pruritus are insect bite hypersensitivity (eg, flea allergy, mosquito bite allergy, fly bite), food allergy, and atopy. Flea allergy dermatitis and insect bite hypersensitivity are ruled out based on response to insect control. Animals that do not have insect bite hypersensitivity but are seasonally pruritic most likely have atopic dermatitis. Animals with year-round allergic pruritus have atopy and/or food allergy. Food allergy is ruled in or out based on response to a diet trial and provocative challenge. Atopy is a clinical diagnosis; in vitro allergy testing and intradermal skin testing show only antigen exposure patterns. These tests are used to determine the contents of an immunotherapy vaccine.

Treatment: Successful therapy depends on identification of the underlying cause. Patients with idiopathic pruritus or those in which treatment of the underlying disease does not eliminate the pruritus (eg, atopic patients) will require medical management of pruritus.

Antihistamines: The efficacy of antihistamines for the treatment of pruritus is highly variable. The most commonly used antihistamines include hydroxyzine hydrochloride (2.2 mg/kg, PO, TID), diphenhydramine (2.2 mg/kg, PO, BID), amitriptyline hydrochloride (2.2 mg, PO, BID), cetirizine (5 mg/cat or 5-10 mg/dog, SID or BID), and fexofenadine (2-3 mg/kg, PO, SID or BID). A 7-10 day therapeutic trial of any one antihistamine is required to see maximum benefit.

Essential Fatty Acids: Essential fatty acids (EFA) are rarely effective as sole antipruritic agents; however, they often act synergistically with antihistamines and/or glucocorticoids. They may enhance the effectiveness of antihistamines or allow a small dose of glucocorticoids to be used. The exact doses of EFA are unknown, but the current recommendation is 180 mg eicosapentaenoic acid/5 kg, PO, SID-BID.

Glucocorticoids: Glucocorticoids are the most effective drugs in the management of pruritus. However, they cannot be used safely for longterm management due to adverse effects (eg, suppression of adrenal function, risk of development of diabetes mellitus, risk of secondary urinary tract infections). In addition, owners can rarely tolerate the common side effects (polydipsia, polyuria, polyphagia, and panting) for long periods of time. Anti-inflammatory dosages range from 0.5-1.0 mg/kg, PO, SID for 5-10 days and then every other day.

Other Systemic Antipruritic Agents: Other effective agents include cyclosporine 5-10 mg/kg, PO, SID), pentoxifylline (10-25 mg/kg, PO, BID-TID), and misoprostol (3-6 μg/kg, PO, TID).

PRINCIPLES OF TOPICAL THERAPY

See also SYSTEMIC PHARMACOTHERAPEUTICS OF THE INTEGUMENTARY SYSTEM, p 2001.

Topical therapy is an important part of veterinary dermatology. It is often beneficial in improving the cosmetic appearance or odor of the animal, pending the final diagnosis. It can be beneficial as an adjunct to systemic therapy. Finally, it may be the preferred method of treatment for some diseases, eg, flea infestations.

The following are some basic guidelines to consider when prescribing topical therapy: 1) As much of the hair coat as possible should be removed when treating skin diseases. Good grooming practices can significantly help shorten the course of disease. In addition, good grooming practices facilitate topical therapy. 2) The cooperation of the owner (and animal) should be evaluated before any topical therapy is prescribed. 3) Animals tend to groom off topical products and may vomit after ingestion. The risk of toxicity is a constant worry for clients. Local ointments, gels, and sprays are best used sparingly, under occlusion, and for specific diseases. Such medications often sting when applied to the skin, especially many of those instilled into the ears. Many agents also may mat the hair. 4) Tepid water is the temperature of choice for bathing animals. 5) The old adage, "If it's wet, dry it and if it's dry, wet it," has some truth to it; however, this advice should not be carried to extremes. Exudative lesions, eg, areas of pyotraumatic dermatitis, heal faster if they are kept clean and covered with an antibiotic ointment or gel; previous recommendations suggested aggressive astringent use. Dry, lichenified skin is often pruritic, and the judicious use of emollients may be beneficial. 6) The animal should be monitored closely for possible development of irritant or allergic contact dermatitis from topical agents. Many topical agents have very similar bases or ingredients, and changing from one to another may just exacerbate the problem. 7) Owners should be given careful and thorough instructions on how to administer the therapy.

Shampoo Therapy: Shampoos are the most commonly used topical treatments. There are 3 broad classes of shampoos: cleansing, antiparasitic, and medicated. **Cleansing shampoos** remove dirt and excess oils from the coat. These products include over-the-counter dog grooming shampoos, flea shampoos, and many mild products for people. These products lather well and must be rinsed from the coat. **Antiparasitic shampoos** are "flea shampoos." In most cases, the amount of insecticide in these products is not adequate to kill all of the fleas in a severe infestation. However, these products are excellent routine cleansing products. **Medicated shampoos** include antimicrobial and antiseborrheic products. The most widely used antibacterial shampoos contain chlorhexidine or benzoyl peroxide. Miconazole and ketoconazole shampoos are usual adjuvant therapy for the treatment of *Malassezia* infections, but not for dermatophytosis. There is little evidence to suggest that the use of those products shortens the course of infection. Antiseborrheic shampoos contain some combination of tar, sulfur, and salicylic acid—ingredients that are keratoplastic and keratolytic. Tar is recommended for oily seborrhea, and sulfur and salicylic acid are recommended for scaly seborrhea. Most animals benefit from products that contain all 3 agents; however, tar products are contraindicated in cats.

When a medicated shampoo is used, the animal should be washed in a cleansing shampoo before the medicated shampoo and rinsed well. Medicated shampoos often are not good cleansing agents, do not lather well, or do not work well in the presence of organic debris. The medicated shampoo should be applied evenly to the hair coat after being prediluted in water. Prediluting the shampoo will facilitate it being rinsed from the coat and minimize the potential for irritant or allergic contact dermatitis. Depending on the shampoo, the concentration of shampoo to water will vary between 1:3 and 1:4. If possible, the medicated shampoo should be allowed to have a contact time of 10 min with the skin and then rinsed thoroughly from the coat. Shampoo residue is a common cause of irritant reactions. Finally, the medicated shampoo should be used often, usually 2-3 times/wk during the early stages of therapy.

CONGENITAL AND INHERITED ANOMALIES OF THE INTEGUMENTARY SYSTEM

Congenital dermatoses of the skin may be genetic or arise during embryogenesis because of nongenetic factors. Genetic mutations that cause skin anomalies may be present at birth or become apparent weeks to months later. These late-onset manifestations are referred to as tardive developmental defects. Both congenital and tardive developmental dermatoses are fairly common in domestic animals of all species, with the greatest number of well-defined defects described in cattle and dogs.

CONGENITAL ANOMALIES OF THE SKIN

Epitheliogenesis imperfecta (aplasia cutis) is a congenital discontinuity of squamous epithelium. It is seen in cattle (autosomal recessive trait), horses, swine, sheep, cats, and dogs. It is rare in the latter 3 species. In cattle, affected breeds include Holstein-Friesian, Hereford, Ayrshire, Jersey, Shorthorn, Angus, Dutch Black Pied, Swedish Red Pied, and German Yellow Pied. It is common in swine, in which large lesions are obvious at birth as glistening red, well-demarcated discontinuities in the skin or mucous membranes. Infection and ulceration is an early consequence. One or more hooves or claws may be deformed or absent; in some affected animals, there are other associated congenital anomalies. The condition is fatal when extensive, but small defects can be surgically corrected. Recent ultrastructural evaluation of this condition in American Saddlebred foals has demonstrated a relationship with junctional epidermolysis bullosa (p 682).

Focal cutaneous hypoplasia and **subcutaneous hypoplasia** are congenital, circumscribed hypoplastic defects of multiple or deeper skin layers in swine. The lesions manifest as skin depressions in which all skin layers or the subcutaneous fat layers fail to develop normally.

A **nevus** is a circumscribed developmental defect of the skin, while a **hamartoma** is a hyperplastic mass formed as a result of a developmental defect in any organ. Both nevi and hamartomas have been described as congenital skin defects, but the problem may not become obvious until later in life. In dogs, sebaceous nevi, pigmented epidermal nevi, inflammatory linear verrucous epidermal nevi, nevi comedonicus, linear organoid nevi, and follicular hamartomas are known to occur. In horses, cannon keratosis and linear epidermal nevi have been described. Doubtless, similar defects occur in all species. Mixed, or organoid, nevi consist of circumscribed collections of densely packed adnexal structures (pilosebaceous nevus and pilosebaceosudoriferous nevus). Collagenous nevi are nodules composed of focal collagen hyperplasia that displace the normal structures of the skin. Most lesions are alopecic, with pigmented, pitted surfaces. When not extensive, nevi can be excised; otherwise there is no known effective treatment.

Dermoid sinuses or cysts occur in Thoroughbred horses and Rhodesian Ridgebacks (in which they are inherited) and occasionally other breeds of dogs. These are cystic structures lined with skin into which exfoliated skin, hair, and glandular debris accumulate. They are caused by failure of complete separation of the neural tube from the epidermis during embryogenesis; they are found on the dorsal midline and are rarely associated with spinal cord neural deficits. They can be removed by surgical excision.

Follicular cysts develop by abnormal hair follicle morphogenesis and by retention of follicular or glandular products. They may be congenital when caused by the failure of the follicular orifice to develop normally. Congenital cysts are most commonly identified in Merino and Suffolk sheep. Periauricular (dentigerous) cysts are seen in horses and, although present at birth, may not be recognized until adulthood. Wattle cysts are seen in Nubian goats; these arise from the bronchial cleft. Porcine wattles are seen fairly frequently in all breeds of swine. These are teat-like growths on the lower jaw.

HEREDITARY ALOPECIA AND HYPOTRICHOSIS

Alopecia is the absence of hair; hypotrichosis, which is much more common, is the presence of less hair than normal. Although these defects can be generalized, they commonly develop in patterns that spare the extremities or correlate with hair color. These ectodermal defects can be congenital or tardive and can be associated with abnormal or absent adnexa, with defects in other ectodermal structures (such as teeth, claws, and eyes), or with skeletal and other developmental defects. There are various modes of inheritance in those instances in which familial occurrence has been studied. X-linked ectodermal dysplasia has been recently reported in German Shepherds. Hairless breeds of dogs (eg, Mexican Hairless, Chinese Crested, American Hairless Terrier) and cats (Sphinx) have been bred for these ectodermal defects. Many sporadic cases of ectodermal defects are described in dogs, most often in males. Many affected dogs, including most of the hairless breeds, have patchy or pattern hypotrichosis as well as associated dental anomalies. All animals with abnormal follicular development are prone to comedone formation, hair follicle infections, and hair foreign-body granulomas.

At least 13 types of **hypotrichosis** have been described in cattle, affecting Angus; Ayrshire; Brangus; Holstein-Friesian; Hereford; polled Hereford; Guernsey; Gelbvieh; Jersey; and Normandy-Maine, Anjou-Charolais, and Simmental crosses. Most have autosomal recessive or sex-linked modes of inheritance. Associated defects include failure of horn development, hypophyseal hypoplasia, macroglossia, dental anomalies, abnormal coat coloration, and death (lethal hypotrichosis). Viable hypotrichosis, hypotrichosis with anodontia, semi-hairlessness, streaked hairlessness, black hair follicle dysplasia (Holstein), and cross-related hypotrichosis (rat tail) are specific types described in cattle.

In sheep, hypotrichosis is rarely reported, with the best known syndrome affecting the Polled Dorset. This involves the hair of the face most severely, but the wool is also of poor quality. In goats, hypotrichosis is associated with congenital goiter. In swine, 2 forms of hypotrichosis are known (Mexican Hairless, German), one of which is associated with goiter and death in the homozygote.

In dogs, there are several tardive **follicle dysplasias**, including color dilution alopecia. This is found in some dogs bearing the coat color genotype dd, which renders black genotypes blue and liver genotypes beige or fawn. This syndrome is best known in Doberman Pinschers but is also commonly seen in color dilute Dachshunds, Italian Greyhounds, Greyhounds, Whippets, Yorkshire Terriers, and tricolor hounds and has now been reported in a German Shepherd. Affected dogs are born with normal hair coats but before 1 yr of age begin to develop folliculitis and hypotrichosis that is progressive and confined to the blue or fawn colored areas. Black hair follicle dysplasia, a similar but earlier developing and more complete hypotrichosis, is seen in black and white piebald dogs. The hypotrichosis develops shortly after birth and affects only the black-colored areas. This syndrome is best known in the Papillon and Bearded Collie. Recent genetic analysis in Large Munsterlanders has indicated an autosomal recessive inheritance in this breed. A similar follicular dysplasia is reported in nonpiebald breeds. Other types of follicular dysplasias that are apparently affected by endocrine and dietary factors are seasonal flank alopecia of Boxers and Airedale Terriers and various woolly syndromes and post-clipping alopecia in Spitz-type breeds. Familial hypotrichosis of Irish Water Spaniels has been shown to be influenced by both dietary factors and sex hormones. The condition formerly known as growth hormone-responsive alopecia in Pomeranians and other breeds is now called alopecia X, reflecting the complexity of factors, hereditary and otherwise, influencing these syndromes.

In cats, follicular dysplasia occurs in the Devon Rex. In horses, both color dilution alopecia and black hair follicle dysplasias are occasionally reported, especially in Appaloosas. Congenital progressive hypotrichosis has been reported in a blue roan Percheron. Reported hair shaft structural abnormalities of dogs and cats include pili torti (American Wirehaired Cat), trichorrhexis nodosa, and spiculosis (Kerry Blue Terrier).

HYPERPLASTIC AND SEBORRHEIC SYNDROMES

Many anomalies affect keratinization; some are associated with hereditary hypotrichoses (*see* above), while others are associated with systemic metabolic derangements. Those for which none of these associations has yet been made are a diverse group of syndromes that may affect localized parts of the epithelium or that may be generalized. Among the latter are included the poorly characterized congenital or familial seborrheic syndromes, the best known of which is idiopathic seborrhea oleosa of Spaniels and Persian cats. **Hereditary congenital follicular parakeratosis** is a newly recognized syndrome of female Rottweilers and Siberian Huskies. It is a severe keratinization defect associated with various noncutaneous abnormalities.

Cutaneous ichthyoses are characterized by abnormal and hypertrophic epithelial proliferation, with accumulation of extensive scale and hyperkeratosis on the skin surface. Cases have been described mostly in cattle and dogs, but chicken and several mouse models are also known, and there is one report in a llama. In cattle, the severity varies; some forms are lethal shortly after birth. Affected breeds include Red Poll, Friesian, Holstein, Brown Swiss, Pinzgauer, and Chianina. Canine ichthyosiform dermatoses are also heterogeneous and occur sporadically in a number of breeds, including Doberman Pinschers, Rottweilers, Irish Setters, Collies, English Springer Spaniels, Cavalier King Charles Spaniels, Golden Retrievers, Labrador Retrievers, and terriers (including Jack Russell Terriers). There is some evidence of a familial inheritance pattern in Jack Russell Terriers and Golden Retrievers. In dogs, the body is covered with large adherent scales that may flake off in large sheets. The planum nasale and digital pads may be markedly thickened in some forms; the latter usually is associated with apparent discomfort. Clinical management is difficult, but signs may be ameliorated with keratolytic shampoos or solutions (eg, selenium disulfides, lactic acid, benzoyl peroxide) and with humectants (eg, lactic acid, urea, propylene glycol, and essential fatty acid preparations). Experimental use of synthetic retinoids has been useful. Control of secondary pyoderma is frequently required.

Psoriasiform-lichenoid dermatosis affects young English Springer Spaniels and is presumed to be genetic. The erythematous, symmetric lesions, which consist of papules and plaques on the pinnae and inguinal region, are covered with scale and become increasingly hyperkeratotic if left untreated. In some affected dogs, the lesions may eventually spread and resemble severe seborrhea oleosa. Spontaneous remissions and a waxing and waning course are recorded. Some dogs respond to antibiotic treatment or to synthetic retinoids, but most are refractory to therapy.

Pityriasis rosea of pigs is a familial disease in which the mode of inheritance is not known. (*See* p 796 for clinical findings, diagnosis, and treatment.) **Dermatosis vegetans** of Landrace pigs is a hereditary, possibly congenital, disorder with an autosomal recessive mode of inheritance. It must be differentiated in the early stages from pityriasis rosea. This is a more serious disease and affects the hooves as well as the skin. Lesions begin as macules and papules and are scaly as in pityriasis rosea. They later become covered with brown-black crusts and are associated with coronitis and hoof deformity. Piglets fail to thrive and eventually develop pneumonia; the disease is not uniformly fatal, but affected survivors are stunted. There is no effective treatment.

Familial footpad hyperkeratosis is reported in Irish Terriers and Dogues de Bordeaux. All pads of all feet are involved from a young age, although the disease is not usually congenital. When hyperkeratosis is severe, horns, fissures, and secondary infection cause pain and lameness. No other skin lesions are present. Treatment is symptomatic, with soaking, keratolytic and emollient treatments, and treatment of bacterial pyoderma. No reports of the use of synthetic retinoids are available.

Granulomatous sebaceous adenitis is an idiopathic disease that destroys the sebaceous glands and, in some breeds of dogs, is associated with a severe seborrheic and alopecic dermatosis. It is hereditary in Standard Poodles and suspected to be familial in Akitas. It first manifests itself in young adults, but inapparent carriers are known in Poodles. Marked hyperkeratosis precedes the development of hair coat abnormalities, which begin as the loss of normal hair kinkiness and progress to patchy alopecia. Akitas tend to have more seborrhea oleosa and less alopecia than Poodles. Response to treatment is inconsistent and incomplete. Mildly affected dogs are treated with antiseborrheic shampoos and treatment of pyoderma as needed. Severely affected dogs have benefited from propylene glycol or hot oil treatments. Some dogs respond to oral supplementation with omega-3 fatty acids, and some to synthetic retinoids. Cases of spontaneous remission have been recorded.

PIGMENTARY ABNORMALITIES

Many associations between skin and coat color and developmental anomalies have been recorded in domestic animals. Some of the associations with hypotrichosis are discussed under hereditary alopecia (p 679).

Albinism appears to be rare in domestic animals. True albinism is always associated with pink or pale irises and with visual defects and increased risk of solar radiation-induced neoplasms of the skin. It has been noted in Icelandic sheep and in Guernsey, Austrian Murboden, Shorthorn, Brown Swiss, and Charolais cattle. Albinism must be differentiated from extreme white spotting or piebaldism and dominant white. Some animals with extreme piebaldism or dominant white have associated neurologic anomalies, deafness, or suffer death in utero. Lethal white foal syndrome is one that results from breeding 2 Overo Paints. In both dogs and cats, dominant white or extreme piebaldism can be associated with unilateral or bilateral deafness, and sometimes with blue irides or iris heterochromia. White cats with bilateral blue eyes have a 75% chance of deafness. In dogs, deafness may also be associated with merle hair coats and is found in Dalmatians, Sealyham Terriers, harlequin Great Danes, Collies, and white Bull Terriers. Cyclic neutropenia (p 51) may be found in gray or pale merle Collies. In Rhodesian Ridgebacks, pale coat color is associated with cerebellar degeneration. In Chédiak-Higashi syndrome (p 51) of cats and cattle (Herefords, Japanese Black, Brangus), coat color dilution (blue smoke in cats) is associated with neutrophil and platelet abnormalities and shortened life span. This is inherited as an autosomal recessive trait. Male tricolor cats (calico and tortoiseshell) are sterile because the gene for orange is X-linked and recessive, and males have the abnormal XXY genotype.

Pigmentary abnormalities may be acquired, and some of these may be hereditary or familial as in **vitiligo**. As a familial disease, vitiligo is best recognized in Arabian horses (Arabian fading syndrome, pinky syndrome); it may also be familial in cattle (Holstein-Friesian), Siamese cats, and in some breeds of dogs (Belgian Tervuren, Rottweiler). Affected animals develop somewhat symmetric macular depigmentation of the skin that occasionally also affects the hair coat and claws or hooves. The onset is usually in young adulthood. Most lesions are on the face, especially the muzzle or planum nasale or around the eyes. Depigmentation may wax and wane. Complete remission may occur but is rare. There is no accompanying systemic or cutaneous pathology. No treatment is available; treatments used in people with vitiligo are unlikely to provide significant cosmetic results in animals.

Lentigo in orange and orange-faced male cats is marked by the development of asymptomatic, pigmented macules. Lesions are first seen on the lips and eyelids at <1 yr of age. Other sites include the planum nasale and gingivae. Lentigines are not precancerous and have no medical consequence.

Acquired aurotrichia of Miniature Schnauzers is a familial syndrome in which hair along the dorsal midline changes to golden from the normal black or gray of this breed. The onset is usually in young adulthood. The change may be associated with thinning in the hair coat but no other cutaneous or systemic signs. In most dogs, coat color reverts to normal within 1-2 yr.

DEFECTS OF STRUCTURAL INTEGRITY

This category includes genetic defects in structural elements responsible for the integrity of the epidermis and dermal-epidermal junction, as well as some dermal structural anomalies.

Cutaneous asthenia (dermatosparaxis, Ehlers-Danlos syndrome) is a group of syndromes characterized by defects in collagen production. This results in a variety of clinical signs, including loose, hyperextensible, fragile skin; joint laxity; and other connective tissue dysfunctions. These collagen defects have been described in cattle (Belgian Blue and White, Charolais, Hereford, Holstein-Freisian, Simmental), a goat, sheep (Norwegian Dala, Border Leicester-Southdown, Finnish-Merino cross, Romney, White Dorper), pigs (Large White-Essex cross), horses (Quarter horse, Arabian cross), rabbits (New Zealand white), cats (Himalayan and domestic shorthair), mink, and dogs (a litter of Garafiano Shepherds, sporadically in several breeds). The mode of inheritance has been demonstrated for Himalayan cats (recessive) and domestic shorthair cats (dominant). Clinical features include fragile skin from the time of birth, wounds that heal with thin scars, delayed wound healing, pendulous skin, and hematoma and hygroma formation. In lambs, rupture of the GI tract and arterial aneurysms are features, and the disease is fatal in lambs and calves. In horses, the onset is later and the lesions are well circumscribed, consisting of hyperextensible and somewhat fragile skin. In dogs and cats, the disease is not fatal, and older animals develop hanging folds of skin and exhibit extensive scarring; some have joint laxity or ocular anomalies. Diagnosis is based on clinical signs and histopathologic studies of the collagen structure, which require age and breed-matched controls. For diagnosis in cats and dogs, a skin extensibility index has been developed. There are anecdotal reports of improvement of affected dogs with vitamin C supplementation. The major differential diagnosis in adult cats is feline hyperadrenocorticism with acquired skin fragility.

The **epidermolysis bullosa syndromes** are a group of congenital and hereditary diseases that result from defects in the dermal-epidermal attachment structures. These are known as mechanobullous diseases because minor cutaneous trauma results in dermal-epidermal separation with formation of flaccid bullae that soon rupture, leaving glistening, flat erosions. Syndromes are classified according to the ultrastructural location of the epidermal-dermal defect: simplex, in the epidermal basal cell layer; junctional, within the basement membrane; and dystrophic, below the basement membrane in the subepidermal anchoring fibrils. In large animals, lesions are most common on the gingivae, palate, lips, tongue, and feet. Some forms of epidermolysis bullosa are scarring, and most are fatal. In large animals, epidermolysis bullosa syndromes are known in calves (Simmental, Brangus), domestic buffalo, lambs (Suffolk, South Dorset Down, Scottish Blackface, Weisses Alpenschaf, Welsh Mountain), and Belgian foals. All 3 forms of epidermolysis bullosa have been characterized in dogs and cats. Epidermolysis bullosa simplex has been described in Collies and Shetland Sheepdogs. Junctional epidermolysis bullosa has been reported in a Toy Poodle, German Shorthaired Pointers, mixed-breed dogs, and Siamese cats, and tentatively identified in Beaucerons. Dystrophic epidermolysis bullosa has been reported in a domestic shorthair cat and a Persian and in Golden Retrievers and Akitas. Lesions may be present at birth or develop within the first weeks of life. The most severe lesions are on the feet, with sloughing of hooves, claws, or footpads, and oral mucous membrane and facial and perigenital skin (erosions). Except for epidermolysis bullosa simplex, these diseases are fatal.

Canine benign familial chronic pemphigus is a mechanobullous disorder that is caused by a defect in cell-to-cell adhesion in the epidermis. This disorder has been described in a family of English Setters. It develops within a few weeks of birth and causes crusting alopecic lesions on the pressure points of the skin that slowly enlarge as the puppies grow. The disease is benign, and no treatment is reported. **Familial acantholysis**, reported in New Zealand Angus calves, is a similar syndrome. This fatal syndrome is reported to be an autosomal recessive trait. Affected calves develop erosions, with collarettes and crusts, in areas subjected to trauma. Some show partial separation of the hooves. Diagnosis in both puppies and calves is established by skin biopsy of newly forming lesions.

Cutaneous mucinosis is thought to be a familial problem in some lines of Chinese Shar-Peis. Normal Shar-Peis have more cutaneous mucin than other dogs, but in some young dogs, cutaneous mucin formation in the dermis is so excessive that the skin exhibits pronounced folding and mucinous vesiculation. Diagnosis is by skin prick of the vesicles and observation of the strings of mucus that have the same appearance as normal joint fluid or, alternatively, by skin biopsy. The syndrome is partially responsive to corticosteroids, but this treatment is contraindicated because of the young age of the affected dogs. As these dogs mature, the severity of the syndrome may abate, but it can be exaggerated by the development of allergic skin disease, which is common in the breed. The major differential diagnosis is hypothyroidism.

CUTANEOUS MANIFESTATIONS OF MULTISYSTEMIC AND METABOLIC DEFECTS

Baldy calf syndrome of female Holsteins, as the name implies, is associated with hypotrichosis. This autosomal recessive trait is lethal to male fetuses. Affected calves appear normal at birth but lose condition and patches of hair beginning 1-2 mo later. The skin then becomes thickened and wrinkled, and the tips of the ears may curl. Calves salivate profusely and become emaciated, and affected female calves die by 6-8 mo of age. The underlying metabolic defect is not known. A similar appearing syndrome, known as **congenital anemia, dyskeratosis**, and **progressive alopecia**, is described in polled Hereford calves of either sex. Anemia and small size are noted at birth and become progressively more severe. Alopecia, abnormal curly hair, and hyperkeratosis begin around the muzzle and ear margins and become more extensive as the calves mature. Later, the skin becomes markedly wrinkled, and neurologic abnormalities develop. Calves have diarrhea and die before 6 mo of age.

Familial vasculopathy has been described in German Shepherds and Jack Russell Terriers. In these dogs, the skin lesions develop shortly after the first set of puppy vaccinations and seem to be exacerbated after subsequent vaccinations. The main cutaneous signs are footpad swelling and depigmentation that may progress to ulceration; all footpads are typically affected. Crusting and ulceration of the ear and tail tips and depigmentation of the planum nasale are also features. As the dogs mature, the disease may resolve, but pad lesions may be so severe that euthanasia is warranted. No known treatment is uniformly effective, although some dogs appear to respond to high dosages of corticosteroids. A severe form of **neutrophilic vasculitis** recently described in young Shar-Peis may be familial.

Familial dermatomyositis is an idiopathic inflammatory disease of the skin and muscles of young Collies and Shetland Sheepdogs. The mode of inheritance is reported to be autosomal dominant in Collies, but there is some evidence of a role for an unidentified infectious agent in the pathogenesis. A vasculopathy is associated with the early inflammatory stages of the disease in the skin and muscle; in both tissues, the eventual sequela is atrophy. The onset is typically at <6 mo of age, although onset in adulthood has been recorded. Progression of lesions is variable, and individual pups within a litter may be affected mildly to severely. Skin lesions appear in areas of increased trauma and are seen on the face, ear tips, tail tips, and lateral surfaces of the extremities. Skin lesions, which consist of erosion, crusting, and alopecia, are exacerbated by heat and sun exposure. The muscles affected most severely are on the head and extremities. Diagnosis is established by evaluation of littermates and family history, skin biopsy, electromyography, and muscle biopsy, which must be performed early in the course of the disease. There are reports of disease amelioration with dosages of corticosteroids, vitamin E, and omega-3 fatty acids, but severely affected dogs rarely respond satisfactorily to treatment.

Hereditary lupoid dermatosis of German Shorthaired Pointers is first noted when the dog is ~6 mo old. It begins with scaling and crusting on the head and dorsum and quickly progresses to generalized scaling with erythema. The dermatopathy appears to be either painful or pruritic. Affected dogs become pyrexic and develop lymphadenopathy. Some develop a poorly characterized enteropathy; most lose condition. As the name implies, skin biopsy specimens reveal features of a lupus-like dermatitis. The disease is progressive and ultimately fatal. No successful treatment has been reported.

Hereditary zinc deficiency syndromes are best known in cattle and have also been described in dogs. In cattle, these syndromes include hereditary parakeratosis, lethal trait A46, edema disease, and hereditary thymic hypoplasia. Affected breeds include Friesian, Shorthorn, Angus, and Black Pied. These syndromes all become apparent within days to weeks of birth and are characterized by symmetric, mostly acral, hyperkeratosis; crusting and unthriftiness; susceptibility to infection; and early death. Affected calves exhibit conjunctivitis, ptyalism, rhinitis, and diarrhea, and often succumb to pneumonia. In most breeds of cattle, the trait appears to be autosomal recessive and associated with intestinal malabsorption of dietary zinc, which is more or less responsive to dietary zinc supplementation. In some breeds, the defect in absorption is absolute, and parenteral administration of zinc is needed to achieve remission. As such manipulations are rarely feasible in food animals, these are lethal traits. Diagnosis is established by ruling out dermatophilosis (p 692) and by skin biopsy (showing mostly parakeratosis), by measuring serum zinc levels, and by necropsy findings that include hypoplasia of thymus and lymph nodes.

In dogs, there are 2 familial zinc deficiency syndromes. In white Bull Terriers, **lethal acrodermatitis** is characterized by retarded growth; progressive, acral, hyperkeratotic dermatitis; and pustular dermatitis around mucocutaneous junctions. These signs are apparent by 10 wk of age and are later accompanied by diarrhea, pneumonia, and death before 2 yr of age. In older dogs, footpad hyperkeratosis and paronychia contribute significantly to morbidity. The severity of the cutaneous disease can be ameliorated somewhat by control of secondary bacterial and *Malassezia* infections and, with aggressive medical treatment, the lives of affected dogs can be prolonged. These dogs do not respond to oral zinc therapy. A **familial zinc-responsive dermatopathy** that is manifest mostly by cutaneous lesions and is responsive to supplemental oral zinc is seen in Alaskan Malamutes, Huskies, and German Shorthaired Pointers. Signs develop at weaning or later in life and consist of crusting and hyperkeratosis of the extremities and mucocutaneous junctions. Often, bitches will develop signs associated with estrus or whelping and lactation. Secondary *Malassezia* infections are common. Diagnosis is established by skin biopsy and response to oral zinc supplementation.

Tyrosinemia has been described in 1 German Shepherd puppy. It was compared to a type of tyrosinemia in humans and thus thought to be hereditary. Clinical manifestations included erosions and ulcerations of the footpads and nose and bullous lesions and depigmentation of the skin, loss of claws, and eye lesions. It must be differentiated from the familial vasculopathy of German Shepherds described above. In the puppy, serum tyrosine levels were 20-30 times above normal levels, and urine specimens contained similar high concentrations.

Porphyria is an inherited defect in the metabolism of hemoglobin and its byproducts. In cattle, accumulation of aberrant porphyrins in the skin increases sensitivity to ultraviolet light. (Porphyria has been described in cats and swine but does not result in photosensitivity.) In cattle, there are 2 types of inherited porphyries. Bovine protoporphyria has been reported in crossbred Limousin cattle and is inherited as an autosomal recessive trait. Signs include photodermatitis and photophobia. Affected calves may die, but mature animals may be less severely affected. Bovine erythropoietic porphyria (p 804) is more common and more severe. It is reported in several breeds (including Shorthorn, Holstein-Friesian, and Hereford) as an autosomal recessive trait. In addition to severe photosensitivity, signs include red-brown discoloration of teeth, bones and urine; regenerative anemia; and stunted growth. Teeth and urine from affected animals fluoresce orange under a Wood's lamp. Skin biopsy is also useful in diagnosis.

Leukocyte adhesion deficiency (p 52) in Holstein cattle is an inherited disease (autosomal recessive) with many manifestations. It is fatal before adulthood. Skin lesions are frequently seen in affected calves and include dermatitis and vasculitis. This disease can be diagnosed by molecular methods with PCR analysis of fresh or fixed tissue providing identification of affected, carrier, and normal cattle.

CONGENITAL AND HEREDITARY NEOPLASMS AND MULTIPLE HAMARTOMAS

Congenital neoplasms are common in large animals. **Mastocytosis, melanocytosis, cutaneous lymphosarcoma**, and **vascular hamartomas** are found in calves. Melanocytomas may also arise shortly after birth in calves and may be hereditary. These are thought to be benign.

Melanomas are seen in Duroc-Jersey and Sinclair miniature pigs as familial traits. These may undergo spontaneous remission or may behave as malignant tumors. Piglets have also been described with vascular hamartomas and with congenital **fibropapillomatosis**, which is likely infectious.

Congenital tumors are rare in dogs and cats. One dog with a giant congenital pigmented nevus had a malignant melanoma develop within the lesion. In cats, familial benign mastocytosis is described in young Siamese cats.

A syndrome of multiple collagenous nevi is seen in some families of German Shepherds and is called **nodular dermatofibrosis**. Affected dogs are adults. Dozens of skin lesions may occur, and those on the feet often ulcerate or cause foot deformities and lameness. This syndrome is a cutaneous marker for renal cystadenocarcinoma and uterine leiomyoma. **Progressive dermal collagenosis** is a similar disease of postpubertal male miniature pigs. It is thought to be hereditary and is characterized by symmetric, firm plaques on the trunk that consist of thick bundles of collagen replacing the normal dermis and panniculus. A connection with internal malignancy has not been reported.

ALLERGIC INHALANT DERMATITIS

(Atopy)

Allergic inhalant dermatitis is a common form of allergy in dogs and cats. It is generally accepted to be a Type I (IgE or IgG) hypersensitivity and is believed to affect ~10% of the canine population. Its incidence in cats has not been reported.

Etiology and Pathogenesis: Animals with atopy are thought to be genetically programmed to become sensitized to allergens in the environment. Allergens are proteins that, when inhaled or absorbed through the skin, respiratory tract, or GI tract, evoke allergen-specific IgE production. These allergen-specific IgE molecules affix themselves to tissue mast cells or basophils. When they come in contact with the specific allergen, mast cell degranulation results in the release of proteolytic enzymes, histamine, bradykinins, and other vasoactive amines, leading to inflammation (erythema, edema, and pruritus). The skin is the primary target organ in dogs and cats, but rhinitis and asthma can also occur in ~15% of affected animals.

Canine Atopy

Clinical Findings: There is no sex predilection. Breeds predisposed to developing atopy include Shar-Peis, Wirehaired Fox Terriers, Golden Retrievers, Dalmatians, Boxers, Boston Terriers, Labrador Retrievers, Lhasa Apsos, Scottish Terriers, Shih Tzus, and West Highland White Terriers. The age of onset is generally between 6 mo and 3 yr. Clinical signs usually occur on a seasonal basis but may be seen year-round with time. Pruritus is the characteristic sign of atopy and may be the only complaint. The feet, face, ears, flexural surfaces of the front legs, axillae, and abdomen are the most frequently affected areas. Lesions develop secondary to self-trauma and include alopecia, erythema, scaling, salivary staining, hemorrhagic crusts, excoriations, lichenification, and hyperpigmentation. Superficial staphylococcal pyoderma, *Malassezia* dermatitis, and allergic otitis externa with secondary infections are common complications. Chronic or recurrent otitis is the only complaint in a small number of animals.

Diagnosis: The diagnosis is based on the signalment, a thorough history, appropriate physical examination findings, and ruling out of other causes of pruritus. Differential diagnoses include food allergy (nonseasonal), flea allergy (seasonal), contact allergy, and scabies. The primary reason for pursuing intradermal or serologic allergy testing is to identify the offending allergens in an animal, and to formulate specific immunotherapy. Allergy testing (intradermal or serologic) is a diagnostic aid that measures elevated levels of tissue-bound or circulating IgE; alone, it is not sufficient to diagnose atopy. Test results are significant only if the offending allergens identified are compatible with the history or seasonality of pruritus.

Treatment and Control: There are 3 therapeutic options available for management of atopy: avoidance of the offending allergen(s), symptomatic therapy to control pruritus, and immunotherapy (ie, hyposensitization, desensitization, allergy vaccine). A good management plan for atopic dermatitis requires the use of several different treatments, clear client education that ensures the owner has reasonable expectations of response, and frequent progress evaluations so that the plan can be adjusted if needed.

Immunotherapy: Hyposensitization or immunotherapy attempts to increase an animal's tolerance to environmental allergens (subjectively measured when an individual is exposed to an identified allergen without developing clinical signs). Although the mode of action is not completely understood, the primary theory states that IgG increases during the first few months of hyposensitization and exerts a blocking effect on circulating allergens by binding them and preventing mast cell degranulation. After an injection, however, allergen-specific IgE levels may also increase when immunotherapy is initiated due to a response to the additional allergen load from the immunotherapy injections. This may result in increased pruritus in some animals. Reducing the amount of allergen given will often alleviate this reaction, and with time, allergen-specific IgE levels decrease. Decreased IgE levels and clinical improvement are not always directly correlated, however.

Immunotherapy is best considered for animals with problematic clinical signs that occur for several months during the year. The animal must also be cooperative enough to receive allergy injections. The criteria for successful hyposensitization include appropriate interpretation of test results, careful selection of allergens, adequate control of secondary infections, control of other allergies (food or flea), systematic administration of immunotherapy injections, and periodic communications between the owner and veterinarian. The longterm commitment needed from both the owner and the veterinarian for successful immunotherapy cannot be overemphasized. The owner must be willing to follow instructions accurately, be patient, and be able to communicate effectively with the veterinarian. The veterinarian must be able to recognize and treat other primary or secondary causes of pruritus (eg, otitis, pyoderma, *Malassezia* dermatitis, insect hypersensitivity) as they occur. Symptomatic therapy is required in almost every case during the induction period and at various times of the year. Symptomatic therapy includes not only antipruritic medications (ie, glucocorticoids, essential fatty acids, antihistamines, oral cyclosporine, topical shampoos and rinses) but also specific antimicrobial therapy.

Vaccine preparation involves selection of individual allergens for a particular animal. The allergen selection is determined by correlating the positive allergens on the test results with the prominent allergens during the time of year when the animal is symptomatic. If the test shows positive results for pollens that have no clinical relevance (eg, high pollen count during a period when the animal has no pruritus, positive reaction to an allergen not in the geographic area), then either the allergic reaction is mild (subthreshold) or it is a false-positive reaction. Either way, the allergen should not be included in the vaccine. Most veterinary vaccines are aqueous extracts. Development and manufacture of allergen extracts has not been standardized; thus, ragweed pollen from one manufacturer is not necessarily equivalent to ragweed pollen from another. Allergen supply companies are required to culture each allergen or vaccine to ensure sterility before release to a veterinarian. To maintain sterility, vaccines are preserved with either phenol or glycerin and are kept refrigerated. Phenol-preserved vaccines lose potency faster than glycerinated vaccines, but glycerin-preserved vaccines can cause local reactions in animals. Most vaccines and antigens today are preserved with phenol. Vaccine concentrations are measured either as protein nitrogen units (PNU) per mL or weight to volume (w/v). Neither accurately measures biologic potency, but the PNU measurement is generally preferred. Allergen extracts should be refrigerated to preserve shelf life. Enough vaccine should be made to last up to 6 mo. The potency of most vaccines is considered inadequate after 1 yr.

The main variables involved with hyposensitization immunotherapy, other than allergen selection, are the frequency of the injections and the dosage of allergens given. Allergens are administered by SC injection. Current practice is to limit the number of allergens in an individual allergy vaccine to 10-12 because too many allergens in 1 vaccine may dilute the concentration of each individual allergen, yielding an inadequate response.

Vaccine protocols vary but usually have induction and maintenance periods. During the induction period, the dosage of allergen gradually increases until an arbitrary maintenance dosage is reached. Once the maximum dosage is given, this maintenance level is continued. The interval between maintenance dosages may vary from 3-4 days to 3 wk. Adjustments in the interval are based on the animal's response. Owners are advised not to expect much response for 6 mo and are asked to commit to at least 1 yr of therapy before deciding the usefulness of immunotherapy. The best assessment of response is to compare the degree of disease or discomfort between similar seasons. Most owners learn to administer the allergy injections very well, while others may need assistance from a capable friend or veterinary staff member.

Feline Atopy

Feline atopy is similar to canine atopy. It is a pruritic disease in which affected cats have a hypersensitivity reaction to inhaled or contacted environmental allergens. The age of onset is variable but generally is before 5 yr. The signs may be seasonal or nonseasonal. Purebred cats may have an increased risk compared with domestic short-haired cats. As in dogs, pruritic cats may have several clinical presentations (eg, miliary dermatitis, symmetric alopecia, eosinophilic granuloma complex, head and neck pruritus) that are consistent with a diagnosis of atopy but that must be differentiated from other diseases with similar clinical signs. Differential diagnoses include dermatophytosis, flea allergy, various mite infestations (eg, *Cheyletiella*, demodicosis, *Notoedres, Sarcoptes, Otodectes*), mosquito bite hypersensitivity, food allergy, autoimmune disease (eg, pemphigus foliaceus), and cutaneous neoplasia. A thorough review of the pet's history and complete dermatologic and physical examination, along with the standard flea combing, skin scrapings, and fungal cultures, are mandatory first steps. The diagnosis of atopy is made when the other differential diagnoses have been eliminated. Response to glucocorticoids is excellent initially but decreases over time.

Intradermal allergy testing and hyposensitization procedures are similar to those used in dogs, but the intradermal test results are more difficult to read because the reactions are less dramatic and dissipate more rapidly in cats. Response to therapy is similar to that in dogs; owners are advised to commit to 1 yr of therapy before deciding its usefulness.

FOOD ALLERGY

Food allergy is ~10% as common as atopy in dogs and about as common as atopy in cats. The history is that of a nonseasonal pruritus, with little variation in the intensity of pruritus from one season to another in most cases. Most reports do not suggest a breed predilection; however, one report indicated an increased relative risk in Labrador Retrievers, West Highland White Terriers, and Cocker Spaniels. Food hypersensitivities have been reported in Soft Coated Wheaten Terriers in association with protein-losing enteropathy and nephropathy. The age of onset is variable, from 2 mo to 14 yr old. One report indicated that most food allergies begin at <12 mo of age.

The distribution of pruritus and lesions varies markedly between animals. Ear canal disease that manifests as pruritus and secondary infection with bacteria (usually *Staphylococcus intermedius, Pseudomonas* spp, *Proteus* spp, or *Escherichia coli*) or yeast (*Malassezia pachydermatis*) are common and may be the only presenting complaint. Other patterns seen include blepharitis, generalized pruritus, generalized seborrhea, a papular eruption, or a distribution pattern that may mimic that of atopy (feet, face, and ventrum) or flea allergy dermatitis (dorsal lumbosacrum and hindlegs). The most common areas of involvement include the ears, feet, inguinal region, axillary area, proximal anterior forelegs, periorbital region, and muzzle. The degree of pruritus is usually moderate to severe. Response to glucocorticoids varies from poor to excellent.

There is no reliable diagnostic test other than a strict food elimination diet. Serologic testing and intradermal testing for food allergens have proved unreliable. The ideal food elimination diet should be balanced and nutritionally complete and not contain any ingredients that have been fed previously to the animal. Many diets contain novel protein or carbohydrate sources (eg, lamb and rice). However, it is often misunderstood that if *any* previously fed ingredient is present in the elimination diet, the animal may be allergic to the novel ingredient and the diet trial will be a failure. The key point in any food elimination diet trial is that only novel food ingredients can be fed.

The trial diet should be fed for up to 3 mo. If marked or complete resolution in the pruritus and clinical signs occurs during the elimination diet trial, food allergy can be suspected. To confirm that a food allergy exists and that the clinical improvement was not just coincidental, the animal must be challenged with the previously fed food ingredients and a relapse of clinical signs must occur. The return of clinical signs after challenge is usually between 1 hr and 14 days, although it is sometimes within 3 days. Once a food allergy is confirmed, the elimination diet should be reinstituted until clinical signs resolve, which usually takes <14 days. At this point, previously fed individual ingredients should be added to the elimination diet for a period of up to 14 days. If pruritus recurs, the individual ingredient is considered positive for having a causative role in the food allergy. If pruritus does not recur the individual ingredient is not considered important in causing the clinical signs.

The number of offending food allergens varies from 1-5 ingredients. The most frequently identified causative allergens in canine food allergy include beef, chicken, eggs, corn, wheat, soy, and milk. Once the offending allergens are identified, control of the food allergy is by strict avoidance. Concurrent diseases (such as atopy or flea allergy) may complicate the identification of underlying food allergies. Infrequently, a dog will react to new food allergens as it ages.

Clinical presentations of food allergy in cats include miliary dermatitis, feline symmetric alopecia, eosinophilic granuloma complex (primarily the eosinophilic plaque), and severe head and neck pruritus. No breed, sex, or age predilection is seen. Age of onset varies from 3 mo to 11 yr. In one study, however, 46% of affected cats became symptomatic at ≤2 yr of age, and Siamese cats represented 30% of the cases.

Response to steroids is variable, but about two-thirds of cats show excellent response initially. Many cats develop a poor response to steroids with repeated treatments. As with canine food allergy, an elimination diet should be fed for up to 3 mo. The elimination diet should not contain any previously fed ingredients. Food elimination diets can be difficult in cats because many cats are reluctant to change diets. Cats should not be starved or forced into eating a new elimination diet due to the serious nature of hepatic lipidosis that may be induced by prolonged anorexia.

Response time to the elimination diets varies from 1-9 wk. Time until relapse of pruritus after challenge with the offending food varies from 15 min to 10 days. The most frequently identified food allergens in cats include fish, beef, and chicken. Avoidance of the offending allergens will control the clinical signs associated with the food allergy.

URTICARIA

(Hives, Nettle rash)

Urticaria is characterized by multiple plaque-like eruptions that are formed by localized edema in the dermis and that often develop and disappear suddenly. It occurs in all domestic animals but most often in horses (*see also* SWEET ITCH, p 717). Allergic urticaria may be exogenous or endogenous. Exogenous hives may be produced by toxic irritating products of the stinging nettle, the stings or bites of insects, medications, or chemicals (eg, carbolic acid, turpentine, carbon disulfide, or crude oil). Nonimmunologic factors such as pressure, sunlight, heat, exercise, psychologic stress, and genetic abnormalities may precipitate or intensify urticaria. Pruritus is not always present.

Sensitive animals, particularly shorthaired dogs and purebred horses, also may exhibit **dermographism**, a phenomenon wherein rubbing or whipping produces urticaria-like skin lesions. It is of no clinical significance.

Endogenous or "symptomatic" urticaria may develop after inhalation or absorption of ingested allergens; it has been seen mostly in horses and dogs. In horses, it has been noted in the course of GI conditions, particularly severe constipation or inflammation of the intestinal mucosa. A unique form of urticaria has been described chiefly in the Channel Island breeds of cattle (Jersey, Guernsey), which become sensitized to the casein in their own milk (*see also* p 648); it occurs in cases of milk retention or unusual engorgement of the udder with milk. Urticaria has been seen in bitches during estrus. In young horses, dogs, and pigs, urticaria may be associated with intestinal parasites. **Angioneurotic edema** is a life-threatening variant of urticaria in which there is diffuse subcutaneous edema, often localized to the head, limbs, or perineum. In horses, dermatophytosis (ringworm) and pemphigus foliaceus may present as urticaria early in the disease.

Clinical Findings: The wheals or plaques appear within a few minutes or hours of exposure to the causative agent. In severe cases, the cutaneous eruptions are preceded by fever, anorexia, or dullness. Horses often become excited and restless. The skin lesions are elevated, round, flat-topped, and 0.5-8 in. (1-20 cm) in diameter; they may be slightly depressed in the center. They can develop on any part of the body but occur mainly on the back, flanks, neck, eyelids, and legs. In advanced cases, they may be found on the mucous membranes of the mouth, nose, conjunctiva, rectum, and vagina. In general, the lesions disappear as rapidly as they arise, usually within a few hours.

In sheep, lesions usually are seen only on the udder and hairless parts of the abdomen. In pigs, eruptions have been seen around the eyes, between the hindlegs, and on the snout, abdomen, and back.

In general, the prognosis is favorable. Fatalities are rare and are probably due to anaphylaxis or associated angioedema involving the respiratory passages.

Chronic urticaria is a diagnostic challenge. All allergens in an environment should be considered potential causes, and elimination of exposure instituted, if possible.

Treatment: Acute urticaria usually disappears spontaneously. The rapid-acting adrenocorticosteroids, eg, hydrocortisone sodium succinate or prednisolone sodium succinate or hemisuccinate are reported to be useful. Dexamethasone (0.1 mg/kg) has been useful in dogs, cats, and horses. Antihistamines are of questionable value and may induce urticaria if given IV. Epinephrine may be given in life-threatening situations. The lesions promptly disappear but return rapidly if the allergen is not eliminated. Usually, local treatment of the lesions is not necessary. In chronic urticaria, antihistamines such as hydroxyzine may be useful. In horses, the approximate dosage is 2-4 mg/5 kg, BID.

DERMATOPHILOSIS

(*Dermatophilus* infection, Cutaneous streptothrichosis, Lumpy wool, Strawberry footrot)

This infection of the epidermis, which is seen worldwide but is more prevalent in the tropics, is also erroneously called mycotic dermatitis. The lesions are characterized by exudative dermatitis with scab formation. *Dermatophilus congolensis* has a wide host range. Among domestic animals, cattle, sheep, goats, and horses are affected most frequently; and pigs, dogs, and cats rarely. It is commonly called cutaneous streptothrichosis in cattle, goats, and horses; in sheep, it is termed lumpy wool when the wooled areas of the body are affected. Infection in camel herds has been related to drought and poverty. Recent isolates from chelonids may represent a new species of *Dermatophilus*. The few human cases reported usually have been associated with handling diseased animals.

Etiology, Transmission, and Epidemiology: *D congolensis* is a gram-positive, non-acid-fast, facultative anaerobic actinomycete. It is the only species in the genus, but a variety of strains can be present within a group of animals during an outbreak. It has 2 characteristic morphologic forms—filamentous hyphae and motile zoospores. The hyphae are characterized by branching filaments (1-5 μm in diameter) that ultimately fragment by both transverse and longitudinal septation into packets of coccoid cells. The coccoid cells mature into flagellated ovoid zoospores (0.6-1 μm in diameter).

The natural habitat of *D congolensis* is unknown. Attempts to isolate it from soil have been unsuccessful, although it is probably a saprophyte in the soil. It has been isolated only from the integument of various animals and is restricted to the living layers of the epidermis. Asymptomatic chronically infected animals are considered the primary reservoir.

Factors such as prolonged wetting by rain, high humidity, high temperature, and various ectoparasites that reduce or permeate the natural barriers of the integument influence the development, prevalence, seasonal incidence, and transmission of dermatophilosis. The organism can exist in a quiescent form within the epidermis until infection is exacerbated by climatic conditions. Epidemics usually occur during the rainy season. Moisture facilitates release of zoospores from preexisting lesions and their subsequent penetration of the epidermis and establishment of new foci of infection. High humidity also contributes indirectly to the spread of lesions by allowing increases in the number of biting insects, particularly flies and ticks, that act as mechanical vectors. Shearing, dipping, or introducing an infected animal into a herd or flock can spread infection.

Dermatophilosis is contagious only in that any reduction in systemic or local skin resistance favors establishment of infection and subsequent disease.

Pathogenesis: To establish infection, the infective zoospores must reach a skin site where the normal protective barriers are reduced or deficient. The respiratory efflux of low concentrations of carbon dioxide from the skin attracts the motile zoospores to susceptible areas on the skin surface. Zoospores germinate to produce hyphae, which penetrate into the living epidermis and subsequently spread in all directions from the initial focus. Hyphal penetration causes an acute inflammatory reaction. Natural resistance to the acute infection is due to phagocytosis of the infective zoospores, but once infection is established, there is little or no immunity. In most acute infections, the filamentous invasion of the epidermis ceases in 2-3 wk, and the lesions heal spontaneously. In chronic infections, the affected hair follicles and scabs are sites from which intermittent invasions of noninfected hair follicles and epidermis occur. The invaded epithelium cornifies and separates in the form of a scab. In wet scabs, moisture enhances the proliferation and release of zoospores from hyphae. The high carbon dioxide concentration produced by the dense population of zoospores accelerates their escape to the skin surface, thus completing the unique life cycle.

Clinical Findings: Dermatophilosis is seen in animals at all ages but is most prevalent in the young, animals chronically exposed to moisture, and immunosuppressed hosts. Lesions on a host can vary from acute to chronic. Age, sex, and breed do not seem to affect host susceptibility. Pruritus is variable. Most affected animals recover spontaneously within 3 wk of the initial infection (provided that chronic maceration of the skin does not occur). In general, the onset of dry weather speeds healing. Uncomplicated skin lesions heal without scar formation. These infections usually have little effect on general health. Animals with severe generalized infections often lose condition, and movement and prehension are difficult if the feet, lips, and muzzle are severely affected; these animals are often sent to slaughter as incurable. Deaths occasionally occur, particularly in calves and lambs, because of generalized disease with or without secondary bacterial infection and secondary fly or screwworm infestation. The primary economic consequences are damaged hides in cattle, wool loss in sheep, and lameness and loss of performance in horses when severely affected around the pastern area.

Lesions: Distribution of the gross lesions on cattle, sheep, and horses usually correlates with the predisposing factors that reduce or permeate the natural barriers of the integument. In cattle, the lesions can be observed in 3 stages: 1) hairs matted together as paintbrush lesions, 2) crust or scab formation as the initial lesions coalesce, and 3) accumulations of cutaneous keratinized material forming wart-like lesions that are 0.5-2 cm in diameter. Typical lesions consist of raised, matted tufts of hair. Most lesions associated with prolonged wetting of the skin are distributed over the head, dorsal surfaces of the neck and body, and upper lateral surfaces of the neck and chest. Cattle that stand for long periods in deep water and mud develop lesions in areas such as skin folds of the flexor surfaces of the joints. Dairy cows may present with papular crusted lesions on the udder. Lesions initiated by biting flies (mechanical vectors) are found primarily on the back, whereas lesions induced by ticks are primarily on the head, ears, axillae, groin, and scrotum.

Chronic lumpy wool infections are characterized by pyramid-shaped masses of scab material bound to wool fibers. The crusts are primarily on the dorsal areas of the body and prevent the shearing of sheep; spiny plants often predispose to lesions on the lips, legs, and feet. Strawberry footrot is a proliferative dermatitis affecting the skin from the coronet to the carpus or hock.

Lesions on horses with long winter hair coats are similar to those of cattle, developing with matted hair and paint-brush lesions leading to crust or scab formation with yellow-green pus present under larger scabs. With short summer hair, matting and scab formation is uncommon; loss of hair with a fine paint-brush effect can be extensive. Persistent wetting of pasterns in wet yards, stables, or at pasture leads to lower limb infection; white legs and the white-skinned areas of the lips and nose are more severely affected. Generalized disease is also associated with prolonged wet weather. Outbreaks occur on farms with previously affected horses.

Histopathologic examination reveals the characteristic branching hyphae with multidimensional septations, coccoidal cells, and zoospores in the epidermis. The organisms are usually abundant in active lesions but can be sparse or absent in chronic lesions.

Diagnosis: Presumptive diagnosis depends largely on the appearance of lesions in clinically diseased animals and demonstration of *D congolensis* in stained smears or histologic sections from scabs. A definitive diagnosis is made by culture and identification. An indirect fluorescent antibody technique and a single dilution ELISA test have been developed for large serologic and epidemiologic surveys. The most practical diagnostic test is cytologic examination of fresh crusts and/or impression smears of the underside of freshly avulsed lesions. Fresh crusts are minced on a glass microscope slide with a sterile scalpel blade in several drops of sterile saline. The slide is allowed to air dry and is then stained with a fast Giemsa stain or Diff-Quik®. The organisms are seen under oil immersion as 2-6 parallel rows of gram-positive cocci that look like railroad tracks. Differential diagnoses include dermatomycoses in most species, warts and lumpy skin disease in cattle, contagious ecthyma and ulcerative dermatosis in sheep, and dermatophytosis and immune-mediated scaling diseases of horses (eg, pemphigus foliaceus).

Treatment and Control: Because acutely infected animals usually heal rapidly and spontaneously, treatment is indicated only for cosmetic reasons in food-producing animals. Treatment is recommended in horses because these lesions interfere with use and are painful. Organisms are susceptible to a wide range of antimicrobials—erythromycin, spiramycin, penicillin G, ampicillin, chloramphenicol, streptomycin, amoxicillin, tetracyclines, and novobiocin.

Usually, chronic infections can be rapidly and effectively cured with a single IM injection of procaine penicillin (22,000 IU/kg) and streptomycin (22 mg/kg). If this fails, the penicillin-streptomycin combination can be administered for 5 days, or a single injection of long-acting oxytetracycline (20 mg/kg) can be substituted.

In horses, the lesions should be gently soaked and removed. Topical antibacterial shampoo therapy is effective as adjuvant therapy. Chlorhexidine and benzoyl peroxide are recommended. In food-producing animals, topical applications of lime sulfur are a cost-effective adjuvant to antibacterial therapy. Insecticides applied externally are frequently used to control biting insects.

Isolating clinically affected animals, culling affected animals, and controlling ectoparasites are methods used to break the infective cycle.

EXUDATIVE EPIDERMITIS

(Greasy pig disease)

Exudative epidermitis is a generalized dermatitis that occurs in 5- to 60-day-old pigs and is characterized by sudden onset, with morbidity of 10-90% and mortality of 5-90%. The acute form usually affects suckling piglets, whereas a chronic form is more commonly seen in weaner pigs. It has been reported from most swine-producing areas of the world.

Lesions are caused by *Staphylococcus hyicus (hyos)*, which can produce an exfoliative toxin but seems unable to penetrate intact skin. Both virulent and avirulent strains exist. Abrasions on the feet and legs or lacerations on the body precede infection. Such injuries are usually caused by fighting or by abrasive surfaces such as new concrete. Other predisposing factors that may affect the severity and progress of the disease include immunity, hygiene, nutrition, and the presence of mange mites or anything that damages the skin. Mature sows that have acquired a high level of immunity from previous exposure will provide protection to piglets via their colostrum. The incidence is often higher in gilt litters and in newly established SPF herds in which the majority of breeders are gilts.

Pigs develop resistance with age, but *S hyicus* may be recovered from the skin of older pigs, the vagina of sows, and the preputial diverticulum of boars. These inapparent carriers serve as a source of contamination for naive herds. Suckling pigs are usually infected by their dams, in some cases during birth from sows with vaginal infections, or from contamination in the farrowing unit. Suckling piglets are the most commonly and severely affected, but cross-infection occurs after mixing at weaning with a morbidity of up to 80%. However, mortality is usually low in this age group. The incidence appears to have increased due to pig production units with high stocking densities and possibly earlier weaning.

Clinical Findings and Lesions: The first signs are listlessness and reddening of the skin in one or more piglets in the litter. Affected pigs rapidly become depressed and refuse to eat. Body temperature may increase early in the disease but thereafter is near normal. The skin thickens, and reddish brown spots (macules) appear around the eyes, nose, lips, and ears from which serum and sebum exude. The lesions increase in size and develop a vesicular or pustular appearance.

The body is rapidly covered with a moist, greasy exudate of sebum and serum that becomes crusty. Accumulation of dirt gives the affected area a black color. Vesicles and ulcers may also develop on the nasal disk and tongue. The feet are nearly always involved, with erosions at the coronary band and heel; the hoof may be shed in rare cases. In the acute disease, death occurs within 3-5 days. In older animals, the chronic form of the disease is seen as thick, crusty lesions over the entire body or as discrete circumscribed lesions that do not coalesce. Mortality is low except in very young suckling piglets. However, recovery is slow and growth is retarded and often associated with diarrhea, emaciation, and dehydration.

Necropsy of severely affected pigs reveals marked dehydration, congestion of the lungs, and inflammation of the peripheral lymph nodes. Distention of the kidneys and ureters with mucus, cellular casts, and debris is common in peracute and acute forms of the disease. The differential diagnosis includes sarcoptic mange, nutritional deficiencies including zinc (parakeratosis), ringworm, and pityriasis rosea.

Treatment: The causative organism is inhibited by many antibiotics, including amoxicillin, ampicillin, erythromycin, lincomycin, penicillin, tylosin, trimethoprim-sulfonamide, the aminoglycosides, and cephalosporins. Successful treatment requires that the antimicrobial be given in high dosages early in the disease and for a period of 7-10 days. Success is greatest when antimicrobial therapy is combined with daily applications of antiseptics to the entire body surface. Treatment is less effective in very young pigs and ineffective in advanced cases. In severe outbreaks, in-contact pigs should also be given antibiotics for several days. Sows due to farrow, and their housing, should be thoroughly disinfected to prevent outbreaks. Hygiene in the weaner accommodation and strategic in-water or in-feed medication for 3-5 days will help control outbreaks after weaning. Other procedures that may decrease the severity of an outbreak include clipping the needle teeth of newborn pigs, providing soft bedding, segregating infected animals, and avoiding mixing of animals to decrease the possibility of skin lesions due to fighting. Autogenous bacterins have been used with some success to reduce the incidence of disease in chronically infected herds.

INTERDIGITAL FURUNCULOSIS

Interdigital furuncles, often incorrectly referred to as interdigital cysts, are painful nodular lesions located in the interdigital webs of dogs. Histologically, these lesions represent areas of nodular pyogranulomatous inflammation—they are almost never cystic.

Etiology: The most common cause is a deep bacterial infection. Many dog breeds (eg, Shar-Pei, Labrador Retriever, English Bulldog) are predisposed to bacterial interdigital furunculosis because of the short bristly hairs located on the webbing between the toes, prominent interdigital webbing, or both. The short shafts of hairs are easily forced backward into the hair follicles during locomotion (traumatic implantation). Hair, ie, keratin, is very inflammatory in the skin, and secondary bacterial infections are common. Less commonly, foreign material is traumatically embedded in the skin.

Demodicosis (p 744) may be a primary cause of interdigital furunculosis. Canine atopy (p 686) is also a common cause of recurrent interdigital furunculosis.

Clinical Findings and Lesions: Early lesions of interdigital furunculosis may appear as focal or generalized areas of erythema and papules in the webbing of the feet that, if left untreated, rapidly develop into single or multiple nodules. The latter usually are 1-2 cm in diameter, reddish purple, shiny, and fluctuant; they may rupture when palpated and exude a bloody material. Interdigital furuncles are most commonly found on the dorsal aspect of the paw, but may also be found ventrally. Furuncles are usually painful, and the dog may be obviously lame on the affected foot (or feet) and lick and bite at the lesions. Lesions caused by a foreign body, eg, a grass awn, are usually solitary and often occur on a front foot; recurrence is not common in these cases. If bacteria cause the interdigital furunculosis, there may be several nodules with new lesions developing as others resolve. A common cause of recurrence is the granulomatous reaction to the presence of free keratin in the tissues.

Diagnosis: This is often based on clinical signs alone. The major differential diagnoses are traumatic lesions and neoplasia, although the latter is rare. The most useful diagnostic tests include skin scrapings for *Demodex* mites, impression smears, or fine-needle aspirates to confirm the presence of an inflammatory infiltrate. Unusual or recurrent lesions should be excised for histopathologic examination. Solitary lesions may require surgical exploration to find and remove foreign bodies such as grass awns.

Treatment: Interdigital furuncles respond best to a combination of topical and systemic therapy. Cephalexin (20 mg/kg, PO, TID, or 30 mg/kg, PO, BID) is recommended for 4-6 wk of initial therapy. However, because the lesions are pyogranulomatous, it may be difficult for antibiotics to penetrate them; therefore, >8 wk of systemic antibiotic therapy may be required for lesions to completely resolve. These lesions are often complicated by concurrent *Malassezia* spp infections. Oral ketoconazole or itraconazole (5-10 mg/kg) for 30 days may be indicated. The presence of *Malassezia* can be documented by cytologic examination of nail bed debris and/or impression smears of the skin. Topical foot soaks in warm water with or without an antibiotic solution (eg, chlorhexidine) and the application of mupiricin ointment are recommended. Some dogs may benefit from antibiotic wraps and bandaging. Antihistamines given for the first several weeks of treatment may partially alleviate pruritus, if present. Glucocorticoids are contraindicated.

Chronic, recurrent interdigital furunculosis is most often caused by inappropriate antibiotic therapy (too short, wrong dose/dosage, wrong drug), concurrent corticosteroid administration, demodicosis, an anatomic predisposition, or a foreign body reaction to keratin. Lesions that recur in spite of therapy can also be a sign of an underlying disease, eg, atopy, hypothyroidism, or concurrent *Malassezia* infection. Lesions in confined dogs are likely to recur unless the dog is removed from wire or concrete surfaces. In some chronic cases, surgical excision or surgical correction of the webbing via fusion podoplasty may be needed. Alternatively, pulse antibiotic therapy (full dosage therapy 2-3 times/wk) or chronic low dosage antibiotic therapy (eg, 500 mg/dog, PO, SID) may help maintain clinical remission and provide pain relief in dogs with chronic lesions. This therapy is recommended only when the inciting cause cannot be identified (eg, idiopathic pyoderma), treated (eg, anatomic predisposition), or resolved (eg, chronic infection caused by foreign body material or keratin).

PYODERMA

Pyoderma literally means "pus in the skin" and can be caused by infectious, inflammatory, and/or neoplastic etiologies; any condition that results in the accumulation of neutrophilic exudate can be termed a pyoderma. Most commonly, however, pyoderma refers to bacterial infections of the skin. Pyodermas are common in dogs and less common in cats.

Bacterial pyodermas are classifed by depth of infection, etiology, and whether or not they are primary or secondary. Bacterial pyodermas limited to the epidermis and hair follicles are referred to as superficial, whereas those that involve the dermis, deep dermis, or cause furunculosis are referred to as deep. Etiologic classification refers to the pathogenic organism involved in the infection (eg, staphylococci, streptococci, etc). Most skin infections are superficial and secondary to a variety of other conditions, most notably allergies (flea allergy, atopy, food allergy), internal diseases (particularly endo-crinopathies such as hypothyroidism or hyperadrenocorticism), seborrheic conditions (including follicular or sebaceous gland diseases), parasitic diseases (eg, *Demodex canis*), or anatomic predispositions (eg, skin folds). Primary pyoderma occurs in other-wise healthy animals, without an identifiable predisposing cause, resolves completely with appropriate antibiotics, and is usually due to *Staphylococcus intermedius* or other staphylococci.

Etiology: Bacterial pyoderma is usually triggered by an overgrowth/overcolonization of normal resident or transient flora. *S intermedius* is the most common etiologic agent isolated from clinical infections. Normal resident bacteria in canine skin also include coagulase-negative staphylococci, streptococci, *Micrococcus* sp, and *Acinetobacter* sp. Transient bacteria in canine skin include *Bacillus* sp, *Corynebacterium* sp, *Escherichia coli*, *Proteus mirabilis*, and *Pseudomonas* sp. These organisms may play a role as secondary pathogens, but often *S intermedius* is required for a pathologic process to ensue. Normal resident bacteria in feline skin include *Acinetobacter* sp, *Micrococcus* sp, coagulase-negative staphylococci, and α-hemolytic streptococci. Transient bacteria in feline skin include *Alcaligenes* sp, *Bacillus* sp, *Escherichia coli*, *Proteus mirabilis*, *Pseudomonas* sp, coagulase-positive and coagulase-negative staphylococci, and α-hemolytic streptococci.

The most important factor in superficial pyodermas that allows a bacteria to colonize the skin surface is bacterial adherence or "stickiness" to the keratinocytes. Warm, moist areas on the skin, such as lip folds, facial folds, neck folds, axillary areas, dorsal or plantar interdigital areas, vulvar folds, and tail folds, often have higher bacterial counts than other areas of skin and are at an increased risk for infection. Pressure points, such as elbows and hocks, are prone to infections, possibly due to follicular irritation and rupture due to chronic repeated pressure. Any skin disease that changes the normally dry, desert-like environment to a more humid environment can predispose the host to overcolonization of the skin with resident and transient bacteria.

Clinical Findings and Lesions: The most common clinical sign of bacterial pyo-derma in both dogs and cats is excessive scaling; scales are often pierced by hairs. Pruri-tus is variable in dogs and cats. In dogs, superficial pyoderma commonly appears as mul-tifocal areas of alopecia, follicular papules or pustules, epidermal collarettes, and serous crusts. The trunk, head, and proximal extremities are most often affected. Shorthaired breeds often present with multiple superficial papules that look similar to urticaria be-cause the inflammation in and around the follicles causes the hairs to stand more erect. These hairs are often easily epilated, an important feature that helps to distinguish su-perficial pyoderma from true urticaria, in which hairs do not epilate. In bacterial pyo-derma, affected hairs epilate and progress to form focal areas of alopecia 0.5-2 cm in diameter. At the margins of the hair loss, mild epidermal collarette formation may be present, but follicular pustules and erythema are often absent in shorthaired breeds, making diagnosis difficult. Collies and Shetland Sheepdogs often have diffuse areas of widespread alopecia with mild erythema and epidermal collarette formation at the lead-ing edge of the expanding area, often mimicking an endocrinopathy. Pustules and crusts are infrequently found.

The hallmarks of deep pyoderma in dogs are pain, crusting, odor, and exudation of blood and pus. Erythema, swelling, ulcerations, hemorrhagic crusts and bullae, hair loss, and draining tracts with serohemorrhagic or purulent exudate may also be seen. The bridge of the muzzle, chin, elbows, hocks, interdigital areas, and lateral stifles are more prone to deep infections, but any area may be involved. Acral lick granulomas and areas of pyotraumatic dermatitis are also clinical manifestations of deep pyoderma. Interdigital furunculosis (p 693) is another manifestation of deep pyoderma. Plant awns, naked keratin from hair shafts or ruptured hair follicles, and other foreign bodies play a significant role in the inflammatory process associated with deep pyodermas.

Superficial pyoderma in cats is often overlooked and underdiagnosed. The most common clinical finding is scaling, particularly over the lumbosacral area; scales pierced by hairs are a common finding. Intact pustules are almost never found. Superficial pyoderma in cats is usually due to *Staphylococcus intermedius*. Miliary dermatitis can be a clinical manifestation of superficial pyoderma. Cats with deep pyodermas often present with alopecia, ulcerations, hemorrhagic crusts, and draining tracts. Eosinophilic plaques are a common clinical presentation of deep pyoderma secondary to an allergic disease. Recurrent nonhealing deep pyoderma in cats can be associated with systemic disease, such as feline immunodeficiency virus or feline leukemia virus, or atypical mycobacteria.

Diagnosis: The diagnosis of superficial pyoderma is usually based on clinical signs—hair loss, scaling, erythema, papules, pustules, and epidermal collarettes. Differential diagnoses for superficial pyoderma include demodicosis, *Malassezia* dermatitis, dermatophytosis, and other causes of folliculitis as well as uncommon crusting diseases such as pemphigus foliaceus. Diagnosis of pyoderma should also include steps to identify any predisposing causes.

Identification of the dermatologic lesions described above allows a tentative diagnosis of superficial pyoderma. Direct impression smears of intact pustules, areas underlying crusts or epidermal collarettes, or moist erythematous areas may reveal cocci, rods, or inflammatory cell infiltrates. Impression smears of areas of hair loss and scaling may only reveal large numbers of exfoliative keratinocytes. One of the most important reasons to do impressions is to determine whether a concurrent *Malassezia* infection or overcolonization is present; there is a symbiotic relationship between *Staphylococcus* and *Malassezia*, and both are found in ~50% of cases. The infection will not resolve without concurrent systemic antimicrobial therapy. Multiple deep skin scrapings are needed to rule out parasitic infections, particularly *Demodex canis*. Dermatophyte cultures should be done to rule out dermatophytosis. Bacterial culture and sensitivity testing is mandatory in cases of deep pyoderma and recurrent superficial pyoderma. Accurate test results are most likely obtained from intact pustules or induced rupture of deep lesions. Caution should be exercised in interpreting culture results from samples submitted from crusted lesions, papules, epidermal collarettes, and fistulous tracts because contamination of the sample is more likely than with samples obtained from a closed lesion. Empiric antibiotic therapy is appropriate in mild, first-time superficial pyodermas with no complicating factors.

The most common underlying triggers of superficial pyoderma include fleas, flea allergy dermatitis, atopy, food allergy, hypothyroidism, hyperadrenocorticism, and poor grooming. Appropriate diagnostic testing and treatment of underlying triggers is mandatory. The most common causes of recurrent bacterial pyoderma include failure to identify an underlying trigger, antibiotic undertreatment (dose too low or duration of therapy too short), concurrent use of glucocorticoids, wrong antibiotic, or wrong dose.

Treatment: The primary treatment of superficial pyoderma is with appropriate antibiotics for ≥21 and preferably 30 days. All clinical lesions (except for complete regrowth of alopecic areas and resolution of hyperpigmented areas) should be resolved for at least 7 days before antibiotics are discontinued. Chronic, recurrent, or deep pyodermas typically require 8-12 wk or longer to resolve completely.

First-time bacterial pyoderma can be treated with empiric antibiotic therapy such as lincomycin, clindamycin, erythromycin, trimethoprim-sulfamethoxazole, trimethoprim-sulfadiazine, chloramphenicol, cephalosporins, amoxicillin trihydrate-clavulanic acid, or ormetoprim-sulfadimethoxine.

Amoxicillin, penicillin, and tetracyline are inappropriate choices for treating superficial or deep pyodermas because they are ineffective in 90% of these cases. Fluoroquinolones should not be used for empiric therapy. Severe deep pyoderma, recurrent pyoderma, or first-time bacterial pyodermas that do not respond to therapy should be treated based on culture and sensitivity.

Topical antibiotics may be helpful in focal superficial pyoderma. A 2% mupiricin oint-ment penetrates skin well and is helpful in deep pyoderma, is not systemically absorbed, has no known contact sensitization, and is not used as a systemic antibiotic that would increase the likelihood of cross-resistance. It is not very effective against gram-negative bacteria. This ointment should not be used in cats with any known or suspected history of renal disease because the preparation contains propylene glycol. Neomycin is more likely to cause a contact allergy than other topicals and has variable efficacy against gram-negative bacteria. Bacitracin and polymyxin B are more effective against gram-negative bacteria than other topical antibiotics but are inactivated in purulent exudates.

Attention to grooming is often overlooked in the treatment of both superficial and deep pyoderma. The hair coat should be clipped in patients with deep pyoderma and a profes-sional grooming is recommended in medium- to longhaired dogs with generalized superfi-cial pyoderma. This will remove excessive hair that can trap debris and bacteria and will facilitate grooming. Longhaired cats usually benefit most from having the hair coat clipped.

Dogs with superficial pyoderma should be bathed 2-3 times/wk during the first 2 wk of therapy and then 1-2 times until the infection has resolved. Dogs with deep pyoderma may require daily hydrotherapy. Medicated shampoos should be prediluted 1:2 to 1:4 prior to application to facilitate lathering, dispersal, and rinsing. Appropriate antibacte-rial shampoos include benzoyl peroxide, chlorhexidine, chlorhexidine-ketoconazole, ethyl lactate, and triclosan. Shampooing will remove bacteria, crusts, and scales, as well as reduce the pruritus, odor, and oiliness associated with the pyoderma. Clinical im-provement in superficial pyodermas may not be evident for a least 14-21 days, and recov-ery may not be as rapid as expected.

CONTAGIOUS ECTHYMA

(Orf, Contagious pustular dermatitis, Sore mouth)

Contagious ecthyma is an infectious dermatitis of sheep and goats that affects primar-ily the lips of young animals. The disease is usually more severe in goats than in sheep. Humans are occasionally affected, and the disease has been reported in dogs that have eaten infected carcasses.

Etiology and Epidemiology: The causal poxvirus (a parapoxvirus) is related to those of pseudocowpox and bovine papular stomatitis. Infection occurs by contact. The virus is highly resistant to desiccation, having been recovered from dried crusts after 12 yr. It is also resistant to glycerol and to ether.

Contagious ecthyma is found worldwide and is most common in late summer, fall, and winter on pasture, and in winter in feedlots. It may occur in young lambs in early spring and occasionally in mature sheep that do not have immunity from natural exposure.

Clinical Findings and Diagnosis: The primary lesion develops on the skin of the lips and frequently extends to the mucosa of the mouth. Occasionally lesions are found on the feet, usually in the interdigital region and around the coronet. Ewes nursing infected lambs may develop lesions on the udder. In young lambs, the initial lesion may develop on the gum below the incisor teeth. The lesions develop as papules and progress through vesicular and pustular stages before encrusting. Coalescence of numerous discrete lesions often leads to the formation of large scabs, and the proliferation of dermal tissue produces a verrucose mass under them. When the lesion extends to the oral mucosa, secondary necrobacillosis (p 1186) frequently develops.

During the course of the disease (1-4 wk), the scabs drop off and the tissues heal without scarring. During active stages of infection, more severely affected lambs fail to eat normally and lose condition. Extensive lesions on the feet lead to lameness. Mastitis may occur in ewes with lesions on the udder.

The lesion is characteristic. The disease must be differentiated from ulcerative der-matosis (p 703), which produces tissue destruction and crateriform ulcers. Ecthyma usually affects younger animals than does ulcerative dermatosis, although this criterion can only be used presumptively. A positive differentiation may be obtained by inoculating susceptible and ecthyma-immunized sheep.

Treatment and Control: Antibacterials may help combat secondary infection. In endemic areas, appropriate repellents and larvicides should be applied to the lesions. The virus is transmissible to humans, and the lesions, usually confined to the hands and face, are more proliferative and occasionally very distressing. Veterinarians and sheep handlers should exercise reasonable protective precautions. Diagnosis in humans is established by transmitting the virus to sheep; a complement-fixation test may be of value.

Sheep that have recovered from natural infection are highly resistant to reinfection. Despite a multiplicity of immunogenic virus strains, the presently used commercial single-strain vaccines have produced fair immunity in all parts of the USA (with an occasional exception). Vaccine breaks appear to be due to the virulence of the infecting strain rather than to differences in antigenicity of the vaccine. Sheep immunized against contagious ecthyma remain susceptible to ulcerative dermatosis.

Vaccines should be used cautiously to avoid contaminating uninfected premises, and vaccinated animals should be segregated from unprotected stock until the scabs have fallen off. A small amount of the vaccine is brushed over light scarifications of the skin, usually on the inside of the thigh. Lambs should be vaccinated when ~1 mo old. For best results, a second vaccination ~2-3 mo later is suggested. Nonimmunized lambs should be vaccinated before entering infected feedlots. Experimental work suggests that parenteral administration of virulent vaccine induces better immunity than does the current procedure.

POX DISEASES

Pox diseases are acute viral diseases that affect many animals, including humans and birds, but not dogs. Typically, lesions of the skin and mucosae are widespread and progress from macules to papules, vesicles, and pustules before encrusting and healing. Most lesions contain multiple intracytoplasmic inclusions, which represent sites of virus replication in infected cells. In some poxvirus infections, vesiculation is not clinically evident, but microvesicles can be seen on histologic examination and, in some, proliferative lesions are characteristic.

Infection is acquired either by inhalation or through the skin (eg, sheeppox). In certain instances (eg, fowlpox, swinepox), the virus is transmitted mechanically by biting arthropods. Infection may be followed by generalized lesions (eg, sheeppox) or remain localized (eg, pseudocowpox). Strains of poxvirus with reduced virulence are used to immunize against some infections, the classic example being the global eradication of smallpox in humans by immunization with strains of live vaccinia virus.

Poxviruses can be classified according to their physicochemical and biologic properties. Immunologically, the viruses of smallpox, cowpox, monkeypox, etc, are closely related to vaccinia virus. The avian poxviruses, the myxoma viruses, and some of the other poxviruses (eg, swinepox) are species-specific. The viruses of orf, pseudocowpox, and bovine papular stomatitis are parapoxviruses.

In Europe, localized skin infections, and in some cases fatal generalized disease, have been reported in cheetahs, lions, and domestic cats infected with cowpox virus (*see* below).

COWPOX

In this mild, eruptive disease of dairy cows, lesions occur on the udder and teats. Although once common, cowpox is now extremely rare and reported only in western Europe (*see also* POXVIRUS INFECTION IN CATS, p 701).

The virus of cowpox is closely related antigenically to vaccinia and smallpox viruses. Indeed, the first two can be differentiated only by sophisticated laboratory techniques.

Before vaccination against smallpox was discontinued, some outbreaks in cows were due to infection with vaccinia from recently vaccinated persons.

The disease spreads by contact during milking. After an incubation period of 3-7 days, during which cows may be mildly febrile, papules appear on the teats and udder. Vesicles may not be evident or may rupture readily, leaving raw, ulcerated areas that form scabs. Lesions heal within 1 mo. Most cows in a milking herd may become affected. Milkers may develop fever and have lesions on the hands, arms, or face.

Cowpox or vaccinia infection may be confused with bovine herpes mammillitis (p 1144); because the lesions are superficially similar, laboratory confirmation is required. Pseudocowpox is a milder disease.

Measures to prevent spread within a herd must be based on segregation and hygiene.

PSEUDOCOWPOX
(Milker's nodes, Paravaccinia)

This common, mild infection of the udder and teats of cows is caused by a parapoxvirus and is widespread worldwide. The virus of pseudocowpox is related to those of contagious ecthyma (p 697) and bovine papular stomatitis (p 173). These parapoxviruses differ morphologically from vaccinia virus and other poxviruses. They have a limited host range and cannot be propagated in fertile eggs, and they will grow in some cell cultures although relatively poorly.

Lesions begin as small, red papules on the teats or udder. These may be followed rapidly by scabbing, or small vesicles or pustules may develop before scabs form. Scabs may be abundant but can be removed without causing pain. Granulation occurs beneath the scabs, resulting in a raised lesion that heals from the center and leaves a characteristic horseshoe or circular ring of small scabs. This stage is reached in ~7-12 days. Some lesions persist for several months, giving the affected teats a rough feel and appearance, and more scabs may form. The infection spreads slowly throughout milking herds, and a variable percentage of cows shows lesions at any time. Cattle may become reinfected in subsequent lactations.

The scabbed lesions may be confused with mild traumatic injuries to the teats and udder. Scabs examined with an electron microscope frequently show characteristic virus particles.

Control of infection within a herd is difficult and depends essentially on hygienic measures, such as teat dipping, to destroy the virus and prevent transmission. Little immunity appears to develop.

Humans may become infected with painless but itchy purplish red nodules that are generally present on the fingers or hands. These lesions cause little disturbance and disappear after several weeks.

LUMPY SKIN DISEASE

Lumpy skin disease is an infectious, eruptive, occasionally fatal disease of cattle characterized by nodules on the skin and other parts of the body. Secondary infection often aggravates the condition. Traditionally, it is found in southern and eastern Africa but, in recent years, has extended northwest through the continent into subSaharan west Africa. It has also been recorded in Israel.

Etiology and Epidemiology: The causal virus is related to that of sheeppox. The prototype strain is known as the Neethling poxvirus. Lumpy skin disease appears epidemically or sporadically. Frequently, new foci of infection appear in areas far removed from the initial outbreak. Its incidence is highest in wet summer weather, but it may occur in winter. It is most prevalent along water courses and on low ground. Because quarantine restrictions designed to limit the spread of infection have failed, biting insects have been suspected as vectors; however, outbreaks have occurred under conditions in which insects practically could be excluded. Because the disease can be transmitted by infected saliva, contact infection must be accepted as a method of spread. African buffalo are suspected of being carriers in Kenya.

Artificial infection can be produced by inoculation of cutaneous nodule suspensions or of blood taken during the early febrile stage, or by feed or water contaminated with saliva from infected animals.

Clinical Findings: A subcutaneous injection of infected material produces a painful swelling and then fever, lacrimation, nasal discharge, and hypersalivation, followed by the characteristic eruptions on the skin and other parts of the body in ~50% of susceptible cattle. The incubation period is 4-14 days.

The nodules are well circumscribed, round, slightly raised, firm, and painful and involve the entire cutis and the mucosa of the GI, respiratory, and genital tracts. Nodules may occur on the muzzle and within the nasal and buccal mucous membranes. The skin nodules contain a firm, creamy-gray or yellow mass of tissue. Regional lymph nodes are swollen, and edema develops in the udder, brisket, and legs. Secondary infection sometimes occurs and causes extensive suppuration and sloughing; as a result, the animal may become extremely emaciated, and euthanasia may be warranted. The nodules either regress in time, or necrosis of the skin results in hard, raised areas ("sit-fasts") clearly separated from the surrounding skin. These areas slough to leave ulcers, which heal and scar.

Morbidity is 5-50%; mortality is usually low. The greatest loss is due to decreased milk yield, loss of condition, and rejection or reduced value of the hide.

Diagnosis: The disease may be confused with **pseudo-lumpy-skin disease**, which is caused by a herpesvirus (bovine herpesvirus 2). These diseases can be similar clinically, although in some parts of the world, the herpesvirus lesions seem confined to the teats and udder of cows, and the disease is called herpes mammillitis (p 1144).

Pseudo-lumpy skin disease is a milder disease than true lumpy skin disease, but differentiation depends essentially on isolation and identification of the virus. Histologic and ultrastructural examination of nodules may be helpful. Poxlike intracytoplasmic inclusion bodies or eosinophilic intranuclear herpesvirus inclusions may be seen in the nodules.

Dermatophilus congolensis also causes skin nodules in cattle (*see* DERMATOPHILOSIS, p 704).

Prevention and Treatment: Quarantine restrictions are of limited use. Vaccination with attenuated virus offers the most promising method of control. Goat poxvirus and sheep poxvirus passed in tissue culture also have been used.

Administration of sulfonamides to control secondary infection and good nursing care are recommended.

SHEEPPOX AND GOATPOX

Sheeppox and goatpox are serious, often fatal, diseases characterized by widespread skin eruption. Both diseases are confined to parts of southeastern Europe, Africa, and Asia. The poxviruses of sheep and goats (capripoxviruses) are closely related, both antigenically and physicochemically. They are also related to the virus of lumpy skin disease (*see* above). Reports on the natural susceptibility of sheep to goat poxvirus and vice versa are conflicting; at least some strains seem capable of infecting both species.

The incubation period of sheeppox is 4-8 days and that of goatpox 5-14 days. The clinical picture is similar in the 2 diseases but is generally less severe in goats. Fever and a variable degree of systemic disturbance develop. Eyelids become swollen, and mucopurulent discharge crusts the nostrils. Widespread skin lesions develop that are most readily seen on the muzzle, ears, and areas free of wool or long hair. Palpation can detect lesions not readily seen. Lesions start as erythematous areas on the skin and progress rapidly to raised, circular plaques with congested borders caused by local inflammation, edema, and epithelial hyperplasia. Although microvesicles are present histologically, vesicles and pustules are not evident clinically. Virus is abundant in skin lesions at this stage. As lesions start to regress, necrosis of the dermis occurs, and dark, hard scabs form, which are sharply separated from the surrounding skin. Regeneration of the epithelium beneath the scabs takes several weeks. When scabs are removed, a star-shaped scar, free of hair or wool, remains. In severe cases, lesions can develop in the lungs. In some sheep and in certain breeds, the disease may be mild or the infection inapparent.

It has been suggested that transmission may be airborne or may occur by direct contact with lesions or mechanically by biting insects.

The disease in either species must be differentiated from the milder infection, contagious ecthyma (orf, p 697), which mainly causes crusty, proliferative lesions around the mouth.

Infection results in solid and enduring immunity. Live, attenuated virus vaccines induce longer immunity than inactivated virus vaccines. Live, attenuated, lumpy skin disease virus also can be used as a vaccine against sheeppox and goatpox.

SWINEPOX

Swinepox is an acute, often mild, infectious disease characterized by skin eruptions that affects only pigs. It is present in the USA, particularly in the midwest, and has been reported from all continents, although the incidence is generally low.

Historically, vaccinia virus was involved in some outbreaks; currently, swinepox virus appears to be the only cause. The disease described here is that caused by the latter. Swinepox virus is distinct from other poxviruses and does not protect against infection with vaccinia virus. It will grow on pig cell cultures but not embryonating eggs. It is relatively heat stable and survives for ~10 days at 37°C.

The disease is most frequently seen in young pigs, 3-6 wk old, but all ages may be affected. After an incubation period of ~1 wk, small red areas may be seen most frequently on the face, ears, inside the legs, and abdomen. These develop into papules and, within a few days, pustules develop, or small vesicles may be seen. The centers of the pustules become dry and scabbed and are surrounded by a raised, inflamed zone so that the lesions appear umbilicated. Later, dark scabs (1-2 cm in diameter) form, giving affected piglets a spotted appearance. These eventually drop or are rubbed off without leaving a scar. Successive crops of lesions can occur so that all are not at the same stage. The early stage of the disease may be accompanied by mild fever, inappetence, and dullness. Few pigs die of uncomplicated swinepox.

Virus is abundant in the lesions and can be transferred from pig to pig by the biting louse (*Haematopinus suis*). The disease also may be transmitted, possibly between farms, by other insects acting as mechanical carriers.

Recovered pigs are immune. There is no specific treatment. Eradication of lice is important.

POXVIRUS INFECTION IN CATS

Poxvirus infection in domestic cats has occurred sporadically in the UK and possibly western Europe. Affected cats usually have multiple skin lesions, although respiratory and other signs also may be seen.

Etiology and Epidemiology: To date, all isolates examined from domestic cats have been indistinguishable from cowpox virus (*see* p 698). Cowpox or infection with other closely related viruses also has been recorded in captive Felidae and in other species (eg, elephants, rhinoceros, and anteaters) in various European zoos. However, the relationship of some of these viruses to established species within the genus is not clear. Cowpox apparently does not occur in the USA, although another orthopoxvirus has been isolated from raccoons. It is possible that this virus may also infect other hosts. Cowpox virus is also infectious to humans, and cat-to-human transmission has been recorded. Owners should be advised accordingly.

Although traditionally described as a disease of cattle, cowpox virus is in fact rare, and it is generally accepted that its reservoir hosts are small wild mammals. Cats, which are now the most commonly recognized host of cowpox virus, are believed to become infected when hunting. Most affected cats come from rural environments and are known to hunt rodents; the initial lesion is often described as having originated as a small bite-like wound. Infection in cats has a marked seasonal incidence, with most cases occurring between September and November. Cat-to-cat transmission can also occur but usually results in only subclinical infection. Rare bovine cases presumably result from direct or indirect contact with the reservoir host, as do some human cases. However, cat-to-human and cow-to-human transmissions are also possible.

The significance of the disease and its relatively recent recognition in cats is an enigma. It may have always been present in the feline population but not recognized. Alternatively, the disease may be increasing in importance, as a result of a change either in the epidemiology of the disease in the reservoir host or (perhaps less likely) in the nature of the dominant biotype of the virus itself.

Pathogenesis: The most common route of entry appears to be through the skin, but oronasal infection is also possible. After local replication and development of a primary skin lesion, the virus spreads to local lymph nodes and a leukocyte-associated viremia develops. The viremic phase may be associated with pyrexia and depression and, during this period, virus can be isolated from various tissues, including the skin, turbinates (and sometimes lungs), and lymphoid organs. Widespread secondary skin lesions appear a few days after the onset of viremia, and new lesions continue to appear for 2-3 days, at which time the viremia subsides.

Clinical Findings: Most affected cats have a history of a single primary skin lesion, usually on the head, neck, or a forelimb. The primary lesion can vary from a small, scabbed wound to a large abscess. About 7-10 days after the primary lesion appears, widespread secondary lesions begin to appear. Over 2-4 days, these develop into discrete, circular, ulcerated papules ~0.5-1 cm in diameter. The ulcers soon become covered by scabs, and healing is usually complete by ~6 wk. Many cats show no signs other than skin lesions, but ~20% may develop mild coryza or conjunctivitis. Some cats may also be pyrexic, depressed, and inappetent during the viremic phase just before and during the early development of secondary lesions. Concurrent bacterial infection, particularly of the primary lesions, may give rise to systemic signs. However, most domestic cats recover uneventfully. More severe pulmonary disease is uncommon in domestic cats but frequently occurs in cheetahs and is often fatal in both species. More severe disease in domestic cats is often associated with immunosuppression, either after treatment with corticosteroids or associated with infection with feline leukemia or immunodeficiency viruses.

Lesions: Because most cats survive, skin biopsies generally are the only tissue available for histologic examination. Early lesions consist of areas of epidermal hyperplasia and hypertrophy with vesiculation of the prickle cell layer. Many of the epidermal cells bordering such vesicles contain characteristic eosinophilic cytoplasmic inclusions. Later, there is ulceration and necrosis of the epidermis and replacement by an eosinophilic coagulum of necrotic cells and fibrin. A heavy, mixed inflammatory cell exudate is present in the dermis surrounding the lesion. As healing ensues, a thin layer of epidermis covers the skin beneath the scabs, early scar tissue is present, and there is a moderate, mainly mononuclear cell infiltrate.

In rarer cases, in which the disease has generalized, lesions may also be present in the liver, lungs, trachea, bronchi, oral mucosa, and small intestine.

Diagnosis: If multiple, well-circumscribed skin lesions are present, and especially if there is a history of hunting or exposure to a rural environment, a presumptive diagnosis may be based on clinical signs. Cowpox virus infection also should be suspected when skin lesions do not respond to antibiotics. Differential diagnoses include miliary dermatitis, feline herpesvirus or calicivirus infection, eosinophilic granuloma, bite wounds, ringworm, and other chronic bacterial or fungal conditions.

Presumptive and rapid diagnosis can be made in most cases from unfixed scab, exudate, or biopsy material examined for characteristic brick-shaped orthopox virions by electron microscopy. A more accurate and sensitive method of diagnosis is isolation of virus in cell culture or on chick chorioallantois. If no virus is isolated, fixed biopsy material for histologic examination and serum for antibody determination also can be sent to the laboratory.

Treatment and Control: In both domestic cats and cheetahs, it is important that cowpox be diagnosed promptly because steroid treatment, which is often used in the therapy of other skin conditions, is contraindicated. Although the disease is often severe in cheetahs, in domestic cats, supportive treatment (broad-spectrum antibiotics, fluid therapy) is generally successful, and mortality low.

Because it seems that infection in domestic cats is mainly sporadic and acquired from chance contact with an infected wildlife reservoir, control measures probably are not indicated. In wildlife parks, where big cats are at risk from contact with small wild rodents, and especially where the disease has already occurred, vaccination may be helpful. Vaccinia virus appears to be of low pathogenicity in domestic cats, and cheetahs appear to be refractive; no trials have yet been done with other orthopoxvirus vaccines. Thus, at present, management of outbreaks among large cats depends on prompt diagnosis and segregation of affected animals to reduce the possibility of cat-to-cat spread. Premises may be disinfected with hypochlorite bleach or detergents. At ambient temperatures, poxviruses are relatively resistant and may remain infective in dried crusts for months.

ULCERATIVE DERMATOSIS OF SHEEP

(Lip and leg ulceration, Venereal balanoposthitis and vulvitis)

Ulcerative dermatosis is an infectious disease of sheep caused by a virus similar to the ecthyma virus. It manifests in 2 somewhat distinct forms, one characterized by formation of ulcers around the mouth and nose or on the legs (lip and leg ulceration), and the other as a venereally transmitted ulceration of the prepuce and penis or vulva.

Clinical Findings: The lesion, regardless of location, is an ulcer with a raw crater that bleeds easily, varies in depth and extent, and contains an odorless, creamy pus; it is covered from the beginning with a scab.

Face lesions occur on the upper lip, between the border of the lip and the nasal orifice, on the chin, and on the nose. In severe cases, the ulcers may perforate the lip. Foot lesions occur anywhere between the coronet and the carpus or tarsus.

Venereal lesions partially or completely surround the preputial orifice and may become so severe as to produce phimosis. Rarely, the ulcers may extend to the glans penis so that the ram becomes unfit for natural breeding. In ewes, edema, ulceration, and scabbing of the lips of the vulva have less serious consequences.

There are no noticeable early systemic reactions. Morbidity rates of 15-20% are usual, although up to 60% of a flock may be infected. Often, the disease remains unrecognized until the lesions are so advanced that signs of lameness or disturbed urination become apparent.

Diagnosis: This depends entirely on recognition of the characteristic ulcerative lesion. Differentiation between this lesion and that of contagious ecthyma (p 697), which is essentially proliferative in character, is fundamental. In most cases, on removal of the scabs, the lesions of ulcerative dermatosis are crateriform or ulcerative, while lesions of contagious ecthyma are proliferative. The question of the similarity of the agents of these 2 conditions is not clearly defined, but inoculation of sheep previously immunized against contagious ecthyma helps in making a diagnosis. It is also difficult, and in some instances impossible, without resorting to sheep inoculation, to differentiate between ulcerative posthitis and vulvitis (p 1147) and ulcerative dermatosis.

Prevention and Treatment: Infected animals should be isolated, and those with genital lesions should not be bred. Recovery takes 2-8 wk and is not greatly influenced by treatment, which therefore is usually not attempted unless the animals are to be bred soon, lip lesions interfere with eating, foot lesions make the animals so lame that they are losing flesh, or secondary bacterial infections become severe.

Treatment consists of removing the scabs and all necrotic tissue from the ulcers and applying any one of the following preparations: silver nitrate (styptic pencil), strong tincture of iodine, 30% copper sulfate solution, 4% formaldehyde, 5% cresol (sheep dip), or sulfa-urea powder. Foot and lower leg lesions can be treated with copper sulfate or formaldehyde solutions in footbath troughs.

DERMATOPHYTOSIS

(Ringworm)

Dermatophytosis is an infection of keratinized tissue (skin, hair, and claws) by one of the 3 genera of fungi collectively called dermatophytes—*Epidermophyton, Microsporum,* and *Trichophyton*. (*See also* FUNGAL INFECTIONS, p 510.) These pathogenic fungi are found worldwide, and all domestic animals are susceptible. In developed countries, the greatest economic and human health consequences come from dermatophytosis of domestic cats and cattle. A few dermatophyte species are soil inhabitants (geophilic), eg, *M gypseum* and *T terrestre,* and cause disease in animals that are exposed while digging or rooting. Other species are host-adapted to humans (anthropophilic), eg, *M audouinii* and *T rubrum,* and infect other animals rarely. The most important animal pathogens worldwide are *M canis, M gypseum, T mentagrophytes, T equinum, T verrucosum,* and *M nanum*. These species can be spread to people, especially *M canis* infections of domestic cats and *T verrucosum* of cattle and lambs. The zoophilic species are transmitted primarily by contact with infected individuals and contaminated fomites such as furniture, grooming tools, or tack. Contact with a dermatophyte does not always result in infection. Whether infection is established depends on the fungal species and on host factors, including age, immunocompetence, condition of exposed skin surfaces, on host grooming behavior, and nutritional status. Infection elicits specific immunity, both humoral and cellular, that confers incomplete and short-lived resistance to subsequent infection or disease.

Under most circumstances, dermatophytes grow only in keratinized tissue, and advancing infection stops on reaching living cells or inflamed tissue. Infection begins in a growing hair or in the stratum corneum, where threadlike hyphae develop from the infective arthrospores or fungal hyphal elements. Hyphae can penetrate the hair shaft and weaken it, which, together with follicular inflammation, leads to patchy hair loss. As the infection matures, clusters of arthrospores develop on the outer surface of infected hair shafts. Broken hairs with associated spores are important sources for spread of the disease. As inflammation and host immunity develop, further spread of infection is inhibited, although this process may take several weeks. Thus, for most healthy adult hosts, dermatophyte infections are self-limiting. In young or debilitated animals and, to some extent, in longhaired breeds of domestic cats, infection may be persistent and widespread.

Dermatophytosis is diagnosed by fungal culture, examination with a Wood's lamp, and direct microscopic examination of hair or skin scale. Fungal culture is the most accurate means of diagnosis. Dermatophyte test medium (DTM) may be used in a clinical setting. Selected lesions should have the hair clipped to a length of ~0.3 cm. The area should be gently patted with an alcohol-moistened sponge and then patted dry to reduce contamination with saprophytic fungi. Hair stubble and skin scale are collected for placement on the agar, which is then lightly covered to prevent drying. Incubation at room temperature is sufficient except when culturing for *T verrucosum* from food and fiber animals, in which case incubation at 37°C is necessary. Dermatophyte growth is usually apparent within 3-7 days but may require up to 3 wk. Dermatophytes growing on DTM cause the medium to change to red at the time of first visible colony formation. Dermatophyte fungi have white to buff-colored, fluffy to granular mycelia. Saprophytic contaminant colonies are white or pigmented and almost never produce an initial color change on DTM. Definitive diagnosis and species identification require removal of hyphae and macroconidia from the surface of the colony with acetate tape and microscopic examination with lactophenol cotton blue stain.

The Wood's lamp is useful in screening examinations for *M canis* infections in cats and dogs. Infected hairs fluoresce yellow-green; however, only 80% of *M canis* infections fluoresce, and other fungal species in animals do not. Therefore, negative Wood's lamp examinations are not meaningful. False-positive examinations may occur and are especially likely in oily, seborrheic skin conditions. Fluorescing hairs should always be cultured to confirm the diagnosis.

Direct microscopic examination of hairs or skin scrapings may allow early diagnosis by demonstration of characteristic hyphae or arthrospores in the specimen. The technique is more useful in diagnosing dermatophytosis in large animals than in small animals. Hairs (preferably white ones) and scrapings from the periphery of lesions are examined for fungal elements in a wet preparation of 20% potassium hydroxide that has been gently warmed or incubated in a humidity chamber overnight.

Cattle

Trichophyton verrucosum is the usual cause of ringworm in cattle, but *T mentagrophytes*, *T equinum*, *Microsporum gypseum*, *M nanum*, *M canis*, and others have been isolated. Dermatophytosis is most commonly recognized in calves, in which nonpruritic periocular lesions are most characteristic, although generalized skin disease may develop. Cows and heifers are reported to develop lesions on the chest and limbs most often, and bulls in the dewlap and intermaxillary skin. Lesions are characteristically discrete, scaling patches of hair loss with gray-white crust formation, but some become thickly crusted with suppuration. Ringworm as a herd health problem is more common in the winter and is more commonly recognized in temperate climates and in English rather than Zebu breeds of cattle.

Many topical treatments have been reported to be successful in cattle, but because spontaneous recovery is common, claims of efficacy are difficult to substantiate. Valuable individual animals should still be treated because this may well limit both progression of existing lesions and spread to others in the herd. Thick crusts should be removed gently with a brush, and the material burned or disinfected with hypochlorite solution. Treatment options depend on the limitations on the use of some agents in animals meant for slaughter. Agents reported to be of use include washes or sprays of 4% lime sulfur, 0.5% sodium hypochlorite (1:10 household bleach), 0.5% chlorhexidine, 1% povidone-iodine, natamycin, and enilconazole. Individual lesions can be treated with miconazole or clotrimazole lotions. An attenuated fungal vaccine is in use in some European countries; it prevents development of severe clinical lesions and also has greatly reduced the incidence of zoonotic disease in animal care workers. Unfortunately, vaccinated animals shed fungal spores for a time after vaccination. No live vaccine is available in North America.

Dogs and Cats

In dogs, ~70% of cases are caused by *Microsporum canis*, 20% by *M gypseum*, and 10% by *Trichophyton mentagrophytes*; in cats, 98% are caused by *M canis*. The Wood's lamp is useful in establishing a tentative diagnosis of dermatophytosis in dogs and cats but cannot be used to rule out this type of infection. Definitive diagnosis is established by DTM culture (*see* above). Detection of infection in asymptomatic carrier animals is facilitated by brushing the coat with a new toothbrush and then inoculating a culture plate by pressing the bristles to the surface of the medium.

The clinical appearance of ringworm in cats is quite variable. Kittens are affected most commonly. Typical lesions consist of focal alopecia, scaling, and crusting; most are around the ears and face or on the extremities. Cats with clinically inapparent infections can still serve as a source of infection to other cats or people. Occasionally, dermatophytosis in cats causes feline miliary dermatitis and is pruritic. Cats with generalized dermatophytosis occasionally develop cutaneous ulcerated nodules, known as dermatophyte granulomas or pseudomycetomas.

Lesions in dogs are classically alopecic, scaly patches with broken hairs. Dogs may also develop regional or generalized folliculitis and furunculosis with papules and pustules. A focal nodular form of dermatophytosis in dogs is the kerion reaction. Generalized ringworm in adult dogs is uncommon and is usually accompanied by immunodeficiency, especially endogenous or iatrogenic hyperadrenocorticism. Differential diagnoses in dogs for classic ringworm lesions include demodicosis, bacterial folliculitis, and seborrheic dermatitis.

Dermatophytosis in dogs and shorthaired cats is usually self-limiting, but resolution can be hastened by treatment. Another primary objective of therapy is to prevent spread of infection to other animals and people. However, whole-body topical therapy is controversial, and recent studies have not confirmed that any currently available topical rinse or shampoo is truly effective. Enilconazole, a rinse not currently available in North America, is most likely to be effective. Local lesions can be treated effectively with topical miconazole or clotrimazole. For chronic or severe cases and for ringworm in longhaired breeds of cats, systemic treatment is indicated. The microsized formulation of griseofulvin can be used in dogs (25-100 mg/kg, SID or divided doses) and in cats (25-50 mg/kg, daily in divided doses). These dosages are higher than those approved by the FDA. The ultramicrosized formulations used in human medicine can be used at lower dosages (10-15 mg/kg). Cats may develop bone marrow suppression, especially neutropenia, at higher doses or as idiosyncratic reactions. In both dogs and cats, GI upset is a fairly common sequela of griseofulvin administration. Alternative and effective treatments include terbinafine (30 mg/kg) or itraconazole (5-10 mg/kg, SID), but neither of these drugs is approved for use in domestic animals. Systemic and topical treatments for dermatophytosis should be continued for 2-4 wk past clinical cure or until a negative brush culture is obtained. This may require treatment for 1-3 mo with griseofulvin or for ≥1 mo with azole antifungals. A killed fungal cell wall vaccine is approved for treatment and prevention of *M canis* ringworm in cats. The vaccine hastens clinical resolution but apparently does not affect time to mycologic cure. It also reduces the severity, but not the frequency, of infection in kittens that are subsequently exposed. Use of the vaccine in management of dermatophytosis in pet cats or multicat facilities remains to be defined. Recent reports of the efficacy of lufenuron in treating ringworm in dogs and cats have not been confirmed in controlled studies.

Horses

Trichophyton equinum and *T mentagrophytes* are the primary causes of ringworm in horses, although *Microsporum gypseum*, *M canis*, and *T verrucosum* have also been isolated. Clinical signs consist of one or more patches of alopecia and erythema, scaling, and crusting, which are present to varying degrees. Early lesions may resemble papular urticaria but progress with crusting and hair loss within a few days. Diagnosis is confirmed by culture. Differential diagnoses include dermatophilosis, pemphigus foliaceus, and bacterial folliculitis. Transmission is by direct contact or by grooming implements and tack. Most lesions are seen in the saddle and girth areas ("girth itch").

Treatment is generally topical because systemic therapy is expensive and of unproven efficacy. Whole-body rinses as described above for cattle may be recommended, and individual lesions treated with clotrimazole or miconazole preparations. Grooming implements and tack should be disinfected, and affected horses should be isolated.

Pigs, Sheep, and Goats

Dermatophytosis in pigs is usually caused by *Microsporum nanum*. Lesions are rings of inflammation or brown discoloration that spread centrifugally up to a diameter of 6 cm. Lesions are fairly asymptomatic in adults, and ringworm in swine is generally of little economic consequence. Zoonotic infections in farm workers are not common. Ringworm is a common, troublesome problem in show lambs but is otherwise uncommon in production flocks of sheep and goats. The infecting species include *M canis*, *M gypseum*, and *Trichophyton verrucosum*. Lesions in lambs are most often noticed on the head, but widespread lesions under the wool may be apparent in lambs sheared for show. Infected lambs should not be issued certificates for transport to show until the infection is cleared. Because there is little evidence that lambs with a functional rumen will absorb griseofulvin to effective levels, treatment is best accomplished with sodium hypochlorite solutions or enilconazole rinses (where available). In healthy lambs, as in other species, these infections are self-limiting, but resolution may not be evident in time to salvage the use of the animal in the show ring.

CATTLE GRUBS

Hypodermosis of cattle in the northern hemisphere is caused by the larvae (cattle grubs or ox warbles) of flies of the genus *Hypoderma* (order Diptera, family Oestridae). *Hypoderma (Oedemagena) tarandi* parasitizes native Cervidae and reindeer in Arctic regions. In Central and South America, larvae (tropical warbles) of *Dermatobia hominis* (order Diptera, family Cuterebridae) are important pests of cattle.

HYPODERMA SPP

Two species of *Hypoderma*, *H bovis* and *H lineatum*, are important pests of cattle. They are found between 25° and 60° latitude in the northern hemisphere in >50 countries of North America, Europe, Africa, and Asia. In North America, *H lineatum*, the common cattle grub, is found in Canada, the USA, and northern Mexico; *H bovis*, the northern cattle grub, is generally found north of the 35th parallel. Occurrence in cattle and American bison is common. Larvae of *Hypoderma* spp also have been reported in horses, sheep, goats, and humans. The prevalence of both *Hypoderma* species has declined dramatically in North America.

Life Cycle: Adult *Hypoderma*, known also as heel flies, are ~15 mm long, hairy, and bee-like in appearance. In late spring or early summer, they attach their eggs on the hair of cattle, particularly on the legs and lower body regions. The eggs hatch in 3-7 days, and first-stage larvae travel to the base of the hair shaft and penetrate the skin. Normally, the first-stage larvae travel through the fascial planes between muscles, along connective tissue, or along nerve pathways. They secrete proteolytic enzymes that facilitate their movement. During fall and winter, larvae migrate toward 2 different regions, depending on the species. *H lineatum* larvae migrate to the submucosal connective tissue of the esophageal wall, where they accumulate for 2-4 mo. *H bovis* larvae migrate to the region of the spinal canal, where they are found in the epidural fat between the dura mater and the periosteum for a similar period.

Beginning in early winter, the larvae arrive in the subdermal tissue of the back of the host where they make breathing holes through the skin. Cysts or warbles form around the larvae, which undergo 2 molts (second and third stage). The warble stage lasts 4-8 wk. Finally, third-stage larvae emerge through the breathing holes, drop to the ground, and pupate. Flies emerge from the pupae in 1-3 mo, depending on weather conditions. Adult flies, which do not feed, live <1 wk. The life cycle is complete in 1 yr.

For the 2 species, seasonal events are similar except that those for *H lineatum* occur ~6-8 wk earlier than those of *H bovis*. These events vary from year to year but correlate with local and regional climatic conditions. Larvae first appear in backs of cattle about mid September in southern USA but not until late January or later in northern USA. Grubs first emerge from the back during the last half of November in Texas and during the first half of March in Montana. When both species are present, grubs may appear in the back for ~5-6 mo; when only one species is present, for ~3-4 mo. The activity of ovipositing (by female flies) is at its height from January to March in southern USA and from May to July in northern USA.

Clinical Findings and Pathogenesis: During periods of sunshine on warm days, cattle may run with their tails high in the air when chased by female heel flies, particularly *H bovis*. Not all stampeding or "gadding" of this kind is the result of heel fly attacks, as this activity has been seen in the absence of heel flies.

In otherwise normal cattle, *H bovis* larvae and their secretions in the epidural fat of the spinal canal are associated with dissolved connective tissue, fat necrosis, and inflammation. Sometimes, the inflammation extends to the periosteum and bone, producing a localized area of periostitis and osteomyelitis. Occasionally, the epineurium and perineurium may become involved. In rare severe cases, paralysis or other nervous disorders may occur. Similarly, *H lineatum* in the submucosa of the esophagus may cause sufficient inflammation and edema in the surrounding tissues to hinder swallowing or eructation. It is unusual, however, for clinical signs of parasitism to be evident during the migratory phase.

Penetration of the skin by newly hatched larvae may produce a hypodermal rash, most often in older, previously infested cattle. The points of penetration are painful and inflamed and usually exude a yellowish serum. Warbles may occur in the back from tailhead to shoulders, and from topline to about one-third the distance down the sides. Usually, the cysts are firm and raised considerably above the normal contour of the skin. In each cyst, there is a breathing hole, ranging in size from a small slit to a round hole (3-4 mm in diameter) for more mature larvae. Generally, secondary infection is depressed; however, cysts may occasionally develop in large, suppurating abscesses.

The emergence of the grub, its forced expulsion, or its death within the cyst usually results in healing of the lesion without complications. Carcasses and hides of cattle infested with cattle grubs show marked evidence of the infestation and are reduced in value.

An infested animal may have 1 to ≥300 warbles but generally <100; infested herds often have individual animals with no grubs. Young animals are most heavily infested.

If migrating *Hypoderma* die in esophageal tissue (*H lineatum*) or near the spinal cord (*H bovis*), they can cause severe reactions that are sometimes fatal. These reactions appear to be related to the numbers of grubs but are rare in any case.

Death of first-stage larvae of *H bovis* in the spinal canal of cattle after systemic insecticide treatment has resulted in stiffness, ataxia, muscular weakness, and paralysis of hindlimbs. Recovery is usually rapid and complete, but occasionally, paralysis may be permanent.

Death of first-stage larvae of *H lineatum* in the submucosal connective tissue of the esophagus causes inflammation of the esophageal wall, dysphagia, drooling, and bloat. Again, recovery is usually rapid and complete (48-72 hr after treatment), but in severe cases, the bloat may be fatal. Rupture of the esophagus may be caused by attempted passage of a stomach tube in an affected animal.

Diagnosis: Third-stage larvae can be easily differentiated. *H bovis* is generally larger and has no spines on the tenth segment and a funnel-shaped spiracular plate; *H lineatum* is smaller and has spines on the tenth segment and typically a flat spiracular plate. In cases of bloat or paralysis, the presence of disintegrating grubs and the associated hemorrhage and tissue damage distinguishes animals that are parasitized from those that are not.

Treatment and Control: Systemic insecticides in various formulations are available for treatment. Pour-on treatments of the organophosphates famphur and fenthion or the macrocyclic lactones doramectin, eprinomectin, ivermectin, or moxidectin are poured evenly along the midline of the back. Fenthion in a 20% formulation is applied to a single spot on the midline. Some products must not be applied when the skin or hair coat are wet or when rain is expected to wet cattle within 6 hr. The application site should be free of skin lesions, mud, or manure.

Doramectin and ivermectin are systemically active against cattle grub larvae when administered as a SC injection. Famphur and ivermectin are also available as an oral paste. The injectable and pour-on systemic treatments are approved for control of *Hypoderma* and other myiasis-causing flies in many countries. Coumaphos may be applied as a whole body spray for control of *Hypoderma*; however, in the USA the practices of dipping or spraying cattle for cattle grub control have been replaced by the pour-on and/or injectable treatment methods.

No organophosphate systemic agent should be used in conjunction with another because their actions may be synergistic. Cattle stressed by castration, overheating, vaccination, or shipping should not be treated. Famphur should not be used to treat Brahman bulls.

Eprinomectin and moxidectin pour-on are approved for treatment of both beef and dairy cattle. Otherwise use of drugs for cattle grub control is prohibited in dairy animals of breeding age. Because residues may be present in cattle for varying periods after treatment, withdrawal times for all treatments must be observed.

In areas where grub numbers are high, cattle, especially calves, should be treated as soon as possible after the end of the heel fly season. They should not be treated later than 8-12 wk before the anticipated first appearance of grubs in the backs because adverse reactions may occur when migrating larvae are killed.

Where systemic insecticides cannot be used, cattle grubs can be controlled by applying stirofos dust to the warbles in the back. The dust should be applied to the animal's back and worked into the grub holes. Because new grubs continue to appear in the back, treatment must be repeated every 30-45 days during the warble season.

On small groups of tractable animals, extraction by instrument or hand expulsion (by squeezing) of the individual grubs is effective. Rarely, when this procedure is performed carelessly, the grub is crushed in its cyst and an anaphylactic reaction results.

DERMATOBIA HOMINIS

The tropical warble fly or torsalo, one of the most important parasites of cattle in Latin America, is distributed between southern Mexico and northern Argentina. Larval stages are found in many hosts, including cattle, sheep, goats, pigs, buffalo, dogs, cats, rabbits, and humans. Cattle and dogs are infected most commonly. *D hominis* is thought to initiate the lesion that gives rise to lechiguana, a recently characterized disease in cattle (*see* below).

Life Cycle: The adult fly is 12-15 mm long and has a short life span (1-9 days). The adult fly fastens its eggs to different types of insects (49 [mostly mosquitos and muscoid flies] have been described as vectors of *D hominis* in Latin America) that then transport them to warm-blooded hosts where they hatch as the insects feed. The larvae penetrate the skin of the animal within a few minutes of hatching and remain in the subcutaneous tissue for 4-18 wk. During this period, the larvae grow within warbles with breathing holes. When mature, the larvae leave the host and drop to the ground, burrow, and pupate. After the pupal period, which lasts 4-11 wk, the flies emerge as adults. The complete life cycle takes 11-17 wk.

Larval penetration of the skin is accompanied by pain and local inflammation, and pus gradually forms. Infested hides are condemned at slaughter, and production of milk and meat is reduced.

Treatment and Control: Different contact and systemic insecticides in various formulations are available for treatment. Generally, torsalo are susceptible to systemic organophosphates and macrocyclic lactone endectocides, which may be approved and available locally.

Lechiguana

Lechiguana is a recently described, sporadic, chronic disease of cattle that, thus far, has been reported only from southern and southeastern Brazil, in areas where infection by *D hominis* is common. It is characterized by large, hard, subcutaneous swellings that develop rapidly, mainly in the scapular and adjacent areas (chest, neck, shoulders, and ribs). Most cattle affected have only 1 swelling, but 2 swellings are occasionally observed. The regional lymph nodes are enlarged.

A new bacterial species, *Mannheimia (Pasteurella) granulomatis*, has been recovered from lesions and is considered causal. The lesion that gives rise to lechiguana is initiated by *D hominis* larvae. *M granulomatis* is consistently recovered from lesions of the clinical disease, and it is thought to be mainly responsible for the characteristic tissue changes. The habitat or source of *M granulomatis* is not known.

Histologically, lesions consist of focal proliferation of fibrous tissue infiltrated by plasma cells, eosinophils, lymphocytes, and sometimes neutrophils. The primary lesion is an eosinophilic lymphangitis, which results in eosinophilic abscesses, with occasional rosettes containing bacteria in their centers. The subcutaneous, tumorous mass produced may attain a size as great as 40×50 cm in 2 mo. Without treatment, death occurs after 3-11 mo.

When well established, the disease is clinically obvious. Diagnosis is confirmed by recovery of *M granulomatis* and observation of the characteristic histopathologic changes in lesions.

Treatment with chloramphenicol (3 g, SID for 5 days) or danofloxacin mesylate (1.25 mg/kg, SID for 3 days) results in rapid reduction of swellings, with almost complete regression in 30 days. Conducting susceptibility tests is advisable before using other antimicrobials.

CUTEREBRA INFESTATION IN SMALL ANIMALS

This opportunistic, parasitic infestation of dogs, cats, and ferrets is caused by the rodent or rabbit botfly, *Cuterebra* spp (order Diptera, family Cuterebridae). Flies are usually host- and site-specific relative to their life cycle. However, rabbit *Cuterebra* are less host-specific and are usually associated with dog and cat infestations. Rarely, cats and dogs may be infested with *Hypoderma* spp or *Dermatobia hominis*. Ferrets housed outside may be infested by *Hypoderma* or *Cuterebra* spp.

Etiology: Adult *Cuterebra* flies are large and bee-like and do not feed or bite. Females deposit eggs around the openings of animal nests, burrows, along runways of the normal hosts, or on stones or vegetation in these areas. A female fly may deposit 5-15 eggs/site and >2,000 eggs in her lifetime. Animals become infested as they pass through contaminated areas; the eggs hatch in response to heat from a nearby host. In the target host, the larvae enter the body through the mouth or nares during grooming or, less commonly, through open wounds. After penetration, the larvae migrate to various species-specific subcutaneous locations on the body, where they develop and communicate with the air through a breathing pore. After ~30 days, the larvae exit the skin, fall to the soil, and pupate. The duration of the pupation varies depending on the environmental factors and winter diapause.

Clinical Findings and Diagnosis: *Cuterebra* lesions are most common in the summer and fall when the larvae enlarge and produce a fistulous swelling ~1 cm in diameter. Dogs, cats, and ferrets are abnormal hosts for this parasite; aberrant migrations can involve the head, brain, nasal passages, pharynx, and eyelids. In the skin, typical lesions are seen around the head, neck, and trunk. The hair is often matted, and a subcutaneous swelling is present beneath the lesions. Cats often groom the area aggressively. Pain at the site is variable and usually associated with secondary infections. Purulent material may exude from the lesion; the most common differential diagnosis is an abscess or foreign body.

Definitive diagnosis is made by finding and identifying a larva. Second instar larvae are 5-10 mm in length and are gray to cream in color. Third instar larvae are dark, thick, heavily spined and are the stage most commonly seen by veterinarians.

Treatment: Suspect lesions should be explored by carefully enlarging and probing the breathing pore or fistula with mosquito forceps. The lesion should not be squeezed because this may rupture the larva and lead to a chronic foreign body reaction and secondary infection. There are anecdotal reports of larval rupture causing anaphylaxis. If possible, the larva should be removed in one piece; recurrent abscesses at the site of previous *Cuterebra* infestation suggest residual infection or remaining pieces of larva. The area should be thoroughly flushed with sterile saline, debrided (if necessary), and allowed to heal by granulation. Healing may be slow.

FLEAS AND FLEA ALLERGY DERMATITIS

There are >2,200 species of fleas recognized worldwide. In North America, only a few species commonly infest dogs and cats: *Ctenocephalides felis* (the cat flea), *C canis* (the dog flea), *Pulex simulans* (a flea of small mammals), and *Echidnophaga gallinacea* (the poultry sticktight flea). However, by far the most prevalent flea on dogs and cats is *C felis*. Cat fleas cause severe irritation in animals and humans and are responsible for flea allergy dermatitis. They also serve as the vector of typhus-like rickettsiae and *Bartonella* sp, and are the intermediate host for filarid and cestode parasites. Cat fleas have been found to infest >50 different mammalian and avian hosts throughout the world. In North America, the most commonly infested hosts are domestic and wild canids, domestic and wild felids, raccoons, opossums, ferrets, and domestic rabbits.

Transmission, Epidemiology, and Pathogenesis: Cat fleas deposit their eggs in the pelage of their host. The eggs are pearly white, oval with rounded ends, and 0.5 mm long. They readily fall from the pelage and drop onto bedding, carpet, or soil, where hatching occurs in ~1-6 days. Newly hatched flea larvae are 1-5 mm long, slender, white, segmented, and sparsely covered with short hairs. Larvae are free-living, feeding on organic debris found in their environment and on adult flea feces, which are essential for successful development. Flea larvae avoid direct light and actively move deep in carpet fibers or under organic debris (grass, branches, leaves, or soil).

Larvae are susceptible to desiccation, with exposures to relative humidity <50% being lethal. The areas within a home with the necessary humidity are limited, and suitable outdoor sites are even rarer. Flea development occurs outdoors only where the ground is shaded and moist (1-20% soil moisture content) and where the flea-infested pet spends a significant amount of time so that adult flea feces will be deposited into the larval environment. In the indoor environment, flea larvae probably survive only in the protected microenvironment deep within carpet fibers, in cracks between hardwood floors in humid climates, and on unfinished concrete floors in damp basements. The larval stage usually lasts 5-11 days but may be prolonged for 2-3 wk, depending on availability of food and climatic conditions.

After completing its development, the mature larva produces a silk-like cocoon in which it pupates. The cocoon is ovoid, ~0.5 cm long, whitish, and loosely spun. Flea cocoons can be found in soil, on vegetation, in carpets, under furniture, and on animal bedding.

Once the pupa has fully developed (1-2 wk), the adult flea emerges from the cocoon when properly stimulated by physical pressure, carbon dioxide, substrate movement, or heat. The preemerged adult (which is a fully formed adult flea) residing in the cocoon is the stage that can extend the longevity of the flea. If the preemerged adult does not receive the proper stimulus to emerge, it can remain quiescent in the cocoon for several weeks until a suitable host arrives. Emergence can be delayed up to 350 days if preemerged adults are protected from desiccation. Newly emerging fleas move to the top of the carpet pile or vegetation, where they are more likely to encounter a passing host. A newly emerged cat flea can survive 24-72 hr before requiring a blood meal. It is the newly emerged unfed fleas that infest pets and bite people. Cat fleas that have found a preferred host (eg, dog, cat, opossum, etc) generally do not leave their host unless forced off by grooming or insecticides.

Depending on temperature and humidity, the entire life cycle of the cat flea can be completed in as little as 12-14 days or can be prolonged for up to 350 days. However, under most household conditions, cat fleas complete their life cycle in 3-6 wk.

Adults begin feeding almost immediately once they find a host. Female cat fleas can consume 13.6 µL of blood daily. After rapid transit through the flea, the excreted blood dries within minutes into reddish black fecal pellets or long tubular coils (flea dirt). Fleas mate after feeding, and egg production begins within 24-48 hr of females taking their first blood meal. Female cat fleas can produce up to 40-50 eggs/day during peak egg production, averaging 27 eggs/day through 50 days, and may continue to produce eggs for >100 days.

Cat fleas are susceptible to cold. No stage of the life cycle (egg, larva, pupa, or adult) can survive exposure to <3°C (37.4°F) for several days. Therefore, cat fleas survive winters in north temperate climates as adults on untreated dogs and cats or on small wild mammals (eg, raccoons or opossums) in the urban environment. As these animals pass through yards in the spring or set up nesting sites in crawl spaces or attics, the eggs laid by surviving female fleas drop off and subsequently develop to adults. Cat fleas may also survive the winter as preemerged adults in microenvironments protected from the cold.

Fleas can cause iron deficiency anemia in heavily infested hosts, particularly in young animals. Fleas in the genus *Ctenocephalides* have been reported to produce anemia in poultry, dogs, cats, goats, cattle, and sheep.

Cat fleas are also involved in disease transmission. Murine typhus, caused by *Rickettsia typhi* and *R felis*, is a mild to severe febrile disease of humans characterized by headaches, chills, and skin rashes, with infrequent involvement of the kidneys and CNS. The disease occurs in humans and many small mammals along the southeastern, southwestern, and

Gulf coasts. In the USA, the principal transmission cycle involves opossums and cat fleas. Cat fleas also serve as the intermediate host of the nonpathogenic subcutaneous filarid nematode of dogs, *Dipetalonema reconditum*. *Dipylidium caninum*, the common intestinal cestode of dogs and cats (and rarely children), develops as a cysticercoid in *C felis*, *C canis*, and *P irritans*. Flea larvae ingest the eggs of the tapeworm, which develop into cysticercoids in the body of the flea. When grooming themselves, dogs and cats may ingest infected fleas, and the cysticercoids are released.

Flea allergy dermatitis (FAD) or flea bite hypersensitivity is the most common dermatologic disease of domestic dogs in the USA. Cats are also afflicted with FAD, which is one of the major causes of feline miliary dermatitis. FAD is most prevalent in the summer, although in warm climates flea infestations may persist throughout the year. In north temperate regions, the close association of pets and their fleas with human dwellings creates conditions that permit a year-round problem. Temperature extremes and low humidity tend to inhibit flea development.

When feeding, fleas inject saliva that contains a variety of histamine-like compounds, enzymes, polypeptides, and amino acids that span a wide range of sizes (40-60 kD) and induce Type I, Type IV, and basophil hypersensitivity. Flea-naive dogs exposed intermittently to flea bites develop either immediate (15 min) or delayed (24-48 hr) reactions, or both, and detectable levels of both circulating IgE and IgG antiflea antibodies. Dogs exposed continuously to flea bites have low levels of these circulating antibodies and either do not develop skin reactions or develop them later and to a considerably reduced degree. This could indicate that immunologic tolerance may develop naturally in dogs continuously exposed to flea bites. Although the pathophysiology of FAD in cats is poorly understood, similar mechanisms may exist.

Clinical Findings: Clinical signs associated with FAD are variable and depend on frequency of flea exposure, duration of disease, presence of secondary or other concurrent skin disease, degree of hypersensitivity, and effects of previous or current treatment. Nonallergic animals may have few clinical signs other than occasional scratching due to annoyance of flea bites. Those that are allergic will typically have a dermatitis that is characterized by pruritus.

In dogs, the pruritus associated with FAD can be intense and may manifest over the entire body. Classic clinical signs are papulocrustous lesions distributed on the lower back, tailhead, and posterior and inner thighs. Dogs may be particularly sensitive in the flanks, caudal and medial thighs, ventral abdomen, lower back, neck, and ears. Affected dogs are likely to be restless and uncomfortable, spending much time scratching, licking, rubbing, chewing, and even nibbling at the skin. Hair may be stained brown from the licking and is often broken off. Common secondary lesions include areas of alopecia, erythema, hyperpigmented skin, scaling, papules, and broken papules covered with reddish brown crusts. The rump and tailhead areas are typically the first, most evident, areas affected. As FAD progresses and becomes chronic, the areas become alopecic, lichenified, and hyperpigmented and the dog develops secondary bacterial and yeast infections.

In extremely hypersensitive dogs, extensive areas of alopecia, erythema, and self-trauma are evident. Traumatic moist dermatitis (hot spots) can also occur. As the disease becomes chronic, the dog may develop generalized alopecia, severe seborrhea, hyperkeratosis, and hyperpigmentation.

In cats, clinical signs vary from minimal to severe, depending on the degree of sensitivity. The primary dermatitis is a papule, which often becomes crusted. This miliary dermatitis is typically found on the back, neck, and face. The miliary lesions are not actual flea bites but a manifestation of a systemic allergic reaction that leads to generalized pruritus and an eczematous rash. Pruritus may be severe, evidenced by repeated licking, scratching, and chewing. Cats with FAD can have alopecia, facial dermatitis, exfoliative dermatitis, and "racing stripe" or dorsal dermatitis.

Diagnosis: A number of factors must be considered in the diagnosis of FAD, including history, clinical signs, presence of fleas or flea excrement, results of intradermal testing, and ruling out other causes of dermatologic disease.

Most cases occur in the late summer, corresponding to the peak of flea populations. In these cases, history can be highly suggestive. Age of onset is also important because FAD does not ordinarily occur before 1 yr of age. Usually, diagnosis is made by visual observation of fleas on the infested pet. Demonstration to the owner of the presence of fleas or flea excrement is helpful. Slowly parting the hair against the normal lay often reveals flea excrement or the rapidly moving fleas. Flea excrement is reddish black, cylindrical, and pellet- or comma-shaped. Placed in water or on a damp paper towel and crushed, the excrement dissolves, producing a reddish brown color.

Extremely hypersensitive animals are likely to be virtually free of fleas due to excessive self-grooming. In these cases, it is usually difficult to find evidence of fleas, thus making it more difficult to convince owners of the problem. Use of a fine-toothed flea comb (32 teeth/in.) facilitates finding of fleas and their excrement. Examination of the pet's bedding for eggs, larvae, and excrement is also useful.

Intradermal skin testing may be used to support a presumptive diagnosis of FAD. Positive immediate reactions are characterized by a wheal 3-5 mm larger in diameter than the negative control. Alternatively, a positive wheal measurement can be defined as a response that is at least equal to the halfway point between the size of positive and negative control reactions. Observations for an immediate reaction (15-20 min) and, if negative, a 24-hr delayed reaction are recommended. The delayed reaction may not occur as a discrete wheal but rather as a diffuse erythematous reaction. A positive reaction does not conclusively indicate that the clinical condition is FAD—it indicates only that the animal is allergic to the flea antigen, either from present or past exposure. The reliability of intradermal skin testing in cats to diagnose FAD has been variable.

Serologic testing of IgE directed against flea-specific salivary antigens can be used to aid in the diagnosis of FAD.

FAD must be differentiated from other causes of dermatologic disease. The presence of fleas or a positive reaction to an intradermal test does not rule out the presence of another dermatologic disease responsible for the clinical signs. In dogs, differential diagnoses include allergic inhalant dermatitis (atopy), food allergy dermatitis, sarcoptic or demodectic mange, other ectoparasites, and bacterial folliculitis. In cats, other conditions that can result in miliary dermatitis include external parasites (cheyletiellosis, trombiculosis, notoedric mange, and pediculosis), dermatophytosis, drug hypersensitivity, food allergy, atopy, bacterial folliculitis, and idiopathic miliary dermatitis.

Treatment and Control: *See also* ECTOPARASITICIDES OF SMALL ANIMALS, p 2165.

Flea control measures have changed dramatically in recent years. Historically, flea control was achieved through repeated application of on-animal products and application of insecticides and insect growth regulators (IGR) on the premises. The difficulty with this approach was achieving consistent compliance with treatment protocols. The recent development of insecticides and IGR with convenient dosage formulations and prolonged residual activity has dramatically improved owner compliance and has helped eliminate recurrent infestations. The goals of flea control are elimination of fleas on pet(s), elimination of existing environmental infestation, and prevention of subsequent reinfestation. The first step is still the elimination of existing pet flea infestations. Elimination of those fleas currently established on the dog or cat is necessary to eliminate pet discomfort. One term commonly employed when discussing flea kill on a pet is rate or speed of flea kill. However, it is important to differentiate between speed of elimination of established infestations and speed of elimination of newly acquired fleas after the product has been applied. When treating a dog or cat with a topically applied formulation, it could take several hours (12-36 hrs) until the compound has spread sufficiently or reached sufficient systemic concentrations to eliminate all existing fleas. If a more rapid rate of kill is needed, a flea spray or nitenpyram may be desirable.

Several currently available insecticides provide excellent elimination of established flea infestations on both dogs and cats; these include fipronil, imidacloprid, nitenpyram, selamectin, and pyrethroids. Orally administered nitenpyram will eliminate fleas within 3-4 hr, while the topically applied residual spot-on formulations containing fipronil, imidacloprid, or selamectin take 12-42 hr.

The second goal is to eliminate existing infestation in the pet's environment. This can be accomplished in several ways: 1) topical application of residual insecticides that kill newly acquired fleas (within 24 hr) before they can initiate reproduction, 2) administration of topical, injectable, or oral IGR to stop flea reproduction, 3) repeated application of insecticides and/or IGR to the premises, or 4) combinations of the above.

Topical application of residual insecticides and administration of topical, injectable, or oral IGR have become the preferred methods of eliminating flea infestations. Several of these new insecticides and IGR have been shown to be extremely effective in controlling fleas on pets living in infested premises. Field studies have shown that fipronil (with or without the addition of (S)-methoprene), imidacloprid, lufenuron (with pyrethroid spray or nitenpyram tablets), and selamectin may be effective in controlling flea infestations, without the need for premise treatment. Flea infestations can be eliminated via chronic use of topical and systemic approaches because most fleas are killed prior to and/or directly inhibited from reproducing.

If residual flea products are applied at the appropriate dose and treatment intervals, there may be adequate residual activity between applications to kill many newly acquired fleas before egg production is initiated. However, flea survival and reproduction may occur prior to the next application for a variety of reasons such as: 1) residual activity <100% within the labeled time frame, 2) rate of flea kill slows during the third or fourth week, 3) delayed or infrequent product reapplication 4) simple under-dosing, and 5) mechanical removal of water-soluble insecticides during bathing or swimming. These problems may result in delays in control or outright treatment failures.

None of the currently available residual flea products is 100% effective against all cat flea strains between labeled reapplication periods due to genetic variability of different flea populations. Many of the factors that allow flea infestations to persist could possibly lead to genetic selection of resistant flea populations. Surviving fleas may be capable of producing viable eggs. Continued reproduction must be halted to prevent persistent flea infestations and selection for resistant fleas. Reproduction can be prevented by administration of topical or systemic IGR, which provide prolonged residual ovicidal activity, interrupting future flea development even after residual activity of an insecticide is diminished. Application of methoprene or pyriproxyfen to the hair coat of dogs and cats rapidly kills developing flea eggs in addition to residual ovicidal activity. The combination of fipronil/(S)-methoprene or other adulticidal/ovicidal products has demonstrated activity against adult fleas and provides prolonged residual ovicidal activity, thus reducing the potential for genetic selection. Not only have topically applied IGR been shown to be ovicidal, but orally administered or injectable (cats only) lufenuron also provides ovicidal activity. While not an IGR, selamectin also demonstrates ovicidal activity in cats.

In cases of massive flea infestations or severe pet or human flea allergy, treatment of the premises with adulticides and IGR may still be necessary. Control may be achieved by using insecticides with residual activity (or by repeated application of short-acting insecticides) in combination with an IGR to prevent the development of flea eggs and larvae. Methoprene and pyriproxyfen are the 2 currently available IGR for premise application. Insecticides and IGR can be applied by broadcast treatment (hand pump sprayers or pressurized aerosols) or with total release aerosols or "foggers." During application, the surface of all rugs and carpets must be treated adequately. Efforts should be directed to areas where flea eggs and larvae accumulate, such as carpets, cracks, grooves in hardwood floors, behind baseboards, under the edge of rugs, beneath furniture (beds, tables, and sofas), and within closets. In severe infestations, a second treatment may be necessary 7-10 days later due to continued emergence of adult fleas from cocoons hidden deep within carpets.

Elimination of fleas in the yard can be an important aspect of flea control. Outdoor treatments (eg, cyfluthrin, fenvalerate) should concentrate on primary areas of flea development, including protected microhabitats such as dog houses, within garages, under porches, and in animal lounging areas beneath shrubs or other shaded areas. Entomopathogenic nematodes that parasitize flea larvae and pupae also can be used in these areas to inhibit the buildup of the flea population. Spraying flea control products over the large expanse of a shade-free lawn generally is not beneficial.

Pet owners should also conduct mechanical control. Helpful procedures include washing pet blankets, throw rugs, and pet carriers; in addition, pet sleeping and resting areas should be vacuumed thoroughly to help remove flea eggs and larvae. Seat cushions and pillows on sofas and chairs should be removed and vacuumed, and special attention should be given to crevices in sofas and chairs and to areas beneath sofas or beds where flea eggs and feces may drop from the pet and accumulate.

Despite the efforts of pet owners, the total elimination of fleas may not be feasible in some situations or may not occur rapidly enough to control clinical signs of FAD. Supportive medical therapy must be instituted to control pruritus and secondary skin disease in hypersensitive animals. Systemic glucocorticoids are often needed to control inflammation and associated pruritus. Short-acting prednisone or prednisolone can be administered initially at a dosage of 0.5-1.0 mg/kg, SID, tapering the dosage and using alternate-day therapy until the lowest dose possible that still controls the pruritus is given. As soon as flea control is accomplished, the glucocorticoid can be discontinued. Anti-inflammatory therapy should never be used as a substitute for flea control.

Secondary bacterial skin infection can be associated with FAD. Systemic antibiotics are commonly used to control the pyoderma and thus reduce the associated inflammation and pruritus. Selection of an appropriate antibiotic should be based on bacterial cultures and results of antibiotic sensitivity tests.

Hyposensitization consists of administering allergens to a hypersensitive animal on a regular basis in an attempt to obtain a state of clinical nonreactivity to flea bites. The effectiveness of currently available whole flea extracts is controversial.

FLIES

Flies belong to the order Diptera, a large, complex order of insects. Most members of this order have 2 wings (1 pair) as adults. However, there are a few wingless dipterans. Dipterans vary greatly in size, food source preference, and in the developmental stage that parasitizes the animal or produces pathology. As adults, dipterans may intermittently feed on vertebrate blood or on saliva, tears, or mucus. These dipterans are referred to as periodic parasites and may serve as intermediate hosts for helminth parasites or for protozoan parasites. They may also serve as vectors for bacteria, viruses, spirochetes, chlamydiae, etc. As larvae, dipterans may develop in the subcutaneous tissues of the skin, respiratory passages, or GI tract of vertebrate hosts and produce a condition known as myiasis.

DIPTERANS WITH BITING MOUTHPARTS

Blood-feeding dipterans can be classified in several ways based on which sexes feed on vertebrate blood and on food preference. In certain species of dipterans, only the females feed on vertebrate blood, which is required for egg laying; these species include black flies, sand flies, biting midges, mosquitos, horse flies, and deer flies. In other species of blood-feeding dipterans, both male and female flies feed on vertebrate blood; these species include stable flies, horn flies, buffalo flies, tsetse flies, sheep keds, and hippoboscid or louse flies.

BLACK FLIES

Members of the family Simulidae are commonly called black flies (although their coloration may vary from black to gray to yellow to olive) or buffalo gnats (because their thorax is humped over the head, giving the appearance of a buffalo's hump). Black flies are the tiniest of the blood-feeding dipterans, 1-6 mm long. They have broad, unspotted wings with prominent veins along the anterior margins. Black flies have compound eyes; eyes of females are distinctly separated, while those of the males are contiguous above the antennae. The palps have five segments. Female black flies have scissor-like mouthparts with serrated edges. The female flies require a blood meal so that they can lay eggs. Males feed on nectar from flowers.

Although there are >1,000 species of black flies, only a few are considered important as pests. Black flies feed on all classes of livestock, wildlife, birds, and humans.

Black flies are distributed throughout the world in areas where conditions permit development of the immature forms. Larvae nearly always are found in swiftly flowing, well-aerated water; shallow mountain torrents are favored breeding places. Some species breed in larger rivers; others live in temporary or semipermanent streams. Black flies are particularly abundant in the north temperate and subarctic zones, but many species are found in the subtropics and tropics where factors other than seasonal temperatures affect their developmental and abundance patterns.

Larval black flies are cylindrical and attach themselves by a large posterior sucker. On the anterior end are the mouthparts and a pair of brush-like organs. The larvae are carnivorous. Just below the mouthparts is an arm-like appendage called the proleg. Larvae attach to rocks or other solid objects in the stream, sometimes clinging to aquatic or emergent vegetation. The mature larva spins a triangular cocoon on the floor of the stream. The oblong pupa has 1 dorsal and 1 ventral respiratory tube, the branches of which float out of the cocoon.

Black flies produce 1-6 generations per year, depending on the species and climatic conditions. Adult female feeding activity may last from 2-3 wk to 3 mo. Adult black flies may fly 8-11 miles (12-18 km) from the swiftly flowing streams; migrating windborne swarms have been known to travel much farther. *Simulium arcticum* may travel ≥90 miles (150 km) in this manner in western Canada. Other species have been reported to travel ≥250 km.

Pathology: Because of their tiny, serrated mouthparts, female black flies inflict painful bites. The ears, neck, head, and abdomen of cattle are favorite feeding sites. In addition to local reactions (redness, itching, wheals) at the bite site, there may be general conditions that vary in intensity with the sensitivity of the animal and the number of bites. Attacks by large numbers of black flies can cause severe damage and high mortality in livestock. Humans may be similarly attacked.

Death from black fly attack apparently results from a toxin in the saliva, which increases the permeability of the capillaries and permits the fluid from the circulatory system to ooze into the body cavity and tissue spaces. The animal rapidly succumbs to a mass attack but can recover quickly if protected from further attacks. Reduced milk, meat, and egg production may result from less extensive attacks. Certain species of black flies sometimes cause losses in poultry, either by direct attack or through transmission of *Leukocytozoon* spp. In Africa, *S damnosum* and *S neavei* are important as vectors of *Onchocerca* spp. *S neavei* is an important vector of *O volvulus*. In Central America, *S ochraceum*, *S metallicum*, *S callidum*, and *S exiguum* are important vectors of *Onchocerca* spp. *S ochraceum* and *S metallicum* also are vicious biters.

Diagnosis: Black flies are most often collected in the field and not found on the animals. Adults flies can be identified by their small size, humped back, prominent venation in the anterior region of the wings, and tiny, serrated mouthparts. Identification of black flies to genus and species is probably best left to an entomologist.

Treatment and Control: If public funds and trained supervisory personnel are available, large-scale control of black flies is possible by treating breeding streams with an approved larvicide. However, black fly control is difficult because of the large number of flowing water breeding sites. Streams can be treated using the natural product, *Bacillus thuringiensis* var *israeliensis*, a product with no mammalian toxicity.

Treatment of streams and rivers involves techniques similar to those used by mosquito abatement programs. As a rule, pesticides should not be used owing to their potential negative effects on the environment. Pesticide treatments involving water surfaces or large land areas are subject to governmental regulation and must be performed with due regard for possible deleterious environmental effects and residues in food products.

Adult black flies are small enough to pass through window screens or may come indoors on or within a pet's hair coat. More often, the adult female flies prefer to feed outdoors and during the daylight hours. Since black flies feed predominantly during the daylight hours, it is wise to limit exposure of pets to swiftly flowing streams. Pet owners concerned about black fly bites may use over-the-counter insect repellents. An herbal treatment has geraniol as an active ingredient.

Because area-wide control of black flies is difficult and expensive, livestock producers frequently resort to the daily use of repellents to protect their animals. Extension entomology personnel should be contacted for the latest approved recommendations.

SAND FLIES

The phlebotomine sand flies, *Phlebotomus* spp (Old World sand flies) and *Lutzomyia* spp (New World sand flies), are members of the family Psychodidae. These flies are confined primarily to the tropical and subtropical regions of the world. Members of these genera are tiny, moth-like flies, ~1.5-4 mm long. The legs are as long as the antennae, comprising 16 segments that often have a beaded, hairy appearance. They are commonly known as sand flies, moth flies, or owl midges. The key morphologic feature for identification is that the body of the sand fly is covered with fine hairs. The females have piercing mouthparts and feed on blood of a variety of warm-blooded animals, including humans. Many species feed on reptiles. Male sand flies suck moisture from any available source and are even said to suck perspiration from people. Sand flies tend to be active only at night and, in contrast to black flies, are weak fliers; their flying is deterred by air currents, even slight ones. During the day, sand flies seek protection in crevices and caves, among vegetation, and within dark buildings. They often seek protection within rodent and armadillo burrows; these mammals can serve as reservoir hosts for *Leishmania* spp. Sand flies breed in dark, humid environments that have a supply of organic matter that serves as food for the larvae. They do not breed in aquatic environments.

Pathology: These tiny flies serve as an intermediate host for *Leishmania* spp, a protozoan parasite that infects the reticuloendothelial cells of capillaries, the spleen, and other organs but may be seen in monocytes, polymorphonuclear leukocytes, and macrophages of humans, dogs, cats, horses, and sheep (*see also* p 643).

Diagnosis: Like black flies, sand flies can most often be collected in the field and are not found on animals. They can be identified by their small size and hairy wings and bodies. Identification of genus and species is probably best left to an entomologist.

Treatment and Control: Insecticide spraying of larval habitat is usually not possible because of the difficulty of accessing their breeding sites. Removal of dense vegetation discourages breeding. Spraying of residual insecticides on surfaces in the home is the main way to control sand flies; however, this is ineffective for species that bite away from the home. Generally speaking, populations of sand flies have been reduced as a result of intense mosquito control programs.

BITING MIDGES

The biting midges, "no-see-ums," or punkies belong to the family Ceratopogondiae. The most common biting midges are *Culicoides* spp. They are associated with aquatic or semiaquatic habitats, eg, mud or moist soil around streams, ponds, and marshes. Biting midges are tiny gnats (1-3 mm long) and, like black flies, inflict painful bites and suck the blood of their hosts, both humans and livestock.

Pathology: *Culicoides* spp are vicious biters and can cause intense irritation and annoyance. In large numbers, they can cause livestock to be nervous and interrupt their feeding pattern. These gnats tend to feed on the dorsal or ventral areas of the host; feeding site preference depends on the species of biting gnat. They fly only in the warm months of the year and are most active before and during dusk. They feed often on the mane, tail, and belly of horses. Horses often become allergic to the bites, scratching and rubbing these areas, causing alopecia, excoriations, and thickening of the skin. This condition has several names, including culicoid hypersensitivity in Canada, Queensland itch in Australia, Kasen in Japan, sweat itch, and sweet itch. Because it is often seen during the warmer months of the year, it is also referred to as summer dermatitis. These flies also serve as the intermediate host for *Onchocerca cervicalis*; the microfilariae of this nematode are found in the skin of horses. Onchocerciasis (p 736) is a nonseasonal dermatosis that is similar to sweet itch but usually is less pruritic and affects the head, neck, and belly. These flies also transmit the bluetongue virus (p 590) in sheep and cattle.

Diagnosis: Like black flies and sand flies, biting midges are most often collected in the field and not found on the animals. In contrast to the clear, heavily veined wings of black flies, the wings of *Culicoides* spp are mottled. Identification is probably best left to an entomologist.

Treatment and Control: Larvae may be attacked in their breeding grounds. Extension entomology personnel should be contacted for the latest approved recommendations.

Bio Kill Stable Spray™, a modified permethrin, is approved for the spraying of stables and horseboxes to aid in the control of biting midges. A backpack or handheld bulk pesticide spray pack, turbo-blower, or fogger should be used. A fine spray should be produced under pressure, in the amount of 500-750 mL per stable (stable size: 3 m × 3.5 m to 4 m × 4 m). All surfaces in the stable should be sprayed. A reapplication 7-10 days later is needed. Thereafter, application every 3-4 wk should provide ample product buildup on the walls.

A fan may be used in the stable to create air movement around the horses, because *Culicoides* spp are poor flyers. Fly repellent ear tags attached to the horse's mane and tail (not approved in the USA); pyrethrum synergized with piperonyl butoxide, applied weekly; butoxypolypropylene glycol 800, applied daily; stable blankets; and fine screens on stable doors and windows have been used with mixed success.

MOSQUITOS

Mosquitos are members of the family Culicidae. Important genera include *Aedes*, *Anopheles*, *Culex*, *Culiseta*, and *Psorophora*. Although they are tiny, fragile dipterans, mosquitos are perhaps some of the most voracious of the blood-feeding arthropods. About 300 species have been described worldwide, with ~150 species found in the temperate regions of North America. Mosquitos are found in such diverse areas as salt marshes of the coastal plains to snow pools above 14,000 ft (4,300 m) to the gold mines of India 3,600 ft (1,100 m) below sea level. The volume of water in which mosquitos will breed varies from that within a can or tree hole to large shallow pools of accumulated, standing water.

Mosquitos lay their eggs either on the surface of standing water (eg, *Aedes* and *Psorophora* spp) or on a substrate (such as damp soil) where the eggs will hatch after inundation from rainfall, irrigation, snow melt, etc. Larval mosquitos are known as wrigglers, while pupal mosquitos are known as tumblers. These stages are always aquatic and are found in a wide variety of habitats. Large numbers of mosquitos can be produced from eggs laid in relatively small bodies of water. Some species have several generations per year. The flight habits of adult mosquitos vary with the species; some *Aedes* spp will migrate many miles for their aquatic, larval habitat. In strong winds, mosquitos may be carried great distances. Some species overwinter as eggs, while others overwinter as adults.

Pathology: Only female mosquitos actively take a blood meal so that they can lay eggs. Males feed on nectar, plant juices, and other liquids. Mosquitos annoy livestock, cause blood loss, and transmit disease. Also, the toxins injected at the time of biting may cause systemic effects. Mosquitos have been known to plague humans and livestock and, like black flies, in swarms, they have been known to keep cattle from grazing or cause them to stampede. The feeding of large numbers of swarming mosquitos can cause significant anemia in domestic animals. Although they are known for spreading malaria, yellow fever, dengue, and elephantiasis in humans, mosquitos are probably best known in veterinary medicine as the intermediate host for the canine heartworm, *Dirofilaria immitis*, and as the vectors of the equine viral encephalitides, including West Nile virus.

Anopheles quadrimaculatus is the intermediate host for malaria (*Plasmodium* spp) in humans and other primates. *Aedes aegypti* is the yellow fever mosquito, transmitting this virus among people. *Psorophora columbiae* is a severe pest of both livestock and humans in the rice fields of Louisiana and Arkansas. *Culex tarsalis* is an important vector of western equine encephalitis and is found in the western, central, and southern USA. *Aedes vexans* is an important nuisance species found in the midwest. *Aedes albopictus* is a recently introduced Asian species that also spreads yellow fever, dengue, and equine encephalitis. Certain *Mansonia* spp are severe pests of livestock in Florida. In Central and South America, the adult female bot fly *Dermatobia hominis* fastens her eggs to a species of *Psorophora* mosquito, which then transmits them to the mammalian host during feeding.

Diagnosis: Adult mosquitos are most often collected in the field and are not found on animals. Adults are 3-6 mm long and slender, with small, spherical heads and long legs. The wing veins, body, head, and legs are covered with tiny, leaf-shaped scales. The long, filamentous antennae have 14-15 segments and are plumose in the males of most species. They also have proboscides designed for lacerating tiny blood vessels and sucking up pooled blood. Identification of the plethora of mosquito species (adult, larval, and pupal stages) is probably best left to an entomologist.

Treatment and Control: Area control of mosquitos usually involves the cooperation of many individuals and can be accomplished successfully by experienced personnel with proper equipment. Areas that can serve as breeding sites for mosquito larvae should be eliminated or reduced. In addition, area programs generally include extensive use of larvicides; however, mosquito larvicides can disrupt the normal ecologic balance within an ecosystem. Recently, the use of various species of fish as biologic controls has been successful. In massive emergence of adult mosquitos, particularly when disease transmission is a concern, application of an insecticide active against the adult may be necessary.

Caution is advised with area treatment programs because many nontarget organisms (eg, fish, shrimp, bees) may be exposed to insecticides. A local extension entomologist should be consulted regarding appropriate materials for use on animals or within premises. Large-scale programs usually are coordinated by mosquito abatement district or other government agencies.

It is difficult for individual producers to protect their animals; residual sprays on the animals do not prevent attachment, and currently available repellents do not confer adequate protection during massive emergence. Protection from adult mosquitos may be provided by ground and, in some cases, aerial application of an insecticide at the time of emergence. Depending on local conditions, this protection may be of short duration. Valuable animals should be housed in closed or screened buildings, and the mosquitos inside killed with a fog or aerosol formulation of an approved insecticide. Temporary relief may be afforded by a spray or "wipe on" of materials commercially available.

Walking pets in the early morning or early evening hours when adult mosquitos are most abundant should be avoided to reduce exposure to mosquito bites. Imidacloprid has been used as a topical prevention and treatment of ticks, fleas, and mosquitos on dogs and puppies 7 weeks of age and older, weighing > 2 lb (0.91 kg). The compound has been shown to repel adult female mosquitos for up to 4 wk. Unfortunately, it cannot be used on cats. Mosquitos are not attracted to light; thus, electrocution devices are not helpful in mosquito control and may actually be detrimental because they may destroy beneficial insects that prey on mosquitos.

HORSE FLIES AND DEER FLIES

Tabanus spp (horse flies) and *Chrysops* spp (deer flies) are large (up to 3.5 cm long), heavy bodied, robust dipterans with powerful wings and very large eyes. They are swift fliers. These flies are the largest in the dipteran group in which only the females feed on vertebrate blood. Horse flies are larger than deer flies; many horse flies are highly colored. Deer flies are medium sized; they have a dark band passing from the anterior to the posterior margin of the wings and a yellow to brown abdomen with black patches and longitudinal bands.

Adult horse flies and deer flies lay eggs in the vicinity of open water. Larval stages are found in aquatic to semiaquatic environments, often buried deep in mud at the bottom of lakes and ponds. Adults are seen in summer, particularly in sunlight.

Pathology: Adult females of both species feed in the vicinity of open water and have reciprocating, scissor-like mouthparts, which they use to lacerate tissues and lap up the oozing blood. They consume 0.1-0.3 mL of blood at a single feeding. Bites are painful and irritating. These flies feed primarily on large animals, such as cattle and horses, which become restless when the flies are present. Site preferences include the underside of the abdomen around the navel, the legs, or the neck and withers. Horse flies and deer flies feed a number of times in multiple feeding sites before they become replete. When disturbed by the animal's swatting tail or by the panniculus reflex, the flies leave the host, yet blood continues to ooze from the open wound. These flies may act as mechanical transmitters of anthrax, anaplasmosis, tularemia, and the virus of equine infectious anemia.

Diagnosis: These flies can be identified by their large size, powerful wings, compound eyes, and lacerating scissor-like mouthparts. Species identification of intact adult and larval horse and deer flies is probably best left to an entomologist.

Treatment and Control: Horse flies and deer flies are the most difficult to control of all of the blood-sucking flies. Many of the adulticide compounds used for other biting flies will kill both horse and deer flies. However, because these flies are intermittent feeders that alight on the host for only a short time, they may not be exposed long enough to be affected. Thus, larger doses of the compounds may be required.

Horse fly traps have been effective when used around cattle confined to manageable areas. For livestock, pyrethroid pour-ons function as limited repellents. Self-application techniques are usually not effective for horse and deer flies.

Manipulation of these flies' aquatic habitat has been attempted by removing unnecessary woody plants from residential areas or draining wet areas. Application of insecticides in the water may have detrimental environmental effects.

STABLE FLIES

The stable fly, *Stomoxys calcitrans*, is often called the biting house fly. It is about the same in size and general appearance as *Musca domestica*, the house fly. It is brownish gray, the outer of 4 thoracic stripes is broken, and the abdomen has a checkered appearance. It has a bayonet-like, needle-sharp proboscis that, when at rest, protrudes forward from the head. The wings, when at rest, are widely spread at the tips. These flies are found throughout the world. In the USA, they are found in the midwestern and southeastern states.

The larval and pupal forms develop in decaying organic matter, including grass clippings and seaweed along beaches. In the midwestern USA, larvae can be found in wet areas around the edges of hay stacks and silage pits. Where cattle are fed hay, breeding can occur at the edge of the feeding area where hay has become mixed with urine and feces. The life cycle in the field can be completed in 2-3 wk, and adults may live ≥3-4 wk.

Pathology: Both male and female stable flies are avid blood feeders, feeding on any warm-blooded animal. Stable flies stay on the host for short periods of time, during which they obtain blood meals. This is an outdoor fly; however, in the late fall and during rainy weather, it may enter barns.

Horses are the preferred hosts. The fly usually lands on the host with its head pointed upward and inflicts painful bites that puncture the skin and bleed freely. It is a sedentary fly, not moving on the host. Stable flies usually attack the legs and ventral abdomen and may also bite the ears. They can be a problem in cattle feedlots in the midwestern USA. The damage inflicted to cattle is caused by the painful bite and blood loss, and the irritation results in a reduced efficiency in converting feed to meat or milk. In pets, stable flies prefer to feed on the tips of the ears of dogs with pointed ears, especially German Shepherds.

Stable flies are mechanical vectors of anthrax, surra, and equine infectious anemia. They are the intermediate host for *Habronema muscae*, a nematode found in the stomach of horses.

Diagnosis: Stable flies are easily identified by their size (about the same as that of the house fly), coloration, and bayonet-like proboscis that protrudes forward from the head.

Treatment and Control: The main consideration in stable fly control is sanitation, which can effect up to 90% control. Areas along fence rows, under feed bunks, or wherever manure and straw or decaying matter can accumulate should be kept clean because these substrates provide the medium in which the larval flies develop. If good sanitation procedures are practiced, chemical control is less likely to be needed. Various insecticides can be sprayed where flies may be resting in barns or on fence rows.

Stable flies feed on the lower portions of cattle, around the legs and belly, including the udder. They usually feed only once or twice daily for short periods, thus minimizing exposure to compounds applied to these areas. Often, insecticides applied to these body regions are rubbed off by contact with dense vegetation and mud or rinsed off when dairy cattle are rinsed prior to milking. Pour-on pyrethroid products are ineffective against stable flies on dairy cattle.

HORN FLIES

The common name of *Haematobia irritans* comes from the fact that these flies often cluster in the hundreds around the base of the horns of cattle. This major pest of cattle is found in most cattle-producing areas of the world. Populations are common in Europe, North Africa, Asia Minor, and the Americas. Throughout North America, horn flies are found almost exclusively on cattle, but they will feed on horses, sheep, goats, and wildlife. Horn flies are found in much larger numbers and for longer periods of time in the southern and southwestern USA.

Adult horn flies spend their entire life on their host, and females leave only to oviposit eggs on fresh cow feces, where larval and pupal development occurs. In the southern USA, the life cycle can be as short as 1 wk, but in cooler climates and in the spring or fall, development can take 2-3 wk. In some warmer areas (south Florida and southernmost Texas), horn flies reproduce actively throughout the year.

When the air temperature is <70°F (21°C), horn flies cluster around the base of the horns of cattle. In warmer climates, the flies often cluster in large numbers on the shoulders, back, and sides; these areas are least disturbed by tail switching. On hot sunny days, horn flies accumulate on the ventral abdomen.

Newly emerged flies seeking their host may travel 7-10 miles (11-15 km) but usually find a host in much shorter distances. Migration seldom occurs over any great distance. In the southern USA, fly populations on individual animals may be in the thousands, especially on bulls not receiving chemical treatment; in the north, they may not exceed 100, although the damage inflicted is similar.

Pathology: Horn flies feed frequently (up to 20 times/day), sucking blood and other fluids; female flies are more aggressive than males. Feeding causes pain, annoyance, and blood loss in cattle. Irritated animals also lose weight because of their less efficient use of feed. Heavy infestations cause lesions along the ventral midline of the animal. Horn flies cause great economic losses annually in the USA; 14% reductions in weight gains on range cattle and losses of 12-14 lb (5-6 kg/head) in weaned calves are common. In dairy cattle, milk production may be reduced 10-20%. These flies also serve as the intermediate host for *Stephanofilaria stilesi*, a filarial parasite that produces plaquelike lesions on the ventral abdomen of cattle.

Diagnosis: Horn flies can be easily identified by their dark color, size (~3-6 mm long, about half the size of a stable fly), and bayonet-like proboscis that protrudes forward from the head.

Treatment and Control: Horn flies are relatively easy to control with whole-animal chemical sprays and with self-treating devices (eg, dust bags or back rubbers) in a forced-use manner. Dust bags are most effective when cattle are required to pass under them daily to reach water or mineral supplements. Dust bags leave a deposit of insecticides along the dorsum, the areas where horn flies spend most of their time. Back rubbers allow cattle to treat themselves as they scratch. The insecticide should be diluted with a good grade of mineral oil according to label instructions. Feed additives pass through the animal to kill larval stages that develop in fresh cow feces. All animals must eat a minimum dose of a feed additive regularly. Insect growth regulators also prevent development of larvae in cow feces. When used according to label directions, insecticide-impregnated cattle ear tags (eg, pyrethroids) release small amounts of insecticides that are distributed over the animal during grooming or rubbing. Animals should be tagged at or near the beginning of fly season, the tags removed at or near the end of fly season, and alternate methods with nonpyrethroid insecticides used near the end of fly season. Pour-on insecticide formulations are also effective against horn flies. These compounds are applied to cattle in measured doses based on body weight. Most of these pour-ons function as contact insecticides.

BUFFALO FLIES

Buffalo flies, *Haematobia irritansexigua*, are similar to horn flies in size and appearance and in feeding and breeding habits. The buffalo fly is a primary pest of cattle and water buffalo but occasionally feeds on horses, sheep, or wildlife. It is distributed throughout northern Australia and New Guinea and is found in parts of southern, southeastern, and eastern Asia as well as Oceania; it is not found in New Zealand. Its life cycle is similar to that of the horn fly; the adult leaves the host long enough to oviposit on fresh manure, where development occurs. The life cycle may take as little as 7-10 days, depending on weather conditions.

Pathology: Buffalo flies irritate and annoy animals, usually biting about the shoulders and withers. Bite wounds may provide a site for screwworm (*Chrysomyia bezziana*) infection. During hot weather, the flies move to shaded parts of the body. Affected animals suffer blood loss and are irritated by the flies; feed efficiency and production may be affected adversely.

Diagnosis: Buffalo flies can be identified by their dark color, size (about half that of a stable fly), and bayonet-like proboscis that protrudes forward from the head.

Treatment and Control: Insecticides should be avoided in the treatment of buffalo fly populations. Many of the chemicals used to treat these flies result in meat residues. Buffalo flies have developed resistance to the synthetic pyrethroids and to some of the organophosphates. Buffalo fly traps have been developed in Australia. The trap consists of a rounded, clear plastic tent through which the cattle walk. The flies are brushed off the cattle within the tent and are then trapped inside where they die of desiccation. These traps remove ~80% of the buffalo flies each time the cattle pass through. When cattle pass through the trap every day or every second day, sufficient fly control is usually achieved.

TSETSE FLIES

The tsetse flies, *Glossina* spp, are important blood-feeding flies found in Africa (latitude 5°N to 20°S). Tsetse flies are narrow bodied, yellow to dark brown, and 6-13.5 mm long. When resting, their wings are held over the back in a scissor-like configuration. The thorax has a dull greenish color with inconspicuous spots or stripes. The abdomen is light to dark brown.

Both sexes are avid blood feeders. One copulation renders a female fly fertile for her lifetime, during which she can produce as many as 12 larvae. She produces 1 larva at a time, retaining it within her uterus; after ~10 days, the larva is deposited on loose, sandy soil, where it digs in and begins pupation within 60-90 min. This pupation period averages ~35 days, after which the adult emerges. Adult flies feed avidly on vertebrate blood about every 3 days.

Pathology: Tsetse flies serve as the intermediate hosts for several species of trypanosomes that cause fatal diseases of both domestic animals (nagana) and humans (African sleeping sickness). Trypanosomes invade the blood, lymph, CSF, and various organs of the body, such as the liver and spleen. Nagana, a related complex in cattle caused by *Trypanosoma brucei*, has occurred over enormous areas estimated to be as great as one quarter of the African continent. The disease is fatal to horses, mules, camels, and dogs.

Cattle, sheep, and goats usually survive, except when parasitized by certain strains. Many wild ungulates native to Africa show no evidence of harm. *See also* TRYPANOSOMIASIS, p 32.

Diagnosis: Tsetse flies can be identified by their honeybee-like appearance, the long proboscis with its onion-shaped bulb at its base, and the unique wing venation with the characteristic cleaver- or hatchet-shaped cell in the center of the wing.

Treatment and Control: Tsetse flies can be controlled by catching and trapping (tsetse traps), bush clearing, fly screens, repellents, insecticides, and sterile male release techniques.

SHEEP KEDS

The sheep ked, *Melophagus ovinus*, is one of the most widely distributed and important external parasites of sheep. There are also keds that parasitize deer in North America (*Lipoptena depressa* and *Neolipoptena ferrisi*).

Keds are wingless dipterans. The adult is ~7 mm long; a brown or reddish color; and covered with short, bristly hairs. The head is short and broad, and the legs are strong and armed with stout claws.

The female gives birth to a single, fully developed larva, which is cemented to the wool and pupates within 12 hr. A young ked emerges after ~22 days. Females live 100-120 days and produce ~10 larvae during this time; males live ~80 days. The entire life cycle is spent on the host. Keds that fall off the host usually survive <1 wk and present little danger of infestation to a flock. Ked numbers increase during the winter and early spring when they spread rapidly through a flock, particularly when sheep are assembled in close quarters for feeding or shelter.

Pathology: To feed, sheep keds pierce the skin with their mouthparts and suck blood. They usually feed on the neck, breast, shoulder, flanks, and rump but not on the back where dust and other debris collect in the wool. Ked bites cause pruritus over much of the host's body; sheep will often bite, scratch, and rub themselves, thus damaging the wool. The fleece becomes thin, ragged, and dirty. The excrement of the keds causes permanent discoloration, which is likely to reduce the value of the wool. Keds also cause a defect in hides called a cockle, which affects the grade and value of the sheep skin. Infested sheep, particularly lambs and pregnant ewes, may lose vitality and become unthrifty. Heavy infestations can considerably reduce the condition of the host and even cause anemia. Keds also transmit *Trypanosoma melophagium*, a nonpathogenic protozoan parasite of sheep.

Diagnosis: Close inspection of the damaged, dirty wool and underlying skin reveals infestation by the unique appearance of these wingless, hairy flies.

Treatment and Control: Shearing removes many pupae and adults. Thus, shearing before lambing and subsequent treatment of the ewes with insecticides to control the remaining keds can greatly reduce the possibility of lambs becoming heavily infested. Sheep are usually treated after shearing, and best results are obtained if an insecticide that has a residual activity of ≥3-4 wk is used. By this means, the keds that emerge from the pupae are also killed. Modern treatments to control lice also control keds.

Dipping is also an effective method of treatment. Completely submerging the sheep in vats ensures the destruction of all keds present but, in most instances, does not kill the pupated larvae; a long-acting insecticide is required to kill newly emerging keds. Large flocks of range sheep should be treated in a permanently constructed dipping vat. Smaller flocks and farm flocks may be successfully treated in portable, galvanized-iron dipping vats or in smaller tanks, tubs, or canvas dipping bags.

Spraying may be as effective as dipping and is more convenient in some areas. Pressures of 100-200 lb/sq in. (7-14 kg/cm^2) for short wool and 300-350 lb/sq in. (21-28 kg/cm^2) for long wool are commonly used.

Shower dipping is also sometimes used; the sheep are held in a special pen and showered from above and below until the fleece is saturated. The run-off is returned for recirculation, and the concentration of insecticide used is the same as for dipping. The concentration of the insecticide can drop rapidly and become ineffective if the instructions for replenishment are not followed explicitly.

Jetting involves the forceful application of the insecticide by means of a hand-held, multiple-jet comb drawn through the short fleece. Although a little slower and less effective than dips or sprays, it may be advantageous for smaller flocks because it is economical and does not require a permanent installation.

Spot-on or pour-on formulations of the newer pyrethroids are easy to apply and very effective.

Powder dusting fits well into management practices at shearing time. It is rapid, economical, and avoids wetting the animals. Various types of equipment for dusting are available commercially.

HIPPOBOSCID OR LOUSE FLIES

The hippoboscid or louse flies, *Pseudolynchia* and *Lynchia* spp, are winged versions of the keds. They infest many song birds, raptors, and pigeons. The pigeon fly, *P canariensis*, is an important parasite of domestic pigeons throughout the tropical and subtropical regions of the world. It is found throughout the southern USA and northward along the Atlantic coast to New England. These dark brown flies have long wings (6.5-7.5 mm) and are able to fly swiftly from the host.

Pathology: Hippoboscid flies move about quickly among the feathers of their avian hosts and bite and suck blood from parts that are not well feathered. They may serve as intermediate hosts for many avian blood protozoans of the genus *Haemoproteus*. Pigeon flies readily attack people who handle adult birds; the bite is said to be as painful as a bee sting, and its effects may persist for ≥5 days.

Diagnosis: Close inspection of the ruffled feathers and underlying skin reveals infestation by the unique appearance of these winged, swiftly flying flies.

Treatment and Control: Any flies on the birds can be killed by spraying the birds with permethrin. Thorough cleaning of the premises and destruction of the debris are essential for control. Spraying the loft with permethrin, when coupled with cleaning, will alleviate the infestation.

DIPTERANS WITH NONBITING MOUTHPARTS

FACE FLIES

Face flies, *Musca autumnalis*, are so named because they gather around the eyes and muzzles of livestock, particularly cattle. They may also be found on the withers, neck, brisket, and sides. Their mouthparts are adapted for sponging up saliva, tears, and mucus. Face flies are usually not considered blood feeders because their mouthparts are not piercing or bayonet-like. However, they follow blood-feeding flies, disturb them during the feeding process, and then lap up the blood and body fluids that accumulate on the host's skin. Face flies are found on animals that are outdoors and usually do not follow animals into barns.

Face flies are found on rangeland cattle throughout southern Canada and most of the USA. The mouthparts consist of sponging labellae, and there are 4 longitudinal stripes on the abdomen. Although similar in appearance to the common house fly, face flies can be differentiated by the closeness and angles of the interior margins of the eyes and by the distinctive coloration of the face and abdomen. Speciation requires the skills of a trained entomologist.

Cattle are the principal host of the face fly in the USA, but face flies will also feed on horses and probably sheep and goats. The face fly is a pest of range cattle; it does not develop in feedlot situations and thus is not a parasite of confined cattle. The eggs are laid in fresh cattle feces in rangeland situations and hatch in ~1 day. The yellowish larvae develop in 2-4 days and, when mature, leave the manure to pupate in the surrounding soil. The complete life cycle from egg to adult requires 12-20 days, depending on climatic conditions. The diapausing adult overwinters within buildings and other protective places.

Pathology: Face flies annoy the host and ultimately interfere with the host's productivity. Females feed on facial secretions, such as tear fluid, nasal mucus, and saliva, to obtain protein for egg development. The irritation around the host's eyes stimulates the flow of tears, which attracts even more flies.

Face flies also feed on other fluid sources, such as blood from wounds and milk on calves' faces. Because face flies have small, rough spines (prestomal teeth) on their sponging mouthparts, only a few flies can cause irritation and mechanical damage to the eye tissue of the host. The feeding activity of face flies enhances transmission of *Moraxella bovis* (*see* INFECTIOUS KERATOCONJUNCTIVITIS, p 412). Face flies can also serve as intermediate hosts for *Thelazia* spp and for *Parafilaria bovicola*.

Diagnosis: Adult face flies are morphologically similar to house flies. These 2 species can be differentiated only by minor differences in eye position and color of the abdomen. Speciation requires the skills of a trained entomologist. In general, if a medium-sized fly is found feeding around the eyes and nostrils of a cow or horse, it is most probably a face fly.

Treatment and Control: Control of face flies is difficult. Much effort has been made using various insecticides and application techniques, such as dust bags, mist sprays, and wipe-on formulations. Also, insecticides and insect growth regulators are used as feed additives. However, results are usually less than satisfactory. The introduction of insecticide-impregnated ear tags has provided somewhat better control, but generally, seasonal face fly reduction of only 70-80% has been achieved, even with 2 tags (1 in each ear) per animal.

HEAD FLIES
(Plantation flies)

Head flies or plantation flies, *Hydrotaea irritans*, are nonbiting flies found in large numbers in northern European countries, especially Denmark and Great Britain, where they are pests of cattle, sheep, and other livestock. This fly resembles the house fly and is ~4-7 mm long. The thorax is black with gray patches, the abdomen is olive green, and the wing bases are orange yellow.

Head flies are a nuisance to domestic animals and humans because they are attracted to the mouth, nose, ears, eyes, and wounds to feed on secretions. Unlike other *Hydrotaea* spp, *H irritans* produces 1 generation per year, with 3 larval instar stages. Eggs deposited in late summer hatch out larvae within a few days. The saprophagous stage is brief, before development to the stage that is predatory on other insect larvae. Overwintering occurs as late-stage larvae. Adults are most active from early June until late September and are common in the vicinity of thickets or woodlands in which they shelter between periods of feeding.

Pathology: In Great Britain, sheep are mainly affected. Large swarms of flies, attracted by the movement of animals, congregate to feed on secretions from the eyes and nose and on the cellular debris at the grown horn base. To alleviate the persistent irritation, the sheep scratch and rub their heads, resulting in raw wounds or "broken heads," especially on the poll. Flies, attracted by the blood, settle on these self-inflicted lesions and extend the margins by their feeding activity. Sheep of all ages are involved, but breeds with horns and without wool on the head are most severely affected.

Head flies also attack humans, deer, horses, cattle, and rabbits. Although no corresponding broken head lesions develop in cattle, the occurrence of summer mastitis (due to *Corynebacterium pyogenes*) and the seasonal activity of head flies are closely associated, especially in Denmark. Head flies may also be involved in the spread of myxomatosis in rabbits.

Treatment and Control: The development, emergence, and congregation of head flies, which occur away from farm areas, preclude the traditional methods of insecticide spraying of generalized breeding sites and resting habitats. Control at the point of contact between the feeding adult insects and the mammalian hosts is also limited in value. With sheep, the retention of organophosphate compounds or pyrethrin derivatives on the susceptible head areas is of short duration, which necessitates impractical reapplications in free-ranging animals. Use of insecticide-impregnated ear tags in cattle decreases the incidence of summer mastitis, presumably by reducing transmission by head flies.

Removal of livestock from infested locations during the fly season is the only completely effective way to prevent damage. Once broken heads have occurred, the housing of sheep is the only successful method of stopping further fly damage.

FILTH-BREEDING FLIES

The following adult dipterans are often referred to as filth-breeding flies: *Musca domestica* (the house fly); *Calliphora, Phaenicia, Lucilia,* and *Phormia* spp (the blow flies or bottle flies); *Sarcophaga* spp (the flesh flies); *Fannia* spp (the little house flies); *Muscina* spp (the false stable flies); and *Hermetia illucens* (the black soldier flies). Large populations of these adult flies are often found around facilities associated with animal feces. Larval stages may be associated with skin wounds contaminated with bacteria or with a matted hair coat contaminated with feces (*see* FACULTATIVE MYIASIS, p 727). The life cycle of *Musca domestica* will be used as a representative example of that of the filth-breeding flies.

The house fly is commonly found around livestock and poultry operations, where it readily breeds in accumulating manure sources. It is a medium-sized (up to 9 mm), grayish fly with 4 dark thoracic stripes and sponging, nonbiting mouthparts designed for sucking semiliquid food (there are no mandibles or maxillae). The labium is expanded into 2 labellae that can transfer fluids and semifluids.

After oviposition, the creamy-white, banana-shaped egg (~1 mm long) hatches in 6-12 hr under optimal conditions. The eggs are not resistant to drying, and few appear to survive temperatures >40°C or <15°C. Larvae may develop in a few days to 3 wk, depending on the temperature and availability of food. When temperature for larval development is optimal (~36°C), the larvae develop to pupae in ~6 hr. Pupae persist 4-5 days in warm weather. After the adults emerge, the flies search for food and copulate after a few days. The life cycle is usually completed in ~3 wk, although it can be completed in as little as 10-14 days under favorable conditions. In temperate climates, it is thought that house flies overwinter as pupae.

Pathology: Even though these flies do not feed on blood, annoyance caused by their movement on and off animals can lead to reduced performance. In addition, they have been implicated in the transmission of numerous pathogens (helminth, protozoan, bacterial, and viral) of humans and other animals. Large populations of these adult flies often are found around poorly managed livestock or poultry facilities and become a public annoyance. These are synanthropic flies, ie, they are often associated with human dwellings. The flies are "vomit drop" feeders and fly from feces to food, spreading bacteria on their feet and within their disgorged stomach contents.

Diagnosis: All adult filth-breeding flies have similar sponging, nonbiting mouthparts, designed for sucking semiliquid food. The identification of adult flies is probably best left to a specialist. House flies are medium sized, grayish flies with 4 dark thoracic stripes. A preliminary identification of blow flies or bottle flies may be made on the basis of the metallic coloring of the adults. Flesh flies are medium sized, grayish flies with a checkerboard abdominal pattern.

Treatment and Control: A thorough sanitation program is necessary to control fly populations in and around livestock and poultry facilities. All manure accumulations should be removed at least twice a week or handled properly, if stored on the premises, to minimize fly breeding. If solid manure management practices are applied, efforts should be made to reduce manure moisture. If a liquid manure pit is used, manure should not be allowed to accumulate above the waterline, either floating or sticking to the sides, because this is an ideal site for fly reproduction. Insecticides should be considered as supplementary to sanitation and management measures aimed at preventing fly breeding. Residual sprays providing 2-4 wk control with 1 treatment may be applied to fly-resting surfaces. Space sprays, mists, or fogs with quick knockdown but no residual action can be used for immediate reduction of high numbers of adult flies. Other measures for control of adult flies include use of insecticide resin strips or various fly baits. These measures also can be applied directly to fly-breeding sources; however, this should be considered only for fly-breeding spots that cannot be eliminated by normal sanitation practices.

EYE GNATS

The eye gnats or the eye flies (*Hippelates* spp) are very small (1.5-2.5 mm long) flies that frequently congregate around the eyes, as well as mucous and sebaceous secretions, pus, and blood.

In the desert and foothill regions of southern California, adult *Hippelates* flies are present throughout the year; they are annoying from April through November. During the peak months, they are noticeable in the early morning and late afternoon. They enjoy the deep shade, such as among densely planted shrubs or in the shade of a dwelling. The eggs are ~0.5 mm long, fluted, and distinctly curved. They are deposited on or below the surface of the soil. The larvae hatch and feed on decaying organic matter, including excrement. The larval stage lasts 7-11 days. During the winter months, the larval and pupal stages may persist for many weeks. Pupation occurs close to the surface of the soil and lasts ~6 days. The entire life cycle lasts ~21 days. The adults are generally strong flyers, flying both with and against the wind.

Pathology: Some species are attracted to the genital organs of mammals; for example, *H pallipes* clusters around a dog's penis. These gnats quietly approach their mammalian hosts. They usually alight some distance from their feeding site and then crawl over the skin, or fly intermittently and alight, thus avoiding annoyance to the host. They are persistent and, if brushed away, quickly return to continue engorging themselves. They are nonbiting flies; however, the labellae have spines that scarify host tissue and allow entrance of pathogenic organisms. *Hippelates* flies often hover around the body orifices of calves, yearlings, pregnant heifers, and lactating cows. They feed on lacrimal fluid, fatty body secretions, milk droplets, and on secretions at the tips of the teats of animals. *Hippelates* flies also serve as vectors for *Arcanobacterium (Actinomyces) pyogenes* (summer mastitis) and *Moraxella bovis* (pinkeye).

Diagnosis: These small flies have sponging type mouthparts. They resemble house flies in form and structure and have short aristate antennae.

Treatment and Control: Repellents, such as those recommended for mosquitos, provide temporary relief from eye gnats. Applications of insecticides on a community-wide basis (as would take place with mosquito abatement) may provide temporary control of adults, but more adults invade the treated area after the insecticide has dissipated.

DIPTERANS THAT PRODUCE MYIASIS

Larval dipterans may develop in the subcutaneous tissues of the skin or organs of many domestic animals, producing a condition known as **myiasis**. There are 2 types of myiases based on degree of host dependence. In **facultative myiasis**, the fly larvae are usually free-living; however, under certain circumstances, these larvae can adapt themselves to a parasitic dependence on a host. In **obligatory myiasis**, the fly larvae are completely parasitic, ie, they depend on the host to complete the life cycle. Without the host, obligatory parasites will die.

FACULTATIVE MYIASIS-PRODUCING FLIES

The following larval dipterans are often referred to as facultative myiasis-producing flies: *Musca domestica* (the house flies); *Calliphora, Phaenicia, Lucilia,* and *Phormia* spp (the blow flies or bottle flies); and *Sarcophaga* spp (the flesh flies). Their adult stages are synanthropic flies, ie, they are often associated with human dwellings and readily fly from feces to food. Larval stages are usually associated with skin wounds of any domestic animal that have become contaminated with bacteria or with a matted hair coat contaminated with feces. In the larval stages, the characteristics of the distinctive posterior spiracular plates and the cephalopharyngeal skeleton are unique for each species and are used for identification.

The life cycle of *Musca domestica* is a representative example of that of the filth-breeding flies (*see* p 726). Several species of blow flies cause myiasis in sheep. Primary flies in the USA and Canada are *Phormia regina* and *Protophormia terraenovae* (the black blow flies) and *Lucilia sericata* (the green bottle fly). *L illustris, Cochliomyia (Callitroga) macellaria* (secondary screwworm), and some others are usually secondary invaders. *L cuprina* is the most important primary fly in Australia and South Africa; *L sericata* in Great Britain; and *L cuprina, L sericata*, and *Calliphora stygia* in New Zealand.

Eggs, usually laid below the tip of the fleece, hatch within 24 hr if conditions are moist. Moisture and nutrients from serum, feces, etc, are necessary for survival of first-stage larvae. Second-stage larvae can abrade the skin with their mouth hooks to obtain food. Once established, strikes can spread rapidly and attract more blow flies, secondary as well as primary. Mild strikes can cause rapid loss of condition, and bad strikes can be fatal. Strikes should be diagnosed early; behavior of sheep is a good indicator of myiasis. Affected animals become depressed, stand with their heads down, do not feed, and attempt to bite the infested areas. Screwworm may be suspected if the larvae are associated with wounds.

Pathology: Under normal conditions, adult flies of these genera lay their eggs in feces or in decaying animal carcasses. In facultative myiasis, the adult flies are attracted to a moist wound, skin lesion, or soiled hair coat. A common site is the breech, where flies may be attracted to wool soaked with urine or feces. As adult female flies feed in these sites, they lay eggs. The eggs hatch, producing larvae (maggots) that move independently about the wound surface, ingesting dead cells, exudate, secretions, and debris, but not live tissue. This condition is known as fly strike or strike. The larvae irritate, injure, and kill successive layers of skin and produce exudates. Maggots can tunnel through the thinned epidermis into the subcutis. This process produces tissue cavities in the skin that measure up to several centimeters in diameter. Unless the process is halted by appropriate therapy, the infested animal may die from shock, intoxication, histolysis, or infection. A peculiar, distinct, pungent odor permeates the infested tissue and the affected animal. Advanced lesions may contain thousands of maggots.

The body of the sheep also may be struck. This is usually associated with soaking rains that cause the development of fleece rot, often characterized by discoloration due to *Pseudomonas* spp or dermatophilosis. Other sites are the horns of rams, wool around the prepuce, sides where feet with footrot come in contact with fleece, and wounds.

As adults, these flies can be pestiferous in veterinary clinics, farms, or poultry operations. The flies are vomit drop feeders and fly from feces to food, spreading bacteria on their feet and from their disgorged stomach contents.

These fly larvae have also been associated with toxic effects in chickens. Botulism (p 2286), also known as limberneck in chickens, has been associated with ingestion of large numbers of larvae of *Lucilia caesar, Phaenicia sericata*, and other species of flies. *Clostridium botulinum* multiplies in carrion, where it may be picked up by fly larvae breeding in that medium and then passed on to chickens that eat the maggots. Dead animals should be speedily and safely disposed of, preferably by incineration.

Diagnosis: The species of myiasis-producing flies can be definitively identified by closely examining the larvae. The caudal ends of several third-stage larvae infesting the wound should be sliced using a scalpel blade. When the sliced caudal ends are placed cut surface down on a glass slide, covered with a coverglass, and examined under a compound microscope, a dichotomous key can be used to identify the genus or genera of flies within the wound. The unique spiracular plates are distinct for a particular genus. Several specimens should be examined because more than one genus may be present within the lesion. The first larvae to hatch in the lesion often create a favorable medium attractive to flies of other genera. Also, the possibility of obligatory myiasis caused by *Cochliomyia hominivorax* (*see* p 729) or *Chrysomyia bezziana* (*see* p 731) should be considered.

Treatment and Control: Blow fly infestation of the breech can be effectively controlled for ~6-8 wk by tagging or crutching (ie, wool is shorn between the legs and around the tail). Complete shearing controls outbreaks involving other parts of the body. Wool removed from around the head and the prepuce can prevent strike in these areas. Urine staining of the crutch of Merino ewes can be virtually eliminated by removal of breech wrinkles (Mules operation), and fecal contamination can be greatly reduced by docking tails at the third joint. Scouring should be controlled. Odors and associated moisture attract flies and stimulate oviposition, particularly during hot, humid weather.

Chemoprophylaxis consists of wetting to complete saturation of susceptible areas with suitable insecticidal and larvicidal preparations, such as the organophosphate insecticides or cyromazine, a specific larvicide in dips and sprays. Jetting is the most efficient procedure—insecticide is forced into the fleece, usually locally to the breech and along the back and head, under high pressure. Protection can last 6-8 wk, but where the primary fly is resistant (eg, *L cuprina* in Australia), it may last only 2-3 wk. Weekly application of agents such as ronnel (2.5%) under pressure to wounds until healed can be highly beneficial, particularly for screwworm infestation. Before suitable agents are applied, all wool should be removed from the struck area and around it.

Burning or deep burying of the carcass may be a valuable general hygienic measure but may have little effect on primary strikes. The main source of primary flies is the struck sheep. A genetic manipulation approach has been used to control a strain of blow fly in Australia; male flies are partially sterile but transmit a gene that causes blindness in female offspring.

Treatment and control measures for myiasis in dogs and cats are limited. If these larvae are detected in small animals, immediate therapy is necessary. The hair coat should be clipped to determine the extent of the lesion and to remove many of the larvae present in the hair. Removing maggots from existing deep tissue pockets may be difficult, and sedating or even anesthetizing the animal may be necessary. The lesion should be examined on successive days; adult flies lay eggs in the wound at different times, and hatching of larvae may not be synchronous.

Depressed, febrile, and prostrate animals should be treated according to their clinical signs. Ideally, culture and sensitivity studies should be performed on samples or scrapings of the wounds. If secondary bacterial or fungal infections are present, administration of broad-spectrum antibiotics is advisable.

With respect to prevention, owners should be educated about the effectiveness of treating all skin wounds. Animals with skins wounds should be confined to fly-free areas. The hair coat should be kept clean of urine or feces and should not be permitted to become matted. Contaminated wounds and matted hair coats soaked in urine or feces rapidly attract adult myiasis-producing flies. The control of adult flies in the field and the destruction of their breeding places are excellent preventive measures. All areas should be free of opened garbage cans and decaying carcasses or carrion.

OBLIGATORY MYIASIS-PRODUCING FLIES

Many dipteran flies produce larvae that lead a parasitic existence and result in obligatory myiasis. Only 1 fly in North America, *Cochliomyia hominivorax*, is a primary invader of fresh, uncontaminated skin wounds of domestic animals. Another species of screwworm, *Chrysomyia bezziana*, is found in Africa and southern Asia, including Papua New Guinea.

Cochliomyia hominivorax
(Primary screwworm, New World screwworm)

Cochliomyia hominivorax is distributed throughout the neoarctic and neotropical regions of the western hemisphere. As a result of massive state, federal, and international eradication programs, extant populations of *C hominivorax* are no longer found in the USA or Mexico; isolated reports are often traced to importation of infested animals from locations where the screwworm is still prevalent. Extant populations are found in Central and South America and in certain Caribbean Islands.

Adult female flies lay batches of 200-400 eggs in rows that overlap like shingles in a mass on the edge of a fresh wound. After 12-21 hr, larvae hatch, crawl into the wound, and burrow into the flesh. The larvae feed on wound fluids and live tissue. After 5-7 days, grown larvae exit from the wound, fall to the ground, and burrow in the soil to pupate. The pupal period varies from 7 days to 2 mo, depending on the temperature. Freezing or sustained soil temperatures <46°F (8°C) kill the pupae. Adults breed only once during their lifetime, a fact used in biologic control. They usually mate when 3-4 days old, and gravid females are ready to oviposit when ~6 days old. In warm weather, the life cycle may be completed in 21 days. Only female flies feed and oviposit on wounds; males and younger, virgin females gather to mate in vegetation, especially flowering vegetation.

Pathology: Newly infested wounds contain screwworm larvae of a single age; older, larger wounds may contain larvae of various ages and of different species of flies. The malodorous, reddish brown fluid produced in the wound usually drains and may stain the hair or wool around or below the wound. As annoyance increases, the infested animal seeks protection by retreating to the densest available shade. Even a small and relatively inconspicuous wound infested with screwworm larvae attracts not only more screwworm flies but also facultative myiasis-producing flies. Necrotic tissues attract even more flies. The wound can become greatly enlarged due to multiple infestation and, unless treated, usually results in death of the animal.

Diagnosis: The parasitic larvae are tapered and have mouth hooks at the narrow end and breathing spiracles at the wide end. Body segments are ringed with spines. Fully grown larvae can be as long as 1.5 cm. Larvae are often identified by their "wood screw" shape and appearance and can be distinguished from the larvae of the facultative myiasis-producing flies by the darkly pigmented tracheal tubes on the dorsal aspect of the posterior end of third-stage larvae. These tubes can be easily visualized through the larval cuticle.

Adult screwworm flies are similar in appearance to other blow flies. They are bluish to bluish green, have a reddish orange head and eyes, and are slightly larger than a house fly. They are difficult to distinguish from other blow flies or bottle flies. Identification of adult screwworms is probably best left to an entomologist.

Treatment and Control: Screwworm infestation must be reported to both state and federal authorities. *C hominivorax* has been eradicated from the USA but occasionally enters the country surreptitiously on imported animals. In the USA, if a wound is thought to be infested with screwworm larvae, appropriate samples should be collected and sent to eradication officials at P.O. Box 969, Mission, TX, 78572.

Screwworms in wounds can be killed by direct application of a wound dressing, called a smear. Such smears, which contain lindane or ronnel, may be difficult to find in the USA because of the eradication program. Smears are best applied with a 1-in (2.5-cm) paint brush and should reach all of the many pockets formed by the burrowing larvae in deep wounds. A thin layer should also be applied to the skin surrounding the wound to protect it from reinfestation. Wounds may also be treated with aerosol, dust, or foam formulations of coumaphos, lindane, or ronnel. To protect animals from infestation and also to kill larvae in small wounds that are difficult to detect, animals can be sprayed thoroughly with ronnel or sprayed with or dipped in coumaphos.

Sterile Male Release Eradication Program: In 1958, the USDA initiated a program in the southeastern states to eliminate screwworms by the sterile male release technique. When reared artificially and exposed to irradiation shortly before they emerge from the pupae, male flies are sterile but able to mate. The female mates only once, and when mated with a sterile male, lays eggs that do not hatch. Therefore, release of sufficient numbers of sterile males in an area over a period of time leads to eradication. By 1959, screwworms had been eliminated from Florida. The program cost ~$11 million, whereas the fly and its treatments had been estimated to cost $200 million annually.

This program was expanded to cover the rest of the area involved in the USA and then, via a joint Mexico-USA agreement, to include most of Mexico. This, along with the use of screwworm attractant and an insecticide system that attracted and killed adults, led to eradication of screwworms from Mexico. There is interest in expanding this area throughout Central America and the Caribbean. However, until this has been achieved, constant vigilance by all who deal with animals in the southern USA and Mexico is necessary to detect an infestation quickly and to eradicate it before the flies reproduce and spread.

Chrysomyia bezziana
(Old World screwworm, Oriental fly, Bezzi's blow fly)

Chrysomyia bezziana is found in Africa, the Indian subcontinent, and southeast Asia from Taiwan in the north to Papua New Guinea in the south. This fly is not indigenous to Australia. Owing to its geography, the most likely potential port of entry for *C bezziana* to the USA is Hawaii.

The adult screwworms are usually not seen in the field. The adult fly has a dark metallic green body with abdominal segments with narrow bands along the posterior margins. The legs are black or partially brown. The face is orange-yellow. The first larval stage probably goes unnoticed because of its small size, up to 3 mm at the time of its molt to the second stage. The second stage is quite similar to the third but is 4-9 mm long. The third-stage larvae are large, up to 18 mm long. The body is composed of 12 segments that have broad encircling bands of spinules. All 3 stages are maggot-like in their appearance and have posterior spiracles that are unique to the species. The posterior end of the larva has its spiracular plate located in a deep cleft at the end of the eighth abdominal segment. The spiracular plates are large and well separated. The peritreme and the 3 breathing slits are wide.

C bezziana produce a particularly vile myiasis. Female flies are attracted to open wounds of humans and domestic and wild animals, laying their eggs in masses of 150-500 at the edge of wounds or near body orifices. Larvae develop to the third stage ~2 days after hatching. They burrow deep into the wound such that only their posterior ends are visible. The entire larval stage lasts 5-6 days. The pupal stage lasts 7-9 days in tropical conditions and longer in cooler environments. The adult flies emerge later to mate, locate a new host, and continue the cycle. Female flies mate only once during their lifetime—a fact paramount in prevention and control. Under favorable conditions, there may be ≥8 generations per year.

Pathology: The larvae of *C bezziana* are obligatory wound parasites, never developing in carcasses or decomposing organic material. Although female flies are attracted to open wounds, occasionally eggs are deposited on the unbroken, soft skin of various parts of the body, especially if contaminated by blood or mucous discharge. When the larvae hatch, they burrow into the flesh of the host, using their hooked mouthparts to scrape away at the tissues and lacerate the fine blood vessels. Larvae are voracious blood feeders. During the blood-sucking phase, only the caudal ends of the maggots with their blackish peritremes remain visible at the surface of the lesion, enabling the larvae to breathe. As many as 300 maggots have been seen in some wounds. In untreated wounds, the destructive activity of the larvae may lead to the death of the animal within a very short time. Secondary infestation with the facultative myiasis-producing flies (*see* p 727) may complicate treatment and control.

Diagnosis: The identification of the rarely observed adult flies and their associated larval stages is best left to an entomologist. A definitive diagnosis can be made only after observation, extraction, and identification of typical larvae. Diagnosis may often be made by residence in or history of travel to an area endemic for *C bezziana*. If a wound is thought to be infested with larvae of *C bezziana*, samples should be collected and sent to appropriate eradication officials.

Treatment and Control: Treatment of screwworm infestation involves killing the larvae in the lesions, promoting healing, and preventing secondary reinfestation with larvae of the facultative myiasis-producing flies. The extent of the lesions is determined by clipping the hair coat and removing as many larvae as possible. The larvae that are removed should be killed to prevent them from pupating and developing into adults. Larvae located deep within tissues must be extracted.

Ivermectin at dosages of 50, 100, and 300 µg/kg administered to infested cattle resulted in 100% larval mortality for at least 6, 12, and 14 days, respectively. Depending on their age, larvae survived in established strikes after treatment at 200 µg/kg. Mortality was 100% in larvae up to 2 days old but less in older larvae. However, many of the larvae that survived ivermectin therapy failed to develop to the adult stage. After treatment with 200 µg/kg, residual protection lasted 16-20 days, 2-3 times that of most insecticide smears.

All wounds on domestic animals should be properly dressed, and all elective surgical procedures avoided during the fly season.

The fact that the female flies mate only once during their lifetime is an important fact to consider in the control of *C bezziana*. Pupal flies exposed to irradiation lead to sterile adults that can be released to breed with wild male and female flies. As a result, no viable offspring are produced in the wild.

Wolves (Warbles) of Small Animals

Larvae of the genus *Cuterebra* are often referred to as wolves, warbles, rabbit bots, or rodent bots. These fly larvae infest the skin of rabbits, squirrels, mice, rats, chipmunks, and occasionally dogs and cats. *See* CUTEREBRA INFESTATION IN SMALL ANIMALS, p 710, for clinical findings, diagnosis, and treatment.

Gray Flesh Fly

The gray flesh fly, *Wohlfahrtia vigil* is responsible for cutaneous myiasis in North America, particularly in southern Canada and the northern part of the USA. The adult flies have been recorded from the New England states to Alaska, but most reports are from eastern sections of Canada and the neighboring northeastern parts of the USA. All reports of infestation are in the skin of healthy animals, particularly the unbroken skin of the young.

All 3 larval stages are maggot-like in their appearance and have posterior spiracles that are unique to the species. The first larval stage is 1.5 mm at hatching and grows to 3.5 mm at the time of its molt to the second stage. The third stage is 7.0-18.5 mm long. Its posterior end is narrow, and it is covered with many irregular rows of small spines that have dark points and are directed posteriorly. This larva is better adapted to maintain an attachment to living tissues. The oral hooks are strongly developed. The posterior end of the larva has its spiracular plate located in a deep pit formed by the margins of the segment. The posterior spiracles have wide slits and a strong peritreme.

The gray flesh fly is larviparous—it deposits larvae instead of eggs on healthy, uninjured skin of suitable hosts, particularly young animals. Larvae penetrate the unbroken skin and form a boil-like (furuncular) swelling. Development to the infective third-larval stage is usually completed in 9-14 days. The parasites then drop to the ground and pupate, ~11-18 days, varying with the season of the year and the temperature. When cold weather approaches, the pupation period is greatly prolonged. Under laboratory conditions, it has been observed to last 7 mo. Parasites survive the winter in pupal form. Adults emerge and mate after ~3-4 days. Female flies begin larviposition ~1 wk later, depositing 6-16 larvae at a time. Female flies live for 35-40 days; males seldom survive >3 wk.

Pathology: Female *W vigil* deposit active larvae near or directly on the host. Although larvae usually penetrate unbroken skin, in small animals, penetration may go deeper than the dermal tissue, even into the coelomic cavity.

The first indication that an animal is infected is exudation of serum and matting of the hair coat over the site of penetration. In light-skinned animals, a small inflammatory area is noticeable in the center or to one side of which a tiny hole is visible. These lesions may be palpated as they develop. On the third or fourth day, the larvae are 1.5-2 cm long and produce abscess-like lesions resembling those of *Hypoderma* spp in cattle. These lesions vary in size, shape, position, and the number of larvae they contain. The hair coat often becomes parted over the summit of the lesions and reveals an opening 2-3 mm in diameter. The posterior aspect of the larva is visible in these openings, through which it breathes. Openings are generally circular and well-defined; however, if several larvae are present in a single lesion, the shape of the opening is quite variable. Small animals infected with ≥5 larvae for several days become emaciated, and the skin becomes dry and loses its luster.

The penetration of the skin by the larvae, their development in the subcutaneous tissues, and secondary bacterial infection produce intense irritation and inflammation. Attempts by the animal to remove the larvae or relieve the irritation tend to aggravate the condition. Young animals may die from exhaustion. It has also been suggested that the larvae may produce toxic secretions. *W vigil* has been isolated from the skin of young children, particularly infants.

Diagnosis: Adult gray flesh flies are nonparasitic and as a result will probably not be seen by owners or veterinarians. They are large grayish flies (~13 mm long), about twice the size of a house fly. The dorsal surface of the thorax is marked with 3 longitudinal bands, while the dorsal surface of the abdomen has 3 well-defined rows of oval black spots that are confluent with one another.

The identification of adult flies and their associated larval stages should be left to an entomologist. The presence of a dermal swelling with a central opening may lead to a tentative diagnosis of myiasis due to *W vigil*. A definitive diagnosis can be made only after extraction and identification of a typical larva. Extensive descriptions and dichotomous keys for the 3 larval stages are available. A tentative diagnosis may often be made by a history of either residence in or travel to a geographic area endemic for *W vigil*.

Treatment and Control: Larvae must be extracted from the skin. Applying heavy oil, liquid paraffin, pork fat, or petrolatum jelly to the opening of the lesions will occlude the airway of the larvae. Applying a small amount of chloroform or ether to the opening may be helpful before removing larvae with forceps. Lidocaine hydrochloride can also be injected into the furuncular lesion to facilitate extraction. Great care should be taken during the extraction process to avoid rupturing larvae in situ, although anaphylaxis has not been reported. Antibiotics should be prescribed.

This parasite often infects young mink. A teaspoon of ronnel can be placed in the bedding of their nest box as a control measure; however, ronnel should not be used in the bedding of kits <3 days old. Protection can be provided by keeping flies out of cages using wire gauze.

African Tumbu Fly
(Mango fly, Skin maggot fly, Ver du Cayor, Worms of Cayor)

The African tumbu fly, *Cordylobia anthropophaga*, is responsible for another boil-like (furuncular) myiasis in both humans and animals in Africa, particularly in the subSaharan regions.

The adult flies are nonparasitic and as a result are not seen by owners or veterinarians. They are stout, compact flies, 6-12 mm long. They are light brown, with diffuse blue-gray patches on the thorax, and dark gray on the posterior part of the abdomen. The face and legs are yellow. The second- and third-stage larvae are the stages usually seen in the animal's skin.

Second-stage larvae are slightly club-shaped and exhibit large, black cuticular spines that are directed posteriorly and distributed irregularly over segments 3-8. Segments 9-11 are almost bare when compared with the preceding segments. The segments have a few rows of small, pale spines posteriorly. Segment 12 is densely covered with these spines. Segment 13 is indistinctly demarcated, lacking spines but possessing 2 pair of short processes. Each tracheal tube opens through 2 slightly bent slits. The second-stage larvae are 2.5-4.0 mm long. The size of advanced second-stage larvae varies greatly, as does the size of third-stage larvae. Fully mature larvae are 1.3-1.5 cm long. The body is cylindrical with 12 identifiable segments. Curved spines that are directed posteriorly are densely arranged at least up to segment 7; the last 5 segments may be either partially or densely covered with spines.

After fertilization, female flies produce 100-500 banana-shaped eggs, usually depositing them in dry, shady, sandy soil that has often been contaminated by urine or feces.

Eggs are never deposited on the skin of the host. Eggs hatch after 1-3 days, and the larvae are initially 0.5-1.0 mm long. Larvae can survive up to 15 days while waiting for a host and can penetrate the host in as little as 25 sec. After penetration, larvae reside in a cavity in the dermis and hypodermis. This cavity communicates to the external environment by means of a central breathing pore, which corresponds to the caudal end of the larva with its spiracles. A single larva is found in each cavity, within which the larva develops to the second and third stages. Larvae require 7-15 days to mature and then emerge through the breathing pore and drop to the ground, where they pupate. Adult flies emerge 10-20 days later, and the cycle begins again.

Rats and dogs are the usual definitive host; however, humans, mice, monkeys, mongooses, squirrels, leopards, boars, antelopes, cats, goats, pigs, rabbits, guinea pigs, and chickens can be infested.

Pathology: Clinically, the infestation is characterized by a small erythematous papule that appears 2-3 days after larval penetration. Within days, the papule enlarges until it becomes a nodule that resembles a boil (furuncle); hence, the description furunculoid myiasis. At the center of the nodule is a pore through which serous fluid oozes. This fluid can be hemorrhagic or purulent and contains larval feces.

Dogs with thin, soft skin seem to be more suitable hosts for larval development than dogs with thick skin. Preferential sites of infestation are the feet, genitals, tail, and axillae. In endemic areas, mild infestations in dogs do not produce clinical distress. Massive infestation may induce marked swelling and edema, especially if larvae are in close proximity to each other. Larvae can penetrate deep into tissues and cause considerable damage and even death.

Diagnosis: The presence of a dermal swelling with a central opening may lead to a tentative diagnosis of myiasis due to *C anthropophaga*. A definitive diagnosis can be made only after extraction and identification of typical larvae. The identification of adult flies and their associated larval stages should be left to an entomologist.

A tentative diagnosis may often be made by a history of either residence in or travel to a geographic area endemic for *C anthropophaga*. However, the parasite has also been diagnosed in travelers and their accompanying pets from geographic areas where the parasite does not exist.

Treatment and Control: Larvae can be removed by coating the breathing pore with a thick, viscous compound, such as heavy oil, liquid paraffin, sticking plaster, pork fat, or petrolatum jelly. Clogging the pore causes the larva to become hypoxic and leave the cavity in search of oxygen. Light pressure at the edge of the lesion also aids in larval removal.

Lidocaine hydrochloride can be injected into the furuncular lesion to facilitate larval extraction with thumb forceps. Surgical excision is usually unnecessary and unwarranted while the larvae are alive but is used to remove dead or decaying larvae. Great care should be taken during the extraction process to avoid rupturing larvae in situ, although anaphylaxis has not been reported. Antibiotics should be prescribed.

Adult flies should be killed if seen indoors. Larvae should be removed from animals entering the house and destroyed. All rats should be killed and burned. Clothes should not be left lying out; they should be ironed and put away. Prevention of an infestation depends on cleanliness and regular disinfection of the animal's sleeping quarters. In the case of valuable animals (eg, Angora rabbits), flies may be kept out of rabbit pens using wire gauze.

Because the adult female flies lay eggs in sandy soil contaminated by feces or urine, the parasite can be controlled in the pet's environment by prompt removal of the pet's feces and by covering urination sites on the premises with a layer of dirt.

PSEUDOMYIASIS

In pseudomyiasis, dipteran larvae have been accidentally ingested and are found within an animal's GI tract, where they are not able to continue their development. Dogs or cats infested with larvae of the facultative myiasis-producing flies in wounds or in the hair coat often ingest larvae while licking or grooming. These larvae pass through the GI tract and appear in the feces undigested. Passage of dipteran larvae in the feces may also occur when a roaming dog or cat ingests carrion that contains maggots; these maggots pass to the external environment undigested.

Pseudomyiasis can also occur if feces submitted for parasitologic examination are not fresh. Adult facultative-myiasis flies may have laid their eggs in these feces, and larval development may have begun.

Eristalis tenax, the rat-tailed maggot, may be seen in the gutter behind cows in dairy barns. These maggots are associated with liquid feces and with feces that have not been removed from the environment. The larvae are known as rat-tailed maggots because their breathing pores are found at the tip of a long, siphon-like breathing tube on their posterior end. Many farmers erroneously assume that the cows defecated these maggots. The adults are nonparasitic, free-living flies.

HELMINTHS OF THE SKIN

CUTANEOUS HABRONEMIASIS
(Summer sores, Jack sores, Bursatti)

Cutaneous habronemiasis is a skin disease of Equidae caused in part by the larvae of the spirurid stomach worms (p 265). When the larvae emerge from flies feeding on pre-existing wounds or on moisture of the genitalia or eyes, they migrate into and irritate the tissue, which causes a granulomatous reaction. The lesion becomes chronic, and healing is protracted. Diagnosis is based on finding nonhealing, reddish brown, greasy skin granulomas that contain yellow, calcified material the size of rice grains. Larvae, recognized by spiny knobs on their tails, can sometimes be demonstrated in scrapings of the lesions. Many different treatments have been used, most with poor results. Symptomatic treatment, including use of insect repellents, may be of benefit, and organophosphates applied topically to the abraded surface may kill the larvae. Surgical removal or cauterization of the excessive granulation tissue may be necessary. Treatment with ivermectin (200 µg/kg) has been effective, and although there may be temporary exacerbation of the lesions (presumably in reaction to the dying larvae), spontaneous healing may be expected. Moxidectin at 400 µg/kg also appears to be active against *Habronema* spp in the stomach. Control of the fly hosts and regular collection and stacking of manure, together with anthelmintic therapy may reduce the incidence.

DRACUNCULUS INFECTIONS

Dracunculus insignis is found mainly in the subcutaneous connective tissues of the legs of raccoons, mink, and other animals, including dogs, in North America and possibly other parts of the world. The females (≥300 cm long) are much longer than the males (~20 mm). They produce ulcers in the skin of their host, through which their anterior end is protruded on contact with water. They lay characteristic long, thin-tailed larvae. Water fleas (*Cyclops* sp) are the intermediate host in which infective larvae develop. Dogs become infected through ingestion of contaminated water or a paratenic host (frogs).

Subcutaneous, serpentine, inflammatory tracts and nonhealing, crater-like, edematous skin ulcers are seen. Infections are rare but are occasionally found in animals that have been around small lakes and bodies of shallow, stagnant water. Treatment is by careful, slow extraction of the parasite. Administration of miridazole or benzimidazole compounds may be useful.

D medinensis, the guinea worm of parts of Africa, Asia, and the Middle East, although primarily a parasite of humans, is also found in dogs and other animals.

ELAEOPHOROSIS
(Filarial dermatosis, "Clear-eyed" blindness, Sorehead)

Elaeophora schneideri is a parasite of mule deer and black-tailed deer found in the mountains of western and southwestern USA; it also has been found in white-tailed deer in the southern and southeastern regions. Adult parasites are 60-120 mm long and usually are found in the common carotid or internal maxillary arteries. The microfilariae, ~275 μm long and 15-17 μm thick, normally are found in skin capillaries on the forehead and face. Development in the intermediate hosts, horse flies of the genera *Tabanus* and *Hybomitra*, requires ~2 wk. Infective larvae invade the host as the horse fly feeds, migrate to the leptomeningeal arteries, and develop to immature adults in ~3 wk. These young adults migrate against the blood flow and establish in the common carotid arteries, where they continue to grow. The parasites reach sexual maturity ~6 mo later and begin producing microfilariae. The life span of adults is 3-4 yr.

Clinical Findings: Clinical disease has not been reported in mule deer and black-tailed deer; therefore, they are considered to be the normal definitive hosts. When horse flies transmit the infective larvae to elk, moose, domestic sheep and goats, sika deer, and possibly white-tailed deer, the larvae develop in the leptomeningeal arteries and cause ischemic necrosis of brain tissue, resulting in blindness, brain damage, and sudden death. Blindness in these animals is characterized by absence of opacities in the refractive media of the eye ("clear-eyed" blindness).

Domestic sheep and goats, especially lambs, kids, and yearlings, may die suddenly 3-5 wk after infection. Death is usually preceded by incoordination and circling and often by convulsions and opisthotonos. Numerous thrombi occur in the cerebral and leptomeningeal arteries. One or more young adult *E schneideri* accompany each thrombus. If sheep or goats survive the early infection, a raw bloody dermatitis on the poll, forehead, or face ("sorehead") develops 6-10 mo later. Lesions occasionally develop on the legs, abdomen, and feet. These lesions are an allergic dermatitis in response to the microfilariae lodged in capillaries. Lesions persist, with periods of intermittent and incomplete healing for ~3 yr, followed by spontaneous recovery. Hyperplasia and hyperkeratosis develop in the epidermis of the parasitized area.

Diagnosis: Differential diagnoses include coenurosis (*Taenia*, p 1035), cerebrocortical necrosis (p 1061), and enterotoxemia (p 493). Elaeophorosis should not be considered unless sheep have been in endemic areas during the summer. Diagnosis in lambs, kids, or elk yearlings or calves usually is made at necropsy; numerous thrombi and parasites are found in the common carotid, internal maxillary, cerebral, and leptomeningeal arteries. Presumptive diagnosis in mature sheep is based on history and location and type of lesion. The skin lesion must be differentiated from that of ulcerative dermatosis (p 703). Confirmation is by recovery of microfilariae from the lesion or by postmortem recovery of the adult parasites. A skin biopsy of the lesion is macerated in isotonic saline solution and allowed to stand ≥6 hr at room temperature. The skin is strained off and the fluid examined for the typical microfilariae.

Treatment: Piperazine salts (220 mg/kg, PO) are effective. Complete recovery occurs in 18-20 days. No treatment is available for the cerebral form of the disease.

ONCHOCERCIASIS

The taxonomic status of the 3 species of *Onchocerca* currently recognized in the USA, and other previously recognized species, is under debate. *O cervicalis* is found in the ligamentum nuchae and possibly other sites in Equidae. In cattle, *O gutturosa* locates in the ligamentum nuchae, and *O lienalis* in the gastrosplenic ligament. Adults are associated with connective tissues and are very thin and 3-60 cm long. Microfilariae are found in the dermis and on rare occasions circulating in peripheral blood. The microfilariae lack a sheath and are 200-250 μm long with a short, sharply pointed tail. *Culicoides* spp are the intermediate hosts for *O cervicalis*, and *Simulium* spp for *O gutturosa* and *O lienalis*.

Clinical Findings: *O cervicalis* has been associated with fistulous withers, poll evil, dermatitis, and uveitis in horses. However, because large numbers of the parasite are common in horses without these diseases, there is some debate about its role in the pathogenesis of these conditions.

Adults in the ligamentum nuchae induce inflammatory reactions ranging from acute edematous necrosis to chronic granulomatous changes, resulting in marked fibrosis and mineralization. Mineralized nodules are more common in older horses. Although lesions are found in these areas, presumably associated with dead parasites, it is generally agreed that fistulous withers and poll evil are not caused by *O cervicalis* infections.

Microfilariae concentrate in the skin of the ventral midline. Large numbers can be found in horses without dermatitis as well as in horses with dermatitis of the face, neck, chest, withers, forelegs, and abdomen. These lesions often include areas of scale, crusts, ulceration, alopecia, and depigmentation; they may be pruritic. The dermatitis may be associated with an immunologic reaction to dead and dying microfilariae. Although the pathogenesis of these lesions is unclear, treatment with microfilaricidal drugs may result in dramatic improvement. Allergic reactions to the bites of small flies may produce similar lesions or exacerbate microfilaria-associated dermatitis. Thus, diagnosis of *Onchocerca*-associated dermatitis may be based on responsiveness to microfilaricidal treatment.

Microfilariae also accumulate in the eyes of horses, but not all agree that a clear association has been made between microfilariae and equine uveitis (p 407) or other ocular lesions in horses.

Diagnosis: The most effective method of diagnosis is by skin biopsy, preferably a full-thickness biopsy ≥6 mm. The tissue is minced and macerated in isotonic saline for several hours. Microfilariae are concentrated and stained with new methylene blue after removal of skin pieces. The microfilariae can be differentiated microscopically from *Setaria* spp, which are found in the blood of cattle and Equidae, by the presence of a sheath around *Setaria*. (*See also* SWEET ITCH IN HORSES, p 717.)

Treatment: No treatment is effective against the adults. Ivermectin (200 µg/kg) and moxidectin (400 µg/kg) are efficacious (>99%) against microfilariae and produce marked clinical improvement in horses with onchocercal dermatitis. A small portion of horses infected with *O cervicalis* react to the treatment with a marked, edematous ventral midline swelling 1-3 days after treatment. Ocular lesions have also been reported. These reactions usually resolve spontaneously, but symptomatic treatment may be necessary.

PARAFILARIA INFECTION

Parafilaria bovicola

This filarial parasite of cattle causes subcutaneous lesions that resemble bruising. It also has been reported from water buffalo (*Bubalus bubalis*). The worm is whitish; adult females are 50-65 mm long, and males 30-35 mm. It is found in Asia (Philippines, Japan, Russia, Pakistan, India), Europe (Bulgaria, Romania, France, Sweden), and Africa (Morocco, Tunisia, Rwanda, Burundi, South Africa, Namibia, Botswana, Zimbabwe). A specimen was recovered in Canada from a bull imported from France, but *P bovicola* does not appear to have established itself on the American continents and has not been reported from Australia.

Parafilaria infection has been identified as a source of considerable economic loss to the beef industries of South Africa and Sweden, despite their climatic differences. The disease occurs primarily in range cattle in the savanna areas of southern Africa, whereas in Sweden, it has emerged as a problem in cattle following spring turnout to pasture after winter housing.

The only external signs of infection in cattle are focal cutaneous hemorrhages ("bleeding spots") that may ooze for some hours before clotting and drying in the matted hair of the coat. Bleeding spots are induced by the female worm, which causes the formation of a small nodule, perforates the skin, and oviposits in the blood dripping from the central wound. The tiny eggs contain the first larval stage (microfilariae) of the parasite. In both the northern and southern hemispheres, bleeding spots are markedly seasonal, being most common in spring and early summer. Most bleeding spots occur along the dorsum of the animal, particularly in the forequarters.

The invertebrate hosts are face flies of the genus *Musca* (subgenus *Eumusca*), which ingest the eggs when feeding at the bleeding spots. *M autumnalis* has been identified as a host in Sweden, *M lusoria* and *M xanthomelas* in South Africa, and *M vitripennis* in Asia. Development to infective third-stage larvae in the fly takes 10-12 days. Transmission to cattle probably occurs when the flies feed on wounds, *Parafilaria* bleeding spots, or ocular secretions.

Because of seasonal bleeding and the cutaneous nodules, severe infections of *P bovicola* have been reported to impair the productivity of working bullocks in India; however, the major importance of *Parafilaria* in beef-producing countries is damage to the subcutaneous tissues. Carcasses of infected animals display irregular, edematous, greenish yellow lesions that resemble bruising. These are usually superficial, but occasionally underlying muscles are extensively involved. Lesions are most severe during the spring and summer.

Trimmed carcasses are often seriously disfigured and consequently downgraded. In severe cases, the carcass may be condemned. Lesions are more common and severe in bulls than in steers, which in turn are less severely affected than female animals.

The seasonal bleeding spots are sometimes confused with those caused by thorns, wire, ticks, or biting insects. For differentiation, either fresh or dried blood should be mixed with water in a test tube and centrifuged. The characteristic eggs are found on microscopic examination of the sediment.

Carcass lesions can be differentiated from bruising by the presence of numerous eosinophils in Giemsa-stained impression smears made from the lesions. In addition, affected tissue has a characteristic, disagreeable, metallic smell.

Usually, only small numbers of worms are present in affected carcasses and are often difficult to find because of their color and the accompanying inflammatory reaction. Affected tissues can be incubated in warm saline to facilitate the recovery of parasites. An ELISA for the detection of antibodies against *P bovicola* has been developed.

Ivermectin (200 µg/kg) or nitroxynil (20 mg/kg) given by SC injection reduces the number and surface area of *Parafilaria* lesions. Animals should be treated at least 70-90 days before slaughter to provide sufficient time for lesions to resolve. The treatment-to-slaughter interval should not be >120 days because unaffected larval forms of the parasite may induce fresh lesions as they mature.

In trials in Sweden, use of pyrethroid-impregnated ear tags gave good control of flies and reduced parafilarial lesions at slaughter by 75%. Ear tagging all cattle in an area resulted in total control of the parasite. The use of residually active, synthetic pyrethroid dips has also been effective in reducing transmission.

It may be possible to screen imported animals with the ELISA to prevent spread of the disease to presently unaffected countries or, in conjunction with residual insecticides and effective anthelmintics, to eradicate new foci of infection.

Parafilaria multipapillosa

P multipapillosa is found in the subcutaneous tissues of horses in various parts of the world; it is especially common in the Russian steppes and eastern Europe. It is similar in size, appearance, life cycle, and development to *P bovicola*. Blood-sucking *Haematobia* spp are thought to be the invertebrate hosts.

In spring and summer, the parasite causes skin nodules, particularly on the head and upper forequarters. These bleed transiently but often profusely ("summer bleeding") and then resolve; other hemorrhaging nodules develop as the parasite moves to a different site. Occasionally, the nodules suppurate. The nodules and bleeding are unsightly and interfere with harnesses of working horses but generally are of little consequence. The clinical signs are pathognomonic.

No satisfactory treatment is available, but fly control may reduce the incidence.

PELODERA DERMATITIS
(Rhabditic dermatitis)

This rare, nonseasonal, acute dermatosis results from invasion of the skin by larvae of the free-living saprophytic nematode *Pelodera (Rhabditis) strongyloides*. The larvae are ubiquitous in decaying organic matter and on or near the surface of moist soil but are only occasionally parasitic. Exposure to the larvae occurs through direct contact with infested material such as damp, filthy bedding. The larvae may not be able to invade healthy skin; preexisting dermatoses or environmental conditions favoring maceration of the skin, eg, constant exposure to mud or damp bedding, may facilitate invasion. *Pelodera* dermatitis has been reported in dogs, cows, horses, sheep, guinea pigs, and humans.

Typically, lesions are confined to body areas in contact with the infested material, such as the extremities, ventral abdomen and thorax, and perineum. Affected skin is erythematous and partially to completely alopecic, with papules, pustules, crusts, erosions, or ulcerations. Pruritus is usually intense but can be moderate or even absent. Differential diagnoses include demodicosis, canine scabies, dermatophytosis, pyoderma, and other rare cutaneous larval infestations such as hookworm dermatitis, dirofilariasis, dipetalonemiasis, and strongyloidiasis.

Diagnosis is confirmed easily by finding live, motile *P strongyloides* larvae in skin scrapings of affected areas. The larvae are cylindrical and ~600 × 38 μm. Histologic examination of skin biopsy specimens reveals larvae in the hair follicles and superficial dermis and usually an inflammatory dermal infiltrate. The larvae are easily cultivated on blood agar plates at 77°F (25°C).

Effective treatment consists primarily of removing and destroying moist, infested bedding material and moving the animal to a clean, dry environment. Usually, spontaneous recovery ensues. It may be desirable to dip or spray the affected animals with an insecticidal preparation at least twice at weekly intervals. Short-term use of corticosteroids may be indicated if pruritus is severe.

STEPHANOFILARIASIS
(Filarial dermatitis of cattle)

Stephanofilaria stilesi is a small filarial parasite that causes a circumscribed dermatitis along the ventral midline of cattle. It has been reported throughout the USA but is more common in the west and southwest. The adult worms are 3-6 mm long and usually are found in the dermis, just beneath the epidermal layer. Microfilariae are 50 μm long and are enclosed in a spherical, semirigid vitelline membrane. The intermediate host for *S stilesi* is the female horn fly, *Haematobia irritans* (p 721). Horn flies feeding on the lesion ingest microfilariae that develop to the third-stage infective larvae in 2-3 wk. The infective larvae are introduced into the skin as the horn fly feeds.

The dermatitis develops along the ventral midline, usually between the brisket and navel. With repeated exposure, the lesion spreads and often involves the skin posterior to the navel. Active lesions are covered with blood or serous exudate, while chronic lesions are smooth, dry, and devoid of hair. Hyperkeratosis and parakeratosis occur in the epidermis of the parasitized area.

Deep skin scrapings are macerated in isotonic saline solution and examined microscopically for adults or microfilariae. The microfilariae must be differentiated from microfilariae of *Onchocerca lienalis*, *O gutturosa*, and *Setaria* spp, which are much larger (200-250 μm), and *Pelodera strongyloides* (*see* above), a small free-living nematode that is occasionally responsible for a moist, superficial dermatitis. The rhabditiform esophagus of *P strongyloides* is not found in filarial nematodes.

No approved treatment is available for *S stilesi*, but topically applied organophosphates (trichlorfon 6-10%, SID or on alternate days for 7 days) have proved effective against other species of *Stephanofilaria*.

LICE
(Pediculosis)

Numerous species of biting or chewing lice (order Mallophaga) and sucking lice (order Anoplura) are obligate ectoparasites of domestic animals. Lice live within the microenvironment provided by the skin and its hair or feathers, and are transmitted primarily by contact between hosts. In temperate regions, lice are most abundant during the colder months and often are very difficult to find in the summer. Lice are largely host-specific, living on one species or several closely related species. Anoplura are parasites of mammals only. However, Mallophaga infest both mammals and birds. (*See also* ECTOPARASITES OF POULTRY, p 2272.)

Etiology: Lice are wingless, flattened insects, usually 2-4 mm long. The claws of the legs are adapted for clinging to hairs or feathers. Mallophaga have ventral chewing mandibles and they feed on epidermal products, primarily skin scales and scurf. The head of the mallophagan is wider than the prothorax. Anoplura are blood feeders. When not in use, their mouthpart stylets are retracted within the head.

Louse eggs or nits are glued to hairs of mammalian hosts near the skin surface and are pale, translucent, and suboval. The 3 nymphal stages, of increasing size, are smaller than adults but otherwise resemble them in habits and appearance. About 3-4 wk are required to complete one generation, but this varies with species.

In temperate climates, cattle may be infested with one species of Mallophaga, the cattle biting louse, *Damalinia (Bovicola) bovis*, and 3 species of Anoplura: the long-nosed cattle louse, *Linognathus vituli*; the little blue cattle louse, *Solenopotes capillatus*; and the shortnosed cattle louse, *Haematopinus eurysternus*. It is not uncommon for cattle, especially young animals, to be infested with 2, 3, or all 4 species. These lice may be found on the head (including the ears), neck, topline, and brisket. In heavy infestations, they may be found over most of the body.

Haematopinus quadripertusus, the cattle tail louse, is a tropical, sucking louse that has extended its distribution into subtopical areas (California, Florida, and Gulf Coast in the USA). The adults and ova are found in the tail switch; nymphs may be found on other parts of the body, including the perineum and vulva. The cattle tail louse is known to parasitize both European and Zebu breeds of cattle.

Haematopinus tuberculatus, the louse of the Asiatic water buffalo, appears to have transferred to cattle in various parts of the world, and is able to maintain itself on cattle in tropical climates. These lice are usually found on the back and hindlegs, although the eggs are usually deposited on the neck, shoulders, and forelegs of the host.

Horses and donkeys may be infested by 2 species of lice, *Haematopinus asini*, the horse sucking louse, and *Damalinia equi*, the horse biting louse. Both species are worldwide in distribution. Normally, *H asini* is found at the roots of the forelock and mane, around the base of the tail, and on the hairs just above the hoof. *D equi* prefers to oviposit on the finer hairs of the body and is found on the sides of the neck, the flanks, and the base of the tail.

Domestic pigs are infested with only one species of louse, *Haematopinus suis*, the hog louse. This very large (5-6 mm) sucking louse is common on domestic swine worldwide. Nymphal lice are normally found on the inside of the ears, often deep inside; on the skin behind the ears; in the folds of the neck; on the inside of the legs, close to the body; and on the inner flanks. All stages may be found under the scurf of the skin elsewhere on the body.

Sheep may become infested with the sheep biting louse, *Damalinia ovis*, and 3 species of sucking louse: the sheep foot louse, *Linognathus pedalis*; the face and body louse, *L ovillus*; and the African blue louse, *L africanus*. Outside the USA, *D ovis* is also referred to as the sheep body louse. The foot louse of sheep is so named because, except in very heavy infestations, it is confined to the hairy parts of the foot. The face louse is usually found on hairy parts of the sheep's skin; as populations increase, they spread to other parts of the body. *L africanus* forms clusters, often on the flanks of coarse-wooled sheep. Slippage of wool is common. *L africanus* has also been reported from a variety of hosts including goats and several species of deer.

Linognathus stenopsis, the goat sucking louse, is found on both shorthaired and Angora breeds of goats. It has been reported from sheep in various parts of the world. *Damalinia caprae*, the goat biting louse, is most frequently found on short-haired goats, whereas chewing lice on Angora breeds are more likely to be *D limbatus* (the Angora goat biting louse) or *D crassipes*.

Dogs are occasionally infested with *Linognathus setosus* (the dog sucking louse), and the biting louse, *Heterodoxus spiniger*. Animals in poor health may become heavily infested. *H spiniger*, which may be quite rare in North America, serves as an intermediate host of the tapeworm *Dipylidium caninum* and of the filarial worm *Dipetalonema reconditum*. The cat louse, *Felicola subrostrata*, is a chewing louse that occasionally parasitizes cats. The louse may be seen more frequently on older, longhaired cats that are unable to groom themselves.

Clinical Findings and Diagnosis: Pediculosis is manifest by pruritus and dermal irritation with resultant scratching, rubbing, and biting of infested areas. A generally unthrifty appearance, rough coat, and lowered production in farm animals are common. In severe infestations, there may be loss of hair and local scarification. Extreme infestation with sucking lice can cause anemia. In sheep and goats, rubbing and scratching often results in broken fibers, which gives the fleece a "pulled" appearance. In dogs, the coat becomes rough and dry and, if lice are numerous, the hair may be matted. Sucking lice cause small wounds that may become infected. The constant crawling and piercing or biting of the skin causes nervousness in hosts.

Diagnosis is based on the presence of lice. The hair should be parted, and the skin and proximal portion of the coat examined with the aid of light if indoors. The hair of large animals should be parted on the face, neck, ears, topline, dewlap, escutcheon, tail base, and tail switch. The head, legs, feet, and scrotum should not be overlooked, particularly in sheep. On small animals, the ova are readily seen. Occasionally, when the coat is matted, the lice can be seen when the mass is broken apart. Biting lice are active and can be seen moving through the hair. Sucking lice usually move more slowly and are often found with mouthparts embedded in the skin.

Pediculosis of livestock is most prevalent during the winter; severity is greatly reduced with the approach of summer. Infestations, particularly of sucking lice, may become severe. In dairy herds, the young stock, dry cows, and bulls may escape early diagnosis and suffer more severely. Young calves may die, and pregnant cows may abort. Effective treatment results in prompt improvement.

Transmission usually occurs by host contact. Lice dropped or pulled from the host die in a few days, but disengaged ova may continue to hatch over 2-3 wk in warm weather. Therefore, premises recently vacated by infested stock should be disinfected before being used for clean stock.

Treatment: Louse control requires treatment with an effective insecticide or drug (*see* ECTOPARASITICIDES, p 2158, and ANTHELMINTICS, p 2124). Products that may be used are determined by government regulations, and users are required to read and follow product labels. Formulations classified for restricted use may be purchased and used only by certified applicators or by persons under their direct supervision. Some product labels direct retreatment in 2 wk to control a particularly refractory infestation.

A few compounds may be applied as a whole-body spray for lice control. A light, mist application of some formulations may be effective, while others may require soaking the hair to the skin.

Zero to very low residue tolerances for pesticides in milk limit the insecticides that may be applied to dairy cattle and dairy goats. Permethrin spray may be applied to these animals for control of lice. Additionally, dairy cattle may be sprayed with permethrin synergized with piperonyl butoxide, coumaphos, tetrachlorvinphos plus dichlorvos, and amitraz. Nonlactating goats may be sprayed with several compounds, including fenvalerate, malathion, or methoxychlor. Beef cattle, sheep, and swine may be sprayed with coumaphos, malathion, methoxychlor, or permethrin. Tetrachlorvinphos, lindane, phosmet, and amitraz spray may be used on beef cattle and swine. Both swine and sheep may be sprayed with fenvalerate. A low-volume spray of fenvalerate is approved for sheep and nonlactating goats. Permethrin synergized with piperonyl butoxide, tetrachlorvinphos, and tetrachlorvinphos plus dichlorvos may be applied to both dairy and beef cattle. Diazinon spray is approved for control of lice on sheep. Horses may be treated with a permethrin spray, and horses not intended for slaughter may be sprayed with coumaphos or malathion.

Many, but not all compounds approved for beef cattle are approved for nonlactating dairy cattle. In lactating dairy cattle, appropriate milk withdrawal times must be observed.

Because of ease of application and reduced stress to the treated animal, the pour-on method has become a popular means of applying a variety of insecticides, both nonsystemic and systemic, for control of lice. Beef cattle, lactating and nonlactating dairy cattle, sheep, and nonlactating goats may be treated with pour-on formulations of permethrin for louse control. A wipe-on formulation of permethrin is available for lice control on horses. Because the percentage of active ingredient in commercial pour-on formulations varies from 1 to 10%, it is important that the formulation is approved for the animals being treated. A permethrin pour-on that is synergized with piperonyl butoxide is also available for lice control on beef cattle, lactating and nonlactating dairy cattle, and sheep. Fenvalerate pour-on is approved for louse control on swine, sheep, and nonlactating goats. Cyfluthrin pour-on is approved for beef cattle and lactating and nonlactating dairy cattle, but l-cyhalothrin is approved only for beef cattle. Fenthion is approved as a pour-on for beef cattle and nonlactating dairy cattle, and amitraz pour-on is approved for swine.

Several systemic insecticides are available as pour-on formulations for control of cattle lice as well as a variety of other parasites. Because these products also control cattle grubs, precautions should be taken to avoid host-parasite reactions (*see* CATTLE GRUBS, p 706). Pour-on formulations of doramectin, eprinomectin, famphur, fenthion, ivermectin, and moxidectin are effective against both chewing and sucking lice of beef cattle. Lactating dairy cattle may be treated with eprinomectin, fenthion, and moxidectin pour-on. Doramectin and ivermectin are also formulated as injectables, and ivermectin is available as an oral paste; however, these are less effective against chewing lice than are the typical pour-ons. A paste formulation of famphur is approved for control of both chewing and sucking lice of cattle. Ivermectin, injectable and premix, is effective against the sucking louse of swine.

Lice on beef cattle can be controlled or suppressed by wintertime use of self-treatment devices, eg, back rubbers, dust bags, and insecticide ear tags, that are used for fly control in the summer. Insecticide ear tags containing a variety of active ingredients (eg, organophosphate insecticides, pyrethroid insecticides, piperonyl butoxide) control or aid in the control of biting and sucking cattle lice. Some tags contain a single active ingredient, while others contain a mixture. All of the tags are approved for use on beef cattle; however, not all are approved for lactating dairy cattle. Louse populations also can be reduced by hand-dusting with coumaphos, methoxychlor, tetrachlorvinphos, or permethrin on beef or dairy cattle; malathion or phosmet on beef cattle and swine; permethrin on swine; and malathion on sheep and goats. For severe infestations, dust formulations of permethrin, tetrachlorvinphos, and coumaphos can be used to treat bedding of swine.

Dogs can be treated with dips, washes, sprays, or dusts. Effective compounds include permethrin, pyrethrins, rotenone, methoxychlor, lindane, diazinon, malathion, or coumaphos. Doses of ivermectin high enough to be effective against lice are not recommended in dogs. On cats, only carbaryl, rotenone, or pyrethrins should be used.

In most countries, regulatory agencies specify tissue residue limits of insecticides and carefully regulate insecticide use on livestock. All such regulations are subject to change; pertinent current local laws and requirements should be determined. The treatment of meat and dairy animals must be restricted to uses specified on the labels, and all label precautions should be carefully observed.

MANGE

(Cutaneous acariasis, Mite infestation)

MANGE IN CATTLE

Sarcoptic Mange (Scabies): This very contagious disease is spread by direct contact or indirectly by fomites. The causative mite, *Sarcoptes scabiei* var *bovis*, can be transmitted to humans and is a reportable disease. Lesions start on the head, neck, and shoulders and can spread to other parts of the body; pruritus is intense. Papules develop into crusts, and the skin thickens and forms large folds. The whole body may be involved in 6 wk. Diagnosis is made by deep skin scrapings, skin biopsy, or response to therapy. Treatment is as for psoroptic mange (*see* below).

Psoroptic Mange: This reportable disease, caused by *Psoroptes ovis*, does not spread to humans. It is seen in range and feedlot beef cattle from the central and western states of the USA, with the largest numbers of outbreaks reported from Texas, New Mexico, Oklahoma, Kansas, Colorado, and Nebraska. Intense pruritus usually begins on the shoulders and rump; papules, crusts, excoriation, and lichenification are seen. Lesions may cover almost the entire body; secondary bacterial infections are common in severe cases. Death in untreated calves, weight loss, decreased milk production, and increased susceptibility to other diseases can occur. Treatment can be done by spray dipping or vat dipping; topical application of nonsystemic acaricides; and oral, topical, or injectable formulations of systemic drugs. Spray dipping is time consuming but useful for small herds, whereas vat dipping is efficient but fairly expensive and difficult to manage (use of large volumes of water, disposal of wash solution). In the USA, 0.5-0.6% toxaphene spray (28-day withdrawal time); 0.3% coumaphos, 2 dippings (no withdrawal time); 0.20-0.25% phosmet, 2 dippings (21-day withdrawal time); or 2% hot lime-sulfur dip, 3 dippings (no withdrawal time) can be used for dipping. Outside the USA, other treatments are available, eg, 0.1% phoxim, 0.075% diazinon, and 0.025-0.050% amitraz. Dippings should be repeated at 10- to 14-day intervals. Only hot lime-sulfur is registered for use on lactating dairy cows. The topical application of flumethrin (2 mg/kg, twice at a 10-day interval) is also available in many countries outside the USA. Injectable formulations of avermectins (ivermectin and doramectin) and milbemycins (moxidectin) are approved for control of psoroptic and sarcoptic mange at 200 µg/kg (not in lactating dairy cattle). Although one treatment is effective, cattle should be isolated for 2 wk after treatment. Eprinomectin is available as a pour-on formulation at 500 µg/kg. It is approved for the control of sarcoptic mange (no withdrawal time).

Chorioptic Mange (Leg Mange): This reportable disease, caused by *Chorioptes bovis*, does not affect humans. It is the most common type of mange in cattle in the USA; it is more prevalent during the winter and often spontaneously regresses in summer. The pastern areas of the legs are preferred sites for the mites. A high proportion of cattle can be infested without showing clinical signs. Lesions start as papules, crusts, and ulcerations on the legs and can spread to the udder, scrotum, tail, and perineal area. Cattle can be treated with 0.25% crotoxyfos spray at high pressure to completely wet the animal; the other dips used for bovine psoroptic scabies are also effective against *Chorioptes*. They should be done twice at 10- to 14-day intervals. Lime-sulfur dip weekly for 4-6 dips is effective. Ivermectin, doramectin, eprinomectin, and moxidectin applied topically as a pour-on at 500 µg/kg are effective against chorioptic mange. With the exception of eprinomectin, these drugs are not approved in lactating dairy cattle.

Demodectic Mange: *Demodex bovis* is transferred from cow to calf while nursing and may cause considerable damage to hides. Pruritus is absent. Lesions consist of follicular papules and nodules, especially over the withers, neck, back, and flanks. Ulceration, abscesses, and fistulae can develop due to follicular rupture or secondary infection. Diagnosis is made by deep skin scrapings. Bovine demodicosis usually is benign, although the course may extend for many months. Recovery is usually spontaneous; consequently, treatment is rarely done. Trichlorfon dips (2%) every other day for 3 treatments have been reported to be curative.

Psorergatic Mange (Itch Mite): *Psorergates bos* has been reported in cattle in the USA, Canada, and South Africa. Affected animals show mild, patchy alopecia and pruritus. The disease does not cause significant economic losses; thus, animals are usually not treated. Several dips and injectable ivermectins and milbemycins are effective in controlling this infestation.

MANGE IN SHEEP AND GOATS

Sarcoptic Mange: *Sarcoptes scabiei* var *ovis* is rare in sheep and is reportable in the USA. It affects the nonwooly skin, usually starting on the head and face. In goats, *S scabiei* var *caprae* is responsible for a generalized skin condition characterized by marked hyperkeratosis. Lesions start usually on the head and neck. In both species, the injectable formulations of ivermectin, doramectin, or moxidectin at 200 µg/kg are efficient treatments.

Chorioptic Mange: *Chorioptes bovis* is common in Europe, New Zealand, and Australia during the winter. It has been eradicated in sheep in the USA and is a reportable disease. The distribution of lesions is the same as that in cattle. *C caprae* is fairly common in goats. Papules and crusts are seen on the feet and legs. If necessary, the animals can be treated using sprays or dips containing organophosphates (diazinon, metrifonate, propetamphos) or pyrethroids (deltamethrin, flumethrin) as permitted.

Psoroptic Mange (Sheep Scab): *Psoroptes ovis* infestation is a reportable disease. No cases have been reported in the USA since 1970, but sheep scab is still present in many countries, including some in western Europe. Large, scaly, crusted lesions develop almost exclusively on wooly parts of the body. Intense pruritus manifests by biting and scratching. Left untreated, sheep often become emaciated and anemic. Mites are sometimes found in the ears. Ivermectin and moxidectin (200 µg/kg) given twice with a 7- or 10-day interval, respectively, are effective. Doramectin (300 µg/kg) given once is also effective. Dipping is most effective if done within 2 wk after shearing and must be repeated after 14 days. Approved treatments for mange in sheep are 0.3% coumaphos, 0.15-0.25% phosmet, 0.03-0.1% diazinon, and 2% hot lime-sulfur. Outside the USA, other sprays or dips such as propetamphos, phoxim, amitraz, or flumethrin are available.

Psoroptic mange (ear mange) in goats, caused by *Psoroptes cuniculi*, usually affects the ears but can spread to the head, neck, and body and cause severe irritation. This occurs particularly in Angora goats, in which the mohair is considerably damaged. The disease in Angora goats is reportable in Texas. Although the course is chronic, the prognosis is good. Any of the acaricides approved for use in sheep will eliminate *P cuniculi* in goats. Lactating dairy goats should be treated only with lime-sulfur solution.

Demodectic Mange: This has been reported in sheep (*Demodex ovis*) and goats (*D caprae*), in which it causes lesions similar to those in cattle. In goats, nonpruritic papules and nodules develop, especially over the face, neck, shoulders, and sides. The nodules contain a thick, waxy, grayish material that can be easily expressed; mites can be found in this exudate. The disease can become chronic. Localized lesions in goats can be incised, expressed, and infused with Lugol's iodine or rotenone in alcohol (1:3). For generalized cases in goats, treatments include ronnel in propylene glycol (180 mL of 33% ronnel in 1 L of propylene glycol) applied to one-third of the body daily until cured, and rotenone in alcohol (1:3) applied to one-fourth of the body daily. Trichlorfon (2%) has been reported to be effective for demodicosis in sheep.

Psorergatic Mange (Itch Mite, Australian Itch): *Psorergates ovis* is a common skin mite of sheep in many parts of the world; it has been eradicated in the USA and is a reportable disease. The disease is characterized by intense generalized pruritus and scaliness, with matting and loss of wool. Because of their small size, the mites are difficult to find in skin scrapings. This disease can cause significant economic losses through weight loss and wool damage. Dipping or spraying with 2-3% lime-sulfur, 0.2% malathion, or 0.3% coumaphos is effective in controlling the disease; 2 treatments with a 14-day interval are needed. Ivermectin and other avermectins/milbemycins given SC have been reported to be curative.

MANGE IN HORSES

Sarcoptic Mange: *Sarcoptes scabiei* var *equi* is rare in the USA but is the most severe type of mange in horses. The first sign is intense pruritus due to hypersensitivity to mite products. Early lesions appear on the head, neck, and shoulders. Regions protected by long hair and lower parts of the extremities are usually not involved. Lesions start as small papules and vesicles that later develop into crusts. Alopecia and crusting spread, and the skin becomes lichenified, forming folds. If untreated, lesions may extend over the whole body, leading to emaciation, general weakness, and anorexia. Negative skin scrapings do not rule out the disease; biopsy may establish a diagnosis. If suspected, sarcoptic mange must be treated. Organophosphate insecticides or lime-sulfur solution can be used by spraying, sponging, or dipping. Treatment should be repeated at 12- to 14-day intervals at least 3-4 times. Alternatively, the oral administration of ivermectin or moxidectin at 200 µg/kg can be attempted. Several treatments are required 2-3 wk apart. It is important to treat all contact animals.

Psoroptic Mange: *Psoroptes equi* is rare in horses; it produces lesions on thickly haired regions of the body, such as under the forelock and mane, at the base of the tail, under the chin, between the hindlegs, and in the axillae. *P cuniculi* can sometimes cause otitis externa in horses and may cause head shaking. Pruritus is characteristic. Lesions start as papules and alopecia and develop into thick, hemorrhagic crusts. Mites are more easily recovered from skin scrapings compared with sarcoptic mange. Treatment is as for sarcoptic mange.

Chorioptic Mange (Leg Mange): Chorioptic mange is common in heavy breeds of horses. Lesions caused by *Chorioptes equi* start as a pruritic dermatitis affecting the distal limbs around the foot and fetlock. Papules are seen first, followed by alopecia, crusting, and thickening of the skin. A moist dermatitis of the fetlock develops in chronic cases. It is a differential diagnosis for "greasy heel" in draft horses. The signs subside in summer but recur with the return of cold weather. The disease course is usually chronic without treatment, but the prognosis is favorable when treated. Topical treatments recommended for other manges are effective.

Demodectic Mange: *Demodex equi* is rare in horses. The mites live in the hair follicles and sebaceous glands; *D equi* lives on the body, and *D caballi* in the eyelids and muzzle. Demodicosis in horses can manifest as patchy alopecia and scaling, or as nodules. Lesions appear on the face, neck, shoulders, and forelimbs. Pruritus is absent. This disease has been reported in association with chronic corticosteroid treatment. No effective treatment regimens have been developed. Amitraz, used in other species, is contraindicated in horses because it can cause severe colic and death.

Trombiculidiasis (Chiggers, Harvest Mite): Trombiculid mites can parasitize the skin of horses, especially during the late summer and fall. The adult mites live on invertebrates and plants; the larvae normally feed on small rodents, but they can opportunistically feed on humans and domestic animals including horses. Lesions consist of severely pruritic papules and wheals. Specific treatment is not required; the pruritus can be controlled with glucocorticoids. Repellents may help prevent infestation.

Straw Itch Mite (Forage Mite): These mites usually feed on organic material in straw and grain and can opportunistically infest the skin of horses. Papules and wheals appear on the face and neck if horses are fed from a hay rack, and on the muzzle and legs if fed from the ground. Pruritus is variable and can be controlled with glucocorticoids.

MANGE IN PIGS

Sarcoptic mange (*Sarcoptes scabiei* var *suis*) is the only form of any importance in pigs. Mange mites are typically introduced to a herd after the purchase of infested breeding stock, and spread after direct contact is rapid. Survival of the mite eggs away from the host is limited; however, exposure as little as 24 hr to pens that have been immediately vacated by previously infested pigs has resulted in infestation. Laboratory experiments indicate that mites did not survive >96 hr at temperatures <25°C or >24 hr at 20-30°C. Survival was <1 hr at temperatures >30°C.

S scabiei suis infestations are negatively correlated with daily weight gains and feed conversion in pigs. The lesions usually start on the head, especially the ears, then spread over the body, tail, and legs. Itching is usually intense and associated with a hypersensitivity reaction to the mites. As the hypersensitivity subsides, usually after several months, the thickened, rough, dry skin is covered with grayish crusts and thrown into large folds. Skin scrapings should be examined to differentiate mange from other skin diseases affecting swine, including ringworm. Pruritus is frequently a better indicator of infestation than mite recovery, especially in sows and nursing piglets. Spraying with lindane (0.05-0.1%) or malathion (0.05%) is effective; chlordane solution (0.25%) also has been used. (Use of some or all of these on food-producing animals is prohibited in some countries.) Ivermectin (300 µg/kg, SC) is also effective, and programs have been developed for elimination of mange on commercial farms. Injectable (300 µg/kg) and feed-grade (100 µg/kg) products are commercially available.

Demodectic mange is also seen in pigs, causing skin lesions similar to those seen in other large animals. There is no reliable treatment.

MANGE IN DOGS AND CATS

Sarcoptic Mange (Canine Scabies): *Sarcoptes scabiei* var *canis* infestation is a highly contagious disease of dogs found worldwide. The mites are fairly host-specific, but animals (including humans) that come in contact with infested dogs can also be affected. Adult mites are 0.3-0.5 mm long, roughly circular in shape, without a distinctive head, and have 4 pairs of short legs. Females are almost twice as large as males. The entire life cycle (17-21 days) is spent on the dog. Females burrow tunnels in the stratum corneum to lay eggs. Sarcoptic mange is readily transmitted between dogs by direct contact; infestation by indirect contact is less frequent but may occur. The incubation period is variable (10 days to 8 wk) and depends on level of exposure, body site, number of mites transmitted, and individuals. Asymptomatic carriers may exist. Intense pruritus is characteristic and is probably due to hypersensitivity to mite products. Primary lesions consist of a papular eruption that, due to self-trauma, develops thick crusts. Secondary bacterial and yeast infections may occur. Typically, lesions start on the ventral abdomen, chest, ears, elbows, and legs and, if untreated, become generalized. Dogs with chronic, generalized disease develop seborrhea, severe thickening of the skin with fold formation and crust buildup, peripheral lymphadenopathy, and emaciation; dogs so affected may even die. "Scabies incognito" has been described in well-groomed dogs; these dogs, infested with sarcoptic mites, are pruritic, but demonstrating the mites on skin scrapings is difficult because the crusts and scales have been removed by regular bathing. Untypical clinical forms that are probably linked to the extensive use of insecticides or acaricides may be observed.

Diagnosis is based on the history of severe pruritus of sudden onset, possible exposure, and involvement of other animals, including humans. Making a definitive diagnosis is sometimes difficult because of negative skin scrapings. Concentration and flotation of several scrapings may increase chances of finding the mites, eggs, or feces. Several extensive superficial scrapings should be done of the ears, elbows, and hocks; nonexcoriated areas should be chosen. Fecal flotation may reveal mites or eggs. Recently, a specific and sensitive ELISA for detection of specific antibodies became commercially available. If mites are not found, but the history and clinical presentation are highly suggestive of sarcoptic mange, trial therapy is warranted. Treatment can be either topical or systemic, and should include all dogs in contact. For topical treatment, hair can be clipped, the crusts and dirt removed by soaking with a good antiseborrheic shampoo, and an acaricidal dip applied. Lime-sulfur is highly effective and safe for use in young animals; several dips 5 days apart are recommended. Phosmet has been successfully used according to label instructions. Amitraz is an effective scabicide, although it is not approved everywhere for this use, and there have been some reports of lack of efficacy. Fipronil spray was reported to be effective but should be considered an aid in the control rather than a primary therapy. Systemic treatments of scabies are based on the administration of macrocyclic lactones. Among them, only selamectin is approved for this use; it is given as a spot-on formulation at 6 mg/kg twice at a 1-mo interval. This drug appears to be safe, even in ivermectin-sensitive Collies, and is the systemic treatment of choice. Other endectocides, such as moxidectin and ivermectin, which are not registered for the treatment of sarcoptic mange in dogs, have been reported to be quite effective depending on the dosage and route of administration. Ivermectin (200 µg/kg, PO or SC, 2 treatments 2 wk apart) is very effective and usually curative. Ivermectin at this dosage is contraindicated in Collies and Collie crosses. Idiosyncratic reactions in other breeds may also occur. Additionally, the heartworm status of the dog should be evaluated before treatment.

Notoedric Mange (Feline Scabies):   This rare, highly contagious disease of cats and kittens is caused by *Notoedres cati*, which can opportunistically infest other animals, including humans. The mite and its life cycle are similar to the sarcoptic mite. Pruritus is severe. Crusts and alopecia are seen, particularly on the ears, head, and neck, and can become generalized. Mites can be found in skin scrapings. Treatment consists of lime-sulfur dips at 10-day intervals. Nonapproved treatments include amitraz at half the concentration used in dogs, selamectin (4 mg/kg, spot on) and ivermectin (200 µg/kg, SC). Sudden death in kittens has been reported with the use of ivermectin.

Otodectic Mange: *Otodectes cynotis* mites are a common cause of otitis externa especially (p 421) in cats but also in dogs. Mites are usually found deep in the external ear canal, but occasionally are seen on the body. Clinical signs include head shaking, continual ear scratching, and ear droop. Pruritus is variable. Purulent inflammation and discharge of the external ear, and possible perforation of the tympanic membrane may be seen in severe cases. Affected animals should receive appropriate parasiticide treatment in the ears and on the whole body for 2-4 wk.

Cheyletiellosis (Walking Dandruff):   *Cheyletiella blakei* infests cats, *C yasguri* infests dogs, and *C parasitovorax* infests rabbits, although cross-infestations are possible. This disease is very contagious, especially in animal communities. Human infestation is frequent. Mite infestations are rare in flea endemic areas, probably due to the regular use of insecticides. These mites have 4 pairs of legs and prominent hook-like mouthparts. They live on the surface of the epidermis, and their entire life cycle (3 wk) is spent on the host. Clinical disease is characterized by scaling, a dorsal distribution, and pruritus, which varies from none to severe. Cats can develop dorsal crusting or generalized miliary dermatitis. Asymptomatic carriers may exist. The mites and eggs may not be easy to find, especially in animals that are bathed often. Acetate tape preparations, superficial skin scrapings, and flea combing can be used to make the diagnosis. Weekly dippings with pyrethrins or lime-sulfur for 6-8 wk are necessary to eradicate the mites. Fipronil and ivermectin are effective, but nonapproved, treatments. The environment should also be treated with a good acaricide, especially in animal communities (eg, breeding colonies, kennels), given the fact that adults may survive off the host for several days or even weeks.

Canine Demodicosis: This skin disease of dogs occurs when large numbers of *Demodex canis* mites inhabit hair follicles and sebaceous   glands. In small numbers, these mites are part of the normal flora of the skin of dogs and cause no clinical disease. The mites are transmitted from dam to puppies during nursing within the first 72 hr after birth. The mites spend their entire life cycle on the host, and the disease is not considered to be contagious. The pathogenesis of demodicosis is complex and not completely understood; evidence of hereditary predisposition for generalized disease is strong. Immunosuppression, natural or iatrogenic, can precipitate the disease in some cases. Secondary bacterial furunculosis or cellulitis may occur, leading to a guarded prognosis.

Two clinical forms (localized and generalized) of the disease exist. Localized demodicosis occurs in dogs <2 yr old, and most of these cases, especially the nummular forms, are thought to resolve spontaneously. Lesions consist of areas of focal alopecia, erythema and/or hyperpigmentation, and comedones. Pruritus is usually absent or weak. A percentage of these cases, especially the diffuse localized forms, progress to the generalized form. Generalized demodicosis is a severe disease with generalized lesions that are usually aggravated by secondary bacterial infections (pyodemodicosis). Accompanying pododermatitis is common. Dogs can have systemic illness with generalized lymphadenopathy, lethargy, and fever when deep pyoderma, furunculosis, or cellulitis is seen. Deep skin scrapings reveal mites, eggs, and larval forms in high numbers. Whenever generalized demodicosis is diagnosed in an adult dog, medical evaluation to identify an underlying systemic disease should be pursued.

Nummular localized demodicosis can be left untreated. The prognosis for this form is usually good, and spontaneous recovery is frequent. In contrast, treatment is required in cases of diffuse localized demodicosis (which can generalize), generalized demodicosis, pyodemodicosis, and pododemodicosis, for which prognosis is always guarded. Hair clipping and body cleansing, especially with benzoyl peroxide shampoo used for its follicular flushing activity, may be required. Whole-body amitraz dips (0.025%) applied every 2 wk is an approved treatment for generalized demodicosis in the USA. Higher concentrations (0.1%) and shorter treatment intervals (1 wk) may be more efficient. Other experimental protocols using daily half-body amitraz dips have been proposed for refractory generalized demodicosis. Among macrocyclic lactones, only milbemycin oxime (0.5-1 mg/kg, PO, SID) is approved for generalized demodicosis in some countries. Other reportedly successful nonlicensed systemic treatments include moxidectin (400 µg/kg, PO, SID) and ivermectin (300-600 µg/kg, PO, SID). For the latter, different therapeutic protocols have been proposed with a gradually increased dosage and thorough monitoring of patients to detect any potentially toxic effect. Ivermectin is contraindicated in Collies and Collie crosses. Local and systemic corticosteroids are contraindicated in any animal diagnosed with demodicosis. Secondary bacterial infections are treated with an appropriate antibiotic. Antiparasitic therapy must be continued not only until clinical signs abate but also until at least 2 consecutive negative skin scrapings are obtained at 1-mo intervals. As the sole prophylactic measure, demodectic dogs should not be used for breeding.

Feline Demodicosis: Two species of mites cause disease in cats. *Demodex cati* is thought to be a normal inhabitant of feline skin. It is a follicular mite, similar to but narrower than the canine mite. The other species of *Demodex* (usually named *D gatoi*) is shorter, with a broad abdomen, and is found only in the stratum corneum. Feline demodicosis is uncommon. In localized demodicosis, there are one or several areas of focal alopecia on the head and neck. In generalized disease, alopecia, crusting, and secondary pyoderma of the whole body are seen. The generalized form has also been associated with other systemic diseases, especially diabetes mellitus. In some cases, ceruminous otitis externa is the only clinical sign. Pruritus is variable; both species can cause similar disease, but cats infested with *D gatoi* are more frequently pruritic. Diagnosis is made by deep skin scrapings, although mite numbers are often small. Medical evaluation is indicated in cats with generalized disease. Dermatophyte cultures are essential, because dermatophytosis and demodicosis can be concomitant conditions. Prognosis of generalized demodicosis is unpredictable because of its potential relationship with systemic disease. Some cases spontaneously resolve. Weekly lime-sulfur dips (2%) are safe and usually effective; amitraz (0.025-0.05%) has been used, but is not approved for use in cats and can cause anorexia, depression, and diarrhea. The use of antiparasitic macrocyclic lactones has been reported but their efficacy is unclear.

Trombiculosis: This common, seasonal noncontagious acariasis is caused by the parasitic larval stage of free-living mites of the family Trombiculidae. It can affect domestic carnivores, other domestic or wild mammals, birds, reptiles, and humans. Two common species found in cats and dogs, *Neotrombicula (Trombicula) autumnalis* and *Eutrombicula alfreddugesi*, are reported in Europe and in America, respectively. Adult (harvest mites) and nymphs look like small spiders and live on rotting detritus. In temperate areas from summer to fall, dogs and cats can acquire the larvae as parasites when lying on the ground or walking in suitable habitat. In warmer regions, infestation occurs throughout the year. The larvae (0.25 mm long) attach to the host, feed for a few days, and leave when engorged. At that time, they are easily identified as ovoid, 0.7 mm long, orange to red, immobile dots, usually found clustering on the head, ears, feet, or ventrum. Pathogenicity is through traumatic and proteolytic activities. Hypersensitivity reactions are suspected in some animals, as pruritus may vary from none to severe. Lesions include erythema, papules, excoriations, hair loss, and crusts. When present, intense pruritus can persist even after the larvae have left the animal.

Diagnosis is based on history and clinical signs. The infestation is a seasonal threat to free-ranging dogs and cats. Differential diagnoses include other pruritic dermatoses, mainly atopy. Diagnosis is confirmed by careful examination of the affected areas. Microscopic examination of samples obtained from skin scrapings may help to identify the larvae, which have an oval-shaped body that is densely covered with setae, 6 long legs, and curved pedipalps terminating in claws.

Management is difficult. The most useful approach, if feasible, consists of keeping pets away from areas known to harbor large numbers of mites to prevent reinfestation during periods of risk. The application of repellents to prevent infestation has yielded variable results. However, lindane, amitraz, fipronil, and pyrethroids could be used, both for prevention and treatment of infested animals. Symptomatic treatment may be required in cases of severe pruritus.

TICKS

Ticks are obligate ectoparasites of most types of terrestrial vertebrates virtually wherever these animals are found. Ticks are large mites and thus are arachnids, members of the subclass Acari. They are more closely related to spiders than to insects. The ~850 described species are exclusively blood-sucking in all feeding stages. Ticks transmit a great variety of infectious agents. Some of these agents are only slightly pathogenic to livestock but may cause disease in humans; others cause diseases in livestock that are of tremendous economic importance. In addition, ticks can harm their hosts directly by inducing toxicosis (eg, sweating sickness [p 546], tick paralysis [p 1073] caused by salivary fluids containing toxins), skin wounds susceptible to secondary bacterial infections and screwworm infestations, and anemia and death. International movement of animals infected with the tick-transmitted blood parasites *Theileria*, *Babesia*, *Anaplasma*, and *Cowdria* spp is widely restricted.

Primary factors in the extensive distribution and prevalence of many tick species and tickborne disease agents are movement of tick-infested livestock over great distances, and introduction of livestock to tick species and tickborne agents that they have not previously experienced and against which they have no immunity or innate resistance. A number of introduced tick species thrive in the vast grazing and browsing environments established during recent centuries of human and livestock population explosions.

Two of the 3 families of ticks parasitize livestock: the Argasidae (argasids, "leathery" or "soft ticks") and the Ixodidae (ixodids, "hard ticks"). Although they share certain basic properties, argasids and ixodids differ in many structural, behavioral, physiologic, ecologic, feeding, and reproductive patterns. Tropical and subtropical species may undergo 1, 2, or rarely 3 complete life cycles annually. In temperate zones, there is often 1 annual cycle; in northern regions and at higher elevations in temperate regions, 2-4 yr are required by most species. There are 4 developmental stages: egg, larva, nymph, and adult. All larvae have 3 pairs of legs; all nymphs and adults, 4. Adults have a distinctive genital and anal area on the ventral body surface. The foreleg tarsi of all ticks bear a unique sensory apparatus—Haller's organ—for sensing carbon dioxide, chemical stimuli (odor), temperature, humidity, etc. Pheromones stimulate group assembly, species recognition, mating, and host selection.

Certain tick species that parasitize livestock can survive several months, and occasionally a few years, without food if environmental conditions permit. Tick host preferences are usually limited to a certain genus, family, or order of vertebrates; however, certain ticks are exceptionally adaptable to a variety of hosts, so each species must be evaluated separately. The larvae and nymphs of most ixodids that parasitize livestock feed on small wildlife such as birds, rodents, small carnivores, or even lizards.

In the Argasidae, the leathery dorsal surface lacks a hard plate (scutum). Male and female argasids appear to be much alike, except for the larger size of the female and differences in external genitalia. The argasid capitulum (mouthparts) arises from the anterior of the body in larvae but from the ventral body surface in nymphs and adults.

In the Ixodidae, the male dorsal surface is covered by a scutum. The scutum of the ixodid female, nymph, and larva covers only the anterior half of the dorsal surface. The ixodid capitulum arises from the anterior end of the body in each developmental stage.

Argasid Parasitism: The Argasidae are highly specialized for sheltering in protected niches or crevices in wood or rocks, or in host nests or roosts in burrows and caves. Some argasid species are known to survive unfed for several years. Most of these leathery parasites inhabit tropical or warm temperate environments with long dry seasons. Hosts are those that either rest in large numbers near the argasid microhabitat, or return from time to time to rest or breed there.

Most of the ~55 *Argas* spp described parasitize birds that breed in colonies in trees or against rock ledges; others parasitize cave-dwelling bats. Few feed on reptiles or wild mammals and none on livestock. Several species have become important pests of domestic fowl and pigeons; among these are the vectors of *Borrelia anserina* (avian spirochetosis) and the rickettsia *Aegyptianella pullorum* (aegyptianellosis). *Argas* spp also cause tick paralysis, and many are vectors of a variety of arboviruses, some of which also infect humans.

The nearly 100 species of *Ornithodoros* shelter in caves, burrows, or dens; under the shade of trees; in the substrate or under stones or debris in ground-level bird breeding colonies; in bird nests in tree holes; or under large stones together with lizards or tenrecs. Different groups of the species parasitize reptiles, birds, or mammals. A few species have adapted to different environments where livestock are confined and also are pests of humans. Certain species are vectors of relapsing fever spirochetes (*Borrelia* spp) and the virus causing African swine fever; some species also cause toxicosis, and one species transmits a spirochete causing epizootic bovine abortion in the western USA. Numerous *Ornithodoros*-transmitted salivary toxins or arboviruses cause irritation or febrile illnesses in humans.

An argasid population typically parasitizes only a single kind of vertebrate and inhabits its shelter area. Argasids use multiple hosts, ie, the larvae feed on one host and drop to the substrate to molt; the several nymphal instars each feed separately, drop, and molt; adults feed several times (but do not molt). Argasid nymphs and adults feed rapidly (usually 30-60 min). Larvae of some argasids also feed rapidly; others require several days to engorge fully. Adult argasids mate off the host several times; afterward, females deposit a few hundred eggs in several batches and feed between ovipositions.

The unique argasid genus *Otobius* is discussed on p 762.

Ixodid Parasitism: The Ixodidae number >650 species, occupy many more habitats and niches than do argasids, and parasitize a greater number of vertebrates in a wider variety of environments. More than 600 ixodid species have a 3-host life cycle; others have a 2-host cycle, and a few have a 1-host cycle. Each ixodid postembryonic developmental stage (larva, nymph, adult) feeds only once but for a period of several days. Males and females of most species that parasitize livestock mate while on the host, although some mate off the host on the ground or in burrows. Males take less food than females but remain longer on the host and may mate with several females. During inactive seasons, few or no females are found feeding, even though males are still attached to the hosts. Such males may continue to transmit pathogens to new susceptible animals by serial interhost transfer. Larval and nymphal population activity generally peaks during the "off seasons" of adults, although in some species, there is overlap in the seasonal dynamics of immatures and adults.

The ixodid males, except those in the genus *Ixodes*, become sexually mature only after beginning to feed, after which they mate with a feeding female. Only after mating does the female become replete and proceed to lay eggs. She then detaches, drops from the host, and over a period of several days, deposits a single batch of many eggs on or near the ground, usually in crevices or under stones or debris. Depending on species and quantity of female nourishment, the egg batch usually numbers 1,000-4,000 but may be >12,000. The female dies after ovipositing. Notably, ixodids (except 1- and 2-host species, which use vertebrate host animals as habitat for much of their life cycle) spend ≥90% of their lifetime off the host, a fact of utmost significance in planning control measures. The several-day feeding process progresses slowly; the balloon shape characteristic of engorged larvae, nymphs, and females develops only during the final half day of feeding and is followed by detaching. The dropping time at certain hours of the day or night is governed by a circadian rhythm closely associated with the activity cycle of the principal host.

It is also important, especially in understanding the epidemiology of tickborne pathogens, to know whether immatures of an ixodid species feed on the same host species as do the adults, or on smaller vertebrates. Where acceptable smaller-sized hosts are scarce, immatures of some ixodid species can feed on the same livestock hosts as adults; immatures of other species seldom or never do so.

The proximity of acceptable hosts, air temperature gradients, and atmospheric humidity during resting and questing periods are among the factors that regulate the development of each stage and, in the case of females, oviposition.

Three-host Ixodids: Most ixodids have a 3-host cycle. The recently hatched larvae quest for a suitable host, usually from vegetation, feed for several days, drop, and molt to nymphs, which repeat these activities and molt to adults. Of the 3-host species that parasitize livestock, a few have immatures and adults that parasitize the same kind of host; these often develop tremendous population densities. The success of ixodid species that require smaller-size hosts for immatures depends on the availability of those hosts in the livestock browsing and grazing grounds. The natural hazards inherent in the 3-host cycle have been compensated for by the benefits afforded adaptable tick species by animal husbandry practices. Only certain ixodids specific for herbivores have adapted to coexistence with livestock, and therein lies the answer to numerous livestock tick problems in Africa, where hosts for adults and immatures are abundant.

Two-host Ixodids: Some ixodids, especially those that parasitize wandering mammals (and also birds in certain cases) in inclement environments of the Old World, have developed a 2-host cycle in which larvae and nymphs feed on one host, and adults on another. As in 3-host species, both hosts may be different or may be the same species. Two-host parasites of livestock thrive in both inclement and clement environments and are difficult to control. This is especially true of 2-host species that feed in the ears and anal areas of livestock.

One-host Ixodids: Among the most economically important ticks are several 1-host species. These parasites evolved together with herbivores that wandered in extensive ranges in the tropics (*Boophilus* spp, *Anocentor nitens*, etc) or in temperate zones (*Dermacentor albipictus*, *Hyalomma scupense*). Larvae, nymphs, and adults feed on a single animal until the mated, replete females drop to the ground to oviposit.

Feeding Sites: Each species has one or more favored feeding sites on the host, although in dense infestations, other areas of the host may be used. Some feed chiefly on the head, neck, shoulders, and escutcheon; others in the ears; others around the anus and under the tail; and some in the nasal passages. Other common feeding sites are the axillae, udder, male genitalia, and tail brush. Immatures and adults often have different preferred feeding sites. Attachment of the large, irritating *Amblyomma* spp is regulated by a male-produced aggregation-attachment pheromone, which ensures that the ticks attach at sites least vulnerable to grooming.

IMPORTANT IXODID TICKS

AMBLYOMMA SPP

Amblyomma ticks are large, 3-host parasites. They have eyes and long, robust mouthparts. They are more or less brightly ornamented and generally confined to the tropics and subtropics. Adults and immatures of 37 of the 102 known species in this genus parasitize reptiles, which together with ground-feeding birds, are often hosts of immature *Amblyomma* ticks that have adapted, in the adult stage, to parasitizing mammals. Their long mouthparts make *Amblyomma* ticks especially difficult to remove manually and frequently cause serious wounds that may become secondarily infected by bacteria or screwworms.

Several African *Amblyomma* spp that infest livestock are vectors of *Cowdria ruminantium*, the rickettsial agent that causes heartwater (p 604).

Amblyomma americanum, the lone-star tick, is abundant in the southern USA from Texas and Missouri to the Atlantic Coast and ranges northward into New Jersey. It is also a notorious pest in Mexico and Central and South America.

The scutum is distinctive because of pale ornamentation in males and a conspicuous, silvery spot ("star") near the posterior margin in females. Larvae, nymphs, and adults are indiscriminate in host choice and parasitize a variety of livestock, pets, and wildlife as well as humans. Activity in the USA continues from early spring to late fall. Feeding sites on domestic and wild mammals are usually skin areas with sparse hair; wounds at these sites predispose livestock to attack by the screwworm fly *Cochliomyia hominivorax*. The lone-star tick transmits the agents that cause tularemia, Rocky Mountain spotted fever, Q-fever, and Lyme disease, and it may cause tick paralysis in humans and dogs. This tick also transmits *Ehrlichia chaffeensis*, which causes nongranulocytic ehrlichiosis in humans, and *E ewingii*, which causes granulocytic ehrlichiosis in dogs. Lone-star virus (Bunyaviridae) has been isolated from *A americanum* in Kentucky.

Amblyomma cajennense, the Cayenne tick, ranges from South America into southern Texas. As with *A americanum*, each active stage is indiscriminate in host choice: livestock and a large variety of avian and mammalian wildlife serve as hosts. People are severely irritated by clusters of *A cajennense* larvae ("seed ticks") in wooded and high-grass areas. Most adults attach on the lower body surface, especially between the legs; some feed elsewhere on the body. Activity continues throughout the year. *A cajennense* is apparently a vector of the rickettsial agent of Rocky Mountain spotted fever and has been experimentally incriminated as a vector of *Cowdria ruminantium*. Wad Medani virus (an orbivirus, Reoviridae), an African virus transported to Caribbean islands by *A variegatum*-infested cattle from Senegal, has been isolated from *A cajennense* in Jamaica.

A maculatum, the Gulf Coast tick, is an important pest of livestock, particularly cattle, from South America to southern USA. Optimal habitats are warm areas with high rainfall, near seacoasts. Immatures usually parasitize birds and small mammals; adults parasitize deer, cattle, horses, sheep, pigs, and dogs. Adult feeding activity is chiefly in late summer and early fall but may begin later after a dry summer. Most adults infest the ears, where the feeding wounds are initial sites of screwworm infestations. Clustered feeding adults also cause much irritation to the upper parts of the neck of cattle and to the humps of Brahman cattle.

A imitator parasitizes livestock from Central America to southern Texas. Occasional pests of livestock in tropical America are *A neumanni* (Argentina), *A ovale* and *A parvum* (Argentina to Mexico), *A tigrinum* (much of South America), and *A tapirellum* (Colombia to Mexico).

A testudinarium inhabits Asian tropical wooded environments from Sri Lanka and India to Malaysia and Vietnam, Indonesia, Borneo, Philippines, Taiwan, and southern Japan. Adults are particularly abundant on wild and domestic pigs and also infest deer, cattle, other livestock, and humans. Immatures parasitize birds and small mammals as well as humans. In India and Sri Lanka, adult *A integrum* and *A mudlairi* also parasitize livestock, wild ungulates, and humans.

A hebraeum, the southern Africa bont tick, inhabits warm, moderately humid savannas of South Africa, Namibia, Botswana, Zimbabwe, Malawi, Mozambique, and Angola. Immatures feed on various small mammals, ground-feeding birds, and reptiles. Adults infest livestock, antelope, and other wildlife. Adults, attached chiefly to body areas with relatively little hair, cause serious wounds that become secondarily infected by bacteria and the screwworm *Chrysomyia bezziana*. Like other African *Amblyomma* ticks (bont ticks) that parasitize livestock, *A hebraeum* is an important vector of *Cowdria ruminantium*, and the larvae transmit *Rickettsia conorii* (tick typhus) to humans.

A variegatum, the tropical African bont tick, is an easily visible, brightly colored parasite found throughout subSaharan savannas southward to the range of *A hebraeum*, and also in southern Arabia and several islands in the Indian and Atlantic Oceans and the Caribbean. Host preferences are similar to those of *A hebraeum* but also include camels. Adults feed chiefly during rainy seasons, immatures during dry seasons. Most adults attach to the underside of the host body, on the genitalia, and under the tail. *A variegatum* injuries to hosts and transmission of *C ruminantium* are similar to those of *A hebraeum* but also include the spread of acute bovine dermatophilosis (p 690). This tick is not considered to be an effective vector of Nairobi sheep disease virus but is a secondary vector of Crimean-Congo hemorrhagic fever virus. Dugbe virus has been isolated from *A variegatum* in 6 countries north of the equator; the Thogoto and Bhanja viruses are also associated with this tick in various areas north of the equator. Notably, yellow fever virus has been isolated from *A variegatum* collected from cattle in the Central African Republic and has been demonstrated to be transovarially transmitted to the progeny of infected females. Jos virus infects *A variegatum* from Ethiopia to Senegal and has been transported in this tick to Jamaica.

A lepidum, the East African bont tick, inhabits xeric savanna environments from northern Tanzania to central Sudan. *A gemma*, the gem-like bont tick, occurs in similar environments of Tanzania, Somalia, Kenya, and Ethiopia. A small variety of the buffalo bont tick, *A cohaerens*, is abundant on cattle in Ethiopian highlands, but from Zaire to Tanzania the larger variety of *A cohaerens* parasitizes chiefly Cape buffalo. Other African *Amblyomma* ticks of Cape buffalo and various other large mammals, including livestock, are *A pomposum* of humid highland forests in Angola, Zaire, Uganda, southern Sudan, Kenya, and Zimbabwe, and *A astrion* of West Africa and Zaire.

BOOPHILUS SPP

Each of the 5 *Boophilus* spp has a 1-host life cycle that may be completed in 3-4 wk and results in a heavy tick burden. Under these conditions, acaricide resistance becomes a major problem in control efforts. Zebu cattle, which have served for centuries as hosts of *B microplus* in the Indian region, have developed resistance to feeding by large numbers of *Boophilus* and are used (purebred or crossbred) in integrated control programs. *B microplus*, considered the world's most important tick parasite of livestock, has been introduced from the bovid- and cervid-inhabited forests of the Indian region to many areas of tropical and subtropical Asia, northeastern Australia, Madagascar, coastal lowlands of southeastern Africa to the equator, and much of South and Central America, Mexico, and the Caribbean. *B microplus* and *B annulatus* were eradicated from the USA after a long, costly control program. Constant surveillance is maintained to prevent their reintroduction. *B annulatus* of southern former USSR, the Near and Middle East, and the Mediterranean area, was introduced with livestock of the early Spanish colonialists into northeastern Mexico but has not spread into Central America. In Africa, south of the Sahara and north of the equator, cattle movements probably account for the many *B annulatus* populations.

B decoloratus, which ranges from southern Africa to the Sahara, is being replaced in the southeastern part of this area by *B microplus*. In more humid West African zones, *B annulatus* mixes with or is totally replaced by *B geigyi*. Scattered *B geigyi* populations are found as far east as southern and central Sudan. In Sri Lanka, an unnamed species infests domestic cattle and buffalo and wild deer. The only boophilid restricted to sheep and goats (and occasionally horses) is *B kohlsi* of Syria, Iraq, Israel, Jordan, western Saudi Arabia, and Yemen. *B microplus* is an experimental vector of *Babesia equi*, and has been collected from the nasal passages of equids in Panama. This tick and *B annulatus* are major vectors of *Babesia bigemina*, *Babesia bovis*, and *Anaplasma marginale*. *B decoloratus* is an efficient vector of *B bigemina* and *A marginale* but does not transmit *B bovis*. This tick apparently does not transmit *B equi*, but it is an experimental vector of *A marginale* to cattle.

DERMACENTOR SPP AND ANOCENTOR SP

Of the 29 *Dermacentor* spp, 19 inhabit temperate zones. Of the 10 tropical species, none is of major veterinary importance, although they may transmit zoonotic infections, and adults may be common on wildlife such as pigs, deer, and antelope. Immatures infest chiefly rodents and lagomorphs. *Dermacentor* spp in cold areas (and *Anocentor nitens* in tropical America) have specialized life cycles and seasonal dynamics of activity, each of which must be considered separately. Otherwise, the *Dermacentor* life cycle is of the typical 3-host pattern.

A nitens, the 1-host tropical horse tick previously assigned to the genus *Dermacentor*, is of considerable veterinary importance. It originally parasitized deer (*Mazama*) in the forests of northern South America. With the introduction of Equidae and other livestock into its habitat, it adapted to these animals. Spending its entire parasitic life deep in the hosts' ears, this parasite was easily spread by human activities to other areas of the Americas, including Florida and Texas. In addition to ear cavities, each active stage may infest nasal passages and the mane, ventral abdomen, and perianal area. *A nitens* transmits *Babesia caballi* transovarially to successive generations and is important in the horse-racing industry. It also is an experimental vector of *A marginale* to cattle.

Another American 1-host species, *D albipictus*, the winter or moose tick, ranges from Canada and northern USA into western USA and Mexico. A brownish form, sometimes called *D nigrolineatus*, is distributed from New Mexico to southern and eastern USA and may merit subspecies if not full-species rank. The larval-nymphal-adult feeding period on a single host (moose, deer, elk, or domestic cattle or horses) extends from fall to spring. Heavily infested hosts may die. *D albipictus* causes the often fatal "phantom moose disease" of Canada, is a secondary vector of Colorado tick fever virus, and an experimental vector of *B caballi*; it is a natural vector of *A marginale* in Oklahoma.

The 6 other American *Dermacentor* spp have 3-host life cycles. The Rocky Mountain wood tick, *D andersoni*, is found from Nebraska westward to the western mountains (Cascades and Sierra Nevadas), in northern New Mexico and Arizona, and in western Canada. The American dog tick, *D variabilis*, is found west of the Cascades and Sierra Nevadas, in Mexico, from Montana to Texas and east to the Atlantic, and in eastern Canada. Both species produce tick paralysis in livestock, wildlife, and humans. They are the chief vectors of *Rickettsia rickettsii*, the agent of Rocky Mountain spotted fever (p 641). *D andersoni* is also the chief vector of Colorado tick fever virus and transmits Powassan virus, *A marginale*, *A ovis*, and the agents of tularemia and Q-fever. *D variabilis* transmits Sawgrass virus, *A marginale*, and agranulocytic ehrlichiosis to dogs and is an experimental vector of *B caballi* and *B equi*. Adults of both species parasitize livestock and wildlife including deer, bison, and elk, but those of *D variabilis* prefer skunk, raccoon, puma, etc, and domestic dogs. Immatures feed on rodents and other small wild mammals. A related, biologically similar species, *D occidentalis*, is restricted to the Pacific lowlands and foothills from Oregon to Baja California and is a natural vector of *A marginale*.

In western USA and Mexico, *D parumapterus*, *D hunteri*, and *D halli* parasitize various hares and rabbits, mountain sheep, and peccaries, respectively. These ticks seldom make contact with livestock. *D hunteri* is an experimental vector of *A marginale* and *A ovis*. In Mexico and Guatemala, *D dissimilis* parasitizes a variety of hosts and may be a 1-host tick on horses. In Costa Rica and Panama, *D latus* infests tapirs.

In Eurasian steppes, forests, and mountains, *D marginatus*, *D reticulatus*, and *D silvarum*, collectively, are vectors of numerous viruses and *Babesia bovis*, *B caballi*, *B equi*, *B canis*, *Theileria ovis*, and *A ovis*, together with the agents of tularemia and Q-fever. *D marginatus* is found in forests, marshes, semideserts, and alpine zones from France to southwestern Siberia, Kazakhstan, Xinjiang Uygur Autonomous Region of China, Iran, and northern Afghanistan. *D reticulatus* ranges from Ireland and Britain to northwestern Siberia and Xinjiang, China, in meadows, floodplains, and deciduous and deciduous-conifer forests. *D silvarum* ranges from central Siberia and northeastern China to Japan in marshes, meadows, shrubby and secondary forests, and farmlands in taiga forest areas. Some males in populations of each of these 3 species remain attached to the host during winter. Adults and immatures may overwinter on the ground. Greatest adult activity is from early spring to summer with a lower peak in fall. Larvae and nymphs are active from spring through fall. The life cycle may be completed in 1 yr or extended by one or more summer or winter diapauses to 2-4 yr.

About 12 other *Dermacentor* spp inhabit certain lowland, mountain steppe, and semidesert areas of temperate Asia. Their adults are commonly taken from camels, cattle, horses, sheep, and goats. In tropical Asia, the several species of the *Dermacentor* subgenus *Indocentor* are parasites of wild pigs; they also infest larger wildlife but seldom if ever feed on livestock.

HAEMAPHYSALIS SPP

Few of the 155 species of *Haemaphysalis* parasitize livestock, but those that do are economically important in Eurasia, Africa, Australia, and New Zealand. Some haemaphysaline parasites of wild deer, antelope, and cattle have adapted to domestic cattle and, to a lesser extent, to sheep and goats. Others, originally specific for various wild sheep and goats, have adapted chiefly to the domestic breeds of these animals. A few African species that evolved together with carnivores now parasitize domestic dogs. Immatures of species that parasitize livestock generally feed on small vertebrates, but there are a few notable exceptions. All *Haemaphysalis* spp have a 3-host life cycle. They are small (unfed adults <4.5 mm long), brownish or reddish, and eyeless. Most have very short mouthparts. Different species produce tick paralysis and are vectors of the agents that cause Q-fever, tularemia, and brucellosis, and of *Theileria orientalis*, *T ovis*, *Babesia major*, *B motasi*, *B canis*, *Anaplasma mesaeterum*, etc.

H punctata is widely distributed where sheep, goats, and cattle feed in certain open forests and shrubby pastures from southwestern Asia (Iran and former USSR) to much of Europe, including southern Scandinavia and Britain. Immatures infest birds, hedgehogs, rodents, and reptiles. In addition to transmitting *Anaplasma* and *Babesia* spp, different *H punctata* populations are infected by tickborne encephalitis virus, Tribec virus, Bhanja virus, and Crimean-Congo hemorrhagic fever virus.

H sulcata adults parasitize livestock (chiefly sheep and goats) from northwestern India and southern former USSR to Arabia, Sinai, and southern Europe. *H parva (otophila)* adults parasitize these hosts from southwestern former USSR and the Near East to the Mediterranean area (but not Egypt). Immature *H sulcata* are especially common on lizards, but the range of hosts of larvae and nymphs of both species is similar to that of *H punctata*.

H longicornis is a parasite of deer and livestock in Japan and northeast Asia; there is a bisexual form (race) in southern areas and a parthenogenetic race in northern areas. The latter has been introduced into Australia, New Zealand, and the Pacific islands, where it preserves this unusual reproductive ability. Immatures usually parasitize small mammals and birds but may also feed on livestock; heavy population densities may become serious pests of deer and livestock. This tick is the chief vector of *Theileria orientalis* and also transmits *Babesia ovata*, *B gibsoni*, and the agents of Q-fever, Powassan encephalitis, and Russian spring-summer encephalitis. Larval feeding causes acute dermatitis in humans.

Other Eurasian haemaphysalines of livestock are *H inermi* (lowlands from northern Iran and southwestern former USSR to central and southeastern Europe to Italy), *H pospelovashtromae* (mountains of southern former USSR and Mongolia), *H kopetdaghicus* (Caspian Sea area, mountains of former USSR, and Iran), and *H tibetensis*, *H xinjiangensis*, and *H moschisuga* (China).

Of the several haemaphysaline species of livestock parasites found chiefly in India, 3 are especially noteworthy: *H bispinosa* ranges to Pakistan, Bangladesh, Nepal, Bhutan, Sri Lanka, and Malaysia, and transmits *Babesia* spp to cattle, sheep, and dogs; *H spinigera* is the chief vector of Kyasanur Forest disease virus in humans in Karnataka state, India; and *H anomala* ranges from the Nepal lowlands to Sri Lanka and the mountains of northwestern Thailand.

In temperate Asia, 18 other haemaphysalines parasitize livestock: 9 high in the Himalayas and outlying mountains, and 9 in northeastern former USSR, Korea, and Japan. Yak and yak-cattle hybrids are among the livestock hosts of Himalayan haemaphysalines. Several Himalayan species appear to prefer sheep and goats.

In subSaharan Africa, 4 haemaphysalines infest livestock in highland forests or lowland, humid, secondary or riparian forests. These are *H parmata* (Ethiopia and Kenya,

Central and West Africa, to Angola), *H aciculifer* (Ethiopia to Cameroon and Zimbabwe, introduced into South Africa), *H rugosa* (southern Sudan and Uganda to Ghana and Senegal), and *H silacea* (Zululand and eastern south Africa).

HYALOMMA SPP

Hyalomma ticks are often the most abundant tick parasites of livestock, including camels, in warm, arid, and semiarid, generally harsh lowland and middle altitude biotopes, and those with long dry seasons, from central and southwest Asia to southern Europe and southern Africa. Of the 30 known *Hyalomma* spp, ≥15 are important vectors of infectious agents to livestock and humans. The 3-host life cycle predominates in this genus, but some species have either a 1- or 2-host cycle. Some 3-host species can develop in 1- or 2-host cycles, a facultative ability unique to this ixodid genus. Hyalommines are mostly moderately large to large ticks with long mouthparts.

In the subgenus *Hyalommasta*, immatures of the single species, *H aegyptium*, parasitize tortoises and small wildlife and livestock from Pakistan to both sides of the Mediterranean basin. Adults are specific for tortoises.

The subgenus *Hyalommina* is found on the Indian subcontinent and Somalia. Each of the 6 species has a 3-host cycle. Immatures parasitize small mammals, especially rodents. Adult host preferences among livestock reflect the wild gazelle, bovine, caprine, or ovine group with which each species evolved. Two species now infest chiefly cattle and the domestic buffalo—*H brevipunctata* (India and Pakistan) and *H kumari* (India, Pakistan, Afghanistan, northwestern Iran, and Tadzhikistan). Three usually parasitize sheep and goats—*H hussaini* (India, Pakistan, Burma), *H rhipicephaloides* (Dead Sea and Red Sea areas), and *H arabica* (Yemen and Saudi Arabia). *H punt* (Somalia and Ethiopia) feeds on antelope, camels, cattle, sheep, and goats.

The subgenus *Hyalomma* contains 15 species of veterinary and public health importance. Three of the 15 species have 2, 3, and 4 subspecies, respectively. Chief among these is the 2-host *H anatolicum anatolicum*, which ranks high among the world's most damaging ticks and has been widely distributed by camels, cattle, and horses in steppe and semidesert environments from central Asia to Bangladesh, the Middle and Near East, Arabia, southeastern Europe, and Africa north of the equator. Immatures and adults generally infest the same kinds of hosts. Nymphs and unfed adults spend the dry and winter season in crevices in stone walls, stables, and weedy or fallow fields. When immatures infest smaller mammals, birds, or reptiles, the life cycle type is 3-host. *H anatolicum anatolicum* transmits *Theileria annulata*, *Babesia equi*, *B caballi*, *Anaplasma marginale*, *Trypanosoma theileri*, and at least 5 arboviruses; it is a significant vector of Crimean-Congo hemorrhagic fever virus to humans.

The numerous *H anatolicum anatolicum* immatures and adults that often parasitize livestock cause unthriftiness. Immatures of the subspecies *H anatolicum excavatum* (a 3-host parasite) infest chiefly burrowing rodents in somewhat different biotopes in the same environments as *H anatolicum anatolicum*. Adults of both subspecies may infest the same animal. Distribution of *H anatolicum excavatum* is somewhat more limited than that of *H anatolicum anatolicum*, but its winter season population densities are often greater. A closely related species, *H lusitanicum*, replaces *H anatolicum anatolicum* from central Italy to Portugal, Morocco, and the Canary Islands; it is associated with equine and bovine babesiosis. In addition to livestock, deer and rabbits serve as hosts.

The *H marginatum* complex consists of 4 subspecies, each apparently invariably 2-host. Adults parasitize livestock and wild herbivores. Immatures primarily parasitize birds. Rodents are rarely, if ever, parasitized. Hares and hedgehogs are secondary hosts. The subspecies are *H marginatum marginatum* (Caspian area of Iran and former USSR to Portugal and northwestern Africa), *H marginatum rufipes* (south of the Sahara to South Africa, also Nile Valley and southern Arabia), *H marginatum turanicum* (Pakistan, Iran, southern former USSR, Arabia, parts of northeastern Africa—introduced with sheep from Iran to Karoo), and *H marginatum isaaci* (Sri Lanka to southern Nepal, Pakistan, northern Afghanistan). *H marginatum* subspecies are important vectors of Crimean-Congo hemorrhagic fever virus and also transmit agents of livestock diseases and other viruses that infect wildlife, livestock, and humans.

The *H asiaticum* complex consists of 3 subspecies with 3-host life cycles and inhabits deserts, semideserts, and steppes from southwestern China, Mongolia, and southern former USSR into the Middle East as far as Iraq. Rodents are the chief hosts of immatures; hares also may be infested. Adults parasitize livestock, particularly camels. The subspecies from east to west, *H asiaticum kozlovi, H asiaticum asiaticum,* and *H asiaticum caucasicum,* are of veterinary and medical importance.

Three additional 3-host *Hyalomma* spp that parasitize camels and other livestock are *H dromedarii* (India to Africa north of the equator), *H schulzei* (eastern Iran to Arabia and northern Egypt), and *H franchinii* (Syria to Tunisia). Immatures parasitize rodents and other small mammals, birds, and reptiles; those of *H dromedarii* also infest livestock. *H dromedarii* is of veterinary and medical importance; the other 2 species have been little investigated.

H detritum, an important vector of *Theileria annulata,* is a 3-host species; both adults and immatures parasitize livestock. Its biotopes are humid areas in steppes, deserts, and semideserts from southern China, Mongolia, and Nepal lowlands to southern Europe and northern Africa. *H impeltatum* ranges from Iran and Arabia to northern Tanzania and Chad. Adults parasitize livestock; immatures feed on rodents and other small mammals, birds, and reptiles.

H scupense, a 1-host parasite of cattle and horses in southwestern former USSR and southeastern Europe, is, (like Canadian strains of *Dermacentor albipictus*) unusual in that it overwinters on the host, which often suffers greatly from the long feeding period of numerous larvae (late fall), nymphs (winter), and adults (spring). *H scupense* is a vector of *Theileria annulata* and *Babesia equi.*

In addition to the several species already mentioned, the African savannas harbor 5 other *Hyalomma* spp of livestock and wildlife: *H truncatum* (southeastern Egypt to southern Africa), *H albiparmatum* (southern Kenya, northern Tanzania), *H erythraeum* (eastern Somalia and Ethiopia, and Yemen), *H impressum* (western Sudan and West Africa), and *H nitidum* (Central African Republic and West Africa). Immatures of these 3-host species generally infest small mammals, less often birds and reptiles. *H truncatum,* which causes bovine sweating sickness and lameness and also human and ovine tick paralysis, is a vector of Crimean-Congo hemorrhagic fever virus, *Coxiella burnetii* (Q-fever), and *Rickettsia conorii* (tick typhus).

IXODES SPP

This, the largest genus of the family Ixodidae, contains ~220 species and is highly specialized both structurally and biologically. So far as is known, all *Ixodes* spp have a 3-host life cycle. Almost all inhabit temperate or tropical forest zones or wooded or shrubby grasslands; fewer are adapted to humid areas in semideserts or to arctic or subantarctic nesting colonies of marine birds. Hosts are a wide variety of birds and mammals and a few reptiles. Most species parasitize burrowing hosts or those that return regularly to caves, dens, or terrestrial or arboreal nesting colonies. The few *Ixodes* spp that parasitize wandering artiodactyls or perissodactyls are exceptionally adaptable; they also parasitize livestock and are important pests or vectors of agents that infect livestock and humans.

The *I ricinus* group of Eurasia, northwestern Africa, and North and South America is especially important. *I ricinus,* the so-called sheep tick and prototype of this group, inhabits relatively humid, cool, shrubby and wooded pastures, gardens, windbreaks, floodplains, and forest through much of Europe to the Caspian Sea and northern Iran, and also northwestern Africa. Its life cycle is 2-4 yr, depending on environmental temperature. (In drier, warmer, eastern Mediterranean biotopes, *I ricinus* is replaced by *I gibbosus,* which completes its life cycle in 1 yr.) *I ricinus* larvae feed on small reptiles, birds, and mammals. Nymphs feed on small and medium-sized vertebrates, and adults feed chiefly on herbivores and livestock. All stages, especially nymphs and adults, parasitize humans. Male *I ricinus* take little or no food but mate on the host while the female feeds. If *I ricinus* is like other campestral species in the genus, unfed adults often mate while on vegetation. Adult activity peaks in spring; in some populations, there is a lower peak of adult activity in the fall. Chief among the numerous arboviral diseases transmitted by

I ricinus are louping ill, tickborne encephalitis, and Crimean-Congo hemorrhagic fever. Other agents transmitted to livestock are *Coxiella burnetii*, *Anaplasma marginale*, *Babesia divergens*, and *Anaplasma phagocytophilum*.

I persulcatus, the taiga tick, is closely related to *I ricinus* and has similar host preferences. It ranges from the central and eastern mountains of Europe through the lowland forests from the Baltic Sea and Karelia eastward through the Siberian taiga to the Seas of Japan and Okhotsk and the northern islands of Japan. The life cycle is completed in 2-4 yr. It is the chief vector of Russian spring-summer encephalitis virus, and it transmits *Babesia* spp and the agents of ovine anaplasmosis and tularemia.

Other Asian representatives of the *I ricinus* group are *I sinensis* of China; *I kashmiricus* of mountainous northern India, Pakistan, and Kyrgyzstan; *I pavlovskyi* of southern Siberian mountains of Russia; and *I kazakstani* of mountain taiga and deciduous forest in Kazakhstan, Kyrgyzstan, and Turkmenistan.

I scapularis (also a member of the *I ricinus* group) is a vector of *Borrelia burgdorferi*, the agent of Lyme disease in northeastern and north central USA and Southern Canada; it is also a vector of *Babesia microti*, the agent of human babesiosis in coastal areas from New York to Massachusetts. This tick also is a vector of human granulocytic ehrlichiosis. The chief hosts of adult *I scapularis* are deer; livestock seldom graze in the wooded zones inhabited by this tick. Adults of *I pacificus* parasitize livestock from Baja California to British Columbia and in inland pockets of Idaho, Nevada, and Oregon. *I pacificus* and *I neotomae* transmit the agents of Lyme disease, tularemia, and a rickettsia of the Rocky Mountain spotted fever group; *I pacificus* also transmits *Ehrlichia equi*, causing granulocytic ehrlichiosis in horses. The tick bites cause slowly healing ulcers. A related species, *I affinis*, ranges from South Carolina and Florida to Argentina. It is recorded chiefly from wildlife and has not been shown to be a vector.

In Africa, only 4 *Ixodes* spp have adapted to livestock. Chief among these is the South African paralysis tick, *I rubicundus*, of humid hill and mountain karoo vegetation in South Africa. Its salivary toxins cause a flaccid tetraplegia in livestock, humans, dogs, and jackals. Immatures parasitize the rock hare, other hares, and elephant shrews. Other parasites of livestock in African highlands are *I drakenbergensis* (Natal), *I lewisi* (Kenya), and *I cavipalpus* (southern Sudan to Zimbabwe and Angola).

MARGAROPUS SPP

Closely related to *Boophilus*, the 3 highly specialized beady-legged, 1-host *Margaropus* spp are restricted to limited areas of Africa. *M reidi* and *M wileyi* are recorded from giraffe in the Sudan and in Kenya and Tanzania, respectively. *M wileyi* is also known to parasitize zebras and gnu. *M winthemi*, a winter-feeding parasite of zebras, horses, and less often other livestock and antelope, is confined to mountains of South Africa and may contribute to loss of condition during winter.

NOSOMMA SP

Adults of the single species in this genus, *N monstrosum*, particularly parasitize wild and domestic buffalo, and also humans, livestock, and wildlife, through much of India, Nepalese lowlands, Bangladesh, Thailand, and Laos. Immatures parasitize chiefly murid rodents.

RHIPICEPHALUS SPP

Rhipicephalid species occur in Eurasia and northern Africa (15 species) and in subSaharan Africa (~55 species). Adults of most species parasitize wild and domestic artiodactyls, perissodactyls, or carnivores. Immatures feed mostly on smaller mammals; however, of those that parasitize rodents or hyraxes, and of those that parasitize artiodactyls, a few feed on the same host as the adults. The rhipicephalid life cycle is typically 3-host, but in the Mediterranean climatic zone (long, warm summer with low rainfall), *R bursa* has a 2-host cycle. In subSaharan Africa with long dry seasons, *R evertsi* and *R glabroscutatum* also have 2-host cycles.

A number of *Rhipicephalus* spp have long been difficult to identify or have been incorrectly identified. Current concepts of tick phylogeny, taxonomy, and nomenclature are being revised and expanded based on molecular analyses. This ongoing work is likely to expand and alter the current understanding of the phylogeny and evolution of the subfamily Rhipicephalinae (as exemplified by the current view that the genus *Rhipicephalus* is probably paraphyletic with respect to the genus *Boophilus*). Problem areas are indicated below.

Tropical Asia is the home of 5 *Rhipicephalus* spp; adults of 2 species parasitize domestic animals. *R haemaphysaloides* infests all types of livestock, and wild antelope, deer, carnivores, and hares in continental southeast Asia (and Taiwan and the Philippines) westward to India, Sri Lanka, Nepal, Pakistan, and western Afghanistan. *R pilans* infests livestock and wildlife in Indonesia and Borneo. Immatures of both species feed chiefly on rodents, also on shrews, hares, and smaller carnivores.

From central Europe to Kazakhstan, *R rossicus*, *R schulzei*, and *R pumilio* are of medical and veterinary importance. In southwestern Europe, *R pusillus* infests dogs as well as European rabbits, foxes, and wild pigs. *R turanicus*, as presently recognized, ranges from China, southern former USSR, India into southern Europe, and Africa as far south as South Africa. A member of the taxonomically difficult *R sanguineus* group, "*R turanicus*" and its various populations, which may represent separate species, requires further studies of its abilities as a vector.

An easily recognized 2-host species, *R bursa*, ranges from the western Mediterranean area of Europe to Iran and Kazakhstan. Adults and immatures parasitize livestock, hares, deer, wild sheep and goats, and humans. It causes ovine paralysis and transmits Crimean-Congo hemorrhagic fever virus and other viruses to humans, and *Babesia*, *Theileria*, and *Anaplasma* spp to livestock.

The best known African rhipicephalid, *R sanguineus*, the kennel tick or brown dog tick, has traveled worldwide with domestic dogs. It is now established in buildings as far north as Canada and Scandinavia and as far south as Australia. In Africa, the Near East, and parts of southern Europe, adults parasitize wild and domestic carnivores, sheep, goats, camels, other livestock, and various wild mammals, especially hares and hedgehogs. Immatures in nature in this area feed on small mammals. However, in urban situations everywhere, dogs are virtually the only hosts of immatures and adults. Humans are rarely attacked. Strains of adult *R sanguineus* that feed on cattle are recorded in parts of Mexico and in Tahiti. This tick is active throughout the year in the tropics and subtropics but only from spring to fall in temperate zones. Newly active adults and nymphs are frequently seen climbing walls from floor-level cracks. *R sanguineus* is a vector of *Babesia canis*, *Ehrlichia canis*, *Rickettsia rhipicephali*, *Rickettsia conorii*, Crimean-Congo hemorrhagic fever virus, and Thogoto virus. In southcentral USA, *R sanguineus* is associated with scattered foci of *Leishmania mexicana*. Implications of this tick as a vector of other infectious agents require confirmation. Certain American populations have become resistant to insecticides. The hymenopteran (chalcid) parasite of ticks, *Hunterellus hookeri*, frequently infests nymphal *R sanguineus* in East Africa.

R appendiculatus, the brown ear tick, is a major pest in cool, shaded, woody and shrubby savannas from southern Sudan and eastern Zaire to Kenya and South Africa. Adults and immatures feed in the ears of cattle, other livestock, and antelope, but also on other areas when the infestation is massive. Immatures may infest small antelope and carnivores, and occasionally rodents. Seasonal activity is closely associated with temperature and rain periods. *R appendiculatus* is the major vector of the *Theileria parva* group of diseases (East Coast fever, Corridor disease, Zimbabwe malignant theileriosis) and Nairobi sheep disease virus, and is also a vector of *Theileria taurotragi*, *Ehrlichia bovis*, *Rickettsia conorii*, and Thogoto virus. Heavy infestations on susceptible *Bos taurus* cattle cause a sometimes fatal toxemia, loss of resistance to various infections, and severe damage to the host's ears.

The closely related *R zambeziensis*, with similar host preferences, is found in drier lowland savannas in Tanzania, Zimbabwe, Zambia, Botswana, and Transvaal; it also is a vector of East Coast fever. Other species closely related to *R appendiculatus* include *R nitens* in the Cape Province of South Africa and *R duttoni* in Angola and Zaire.

The ivory-ornamented *R pulchellus*, a parasite of zebras, also infests livestock and game animals in savanna habitats east of the Rift Valley from southern Ethiopia to Somalia and northeastern Tanzania. Adults and immatures generally infest the same host; however, immatures also feed on hares, and larvae ("seed ticks") are notoriously annoying pests of humans. *R pulchellus* feeds in the ears and on the lower abdomen, chiefly during wet seasons. This tick is a vector of *Babesia equi* (among zebra), *Theileria* spp, *Trypanosoma theileri*, *Rickettsia conorii*, several Bunyaviridae (Crimean-Congo hemorrhagic fever virus; Nairobi sheep disease; and Kajiado, Kismayo, and Dugbe viruses), and Barur virus.

The 2-host African rhipicephalids are *R evertsi* subspecies and *R glabroscutatum*. *R evertsi evertsi*, a large, beady-eyed, red-legged tick, a parasite of the East African zebra, parasitizes all types of herbivorous wildlife and livestock (but seldom pigs). Immatures and adults infest the same hosts; immatures are also recorded from hares. It ranges from South Africa through eastern Africa east of the Nile to southern Sudan and is established in the mountains of Yemen. Scattered foci, introduced by domestic animals, occur west of the Nile. Immatures feed in the ear canal; adults feed mostly around the anus and under the tail but also in the axillae and groin and on the sternum. Large numbers on a single host are common on Equidae and are difficult to control because of their concentrations in difficult-to-reach feeding sites. The life cycle continues through the year but slackens in cooler seasons. *R evertsi evertsi* transmits *Babesia equi*, *Theileria parva* (secondary vector), *Borrelia theileri*, *Rickettsia conorii*, and Kerai, Wad Medani, and Thogoto viruses. The banded-legged (*Hyalomma*-like) western subspecies, *R evertsi mimeticus*, found from western Botswana to Namibia, Angola, and Zaire, is like the nominate subspecies in host preferences, feeding sites, and life cycle.

The tiny *R glabroscutatum* has become a common pest of sheep, goats, and other livestock in the arid, small-shrub savanna of southeastern Cape Province, South Africa. Kudu and other small antelope are also infested. The few records of immatures are from rodents.

The *R pravus* group, presently under taxonomic study, consists of 4 or more species of which the adults feed on livestock and herbivorous wildlife (including hares); immatures feed on elephant shrews (insectivores), hares, and other small mammals. *R pravus*, a brown, convex-eyed tick, occurs in shrubby and wooded savannas in east Africa. It is infected by Kadam virus. The closely related *R occulatus*, a parasite of hares, and another related, unnamed parasite of livestock are found in southern Africa.

The difficult-to-classify *R punctatus* group of parasites of livestock and wild artiodactyls consists of *R punctatus* (Angola, Mozambique, Tanzania), *R kochi (neavi)* (Botswana to Kenya and Zaire), and an as yet unnamed species from Zimbabwe and South Africa.

The *R capensis* group is also under study. Originally parasites of the Cape buffalo, these species now parasitize livestock and wildlife in Namibia and South Africa (*R capensis*, including the possibly synonymous *R gertrudae*), East Africa (*R compositus* and *R longus*), and West Africa to southwestern Sudan (*R cliffordi*).

Above 5,900 ft (1,800 m) altitude in East African forest and shrub zones, *R hurti* and *R jeanelli* infest livestock and Cape buffalo and other large game animals. *R hurti* also inhabits mountains in Zaire. Both species feed chiefly in the hosts' ears; *R jeanelli* also feeds in the tailbrush.

R simus, the prototype of the *R simus* group and long considered to be a well-established species, is now divided into several species. In the new classification, *R simus sensu stricto* is found through central and southern Africa, roughly south of latitude 8°S, where it is a competent experimental vector of *Anaplasma marginale* and *A centrale*. In eastern and northern Africa, *R simus* is replaced by a less punctate species, *R praetextatus*, which ranges from central Tanzania to Egypt. Adults of both species parasitize livestock, dogs, wild carnivores, large and medium-sized game animals, and humans. Occurrence and densities on livestock are inexplicably erratic. Immature stages feed on the common burrowing rodents in savannas. Both species cause tick paralysis of humans and transmit *Rickettsia conorii* and *Coxiella burnetii*. In Kenya, *R praetextatus* is a vector of Thogoto virus and may be a secondary vector of Nairobi sheep disease virus. West of the Nile, these species are replaced by *R senegalensis* and *R muhsamae*.

Much literature regarding *R tricuspis* (Tanzania to South Africa) and *R lunulatus* (West Africa to Ethiopia and Tanzania) has been incorrect. The chief feeding site of both on livestock and wildlife is the tailbrush, but other parts of the host are also feeding sites.

R sanguineus and *R turanicus* of the *R sanguineus* group are described above. Related species are *R camicasi* and *R bergeoni* of northeastern Africa, *R guilhoni* and *R moucheti* of West Africa, and 2 widely distributed "forms" of *R sulcatus*, which are under study.

Two quite distinctive species often confused with *R appendiculatus* are *R supertritus* (Natal to southern Sudan) and *R muhlensi* (Kenya and southern Sudan to Central Africa). Adults of both species parasitize cattle, Cape buffalo, antelope, and big game animals; *R supertritus* also is found on carnivores.

IMPORTANT ARGASID TICKS

ARGAS SPP

Most of the 56 known *Argas* spp are specific for birds or bats; a few parasitize wild terrestrial mammals or Galapagos giant tortoises. The species of importance in transmitting *Aegyptianella pullorum* and *Borrelia anserina* to poultry are *A persicus* (many tropical and subtropical areas of the world), *A arboreus* (much of Africa, including Egypt), *A africolumbae* (tropical Africa), *A walkerae* (southern Africa), and *A miniatus* (South and Central America). Other species that infest poultry appear to transmit both *A pullorum* and *B anserina*. (*See also* FOWL TICKS, p 2273.) Tick paralysis is caused by feeding *A persicus*, *A arboreus*, *A walkerae*, *A miniatus*, *A radiatus*, and *A sanchezi* (USA). These and other *Argas* spp can cause great irritation when feeding on humans.

ORNITHODOROS SPP

Most of the ~100 *Ornithodoros* spp inhabit protected niches in burrows, caves, dens, cliffsides, and bird colonies. Among the few that parasitize livestock, *O savignyi* and *O coriaceus* are exceptional because they have eyes and because they rest just below or above ground level under the shade of trees and rocks where livestock and game animals rest and sleep. *O savignyi*, the sand tampan, lives in semiarid areas from Namibia to India and Sri Lanka and is often tremendously abundant. Humans and tethered livestock suffer severe irritation and toxicosis from sand tampan bites, and paralysis and death of animals are recorded. *O coriaceus*, the "pajaroello" of hillside scrub oak habitats from northern California and Nevada to Chiapias, Mexico, occupies deer beds under trees and near large rocks. It is well-known for irritating deer and cattle, and, in humans, its bite produces a severe skin reaction. Epizootic bovine abortion, caused by *Borrelia crocidurae*, appears to be transmitted only by *O coriaceus*. *O guerneyi* shelters in tree-shaded soil in arid zones of Australia where kangaroos and humans rest; livestock are rare or absent in these habitats.

Among the numerous *Ornithodoros* spp that inhabit burrows, several species are either naturally infected with African swine fever (ASF) virus in Africa, or have the laboratory-confirmed ability to harbor and transmit the agent in Europe and the Americas. The natural reservoir and vector of ASF virus is *O porcinus porcinus* (*O moubata porcinus*), which is abundant in burrows of tropical African pigs and also of antbears and porcupines. Domestic pig populations in the vicinity of infected wild pigs can be decimated by ASF. Wild and domestic pigs are not involved in the epidemiology of *Borrelia duttoni*, the agent of human African relapsing fever, which is transmitted by *O moubata*. ASF virus has been transported in infected meat to Spain where *O marocanus* (*erraticus*), an inhabitant of rodent burrows and pig sties, is an efficient vector. *O marocanus* is also a reservoir and vector of *Borrelia hispanica*, the agent of Spanish-northwest African human relapsing fever. ASF has likewise been introduced in Brazil, Haiti, the Dominican Republic, and Cuba. The American *O puertoricensis*, *O turicata*, *O talaje*, *O dugesi*, and *O coriaceus* are potential vectors of ASF virus.

O tholozani (*O papillipes*, also *O crossi*) infests burrows, caves, stables, stone and clay fences, and human habitations in semidesert, steppe, and long dry-season environments from China, southern former USSR, northwestern India, and Afghanistan to Greece, northeastern Libya, and eastern Mediterranean islands. Numerous rodents, hedgehogs, porcupines, and domestic animals support *O tholozani* populations. Humans develop severe, sometimes fatal, Persian relapsing fever when bitten by *O tholozani* infected with *Borrelia persicus*.

O lahorensis, originally a parasite of wild sheep resting in the lee of cliffsides, is an important pest of stabled livestock in lowlands and mountains of Tibet, Kashmir, and southern former USSR to Saudi Arabia and Turkey, Greece, Bulgaria, and Yugoslavia. The 2-host life cycle and long wintertime attachment of *O lahorensis* is biologically remarkable. It is deleterious to livestock held for much of the winter in heavily infested stables; it may cause paralysis, anemia, and toxicosis, and it transmits the agents of piroplasmosis, brucellosis, Q-fever, and tularemia. In Iran and Turkmenistan, the seldom studied *O canestrini* also parasitizes livestock in caves and stables.

O turicata parasitizes rodents that live in burrows, crevices, or caves; owls; snakes; tortoises; and also domestic pigs and other livestock in southern USA and Mexico. Contrary to most *Ornithodoros* feeding patterns, immature *O turicata* engorge in ≤30 min, but adults may attach for up to 2 days. *O turicata* has been associated with diseases of pigs, and serious toxic reactions and secondary infections can result when humans are bitten.

O furucosus parasitizes humans and livestock in houses and stables in northwestern South America. Other South American pests of livestock and humans, probably originally parasites of the peccary, are *O braziliensis* and *O rostratus*.

OTOBIUS SPP

Otobius megnini, which is exceedingly specialized biologically and structurally, infests the ear canals of pronghorn antelope, mountain sheep, and Virginia and mule deer in low rainfall biotopes of western USA and in Mexico and western Canada. Cattle, horses, goats, sheep, dogs, and humans are similarly infested. This well-concealed parasite has been transported with livestock to western South America, Galapagos, Cuba, Hawaii, India, Madagascar, and southeastern Africa. Notably, adults have nonfunctional mouthparts and remain nonfeeding on the ground but may survive for almost 2 yr. Females can deposit up to 1,500 eggs in a 2-wk period. Larvae and 2 nymphal instars feed for 2-4 mo, mostly in winter and spring. There can be 2 or more generations per year. Humans and other animals may suffer severe irritation from ear canal infestations, and heavily infested livestock lose condition during winter. Tick paralysis of hosts and secondary infections by larval screwworms are reported. *O megnini* is infected by the agents of Q-fever, tularemia, Colorado tick fever, and Rocky Mountain spotted fever. The second *Otobius* sp, *O lagophilus*, feeds on the heads of jackrabbits (hares) and rabbits in western USA.

TICK CONTROL

The main reasons for tick control are to protect hosts from irritation and production losses, formation of lesions that can become secondarily infested, damage to hides and udders, toxicosis, paralysis, and of greatest importance, infection with a wide variety of disease agents. Control also prevents the spread of tick species and the diseases they transmit to unaffected areas, regions, or continents.

Cultural and Biologic Control: These measures can be directed against both the free-living and parasitic stages of ticks. The free-living stages of most tick species, both ixodid and argasid, have specific requirements in terms of microclimate and are restricted to particular microhabitats within the ecosystems inhabited by their hosts. Destruction of these microhabitats reduces the abundance of ticks. Alteration of the environment by removal of certain types of vegetation has been used in the control of *Amblyomma americanum* in recreational areas in southeastern USA and in the control of *Ixodes rubicundus* in South Africa. Control of argasid ticks such as *Argas persicus* and *A walkerae* in poultry can be achieved by eliminating cracks in walls and perches, which provide shelter to the free-living stages.

The abundance of tick species can also be reduced by removal of alternate hosts or hosts of a particular stage of the life cycle. This approach has occasionally been advocated for the control of 3-host ixodid ticks such as *Rhipicephalus appendiculatus*,

Amblyomma hebraeum and *Ixodes rubicundus* in Africa, and *Hyalomma* spp in southeastern Europe and Asia.

Rotation of pastures or pasture spelling has been used in the control of the 1-host ixodid tick *Boophilus microplus* in Australia. The method could also be applied to other 1-host ticks, in which the duration of the spelling period is determined by the relatively short life span of the free-living larvae. However, it has minimal application to multihost ixodid ticks or argasid ticks because of the long survival periods of the unfed nymphs and adults.

Predators, including birds, rodents, shrews, ants, and spiders, play a role in some areas in reducing the numbers of free-living ticks. In the New World, fire ants (*Pheidole megacephala*) are noteworthy tick predators. Engorged ticks may also become parasitized by the larvae of some wasps (Hymenoptera), but these have not significantly reduced tick populations.

Zebu (*Bos indicus*) and Sanga (a *B taurus, B indicus* crossbreed) cattle, the indigenous breeds of Asia and Africa, usually become very resistant to ixodid ticks after initial exposure. In contrast, European (*B taurus*) breeds usually remain fairly susceptible. The tick resistance of Zebu breeds and their crosses is being increasingly exploited as a means of control of the parasitic stages. The introduction of Zebu cattle to Australia has revolutionized the control of *B microplus* on that continent. Use of resistant cattle as a means of tick control is also becoming important in Africa and the Americas. In Africa, infestations of ixodid ticks on livestock and wild ungulates may also be reduced by oxpeckers (*Buphagus* spp), which are birds that feed on attached ticks.

Chemical Control: *See also* ECTOPARASITICIDES, p 2158. Control of ticks with acaricides may be directed against the free-living stages in the environment or against the parasitic stages on hosts. Control of ixodid ticks by acaricide treatment of vegetation has been done in specific sites (eg, along trails) in recreational areas in the USA and elsewhere, to reduce the risk of tick attachment to people. This method has not been recommended for wider use because of environmental pollution and the cost of treatment of large areas. Dog kennels, barns, and human dwellings may also require periodic treatment with acaricides to control the free-living stages of ixodid ticks such as the kennel tick, *Rhipicephalus sanguineus.*

The free-living stages of argasid ticks, which infest specific foci such as fowl runs, pigeon lofts, pig sties, and human dwellings, are more frequently and more effectively treated with acaricides.

Treatment of hosts with acaricides to kill attached larvae, nymphs, and adults of ixodid ticks and larvae of argasid ticks has been the most widely used control method. In the first half of the century, the main acaricide was arsenic trioxide. Subsequently, organochlorines, organophosphates, carbamates, amidines, pyrethroids, and avermectins have been used in different parts of the world. The introduction of new compounds, such as the phenylpyrazoles, has been necessary because of the development of resistance in tick populations.

Acaricides are most commonly applied to livestock by use of dips or sprays, with dips being considered the more effective. In recent years, several other means of acaricide application have been developed, including slow release of systemics from implants and boluses, slow release of conventional acaricides from impregnated ear tags, pourons (which are applied on the back and spread rapidly over the entire body surface), and spot-ons (which are similar but have less ability to spread). On fowl, acaricides are usually applied as dusts; on cats as dusts or washes; and on dogs as dusts.

For many years, pyrethroids and organophosphates formulated as dusts, dips, or collars were used on dogs and cats to control ticks. With the advent of the phenylpyrazoles, long-lasting spray and convenient spot-on formulations were introduced. Recently, pyrethroids have been introduced as highly concentrated spot-on products that are labeled only for dogs due to their toxicity in cats. The use of these concentrated pyrethroids is not advised on dogs if a cat is even in the same household.

Vaccines: A recent advance of potentially great importance has been the production, using biotechnology, of a promising vaccine against *B microplus.* The immunizing agent is a concealed tick antigen, not normally encountered by the host. The immune mechanism that it stimulates is different from that stimulated by exposure to ticks (ie, tick feeding). The antigen was derived from a crude extract of partially engorged adult female ticks. It stimulates the production of an antibody that damages tick gut cells and kills the ticks or drastically reduces their reproductive potential. Prospects of developing similar vaccines against other ixodid tick vectors of cattle diseases of major veterinary importance are not clear. *Boophilus* ticks are good candidates for such vaccines in that they are 1-host ticks and show a marked preference for bovine hosts, which act as the principal reservoir of perhaps the most important group of disease agents (*Babesia* spp) that *Boophilus* ticks transmit. By contrast, most other tick vector species of agents that cause important cattle diseases (eg, anaplasmosis, heartwater, theileriosis) are 3-host ticks, which infest not only cattle but also wild ungulate species, for which vaccination is not feasible. Moreover, many wild ungulate hosts of the vector ticks serve as reservoirs of these disease agents. For these reasons, vaccines against nonboophilid vector ticks may be unable either to eradicate the ticks or to eliminate important sources of the disease agents they transmit.

Control Strategies: Initially the main uses of acaricides were tick eradication, prevention of spread of ticks and tickborne diseases (quarantine), and eradication and control of tickborne diseases. The eradication programs were successful in some ecologically marginal subtropical areas, such as southern USA and central Argentina where *Boophilus* spp and babesiosis were eradicated, and southern Africa where East Coast fever (caused by *Theileria parva parva*) was eradicated. The programs were less successful in the ecologically more favorable tropical areas of northeastern Australia, Central America, the Caribbean Islands, and East Africa.

In the areas where eradication was not achieved, the costs of maintaining intensive tick control programs often have become prohibitive. For this reason, integrated biologic and chemical control strategies are being adopted. The effectiveness of these cost-containment strategies requires better knowledge of the dynamic associations among the disease agents, their vertebrate hosts, the tick vectors, and the environment. Strict quarantine measures to prevent reintroductions are enforced in countries from which ticks and tickborne diseases have been eradicated. Climate-matching models, geographic information systems, and expert systems (models based on expert knowledge and artificial intelligence) are being used to identify unaffected areas in which tick pests could become established if introduced.

Control of these diseases will require using the principles of endemic stability and developing improved recombinant vaccines. A current, promising strategy is the identification of receptor sites on the midgut of vector ticks, and the development of antibodies that bind with these sites, thereby blocking tick-ingested tickborne pathogens from infecting the tick. Cattle injected with receptor-site antigens may produce antibodies that feeding ticks ingest.

TUMORS OF THE SKIN AND SOFT TISSUES

Cutaneous tumors are the most frequently diagnosed neoplastic disorders in domestic animals, in part because they can be identified easily and in part because the constant exposure of the skin to the external environment predisposes this organ to neoplastic transformation. Chemical carcinogens, ionizing radiation, and viruses all have been implicated, but hormonal and genetic factors may also play a role in development of cutaneous neoplasms.

The skin is a complex structure composed of various epithelial (epidermis, adnexa), mesenchymal (fibrous connective tissues, blood vessels, adipose tissue), and neural and neuroectodermal tissues (peripheral nerve, Merkel cells, melanocytes), all with the potential of developing distinctive tumors. Because cutaneous tumors are so diverse, their classification is difficult and often controversial. There is also controversy regarding the criteria used to define whether a lesion that arises in the skin or soft tissues is neoplastic and, if so, whether it is benign or malignant. To avoid confusion, the following terms are used in this discussion: A **hamartoma (nevus)** is a localized developmental defect associated with enlargement of one or more elements of the skin. A sebaceous hamartoma, for example, refers to a localized region of the skin where sebaceous glands are extremely prominent and sometimes malformed. Although by strict definition, hamartomas are present at birth, they may occasionally take a long time to reach a size when they are clinically apparent and may not be diagnosed until an animal is mature. To confuse matters further, some lesions with clinical and histologic features of congenital hamartomas may develop in adult animals. Such "acquired" hamartomas are difficult to separate from benign epithelial and mesenchymal neoplasms. In human medical literature and some veterinary texts, the term "nevus" is used synonymously with hamartoma. A **benign neoplasm** is localized, noninfiltrative, and because it is surrounded by a capsule, easily excisable. A **neoplasm of intermediate malignancy** is locally infiltrative and difficult to excise but does not metastasize. A **malignant neoplasm** is infiltrative with metastatic potential.

Although cutaneous neoplasms characteristically are nodular or papular, they also can occur as localized or generalized alopecic plaques, erythematous and pigmented patches and plaques, wheals, or nonhealing ulcers. The variability in clinical presentation can make distinguishing a neoplasm from an inflammatory disease difficult; furthermore, distinguishing a benign tumor from a malignant tumor is even more subjective because sarcomas or carcinomas early in their development may palpate as discrete, encapsulated masses. To establish a definitive diagnosis, histopathology is generally required. Cytologic evaluation can also be useful and, for some neoplasms (eg, round cell tumors), can rival or even surpass the value of histologic examination.

Therapy depends largely on the type of tumor, its location and size, and signalment of the animal. For benign neoplasms associated with neither ulceration nor clinical dysfunction, no therapy may be the most prudent option, especially in aged dogs. For more aggressive neoplastic diseases or benign tumors that inhibit normal function or are cosmetically unpleasant, there are several therapeutic options. For most, surgical intervention with complete excision provides the best chance of a cure at least cost and often with the fewest side effects. Lumpectomy is adequate for benign lesions, but if a malignancy is suspected, the lesion should be removed with wide (3 cm) surgical margins. For tumors that cannot be completely excised, partial removal or debulking may prolong the life of the animal and increase the effectiveness of radiation or chemotherapy. Cryosurgery is also an option, although it is more effective for benign, superficial lesions than for malignant cutaneous neoplasms. Radiation therapy is of most value for infiltrative neoplasms that are not surgically resectable, or when surgical intervention would cause unacceptable physical impairment. Chemotherapy can be used either as a primary method for treatment of malignant neoplasms or as an adjunct to surgery or radiotherapy. In the skin, it is most commonly used to treat round cell tumors (eg, lymphosarcomas, mast cell tumors, transmissible venereal tumors, etc) or solid tumors that cannot be excised completely. Although generally palliative, long remissions may sometimes be obtained. Other forms of therapy include hyperthermia, laser therapy, photodynamic therapy, antiangiogenic therapy, gene therapy, and immunotherapy.

EPIDERMAL AND HAIR FOLLICLE TUMORS

Ceruminous gland tumors are discussed in TUMORS OF THE EAR CANAL (p 426).

Benign, Nonvirus-associated Papillomatous Lesions

For a discussion of papillomas (viral warts), the most common viral-induced neoplasms of the skin, *see* p 774. Benign, proliferative lesions not associated with papilloma virus infection can have a similar gross morphology to that of papillomas.

Epidermal hamartomas (nevi) are rare proliferations identified only in dogs, most often in the young. The disease may be heritable in Cocker Spaniels. Grossly, epidermal nevi appear as pigmented, hyperkeratotic, vaguely papillated papules and plaques that are occasionally arranged in a linear pattern. Some forms are associated with pustules and acantholytic cells. They are benign, but their appearance is unpleasant, and the extensive hyperkeratosis is prone to secondary bacterial infection. Localized lesions can be excised; dogs with multiple lesions or lesions too large to be surgically removed may be responsive to isotretinoin or etretinate. Hyperkeratosis may be transiently controlled by use of topical keratolytic shampoos and emollients.

Congenital papillomas of foals are rare and probably a developmental defect rather than a result of papilloma virus infection. They are found anywhere on the body but most commonly on the head. Thoroughbreds may be predisposed. Present at birth, the lesions are often several centimeters in diameter, hairless, pedunculated, and exophytic, with a papillated surface reminiscent of a cauliflower. They are benign, and excision is curative.

Canine warty dyskeratomas are rare, benign neoplasms of uncertain derivation but with histologic features of follicular or apocrine neoplasms (or both). They appear grossly as verrucous papules or nodules with a keratotic, umbilicated center. Excision is curative.

Basal Cell Tumors and Basal Cell Carcinomas
(Basal cell epitheliomas, Basaliomas, Trichoblastomas, Basosquamous cell carcinomas)

Basal cell tumors represent a heterogeneous group of cutaneous epithelial neoplasms recognized commonly in dogs and cats, occasionally in horses, and seldom in other domestic animals. These neoplasms are composed of a proliferation of small basophilic cells that exhibit morphology reminiscent of the progenitor cells of the epidermis and adnexa. As these tumors have been examined more closely, evidence of differentiation (follicular, sebaceous, etc) has been discovered, giving justification for reclassification. For example, in dogs, what in the past was called a basal cell tumor is best characterized as a **trichoblastoma**, a tumor of hair bulb (the site of the follicle that produces the hair shaft) origin. Some reclassification schemes have suggested that the use of the term basal cell tumor be restricted to a benign neoplasm in cats (the derivation of which has yet to be defined). Because this revised terminology is being adopted by pathologists and clinicians slowly, traditional terminology will be used herein. That is, a benign proliferation of basal cells will be called a basal cell tumor; a malignant proliferation will be called a basal cell carcinoma. In domestic animals, most basal cell tumors are benign and originate in the mid to deep dermis, indicating probable adnexal derivation. These features distinguish basal cell tumors in domestic animal from those in humans, the latter being locally invasive (ie, they are true carcinomas) and originating in the epidermis. In addition, solar injury is a common cause of neoplasms derived from basal cells in humans, but its role in inducing basal cell tumors of other animals remains to be defined.

Canine basal cell tumors most commonly develop in middle-aged to older dogs. Many breeds are predisposed, especially Wirehaired Pointing Griffons and Kerry Blue and Wheaten Terriers. These tumors are found most commonly on the head (especially the ears), the neck, and forelimbs. In cats, basal cell tumors also develop in older animals. Domestic longhair, Himalayan, and Persian are the breeds most at risk, and tumors may develop almost anywhere on the body. In both dogs and cats, these tumors generally appear as firm, solitary, encapsulated, and often hairless or ulcerated nodules that may be pedunculated; they vary in size from <1 cm to >10 cm in diameter. In cats more often than dogs, these tumors are often densely pigmented, and on cut section, they can be difficult to distinguish from dermal melanocytomas. Cystic variants are also more common in cats. Although basal cell tumors are benign, they are expansive neoplasms and may be associated with extensive ulceration and secondary inflammation. Complete excision is curative.

Basal cell carcinomas are more frequently recognized in cats than in dogs. In cats, they develop most frequently in aged animals. Persians are predisposed. They often appear as ulcerated plaques on the head, extremities, or neck. Unlike benign basal cell tumors, these carcinomas generally have continuity with the epidermis, are locally invasive, and may be multicentric. Although evidence of vascular invasion may be identified on histologic sections, local or systemic metastasis rarely occurs. Consequently, surgical excision is the treatment of choice. In dogs, most basal cell carcinomas have histologic evidence of cornification, a feature they have in common with squamous cell carcinomas. Therefore, they are generally called **basosquamous cell carcinomas**. These tumors are generally recognized in older dogs. Saint Bernards, Scottish Terriers, and Norwegian Elkhounds are most at risk. Unlike canine basal cell tumors, basosquamous cell carcinomas do not have a tendency to develop on the head and can be found almost anywhere on the body where they have continuity with the epidermis and appear as exoendophytic nodules or plaques. These tumors are locally invasive but seldom metastasize. Surgical excision is the treatment of choice.

Intracutaneous Cornifying Epitheliomas
(Keratoacanthoma, Infundibular keratinizing acanthoma)

Intracutaneous cornifying epitheliomas are benign neoplasms of dogs and possibly cats. As in human keratoacanthomas, these lesions most likely arise from the hair follicle and not from the interfollicular epidermis. They can develop anywhere on the body, with the back, tail, and extremities the most common sites. Intracutaneous cornifying epitheliomas are tumors of middle-aged dogs. Norwegian Elkhounds, Belgian Sheepdogs, Lhasa Apsos, and Bearded Collies are most likely to develop these tumors, with Norwegian Elkhounds and Lhasa Apsos at risk for developing generalized lesions. The most characteristic presentation is a papule or nodule with a central cornified pore that may protrude above the epidermal surface, giving the appearance of a horn; however, many of these tumors never have continuity with the epidermis and may appear solely as cornified cysts. These tumors are benign and treatment is optional, provided a definitive diagnosis has been established and there is no self-trauma, ulceration, or secondary infection. Excision is curative; however, dogs are prone to develop additional tumors over time. For animals with a generalized form of the disease, oral retinoids (eg, isotretinoin or etretinate) may be of therapeutic benefit.

Squamous Cell Carcinomas
(Epidermoid carcinomas, Prickle cell carcinomas)

Thought to arise from either the epidermis or the epithelium of the superficial (infundibular) regions of the outer root sheath of the hair follicle, squamous cell carcinomas have been recognized in all domestic animals. Although most arise without antecedent cause, in many species, especially in white cats, prolonged exposure to sunlight is a major predisposing factor. The grooming habits of cats also expose them to particulate carcinogens from cigarette smoke and flea collars. In addition, a unique form of feline squamous cell carcinoma associated with papilloma virus infection has been described (*see* below).

In dogs, these are the most frequently diagnosed carcinomas arising in the skin. Two forms are recognized—cutaneous and subungual. **Cutaneous squamous cell carcinomas** are tumors of older dogs, with Bloodhounds, Basset Hounds, and Standard Poodles at greatest risk. Lesions commonly arise on the head, distal extremities, ventral abdomen, and perineum. Most cutaneous squamous cell carcinomas appear as firm, raised, frequently ulcerated plaques and nodules; sometimes they can be extremely exophytic and have a surface reminiscent of a wart. The etiology of most of these tumors is undefined; however, some are induced by prolonged solar injury. These usually develop on ventral abdominal, preputial, scrotal, and inguinal skin in white-skinned, shorthaired breeds such as Dalmatians, Bull Terriers, and Beagles. They develop in a ventral location because the poorly haired skin offers minimal shielding from ultraviolet radiation, many animals sun themselves lying on their backs, and perhaps because solar radiation reflects from the ground. Before a carcinoma develops, animals acquire focal zones of lichenification, hyperkeratosis, and erythema known as **solar keratosis** (solar dermatosis, actinic keratosis, senile keratosis).

Subungual squamous cell carcinomas are most commonly found in Giant and Standard Schnauzers, Gordon Setters, Briards, Kerry Blue Terriers, and Standard Poodles.

Generally, all are darkhaired breeds, and a dark coat color has been associated with the development of subungual squamous cell carcinomas arising on multiple digits, often on different extremities. Females have a slight predilection and both fore- and hindlimbs are equally predisposed to tumor development.

In cats, cutaneous squamous cell carcinomas most commonly develop in conjunction with chronic solar injury. Consequently, they usually develop on the pinnae, frontal ridges, eyelids, nose, or lips of cats that have white skin in these regions. There is no breed or sex predilection. As in dogs, solar keratosis or carcinoma in situ (early superficial stage), often precedes development of a malignant tumor. Recently, coat-associated particulate carcinogens from exposure to cigarette smoke and flea collars have been identified as risk factors for cats with oral squamous cell carcinoma. Lesions not caused by sun exposure most commonly develop on the digits, but subungual forms are uncommon.

Cutaneous squamous cell carcinomas are the most common malignant neoplasm in horses. They generally develop in adult or aged horses with white or part-white coats; breeds at risk include Appaloosa, Belgian, American Paint, and Pinto. Although they can arise anywhere on the body, these tumors most commonly arise in nonpigmented, poorly haired areas near mucous membranes. Thus, the periorbital regions, lips, nose, anus, and external genitalia (especially the penile sheath) are sites most likely to be affected.

In cattle, these tumors are most common in breeds with white hair and poorly pigmented skin (especially Holsteins and Ayrshires) and, as in horses, develop around the mucous membranes, usually at the mucocutaneous junctions, particularly the periocular and vulvar regions. In India, squamous cell carcinomas of the horn core are common in aged bullocks. The most common cause is actinic injury. Solar keratoses often precede development of an invasive tumor; genetic factors, immunodeficiency, and viruses may also play a role.

In sheep, squamous cell carcinomas are of economic significance in some parts of the world. In a study in Australia, they were responsible for more than one-third of all condemnations before slaughter. The Merino breed is most at risk, and females more so than males. The most common sites are the poorly haired skin of the ears, lips, muzzle, and the vulvar lips after they have been externalized by Mules operation to prevent fly strike. Tumors at these sites develop in conjunction with solar injury, which is heightened when animals ingest photosensitizing plants. Tumors of the ears also occur more frequently after a procedure such as ear tagging. Squamous cell carcinomas can develop from follicular cysts on sites not commonly exposed to sunlight.

In goats, squamous cell carcinomas develop most frequently in females, in which tumors develop on the perineal and vulvar regions and on the skin of the teats and udders. Both males and females can develop sun-induced tumors on the ears. Although Angoras are most at risk, Saanan goats occasionally develop squamous cell carcinomas on the udder in association with papillomas. The role papilloma viruses play in tumor progression is undefined.

Squamous cell carcinomas are extremely uncommon in swine.

Most squamous cell carcinomas are solitary lesions; however, multiple tumors may develop in conjunction with solar injury. They appear as endophytic or exo-endophytic lesions, the former as raised, irregular dermal masses with an ulcerated surface, and the latter as raised, irregular dermal masses covered by a papillated epidermis. Cats initially exhibit small crusting facial sores that do not heal. The lesions are often allowed to persist for months before defects appear on the ear tips, nares, and eyelids. Subungual squamous cell carcinomas of dogs are first identified by lameness or malformation, an infection that mimics chronic osteomyelitis, or loss of the claw of the affected digit. In cattle with involvement of the horn, the first sign is distorted growth.

Squamous cell carcinomas are characteristically invasive into adjacent soft and bony tissues. Infrequently, in cattle, they regress spontaneously. In small animals, longterm survival and the likelihood of metastasis are correlated with histologic differentiation. Well-differentiated tumors are slowly progressive or remain localized; undifferentiated tumors are more likely to metastasize or recur within 20 wk of excision. In general, failure of treatment is due to late diagnosis and lack of control of local disease rather than metastasis.

For dogs and cats, surgical excision, such as amputation of the involved digit or pinnae or nosectomy, is the treatment of choice, and margins of at least 2 cm are recommended. One review of 117 digit masses in dogs found that 25% of the lesions were squamous cell carcinomas and 66% were subungual lesions. These had a 95% 1-yr survival after amputation; however if the lesion originated in other parts of the digit, the 1-yr survival was 60%. Excision may be combined with radiation or chemotherapy. Feline squamous cell carcinomas are more radiosensitive than their canine counterparts. Still, the 1-yr survival rate is <10% for invasive neoplasms. Cryosurgery and hyperthermia may be helpful for local therapy especially in early (carcinoma in situ) lesions, but controlled studies have not been done to determine their effectiveness. Intralesional implant chemotherapy with 5-fluorouracil, cisplatin, or carboplatin along with retinoids and photodynamic therapy has been used with variable success. Intratumoral injection of nasal plane squamous cell carcinomas in cats using carboplatin in a water-sesame seed oil emulsion resulted in a 70% general response with 1-yr progression-free survival rate of ~50%. In dogs with multiple ventral actinic keratoses, topical dinitrochlorbenzene or 5-fluorouracil (5%) may be of benefit. Limiting exposure to ultraviolet radiation may help prevent solar-induced squamous cell carcinomas in dogs and cats. This may be accomplished by using UV window screens, sunscreen, and keeping the animals indoors during hours of peak sunlight. Tattoos, magic markers, and sunscreen are used with variable success. In horses, radiotherapy using surface or interstitial brachytherapy is the treatment of choice for squamous cell carcinomas. Other options include ^{90}Sr or ^{192}Ir implants, wide surgical excision (especially for neoplasms of the third eyelid, penis, and prepuce), and cryosurgery. Immunotherapy, with either an autogenous vaccine made from the tumor tissue suspended in Freund's adjuvant, or nonspecific immunomodulation using *Corynebacterium parvum*, has had some success in treating ocular or horn core squamous cell carcinomas in cattle.

Feline multicentric squamous cell carcinoma in situ (feline Bowen's disease) is a disease of aged (>10 yr old) cats may be associated with immunosuppression. There is no defined breed or sex predilection. Clinically, lesions appear as multiple discrete, erythematous, black or brown hyperkeratotic plaques and papules. Lesions are nonpruritic, and ulceration is uncommon. Their development is associated with the presence of a papilloma virus. The term in situ refers to a malignant proliferation of epidermal and follicular outer sheath cells that are not invasive into the underlying dermis. Unfortunately, lesions may progress over time into an invasive carcinoma. Metastasis is extremely uncommon. These lesions usually develop in systemically ill or immunosuppressed cats and are believed to be virally induced; they have not been amenable to therapy.

Keratinized Cutaneous Cysts

Most of these are malformations of the hair follicle. They are common in dogs; occasionally identified in cats, horses, goats, and sheep; and rare in cattle and pigs. Excision is the treatment of choice. Vigorous squeezing of these lesions is contraindicated because it often incites a severe foreign body inflammatory response.

Infundibular follicular cysts (epidermoid cysts, epidermal inclusion cysts, erroneously called sebaceous cysts) are the most common. They are a cystic dilatation of the upper portion of the outer sheath of the hair follicle (the infundibulum) lined by a layer of stratified cornifying epithelial cells that are indistinguishable from the epidermis. These cysts vary in size from 2 mm to >5 cm (lesions <5 mm in diameter are often called milia). The only domestic animals identified at risk are Merino sheep, in which these cysts are often multiple and may progress to squamous cell carcinomas. As with all follicular cysts, these are usually solitary, papular to nodular lesions that are freely movable. They are generally partially compressible on palpation and occasionally have a small opening through the epidermis from which the cystic contents can be extruded. On cut surface, they are filled with a gray, brown, or yellowish, granular, "cheesy" material that is lumenal keratin.

Isthmus catagen cysts (trichilemmal cysts, pilar cysts, cystic intracutaneous cornifying epithelioma) are follicular cysts that have the keratinization pattern of the lower portion of the outer root sheath. They have been definitively identified only in dogs and rarely in cats.

Matrix cysts are follicular cysts in which the wall resembles the epithelium of the hair bulb (the matrix portion of the hair follicle) and the inner root sheath. They occur predominantly in dogs and cats. Many progress to pilomatricomas (*see* below).

Hybrid cysts (panfollicular cysts) are follicular cysts that have a combination of the characteristics of epidermal inclusion, trichilemmal, and matrix cysts and that are found predominantly in dogs and cats. Many progress to trichoepitheliomas (*see* below).

Dermoid cysts are congenital malformations found most commonly on the dorsal midline of the head or along the vertebral column. They are most commonly identified in Boxers, Kerry Blue Terriers, and Rhodesian Ridgeback dogs; Thoroughbred horses; and possibly Suffolk sheep. Typically multiple, they differ from other follicular cysts in that on cut surface they contain fully formed hair shafts. They are arguably the only true epidermal inclusion cysts because they most likely represent an embryonal invagination of the epidermis with associated adnexa. These adnexa are responsible for the hair shafts within the cyst lumens.

Keratomas are cystic lesions in the hoof wall of the toe or, less frequently, the quarter or heel in simple or cloven-hoofed animals. They often occur secondary to a traumatic injury. Although often asymptomatic, they commonly induce lameness and deformity of the hoof wall or sole and may be associated with distal phalangeal lysis. Keratomas are seldom >5 cm in diameter and contain white to brown laminated keratin, often with a necrotic center associated with secondary inflammation. When lameness is present, surgical excision and curettage of the underlying bone, if affected, is the treatment of choice.

Dilated pores of Winer are rare, hair-follicle neoplasms recognized only in aged cats. Males may be predisposed. These lesions most often develop on the head. Clinically, they appear as solitary, dome-shaped lesions with the appearance of a giant comedo. Compact keratin may protrude through (above) the surface, giving them the appearance of a cutaneous horn. These lesions are benign, and complete excision is curative.

Tumors of the Hair Follicle

The hair follicle is a complex structure composed of 8 different epithelial layers. Hair-follicle tumors display a similar complexity, and much work needs to be done to characterize them further. They are most common in dogs, less frequent in cats, and rare in other domestic animals.

Tricholemmomas are rare, benign, hair-follicle neoplasms of dogs, most commonly found on the head. Poodles may be predisposed. These tumors are derived from the lower portion of the outer root sheath and often have areas of transition into basal cell tumors. They have little in common with a tumor of the same name in humans that represents an old wart. They appear as firm, ovoid masses, 1-7 cm in diameter, that are encapsulated but expand over time. Excision is curative.

Trichofolliculomas are extremely rare follicular tumors of dogs composed of the inferior and isthmic regions of multiple abortive follicles that extrude their lumenal contents into a dilated abnormal cystic infundibulum. Too few have been recognized to determine age, breed, or sex predilection. Considered by some to be more a hamartoma than a true neoplasm, these tumors are benign, and complete surgical excision is curative.

Trichoepitheliomas are cystic hair follicle neoplasms of dogs and, less commonly, cats, in which all elements of the hair follicle (infundibulum, isthmus, and inferior portions) and the patterns of cornification they produce are represented. The epithelium and cornification of the infundibular and isthmic portions predominate. Benign and malignant forms are recognized. In dogs, these lesions can occur at any age but are found most commonly during late middle age. Many breeds are predisposed, including Basset Hounds, Bull Mastiffs, Irish Setters, Standard Poodles, English Springer Spaniels, and Golden Retrievers. There is no defined sex predilection. Tumors can develop anywhere on the body but most commonly on the trunk in dogs and on the head, tail, and extremities in cats. Benign forms appear as palpably encapsulated cystic nodules (1-5 cm in diameter) in the dermis and subcutaneous fat. Expansion of cysts or self-trauma may induce ulceration associated with extrusion of lumenal keratin that appears as a condensed, yellow, granular, "cheesy" material. Excision is curative; however, animals that develop one such tumor are prone to develop additional lesions at other sites. This is especially true for Basset Hounds and English Springer Spaniels. **Malignant trichoepitheliomas** are much less common than benign trichoepitheliomas and are differentiated by their local invasiveness; continuity with the epidermis; and association with extensive inflammation, necrosis, and fibrosis. Metastasis is uncommon. Wide surgical excision is the treatment of choice and is often curative in those tumors that are invasive but have minimal metastatic potential.

Pilomatricomas (hair matrix tumors, calcifying epitheliomas [of Malherbe]) are cystic hair follicle neoplasms that are recognized almost exclusively in dogs. Unlike trichoepitheliomas, in which all elements of the follicle are represented, in pilomatricomas only the cells of the matrix region of the inferior part of the hair follicle and the cornification patterns they produce (hair shaft and inner root sheath) are present. Benign and malignant forms are recognized. Benign tumors are most common on the trunk of middle-aged dogs. Kerry Blue and Wheaten Terriers, Bouviers des Flandres, Bichons Frise, and Standard Poodles are most at risk. Grossly, these tumors are indistinguishable from trichoepitheliomas, but their cystic contents are often gritty due to mineralization. Excision is the treatment of choice. As in trichoepitheliomas, when one such lesion develops, additional lesions often develop over time. **Malignant pilomatricomas** (malignant hair matrix tumor, matrical carcinoma) are rare and have been identified most often in dogs. They are a tumor of old dogs and grossly characterized as solitary or multinodular, variably cystic tumors that are often firmly attached to subjacent soft tissues. Because they are invasive, they are difficult to excise, and recurrence is common after attempts at surgical excision. They often metastasize to draining lymph nodes and internal organs, especially the lungs. Aggressive surgery is recommended. It is unknown whether they respond to radiation or chemotherapy.

Cutaneous Apocrine Gland Tumors

Sweat glands are of two types: apocrine and eccrine. Apocrine glands are tubular glands with a coiled secretory portion and a long straight duct that empty into the follicular infundibulum. In domestic animals, all hair follicles have apocrine glands. Apocrine glands in dogs and cats are also present in association with the anal sac, and modified apocrine glands, known as ceruminous glands, are present in the external auditory meatus. In most mammals, apocrine glands produce an odiferous, oily compound that is a sexual attractant, a territorial marker, and a warning signal. In horses and cattle, these glands play a role in thermoregulation by producing sweat.

Apocrine gland tumors and malformations are most common in dogs and cats. Three diseases of apocrine glands of haired skin have been characterized.

Cystic apocrine gland dilations (apocrine gland cysts, cystic apocrine gland hyperplasia, apocrine cystomatosis) are best characterized as hamartomas. Two forms exist: a cystic form in which one or more cysts develop in the mid to upper dermis with a poor association with hair follicles, and a more diffuse form characterized by cystically dilated apocrine glands associated with multiple hair follicles in nontraumatized skin. Both are found in middle-age or older dogs and, less commonly, cats. The head and neck are the most common sites where these lesions develop. In both species, lesions appear as fluctuant dermal cysts or as translucent bullae. Complete excision is curative; however, this may be difficult to accomplish in the more diffuse form.

Apocrine gland adenomas are diagnosed almost exclusively in dogs, cats, and rarely horses. Two types are recognized based on whether their histologic appearance primarily resembles the secretory or ductular portion of the apocrine gland. **Apocrine adenomas** resemble the secretory region of the apocrine glands. They are found in older dogs and cats. Great Pyrenees, Chow Chows, and Alaskan Malamutes are the most commonly affected breeds. The head, neck, and extremities are the most frequent sites of development. In cats, apocrine adenomas are more likely to occur in males, and no breed appears at greater risk than any other. The vast majority occur on the head, especially the pinnae. In horses, no age, sex, or breed association is known. The pinnae and vulva are the most likely regions to develop these tumors. In all species, these tumors appear as firm to fluctuant cysts, seldom >4 cm in diameter. They contain varying amounts of clear to brownish fluid. In cats, the luminal fluid may be darkly pigmented, and apocrine cysts can be confused clinically with melanocytomas, especially when present on the inner aspect of the ears. **Apocrine ductular adenomas** are less common. They are found in older dogs and cats and are putatively derived from or show differentiation toward apocrine ducts. In dogs, these tumors are most commonly recognized in Peekapoos, Old English Sheepdogs, and English Springer Spaniels. They are often smaller, firmer, and less cystic than apocrine adenomas. Because they often consist of a large population of basal cells and because evidence of ductular differentiation can be extremely subtle, these tumors are often diagnosed histologically as basal cell tumors (*see* p 766). Apocrine adenomas and apocrine ductular adenomas are benign, and complete surgical excision is curative.

Apocrine gland adenocarcinomas of haired skin are rare in all domestic animals but most frequently identified in older dogs and cats. In dogs, Treeing Walker Coonhounds, Norwegian Elkhounds, German Shepherds, and mixed-breed dogs are most at risk; in cats, Siamese may be predisposed. In both species, this tumor most commonly arises in axillary and inguinal regions—sites that allow it to be easily confused clinically and histologically with mammary gland ductular adenocarcinomas. Apocrine gland adenocarcinomas generally are larger than adenomas and have a variable clinical appearance ranging from fibrotic dermal nodules to ulcerated plaques. They are locally invasive and frequently metastasize to draining lymph nodes. Less commonly, skin and lung metastasis may occur. Complete surgical excision is the treatment of choice. Little is known about response to adjunct chemotherapy.

Apocrine Gland Tumors of Anal Sac Origin

These have been definitively identified only in dogs, although anecdotal reports suggest they may also occur in cats. Older English Cocker and Springer Spaniels, Dachshunds, Alaskan Malamutes, German Shepherds, and mixed-breed dogs are most at risk. Unlike hepatoid gland tumors (*see* p 773), there is no sex predilection. They most commonly appear as deep, firm, nodular masses near the anal sac. As these lesions grow, they may compress the rectum and induce constipation. Some of these tumors are associated with a paraneoplastic syndrome that is characterized by hypercalcemia and results in anorexia, weight loss, polyuria, and polydipsia. They are often highly infiltrative into the pelvic canal and commonly (90%) metastasize to the sublumbar lymph nodes or to distant internal organs (40%). Wide surgical excision, including involved lymph nodes, is the treatment of choice. Even if the tumor cannot be totally resected, debulking can be of value in dogs with pseudohyperparathyroidism because the hypercalcemia is related to the total tumor mass. Adjunct chemotherapy and radiation therapy may also be of benefit, but few dogs live >1 yr after the tumor has been recognized.

Eccrine Gland Tumors

Eccrine glands are the coiled, tubular, sweat glands present on the footpads of carnivores, the frog of ungulates, the carpus of pigs, and the nasolabial region of ruminants. Tumors derived from these glands are extremely rare and have been identified only on the footpads of dogs and cats. Most are malignant and invasive. These tumors are reported to have a high potential to metastasize to draining lymph nodes.

Sebaceous Gland Tumors

Tumors and tumor-like conditions of sebaceous glands are common in dogs, infrequent in cats, and rare in other domestic animals. Based on morphologic more than on behavioral features, 4 categories of benign sebaceous gland proliferations have been described. In humans, in which a roughly similar classification scheme is traditionally used, it has been proposed that all benign sebaceous gland tumors be called sebaceomas.

Sebaceous gland hamartomas are solitary lesions reported only in dogs. These lesions are distinguished from sebaceous gland hyperplasias and adenomas because they are linear or circumscribed, several centimeters in length or diameter, and are usually identified shortly after birth.

Sebaceous gland hyperplasias (senile sebaceous hyperplasias) represent a senile change in dogs and cats. In dogs, Manchester, Wheaten, and Welsh Terriers are at greatest risk. In cats, there is no breed predilection, but females develop these lesions more frequently than males. In both species, the head and abdomen are affected most commonly. Sebaceous hyperplasias commonly appear as papillated masses seldom >1 cm in diameter often with a shiny, keratotic surface.

Sebaceous gland adenomas are seen in all domestic animals but are so common in older dogs and cats, they can be considered primarily a small animal neoplasm. Coonhounds, English Cocker Spaniels, Cocker Spaniels, Huskies, Samoyeds, and Alaskan Malamutes are the canine breeds most likely to develop these tumors; Persians are the feline breed most predisposed. In dogs, these tumors frequently are clinically indistinguishable from sebaceous hyperplasias, but they tend to be larger (typically >1 cm). They are often multiple and may occur anywhere on the body but are commonly found on the head. Sebaceous adenomas may be covered with a serocellular crust and exhibit pleocellular inflammation and superficial pyoderma. **Sebaceous gland epitheliomas** are a variant of sebaceous adenoma distinguished by lobules composed primarily of basal progenitor cells rather than mature sebocytes. Because they often have irregular lobules that extend into the deep dermis, they can occasionally be confused with sebaceous carcinomas. These tumors are found in older dogs and rarely cats. They appear as ulcerated nodules that may be several centimeters in diameter. A papillated epidermal surface and pigmentation are variable findings.

Sebaceous gland adenocarcinomas are rare in domestic animals. They are recognized almost exclusively in dogs and cats, generally in middle-aged or older animals. Cavalier King Charles Spaniels, Cocker Spaniels, and Scottish, Cairn, and West Highland White Terriers are most at risk. Male dogs and female cats may be predisposed. These lesions are often ulcerated and may be indistinguishable from sebaceous epitheliomas or other cutaneous carcinomas. They are locally infiltrative and may metastasize to regional lymph nodes late in the disease.

Once a diagnosis is established, treatment is optional for benign sebaceous gland tumors unless they are secondarily inflamed and infected. For malignant adenocarcinomas, excision is the treatment of choice, but complete removal can be difficult due to the infiltrative nature of this tumor; adjunct radiotherapy may be required. Even benign sebaceous gland growths recur if remnants are left at the surgical site. In addition, animals that develop one sebaceous gland hyperplasia or adenoma often develop new lesions at other sites over time. No established protocol of chemotherapy for any of these lesions has been defined. Oral retinoids may prevent recurrence of sebaceous hyperplasia, but their use remains poorly defined and consultation with a veterinary oncologist or dermatologist is strongly recommended.

Hepatoid Gland Tumors
(Perianal gland tumors, Circumanal gland tumors)

These common neoplasms arise from modified sebaceous glands that are most abundant in the cutaneous tissues around the anus but may also be present along the ventral midline from the perineum to the base of the skull, the dorsal and ventral tail, and in the skin of the lumbar and sacral regions. Because androgens stimulate the development of hepatoid glands, the incidence of proliferative lesions of hepatoid glands in intact, male dogs is 3 times that in females.

Benign hepatoid gland tumors are divided into hepatoid gland hyperplasias and adenomas; however, as with benign sebaceous gland tumors, there is a continuum from hyperplasia to adenoma. Here, they will be considered as a single entity. Hepatoid gland adenomas are most common in aged dogs. Siberian Huskies, Samoyeds, Pekingese, and Cocker Spaniels are most commonly affected. Tumors may develop at any site where hepatoid glands are present, but 90% occur in the perianal region. Grossly, they appear as one or (more commonly) multiple intradermal nodules 0.5-10 cm in diameter. Larger lesions commonly ulcerate, and hemorrhagic, keratinaceous material can often be extruded with local pressure. Large tumors can compress the anal canal and make defecation difficult. Up to 95% of male dogs respond completely to castration; in those that do not, the pituitary-adrenal axis should be evaluated and, if no abnormality is detected, the dog should be reevaluated for the presence of a low-grade hepatoid gland adenocarcinoma. Excision may be used concurrently to remove extremely large or ulcerated tumors that have become secondarily infected. Surgery is the treatment of choice for females with hepatoid gland adenomas but may need to be repeated because recurrence is common. Radiation therapy is also an option and has a 2-yr cure rate of 69% for benign tumors. Cryosurgery is another therapeutic alternative, but because of the complication of fecal incontinence, should be used only when tumors are not amenable to surgical intervention. Diethylstilbestrol has been used in the past as an alternative to castration, but because of severe side effects, including aplastic anemia and cystic prostatic hyperplasia, it should be used with extreme caution, if at all.

Hepatoid gland adenocarcinomas are uncommon canine neoplasms that generally appear as nodular lesions affecting the perianal region. These tumors are found in male dogs 10 times more commonly than in females. Siberian Huskies, Alaskan Malamutes, and Bulldogs are most likely to develop this tumor. Histologic evaluation is the best means of diagnosis; however, there is debate about how to distinguish low-grade malignant tumors from hepatoid adenomas because well-differentiated forms can be confused with adenomas, and anaplastic forms can be confused with apocrine gland adenocarcinomas of anal sac origin. These tumors have metastatic potential and often spread to regional lymph nodes. Treatment consists of wide surgical excision including involved lymph nodes and, possibly, subsequent radiation. These tumors are generally not responsive to castration or to estrogen therapy, and it is unknown whether chemotherapy is of benefit for metastatic disease. The prognosis is guarded.

Primary Cutaneous Neuroendocrine Tumors
(Merkel cell tumors, Atypical histiocytomas, Trabecular carcinomas, Extramedullary plasmacytomas)

In veterinary medicine, the diagnosis of tumors derived from Merkel cells (tactile, neurosecretory cells of epithelial derivation present in the basal cell layer of the epidermis) has fallen in disfavor, and most pathologists consider this tumor to be an extramedullary plasmacytoma. Merkel cell tumors most likely develop in animals but are not recognized as such.

Papillomas
(Warts)

Papilloma viruses are small, double-stranded DNA viruses of the Papovaviridae family. Some mammals have several distinct papilloma viruses—humans have >20; cattle, 6; dogs, 3; and rabbits, 2. Different papilloma viruses often have considerable species, site, and histologic specificity. The virus is transmitted by direct contact, fomites, and possibly by insects. Papillomas have been reported in all domestic animals, birds, and fish. Multiple papillomas (papillomatosis) of skin or mucosal surfaces generally are seen in younger animals and are usually caused by viruses. Papillomatosis is most common in cattle, horses, and dogs. Single papillomas are more frequent in older animals, but they may not always be caused by viral infection.

When lesions are multiple, they may be sufficiently characteristic to confirm the diagnosis; however, there are many simulants of warts, and a definitive diagnosis requires identification of the virus or its cytopathic effects on individual cells—a change known as koilocytic atypia or koilocytosis.

In cattle, warts commonly are found on the head, neck, and shoulders, and occasionally on the back and abdomen. The extent and duration of the lesions depend on the type of virus, area affected, and degree of susceptibility. Warts appear ~2 mo after exposure and may last ≥1 yr. Papillomatosis becomes a herd problem when a large group of young, susceptible cattle become infected. Immunity usually develops 3-4 wk after initial infection, but papillomatosis occasionally recurs, probably due to loss of immunity.

Although most warts appear as epidermal proliferations that have a keratotic surface resembling a cauliflower (verruca vulgaris), some bovine papilloma viruses (bovine papilloma types 1 and 2) involve dermal fibroblasts and keratinocytes and appear as a papulonodule with a warty surface. Such fibropapillomas may involve the venereal regions where they can cause pain, disfigurement, infection of the penis of young bulls, and dystocia when the vaginal mucosa of heifers is affected.

A form of persistent cutaneous papillomatosis with smaller numbers of papillomas may be seen in herds of older cattle. A bovine papilloma virus has been demonstrated in bladder tumors associated with bracken fern ingestion (p 2349) and in upper GI tract papillomas of cattle in Scotland. It is believed that the papilloma virus acts as a co-carcinogen. When bovine papilloma virus type 1 or 2 is injected into the skin of horses, a dermal tumor similar to equine sarcoid develops.

In horses, small, scattered papillomas develop on the nose, lips, eyelids, distal legs, penis, vulva, mammary glands, and inner surfaces of the pinnae, often secondary to mild abrasions. They can be a herd problem, especially when young horses are kept together, but regress in a few months, as a foal's immune system matures. When they develop in older horses, they often persist for >1 yr. So-called aural plaques are also thought to be a flat form of papilloma (verruca planum). Equine papillomas are disfiguring but benign. They need to be distinguished from verrucous equine sarcoid (p 777).

In dogs, 3 clinical presentations of canine papilloma virus infection have been described. The first is **canine mucous membrane papillomatosis**, which primarily affects young dogs. It is characterized by the presence of multiple warts on oral mucous membranes from lips to (occasionally) the esophagus and on the conjunctival mucous membranes and adjacent haired skin. When the oral cavity is severely affected, there is interference with mastication and swallowing. A viral etiology has been clearly established for these lesions. The second presentation is **cutaneous papillomas**, which are indistinguishable from the warts that develop on or around mucous membranes. However, they are more frequently solitary and develop on older dogs. Cocker Spaniels and Kerry Blue Terriers may be predisposed. A definitive viral etiology has not been established, and lesions may be confused with cutaneous tags. Recently, a syndrome characterized by papillomatosis of one or more footpads has been described. Clinically, lesions appear as multiple, raised keratin horns. A viral etiology has been suggested but not proven. The third presentation is **cutaneous inverted papillomas**, which have more in common clinically with intracutaneous cornifying epitheliomas. In this disease of young, mature dogs, lesions most commonly develop on the ventral abdomen where they appear as raised papulonodules with a keratotic center. Infrequently, viral papillomas in dogs may progress to invasive squamous cell carcinomas.

In cats, papilloma virus infection appears most commonly as a multicentric squamous cell carcinoma (p 767). The typical warty lesions associated with papilloma virus infection in most species are not present. Papillomas may affect the skin of goats, and infection on the teats has been reported to induce malignant transformation. In sheep, papillomas are rare and most commonly appear as fibropapillomas. In pigs, they are very rare and when present are identified as solitary or multiple lesions on the face or genitalia. For discussion of papillomatosis in rabbits, *see* p 1583.

A cutaneous fibroma occurs in white-tailed, black-tailed, and mule deer, and in antelope, moose, and caribou. It is caused by a papilloma virus that resembles a bovine papilloma virus and is found only in the epithelium that covers the tumors.

Infectious papillomatosis is a self-limiting disease, although the duration of warts varies considerably. A variety of treatments have been advocated without agreement on efficacy. Surgical removal is recommended if the warts are sufficiently objectionable. However, because surgery in the early growing stage of warts may lead to recurrence and stimulation of growth, the warts should be removed when near their maximum size or when regressing. Affected animals may be isolated from susceptible ones, but with the long incubation period, many are likely to have been exposed before the problem is recognized.

Vaccines are of some value as a preventive but are of little value in treating cattle that already have lesions. Because wart viruses are mostly species-specific, there is no merit in using a vaccine derived from one species in another.

When the disease is a herd problem, it can be controlled by vaccination with a suspension of ground wart tissue in which the virus has been killed with formalin. Autogenous vaccines may be more effective than those commercially available. It may be necessary to begin vaccination in calves as early as 4-6 wk of age with a dose of ~0.4 mL intradermally given at two sites. The vaccination is repeated in 4-6 wk and at 1 yr of age. Immunity develops in a few weeks but is unrelated to whatever mechanism is involved in spontaneous regression. If the animal was exposed to the virus before vaccination, immunity may develop too late to prevent warts. A vaccination program must be in effect for ~3-6 mo before its preventive value will be evident. Vaccination should be continued for ≥1 yr after the last wart disappears because the premises may still be contaminated. Stalls, stanchions, and other inert materials can be disinfected by fumigating with formaldehyde.

CONNECTIVE TISSUE TUMORS

Benign Fibroblastic Tumors

Collagenous nevi are benign, focal, developmental defects with increased deposition of dermal collagen. They are common in dogs, uncommon in cats, and rare in large animals. They generally are found in middle-aged or older animals, most frequently on the proximal and distal extremities, head, neck, and areas prone to trauma. They are sessile to raised, dermal nodules, often with a papillated surface. Two forms are seen; one develops in the interfollicular dermis or subcutaneous fat that is not accompanied by adnexal involvement, and one incorporates adnexa and induces enlarged, often malformed follicles, sebaceous glands, and apocrine glands. This latter form has been called **focal adnexal dysplasia**. Excision of both forms is generally curative although, infrequently, expansive forms have been identified that may grow too large to be surgically removed.

Generalized nodular dermatofibrosis (dermatofibromas), recognized rarely in German Shepherds (believed to be an inherited, autosomal dominant trait) and even less commonly in other canine breeds, is a syndrome in which multiple collagenous nevi are associated with renal cystadenocarcinomas and, in females, multiple uterine leiomyomas. Skin lesions, first recognized when animals are 3-5 yr old, are characterized by the development of multiple collagenous nevi varying from barely palpable to large and nodular, generally on the limbs, feet, head, and trunk. They may be symmetrically distributed. Renal disease develops ~3-5 yr after the skin lesions are recognized. No known therapy can prevent development of the renal and uterine neoplasms.

Acrochordons (cutaneous tags, soft fibromas, fibrovascular papillomas) are distinctive, benign, cutaneous lesions of older dogs. These lesions are common, may be single or multiple, and can develop in any breed, although large breeds may be at increased risk. Most commonly, they appear as pedunculated exophytic growths, often covered by a verrucous epidermal surface. Treatment is optional, but a biopsy is recommended to confirm the diagnosis. Acrochordons are amenable to excision, electrosurgery, and cryosurgery, but dogs that develop one are prone to develop others over time.

Fibromas are discrete, generally cellular proliferations of dermal fibroblasts. Histologically, they resemble collagenous nevi or cutaneous tags. Fibromas occur in all domestic species but are primarily a tumor of aged dogs. Doberman Pinschers, Boxers (predisposed to developing multiple tumors), and Golden Retrievers are most at risk. The head and extremities are the most likely sites. Clinically, the lesions appear as discrete, generally raised, often hairless nodules originating in the dermis or subcutaneous fat. They palpate as either firm and rubbery (**fibroma durum**) or soft and fluctuant (**fibroma molle**). These lesions are benign, and treatment is optional; however, complete excision is recommended because they may grow quite large.

Soft-tissue Sarcomas

This group of malignancies includes equine sarcoids, fibromatoses, fibrosarcomas, malignant fibrous histiocytomas, neurofibrosarcomas, leiomyosarcomas, rhabdomyosarcomas, and variants of liposarcomas, angiosarcomas, synovial cell sarcomas, mesotheliomas, and meningiomas. As a group, sarcomas are widely recognized, yet poorly characterized neoplasms. The confusion stems in part from the fact that spindle-cell sarcomas demonstrate much greater morphologic heterogeneity than carcinomas; often, features of one sarcoma are intermixed with features of another. Consequently, it is widely accepted that the cell of origin of all soft-tissue sarcomas is a primitive mesenchymal cell that can differentiate in many different directions. This makes it difficult to define histopathologic criteria necessary for making an unequivocal diagnosis of specific spindle-cell sarcomas. In addition, comparing neoplastic mesenchymal cells with the normal cell they most closely resemble does not imply origin from those cells. A second cause for the confusion stems from the difficulty in determining whether these are benign or malignant or what their biologic behavior will be in certain locations or breeds. Most spindle-cell sarcomas of domestic animals are locally infiltrative, difficult to excise, and yet seldom metastasize. Because, by definition, only malignant tumors have metastatic potential, these tumors should be considered benign; however, again by definition, benign neoplasms are not infiltrative, and those tumors should be considered malignant and treated aggressively from the start. In human pathology, infiltrative but nonmetastasizing mesenchymal spindle-cell tumors have been defined as sarcomas of intermediate malignancy, a concept used below.

Clinically, 4 general principles relate to spindle-cell sarcomas and soft-tissue sarcomas: The more superficial the location, the more likely the tumor is to be benign (deep tumors tend to be malignant). The larger the tumor, the more likely it is to be malignant. A rapidly growing tumor is more likely to be malignant than one that develops slowly. Benign tumors are relatively avascular, whereas most malignancies are hypervascular.

Excision is the treatment of choice; wide excision or amputation should be performed when anatomically feasible because spindle-cell sarcomas often infiltrate along fascial planes, making it difficult to determine from gross examination the peripheral margins of the tumor. The best, if not only, opportunity to completely remove a spindle-cell sarcoma is during the first surgical attempt. A presurgical biopsy should be performed and a clear surgical plan formulated that includes the intention of complete removal with biopsy samples submitted for margin determinations. Those sarcomas that recur have a greater potential for metastasis, and the time between recurrence often shortens with each subsequent attempt at excision. In addition, many soft-tissue tumors have a pseudocapsule, which on gross examination gives the impression of complete encapsulation; these tumors should not be "shelled out" because neoplastic cells are usually present in the pericapsular connective tissues. Many sarcomas are shaped like an octopus, with tentacles that extend deeply into the tumor bed. Except for equine sarcoids, cryosurgery is usually not used for these tumors because some types, most notably fibrosarcomas, are resistant to freezing. Spindle-cell sarcomas generally do not respond well to conventional doses of radiation; however, higher doses have been reported to control ~50% of them for 1 yr. Surgical debulking followed by radiation is also an option for local control. Chemotherapeutic protocols for sarcomas have become more accepted as a means of treatment. Most involve the use of adriamycin often in combination with other agents, including cyclophosphamide, vincristine, dacarbazine, and methotrexate. Some clinicians use carboplatin and will often rotate it with adriamycin. Although chemotherapy may improve the quality and prolong the life of an affected animal, it is seldom curative.

Equine sarcoids are the most frequently recognized neoplasm in horses. A viral etiology is suspected, and both papilloma virus and retrovirus particles have been identified on ultrastructural examination of sarcoids. In addition, cell-free extracts of bovine papilloma virus can induce a transient form of equine sarcoid when injected into horses. Evidence also suggests that sarcoids are transmissible by direct contact or via arthropod vectors or fomites, eg, contaminated brushes and needles. Sarcoids occur in horses, donkeys, or mules, most commonly in those <4 yr old. Although there is a tendency for sarcoids to develop in families, no breed, sex, or coat color predisposition has been defined. Sarcoids may be found anywhere on the body, and up to 84% of affected horses have multiple lesions. The most common site varies with geographic area; in the UK, the penis is the most commonly reported site, while in the northwest USA, the limbs are affected most frequently. Sarcoids are highly variable in appearance, and 4 manifestations are recognized: 1) verrucous, which may be confused with squamous papillomas or squamous cell carcinomas; 2) fibroblastic, which may be confused with granulation tissue or fibromas; 3) sessile or flat, which may be confused with flat warts (verruca plana); and 4) mixed verrucous and fibroblastic, which may be confused with fibropapillomas. They should be considered sarcomas of intermediate malignancy—they do not metastasize but are locally invasive. The fibroblastic and sessile forms are generally the most aggressive.

Cryosurgery, after surgical debulking of larger lesions, is the treatment of choice. Two freeze-thaw cycles are generally used. A 1-yr remission rate of ~90% has been reported. Also, nontreated lesions may regress spontaneously, although ≥50% of equine sarcoids recur after surgery. Radiation therapy using iridium may control up to 85% of equine sarcoids. This treatment is most commonly used when sarcoids develop in locations not amenable to cryosurgery or excision. Immunotherapy with inoculations of bacillus Calmette-Guérin (BCG) or cell wall extract of *Mycobacterium bovis* remains controversial; some reports indicate ~50% of tumors can be controlled with such immunomodulating therapies. Tumors so treated may take several months to regress. Treatment with flunixin meglumine and prednisolone 30 min before BCG inoculation is recommended. Lastly, BCG therapy should not be used when treated horses could be exposed to cattle because BCG can induce a positive tuberculin reaction in the latter.

Fibromatosis (aggressive fibromatosis, extra-abdominal desmoids, desmoid tumors, low-grade fibrosarcomas, nodular fasciitis) is a sclerosing and infiltrative proliferation of well-differentiated fibroblasts derived from aponeuroses and tendon sheaths. They are generally seen on the heads of dogs, especially Doberman Pinschers and Golden Retrievers, where they are commonly diagnosed as nodular fasciitis. In veterinary medicine, the term nodular fasciitis is applied to 2 different diseases—one that behaves as a fibromatosis and one that commonly affects the periocular tissues (known as canine fibrous histiocytoma [*see* below]). Fibromatoses are infrequently diagnosed in cats and horses. Grossly, fibromatoses are generally indistinguishable from infiltrative fibrosarcomas; however, they can be differentiated on histologic examination. Focal lymphoid nodules are scattered throughout the tissues. The fibromatoses are locally infiltrative with essentially no metastatic potential. If feasible, excision is the treatment of choice. Recurrence is common, and radiation therapy may be of value for local control.

Fibrosarcomas are aggressive mesenchymal tumors in which fibroblasts are the predominant cell type. They are the most common soft-tissue tumors in cats and are also common in dogs but are rare in other domestic animals. In dogs, these tumors are most common on the trunk and extremities. Gordon Setters, Irish Wolfhounds, Brittany Spaniels, Golden Retrievers, and Doberman Pinschers may be predisposed. Fibrosarcomas vary markedly in their appearance and size. Neoplasms arising in the dermis may appear nodular. Those arising in the subcutaneous fat or subjacent soft tissues may require palpation to identify. They appear as firm, fleshy lesions involving the dermis and subcutaneous fat and often invade musculature along fascial planes. When tumors are multiple, they are usually found within the same anatomic region. Fibrosarcomas with abundant interstitial proteoglycans (connective tissue mucins) are called **myxosarcomas** or **myxofibrosarcomas**. Myxosarcomas remain poorly defined in veterinary medicine, and many of them could be characterized as variants of liposarcomas or malignant fibrous histiocytomas. Fibrosarcomas in dogs are invasive tumors; ~10% metastasize. Factors that affect whether a fibrosarcoma can be completely excised include the surgeon's skill, intent of the surgical plan, rate of growth (as defined by the mitotic index and quantity of necrosis), degree of cellular atypia, and the tumor's infiltrative nature, size, and location (which may require imaging to define properly).

Three forms of fibrosarcoma are recognized in cats: a multicentric form in the young (generally <4 yr old) caused by the feline sarcoma virus (FSV); a solitary form in the young or old, in which FSV has not been implicated; and a fibrosarcoma that develops in the soft tissues where cats are commonly vaccinated. This latter neoplasm is being recognized with increasing frequency in the USA (*see also* p 1745). An association with rabies and feline leukemia virus vaccinations is better defined than with vaccinations for other viral or bacterial diseases. Aluminum (commonly used in adjuvants) has been identified in vaccine-induced fibrosarcomas, and a prolonged proliferation of fibroblasts in response to the adjuvant may predispose them to undergo neoplastic transformation. These tumors appear as nodules or plaques between the shoulder blades, in the soft tissues of the proximal hindlimbs, or less commonly, over the lumbar areas. Although commonly classified as fibrosarcomas, vaccination-site sarcomas are extremely heterogeneous and may be appropriately called malignant fibrous histiocytomas (giant cell tumors), liposarcomas, osteosarcomas, or chondrosarcomas.

Wide and deep surgical excision is the treatment of choice for fibrosarcomas, but because most practitioners underestimate the necessary margin extent, recurrence is common (>70% within 1 yr of the initial surgery). The rate of recurrence is >90% for vaccine-associated sarcomas. Even when surgical excision is clinically and histologically complete, recurrence is still the rule. Chemotherapy with carboplatin, doxorubicin and cyclophosphamide, or dacarbazine has been recommended for nonresectable tumors. Initial results using a biologic response modifer (used intratumorally before excision and followed by radiation therapy) appears promising. Further work suggests that its effectiveness as an adjunct to surgery and radiation may increase tumor-free intervals up to 20% compared with historical controls.

Fibrohistiocytic Tumors

These pleomorphic, mesenchymal tumors composed of fibroblasts and histiocytic cells (often present as multinucleated giant cells) remain poorly defined in veterinary medicine. A lesion called **canine fibrous histiocytoma** (nodular granulomatous episclerokeratitis, nodular fasciitis, proliferative keratoconjunctivitis, conjunctival granuloma, Collie granuloma) is recognized at the episcleral junction and cornea primarily in young to middle-aged (2-4 yr old) Collies, but the histologic features are more suggestive of a granulomatous inflammatory response than a neoplasm. As might be expected for a noninfectious inflammatory process, these are generally responsive to sublesional injections of 10-40 mg of methylprednisolone.

Malignant fibrous histiocytomas (extraskeletal giant cell tumors, giant cell tumors of soft parts, dermatofibrosarcomas) are most frequently found in the skin and soft tissues of cats, occasionally found in horses and mules, and rarely in the skin of other domestic species, including dogs. In cats, malignant fibrous histiocytomas are most common on the distal extremities or ventral cervical regions of the aged but may also be diagnosed at vaccination sites. In horses and mules, these have been described as giant cell tumors of soft parts. Occurring in young adult to middle-aged Equidae, they are firm, nodular to diffuse swellings that are white on cut surface, with variable hemorrhage. Malignant fibrous histiocytomas are sarcomas of intermediate malignancy. They are locally invasive and tend to recur after attempts at complete excision but seldom metastasize. Radical excision is recommended.

Peripheral Nerve Sheath Tumors

Amputation neuromas (traumatic neuromas) are non-neoplastic, disorganized proliferations of peripheral nerve parenchyma and stroma that form in response to amputation or traumatic injury. They are most commonly identified after tail docking in dogs or neurectomy in the distal extremities of horses. The most common clinical presentation is a young dog that continuously traumatizes its docked tail. In horses, such a lesion appears as a firm, often painful swelling at a neurectomy surgery site. Excision is curative.

Neurofibromas and **neurofibrosarcomas** (perineuromas, neurilemmomas, nerve sheath tumors, hemangiopericytomas, neurothekomas, schwannomas) are spindle-cell tumors that arise from the connective tissue components of the peripheral nerve.

They are believed to arise from Schwann cells, but they could also arise from mesenchymal cells, which produce the nonmyelinated connective tissues that surround the myelinated nerve fiber. In dogs, forms of this tumor can be virtually indistinguishable from hemangiopericytomas and may be the same tumor.

In dogs and cats, peripheral nerve sheath tumors of the skin are found in older animals. In cattle, they have a suspected genetic basis, may be multiple, can develop in both the young and old, and are generally an incidental finding at slaughter; they arise from the deep nerves of the thoracic wall and viscera, and cutaneous involvement is rare. Regardless of the species, these tumors appear as white, firm, nodules. Attachment to a peripheral nerve may occasionally be noted. Both benign and intermediate-grade malignant variants are recognized. Benign tumors are most common in cattle in which, due to their indolent nature, treatment is optional; also, additional tumors often develop spontaneously at other sites over time. In dogs, cats, and horses, most are locally infiltrative but do not metastasize. Complete excision is the treatment of choice. Where margins are narrow or insufficient, followup radiation therapy may increase the tumor-free interval.

Adipose Tissue Tumors

Lipomas are benign tumors of adipose tissue, perhaps more accurately characterized as hamartomas. They are common in dogs, occasionally identified in cats and horses, and rare in other domestic species. In dogs, they generally occur in older, obese females, most commonly on the trunk and proximal limbs. The breeds most at risk are Doberman Pinschers, Labrador Retrievers, Miniature Schnauzers, and mixed-breed dogs. Older, neutered male, Siamese cats are predisposed, and tumors are most commonly found on the ventral abdomen. Obesity does not appear to be a factor in the development of lipomas in cats. Affected horses are generally <2 yr old. Lipomas typically appear as soft, occasionally pedunculated, discrete nodular masses, and most are freely movable. In dogs and cats, >5% are multiple. In general, these tumors float when placed in formalin. A rare variant of this tumor, **diffuse lipomatosis**, has been identified in Dachshunds, in which virtually the entire skin is affected, resulting in prominent folds on the neck and truncal skin. Many lipomas merge imperceptibly with the adjacent nonneoplastic adipose tissue, making it difficult to determine when the entire lesion is excised. Lipomas with an abundant connective tissue stroma (fibrolipomas), cartilaginous stroma (chondrolipomas), or a prominent vascular component (angiolipomas) are also recognized. Despite their benign nature, lipomas should not be ignored because they tend to enlarge over time, and their gross presentation may be indistinguishable from that of infiltrative lipomas or liposarcomas (*see* below). Excision is curative. In dogs, dietary restriction several weeks before surgery may allow for better definition of the surgical margins of the tumor.

Infiltrative lipomas (intra- and intermuscular lipomas) are rare in dogs and even less common in cats and horses. In dogs, they are most common in middle-aged females, usually on the thorax and limbs. The breeds (dogs) most at risk are the same as those for lipomas. These tumors are poorly confined, soft, nodular to diffuse swellings that typically involve the subcutaneous fat and underlying muscle and connective tissue stroma. Infiltrative lipomas, which dissect along fascial planes and between skeletal muscle bundles, are considered sarcomas of intermediate malignancy. They rarely metastasize. Aggressive excision is recommended, and amputation may be necessary.

Liposarcomas are rare neoplasms in all domestic animals. Most are recognized in older male dogs in which they usually develop on the trunk and extremities; Shetland Sheepdogs and Beagles may be predisposed. In cats, feline leukemia virus infection has been infrequently associated with their development; whether this is a coincidence or such infections play a causative role remains undefined. Liposarcomas are nodular and soft to firm. They may exude a mucinous fluid when sectioned. Many have palpable, partially encapsulated areas, but these zones should not be construed as evidence of a benign tumor. Liposarcomas are malignant neoplasms that have a low metastatic potential but are frequently pseudoencapsulated. Wide excision is recommended. Recurrence is common, so followup radiation therapy is indicated in cases with insufficient margins.

Vascular Tumors

Hemangiomas of the skin and soft tissues are benign proliferations that closely resemble blood vessels. Whether these are neoplasms, hamartomas, or vascular malformations remains undefined, and no clear criteria exist that allow for their separation. They are most commonly identified in dogs, occasionally in cats and horses, and rarely in cattle and pigs; they are an exceptional finding in other domestic animals. In dogs, they are tumors of adult dogs and most commonly develop on the trunk and extremities. Many canine breeds (including Gordon Setters; Boxers; and Airedale, Scottish, and Kerry Blue Terriers) are considered to be at risk. Cats most frequently develop hemangiomas when they are adults. Lesions are most common on the head, extremities, and abdomen. In horses, they are most common on the distal extremities of young (<1 yr old) animals. In cattle, they may be seen as congenital lesions or in older animals. Dairy cattle are predisposed to developing disseminated hemangiomas (angiomatosis) in the skin and internal organs. In pigs, these lesions generally develop in the scrotal or perineal skin of Yorkshire, Berkshire, and less commonly Chester White boars. In the first 2 breeds, the disease is believed to be genetically transmitted. Hemangiomas are single to multiple, circumscribed, often compressible, red to black nodules. The lining epidermis may be unaffected or ulcerated or papillated. Small, superficial hemangiomas that often appear as a "blood blister" are known as angiokeratomas. When erythrocytes are sparse or absent within vascular lumens, the term lymphangioma is applied. Hemangiomas are benign, but their tendency to ulcerate and grow quite large, along with the importance of confirming the diagnosis to make a prognosis, indicate removal. Excision is the treatment of choice; however, in large animals in which the lesions may be large and involve the distal extremities, this may be difficult. In these cases, cryosurgery or radiation therapy may be necessary. Except in dairy cattle with angiomatosis, development of additional tumors at new sites after complete excision is uncommon.

Hemangiopericytomas (canine spindle-cell sarcoma, canine malignant fibrous histiocytoma, canine neurofibrosarcoma, canine perineuroma) are common in dogs and rare in cats (if they occur at all). This tumor was initially named because it was thought to be derived from fibroblastic cells that surround small vessels; however, the appropriateness of the name remains a topic of debate. These tumors develop most commonly on the distal extremities and thorax of older dogs. Females appear to be predisposed, and Siberian Huskies, mixed-breed dogs, Irish Setters, and German Shepherds are most at risk. Hemangiopericytomas typically present as firm, multilobulated, solitary lesions with irregular borders, most commonly in the subcutaneous fat but sometimes in the dermis. They are of intermediate malignancy and have limited metastatic potential. Complete excision is the treatment of choice but, due to their infiltrative nature, ~30% recur. If the first excision of any sarcoma is not adequate, followup surgery to completely remove the tumor bed is indicated. At surgery, intralesional chemotherapy with carboplatin and intraoperative radiation therapy may improve the tumor-free interval. Followup external beam radiation therapy may also be considered as an option to control local recurrence following incomplete excision or narrow margins.

Angiosarcomas, arguably the most aggressive of all soft-tissue tumors, are composed of cells that have many functional and morphologic features of normal endothelium. Although these tumors are often divided into hemangiosarcomas (of purported blood vessel origin) and lymphangiosarcomas (of lymphatic vessel origin), such a distinction is arbitrary. The term **angioendothelioma** is also used. These tumors generally arise spontaneously, but in dogs with short, often white coats, chronic solar injury has induced a change in the superficial vascular plexus, which initially appears as a hemangioma and then progresses to a malignant vascular tumor. The breeds prone to actinically induced angiosarcomas are Whippets, Italian Greyhounds, White Boxers, and Pit Bulls. Pathologists will often diagnose these lesions as cutaneous hemangiosarcomas.

Angiosarcomas of the skin and soft tissues are seen in all domestic animals but are most common in dogs, generally in adult or aged animals. In dogs, they most frequently develop on the trunk, hip, thigh, and distal extremities. In addition to the breeds prone to actinically induced angiosarcomas, Irish Wolfhounds, Vizslas, Golden Retrievers, and German Shepherds are also at risk. In cats, this tumor is seen most commonly in older, neutered males, on the extremities and trunk. Cats with skin, subcutaneous, or visceral involvement develop distant metastasis. Angiosarcomas can vary markedly in appearance. Most commonly, they appear as one or more erythematous nodules present anywhere in the skin or underlying soft tissues. Less frequently, they appear as a poorly defined bruise. All grow rapidly, often are associated with large zones of necrosis and thrombosis, and typically are red to black on cut section. Tumors often diagnosed as lymphangiosarcomas may have much less lumenal blood, and the vascular spaces are typically filled with serum. Characteristically, angiosarcomas create their own vascular space by dissecting through soft tissues. Distant metastasis, especially to the lungs and liver, is common. In other domestic animals, these tumors do not appear to behave as aggressively, and postexcisional recurrence rather than metastasis is more common. For all species, wide excision is the treatment of choice. Solar-induced canine cutaneous hemangiosarcomas generally do not have an aggressive biologic behavior, although numerous lesions may continue to appear over a period of several years. Superficial lesions are easily controlled with topical cryotherapy as needed. Avoidance of further sun injury may reduce the development of new lesions. Recently, adjuvant chemotherapy consisting of vincristine, doxorubicin, and cyclophosphamide has been reported to shrink angiosarcomas; however, the effects of chemotherapy for systemic control or radiation therapy for local control and longterm survival remain to be defined. The role of NSAID such as thalidomide and piroxicam are still not completely understood and may vary from drug to drug. Investigators are hoping to use antiangiogenic or angiostatic compounds such as canine canstatin that attack the blood supply of tumors to control and prevent metastases; however, results of clinical trials are pending.

Cutaneous Smooth Muscle Tumors

Because they either are not recognized or do not occur with any regularity in domestic animals, cutaneous smooth muscle tumors (leiomyomas or leiomyosarcomas) are diagnosed rarely. Those reported generally have been malignant and found in dogs and cats. Usually, they are firm cutaneous masses. Leiomyomas are small and tend to be limited to the dermis, whereas leiomyosarcomas are larger and most arise from (or extend into) the subcutaneous fat. The behavior of malignant smooth muscle tumors remains poorly defined. Complete excision is the treatment of choice for both leiomyomas and leiomyosarcomas.

UNDIFFERENTIATED AND ANAPLASTIC SARCOMAS

These malignant mesenchymal tumors are difficult to characterize microscopically. Undifferentiated sarcomas lack distinctive features (eg, architectural patterns, cytoplasmic and nuclear features, cell products). Anaplastic sarcomas have most of the following features: variations in size and shape of nuclei, nuclear hyperchromasia, striking irregularity of chromatin pattern, abnormal mitotic figures, and large numbers of mitotic figures. As such, anaplastic sarcomas are generally undifferentiated, but undifferentiated sarcomas do not have to be anaplastic. In both cases, wide excision is indicated; however, the prognosis is generally poorer for anaplastic sarcomas than for undifferentiated sarcomas.

LYMPHOCYTIC, HISTIOCYTIC, AND RELATED CUTANEOUS TUMORS

Lymphoid Tumors of the Skin

Canine extramedullary plasmacytomas (atypical histiocytomas, cutaneous neuroendocrine tumors [p 774], reticulum cell sarcomas, cutaneous nodular amyloidosis) are relatively common cutaneous tumors. Although their derivation was long debated, neoplastic cells characteristically express cytoplasmic immunoglobulin and may produce primary amyloid, leaving little doubt as to their lymphoplasmacytic origin. These tumors of dogs and, rarely, cats are most frequently identified on the head (including ears, lips, and oral cavity) and extremities of mature to aged animals.

Cocker Spaniels, Airedales, Scottish Terriers, and Standard Poodles are most at risk. The tumors are generally small (<5 cm) and sometimes pedunculated. Most of these tumors are locally confined, and complete but conservative surgical excision is the treatment of choice. Infrequently, extracutaneous plasmacytomas may be locally invasive or multiple (or both), especially when they occur in the oral cavity. Recurrence has also been correlated with the presence of amyloid (p 478). Treatment for these tumors remains poorly defined. For recurrent, invasive tumors, more aggressive attempts at excision may be required. When tumors are multiple or surgical excision is not feasible, radiation therapy appears to be the best secondary treatment. For tumors resistant to radiation, chemotherapeutic agents, including melphalan, cyclophosphamide, and glucocorticoids, have been recommended.

Cutaneous lymphosarcoma may occur as a disease in which the skin is the initial and primary site of involvement, or it may be secondary to systemic, internal disease. (*See also* CANINE MALIGNANT LYMPHOMA, p 35, BOVINE LEUKOSIS, p 593, and FELINE LEUKEMIA VIRUS AND RELATED DISEASES, p 631.) Cutaneous lymphosarcoma is uncommon but has been identified in all domestic species. In general, 2 distinct forms are recognized—an epitheliotropic form (in which there is infiltration by malignant lymphocytes into the epidermis and adnexa) and a nodular, nonepitheliotropic form. Both usually express surface and cytoplasmic antigens characteristic of T cells; this, along with the frequent identification of at least small foci of epitheliotropism in many cases of "nonepitheliotropic" forms in dogs and cats, suggest they may be different variants of the same tumor.

Epitheliotropic cutaneous lymphosarcoma (ECL, mycosis fungoides) is the most frequently recognized form of cutaneous lymphosarcoma in dogs and arguably cats. It is a disease of middle-aged and older dogs, and Poodles and Cocker Spaniels may be predisposed. Classically, the lesions progress from patch to plaque to tumor; however, one or any combination of these 3 primary lesions may be present. For example, a form of ECL known as pagetoid reticulosis has minimal to no dermal involvement, and cutaneous lesions always appear as erythematous patches. Another common feature of the disease in dogs is the presence of areas of alopecia due to follicular atrophy caused by infiltration of neoplastic cells into the outer sheath and lumen of hair follicles. Although most cases are associated with diffuse cutaneous involvement, forms limited primarily to mucous membranes or the footpads have been identified. Because of the variable clinical appearance of this tumor, diagnosis based on clinical features can be very difficult, and early stages can be confused with allergic, autoimmune, endocrine, infectious, or seborrheic diseases. Most cases are limited to the cutis until late in the course of the disease. ECL with concurrent leukemia is known as Sézary syndrome.

In dogs, ECL is a slow to moderately progressive disease for which a number of therapies have been attempted. To date, all appear more effective in improving the clinical features of the disease than in prolonging an affected dog's life. Methchlorethamine (nitrogen mustard) has been used in the past as a topical therapy, but because large areas of a dog's body may be affected (including the mucous membranes) and because of its sensitizing potential in humans, it is infrequently used. The disease is often transiently responsive to steroids. Chemotherapeutic agents, such as combinations of adriamycin, chlorambucil, cyclophosphamide, doxorubicin, and vincristine, are variably effective. Retinoids with and without glucocorticoids may also achieve partial or complete remission.

In cats, ECL tends to develop in older animals. Lesions often follow a defined progression, appearing initially as a crusty plaque that is variably pruritic. Biopsies of early lesions are often diagnosed as lymphocytic mural folliculitis. In many cases in which this diagnosis is applied, the lesions evolve into unequivocal cutaneous lymphosarcoma. In contrast to ECL in dogs, epitheliotropism is often extremely subtle in cats. Little is known about therapy or whether therapy used in dogs would be effective if used in cats.

Nonepitheliotropic cutaneous lymphosarcoma (NECL) is the most recognized form of cutaneous lymphosarcoma in all domestic animals but dogs and cats. In dogs, NECL is most common in middle-aged or older animals. Lesions are nodules or plaques that most commonly develop on the trunk. They generally are multiple, although solitary lesions may be noted, especially in cats. In many cases, NECL is grossly indistinguishable from the tumor stage of ECL. A definitive diagnosis is important because NECL in dogs is generally more aggressive than ECL, and systemic involvement occurs commonly and early in the course of the disease. Various modes of therapy, including excision, chemotherapy, and less frequently radiotherapy, have been used both singly and in combination. Excision is the choice when the disease is limited to a solitary tumor, and complete cures have occasionally been obtained. Excision or cryosurgery in more diffuse forms infrequently elicit longterm remissions. Chemotherapy or chemoimmunologic protocols used for other forms of canine lymphosarcoma should be considered as palliative. The average remission time is ~8 mo.

In cats, NECL is a disease of middle-aged or older animals. The role of feline leukemia virus remains undefined. The lesions are plaques or nodules that may be solitary or multiple, alopecic or haired, and ulcerated or lined by an intact epidermis. Feline NECL is aggressive; even when complete excision of a solitary nodule is attempted, recurrence is common. To date, no therapy is known. It is unknown whether chemotherapeutic protocols used in treating other forms of feline lymphosarcoma are of value in NECL.

In horses, NECL (nodular lymphosarcoma, subcutaneous lymphosarcoma, lymphohistiocytic lymphosarcoma) may be recognized at any age but is most common in young and middle-aged animals. Firm, nonulcerated nodules are most common in the subcutaneous fat of the ventral body surface. Microscopically, 2 types of nodular lymphosarcoma are recognized in horses. The most common consists of a mixture of histiocytes and small, well-differentiated lymphocytes, occasionally with plasmacytoid features; the second consists of a monomorphic population of large atypical lymphocytes, with only occasional histiocytic cells. Differentiation between these 2 forms is important because most cases of cutaneous lymphosarcoma in horses with a monomorphic pattern of cells have internal involvement, and the disease progresses rapidly. In contrast, the lymphohistiocytic form seldom is associated with internal involvement, and affected horses may live for years. As the lymphohistiocytic form progresses, the nodules tend to become more frequent on the ventral cervical regions. In many cases, euthanasia may be warranted when pharyngeal involvement induces dyspnea. Because of the expense of cytotoxic drugs, therapy is generally limited to glucocorticoids administered orally or intralesionally; remission, if induced, is usually short term.

In cattle, cutaneous lymphosarcoma is a disease of young animals (generally <4 yr old). It is infrequently associated with bovine leukemia virus infection (p 593). The lesions are typically nodular, involve the dermis or subcutaneous fat, and are often ulcerated. There is no known therapy.

Cutaneous Mast Cell Tumors
(Mastocytomas, Mast cell sarcomas)

These tumors are the most frequently recognized malignant or potentially malignant neoplasms of dogs. In addition, leukemic and visceral forms can occur. A viral etiology has been speculated but remains controversial. Tumors may be seen in dogs of any age (average 8-10 yr). They may develop anywhere on the body surface as well as in internal organs, but the limbs (especially the posterior upper thigh), ventral abdomen, and thorax are the most common sites; ~10% are multicentric. Location on mucocutaneous junctions or on the ventral surface of the body is associated with a more aggressive biologic behavior. Many breeds appear to be predisposed, especially Boxers and Pugs (in which tumors are often multiple), Rhodesian Ridgebacks, and Boston Terriers. The tumors vary markedly in size, and clinical appearance alone cannot establish a diagnosis. Most commonly, they appear as raised, nodular masses that may be soft to solid on palpation. Although they often seem encapsulated, mast cell tumors in dogs are seldom discrete. Rather, they consist of a highly cellular center surrounded peripherally by a halo of smaller numbers of mast cells that palpate as normal skin. Dogs can also develop clinical signs associated with the release of vasoactive products from the malignant mast cells. Most common is gastroduodenal ulceration that may be present in up to 25% of cases. Cytologic evaluation of Wright-stained, fine-needle aspirates or impression smears can be used to establish the diagnosis of mast cell tumors in dogs. All skin tumors should be examined by fine needle aspiration cytology prior to excision to rule out mast cell cancer.

If the surgeon is aware that the tumor is a mast cell, a surgical plan for wide and deep excision will yield the best results. All mast cell tumors need to be submitted for biopsy to determine margins and grade because cytology is not a substitute for histopathology—only the latter has been correlated with prognosis. Two systems of histopathologic grading have been defined, and to avoid confusion, it is essential to know which system is being used.

Although there is believed to be a benign variant of canine mast cell tumor, there is no clinical or microscopic means of identifying it. In addition, small mast cell tumors may remain quiescent for long periods before becoming aggressive. Thus, all should be treated as at least potential malignancies.

Treatment depends on the clinical stage of the disease and the predicted aggressive biologic behavior. For Stage I tumors (a solitary tumor confined to the dermis without nodal involvement), the preferred treatment is complete excision with a wide margin; at least 3 cm of healthy tissue surrounding all palpable borders should be removed in an attempt to excise both the nodule and its surrounding halo of neoplastic cells. Intraoperative cytology (examination of impression smears at the excised tissue margins) can guide the surgeon, who should continue to remove tissue until the margins are free of mast cells. If histologic evaluation suggests that the tumor extends beyond the surgical margins, reexcision should be attempted. Alternatively, because mast cells are sensitive to radiation, intraoperative radiation therapy or followup external beam radiation therapy may be curative if the remaining tumor is small or can only be seen microscopically. Combined radiation and hyperthermia may be more effective than radiation alone.

At present, there is no agreed upon mode of therapy for Stage II-IV mast cell tumors. For Stage II tumors (a solitary tumor with regional lymph node involvement), options include excision of the mass and the affected regional node (if feasible), prednisolone, and radiotherapy, used either singly or in combination. Intracavitary injections of triamcinolone or medroxyprogesterone acetate in a sesame seed oil or safflower oil emulsion placed evenly into the open tumor bed at the time of surgery may also help, especially when combined with intraoperative radiation therapy and followup external beam therapy. Treatment of Stage III (multiple dermal tumors with or without lymph node involvement) or Stage IV (any tumor with distant metastasis or recurrence with metastasis) tumors is generally palliative. One recommended therapy is prednisolone (2 mg/kg, PO, for 5 days, followed by a maintenance dose of 0.5 mg/kg, SID) or intralesional injections of triamcinolone (1 mg/cm diameter of tumor, every 2 wk). Treatment with H_1- and H_2-receptor antagonists for the peripheral and gastric effects of histamine, respectively, may be indicated for animals with systemic disease or clinical signs referable to histamine release. Chemotherapy with vinca alkaloids (vincristine, vinblastine), L-asparaginase, and cyclophosphamide has also been used with some effectiveness. Prednisone and vinblastine used as adjuvant chemotherapy to incomplete surgical resection conferred an apparent improvement over historical survival data employing surgery alone, yielding a 57% 1- and 2-yr disease-free state and a 45% survival at 1 and 2 yr for dogs with Grade III tumors. In 19 dogs on a high dose of lomustine given every 21 days, 42% of mast cell tumors showed measurable responses, ranging from stable to partial with one complete response. Neutropenia appears 7 days after treatment with neutrophil counts of 1,500 cells/μL.

In cats, cutaneous mast cell tumors are common. In addition to cutaneous tumors, systemic, leukemic, and GI forms have been recognized. Two distinct variants of the form occur—a mast cell type analogous to, but not identical with, cutaneous mast cell tumors in dogs, and a histiocytic type unique to cats.

The mast cell type is most common. It is found primarily in cats >4 yr old and may develop anywhere on the body but most commonly on the head and neck. The tumors are single, alopecic nodules, generally 2-3 cm in diameter, that occasionally extend into the subcutaneous fat. Lymphoid nodules are common; eosinophils are rare. Unlike mast cell tumors in dogs, those in cats are benign, and generally, atypia and clinical behavior are poorly correlated. Surgical excision is the treatment of choice; <20% of tumors recur after surgery and of those that do, considerably fewer metastasize. Cryotherapy may be a good option to treat multiple recurrent small lesions while avoiding anesthesia.

The histiocytic type of cutaneous mast cell tumor in cats is recognized primarily in Siamese cats <4 yr old. Lesions may develop anywhere on the body and appear as multiple, small (generally 0.5-1 cm in diameter), firm, subcutaneous papulonodules. Usually, the older the cat, the fewer the lesions. This variant may be difficult to distinguish morphologically from a granulomatous inflammatory response. Because these tumors are reported to resolve spontaneously, no treatment is necessary.

In horses, mast cell tumors are uncommon, benign tumors. There is debate as to whether they are actually a neoplastic process or an unusual inflammatory response. Lesions may develop anywhere on the body but are most common on the head and legs. Typically, there is a single, solitary mass in the dermis or subcutaneous fat that may expand to involve the underlying musculature. The tumor begins as a nodule composed of a generally monomorphic proliferation of mast cells. As the lesion evolves, the mast cells are limited to aggregates in a fibrous stroma that surrounds large foci of liquefactive necrosis containing numerous eosinophils. In the late stages, the necrotic foci undergo dystrophic mineralization, and mast cells may be very difficult to identify. Once mineralization occurs, the lesion is gritty on sectioning. Alopecia and ulceration are variable features. Excision is the treatment of choice. These lesions do not metastasize. A variant of cutaneous mast cell tumor is seen in newborn foals, in which the lesions may become generalized but regress over time, suggesting an equine equivalent of urticaria pigmentosa in humans.

In pigs and cattle, mast cell tumors are rare. In pigs, most appear as discrete, solitary, cutaneous nodules. Most are benign but disseminated, and leukemic variants do occur. In cattle, most are malignant and characterized by multiple cutaneous nodules often accompanied by systemic involvement; purely cutaneous forms have been recognized occasionally.

Tumors with Histiocytic Differentiation

These comprise a group of poorly defined skin diseases all characterized by a proliferation of histiocytes (tissue macrophages) in the absence of any known stimulus.

Cutaneous histiocytomas are common in dogs and rare in goats and cattle; it is debatable whether they are found in cats. Strong immunohistochemical evidence suggests that in dogs they are derived from Langerhans (intraepidermal antigen processing) cells. These tumors are typically seen in dogs <3.5 yr old but can occur at any age. English Bulldogs, Scottish Terriers, Greyhounds, Boxers, and Boston Terriers are most at risk. The head (including the pinnae) and limbs are the most common sites of involvement, where the tumors appear as solitary, raised, generally ulcerated nodules that are freely movable. Although a common neoplasm, histiocytomas are not always easy to diagnose histologically and can be confused with granulomatous inflammation, mast cell tumors, plasmacytomas, and cutaneous lymphosarcomas. Canine histiocytomas should be considered benign, and most resolve spontaneously within 2-3 mo without treatment. Surgical excision is optional once the diagnosis is established (which can often be made via cytology).

In goats and cattle, histiocytomas are extremely rare and behave the same as those in dogs. Histiocytomas have also been reported in young cats; however, they most likely represent the histiocytic form of mast cell tumor in cats.

Cutaneous histiocytosis is associated with development of numerous plaques and nodules involving the dermis or subcutaneous fat. It is rare in dogs and can develop at any age but is most common in young adults. Shar Peis and German Shepherds may be predisposed. The nodules and plaques tend to wax and wane, and the extremities and trunk are involved most commonly. Lesions are nonpruritic, and larger lesions may ulcerate. Cutaneous histiocytosis seldom involves internal organs, but its diffuse nature and the unsightly appearance often force the owner to consider euthanasia. Various forms of therapy have been tried, including systemic glucocorticoids and a combination of glucocorticoids and chemotherapy. Response is variable; the lesions in some dogs respond rapidly and permanently, whereas in others, lesions are either transiently improved or unchanged.

The **histiocytoses of Bernese Mountain Dogs** are systemic, familial disorders of unknown etiology with 2 manifestations—a more indolent and generally cutaneous form known as systemic histiocytosis and a more aggressive form in which skin lesions are rare, known as malignant histiocytosis. Malignant histiocytosis has been infrequently identified in other canine breeds. In systemic histiocytosis, males (mean age at onset 4 yr) are affected more often than females. There are multiple cutaneous nodules, papules, and plaques involving the skin (especially of the scrotum), nasal mucosa, and eyelids. The lesions are poorly circumscribed and variably alopecic and may be ulcerated; they develop in waves and slowly regress, only to recur several months later. The clinical disease tends to become more severe with each new wave of eruptions. Although the skin is the primary target organ, lesions may also develop in other organs, including lymph nodes, spleen, and bone marrow. The disease may be episodic in its clinical presentation, but it is progressive and eventually fatal.

Malignant histiocytosis is seen in male Bernese Mountain Dogs (mean age at onset 7 yr) and, less frequently, in other canine breeds. The lungs, lymph nodes, and liver are the most common organs affected, and the disease tends to spare the skin. Grossly, the lesions appear as large, solitary, firm masses that may efface large portions of affected internal organs. The disorder is rapidly progressive and does not wax and wane as does systemic histiocytosis. Few dogs survive >6 mo.

Various chemotherapeutic regimens have been used to treat both forms. Bovine thymosin fraction 5 may be of benefit in inducing remissions, especially in the systemic form. However, both forms of the disease are ultimately fatal.

Transmissible Venereal Tumors

See TRANSMISSIBLE CANINE VENEREAL TUMOR, p 1165. These can also develop initially on haired skin due to inoculation via cutaneous injuries.

TUMORS OF MELANOCYTIC ORIGIN

These tumors are most common in dogs, gray horses, and miniature pigs; uncommon in goats and cattle; and rare in cats and sheep. The terminology used to describe melanocytic lesions in veterinary medicine is different from that used in human dermatology. In animals, the terms melanocytoma and malignant melanoma are used to describe benign and malignant melanocytic proliferations, respectively. In humans, a benign melanocytic proliferation (whether congenital or acquired) is called a nevus, and the term melanoma by definition refers to a malignancy (ie, in people, there are no benign melanomas). In addition, although solar injury is a common cause of melanocytic tumors in humans, actinic damage is seldom associated with the development of analogous tumors in domestic animals.

Dogs: Melanocytomas of the skin are diagnosed much more frequently than malignant melanomas. They most commonly develop on the head and forelimbs in middle-aged or older dogs. There may be a predilection for males. Miniature and Standard Schnauzers, Doberman Pinschers, Golden Retrievers, Irish Setters, and Vizslas are the breeds in which these tumors are most commonly recognized. They can appear as macules or patches; as papules or plaques; or as elevated, occasionally pedunculated masses. Most have a pigmented surface. Although generally solitary, lesions may be multiple, especially in the breeds at risk. These tumors are benign, and complete excision is curative.

Malignant melanomas most commonly develop in dogs somewhat older than those that develop melanocytomas. Miniature and Standard Schnauzers and Scottish Terriers are most at risk. The mucocutaneous junctions of the lips, in the oral cavity (p 308), and in the nail beds are the most common sites of development. Malignant melanomas of haired skin are rare, and most arise on the ventral abdomen and the scrotum. Males are affected more commonly than females. Most malignant melanomas appear as raised, generally ulcerated nodules that are variably pigmented. When present on the mucocutaneous regions of the lip, the tumors may be pedunculated with a papillated surface; when present in the nail bed, they appear as swellings of the digit, often with loss of the nail and destruction of underlying bone, mimicking osteomyelitis. Whenever a toe is festering in an older dog, radiographs and a deep punch biopsy are indicated for diagnosis. Canine malignant melanomas are aggressive and have considerable metastatic potential.

Treatment generally consists of complete excision; however, the infiltrative nature of the tumor may make this difficult. When present on the digits, amputation is indicated; when present on the mandible, a hemimandibulectomy may allow for complete excision and an acceptable postsurgical cosmetic appearance and survival. Lesions at rostral locations on the maxilla or mandible showed the best survival times of 10.9 mo in 1 study. Melanomas are generally considered insensitive to radiation therapy, and there is no established chemotherapeutic protocol shown to be highly effective. Survival times range from 1-36 mo, indicating that individual variations in host defense mechanisms and the aggressiveness of the tumor may play a role in establishing a prognosis. In one study of 117 dogs with digit masses, 24 had melanoma and a median survival time of 12 mo with 42% alive at 1 yr and 13% alive at 2 yr. Gene therapy vaccinations of plasmid DNA encoding human tyrosinase can produce antibody and cytotoxic T-cell responses and has shown potential therapeutic value for dogs with advanced melanoma in preclinical trials.

Cats: Cutaneous melanocytic neoplasms are uncommon and most often identified on the head (especially the pinnae), neck, and distal extremities in middle-aged or older cats. An association with the oral cavity and subungual regions is less well defined than in dogs, and a higher percentage are malignant. Excision is the treatment of choice.

Horses: Most melanocytic neoplasms are in gray horses, in which the coat turns gray (or white) with age. They are especially common in Lipizzaners, Arabians, and Percherons, and 80% of gray or white horses of these breeds may be affected. They are generally recognized in older horses but usually begin their development when animals are 3-4 yr old. The perineum and the base of the tail are the most common sites of development, but these tumors may develop in any location, including the parotid area. The tumors are often multiple and may appear as coalescent, frequently pedunculated nodules that often extend in a linear arrangement up the tail base. They increase in size and number over time. Although most are benign, invasive variants, some with metastatic potential, can develop. Most are black on cross-section. Many gray horses have evidence of lymph node involvement; however, there is debate as to whether this represents metastasis or whether the intranodal melanocytes and melanophages represent a stimulation of extracutaneous melanocytes that are normally present in the lymph node. Treatment consists of surgical or cryosurgical removal; however, affected animals are predisposed to develop additional tumors over time. Little is known about the use of radiation or chemotherapy for the treatment of equine melanocytoma or malignant melanoma. Early reports suggesting that cimetidine may be of value in controlling recurrence have not been supported by followup studies. Intralesional chemotherapy with cisplatin or carboplatin after surgical debulking may be of benefit in the treatment of large or inoperable masses. Recurrent tumors do not develop resistance to cisplatin, and they can be treated a second time, sometimes with good results.

Melanocytic neoplasms of nongray horses are rare tumors usually found on the trunk and extremities of young (often <2 yr old) horses. They may represent expansion of a congenital lesion. Masses characteristically appear as solitary nodules. Most are benign; however, congenital malignant melanomas may infrequently develop. Such tumors are invasive, with little metastatic potential. Surgical excision or cryosurgery is the treatment of choice. If the tumors are benign and surgically extirpated, the prognosis is excellent. For invasive tumors, the prognosis is guarded.

Pigs: Melanocytic neoplasms of pigs are seen as congenital lesions and sporadically in adults of the Sinclair (Hormel) miniature pigs and Duroc and Duroc crosses. Selective breeding in these strains has increased the prevalence of tumors. These tumors develop both pre- and postnatally, anywhere on the body. Generally multiple, they can appear as pigmented macules or patches with smooth borders; as raised, often ulcerated pigmented lesions; or as deeper, slightly raised, blue masses. Deeply invasive melanomas are often associated with metastatic disease. The lymph nodes and lungs are the most common sites of metastasis. Not all of these tumors become invasive, and many undergo spontaneous regression associated with an intense lymphocytic infiltrate. Melanocytic lesions in pigs are not treated; because of the heritable nature of the disease, prevention by selective breeding is recommended if lesions are frequently recognized in a herd.

Cattle: Melanocytic neoplasms in cattle develop infrequently anywhere on the body. They can be found at any age but are most commonly recognized in young animals; congenital forms have been recognized. Angus cattle appear to be predisposed. Most commonly, the tumors are large nodular masses, densely pigmented on cut surface, and benign. Excision is curative for most; however, rare malignant variants have been recognized with distant metastasis.

Sheep: Melanocytic neoplasms in sheep are most common in middle-aged or older animals but have been recognized in neonates. They are most common in Suffolks and Angoras, in which they appear as multiple, densely pigmented dermal or subcutaneous masses. They should be considered malignant; metastasis is common.

Goats: Melanocytic tumors in goats are rare. They are most common in middle-aged or older animals and possibly in Angoras. There may be a site predilection for the coronary band and udder. Lesions are seen as solitary or multiple masses with variable pigmentation on cut surface. Most tend to grow rapidly, and metastasis is common.

METASTATIC TUMORS

The spread of a primary neoplasm to the skin is unusual in domestic animals. It is occasionally identified in dogs; less commonly in cats; and rarely in horses, cows, sheep, goats, and pigs. Although all malignant neoplasms are capable of secondary cutaneous involvement, metastatic potential is greatest in mammary gland adenocarcinomas, squamous cell carcinomas, transitional cell carcinomas, transmissible venereal tumors, pulmonary adenocarcinomas, and angiosarcomas. Although appearance is variable, the lesions most commonly are multiple, ulcerated papulonodules. Early cutaneous metastasis is characterized by aggregates of neoplastic cells within superficial and deep dermal vessels. As these lesions evolve, they extend into the dermis and are associated with effacement of adnexa. Generally, it is difficult to distinguish the primary neoplasm based on the morphologic features of a metastatic site. This is because only a small population of cells in the primary tumor have the potential for metastasis, and these cells may have different microscopic features. In cats, pulmonary adenocarcinomas appear to preferentially metastasize to the distal extremities, and when carcinomas are diagnosed on multiple feet, examination for a lung tumor should be performed. Cutaneous metastasis is usually a feature of aggressive tumors and is associated with a guarded prognosis.

ACANTHOSIS NIGRICANS

Acanthosis nigricans describes a clinical reaction pattern in dogs characterized by axillary and inguinal hyperpigmentation, lichenification, and alopecia.

Etiology and Clinical Findings: Acanthosis nigricans is a clinical sign, not a diagnosis. The pathogenesis is poorly understood, but clinical signs are invariably a result of inflammation due to constant friction and the resultant dermatitis. It can be primary (idiopathic) or secondary. Primary acanthosis nigricans is rare, occurs almost exclusively in Dachshunds, and has no sex predilection; it is considered a genodermatosis. Clinical signs are usually evident by 1 yr of age. Secondary acanthosis nigricans is relatively common and can occur in any breed of dog, most commonly those breeds predisposed to the following common underlying causes: conformational abnormalities, obesity, endocrinopathies (eg, hypothyroidism, hyperadrenocorticism, sex hormone abnormalities), axillary and inguinal pruritus associated with atopy, food allergy, contact dermatitis, and skin infections (eg, staphylococcal pyoderma, *Malassezia* dermatitis).

Clinical signs typically consist of bilaterally symmetric axillary or inguinal hyperpigmentation and lichenification. The edges of these lesions are often erythematous; this is a sign of secondary bacterial and/or yeast pyoderma. With time, lesions may spread to the ventral neck, groin, abdomen, perineum, hocks, periocular area, and pinnae. Pruritus is variable and may be caused by the underlying disease or a secondary infection. As the lesions progress, secondary alopecia, seborrheic dermatitis, and infections (staphylococcal or *Malassezia* dermatitis) develop.

Diagnosis: The physical findings compatible with a clinical diagnosis of acanthosis nigricans are not difficult to recognize. Primary acanthosis nigricans is a diagnosis of exclusion; acanthosis nigricans in a juvenile Dachshund is not always caused by a genodermatosis. A careful history and physical examination should be performed to identify an underlying cause. Skin scrapings should be performed to rule out demodicosis, especially in young dogs. Impression smears are useful to identify bacterial and *Malassezia* infections. Depending on the nondermatologic signs, endocrine function tests for thyroid and adrenal disease may be useful; endocrine skin diseases are not pruritic unless accompanied by secondary skin infections. Intradermal skin testing, a food trial, or both may be necessary. Skin biopsies are usually nondiagnostic but may be helpful in some cases to identify secondary bacterial infections not previously recognized. The presence of such infections is common but often overlooked. In most cases, it is useful to treat the secondary bacterial and/or *Malassezia* infections before proceeding with other diagnostic tests.

Treatment: Primary acanthosis nigricans in Dachshunds is not curable. Early cases may respond to shampoo therapy and local topical glucocorticoids, eg, betamethasone valerate ointment. As lesions progress, more aggressive systemic therapy may be useful. The following systemic therapies have been used, alone or in combination, with varying degrees of success: vitamin E, 200 IU, PO, BID, for 2-3 mo; systemic glucocorticoids, 1 mg/kg, PO, SID for 7-10 days, then on alternate days; melatonin, 2 mg/dog, SC, SID for 3-5 days, then weekly or monthly as needed. The concurrent treatment of secondary bacterial or *Malassezia* infections is helpful and is required before systemic glucocorticoids are administered; antimicrobial therapy is compatible with the other therapies. Antiseborrheic shampoos are often beneficial for removing excess oil and odor.

In secondary acanthosis nigricans, the lesions will spontaneously resolve after identification and correction of the underlying cause. However, this will not occur if secondary bacterial and yeast pyodermas are not treated appropriately. Cephalexin (30 mg/kg, PO, BID) and concurrent itraconazole or ketoconazole (5-10 mg/kg, PO, SID) is an effective treatment regimen. Affected dogs benefit greatly from appropriate antimicrobial therapy and antiseborrheic shampoos (2-3 times/wk).

Clinical signs resolve slowly, possibly over months.

EOSINOPHILIC GRANULOMA COMPLEX

The etiology of this group of diseases that affects cats, dogs, and horses has focused on an underlying hypersensitivity reaction. This is particularly true in cats and horses. Insect, environmental, and dietary hypersensitivities have been documented in cats, while insect hypersensitivity has been seen in some equine cases and in a smaller number of canine cases. Genetic predisposition and bacterial infections have also been seen in cats. In all species, idiopathic cases exist.

Clinical Findings and Diagnosis: In **cats**, 3 disease entities have been grouped in the complex.

Eosinophilic Ulcer: This well-circumscribed, erythematous, ulcerative lesion, usually not painful or pruritic, is usually found on the upper lip. Although reported to occur, progression to squamous cell carcinoma is extremely rare. Histology shows an ulcerative dermatitis, with a cellular infiltrate of neutrophils, plasma cells, and mononuclear cells predominating. Mild to moderate fibroplasia is common. Tissue or peripheral eosinophilia is uncommon.

Eosinophilic Plaque: This well-circumscribed, erythematous, raised lesion is most commonly found in the medial thigh and abdominal regions; it is extremely pruritic. Regional lymphadenopathy can be seen. Histology shows a diffuse eosinophilic dermatitis, with marked inter- and intracellular edema and vesicles containing eosinophils in the epidermis and dermis. Mast cells may also be present. Peripheral eosinophilia is common.

Eosinophilic Granuloma: These typically raised, well-circumscribed, yellowish to pink lesions may be found anywhere on the body but are most common on the head, face, bridge of the nose, pinnae, pads of the feet, perineal region, lips, chin, oral cavity, and caudal thighs. The caudal thigh location is usually distinctly linear. Linear lesions have been seen on other body locations, but more commonly these are papular, nodular or diffusely swollen, and firm. Histologically, a granulomatous inflammatory response surrounds degenerative collagen. Tissue and peripheral eosinophilia are marked when the lesions are in the mouth but vary when lesions are on the skin.

In **dogs**, the lesions reported as eosinophilic granulomas histologically resemble the eosinophilic granuloma of cats, with marked collagen degeneration surrounded by a granulomatous and eosinophilic infiltrate. These lesions may be seen as ulcerated or vegetative masses in the oral cavity or, less commonly, as plaques, nodules, or papules on the lips and other areas of the body. Any breed may be affected, but Siberian Huskies may be at greater risk.

In **horses**, the disease has been termed equine eosinophilic granuloma with collagen degeneration, nodular necrobiosis of collagen, and collagenolytic granuloma. The lesions are nodular, nonulcerative, and nonpruritic. They often are found in the saddle, central truncal, and lateral cervical areas and may have a gray-white central core. Older lesions may become mineralized. Both insect bites and trauma have been suggested as etiologies, although the occasional onset during winter in cold climates and in noncontact saddle or tack areas suggests multifactorial causes. Histology reveals multifocal areas of collagen degeneration surrounded by granulomatous inflammation containing eosinophils. Thus, histologically, this lesion is similar to eosinophilic granuloma of cats and dogs.

Treatment: In **cats**, hypersensitivity disorders (allergy to fleas, food, or inhalants) should be investigated by allergy testing (intradermal or in vitro) and dietary elimination trials. Hyposensitization, insect control, and dietary management should be instituted when appropriate. Antibiotic therapy (amoxicillin-clavulanate, cefadroxil, or fluoroquinolones) should always be tried empirically, especially in refractory cases. If no underlying cause can be determined and the condition is refractory, corticosteroids, such as methylprednisolone acetate (4 mg/kg, IM, once every 2 wk for 2-3 injections), oral prednisolone (2-4 mg/kg/day), or oral triamcinolone (0.8 mg/kg/day), can be tried. Oral corticosteroids should be tapered to alternate days (or to every third day in the case of triamcinolone), and dosages reduced when used for longterm management. Long-acting injectable methylprednisolone acetate should not be used more often than every 6-12 wk due to the potential for inducing hyperadrenocorticism. Aurothioglucose (gold salts) at 1 mg/kg, IM, weekly for 6-14 wk, may also be effective. If responses are seen, the dosage and frequency can be reduced or discontinued. Chlorambucil at 0.2 mg/kg, 3 times/wk, has also been used in refractory cases and requires more extensive blood monitoring due to its bone marrow suppressive properties; 6-12 wk may be needed before a response is seen and, like gold salts, the dosage and frequency should be reduced if response is seen. Recently, cyclosporine (5 mg/kg/day) has been used in refractory cases. This requires monthly laboratory monitoring for metabolic (eg, renal) changes. Other methods of treatment include radiotherapy, cryosurgery, laser, surgical excisions, interferon, and levamisole. Progestational drugs, such as megestrol acetate or medroxyprogesterone acetate, have also been effective; however, they are not recommended because of their potential side effects.

In **dogs**, antibiotics should also be tried initially. Many lesions seem much more responsive to corticosteroids, and therapy is usually oral prednisone or prednisolone (0.5-2 mg/kg/day initially, tapering the dosage over 20-30 days). Lesions recur in some dogs, in which case low-dose, every-other-day corticosteroid therapy is indicated.

In **horses**, solitary lesions may be treated with systemic antibiotics, surgical excision, or sublesional corticosteroid injections. Mineralized lesions require excision. Triamcinolone acetonide (3-5 mg/lesion) or methylprednisolone acetate (5-10 mg/lesion) is effective. No more than 20 mg triamcinolone acetonide should be administered sublesionally because of the potential to induce laminitis. Horses with multiple lesions may be treated with oral prednisone or prednisolone at 1.1 mg/kg, SID, for 2-3 wk. In horses with recurrent lesions, intradermal allergy testing, particularly with insect antigens, is recommended. Hyposensitization and insect control can be palliative in some cases.

HYGROMA

A hygroma is a false bursa that develops over bony prominences and pressure points, especially in large breeds of dogs. Repeated trauma from lying on hard surfaces produces an inflammatory response, which results in a dense-walled, fluid-filled cavity. A soft, fluctuant, fluid-filled, painless swelling develops over pressure points, especially the olecranon. If longstanding, severe inflammation may develop, and ulceration, infection, abscesses, granulomas, and fistulas may occur. The bursa contains a clear, yellow to red fluid.

If diagnosed early and if still small, hygromas can be managed medically via aseptic needle aspiration, followed by corrective housing. Soft bedding or padding over pressure points is imperative to prevent further trauma. Surgical drainage, flushing, and placement of Penrose drains are indicated for chronic hygromas. Areas with severe ulceration may require extensive drainage, extirpation, or skin grafting procedures. Use of intrahygromal corticosteroids is not recommended.

MISCELLANEOUS SYSTEMIC DERMATOSES

A number of systemic diseases produce various lesions in the skin. Usually, the lesions are noninflammatory, and alopecia is common. In some instances, the cutaneous changes are characteristic of the particular disease. Often, however, the dermatosis is not obviously associated with the underlying condition and must be carefully differentiated from primary skin disorders. Some of these secondary dermatoses are mentioned briefly below and are also described in the chapters on the specific disorders.

Dermatosis may be associated with nutritional deficiency, especially of proteins, fats, minerals, some vitamins, and trace elements. However, this is uncommon in dogs and cats fed modern, balanced diets. Siberian Huskies, and occasionally other breeds, may develop a disease similar to parakeratosis in pigs and require additional zinc in their diet (2-3 mg/kg elemental zinc per day). Zinc-responsive dermatoses also have been reported in cattle, sheep, goats, and llamas and are associated with a higher individual requirement, not a dietary deficiency.

Dermatitis is sometimes seen in association with disorders of internal organs, such as the liver, kidneys, or pancreas. Hepatic parenchymal dysfunction has been associated with superficial necrolytic dermatitis (hepatocutaneous syndrome, diabetic dermatosis) in old dogs and rarely in cats. This has been associated with hypoaminoacidemia. The cutaneous lesions include erythema, crusting, oozing, and alopecia of the face, genitals, and distal extremities, as well as hyperkeratosis and ulceration of the footpads. The skin disease may precede the onset of signs of the internal disease. Histopathologic findings are diagnostic and include superficial perivascular to lichenoid dermatitis, with marked diffuse parakeratotic hyperkeratosis and striking inter- and intracellular edema limited to the upper half of the epidermis. Hyperglucagonemia has also been documented in dogs with this syndrome; however, dogs tend to have hepatic parenchymal dysfunction more commonly than glucagonomas. In dogs, therapy relies on IV amino acid infusion or surgical removal of the glucagonoma. Skin fragility syndrome (excessive skin friability) in cats has been seen in association with pancreatic neoplasia, hepatic lipidosis, or adrenal dysfunction. Pancreatic neoplasia has also been associated with crusting of the footpads and alopecia in cats. A generalized nodular dermatofibrosis syndrome in German Shepherds, and occasionally other breeds, associated with renal cystadenomas, cystadenocarcinomas, or renal epithelial cysts has been reported. Histopathologic examination of the skin nodules reveals dense collagen fibrosis.

Poisoning by thallium sulfate (rat poisons, p 2512), ergot (p 2414), mercury (p 2405), and iodides may cause various skin changes. Hyperkeratosis in cattle can be caused by chlorinated naphthalene toxicity.

In dogs, dermatosis can develop as a result of endocrine dysfunction (*see also* THE ENDOCRINE SYSTEM, p 429 et seq). In males with Sertoli cell tumors, bilateral alopecia and occasional pruritus with a papular eruption may be seen. Intact female dogs with hormonal imbalances are usually pruritic and have a papular eruption, mammary tissue enlargement, and frequent estrous cycles. The skin lesions of both disorders may begin in the inguinal or flank region and progress cranially. Dermatosis due to neutering is not common in dogs and cats; when it does occur, it is generally nonpruritic, with mild alopecia in the perineal or inguinal areas.

Dermatoses have been seen in hypothyroidism (p 461). The skin lesions are characterized by diminished hair growth and bilaterally symmetric alopecia. The skin is dry, scaly, thickened, and folded. Pyoderma and seborrhea may occur. The margins of the pinna may develop excess scale. In rare cases, cutaneous myxedema develops.

Faulty production of hypophyseal hormones may rarely cause dermatoses. Hypopituitarism is characterized by alopecia, especially in the axillary regions and on the lateral thorax and abdomen. Hyperadrenocorticism also is manifest by skin changes such as hyperpigmentation, alopecia, seborrhea, calcinosis cutis, and secondary pyoderma. In cats, the skin becomes extremely friable. In diabetes mellitus, pruritus and secondary infection rarely occur.

Treatment of all these conditions depends on a specific etiologic diagnosis. Once this is established and managed, the skin lesions usually need only symptomatic care (eg, control of scratching) until they resolve with resolution of the primary disease.

NASAL DERMATOSES OF DOGS

(Collie nose, Nasal solar dermatitis)

Nasal dermatoses of dogs may be caused by many diseases. Lesions may affect the bridge of the nose, the planum nasale, or both. In pyoderma, dermatophytosis, and demodicosis, the haired portions of the nose are affected. In systemic lupus erythematosus or pemphigus, the whole muzzle is often crusted (with occasional oozing of serum) or ulcerated. In systemic and discoid lupus, and occasionally in pemphigus and cutaneous lymphoma, the planum nasale is depigmented, erythematous, and eventually may ulcerate. Nasal dermatosis due to solar radiation probably is a rare disease and may often be a misdiagnosis for the lupus variants. In true nasal solar dermatitis, the nonpigmented areas of the planum nasale are affected first, and occasionally the bridge of the nose may become inflamed and sometimes ulcerated. The lesions are worse in the summer, although lupus and pemphigus may also show this seasonal variation. Any of the above diseases may affect the periocular areas. (See also SYSTEMIC LUPUS ERYTHEMATOSUS, p 654, and PEMPHIGUS, p 653.) The sudden onset of nasal swelling, erythema, and exudation is often eosinophilic furunculosis; this is thought to be caused by an arthropod sting or bite. The protozoal disease leishmaniasis may cause depigmentation of the nasal planum.

Treatment depends on etiology. Diagnostic tests should include skin scrapings, bacterial and fungal cultures, and biopsies for both histopathology and immune testing. If the diagnosis is nasal solar dermatitis, a topical corticosteroid lotion (betamethasone valerate, 0.1%) may help relieve inflammation. Exposure to sunlight must be severely curtailed. Topical sunscreens may be effective but need to be applied at least twice daily. Treatment for eosinophilic furunculosis is systemic corticosteroids, prednisone or prednisolone at 1 mg/kg, BID, for 1 wk, after which the dosage should be gradually decreased.

PARAKERATOSIS

Parakeratosis is a nutritional deficiency disease of 6- to 16-wk-old pigs characterized by lesions of the superficial layers of the epidermis. It is a metabolic disturbance resulting from a deficiency of zinc (see also p 1886) or inadequate absorption of zinc due to an excess of calcium, phytates, or other chelating agents in the diet. Predisposing factors include rapid growth, deficiency of essential fatty acids, or malabsorption due to GI diseases.

Signs are limited to the skin, although mild lethargy, anorexia, and growth depression may be seen in severe cases; there is little if any pruritus. The outstanding lesions are symmetrically distributed areas of excessive and abnormal keratinization of the epidermis with the formation of horny scale and fissures. Brown spots or papules are first seen on the ventrolateral areas of the abdomen and inner thigh, pastern, fetlock, hock, and tail regions. These lesions coalesce to involve larger areas until the entire body may be covered. The scale is horny, dry, and usually easily removed. Occasionally, secondary infection of the cracks and fissures causes them to fill with dark, sticky exudate and debris, which may resemble exudative epidermitis (p 692); however, this usually occurs in younger piglets. Chronic sarcoptic mange and deficiencies of B vitamins or iodine must also be considered in a differential diagnosis. Clinical signs, skin biopsy, and low serum levels of zinc and alkaline phosphatase will help to confirm a diagnosis.

Highly satisfactory results can be obtained by adjusting the intake of calcium or zinc, or both. Pig starter diets should contain 0.9% calcium and 125 ppm zinc. Grower diets should contain 0.60-0.65% calcium and 75 ppm zinc, while finisher diets should contain 0.45 to 0.50% calcium and 50 ppm zinc. Sow and boar diets should contain 0.9% calcium and 150 ppm zinc. Correction of the deficiency results in rapid recovery.

PHOTOSENSITIZATION

Photosensitization is a clinical condition in which skin (areas exposed to light and lacking significant protective hair, wool, or pigmentation) is hyperreactive to sunlight due to the presence of photodynamic agents. Molecules of photosensitizing agents present in the skin are energized by light. When the molecules return to the less energized state, the released energy is transferred to receptor molecules that quickly initiate chemical reactions in various skin components. Tissue injury is thought to result from the production of reactive oxygen intermediates or from alterations in cell membrane permeability. Photosensitization can be difficult to differentiate clinically from actual sunburn.

Photosensitization is often classified according to the source of the photodynamic pigment. These categories are primary or type I photosensitivity, aberrant endogenous pigment synthesis or type II photosensitivity, and type III or secondary (hepatogenous) photosensitivity. Sometimes a fourth category has been identified, labeled idiopathic type IV photosensitivity. (See also CONGENITAL ERYTHROPOIETIC PORPHYRIA, p 804, and PROTOPORPHYRIA, p 685.)

A wide range of chemicals, including some that are fungal and bacterial in origin, may act as photosensitizing agents. However, most compounds that are important causes of photosensitivity in veterinary medicine are plant-derived. Photosensitization occurs worldwide and can affect any species, but is probably most commonly seen in cattle, sheep, goats, and horses.

Primary Photosensitization: Primary photosensitization occurs when the photodynamic agent is absorbed either through the skin or from the GI tract unchanged, reaching the skin in its native form. Examples of primary photosensitizers are hypericin (from *Hypericum perforatum* [St. John's wort]) and fagopyrin (from *Fagopyrum esculentum* [buckwheat]). Plants in the families Umbelliferae and Rutaceae contain photoactive furocoumarins (psoralens), which cause photosensitization in livestock and poultry. *Ammi majus* (bishop's weed) and *Cymopterus watsonii* (spring parsley) have produced photosensitization in cattle and sheep, respectively. Ingestion of *A majus* and *A visnaga* seeds has produced severe photosensitization in poultry. Species of *Trifolium*, *Medicago* (clovers and alfalfa), *Erodium*, *Polygonum*, and *Brassica* have been incriminated as primary photosensitizers. Many other plants have been suspected, but the toxins responsible have not been identified (eg, *Cynodon dactylon* [bermudagrass]). Additionally, some coal tar derivatives, phenothiazine, sulfonamides, and tetracyclines have induced primary photosensitivity.

Aberrant Pigment Metabolism: Type II photosensitivity due to aberrant pigment metabolism is known to occur in both cattle and cats. In this syndrome, the photosensitizing porphyrin agents are endogenous pigments that arise from inherited or acquired defective functions of enzymes involved in heme synthesis. Bovine congenital erythropoietic porphyria (p 804) and bovine erythropoietic protoporphyria are the most commonly reported diseases in this category.

Secondary (Hepatogenous) Photosensitization: Secondary or type III photosensitization is by far the most frequent type of photosensitivity observed in livestock. The photosensitizing agent, phylloerythrin (a porphyrin), accumulates in the plasma due to impaired hepatobiliary excretion. Phylloerythrin is derived from the breakdown of chlorophyll by microorganisms present in the GI tract. Phylloerythrin, but not chlorophyll, is normally absorbed into the circulation and is effectively excreted by the liver into the bile. Failure to excrete phylloerythrin due to hepatic dysfunction or bile duct lesions increases the amount in the circulation. Thus, when it reaches the skin, it can absorb and release light energy, initiating a phototoxic reaction.

Phylloerythrin has been incriminated as the phototoxic agent in the following conditions: common bile duct occlusion; facial eczema (p 2417); lupinosis (p 2420); congenital photosensitivity of Southdown and Corriedale sheep (*see* p 796); and poisoning by numerous plants including *Tribulis terrestris* (puncture vine), *Lippia rehmanni*, *Lantana camara*, several *Panicum* spp (kleingrass, broomcorn millet, witch grass), *Cynodon dactylon*, *Myoporum laetum* (ngaio), and *Narthecium ossifragum* (bog asphodel).

Photosensitization also has been reported in animals that have liver damage associated with various poisonings: pyrrolizidine alkaloid (eg, *Senecio* spp, *Cynoglossum* spp, *Heliotropium* spp, *Echium* spp; p 2506), cyanobacteria (*Microcystis* spp, *Oscillatoria* spp), *Nolina* spp (bunch grass), *Agave lechuguilla* (lechuguilla), *Holocalyx glaziovii*, *Kochia scoparia*, *Tetradymia* spp (horse brush or rabbit brush), *Brachiaria brizantha*, *Brassica napus*, *Trifolium pratense* and *T hybridum* (red and alsike clover), *Medicago sativa*, *Ranunculus* spp, phosphorus, and carbon tetrachloride. Phylloerythrin is likely the phototoxic agent in many of these poisonings.

Type IV Photosensitivity: Photosensitivity where the pathogenesis is unknown is classified as type IV. Examples include winter wheat (cattle), *Medicago* spp (alfalfa), *Brassica* spp (mustards), and *Kochia scoparia* (fireweed). Many plants that fall in this category may perhaps be type I photosensitizers.

Clinical Findings and Lesions: The clinical signs associated with photosensitivity are similar regardless of the cause. Photosensitive animals are photophobic immediately when exposed to sunlight and squirm in apparent discomfort. They scratch or rub lightly pigmented, exposed areas of skin (eg, ears, eyelids, muzzle). Severe phylloerythrinemia and bright sunlight can induce typical skin lesions, even in black-coated animals. Erythema develops rapidly and is soon followed by edema. If exposure to light stops at this stage, the lesions soon resolve. When exposure is prolonged, serum exudation, scab formation, and skin necrosis are marked. In cattle, and especially in deer, exposure of the tongue while licking may result in glossitis, characterized by ulceration and deep necrosis.

Depending on the initial cause of the accumulation of the photosensitizing agent, other clinical signs may be seen. For example, if the photosensitivity is hepatogenous, icterus may be present. In bovine congenital erythropoietic porphyria, discoloration of dentin, bone (and other tissues), and urine often accompanies the skin lesions. Photodermatitis is the sole manifestation observed in bovine erythropoietic protoporphyria.

Diagnosis: Clinical signs are easily recognized in cases of marked photosensitivity but are similar to the primary actinic effects of sunburn in early or mild cases. Reference to the specific diseases in which photosensitization is an objective sign may assist in diagnosis of the underlying disease. Evaluation of serum liver enzymes and liver biopsies may be necessary to confirm the presence of hepatic disease. Examination of blood, feces, and urine for porphyrins can also be performed.

Treatment: Treatment involves mostly palliative measures. While photosensitivity continues, animals should be shaded fully or, preferably, housed and allowed to graze only during darkness. The severe stress of photosensitization and extensive skin necrosis can be highly debilitating and increase mortality. Corticosteroids, given parenterally in the early stages, may be helpful. Secondary skin infections and suppurations should be treated with basic wound management techniques, and fly strike prevented. The skin lesions heal remarkably well, even after extensive necrosis.

The prognosis and eventual productivity of an animal is related to the site and severity of the primary lesion and/or hepatic disease, and to the degree of resolution.

Congenital Photosensitization in Sheep

Southdown and Corriedale sheep may inherit a hepatobiliary incompetence that results in photosensitization.

In mutant Southdown sheep, the inherited defect is in hepatic uptake of unconjugated bilirubin and organic anions. Plasma levels of unconjugated bilirubin are consistently increased and, because bilirubin is partially excreted, icterus is not a clinical feature. Phylloerythrin is less effectively excreted, and affected lambs become photosensitized when they first begin grazing green plant material. Unless chlorophyll is excluded from the diet, or exposure to sunlight is prevented, the lesions and stress of photosensitization result in death within weeks. Mutant sheep so protected develop progressive renal lesions in which radial, fibrous bands form in the medulla, along with increasing numbers of cystic tubules. The changes ultimately result in renal insufficiency and death. The liver is small, with pericanalicular deposits of lipofuscin. This semilethal trait appears to be inherited as a simple recessive trait. Elimination of carriers is the only feasible control.

In mutant Corriedale sheep, the hepatocellular incompetence is in the excretion of conjugated bilirubin and other conjugated metabolites. There is no obvious icterus, but phylloerythrin excretion is sufficiently impaired to produce photosensitization. Hepatic pigmentation is an obvious gross feature. Brown-black, melanin-like pigment is confined to centrilobular parenchymal cells. This is transmitted as an autosomal recessive trait. Control is by detection and removal of carriers.

PITYRIASIS ROSEA IN PIGS

(Porcine juvenile pustular psoriaform dermatitis)

Pityriasis rosea is a sporadic disease of unknown etiology of pigs, usually 8-12 wk old, but occasionally as young as 2 wk and very rarely in pigs up to 10 mo. One or more pigs in a litter may be affected. The disease is mild, but transient anorexia and diarrhea have been reported. The initial skin lesions are characterized by small erythematous papules, which rapidly expand to form a ring (collarette) with distinct raised and reddened borders. The lesions enlarge at their periphery, and adjacent lesions may coalesce. The center of the lesion is flat and covered with a bran-like scale overlaying normal skin. The lesions are found predominantly on the ventral abdomen and inner thighs but occasionally may be seen over the back, neck, and legs. Characteristically, there is no pruritus, and recovery is spontaneous in 6-8 wk. Treatment is generally considered unnecessary. Diagnosis can usually be made from the characteristic lesions, but laboratory tests, culture, and biopsy may be used to differentiate from dermatomycosis, exudative epidermitis, dermatosis vegetans, and swinepox.

The disease is considered to be partially hereditary, pigs of the Landrace breed being most commonly affected, but the mode of inheritance is uncertain. The disease does not resemble pityriasis rosea in humans clinically or pathologically.

Lesions appear to be more extensive in pigs reared in high stocking densities with high ambient temperatures and high humidity. Under these conditions, secondary bacterial infection (eg, *Staphylococcus hyicus*) is common. Treatment is of little value and does not affect the course of the disease; however, treatment aimed at controlling secondary infections may be warranted.

SADDLE SORES

(Collar galls)

The area of riding horses that is under saddle, or the shoulder area of those driven in harness, is frequently the site of injuries to the skin and deeper soft and bony tissues. Clinical signs vary according to the depth of injury and the complications caused by secondary infection. Sores affecting only the skin are characterized by inflammatory changes that range from erythematous to papular, vesicular, pustular, and finally necrotic. Frequently, the condition starts as an acute inflammation of the hair follicles and progresses to a purulent folliculitis. Affected areas show hair loss and are swollen, warm, and painful. The serous or purulent exudate dries and forms crusts. Advanced lesions are termed "galls." When the skin and underlying tissues are damaged more seriously, abscesses may develop. They are characterized by warm, fluctuating, painful swellings from which purulent and serosanguineous fluid can be aspirated. Severe damage to the skin and subcutis or deeper tissues results in dry or moist necrosis. Chronic saddle sores are characterized by a deep folliculitis/furunculosis (boils) with fibrosis or a localized indurative and proliferative dermatitis. Lesions are usually caused by poorly fitting tack.

Identification and elimination of the offending portion of tack is more important than any other treatment. Excoriations and inflammation of the skin of the saddle and harness regions are treated as any other dermatosis. Absolute rest of the affected parts is necessary. During the early or acute stages, astringent packs (Burow's solution) are indicated. Chronic lesions and those superficially infected may be treated by warm applications and topical or systemic antibiotics. Hematomas should be aspirated or incised. Necrotic tissue should be removed surgically. In severe folliculitis and furunculosis, antibiotics are always indicated.

SEBORRHEA

Seborrhea is a skin disease in dogs that is characterized by a defect in keratinization or cornification. Clinically, it results in increased scale formation, occasionally excessive greasiness of the skin and hair coat, and often secondary inflammation and infection.

Etiology, Clinical Findings, and Diagnosis: Primary seborrhea is an inherited skin disorder characterized by faulty keratinization or cornification of the epidermis, hair follicle epithelium, or claws. It is seen more frequently in American Cocker Spaniels, English Springer Spaniels, Basset Hounds, West Highland White Terriers, Dachshunds, Labrador and Golden Retrievers, and German Shepherd dogs. There is usually a familial history of seborrhea, suggesting genetic factors are involved. The disease begins at a young age (usually <18-24 mo) and progresses throughout the dog's life. A diagnosis of generalized primary idiopathic seborrhea should be reserved for dogs in which all possible underlying causes of seborrhea have been ruled out.

Most seborrheic dogs have secondary seborrhea, in which a primary underlying disease predisposes to excessive scale, crusting, or oiliness, often accompanied by superficial pyoderma, *Malassezia* infection, and alopecia. The most common underlying causes are endocrinopathies and allergies. The goal is to identify and treat any underlying cause of the seborrhea. Palliative therapies that do not compromise the diagnostic evaluation should be instituted concurrently to provide as much immediate relief as possible for the dog.

Underlying diseases may present with seborrhea as the primary clinical problem. The signalment (age, breed, sex) and history may provide clues in diagnosing the underlying cause. Allergies are more likely to be the underlying cause if the age of onset is <5 yr, whereas an endocrinopathy or neoplasia is more likely if the seborrhea begins in middle-aged or older dogs.

The degree of pruritus should also be noted. If pruritus is minimal, endocrinopathies, other internal diseases, neoplasia, or certain diseases limited to the skin (eg, demodicosis or sebaceous adenitis) should be ruled out. If pruritus is significant, allergies and pruritic ectoparasitic diseases (eg, scabies, fleas) should be considered. The presence of pruritus does not rule out nonpruritic disease as the underlying cause, because the presence of a pyoderma or the inflammation from the excess scale can cause significant pruritus. However, a lack of pruritus helps to rule out allergies, scabies, and other pruritic diseases as the underlying etiology.

Other important considerations include the presence of polyuria, polydipsia, or polyphagia; heat-seeking behavior; abnormal estrous cycles; occurrence of pyoderma; the influence of seasonality; diet; response to previous medications (including corticosteroids, antibiotics, antihistamines, or topical treatments); zoonosis or contagion; and the environment. The duration and severity of disease as well as level of owner frustration are important factors in determining the aggressiveness of the diagnostic plan.

A thorough physical examination, including internal organ systems and a comprehensive dermatologic examination, is the first step in identifying the underlying cause. The dermatologic examination should document the type and distribution of the lesions; the presence of alopecia; and the degree of odor, scale, oiliness, and texture of the skin and hair coat. The presence of follicular papules, pustules, crusts, and epidermal collarettes usually indicates the existence of a superficial pyoderma. Hyperpigmentation indicates a chronic skin irritation (such as pruritus, infection, or inflammation), and lichenification indicates chronic pruritus. Yeast (*Malassezia* spp) infection should always be considered when evaluating a seborrheic dog.

Secondary infection plays a significant role in most seborrheic dogs. The sebum and keratinization abnormalities that are common in seborrheic dogs frequently provide ideal conditions for bacterial and yeast infections. The self-trauma that occurs in pruritic animals increases the likelihood of a secondary infection. Often, coagulase-positive *Staphylococcus* spp or *Malassezia* spp are present. The infections add to the pruritus and are usually responsible for a significant amount of the inflammation, papules, crusts, alopecia, and scales.

One of the first diagnostic steps is to obtain superficial cytology of the affected areas to identify the quantity and type of bacteria or yeast present. If numerous cocci and neutrophils are present, pyoderma is likely. In addition to systemic therapy, topical shampoos will aid in the treatment of secondary infections. In a seborrheic dog with pruritus, the infection may cause all or most of the pruritus. Instead of considering allergies as the underlying disease in these dogs, nonpruritic diseases (eg, endocrinopathies) may be uncovered by addressing the infections.

After the infections have been addressed, other diagnostic tests that should be considered include multiple deep skin scrapings, dermatophyte culture, impression smears, trichograms, and flea combing. If these are negative or normal, a CBC, serum biochemical profile, and complete urinalysis will complete the minimum database. Examples of diagnostic clues include increased serum alkaline phosphatase (which may suggest hyperadrenocorticism or previous steroid therapy), cholesterol (which may suggest hypothyroidism), blood glucose (which suggests diabetes mellitus), and BUN or creatinine (which may suggest renal disease).

Treatment: Palliative therapy is needed to keep the dog comfortable while the underlying cause is identified and secondary skin diseases are corrected. For treatment of pyoderma, an antibiotic with known sensitivity against *Staphylococcus intermedius* should be appropriate. *Malassezia* may be treated systemically with ketoconazole. In addition to addressing any secondary infections, antipruritic therapy and shampoo therapy are usually needed to help control the seborrhea and speed the return of the skin to a normal state. Shampoo therapy can decrease the number of bacteria and yeast on the skin surface, the amount of scale and sebum present, and the level of pruritus; it also helps normalize the epidermal turnover rate.

In the past, seborrhea has been classified as seborrhea sicca (dry seborrhea), seborrhea oleosa (oily seborrhea), or seborrheic dermatitis (inflammatory seborrhea). This scheme can still be used in determining the type of shampoo needed; however, most seborrheic animals have varying degrees of all 3 of these classifications of seborrhea.

Most products contained in shampoos can be classified based on their effects as keratolytic, keratoplastic, emollient, antipruritic, or antimicrobial. **Keratolytic products** include sulfur, salicylic acid, tar, selenium sulfide, propylene glycol, fatty acids, and benzoyl peroxide. They remove stratum corneum cells by causing cellular damage that results in ballooning and sloughing of the surface keratinocytes. This reduces the scale and makes the skin feel softer. Shampoos containing keratolytic products frequently exacerbate scaling during the first 14 days of treatment, due to the sloughed scales getting caught in the hair coat. The scales will be removed by continued bathing, but owners should be warned that the scaling often worsens initially. **Keratoplastic products** help normalize keratinization and reduce scale formation by slowing down epidermal basal cell mitosis. Tar, sulfur, salicylic acid, and selenium sulfide are examples of keratoplastic agents. **Emollients** (eg, lactic acid, sodium lactate, lanolin, and numerous oils, such as corn, coconut, peanut, and cottonseed) are indicated for any scaling dermatosis because they reduce transepidermal water loss. They work best after the skin has been rehydrated and are excellent adjunct products after shampooing. **Antibacterial agents** include benzoyl peroxide, chlorhexidine, iodine, ethyl lactate, and triclosan. **Antifungal ingredients** include chlorhexidine, sulfur, iodine, ketoconazole, and miconazole. Boric and acetic acids are also used as topical antimicrobials.

It is important to know how individual shampoo ingredients act, as well as any additive or synergistic effects they have, because most shampoos are a combination of products. The selection of appropriate antiseborrheic shampoo therapy is based on hair coat and skin scaling and oiliness, of which there are 4 general presentations: 1) mild scaling and no oiliness, 2) moderate to marked scaling and mild oiliness (the most common), 3) moderate to marked scaling and moderate oiliness, 4) mild scaling and marked oiliness. These categories are intended to guide the type of shampoo therapy necessary; however, all factors for each individual dog should be considered.

Dogs with mild scaling and no oiliness need mild shampoos that are gentle, cleansing, hypoallergenic, or moisturizing. These shampoos are indicated for dogs that have mild seborrheic changes or that are irritated by medicated shampoos, or for owners that tend to bathe the dog too often. These products often contain emollient oils, lanolin, lactic acid, urea, glycerin, or fatty acids. Emollient sprays or rinses are often used in conjunction with these shampoos.

Dogs with moderate to marked scaling and mild oiliness should be bathed with shampoos that contain sulfur and salicylic acid. Both agents are keratolytic, keratoplastic, antibacterial, and antipruritic. In addition, sulfur is antiparasitic and antifungal. Some of these shampoos also contain ingredients that are antibacterial, antifungal, and moisturizing, which can help control secondary pyoderma, *Malassezia* spp, and excessive scaling. Shampoos that contain ethyl lactate lower the cutaneous pH (which has a bacteriostatic or bactericidal action by inhibiting bacterial lipases), normalize keratinization, solubilize fats, and decrease sebaceous secretions. These actions also result in potent antibacterial activity.

Dogs with moderate to severe scaling and moderate oiliness often benefit most from tar-containing shampoos. Tar exerts potent keratoplastic effects by slowing basal epidermal cell DNA synthesis. It is often combined with sulfur and salicylic acid. Wood and coal are distilled to produce a tremendous variety of products called crude coal tars. Because of the variation in agents and techniques used, exact comparisons of shampoos are difficult. More refined tars are usually less irritating and more stable but are more expensive to produce. More tar is not necessarily better. Only those tar products from reputable companies should be used. Tar shampoos usually have a distinct and unpleasant odor that lessens as the hair coat dries. Owner compliance is often diminished for products that have a prominent odor.

In dogs with severe oiliness and minimal scaling, profound odor, erythema, inflammation, and a secondary generalized pyoderma or *Malassezia* dermatitis are often present. This group requires the most aggressive topical therapy. Shampoos that contain benzoyl peroxide provide strong degreasing actions along with potent antibacterial and follicular flushing activities. Because benzoyl peroxide shampoos are such strong degreasing agents, they can be irritating and drying. Other antibacterial shampoos are better suited in dogs that have superficial pyoderma without significant oiliness. As with tar, benzoyl peroxide has critical production requirements, and only refined products from reputable companies should be used. Most human products contain 5-10% benzoyl peroxide and should not be used because they are irritating to dogs. The follicular flushing action of benzoyl peroxide makes it ideal for dogs with numerous comedones or with demodicosis. Benzoyl peroxide gels (5%) are good choices when antibacterial, degreasing, or follicular flushing actions are desired for focal areas, such as in localized demodicosis, canine acne, or Schnauzer comedone syndrome. However, these gels may be irritating.

METABOLIC DISORDERS

METABOLIC DISORDERS INTRODUCTION

Metabolic diseases may be inherited or acquired, the latter being more common and significant. Metabolic diseases are clinically important because they affect energy production or damage tissues critical for survival.

Metabolic Storage Disorders and Inborn Errors of Metabolism

Storage diseases and inborn errors of metabolism are classified as either genetic or acquired. These diseases are characterized by the accumulation or storage of specific lysosomal enzyme substrates or byproducts within cells because of partial or complete deficiency of those enzymes. Although lysosomal storage diseases are often widespread throughout the body, the majority of clinical signs are due to the effects on the CNS.

Genetic storage diseases are named according to the specific metabolic byproduct that accumulates in the lysosomes. Animals are typically normal at birth, then manifest clinical signs within the first weeks to months of life. These diseases are progressive and usually fatal, as specific treatments do not exist. In small animals the gangliosidoses (GM_1 and GM_2) are seen in Siamese, Korat, and domestic cats, and in Beagle crosses, German Shorthaired Pointers, and Japanese Spaniels. Sphingomyelinosis is seen in German Shepherds and Poodles, and in Siamese and domestic shorthaired cats. Glucocerebrosidosis is seen in Australian Silky Terriers and Dalmatians. Ceroid lipofuscinosis is seen in English Setters, Cocker Spaniels, Dachshunds, Chihuahuas, Salukis, Border Collies, and domestic cats. Mannosidosis is seen in Persian and domestic cats. Glycogenosis is seen in Silky Terriers, and in domestic shorthaired and Norwegian forest cats. Globoid cell leukodystrophy (Krabbe's disease) is seen in Cairn Terriers, West Highland White Terriers, Beagles, Bluetick Hounds, Poodles, and domestic shorthaired cats. Mucopolysaccharidosis type I is seen in Siamese, Korat, and domestic shorthaired cats; type IV is seen in Siamese cats. In dogs, mucopolysaccharidosis is seen in Miniature Pinschers, Plott Hounds, and mixed-breed dogs and is associated with lameness. Diseases associated with decreased RBC survival and anemia include pyruvate kinase deficiency in Basenjis, Beagles, and West Highland White and Cairn Terriers; phosphofructokinase deficiency in English Springer and American Cocker Spaniels; and porphyria in Siamese and domestic shorthaired cats.

In large animals, α-mannosidosis occurs in Angus, Murray Grey, Simmental, Galloway, and Holstein cattle. β-mannosidos is seen in Saler cattle and Nubian and Nubian-cross goats. Generalized glycogenosis (GM_1) is seen in Holstein cattle and Suffolk sheep. Generalized glycogenosis (GM_2) is seen in Shorthorn and Brahman cattle, and in pigs. Globoid cell leukodystrophy is seen in polled Dorset sheep. Other identified diseases that are manifest by neurologic signs and appear to be inherited include neuronal lipodystrophy in Angus and Beefmaster cattle, shaker calf syndrome of horned Hereford cattle, maple syrup urine disease of Hereford and polled Shorthorn cattle, and hereditary neuraxial edema of polled and horned Hereford and Hereford-Friesian cross cattle. There have been no reports of lysosomal storage diseases in horses; however, inherited diseases manifest by neurologic signs include inherited myoclonus of Peruvian Paso foals and congenital encephalomyelopathy in Quarter Horses.

Other inherited diseases that involve basic errors of metabolism in various tissues include goiter of sheep and goats, inherited parakeratosis (edema disease) of cattle, osteogenesis imperfecta of sheep and cattle, and possibly cardiomyopathy of cattle, the hypotrichoses, baldy calves, photosensitization of sheep (p 794), dermatosis vegetans and porcine stress syndrome (p 832) of pigs, dermatosparaxia and Ehlers-Danlos syndrome of cattle, hemochromatosis of cattle (p 297), and Marfan syndrome in cattle. Many other inherited defects, especially those based on abnormal growth of collagen, cartilage, and bone, also are likely to have basic errors of metabolism of structural tissues. Many disorders of metabolism have been described involving dysfunctions of the immune system.

Acquired storage diseases are caused by the ingestion of plants that contain inhibitors of specific lysosomal catabolic enzymes. Chronic ingestion of locoweed plants (*Astragalus* or *Oxytropis* spp) results in an acquired neurologic storage disease. Several toxic components including locoine, swainsonine n-oxide, and indolizidine alkaloids interfere with α-mannosidase activity. Horses are most susceptible to intoxication; however, cattle, sheep, and goats can also be affected. (*See also* PLANTS POISONOUS TO ANIMALS, p 2432.)

Production-related Metabolic Disorders

While the development of the following diseases is largely related to production or management factors, the pathogenesis of each disease is primarily related to alterations in metabolism. In most cases the basis of disease is not a congenital or inherited error in metabolism, but rather an increased demand for a specific nutrient that has become deficient under certain conditions. Diseases such as hypocalcemia, hypomagnesemia, and hypoglycemia are augmented by management practices that are directed toward improving and increasing production. They are therefore correctly considered production diseases. However, they are also metabolic diseases because management of the animal is directed at production, which at its peak, is beyond the capacity of that animal's metabolic reserves to sustain a particular nutrient at physiologic concentrations. For example, parturient paresis of cows (p 806) occurs when the mass of calcium in the mammary secretion is greater than the cow's diet or its skeletal reserves can supply. Comparable situations occur with magnesium and glucose metabolism, and with phosphorus in relation to postparturient hemoglobinuria (p 814).

Most production-induced metabolic diseases result from a negative balance of a particular nutrient. In some cases, dietary intake of the nutrient is rapidly reduced because of an ongoing, high metabolic requirement for that nutrient. Examples include pregnancy toxemia of ewes (p 828), protein-energy malnutrition in beef cattle (p 1812), fat cow syndrome in dairy cattle (p 824), and hyperlipemia in ponies (p 294). Furthermore, some diseases may be precipitated when producers, primarily due to economic concerns, are compelled to not supplement animals that already have a substandard nutritional plane.

Exertional rhabdomyolysis of horses (p 951) is another production-induced metabolic disease. In this case, the production activity (draft or racing) is maintained by and matched to a level of caloric intake. Management decisions not to work or race these horses without a concomitant decrease in caloric intake may result in accumulation of muscle glycogen to dangerous levels. Disease results when work is resumed and the production of lactate exceeds its metabolism.

The difference between production-related metabolic diseases and nutritional deficiencies is often subtle. Typically, nutritional deficiencies are longterm, steady state conditions that can be corrected through dietary supplementation. Metabolic diseases are generally acute states that dramatically respond to the systemic administration of the deficient nutrient or metabolite, although affected animals may require subsequent dietary supplementation to avoid recurrence. An important aspect of dealing with production-induced metabolic diseases is accurate and rapid diagnosis. Ideally, diagnostic tests can be used to predict the occurrence of disease before its clinical onset.

CONGENITAL ERYTHROPOIETIC PORPHYRIA

(Porphyrinuria, Pink tooth, Osteohemochromatosis)

Congenital erythropoietic porphyria is a rare hereditary disease of cattle, pigs, cats, and humans in which defective hemoglobin formation results in production of an excess of Type I porphyrins in the nuclei of developing normoblasts. The defect in cattle is inherited as a simple autosomal recessive and is usually confined to herds in which inbreeding or close line-breeding is practiced. The condition has been recognized in the USA, Canada, Denmark, Jamaica, England, South Africa, Australia, and Argentina. This broad geographic distribution indicates that the disease likely occurs worldwide and probably affects all meat-producing animals, especially cattle, swine, and sheep.

Heterozygous animals seem to be normal, but homozygous recessive animals are affected at birth with reddish brown discoloration of the teeth, bones, and urine that persists for the life of the animal. The inherited enzymatic defect causes deficient activity of uroporphyrinogen III synthase—an essential part of porphyrin-heme biosynthesis. Uroporphyrinogen III cosynthetase is the enzyme that is deficient. The urine contains an excess of coproporphyrin I and uroporphyrin I; in affected animals, the color is amber or reddish brown. Bones, urine, and teeth (especially the deciduous teeth) fluoresce pink when irradiated with near-ultraviolet light. Prolonged exposure to sunlight causes typical lesions of photosensitization with hyperemia, vesicle formation, and superficial necrosis of unpigmented portions of the skin. The severity of the skin lesions depends on the intensity of the solar radiation and the extent of cutaneous pigmentation occurring in specific families of animals. A normochromic, hemolytic anemia with macrocytes and microcytes and marked basophilic stippling develops. Splenomegaly eventually occurs. The texture of bones is not altered except in cases in which bones have increased fragility due to a diminished cortex. Affected animals are generally of medium to good condition unless solar injury has occurred. Some animals become progressively unthrifty unless protected from sunlight. A similar disease, bovine protoporphyria (p 683), causes photosensitivity only in Limousin cattle and humans.

In humans, a series of porphyrias caused by defective functions of enzymes in porphyrin-heme biosynthesis have been described and grouped according to their presenting clinical signs. These vary broadly and may include severe cutaneous lesions on exposed areas of the body, acute photosensitivity reactions, serious liver damage, and acute attacks of neurologic dysfunction. In animals, the recognized diseases are commonly classified as either congenital erythropoietic porphyria, congenital erythropoietic protoporphyria, or porphyria. It is likely that all of the syndromes described in humans also occur in animals and that a broader classification could be used.

The defect in pigs and cats is extremely rare and differs from the condition in cattle in that photosensitization is not a feature. In pigs and cats, the disease is transmitted as an autosomal dominant. In pigs, even with high levels of porphyrins in the blood, photodynamic dermatitis does not occur. The disease has been reported only in Denmark and New Zealand; in cats, it has been recognized only in the USA.

Diagnosis should be based on the excretion of abnormal uroporphyrins, the brown discoloration of the teeth (which fluoresce when irradiated with near-ultraviolet light), the appearance of discolored urine, and hemolytic anemia.

The recessive genetic character is widely distributed in cattle, but the clinical condition is comparatively rare. Clinically normal heterozygotes have lower levels of uroporphyrinogen III cosynthetase than do normal animals, but laboratory identification of the carrier state is impractical due to the relatively low incidence of the disease and is not widely used. Morbidity can be controlled by keeping affected animals indoors and out of direct sunlight.

DISORDERS OF CALCIUM METABOLISM

HYPOCALCEMIC TETANY IN HORSES
(Transport tetany, Lactation tetany, Eclampsia)

Hypocalcemic tetany in horses is an uncommon condition associated with acute depletion of serum ionized calcium and sometimes with alterations in serum concentrations of magnesium and phosphate. It occurs after prolonged physical exertion or transport (transport tetany) and in lactating mares (lactation tetany). Signs are variable and relate to neuromuscular hyperirritability.

Etiology: Mechanisms of hypocalcemia include decreased absorption from the intestines; increased loss of calcium from the kidneys, sweat, or milk; or inhibition of osteolysis due to alterations in parathyroid hormone, calcitonin, or vitamin D. In lactating mares, high milk production and grazing of lush pastures appear to be predisposing factors. Hypocalcemia after prolonged physical activity (eg, endurance rides) results from sweat loss of calcium, increased calcium binding during hypochloremic alkalosis, and stress-induced high corticosteroid levels. Corticosteroids inhibit vitamin D activity, which leads to decreased intestinal absorption and skeletal mobilization of calcium. Stress and lack of calcium intake have been associated with transport tetany. Occasionally, hypocalcemic tetany may be precipitated by hypocalcemia after blister beetle ingestion (see CANTHARIDIN POISONING, p 2351).

Clinical Findings: The severity of clinical signs corresponds with the serum concentration of ionized calcium. Increased excitability may be the only sign in mild cases. Severely affected horses may show synchronous diaphragmatic flutter, anxious appearance, and signs of tetany including increased muscle tone, stiffness of gait, muscle tremors, prolapse of the third eyelid, inability to chew, trismus, salivation, recumbency, convulsions, and cardiac arrhythmias. In lactating mares, if not treated, the disease may take a progressive and sometimes fatal course over 24-48 hr.

Differential diagnoses include tetanus, endotoxemia, colic, exertional rhabdomyolysis or other muscle disorder, seizure disorder, laminitis, and botulism.

Diagnosis: A tentative diagnosis is based on clinical signs, history, and response to treatment. Definitive diagnosis requires demonstration of low serum levels of ionized calcium. Most laboratories measure only total (protein-bound and free) serum calcium, which is an acceptable diagnostic test in most cases. However, discrepancies may arise in alkalotic and hypoalbuminemic horses. Alkalosis increases albumin binding of calcium, which results in a decreased concentration of ionized calcium. Thus, alkalotic horses may have normal total serum calcium while exhibiting signs of hypocalcemia. Likewise, hypoalbuminemic or acidotic horses may have decreased total serum calcium without developing signs of hypocalcemia. Total serum calcium can be adjusted for albumin concentration by the following formula:

$$\text{adjusted } Ca^{2+} = \text{measured } Ca^{2+} - \text{serum albumin concentration} + 3.5$$

Treatment: IV administration of calcium solutions, such as 20% calcium borogluconate or solutions recommended for treatment of periparturient paresis in cattle, usually result in full recovery. These solutions should be administered slowly (over 20 min) at

250-500 mL/500 kg, diluted at least 1:4 in saline or dextrose, and the cardiovascular response should be closely monitored. An increased intensity of heart sounds is expected. If arrhythmias or bradycardia develop, the IV treatment should be discontinued immediately. Once the heart rate has returned to normal, the infusion may be resumed at a slower rate. If the horse does not improve within 1-2 hr of the initial infusion, a second dose may be given, although laboratory verification of hypocalcemia is indicated. Some horses require repeated treatments over several days to recover from hypocalcemic tetany. Mildly affected horses may recover without specific treatment. If the tetany is associated with physical exertion, incorporating magnesium into the solution may be advisable.

Prevention: A balanced feed ration should be provided to supply adequate amounts and ratios of calcium and phosphorus throughout gestation. In times of increased calcium demand such as lactation, fasting should be avoided and high-quality forage such as alfalfa or calcium-containing mineral mixes should be provided. Stress and fasting during transport should be minimized. In endurance horses, water and electrolyte deficits associated with prolonged exercise and sweating may be prevented by provision of a sufficient water supply and electrolyte supplementation.

PARTURIENT PARESIS IN COWS
(Milk fever, Hypocalcemia)

Parturient paresis is an acute to peracute, afebrile, flaccid paralysis of mature dairy cows that occurs most commonly at or soon after parturition. It is manifest by changes in mentation, generalized paresis, and circulatory collapse.

Etiology: At or near the time of parturition, the onset of lactation results in the sudden loss of calcium into milk. Serum calcium levels decline from a normal of 10-12 mg/dL to 2-7 mg/dL. Commonly, serum magnesium is increased, serum phosphorus is decreased, and cows are hyperglycemic. The disease may be seen in cows of any age but is most common in high-producing dairy cows >5 yr old. Incidence is higher in the Jersey breed.

Clinical Findings and Diagnosis: Parturient paresis usually occurs within 72 hr of parturition. The disease can contribute to dystocia, uterine prolapse, retained fetal membranes, metritis, abomasal displacement, and mastitis.

There are 3 discernible stages of parturient paresis. During stage 1, animals are ambulatory but show signs of hypersensitivity and excitability. Cows may be mildly ataxic, have fine tremors over the flanks and triceps, and display ear twitching and head bobbing. Cows may appear restless, shuffling their rear feet and bellowing. If calcium therapy is not instituted, cows will likely progress to the second, more severe stage.

Cows in stage 2 are unable to stand but can maintain sternal recumbency. Cows are obtunded, anorectic, and have a dry muzzle, subnormal body temperature, and cold extremities. Auscultation reveals tachycardia and decreased intensity of heart sounds. Peripheral pulses are weak. Smooth muscle paralysis leads to GI stasis, which can be manifest as bloat, failure to defecate, and loss of anal sphincter tone. An inability to urinate may be manifest as a distended bladder on rectal examination. Cows often tuck their heads into their flanks, or if the head is extended, an S-shaped curve to the neck may be noted.

In stage 3, cows lose consciousness progressively to the point of coma. They are unable to maintain sternal recumbency, have compete muscle flaccidity, are unresponsive to stimuli, and can suffer severe bloat. As cardiac output worsens, heart rate can approach 120 bpm, and peripheral pulses may be undetectable. If untreated, cows in stage 3 may survive only a few hours.

Differential diagnoses include toxic mastitis, toxic metritis, other systemic toxic conditions, traumatic injury (eg, stifle injury, coxofemoral luxation, fractured pelvis, spinal compression), calving paralysis syndrome (damage to the L6 lumbar roots of sciatic and obturator nerves), or compartment syndrome. Some of these diseases, in addition to aspiration pneumonia, may also occur concurrently with parturient paresis or as complications. (*See also* PROBLEMATIC BOVINE STERNAL RECUMBENCY, p 957.)

Treatment: Treatment is directed toward restoring normal serum calcium levels as soon as possible to avoid muscular and nervous damage and recumbency. Recommended treatment is IV injection of a calcium gluconate salt, although SC and IP routes are also used. A general rule for dosing is 1 g calcium/45 kg (100 lb) body wt. Most solutions are available in single-dose, 500 mL bottles that contain 8-11 g calcium. In large, heavily lactating cows, a second bottle given SC may be helpful because it is thought to provide a prolonged release of calcium into the circulation. SC calcium treatment alone may not be adequately absorbed due to poor peripheral perfusion and should not be the sole route of therapy. No matter what route is used, strict asepsis should be employed to lessen the chance of infection at the injection site. Solutions containing formaldehyde or >25 g dextrose/500 mL are irritating if given SC. Many solutions contain phosphorus and magnesium in addition to calcium. Although administration of phosphorus and magnesium is not usually necessary in uncomplicated parturient paresis, detrimental effects of their use have not been reported. Magnesium may protect against myocardial irritation caused by the administration of calcium. Most products available to veterinarians contain phosphite salts as the source of phosphorus. However, phosphorus found in blood and tissues of cattle is primarily in the form of the phosphate anion. Because no pathway exists for the conversion of phosphite to the usable phosphate form, it is unlikely that these solutions are of any benefit in addressing hypophosphatemia.

Calcium is cardiotoxic; therefore, calcium-containing solutions should be administered slowly (10-20 min) while cardiac auscultation is performed. If severe dysrhythmias or bradycardia develop, administration should be stopped until the heart rhythm has returned to normal. Endotoxic animals are especially prone to dysrhythmias caused by IV calcium therapy.

Administration of oral calcium avoids the risks of cardiotoxic side effects and may be useful in mild cases of parturient paresis. Calcium propionate in propylene glycol gel or powdered calcium propionate (0.5 kg dissolved in 8-16 L water administered as a drench) is effective and avoids the potential for metabolic acidosis caused by calcium chloride. Oral administration of 50 g of soluble calcium results in ~4 g calcium being absorbed into the circulation.

Hypocalcemic cows typically respond to therapy immediately. Tremors are seen as neuromuscular function returns. Improved cardiac output results in stronger heart sounds and decreased heart rate. Return of smooth muscle function results in eructation, defecation, and urination once the cow rises. Approximately 75% of cows stand within 2 hr of treatment. Animals not responding by 4-8 hr should be reevaluated and retreated if necessary. Of cows that respond initially, 25-30% relapse within 24-48 hr and require additional therapy. Incomplete milking has been advised to reduce the incidence of relapse. Historically, udder inflation has been used to reduce the secretion of milk and loss of calcium; however, the risk of introducing bacteria into the mammary gland is high.

Prevention: Historically, prevention of parturient paresis was approached by feeding low-calcium diets during the dry period to stimulate intestinal absorption and enhance skeletal resorption prior to the sudden demand for calcium at the onset of lactation. While mobilization of calcium is somewhat enhanced, it is now known that feeding low-calcium diets is not as effective as initially believed. Furthermore, it is difficult to formulate diets that are low enough in calcium. Alternative methods for prevention of hypocalcemia include delayed or incomplete milking after calving, which maintains pressure within the udder and decreases milk production. This practice may aggravate latent mammary infections and increase incidence of mastitis. Prophylactic treatment of susceptible cows at calving may help reduce parturient paresis. Cows are administered either SC calcium on the day of calving or oral calcium gels at calving and 12 hr later.

Most recently, the prevention of parturient paresis has been revolutionized by the use of the dietary cation-anion difference (DCAD), which decreases the blood pH of cows during the late prepartum and early postpartum period. This method is more effective and more practical than lowering prepartum calcium in the diet. The DCAD approach provides an excess of anions over cations in the diet by adjusting the components of the diet, adding anionic salts to the ration, or both. Adding excess anions to the diet is believed to enhance calcium resorption from bone and absorption from the GI tract.

An important strategy for decreasing blood pH in periparturient cattle is reducing the potassium content of the diet. Including corn silage as a major portion of the dry cow's diet is essential as it tends to have the lowest content potassium of available forages. Alfalfa is another forage source that may prove beneficial in maintaining proper blood pH. In the past, including alfalfa in a dry cow ration was not considered ideal due to the high calcium content. However, it has since been determined that calcium has little effect on the alkalinity of cow's blood. Withholding potassium fertilizers on fields used to grow dry cow forages is another means of decreasing potassium levels in hay fed to dry cows. Alternatively, anionic salts can be added to counteract the effects of high cation levels (potassium and sodium) in the diet. Anionic salts to consider include calcium chloride, magnesium chloride, magnesium sulfate, calcium sulfate, ammonium sulfate, and ammonium chloride. Recent research evaluating the acidifying activity of different anionic salts has resulted in the following equation that describes the ion balance in rations:

$$\text{Ion balance (mEq/g)} = (0.15\ Ca^{2+} + 0.15\ Mg^{2+} + Na^+ + K^+) - (Cl^- + 0.25\ S^- + 0.5\ P^-)$$

This equation suggests the major ions determining blood pH are sodium, potassium, and chloride. The target value for close-up dry cow rations is +200 to +300 mEq/kg. An important drawback to feeding anionic salts is poor palatability, which can be overcome by using a mixture of anionic salts within a moist, palatable ration such as corn silage, brewer's grain, distiller's grain, or molasses. While sulfate salts are more palatable than chloride salts, they are less effective in acidifying the blood.

Administration of vitamin D_3 and its metabolites is effective in preventing parturient paresis. Large doses of vitamin D (20-30 million U, SID), given in the feed for 5-7 days before parturition, reduces the incidence. However, if administration is stopped more than 4 days before calving, the cow is more susceptible. Dosing for periods longer than those recommended should be avoided due to potential toxicity. A single injection (IV or SC) of 10 million IU of crystalline vitamin D given 8 days before calving is an effective preventive. The dose is repeated if the cow does not calve on the due date. Newer compounds used (where available and approved) in lieu of vitamin D and less likely to cause hypervitaminosis include 25-hydroxycholecalciferol, 1,25-dihydroxycholecalciferol, and 1α-hydroxycholecalciferol. After calving, a diet high in calcium is required. Administering large doses of calcium in gel form (PO) is commonly practiced. Doses of 150 g of calcium gel are given 1 day before, the day of, and 1 day after calving.

Use of synthetic bovine parathyroid hormone (PTH) may prove to be superior to administration of vitamin D metabolites. Vitamin D metabolites enhance GI calcium absorption, whereas PTH enhances GI calcium absorption and stimulates bone resorption. PTH is administered either IV 60 hr before parturition, or IM 6 days before parturition. Drawbacks to the use of PTH include increased labor requirements for administration, as well as the availability of such compounds.

PARTURIENT PARESIS IN SHEEP AND GOATS
(Milk fever, Hypocalcemia)

Parturient paresis in pregnant and lactating ewes and does is a disturbance of metabolism characterized by acute hypocalcemia and rapid development of hyperexcitability, ataxia, paresis, coma, and death.

Etiology: The exact cause is unknown, but the conditions under which field outbreaks occur are fairly well defined. Low concentrations of serum calcium are found in heavily lactating animals or those with multiple fetuses. Some cases are also complicated by hypophosphatemia and hyper- or hypomagnesemia. The disease occurs at any time from 6 wk before parturition to 10 wk after. Due to calcification of fetal bones, the greatest demand for calcium for nondairy animals occurs 3-4 wk prepartum, particularly if >1 fetus is present in utero. Whenever an abrupt calcium demand occurs, the body requires 24-72 hr to activate the metabolic machinery necessary to mobilize stored calcium. High intake of calcium, phosphorus, or some cations (potassium, sodium) may decrease the production of parathyroid hormones. During decreased parathyroid function, less 1,25-dihydroxycholecalciferol is produced, resulting in lowered absorption and mobilization of calcium from the intestines and bones, respectively.

Clinical Findings and Diagnosis: Characteristically, the disease occurs in outbreaks with more cases in late gestation. The incidence is usually <5%, but in severe outbreaks, 30% of the flock may be affected at one time. The onset is sudden and almost invariably follows—within 24 hr—an abrupt change of feed, a sudden change in weather, or short periods of fasting imposed by circumstances such as shearing, crutching, or transportation (*see also* TRANSPORT TETANY IN RUMINANTS, p 834). In early hypocalcemia, a stiff gait or ataxia, tremors, tetany, constipation, and/or depressed rumen motility are seen. As the disease progresses, signs include increased heart and respiratory rates, regurgitation of rumen contents, bloat, depression, and eventually, if untreated, opisthotonos and/or death.

Diagnosis is based on the history and clinical signs. In outbreaks occurring before lambing, pregnancy toxemia (p 828) is the main differential diagnosis. These diseases may also occur concurrently. A tentative diagnosis of acute hypocalcemia can be confirmed readily by a dramatic and usually lasting response to calcium therapy.

Treatment and Prevention: Treatment should be initiated immediately, usually as IV calcium borogluconate (50-150 mL of a 23% solution). Oral administration of a calcium gel or the SC administration of calcium solutions helps prevent relapse. During treatment, the heart should be monitored, and therapy slowed or stopped if arrhythmias occur. An alternative mode of therapy would be to add 50-150 mL of a 23% calcium borogluconate or gluconate solution to 1 L of a 5% dextrose solution. The more hypocalcemic an animal is (ie, the worse the clinical signs are), the more cardiotoxic the intravenously administered calcium becomes. Dietary modifications useful for the prevention of milk fever in dairy cattle may be of value in dairy sheep and goats. Therefore, reducing or eliminating diets rich in cations (alfalfa), clovers, or supplemental calcium and phosphorus in the late dry period may aid in prevention. Immediately after parturition the calcium levels in the diet should be increased. Movement, periods of inadequate dietary intake, heavy parasite burdens, or other forms of stress should be minimized in sheep during the final 8 wk of gestation.

PUERPERAL HYPOCALCEMIA IN SMALL ANIMALS
(Postpartum hypocalcemia, Periparturient hypocalcemia, Puerperal tetany, Eclampsia)

Puerperal hypocalcemia is an acute, life-threatening condition usually seen at peak lactation, 2-3 wk after whelping. Small-breed bitches with large litters are most often affected. Hypocalcemia may also occur during parturition and may precipitate dystocia.

Etiology and Pathogenesis: Hypocalcemia most likely results from the loss of calcium into the milk and from inadequate dietary calcium intake. This imbalance in calcium metabolism occurs because calcium mobilization from bone into the serum pool is insufficient to maintain the efflux of calcium leaving through the mammary glands. Heavy lactational demands from large neonates or a large litter are often noted. The incidence is increased in small breeds of dogs, although puerperal hypocalcemia can occur in any breed of dog, with any size litter, and at any time during lactation. Rarely, it occurs during late gestation in bitches. Although uncommon in queens, it may occur during early lactation.

Inadequate production of parathyroid hormone (PTH) during the hypocalcemic crisis is not responsible for eclampsia. In dairy cows with a similar condition (*see* PARTURIENT PARESIS IN COWS, p 806), production of PTH is adequate, but the pool of osteoclasts for PTH to stimulate is not. The small osteoclast pool results from feeding a high level of dietary calcium during the nonlactating period, which suppresses parathyroid gland secretion of PTH and stimulates C-cell secretion of calcitonin. In dogs, supplementation with oral calcium during pregnancy may predispose to eclampsia during peak lactation, because excessive calcium intake during pregnancy causes downregulation of the calcium regulatory system and subsequent clinical hypocalcemia when calcium demand is high.

The paresis seen in cattle, rather than the tetany seen in dogs, is probably the result of a combination of factors. Cows often have concurrent mild hypermagnesemia and fail to release acetylcholine at neuromuscular junctions, have increased volatile fatty acids (which are inhibitory at neuromuscular synapses), and have a higher threshold for firing of neuromuscular junctions than do dogs. In dogs, hypocalcemia has an excitatory effect on nerve and muscle cells. Excitation-secretion coupling is maintained at the neuromuscular junction in dogs with hypocalcemia. Tetany occurs as a result of spontaneous repetitive firing of motor nerve fibers. As a result of the loss of stabilizing membrane-bound calcium, nerve membranes become more permeable to ions and require a stimulus of lesser magnitude to depolarize. Hypoglycemia can occur concurrently.

Clinical Findings: Panting and restlessness are early clinical signs. Mild tremors, twitching, muscle spasms, and gait changes (stiffness and ataxia) result from increased neuromuscular excitability. Behavioral changes such as aggression, whining, salivation, pacing, hypersensitivity to stimuli, and disorientation are frequent. Severe tremors, tetany, generalized seizure activity, and finally coma and death may be seen. Hyperthermia may occur in severe cases. Prolonged seizure activity may cause cerebral edema. Tachycardia, hyperthermia, polyuria, polydipsia, and vomiting are sometimes seen. Historically, the bitch has been otherwise healthy and the neonates have been thriving.

Although hypocalcemia usually occurs postpartum, clinical signs can appear prepartum or at parturition. Hypocalcemia, with a serum calcium concentration >7 mg/dL but below the low normal level, may contribute to ineffective myometrial contractions and slow the progression of labor without causing any other clinical signs. Heavy panting may produce a respiratory alkalosis. Ionized calcium concentration is affected by protein concentration, acid-base status (alkalosis favors protein binding of serum calcium and exacerbates hypocalcemia), and other electrolyte imbalances. Thus, the severity of clinical signs may not correlate with the total calcium concentration.

Diagnosis: Diagnosis is often made from the signalment, history, clinical signs, and response to treatment. A pretreatment serum calcium concentration <7 mg/dL (<6 mg/dL in cats) confirms the diagnosis. (IV therapy with calcium is often started, however, before serum calcium concentration is determined.) A serum chemistry profile is useful to rule out concurrent hypoglycemia and other electrolyte imbalances. Prolongation of the QT interval and ventricular premature contractions may be seen on the ECG.

Differential diagnoses include other causes of seizures such as hypoglycemia, toxicoses, and primary neurologic disorders such as idiopathic epilepsy or meningoencephalitis. Other causes of irritability and hyperthermia such as metritis and mastitis should also be ruled out.

Treatment and Prevention: Slow IV administration of 10% calcium gluconate is given to effect (0.5-1.5 mL/kg over 10-30 min; 5-20 mL is the usual dose). This usually results in rapid clinical improvement within 15 min. Muscle relaxation should be immediate.

During administration of calcium, heart rate should be carefully monitored for bradycardia or arrhythmia by auscultation or by ECG. Signs of toxicity from too rapid administration of calcium include bradycardia, shortening of the QT interval, and premature ventricular complexes. If an arrhythmia develops, calcium administration should be discontinued until the heart rate and rhythm are normal; then administration is resumed at half the original infusion rate.

It is important to calculate the dosage of calcium based on elemental (available) calcium, because different products vary in the amount of calcium available. The dosage of elemental calcium for hypocalcemia is 5-15 mg/kg/hr. Calcium gluconate, 10%, contains 9.3 mg of elemental calcium/mL. Calcium chloride, 27%, contains 27.2 mg of elemental calcium/mL. Thus, for 10% calcium gluconate, the dosage is 0.5-1.5 mL/kg/hr, IV, and for 27% calcium chloride the dosage is 0.22-0.66 mL/kg/hr, IV. Calcium gluconate, as a 10% solution, is recommended because unlike calcium chloride, calcium gluconate extravasation is not caustic.

Once the animal is stable, the dose of calcium gluconate needed for initial control of tetany may be diluted in an equal volume of normal (0.9%) saline and given SC, TID, to control clinical signs. (Calcium chloride cannot be given SC.) Alternatively, 5-15 mg of elemental calcium/kg/hr can be continued IV. This protocol effectively supports serum calcium concentrations while waiting for oral vitamin D and calcium therapy to have effect. Ideally, serum calcium concentration should be maintained >8 mg/dL. Serum calcium concentrations at <8 mg/dL indicate the need to increase the dose of parenteral calcium, whereas concentrations >9 mg/dL suggest that it be reduced. The aim of longterm therapy is to maintain the serum calcium concentration at mildly low to low-normal concentrations (8-9.5 mg/dL).

The bitch may remain nonresponsive after correction of hypocalcemia if cerebral edema has developed. Cerebral edema, hyperthermia, and hypoglycemia should be treated if present. Fever usually resolves rapidly with control of tetany, and specific treatment for fever may result in hypothermia.

It is best not to let the puppies or kittens nurse for 12-24 hr. During this period, they should be fed a milk substitute or other appropriate diet; if mature enough, they should be weaned. If tetany recurs in the same lactation, the litter should be removed from the bitch and either hand raised (<4 wk of age) or weaned (>4 wk of age).

After the acute crisis, 25-50 mg of elemental calcium/kg/day in 3 or 4 divided doses is given PO for the remainder of the lactation. Again, the dose of calcium is based on the amount of elemental calcium in the product (ie, calcium carbonate tablets contain 295 mg elemental calcium/1 g tablet). In dogs, the dosage is usually 1-4 g/day, in divided doses. In cats, the dosage of calcium is approximately 0.5-1 g/day, in divided doses. Longterm maintenance therapy with oral vitamin D and oral calcium supplementation usually requires a minimum of 24-96 hr before an effect is achieved. Hypocalcemic animals should, therefore, receive parenteral calcium support during the initial post-tetany period. Calcium carbonate is a good choice because of its high percentage of elemental calcium, ready availability in drugstores in the form of antacids, low cost, and lack of gastric irritation. The dose of calcium can be gradually tapered to avoid unnecessary therapy; there is usually sufficient calcium in commercial pet food to meet the needs of dogs and cats. However, to avoid acute problems of hypocalcemic tetany, oral calcium supplementation should continue throughout lactation.

Vitamin D supplementation is used to increase calcium absorption from the intestines. The concentration of serum calcium should be monitored weekly. The dosage of 1,25-dihydroxyvitamin D_3 (calcitriol) is 0.03-0.06 µg/kg/day. Calcitriol has a rapid onset of action (1-4 days) and short half-life (<1 day). Iatrogenic hypercalcemia is a common complication of this therapy. If hypercalcemia results from overdosage, it can be rapidly corrected by discontinuing calcitriol. The toxic effects resolve in 1-14 days. This is a much briefer period than that seen with dihydrotachysterol (1-3 wk) or ergocalciferol (vitamin D_2; 1-18 wk).

Corticosteroids lower serum calcium and, therefore, are contraindicated. They may interfere with intestinal calcium transport and increase urinary loss of calcium.

Owners should be warned that this condition is likely to recur with future pregnancies. Steps to consider to prevent puerperal hypocalcemia in the bitch include feeding a high-quality, nutritionally balanced, and appropriate diet during pregnancy and lactation, providing food and water ad lib during lactation, and supplemental feeding of the puppies with milk replacer early in lactation and with solid food after 3-4 wk of age. Oral calcium supplementation during gestation is not indicated and may cause rather than prevent postpartum hypocalcemia. Calcium administration during peak milk production may be helpful in bitches with a history of puerperal hypocalcemia.

DISORDERS OF MAGNESIUM METABOLISM

Magnesium (Mg) homeostasis is not under direct hormonal control but is mainly determined by absorption from the GI tract; excretion by the kidneys; and the varying requirements of the body for pregnancy, lactation, and growth. Magnesium in the extracellular fluids represents ~1% of total body Mg, bone contains 50-70%, and the remainder is in the intracellular compartment. Therefore, plasma Mg does not provide an indication of intracellular or bone Mg stores. Intracellular Mg is required for activation of enzymes involving phosphate compounds such as ATPases, kinases, and phosphatases; synthesis of RNA, DNA, or protein; and stabilization of membranes. Extracellular Mg is involved in the regulation of membrane channels as well as in excitation-contraction coupling in skeletal muscle. Low ionic Mg concentrations accelerate the transmission of nerve impulses.

Ruminants are more prone to hypomagnesemia than nonruminant and monogastric animals. The variation in Mg metabolism between species is due mainly to anatomic and physiologic differences in digestive tracts. Ruminants absorb Mg less efficiently than nonruminants (35% vs 70% of intake). The rumen is the main site of absorption, and there are active transport mechanisms. Absorption from the large intestine occurs with high Mg intakes. In nonruminants, the small intestine is the main site of absorption. Differences in Mg metabolism within some species are attributable to variation in absorption efficiency of Mg from the gut, and in others to variation in reabsorption of Mg by the kidney tubules.

HYPERMAGNESEMIA

Hypermagnesemia (plasma Mg concentration >2 mg/dL [1.1 mmol/L]) is a rare condition that has been reported only in monogastric animals. Horses show signs of sweating and muscle weakness within 4 hr of receiving excessive oral doses of magnesium sulfate for constipation. This is followed by recumbency, tachycardia (120 bpm), and tachypnea (60 breaths/min). Signs subside following treatment with slow IV infusion of calcium gluconate (23% solution). Hypermagnesemia has been reported in cats with renal failure that were receiving IV fluid therapy. As plasma Mg concentrations exceed 2.5 mmol/L, there may be ECG changes with prolongation of the PR interval; at 5 mmol/L deep tendon reflexes disappear, followed by hypotension and respiratory depression. Cardiac arrest may occur with blood Mg levels >6.0-7.5 mmol/L.

HYPOMAGNESEMIC TETANY IN ADULT CATTLE AND SHEEP
(Grass tetany, Grass staggers)

Hypomagnesemic tetany is a complex metabolic disturbance characterized by hypomagnesemia (plasma Mg <1.5 mg/dL [<0.65 mmol/L]) and a reduction in the concentration of Mg in the CSF (<1.0 mg/dL [0.5 mmol/L]), which lead to hyperexcitability, muscular spasms, convulsions, respiratory distress, collapse, and death. Adult lactating animals are most susceptible due to the loss of Mg in milk. Hypomagnesemic tetany occurs mainly when animals are grazed on lush grass pastures or green cereal crops, but can occur in lactating beef cows fed silage indoors. It is rare in nonlactating cattle but has occurred when undernourished cattle were introduced to green cereal crops.

Etiology: The disorder occurs after a decrease in plasma Mg concentration when absorption of dietary Mg is unable to meet the requirements for maintenance (3 mg/kg body wt) and lactation (120 mg/kg milk). This can arise after a reduction in food intake during inclement weather, transport, or when cows graze short-grass dominant pastures containing <0.2% Mg on a dry-matter basis. Low herbage availability (<1,000 kg dry matter/hectare) results in liveweight losses during lactation, and plasma Mg decreases because insufficient Mg is obtained from body tissues mobilized during loss of liveweight to support lactation.

Mg absorption from the rumen may be reduced when potassium and nitrogen intakes are high and sodium and phosphorus intakes are low. Soils that are naturally high in potassium and those fertilized with potash and nitrogen are high-risk areas for hypomagnesemic tetany. The more complex mineral interactions are likely to be involved in herds in which hypomagnesemic tetany occurs in first- and second-calving cows as well as in older cows.

Cows often do not develop signs of hypomagnesemic tetany until blood calcium concentrations are <8 mg/dL (2.0 mmol/L), which commonly occurs in cattle grazing green cereal crops. The hypocalcemia arises from either a reduction in calcium intake or absorption, or both. Lush grass pastures and green cereal crops may predispose cattle to metabolic alkalosis (urine pH >8.5) with a reduced available pool of calcium, thereby increasing the risk of hypocalcemia. Urine Mg concentrations are a useful guide to Mg status and are undetectable in cows with hypomagnesemia.

Clinical Findings: In the most acute form, affected cows, which may appear to be grazing normally, suddenly throw up their heads, bellow, gallop in a blind frenzy, fall, and exhibit severe paddling convulsions. These convulsive episodes may be repeated at short intervals, and death usually occurs within a few hours. In many instances, animals at pasture are found dead without observed illness, but an indication that the animal had convulsions before death may be seen from marks on the ground. In less severe cases, the cow is obviously ill at ease, walks stiffly, is hypersensitive to touch and sound, urinates frequently, and may progress to the acute convulsive stage after a period as long as 2-3 days. This period may be shortened if the cow is transported or driven to a fresh pasture. When animals have hypocalcemia and hypomagnesemia, the signs shown depend on which predominates. With hypomagnesemia, tachycardia and loud heart sounds are characteristic signs.

Clinical signs of hypomagnesemic tetany in sheep occur when hypomagnesemia (plasma Mg <0.5 mg/dL [0.2 mmol/L]) occurs concomitantly with hypocalcemia (plasma Ca <8 mg/dL [2.0 mmol/L]). The disease in lactating ewes occurs under essentially the same conditions and has the same clinical signs as in cattle.

Diagnosis: Diagnosis is usually confirmed by response to treatment, followed by confirmation of hypomagnesemia in samples taken prior to treatment. Tetany usually occurs when plasma Mg is <1.2 mg/dL (0.5 mmol/L) in cattle and <0.5 mg/dL (0.2 mmol/L) in sheep. Urine Mg is usually undetectable in cows with hypomagnesemic tetany. Mg concentrations <1.8 mg/dL (0.75 mmol/L) in the vitreous humour of the eye removed from animals within 24 hr after death are indicative of hypomagnesemic tetany.

Treatment: Animals showing clinical signs require treatment immediately with combined solutions of calcium and Mg, preferably given slowly IV while monitoring the heart (*see* PARTURIENT PARESIS IN COWS, p 806). The response to treatment is slower in animals with hypomagnesemic tetany than in animals with hypocalcemia alone, due to the time it takes to restore Mg in the CSF. The animal should not be stimulated during treatment, as this could trigger fatal convulsions. Additional Mg sulfate (200 mL of a 50% solution/cow) can be given SC. After treatment, cows should be left to respond without stimulation, and then moved off the tetany-prone pasture, if possible. Animals must be provided with hay treated with 2 oz (60 g) of Mg oxide daily; if this is not done, the condition can recur within 36 hr after therapy.

Prevention: Mg has to be given daily to animals at risk because the body has no readily available stores. Daily oral supplements of Mg oxide (2 oz [60 g] to cattle and 1/3 oz [10 g] to sheep) should be given in the danger period. Most Mg salts are unpalatable and must be combined with other palatable ingredients such as molasses, concentrates, or hay. Feeding hay alone may be all that is required to prevent hypomagnesemic tetany in herds in which only old cows (>6 yr) are affected. If slow-release intraruminal Mg devices are administered, it is recommended that the animals also be provided with hay. Fertilizers containing Mg are effective in increasing herbage Mg only on certain soil types. Herbage may be dusted with powdered Mg oxide (500 g/cow), or sprayed with a 2% solution of Mg sulfate at intervals of 1-2 wk. If rainfall exceeds 40-50 mm within 2-3 days of dusting, the herbage will require another dusting.

Out-wintered stock should be protected from wind and cold and provided with supplementary food. Sheep and cattle should have access to hay, particularly when grazing either green cereal crops or pastures fertilized with potassium or nitrogen (or both).

HYPOMAGNESEMIC TETANY IN CALVES

Etiology and Pathogenesis: Magnesium absorption efficiency in calves fed milk falls from 87% at 2-3 wk to 32% at 7-8 wk of age. Hypomagnesemic tetany occurs in 2- to 4-mo-old calves being fed milk only, or in younger calves with chronic scours while being fed milk replacer.

Clinical Findings: Clinical signs are similar to those of hypomagnesemic tetany in adult cattle (*see* above) and include hyperexcitability, muscular spasms, convulsions, and death.

Diagnosis: Hypomagnesemic tetany in calves must be differentiated from acute lead poisoning (p 2404), tetanus (p 495), strychnine poisoning (p 2521), polioencephalomalacia (p 1061), and enterotoxemia caused by the toxin of *Clostridium perfringens* (p 493). Analysis of bone aids diagnosis—normal bone has a calcium:Mg ratio of 70:1; in hypomagnesemic calves, the ratio may be ≥90:1.

Treatment, Prevention, and Control: Affected calves require prompt treatment with a 10% solution of magnesium sulfate (100 mL, SC) followed by 10 g Mg oxide, PO, SID. Provision of good-quality legume hay and a starter ration from 2 wk of age prevents the disorder.

DISORDERS OF PHOSPHORUS METABOLISM

Chronic Phosphorus Deficiency/Hypophosphatemia

Phosphorus is essential for many intracellular processes, notably glycolysis, membrane maintenance, oxygen transport, muscle contraction, and protection from oxidative damage. It is also an important component of bones, teeth, milk, and ruminant saliva. Deficiency is usually primary and results in multiorgan system dysfunction and eventually progressive demineralization of bone.

Etiology: Phosphorus is supplied by the diet. Soil and pasture plants are naturally deficient in many parts of the world. Fertilization is used to increase plant phosphorus content, but inadequate or poor-quality fertilizer application, interference in uptake by other minerals, soil retention, leaching by rain, soil depletion through repeated crop or grass harvesting, and poor growth of plants during periods of drought may still result in phosphorus-deficient forage.

Vitamin D promotes intestinal uptake of phosphorus, but secondary deficiency related to hypovitaminosis D is uncommon in herbivores without at least marginal concurrent dietary deficiency. Secondary deficiency appears to be most common in areas with limited sunlight during critical skeletal growth periods, and is seen most frequently in young, growing animals.

Ruminants secrete large quantities of phosphorus in saliva. In times of need, this is recycled through the intestine; in times of sufficiency, fecal loss is the primary mode of excretion.

Clinical Findings: Most clinical manifestations of phosphorus deficiency arise only after several months of deficient intake. Poor growth, dull hair coat, subnormal milk production, and poor reproductive performance are among the earliest signs. Most animals in the herd are affected to some degree. Pica, including osteophagia, follows, with possible complications of botulism or traumatic reticulitis. Atypical shifting-leg lameness, swollen joints, and spontaneous fractures occur after longer periods of deficiency. Fractures occur most commonly in the ribs, pelvis, or vertebral bodies. With secondary deficiency, osteodystrophic signs, including stiff-legged lameness, hunched posture, widened and painful growth plates and costochondral junctions, shortened long bones, and angular limb deformities, are seen earlier in the course of the disease.

With multigenerational deficiency, cattle develop a characteristic appearance, including a rough hair coat, narrow girth with a small pelvis, and thin, breakable ribs. The thinness of the trunk imparts a "leggy" appearance to the cow.

Acute manifestations of phosphorus deficiency are rare. Recumbency due to apparent muscle weakness without hemolysis or mental dullness is occasionally seen in dairy cattle in late gestation or early lactation. Intravascular hemolysis with hemoglobinuria may also occur in postparturient dairy cattle (see below). These acute syndromes are seen exclusively in dairy cattle. It is postulated that the abrupt increase in phosphorus demand for fetal bone and maternal colostrum and milk production lead to rapid depletion of the circulating pool. High oxidant challenge and lack of sufficient antioxidant compounds may also contribute to clinical disease.

Lesions: Necropsy findings are not generally remarkable unless osteomalacia is significant, or fractures or hemolysis have occurred. Growth plates may appear wide and irregular in younger animals, with lack of mineralization.

Diagnosis: Diagnosis of phosphorus deficiency can be difficult and often requires exclusion of other causes of ill-thrift and poor reproductive performance, including selenium deficiency, protein-calorie malnutrition, and parasitism. Feed analysis with particular emphasis on phosphorus form and content is the most direct way of diagnosing a deficiency. In chronic deficiency syndromes, serum phosphorus concentrations may be low, but more commonly are maintained within reference ranges by liberation of bone mineral. Diurnal variation makes systematic sampling necessary. Bone resorption can be estimated by measuring serum hydroxyproline, an amino acid liberated from collagen, or by measuring the ratio of bone ash to organic matrix in a core biopsy. Fecal phosphorus provides an indirect measure of dietary sufficiency.

In acute syndromes, serum phosphorus concentrations are often low for affected cattle, but are within reference ranges for unaffected herdmates, even ones that later develop clinical signs. Feed phosphorus is usually low.

Treatment: Chronic syndromes can often be reversed by placing the animal on an adequate diet. Reproductive performance can improve in as little as a month; remodeled bone takes longer and, in severe cases, may not completely correct. Oral supplements usually come in the form of dicalcium phosphate, rock phosphate, or bone meal. Mono-, di-, or trisodium phosphate, ammonium phosphate, phosphoric acid, and superphosphate may be used, but these must be handled carefully to avoid phosphorus toxicosis.

Acute syndromes require more immediate correction. There are no phosphorus-only compounds labeled by the FDA for parenteral use in cattle, and multiple mineral (predominately calcium) preparations contain a form of phosphorus with low bioavailability. Thus, all parenteral supplementation is extra-label. Monosodium phosphate, sodium acid phosphate, and diluted phosphate enema solutions all have been used IV to rapidly correct hypophosphatemia. Licensed oral gel preparations provide a large dosage over a longer period of time, and are useful in less severe cases and to maintain blood concentrations after IV correction.

Prevention: Phosphorus deficiency is best prevented by ensuring adequate dietary intake. Recommendations vary with area, age, and use of the cow. Maintaining at least 0.042% dietary phosphorus in dairy cattle appears to be adequate to prevent acute disease in most herds. Total mixed rations, mineral supplements, top-dressed feeds, and supplemented drinking water all have been used successfully. The ratio of calcium:phosphorus in the diet should not be <2:1.

Postparturient Hemoglobinuria

Cows affected with this disease of rapid intravascular hemolysis develop severe anemia and weakness, and milk production drops markedly. The disease is seen worldwide. The exact cause is unknown, but the most likely predisposing factors are phosphorus deficiency (*see* above), which increases osmotic fragility of erythrocytes, and copper deficiency (in New Zealand), which increases susceptibility of erythrocytes to oxidative injury. Hemolytic or oxidative plant toxins (often from *Brassica* spp, sugar beets, or green forage), selenium deficiency, and ketoacidosis probably contribute. In North America, the disease is sporadic and common in older, high-producing dairy cows, while in New Zealand, herd outbreaks occur involving cows of all ages. Most affected cattle are in week 2-5 of lactation. Beef and nonlactating cattle are rarely affected.

Clinical disease is rare but, when it occurs, the case fatality rate is high (10-30%). The incidence of subclinical disease is unknown; many postparturient dairy cows have blood or hemoglobin in their urine, and the source is rarely established. With clinical disease, rapid intravascular hemolysis leads to severe anemia, tachycardia, weakness, hemoglobinuria with dark brown or red urine, and pallor over several days. Milk production drops rapidly over sequential milkings. Affected cows also may have fever, diarrhea, and tachypnea. Cows that survive the hemolytic crisis may take several months to recover completely. Convalescent cows and cows with subclinical disease develop icterus and evidence of increased erythrogenesis.

Diagnosis is usually made by recognition of clinical signs, particularly dark urine and anemia. Hemoglobinuria may best be diagnosed by noting failure of the urine to clear with centrifugation (ruling out hematuria) and presence of concurrent severe anemia (making hemoglobinuria more likely than myoglobinuria [*see* TABLE 1]). Intravascular hemolysis caused by *Babesia* (p 20) or *Theileria* (p 30) may be ruled out by blood film analysis, and standard laboratory methods can be used to rule out leptospirosis (p 525) or bacillary hemoglobinuria (p 487). Diagnostic testing and feed or pasture analysis can be performed to identify toxic plants and deficiency of phosphorus, copper, and other antioxidants.

Transfusion of large quantities of whole blood is the best treatment for severely affected cows. Crystalloid fluids may be beneficial if blood is not available and may protect the kidneys against toxic and anoxic damage. Treatment with sodium acid phosphate (60 g in 300 mL of sterile water, IV followed by SC, every 12 hr) or copper glycinate (120 mg available copper) may halt hemolysis. Use of these products is not approved in lactating cows. Correction of mineral deficiencies and elimination of plant toxins from the diet may help prevent recurrence.

TABLE 1. Common Causes of Red Urine in Cattle

Hematuria*	Hemoglobinuria†
Clostridial infections	Postparturient hemoglobinuria
Malignant catarrhal fever	Leptospirosis
Anticoagulant poisoning	Water or salt poisoning
Urolithiasis	*Brassica* or onion intoxication
Cystitis	Chronic copper intoxication
Enzootic hematuria (bracken fern poisoning)	
Facial eczema (sporidesmin poisoning)	
Oxalate poisoning (ethylene glycol)	
Babesiosis	

*Clears with centrifugation
†Does not clear with routine centrifugation

FATIGUE AND EXERCISE

Muscular fatigue during exercise results in a decrease in the ability of muscle to produce force. Fatigue can occur during both submaximal and maximal intensities of exercise. The mechanisms of fatigue in events of different intensity and duration have been subject to much research, but no single cause of fatigue has been identified; fatigue is therefore usually referred to as multifactorial. Fatigue during exercise is a common presenting complaint in veterinary clinical practice. It can be caused by many diseases and dysfunction of many body systems, and these problems are discussed in other chapters. This chapter focuses on fatigue during exercise in healthy animals.

Fatigue is a normal consequence of exercise that is continued at high intensity or for prolonged periods of time. The decrease in force production can be regarded as a safety mechanism. If fatigue did not occur, or were delayed greatly, structural damage to muscle cells and supportive tissues could occur during intense exercise. Most knowledge concerning fatigue in animals has been described in horses because of the ease of studies in laboratories with high-speed treadmills that enable investigation of the respiratory, cardiovascular, and metabolic responses during exercise, and of collection of muscle biopsies before and after exercise. Fatigue in these studies is usually defined as inability or unwillingness of the horse to maintain the same velocity as the treadmill during tests in which velocity is increased every 1-2 min. Fatigue during intense treadmill exercise is associated with changes in gait, including increases in stride length and decreases in stride frequency. More dramatic changes are seen in the movement of the fetlock joint during fatigue. These gait and biomechanical changes may be an important influence on certain types of injury to the locomotor system of racehorses. The results suggest that training of racehorses should avoid exercise intensities and durations that result in locomotor changes due to fatigue.

Fatigue has been classified into 2 types—peripheral and central. Peripheral fatigue has been described as fatigue due to altered muscle function. Studies of muscle metabolism after exercise have relied mainly on muscle biopsies and measurement of the concentrations of muscle glycogen and creatine phosphate, ATP, ADP, inosine monophosphate (IMP), inorganic phosphate, glycolytic intermediary products, protons, and other metabolites. The fundamental problem in muscular fatigue is failure of ATP resynthesis and accumulation of ADP and inorganic phosphate ions. Central fatigue is attributed to signals arising from the CNS, directing a decrease in performance via a change in the frequency of action potentials in motor neurons. It may occur secondary to pain, dyspnea, perceptions of exertion, hypoglycemia, hyperthermia, ammonia accumulation, and altered amino acid metabolism. However, central fatigue in response to these stimuli is probably highly variable. For example, some horses can continue endurance exercise despite severe hyperthermia, dehydration, and plasma electrolyte disturbances.

Fatigue during High-intensity Exercise

In general, the cause of fatigue during exercise depends greatly on the duration and energy demands of the event. Some events last ~20 sec (eg, Quarter Horse races, some Greyhound races), and energy demands may be >90% anaerobic; other events last many hours (eg, endurance races for horses, camels, and dogs), and energy demands are >90% aerobic. During intense exercise at maximal speeds lasting 20 sec to 3 min, as in Quarter Horse, Standardbred, and Thoroughbred horse races, energy supply is both anaerobic and aerobic. It has been estimated that energy supply is probably >50% aerobic in horse races that last >1 min. Intramuscular stores of ATP decrease by 50% in racehorses after such exercise. Superior racing performance in Thoroughbreds and Standardbreds has been correlated with high rates of oxygen transport and low rates of accumulation of lactate in the blood during submaximal exercise tests.

Catabolism of ATP, creatine phosphate, and glycogen is the anaerobic source of energy during high-intensity exercise. Such exercise at an individual animal's highest attainable speed cannot be maintained for more than ~30-40 sec. Thereafter, fatigue occurs and the animal slows down. Mean ATP loss reported after repeated fast gallops in Thoroughbred horses was 32%, but the ATP content in some individual muscle cells after fast exercise in horses may be negligible. Fatigue during intense exercise is also usually attributed to depletion of stores of creatine phosphate and to accumulation of ADP and inorganic phosphate, and to accumulation of lactate anions and protons in active muscle cells. Intracellular acidosis has a negative feedback effect on glycolytic enzymes such as phosphofructokinase, and reduces the efficiency of the muscle contraction by interfering with the binding of calcium with troponin C, a vital step in excitation-contraction coupling. Recent research suggests that calcium accumulates in the sarcoplasm in such conditions, rather than being recycled through the sarcoplasmic reticulum (a process that requires ATP). Potassium ions accumulate in the extracellular fluid during fatigue after intense exercise, probably as a result of the decrease in intracellular ATP. Changes in the ratio of intracellular to extracellular potassium alter the resting membrane potential and action potential of muscle cells.

The decline in intramuscular ATP is correlated with the accumulation of lactate and the appearance of ammonia in the muscle. It has been postulated that ammonia accumulation in plasma may also contribute to fatigue. Increased ADP concentration also results in accumulation of AMP, IMP, allantoin, ammonia, and uric acid in horses. In treadmill studies, the decrease in muscle ATP during intense exercise is correlated with the increase in plasma uric acid concentration 30 min after exercise. Running time during the treadmill tests is correlated with uric acid concentrations after exercise. Significant but low correlations have also been found between racing performance of Standardbred pacers and uric acid concentrations after the race. Infusion with ammonium acetate during a treadmill exercise to fatigue did not significantly affect the time to fatigue in horses, suggesting that plasma ammonia levels do not have a role in fatigue during intense exercise.

Electrolyte disturbances in muscle may also play a role in fatigue after intense exercise. During intense exercise, water moves into muscle cells, and intracellular concentrations of potassium decrease. This decrease, along with an increase in concentration of potassium in the extracellular fluid and accumulation of sodium in the sarcoplasm, tends to depolarize sarcolemma and t-tubule membranes and decrease the strength of muscle contractions. It has been suggested that accumulation of calcium and depletion of ATP in muscle cells during exercise induces more rapid potassium efflux from muscle cells. This may inactivate the sarcolemma and t-tubule membranes and prevent tension development.

Synchronous diaphragmatic flutter (SDF, p 77) is sometimes seen after races in Thoroughbreds and Standardbreds, although it is more usually associated with fatigue during prolonged exercise in horses. Its occurrence in horses after races of 2-3 min duration suggests that it may be related to electrolyte disturbances. SDF can occur in Standardbred horses after a particularly strenuous race, and it often resolves within 30-60 min without treatment.

Highly intense exercise training over many weeks can result in a form of chronic fatigue, referred to as overtraining. This condition causes decreased performance during intense exercise, which is not reversed by 1-2 wk of rest. The syndrome has been associated with a decrease in the plasma cortisol response to intense exercise, suggesting that overtraining is associated with dysfunction of the hypothalamic-pituitary-adrenal axis. Overtraining with poor race performance has been associated with a syndrome of red cell hypervolemia in Swedish trotters. However, reversal of the red cell hypervolemia did not increase performance. Instead, removal of 36 mL/kg body wt of blood resulted in decreased oxygen transport and uptake during intense exercise, and run time to fatigue was shorter after the exsanguination, suggesting that red cell hypervolemia is not the mechanism of poor performance in overtrained horses. A longitudinal treadmill study of overtraining also found no evidence of red cell hypervolemia in Standardbred horses. Furthermore, prolonged training with onset of overtraining syndrome was not associated with any significant changes in resting hematology or biochemistry values. Use of these methods to monitor fitness or the "stress" of training has no scientific basis.

Fatigue during intense exercise is influenced by environmental conditions. Intense exercise in hot conditions is associated with earlier onset of fatigue. In such conditions, blood flow decreases to the skin and working muscles in horses. Earlier onset of fatigue in hot conditions could be a protective response to avoid heat stroke; the fatigue could be due to decreased blood flow and oxygen transport to muscle and to high brain temperature.

Fatigue during Prolonged Exercise

During prolonged exercise lasting many hours, heat generated in the course of mainly aerobic ATP resynthesis imposes a thermoregulatory demand on the animal. Responses include sweating and/or panting to remove heat from the body. The result is dehydration and acid-base and electrolyte disturbances. These factors are usually implicated in the fatigue, exhaustion, and even death that can occur after such exercise in horses. Fatigue during prolonged exercise has also been associated with depletion of muscle and liver glycogen stores and hypoglycemia. Studies of fatigue during prolonged exercise are difficult in horses because they will continue to perform treadmill exercise in the presence of severe, life-threatening hyperthermia and dehydration.

Horses occasionally die at endurance events, despite current practices of evaluation of recovery at rest stops. Horses that have competed in 3-day events or endurance rides may present with exhaustion, a life-threatening condition. Horses may lose fluids at 10-15 L/hr by sweating during prolonged exercise, and urgent treatment of fluid and electrolyte deficits and hyperthermia (rectal temperatures >40.5°C) may be required. Affected horses may lose ≥10-20 L of body water; many have body fluid deficits of 40 L. Sodium and potassium deficits may be 4,000 and 1,600 mmol, respectively. Affected horses show signs of depression, fatigue, dehydration, elevated heart and respiratory rates, and hyperthermia. Hyperthermic horses should be continuously hosed with cold water, stood in the shade and, if possible, placed in a cooling breeze. Washing the horse water that is extremely cold (an "ice slurry") is a more aggressive and more effective form of cooling a hyperthermic horse. Isotonic balanced electrolyte solutions can be administered PO and IV for dehydration. Horses can be given 8 L, PO, initially, with subsequent administration of 4-8 L every 1-2 hr if needed. Numerous commercial electrolyte mixtures are available for oral administration. Hypertonic, hypotonic, and alkaline solutions should not be used. In severe cases, IV treatment is preferred. Up to 50 L may be required, which can be given at 5-10 L/hr. About 30 L of Ringer's solution is required to replace a sodium deficit of 4,000 mmol.

Environmental temperature and humidity have a major impact on the degree of disturbance to body fluids during prolonged exercise. It is particularly important to ensure adequate hydration before the event and to provide access to fluids during and after the event to reduce the likelihood of exhaustion. Administration of supplementary water, electrolytes, and glucose to horses before and during competition may reduce the incidence of exhausted horse syndrome.

Prevention of Fatigue

Physical training is the most effective way of reducing fatigue and increasing the capacity for exercise. Many physiologic responses to training contribute to increased exercise capacity. The maximal rate of oxygen transport increases. There are increases in stroke volume, capillary density in muscle, blood volume, and total blood hemoglobin content. Hypertrophy of muscle cells occurs, coupled with increases in concentrations of mitochondria, glycogen, and enzymes concerned with energy production. Sprint training can result in decreased proportions of slow-twitch fibers, and endurance training can result in increased oxidative capacity of fast-twitch fibers. Sprint training also affects the uptake of calcium by the sarcoplasmic reticulum in skeletal muscle cells. Exercise results in decreased calcium uptake rate and Ca^{2+}-ATPase activity, but these decreases are moderated by training.

Adaptations to training in skeletal muscle depend on the training intensity. Horses trained at intensities >80% of their maximal oxygen uptake (VO_2max) had an increase in their percentage of fast-twitch, high oxidative fibers and an 8% increase in the buffering capacity of exercised muscle, but these responses did not occur in horses trained at 40%

VO_2max. Heart rate meters can be used to guide the intensity of training. Heart rates that result in 80% VO_2max are ~90% of maximal heart rate. Maximal heart rates range from ~210-240 bpm in horses. To promote greater muscle adaptation to training, it is appropriate to use heart rate meters to measure an individual horse's heart rates during slow and fast exercise and to calculate the exercise velocities that result in heart rates of 90% of the maximal heart rate. Blood lactate after exercise can also be used to measure the appropriate training intensity. At an exercise intensity of 80% VO_2max, plasma lactate concentrations during treadmill exercise are in the range of 4-10 mmol/L. Warmup before exercise significantly increases the time to fatigue during intense exercise in racehorses. Warmup increases muscle temperature before exercise and the peak oxygen uptake during exercise. The oxygen deficit at the beginning of intense exercise and the rate of glycogen metabolism during exercise are also lower after prior warmup. In one report, the effects of a low-intensity warmup (10 min at 50% of VO_2max) and high-intensity warmup (7 min at 50% VO_2max) and brief exercise at high intensities (including 45 sec at 100% VO_2max) were not different. The practical importance of this finding is that a 10-min warmup before competition involving intense exercise is likely to reduce fatigue in Quarter Horse, Thoroughbred, and Standardbred races.

It has been suggested that fatigue during intense exercise may be delayed by manipulation of acid-base status before exercise. Although some trainers have administered sodium bicarbonate before races, this practice is now banned by many racing administrations. The treatment does alter blood pH and lactate concentrations during exercise. However, the effect of alkalinizing solutions on equine performance is equivocal, and recent treadmill studies using sodium bicarbonate at a dosage of 0.6 g/kg have not shown an effect on the time at which fatigue occurs. In addition, administration of sodium bicarbonate before intense treadmill exercise did not have any significant effect on the muscle metabolic response to exercise. In Greyhounds, a dose of sodium bicarbonate at 0.4 g/kg did not have a significant effect on race times in races >400 m long. However, there may be an ergogenic effect when sodium bicarbonate is used at high dosages. Sodium bicarbonate at a dosage rate of 1 g/kg (by nasogastric tube) increased the time to fatigue in horses, and it was concluded that the treatment affected performance.

Manipulation of energy supply and hydration are frequently used in human athletics to limit fatigue during endurance exercise. Dehydration before exercise results in higher core temperatures during exercise in horses. It would be inappropriate for an animal to begin endurance exercise with suboptimal hydration or glycogen concentrations in liver and muscle. Horses are more susceptible to hyperthermia during prolonged exercise because of their high body mass to surface area ratio. Equine thermoregulation results in extreme perturbations of body fluid status, and there is increasing interest in ways of limiting these responses to exercise by pre-exercise fluid administration. Hyperhydration by administration of saline solutions orally before exercise results in expansion of the blood volume during exercise. Recent studies suggest that hyperhydration before prolonged exercise does help conserve plasma volume during exercise, but does not result in lower body temperatures. Horses should be acclimated to hot environments before competition. Horses that are not acclimated could be expected to have higher body temperatures during exercise and earlier fatigue.

Horses should not be given large meals 1-2 hr before competition, because plasma volume is decreased for at least 1 hr after a large meal. Feeding small portions every 4 hr does not result in changes to plasma volume. A decreased volume of water in the GI tract could decrease fatigue during intense exercise because it would decrease the oxygen needed for locomotion. Reduced fiber intake before racing is a strategy to reduce water volume in the hindgut. Excessive fatness is also likely to cause earlier fatigue because it could contribute to higher body temperatures during exercise.

Glucose supplementation may be important in limiting fatigue in equine endurance exercise. Endurance time during treadmill running was prolonged by the IV infusion of glucose solution during exercise. Plasma glucose was higher during exercise in the horses receiving glucose, and plasma lactate and body core temperatures were lower at fatigue. Plasma volume decreased more slowly in treated horses. These results suggest that supplemental glucose during exercise prolongs performance time in horses. This increase may be due to increased glucose availability, reduced reliance on anaerobic energy production, lower core temperature, and better maintenance of plasma volume.

Glycogen concentration in skeletal muscle prior to performance is relevant to fatigue during both short-term/intense and prolonged exercise. Depletion of muscle glycogen causes a decrease in anaerobic power generation and capacity for high-intensity exercise. Horses should not be depleted of glycogen before short-term or endurance events. Intense or prolonged exercise depletes the muscle glycogen stores, and it is sensible to allow at least 48 hr for adequate postexercise glycogen resynthesis in horses. No method of glycogen loading using adjustments to normal feeding has been described in horses. Use of glucose or other carbohydrate solutions prior to racing to promote performance in Standardbred and Thoroughbred racehorses has no scientific basis.

Feeding fat can increase performance during prolonged exercise. Elevation of free fatty acid concentrations in blood prior to endurance exercise results in an increased use of fat as an energy source during low-intensity exercise, and in higher blood glucose concentrations during exercise. The shift to greater use of fat as a fuel results in lower respiratory demands for the exercise, because less carbon dioxide must be expired when more fat is used for energy. Fat adaptation appears to facilitate the metabolic regulation of glycolysis by sparing glucose and glycogen at low-intensity work and by promoting glycolysis when power is needed for high-intensity exercise. Adding fat to the diet affects the metabolic and thermoregulatory responses to exercise. Feeding vegetable oil at a rate of 100-120 g/kg has been suggested as ample.

Creatine has been used in horses as an ergogenic aid, but there is no evidence for its efficacy. Horses receiving 25 g creatine monohydrate twice daily for 6.5 days did not have significantly different run times to fatigue compared with controls. The supplementation also had no significant effect on muscle or blood creatine concentrations at rest or after exercise.

An association between vitamin E concentration and performance has been described in sled dogs. Dogs with higher prerace vitamin E concentrations were more likely to finish the race and were less likely to be withdrawn during the race for poor health, fatigue, or other reasons. This result needs to be followed up by other studies that investigate if the reduced fatigue is caused by higher vitamin E concentrations in blood.

Performance of horses in a 160-kilometer endurance ride was associated with diet and training strategies in a survey of 52 owners of 54 horses. Horses that were eliminated from the race for metabolic reasons were more likely to be trained hard without a concomitant increase in energy intake, compared with horses that completed the ride. Suboptimal energy intake during training was associated with feeding of more roughage. Provision of more protein and vitamins did not confer an advantage.

Recovery

Recovery of horses after endurance rides is influenced by the rehydration strategy used. After prolonged treadmill exercise and furosemide-induced dehydration, horses offered a saline solution (NaCl, 0.9%) as the initial rehydration fluid maintained an elevated plasma sodium concentration, and recovery of body weight was more rapid than in horses offered water. Horses may need to be trained to drink a saline solution. Use of saline solutions should be encouraged, especially in horses that are required to compete in events on consecutive days, such as endurance and 3-day events.

FEVER OF UNKNOWN ORIGIN

In both veterinary and human patients, fever may indicate infectious, inflammatory, immune-mediated, or neoplastic disease. In most cases, the history and physical examination reveal the cause of the fever, or the fever resolves spontaneously or in response to antibiotic therapy. However, in a small percentage of patients, the cause of fever is not readily apparent, and the problem becomes persistent or recurrent. These patients are said to have fever of unknown origin (FUO).

In human medicine, classical FUO is defined as fever >101°F (38.3°C) on several occasions over a period >2-3 wk with no diagnosis established after 3 outpatient visits or 3 days in the hospital. There is no recognized definition of this syndrome in veterinary medicine, making it difficult to determine its true prevalence. FUO is probably less prevalent now than 20 years ago due to improved diagnostic technology (eg, imaging, laboratory tests).

Body Temperature Regulation: Body temperature is regulated by the hypothalamus. This area of the brain acts as a thermostat to maintain temperature as close as possible to a normal set-point. The hypothalamus receives input from internal and external thermoreceptors, and it activates physiologic and behavioral activities that influence heat production, heat loss, and heat gain.

Hyperthermia refers to any increase in body temperature above the normal range. Fever is a particular form of hyperthermia in which the heat loss and heat gain mechanisms are adjusted to maintain body temperature at a higher hypothalamic set-point; thus, fever is essentially a regulated hyperthermia. In nonfebrile cases of hyperthermia (eg, heat stroke, exercise-induced hyperthermia, malignant hyperthermia, seizure), body temperature is elevated by abnormal and unregulated heat loss, heat gain, or heat production, and the hypothalamic set-point is not altered. Depending on their severity, these conditions can potentially result in body temperatures ≥106°F (41.1°C). In comparison, most patients with true fever have body temperatures in the range of 103-106°F (39.5-41.1°C).

Elevation of the hypothalamic set-point may be initiated by exogenous pyrogens, which include drugs, toxins, and viral or bacterial products (eg, endotoxin). These pyrogenic stimuli lead to the release of cytokines, termed endogenous pyrogens, from inflammatory cells. Ultimately, locally synthesized prostaglandin E_2 in the hypothalamus is responsible for elevating the set-point, resulting in fever.

Etiology and Pathogenesis: FUO may be defined as fever that does not resolve spontaneously in the period expected for self-limited infection and for which a cause cannot be found despite considerable diagnostic effort. This excludes patients that respond to antibiotic therapy (and do not relapse) and patients in which the cause of fever is determined from initial history, physical examination, or laboratory tests, or in which fever resolves spontaneously.

Infectious, immune-mediated, and neoplastic disease are the most common causes of FUO in dogs. In a study of 101 dogs with fever, 22% had immune-mediated diseases, 22% primary bone marrow abnormalities, 16% infectious diseases, 9.5% neoplasia, 11.5% miscellaneous conditions, and 19% had genuine FUO. In cats, the cause is more likely to be infectious, but there are fewer published data on feline cases compared with canine cases. In a case series of horses with FUO, 43% had infectious disease, 22% had neoplasia, 6.5% had immune-mediated disease, 19% had miscellaneous causes, and in 9.5% the cause was not determined. In farm animals, the most likely causes of FUO are infectious or inflammatory diseases such as pneumonia, peritonitis, abscesses, endocarditis, metritis, mastitis, polyarthritis, and pyelonephritis.

Diagnosis: The key to diagnosis of FUO is to develop and follow a systematic plan that allows for the detection of both common and uncommon causes of fever. Clients should be informed that diagnosis of FUO may require considerable time and patience and may demand more advanced or expensive diagnostic tests. Nevertheless, simple and inexpensive tests may also reveal diagnostic clues that eventually point to the cause of the fever.

A staged or tiered approach to diagnosis can assist in choosing appropriate tests. The first stage should include history, physical examination, ophthalmic and neurologic examinations, CBC, fibrinogen, serum chemistry profile, urinalysis and urine culture, feline leukemia virus and feline immunodeficiency virus tests (cats), and usually thoracic and abdominal radiographs in small animals. In the second stage, some first-stage tests may be repeated (particularly the physical examination) and additional specialized tests are performed. These may be dictated by abnormal findings in the first stage of testing or may be determined by consideration of the most common known causes of FUO.

Tests included in this stage include blood cultures, arthrocentesis, abdominal ultrasound, lymph node aspiration, aspiration of other organs or masses, analysis of body fluids (eg, fluid from body cavities, milk samples, reproductive tract secretions), fecal culture, echocardiography (in the presence of a murmur), long-bone and joint radiographs, contrast radiographs, and serology. The third stage again may repeat earlier tests, as well as additional specialized procedures. These procedures are most likely to be chosen on the basis of previous findings, but may also be considered when all previous testing has been unrewarding. Examples include echocardiography (in the absence of a murmur), dental radiographs, bone marrow aspiration, bronchoscopy and bronchoalveolar lavage, CSF analysis, computed tomography (CT), MRI, laparoscopy, thoracoscopy, biopsies, exploratory surgery, or trial therapy.

History and Physical Examination: Epidemiologic characteristics such as vaccination, parasite control, and travel history should always be reviewed. The response to previous medications should be determined, as well as the presence of illness in other animals or humans. Clients should be questioned carefully about specific clinical signs as these may help localize the source of the fever. The physical examination should be detailed and repeated frequently.

CBC and Serum Chemistry Profile: The CBC and chemistry changes in FUO patients are often nonspecific, but may suggest further diagnostic tests. The CBC should always be accompanied by blood smear evaluation to detect parasites or morphologic changes.

Urine Culture: This test is always indicated to evaluate FUO in small animals, regardless of the appearance of the urine sediment.

Radiography and Advanced Imaging: Thoracic and abdominal radiographs are useful screening tools for the early localization of fever. Skeletal radiographs and contrast radiographs may subsequently be considered, depending on initial findings. For example, myelography may be used to investigate back pain. The use of advanced techniques such as CT and MRI is determined by the results of initial diagnostic testing or by consideration of the body system of interest, eg, MRI is particularly useful for evaluating the CNS.

Ultrasonography and Echocardiography: Abdominal ultrasound may reveal a source of fever in the abdomen, such as neoplasia, peritonitis, pancreatitis, or abscesses. The thoracic cavity, limbs, and retrobulbar areas may also be examined by ultrasound. Echocardiography is indicated at the early stages of evaluation of the FUO patient with a murmur. This may aid in the detection of endocarditis, although this diagnosis should also be based on signalment, onset of the heart murmur, and blood culture results.

Bone Marrow Evaluation: Bone marrow cytology and histology should be evaluated in any patient with unexplained CBC abnormalities. Bone marrow disease is a common cause of FUO in small animals; therefore, bone marrow aspiration should also be included in the second stage of diagnostic testing in these patients.

Arthrocentesis: Because immune-mediated polyarthritis is a common cause of FUO in dogs, arthrocentesis is included in the second stage of diagnostic testing in this species, even if the joints are normal on palpation. Some dogs with steroid-responsive meningitis-arteritis also have concurrent immune-mediated polyarthritis; therefore, arthrocentesis should be performed in dogs with spinal pain. Infectious polyarthritis is more commonly recognized in large animals, in which arthrocentesis is an important diagnostic test.

Blood Culture: Blood cultures are recommended in all patients with unexplained fever. The techniques used should allow the collection of adequately large volumes of blood under aseptic conditions. If the size of the patient allows collecting more than one blood culture set, using appropriately sized aerobic and anaerobic bottles increases the sensitivity and specificity of the test.

Serology: Serologic tests are available for the diagnosis of many infectious diseases and some immune-mediated disorders. Selection should be based on the signalment, clinical signs, and epidemiologic characteristics of the patient. Interpretation of test results requires an understanding of disease prevalence, vaccination history, and sensitivity and specificity of the test. The use of immune panels or autoantibody screens in small animal patients with FUO is discouraged. Neither antinuclear antibody or rheumatoid factor titers alone are sensitive or specific enough to diagnose systemic lupus erythematosus or rheumatoid arthritis, respectively.

Microbiology, Cytology, and Histology: Fine-needle aspirates are safe and simple to obtain from effusions, masses, nodules, organs, tissues, and body fluids. Fluids should be examined cytologically and also submitted for microbiologic testing. Tissue biopsies are generally obtained in the second or third stages of diagnostic testing, after clinical signs or initial diagnostic tests have localized the fever. When biopsies are obtained, sufficient samples should be submitted for histopathology, appropriate culture (aerobic and anaerobic, fungal, mycoplasmal, mycobacterial, etc), and special stains. If exploratory surgery is performed, biopsies should be obtained from several sites.

Treatment: In some FUO cases a specific diagnosis is not reached, or diagnostic testing is discontinued, leading to consideration of therapy in the absence of a diagnosis. Options include antibiotics, antifungal agents, and anti-inflammatory or immunosuppressive therapy (usually with corticosteroids). Trial therapy may resolve the patient's clinical signs or may confirm a presumptive diagnosis, but it is also associated with significant risk. Before pursuing a therapeutic trial, the client should be informed of the potential risks and should be committed to careful monitoring of the patient for an appropriate length of time. The therapeutic trial should be based on a tentative diagnosis and should define the parameters to be followed and the criteria used to determine treatment success or failure.

In true fever, the elevation in body temperature is regulated; therefore, cooling methods such as water baths work against the body's own regulatory mechanisms. It is also likely that fever itself has some beneficial effects, particularly in infectious diseases. However, fever can lead to anorexia, lethargy, and dehydration. Thus, FUO patients may benefit from IV fluid therapy or from the use of antipyretic medications. Examples include NSAID such as aspirin, carprofen, ketoprofen, and meloxicam (small animals) and flunixin meglumine or phenylbutazone (large animals).

HEPATIC LIPIDOSIS

FATTY LIVER DISEASE OF CATTLE

Fatty liver is most common in periparturient cattle. Although often considered a postpartum disorder, it usually develops prior to and during parturition. Endocrine changes associated with parturition and lactogenesis contribute to the development of fatty liver; however, inappetence almost always accompanies severe cases. Cows that are overconditioned at calving are most likely to develop fatty liver. The disease can develop whenever there is a decrease in feed intake and may occur secondary to the onset of another disorder. Cows that develop fatty liver at calving are more susceptible to ketosis.

Etiology: Fatty liver occurs during periods when blood nonesterified fatty acid concentrations (NEFA) are elevated. The most dramatic elevation occurs at calving when plasma concentrations are often >1,000 µEq/L. Concentrations can reach that level if the animal goes off feed. Uptake of NEFA by the liver is proportional to NEFA concentrations in the blood. NEFA taken up by the liver can either be oxidized or esterified. The primary esterification product is triglyceride, which can either be exported as part of a very low density lipoprotein, or be stored. In ruminants, export occurs at a very slow rate relative to many other species. Therefore, under conditions of elevated hepatic NEFA uptake and esterification, triglycerides accumulate. Oxidation of NEFA leads to the formation of CO_2 and ketones, primarily acetoacetate and β-hydroxybutyrate. Ketone formation is favored when blood glucose concentrations are low. Conditions that lead to low blood glucose and insulin also contribute to fatty liver because insulin suppresses fat mobilization from adipose tissue.

The greatest increase in liver triglyceride typically occurs at calving. The extent of feed intake depression before and after calving or during disease moderates the degree of triglyceride infiltration. Fatty liver can develop within 24 hr of an animal going off feed. Because of the slow rate of triglyceride export as lipoprotein, once fatty liver has developed, it will persist for an extended period. Depletion usually begins when the cow reaches positive energy balance and may take several weeks to fully subside.

Fatty liver is a consequence of negative energy balance, not positive energy balance. Energy consumption above requirements for maintenance and productive purposes will not directly result in deposition of triglyceride in hepatic tissue. Triglyceride deposition will occur only if the animal becomes overconditioned and consequently reduces feed intake.

Clinical Findings and Diagnosis: There are no known clinical signs that are unique to cows with fatty liver. Fatty liver has been associated with low milk production, increased clinical mastitis, and poor reproductive performance. However, cause and effect has not been established. Metabolic consequences of triglyceride accumulation in the liver include reduced gluconeogenesis, ureagenesis, hormone clearance, and hormone responsiveness. Consequently, hypoglycemia, hyperammonemia, and altered endocrine profiles may accompany fatty liver.

Fatty liver is likely to develop concurrently with another disease, typically disorders that are seen at or shortly after calving. These include metritis, mastitis, displaced abomasum, acidosis, and hypocalcemia. Field observations suggest that response to treatment of concurrent disorders is poor if cows have extensive triglyceride infiltration of the liver. Cows that are slow to increase in milk production and feed intake after calving are likely to have fatty liver. However, fatty liver is probably the result rather than the cause of poor feed intake. Cows with fatty liver are more prone to develop ketosis. Fatty liver is often associated with obese cows and downer cows (p 957). Overconditioned cows exhibit poor feed intake prior to and after calving and, therefore, are susceptible to fatty liver. Although overconditioned cows are likely candidates to develop fatty liver, it is not restricted to obese cows. Similarly, obese cows do not necessarily have fatty liver. It is unlikely that triglyceride accumulation in the liver is a direct cause of downer cow syndrome.

Diagnosis: Diagnostic tools for fatty liver are of limited value. Fatty liver is usually diagnosed after the animal has been off feed or has died due to another complication. A positive diagnosis does not mean that clinical signs of illness are the result of fatty liver, and misinterpretation of a positive diagnosis is common.

Liver biopsy is the only reliable method to determine severity of fatty liver in dairy cattle. Measurement of total lipid or triglyceride content by gravimetric or chemical methods following extraction from tissue by organic solvents is necessary for quantitative assessment; however, these assays are not routinely conducted in commercial laboratories. Estimation of triglyceride content by flotation characteristics of the tissue in copper sulfate solutions of varying specific gravity is rapid, easy, and available for use under field conditions.

Blood and urine metabolites or blood enzyme activity have been proposed as diagnostic tools. Blood glucose concentrations are low and blood NEFA and β-hydroxybutyrate concentrations are high when conditions are conducive to the development of fatty liver. Blood cholesterol concentration is usually low when fatty liver occurs, which may reflect an impaired ability of the liver to secrete lipoproteins. AST, ornithine decarboxylase, and sorbitol dehydrogenase are hepatic enzymes that may be positively associated with liver triglyceride and liver damage. Blood metabolites or enzymes are often unreliable indices of fatty liver because baseline (normal) concentrations vary tremendously among animals. The same problem exists when attempting to determine liver function by measuring sulfobromophthalein clearance from blood.

Measurement of plasma NEFA is a popular diagnostic tool for identifying herds that may be at risk for fatty liver. In addition to extreme variations in plasma NEFA concentrations among animals, there is extreme variation in a single individual, as concentrations increase dramatically immediately before and after calving. Therefore, a large number of animals must be sampled at a consistent time relative to calving. Care must be taken not to excite animals prior to sampling blood because NEFA increase rapidly in response to stress. The plasma NEFA concentrations at which triglyceride accumulates in the liver have not been established, but are probably ~600 µEq/L and above. These concentrations are common within 24-48 hr of parturition. However, prolonged exposure of the liver to concentrations >600 µEq/L will likely lead to fatty liver. Primiparous cows are less susceptible to fatty liver during periods of elevated plasma NEFA. Therefore, mature animals should be sampled when using plasma NEFA as a predictor of fatty liver.

Microscopic evaluation can be used to estimate the volume of the tissue occupied by fat. Estimates obtained by this method agree fairly well with chemical determination of triglyceride when expressed as a percentage of tissue dry weight. Mild, moderate, and severe fatty liver are often defined as <20%, 20-40%, and >40% fat (percentage of cell volume) respectively, but these values have little meaning relative to impact on physiologic function or clinical signs of the animal. Use of ultrasound as an alternative noninvasive procedure is being developed for determining the severity of fatty liver.

Prevention and Treatment: Reducing severity and duration of negative energy balance is crucial in the prevention of fatty liver. This can be achieved by avoiding overconditioning cattle, rapid diet changes, unpalatable feeds, periparturient diseases, and environmental stress. Cows within a herd should enter the dry period with an average body condition score of 3-3.5 (scale 1 = thin, 5 = obese). Thin cows (body condition score of ≤2.5) can be fed additional energy during the dry period to replenish condition without fear of causing fatty liver. Overconditioned cattle (body condition score of ≥4.0) should not be feed restricted as this will promote fat mobilization from adipose tissue and elevate blood NEFA and liver triglyceride.

The critical time for the prevention of fatty liver is ~1 wk prior to calving through 1 wk after parturition. This is when cows are most susceptible to development of fatty liver. Cows that are candidates for preventive measures are those that are overconditioned or are starting to go off feed. Glucose or compounds that can be converted to glucose by the liver can be administered IV. Propylene glycol, 10-30 oz, given as an oral drench, SID, during the final week prepartum has been effective in reducing plasma NEFA and the severity of fatty liver at calving. Propylene glycol can be fed, but feeding may not be as effective if the full dose is not consumed in a short period of time. Glycerin may be a less expensive alternative to propylene glycol. Sodium propionate is also a glucose precursor, but feeding can cause a depression in feed intake and reduce efficacy.

Glucose or glucose precursors are effective because they may cause an insulin response. Insulin is antilipolytic, ie, it decreases lipid mobilization from adipose tissue. Slow-release insulin compounds are available. A single 100 IU IM dose of a 24-hr slow-release insulin immediately after calving may be prophylactic. Higher doses may cause severe hypoglycemia and should not be used without concurrent glucose administration. Glucagon stimulates glycogenolysis, gluconeogenesis, and insulin production. In contrast to nonruminants, there is a negligible lipolytic effect of glucagon in ruminants. Glucagon (10 mg/day, IV, for 14 days) is effective at reducing liver triglyceride. A more practical protocol for use of glucagon to prevent fatty liver has not been established. Niacin is an antilipolytic agent that may have potential for prevention of fatty liver, but feeding 12 g/day beginning prepartum was not effective. Larger doses may be required; however, feed intake may be compromised when diet is the method of delivery.

Minimizing stress is important for prevention of fatty liver. Sudden changes in environment should be avoided. For example, changes in ration, housing, temperature, herdmates, etc may cause a reduction in feed intake and trigger catecholamine-mediated increases in fat mobilization.

Besides longterm IV infusion of glucagon, there is no proven treatment for fatty liver. In theory, effective treatments would be those that enhance lipoprotein triglyceride export from the liver. However, compounds that are known lipotropic agents in nonruminants have not been proved to be effective in ruminants. IV administration of choline, inositol, methionine, and vitamin B_{12} are often suggested as treatments, but scientific data are insufficient to support their use. Oral administration of these compounds is not effective because they are degraded in the rumen. In essence, treatment is the same as prevention; attempts should be made to avoid negative energy balance and to minimize fatty acid mobilization from adipose tissue. Once positive energy balance is attained, liver triglyceride can be reduced significantly in 7-10 days.

PREGNANCY TOXEMIA IN COWS

Pregnancy toxemia in cows is similar to the condition in small ruminants and is the result of fetal carbohydrate or energy demand exceeding maternal supply during the last trimester of pregnancy. It is precipitated by large or multiple fetuses, feed low in energy or protein, and health conditions that increase energy demand or decrease ability to take in nourishment (eg, lameness and oral diseases). The fetoplacental unit uses carbohydrate for energy and removes these compounds from the blood in an insulin-independent fashion. When this demand exceeds maternal supply, adipose tissue is mobilized to supply energy as acetate or ketone bodies, sparing carbohydrate consumption by other maternal tissues. However, only a small amount of new carbohydrate is generated from fat metabolism (from glycerol). This condition is more severe than ketosis (p 830) because fetal demand increases during pregnancy, while milk demand can decline in response to negative energy balance.

Although the mechanism is unknown, clinical disease develops in some cows with negative energy or carbohydrate balance. Proposed mediators of clinical disease include glucose deficiency with intermittent hypoglycemia, ketone body accumulation with metabolic acidosis or appetite suppression, and death of the fetus with secondary infection and toxemia. Individual cows of any breed can be affected, but herd problems are most common in beef cattle, which frequently are managed so that late pregnancy coincides with the poorest availability of feed. Both thin and fat cows can be affected, but the first noted abnormality often is loss of body condition over 1-2 wk. Decreased appetite, rumination, fecal production, and nose-licking are general signs of illness. With time, affected cows become markedly depressed, weak, ataxic, and recumbent. Opisthotonos, seizures, or coma may be seen terminally. Ketonuria is present from the early stage of disease and is the most specific finding; even mild ketonuria should not be found in normal pregnant cows until a few days before calving. Hypoglycemia is also common, but excited or seizuring cows may have hyperglycemia. With more advanced disease, there may be variable increases in serum activities of muscle or liver enzymes, as well as clinicopathologic evidence of infection, metabolic acidosis, internal organ dysfunction or failure, and circulatory collapse. Hepatic lipidosis in conjunction with large or multiple fetuses is a common necropsy finding; evidence of muscle pressure necrosis and toxemia may also be found.

Successful treatment requires early identification of the disease. There are few differential diagnoses, and pregnancy toxemia must be considered a factor in any disease that affects cattle in late gestation. Cattle that have lost weight but are still eating may be managed by feeding concentrate or propylene glycol (0.5-1 g/kg/day). Anorectic cattle must be treated aggressively, because the decrease in energy intake causes the disease to progress rapidly. Propylene glycol can be force-fed, or dextrose given IV (0.5 g/kg). Cattle with dehydration, organ dysfunction, or metabolic acidosis should be treated with large volumes (20-60 L/day, PO or IV) of electrolyte fluids; if IV fluid administration is practical, continuous dextrose infusion (5%) is recommended. Protamine zinc insulin (200 U, SC, every 48 hr) may be given after dextrose administration to suppress ketogenesis. Insulin is not approved for use in cattle, however. Recumbent cattle may benefit from good nursing care (see PROBLEMATIC BOVINE STERNAL RECUMBENCY, p 957) but rarely respond to treatment. To decrease the energy drain of any cow with pregnancy toxemia, induction of parturition or removal of the fetus by cesarean section should be considered.

On the herd level, the disease can be prevented by adequate attention to nutrition and health care of cattle in late gestation. For the individual cow, recognition of the precarious state of energy and carbohydrate balance during late gestation dictates careful monitoring of energy intake, attitude, and fat mobilization, especially during times of illness or other stress.

PREGNANCY TOXEMIA IN EWES
(Twin lamb disease, Pregnancy ketosis, Sleeping ewe disease)

Pregnancy toxemia in ewes is a disease affecting sheep during late gestation, characterized by feed refusal and neurologic dysfunction progressing to recumbency and death. It is seen more often in older ewes and those carring multiple fetuses. Pregnancy toxemia is almost never observed in replacement ewe-lambs or yearlings lambing for the first time.

Epidemiology and Pathogenesis: The primary predisposing cause of pregnancy toxemia is inadequate nutrition during late gestation, usually due to insufficient energy density of the ration and decreased rumen capacity as a result of fetal growth. In the last 4 wk of gestation, metabolizable energy requirements rise dramatically. For example, ewes pregnant with twin lambs need ~1.8-1.9 times more energy and protein than maintenance requirements.

In late gestation the liver increases gluconeogenesis to facilitate glucose availability to the fetuses. Each fetus requires 30-40 g of glucose/day in late gestation, which represents a significant percentage of the ewe's glucose production and which is preferentially directed to supporting the fetuses rather than the ewe. Mobilization of fat stores is increased in late gestation as a method of assuring adequate energy in the face of increased demands of the developing fetus(es) and impending lactation. However, in a negative energy balance, this increased mobilization may overwhelm the liver's capacity and result in hepatic lipidosis with subsequent impairment of function.

Ewes with a poor body condition score (BCS ≤2.0) or that are overconditioned (BCS ≥4.0) and carrying >1 fetus are most at risk of developing pregnancy toxemia, although it can occur even in ideally conditioned ewes on an adequate ration. Susceptible thin ewes develop ketosis due to a chronically inadequate ration being offered and, in the face of increasingly insufficient energy to meet increasing fetal demands, the ewe mobilizes more body fat with resultant ketone body production and hepatic lipidosis. Overconditioned ewes may have depressed appetites, and adipose mobilization quickly overwhelms the liver's capacity resulting again in hepatic lipidosis. In addition, there may be a population of sheep that are less responsive to insulin production in the face of inadequate nutrition. Ewes fitting these criteria may quickly shift from subclinical ketosis to clinical pregnancy toxemia if feed intake is acutely curtailed by such events as adverse weather, transport, handling for shearing or preventive medication, or other concomitant disease (footrot, pneumonia, etc). These variants of pregnancy toxemia have been termed primary pregnancy toxemia (thin ewes and inadequate nutrition), estate ketosis (fat ewes), and secondary pregnancy toxemia (ewes suffering from other disease).

Clinical Findings: Early clinical signs can be detected by an observant shepherd. Most cases develop within 1-3 wk of lambing. Onset earlier than day 140 of gestation is associated with more severe disease and increased risk of mortality. Decreased aggressiveness at feeding, particularly with grain consumption, indicates a problem. Ewes may also show signs of listlessness, aimless walking, muscle twitching or fine muscle tremors, opisthotonos, grinding of the teeth, and as the disease progresses (generally over 2-4 days), blindness, ataxia, and finally sternal recumbency, coma, and death. Cerebral hypoglycemia coupled with ketosis, ketoacidosis, and reduced hepatic and renal function lead to the clinical signs and fetal death. Blood glucose levels may return to normal or even become high terminally, possibly indicating death of the fetus(es). Septicemia develops in the ewe after fetal death.

Lesions: Postmortem changes demonstrate varying degrees of fatty liver, enlarged adrenal glands, and often include multiple fetuses in a state of decomposition indicating premortem death. Very thin ewes may appear starved (eg, serous atrophy of the kidney and heart fat). However, these signs alone are not pathognomonic for death due to pregnancy toxemia. Postmortem samples of aqueous humor or CSF can be analyzed for β-hydroxybutyrate (BHB). Levels >2.5 and 0.5 mmol/L, respectively, are consistent with a diagnosis of pregnancy toxemia.

Diagnosis: Laboratory findings in individual ewes may include hypoglycemia (often <2 mmol/L), elevated urine ketone levels (evaluated by commercial qualitative test tablets), elevated BHB levels (normal <0.8 mmol/L, subclinical ketosis >0.8 mmol/L, and clinical disease >3.0 mmol/L), and frequently hypocalcemia and hyperkalemia due to severe ketoacidosis. Hypoglycemia is not a consistent finding, with up to 40% of cases having normal glucose levels and up to 20% having hyperglycemia. If the diagnosis needs further confirmation, CSF glucose levels may be more accurate than blood; they remain low even when serum glucose rebounds in advanced cases after fetal death. BHB is a more reliable indicator of disease severity than are blood glucose levels. Nonesterified fatty acids can also be elevated above 0.4 mmol/L, indicating likely hepatic lipidosis resulting in impaired hepatic function.

While hypocalcemia is common in cases of pregnancy toxemia, it should also be considered when formulating hypotheses regarding recumbent late gestational sheep. This is similarly true with hypomagnesemia, which is a common finding in cases of pregnancy toxemia but should also be considered as a differential diagnosis for periparturient CNS disease. Other CNS diseases to be considered include polioencephalomalacia, pulpy kidney disease, rabies, lead poisoning, chronic copper toxicity, and listeriosis. These can be differentiated based on clinical and laboratory findings.

Treatment: Treatment of advanced cases of pregnancy toxemia is frequently unrewarding. If a ewe is already comatose, treatment should focus on the rest of the flock. However, if the ewe or lambs are valuable, then aggressive therapy should be directed against the ketoacidosis and hypoglycemia. Before starting this therapy, it should be determined whether the fetuses are alive (eg, real time or Doppler ultrasound). If the fetuses are alive and within 3 days of a calculated due date (gestation length 147 days), then an emergency cesarean section may be considered but is often economically unfeasible. If the fetuses are dead or too premature to survive a cesarean section, it is less stressful to the ewe to induce early lambing with dexamethasone (15-20 mg, IV or IM). Prophylactic antibiotics (usually procaine penicillin G at 20,000 IU/kg, SID) are appropriate if the fetuses are thought to be dead.

Ketoacidosis can be corrected by administering sodium bicarbonate solution IV, followed by balanced electrolyte solution. Hypoglycemia can be treated by a single injection of 60-100 mL 50% dextrose IV, followed by balanced electrolyte solution with 5% dextrose. IV drips and lower dextrose levels in solution might cause less of a diuretic effect; however, this is often impractical in a field setting. Repeated boluses of IV glucose should be avoided as they may result in a refractory insulin response. Insulin can be administered (20-40 IU protamine zinc insulin, IM, every other day). Calcium (50-100 mL of a commercial calcium gluconate or borogluconate solution, SC) can be given safely without serum biochemistry data. If serum biochemistry demonstrates hypocalcemia, ~50 mL of a commercial calcium solution can be given by slow IV injection while monitoring the heart. Oral potassium chloride (KCl) can be given as well in cases of severe ketoacidosis. In trials using recombinant bovine somatotropin, treated ewes had fewer days to clinical recovery than untreated ewes (6.5 vs 7.8 days). While aggressive therapy and intensive nursing care may be successful, it is not unusual to see case fatality rates >40%. Given the cost, it is prudent to share the guarded prognosis with owners prior to undertaking treatment.

Ewes in the early stages can often be treated successfully with propylene glycol (60 mL, BID for 3 days). Adding oral calcium (12.5 g calcium lactate), oral potassium (7.5 g KCl), and insulin (0.4 IU/kg, SC, SID) has increased survival rates. Oral commercial calf electrolyte solutions containing glucose may also be given by stomach tube at a dose of 3-4 L, QID, or drenched as a concentrated solution. The contributing factors (eg, nutrition, housing, other stressors) should be corrected for the group and feeding management assessed (eg, adequate feeder space, feeding frequency, protection from adverse weather).

A sample of late-gestation ewes can be tested for BHB levels to determine the extent of the risk in the rest of the flock. Generally 10-20 ewes should be sampled (3-20% of the pregnant flock). The risk of the flock can be determined based on the mean value of these results: normal (low risk) 0 to 0.7; moderate underfeeding (moderate risk) 0.8-1.6; and severe underfeeding (high risk) 1.7-3.0 mmol/L. Other diseases should be treated (eg, contagious footrot). Ewes off feed should be separated from the group and hand fed, keeping in mind that ewes should be able to see the group to feel comfortable.

Prevention: Ewes should not enter the last 6 wk of gestation with a BCS <2.5; this can be prevented by good feeding management and ration formulation. During the last 6 wk of gestation, grain is required as a source of carbohydrates in the ration to maintain the health of multiple-bearing ewes. Amount varies depending on forage quality, adult body weight and condition score, and number of fetuses, but protein must also be balanced for rumen microbes to make optimal use of available carbohydrates.

Producers should ideally assess BCS at breeding and midgestation so that thin ewes can be fed as a separate group. If B mode ultrasound scanning allows for fetal number determination, then ewes should also be managed based on fetal numbers. Producers may find it convenient to feed pregnant ewe-lambs with twin-bearing ewes and thin single-bearing ewes (due to the added energy ewe-lambs need for growth). With prolific breeds, triplet-bearing ewes and thin twin-bearing ewes can be fed together. Overconditioned ewes are not as common but may be seen in small hobby flocks. Fat ewes are much less responsive to therapy, and owners should be advised on how to avoid the problem through proper feeding management. However, late pregnancy is not the time to reduce BCS in overconditioned ewes. BHB serum levels can be used as a flock screening test to detect flocks at risk of pregnancy toxemia. In flocks with values ranging from >0.80 to 3.0 mmol/L, feeding management should be corrected quickly to avoid clinical disease.

Recently, considerable research has supported the use of ionophores, particularly monensin, in transition dairy cows to prevent subclinical ketosis and other early post-partum diseases. Ionophores improve feed efficiency by changing microflora populations in the rumen, resulting in increased feed efficiency and production of proprionic acid, followed by improved gluconeogenesis. There is some evidence that monensin may be beneficial for late-gestation ewes. It has improved feed efficiency by lowering feed intake. Treated ewes also showed lower serum BHB in late gestation, with no adverse effects on lamb birth weights. Lasalocid has been similarly studied. Again, feed intake was suppressed but lamb survival was better in the treatment group. More work needs to be done with both drugs to assess their use in preventing pregnancy toxemia in prolific ewes.

KETOSIS IN CATTLE

(Acetonemia, Ketonemia)

Ketosis is a common disease of adult cattle. It typically occurs in dairy cows in early lactation and is most consistently characterized by partial anorexia and depression. Rarely, it occurs in cattle in late gestation, at which time it resembles pregnancy toxemia of ewes. In addition to inappetence, signs of nervous dysfunction, including pica, abnormal licking, incoordination and abnormal gait, bellowing, and aggression are occasionally seen. The condition is worldwide in distribution, but is most common where dairy cows are bred and managed for high production.

Etiology and Pathogenesis: The pathogenesis of bovine ketosis is incompletely understood, but it requires the combination of intense adipose mobilization and a high glucose demand. Both of these conditions are present in early lactation, at which time negative energy balance leads to adipose mobilization and milk synthesis creates a high glucose demand. Adipose mobilization is accompanied by high blood serum concentrations of nonesterified fatty acids (NEFA). During periods of intense gluconeogenesis, a large portion of serum NEFA is directed to ketone body synthesis in the liver. Thus, the clinicopathologic characterization of ketosis includes high serum concentrations of NEFA and ketone bodies and low concentrations of glucose. In contrast to many other species, cattle with hyperketonemia do not have concurrent acidemia. The serum ketone bodies are acetone, acetoacetate, and β-hydroxybutyrate (BHB).

There is speculation that the pathogenesis of ketosis cases occurring in the immediate postpartum period is slightly different than that of cases occurring closer to the time of peak milk production. Cases of ketosis in very early lactation are usually associated with fatty liver. Both fatty liver and ketosis are probably part of a spectrum of conditions associated with intense fat mobilization in cattle. Ketosis cases occurring closer to peak milk production, which usually occurs at 4-6 wk postpartum, may be more closely associated with underfed cattle experiencing a metabolic shortage of gluconeogenic precursors than with excessive fat mobilization.

The exact pathogenesis of the clinical signs is not known. They do not appear to be associated directly with serum concentrations of either glucose or ketone bodies. There is speculation that they may be due to metabolites of the ketone bodies.

Epidemiology: All dairy cows in early lactation (first 6 wk) are at risk of ketosis. The incidence in lactation is estimated at 5-16%, but incidence in individual herds varies substantially. Ketosis occurs in all parities (although it appears to be less commin in primiparous animals) and does not appear to have a genetic predisposition, other than being associated with dairy breeds. Cows with excessive adipose stores (body condition score ≥3.75 out of 5.0) at calving are at increased risk of ketosis, compared with those with lower body condition scores. Lactating cows with hyperketonemia (subclinical ketosis— serum BHB concentrations >12 mg/dL) are at increased risk of developing clinical ketosis, compared with cows with lower serum BHB concentrations.

Clinical Findings: In cows maintained in confinement stalls, reduced feed intake is usually the first sign of ketosis. If rations are offered in components, cows with ketosis often refuse grain before forage. In group-fed herds, reduced milk production, lethargy, and an "empty" appearing abdomen are usually the signs of ketosis noticed first. On physical examination, cows are afebrile and may be slightly dehydrated. Rumen motility is variable, being hyperactive in some cases and hypoactive in others. In many cases there are no other physical abnormalities. CNS disturbances are noted in a minority of cases. These include abnormal licking and chewing, with cows sometimes chewing incessantly on pipes and other objects in their surroundings. Incoordination and gait abnormalities occasionally are seen, as are aggression and bellowing. These signs occur in a clear minority of cases, but because the disease is so common, finding animals with these signs is not unusual.

Diagnosis: The clinical diagnosis of ketosis is based on presence of risk factors (early lactation), clinical signs, and ketone bodies in urine or milk. When a diagnosis of ketosis is made, a thorough physical examination should be performed because frequently ketosis occurs concurrently with other peripartum diseases. Especially common concurrent diseases include displaced abomasum, retained fetal membranes, and metritis. Rabies and other CNS diseases are important differential diagnoses.

Cow-side tests for the presence of ketone bodies in urine or milk are critical for diagnosis. Caution should be exercised in the use of such tests within 48 hr after calving. Due to the large surge in plasma NEFA at calving, a positive test for ketones is very common during this period. The majority of commercially available test kits are based on the presence of acetoacetate or acetone in milk or urine. Dipstick tests are convenient, but those designed to detect acetoacetate or acetone in urine are not suitable for milk testing. All of these tests are read by observation for a particular color change. In a given animal, urine ketone body concentrations are always higher than milk ketone body concentrations. Trace to mildly positive results for the presence of ketone bodies in urine do not signify clinical ketosis. Without clinical signs, such as partial anorexia, these results indicate subclinical ketosis. Milk tests for acetone and acetoacetate are more specific than urine tests. Positive milk tests for acetoacetate and/or acetone usually indicate clinical ketosis. A dipstick designed to detect BHB in milk, available in Japan and Europe, is more sensitive than milk tests for acetone and acetoacetate and may be useful for monitoring incidence of subclinical ketosis.

Treatment: Treatment is aimed at reestablishing normoglycemia and reducing serum ketone body concentrations. Bolus IV administration of 500 mL of 50% dextrose solution is a common therapy. This solution is very hyperosmotic and, if administered perivascularly, results in severe tissue swelling and irritation, so care should be taken to assure that it is given IV. Bolus glucose therapy generally results in rapid recovery, especially in cases occurring near peak lactation. However, the effect frequently is transient and relapses are common. Administration of glucocorticoids including dexamethasone or isoflupredone acetate at 5-20 mg/dose, IM, generally results in a more sustained response. Glucose and glucocorticoid therapy may be repeated daily as necessary. Propylene glycol (250-400 g/dose, PO, [~8-14 oz]) acts as a glucose precursor and may be effective as ketosis therapy, especially in mild cases or in combination with other therapies. This dose may be administered twice per day. Overdosing propylene glycol leads to CNS depression.

Ketosis cases occurring within the first 1-2 wk after calving frequently are more refractory to therapy than those cases occurring nearer to peak lactation. In these cases, a long-acting insulin preparation given IM at 150-200 IU/day may be beneficial. Insulin suppresses both adipose mobilization and ketogenesis, but should be given in combination with glucose or a glucocorticoid to prevent hypoglycemia. Use of insulin in this manner is an extra-label, unapproved use. Other therapies that may be of benefit in refractory ketosis cases are continuous IV glucose infusion and tube feeding. (*See also* FATTY LIVER DISEASE OF CATTLE, p 824.)

Prevention and Control: Prevention of ketosis is via nutritional management. Body condition should be managed in late lactation, when cows frequently become too fat. The dry period is generally too late to reduce body condition score. Reducing body condition in the dry period may even be counterproductive, resulting in excessive adipose mobilization prepartum. A critical area in ketosis prevention is maintaining and promoting feed intake. Cows tend to reduce feed consumption in the last 3 wk of gestation. Nutritional management should be aimed at minimizing this reduction. Controversy exists over the optimal dietary characteristics during this period. It is likely that optimal energy and fiber concentrations in rations for cows in the last 3 wk of gestation vary from farm to farm. Feed intake should be monitored and rations adjusted to maximize dry matter and energy consumption in late gestation. After calving, diets should promote rapid and sustained increases in feed and energy consumption. Rations should be relatively high in nonfiber carbohydrate concentration, but contain enough fiber to maintain rumen health and feed intake. Neutral-detergent fiber concentrations should usually be in the range of 28-30% with nonfiber carbohydrate concentrations in the range of 38-41%. Dietary particle size will influence the optimal proportions of carbohydrate fractions. Some feed additives, including niacin, calcium propionate, sodium propionate, propylene glycol, and rumen-protected choline, may be beneficial in preventing and managing ketosis. To be effective, these supplements should be fed in the last 2-3 wk of gestation, as well as during the period of ketosis susceptibility.

MALIGNANT HYPERTHERMIA

(Porcine stress syndrome)

Malignant hyperthermia (MH) is a hypermetabolic syndrome involving skeletal muscle characterized by hyperthermia, tachycardia, tachypnea, increased oxygen consumption, cyanosis, cardiac dysrhythmias, metabolic acidosis, respiratory acidosis, muscle rigidity, unstable arterial blood pressure, and death. There also may be electrolyte abnormalities, myoglobinuria, CK elevation, impaired blood coagulation, renal failure, and pulmonary edema.

Although MH was initially recognized as a fatal syndrome in humans, the term describing its occurrence in swine is **porcine stress syndrome**. MH is most prevalent in swine, but this syndrome has also been reported in dogs (especially Greyhounds), cats, and horses.

MH is a heritable disease in people and may manifest as unexplained anesthetic deaths. Questions regarding unexplained anesthetic deaths are part of the family history questionnaire filled out by human patients and should be included on history forms for veterinary patients as well. In addition, whenever a suspected case of MH occurs, it is prudent for veterinarians to notify owners of siblings and breeders if applicable. However, MH can occur sporadically without any pedigree history. Many times, MH has occurred following a previous anesthetic procedure, but because of subtle signs that might go unrecognized, the syndrome was not suspected or diagnosed.

Porcine stress syndrome has been reported in most swine breeds. Prevalence varies, with incidence >90% in some strains. Incidence is higher in lean, heavily muscled breeds, eg, Pietrain, Poland China, Landrace, Duroc, and Large White. Mortality in finishing pigs was reported to be 3.2% but could be considerably higher in susceptible herds.

Etiology: An autosomal recessive gene that has variable penetrance determines susceptibility to MH. The causative mutation has been localized to a C-to-T transition in the gene that controls the Ca^{2+} release channel (ryanodine receptor) of sarcoplasmic reticulum in skeletal muscle. Loss in regulation of muscle cell Ca^{2+} is believed to be the primary etiologic event for induction of MH. It is consistently triggered in genetically susceptible animals by excitement, apprehension, exercise, or environmental stress. This is particularly true in pigs, but exercise-induced MH has also been reported in dogs, suggesting the existence of canine stress syndrome. Exposure to volatile anesthetics or depolarizing neuromuscular blocking agents will consistently trigger MH in susceptible animals. In fact, testing with halothane can be used as a screening method.

Subsequent to the initial challenge or stress, the hypersensitive ryanodine receptor floods the myoplasm of skeletal muscle with Ca^{2+}. Muscle contracture and hypermetabolism develop rapidly as a direct result of this uncontrolled and sustained increase in myoplasmic Ca^{2+}. ATP in skeletal muscle is depleted as energy requirements for contracture exceed supply. Increased aerobic and anaerobic metabolism results in excessive CO_2 and lactic acid production, while thermogenesis and peripheral vasoconstriction increase core body temperature. As the MH episode progresses, the combination of increased temperature, acidosis, and ATP depletion leads to rhabdomyolysis. Myoplasmic enzymes and electrolytes are released from the cells, and additional Ca^{2+} enters the myoplasm. Contracture and its subsequent energy requirements are further enhanced and eventually, due to temperature and pH changes, contracture proceeds independently of myoplasmic Ca^{2+} levels. Death occurs due to an increase in serum K^+, which causes cardiac dysrhythmia and arrest.

Clinical Findings: The rapidity with which clinical signs develop varies. Signs include muscle stiffness or fasciculations that progress to muscle rigor. Ventricular tachycardia develops early and continues until serum K^+ reaches cardiotoxic levels. In unanesthetized animals, open-mouthed breathing, tachypnea, and hyperventilation may progress to apnea. Blanching and erythema followed by blotchy cyanosis are seen in the skin of light-colored animals. Core body temperature rapidly increases and can reach 113°F (45°C) antemortem. In anesthetized animals, the CO_2 absorbant is rapidly depleted, and the breathing circuit canister is hot to touch. Because hypothermia is an expected consequence during general anesthesia, detection of hyperthermia is a key sign, along with the presence of tachycardia and tachypnea. The disease is usually fatal. Rigor mortis develops within minutes, and muscle temperature is significantly increased. Affected muscles from an animal that dies acutely are pale and soft and appear exudative or wet. Pale, soft exudate pork syndrome is often linked to MH.

Diagnosis: Clinical diagnosis is based on development of clinical signs in an animal exposed to a volatile anesthetic and/or stressful event. The acute nature of the disease and its relationship to a stressor enables differentiation of MH from other fatal disorders. Numerous laboratory tests have been developed to aid in the identification of

MH-susceptible animals, but none enables rapid diagnosis of MH in an acute situation. Most screening tests lack the sensitivity and specificity to identify MH-susceptible animals or carriers. The caffeine contracture test involves in vitro exposure of extracted muscle tissue to caffeine and halothane. Muscle from MH-susceptible subjects will contract when exposed to lower concentrations of caffeine and halothane, compared with normal muscle. This test has limited application in animals because special laboratory facilities are required and the test must be run within minutes after the specimen is obtained. A molecular genetic test is specific for the MH gene. This DNA-based assay is performed on a small sample of anticoagulated blood to detect mutation in the ryanodine receptor gene and can identify homozygous MH-resistant and MH-susceptible animals as well as heterozygous carriers. It has been reported to more accurately predict both the homozygous and heterozygous forms of the MH gene than does the halothane challenge test.

Treatment: Often, MH episodes are not treated in the field. During anesthesia, early detection is essential for a successful outcome. Exposure of the animal to the volatile anesthetic must stop. Breathing tubes and CO_2 canisters must be changed, and dantrolene sodium given at 4-5 mg/kg, IV. It is essential that dantrolene be administered early in the course of the disease because muscle blood flow is significantly reduced as the disease progresses. Additional doses of dantrolene may be given as needed. Supportive treatment includes fluid therapy and management of acidosis through ventilatory support and administration of sodium bicarbonate. Increases in core body temperature can be managed by surface cooling and/or chilled saline lavages. If an MH anesthetic event is detected in cold climates, moving an animal outside and to a snow bank may be a lifesaving maneuver. Other supportive measures include oxygen enrichment of inspired gases and treatment of cardiac dysrhythmias.

Control: Reducing the prevalence of MH within the swine population requires genetic selection against the trait. With the advent of DNA-based assays, it is possible to cull MH-susceptible animals and carriers. However, the industry and individual producers must decide whether the economic benefits of eliminating MH from the swine population outweigh the costs associated with reduced performance characteristics. There is concern that some breeds may, in fact, not be sustained if there were an active selection program to eliminate MH from the population. At this time, prevention of MH episodes in individual animals requires that management practices to minimize stress be followed.

If a documented MH survivor or a suspected susceptible animal requires anesthesia and surgery, dantrolene should be given at 3-5 mg/kg, PO, 1-2 days before anesthesia. A tranquilizer-opioid combination can be given as preanesthetic medication and propofol used to induce anesthesia. Acepromazine and droperidol inhibit development of MH, and propofol has not been reported to trigger MH. Volatile anesthetic agents must be avoided. The CO_2 absorber should be cleaned, and new absorbant used along with a new breathing circuit and endotracheal tube. Amide local anesthetics are safe to use in MH-susceptible animals. Finally, the procedure must be kept as short as possible because MH happens most often when anesthesia lasts >1 hr. All of these maneuvers help reduce the possibility of but may not prevent an MH crisis.

TRANSPORT TETANY IN RUMINANTS

(Railroad disease, Railroad sickness, Staggers)

Transport tetany occurs after the stress of prolonged transport, typically in cows and ewes in late pregnancy, although it is also seen in lambs transported to feedlots and in cattle and in sheep transported to slaughter. Crowded, hot, poorly ventilated transport vehicles (railroad cars or trailers) with minimal or no access to feed or water appear to predispose animals to the condition; however, prolonged travel by foot is also a risk factor. The disease is characterized by recumbency, GI stasis, and coma, and is generally fatal.

Although cows in late gestation are most commonly affected, the disease is also seen in cows that have recently calved, as well as in bulls, steers, and dry cows. Risk factors include heavy feeding prior to shipment, deprivation of feed and water for >24 hr during transit, and unrestricted access to water and exercise immediately after arrival. Exposure to hot environmental conditions is also associated with an increased incidence. While the specific cause of tetany is unknown, the condition may be a form of acute hypocalcemia precipitated by late pregnancy and early lactation, or by fasting before or during transit. Physical stress is undoubtedly related. Hypomagnesemia may be a precipitating factor in cattle and a contributing factor in sheep.

Clinical signs in cattle may occur while in transit or up to 48 hr after arrival. Early clinical signs include restlessness and excitement, trismus, and grinding of teeth. A staggering gait may be observed and later, if recumbent, cattle often demonstrate paddling of the hindlegs. Rumen motility and GI stasis is observed and animals become completely anorectic. Tachycardia and rapid, labored respiration may be observed. Abortion may be a complication. Cattle that do not recover gradually become more obtunded to the point of coma and die within 3-4 days. Moderate hypocalcemia and hypophosphatemia may be observed in cattle. Some sheep are hypocalcemic and hypomagnesemic or hypoglycemic; however, some show no measurable biochemical abnormalities. No specific lesions are observed at necropsy aside from lesions associated with prolonged recumbency. Ischemic muscle necrosis is the most common of these. In lambs, early signs include restlessness, staggering, and partial hindlimb paralysis followed by lateral recumbency. Death can occur rapidly or after 2-3 days of recumbency. In lambs, mild hypocalcemia may be noted. Recovery rates are fair even with treatment. The relationship of clinical signs with transport or forced, prolonged exercise is diagnostic.

Some animals respond to treatment with combinations of parenteral calcium, magnesium, and glucose. IV injections of calcium borogluconate (25% solution at 400-800 mL/cow or 100 mL/ewe) or calcium borogluconate with magnesium sulfate (5% solution, same volumes) can be administered slowly. A dose of 50 mL can be given SC, SID, to affected lambs in feedlots. Repeated injections may be warranted, but failure to respond is common (50%) and most likely due to concurrent muscle necrosis. Additional treatment considerations include IV administration of large volumes of polyionic fluids such as lactated Ringer's solution. Animals should be offered good quality feeds (eg, alfalfa hay), fresh water, and soft bedding with good footing underneath. Sedation may be necessary if animals are hyperexcitable or convulsing.

If prolonged transport times of cows or ewes in advanced pregnancy is unavoidable, animals should be fed a restricted diet several days prior to shipment, then provided adequate feed, water, and rest periods during transport. Administration of ataractic agents (unless transport is to slaughter) such as promazine hydrochloride before loading is recommended, especially for nervous animals. Upon unloading at the destination, animals should be allowed limited access to water for the first 24 hr and minimal exercise for 2-3 days.

■ ■ ■

LAMENESS IN GOATS 893

MUSCULOSKELETAL SYSTEM INTRODUCTION

The musculoskeletal system consists of the bones, cartilage, muscles, ligaments, and tendons. Primary functions of the musculoskeletal system include support of the body, provision of motion, and protection of vital organs. The skeletal system serves as the main storage system for calcium and phosphorus and contains critical components of the hematopoietic system. Because many other body systems, including the nervous, vascular, and integumentary systems, are interrelated, disorders of one of these systems may also affect the musculoskeletal system and complicate diagnosis.

Diseases of the musculoskeletal system most often involve motion deficits or functional disorders. The degree of impairment depends on the specific problem and its severity. Skeletal and articular disorders are by far the most common; however, primary muscular diseases, neurologic deficits, toxins, endocrine aberrations, metabolic disorders, infectious diseases, blood and vascular disorders, nutritional imbalances or deficits, and occasionally congenital defects are diagnosed as well.

Disorders of muscles that are part of another body system may induce specific aberrations such as impairment of ocular motion and control, respiratory dysfunction, bladder malfunction, lack of penile retraction, and impairment of mastication and deglutition. Complete paralysis, paresis, or ataxia may be caused by primary muscular dysfunctions of infectious, toxic, or congenital origin; however, in most instances the primary disorder can be attributed to the nervous system (eg, tetanus, rhinopneumonitis, canine distemper, protozoal myelitis), with the muscular system merely representing the effector organ.

The structural and functional unit of skeletal muscle is the motor unit. It consists of a ventral motor neuron with its cell body in the central horn of the spinal cord and its peripheral axon, the neuromuscular junction, and the muscle fibers innervated by the neuron. Each of these components must be functionally intact for the muscle to contract properly. The ventral motor neuron is the final common pathway conducting neural impulses from the CNS to the muscle.

The transmission of a nerve impulse at the neuromuscular junction involves massive release of acetylcholine from small synaptic vessels, where it is stored. The acetylcholine fills the synaptic cleft between the nerve terminal and the muscle fiber membrane, where most of it is destroyed by cholinesterase within a fraction of a second. This short period of activity is sufficient to excite the muscle fiber membrane, which results in a significant increase in membrane permeability to sodium ions and allows rapid influx of sodium into the muscle fiber. The sodium ion increases the endplate potential, which elicits electrical currents that spread to the interior of the fibers where they cause a release of calcium ions from the sarcoplasmic reticulum. The calcium ions initiate, in turn, the chemical events of the contractile process. When this occurs in all the muscle fibers innervated by each motor neuron (possibly thousands), muscle contraction results.

Normal muscle, comprising many motor units, is dynamic, and its function and structure can be influenced by many diseases. Disorders that affect the neuromuscular junction (eg, myasthenia gravis, hypocalcemia, hypermagnesemia) can result in muscle fatigue, weakness, and paralysis. The neuromuscular junction can also be affected by muscle-relaxing drugs (eg, curare, succinylcholine, M99), certain antibiotics, and toxins (eg, botulism, tetanus, venoms).

Disorders primarily of the muscle membrane and, to some extent, of the actual muscle fibers are called myopathies. Muscle membrane disorders may be hereditary (eg, myotonia congenita in goats) or acquired (eg, vitamin E and selenium deficiencies, hypothyroidism, and hypokalemia). Myopathies involving the actual muscle fiber components include muscular dystrophy, polymyositis, eosinophilic myositis, white muscle disease, and exertional rhabdomyolysis. Various laboratory tests, eg, histopathologic examination, determination of serum enzyme levels, electromyographic studies, thermography, and determinations of conduction velocity, are very useful in confirmation of a specific diagnosis.

Tendons act as bridging and attachment structures for the muscles; some bridge long gaps between the muscle bellies and target bone and, therefore, are prone to injury themselves, especially because they are often loaded to the extreme and are only minimally capable of elastic elongation. A prime example is the superficial flexor tendon of horses, which is frequently injured by partial tearing that leads to tendinitis. Another acquired injury of tendons involves traumatic disruptions. Due to the relatively poor blood supply of both tendons and ligaments, healing is delayed and frequently poor. Management of injuries to ligaments and tendons requires patience and prudent long-term rehabilitation.

Bone diseases are generally congenital or hereditary, nutritional, or traumatic. Congenital disorders include in utero malformations and atavisms, such as polydactyly or persistent ulnae or fibulae in foals; examples of genetic defects are atlanto-occipital malformations in Arabian horses or certain cases of spinal ataxia (see WOBBLER SYNDROME, p 999), canine hip dysplasia, and abnormal bone formation such as that caused by parathyroid hypoplasia.

Bone defects due to nutrition are caused primarily by imbalances or deficiencies in minerals, particularly the trace minerals such as copper, zinc, and magnesium. Calcium and phosphorus concentrations must also be present in the correct ratio. Osteomalacia represents the classic example of imbalanced or deficient calcium and phosphorus intake. Other nutritional disorders are caused by excessive protein intake of growing animals. Either deficiency or excess intake of certain vitamins, particularly vitamins A and D, may influence growth and development of bone. Aseptic physitis or special osteochondrotic conditions of the physes may be caused by zinc toxicity or copper deficiency.

Traumatic causes of bone disorders represent the vast majority of cases and include fractures, fissures, periosteal reactions as a result of trauma, sequestrum formation, and insertion desmopathies or tendinopathies, respectively. Lack of weight bearing, reduced motion, instability, pain, heat, or swelling usually accompany these disorders. Diagnostic procedures include inspection, manual palpation, diagnostic imaging (such as radiography, ultrasonography, or thermography, and increasingly scintigraphy, computed tomography, or MRI), and diagnostic anesthesia to determine the specific anatomic structure or region involved in the problem.

Articulations are divided into synarthroses, in which the osseous components are united by fibrous tissue or cartilage, and diarthroses, in which the opposing bone ends are covered with hyaline cartilage and are separated by a joint cavity filled with synovial fluid. Synarthroses are practically immovable and are rarely associated with joint disease other than fractures. In most cases, diarthroses are movable joints, with a variable degree of mobility depending on the anatomic location of the joint. Diarthroses are frequently involved in pathologic changes involving any of their anatomic structures: the fibrous joint capsule, synovial membrane, hyaline articular cartilage, subchondral bone, and intra-articular ligaments (and also the menisci in the stifle joint). Joint disorders may be caused by trauma (acute, sharp, or blunt), chronic inflammation, developmental factors, or infections. Acute trauma frequently results in luxation, subluxation, fracture, or distortion of a joint. Direct articular trauma may also lead to septic arthritis or rupture of a collateral ligament or the joint capsule.

Developmental defects include osteochondritis dissecans, equine ataxia, and lumbar disk syndrome in certain breeds of dogs. Extension of physitis into the adjacent joint and damage due to continuous abnormal weight bearing in animals with angular limb deformities are other inciting causes of joint disease. Bacterial and fungal infections involving joints and other synovial structures, such as tendon sheaths, are usually quite clearly recognizable and require immediate and aggressive treatment.

Chronic inflammation of joints and surrounding structures is most common in articulations associated with locomotion, although other joints, such as the temporomandibular, may occasionally be affected. Normal synovial fluid lubricates the synovial tissues in a joint through boundary lubrication, including a glycoprotein expressed from the cartilage during weight bearing. The synovial fluid also nourishes the articular cartilage. Any joint injury alters the volume and composition of the synovial fluid (as a result of an increased permeability of the inflamed synovial membrane relative to blood components) and increases the intraosseous pressure in the involved bones. The increased WBC count leads to an increased concentration of proteolytic enzymes within the synovial fluid, which leads to proteoglycan washout and eventually cartilage destruction.

Diagnostic procedures to determine the nature, extent, and exact location of the joint disorder include inspection, manual palpation and manipulation, diagnostic imaging techniques, local or intra-articular anesthesia, diagnostic arthroscopy, and laboratory examination of synovial fluid or biopsy of synovial membrane.

The diagnostic and therapeutic options for management of musculoskeletal disorders have greatly expanded during the last few years and allow a return to a useful life for most animals if done early in the disease process.

CONGENITAL AND INHERITED ANOMALIES OF THE MUSCULOSKELETAL SYSTEM

Congenital and inherited anomalies can result in the birth of diseased or deformed neonates. Congenital disorders can be due to viral infections of the fetus or to ingestion of toxic plants by the dam at certain stages of gestation. The musculoskeletal system can also be affected by certain congenital neurologic disorders.

MULTIPLE SPECIES

Contracted Flexor Tendons

Contracted flexor tendons are probably the most prevalent abnormality of the musculoskeletal system of newborn foals and calves. An autosomal recessive gene causes this condition. In utero positioning may also affect the degree of disability.

At birth, the pastern and fetlocks of the forelegs and sometimes the carpal joints are flexed to varying degrees due to shortening of the deep and superficial digital flexors and associated muscles. A cleft palate may accompany this condition in some breeds. Slightly affected animals bear weight on the soles of the feet and walk on their toes. More severely affected animals walk on the dorsal surface of the pastern and fetlock joint. If not treated, the dorsal surfaces of these joints become damaged, and suppurative arthritis develops. Rupture of the common digital extensor can occur as a sequela. This condition should be differentiated from arthrogryposis.

Mildly affected animals recover without treatment. In moderate cases, a splint can be applied to force the animal to bear weight on its toes. The pressure from the splint must not compromise the circulation, or the foot may undergo ischemic necrosis. Frequent manual extension of the joints, attempting to stretch the ligaments, tendons, and muscles, aids in treating these intermediate cases. Severe cases require tenotomy of one or both flexor tendons. A plaster-of-Paris cast may also be indicated in some cases. Extreme cases may not respond to any treatment. (*See also* FLEXION DEFORMITIES, p 931.)

Dyschondroplasia

Dyschondroplasia of genetic origin is seen in most breeds of cattle. The forms range from the so-called Dexter "bulldog" lethal, in which the calf is invariably stillborn, to those animals that are mildly affected.

The **brachycephalic dwarfs** that were common in Hereford cattle in the 1950s largely have been eliminated through genetic selection. Short faces, bulging foreheads, prognathism, large abdomens, and short legs are characteristic. They are approximately half normal size. The **dolichocephalic dwarf**, most commonly seen in Angus cattle, is of the same general body conformation as the brachycephalic dwarf, except that it has a long head and does not have either a bulging forehead or prognathism. The short-faced calves are frequently referred to as "snorter" dwarfs because of their labored and audible breathing. Both types are of low viability and susceptible to bloat. Their carcasses are undesirable, and they are rarely kept except for research purposes.

Dyschondroplasia of the appendicular and axial skeletons also is seen in dogs. The former is reported in Poodles and Scottish Terriers, the latter in Alaskan Malamutes, Basset Hounds, Dachshunds, Poodles, and Scottish Terriers. In some breeds (Bassets, Dachshunds, Pekingese), the appendicular dyschondroplastic characteristics are an important feature of breed type. In Malamutes, the condition is accompanied by anemia.

Dystrophy-like Myopathies

Numerous examples of progressive myopathies have been described in animals; many are heritable, and many resemble various types of muscular dystrophy in humans. Affected muscles have a variety of degenerative and atrophic changes. In Meuse-Rhine-Yssel cattle of Holland, a progressive fatal myopathy of the diaphragm and intercostal muscles has been described. Another dystrophy in cattle is weaver syndrome in Brown Swiss. Hyperplasia, commonly called double muscling (p 849), is a congenital myopathy found in some European breeds of cattle. Progressive myopathies have been reported in Merino sheep in Australia (an inherited autosomal recessive), in Pietrain pigs (Pietrain creeper syndrome), and in dogs, cats, chickens, turkeys, and mink. Inherited muscular dystrophy of mice and hamsters has been studied extensively; the hamsters have severe myocardial lesions and serve as a model for studies of cardiomyopathy.

Several types of muscular dystrophy are seen in dogs. An X-linked Duchenne-like muscular dystrophy is reported in Golden Retrievers in the USA and in Irish Terriers in Europe. Affected dogs, generally males, develop progressive muscular weakness, dysphagia, stiffness of gait, and muscular atrophy. Microscopically, the distinctive alteration is lack of dystrophia, a protein concentrated in the sarcolemma and essential for normal membrane function. Some dogs die with accompanying cardiomyopathy. A similar X-linked dystrophy with a lack of dystrophia is described in cats. A second type of dystrophy involves Labrador Retrievers in North America, Europe, and Australia. Clinical signs, which include stiffness, exercise intolerance, and muscular atrophy, develop by 6 mo of age. Autosomal recessive inheritance is implicated. A further dystrophy was described in dysphagic Bouviers in Europe.

Glycogen Storage Disease
(Glycogenosis)

Progressive muscular weakness and inability to rise properly may be seen in animals with glycogen storage diseases. To date, 5 of the 8 types of glycogen storage diseases characterized in humans have been identified in animals (types I, II, III, VII, and VIII). Affected species include cattle, sheep, dogs, cats, horses, Japanese quail, rats, and mice. Type II glycogenosis in Shorthorn and Brahman cattle has been well documented and is inherited as an autosomal recessive disorder. Affected cattle develop muscular weakness and die at 9-16 mo of age, often with accompanying cardiomegaly and congestive heart failure. Morphologic and biochemical study reveals extensive intralysosomal and cytoplasmic glycogen deposits. Corriedale sheep and Lapland dogs also develop type II glycogenosis.

Myophosphorylase deficiency (type V glycogenosis) is an autosomal recessive disorder in Charolais cattle. Affected cattle show exercise intolerance and may have increased serum activities of skeletal muscle-origin enzymes.

Muscular Steatosis

In muscular steatosis, which has been seen occasionally in cattle, sheep, and pigs at slaughter, fat replaces muscle fibers. No clinical disease results, and the cause is unknown. The gross lesions are symmetric, pale areas in affected muscles, especially of the back, neck, and upper limbs. Microscopically, many muscle fibers are replaced by fat cells.

Myopathy Associated with Congenital Articular Rigidity
(Arthrogryposis)

This syndrome, one of the more common congenital defects of calves, is characterized by rigid fixation of the limbs in abnormal postures; it often produces dystocia. Affected animals may have other anomalies, including hydrocephalus, palatoschisis, and spinal dysraphism. The condition may be lethal, but some mildly affected animals recover completely. The muscle lesions may be primary in some types of the disease, but the neural lesions generally are primary, and the muscular alterations represent denervation atrophy. Congenital articular rigidity is seen in cattle, sheep, horses, and pigs. Numerous etiologic factors have been recognized. In cattle, these include viral (Akabane virus [p 501], bluetongue virus [p 590]) and plant (*Lupinus* sp [p 2423]) teratogens, and a heritable recessive trait in Charolais (*see* ARTHROGRYPOSIS, p 849). In sheep, plant (locoweed) and viral (Akabane, Wesselsbron [p 624] teratogens, Rift Valley fever [p 617]), parbendazole exposure, and inherited autosomal recessive primary myopathies of Merino and Welsh Mountain lambs may cause congenital articular rigidity. In pigs, the condition may be inherited as an autosomal recessive, or result from deficiency of vitamin A or manganese or from exposure of pregnant sows to plant toxins (eg, tobacco, thornapple, hemlock, and black cherry).

Osteochondrosis

Osteochondrosis is a disturbance in endochondral ossification that is sometimes classified as dyschondroplasia. The immature articular cartilage may separate from the underlying epiphyseal bone, which sometimes dissects completely free and floats loose in the synovial cavity, resulting in accompanying synovitis or the retention of pyramidal cores of physeal cartilage projecting into the metaphysis. Often, these two lesions are seen simultaneously in the same bone. The disease develops during maximal growth when the biomechanical stresses are greatest in the immature skeleton (4-8 mo in dogs, 80-120 lb [36-54 kg] in pigs). It is most common in large and giant breeds of dogs (p 963) and in rapidly growing pigs, horses (p 929), turkeys, and chickens.

Osteogenesis Imperfecta

Osteogenesis imperfecta is a generalized, inherited bone defect in cattle, dogs, and cats, characterized by extreme fragility of bones and joint laxity. The long bones are slender and have thin cortices. Calluses and recent fractures may be present. The sclera of the eyes may be bluish. The inheritance is most likely polygenic.

Osteopetrosis

Osteopetrosis is a rare disease that appears to be inherited as a simple autosomal recessive trait in Angus, Simmental, and Hereford cattle. It is also seen in dogs and foals. It is characterized by premature stillbirth 10 days to 1 mo before term, brachygnathia inferior, impacted molar teeth, and easily fractured long bones. Bone marrow cavities are absent and replaced by primary spongiosa. The fetal-like abnormal intramedullary bone consists of chondro-osseous tissue. Foramina of the skull and long bones are hypoplastic or aplastic. The cranium is thickened and compresses the brain. Extensive mineralization is present in vessel walls and neurons of the brain. Diagnosis is confirmed by a longitudinal bisection of long bones revealing the diaphyses filled with a plug of bone instead of marrow.

Syndactyly and Polydactyly

Syndactyly or mule foot is the partial or complete fusion of the digits of one or more feet. Reported in numerous cattle breeds, it is most prevalent in Holsteins and is inherited as a simple autosomal recessive condition. The forefeet are affected most often but 1 or all 4 feet may be affected. Animals affected with syndactyly walk slowly, usually have a high-stepping gait, and may be more prone to hyperthermia.

Polydactyly is a genetic defect of cattle, sheep, pigs, and occasionally horses. In its most common form, the second digit is developed but the medial dewclaw is missing. The toes may be fused to give rise to polysyndactyly. Rarely 1 or all 4 limbs have the condition. Polydactyly in cattle appears to be polygenic with a dominant gene at one locus and a homozygous recessive at another.

CATTLE

Arthrogryposis

Arthrogryposis is ankylosis of the limbs, usually combined with a cleft palate and other growth deformities. It is seen in all breeds of cattle, particularly Charolais. At birth, affected calves exhibit joints fixed in abnormal positions and frequently have scoliosis and kyphosis. They are usually unable to stand or nurse. Muscle changes, notably atrophy, have also been seen. In the spinal cord, necrosis of neurons and lesions of the white matter may be seen. Arthrogryposis has more than one etiology and pathologic entity. The arthrogryposis syndrome in Charolais is caused by an autosomal recessive gene with complete penetrance in the homozygous state. Teratogens identified as causing arthrogryposis include plants such as lupines (anagyrine as the toxic agent) that are ingested by pregnant cows between day 40 and 70 of gestation. Prenatal viral infections with the Akabane (p 501) or bluetongue (p 590) virus can also cause arthrogryposis.

Brown Atrophy
(Xanthosis, Lipofuscinosis)

In dairy cattle with brown atrophy, the skeletal muscles and myocardium are yellow-brown to bronze. The masseter muscles and the diaphragm are affected most frequently. No clinical disease results. Microscopically, brown lipofuscin pigment granules accumulate under the sarcolemma or centrally in the muscle fibers. A genetic cause is presumed because certain breeds (eg, Ayrshire) are more predisposed than others.

Double Muscling

Double muscling is an overdevelopment of the musculature in the neonate. The condition is seen in various beef breeds including Charolais, Santa Gertrudis, South Devon, Angus, Belgian Blue, Belgian White, and Piedmontese. The muscles of the shoulder, back, rump, and hindquarters are separated by deep creases, particularly between the semitendinosus and biceps femoris, and between the longissimus dorsi muscles of either side. Necks of double-muscled cattle are shorter and thicker, and their heads appear smaller. Associated disorders include hypoplastic reproductive tracts, delayed reproductive age of maturity, and lengthened gestation and increased birth weights combined with dystocia. Double muscling is caused by a pair of incompletely recessive genes that result in various degrees of the condition. Succinic dehydrogenase activity is significantly decreased in affected calves.

Limber Leg

Limber leg is a hereditary condition of Jersey cattle, apparently controlled by a simple recessive gene. Some affected calves are born dead. Living calves appear normal at birth but are unable to stand because of incompletely formed muscles, ligaments, tendons, and joints. The shoulder and hip joints can be rotated in any direction without apparent discomfort. Diagnosis is based on signs, necropsy findings, and identification of carrier animals.

HORSES

Angular Limb Deformities

In these congenital or acquired skeletal defects, the distal portion of a limb deviates laterally or medially early in neonatal life. In utero malposition, hypothyroidism, trauma, poor conformation, excessive joint laxity, and defective endochondral ossification of the carpal or tarsal and long bones have been implicated. One to 4 limbs may be affected, depending on the severity of the condition.

The carpus is affected most frequently, but the tarsus and fetlocks are occasionally involved. The deviation is obvious but varies in severity. A lateral deviation (valgus) of up to 6° of the distal portion of a limb may be regarded as normal. Most foals are asymptomatic, but lameness and soft-tissue swelling can accompany severe deviations. Outward rotation of the fetlocks invariably accompanies carpal valgus. Foals with defective ossification of the carpal cuboidal bones or excessive joint laxity are frequently lame as the legs become progressively deviated. Affected limbs must be palpated carefully to detect ligament laxity and specific areas that may be painful.

Diagnosis should include a precise determination of the site and cause for the deviation. The distal radial metaphysis, physis, epiphysis, or cuboidal bones may be the site of deviation. Radiography is helpful in detecting physeal flaring, epiphyseal wedging, and deformation of carpal bones. Mildly affected foals frequently improve spontaneously without treatment.

Treatment depends on the severity of the condition and tissues affected. Excessive joint laxity, with or without cuboidal carpal bone involvement, requires tube casts or splints. The fetlock and phalangeal region should not be included in the casts, which should protect the weak joint from trauma but allow restricted exercise to maintain tendon and ligament tone. Such limb support may be required for up to 6 wk.

Physeal and epiphyseal growth disturbances are also amenable to surgical correction through hemicircumferential transection and periosteal elevation of the distal radius on the concave side of the defect or through transphyseal bridging of the physis on the convex side. These surgeries must be performed before the physeal growth plates close (as early as 2-4 mo of age), and success depends on continued growth and development of the bones. Sequential examinations and radiographs are necessary to follow spontaneous improvement or to establish a need for surgery.

Without treatment, the prognosis for severe carpal valgus is poor. The conformational anomaly leads to early degenerative joint disease. Likewise, deformity of the cuboidal carpal bones contributes to a poor prognosis. However, with early detection, careful evaluation, and proper surgical treatment, most foals respond favorably.

Defects of the Spine

Defects of the spine include scoliosis, synostosis, and lordosis. Although all of these conditions are uncommon in foals, congenital scoliosis is encountered most frequently.

On clinical examination, it is often difficult to assess the severity. A better appreciation of the condition can be obtained by radiographic examination. In mild cases, improvement is spontaneous and may be complete. Even in the more severe cases, there is rarely any obvious abnormality in gait or maneuverability. However, these foals frequently are not raised because they appear unlikely to be able to withstand being ridden or worked.

Another occasional congenital deformity is that of synostosis (fusion of vertebrae), which may be associated with secondary scoliosis. Radiography is necessary for confirmation.

Congenital lordosis (swayback) is associated with hypoplasia of the intervertebral articular processes. In adult horses, degrees of acquired lordosis and kyphosis (roachback) are occasionally seen, which contribute to back weakness. Diagnosis is based on the clinical appearance and can be confirmed by radiography, which reveals an undue curvature of the vertebral column, usually in the cranial thoracic region (T5-10) in lordosis and in the cranial lumbar region (L1-3) in kyphosis.

Hyperkalemic Periodic Paralysis

Hyperkalemic periodic paralysis (HPP) is a hereditary condition of Quarter Horses that is the result of a genetic mutation in the skeletal muscle sodium channel gene. It is inherited as an autosomal dominant trait. Most affected horses are heterozygotes. (*See* HYPERKALEMIC PERIODIC PARALYSIS, p 954.)

Polysaccharide Storage Myopathy

See CHRONIC EXERTIONAL RHABDOMYOLYSIS, p 952.

Glycogen Branching Enzyme Deficiency

Glycogen branching enzyme (GBE) deficiency may be a common cause of neonatal mortality in Quarter Horses that is obscured by the variety of clinical signs that resemble other equine neonatal diseases. Clinical signs of GBE deficiency may include transient flexural limb deformities, stillbirth, seizures, respiratory or cardiac failure, and persistent recumbency. Leukopenia, high serum CK, AST, and γ-glutamyl transferase are present in most affected foals. Gross postmortem lesions are inconclusive. Muscle, heart, or liver samples contain abnormal periodic acid-Schiff-positive globular or crystalline intracellular inclusions in amounts proportional to the foal's age at death. Accumulation of an unbranched polysaccharide in tissues is suggested by a shift in the iodine absorption spectra of polysaccharide isolated from the liver and muscle of affected foals. Skeletal muscle total polysaccharide concentrations are reduced, but liver and cardiac muscle glycogen concentrations are normal. Several glycolytic enzyme activities are normal, whereas GBE activity is virtually absent in cardiac and skeletal muscle, as well as in liver and peripheral blood cells. GBE activities in peripheral blood cells of dams of affected foals and several of their half-siblings or full siblings are ~50% of controls. GBE protein in liver is markedly reduced to absent in affected foals. Pedigree analysis supports an autosomal recessive mode of inheritance.

SHEEP

Spider Lamb Syndrome

Hereditary chondrodysplasia, or spider lamb syndrome, is an inherited, semilethal, musculoskeletal disease affecting lambs primarily of Suffolk or Hampshire breeds. Lambs have pronounced medial deviation of the carpus and hock and are unable to stand without distress. Pathologic changes in the skull reveal a rounding of the dorsal silhouette, producing a "Roman nose" appearance and a narrowed elongation of the occipital condyles. The thoracic and lumbar vertebrae are moderately kyphotic, which causes a dorsal rounding of the backline. The sternebrae are dorsally deviated, leading to a flattening of the sternum. The forelimbs have a medial deviation of the carpal joints with a bowed radius and ulna and irregular thickening of the growth plate cartilage. The hindlimbs have medially deviated hocks and bowed tibiae, which also have thickened, irregular growth plates. Muscle atrophy is also predominant. The regulation of liver insulin-like growth factor (IGF) and the IGF-binding proteins may be involved in the physical manifestations of this disorder. It is suggested that the condition is inherited in a simple autosomal recessive pattern.

PIGS

Splayleg
(Spraddleleg, Myofibrillar hypoplasia)

In this condition of neonatal pigs, the hindlegs are spread apart or extended forward due to weakness of the adductor muscles relative to the abductors. Affected pigs are susceptible to overlaying, starvation, and chilling because of poor mobility. Mortality may reach 50%. Genetic influence has been demonstrated. There are significant differences in the incidence among litters of different sires and breeds. It is seen more frequently in males than females and in pigs of lower birthweight. The syndrome also may be produced if glucocorticoids are administered during pregnancy, and it appears possible that stress-sensitivity of the heavily muscled parent(s) may be a contributing factor. However, any cause of stretching of the adductor muscles increases the incidence. Stretching can result from slippery or sloping floors, struggling while legs are caught in cracks in the floor, or as the result of damage to nerve pathways from intrauterine viral infections. Mycotoxins have been suggested to play a role in some cases. The general nutrition of the sow (choline, methionine, and vitamin E levels) may influence the incidence, but benefits from feeding supplements to sows is questionable.

The clinical signs are distinctive. In utero infections with hemagglutinating encephalitis virus, enteroviruses, other viruses, and postpartum bacterial meningeal infection and trauma should be considered. The affected muscles are generally hypoplastic, and the small muscle fibers contain few myofibrils, as would be found in muscles of normal fetuses nearing parturition. Frequently affected muscles include the semitendinosus, longissimus dorsi, and triceps.

Dry, nonslippery floors should be provided, with no cracks in which the legs can become trapped, especially for the first 2 days. Pigs should be protected from injury by the sow, and adequate suckling should be ensured. In affected piglets, the hindlegs should be secured together above the hocks with a loose "figure 8" of adhesive tape for 2-4 days. Appropriately treated pigs usually recover within a week, although few recover if the front legs are also affected. Glucocorticoids should not be administered late in gestation. Highly susceptible blood lines should be eliminated.

DYSTROPHIES ASSOCIATED WITH CALCIUM, PHOSPHORUS, AND VITAMIN D

The principal causes of osteodystrophies are deficiencies or imbalances of dietary calcium, phosphorus, and vitamin D. Their interrelationships are not easily defined, and their interrelationship with the parathyroid gland must also be considered. Deficiencies of any of the 3 may be absolute or relative and must be assessed in relation to availability and growth rate.

The primary source of calcium and phosphorus is the diet. These elements are absorbed in amounts depending on the source of the minerals, intestinal pH, and dietary levels of vitamin D, calcium, phosphorus, iron, and fat. If vitamin D or its activity is decreased, calcium and phosphorus absorption are reduced. Vitamin D is obtained either through the diet or by production when the skin is exposed to sunlight (ultraviolet radiation). Before vitamin D can be used, it must be processed into its metabolically active form by the liver and kidney. Vitamin D_3 (cholecalciferol) acts primarily on the GI tract to increase absorption but also affects the bone, thereby increasing availability of elemental calcium.

Parathyroid hormone (PTH) is secreted in response to a low circulating calcium ion concentration. In general, it plays a role in increasing available calcium. The 3 target organs of PTH are the kidneys, bones, and intestines. In the kidneys, PTH promotes renal tubular absorption of calcium while enhancing renal excretion of phosphorus, thereby maintaining an appropriate calcium:phosphorus ratio. In the intestine, PTH promotes absorption of calcium. PTH also facilitates mobilization of calcium from bone by allowing utilization of calcium from the osteoid matrix.

Specific bony lesions are associated with abnormalities in absolute or relative amounts of vitamin D, calcium, phosphorus, and PTH. Often, in addition to the deficiency or excess in one element, this also causes a secondary pathology due to feedback mechanisms, altered ratios, or concomitant metabolic deficiencies. Specific disease syndromes can be classified as nutritional or metabolic in nature.

Abnormal levels of calcium and phosphorus may also cause secondary disease. In general, diseases to which dogs are genetically predisposed can be increased in incidence by oversupplementation of calcium and phosphorus. Specifically, osteochondritis dissecans and hypertrophic osteodystrophy are more frequent in giant-breed dogs fed excess calcium.

NUTRITIONAL OSTEODYSTROPHIES

RICKETS

Rickets is a disease of young, growing animals. The most common causes are dietary insufficiencies of phosphorus or vitamin D. Calcium deficiencies can also cause rickets, and while this rarely occurs naturally, poor balanced diets that are deficient in calcium have been said to cause the disease. As in most diets causing osteodystrophies, the abnormal calcium:phosphorus ratio is most likely the cause.

Clinical Findings and Lesions: The characteristic lesions of rickets are failure of both vascular invasion and mineralization in the area of provisional calcification of the physis. This pathology is most obvious in the metaphyses of the long bones. There may be a wide variety of clinical signs, including bone pain, stiff gait, swelling in the area of the metaphyses, difficulty in rising, bowed limbs, and pathologic fractures. On radiographic examination, the width of the physes is increased, and the nonmineralized physeal area is distorted. In advanced cases, angular limb deformity can be seen due to asynchronous bone growth.

Animals fed all-meat diets are commonly affected. Kittens that are fed beef heart exclusively develop locomotor disturbances within 4 wk, even though the high content of digestible protein (>50% on a weight basis) and fat promotes rapid growth, the animals appear well nourished, and their coat maintains a good luster. The predominant clinical signs are reluctance to move, posterior lameness, and ataxia. The kittens often stand with characteristic deviation of the paws. The skeletal disease becomes progressively more severe after 5-14 wk. The kittens become quiet and reluctant to play; they assume a sitting position or sternal recumbency with the hindlimbs abducted. Normal activities may result in the sudden onset of severe lameness due to incomplete or folding fractures of 1 or more bones. Lameness is the initial functional disturbance in growing dogs and may vary from a slight limp to inability to walk. The bones are painful on palpation, and folding fractures of long bones and vertebrae are common.

Rickets and other bone pathologies have been reported in young pigs housed indoors and fed processed feed. Processing of the feed removes natural vitamin D and other fat-soluble vitamins. Without vitamin supplementation, nutritional osteodystrophy may result.

Diets with excessive amounts of calcium (3 times normal concentrations) have caused ricket-like signs in growing Great Danes. Several other bone pathologies such as retained cartilaginous cores, osteochondrosis, and stunted growth were seen in these dogs as well.

Treatment: Correction of the diet is the primary treatment. The prognosis is good in the absence of pathologic fractures or irreversible damage to the physes. If the animals are housed, exposure to sunlight (ultraviolet radiation) will also increase the production of vitamin D_3 precursors.

Recent studies show that many homemade diets for dogs are deficient in minerals and have altered calcium:phosphorus ratios. Therefore a high-quality commercial food, or one designed by a credentialed veterinary nutritionist, is recommended.

OSTEOMALACIA
(Adult rickets)

Osteomalacia has a pathogenesis similar to that of rickets but it is seen in mature bones. Because bones mature at different rates, both rickets and osteomalacia can be seen in the same animal. Osteomalacia is characterized by an accumulation of excessive unmineralized osteoid on trabecular surfaces.

Clinical Findings: Affected animals are unthrifty, may have abnormal estrus, and may exhibit pica. Nonspecific shifting lamenesses are common. Fractures can be seen, especially in the ribs, pelvis, and long bones. Spinal deformation such as lordosis or kyphosis may be seen.

In horses, nutritional osteodystrophy is known as **bran disease**, **miller's disease**, and **"big head."** The diet of pampered horses is often too high in grains and low in forage; such a diet is high in phosphorus and low in calcium. Many of the obscure lamenesses of horses have been attributed to nutritional osteodystrophy. The pathologic changes are similar to those in other species, with the provisos that the bones of the head are particularly affected in severe cases and that gross or microscopic fractures of subchondral bone (with consequent degeneration of articular cartilage and tearing of ligaments from periosteal attachments) are dominant clinical signs. Unilateral facial deformity due to secondary (nutritional) hypoparathyroidism was recently reported in a 1-yr-old filly.

Nutritional osteodystrophy is uncommon in cattle and sheep but is seen occasionally in feedlots. Marrow fibroplasia is not a feature of the condition in these species. Osteoporosis is the dominant lesion, but "big head" may be seen in goats. Bone deformities in recovered animals can cause obstipation or dystocia.

Diagnosis: To establish a firm diagnosis, the diet should be evaluated for calcium, phosphorus, and vitamin D content. There is radiographic evidence of generalized skeletal demineralization, loss of lamina dura dentes, subperiosteal cortical bone resorption, bowing deformities, and multiple folding fractures of long bones due to intense localized osteoclast proliferation. Laboratory values used to assess renal function should be within normal limits in animals with nutritional osteodystrophy.

Treatment: Affected animals should be confined for several weeks after initiation of the supplemental diet. Response to therapy is rapid; within 1 wk the animals become more active, and their attitude improves. Jumping or climbing must be prevented because the skeleton is still susceptible to fractures. Restrictions can be lessened after 3 wk, but confinement with limited movement is indicated until the skeleton returns to normal (response to treatment should be monitored radiographically).

ENZOOTIC CALCINOSIS
(Enteque seco, Enteque ossificans, Espichamento, Espichacao, Manchester wasting disease, Naalehu disease, Weidektankheit)

Enzootic calcinosis is a disease complex of ruminants and horses caused by plant poisoning or mineral imbalances and characterized by extensive calcification of soft tissues. The prevalence of the disease in cattle varies widely (10-50%) in areas of Argentina, Brazil, Papua-New Guinea, Jamaica, Hawaii, and Bavaria. It is said to cause up to 60% mortality and affect 17% of the sheep in southern Brazil and Mattewara (India), respectively. Incidence elsewhere (Australia, Israel, South Africa, and southern USA) is less well documented, and in many areas enzootic calcinosis is rare or nonexistent.

Etiology and Pathogenesis: Known causes fall into 2 categories: plant poisonings and mineral imbalances in the soil, the first probably being the more important. *Cestrum diurnum* (wild jasmine, day-blooming jessamine, king-of-the-day), *Trisetum flavescens* (golden oats or yellow oat grass), *Nierembergia veitchii*, *Solanum esuriale*, *S torvum*, and *S malacoxylon (glaucophyllum)* contain 1,25-dihydroxycholecalciferol (calcitriol) glycoside or a substance that mimics its calcinogenic action. Studies indicate that *S malacoxylon* has the required enzyme systems for the synthesis of calcitriol from vitamin D_3. No concrete evidence incriminating other plants is available.

The imbalance of minerals in certain soils in Hawaii, India, Austria, and possibly elsewhere has been thought to be the main etiologic factor; dietary mineral imbalance may contribute to the calcification chiefly associated with plant poisoning. Excessive phosphate or calcium, absolute or conditioned magnesium deficiency, and deficiency of potassium and nitrogen have all been incriminated or suspected.

Osteodystrophy of bulls after prolonged intake of excessive calcium is a similar condition; calcification of the cardiovascular system associated with aging and such cachectic diseases as tuberculosis is not identical. Excessive vitamin D_3 and normal or excessive calcium intake induces aortic calcification and atherosclerosis in ruminants.

Normally, the conversion of 25-hydroxycholecalciferol (calcifediol) to calcitriol in the kidney is controlled by a feedback mechanism. The calcitriol-like factor in the leaves of plants bypasses this mechanism, and more calcium is absorbed than can be accommodated physiologically. Hypercalcemia promotes calcitonin production, calcinosis, and osteoporosis.

Changes in plasma calcium, phosphorus, and magnesium are different in different species. Horses develop hyperphosphatemia; plasma calcium remains normal but rises with excess doses of calcitriol. Frequently, both serum calcium and inorganic phosphorus are increased in cattle. Hypomagnesemia also may be present.

Clinical Findings: The disease is progressive and chronic, extending over weeks or months. The earliest signs are stiffened and painful gait, which is most pronounced when the animal rises after prolonged rest. Forelimbs are particularly affected, and some animals even walk or graze on their knees. When standing, the forelimbs bow forward because the joints cannot be extended completely. The animal shifts weight to the forepart of the hooves or, alternatively, to each forelimb to ease stress on the carpus, which is thickened and painful. The distal joints become abnormally straight. When affected animals are forced to walk, their gait is awkward, stiff, and slow, and their steps are short. After walking only short distances, breathing becomes shallow and diaphragmatic, the nostrils are flared, and the head and neck are extended. Varying degrees of heart murmur are detectable, usually as a double or blurred second sound; these are exaggerated after exercise. Pulse rate is increased after slight exercise. Jugular pulse is prominent in some cases.

As the disease progresses, the animal loses weight and becomes weak and listless. The coat becomes shaggy, dull, and faded, particularly in cattle. There is wasting of muscles, a prominent skeleton, tucked up abdomen, kyphosis, and raised tailhead. Ovarian function is impaired. Appetite is usually unimpaired but sometimes becomes depraved. Calcification of vessels is palpable on rectal examination.

Osteodystrophy is seen in calcinosis due to *T flavescens* and *C diurnum* toxicities in Bavarian cattle and Florida horses, respectively. Severely affected horses stand with forelimbs somewhat abducted and luxated caudally at the shoulder joints. The flexor tendons, particularly the suspensory ligaments, are painful. Fetlock joints are overextended to varying degrees.

Lesions: Degeneration and calcification of soft tissues are seen, with emaciation and varying amounts of excess fluid in the thoracic and abdominal cavities and pericardial sac. The cardiovascular system is the first to be involved, followed by lung, kidney, and tendons. The heart and aorta show the most marked effects. The left side of the heart is more affected than the right. In extreme cases, calcified foci are seen on valves and chordae tendinae. White, elevated plaques of irregular size and shape are seen on the luminal surface; in advanced cases, these are seen throughout the length of the aorta and its main branches.

Mineral deposits are found on the pleura, on the surface and edges of the diaphragmatic and apical lobes of lungs, in the renal artery and pelvis of the kidney, and on the ligaments and tendons (particularly of the forelimbs). Capsular thickening and irregular erosions of articular surface of cartilage and joints are seen, especially of the carpus and hock.

The basic histologic evidence is necrosis and calcification of connective tissue, followed by cellular proliferation in the affected area.

Diagnosis: This is usually based on the history, signs, and lesions but may be difficult at early stages. Radiography and electrocardiography may be helpful.

Control: Removal of the causal factor(s) is essential, but when the disease is associated with the mineral content of the soil, control may be difficult. Change of pasture, forage, and environment may effect clinical improvement and even diminish the soft-tissue mineral deposits. Experimentally, daily administration of 15 g of aluminum hydroxide, PO, prevented the development of calcinosis in sheep fed *T flavescens*.

METABOLIC OSTEODYSTROPHIES

FIBROUS OSTEODYSTROPHY
(Rubber jaw syndrome)

Primary Hyperparathyroidism

In primary hyperparathyroidism (p 446), there is excess production of parathyroid hormone (PTH) by an autonomous functional lesion in the parathyroid gland. The normal control mechanisms for PTH secretion by the concentration of blood calcium are lost, and the parathyroid produces excess PTH despite increased levels of blood calcium. This disease is encountered infrequently in older dogs, and it does not appear to be a sequela of renal secondary hyperparathyroidism (*see* p 858).

PTH acts on cells of the renal tubules initially to promote the excretion of phosphorus and retention of calcium. A prolonged increased secretion of PTH results in accelerated osteocytic and osteoclastic bone resorption. Mineral is removed from the skeleton and replaced by immature fibrous connective tissue. Fibrous osteodystrophy is generalized throughout the skeleton but is accentuated in local areas such as the cancellous bone of the skull. The increased PTH levels also inhibit the renal tubular resorption of phosphorus.

The lesion in the parathyroid gland in dogs is usually an adenoma, occasionally a carcinoma, composed of active chief cells. Usually, adenomas are single, light brown-red, and located in the cervical region near the thyroid gland.

Clinical Findings: Lameness follows severe osteoclastic bone resorption, and fractures of long bones occur after minor physical trauma. Compression fractures of weakened vertebral bodies may exert pressure on the spinal cord and nerves, resulting in motor and sensory dysfunction.

Facial hyperostosis with partial obliteration of the nasal cavity (by poorly mineralized woven bone and highly vascular fibrous connective tissue) and loss or loosening of teeth has been seen in dogs. This may result in an inability to close the mouth properly and development of gingival ulcers. The maxillae and rami of the mandibles often are coarsely thickened by the excess woven bone. Bones of the skull are markedly thinned by the increased resorption and have a characteristic "moth-eaten" appearance radiographically. In advanced cases, the mandible can be twisted gently due to loss of osteoid and severe fibrous osteodystrophy—hence the name "rubber jaw" syndrome.

Lesions: Histologic demonstration of a rim of normal tissue and a partial to complete fibrous capsule in an enlarged parathyroid suggests an adenoma rather than focal hyperplasia. Chief-cell carcinomas tend to be larger than adenomas and fixed to the underlying tissues due to local infiltration of neoplastic cells.

Diagnosis: Although other laboratory findings may be variable, hypercalcemia is consistent and results from accelerated release of calcium from bone. The blood calcium in normal dogs is ~10 ± 1 mg/dL, depending on age and diet (and assay method). Serum calcium values consistently >12 mg/dL indicate hypercalcemia. Dogs with primary hyperparathyroidism usually have a serum calcium of ≥12-20 mg/dL. The blood phosphorus is low or in the low-normal range (≤4 mg/dL). The urinary excretion of phosphorus, and often of calcium, is increased and may result in nephrocalcinosis and urolithiasis. Accelerated bone matrix metabolism is reflected by increased urinary excretion of hydroxyproline. Serum alkaline phosphatase activity may be increased in animals with overt bone disease. Demonstration of increased levels of PTH by a species-specific assay in an adult to aged dog with hypercalcemia, hypophosphatemia, and evidence of generalized bone disease provides conclusive evidence of primary hyperparathyroidism. PTH can be measured by sensitive radioimmunoassays or immunoradiometric assays.

The intact PTH assay or dual-site assays can be performed using either serum (preferred) or plasma that has been separated and frozen (-70°C in either glass or plastic tubes) as soon as possible after collection. Using this method, circulating levels of PTH in most animals are near 20 pg/mL (dogs, 20 ± 5 pg/mL; cats, 17 ± 2 pg/mL), with levels in nonhuman primates being slightly lower (normal values also vary among laboratories). PTH assays that use antibody generated against the carboxy terminal end of the human molecule usually give less consistent results in animals other than humans.

Differential diagnoses include other causes of hypercalcemia, such as vitamin D intoxication (overdosage), enzootic calcinosis (see above), malignant neoplasms with osseous metastasis, and humoral hypercalcemia of malignancy (see also p 444). The hypercalcemia of hypervitaminosis D may be as high as that in primary hyperparathyroidism but is accompanied by varying degrees of hyperphosphatemia and normal serum alkaline phosphatase activity. Skeletal disease usually is absent, because the increased concentrations of blood calcium and phosphorus are derived principally from augmented intestinal absorption rather than from bone resorption.

Malignant neoplasms with osseous metastases may cause moderate hypercalcemia and hypercalciuria, but the alkaline phosphatase activity and serum phosphorus level usually are normal or only slightly increased. These changes are believed to be due to the release of calcium and phosphorus into the blood from areas of bone destruction at rates greater than can be cleared by the kidneys and intestine. Bone involvement is more sharply demarcated and localized to the area of metastasis. Osteolysis associated with tumor metastases results not only from a physical disruption of bone by proliferating neoplastic cells but also from local production of humoral substances that stimulate bone resorption, such as prostaglandins and interleukin-1.

Primary parathyroid hyperplasia has been described in German Shepherd pups. The condition was associated with hypercalcemia, hypophosphatemia, increased immunoreactive PTH, and increased fractional clearance of inorganic phosphorus in the urine. Clinical signs include stunted growth, weakness, polyuria, polydipsia, and a diffuse reduction in bone density. IV infusion of calcium fails to suppress the autonomous secretion of PTH by the diffuse hyperplasia of chief cells in all parathyroids. Lesions include nodular hyperplasia of thyroid C cells and widespread mineralization of the lungs, kidneys, and gastric mucosa. The disease is inherited as an autosomal recessive.

Hypercalcemia also may be associated with multifocal osteolytic lesions associated with septic emboli, complete immobilization, osteosarcoma, hypoadrenocorticism (Addison's-like disease), hypocalcitoninism due to a destructive thyroid lesion, chronic renal disease, hemoconcentration, or hyperproteinemia. Hypercalcemia is detected occasionally in dehydrated animals but usually is mild. It is attributed to fluid volume contraction that results in hyperproteinemia and increased concentrations of ionized and nonionized calcium; it resolves rapidly after fluid therapy.

Treatment: The objective is to eliminate the source of excessive PTH production. An attempt should be made to identify all 4 parathyroid glands before excising any tissue. Single or multiple adenomas should be removed in toto. If all identifiable parathyroids in the cervical region appear to be of normal or smaller size, and the diagnosis is reasonably certain, surgical exploration of the thorax near the base of the heart may be necessary to localize the parathyroid neoplasm.

Removal of the functional parathyroid lesion results in a rapid decrease in circulating PTH levels because the half-life of PTH in plasma is <15 min. Because plasma calcium levels in animals with overt bone disease may decrease rapidly and be subnormal within 12-24 hr after surgery, they should be monitored frequently. Postoperative hypocalcemia (≤6 mg/dL) can result from the following: 1) depressed secretory activity of chief cells due to suppression by the chronic hypercalcemia or injury to the remaining parathyroid tissue during surgery, 2) abruptly decreased bone resorption due to lowered PTH levels, and 3) accelerated mineralization of osteoid matrix formed by the hyperplastic osteoblasts, which was previously prevented by the increased PTH levels (known as "hungrybone syndrome"). Infusions of calcium gluconate to maintain the serum calcium between 7.5 and 9 mg/dL, plus feeding high-calcium diets and supplemental vitamin D therapy, corrects this serious postoperative complication. If hypercalcemia persists for ≥1 wk after surgery, or recurs after initial improvement, a second adenoma or metastases from a carcinoma should be suspected.

Renal Secondary Hyperparathyroidism

Renal secondary hyperparathyroidism is a complication of chronic renal failure characterized by increased endogenous levels of parathyroid hormone (PTH). It is more common than primary hyperparathyroidism. In contrast to primary hyperparathyroidism, renal secondary hyperparathyroidism tends not to be autonomous. It is seen frequently in dogs, occasionally in cats, and rarely in other species.

With progressive renal disease, serum hyperphosphatemia develops as the glomerular filtration rate decreases. Hyperphosphatemia leads to lower serum concentration of ionized calcium. Renal synthesis of calcitriol is also reduced. Calcitriol normally acts on the intestine and kidneys to maintain normal calcium levels. Decreased ionized calcium and calcitriol concentrations cause an increase in serum PTH concentrations. As glomerular filtration rate decreases with advancing renal disease, PTH concentrations progressively increase, leading to the clinical manifestations of renal secondary hyperparathyroidism.

Clinical Findings: The predominant signs of renal insufficiency (eg, vomiting, dehydration, polydipsia, polyuria, and depression) are usually present. Skeletal lesions range from minor changes with early (or mild) renal disease to severe fibrous osteodystrophy of advanced renal failure. The volume of affected bones usually is normal (isostotic), particularly in older dogs because of the slow onset of renal failure and lower metabolic activity of bones. Hyperostotic bone lesions, such as facial swelling, may be seen in younger dogs in which deposition of unmineralized osteoid by hyperplastic osteoblasts and production of fibrous connective tissue exceed the rate of bone resorption.

Skeletal involvement is generalized but not uniform. Lesions become apparent earlier and reach a more advanced stage in certain areas, such as cancellous bones of the skull. Resorption of alveolar bone occurs early and results in loose teeth, which may be dislodged easily and interfere with mastication. As a result of accelerated resorption of cancellous bone of the maxilla and mandible, bones become softened and pliable ("rubber jaw" syndrome), and the jaws fail to close properly. This often results in drooling and protrusion of the tongue. Severely demineralized mandibles are predisposed to fractures and displacement of teeth from alveoli. Long bones are less dramatically affected. Lameness, stiff gait, and fractures after minor trauma may result from increased bone resorption.

Lesions: All parathyroid glands are enlarged, initially due to hypertrophy of chief cells and subsequently by compensatory hyperplasia. Although the parathyroids are not autonomous, the concentration of PTH in the peripheral blood often exceeds that of primary hyperparathyroidism. Changes such as osteoclastosis, marrow fibrosis, and a higher concentration of woven osteoid may be seen histologically. Severe hypercalcemia, hyperphosphatemia, and high concentrations of PTH seen in advanced disease may cause osteosclerosis.

Diagnosis: Renal secondary hyperparathyroidism is diagnosed by laboratory abnormalities consistent with renal insufficiency accompanied by an increase in serum PTH. Radioimmunoassay of PTH can be performed at various diagnostic laboratories. Assays that measure fragments of the PTH molecule should not be used because the concentration of biologically inactive metabolites of PTH increases with renal failure.

Treatment: Treatment options include dietary modification, calcitriol supplementation, and phosphate binders, as well as management of the underlying renal disease. Prescription diets with restricted dietary phosphorus are available. Oral calcitriol (1.5-3.5 ng/kg/day) has reversed hyperparathyroidism of chronic renal failure, but calcitriol therapy is contraindicated with hyperphosphatemia or hypercalcemia. (Special compounding of calcitriol is needed because the dosages currently available commercially are much larger than those needed clinically.) Dietary phosphorus binders are used to decrease the amount of phosphorus absorbed in the intestines and should be administered with meals. This therapy is especially important during calcitriol supplementation because calcitriol increases the absorption of phosphorus as well as calcium.

HYPOPARATHYROIDISM

In hypoparathyroidism (p 449), either subnormal amounts of parathyroid hormone (PTH) are secreted, or the hormone secreted is unable to interact normally with target cells. It has been recognized primarily in dogs, particularly in smaller breeds such as Miniature Schnauzers, but other breeds may be affected.

Various pathogenic mechanisms can result in inadequate secretion of PTH. Parathyroid glands may be damaged or inadvertently removed during thyroid surgery. After damage to the glands or their vascular supply, adequate functional parenchyma often regenerates and clinical signs subsequently disappear.

Idiopathic hypoparathyroidism in adult dogs usually is the result of diffuse lymphocytic parathyroiditis that causes extensive degeneration of chief cells and replacement by fibrous connective tissue. Other possible causes of hypoparathyroidism include destruction of parathyroids by primary or metastatic neoplasms in the anterior cervical area, and atrophy of parathyroids associated with chronic hypercalcemia. The presence of numerous distemper virus particles in chief cells of the parathyroid gland may contribute to the low blood calcium in certain dogs with this disease. Agenesis of the parathyroids is a rare cause of congenital hypoparathyroidism in pups. Certain cases of idiopathic hypoparathyroidism in animals (including humans) with histologically normal parathyroids may be due to lack of the specific enzyme in chief cells that converts the pro-PTH molecule to the biologically active PTH secreted by the gland. In other cases, an immune-mediated mechanism may be involved, because a similar destruction of secretory parenchyma and lymphocytic infiltration has been produced experimentally in dogs by repeated injections of parathyroid tissue emulsions.

Pseudohypoparathyroidism is a variant that is seen in humans, but it is uncertain whether it is seen in other animals. Target cells in kidney and bone are unable to respond to normal or increased amounts of PTH, and severe hypocalcemia develops even though the parathyroid glands are hyperplastic.

Clinical Findings and Lesions: The functional disturbances and clinical manifestations of hypoparathyroidism primarily are the result of increased neuromuscular excitability and tetany. Bone resorption is decreased because of the lack of PTH, and blood calcium levels diminish progressively (4-6 mg/dL). Affected dogs are restless, nervous, and ataxic, with weakness and intermittent tremors of individual muscle groups that progress to generalized tetany and convulsions. Blood phosphorus levels are increased substantially, owing to increased renal tubular reabsorption. Calcification of microvasculature, intracerebral calcification, decreased mental function, cataracts, osteopenia, and ligamentous ossification have been associated with chronic hypoparathyroidism.

In the early stages of immune-mediated lymphocytic parathyroiditis in dogs, there is infiltration of the gland with lymphocytes and plasma cells and nodular regenerative hyperplasia of remaining chief cells. Later, the parathyroid gland is replaced by lymphocytes, fibroblasts, and capillaries, with only an occasional viable chief cell.

Diagnosis: This is based on clinical signs of increased neuromuscular excitability, severe hypocalcemia, and often moderate hyperphosphatemia in a nonparturient animal, as well as on the response to therapy. Some of the signs (eg, tetany) and laboratory data (eg, hypocalcemia) are similar to those of puerperal hypocalcemia (p 809). However, puerperal hypocalcemia usually is accompanied by hypophosphatemia and a low-normal or subnormal blood glucose concentration as a result of the associated intense muscular activity.

Treatment: The neuromuscular tetany should be treated initially by restoring blood calcium levels to near normal by IV administration of calcium gluconate. One recommended therapeutic regimen is 10 mL of 10% calcium gluconate in 250 mL of 0.9% saline administered at 2.5 mL/kg/hr for 8-12 hr. Care must be taken not to administer the calcium too rapidly due to its cardiotoxic properties. Longterm maintenance of blood calcium levels in the absence of normal PTH secretion should be attempted by feeding diets that are high in calcium and low in phosphorus and that are supplemented with calcium (gluconate or lactate) and vitamin D_3.

Large doses of vitamin D_3 ($\geq$25,000-50,000 U/day, depending on the weight of the dog) may be required initially to increase the blood calcium level in hypoparathyroid animals because the lack of PTH diminishes the rate of formation of the biologically active vitamin D metabolite in the kidney. To prevent hypercalcemia and extensive soft-tissue mineralization, the dosage of vitamin D should be carefully adjusted after frequent determination of the serum calcium level. After adjusting the dose of vitamin D, a 4- to 5-day interval should precede the next blood calcium determination. Once the blood calcium has returned to normal, substantially lower doses of vitamin D are indicated for longterm maintenance; in some dogs, only dietary calcium supplementation is required for longterm stabilization.

ARTHROPATHIES IN LARGE ANIMALS

See also LAMENESS IN CATTLE, p 867; HORSES, p 904; SHEEP, p 942; GOATS, p 893; and PIGS, p 932.

ARTHRITIS

Arthritis is a nonspecific term denoting inflammation of a joint. All joint diseases of large animals have an inflammatory component to varying degrees. Arthritic entities of importance include traumatic arthritis, osteochondritis dissecans, subchondral cystic lesions, septic (or infective) arthritis, and osteoarthritis (also called degenerative joint disease).

Traumatic Arthritis

Traumatic arthritis includes traumatic synovitis and capsulitis, intra-articular chip fractures, ligamentous tears (sprains) involving periarticular and intra-articular ligaments, meniscal tears, and osteoarthritis. Traumatic arthritis is seen in all breeds of horses worldwide.

Clinical Findings and Diagnosis: Traumatic synovitis and capsulitis is inflammation of the synovial membrane and fibrous joint capsule associated with trauma. Typically, the horse is an athlete and presents with synovial effusion in the acute stage, along with general thickening and fibrosis in the more chronic stage. Lameness varies from a mild gait change to severe lameness. Traumatic synovitis and capsulitis is differentiated from other traumatic entities by use of radiography to exclude osteochondral fractures or disease. Tearing of ligaments or menisci (in femorotibial joints) can often be excluded only by diagnostic arthroscopy. Osteochondral fractures are diagnosed with radiographs. Osteoarthritis is diagnosed with radiographs when the changes are sufficiently severe to demonstrate loss of joint space (associated with articular cartilage loss), subchondral sclerosis, and osteophyte or enthesophyte formation. Lesser degrees of osteoarthritis can be defined only with diagnostic arthroscopy. Clinical signs of osteochondral fractures are similar to those of synovitis and capsulitis, as well as those of osteoarthritis; differential diagnosis of these entities is based on radiographs and, in some cases, arthroscopy.

Arthritis generally results in pain and altered function of the joint. If the process is active or acute, there is usually synovial effusion, and the surrounding tissues are swollen and warm. In more severe cases, manipulation of the joint causes pain. In more subtle cases, flexion tests are required to elicit lameness. As the disease process becomes chronic, the range of motion is reduced with fibrous thickening of the joint capsule. Radiographic evaluation is necessary for positive confirmation of a number of disease entities. Arthroscopy is used to accurately assess the amount of damage to the articular cartilage and to establish a prognosis.

Treatment: Treatment of acute traumatic synovitis and capsulitis includes rest and physical therapy regimens such as cold water treatment, ice, passive flexion, and swimming. NSAID (usually phenylbutazone) are used routinely. In more severe cases, the joint is lavaged to remove inflammatory products produced by the synovial membrane, as well as articular cartilage debris that exacerbates the synovitis. Joint drainage alone, without lavage or injection of medication, provides only short-term relief. Various intraarticular medications have been used. Corticosteroids are the most potent anti-inflammatory agents and are effective in acute traumatic arthritis. However, there are differences in the side effects between various corticosteroids and various dosages. Betamethasone products and triamcinolone acetonide are effective with no deleterious side effects. Methylprednisolone acetate is more potent and longer acting than the other 2 drugs, but excessive use could lead to degenerative changes in the articular cartilage. Intra-articular sodium hyaluronate has been used effectively for mild to moderate synovitis but has minimal effect when there is articular cartilage damage or when intra-articular fractures are present. Use of an IV formulation of hyaluronic acid (systemic dose 40 mg) in clinical cases appears to be effective, and this is supported by research data in a controlled model of arthritis in horses. Polysulfated glycosaminoglycans (PSGAG) are also used frequently for traumatic arthritis entities. PSGAG have chondroprotective properties and are indicated to prevent ongoing degeneration of articular cartilage. Although effectiveness of PSGAG when used intra-articularly (250 mg) has much scientific support, effectiveness when used IM (500 mg) is less certain.

Horses with osteochondral chip fragmentation (most commonly seen in the carpus and fetlock joints) are treated with arthroscopic surgery to minimize the ongoing development of osteoarthritis. Fragments are removed, and defective bone and cartilage debrided. Rest periods of 2-6 mo follow, and physical therapy regimens are instituted in the convalescent period. The success rate in returning horses to previous performance level is high when secondary osteoarthritic changes are minimal at the time of surgery. Osteochondral chip fragments amenable to arthroscopic surgery and that have successful results include those associated with the distal radius or carpal bones; dorsoproximal first phalanx; proximal palmar/plantar first phalanx; apical, abaxial, and basilar fragments of the proximal sesamoid bones; fragmentation of the distal patella and the femoropatellar joint; chip fragments of the tibiotarsal joint; and fragments of the extensor process of the distal phalanx (coffin joint).

Osteochondritis Dissecans

For complete discussion of equine osteochondrosis, *see* p 929.

In osteochondritis dissecans (OCD), a focal area of the immature articular cartilage is retained, and the matrix in the basal area of this region becomes chondromalacic and acellular. The immature articular cartilage separates from the underlying trabecular bone. The chondral fracture extends horizontally and vertically until a flap is formed. Synovial fluid gains entrance to the underlying medullary space, and subchondral cysts may form (usually only in larger animals). The flap of immature articular cartilage may break away completely ("joint mice") or may reattach by endochondral ossification to the underlying bone, especially in pigs, and result in a wrinkled articular surface. The latter occurs only if the joint is rested or protected, which permits reestablishment of the circulation necessary for endochondral ossification. If the flap is torn free by joint motion, it may be ground into smaller pieces during locomotion and disappear, while the larger plaques may become attached to the synovial membrane, become vascularized, and ossify. The resultant articular defect, in time, fills with fibrocartilage.

Etiology: The exact cause is unknown but is assumed to be multifactorial. Factors include genetic predisposition, fast growth, high caloric intake, low copper and high zinc levels, and endocrine factors.

Clinical Findings: The most common sites of OCD, which usually is seen in young animals, are the femoropatellar joint, tibiotarsal (tarsocrural) joint, fetlock (metacarpophalangeal and metatarsophalangeal) joints, and the shoulder.

Animals with OCD of the shoulder usually present when <1 yr old with severe forelimb lameness and possibly some muscular atrophy. Animals with osteochondrosis in the other joints usually present with synovial effusion and varying degrees of lameness. Diagnosis is confirmed with radiographs.

Diagnosis: The history, age, breed, sex, and clinical signs provide useful information; however, radiographs are required to substantiate the diagnosis.

Treatment: The treatment of OCD depends on the location and degree of involvement. Femoropatellar joint lesions are associated with the lateral trochlear ridge of the femur, medial trochlear ridge of the femur, or distal patella. They are amenable to arthroscopic surgery, which is recommended in all cases except early lesions characterized by flattening (without fragmentation) <2 cm long on the lateral trochlear ridge. In the tarsocrural joint, OCD lesions are seen in decreasing frequency on the intermediate (sagittal) ridge of the tibia, lateral trochlear ridge of the talus, medial malleolus of the tibia, and medial trochlear ridge of the talus. All lesions are amenable to arthroscopic surgery, and the prognosis is usually good. Surgery is recommended when synovial effusion is present. Lesions without fragmentation in the metacarpophalangeal or metatarsophalangeal joints can be treated conservatively, and most affected animals recover well. If a fragment is present, arthroscopic surgery is recommended. In the shoulder, surgery is always recommended, but the prognosis is less favorable than in the other joints.

Subchondral Cystic Lesions

Subchondral cystic lesions are seen in the femorotibial joint and in the fetlock, pastern, elbow, shoulder, and distal phalanx. The diagnosis is usually made on the basis of localization of lameness with intra-articular analgesia (synovial effusion is variable) and confirmed with radiographs.

Subchondral cystic lesions are most frequent in the femorotibial joint. Surgery (arthroscopic) is currently recommended in the femorotibial joint whenever a complete cystic lesion is present. Smaller, dome-shaped or flattened lesions are treated conservatively in the initial period. Athletic soundness is achieved in 65-70% of these horses. More recently, some horses have been treated with intralesional injection of corticosteroids under arthroscopic visualization. Surgery is usually recommended for subchondral cystic lesions of the distal metacarpus in the fetlock. Single lesions associated with the pastern and elbow joint are treated conservatively and have a fair prognosis. If possible, surgery is recommended for cystic lesions of the distal phalanx (results with conservative treatment are very poor).

Septic Arthritis
(Infective arthritis)

Etiology and Epidemiology: Septic or infective arthritis results from sequestration of bacterial infection in a joint. Infection of a joint develops in 3 main ways: 1) hematogenous infection, which is common in foals, calves, and lambs (commonly referred to as navel ill); 2) traumatic injury with local introduction of infection; 3) iatrogenic infection associated with joint injection or surgery (usually in horses). Navel ill is only one example of a hematogenous route of infection, which can also be gained from GI or pulmonary sources.

Clinical Findings and Diagnosis: Septic arthritis is usually characterized by severe lameness and distention of the joint with cloudy, turbid synovial fluid that contains >30,000 WBC/mm^3 and a total protein level of >4 g/dL. In foals, hematogenous osteomyelitis often accompanies septic arthritis. Septic arthritis in foals has been classified into type S (septic joint only), type P (involving osteomyelitis of the adjacent growth plate as well), or type E (involving osteomyelitis of the epiphyseal and subchondral bone). Various organisms may be involved. In young lambs, *Actinobacillus seminis* causes polyarthritis, as do *Chlamydophila (Chlamydia) psittaci* and *Erysipelothrix insidiosa*. The latter can follow docking, castration, or navel infection. Viruses and mycoplasma may also be etiologic agents in food-producing animals. In mature goats, caprine arthritis and encephalitis virus (p 598) is an important cause of infective arthritis. In young goats, *C psittaci* and *Mycoplasma mycoides* are frequent causes. Bacterial (including *Mycoplasma*) arthritides are seen in young pigs. In newborn pigs, septic arthritis usually is due to intrauterine or navel infection with *Escherichia coli, Corynebacterium, Streptococcus,* or *Staphylococcus* spp. Control is best directed toward reducing the possibility of infection from the environment. Older pigs sometimes develop arthritis as a sequela of infection with *Haemophilus, Erysipelothrix,* or *Mycoplasma* spp. Although diagnosis in the early stages is not difficult, the more chronic stages can be confused with articular lesions produced by dietary hypervitaminosis A.

Treatment: Septic arthritis requires prompt treatment to avoid irreparable damage. Systemic broad-spectrum antibiotics are indicated; the initial choice is based on the most likely pathogen but is subject to change based on culture and sensitivity tests. Systemic antibiotic treatment is often combined with intra-articular antibiotics (to achieve more effective sterilization of the joint) and other local therapy, including joint lavage (initially) and arthroscopic debridement and drainage. Adjunctive treatment with NSAID (eg, phenylbutazone) is also done. The effectiveness of treatment is monitored carefully with clinical signs and repeat synovial fluid analyses.

Osteoarthritis

(Degenerative joint disease)

Etiology and Epidemiology: Osteoarthritis is a progressive degradation of articular cartilage and represents the end stage of most of the other diseases discussed above if treatment is ineffective or the initial problem is too severe. For this reason, prompt diagnosis and correct management of traumatic synovitis and capsulitis, intra-articular fractures or traumatic cartilage damage, osteochondritis dissecans, subchondral cystic lesions, and septic arthritis are critical.

Clinical Findings and Diagnosis: Lameness can be localized with analgesia to the affected joint. There are varying degrees of synovial effusion, joint capsule fibrosis, and restricted motion (decreased flexion). Radiographic signs of osteoarthritis include decreased joint space, osteophytosis, enthesitis, and subchondral sclerosis. In less severe cases, articular degradation requires definition with arthroscopy.

Treatment: Treatment of osteoarthritis is most commonly palliative and includes the use of NSAID, polysulfated glycosaminoglycans, intra-articular corticosteroids, and IV hyaluronic acid. Physical therapy regimens may prove helpful. In advanced cases, surgical fusion (arthrodesis) may be performed on selected joints. Surgical fusion of the proximal interphalangeal joint (pastern) or distal tarsal joints can effect athletic soundness. Fetlock arthrodesis is also done in valuable animals and makes them very comfortable and capable of breeding. Treatment is usually unsuccessful in chronic cases in bulls and cows, but restricted exercise and careful feeding and nursing prolong the life of and can be worthwhile for valuable breeding animals.

BURSITIS

Bursitis is an inflammatory reaction within a bursa that can range from mild inflammation to sepsis. It is more common and important in horses. It can be classified as true or acquired. True bursitis is inflammation in a congenital or natural bursa (deeper than the deep fascia), eg, trochanteric bursitis and supraspinous bursitis (fistulous withers, see below). Acquired bursitis is development of a subcutaneous bursa where one was not previously present or inflammation of that bursa, eg, capped elbow over the olecranon process, shoe boil over the point of the elbow, and capped hock over the tuber calcaneus.

Bursitis may manifest as an acute or chronic inflammation. Examples of acute bursitis include bicipital bursitis and trochanteric bursitis in the early stages. It is generally characterized by swelling, local heat, and pain. Chronic bursitis usually develops in association with repeated trauma, fibrosis, and other chronic changes (eg, capped elbow, capped hock, and carpal hygroma). Excess bursal fluid accumulates, and the wall of the bursa is thickened by fibrous tissue. Fibrous bands or a septum may form within the bursal cavity, and generalized subcutaneous thickening usually develops. These bursal enlargements develop as cold, painless swellings and, unless greatly enlarged, do not severely interfere with function. Septic bursitis is more serious and is associated with pain and lameness. Infection of a bursa may be hematogenous or follow direct penetration.

The pain in acute bursitis may be relieved by application of cold packs, aspiration of the contents, and intrabursal medication. Repeated injections may result in infection. Treatment of chronic bursitis is surgical. In infected bursitis, systemic antibiotics as well as local drainage are required.

Capped Elbow and Hock

Capped elbow and hock are inflammatory swellings of the subcutaneous bursae (acquired bursitis) located over the olecranon process and tuber calcaneus, respectively, of horses. Trauma from lying on poorly bedded hard floors, kicks, falls, riding the tailgate of trailers, iron shoes projecting beyond the heels, and prolonged recumbency are frequent causes.

Circumscribed edematous swelling develops over and around the affected bursa. Lameness is rare in either case. The affected bursa may be fluctuating and soft at first but, in a short time, a firm fibrous capsule forms, especially if there is a recurrence of an old injury. Initial bursal swellings may be hardly noticeable or quite sizable. Chronic cases may progress to abscessation.

Acute early cases may respond well to applications of cold water, followed in a few days by aseptic aspiration and injection of a corticosteroid. The bursa may also be reduced in size by application of a counterirritant or by ultrasonic or radiation therapy. Older encapsulated bursae are more refractory. Surgical treatment (usually curettage and drainage) is recommended for advanced chronic cases or for those that become infected. A shoe-boil roll should be used to prevent recurrence of a capped elbow if the condition has been caused by the heel or the shoe. With capped hock, behavioral modification so the horse does not kick the stall offers the only hope of permanently resolving the problem.

Fistulous Withers and Poll Evil

Fistulous withers and poll evil are rare, inflammatory conditions of horses that differ essentially only in their location in the respective supraspinous or supra-atlantal bursae. This discussion is of fistulous withers but, except for anatomic details, also applies to poll evil. In the early stage of the disease, a fistula is not present. When the bursal sac ruptures or when it is opened for surgical drainage, and secondary infection with pyogenic bacteria occurs, it usually assumes a true fistulous character.

Etiology: The condition may be traumatic or infectious in origin. Agglutination titers support an infectious etiology. *Brucella abortus* and occasionally *B suis* can be isolated from the fluid aspirated from the unopened bursa, and outbreaks of brucellosis in cattle (p 1110) have followed contact with horses with open bursitis. A *Brucella* titer should always be evaluated in these cases; if significant, the owners should be made aware of the public health significance.

Clinical Findings: The inflammation leads to considerable thickening of the bursa wall. The bursal sacs are distended and may rupture when the sac has little covering support. In more chronic, advanced cases, the ligament and the dorsal vertebral spines are affected, and occasionally these structures necrose.

In the early stage, the supraspinous bursa distends with a clear, straw-colored, viscid exudate. The swelling may be dorsal, unilateral, or bilateral, depending on the arrangement of the bursal sacs between the tissue layers. It is an exudative process from the beginning, but no true suppuration or secondary infection occurs until the bursa ruptures or is opened.

Treatment and Prevention: The earlier treatment is instituted, the better the prognosis. The most successful treatment is complete dissection and removal of the infected bursa. The expense of the protracted treatment required in chronic cases often exceeds the value of the animal, and the public health aspects (in cases in which *Brucella* spp are involved) should be carefully considered. *Brucella* vaccines have not proved helpful. Sodium iodide therapy is of limited value. It is reasonable to keep horses separate from *Brucella*-infected cattle, and cattle separate from horses with discharging fistulous withers.

CHLAMYDIAL POLYARTHRITIS-SEROSITIS
(Transmissible serositis)

This infectious disease affects sheep, calves, goats, and pigs. Chlamydial polyarthritis of sheep was first described in Wisconsin and has since been recognized in the western USA, Australia, and New Zealand. The disease was identified in calves from the USA, Australia, and Austria, and in pigs from Austria, Bulgaria, and the USA.

Etiology and Epidemiology: Strains of the causal agent, *Chlamydophila (Chlamydia) psittaci*, isolated from affected joints of sheep and calves are identical, but strain-specific antigens in their cell walls distinguish them from those that cause abortions in sheep and cattle (p 1098).

The GI tract is of prime importance in the pathogenesis of chlamydial polyarthritis (*see* INTESTINAL CHLAMYDIAL INFECTIONS, p 155). The disease has been reproduced experimentally by oral inoculation. Because chlamydiae can be recovered from the feces of clinically normal calves and lambs, it is most likely the GI tract wherein the host and parasite stay frequently in balance. If there is a shift in favor of the chlamydiae, then a systemic infection and chlamydemia ensues; the ultimate site of replication is the synovial membrane. The GI tract also has been infected after experimental intra-articular inoculations. Chlamydiae are excreted in the feces and urine and transmitted via ingestion or, in some cases, inhalation.

Clinical Findings: Chlamydial polyarthritis is seen in lambs on range, on farms, and in feedlots. Morbidity may be 5-75%. Rectal temperatures are 102-107°F (39-41.5°C). Varying degrees of stiffness, lameness, anorexia, and a concurrent conjunctivitis (p 406) may be seen. Affected sheep are depressed, reluctant to move, and often hesitate to stand and bear weight on one or more limbs, but they may "warm out" of stiffness and lameness after forced exercise. Incidence of the disease in sheep on range is highest between late summer and early winter.

The disease affects cattle of all ages but calves 4-30 days old are affected more severely. Calves may have fever, are moderately alert, and usually nurse if carried to the dam and supported while sucking. They invariably also have diarrhea, which can be severe. Affected calves assume a hunched position while standing; their joints usually are swollen, and palpation causes pain. Navel involvement and nervous signs are not seen.

Chlamydial polyarthritis has been recognized in older pigs as well as in young piglets. The affected piglets become febrile and anorectic and may develop nasal catarrh, difficulties in breathing, and conjunctivitis. This condition has not been clearly differentiated from other infections that lead to polyserositis and arthritis in pigs.

Lesions: The most striking tissue changes are in the joints. In lambs, enlargement of the joints is not often noticed, but in chronic advanced cases, the stifle, hock, and elbow may be slightly enlarged. In calves, periarticular subcutaneous edema along tendon sheaths and fluid-filled, fluctuating synovial sacs contribute to enlargement of the joints. Most affected joints of lambs or calves contain excessive, grayish yellow, turbid synovial fluid. Fibrin flakes and plaques in the recesses of the affected joints may adhere firmly to the synovial membranes. Joint capsules are thickened. Articular cartilage is smooth, and erosions or evidence of marginal compensatory changes are not present. Tendon sheaths of severely affected lambs and calves may be distended and contain creamy, grayish yellow exudate. Surrounding muscles are hyperemic and edematous, with petechiae in their associated fascial planes.

Diagnosis: The history and careful examination of the pathologic changes in the joints and other organs can be of diagnostic value. Cytologic examination of synovial fluids or tissues may reveal chlamydial elementary bodies or cytoplasmic inclusions. Isolation and identification of the causative agent from affected joints confirms the diagnosis. Bacteriologic cultures of affected joints are usually negative, but *Escherichia coli* or streptococci occasionally may be isolated. If the joints of young calves are arthritic, and navel lesions are absent, chlamydial polyarthritis should be considered.

Clinical and pathologic features distinguish chlamydial polyarthritis from most other conditions that cause stiffness and lameness in lambs. Lambs with mineral deficiency or osteomalacia usually are not febrile. The abnormal osteogenesis in these 2 conditions and the distinct lesions of white muscle disease are virtually pathognomonic. In arthritis caused by *Erysipelothrix rhusiopathiae*, there are deposits on and pitting of articular surfaces, periarticular fibrosis, and osteophyte formation. Laminitis due to bluetongue virus infection can be differentiated clinically and etiologically. Detailed microbiologic investigations are required to differentiate chlamydial arthritis from mycoplasmal arthritis.

Treatment and Prevention: If begun early, therapy with long-acting penicillin, tetracyclines, or tylosin appears to be beneficial. More advanced lesions do not respond satisfactorily. Feeding chlortetracycline at 150-200 mg/day to affected lambs in feedlots reduces the incidence of chlamydial polyarthritis. No approved vaccines are available.

TENDINITIS
(Bowed tendon)

Inflammation of a tendon can be acute or chronic, with varying degrees of tendon fibril disruption. Tendinitis is most common in horses used at fast work, particularly racehorses. The problem is seen in the flexor tendons and is more common in the forelimb than in the hindlimb. In racehorses, the superficial flexor is involved most frequently. The primary lesion is a rupture of tendon fibers with associated hemorrhage and edema.

Etiology: Tendinitis usually appears after fast exercise and is associated with overextension and poor conditioning, fatigue, poor racetrack conditions, and persistent training when inflammatory problems in the tendon already exist. Improper shoeing may also predispose to tendinitis. Poor conformation and poor training also have been implicated.

Clinical Findings and Diagnosis: During the acute stage, the horse is severely lame and the involved structures are hot, painful, and swollen. In chronic cases, there is fibrosis with thickening and adhesions in the peritendinous area. The horse with chronic tendinitis may go sound while walking or trotting, but lameness may recur under hard work. Ultrasonography delineates many defects and injuries that are ill-defined or undetectable by palpation.

Treatment: Tendinitis is best treated in the early, acute stage. The horse should be stall-rested, and the swelling and inflammation treated aggressively with cold packs and systemic anti-inflammatory agents. Some degree of support or immobilization should be used, depending on the amount of damage to the tendon. Intratendinous corticosteroid injections are contraindicated. When a distinct hypoechoic or anechoic core lesion is present on ultrasound examination, tendon splitting is recommended (the rationale is to decrease intratendinous pressure due to serum or hemorrhage). Recently, the use of bone marrow injection of the core lesion (to introduce stem cells and growth factors) has been done with encouraging results. The horse should be rehabilitated using a regimen of increasing exercise. Superior check ligament desmotomy has been used as an adjunctive treatment to minimize recurrence of the problem when the horse is returned to training.

Other treatments for chronic tendinitis have included superficial point firing (of questionable benefit), percutaneous tendon splitting, and carbon fiber implantation. Annular ligament desmotomy is also used when tendinitis involves the area of the digital tendon sheath.

The prognosis for a racehorse to return to racing after a bowed tendon is guarded, regardless of treatment.

TENOSYNOVITIS

Tenosynovitis, an inflammation of the synovial membrane and usually the fibrous layer of the tendon sheath, is characterized by distention of the tendon sheath due to synovial effusion. It has a number of possible causes and clinical manifestations. The various types of tenosynovitis include idiopathic, acute, chronic, and septic (infectious). Idiopathic synovitis refers to synovial distention of tendon sheaths in young animals, in which the cause is uncertain. Acute and chronic tenosynovitis are due to trauma. Septic tenosynovitis may be associated with penetrating wounds, local extension of infection, or a hematogenous infection.

Clinical Findings and Diagnosis: There are varying degrees of synovial distention of the tendon sheath and lameness, depending on the severity. Horses are markedly lame in septic tenosynovitis. Chronic tenosynovitis is common in horses in the tarsal sheath of the hock (thoroughpin) and in the digital sheath (tendinous windpuffs). These 2 entities must be differentiated from bog spavin and synovial effusion of the fetlock.

Treatment: In idiopathic cases, no treatment is initially recommended. Acute cases with clinical signs may be treated symptomatically with cold packs, NSAID, and rest. Application of counterirritants and bandaging has been used in more chronic cases. Radiation therapy is helpful. Septic tenosynovitis requires systemic antibiotics and drainage. If adhesions develop between the tendon sheath and the tendon, persistent effusion and lameness is the rule.

LAMENESS IN CATTLE

Lameness is the third most important problem on many modern dairy farms after mastitis and reproductive failure. The considerable economic losses are attributable to the cost of treatment, decreased milk production, decreased reproductive performance, and increased culling. The incidence of lameness has steadily increased over the past 20 yr, and on some farms over half of the animals become lame at least once each year. The 2 most troublesome causes of lameness are diseases associated with subclinical laminitis and digital dermatitis.

DIAGNOSTIC PROCEDURES

Physical Examination

Visual Appearance of the Standing Animal: The first step of the lameness examination is evaluation of the animal for any obvious signs of disease. Some signs, such as a change in hair coat that might indicate zinc or copper deficiency, would be present in several animals in a herd. Abrasions or swellings suggest a prior traumatic event. Decubital lesions might indicate prolonged periods of recumbency or difficulty experienced by the animal when rising and suggests examination of the design and management of the free stalls. Muscular atrophy, particularly noticeable in the gluteal region, can be associated with a painful condition of some duration. However, animals experiencing extreme pain can lose body condition rapidly.

In normal stance, the point of the hock lies directly beneath the pin bone when viewed either from the side or from behind. Approximately 60% of the body weight is borne by the forelimbs compared with the hindlimbs. Weight is distributed evenly between the 2 claws on each foot. A lame animal assumes a different stance or posture because of some abnormal influence or to relieve pain. A painful abscess in a lateral hindclaw causes the animal to abduct that limb. If the horn of the sole beneath the heel of a lateral claw increases in thickness (overburdened), the animal assumes a "cow hocked" posture. Some abnormal postures can be confused with abnormal conformation. An animal is said to be "camped forward" when the limb is protracted forward more than is normal. This posture is associated with pain in the apex (toe) of the claw. In the hindlimb, this can be confused with "sickle hock," a conformation in which the angle of the hock is <160°. By contrast, when there is pain in the heel region, the limb is retracted or held further back than is normal, and the animal is said to be standing "camped back." This posture may be confused with "post leg," a conformation in which the angle of the hock is >180°. When the hindfeet are held closer together than normal (adducted), pain in the medial claw is indicated. The animal is said to be "standing narrow." This posture is often confused with the conformation called "bow leg."

Evaluation of Gait: Characteristics of abnormal gait are comparable to those of abnormal posture. For example, if there is pain in the toe, the retraction phase of the stride (when the foot passes behind the phase of vertical weight bearing) is reduced considerably. In contrast, if there is pain in the heel, the protraction phase of the stride is reduced or the foot is not carried as far forward as is normal. Usually the gait of one limb can be compared with that of the contralateral limb when viewed from the side. However, lameness that is simultaneously present in contralateral limbs tends to appear less severe than is actually the case. It is not unusual in cases of subacute laminitis for all limbs to be affected more or less equally. In these cases, no specific gait change is seen, but the animals tend to place their feet at each step with care; they are said to "plod" or have a stilted gait.

Examination of the Claw: The axial surfaces of the claws should be equally concave. If they are not in young animals (2 yr old), this could indicate a predisposition to abnormality in later life, particularly in bulls. If the animal has been exposed to concrete surfaces, the sole will probably be worn flat. To facilitate examination, the surface of the sole should be washed and examined carefully for black marks, which should be explored with a hoof knife. In cows kept on concrete, the lateral hindclaw usually becomes wider than the medial. If the sole is heavily caked with mud and manure (eg, animals at pasture or confined in corrals or straw wards), it is quicker and easier to cut off a layer of superficial horn together with the caked material to expose fresh horn beneath. Particular attention should be paid to the abaxial white line area. Removal of large amounts of sole horn is contraindicated in the diagnostic phase of an examination. The interdigital space should be evaluated by separating the claws and examining carefully for evidence of a foreign body, fibroma, footrot, interdigital dermatitis, or digital dermatitis.

Differential diagnosis can be aided by selective anesthesia of the nerves of the digit.

Radiography

Radiography of the Digital Region: The cause of >90% of lameness is located in the digital region. Radiography can help identify the site of lameness and provide information about the stage to which the pathology has developed to determine the most advantageous treatment. When pathologic changes are seen in the region of the distal interphalangeal joint, tissue damage is often rapid and severe.

Before a radiograph is taken, the interdigital space and both claws should be cleansed thoroughly, and both claws should be lightly trimmed. If this is not done, false images or shadows may mask abnormalities present in the claws. The digits can be viewed radiographically using 4 angles or projections.

In the **dorsopalmar/plantar projection**, the image produced shows all of the major bones and joints without overlap. This view allows diagnosis of many diseases of the bovine foot.

In the **oblique projection**, the plate is positioned beneath the claw and the head of the machine is placed dorsad to the digits and rotated backward at a 45° angle. Because cattle have 2 digits that overlap one another when viewed radiographically from the side, the clarity of an abnormality may be obscured. The oblique view allows the digit to be viewed from such an angle that 1 claw appears to be behind the other, which gives a much clearer picture than can be obtained when the digits are superimposed. Because each digit is projected differently on an oblique view, it is best to compare 2 radiographs of oblique views taken at comparable but opposite angles.

The **lateromedial or mediolateral projection** is generally of much less value than the oblique view. However, because positioning is relatively easy, this view is useful for evaluating fractures, fracture repairs, and luxations.

In the **axial projection**, a lateromedial or mediolateral view of a single claw is accomplished by placing a nonscreen film (eg, a paper "cassette") between the digits. This view produces a good image of the affected distal phalanx and, if interdigital soft-tissue swelling is not too great, the distal interphalangeal joint.

Radiographic Analysis and Interpretation: A number of factors should be considered in radiographic analysis and interpretation. Age differences can be seen radiographically as differences in skeletal development. In calves, physes are present in the distal metacarpus and metatarsus and at the proximal ends of the proximal and middle phalanges. In a very young calf, the distal phalanges may be incompletely ossified so that the bones appear small, and their distal ends are rounded and indistinct. The subchondral bone may appear indistinct and finely irregular; this should not be mistaken for the subchondral bone lysis that is seen in septic arthropathy.

Diseases stimulating periosteal new bone in cattle (such as corkscrew claw and post-recovery septic arthritis) can cause marked changes in bone contour and increased bone opacity.

Slight bony changes at articular margins and musculotendinous attachments are commonly seen on radiographs of older cattle. Roughening of the distal surface of the distal digit is a normal sign of aging. Changes that occur during the normal aging process should not be confused with active bony changes.

Reactive new bone (osteophyte, enthesiophyte, or exostosis) that has been present for some time has a distinct border and a rough outline, and the opacity is normally even. Active new bone has an indistinct border and a rough outline, and the opacity is uneven.

Diffuse loss of bone opacity occurs in subacute laminitis, nutritional bone disease, and after limb immobilization. Focal or localized loss of bone opacity occurs in bone infection (osteomyelitis) or inflammation (osteitis), early fracture healing, and with defects in endochondral ossification (osteochondrosis).

Increase in joint width is caused by the presence of increased fluid in the joint. However, this is less evident if the animal is bearing weight at the time the radiograph is taken. To confirm that the joint is in fact wider than normal, it may be compared with the contralateral joint.

Indistinctness and loss of opacity of the subchondral bone is often associated with joint infections. Loss of opacity is often irregular. For this reason, a single radiograph is unlikely to detect this pathology; therefore, several radiographs taken from different angles are usually advised. Comparison between suspect and known normal joints is recommended. Subchondral bone may be indistinct in a young animal.

Radiography is important for evaluating the progress of a fracture repair. A radiograph taken immediately after a fracture has been realigned is the basis for future evaluations, and subsequent radiographs are essential if nonunion or bone infection is suspected.

Loss of bone opacity is difficult to recognize with certainty in metabolic and nutritional diseases. Because all of the bones in the body may be equally affected, it is not helpful to compare one bone with another. In an adult animal, cancellous regions in the bone ends may become coarser or "granular" in appearance as smaller bone trabeculae are resorbed. In the diaphysis of a normal bone in both immature and adult animals, the cortex is thickest at midshaft and becomes thinner toward both ends. If the cortex at midshaft approaches the thinness of the proximal and distal diaphyses, generalized osteopenia must be suspected.

Soft-tissue swelling can be demonstrated on radiographs only in the early stages of a septic disease. The characteristics of a soft-tissue swelling may indicate the location of a lesion and the tissues involved, muscle or tendon disease, cellulitis or edema, or dark gas shadows (eg, a sinus or a cap of an abscess).

Ultrasonography: Ultrasonography has not been an important practical application for the diagnosis of lameness in cattle. However, ultrasonography can be used to evaluate injuries to the tendons and ligaments, and it may prove of value in identifying radiolucent foreign bodies and in tracing sinus tracts and deep abscesses, particularly within large muscle masses.

Electromyography: Electromyography (EMG) can be used to detect failure in the nerve supply to muscles. Portable equipment is available for use on the farm, but detailed studies are best conducted in a referral facility. EMG examination can detect the degree of lower motor neuron disease before clinical signs appear. Active myositis gives a positive EMG response. Degenerative muscle disorders (eg, white muscle disease) are usually negative on EMG examination. Estimates of rate of recovery can be made before there is any clinical evidence of such.

Regional Analgesia

The selective use of **spinal analgesia** may be indicated under extreme field conditions, eg, splinting a limb before transportation. Spinal analgesia may also be used to facilitate the replacement of a dislocated hip. However, for surgical procedures such as amputation of a digit, regional analgesia is needed. Spinal analgesia is more applicable for use in beef cattle at pasture than for dairy cattle on concrete.

The dose of 2% lidocaine required for complete immobilization of the posterior extremities of a 450-kg cow is ~60 mL injected into the epidural space. Lower dosages can result in ataxia, which may be counterproductive. Xylazine is a potent sedative and analgesic as well as a local anesthetic; therefore, it can be injected into the epidural space alone or combined with lidocaine. Ten mL of 2% lidocaine combined with xylazine at 0.07 mg/kg causes mild sedation and satisfactory analgesia.

A **high nerve block of a pelvic limb** is appropriate for treating injuries proximal to the digits. Only 2 nerves—the peroneal and tibial nerves—have to be perfused. The peroneal nerve can be palpated in thin-skinned animals at the posterior edge of the lateral condyle of the femur. In a mature cow, ~20 mL of 2% lidocaine should be used. The tibial nerve can be palpated just beneath the deep flexor and gastrocnemius tendons. It should be infiltrated with 15-29 mL of 2% lidocaine on each side (medial and lateral).

For **distal digital analgesia** (used for surgical or diagnostic procedures), the dorsal site is located on the dorsal axis proximal to the interdigital space close to the metacarpal or metatarsal phalangeal joint. The needle should be placed with care (because the proper digital artery can be found at the dorsal site), and 10 mL of 2% lidocaine injected. If the needle is inserted deep into the interdigital space, the nerves of the flexor surface can be reached. This obviates the necessity of a flexor site block for simple procedures. The distribution of the nerve supply to the axial face of the digits of the forelimb is not constant, which makes this technique unreliable for digital analgesia of the forelimb.

The preferred flexor site is a little lower than the dorsal site because it is difficult to pass a needle through the partially cartilaginous palmar/plantar ligament. The medial and lateral sites are located at the level of the dewclaws, and the needle is inserted dorsally (horizontal in the standing animal) from a point 2.5 cm slightly proximal to the dewclaws. For the flexor site and the medial and lateral sites, ~5-8 mL of 2% lidocaine is injected. For surgery of the digit (eg, amputation), the dorsal, palmar/plantar, and medial or lateral sites are used, depending on the claw. For interdigital surgery (eg, removal of corns), both the dorsal and palmar/plantar sites are used.

Intravenous regional analgesia is the method of choice of analgesia for most digital surgical procedures. The animal should be sedated and, if possible, placed in lateral recumbency. The limb should be restrained.

A tourniquet is applied distal to the tarsus or carpus within working distance of the surgical site. The enlarged veins can be palpated distal to the tourniquet, and the site should be prepared as for sterile surgery. One or more gauze rolls (depending on the site and number of veins) placed beneath the tourniquet and directly over the vein being injected improves hemostasis and promotes retrograde movement of the lidocaine and contact with nerve endings. In adult cattle, a 20- to 22-gauge needle should be used. Butterfly trocars can be used for prolonged procedures or antibiotic infusions. The amount of lidocaine (2%) without epinephrine needed to produce analgesia, which develops in ~10 min, varies from 10-30 mL (the total dose should not exceed 9 mg/kg). After the surgery is completed, the tourniquet is released slowly and then retightened. If antibiotics are used, they should be introduced at this point, and the tourniquet released a few minutes later. It is inadvisable to keep a tourniquet in place for >1 hr.

Arthroscopy and Arthrocentesis

Arthroscopy enables visualization of the interior surfaces of a joint for diagnostic or surgical purposes. Arthrocentesis is a procedure by which synovial fluid may be removed from a joint for examination. Local anesthetic can be introduced to ascertain if painful lesions are present in the joint. Intra-articular therapy permits medication to be deposited into the joint.

Joint Entry Sites: For the distal interphalangeal (coffin) joint, the needle is inserted lateral to the common or long extensor tendon, which inserts into the extensor process of the distal phalanx. The entry point is just proximal to the coronary band. For the pastern joint (proximal interphalangeal joint), the needle is inserted lateral to the extensor tendon. For the fetlock joint (metacarpophalangeal or metatarsophalangeal joint), the needle is directed downward close to the bone and between it and the interosseous (suspensory) ligament. Because this procedure may be painful, a nerve block at a higher level is recommended. The joint can also be entered from the dorsal surface in a similar manner to the distal joints; however, the flexor pouch is more capacious than the dorsal one. For the digital synovial sheath (sheath of the deep flexor tendon), the needle is directed downward behind the interosseous ligament.

For the stifle joint, it is advisable to use 2 sites because the lateral femorotibial compartment in some animals may not communicate with the rest of the joint. The first site is close behind the lateral patellar ligament (lateral femorotibial compartment), and the needle should be directed caudally. The needle is inserted in the second site between the medial and middle patellar ligaments and directed slightly down and toward the large medial lip of the trochlea (femoropatellar and medial femorotibial compartments).

For the hip joint, the needle should be directed caudally and medially in front of the trochanter major and just in front of the insertion of the middle gluteus.

PREVENTIVE PROCEDURES

Pain Management

Surgery, injury to tissues, and swellings caused by infection result in pain. The stress response to pain increases the nutritional requirement of the animal (particularly zinc intake) and, if prolonged, can cause debility. Pain-related stress may also increase susceptibility to disease. Measures to control pain (eg, use of analgesics) promote healing and recovery. Analgesic drugs should be administered to effect, but the following dosages can be used as guidelines: morphine, 0.2-0.4 mg/kg, IM; meperidine, 1-2 mg/kg, IM; oxymorphone, 0.05-0.1 mg/kg, IM; pentazocine, 1-2 mg/kg, IM; butorphanol, 0.1-0.2 mg/kg, IM or IV; and buprenorphine, 0.005-0.008 mg/kg, IM or IV.

The use of corticosteroids and NSAID is controversial, but the latter are useful in counteracting substances such as prostaglandins from injured and inflamed tissues. NSAID are valuable for treating pain due to inflammatory reactions or joint diseases, but their use for long periods should be avoided because of adverse side effects. For example, phenylbutazone should not be administered more often than once every 36-48 hr and not repeated more than 2-3 times. The following NSAID are commonly used: aspirin, 100 mg/kg, PO, BID; flunixin meglumine, 1.1-2.2 mg/kg, IV or IM; phenylbutazone, 10 mg/kg, IV or PO, every 48 hr; and dipyrone, 20 mg/kg, IV, IM, or SC, BID-TID. Dimethyl sulfoxide is a topical anti-inflammatory agent that can be applied over the affected area.

Functional Claw Trimming

Under normal circumstances, horn growth keeps pace with wear, and the growth/wear rate at the heel is greater than it is at the toe. Horn that is dry tends to be extremely resistant to wear and may grow longer than normal. The claws of cattle maintained in straw yards tend to become overgrown. Conversely, the claws of cattle maintained in extremely wet conditions are softer than normal and more prone to wear. If the animals are housed on concrete surfaces the lateral hindclaw tends to wear less than the medial.

It has been reported that if claws are correctly trimmed at least once each year, longevity of the herd may be extended by 1 yr. However, unskilled claw trimming has a negative effect on the claw health of a herd. In many countries, claw trimming is performed by a professional claw trimmer rather than a veterinarian. In these cases, collaboration is recommended in which the role of each party is clearly defined, eg, the claw trimmer would keep extensive records for epidemiologic investigation by the veterinarian.

Functional claw trimming (the "Dutch" method) aims to restore the foot to its normal function. It is based on the concept that correct trimming will reestablish the stability of unbalanced claws. Normally, both claws should bear weight equally, but when cows walk on concrete, the lateral claw tends to slip and grow faster than it wears. Thus, when standing, the lateral claw bears much more weight than the medial claw.

All claws should be evaluated before trimming. On average, the front (dorsal flexure) wall of a claw measures ~7.5 cm long from apex to hair line. When the dorsal surface increases in length, the toe buckles like the instep of a human shoe causing more pressure to be exerted in the region of the heel. This increases pressure on the flexor process of the distal phalanx, the point beneath which sole ulcers develop. In addition, the longer the toe, the greater the stress on the flexor system. In all cases, the angle between the wall and the ground surface should be >45° at the toe. When the claws are short and the dorsal wall is <7.5 cm, there is considerable risk that the thickness of the sole at the apex will be less than the desirable 7 mm. Thinning of the apex of the sole of short-clawed animals should be avoided.

The Dutch method of claw trimming consists of 5 steps. In every case of lameness in which there is a lesion in the sole, the first 3 steps must be performed before attention is turned to the lesion itself.

In step 1, the length of the dorsal wall of the medial claw should be cut back to 7.5 cm. The thickness of the sole at the apex should be ~5-7 mm. The horn beneath the bulbs should not be trimmed at this stage.

In step 2, both the sole and the heel of the lateral claw should be shortened to match the medial claw. This may not be possible if the medial claw is already <7.5 cm long. When the heel of the lateral claw is significantly thicker than that of the medial claw, trimming should continue. The thickness of the sole anterior to the heel/sole junction should measure about 15 mm. If slight resilience is detectable on thumb pressure, no more horn should be removed. The claw should be left flat from apex to bulb with a slight slope from abaxial to axial border. Lack of attention to these principles may result in too much sole being left in the center of the prebulbar region, in which case sole ulcers can develop. A common error is to reduce the bearing surface of the wall at the level of the axial groove—a procedure that may transfer weight bearing to the center of the sole.

In step 3, the central quadrant to the axial border of the sole is shaped to a gentle concave slope.

In step 4, because >90% of lesions causing lameness are found in the sole of the lateral hindclaw, the strategy is to transfer weight to the medial claw by leaving it untouched while the thickness of the sole of the lateral claw is reduced as much as is reasonable in the prebulbar and bulbar regions.

In step 5, rough fragments of sole horn should be removed. If cows with problem claws are encountered during the annual herd trimming, the claws should be trimmed twice each year thereafter. It is preferable for claw trimming to be done when cows are not heavily pregnant or during peak lactation.

Footbaths

Using a footbath is not a substitute for either good hygiene or claw trimming. Permanent, concrete foot baths may measure 10 ft in length and be at least 3 ft wide. The sides of the bath should slope inward to a maximum depth of 6 in. Ideally, 2 baths should be built in sequence. The first bath would contain a foot-washing solution, the second would be medicated. Both should have drainage pipes. Portable baths constructed from fiberglass are available. A hoof mat, consisting of a sheet of foam plastic encased in a perforated plastic cover, is also available. The foam is soaked in medication that squirts up between the claws when the cow walks on the mat.

Formalin (3-5%) is the least expensive footbath solution. It controls interdigital dermatitis and is of some value in the prevention of footrot. Formalin may be used alternately with antibiotics in the control of digital dermatitis. The solution should be changed after the passage of 500-600 cows, more frequently if the bath is heavily contamined with manure. Formalin has good bacteriostatic activity and some potential for hardening the epidermis. However, the fumes irritate the lungs of milkers and, under certain conditions, milk can be tainted. In many areas, local laws prohibit the use of formalin. Formalin is also ineffective at temperatures <13°C.

The stronger the formalin solution used, the more effective it is, but the danger of a chemical burn on the cow's skin is also greater. Therefore, the status of the hair around the claw should be carefully monitored. If the hair appears to be standing on end or the skin is pink, treatment should be suspended. Normally, cows can tolerate twice daily baths for 3 days using a 3% solution. The treatment should be repeated every 3 wk. Higher concentrations should be used for the most resistant conditions.

Footbathing with a 5% solution of copper and zinc sulfate controls interdigital dermatitis and is of some value in controlling footrot (interdigital phlegmon). The sulfates are quite rapidly deactivated by combining with the proteins in manure. Prewashing of the cow's feet is advised, and the solution should be changed after the passage of 200 cows.

The use of antibiotics in footbaths is a popular strategy for the treatment, control, and prevention of digital dermatitis. The cost can be reduced by using a "minimal fluid footbath." The type of antibiotic used in footbaths should be changed at intervals of <6 mo to avoid development of resistant strains of the causal organisms. However, treatment may be given for 2 or 3 days and repeated once after 7 days. Formalin footbaths may be added if more aggressive treatment is necessary. Antibiotics used in a footbath do not result in detectable levels of the drug in the bloodstream.

A new generation of chemical agents has been developed for use in footbaths, but the claims for these products have not yet been adequately substantiated in controlled trials.

LAMINITIS

Laminitis is a pathophysiologic disturbance of the microvasculature of the corium that compromises the function of the tissues, particularly those of the horn-producing cells. Laminitis can be subclinical, acute, or chronic, depending on the severity of the several causative variables.

Acute or Subacute Laminitis

Acute laminitis is not common in cattle and usually is seen in a single animal or a group that has accidentally engorged on large quantities of grain. The incidence of acute laminitis in dairy cattle probably varies from 0.6-1.2%. Subacute laminitis may be seen in young beef bulls on feeding trials and in feeder calves that have been fed rations rich in carbohydrates.

Clinical Findings: Acute and subacute laminitis have a rapid onset. In the most acute cases, there may be fever and an increased respiratory rate. In the initial phases, the claws may be warm to the touch, and a pronounced digital pulse will be perceptible. Pain may be detected in the claws with the use of hoof testers.

Treatment: If the cause is obvious, such as grain overload, it should be corrected. Keeping the animal moving and the claws cool are helpful. Antihistamines may be useful if given within the first 48 hr after a known insult. Anti-inflammatory drugs may be useful if given before the onset of acute signs. However, caution should be exercised in using corticosteroids later than 24 hr after signs appear.

Control: Because acute laminitis usually develops as the result of an accident, little can be done to prevent the condition.

Chronic Laminitis

See SLIPPER FOOT, p 881.

Chronic laminitis is recognized by the bent, flat, square-toed, and heavily ridged appearance of the claw (slipper foot). It is the result of a prolonged process, and is assumed to be caused by a series of laminitic insults. It is most common in dairy cows >5 yr old.

Subclinical Laminitis

This form of laminitis is of considerable economic importance to the dairy industry as it predisposes mature cows to sole and toe ulcer, white line disease, and double sole. It has been seen in dairy cows in most developed countries and is of greatest concern in intensively managed herds.

Etiology: The classic hypothesis for the etiology of laminitis in cattle is comparable to that of laminitis in horses (p 873). High levels of carbohydrate in the rumen invoke an increase of *Streptococcus bovis* and *Lactobacillus* spp, which in turn lead to a state of acidosis in the rumen. It is further hypothesized that this environment is unfavorable for gram-negative organisms and, as they die, vasoactive endotoxins are released. Rumenitis is frequently associated with ruminal acidosis and a high incidence of liver abscesses. High levels of histamine in the blood have been found in the early stages of the disease. Fiber and the frequency of feeding are extremely important factors.

A second hypothesis involves the receptors for epidermal growth factor (EGF) that are present in the corium of the claw. Because EGF is liberated in large quantities from the GI tract that has been damaged, it could be involved in the pathogenesis of laminitis. In addition to its mitogenic effect, EGF can inhibit the differentiation of keratinocytes in vitro. Inhibited differentiation of keratinocytes of the hoof matrix is a dominant morphologic feature in the early stages of laminitis. This hypothesis might account for the irregularities in horn production that are seen in some cases of laminitis.

Recent investigations have studied the role of matrix metalloproteinase activity in the pathophysiology of laminitis. The results support the hypothesis that laminitis histopathology results from an inadequate regulation of gelatinase activity, resulting in selective degradation of basement membrane components, leading to laminitis due to failure of the basement membrane-epidermis attachment.

In cattle, nutritional mismanagement leading to acute acidosis is still considered to be the primary cause of the condition. However, stress arising from the effects of other risk factors causes variations in the signs of the disease and must be considered when devising control protocols.

Pathogenesis: The pathophysiologic process causing laminitis may be summarized as a toxic influence on capillary walls that results in insufficient nutrient supply to the keratin-producing cells and synthesis of structurally incompetent keratin. It is believed that when vasoactive toxins reach the corium, the arteriovenous shunts are paralyzed. Pressure inside the claw rises, and the vessels are damaged, which allows blood or blood fluids to escape and soak into the horn claw staining it either pink or yellow. Hemorrhagic staining of the horn tubules of the sole give a "brush mark" appearance. Increased blood pressure inside the claw (intraungular pressure) and the associated reduced blood flow is usually followed by thrombus formation. This is a characteristic feature of laminitis. Thrombi form as fine layers inside the walls (mural thrombi) of the vessels. Because of reduced blood flow, fewer nutrients reach horn-producing tissues, and horn quality deteriorates. The blood vessels can eventually become completely blocked, causing ischemic changes followed by scar tissue formation.

Frequently, young animals appear to recover from laminitis. This may be because new blood vessels develop to form collateral circulation and take over the function of those that have been damaged. Nevertheless, each time an animal has a bout of laminitis, more scar tissue is formed and the animal is less able to recover from the next insult.

Clinical Findings: Some animals appear to walk in a deliberate, careful manner. Hemorrhages in the sole and/or white line are consistent findings but they are not present until several weeks after the start of the nutritional insult. In the long term, the appearance of sole and toe ulcers, white line disease, and double sole confirm the suspicion that subclinical laminitis is present. If the annual incidence of these diseases collectively exceeds 10% in the multiparous cows in a herd, it may be assumed that subclinical laminitis exists.

Erythema and edema (puffy heel) of the skin above the coronary band and around the dewclaws in freshly calved cows may be an indication that a transitory laminitis-like insult is occurring. A prevalence of 10% is probably an indication that the cows are being introduced to concentrate too rapidly.

Treatment and Control: Treatment for subclinical laminitis is impractical because diagnosis in an individual animal is not possible at the time of the causative insult(s). Control depends on epidemiologic study (to determine the age of animals most severely affected and the time when the main insults are occurring) and on minimizing environmental risk factors that exacerbate the disease. The most important risk factors are: 1) The quantity and digestibility of the carbohydrate being fed—some carbohydrates, eg, barley and wheat, are more digestible than others, eg, corn (maize). Finely ground or moist grains are more digestible than dry, cracked grain. 2) Changes in diet—slug feeding once a day is contraindicated, and the more frequently concentrates are fed the better. Sudden changes in the diet or formulation of the diet are extremely dangerous. Component-fed cows should be given ≤7.5% of their body wt in concentrates around calving. After calving, it is safest if rations are not increased by more than 0.25 kg/day for multiparous cows and by 0.20 kg/day for primiparous cows to a maximum of 14-16 kg (30-36 lbs). 3) The quality and quantity of fiber fed—this is probably more important than the carbohydrate component of the diet. If the carbohydrate:fiber ratio is >50% carbohydrate, the animal is increasingly at risk of rumenal acidosis. If the percentage of acid detergent fiber for the complete ration is <20%, risk of ruminal acidosis also increases. If the particle length of silage is cut too short (25% cut <5 cm long), the contribution of effective fiber is reduced. If corn silage is fed, considerable care must be taken to ensure that the energy level derived from the silage is not underestimated. The energy level varies according to stage of growth when the corn was harvested and mode of conservation. The manure should not contain fiber particles >1 cm or undigested grain. Feces should not contain mucin/fibrin casts, be foamy, or contain gas bubbles. The feces in the same feeding group should not vary from firm to diarrhea. 4) The Cow Comfort Index (CCI)—this is measured 1 hr before milking as the proportion of animals standing. If the CCI is >20%, risk factors affecting cow comfort should be reviewed. These include stall size, adequacy of bedding and bunk space, placement of water sources, and alley widths sufficient to avoid congestion or queuing. Time spent ruminating should be normal; rumen stasis and hypermotility should not be detectable. 5) Lack of producer knowledge and skill—a producer is 2.5 times more likely to underestimate the incidence of lameness in a herd than a skilled observer. It is critical that producers learn to recognize the major lesions and characteristics of diseases that cause lameness and keep accurate records of the incidence and causes of lameness. 6) The availability of micronutrients from forage or pasture—this should be evaluated in herds with a lameness problem. Some minerals may be available only at marginal levels. The presence of high levels of sulfates or iron in the drinking water antagonizes the absorption of some micronutrients. 7) The level of protein, fiber, and energy content of pasture grasses—these vary considerably depending on the species of grass, the stage of its maturity, ambient temperature, and rainfall. Sudden changes in nutrient intake are seen when cattle are introduced to fresh pasture, particularly when rotational grazing is practiced. These changes can result in grass founder. Particular attention should be paid when changing from a housing system to a pastoral system and vice versa.

DISORDERS OF THE CLAW CAPSULE

Sole Ulcer
(Pododermatitis circumscripta)

A sole ulcer is a lesion located in the region of the sole/bulb junction, usually nearer the axial than abaxial margin. Damage to the dermis is associated with a circumscribed zone of localized hemorrhage and necrosis. Sole ulcers commonly affect 1 or both lateral hindclaws, predominantly in heavy, high-yielding dairy cattle kept under confined conditions. Sole ulcers are common in dairy herds in which animals are managed in loose-housing systems, particularly if conditions are unhygienic as is often the case during winter months. The incidence is variable, but in some herds, >50% of the mature cows can be affected.

Etiology and Pathogenesis: It is now believed that subclinical laminitis is a major predisposing factor. Laminitis damages horn-producing tissues, resulting in softer than normal sole horn. The horn is further softened if it is exposed to moisture, while the chemical agents in slurry are thought to disrupt the integrity of the horn. Excess wear of the softened sole horn flattens and thins the sole. Weightbearing beneath the flexor process of the distal phalanx causes the sole to squeeze the corium in the region and leads to an ischemic necrosis developing over a small area. Horn production ceases in this specific area, and as the surrounding horn continues to grow, the damaged area persists as a perforation. As the damaged corium undergoes repair, a red knob of granulation tissues erupts through the sole.

Poor claw trimming technique can also transfer pressure to the sole region beneath the flexor process. This is particularly likely if too much of the bearing edge of the abaxial wall is removed. Sometimes, displaced pads of horn move over to the vulnerable area, causing abnormal pressure onto the flexor process of the distal phalanx. Another potential cause of a sole ulcer is severe heel erosion. Normally, weight is borne by the bulb of the heel, but if heel erosion occurs, the weightbearing function is transferred forward to the region beneath the flexor process.

Clinical Findings: The progress and severity of lameness are variable and often masked in bilateral cases, depending on size of the lesion and extent of the secondary infection. Because the lateral digit is usually involved, the limb is often held slightly abducted with weight bearing on the unaffected medial digit. In tie stalls, the hind toes may be rested on the edge of a curb in an attempt to relieve pressure on the heel-sole junction. On flat surfaces, an affected animal stands with the hindlimbs camped back. Some cows may shake the affected foot frequently, and those with bilateral lesions may continually shift weight from limb to limb and frequently lie down.

Grossly, the lesion varies from a soft, slightly discolored area that may be painful under pressure to an obvious circumscribed perforation. This is often the stage at which the lameness becomes severe enough to be noticed. In later stages, granulation tissue protrudes through the sole defect. Infection of the exposed corium may cause varying degrees of separation of the sole. Once the corium is exposed, infection can invade the deeper structures of the claw and spread proximally to involve the navicular bursa, resulting in necrosis of the flexor tendon and ligaments of the navicular bone. A retroarticular abscess may develop, which may be further complicated by infection of the distal interphalangeal joint. Rupture of the flexor tendon leads to dorsal rotation (upward) of the toe ("cocked toe"). In complicated cases, infection may progress up the deep flexor tendon sheath.

Treatment: Treatment is aimed at removing pressure from the affected area. Skillful therapeutic claw trimming is highly effective. This procedure lowers the entire bearing surface of the lateral claw, which transfers weight bearing to the sound medial claw. Applying a "lift" has become the accepted treatment for this condition. The simplest form of lift is a wooden or rubber block that is glued or nailed to the unaffected medial claw, thereby removing all weight bearing from the ulcer region. Recently, various models of easier-to-apply plastic slippers have been developed. Care must be taken when applying either a block or a slipper to avoid the sharp hard rear edge of the device from causing pressure under the sole. Blocks should be removed after ~1 mo to avoid causing damage to the sole.

Protruding granulation tissue should not be excised or treated with any caustic agent, as this can retard healing. Bandages should not be applied because this results in continued weight bearing at the ulcer site; furthermore, covering the lesion causes it to remain moist and promotes maceration and bacterial infection.

Many ulcers never fully resolve; and affected cows may have chronic low-grade lameness and need corrective foot trimming 2-4 times/yr for their productive lives.

Prevention and Control: Because the development of sole ulcers is intimately related to subclinical laminitis, the latter should be investigated and appropriate control measures instituted.

White Line Disease

White line disease is characterized by the separation (avulsion) of the fibrous junction between the sole and wall on the abaxial border of the sole at the heel-sole junction. The corium becomes infected through this opening and tracks of infection may localize as an abscess or may penetrate deeper to form a retroarticular abscess. White line disease is a major cause of lameness, particularly when cattle are housed and fed concentrates. The incidence in multiparous cows can be as high as 35%.

Etiology and Pathogenesis: The white line is as deep as the contiguous sole and is the softest part of the horn capsule. It is composed of extensions of the lamellae around which a keratinous matrix is formed. Exposure to moisture softens the zone still further. Rupture of the white line is exacerbated by the impact of locomotion, particularly among animals housed on concrete. The abaxial region of the wall of the hindlimb is the area of the claw that absorbs concussion first and in which horn growth and wear is maximal.

Solid foreign bodies may lodge in the softened, widened zone. They may push through to the corium beneath and introduce infection; however, the presence of a foreign body is not essential for the lesion to develop. There are 3 possible sequelae of localized infection: 1) a localized abscess may develop; 2) infection may be forced proximally along the spaces between the lamellae to form a track that may discharge at the coronary band; 3) the infected track may, as it forces its way proximally, infect other structures, depending on the site of the initial infection. The most anterior tracks can infect the distal interphalangeal joint directly. Tracks forming closer to the heel are likely to cause infection of the bursa of the deep flexor tendon. Invariably, the bursa ruptures into the retroarticular space, and an abscess develops in this location. Infection of the distal interphalangeal joint and the tendon sheath of the deep flexor tendon may follow. Necrosis and avulsion of the insertion of the deep flexor tendon into the distal phalanx is a frequent complication.

When this condition is associated with subclinical laminitis, the first indication may be hemorrhage into the white line, which may become apparent ~10 wk after calving.

Clinical Findings: The lateral claw of the hindfoot (often both) is usually involved. If bilateral, the disease may remain unnoticed until lameness is more pronounced in one limb than the other. Because the outer hindclaw is affected, the limb is swung away from the body during each stride. The animal may stand with the medial claw bearing weight.

White line separation without complications is frequently seen at claw trimming. The degree of pain and lameness depends on the rate of development and extent of the sub-solar abscess. Routine examination of the sole must include the complete exploration of the abaxial white line region. Black marks must be explored with the tip of a hoof knife as potential sites for track formation. Discharge of pus from the skin/horn junction above the abaxial wall is always reason to suspect a white line lesion. In these cases, the white line must always be examined very carefully.

Swelling of the heel bulb represents the most advanced form of this condition; it is frequently misdiagnosed as footrot (often presented as a case of footrot that is resistant to treatment). Footrot causes the foot to swell evenly to the fetlock; in contrast, a ret-roarticular abscess leads to enlargement of only one heel bulb.

When the deep flexor tendon is infected (and becomes necrotic), the insertion of the tendon into the distal phalanx usually avulses, and the toe of the affected digit hyperex-tends with each step and eventually ankyloses in a "cocked-up" position.

Treatment: For a local abscess, removal of an elliptical segment of the wall adjacent to the lesion aids free drainage by providing a self-cleansing abaxial opening.

Abscessation with sinus formation at the coronary band requires the removal of a segment of the abaxial wall (~0.75 cm wide) from the white line to the coronary band. This procedure is best performed with the cutting disc of a grinding tool under local anesthesia. Often, a plug of necrotic debris is found in the track.

Retroarticular abscesses are usually quite large and surrounded by a mass of fi-broelastic tissue that inhibits drainage. Drainage is accomplished by passing a probe through the abscess from the lesion on the abaxial wall until it can be palpated under the skin on the axial surface of the bulb. An incision is made onto the probe and a drainage tube is drawn through the abscess. Continuous irrigation of the lesion for several days with saline is indicated. The application of a lift to the sound claw is helpful, as is com-plete immobilization of the digit. Immobilization of the joint reduces the risk of perma-nent deformity due to avulsion of the deep flexor tendon.

Toe Ulcer

A toe ulcer is a hemorrhage or separation of the white line in the toe region. This lesion is being reported more frequently now than 5 yr ago. It is generally thought to be associated with subclinical laminitis.

Etiology and Pathogenesis: This phenomenon probably results from congestion of the circumferential artery in the toe after sudden introduction to high-energy feed. The increased intraungular pressure is believed to cause depression of the distal phalanx and rupture of the white line in the toe. Many animals with a rotated digit also have a ridge (the reaction ridge) running around the wall. The ridge is similar in location to a hardship groove and is displaced distally in a similar manner. Osteomyelitis of the distal phalanx can be seen in complicated cases.

Clinical Findings: In many cases, the white line in the toe region may be stained with serum or blood. In more advanced cases, a prolapse of the sole may occur with associ-ated infection.

Treatment and Control: If perforation at the toe has occurred, the longterm progno-sis is poor. However, if treatment is attempted, aggressive systemic antibiotic therapy should be instituted immediately. The lesion should be packed with a hygroscopic mix-ture (50% magnesium sulfate and 50% glycerin) and left bandaged for a maximum of 24 hr. The lesion should be thoroughly dried, dressed with antibiotic powder, and closed with methyl methacrylate. A block should be applied to the unaffected claw to relieve undue flexor influence on the rotated phalanx. If there is evidence of sloughing of black necrotic tissue, the apex of the toe can be amputated to remove dead tissue and bone. After a few days of topical and systemic antibiotic therapy, the wound can be closed with methyl methacrylate.

Control of subclinical laminitis is likely to lower the incidence of toe ulcer.

Toe Abscess

Toe abscess is similar clinically to toe ulcer but is seen in yearling calves soon after they enter the feedlot. The cause is unclear but may be related to aggressive handling of excitable animals that causes them to abrade the tips of their claws during procedures such as being loaded into a wagon. Recent evidence suggests that this lesion has a laminitis-like etiology. For this reason, it would be prudent to explore nutritional causes.

Treatment has so far been reported to be unsuccessful. Many cases become recumbent and succumb to conditions such as pneumonia. Control measures should concentrate on reducing stress during transportation and providing stringent measures to acclimate the animals to nutritional changes.

Double Sole

In a double sole, a superficial sole is separated by a space from a second sole that is attached directly to the dermis.

Etiology and Pathogenesis: A double sole may result from a short-term nutritional insult. A sudden disturbance in the microcirculation of the dermis probably results in an effusion of serum that separates the dermis from the epidermis. Double sole has been seen in animals suddenly changed from a mainly forage diet to one rich in concentrates and in beef cattle turned out in the spring on lush grass after a winter ration of forage. The etiology is similar to that causing toe ulcer or digit rotation, but it is not known why one manifestation is seen in one group of animals and a different one in another group. Double sole can be confused with underrunning of the heel, which has a traumatic etiology (*see* FOREIGN BODIES IN THE SOLE, below).

Treatment and Control: Treatment is simple unless mismanaged. The abaxial wall must remain completely intact and only a portion (≤30%) of the sole covering the bulb cut away. The sole beneath is extremely soft and vulnerable to damage; therefore, the animal should be confined to a well-strawed loose stall until the new horn has hardened, after which more of the sole may be removed.

Sudden changes in the quality of the forage should be avoided. Double sole has been observed after feeding moldy hay.

Foreign Bodies in the Sole

Occasionally, a foreign body such as a stone, chip of glass, or nail becomes embedded in the sole. Even if the material does not penetrate to the corium, localized pressure causes pain and lameness. Removal of the foreign body usually resolves the lameness without incident.

If the foreign body penetrates through to the corium, infection is introduced to the dermal level and an abscess develops. The rapidity of onset and severity of the lameness depends to some extent on the location of the sole penetration.

In the apical and subapical region, the abscess is located between the distal phalanx and the nonresilient sole. As the abscess develops, interungular pressure increases rapidly. Thus, the onset of lameness is rapid and the degree of pain very severe. Acute lameness may cause the animal to stand with the foot off the ground or with the toe lightly touching. A differential diagnosis is fracture of the distal phalanx.

Treatment consists of removing the foreign body and coring out the track to the corium with a fine-pointed hoof knife. Creating a large hole is inappropriate. Pus is often released under considerable pressure. Antibiotic should be squeezed into the cavity, which closes rapidly. The opening should not be plugged but covered with elastic waterproof material to prevent blockage with mud or manure.

In the sub-bulbar region, the corium is located between the digital cushion (a flexible structure) and the soft resilient horn of the bulb.

The onset of lameness is relatively slow, and the pain generated is significant but not severe. The pus in the abscess tends to spread over a wide area through the fascial plane and to cause separation of the skin-horn junction at the heel. A moist discharge from this area may be the first indication of the lesion. This is referred to as **underrunning of the heel**, a condition that can be confused with double sole.

Treatment consists of removing the foreign body if still present. The detached horn should not be stripped off in its entirety. Part of the detached horn may be removed, but the abaxial wall must be left intact to bear weight and spare the exposed newly forming sole. Bandaging may not be required, but the animal should be housed in a well-strawed area for a few days.

Sandcracks
(Vertical fissures)

Sandcracks are vertical fissures or cracks in the wall of the claw. They account for ~0.2% of lesions of the claws of dairy cows. In western Canada, the average incidence in mature beef cows is ~20%. In individual herds, the incidence can be as high as 60%. No breed differences have been recorded.

Etiology: The etiology remains uncertain. Most fissures develop in the front outside claw. The incidence is highest in mature, heavy cows.

Sandcracks are classified into 5 types. Type I fissures are confined to the coronary band and are mostly caused by traumatic injury. Type II fissures run from the coronary band to the center of the dorsal wall, and type III fissures involve the whole of the wall. Types II and III sandcracks are frequently associated with horizontal fissures (*see* below). A horizontal fissure becomes a point of structural weakness around which the claw will bend once it has grown to a point halfway between the coronary band and the apex of the toe. The stability of the wall is compromised, and vertical fissures apparently result from mechanical stress. Type IV fissures are quite rare. They run from the center of the wall to the bearing surface and probably represent the resolving stages of type II or III fissures. Type V fissures involve only the central region of the claw.

Treatment: Most sandcracks are not painful and require no treatment. However, if the origin of the lameness can be traced to a claw in which a sandcrack is present, routine treatment of the crack is appropriate.

Type I fissures are dangerous only if they are located on the coronary band abaxial to the extensor process of the distal phalanx. At this location, the dorsal pouch of the distal interphalangeal joint lies immediately beneath. If such a fissure is infected, the risk of a septic joint is considerable. In these cases, a small segment of horn should be dissected from either side of the fissure, and the cavity dressed with antibiotic powder. A tightly rolled gauze bandage should be applied to the wound and held in place with a 1 in. (2.5 cm) adhesive bandage applied around the coronary band.

Types II and III fissures often have ragged edges that may be twisted and gape open. Cosmetic treatment may be requested in the case of show animals. The axial wall at the tip of the claw should be cut back so that the weight is borne only by the abaxial portion of the wall. The ragged edges of the fissure should be trimmed, ideally with the cutting disk of a grinding tool. In selected cases, a fissure can be immobilized with an application of methyl methacrylate after the 2 edges of the fissure have been laced together with steel wire.

Horizontal Fissures

Horizontal fissures result from disruption of horn production at the dermis beneath the coronary band, leading to a defect in the integrity of the wall. These fissures run parallel to the coronary band. The defect varies in severity from a shallow groove (hardship groove) to a complete fracture (fissure) of the wall. A comparable anomaly is seen as a band of horn differing in appearance from the remainder of the claw. One form of the band is seen in animals stressed following weaning (weaning groove) or during a period of nutritional deprivation. The fissure moves distally as the claw grows, and the distal portion becomes progressively more mobile (thimble) until it fractures, leaving a "broken toe." A series of grooves can destabilize the vertical strength of the dorsal wall causing it to bend (buckled toe).

Etiology: Fissures are believed to be caused by a wide variety of stressors, including an acute febrile disease or a sudden, relatively short-term but significant change in nutrition (*see also* LAMINITIS, p 873).

Clinical Findings: The horizontal groove or fissure is an important indicator of metabolic disturbance. The date on which the causal insult occurred can be calculated by measuring the distance from the hair line to the fissure and dividing that number by the growth rate of the claw. In mature dairy cows, the rate of growth of the wall measured along the dorsal flexure of the claw is ~0.5 cm/mo. Growth rates are more rapid in young animals, in animals on intensive feed, and during the summer months.

Treatment: Most cases require no treatment. Very deep fissures may eventually result in the formation of a thimble, which is extremely painful. In these cases, the loose horn should be removed with pincers; regional anesthesia may be needed.

Corkscrew Claw

A corkscrew claw is twisted throughout its length in a configuration that displaces the abaxial wall 360°. One or both lateral hindclaws may be affected in cows >4 yr old. Although corkscrew claws are rarely seen in bulls, many believe there is a heritable component.

Bone molding is seen in the distal and intermediate phalanges, but it is not known if this is a matter of cause or effect. Periarticular exostoses develop around the distal interphalangeal joint. Pressure from the exostosis on the dermis of the wall may account for the excessive growth of the wall.

Correctly trimming a corkscrew claw requires much skill. The horn formation is extremely hard and difficult to cut. The abnormally narrow shape of the distal phalanx makes it difficult to pare the claw without causing bleeding at the toe. The strategy is to shorten the claw as much as possible without causing bleeding. Next, the horn wall that is displaced beneath the claw is cut away. Then, so far as is possible, the horn is shaped to approximate normal. Trimming helps the animal get around for a while but does not "cure" the condition, and affected animals should ultimately be culled.

Slipper Foot

A slipper foot is named for its alleged likeness to a Persian slipper. The claw is flat and curled upward to form a square end. The horn is heavily ridged and has lost its shine, and the coronary band is rougher and darker than normal. Although there is no objective evidence to support the theory, the slipper foot is probably synonymous with chronic laminitis and may be a sequela of either acute or subclinical laminitis. Treatment is always disappointing. The claw can be shaped to approximate normal, but invariably it collapses and serious sequelae follow. Animals with slipper foot should be culled as soon as economically appropriate.

Heel Erosion

Heel erosion is an aberration in the appearance of the surface of the bulb of the heel. The prevalence of heel horn erosion ("slurry heel") is highest during the winter, particularly when the claws are exposed to an unhygienic, moist environment (such as exists in intensively managed dairy units). Because heel erosion does not cause lameness per se, the true incidence is unknown. However, subjective observations suggest that once cows have been exposed to copious slurry, the incidence of heel erosion rapidly approaches 100%. In some animals, heel erosion advances to a point at which complications develop and lameness may be apparent.

Etiology and Pathogenesis: Heel erosion can manifest in several forms, depending on the relative significance of several factors. Therefore, the etiology is complex and best considered as occurring in phases, within which one or more separate processes may be active.

In intensively managed herds, in which subclinical laminitis is often present, the soft horn covering the bulb becomes vulnerable to direct bacterial attack. This may account for the pitted appearance of some claws. Hemorrhagic layers in the sole terminate in concentric grooves that form around the bulbs, and bacterial invasion into these grooves results in massive destruction of the horn of the heel. In some cases, ridges, layers, and deep grooves are seen in the heels.

Claws exposed to slurry appear to have a higher incidence of erosions than those that are kept clean and dry. Moisture undoubtedly softens horns, and slurry contains a huge bacterial burden as well as an undetermined number of irritants.

In the secondary phase, it is thought that the distribution of weightbearing changes as the result of heel horn loss. This in turn causes an increase in the rate of horn produced beneath the heel. The excessive horn growth is often more pronounced in the lateral claw and causes the hock to turn in (cow-hocked stance). This stance resolves after correct therapeutic claw trimming. Generally, the condition is progressive unless corrected. The disturbance interferes with shock absorption, and the animal throws more and more weight further forward. A common concurrent lesion is a sole ulcer.

Clinical Findings: Lameness is not obvious until the destructive phase is advanced. The most typical lesions are the deep, black V and the concentric grooves. In the secondary phase, the appearance of the heel can be quite variable. Loss of horn tends to be greatest in the axial part of the bulbs, which can appear to be completely denuded of horn.

Treatment and Control: Both heels should be reduced to the same height by paring away excess horn. Careful attention must be paid to maintaining the bearing function of the abaxial wall and sloping the sole toward the axial border.

Attention to hygiene and the reduction of slurry is essential. The claws of dairy cows should be trimmed regularly, and a weekly footbath (where permitted, 3-5% formalin), starting no later than October in the northern hemisphere, provided.

DISORDERS OF THE INTERDIGITAL SPACE

The digital lesions of foot-and-mouth disease can, in some instances, be confused with other diseases causing lesions of the interdigital space (*see* FOOT-AND-MOUTH DISEASE, p 507; VESICULAR STOMATITIS, p 555).

Footrot
(Interdigital phlegmon, Foul in the foot)

Footrot is a subacute or acute necrotic infection originating from a lesion in the interdigital skin that leads to a cellulitis in the digital region. Pain, severe lameness, fever, anorexia, loss of condition, and reduced milk production are major signs of the disease. Footrot has a worldwide distribution and is usually sporadic but may be endemic in intensive beef or dairy cattle production units. The incidence varies according to weather, season of year, grazing periods, and housing system. On average, footrot accounts for ~15% of claw diseases.

Etiology and Pathogenesis: Injury to the interdigital skin provides a portal of entry for infection. Maceration of the skin by water, feces, and urine may predispose to injuries. *Fusobacterium necrophorum* is considered to be the major cause of footrot. It can be isolated from feces, which may explain why control is difficult. Other organisms, such as *Staphylococcus aureus*, *Escherichia coli*, *Arcanobacterium (Actinomyces) pyogenes*, and possibly *Bacteroides melaninogenicus*, can also be involved.

Clinical Findings: The fore- or, more commonly, the hindlimbs can be affected, but more than one foot is rarely involved at the same time in mature cows. However, footrot can occasionally develop in several feet in calves. The first sign is swelling and erythema of the soft tissues of the interdigital space and the adjacent coronary band. The inflammation may extend to the pastern and fetlock. Typically, the claws are markedly separated, and the inflammatory edema is uniformly distributed between the 2 digits. The onset of the disease is rapid, and the extreme pain leads to increasing lameness. In severe cases, the animal is reluctant to bear weight on the affected foot. Fever and anorexia are seen. The skin of the interdigital space first appears discolored; later, it fragments with exudate production. As necrosis of the skin progresses, sloughing of tissue is likely to follow. A characteristic foul odor is produced.

If the disease proceeds unchecked, weight loss is severe and milk yield is significantly reduced. Milk production may not recover during the current lactation. Open lesions can be infected with secondary invaders. If the necrotic lesion is located in the anterior region of the interdigital space, the distal interphalangeal joint can become infected because of its proximity.

Hematogenous infection of the tissues of the interdigital space may account for peracute cases of footrot, which are referred to as either "blind" or "super foul." This form of footrot is characterized by the initial absence of a skin lesion, extreme pain, and the tendency to progress despite aggressive therapy.

Diagnosis: It is frequently assumed that every cow with a swollen foot has footrot. However, many other conditions, such as infected sandcracks, white line disease, retroarticular abscesses, foreign bodies in the interdigital space, and infection of the distal interphalangeal joint can have a similar appearance if viewed from a distance. Despite the difficulties encountered in lifting a hindlimb, a detailed examination should be performed in every case. An incorrect diagnosis can have disastrous results.

Treatment: Most treated animals recover in a few days. Good results are obtained with penicillin G, IM, for 3 days. Treatment should be administered as soon as signs are observed. However, the label dosage may be inadequate to effect a rapid resolution, and increased dosages may be needed, requiring increased withdrawal times. Treatment of "super foul" must be particularly aggressive. Early cases respond well to single doses of long-acting oxytetracycline.

Sodium sulfadimidine solution IV or trimethoprim/sulfadoxine IV or IM, BID for 3 days, can also be used. A single oral administration of a long-acting bolus containing baquiloprim/sulfadimidine may be suitable for treating beef cattle.

High concentration of an agent in the target tissues can be achieved by a regional IV injection. Positive results have been obtained with penicillin or oxytetracycline.

Local treatment is essential for some longstanding cases and in all instances in which the anterior region of the interdigital space has been compromised. The animal must be adequately restrained and the lesion cleansed. It is inadvisable to curette or otherwise remove necrotic tissue surgically. The dorsal pouch of the distal phalangeal joint is very superficial at this point. A nonirritant bacteriostatic agent (such as nitrofurazone or a sulfa preparation) should be applied as a topical dressing. The application of gauze, cotton batting, or bandages is contraindicated. However, the lesion can be protected and immobilized by binding the digits together with a bandage. The entire digital region can be protected from contamination if it is enclosed in a plastic bag that is fixed in place with an adhesive bandage. However, prolonged protection is not advocated because the enclosed lesion tends to macerate further. Bandages, if used, should be replaced daily.

Prevention and Control: Animals that are actively shedding infectious organisms should be isolated until signs of lameness have disappeared. If this is not possible, a waterproof dressing or protective boot should be applied; however, animals wearing protective boots should be monitored carefully to avoid additional damage. Boots should be disinfected between use.

Because busy traffic areas are invariably heavily contaminated, steps should be taken to ensure that areas around drinking troughs, gateways, and tracks are adequately drained. Animals at pasture might be moved to a clean, dry area, or possibly housed during periods of heavy rainfall. Contaminated concrete must be frequently cleaned and scraped free of manure.

Preventive use of a footbath with an antiseptic and astringent solution (eg, copper or zinc sulfate [7-10% in water]) has given beneficial results. Formaldehyde solution (3-5% in water) can also be used, but in some areas it is considered to be an environmental hazard if discharged into natural waterways.

Ethylenediamine dihydroiodide has been used as a feed supplement for prevention, but the results are extremely uncertain. Vaccines against *F necrophorum* have failed because of the weak immune response to the bacterium. High levels of zinc fed as a supplement have a beneficial effect by improving epidermal resistance to bacterial invaders.

Interdigital Dermatitis
(Stable footrot, Slurry heel, Scald)

Interdigital dermatitis is a low-grade infection of the interdigital epidermis that causes a slow erosion of the skin with discomfort but no lameness unless the lesion becomes complicated. It is seen worldwide but is most prevalent under poor hygienic conditions in intensive dairy production. Morbidity is usually high in housed animals, particularly toward the end of the winter. When animals in such herds are examined, it is not unusual for 100% to have lesions of varying degrees of severity. The prevalence of heel horn erosion may increase in herds that have a high prevalence of interdigital dermatitis, suggesting a close relationship between the 2 diseases.

In tied systems, the hindlegs are affected more often than the forelegs. In loose housing systems, the distribution between fore- and hindlegs is about equal. Animals on slatted floors are affected less often than animals on solid floors.

Etiology and Pathogenesis: Interdigital dermatitis is caused by a mixed bacterial infection, but *Dichelobacter nodosus* has been considered to be the most active component. The disease is most commonly seen when humidity is high, in temperate climates, and under poor hygienic conditions, especially in housed dairy cattle. The source of the infection is the cow itself, and the infection spreads from infected to noninfected animals through the environment. *D nodosus* cannot survive >4 days on the ground but can persist in filth that is caked onto the claws. The bacteria invade the epidermis, but the organisms do not penetrate to the dermal layers. As the condition progresses, the border between the skin and soft heel horn disintegrates, producing lesions similar to ulcers or erosions. At this stage, the lesions cause discomfort.

Clinical Findings: The first stage of the condition appears to be an exudative dermatitis. The exudate oozes to the commissures of the interdigital space and forms a crust or scab, which may be observed occasionally on the dorsal surface of the digits. As the condition progresses, the animal shows discomfort by "paddling," ie, constantly moving from one foot to the other. If the heels of the hindfeet are especially painful, the limbs are held further back than normal. True lameness does not develop until a complicating lesion is present. After a prolonged period, during which the animal has avoided bearing weight on the heel, the horn beneath the heel increases in thickness and some aberrations of gait result. In dairy cows, interdigital hyperplasia (corns, fibroma) may be caused by the chronic irritation of the interdigital space. Often, the fibroma develops on one side of the interdigital space.

The primary differential diagnosis is digital dermatitis (*see* below). The most obvious differences between the 2 diseases are the clinical signs and the highly contagious nature of digital dermatitis. Some systemic viral infections (foot-and-mouth disease, mucosal disease, and malignant catarrhal fever) also give rise to local lesions resembling those of interdigital dermatitis.

Treatment: Systemic therapy, including the use of antibiotics, is not cost effective. In severe cases, the lesions should be cleaned and dried, after which a topical bacteriostatic agent is applied, eg, a 50% mixture of sulfamethazine powder and anhydrous copper sulfate. Alternatively, an animal can be confined in a footbath for 1 hr, BID for 3 days.

Control: Good management and housing systems to keep claws dry and clean are most important. Regular foot trimming helps avoid complications. Foot bathing, beginning in late fall and before clinical cases can be identified during high-risk periods, is essential in herds known to be infected. Weekly foot bathing may be sufficient in the late fall, but the frequency may have to be increased in late winter.

Digital Dermatitis
(Hairy warts, Papillomatous digital dermatitis)

Digital dermatitis is a highly contagious, erosive, and proliferative infection of the epidermis proximal to the skin-horn junction in the flexor region of the interdigital space. Morbidity within a herd can be >90%. It can affect any breed or age group, although young animals with a poor immune response are most susceptible. It spreads rapidly from newly acquired animals, or it may be introduced by any mechanical vector, eg, boots or hoof trimming instruments.

The condition was first seen in European countries, but during the last decade it has spread across the dairy-producing areas of the USA. The incidence in beef cattle appears to be minimal. The incidence is highest in loose-housed herds that are not kept clean. The prevalence is highest in the fall and winter and is lowest if the animals are pastured.

Etiology and Pathogenesis: Two main types of lesions are seen, one is erosive/reactive, the other is proliferative or wart-like. Both forms cause varying degrees of discomfort and may give rise to severe lameness. Sometimes, one particular form predominates in one area, but both forms can be seen in the same animal. The 2 forms likely represent different stages of the disease process. Some of the variation may be due to concurrent interdigital dermatitis (*see* above).

Deep in the epidermis of erosive/reactive lesions, 2 types of spirochetes can be demonstrated using Warthin-Starry stain. One is a long, spiral, filamentous organism 12×0.3 μm, and the other is a shorter, thicker spirochete $5\text{-}6 \times 0.1$ μm. However, it is thought that there is a multifactorial etiology with multiple organisms involved. *Dichelobacter nodosus* is likely to be implicated. Strong circumstantial evidence suggests that a virus plays a part in the pathogenesis of the disease, but to date, none has been isolated.

Clinical Findings: Lesions are most common in the region of the flexor commissure of the interdigital space. Less typically, lesions have been seen on the dorsal surface of the foot as well as around the dewclaws. One or both hindfeet are most commonly involved, although both hind- and forefeet can be affected.

Small, early lesions are clearly separated from surrounding healthy skin and are very similar in appearance to early digital dermatitis lesions. They develop into a round or oval lesion ~0.5-2.0 cm in diameter. The surface of the lesion may be flat or concave, raw, moist, and red, yellow, or gray with a finely tufted or granular surface. As it develops, the lesion is often referred to as "strawberrylike" and may be surrounded by a "halo" of white tissue. Mature lesions are usually raised by as much as 2-4 cm, with the surface covered by gray, brown, or black hair-like papillary growths. The lesions are usually extremely tender to the touch. An affected animal may hold its foot off the ground or walk on its toes.

Digital dermatitis is distinctly different in appearance from footrot because swelling and fever are normally absent.

Treatment: Herd outbreaks are best treated with a footbath containing oxytetracycline or lincomycin-spectinomycin. For optimal effect, the heels of the cows should be washed thoroughly before entering the footbath. Repeat treatments may be needed after 4-6 wk, depending on the extent of the environmental challenge. Results of footbaths containing copper sulfate, zinc sulfate, or formalin have been poor to inconclusive. However, these footbaths may have a beneficial effect in reducing the prevalence of interdigital dermatitis, thus decreasing the susceptibility for digital dermatitis.

In advanced cases, individual treatment is necessary. The foot, especially the interdigital area, should be thoroughly cleansed to remove the prolific population of spirochetes. A single dressing of 36% muriatic acid can be applied carefully to the infected tissue and protected by a waterproof bandage. Repeated dressing with the caustic preparation is not advisable.

Topical dressing of the lesion and surrounding surfaces with soluble oxytetracycline or lincomycin-spectinomycin (66 g and 132 g/L of water, respectively) produces the best results. More than 1 treatment will probably be necessary. Topical dressings should be protected by waterproof bandages or a reinforced nylon device that can be affixed with Velcro® closures. Oxytetracyline treatment has not resulted in detectable residual levels of the antibiotic in blood or milk. Extremely high parenteral antibiotic doses have been reported to help resolve severe lesions.

Topical sprays can be applied when the cows are recumbent. The nozzle of the wand of a portable unit can be applied directly to the lesion. This is a useful followup technique to either foot bathing or direct application of medication. With extreme care, formalin may also be used to reinforce antibiotic therapy.

Control: Digital dermatitis is exacerbated by filthy, wet conditions. Slurry removal and improved standards of hygiene are essential for control. In herds in which this condition is not a problem, animals should be isolated for 1 mo before being added to the herd. Effective vaccines are not available.

Interdigital Hyperplasia
(Corns)

Interdigital hyperplasia is a firm, tumor-like mass located in the interdigital space. It is not common, except in certain breeds (eg, Herefords, in which it is considered to be heritable).

Etiology and Pathogenesis: In heavy beef breeds, the condition is thought to result from stretching of the insertions of the distal interphalangeal ligament. The claws splay, and the interdigital skin is stretched. When not involved in weight bearing, the skin folds outward and subcutaneous scar tissue develops. In these cases, the mass tends to develop in the axis of the interdigital space. The mass may become so large that it touches the ground and may become necrotic. In dairy cows, in which the feet are continually exposed to slurry, chronic irritation or dermatitis in the interdigital region is seen, which accounts for the development of masses close to the skin line on the dorsal commisure of the space.

Clinical Findings: Interdigital hyperplasia can be found in one or more limbs, although hindlimbs tend to be affected more frequently than forelimbs. Lameness results more often than not. As the lesion becomes larger, its surface may become excoriated, sore, and infected.

Treatment: In simple cases, treatment may be unnecessary. For surgical removal, the animal should be sedated, and dorsal and flexor regional nerve blocks performed. Surgery can be performed with the animal standing or in lateral recumbency. After preparation of the surgical site, a tourniquet is applied and the claws separated manually or with retractors. The mass is removed, leaving as much of the interdigital skin as possible. If any fat protrudes when the claws are pressed together, it should be removed. Care must be taken to avoid cutting deep structures such as the distal interphalangeal ligament. After surgery, the wound should be dressed with an antibiotic powder and the claws bandaged closely together. Some field reports suggest considerable success with wiring the toe together. Movement of the wound or separation of the claws must be avoided until ~10 days after surgery. Cryosurgery is also an option.

DISORDERS OF THE BONES AND JOINTS

Ankylosing Spondylosis

In ankylosing spondylosis, exostoses develop on the ligament of the ventral aspect of the lumbar vertebrae, primarily in older bulls. Fracture of the exostosis and associated vertebrae causes pressure on the spinal cord, which results in severe ataxia or paralysis. There is no treatment.

Degenerative Arthropathy

This nonspecific condition affecting mainly the hip and stifle is characterized by degeneration of articular cartilage and eburnation of subchondral bone, joint effusion, fibrosis with calcification of the joint capsule, and osteophytes.

Etiology: Many causes and predisposing factors probably influence the development, age of onset, and severity. Inherited predisposition to degenerative arthropathy is a factor. Certain conformations, eg, straight hocks in beef bulls, are incriminated. Joint instability after trauma is a common cause. Nutritional factors involved in some cases are rations high in phosphorus and low in calcium, which probably influence the strength of subchondral bone. Copper deficiency or fluoride poisoning also may act similarly. Forced traction of a calf in breech presentation can impede the blood supply to the hip joint, and arthritis may result. The role of infection is unclear. Infectious arthritis in calves usually produces severe changes in the hock, but degenerative arthropathy rarely involves this joint.

Bulls fed high-grain diets for show may become lame when as young as 6-12 mo, but most cases are first noticed at 1-2 yr.

Clinical Findings: Onset is gradual, and both hip joints are usually affected; stifle involvement is rare. Signs progress concomitantly with degeneration of cartilage and development of osteophytes. Lameness to the point of incapacitation, with crepitation of degenerate joints, may develop in a few months; however, correlation between pathologic changes and clinical signs is poor. The earliest changes occur in the acetabulum and on the dorsomedial surface of the femoral head.

In cows, the stifle is affected most often, and the medial condyle of the femur shows the earliest changes. Onset of signs is later than in bulls, usually seen in adults. Because degenerative arthropathy may result from any of several initiating factors, a specific diagnosis may be difficult. Radiographic, cytologic, and microbiologic evaluation of the synovial fluid are useful diagnostic aids. Arthroscopy of articular surfaces and ligaments may help attain a definitive diagnosis and prognosis.

Treatment: Changes in the joints are usually irreversible by the time of diagnosis. Palliative treatment in valuable breeding animals should be undertaken with the knowledge that the condition or predisposing factors may be inherited. The diet should be carefully analyzed and, if necessary, corrected. This is especially important in fast-growing animals, in which adequate exercise is indicated and overfinishing should be avoided.

Dislocations

Coxofemoral Luxation: Luxation of the coxofemoral joint is usually upward. It is seen in bulls serving cows confined on a slippery surface and in cows riding each other. The affected limb appears shorter than the contralateral limb. The hock is turned inward and, when trying to walk, the animal appears to be dragging one foot behind the other.

Resolution is possible, provided that the head of the femur or the rim of the acetabulum has not been fractured. The animal should be deeply sedated to the level of recumbency. A rope should be looped around the groin of the affected limb, which should be uppermost. The free ends of the rope should be tied around a tree or some other fixed object, and traction should be applied to forcibly extend the limb. Downward pressure should be applied to the hock, which should be strongly rotated outward (upward) until the head of the femur slips back into the acetabulum. Traction should be applied at several angles until the head of the femur clicks back into the acetabulum. If the head of the femur or the rim of the acetabulum is fractured, there will be considerable crepitation and the limb will displace as soon as traction is stopped.

Patellar Luxation: Intermittent fixation of the patella on the upper part of the femoral trochlea results in a characteristic jerky action of one or both hindlimbs. The limb remains in caudal extension for a longer period than normal and may even be dragged for a few steps before clicking forward to a normal posture. In young animals, the condition may resolve spontaneously. For luxations that do not resolve, medial patellar desmotomy should be performed.

Dislocation of the Fetlock: This is seen frequently in young cattle when they cross cattle guards (grillwork laid over a pit as a gate substitute). Tranquilization or light anesthesia facilitates replacement of dislocated structures. A padded fiberglass cast maintained in place for 3 wk usually promotes a satisfactory recovery.

Hip Dysplasia: This bilateral malformation of the hip joint is often associated with secondary osteoarthritis. It may be present at birth. However, abnormal gait may develop in rapidly growing animals. Usually, it is possible to rock the hindquarter to produce a click as the head of the femur pops in or out. Radiography may confirm the diagnosis in young animals. There is no treatment.

Fractures

Bone fractures occur in cattle of all ages, but they are most common in those <1 yr old. Corrective procedures may be justified economically in this age group, provided that joints are not involved. External fixation techniques or Thomas splints have been used successfully. In selected cases, percutaneous transfixation or internal fixation may be attempted.

Fractures of major long bones in adult cattle usually are not treated. The tuber coxae may fracture when cattle are hurried through narrow doorways. In these cases, spicules of bone may penetrate the skin, or unsightly distortions of the flank can result. Fractures of the proximal and intermediate phalanges may be considered for treatment in tractable, young adult cattle.

Fracture of the distal phalanx is relatively common in adult cattle. Onset of lameness is rapid, and the pain is usually severe. If the medial digit is involved, the animal may seek relief from the pain by crossing its legs. Natural recovery is prolonged, and because most such fractures extend into the distal interphalangeal joint, a debilitating arthritis may develop at the fracture site. If treatment is undertaken, the sound digit should be elevated on a wooden block, and the affected digit immobilized in a flexed position to the block using methyl methacrylate adhesive.

The risk of fractures is minimized if the most common causes are avoided. Slippery surfaces are hazardous, particularly to animals in estrus. Narrow doorways should be widened so that several animals can pass through them.

Septic Arthritis of the Distal Interphalangeal Joint

Etiology: Infection enters the distal interphalangeal joint via 3 possible main sites: 1) the dorsal commissure of the interdigital space, via penetrating trauma or complicated footrot (interdigital phlegmon); 2) sandcracks; or 3) white line disease or retroarticular abscess.

Clinical Findings: Most frequently, one of the causal lesions is present and the transition from the initial lesion to the joint infection is readily apparent. However, when a swollen foot is treated before the cause has been established, a joint infection may have been ongoing for weeks before the true nature of the condition is diagnosed. If aggressive treatment of a footrot case does not lead toward resolution within 3 days, septic arthritis should be suspected. Increased pain, together with swelling of the anterior region of the coronary band in cases of sandcrack and white line disease, is suggestive of joint infection. Using regional analgesia and strict aseptic technique, an aspirate of the joint can be collected and examined for infection. A radiograph may indicate an abnormal separation of the joint surfaces.

Treatment: Digital amputation is indicated in animals that have a limited life expectancy, eg, old or poor-producing animals. The procedure is simple, quick, can be performed in standing animals under regional analgesia, and in most cases, produces rapid relief. Amputation is performed through the skin with an embryotomy wire placed as close to the skin-horn junction as possible. Hemorrhage is arrested by means of a tight bandage.

Arthrodesis fuses the distal and middle phalanges and is used to extend the functional life of valuable animals. General anesthesia is recommended. A 1-cm canal is drilled through the abaxial wall into the joint, and a second canal is drilled from the causal lesion into the joint. The joint cavity is enlarged by curettage, and a drainage tube drawn through. Continuous irrigation with sterile saline should be performed for 2-3 days. A wooden block is then applied to the sound claw, and the affected digit immobilized by fixing it to the block with methyl methacrylate. Immobilization is further facilitated by encasing the digital region in a cast. The cast is removed after 4 wk.

Serous Tarsitis
(Bog spavin, Puffy hock)

Serous tarsitis is characterized by 3 soft, fluctuating swellings between the ligaments of the femorotarsal joint and is often seen in related animals. It does not cause pain or lameness. In later life, there may be a predisposition to arthritis. The condition is diagnosed by depressing the swelling of the joint capsule at one location and palpating the fluctuation that is seen at another. There is no successful treatment.

NEUROLOGIC DISORDERS CAUSING LAMENESS

See also PROBLEMATIC BOVINE STERNAL RECUMBENCY (DOWNER COW), p 957, and LIMB PARALYSIS, p 1040.

Suprascapular Paralysis

This rare condition results from paralysis of the supraspinatus and infraspinatus muscles caused by damage to the sixth and seventh cranial nerves. Acute trauma to the prescapular area (eg, struggling into a head gate) produces a nonspecific ataxia immediately after the injury. Several days after the injury, the muscles may show signs of wasting, indicating the possibility of permanent damage.

Chronic injury to the nerves causes marked wasting of the muscles within weeks. A specific gait aberration develops. The stride is shorter than normal; when weight is borne on the limb, it tends to swivel. In some cases, the cause may be nerve compression in or around the vertebrae (eg, an abscess or fracture), which may be identified on radiographs.

If the trauma is complicated, primary treatment must be directed toward resolving the immediate problem. However, if the clinical presentation suggests that the injury is localized to the nerve, immediate treatment with steroids or other anti-inflammatory agents is appropriate.

Radial Paralysis

Distal radial paralysis results in an inability to extend the carpus and digit. Proximal radial paralysis prevents the animal from extending the elbow, carpus, and fetlock to bear weight.

Etiology: The proximal radial nerve may be injured by stretching close to the brachial plexus, in which case the triceps muscles as well as the extensors of the carpus and digits may be compromised. The damage is frequently associated with casting an animal with ropes or with any situation in which the forelimb is accidentally restrained and the animal struggles violently to free itself. Either distal or proximal radial paralysis can result from prolonged recumbency in very heavy animals.

The distal radial nerve is vulnerable to injury in the musculospiral groove of the humerus, either from fractures or deep soft-tissue trauma. A lesion of the nerve proximal to the sulcus for the brachial muscle causes proximal radial paralysis.

Clinical Findings and Diagnosis: In proximal radial paralysis, the elbow drops, the carpus and fetlock are in partial flexion, and the limb is usually dragged. In distal radial paralysis, because the triceps muscles remain functional, dropping of the elbow is minimal. However, paresis affecting carpal and fetlock position is present.

Treatment: Rapid improvement can be expected in most cases. Animals should be confined in a generously bedded stall. Anti-inflammatory drugs may be helpful, particularly in the early hours after the initial trauma. If skin sensation in the forelimb has been completely lost, the prognosis is guarded. When the condition persists for ≥2 wk, damage is likely permanent and the prognosis is grave.

Ischiatic Paralysis
(Sciatic paralysis)

Damage to the ischiatic and obturator nerves after intrapelvic parturient trauma may cause recumbency after calving. It may be a component of the downer cow syndrome (p 957). The tibial and peroneal nerves are branches of the ischiatic nerve that can be damaged at extrapelvic sites.

Obturator Paralysis

Passage of a calf through the pelvis exerts pressure on the obturator nerve. The close association of the obturator nerve with the origin of the ischiatic nerve can complicate the interpretation of clinical signs.

Clinical Findings: Because the adductors are innervated by the obturator nerve, an animal adopts a base-wide stance or, in recumbency, a sitting position with both hind-limbs extended forward. There is considerable risk that the adductor muscles will be damaged and that permanent recumbency will result. In addition to the base-wide stance, knuckling of the fetlock may be present. This indicates injury of the ischiatic nerve. Both conditions may contribute to the downer cow syndrome (p 957).

Treatment: If obturator paralysis is recognized early enough, vigorous measures should be adopted to prevent complications involving the adductor muscles. The animal should be immediately transferred to a site where there is good footing (eg, a base of tenacious manure over which clean straw has been spread) to prevent slippage when the animal attempts to rise. The hindlimbs can be tied together with a soft nylon strap fixed below the hocks. The limbs are restrained from "spreading" >3 ft (1 m) apart.

Femoral Paralysis

In femoral paralysis, paralysis of the quadriceps muscles, which extend the stifle, and partial paralysis of the psoas major muscle, which flexes the hip, are seen.

Clinical Findings and Diagnosis: Femoral nerve paralysis is seen in large, newborn calves (eg, Charolais, Simmental) after the use of mechanical force during an assisted birth. Reduced quadriceps tonicity reduces tension on the patella with the result that a lateral patellar luxation may develop. Atrophy of the quadriceps soon becomes obvious and, although the patella can be replaced easily, the animal has extreme difficulty in walking. The condition may affect one or both limbs. The prognosis is related to the severity of the clinical signs.

Treatment: Despite a fair or good prognosis, the animal may be unable to suckle unaided. The animal should be maintained in a well-bedded area, and colostrum should be given as soon as possible after birth. A radiographic study should be done to exclude fractures. The administration of anti-inflammatory drugs may be useful.

Peroneal Paralysis

Peroneal paralysis results in paralysis of the muscles that flex the hock and extend the digits.

Clinical Findings: The peroneal nerve is the cranial division of the ischiatic nerve. It passes superficially over the lateral femoral condyle and the head of the fibula, which makes it vulnerable to external trauma or pressure from recumbency. An affected animal stands with the digit knuckled over onto the dorsal surface of the pastern and fetlock. The hock may appear to be overextended. In mild cases, the fetlock tends to knuckle over intermittently during ambulation; however, this may also occur if the animal is experiencing pain in the heels.

In severe cases, the dorsal surface of the hoof may be dragged along the ground, and sensation to the dorsum of the fetlock is often decreased. Testing of reflexes may demonstrate that hock flexion is absent, but stifle and hip flexion are normal. This would not be the case if the ischiatic nerve was involved.

Treatment: Most cases resolve naturally. However, if the condition is associated with long periods of recumbency, care must be taken to avoid exacerbation of the initial injury.

Tibial Paralysis

In tibial paralysis, there is paralysis of the extensors of the hock and flexors of the digits.

Etiology: The tibial nerve is the caudal branch of the ischiatic nerve, which, in its proximal course, is well protected by the gluteal muscles. Distally, it progresses beneath the tendon of the gastrocnemius muscle and can be damaged when the tendon is traumatized.

Clinical Findings: The hock joint is overflexed (dropped hock syndrome) and the fetlock is partially flexed. The gastrocnemius appears to be longer than normal and gives the impression that it or its tendon could be ruptured. The fetlock tends to be buckled, but the animal can walk and bear weight, although its attempts to do so are awkward. Compared with that seen in peroneal nerve injury, the gait disturbance is mild, but the postural disturbance could be permanent.

Treatment: The use of anti-inflammatory drugs may be of value in the early stages. However, the primary efforts should be directed toward ensuring that the animal does not injure itself further, by maintaining it on surfaces with good footing.

Spastic Syndrome
(Progressive hindlimb paralysis)

Episodic, involuntary muscle contractions or spasms involving the hindlimbs are associated with postural and locomotor disturbances as well as spasticity. The condition may progress to posterior paresis or hindlimb paralysis. It is seen most frequently in Holstein and Guernsey cattle 3-7 yr old. Spastic syndrome is regarded as a genetic disease, possibly due to an autosomal dominant gene with incomplete penetrance. The pathology and pathophysiology remain obscure.

Clinical Findings: Clinical signs may vary in severity, duration, and frequency. Usually, some stimulus provokes the onset of clinical signs, such as the effort associated with rising or any factor that induces a significant emotional reaction. Pain, particularly in the feet or joints, may precipitate an attack. During an attack, the animal may be unable to move forward, stands trembling, and characteristically extends its hindlimbs backward. Between episodes, the animal can ambulate normally.

Treatment: Spastic syndrome is progressive, and because of the possibility of genetic transmission, animals (particularly bulls used for artificial insemination) are best eliminated as soon as a positive diagnosis is made. Palliative treatment for animals in the peak of production may be helpful. Mephenesin (30-40 mg/kg, PO, for 2-3 days) may be given during an episode. Phenylbutazone may also have beneficial effects.

Spastic Paresis
(Elso heel)

Spastic paresis is a progressive unilateral or bilateral hyperextension of the hindlimb(s). It is seen sporadically in most breeds of cattle. Post-legged cattle are most frequently affected. Attempts to move are believed to simultaneously trigger contractions of both extensors and flexors of the limb. Spastic paresis is currently considered to be inherited via a recessive gene(s) with incomplete penetrance.

Clinical Findings: The disease may be seen within the first 6 mo of life. As the animal ages, the gastrocnemius muscles gradually contract. The hock and stifle become increasingly extended. Over a period of months, the hindlimbs become so stiff that the animal walks with short pendulum-like steps. If only one limb is affected, the animal stands with the affected limb camped back and the sound limb held toward the midline to maintain balance. If both hindlimbs are affected, the animal may attempt to bear more weight on the forelimbs by holding them well back and simultaneously arching its back.

Treatment: There is no successful medical treatment. Because spastic paresis is heritable, affected animals (especially breeding bulls) should be eliminated from the herd. Palliative surgical treatment may be attempted, although ethical issues should be considered when breeding stock is involved. The procedures, usually performed on calves, include complete tenotomy of the gastrocnemius tendon, which results in a dropped hock; complete tibial neurectomy, which results in sufficient relief to permit a steer to be finished for slaughter; and partial tenectomy of the 2 insertions of the gastrocnemius muscle and the calcanean tendon sheath, which overcomes the problem of the dropped hock.

SOFT-TISSUE DISORDERS CAUSING LAMENESS

Carpal Hygroma

Carpal hygroma is a localized swelling of tissues, including the precarpal bursa, dorsal to the carpal joint. It results from intermittent mild trauma to the precarpal area caused by lack of bedding or a poorly designed manger. *Brucella abortus* may be isolated from the false bursa of some cases in countries where this organism has not been controlled. The lesion is a firm swelling, possibly fluctuating and up to several inches in diameter, located over the dorsal aspect of the carpus. The hygroma is a lesion that is very difficult to resolve. The first step is to ascertain radiographically if there is more than one cavity. Each cavity should be drained and infiltrated with a long-acting corticosteroid preparation. Surgical removal is messy, with little guarantee of a successful outcome. Introducing irritant materials into the cavity has had uncertain results. If the animal is milking and eating well, hygromas should be left untreated.

Frostbite

A calf born into an environment of <0°F (-18°C) with a high wind chill factor is at risk of hypothermia. A weak calf, born to an exhausted cow after a long labor in a cold and windy environment (eg, a temperature of 20°F [-7°C] and a wind of 30 mph [50 km/hr]) can suffer frostbite of the feet and other extremities. After several days, the calf becomes reluctant to follow its dam or to stand but has a normal appetite. A severely affected calf has a crusted muzzle, devitalized ear tips and tail end, and cold hindfeet. (The forefeet are generally placed under the body when the calf lies down and, therefore, are protected from the cold by body heat.) Several days to weeks later, the devitalized tissue (including the hooves) begins to slough, and the calf refuses to stand.

The major diagnostic problem is differentiation from fescue or ergot toxicity. Age of the animal and temperature and wind chill on the day of birth help to verify the diagnosis. Treatment is often unsuccessful.

Hematoma

A hematoma is a collection of blood, frequently clotted, beneath the skin or in a deep muscle mass (most frequently of the thigh). Hematomas are caused by trauma, most frequently from one animal butting another in confined quarters or from 2 animals attempting to rush through a narrow doorway at the same time.

In some locations, a hematoma can be confused with an abdominal hernia or a large abscess. Aspiration of fluid using a strict aseptic technique should precede any attempts to open a swelling. Hematomas should not be opened because the hemorrhaging vessel is almost impossible to locate and will continue to bleed until pressure within the hematoma equals that in the vessel. Bleeding from beneath a clot rarely stops spontaneously until either the blood pressure falls or the clot begins to organize. Eventually, this process occurs, and most of the clot will be resorbed. However, it is quite usual for an unsightly irregular lump to remain.

Rupture of the Gastrocnemius Muscle or Tendon

Rupture of the gastrocnemius muscle is relatively rare. It is most likely to be associated with deficiencies of calcium, phosphorus, and vitamin D. Prolonged recumbency, with resulting myositis and struggling to rise, occasionally precipitates rupture of one or both of these muscles. Occasionally, the condition has been associated with pyelonephritis, which presumably caused a myositis, weakening the muscle enough to permit rupture. Injections of irritating medicaments into the gastrocnemius muscle may cause necrosis and rupture.

The hock remains flexed. When the muscle is completely ruptured, the standing animal rests the hock and distal portion of the limb on the ground or walking surface, which is diagnostic, although rupture of the Achilles tendon may produce an identical gait.

Successful treatment is extremely unlikely in heavy adult animals. A leg cast or splint that maintains the hock in extension, supplying adequate vitamins and minerals, and proper nursing may be successful, but a long recovery period is required.

Rupture of the Achilles tendon is usually traumatic. The clinical signs are similar to those of rupture of the muscle.

Rupture of the Peroneus Tertius Muscle

The peroneus tertius muscle can be forcibly avulsed from its insertion by accidents associated with mounting or, more frequently, by the inexperienced use of ropes to restrain a hindlimb.

The hock is abnormally extended, while the stifle remains flexed. The limb cannot be advanced normally, the calcanean tendon is flaccid, and the hooves may be dragged. The site of avulsion may be painful to the touch. A specific diagnostic feature is that the limb can be pulled backward without any resistance from the animal.

The condition may improve slowly if the animal is confined in a stall (loose) for several months.

Tarsal Cellulitis

Tarsal cellulitis is a false bursa characterized by a firm, subcutaneous swelling on the lateral aspect of the hock that has little effect on joint mobility. It is caused by severe abrasion of the skin and subcutaneous tissue overlying bony prominences. The skin may be excoriated by contact with concrete and particularly sharp curbs. Superficial abscesses must be drained extremely cautiously because there is considerable danger of entering the joint. Padding and bandages should always be applied. Poultices rapidly reduce acute swelling.

LAMENESS IN GOATS

Abnormality of gait is a sign common to many diseases and conditions. A complete history is important for diagnosis and should include incidence and duration in the herd, nutrition, feed changes, method of rearing, and recent introductions to the herd. (*See also* HEALTH-MANAGEMENT INTERACTION: GOATS, p 1731.)

Some causes of lameness may be associated with systemic disease. Therefore, a thorough physical examination should always be performed, followed by a specific assessment of gait and mobility in an attempt to localize locomotor problems and by a detailed examination of the limbs. In goats, as in other species, locomotor difficulties usually involve the musculoskeletal system directly, but conditions of the nervous system can mimic musculoskeletal disease and should be considered during the clinical examination.

The hoof of the affected leg(s) should be examined, and excess horn material removed to leave a level weight-bearing surface. If the feet have not been trimmed for a long period, or the goats have been on soft ground or bedding, excess horn commonly overgrows from the walls, toes, and heels, and folds over the sole. With severe neglect, "sled-runner"- or "Turkish slipper"-type hooves (elongated toes) may cause the goat to walk on its heels. The following should be noted during foot paring: any portion of the horn that is abnormally thickened, any underrunning of the heel or sole, any abnormal wear of one claw, or any abnormal or necrotic smell.

After paring, the feet should be scrubbed clean and inspected for puncture wounds, foreign bodies (eg, stones or clover burrs caught in the interdigital area), or pus from a discharging abscess—especially about the coronet.

The rest of the leg should be palpated carefully, including the bones, tendons, and muscles. Any muscle atrophy or restriction of movement should be noted. The joints also should be checked for heat, swelling, or pain. Contralateral limb structures should be compared for signs of asymmetry.

If the clinical examination suggests joint involvement, it may be necessary to aseptically collect some joint fluid from an affected joint (usually the carpus) for visual examination, cytology, Gram's stain, and culture and sensitivity tests. Joint fluid containing pus alone, or gram-positive bacteria, indicates joint-ill; fibrin and pus combined suggest *Mycoplasma* spp; clear or cloudy joint fluid with many mononuclear cells suggests caprine arthritis and encephalitis virus (CAE, *see* below).

A blood or serum sample may also be useful in establishing the underlying cause of lameness. In joint-ill, the WBC count is high, with neutrophilia. Blood calcium, phosphorus, and vitamin D levels may help diagnose bent leg or rickets, although blood levels often return to normal before the affected goat is examined. If CAE is suspected, the presence of antibody can be checked; however, false negatives may be seen during severe stress, and positive tests may be coincidental to another cause of lameness if seroprevalence is high in the herd of origin.

Radiography may be helpful. In "bent leg," the growth plates should be checked; there is also lateral deviation of the radii and occasionally thinness of the bone. In CAE virus infection, the initial swelling of the soft tissue surrounding the affected joint is followed by calcium deposits in the swollen periarticular tissue, joint capsule, ligaments, tendons, tendon sheaths, and finally the muscle bellies. Later changes consist of mild periarticular osteophyte production, "joint mice," and rough extensions of the periarticular bone proximally and distally.

Some of the more important conditions that cause lameness in goats are discussed below. The differential diagnosis in any case of lameness is influenced by geographic location, herd history, management practices, and other relevant factors.

BENT LEG
(Epiphysitis)

Bent leg is the result of a calcium:phosphorus imbalance. It is seen in young, rapidly growing kids (more often in males than in females) and in young does in the later stages of their first pregnancy or in the early stages of their first lactation. These does are either young (eg, 12 mo), extremely heavy milkers, or carrying twins or triplets. Bent leg is sometimes compounded by rickets (p 853).

Clinical Findings and Diagnosis: Bent leg starts with lateral or medial bowing of one or both radii. Later changes may consist of lateral deviation of the digits on the fore- or hindfeet; lameness and reluctance to walk; an arched back; and soft swelling and pain in the carpal, metacarpophalangeal, tarsal, and metatarsophalangeal joints. Diagnosis can be confirmed with radiography.

Conditions that have been implicated in the cause include an excess of dietary calcium with a calcium:phosphorus ratio of >1.4:1 (generally >1.8:1), excess protein intake (has caused epiphysitis in other species), excess dietary iron (has reduced serum phosphorus levels in lambs by decreasing vitamin D metabolite formation), and housing of kids or lack of vitamin D caused by prolonged overcast weather and low vitamin D levels in the feed. Carotene has an antivitamin D effect. Vitamin D has poor stability in prepared feed, especially when mixed with minerals. Alfalfa is high in calcium (1.4% calcium to 0.2% phosphorus) and protein. Owners frequently keep kids on fresh milk for prolonged periods because often no commercial outlet for the milk is available.

Treatment and Control: Once the probable cause(s) is identified, the diet should be corrected and the appropriate supplement given—usually injectable vitamin D and phosphorus or oral balanced calcium/phosphorus supplements (or both).

Predisposing factors also must be corrected. The diet of growing kids should be changed to slow their growth rates. The mating of very young does should be discouraged. Buck kids should be separated from doe kids when 3-4 mo old. Young does in milk with limb deformities should be managed so that full lactation is discouraged, eg, by not milking out fully and drying off as early as possible.

Treatment stops limb deformities from worsening and should improve them to a great extent. However, a return to completely normal limbs is rare.

CAPRINE ARTHRITIS AND ENCEPHALITIS

Caprine arthritis and encephalitis (p 598) virus infection has emerged over the last 20 yr as a major cause of disease, primarily in European breeds of dairy goats throughout the world, and particularly under intensive management conditions in Europe and North America. Two distinct forms of locomotor problems are seen. A neurologic form of the disease is seen in young goats, usually 2-4 mo old but up to 1 yr of age. It produces a progressive paresis with incoordination leading to paralysis, usually involving the hindlimbs but sometimes affecting the forelimbs as well. In older, adult goats, the virus infection manifests as a chronic, progressive arthritis involving one or more joints and usually involving the carpal joints. The initial sign is usually swelling of the affected joint(s), followed by progressive degeneration of articular and periarticular tissues with calcification, leading to decreased range of motion, ankylosis, and overt loss of mobility.

CONTRACTED TENDONS IN KIDS

Contracted tendons in newborn kids are seen sporadically in goats of all breeds throughout the world, usually with unexplained causation. However, there are 2 specific, inherited conditions of goats that result in contracted tendons of newborns, discussed below.

A usually bilateral, congenital condition that is a genetic defect is seen in Angoras in Australasia. It is due to a recessive autosomal allele that must reach a certain level before affected animals appear; the time between purchase of a carrier buck and appearance of affected kids may be 5-6 generations. Either the fore- or hindlimbs are affected. In rare cases, only 1 forelimb is twisted. In severe cases, the kid is either unable to stand or walks on its fetlocks. In less severe cases, it may move relatively easily with fetlocks that are permanently partly flexed. In mild cases, the limbs may gradually be splinted straighter and straighter until the kid is able to bear weight on its feet.

Anglo-Nubians in the USA, Canada, Australia, and New Zealand can have a genetic condition called β-mannosidosis. At birth, affected kids have varying degrees of fixed flexion of the forelimbs and fixed extension of the hindlimbs. They can see and bleat and suckle if held up to the teat. Their withdrawal reflexes are normal or depressed, and there is intention tremor, especially of the head. There may be nystagmus, deafness, and facial abnormalities. At necropsy, cutting the tendons allows free movement of the limbs. Histologic examination reveals typical lesions of lysosomal storage disease characterized by cellular vacuolation. Affected kids have no plasma levels of β-mannosidase, and both parents have levels half the normal range.

COPPER DEFICIENCY

Copper deficiency may cause locomotor difficulties in goats in 2 distinct ways. Abnormal bone growth with increased bone fragility can predispose to fractures of long bones. Independently, a neurologic condition known as enzootic ataxia or swayback develops, in which copper deficiency of kids in utero or after birth results in myelin degeneration in the spinal cord leading to progressive incoordination and paralysis with failure of mobility. Clinically, this appears similar to the neurologic form of caprine arthritis and encephalitis virus (*see* above) infection in young kids. Copper status of the ration needs to be evaluated, and copper supplementation provided as necessary.

FOOTROT AND FOOT SCALD

Footrot and foot scald are serious problems of goats and other species (*see* p 944 and p 882).

JOINT-ILL

Several joints of kids can be involved in this nonspecific bacterial infection. Bacteria that have been incriminated are mainly gram positive and include staphylococci, streptococci, *Corynebacterium* spp, *Actinomyces* spp, and coliforms. *Erysipelothrix rhusiopathiae* is an uncommon cause of joint-ill in goats relative to sheep, and when it is seen, it is mainly in kids 3-4 mo old.

Environmental bacteria gain entry to the neonate's circulation, usually via the umbilical cord. Other methods of entry include contamination of breaks in the skin or via the GI or respiratory tract. Predisposing factors include lack of routine dipping of the umbilical cord; poor sanitation in the kidding pens; or does kidding in overcrowded, dirty conditions. *E rhusiopathiae* are soil-living bacteria that may persist on farms or in pens used by sheep or pigs. Mycoplasma infection is also a differential diagnosis (*see* below).

Clinical Findings: More than 1 joint is hot, swollen, and painful. Often, the affected limb(s) cannot bear weight. Kids with more than 1 leg affected may be unable to stand. The more commonly affected joints are the carpus, shoulder, hock, and stifle. Generally, there is a fever but no reduction in appetite. Sometimes the navel area is inflamed, but often there is no visible abnormality. An abscess may form on the navel long after the kid has recovered. The WBC count may be increased with a left shift.

If the condition becomes chronic, the limbs are stiff, some joints may be ankylosed, and overall growth is poor. At this stage the temperature is normal.

Treatment: To be successful, treatment must be given early and, when possible, antibiotic selection should be based on culture and sensitivity testing. Frequent injections of high doses of parenteral antibiotics given for ~1 wk often effect a cure if combined with careful nursing. Joint lavage with saline and antibiotic solutions may enhance therapeutic outcome in selected cases. Complications should be prevented by providing soft bedding, frequently turning any kid unable to stand, and massaging the affected joints. If ankylosis starts to develop, the kid should be supported in a sling for short periods as frequently as possible.

In large commercial herds, treating severely affected kids may not be economically justified. Many that do recover remain unthrifty for the rest of their lives.

Control: Hygiene at parturition is essential. A deep bed of clean sawdust, wood shavings, or straw should be provided; it is often better to allow the doe to kid on fresh pasture if the weather is warm.

The umbilical cords of newborn kids should be dipped several times in a strong antiseptic, eg, 7% tincture of iodine or iodophor teat dip. Cords should be dipped each time the kid is handled in the first 24-48 hr. Owners should clean their footwear before entering kidding pens.

LAMINITIS

(Founder)

Laminitis in goats is seen worldwide, but the incidence is lower than that in dairy cattle and horses. Predisposing causes include overeating or sudden access to concentrates, high-grain and low-roughage diets, or high-protein diets. Laminitis can also develop as a complication of acute infections such as mastitis, metritis, or pneumonia, especially after kidding.

When laminitis is severe, the affected goat is lame and reluctant to move; there is a fever, and all 4 feet are hot to the touch. Touching the coronet elicits a severe pain reaction.

In less severe cases, only the forefeet are affected. Laminitis can become chronic if the initial phase is not diagnosed or treated successfully. The onset is insidious, but eventually the goat is seen walking on its knees, with "sled-runner" deformities of its hooves.

In acute laminitis, the predisposing condition, if identifiable, must be corrected promptly. The laminitis is treated with analgesics (eg, phenylbutazone at 2-4 mg/kg, flunixin meglumine at 1.1 mg/kg, or aspirin at 30-100 mg/kg) daily; hosing or soaking the affected feet is also useful. Although antihistamines are frequently used, their effectiveness in treatment of laminitis in goats remains unproved. Similarly, the use of corticosteroids is controversial because they may contribute to laminitis in horses. Regardless, they should not be used in pregnant does due to risk of abortion. Chronic laminitis with deformed hooves is treated by routine vigorous foot trimming.

MYCOPLASMOSIS

See also p 1114 and p 1229. Kids infected with *Mycoplasma mycoides mycoides* (large colony variant) or other *Mycoplasma* spp may show severe lameness with multiple hot swollen joints, weight loss, pyrexia, and poor coats. Some have diarrhea, and some have increased lung sounds and respiratory rates. Affected kids are generally 2-4 wk old. Morbidity and mortality rates of 90% and 30%, respectively, have been reported. Adult does with *Mycoplasma* infection may have mastitis and polyarthritis. Treatment is with tetracycline, tylosin, or tiamulin, but prognosis for complete recovery is guarded.

TRAUMA

Goats, in general, are agile creatures, but if frightened they may attempt impossible jumps, with resultant fractures or other injuries. Yards designed for goats that are infrequently handled should have a visual as well as physical barrier. Chain-link fences are often associated with limb fractures when used for goat enclosures. Fortunately, most fractures of the lower limbs heal rapidly with normal casting. Shearing of Angoras is a source of potential problems, eg, when the shearer's comb cuts into or through the Achilles tendon. Orthopedic procedures suitable for large dogs can be used.

Some IM injections can cause problems. For example, mixed clostridial vaccines can cause severe soft-tissue swelling and lameness for ≥48 hr. Irritant drugs can damage nearby nerves and cause lameness, particularly when thin or young goats are injected in the thigh muscles and the sciatic nerve is affected. In some cases of severe mastitis, especially gangrenous, there is a hindlimb lameness on the affected side as the doe changes her gait due to the swelling and pain in the udder.

WHITE MUSCLE DISEASE

See also p 948. Most affected kids have been in good condition and are 2-3 mo old (range 1 wk to 4 mo). Commonly, sudden death is associated with cardiac muscle damage. Other kids are depressed, reluctant to move, and appear stiff with a "sawhorse" stance. Muscles, especially of the hindlimbs, are firm and painful to the touch. Treatment is with selenium and vitamin E injection in acute cases.

LAMENESS IN HORSES

Lameness is the result of a change from normal stance and gait caused by either a structural or a functional disorder of one or more of the limbs, the neck, or the trunk. It is not a disease, but a manifestation of either pain caused by an impediment in the musculoskeletal system or, if pain is not involved, of a mechanical lameness, although a combination of the two frequently exists. Mechanical lameness is best typified by fibrotic myopathy with its characteristic gait abnormality, but can also be the result of a restriction (eg, tendon sheath restriction in annular ligament syndrome). It is important to correctly distinguish the type of mechanical lameness, eg, fibrotic myopathy from stringhalt. In fibrotic myopathy, the affected limb is pulled back and down before the end of the protraction phase, resulting in a lengthened weightbearing phase and a shortened cranial phase. The signs are most obvious at the walk. In stringhalt, the affected limb is hyperflexed during the cranial or swing phase, while the stepwise caudal jerking movement before foot contact does not occur.

Pain-related lameness can be classified as weightbearing (supporting leg) or non-weightbearing (swinging leg) lameness, although lameness most often is composed of both. A supporting leg lameness is seen when the horse attempts to reduce the amount of time a particular limb is bearing weight. The horse elevates its head and shifts its weight away from a particular limb during weightbearing for a forelimb lameness, whereas the opposite is true for a hindlimb lameness. Hindlimb lamenesses should be assessed from the side as well as from behind, because this provides an opportunity to assess arc of flight, duration of protraction and retraction phases, and length of weightbearing phase. In milder cases, the horse might fail to make a circle when lunged because it is trying to redistribute its weight to offload the lame leg, most commonly seen when the lame limb is the outside limb on a circle. A supporting leg lameness may originate from anywhere in the limb (proximal or distal), while a swinging leg lameness, although often believed to represent a proximal problem, may originate either proximally or distally.

Factors that predispose to lameness include physical immaturity (eg, bones that are anatomically normal but biomechanically weak due to the age of the horse at the onset of training or bone that is abnormally weak due to developmental orthopedic disease), and monotonous repetitive stresses on bones (eg, stress fractures in racehorses continuously training around left-handed bends, or chronic imbalance of the feet resulting in repeated abnormal loading of a particular limb). Inciting factors in lameness include direct or indirect trauma, incoordination of muscle action following fatigue in racehorses racing over long distances, or inflammation—more often than not without infection—of joints, tendons, and ligaments in particular.

Lameness in one part of a limb likely results in at least some secondary soreness from another area of the same limb as well as a small degree of lameness in the contralateral fore- or hindlimb. The former is regularly proved by the complexity in step-by-step elimination of lameness in the distal limb in particular, the latter by the almost invariable switch of lameness, often of a much lesser degree, to the contralateral limb. One dramatic example of this is the development of traumatic inflammation and occasionally rotation or sinking of the distal phalanx in the contralateral limb to a severe, nonweightbearing lameness (eg, a fracture).

THE LAMENESS EXAMINATION

A systematic investigation of a lame horse is time consuming. The examination also benefits from standardized facilities such as a level, firm running-up track and ideally both a firm, nonslippery surface and a softer area for lunging or riding the lame horse.

The examination begins with a comprehensive medical history; type, age, and training regimen may give important clues to the lameness as will the time since onset of lameness and interim management. The interval since the last shoeing should be noted, as well as any suggestions that the lameness may improve with either rest or exercise. Response to anti-inflammatory or analgesic medications may provide useful information. Results of hematologic and biochemical analyses may shed light on other problems that influence overall performance. Anemia may be associated with muscle fatigue, while enzymes such as AST and CK in combination are reasonably muscle-tissue specific; they rise as the result of severe muscle cell damage and may not be elevated in cases of moderate sprain of a single muscle, in particular if the pathology affects the connective tissues of the musculo-tendinous junction rather than the muscle fiber itself.

In cases of chronically elevated muscle-related enzymes suggestive of equine rhabdomyolysis, a muscle biopsy may be useful to check for subgroups such as polysaccharide storage myopathies (p 951).

Although valuable, modern diagnostic imaging techniques are no substitute for detailed visual inspection and thorough manual palpation of the limbs in weightbearing and nonweightbearing positions. The high degree of variation between horses should be remembered, and comparision with the contralateral limb should always take place, although the latter may not necessarily be a useful control. Any heat, joint distention, or abnormal tissue tension should be noted, as well as the reaction of the horse and range of flexion and extension of all joints. Specific areas of muscle wastage may also provide useful information. The feet should be thoroughly examined, including compression of the walls and sole with hoof testers. Wear patterns of shoes and feet should be noted. A number of abnormalities such as broken toe/pastern axis; mismatched hoof angles; under-run, contracted, and sheared heels, and disproportionate hoof size are seen more frequently in lame than in sound horses. Shoes should be left on, as removing them at this stage might make the horse footsore and thereby preclude further examination. However, occasionally it may prove useful to remove the front shoes to demonstrate that the shoeing was the cause of the lameness.

The back and neck should be thoroughly examined with the horse restrained and standing square on a level surface. The neck should be assessed for range of movement in all planes and for evidence of muscle asymmetry and pain. The dorsal midline of the back should be straight, and equal tone should be present in the paravertebral musculature on either side of the midline. The same should be true of the gluteal musculature and the hamstrings. The definitive diagnosis of a strained or torn muscle can be extremely difficult, especially in more chronic cases. Spatial alignment of the tubera coxae and sacrale should also be observed. Flexibility and extensibility of the back can be checked by alternately pinching the midline in the midthoracic and sacrococcygeal regions, while lateral flexion can be checked by turning the horse short around its own axis.

Examination during exercise becomes an option only if the degree of lameness is minor and chronic. If lameness is major and acute (eg, suspected fracture), additional exercise could result in a catastrophic breakdown with dire consequences for the horse. It is important to check whether the horse may have been given analgesic medication prior to the lameness examination.

A firm, nonslippery surface (eg, hardcore fine gravel) is ideal for trotting on a straight line and for lunging on a firm surface. It also provides an opportunity to listen to the footfall and consider this information along with the visual appraisal. However, feet of different shapes make slightly different impact sounds, which may be confusing. Although a horse may be regular in its stride, it may have a slightly weaker limb, particularly if recovering from a previous problem. Lunging on tarmac (asphalt) or concrete increases the risk of the horse slipping. It also generally alters the gait so much that it has little value in lameness examination. Leading the horse on a circle at a trot also tends to alter the horse's stride too much; the horse cannot move its neck and instead "sets" its head on the leader's hand. Assessing the horse at a canter, which requires a softer surface, is always important. A surprising number of horses with lower back pain may appear normal at a trot but are unable to maintain a normal 3-beat canter rhythm or may canter disunited.

Flexion tests are useful diagnostic tools. The range of movement and response to passive flexion, along with any suggestion of increased lameness or onset of lameness following flexion, should be observed. The distal phalanges in both forelimbs and hindlimbs should be flexed independently of carpus and hock to obtain maximal information. However, results of recent studies have suggested that "false-positive" results may be seen if excessive forces are applied. Consistency should always be applied, and individual experience used. A single positive flexion test without associated lameness may not be of significance and in some horses has proved to be a lifelong observation.

To establish consistency, the entire examination should involve the same handler, the same bitting, and the same surfaces under foot. The horse should be controlled so that it is trotting at a useful, repeatable pace to evaluate the lameness (eg, trotting in a straight line with the horse straight through its neck and trunk). This "correct" pace varies between horses. Correct bitting, eg, using a Chifney bit, is important but can be confusing due to an altered posture when lunging and should be avoided if possible. Very slight sedation (eg, 0.3 mL romifidine [10 mg/ml]) may also result in a horse with a more relaxed outline and allow a better assessment without seemingly influencing the degree of lameness. Slowing down the pace at the trot often illustrates a subtle lameness better because the horse loses its momentum and struggles with suspension in the affected limb(s).

A ridden assessment of the horse is often necessary, particularly with a subtle lameness or a horse that is unwilling to perform certain movements (eg, a dressage horse). A multilimb lameness without an obvious single-limb lameness may also be involved. The clinical signs may be minor (eg, signs of aversion as opposed to lameness). Subtle signs include an unwillingness to take a strong contact with the rider's hand, a slight heat tilt, and tail swishing. Seeing the horse and rider at work is necessary to look for subtle lamenesses. However, a good rider can, often inadvertently, hide a problem by his or her inherent expertise and ability to "correct" difficulties. Similarly, a bad rider can make a sound horse look lame ("bridle lame"). Deliberately riding on the wrong diagonal frequently helps illustrate a problem, especially those involving the back. A change of rider may occasionally be required to highlight a particular problem. Occasionally a horse appears to be sound when lunged and ridden, but the rider feels that the performance is impaired. In such cases it may be worth working the horse on concomitant analgesic or anti-inflammatory medication at therapeutic levels for an adequate period (eg, phenylbutazone 2-3 g/day, PO for 7-14 days) to assess whether improvement occurs. If so, medication should be withdrawn and diagnostic anesthesia used beginning in an arbitrary limb, most often a forelimb. In this way, multiple limb lamenesses (as many as 4), often mimicking the clinical picture associated with back pain, can be evaluated and treated. Some veterinarians choose to ride the horse as part of the lameness examination; however, in most cases time spent on the ground observing the horse on different surfaces and in different training situations is time better spent.

Because lameness may indicate a peripheral nerve dysfunction, a neurologic examination should always be part of the lameness examination and might include observing the horse execute "complicated" movements such as turning short, backing, "hopping" on one forelimb (with the other forelimb held up), and negotiating a curb. These tests help determine whether reduced proprioception, weakness, or spasticity are present or suggest abnormalities in the motor function of the major muscle groups that flex and extend the limbs. In acute traumatic injuries of the nerves to the limbs, the presence of these gait deficits relative to the major muscle groups provide the key to diagnosis. Long-standing peripheral neuropathies also give rise to denervation atrophy of the innervated muscles as seen in suprascapular nerve trauma ("sweeney"), in which atrophy of both the infraspinatus and supraspinatus muscle develops.

IMAGING TECHNIQUES

Imaging techniques provide important pathologic and physiologic information necessary to treat specific conditions. Imaging can be divided into anatomic and physiologic methods. Anatomic imaging methods include radiology, ultrasonography, computed tomography, and MRI. Physiologic imaging methods include scintigraphy and thermography. When diagnostic analgesia has failed to eliminate the lameness, the lameness is too subtle for localization by diagnostic analgesia, or the horse is not amenable to handling or injection, physiologic imaging techniques may help narrow the problem to a specific region. Anatomic imaging methods can then be used to evaluate those areas. Imaging may also help prevent injury. This requires early detection of the physiologic changes associated with injury. Although frequent use of an anatomic imaging method can detect change in one region, physiologic imaging allows assessment of the entire horse on a routine basis.

Anatomic Imaging Techniques

Radiologic techniques are the methods most commonly used to evaluate lameness in horses. Plain film radiography requires multiple projections to evaluate any area. It allows assessment of bony tissues and reflects chronic changes. Occasionally, radiographic techniques that provide more information are needed. Contrast radiography provides information about articular cartilage and surfaces and is of particular value in determining whether subchondral cysts communicate with the joint and in delineating subcutaneous tracts. Pathologic diagnoses are usually made by radiography in conjunction with clinical examination. The future of radiography lies in digital techniques such as computed radiography (CR) and digital radiography (DR). CR uses a special plate that is read by the computer. Advantages of CR include fewer retakes, a lower radiation requirement, and postprocessing techniques that eliminate contrast problems. DR also uses a special plate, but the computer reads the radiation directly from the cassette to produce the image. It has the same advantages as CR but is faster.

Ultrasonographic examination can be used to assess any soft tissues. The deeper the tissue that needs to be evaluated, the lower the wavelength of the probe used. Ultrasonography is most useful in the evaluation of tendons and ligaments but can also be used to evaluate muscle and cartilage. It can also help determine whether a lesion is active or chronic.

Assessment of anatomic changes serves as the basis for any pathologic diagnosis, as well as being important in determining prognosis. For these purposes, radiography and ultrasonography are complementary. Radiography provides information regarding bony tissues, while ultrasonography provides information about the soft tissues that connect bone or provide support.

MRI and computed tomography are high-detail anatomic imaging tools. They are not currently used in clinical practice but may be useful in research.

Physiologic Imaging Techniques

These techniques provide images that reflect physiologic processes. Unlike anatomic imaging, which reflects structure, physiologic imaging techniques assess metabolism or circulation. Thermography and scintigraphy allow examination of the entire horse. When combined with a thorough clinical examination, these methods are useful for identifying injuries that may otherwise go undetected.

Thermography is the pictorial representation of the surface temperature of an object. It is a noninvasive technique that measures emitted heat and is useful for detecting inflammatory changes that may contribute to lameness. Relative blood flow dictates the thermal pattern; normal thermal patterns can be predicted based on vascularity and surface contour. Skin overlying muscle is also subject to temperature increase during muscle activity. Circulation is invariably altered in injured or diseased tissues. Thermographically, the "hot spot" associated with the localized inflammation generally is seen in the skin directly overlying the injury. However, diseased tissues may have a reduced blood supply due to swelling, vessel thrombosis, or tissue infarction. With such lesions, the area of decreased heat is usually surrounded by increased thermal emissions, probably due to shunting of blood.

During scintigraphy, polyphosphonate radiopharmaceuticals are given IV. Their distribution is then measured by a gamma camera. The polyphosphonates bind rapidly to exposed hydroxyapatite crystal, generally in areas where bone is actively remodelling. Because inflammation causes an increase in blood flow, capillary permeability, and extracellular fluid volume, inflamed tissues accumulate high levels of radiopharmaceutical during the soft-tissue phase of scintigraphy, allowing evaluation of soft-tissue injuries. During the bone phase, the radiopharmaceutical accumulates in areas of increased remodelling or vascularity. Because injured bone is remodelled more rapidly, scintigraphy is useful for detecting lesions in bone and ligaments, particularly in identifying enthesopathy (damage to the insertions of tendons and ligaments on bone).

ARTHROSCOPY
(Tenoscopy, Bursoscopy)

Arthroscopy is the ultimate way of assessing the soft tissues of a joint. It often combines diagnosis with therapy (surgery), with one procedure often following the other during the same anesthetic procedure. Arthroscopy provides the only option for examining all the soft tissues of the joint interior and enables minimally invasive surgical techniques, ensuring rapid healing of soft tissues, as only minute stab incisions are required. It enables access to parts of joints not accessible during an arthrotomy and allows for detailed magnified images to be stored and reproduced. Arthroscopy also provides increased cosmetic and functional advantages and has lower postsurgical morbidity, while decreasing convalescence time and ensuring an earlier return to work. It allows much improved mechanical lavage of joints (eg, use of 10-20 L of saline under up to 300 mm Hg).

Most equine joints of the appendicular skeleton are large enough to allow arthroscopy using a rigid endoscope of 2.5-5 mm diameter, inserted through a rigid sleeve. Camera attachments transmit the images to a monitor from which still or video images can be obtained.

Although a technique for arthroscopic removal of proximal P_1 fragments in standing horses has recently been described, most diagnostic and surgical arthroscopies take place with the horse under general anesthesia. The majority of procedures are performed with the horse in dorsal recumbency to ensure that triangulation techniques can be applied. Dorsal recumbency also permits good hemostasis and enables surgery of multiple joints or limbs.

Diagnostic and surgical arthroscopy requires good knowledge of joint anatomy and good hand-eye coordination and spatial awareness. Diagnostic arthroscopy provides a unique opportunity for evaluating the synovial membrane, articular cartilages, and intra-articular structures such as menisci, plicae, and villi. Classification of soft-tissue changes has been established for reference. Arthroscopy also enables intra-articular biopsies.

Diagnostic and surgical tenoscopy and bursoscopy are also used, often for cases of sepsis of synovial structures. Bursoscopy of the navicular bursa has almost eliminated the "streetnail procedure" for surgical treatment of sepsis, as has calcaneal tenoscopy for infections that often follow kicks to the hock. The minimal soft-tissue trauma described with tenoscopy is invaluable in restoring the normal intrasynovial environment and has revolutionized the recovery rate from septic tenosynovitis.

Surgical arthroscopy most commonly involves the removal of osteochondral fragments; debridement of damaged articular surfaces, menisci, and intra-articular ligaments (eg, palmar intercarpal ligaments); synovectomy; and repair of intra-articular fractures.

REGIONAL ANALGESIA

Diagnostic local analgesia is an important component of the equine lameness examination if the site of pain is uncertain after a thorough clinical examination. The appendicular nervous system is quite consistent, and there are few indications for ringblocks. It should be used with care in horses with severe lameness as, for example, a simple fracture may become comminuted if the protective effect of pain is lost. Common conditions in which regional analgesia is important in determining an accurate diagnosis include superficial foot pain, navicular disease, traumatic joint disease, and proximal suspensory desmitis.

Perineural analgesia should start distally and progress proximally. Intrasynovial analgesia may start proximally if indicated by clinical findings, as this does not preclude subsequent distal analgesia. Intrasynovial analgesia is more specific and localized than perineural analgesia and may be performed once a nerve block has worn off (allow at least 2 hr and preferably more) to give a more accurate localization of the painful site.

Technique: The horse should be consistently lame—enough that any improvement can be detected. A subtle lameness may be exacerbated by lunging or riding. Good restraint of the horse is necessary, and the use of a bridle and twitch is recommended. Distal limb blocks are often more safely performed with the leg held up. For the proximal limb, or some distal intrasynovial blocks, the limb should be weight bearing; holding the opposite leg may help. Good, quick, accurate technique, based on a thorough knowledge of the anatomy and different approaches, is essential in fractious animals. Occasionally, short-acting sedatives, eg, xylazine, may be necessary. For more proximal blocks, in which larger needles are used, desensitization of the skin with 1-2 mL of local anesthetic placed with a fine needle may be helpful. Mepivacaine is the local anesthetic of choice because of low tissue reactivity, but lignocaine and prilocaine are less expensive.

For perineural anesthesia, the site must be clean. Swabbing with alcohol alone is usually sufficient in fine-coated horses. Strict asepsis is recommended for intrasynovial analgesia. The site should be clipped, surgically scrubbed, and sterile gloves worn to draw up the local anesthetic and perform the injection. With intrasynovial analgesia, the retrieval of synovial fluid and free injection of local anesthetic confirm placement within the synovial cavity.

The effectiveness of a nerve block is assessed by checking loss of skin sensation in the appropriate area with a blunt object such as a ballpoint pen. Analgesia may begin in 5-10 min for a perineural block but can take up to 30-40 min to be fully effective. The effectiveness of intrasynovial analgesia cannot be assessed other than by a positive response. Initially, 5 min are allowed; the response is further assessed at 15 and 30 min.

Perineural Analgesia: Distal blocks are performed most commonly because the majority of lameness originates in the distal limb. Sequential blocks are started distally. Blocks up to low 4/6-point level are easy to perform, but the more proximal blocks require more technical precision and are less frequently performed in general practice. The commonly performed blocks in the forelimb are: 1) palmar digital nerve block—desensitizes the palmar third of the foot; 2) abaxial sesamoid nerve block—blocks the palmar nerves at the level of the fetlock and desensitizes the whole of the foot and the majority of the pastern; 3) low 4-point nerve block—blocks the palmar and palmar metacarpal nerves in the distal metacarpal region, desensitizing the fetlock; 4) subcarpal nerve block—desensitizes the origin of the suspensory ligament; and 5) median and ulnar nerve blocks—desensitizes the carpus. Commonly performed blocks in the hindlimb are: 1) abaxial sesamoid nerve blocks—as for forelimb; 2) low 6-point nerve block—as for forelimb but also blocks the dorsal metatarsal nerves; 3) subtarsal nerve block—as for forelimb; and 4) tibial and peroneal nerve blocks—desensitizes the tarsus.

Intrasynovial Analgesia: All synovial structures can be blocked with an appropriate knowledge of the different approaches, but radiographic guidance is commonly used for injecting the navicular bursa. Joints that can be considered as single spaces from the point of view of diagnostic analgesia include the coffin, pastern, fetlock, radiocarpal, elbow, shoulder, and hip. The carpometacarpal and intercarpal joints and the tibiotarsal and proximal intertarsal joints communicate in all horses and thus do not need to be blocked separately. The tarsometatarsal and distal intertarsal joints may communicate in some cases, but this is not consistent and both joints should be blocked separately. There is variable communication between the femoropatellar and medial and lateral femorotibial joints. Thus, the individual blocks may not be specific, and interpretation can be easier if all 3 compartments of the stifle are blocked at once. The joints that are blocked most commonly include the coffin, fetlock, carpal, tarsal, and stifle joints.

Interpretation: The degree of lameness should be objectively assessed after each block. The lameness is significantly improved, rather than completely abolished, in many cases. A positive response is considered to be ≥75% improvement with a perineural block, and ≥50% for an intrasynovial block. A horse may appear to improve as it "warms up," leading to the false impression of a positive response. Contralateral limb lameness may become apparent following successful blocking of one limb, or there may be more than one problem in the same limb.

In the majority of cases, interpretation of the results is fairly straightforward. There are, however, many reasons for an unexpected response to local analgesia. Severe pain, eg, that from a subsolar abscess, does not always block well. Only lameness from pain is improved, whereas mechanical and neurologic lamenesses generally do not respond. There may be variation in the precise course of nerves between horses. Deep-seated joint pain may not respond to intra-articular analgesia. There may be diffusion of local anesthetic over a relatively large area, so that more proximal structures are blocked (eg, an abaxial sesamoid nerve block may desensitize the fetlock joint). Communications between individual joints, as discussed above, must be considered. There may also be diffusion between adjacent synovial structures (eg, distal interphalangeal joint to navicular bursa, between distal tarsal joints, between separate compartments of the stifle). There may also be false-positive results from nerves overlying, or adjacent to, synovial cavities. Thus, a subcarpal block may inadvertently desensitize the intercarpal joint, and conversely, a block of that joint may desensitize the origin of the suspensory ligament. Local anesthetic injected into the distal interphalangeal joint can block solar pain. Overall, regional analgesia remains an invaluable tool in equine orthopedics, but diagnostic accuracy is improved by good technique and a thorough knowledge of the nuances of interpretation.

DISORDERS OF THE FOOT

BONE CYST IN PEDAL BONE

A large cyst in the pedal bone results in a chronic lameness that may be severe and is unresponsive to anti-inflammatory medication. This uncommon condition may be seen in any foot but is seen more often in a hindfoot. There is no apparent age, breed, or sex predisposition. It is assumed to be traumatic in origin and not part of the osteochondrosis syndrome (p 929). Cystic demineralization can accompany prolonged subsolar abscesses. The cyst may communicate with the distal phalangeal (coffin) joint. Multiple cysts are sometimes present; they may enlarge and eventually involve a large part of the pedal bone. Diagnosis is confirmed by volar nerve block and radiography. Differential diagnoses include keratoma, navicular disease, pedal osteitis, and pedal bone abscess. Surgical treatment is not always successful because of the site and size of the lesion. Secondary fracture of the pedal bone can occur due to progressive weakening of the bone. Some horses return to performance status, while others are salvaged for alternative uses such as breeding.

BRUISED SOLE AND CORNS

Bruising on the volar surface of the foot usually is caused by direct injury from stones, irregular ground, or other trauma. Poor shoeing, especially in horses with flat feet or dropped soles, predisposes to bruising, usually around the periphery of the sole. Bruising may or may not be associated with lameness, but if it becomes chronic, the affected area can become infected. Persistent, nonresponsive bruised sole suggests pedal osteitis.

A "corn" is a specific type of bruising that is seen in the sole at the buttress (ie, the angle between the wall and the bar). It is most common in the forefeet on the inner buttress and is usually associated with the heel of a shoe that was improperly placed or left on too long and caused pressure on the sole. Shoes that have been fitted too closely at the quarters can also cause corns. Faulty foot conformation, straight walls that tend to turn in at the quarters, or contracted feet may predispose to corns. Other causes include excess trimming of the sole (which exposes the sensitive tissue to contusion) or neglect of the feet to the extent that they become long and irregular.

Corns are described as dry when only mild inflammatory changes exist, as moist when there is excess inflammatory exudate, and as suppurative once they become secondarily infected. When the foot is raised and the solar surface freed of dirt and loose horn, a discoloration, either red or reddish yellow, is noted. Supporting-leg lameness is an early sign, but lameness is not always seen. Tapping with a light hammer over the area or applying pressure with a hoof tester usually causes discomfort. If infection is present, pain is pronounced when pressure is applied with hoof testers; if not promptly treated, a tract may extend through the coronet to produce a suppurating sinus.

The prognosis is favorable. In uncomplicated dry corns, relief from pressure on the affected area is the first consideration. This can be achieved by shortening the toe if it is too long and by applying a bar shoe to promote frog pressure. A three-quarter-bar shoe may be of value in relieving pressure.

If the corn is suppurating, it should be drained immediately by a surgical opening directly through the sole. After drainage, the foot should be dressed to permit drainage. Hot foot baths and poultices may be helpful. The horse should be kept in a dry, clean box stall. After infection is controlled, the cavity can be packed with sterile gauze and topical antibiotic ointment, and a metal, rubber, or leather sole placed between the shoe and the foot. Parenteral antibacterial therapy is of questionable value unless systemic illness is present.

CANKER

Canker is a chronic hypertrophy and apparent suppuration of the horn-producing tissues of the foot, involving the frog and the sole. The cause is unknown. Primarily a disease of the heavy draft horse, canker is seldom seen today, although it has been seen frequently in certain stables of light horses in the southern USA. It is most often found in the hindfeet and is frequently well advanced before detection. The frog may appear to be intact but has a ragged, oiled appearance. The horn tissue of the frog loosens easily and reveals a swollen, foul-smelling corium covered with a caseous exudate. The surface of the corium is irregular with a characteristic vegetative growth. The disease process may extend to the sole and even to the wall, showing no tendency to heal.

The prognosis is guarded. Treatment must be radical and intensive. All loose horn and affected tissue should be removed, and an antiseptic or antibiotic dressing applied daily. A clean, dry wound environment must be maintained to allow healing, which may take weeks or months. Waterproof materials and plastic boots are used for such purposes. If the horse is not lame, it can be returned to work during the period of healing by use of a special shoe with a removable sole plate to maintain the dressing.

CONTRACTED HEELS

Contracted heels are seen principally in the forefeet of light horses. It may be caused by improper shoeing that draws in the quarters, which prevents hoof expansion and adequate frog pressure. Dry hooves, excess rasping of the wall, and trimming of the bars are predisposing factors. The condition may follow the use of a hoof-immobilizing shoe, as used for fracture of the third phalanx.

The frog is narrow and shrunken, the bars may be curved or almost parallel to each other, and the quarters and heels are markedly contracted and drawn in. The hoof horn is dry and hard. Lameness is evident when the horse is worked at speed. The length of stride is shortened, and heat may be noticed around the heels and quarters.

The prognosis is guarded; recovery in advanced cases takes 6-12 mo. The most important factors in treatment are to moisturize the hooves and to promote expansion. This can be achieved by soaking the feet in water daily for 10-14 days followed by corrective shoeing. Hoof-moisturizing products that contain oils or waxy substances should be used with caution because they can seal the water out of the hoof. Slipper shoes with no more than three nails in each branch promote hoof expansion. Quarter clips and the fourth nail must be avoided.

Thinning the wall of the quarters just below the coronary band with a rasp, or grooving the walls parallel to the coronet, $^3/_4$ in. (2 cm) below the hairline from the heel halfway to the toe, aids in expanding the heels; the second and third grooves should be $^1/_2$ in. (1.2 cm) apart and parallel to the first. As the quarters grow out, the procedure may need to be repeated until the heels and quarters are expanded normally.

FRACTURE OF NAVICULAR BONE

This may occur as a result of trauma or concussion to the foot or as a sequela of navicular disease (p 909). It is much less common than pedal bone fracture but may be seen in fore- or hindfeet. Although pain is variable, hoof testers usually indicate the general site. Lameness is persistent and can be eliminated by palmar digital nerve block. Radiography confirms the diagnosis; however, care should be taken with interpretation because congenital bipartite navicular bones can be confused with fractures.

Treatment is prolonged rest and corrective trimming to alleviate tendon adhesions, but a satisfactory bony union at the fracture site seldom occurs. Surgical repair by lag screw has been described. Prognosis is guarded to poor. Although this is the type of malunion fracture that might respond to low-intensity magnetic field therapy, supportive evidence is lacking.

FRACTURE OF PEDAL BONE
(Fracture of third phalanx, os pedis, or distal phalanx)

Fracture of the pedal bone is not an uncommon injury. It occurs due to concussion and produces a sudden onset of lameness during exercise or a race. Most fractures are through the lateral wing of the pedal bone and often extend into the distal phalangeal joint.

Acute weight-bearing lameness is seen, and usually there is pain on compression of the foot with hoof testers. Lightly tapping the hoof with a hammer also may elicit pain. Lameness is exacerbated by turning the horse or making it pivot on the affected leg. If the fracture does not extend into the joint, the lameness may improve considerably after 48 hr of stall rest.

The clinical signs may be suggestive, but the diagnosis is confirmed by distal palmar nerve block and radiography. Often, more than two views are required before the fracture line is evident. Radiographic confirmation may be difficult immediately after the injury because the fracture is only a hairline at this stage. Repeating the radiography 48-72 hr later and using oblique views may be necessary to confirm the presence and exact site of the fracture. Determining whether the fracture extends into the distal phalangeal joint is important.

Conservative treatment of 6-9 mo rest is usually all that is required for fractures that do not involve the joint. Fractures often heal with a fibrous union, so that even though the horse returns to soundness, radiographic evidence of the fracture remains. It is usual to fit a plain bar shoe with a clip well back on each quarter to limit expansion and contraction of the heels. In young horses (<3 yr old), fractures into the joint usually heal satisfactorily, provided a 12-mo rest period is given. Older horses (>3 yr old) have a much less favorable prognosis, and insertion of a cortical bone screw using interfragmentary compression across the fracture site is indicated. However, infection is a frequent complication. Many fractures heal in the presence of infection, but the screw must be removed at a second surgery to restore the horse to complete working soundness. Palmar digital neurectomy of racehorses with wing fractures has been used to allow return to competition without the delay for complete healing.

KERATOMA
(Keraphyllocele)

A keratoma is hypertrophy of the horn on the inner aspect of the wall, usually at the toe. It is believed to follow a chronic inflammatory process of the laminar matrix caused by "nail bind," mechanical injury to the wall or coronet, or hoof-grooving. The condition may be difficult to detect until the growth is well advanced. Examination of the palmar surface shows that the growth, commonly cylindrical, has pushed the white line in toward the center of the sole. Pressure atrophy of the pedal bone commonly follows in severe cases. Surgical removal of the mass is indicated. In mild cases, corrective shoeing may give some temporary relief. The prognosis is guarded.

LAMINITIS
(Founder, Fever in the feet)

Traditionally defined as inflammation or edema of the sensitive laminae of the hoof, laminitis is now thought to be a transient ischemia associated with coagulopathy that leads to breakdown and degeneration of the union between the horny and sensitive laminae. In refractory cases, rotation of the pedal bone is a common sequela that may progress to perforation of the sole. The disease is a local manifestation of a more generalized metabolic disturbance, and the hoof problems are classified as acute, subacute, or chronic. It can develop in the forefeet, all four feet, or occasionally only in the hindfeet. Biomechanical laminitis can be seen in a single foot, usually as a complication of a severe lameness or orthopedic disease in the contralateral limb.

Etiology: The most common causes of laminitis are ingestion of excess carbohydrate (grain overload), grazing of lush pastures (especially in ponies), and excess exercise and concussion in an unfit horse. It also may develop secondary to postparturient metritis, endotoxemia, colic and enteritis, or administration of an excess of corticosteroid or some other medicament. The risk is higher in ponies and in horses that are overweight and unfit. Incidence of the acute and subacute forms is higher whenever there is a flush of new grass.

The initial change in acute laminitis is ischemia of the lamellar arterioles and venules. The arterial blood is then shunted to the venous return via the many anastomotic blood vessels in the foot (especially at the coronary band) and bypasses the corium; the result is stagnation of blood and functional congestion and thromboembolism of the capillary beds. Laminar necrosis contributes to rotation.

These disturbances in the circulation to the foot, which initially are reversible, probably cause the exhibited pain. However, if the condition becomes protracted and there is chronic hypoxia and a lack of essential sulfur-containing amino acids for the corium, then keratinization slows or stops between the stratum germinativum and the keratogenous zone. The end result, in mild cases, is production of "laminitic rings"; in severe cases, pedal rotation or complete separation of the hoof from the underlying tissues occurs. The separation of the horny and sensitive laminae is due to ischemia, faulty keratinization, and the constant pull of the deep flexor tendon on the pedal bone, along with the upward push of the toe as the horse stands. There is some support at the back of the pedal bone from the deep digital flexor tendon and the digital cushion; however, these supportive structures may serve as a fulcrum, resulting in pedal bone rotation. If the separation occurs rapidly, the pedal bone may "sink" within the hoof. In chronic cases, the corona of the pedal bone may penetrate the sole just in front of the frog. The prognosis in severe cases is poor because the changes become irreversible, and secondary infection is common. In subacute and chronic cases, the rotation of the pedal bone occurs relatively slowly. The sole tends to become convex and thicken, and the hoof alters shape to accommodate the new position.

Clinical Findings: In acute laminitis, the horse is depressed and anorectic and stands reluctantly. Resistance to any exercise is marked, and the normal stance is altered in attempts to relieve the weight borne by the affected feet. If forced to walk, the horse shows a slow, crouching, short-striding gait. Each foot, once lifted, is set down as quickly as possible.

Usually, heat is apparent in the whole hoof, especially near the coronary band. An exaggerated and bounding pulse can be palpated and may be visible in the digital arteries. Pain can cause muscular trembling, and a fairly uniform tenderness can be detected when pressure is applied to the feet. The pedal bone may rotate during or after the acute stage if efficacious treatment is not given rapidly. Radiographic evidence of rotation can be present as early as the third day. The visible mucosae are often injected, with increased body temperature (104-106°F [40-41°C]), pulse rate (80-120/min), and respiratory rate (80-100/min). In exceptionally severe cases, for which the prognosis is unfavorable, a blood-stained exudate may seep from the coronary bands.

Subacute cases may exhibit any or all of the above clinical signs but to a lesser degree. Often, there is only a mild change in stance, with reluctance to walk and some increased sensitivity to concussion on the soles of the affected feet. There may be no demonstrable heat in the coronary band or increase in digital pulse. The acute and subacute forms of laminitis tend to recur at varying intervals and may develop into the chronic form.

Chronic laminitis is characterized by changes in the shape of the hoof and usually follows one or more attacks of the acute form. Bands of irregular horn growth (laminitic rings) may be seen in the hoof, close at the toe and diverging at the heel. The hoof itself becomes narrow and elongated, with the wall almost vertical at the heel and horizontal at the toe.

As the condition progresses, the sole becomes thickened and either flattened or somewhat convex in outline. The gait is similar to that already described, and when standing, the body weight is continually shifted from one foot to the other. Radiography reveals rotation and some osteoporosis of the pedal bone. The corona of the bone is forced downward and presses on the horny sole. In severe cases, it may penetrate the sole just in front of the point of the frog.

Diagnosis: In acute and severe laminitis, diagnosis is based on the history (eg, grain overload) and posture of the horse, increased temperature of the hooves, a hard pulse in the digital arteries, and reluctance to move. Mild cases with no visible hoof deformity can be identified via radiography of the affected feet, which show a lack of parallelism on the lateral projection between the hoof wall and cranial face of the third phalanx. Divergence of ≥11° indicates a guarded to unfavorable prognosis for return to performance.

Treatment: Acute laminitis constitutes a medical emergency because pedal rotation can occur rapidly. Despite prompt therapy, the prognosis is guarded until recovery is complete and it is evident that the hoof architecture is not altered. In acute laminitis, especially in cases of grain overload, mineral oil is indicated; 1 gal. (4 L), PO, acts as a laxative and tends to prevent absorption of toxic material from the GI tract. Purgation should not be done in the acute phase because most horses tend to be dehydrated.

Traditionally, cold packs or ice packs applied to the affected feet have been advocated, but recent evidence suggests that hot packs used early in the course of the disease may be more beneficial. Antihistamines are of doubtful value during acute lameness, but isoxsuprine hydrochloride paste, a peripheral vasodilating agent, may be of value. Heparin (40 u/kg, TID for 3 days) has been used because of the suspected accompanying coagulopathy and thromboembolism; however, heparin therapy in horses has been associated with RBC clumping which, in a dehydrated animal, could aggravate dynamics of local blood flow in the feet.

Flunixin meglumine and phenylbutazone are the preferred anti-inflammatory agents, and meclofenamic acid also has been of value; however, all three may be toxic. These NSAID should be used according to label instructions and, if used in combination, the dosage of each should be reduced accordingly.

Phenoxybenzamine hydrochloride (0.66 mg/kg, IV, in 500 mL saline), which is an α-adrenergic blocker that causes vasodilation for up to 24 hr, has been used in severe and acute cases of laminitis. However, it may cause depression and should be avoided in horses in shock.

Heart-bar shoes have been used in acute cases in an attempt to diffuse sole pressure and avoid pedal rotation. Because an improperly fitted heart-bar shoe aggravates the pain, correct fitting is essential.

Administration of corticosteroids is contraindicated because serious cellular catabolism and inhibition of the immune responses often result in muscular wasting and worsening of the laminitis. Because gram-negative endotoxins due to carbohydrate overload have been implicated in laminitis, it is especially important to preserve the normal immune responses during treatment.

Experimentally, a combination vaccine consisting of a killed *Salmonella* mutant bacterin, an endotoxoid, and an aluminum hydroxide adjuvant has been effective in reducing the endotoxin-related complications of laminitis.

Digital nerve blocks in the early stages of the disease permit the horse to be walked, which increases the arterial blood flow through the terminal arch. However, nerve blocking and walking are contraindicated once pedal rotation has begun. Because of its value in hoof keratinization, methionine has been used at dosages of 10 mg/lb (22 mg/kg), daily for 1 wk followed by 5 mg/lb for the second week and 2.5 mg/lb for the third.

Treatment of chronic laminitis has consisted of attempting to restore the normal alignment of the rotated coffin bone and encouraging frog pressure by lowering the heels, removing excess toe, and protecting the dropped sole. This requires corrective hoof trimming and the use of full leather pads or a heart-bar shoe. Acrylic compounds are useful in conjunction with proper trimming to build up the toe and to protect the sole. The hoof should be trimmed and the shoe reset at 4- to 6-wk intervals. This approach can be successful in selected cases but is expensive, labor intensive, and prolonged.

Resection of the separated hoof wall may also be indicated and has been used in acute and chronic cases, particularly those with seedy toe or infection. This surgical procedure carries risk and should follow consultation between the veterinarian and farrier.

NAVICULAR DISEASE
(Podotrochlosis, Podotrochlitis)

Navicular disease is essentially a chronic degenerative condition of the navicular bursa and navicular bone that involves damage to the flexor surface of the bone and the overlying deep digital flexor tendon with osteophyte formation on the lateral and proximal borders of the bone. Thus, it is a syndrome with a complex pathogenesis rather than a specific disease entity. It is one of the most common causes of chronic forelimb lameness in horses but is essentially unknown in ponies and donkeys.

Etiology: The exact cause is unknown, but it is likely to be multifactorial involving the navicular bone and its blood supply, the suspensory ligament, the distal phalangeal joint, the navicular bursa, and the deep digital flexor tendon. It is considered to be a disease of the more mature riding horse, but radiographic signs have been seen in 3-yr-olds. It may be partially hereditary; it is certainly associated with upright conformation of the forefoot. The conformation of the foot in chronic cases becomes abnormal; it is upright and narrow and has a small frog. Defective shoeing that inhibits the action of the frog and the quarters may be contributory. Concussion between the flexor tendon and the navicular bone can cause a local bursitis that leads to hyperemia and rarefaction of the bone with resultant alteration of the flexor surface of the bone.

Clinical Findings and Diagnosis: Usually, the disease is insidious in onset. Attention is first directed to the affected foot or feet by the attitude of the horse when at rest. The horse relieves the pressure of the deep digital flexor tendon on the painful area by pointing or advancing the affected foot with the heel off the ground. If both forefeet are affected, they are pointed alternately. An intermittent lameness is manifest early in the course of the disease. The stride is shortened, and the horse may tend to stumble. A flexion test involving the distal forelimb usually produces a transient exacerbation of lameness. There may be soreness in the brachiocephalic muscles secondary to the changes in posture and gait, thus the frequent complaint of "shoulder lameness."

Clinical diagnosis is reasonably straightforward and is based on a complete history and careful physical examination. The lameness can be eliminated by palmar digital nerve block. Radiographic changes include a range of degenerative changes involving the navicular bone. These include marginal osteophytes, bone remodeling, enlarged synovial fossae (so-called vascular channels), and flexor cortex changes. These lesions may result from navicular disease or natural aging and must be interpreted in light of the history and clinical findings.

Treatment: Because the condition is both chronic and degenerative, it can be managed in some horses but not cured. With severe lameness, rest is indicated. Foot care is directed to trimming and shoeing that restores normal phalangeal alignment and balance. Thinning the quarters with a rasp and proper hoof moisturization may relieve hoof contraction. Slippered branches and a wedge pad assist hoof expansion, but the normal angle must be maintained and only three nails used in each branch; a fourth nail in the heel will nullify the slipper effect. Toes should be rounded to facilitate the "break-over." NSAID such as phenylbutazone, along with proper foot management, extend serviceable soundness in some horses. Intrabursal injection of corticosteroid also is more palliative than curative. Another therapy is isoxsuprine hydrochloride (0.27 mg/lb [0.6 mg/kg], PO, BID for 6-14 wk) in a paste form, which acts as a peripheral vasodilator, but recurrences follow cessation of therapy.

Palmar digital neurectomy may render relief from pain and prolong the usefulness of the horse, but no neurectomy should be considered curative. Digital neurectomy can be accompanied by severe complications such as painful neuroma formation. Volar and higher neurectomy should never be done.

A technique of desmotomy of the collateral sesamoidean ligament has also been described. By cutting this ligament, the concussive forces between the navicular bone and the deep digital flexor tendon are thought to be reduced. The results are preliminary and unsubstantiated.

Although the prognosis is guarded to poor, a carefully designed therapeutic regimen can prolong the usefulness of most horses, and the competitive status of many. Over months or years, all affected horses reach a point of nonresponsiveness to treatment.

PEDAL OSTEITIS

Pedal osteitis is an inflammation of the sensitive structures of the volar aspect of the forefeet, associated with osteitis and demineralization of the coffin bone. Repeated concussion, laminitis, persistent corns, and chronic bruised sole have been implicated as causes. Pedal osteitis is common in performance horses and usually is associated with work on hard tracks. Lameness may not be obvious because usually both forelimbs are affected. There may be a stilted or shuffling action in front, with signs of discomfort in the hoof region. Percussion and pressure from hoof testers usually reveal tenderness over the whole of the sole. Radiography is helpful in diagnosis and in differentiation between navicular disease.

Treatment involves prolonged rest, anti-inflammatory medication, and careful shoeing to relieve sole pressure. Prognosis is guarded, but the serviceable soundness of many horses can be extended by proper management.

PUNCTURE WOUNDS OF THE FOOT
(Pricked foot, Nail bind, Nail prick, Subsolar abscess)

Puncture wounds are usually the result of poor farriery technique but can occur when a horse steps on a penetrating foreign body. "Nail bind" implies that a nail has been driven close to the sensitive structures of the foot, causing acute pain. "Nail prick" means the corium has been penetrated.

Puncture of the sole by a foreign body is associated with introduction of pathogenic microorganisms. Lameness is usually severe, especially when bearing weight; the degree may be similar to that of a fracture. The horse may stand pointing the affected foot. There is increased heat and pain in the foot, which progress to the coronary band as abscess formation proceeds. Subsequently, there is edematous swelling of the pastern and fetlock areas. In neglected cases, there is draining at the coronary band after 2-3 wk. Diagnosis is made by confirming the site of pain by pulling the shoe, using hoof testers, and paring the suspect area to locate the foreign body or its track.

Prompt treatment with disinfectants and poultices is important for nail bind and nail prick. Ensuring adequate drainage from the site helps prevent abscess formation. In pricked foot, the prognosis is good, provided diagnosis is made and therapy begun early. If a chronic subsolar abscess has developed, treatment may be prolonged and the prognosis guarded. If infection spreads to the distal interphalangeal joint, the prognosis is unfavorable.

If present, foreign bodies must be found and removed, and the infected area pared with a hoof knife to establish adequate drainage. The foot should then be kept in a rubber or plastic boot for 3-5 days with a cotton pad soaked in saturated magnesium sulfate solution or other suitable poultice. All horses with puncture wounds should be immunized against tetanus. If pain is severe, a palmar nerve block provides temporary relief. Local and systemic antibiotic therapy are not necessary, provided the infection is localized and good drainage has been achieved. Deep punctures of the foot that involve the deep digital flexor tendon, navicular bursa, navicular bone, or third phalanx are surgical emergencies.

PYRAMIDAL DISEASE
(Extensor process disease, Buttress foot)

Once classified as a type of low ringbone (p 914), pyramidal disease arises from a traumatically induced periostitis or an avulsion fracture of the extensor process of the third phalanx caused by excess tension at the tendon insertion. The close association of the extensor process with the distal phalangeal joint means secondary arthritis is a likely complication. In early cases, heat and pain on pressure may be manifest. An enlargement of the toe region just above the coronet is usually present, which results in the "buttress foot" appearance. Systemic anti-inflammatory medication may be beneficial. Surgery has been successful for avulsion fractures.

QUITTOR
(Coronary sinus)

Quittor is a chronic, purulent inflammation of the cartilage of the third phalanx characterized by necrosis of the cartilage and one or more sinus tracts extending from the diseased cartilage through the skin in the coronary region. It is seldom encountered today but used to be common in working draft horses. Quittor follows injury to the coronet or pastern over the region of the cartilage, by means of which infection is introduced into the deep tissues to form a subcoronary abscess, or it may follow a penetrating wound through the sole. The first sign is an inflammatory swelling over the region of the alar cartilage, which is followed by abscessation and sinus formation. During the acute stage, lameness occurs.

Surgery to remove the diseased tissue and cartilage is usually successful. Local or parenteral therapy (or both) without surgery is likely to fail. In the absence of any therapy, poor drainage, cartilage necrosis, and recurrent abscessation lead to chronic lameness and extension to deep structures. If damage is extensive and the distal interphalangeal joint has been invaded, the prognosis is unfavorable.

SANDCRACK
(Toe crack, Quarter crack)

In sandcrack, cracks in the wall of the hoof begin at the coronet and run parallel to the horn tubules. They are most common in racehorses. Excess drying of the hoof is predisposing, but trauma or conformational factors are cited as the most likely causes. Extensive injury to the coronet may give rise to a crack in the wall characterized by buildup and overlapping of the hoof wall at the site of injury. This latter condition is referred to as false quarter.

A crack in the horn emanating from the coronet is the most obvious sign. Lameness is usually not seen. If infection is established, there may be a bloody or purulent discharge and signs of inflammation and lameness. Therapy involves surgery and corrective shoeing to change the distribution of weight on the hoof. Growth of new horn may be encouraged by application of a counterirritant (eg, tincture of iodine) to the coronet over the crack. Iodine should be used with caution on light-colored or white skin. If the crack has become infected, an antiseptic pack is indicated. Patching techniques using acrylics or fiberglass are useful if properly and judiciously applied. Complete stripping of the wall caudal to the crack, being careful not to damage the coronet, is often the treatment of choice in early and severe quarter cracks, or when a hoof spur has formed. The hoof is then bandaged until new horn formation is evident. The horse is then shod with a three-quarter or three-quarter-bar shoe to relieve any pressure over the stripped portion of the wall.

SCRATCHES
(Greasy heel, Dermatitis verrucosa)

Scratches is a chronic, seborrheic dermatitis characterized by hypertrophy and exudation on the caudal surface of the pastern and fetlock. It often is associated with poor stable hygiene, but no specific cause is known. Heavy horses are particularly susceptible, and the hindlimbs are affected more commonly. Standardbreds frequently are affected in the spring when tracks are wet. The common use of limestone on racetracks has been associated with scratches.

Scratches may go unnoticed if hidden by the "feather" at the back of the pastern. The skin is itchy, sensitive, and swollen during the acute stages; later, it becomes thickened and most of the hair is lost. Only the shorter hairs remain, and these stand erect. The surface of the skin is soft, and the grayish exudate has a fetid odor. The condition can become chronic, with vegetative granulomas. Lameness may or may not be present; it can be severe and associated with generalized cellulitis of the limb. As the condition progresses, there is thickening and hardening of the skin of the affected regions, with rapid hypertrophy of subcutaneous fibrous tissue.

Persistent and aggressive treatment is usually successful. This consists of removing the hair, regular washing and cleansing with warm water and soap to remove all soft exudate, drying, and applying an astringent dressing. If granulomas appear, they should be cauterized. Cellulitis requires systemic antibiotic therapy and tetanus prophylaxis.

SEEDY TOE
(Hollow wall, Dystrophia ungulae)

Seedy toe is a condition of the hoof wall in the toe region, characterized by loss of substance and change in character of the horn. It is most often a sequela of mild chronic laminitis. The outer surface of the wall appears sound, but on dressing the palmar surface of the hoof, the inner surface of the wall is mealy, and there may be a cavity due to loss of horn substance. Tapping on the outside of the wall at the toe elicits a hollow sound over the affected portion. The disease may involve only a small area or nearly the entire width of the wall at the toe. Lameness is infrequent but accompanies the occasional infection and abscessation.

The prognosis is usually good. The diseased portion should be cleaned and packed with juniper tar and oakum. In the absence of lameness, shoeing and work can continue. If the condition is extensive, the outer wall may need to be removed over the affected area.

SHEARED HEELS

In sheared heels, there is severe acquired imbalance of the foot with asymmetry of the heels. The imbalance results in one side of the heel contacting the ground before the other, which creates a shearing force at the bulbs of the heel, asymmetrical growth of the toe, and severe overriding contraction of the heels. There is chronic heel soreness indistinguishable from that of navicular disease. The asymmetrical foot must be viewed carefully from all angles, and the gait observed at a slow walk to detect the abnormal weight bearing and shearing stresses in the central sulcus region. Hoof cracks, deep fissuring between the bulbs of the heel, and thrush frequently accompany the problem. Navicular disease may be concurrent.

Corrective trimming and shoeing to restore proper heel alignment and foot balance are required. A full bar shoe with a reinforcing diagonal bar to support the affected quarter and heel is used. Several shoe resettings are required before improvement is evident. The prognosis is good in uncomplicated cases if the corrective measures are consistently applied until new hoof growth occurs.

SIDEBONE

Sidebone is ossification of the cartilages of the third phalanx. It is most common in the forefeet of heavy horses working on hard surfaces. It also is frequent in hunters and jumpers but rare in racing Thoroughbreds. Repeated concussion to the quarters of the feet is probably the essential cause. Predisposition may be inherited, but this has not been confirmed. Improper shoeing that inhibits normal physiologic movement of the quarters is also predisposing. Some cases arise from direct trauma.

Loss of flexibility on digital palpation of either one or both cartilages is indicative of sidebone. Because the rigidity of the cartilages is accompanied by ossification, the cartilages may protrude prominently above the coronet. Lameness may be a sign, depending on the stage of ossification, the amount of concussion sustained by the feet, and the character of the terrain. Lameness is most likely when sidebone is associated with a narrow or contracted foot or an accompanying condition such as navicular disease. The stride may be shortened, and walking the horse across a slope may exaggerate the soreness. Mules often have prominent sidebones, yet seldom show any lameness.

Sidebone may be suspected after palpation and observation, but radiographic examination is essential for confirmation. It should be remembered that ossification of the cartilages commonly develops without signs of lameness. When lameness is present, corrective shoeing to promote expansion of the quarters and to protect the foot from concussion is often of value. Grooving the hooves, along with applying a counterirritant (eg, tincture of iodine) to the coronary region to promote hoof growth, also may promote expansion of the wall.

THRUSH

Thrush is a degeneration of the frog with secondary bacterial infection that begins in the central and collateral sulci. It results from poor management and hygiene that permit horses to stand in wet conditions for prolonged periods and from failure to clean the hooves regularly. It is more common in the hindfeet. The affected sulcus is moist and contains a black, thick discharge with a characteristic foul odor. These signs alone are sufficient to make the diagnosis.

Treatment should begin by providing dry, clean standings and cleaning out the hoof with removal of all macerated horn. An astringent lotion, used with daily hoof cleaning, aids recovery after removal of the diseased tissue. Use of a bar shoe after the disease process has been arrested may help in the regeneration of the frog. The prognosis is usually favorable, but if the corium of the frog has been damaged, all diseased frog tissue must be removed.

DISORDERS OF THE FETLOCK AND PASTERN

FRACTURE OF PHALANGES AND PROXIMAL SESAMOIDS

Fractures of the first phalanx are not uncommon in racehorses. They may be small "chip" fractures along the dorsal margin of the proximal joint surface, longitudinal fractures (split pastern), or comminuted. Another category, seen exclusively in Standardbreds, involves chip or avulsion-type fractures of the palmar or plantar proximal aspect of the first phalanx (so-called Birkeland fractures).

Signs of longitudinal fractures involve acute weightbearing lameness after work or a race. There may be little or no swelling initially, but there is intense pain on palpation or flexion of the fetlock. Lameness may be less pronounced with chip or avulsion fractures, but flexion of the joint exacerbates the problem.

Diagnosis is confirmed by radiography, although a number of oblique views may be necessary to ensure visibility of the fracture line, which may be seen initially as a fine fissure extending from the fetlock joint into the distal cortex.

Chip and avulsion fractures can be removed by arthroscopic surgery. Longitudinal fractures can be repaired by internal fixation using two or more cortical bone screws by the technique of interfragmentary compression. Conservative treatment of severely comminuted fractures involves immobilization with a plaster or fiberglass cast for up to 12 wk. However, complications include poor alignment at the fracture site and secondary arthritis.

Fractures of the second phalanx are similar to those of the first phalanx but less common. Treatment and prognosis are similar.

Fractures of the proximal sesamoid bones are relatively common. They are caused by overextension and often are associated with suspensory ligament damage, as in the forelimb of Thoroughbreds. The lateral proximal sesamoid in the hindlimb of Standardbreds may be fractured as a result of torque forces induced by shoeing with a trailer-type shoe. The fractures may be apical, middle, basal, or multiple; they may involve one or both sesamoids. Clinical signs include heat, pain, and acute lameness, which is exacerbated by flexion of the fetlock. There is hemarthrosis and synovial effusion of the fetlock joint. Diagnosis is confirmed radiographically. The prognosis is fairly good if small fragments are promptly surgically removed. Standardbreds respond more favorably than Thoroughbreds because of their 2-beat, symmetrical gait. The prognosis in large basilar fractures is poor, regardless of surgical approach. Complete disruption of the suspensory apparatus, including fractures of both sesamoid bones, is a catastrophic injury accompanied by vascular compromise of the foot; however, some horses can be salvaged for breeding by surgical arthrodesis of the fetlock joint.

OSSELETS
(Osslets, Periostitis and serous arthritis)

Osselets refer to an inflammation, usually bilateral, of the periosteum on the dorsal distal epiphyseal surface of the third metacarpal bone and the associated capsule of the fetlock joint. The proximal end of the first phalanx may also be involved. Hence, osselets constitutes a form of periostitis and serous arthritis that may progress to degenerative joint disease. The exciting cause is the strain and repeated trauma of hard training in young horses and is recognized as an occupational hazard of the young Thoroughbred.

The gait is short and choppy. Palpation and flexion of the fetlock joint produce pain, and examination reveals a soft, warm, sensitive swelling over the front and sometimes the side of the joint. Radiography in the initial stages may show no evidence of new bone formation, in which case the condition is called "green osselets." Later, enthesopathy may be seen in the area of attachment of the fetlock joint capsule to the large metacarpal bone and first phalanx. New bone or spur formation may break off and appear as "joint mice."

Rest is very important and can be curative for early cases. The inflammation may be relieved by the application of cold packs for several days. Systemic anti-inflammatory drugs such as phenylbutazone may also be used. Corticosteroid can also be injected intra-articularly; however, this and other forms of anti-inflammatory medication, if used along with continued training or racing, inevitably lead to destruction of the joint surfaces. Intra-articular sodium hyaluronate is useful to reestablish normal synovial viscosity.

RINGBONE

Ringbone is a periostitis or osteoarthritis of the phalanges that leads to exostoses. Faulty conformation, improper shoeing, or repeated concussion through working on hard ground are causative; trauma and infection, especially wire-cut wounds, are also incriminated. In light horses, the strain of ligaments and tendinous insertions in the pastern region are frequent causal factors. It may be a part of the osteochondrosis syndrome (p 929) in young, rapidly growing horses.

There is a characteristic bell-shaped appearance to the pastern region. Lameness due to periostitis is seen initially. Once bone proliferation has occurred, lameness may not be present, particularly if there is no involvement of the articular surfaces. However, lameness usually persists if the joint surfaces are involved, and this may progress to ankylosis.

Clinical diagnosis is based on visualization and palpation of soft-tissue thickness and new bone proliferation in the pastern region. Usually, the range of joint movement is restricted, and there is pain on forced flexion of the involved articular surfaces. Regional nerve blocks identify the pastern region as the site of pain. Radiography confirms the diagnosis.

Complete rest is the most important requirement for treatment. Cold and astringent applications as well as radiation therapy in the early stages may be beneficial. Anti-inflammatory medication may relieve the signs of lameness. Surgical arthrodesis of the pastern joint is curative and is used successfully to restore the performance future of young horses with osteochondrosis.

SESAMOIDITIS

The sesamoid bones are maintained in position by the suspensory ligament proximally and by a number of sesamoidean ligaments distally. Due to the great stress placed on the fetlock during fast exercise, the insertion of some of these ligaments can tear, which results in sesamoiditis.

The clinical signs are similar to, but less severe than, those resulting from sesamoid fracture. Depending on the extent of the damage, there are varying degrees of lameness and swelling. Reduced speed may be the only manifestation of lameness. Pain and heat are evident on palpation and flexion of the fetlock joint. The radiographic features include periosteal new bone proliferation or osteolytic lesions (or both), particularly on the abaxial surface of the affected sesamoid, and radiolucent lines, which look similar to fracture lines except there is no fragment distraction, running obliquely across the bone.

These lines are prominent vascular channels. Oblique radiographic views are essential for accurate diagnosis and evaluation.

Despite various treatments, the prognosis is guarded or poor. Even after 9-12 mo rest, many horses become lame 6-8 wk after resuming training. The recommended treatment is a 2- to 3-wk course of phenylbutazone. For mild sesamoiditis, ≥6 mo rest is required; for severe cases, 9-12 mo.

VILLONODULAR SYNOVITIS

The cause of this inflammation of the synovial membrane of the dorsoproximal aspect of the forelimb fetlock joints is unknown. Affected horses are 2-18 yr old. Incidence is slightly higher in males. Bilateral involvement has been reported. The intra-articular nodules are usually attached by a broad stalk to the dorsal portion of the dorsal proximal pouch of the fetlock joint, are firm and grayish white, and may be circumscribed or lobulated. Erosive bone lesions are typically associated with the mass and, in some cases, may extend to erosion of the articular surface. Microscopically, the lesions consist of dense, well-collagenized stroma lined by synovial cells. Vascularization is prominent, and hyaline change in the stroma and osseous metaplasia are occasionally seen.

Diagnosis can be suspected by palpation and confirmed radiographically. Treatment is by surgical excision of the lesion. Smaller masses are amenable to arthroscopic surgery. Radiation therapy appears to help prevent recurrences after surgical excision.

WINDGALLS
(Windpuffs)

These puffy, fluid-filled swellings around the fetlock joints (of either or both fore- and hindlimbs) usually are not accompanied by heat, pain, or lameness. They are said to be associated with trauma and hard exercise, but the exact pathogenesis is uncertain. Although usually benign, windgalls should be regarded with suspicion in the presence of lameness. Some horses, particularly heavy ones, seem to be more susceptible. Treatment is problematic; in the absence of lameness, it is unwarranted. Windgalls may disappear spontaneously or respond to periods of rest, bandaging, and exercise. Recurrence is common.

DISORDERS OF THE CARPUS AND METACARPUS

The carpus involves 3 articulations—the radiocarpal (antebrachial carpal), intercarpal (midcarpal), and carpometacarpal joints. Problems are localized to the carpal area based on lameness examination (including characteristic gait), swelling, synovial effusion and pain on palpation, and responses to flexion and diagnostic analgesia. The only clinical evidence of carpal problems may be synovial effusion and minor gait deficits. Visualization and palpation are important to determine the site of swelling in the carpus (eg, synovial fluid in the joint or tendon sheath or swelling in the subcutaneous space). Light palpation with fingers with the horse standing is useful initially. Synovial fluid accumulations tend to be more difficult to ascertain when the leg is picked up. Knowledge of the normal anatomic boundaries of the structures is important. The individual carpal bones can be assessed with the carpus flexed; direct palpation of lesions often elicits pain and the degree of carpal flexion possible may be noted.

Diagnostic analgesia of the carpal joints is usually done intra-articularly. The radiocarpal and intercarpal joints can be injected easily. The carpometacarpal joint communicates with the intercarpal joint; therefore, local analgesia in the intercarpal joint provides analgesia to the carpometacarpal joint. There is considerable distal outpouching of the carpometacarpal joint, and with time, analgesia will diffuse into the area of the proximal suspensory ligament.

Radiography of the carpus is critical for specific diagnosis of intra-articular fractures, osteochondrosis, subchondral cystic lesions, osteoarthritis, septic arthritis, and osteochondroma of the distal radius.

BUCKED SHINS
(Sore shins, Saucer fractures)

Bucked shins is a painful, acute periostitis on the cranial surface of the large metacarpal or metatarsal bone. It is seen most often in the forelimbs of young Thoroughbreds (2- to 3-yr-olds) in training and racing, and less commonly in Standardbreds and Quarter Horses.

This injury is generally brought about by strains placed on the dorsal cortex during high-speed exercise in young horses in which the bones are not fully conditioned. Microfractures (ie, stress fractures) are believed to be involved. It may progress to a cortical saucer fracture or even incomplete longitudinal fracture. In mild cases, subperiosteal hematoma formation and thickening of the superficial face of the cortex may be all that is clinically apparent. There is a warm, painful swelling on the cranial surface of the affected bone. The horse is usually lame initially, the stride is short, and the severity of the lameness increases with exercise.

Rest from training is important until the soreness and inflammation resolve. The acute inflammation may be relieved by anti-inflammatory analgesics and application of cold packs. Screw fixation of fissure fractures may be indicated in older horses with dorsal cortical fractures that fail to respond to conservative treatment.

DEGENERATIVE SUBCHONDRAL LESIONS OF THE CARPAL BONES

Degeneration and necrosis of the proximal surface of the third carpal bone is considered to be a consequence of cyclic trauma and probably precedes most intra-articular fractures. Recently, the presence of subchondral bone disease in other locations in the carpus has been recognized. Cases on the third carpal bone can be diagnosed radiographically with a skyline view. Other locations are often not seen until arthroscopic examination is done. The treatment is surgical debridement, and the prognosis is relatively good.

DESMITIS OR SPRAIN OF THE INFERIOR CHECK LIGAMENT

Inferior check ligament desmitis is a commonly made diagnosis and is often confused with desmitis of the proximal suspensory ligament. Before the use of diagnostic ultrasound, the differentiation was difficult. The primary clinical sign is lameness that is alleviated by infiltration of anesthetic behind the proximal aspect of the metacarpus. Anesthetic injected in this area, however, may infiltrate outpouchings of the carpometacarpal joint in >30% of horses, leading to analgesia of both the carpometacarpal and intercarpal joints. Therefore, a local block of the proximal aspect of the palmar metacarpal nerves is preferable. This condition has been treated conservatively in the past, but sectioning of the ligament has been performed more recently with good results.

FRACTURE OF THE CARPAL BONES

Intra-articular Osteochondral Chip Fragments of the Carpus

These are the most common fractures in the carpal joints of racehorses. They occur less commonly in working Quarter Horses and sport horses. The primary etiologic factor is trauma, usually associated with fast exercise. Chips may occur on the dorsal aspect of all the carpal bones. In the intercarpal joint, the most frequent site is the distal radial carpal bone, followed by the distal intermediate carpal bone and the proximal third carpal bone. In the radial carpal joint, the most common location is the proximal intermediate carpal bone, followed by the proximal radial carpal bone, distal medial radius, and the distal lateral radius. The diagnosis is based on clinical signs of synovitis and capsulitis and radiographic demonstration of chip fragments. Arthroscopic surgery is the treatment of choice. The overall prognosis is excellent, but the percentage chance of the horse returning to previous performance levels decreases with chronicity and consequent excessive loss of articular cartilage and subchondral bone.

Carpal Slab Fractures

Slab fractures extend from one articular surface to another articular surface. In the carpus, slab fractures occur in both frontal and sagittal planes. The most common fracture is a frontal fragment of the radial facet of the third carpal bone, followed by fractures of the intermediate facet and both facets of this bone. When a frontal slab fracture of the third carpal bone occurs without joint collapse, it is considered to be "routine." The treatment is lag screw fixation (done arthroscopically), and many of these horses return to full athletic activity.

Collapsing slab fractures also occur in the carpal bones. The fracture typically involves the third carpal bone, but there is displacement and comminution to the extent that one row of carpal bones tends to collapse. If untreated, the leg progresses to a carpal varus conformation and laminitis develops in the opposite forelimb. Collapsing slab fractures require internal fixation, augmented with cast fixation for up to 6 wk, to minimize later collapse of the joint.

Accessory Carpal Bone Fractures

These are less common than other fractures in the carpus. Lameness generally is seen, and there may be synovial effusion in the carpal canal. Radiographs confirm the diagnosis. These fractures are treated conservatively. Union will occur in some cases. Fibrous union may enable a horse to return to athletic activity.

FRACTURES OF THE SMALL METACARPAL AND METATARSAL (SPLINT) BONES

Fractures of the second and fourth metacarpal and metatarsal (splint) bones are not uncommon. The cause may be from direct trauma, such as interference by the contralateral leg, but splint fractures more often follow a suspensory desmitis (*see* p 919) and the resulting fibrous tissue buildup and encapsulation of the distal, free end of the bone. The usual site of these fractures is through the distal end, ~2 in. (5 cm) from the tip. Immediately after the fracture occurs, acute inflammation is present, usually involving the suspensory ligament. A supporting-leg lameness is noted, which may recede after several days rest and recur only after work.

Chronic, longstanding fractures cause a supporting-leg lameness at speed. Thickening of the suspensory ligament at and above the fracture site results. The fracture may show a considerable buildup of callus at the fracture site but little tendency to heal.

Diagnosis is confirmed by an oblique radiograph. Surgical removal of the fractured tip and callus is the treatment of choice. The prognosis is based on severity of the associated suspensory desmitis, which has a greater bearing on future performance than the splint fracture itself.

FRACTURE OF THE THIRD METACARPAL (CANNON) BONE

A transverse fracture in the midmetacarpal region can result from direct trauma, usually from a kick. The stress of racing on a hard surface may result in a longitudinally oblique (ie, condylar) fracture that progresses up the metacarpal shaft from the fetlock and sometimes also involves the proximal sesamoids. Incomplete fractures of the dorsal cortex of the midmetacarpal region can occur as stress-type fractures. Diagnosis is confirmed by radiography; the fissure fractures can be difficult to demonstrate, and a range of oblique views may be necessary.

Midmetacarpal fractures may heal with just a cast, although prolonged immobilization may be necessary because union is often delayed. Malunion and the encroachment of callus on surrounding tendons and ligaments cause further problems. Internal fixation with dynamic compression plates and screws is the treatment of choice. Condylar fractures can be treated conservatively by casting, but such articular injuries are best managed by screw fixation using interfragmentary compression if osteoarthritis is to be minimized or avoided. Fissure fractures also may show delayed union unless a cortical bone screw is applied. (*See also* BUCKED SHINS, p 916.)

HYGROMA

A hygroma is inflammation of an acquired bursa (one that develops as a result of trauma where normally there is no bursa) over the dorsal aspect of the carpus. There is accumulation of excessive bursal fluid and thickening of the bursal wall by fibrous tissue. Lameness is not usually present. The diagnosis is made by palpation and visualization. Hygromas can be treated in the early stage with drainage, steroid injections, and bandaging. Later, the implantation of drains is required.

OSTEOARTHRITIS (DEGENERATIVE JOINT DISEASE)

In the carpus, osteoarthritis typically appears with chronic thickening of the joint, usually associated with capsular fibrosis. There is a decreased range of motion and sometimes a history of treatment of an acute problem. Radiographic changes develop slowly, and usually the degree of articular cartilage compromise is severe. Cases that can possibly lead to osteoarthritis should be treated aggressively and correctly. Treatment of severe osteoarthritis is largely palliative, but debridement and lavage, followed by intra-articular and systemic therapy, may help. (*See also* OSTEOARTHRITIS, p 863.)

OSTEOCHONDROSIS

Osteochondrosis of the carpal joints is rare. The typical presentation is a yearling with synovial effusion. Lameness is usually present and can be exacerbated by carpal flexion. Radiographs show the presence of subchondral lucencies typical of osteochondrosis, commonly in the distal radius. Treatment is arthroscopic surgery, but refragmentation and development of osteoarthritis has been seen. The prognosis is guarded. (*See also* OSTEOCHONDROSIS, p 929.)

OSTEOCHONDROMA OF THE DISTAL RADIUS (SUPRACARPAL EXOSTOSIS)

Osteochondroma formation at the distal end of the diaphysis and metaphysis of the radius is usually seen in young animals. The typical clinical history is swelling of the carpal canal sheath cranial to the ulnaris lateralis after exercise (often resolving in a few hours). At exercise, these horses exhibit moderate lameness. Deep palpation may elicit tenderness and a withdrawal response. Pain is usually elicited with rapid flexion. Diagnosis is generally made by radiography, but ultrasonic examination may be necessary to define the presence of the osteochondroma. The condition can be treated successfully via arthroscopic surgery. The protruding osteochondroma is removed and any concomitant damage to the deep flexor tendon debrided.

RUPTURE OF THE COMMON DIGITAL EXTENSOR TENDON

This developmental problem is present at birth or is seen shortly after. Foals usually show a carpal flexure deformity or a fetlock flexural deformity. If the condition is not noticed immediately, secondary contracture of the flexor muscle-tendon unit develops. The condition is confirmed by palpation of the swollen disrupted ends of the extensor tendon within the tendon sheath over the carpus. Management involves preventing secondary tendon contracture with the use of PVC splints to prevent knuckling, if appropriate. Healing will occur.

SPLINTS
(Metacarpal exostosis)

Splints primarily involve the interosseous ligament between the large (third) and small (second) metacarpal (less frequently the metatarsal) bones. The reaction is a periostitis with production of new bone (exostoses) along the involved splint bone. Trauma from concussion or injury, strain from excess training (especially in the immature horse), faulty conformation, imbalanced or overnutrition, or improper shoeing may be contributory factors.

Splints most commonly involve the medial rudimentary metacarpal bones. Lameness is seen only when splints are forming and is seen most frequently in young horses.

Lameness is more pronounced after the horse has been worked. In the early stages, there is no visible enlargement, but deep palpation may reveal local painful subperiosteal swelling. In the later stages, a calcified growth appears. After ossification, lameness disappears, except in rare cases in which the growth encroaches on the suspensory ligament or carpometacarpal articulation. Radiography is necessary to differentiate splints from fractured splint bones.

Complete rest and anti-inflammatory therapy is indicated. Intralesional corticosteroids may reduce inflammation and prevent excessive bone growth. Their use should be accompanied by counterpressure bandaging. In Thoroughbreds, it has been traditional to point-fire a splint, the aim being to accelerate the ossification of the interosseous ligament; however, in most cases, irritant treatments are contraindicated. If the exostoses impinge against the suspensory ligament, surgical removal may be necessary.

SUBCHONDRAL CYSTS AND SEPTIC ARTHRITIS

Subchondral cysts (p 862) may be seen in both the distal radius and the carpus. Many, particularly when bilateral and in the ulnar carpal bone, are normal. However, they are commonly symptomatic in the distal radius. They are diagnosed by radiography, and if conservative treatment does not solve the problem, arthroscopic debridement is done.

Infectious (septic) arthritis of the carpal joints is relatively rare. The most common cause is iatrogenic, in association with intra-articular injections. Horses show severe lameness and marked synovial effusion, as well as more peripheral swelling in the joint. Heat, pain, and synovial fluid changes are obvious. Synovial fluid WBC counts >30,000 and usually 100,000 cells/mm^3, protein levels of 4-6 g/dL in the presence of low viscosity, and a serosanguineous appearance are typical findings. For treatment, see SEPTIC ARTHRITIS, p 966.

SUSPENSORY DESMITIS

Injuries of the suspensory ligament (superior sesamoidean ligament or interosseous muscle) are common injuries in both forelimbs and hindlimbs of horses. Lesions are frequently restricted to the proximal one-third of the ligament, to the body or middle one-third, or to one or both branches.

Proximal Suspensory Desmitis: The term proximal suspensory desmitis is restricted to lesions confined to the proximal one-third of the metacarpus (or metatarsus). It is relatively common and affects both forelimbs and hindlimbs of horses of all ages. In contrast to lesions involving the body or branches (or both) of the suspensory ligament, there is usually associated lameness, poor performance, or poor action. The condition may be unilateral or, less commonly, bilateral. It sometimes is seen in association with more distal limb pain (eg, navicular disease) and is frequently seen in horses with poor mediolateral or dorsopalmar foot balance. Straight hock conformation or hyperextension of the metatarsophalangeal joints may predispose to this type of injury.

Lameness can vary in degree from mild to severe and, in early cases, is generally exacerbated by work and improved by rest. Forelimb lameness may be accentuated by flexion of the fetlock and interphalangeal joints but is generally unaffected by carpal flexion, whereas hindlimb lameness may be increased by flexion of the fetlock and interphalangeal joints or by flexion of the hock and stifle joints.

In acute cases, there may be localized heat in the proximal metacarpal (or metatarsal) region with or without periligamentous soft-tissue swelling. In more chronic cases, frequently no palpable abnormality can be detected.

Diagnosis is made by local anesthesia and ultrasonographic examination, which usually demonstrates diffuse or central hypoechoic areas with hyperechogenic foci in chronic cases. Treatment is stall rest, followed by a graduated program of exercise combined with correction of foot imbalance.

Desmitis of the Body of the Suspensory Ligament: This is principally an injury of racehorses. Injuries usually affect the forelimb of Thoroughbreds, and both forelimbs and hindlimbs in Standardbreds. Soreness on palpation of the forelimb suspensory ligament is quite common in horses with lameness associated with a more distal limb problem; however, only rarely is any structural abnormality of the ligaments identifiable ultrasonographically. The clinical signs vary and involve enlargement of the ligament, local heat, swelling, and pain. Diagnosis is usually based on clinical signs and can be confirmed ultrasonographically. Treatment is aimed at reducing inflammation by systemic NSAID, hydrotherapy, and controlled exercise.

Desmitis of the Medial or Lateral Branch of the Suspensory Ligament: This relatively common injury is seen in all types of horses in both forelimbs and hindlimbs. Usually only a single branch in a single limb is affected, although both branches may be affected, especially in hindlimbs. Foot imbalance is often recognized in affected horses, and this may be a predisposing factor.

The clinical signs depend on the degree of damage and the chronicity of the lesion(s) and include localized heat and swelling. Swelling is often due to local edema of the affected branch. Pain is usually elicited either by direct pressure applied to the injured branch or by passive flexion of the fetlock. Lameness is variable and may be absent.

Diagnosis is based on clinical signs and ultrasonographic examination. Only rarely are local analgesic techniques required. Ultrasonography can detect a range of abnormalities, including enlargement, alteration of shape, and alterations in echodensity.

Management depends on the severity of the signs and on the breed and use of the horse. Prognosis is guarded. The lesions frequently resolve slowly, and the clinical signs may take many months (≥6) to improve. The condition may recur.

SYNOVIAL HERNIA AND GANGLION AND SYNOVIAL FISTULAE

These conditions are relatively uncommon, but are important in the differential diagnosis of fluid-filled swellings over the dorsal aspect of the carpus. A synovial hernia is a cyst arising from herniation of synovial membrane through a defect in the fibrous joint capsule or fibrous sheath of a tendon. Diagnosis of these conditions is confirmed with contrast radiography; if accessible, the hernia or fistula is surgically repaired.

TEARING OF THE MEDIAL PALMAR INTERCARPAL LIGAMENT

This injury, first described in 1990, most commonly involves the medial palmar intercarpal ligament but may involve the lateral palmar intercarpal ligament. A typical presentation is synovitis and capsulitis unresponsive to therapy or the presence of carpal chip fragments with an untoward amount of lameness. Diagnosis is made arthroscopically, and the treatment is arthroscopic debridement of the torn fibers. The prognosis is excellent in horses with <50% tearing.

TENOSYNOVITIS OF THE TENDON SHEATHS ASSOCIATED WITH THE CARPUS

There are several forms of tenosynovitis, including idiopathic, acute traumatic, chronic traumatic, and septic. In the idiopathic form, there is no lameness and synovial effusion localized to the tendon sheath is the only manifestation. It may be seen in the common digital extensor tendon sheath or the extensor carpi radialis tendon sheath; these can be differentiated by knowledge of anatomy. Traumatic forms of tenosynovitis are seen in older animals. In the acute stage, there is fluid distention; in the chronic stage, fibrosis may be present as well. Treatment consists of systemic and local anti-inflammatory therapy (eg, phenylbutazone therapy for 5-7 days). DMSO can be applied topically to the injured area for 7-10 days. In chronic cases in jumpers, surgical debridement may be helpful. Septic tenosynovitis of the carpus is rare. When it is seen, there are acute signs of lameness, heat, and swelling as seen in septic arthritis.

TRAUMATIC SYNOVITIS AND CAPSULITIS

Traumatic synovitis and capsulitis is inflammation of the synovial membrane and fibrous capsule with no apparent radiographic involvement of bone or other structures. Soft tissues involved can include synovial membrane, fibrous joint capsule, and intra-articular ligaments. Synovitis and capsulitis of the carpus is a common primary clinical condition but also may be accompanied by radiographically unapparent osteochondral damage. The cause is usually considered to be cyclic trauma.

Clinical signs include varying degrees of lameness with local heat and swelling. In chronic synovitis and capsulitis, radiographs may show enthesophytes or osteophytes, but in many instances there are no significant radiographic changes. Treatment is as described under osteoarthritis (see p 918). The most common treatments are intra-articular corticosteroids, alone or in combination with hyaluronic acid, as well as systemic NSAID. If carpal synovitis and capsulitis do not respond to intra-articular therapy, diagnostic arthroscopy is indicated to eliminate medial palmar intercarpal ligament tearing, osteochondral fragmentation not visible on radiographs, or osteochondral degenerative disease.

DISORDERS OF THE SHOULDER AND ELBOW

ARTHRITIS OF THE SHOULDER JOINT

Inflammation of the structures of the shoulder joint is uncommon. It is secondary to changes in the joint capsule or, more frequently, to bony changes of the articular surfaces of the humerus or scapula (such as might be caused by osteochondrosis). Occasionally, fractures involving the articular surfaces are present. Trauma to the point of the shoulder is a frequent cause. Bacterial infection of the joint from puncture wounds or of hematogenous origin (pyosepticemia) in foals results in a purulent arthritis.

A swinging- and supporting-leg lameness are present in severe cases. In milder cases, only the swinging-leg lameness may be noted. The forward phase is shortened, the toe may be worn, and the leg is often circumducted to avoid flexion of the joint. Forced extension of the leg, which pulls the shoulder forward, often causes pain. Radiographs of the shoulder joint, preferably taken with the horse in lateral recumbency, may demonstrate the arthritic changes.

Often, treatment is ineffective because of severe arthritic changes. Intra-articular injections of a steroid may be of some benefit. Systemic steroids or phenylbutazone may relieve signs of pain. Hyaluronic acid, because of its apparent benefit in cases of degenerative disease in other joints, may be considered.

BICIPITAL BURSITIS

Bicipital bursitis is an inflammation of the bursa between the tendon of the biceps and the bicipital groove of the humerus. The usual cause is direct trauma to the point of the shoulder.

Essentially, bicipital bursitis results in a swinging-leg lameness with the forward phase being shortened. The horse may stumble because the toe is not being lifted sufficiently to clear the ground. In severe cases, a supporting-leg lameness is also present; the horse rests the limb in a characteristic semiflexed position. Forced extension of the leg usually causes a pain reaction, as can deep digital pressure over the bursa and the tendon of the biceps. Ultrasonography can demonstrate the excess fluid and associated lesions of the biceps tendon. In chronic cases, radiographs may show calcification of the bursa, which is a common sequela.

Prolonged rest is indicated (>6 mo), particularly in acute cases. Intrabursal injection of hyaluronic acid or steroids may be successful. Phenylbutazone and oral steroids may also be helpful. The prognosis is guarded.

FRACTURES OF THE ELBOW

Fractures of the elbow are not uncommon orthopedic injuries in horses, the most frequent being fracture of the ulna. They occur at any age as a result of a kick or fall. In foals (<12 mo old), they involve the physeal plate of the olecranon. Onset of lameness is sudden, and there is pain and swelling of the elbow. The fracture is usually transverse, extending through the semilunar notch, and is frequently articular. The olecranon is distracted by the pull of the triceps tendon of insertion; the elbow is dropped and cannot be extended, which produces signs similar to those of radial nerve paralysis. The carpus and fetlock are flexed, with the toe resting on the ground. Diagnosis must be confirmed radiographically.

Treatment may be conservative or surgical. In nonarticular and nondisplaced fractures, full-leg splinting and stall rest are successful. Otherwise, open reduction and internal fixation using a tension band plate is the method of choice. The prognosis is favorable with proper treatment.

FRACTURES OF THE SHOULDER

Fractures of the distal scapula (tuber scapulae) and proximal humerus (lateral tuberosity) are the most common shoulder fractures. They usually result from falls or kicks. Lameness is severe and sudden in onset. Often, there is much local soft-tissue swelling and hematoma formation. Diagnosis is confirmed radiographically. Conservative treatment by prolonged stall rest often results in improvement. Surgical treatment can be successful in selected cases. Unless treated surgically, both types of fractures heal with fibrous union. The prognosis is poor if the articular surfaces are involved.

SWEENEY
(Shoulder atrophy, Slipped shoulder)

Sweeney is disuse or neurogenic atrophy of the supraspinatus and infraspinatus muscles. Disuse atrophy, sometimes involving the triceps also, follows any lesion of the limb or foot that leads to prolonged diminished use of the limb. Neurogenic atrophy is due to damage to the suprascapular nerve, which supplies the supraspinatus and infraspinatus muscles. Polo ponies are occasionally affected because of collision during competition.

If trauma is not evident, pain may be absent, and lameness may be difficult to detect until atrophy develops. If injury is evident, there is usually some difficulty in extending the shoulder. As atrophy progresses, there is a noticeable hollowing on each side of the spine of the scapula, especially in the infraspinous area, resulting in prominence of the spine. Because the tendons of insertion of the two affected muscles act as lateral collateral ligaments to the humeroscapular joint, atrophy of the muscles leads to a looseness in the shoulder joint. Abduction of the shoulder follows and, in severe cases, is sometimes erroneously diagnosed as a dislocation. The affected limb, when advanced, takes a semicircular course and, as weight is borne by the limb, the shoulder joint moves laterally (shoulder slip). At rest, along with abduction of the shoulder, there is an apparent abduction of the lower part of the limb.

Treatment for disuse atrophy consists of removing the cause of the failure to use the limb. For neurogenic atrophy, massage with stimulating liniments or by an electrical vibrator may be of benefit. Rhythmic muscular contractions by faradism have maintained muscle bulk until the nerve regenerates. Surgical release of the suprascapular nerve from scar tissue impingement, by "notching out" the rostral border of the scapula, has also been recommended. For best results, the surgery should be performed before looseness and slipping of the shoulder joint are advanced.

The prognosis for cases of disuse atrophy depends on removal of the primary cause. In neurogenic atrophy, the prognosis is guarded; mild cases should recover in 6-8 wk. When damage to the nerve has been severe, spontaneous recovery may take many months, if it occurs at all. Such cases are candidates for surgical release. If the nerve has been severed, recovery is unlikely.

DISORDERS OF THE TARSUS

See also FRACTURE OF THE SMALL METACARPAL AND METATARSAL (SPLINT) BONES, p 917.

BOG SPAVIN
(Tarsal hydrarthrosis)

Bog spavin is a chronic synovitis of the tibiotarsal joint characterized by distention of the joint capsule. Faulty conformation may lead to weakness of the hock joint and increased production of synovia. In such cases, both limbs are affected. The unilateral case is more likely to be a sequela of a sprain or some underlying problem within the joint (eg, osteochondrosis).

The horse usually is not lame unless the condition is complicated by bone involvement. The primary distention of the joint capsule is on the dorsal medial surface of the hock, while smaller swellings develop on each side of the proximal caudal aspect. Uncomplicated bog spavin rarely interferes with the usefulness of the horse but is an unsightly blemish and indicates the need for radiographic evaluation. The distention may spontaneously appear and disappear in weanlings and yearlings.

The excess fluid within the joint capsule may be aspirated. Intra-articular corticosteroids provide variable and transient relief. The procedure may be repeated 3 wk later if necessary. Arthroscopy should be done when osteochondral involvement is suspected. Bog spavin tends to recur, especially if poor conformation is a factor.

BONE SPAVIN

Bone spavin is osteoarthritis or osteitis of the hock joint, usually the distal intertarsal and tarsometatarsal articulations, and occasionally the proximal intertarsal joint. Lesions involve degenerative joint disease, particularly on the craniomedial aspect of the hock with periarticular new bone proliferation, which eventually leads to ankylosis. Although bone spavin usually causes lameness, this may be obscured if the lesions are bilateral. Theories advanced to explain this condition include faulty hock conformation, excessive concussion, and mineral imbalance. All breeds can be affected, but it is most prevalent in Standardbreds and Quarter Horses.

The lame horse tends to drag the toe. The forward flight of the hoof is shortened, and hock action is decreased. The lameness sometimes is continuous because the bone lesions involve the articular surfaces. The heel may become elongated. Standardbreds develop soreness in the gluteal musculature (so-called trochanteric bursitis, p 928) secondary to spavin. In advanced cases, the bony proliferation may be visible on the distal craniomedial aspect of the hock (seat of spavin). When standing, the horse may rest the toe on the ground with the heel slightly raised. The lameness often disappears with exercise and returns after rest. The spavin test (ie, trotting after limb flexion for ~60 sec) may be a useful aid to diagnosis but is not specific for this condition or even this joint. In so-called occult spavin, there are no visible or radiographic exostoses. Local anesthesia of the individual tarsal joints is necessary to localize the exact site of pain responsible for the lameness.

The disease is self-limiting, ending with spontaneous ankylosis of the affected joint(s) and a return to soundness. In the early stages, intra-articular injection of corticosteroids or sodium hyaluronate (or both) may be beneficial. NSAID (eg, phenylbutazone) eliminate or reduce the clinical signs. Working the horse after this treatment is aimed at accelerating ankylosis and resolution of lameness. Surgical arthrodesis is another means of accelerating ankylosis of the affected joint. Cunean tenotomy is commonly used but of questionable value by itself. Deep-point firing used to be advocated for hastening ankylosis, but it is very doubtful that it has any beneficial effect beyond encouraging rest. Corrective shoeing by raising the heels and rolling the toe may help but is unlikely to eliminate lameness on its own.

CURB

Curb is a thickening or bowing of the plantar tarsal ligament due to strain. This ligament may become inflamed and thickened after falling, slipping, jumping, or pulling. It is most common in Standardbreds, in which poor conformation of the hock is a predisposing factor. There is an enlargement over the caudal surface of the fibular tarsal bone ~4 in. (10 cm) below the point of the hock. It is easily seen when observing the horse from the side. A recently formed curb is associated with acute inflammation and lameness. The horse stands and favors the limb with the heel elevated. In chronic cases, there is rarely any lameness or pain.

If the curb is due to acute inflammation, cold packs and rest are indicated. Little can be done to overcome the curb that is secondary to poor conformation. Fortunately, the problem seems to be self-limiting, without lasting effects on performance.

DISPLACEMENT OF SUPERFICIAL FLEXOR TENDON FROM THE POINT OF THE HOCK

Damage to the medial attachment of the superficial flexor tendon as it passes over the tuber calcaneus can cause a lateral luxation of the tendon. The injury occurs due to sudden flexion of the hock, and the tendon can occasionally slip to the medial aspect of the hock. Initially, there is lameness in the limb, with local heat and swelling. Treatment involves rest for ≥3 mo, possibly with application of a cast. The lameness improves, but the horse may be left with a permanently displaced flexor tendon and a rather jerky hock action. There is usually no difficulty during fast exercise or jumping, but dressage movements may be affected. Surgical treatment has been reported in a limited number of cases. The results have not been very successful, particularly in larger horses.

FRACTURE OF THE TARSUS

Fractures of the tarsus or hock occur as a result of trauma or as a secondary complication of degenerative joint disease. The hock is a complex joint that comprises eight bones. As in the carpus, a wide range of locations and types of fractures can occur. Specific diagnosis depends on careful radiographic examination.

Some of the more common fractures involve chips of the tibiotarsal bone and the medial or lateral malleolus of the tibia. Slab fractures of the central and third tarsal bones are also seen, particularly in Standardbreds. Because these often are quite small and may not cause lameness, it is important to use local anesthesia to positively identify the site of lameness. In many instances, a rest period (3-6 mo) is all that is required for full recovery, although with large chip fragments, surgical removal may be better. The tibiotarsal joint is amenable to arthroscopy and surgery, with most involved areas being accessible. Slab fractures are amenable to lag screw fixation.

HINDLIMB TENDON RUPTURES

Laceration of the entire Achilles tendon involving both the gastrocnemius and superficial flexor tendons is rare. The hock drops to the ground and is unable to bear weight. The prognosis is grave.

Gastrocnemius muscle rupture is more common and can result from excess stress applied to the hock (eg, sudden stopping). It can be bilateral and weight can be borne, but there is excess flexion of the hock, which makes walking difficult. There is no satisfactory treatment. Splinting the limb and slinging the horse have been attempted but are usually unsuccessful.

Injuries to the extensor tendons, the long and lateral digital extensors, frequently accompany hindlimb lacerations. If one tendon is involved, the prognosis is usually good. If both extensor tendons are severed, the horse may be left with a gait deficit for performance, but it may be useful for slow speeds or for breeding. Conservative treatment leads to wound healing, but surgical repair and casting should be considered if both tendons are severed or if performance status is desired.

The superficial and deep flexor tendons sometimes rupture as a racing injury or accompany lacerations. These are serious injuries with marked lameness and varying degrees of overextension of the fetlock and pastern. Treatment involves surgical repair with splinting and casting the limb, but the prognosis is poor for future performance.

RUPTURE OF THE PERONEUS TERTIUS MUSCLE

Injury to the peroneus tertius muscle affects the stay apparatus of the hindlimb and disrupts the reciprocal action of the stifle and hock joints. The most characteristic diagnostic feature is the ability to extend the hock and flex the stifle simultaneously. The horse is lame but usually able to bear weight on the limb. The affected hindlimb exhibits a jerking motion as it is brought forward. Conservative treatment consisting of prolonged rest (usually 4 mo) is indicated; the prognosis is favorable.

STRINGHALT
(Springhalt)

Stringhalt is a myoclonic affliction of one or both hindlimbs seen as spasmodic overflexion of the joints. The etiology is unknown, but lesions of a peripheral neuropathy have been identified in the sciatic, peroneal, and tibial nerves. Severe forms of the condition have been attributed to lathyrism (sweet pea poisoning) in the USA and possibly to flat weed intoxication in Australia. Horses of any breed may be affected; it is rare in foals.

All degrees of hyperflexion are seen, from the mild, spasmodic lifting and grounding of the foot, to the extreme case in which the foot is drawn sharply up until it touches the belly and is then struck violently on the ground. In severe cases, there is atrophy of the lateral thigh muscles. In Australian stringhalt and lathyrism, the condition may be progressive, and the gait abnormality may become so severe that euthanasia is warranted.

Mild stringhalt may be intermittent. The signs are most obvious when the horse is sharply turned or backed. In some cases, the condition is seen only on the first few steps after moving the horse out of its stall. The signs are often less intense or even absent during warmer weather. Although it is regarded as unsoundness, stringhalt may not materially hinder the horse's ability to work, except in severe cases when the constant concussion gives rise to secondary complications. The condition may also make the horse unsuitable for equestrian sports (eg, dressage).

Diagnosis is based on clinical signs but can be confirmed by electromyography. If the diagnosis is in doubt, the horse should be observed as it is backed out of the stall after hard work for 1-2 days. False stringhalt sometimes appears as a result of some temporary irritation to the lower pastern area or even a painful lesion in the foot. The occasional horse with momentary upward fixation of the patella may exhibit a stringhalt-like gait.

When intoxication is suspected, removal to another paddock may be all that is required. Many of these cases apparently recover spontaneously. In chronic cases, tenectomy of the lateral extensor of the digit, including removal of a portion of the muscle, has given best results. Improvement may not be evident until 2-3 wk after surgery. Prognosis after surgery is guarded—not all cases respond. This is not surprising because the condition is a distal axonopathy. Other methods of treatment include large doses of thiamine and phenytoin.

THOROUGHPIN

Thoroughpin is a distention of the tarsal sheath of the deep digital flexor tendon just above the hock. It is characterized by plantar fluid-filled swellings visible on both medial and lateral sides proximal to the tibiotarsal joint, which distinguish it from bog spavin (p 889). It is usually unilateral and varies in size. The lesion is referred to as a tenosynovitis of traumatic origin, but it may not be associated with any detectable inflammation, pain, or lameness. It essentially constitutes a blemish and so is of major clinical importance in show horses. Treatment is by withdrawal of the fluid and injection of hyaluronic acid or a long-acting corticosteroid, which may need to be repeated until the swelling does not recur. Radiation therapy also helps reduce the secretory property of the tendon sheath.

DISORDERS OF THE STIFLE
FRACTURE OF THE STIFLE

Severe fractures of the stifle involving either the distal femur or proximal tibia are uncommon. The associated damage to the femorotibial joint, ligaments, and menisci, and marked soft-tissue swelling make treatment in adult horses difficult or impossible. Fractures of the patella usually cause much less severe lameness and swelling. Radiography is necessary to confirm the diagnosis. Patellar fractures may respond to conservative treatment or, if a large bone fragment is involved, require surgical repair. Fracture of the tibial crest also occurs occasionally and requires surgical repair.

GONITIS

Gonitis is an inflammation of the stifle leading to degenerative joint disease. The joint is complex, and gonitis may be precipitated by multiple causes, including osteochondrosis, persistent upward fixation of the patella, injuries to the medial or lateral collateral ligaments, injuries to the cruciate ligaments or the menisci, erosions of the articular cartilage, or bacterial infection of the joint from puncture wounds or of hematogenous origin (eg, pyosepticemia).

Signs vary with the cause and extent of the pathologic changes. The femoropatellar capsule is distended just below the patella. A swinging-leg lameness is noted as a shortening of the forward phase. At rest, the fetlock is flexed with only the toe touching the ground. In moderately severe cases, both a supporting- and a swinging-leg lameness are noted. In severe cases, the leg may be carried in a flexed position. Crepitation may be noted if the menisci, cruciate ligaments, or the collateral ligaments of the joint have ruptured. Radiographs are of value in confirming osteochondral involvement, whereas ultrasonography is of value for evaluating ligaments, menisci, and soft tissue.

Prolonged rest is indicated. Repeated intra-articular injections of steroids or hyaluronic acid may be useful. Phenylbutazone and systemic steroids may relieve the lameness in less severe cases. Those cases due to rupture of ligaments or damage to the menisci rarely respond satisfactorily and rapidly progress to secondary arthritis. The prognosis is poor if the condition is chronic or if severe injuries to the articular surface, ligaments, or the menisci have occurred.

PATELLAR LUXATION

True dislocation of the patella is uncommon in horses. When it does occur, it is usually a serious injury and the lateral luxation is readily apparent. In some breeds, a congenital form of lateral luxation is seen similar to that in small dogs (p 963). The most frequent problem involving the patella is upward fixation or locking of the medial patellar ligament over the proximal part of the medial femoral trochlear ridge. Some pony breeds may have a hereditary predisposition, but patellar luxation is also seen in immature animals with poorly developed thigh muscles. It may be uni- or bilateral. The classical signs are of an intermittent locking of the limb in extension followed by a sudden jerk or hyperflexion as the patellar ligament becomes freed from the medial trochlear ridge. The signs are most frequently seen after standing still for any period (eg, overnight in the stable, or after travelling in a trailer). However, the clinical signs are often much less dramatic, which makes diagnosis difficult. There may simply be a lack of hindlimb impulsion associated with a rather jerky patellar action.

In many cases, a general improvement in fitness and muscle tone of the hindquarters effects a cure. In the more severe and persistent cases, desmotomy of the medial patellar ligament is indicated. However, desmotomy, which has been commonly used in the past, is currently in disfavor. A fragmentation of the distal extremity of the patella is believed to follow the surgery, particularly if postoperative exercise is initiated early. When surgery is done, rest should be sufficient (eg, 4-6 wk) to permit complete healing before training is resumed.

SUBCHONDRAL BONE CYST
(Osseous cyst-like lesion)

Large, radiolucent, cyst-like structures may be seen in various sites in the body, particularly in the stifle. Their pathogenesis is not completely understood, but they may arise after trauma to the articular cartilage or as a result of an osteochondrotic lesion. They seem to appear at a point of load-bearing; the common sites are the medial condyle of the femur, the third phalanx, the shoulder, the fetlock, and the carpus.

In the stifle, cysts are most common in young Thoroughbreds (1-2 yr olds); usually, lameness is first noticed when breaking-in or training begins. Although femoropatellar joint distention is characteristic, these cystic lesions can cause quite severe lameness without joint distention or pain on palpation. They are readily diagnosed radiographically. Some horses respond to rest for 4-6 mo and treatment with phenylbutazone.

When this conservative treatment fails, particularly in more mature animals, surgery is indicated. This involves drilling and curetting the cyst lining and packing the space with an autogenous bone graft. Because of the favorable results, surgery may be considered before more conservative treatment. Both arthroscopy and arthrotomy are being used.

DISORDERS OF THE HIP

COXITIS
(Osteoarthritis of the hip)

Coxitis is inflammation of the hip that leads to osteoarthritis of the coxofemoral joint. Most cases are traumatic in origin, secondary to falls or being cast (within a stall) in recumbency; however, tears of the rim of the acetabulum or fractures through the acetabulum, and localization of a systemic infection, particularly pyosepticemia in young animals, have been seen.

Both a supporting- and a swinging-leg lameness are noted. In severe cases, the leg may be carried. In less severe cases, the gait is rolling, ie, the affected quarter is elevated as weight is borne on the leg. The limb is advanced in a semicircular manner with the forward phase of the stride shortened. The toe may be worn from dragging. The horse often stands with the limb partially flexed, the stifle turned out, and the point of the hock turned inward. The muscles of the quarter atrophy in chronic cases. Rectal palpation may reveal an enlargement over the acetabulum, particularly if a fracture through it has occurred. Radiography of the joint confirms the diagnosis.

The prognosis is poor. Rest is indicated, and intra-articular steroids may relieve the lameness temporarily in milder cases. Phenylbutazone is useful, but many horses are too painful for the drug to have a beneficial effect.

DISLOCATION OF THE HIP

Dislocation of the hip can occur in association with rupture of the round (teres) ligament, accessory ligament, or joint capsule. This type of injury is secondary to trauma but is quite uncommon. Fracture of the dorsal acetabular rim frequently accompanies the dislocation. Dislocation with dorsal displacement of the femoral head is accompanied by upward fixation of the patella.

Rupture of the round ligament of the hip joint is associated with a typical appearance of the hindlimb in which the stifle and toe rotate outward and the hock rotates inward. Dislocation of the hip joint is not always complete; when it is, there is a marked effect on gait, with a reluctance to bear weight. The femur is rotated outward, and the greater trochanter is more prominent than usual.

Relocation of the hip joint may be attempted under general anesthesia, but the long-term results are usually poor.

PELVIC FRACTURE

Pelvic fractures can occur at any age but are most prevalent in horses 6 mo to 2 yr old. Almost any part of the pelvic girdle may be involved. The site and extent of soft-tissue damage affect the ultimate prognosis. There is sudden onset of hindlimb lameness with considerable pain. Crepitus may be difficult to appreciate initially. A pelvic fracture can usually be confirmed by rectal examination, especially if the fragments are displaced. If the lameness is not too severe, but a fracture is suspected, it is better to rest the horse for 4-6 wk before giving a general anesthetic for radiographic examination.

In more chronic cases, the lameness is associated with atrophy of the gluteal muscles. Radiography can demonstrate the site and assist with the prognosis. Fractures of the tuber coxae, wing of the ilium, tuber ischii, and ischial shaft have a hopeful prognosis, particularly in young horses. Rest (9-12 mo) is usually the only treatment necessary. Fractures of the acetabulum, shaft of the ilium, and pubis have a much more guarded prognosis.

TROCHANTERIC BURSITIS

("Whirlbone" lameness)

Trochanteric bursitis is an inflammation of the tendon of the middle gluteal muscle, of the bursa between this tendon and the trochanter major, or of the cartilage of the trochanter major. It is most common in Standardbreds, in which bursitis and gluteal myositis are secondary to hock problems.

The weight is placed on the medial wall of the foot so that it is worn more than the lateral wall. The stride of the affected leg is shorter, and the leg is rotated inward. The horse tends to carry the hindquarters toward the sound side. In chronic cases, the muscles between the external and internal angles of the ilium are atrophied, giving the croup a flat appearance. Pressure over the greater trochanter results in evidence of pain.

If the inflammation is acute, the horse should be rested and hot packs applied over the affected area. Injection of corticosteroid into the bursa temporarily relieves the inflammation. In chronic cases, the injection of 1 mL of 5% Lugol's solution diluted with equal parts of distilled water into or around the bursa as a counterirritant has been recommended.

DISORDERS OF THE BACK

FRACTURES

Multiple fractures of the summits of the dorsal spinous processes of T4-10 are sometimes seen in young horses that have reared up and fallen over backward. The tips of the summits and centers of ossification are fractured and displaced laterally. After the initial pain and local reaction have subsided, recovery is satisfactory. Usually, there is no permanent effect on performance, but a persistent swelling over the withers may require use of a special saddle. Occasionally, other fractures of individual spinous processes occur, and their presence can be confirmed by radiography. The clinical signs in these cases are variable.

Fractures of the vertebral bodies are more serious. There is often a history of a bad fall entailing a somersault. Complete or partial paraplegia results from damage to the spinal cord. The prognosis is grave.

MUSCLE AND LIGAMENT STRAIN

See also MYOPATHIES AND MYOSITIDES, p 947.

Damage to the soft tissues is undoubtedly the most common cause of back soreness in the horse. This mostly involves the longissimus dorsi complex of muscles, which act to extend (dorsiflex) and laterally flex the spine. All or part of the longissimus muscles usually are strained during ridden exercise, and clinical signs are associated with altered performance and back pain of acute onset. The principal sites of damage are the caudal withers and cranial lumbar regions (just in front of and behind the saddle area). Most of these injuries respond to rest and physiotherapy, although several weeks may be needed for full recovery.

Another fairly common site of soft-tissue damage is the supraspinous ligament, which runs down the middle of the back and is adherent to the summits of the thoracic and lumbar dorsal spinous processes. It is made up of the multiple tendinous insertions of the various parts of the longissimus dorsi complex and, therefore, is subject to the same strains as the muscles. The clinical signs usually persist longer, and the chances of complete recovery are not as good as for the uncomplicated muscle strains.

There is considerable controversy over the diagnosis and treatment of back problems in horses. Much credit is given to the value of physiotherapy, particularly chiropractic and osteopathic manipulation, but there are no substantiated reports of their efficacy.

OSSIFYING SPONDYLOSIS

Spondylitic lesions of the vertebral bodies of the mid to caudal thoracic region are uncommon in working horses. However, when they are seen, they have serious effects, and little permanent treatment can be done to keep the horse working.

Osteoarthritic lesions of the transverse and articular processes of the lumbar vertebrae are much more common, especially in older horses. However, they appear to cause little inconvenience to the horse because this part of the spine is kept particularly rigid even when the horse is jumping.

OVERRIDING OF THE DORSAL SPINOUS PROCESSES
(Kissing spines syndrome)

Impingement of the summits of the dorsal spines beneath the saddle area predisposes to back pain in some horses. Pressure points between adjacent overriding spines are shown by local periosteal reaction, small bone cysts, and false joint formation. Radiographic lesions of this type are sometimes seen in horses that do not suffer from back trouble, although incidence is lower and lesions are less severe. Diagnosis can be aided by injection of local anesthetic into the affected interspinous spaces. Many cases respond to rest and physiotherapy, but treatment in persistent cases is by resection of one or more of the summits to relieve the crowding of the spines.

SACROILIAC INJURY
(Sacroiliac subluxation, Sacroiliac strain, Sacroiliac arthrosis, Hunter's bumps)

Acute and severe strain of the sacroiliac ligaments is associated with a history of injury and of severe pain in the pelvic or sacroiliac region, often with marked hindlimb lameness. Subacute or chronic sacroiliac strain is low-grade damage that causes typical back soreness. It represents incomplete healing or reinjury of an acute strain. There may be a history of poor performance with an intermittent, often shifting, hindlimb lameness. This may be associated with some restriction in hindlimb action and dragging of the toe of one or both hooves. There usually is prominence or asymmetry of the sacral tuber. Rectal palpation helps identify crepitation or shifting in the sacroiliac region.

Sacroiliac injury is common in Standardbreds and hunter-jumper horses and has been confused with chronic stifle problems. Usually, there is rather poor muscling of the gluteal masses and, when viewed from behind, some asymmetry of the croup. This may be due to some tilting or rotation of the pelvis or muscle wastage of one quarter, or both. The tail may be held slightly to the side. Pain in the early stages may be evinced when pressure is applied to the midline in front of the tuber coxae, and usually there is a reluctance to ventroflex the back. If diagnosis is made early and the horse rested sufficiently for complete healing of the damaged ligaments (6-9 mo), recovery can occur. However, Standardbreds usually do not then compete well. Chronically affected horses continue to perform poorly despite rest and anti-inflammatory medication.

DEVELOPMENTAL ORTHOPEDIC DISEASE

Developmental orthopedic diseases of horses constitute an important group of conditions that includes osteochondrosis, physeal dysplasia, acquired angular limb deformities, flexion deformities, and cuboidal bone malformations.

OSTEOCHONDROSIS
(Osteochondritis dissecans, Dyschondroplasia)

Osteochondrosis (*see also* p 918) is one of the most important and prevalent developmental orthopedic diseases of horses. Although its specific etiology is not known, it is considered to arise from a focal disturbance in endochondral ossification. The term osteochondrosis is currently used to describe the clinical manifestation of the disorder; however, the term dyschondroplasia is preferred when referring to early lesions because primary lesions are seen in cartilage.

Osteochondrosis has a multifactorial etiology that includes rapid growth, overnutrition, mineral imbalance, and biomechanics (ie, trauma to cartilage). Genetics has been implicated in some breeds (eg, Standardbred and Swedish Warmblood). The condition mainly affects articular growth cartilage, but the metaphysis may also be involved. If the physeal metaphyseal cartilage is affected, bone contours and longitudinal growth are disturbed (see PHYSITIS, p 931). Involvement of articular cartilage at the periphery of joint surfaces leads to regressive changes at the joint margins, dissecting lesions, and the formation of flaps (osteochondrosis). Central articular lesions, because of weight-bearing effects, involve focal retention of cartilage within the subchondral bone (see SUBCHONDRAL CYSTS, p 862). Axial skeletal involvement includes vertebral articular facets, and this may lead to stenosis of the vertebral canal and, ultimately, ataxia and proprioceptive deficits (ie, wobbler syndrome).

Clinical Findings: The clinical signs of equine osteochondrosis are difficult to characterize specifically because of the wide range of lesions and sites involved. In severe cases, other signs of developmental orthopedic disease also may be apparent. Furthermore, lesions of dyschondroplasia do not always progress to osteochondrosis and produce clinical signs. These signs may begin with mild stiffness or lameness, but if there is superimposed biomechanical trauma, the joint damage progresses to pain and lameness or loss of performance.

The most common sign of osteochondrosis is a nonpainful distention of an affected joint (eg, gonitis, bog spavin). Clinical signs may be divided broadly into two categories; those seen in foals <6 mo old and those seen in older animals. Often the first sign noted in foals is a tendency to spend more time lying down. This is accompanied frequently by joint swelling, stiffness, and difficulty keeping up with other animals in the paddock. An accompanying sign may be the development of upright conformation of the limbs, presumably as a result of rapid growth. Fetlock osteochondrosis is particularly seen in younger foals (<6 mo old).

Marked lameness is not usually a feature of equine osteochondrosis, although it is seen with damage in some sites. For example, lesions in the shoulder frequently result in moderate to severe lameness, muscle atrophy, and pain on joint flexion. In the stifle, some horses with subchondral bone cysts in the medial femoral condyle present with lameness severe enough that a fracture may be suspected but without a discernible site of pain or any joint swelling. The true origin of pain in osteochondrosis is unknown. Horses often exhibit severe pathologic changes without showing much pain or distress in contrast to some situations seen in some other species and sites (eg, canine elbow).

The main signs in yearlings or older horses are stiffness of joints, flexion responses, and varying degrees of lameness. These signs are usually associated with the onset of training and, therefore, suggest a biomechanical influence and an activation of subclinical or "silent" lesions.

Diagnosis: Clinical diagnosis can often be made on the basis of signalment and signs. More definitive diagnosis requires the use of some specific clinical aids. Radiographic examination has been the traditional method of confirming diagnosis; however, early lesions involving cartilage without significant subchondral bone damage will not be visualized. In the distal limb, oblique views may be helpful; in the hock, because the most common site of a lesion is the distal intermediate ridge of the tibia, the best view is a plantarolateral/dorsomedial oblique. Ultrasonographic examination of the swollen joints can also be helpful and can delineate articular damage and "joint mice." The most accurate way to confirm diagnosis is by arthroscopy, and most of the predilection sites are accessible except for the cervical articulations.

Other aids include nuclear imaging (scintigraphy), which usually has negative results unless there is active secondary bone damage. Magnetic resonance imaging is ideal for diagnosis of both early and late lesions but is not widely available. Clinical pathology and the evaluation of synovial fluid may be helpful but is used largely to eliminate inflammatory causes of swollen joints.

Treatment and Management: Management of osteochondrosis depends on the site and severity of signs. Mild cases recover spontaneously, and a conservative approach may be appropriate. In young animals (<12 mo old), this involves restricted exercise for some weeks combined with a reduction in feed intake to slow the growth rate. Particular care should be taken to ensure appropriate mineral supplementation (eg, suspected copper deficiency). It is controversial whether correcting the diet, once signs have developed, will actually assist resolution, but it may help limit or prevent further cases on stud farms. Intraarticular medication with hyaluronic acid may be beneficial, and injection of long-acting corticosteroids may help reduce swelling and improve any associated synovitis.

Those cases considered for surgery are mainly treated arthroscopically. This technique has been successful in most affected sites, particularly the hock, stifle, and fetlock. In addition to removing damaged cartilage and loose pieces of subchondral bone (ie, "joint mice"), the bone overlying the lesion is curetted and the joint flushed extensively. Prognosis should be good in all but those cases with severe joint disruption or secondary arthrosis (degenerative joint disease).

Treatment of osteochondrotic lesions in the shoulder are often more problematic to treat surgically because arthroscopic access is more difficult, and there is usually more extensive subchondral bone damage, often with formation of multiple cysts. Therefore, the prognosis is always rather guarded.

PHYSITIS
(Epiphysitis, Physeal dysplasia, Dysplasia of the growth plate)

Physitis involves swelling around the growth plates of certain long bones in young horses. It can be a component of osteochondrosis. Suggested causes include malnutrition, conformational defects, faulty hoof growth, compression of the growth plate, and toxicosis. The most acceptable hypothesis at this time appears to be the compression theory. However, the changes seen in physitis also occur in clinically normal horses; the condition is seen frequently in well-grown, fast-growing, heavy-topped foals during the summer when the ground is dry and hard, and on stud farms where the calcium:phosphorus ratio in the diet is imbalanced.

Physitis most commonly involves the distal extremities of the radius, tibia, third metacarpal or metatarsal bone, and the proximal aspect of the first phalanx. It is characterized by swelling at the level of the growth plate, giving a typical "boxy" appearance to the affected joints. Radiographs aid the clinical assessment. Microscopically, the physeal cartilage appears crushed and thinned, and new bone is formed.

Treatment consists of reducing food intake to reduce body weight or at least growth rate; confining exercise to a yard or a large, well-ventilated loose box with a soft surface (eg, peat moss, deep straw, shavings, or sand); ensuring that the feet are carefully and frequently trimmed; and correcting the diet if necessary. The calcium:phosphorus ratio should be adjusted to 1.6:1, and protein content limited to <10% of dry matter. In general terms, bran should not be fed, and dicalcium phosphate or bone flour (10-30 g daily) should be added to the diet. Vitamin D supplements (PO or parenteral) are indicated, but the dosage must be monitored closely to avoid hypervitaminosis D.

As a preventive measure, the older foal or yearling that is fat or heavy-topped should be watched carefully for clinical signs, especially when the ground is hard and dry. When these conditions prevail, feed rations and exercise should be restricted.

FLEXION DEFORMITIES
(Contracted tendons, Club foot, Knuckling)

Flexor tendon disorders are associated with postural and foot changes, lameness, and debility. There are congenital and acquired causes. Uterine malposition, teratogenic insults (arthrogryposis, p 849), and genetic defects have been either implicated or proved to cause contracted limbs in newborn foals. Chronic pain is the most common cause of acquired tendon contracture. Pain can arise from physitis, osteochondrosis, degenerative joint disease, or soft-tissue wounds and infection. Pain induces the withdrawal reflex with shortening of the musculotendinous units. Flexors are stronger than extensors, so the horse walks on its toes or knuckles in the fetlocks. Nutritional errors referable to problems associated with bone growth (ie, osteochondrosis and physitis) are intimately associated with the syndrome and must be addressed as a part of the treatment. (See also p 850 and p 846.)

Clinical Findings: Signs vary widely in newborn foals. Some cannot stand, some attempt to walk on the dorsum of their fetlocks, and others can stand but knuckle in the fetlocks or carpi. One foal may improve spontaneously, yet another, seemingly healthy at birth, may become progressively worse. Onset may be rapid in sucklings and weanlings 3-12 mo old; such animals may walk around on their toes with their heels off the ground. A slower onset is characterized by a "boxy" hoof with an elongated heel and concave toe. Physitis frequently is evident in these horses. Involvement of both forelimbs is the rule, with a tendency to be worse in one leg. Toe abscesses are a frequent complication of the hoof and locomotion changes, and they add to the pain and deformity.

Older horses (1-2 yr old) commonly knuckle in the metacarpophalangeal joints, which are swollen and enlarged. These horses are upright and straight-legged in both fore- and hindlimbs with flexor tendon and suspensory ligament involvement. Yearlings usually are more severely affected and more difficult to treat than younger animals. The specific diagnosis of tendon involvement is not difficult if a complete examination is performed, and careful judgement applied. The associated or underlying bone or joint disease and nutritional mismanagement must be identified and corrected.

Treatment: Various types of splints and casts are used for foals with contracted tendons. Forced extension of the limbs induces the inverse myotatic reflex with relaxation of the flexor muscles. Early cases in sucklings and weanlings can be managed conservatively with nutritional correction, proper hoof trimming, and analgesia. Surgical treatment can be simple or complex, depending on the degree of involvement. Desmotomy of the accessory ligament of the deep digital flexor tendon (inferior check desmotomy) is the most successful and commonly used procedure and does not interfere with future performance. Other types of surgery, including tenotomy and tendon lengthening, tend to be less successful. Joint capsule contracture, collateral ligament malformation, and bone involvement are complications in chronic cases that preclude a successful outcome. Nutritional correction, proper foot trimming, and analgesia are integral to recovery, even when surgery is indicated. The prognosis is fair to good for horses that are diagnosed early and managed properly.

LAMENESS IN PIGS

Lameness in pigs is often a problem in individual herds. Musculoskeletal problems are the second highest cause of culling in grower/finisher pigs and sows; in herds with lameness problems, sow mortality is likely to be >5%. Therefore, veterinarians and swine producers must continuously evaluate the importance of lameness on productivity or on the efficiency of production. Problems may be seen in pigs of any age, but the greatest impact in a commercial herd may be related to interference with the production cycle due to inadequate performance of lame gilts and boars.

If piglets become lame because they are injured by the sow or develop joint infections when they are in the crate, their chances of survival or vigorous growth are reduced. Problems in growing or finishing pigs can be more subtle. With the selection of lines of fast-growing pigs and trends toward least-cost rations, each batch of feedstuff should be adequate in terms of both macro- and micronutrients. Although a nutrient deficiency or excess may be temporary, it could have a long-lasting effect on the development of the fast-growing skeleton or other components of the musculoskeletal system. In maturing gilts, boars, and barrows, the specific causes of osteochondrosis and osteoarthrosis should be identified so that preventive measures can be instituted.

History: A thorough history is essential and should include information on morbidity, mortality, age of onset, number of groups affected, typical clinical signs, and the progression of the lameness. A vaccination history and the frequencies of treatments for lameness and culling due to unsoundness should be determined. Data relating to condemnations at slaughter plants due to periarticular abscesses, septic arthritis, fractured bones, bruises, and damaged or pale muscles is also useful.

Often, evaluations of lameness in pigs are limited to those methods that can be used on the farm. Occasionally, selected crippled pigs are submitted for necropsy at diagnostic laboratories. Diseases that affect bones, joints, or feet also may be found incidentally when pigs are submitted for diagnosis of an unrelated problem.

Evaluation: A thorough, systematic approach for evaluating all components of the locomotor system is essential. In addition to the skeleton (including the joints), the feet, muscles, and nervous system should each be considered in determining a diagnosis.

When examining a herd with a locomotor problem, the focus should not be solely on 1 group of affected pigs. Younger pigs should be evaluated to identify potential underlying causes or any predisposition to the problem under investigation. Other groups of pigs of similar ages and more mature pigs that are housed in other pens or buildings should also be evaluated to determine if they have similar or different problems. The conditions potentially causing the problem should not be assumed to be restricted to those most often associated with one particular age group.

Pigs should be moved around in groups in their pens to assess gait and body conformation and condition. Then, individual pigs should be examined more closely. A general physical examination of affected pigs is important, including palpation and manipulation of limbs and joints using minimal restraint. A systematic approach to palpating and manipulating the limbs should be adopted, eg, thoracic limbs (foot to shoulder), followed by pelvic limbs, and then the pelvis and spine. Auscultation may be helpful in locating crepitus in joints or fractured long bones.

The feet should be carefully examined with the pig standing or walking, so that the gait, position of the toes, and condition of the coronary band and the wall can be noted. All 4 feet should be examined individually; this can be done more easily on an open, clean, dry, level concrete surface than on dirt lots. The feet of sows in gestation or farrowing crates can be readily examined while the sows are lying down. The number of sows with each type of foot problem should be recorded to accurately assess the extent of the herd problem. All soiled feet should be hosed and cleaned before examination. The soles of the feet must be evaluated. If the pig is tractable, it may be possible to lift a foot with minimal restraint; if not, the pig can be restrained with a snare, and a lariat rope used to lift the foot.

The size, tonicity, symmetry, uniformity, and temperature of muscle masses can be determined as muscles are visualized and palpated. In modern, muscular, hybrid pigs, the contours of muscle masses are more clearly defined, making them easier to locate.

Neurologic examination should be performed in a similar fashion to that used for dogs, cows, and horses (*see* p 984). The pig should be observed to determine its mental state, degree of sensory perception, posture and gait, and whether reflex activity is normal (eg, the lack of involuntary movements). Cranial nerves can be evaluated with the pig confined in a small pen that can be darkened. Disorders of the spinal cord and peripheral nerves can be assessed using such techniques as downward pressure over the spinal column in standing pigs and withdrawal and patellar reflexes in recumbent pigs.

Unlike examinations for soundness in horses or cattle, a simpler system for grading gait abnormalities can be adopted in pigs, with 3 or 4 categories used to define clinical signs. The willingness to stand, the positioning of the feet and limbs, and the degree of weight bearing by individual limbs must be considered. Radiographic and ultrasonographic imaging can be used to identify bony changes or cartilaginous flaps and other soft-tissue changes in and around joints. However, these techniques are usually restricted to research applications. Any abnormalities should be recorded.

Environment and Management: The environment should be evaluated, particularly the type, condition, dampness, and cleanliness of the flooring. Footrot is associated with wet floors. Intensive farming systems and artificial floors have increased lameness problems in pigs. There is no ideal floor for all pigs and, at best, efforts to produce comfortable yet supportive floors have been only partially successful. Rough, irregular, or "green" solid concrete; concrete slats (particularly if they have chipped, sharp edges, rather than pencil edges); and aluminum slats have predisposed growing/finishing pigs to more severe lesions or to a greater frequency of foot lesions. Nursery pigs are prone to injury when the openings of slatted floors are too wide, enabling the foot to fall between the slats. Although piglets prefer plastic-coated expanded metal over expanded metal, molded plastic, fiberglass slats, or woven wire, these floors are less than ideal for sows if they slip and injure their feet and limbs. Slippery breeding pens cause joint injuries to sows and boars. Gestation stalls increase the likelihood of osteochondrosis in gilts. The use of bedding is likely to be more acceptable in Europe than in the USA.

Behavior patterns among the pigs, stocking density, and the way the pigs are handled on the farm also may be important in some musculoskeletal disorders. For example, poor techniques (eg, trauma or rough handling of pigs when they are moved, inadequate hygiene with needles when pigs are injected) can cause lameness and sepsis.

Management systems such as medicated early weaning and segregated early weaning or the more rigorous practice of "all-in/all-out" may help to reduce the frequency of lameness caused by infectious agents in young pigs. However, pigs reared under such conditions tend to grow faster and may, therefore, be more prone to growth-related disorders.

Nutrition: Skeletal development may be affected by relatively short-term nutritional deficiencies, especially considering expectations for rapid growth and muscle development in modern hybrid pigs. Problems early in the production cycle may be reflected as abnormal bone growth in nursery or growing pigs, whereas recurrent deficiencies or those seen later in the finishing phase may result in weak bones in slaughter pigs or replacement breeding stock. During the growing phase, the goal of the nutritional program should be to ensure the development of a strong skeleton so that incidence of spontaneous bone fractures during the slaughter process is low, thus preventing large numbers of partial or complete condemnations of carcasses. Fractures of the femur, humerus, ribs, or vertebrae may be induced by strong muscle contractions during the slaughter process; however, if the problem is seen frequently, it may be a reflection of the overall integrity of the skeleton and warrants further evaluation of the minerals and vitamins in the ration.

Nutritional programs used on the farm should be reviewed, and the nutrient requirements of rapidly growing, modern hybrid pigs should be continually reviewed and reassessed (*see also* NUTRITION: PIGS, p 1889). The content of rations should be considered, and ration analysis performed. The milling equipment should be inspected, the mixing process watched, and the adequacy of on-farm feed storage determined. A sufficient supply of clean, uncontaminated water is essential. For some vaguely defined locomotor disorders, contamination of food or water by toxins is a possibility.

Necropsy: The necropsy of lame pigs is required to reach a definitive diagnosis for a herd lameness problem. This is particularly true of sow lameness problems, which are economically costly to producers. Evaluation of affected or cull pigs at a slaughter plant is inadequate. The lines at packing plants are often too fast for adequate evaluation of all the elements of the musculoskeletal system (unless a carcass is condemned and is accessible) and all joints cannot be thoroughly examined. If pigs are to be submitted to a diagnostic laboratory, appropriate pigs must be selected and delivered, accompanied by an adequate history and a list of differential diagnoses. Adequate numbers of representative, lame, untreated pigs are essential.

PIGS IN FARROWING HOUSES

Hereditary and Congenital Disorders: These can affect locomotion, prevent the pig from nursing, or predispose to problems such as neonatal polyarthritis. Congenital tremors cause pigs to shake when awake and remain still when sleeping. Either heredity or viral infections may cause the problem. Congenital tremors usually last for 1 wk and make it difficult for pigs to nurse. Affected pigs must be assisted with nursing until the tremors subside. Mycotoxins in the sow's feed can cause arthrogryposis, which involves deformity of limb bones, but the primary effect may be on the neuromuscular system. Pigs affected by hereditary hyperostosis have thickened thoracic limbs and a domed forehead and generally do not survive.

Joint-ill and Localized Infections: Neonatal septic arthritis (joint-ill) causes death of up to 1.5% in pigs. Joint-ill is caused by various organisms, both facultative and specific pathogens. Microorganisms gain entry to the circulatory system via the tonsils, oropharynx, or a damaged integument, or as a result of an ascending omphalophlebitis. Suckling pigs typically "paddle" with their legs, abrading the skin of the carpuses or coronary bands. A localized infection soon becomes established. Poor hygiene when pigs undergo tail-docking, ear-notching, or castration, and careless clipping of needle teeth also can result in localized infections. Separate instruments should be used for teeth and tails, and the instruments should be put in a disinfectant solution between pigs. Castration equipment must be kept clean and sharp. If teeth are not clipped or if there are sharp remnants of clipped teeth, pigs that suckle aggressively can lacerate the faces of other pigs, which results in pyoderma. Regardless of cause of a local infection, if a bacteremia ensues, polyarthritis is likely to develop. Pigs with exudative epidermitis (p 692) are also prone to polyarthritis.

Polyarthritis: Affected pigs are lethargic and may fail to suckle. Joints are warm, painful, and swollen, and lameness is severe. With time, the soft, fluctuating swellings become firm. The umbilicus should be examined to see if it is hard and swollen. Ultimately, untreated, affected pigs become runts. At necropsy, cream or green pus is found in and around swollen joints (particularly the elbows, carpuses, stifles, and hocks), in the umbilical stalk, and sometimes over the meninges. Organisms isolated from baby pigs have included streptococci (including *Streptococcus suis*), staphylococci, *Actinobacillus suis*, *Arcanobacterium (Actinomyces) pyogenes*, and occasionally *Erysipelothrix rhusiopathiae* or *Haemophilus* spp.

Treatment must be based on a bacterial culture and an antimicrobial sensitivity profile. Antimicrobial therapy must be initiated early in the course of the disease if it is to be effective, and treating all pigs in the group at risk may be prudent. Penicillin and lincomycin have been the drugs of choice, but increased numbers of penicillin-resistant *S suis* isolates have recently been identified.

Prevention is based on selecting flooring that minimally abrades and contaminates the feet and skin. The lesions are associated with worn floor surfaces and with floors that have solid floor surfaces adjoining perforated surfaces. Plastic-covered woven wire provides a smooth, self-cleaning flooring; plain woven wire is similar. An "all-in/all-out" flow of pigs is important, and scrupulous hygiene in farrowing crates helps to reduce the frequency of neonatal polyarthritis. Rough flooring can cause bruising in the soft tissue below the hoof wall or sole; if spaces are large, the digits can be entrapped, and the pig can become lame because of bruising or damage and infection at the coronary band. Pigs on expanded metal floors have incurred heel and wall injuries and have lost accessory digits. Second and third digits were damaged as the pigs thrust with their feet during suckling and caught their toes against sharp metal edges. Sharp spicules on woven wire lacerate the feet of pigs and predispose to infectious laminitis. Crossfostering within 24 hr of birth to reduce large litter sizes reduces competition at the udder. Large litters are prone to lesions on the faces and the forelimbs. Piglets nursing sows with hypogalactia spend more time nursing, leading to more forelimb lesions. Piglet processing techniques should be reviewed to ensure appropriate use; lack of equipment maintenance often leads to polyarthritis. Hemorrhages in the wall and sole of feet of newborn pigs from sows fed high concentrations of selenium have been reported, but there was no indication of the longterm effect of these lesions. Infectious conditions can be controlled by improving floors and the environment, and antimicrobial therapy must be initiated before abrasions become infected. Litters of gilts are more prone to neonatal polyarthritis; colostral protection against this syndrome and other infectious diseases of baby pigs may increase as the sows age.

Splayleg or Spraddleleg: This lameness is precipitated by weakness and immaturity of skeletal muscles at birth. Unless affected pigs are carefully managed and pelvic limbs are temporarily hobbled, skin and foot abrasions develop rapidly, predisposing to arthritis, polyarthritis, or pododermatitis and osteomyelitis of the digits. These pigs may require assistance to suckle colostrum and milk for the first few days of life.

Neurologic Disorders: Meningoencephalocoele and cerebellar hypoplasia interfere with locomotion in affected pigs, as can infections with *Listeria monocytogenes* and *S suis*. Thus, *S suis* can cause locomotion problems as a result of meningitis and neurologic signs, or a suppurative arthritis can be the primary complaint.

PIGS IN NURSERIES

By the time pigs are weaned, diseases that affected the locomotor system during the nursing phase most likely will have resolved spontaneously, responded to aggressive therapy, or resulted in death, or the pig may have been culled. Because pigs that survive episodes of polyarthritis generally remain lame, have ≥1 swollen "knotty" joints, and are in poor condition, they should be culled.

Infectious Arthritis or Polyarthritis: Causes include *Mycoplasma hyorhinis, Haemophilus parasuis, Streptococcus suis,* or *Erysipelothrix rhusiopathiae,* which are found sporadically among groups of pigs or herds. As with many infectious diseases, management or environmental factors that stress the pig or depress the immune response can precipitate infectious arthritis. Moving and mixing pigs; overcrowding; cold, damp, or drafty environments; or changing rations are major stresses and can lead to the development of infectious arthritides. In addition, active infection due to porcine reproductive and respiratory syndrome virus (p 581) often predisposes groups of nursery pigs to these infectious causes of polyarthritis.

The clinical signs seen in infections caused by *M hyorhinis, S suis* (p 585), and *H parasuis,* (Glässer's disease, p 576) are similar, because these organisms cause polyarthritis and polyserositis. The upper respiratory tract of the sow is the source of the organism for the baby pig and, presumably, some older pigs are also carriers. Infection with *M hyorhinis* usually results in moderate morbidity and low mortality, but *H parasuis* and *S suis* can cause infection in 50-75% of pigs and mortality of up to 10%. Outbreaks of Glässer's disease have been particularly severe in SPF herds. Fever is associated with both conditions but can be highest in Glässer's disease (>107°F). A shifting-leg lameness occurs, and joints are warm and swollen. Pneumonia develops with all 3 conditions, and sometimes *H parasuis* and *S suis* cause neurologic signs. Susceptible, stressed, adult pigs can succumb to *M hyorhinis* with a higher fever and a more severe lameness than is seen in nursery pigs. Boars may develop scrotal edema and discomfort.

At necropsy, polyarthritis and polyserositis are seen with both mycoplasmal arthritis and Glässer's disease, and pneumonia may have developed. In Glässer's disease and *S suis,* there may also be a meningitis. However, whereas the exudative response is usually serous or serofibrinous with a mycoplasmal infection, typically it is fibrinous or fibrinopurulent with Glässer's disease and *S suis.* Hence, *M hyorhinis* causes a mild synovitis with villous hypertrophy and hyperplasia; an excess of clear, yellow, or brown synovia; and a serofibrinous pericarditis, pleuritis, and peritonitis. *H parasuis* initiates a fibrinopurulent synovitis with periarticular edema and a fibrinopurulent meningitis and polyserositis with pseudomembranes. The articular surface is usually unaffected in either condition. Stunted pigs in the grower/finisher group that have chronic, severe, fibrinous, fibrinopurulent, or fibrous pleuritis, peritonitis, and arthritis could have been affected by either condition earlier in their lives and are best culled rather than kept as a source of infection for other pigs. They are unlikely to reach market weight.

Diagnosis is based on clinical signs, necropsy findings, and the isolation of the organism; however, if any treatment has been instituted, the chances of finding the organisms are reduced. Treatment for either disease must be aggressive and start soon after the onset of clinical signs. The effectiveness of treating *M hyorhinis* infections with tylosin (not labeled for this use), tetracycline, or lincomycin has been variable. Provided that the organism is susceptible to an antimicrobial compound, treatment of *S suis* and Glässer's disease with penicillin, ampicillin, streptomycin, tetracyclines, ceftiofur, or sulfa drugs has been more successful. Penicillin is the only drug labeled for use against arthritis caused by *S suis* or Glässer's disease. Appropriate changes in management to reduce stress, strict "all-in/all-out" housing, and control of porcine reproductive and respiratory syndrome help to minimize the impact of these diseases. Herds that maintain an SPF status may be free of both *M hyorhinis* and *H parasuis*, but if outbreaks of Glässer's disease occur in these herds, morbidity and mortality are high and production is decreased. Vaccination with *Haemophilus* bacterin may alleviate the problem in SPF herds, and it is important to vaccinate SPF pigs that are to be shipped to conventional herds. Vaccination of sows against *H parasuis* reduces the prevalence of the problem in nursery pigs through passive immunity.

Erysipelas: Although acute erysipelas can be seen in nursery pigs, it may be more typical of growing/finishing pigs (*see* below). If the acute form of the disease affects nursery pigs and is not treated appropriately, the subsequent progression of the disease to the chronic form is seen in the grower/finisher pigs anyway. (*See also* p 505.)

Vertebral Deformities: Kyphosis or lordosis and cuneiform deformities of vertebrae have been seen in weaned pigs, but a cause has not been identified. "Humpy back" pigs are seen sporadically in some herds; the spine is curved in the vertical plane such that the lumbar vertebrae are higher than the thoracic vertebrae, and there is a "kink" between the 2 segments. However, grossly, there is not always evidence of incomplete or deformed vertebrae. The condition may have a genetic predisposition, but multiple fractured ribs found in the same pig increase suspicion of an underlying or aggravating, perhaps intermittent, nutritional deficiency, such as that which can cause rickets. Rickets is usually not seen clinically until the grower phase, but lesions must have begun to develop earlier.

PIGS IN GROWER/FINISHER AREAS

Arthritis: Arthritis caused by *Mycoplasma hyosynoviae* and *Erysipelothrix rhusiopathiae* emerge as important causes of lameness in pigs that have been moved to the growing and finishing areas. Again, mixing and moving groups of pigs; overcrowding; cold, drafty environments; or changes in management and feed may precipitate outbreaks of lameness.

In the case of *M hyosynoviae*, the upper respiratory tract of sows and older pigs in peer groups is the likely source. As colostral immunity wanes at 6-8 wk of age, pigs become susceptible to infection. Morbidity may be low to moderate, but mortality is very low. An acute, afebrile lameness, lasting up to 10 days, develops in groups of grower/finisher pigs or selected replacement stock. Arthritis may be exacerbated by trauma or stress, and pigs exhibit pain in major joints (eg, elbows and stifles) that may develop fluctuating swellings. On necropsy, lesions are restricted to the joints, especially the stifles, and include an excess of clear, yellow synovial fluid that may have fibrin flakes, and yellow synovium with obvious villous hypertrophy. Articular surfaces and periarticular tissues usually are unaffected.

Diagnosis is based on the age of onset of clinical disease and clinical signs that exclude fever or evidence of pneumonia, pleuritis, and peritonitis. If a definitive diagnosis is to be made based on isolation of the organism, samples of synovium and synovial fluid should be collected from untreated pigs within 3-4 days of the onset of clinical signs. However, *M hyosynoviae* can be cultured from normal joints and is not always recovered from affected joints. Unlike polyarthritis caused by *M hyorhinis*, response to treatment with tylosin and lincomycin is generally good, and tiamulin, tetracycline, and enrofloxacin may be effective. (Of these, only lincomycin is labeled for use against arthritis in swine.) Concurrent treatment with corticosteroids may be used to curtail the inflammatory response and to alleviate the discomfort. Isoflupredone is labeled for use in food-producing animals. Reduction of any stresses such as mixing and moving batches of pigs helps prevent the problem, and SPF herds can be kept free of the condition. Mycoplasmal arthritis may exacerbate clinical signs associated with degenerative joint disease and osteoarthrosis and vice versa.

Erysipelas: *Erysipelothrix rhusiopathiae* is acquired from healthy carrier pigs or the environment, in which the organism can survive for weeks. Erysipelas can be peracute, acute, or chronic. In the peracute form, pigs are found dead without prior clinical signs. In the acute form, pigs become moderately febrile, lethargic, unwilling to rise because of painful joints, anorectic, and cyanotic in their extremities; after 2-3 days, the classic "diamond" (focal, urticarial) skin lesions develop over the body surface. In some outbreaks, lameness is seen without the skin lesions. In the chronic form, the arthritis progresses such that the carpuses and hocks become swollen and firm, and skin necrosis can result in extensive sloughing of portions of the integument. In chronic cases, diskospondylosis also may develop. As the arthritis progresses and joints fuse, pain in the lumbar vertebrae may reduce the libido of a boar.

If the chronic form of erysipelas is investigated as a lameness problem and pigs are necropsied, early changes in the disease process (eg, hemorrhages in lymph nodes, kidneys, and muscles) may be less obvious. An excess of synovial fluid accumulates during the acute phase, but in chronically affected joints, there is villous hypertrophy and hyperplasia, hyperemia, and periarticular fibrosis. If a pannus has formed, the articular surface becomes disrupted. Raised, focal skin lesions progress to sloughed areas and, in extreme cases, the ears and tail may also slough. Vegetative endocarditis is a frequent change.

Diagnosis is based on the clinical signs, of which the "diamond" skin lesions are most consistently useful. All 3 forms of the disease may be seen in the same herd if the problem has not been investigated and treatment has been delayed. Isolation of the causal organism is important for a definitive diagnosis and is most successful if acutely affected, untreated pigs are necropsied. A bacterial culture with an antibiotic sensitivity pattern is useful during treatment of the herd. Sometimes, a rapid response of the acute condition to penicillin is a diagnostic aid.

Vaccination with either modified live or killed organisms is effective in controlling erysipelas in a herd, and outbreaks may be related to noncompliance with vaccination protocols rather than to changes in the virulence of the causal organism or the nature of the disease. Therefore, any investigation of the problem should begin with a detailed vaccination history. However, in some herds, sow vaccination is not sufficient to control the infection in grower/finisher pigs. On these farms, growers must be vaccinated as well as the sows. In the face of an outbreak, concurrent use of killed vaccine and antibiotic is likely to be the most effective control measure. Affected pigs are individually treated with penicillin IM. (*See also* p 505.)

Osteomyelitis: This can be seen in pigs of any age. If the integument is damaged, sepsis develops and a suppurative lesion extends to the periosteum and bone. Alternatively, organisms can invade bone from the synovium and infected joints. Poor processing or injection techniques can initiate abscesses that can extend into adjacent bone. Disruption of the integrity of the hoof wall initiates cellulitis and osteomyelitis of one or more phalanges. Ear and flank biting wounds are other foci of infection. Tail biting leads to spinal abscesses that either affect vertebral bodies directly or start as epidural abscesses. Lesions and clinical signs may develop slowly.

Clinical signs vary with both the site and nature of the lesion. If bones or joints of a limb are affected, the condition is usually chronic and the pig becomes 3-legged lame. Young pigs cease to grow. With tail biting, the pig becomes lame or paralyzed in the hind end.

At necropsy, cream or green, caseous pus is seen at the site of the lesion. If *Arcanobacterium (Actinomyces) pyogenes* is involved, there are abundant pockets of green, semiliquid pus. Other organisms isolated from the abscesses include streptococci, staphylococci, and enterobacteria. Treatment is not usually feasible, and pigs should be culled for humane reasons. However, when applicable, hygiene should be improved and vices such as tail biting controlled or prevented.

Osteochondrosis and Osteoarthrosis: Lameness associated with these problems may become clinically relevant by the time the pigs are 4-6 mo old, but the major ramifications are in gilts, sows, and boars (*see* below). The importance of these problems increases if affected replacement breeding stock is brought into a herd that was previously free of either condition.

Rickets: Although now uncommon, rickets (p 853) is occasionally seen. Rickets affects rapidly growing young pigs with a clinical onset at ~10 wk of age. Morbidity is high, and affected pigs become crippled, anorectic, and unthrifty. Limbs are stunted and bowed, joints are swollen, and the head may seem disproportionately large. Long bones of the limbs or ribs can spontaneously fracture so that the pig becomes immobile. Some pigs develop posterior paresis and sit on the ground. Absolute deficiencies of calcium, phosphorus, or vitamin D, or an imbalance of the calcium:phosphorus ratio cause cessation of mineralization at the metaphysis and thickening of the growth plate and epiphyseal growth cartilage.

On necropsy, bones should be dissected to determine if there are any fractures or healing fractures, particularly in the ribs, humeruses, and femurs. The costochondral junctions of most ribs are enlarged to form a rachitic rosary, and ribs may bend. Bone remodelling is inadequate and, radiographically, bones are poorly mineralized. Failure of calcification and endochondral ossification results in thickened, irregular growth plates and epiphyseal growth cartilages in which hemorrhages may be seen grossly. A generalized dietary fibrous osteodystrophy may develop, and bones are easily cut with a knife. Ration analysis is useful, but current batches of feed may have been mixed correctly or with different batches of ingredients, thus making it difficult to relate cause and effect. Keeping samples of each batch of feed for retrospective analysis may be a good practice.

Although rations can be corrected and vitamin D given parenterally, there is no effective treatment, and attempts to rear large numbers of affected pigs have been economically disastrous.

Foot Disorders: On occasion, grower/finisher pigs have overgrown claws or bruises and cracks in the wall or sole of the hoof. The type of the floor is perhaps the single greatest factor in determining if lesions develop or resolve. Floors with wide slots enable feet to fall between the slats, causing damage. If the floor is too smooth, the balance between growth and wear of the horn is lost; if it is too rough, the hoof wall, coronary band, or skin above the hoof is damaged so that infectious agents can penetrate the foot or adjacent joints. Footrot then develops.

GILTS, SOWS, AND BOARS

Many diseases that affect grower/finisher pigs (*see* above) can also affect young gilts and boars that have been selected as breeding stock. Lameness caused by *Mycoplasma hyosynoviae*, or acute or chronic erysipelas can cause an incapacitating lameness. Polyarthritis and polyserositis caused by *M hyorhinis* are seen occasionally in these older pigs. If rickets or skeletal weakness has been a problem, pigs that could have been affected should not be retained as breeding stock. Ambulation should be assessed as a component of breeding stock selection. Pigs with conformational abnormalities should be culled. Gilts with buck-kneed forelegs, swaying hindquarters, or a "standing-under" position of the hindlegs are likely to be culled for lameness early in their reproductive life. Feet should be evaluated for uniformity among and angulation of the digits and for integrity of the wall, sole, and heel.

Lame breeding pigs result in the following: 1) continuous replacement of breeding stock and increased risk of disease introduction; 2) an inability to maintain a breeding schedule due to an unreliable pool of breeding pigs; 3) increased cost of maintaining additional breeding stock; 4) poorer reproductive performance due to regular replacement of lame sows; 5) increased preweaning mortality due to clumsy, lame sows; and 6) reduced fertility in sound boars that are overworked.

Rickets, Osteomalacia, and Osteoporosis: These syndromes can affect one or more age groups of pigs with various clinical outcomes. Most pigs, including breeding stock, are slaughtered before their skeleton has fully matured; however, some growth plates are functional up to 3.5 yr of age and, therefore, are susceptible to rachitic and other changes.

Osteomalacia is characterized by an excess of unmineralized or poorly mineralized osteoid that forms as bone remodeling occurs (or does not occur). Rickets (*see* above) is the component of osteomalacia that affects the growth plate. The pathogenesis of osteoporosis is different from that of either rickets or osteomalacia. Established bone loses mineral and mass by a process of osteolysis. Consequently, particularly in sows late in gestation, during lactation, or soon after weaning, bones become weaker and are susceptible to fractures.

A gilt selected for breeding stock that has had clinically normal skeletal development must meet the needs of her own skeleton and that of the growing fetuses. This may result in development of osteomalacia, which is compounded by secretion of mineral in her milk when lactation begins. The gilt may soon draw on her skeletal reserves and become osteoporotic. Because sows can become pregnant within 7 days of weaning, there is little time for recovery of skeletal mass between one breeding cycle and the next, so the skeleton becomes progressively weaker. Therefore, it is not surprising that considerable numbers of first- and second-litter sows are culled due to fractures and lameness.

Factors that may lead to bone fractures include entrapment of a limb in or under the bars of a farrowing crate, activity as sows are moved from their farrowing crates, and fighting as new groups of weaned sows reestablish a social order in the breeding or gestation area. Sows mounted by other sows that are in estrus are also prone to injury. The most frequent sites of fractures are the humerus, femur, lumbar vertebrae, and occasionally ribs. Multiple vertebral body fractures have been described in gilts that were considered to have been exposed to stray electrical voltage (p 1697). Whatever the factors that precipitate the fractures, affected sows are in pain and are either severely lame and unwilling to move or paraplegic.

Diagnosis is based on a history of acute lameness or paraplegia in pregnant, lactating, or recently weaned gilts or sows. Sometimes, crepitus can be detected in affected limbs. A neurologic examination can aid in locating spinal lesions. Affected sows should be culled after an early diagnosis, but they have little salvage value. Prevention through adequate nutrition and exercise for gilts and sows is the best (and only) way to curtail the problem.

Osteomyelitis and Spinal Abscesses: In addition to the causes discussed under grower/finisher pigs (above), osteomyelitis may also develop secondary to a vertebral fracture or an epiphyseal separation. It is reasonable to assume that occasional "showering" with organisms from superficial wounds, abscesses, or the respiratory or GI tracts can be a source of infection. *Arcanobacterium (Actinomyces) pyogenes* seems to be a frequent cause of the suppuration and abscessation. Osteomyelitis of the ulnar epiphysis in young boars and sows has been reported.

Vertebral osteomyelitis and epidural abscesses can cause a variety of signs, including lameness or bilateral flaccid paralysis of the pelvic limbs, and hypermetria or ataxia. Except for the temporal nature of the infectious process, clinically, it is difficult to differentiate a destructive or space-occupying abscess from a fracture. Regardless of underlying cause, recovery is unlikely, and the pig should be culled.

Degenerative Joint Disease (Osteochondrosis Dissecans, Osteoarthritis, Osteoarthrosis), Dyschondroplasia (Osteochondrosis), and Leg Weakness: These syndromes are the most important causes of lameness and culling for lameness in breeding stock animals and cause major losses in commercial pig herds. They are more important than ever given the increased scale of production in many herds and the shift toward pigs that grow faster, are more muscular, and finish heavier.

Osteochondrosis and osteoarthritis are seen in all the major breeds of commercial pigs; they are particularly important and common because they are not eliminated by crossbreeding. In addition, epiphyseolysis and epiphyseal separation may be precipitated by weakening of underlying growth plates if they are affected by osteochondrosis. Degenerative joint disease (DJD) can also decrease growth rate in lame finishing pigs, and there is a risk of partial carcass condemnations if affected joints are swollen.

Although lesions that precede or develop into DJD or result in limb deformities begin to develop in younger pigs, clinical problems are not usually seen until pigs are >4-8 mo old. Frequently the fastest growing, most muscular, heaviest pigs are affected. Given time, some pigs (if not culled) recover from episodes of lameness, but deformities remain. Clinical signs vary with the site and extent of lesions and can range from stiffness and a shortened stride or a stride affected by an angular limb deformity to a 3-legged lameness or an inability to stand. Most commonly, these animals have a weightbearing, shifting lameness due to the bilateral lesions that affect multiple joints in the same pig.

Lesions of the ischial tuberosity cause a tendency to slip. Pigs that "walk" on flexed carpuses usually have severe DJD in the elbows, and pigs that "tuck" their pelvic limbs under their abdomen or develop kyphosis often have DJD that affects stifles, tibial tarsal bones, or joints on intervertebral processes.

If epiphyseal separation of the femoral head has occurred, the pig has difficulty in standing and initially will not use the affected limb. A pig that has unilateral separation of the ischiatic tuberosity also has difficulty standing; if both tuberosities are affected, the pig has a hopping gait for a few steps and then collapses. The severity of clinical signs in any of these conditions varies individually, and seemingly less severely affected joints may be protected by the gait if they are more painful than other degenerating joints. Severe joint lesions have been seen in pigs that did not appear to be lame.

In pigs that have limb deformities (eg, osteochondrosis affecting the distal ulnar growth plate), thickened, irregular growth plates are seen on radiographs or at necropsy. In degenerating joints, there is an excess of yellow synovia, and synovial villi may have proliferated. There are various irregularities of the articular surface, including folds in the cartilage, clefts, flaps of cartilage, and in severe cases, craters and exposed subchondral bone. In chronic cases, osteophytes develop, detached fragments of cartilage become embedded in the synovium and start to ossify, and craters fill with fibrocartilage. If vertebral joints are affected, vertebrae eventually fuse. Growth plates that are most severely affected by dyschondroplasia are those of the distal part of the ulna and the ribs, whereas sites most often affected by DJD include the elbow, stifle, hock, and intervertebral synovial joints.

The pathogenesis of lesions is poorly understood, but foci of poorly mineralized cartilage persist in the metaphyses and epiphyses (and may be points of weakness), or foci of necrotic chondrocytes develop in the middle region of the articular-epiphyseal cartilage complex. It is postulated that there is failure of the vasculature that supplies or penetrates the sites where lesions develop or that chondrocytes are not functioning normally to maintain the homeostasis of the cartilage or to promote endochondral ossification.

Many potential causes of DJD or osteochondrosis have been investigated. Breeds and lines of pigs that are heavy and well muscled, particularly in the hams, are commonly affected; therefore, crossbreeding for hybrid vigor does not solve the problem. The fastest growing pigs in a group seem to have a greater propensity for lesions developing in either growth plates or joints, but once slower growing pigs reach the body weight of their faster growing peers, lesions are comparable. Growth hormone may affect chondrocyte metabolism and thereby influence the onset of articular lesions. Overgrown claws predispose gilts to osteochondrosis. Mechanical stress to joints also leads to an increased prevalence of this condition in breeding stock. This occurs during transport or when animals are housed on slippery floors.

Research into manipulating the energy and protein concentrations of the ration in an attempt to influence the development of lesions has been inconclusive. None of the imbalances or deficiencies of nutrients that typically are associated with lesions of cartilage or bone (calcium, phosphorus, and vitamins A, C, and D) seemed to exacerbate DJD or osteochondrosis. Deficiencies of zinc and manganese may be causal factors in DJD.

The stress of mixing pigs appears to have little impact on the frequency of DJD. The culling rate due to lameness for sows kept on solid floors is less than that for those kept on slats. Pigs with DJD placed on dirt lots or pasture usually become clinically sound within 6 wk.

Because osteochondrosis and DJD interfere with production efficiency, the prognosis for affected pigs is poor. Downgrading carcass characteristics by using genetic selection or reducing growth rates by controlling protein and energy intake is counter to the goals of modern swine production for providing quality pork. The use of drugs may alleviate clinical signs but mask the real incidence. At best, the following practices are recommended: selecting against replacement pigs that are lame or have poor conformation, providing adequate rations for the growth of a strong skeleton, and housing gilts in pens with ≥12 sq ft (1.1 sq m) per animal, promoting exercise on nonslip floors. In problem herds, providing a "hardening off" period for gilts is encouraged. This includes purchasing gilts at <75 kg live weight, restricting their feed intake to slow their growth rate, providing ≥1.1 sq m per animal in pens with solid or only partially slatted floors, waiting to breed gilts until they are 8-10 mo of age, and housing gilts in pens until they farrow. When these practices are not followed, suitable breeding stock must be selected and inferior pigs rejected at the time of arrival at the farm.

Footrot or Septic Laminitis: This can develop in any age pig but causes serious losses in breeding pigs. Footrot is seen in both confinement and semiconfinement systems, with morbidity of 20-68%. Often a single limb is affected, and the lameness progresses to the point that the pig is 3-legged lame.

Lesions usually develop gradually, and the foot becomes swollen. Lesions vary in severity and can include heel erosions, separation along the white line, toe erosions, sole erosions, false sandcracks, deep necrotic ulcers, sinuses at the coronary band, and chronic fibrosis. A mixture of organisms has been isolated from the lesions or identified in smears from lesions and tissue sections. These included *Arcanobacterium (Actinomyces) pyogenes, Fusobacterium necrophorum, Borrelia suilla,* and a mixture of gram-negative and gram-positive cocci and rods.

A diagnosis is made from the clinical signs and a thorough evaluation of the feet. If there is a herd problem, all sows in crates should be examined and their feet evaluated at the slaughterhouse. To ensure that lesions are severe enough to be the cause of the lameness, it is advisable to section feet parallel with the sole to determine if the soft tissues and bones within the foot are infected.

Treatment with penicillin has proved effective (200,000 U into the lesion or 600,000 U, IM), but success decreases with chronicity of the lesion. Prevention involves improving the nature and cleanliness of the flooring, reducing moisture, and removing abrasive areas. As replacement gilts mature, biotin supplementation seems to enhance the quality of the hoof wall. Foot baths that include copper sulfate, formalin, or oxytetracycline and paraffin help to prevent or alleviate lesions. Success in increasing longevity of pigs with amputated digits has been variable.

Trauma: Trauma associated with overexertion was considered to have caused detachment of muscle tendons and a proliferative osteitis on the medial humeral epicondyle and the greater trochanter of the femur in sows. Mixing gilts or sows after breeding or at weaning is a common source of trauma. This can lead to osteochondrosis (*see* above), epiphysiolysis, fractures, or skin abrasions that may cause secondary bacterial infections.

Sows housed in stalls with concrete slats may tear their dewclaws when they attempt to stand. Affected animals must be moved to a pen to avoid repeated trauma to the injured foot. Treatment with a broad-spectrum antibiotic and penned housing enable the lesion to heal.

LAMENESS IN SHEEP

Lameness in sheep may be caused by a number of systemic diseases. The more common conditions, listed by age group usually affected, are as follows: lambs—joint-ill, tetanus, white muscle disease, enzootic ataxia (copper deficiency), polyarthritis (chlamydial), rickets, poisonous plant intoxication (eg, sneezeweed), and contagious ecthyma (orf); adults—mastitis, epididymitis, and mineral and trace element imbalances; any age—erysipelas (one of the more important, p 504), laminitis, bluetongue, ulcerative dermatosis, foot-and-mouth disease, and dermatophilosis. Additional information on differential diagnosis, treatment, and prevention can be found under the specific topics (*see*, eg, THE MUSCULOSKELETAL SYSTEM, p 837, and THE NERVOUS SYSTEM, p 977).

Many lamenesses are due to injuries. The general principles of treatment and prevention of these are the same for sheep as for other species.

In addition to systemic diseases and injuries, lameness can be caused by a group of infections specific to the feet. These are mixed infections with combinations of bacteria, including *Fusobacterium necrophorum*. The skin between the claws is the primary site of invasion, but this usually does not occur when the stratum corneum is dry and intact.

Predisposing causes are damage by water, maceration, frostbite, or mechanical trauma. Epidermal penetration by *F necrophorum* and *Arcanobacterium (Actinomyces) pyogenes* induces a transient condition, ovine interdigital dermatitis; when there is concurrent invasion by *Dichelobacter nodosus*, footrot results. This may be benign or virulent, depending on the strain of *D nodosus*. When the dermal and subdermal invasion by *F necrophorum* and *A pyogenes* involves the distal interphalangeal tissues and joint, foot abscess develops. Infection of the hoof matrix with these organisms results in septic laminitis. These 5 distinct but related conditions are discussed below.

FOOT ABSCESS
(Infective bulbar necrosis, Heel abscess, Bumblefoot)

A foot abscess is a necrotizing or purulent infection involving the distal interphalangeal tissues and sometimes the joint. The incidence is usually sporadic, but up to 15% of the flock may be affected.

The 2 organisms most consistently recovered from foot abscess are *Fusobacterium necrophorum* and *Arcanobacterium (Actinomyces) pyogenes*. Most commonly, foot abscesses develop as a complication of ovine interdigital dermatitis (*see* below) by extension of the necrotic process into the subcutis and then into the distal interphalangeal joint. This joint is vulnerable to infection on the interdigital aspect where the joint capsule protrudes above the coronary border as the dorsal and volar pouches. At these 2 sites, the joint capsule is protected only by the interdigital skin and a minimal amount of subcutaneous tissue. Sporadic cases of foot abscess may also develop after penetration by sharp objects (eg, crusted snow, the stiff stubble of cut alfalfa fields) or careless paring of the hoof.

Foot abscesses develop most often when the soil and pastures are wet. The disease causes an acute lameness that is usually restricted to one foot. In the early stages, it may be possible to express necrotic material through an opening in the interdigital skin via the channel caused by the bacterial invasion. Later, the sinuses may extend to break out at one or more points above the coronet. In ~50% of the cases, movement of the affected digit is exaggerated, which indicates that the ligaments about the distal interphalangeal joint have ruptured; displacement of the digit during locomotion and permanent deformity are likely.

Acute lameness, swelling of one digit, and discharging sinuses distinguish foot abscess from footrot. Radiographs can help determine the extent of joint damage.

Early treatment with parenteral antibiotics is often effective and may prevent joint infection. Once the infection becomes established in the joint, treatment is of limited value. Therapy should be aimed at maintaining the integrity of the joint ligaments by draining the abscess, bandaging to reduce stress on the ligaments, and countering the bacterial infection with antibiotics or sulfonamides. Although the prognosis for complete recovery is poor, in most cases the foot heals sufficiently to allow adequate locomotion after ~2 mo. Control depends on early treatment and avoidance of the conditions that lead to ovine interdigital dermatitis. Although *F necrophorum* vaccines are available, they have not proved to be entirely satisfactory.

OVINE INTERDIGITAL DERMATITIS
(Foot scald)

Ovine interdigital dermatitis is a necrotizing condition of the interdigital skin caused by a mixed infection with *Fusobacterium necrophorum* and *Arcanobacterium (Actinomyces) pyogenes*. It often precedes or accompanies footrot. In Australia, it is considered to be caused by less virulent strains of *Dichelobacter nodosus* and is termed benign footrot (*see* below). Cold weather and damp pastures are predisposing factors. A similar condition has been attributed to mechanical damage inflicted by short, stiff stubble. These lesions often result in foot abscess (*see* above). Similar injuries to the interdigital epithelium frequently result from "clay balling," a condition in which balls of clay, molded into the shape of the interdigital space, harden and become difficult to dislodge, causing constant irritation and enhancing bacterial invasion.

Lameness may be seen in 90% of sheep, and all 4 feet may be affected. In milder cases, the interdigital skin is red and swollen and covered by a moist film of whitish necrotic material. In severely affected cases, the interdigital skin is necrotic and eroded, and subcutaneous tissues are exposed. Suppuration and swelling of the deeper interdigital tissues may develop. The sole and wall of the hoof does not separate from the underlying tissue, and the characteristic odor associated with virulent *D nodosus* infections is not present. Under dry conditions, the disease often is transient but may persist or recur while pastures remain wet.

The clinical appearance is characteristic, but similar conditions such as benign or virulent footrot must be excluded. Dermatophilosis (strawberry footrot, p 690) affects the hairy skin of the coronet and pastern. Viral diseases such as ulcerative dermatitis, contagious ecthyma, and foot-and-mouth disease may be excluded by flock history, clinical signs, and serology. *F necrophorum* may also infect the lesions caused by these diseases. Most lesions heal rapidly with the advent of dry conditions or removal to drier pastures. When the disease is associated with stubble, improvement usually follows removal to ordinary pastures. External application of disinfectants such as 5% formaldehyde or 10% zinc sulfate may help. In severe cases, housing in dry conditions may be appropriate.

FOOTROT

Benign Footrot

In benign footrot, the infection is confined largely to the interdigital skin, with minimal underrunning of the adjacent horn. Clinically, it is similar to ovine interdigital dermatitis (*see* above), but *Dichelobacter nodosus* is involved. Lameness is common but less severe than in virulent footrot (*see* below). The etiology and pathogenesis are the same, but the causal strains of *D nodosus* are less virulent and lack the hoof-invasive properties of the strains that cause virulent footrot. *D nodosus* isolated from cattle usually causes only the benign form of footrot in sheep. The economic effect of benign footrot is much less than that of virulent footrot. Foot baths with 10% zinc sulfate or 5% formaldehyde solution are usually adequate for control.

Virulent Footrot
(Malignant footrot, Contagious footrot)

Virulent footrot is a specific, chronic, necrotizing disease of the epidermis of the interdigital skin and hoof matrix that begins as an interdigital dermatitis and extends to involve large areas of the hoof matrix. Because the infected tissue is destroyed, the hoof corium (or horny hoof) loses its anchorage to the basal epithelium and becomes detached. Footrot is contagious and, under suitable conditions, morbidity may approach 100%. The infection is also found in goats and deer but rarely in cattle. The potential for genetic selection for increased resistance to footrot has been established.

Etiology: Virulent footrot is due to a mixed infection of 2 gram-negative, anaerobic bacteria. *Fusobacterium necrophorum* is a normal resident of the sheep's environment, but infection depends on the presence of *Dichelobacter nodosus*, which does not survive for more than 2 wk in the soil or pastures. Because the longterm presence of *D nodosus* depends on the presence of infected animals, it is regarded as the transmissible and specific causal agent, although its contribution to the disease process is not necessarily greater than that of *F necrophorum*. Several different strains of *D nodosus*, with varying pathogenicity, have been identified.

The transmission of footrot to healthy animals requires a warm, moist environment. Under these conditions, the interdigital stratum corneum becomes macerated; filaments of *F necrophorum* invade the superficial epidermis and induce ovine interdigital dermatitis (*see* above). If *D nodosus* is in contact with the skin at this stage, virulent footrot results. Injuries to the feet enhance transmission, although it usually does not occur when the soil temperature is <40°F (4.5°C).

Clinical Findings: The most obvious sign is lameness, which may be severe. Some sheep remain recumbent or on their brisket and knees, which tend to become hairless and ulcerated. Affected sheep lose body condition. Rams infected in the hindfeet may be unable to serve, and ewes with hindfeet lesions may be unable to bear the weight of a ram at service. Wool production is reduced. In early cases, examination of the feet may reveal nothing more than dermatitis similar to ovine interdigital dermatitis. In slightly more advanced cases, in which the infection has begun to extend into the hoof matrix, there is slight detachment of areas of the hoof. As the disease progresses, the epidermal necrosis and separation of the horn spread further under the heel and sole, and finally the outer wall, so that the horny hoof may eventually be attached only at the coronet. The necrotic tissue has a characteristic odor. Myiasis is a common sequela and may extend to the sides of the sheep at sites where the infected feet are placed when the sheep lie down. The disease persists for months in some sheep. Infection may be hidden in small pockets within the foot where it is detectable only on extensive paring; these sheep act as subclinical carriers. These small pockets may become active within the foot, or open and contaminate the soil when favored by a moist external environment. Recovery occurs but is not followed by appreciable immunity.

Diagnosis: Early cases confined to the interdigital space may be confused with ovine interdigital dermatitis or benign footrot, and advanced ones with foot abscess (*see* above). In flocks affected with virulent footrot, underrunning and separation of the hard horn of the hoof, usually of more than one foot, are characteristic. In foot abscess, there is a deeper invasion and discharge of necrotic and purulent material; usually, only one foot is affected. *D nodosus* usually can be identified in smears of stained necrotic material from footrot, although other bacteria predominate.

Treatment: Treatment efforts may be directed toward temporary control of the disease or eradication from the flock. At certain times, eg, during a wet season, temporary control may be the only realistic goal.

Treatment may be topical or parenteral. Topical treatment requires careful hoof paring to remove all underrun horn and to expose necrotic tissue. Bactericidal solutions are then applied by aerosol spray, footbathing, or footsoaking. Common footbathing solutions are 10% zinc sulfate, 10% copper sulfate, or 5% formaldehyde. The solutions used as aerosol sprays include those used for footbathing as well as 20% cetrimide and 1.3% oxytetracycline in water and alcohol.

For footsoaking, the sheep are kept standing for 1 hr in a solution of 10% zinc sulfate and 0.2% v/v of laundry detergent containing nonionic surfactants or the surfactant sodium lauryl sulfate. In moist conditions, or with mild to moderate underrunning, it is not necessary to pare the feet previously; if the feet are dry and hard, or with severe underrunning, paring improves the recovery rate. The footsoaking should be repeated every 5-10 days for 3 treatments.

Parenteral treatment consists of injections of penicillin and dihydrostreptomycin at 50,000-70,000 U/kg and 50-70 mg/kg, respectively (this dosage exceeds by 2-3 times the approved dosage in most countries); erythromycin at 22 mg/lb (10 mg/kg); oxytetracycline; benzathine penicillin G (not an approved use in all countries); or a combined lincomycin and spectinomycin product. The problems with parenteral treatment are the expense and the short duration of benefit. Injections of long-acting antibiotics have been successful in Australia; however, the sheep must be kept in a completely dry area for at least 24 hr after treatment. Even dew on grass greatly reduces the efficacy of this treatment.

The success rate for either topical or parenteral treatment is substantially improved if the treated sheep are kept in a dry environment after treatment (even for 24 hr). This is essential when parenteral treatment is used. The feet of treated sheep should be examined every 1-2 wk to identify those not responding to treatment or those needing further paring.

Reports from several countries indicate an improved response from the use of oral zinc sulfate along with vitamin A. However, this response apparently is seen only in flocks that are deficient in these nutrients. Laser therapy has been successfully used experimentally.

Combining both topical and parenteral methods of treatment does not immediately eradicate virulent footrot. Time is necessary to identify the subclinical or relapsing cases.

Prevention and Control: Flocks may be kept free of virulent footrot by preventing the introduction of *D nodosus*. Any sheep to be added to the flock should be examined, isolated for 1 mo, and then reexamined. Any vehicles or facilities in which unknown or infected sheep have been held must be cleaned and disinfected before placing uninfected sheep in them.

During periods of the year that favor transmission of virulent footrot, footbaths may provide some control for affected flocks, along with individual treatment (either topical or parenteral) of severely affected sheep.

D nodosus vaccines accelerate healing in affected sheep and aid in protecting unaffected ones. Their effectiveness may depend on the strain(s) causing the infection and those present in the vaccine. Alum-precipitated vaccines require 2 doses 4-6 wk apart to establish effective immunity, which persists for ~2 mo. Lesions heal within 4-6 wk if immunity is established. Oil-emulsion vaccines induce immunity within 3 wk of the initial dose and may persist for 3-4 mo. In endemic areas, revaccination is recommended at intervals of 3-6 mo. Vaccines for *F necrophorum* have been of some benefit in both treatment and prevention. Vaccination alone usually does not provide complete control or eradication and is most beneficial when used in conjunction with other control and treatment measures, such as hoof paring and footbaths. Some vaccines may cause lumps or abscesses at the injection sites.

Eradication: Eradication may be achieved only by eliminating all cases of virulent *D nodosus* infection and preventing its reintroduction. This can be done by replacing the affected flock with disease-free sheep or by rigorously treating all new infections and culling affected sheep that do not respond readily to treatment. Affected sheep are identified by clinical examination; no other diagnostic tests are practical under such circumstances. Subclinical cases constitute a major problem because they may relapse during the next 2-3 mo and transmit infection. Other ruminants (goats, deer, cattle) are potential sources of *D nodosus* and should be considered in eradication programs.

Eradication should be undertaken only when the environment is dry; at other times, treatments should be directed toward control within the flock. A successful eradication program requires planning, commitment, and an investment of time and money; however, it is usually well worth the effort and expense when compared with managing a permanently infected flock.

Before eradication is attempted, prevalence should be reduced to <15% by use of chemotherapy, parenteral antibiotics, or vaccination. Once this is achieved, or if the prevalence is already low, the feet of all sheep in the flock should be examined, and the flock divided into affected and unaffected groups. Sheep with no visible lesions are isolated, undergo footbathing, and placed on clean, dry ground. This group should receive footbaths weekly during the next 2-3 mo, and any lame sheep should be removed immediately. The sheep with virulent footrot lesions are either culled or, after careful and extensive hoof paring, medicated topically (and parenterally if desired) and then kept separate from the group with no lesions. Sheep in the affected group should undergo footbathing or be medicated topically every 3-4 days; their feet should be examined and hooves pared every 1-2 wk. Eventually, a potentially clean group can be formed from those appearing to respond to treatment. This group must be monitored for 1-3 mo or through a period conducive to the spread of footrot to detect and isolate (again) any subclinical cases that relapse. Eventually, this group may be placed with the clean flock. Those sheep that remain affected (after 4-6 wk of treatment) or that relapse should be culled. An alternative eradication program involves footsoaking (in zinc sulfate and surfactant) for 1 hr every 7 days for 3 treatments. Hoof paring is done only for diagnostic purposes.

Most affected sheep recover with adequate treatment and time. However, placing a single active or subclinical case in the clean flock may lead to failure of the eradication program.

Australia has implemented an effective eradication program over a wide area, involving many flocks. The program has 3 phases. The **control phase** is used during periods of active spread or to reduce the number infected. During this phase, vaccination, footbathing, and parenteral antibiotics can all be used. The **eradication phase** must take place during the dry season and cannot begin until several weeks after the use of all medications has been stopped and 10-12 wk after vaccination. Footbathing and vaccination tend to mask the presence of infection. During this phase, every foot of every sheep is inspected every 3-4 wk. Infected sheep can be treated with parenteral antibiotics at the first inspection only. After this, all infected sheep are culled at each inspection. This continues until there are 2 completely negative, consecutive flock tests. In the **surveillance phase**, all lame sheep in the flock are examined immediately. If footrot is present, the flock goes back to phase 2 or 1 again.

IMPACTED OR INFECTED OIL GLAND

Sheep have a sebaceous (oil) gland in the skin of the digit. An oily, glandular secretion is stored in a small pouch lying between the phalanges and is discharged to the skin surface through a duct in the skin. Occasionally, the duct may be occluded and cause impaction and distention of the oil pouch, which may cause lameness. The interdigital tissues may appear distorted. The oil sac also may become infected and result in a local cellulitis or abscess. Expression of the contents by manual pressure relieves impaction. Infected glands can then be treated with local or systemic antibiotics or both, depending on the extent and severity of the infectious process.

INTERDIGITAL FIBROMA

An interdigital fibroma is a mass of fibrous tissue between the toes that may resemble a papilloma. If not removed, it grows upward between the first phalanges and may cause severe lameness. If it is detected early, surgical removal (cryosurgery and electrocautery) is successful.

SEPTIC LAMINITIS
(Lamellar suppuration, Toe abscess)

Septic laminitis is an acute bacterial infection of the laminar matrix of the hoof that is usually restricted to the toe and abaxial wall. The disease is sporadic and the etiology variable, but cases due to *Fusobacterium necrophorum* and *Arcanobacterium (Actinomyces) pyogenes* usually are more severe and extensive than those involving streptococci or other organisms. The organisms probably enter through fissures between the wall and sole and through vertical and horizontal fractures of horn. Sometimes, infection is enhanced by impaction with mud and feces, by overgrowth of the hoof, or by separation of the wall after laminitis.

Front feet are affected more commonly. Lameness is severe, and the affected digit hot and tender. There may be a sinus above the lesion at the coronet. Affected sheep usually recover rapidly after paring of the horn to provide dependent drainage.

MYOPATHIES AND MYOSITIDES

Diseases that produce primary damage to the skeletal muscle fiber, excluding those of inflammatory origin and those secondary to neural lesions, are considered myopathies. Many myopathies are seen in animals; some are of much economic importance (eg, the nutritional and exertional myopathies), and others are important models of human diseases. For discussion of congenital myopathies, *see* CONGENITAL AND INHERITED ANOMALIES, p 846.

The myositides are diseases producing a predominantly inflammatory reaction in muscle. Major examples are *Clostridium* spp infections (blackleg, malignant edema), parasitic diseases (sarcocystosis, trichinellosis, and cysticercosis), and an immune-mediated condition (purpura hemorrhagica).

NUTRITIONAL MYOPATHIES

The most common and economically important myopathies of food animals are those due to deficiency of selenium or vitamin E, or both. Characteristically, these are acute diseases and most often, but not exclusively, affect young animals of suckling age. The clinical signs vary widely, depending on the distribution and severity of muscle damage. Frequently, they include stiffness or inability to stand as a result of symmetric damage to the girdle muscles or the large muscles of the limbs. Complications, such as bronchopneumonia or inability to nurse, may lead to prostration and death within a few days to ~1 wk after onset. Acute cardiac failure is often the precipitating cause of death, especially in calves.

The lesions in heart or skeletal musculature are almost always bilaterally symmetric and vary from diffuse, light-colored areas to well-defined white streaks or patches. Most muscles can be involved, but macroscopic lesions are most common in the heart or in the large muscles of the shoulder girdle, back, and thighs; the diaphragm and tongue also may be affected. Examples have been described under various names in most domestic and laboratory animals, including muscular dystrophy, white muscle disease, nutritional muscular dystrophy, stiff lamb disease, late-lactation paralysis, white flesh, fish flesh, waxy degeneration, paralytic myoglobinuria, and selenium-responsive myopathy.

Pathologic changes in other tissues often occur in association with some of the myopathies. These include liver necrosis, subcutaneous and pulmonary edema with exudation into the body cavities, steatitis, gastric ulceration, pancreatic necrosis, gizzard myopathy, anemia, intestinal lipofuscinosis, testicular degeneration, embryonic death and resorption, and encephalomalacia and other nervous system lesions. In some cases, the lesions in other tissues predominate or appear to constitute the sole pathology (eg, exudative diathesis and encephalomalacia in the chick; necrosis of heart, liver, muscle, and kidney in the mouse; dietary liver necrosis in the rat). Some, but not all, reports have also attributed a causative role to selenium and vitamin E deficiency in the development of mastitis, metritis, placental retention, cystic ovaries and impaired reproductive performance in dairy cattle, and in immunosuppression in calves.

In addition to structural changes in the various myopathies, chemical changes may be detected in muscle tissue, blood, and urine. Concentrations of muscle creatine are generally decreased, with increased calcium and sodium and decreased potassium. Serum from myopathic animals has decreased levels of selenium and glutathione peroxidase and increased levels of lactic dehydrogenase, AST, and CK. The urine frequently has an increased creatine to creatinine ratio as a result of increased creatine excretion.

For discussion of equine polysaccharide storage myopathy, *see* CHRONIC EXERTIONAL RHABDOMYOLYSIS, p 952.

NUTRITIONAL MYOPATHY OF CALVES AND LAMBS
(White muscle disease, Stiff lamb disease, Enzootic muscular dystrophy)

A myodegeneration frequently develops in calves and lambs of dams that received selenium-deficient feed during or before gestation. Legume forages grown in certain areas where selenium is either deficient or unavailable in the soil seem to be particularly involved and appear to be less effective in taking up selenium from the soil than are grasses. When the diet is restricted to such feeds, as in range cattle or sheep production, the cows and ewes may receive inadequate selenium. This condition has been recorded in many countries and has been produced experimentally in several species by restricting intake of selenium and vitamin E. A similar myopathy is seen naturally in yearling and young adult cattle, goats, deer, foals, adult horses, dogs, rabbits, poultry, fish, and various laboratory and wild animals.

Etiology: Some myopathies (especially in herbivores) and some of the related conditions listed above have been attributed to a deficiency of vitamin E, which may be caused by large amounts of unsaturated fatty acids and other peroxide-forming substances in the diet. For example, continuous supplementation with cod liver oil has induced cases of vitamin E deficiency. White muscle disease in pastured cattle after spring turnout has been attributed to absorption of the portion of polyunsaturated fatty acids in lush grasses that escapes ruminal hydrogenation. In many cases of nutritional myopathy, selenium deficiency is present. This may be a simple deficiency caused by animals eating forage grown on selenium-deficient soils, or it may be precipitated by antagonistic effects of various metals (eg, silver, copper, cobalt, cadmium, mercury, tin). High dietary intake of phosphorus has enhanced the severity of the disease and resulted in decreased hepatic selenium content in sheep. Application of sulfur to pasture soils, as elemental sulfur or gypsum, may interfere with uptake of selenium by forage plants and precipitate the disease in grazing ruminants.

Some myopathies and related conditions respond only to selenium, some only to vitamin E, others to either. While vitamin E cannot completely satisfy the need for selenium, it can reduce the amount required to protect against exudative diathesis. The converse is also true. A vitamin E deficiency in chicks (p 2329) apparently leads to development of encephalomalacia and muscular dystrophy even in the presence of selenium sufficient to protect against exudative diathesis (on a low-methionine, low-cystine diet). Similarly, selenium cannot replace vitamin E to prevent the sterility and myopathy in some experimental animals (rabbits) or encephalomalacia in chicks produced by diets deficient in vitamin E. Conversely, a naturally occurring infertility in ewes, apparently related to fetal deaths and sometimes associated with a high incidence of white muscle disease in lambs receiving adequate vitamin E, responds remarkably to minute supplements of selenium, as does alopecia in rats and primates. The hepatic necrosis seen in rats and pigs appears to respond to either nutrient.

Clinical Findings: The congenital type of white muscle disease may result in sudden death within 2-3 days of birth, usually with involvement of the myocardium. The delayed type is associated with cardiac or skeletal muscle involvement and may be precipitated by vigorous exercise. Affected animals may move stiffly with an arched back and frequently become recumbent. If the condition is severe enough to prevent nursing, either from dysfunction of the muscles of the legs or the tongue, death may result from starvation. Sometimes, there is profuse diarrhea. In chronic cases, there may be relaxation of the shoulder girdle and splaying of the toes. In progressive cardiac failure, dyspnea results. Signs vary with dietary selenium status; in some areas, general unthriftiness may be the only sign associated with selenium deficiency.

Lesions: Generally, skeletal muscle lesions are bilaterally symmetric and may affect one or more muscle groups. Grossly, the affected muscle is pale and dry. It usually shows distinct longitudinal striations or a pronounced chalky whiteness due to abnormal calcium deposition, but sometimes the involvement may be diffuse. Cardiac lesions are well-defined subendocardial plaques that often are more pronounced in the right ventricle in lambs and in the left ventricle in calves. Microscopically, evidence has been established for sequential changes in damaged muscle progressing from mitochondrial swelling and myofibrillar lysis to either hyaline or granular necrosis. When the heart is involved, cardiac muscle cells and Purkinje fibers may be damaged. Pleural, pericardial, and peritoneal effusions with pulmonary congestion and edema are not uncommon.

Diagnosis: In lambs, outbreaks of infectious, nonsuppurative arthritis result in a clinical syndrome similar to that of white muscle disease, and sudden deaths from heart failure might be confused with enterotoxemia. The history and necropsy findings, however, are usually characteristic. In mild cases and in very young lambs, laboratory studies such as histologic examination and levels of glutathione peroxidase, AST, and CK may be necessary.

In calves, the typical syndrome and lesions are reasonably definitive. In mild cases—and particularly in older animals—diagnosis can be difficult, and laboratory studies (as with lambs) may be necessary.

Prevention: To prevent white muscle disease within 4 wk after birth, ewes are given 5 mg and cows 15 mg of selenium, PO or SC, usually as sodium selenite 4 wk before expected parturition. To prevent the delayed type, lambs are given 0.5 mg and calves 5 mg of selenium at 2-4 wk of age and twice more at monthly intervals. A selenium and vitamin E mixture is advocated in some areas. Other procedures for selenium supplementation include administration of intraruminal selenium pellets, use of selenium-fortified salt or mineral mixtures, SC implantation of selenium pellets, or soil application of selenium at 4 g/acre (10 g/hectare) in fertilizer.

Adding selenium to feed for breeding animals or their young is useful in areas of known deficiency. The recommended supplemental level is 0.3 ppm selenium, calculated on the basis of total dry-matter intake. It is added as sodium selenite, which contains 45.65% selenium. Because of the minute quantities involved and the toxicity of excess intake, premixing and thorough subsequent mixing is necessary. In some countries, including the USA, addition of selenium to feeds is controlled by law, and appropriate authorities should be consulted; in all areas, caution in the use of selenium is indicated.

Treatment: Lambs and calves may be given sodium selenite and vitamin E in sterile emulsion, SC or IM, at 1 mg selenium and 50 mg (68 IU) of vitamin E per 18 kg (40 lb) body wt. This may be repeated after 2 wk, but no more than 4 doses should be given. Larger dosages are sometimes advocated, but caution is advised because they approach the toxic level. In practice, several products are available for use with designated animal species. When simple vitamin E deficiency is apparent, dietary supplementation with α-tocopherol or substances rich in vitamin E should be instituted. Minimum dosages have not been established. However, cures have been reported after daily doses of 5 mg of α-tocopherol to rabbits; 500 mg initially, followed by 100 mg on alternate days to lambs; and 600 mg initially, followed by daily doses of 200 mg to calves. When the causative diet contains substances antagonistic to vitamin E, such as unprotected, polyunsaturated fats, these must be removed or stabilized by addition of an appropriate antioxidant. Dry concentrates of vitamins A and D may substitute for cod-liver oil, thus removing a potential source of oxidative damage.

NUTRITIONAL MYOPATHY OF PIGS
(Hepatosis dietetica, Mulberry heart disease)

There are several specific diseases of pigs in which muscle degeneration may be extensive (eg, mulberry heart disease) and others in which the degeneration is frequently less conspicuous (eg, hepatosis dietetica). Yellow fat disease (p 968) may be seen with accompanying myopathy.

Etiology: Mulberry heart disease and hepatosis dietetica are associated with diets low in selenium or vitamin E. Administration of iron dextran to piglets having low vitamin E status may precipitate a severe myopathy (p 2403) with lesions identical to those of selenium or vitamin E deficiency. Other factors that may increase the selenium requirement include diets with low concentrations of protein (especially sulfur-containing amino acids), diets with an excess of selenium antagonistic compounds, and possibly genetic influences on selenium metabolism. Vitamin E may be less available in diets with high concentrations of polyunsaturated fatty acids, vitamin A, or mycotoxins.

Clinical Findings: These conditions have certain characteristics in common. Losses tend to occur sporadically, and rapidly growing pigs 2-16 wk old are affected. Death almost invariably occurs suddenly and is often precipitated by exercise.

Lesions: In mulberry heart disease, the characteristic lesions are a pericardial sac grossly distended with straw-colored fluid that contains fibrin strands, and extensive hemorrhage throughout the epicardium and myocardium. Microscopically, the heart shows both vascular and myocyte lesions; in addition to interstitial hemorrhage, there is usually extensive myocardial necrosis together with fibrin thrombi in capillaries. If pigs survive for a few days, nervous signs may be seen as a result of focal encephalomalacia.

In hepatosis dietetica, there is often subcutaneous edema and varying amounts of transudate in serous cavities. Fibrin strands adhere to the liver, which has a characteristic mottled appearance caused by irregular foci of parenchymal necrosis and hemorrhage. Acute lesions may appear as scattered, red, swollen lobules and edema of the gallbladder wall. Focal lesions of myocardial necrosis and, less frequently, skeletal myonecrosis may be apparent.

Many pigs that die with selenium or vitamin E deficiency have esophagogastric ulceration or preulcerative changes.

Diagnosis: The history and gross necropsy findings may be distinctive, but histology to demonstrate specific cardiac and skeletal muscle lesions may be necessary. Differential diagnoses for mulberry heart disease include acute septicemic diseases (eg, salmonellosis, erysipelas, and streptococcosis), pericarditis, polyserositis, and edema disease. For hepatosis dietetica, pitch poisoning and gossypol toxicosis should also be considered, as should porcine stress syndrome for pigs with prominent skeletal muscle lesions. Cases of selenium or vitamin E deficiency in pigs can be identified, as in other species, by decreased levels of selenium, vitamin E, and glutathione peroxidase in the serum and tissues and by increased levels of CK and AST in the serum.

Prevention and Treatment: Rations may be supplemented with selenium or vitamin E, or both (as for ruminants). Affected pigs and their herdmates may be given injections of selenium/vitamin E to increase tissue levels rapidly. Injection of sows in late gestation increases tissue levels in newborn piglets.

NUTRITIONAL MYOPATHY OF EQUIDS

Myodegeneration, associated with selenium or vitamin E deficiency, can be seen in adult horses, donkeys, and mules. The disease in adult equids may manifest in the acute form by sudden unexpected death or in the subacute form by staggering gait, myoglobinuria, dysphagia with swelling of the masseter and lingual muscles, dyspnea, and tachycardia. Lesions involve the skeletal muscles and myocardium. Diagnosis and treatment are as for ruminants (p 948) and pigs (p 950). In foals, a myopathy that appears similar to the vitamin E/selenium-responsive disorders of other species may be seen at birth or shortly thereafter and may be accompanied by steatitis or "yellow fat" (p 968). Stiffness and pain on palpation of subcutaneous fat masses are noticeable, and severely affected foals may be unable to suckle. Selenium and glutathione peroxidase levels in affected foals may be no different than in healthy ones. Treatment with vitamin E appears more effective than with selenium.

EXERTIONAL MYOPATHIES
EXERTIONAL MYOPATHIES IN HORSES

Exertional myopathies in horses are a syndrome of muscle fatigue, pain, or cramping associated with exercise. Most exercise-associated myopathies result in necrosis of striated skeletal muscle and are therefore termed exertional rhabdomyolysis. Although exertional rhabdomyolysis was previously considered a single disease described as azoturia, tying-up, or cording up, it is now known to comprise several different myopathies, which, despite similarities in clinical presentation, differ significantly in etiopathology.

Clinical signs usually are seen shortly after the onset of exercise. Excessive sweating, tachypnea, tachycardia, muscle fasciculations reluctance or refusal to move, and firm, painful lumbar and gluteal musculature are common signs. Episodes range from subclinical to severe episodes of muscle necrosis with recumbency and myoglobinuric renal failure. The severity varies extensively between individuals and to some degree within the same individual. A diagnosis of exertional rhabdomyolysis is based on demonstration of abnormal elevations in serum CK, lactate dehydrogenase, and AST.

Differential diagnoses for reluctance to move, acute recumbency, and discolored urine include lameness, colic, laminitis, fracture, pleuropneumonia, tetanus, aortoiliac thrombosis, neurologic diseases resulting in recumbency or reluctance to move, intravascular hemolysis, and bilirubinuria. Causes of non-exercise-associated rhabdomyolysis include infectious and immune-mediated myopathies (eg, *Clostridium* sp, influenza, *Streptococcus equi*, *Sarcocystis*), nutritional myodegeneration (vitamin E or selenium deficiency), traumatic or compressive myopathy, idiopathic pasture myopathy, and toxic muscle damage from the ingestion of ionophores (eg, monensin, lasalocid, rumensin). Plants, including white snake root and vitamin D-stimulating species, should also be considered (TABLE 1).

Exertional rhabdomyolysis can be either sporadic, with single or very infrequent episodes of muscle necrosis with exercise, or chronic, with repeated episodes of rhabdomyolysis and increased muscle enzyme activity, often with mild exertion. All breeds of horses are susceptible to sporadic exertional rhabdomyolysis.

Sporadic Exertional Rhabdomyolysis

The most common cause of sporadic tying-up is exercise that exceeds the horse's underlying state of training. The incidence of muscle stiffness also has increased during an outbreak of respiratory disease. Deficiencies of sodium, calcium, vitamin E, or selenium in the diet may also be contributory factors.

A diagnosis of sporadic exertional rhabdomyolysis is made on the basis of a horse with no previous history of exertional rhabdomyolysis, signs of muscle cramping and stiffness following exercise, and moderate to marked elevations in serum CK and AST. Immediately on detection of signs of exertional rhabdomyolysis, exercise should cease and the horse should be moved to a well-bedded stall with access to fresh water. The objectives of treatment are to relieve anxiety and muscle pain, as well as to correct fluid and acid-base deficits. Tranquilizers, opioids, or NSAID may be given. Most horses are relatively pain free within 18-24 hr.

Severe rhabdomyolysis can lead to renal compromise due to ischemia and the combined nephrotoxic effects of myoglobinuria, dehydration, and NSAID therapy. The first priority in horses with hemoconcentration or myoglobinuria is to reestablish fluid balance and induce diuresis. In severely affected animals, regular monitoring of BUN and/or serum creatinine is advised to assess the extent of renal damage. Diuretics are contraindicated in the absence of IV fluid therapy and are indicated if the horse is in oliguric renal failure.

Horses should be stall rested on a hay diet for a few days. For horses with sporadic forms of tying-up, rest with regular access to a paddock should continue until serum muscle enzyme concentrations are normal. Because the inciting cause is usually temporary, most horses respond to rest, a gradual increase in training, and dietary adjustment. Endurance horses should be encouraged to drink electrolyte-supplemented water during an endurance ride and monitored particularly closely during hot, humid conditions.

Chronic Exertional Rhabdomyolysis

Some horses have recurrent episodes of rhabdomyolysis, even with light exercise. Two forms of chronic tying-up have been identified using muscle biopsies—polysaccharide storage myopathy (PSSM) and recurrent exertional rhabdomyolysis.

Polysaccharide storage myopathy is seen frequently in Quarter Horse-related breeds, Warmbloods, and draft horses. It is an inherited muscle disorder in Quarter Horse-related breeds. Light-breed horses with PSSM often develop episodes of rhabdomyolysis at a young age with little exercise. Rest for a few days prior to exercise is a common triggering factor. Episodes are characterized by a tucked-up abdomen, a camped-out stance, muscle fasciculations, sweating, gait asymmetry, hindlimb stiffness, and reluctance to move. Some horses paw or roll resembling colic. Serum CK and AST are increased during an episode (usually >10,000 U/L) and, unlike in other forms of rhabdomyolysis, subclinical episodes characterized by persistently abnormal CK are common. Clinical signs in draft horses may include loss of muscle mass, difficulty standing with one hindleg raised, difficulty backing without shaking a hindlimb, progressive weakness, and recumbency. CK and AST may be normal in draft horses with this syndrome.

Recurrent exertional rhabdomyolysis is seen frequently in Thoroughbreds, Standardbreds, and Arabian horses. It is likely due to abnormal regulation of intracellular calcium in skeletal muscles. It appears there is intermittent disruption of muscle contraction, particularly when horses susceptible to the condition are fit and have a nervous temperament. In Thoroughbreds, it is likely inherited as an autosomal dominant trait.

TABLE 1. Differential Diagnoses of Equine Myopathies

Non-exercise-associated Rhabdomyolysis

Inflammatory myopathies
  Clostridial myositis
  Influenza myositis
  Sarcocystis myositis
  Immune-mediated myopathy
Nutritional myopathy
  Vitamin E and selenium deficiency
Toxic myopathy
  Ionophore toxicity
  Pasture myopathies
    Rayless goldenrod/white snakeroot
    Cassia occidentalis
  Atypical myoglobinuria
Traumatic myopathy
  Compressive anesthetic myopathy
  Trauma
Metabolic myopathy
  Glycogen branching enzyme deficiency in Quarter Horses

Exertional Rhabdomyolysis

Focal muscle strain
Sporadic tying-up (overexertion)
Chronic tying-up
  Dietary imbalances, vitamins, minerals, electrolytes
  Polysaccharide storage myopathy (biopsy diagnosis)
  Recurrent exertional rhabdomyolysis (biopsy diagnosis)
  Idiopathic chronic exertional rhabdomyolysis

Exertional Myopathy with Normal CK

Mitochondrial myopathy

Muscle Atrophy

Myogenic atrophy
  Severe rhabdomyolysis
  Disuse
  Cushing's disease
  Immune-mediated myositis (rapid atrophy)
Neurogenic atrophy
  Equine protozoal myelitis
  Local nerve trauma
  Equine motor neuron disease

Muscle Fasciculations

Pain, fear
Electrolyte abnormalities
Equine motor neuron disease
Hyperkalemic periodic paralysis
Hypokalemia
Otobius megnini (ear tick) infestation
Myotonic dystrophy
Stiff horse syndrome

Diagnostic tests to determine the cause of chronic tying-up include a CBC, serum chemistry panel, blood vitamin E and selenium concentrations, urinalysis to determine electrolyte balance, dietary analysis, exercise testing, and muscle biopsy. An exercise challenge test is useful to detect subclinical cases. In addition, quantifying the extent of exertional rhabdomyolysis during mild exercise is helpful in deciding how rapidly to reinstate training.

A diagnosis of PSSM is based on the presence of muscle fibers with subsarcolemmal vacuoles, dark periodic acid-Schiff (PAS) staining for glycogen, and most notably, amylase-resistant abnormal complex polysaccharide accumulation. Diagnosis of recurrent exertional rhabdomyolysis is based on history, clinical signs, elevations in serum CK and AST, and muscle biopsy.

Quarter Horses with PSSM have enhanced sensitivity to insulin, resulting in high muscle glycogen concentrations. When fed a starch meal, these horses store a higher proportion of the absorbed glucose in their muscles compared with healthy horses. Thus, the ideal diet for PSSM is based on feeding forage at a rate of 1.5-2% of body weight, providing >15% of digestible energy as fat and limiting starch to <10% of daily digestible energy by limiting grain or replacing it with a fat supplement. Caloric needs should be assessed first to prevent horses becoming obese on a high-fat diet. Improvement in signs of exertional rhabdomyolysis for horses with PSSM requires both dietary changes and gradual increases in the amount of daily exercise and turn-out.

Management of recurrent exertional rhabdomyolysis is aimed at decreasing the triggering factors for excitement and pharmacologic alteration of intracellular calcium flux with contraction. Management changes that may decrease excitement include minimizing stall confinement by using turn-out or a hot walker, exercising and feeding horses with recurrent exertional rhabdomyolysis before other horses, providing compatible equine company, and the judicious use of low-dose tranquilizers during training. A high-fat, low-starch diet is beneficial, possibly by decreasing excitement. In contrast to PSSM, horses that have recurrent exertional rhabdomyolysis often require higher caloric intakes (>24 Mcal/day). At these high caloric intakes, specialized feeds designed for exertional rhabdomyolysis are necessary, as additional vegetable oil or rice bran cannot supply enough calories for athletes in intense training. Hay should be fed at 1.5-2% of body weight and high-fat, low-starch concentrates should be selected that provide ≤20% of daily digestible energy as nonstructural carbohydrate and 20-25% of digestible energy as fat.

Dantrolene (4 mg/kg, PO) given 1 hr before exercise to horses that are not fed prior to exercise may decrease the release of calcium from the calcium release channel. Phenytoin (1.4-2.7 mg/kg, PO, BID), has also been advocated as a treatment for horses with recurrent exertional rhabdomyolysis. Therapeutic levels vary, so oral dosages are adjusted by monitoring serum levels to achieve between 8 µg/mL and 12 µg/mL. Longterm treatment with dantrolene or phenytoin is expensive, however.

Hyperkalemic Periodic Paralysis

Hyperkalemic periodic paralysis (HyPP) is an autosomal dominant trait affecting Quarter Horses, American Paint horses, Appaloosas, and Quarter Horse crossbreeds worldwide. A point mutation that results in a phenylalanine/leucine substitution in the voltage-dependent skeletal muscle sodium channel a subunit is responsible. The prevalence in Quarter Horses is ~4%.

Clinical signs range from asymptomatic to intermittent muscle fasciculations and weakness and are first identified from foals to 3 yr of age. Homozygous horses are often more severely affected and may be identified at a younger age than heterozygotes. A brief period of myotonia is often observed initially, with some horses showing prolapse of the third eyelid. Muscle fasciculations beginning on the flanks, neck, and shoulders may become more generalized. While most horses remain standing during mild attacks, weakness with swaying, staggering, dogsitting, or recumbency may be seen, with severe attacks lasting 15-60 min or longer. Heart and respiratory rates may be elevated, but horses remain relatively bright and alert. Respiratory distress occurs in some horses as a result of upper respiratory muscle paralysis. Once episodes subside, horses regain their feet and appear normal with absent or minimal gait abnormalities. Young horses that are homozygous for the HyPP trait may have respiratory stridor and periodic obstruction of the upper respiratory tract.

Common factors that trigger episodes include sudden dietary changes or ingestion of diets high in potassium (>1.1%), such as those containing alfalfa hay, molasses, electrolyte supplements, and kelp-based supplements. Fasting, anesthesia or heavy sedation, trailer rides, and stress may also precipitate clinical signs. The onset of signs, however, is often unpredictable. Exercise per se does not appear to stimulate clinical signs; serum CK shows no or minimal increases during episodic fasciculations and weakness.

Descent from the stallion Impressive in a horse with episodic muscle tremors is strongly suggestive of HyPP. Hyperkalemia (6-9 mEq/L), hemoconcentration, and hyponatremia are seen during clinical episodes, but a definitive diagnosis requires DNA testing of mane or tail hair. Electromyographic examination of affected horses between attacks reveals abnormal fibrillation potentials and complex repetitive discharges, with occasional myotonic potentials and trains of doublets between episodes. Differential diagnoses for hyperkalemia include delay before serum centrifugation, hemolysis, chronic renal failure, and severe rhabdomyolysis.

Many horses recover spontaneously from HyPP episodes. Owners may abort early mild episodes using low-grade exercise or feeding grain or corn syrup to stimulate insulin-mediated movement of potassium across cell membranes. In severe cases, administration of calcium gluconate (0.2-0.4 mL/kg of a 23% solution diluted in 1 L of 5% dextrose) or IV dextrose (6 mL/kg of a 5% solution), alone or combined with sodium bicarbonate (1-2 mEq/kg), often provides immediate improvement. With severe respiratory obstruction, a tracheostomy may be necessary. Acute death is common, especially in homozygous animals.

Prevention requires decreasing dietary potassium to 0.6-1.1% total potassium concentration and increasing renal losses of potassium. High-potassium feeds such as alfalfa hay, brome hay, canola oil, soybean meal or oil, sugar molasses, and beet molasses should be avoided. Optimally, later cuts of timothy or bermuda grass hay; grains such as oats, corn, wheat, and barley; and beet pulp should be fed in small meals several times a day. Regular exercise and/or frequent access to a large paddock or yard are also beneficial. Pasture is ideal for horses with HyPP because the high water content of pasture grass makes it unlikely that horses will consume large amounts of potassium in a short period of time. Complete feeds for horses with HyPP are commercially available. For horses with recurrent episodes even with dietary alterations, acetazolamide (2-4 mg/kg, PO, BID-TID) or hydrochlorothiazide (0.5-1 mg/kg, PO, BID) may be helpful. Breed registries and other associations have restrictions on the use of these drugs during competitions.

CAPTURE MYOPATHY OF WILD ANIMALS

This syndrome often develops after restraint of wild animals. Affected animals may die acutely from lactic acidosis or may live several days and show muscular stiffness or become recumbent. Severe skeletal muscle lesions with myocardial necrosis and myoglobinuric nephrosis may be present. Careful handling and reduction of stress are useful; IV fluids and sodium bicarbonate may help. If the animals are from areas considered to be deficient in selenium, the condition may be an exercise-induced myopathy that is responsive to selenium or vitamin E. (*See also* FATIGUE AND EXERCISE, p 817.)

TOXIC MYOPATHIES

IONOPHORE TOXICITY

Monensin, lasalocid, salinomycin, maduramicin, and narasin may cause myopathy. Horses are highly susceptible, and toxicity has also been reported in cattle, sheep, pigs, dogs, chickens, turkeys, and guinea fowl. Toxicity generally results from exposure to undiluted premixes or from mixing errors. Toxicosis may be potentiated by various antibiotics and sulfonamides incorporated into feeds in combination with ionophores. Affected horses and cattle may develop anorexia, cardiac failure with tachycardia, dyspnea, diarrhea, stiffness, muscular weakness, recumbency, and myoglobinuria. At necropsy, pale areas of myocardial necrosis and pulmonary congestion are usually prominent in horses and cattle. Pigs and sheep tend to have mainly skeletal muscle lesions that appear quite similar grossly and histologically to those of nutritional myopathy. Diagnosis requires history of exposure with development of characteristic clinical and pathologic alterations.

PLANT INTOXICATION

Degeneration of skeletal and cardiac muscles results when cattle and some other animals, notably goats, consume the fruit or beans of certain plants. *Karwinskia humboldtiana* (coyotillo) and *Cassia* spp (sennas) have been incriminated, but other species also may cause similar damage. Affected animals show weakness and gait abnormalities, and there is pallor of severely degenerated muscles in severely affected animals with recumbency. Microscopic lesions consist of hyaline necrosis and granular degeneration. Some serum enzymes are increased, and myoglobinuria may be seen. Treatment consists of supplemental feeding and removal of animals from offending range.

Pigs fed excessive amounts of cottonseed meal develop gossypol toxicosis with lesions in skeletal muscle, myocardium, liver, and lungs. (*See* GOSSYPOL POISONING, p 2365.)

CIRCULATORY DISTURBANCES

ISCHEMIC MYOPATHY

Thrombosis of the iliac artery in horses results in extensive ischemic necrosis of the musculature of the hindlimb. In cattle, massive necrosis of the thigh muscle may be present in downer cows (p 957) and probably is due to the effects of both ischemia and physical trauma associated with prolonged recumbency and abortive attempts to rise.

POSTANESTHETIC MYOPATHY (MYONEUROPATHY) IN HORSES

Complications of general anesthesia in horses may cause muscle lesions due to regional ischemia from arterial hypotension induced by gas anesthesia. This syndrome may be seen as a localized form in muscle groups in contact with the surgery table or as a generalized form with features similar to those of azoturia.

MISCELLANEOUS MYOPATHIES AND MYOSITIDES

EOSINOPHILIC MYOSITIS IN CATTLE AND SHEEP

This focal myonecrosis is associated with large numbers of eosinophilic granulocytes. Sudden deaths in cattle and sheep may involve concurrent myocarditis. The cause is unknown in some instances, but the presence of degenerate *Sarcocystis* spp (p 974) in the center of some of the necrotic lesions suggests that they may be implicated. This condition is seen at slaughter as focal, greenish gray discolorations in skeletal and, occasionally, cardiac musculature that fade when exposed to air.

OTHER GENERALIZED DISEASES WITH MYOSITIS

Various clostridial diseases and parasitic diseases have prominent skeletal muscle lesions. *See* CLOSTRIDIAL DISEASES, p 486; SARCOCYSTOSIS, p 974; TRICHINELLOSIS, p 589; and CYSTICERCOSIS, p 1035.

FIBROTIC AND OSSIFYING MYOPATHY IN QUARTER HORSES

This uncommon condition is seen chiefly in working Quarter Horses as a result of trauma to the semimembranosus, semitendinosus, and gracilis muscles. Usually, it is unilateral and involves a progressive fibrosis with local adhesions of the affected muscles, which eventually ossify. The gait is fairly characteristic; the forward phase of the stride is jerky, and the foot is jerked back a short distance before being placed on the ground. The action is appreciably different from that of stringhalt (p 925) and upward patellar fixation. The hardening of the muscles can be palpated in some cases. Radiography and ultrasonography help to establish the degree of involvement. Treatment involves surgery to excise the fibrotic lesion or to incise the medial ligament of the semitendinosus at the stifle.

IMMUNE-MEDIATED MYOSITIS

Hemorrhagic necrosis of skeletal muscle accompanied by vascular injury may be an immune-mediated sequela of equine respiratory diseases associated with *Streptococus equi*. (*See* DISEASES INVOLVING IMMUNE COMPLEXES, p 654.)

MYOTONIA IN GOATS

See **myotonia congenita** under LARGE ANIMALS, p 1003.

MYOSITIS OSSIFICANS

(Fibrodysplasia ossificans progressiva)

Ossification of muscle represents heterotopic bone formation in muscle and may follow trauma. A generalized form of the condition of suspected heritability has been described in pigs. (*See also* p 969.)

PROBLEMATIC BOVINE RECUMBENCY

(Downer cow)

The term "downer cow" is frequently applied to a mature dairy cow that is still recumbent 3 hr after calving despite treatment for hypocalcemia (*see* PARTURIENT PARESIS IN COWS, p 806). A second type of involuntary sternal recumbency is encountered less commonly in cattle of any age under conditions not associated with parturition and for which the most likely etiology is trauma. Downer cows that are able to actively crawl are often referred to as "creepers" and are considered to have a more favorable prognosis than inactive animals. The cause of the recumbency is, more often than not, elusive even to an experienced clinician. Furthermore, inexperienced clinicians may miss an obvious cause if they do not adopt a systematic approach to diagnosis.

Vigorous intervention is most likely to be successful within 12 hr of initial recumbency. After 12 hr, some musculoskeletal changes may become irreversible. While some downer cows will rise after >14 days of recumbency, this is the exception. The cow should be thoroughly evaluated at the first visit and a routine protocol of activities performed within the first 12 hr.

Etiology, Clinical Findings, and Diagnosis: A routine evaluation of the clinical signs of recumbent cows should be conducted. The following steps help identify possible etiologic factors.

Assessment of Demeanor, Type of Recumbency, and Animal Environment: The cow may be found in lateral recumbency, which may indicate an unresolved metabolic problem such as hypocalcemia, a psychosomatic problem, or simply ignorance on the part of the dairyman regarding the importance of maintaining sternal recumbency. Signs that the cow has been thrashing with the hind limbs may indicate hypomagnesemia or tetanus. Although rare in cattle, tetanus is often associated with parturition. Inquiries into the severity and duration of parturition may suggest that the recumbency is at least partially due to exhaustion. In involuntary sternal recumbency, some cows may have a dull, listless appearance. This may indicate hypocalcemia in periparturient mature cows. The second most likely cause of depression is toxemia, the cause of which is most commonly found in the genital tract or mammary gland. Other cows found in involuntary sternal recumbency may be bright and alert in appearance—the most typical demeanor of the true problem downer cow. If the animal is young or not pregnant, the cause is likely to be either physical damage or from a rare condition, either of which requires careful, detailed examination.

The environment of the animal can have a bearing on the etiology. If the footing is slippery, physical damage to the musculoskeletal system should be suspected. This is much less likely among cows in open space with a dirt or well-bedded surface. A psychosomatic component should be suspected if there is evidence that the cow has been struggling to rise and/or is showing signs of exhaustion. The probability of a psychosomatic cause is higher if the bedding is dry, slippery straw or if the cow is found with her head in a corner.

The positioning of the hindlimbs may indicate the cause of the recumbency. Limbs splayed out behind the animal may indicate obturator paralysis. Sometimes the upper limb is extended sideways in such a manner that a crease is formed in the skin. This sign is most suggestive of rupture of the adductor muscles and may occur when the cow struggles to rise on a slippery surface.

Recumbency of animals, particularly Brown Swiss cattle <2 yr of age, may be caused by the weaver syndrome (*see* p 999).

Physical Examination: A routine examination should be performed when the cow is first presented. Covert factors such as shock, toxemia, dehydration, or fever may be difficult to assess. The rectal temperature should be within the normal range. If it is lower than normal, some level of shock might be present. The persistence of a skin fold for >6 sec indicates dehydration. Pallor of the mucous membranes suggests toxemia, in which case a weak pulse and tachycardia may be present. The respiration of a recumbent cow may be labored by virtue of the pressure of the abdominal contents on the diaphragm. This quality of respiration should not be confused with a more advanced stage of hypostasis and pulmonary congestion with edema. In these cases, pulse and heart rates may be elevated, and the nasal mucosa bright red or cyanotic. Early pneumonia or anaphylaxis might be suspected.

Special Examinations: **Vaginal exploration** is mandatory in every peripartum, recumbent cow and may lead to discovery of a decomposing second fetus. Damage to and infection of the wall of the vagina is common. Metritis and an associated toxemia can contribute to postpartum recumbency.

Rectal exploration is essential for differential diagnosis. The degree of uterine involution should be appropriate to the number of days postpartum. Ballottement of fluid in the organ or lack of tonicity should be noted. Unexpected anomalies may be palpated. Adhesions, lumps of necrotic fat, and enlargement or turgidity of the cervix or vaginal wall are all sequelae of a difficult birth. Fracture of the pelvis may be palpated per rectum, particularly if an assistant manipulates the limb. Traumatic injuries to the pelvis occur as the result of an animal slipping on concrete or icy surfaces. This can occur when cows ride one another during estrus. Movement of the head of the femur in the obturator foramen may also be detected. Upward dislocation of the hip or fracture of the femoral neck can be confirmed if the affected limb appears shorter than the contralateral limb. To confirm that the contralateral limb is not injured, rolling the cow over to expose the limb on which she has been lying should be done to accommodate a repeat examination. Pelvic fractures can be associated with sciatic nerve paralysis, while upward hip dislocation may be associated with some degree of obturator paralysis. If either condition is suspected, the sensory state of the limbs should be evaluated. Involuntary sternal recumbency may be associated with vertebral lymphosarcoma, abscesses, or bizarre traumatic injuries.

Mammary gland examination should always be performed on recumbent cows. A toxic infection of the udder with an organism such as *Escherichia coli* can be a primary cause of recumbency. However, such an infection may be precipitated by the recumbency, especially if the udder is engorged and remains unmilked.

Blood samples are not usually taken when treating routine cases of hypocalcemia. However, the biochemical status of a cow unresponsive to calcium therapy should always be evaluated. Plasma mineral levels may be inconsistent. Some cows persistently have lower than normal levels. Hypokalemia and hypophosphatemia are commonly quoted causes of creeper cows. True downer cows may show normal plasma mineral levels. Elevated CK is a specific indicator of muscle damage. However, CK levels peak shortly after the start of muscle damage and decline noticeably within 4 hr. CK levels should be monitored at every visit. Plasma AST is also elevated in muscle-damaged cows. However, AST is also elevated when cardiac muscle is damaged. In muscle-damaged cows, the urine may contain myoglobin as well as higher than normal levels of protein. Ketonuria and bilirubinuria may be detected but are associated with lowered feed intake. Serum glutamic oxaloacetic acid levels are usually markedly elevated 18-24 hr after the onset of recumbency.

Lesions: Traumatic injuries to nerves are found in 25% of downer cows. Damage to intrapelvic nerves such as the sciatic and obturator account for most cases. However, evidence of decubital injuries to the lateral aspect of the stifle can be associated with damage to the peroneal nerve. Ischemic necrosis of the adductor muscles is a common finding. Hemorrhage and rupture of these muscles may be seen if the animal "spread-eagled" itself while struggling to rise on a wet or icy concrete surface.

Treatment: Downer cows are often hypocalcemic. If an apparently hypocalcemic cow does not respond to calcium therapy, phosphorus, magnesium, and potassium should be given as additional treatments pending the results of laboratory tests. Monitoring the blood mineral status is an important part of downer cow management.

In most cases, recovery depends on the quality of recumbency management and nursing care. Lateral recumbency must be corrected immediately to avoid regurgitation and inspiration of stomach contents. The animal should be rolled into sternal recumbency. However, if this posture is to be maintained, the limb on which the animal has been lying should be drawn from under the body. In other words, if the animal was presented in lateral recumbency on its left side, it should be rolled into sternal recumbency on its right side. Support (eg, straw bale) placed under the shoulder may be required for some animals to maintain sternal recumbency.

Attempting to stabilize a recumbent cow on a concrete surface is highly undesirable but sometimes unavoidable. Bedding the area around and under the cow with wet, sticky manure to a depth ≥6 in. is a common practice. At least 10 in. of dry straw should be distributed over the wet mass. If the cow struggles and scrapes the wet manure, exposing concrete, more manure must be added. The so-called manure pack provides good footing but also may soil the skin with urine and manure. Dermatitis can result, and comfort of the cow is reduced. More seriously, the risk of mastitis resulting from the contaminated environment is very high. A bed of sand ≥10 in. deep is more effective. This usually drains well, and good hygiene can be maintained if the manure is removed several times each day.

Hobbling of the cow may be considered to prevent overabduction that can lead to muscular damage. Ropes should never be used for this purpose. A soft nylon strap may be wrapped twice around the middle of each metatarsus, allowing a distance of at least 3 ft between the legs.

Attempts to Cause the Cow to Rise: On every day of the recumbency, an attempt should be made to bring the cow to its feet. Several simple but effective techniques can be tried. In one method, the clinician stands with feet pressed under the cow at a point below the scapulohumeral joint. A sharp blow is delivered by driving the knees into the muscle mass below and caudal to the scapula. This method must not be used on the thoracic wall unprotected by the muscle mass to avoid fracturing the ribs. If the animal struggles to rise, an assistant should grasp the root of the tailhead with both hands and lift. Lifting on any other part of the tail may cause damage. Recently calved cows can be motivated to rise if they hear their own calf bawling with hunger. The calf is best restrained close to the cow but out of her sight. Some workers use electric goads and various anecdotal or traditional methods of inflicting pain to stimulate a cow to rise. These measures have a low success rate in inexperienced hands.

The value of hip clamps is controversial. Their proper use requires experience, skill, and a delicate touch. Continual use causes trauma and pain that is counterproductive. The forelimbs support 60% of a cow's weight and, therefore, the use of a canvas sling under the sternum is almost mandatory for consistent success. A chest band is required to prevent the sling from slipping backwards. If the sling is suspended from the tine at one end of a fork lift, and the hip clamps from a tine at the other end, minimal trauma results. If a fork lift is not available, a T-bar suspended by a pulley from an overhead beam (or a tripod for animals at pasture) will serve. The jaws of the clamps must be well protected with synthetic foam or rubber secured in place with a wrap of duct tape.

Hip clamps should not be applied too tightly and should lift the cow slowly to allow time for the circulation of the limbs to become reestablished. The device is lifted until the hindfeet just touch the ground. Often, the cow will hang with the limbs slightly flexed. This should not be confused with unilateral flexion, which indicates peroneal paralysis. Next, one assistant on each side of the cow presses a shoulder into the paralumbar fossa while facing the hindlimb. The device is slowly lowered as the assistants attempt to force each hindlimb into a weightbearing posture and to reduce the flexion by manipulating the stifle and hock. As soon as any weight is supported by the 2 limbs, the device should be lowered 1-2 in. This process may have to be repeated several times.

Even if the cow does not stand, the lifted position provides an opportunity to manipulate the limbs, auscultate for crepitation, and perform vaginal and rectal examinations.

Moving a Recumbent Cow: The chances of resolution are considerably enhanced by moving the cow to space with an earthen floor. In warm, relatively dry weather, the very best location for a recumbent cow is grassy pasture. Otherwise, the location selected should have a roof and some protection from the elements. These conditions often exist in a hay barn or implement shed.

Moving the cow requires rolling her into lateral recumbency. The cow can then be slid over dry straw for a short distance (~15 ft) by pulling on a rope attached to a lower forelimb and a halter rope. Transportation over longer distances can be accomplished using a suitably prepared farm gate hauled by tractor. The longest dimension of farm gate is closely applied to the back of the cow still in lateral recumbency. A tarpaulin is placed on the gate to protect the cow from contact with the ground. Dry straw is spread on the tarpaulin, and the cow is rolled over onto the makeshift stretcher. The halter should be tied to the gate to minimize struggling, and a sack placed over the eyes to minimize alarm while the cow is being moved. The tail is best tied to the hock of the upper limb. Once moved, the cow should be restored to sternal recumbency. A few cows, particularly if <12 hr postpartum, will rise immediately.

Supportive Care Cows: It is vital that recumbent cows be provided with clean water at all times. A shallow rubber feed bowl prevents spillage. If the cow does not drink, she must be given fluid therapy either by drench or parenterally. Every effort must be made to roll the cow from one side onto the other every 3 hr. If this is not done, the weight of the cow results in ischemia in the muscles of the hindlimb. This pathology precedes various myopathies and may precipitate the compartment syndrome.

Protection from the elements is essential. Rain and wind can reduce body temperature considerably and worsen shock if present. A windbreak of straw bales is vital. Straw bedding should be provided to help insulate the cow from the ground. A recumbent cow does not require a warm environment; however, in a cold environment, an inactive animal can gradually succumb to hypothermia.

The downer cows most difficult to treat are those that do not try to eat. A cow that salivates on its feed will not eat it later. Rather than being offered large amounts of feed, the cow should be tempted with sweet hay. This should be cleared away every 30 min if not accepted. Placing bitter-tasting weeds such as ivy or dandelion in the mouth may provoke salivation and an interest in eating. Lettuce and cabbage leaves are accepted by some cows. In extreme cases, the cow can be drenched with rumen contents. Sometimes drenching with a thin gruel to which powdered ginger and/or gentian has been added can be helpful.

Prevention: All mature dairy cows must be monitored closely during the postpartum period for signs of parturient paresis (p 806). The elapse of several hours from the commencement of clinical signs of milk fever until treatment seems to be the critical issue. The use of television surveillance of recently calved cows may be a prudent measure. Every cow that has been successfully treated for hypocalcemia should, if necessary, be moved to a location with a good footing and remain there for 48 hr.

The recommended size of maternity pens is 12×12 ft or 10×14 ft (3.6×3.6 or 3×4.2 m, respectively). These dimensions are adequate for managing normal parturition, but to reduce the risk of downer cows, the size should be increased by $\geq 50\%$. One side of the pen should consist of a 10 ft gate to facilitate the translocation of downer cows. The floor of the pen should be deeply scored with grooves formed in a diamond-shaped pattern 2 in. wide and $^{1}/_{2}$ in. deep. Carborundum or aluminum oxide chips should be troweled into the surface. A 5% slope should be provided in the direction of the gate. If the floor cannot be custom prepared, the use of a sand base should be considered. Straw over sand provides good insulation and good footing.

Animal Welfare Considerations: Although as stated above, a cow may rise after being recumbent for ≥14 days, this does not imply that a cow should be left for this period. So long as the cow looks bright, occasionally struggles to rise, and continues to eat and drink, recovery is a possibility. However, if the cow becomes listless, shows no interest in feed, or has decubital lesions or starts to lose condition, slaughter on humane grounds must be considered irrespective of how long she has been recumbent. A cow that has decubital lesions or shows signs of wasting is unsuitable for salvage slaughter. Attempting to send animals in this condition to the slaughterhouse may be interpreted as an act of cruelty in some countries.

In some countries "dragging" animals may be illegal. Both veterinarians and clients must be aware of the legal interpretation of the word dragging. Access to some locations may be so restricted that rolling the animal onto an improvised sled may be impossible. At all times, even when using a sled, great care must be taken to avoid injury to dependent parts of the animal such as the udder, ears, and tail. Blindfolding may also be required for some excitable animals.

LAMENESS IN SMALL ANIMALS

Signs of musculoskeletal disorders include weakness, lameness, limb swelling, and joint dysfunction. Motor or sensory neurologic impairment may develop secondary to neuromuscular lesions. Abnormalities of the musculoskeletal system may also affect other organs of the endocrine, urinary, digestive, hemolymphatic, and cardiopulmonary systems. Evaluation of musculoskeletal disease is aimed at localizing and defining the lesion(s). Diagnosis requires accurate review of the signalment, history, and physical status of the animal. A lameness examination is critical in determining a diagnosis. Useful ancillary tests include radiography, ultrasonography, arthrocentesis, arthroscopy, arthrography, electromyography, and tissue biopsy and histopathology. For subtle lesions, advanced imaging such as bone scan, computed tomography (CT), or MRI may be needed.

The Lameness Examination

The lameness examination is a key feature in identifying musculoskeletal lesions. Evaluation is performed with the animal at rest, rising, and during locomotion on flat or inclined surfaces. Single or multiple limb lameness is noted, and the severity related to the type of activity. With a forelimb lameness, the head is elevated during weightbearing on the unsound limb. The stride is also shortened on the affected side. For hindlimb lameness, the head is dropped during weight bearing of the affected limb. Limbs should be assessed from a distal to proximal manner, and bones, joints, and soft tissue should be palpated. Abnormalities that should be noted include swelling, pain, instability, crepitation, reduced range of motion, and muscle atrophy. In evaluation of a subtle or obscure lameness, serial examinations before and after exercise may be necessary. For fractious animals, sedation may be required; palpation, radiography, and arthrocentesis can often be performed while an animal is sedated with IV butorphanol and acepromazine, propofol, or a combination of ketamine, diazepam, and acepromazine.

Imaging Techniques: Imaging procedures that are helpful in diagnosing lameness include survey and contrast radiography, ultrasonography, nuclear scintigraphy, CT, and MRI. Animals undergoing these evaluations should be heavily sedated or anesthetized. Survey radiography of affected limbs or the spine requires multiple, orthogonal views. Subtle lesions are often identified following comparison with the contralateral normal limb. The most frequent contrast studies used to evaluate lame animals are arthrograms for joint diseases and myelography for spinal canal disorders. Ultrasonography is useful for evaluating musculotendinous injuries such as bicipital tenosynovitis and muscle contracture. Nuclear scintigraphy, CT, and MRI studies are usually available at large referral centers. Nuclear scintigraphy involves IV injection of a radioactive compound that localizes and highlights periosseous soft tissue and bone lesions. CT imaging permits high contrast and resolution of osseous structures, while MRI is helpful for delineating soft tissue and joint injuries.

Arthroscopy: Arthroscopy is a minimally invasive tool used for diagnosis and therapy of lame animals. Advantages of the technique include improved visualization and diagnosis of joint pathology, ability to treat injuries by removal of damaged cartilage or ligament, and reduced surgical dissection. Disadvantages are costs of equipment and a prolonged learning curve. Common conditions that can be diagnosed or treated by arthroscopy include osteochondrosis, bicipital tenosynovitis, joint fractures, and cranial cruciate ligament and medial meniscal injuries.

Pain Management

Control of pain in lame or operative animals involves broad classes of compounds such as NSAID and opioids (*see also* PAIN MANAGEMENT, p 1691). Delivery of analgesia can be via oral, parenteral, epidural, local, or transdermal routes. Nonpharmacologic pain management strategies include acupuncture therapy, massage, and diet. Commonly used NSAID include firocoxib (5 mg/kg, PO, SID), meloxicam (0.1 mg/kg, IV, SC, PO, SID), carprofen (2.2 mg/kg, PO, BID), ketoprofen (1.0 mg/kg, PO, IV, SC, IM, SID), etodolac (12.5 mg/kg, PO, SID), and aspirin (22 mg/kg, PO, BID in dogs; 10 mg/kg, PO, every 48 hr in cats). The use of NSAID is contraindicated in animals with hepatic or renal insufficiency, gastroenteritis, coagulopathy, or in animals receiving concurrent corticosteroid therapy. Opioid analgesics bind to μ, κ, and δ receptors in the CNS to provide pain relief. Commonly used opioids include morphine (0.1 mg/kg, IV, SC, IM, every 3-4 hr), oxymorphone (0.05 mg/kg, IV, IM, SC, every 3-4 hr), hydromorphone (0.1 mg/kg, IV, IM, SC, every 2-4 hr), butorphanol (0.1 mg/kg, IV, IM, SC, every 3-4 hr), and buprenorphine (10 μg/kg, IV, IM, SC, TID). Opioid narcotics can be given with sedatives such as acepromazine (0.5 mg/kg, IV, IM, SC, every 4-6 hr) for enhanced efficacy of analgesia and sedation. Oxymorphone, hydromorphone, and butorphanol are more potent than morphine. Buprenorphine has the longest duration of action. Another opioid, fentanyl, is most frequently administered via transdermal patches applied for 3 days on shaved areas. Oral opioids used for pain relief include butorphanol (1.0 mg/kg, TID), hydromorphone (0.5 mg/kg, TID), and oxycodone (0.3 mg/kg, TID). Local administration of analgesics involves joint injections with morphine (1 mg diluted in 5 mL of saline) or bupivicaine (1 mL/20 kg body wt) before joint surgery as a preemptive block of intracapsular pain receptors. Epidural morphine (0.1 mg/kg) in the lumbosacral space is also a useful adjunct for postoperative pain relief in the hindlimbs and for reduced anesthetic requirements. Corticosteroids are considered weak analgesic adjuncts because they indirectly reduce pain by their primary action as local anti-inflammatory agents at the site of injury. Drugs used include prednisone or prednisolone (1-2 mg/kg, PO, SID) or dexamethasone (1-2 mg/kg, IV, SID). Their use is contraindicated during concurrent treatment with NSAID.

ARTHROPATHIES AND RELATED DISORDERS IN SMALL ANIMALS

Many arthropathies are developmental, including aseptic necrosis of the femoral head, patellar luxation, osteochondrosis, elbow dysplasia, and hip dysplasia. Other arthropathies are degenerative, infectious or septic, immune-mediated, or due to neoplasia or trauma.

ASEPTIC NECROSIS OF THE FEMORAL HEAD
(Legg-Calvé-Perthes disease)

This deterioration of the femoral head seen in young miniature and small breeds of dogs is associated with ischemia and avascular necrosis of the bone. The exact cause is unknown, although there may be a hereditary component in Manchester Terriers. Infarction of the bone leads to collapse of the femoral head and neck, followed by revascularization, resorption, and remodeling. The lesion is often bilateral.

Clinical signs include hindlimb lameness, atrophy of the thigh muscles, and pain during manipulation of the hip joint. Radiography reveals irregular bone density of the femoral head and neck, collapse, and fragment of the bone. Chronic cases have evidence of degenerative joint disease.

Treatment involves surgical excision of the affected femoral head and neck and early postoperative physical therapy to stimulate limb usage. Prognosis for recovery is good.

PATELLAR LUXATION

This hereditary disorder in dogs and cats is characterized by ectopic development of the patella medial or lateral to the trochlear groove of the femur. Patellar luxation is often associated with multiple deformities of the hindlimb, involving the hip joint, femur, and tibia. Medial patellar luxations can be involved with a reduced coxofemoral angle (coxa vara), lateral bowing of the femur, internal rotation of the tibia, shallow trochlear groove, and hypoplasia of the medial femoral condyle; lateral luxations cause the reverse changes.

Clinical signs are variable and based on the severity of luxation. Animals of any age may be affected. In general, cats and small and miniature breeds of dogs have a medial luxation, and large dogs have a lateral luxation. Affected animals are lame or ambulate with a skipping gait. Palpation of the stifle joint reveals displacement of the patella. In Grade I, clinical signs are mild and infrequent, and the patella can be manually luxated but easily returns to the trochlear groove. In Grade II, the patella luxates during flexion of the joint and is repositioned during extension, thus causing animals to have a resolvable skipping lameness. In Grade III, the dislocated patella is more frequently out of than in the trochlear groove, and lameness is consistent. Bone deformities are evident in these animals. In Grade IV, lameness and limb deformations are most severe. Radiography of affected animals reveals various degrees of limb changes based on the grade of the luxation.

The type of surgery is based on the severity of the luxation and can include both orthopedic and soft-tissue procedures. Useful surgeries involve fascial releasing incisions (on the side of the luxation), joint capsule imbrication (on the side opposite the luxation), deepening of the trochlear groove, tibial crest transposition, and fabella to tibial tuberosity derotation sutures. Severe deformations may require femoral or tibial osteotomies, stifle joint arthrodesis, or limb amputation.

Prognosis for recovery is good in mild or moderately affected animals. Concurrent cranial cruciate ligament and medial meniscal injuries should be identified and treated. Cats are less severely affected than dogs and have an excellent prognosis.

OSTEOCHONDROSIS

Osteochondrosis is a developmental disorder of medium and large rapidly growing dogs that is characterized by abnormal endochondral ossification of epiphyseal cartilage in the shoulder, elbow, stifle, and hock joints. *See also* p 918. Although the exact cause is unknown, excessive nutrition, rapid growth, trauma, and a hereditary component are suspected to be contributing factors. As a result of abnormal maturation and vascularity, basal cartilage cells thicken and weaken, thus leading to cartilage cracks, fissures, and flap formation (osteochondritis dissecans) after minor trauma or normal pressure to the joint. Abnormal cartilage congruency and joint debris lead to a synovitis and subsequent arthritis and continued cartilage breakdown. Cartilage flaps can break loose and attach to the joint capsule or migrate and deleteriously affect joint motion.

Clinical signs are lameness, joint effusion, and reduced range of motion in affected joints or limbs. Locations of the lesions include the head of the humerus (shoulder joint), the medial aspect of the humeral condyle (elbow joint), the femoral condyles (stifle joint), and the trochlear ridges of the talus (hock joint). Additionally, fragmented medial coronoid process and ununited anconeal process in the elbow joint may be related conditions. Radiography is useful in identifying joint lesions; changes may include flattening of joint surfaces, subchondral bone lucency or sclerosis, osteophytosis, joint effusion, and "joint mice." Arthrography can be used to delineate cartilage flaps, and arthroscopy can also be performed to identify cartilage or joint lesions.

Treatment involves surgical excision of cartilage flaps or free-floating fragments and curettage of subchondral bone to stimulate fibrocartilage formation. Animals with degenerative joint disease may benefit from NSAID, eg, aspirin (10 mg/kg, PO, BID), carprofen (2.2 mg/kg, PO, BID), or etodolac (12.5 mg/kg, PO, SID). Joint fluid modifiers such as polysulfated glycosaminoglycan (4.4 mg/kg, IM, twice a week for 4 wk) may also help prevent cartilage degeneration. Prognosis for recovery is excellent for the shoulders, good for the stifle joint, and fair for the elbow and tarsal joints. Concomitant signs of degenerative joint disease, other joint conditions, or instability (hock joint) deleteriously affect recovery.

ELBOW DYSPLASIA

(Ununited anconeal process, Fragmented medial coronoid process, Osteochondrosis of the humeral condyle)

Elbow dysplasia is a generalized incongruency of the elbow joint in young, large, rapidly growing dogs that is related to abnormal bone growth, joint stresses, or cartilage development. One or more of the following lesions may be present in the joint: an ununited anconeal process of the ulna, fragmentation of the medial coronoid process of the ulna, and osteochondrosis of the medial aspect of the humeral condyle. Radiographic grading of dysplastic elbow joints is performed by the Orthopedic Foundation for Animals in the USA and in Scandinavian and European kennel clubs.

Ununited Anconeal Process: This results when there is separation of the ossification center of the anconeal process from the proximal ulnar metaphysis. Fusion should be completed by 5-6 mo of age. The fracture is postulated to result from a biomechanical imbalance of force and movement in the rapidly growing elbow. Initially, the anconeal process is connected to the ulna by a bridge of fibrous tissue, which fragments to form a pseudoarthrosis, and the elbow becomes unstable. This joint laxity continues to damage the articular cartilage, and secondary osteoarthritis results. A hereditary basis has been implicated but not proved.

Lameness develops insidiously between 4 and 8 mo of age; however, some bilateral cases may not be diagnosed until the dogs are >1 yr old. Affected elbows may deviate laterally, and the range of motion is restricted. Advanced cases have osteoarthritis, joint effusion, and crepitus. Clinical signs are suggestive, and the diagnosis is confirmed by radiography. A lateral radiograph of the elbow in the flexed position allows visualization of the ununited process. Both elbows should be examined because the condition can be bilateral.

Fragmentation of the Medial Coronoid Process: This is a condition of the medial compartment of the canine elbow, in which the coronoid process fails to unite, either partially or totally, with the ulnar diaphysis and, thus, does not become a part of the articular surface of the trochlear notch. Joint laxity, irritation, and finally osteoarthritis result. This condition and osteochondrosis of the medial humeral condyle are considered to be the most common causes of osteoarthritis of the canine elbow. Before the onset of osteoarthritis in this condition, the fragments can be demonstrated radiographically.

Osteochondrosis of the Medial Humeral Condyle: This results from a disturbed endochondral fusion of the epiphysis of the medial epicondyle with the distal end of the humerus. The exact cause is unknown, but because the carpal and digital flexors originate from the ventral aspect of this structure, it may represent an epiphyseal avulsion. It results in pain on flexion of the elbow or deep digital palpation and is accompanied by soft-tissue swelling. Radiographically, radiodense structures have been seen caudal and distal to the area of the medial epicondyle.

Treatment: Early surgical treatment is recommended before degenerative joint disease develops. For fragmentation of the medial coronoid process, a medial arthrotomy or arthroscopy is performed and the fragmented process removed. For ununited anconeal process, either a lateral arthrotomy is performed and the ununited process removed, or a midshaft ulnar osteotomy is performed to relieve asynchronous growth and result in union of the process. Reattachment of the process by screw fixation is also an option. For osteochondrosis, the subchondral bone lesion is curetted to stimulate fibrocartilage formation. Prognosis after surgery is good if degenerative joint disease has not developed in the joint. Aspirin or NSAID (eg, carprofen, etodolac, meloxicam) can be used to reduce pain and inflammation. Joint-fluid modifiers (glycosaminoglycans, hyaluronic aid) may be useful.

HIP DYSPLASIA

Hip dysplasia is a multifactorial abnormal development of the coxofemoral joint in large dogs that is characterized by joint laxity and subsequent degenerative joint disease. Excessive growth, exercise, nutrition, and hereditary factors affect the occurrence of hip dysplasia. The pathophysiologic basis for hip dysplasia is a disparity between hip joint muscle mass and rapid bone development. As a result, coxofemoral joint laxity or instability develops and subsequently leads to degenerative joint changes, eg, acetabular bone sclerosis, osteophytosis, thickened femoral neck, joint capsule fibrosis, and subluxation or luxation of the femoral head.

Clinical signs are variable and do not always correlate with radiographic abnormalities. Lameness may be mild, moderate, or severe, and is pronounced after exercise. A "bunny-hopping" gait is sometimes evident. Joint laxity (Ortolani sign), reduced range of motion, and crepitation and pain during full extension and flexion may be present. Radiography is useful in delineating the degree of arthritis and planning of medical and surgical treatments. Standard ventrodorsal views of sedated or anesthetized animals can be graded by the Orthopedic Foundation for Animals, or stress radiographs performed and joint laxity measured (Penn Hip). A dorsal acetabular rim view is used by some surgeons to evaluate the acetabulum before reconstructive surgery. Modified ventrodorsal and dorsoventral projections have also been proposed in an effort to mimic the normal standing posture of dogs.

Treatments are both medical and surgical. Mild cases or nonsurgical candidates (due to health or owner constraints) may benefit from weight reduction, restriction of exercise on hard surfaces, controlled physical therapy to strengthen and maintain muscle tone, anti-inflammatory drugs (eg, aspirin, corticosteroids, NSAID), and possibly joint fluid modifiers. Surgical treatments include pectineal myotenectomy to reduce pain, triple pelvic osteotomy to prevent subluxation, pubic fusion to prevent subluxation, joint capsule denervation to reduce pain, dorsal acetabulum reinforcement to reduce subluxation, femoral head and neck resection to reduce arthritis, and total hip replacement for optimal restoration of joint and limb functions. Additionally, femoral corrective osteotomies can be performed to reduce femoral head subluxation, although degenerative arthritis may persist.

Prognosis is highly variable and depends on the overall health and environment of the animal. In general, if surgery is indicated and performed correctly, it is beneficial. Animals on which surgery is not performed may require an alteration in lifestyle to lead a comfortable existence.

DEGENERATIVE ARTHRITIS
(Degenerative joint disease, Osteoarthritis)

Progressive deterioration of articular cartilage in diarthrodial joints is characterized by hyaline cartilage thinning, joint effusion, and periarticular osteophyte formation. Joint degeneration can be caused by trauma, infection, immune-mediated diseases, or developmental malformations. The inciting cause initiates chondrocyte necrosis, release of degradative enzymes, synovitis, and continued cartilage destruction and inflammation. Abnormal cartilage congruency and joint capsule anatomy can further lead to alteration in normal joint biomechanical function. Pain and lameness develop secondary to joint dysfunction or muscle atrophy and to limb disuse. Although more common in dogs, joint degeneration may also be seen in cats.

Clinical signs of degenerative joint disease include lameness, joint swelling, muscle atrophy, pericapsular fibrosis, and crepitation. Radiographic changes in the joint include joint effusion, periarticular soft-tissue swelling, osteophytosis, subchondral bone sclerosis, and possibly narrowed joint space. Arthrocentesis may be unremarkable or yield minor changes in color, turbidity, or cell counts of synovial fluid.

Treatments can be medical or surgical. Nonsurgical therapies include weight reduction, controlled exercise on soft surfaces, and therapeutic application of warm compresses to affected joints. NSAID (eg, aspirin, phenylbutazone, etodolac, carprofen, deracoxib, meloxicam, firocoxib) reduce pain and inflammation. Caution is advised in longterm NSAID usage in dogs. The most frequently cited adverse effects include GI problems such as inappetence, vomiting, and hemorrhagic gastroenteritis. A carprofen-associated hepatopathy in Labrador Retrievers has also been reported. Corticosteroids also suppress prostaglandin synthesis and subsequent inflammation, but short-term use is advised to prevent iatrogenic Cushing's syndrome, cartilage degeneration, and intestinal perforation. Joint-fluid modifiers such as glycosaminoglycans or sodium hyaluronate may prevent cartilage degradation. Surgical options include joint fusion (arthrodesis), most frequently performed on the carpus and tarsus; joint replacement, such as total hip replacement; joint excision, such as femoral head and neck osteotomy; and amputation. Prognosis is variable and depends on the location and severity of the arthropathy.

SEPTIC ARTHRITIS

Infectious arthritis is most frequently associated with bacterial agents such as staphylococci, streptococci, and coliforms. Causes include hematogenous spread or penetrating trauma, including surgery. Other agents producing a septic arthritis include rickettsia (Rocky Mountain spotted fever, ehrlichiosis) and spirochetes (borreliosis).

Clinical signs of septic arthritis include lameness, swelling, pain of affected joint(s), and systemic signs of fever, malaise, anorexia, and stiffness. Radiography may reveal joint effusion in early cases and degenerative joint disease in chronic conditions. Arthrocentesis reveals increased WBC, especially neutrophils. The synovial fluid may be grossly purulent. Bacterial culture and antimicrobial sensitivity testing may confirm the diagnosis. Serologic testing is used for nonbacterial agents. Treatment is with appropriate IV and oral antibiotics, joint lavage, and surgical debridement in severe cases.

IMMUNE-MEDIATED ARTHRITIS

Inflammatory polyarthritis secondary to deposition of immune complexes can produce erosive (destruction of articular cartilage and subchondral bone) or nonerosive (periarticular inflammation) forms of joint diseases. Rheumatoid arthritis, Greyhound polyarthritis, and feline progressive polyarthritis are examples of erosive arthritides. Systemic lupus erythematosus (SLE) is the most common form of nonerosive arthritis.

Clinical signs are lameness, multiple joint pain, joint swelling, fever, malaise, and anorexia. Clinical signs commonly wax and wane.

Diagnosis is aided by radiography, biopsy, arthrocentesis, and serologic testing. Radiography reveals periarticular swelling, effusion, and joint collapse plus subchondral bone destruction in erosive conditions. Arthrocentesis reveals synovial fluid with reduced viscosity and increased inflammatory cell counts. Biopsy of synovial tissue reveals mild to severe inflammation and cellular infiltrates. Serologic testing is performed for rheumatoid factor and antinuclear antibodies.

Treatment involves anti-inflammatory medications (eg, corticosteroids) and chemotherapeutic agents (eg, cyclophosphamide, azathioprine, or methotrexate). Prognosis is guarded due to relapses and inability to determine the inciting cause of the autoimmune reactions.

NEOPLASTIC ARTHRITIS

Synovial cell sarcoma is the most common malignant tumor involving the joints. The tumor arises from primitive mesenchymal cells outside the synovial membrane. Clinical signs include lameness and joint swelling. Radiography reveals soft-tissue swelling and a periosteal reaction. Pulmonary metastasis is detected in ~25% of animals at initial examination. Biopsy reveals evidence of a soft-tissue tumor. Limb amputation is the treatment of choice.

JOINT TRAUMA

Cranial Cruciate Ligament Rupture

Rupture of the cranial cruciate ligament is most frequently due to excessive trauma and a possibly weakened ligament secondary to degeneration, immune-mediated diseases, or conformational defects (straight-legged dogs). Most injuries involve a midsubstance tear, although bone avulsion at the origin of the ligament is possible. Instability of the stifle joint after rupture of the cranial cruciate ligament can lead to medial meniscal injury, joint effusion, osteophytosis, and joint capsule fibrosis.

Clinical signs involve lameness, pain, medial joint swelling, effusion, crepitation, excessive cranial laxity of the tibia relative to the femur (drawer sign), and increased internal tibial rotation. Partial cranial crucial ligament tears are characterized by a reduced cranial laxity, usually more pronounced in flexion. Medial meniscal injury may be identified by a clicking sound during locomotion or flexion and extension. A tibial compression test (flexion of the hock and cranial displacement of the tibial tuberosity) can also be used to demonstrate laxity of the cranial cruciate ligament. Radiography reveals joint effusion and signs of degenerative joint disease in chronic injuries. Arthrocentesis may reveal mild cellular increases and hemarthrosis. Arthroscopy can confirm the diagnosis but requires specialized equipment.

Treatments include medical and surgical therapies. Weight reduction, controlled physical therapy, and NSAID alleviate pain and discomfort from inflammation and degenerative joint disease. Surgical stabilization of the stifle joint is recommended for active dogs. Extracapsular techniques include fascial suturing, fabella to tibial tuberosity imbrication sutures, cranial transposition of the fibular head, and leveling of the tibial plateau. Intracapsular techniques include fascia lata or patellar tendon grafts sutured over the top of the lateral femoral condyle or use of synthetic grafts. Medial meniscal injury requires removal of damaged avascular tissue. Postoperative physical therapy is critical for clinical recovery. Prognosis after surgery is good as long as degenerative joint disease is not advanced.

Joint Fractures

Traumatic fractures frequently involve the shoulder, elbow, carpal, hip, stifle, and tarsal joints. In immature animals, the weakness of the physis compared with adjacent bones, ligaments, and joint capsule predisposes this area to injury. A Salter-Harris classification scheme (I-V) is often used to describe the location of the fracture relative to the physis and joint. Specific common sites of injury include the greater tubercle and condyle of the humerus, distal ulnar physis, and the head and condyles of the femur. The humeral condyle is also frequently injured in mature Spaniel breeds and characterized by Y or T fracture configurations.

Clinical signs of joint fractures include lameness, pain, and joint swelling. Chronic injuries may be characterized by angular limb deformities if the injury affected an open growth plate. Radiography is useful in delineating the fracture.

The goal of joint fracture treatment is stable anatomic reconstruction to maintain joint congruency and joint and limb functions. Internal fixation with pins, wires, or screws is performed to achieve stable fixation. Prognosis for recovery is good if proper surgical technique has been used and joint trauma has not been excessive.

Palmar Carpal Breakdown

This hyperextension injury secondary to falls or jumps produces excessive force on the carpus, which leads to collapse of the proximal, middle, and/or distal joints secondary to tearing of the palmar carpal ligaments and fibrocartilage. Clinical signs include lameness, carpal swelling, and a characteristic plantigrade stance. External splints or casts may be attempted in mild cases, although surgical treatment is usually required to restore limb function. Surgery involves fusion (arthrodesis) of the affected joints using a bone plate and screws, pins and wires, or external skeletal fixation. A cancellous bone graft is used to enhance bone union, and postoperative support is necessary. Prognosis for recovery is good.

Hip Luxation

Traumatic dislocation of the hip is most frequently a craniodorsal displacement of the femoral head relative to the acetabulum. Clinical signs include lameness, pain during manipulation of the hip joint, and a shortened limb due to dorsal displacement of the femur. Radiography is useful in confirming the luxation and delineating the presence of other fractures in the femoral head or acetabulum. Treatment involves either closed manipulation and postoperative slings to maintain the reduction or open surgical stabilization using sutures or pins. Femoral head and neck resection or total hip replacement can be performed after failed reductions. Prognosis for recovery is usually excellent.

MYOPATHIES IN SMALL ANIMALS

Myopathies can be congenital, idiopathic, inflammatory, or metabolic, or due to nutritional imbalances, muscular trauma, or neoplasia. *See also* MYOPATHIES AND MYOSITIDES, p 947.

YELLOW FAT DISEASE
(Nutritional steatitis, Nutritional panniculitis)

Yellow fat disease is characterized by a marked inflammation of adipose tissue and deposition of "ceroid" pigment in fat cells. It may be seen alone in cats or with accompanying myopathy in rats, mink, foals, and pigs.

It is believed that an overabundance of unsaturated fatty acids in the ration, together with a deficiency of vitamin E or other antioxidants, results in lipid peroxidation and deposition of "ceroid" pigment in the adipose tissue. Most naturally occurring and experimentally induced cases have been in animals that have had fish or fish byproducts as all or part of the diet. The specific cause is believed to be related jointly to the high unsaturation of the fish oil fatty acids and their lack of protection with vitamin E or other antioxidants.

Affected cats are frequently obese, usually young, and of either sex. They lose agility, are unwilling to move, and resent palpation of the back or abdomen. In advanced disease, even a light touch causes pain. Fever is a constant finding, and anorexia may be present.

In mink, kits may be affected with steatitis shortly after weaning and, if untreated, losses may continue to pelting time. Signs appear suddenly; the kits may refuse a night feeding and be dead by morning. Affected mink may refuse their feed and show a peculiar, unsteady hop, followed by complete impairment of locomotion and coma. At pelting, survivors show yellow fat deposits and hemoglobinuria.

The typical laboratory finding is an increased WBC count, with neutrophilia and sometimes eosinophilia. Biopsy of the subcutaneous fat shows it to be yellowish brown and firm. Histologic examination reveals severe inflammatory changes and associated ceroid pigment.

The offending excessive fat source must be removed from the diet. Administration of vitamin E, in the form of α-tocopherol, at least 30 mg daily for cats, or 15 mg daily for mink, is necessary. Antibiotics are of doubtful value, despite the fever and leukocytosis.

Parenteral use of fluids is not advisable unless dehydration exists. Because of associated pain, affected animals should be handled as little as possible.

TYPE II MUSCLE FIBER DEFICIENCY

Type II muscle fiber deficiency is a congenital myopathy that has been described in Labrador Retrievers. The cause is unknown. Clinical signs are seen at <5 mo of age and include skeletal muscle atrophy, stunted growth, and weakness. Signs are progressive until the animal reaches maturity, when they stabilize. Animals may have a normal life span. Diagnosis is by creatinuria, muscle biopsy, and electromyography. Histology reveals increased connective tissue around muscle fibers and staining deficiency of type II fibers. Myotonic discharges are seen with an electromyography. There is no effective treatment.

FIBROTIC MYOPATHY

Fibrotic myopathy is a chronic, progressive, idiopathic, degenerative disorder affecting the semitendinosus, gracilis, quadriceps, infraspinatus, and supraspinatus muscles, primarily in dogs. The cause is unknown. Affected muscles are characterized by contracture and fibrosis. Normal tissues are replaced by dense collagenous connective tissue. Clinical signs include a nonpainful, mechanical lameness. Neurologic function is normal. Surgical release of affected tissues via tenotomy, myotenotomy, Z-plasty, or complete resection produces inconsistent results. Prognosis is guarded due to recurrence.

MYOSITIS OSSIFICANS

Myositis ossificans is an idiopathic non-neoplastic form of heterotopic ossification of fibrous connective tissue and muscle that frequently affects tissues near the hip joint in Doberman Pinschers. It may be related to a bleeding disorder (von Willebrand's disease) in these dogs. Surgical resection of the mineralized mass is usually rewarding.

POLYMYOSITIS

Polymyositis is a systemic, noninfectious, possibly immune-mediated, inflammatory muscle disorder in adult dogs. It may be acute or chronic and progressive. Clinical signs include depression, lethargy, weakness, weight loss, lameness, myalgia, and muscle atrophy. CK may be increased, and electromyography reveals abnormal spontaneous muscle activity. Muscle biopsy reveals myonecrosis, lymphocytic-plasmacytic perimuscular infiltration, phagocytosis, and fiber regeneration. Polymyositis may be associated with megaesophagus and immune-mediated disorders (myasthenia gravis, lupus erythematosus, polyarthritis). Oral corticosteroids (1-2 mg/kg, BID for 3-4 wk) are the treatment of choice; other immunosuppressive agents such as azathioprine or cyclophosphamide can also be used. Prognosis is favorable, although relapses are not uncommon.

MASTICATORY MYOSITIS
(Eosinophilic myositis)

Masticatory myositis is an immune-mediated, inflammatory condition that affects the muscles of mastication. The exact cause is unknown. Specific autoantibodies directed against type II muscle fibers have been detected in affected animals. In acute cases, muscles are swollen and there is difficulty in opening the jaw. In chronic cases, there is anorexia, weight loss, difficulty in opening the jaw, and muscle atrophy. Diagnostic hematologic values include eosinophilia and increased levels of globulin and muscle enzymes. Electromyography reveals abnormal spontaneous electrical activity in affected muscles. A biopsy sample of the temporalis muscle is usually taken; histologic changes include lymphocytic-plasmacytic cellular infiltrates, muscle atrophy, and fibrosis. Although spontaneous regression can occur, treatment with oral corticosteroids (gradually decreasing the dosage) is usually effective. Relapses are common, and longterm medication may be required.

FELINE HYPOKALEMIC POLYMYOPATHY

Feline hypokalemic polymyopathy is a generalized metabolic muscle weakness disorder in cats secondary to hypokalemia associated with excessive urinary depletion or inadequate dietary intake. Extracellular hypokalemia causes muscle cell membrane hyperpolarization and secondary excessive permeability to sodium. This leads to hypopolarization of the muscle cell and subsequent weakness.

Clinical signs include generalized weakness, ventroflexion of the neck, abnormal gait, anorexia, and muscle pain. The neurologic examination is normal. Serum chemistries reveal hypokalemia (<3.5 mEq/L) and increased creatinine and CK. The urine has a low specific gravity, and potassium excretion is increased. Treatment is by potassium supplementation, given PO (5-8 mEq/day) or IV in cats with profound hypokalemia. Prognosis is excellent with early diagnosis and treatment.

MALIGNANT HYPERTHERMIA

Malignant hyperthermia (see also p 832) is a hypermetabolic disorder of skeletal muscle characterized by catabolism and contracure usually secondary to inhalant anesthetic agents and stress. It is seen most frequently in heavily muscled dogs. Abnormal calcium regulation, glycogenolysis, and contractile protein activity result in production of heat, CO_2, and lactic acid.

Clinical signs include tachycardia, tachypnea, pyrexia, muscle rigidity, and cardiopulmonary failure. Signs develop 5-30 min after exposure to the anesthetic agent. Treatment consists of immediate cessation of anesthesia and hyperventilation with oxygen. IV fluid therapy, corticosteroids, and ice packs are also used. Dantrolene, a muscle relaxant, may be given at 2-5 mg/kg, IV. Prognosis is poor in severe cases. Urinary output, serum potassium levels, and cardiac function should be monitored.

EXERTIONAL MYOPATHY

(Rhabdomyolysis, Tying-up, Monday morning disease)

This acute exertional myopathy of racing Greyhounds and working dogs is characterized by muscle ischemia secondary to exercise or excitement. Avascularity and lactic acidosis cause muscular lysis, myoglobin release, and a nephropathy.

Clinical signs include muscle pain and swelling 24-72 hr after racing. Severe cases are characterized by stiffness, hyperpnea, collapse, myoglobinemia, and acute renal failure. Urinalysis reveals myoglobinuria; serum potassium, phosphorus, and muscle enzymes are increased. Treatment includes supportive care such as IV fluids, bicarbonate, body cooling, rest, and muscle relaxants (eg, diazepam). Prognosis depends on severity. (See also EXERTIONAL MYOPATHIES IN HORSES, p 951.)

MUSCULAR TRAUMA

Infraspinatus Contracture: Infraspinatus contracture is a uni- or bilateral fibrotic myopathy of the infraspinatus muscle that is usually secondary to trauma in hunting or working dogs. Clinical signs include an acute lameness, pain, and swelling in the shoulder region. The lameness subsides, but a gait abnormality develops 2-4 wk after injury as muscle fibrosis and contracture progress. Clinical signs include a characteristic adduction of the elbow, abduction of the foreleg, and external rotation of the carpus and paw. The limb is circumducted with each stride of the leg. Palpation of the shoulders reveals outward rotation of the humerus as the elbow is flexed. Treatment consists of resection of the fibrous musculotendinous portion of the muscle, including tenotomy of the tendon of insertion. Limb and joint functions are immediately improved, and prognosis for full recovery is excellent.

Tenosynovitis of the Biceps Brachii Tendon: This inflammation of the biceps brachii tendon of origin and associated synovial sheath can be uni- or bilateral. It usually affects mature, large dogs. The mechanism of injury can be direct, indirect, overuse, or migration of osteochondral fragments ("joint mice") from humeral osteochondrosis lesions.

Clinical signs include a progressive or chronic, intermittent lameness that worsens after exercise and improves with rest. The range of motion of the shoulder joint is reduced, and atrophy of the shoulder muscles may be apparent. Acute pain can be elicited by applying digital pressure to the biceps tendon during flexion and extension of the shoulder joint.

Diagnosis can be confirmed by radiography of the shoulder, which reveals dystrophic calcification of the tendon, osteophytes in the intertubercular groove or mineralized fragments within the tendon sheath. Contrast arthrography may demonstrate filling defects and irregularities of the synovial sheath. Ultrasonography of the damaged biceps tendon and sheath is also helpful for diagnosis. Arthroscopy can be used to visualize tendon injury. Arthrocentesis may be inconclusive. Diagnosis can also be performed by exploration of the tendon and associated sheath.

Acute, mild cases can be treated with rest and oral NSAID (eg, aspirin, carprofen). Acute, severe cases can be treated with intralesional injections of methylprednisolone acetate (20-40 mg, every 2 wk) and rest. Chronic cases refractory to multiple corticosteroid injections or cases involving identifiable "joint mice" are treated by tenodesis (resection and attachment of the tendon to the proximal humerus) and osteochondral fragment removal. Prognosis for recovery is good, although severe degenerative changes in chronic cases may cause a residual lameness.

Quadriceps Contracture (Quadriceps Tie-down, Stiff Stifle Disease): This serious fibrosis and contracture of the quadriceps muscles develops secondary to distal femoral fractures, inadequate surgical repair, and excessive dissection in young dogs. Adhesions develop between the bone, periosteal tissue, and quadriceps muscles, which lead to limb extension, disuse, osteoporosis, degenerative joint disease, and bone and joint deformations. Clinical signs include hyperextension and cranial displacement of the affected limb. Surgery is usually required to resect fibrous tissues and increase motion of the stifle joint. Bone and soft-tissue reconstructions along with postoperative flexion bandages and physical therapy are required to recover limb function. Prognosis is guarded. Prevention of the condition by accurate, biologic stable repairs of bone fractures is preferred.

Achilles Tendon Disruption (Dropped Hock): This acute, traumatic injury to the common calcaneal tendon (gastrocnemius, superficial digital flexor, biceps femoris, semitendinosus, and gracilis muscle tendons) is seen primarily in mature working and athletic dogs. The common tendon can be ruptured or avulsed from the tuber calcanei of the talus. Ruptures may be partial or complete, and the gastrocnemius tendon component is most frequently affected. Clinical signs include a severe nonweightbearing lameness, tarsal hyperflexion, and a plantigrade stance. Palpation reveals swelling, pain, and torn or fibrotic tendon ends. Radiography may reveal avulsed bone fragments. Treatment is by surgical repair of torn ends and reattachment of tendinous tissue to the tuber calcanei. External splints or fixators should be used to protect the repair for 4 wk. Prognosis is variable and based on chronicity of the injury, success of the surgery, and expected performance of the dog.

MUSCLE TUMORS

Primary skeletal muscle tumors can be benign (rhabdomyoma) or malignant (rhabdomyosarcoma). Secondary tumors involved with metastatic spread include lymphosarcoma, hemangiosarcoma, and adenocarcinomas. Local tumors (fibrosarcoma, osteosarcoma, mast cell tumors) can also invade adjacent muscle.

Clinical signs include localized swelling and lameness. Diagnosis is confirmed by biopsy and histologic evaluation of the samples. Treatment is by surgical excision or limb amputation; chemotherapy and radiation may be used depending on the type of tumor.

OSTEOPATHIES IN SMALL ANIMALS

Osteopathies can be developmental, infectious (osteomyelitis), idiopathic (eg, hypertrophic osteopathy), nutritional, or due to bone tumors or trauma.

DEVELOPMENTAL OSTEOPATHIES

Angular Deformity of the Forelimb
(Radial and ulnar dysplasia)

Abnormal development of the radius and ulna can occur secondary to distal physeal injury or hereditary breed characteristics (Bulldogs, Pugs, Boston Terriers, Basset Hounds, Dachshunds). Asynchronous growth of the 2 bones leads to shortened limbs, cranial bowing of the bones, elbow joint subluxation, and valgus or varus deformities in the carpus.

Clinical signs include lameness and reduced painful motion in the elbow or carpal joints. Radiography reveals the bone deformations and closed physes.

Treatment is based on correcting angulation and length of the limb, and reestablishing joint congruity. Surgical procedures include corrective osteotomy and stabilization with internal or external implants, and tension-releasing osteotomies. Prognosis is good for animals without severe limb deformations.

Craniomandibular Osteopathy

Craniomandibular osteopathy is a non-neoplastic, proliferative bone disorder of growing dogs that affects the mandible and tympanic bullae of Terrier breeds. The cause is unknown, but a genetic basis is suspected. The bone lesion is characterized by cyclical resorption of normal bone and replacement by immature bone along endosteal and periosteal surfaces.

Clinical signs vary in severity and include oral discomfort, weight loss, fever, and painful palpable enlargement of the mandible. Radiography reveals bilateral bone proliferation in the mandibles and tympanic bullae.

Therapy is symptomatic and consists of aspirin or corticosteroids to reduce inflammation and discomfort, and a soft-food diet. Prognosis is good because bone proliferation ceases when the animal matures.

Hypertrophic Osteodystrophy

Hypertrophic osteodystrophy is a developmental disorder of the metaphyses in long bones of young, growing dogs, usually of a large or giant breed. The exact etiology is unknown, although excessive dietary supplementation is suspected. The pathophysiology is based on metaphyseal vascular impairment leading to a failure in ossification and trabecular necrosis and inflammation.

Clinical signs include bilateral metaphyseal pain and swelling in the distal radius and ulna, fever, anorexia, and depression. Clinical signs may be periodic. Angular limb deformities may develop in severely affected dogs. Radiography reveals metaphyseal bone lucencies and circumferential periosteal bone formation.

Therapy is symptomatic and aimed at relieving pain (eg, NSAID), reducing dietary supplementation, and providing supportive fluid care.

Multiple Cartilaginous Exostoses
(Osteochondromatosis)

Multiple cartilaginous exostoses is a proliferative disease of young dogs and cats characterized by multiple ossified protuberances arising from metaphyseal cortical surfaces of the long bones, vertebrae, and ribs. Animals may be asymptomatic, and diagnosis is confirmed by palpation and radiography. Surgical excision of the masses is recommended if clinical signs such as lameness or pain develop.

Panosteitis

Panosteitis is a spontaneous, self-limiting disease of young, rapidly growing, large and giant dogs that primarily affects the diaphyses and metaphyses of long bone. The exact etiology is unknown, although genetics (in German Shepherds), stress, infection, and metabolic or autoimmune causes have been suspected. The pathophysiology of the disease is characterized by intramedullary fat necrosis, excessive osteoid production, and vascular congestion. Endosteal and periosteal bone reactions occur.

Clinical signs are acute, cyclical, and involve single or multiple bone(s) in dogs 6-16 mo old. Animals are lame, febrile, inappetent, and have palpable long bone pain. Radiography reveals increased multifocal, intramedullary densities and irregular endosteal surfaces along long bones. Therapy is aimed at relieving pain and discomfort; oral NSAID or corticosteroids can be used during periods of illness. Excessive dietary supplementation in young, growing dogs should be avoided.

Retained Ulnar Cartilage Cores

Retained ulnar cartilage cores is a developmental disorder of the distal ulnar physis in young, large, and giant dogs characterized by abnormal endochondral ossification. As a result, progressive physeal calcification ceases, and forelimb bone growth is restrained. The exact etiology is uncertain, although dietary causes are suspected.

Clinical signs include lameness and angular limb deformities. Radiography reveals a radiolucent cartilage core in the center of the distal ulnar physis. Treatments include cessation of dietary supplements and osteotomy or ostectomies of the bone to reduce limb deformation. Prognosis is based on the severity of the condition.

Scottish Fold Osteodystrophy

This heritable condition of Scottish Fold cats is characterized by skeletal deformations of the vertebrae, metacarpal and metatarsal bones, and phalanges secondary to abnormal endochondral ossification. Affected cats are lame, and affected bones are deformed and swollen. Treatment is by removal of exostoses. Prognosis is guarded.

OSTEOMYELITIS

Inflammation and infection of the medullary cavity, cortex, and periosteum of bone are most frequently associated with bacteria such as *Staphylococcus* spp, *Streptococcus* spp, *Escherichia coli*, *Proteus* spp, *Pasteurella* spp, *Pseudomonas* spp, and *Brucella canis*. Anaerobic bacteria are less frequently isolated and may be part of a polymicrobial infection. Fungal diseases are based on geographic distributions and include *Coccidioides immitis* (southwestern USA), *Blastomyces dermatitidis* (southeastern USA), *Histoplasma capsulatum* (central USA), *Cryptococcus neoformans*, and *Aspergillus* spp (worldwide). Factors contributing to infection include ischemia, trauma, focal inflammation, bone necrosis, and hematogenous spread.

Clinical signs may be acute or chronic. Animals may have lameness, pain, abscessation at the wound site, fever, anorexia, and depression. Radiography can reveal bone lysis, sequestration, irregular periosteal reaction, loosening of implants, and fistulous tracts. Deep, fine-needle aspiration, cytology, and blood cultures may also reveal evidence of infection.

Treatment includes both medical and surgical therapies. Longterm oral or injectable antibiotics such as cephalexin (30 mg/kg, BID), clindamycin (11 mg/kg, BID), enrofloxacin (15 mg/kg, BID), amikacin (15 mg/kg, BID), or oxacillin (22 mg/kg, TID) are used. Additionally, wound debridement, lavage, and removal of loose implants are recommended. Open or closed wound drainage and delayed autogenous, cancellous bone grafting can also be performed. In chronic, refractory cases, limb amputation may be warranted. Prognosis is variable and based on the severity and chronicity of the infection. Appropriate antimicrobial therapy based on bacterial culture and antibiotic sensitivity testing is mandatory for successful results.

HYPERTROPHIC OSTEOPATHY

Hypertrophic osteopathy is a diffuse periosteal proliferative condition of long bones in dogs secondary to neoplastic or infectious masses in the thoracic or abdominal cavity. The exact pathogenic mechanism is unknown, but periosteal vascularity is reduced.

Clinical signs include lameness, long-bone pain, and signs secondary to body cavity masses. Radiography reveals the primary masses and peripheral bone reactions.

Treatment includes thoracic or abdominal surgery to remove masses and unilateral vagotomy to block the neurovascular reflex associated with bone changes.

NUTRITIONAL OSTEOPATHIES

See also DYSTROPHIES ASSOCIATED WITH CALCIUM, PHOSPHORUS, AND VITAMIN D, p 852.

Reduced bone mass, bone deformities, exostoses, pathologic fractures, and loose teeth (rubber jaw) are skeletal manifestations of nutritional derangements that affect parathyroid hormone function and calcium and vitamin metabolism. Specific causes such as secondary nutritional or renal hyperparathyroidism, hypovitaminosis D, and hypervitaminosis A can produce lamenesses. Diagnosis is by serum chemistry analyses, radiography, and identification of underlying nutritional deficiencies. Treatment is aimed at reversing the specific etiology. Surgery is rarely indicated.

BONE TUMORS

Skeletal tumors can be benign or malignant and primary or secondary to metastases or adjacent soft-tissue structures. The most common primary bone tumor is osteosarcoma that affects the distal radius, proximal humerus, distal femur, or proximal tibia.

Clinical signs include lameness, bone swelling, and an acute, nontraumatic pathologic fracture of the bone. Radiography reveals osteolysis, proliferation, and soft-tissue swelling; thoracic radiographs should be performed to delineate metastatic masses. Bone biopsy using a Michelle bone trephine or Jamshidi biopsy needle is imperative in confirming the diagnosis. Less frequently identified tumors include chondrosarcoma, fibrosarcoma, and hemangiosarcoma. Treatment includes limb amputation and chemotherapy with carboplatin, cisplatin, or doxorubicin. Prognosis is guarded. Untreated animals rarely live more than several months. Amputation and chemotherapy effectively double the survival times. Median survival times after amputation are 5 mo in dogs and 4 yr in cats. Advanced procedures such as limb sparing and excision of metastases are infrequently performed.

BONE TRAUMA

Bone fractures are frequently caused by vehicular accidents, firearms, fights, or falls. Fractures can be open or closed and involve single or multiple bones. Characteristics of the fracture—such as simple, comminuted, oblique, transverse, or spiral—are based on disruptive trauma forces (bending, compression, tension, and rotation).

Clinical signs invariably include lameness, pain, and swelling. Radiography is useful in delineating the fracture pattern. Treatments are based on the type of fracture, age and health of the animal, owner finances, and technical expertise of the surgeon.

Young, healthy dogs with incomplete fractures can be treated with external splints or casts. Other injuries are treated with internal or external devices, such as bone plates, screws, orthopedic wires, and pins. Frequently, cortical or cancellous bone grafts are used to augment healing. Antibiotics are given for open fractures or prolonged repairs. Perioperative analgesics (eg, epidural morphine, narcotic skin patches, systemic narcotics, oral NSAID) are used to alleviate discomfort.

Prognosis for recovery is usually good depending on the nature of the injury and success of repairs; successful wound therapy and monitoring of cardiopulmonary and urologic functions are essential. Followup care includes radiographic and clinical assessments of fracture healing. Internal implants may not need to be removed unless complications such as stress protection, infection, and soft-tissue irritation develop.

SARCOCYSTOSIS

(Sarcosporidiosis)

In sarcocystosis, the endothelium and muscles and other soft tissues are invaded by protozoans of the genus *Sarcocystis*. As the name implies, *Sarcocystis* spp form cysts in various intermediate hosts—humans, horses, cattle, sheep, goats, pigs, birds, rodents, camelids, wildlife, and reptiles. The cysts vary in size from a few micrometers to several centimeters, depending on the host and species.

Etiology, Transmission, and Pathogenesis: *Sarcocystis* spp normally develop in 2-host cycles consisting of an intermediate host (prey) and the final host (predator). Species-specific prey-predator life cycles have been demonstrated for cattle-dog (*S cruzi*), cattle-cat (*S hirsuta*), cattle-human (*S hominis*), sheep-dog (*S capracanis, S hircicanis*), sheep-cat (*S gigantea, S medusiformis*), goat-dog (*S capracanis, S hircicanis*), goat-cat (*S moulei*), pig-dog (*S meischeriana*), pig-human (*S suihominis*), pig-cat (*S porcifelis*), and others. Some wildlife may serve as intermediate hosts (such as raccoons) or final hosts (coyotes) for some species of *Sarcocystis*.

About 1 wk after ingesting muscle tissue that contains *Sarcocystis* cysts (sarcocysts), the final host begins to shed infective sporocysts in the feces; shedding continues for several months. After ingestion of sporocysts by a suitable intermediate host, sporozoites are liberated and initiate development of schizonts in vascular endothelia. Merozoites are liberated from the mature schizonts and produce a second generation of endothelial schizonts. Merozoites from this second generation subsequently invade the muscle fibers and develop into the typical sarcocysts. Initially, sarcocysts contain only a few metrocytes—round, noninfective parasites that give rise to the banana-shaped infective zoites found in mature cysts beginning 2-3 mo after infection. Sarcocysts of some species grow so large that they are easily visible with the unaided eye. The presence of such sarcocysts can cause condemnation of the carcass during meat inspection. *S cruzi* is probably most important in condemnation of beef cattle for human consumption. However, *S hirsuta* has been primarily responsible for dairy cattle condemnation for visible sarcocysts. *S meischeriana* is usually the species responsible for sarcocyst condemnation of pork and may affect meat quality. Sarcocysts are easily recovered from esophagus, diaphragm, and heart muscle. Sarcocysts of some species remain microscopic even though tremendous numbers of cysts may be present in the muscles.

Sarcocystis spp were considered of doubtful pathogenicity until induced infection with *S cruzi* sporocysts from canine feces caused acute disease in calves; eosinophilic myositis in cattle; and abortions, stillbirths, and deaths in pregnant cows. Two cases of necrotic encephalitis in heifers have been reported. Similar pathogenicity has been demonstrated for *S tenella* in lambs and ewes. An outbreak of myositis affecting 20 ewes with flaccid paralysis was a result of heavy *Sarcocystis* infection. Immune status of the host and the dose of cysts may be the most important factors for the development of clinical disease. Immunosuppression may be responsible for tissue invasion of final hosts (eg, dog and cat). Pathologic changes in myocardium and skeletal muscles were more pronounced in cows with lymphatic leukemia. "Immunization" using small doses of sporocysts appears to prevent development or reduce severity of clinical disease in sheep when challenged with large doses later (premunitive immunity). In dogs, a longer prepatent period and shortened patent period resulted after repeated infection. Pigs can also have persistent acquired immunity after immunization infections.

Humans may also serve as intermediate hosts and suffer myositis and vasculitis, but this tissue phase is rare, and the source of such human infection has never been determined. Human intestinal illness, with clinical signs of nausea, abdominal pain, and diarrhea that lasted up to 48 hr, has followed ingestion of sarcocysts of *S suihominis* in uncooked pork and *S hominis* in uncooked beef. The extent of human illness from ingestion of infected meat has not been documented.

Clinical Findings: *Sarcocystis* spp infections are quite prevalent in farm animals; however, there have been few outbreaks of clinical disease. Most animals are asymptomatic, and the parasite is discovered only at slaughter. In cattle severely affected by *S cruzi*, the signs include fever, anorexia, cachexia, decreased milk yield, diarrhea, muscle spasms, anemia, hyperexcitability, weakness, prostration, and death. Cows infected in the last trimester of pregnancy may abort. *Sarcocystis* sp infection was associated with the loss of tailswitch hair in a group of feedlot cattle. After recovery from acute illness, calves failed to grow well and eventually died in a cachectic state. Anemia, hepatitis, and myocarditis were the primary lesions in acute ovine sarcocystosis after experimental challenge with *S tenella* sporocysts. Cases of encephalomyelitis in sheep were associated with a *Sarcocystis* sp infection. After recovery from acute illness, some sheep may lose their wool. At necropsy, acutely affected animals have hemorrhage of the serous membranes of the viscera and myocardium. *Sarcocystis* spp infections are probably most important in growing ruminants and swine, in which they can result in subclinical anemia and reduced weight gain. *Sarcocystis* spp may also induce abortion in sheep.

Equine protozoal myeloencephalitis (EPM, p 1031) is now considered to be caused by *S neurona*. An experimental DNA probe appears promising as a diagnostic tool. Only asexual stages of this parasite have been found, and they may be located in neurons and leukocytes of the brain and spinal cord. Horses may also develop a myopathy. Multifocal myositis has been reported and is possibly due to *S fayeri*. Clinical signs in horses include gait abnormalities such as ataxia, knuckling, and crossing over. Muscle atrophy, which is usually unilateral, is possible. The lesions are typically focal, and brain-stem involvement is common. Depression, weakness, head tilt, and dysphagia are other possible signs. EPM can mimic many neurologic diseases.

Control: Livestock become infected by sporocysts from the feces of carnivores. Because most adult cattle, sheep, and many pigs harbor cysts in their muscles, dogs and other carnivores should not be allowed to eat raw meat, offal, or dead animals. Supplies of grain and feed should be kept covered; dogs and cats should not be allowed in buildings used to store feed or house animals. Amprolium (100 mg/kg, SID for 30 days), fed prophylactically, reduced illness in cattle inoculated with *S cruzi*. Prophylactic administration of amprolium or salinomycin also protected experimentally infected sheep. Therapeutic treatment of cattle and sheep has been ineffective. Vaccines are not available. Experimental work demonstrated that infected pork could be made safe for consumption by cooking at 70°C for 15 min or by freezing at -4°C for 2 days or -20°C for 1 day.

■ ■ ■

NERVOUS SYSTEM

NERVOUS SYSTEM INTRODUCTION

The nervous system is composed of billions of neurons with long, interconnecting processes that form complex integrated electrochemical circuits. It is through these neuronal circuits that animals experience sensations and respond appropriately.

Neuronal processes that transmit electrical alterations to the cell body are called **dendrites**. Dendrites have receptor sites that receive stimulation or inhibition from outside sources. If electrical stimulation of the cell body reaches a critical threshold, an electrical discharge called an **action potential** develops. The action potential spontaneously travels away from the cell body along an outgoing process called an **axon**. When the action potential reaches the terminal branches of the axon, chemicals called **neurotransmitters** are released. Neurotransmitters either stimulate or inhibit receptor sites on other neurons, muscles, or glands. Although neurons may have a variety of shapes, each one has dendrites, a cell body, and an axon, and releases neurotransmitters.

Basic Sensory and Motor Functions: The **peripheral nervous system** (PNS) is formed by neurons of the cranial and spinal nerves. The **central nervous system** (CNS) is formed by neurons of the spinal cord, brain stem, cerebellum, and cerebrum.

Groups of neuronal cell bodies in the PNS are called ganglia, while those in the CNS are called nuclei. Nuclei form the CNS gray matter. Groups of axons in the CNS form the white matter and are arranged into tracts. The tracts are usually named after their site of origin and termination (eg, the spinocerebellar tract begins in the spinal cord and ends in the cerebellum).

PNS sensory or afferent neurons carry information such as nociception, proprioception, touch, temperature, taste, hearing, equilibrium, vision, and olfaction to the spinal cord or brain stem. CNS sensory neurons carry information to the cerebellum, brain stem, and cerebrum for further interpretation. Important spinal cord and brain-stem sensory tracts include several spinocerebellar, spinothalamic, and spinoreticular tract systems. The spinoreticular tracts begin in the spinal cord and terminate in the reticular formation of the medulla. The fasciculus gracilis and cuneatus of the spinal cord and the medial and lateral lemniscus of the brain stem are also important sensory tracts. In animals, these sensory tracts may carry fibers from many sensory modalities such as proprioception, nociception (pain), and touch, which allows them to compensate for sensory deficits after CNS injury. An alteration in sensation may be due to either CNS or PNS disease.

Reactions to sensory inputs are initiated by efferent or motor neurons in the cerebrum and brain stem called **upper motor neurons** (UMN). The UMN axons descend to brain stem and spinal cord segments in tracts named after their site of origination and termination.

The UMN of the reticulospinal tracts (from midbrain, pons, and medulla oblongata reticular formation) and the rubrospinal tract (from midbrain) are important for voluntary movements of skeletal muscles in domestic animals. The corticospinal tracts (cell bodies in the cerebral cortex) are most important for voluntary movement in primates. Domestic animals with severe cerebrocortical disease may suffer only transient loss of voluntary movements because the corticospinal tract has limited influence.

The reticulospinal and vestibulospinal tracts (from vestibular nuclei of the medulla oblongata) supply extensor skeletal muscle activity used to support the body. Knowledge of location and function of sensory and motor brain stem and spinal tracts is essential for localizing nervous system lesions and determining their severity. Mild spinal cord compression affects the superficial spinal cord tracts, ie, spinocerebellar and vestibulospinal tracts, so initial signs include ataxia and extensor weakness. Important voluntary motor tracts are located in the lateral portions of the spinal cord deep to the spinocerebellar tracts, and paresis or paralysis develops with moderate spinal cord compression. Because many tracts are involved, loss of nociception from the periosteum of the toes and tail (deep pain) occurs when spinal cord lesions are bilateral and severe.

Motor neurons with cell bodies in the brain stem, and spinal cord gray matter and axons that travel in the PNS cranial and spinal nerves, respectively, are referred to as **lower motor neurons** (LMN). Injury to either the UMN or LMN results in paresis or paralysis. Brain-stem and spinal cord reflexes are the phylogenetically oldest responses of the nervous system. When the eyelid is touched, it closes; when the toe is pinched, the limb withdraws before conscious perception intervenes. Only a sensory neuron in the PNS, a connector (internuncial) neuron in the CNS, and a LMN are necessary for a reflex to be present. In a monosynaptic reflex (eg, patellar reflex), only a sensory neuron and LMN are present. During the neurologic examination (p 984), testing brain-stem and spinal reflexes is helpful to localize CNS and PNS lesions to specific areas. If a reflex is depressed or absent, a lesion involves the sensory nerve, internuncial neuron, or LMN at that particular site.

The autonomic nervous system is divided into sympathetic and parasympathetic portions and controls activity in smooth and cardiac muscles and glands. Visceral afferent (sensory) neurons travel in cranial and spinal nerves and sensory spinal cord tracts to the thalamic and hypothalamic regions of the brain stem. UMN in the hypothalamus descend to LMN cell bodies of the brain-stem nuclei and to the intermediolateral gray matter of the spinal cord.

LMN of the sympathetic nervous system exit through thoracolumbar spinal nerves (T1 to L4) to affect smooth muscles associated with the pupils, eyelids, orbits, hair follicles, blood vessels, and thoracic and abdominal viscera. **Horner's syndrome** (ptosis, miosis, and enophthalmos) is a common finding associated with loss of sympathetic innervation to the eye.

LMN of the parasympathetic nervous system exit cranial nerve (CN) III to innervate smooth muscle of the pupils and eyelids, CN VII to the lacrimal and salivary glands, CN IX to salivary glands, and CN X to cardiac muscles and glands and to smooth muscles of all the thoracic and abdominal viscera to the transverse colon. LMN of the parasympathetic nervous system also exit through the sacral segments to all the viscera of the caudal abdomen, including the bladder and colon. Sacral lesions commonly result in loss of the urinary bladder reflex.

Divisions and Effects of Lesions: *See also* THE NEUROLOGIC EXAMINATION, p 984. The PNS consists of 26 or more pairs of spinal nerves that correspond to each spinal cord segment and 12 pairs of cranial nerves that correspond to specific brain and brain-stem segments.

The PNS spinal nerves form the brachial plexus to the thoracic limb; the lumbosacral plexus to the pelvic limb; and the cauda equina to the bladder, anus, and tail. Brachial or lumbosacral plexus lesions cause paresis or paralysis of a thoracic or pelvic limb, respectively, with reduced or absent spinal reflexes and sensation of the limb. (*See also* p 1040.) Cauda equina lesions result in an atonic bladder; a dilated, unresponsive anus; and a flaccid, paralyzed tail.

Lesions of all spinal nerves (eg, acute polyradiculoneuritis) result in paresis or paralysis of all 4 limbs (quadriparesis or quadriplegia, respectively) with depressed or absent spinal reflexes and altered sensation of the limbs. Lesions restricted to PNS cranial nerves result in deficits associated with dysfunction of that particular nerve and no signs of dysfunction in the limbs or other parts of the nervous system.

The spinal cord of dogs and cats is divided into 8 cervical, 13 thoracic, 7 lumbar, 3 sacral, and 5 or more caudal segments. Horses and cows have 6 lumbar and 5 sacral segments, and pigs have 6-7 lumbar and 4 sacral segments. Spinal cord lesions from T2 to L7 (L6 in horses, cattle, and pigs) produce paresis or paralysis of the pelvic limbs (paraparesis and paraplegia, respectively). Lesions from T2 to L3 cause pelvic limb ataxia, conscious proprioceptive deficits, and paresis and paralysis with normal or exaggerated spinal reflexes (UMN signs). Pelvic limb sensation caudal to the lesion may also be depressed or absent.

Spinal cord lesions from L4 to S2 cause pelvic limb ataxia, conscious proprioceptive deficits, and paresis or paralysis with depressed or absent spinal reflexes and muscle tone (LMN signs). Sensation may also be depressed or absent below the lesion.

Spinal cord lesions from C1 to T2 cause hemiparesis or hemiplegia (paresis or paralysis of the limbs on one side), or quadriparesis. Spinal reflexes in all 4 limbs are often preserved. In intramedullary spinal cord lesions extending from C6 to T2, thoracic limb spinal reflexes are depressed or absent. Severe lesions cause quadriplegia and may cause respiratory distress or arrest due to involvement of the UMN to respiratory muscles.

The brain stem is divided from caudal to rostral into 4 segments: the medulla oblongata (myelencephalon), the pons (metencephalon), the midbrain (mesencephalon), and the thalamus and hypothalamus (diencephalon).

Lesions of the medulla oblongata cause conscious proprioceptive deficits and weakness on the same side (ipsilateral) or both sides with normal or hyperactive limb reflexes similar to cervical spinal cord lesions. However, involvement of CN nuclei IX, X, XI, or XII localizes the lesion to the caudal medulla oblongata. Involvement of CN nuclei VI, VII, or VIII localizes the lesion to the rostral medulla oblongata. It is rare to have a lesion of the medulla oblongata that does not affect one or more of the cranial nerves as well as sensory and motor tracts.

Pontine lesions cause ipsilateral conscious proprioceptive deficits, hemiparesis or quadriparesis with normal or hyperactive limb reflexes, mental depression from involvement of the ascending reticular activating system (ARAS), and CN V deficits.

Caudal midbrain lesions cause ipsilateral conscious proprioceptive deficits and hemiparesis. Rostral midbrain lesions cause contralateral (on the side opposite the lesion) conscious proprioceptive deficits and hemiparesis. CN III nucleus involvement is present on the ipsilateral side and localizes the lesion to the midbrain. In large midbrain lesions, the ARAS is affected, and the animal will be stuporous or comatose. If the sympathetic UMN and parasympathetic LMN are both affected in the midbrain, the pupils will be midrange size and unresponsive to light.

Diencephalic lesions can be difficult to differentiate from cerebral cortical lesions, because many tracts going to and from the cerebrum pass through the diencephalon. The thalamus, hypothalamus, and subthalamus of the diencephalon have many important structures that alter feeding, drinking, sexual, sleeping, and other behaviors, as well as regulate body temperature. The pituitary gland, which controls many hormonal functions of the body, is connected to the hypothalamus. The ARAS projects through the subthalamus area, in which lesions also produce stupor or coma.

The cerebellum is part of the metencephalon and is attached to the dorsal surface of the pons and medulla by rostral, middle, and caudal cerebellar peduncles. The cerebellum coordinates all muscle activity and establishes muscle tone. The flocculonodular lobe of the cerebellum has equilibrium functions. Unilateral lesions of the cerebellum cause ipsilateral dysmetria (hypermetria or hypometria) and a contralateral head tilt. Bilateral lesions of the cerebellum cause generalized incoordination of the head and limbs, head tremors, and generalized disequilibrium.

The telencephalon, also called the cerebral cortex, is divided into the neocortex, paleocortex, and archicortex. The paleocortex and archicortex include the olfactory and limbic regions, which provide smell and emotional reactions to all stimuli. The neocortex is divided into the frontal, parietal, occipital, and temporal lobes. The frontal cortex functions include intelligence and fine motor skills (corticospinal tract). Lesions in this area cause dementia, lack of recognition of the owner, difficulty in training, compulsive pacing, circling toward the lesion (adversion syndrome), and motor seizures with contralateral involuntary muscle twitching. Contralateral hopping and placing deficits are also found with frontal lobe lesions. Ascending and descending tracts to and from the frontal lobe form the internal capsule through the region of the basal nuclei and diencephalon. Lesions of the internal capsule can produce the same signs as frontal lobe lesions. Because few neurologic signs are associated with parietal lobe lesions in animals, cerebral biopsies may be obtained from this site.

Occipital lobe and optic radiation lesions result in blindness with pupils that respond normally to light. Unilateral occipital lobe and optic radiation lesions result in some degree of visual loss in the contralateral eye depending on the percentage of crossover of the optic nerve fibers in the optic chiasm of the species (65% in cats; 75% in dogs; 80-90% in cattle, horses, pigs, and sheep). The pupils still respond normally to light. Blindness with pupils that do not respond to light is associated with lesions of the retina, optic nerve, optic chiasm, or rostral optic tract.

Difficulty in localizing sound may occur with temporal lobe lesions, as may psychomotor seizures characterized by hysterical running. "Fly-biting" hallucinations are suspected to occur with lesions in the temporal-occipital region. Aggression occurs when the pyriform area (paleocortex) of the temporal lobe and the underlying amygdaloid nucleus are affected. Aggression can also occur with hypothalamic lesions.

Lesions of the olfactory region may alter feeding or sexual behavior. Slow-growing lesions of the cerebrum and diencephalon often result in few clinical signs due to the adaptability of functions in these areas in animals.

Mechanisms of Disease: Disease processes affecting the nervous system may be congenital or familial, infectious or inflammatory, toxic, metabolic, nutritional, traumatic, vascular, degenerative, neoplastic, or idiopathic.

Congenital disorders may be obvious at birth or shortly after (eg, an enlarged head from hydrocephalus or an incoordinated gait from an underdeveloped cerebellum). Some familial disorders (eg, lysosomal storage diseases) cause a progressive degeneration of neurons in the first year of life, while others (eg, inherited epilepsy) may not manifest for 2-3 yr. (*See also* CONGENITAL AND INHERITED ANOMALIES OF THE NERVOUS SYSTEM, p 995.)

Infections of the nervous system are due to specific viruses, fungi, protozoa, bacteria, rickettsia, prions, and algae. Nonspecific inflammations such as steroid-responsive meningoencephalomyelitis and granulomatous meningoencephalomyelitis may be immune-mediated.

Toxicity of the nervous system is most frequently caused by organophosphates (p 2398), pyrethrins (p 2398), carbamates (p 2394), bromethalin (p 2509), metaldehyde (p 2510), ethylene glycol (p 2357), metronidazole (p 2097), theobromines (p 2362), and sedatives. Botulinum, tetanus, and tick toxins, as well as coral and tiger snake venom intoxication, cause neurologic signs.

Metabolic alterations of nervous system function most commonly result from hypoglycemia, hypoxia or anoxia, hepatic dysfunction, hypocalcemia, hypomagnesemia, hypernatremia, hypokalemia, and uremia. Hypothyroidism, hyperthyroidism, hypoadrenocorticism, and hyperadrenocorticism are endocrine disorders that can cause neurologic dysfunction.

Thiamine deficiency results in ataxia, stupor, and coma or seizures in dogs, cats, and cattle. Deficiency of vitamin B_6 may cause seizures.

Trauma to the PNS and CNS causes focal and multifocal neurologic signs from physical damage, hemorrhage, edema, and progressive formation of oxygen-containing free radicals and nervous system destruction that is usually complete in 24-48 hr.

Vascular lesions of animals are usually due to septicemia and bacterial embolization of the CNS. Fibrocartilaginous embolization of the spinal cord is common in dogs. Arteriovenous malformations occur occasionally and cause spontaneous hemorrhages. Cerebrovascular disease from arteriosclerosis and hypertension are rare in domestic animals.

Familial degeneration of neurons occurs in lysosomal storage disorders. Degeneration of intervertebral disks that subsequently herniate into the vertebral canal often produces paresis and paralysis in dogs.

Neoplasms of the CNS and PNS are most common in dogs and cats. Astrocytes, oligodendrocytes, and microglia, some of the cells of the nervous system that support proper neuronal function, can become neoplastic and form astrocytomas, oligodendrogliomas, and gliomas. Ependymal cells and the choroid plexus, which line the internal cavities of the CNS and produce CSF, also can become neoplastic and form ependymomas and choroid plexus papillomas. Meningeal cells of the dura, arachnoid, and pial membranes form meningiomas, which are common in dogs and cats. Neurofibrosarcomas are common tumors of the nerve sheaths of peripheral nerves in dogs. Lymphosarcoma is a common metastatic tumor of the PNS and CNS in dogs, cats, and cattle. (*See also* NEOPLASIA OF THE NERVOUS SYSTEM, p 1047.)

The idiopathic mechanism of disease is reserved for described syndromes with characteristic clinical signs, predictable outcomes, and no known necropsy findings.

THE NEUROLOGIC EVALUATION

An accurate history and thorough physical and neurologic examinations are necessary to evaluate a problem involving the nervous system. An understanding of functional neuroanatomy, neurophysiologic concepts, and mechanisms of disease is a prerequisite for accurate interpretation of clinical findings. Based on the initial clinical assessment, the problem may be defined as diffuse, multifocal, or focal; symmetric or asymmetric; painful or nonpainful; progressive, regressive, or static; and mild, moderate, or severe. In addition, the anatomic locations can be determined. The potential mechanisms of disease must also be considered in determining differential diagnoses. Further diagnostic tests include clinicopathologic tests (on serum, blood, urine, feces, and CSF), diagnostic imaging (including plain and contrast radiography and other imaging techniques), and electrodiagnostic testing.

HISTORY

Neurologic diseases tend to have a species, age, breed, and occasionally a sex predilection. The primary complaints for neurologic problems often include behavioral changes, seizures, tremors, cranial nerve deficits, ataxia, and paresis or paralysis of one or more limbs. Information about the onset, course, and duration of the primary complaint can be used to determine the most probable disease mechanisms. Congenital and familial disorders are most common in purebred animals at birth or within the first few years of life. Inflammatory, metabolic, toxic, and nutritional disorders can be seen in any species, breed, or age; tend to have an acute or subacute onset; and are usually progressive. Vascular and traumatic disorders have an acute onset and rarely progress after 24 hr. Most degenerative and neoplastic disorders tend to occur in older animals (except for familial neuronal degeneration) and have a chronic onset and progressive course. Many idiopathic disorders begin acutely and improve over a short time. Information about similar familial problems, concurrent or recent systemic disease, vaccination status, other affected animals, diet, possible exposure to toxins or trauma, and past neoplastic disorders may be useful to further support certain mechanisms of disease.

PHYSICAL AND NEUROLOGIC EXAMINATIONS

Evidence of disease in other body systems may be associated with inflammatory, metabolic, toxic, or metastatic neoplastic disorders of the nervous system. External signs of traumatic or toxic exposure may support these mechanisms of disease.

The neurologic examination consists of evaluation of the following: 1) the head, 2) the gait, 3) the neck and thoracic limbs, and 4) the trunk, pelvic limbs, anus, and tail. Initially, an attempt should be made to relate all deficits to a focal anatomic lesion.

If abnormalities are found on evaluation of the head, then an initial attempt should be made to explain all limb abnormalities by a lesion above the foramen magnum (C1). If no abnormalities are found on evaluation of the head, but thoracic limb abnormalities are present, then an attempt should be made to explain the abnormalities by a cervical lesion (C1-T2). Paralysis or paresis of all 4 limbs with loss of all spinal reflexes (with or without cranial nerve deficits) is often associated with diffuse peripheral nerve or neuromuscular junction disease (*see also* p 1010).

Knowledge of specific diseases within a certain mechanism for a given species, age, breed, and sex of animal enables an accurate list of differential diagnoses and a diagnostic plan to be formulated after the history and physical and neurologic examinations are completed. Toxic, metabolic, and nutritional mechanisms rarely produce asymmetric neurologic deficits. The other mechanisms of disease may result in symmetric or asymmetric deficits.

Evaluation of the Head

The mentation, head posture and coordination, and cranial nerve functions are observed during evaluation of the head. Abnormal findings are due to lesions above the level of the foramen magnum in the cerebrum, the brain stem (diencephalon, midbrain, pons, or medulla oblongata), or the cerebellum. Dementia, compulsive pacing, or other behavioral abnormalities and seizures are frequently due to lesions in the cerebrum or diencephalon. Depression, semicoma, or coma may be due to lesions of the cerebrum, diencephalon, or midbrain. A head turn or compulsive circling without a head tilt is also associated with a cerebral or diencephalic lesion on the side toward which the animal turns. A head tilt is due to vestibular system disease (CN VIII, rostral medulla oblongata, or cerebellum). Abnormal head coordination, bobbing, and tremors result from cerebellar dysfunction.

The **cranial nerves** consist of 12 left and right pairs and are located at specific brainstem segments; they are simple to test, and results can localize disease to that segment. Abnormal findings are produced by lesions of the peripheral cranial nerve or cranial nerve brain-stem nuclei. If a brain-stem lesion is present, abnormalities are seen in the gait, the thoracic or pelvic limbs, and at times the mental status. If only a peripheral cranial nerve is affected, the other 3 parts of the examination are normal. Cranial nerve lesions of one side produce ipsilateral deficits except for lesions of the trochlear nerve, which crosses in the midbrain.

I. Olfactory: The olfactory nerves transmit smell.

Tests: The animal's ability to find food or the reaction to chemicals (such as cloves, benzene, or xylol) should be observed. Substances that irritate the nasal mucosa and the trigeminal nerve endings (eg, camphor or phenol) should not be used.

Signs of Dysfunction: Inability to find food or respond to nonirritating chemicals is found with disease of the cribriform plate, olfactory bulbs, and olfactory region.

II. Optic: The optic nerves are necessary for vision and also carry the afferent fibers of the pupillary light reflex to the midbrain.

Visual Tests: Cotton balls can be dropped and the animal observed watching them fall to the floor. The menace response is tested by making a threatening gesture toward each eye and causing the animal to blink. Excessive air currents or touching the eyelashes should be avoided because this will test response to touch, rather than to vision. Obstacle testing may be necessary when visual acuity is in doubt. It is useful to blindfold one eye at a time to detect blindness of either eye.

Pupillary Light Reflex: A bright focal light is directed into each pupil toward the temporal retina, and the pupil observed for immediate constriction. The opposite pupil should constrict consensually.

Ophthalmoscopic Examination: This detects local eye diseases. Chorioretinitis or papilledema may be associated with central or peripheral nervous system diseases.

Signs of Dysfunction: Unilateral optic nerve dysfunction results in a decrease or loss of vision and pupillary light reflexes on the affected side. Consensual pupillary constriction of the affected eye should still occur when the other eye is stimulated with light. Unilateral lesions of the optic tract, optic radiation, thalamus (lateral geniculate nucleus), or occipital cortex usually produce a contralateral visual deficit with normal pupillary light reflexes (*see* above).

III. Oculomotor: These nerves carry efferent parasympathetic fibers from the pupillary light reflex center of the midbrain to the fibers of the ciliary ganglion, which innervate the constrictor muscle of the pupils. They are also efferent to the levator palpebrae muscles; the dorsal, medial, and ventral rectus muscles; and the ventral oblique muscles of the eye.

Tests: The pupillary light reflex test should be performed as for the optic nerves, and constriction of the pupils to light observed. The presence or absence of ptosis of the upper eyelid as well as ventrolateral strabismus should be noted.

IV. Trochlear: These are the motor nerves to the dorsal oblique muscles of the eye.

Test: The eyeballs should be observed for dorsomedial strabismus (easiest to see in species with a horizontal or vertical shaped pupil).

Signs of Dysfunction: Trochlear nerve or midbrain lesions may result in ipsilateral dorsomedial strabismus.

V. Trigeminal: These nerves have 3 branches. The mandibular branch is the motor nerve to the muscles of mastication and the sensory nerve to the floor of the oral cavity, ventral arcade, and the skin of the ventrolateral head. The ophthalmic and maxillary branches are sensory to the skin of the dorsolateral head; mucous membranes of the roof of the oral cavity, the dorsal arcade, and the nasal cavity; and the eyeball, including the cornea (pain).

Tests: Jaw tone and masticatory movements should be evaluated, and the masseter and temporalis muscles palpated for atrophy to evaluate the motor component of the trigeminal nerve. The sensory function can be evaluated by touching the medial and lateral canthi of the eyelid, which elicits the **palpebral reflex** and closure of the eyelids. Stimulation of the cornea results in globe retraction. In stoic animals, sensation is tested by a pinprick to the nasal mucosa (an avoidance response will be seen).

Signs of Dysfunction: Lesions of the trigeminal nerves or pons produce temporal and masseter muscle atrophy and/or loss of sensation to the face, cornea, and nasal mucosa. A bilateral lesion of the trigeminal motor nerves produces a dropped jaw.

VI. Abducent: These are the motor nerves to the lateral rectus and retractor bulbi muscles of the eye.

Tests: The eyeballs should be observed for medial strabismus. The corneal reflex should be elicited with the eyelids held open, and the eyeball observed for retraction and the third eyelid observed for prolapse.

Signs of Dysfunction: Lesions of the abducent nerves or rostral medulla oblongata result in medial strabismus and lack of globe retraction.

VII. Facial: These are the motor nerves to the muscles of facial expression (ear, eyelids, nose, and mouth).

Tests: The menace and palpebral reflexes should be elicited to test orbicularis oculi muscle function. The nose should be examined for deviation (with unilateral lesions). The lip should be pinched to see if it retracts. The ear should be tickled to see if it moves. A Schirmer tear test should be performed to evaluate parasympathetic innervation of tear glands.

Signs of Dysfunction: A facial nerve lesion results in an inability to blink the eyelid or move the lips or nose; acutely it produces a droopy face, and food accumulates in the affected cheek. Tear and saliva production may be reduced on the side of the lesion. Later, facial muscle contractures are observed.

VIII. Vestibulocochlear: There are 2 main divisions of these nerves. The first division, the cochlear nerve, transmits auditory stimuli. The second division, the vestibular nerve, functions to maintain posture, muscle tone, and equilibrium.

Tests: Deafness is detected when loud noises do not evoke a response from an awake or sleeping animal. Unilateral deafness is best detected with a brain stem auditory evoked response (BAER) test. Head tilt, disequilibrium, and a tendency to circle, fall, or roll to one side develop with unilateral or asymmetric vestibular lesions. The animal should be examined for the presence of spontaneous nystagmus with the head held in a normal position and in a deviated position (positional nystagmus), as well as for abnormal eye position with the head elevated (positional strabismus). Normal vestibular nystagmus is seen as a few beats to the left as the head is turned to the left, and to the right as the head is turned to the right.

Signs of Dysfunction: Unilateral lesions of the vestibulocochlear nerves or rostral medulla oblongata produce disequilibrium with a head tilt toward the side of the lesion. A spontaneous or positional horizontal and rotary nystagmus is often present. A bilateral vestibular lesion results in disequilibrium on both sides, wide side-to-side excursions of the head (often with no head tilt), loss of normal vestibular nystagmus, and deafness. Occasionally, a rostral medulla oblongata lesion will result in a head tilt away from the lesion, but conscious proprioceptive deficits and hemiparesis will be ipsilateral. A unilateral cerebellar lesion results in a head tilt away from the side of the lesion with hypermetria of limbs on the ipsilateral side.

IX. Glossopharyngeal and X. Vagus: The glossopharyngeal nerves provide sensory and motor control of the pharynx and larynx, and the vagus nerves, of the viscera.

Tests: The hyoid bones should be pinched to elicit a gag reflex. The animal should be observed for normal phonation and respiratory sounds.

Signs of Dysfunction: Lesions of the glossopharyngeal and vagus nerves or caudal medulla oblongata result in dysphagia. Megaesophagus, laryngeal paresis or paralysis, and a change in phonation also occur with vagus nerve and nucleus lesions.

XI. Spinal Accessory: These nerves innervate the trapezius, sternocephalic, and brachycephalic muscles.

Tests: The muscles should be palpated.

Signs of Dysfunction: Lesions of the cranial cervical spinal cord or caudal medulla oblongata may result in muscle atrophy.

XII. Hypoglossal: These are the motor nerves to the tongue and geniohyoid muscles.

Tests: The tongue should be observed for muscular control during licking and lapping of water. The tongue curls under to lap water in dogs and cats.

Signs of Dysfunction: Lesions of the hypoglossal nerves or caudal medulla oblongata may result in deviation or atrophy of the tongue.

Evaluation of the Gait

The gait is observed while the animal walks, trots, gallops, turns, sidesteps, and backs. In large animals, ambulation up and down a grade, on and off a curb, and while blindfolded may accentuate subtle gait deficits. Evaluation of gait is especially important in ambulatory large animals because postural reactions are difficult to obtain due to size and because spinal reflexes usually are not tested unless the animals are recumbent. In small animals, subtle deficits may be detected by postural reaction testing of the limbs (*see* below) and by hemistanding and hemiwalking (standing or walking on one side). Animals with chronic lesions in the cerebral cortex and diencephalon usually have a relatively normal gait but may circle compulsively. Animals with lesions of the midbrain, pons, and medulla oblongata have paresis or paralysis of the limbs, with deficits often more severe on the side of the lesion. Cerebellar lesions produce ataxia and dysmetria. Vestibular dysfunction causes ipsilateral falling, rolling, or circling. If no abnormalities are found on evaluation of the head, but the gait is abnormal, a lesion most likely is located in the spinal cord, peripheral nerves, or muscles.

Evaluation of the Neck and Thoracic Limbs

The neck is examined for pain and, in large animals, atrophy and desensitization to pinprick, which indicate a lesion of the cervical spinal cord. Wheelbarrowing, tonic neck and eye, conscious proprioceptive positioning, placing, hopping, and righting are postural reactions that detect subtle lesions.

Wheelbarrow: The pelvic limbs of small animals are lifted slightly off the ground while keeping body posture as normal as possible, and the animal is evaluated while walking on the thoracic limbs. This test is used to detect subtle deficits of the thoracic limbs. Normal animals should not stumble or knuckle over on the toes as they walk.

Tonic Neck and Eye: With the dog or cat standing, the nose is elevated and the eyes observed to see if they coordinately adjust to the center of the palpebral fissures. In vestibular dysfunction, the eyeball on the affected side will rotate downward (positional strabismus or eye drop). Simultaneously, the thoracic limbs should extend with no tendency to knuckle or collapse, and the pelvic limbs should flex. If neck pain is present, a lesion in this area should be considered.

Conscious Proprioceptive Positioning: Each foot is displaced by turning it onto its dorsum or by abducting or adducting the limb widely. The animal should immediately replace the leg to a normal position. Lesions of the nervous system often affect conscious proprioception first.

Placing: Small animals may be carried toward a table top; on seeing the table, a normal animal anticipates placing its forepaws on the surface. If blindfolded, the animal should place the forepaws on the table only when the limbs contact the edge of the table. A loss of placing response may be present in subtle dysfunction even when the gait is normal.

Hopping: In small animals, 3 legs can be held off the ground with normal posture maintained, and the animal forced to move or hop (by being pushed laterally and forward) on the fourth limb. For large dogs and other large animals, one pelvic or thoracic limb opposite the side to be tested is held off the ground. When the animal is pushed toward the side to be tested, it should hop on the limb. Motor and proprioceptive loss, cerebellar incoordination, and cerebrocortical deficiency may be detected.

Righting: The animal is observed to see if it can right itself from lateral recumbency. A small animal suspended upside down by the hips attempts to hold its head up when the trunk is rotated from side to side and extends its forelimbs to support weight when lowered to the ground. With vestibular dysfunction, the animal twists toward the side of the lesion or curls its head under (bilateral vestibular lesions).

Spinal Reflexes: The spinal reflexes are tested with the animal in lateral recumbency and the limbs relaxed. When the toes or skin of the distal limb are pinched, that limb should withdraw and the opposite limb usually does not move. This is the **flexor or withdrawal reflex**; it is present if spinal cord segments C6 to T2 and nerves of the brachial plexus are intact. Intramedullary spinal cord lesions at C6 to T2 usually depress or abolish the reflex, but mild extramedullary lesions may produce no change. With lesions cranial to C6, a simultaneous extension of the opposite limb (the **crossed extensor reflex**) may occur when the tested limb flexes.

Other tendons (biceps and triceps) and muscles (extensor carpi radialis) may be tapped with a percussion hammer and the response evaluated to test C6-C7 or the musculocutaneous nerve, and C7 to T2 or the radial nerve, respectively. These reflexes can be difficult to obtain in normal animals, so a reduced response should be interpreted with caution. All reflexes may be normal or exaggerated with lesions above C6.

Muscle Atrophy: Focal muscle atrophy of the limbs or neck localizes the lesion to the cell body in the spinal cord, ventral spinal nerve root, or peripheral axon of the nerve that innervates that muscle.

Sensation: Conscious perception of superficial (skin) or deep (osseous) pain is tested by applying forceps to the skin or bone, respectively, and observing a behavioral response. Such a response indicates that the peripheral sensory nerve and spinal cord, as well as the pathways through the brain stem to the cortex, are intact.

If the evaluation of the head is abnormal, an initial attempt should be made to explain any thoracic limb abnormalities by a lesion above the foramen magnum. If the thoracic limb abnormalities cannot be explained by a lesion in the head, then a multifocal or diffuse disease process (such as an inflammatory, toxic, metabolic, nutritional, traumatic, or metastatic neoplastic disorder) must be present.

If there are no abnormalities on evaluation of the head, and the thoracic limbs are abnormal, then a lesion of the cervical spinal cord or brachial plexus is present. In lesions of the cervical spinal cord, the gait of the thoracic and pelvic limbs is abnormal, and pelvic limb spinal reflexes are normal or exaggerated.

If no abnormalities are found on evaluation of the head and thoracic limbs, then a lesion, if it exists, must be below the T2 spinal cord segment.

Evaluation of the Trunk, Pelvic Limbs, Anus, and Tail

The trunk of the animal is observed for abnormal posture or deviation of the vertebral column, pain, desensitization or hyperesthesia to light pinpricking, and focal muscle atrophy.

Cutaneous Trunci and Panniculus Reflex: Pinpricks applied to the skin of the thorax and abdomen result in contraction of the cutaneous trunci muscle. This reflex arc includes the afferent cutaneous branches of the lumbar and thoracic spinal nerves, a spinal cord tract that ascends to T2, and the LMN in the lateral thoracic nerve to cutaneous trunci muscles. The reflex is used to localize spinal cord lesions between the site of afferent stimulation and T2.

Postural Reactions: Wheelbarrowing, proprioceptive positioning, placing, and hopping are evaluated on the pelvic limbs in a manner similar to that used for the thoracic limbs. As with the thoracic limbs, these tests require complete integrity of the brain, spinal cord, and peripheral nerves; thus, they are not useful for localizing lesions but are useful in detecting subtle deficits that support the presence of a neurologic lesion.

Spinal Reflexes: The pelvic limb spinal reflexes are more reliable for localizing thoracolumbar lesions than are the thoracic limb reflexes. Spinal reflexes are normal or exaggerated with lesions above the reflex arc and are depressed or absent with lesions at the level of the reflex. Percussion of the patellar tendon should cause the stifle to extend if L4-L5 spinal cord segments and the femoral nerve are intact. Percussion of the gastrocnemius and cranial tibial muscles causes the hock to extend or flex, respectively, and tests the tibial and peroneal nerves, lumbosacral plexus, and L6 to S2 spinal cord segments. A crossed extensor reflex may be associated with lesions above L6. When the anus is pinched or pricked with a pin, the sphincter tightens and the tail pulls down if S1-S3 (anus) and caudal (Cd) tail segments and nerves are intact. An atonic (areflexic) bladder, anus, and tail are seen with lesions affecting S1 to Cd5 or the cauda equina.

Muscle Atrophy: Focal muscle atrophy of the trunk or pelvic limb localizes a lesion to the nerve that innervates that muscle.

Sensation: In moderate to severe spinal cord lesions, superficial sensation may be absent from the cranial aspect of the lesion caudally. In severe spinal cord lesions, deep pain is absent from the periosteum of all toes and the tail.

Schiff-Sherrington Phenomenon: In some animals with acute, severe lesions of the spinal cord between T2 and L3, the pelvic limb paralysis is accompanied by an extensor rigidity of the thoracic limbs when the animal is in lateral recumbency. Although a severe lesion produces this syndrome, the prognosis is probably not hopeless if deep pain can be elicited.

CLINICAL PATHOLOGY

Abnormalities of serum glucose, liver enzymes, BUN, bile acids, ammonia, electrolytes, or blood gases can occur with metabolic dysfunctions. Serum cholinesterase is decreased in acute organophosphate toxicity, and serum lead determinations are increased in lead toxicity. Serum thyroid and cortisol determinations and stimulation tests are useful to detect endocrinopathies. Serum titers for viral, fungal, protozoal, and rickettsial organisms can be evaluated. Serum muscle enzymes, especially creatine kinase, may be increased in myopathies. Serum muscle receptor antibodies can be detected in dogs and cats with myasthenia gravis. Muscle and nerve biopsies are essential for diagnosis and characterization of neuromuscular disorders. In some cases, brain biopsy is necessary to confirm and characterize an inflammatory or neoplastic process so that proper antimicrobial therapy, chemotherapy, or radiation therapy can be administered.

CEREBROSPINAL FLUID ANALYSIS

The analysis of CSF may further aid in determining the mechanism of a CNS disorder (especially inflammation). The technique of collection is simple and safe with practice. Analysis of CSF requires minimal special equipment. Cell counts and identification should be performed within 30 min after collection because cells begin to degenerate after that time. Several techniques are available to concentrate cells so that a differential cell count can be obtained.

CSF is collected from the cerebellomedullary cistern or the subarachnoid space in the lumbar region. An increase in protein is often associated with encephalitis, meningitis, neoplasia, or spinal cord compression. Cellular content increases most frequently with inflammation of the CNS. Neutrophils are indicative of bacterial infections, subarachnoid hemorrhage (RBC are also present), brain abscess or a steroid-responsive suppurative meningoencephalitis, or in some cases, necrosis within a tumor. Increased numbers of lymphocytes, monocytes, and neutrophils are most common in steroid-responsive nonsuppurative meningoencephalitis, granulomatous meningoencephalitis, fungal infections, toxoplasmosis, and neosporosis. Cultures of CSF may demonstrate the causative agent in bacterial and fungal infections. Paired serum and CSF immunoassays for canine distemper virus, cryptococcosis, toxoplasmosis, neosporosis, Rocky Mountain spotted fever, ehrlichiosis, and borreliosis can assist in diagnosis of these infections.

RADIOGRAPHY

Plain radiographs of the skull and vertebral column are useful to detect fractures, subluxation, infection, or neoplasia of osseous structures. In most infections or neoplastic processes of the brain and spinal cord, plain radiographs are normal. Myelography is used to detect compressive or expansive spinal cord lesions, including herniated or protruded intervertebral disks and spinal cord tumors. Computed tomography (CT) and magnetic resonance imaging (MRI) scans are useful to evaluate lesions of the brain and spinal cord in small animals. CT scans are helpful to detect changes in bone, acute hemorrhage, and CNS neoplasia. MRI scans can demonstrate neoplasia, abscesses, inflammation, and hemorrhage. Magnetic resonance angiography can be used to evaluate vascular changes in the CNS.

ELECTRODIAGNOSIS

An electroencephalogram (EEG) is a recording of the electrical activity of the cerebral cortex, which is influenced by subcortical structures. The EEG is consistently abnormal in hydrocephalus, meningoencephalitis, head trauma, and cerebral neoplasia. An EEG may determine whether seizure discharges are focal or diffuse. The EEG is often normal in idiopathic epilepsy, unless seizures are not well controlled and interictal spikes are present.

An electromyogram (EMG) is a recording of the electrical activity of muscles and is used to evaluate the health of the peripheral nerve, neuromuscular junction, and skeletal muscle. The peripheral nerve can be stimulated, and motor and sensory nerve conduction velocities calculated. Repetitive nerve stimulation may lead to a reduction of the evoked potential in myasthenia gravis and distal axonopathies. Abnormalities of late waves may be associated with disorders of nerve roots.

The brain stem auditory evoked response (BAER) is a recording of electrical activity in the auditory pathway from the inner ear receptors through the brain stem to the cerebral cortex. No response is seen in auditory nerve disorders associated with hearing loss. Brain-stem disorders may also alter the BAER.

Spinal cord evoked potentials and motor evoked potentials can be used to evaluate spinal cord integrity.

PRINCIPLES OF THERAPY

See also SYSTEMIC PHARMACOTHERAPEUTICS OF THE NERVOUS SYSTEM, p 2014.

Seizure Control: Status epilepticus (continuous or cluster seizures) in dogs and cats may be interrupted by diazepam, given at 0.5 mg/kg (not to exceed 10 mg at one time), IV. Sodium pentobarbital to effect, not to exceed 3-15 mg/kg, IV, may also be used, followed by phenobarbital at 2-4 mg/kg, IM, every 6 hr. Diazepam given at 0.1-2 mg/kg/hr, IV, may be used to control persistent status epilepticus. Oral anticonvulsants should be resumed as soon as possible if currently being given.

Recommended maintenance anticonvulsant therapy in dogs and cats is phenobarbital at 2-4 mg/kg, PO, BID-TID as needed to control seizures or to maintain serum levels at 25-30 μg/mL. Dogs can be treated with potassium bromide (KBr), 22 mg/kg, BID with food until the serum level is 1,500-4,000 μg/mL 3 mo after initiation of therapy. Phenobarbital is good for animals with seizures multiple times weekly as it may become clinically effective in 72 hr, whereas KBr may take several weeks. KBr bypasses the liver so it is better than phenobarbital in animals with liver disease. Phenobarbital and KBr may be given in combination. KBr may cause asthma in cats. Since KBr is not commercially available, it may be prepared by a compounding pharmacist by mixing chemical grade KBr crystals in water at a concentration of 125 mg/mL or 250 mg/mL. Once the effective dose is obtained, the crystals may be packed in gelatin capsules. Because KBr is toxic to people, owners are advised to wear gloves while medicating the dog. KBr serum levels are affected by the salt content of the diet, so the diet should be consistent. KBr has proved more efficacious in dogs with cluster seizures than phenobarbital. Other oral anticonvulsants are rarely used because of side effects, ineffectiveness, or expense. Diazepam at 0.5-1 mg/kg, PO, BID, may be used in cats with uncontrolled seizures on phenobarbital; it is not an effective oral anticonvulsant in dogs. A compounding pharmacist can prepare rectal suppositories containing diazepam 0.5-2 mg/kg for use at home in dogs with cluster seizures. Acupuncture may be useful to control seizures in all species.

Acute Spinal Cord Injury: Acute spinal cord injury from trauma, intervertebral disk herniation, or fibrocartilaginous embolization resulting in paraplegia must be treated aggressively in dogs to ensure the best chance for recovery. Methylprednisolone sodium succinate or prednisolone sodium succinate is given at 30 mg/kg, IV, followed by 15 mg/kg in 2 and 6 hr, then 2.5 mg/kg/hr as a constant IV infusion. Dexamethasone is not rapid-acting enough to use. Oral famotidine at 0.5-1 mg/kg, SID or BID, cimetidine at 5-10 mg/kg, BID, or misoprostol at 3 μg/kg, BID, can be used to protect the GI tract. For maximum benefit, decompressive spinal surgery should be performed as soon as possible, usually within 24 hr, when indicated.

Anti-inflammatory Drugs: For control of CNS inflammation in dogs and cats unassociated with a virus or other agent, either prednisone at 2 mg/kg or dexamethasone at

0.2 mg/kg may be given PO, SID. Oral famotidine at 0.5-1 mg/kg, SID or BID; cimetidine at 5-10 mg/kg, BID; or misoprostol at 3 µg/kg, BID, is given to prevent GI irritation. If GI ulcers develop and melena is detected, sucralfate (500 mg for cats and dogs <20 kg; 1 g for dogs >20 kg), PO, TID-QID, is given 2 hr apart from other drugs. Phenylbutazone, carprofen, etodolac, or aspirin should never be given in conjunction with steroids as GI ulceration is common. The dosages of all steroids given should be slowly tapered; abrupt withdrawal should be avoided. Prednisone can be used as longterm maintenance therapy on alternate days to avoid complete suppression of adrenal function.

Antiedema Drugs: After cranial surgery and in animals with brain tumors or head injuries causing a declining neurologic status, 20% mannitol, 1-2 g/kg, may be given slowly IV. Mannitol is not given in spinal cord injuries. Use of methylprednisolone sodium succinate as described above for acute spinal cord injury reduces edema as well.

Muscle Relaxants: Diazepam at 0.5 mg/kg or methocarbamol at 40 mg/kg, PO, TID-QID, relieves muscle spasms from intervertebral disk protrusion and other sources of nerve root irritation.

Antimicrobial Therapy: Refer to discussions of specific infections for antimicrobial therapy recommendations.

Nursing Care: Animals with paraplegia and quadriplegia need intensive nursing care. The animal should be maintained on padding and turned every 4-6 hr to avoid decubital ulcers. The bladder must be expressed or catheterized every 6-8 hr. Urine must be monitored for evidence of cystitis. The skin must be kept clean and free of urine and feces to prevent dermatitis. Quadriplegic animals may need to be hand fed nutritious food and given plenty of water. Manual extension and flexion of joints and muscle massage will help delay contractures and muscle atrophy in paralyzed limbs.

BOVINE SPONGIFORM ENCEPHALOPATHY

Bovine spongiform encephalopathy (BSE) is a progressive, fatal, neurologic disease of adult domestic cattle that resembles scrapie of sheep and goats (p 1071). It was first diagnosed in Britain in 1986.

BSE has been transmitted experimentally to mice, pigs, sheep, goats, cattle, mink, Macaque monkeys, and marmosets. During the epidemic of BSE in Great Britain, small numbers of cases of spongiform encephalopathy were seen in several species of captive bred ungulates (nyala, gemsbok, eland, arabian oryx, kudu, scimitar oryx, ankole cow, and bison) and in 5 species of felids (puma, cheetah, ocelot, lion, and tiger) either kept in or originating from British zoologic collections. A low incidence has been seen in domestic cats in the British Isles, with one isolated case in Norway. The ungulates were infected from the same foodborne source as cattle (*see* below), and all species of felids were most likely infected by consuming infected bovine tissues.

Only the UK has experienced a significant epidemic that, at its peak at the end of 1992, represented an annual incidence of ~1% of adult cattle. Lower incidences have been seen in indigenous cattle in Ireland, France, Switzerland, the Netherlands, Portugal, Germany, Denmark, Italy, Spain, Austria, Belgium, the Czech Republic, Finland, Greece, Israel, Japan, Liechtenstein, Luxembourg, Poland, Canada, Slovakia, and Slovenia. BSE has been detected in the majority of these countries as a result of active surveillance (*see* below). Cases in animals exported from Great Britain have been seen in Canada, the Falkland Islands, and the Sultanate of Oman. Cattle populations in other countries may have become infected as a result of the importation of cattle and/or ruminant-derived meat and bone meal from countries with the disease.

Etiology: The molecular nature of the agent causing BSE is uncertain. The disease is associated with an abnormal form of a membrane protein, PrP (prion protein). This has led to the prion hypothesis for which this abnormal protein is assumed to be the infectious agent. These agents, in addition to causing scrapie in sheep, cause transmissible mink encephalopathy (p 1547), chronic wasting disease of deer and elk (p 993), and kuru and Creutzfeldt-Jakob disease, Gerstmann-Sträussler-Scheinker syndrome, and fatal familial insomnia in humans.

Transmission, Epidemiology, and Pathogenesis: BSE develops as a result of food-borne exposure to a scrapie-like agent via contaminated meat and bone meal included in cattle rations. There is no evidence that transmission occurs naturally between cattle; however, there is some evidence suggesting a maternally-associated risk for calves born to affected cows.

There is no sex or breed predisposition, and no genotypic variation in susceptibility as there is in sheep to the scrapie agent. The modal age at onset is 5 yr, with a range from 2 yr to the extent of the commercial lifespan of cattle. The incidence within affected herds is generally low; in the peak year of the epidemic in Britain, an average of 2% of cattle developed clinical disease in affected herds.

The details of pathogenesis are unknown, but studies indicate that after oral exposure the agent replicates in the Peyer's patches of the ileum followed by migration, via peripheral nerves, to the CNS.

Clinical Findings: Initial clinical signs are subtle and behavioral in nature. The spectrum increases and progresses over weeks to months, with most animals reaching a terminal state by 3 mo after clinical onset. With repeated examinations, a reduced time spent ruminating can be detected by an experienced clinician; an increased frequency of nose licking, sneezing or snorting, nose wrinkling, head rubbing and tossing, and tooth grinding are all indicative of a disturbance of the trigeminal sensory nerve. Restrained animals exhibit exaggerated responses to the menace reflex, the corneal reflex, and sensation of nasal mucosae; frenzy, head shyness, and kicking also occur. Unrestrained animals in familiar environments demonstrate an increased startle response to unexpected visual, auditory, or tactile stimuli. If undisturbed, animals with advanced disease appear to have general hypokinesis, with long periods spent standing or idling with a low head carriage and a fixed, staring facial expression. Locomotory signs of gait ataxia, hypermetria, falling, and generalized paresis eventually become dominant. Weight loss and decreased milk production are common. Tremors and muscle fasciculations occur, but intense pruritus of the trunk, as seen in sheep scrapie, is rare. Euthanasia is advisable as soon as there is some certainty of the clinical diagnosis because animals become unmanageable and their welfare is at risk.

Lesions: Lesions are confined to histologic changes in the CNS and comprise bilateral, usually symmetric, vacuolation of gray matter neuropil (spongiosis) and neurons, similar to the lesions seen in scrapie. Gross pathologic changes associated with falling and recumbency may be present.

Diagnosis: Repeated clinical examinations do not provide a definitive diagnosis. The accepted international confirmatory diagnostic methods on the hindbrain are histopathology, immunohistochemistry (IHC), and electron microscopy, after detergent extraction, for scrapie-associated fibrils to detect abnormal PrP. The last 2 methods can be used on autolyzed brain tissue and IHC positivity precedes morphologic, vacuolar changes. Two specific ELISA methods and a Western immunoblot method are available for active surveillance of cattle populations.

The furious form of rabies (p 1067) has clinical similarities, but the clinical course of BSE is more protracted. Other differential diagnoses include encephalitic listeriosis (p 531), hypomagnesemia (p 812), lead poisoning (p 2404), downer cow syndrome (p 957), nervous ketosis, intracranial abscess or tumors, lesions in the CNS, and trauma to the spinal column. The protracted clinical course of the disease is helpful in differentiation, but in a small proportion of cases the clinical duration is short (days or weeks), and the extent that animals have been observed needs to be considered.

Treatment and Control: Treatment is ineffective. Control has been effected in Britain and other European countries by the statutory prohibition of the use of mammalian-derived protein in the rations for all farm animal species. The USA has also banned the use of such proteins as a preventive measure.

Zoonotic Risk: A novel variant of Creutzfeldt-Jakob disease (vCJD) in the human population in Great Britain, initially seen in 1996, has been associated with the emergence of the BSE agent. Cases of vCJD have been seen outside Britain. A proportion of the affected individuals had been living in Britain, but cases have been seen in Italy and France among people who had not visited Britain. Infection of humans is presumed to result from eating infected bovine tissues. As a result, BSE-affected countries have introduced the statutory removal of high-risk bovine tissues from the human food chain. No cases of vCJD have been seen in laboratory workers, but appropriate safety precautions for handling the BSE agent and conducting necropsies of cattle suspected of being infected are recommended. Safety precautions should primarily be aimed at avoiding accidental ocular or oronasal exposures.

CHRONIC WASTING DISEASE

Chronic wasting disease (CWD) is a contagious disease of captive and free-ranging deer and elk that causes progressive, fatal CNS disease in adult animals. It is a member of the transmissible spongiform encephalopathy (TSE) family of diseases that includes bovine spongiform encephalopathy of cattle; scrapie of sheep and goats; transmissible mink encephalopathy of farmed mink; and kuru, Creutzfeldt-Jakob disease (CJD), and variant CJD of humans. CWD was first identified as a clinical syndrome in the late 1960s among captive mule deer in Colorado; a decade later, it was recognized to be a spongiform encephalopathy with characteristics similar to those of scrapie. It is found in free-ranging populations of mule deer, white-tailed deer, and elk (wapiti) in southeastern and southcentral Wyoming, northern Colorado, northwestern Nebraska, and southwestern South Dakota and in a population of white-tailed deer in southcentral Wisconsin. Small numbers of free-ranging deer in other states have been identified by intensive testing; it is not yet known if these represent endemic foci. CWD has also been found in farmed elk and white-tailed deer in a number of western states and Canadian provinces and a few midwestern states. CWD has been identified outside of North America only once; a few elk imported into Korea from Canada had CWD. Many states and provinces have developed regulations for control and management of CWD in farmed populations, federal regulations are in place in Canada, and federal regulations for CWD are pending in the USA. It is a reportable disease in some jurisdictions.

Etiology: The etiology of CWD, as with the other TSE, is thought to be a protein with abnormal conformation (ie, protease-resistant prion protein). These disease-associated proteins are derived from normal host cell surface glycoproteins (designated cellular prion protein or PrP^C). Disease-associated proteins cause PrP^C to assume an abnormal conformation that is rich in β-pleated sheets and highly resistant to cellular processes that break down normal proteins. Thus it accumulates, primarily in the CNS and, in some TSE, in lymphoid tissue.

CWD is known to naturally affect only mule deer, white-tailed deer, and elk. Experimentally, CWD can be transmitted by intracerebral inoculation to cattle, sheep, goats, domestic ferrets, mink, mice, hamsters, and squirrel monkeys. A large study to investigate susceptibility of cattle by the more natural route of oral or contact exposure began in 1997; as of January 2004, there was no evidence of CWD in the experimental animals. The origin of the disease, however, is unknown.

Transmission, Epidemiology, and Pathogenesis: CWD is transmitted horizontally either directly from an affected animal or via indirect environmental contamination. While maternal transmission cannot be ruled out, it does not appear to be important. The exact mechanisms of transmission are still being studied. The agent probably enters a susceptible host via ingestion and is taken up by lymphoid tissues associated with the alimentary tract. The agent most likely arrives in the brain by retrograde movement up the vagus nerve and its roots to the dorsal motor nucleus of the vagus at the obex region of the medulla oblongata. It continues to accumulate in the brain, involving more areas, and in the lymphoid tissues throughout the body during the incubation period. Spongiform lesions in the brain develop first in the vagal nucleus at about the time of onset of clinical disease. This occurs naturally with an incubation period of ~1.5-3 yr, although maximum incubation periods have yet to be determined. Prevalence in captive herds of deer and elk may reach nearly 100% in heavily contaminated facilities; prevalence in free-ranging cervids is extremely variable from <1% to ~30%. It is not known how the CWD agent exits an infected animal, but excretions and secretions are thought to be important. Research is focusing on the potential role of feces in transmission, although other routes are possible. Because all prions are highly resistant to environmental and chemical inactivation, they may accumulate in the environment and thus be available to infect susceptible cervids. Environmental contamination may be important in CWD. In free-ranging populations, decomposing carcasses may provide a source of infectivity to susceptible animals.

The movement of CWD in populations of free-ranging deer and elk follows natural migration routes, often along waterways and natural corridors. In the past, movement of CWD in farmed deer and elk in commerce was through human-facilitated transportation of animals incubating CWD. Now that programs and regulations are in place in most jurisdictions, movement of CWD in live animals should be curtailed. Surveillance, however, should continue.

Clinical Findings: Animals with clinical CWD are >16 mo of age and show a spectrum of signs. The earliest and most difficult to appreciate are subtle changes in behavior and weight loss. These changes are often detectable only by animal caregivers familiar with the individual animal. As the disease progresses, behavioral changes may include alterations in how the animal interacts with herdmates and caregivers, loss of wariness, somnolence, persistent walking, polydipsia and polyuria, and hyperexcitability when handled. Affected animals may show variable locomotor signs including ataxia (especially posterior ataxia) and head tremors. Late in the disease, animals may have a low head carriage, drooped ears, and fixed staring gaze; they may hypersalivate and grind their teeth. Death following routine chemical immobilization has been noted. Aspiration pneumonia may be the only presenting clinical sign; CWD should be suspected in any adult cervid with aspiration pneumonia. Weight loss is progressive throughout the course of disease, even when adequate feed is present, but it is important to recognize that CWD may be present in cervids that are not emaciated. Death of CWD-affected animals may be precipitated by cold weather or other acute stressors.

Lesions: Some animals may die of CWD without gross lesions. When present, gross lesions are nonspecific and reflect the clinical signs. The most common are poor body condition, watery rumen contents, and dilute urine. Aspiration pneumonia in farmed cervids is often the proximal cause of death. Samples should be, and in many jurisdictions are required to be, submitted to certified laboratories to be tested for evidence of CWD. It is good practice either to send the carcass to the diagnostic laboratory or to collect a wide variety of samples so that if diseases other than CWD are present they will be identified. At a minimum, samples for CWD testing should include brain and retropharyngeal lymph nodes. Many laboratories accept whole heads from cervids for testing. Surveillance programs for free-ranging cervids vary depending on the jurisdiction and are usually conducted by the local wildlife management agency, which should be consulted if CWD is suspected in a free-ranging deer or elk.

Diagnosis: Diagnosis of CWD is by detecting disease-associated PrP in CNS or lymphoid tissues. Detection of spongiform encephalopathy by routine histopathology has been supplanted by more sensitive and specific tests, which include immunohistochemistry or ELISA on brain and/or lymph nodes. In the USA, these tests are run only at USDA-certified laboratories. In mule deer and white-tailed deer, the CWD PrP accumulates in the retropharyngeal lymph node prior to arriving in the brain; thus, it is considered to be the most important tissue to collect for testing. Both brain and lymph node samples should be collected from elk. The correct portion of the brain (ie, the obex, at the caudal end of the fourth ventricle below the cerebellum) must be collected for a meaningful test. The laboratory should be consulted to determine if the samples must be fixed in 10% buffered formalin, chilled or frozen, or if portions of the samples should be sent both fixed and frozen. ELISA is used as a screening test, and immunohistochemistry, which is considered the preferred test, is used to confirm positive ELISA.

Differential diagnoses for animals suspected of CWD include brain abscesses, traumatic injuries, meningitis, encephalitis, peritonitis, pneumonia, arthritis, starvation and nutritional deficiencies, dental attrition, and anesthetic deaths.

Treatment and Control: There are no treatments available for any TSE. Control in farmed cervids is by depopulation with indemnity and development of herd plans. These plans typically require 5 yr of monitoring to achieve the highest status. The bases for CWD control programs in the farmed cervid industry are individual animal identification, CWD testing in all animals in the herd that die over a certain age, and limiting new herd additions to animals from herds of comparable or higher CWD status.

Control of CWD in free-ranging populations is extremely difficult and varies depending on the location. All jurisdictions have banned movement of live cervids from endemic areas for translocations, and many have regulations on movement of parts of hunted deer and elk. In areas where CWD occurs, attempts at control have included population reduction, test and removal, and intensified surveillance.

Only a few disinfectants and methods of disposal inactivate prions. Fresh household bleach at 50% concentration for 30-60 min will inactivate the agent and is inexpensive and readily available, but it may be corrosive to some surfaces and instruments. Additional disinfectants are being considered for general use but are not yet approved. Incineration in a medical incinerator, alkaline digestion in specially designed equipment, and disposal in municipal landfills are used for disposal of tissues and carcasses of animals with CWD.

Zoonotic Risk: Although CWD has been present in hunted populations of deer and elk for >30 yr, no case of human CWD has been identified. The risk to humans appears to be minimal. However, public health authorities and wildlife management agencies suggest the following precautions for hunters and people handling cervids in the areas where CWD is found to further reduce risk of human exposure: do not harvest deer or elk that appear to be sick or abnormal; wear rubber, plastic, or latex gloves when dressing the carcass; avoid contact with brain, spinal cord, and lymphoid tissues; debone the meat when processing; disinfect knives, saws, and tables with 50% bleach; and have the animal tested for CWD. All pubic health authorities recommend that animals positive for any TSE not be consumed by humans or other animals.

CONGENITAL AND INHERITED ANOMALIES OF THE NERVOUS SYSTEM

Congenital defects of the CNS are, by definition, present at birth. Some congenital defects are known to be inherited, others are caused by environmental factors (toxic plants, nutritional deficiencies, viral infections); for many, the cause is unknown. In those animals born with a well-developed nervous system (foals, calves, lambs, pigs), the clinical signs of a congenital neurologic disorder may actually be recognizable at birth. Kittens and puppies are born with a less well-developed nervous system, and in those species, neurologic signs may not be apparent until they begin to walk. In some instances, clinical signs of an inherited disorder are not seen until the animal is an adult, even though the defect has obviously been present since birth.

Congenital lesions can be categorized according to the primary region of the CNS affected: **Forebrain disorders** (cerebrum and thalamus) primarily result in clinical signs such as visual disturbances, changes in mental status or behavior, abnormal movements or postures, and seizures. **Cerebellar disorders** usually result in an intention tremor and incoordination (dysmetria) of both the head and limbs. **Spinal cord disorders** do not affect cerebral function and normal coordination of head movement but produce motor dysfunction or proprioceptive deficits, including either dysmetria or reduced paw position sense in more than one limb. (*See also* DISEASES OF THE SPINAL COLUMN AND CORD, p 1017.) **Peripheral nerve and muscle disorders** can result in signs of weakness and ataxia similar to those seen in spinal cord disease. In addition, they often cause widespread disturbance of reflex function, pain sensation, or marked muscle atrophy. **Multifocal disorders** result in combinations of signs from more than one of these categories of neurologic deficits.

CEREBRAL DISORDERS

Large Animals

Anencephaly means that the brain is largely absent at birth. It is a rare disorder but is seen sporadically in calves; the cause is unknown. Because the pituitary gland may also be absent, prolonged gestation (p 1137) of affected calves can occur. Signs include profound lethargy, head pressing, and blindness with normal pupillary reflexes. Cerebral aplasia in calves is usually associated with complete absence of both cerebral hemispheres, and CSF may leak out of a small opening on the midline between the frontal bones.

Exencephaly means that the brain is exposed through a large defect in the skull (cranium bifida). The brain (encephalocele), meninges (meningocele), or both (meningoencephalocele) may protrude through this opening. Encephalocele and meningocele are inherited in pigs.

In **hydranencephaly**, there is a marked loss of cerebral cortical tissue (primarily the neocortex) within a cranial vault of normal conformation. The resultant cavity communicates with the ventricular system, has an incomplete ependymal cell lining, and is filled with CSF. Hydranencephaly develops as a result of the destruction of developing neural tissues and is sometimes accompanied by cerebellar hypoplasia and arthrogryposis. Hydranencephaly is seen sporadically or as an epidemic in calves, lambs, and less commonly in piglets. Known causes include infection in utero with a number of viruses, including Akabane virus (p 501) in ruminants in Australia, Japan, and Israel; bluetongue virus (p 590) in sheep and cattle in North America; Rift Valley fever virus (p 617) and the virus of Wesselsbron disease (p 624) in sheep and cattle in Africa; the Cache Valley virus in sheep in the USA; and the Chuzan virus in calves in Japan. Rarely, bovine viral diarrhea (p 220) and Border disease virus (p 503) produce hydranencephaly in lambs and calves. Hydranencephaly and porencephaly (cystic cavities in the cerebrum) are seen sometimes in lambs with in utero copper deficiency (swayback). It also is seen in a syndrome of prolonged gestation in sheep in Scotland (cause unknown). Clinical signs may include lethargy, propulsive circling, head pressing, and blindness.

Hydrocephalus, an increase in volume of the CSF, can appear similar to hydranencephaly, but in hydrocephalus the ventricles retain a complete ependymal lining. There may be extensive expansion of the lateral ventricles in the frontal lobes. Hydrocephalus is seen sporadically in all large animals, although it is relatively common in calves, in which inheritance and vitamin A deficiency have been implicated.

Cyclopia is characterized by a single orbital fossa. One cause in lambs is ingestion by the gestating dam of plant alkaloids from *Veratrum californicum*. This malformation also is seen in pigs.

Idiopathic or familial epilepsy has been described in many species. Benign epilepsy is seen in young foals, particularly Arabians, up to 12 mo of age. The foal may present either for seizures, or for head injuries or postictal blindness. Foals usually recover spontaneously within a few months, but anticonvulsant therapy (phenobarbital, 100-500 mg, PO, BID, for a 50-kg foal) is probably advisable for 1-3 mo, followed by withdrawal over 2 wk. Epilepsy beginning by 1 yr of age has been recorded in Brown Swiss and Swedish Red cattle. Seizures are also seen in young Aberdeen Angus calves; if these calves survive, they show cerebellar signs but become clinically normal by 2 yr of age.

Metabolic disorders and lysosomal storage disorders often cause signs of forebrain dysfunction, along with other neurologic deficits, and are discussed further under multifocal disorders (p 1006). Cerebral signs seem to be most prominent in citrullinemia.

Citrullinemia is a fatal hereditary metabolic defect of Holstein-Friesian calves (mainly in Australia and New Zealand) associated with cerebral cortical edema. It is due to increased citrulline in plasma, caused by deficiency of the urea cycle enzyme argininosuccinate synthetase. Affected calves appear healthy at birth but die of acute neurologic disease in 1-4 days. Signs are sudden in onset and consist of depression, aimless wandering, blindness, seizures, opisthotonos, and recumbency.

Narcolepsy, a disorder of sleep-wake control (typically characterized by excessive sleepiness or sudden paroxysmal attacks of flaccid paralysis with conservation of consciousness), has been reported in several equine breeds, particularly Shetland ponies. The animal is otherwise healthy. During narcoleptic episodes, rapid eye movements occur, and at the same time, the animal may also show cataplexy or sudden loss of muscle tone with collapse.

Small Animals

The same structural anomalies of the brain as described for large animals (see above) are also found in small animals.

Hydranencephaly has been described mainly in kittens after in utero exposure to feline panleukopenia virus/parvovirus (p 635). Brain stem malformations and cerebellar hypoplasia may be seen concomitantly.

Hydrocephalus is most common in dogs, particularly in toy and brachycephalic breeds. It can be classified as communicating (nonobstructive), in which CSF can flow freely into the subarachnoid space, or noncommunicating (obstructive). Known causes of noncommunicating hydrocephalus include atresia of the mesencephalic aqueduct, perinatal encephalitis, or adhesions caused by intraventricular hemorrhage at birth. Clinical signs of hydrocephalus usually indicate cerebral dysfunction and often progress, although some animals may remain asymptomatic. The fontanelles are often patent, and affected animals may have ventrolateral strabismus. Blindness due to polymicrogyria (excessive number of smaller gyri) and asymmetric dilatations of the lateral ventricles have been described in Standard Poodles. Hydrocephalus has been observed in Saint Bernard puppies in association with aphakia (absence of the lens) and multiple ocular defects. Imaging by ultrasonography (through the fontanelle), computed tomography, or MRI can provide the diagnosis, and CSF analysis should identify encephalitis. Treatment relies on either corticosteroids or surgery to shunt CSF into the peritoneum.

Lissencephaly, an absence or reduction of cerebral gyri, is a rare disorder that is seen in Lhasa Apsos. It is also seen in association with cerebellar hypoplasia in Irish Setters, Wirehaired Fox Terriers, and Samoyeds and in Korat cats with microencephaly. The clinical signs of lissencephaly consist of mild behavioral abnormalities and seizures.

Pug encephalitis is an ultimately fatal disease that may have a familial basis. Dogs show behavioral changes, seizures, and CSF pleocytosis. A similar nonsuppurative, necrotizing encephalitis has been reported in both Yorkshire Terriers and Maltese Terriers.

Idiopathic epilepsy may be inherited in certain breeds, including Beagles, Keeshonden, Irish Setters, Belgian Tervurens, Siberian Huskies, Springer Spaniels, Labrador Retrievers, Golden Retrievers, and German Shepherds. A specific type of seizure known as temporal lobe epilepsy appears to be familial in Cavalier King Charles Spaniels and is characterized by behavioral manifestations such as fly biting. The diagnosis of idiopathic epilepsy depends on eliminating other causes of seizures, particularly structural brain abnormalities (such as hydrocephalus), encephalitis, or metabolic causes (such as hepatic encephalopathy).

Hepatic encephalopathy is usually caused by a congenital portosystemic shunt. The shunt may be a single large vessel, or there may be microscopic shunting of blood within the liver. Breeds often affected include Miniature Schnauzers, Yorkshire Terriers, Cairn Terriers, Australian Cattle Dogs, Old English Sheepdogs, and Maltese Terriers. The clinical signs are usually noticed before 6 mo of age and primarily reflect cerebral dysfunction, including staring into space, inappropriate vocalizing, aggression, and agitation. Advanced neurologic alterations can cause depression, blindness, myoclonus, stupor, coma, or seizures. In cats, these signs are often accompanied by excessive salivation. A rare cause of hepatic encephalopathy is a deficiency of hepatic urea cycle enzymes. Diagnosis may be facilitated by use of radiographic imaging techniques, such as positive contrast portography, computed tomography, transcolonic portal scintigraphy, or diagnostic gray-scale ultrasonography.

Lysosomal storage disorders that commonly cause seizures include ceroid lipofuscinosis and fucosidosis (see MULTIFOCAL DISORDERS, p 1006).

Puppy hypoglycemia is an idiopathic syndrome in toy breeds of dogs that is seen in the first 6 mo of life. It seems to relate to a relative immaturity of the liver and can usually be managed by providing frequent meals of a commercial puppy diet. The problem usually resolves as the animal matures.

Narcolepsy or cataplexy is inherited in Doberman Pinschers, Labrador Retrievers, and Dachshunds and has been described in additional canine breeds. It is rare in cats. It must be differentiated from various types of syncope. Physostigmine (0.025-0.1 mg/kg, IV) potentiates the frequency and severity of cataleptic attacks. Imipramine (0.5-1.0 mg/kg, PO, TID) can be used to control the severity of the cataplexy.

CEREBELLAR DISORDERS

Large Animals

Arnold-Chiari malformation is a complex malformation of the caudal brain stem and cerebellum, and typically consists of herniation of cerebellar tissue through the foramen magnum into the cervical spinal canal. It may be associated with spina bifida, hydrocephalus, or meningomyelocele. It is rare in domestic animals, and the cause is unknown. In calves, it may be seen with bilateral elongation and extension of the occipital lobes.

Cerebellar hypoplasia has been described in many species. In utero viral infection (bovine viral diarrhea [p 220], bluetongue virus [p 590], and swine fever virus [p 570]) during midgestation is the most common cause. Cerebellar lesions may also be seen with bovine fetuses infected with Akabane or Wesselsbron viruses. Clinical or subclinical hydranencephaly and arthrogryposis may accompany the cerebellar disease. The pathologic features include destruction or loss of one or more layers of the cerebellar cortex, particularly the granule and Purkinje cell layers. Prophylactic vaccination of the dam before breeding can prevent the problem. A hereditary cerebellar hypoplasia/dysplasia is seen in Hereford, Shorthorn, Ayrshire, and Angus calves. Cerebellar hypoplasia is present at birth and is nonprogressive, in distinction to the abiotrophies.

Cerebellar abiotrophies have been reported in many species. In abiotrophies, the cerebellar development proceeds normally, and the animal remains unaffected for a period of months or even years before cerebellar neurons begin to die off prematurely. This is in contrast to the cerebellar hypoplasias, in which developing cerebellar germinal cells and neurons are destroyed in utero. In Aberdeen-Angus calves, clinical signs of abiotrophy start early and are accompanied initially by seizures. In Arabian foals and Swedish Gottland ponies, the onset of signs is from birth to 9 mo; in Yorkshire and Large White piglets, 1-3 mo; in Holstein calves, 3-8 mo; and in Merino sheep, 3-6 yr. Most abiotrophies are probably inherited (eg, recessive inheritance for affected Hereford cattle and Welsh Mountain and Corriedale sheep), but toxic etiologies should also be considered. The latter include locoweed, methylmercury, and exposure to organophosphates in utero (p 2398). Use of trichlorfon during pregnancy can cause a congenital tremor in piglets due to both cerebellar hypoplasia and hypomyelination.

Hypomyelinogenesis congenita, in which myelination is delayed throughout the CNS, can resemble cerebellar disease due to the severe head and body tremor that usually develops. In contrast to pure cerebellar disease, a persistent fine tremor at rest is usually present as well as a marked intention tremor. Newborn lambs, piglets, and occasionally calves are affected. The condition can be associated with in utero infection by viruses such as the virus of Border disease (p 503) or swine fever virus (p 570) or exposure to trichlorfon (p 2400). Affected lambs are often called "hairy shakers." The condition is inherited in Saddleback and Landrace pigs, and in Jersey and Shorthorn cattle. Signs are usually nonprogressive or may resolve completely if myelination has only been delayed.

Swayback or enzootic ataxia is largely due to copper deficiency, although there may be a familial predisposition. Hypomyelinogenesis can occur in utero, and cause obtundation, blindness/deafness, falling or lying prostrate, and head tremor in lambs. The condition can be prevented by treating affected ewes in pregnancy. Kids, piglets, and perhaps calves may also be affected.

Small Animals

Cerebellar hypoplasia is seen in kittens after in utero infection with feline panleukopenia virus (p 635). The condition is nonprogressive, and affected animals may make suitable pets. Diagnosis can be obtained antemortem using MRI. Concomitant hydrocephalus or hydranencephaly may also be seen. Cerebellar hypoplasia has also been reported in Chow Chows and is seen in association with lissencephaly in Irish Setters and Wirehaired Fox Terriers. A selective hypoplasia of the cerebellar vermis is also seen in dogs, and when combined with hydrocephalus and cyst-like dilatation of the fourth ventricle, the condition has been termed the Dandy-Walker syndrome, which may have a familial basis.

Cerebellar abiotrophies have been described in a number of breeds of dogs. In Samoyeds and Beagles, the signs are apparent at the onset of ambulation; in Australian Kelpies, Rough-coated Collies, and Kerry Blue Terriers, the clinical signs are seen in puppies from 4-16 wk of age; and in Brittany Spaniels, Old English Sheepdogs, and Gordon Setters, the signs appear in young or mature adults.

Congenital hypomyelination is seen as a familial/inherited disorder in Springer Spaniels, Chow Chows, Weimaraners, and Bernese Mountain Dogs, usually with signs developing around 2-8 wk of age. In the latter 3 breeds, it is often termed dysmyelination because the clinical signs of whole body tremor usually resolve spontaneously with time. The disorder is rare in cats. The diagnosis can be confirmed using MRI. (*See also* p 1009.)

SPINAL CORD DISORDERS

See also DISEASES OF THE SPINAL COLUMN AND CORD, p 1017.

Large Animals

Spinal muscular atrophy is 1 of 3 inherited disorders of Brown Swiss calves (*see also* bovine progressive degenerative myeloencephalopathy [BPDME] and spinal dysmyelination, below). The first clinical sign of spinal muscular atrophy is weakness of the pelvic limbs at 2-6 wk of age; calves (the majority are female) have difficulty getting up and then become recumbent. The characteristic sign is severe muscle atrophy, especially of the pelvic limbs. Histopathologic examination reveals degeneration and loss of motor neurons in the ventral horns of the spinal cord. Neurogenic atrophy of muscles is a consistent lesion. A similar disorder is seen in red Danish calves of American Brown Swiss lines. It is possible that spinal muscular atrophy and BPDME are in some way related because they can be seen in the same blood lines, but the onset of BDPME occurs after 5 mo of age, and it causes ataxia and dysmetria rather than weakness and muscle atrophy. A motor neuron disease with neurofilament accumulation is seen in horned Hereford cattle in Canada with signs appearing soon after birth that are characterized by general tremors, incoordination, difficulty standing, and hyperesthesia to tactile stimulation. A suspected hereditary lower motor neuron disease with accumulation of neurofilaments also is seen in Yorkshire pigs around 5 wk of age, characterized by pelvic limb paresis progressing to recumbency. There is degeneration and loss of motor neurons throughout the spinal cord and brain stem. A similar condition is seen in young Hampshire pigs.

Bovine progressive degenerative myeloencephalopathy (BPDME, weaver syndrome) is a neurodegenerative disorder of Brown Swiss cattle that is seen in the

USA, Canada, and Europe. Four basic criteria are required to establish a clinical diagnosis: 1) onset of bilateral pelvic limb ataxia and dysmetria at 5-8 mo of age; 2) deficient proprioceptive responses, ataxia in all 4 limbs, and progressive paraparesis; 3) normal spinal reflexes and cranial nerve function and absence of dramatic muscle atrophy; and 4) a familial relationship. The disease was initially described as "weaver" because of the peculiar weaving gait. The histopathologic changes are primarily in the sensory nervous system, in contrast to those of spinal muscular atrophy (see above). Spinal dysmyelination causes congenital lateral recumbency and opisthotonos, but spinal reflexes and alertness are normal.

Simmental encephalomyelopathy, which is seen in association with behavioral change (eg, aggression or dullness), has an onset in Simmental and Simmental-cross calves between 5-12 mo of age. The gait abnormality progresses from pelvic limb ataxia to recumbency with opisthotonos, and death occurs within 6 mo. It has been reported in the USA, UK, Australia, and New Zealand. Characteristic lesions consist of symmetric necrosis in the caudate nuclei and in other areas of the brain and spinal cord. Similar multifocal lesions are seen in 1- to 4-mo-old Limousin and Limousin-cross calves (with additional signs of blindness) in Australia and England, and in Angus calves in Australia and the USA.

Progressive myelopathy of Murray Grey cattle in Australia is inherited (autosomal recessive), and calves usually show spastic paraparesis and ataxia at birth. Neuronal degeneration is widespread in the brain and spinal cord; primary demyelination also develops in the cord.

Progressive ataxia of Charolais cattle has been reported in the UK and North America. It causes clinical signs that are first noticed between 6 and 36 mo of age and progress over 1-2 yr from slight ataxia involving all 4 limbs to recumbency. Female cattle typically manifest a rhythmic pulsatile pattern of urination. Histologic lesions consist of eosinophilic plaques and myelin breakdown in the white matter of the cerebellum and spinal cord.

Neuraxonal dystrophy (NAD) appears to be inherited in sheep and causes an unsteady, stiff, and swaying gait that progresses to paraparesis and finally tetraparesis. Suffolk and New Zealand Coopworth sheep are affected as lambs 1-6 mo old; Romney sheep are affected at 6-18 mo of age. Merinos develop a very similar disease at 1-4 yr of age. NAD has also been seen in 4- to 7-mo-old Merino lambs. Axonal swellings (spheroids) are typically found in gray matter of brain stem and spinal cord, although in the older Merino sheep, axonal spheroids mainly develop in large white matter tracts of the CNS. NAD of Morgan horses affecting the lateral (accessory) cuneate nucleus usually develops at 6-12 mo of age and causes spastic paraparesis and pelvic limb ataxia. It is presumed to be inherited. NAD affecting several brain-stem nuclei and causing mild pelvic limb ataxia has also been reported in 4-mo-old Hafflinger horses in Germany.

Equine degenerative encephalomyelopathy has been mainly associated with vitamin E deficiency, but it may have a familial basis in Appaloosa horses and other breeds, based on occurrence of clusters of cases. Degeneration of the spinocerebellar tracts results in a slowly progressive, symmetric ataxia and paresis of all 4 limbs that starts as early as 7 mo of age. *See also* DEGENERATIVE DISEASES OF THE SPINAL COLUMN AND CORD, p 1017.

Progressive paresis in Angora goats has been reported in Australia and may have a heritable basis. Clinical signs of spastic paresis and ataxia appear from birth to 4 mo of age and progress to recumbency within a few weeks. Widespread (multisystem) neuronal degeneration is seen at necropsy.

Generalized glycogenosis in Shorthorn (type II) and Brahman (type IIb) cattle and in Corriedale sheep (resembling type II) is a lysosomal storage disease that causes ill thrift, respiratory signs, paraparesis, ataxia, and muscle weakness at 3-9 mo of age.

Cervical stenotic myelopathy (wobbler syndrome) almost certainly has some familial basis in young, rapidly growing horses, particularly Thoroughbreds, with males being more commonly affected than females. Overnutrition is an important contributory factor, and the clinical signs often can be reversed in animals <9 mo old by reducing caloric intake and restricting exercise. Clinical signs usually become apparent between

6 mo and 3 yr of age and include cervical myelopathy, with the pelvic limbs usually affected more severely. Survey radiography and myelography can be used to identify stenotic or proliferative lesions causing spinal cord compression in the midcervical spine. Treatment usually requires surgical decompression of the spinal cord or vertebral stabilization. Prognosis is guarded.

Occipitoatlantoaxial malformation is an inherited disorder (autosomal recessive) in Arabian foals and may also be seen in Miniature horse foals, Holstein calves, and lambs. Clinical signs are progressive ataxia, tetraparesis, and an extended neck posture. Affected foals are usually tetraparetic at birth, although neurologic deficits may not develop for several years. Diagnosis is by radiography. Laminectomy has been reported to be successful in some cases.

Spina bifida is seen in most species and usually results in dysfunction of the tail and anus, incontinence, and sometimes pelvic limb weakness (*see also* SPINAL DYSRAPHISM, below).

Small Animals

Spinal muscular atrophy is an inherited lower motor neuron (LMN) disorder in Brittany Spaniels that can have an early (by 1 mo), intermediate (by 4-6 mo), or delayed (>1 yr old) onset. Rottweilers can also develop an early form of spinal muscular atrophy that is referred to as a motor neuron disease. Swedish Lapland puppies are affected at 5-7 wk of age, Stockard's paralysis (seen in Great Danes crossed with Bloodhounds or Saint Bernards) has an onset at 11-14 wk, and English Pointers are affected when ~5 mo old. LMN disease also is seen in puppies of other breeds, including Doberman Pinschers and Briquet Griffon Vendéens; a focal form involving the thoracic limb(s) is seen in German Shepherds. Paraparesis or tetraparesis with neurogenic muscle atrophy are the main clinical features. The severe, generalized LMN disease in spinal muscular atrophy closely resembles the signs of a peripheral neuropathy. Loss of motor neurons in the spinal cord is the most striking feature on necropsy. There is no treatment.

Demyelination of miniature Poodles is presumed to be an inherited disorder involving primarily the spinal cord. This rare condition causes paraparesis at 2-4 mo of age that rapidly progresses to tetraplegia. There is no treatment.

Ataxia of Jack Russell and Smooth-haired Fox Terriers causes ataxia and dysmetria of the pelvic limbs at <6 mo of age. Signs progress over 1-2 yr. Many cases manifest seizures. Spinal cord demyelination is found on necropsy. Clinical signs may stabilize after several months, and some affected animals are able to live a relatively normal life, in spite of the abnormal movements.

Afghan Hound myelopathy is an inherited disorder that causes both demyelination and necrosis of the spinal cord. Paraparesis develops some time during the first year of life and progresses to paraplegia within 1 wk. The thoracic limbs become involved over the next 1-2 wk. A similar condition is seen in young Kooiker dogs (Dutch Decoy dogs), of either sex, with signs beginning from 3-12 mo of age. Prognosis is poor in both breeds.

Neuraxonal dystrophy is described in both cats and dogs but primarily in Rottweiler dogs (autosomal recessive inheritance). In Rottweilers, the onset is between 3-24 mo of age, and the disorder progresses slowly over several years. Signs include cerebellar dysfunction and dysmetria in all 4 limbs, but with preservation of paw position sense, which should distinguish it from leukoencephalomyelopathy (*see* below) and from advanced motor neuron disease in the same breed. Collie dogs in Australia and New Zealand develop similar clinical signs at 2-4 mo of age. There is also early onset in Papillons and Chihuahuas and in cats (autosomal recessive in Domestic Tricolored cats). Axonal spheroids, often in specific regions of the brain and spinal cord, are the characteristic pathologic finding of these conditions.

Leukoencephalomyelopathy of Rottweilers has a later onset than neuraxonal dystrophy (*see* above), usually at ~2-3 yr of age. It is possible that the disorders have a similar basis because animals occasionally may show histopathologic features of both conditions. In leukoencephalomyelopathy, there is no head tremor and paw position sense is delayed. Bilaterally symmetric areas of spinal cord demyelination are the predominant findings on necropsy.

Calcium phosphate deposition in Great Danes causes mineralization of soft tissues and bone deformity, with dorsal displacement of C7. The resultant compressive myelopathy is seen in puppies 1-2 mo old. This condition is distinct from caudal cervical spondylomyelopathy (*see* below).

Progressive axonopathy of Boxer dogs is an autosomal recessive disorder that causes patellar hyporeflexia, severe dysmetria, loss of paw position sense, and spastic paresis at 1-7 mo of age. Axonal spheroids are widespread in both the central and peripheral nervous system on necropsy. Although this condition does cause loss of the patellar reflex, in general, the signs are more suggestive of spinal cord disease than of a peripheral neuropathy. There is no treatment, but affected dogs can live relatively comfortably for a considerable time.

Breed-associated aseptic meningitis (steroid-responsive meningitis-arteritis) has been reported in Beagles, Bernese Mountain Dogs, Boxers, German Shorthaired Pointers, and sporadically in other breeds. The main signs are neck pain, pyrexia, and dramatic pleocytosis in the CSF in young dogs. Prognosis is guarded to favorable, especially in dogs with acute disease that are treated promptly using immunosuppressive doses of corticosteroids.

Congenital vertebral malformations include **hemivertebrae** (shortened or misshapen vertebrae), block (fused) vertebrae, and butterfly vertebrae (having a sagittal cleft). Hemivertebrae are most common in screw-tailed dog breeds and are inherited in German Shorthaired Pointers. Decompressive surgery can be very successful but sometimes needs to be combined with spinal stabilization. **Multiple cartilaginous exostosis** is a benign proliferation of cartilage or bone that can affect the ribs, long bones, or vertebrae and may have a familial basis. **Transitional vertebrae** are often clinically associated with lumbosacral stenosis. Myelography or specialized imaging techniques (eg, computed tomography) are usually required to confirm spinal cord compression in these congenital conditions. Treatment consists of surgical removal.

Caudal cervical spondylomyelopathy (wobbler syndrome) may have a heritable basis in Borzois (5-8 yr) and Basset Hounds (<8 mo) and probably also Doberman Pinschers (≥2 yr) and Great Danes (<2 yr). Neurologic deficits range from mild ataxia of the pelvic limbs to tetraplegia. Affected dogs often keep their neck flexed ventrally, and there may be caudal cervical pain. Spinal radiographs may show malalignment or remodeling of the vertebrae, narrowing of one or more disk spaces, or spondylosis deformans. Myelography usually reveals a marked stenosis at the cranial orifice of the midcervical or caudal cervical vertebrae. Several surgical techniques can provide stabilization of the vertebrae or decompression of the spinal cord.

Atlantoaxial subluxation is most commonly seen as a congenital disorder in young toy or miniature breeds of dogs and occasionally as a congenital disorder in several large breeds, including Rottweilers and Doberman Pinschers. Signs usually develop within the first few years of life and consist of an acute or slowly progressive onset of neck pain or gait dysfunction, ranging from ataxia to tetraplegia. Radiographic confirmation of diagnosis should be followed by stabilization using ventral lag screw fixation. The prognosis is guarded.

Arachnoid cysts (meningeal cysts, leptomeningeal cysts, subarachnoid cysts) cause accumulations of CSF and a focal myelopathy in young dogs. The etiology is unknown, but some cysts may have a congenital origin. Signs consist of progressive ataxia and weakness. Diagnosis is made by myelography and/or computed tomography. Prognosis may be favorable following surgical excision, although recurrence is possible.

Spinal dysraphism or myelodysplasia includes anomalies of the skin, vertebrae, and spinal cord that are secondary to faulty closure of the neural tube. Spinal dysraphism is inherited in Weimaraners. Neurologic deficits are evident by 4-6 wk of age and include paraparesis and a symmetric "bunny-hopping" gait in the pelvic limbs. There is a bilateral flexor reflex; pinching one paw elicits flexion of both pelvic limbs. There may be scoliosis or abnormal hair streams on the dorsal aspect of the neck. Diagnosis is based on clinical signs and imaging techniques such as myelography and computed tomography. There is no treatment, but neurologic deficits usually do not progress. Similar malformations have been seen in other breeds of dogs and in calves, foals, and lambs.

Syringomyelia is the development of one or more fluid-filled cavities within the spinal cord. **Hydromyelia** is accumulation of fluid within an enlarged central canal of the spinal cord. It is often difficult to differentiate between syringomyelia and hydromyelia, so the term **syringohydromyelia** is often used. Syringohydromyelia causes progressive ataxia and paresis; scoliosis and spinal pain is possible. Causes include trauma, neoplasia, inflammatory conditions, and developmental malformations. The most important is Chiari I malformation, an underdeveloped occipital bone that induces overcrowding of the caudal fossa. This interferes with the circulation of spinal fluid and can result in hydrocephalus and/or syringohydromyelia of the cervical spinal segments. Syringohydromyelia associated with Chiari I malformation is most common in small-breed dogs, especially Cavalier King Charles Spaniels. Any age dog can be affected. Signs consist of ataxia and tetraparesis, neck pain, and persistent scratching at the base of the head or shoulder. Radiography and myelography are usually normal. MRI can identify the cavitation in the spinal cord and any caudal fossa malformations. Treatment is directed at the underlying cause, if possible. Signs may improve with corticosteroids (prednisone at 1 mg/kg, SID). Surgery to decompress the caudal fossa can be helpful for Chiari I malformations.

Spina bifida occulta is a failure of the neural arch to fuse; if the spinal cord is also involved, it is called **spina bifida manifesta**. The most likely clinical signs of spina bifida are LMN signs in the pelvic limbs and urinary or fecal incontinence. The prognosis for animals with substantial neurologic deficits is poor. Spina bifida can also accompany the **sacrocaudal dysgenesis** that is inherited as an autosomal dominant trait in Manx cats.

Pilonidal sinus (dermoid sinus, dermoid cyst) is another consequence of faulty neural tubulation that appears to be inherited (autosomal recessive) in Rhodesian Ridgeback dogs. The sinus is lined by skin and may communicate with the subarachnoid space, causing possible meningitis or myelitis. Treatment consists of antibiotics and surgical excision of the sinus.

Epidermoid cysts are rare lesions that arise from entrapment of epithelial cells during closure of the neural tube. Myelography will reveal an intramedullary lesion in a young dog with progressive neurologic deficits.

PERIPHERAL NERVE AND MUSCLE DISORDERS

See also DISEASES OF THE PERIPHERAL NERVE AND NEUROMUSCULAR JUNCTION, p 1010.

Large Animals

Spastic paresis is seen in many breeds of cattle and has been referred to as "contraction of the Achilles tendon," "straight hock," and "Elso heel." (*See also* LAMENESS IN CATTLE, p 867.) It can be divided into 2 syndromes, one that affects calves and one that affects adults. In calves, the condition appears to be familial and can be seen in many breeds, with signs beginning between 1 wk and 1 yr of age. It is characterized by extension of the stifle and tarsus and by spastic contracture of the muscles of one or both pelvic limbs. Spasticity primarily affects the gastrocnemius and superficial flexor muscles; in some cases, other muscles of the pelvic limb are involved. The leg is usually held in extension behind the calf and does not touch the ground during walking. The disease is progressive but usually responds to neurectomy of the tibial nerve. The etiology is unknown. No lesions are seen in peripheral nerves, and the condition is thought to involve excessive activity of the neuromuscular spindle reflex arc. Adult cattle are affected at 3-7 yr of age. Extensor muscles of the back and pelvic limbs are affected, causing lumbar lordosis and caudal extension of the limbs. This condition is also thought to be familial and is usually progressive. Mephenesin (30-40 mg/kg, PO, for 2-3 days) may produce variable control of signs. Quadriceps muscle hypoplasia as a cause of congenital lameness has been described in Holstein calves. Reduced numbers of spinal cord motor neurons suggest that there is failure to innervate the muscle on the affected side.

Hyperkalemic periodic paralysis is seen in Quarter Horses 2-3 yr old and is due to an inherited mutation of the sodium channel. It causes episodes of muscle tremor and sometimes recumbency, both of which may be precipitated by exercise. Hyperkalemia is usually present during an attack, and electromyography can also be helpful for diagnosis. Acetazolamide (0.5-2.2 mg/kg, PO, BID) and hydrochlorthiazide (0.5 mg/kg, PO, BID) may lessen the frequency and severity of attacks.

Myotonia congenita is an inherited/familial disorder in goats and Shropshire lambs and is occasionally seen in horses. It causes muscle rigidity; marked dimpling on percussion of the muscle belly; and a stiff, stilted gait. Electromyography is a useful aid to diagnosis. This disease results from a mutation in a chloride channel.

Muscular dystrophy is an inherited disease in Merino sheep. It results in a slowly progressive stiffness that affects the limbs and neck from 3-4 wk of age onwards. Clinically affected sheep have high resting and postexercise concentrations of serum CK and lactic dehydrogenase.

Porcine stress syndrome or malignant hyperthermia (p 832) is a hypermetabolic and hypercontractile syndrome that, when triggered by anesthesia or stress, produces a sustained increase of intracellular calcium levels within skeletal muscle fibers. This in turn causes muscle stiffness, hyperventilation, hyperthermia, and pale exudative pork. It results from a mutation in a calcium-channel gene that is inherited as an autosomal dominant trait, usually in Landrace pigs.

Small Animals

Hypertrophic neuropathy of Tibetan Mastiff dogs is an autosomal recessive disease that has been recognized in the USA, Switzerland, and Australia. It causes paraparesis by 8 wk and may progress to tetraparesis. Hyporeflexia is marked, but sensory function is preserved. Demyelination and remyelination are seen on nerve biopsy. Prognosis is guarded. Some puppies regain the ability to walk but remain weak. There is no treatment.

Alaskan Malamute polyneuropathy affects Alaskan Malamutes 10-18 mo old. There is exercise intolerance, paraparesis progressing to tetraparesis, muscle atrophy, hyporeflexia, and, in some cases, laryngeal paralysis. Electromyography shows diffuse fibrillation potentials and positive sharp waves. On nerve biopsy, there is axonal necrosis with demyelination. There is no effective treatment, although clinical signs stabilize in some patients. In most affected dogs, however, progressive disability leads to euthanasia.

Congenital laryngeal paralysis is seen in Bouvier des Flandres (autosomal dominant) and Siberian Huskies, Rottweilers, and Bull Terriers <1 yr old. It results in exercise intolerance and inspiratory dyspnea. Diagnosis is confirmed by visualization on laryngoscopy. Congenital laryngeal paralysis with diffuse peripheral neuropathy is seen in several breeds, including Dalmatians, Rottweilers, and Pyrenean Mountain Dogs. Prognosis is guarded to poor.

Primary hyperoxaluria (L-glyceric aciduria) is a rare inherited (autosomal recessive) neurofilament disorder of domestic shorthaired cats that results in renal disease and also produces weakness due to a peripheral neuropathy. Signs develop at 5-9 mo of age. A plantigrade stance is the most prominent sign, and spinal reflexes are sometimes reduced. Urine contains increased oxalate and L-glycerate levels. There is no treatment.

Neuropathy of hereditary hyperchylomicronemia (hyperlipidemia) is a suspected autosomal-recessive disorder that causes a generalized peripheral neuropathy in cats. Clinical signs do not develop until at least 8 mo of age. The hyperlipidemia results in deposition of lipid granules within nerves, and there is evidence that the clinical signs can be controlled by a low-fat diet. Blood samples from affected cats have the appearance of "cream of tomato soup."

Sensory neuropathy of longhaired Dachshunds (probably autosomal recessive) causes pelvic limb ataxia at 8-12 wk of age. Urinary and GI function may also be disturbed. Paw position sense, spinal reflexes, and pain sensation are depressed, and self-mutilation can occur. There is a loss of myelinated fibers in sensory nerves and in selected areas of the spinal cord. There is no treatment, but affected dogs may have a relatively normal quality of life provided self-mutilation does not develop.

Sensory neuropathy in Pointers is seen in English Pointers (autosomal recessive) in the USA and Shorthaired Pointers in Europe. Self-mutilation of the digits is the main clinical sign, and the disease onset is before 6 mo of age. Pain perception is absent in the pelvic limbs and depressed in the thoracic limbs. There is neuronal loss in dorsal root ganglia. Prognosis is poor. There is no treatment.

Congenital myasthenia gravis (autosomal recessive) has been described in Jack Russell Terrier, Smooth-haired Fox Terrier, and Springer Spaniel puppies. It is due to either a deficiency or dysfunction of the acetylcholine receptor, and there is none of the circulating antireceptor antibody seen in the more common acquired form of the disease. Clinical signs usually start at 5-10 wk of age. The characteristic finding is an exercise-induced weakness, often associated with megaesophagus. The prognosis is more guarded than in acquired myasthenia gravis. The congenital disease has also been described in cats. A presynaptic form is seen in 12- to 16-wk-old Gammel Dansk Hønsehund dogs (autosomal recessive). Treatment consists of anticholinesterase drugs.

Scotty cramp (autosomal recessive) causes episodes of muscular hypertonicity in Scottish Terrier puppies. These episodes are exacerbated by excitement, exercise, stress, and poor health and are characterized by a hypermetric gait and arching of the spine, which can cause the dog to somersault when it runs. The disorder seems to be related to faulty serotonin metabolism. Diazepam and promazines help to relieve signs.

Congenital myoclonus of Labrador Retrievers (familial reflex myoclonus) causes muscle spasms/hypertonicity from an early age. Puppies may be unable to walk or even maintain a sternal position due to extensor rigidity. The prognosis is very poor.

Hypokalemic myopathy of Burmese cats (autosomal recessive) causes periodic paralysis or weakness with ventral flexion of the neck. Cats are affected at 3-4 mo of age. Serum CK is markedly increased. Dietary supplementation of oral potassium usually produces a favorable response (eg, potassium gluconate solution at 2-4 mEq or mmol/cat, PO, SID, until serum potassium levels are stable).

Myotonia congenita is seen in Chow Chows, Staffordshire Terriers, Great Danes, and Miniature Schnauzers (autosomal recessive) and causes signs similar to those seen in myotonic goats. There is often a degree of muscle hypertrophy, and marked stiffness is seen when dogs first rise. Dimpling is seen on percussion of several muscles, including the tongue. Diagnosis can usually be confirmed by electromyography (characteristic "dive bomber" sound); muscle biopsy changes are mild and nonspecific. Prognosis is guarded, although membrane-stabilizing drugs (procainamide, mexiletine) result in significant improvement.

X-linked muscular dystrophies have been described in Irish Terriers, Golden Retrievers, Miniature Schnauzers, Rottweilers, Samoyeds, German Shorthaired Pointers, Groenendaeler Belgian Shepherds, Brittany Spaniels, Rat Terriers, Labrador Retrievers, Japanese Spitz dogs, and also in cats. All are due to mutations in the dystrophin gene. Males show muscle stiffness, dysphagia, and weakness at an early age, along with a plantigrade stance and muscle atrophy as the animal gets older. Initial muscle hypertrophy may be marked, particularly in cats. Diagnosis is facilitated by the initial massive increases in serum levels of CK and by demonstration of hyalinized and mineralized muscle fibers on biopsy. Prognosis is guarded to poor. At present, there is no treatment. A novel congenital muscular dystrophy has recently been reported in cats associated with deficiency of merosin (laminin α_2), in which degenerative changes occur in both muscles and peripheral nerves.

Labrador Retriever myopathy (autosomal recessive) causes a stiff gait and marked muscle atrophy in puppies of both sexes. Signs worsen with cold, stress, or exercise, and affected dogs may be unable to keep their heads elevated in a normal position from as early as 3 mo of age. Tendon reflexes are usually absent. Signs stabilize by 6-8 mo of age, and the prognosis is favorable so that affected dogs can make good pets. There is preferential atrophy of type II muscle fibers.

Dermatomyositis of Collies and Shetland Sheepdogs (inherited as a dominant trait with variable expressivity) causes atrophy and weakness of the masticatory and distal limb muscles from a few months of age, sometimes associated with trismus and megaesophagus. These signs are combined with a dermatitis over the face and extremities. The clinical signs may wax and wane and, in general, do not become severely debilitating. Polymyositis and dermatitis are evident on histopathologic examination. This disorder has also been seen in Beauceron Shepherds, Pembroke Welsh Corgis, Australian Cattle Dogs, Lakeland Terriers, Chow Chows, German Shepherds, and Kuvasz dogs.

Glycogen storage diseases can cause muscle weakness and exercise intolerance in young dogs and cats. Examples include glycogenosis types II (Lapland dogs), III (German Shepherds and Akitas), IV (autosomal recessive in Norwegian Forest cats), and VII (English Springer Spaniels).

Mitochondrial myopathy has been described in Clumber and Sussex Spaniels and in Old English Sheepdogs. Mitochondrial myopathies result in exercise intolerance and collapse, and blood lactate and pyruvate levels are often increased after exercise. Ragged red fibers, indicating increased numbers of mitochondria, may be seen on muscle biopsy. Inherited disorders of carnitine metabolism are another cause of mitochondrial myopathy; they may cause accumulation of lipid vacuoles within muscle fibers.

Nemaline rod myopathy (probable autosomal recessive) in cats causes weakness and later a hypermetric gait at 6-18 mo of age. Patellar reflexes are depressed, and muscle atrophy develops progressively. Large numbers of nemaline rods are found in skeletal muscle fibers. The prognosis is poor. A similar disorder is seen sporadically in young dogs.

Central core myopathy has been described as a cause of weakness, muscle atrophy, and exercise intolerance/collapse in young Great Danes in the UK. Signs begin around 6 mo of age. Prognosis is poor.

Congenital megaesophagus is inherited in Wirehaired Fox Terriers and Miniature Schnauzers, and possibly also in German Shepherds, Great Danes, Irish Setters, Newfoundlands, Shar-Peis, Greyhounds, and Siamese cats. Clinical signs include regurgitation and aspiration pneumonia. Prognosis is guarded.

Devon Rex cat hereditary myopathy (autosomal recessive) is seen in kittens around 4-7 wk old and is characterized by exercise intolerance and passive ventroflexion of the head and neck, which is especially noticeable during locomotion, urination, or defecation. Some cats assume a "dog-begging" position. Megaesophagus is present. Prognosis is guarded.

MULTIFOCAL DISORDERS

Large Animals

Hereditary neuraxial edema with congenital myoclonus (probable autosomal recessive) was first reported in neonatal Herefords. The calves are alert but unable to rise; they are incoordinated and have coarse, tonic muscular contractions. Sudden stimuli cause vigorous extension of the legs and neck.

Shaker calf syndrome is a neurodegenerative disorder that is seen in Hereford calves. Affected animals show a marked tremor within hours of birth, difficulty in rising, a stiff gait, and loss of voice; signs progress to spastic paraplegia. There is excessive accumulation of neurofilaments within neurons of the central, peripheral, and autonomic nervous systems.

Vitamin A deficiency of sows can cause incoordination, head tilt, pelvic limb paralysis, paddling, and ocular lesions in piglets. Similar signs are seen in congenitally affected calves born from deficient dams.

Generalized Metabolic and Lysosomal Storage Disorders: Maple syrup urine disease is a genetic amino aciduria (consistent with a branched-chain ketoacid decarboxylase deficiency) in Hereford calves. Affected calves are dull, become recumbent in 2-4 days, and terminally have opisthotonos. The histologic lesions are severe and consist of generalized status spongiosus in the CNS.

GM_1 gangliosidosis is seen in inbred Friesian calves. Clinical signs become evident during the first week of life and include depression, swaying of the hindquarters, reluctance to move, and stiffness. Death occurs in 6-8 mo.

GM_2 gangliosidosis causes hypermetria and weakness in Yorkshire piglets within the first 3 mo of life. Death occurs in 4-6 mo.

α-Mannosidosis (autosomal recessive) is seen in Angus, Murray Grey, and Galloway breeds. It produces ataxia, head tremor, aggression, and failure to thrive. There may also be abortions and neonatal death. Most affected calves die within the first year, sometimes shortly after birth. Affected (homozygous) calves have an absolute deficiency of α-mannosidase, and heterozygotes are partially deficient. Mannosidosis can be controlled by identifying and eliminating heterozygotes on the basis of biochemical testing.

β-**Mannosidosis** causes recumbency and cerebellar signs in newborn Nubian goats and Salers calves.

Ceroid lipofuscinosis is seen in sheep, cattle, and goats. Young Nubian goats show cerebellar signs. Rambouillet sheep show blindness and decreased mentation from 8 mo of age. South Hampshire lambs 9-12 mo old show blindness, depression, head and thoracic limb tremor, and facial twitching, and die by 30 mo of age. Devon cattle become blind and weak by 14 mo and die by 4 yr of age.

Globoid cell leukodystrophy has been reported in polled Dorset sheep 4-18 mo old. Exaggerated tendon reflexes, ascending paralysis, and cerebellar signs may be seen.

Small Animals

Multisystemic chromatolytic neuronal degeneration in Cairn Terriers causes paraparesis in young puppies that progresses rapidly to produce cerebellar involvement with bouts of cataplectic collapse. Degeneration of neurons is widespread in the brain, spinal cord, and sensory ganglia.

Multisystemic neuronal degeneration has also been reported in red-haired Cocker Spaniels and causes abnormal behavior and cerebellar signs. Neuronal changes are found in various brain-stem nuclei. A similar condition is seen in Miniature Poodles (3-4 wk) with signs characterized by rolling from side to side, inability to stand or right into sternal position, periodic opisthotonos, intention tremors, and lack of a menace response associated with neuronal degeneration in the cerebral cortex and cerebellum.

Hydrocephalus in Bull Mastiffs is an inherited disorder that is also associated with abnormal myelin. It results in blindness, abnormal behavior, and cerebellar signs. Bilaterally symmetric spongiform lesions are found in the deep cerebellar nuclei.

Dalmatian leukodystrophy is a rare inherited condition that causes visual deficits with progressive ataxia and tetraparesis at 3-6 mo of age. There is dilatation of ventricles, cavitation of cerebral white matter, and widespread loss of myelin.

Fibrinoid leukodystrophy has been described in two 8-mo-old Labrador Retrievers, a 9-mo-old male Scottish Terrier, a 6-mo-old female Miniature Poodle, and a 13-wk-old Bernese Mountain Dog. It results in progressive ataxia and tetraparesis with personality changes, starting at 6 mo of age. Rosenthal fibers are found around blood vessels of the CNS, and the cause seems to be a disorder of astrocyte function. Prognosis is poor.

Spongiform degenerative conditions have been described in young dogs and cats (breeds include Labrador Retriever, Shetland Sheepdog, Samoyed, Silky Terrier, Bull Mastiff, Saluki, Cocker Spaniel, Malinois-Shepherd crosses, Rottweiler, and Egyptian Mau and Burmese kittens) and are often associated with signs of ataxia/hypermetria, head tremors, intermittent contractures, postural abnormalities, and behavioral changes. The underlying pathology relates to spongy degeneration of either white or gray matter. The pathogenesis of these disorders remains uncertain. Prognosis is poor.

Hereditary quadriplegia and amblyopia in Irish Setters produces signs of head tremor, visual impairment, nystagmus, inability to stand, and seizures beginning at birth.

Lysosomal Storage Disorders: This clinically rare group of conditions results from deficiency of an enzyme that is essential for the metabolism of a protein, carbohydrate, or lipid substrate. Clinical signs usually appear early in life, although occasionally the onset is delayed. Specific diseases have been associated with a particular breed, but in theory, any breed could develop any one of these disorders, and many have been described in more than one breed. Considerable phenotypic variation should be expected beyond the classic signs described below. Prognosis is poor for all of these disorders, although gene replacement therapies are being actively investigated.

Fucosidosis of English Springer Spaniels has been reported in Australia, New Zealand, the UK, and North America. It is characterized by clinical signs of ataxia, personality change, dysphonia, dysphagia, hearing/visual deficits, and seizures. Signs tend to progressively develop from 6 to >24 mo of age. A high proportion of peripheral lymphocytes may show cytoplasmic vacuolation. A DNA-based blood test is available for diagnosis. Prognosis is poor, and there is no effective treatment.

GM_1 **gangliosidosis** is seen primarily in cats, particularly Oriental breeds, and in Beagles, Portuguese Water Dogs, English Springer Spaniels, Alaskan Huskies, and Shibas. Signs of cerebellar dysfunction predominate, and corneal clouding may develop.

GM_2 **gangliosidosis or familial amaurotic idiocy** has been seen in German Short-haired Pointers, Japanese Pointers, mixed-breed cats, and Korat cats. Clinical signs seen at 6 mo of age include behavioral change and visual disturbances. Progressive ataxia and dementia develop later. Clinical signs of ataxia, hypermetria, head tremor, and corneal opacity develop in kittens at ~3 mo of age.

Niemann-Pick disease affects cats and causes cerebellar dysfunction with an associated abdominal enlargement due to hepatosplenomegaly. The neurologic deficits tend to vary with the 6 subtypes of this disease, ranging from severe cerebellar-like signs (types A and C) to neuropathic signs (type A variant).

Glucocerebrosidosis (Gaucher's disease) is a rare disorder of Australian Silky Terriers that produces mainly cerebellar signs at 4-6 mo of age.

α-**Mannosidosis** has been seen mainly in cats and may cause retinal and skeletal abnormalities as well as neurologic deficits. Cerebellar signs are the most consistent feature of the otherwise somewhat variable neurologic deficits.

Mucopolysaccharidosis is primarily a disorder of cats that is associated with a flattening of the face, corneal clouding, and multiple bone dysplasias. Plott hounds can also be affected. Several types of this disease are reported; type VI is often associated with progressive paraparesis secondary to focal bony protrusions into the vertebral canal. The skeletal changes are nonprogressive after 9 mo of age, and decompressive surgery may improve the neurologic deficits.

Ceroid lipofuscinosis is characterized by reduced vision, personality change, ataxia, and seizures when animals are 12-24 mo old. The condition is an autosomal recessive trait in English Setters, Tibetan Terriers, and Border Collies. It has been reported in many additional breeds of dogs, as well as in Siamese cats. The phenotype and age of onset are variable, and signs tend to slowly evolve over several years.

Globoid cell leukodystrophy (Krabbe's disease) is seen mainly in Cairn and West Highland White Terriers. Several other breeds of dogs, as well as cats, may be affected. Clinical signs are variable, and either an ascending paralysis is seen by itself or combined with a cerebellar disturbance. Death occurs 2-3 mo after the onset of signs. Total protein content of CSF may be increased. Large globoid cells are distributed throughout the white matter of the spinal cord and brain.

MISCELLANEOUS CONGENITAL DISORDERS

Large Animals

Pendular nystagmus is seen in various breeds of dairy cattle but appears to have little clinical significance.

Congenital deafness has been reported in horses.

Small Animals

Congenital vestibular disease has been described in a number of breeds, including English Cocker Spaniels, German Shepherds, and Doberman Pinschers, and also in Oriental breeds of cats. Vestibular dysfunction is manifest by varying degrees of head tilt, nystagmus, circling, and rolling at an early age. In some animals, the signs may resolve spontaneously.

Congenital deafness is primarily associated with Dalmatians but has also been recorded in a number of breeds including Australian Blue Heelers and Shepherds, English Setters, Boston Terriers, and Old English Sheepdogs. It is linked to blue eye color in white cats. The brain stem auditory evoked response is a useful diagnostic test primarily used to identify carriers in a litter of affected animals. (*See also* DEAFNESS, p 416.)

DEMYELINATING DISORDERS

Hypomyelination and dysmyelination are developmental disorders of myelination characterized by axons with thin myelin sheaths, or by axons that are nonmyelinated or with abnormal myelin. There appears to be 2 possible pathologic classifications: 1) thinly myelinated axons with predominantly normal myelin and occasional nonmyelinated axons, or 2) thinly myelinated axons with predominantly abnormal myelin and mainly nonmyelinated axons. These categories have been called hypomyelinating and dysmyelinating disease, respectively, and are characteristic of the congenital myelin disorders seen in young animals. These pathologic changes should not be confused with demyelination in which there is a breakdown and loss of previously normal myelin. In general, demyelinating diseases do not present clinically as congenital problems.

Etiology and Epidemiology: Demyelinating disorders have been reported worldwide in humans, mice, pigs, cattle, hamsters, rats, sheep, Siamese kittens, and a number of dog breeds, including Chow Chow, Springer Spaniel, Dalmatian, Samoyed, Golden Retriever, Lurcher, Bernese Mountain Dog, Vizsla, Weimaraner, Australian Silky Terrier, and mixed breeds.

In utero infection and heredity are the general causes of hypomyelination. The viruses of classical swine fever, border disease, and bovine viral diarrhea have been incriminated, but mechanisms responsible for the hypomyelination have not been defined; these 3 pestiviruses are closely related members of the family Togaviridae and are transmitted both vertically and horizontally. Most toxins that affect myelin cause demyelination. One in particular, trichlorfon, is an organophosphate (p 2398) with a unique toxicity that causes Type A-V porcine congenital tremor syndrome. Pregnant sows treated with trichlorfon during mid and late gestation (days 45-77) produce litters in which up to 90% of the piglets develop a marked tremor syndrome secondary to cerebellar hypoplasia and hypomyelinogenesis. The mortality rate is high.

Other disorders resulting in hypomyelination are hereditary. Almost all of these disorders result in CNS hypomyelination, except in Golden Retrievers, in which hypomyelination of the peripheral nervous system (PNS) has been reported. In CNS hypomyelination, the basic defect involves interference with the functional maturation of oligodendrocytes. The exact mechanisms for the defect are not known, but a point mutation on a critical gene has been found in Springer Spaniels. In PNS hypomyelination, the defect involves Schwann cells.

The genetic basis for the inherited hypomyelination syndromes is not fully defined, but in most instances, males are affected more often and more severely affected than females. This supports a sex-linked recessive trait or mode of inheritance.

Clinical Findings: Clinical signs from hypomyelination of the CNS can be seen as early as 10-12 days of age and certainly by the time of weaning. Signs include, most notably, a gross whole body tremor that involves the limbs, trunk, head, and eyes. The tremor lessens or disappears when the animal is resting or sleeping but reappears on arousal and increases with excitement. The tremors are very noticeable when the animal is eating and are a severe form of intention tremor. In addition, some animals may have difficulty standing and ambulating and may have weakness in the limbs. Secondary to this, postural test reactions may be deficient. Affected animals appear to have vision and other cranial nerve function, but occasionally a pendular nystagmus or a jerk nystagmus is seen when the globes are voluntarily moved. These neurologic deficits may be so severe in some animals that euthanasia is warranted. In some breeds of dogs, such as Chow Chows, the signs slowly dissipate over the first year of life, and the dogs are normal by 12-18 mo of age.

In Golden Retrievers with PNS hypomyelination, the clinical signs include ataxia, paresis, muscle atrophy, and hyporeflexia to areflexia. There is no evidence of CNS hypomyelination in this breed, and tremors are not present.

Lesions: In CNS hypomyelination, gross pathology reveals pallor of the white matter of the brain and spinal cord and possibly a gelatinous appearance. In PNS hypomyelination, the gross changes are minimal and there is no evidence of CNS changes. In CNS hypomyelination, the microscopic changes include lack of myelin (which is usually severe but not absolute), fewer oligodendrocytes, astrocytes outnumbering oligodendrocytes, oligodendrocytes that differ in appearance from those in healthy animals, and abnormal types of glial cells. In PNS hypomyelination, the microscopic changes consist of paucity of myelinated fibers, fibers with inappropriately thin myelin sheaths relative to the caliber of their enclosed axons, occasional fibers with poorly compacted myelin, Schwann cells with larger than normal cytoplasmic volume, and increased numbers of Schwann cell nuclei.

Diagnosis: The diagnosis of CNS hypomyelination is made primarily from the spectrum of neurologic deficits and signs and the early age of onset. Unfortunately, histopathology is the only definitive method to confirm a diagnosis. In cases with a heritable basis, pedigree evaluation may be helpful. In cases with a viral etiology, confirmation may involve immunofluorescent antibody staining techniques or virus isolation from nervous tissue (or both). In cases of PNS hypomyelination, biopsy of peripheral nerves is beneficial.

Differential diagnoses include disorders that could cause tremors in young animals. The possibilities are numerous, but some of the more common include glycogen storage disease, lysosomal storage disease, cerebellar hypoplasia, encephalitis, hypocalcemia, hypoglycemia, hyperammonemia, toxins (eg, metaldehyde, organophosphates, chlorinated hydrocarbons, fluoroacetate, strychnine, hexachlorophene, bromethalin), and mycotoxins (eg, penitrem-A).

Treatment, Control, and Prevention: There is no specific treatment for hypomyelination. The only means of control and prevention are selective breeding (for heritable syndromes) and immunization (for viral-induced syndromes). If given the time to develop normal or further myelin, some animals with congenital hypomyelination syndromes become normal by the age of 12-18 mo.

DISEASES OF THE PERIPHERAL NERVE AND NEUROMUSCULAR JUNCTION

Diseases of the peripheral nerve and neuromuscular junction include degenerative diseases, inflammatory diseases, metabolic disorders, neoplasia, nutritional disorders, toxic disorders, trauma, and vascular diseases. See CONGENITAL AND INHERITED ANOMALIES, p 995, for a discussion of congenital disorders.

DEGENERATIVE DISEASES

Acquired laryngeal paralysis (p 1180) is common in middle-aged and older dogs. Large breeds, such as Labrador Retrievers, Golden Retrievers, and Saint Bernards, are predisposed, but small breed dogs and cats can be affected. In the majority of cases, no underlying cause is identified and the disease is classified as idiopathic. A few cases are due to trauma or neoplasia affecting the neck or mediastinum. Hypothyroidism (p 461) is also a potential cause. Clinical signs consist of voice change, laryngeal stridor, and a dry cough. In severe cases, exercise intolerance and episodes of respiratory—especially inspiratory—distress and cyanosis occur. Some affected animals have signs of a more generalized polyneuropathy, such as weakness and proprioceptive deficits. Diagnosis is based on laryngoscopy with the animal lightly anesthetized. There is a unilateral or bilateral lack of abduction of the arytenoid cartilages and vocal folds during inspiration. Management consists of identifying and treating any underlying disorder. Treatment of idiopathic laryngeal paralysis consists of surgery, such as laryngeal tie back. Surgery does not restore normal laryngeal function but is usually successful in diminishing severe inspiratory dyspnea. A potential complication of surgery is aspiration of food or liquid.

For **equine laryngeal paralysis**, see LARYNGEAL HEMIPLEGIA, p 1216.

Dancing Doberman disease is a neuromuscular disease of Doberman Pinschers of either sex, 6 mo to 7 yr old. Initially, affected dogs intermittently flex the hip and stifle of one pelvic limb while standing. Within several months, most dogs alternately flex and extend both pelvic limbs in a dance-like fashion. They often prefer to sit rather than stand. The condition slowly progresses to mild paraparesis, decreased proprioception, and atrophy of the gastrocnemius muscles. The thoracic limbs are not affected. The etiology is unknown. Pathologic changes have been reported in pelvic limb muscles as well as peripheral nerves, and whether this is a primary muscle or nerve disease remains to be clarified. There is no treatment, and signs do not resolve. However, the disease usually does not result in severe disability and does not appear to be painful.

Distal denervating disease is a common polyneuropathy of dogs in the UK but has not been reported elsewhere. The cause is unknown. Any age and breed of dog may be affected. The onset of signs varies from a few days to several weeks. There is progressive tetraparesis, hyporeflexia, and atrophy of proximal skeletal muscles. Sensory deficits are not apparent. Electrodiagnostic evaluation typically shows denervation of limb muscles, relatively normal nerve conduction velocity, and markedly reduced amplitude of M waves. Peripheral nerve biopsies are usually normal, but examination of intramuscular nerves may be diagnostic; distal intramuscular axons degenerate with collateral axonal sprouting. Treatment is supportive, and the prognosis is excellent with recovery in 4-6 wk. Relapse has not been reported.

Distal polyneuropathy of Rottweilers is characterized by paraparesis that slowly progresses to tetraparesis, hyporeflexia, and muscle atrophy. Male and female Rottweilers 1-4 yr old have been affected. The cause is unknown. Electrodiagnostic testing shows denervation in distal muscles of the limbs and decreased motor nerve conduction velocity. Nerve biopsy changes consist of axonal necrosis and demyelination, often with infiltrates of macrophages, most severe in distal nerve fibers. Prognosis is poor, although some dogs may temporarily improve with corticosteroid treatment.

Idiopathic facial paralysis is a common disorder resulting in unilateral or bilateral paresis or paralysis of the facial muscles in dogs and cats. Cocker Spaniels, Pembroke Welsh Corgis, Boxers, English Setters, and domestic longhaired cats are at increased risk. There is acute onset of unilateral or bilateral inability to blink, drooping ear, drooping upper lip, and drooling from the corner of the mouth. Facial sensation (mediated via the trigeminal nerve) remains intact. Diagnosis is based on clinical features and exclusion of other causes of facial paralysis, including ear disease, trauma, and brain-stem lesions. Pathologic findings consist of degeneration of myelinated axons in the facial nerve. There is no inflammation. The cause is unknown, and there is no specific treatment. Artificial tears are often helpful in preventing corneal damage. Partial improvement may occur in a few weeks, but persistent dysfunction is common.

Stringhalt (p 925) in horses is characterized by brisk, involuntary flexion of one or both pelvic limbs during the protraction phase of the gait. Severity ranges from a mild jerk in the limb to flexion so severe that the affected horse can hardly walk. There may be atrophy of the muscles in the distal aspect of the affected limb(s). Stringhalt is seen in 2 forms. Ordinary or classic stringhalt is seen sporadically throughout the world, usually as a unilateral problem in individual horses. The cause is unknown. Some cases resolve spontaneously, while long digital extensor tenectomy is effective in others. Australian stringhalt is seen in outbreaks that affect multiple horses in a region and often affects both pelvic limbs. Horses in Australia, New Zealand, and the USA have been affected, usually in late summer or autumn. Australian stringhalt is associated with ingestion of Australian dandelion, European dandelion, and mallow, perhaps due to mycotoxins affecting these plants. Pathologically, the distal aspect of axons in the peroneal and tibial nerves degenerates. Horses with Australian stringhalt usually recover spontaneously when removed from offending pastures.

INFLAMMATORY DISORDERS

Acquired myasthenia gravis is failure of neuromuscular conduction due to reduction in number of acetylcholine receptors at the neuromuscular junction. It is caused by the development of circulating antibodies directed against the acetylcholine receptors at the neuromuscular junction. It is fairly common in mature dogs, especially German Shepherds, Golden Retrievers, and Labrador Retrievers, but is uncommon in cats. The classic presentation is exercise-induced stiffness, tremors, and weakness that resolve with rest. However, weakness is not always associated with exercise. Facial, pharyngeal, or esophageal weakness is common, and in many cases there is megaesophagus without generalized weakness (focal myasthenia). Regurgitation and aspiration pneumonia are frequent complications. Generalized weakness often resolves quickly after IV administration of edrophonium chloride (0.1-0.2 mg/kg), which is often used as a diagnostic test. Definitive diagnosis is based on the detection of antibodies in serum. Treatment consists of anticholinesterase drugs, eg, pyridostigmine (1-3 mg/kg PO, BID-TID) or neostigmine (0.04 mg/kg, SC, QID). Immunosuppressive dosages of prednisone are recommended in animals that do not respond to anticholinesterase therapy. The prognosis is generally good, and many dogs will undergo spontaneous remission, evident by a decrease in antibody titer. The prognosis is guarded for animals with aspiration pneumonia or persistent weakness.

Acute idiopathic polyradiculoneuritis is a common inflammatory disease primarily affecting the ventral nerve roots and peripheral nerves. It is common in dogs and rare in cats. Clinical signs often develop 7-14 days after a raccoon bite or scratch (**Coonhound paralysis**); however, other affected animals have no exposure to raccoons. A similar syndrome can develop in dogs and cats within 1-2 wk of vaccination. An immune-mediated reaction to raccoon saliva or other antigen is suspected. Typically, flaccid paresis begins in the pelvic limbs and progresses within 1-2 days to tetraparesis and, in some cases, facial and laryngeal weakness. Occasionally, the thoracic limbs are initially affected. Death from respiratory paralysis can occur in severe cases. Spinal cord reflexes are weak to absent, and severe muscle atrophy is evident within 10-14 days. Pain perception is intact and some dogs may appear hyperesthetic. Mentation and appetite are not affected. Urination, defecation, and tail movement usually remain normal. Analysis of CSF collected from the lumbar subarachnoid space shows increased protein with a normal cell count. Electromyography shows denervation, and nerve conduction studies show marked dispersion and prolonged latency of F-waves, indicative of slowed conduction in the ventral roots. There is no effective treatment other than nursing care, and corticosteroids are not helpful. Most affected animals begin to improve spontaneously within 3 wk, with complete recovery by 2-6 mo. Animals with severe signs and marked muscle atrophy may recover incompletely. Relapses can occur, especially in hunting dogs that frequently encounter raccoons. Pathologically there is inflammation, demyelination, and varying degrees of axonal degeneration in the ventral nerve roots and peripheral nerves.

Chronic relapsing idiopathic polyradiculoneuritis is a rare disease associated with inflammation of the nerves and nerve roots. It affects mature dogs and cats. Exercise intolerance, ataxia, and weakness develop slowly over several months. Some animals have spontaneous temporary remissions. Spinal cord reflexes are decreased, and cranial nerves may be affected. In severe cases, decreased sensation is evident. Diagnosis is based on nerve biopsy. There is nonsuppurative inflammation; axonal degeneration; and demyelination of nerves, nerve roots, and, in some cases, dorsal root ganglia. The cause is unknown, although immune-mediated mechanisms are suspected. Corticosteroids are helpful in some cases, but the disease tends to slowly wax and wane, gradually becoming more severe over months to years.

Chronic inflammatory demyelinating polyneuropathy is fairly common in adult dogs and cats. Onset of tetraparesis with hyporeflexia is insidious and is sometimes accompanied by cranial nerve dysfunction. Electromyography is usually normal, but nerve conduction velocities are slowed with temporal dispersion. Nerve biopsy shows multifocal paranodal demyelination. Clinical signs usually improve with the administration of corticosteroids (eg, prednisone 1-2 mg/kg/day), although signs may relapse when therapy is stopped. The etiology is unknown.

Polyneuritis equi (neuritis of the cauda equina) is characterized by inflammation of the sacrocaudal nerves, and occasionally other nerves. It is seen in adult horses of all breeds in Europe and North America. The cause is unknown, although an immunologic reaction incited by a viral infection is possible. Affected horses have circulating antibodies against P2 myelin protein. The most consistent clinical signs reflect involvement of the sacrocaudal nerves and include urinary and fecal incontinence, tail paralysis, perineal paresthesia or analgesia, and mild pelvic limb ataxia. Affected horses may rub the tail. The thoracic limbs and cranial nerves may also be affected. CSF may be xanthochromic with elevated protein content and mononuclear pleocytosis. Diagnosis can usually be based on clinical findings. Sacral fracture should be excluded by rectal examination and radiography. There is no treatment, and the prognosis for recovery is poor. Pathologically, there is granulomatous inflammation primarily affecting the extradural portions of the sacrocaudal nerves.

Protozoal polyradiculoneuritis occurs in dogs, especially puppies, and is caused by infection with *Toxoplasma gondii* (p 547) or *Neospora caninum* (p 535). Inflammation of nerve roots, peripheral nerves, and skeletal muscle results in progressive paralysis and rigidity of the pelvic limbs. Serum CK concentration is often increased. Analysis of CSF usually shows elevated protein and leukocytes (both neutrophils and mononuclear cells). Serum or CSF antibodies or identification of the organism on muscle biopsy are helpful in diagnosis. Early treatment with clindamycin (15-20 mg/kg, IM, PO, BID) or trimethoprim/sulfadiazine (15 mg/kg, BID) and pyrimethamine (1 mg/kg/day) may be effective. The prognosis is poor in dogs with pelvic limb rigidity.

Trigeminal neuritis (idiopathic trigeminal neuropathy) is common in dogs and uncommon in cats. It is characterized by acute onset of flaccid jaw paralysis. Affected animals cannot close the mouth and have difficulty eating and drinking. Horner's syndrome, facial paresis, and decreased facial sensation are also possible. The cause is unknown. Pathologically, there is bilateral nonsuppurative inflammation and demyelination in the motor branches of the trigeminal nerve. Affected animals usually recover spontaneously within 3-4 wk. Fluid and nutritional support may be necessary.

METABOLIC DISORDERS

Diabetic neuropathy is an uncommon complication of diabetes mellitus (p 439) in cats and rarely dogs. Signs include weakness, ataxia, and muscle atrophy. Affected cats often have unilateral or bilateral tibial nerve dysfunction, evident as a plantigrade stance. There are several proposed pathophysiologic mechanisms, but prolonged hyperglycemia seems to be the important underlying factor. Pathologic findings in nerves consist of demyelination with remyelination, axonal degeneration, or both. Diagnosis is based on clinical findings, laboratory evidence of diabetes mellitus, and nerve biopsy. The prognosis is guarded, but partial or complete recovery can occur with insulin therapy.

Hypothyroid neuropathy is a common neuropathy in dogs with hypothyroidism (p 461). Mature dogs, especially large-breed dogs, are predisposed. Several syndromes have been reported, including tetraparesis with proprioceptive deficits and hyporeflexia, vestibular dysfunction, megaesophagus, and laryngeal paralysis. In some cases, classic signs of hypothyroidism (eg, obesity and dermatopathy) are absent, and neurologic dysfunction is the only sign of illness. Pathologic findings in peripheral nerves consist of demyelination or remyelination and axonal degeneration. The pathophysiology is poorly understood and, in some affected dogs with motor deficits, a myopathy may also be present. Diagnosis is based on clinical features, laboratory assessment of thyroid function, and response to thyroid supplementation. In some, but not all, cases, signs resolve within several months of starting thyroid replacement therapy.

NEOPLASIA

Nerve sheath tumors include those tumors referred to as schwannomas, neurilemmomas, and neurofibromas. They are seen in most domestic animals but are most common in dogs and cattle. In dogs, tumors often arise in the nerves of the brachial plexus, initially causing unilateral thoracic limb lameness and pain that may be confused with musculoskeletal disease. Pain may be elicited on palpation of the axilla or abduction of the limb; large tumors can be palpated. Muscle atrophy and monoparesis eventually develop. The spinal cord may become compressed by the invasive tumor, causing neurologic deficits in other limbs. The trigeminal nerve is the most frequently affected cranial nerve. This results in unilateral atrophy of the temporalis and masseter muscles and facial dysesthesia or anesthesia. Eventually, brain-stem compression can develop. Early surgical excision may be curative, although recurrence at the proximal stump of the resected nerve(s) is common. In cattle, nerve sheath tumors are often recognized incidentally in old animals at slaughter. Often, multiple nerves, especially autonomic nerves and cranial nerve VIII, are affected. Peripheral nerves may also be affected by other tumors, including lymphoma and leukemia. (*See also* p 1047 and p 779).

Paraneoplastic neuropathy (p 1060) refers to neuropathy associated with neoplasia unrelated to tumor infiltration of nerves. It is most common in dogs with insulinoma but has been associated with a variety of tumors, including bronchogenic carcinoma, multiple myeloma, sarcoma, and adenocarcinoma. The pathogenesis is not well understood but may be related to an immune response directed against the tumor that crossreacts with nerve components. Clinically, there is paraparesis or tetraparesis that progresses over several weeks with decreased spinal reflexes and muscle atrophy. Diagnosis is based on identifying the underlying tumor, clinical and electrodiagnostic findings of neuropathy, and in some cases, nerve biopsy. Signs may improve with successful treatment of the underlying tumor.

NUTRITIONAL DISORDERS

Pantothenic acid deficiency may develop in animals (particularly pigs) on rations of corn. Clinical signs include pelvic limb ataxia and a "goose-stepping" gait in which the stifles remain extended and the hips flex to lift the limbs off the ground. Pathologic findings consist of degeneration of myelinated fibers in peripheral nerves and chromatolysis and loss of sensory neurons in spinal ganglia.

Riboflavin deficiency in chickens (curled toe paralysis, p 2334) can develop if feed is not formulated properly. Affected chicks show poor growth, diarrhea, and weakness. There is inability to extend the hocks and progressive inward curling of the toes so that chicks rest and walk on their hocks. Mortality is high by the third week. At necropsy the peripheral nerves, especially the sciatic nerves, are swollen. Histopathologically, there is hypertrophy of Schwann cells, demyelination, and minimal axonal degeneration. Chickens often recover with riboflavin supplementation unless the curled-toe deformity is longstanding.

TOXIC DISORDERS

Botulism is intoxication with a neurotoxin produced by *Clostridium botulinum*. It is seen in horses, cattle, sheep, and birds worldwide. (*See also* BOTULISM, p 490 and p 2286). It is uncommon in dogs and pigs. Botulism is usually the result of ingestion of the preformed toxin, often in carrion that has contaminated the feed. Proliferation of *C botulinum* is also possible in decaying vegetation, eg, rotting hay or silage. Multiple animals may be affected. Toxicoinfectious botulism is seen in horses, especially foals in the eastern USA, when the organism grows in the GI tract with subsequent in vivo production of toxin (shaker foal syndrome). It can also develop from wound infection. There are 8 types of antigenically distinct botulism toxins (types A, B, C_a, C_b, D, E, F, G). Intoxication in dogs is almost always due to type C toxin, and most cases in large animals are due to types B, C, or D. The toxin inhibits release of acetylcholine at the neuromuscular junction, resulting in rapidly progressing flaccid tetraparesis and hyporeflexia. Cranial nerve dysfunction is common. Autonomic dysfunction has also been reported. Mentation and sensory perception remain normal. Mortality is high in large animals and is due to respiratory paralysis. Definitive diagnosis requires identifying the toxin in the feed, blood, vomitus, or feces. There are no specific pathologic findings. Treatment is generally supportive. Gastric lavage and purgatives may remove unabsorbed toxin from the GI tract. Antitoxins are available that neutralize circulating toxin, but they are not effective after the toxin has entered the nerve terminals, which occurs soon after the toxin is absorbed into the circulation. Toxicoinfectious botulism should be treated with penicillin. Most affected dogs recover within 14 days. The prognosis is poor for recumbent large animals. To help prevent botulism, feed should be kept dry and free of contamination by rodent carcasses. A vaccine is available for horses and cattle in endemic areas.

Ionophore toxicity (p 955) has been seen in cattle, sheep, pigs, dogs, cats, and poultry; horses are particularly susceptible. Lasalocid-contaminated food has caused flaccid tetraparesis with hyporeflexia in dogs. In 1995, cat food contaminated with sialinomycin caused an outbreak of polyneuropathy in ~850 cats in the Netherlands and Switzerland. Affected cats suffered an acute onset of tetraparesis, hyporeflexia, dysphagia, respiratory weakness, and eventual muscle atrophy. Histopathologic findings consisted of degeneration of distal sensory and motor axons. Affected animals usually recover with supportive care and removal of the offending food.

Organophosphate poisoning (p 2398) can cause 3 syndromes. The **acute form** is due to irreversible inhibition of acetylcholinesterase, resulting in increased acetylcholine activation of the nicotinic and muscarinic receptors in the parasympathetic nervous system, nicotinic receptors at the neuromuscular junction, nicotinic receptors of the sympathetic nervous system, and cholinergic pathways within the CNS. Clinical signs of acute toxicity include muscarinic signs (eg, vomiting, diarrhea, salivation, bronchoconstriction, increased bronchial secretions), nicotinic signs (eg, muscle tremor and twitching), and CNS signs (eg, behavioral change, seizures). The **intermediate form** is primarily manifest as generalized muscle weakness due to accumulation of acetylcholine at the nicotinic neuromuscular junction, causing a depolarizing block. Cats are especially prone to this form of toxicity, most commonly due to chlorpyrifos. Affected cats often do not have obvious signs of acute toxicity, instead developing tetraparesis and ventroflexion of the neck several days after exposure. Mydriasis is common. Diagnosis is based on a history of exposure and the presence of typical clinical signs. Decreased cholinesterase activity in whole blood is supportive. Treatment of acute or subacute toxicity should include administration of atropine (0.2 mg/kg, IM) if dyspnea due to bronchial secretions and bronchoconstriction is present. Atropine will not relieve the nicotinic signs of tremors and weakness, which should be treated with pralidoxime chloride (20 mg/kg, IM or SC, BID). Diphenhydramine (4 mg/kg, IM or PO, BID) may help alleviate muscle weakness. Treatment for several weeks may be necessary. The **delayed form** of toxicity is associated with degeneration of distal axons in the peripheral and central nervous systems. It is unrelated to inhibition of acetylcholinesterase and is seen only with certain organophosphates. Signs develop several weeks after exposure and are characterized by weakness and ataxia of the pelvic limbs. In horses, laryngeal paralysis has also been reported. There is no specific treatment.

Tick paralysis (p 1073) is characterized by rapidly progressing paralysis caused by several species of ticks. Some female ticks produce a salivary toxin that interferes with acetylcholine release at the neuromuscular junction. In North America, *Dermacentor variabilis* and *D andersoni* may affect dogs, sheep, and cattle. In Australia, *Ixodes holocyclus* causes an especially severe form of tick paralysis in dogs, cats, and sheep. In Africa, the major tick associated with paralysis is *I rubicundus*, with cattle, sheep, goats, and rarely dogs, being affected. A wide variety of ticks affect animals in Europe and Asia. Clinical signs consist of paraparesis that progresses within 24-72 hr to flaccid tetraplegia, with weak to absent spinal cord reflexes. Sensory perception and consciousness remain normal. Dysphagia, facial paralysis, masticatory muscle weakness, and respiratory paralysis may develop in severe cases. Treatment consists of removal of the tick and application of a topical acaricide to kill any hidden ticks. For all except *I holocyclus* paralysis, prognosis is good and recovery occurs within 1-2 days. A hyperimmune serum is available for treatment of *I holocyclus* paralysis, but prognosis is guarded as death from respiratory paralysis may occur despite treatment.

TRAUMA

Brachial plexus avulsion occurs in dogs, cats, and birds due to traumatic injury to the C6 to T2 nerve roots that innervate the thoracic limb. With severe extension or abduction of the limb, the nerve roots stretch or tear from their attachment to the spinal cord. Clinical signs vary with the extent of root involvement. Complete avulsion results in flaccid paralysis of the limb, anesthesia distal to the elbow, ipsilateral Horner's syndrome, and ipsilateral loss of the cutaneous trunci (panniculus) reflex. The injured animal bears little or no weight on the limb and drags the dorsal surface of the paw on the ground. Sensation to the ventral surface of the paw is spared if only the cranial nerve roots are affected. Avulsion of the caudal nerve roots causes loss of sensation on the caudal surface of the limb with variable loss on the cranial surface. There is no treatment, and the prognosis for complete avulsion is poor. Amputation of the limb may be necessary because of damage from dragging or self-mutilation. Recovery is possible in mild cases in which the roots are contused rather than avulsed.

Peripheral nerve injuries are some of the most common neuropathies in animals. The **sciatic nerve** or its branches may be injured by pelvic fractures, during or after retrograde placement of intramedullary pins in the femur, or by injections of irritative substances in or near the nerve. Damage to the proximal aspect of the sciatic nerve causes monoparesis with inability to flex the stifle. The hock and digits cannot flex or extend, and weight is supported on the dorsal surface of the foot with the hock excessively flexed. There may be loss of sensation below the stifle except for the medial aspect, which is innervated by a branch of the femoral nerve. Injury to the **tibial nerve** results in inability to extend the hock or flex the digits and reduced sensation over the plantar surface of the foot. Injury to the **peroneal nerve** results in inability to flex the hock or extend the digits and decreased sensation over the craniodorsal surface of the foot, hock, and stifle. The **femoral nerve** may be injured in calves and foals during dystocia if excessive traction stretches or otherwise damages it. This results in an inability to bear weight on the limb because of an inability to extend the stifle. The patellar reflex is weak or absent. Sensation is lost along the medial surface of the limb (saphenous nerve). The **suprascapular nerve** is most commonly injured in large animals secondary to trauma of the shoulder region. This results in atrophy of the supraspinatus and infraspinatus muscles and instability of the shoulder joint (sweeney, p 922). In horses, the nerve may be entrapped by connective tissue that develops in the region of the supraspinous fossa.

Calving paralysis is seen in heifers with oversized fetuses. It has previously been attributed to bilateral compression of the obturator nerve, but damage to the sixth lumbar nerve root, which contributes to the obturator and sciatic nerve, probably accounts for most of the paralysis. Ischemic necrosis of muscles secondary to compression, and ruptures of muscles during attempts to rise, also contribute to the paraparesis. Additionally, metabolic derangements, such as hypocalcemia, may complicate the syndrome. (*See also* PROBLEMATIC BOVINE STERNAL RECUMBENCY, p 957.)

Facial nerve trauma is most common in large animals that become recumbent with subsequent compression of the side of the face. It can be caused by pressure from a halter in horses after general anesthesia. There is ipsilateral lip paralysis, deviation of the muzzle to the contralateral side, and weak to absent palpebral reflex. A drooping ear can result from injuries to the proximal aspect of the nerve.

The immediate effect of injury of a peripheral nerve is a variable degree of dysfunction, depending on the severity of the injury. The mildest form of injury is neuropraxia, which temporarily disrupts function with minimal morphologic alterations in the nerve. Axonotmesis is disruption of axons without disruption of the surrounding connective tissue of the nerve. The most severe form of injury is neurotmesis, which is complete severance of the nerve. With both axonotmesis and neurotmesis, there is subsequent degeneration of the axons distal to the injury site and in a portion of the nerve proximal to the injury site.

Diagnosis of peripheral nerve injuries is based on the history and clinical assessment of the motor and sensory function of the affected nerve(s). Electromyography is often helpful in identifying denervated muscles 5-10 days after injury. Nerve conduction studies may also be useful in diagnosis.

Prognosis is guarded. With neuropraxia, complete recovery usually occurs within 3 wk. For function to return after axons are disrupted (axonotmesis, neurotmesis), the nerve must regenerate from the point of injury all the way to the innervated muscle. The growth rate of regenerating axons in the distal stump is 1-3 mm/day. Recovery is unlikely if the severed axons are substantially separated or if scar tissue interferes with axonal growth. Although various anti-inflammatory drugs have been recommended for traumatic nerve injuries, there is little evidence of benefit. Surgery to appose the nerve stumps should be performed promptly in cases in which the nerve has been sharply transected. In instances of blunt trauma, surgical exploration and excision of scar tissue may help. Surgery is often successful in horses with fibrous compression of the suprascapular nerve. Longterm management consists of physical therapy to minimize muscle atrophy and decreased mobility of joints. Bandages or splints may be necessary to help protect the affected limb.

VASCULAR DISEASES

Ischemic neuromyopathy is most common in cats with arterial thromboembolism secondary to myocardial disease. It also is seen in dogs with a variety of underlying conditions including hyperadrenocorticism, hypothyroidism, renal disease, cancer, and heart disease. Occlusion occurs most commonly at the distal aortic trifurcation, resulting in ischemia of muscles and nerves in the pelvic limbs. There is acute, painful paraparesis and an inability to flex or extend the hock. The flexor reflex and, in some cases, the patellar reflex are lost. Sensation distal to the hock is decreased. The gastrocnemius and cranial tibial muscles are often firm and painful. The nails may be cyanotic, and the femoral pulses are weak or absent. Diagnosis can usually be made based on clinical features. Serum CK is often elevated. Doppler ultrasonography is useful in evaluating blood flow in the distal aorta and femoral arteries. Pathologic changes are present distal to the level of the middle to lower thigh and are characterized as focal muscle necrosis and degeneration of the central portions of the sciatic nerve and its branches. Management consists of diagnosis and treatment of any underlying disease (eg, cardiomyopathy) and anticoagulant or antiplatelet-aggregating drugs. Neurologic deficits may improve within 2-3 wk, but 6 mo may be required for complete recovery. Permanent deficits are possible. The longterm prognosis is guarded because of the underlying heart disease and high risk for recurrence of thromboembolism.

DISEASES OF THE SPINAL COLUMN AND CORD

Diseases of the spinal column and cord include congenital disorders, degenerative diseases, inflammatory and infectious diseases, neoplasia, nutritional diseases, trauma, toxic disorders, and vascular diseases. *See* CONGENITAL AND INHERITED ANOMALIES, p 995, for a discussion of congenital disorders related to the spinal column and cord.

DEGENERATIVE DISEASES

Degenerative lumbosacral stenosis is narrowing of the lumbosacral vertebral canal that results in compression of the cauda equina or nerve roots. It is most common in large breeds of dogs, especially German Shepherds, and is rare in cats. It results from degeneration and protrusion of the L7 to S1 disk, hypertrophy of the ligamentum flavum, or rarely subluxation of the lumbosacral joint. The cause is unknown, although German Shepherds with congenital transitional vertebrae are at increased risk. Clinical signs typically begin at 3-7 yr of age and may include difficulty using the pelvic limbs, pelvic limb lameness, tail weakness, and incontinence. Pain on palpation or extension of the lumbosacral joint is the most consistent finding. There may be proprioceptive deficits, muscle atrophy, or a weak flexor reflex in the pelvic limbs. Plain radiographs may show degenerative changes, but definitive diagnosis requires MRI, computed tomography, or epidurography. Dogs in which mild pain is the only sign may improve with 4-6 wk of rest. Treatment consists of surgical decompression of the cauda equina and spinal nerves. Prognosis for recovery is good, although urinary incontinence may not resolve.

Degenerative myelopathy of dogs (chronic degenerative radiculomyelopathy) is a slowly progressive, noninflammatory degeneration of the axons and myelin in the white matter of the spinal cord. It is most common in German Shepherds and Welsh Corgis, but is occasionally recognized in other breeds. The cause is unknown, although genetic factors are suspected. Pathologically, there is noninflammatory degeneration of axons in the white matter of the spinal cord, which is most severe in the thoracic region. Affected dogs are usually >5 yr old and develop an insidious onset of nonpainful ataxia and weakness of the pelvic limbs. Spinal reflexes are usually normal or exaggerated, but in ~10% of cases, patellar reflexes are weak, reflecting involvement of lumbar dorsal nerve roots. Early cases may be confused with orthopedic disorders; however, proprioceptive deficits are an early feature of degenerative myelopathy and are not seen in orthopedic disease. Signs slowly progress to paraplegia over 6-36 mo, although signs may fluctuate. Myelography or MRI and CSF analysis are essential to rule out compressive and inflammatory diseases. Treatment with aminocaproic acid (500 mg, PO, TID), vitamin supplements, and exercise has been recommended, but the safety and efficacy of this treatment has not been documented. The longterm prognosis is poor; most animals are euthanized within 1-3 yr of diagnosis.

Equine degenerative encephalomyelopathy is a progressive neurologic disorder of horses and zebras characterized by diffuse degeneration of axons, myelin, and neurons in the spinal cord and, to a lesser degree, the brain stem. It has been reported in many equine breeds in North America, Australia, and England. The etiology is incompletely understood, but a vitamin E deficiency and genetic factors are suspected. Clinical signs usually become apparent during the first year of life and consist of ataxia and weakness in all 4 limbs, although the hindlimbs may be more severely affected. Clinical signs may stabilize or slowly progress. Myelography and CSF analysis are normal. Vitamin E supplementation is preventive in some cases, and affected horses may improve with supplementation.

Intervertebral disk disease is degeneration and protrusion of the intervertebral disk that results in compression of the spinal cord, spinal nerve, and/or nerve root. It is a common cause of spinal disease in dogs. Clinical signs due to disk disease are rare in cats and horses. Chondrodystrophoid breeds of dogs (eg, Dachshund, Beagle, Shih Tzu, Lhasa Apso, and Pekingese) are most commonly affected. In these breeds, there is chondroid degeneration of the disks within the first few months of life. Disk extrusion can occur as early as 1-2 yr of age, and clinical signs are often acute and severe. In contrast, fibroid disk degeneration typically occurs in large breeds of dogs >5 yr old and causes slowly progressive clinical signs. The most common sites of disk extrusion are the cervical and thoracolumbar regions. The predominant sign of cervical disk extrusion is neck pain, manifested as cervical rigidity and muscle spasms. There may be thoracic limb lameness or neurologic deficits, ranging from mild tetraparesis to tetraplegia. In thoracolumbar disk extrusion, there may be back pain, evident as kyphosis and reluctance to move. Neurologic deficits are usually more severe than those seen in cervical disk disease and range from pelvic limb ataxia to paraplegia and incontinence. In paraplegic animals, the most important prognostic finding is whether or not there is deep pain perception caudal to the lesion. This is assessed by pinching the toe or tail and observing whether or not there is a behavioral response, such as a bark or turn of the head. Reflex flexion of the limb must not be mistaken for a behavioral response.

Definitive diagnosis of disk extrusion is based on radiography and myelography. Dogs with pain and minimal to moderate neurologic deficits often recover with 2-3 wk of cage rest. A short course of prednisone (1 mg/kg/day for 3 days) is often helpful in relieving pain. The use of anti-inflammatory or analgesic medication without concurrent cage rest is contraindicated because an increase in the dog's activity may lead to further disk extrusion and worsening of spinal cord compression. Clinical signs recur after conservative therapy in 30-40% of cases.

In animals with severe neurologic deficits, methylprednisolone sodium succinate may improve recovery of severe spinal cord injuries if given within 8 hr of injury (*see* TRAUMA, p 1024). Medical therapy, however, is not a substitute for surgery, which should be performed promptly to decompress the spinal cord in animals with substantial neurologic deficits. Other indications for surgery are failure of conservative therapy and recurrent episodes. The prognosis is good for dogs with intact deep pain perception that are treated surgically. If surgery is performed within 24 hr of the loss of deep pain perception, the chance of recovery is ~50%. If surgery is delayed for >48 hours after deep pain perception is lost, the prognosis is poor. Progressive myelomalacia develops in a small percentage of dogs with paraplegia and loss of deep pain perception caused by acute disk extrusion.

Equine motor neuron disease is a progressive, noninflammatory degeneration of motor neurons in the spinal cord and brain stem of horses. It is most common in the northeastern USA but has been reported in several areas of North and South America, Europe, and Japan. The etiology is unknown, although low plasma concentrations of vitamin E have been detected in affected horses. Adult horses of any age and breed can be affected, although Quarter Horses are affected most commonly. It is more common in horses without access to pasture grass. Clinical signs consist of generalized symmetric weakness, trembling, and muscle atrophy. Affected horses often stand with their head held low and their feet camped under their body, frequently shifting their weight from one limb to another. Ataxia is not a feature of this disease, in contrast to most spinal cord diseases. Many affected horses have retinal abnormalities, including a distinct reticulated pigment pattern and areas of hyper-reflectivity. Electromyography and biopsy of the spinal accessory nerve or the sacrodorsalis caudalis muscle are useful in the diagnosis. There is no specific treatment, but some horses improve partially after 2-3 mo of illness.

Degeneration of motor neurons is seen as an inherited or sporadic disease in Brittany Spaniels, Pointers, German Shepherds, Doberman Pinschers, and Rottweilers; cats; Hereford, Brown Swiss, and red Danish cattle; Yorkshire pigs; and goats.

Metabolic storage disorders are rare, usually inherited, metabolic disorders that can affect the CNS, including the spinal cord. *See also* CONGENITAL AND INHERITED ANOMALIES OF THE NERVOUS SYSTEM, p 995.

Spondylosis deformans is a noninflammatory, degenerative disease characterized by production of osteophytes along the ventral and lateral aspects of the vertebral bodies. In advanced cases, the osteophytes may appear to bridge the intervertebral disk space. It is seen in dogs, cats, and bulls, and the incidence increases with age. The cause is breakdown of the outer fibers of the annulus fibrosis and stretching of the longitudinal ligament. The increased stress at the vertebral attachment of the longitudinal ligament incites osteophyte production. It is usually an incidental radiographic finding. Rare cases cause spinal hyperesthesia, which should be treated with analgesics.

INFLAMMATORY AND INFECTIOUS DISEASES

Infectious and inflammatory diseases of the spinal column and spinal cord include bacterial, rickettsial, viral, fungal, protozoal, and parasitic infections and idiopathic inflammatory disease. Many of these diseases can also affect the brain (*see* MENINGITIS AND ENCEPHALITIS, p 1044). Some of the more common infectious and inflammatory diseases in which involvement of the spinal column or cord is a prominent feature are discussed below.

Bacterial Diseases

Diskospondylitis is inflammation of the intervertebral disk and adjacent vertebral bodies. **Vertebral osteomyelitis** is inflammation of the vertebra without concurrent disk infection. Both diseases are usually caused by hematogenous spread of bacterial or fungal infection. Immunosuppression may play a role in some infections. Diskospondylitis is most common in dogs, especially larger breeds. Osteomyelitis of the lumbar vertebrae can develop in dogs secondary to migration of plant awns. In cats, it is rare and usually due to direct spread of infection from an adjacent wound. Diskospondylitis and vertebral osteomyelitis have also been reported in horses, ruminants, and pigs, especially neonates. Infection may be seen at any disk space, and multiple lesions may be seen.

In canine diskospondylitis, the most commonly isolated organisms are *Staphylococcus* spp. Other organisms include *Brucella canis, Streptococcus* spp, *Escherichia coli,*

Proteus spp, *Corynebacterium diphtheroides*, *Nocardia* spp, and *Aspergillus* spp. Spinal pain is the most consistent clinical finding. Systemic signs, such as fever, depression, and weight loss, are seen in a few dogs. Neurologic deficits may develop due to spinal cord compression caused by proliferative tissue or, rarely, spread of infection to the spinal cord or pathologic fracture. Early radiographic findings consist of destruction of the adjacent vertebral end plates and collapse of the disk space. More advanced lesions also have variable degrees of osteophyte formation. Blood and urine cultures are often effective in identifying the causative organism. Affected dogs should be tested for brucellosis (p 1159). Although clinical signs usually resolve within 5 days of treatment with an appropriate antibiotic, treatment should be continued for at least 8 wk. First-generation cephalosporins for presumed *Staphylococcus* spp are a good choice if cultures are negative. Surgery to decompress the spinal cord may be necessary in animals with neurologic deficits refractory to antibiotic therapy.

Rickettsial Diseases

Neurologic abnormalities, including signs of spinal cord dysfunction, are sometimes seen in dogs with rickettsial infection. Dogs with **Rocky Mountain spotted fever** (*Rickettsia rickettsii*, p 641) often have thrombocytopenia, leukocytosis, and a neutrophilic pleocytosis and mildly increased protein on CSF analysis. Diagnosis is based on a 4-fold increase in serum antibody concentration. Dogs with **ehrlichiosis** (*Ehrlichia canis*, p 638) often have thrombocytopenia, anemia, leukopenia, hyperglobulinemia, and mononuclear pleocytosis and marked increase in protein on CSF analysis. A single serum antibody titer is usually sufficient for diagnosis of *E canis*. Treatment of rickettsial myelitis consists of doxycycline or chloramphenicol for 14-21 days. Prognosis is good with early treatment, although neurologic deficits occasionally progress despite treatment.

Viral Diseases

Canine distemper encephalomyelitis (p 625), caused by a Morbillivirus, remains one of the most common CNS disorders in dogs worldwide. Onset of neurologic deficits may be acute or slowly progressive, reflecting the location of the lesion(s) within the CNS. The brain stem and spinal cord are the regions most commonly affected in mature dogs. Neurologic signs are usually not preceded by, nor coincident with, the systemic illness seen in young dogs. Definitive antemortem diagnosis is difficult. There may be active or inactive chorioretinitis on fundoscopy. A mononuclear pleocytosis with increased protein concentration is the most common finding on CSF analysis. The finding of canine distemper antigen or antibodies in the CSF is suggestive, although false negatives are common. There is no specific treatment, and the prognosis is poor for severely affected dogs. Vaccination is usually successful in preventing the systemic form of distemper, but previously vaccinated dogs can be affected by the neurologic form.

Caprine arthritis and encephalomyelitis (p 598) is caused by a lentivirus that can also cause pneumonitis and arthritis. It has been reported in North America, Europe, Australia, and New Zealand. CNS disease is most common in goats 2-4 mo old, although older animals may also be affected. There is an acute onset of slightly asymmetric spastic paraparesis that may progress to tetraplegia with exaggerated reflexes. A mononuclear pleocytosis and increased protein in the CSF are present in ~50% of the cases. Serologic testing is helpful in detecting infection, but false negatives can be seen. There is no treatment, and recovery is unlikely. Histologically, there is severe nonsuppurative inflammation with demyelination or necrosis, most prominent in the white matter of the spinal cord.

A related lentivirus is a rare cause of chronic encephalomyelitis in sheep (**maedi**, p 1233). Affected sheep are usually >2 yr old and suffer an insidious onset of progressive ataxia, paraparesis, or tetraparesis.

Equine infectious anemia (p 559) occasionally produces encephalomyelitis in horses. Neurologic deficits are usually referable to spinal cord disease and include ataxia and weakness in the hindlimbs. The protein concentration of and the number of lymphocytes in the CSF are often increased. Diagnosis is by positive agar gel immunodiffusion testing. There is no treatment, and affected horses are usually euthanized to prevent spread of the disease.

Equine herpesvirus 1 (EHV-1) encephalomyelopathy is a neurologic disorder that affects horses worldwide. The EHV-1 virus infects vascular endothelial cells, particularly those within the CNS. It causes an immune-mediated vasculitis with secondary infarction and hemorrhage throughout the brain and spinal cord. The EHV-1 virus has also been associated with meningoencephalitis in alpacas and llamas. In horses, neurologic signs may be seen as the primary disease or follow rhinopneumonitis or abortion. Any age animal may be affected. Neurologic deficits have an abrupt onset, vary from mild hindlimb ataxia to paraplegia, and usually do not progress after 24 hr. Urine dribbling, fecal retention, and sensory deficits in the perineum and tail are common. The CSF is often xanthochromic with increased protein content and normal numbers of cells. Diagnosis is based on clinical findings and an increase in antibody concentration in paired serum samples. There is no specific treatment, but mildly affected horses often recover with supportive care. Even recumbent horses can eventually recover. Vaccination does not protect from the neurologic form of this disease. (*See also* p 1203.)

Feline infectious peritonitis (p 628) is a disease of domestic cats caused by an immune-mediated response to a coronavirus. Involvement of the CNS is usually associated with the parenchymatous (dry) form rather than with the effusive (wet) form. There are pyogranulomatous lesions involving the neural parenchyma, choroid plexuses, ependyma, and leptomeninges. Clinical signs of spinal cord involvement include spinal hyperesthesia and paraparesis or tetraparesis. Hyperglobulinemia and involvement of other organs, especially the eyes, are common. Serum antibody tests that are currently available are nonspecific and often negative. A mixed (neutrophilic and mononuclear) pleocytosis with increased protein concentration is the most common finding on CSF analysis. There is no effective treatment, and the prognosis is poor.

Feline leukemia virus-associated myelopathy is seen in some cats infected with the feline leukemia virus (FeLV, p 631) for ≥2 yr. Ataxia and weakness of the pelvic limbs progresses to paraplegia within 1 yr. Other signs include diffuse spinal pain and abnormal behavior. Diagnosis is based on clinical features, FeLV serology, and exclusion of other causes, such as spinal lymphoma and myelitis due to toxoplasmosis or fungal infection. There is no treatment; affected cats are eventually euthanized because of disability. Pathologic findings consist of white matter degeneration, swollen axons, and dilation of myelin sheaths in the spinal cord and brain stem. FeLV antigen is present in the nervous system, indicating that the lesions are due to viral infection.

Porcine enteroviral encephalomyelitis (p 1064), also called Teschen disease, Talfan disease, poliomyelitis suum, and benign enzootic paresis, is caused by a neurotropic teschovirus that was previously classified as an enterovirus. All ages of pigs may be affected, but disease is most common in suckling and weanling pigs. There is a peracute or subacute onset of hindlimb ataxia and paresis with hyporeflexia, depression, seizures, and death. Definitive antemortem diagnosis is difficult. Histologically, there is neuronal degeneration, glial nodules, and lymphocytic perivascular cuffing, most prominent in the spinal cord. Older pigs may survive, but mortality is high in young pigs.

Porcine hemagglutinating encephalomyelitis virus is a coronavirus that causes both vomiting and wasting disease (p 577) and an encephalomyelitis. It is most common in piglets <3 wk old, and there is some overlap of these syndromes. The CNS disease starts with several days of vomiting, which is followed by hyperesthesia, muscle tremors, ataxia, paresis, opisthotonos, coma, and death. Pathologically, there is diffuse nonsuppurative encephalomyelitis, primarily involving gray matter. Diagnosis is based on necropsy or an increase in antibody titer in paired sera. There is no treatment.

Rabies (p 1067) is caused by a neurotropic rhabdovirus that reaches the CNS via peripheral nerves. It produces multifocal, nonsuppurative polioencephalomyelitis in all domestic mammals. Rabies is endemic on all continents except Australia, although it is excluded from some islands, including Great Britain, New Zealand, Iceland, and Hawaii. Initial clinical signs are extremely variable, and rabies should be considered in any unvaccinated animal with acute neurologic dysfunction. Signs of spinal cord involvement include ataxia and progressive paralysis, usually with absent reflexes. Affected animals typically, but not invariably, die with progressive neurologic signs within 2-7 days of illness. There is no treatment. Definitive diagnosis is based on fluorescent antibody testing of the brain. Prevention is by vaccination.

Fungal Diseases

Cryptococcus neoformans is the most common fungus to involve the CNS in animals. Infection is most common in dogs and cats and occurs occasionally in horses. Other fungal organisms may invade the CNS, including *Blastomyces dermatitidis, Histoplasma capsulatum, Coccidioides immitis, Aspergillus* spp, and phaeohyphomycoses. Affected animals often have involvement of other organs, such as the lungs, eyes, skin, or bones. Signs of spinal cord involvement include paresis or paralysis and spinal hyperesthesia. Diagnosis is based on serology, culture, or identifying the organism in CSF or extraneural tissue. Fluconazole is often effective for cryptococcosis and coccidioidomycosis. Itraconazole or amphotericin B are recommended for histoplasmosis and blastomycosis, but the prognosis is guarded to poor. (*See also* FUNGAL INFECTIONS, p 510.)

Protozoal Diseases

Equine protozoal myeloencephalitis (p 1031) is a common disease of horses that produces a nonsuppurative, often necrotizing, meningoencephalomyelitis. Horses are an aberrant host for the causative organism, usually *Sarcocystis neurona*, but less commonly, other protozoa cause the disease. Any age horse can be affected. Neurologic signs are extremely variable and often asymmetric, reflecting involvement anywhere in the CNS. Ataxia and paresis are common. Other potential signs include obscure lameness, focal muscle atrophy, and cranial nerve dysfunction. Diagnosis is based on neurologic signs, exclusion of other potential causes, detection of antibodies to *S neurona* in the CSF, and response to treatment. Treatment protocols include ponazuril (5 mg/kg/day, PO for 28 days) or pyrimethamine (1 mg/kg/day, PO) and sulfadiazine (20 mg/kg/day, PO) for 90-180 days. Many horses recover with treatment, but permanent neurologic deficits are possible. Prevention is difficult but involves reducing access of opossums (the definitive host) to horses, feed, and water. A vaccine is also available.

Neosporosis (p 535) is caused by *Neospora caninum*, a protozoan that can cause a nonsuppurative encephalomyelitis, most commonly in dogs. The life cycle of this organism has not been defined. Many previously reported cases of toxoplasmosis in dogs were probably neosporosis. Infection in young puppies typically causes ascending paralysis with rigid contraction of the muscles of one or both pelvic limbs. Other organs, including muscle, liver, and lungs, can be affected. Diagnosis is based on serology or identification of the organism in tissue samples. Early treatment with clindamycin or sulfadiazine and pyrimethamine may be effective, but the prognosis is poor.

Toxoplasmosis (p 547) is caused by *Toxoplasma gondii* and can occasionally cause a nonsuppurative encephalomyelitis in dogs and cats. Infected cats often have evidence of disease in other organs, such as uveitis, pancreatitis, and respiratory disease. Dogs with toxoplasmosis often also have other diseases, such as canine distemper. Diagnosis is based on identifying the organism in tissue or a 4-fold increase in IgG antibody in paired sera. In cats, a high concentration of IgM antibody in serum or CSF is supportive. Clindamycin or sulfadiazine and pyrimethamine are recommended for treatment.

Parasitic Diseases

Verminous myelitis is inflammation of the spinal cord caused by parasite migration. Organisms include *Parelaphostrongylus tenuis* in sheep, goats, and llamas; *Hypoderma bovis* in cattle; *Strongylus vulgaris, Halicephalobus (Micronema) deletrix,* and *Setaria* spp in horses; *Stephanurus dentatus* in pigs; *Cuterebra* spp in cats; and *Baylisascaris procyonis* in dogs. Signs of spinal cord involvement are usually acute, often asymmetric, and may be progressive. Antemortem diagnosis is difficult. Increased eosinophils in the CSF is suggestive, but CSF findings are variable. Treatment with fenbendazole, thiabendazole, or ivermectin is recommended, but the prognosis is guarded. (*See also* CNS DISEASES CAUSED BY HELMINTHS AND ARTHROPODS, p 1034.)

Idiopathic Inflammatory Diseases

Feline nonsuppurative meningoencephalomyelitis (feline polioencephalomyelitis, staggering disease) is a slowly progressive, inflammatory disease of the CNS in domestic cats. It has been reported in North America, Europe, and Australia. The cause is unknown, but an infectious agent, probably a virus, is strongly suspected. The disease causes neuronal degeneration, axonal loss, and demyelination with mononuclear inflammation, most severe in the thoracic segments of the spinal cord. The clinical course is marked by progressive paraparesis of 1-2 mo duration, often with focal hyperesthesia, head tremor, and behavioral changes. Antemortem diagnosis is difficult. There is no treatment, and the prognosis is poor.

Granulomatous meningoencephalomyelitis (GME) is an inflammatory disease of the CNS in dogs worldwide. The cause is unknown, although an infectious agent, most likely a virus, is suspected. In the disseminated form, previously called inflammatory reticulosis, there are perivascular accumulations of mononuclear cells and neutrophils. In the focal form, previously called neoplastic reticulosis, there are granulomatous lesions containing primarily reticulohistiocytic cells. Adult dogs of any breed can be affected, but female, small-breed dogs, especially Poodles, may be predisposed. Clinical signs are variable and may indicate focal or multifocal brain or spinal cord dysfunction. Cervical pain and tetraparesis are the most common signs of spinal cord involvement. Signs are often acute, but the focal form of GME can cause neurologic deficits that slowly progress over the course of several months. The CSF usually has increased protein and pleocytosis, with either mononuclear cells or neutrophils predominating. Tentative diagnosis is based on clinical findings and CSF analysis and exclusion of other possible diseases. Dogs often improve temporarily with immunosuppressive doses of corticosteroids, but the longterm prognosis is poor.

NEOPLASIA

See also NEOPLASIA OF THE NERVOUS SYSTEM, p 1047.

In **dogs**, neoplasms commonly affecting the spinal cord include osteosarcoma, fibrosarcoma, meningioma, nerve sheath tumor, and metastatic neoplasia. A tumor resembling nephroblastoma is seen in young dogs (5-36 mo of age), with German Shepherds affected most commonly. This tumor is consistently located within the dura mater between T10 and L2, causing progressive paraparesis. Diagnosis of spinal neoplasia is based on radiography, myelography, and surgical biopsy. Surgical excision is possible in some cases, but in general, the prognosis is poor.

In **cats**, lymphoma is the most common neoplasia to affect the spinal cord. Adult cats of any age can be affected. There is an acute or slowly progressive onset of signs referable to a focal, often painful, lesion of the spinal cord. About 85% of affected cats have positive test results for feline leukemia virus (p 631), and many have leukemic bone marrow. Myelography shows extradural compression. Treatment consists of combination chemotherapy, such as prednisone, vincristine, and cyclophosphamide. Remission is possible in many cases, but the longterm prognosis is poor.

In **cattle**, lymphosarcoma may develop in the epidural space at any level, causing spinal cord compression. Often, there is an acute onset of paraparesis or recumbency. Usually, there is other evidence of bovine leukosis (p 593). Definitive diagnosis is based on histopathologic examination.

Neoplasia is a rare cause of spinal cord disease in horses, pigs, sheep, and goats.

NUTRITIONAL DISORDERS

Copper deficiency causes CNS disease in sheep, goats, and pigs. **Swayback** is the congenital form in lambs and is characterized by degeneration and necrosis of the cerebrum. The acquired form, **enzootic ataxia**, affects lambs, kids, and pigs. Affected animals appear normal at birth but develop progressive paraparesis with hyporeflexia and muscle atrophy within the first few months of life. Other signs include diarrhea and unthriftiness and, in lambs, abnormal fleece. Histologically, there is chromatolysis and loss of neurons and degeneration of axons, primarily in the spinal cord and caudal aspect of the brain stem. Animals may improve with copper supplementation, but permanent neurologic deficits are likely in severely affected animals.

Hypervitaminosis A develops in cats fed excess vitamin A, usually diets consisting largely of liver. This results in extensive exostoses, most prominent in the cervical and thoracic spine. Clinical signs include neck pain and rigidity and forelimb lameness. Vertebral lesions are evident on radiographs. Reduction of dietary vitamin A prevents further exostosis but does not significantly reduce the lesions already present.

TRAUMA

Acute spinal cord injuries are commonly associated with spinal fracture or luxation. Common causes in dogs and cats are automobile accidents, bite wounds, and gunshot wounds. Falls are common causes in horses. Cattle are susceptible to injuries from breeding. Pathologic fractures are common in cattle, sheep, and pigs with malnutrition or vertebral osteomyelitis. Damage to the spinal cord is caused not only by the primary mechanical injury, but also as a result of secondary pathologic changes, including edema, hemorrhage, demyelination, and necrosis. These secondary changes are due to biochemical factors, including the release of free radicals, leukotrienes, and prostaglandins that cause further injury to nervous tissue and compromise blood flow to the spinal cord. In a small percentage of severe injuries, these secondary events lead to progressive ascending and descending necrosis of the spinal cord, termed **progressive myelomalacia** or **hematomyelia**.

Signs of spinal trauma are typically acute and may progress in instances of unstable fractures or luxations. Severe thoracolumbar spinal cord injury may cause paraplegia with increased extensor tone in the thoracic limbs (**Schiff-Sherrington phenomenon**). Progressive myelomalacia causes ascending and descending flaccid paralysis that typically progresses over several days and leads to death from respiratory paralysis. Radiographs usually demonstrate vertebral fractures and luxations. Treatment with methylprednisolone may be helpful if instituted within the first few hours of injury. One protocol is 30 mg/kg, IV, followed 2 hr later by 15 mg/kg, IV, followed 6 hr later by 15 mg/kg, IV, every 6 hr for a total of 24 hr of treatment. Dexamethasone is less effective and is associated with an increased risk of GI ulceration and pancreatitis. NSAID have minimal benefit in acute spinal cord injury and increase the risk of complications, especially if used in conjunction with corticosteroids. DMSO (0.5-1.0 g/kg/day of a 10-20% solution, given slowly IV for 3 days) is recommended in horses with acute spinal cord injury. Animals with mild neurologic deficits often recover with 4-6 wk of cage or stall rest. Surgical reduction and stabilization is indicated for unstable vertebral injuries causing severe neurologic dysfunction. The prognosis is guarded for recumbent horses and cattle. In animals that have lost deep pain perception caudal to the lesion, the prognosis for return of neurologic function is poor.

TOXIC DISORDERS

Arsenic poisoning (p 2346) can be seen in swine due to an overdose of organoarsenicals, which are often used as feed additives to promote growth and to control swine dysentery. With 3-nitro-4-hydroxyphenylarsonic acid ("3-nitro") poisoning, there is degeneration of the spinal cord, optic nerve, and peripheral nerves. Clinical signs consist of tremors and paraparesis. Mildly affected animals can recover after withdrawal of the offending feed.

Delayed organophosphate intoxication can be seen after oral or topical administration of organophosphate-containing insecticides or anthelmintics, including haloxon. In addition to the acute signs, delayed paralysis can develop 1-4 wk after exposure. Suffolk sheep have an inherited predisposition to this neurotoxicity because they have low levels of plasma arylesterase activity. Affected animals have progressive, symmetric paraparesis and occasionally become tetraplegic. Diagnosis is based on clinical signs and history of exposure. The prognosis for severely affected animals is poor. On histopathologic examination, there is Wallerian degeneration, most prominent in the spinal cord and brain stem. (*See also* ORGANOPHOSPHATES, p 2398.)

Sorghum spp, such as Sorghum, Sudan, and Johnson grass, can cause degeneration of the spinal cord in horses and occasionally in cattle and sheep. The pathogenesis may be related to the high content of hydrocyanide in these grasses. There is ataxia and weakness of the pelvic limbs and incontinence. Urine retention often leads to cystitis and hematuria. Diagnosis is based on clinical features and a history of exposure. Signs may improve with removal of the offending feed, although persistent deficits are possible. (*See also* SORGHUM POISONING, p 2520.)

Tetanus (p 495) is caused by toxins produced by the vegetative form of *Clostridium tetani*. Susceptibility varies markedly among species; dogs and cats are fairly resistant compared with horses. Clinical signs usually develop within 5-10 days of infection. These include localized or generalized muscle stiffness and extensor rigidity, dysphagia, protrusion of the third eyelid, and contracted masticatory (lockjaw) and facial (risus sardonicus) muscles. In severe cases, the animal may be recumbent with opisthotonos and reflex muscle spasms. Diagnosis is based on characteristic clinical features. Treatment consists of wound care, antibiotics to kill any remaining organisms, and tetanus antitoxin. In mild cases, prognosis is good with early treatment. In severe cases, death may occur due to respiratory paralysis.

VASCULAR DISEASES

Fibrocartilagenous embolism results in ischemia and infarction of the spinal cord. The cause is occlusion of spinal cord arteries or veins (or both) with fragments of fibrocartilage, believed to arise from the intervertebral disks. It is seen primarily in adult dogs, especially large and giant breeds. Miniature Schnauzers and Shetland Sheepdogs also may be predisposed. It is rare in cats, horses, and pigs. Affected dogs have an abrupt onset of gait dysfunction, often occurring during activities such as running or jumping. Deficits are referable to a focal, often asymmetric, lesion in the spinal cord and rarely progress beyond 12 hr. Spinal pain is typically absent. Diagnosis is based on clinical findings and exclusion of compressive lesions with myelography. In the acute stage, the CSF may have a mild increase in neutrophils and protein concentration. Mildly affected dogs often improve substantially within 1-2 wk. Prognosis is poor if deep pain perception is absent or if there is no improvement within several weeks.

Postanesthetic hemorrhagic myelopathy in horses is a rare complication of general anesthesia in dorsal recumbency. The cause may be related to impaired venous drainage of the spinal cord due to compression of the caudal vena cava or azygous vein because of the weight of abdominal viscera. There is paraplegia immediately after recovery from anesthesia. Pathologic findings consist of hemorrhagic necrosis of the thoracolumbar spinal cord segments. The prognosis is poor. Positioning the horse slightly tilted off the perpendicular and maintaining adequate blood pressure may help prevent this complication.

DYSAUTONOMIA

FELINE DYSAUTONOMIA

Feline dysautonomia is characterized by widespread dysfunction of the autonomic nervous system. All breeds and age groups are susceptible. Feline dysautonomia was first reported in 1982 and initially became widespread in the UK; the incidence declined considerably but recently seems to have risen again, although the condition is in a somewhat attenuated form. Cases have been reported throughout Europe, a few have been documented in North America, and sporadic cases have been seen in Dubai, New Zealand, and Venezuela. The etiology is unknown. Dysautonomias in horses, dogs, rabbits, and hares share striking similarities to the condition in cats.

Clinical Findings: Affected cats initially are mildly obtunded and anorectic and often have upper respiratory signs or transient diarrhea. The onset of more definite signs varies from peracute to chronic. The most common of these signs are dilated, nonresponsive pupils, ptosis, and third eyelid protrusion; a dry rhinarium; reduced lacrimal secretion; esophageal dysfunction with regurgitation; and constipation. Other signs include dry oral mucous membranes, prolapse of the nictitating membrane, bradycardia, and urinary or fecal incontinence. These signs reflect both sympathetic and parasympathetic dysfunction, and there is a wide range in the severity of presenting signs. Somatic signs include anal areflexia. Pelvic limb proprioceptive deficits have been reported but should be carefully differentiated from paresis—ataxia is not a feature of dysautonomia in other species. Clinical pathology findings are nonspecific.

Lesions: Necropsy may show megaesophagus, diphtheritic mucous membranes, an atonic bladder, and retention of fecal material. During the first few weeks after onset, chromatolysis and neuronal degeneration of pre- and postganglionic sympathetic and parasympathetic neurons is typical. A very specific distribution of chromatolytic autonomic and somatic lower motor neurons is found in the brain stem and spinal cord. Chronic cases can be difficult to confirm because surviving neurons appear normal, and diagnosis depends on an assessment of their numbers relative to surrounding stromal cells.

Diagnosis: Definitive diagnosis depends on histopathologic examination of autonomic ganglia. Clinical confirmation may be aided by contrast radiography (including fluoroscopy) of the esophagus and by reduced lacrimal secretion (<5 mm/min when measured by the Schirmer tear test). Pilocarpine (0.1%) applied to the cornea causes profound miosis within 10-15 min due to denervation hypersensitivity but has no effect on a healthy cat. Dilute (0.5%) phenylephrine reverses the ptosis and protruding third eyelid. Although feline leukemia virus (FeLV, p 631) infection can cause both anisocoria and urinary incontinence, cats with dysautonomia usually show other clinical signs and are FeLV-negative.

Treatment and Prognosis: The main aim of therapy is first to rehydrate the cat and then to maintain adequate fluid balance. Total parenteral nutrition is useful initially but later can be replaced by gastrostomy or nasogastric tube feeding when regurgitation resolves. Maintaining an upright posture after oral intake is important because the main complication of this condition is inhalation pneumonia. Thrice daily evacuation of the bladder, provision of warmth, use of artificial tears and steam inhalation, and assistance with grooming are all important nursing considerations. Liquid paraffin PO is helpful for constipation but increases the risk of aspiration; danthron (5 mg, PO, daily) is a safer laxative. Other parasympathomimetics, such as bethanechol (1.0-2.5 mg, PO, BID or TID), may be of use; however, their effect is crude, and overdosage requires treatment with atropine. Metoclopramide (0.1 mg/kg, IV, or 0.3 mg/kg, SC, TID) may improve gastric emptying.

A small proportion of cats have recovered, and others are able to cope with residual autonomic deficits. Such improvements often require up to 1 yr. In general, the prognosis is poor for severely affected cats.

CANINE DYSAUTONOMIA

Cases have been reported from both Europe and the USA, where canine dysautonomia is seen primarily in the midwest. Pupillary light responses tend to be absent, with normal vision. Pupil size is variable, and elevated third eyelids, ptosis, and enophthalmos are often present. Dysuria has been noted. Decreased anal sphincter tone and rhinitis sicca are present in most dogs. Secondary effects of autonomic dysfunction, such as aspiration pneumonia and lethargy may develop. Weight loss is often dramatic. Laboratory findings are nonspecific. Pharmacologic testing of the pupils is probably the best single test for confirming the diagnosis. Dilute pilocarpine (0.05% ophthalmic solution) results in rapid pupillary constriction in dogs with dysautonomia. The prognosis is grave.

LEPORINE DYSAUTONOMIA

This disease occurs in wild hares, and fatal cases have been reported in the UK. Gross lesions are similar to those of equine dysautonomia, including gastric distention, colonic impaction, and weight loss; histopathologic changes in the central and peripheral nervous systems are almost identical.

EQUINE DYSAUTONOMIA
(Grass sickness)

A fatal dysautonomia of unknown etiology, equine grass sickness causes marked reduction of GI motility due to widespread degeneration within the autonomic nervous system. It is seen throughout northern Europe, and a few cases have recently been diagnosed in the USA in the same geographic area (midwest) that has a high prevalence of canine dysautonomia.

Grass sickness is seen at any age after weaning and at any time of year, but the incidence is highest in spring and in horses 2-7 yr old. Although associated with recently acquired horses kept solely at grass, the condition has very rarely been seen in housed stock. All Equidae appear susceptible. Peracute, acute, subacute, and chronic forms are recognized. Death occurs within 24 hr, 7 days, and >1 wk, respectively, for the first 3 forms. Chronic cases can survive for weeks or months; a few cases have recovered. The exact etiology is unknown, but the causal agent is thought to be associated with grazing. A *Clostridium botulinum* toxin may be involved.

Clinical Findings: Horses are afebrile and show obtundation, tachycardia, ileus, and colic. Patchy sweating and fine muscular fasciculations are often seen over the shoulders and flanks, and penile prolapse may develop. In contrast to feline dysautonomia, pupillary light reflexes and tear production are normal. Ptosis, with "droopy" eyelashes, tends to be prominent. Affected horses often have dysphagia and esophageal dysfunction, which cause drooling, difficulty passing a stomach tube, nasal reflux of gastric contents, and pooling of barium contrast in the thoracic esophagus. A "tucked-up" stance (similar to that seen in equine motor neuron disease), with thoracic and pelvic limbs held close together, may be noted. On rectal palpation, the mucosa is dry and tacky, and feces are scant and hard. Distended loops of small intestine and an impacted large colon are seen in the more acute cases. Secondary ileal dilation/impaction and displacement of the large colon can be confusing features. Cachexia can be profound in chronic cases.

Lesions: In acute cases, the stomach and small intestine are markedly distended with fluid (which can result in gastric rupture), and the large intestine is impacted. In chronic cases, the GI tract is usually empty. All forms may show splenomegaly; linear ulceration of the esophagus; and hard, tarry fecal balls. Neuronal degeneration of pre- and postganglionic sympathetic and parasympathetic neurons is common. A specific distribution of chromatolytic autonomic and somatic lower motor neurons is found in the brain stem and spinal cord.

Diagnosis: No reliable in vivo diagnostic test is available, but dysphagia, tachycardia despite few signs of pain, decreased GI tract motility, a tucked-up stance (chronic cases), and ptosis are useful features. Administration of dilute (0.5%) phenylephrine to one eye should, within 30 min, result in marked decrease in ptosis (most easily seen as a decrease in the angle of the eyelashes to the head when viewed from the front). Confirmation of diagnosis depends on histopathologic examination of autonomic ganglia. Other causes of intestinal distention and ileus must be ruled out. Other causes of emaciation should be considered in the chronic form, including equine motor neuron disease (p 1017).

Treatment: A proportion of mildly affected (chronic) cases can survive with dedicated nursing care; a wide variety of feeds should be offered to encourage feed intake. Acute and subacute cases have not survived and should be euthanized on humane grounds. Stabling at-risk stock for part of the day has been recommended.

EQUINE ENCEPHALOMYELITIS

(Equine encephalitis)

The equine encephalitides are clinically similar and are characterized by signs of CNS dysfunction and moderate to high mortality. Arboviruses are the most common cause of equine encephalitis, but *Sarcocystis neurona* (p 974) and *Neospora* sp (p 535) may also cause encephalitis. Arboviruses are transmitted by mosquitos or other hematophagous insects and infect a variety of vertebrate hosts, sometimes including humans, and may cause serious disease. In the western hemisphere, most pathogenic arboviruses use a mosquito to bird or rodent cycle.

Etiology and Epidemiology: The most pathogenic viruses for horses are alphaviruses of the family Togaviridae. These species include Eastern, Western, Highlands J, and Venezuelan viruses. Other alphaviruses associated occasionally with equine encephalitis are Semliki Forest, Ross River, and Una viruses. These viruses are not found in North America and only infrequently cause clinical disease. The Eastern equine encephalomyelitis (EEE) virus, although one virus, has 2 distinct antigenic variants that function as separate viruses. The North American variant is the most pathogenic and the most antigenically homogenous. It is found in eastern Canada; all states within the USA east of the Mississippi River and in Arkansas, Minnesota, South Dakota, and Texas; and in the Caribbean Islands. The South American virus is less pathogenic and more heterogeneous and is found in central and South America. Subtypes of the Western equine encephalomyelitis (WEE) group consist of WEE, Sindbis, Aura, Ft. Morgan, and Y 62-33. WEE is found in western Canada, states in the USA west of the Mississippi, and in Mexico and South America. The Highlands J (HJ) virus was originally classified as a subgroup of WEE but has subsequently been shown to be a distinct alphavirus. WEE previously isolated in the eastern USA has been shown to belong to the HJ virus serogroup. Venezuelan equine encephalomyelitis (VEE) has 6 antigenically related subtypes: subtype I (VEE), Everglades, Mucambo, Pixuna, Cabassou, and AG80-663. Within subtype I are 5 serovars. Until 1993, only subtype I, serovars A/B and C, caused sporadic epizootics in horses; other subtypes and variants cause enzootic or sylvatic cycles and appear to be nonpathogenic to equids. In 1993, however, an epizootic in Mexico was caused by subtype I, serovar E. Sylvatic or enzootic subtypes of VEE are found annually in tropical and subtropical areas of the USA, Mexico, and Central and South America. Sylvatic subtype II (Everglades) has been isolated from humans and mosquitos in Florida; subtype III has been isolated in the Rocky Mountains and northern plains states. Epizootic strains are not generally found in the USA, although there was an epizootic of VEE in 1971.

The principal means of transmission and amplification of EEE is a mosquito-vertebrate-mosquito cycle. EEE has been isolated from 27 different mosquitos in the USA. The primary mosquito vector for the enzootic or sylvatic cycle of EEE is *Culiseta melanura*. Population densities of *C melanura* are highest deep in the interior of swamp habitats, where most of the enzootic transmission of EEE occurs. During late summer and early fall, mosquitos leave the swamp breeding sites and move to drier, upland forested habitats. Epizootics in equids, epornitics in pheasant and quail, and human cases are seen when virus infection rates are high in birds. *Aedes vexans* and *A canadensis* mosquitos (which breed in containers) are believed to be responsible for bird to mammal transmission. The identification of vectors in epidemics is difficult because no single species is consistently associated with the transmission of the virus to horses and people.

Seasonal changes in *C melanura* biology and their relationship to EEE virus transmission vary with the geographic location and its associated climate. In subtropical areas (eg, Florida), transmission occurs throughout the year with a peak in summer. In more temperate regions, there is a distinct transmission season. The virus is not detected until midsummer and can remain active until the first heavy frost. Virus is isolated most often in late August through November. The mechanism of viral persistence during the winter in temperate areas, where transmission is not continuous, remains unknown. It is possible that sporadic epizootics result from adult mosquitos surviving periods of inactivity, long distance movement of infected vectors by wind currents occurs, or migration of infected hosts (birds), and subsequent climactic conditions favorable to mosquito proliferation. In South America, serologic studies suggest that forest-dwelling rodents and marsupials are the vertebrate hosts. EEE is readily recovered from sentinel mice and hamsters.

WEE is transmitted by mosquito vectors (primarily *C tarsalis*) that breed in sunlit marshes and in pools of irrigation water in pastures and by the tick *Dermacentor andersoni*.

Epizootics of WEE are associated with increased rainfall in early spring followed by warmer than normal temperatures.

Sylvatic VEE viruses are found throughout North, Central, and South America in jungle or swampy environments with persistent fresh or brackish water. The mosquitos that serve as the primary vectors for the bird- or rodent-mosquito life cycle are members of the subgenus *Culex*.

All subtypes of the VEE virus are serologically related and provide cross-protection against infection with epizootic VEE virus. The origin of epizootic strains is unknown and does not appear to have any relationship with the sylvatic subtypes. No single vector has been associated with transmission of the epizootic VEE virus—many mosquitos and other hematophagous insects have been incriminated. Epizootics of VEE appear sporadically in Central and South America. In 1993, an epizootic occurred in Chiapas, Mexico, caused by VEE subtype I, serovar E, which had not previously been associated with clinical disease outbreaks.

Viruses belonging to the family Flaviviridae and Bunyaviridae are less pathogenic than the Togaviridae. Flaviviruses present in the USA prior to 1999 that have been associated with encephalitis in horses are the St. Louis encephalitis virus and the Japanese B virus. The former is primarily a human pathogen found from central Canada to Argentina and is transmitted among birds by *Culex* mosquitos. Encephalitis can be produced experimentally in horses, but most naturally occurring infections in horses are asymptomatic. Japanese B virus is found throughout the Far East and is associated with clinical disease, although mortality is low.

In 1999, clinical disease caused by West Nile virus (WNV, p 1077), which is antigenically related to Japanese B virus, was seen in the USA in New York state in horses and humans as well as in birds, the primary vertebrate host. Since then, the virus has been found in 27 different species of mosquitos and >150 species of birds in the USA in 48 states and is now considered endemic. The viral strain of WNV in the USA is more pathogenic than the endemic strains found in Africa, Asia, and the Middle East, which is thought to result from a change in viral biology. WNV infection follows the pattern of EEE, occuring seasonally in temperate regions and throughout the year in subtropical areas.

Cache Valley virus (transmitted by mosquitos and *Culicoides* sp among rabbits), Maindrain virus (transmitted by *Culicoides varipennis* to hares and rodents in the western USA), and Snowshoe hare virus (transmitted by *Culiseta* and *Aedes* mosquitos among rabbits in southern Canada and northern USA) have all been identified, although infrequently, as the cause of encephalitis in horses.

Pathogenesis and Clinical Findings: The pathogenesis and clinical signs are similar for the alphaviruses. After inoculation by the vector, the virus travels via the lymphatics to lymph nodes and replicates in macrophages and neutrophils, resulting in lymphopenia, leukopenia, and fever. Subsequent replication occurs in other organs and is associated with viremia. Initially, horses are quiet and depressed with clinical neurologic signs generally occurring 5 days after infection. Any and all signs attributable to cortical and thalamic lesions may be seen, as well as brain-stem deficits as the neurologic signs progress. The lesions are not necessarily symmetrically distributed; therefore, neurologic deficits may be asymmetric. Clinical signs include altered mentation, impaired vision, aimless wandering, head pressing, circling, inability to swallow, irregular ataxic gait, paresis and paralysis, convulsions, and death. Most deaths occur within 2-3 days after onset of clinical signs.

In contrast, neurologic lesions in WNV are more prevalent in the brain stem than the cortical and thalamic regions, with lesions often increasing in number in the spinal cord. Thus, horses with WNV may present with signs of spinal cord ataxia, hyperesthesia, and muscle fasiculations without cortical signs. Fever occurs in <25% of horses with clinical disease from WNV.

Horses infected with the EEE virus have a transient but significant viremia and may, under circumstances of a large vector population and a large population of nearby horses, provide transient amplification of the virus. Horses infected with WEE and WNV do not have a significant viremia; therefore, they do not amplify the virus and are true dead-end hosts. Horses infected with the sylvatic subtypes of VEE are also dead-end hosts; however, horses infected with epizootic strains of VEE have a persistent and significant viremia that results in virus shedding in body fluids. Infection may pass from horse to horse via aerosolized respiratory secretions or direct contact. Horses infected with the epizootic strains of VEE are systemically ill, and many die without showing neurologic signs. Asymptomatic infections may occur with all viruses. Mortality of horses showing clinical signs from WEE is 20-50%, from EEE 50-90%, from VEE 50-75%, and from WNV 20-40%. Horses with clinical neurologic signs from alphavirus infection that recover have a high incidence of residual neurologic deficits, whereas many horses that recover from WNV have been reported to have no residual neurologic deficits.

Diagnosis: A presumptive diagnosis may be made on the basis of clinical signs, the location of the affected horse(s), and season of the year. A specific diagnosis can be made only by virus isolation and identification or by detecting a specific increase in antibody titer between paired acute and convalescent sera. CSF from arbovirus-infected horses has an increased nucleated cell count (>50 cells/μL) that consists primarily of mononuclear cells and an increased protein concentration (>70 mg/dL). The virus may be isolated from the CSF of horses with acute infections. By the time neurologic signs are seen, viremia has ended; thus, virus isolation from blood is best attempted from febrile herdmates.

Serologic tests for acute and convalescent sera consist of hemagglutination inhibition, complement fixation, virus neutralization (PRNT), and antibody capture ELISA for IgM. Hemagglutination inhibition antibody cross-reacts among EEE, WEE, and VEE, but virus neutralizing antibody does not. By performing all 3 serologic tests, it is possible to differentiate between viruses. Antibody capture ELISA for IgM is specific for EEE and can be used to differentiate EEE from WEE; however, it will not distinguish between vaccinated and infected animals. WNV antibodies develop early after infection but not after vaccination; thus, IgM capture ELISA for these antibodies may be used to determine recent infection. Caution should be used in diagnosing VEE in regions where the sylvatic subtypes of the virus are found, as subtypes cross-react in serologic tests. Because virus neutralizing antibodies appear at the end of viremia and may precede the appearance of neurologic signs, paired samples may not show a 4-fold increase in horses with neurologic signs. Paired samples from febrile herdmates may be more diagnostic. Maternal antibodies may interfere with serodiagnosis in young foals.

In dead animals, the brain should be examined microscopically for the presence of nonsuppurative meningoencephalitis. Virus isolation should also be attempted from the brain (and from the spinal cord if WNV is suspected) of dead animals. Antigen capture ELISA for EEE and WNV may be used to help identify the virus in brain tissue. Immunohistochemistry and PCR may also be used to identify virus in neurologic tissue.

Differential diagnoses include rabies, hepatoencephalopathy, leukoencephalomalacia, protozoal encephalomyelitis, equine herpesvirus 1, verminous meningoencephalomyelitis, cranial trauma, botulism, and meningitis. Differential diagnoses for horses suspected to have WNV infection include hypocalcemia, tremorgenic toxicities, and compression of the spinal cord.

Treatment: There is no specific therapy for viral encephalitis. Supportive care includes fluids if the horse is unable to drink, judicious use of anti-inflammatory agents, and anticonvulsants if necessary. Good nursing care is essential.

Prevention: Susceptible horses should be vaccinated with formalin-inactivated viral vaccines for EEE, WEE, and VEE. Vaccines are commercially available in the mono-, bi-, or trivalent form. The viral strain of VEE in vaccines is TC-83, which was originally developed as a modified live inoculation to protect laboratory workers investigating VEE. The modified live vaccine was used in the 1971 outbreak of VEE in the USA and conferred immunity as soon as 3 days after inoculation. Horses vaccinated with this agent developed a transient viremia and often showed mild signs of illness. To address concerns that the virus would revert to the wild type, this strain is now inactivated in currently available vaccines. The initial vaccination protocol consists of 2 injections

30 days apart, followed by an annual or biannual booster depending on the geographic location of the horses.

Colostral antibodies at a titer >1:10 interfere with vaccination. Consequently, foals should be immunized at 3, 4, and 6 mo of age and then according to the protocol for adults. Mares should be vaccinated 3-4 wk before foaling.

An inactivated monovalent vaccine for WNV was licensed provisionally in 2001 and received full licensure in 2003. The vaccination protocol specifies 2 doses given IM, 3-6 wk apart, in adult horses. In foals, an initial series of 3 doses is required; the vaccination schedule should be similar to that for EEE and WEE. For the first million doses administered, adverse reactions to the virus were no different than those known to occur following alphavirus immunization. Efficacy studies are currently in progress. A recombinant canarypox vaccine was also licensed in 2003.

Vector suppression by elimination of breeding sites and control of mature insects, as well as protection of the hosts from insect predation, increase the success of preventive measures, particularly during epizootics. Horses may be partially protected from insect feeding by using repellents and by stabling with fans and screens to limit insect access.

Zoonotic Risk: People may be infected by all 4 of the arboviruses that commonly cause viral encephalitis in horses. Clinical signs in humans vary from mild flu-like symptoms to death. Children, the elderly, and immunosupressed people are the most susceptible. People with neurologic disease due to arboviruses usually have permanent neurologic impairment on recovery. Human disease is reported infrequently and generally follows equine infections by ~2 wk. Veterinarians should be aware of the possibility of human infection and use repellents and other procedures to protect themselves from hematophagous insects when working in sylvatic virus habitats or handling viremic horses.

EQUINE PROTOZOAL MYELOENCEPHALITIS

Equine protozoal myeloencephalitis (EPM) is a common neurologic disease of horses in the Americas; it has been reported in most of the contiguous 48 states of the USA, southern Canada, and several countries in Central and South America. In other countries, EPM is seen sporadically.

Etiology and Epidemiology: Most cases of EPM are caused by an Apicomplexan protozoan, *Sarcocystis neurona*. Horses are infected by ingestion of *S neurona* sporocysts in contaminated feed or water. The organism is assumed to undergo early asexual multiplication (schizogony) in extraneural tissues before parasitizing the CNS. Because infectious sarcocysts are not formed, the horse is considered an aberrant, dead-end host for *S neurona*. All *Sarcocystis* spp have an obligate predator-prey life cycle. The definitive (predator) host for *S neurona* is believed to be the opossum (*Didelphis virginiana*). Opossums are infected by eating sarcocyst-containing muscle tissue from an infected intermediate (prey) host and, after a brief prepatent period (probably 2–4 wk), infectious sporocysts are passed in the feces. Nine-banded armadillos, striped skunks, raccoons, sea otters, Pacific harbor seals, and domestic cats have all been implicated as intermediate hosts; however, the importance in nature of each of these species is unknown. A few cases of EPM, both in the Americas and Europe, are associated with *Neospora hughesi*, an organism that is closely related to *S neurona*. The natural host(s) of this organism have not yet been identified.

Clinical Findings: Because the protozoa may infect any part of the CNS, almost any neurologic sign is possible. The disease usually begins insidiously but may present acutely and be severe at onset. Signs of spinal cord involvement are more common than signs of brain disease. Horses with EPM involving the spinal cord have asymmetric or symmetric weakness and ataxia of one to all limbs, sometimes with obvious muscle atrophy. When the caudal spinal cord is involved, there are signs of cauda equina syndrome. EPM lesions in the spinal cord also may result in demarcated areas of spontaneous sweating or loss of reflexes and cutaneous sensation. The most common signs of brain disease in horses with EPM are depression, head tilt, and facial paralysis. Any cranial nerve nucleus may be involved, and there may be seizures, visual deficits including abnormal menace response, or behavioral abnormalities. Without treatment, EPM often progresses to cause recumbency and death. Progression to recumbency occurs over hours to years and may occur steadily or in a stop-start fashion.

Lesions: There is focal discoloration, hemorrhage, and/or malacia of CNS tissue. Histologically, protozoa are found in association with a mixed inflammatory cellular response and neuronal destruction. Schizonts, in various stages of maturation, or free merozoites commonly are seen in the cytoplasm of neurons or mononuclear phagocytes. Also parasitized are intravascular and tissue neutrophils and eosinophils and, more rarely, capillary endothelial cells and myelinated axons. Merozoites may be found extracellularly, especially in areas of necrosis. In at least 75% of cases, protozoa are not seen on H&E-stained sections, and the diagnosis is made on the basis of characteristic focal or multifocal inflammatory change.

Diagnosis: Postmortem diagnosis is confirmed by demonstration of protozoa in CNS lesions. An immunoblot (Western blot) test for *S neurona* is used as an aid to antemortem diagnosis. In horses with neurologic signs, demonstration of specific antibody in CSF (by immunoblot) is highly suggestive of EPM. A positive immunoblot test in serum only indicates exposure to *S neurona*. Conversely, a negative immunoblot result, in either serum or CSF, tends to exclude the diagnosis of EPM. In a few horses with EPM, CSF analysis reveals abnormalities such as mononuclear pleocytosis and increased protein concentration.

Depending on the clinical signs, differential diagnoses may include cervical stenotic myelopathy, trauma, aberrant metazoan parasite migration, equine degenerative myeloencephalopathy, myeloencephalopathy caused by equine herpesvirus 1, equine motor neuron disease, neuritis of the cauda equina, arboviral (Eastern or Western equine, West Nile) encephalomyelitis, rabies, bacterial meningitis, and leukoencephalomalacia.

Treatment and Control: The only FDA-approved treaments for EPM are ponazuril (5 mg/kg, PO, SID for 28 days) and nitazoxanide (50 mg/kg, PO, SID for 28 days), both as paste formulations. An alternative approach is the use of antifolate drugs, eg, sulfadiazine, or sulfamethoxazole (15-25 mg/kg, PO, SID-BID) in combination with pyrimethamine (1 mg/kg, PO, SID). The sulfonamide can be given with or without trimethoprim. Pyrimethamine must be given at least 1 hr before or after hay is fed. Treatment is usually continued for 6 mo. Anemia may develop after prolonged treatment with antifolate drugs and is best prevented by provision of high quantities of green forage. At least 60% of horses improve with treatment, but <25% recover completely. Relapses are common in horses that remain positive on immunoblot and rare in those that become negative.

No proven preventive is available. A conditionally approved vaccine is marketed, and its efficacy continues to be evaluated. There is interest in using antiprotozoal drugs for prevention; however, evidence-based protocols are not yet available. The source of infective sporocysts is probably opossum feces, so it is prudent to prevent access of opossums to horse-feeding areas. Horse and pet feed should not be left out; open feed bags and garbage should be kept in closed galvanized metal containers, bird feeders should be eliminated, and fallen fruit should be removed. Opossums can be trapped and relocated. Because putative intermediate hosts cannot be directly infective for horses, it is unlikely that control of these populations will be useful in EPM prevention.

FACIAL PARALYSIS

Asymmetry of facial expression is common with unilateral lesions of the facial nucleus or nerve in most species. Bilateral facial paralysis may be more difficult to recognize, but affected animals drool and have a dull facial expression. Complete facial paralysis is an inability to move the eyelids, ears, lips, or nostrils. Facial paresis is reduced movement of the muscles of facial expression and indicates milder nucleus or nerve involvement.

The nucleus of the facial nerve is located in the rostral medulla oblongata of the brain stem. The facial nerve, cranial nerve VII, exits the brain stem near the vestibulocochlear nerve, passes through the petrous temporal bone, and then exits the skull through the stylomastoid foramen and splits into auricular, palpebral, and buccal branches.

Clinical Findings and Location of Lesions: Clinical signs of facial paralysis vary with the location, severity, and chronicity of the lesion. If a unilateral lesion is located in the facial nucleus or proximal portion of the facial nerve, paresis or paralysis of the eyelids, ears, lips, and nostrils on that side are seen. A lesion of the auriculopalpebral branch of the facial nerve, near the zygomatic arch, results in paresis or paralysis of the eyelids and ear only. A lesion of the palpebral branch of the facial nerve, crossing the zygomatic arch, results in paresis or paralysis of the eyelids only. A lesion of the buccal branch of the facial nerve, as it courses along the surface of the masseter muscles, results in paresis or paralysis of the lips and nostrils only.

In small animals with facial paralysis, the palpebral fissure may be slightly larger on the affected side; in horses and food animals, the palpebral fissure is slightly smaller owing to a loss of tone in the frontalis muscles above the eyelid. When the medial or lateral canthus of the eyelids or cornea are touched, the eyelids do not close, but the eyeball will retract into the orbit (if the trigeminal and abducent nerves are functioning properly). The third eyelid will passively elevate as the globe retracts. If both eyes are tested simultaneously, movement on each side can be compared. When the animal is unable to blink the eye, corneal irritation may result in excessive tear production. In acute denervation, the ear carriage is often lower on the side of the lesion in all species, but in chronic denervation with muscle fibrosis, the ear carriage may be higher. The fibrosis of the auricular muscles can be palpated, and the ear becomes adhered in the abnormal position. In acute lesions, the lips on the paralyzed side may hang loosely, exposing mucosa. When the animal eats or drinks, food and fluids may fall from the lips. The animal may drool excessively, and food may collect between the lips and teeth. In chronic lesions, fibrosis of the lip muscles can be palpated, and the lip on the affected side is higher than the normal side. In acute, unilateral lesions, the nose deviates away from the side of the lesion, owing to a loss in muscle tone on the affected side. In horses, the affected nostril is unable to dilate on inspiration. In chronic lesions, muscle fibrosis and contracture cause the nose to deviate toward the lesion, and the muscles feel firm and inflexible.

Often the parasympathetic portion of the facial nerve is also affected, and tear and saliva production on the side of the lesion is reduced or absent. Reduced or absent tear production, with eyelid paresis or paralysis, can result in corneal ulceration. In cases of facial nerve paralysis, a Schirmer tear test can be used to determine if administration of artificial tears is needed. Reduced saliva production can result in dry mucous membranes, and food may collect in the buccal folds. Dryness on the side of the lesion can be detected by simultaneously palpating the mucous membranes on both sides and comparing the degree of moisture.

Other concomitant neurologic deficits can further localize the facial nerve lesion. If the animal has ataxia, hemiparesis, quadriparesis, or conscious proprioceptive deficits associated with facial nerve paralysis, a brain-stem lesion is probable. If the animal has facial paralysis with a head tilt, nystagmus, or other evidence of vestibular deficits, but no hemiparesis, quadriparesis, or conscious proprioceptive deficits, then a lesion of the facial nerve exists as it exits the brain stem or passes through the petrous temporal bone. If a small animal has facial paralysis with ptosis, miosis, and enophthalmos (Horner's syndrome), a lesion of the middle ear is likely.

Diagnosis and Treatment: Trauma is a common cause of facial paralysis in all species. In horses, halter injuries and prolonged lateral recumbency may injure the buccal branches of the facial nerve on the side of the jaw and cause unilateral or bilateral paresis or paralysis of the lips and nostrils. Cattle that struggle in stanchions may injure the palpebral branch of the facial nerve as it crosses the zygomatic arch, causing unilateral or bilateral paresis or paralysis of the eyelid(s). Small animals may incur peripheral facial nerve injuries from rough handling, automobile accidents, or surgery in the area.

Electromyography, including electrical stimulation of the facial nerve, can be used to determine the location and severity of the injury.

There is no specific therapy for injury except massage and heat of denervated muscles for 15 min, BID-TID. The facial nerve can regenerate ~1-4 mm/day, so serial neurologic examinations can also help determine the prognosis. If there has been no improvement after 6 mo, the chance for recovery is poor. Horses with collapsing nostrils may require corrective surgery. Species that need the lips for drinking and prehending food must be given deep water containers and wet bulky mashes.

Otitis media is another common cause of facial paralysis in all species, especially in dogs with chronic dermatitis. Otitis externa and a ruptured or diseased tympanic membrane are often seen on otoscopic examination under general anesthesia. Skull radiographs, computed tomography, and MRI may be necessary to confirm otitis media. The prognosis can be good, if the diagnosis is made early and the animal treated for 4-6 wk with the appropriate antibiotic, determined by culture and sensitivity. Corticosteroids should be avoided because they may encourage osteomyelitis (*see also* OTITIS MEDIA AND INTERNA, p 425). The facial nerve paralysis can be permanent, and longterm administration of artificial tears may be necessary. Guttural pouch infections (p 1221) can produce facial paralysis in horses. Lesions of the facial nerve nucleus can result in facial nerve paralysis in equine protozoal myeloencephalitis (EPM, p 1031). CSF analysis and titers for EPM are essential for diagnosis and institution of appropriate therapy.

Idiopathic facial nerve paralysis is common in dogs and is diagnosed by ruling out other diseases. Otitis media must be ruled out with examination and radiographs. Because hypothyroidism (p 461) can cause facial nerve paralysis, levels of thyroxine (T_4) and thyroid-stimulating hormone should be determined in all dogs with facial paralysis. Thyroid replacement therapy results in resolution of the facial paralysis in hypothyroid dogs. If there is no infection, thyroid function is normal, and there has been no known trauma, the diagnosis of idiopathic facial paralysis is made. There is no therapy. Artificial tear administration may be necessary. Facial paralysis can be unilateral or bilateral and can resolve spontaneously or be permanent. It can occur on one side, resolve, and then occur on the other side at a later time. Permanent paralysis may be disfiguring but does not affect the quality of life in dogs.

Primary neoplasia of the facial nerve is rare, but dogs and cats can develop a neoplastic process that affects middle ear structures, including the facial nerve. Squamous cell carcinoma and polyps of the middle ear are most common in cats. Otoscopy of the external ear canal under anesthesia with biopsy and histologic examination of abnormal tissue can assist with the diagnosis. Computed tomography and MRI of the osseous bulla are necessary to determine the extent of the lesion before surgery. Early radical excision of the tumor and radiation, if indicated, may afford a good longterm prognosis depending on tumor type.

CNS DISEASES CAUSED BY HELMINTHS AND ARTHROPODS

A number of metazoan parasites (helminths and arthropods) are associated with pathology in the CNS and may be categorized as described below.

Immature (larval) stages of parasites of carnivorous animals: These developmental stages may induce behavioral changes in the intermediate host that are likely to enhance transmission to the definitive host by means of predation. For example, *Taenia multiceps multiceps* is acquired by the canine definitive host when the dog ingests the infective larval stages of the tapeworm *Coenurus cerebralis* in the brain and spinal cord of the ovine intermediate host. In sheep, *C cerebralis* causes ataxia, which allows the dog (a carnivore) to more easily prey upon the sheep.

Immature stages of parasites exhibiting a neurotropic affinity: These developmental stages require conditions provided by the host's CNS for their growth and development. For example, *Hypoderma bovis* in cattle must migrate through the spinal cord and adjacent tissues to reach its predilection site, the dorsum of the back.

Erratic or aberrant parasites: These parasites are normally found in non-neurologic, predilection sites within the definitive host but, on occasion, may wander erratically into some portion of the CNS. For example, larvae of *Cuterebra* spp are normally found in subcutaneous sites in the dog or cat but may also aberrantly wander into the CNS and localize in the cerebrum or cerebellum.

Incidental parasites: These parasites are found in a different host than that in which they normally are found. For example, *Parelaphostrongylus (Pneumostrongylus) tenuis* normally is found in neurologic sites within the definitive host, white-tailed deer, in which the parasite is nonpathogenic. However, in an incidental host, such as moose, elk, or llama, the parasite produces an often fatal neurologic disease.

Facultative parasites: These parasites are normally free-living but, on occasion, can develop into a parasitic existence. For example, *Halicephalobus (Micronema) deletrix*, a saprophytic soil nematode that is found free-living in nature, has been reported to produce pathology in the CNS of horses.

Successful chemotherapeutic treatment for cerebrospinal nematodiasis has been reported with diethylcarbamazine at 100 mg/kg (45 mg/lb). Ivermectin and organophosphates kill larval bots and at least some nematodes, but killing parasites in the CNS may provoke additional tissue damage.

Before implementing therapy for a pathogenic helminth or arthropod, other possible etiologies for neuropathology should be carefully considered. In particular, rabies should always be included in the differential diagnoses. The animal's age, vaccination status, exposure status, and history are factors that should be considered when rendering a diagnosis.

CESTODES

Coenurosis: *Taenia multiceps multiceps* is an intestinal parasite of canids (especially dogs, foxes, and jackals) and humans. Its intermediate hosts include sheep, goats, deer, antelope, chamois, rabbits, hares, horses, and less commonly cattle, which acquire the eggs while grazing. Some oncospheres reach the brain and develop by endogenous budding into a metacestode (larval) stage known as *Coenurus cerebralis*. Initial invasion and development of the oncospheres may be responsible for acute suppurative meningoencephalitis. The fully developed coenurus may be 5-6 cm in diameter and cause increased intracranial pressure, which results in ataxia, hypermetria, blindness, head deviation, stumbling, and paralysis. This clinical condition is known as gid, sturdy, or staggers. In sheep, palpation of the skull caudal to the horn buds may reveal refraction; surgery to remove the cyst, including its wall, has a reasonable chance of success and is justified in valuable animals. Dogs associated with sheep and other livestock should not be fed the brain or spinal cord from infected animals and should be dewormed regularly.

Cysticercosis: *Taenia solium* is a tapeworm found in the small intestine of humans. Its metacestode (larval) stage, a cysticercus, is a large fluid-filled cavity or vesicle or bladder found in the musculature of pigs. This larval stage was once regarded as a separate parasite, and it still retains the scientific name *Cysticercus cellulosae*. In humans, this larval stage may also develop in subcutaneous sites and musculature but may be found in nervous tissues, eg, the brain and ocular tissues. Infection in humans stems from ingestion of tapeworm eggs in contaminated foods or from dirty hands. In the brain, the parasite usually develops in the ventricles and becomes proliferative. Infection causes pain, paralysis, epileptiform seizures, locomotor disturbances, and possibly death. The coenuri commonly localize on the meninges and in the neuropil. Treatment of human cysticercosis is by surgical removal of the lesion; however, the prognosis is not good.

Echinococcosis: *Echinococcus granulosus* is a tapeworm found in the small intestine of the canid definitive host. Its eggs are ingested by the intermediate hosts, wild and domestic herbivores, eg, sheep, cattle, and moose. Humans can also serve as intermediate hosts. After hatching in the intestine of the intermediate host, the oncospheres invade the circulatory system and lodge in various organs (the liver and lungs), where they develop into large, thick-walled, unilocular hydatid cysts that bud protoscolices endogenously. Hydatids have been rarely reported in the CNS of domestic animals and are rare in humans, in which they produce symptoms similar to those of a brain tumor.

Foxes are the definitive host for a related species, *Echinococcus multilocularis*. Microtine rodents (such as voles) are the intermediate host. This parasite has been rarely found in the brain of humans, in which the invasive, thin-walled multilocular hydatid cyst do not produce scolices. Surgical intervention is more successful in removing hydatid cysts of *E granulosus*.

TREMATODES

Paragonimiasis: *Paragonimus westermani* and *P kellicotti*, the lung flukes, have been reported to migrate aberrantly and produce cysts in the brain and spinal cord of pigs, dogs, cats, rats, and humans. Flukes in these extrapulmonic sites in dead-end hosts do not produce patent infections.

Schistosomiasis: Schistosomes, or blood flukes, normally deposit their eggs in the small vessels of the gut and urinary bladder, from which they pass into the external environment via the feces or urine. Some eggs, however, may get into the general circulation and may reach the CNS where they become encapsulated. This condition has been noted in humans and domestic animals.

Troglotremiasis: *Troglotrema acutum* inhabits the frontal and ethmoidal sinuses of foxes and mustelids in Europe. Flukes live in pairs in cysts in these sinuses. These parasites cause decalcification and atrophy of the bony walls of the sinuses and eventually result in perforation into the cranial cavity. Microorganisms enter the cranial vault, leading to fatal, purulent meningitis. Treatment for this condition is not known.

NEMATODES

Ascarids

The larvae of some ascarid roundworms, including *Toxocara* spp of dogs and cats and *Baylisascaris* spp of mustelids, can cause CNS disease.

Nervous disorders, frequently associated with ascarid infection in dogs, may be due to focal lesions in the CNS due to the death of aberrant arrested larvae of *T canis*. *Toxocara* larvae may also invade the eye and cause ocular larva migrans in humans.

Baylisascaris procyonis is the ascarid found in the small intestine of raccoons. It causes larva migrans in both wild and domestic animals in North America and is usually associated with the production of clinical CNS disease. More than 90 species of wild and domesticated animals have been identified as infected with *B procyonis* larvae. Some species, including opossums, skunks, cats, pigs, sheep, and goats, appear to be marginally susceptible or resistant to the migration. The parasite has been associated with the production of cerebrospinal nematodiasis in humans, particularly children; it also has been implicated as a cause of ocular larva migrans.

Filarids

Dirofilaria immitis is often referred to as the canine heartworm but can also infect cats and ferrets. As adults, these parasites usually infect the right ventricle and the pulmonary artery and its fine branches. *D immitis* has been recovered from a variety of aberrant sites, including the CNS of its definitive hosts and the anterior chamber of the eye. (*See also* HEARTWORM DISEASE, p 100.)

Elaeophora schneideri, a filarid of the carotid arteries and its branches, is common in mule deer, primarily in western North America. Microfilariae accumulate in the skin of the head and face; intermediate hosts are tabanid horseflies. Larvae develop in arteries of the leptomeninges before migrating to the carotids. Infection is usually asymptomatic in normal definitive hosts. In wapiti, moose, white-tailed deer, sheep, and goats, worms in the arteries cause degeneration and loss of the endothelium and accumulation of plasma proteins and platelets on and within the intima. Thrombosis, infiltration of the intima, and fibroblastic proliferation may eventually result in occlusion and ischemic necrosis in associated tissues. Necrotic lesions associated with occlusion of lepto-meningeal arteries are commonly found in the brain. Neurologic signs include blindness, head deviation, circling, ataxia, and paralysis (*see also* ELAEOPHOROSIS, p 735).

Setaria digitata is found in Asia and is a common parasite of the peritoneal cavity. Microfilariae are found in the blood; mosquitos are intermediate hosts. Details of development in the normal host are unknown. In cattle, clinical signs do not appear to develop. In horses, goats, and sheep, the developing worms invade the CNS and cause motor weakness, ataxia, lameness, drooping eyelids or ears, and lumbar paralysis. Lesions include focal malacia and degeneration of axis cylinders and myelin sheath in all regions of the CNS.

Setaria cervi (Elaphostrongylus altaica) has been reported on the leptomeninges of deer in Europe and in the former USSR, often in association with *E cervi. Setaria* spp have also been found in the CNS of horses. The significance of these findings is unclear.

Filarids may also parasitize avian species. *Splendidofilaria quiscula* is found in the cerebral hemispheres of grackles (*Quiscalus quiscua*) and other birds in North America. *Paronchocerca helicina* is found in the cranial leptomeninges of the snake bird (*Anhinga anhinga*) in the USA.

Metastrongyles

Angiostrongylus cantonensis is a common parasite of the pulmonary arteries of rats in southeast Asia and the south Pacific. Terrestrial, aquatic, and amphibious snails and slugs are intermediate hosts. Paratenic hosts are freshwater prawns, land crabs, coconut crabs, and planarians. Larvae invade the cerebrum and develop in the neural parenchyma for ~2 wk, then enter the subarachnoid space and migrate, ~1 mo after infection, to the pulmonary arteries via the venous system. Neurologic signs are rare in rats with light to moderate infections, but circling, cannibalism, and paraplegia may develop in heavy infections. In endemic areas, humans frequently acquire infections by consuming raw or undercooked intermediate or paratenic hosts. In humans, this parasite may produce a fatal eosinophilic meningoencephalitis. In Australia, *A cantonensis* has produced an ascending paralysis in puppies. It may be an incidental parasite in dogs.

Gurlita paralysans is found in the spinal veins of cats and has reportedly produced a high incidence of paralysis. It may be an incidental parasite in cats.

Elaphostrongylus cervi (rangiferi) is a common parasite of the skeletal musculature of *Rangifer* and *Cervus* spp (reindeer and elk) in the holarctic region, especially Eurasia. It is transmitted through terrestrial snails and slugs and apparently develops for a time in the CNS before migrating to the muscles. Infection is associated with lumbar weakness, paresis, and paralysis in cervids in Sweden and in the former USSR.

Parelaphostrongylus (Pneumostrongylus) tenuis is found in the subdural space and venous sinuses of the cranium of white-tailed deer in eastern North America. Eggs reach the lungs in the venous blood and develop into larvae, which pass up the bronchial tree and out with the feces. Infective larvae, acquired from terrestrial snails and slugs as the deer feeds, invade the spinal cord and develop for several weeks in the dorsal horns of the gray matter; then, they invade and mature in the subdural space. The infection is usually asymptomatic in white-tailed deer. However, *P tenuis* will produce pathology in the CNS of various cervids (moose, caribou, wapiti) and antelope, llamas, sheep, and goats. In these hosts, the parasite produces considerable trauma in the CNS. In addition, eggs deposited in the neural tissue provoke marked inflammatory reactions. Clinical signs consist of lumbar weakness, ataxia, lameness, stiffness, circling, abnormal positions of the head, and paralysis. Signs vary in onset and character in individual animals. Temporary remissions are typical.

Skrjabingylus nasicola and *S chitwoodorum* are found in the frontal sinuses of mustelids, especially mink, weasels, and skunks. Larvae acquired from terrestrial snails and slugs develop for a time in the gut wall, then migrate to the spinal cord. They move on to the leptomeninges to the brain and along the olfactory tracts to the cribriform plate, which they penetrate to reach the frontal sinuses. Their presence on the leptomeninges elicits hemorrhage and leptomeningitis. In heavy infections, some subadult worms may invade the brain and cause neurologic signs, including paralysis.

Rhabditorids

Halicephalobus (Micronema) deletrix is a free-living soil rhabditiform associated with soil and decaying vegetation. This nematode has been reported in the CNS of both horses and humans. It may reach the CNS through wounds contaminated by soil that contain these nematodes or through abscesses in the oral and nasal cavities. The nematode multiplies in the CNS and is highly destructive of neural tissues. Pathogenicity in the CNS can be attributed to trauma caused by activities of the parasites; the role of excretory and secretory products is unknown. Also, the parasites may transport pathogenic microorganisms to the CNS. Clinical signs are related to the location of the parasite and the lesions produced by it. Signs resemble viral encephalitis and include motor weakness, ataxia, head deviation, circling, depression, blindness, drooping of the ear or eyelid, loss of the herding instinct, and paralysis. Lesions consist of vasculitis, hemorrhagic necrosis, and malacia.

Miscellaneous Nematodes

Migrating larvae of strongyles (perhaps *Strongylus vulgaris*) have been reported in the CNS of horses. Larvae of *Stephanurus dentatus* rarely invade the CNS of pigs. Larvae of *Trichinella spiralis* were found in the brain in a fatal case of trichinosis in a human. Larvae of *Strongyloides stercoralis* may invade the brain of experimentally infected animals. *Gnathostoma spinigerum* has been found rarely in the CNS of humans. *Eustrongylides ignotus* implanted subcutaneously in rats and chickens migrated to the CNS and caused death of the host.

ARTHROPODS

Myiasis is the development of larval dipteran flies (bots and warbles) within the tissues or organs of humans and other domestic or wild animals. Myiasis involving the CNS is rather uncommon except for the larval stages of *Hypoderma bovis*, the cattle heel fly. Its larvae normally burrow between the periosteum and dura mater of the bovine spinal cord during migration to the subcutaneous tissues of the back. Neurologic signs, varying from a transient, stiff, unsteady gait to paralysis, may be seen in cattle given systemic insecticides when the larvae are present in the spinal canal. (*See also* CATTLE GRUBS, p 706.)

The larvae of *Oestrus ovis*, the nasal bot fly of sheep (p 1231), are normally found in the nostrils and paranasal sinuses. They rarely penetrate the ethmoid bone and reach the forebrain. However, it is possible that other factors facilitate entry of larvae into the brain. The bones of the skull may erode. If the brain is injured, clinical signs, such as a high-stepping gait and incoordination, may mimic infection with *Coenurus cerebralis*. This condition is often referred to as false gid. Surgical intervention may be useful but can prove difficult if the larvae are difficult to reach.

Larval *Cuterebra* spp, which are normally found in subcutaneous sites in dogs or cats, have been known to wander into the CNS and localize in the cerebrum or cerebellum. (*See also* p 710.) Intracranial migrations by larvae of dipteran flies have been reported in humans (*Dermatobia hominis*), cattle (*Hypoderma bovis*), and horses (*Hypoderma* spp).

Bots and warbles may move rapidly after death of the host and migrate into tissues far from the site of origin.

Treatment of intracranial myiasis is currently experimental. Surgical and medical therapies for alleviating intracranial myiases have been considered. The efficacy of systemic organophosphates against migrating larvae of *Hypoderma* suggest that organophosphates may be effective in eliminating certain dipteran larvae from the nervous system. Parenteral corticosteroids are also recommended to prevent additional inflammatory damage and intracranial pressure throughout the treatment period. Ivermectin (300 μg/kg on alternate days) used in conjunction with corticosteroids should be considered experimental therapy for intracranial cuterebrosis in cats; it is not approved by the FDA for this use.

HYPOXIC ISCHEMIC ENCEPHALOPATHY

(Neonatal maladjustment syndrome, Peripartum asphyxia, Barker, Wanderer, Dummy)

Hypoxic ischemic encephalopathy (HIE) is a term used to describe a variety of behavioral disturbances in the newborn foal.

Pathogenesis: HIE is noninfectious and thought to result from some degree of asphyxia (decreased oxygen delivery to tissues) during birth. The resulting hypoxia causes varying degrees of CNS tissue damage, depending on the age of the fetus and the severity and duration of the hypoxia. Partial prolonged asphyxia may be associated with the development of cerebral edema, focal hemorrhage, and necrosis. It has been proposed that fetal asphyxia may result in accumulation of toxic concentrations of excitatory neurotransmitters (eg, glutamate, aspartate), which allows intracellular influx of sodium and chloride and passive flow of water, leading to neuronal swelling. The production of oxygen free radicals as well as reperfusion injury may also play a role in the pathogenesis of HIE. Perinatal asphyxia may be strongly suspected in cases of dystocia or generalized placental pathology, but could remain unidentified if in utero placental separation occurs.

Clinical Findings: Many different abnormal behaviors may be grouped under the diagnosis of HIE. Signs range from a slow suckle response at birth to hyperexcitability, aimless wandering, depression, recumbency, generalized hypotonia, and seizures. This may reflect different degrees of asphyxia and CNS pathology. In the classic syndrome, the foal appears normal at birth and progressively loses interest in its dam, loses its suckle reflex, becomes recumbent, develops clonic seizures, and may start vocalizing. The vocalization has been described as that of a barking dog, hence the term "barker" foal.

Diagnosis: Because the signs of HIE are seen soon after birth, it is often associated with failure of passive transfer of antibodies, which can lead to septicemia. There are no definitive blood chemistry or WBC abnormalities that aid in diagnosis, but these tests are helpful in eliminating other causes of the clinical signs. Other clinical syndromes that can present with similar signs and must be differentiated from HIE include hypoglycemia, electrolyte and acid-base derangements, septic meningitis, head trauma, cerebral bleeding, and congenital CNS defects.

Treatment: The management of HIE is supportive. Providing warmth and nutrition is essential. If the foal does not have a suckle response, an indwelling nasogastric tube should be placed and the foal fed mare's milk or a mare milk substitute at 15-25% of its body weight over each 24-hr period. Lactated Ringer's solution plus 5% dextrose IV will ensure hydration and adequate glucose levels. If the foal did not receive adequate colostrum, a plasma transfusion is indicated. Although HIE is not infectious, foals should receive antibiotics to prevent secondary infections.

Seizure control is imperative. Diazepam (0.11-0.44 mg/kg) is usually effective. This dosage can be repeated as needed, but if longterm control is required, phenobarbital (2-10 mg/kg, IV, BID-TID) can be given. Dimethyl sulfoxide (1 g/kg in a 10% solution, IV) may be used as an adjunct to decrease cerebral edema. Mannitol (1 g/kg as a 20% solution, IV) has been proposed for similar reasons, but it should be used with caution due to the common presence of subdural hemorrhage in these foals.

Self-trauma can be a problem during seizures and can be prevented by providing a protected or padded environment and a human holder to cradle the animal. These foals are especially susceptible to eye trauma and corneal ulceration during their seizures; fluorescein staining and subsequent ocular treatment are often important.

Prognosis for HIE is fair to good if uncomplicated by sepsis; ~75% of HIE foals recover and grow to be normal adults. Generally, improvement is seen each day. The more severely affected foals may take 5-7 days before they are able to recognize their dam and suckle. Less severely affected foals may recover in 48 hr.

LIMB PARALYSIS

Paralysis of one limb is referred to as monoplegia and is most often associated with diseases of the peripheral spinal nerves. Paralysis of the thoracic limb is usually associated with a lesion of the C6 to T2 nerve roots; brachial plexus; or musculocutaneous, radial, median, or ulnar nerve. Paralysis of the pelvic limb is usually associated with a lesion of the L4 to S2 nerve roots; lumbosacral plexus; or femoral, sciatic, peroneal (fibular), or tibial nerve.

Clinical Findings and Location of Lesions: Evaluation of the posture and gait, spinal reflexes, superficial and deep nociception, and muscle mass of the affected limb can localize the lesion to the nerve roots or plexus or to a specific nerve branch. The closer a nerve injury is to the muscle to be reinnervated, the better the prognosis for recovery. Determining the exact location of the lesion is important for an accurate prognosis. In general, nerve root or plexus lesions have a poorer prognosis than do peripheral nerve lesions.

Muscle atrophy from denervation develops within a few days and is more severe than disuse atrophy. With disease of the suprascapular nerve, the supraspinatus and infraspinatus muscles are atrophied, but little gait deficit is noted. If the musculocutaneous nerve is affected, the animal is unable to flex the elbow, and the biceps muscle is atrophied. With radial nerve disease, the elbow is dropped, the digits are knuckled onto their dorsal surface, and the limb is unable to bear weight. The thoracic limb flexor reflex is depressed or absent with lesions of the radial nerve (sensory portion), axillary nerve (shoulder flexion), musculocutaneous nerve (elbow flexion), or median and ulnar (carpal and digit flexion) nerves. The triceps and carpal extensor muscles may also atrophy in radial nerve disease. Superficial and deep digital flexor muscles atrophy with lesions of the median and ulnar nerves.

Superficial sensation is tested by observing a behavioral response (such as looking, wincing, crying, or biting) when the skin is pinched with hemostatic forceps or pricked with a needle. Regions of skin sensation associated with specific nerves are less distinct in equine and food animal species than in small animals. A loss of sensation on the anterior skin surface of the thoracic limb from the elbows to the paws indicates radial nerve disease. The skin of the caudal aspect of the limb, from the elbow to the pads, is desensitized in median and ulnar nerve disease. **Deep pain** is tested by applying hemostatic forceps to the bones of the digits or hoof testers to the hoof and observing a behavioral response. The presence of deep pain from the fifth digit in small animals indicates integrity of the ulnar nerve. The presence of deep pain from the other digits of the thoracic limb indicates integrity of the radial, median, and ulnar nerves.

The eye on the side of the thoracic limb paralysis will show Horner's syndrome (ptosis, miosis, and enophthalmos) when the lesion involves the T1 to T2 nerve roots as they exit the spinal cord. Horner's syndrome is manifest in horses by ocular changes and ipsilateral sweating of the face and neck and in cattle by ocular changes and a unilateral loss of moisture on the muzzle.

Inability to extend the stifle to support weight in the pelvic limb is seen with L4 to L5 nerve root or femoral nerve disease; the patellar reflex is reduced or absent, the quadriceps muscle is atrophied, and sensation of the skin is reduced or absent on the medial surface of the limb. Inability to actively flex the stifle, hock, and digits or to extend the hock and digits is seen with lesions of the sciatic nerve. The animal will support some weight if the femoral nerve is spared, but will stand knuckled onto the dorsum of the paw or hoof with the hock excessively flexed. If only the peroneal branch of the sciatic nerve is affected, the hock will be overextended and the digits knuckled. If only the tibial branch of the sciatic nerve is affected, the hock will be overflexed and the digits overextended. The prognosis for tibial or peroneal nerve lesions may be better than that for sciatic lesions, so differentiation is important.

The pelvic limb flexor reflex is diminished or absent with sciatic nerve lesions. The gastrocnemius reflex is diminished or absent with lesions of the sciatic or tibial nerve. The cranial tibial muscle reflex is diminished or absent with lesions of the sciatic or peroneal nerve. The distribution of denervation muscle atrophy can indicate whether the sciatic or only one of its branches are involved. Atrophy of gluteal, semimembranosus, semitendinosus, and all muscles below the stifle indicates a lesion of the L6 to S2 nerve roots as they exit the spinal cord. If the gluteal muscles are normal but the others are atrophied, then a lesion of the sciatic nerve is located at the sciatic notch or the proximal two-thirds of the femur. Atrophy of the cranial tibial or gastrocnemius muscles alone indicates a lesion of the peroneal or tibial nerve, respectively. If superficial sensation is reduced or absent on the cranial and caudal aspects of the limb and in the perineal region on the same side, then a lesion of the L6 to S2 nerve roots is likely. With peroneal nerve lesions, superficial sensation on the cranial surface of the hock and tibia and on the dorsal aspect of the foot is reduced or absent. With tibial nerve lesions, superficial sensation of the caudal surface of the hock and tibia and plantar surface of the paw is reduced or absent. Sciatic nerve lesions cause a loss of superficial sensation in the cranial, caudal, dorsal, and plantar regions. A loss of deep pain may be associated with sciatic nerve lesions.

Electromyography can be used 7-10 days after a nerve insult to detect denervation in muscles and to outline the distribution of the nerve lesion. Denervation of limb and paravertebral muscles indicates nerve root lesions. Denervation of a specific muscle group indicates a lesion in its respective nerve. Electrical stimulation of the nerve can be used to determine nerve integrity. If some nerve integrity is present, the prognosis is better if motor nerve conduction velocity is normal than if it is slowed.

Diagnosis and Treatment: Trauma is the most common cause of acute monoplegia. Traumatic loss of nerve function may be due to neurapraxia, axonotmesis, axonostenosis, or neurotmesis. **Neurapraxia** is a temporary nerve conduction dysfunction that can last several weeks, but recovery is complete. **Axonotmesis** is rupture of some axons within the nerve, but with an intact nerve sheath. Most closed nerve injuries from stretch or compression are a combination of neurapraxia and axonotmesis. Ruptured axons regenerate 1-4 mm/day, but functional recovery depends on the integrity and diameter of the nerve sheath and on the distance between injury and reinnervation sites. Nerves injured >180 mm from their respective muscles may be unable to make anatomic contact. If anatomic contact is made, the nerve sheath contracture, which develops over time, may not leave enough room to develop sufficient myelin to conduct an effective electrical impulse. **Axonostenosis** or narrowed nerve sheaths with reduced nerve function may be a sequela of nerve injuries. **Neurotmesis** is total nerve rupture, and surgical reattachment is required for regeneration. If no nerve function is found on the initial neurologic examination, neurapraxia, axonotmesis, and neurotmesis can be difficult to differentiate. Electrical stimulation of a nerve with neurapraxia is usually normal and the prognosis is good, regardless of the findings of the initial neurologic examination. If the affected nerve does not respond to electrical stimulation distal to the site of the lesion ≥3 days after injury, the prognosis for recovery is guarded. Serial neurologic examinations over a 6-mo period are necessary if electromyographic evaluation is not performed.

Injury to the **brachial plexus** or the C6 to T2 nerve roots is common in most species from direct shoulder trauma or abnormal shoulder abduction (eg, in small animals hit by automobiles). Horses and cattle cast on hard surfaces for foot or other surgeries may develop a brachial plexus injury. If Horner's syndrome is present on the same side as a thoracic limb that has lost sensation and is areflexic and paralyzed, a brachial plexus avulsion is likely, and the prognosis for recovery grave. With brachial plexus avulsion, the nerve roots are torn from the spinal cord and cannot be repaired. If there is also no response to radial nerve stimulation, recovery is hopeless. If the limb drags on the ground, it can be held up with a neck sling or amputated in small animals to avoid laceration of the dorsal surface of the paw. Three-legged dogs and cats generally have a good quality of life. If no Horner's syndrome is present with thoracic limb paralysis, the prognosis for recovery may be better.

Lumbosacral plexus injuries are less common than brachial plexus injuries but can be associated with automobile accidents or extreme limb abduction. Fractures of long bones can injure peripheral nerves locally. Surgical intervention for pelvic and hip disease and injection injuries are common causes of sciatic nerve injuries. Sustained pressure on the lateral aspect of the stifle can cause peroneal nerve injury. Heat application, massage, and stretching of tendons should be performed for 15 min 2-3 times/day to keep muscles, tendons, and joints healthy while the nerve is regenerating. A light bandage may prevent damage to the foot from dragging, but reduction of circulation should be avoided. There is no specific therapy currently available to assist nerve regeneration. Small animals may be given oral prednisone at 2 mg/kg/day, reduced by 25% every 3 days for 3 times, then given every other day for 3 times, and then discontinued to reduce edema, which can compromise circulation to the nerve. NSAID can be given to horses to reduce edema. If voluntary movement, nociception, and spinal reflexes improve over 1-2 mo, the prognosis is good. Limb mutilation can be transient in recovering nerve injuries and may be prevented by temporary use of an elizabethan collar. If nerve injury is suspected to be permanent and the animal is mutilating the limb, amputation is recommended in small animals.

Neoplasia of nerve roots and peripheral nerves can cause a chronic, progressive, often painful paresis of a thoracic or pelvic limb. (*See also* p 1013 and p 1047.) Nerve sheath tumors are common in dogs. Lymphosarcoma of the brachial or lumbosacral plexus is seen in dogs, cattle, and cats. If the nerve roots within the spinal canal are affected, an extramedullary spinal cord mass may be visualized with a myelogram, computed tomography, or MRI in dogs and cats. Surgical exploration and removal or biopsy are essential to determine diagnosis or prognosis. The longterm prognosis for nerve sheath tumors is poor, even after attempted surgical removal and limb amputation. Nerve sheath tumors often affect multiple nerve roots, and the tumor is difficult to completely remove. If appropriate chemotherapy is instituted for lymphosarcoma, the length and quality of life may be improved.

Horses with equine protozoal myeloencephalitis (EPM, p 1031) may develop monoparesis and focal muscle atrophy. CSF analysis and CSF and serum EPM titers should be evaluated so appropriate therapy can be administered.

LOUPING ILL

(Ovine encephalomyelitis)

Louping ill is an acute, tick-transmitted viral disease of the CNS that primarily affects sheep, but cattle, goats, horses, dogs, pigs, red deer, roe deer, red grouse, and people also can be affected; humans can be infected by tick bites or exposure to tissues or instruments contaminated with virus. The disease is seen throughout the rough hill grazings of the British Isles wherever the vector tick, *Ixodes ricinus*, is prevalent. Diseases of sheep indistinguishable from louping ill and caused by similar viruses have been reported in Norway, Spain, Turkey, and Bulgaria, which suggests that the condition may not be restricted to the British Isles.

Etiology and Transmission: The virus belongs to the Flaviviridae family, is distributed throughout the northern temperate regions, and is part of an antigenically closely related complex of viruses known as the tickborne encephalitides, which are primarily associated with disease in humans. Infection is transmitted trans-stadially by the tick vector; transovarial transmission does not appear to occur. In sheep, mortality ranges from 60% in newly introduced stock to 5-10% in sheep acclimatized to the pasture. On farms where the disease is endemic, losses are mainly confined to animals <2 yr old; adults tend to be immune as a result of previous infection, and lambs are protected in their first season by colostral antibody. However, when the disease appears for the first time, or after a lapse of several years, all ages of sheep are susceptible. Mortality is variable in other species but tends to be high in red grouse. All species of vertebrates that come in contact with questing ticks may become parasitized and infected with louping-ill virus, but only sheep and grouse develop titers of viremia sufficient to pass the infection to the vector tick. Infection also can be spread through contact with contaminated instruments or tissues. Infected lactating goats can excrete high titers of virus in their milk, which may cause fatal infection of their kids and be a potential human health hazard.

Pathogenesis, Clinical Findings, and Lesions: The course of infection in all species is similar, and varies only in the intensity of viremia and frequency with which clinical signs develop. After inoculation by an infected tick, virus initially replicates in lymphoid tissues, which gives rise to viremia that lasts 1-5 days. Only animals that develop high titers can transfer the virus to ticks. During viremia, a febrile reaction may be seen, but overt clinical signs are generally absent until the virus enters the CNS and begins replication, even though the immune response has eliminated the virus from the extraneuronal tissues. The extent of neuronal damage consequent to viral replication determines the severity of signs, from none (subclinical) through varying degrees of neurologic dysfunction to sudden death. Histologic lesions may be present whether or not signs develop. Signs include fine muscular tremors, nervous nibbling, ataxia (particularly of the hindlimbs), weakness, and collapse; death may occur 1-3 days after onset of signs. Peracute deaths may also occur. In some recovered animals, residual paresis or torticollis may persist. All recovered animals are solidly immune for life.

The severity of clinical disease in animals recently infected with *Anaplasma phagocytophilum* (the cause of tickborne fever [p 620]) is markedly increased, presumably due to the immunosuppressive effect of this organism. The accompanying pathology may be complex and may account for the high mortality experienced when naive flocks are introduced to tick-infested pasture.

No specific gross lesions are present, although secondary pneumonia may develop. Histologic examination of the CNS usually shows a nonsuppurative polioencephalomyelitis with lesions predominantly in the brain stem.

Diagnosis: The disease normally is seen only in animals that have had access to tick-infested pasture; however, the variable clinical picture necessitates differentiation from other conditions that cause locomotor or neurologic dysfunction. Confirmation is by histologic examination of the brain, virus isolation from CNS tissue, and serology. As much of the brain and brain stem as possible should be fixed in formaldehyde solution (10% in saline), and sections examined for the characteristic lesions, which can be useful in reaching a presumptive diagnosis. A definitive diagnosis requires virus isolation. Brain stem (1 cm^3) should be collected aseptically into 50% glycerol saline for isolation of the virus by mouse or tissue-culture inoculation, and subsequent identification by fluorescent antibody tests or neutralization with specific antibodies. Measurement of serum neutralizing and hemagglutination inhibition antibodies also can be useful in reaching a diagnosis and for surveys. The presence of IgM antibody in cattle and sheep, detected by the hemagglutination inhibition test, provides good evidence that the animal was infected within the preceding 10 days.

Treatment and Control: No specific treatment is available, but nursing, hand-feeding, and sedation may be helpful. An inactivated, tissue-culture-propagated vaccine is available and has successfully protected sheep, cattle, and goats. A single injection induces an antibody response that provides protection for >2 yr. Colostrum from the vaccinated ewe prevents infection of lambs in their first months. Generally, all animals to be retained for breeding are vaccinated at 6-12 mo of age. Use of insecticidal dips to protect against exposure to ticks generally is inadequate, although pour-on preparations reduce exposure and their systematic use may be effective in reducing the abundance of ticks.

Zoonotic Risk: Louping-ill virus infection of humans can cause severe encephalomyelitis. Symptoms are biphasic; the initial flulike symptoms are replaced 4-5 days later with signs of encephalitis. People become infected through the bite of infected ticks or through contact with infected carcasses, sharp instruments, or aerosol. Only a few cases of natural transmission have been reported, most occurring in laboratory workers. Those engaged in the diagnosis or research of this virus should be vaccinated with a human vaccine against tickborne encephalitis virus. As goats can excrete high titers of virus in their milk, goats kept for milk production in endemic areas must be vaccinated.

MENINGITIS AND ENCEPHALITIS

Inflammation of the meninges (meningitis) and inflammation of the brain (encephalitis) often are seen simultaneously (meningoencephalitis) in the same animal, although either can be seen separately. In animals with meningoencephalitis, the clinical signs of meningitis often precede the clinical signs of encephalitis and may remain the predominant feature of the illness. Causes of meningitis, encephalitis, and meningoencephalitis include bacteria, viruses, fungi, protozoa, rickettsia, parasite migrations, chemical agents, and idiopathic or immune-mediated diseases. In ruminants, generally bacterial infections are more common than other causes of meningitis or encephalitis. In species other than ruminants, especially adult animals, viruses, protozoa, rickettsia, and fungi are as frequent or more frequent causes of meningitis or encephalitis than are bacteria. Some causes of meningitis or encephalitis, eg, certain rickettsia and bacteria, are seasonal.

Etiology and Pathogenesis: The incidence of meningitis and encephalitis is fairly low compared with that of infections of other organs. This appears to result from the better protection offered to the nervous system by its barriers, rather than to a scarcity of infectious agents that can attack the nervous system. Infections of the nervous system often are the result of some injury to its protective barriers. In all species, direct extension of bacterial or mycotic infections to the CNS can develop from sinusitis, otitis media or interna, vertebral osteomyelitis, or diskospondylitis; these infections can also be secondary to migrating grass awns or other foreign bodies, deep bite wounds, or traumatic injuries adjacent to the head or spine. Iatrogenic infections are possible from contaminated spinal needles or surgical instruments. Infections may develop if CSF taps are performed in animals with bacteremia. Brain abscesses also can arise from direct infections or by septic embolism of cerebral vessels. Pituitary abscesses in ruminants are thought to originate from bacterial invasion of the rete mirabile surrounding the pituitary gland. In chronic brain abscesses, an adjacent or occasionally diffuse fibrinous leptomeningitis may develop. A spontaneous bacterial meningitis or meningoencephalitis can develop in dogs (although less commonly than in farm animals) from which various aerobic bacteria (*Pasteurella multocida, Staphylococcus* spp, *Escherichia coli, Streptococcus* spp, *Actinomyces* spp, and *Nocardia* spp) and anaerobic bacteria (*Bacteroides* spp, *Peptostreptococcus anaerobius, Fusobacterium* spp, *Eubacterium* spp, and *Propionibacterium* spp) have been isolated. Bacterial endocarditis and septicemia are important sources of CNS infection in dogs. When bacterial infections do occur, they are more likely to be sporadic than epidemic.

Bacterial meningoencephalitis often affects neonatal farm animals as a sequela of septicemia caused by *E coli* (p 600) or streptococci; *Actinobacillus equuli* infection is an important cause of meningoencephalitis in foals. Failure of passive transfer of immunoglobulins is the single most important factor predisposing neonates to omphalophlebitis or enteritis, with subsequent hematogenous spread of the infection to the CNS. In older or adult animals, well-recognized disease entities, such as histophilosis of cattle (*Histophilus somni,* p 606), Glässer's disease of pigs (*Haemophilus parasuis,* p 576), and *Haemophilus agni* septicemia in feeder lambs, also cause meningoencephalitis by the hematogenous route. Listeriosis (p 531), which is caused by *Listeria monocytogenes* and is a common infection in cattle, sheep, and goats, is an example of a multifocal brainstem meningoencephalitis that ascends to the CNS via transaxonal migration in cranial nerves. *Mannheimia haemolytica* and *Pasteurella multocida,* although usually resulting in fibrinous pneumonia and hemorrhagic septicemia in ruminants, occasionally produce a localized fibrinopurulent leptomeningitis. Meningoencephalitis due to *M haemolytica* has also been reported in horses, donkeys, and mules. *Actinomyces, Klebsiella,* and *Streptococcus* spp are sporadic causes of meningitis in adult horses.

Other agents that can cause meningoencephalitis, especially in dogs and occasionally cats and other species, include protozoa such as *Toxoplasma gondii, Neospora caninum, Sarcocystis neurona, Encephalitozoon cuniculi,* and *Trypanosoma* spp; fungi such as *Cryptococcus neoformans, Blastomyces dermatitidis, Histoplasma capsulatum, Aspergillus* spp, and *Coccidioides immitis*; the rickettsial organisms that cause Rocky Mountain spotted fever, salmon poisoning, and ehrlichiosis; and *Acanthamoeba* spp. Rarely, other fungi, such as *Candida* spp, *Cladosporium trichoides, Paecilomyces variotii, Chryseobacterium (Flavobacterium) meningosepticum,* and *Geotrichum candidum,* cause meningoencephalitis. Aseptic suppurative or eosinophilic meningoencephalitis associated with aberrant migration of parasites into the CNS can develop in number of species, especially *Parelaphostrongylus tenuis* in goats and llamas. Viruses such as those of canine distemper, canine parvovirus, feline infectious peritonitis, malignant catarrhal fever in ruminants, and sporadic bovine encephalomyelitis also produce meningitis in addition to encephalitis. Eosinophilic meningoencephalitis is an unusual inflammatory response to salt poisoning in pigs. Unicellular plants, *Prototheca wickerhamii* and *P zopfii,* can also produce an eosinophilic meningoencephalomyelitis in dogs.

Several idiopathic meningoencephalitides are recognized in dogs. A **pyogranulomatous meningoencephalomyelitis** is seen in mature Pointer dogs. It has been reported as an acute, rapidly progressive disorder. The lesions consist of extensive mononuclear cells and neutrophils infiltrating the leptomeninges and parenchyma, especially in the cervical spinal cord and brain stem. An etiologic agent has not been identified. **Granulomatous meningoencephalomyelitis** (GME, p 1023) is a more common CNS disease of dogs that most often affects young to middle-aged small-breed females. A necrotizing meningoencephalitis of unknown etiology has been reported in young, adult Pug dogs (**Pug encephalitis**), as well as in Yorkshire Terriers and Maltese dogs. A steroid-responsive suppurative meningitis affecting mainly young (<2 yr), large-breed dogs and a severe **necrotizing vasculitis and meningitis** syndrome in Beagles, Bernese Mountain Dogs, and German Shorthaired Pointers have both been identified as possible immunologic disorders with a hereditary predisposition. (*See also* CONGENITAL AND INHERITED ANOMALIES OF THE NERVOUS SYSTEM, p 995.) An eosinophilic meningoencephalitis that has been described in adult dogs is believed to have an immunologic basis.

Clinical Findings: The usual signs of meningitis are fever, hyperesthesia, neck rigidity, and painful paraspinal muscle spasms. Dogs and occasionally horses display this syndrome acutely and sometimes chronically without clinical signs of brain or spinal cord involvement. However, in diffuse meningoencephalitis due to any agent, depression, blindness, progressive paresis, cerebellar or vestibular ataxia, opisthotonos, cranial nerve deficits, seizures, dementia, agitation, and depressed consciousness (including coma) can develop, depending on the rapidity of onset, pathology, and location of the lesions. In neonatal infections, omphalophlebitis, polyarthritis, and ophthalmitis with hypopyon can accompany the CNS inflammation. Because of its unusual pathogenesis, listeriosis often causes asymmetric vestibular dysfunction, with head tilt and circling, in addition to other cranial nerve deficits such as facial and pharyngeal paralysis. In histophilosis of cattle, the nervous signs tend to be peracute, with sudden collapse and profound depression of consciousness (stupor or coma); fever and limb stiffness may be the only signs detectable in the prodromal stages. Clinical signs of pyogranulomatous meningoencephalomyelitis include neck rigidity, kyphosis, inability to raise the head, reluctance to move (eggshell gait), and limb incoordination (ataxia). Sometimes, bradycardia, vomiting, and in chronic cases, atrophy of cervical muscles may be seen. Cranial nerve signs may include Horner's syndrome and paralysis of any cranial nerve but most commonly the trigeminal and facial nerves. The signs of GME in dogs vary with the distribution of the lesions. The ocular form of GME is characterized by acute loss of vision with dilated, unresponsive pupils. Visual deficits, neck pain, seizures, behavioral disturbances, ataxia, weakness, cranial nerve deficits, and depression may be seen in either the focal or disseminated form of the CNS disease. The focal form of GME typically progresses insidiously over many months to years. The disseminated form of GME has a shorter, more fulminating course, with death typically occurring within weeks to months. The necrotizing encephalitis of Pugs and Maltese dogs causes forebrain signs, such as seizures, behavioral changes, visual deficits, and circling, while the condition in Yorkshire Terriers may manifest with either forebrain or brain-stem dysfunction. The latter is characterized by depression of consciousness, limb weakness, and cranial nerve deficits.

Lesions: Pathologic changes characteristic of meningitis include diffuse infiltration of leukocytes into the leptomeninges. Frequently, the entire subarachnoid space of the brain and spinal cord is inflamed. Vasculitis of meningeal vessels and CNS arterioles may also be apparent. In meningoencephalitis, the inflammation extends into the CNS parenchyma, resulting in leukocyte infiltration with large areas of perivascular cuffing. Necrosis and malacia of the CNS may be seen, with infiltrations of macrophages, neutrophils, and plasma cells. Listeriosis uniquely causes microabscesses deep within the CNS parenchyma, which consist of accumulations of neutrophils and microglial cell reaction with central liquefactive necrosis.

Diagnosis: The analysis of CSF is the most reliable and accurate means of identifying meningitis or meningoencephalitis. CSF should be collected whenever history or species or breed predisposition suggests meningitis or encephalitis, or whenever clinical signs indicate a disseminated or multifocal CNS disorder. Without CSF analysis, an animal exhibiting back or neck pain and perhaps a mild fever may be misdiagnosed. In the early stages, meningitis can easily be mistaken for intervertebral disk extrusion, polyarthritis, pleuritis, pancreatitis, or pyelonephritis. Dogs with bacterial meningitis and encephalitis, steroid-responsive suppurative meningitis, and vasculitis and meningitis typically have a marked neutrophilic pleocytosis in the CSF, with cell counts in the hundreds to thousands. The protein content of the CSF is usually also significantly increased (>100 mg/dL), with an increase in the globulin component of CSF. Occasionally, bacteria are seen on cytologic examination of the CSF and identified with Gram's stain. Successful culture of bacteria from CSF is more likely in large animals than in dogs. In some cases, serial blood cultures are more successful for isolation of the causative organism. Viral infections and listeriosis typically produce a mild to moderate mononuclear pleocytosis in CSF, with an associated increase in protein levels. Feline infectious peritonitis is an exception to this, and classically results in a neutrophilic pleocytosis with a protein concentration >200 mg/dL. Rickettsial infections most often cause a mild to moderate mononuclear pleocytosis, although Rocky Mountain spotted fever can cause neutrophilic inflammation secondary to vasculitis. Granulomatous inflammations usually induce moderate to high cell numbers and increased protein in the CSF. The cell population is predominately mononuclear or a mixed population of neutrophils and mononuclear cells. Distinguishing a granulomatous infection due to a fungal or protozoal organism from GME is often difficult. Eosinophilic inflammation can be seen with some fungal (especially *Cryptococcus*) and protozoal infections. Cryptococci and occasionally protozoa have been identified in CSF, but usually serology is necessary to confirm mycotic and protozoal infections in vivo. The necrotizing encephalitides typically cause a mild increase in CSF mononuclear cells and protein concentration.

Treatment: Other than for animals with the probable immune-mediated, steroid-responsive inflammatory CNS diseases and animals with meningoencephalitis caused by rickettsia and certain bacteria, the prognosis is guarded and treatment often of little benefit. The case fatality rate in calves with bacterial meningitis has been reported to be 100%.

Appropriate use of antibiotics, according to culture or serology results, is basic to successful therapy. Relapses are common, and prolonged therapy is often necessary. Correction of any immunodeficiency is critical in neonatal large animals. Broad-spectrum antibacterials that can penetrate the blood-brain barrier should be selected, and bactericidal drugs are preferred over those that are bacteriostatic. Recommended drugs include ampicillin, metronidazole, tetracyclines, trimethoprim-sulfas, fluoroquinolones, and third-generation cephalosporins; higher than normal dosages may be necessary to achieve and maintain adequate concentrations in the CNS. In farm animals, selection of drugs must be based not only on drug efficacy but also on whether the available drug is appropriate for use in a food animal.

Mycotic infections of the CNS have been treated successfully in humans, but results in veterinary medicine are less promising. Treatment with itraconazole or fluconazole may be of benefit, but longterm therapy is required and relapses are frequent. Protozoal infections (eg, toxoplasmosis, neosporosis, sarcocystosis) may respond to a sulfa/pyrimethamine combination or to clindamycin therapy. However, relapse may occur due to the inability to clear encysted organisms from the CNS. Glucocorticoids are usually contraindicated in animals with meningitis or meningoencephalitis with an infectious etiology; however, a high-dose, short-term course of dexamethasone or methylprednisolone may control life-threatening complications such as acute cerebral edema and impending brain herniation. Immunosuppressive doses of corticosteroids are required for successful therapy of the idiopathic CNS inflammations seen in dogs. Radiation therapy and immunomodulatory drugs have been used in the treatment of GME. Supportive care should be specific for the needs of the individual animal and may include analgesics, anticonvulsants, fluids, nutritional supplementation, and physical therapy.

MOTION SICKNESS

Motion sickness is characterized by nausea, excessive salivation, and vomiting, and affected animals may have other signs referable to stimulation of the autonomic nervous system. Animals may yawn, whine, and show signs of uneasiness or apprehension; severely affected ones may also have diarrhea. Motion sickness is usually seen during travel by land, sea, or air, and signs usually disappear when vehicular motion ceases. Many animals, including people, may be affected. The principal causative mechanism involves stimulation of the vestibular apparatus in the inner ear, which has connections to the emetic center in the brain stem. The chemoreceptor trigger zone (CRTZ) and H_1-histaminergic receptors are involved in this pathway in dogs, but apparently are less important in cats. Fear of the vehicle may be a contributory factor in dogs and cats, and signs may be seen even in a stationary vehicle.

In some cases, motion sickness can be overcome by conditioning the animal to travel. In others, ataractic and antinausea drugs can be used with good results. Antihistamines (such as diphenhydramine hydrochloride, dimenhydrinate, meclizine, and promethazine hydrochloride) prevent motion sickness, provide sedation, and inhibit drooling. The centrally acting phenothiazine derivatives (such as triethylperazine, chlorpromazine, prochlorperazine, and acepromazine maleate) have antiemetic as well as sedative effects. Cats have no histamine receptors in the CRTZ; therefore, antihistamines are ineffective in treating motion sickness in this species. Motion sickness in cats probably is best treated with an α-adrenergic antagonist (eg, chlorpromazine) instead of a pure H_1-histaminergic antagonist. Phenobarbital and diazepam have been used to produce a general sedative effect. Oral administration of one of these drugs several hours before departure should reduce or eliminate the signs of motion sickness. (*See also* DRUGS TO CONTROL VOMITING, p 1981.)

NEOPLASIA OF THE NERVOUS SYSTEM

Neoplasia of the nervous system is common in cats and dogs. In dogs, the incidence of canine nervous system tumors is 1-3% at necropsy. In cats, nervous system tumors are less common and are mainly meningiomas and lymphomas. Primary nervous system tumors originate from neuroectodermal, ectodermal, and/or mesodermal cells normally present in (or associated with) the brain, spinal cord, or peripheral nerves. Secondary tumors affecting the nervous system may originate from surrounding structures such as bone and muscle or from hematogenous metastasis of a primary tumor in another organ. Tumor emboli can lodge and grow anywhere in the brain, meninges, choroid plexus, or spinal cord. Dissemination or metastasis of CNS tumors is rare but may occur via the CSF pathways, especially if the tumors are located close to the subarachnoid space or ventricular cavities (eg, choroid plexus papilloma, ependymoma, medulloblastoma, neuroblastoma, pinealoblastoma), or via a hematogenous route such as the dural sinus, with later development of remote metastasis, most often in the lung. Tumors may also spread by direct extension to surrounding tissues, especially bone. The osseous tentorium may be used as a reference point for localizing different areas of the brain within the cranial vault. Thus, tumors in the cerebral hemispheres are often referred to as supratentorial or anterior fossa tumors, while those in the brain stem or cerebellum are called infratentorial or posterior fossa tumors.

Classification: Classification of nervous system tumors in animals follows the criteria used for tumors in people and is based primarily on the characteristics of the constituent cell type, its pathologic behavior, topographic pattern, and secondary changes seen within and around the tumor (TABLE 1).

Immunocytochemical studies and imaging techniques may aid classification. Primary tumors typically grow slowly, while secondary, highly malignant, metastatic tumors and bone tumors generally progress more rapidly. Many animal tumors have characteristics analogous to corresponding human neoplasms; however 15-20% of neuroectodermal tumors (especially gliomas) remain unclassified. Many of these are related topographically to the ventricular system and/or subependymal cell nests. Up to 26% of neuroectodermal brain tumors are undifferentiated, as shown by immunocytochemical staining. While brain tumors are occasionally reported in animals <1 yr old, most are found in mature and aged animals. No sex predilection for nervous system tumors has been identified.

Incidence: The reported incidence of nervous system neoplasia in animals varies. However, such tumors are reported more often in dogs than in other domestic animals. In one survey, 2.83% of 6,175 dogs examined at necropsy had intracranial neoplasia. In another report, incidence of intracranial neoplasia was 14.5/100,000 dogs at risk. A retrospective study of young dogs (<6 mo old) indicated that the 3 most common sites for neoplasia (in decreasing order) were the hematopoietic system, brain, and skin. Brachycephalic breeds are at increased risk for some neuroectodermal tumors. (*See* below.)

Brain Tumors: In dogs and cats, the brain is a more common site of primary tumors of the nervous system than the spinal cord or peripheral nerves. Meningiomas, gliomas (eg, astrocytomas, oligodendrogliomas), undifferentiated sarcomas, pituitary tumors, and ventricular tumors (eg, choroid plexus papillomas, ependymomas) are commonly reported primary brain tumors in dogs. Neoplastic reticulosis (considered to be the malignant form of granulomatous meningoencephalomyelitis), also described as gliomatosis and microgliomatosis, is reported sporadically. More recently, the condition has been equated with malignant histiocytosis. Other primary brain tumors (eg, malformation tumors), tumors of nerve cells (eg, neuroblastoma, ganglioneuroblastoma, and ganglioneuroma), pinealomas, craniopharyngiomas (a suprasellar ectodermal tumor that may destroy the pituitary gland), spongioblastomas (embryonal glioma), and medulloblastomas are rare. Adult dogs of several related brachycephalic breeds—Boxers, English Bulldogs, and Boston Terriers—are often cited as having the highest incidence of brain tumors among domestic animals; glial tumors, including unclassified gliomas, are the most numerous tumors in these breeds. A more recent study of 97 dogs indicated that Golden Retrievers also have a high incidence of brain tumors (especially meningiomas).

Primary nasal cavity tumors may extend into the cranial vault. In some cases, the only clinical signs are neurologic abnormalities such as behavioral changes, circling, paresis, seizures, or visual deficits. Respiratory signs such as epistaxis, nasal discharge, sneezing, dyspnea, stertor, or mouth breathing may develop after neurologic signs or may be absent. Nasal tumor types include adenocarcinoma, anaplastic chondrosarcoma, epidermoid carcinoma, esthesioneuroblastoma, neurofibrosarcoma, neuroendocrine carcinoma, and squamous cell carcinoma. Unlike nasal cavity tumors, those that originate in middle or inner ear structures rarely extend into the brain. Secondary tumors extending into the brain from the nasal sinuses are relatively common in dogs, as are metastatic brain tumors (*see* below). Middle or inner ear tumors rarely extend into the brain. In cats, metastases most frequently originate from mammary carcinomas and lymphosarcomas.

Astrocytomas are probably the most common neuroectodermal brain tumor in dogs. They are usually found in adult dogs, but they have been reported in dogs <6 mo old. They are common in brachycephalic breeds but can be seen in any breed. Astrocytomas are uncommon in cats. In one report of 4 cats, the tumors invaded the third and lateral ventricles. Astrocytomas consist of relatively large, protoplasmic-rich cells, or smaller cells with many processes. The cells tend to be arranged around blood vessels. There are several variants (eg, anaplastic, fibrillary, gemistocytic, protoplasmic, and pilocytic), most of which stain positively for glial fibrillary acidic protein (GFAP), the chemical subunit of the intracytoplasmic intermediate filaments of astrocytes. Regressive changes found histologically include necrosis, mucinoid degeneration, cyst formation, vascular proliferation (often in the form of glomeruloid nests), and multinucleated giant cells. Hemorrhage is rare, but is more common in oligodendrogliomas. Malignant astrocytomas display nuclear polymorphism, mitotic figures, and small cells with dense, hyperchromatic nuclei. In one study using computed tomography (CT), astrocytomas and oligodendrogliomas appeared similar to one another because both tumors had ring-like, irregular enhancement and poorly defined margins. Differentiating oligodendrogliomas from malignant astrocytomas with MRI has been difficult. In some instances, however, MRI is considered superior to CT in defining diffuse leptomeningeal and low-grade cerebral astrocytomas.

Choroid plexus papillomas are common tumors in dogs, with reported frequency similar to that of glioblastomas (~12% of neuroglial tumors). Developmentally, the choroid plexus epithelium differentiates from the primitive medullary epithelium and is related to the ependymal cells. These tumors are reddish, papillary growths that may bleed. Histologically, they are well defined, grow by expansion, and have a granular papillary appearance. Tumor papillae consist of vascular stroma lined by one layer of cuboidal or cylindrical epithelium. Immunocytochemical studies reveal that these tumors express epithelial but not glial differentiation, based on absence of staining with GFAP. Keratin may be expressed from some of these tumors. In both benign and malignant variants of choroid plexus papillomas, dissemination to other areas of the brain or spinal cord via the CSF pathways may occur following exfoliation. Obstructive hydrocephalus may occur. Meningeal carcinomatosis may follow spread of the tumor in the subarachnoid space. Choroid plexus tumors are seen as well-defined, hyperdense masses with marked, uniform contrast enhancement on CT scans. Marked enhancement, potentially including hemorrhage and mineralization, is also seen with MRI. Choroid plexus papillomas have no apparent predilection for brachycephalic breeds and are rare in cats.

Ependymomas originate from the epithelium lining the ventricles and central canal of the spinal cord. They are rare, but have been reported most frequently in brachycephalic breeds. The gray to reddish, soft, lobular masses tend to invade the ventricular system and meninges, which may result in obstructive hydrocephalus. Mestastases within the CSF system may be observed. Ependymomas of the fourth ventricle may encircle the brain stem. Both epithelial and fibrillary varieties have been described. Histologically, cells are isomorphic with pale or transparent cytoplasm and round, chromatin-rich nuclei. Nucleus-free zones around blood vessels are characteristic. Some ependymomas appear hemorrhagic, with mucinoid degenerative changes and cyst formation. Malignant or anaplastic ependymomas have moderate degrees of pleomorphism and necrosis and may merge into glioblastoma multiforme. In one study, only 1 of 9 ependymomas was positive for GFAP. In a CT study of brain tumors, ependymomas had no definitive distinguishing features.

Gangliocytomas are rare intracranial tumors reported in adult dogs of several breeds. Histologic findings include mature, neuronal-like cells with multiple processes, a

TABLE 1. Tumors of the Nervous System in Dogs and Cats

Tumor Origin	Predilection Sites	Species	Incidence
Primary Tumors			
Nerve cells			
Ganglioneuroma (gangliocytoma) Ganglioneuroblastoma Neuroblastoma	Variable, eg, cerebellum, cranial nerve roots, eye, cervical ganglion	Dogs	Rare
Neuroepithelium			
Ependymoma	Third and lateral ventricles	Dogs, cats	Uncommon
Nephroblastoma	Meninges, thoracolumbar spinal cord	Dogs (German Shepherd)	Uncommon
Choroid plexus papilloma	Fourth ventricle	Dogs	Common
Neuroglia			
Astrocytoma	Piriform area, convexity of cerebral hemispheres, thalamus, hypothalamus	Dogs (brachycephalic), cats	Common
Oligodendroglioma	Cerebral hemispheres	Dogs (brachycephalic)	Common
Glioblastoma	As for astrocytoma	Dogs (brachycephalic)	Uncommon
Spongioblastoma	Variable, eg, ependymal surfaces, cerebellum, optic nerve and tracts	Dogs (brachycephalic)	Rare
Medulloblastoma	Cerebellum	Dogs, cats	Uncommon
Gliomas (unclassified)	Periventricular areas, especially in cerebral hemispheres	Dogs	Common
Peripheral nerves and nerve sheaths			
Nerve sheath tumors (schwannoma, neurofibroma, neurinoma)	Peripheral nerves	Dogs, cats	Common
Meninges, vessels, and other mesenchymal structures			
Meningiomas	Convexities of cerebral hemispheres and floor of the vault	Dogs (dolicocephalic), cats	Common
Angioblastoma	Variable	Dogs, cats	Rare
Sarcoma	Variable	Dogs, cats	Common

TABLE I. *(continued)*

Tumor Origin	Predilection Sites	Species	Incidence
Focal granulomatous meningoencephalomyelitis (reticulosis)	Cerebral hemispheres and brain stem	Dogs, cats	Common (in dogs)
Pineal gland, pituitary gland, and craniopharyngeal duct			
Pinealoma	Pineal body	Dogs	Rare
Pituitary adenoma	Pituitary gland	Dogs (brachycephalic), cats	Common
Craniopharyngioma	Hypophyseal-infundibular areas	Dogs	Rare
Heterotopic tissues (malformation tumors)			
Epidermoid, dermoid, teratoma, teratoid, intra-arachnoid cyst	Variable (fourth ventricle and cerebellopontine angle for epidermoid, quadrigeminal cistern for intra-arachnoid cyst)	Dogs	Rare
Germ cell tumors	Base of brain above sella turcica	Dogs	Rare
Hamartoma	Variable (eg, hypothalamus)	Dogs	Rare
Secondary Tumors			
Metastatic tumors			
Mammary gland adenocarcinoma, pulmonary carcinoma, prostatic carcinoma, chemodectoma, malignant melanoma, lymphosarcoma, salivary gland adenocarcinoma, hemangiosarcoma, etc	Variable	Dogs, cats	Relatively common
Primary tumors from surrounding tissues			
Osteosarcoma, lipoma, Osteochondroma, chondrosarcoma, fibrosarcoma, nasal adenocarcinoma, hemangiosarcoma, multiple myeloma, calcifying aponeurotic fibromatosis, epidermoid cyst, etc	Variable	Dogs, cats	Relatively common

central nucleus, and a nucleolus. Neuroblast-like immature cells may also be seen, and occasionally, newly formed myelin sheaths. They seem to be seen most often in the cerebellum. Pure gangliocytomas have no glial elements and do not express GFAP. Mineralization and extensive necrosis accompanied by edema and capillary proliferation may also develop.

Suprasellar **germ cell tumors** are located dorsal to the sella turcica at the base of the brain. They are often intimately associated with the pituitary gland, which may be trapped within or replaced by the germ cell tumor. They are thought to result from extensive migration of germ cells during embryogenesis. Neurologic signs may be acute in onset and may include lethargy; depression; bradycardia; dilated, nonresponsive pupils; ptosis; visual deficits; and blindness. Germ cell tumors may be large—extending from the olfactory peduncles to the pons and pyriform lobes—and may envelop other cranial nerves (eg, nerves III-VII). Histologically, the tumors usually contain a mixture of primitive germ cells, cords resembling hepatocytes, and acini and tubules of tall columnar epithelial cells. They may stain positively for fetoprotein. Affected animals are usually 3-5 yr old; Doberman Pinschers may be at higher risk than other breeds. Some germ cell tumors have been misdiagnosed as pituitary tumors or craniopharyngiomas.

Glioblastoma multiforme, considered to be equated with the more malignant forms of astrocytomas, has been reported with varying frequency in dogs. In one study, the incidence was 12% of 215 neuroglial tumors. Most are large and found in the cerebrum. The tumor cells consist of medium-sized, round or fusiform cells with isomorphic nuclei. Some glioblastomas display considerable pleomorphism, with small and large mononucleated and multinucleated cells. They are locally invasive and destructive, well vascularized, and often contain necrotic zones. Glioblastomas sometimes express GFAP and are most common in brachycephalic breeds.

Hamartomas are formed by disorderly overgrowth of tissues normally present at a site. They are focal malformations resembling neoplasms and have been reported only rarely in dogs, usually as a subclinical finding.

Hematogenous metastatic brain tumors commonly originate from extracranial sites. In dogs, they often develop from carcinomas of the mammary glands, thyroid, bronchopulmonary epithelium, kidneys, chemoreceptor cells, nasal mucosa, squamous epithelium of the skin, prostate, pancreas, adrenal cortex, and salivary glands. Brain metastasis from a transmissible venereal tumor has been reported in a 5-yr-old male mixed breed dog. Common sarcoma metastases in dogs include fibrosarcomas, hemangiosarcomas, lymphosarcomas, and melanoblastomas. Brain metastases may accompany intramedullary spinal cord metastasis in dogs with lymphosarcomas or hemangiosarcomas. In cats, metastases stem most often from mammary carcinomas or lymphosarcomas. Most CNS lymphomas, especially in dogs, are one part of a multicentric disease, with extensive infiltration of the choroid plexus and leptomeninges a common finding. Neoplastic angioendotheliomatosis in dogs is thought to be an angiotropic lymphoma, possibly of the B-cell line. Extraneural tumor cells sometimes localize in the meninges (eg, meningeal carcinomatosis), often in association with intestinal carcinoma or mammary adenocarcinoma.

Intracranial intra-arachnoid cysts have been reported in dogs. These rare malformation tumors seem to develop most often in the quadrigeminal cistern. Of the 6 dogs in one report, 3 were <1 yr old, 4 were males, and 5 of the 6 dogs weighed <11 kg. One dog had additional developmental anomalies (abnormal corpus callosum and block vertebrae). On CT scans and MRI the cysts were extra-axial, had sharply defined margins, contained fluid isodense to CSF, and did not show contrast enhancement.

Malformation tumors, including epidermoid and dermoid cysts and teratomas, originate from heterotopic tissue and are rare tumors in dogs. They typically lie close to embryonal lines of closure. Epidermoid and dermoid cysts result from inclusion of epithelial components of embryonal tissue at the time of closure of the neural tube. They reportedly have a predilection for young dogs (eg, 3-24 mo old), although cysts have been found in older dogs. They usually involve the cerebellopontine angle, fourth ventricle, or both. Cysts within the fourth ventricle may secondarily compress the medulla oblongata and cerebellum. Some epidermoid cysts are incidental findings at necropsy.

Histologically, epidermoid cysts may have a multilocular structure; most are lined by stratified squamous epithelium and contain keratinaceous debris, desquamated epithelial cells, and occasional inflammatory cells. In contrast, dermoid cysts contain adnexal structures such as hair follicles, sebaceous glands, and sweat glands. Cysts may measure up to 2.5 cm in diameter. Because of the tumor's location, dogs may show signs of a pontomedullary syndrome (eg, trigeminal, facial, cerebellar, and/or vestibular dysfunction). Teratomas are well-differentiated germ cell tumors (see above) arising from several embryonic germ cell layers.

Malignant histiocytosis, which has focal and diffuse forms, is rarely reported in dogs. Proliferation and/or infiltration of neoplastic histiocytes in the basiarachnoidal and ventricular areas (bilateral) is a characteristic feature. These cells may also infiltrate the spinal dura mater, arachnoidal space, leptomeninges, and spinal nerve roots. Histologically, the cells may have characteristic histiocytic morphology but exhibit moderate pleomorphism and numerous mitotic figures. The pathologic features of malignant histiocytosis appear similar to those seen in the neoplastic form of primary reticulosis.

Medulloblastomas are highly malignant, uncommon neuroectodermal canine tumors that almost always develop in the cerebellum. The tumors tend to bulge into the fourth ventricle, often replacing part of the cerebellar vermis and compressing the midbrain rostrally and the brain stem ventrally. They may infiltrate the meninges, metastasize within the CSF pathways, and cause obstructive hydrocephalus. Histologically, these tumors include sheets of densely packed cells with pale cytoplasm and oval or carrot-shaped nuclei with coarse, granular chromatin. Mitotic figures are common. Regressive changes include pyknosis and karyorrhexis. While most cases are seen in young dogs, a cerebellar medulloblastoma with multiple differentiation was recently noted in a 4-yr-old Border Collie.

Meningioangiomatosis is a rare, benign malformation of CNS blood vessels, characterized by proliferation of the vessels and spindle-shaped, perivascular meningothelial cells in the cerebral cortex and brain stem of juvenile and adult dogs. The meningothelial cells stain positively for vimentin, which, along with the presence of mucopolysaccharides and collagen among proliferating cells, suggests a mesenchymal and fibroblastic origin.

Meningiomas are extra-axial tumors. They arise from elements of the dura within the cranial and spinal spaces and are the most commonly reported brain tumors in cats. They are also one of the most common intracranial tumors in dogs, with a reported incidence of 30-39%. In most studies, meningiomas are seen in dogs >7 yr old and in cats >9 yr old, although they have been observed in young cats (<3 yr old) with mucopolysaccharidosis type I, and in dogs <6 mo old. They are often found in dolichocephalic breeds, especially Golden Retrievers. Canine and feline meningiomas have estrogen, progesterone, and androgen receptors. These usually benign tumors tend to grow slowly under the dura mater, although direct brain invasion has been reported. Pathologic findings include globular, irregular, lobulated, nodular, ovoid, or plaque-like masses ranging in diameter from a few millimeters to several centimeters. Meningiomas are typically discrete and often are firm, rubbery, and encapsulated. They may contain granular calcifications known as psammoma bodies. In addition, there may be focal or massive calcification of the tumor. A substantial proportion of basal and plaque-like meningiomas involve the floor of the cranial cavity, especially when located near the optic chiasm or suprasellar area. They also commonly are found over the convexities of the cerebral hemispheres, less often in the cerebellopontomedullary region, and infrequently in the retrobulbar space (arising from the optic nerve sheath). In cats, common locations include the tela choroidea of the third ventricle and the supratentorial meninges. Cats also have a high incidence of multiple meningiomas. Hyperostosis, a thickening of bone adjacent to the meningioma, may develop, especially in cats. Meningiomas rarely metastasize outside the brain, but may extend into paranasal regions and lungs or be seen as primary extracranial masses as a result of embryonic displacement of arachnoid cells or meningocytes. Those in extracranial locations differ from intracranial meningiomas primarily in their more aggressive behavior and anaplastic/malignant nature. Meningiomas may be distinguishable from tumors within the brain parenchyma on contrast CT scans by their appearance as broad-based, peripherally located masses. Cystic and edematous meningiomas have been detected using CT scans and MRI. When a dural tail (a linear enhancement of thickened dura mater adjacent to an extra-axial mass) is detected by MRI, a meningioma is the most likely cause. The histologic classification of canine meningiomas includes angioblastic, fibroblastic, meningothelial or syncytial, psammomatous, and transitional. Papillary and microcystic forms may also be seen. The tumors usually consist of large meningothelial cells or fusiform cells arranged in whorls, nests, islands, or stream-like patterns. Cell boundaries are typically ill defined and the nuclei contain little chromatin. Canine meningiomas commonly have vimentin intermediate filaments. Regressive changes may include cavernous vascular formations, hemorrhage, hyalinization of connective tissue, and deposits of fat, lipopigments, or cholesterol. Many have evidence of focal necrosis with suppuration. This is the likely cause of the reported predominance of polymorphonuclear cells in CSF in many dogs with meningioma. The majority of feline epitheliomas are meningotheliomatous or psammomatous, often with cholesterol deposits.

In **meningeal sarcomatosis**, sarcomas cause diffuse thickening of the meninges; extensive hemorrhages are common. These rare tumors tend to infiltrate nervous tissue and run along blood vessels. Cell types include lymphoid, plasmacytoid, mature plasma cells, immunoblastic cells, and multinucleate giant cells.

Oligodendrogliomas are common tumors in dogs, particularly in brachycephalic breeds. In one report, they comprised 28% of neuroectodermal tumors. These tumors consist of chromatin-rich, densely packed, round cells with perinuclear halos. Most grow by infiltration and destroy invaded tissue. Capillaries tend to proliferate within these tumors, producing glomerulus-like structures. Regressive changes are similar to those seen in astrocytomas (*see* above). Necrosis and extensive calcification are uncommon. These tumors do not stain with GFAP; in one study, 3 of 11 oligodendrogliomas reacted with myelin-associated glycoprotein, while none reacted with myelin basic protein. Many canine oligodendrogliomas are mixed tumors with areas of astrocytic and, in some cases, ependymal differentiation. The MRI features are similar to those seen with high-grade (malignant) astrocytomas. Oligodendrogliomas are rare in cats.

Pituitary tumors are common in dogs, with an apparent predilection for brachycephalic breeds. They are infrequent in cats. Tumors may be functional or nonfunctional. Either type may cause hypopituitarism by mechanical or functional impairment of remaining pituitary tissue, although this effect is uncommon. Nonfunctional canine pituitary tumors are common and are usually chromophobe adenomas, although adenocarcinomas have also been reported. Functional pituitary tumors associated with the adenohypophysis are typically characterized by pituitary-dependent hyperadrenocorticism (PDH). (*See also* p 435.) Of the cases of pituitary Cushing's disease, ≥80% are reportedly associated with a pituitary tumor. In dogs, these tumors may stem from the pars distalis (80%) or the pars intermedia (20%), because both regions contain cells that can produce adrenocorticotropic hormone. The tumors are generally chromophobic microadenomas (<1 cm in diameter) that do not produce neurologic signs. MRI studies suggest that up to 60% of dogs with PDH and no neurologic signs have pituitary tumors 4-12 mm in diameter. As many as 50% of dogs with PDH have large chromophobic macroadenomas (<1 cm in diameter), but may not show clinical signs related to an intracranial mass. In 1 study, 7 of 8 dogs with pituitary neoplasia that had been treated for PDH for varying periods of time between 1-2 yr developed neurologic signs, including abnormal behavior (eg, head pressing, lethargy, hiding, wandering, pacing, tight circling, and trembling), seizures, and positional nystagmus. Most pituitary tumors, especially those derived from the pars distalis, tend to grow dorsocaudally because the diaphragma sella is incomplete. Chromophobic canine tumors from the pars intermedia are smaller and less destructive. Dorsal extension of pituitary tumors may lead to compression and obliteration of the infundibulum, ventral portion of the third ventricle, hypothalamus, and thalamus and may eventually impinge on the internal capsule and optic tract. Hypothalamic or median eminence involvement may cause central diabetes insipidus (especially in middle-aged and older dogs with neurologic signs), as well as polyuria, polydipsia, and isosthenuria or hyposthenuria. Alteration in water balance results from interference with the synthesis of antidiuretic hormone (ADH) in the supraoptic nucleus or release of ADH into capillaries of the pars nervosa. Although pituitary tumors generally do not lead to visual impairment, acute blindness and dilated, nonresponsive pupils have been noted in 7 dogs and 1 cat with pituitary masses that compressed the optic chiasm. Approximately 80% of cats diagnosed with Cushing's disease have PDH; tumor types include pituitary microadenomas, macroadenomas, and adenocarcinomas. Pituitary acidophil adenomas, especially the large variety, have been associated with acromegaly and nervous system signs (eg, circling, seizures) in cats, accompanied by insulin-resistant diabetes mellitus and high serum growth hormone concentrations.

Histologically, pituitary tumors include polygonal, round, and cylindrical cells arranged in close contact with blood vessels or formed into islands of cells divided by connective tissue. The cell pattern may be uniform, resembling normal pituitary tissue. Many pituitary tumors contain both chromophobic and chromophilic cells. Regressive changes include cyst formation, necrosis, and hemorrhage. MRI with contrast enhancement is extremely helpful for visualizing microtumors (3-10 mm in diameter) and macrotumors (≥24 mm) in dogs with PDH, regardless of neurologic signs. MRI and CT scans of pituitary tumors reveal minimal peritumoral edema, uniform contrast enhancement, and well-defined margins; however, tumors <3 mm in diameter may not be visible. Adrenal and pituitary tumors may coexist in dogs with hyperadrenocorticism, complicating test results and making diagnosis and treatment more difficult.

Primary skeletal tumors do not typically cause neurologic signs. Multilobular osteochondroma originates in the flat bones of the skull, usually in older medium- or large-breed dogs and appears as a firm, fixed mass. It may erode the cranium and compress, rather than infiltrate, underlying brain tissues. Radiographically, the tumor contains nodular or stippled areas of mineralization, resulting in a characteristic "popcorn ball" appearance. Microscopically, the tumor contains multiple lobules of osseous and chondroid tissue. Local recurrence and metastasis are common. Vertebral osteochondroma is the spinal cord counterpart.

Vascular malformations are considered developmental lesions rather than true neoplasms and are uncommon in both dogs and cats. They may be located in the cingulate gyrus, pyriform-hippocampal area of the temporal lobe, basal ganglia, cerebellum, occipital lobe, or septum pellucidum and fornix and comprise variable combinations of arteries, veins, and capillaries. The vessels tend to be dilated, sinusoidal in shape, and accompanied by hemorrhages.

Spinal Cord Tumors: Spinal cord tumors are relatively common in cats and dogs. They are generally classified according to their relationship with the spinal cord and meninges as extradural, intradural-extramedullary, or intramedullary. Depending on tumor location, any of the 4 spinal cord syndromes may be anticipated (eg, cervical, cervicothoracic, thoracolumbar, or lumbosacral syndromes). Regardless of type, the mean age of most dogs with spinal tumors is ~6 yr, and tumors appear to be more common in medium and large breeds. Cats with lymphosarcoma tend to be younger (mean age of ~3.5 yr), possibly due to the infectious etiology of most cases (eg, feline leukemia virus). However, age alone does not preclude a diagnosis of spinal tumor. The clinical course for the various tumor types and locations is not clearly defined. In one study, the rate of progression was fastest with intramedullary tumors (1.7 wk), followed by extradural tumors (3.4 wk), and intradural-extramedullary tumors (5.5 wk).

Extradural tumors are found outside the dura mater and cause spinal cord compression. They are the most common spinal tumors in both cats and dogs. The most frequent types of canine spinal cord tumors are primary, malignant bone tumors (chondrosarcoma, fibrosarcoma, hemangiosarcoma, hemangioendothelioma, multiple myeloma, osteochondromas or multiple cartilaginous exostoses, and osteosarcoma) and tumors metastatic to bone and soft tissue. Reports of secondary vertebral tumors in dogs include anaplastic tumors, aortic body tumors, bronchogenic carcinoma, chemodectoma, fibrosarcoma, ganglioneuroma, hemangiosarcoma, lymphosarcoma, malignant melanoma, mammary carcinoma, osteosarcoma, pancreatic adenocarcinoma, perianal gland carcinoma, prostatic carcinoma, rhabdomyosarcoma, Sertoli cell carcinoma, squamous cell carcinoma, transitional cell carcinoma, thyroid carcinoma, and tonsillar carcinoma.

An extradural ganglioneuroma and its undifferentiated counterpart, ganglioneuroblastoma, have also been reported in dogs. Primary vertebral tumors are rare in cats, with osteosarcoma being the most frequently reported. Metastatic, extradural spinal cord tumors are unusual in dogs, but extradural lymphosarcoma is the most common feline spinal tumor. In most cases, these tumors are secondary to lymphosarcoma elsewhere in the body, although primary spinal cord lymphosarcomas have been reported sporadically in dogs. In one study in cats, extraneural involvement was not found in ~50% of the cases, and the tumors were solitary in 22 of 23 cats. A predilection for the thoracic and lumbar vertebral canal was seen, but the tumors may be seen in any spinal region. Three of the tumors affected the brachial plexus cervical roots (*see* PERIPHERAL NERVE TUMORS, below). Feline spinal lymphomas may extend over multiple vertebral bodies and involve more than 1 level of the spinal cord. Leptomeningeal spinal cord involvement is not common in cats. A tumor termed myxoma-myxosarcoma has been described in 4 dogs. These malignant tumors resembled soft tissue myxomas, with polygonally shaped cells with gray, vacuolated cytoplasm that stained positive for S-100 protein antibody. The masses were extradural in 3 cases and intradural-extramedullary in the other.

Intradural-extramedullary tumors are found in the subarachnoid space and are estimated to account for ~35% of all spinal cord tumors. They are most commonly meningiomas or nerve sheath tumors (eg, neurofibromas, neurilemmomas, and schwannomas) that grow into the vertebral canal and compress the spinal cord. About 14% of CNS meningiomas in dogs (but only 4% in cats) reportedly involve the spinal cord. Tumors may be seen in the cervical, lumbar, or thoracic cord regions. In a report of spinal cord tumors in 29 dogs, nerve sheath tumors were the second most common type after vertebral tumors. In another review of canine spinal tumors, 39 of 60 nerve sheath tumors involved the spinal cord. Nerve sheath tumors often affect the brachial plexus (*see* PERIPHERAL NERVE TUMORS, below).

A primary intradural-extramedullary tumor with a predilection for T10-L2 spinal cord segments in young dogs, particularly retrievers and German Shepherds, has been variously diagnosed as ependymoma, medulloepithelioma, nephroblastoma, or neuroepithelioma. The origin of this tumor is uncertain, and immunocytochemical studies have not supported a neuroectodermal origin. Monoclonal antibody studies suggest it may be a nephroblastoma. Most cases are seen in dogs 5-36 mo old, with males and females affected equally. Clinical signs include a thoracolumbar syndrome. CSF is usually normal, although an elevated protein level was found in 1 dog. The extramedullary masses are a tan to grayish white color and 1-3 cm long. They are generally found dorsal and lateral to the spinal cord, may entrap the spinal roots, and may be accompanied by areas of hemorrhage and severe spinal cord compression. Histologic findings include solid sheets of ovoid to fusiform cells interspersed with areas of acinar and tubular differentiation, rudimentary glomeruli, and focal squamous metaplasia.

Intramedullary tumors are the least common of the 3 categories of spinal cord tumors, with a reported frequency of 15-24%. Primary glial tumors (eg, astrocytoma, choroid plexus papilloma, ependymoma, oligodendroglioma, and undifferentiated sarcoma) are the most commonly diagnosed. Intramedullary spinal cord metastasis is an uncommon complication of systemic malignancy in dogs, and neurologic signs may be the first indication of systemic malignancy. The mean age of affected dogs is ~6 yr, any part of the spinal cord may be involved, and there may be accompanying brain metastasis. Spinal cord malignancy associated with granulomatous meningoencephalomyelitis is reported sporadically.

Malformation tumors rarely affect the spinal cord. In one report, a 2-yr-old, female Rottweiler presenting with a thoracolumbar syndrome had an intramedullary epidermoid cyst. The gray to off-white cyst was ~2 cm long, 1 cm in diameter, and extended from T13-L2 spinal cord segments. The empty lumen was lined by simple stratified squamous epithelium or, in a few regions, by desquamating keratinized epithelium containing keratohyaline granules. The spinal cord was severely compressed. These cysts may arise from growth of primordial epithelial cells entrapped during closure of the neural tube.

Peripheral Nerve Tumors: Tumors of cranial and spinal nerves and nerve roots are common in dogs, cattle, and horses but are rarely seen in cats. In one report, peripheral nerve tumors accounted for ~27% of canine nervous system tumors. Differing opinions on the cell of origin have led to confusion over the terminology used to describe these tumors. While schwannoma, neurilemmoma, and neurofibroma are common, interchangeable designations, the term malignant peripheral nerve sheath tumors (MPNST) is recommended because many of these tumors are malignant (based on cytologic criteria) and determining the cell of origin is usually impossible. Mid to caudal cervical and/or rostral thoracic nerve roots, especially ventral roots, are the most common sites for MPNST. These tumors frequently involve nerves of the brachial plexus, often appearing as bulbous or fusiform thickenings of one or more nerves. They can spread to other nerves once they advance to the common brachial plexus bundle. The tumors typically result in slow, progressive, unilateral thoracic limb lameness and muscle atrophy, often involving the infraspinatus and supraspinatus muscles. Affected animals may display a unilateral Horner's syndrome, pain on leg movement, axillary pain on palpation (an axillary mass may be palpable), and may lick or chew at the foot or carpus of the affected limb. Intradural-extramedullary spinal cord compression is most common with tumors located at the spinal nerve roots, although more peripherally located tumors occasionally may invade the vertebral canal. The trigeminal is the cranial nerve most often affected by MPNST, producing signs of unilateral trigeminal nerve dysfunction (eg, unilateral atrophy of the masseter and temporalis muscles). Brain-stem compression and local vertebral erosion have been reported.

Peripheral nerves may also be affected by other tumor types (eg, giant cell sarcoma with cervical involvement, a malignant tumor of the apocrine sweat glands, and sarcoma extending into the brachial plexus have been described in dogs). Peripheral tumors of neuronal origin, such as ganglioneuromas and their more undifferentiated counterpart, ganglioneuroblastomas, are extremely rare, but have caused extradural spinal cord compression in dogs. Sympathetic ganglia are thought to be the source of ganglioneuromas. Lymphosarcomas may involve cranial and spinal nerves and nerve roots in cats and dogs and may extend intracranially. Myelomonocytic neoplasia of the trigeminal nerve and ganglia, leading to a dropped mandible and symmetric atrophy of masticatory muscles, has been reported in dogs. Tumors of the ear canal (eg, ceruminous adenocarcinoma, fibrosarcoma, and squamous cell carcinoma), as well as osteosarcoma of the skull, may affect the facial nerve or one of its branches. Neurofibromas rarely involve the vestibulocochlear nerve. Cranial nerves may be compressed by meningiomas located on the floor of the cranial vault. The vagosympathetic trunk may be compressed by aortic body tumors.

See also DISEASES OF THE PERIPHERAL NERVE AND NEUROMUSCULAR JUNCTION, p 1010.

Clinical Findings: Some of the clinical signs and syndromes associated with various CNS tumors have already been mentioned. Cerebral, hypothalamic/diencephalic, midbrain, cerebellar, pontomedullary, and vestibular syndromes associated with focal discrete intracranial masses might be expected, depending on tumor location. Accurate anatomic localization is possible in many cases, especially in the early stages of tumor growth. However, correlation of clinicopathologic signs with tumor location may be impossible, because tumor location may be masked by secondary changes (eg, brain herniation, cerebral edema, hemorrhage, obstructive hydrocephalus, tissue necrosis, and tumor spread within the brain) that independently cause clinical signs. Partial brain herniation may result from increased intracranial pressure and/or shifts in the brain caused by the tumor.

Several types of herniation have been described. **Cingulate gyrus herniation** under the falx cerebri toward the unaffected hemisphere leads to compression of the opposite cingulate gyrus. **Occipital or temporal lobe herniation** (primarily the parahippocampal gyrus) under the tentorium cerebelli (caudal transtentorial herniation) often causes dorsoventral and lateral compression of the midbrain at the rostral colliculi and partial occlusion of the mesencephalic aqueduct. Caudal displacement of the diencephalon and midbrain may also occur. Clinical signs include initial pupillary constriction, often followed by mydriasis, tetraplegia, and coma. **Rostral cerebellar vermis herniation** under the tentorium cerebelli (rostral transtentorial herniation) may lead to flattening of the rostral cerebellum, marked compression and rostral displacement of the brain stem, and compression of the temporal cortex. Despite the gross pathology, clinical deficits may be absent. **Cerebellar herniation** (especially the caudal lobe of the cerebellar vermis) through the foramen magnum compresses the underlying medulla oblongata, and may be malacic and hemorrhagic. Apnea, hypoxia-induced coma, and tetraplegia may be observed. Concurrent foramen magnum and caudal transtentorial herniation may cause dysfunction in both the midbrain and medulla oblongata. Herniation combined with attenuation of the ventricular system, especially at the level of the mesencephalic aqueduct, can create obstructive hydrocephalus. The elevated intracranial pressure may lead to ischemic necrosis of the herniated tissue.

Initially, seizures and behavioral changes may be the only abnormalities associated with tumors involving the rostral cerebrum (eg, olfactory and frontal lobes). Lesions of the frontal and prefrontal lobes may result in no clinical signs. Acute blindness may be the initial clinical sign in animals with tumors in the region of the optic chiasm (eg, pituitary tumors, paranasal sinus carcinoma, polycentric lymphosarcoma, and suprasellar germ cell tumors). Papilledema (often bilateral) is thought to result from a generalized increase in intracranial pressure. A variety of causes (eg, multiple small metastatic masses from extracranial tumors, especially with malignant melanoma and hemangiosarcoma) may lead to multifocal clinical signs associated with CNS tumors. Other tumors, such as carcinomas (pulmonary or mammary) tend to produce fewer, larger metastases. The cerebrum, hippocampus, and cerebellar cortex are common sites for hematogenous metastases. Extraneural tumor cells sometimes localize in the meninges (eg, meningeal carcinomatosis associated with mammary adenocarcinoma or intestinal carcinoma). Multifocal syndromes may also result from primary CNS tumors in multiple sites, extension of an original tumor to another site, or metastasis via the CSF.

Choroid plexus papillomas and ependymomas tend to obstruct cerebrospinal pathways because of their ventricular orientation, especially when they arise in the fourth ventricle. Neurologic signs associated with ventricular tumors result from the tumor location and the degree of ventricular dilation caused by obstructive hydrocephalus. Clinical signs often are insidious with either of these tumors; the clinical course generally is protracted, ranging from months to years. Extraneural immunoproliferative diseases in dogs and cats (eg, multiple myeloma and macroglobulinemia-associated lymphocytic leukemia) may also result in a range of intermittent cranial neurologic signs, including disorientation, ataxia, intention tremor of the head, visual impairment, circling, and staggering or falling. Intravascular erythrocyte aggregation impairs blood flow in the affected areas and probably leads to the transient signs.

Pituitary tumors are associated with various endocrine signs, including acromegaly, abnormal hair coat, gonadal atrophy, polydipsia, polyuria, and obesity. (*See also* THE PITUITARY GLAND, p 451). Behavioral changes, circling, paresis, seizures, or visual deficits may result from extension of primary nasal cavity tumors into the cranial vault. Respiratory signs such as dyspnea, epistaxis, nasal discharge, sneezing, stertor, or mouth breathing may follow neurologic signs, or may not occur at all.

Diagnosis: A variety of diagnostic aids, including plain-film radiography, contrast radiography (eg, myelography), and specialized radiographic techniques such as radionuclide imaging (scintigraphy), CT scans, and MRI are used to diagnosis nervous system tumors. These techniques provide information (eg, axial origin, location, shape, pattern of growth, and edema) that can be important when determining prognosis, therapy, and outcome. Bone neoplasia may be observed with plain-film radiography. Intracranial tumors are better evaluated with MRI. While definitive diagnosis of intracranial tumors requires a biopsy, some indices of malignancy (eg, edema, extension of growth across the midline, poor margin definition, and tissue invasion) have been defined using MRI.

Signs of extradural, intradural-extramedullary, and intramedullary tumors vary on myelography. Extradural lesions are located outside the dura mater, resulting in attenuation of the dural tube and spinal cord. Deflection of the contrast column away from the vertebral canal, resulting in a widened epidural space, confirms an extradural lesion. Intramedullary-extramedullary lesions develop in the subarachnoid space, where they act as wedges, displacing the dura mater toward the bony vertebral canal and the spinal cord toward the contralateral vertebral canal. Contrast material abuts the cranial and caudal margins of the tumor, resulting in a characteristic cup or golf tee appearance. In contrast, intramedullary tumors displace the spinal cord material from within, enlarging the circumference of the spinal cord and attenuating the contrast material in the subarachnoid space surrounding the tumor.

Results from one study suggest that CT is better than survey radiographs for visualizing bony changes associated with extradural lesions, but that myelography is better than CT for classifying spinal cord lesions. In another canine study, MRI was used to determine tumor location in all dogs and bone infiltration in all but one. Localization of tumors in the intradural-extramedullary space was not always possible, however. Myelographic interpretation of intramedullary spinal cord metastasis may be difficult; intramedullary tumors must be differentiated from hemorrhage and spinal cord edema. Classically, myelograms of intramedullary masses reveal widening of the spinal cord shadow and tapering and attenuation of contrast in both lateral and ventrodorsal views.

Electrodiagnostic techniques (eg, electromyography, nerve conduction velocity determination), in conjunction with myelography and imaging techniques, can facilitate diagnosis of peripheral nerve tumors. Myelograms reportedly often are negative in animals with cervical MPNST.

Analysis of CSF may reveal moderate increases in total protein content, total white cell count, and CSF pressure. There is a low frequency of tumor cells in CSF from animals with brain or spinal cord neoplasia, but malignant cells have been reported in dogs and cats with intracranial and spinal cord (extradural and intramedullary) lymphosarcomas.

Prognosis and Treatment: The prognosis for animals with nervous system tumors is generally guarded to poor, but depends on the extent of tissue damage, tumor location, surgical accessibility, and rate of tumor growth. Recent improvements in treatment have centered mainly on surgical resection, radiation therapy, and chemotherapy, based on more accurate tumor localization and identification using imaging techniques, such as CT scans and MRI. Better identification and characterization of tumors from tissue biopsies obtained via stereotactically guided biopsy devices may lead to additional improvement. While success rates for different tumor types and locations are not currently known, cerebral tumors (including meningiomas and ependymomas) without brain-stem signs appear to have the best prognosis, especially in cats. Radiation therapy may be the most successful treatment for a range of intracranial tumors and, if surgery is performed, postoperative radiation therapy may prolong survival times. Radiation therapy is beneficial for inoperable tumors and may be better than surgery for dogs with infiltrative masses. A retrospective study of 86 dogs with brain tumors showed that dogs treated with ^{60}Co radiation, with or without other combinations of therapy, lived significantly longer that dogs that underwent surgery (some with ^{125}I implants) or dogs that received symptomatic treatment. Dogs with a solitary site of involvement had a better prognosis. Longterm control of brain tumors using cytotoxic chemotherapy alone is poor; symptomatic treatment (eg, use of anticonvulsants and/or anti-inflammatory doses of corticosteroids) is palliative at best. Corticosteroids may relieve signs by reducing edema near the tumor and by causing temporary regression of lymphoid and reticulohistiocytic tumors. The treatment of choice for meningioma in dogs is surgery. In a report of meningiomas treated by surgery alone, mean survival times were 198 days in dogs and 485 days in cats, with 1-yr survival rates of 30% for dogs and 50% for cats. Addition of cytotoxic drugs and/or irradiation may lengthen survival time.

Most extradural spinal tumors are primary bone tumors and removal often causes decreased spinal stability, pathologic fractures, or spinal subluxation. In a study of canine malignant extradural tumors, postsurgical survival times were low. A recent report of 20 vertebral tumors (primary or metastatic fibrosarcomas or osteosarcomas) in dogs treated with combinations of surgery, radiation, and chemotherapy supports a guarded prognosis for dogs with vertebral neoplasia. Median survival time was 135 days, with a range of 15-600 days. Survival time following surgical resection of spinal lymphoma and myxosarcoma in dogs was 560-1,080 days in another report, although some dogs received postsurgical radiotherapy and chemotherapy. Methods recommended for treating spinal lymphosarcoma in cats include focal radiotherapy, surgical cytoreduction, and systemic chemotherapy, including L-asparaginase, cyclophosphamide, vincristine, and prednisone. Longterm results are poor.

Animals with MPNST have a generally poor prognosis, because only a small percentage of these tumors can be completely resected and their recurrence rate is high. Metastasis, often to the lungs, is another complication. Early diagnosis of MPNST may lead to better results. Mean survival of 180 days was reported in one study following surgical resection. Many intradural-extramedullary tumors (eg, lipomas and meningiomas) can be successfully removed, with long postsurgical survival. However, intradural-extramedullary tumors that involve spinal cord segments of an intumescence, are ventrally located, or invade adjacent neural parenchyma have a poor prognosis.

Surgical resection is rarely possible for intramedullary masses. However, there are successful reports of removal of a thoracolumbar intramedullary ependymoma and a tumor resembling a nephroblastoma (by exploratory laminectomy, followed by durotomy and myelotomy). Prognosis for dogs with intramedullary spinal cord metastasis is poor due to the frequent presence of disseminated disease, although corticosteroid therapy may lead to temporary improvement.

Peripheral nerve and nerve root tumors can be successfully resected, but may necessitate removal of the affected nerve and nerve root. Recurrence is common following resection of peripheral tumors, with average time to recurrence of 5 mo in one report. If atrophy of all muscle groups is extreme—as may develop with tumors involving multiple nerves of the brachial plexus—or if more than 1 root is involved, complete amputation of the limb may be required.

PARANEOPLASTIC DISORDERS OF THE NERVOUS SYSTEM

Paraneoplastic syndromes are nonmetastatic complications of cancer. They can affect all parts of the nervous system, including the brain, cranial nerves, spinal cord, dorsal root ganglia, peripheral nerves, and the neuromuscular junction. They are thought to be immunologically mediated and are unrelated to metabolic or nutritional disorders, infection, stroke, or complications of therapy (eg, chemotherapy). Although the exact pathogenesis is unclear, similarities between antigens expressed by tumors and neural tissues may lead to effects against neural tissue by immune cells targeting the tumor.

Paraneoplastic syndromes affecting the CNS are rare in animals, but lack of awareness may have led to a low detection rate. A case involving the spinal cord was recently described in an 8-yr-old, male German Shepherd with a history of acute pelvic limb paralysis. Clinical signs included progressive loss of motor function, conscious proprioceptive deficits, loss of superficial and deep pain sensation over the trunk and pelvic limbs, and Schiff-Sherrington-like hyperextension in the thoracic limbs. Hepatocellular carcinoma with metastasis to the lungs, liver, spleen, and lymph nodes was found on necropsy. Severe necrotizing myelopathy was present throughout the gray and white matter of the thoracic spinal cord, including spongy degeneration, gliosis, demyelination, axonal swelling and degeneration, and neuronal necrosis. In a second case, a range of neurologic deficits in a 17-mo-old, male Poodle was attributed to hyperviscosity syndrome secondary to macroglobulinemia-associated lymphocytic leukemia.

Dogs with thymoma may develop paraneoplastic myasthenia gravis (MG). In a recent review of canine thymoma, 47% of the dogs had MG, 33% had nonthymic cancer (including pheochromocytoma, mammary adenocarcinoma, or pulmonary adenocarcinoma), and 20% had signs of polymyositis. Dogs with thymoma-associated MG may also produce autoantibodies to several neuromuscular antigens, including ryanodine (a skeletal muscle calcium-release channel receptor) and the muscle protein titin.

An association between myositis (eg, dermatomyositis and polymyositis) and malignant neoplasia in people has been well established. Dogs with malignant tumors such as bronchogenic carcinoma, myeloid leukemia, or tonsillar carcinoma may also have muscular necrosis and low-grade myositis, but the frequency of this potentially paraneoplastic association is unknown.

While the frequency of peripheral neuropathy in animals with cancer is also uncertain, certain types of cancer, such as bronchogenic carcinoma, mammary adenocarcinoma, malignant melanoma, insulinoma, osteosarcoma, lymphoma, thyroid adenocarcinoma and mast cell tumor, may facilitate development of peripheral nerve lesions. Histopathologic findings can include paranodal-segmental demyelination, remyelination, axonal degeneration, and myelin globules. The incidence of neuropathy may vary with the type of malignancy. Dogs with multiple myeloma may also develop peripheral neuropathy.

The pathogenesis of paraneoplastic neuropathies is uncertain, although some forms may be related to molecular mimicry. Clinical signs may include reduced or absent spinal or cranial reflexes, flaccid weakness, reduced muscle tone, paralysis of limb or head muscles, and, after 1-2 wk, neurogenic muscle atrophy. Dysphonia may also be present.

Dogs and cats with clinical signs of nervous system disease (or with myositis or necrotizing myopathy confirmed by histopathology) that fail to respond to therapy or that relapse should be carefully checked for malignancy. Testing may include chest radiography, sonography, computed tomography, or MRI as indicated. Such vigilance may detect tumors at a more treatable stage.

POLIOENCEPHALOMALACIA

(Cerebrocortical necrosis)

Polioencephalomalacia (PEM) is an important neurologic disease of ruminants that is seen worldwide. Cattle, sheep, goats, deer, and camelids are affected. The term PEM denotes a lesion with certain gross and microscopic features that are not specific for a particular etiology or pathogenesis. Historically, PEM has been associated with altered thiamine status, but more recently an association with high sulfur intake has been observed. Other toxic or metabolic diseases (eg, acute lead poisoning, sodium toxicosis/water deprivation) can result in PEM as well.

Etiology, Pathogenesis, and Epidemiology: The disease is seen sporadically or as a herd outbreak. In general, younger animals are more frequently affected than adults. Animals on high concentrate diets are at higher risk, but pastured animals also develop PEM. Cattle fed rations with added sulfate to limit intake or with byproducts of corn or sugar cane processing are at higher risk. The patterns of PEM occurrence depend on the etiologic factors involved.

PEM has been associated with 2 types of dietary risks: altered thiamine status and high sulfur intake. Thiamine inadequacy in animals with PEM has been suggested by several types of observations, including decreased concentrations of thiamine in tissues or blood and deficiency-induced alterations of thiamine-dependent biochemical processes (decreased blood transketolase activity, increased thiamine pyrophosphate effect on transketolase, and increased serum lactate). Unfortunately, many of these biochemical features of altered thiamine status are inconsistently observed in cases of PEM.

Thiamine inadequacy can be caused by such factors as acute dietary deficiency of thiamine or ingestion of plant thiaminases or thiamine analogs. A potential mechanism of thiamine inadequacy is the action of thiaminases on thiamine in the GI tract. Thiaminases can be produced by gut bacteria or ingested as preformed plant products. They can either destroy thiamine or form antimetabolites that interfere with thiamine function. Thiaminase I, produced by *Bacillus thiaminolyticus* and *Clostridium sporogenes*, and thiaminase II, produced by *B aneurinolyticus*, catalyze the cleavage of thiamine. The latter microorganism proliferates under conditions of high grain intake.

A neurologic disorder in Australia has been associated with the Nardoo fern (*Marsilea drummondii*), which may contain high levels of a thiaminase I enzyme. Other ferns such as bracken (*Pteridium aquilinum*) and rock fern (*Cheilanthes sieberi*) contain a similar thiaminase I. Although PEM has been produced experimentally by feeding high doses of extracts of such plants, field cases are uncommon because these plants are unpalatable (*see also* p 2349).

Overall, there is not a linear relationship among the presence of ruminal and fecal thiaminase, decreased concentrations of tissue and blood thiamine, and development of disease.

A beneficial response to thiamine therapy by PEM-affected animals is sometimes considered evidence of thiamine inadequacy. This thiamine-responsiveness is often seen if treatment is initiated early in the course of the disease. The assumption that this response indicates that deficiency of thiamine is the true etiology should be viewed with caution, however. Large doses of thiamine, beyond maintenance needs, may have nonspecific, beneficial effects in the energy-impaired brain.

PEM associated with high sulfur intake is recognized with increasing frequency. The basis of sulfur-related PEM appears to be the production of excessive ruminal sulfide due to the ruminal microbial reduction of ingested sulfur. Hydrogen sulfide (H_2S) gas, which has the odor of rotten eggs, accumulates in the rumen gas cap. Concentrations can be demonstrated with commercially available H_2S detection tubes via percutaneous gas sampling. While nonreduced forms of sulfur, such as sulfate and elemental sulfur, are relatively nontoxic, H_2S and its various ionic forms are highly toxic substances that interfere with cellular energy metabolism. The CNS, by virtue of its dependence on a high and uninterrupted level of energy production, is likely to be significantly affected by energy deprivation. When cattle undergo a transition to high sulfur intake, ruminal sulfide concentrations peak 1-4 wk after the change. This pattern is probably due to alterations in ruminal microflora. PEM peaks during the time period when ruminal sulfide concentrations are the highest.

A variety of sulfur sources can result in excessive sulfur intake, including water, feed ingredients, and forage. Many geographic areas have surface and deep waters high in sulfate. When evaporation occurs, water sulfate concentrations increase. Water consumption by cattle is temperature dependent and increases greatly at high temperatures, leading to increased sulfur intake due to concurrent increases in water consumption and sulfate concentrations in water. Alfalfa, by virtue of its high protein and sulfur-containing amino acid content, can serve as a significant source of sulfur. Although grasses tend to be low in sulfur, some circumstances can result in high sulfate concentrations. Certain weeds, including Canada thistle (*Cirsium arvense*), kochia (*Kochia scoparia*), and lambsquarter (*Chenopodium* spp) can accumulate sulfate in high concentration. Cruciferous plants normally synthesize sulfur-rich products and serve as important sources of excess sulfur. These include turnips, rape, mustard, and oil seed meals. Byproducts of corn, sugar cane, and sugar beet processing commonly have a high sulfur content, apparently due to the addition of sulfur-containing acidifying agents. PEM has been associated with the use of these types of byproducts as feed ingredients. A high molasses-urea diet has been associated with a form of PEM that lacks altered thiamine status.

Clinical Findings: PEM may be acute or subacute. Animals with the acute form manifest blindness, recumbency, tonic-clonic seizures, and coma. Those with a longer duration of acute signs have poorer responses to therapy and higher mortality. Animals with the subacute form initially separate from the group, stop eating, and display twitches of the ears and face. The head is held in an elevated position and there is a staggering, sometimes hypermetric gait. As the disease progresses, there is cortical blindness with a diminished menace response and unaltered palpebral and pupillary responses. Dorsomedial strabismus may develop. Head pressing, opisthotonos, and grinding of the teeth may be observed. The subacute form of PEM is frequently followed by recovery with only minor neurologic impairment. However, in a few cases, the subacute form may progress to a more severe form with recumbency and seizures. Animals that survive the acute form or advanced subacute form often manifest significant neurologic impairment that necessitates culling.

Lesions: Gross lesions are inconsistent and frequently subtle, especially early in the disease. Acutely affected animals may have brain swelling with gyral flattening and coning of the cerebellum due to herniation into the foramen magnum. Slight yellowish discoloration of the affected cortical tissue may be present. The brains of acutely affected animals may also have autofluorescent bands of necrotic cerebral cortex evident on meningeal and cut surfaces of the brain when viewed with ultraviolet illumination. As the pathologic process progresses, the affected cerebrocortical tissue has macroscopically evident cavitation, sometimes sufficient to result in apposition of the pia meninges to the white matter.

The initial histologic lesions are necrosis of cerebrocortical neurons. The neurons are shrunken and have homogeneous, eosinophilic cytoplasm. Nuclei are pyknotic, faded, or absent. Cortical spongiosis is sometimes present in the early phases of the acute form. Vessel cells undergo hypertrophy and hyperplasia. At later stages, the affected cortical tissue undergoes cavitation as macrophages infiltrate and necrotic tissue is removed. A pattern observed in brains of cattle with early, severe, acute sulfur-related PEM features multifocal vascular necrosis, hemorrhage, and parenchymal necrosis in deep gray matter including the striatum, thalamus, and midbrain.

Diagnosis: The pattern of clinical signs should arouse suspicion of PEM. At necropsy, macroscopically evident cerebrocortical autofluorescent areas under ultraviolet illumination provide a presumptive diagnosis of PEM. Characteristic histologic lesions are confirmatory.

Differential diagnoses for cattle include acute lead poisoning, water deprivation/sodium toxicosis, *Histophilus* meningoencephalitis, rabies, coccidiosis with nervous involvement, and vitamin A deficiency. Differential diagnoses for sheep include pregnancy toxemia, type D clostridial enterotoxemia (focal symmetric encephalomalacia), and listeriosis.

Confirmation of etiology or pathogenesis requires laboratory testing of samples from affected animals or their environment. Assessment of thiamine status is difficult and results should be interpreted with caution. Few laboratories are capable of measuring thiamine content of blood and tissues, transketolase activity, or the thiamine pyrophosphate effect on transketolase. Demonstration of clinical improvement after thiamine therapy is not adequate evidence for a specific diagnosis. The possibility of sulfur-associated PEM can be assessed by measuring the sulfur content of the water and dietary ingredients and then estimating the total sulfur intake on a dry-matter basis. The maximal tolerated concentration of sulfur is considered to be 0.4% dry matter. Because multiple factors are involved in determining the actual risk of developing PEM, this concentration should not be considered an absolute maximum. Many cattle adapt adequately to sulfur intake levels >0.4%, although negative effects, possibly subclinical, on performance may occur.

Treatment and Prevention: The treatment of choice regardless of cause is thiamine. Therapy must be started early in the disease course for benefits to be achieved. If brain lesions are particularly severe or treatment is delayed, full clinical recovery may not be possible. The dosage of thiamine is 10-20, mg/kg, IM or SC, TID. Initial treatment may be administered IV. Beneficial effects are usually observed within 24 hr and sometimes sooner; however, if there is no initial improvement, treatment should be continued for ≥3 days. Reduction of cerebral edema can be attempted with administration of dexamethasone at a dosage of 1-2 mg/kg, IM or SC. Symptomatic therapy for convulsions may be necessary.

Dietary supplementation of thiamine at 3-10 mg/kg feed has been recommended for prevention, but the efficacy of this approach has not been carefully evaluated. During a PEM outbreak, sufficient roughage should be provided. When the problem could be associated with high sulfur intake, all possible sources of sulfur, including water, should be analyzed and the total sulfur concentration of the consumed dry matter estimated. Dietary ingredients or water with high sulfur concentration should be avoided; if this is not possible, then more gradual introduction to the new conditions can improve the chances of successful adaptation.

PORCINE ENTEROVIRAL ENCEPHALOMYELITIS

(Teschen disease, Talfan disease, Porcine polioencephalomyelitis)

Porcine enteroviral encephalomyelitis is analogous to human poliomyelitis. Severe disease is now rare; it is seen in eastern Europe and Madagascar but was last reported in western Europe from Austria in 1980. In other countries, sporadic mild disease is reported, or the disease is unrecognized.

Etiology, Epidemiology, and Pathogenesis: Until recently, viruses causing this disease were classified within the genus Enterovirus (family Picornaviridae). However, analyses of their complete genome sequences have revealed them to be very different from the enteroviruses, and they have been reclassified in a new genus, Teschovirus, as the species porcine teschovirus (PTV, derived from Teschen disease). Originally, 11 porcine enterovirus (PEV) serotypes were defined by virus neutralization. Of these, PEV 1-7 and 11-13 have been renamed PTV 1-10. An additional serotype (PTV 11) has also recently been described. PEV types 8-10, which have not been associated with neurologic disease, are distinct from the teschoviruses and remain in the Enterovirus genus. PTV are ubiquitous in swine populations throughout the world. Many strains are nonpathogenic, but most neurotropic strains belong to one of the first 3 serotypes; serotype 1 includes not only the highly virulent but also many of the less virulent neurotropic strains. Although antigenic subtypes are recognized, they do not distinguish between more or less virulent strains of virus. PTV can survive in the environment for months.

Transmission is by direct or indirect contact with infected pigs. The virulent serotype 1 strain of classic Teschen disease results in high morbidity and mortality in all ages of pigs but apparently has remained confined to certain geographic areas. Mild, sporadic disease is seen elsewhere. Conventional herds are usually endemically infected, and exclusion of teschoviruses from SPF herds is difficult to maintain. Infection is mainly inapparent, and pigs usually become infected at weaning with the decline of passive maternal immunity and mixing of groups. Sporadic clinical cases of nervous disease are seen mainly around this time, although disease is more common in unweaned piglets after introduction of a serotype to which the herd has not been exposed.

Ingested virus replicates in the GI tract and associated lymphoid tissue. There is no destruction of gut epithelium, but virus is shed from multiplication sites into the feces for several weeks. In some pigs, especially those infected with virulent strains, viremia ensues and results in spread of infection to the CNS (*see also* p 1020).

Clinical Findings: In acute virulent infection, clinical signs appear 1-4 wk after exposure in pigs of all ages. Ataxia is often seen first, followed by fever, lassitude, and anorexia. Seizures, nystagmus, opisthotonos, and coma may occur. Paralysis, initially evident as paraplegia but progressing to quadriplegia, is frequent in severe cases. Death is common within 3-4 days of onset of signs.

In mild disease, signs are essentially ataxia and paresis, the latter more rarely progressing to paralysis. Only young pigs (unweaned or weaned) are susceptible, and recovery is frequent.

Lesions: There are no gross lesions. Microscopic changes are most prominent in the gray matter of the brain stem, cerebellum, and spinal cord. The nonsuppurative encephalitis is characterized by neuronal necrosis, neuronophagia, glial foci, and perivascular lymphocytic cuffing. Meningitis is often present over the cerebellum.

Diagnosis: The clinical signs (especially those of locomotor disturbance), epidemiology, and absence of specific gross necropsy findings offer a presumptive diagnosis. The nature and distribution of histologic lesions provide supportive evidence. Acute and convalescent serum samples, taken ≥2 wk apart, may demonstrate a rise in neutralizing or complement-fixing antibodies. Virus isolation from the CNS is required to confirm the diagnosis. Differentiation of severe and milder forms of the disease can be based only on serologic, clinical, and epidemiologic evidence.

Differential diagnoses include the many other viral encephalitides of pigs, particularly classical swine fever, African swine fever, pseudorabies, rabies, and the encephalopathies of edema disease and water deprivation/salt intoxication. The prominent locomotor signs in porcine enteroviral encephalomyelitis also can be confused with several toxic and nutritional neuropathies.

The different serotypes are identified either by virus neutralization, complement fixation, or ELISA using specific antisera. With the recent availability of genome sequence data for all the PTV serotypes, molecular diagnosis is a possibility; however, no validated protocols are currently available.

Treatment and Control: There is no treatment. Live attenuated vaccine is used for control in areas experiencing severe endemic disease. In the past, eradication measures in central Europe involved ring vaccination and slaughter, and restrictions on importation of pigs and pork products. In many countries, suspected disease must be reported to regulatory authorities. In herds with endemic mild clinical disease, introduction of new breeding stock ≥1 mo before breeding should enhance passive immunity in offspring.

PSEUDORABIES

(Aujeszky's disease, Mad itch)

Pseudorabies is an acute, frequently fatal disease with a worldwide distribution that affects swine primarily and other domestic and wild animals incidentally. The pseudorabies virus has emerged as a significant pathogen in the USA since the 1960s, probably because of the increase in confinement swine housing or perhaps because of the emergence of more virulent strains. Clinical signs are similar to those of rabies, hence the name "mad itch." Pseudorabies is a reportable disease and has been successfully eradicated from the vast majority of the USA.

Etiology: Pseudorabies virus is a DNA herpesvirus. Although the pig is the only natural host, the virus can infect cattle, sheep, cats, dogs, and goats as well as wildlife, including raccoons, opossums, skunks, and rodents. Experimental studies in nonhuman primates indicate that rhesus monkeys and marmosets are susceptible but chimpanzees are not. Reports of human infection are limited and are based on seroconversion rather than virus isolation. Infections in horses are rare. Only one serotype of pseudorabies virus is recognized, but strain differences have been identified using monoclonal antibody preparations, restriction endonuclease assays, and heat and trypsin inactivation markers.

Epidemiology: The virus can be transmitted via nose-to-nose or fecal-oral contact. Indirect transmission commonly occurs via inhalation of aerosolized virus. Infectious virus can persist for up to 7 hr in air with a relative humidity of ≥55%. Data from England indicate that virus may travel via aerosols for up to 2 km in certain weather conditions. Other studies have demonstrated that the virus can survive for up to 7 hr in nonchlorinated well water; for 2 days in anaerobic lagoon effluent and in green grass, soil, feces, and shelled corn; for 3 days in nasal washings on plastic and pelleted hog feed; and for 4 days in straw bedding. The virus is enveloped and, therefore, is inactivated by drying, sunlight, and high temperatures (≥37°C). Dead-end hosts, such as dogs, cats, or wildlife, can transmit the virus between farms, but these animals survive only 2-3 days after becoming infected. The potential role of insects as vectors is being investigated. Birds do not seem to play a role in transmission.

Clinical Findings and Pathogenesis: The clinical signs depend on the age of the affected animal. Young swine are highly susceptible, and losses may reach 100% in piglets <7 days old. In general, signs of CNS disease (eg, tremors and paddling) are seen. If weaned pigs are infected, respiratory disease is the primary clinical problem, especially if complicated by secondary bacterial pathogens. Pseudorabies virus has been reported to inhibit the function of alveolar macrophages, thereby reducing the ability of these cells to process and destroy bacteria. A generalized febrile response (41-42°C), anorexia, and weight loss are seen in infected pigs of all ages. Mortality can be very low (1-2%) in grower and finisher pigs but may reach 50% in nursery pigs. Sneezing and dyspnea are frequently seen, and CNS involvement is reported occasionally.

After natural infection, the primary site of viral replication is nasal, pharyngeal, or tonsillar epithelium. The virus spreads via the lymphatics to regional lymph nodes, where replication continues. Virus also spreads via nervous tissue to the brain, where it replicates, preferentially in neurons of the pons and medulla. In addition, virus has been isolated from alveolar macrophages, bronchial epithelium, spleen, lymph nodes, trophoblasts, embryos, and luteal cells.

Viral excretion begins ~2-5 days after infection, and virus can be recovered from nasal secretions, tonsillar epithelium, vaginal and preputial secretions, milk, or urine for >2 wk. A latent state, in which virus is harbored in the trigeminal ganglia, may exist. In swine with latent infections, shedding may resume after periods of stress such as farrowing, crowding, or transport. Experimentally, corticosteroid injections (dexamethasone, 2 mg/kg, IM) for 5 consecutive days have induced recrudescence.

Lesions: Gross lesions of pseudorabies virus infection are often undetectable. Serous rhinitis, necrotic tonsillitis, or hemorrhagic pulmonary lymph nodes may be seen. Pulmonary edema, as well as pneumonic lesions of secondary bacterial pathogens may be present. Necrotic foci (2-3 mm in diameter) may be scattered throughout the liver. Such lesions are typically found in young (<7 days old) piglets.

Microscopically, nonsuppurative meningoencephalitis is a characteristic lesion that can be present in gray and white matter. Mononuclear perivascular cuffing and neuronal necrosis may also be present. The meninges are thickened as a result of mononuclear cell infiltration. Necrotic tonsillitis with the presence of intranuclear inclusion bodies, as well as necrotic bronchitis, bronchiolitis, and alveolitis are commonly seen. Focal areas of necrosis are often found in the liver, spleen, lymph nodes, and adrenal glands of macerated fetuses.

Diagnosis: In addition to the gross and microscopic lesions, other diagnostic aids include virus isolation, fluorescent antibody testing, and serologic testing. Brain, spleen, and lung are the organs of choice for virus isolation. Nasal swabs can be used for isolation of virus from acutely infected animals. The nasal specimens must be stored and transported in cold, sterile saline with antibiotics to suppress bacterial growth. The fluorescent antibody test can be performed using tonsil or brain.

Many serologic tests are now available, including serum neutralization, ELISA, and latex agglutination. Serum neutralization, which is the standard test, requires 48 hr to complete. An ELISA has been developed as a screening assay for large volumes of sera; however, specificity may be poor. False-positive results are typically reassessed using the serum neutralization test. The latex agglutination test, although highly sensitive and rapid, may also have poor specificity. After infection, antibodies can be detected within 6-7 days using the latex agglutination test, within 7-8 days using the ELISA, and within 8-10 days using the serum neutralization test.

A differential ELISA has recently been used to differentiate antibodies produced as a result of vaccination from those produced as a result of natural infection. The vaccines used in swine are based on the deletion of certain genes (gI, gIII, or gX) from the vaccine virus. Swine vaccinated with a gene-deleted vaccine do not mount an antibody response to the protein coded for by the deleted gene. In contrast, infection with field virus results in antibodies against these proteins.

Colostral antibodies to pseudorabies virus may be present until the pig is 4 mo old (similar to porcine parvovirus). Therefore, paired samples or serologic profiles may be necessary in grower and finisher pigs to assess decreasing levels of maternal antibody and to ensure that pigs are vaccinated at the appropriate time.

Treatment and Control: Although there is no specific treatment for acute infection with pseudorabies virus, vaccination can alleviate clinical signs in pigs of certain ages. Typically, mass vaccination of all pigs on the farm with a modified live virus vaccine is recommended. Intranasal vaccination of sows and neonatal piglets 1-7 days old, followed by IM vaccination of all other swine on the premises, helps reduce viral shedding and improve survival. The modified live virus replicates at the site of injection and in regional lymph nodes. Vaccine virus is shed in such low levels that mucous transmission to other animals is minimal. In gene-deleted vaccines, the thymidine kinase gene has also been deleted; thus, the virus cannot infect and replicate in neurons. It is recommended that breeding herds be vaccinated quarterly, and that finisher pigs be vaccinated after levels of maternal antibody decrease. Regular vaccination results in excellent control of the disease. Concurrent antibiotic therapy via feed and IM injection is recommended for controlling secondary bacterial pathogens.

Numerous programs have been developed for eradication of pseudorabies virus and include whole-herd depopulation, a test and removal strategy, and offspring segregation. Although effective, whole-herd depopulation is costly and time consuming. Usually, problems other than pseudorabies virus (eg, genetic improvement) need to be resolved before whole-herd depopulation can be cost effective.

The test and removal strategy consists of blood testing all breeding swine, culling all positive animals, and repeating this procedure until the population tests negative. Naturally infected animals can be culled when such a strategy is used in conjunction with a differential vaccination program. A test and removal strategy can be effective, but it is laborious, and latently infected animals that do not exhibit an antibody response on serologic testing may potentially resume shedding the virus at a later time.

In an offspring segregation program, young piglets (18-21 days old) are removed from vaccinated sows and raised to adulthood at another site. If enough gilts and boars are raised in this manner, the original breeding herd may be depopulated and subsequently repopulated with seronegative replacements. This method also allows seedstock producers to sell animals, even though the breeding herd is infected. In this case, however, all offspring must be individually tested using the serum neutralization test and have negative results before being sold.

RABIES

Rabies is an acute viral encephalomyelitis that principally affects carnivores and bats, although it can affect any mammal. It is invariably fatal once clinical signs appear. Rabies is found throughout the world, but a few countries claim to be free of the disease due either to successful elimination programs and/or to their island status and enforcement of rigorous quarantine regulations.

Etiology and Epidemiology: Rabies is caused by lyssaviruses in the Rhabdovirus family. Lyssaviruses are usually confined to 1 major reservoir species in a given geographic area, although spillover to other species is common. Identification of different virus variants by laboratory procedures such as monoclonal antibody analysis or genetic sequencing has greatly enhanced understanding of rabies epidemiology. Generally, each virus variant is responsible for rabies transmission between members of the same species in a given geographic area. From an epidemiologic perspective, it is preferable to use the name of the species acting as the reservoir as an adjective: rabies maintained by dog-to-dog transmission is termed canine rabies, whereas rabies in a dog as a result of infection with a variant from a different reservoir, eg, skunk (or fox), should be referred to as skunk (or fox, etc) rabies in a dog.

In North America, distinct virus variants are responsible for rabies in dogs and coyotes in Mexico and south Texas, red and Arctic foxes in Canada and Alaska, raccoons along the eastern seaboard, gray foxes in Texas and a closely related variant in gray foxes in the southwestern USA. Two different variants are responsible for rabies in striped skunks, one in the south central states and the other in the north central states. Another skunk rabies virus variant is seen in California. The epidemiology of rabies in bats is complex, but in general, each variant found in bats may be assigned to a predominant bat species. Spillover from bats to terrestrial animals is seen infrequently. Most human cases of rabies in the USA in the past decade have been caused by bat rabies virus variants (especially the variant associated with *Lasionycteris noctivagans*, the silver-haired bat, and *Pipistrellus subflavus*, the Eastern Pipistrelle).

Reservoirs of rabies vary throughout the world. Canine rabies predominates in Africa, Asia, Latin America, and the Middle East. In North America and Europe, where canine rabies has been practically eliminated, rabies is maintained in wildlife. For many years, skunks were the most commonly reported rabid animal in the USA, but since 1990, rabid raccoons have been the most numerous. Canine rabies became established in coyotes (*Canis latrans*) in southern Texas and Mexico, with the potential to spread throughout much of the USA and Canada. Skunk, raccoon, and fox rabies are each found in fairly distinct geographic regions of North America, although some overlap occurs. Bat rabies is distributed throughout the USA and Central and South America. In Europe, red fox rabies predominates. In parts of northern and eastern Europe, rabies in raccoon dogs is of increasing concern. Rabies in insectivorous bats may be widely distributed in Europe. The vampire bat is an important reservoir in Mexico, Central and South America, and is the source of outbreaks in cattle. Other wild species play an important role in the transmission of rabies in certain areas, including mongooses in the Caribbean, southern Africa, and parts of Asia; jackals in certain parts of Africa; and wolves in parts of northern Europe.

No cat-to-cat transmission of rabies has been recorded, and no feline rabies virus variant is known. However, cats are the most commonly reported rabid domestic animal in the USA. Virus is present in the saliva of rabid cats, and people have developed rabies after being bitten by a rabid cat. Reported cases in domestic cats have outnumbered those in dogs in the USA every year since 1988.

Transmission and Pathogenesis: Transmission is almost always by introduction of virus-laden saliva into the tissues, usually by the bite of a rabid animal. Although much less likely, it is possible for virus from saliva, salivary glands, or brain to cause infection by entering the body through other fresh wounds or through intact mucous membranes. Usually, saliva is infectious at the time that clinical signs occur, but it is possible for dogs and cats to shed virus for several days before onset of clinical signs. Viral shedding in skunks has been reported for up to 8 days prior to onset of signs. Rabies virus has not been isolated from skunk musk (spray).

The incubation period is both prolonged and variable; typically, the virus remains at the inoculation site for a considerable time. The unusual length of the incubation period helps to explain how postexposure treatment, including in humans the practice of locally infiltrating hyperimmune serum, is effective. Most cases in dogs develop within 21-80 days after exposure, but the incubation period may be shorter or considerably longer. One reliably recorded case of rabies in a human had an incubation period >6 yr.

The virus travels via the peripheral nerves to the spinal cord and ascends to the brain. After reaching the brain, the virus travels via peripheral nerves to the salivary glands. If an animal is capable of transmitting rabies via its saliva, virus will be detectable in the brain. Virus is shed intermittently in the brain.

Hematogenous spread does not occur. Under most circumstances, there is no danger of aerosol transmission of rabies. However, aerosol transmission has occurred under very specialized conditions in which the air contains a high concentration of suspended particles or droplets carrying viral particles. Such conditions have been responsible for laboratory transmission under less than ideal containment situations. There has also documented aerosol transmission in 1 bat cave. Oral and nasal secretions containing virus were probably aerosolized from tens of millions of bats. Aerosol infection may occur via direct attachment of the virus to olfactory nerve endings.

Clinical Findings: Clinical signs of rabies are rarely definitive. Rabid animals of all species usually exhibit typical signs of CNS disturbance, with minor variations among species. The most reliable signs, regardless of species, are acute behavioral changes and unexplained progressive paralysis. Behavioral changes may include sudden anorexia, signs of apprehension or nervousness, irritability, and hyperexcitability (including priapism). The animal may seek solitude. Ataxia, altered phonation, and changes in temperament are apparent. Uncharacteristic aggressiveness may develop—a normally docile animal may suddenly become vicious. Commonly, rabid wild animals may lose their fear of humans, and species that are normally nocturnal may be seen wandering about during the daytime.

The clinical course may be divided into 3 phases—prodromal, excitative, and paralytic/endstage. However, this division is of limited practical value because of the variability of signs and the irregular lengths of the phases. During the prodromal period, which lasts ~1-3 days, animals show only vague CNS signs, which intensify rapidly. The disease progresses rapidly after the onset of paralysis, and death is virtually certain. Some animals die rapidly without marked clinical signs.

The term "furious rabies" refers to animals in which aggression (the excitative phase) is pronounced. "Dumb or paralytic rabies" refers to animals in which the behavioral changes are minimal, and the disease is manifest principally by paralysis.

Furious Form: This is the classic "mad-dog syndrome," although it may be seen in all species. There is rarely evidence of paralysis during this stage. The animal becomes irritable and, with the slightest provocation, may viciously and aggressively use its teeth, claws, horns, or hooves. The posture and expression is one of alertness and anxiety, with pupils dilated. Noise invites attack. Such animals lose caution and fear of other animals. Carnivores with this form of rabies frequently roam extensively, attacking other animals, including people, and any moving object. They commonly swallow foreign objects, eg, feces, straw, sticks, and stones. Rabid dogs may chew the wire and frame of their cages, breaking their teeth, and will follow a hand moved in front of the cage, attempting to bite. Young pups can seek human companionship and are overly playful, but bite even when petted, usually becoming vicious in a few hours. Rabid skunks may seek out and attack litters of puppies or kittens. Rabid domestic cats and bobcats can attack suddenly, biting and scratching viciously. As the disease progresses, muscular incoordination and seizures are common. Death results from progressive paralysis.

Paralytic Form: This is first manifest by paralysis of the throat and masseter muscles, often with profuse salivation and inability to swallow. Dropping of the lower jaw is common in dogs. Owners frequently examine the mouth of dogs and livestock searching for a foreign body or administer medication with their bare hands, thereby exposing themselves to rabies. These animals may not be vicious and rarely attempt to bite. The paralysis progresses rapidly to all parts of the body, and coma and death follow in a few hours.

Species Variations: Cattle with furious rabies can be dangerous, attacking and pursuing humans and other animals. Lactation ceases abruptly in dairy cattle. The usual placid expression is replaced by one of alertness. The eyes and ears follow sounds and movement. A common clinical sign is a characteristic abnormal bellowing, which may continue intermittently until shortly before death.

Horses and mules frequently show evidence of distress and extreme agitation. These signs, especially when accompanied by rolling, may be interpreted as evidence of colic. As in other species, horses may bite or strike viciously and, because of their size and strength, become unmanageable in a few hours. People have been killed outright by such animals. These animals frequently suffer self-inflicted wounds.

Rabid foxes and coyotes often invade yards or even houses, attacking dogs and people. The abnormal behavior that can occur is demonstrated by the fox that attacks a porcupine; finding a fox with porcupine quills can, in most cases, support a diagnosis of rabies.

Rabid raccoons and skunks typically show no fear of humans and are ataxic, frequently aggressive, and active during the day, despite their often crepuscular nature. In urban areas, they may attack domestic pets.

In general, rabies should be suspected in terrestrial wildlife acting abnormally. The same is true of bats that can be seen flying in the daytime, resting on the ground, attacking people or other animals, or fighting.

Rodents and lagomorphs rarely constitute a risk for rabies exposure. However, each incident must be evaluated individually. Reports of laboratory-confirmed rabies in woodchucks are not uncommon in association with the raccoon rabies epizootic in the eastern USA.

Diagnosis: Clinical diagnosis is difficult, especially in areas where rabies is uncommon and should not be relied on when making public health decisions. In the early stages, rabies can easily be confused with other diseases or with normal aggressive tendencies. Therefore, when rabies is suspected and definitive diagnosis is required, laboratory confirmation is indicated. Suspect animals should be euthanized and the head removed for laboratory shipment.

Rabies testing should be done by a qualified laboratory, designated by the local or state health department in accordance with established national standardized protocols for rabies testing. Immunofluorescence microscopy on fresh brain tissue, which allows direct visual observation of a specific antigen-antibody reaction, is the test of choice. When properly used, it can establish a highly specific diagnosis within a few hours. Brain tissues examined must include medulla oblongata and cerebellum (and should be preserved by refrigeration with wet ice or cold packs). The mouse inoculation test or tissue culture techniques using mouse neuroblastoma cells may be used for indeterminate fluorescent antibody results, but it is no longer in common use in the USA.

Control: Comprehensive guidelines for control in dogs have been prepared by the World Health Organization and include the following: 1) notification of suspected cases, and euthanasia of dogs with clinical signs and dogs bitten by a suspected rabid animal; 2) reduction of contact rates between susceptible dogs by leash laws, dog movement control, and quarantine; 3) mass immunization of dogs by campaigns and by continuing vaccination of young dogs; 4) stray dog control and euthanasia of unvaccinated dogs with low levels of dependency on, or restriction by, humans; and 5) dog registration.

The Compendium of Animal Rabies Control, compiled and updated annually by the National Association of State Public Health Veterinarians (NASPHV), summarizes the most current recommendations for the USA and lists all USDA-licensed rabies vaccines that are marketed in the USA. Many effective vaccines, such as modified-live virus, recombinant, and inactivated types, are available for use throughout the world; in the USA, no modified-live rabies virus vaccines are currently marketed (for any species). Recommended vaccination frequency is every 3 yr, after an initial series of 2 vaccines 1 yr apart. Several vaccines are also available for use in cats, and a few for use in ferrets, horses, cattle, and sheep. Because of the increasing importance of rabies in cats, vaccination of cats is extremely important. No vaccine is approved for use in wildlife kept as pets (including wolf hybrids), and protective immunity from the commercially available vaccines for domestic species has not been demonstrated in these species.

Until recently, the control of rabies in wildlife populations relied on the destruction of wildlife in an attempt to reduce the contact rate between susceptible animals; however, this proved difficult and often not publicly acceptable or effective. In Europe and Canada, use of oral vaccines distributed in baits to control fox rabies is widespread and effective. The disease in foxes has been eliminated from most of western Europe and curtailed significantly in Ontario. Use of a vaccinia-rabies glycoprotein recombinant virus vaccine in the USA has successfully controlled coyote rabies in southern Texas and appears to be limiting the western expansion of raccoon rabies from the eastern USA. The USDA license limits use of the vaccine to state or federal rabies programs; it is not available to private veterinarians or for individual animal use. It is also being used to assist in the control of dog rabies in developing countries.

Management of Suspected Rabies Cases—Exposure of Pets: Where terrestrial wildlife or bat rabies is known to occur, any animal bitten or otherwise exposed by a wild, carnivorous mammal (or a bat) not available for testing should be regarded as having been exposed to rabies. The NASPHV recommends that any unvaccinated dog, cat, or ferret exposed to rabies be euthanized immediately. If the owner is unwilling to do this, the animal should be placed in strict isolation (ie, no human or animal contact) for 6 mo and vaccinated against rabies 1 mo before release. If an exposed animal is currently vaccinated, it should be revaccinated immediately and closely observed for 45 days.

Zoonotic Risk: When a person is exposed to an animal suspected of having rabies, the risk of rabies transmission should be evaluated carefully. Risk assessment should include consideration of the species of animal involved, the prevalence of rabies in the area, whether exposure sufficient to transmit rabies occurred, and the current status of the animal and its availability for diagnostic testing. Wild carnivores and bats present a considerable risk where the disease is found, regardless of whether abnormal behavior has been observed. Insectivorous bats, though small, can inflict a wound with their teeth and should never be caught or handled with bare hands. Because bat bites often go unnoticed, direct contact with bats could be considered a risk for exposure. Any wild carnivore or bat suspected of exposing a person to rabies should be considered rabid unless proved otherwise by laboratory testing; this includes bats found in rooms with sleeping or otherwise unaware persons. Although some people make "pets" of wildlife, if one of those animals exposes a human or domestic animal, the wild animal should be managed like free-ranging wildlife. Any healthy domestic dog, cat, or ferret, whether vaccinated against rabies or not, that exposes (bites or deposits saliva in a fresh wound or on a mucous membrane) a person should be confined for 10 days; if the animal develops any signs of rabies during that period, it should be euthanized and its brain promptly submitted for rabies diagnosis. If the dog, cat, or ferret responsible for the exposure is stray or unwanted, it may be euthanized as soon as possible and submitted for rabies diagnosis. Since the advent of testing by immunofluorescence microscopy, there is no value in holding such animals to "let the disease progress" as an aid to diagnosis.

Pre-exposure immunization is strongly recommended for all people in high-risk groups, such as veterinary staff, animal control officers, rabies and diagnostic laboratory workers, and travelers working in countries in which canine rabies is endemic or epizootic. Vaccine is administered on days 0, 7, and 21 or 28. However, pre-exposure prophylaxis cannot be absolutely relied on in the event of subsequent rabies exposure and must be supplemented by a limited postexposure regimen (2 doses of vaccine IM on days 0 and 3).

SCRAPIE

(Tremblante du mouton, Rida)

Scrapie is a fatal neurologic disease that produces subacute spongiform encephalopathy in adult sheep. Similar diseases are found naturally in goats and with an increasing incidence in indigenous populations of deer and elk in North America (*see* CHRONIC WASTING DISEASE, p 993). Feedstuff derived from sheep meat and bonemeal that had been inadequately treated during manufacture was formerly thought to be the source of bovine spongiform encephalopathy (BSE, p 991) and the newly recognized transmissible spongiform encephalopathies seen in captive wild ruminants, domestic cats, and captive wild Felidae.

Etiology, Transmission, and Pathogenesis: Two possible structures for the causal neuropathogen have been proposed: 1) the prion—a small exogenous particle consisting of prion protein (PrP), which is an abnormal, proteinase-resistant form of a host cellular protein, that can act as a catalyst to convert more of the host's protein to the abnormal form, and 2) the virino—a hybrid particle consisting largely of a small agent-specific core of nontranslated nucleic acid (which exists only to replicate itself) associated with host cellular proteins (which may include PrP). Whatever the nature of the infectious agent, one of its most striking features is its resistance to conventional physical and chemical treatments that destroy bacteria, spores, fungi, and viruses.

In the course of the disease, the cellular form of PrP undergoes a conformational change, resulting in increased β-sheet folding and subsequent appearance of scrapie-associated fibrils (SAF). Amino acid substitutions in 3 regions of the host PrP gene govern disease susceptibility and influence how rapidly the disease progresses.

Scrapie is frequently transmitted in family lines in flocks, which indicates that some form of maternal transmission may occur at a pre- or postnatal stage. The infected placenta may also be eaten by other sheep or contaminate pastures, which may account for horizontal transmission. In some cases, abnormal PrP can be detected in biopsied tonsils in sheep ≤6 mo old. Subsequently, the agent is detectable at increasing titers in lymphoreticular tissues and after ~2 yr in the CNS, where lesions develop; clinical signs follow typically at $3\frac{1}{2}$ yr.

Clinical Findings: The onset is insidious. Behavioral changes may include increased excitability, nervousness, or aggressiveness, particularly elicited by sudden noise or movement. Fine tremors of the head and neck (tremblante du mouton) and occasional convulsions may be seen. Lack of limb coordination with a tendency to move at a trot or hop like a rabbit is characteristic.

Water metabolism is altered; affected sheep drink small quantities frequently, and urination may be abnormal with voiding of small quantities of urine. Intense pruritus, which often begins over the rump and can also include the head, is common although it is not seen in all cases. The fleece is dry, separable, and brittle, resulting in loss of fleece over large areas. Other areas may be rubbed raw. In some cases, the pruritus makes it difficult for the animal to feed and rest normally, which is a major factor in emaciation and weakness. In less well-defined cases, pressure to the base of the tail can often elicit a nibbling response. Different breeds of sheep may not show the full range of clinical signs, and sheep may die without clinical signs.

Lesions: Pathologic lesions are restricted to microscopic changes in the CNS. Single or multiple vacuoles surrounded by a zone of cytoplasmic degeneration may be present in neurons of the medulla, pons, midbrain, and spinal cord. Spongiform changes may also affect the surrounding neuropil. In scrapie-affected brains, abnormal PrP accumulates in various patterns, including deposits in the cytoplasm and cell membrane of neurons and astrocytes in the medulla oblongata and pons, with amyloid staining in the walls of blood vessels and perivascularly in the thalamus of many infected sheep. The medulla at the level of obex is the earliest site of accumulation, and deposits in the dorsal motor nucleus of the vagus suggest that the agent gains access to the brain from the peripheral innervation of the GI tract.

Diagnosis: This is based on clinical signs and microscopic examination of the CNS. Further confirmation is provided by immunoblotting to detect abnormal PrP or by electron microscopy to detect abnormal SAF. Subclinical disease can also be detected from biopsied tonsils, which can be positive for abnormal PrP in sheep <1 yr old incubating the disease.

Epidemiology and Control: The prevalence of scrapie in sheep is unknown. However, the incidence is probably moderate in Great Britain and lower in most other countries in Europe and North America.

There is no treatment, although the disease was eradicated from Australia and New Zealand by compulsory slaughter of imported sheep and flockmates shortly after release from quarantine. After the disease first appeared in the USA (in 1947), the Scrapie Eradication Program was established. This involved identification of affected animals and destruction of all sheep in the flock as well as other exposed flocks. This procedure was modified in 1983 to destroy mainly bloodline animals because of the strong familial occurrence of the disease. The current program in the USA is based on active, passive, and slaughter surveillance with removal of genetically susceptible sheep from flocks in which scrapie is detected. An eradication scheme has begun in the UK based on PrP gene susceptibility. It aims to replace scrapie-susceptible PrP alleles with more resistant ones, thereby controlling and eventually eliminating the disease from the national flock.

Goats can be infected by contact with scrapie-infected sheep, either directly or by exposure to contaminated pastures.

SPORADIC BOVINE ENCEPHALOMYELITIS
(Chlamydial encephalomyelitis)

Outbreaks of sporadic bovine encephalomyelitis (SBE) have occurred in various parts of the world. Reports indicate that chlamydiae can also cause infections of the brain in humans, opossums, dogs, and several avian species.

Etiology and Epidemiology: SBE is caused by the species *Chlamydophila pecorum.* Subclinical intestinal infections in cattle and other animals are probably much more common than reported and may well be the source of infection in SBE. It is not understood why, in sporadic cases, chlamydiae leave a balanced host-parasite relationship in the intestine, penetrate the intestinal barrier, establish a blood-infectious phase, and infect the brain as the target organ.

The disease is most often seen in cattle 3 mo to 3 yr old. Morbidity rates are usually low but can reach 50%; many sick calves die if not treated at an early stage.

Clinical Findings: The incubation period in experimentally infected calves is 6-30 days. The first sign in natural and experimental cases is fever (104-107°F). The temperature remains increased until shortly before death or recovery. Appetite remains good for the first 2-3 days despite the fever. Afterward, depression, excess salivation, diarrhea, anorexia, and weight loss occur. Calves are incoordinated and stagger or fall over objects. Head pressing and blindness are not seen. In the terminal stage, calves are frequently recumbent and may develop opisthotonos. The course of the disease is usually 10-14 days.

Lesions: Lesions are not limited to the brain; vascular damage can be seen in many different organs. Serofibrinous peritonitis, pleuritis, and pericarditis are common and are especially pronounced in more chronic cases. Microscopic lesions in the brain consist of perivascular cuffs and inflammatory foci in the parenchyma composed primarily of mononuclear cells.

Diagnosis: A tentative diagnosis can be based on clinical signs and particularly on the presence of a serofibrinous peritonitis in the absence of other causes of peritonitis such as intestinal volvulus, intussusception, traumatic perforation of the reticulum, perforated abomasal ulcer, or displaced organs. Differential diagnoses also include rabies, infectious bovine rhinotracheitis with encephalitis, listeriosis, thromboembolic encephalomyelitis, polioencephalomalacia, pseudorabies, and malignant catarrhal fever. A diagnosis of SBE is confirmed by isolation of the organism from brain tissue in either developing chicken embryos or cell cultures, by histologic changes in brain sections, by evaluation of tissue impression smears after Giemsa or immunofluorescent staining, or by demonstration of *Chlamydophila* DNA via PCR testing.

Treatment: The antibiotics of choice are tetracyclines, oxytetracyclines, and tylosin. For treatment to be effective, it must be given as early as possible in high doses (eg, oxytetracyclines at 20-50 mg/kg/day) and for ≥1 wk. If treatment is effective, the fever should drop significantly within 24 hr. Vaccines are not available.

TICK PARALYSIS

Tick paralysis is an acute, progressive, ascending motor paralysis caused by a salivary neurotoxin produced by certain species of ticks. Humans (especially children), a wide variety of other mammals, and birds may be affected. Human cases of tick paralysis caused by the genera *Ixodes, Dermacentor,* and *Amblyomma* have been reported from

Australia, North America, Europe, and South Africa; these 3 plus *Rhipicephalus*, *Haemaphysalis*, *Otobius*, and *Argas* have been associated with paralysis in animals.

Etiology, Epidemiology, and Pathogenesis: The potential for inducing paralysis has been demonstrated, described, or suspected in 64 species of ticks belonging to 7 ixodid and 3 argasid genera. On the eastern coast of Australia, the Australia paralysis tick *I holocyclus* (and to a lesser extent *I cornuatus* and *I hirstii*) causes the most severe form of tick paralysis. In North America, *D andersoni* (the Rocky Mountain wood tick) and *D variabilis* (the American dog tick) are the most common causes, but *D albipictus*, *I scapularis*, *Amblyomma americanum*, *A maculatum*, *R sanguineus*, and *O megnini* may cause paralysis. In fowls, *Argas radiatus* and *A persicus* have caused paralysis. In Africa, *I rubicundus* (Karoo tick paralysis) and *R punctatus* in South Africa, *R evertsi evertsi* and *Argas walkerae* in subSaharan Africa, and *R evertsi mimeticus* in Namibia can cause the disease. In North America, *D andersoni* and *D variabilis* affect dogs most commonly, but sheep, cattle, and humans have also been paralyzed. Cats appear to be resistant to the disease caused by these ticks. Clinical signs of ascending flaccid paralysis are seen 5-9 days after tick attachment, and progress from hindlimb weakness to quadriplegia over the next 24-72 hr. If ticks are not removed, death may occur from respiratory paralysis in 1-5 days. Removal of all ticks usually results in improvement within 24 hr and complete recovery within 72 hr.

I holocyclus in Australia cause a more severe disease than that seen in North America. Dogs and cats are affected, as well as sheep, calves, foals, pigs, flying foxes, poultry, and humans. The natural hosts (marsupials) are rarely affected, presumably acquiring immunity at an early age. Clinical signs in dogs and cats appear usually 5-7 days (occasionally up to 14 days or more) after attachment, and progress rapidly over the following 24-48 hr. Removal of ticks does not immediately halt progression of the disease once clinical signs are apparent. Death from respiratory failure is likely within 1-2 days of onset of signs. Appropriate and timely treatment saves ~95% of affected animals.

Host factors influencing epidemiology include sensitivity to toxin, age, immunity, behavior, reactivity, and population density. Antitoxic immunity, starting at least 2 wk after primary tick exposure and lasting a few weeks, can be boosted by further infestations. Tick factors include the dynamics and virulence of paralysis-inducing capability, sexual activity, rate of infestation, and the sucking phase. The maximal incidence of tick paralysis is associated with seasonal activity of female ticks, mainly in spring and early summer, but in some areas tick activity continues throughout the year. Environmental factors such as temperature and humidity also play a role. Modern rapid transport of ticks attached to people, animals, plant material, etc can give rise to isolated cases of tick paralysis far removed from the particular geographic area where the ticks are naturally found.

Toxicity follows secretion of toxin in tick saliva and its injection into the host animal. Usually this is caused by the adult female ixodid tick during its period of rapid engorgement (days 5-7), although large numbers of larval or nymphal ticks may also cause paralysis. Tick paralysis affects mainly motor pathways. There appears to be some effect on autonomic and possibly on sensory pathways. The neurotoxin interferes with acetylcholine release at the neuromuscular junction, producing a neuromuscular blockade. This manifests primarily as an ascending flaccid paralysis varying from paraparesis (hindleg weakness) to quadriplegia.

I holocyclus causes reversible myocardial depression and diastolic failure, leading to cardiogenic pulmonary edema. In severe cases, increased PCV reflects a fluid shift from the circulation to the lungs. Progressive pulmonary dysfunction appears to be primarily due to edema, leading to hypoxia, hypercarbia, respiratory acidosis, and eventually death. Other factors contributing to pulmonary failure include bronchoconstriction (especially in cats), paralysis and fatigue of respiratory muscles, and aspiration of esophageal or gastric contents.

Paralysis of esophageal muscles develops in most dogs, with or without esophageal dilatation (megaesophagus). Saliva and ingested food or fluid pool in the esophagus, and are regurgitated into the pharynx and mouth. Loss of the gag reflex makes it difficult for the animal to clear this material from the airway, which may result in aspiration pneumonia. Vomiting may occur in *I holocyclus* paralysis, but is not common. A central action of toxin on the vomiting center has been suggested. Most cases of "vomiting" reported by clients are probably regurgitation, although drug-induced vomition may be a complication.

Clinical Findings: Early signs may include change or loss of voice (due to laryngeal paresis), hindlimb incoordination, change in breathing rate and effort, gagging or coughing, regurgitation or vomiting, and pupillary dilation. Hindlimb paralysis begins as slight to pronounced incoordination and weakness. As paralysis ascends, the animal becomes unable to move hindlimbs and forelimbs, stand, sit, or lift its head. Sensation usually is preserved. Breathing abnormality is of greater prognostic importance than limb paralysis. Respiratory rate may initially increase but, as the disease progresses, becomes slower and obviously labored, especially on expiration. Regurgitation of esophageal contents, saliva pooling, depression of the gag reflex, and attempts to clear the throat may produce a characteristic harsh, groaning respiratory sound. Temperature is normal in the early stages. Paralyzed animals with low body mass (especially cats) may become hypothermic. Conversely, animals kept at high ambient temperatures may need to cool themselves by panting, adding to respiratory difficulty.

Blood and fluid values are unchanged in the early stages. Increased PCV indicates a fluid shift into the lungs and a poor prognosis. Other changes may include increased blood glucose, cholesterol, phosphate, and CK, and a decrease in blood potassium. In electrophysiologic studies, motor nerve conduction velocities, nerve compound action potentials, and compound potentials from the corresponding muscles are all decreased. The electroencephalogram is normal.

Diagnosis: The presence of a tick in conjunction with the sudden (12-24 hr) appearance of leg weakness and/or respiratory impairment is diagnostic. The offending tick may no longer be attached, but a tick "crater" (a small hole surrounded by a slightly raised and inflamed area) in the skin confirms the diagnosis. In Australia these animals require treatment. Sometimes neither tick nor crater can be found, but with the appropriate clinical signs in a known tick area, treatment is indicated. Recovery following treatment confirms the provisional diagnosis. Specific laboratory diagnostic techniques are not available. Procedures that may be helpful include a PCV and a lateral thoracic radiograph to assess presence and degree of pulmonary edema, megaesophagus, and any pneumonia due to aspiration.

Botulism, polyradiculoneuritis, acute peripheral neuropathies, and snakebite are differential diagnoses. In regions where ticks are endemic, tick paralysis is usually high on the list of differential diagnoses for any flaccid ascending motor paralysis. It should also be considered in the differential diagnosis of megaesophagus, unexplained vomiting, acute left-sided congestive heart failure (dogs), or asthma (cats).

Treatment: Removal of the tick(s) is necessary. Frequently, multiple ticks are attached to an animal. The entire integument should be searched diligently and repeatedly, especially on long-haired animals. Most ticks are found around the head or neck, but can be anywhere on the body. Some practitioners prefer to kill the tick before removal, using a suitable acaricide.

In North America, removal of all ticks usually results in obvious improvement within 24 hr. Failure to recover indicates that at least one tick may be still be attached, or that the diagnosis should be reviewed.

In Australia, the disease commonly continues to progress after removal of ticks, and treatment is indicated for animals with motor or respiratory impairment. In cases in which an adult female *I holocyclus* has been removed but the animal shows no adverse clinical signs, the owner should monitor the animal for 24 hr and return for treatment if signs of tick paralysis develop.

Canine tick hyperimmune serum, also called tick antiserum (TAS), is the specific treatment for *I holocyclus*-induced tick paralysis. This should be given as early in the disease as possible; subsequent "top up" doses are not very effective. For dogs, a minimal dosage of 0.5-1.0 mL/kg, warmed to room temperature, is given slowly IV. Animals with multiple ticks or in the acute stages of paralysis should receive a higher dose. Some debate exists about the required dose of TAS. It has been suggested that a standard dose should be given, based on the amount needed to neutralize the toxin from one tick, not on the weight of the dog. On this basis, a minimal dose of 10 mL is recommended for dogs, but increased for multiple ticks or severely affected animals. Atropine (0.1-0.2 mg/kg, SC) is recommended before giving TAS; this reduces the incidence of an adverse effect that is seen in some small dogs soon after the injection is given—a temporary collapse with profound hypotension and bradycardia lasting several minutes, associated with the Bezold-Jarisch reflex.

TAS is given to cats at 1.0 mL/kg; 5 mL is the usual minimal dose. Giving canine serum IV to a cat involves a risk of anaphylaxis. This risk is minimized by routine SC injection of 3 mL of 1:10,000 epinephrine 3-4 min before administration of the TAS.

Minimization of stress and anxiety cannot be overemphasized. Acepromazine may be given SC before any other medication or handling that may upset the animal. However, acepromazine should be avoided or given at a reduced dose if the animal is depressed or hypothermic. Opiates are an alternative. Any procedure (eg, IV injection, searching for ticks) that may excite the animal should be postponed until the animal settles.

The animal's condition can be expected to deteriorate for the next 24 hr after ticks are removed. Hospitalization, with monitoring and good nursing care, is advised during this period. The animal should be kept in a quiet, dark, comfortable place. Sternal recumbency should be maintained if comfortable; otherwise, the animal should be positioned in lateral recumbency with its shoulder being the highest point. Eye protectants should be used to prevent corneal ulceration or dry eyes, and the bladder expressed once or twice daily. Suction of the pharynx, larynx, and proximal esophagus minimizes respiratory distress caused by saliva pooling and esophageal dysfunction. An esophageal tube may be inserted to provide drainage. General anesthesia may be indicated in animals that are severely dyspneic to allow administration of oxygen, esophageal suction, and pulmonary drainage. Mechanical or manual ventilation may be required for ≥24 hr.

Nothing should be given PO until paralysis has resolved. IV fluid support is not routinely needed during the first 48 hr of hospitalization. IV fluids may add to pulmonary edema, so they should be used slowly and minimally. If the PCV is >50%, colloid or heta/penta starch fluids should be considered rather than crystalloids. Furosemide can be given IV to help reduce pulmonary edema.

During hospitalization, regular searches for attached ticks should be done. Long or matted hair should be clipped. Application of an acaricide may kill ticks missed in searching. However, the stress of clipping or bathing can be detrimental in severely affected or nervous animals and may increase hypothermia.

About 5% of animals are likely to die despite all treatment efforts, especially those with advanced paralysis and dyspnea. Older animals or those with pre-existing cardiopulmonary disease are at greatest risk.

For animals that recover, owners should be advised to continue searching for ticks, use appropriate preventive methods to avoid reattachment of ticks, and avoid stressing or strenuously exercising the animal over the next 2 mo.

Control: Owners should not rely wholly on chemical control to prevent tick infestation. They should be advised about when and where their pets will be at risk; encouraged to search the coat daily; keep the coat short if possible; and understand the appropriateness, safety, and limitations of available preventive products. Products recommended for tick control in dogs include fipronil (as a topical spray or spot-on), permethrin (spray or rinse), cythioate (given orally), and amitraz (in an impregnated collar). All have limitations but are useful if used correctly. Fipronil is one of the few products approved for use in cats in several countries, including Australia (spray only) and the USA, for tick control.

Attempts to produce an effective vaccine against the *I holocyclus* toxin have so far been unsuccessful.

WEST NILE ENCEPHALOMYELITIS

See also WEST NILE VIRUS INFECTION IN POULTRY, p 2289.

West Nile virus (WNV) is a member of the Japanese encephalitis virus serocomplex in the genus Flavivirus. WNV was first identified in the blood of a woman in Uganda in 1937. By the 1950s, WNV was recognized as a virus that cycled between birds and ornithophilic mosquitos. WNV has the widest geographic distribution of all of the Flaviviruses. Prior to 1999, WNV was recognized in Africa, the Middle East, Asia, and occasionally in European countries. In 1999, WNV infection was first recognized in North America. Since then, the virus has spread throughout the USA and parts of Canada and Mexico. WNV isolated from the outbreak in New York in 1999 appears to be closely related to an isolate recovered from geese in Israel in 1998.

Etiology and Epidemiology: WNV is maintained in an enzootic transmission cycle between wild birds and *Culex* mosquitos. WNV has been recovered from a wide range of North American mosquito species, with *Culex* spp thought to play the largest role in natural transmission. In the eastern and midwestern regions of the USA, *C pipiens* is one of the major vectors, while in the panhandle region and western regions of the USA, *C tarsalis* is thought to be one of the major vectors. WNV activity is based on the presence of competent vectors as well as bird hosts. Both wetland and terrestrial birds may be involved in the natural cycle of WNV. Migratory birds are thought to introduce the virus into a geographic region. A wide range of birds can be infected with WNV; many have high and sustained viremia but show little or no clinical disease. However, during the outbreak of WNV in the USA, fatal infections were common among corvids (eg, crows, blue jays, and magpies). The house finch may be one of the most efficient reservoirs of the virus due to the large numbers of this type of bird in the USA, the high viremia that these birds develop, and the fact that these birds have little or no disease associated with the infection. Ticks have been demonstrated to be infected with WNV, but their role in the natural transmission of WNV is unknown. Recently, other routes of exposure to WNV have been documented, including transplacental infection of one human infant. Experimentally, transmission has been documented between cohabitating birds and from oral exposure to WNV in drinking water in birds. Cats have become infected with WNV from consumption of infected mice.

Since the introduction of WNV into the USA, WNV antibodies have been detected in >150 species of birds, a large array of mammals, and in a few amphibians and reptiles. However, disease has been primarily observed in humans, equids, and corvids. Since 1999, illness due to WNV infection has been seen in a limited number of dogs, a cat, camelids, and a few sheep. Oral transmission is highly efficient in cats; therefore infected prey animals may serve as an important source of infection to carnivores. There have been clusters of WNV-induced illness and death in wild squirrels and farmed alligators. There has also been a report of WNV-induced disease in crocodiles. Whether or not this increased range of species susceptible to WNV-induced disease is due to increased scrutiny and monitoring, the level of viral challenge in the USA, or some other reason is unknown.

Encephalomyelitis due to WNV infection in horses has been called Near Eastern equine encephalitis or lordige in France. The frequency of inapparent infection in association with clinical disease is difficult to determine. Experimental induction of the disease in horses has been difficult; experimental challenges have not induced the severity of disease noted under field conditions with any of the models other than viral injection into the CSF. In the USA, ~10-39% of infected horses develop clinical disease. Once horses show clinical signs of WNV, the case fatality rate is ~30% in the USA. Recent outbreaks of WNV in horses in Italy and Morocco had case fatality rates of 43% and 45%, respectively. Outcome of disease could be based on multiple factors, such as host susceptibility, amount of the viral challenge, virulence of the virus, and treatment.

The spread of WNV across the USA since its introduction in 1999 has been remarkable. In 1999, there were 25 equine cases in a limited area around New York city. By 2002, there were >15,000 equine cases from 41 states. In late 2002, WNV was reclassified as an endemic disease agent in the USA. The number of equine WNV cases declined in 2003 for the first time since the virus was recognized in the USA. This decline could be due to several factors, including an increasing percentage of the equine population protected from disease due to vaccination or natural exposure to the virus, increased mosquito control efforts, lower viral challenge due to increasing immunity among bird populations, less frequent testing of suspect cases due to better recognition of the disease syndrome, and increased cost of testing for the disease. The virus appears to have found a niche wherever it has been introduced. It has been postulated that WNV has spread to new geographic regions through the migration of birds carrying the virus. The virus can be spread by multiple types of mosquitos, based on experimental studies. Horses and humans do not appear to develop adequate viral loads to act as a source of the virus for mosquitos. Cats appear to develop the highest viremia among domestic animals, but compared with birds the level of viremia in cats is relatively low. Thus, cats and dogs are unlikely to play an epidemiologic role as amplifying hosts.

Animals used as plasma or whole blood donors should be protected from WNV infection. Although horses do not develop adequate viremia to be a source of WNV for insect vectors, if several liters of infected blood or plasma were to be transfused into another horse, it could theoretically pose a risk to the recipient horse. No transfusion-induced WNV infection has been reported in horses, but it is recognized as a risk in human medicine.

Clinical Findings: All equids appear equally susceptible to WNV encephalomyelitis (WNE), with biases in breed reflecting regional or hospital variations. Horses of all ages (range 4 mo to >30 yr) can be affected. Adult horses (12-14 yr) represent the mean age of most field populations of affected horses; however, in 2 referral hospital studies, 6-7 yr was the mean age.

The clinical signs and course of disease are highly variable in WNE. There are 2 lineage groups into which isolates of WNV can be placed, based on genetic sequencing. Horses are susceptible to lineage type I WNV, while demonstrating little disease to most African lineage type II WNV. Presenting complaints most often include neurologic abnormalities; other common initial complaints include colic, lameness, anorexia, and fever. Initial systemic signs include a mild low-grade fever, feed refusal, and depression. Neurologic signs are also highly variable, but spinal cord disease and moderate mental aberrations are most consistent. Spinal cord disease manifests as asymmetric, multifocal or diffuse ataxia and paresis. Severe manifestations may occur independently in the front or hindlimbs, unilaterally, or in a single limb. In all clinical studies published to date, >90% of affected horses developed some type of spinal cord signs, while 60% developed behavioral changes characterized by periods of hyperesthesia, ranging from mild apprehension to overt hyperexcitability with fractious reactions to aural, visual, and tactile stimuli. Some horses have periods of cataplexy or narcolepsy that may render them temporarily or permanently recumbent. Coma, blindness, head pressing, and other signs of forebrain disease are seen, but are not as common as in alphavirus encephalitides. Fine and coarse tremors of the face and neck muscles are common and are described in 60-90% of horses. Cranial nerve deficits also are seen in 40-60% of clinically affected horses; these include most cranial nerves with cell bodies located in the mid- and hindbrains. Weakness and/or paralysis of the face and tongue are most frequent. Horses with facial and tongue paresis can be dysphagic, and overt signs of quidding or even esophageal choke can develop. Many horses with severe mental depression and facial paresis will keep their heads low, resulting in severe facial edema. Occasionally, head tilt may be seen. Infrequently, urinary dysfunction ranging from mild straining to stranguria has been reported. After initial signs abate, severity of clinical signs increases within the first 7-10 days of onset in about one-third of cases. This resumption of clinical signs ranges from temporary and mild to progressive full paralysis.

The case fatality rate is generally 30-40%. In horses that progress to complete paralysis of one or more limbs, mortality rates are ~60-80%. Most of these horses are euthanized due to humane reasons, but spontaneous death does occur. Overt clinical signs in horses that recover can last from 1 day to several weeks, with improvement usually occurring within 7 days of the onset of clinical signs. While 80-90% of owners report that the horse returns to normal function 1-6 mo after disease, at least 10% of owners report longterm deficits that limit athletic potential and resale value. Deficits include residual weakness or ataxia in one or more limbs, fatigue with exercise, focal or generalized muscle atrophy, and changes in personality and behavioral aberrations.

Many horses are euthanized due to sequelae. During the neurologic phase, horses frequently thrash and injure themselves. Sepsis from trauma in recumbent horses also occurs. Prolonged recumbency leads to pulmonary infections, especially in foals, in which a long duration of slinging and treatment may be pursued more frequently than in large, recumbent animals. Dysphagia leads to decreased water intake, and renal damage due to concurrent NSAID use can occur. Skin and muscle necrosis are common in recumbent horses. Life-threatening trauma can also occur, including ruptured diaphragm, broken limbs, broken cervical vertebra, and skull fractures.

No consistent changes in clinical pathology have been found in WNE in horses, although peripheral lymphopenia is common. Hyponatremia is seen and is thought to be due to inappropriate antidiuretic hormone secretion. Horses are also frequently azotemic. While some reports demonstrate little value of CSF analysis, reports in larger groups of horses show abnormalities (primarily mononuclear pleocytosis and increased total protein) in up to 70% of horses tested. Lumbosacral samples have significantly higher proteins and cell counts.

Lesions: Gross lesions in WNE are rare and are limited to small multifocal areas of discoloration and hemorrhage throughout the midbrain, brain stem and spinal cord. There may be congestion in the meninges of acutely affected animals. Microscopically, there is a non-necrotizing lymphohistiocytic poliomeningoencephalitis. Slight to severe inflammation, characterized by perivascular cuffing of lymphocytes and monocytes, is present. In the neuropil, dying neurons often are surrounded by microglial cells. Immunohistochemistry reveals positive staining for WNV in neural cytoplasm.

Diagnosis: Serology is the key test for antemortem diagnosis of WNE in horses. IgM rises sharply and falls during the first 6-8 wk after exposure to WNV. Neutralizing antibody titers (primarily IgG) develop slowly during this time and stay elevated for several months. The IgM capture ELISA is the test of choice for detection of recent exposure to the virus. In most states, a veterinarian must submit the test, and any horse demonstrating clinical signs of encephalomyelitis must be reported to the state regulatory services.

Several postmortem diagnostic assays are available and, while specific, vary in sensitivity. Although WNV may cause severe clinical signs, viral levels in equine neural tissues are low. Immunohistochemistry provides confirmatory diagnosis; however, multiple sections of brain and spinal cord must be examined. This test is positive in 60-80% of horses that test positive for WNV by serology. Detection of viral nucleic acids also varies in sensitivity and depends on testing portions of the brain and spinal cord where higher titers of virus may be present. Either nested reverse transcriptase (rt)-PCR or real-time rt-PCR on the medulla oblongata and lumbar spinal cord is recommended. Viral culture of the brain is sensitive only in ~20-30% of clinical cases that test positively by serology.

Both infectious and noninfectious causes of brain and spinal cord diseases should be considered as differential diagnoses. Infectious causes include alphaviruses, rabies, equine protozoal myeloencephalitis (EPM), and equine herpesvirus 1; less likely causes are botulism and verminous meningoencephalomyelitis (eg, *Halicephalobus gingivalis*, *Setaria*, *Strongylus vulgarus*). Noninfectious causes include hypocalcemia, tremorigenic toxicities, hepatoencephalopathy, and leukoencephalomalacia.

Treatment: Treatment of WNE is supportive, as there is no specific antiviral therapy against flaviviruses. As with any of the viral encephalitides, management is focused on controlling pain and inflammation, preventing injuries associated with ataxia or recumbency, and providing supportive care. The treatment of horses with clinical signs has primarily focused on anti-inflammatory drug administration. Flunixin meglumine (1.1 mg/kg, IV, BID) early in the course of the disease decreases the severity of muscle tremors and fasciculations within a few hours of administration. Steroids and NSAID have been given to many horses with WNV-induced disease. Some horses show immediate improvement with anti-inflammatory treatment (eg, a reduction in muscle fasciculations and a return to a more normal attitude), while others do not show any improvement. Recumbent horses are mentally alert and frequently thrash, causing self-inflicted wounds and posing a risk to personnel. Therapy of recumbent horses is generally more aggressive and includes dexamethasone (0.05-0.1 mg/kg, IV, SID) and mannitol (0.25-2.0 g/kg, IV). In a study of equine WNV cases in Colorado and Nebraska from 2002, the majority received some form of anti-inflammatory drug. Flunixin meglumine was the most common treatment, with ~50% receiving steroids and/or dimethyl sulfoxide. Steroid use was not found to be associated with the survival rate. Detomidine (0.02-0.04 mg/kg, IV or IM) is effective for prolonged tranquilization. Low dosages of acepromazine (0.02 mg/kg, IV, or 0.05 mg/kg, IM) provide excellent relief from anxiety in both recumbent and standing horses. Diazepam and butorphanol appear to increase anxiety and tremors and should be avoided. Phenobarbital to effect is appropriate for seizures. A sling and hoist may be used to assist horses that are recumbent and have difficulty rising. Some horses may require fluid and nutritional support. Treatment with antioxidants, such as vitamin E, may also be indicated.

Until EPM is ruled out, prophylactic antiprotozoal medications may be instituted. Other supportive measures (eg, oral and parental fluids and nutrition for dehydrated and dysphagic horses) are also important parts of therapy. Broad-spectrum antibiotics should be given for treatment of wounds, cellulitis, and pneumonia. Slinging of recumbent horses is essential to assess the degree of recumbency. Horses with intermittent or focal neuropathies have a better prognosis than those with complete flaccid paralysis. Slinging also maintains strength and decreases pulmonary and traumatic sequelae. Efficacy of specific antiviral agents for the treatment of naturally occurring WNV infection is unknown, even in humans. Interferon α-2b has been used in the treatment of WNV infection in horses, but the efficacy is unknown.

Equine serum and plasma antibody-containing products are available for treatment. Theoretically, these products may inactivate circulating WNV in horses showing signs of the disease and may protect horses exposed to the virus. One serum product was licensed by USDA in 2003 and another has a conditional license. Results of challenge studies or case-control field studies evaluating these products are not currently available.

Prevention and Control: Options for prevention of WNV in equids include immunization, vector abatement, and optimization of overall health. Vaccines against alphaviruses that cause EEE, WEE, or Venezuelan equine encephalitis offer no cross-protection against WNV infection. A killed, adjuvanted, whole WNV vaccine was given limited approval in 2001 and was used in regions with WNV activity. The vaccine received full licensure in 2003 and has been used extensively to help prevent WNV infection in equids in the USA. The vaccine is approved for use in the prevention of viremia from WNV. A series of 2 vaccinations given 3-6 wk apart, prior to the period when vectors are active, is recommended in adult horses. In foals, an initial series of 3 immunizations is required and should follow a schedule of vaccination similar to that for EEE and WEE. Foals born to immunized mares or those that have had WNV infection should not be vaccinated until they are 6 mo of age. It appears that ~10% of properly immunized horses do not produce neutralizing antibodies to WNV and that 2.3-3% of equine WNV cases are seen in fully vaccinated horses. The duration of immunity from vaccination with the killed, adjuvanted WNV vaccine is unknown. It has been recommended that a booster be given every 3-4 mo in regions where the virus is active >3-4 mo/yr. A recombinant canarypox vaccine carrying protective prM/E genes of WNV was also licensed in 2003, but has not yet been scrutinized under field conditions. In initial experimental trials, all of the immunized horses (28) developed a detectable neutralizing antibody response. In a second study that involved a WNV-infected mosquito challenge of vaccinated and control horses, neither developed clinical signs of disease. All of the vaccinated horses were protected from viremia 2 wk after the primary vaccination and 1 vaccinated horse developed viremia when challenged 1 yr after the initial series, while 80% of the control horses developed a detectable viremia.

Protection of horses from WNV infection must also include efforts to minimize exposure to WNV-infected mosquitos. Briefly, mosquito mitigation includes applying an insect repellent that contains pyrethrin on the horse at least daily during vector season, especially at times of day when mosquitos may be most active. Fans that blow over horses housed in stalls can reduce mosquito feeding. Environmental management is also essential and includes keeping the barn area, paddocks, and pastures cleared of weeds and organic material, such as feces, that might harbor adult mosquitos. Cleaning water tanks and buckets at least weekly will reduce mosquito breeding areas. Removal of other containers such as flower pots and used tires that may hold stagnant water is essential for reducing the number of mosquitos in the area.

Options for control of WNV infection in other animals emphasize reducing exposure. In dogs and cats, keeping them indoors or in a screened area, especially during the time when mosquitos are most active, reduces exposure. Disposal of dead birds or other small prey that might be eaten may reduce the chances of oral exposure. Because very few cases of WNV have been documented in dogs and cats, inconveniences associated with these prevention strategies should be weighed against the risk of WNV infection. The killed adjuvanted vaccine marketed for use in horses has been used in camelids without any reports of major adverse effects. Studies of the immunologic response in horses and camelids immunized with this vaccine are ongoing.

Zoonotic Risk: Asymptomatic infection is the most common outcome of human exposure to WNV by a bite from an infected mosquito. The severe form of disease caused by infection occurs in ~1/150 persons exposed to the virus and is most common in the elderly. West Nile fever, a syndrome characterized by fever, headache, and malaise, is seen in ~20% of people infected with WNV.

Veterinarians should take biosecurity precautions when performing necropsies, especially on birds. Live birds infected with WNV may also pose a handling risk due to the very high viral load in cloacal fluid in some species. Appropriate barrier precautions are indicated.

■ ■ ■

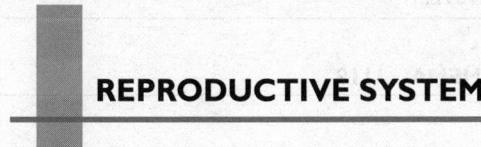

REPRODUCTIVE SYSTEM

REPRODUCTIVE SYSTEM
INTRODUCTION

All functions of the reproductive system must be considered when resolving reproductive problems. The differences in the reproductive system between the sexes and among species are complex. In both sexes, there are primary sex organs and primary regulatory centers. Gonads and function-adapted, tubular, genital organs constitute primary sex organs in both sexes. The pituitary gland and the hypothalamus are the primary regulatory centers; thus, the regulatory function is, in part, neuroendocrine in nature. In pregnant females, the fetoplacental unit has a significant role in maintaining and terminating pregnancy. The temporal and physiologic features of the reproductive cycle vary greatly among species (TABLE 1, TABLE 2, and TABLE 3).

THE GONADS AND TUBULAR GENITAL TRACT

Both sexes have a pair of gonads (ovaries or testes), the main functions of which are gametogenesis and steroidogenesis. Both functions are regulated primarily by gonadotropins released by the anterior pituitary gland under the influence of the hypothalamus. The latter is mediated by a peptide, gonadotropin-releasing hormone (GnRH); the secretion and release of GnRH are governed by CNS stimuli and, through a feedback mechanism, by hormones produced by other endocrine organs such as the gonads, pituitary, thyroid, and adrenal glands. (*See also* THE ENDOCRINE SYSTEM, p 429 et seq.)

The Ovaries: The size and location of the ovaries vary with the species. The ovaries can be directly examined by rectal palpation only in cows and mares. Once puberty is reached (*see* TABLE 3) and an animal starts cycling, the size and form of the ovaries are altered by cyclic functional structures, namely corpora lutea (CL) and follicles. Follicle-stimulating hormone (FSH) is responsible for development of follicle(s) and synthesis of estrogens by the theca cells. Once a certain estrogen level is attained, luteinizing hormone (LH) is released from the anterior pituitary gland in spontaneously ovulating species. This LH peak triggers ovulation, which is followed by development of a new CL. The increase of luteal cells parallels an increase in progesterone output. In nonpregnant polyestrous and seasonally polyestrous females, the functional and morphologic life of the CL is terminated by endogenous prostaglandin (PG) $F_2\alpha$ from the uterus. As the CL regresses, a new ovulatory follicle(s) develops, which completes the estrous cycle. The hormonal changes during the estrous cycle can be monitored by radioimmunoassay and ELISA of hormones in blood, milk, or other body fluids. Estrual cycling is continuous after puberty unless interrupted by pregnancy and, in some species, by season or lactation during the immediate postpartum period. Cycling is also blocked by pathologic conditions of the ovaries (eg, nutritional and stress atrophy, ovarian cysts) and by uterine disease (eg, pyometra, severe endometritis), which may result in persistent CL. Estrogens and progesterone act locally, affecting target organs such as the tubular genital tract, and distally, regulating gonadotropin release by a feedback mechanism on both the hypothalamus and anterior pituitary. In addition, they are responsible for sex characteristics, behavior, and lactation.

The Testes: The testes function in both spermatogenesis and secretion of steroid hormones. Spermatogenesis is stimulated by FSH and augmented by androgens, primarily testosterone. Leydig cells, under the influence of LH, produce testosterone and, in some species (eg, horses), estrogens. Testosterone is required for development and function of accessory glands, copulatory organs, male sex characteristics, and behavior. For optimal spermatogenesis, mammalian testes must descend into the scrotal cavity; however, steroidogenesis occurs in testes that remain within the abdomen, and the libido of cryptorchid males is usually not impaired. Photoperiod affects both sperm cell formation and steroidogenesis in males of species with a seasonal reproductive pattern. Semen quality, libido, and mating ability are reduced during the seasonally anestrous period of females. Testicular function can be assessed by evaluation of representative semen samples and

TABLE I. Approximate Gestation Periods[*]

Domestic Animals	Days	Wild animals	Days
Cat	63	Bear (black)	210
Cattle[†]		Bison	270
Angus	281	Camel	410
Ayrshire	279	Chimpanzee	236
Brahman	292	Coyote	63
Brown Swiss	290	Deer (Mule and White-tailed)	200
Charolais	289	Elephant	660
Guernsey	283	Elk, Wapiti	255
Hereford	285	Giraffe	425
Holstein	279	Gorilla	270
Jersey	279	Hare	36
Limousin	289	Hippopotamus	240
Shorthorn	282	Leopard	95
Simmental	289	Lion	108
Dog	58-72[‡]	Marmoset	150
Donkey	365	Monkey (Macaque)	180
Goat	150	Moose	240
Horse	330	Muskox	255
Llama	350	Opossum	12
Pig	114	Panther	90
Sheep	150	Porcupine	210
Fur Animals	**Days**	Pronghorn	230
Chinchilla	111	Raccoon	63
Ferret	42	Reindeer	225
Fox	52	Rhinoceros (African)	480
Mink		Seal	330
European	41	Shrew	20
American	40-75	Skunk	63
Muskrat	29	Squirrel (gray)	40
Nutria, Coypu	130	Tapir	390
Otter	270-300[§]	Tiger	103
Rabbit	31	Walrus	450
Wolf	63	Whale (sperm)	450
		Woodchuck	31

[*]*See also* SELECTED PHYSIOLOGIC DATA OF LABORATORY ANIMALS, p 1520.

[†]Individuals may range ±7-10 days from these averages

[‡]Gestation period is 58-72 days from breeding at unknown stage of estrus; from day of ovulation (which can be determined by progesterone or LH monitoring), gestation period is 62-64 days.

[§]180+ days due to delayed implantation

TABLE 2. Approximate Incubation Periods

Domestic Birds	Days	Caged and Game Birds	Days
Chicken	21	Budgerigar	18
Duck	28	Finch	14
Muscovy duck	35	Parrot	26
Goose	28	Pheasant	24
Guinea fowl	28	Pigeon	18
Turkey	28	Quail	16
		Swan	35

TABLE 3. Features of the Reproductive Cycle ▶

Species	Age at Puberty	Cycle Type	Cycle Length	Duration of Estrus
Cattle	4-18 (12) mo, usually first bred ~15 mo	Polyestrous all year	21 days (18-24)	18 hr (10-24)
Sheep	7-12 (9) mo	Seasonally polyestrous, early fall to winter; prolonged seasons in Dorsets and Merinos	16½ days (14-20)	24-48 hr
Goat	4-8 (5) mo	Seasonally polyestrous, early fall to late winter	18-21 days (19)	2-3 days
Pig	4-9 (7) mo	Polyestrous all year	21 days (16-24)	2-3 days
Horse	10-24 (18) mo	Seasonally polyestrous, early spring through summer	Variable, ~21 days (19-26)	6 days (2-10)
Dog	5-24 mo; earlier in smaller breeds, later in larger breeds	Unseasonally monestrous	3½-13 mo	2-21 days (6-12 typical)
Cat	4-12 (10) mo; 12-18 mo in Persians	Induced ovulation, seasonally polyestrous spring and early fall	14-21 days	6-7 days
Fox	10 mo	Monestrous December to March but mostly late January to February		2-4 days
Mink	10 mo	Induced ovulation, seasonally polyestrous mid-February to early April	Waves of follicles at intervals of 7-10 days	2 days

hormone assays. Palpation and measurement of the testicles help predict potential sperm output and may reveal pathologic conditions.

The Female Tubular Genital Tract: Except for the vestibulum, which develops from the urogenital sinus, the female genital tract is derived from the embryonic paramesonephric (müllerian) ducts. Each of the segments is adapted to fulfill its function. Thus, the oviduct, through its motility, acquires the egg(s) and moves the zygote(s) into the uterus, while its secretion provides a proper environment for survival of gametes, fertilization, and the first few critical days of embryonic life. Interference with motility or secretion leads to infertility. Species variation of the bicornual, Y-shaped uterus involves the size of the body and length of horns, which are adapted to accommodate species-specific number and form of fetus(es). The cervix provides a protective barrier that is relatively effective against ascending infections. Morphologic and functional integrity of

◄ **TABLE 3.   Features of the Reproductive Cycle (continued)**

Best Time to Breed	First Estrus After Parturition	Comments
Insemination from midestrus until 6 hr after end of estrus	Varies,* best to breed at 60-90 days	Ovulation 10-12 hr after end of estrus. Uterine bleeding ~24 hr after ovulation in most but may require vaginal examination for detection.
18-20 hr after onset of estrus	Next fall	Ovulation near end of estrus.
Daily during estrus	Next fall	Many intersexes born in hornless strains.
~24 hr after onset of estrus	4-10 days after weaning	Ovulation usually ~40 hr after beginning of estrus.
Last few days of estrus; should be bred at 2-day intervals	4-14 (9) days	Ovulation usually 1-2 days before end of estrus. Double ovulation occurs in ~20% of estrous periods, but twins rarely progress to term.
From day 2 of estrus and on alternate days thereafter until end of estrus	Few months (2- to 3½-mo period of metestrus, followed by a highly variable period of anestrus)	Proestrous bleeding 7-10 days. Ovulation usually 1-3 days after first acceptance. Ova shed before first polar body has been extruded. Pseudopregnancy usually ends between 60 and 70 days.
Daily from day 2 of estrus	4-6 wk	Ovulation 24-48 hr after coitus. Pseudopregnancy lasts 36 days. Infertile matings prolong onset of next cycle ~45 days.
	Next winter	Ovulation usually on first or second day of receptivity. Ova shed before first polar body has been extruded. No proestrous bleeding.
Induced ovulator	Next spring	Ovulation begins 36-48 hr after coitus, which must last ≥30 min.

(continued)

TABLE 3.   Features of the Reproductive Cycle (*continued*)

Species	Age at Puberty	Cycle Type	Cycle Length	Duration of Estrus
Chin-chilla	6-8½ mo (400-600 g)	Polyestrous, intense November to May	30-50 days (41)	Vagina perforated ½-6 days during estrus; mate at night
Nutria	5-8 mo	Polyestrous	24-29 days	2-4 days
Rabbit	5-9 mo; range 4-12 mo for most breeds	Induced ovulation; breed all year, more or less; may show seasonal anestrus	No regular estrous cycles	Up to 1 mo
Rhesus monkey	3 yr	Polyestrous all year; tendency to anovulatory cycles in summer in USA	27-28 days (23-33)	~3 days
Rat	37-67 days, varies with strain; body length at puberty 148-150 mm	Polyestrous all year	4-5 days	~14 hr (12-18), usually begins ~7 pm
Mouse	35 days (28-49)	Polyestrous all year	Usually 4 or 5 days	A few hours beginning in evening
Guinea pig	55-70 days	Polyestrous all year	16½ days	6-11 hr, usually begins in evening
Hamster	4-6 wk	Polyestrous all year; few pregnancies in winter	4-5 days	12 hr, one night
Gerbil (Mongolian)	9-12 wk	Polyestrous	4-6 days	12-15 hr

*Under optimal management conditions, many cows ovulate as early as 20 days after parturition, with or without detectable signs of estrus.

the uterus and cervix are required for establishing and maintaining pregnancy and for parturition. Infections contracted at mating and during parturition and puerperium (and their sequelae) are common causes of female infertility. They interfere with normal uterine function, including release of $PGF_{2\alpha}$. Applicability of diagnostic methods for detection of uterine and cervical abnormalities depends on species, size of the animal, and anatomy of the cervix. Clinical diagnosis is by rectal and abdominal palpation, vaginoscopy and fiberoptic hysteroscopy, radiography, and transrectal ultrasonography. Laboratory diagnostic aids include microbiologic and cytologic examination of exudate or secretion, histologic examination of biopsies, endometrial cytology, and hormone assays.

The posterior tract, consisting of the vagina, vestibulum, and vulva, serves as the copulatory organ and as the last segment of the birth canal. It also provides a pathway for ascending infections, particularly when effectiveness of the sphincter of the vulva is lost or reduced due to trauma or relaxation. Puerperal infections commonly involve the entire tubular tract. In addition, vestibulovaginal infection perpetuated by urovagina and pneumovagina may sustain chronic infection of the uterus. However, the vestibulum and vagina

◀ **TABLE 3.** Features of the Reproductive Cycle (*continued*)

Best Time to Breed	First Estrus After Parturition	Comments
Mate on second night, rarely on third night	2-48 hr, ovulation on second night	
	48 hr	
When vulva is enlarged and hyperemic	Immediately, but blastocysts die if doe suckles large litter	In USA, do not breed well in summer. Ovulation $10^1/_2$ hr after coitus. Pseudopregnancy lasts 14-16 days.
Near ovulation, day 10-13 of cycle	After weaning of previous young	Menstruation lasts 4-6 days. Ovulation usually ~13 days after onset.
Near ovulation	Within 24 hr	Ovulation soon after midnight. Stimulation of the cervix causes pseudopregnancy lasting 12-14 days.
Most receptive during first 3 hr	Within 24 hr	Ovulation soon after midnight. Stimulation of cervix causes pseudopregnancy lasting 10-12 days.
Midestrus on	Usually immediately	Ovulation ~10 hr after onset of estrus.
Midestrus	After weaning	Ovulation 8-12 hr after onset of estrus. Pseudopregnancy lasts 7-13 days.
Midestrus	1-3 days	Ovulation spontaneous 6-10 hr after mating.

can be inflamed, even when the uterus is normal or pregnant. Conversely, in closed-cervix pyometras in cows and bitches, the vagina and vestibulum may be essentially normal.

The Male Tubular Genital Tract: In males, the tubular tract provides a pathway for sperm cells and semen. On each side, it begins as the efferent ductules of the testes; includes the head, body, and tail of the epididymis; and continues as the ductus deferens. The ductus deferens ascends into the abdominal cavity via the inguinal ring and passes over the dorsal aspect of the bladder to enter the pelvic urethra. The pelvic and penile urethras are shared as an outlet for semen and urine. Along this pathway, certain segments of the tract have evolved morphologically and functionally to perform additional specific functions. The epididymides are involved in sperm cell maturation and storage and in selective absorption of abnormal spermatozoa. Ampullae and accessory sex glands (ie, seminal vesicles, prostate, bulbourethral glands) contribute to the formation of seminal plasma. The size, form, and function of the accessory sex glands vary among species. The seminal vesicles and the bulbourethral (Cowper's) glands are absent in dogs. In bulls, the epididymides and seminal vesicles are common sites of infection. Epididymitis is also common in rams. Prostate hypertrophy and malignancy are found primarily in dogs. Pathologic conditions of the epididymides, eg, various forms of inflammation, cystic dilatation (spermiostasis), and segmental aplasia, can be diagnosed by scrotal palpation in most animals. Other diseases or functional disturbances may require evaluation of one or several semen samples. The seminal vesicles can be assessed by palpation and ultrasonography in animals large enough for rectal palpation.

INFERTILITY

Interaction of the CNS, hypothalamus, pituitary gland, gonads, and their target organs results in finely coordinated sequences of physiologic events that lead to estrus and ovulation in females and to ejaculation of fertile semen by males. For optimal results, ovulation and deposition of semen into the female genital tract must be closely synchronized. Failure of any single functional event in either sex leads to infertility or sterility.

The ultimate manifestation of infertility is failure to produce offspring. In polyestrous animals, a subnormal number of offspring also constitutes infertility. In females, infertility may be due to failure to cycle, aberrations of the estrous cycle and period (caused by dysfunction of the ovaries or the hypothalamus-pituitary axis), failure to conceive, or prenatal and perinatal death. Major infertility problems in males are caused by disturbances of the production, transport, or storage of spermatozoa; aberration of libido; and partial or complete inability to mate.

Most (if not all) major infertility problems have a complex etiology, and several factors, singly or in combination, can cause reproductive failure. Pathogenesis may be equally complex.

Diagnostic Approach: Because the female bears the offspring, she reflects either success or failure of reproduction. However, especially in naturally mated animals but also with artificial insemination, the first diagnostic step (regardless of the complaint) is to establish the etiologic role of the female and the male. Also, each point of human involvement in the reproductive process (such as observation of estrus, preservation of semen, and insemination) is a potential source of error. Such human errors can be detected or ruled out by assessment of performance with the main emphasis on techniques and procedures and their adequacy and quality.

Diagnostic methods have been developed to test the anatomic and functional soundness of both sexes. These include clinical examination, supported by diagnostic aids such as endoscopy and ultrasonography, and laboratory tests (eg, hormone assays, microbiology, cytology, serology, cytogenetic examination, semen evaluation, etc). The choice of diagnostic methods is determined by the species and size of the animal. Decisions with regard to type and extent of laboratory tests are based on history and information gained during the course of clinical examination. The diagnostic plan should provide evidence for establishing the role of the female, the male, and the manager in each case of reproductive failure. Reproductive problems are seldom accompanied by alarming signs of disease. Furthermore, there is a time interval between when a failure occurs and when it becomes apparent. Examples are intervals between unsuccessful service and return to estrus or failure to give birth. This lag period may allow recovery, yielding negative results on examination. Interpretation of results also must account for species differences and, in species with a seasonal reproductive pattern, that infertility may be physiologic during certain periods of the year.

PRINCIPLES OF THERAPY

See also SYSTEMIC PHARMACOTHERAPEUTICS OF THE REPRODUCTIVE SYSTEM, p 2031, and MANAGEMENT OF REPRODUCTION for the various species, p 1747 et seq.

The increasing demands for production efficiency, along with changing environments (eg, housing and management systems) and, in many instances, the successful eradication of specific infections (eg, brucellosis, tuberculosis, campylobacteriosis), have caused a shift in therapeutic strategies in several domestic species. Especially for food animals, and to some extent for horses, the therapeutic approach of choice often is a combination of pharmacologic agents and correction of management problems. Prevention through vaccination and treatments on a herd basis also have become more important, especially in light of the need for cost effectiveness, eg, the increased use of pharmacologic agents in reproductive management such as synchronization of estrus, superovulation, induction of parturition, and treatment of anestrus and subestrus. Other therapeutic trends in food animals are the result of an increasing awareness of the possible hazards of antimicrobial and hormone residues in tissues and milk; alternatives to antibiotic therapy warrant increased attention.

In small animals, therapeutic strategy has not changed as much as in large animals. The individual animal is still the focus of therapeutic efforts, and the environment of these species has not undergone the same changes as that of large animals. However, diagnostic techniques and treatments have become more sophisticated. More effective therapy may actually propagate hereditary predisposition for lowered fertility by curing diseases that previously were selected against naturally; this should be considered when dealing with fertility problems.

Pharmacologic Control of Reproduction: Control of the estrous cycle—most commonly synchronization of estrus—usually is based on agents that act directly on the ovaries (eg, FSH, LH, or preparations with similar effect, such as equine chorionic gonadotropin [eCG] or human chorionic gonadotropin [HCG], and prostaglandins) or on agents that act mainly at the pituitary-hypothalamic level (GnRH, progesterone, progestins). Superovulation, which has become an essential part of embryo transfer (p 1804), usually is achieved by hormonal treatment during a certain stage of the cycle with FSH or agents with FSH effect (eg, eCG) combined with a product with LH effect (eg, HCG). In ruminants, $PGF_{2\alpha}$ or its analogs are used to lyse the CL and control estrus after FSH stimulation of multiple follicle development.

Pathologic conditions of the ovaries (eg, cystic ovaries, delayed ovulation) are often treated with preparations with LH effect (eg, HCG) or GnRH. For persistent CL, as in cases of bovine pyometra, prostaglandins have become the treatment of choice. Postpartum ovarian inactivity (postpartum anestrus) has been experimentally treated with pulses of FSH or GnRH repeated over time. However, practical delivery systems for these products are currently unavailable, and conditions such as lactation anestrus remain difficult to treat. Delayed puberty in some species (eg, pigs) may respond to treatment with a product that has follicle-stimulating effect (FSH, eCG, or a combination of eCG and HCG).

Other areas in which exogenous hormones can play a role in the control of reproduction are pregnancy and parturition. Estrogens are used as abortifacients in some species (eg, bovine), but prostaglandins are usually more effective. Estrogens have been used for prevention of pregnancy after undesired mating (eg, canine). Progesterone or various progestogens can be used for suppression of estrus to prevent mating in all species. Induction of parturition has become an important management tool in some species (eg, horses, pigs, and cattle). Corticosteroid treatment or $PGF_{2\alpha}$, or a combination thereof, is used in cattle. Dams with a dead fetus usually do not respond well to corticosteroids. In pigs, it appears that either $PGF_{2\alpha}$ or a combination of $PGF_{2\alpha}$ and oxytocin is best. In mares, oxytocin is most effective. It is important in all species that the animal is prepared for parturition. The less prepared the reproductive tract (ie, cervix, fetoplacental unit, and mammary glands), the higher the risk of complications.

For conditions such as prolonged gestation, the same agents are used as for induction of parturition in normal animals. In uterine disorders (pyometra, retained placenta, and endometritis), the best nonantibiotic agents are those that can cause myometrial contractions, increase uterine blood flow, and mobilize defense mechanisms to the uterus. This can be achieved with estrogens and oxytocin. Prostaglandins have a strong stimulus on myometrial contractions in dogs but not in postpartum cows. Pyometra in cows is best treated with $PGF_{2\alpha}$ because the condition is defined as including presence of a functional CL.

Antimicrobial Treatment: Antimicrobial agents, most commonly antibiotics, are used for treatment of infections of the reproductive tract in all species (*see also* ANTIBACTERIAL AGENTS, p 2056, et seq). Drug selection should be based, if feasible, on microbiologic culture and sensitivity tests. The dosage, route of administration, and interval between treatments vary among species and with microbiologic status, blood and tissue distribution, etc. Systemically administered antibiotics penetrate the reproductive tract tissues better than those administered locally by intrauterine infusion.

Nonantibiotic Alternatives: Unsatisfactory results with antibiotics and increased concern about bacterial resistance and tissue residues (for food animals) emphasize the need for nonantibiotic alternatives for treatment of reproductive infections. In general, there are 2 desirable effects of nonantibiotics on the reproductive tract: the contractile effect that causes the evacuation of the tubular tract and the positive effect on the cellular and humoral local defense. Drugs of primary interest for evacuation of the uterus are oxytocin, ergonovine, estrogens, and in some species (eg, dogs), $PGF_{2\alpha}$. Of these drugs, estrogens and $PGF_{2\alpha}$ may have a dual beneficial effect, stimulating both the contractions of the uterus (eg, in cases of retained lochia or placenta, or postpartum metritis) and the local cellular defense. In addition to its contractile effect on the myometrium, $PGF_{2\alpha}$ causes regression of the CL in several species. This allows estrus to occur, which reinforces the effect on the myometrium and produces endogenous estrogen. In pyometra, these effects may work synergistically. Drugs that stimulate either contractions of the tubular tract or local defense mechanisms are used in combination with antibiotics or as the only treatment in cases of retained placenta, metritis, delayed uterine involution, retention of lochia, metrorrhagia, uterine prolapse, pyometra, etc. Oxytocin is commonly used to stimulate milk ejection in mastitis in some species (cattle, horses, dogs, and pigs).

In the past, use of disinfectant douches (eg, Lugol's solution, chlorhexidine, hydrogen peroxide, various iodophors, etc) was common for certain infections. They are still used for that purpose, especially in large animals; however, some of these substances are irritating, and there are indications that the local use of disinfectants may disturb the local immune defense (eg, the phagocytic ability of the WBC). A major reason for the interest in disinfectants and other alternatives to antibiotics is to avoid the problem of antibiotic residues in milk; however, any substance infused into the uterus is likely to also be passed into the milk. Because the beneficial effects have not been confirmed, this type of treatment is now less frequently recommended. It might still have a place among possible treatments for certain purposes such as inducing premature estrus in cows during a certain stage of the cycle. However, the beneficial effect in such cases is associated more with the induction of endogenous $PGF_{2\alpha}$ and estrogen production than with the antimicrobial effect of the drug.

CONGENITAL AND INHERITED ANOMALIES OF THE REPRODUCTIVE SYSTEM

Cryptorchidism is a failure of one or both testicles to descend into the scrotum and is seen in all domestic animals. It is common in stallions and boars and is the most common disorder of sexual development in dogs (13%). Predisposing factors include testicular hypoplasia, estrogen exposure in pregnancy, breech labor compromising blood supply to the testes, and delayed closure of the umbilicus resulting in an inability to increase abdominal pressure. Bilateral cryptorchidism results in sterility. Unilateral cryptorchidism is more common, and the male is usually fertile due to sperm production from the normally descended testicle. The undescended testicle may be located anywhere from just caudal of the kidney to within the inguinal canal. Abdominal testicles produce male hormones, and cryptorchid animals have normal secondary sex characteristics and mating behavior. Because of the inherited nature of the condition, unilateral cryptorchids should not be used for breeding. After puberty the retained testis becomes hypoplastic, degenerate, and fibrotic. Affected animals should be castrated as sertoliomas, seminomas, and interstitial cell tumors tend to develop within cryptorchid testicles and because of the heritability of the condition.

Some cases of **hereditary hypoplasia of the ovaries and testes** are associated with a single recessive gene with incomplete penetrance. It has been described in Swedish Highland cattle and has marked association with white coat color; the incidence has been much reduced by a controlled breeding program. Bilateral, unilateral, partial, or total hypoplasia may be seen. A condition similar to the human Turner's syndrome, with severe bilateral ovarian hypoplasia associated with chromosomal abnormalities, absence of follicles, and fibrosis with consequent infertility has been described in grade mares and in Thoroughbreds, Arabians, Welsh Ponies, Tennessee Walking Horses, Standardbreds, American Saddlebreds, Paso Finos, Belgians, Quarter Horses, and Appaloosas. Affected mares may be smaller than average and show either an absence of estrous cycles or only occasional estrus. They have a small flaccid uterus, a flaccid cervix with an open os, and small to very small ovaries. The ovaries are smooth and firm and have no follicles or corpora lutea. Cytogenetic studies may be indicated in infertile mares that show some or all of the above signs. The most common chromosomal abnormality in these mares is an absence of one of the sex chromosomes, and these animals are designated XO. There is no treatment.

Prolapse of the prepuce is a common defect in bulls, particularly in *Bos indicus* cattle. In *B taurus* cattle, it is common in polled beef breeds. A long, pendulous sheath, a large preputial orifice, and absence or poor development of the retractor prepuce muscles are predisposing inherited anatomic abnormalities. Prolapse of the prepuce predisposes the animal to injury, which can lead to abscess formation, scarring, adhesions, or phimosis. Surgical correction of the prolapse is possible, but as genetic predisposition may play a role, castration should be carefully considered.

Penile deviation is a common cause of copulatory failure in bulls. Two types of penile deviation are described—premature spiral deviation of the penis (corkscrew penis) and ventral deviation of the penis. Both conditions are caused by insufficiency of the dorsal apical ligament of the penis. Trauma is rarely involved. Premature spiral deviation of the penis is the most common penile defect in polled beef bulls and has been reported in most beef and dairy breeds. Spiral deviation is abnormal when it occurs prematurely and prevents intromission on more than one occasion. In affected bulls, the condition can be mild to severe, and premature spiral deviations of the penis may range from <25% to >75% of all services attempted. This may occur within one mating season or over several seasons. Most affected bulls develop the defect between 3 and 6 yr of age. In ventral deviation of the penis, the free part of the penis curves downward and prevents intromission. Deviations of the penis are diagnosed by careful observation of bulls at the time of service or during test mating. Surgical correction can be done, but should not be performed if inheritance is possible.

The opening of the penile urethra may be dislocated on the ventral surface of the penis (**hypospadias**) or on the dorsal surface (**epispadias**).

Persistent penile frenulum is not uncommon and is regarded as an inherited defect. Affected bulls are unable to protrude the penis from the sheath and, in most cases, cannot achieve intromission. Attachment can be minimal (eg, 0.5 cm), or the preputial mucosa can be attached the full length of the ventral raphe of the free part of the penis. Surgical correction should not be performed in bulls intended for seedstock breeding. Many male foals may appear to have a persistent frenulum at birth, but the condition resolves within a few days. If the condition persists, correction should not be attempted until the foal is at least 1 mo old.

Short retractor penis muscle may occur congenitally or after injury to the penis or prepuce. Affected bulls have normal libido, but during attempted service the penis is only partially protruded from the sheath and the ejaculatory thrust does not occur. Failure of erection in bulls may be a congenital condition but is generally a sequela of trauma and/or hematoma of the penis.

Hermaphroditism or intersexuality is occasionally described in goats and pigs. True hermaphrodites are rare and have both ovarian and testicular tissue and exhibit anomalies of the external genitalia. The chromosomal makeup is variable and may be a chimera: mosaic, XX, with or without the SRY gene, or unknown. Pseudohermaphrodites are more common; they have one or the other type of gonad and an anomaly of the external genitalia that resembles, to some degree, that of the opposite sex. The most common intersex condition, the male pseudohermaphrodite, has testicular tissue in the abdominal cavity or beneath the skin in the scrotal region, and external genital organs that resemble those of females. Miniature Schnauzers, Basset Hounds, and, rarely,

Persian cats may present with pseudohermaphroditism when affected by persistent paramesonephric (müllerian) duct syndrome. Undescended testes are attached to the uterine horns and the vasa deferentia are located in the wall of the uterus. There are bilateral oviducts, a complete uterus with a cervix, and a cranial portion of the vagina. Bilateral scrotal testes or unilateral or bilateral cryptorchidism may be present. Affected animals can present clinically with pyometra, urinary tract infection, prostate infection, or Sertoli cell tumor. The diagnosis is confirmed by presence of a 78, XY chromosome constitution, bilateral testes, and the presence of all paramesonephric (müllerian) duct derivatives. Androgen-dependent masculinization is that of a normal male. Treatment is limited to castration and hysterectomy. The defect is inherited as an autosomal recessive trait in Miniature Schnauzers, and both females and males can be carriers. Homozygous affected dogs with a descended testis are generally fertile and capable of transmitting the trait to all offspring.

The paramesonephric ducts are paired embryonic ducts that develop into the anterior vagina, cervix, uterus, and oviducts. **Segmental aplasia of the paramesonephric ducts** results in anomalies of those organs. Ovarian development is normal. Accumulation of secretions proximal to the obstruction occurs secondarily. Variable degrees of persistence of the hymen is the most commonly reported paramesonephric duct anomaly; it may result in development of a fluctuating swelling caused by the accumulation of uterine secretions that is palpable per vagina. Segmental aplasia of the cervix may result in either mucometra, hydrometra, or cystic enlargement of the cervix. Segmental aplasia of the uterus may involve one horn (resulting in a condition called uterus unicornis), both horns, or only part of one horn (which may result in cystic dilatation of the uterine horn anterior to the area of dilatation). Developmental anomalies involving the paramesonephric tracts occur in all breeds, but the hymenal defects are most common in white Shorthorn cattle (white heifer disease).

Double external os of the cervix is due to a failure of the paramesonephric ducts to fuse. It may present as a band of tissue caudal to, or in, the external os of the cervix. In other cases, there is a true double external os opening into a single caudal part of the cervical canal. Affected cows usually conceive normally. Rarely, a true double cervix, with a complete septum between the two cervical canals, each opening into its respective uterine horn (uterus didelphys), occurs.

Gartner's ducts, located beneath the mucosa of the floor of the vagina, may develop multiple cysts, which are generally of no clinical significance.

Freemartins are sterile females born twin to a male. In cattle with multiple conceptions, the chorionic placental blood vessels form a common circulation between the fetuses prior to sexual differentiation, allowing antimüllerian duct hormone and testosterone secreted by the male to inhibit development of the female tract. In ~92% of cases of mixed-sex twins, the females are sterile. The tubular genital organs in affected animals range from cordlike bands to near normal uterine horns. Freemartins have a short vagina that ends blindly without communication with the uterus. The cervix is absent. The ovaries usually fail to develop and remain small. Normal and freemartin cattle can be differentiated on the basis of length of the vagina and on presence or absence of a cervix. In calves (1-4 wk old), the normal vaginal length is 13-15 cm, while in a freemartin vaginal length is 5-6 cm. Vaginal length is easily measured by gently inserting a well-lubricated probe with a blunt end into the vagina. Cytogenetic examination can demonstrate XX and XY chromosome patterns in freemartins. The interchange of cells that occurs in the placental circulation between the fetuses can also be demonstrated by detecting 2 different blood types in a single animal.

Rectovaginal constriction is a simple autosomal recessive defect of Jersey cattle resulting in a severe stenosis or constriction of the anus or vestibule. In females, it is characterized by inelastic constrictions at the junction of the anus, rectum, vestibule, and vulva. Males may have anal stenosis. Affected cattle can copulate and defecate, but rectal examinations are difficult to perform and the vaginal constriction can lead to severe dystocia. In addition, affected cows are prone to develop udder edema at calving, frequently followed by severe mastitis.

ABORTION IN LARGE ANIMALS

Abortion is the termination of pregnancy after organogenesis is complete but before the expelled fetus can survive. If pregnancy ends before organogenesis, it is called early embryonic death. A dead full-term fetus is a stillbirth (its lungs are not inflated). Many etiologies of abortion also cause stillbirths, mummification, and weak or deformed neonates.

The etiologic diagnosis of abortion in livestock is a difficult and often frustrating task. The diagnostic success rate is relatively low: 30-40% for bovine, 60-65% for ovine, and 35-40% for porcine abortion cases submitted to diagnostic laboratories. Numerous factors complicate diagnosis. Often, abortion follows initial infection by weeks or months so that the causative agent is no longer apparent by the time abortion occurs. Expulsion may follow fetal death by hours or days, with lesions obscured by autolysis. Fetal membranes and the aborted fetus are usually contaminated by environmental agents before examination. Many sporadic abortions are likely the result of noninfectious (ie, toxic or genetic) causes about which much less is known in comparison to infectious causes; many diagnostic laboratories are not equipped or staffed to deal with these causes of abortion.

Another problem in determining the cause of abortions is improper or inadequate specimen selection and handling. The best specimen is the complete fetoplacental unit in fresh condition, along with maternal serum. The placenta and fetus should be cleaned with water or saline, packed in clean plastic bags, chilled (but not frozen), and rapidly transported to the diagnostic laboratory. In most cases, autolysis proceeds at a much slower rate in fetuses than in carcasses of animals born alive. If chilled as soon as possible, most fetuses will be suitable for examination, even if they do not reach the laboratory for 1-2 days. Fetal pigs, sheep, and goats are usually small enough to transport or ship the entire fetus and its placenta. If there are multiple fetuses, 3-5 should be submitted with their placentas. It is best to submit calves and foals whole, but in many cases it is more convenient to perform a necropsy and collect samples for submission. The specimens that are routinely used for testing vary somewhat between diagnostic laboratories, but a basic set of samples that will allow thorough examination includes stomach or abomasal contents; heart blood or fluid from a body cavity; lung, liver, kidney, and spleen (some labs also request tissues such as thyroid glands, thymus, heart, brain, abomasum, and stomach; placenta (if available); and dam's serum. These should be submitted in sterile containers to allow for microbiologic cultures. Because they are always contaminated, placentas should not be mixed with other tissues.

Representative samples of the following should also be submitted in 10% buffered formalin for histopathologic examination: lung, liver, heart, kidney, spleen, brain, skeletal muscle, thyroid, adrenal, intestines, and placenta (*see* p 1333). In a large majority of cases, gross lesions other than signs of autolysis (increased pleural and peritoneal fluid and blood-tinged subcutaneous edema) are not present. However, if lesions are found, fresh and formalin-fixed samples of affected tissues should be included.

Most agents, especially bacteria and fungi, infect the placenta and thus gain entry into the aminiotic fluid, which is swallowed by the fetus. Stomach contents can be obtained aseptically, making it the best specimen for detection of fungi and most bacteria. Isolation from the stomach contents is much easier than from the placenta, which is always heavily contaminated. Lungs, liver, spleen, and kidneys are also good for culture. Several agents (eg, fungi, *Chlamydophila*, *Coxiella*) primarily affect the placenta; failure to include placenta decreases the probability that they will be identified. Fetuses sometimes produce antibodies to certain agents (eg, bovine viral diarrhea virus, *Neospora*, *Leptospira*) and fetal serum or fluid from a body cavity can be tested for antibodies. The presence of precolostral antibodies is evidence of in utero exposure.

A single antibody titer in the dam rarely provides evidence of abortion caused by a particular agent unless background herd titer levels are known. High maternal titers may as likely be the reason an animal did not abort due to that agent, but absence of a titer can be used to rule out an agent. Antibody titers to agents with control programs (eg, *Brucella abortus*, pseudorabies virus) are always significant, even if the abortion was caused by something else. Demonstration of a 4-fold increase in antibody titer is required to prove active infection by a specific agent. Often, abortion occurs weeks or months after initial infection of the dam, and her titer is stable or declining at the time of abortion. Paired serum samples obtained 2 wk apart from 10% of the herd or a minimum of 10 animals often demonstrate seroconversion and provide evidence of active infection in the herd.

ABORTION IN CATTLE

See also MANAGEMENT OF REPRODUCTION: CATTLE, p 1747.

Given the low diagnostic success rate, the high cost of laboratory work, and the low profit margin in both the beef and dairy industries, veterinarians should not attempt to make an etiologic diagnosis in every abortion. Instead, veterinarians should become concerned if fetal loss is >3-5% per year or per month.

Noninfectious Causes

The actual incidence of abortions in cows due to genetic factors is unknown. Some genetically caused abortions may not have phenotypically recognizable lesions. Most lethal genes cause early abortion or early embryonic death.

Vitamins A and E, selenium, and iron have been implicated in bovine abortions, but documentation based on experiments is available only for vitamin A.

Heat stress causes fetal hypotension, hypoxia, and acidosis. High maternal temperature due to pyrexia may be more important than environmentally induced heat stress.

While severe trauma may rarely result in abortion (the bovine fetus is well protected by the amniotic fluid), farmers undoubtedly blame too many abortions on the cow "getting bumped."

A number of toxins can cause abortion in cows. Ponderosa pine needles can cause abortion if ingested in the last trimester; the cows may become moribund after delivery and hemorrhage excessively. The toxic factor is believed to be estrogenic. Locoweed (*Oxytropis* or *Astragalus* sp) contains an indolizidine alkaloid that can affect the corpus luteum, chorioallantois, and neurons, resulting in abortion or deformities. Broomweed (*Guttierrezia microcephala*) ingestion can also cause abortion, as can coumarins from rat poison, many grasses, or moldy sweet clover. Sodium iodide, IV, has been contraindicated in pregnant cows, but no abortions or adverse effects occurred in pregnant cows treated with a single high dose in recent studies. Mycotoxins, especially those with estrogenic activity, have been implicated in bovine abortions. Nitrates or nitrites have also been incriminated, but experimental evidence is controversial.

Infectious Causes

Neosporosis: *Neospora caninum* is found worldwide and is the most common cause of abortion in dairy cattle in many parts of the USA. *Neospora* abortion is less common in beef cattle, but it is still economically significant. Abortion can occur any time after 3 mo of gestation, but is most common between 4 and 6 mo of gestation. *Neospora* can be associated with sporadic abortions or abortion storms, and repeat abortions in cows have been reported. Some infected calves survive and are born with paralysis or proprioceptive deficits. Dogs are the definitive host for *Neospora* and can be the source of infection. The role of wild canids is unknown. Cows are not clinically ill, and placental retention is not common. The fetus is usually autolyzed and rarely has gross lesions. Microscopically, nonsuppurative inflammation is common in the brain, heart, and skeletal muscles. Organisms can be identified in these tissues and the kidneys by immunohistochemical staining. Many late gestation fetuses have precolostral antibodies. Infected calves may be born alive and clinically normal. They remain infected for years and possibly for life. During pregnancy, *Neospora* organisms can become activated and infect the fetus. This is thought to be the most common source of infection. There is no treatment. Strict hygiene to prevent fecal contamination of feed by dogs may aid in prevention. A commercial vaccine is available. *See also* p 535.

Bovine Viral Diarrhea (BVD): In several surveys, BVD was the most commonly diagnosed virus in bovine abortion cases. The pathology of BVD in the developing fetus is complex. Infection of the fetus before 125 days of gestation can cause fetal death and abortion, resorption, mummification, developmental abnormalities, or fetal immunotolerance and persistent infection. After 125 days of gestation, BVD may cause abortion, or the fetal immune response may clear the virus. Diagnosis is by identification of BVD virus by isolation, immunologic staining, PCR, or detection of precolostral antibodies in aborted calves. The virus is present in a wide variety of tissues, but the spleen is the tissue of choice. Rising antibody titers to BVD in aborting animals or herdmates is diagnostic of recent infection. BVD virus is immunosuppressive and is found in many fetuses infected by other agents. Outbreaks of abortions by organisms that normally cause sporadic abortion should raise suspicion of possible concurrent BVD virus infection. Prevention should focus on removal of persistently infected cattle and herd vaccination. *See also* p 220.

Infectious Bovine Rhinotracheitis (IBR, Bovine Herpesvirus 1): IBR is a major cause of viral abortion in the USA, with abortion rates of 5-60% in nonvaccinated herds. The virus is widespread and can recrudesce; therefore, any cow with a positive IBR titer is a possible carrier. The virus is carried to the placenta in WBC; over the next 2 wk to 4 mo, it causes a placentitis, then infects the fetus and kills it in 24 hr. Abortion can occur any time but usually is from 4 mo to term. Autolysis is consistently present. Occasionally there are small foci of necrosis in the liver, but in a large majority of cases there are no gross lesions in the placenta or fetus. Microscopically, small foci of necrosis with minimal inflammation are consistently present in the liver. Necrotizing vasculitis is common in the placenta. Diagnosis can be made by immunologic staining of the kidney and adrenal glands. IBR virus can be isolated from ~50% of infected fetuses (most successfully from the placenta). In most cases, maternal titers have peaked by the time of abortion. In abortion storms, rising titers can often be demonstrated in herdmates. Control is by herd vaccination; intranasal, modified live virus, and killed vaccines are available. *See also* p 1193.

Leptospirosis: *Leptospira interrogans,* serovars *grippotyphosa, pomona, hardjo, canicola,* and *icterohaemorrhagiae* usually cause abortions in the last trimester, 2-6 wk after maternal infection. Although dams may show clinical signs of leptospirosis, most abortions are in otherwise healthy cattle. Abortion rates vary from 5-40% or more. The leptospires cause a diffuse placentitis with avascular, light tan cotyledons and edematous, yellowish intercotyledonary areas. The fetus usually dies 1-2 days before expulsion and therefore is autolyzed. Occasionally calves are born alive but weak. There are no specific lesions, but placenta and fetus should be submitted to the laboratory for fluorescent antibody staining or PCR testing for *Leptospira.* Although maternal titers are probably waning by the time of abortion, an initial titer of >1:800 may be suspicious. Approximately one-third of cows aborting because of *L hardjo* have titers of <1:100 at the time of abortion. The dam's urine can be cultured or examined for leptospires within 2 wk of abortion. For control, sources of infection (such as feed or water contaminated by dogs, rats, or wildlife) should be identified and eliminated. Cattle may be lifelong carriers of *L hardjo* and are a source of infection for herd additions. Vaccination with a 5-way bacterin is recommended every 6 mo. Leptospirosis is zoonotic, and urine and milk of dams may be infective for up to 3 mo. (*See also* p 525.)

Brucellosis: Brucellosis (Bang's disease) is a threat in most countries where cattle are raised. In the USA, active control programs, including test, slaughter, and heifer vaccination, have greatly decreased its incidence. Brucellosis causes abortions in the second half of gestation (usually ~7 mo), and ~80% of unvaccinated cows in later gestation will abort if exposed to *Brucella abortus*. The organisms enter via mucous membranes and invade the udder, lymph nodes, and uterus, causing a placentitis, which may be acute or chronic. Abortion or stillbirth occurs 2 wk to 5 mo after initial infection. Affected cotyledons may be normal to necrotic, and red or yellow. The intercotyledonary area is focally thickened with a wet, leathery appearance. The fetus may be normal or autolytic with bronchopneumonia. Diagnosis can be made by maternal serology combined with fluorescent antibody staining of placenta and fetus or isolation of *B abortus* from placenta, fetus, or uterine discharge. Prevention is by calfhood vaccination of heifers.

Brucellosis is a serious zoonosis and a reportable disease, and the appropriate authorities should be contacted. (*See also* p 1110.)

Mycotic Abortion: Fungal placentitis due to *Aspergillus* sp (septic fungi, 60-80% of cases), or to *Mucor* sp, *Absidia*, or *Rhizopus* sp (nonseptate fungi) is an important cause of bovine sporadic abortion. Abortions occur from 4 mo to term and are most common in winter. It is believed the fungi gain entry through the oral or respiratory tracts and travel hematogenously to the placenta. Placentitis is severe and necrotizing. Cotyledons are enlarged and necrotic with turned-in margins. The intercotyledonary area is thickened and leathery. Adventitious placentation is common. The fetus seldom is autolyzed, although it may be dehydrated; ~30% have gray ringworm-like skin lesions principally involving the head and shoulders. The diagnosis is based on the presence of fungal hyphae associated with necrotizing placentitis, dermatitis, or pneumonia. Fungi can also be isolated from the stomach contents, placenta, and skin lesions. Isolation must be correlated with microscopic and gross lesions to rule out post-abortion contamination.

For control, moldy feed should be avoided. (*See also* p 2408.)

Arcanobacterium pyogenes: *Arcanobacterium (Actinomyces) pyogenes* causes sporadic abortion at any stage of pregnancy. Rarely, the incidence in a herd may reach epizootic levels. The bacterium is present in the nasopharynx of many normal cows and in abscesses. It is not normally present, even as a contaminant, in fetuses or fetal membranes, and isolation is almost always significant. It gains entry to the bloodstream and causes an endometritis and placentitis, which is diffuse with a reddish brown to brown color. The fetus is usually autolyzed, with fibrinous pericarditis, pleuritis, or peritonitis possible.

Bronchopneumonia may be evident on histopathology, but *A pyogenes* is best cultured from placenta or abomasal contents. Abortion is usually sporadic, and no effective bacterin is available.

Trichomoniasis: *Tritrichomonas (Trichomonas) foetus* infection causes a venereal disease that usually results in infertility but occasionally causes abortion in the first half of gestation. Placentitis is relatively mild with hemorrhagic cotyledons and thickened intercotyledonary areas covered with flocculent exudate. The placenta is often retained, and there may be pyometra. The fetus has no specific lesions, although *T foetus* can be found in abomasal contents, placental fluids, and uterine discharges. Trichomoniasis can be prevented by artificial insemination using noninfected bulls. (*See also* p 1142.)

Campylobacteriosis: *Campylobacter fetus venerealis* causes venereal disease that usually results in infertility but occasionally causes abortion between 5 and 8 mo of gestation. *C fetus fetus* and *C jejuni* are transmitted by ingestion and subsequent hematogenous spread to the placenta. Both cause sporadic abortions, usually in the last half of gestation. The fetus can be fresh with partially expanded lungs or severely autolyzed. Mild fibrinous pleuritis and peritonitis may be noted, as well as bronchopneumonia. Placentitis is mild with hemorrhagic cotyledons and an edematous intercotyledonary area. *Campylobacter* spp can be identified by darkfield examination of abomasal contents or culture of placenta or abomasal contents. Isolation and identification of the species involved is important if vaccination is to be instituted. Venereal campylobacteriosis can be controlled by artificial insemination and vaccination. (*See also* p 1108.)

Listeriosis: *Listeria monocytogenes* can cause placentitis and fetal septicemia. Abortions are usually sporadic but may affect 10-20% of a herd. Abortion is at any stage of gestation, and the dam may have fever and anorexia before the abortion; retained placenta is common. The fetus is retained for 2-3 days after death, so autolysis may be extensive. Fibrinous polyserositis and white necrotic foci in the liver and/or cotyledons are common. Diagnosis is by culture of *Listeria* from fetus or placenta. There is no available bacterin. Listeriosis is a reportable disease in many areas and is a serious zoonosis with spread possible through improperly pasteurized milk. (*See also* p 531.)

Chlamydophilosis (Chlamydiosis): *Chlamydophila abortus* (*Chlamydia psittaci* serotype 1), the cause of enzootic abortion of ewes, causes sporadic abortion in cattle. Most abortions occur near the end of the last trimester, but they can occur earlier. Placental lesions consist of thickening and yellow-brown exudate adhered to the cotyledons and intercotyledonary areas. Histologically, placentitis is consistently present, and pneumonia and hepatitis can be found in some cases. *C abortus* can be identified by examination of stained smears of the placenta or by ELISA, fluorescent antibody staining, PCR, or isolation in embryonated chicken eggs or cell culture. Organisms can often be identified in the lungs and liver, but not as consistently as in the placenta. There are no vaccines for cattle, although they are produced for sheep (*see* ENZOOTIC ABORTION OF EWES, below). The bacterium is zoonotic, occasionally producing life-threatening disease and abortion in pregnant women.

Ureaplasma diversum Infection: *Ureaplasma diversum* is a common inhabitant of the vagina and prepuce of cattle that also causes abortions. Abortions are usually single, but severe outbreaks occur on occasion. Most fetuses are aborted in the third trimester and are well preserved. The cows are not sick, but retained placentas are common. The intercotyledonary areas are usually thickened and sometimes contain areas of fibrin deposition and hemorrhage. There are no gross lesions in the fetus. Microscopically, there is nonsuppurative placentitis and pneumonia characterized by accumulations of lymphocytes around bronchi and by diffuse alveolitis. Diagnosis is by isolation of *U diversum* from the placenta, lungs, and/or abomasal contents.

Epizootic Bovine Abortion (Foothill Abortion): Epizootic bovine abortion (EBA) is localized to the foothill region surrounding the Sacramento/San Joaquin Valley and the Eastern Sierra Nevada range of California and parts of Nevada, although disease clusters may exist in neighboring states. EBA usually causes a protracted abortion storm affecting primarily heifers or cows recently introduced to the geographic region; however, abortion can occur 3-5 mo after leaving the endemic area. Abortion is usually in the last trimester, and rates may be as high as 60%. The animals abort without illness, and the fetus is seldom autolyzed. While the etiologic agent has not been definitively determined, the vector appears to be the argasid tick *Ornithodoros coriaceus.* The aborted fetus may have hepatomegaly, splenomegaly, and generalized lymphomegaly. Microscopically, there is marked lymphoid hyperplasia in the spleen and lymph nodes and granulomatous inflammation in most organs. Fetal IgG is increased. Cows seldom abort in subsequent pregnancies, and heifers are often exposed to endemic areas before breeding age in an effort to prevent abortions.

Other Causes of Abortion: Bluetongue virus and Akabane virus (where present) cause abortion and fetal anomalies. Parainfluenza-3 virus causes abortion in experimentally inoculated seronegative cattle, but is seldom, if ever, diagnosed in field cases of abortion. Occasionally, *Salmonella* spp cause abortion storms. The cows are usually sick and the fetuses and placentas are autolyzed and emphysematous. Salmonellae can be isolated from the abomasal contents and fetal tissues. *Mycoplasma* spp, *Histophilus somni* (*Haemophilus somnus*), and a wide variety of other bacteria can also cause sporadic abortions in cattle.

ABORTION IN SHEEP

See also MANAGEMENT OF REPRODUCTION: SHEEP, p 1780.

Abortion in ewes, as in cows, is not always easily diagnosed. While many of the toxins that cause abortion in cows also cause problems in ewes, others such as *Veratrum californicum* and kale seem unique to the ewe. The major infectious agents causing abortions in sheep are *Campylobacter, Chlamydophila, Toxoplasma, Listeria, Brucella, Salmonella,* border disease virus, and Cache Valley virus.

***Campylobacter* spp Infection (Vibriosis):** Infection with *Campylobacter fetus fetus* and *C jejuni* results in abortions in late pregnancy or stillbirths. Ewes may develop metritis after expelling the fetus. Placentitis occurs with hemorrhagic necrotic cotyledons and edematous or leathery intercotyledonary areas. The fetus is usually autolyzed, with 40% having orange-yellow necrotic foci (1-2 cm diameter) in the liver. Diagnosis relies on finding *Campylobacter* organisms in darkfield or fluorescent antibody preparations from abomasal or placental smears or in uterine discharge. Identification of the species involved is important because in some areas *C jejuni* is as common as *C fetus*, and some vaccines do not include *C jejuni*. Strict hygiene is necessary to stop an outbreak. Use of tetracyclines may help prevent exposed ewes from aborting. The disease tends to be cyclical, with epizootics occurring every 4-5 yr; therefore, vaccination programs, which help prevent outbreaks, should be consistently practiced.

Enzootic Abortion of Ewes (EAE): *Chlamydophila abortus (Chlamydia psittaci* serotype 1) is the cause of EAE, which is characterized by late term abortions, stillbirths, and weak lambs. *C pecorum* is the cause of chlamydial arthritis and conjunctivitis of sheep. Except for Australia and New Zealand, EAE occurs worldwide and is most important in intensively managed sheep. Abortions occur during the last 2-3 wk of gestation regardless of when infection occurs, and the fetuses are fresh with minimal autolysis. There is placentitis with necrotic, reddish brown cotyledons and thickened brown intercotyledonary areas covered by exudate. Chlamydial elementary bodies can be found by examination of appropriately stained smears of the placenta or vaginal discharge, but the organisms cannot be differentiated from *Coxiella burnetii*, which occasionally causes abortion in sheep. Definitive diagnosis is by identification of *C abortus* by ELISA, fluorescent antibody staining, PCR, or isolation. Ewes seldom abort more than once, but they remain persistently infected and shed *C abortus* from their reproductive tract for 2-3 days before and after ovulation. Rams can be infected and transmit the organism venereally. Control consists of isolating all affected ewes and lambs and treating incontact ewes with long-acting oxytetracycline or oral tetracycline. *C abortus* bacterins are available and are effective in reducing abortions. In parts of Europe, a modified live vaccine is available for use.

C abortus is zoonotic but human cases are rare. All have involved pregnant women, who developed life-threatening illness. Only in a few cases in which the fetus was delivered by cesarean section did the infant survive. Pregnant women should not work with pregnant sheep, especially if abortions are occurring.

Border Disease: Border disease occurs worldwide and is an important cause of embryonic and fetal deaths, weak lambs, and congenital abnormalities. It is caused by a pestivirus closely related to bovine viral diarrhea (BVD) virus and classical swine fever (hog cholera) virus. Abortion can occur at any stage of gestation. There are no clinical signs in the dam. Live infected fetuses usually are undersized, and they often have congenital tremors and an abnormally hairy coat (hairy shaker lambs). Diagnosis is by identification of border disease virus in the placenta or fetal tissues (kidneys, lungs, spleen, thyroid glands, abomasum) by fluorescent antibody staining, virus isolation, or demonstration of precolostral antibodies. There are no vaccines available. Inactivated BVD virus vaccines are sometimes used on sheep, but their effectiveness is unproved. (*See also* p 503.)

Cache Valley Virus: Cache Valley virus is a mosquito-transmitted cause of infertility, abortions, stillbirths, and multiple congenital abnormalities in sheep. The virus is endemic in most parts of the USA, Canada, and Mexico. Often there are epizootics affecting sheep over a wide geographic area that can include several states. The most noticeable effects are stillborn lambs and the birth of live lambs with congenital abnormalities affecting the CNS and musculoskeletal system. Hydranencephaly, hydrocephalus, cerebral and cerebellar hypoplasia, arthrogryposis, scoliosis, torticollis, and hypoplasia of skeletal muscles are common. At the time of abortion or birth the virus is usually no longer viable, and diagnosis is by demonstration of antibodies in precolostral serum or body fluids. Vaccines are not available.

Toxoplasmosis: If ewes become infected with *Toxoplasma gondii* early in gestation, resorption or mummification results; if ewes contract the disease late in gestation, abortions or perinatal deaths occur. Ewes do not usually appear sick. In an outbreak, there is usually a wide range in gestational age of aborted fetuses. In most cases there are no gross lesions, but in a few cases there are distinct small white foci, 1-3 mm in diameter, in some cotyledons. The fetal brain often has focal areas of nonsuppurative inflammation on histology. Fetal serology (indirect hemagglutination inhibition, latex agglutination, or fluorescent antibody) may also be used. Once infected, ewes are immune, so running unbred ewes with aborting ones may allow them to develop immunity. Preventing contamination of feed by cat feces may help reduce exposure. Toxoplasmosis is a zoonosis. (*See also* p 547.)

Listeriosis: Abortion caused by *Listeria monocytogenes* in ewes usually occurs in late gestation. There is some necrosis of cotyledons and the intercotyledonary areas, and the fetus is usually autolyzed. The fetal liver (and possibly lung) may have necrotic foci, 0.5-1 mm in diameter. Diagnosis is by culture. (*See also* p 531.)

Brucellosis: The major importance of *Brucella ovis* is as a cause of epididymitis in rams, but it also causes late-term abortions, stillbirths, and birth of weak lambs. *B melitensis* is rare in the USA but causes abortion in areas where it is found. *B abortus* occasionally causes abortion in sheep. *Brucella* abortions occur late in gestation, resulting in placentitis with edema and necrosis of the cotyledons and thickened, leathery intercotyledonary areas. Many fetuses aborted due to *B ovis* are alive at the beginning of parturition, although fetuses can be mummified or autolyzed. Most fetuses aborted due to *B melitensis* or *B abortus* are autolytic. Culture of the placenta, abomasal contents, and the dam's vaginal discharge are diagnostic. A vaccine for *B melitensis* is available in some countries. *B melitensis* and *B abortus* are zoonotic. (*See also* p 1110.)

Salmonellosis: *Salmonella abortus ovis*, *S dublin*, *S typhimurium*, and *S arizona* have caused abortions in sheep. *S abortus ovis* is endemic in England and Europe but has not been reported in the USA. The other serotypes occur worldwide. Most ewes are sick and febrile before aborting. There are no specific placental lesions, and the fetus is autolyzed. Diagnosis is by culture of placenta, fetus, or uterine discharge. *See also* p 156.

Other Causes of Abortion: Bluetongue virus and Akabane virus (where present) cause abortion and congenital anomalies in sheep and are differential diagnoses for Cache Valley virus infection. *Coxiella burnetii* causes occasional abortion storms in sheep, with the clinical syndrome and fetal pathology being the same as for goats (*see* ABORTION IN GOATS, below). *Neospora caninum* has been reported to cause occasional abortions in sheep with the lesions resembling those of *Toxoplasma gondii*.

ABORTION IN GOATS

See also MANAGEMENT OF REPRODUCTION: GOATS, p 1757.

Noninfectious causes of abortion in goats include plant toxins, such as broomweed or locoweed poisoning; dietary deficiencies of copper, selenium, vitamin A, or magnesium; and certain drugs such as estrogen, glucocorticoids, phenothiazine, carbon tetrachloride, or levamisole (in late gestation).

Major infectious causes of abortion in goats are chlamydophilosis, toxoplasmosis, leptospirosis, brucellosis, *Coxiella burnetii*, and listeriosis. *Campylobacter* causes abortions but is not nearly as important in does as in ewes.

Chlamydophilosis (Chlamydiosis, Enzootic Abortion): *Chlamydophila abortus* (the agent of enzootic abortion of ewes) is the most common cause of abortion in goats in the USA. In naive herds, up to 60% of pregnant does can abort or give birth to stillborn or weak kids. Abortions can occur at any stage of pregnancy, but most are in the last month. Reproductive failure is usually the only sign of *C abortus* infection, but occasionally there is concurrent respiratory disease, polyarthritis, conjunctivitis, and retained placentas in the flock. Aborted lambs are usually fresh with no gross pathology. Placentitis is usually present and consists of reddish-brown exudate covering cotyledons and intercotyledonary areas. Microscopically, necrotizing vasculitis and neutrophilic inflammation are present in the placenta. Chlamydial organisms can be visualized in appropriately stained placental smears, but they cannot be differentiated from *Coxiella burnetii*. Fluorescent antibody or immunohistochemical staining, ELISA, PCR, or culture can be used to definitively identify *C abortus*. The placenta is the specimen of choice, but sometimes the diagnosis can be made by testing liver, lung, and spleen. During an outbreak, aborting does should be isolated and tetracyclines given orally or parentally. There is no chlamydial vaccine for goats, but the vaccine for sheep is relatively effective. Like sheep, goats that abort are immune. Sheep that abort due to *C abortus* remain infected for years, if not life, and shed the organism at the time of ovulation; whether or not this occurs in goats is not known. *C abortus* is zoonotic, occasionally causing serious disease in pregnant women.

Toxoplasmosis: Toxoplasmosis is a common cause of abortion in goats in the USA, and toxoplasmal abortion in goats is similar to the syndrome in ewes (*see* above).

Leptospirosis: The most common serovars of *Leptospira interrogans* involved in caprine abortion are *grippotyphosa* and *pomona*. While sheep are relatively resistant to leptospirosis, goats are susceptible, with abortions occurring at the time of leptospiremia. Some does have anemia, icterus, and hemoglobinemia; others are afebrile and are not icteric. Diagnosis is by serology or identification of *Leptospira* spp in the dam's urine, the placenta, or fetal kidney. (*See also* p 525.)

Brucellosis: *Brucella melitensis* is the principal organism, with occasional abortions due to *B abortus*. Abortion may be accompanied by mastitis and lameness and is most common in the fourth month. The placenta is grossly normal, but does may develop chronic uterine lesions. Infection in adults is lifelong with organisms shed in the milk (*B melitensis* is zoonotic but rare in the USA). In the USA, control is by test and slaughter. Tube agglutination and card tests can be used as screening tests. (*See also* p 1110.)

***Coxiella burnetii* Infection:** *Coxiella burnetii* is increasingly recognized as an important cause of caprine abortion, especially in the western USA. Occasional outbreaks also occur in sheep. Late-term abortions, stillbirths, and weak lambs are the common presentations. Up to 50% of the flock may be involved. The placenta is covered by gray-brown exudate and the intercotyledonary areas are thickened. Microscopically, there is a necrotizing vasculitis in the placenta, and many chorionic epithelial cells are distended by small, coccobacillary organisms <1 μm in diameter. Infection involves only the placenta; without it, the diagnosis usually cannot be made. Diagnosis is by identification of *C burnetii* by immunologic staining methods or by isolation. *Coxiella* is zoonotic, causing Q fever in humans.

Listeriosis: *Listeria monocytogenes* is a common pathogen in goats and causes sporadic abortions. There are no specific fetal lesions, and the fetus is often autolyzed. The doe usually shows no signs before abortion but may develop severe metritis after abortion. Diagnosis is by isolation from the placenta, abomasal contents, or uterine discharge. In the rare case of a herd outbreak, preventive treatment with tetracycline is recommended. (*See also* p 531.)

ABORTION IN PIGS

See also MANAGEMENT OF REPRODUCTION: PIGS, p 1771.

Many agents that cause reproductive failure in sows produce a broad spectrum of sequelae, including abortions and weak neonates, as well as stillbirth, mummification, embryonic death, and infertility. Mummification is seen more frequently in swine than in many other species due to the large litter size. If only a few fetuses die, abortion rarely occurs; instead, mummies are delivered at term, along with live piglets or stillbirths.

Noninfectious Causes

High ambient temperature (>32°C) is associated with increased returns to estrus, increased embryonic mortality, decreased farrowing rates, and small litters. The effect is greatest if heat stress occurs at the time of breeding or implantation. Increased embryonic mortality and increased irregular return to estrus are seen in pigs bred during the summer. High ambient temperature may play a role, but there is evidence that seasonal low progesterone levels are a major factor.

The estrogenic mycotoxins zearalenone and zearalenol interfere with conception and implantation causing infertility, embryonic death, and reduced litter size, but rarely, if ever, abortion. Another class of mycotoxins, the fumonisins, causes acute pulmonary edema in swine; sows that recover from the acute disease often abort 2-3 days later.

Other toxic causes of abortions or stillborn pigs include cresol sprays (used for mange and louse control), dicumarol, and nitrates. Nutritional causes of reproductive failure are not well defined. Vitamin A deficiency can cause congenital anomalies and possibly abortions. Riboflavin deficiency can cause early premature births (14-16 days), and calcium, iron, manganese, and iodine deficiencies have been associated with stillbirths and weak pigs.

Carbon monoxide toxicity due to faulty propane heaters has been associated with increased numbers of stillbirths and autolyzed full-term fetuses. Fetal tissues are cherry red; the sows do not appear affected.

Infectious Causes

The major infectious causes of reproductive failure in pigs include porcine reproductive and respiratory syndrome virus, porcine parvovirus, pseudorabies virus, Japanese B encephalitis virus, classical swine fever (hog cholera) virus, *Leptospira* spp, and *Brucella suis*.

Porcine Reproductive and Respiratory Syndrome (PRRS): PRRS is caused by an arterivirus. It is the most important disease of pigs in the USA and is of major importance throughout most of the world. Most PRRS strains do not cross the placenta until after 90 days of gestation. Consequently, most abortions are near the end of gestation. Affected litters contain fresh and autolyzed dead pigs, weak infected pigs, and healthy, uninfected pigs that often develop respiratory disease within a few days of birth. The sows are often anorectic and feverish a few days before aborting. Concurrent respiratory disease and increased numbers of bacterial infections in the herd are common. Hemorrhage in the umbilical cord, when present, is the only gross lesion associated with PRRS abortions. Not all fetuses are infected, so multiple fetuses should be sampled. Viral antigen is most consistently present in the fetal thymus and in fluid collected from the fetal thoracic cavity. PCR testing of pooled thoracic fluid from 3-5 fetuses is the most reliable means of diagnosis. Herd management is important in control and prevention. Inactivated and modified live virus vaccines are available. (*See also* p 581.)

Porcine Parvovirus: Porcine parvovirus is ubiquitous in pigs in the USA and most of the world. Almost all females are naturally infected before their second pregnancy, and immunity is lifelong. Consequently, it is a disease of first parity pigs. Fetal infection before 70 days of gestation can result in death of the fetus. Not all fetuses are infected at the same time, and death at different stages of pregnancy is typical. Some fetuses survive and are born alive but persistently infected. Most fetuses infected after 70 days of gestation mount an immune response, clear the virus, and are healthy at birth. Infected litters are carried to term. Litters with dead fetuses of varying sizes, including mummified fetuses, along with stillborn and healthy pigs born to first parity sows are the hallmark of porcine parvovirus. Diagnosis is by fluorescent antibody testing, virus isolation using lung from mummified fetuses, or demonstration of precolostral antibody in stillborn pigs. Boars shed virus by varying routes, including semen, for a couple of weeks after acute infection and can introduce the virus into a herd. Effective inactivated vaccines are available.

Pseudorabies (Aujeszky's Disease, Porcine Herpesvirus 1): Pseudorabies is a cause of CNS and respiratory diseases. Infection results in latency, and seropositive animals are considered infected. Infection early in pregnancy can result in embryonic death and resorption of the fetuses. Infection later in pregnancy can result in abortion and birth of stillborn and weak pigs. Mummification can occur but is uncommon. There are no gross lesions in most aborted pigs, but a few have pinpoint white foci of necrosis in the liver and tonsils. Diagnosis is by virus isolation or fluorescent antibody staining. Gene-deleted vaccines that allow serologic differentiation of vaccinated and naturally infected pigs are available and effective. There is a federal eradication program in the USA, and future outbreaks will probably be controlled by slaughter of infected pigs. State and federal authorities should be consulted before vaccinating. (*See also* p 1065.)

Japanese B Encephalitis Virus: Japanese B encephalitis is an arthropod-borne disease that causes reproductive failure in pigs and encephalitis in humans. Infected litters can contain dead pigs of various sizes (including mummies), stillborn pigs, weak pigs, and pigs with CNS signs. Hydrocephalus and subcutaneous edema are the most common gross lesions. Pigs are the primary amplifying host for the virus and are vaccinated not only to prevent reproductive failure, but also to prevent human infection.

Classical Swine Fever (Hog Cholera): Classical swine fever is caused by a pestivirus that has been eradicated from the USA but is a serious problem throughout much of the world. With highly virulent strains that cause serious maternal illness, abortion is common. With strains of moderate or low virulence, birth of mummified and stillborn pigs, weak pigs, and persistently infected pigs are more common. Fluorescent antibody staining and virus isolation are used for diagnosis. Both killed and modified live vaccines are available, but their use in the USA is prohibited. (*See also* p 570.)

Leptospirosis: *Leptospira interrogans* (especially serovar *pomona*) is a major cause of reproductive failure in swine. Although acute leptospirosis occurs in adult swine, most cases are asymptomatic. Abortion occurs 1-4 wk after infection, so the abortuses are autolyzed. Mummification, maceration, stillbirths, and weak pigs are also seen. Diagnosis is based on demonstration of leptospires in fetal tissues or stomach contents. Vaccination with a multivalent bacterin every 6 mo helps prevent the disease. The carrier state can be eliminated by administration of streptomycin at 25 mg/kg. A similar dosage can be given to pregnant sows during an outbreak to control abortions. (*See also* p 525.)

Brucellosis: Brucellosis in swine (*Brucella suis*) has become rare in the USA as a result of state and federal control programs. Infected sows can abort at any stage of gestation, and abortions are not always accompanied by illness. Abortion is probably due to endometritis and fetal infection. There are few fetal or placental lesions, although some fetuses may be autolyzed. Diagnosis is by serology and isolation from the placenta and fetal tissues. No treatment has been uniformly effective. Control is based on test and slaughter. Brucellosis is one of the few venereal diseases recognized in swine. *B suis* causes a serious zoonotic disease. (*See also* p 1110.)

Other Infectious Causes of Abortion: Porcine circovirus 2 (PCV-2) has been associated with abortion and increased stillborn pigs in gilts. Affected pigs had signs of congestive heart failure and myocarditis. The importance of PCV-2 as a cause of reproductive failure remains to be determined. Pigs with foot-and-mouth disease (p 507) and African swine fever (p 568) often abort, but they and their herdmates also have clinical signs of those diseases. Enteroviruses and encephalomyocarditis virus have been reported to cause fetal losses in pigs, but they are not considered economically important. Blue eye paramyxovirus is an important cause of abortion, stillbirths, and mummified fetuses in parts of Mexico. Bacteria that cause sporadic abortions include *Staphylococcus aureus*, *Streptococcus* spp, *Erysipelothrix rhusiopathiae*, *Salmonella* spp, *Pasteurella multocida*, *Arcanobacterium (Actinomyces) pyogenes*, *Listeria monocytogenes*, and *Escherichia coli*.

ABORTION IN HORSES

See also MANAGEMENT OF REPRODUCTION: HORSES, p 1759.

Noninfectious Causes

The most common noninfectious cause of abortion in horses is **twinning**. Most abortions related to twinning occur at 8-9 mo of gestation and may be preceded by premature lactation. Placental insufficiency ultimately causes abortion of twins. **Umbilical cord abnormalities**, such as torsion due to abnormal length, have been incriminated in abortions. Diagnosis of abortion due to cord torsion requires evidence of localized swelling or hemorrhage because torsions occur in some normal births. **Ectopic pregnancy** is rare but may result in abortion at 7-10 mo of gestation.

Mare Reproductive Loss Syndrome (MRLS): Starting in spring 2001, there was an explosive increase in abortions affecting all breeds of horses in central Kentucky. Both mares in late gestation and mares bred 35-90 days previously were affected. Foals aborted late in gestation were dead or weak, dehydrated, and often septic. Foals in the first trimester of gestation usually died in utero before being aborted. An infectious cause is not thought to be responsible. The outbreak occurred after a colder than normal March, followed by above normal temperatures in April. During the third week of April, there was a freeze followed by warm weather. Abortions increased after similar weather patterns in 1980 and 1981, but not to the extent seen in 2001. The warm weather in early April resulted in rapid plant growth and unusually high numbers of eastern tent caterpillars. An absence of eastern tent caterpillars and feeding hay to mares on pasture were associated with few or no abortions. Recently, early- and late-term abortions have been caused by intragastrically inoculating pregnant mares with crushed caterpillars in water. Current recommendations for control of MRLS consist of controlling tent caterpillars and removing wild cherry trees (the principal food source for the caterpillars), frequently mowing pastures used by pregnant mares, and feeding hay to mares on pasture. Secondary measures include increasing the ratio of grass-to-clover in pastures (the presence of higher than average amounts of clover was also associated with increased incidence of MRLS) and reducing the time mares spend on pasture when a hard freeze following a warm spell is expected.

Fescue Grass Toxicosis: Ingestion of fescue infected by the endophyte *Acremonium* causes prolonged gestation, agalactia, and perinatal death. The placenta is thickened and edematous and does not rupture normally at the cervical star. The chorioallantois precedes the foal through the birth canal instead of remaining attached to the uterus, resulting in anoxia and death of the fetus. The source of the infected fescue can be pasture, hay, or bedding. (*See also* p 2418.)

Infectious Causes

Infectious causes of abortion include viral diseases (such as equine rhinopneumonitis and equine viral arteritis) as well as bacterial and fungal infections.

Equine Rhinopneumonitis (Equine Herpesvirus 1): This is the most important viral cause of abortion in horses. Abortion is usually after 7 mo of gestation and is not preceded by maternal illness. The placenta may be edematous or normal. Gross fetal lesions include subcutaneous edema, jaundice, increased volume of thoracic fluid, and an enlarged liver with yellow-white lesions ~1 mm in diameter. Histologically, these lesions represent areas of necrosis containing intranuclear inclusions. Inclusion bodies are also found in necrotic lymphoid tissues. There is often a necrotizing bronchiolitis. Diagnosis is by fluorescent antibody or virus isolation from fetal tissues. Prevention is based on vaccinating at 5, 7, and 9 mo of gestation as well as preventing exposure of pregnant mares to horses attending shows or other equine events. (*See also* p 1203.)

Equine Viral Arteritis (EVA): Abortion may follow clinical cases of EVA by 6-29 days. Arteritis may be found in the fetal myocardium or placenta, but usually there are no fetal lesions. Stallions can be persistently infected, and EVA can spread venereally or by aerosol. Diagnosis is by a history of EVA shortly before abortion, virus isolation from the fetus, or by seroconversion of the dam. Vaccines are available on a limited basis in some states. (*See also* p 560.)

Bacterial Abortion: Potomac horse fever (p 236) caused by *Ehrlichia risticii* may be followed by abortion in mid to late gestation. There is placentitis and the placenta is often retained. The organism has been isolated from fetal lymphoid tissues after abortion. Histologically, there is fetal colitis. Identification of this colitis provides a presumptive diagnosis. There is a vaccine for Potomac horse fever, but its efficacy in preventing abortion is not known.

Leptospirosis has recently been recognized as an important cause of sporadic equine abortion in Kentucky, Northern Ireland, and England. Most fetuses are aborted after 6 mo of gestation and the mares are usually healthy. Infection does not appear to spread horse-to-horse, and often only a single mare on a farm aborts. There are no gross lesions in the fetus or placenta, but microscopically there is suppurative placentitis. Diagnosis is by fluorescent antibody staining of placenta or fetal kidney, liver, or lung and by fetal serology. A large majority of the cases in Kentucky are caused by *Leptospira interrogans* serovar *pomona* type *kennewicki*, although other serovars have also been identified.

Abortion due to *Streptococcus zooepidemicus*, other *Streptococcus* spp, *Salmonella*, *Escherichia coli*, *Pseudomonas*, *Klebsiella*, or other bacteria usually is caused by an ascending infection through the cervix that results in placentitis. The placenta is edematous with brown fibrinonecrotic exudate near the cervical star. Chronic placentitis results in retardation of fetal growth. The fetus may be severely autolyzed when expelled. Organisms can be recovered from aseptically obtained stomach contents.

Equine Mycotic Placentitis: Mycotic placentitis in horses is also due to an ascending infection that causes a thickened chorioallantois with variable exudate. Causative agents include *Aspergillus*, *Mucor*, and *Candida*. Fetuses aborted in late gestation may be fresh, with evidence of growth retardation. A pale, enlarged liver or a dermatitis may be found. Hyphae are found in the placenta, liver, lungs, or stomach contents.

BOVINE GENITAL CAMPYLOBACTERIOSIS

Bovine genital campylobacteriosis is a venereal disease of cattle characterized primarily by early embryonic death, infertility, a protracted calving season, and occasionally abortion. Distribution is probably worldwide.

Etiology and Epidemiology: The cause is the motile, gram-negative, curved or spiral, polar flagellated, microaerophilic bacteria *Campylobacter fetus venerealis* or *C fetus fetus*. For many years, it was thought that *C fetus fetus* was generally an intestinal organism, only occasionally caused abortion in cattle, and was not a cause of infertility. However, *C fetus fetus* can also be a significant cause of the classic infertility syndrome usually attributed to *C fetus venerealis*. There are several strains of *C fetus fetus*, and the only way to determine if a strain is a cause of infertility is to test that possibility in a group of heifers. *Campylobacter* spp are very labile and are destroyed quickly by heating, drying, and exposure to the atmosphere. Unless cultured quickly after collection from the animal and grown under microaerophilic or anaerobic conditions, campylobacters will not grow.

C fetus is transmitted venereally and also by contaminated instruments, bedding, or by artificial insemination using contaminated semen. Individual bulls vary in their susceptibility to infection; some become permanent carriers, while others appear to be resistant to infection. The primary factor associated with this variability seems to be the age-related depth of the preputial and penile epithelial crypts. In young bulls (<3-4 yr of age), in which the crypts have not yet developed, infection tends to be transient, with transmission apparently relying on sexual contact with a noninfected cow within a matter of minutes to days following the initial breeding of an infected cow. Spontaneous clearance in these younger bulls does not seem to be related to any immune response, so reinfection can readily occur. In bulls >3-4 yr old, the deeper crypts may provide the proper microaerophilic environment required for the establishment of chronic infections. In cows, the duration of the carrier state is also variable; some clear the infection rapidly, while others can carry *C fetus* for ≥2 yr. IgA antibodies are shed in cervical mucus in significant amounts in ~50% of cows for several months after infection and are useful diagnostically. Although most of the genital tract may be free of infection when a cow eventually conceives, the vagina may remain chronically infected through pregnancy.

Clinical Findings: Cows are systemically normal, but there is a variable degree of mucopurulent endometritis that causes early embryonic death, prolonged luteal phases, irregular estrous cycles, repeat breeding and, as a result, protracted calving periods, assuming the breeding season is long enough to allow for complete clearance and a successful rebreeding. Observed abortions are not common. In herds not managed intensively, disease may be noticed only when pregnancy examinations reveal low or marginally low pregnancy rates but, more importantly, great variations in gestation lengths, especially when the disease has recently been introduced to the herd. In subsequent years, infertility is usually confined to replacement heifers and a few susceptible cows. Bulls are asymptomatic and produce normal semen.

Diagnosis: Campylobacteriosis and trichomoniasis (p 1142) are similar syndromes, and investigations should be directed at both diseases. Systemic antibody responses are not helpful because they are often due to nonpathogenic *Campylobacter* spp. A vaginal mucus agglutination test (VMAT) is useful, but due to variability in individual responses, at least 10% of the herd or at least 10 cows should be sampled. An ELISA test has been developed for use on vaginal mucus and is said to be more sensitive and able to detect a wider range of antibody responses than the VMAT. Vaginal culture immediately after abortion or infection can be used for diagnosis, but the number of organisms may be low; in addition, because *C fetus* is labile and requires special techniques for isolation, success is limited. An accurate diagnostic method is to test-breed heifers and then examine them for infection, but this is seldom practical. More often, the preputial cavity and fornix are either scraped and aspirated with an infusion pipette or infused with buffered sterile saline, and the prepuce is massaged vigorously in the area of the fornix. The aspirate or sheath washing is then examined using a fluorescent antibody test and culture. *C fetus* will survive for only 6-8 hr after collection, but inoculation into Clark's or similar media will allow survival for >48 hr. For maximum accuracy, bulls should be sampled twice, ~1 wk apart. Caution should be exercised when *Campylobacter* spp are isolated from the placenta because of the possibility of contamination by nonpathogenic fecal *Campylobacter* spp. Conversely, failure to successfully isolate *C fetus* from an infected aborted fetus or placenta often results from overgrowth of the colonies by contaminating organisms or the lethal effects of atmospheric oxygen.

Treatment and Control: Vaccination should start as soon as genital campylobacteriosis is diagnosed. Both infected cows and cows at risk should be vaccinated. Vaccination of infected cows hastens the elimination of *C fetus* and, although cows may remain carriers, fertility is greatly improved. In routine use, the vaccine should be given once, ~4 wk before breeding starts; because antibody responses are short-lived, cows should be revaccinated halfway through the breeding season. Bulls are vaccinated for the same reason as cows (ie, for treatment as well as for prophylaxis) but are given twice the dose used for cows, 3 wk apart. The infection can also be eliminated in bulls by treatment with streptomycin (20 mg/kg, SC, 1-2 treatments) together with 5 g of streptomycin in an oil-based suspension applied to the penis for 3 consecutive days. For practical reasons, cows are not usually treated for genital campylobacteriosis. When practical, artificial insemination is an excellent way to prevent or control genital campylobacteriosis. Because *C fetus* has been isolated from cows for >6 mo after the end of pregnancy, it has been suggested that artificial insemination should continue until all the cows in a herd have been through at least 2 pregnancies.

BRUCELLOSIS IN LARGE ANIMALS

Brucellosis is caused by bacteria of the genus *Brucella* and is characterized by abortion, retained placenta, and to a lesser extent, orchitis and infection of the accessory sex glands in males. The disease is prevalent in most countries of the world. It primarily affects cattle, buffalo, bison, pigs, sheep, goats, dogs (p 1159), elk, and occasionally horses. The disease in humans, sometimes referred to as undulant fever, is a serious public health problem, especially when caused by *B melitensis*.

BRUCELLOSIS IN CATTLE
(Contagious abortion, Bang's disease)

Etiology and Epidemiology: The disease in cattle, water buffalo, and bison is caused almost exclusively by *B abortus*; however, *B suis* or *B melitensis* is occasionally implicated in some cattle herds. *B suis* does not appear to be contagious from cow to cow. Infection spreads rapidly and causes many abortions in unvaccinated cattle. In a herd in which disease is endemic, an infected cow typically aborts only once after exposure; subsequent gestations and lactations appear normal. After exposure, cattle become bacteremic for a short period and develop agglutinins and other antibodies; some resist infection and a small percentage of infected cows recover. A positive serum agglutination test usually precedes an abortion or a normal parturition but may be delayed in ~15% of cows. The incubation period may be variable and is inversely related to stage of gestation at time of exposure. Organisms are shed in milk and uterine discharges, and the cow may become temporarily infertile. Bacteria may be found in the uterus during pregnancy, uterine involution, and infrequently, for a prolonged time in the nongravid uterus. Shedding from the vagina largely disappears with the decrease of fluids following parturition. Some infected cows that previously aborted shed brucellae from the uterus at subsequent normal parturitions. Organisms are shed in milk for a variable length of time—in most cattle for life.

Natural transmission occurs by ingestion of organisms, which are present in large numbers in aborted fetuses, fetal membranes, and uterine discharges. Cattle may ingest contaminated feed and water, or lick contaminated genitals of other animals. Venereal transmission by infected bulls to susceptible cows appears to be rare. Transmission may occur by artificial insemination when *Brucella*-contaminated semen is deposited in the uterus but, reportedly, not when deposited in the midcervix. Brucellae may enter the body through mucous membranes, conjunctivae, wounds, or intact skin.

Brucellae have been recovered from fetuses and from manure that has remained in a cool environment for >2 mo. Exposure to direct sunlight kills the organisms within a few hours.

Clinical Findings: Abortion is the most obvious manifestation. Infections may also cause stillborn or weak calves, retained placentas, and reduced milk yield. Usually, general health is not impaired in uncomplicated abortions.

Seminal vesicles, ampullae, testicles, and epididymides may be infected in bulls; therefore, organisms are present in the semen. Agglutinins may be demonstrated in seminal plasma from infected bulls. Testicular abscesses may occur. Longstanding infections may result in arthritic joints in some cattle.

Diagnosis: Diagnosis is based on bacteriology or serology. *B abortus* can be recovered from the placenta but more conveniently in pure culture from the stomach and lungs of an aborted fetus. Most cows cease shedding organisms from the genital tract when uterine involution is complete. Foci of infection remain in some parts of the reticuloendothelial system, especially supramammary lymph nodes, and in the udder. *B abortus* can frequently be isolated from secretions of nonlactating udders.

Serum agglutination tests have been the standard diagnostic method. Agglutination tests may also detect antibodies in milk, whey, semen, and plasma. An ELISA has been developed to detect antibodies in milk and serum. When the standard plate or tube serum agglutination test is used, complete agglutination at dilutions of 1:100 or more in serum samples of nonvaccinated animals, and of 1:200 of animals vaccinated between 4 and 12 mo of age, are considered positive, and the animals are classified as reactors. Other tests that may be used are complement fixation, rivanol precipitation, and acidified antigen procedures.

Screening Tests: 1) *Brucella* milk ring test (BRT): In official control and eradication programs on an area basis, the BRT has been effective in locating infected dairy herds, but there is a high percentage of false positive tests. The brucellosis status of dairy herds in any area can be monitored by implementing the BRT at 3- to 4-mo intervals. Milk samples from individual herds are collected at the farm or milk processing plant. Cows in herds with a positive BRT are individually blood tested, and reactors are slaughtered.

2) Market cattle testing: Nondairy and dairy herds in an area may also be screened for brucellosis by testing serum samples collected from cattle destined for slaughter or replacements through intermediate and terminal markets, or at abattoirs. Reactors are traced to the herd of origin, and the herd is tested. The cost of identifying reactors by this method is minimal compared with that of testing all cattle in all herds. Screening tests, including the brucellosis card (or rose bengal) test and plate test, may be used in markets and laboratories to identify presumptively infected animals, thus reducing the number of more expensive and laborious diagnostic tests.

Brucellosis-free areas can be achieved and maintained, effectively and economically, by using the BRT on dairy herds and through market cattle testing.

Supplemental tests using sensitive screening methods may be used in cattle in which the brucellosis status is unclear. Use of a battery of these tests improves the probability of detecting infected cattle that have remained in some herds as possible reservoirs of infection. Supplemental tests are also used to clarify the results of plate or card tests, especially in serum samples from vaccinated cattle. These tests, which include complement fixation and rivanol precipitation, are designed to detect primarily the antibodies specifically associated with *Brucella* infection. Another supplemental diagnostic procedure is testing milk samples from individual udder quarters by serial dilution BRT, which can be used to detect chronic infection in udders of cows that may have equivocal serum test reactions.

Control: Efforts are directed at detection and prevention because no practical treatment is available. Eventual eradication depends on testing and eliminating reactors. The disease has been eradicated from many individual herds and areas by this method. Herds must be tested at regular intervals until 2 or 3 successive tests are negative.

Noninfected herds must be protected. The greatest danger is from replacement animals. Additions should be vaccinated calves or nonpregnant heifers. If pregnant or fresh cows are added, they should originate from brucellosis-free areas or herds and be seronegative. Replacements should be isolated for ~30 days and retested before being added to the herd.

Vaccination of calves with *B abortus* Strain 19 or RB51 increases resistance to infection. Resistance may not be complete, and some vaccinated calves may become infected, depending on severity of exposure. A small percentage of vaccinated calves develop antibodies to Strain 19 that may persist for years, which may confuse diagnostic test results. To minimize this problem, calves in the USA are vaccinated with a vaccine that contains 3-10 billion viable *B abortus* Strain 19 organisms per 2 mL dose. Strain RB51 has largely replaced Strain 19. It is a rough attenuated strain and does not cause production of antibodies, which are detected by most serologic tests.

Whole-herd adult cattle vaccination using Strain 19 or RB51 has been practiced in certain high-incidence areas and selected herds in the USA with much success.

Vaccination as the sole means of disease control has been effective. Reduction in the number of reactors in a herd is directly related to the percentage of vaccinated animals. However, when proceeding from a control to an eradication program, a test and slaughter program is necessary. The low prevalence of brucellosis in cattle in the USA has resulted in reduced use of vaccines and current emphasis on depopulation of infected herds.

Brucellosis is endemic in some nondomesticated bison and elk herds in the USA. Transmission of *B abortus* to domestic cattle herds is rare. Nevertheless, many controversies have developed concerning possible control methods. Vaccination of some elk populations has been practiced.

BRUCELLOSIS IN GOATS

The signs of brucellosis in goats are similar to those in cattle. The disease is prevalent in most countries where goats are a significant part of the animal industry. It is rare in the USA. The causal agent is *B melitensis*. Infection occurs primarily through ingestion of the organisms. The disease causes abortion about the fourth month of pregnancy. Arthritis and orchitis may occur. Diagnosis is made by bacteriologic examination of milk or an aborted fetus or by serum agglutination tests. The disease can be eliminated by slaughter of the herd. In most countries where *B melitensis* is endemic, vaccination with the Rev. 1 strain is common. Rev. 1 is an attenuated strain of *B melitensis* and is administered by SC or intraconjunctival routes.

BRUCELLOSIS IN HORSES

Horses can be infected with *Brucella abortus* or *B suis*. Suppurative bursitis, most commonly recognized as fistulous withers or poll evil (p 864), is the most common condition associated with brucellosis in horses. Occasionally, abortion has been reported. It is unlikely that infected horses are a source of the disease for other horses, other animal species, or humans.

BRUCELLOSIS IN PIGS

Clinical manifestations of brucellosis in pigs vary but are similar to those seen in cattle and goats. Although the disease is often self-limiting, it remains in some herds for years. Brucellosis caused by *Brucella suis* rarely occurs in other domestic animals. Epidemics of brucellosis in humans have been reported among packing-house workers, and the usual source is infected pigs. The prevalence in the USA is highest among feral pigs. The incidence of swine brucellosis among domesticated animals in the USA is very low.

Etiology and Transmission: *B suis* is usually spread mainly by ingestion of infected tissues or fluids. Infected boars may transmit the disease during service; the organism can be recovered from semen.

Pigs raised for breeding purposes are sources of infection. Suckling pigs may become infected from sows, but most reach weanling age without becoming infected.

Clinical Findings: After exposure to *B suis*, pigs develop a bacteremia that may persist for up to 90 days. During and after the bacteremia, localization may occur in various tissues. Signs depend considerably on the site(s) of localization. Common manifestations are abortion, temporary or permanent sterility, orchitis, lameness, posterior paralysis, spondylitis, and occasionally metritis and abscess formation.

The incidence of abortion may be 0-80%. Abortions may also occur early in gestation and be undetected. Usually, sows or gilts that abort early in gestation return to estrus soon afterward and are rebred.

Sterility in sows, gilts, and boars is common and may be the only manifestation. Before attempting treatment for other diseases, it is logical to test for brucellosis in herds in which sterility is a problem. Sterility in sows is more frequently temporary but may be permanent. In boars, orchitis, usually unilateral, may occur, and fertility appears to be reduced.

Diagnosis: The principal means of diagnosis in pigs is the brucellosis card test; however, various other serum agglutination tests or complement fixation tests have been used. It is generally accepted that the tests have limitations in detecting brucellosis in individual pigs. Thus, entire herds or units of herds, rather than individual pigs, must be tested in any control program. Low agglutinin titers are seen in almost any size herd, regardless of infection status, and a few infected pigs may have no detectable titer. The card test is usually more accurate than conventional agglutination tests. Supplemental tests designed for cattle may also be used for pigs.

Prevention and Control: Caution should be followed in the purchase of individual pigs that exhibit a low agglutinin titer unless the status of the entire herd of origin is known. Pigs should be isolated on return from fairs or shows before re-entering the herd. Replacements should be purchased from herds known to be free of brucellosis, or they should be tested and isolated for 3 mo and retested before being added to the herd. There is no vaccine for brucellosis in swine, and no practical recommendations can be made for treatment. Control is based on test and segregation, and slaughter of infected breeding stock.

BRUCELLOSIS IN SHEEP

Brucella melitensis infection in certain breeds of sheep causes clinical disease similar to that in goats (*see* p 1112). However, *B ovis* produces a disease unique to sheep, in which epididymitis and orchitis impair fertility—the principal economic effect. Occasionally, placentitis and abortion are seen, and there may be perinatal mortality. The disease was first described in New Zealand and Australia and has since been reported from many sheep-raising areas of the world.

Rams as young as 8 wk have been infected experimentally by various nonvenereal routes. The disease can be transmitted among rams by direct contact. Active infection in ewes is unusual but has developed after mating with naturally infected rams. Contaminated pastures do not appear to be important in spread of the disease. Infection frequently persists in rams, and a high percentage shed *B ovis* intermittently for several years.

Primary manifestations are lesions of the epididymis, tunica, and testis in rams; placentitis and abortion in ewes; and occasionally perinatal death in lambs. Lesions may develop rapidly. In rams, the first detectable abnormality may be a marked deterioration in semen quality associated with the presence of inflammatory cells and organisms. An acute systemic phase is rarely seen in naturally occurring infections. After regression of the acute phase—which may be so mild as to go unobserved—lesions may be palpated in the epididymis and scrotal tunics. Epididymal enlargement may be unilateral or bilateral. The tail of the epididymis is involved more frequently than the head or body, and the most prominent lesion is spermatoceles of variable size containing partially inspissated spermatic fluid. The tunics frequently become thickened and fibrous, and extensive adhesions develop between them. The testes may show fibrous atrophy; these lesions are usually permanent. In a few cases, palpable lesions are transient, while in others, organisms may be present in semen over long periods without clinically detectable lesions.

Because not all infected rams show palpable abnormalities of scrotal tissues (and not all cases of epididymitis are due to brucellosis), the remaining rams must be examined further. Rams shedding organisms, but having no lesions, must be identified by culture of semen. Repeated examinations may be necessary to identify intermittent shedders. Microscopic examination of stained semen smears may also be helpful; fluorescent antibody examination is a highly specific diagnostic aid. Serologic tests used for eradication of disease and certification of animals include ELISA, complement fixation, hemagglutination inhibition, indirect agglutination, and gel diffusion.

Incidence and spread of the disease may be reduced by regular examination of rams before the breeding season and culling of those with obvious genital abnormalities. Because susceptibility in rams increases markedly with age, it is advantageous to keep a young ram flock and isolate noninfected rams from older, possibly infected rams.

Immunization of rams has been practiced extensively in New Zealand using 2 doses of killed *B ovis* cells in adjuvant. Immunization of weaner rams with attenuated (Rev. 1) *B melitensis* has been recommended in other countries. Because infection in ewes apparently originates almost exclusively from service by infected rams, lamb losses through infection of ewes may be controlled economically by restricting vaccination to rams. There is no recommended vaccination in the USA.

Chlortetracycline and streptomycin used concurrently have effected bacteriologic cures. However, treatment is not economic except in especially valuable rams, and even if infection is eliminated, fertility may remain impaired.

CONTAGIOUS AGALACTIA AND OTHER MYCOPLASMAL MASTITIDES OF SMALL RUMINANTS

Known for nearly 200 years, contagious agalactia is primarily a disease of dairy sheep and goats. In lactating female animals, it is characterized by mastitis. Males, young animals, and nonlactating females develop arthritis, keratoconjunctivitis, and respiratory problems. Pregnant females can abort. It is mainly caused by *Mycoplasma agalactiae* but in recent years, *M capricolum capricolum* (*Mcc*), *M mycoides mycoides* LC (*Mmm* LC), and *M putrefaciens* have also been isolated in many countries. The clinical signs of these infections are sufficiently similar to those of contagious agalactia for the OIE to include them as causes of this list B disease.

Etiology and Epidemiology: Sheep and goats are equally susceptible to *M agalactiae*, but goats are additionally affected by *Mcc*, *Mmm* LC, and *M putrefaciens*. Reports from north Africa indicate that *Mcc* may also be a problem in sheep. In general, clinical disease is more pronounced in goats. Antibodies to *Mmm* LC and *Mcc* have been detected in South American camelids, but no mycoplasmas have yet been isolated. As alpacas, llamas, and vicunas develop polyarthritis, pneumonia, and pleuritis, it is likely that mycoplasmas may eventually be found. *Mmm* LC have also been isolated from cattle, although its role in disease in this species is not clear.

Contagious agalactia has been reported in southern Europe, in particular France, Portugal, Spain, Greece, and Italy; Turkey and many parts of the Middle East; India; USA; South America; and north central, and eastern Africa. Recently *Mmm* LC has also been reported in arthritic goats and cattle in New Zealand and in goat kids with polyarthritis in Hungary.

The disease predominantly affects milking sheep and goats. It often appears in a herd soon after lactation begins in the spring, and probably represents the activation of latent infection. Young ruminants become infected directly while suckling; adults are contaminated via the milker's hands, milking machines, or by bedding, which often provides a rich source of mycoplasmas. Transmission by aerosol in infective exudates over short distances and ingestion of contaminated water may also lead to infection. Organisms can persist for >1 yr after clinical recovery in infected animals. The introduction of such carriers into a susceptible flock can cause high morbidity (30-60%) and mortality, especially in lambs and kids (40-70%).

M putrefaciens is common in milking goat herds in western France where it can be isolated from animals with and without clinical signs, although milk production is usually severely affected. It has also been associated with a large outbreak of mastitis and agalactia leading to severe arthritis in goats accompanied by abortion and death in California. *M putrefaciens* was the major finding in an outbreak of polyarthritis in kids in Spain.

Clinical Findings and Lesions: The course of disease is more likely to be chronic with *M agalactiae*, while in goats, *Mmm* LC, *Mcc*, and *M putrefaciens* usually produce acute or hyperacute infection, often with respiratory complications. Animals in the early acute stage of disease show a general malaise that corresponds to septicemia. In <1 wk, animals can become hyperthermic (>41°C), prostrated, and show inappetence. Pregnant females near term may abort. While some animals die without showing any other signs, most develop severe mastitis followed by arthritis and keratitis. An unusual feature of outbreaks caused by *M putrefaciens* is the lack of fever in affected does and kids.

The main target organ of contagious agalactia is the mammary gland, in which a fall in or complete loss of milk production, sometimes within 2-3 days, can be seen. The milk may appear yellow and granular and take on a thick consistency with milk clots that may obstruct the teat duct. The causative mycoplasmas can be isolated from milk when mastitis is present. The udder may become hot, swollen, and tender. In the later stages, the udder atrophies due to extensive fibrosis of the secretory tissue. The severity of arthritis/polyarthritis may range from joint stiffness to severe lameness in which joints—typically the tarsus, carpus, and hock—are swollen with accumulations of synovial fluid. This fluid can be a rich source of specific antibody (often at a higher titer than in the serum) and the causative mycoplasmas themselves. Ocular lesions begin with conjunctivitis and congestion, lacrimation, and photophobia, followed by vascularization of the cornea, inflammatory foci, and parenchymatous keratitis. Severe cases can lead to blindness. Pneumonia has also been reported in cases of contagious agalactia, especially in young animals in which it may represent the only external sign.

Diagnosis: Clinical diagnosis in a severely infected flock is easy as the 3 major signs—mastitis, arthritis, and keratoconjunctivitis—are present within a flock, though rarely in the same animal. However, an acute form, in which there is septicemia without specific local signs, can confuse the diagnosis.

Laboratory diagnosis is the only means of confirmation. Preferred samples from living animals include nasal swabs and secretions, milk from mastitic does or from apparently healthy does when there is a high rate of mortality and morbidity in kids, joint fluid from arthritic cases, eye swabs from cases of ocular disease, and blood for antibody detection from affected and nonaffected animals. The ear canal is a rich source of pathogenic mycoplasmas. Mycoplasmas may be isolated from blood during the acute stage of the disease. Samples from dead animals should include udder and associated lymph nodes, joint fluid, lung tissue (at the interface between diseased and healthy tissue), and pleural or pericardial fluid. Samples should be kept moist and cool and sent promptly to a diagnostic laboratory. PCR tests, which can be performed directly on clinical samples, including milk, can be used to confirm the diagnosis.

Detection of antibodies in serum by complement fixation test or ELISA provides rapid diagnosis but may not be very sensitive in chronically affected herds and flocks. Indirect ELISA, some of which are commercially available, have been used routinely in control programs to screen herds for *M agalactiae* but less so for *Mmm* LC and *Mcc*. Confirmation of infection by isolation and identification is usually necessary in areas believed to be free of contagious agalactia. Serologic tests are not widely available for *M putrefaciens*.

A number of other mycoplasmas such as *M arginini*, *M* serogroup 11, and *M bovis* have occasionally been isolated from mastitic milk, eye swabs, and joint fluids, but their pathogenicity is unknown. Other bacteria causing mastitis include staphylococci, streptococci, *Escherichia coli*, and *Klebsiella*; caprine arthritic encephalomyelitis virus and *Erysipelothrix rhusiopathiae* should also be considered in cases of arthritis.

Treatment, Control, and Prevention: Antibiotics, such as the penicillins, that inhibit cell wall synthesis are not effective against contagious agalactia. Tetracyclines and macrolides can sometimes bring about clinical improvement, but there is always the danger of creating inapparent carriers. Furthermore, erythromycin and tylosin can cause destruction of milk-producing tissue in small ruminants. In many disease-free countries and regions, a confirmed infected herd would be slaughtered.

Regular laboratory monitoring of flocks/herds and replacement animals may help to prevent spread or introduction of disease and can be done on serum and/or milk (including bulk tank milk) by serology, culture, or PCR. Culling or isolation of infected animals is generally advised because udder damage is considered permanent. When this is not possible, hygienic measures, such as improved milking hygiene and pasteurizing milk before feeding to the young, should be implemented.

In countries bordering the Mediterranean, both attenuated and inactivated vaccines have been used with mixed success. Some have provided protection from clinical disease and have been useful in endemic areas; however, they do not prevent transmission of the mycoplasmas. Generally, the duration of immunity, particularly to the formalinized, inactivated vaccines that are used in Europe, is short. New developments with recombinant vaccines and improved adjuvants may eventually help to improve control.

CYSTIC OVARY DISEASE

Among domestic animals, cystic ovary disease is most common in cattle, particularly the dairy breeds, but it occurs sporadically in dogs (p 1153), cats, pigs, and perhaps mares. When diagnosing the reproductive status of mares, it must be remembered that normal follicle size during estrus is 4-6 cm in diameter. Ovulation failure can also be found in mares that are having irregular estrous cycles during the spring or fall transition phases of the reproductive cycle, but this situation is not treated in the same way as the cystic ovary disease condition of cattle. The granulosa cell tumor condition in mares causes marked enlargement of one ovary but differs from cystic ovary disease of cattle (see MANAGEMENT OF REPRODUCTION: HORSES, p 1759).

Three ovarian structures in cattle include the term cyst: follicular cysts, luteal cysts, and cystic corpus luteum (CL). In contrast to the other 2, the structure described as a cystic CL arises after normal ovulation. Cystic CL are known to be a normal stage or variation of CL development because they are found in normally cycling and pregnant cows without concurrent abnormal reproductive performance. Cystic CL have a soft, mushy core area, due to presence of fluid from a degenerating blood clot, compared with the homogeneous, liver-like consistency of the base of a typical CL. Cystic CL are most often detected 5-7 days after estrus when the structure is nearing the end of the corpus hemorrhagicum or growth phase. The cystic CL as well as the typical CL may or may not have an ovulation crown or papilla at its apex. Absence of this ovulation crown or papilla should not be considered diagnostic of the cystic condition because 10-20% of functional, normal CL fail to develop this feature. The two pathologic forms of bovine cystic ovary disease, follicular cysts and luteal cysts, are etiologically and pathogenetically related but differ clinically.

FOLLICULAR CYSTIC OVARY DISEASE
(Follicular cysts, Cystic follicles, Nymphomania, "Bulling")

Behavioral and conformational manifestations of follicular cystic ovary disease vary considerably, as does the overall clinical picture. However, all the signs relate to the focal primary lesions, namely, thin-walled cysts in the ovary and the disruption of the normal endocrine events of the estrous cycle—especially absence of the negative feedback of progesterone from the CL on the hypothalamus and pituitary.

Cystic ovary disease primarily affects dairy cattle, although it has been reported occasionally in beef cattle. This difference is due to the more intensive management and treatment of individual dairy cows. The disease is more common among certain family lines within breeds, which implicates hereditary factors in the etiology.

The cystic ovary syndrome is commonly thought to be caused by high milk production. The observation is biased, however, because higher-producing cows are more likely to be examined, more likely to be treated if found to have cystic ovary disease, and more likely to be allowed to remain in the herd despite some decrease in reproductive performance. Evidence indicates that cystic ovary disease causes cows to produce more milk rather than that high production causes cows to develop cystic ovary disease. Incidence increases with age. Most cases occur within 3-8 wk of parturition at the first attempted postpartum ovulation, coinciding with peak daily milk production and rapidly decreasing body condition. The reported herd incidence is 5-25% per lactation, or higher in some problem herds, and can be influenced by herd-health programs in which examination and detection are emphasized.

Etiology and Pathogenesis: Hereditary predisposition has been implicated in dairy cattle; eg, daughters of previously cystic cows had a higher incidence of cystic ovary disease than did daughters of unaffected cows. Periparturient stress apparently serves as a trigger. The mechanism by which stress elicits the hypothalamic and pituitary defects in genetically predisposed cows is most commonly thought to be a relative deficiency in the release of luteinizing hormone (LH) at estrus. This may be a reflection of failure of hypothalamic release of gonadotropin-releasing hormone (GnRH). Another mechanism that can exist in some cows with cysts is a deficiency of LH and follicle-stimulating hormone receptors in developing follicles.

During normal proestrus, regression of the CL coincides with development of a selected follicle, while the growth of any additional follicles is inhibited. In animals developing cystic ovary disease, ovulation fails to occur and the dominant follicle continues to enlarge. Moreover, other follicles may grow and form multiple cysts either bilaterally or unilaterally. Grossly, follicular cysts resemble enlarged follicles, varying in size from 2.5 to 5-6 cm in diameter. The size and form of an affected ovary depends on the number and size of cysts present. The cystic ovary is capable, at least initially, of steroidogenesis, and its products vary from estrogens to progesterone to androgens. The actions of the various hormones produced or the absence of the stabilizing action of high progesterone from the normal CL during ~75% of the estrous cycle (or both) are responsible for the changes seen in the genital tract, body conformation, and general behavior.

Clinical Findings: Behavioral aberrations range from anestrus to frequent, intermittent estrus with exaggerated monosexual drive to bull-like behavior, including mounting, pawing the ground, and bellowing. This behavior often is accompanied by masculinization of the head and neck. Relaxation of the vulva, perineum, and the large pelvic ligaments, which causes the tail head to be elevated, is common in chronic cases. Some affected cows show these signs, but others may be sexually quiescent. This variation is due to the duration of the condition and the nature of the hormone signals or lack thereof from the diseased ovary. The affected ovaries generally are enlarged and rounded, but their size varies, depending on the number and size of cysts. Their surface is smooth, elevated, and blister-like, particularly when cysts exceed 2.5-3 cm in diameter. Cysts frequently are multiple and may approach 4-6 cm in diameter. Under the influence of hormones produced by the cystic ovary or the lack of hormones (especially progesterone) normally present during estrous cycles, the uterus undergoes palpable changes, which in turn vary with the duration of the cystic condition. Thus, during the first week, the uterine wall is thickened and edematous as an extension of the preceding estrus. Toward the end of the first week, the uterine wall develops a sponge-like consistency. In chronic cases, atony and atrophy of the uterine wall are common. Occasionally, the uterine horns become markedly shortened. Some degree of mucoid to mucopurulent vaginal discharge is common. Hydrometra, a fluid-filled, extremely thin-walled uterus, is seen occasionally.

Diagnosis: Larger, multiple cysts are easily identified by rectal palpation. History, conformation, and uterine changes, when present, provide supplemental diagnostic evidence. Palpation of the uterus is helpful for differentiation between a single follicular cyst and a mature graafian follicle; only the estrous cow has a coiled, extremely turgid uterus. Ultrasound technology per rectum can be used in differentiating cysts from corpora lutea and may be helpful in diagnosing cyst type (ie, follicular vs luteal).

Prognosis: From one viewpoint, the disease responds readily to treatment, be it mechanical (manual rupture) or hormonal. The success rate of manual rupture, when measured in terms of conceptions within 24 days, is ~50%; hormone therapy (*see* below) may be somewhat more successful but is more expensive. Aberrant behavior ceases soon after successful therapy. This is followed by normal conformation of the ovary; a normal, fertile estrus can be expected in 4-7 or 15-25 days after manual rupture and in 15-30 days after LH-type hormonal therapy. With GnRH therapy, 25% of cases required a second treatment, and 5% required a third. One-third of the cases treated for the third time failed to respond. Spontaneous recovery is possible and is most common in cases arising during the first 50 days after calving. That, and the observation that spontaneous recovery involves the same sequence of events as recovery in response to hormonal therapy, suggests caution in evaluating therapeutic efficiency. Each successfully treated cow is more likely to require treatment after the next parturition than are previously unaffected cows. Likewise, successful treatment encourages perpetuation of the disease in the herd if the offspring are used for breeding. While the cystic ovary condition in cattle clearly has a genetic component, it is unlikely that a single farm using artificial insemination can significantly influence the incidence. In Sweden, progress has been made in reducing the condition through culling and selection procedures for bulls used in artificial insemination, but affected cows are still treated.

Treatment: The oldest and least expensive treatment is manual rupture—the ovary is grasped and moderate pressure applied with finger pads, not tips, against the palm until the cyst bursts. After successful rupture, some have recommended that the ovary be compressed briefly to minimize hemorrhage; however, hemorrhage is rarely a sequela of rupture of correctly diagnosed follicular cysts. Hemorrhage probably occurs most often when the condition is misdiagnosed, and rupture of a CL or corpus hemorrhagicum is attempted. The potential danger of traumatizing the ovary and causing hemorrhage with subsequent local adhesions should not be overlooked, but manual rupture has been used often without problems. This method should be weighed against the cost of hormone therapy.

Of several hormone preparations recommended and used in the past, human chorionic gonadotropin (HCG) remains the only one still available and commonly used. It is most efficacious at 10,000 USP units IM, although success with lower doses given IM or IV has also been reported.

Newer hormone therapy includes GnRH or LH-releasing hormone products, which are efficacious at 100 μg, IM. GnRH products are equally effective but less antigenic than HCG. The 2 products may be alternated when retreatment is necessary. To hasten the onset of the first estrus after treatment, prostaglandins can be administered 9-10 days after HCG or GnRH. The claim that breeding on the first estrus is prone to produce twins has not been substantiated. In fact, breeding on the first estrus reduces danger of recurrence by establishing pregnancy as soon as possible.

Progesterone (or its analogs) has been given parenterally and PO to cows that do not respond to HCG and GnRH therapy, but in the USA these products have been removed from the cattle market or are not approved for use in lactating dairy cows. Progesterone treatment has been continued at least 10-12 days, if not 20, in expectation of a normal estrus on withdrawal.

Cystic Ovary Disease as a Herd Problem

Occasionally, individual herds experience exceptionally high rates (~50%) of cystic ovary disease over a period of months. Determining the cause of these episodes is not easy, but the following questions should be addressed: 1) Is the diagnosis accurate, ie, are the structures being identified as cysts really cysts? This can be established via second opinion diagnoses, determination of milk or plasma progesterone levels, ultrasound examination of the ovaries in suspected cases, observing ovarian changes and time of estrus activity after treatment with prostaglandin products, and/or improving diagnostic skills by continuing education. 2) Has the palpation examination schedule for the herd changed? Initiating routine postpartum examinations for all cows and increasing frequency of herd visits can result in an increased apparent incidence. 3) Has the herd incidence of periparturient complications and stress increased? Cows having problems around calving (such as twins, milk fever, dystocia, retained placenta, ketosis, etc) are much more likely to develop cysts. Attempts to reduce these complications are indicated. 4) Have herd genetics been considered? It is well accepted that ovarian cysts are more common in certain lines. 5) Has the nutritional program of the herd been evaluated? Nutritional problems are frequently implicated as causing cows to develop cysts, but rarely have these concerns been confirmed in controlled studies. Inadequacies or imbalances involving calcium and phosphorus, vitamin E and selenium, and energy are most often implicated. Moldy feed or roughages that contain high concentrations of estrogenic substances are also frequently suspected, but better testing methods are needed. Proper nutritional management of dairy herds is always warranted. Monitoring the effects of the nutritional program via a body condition scoring program should be used as part of the effort to reduce ovarian cysts in problem herds.

LUTEAL CYSTIC OVARY DISEASE
(Luteal cysts)

Luteal cystic ovary disease is characterized by enlarged ovaries with one or more cysts, the walls of which are thicker than those of follicular cysts because of a lining of luteal tissue. Incidence ratios of follicular versus luteal cysts vary greatly due to diagnostic tendencies of individual veterinarians. The apparent incidence of luteal cysts has risen in recent years. Some veterinarians now use a much more liberal definition of luteal cysts, including any variation from the classical corpus luteum (CL) type structure. This trend is probably a consequence of the commercial availability and widespread acceptance of the prostaglandin (PG) $F_{2\alpha}$ products in cattle for their luteolytic properties. The incidence pattern is similar to that of follicular cysts.

Etiology and Pathogenesis: The basic causes of true luteal cysts are believed to be the same as for follicular cysts. The release of luteinizing hormone (LH) may be somewhat greater than that occurring when follicular cysts develop, and sufficient to initiate luteinization of follicles but inadequate to cause ovulation. Luteal cysts are an extension of follicular cysts such that the nonovulatory follicle is partially luteinized spontaneously or in response to hormonal therapy.

Clinical Findings: Luteal cysts are accompanied by normal conformation and anestrous behavior. Rectal palpation reveals a quiescent uterus characteristic of the luteal phase of the estrous cycle. Luteal cysts are recognized as smooth, fluctuant domes protruding above the surface of the ovary. Usually, they are single structures. Luteal cysts are differentiated from follicular cysts on the basis of palpable characteristics of both the structure and the uterus and, to some extent, on the cow's behavior. Progesterone assay and ultrasonography can help differentiate between follicular and luteal cysts, although with either method a final diagnostic decision remains somewhat subjective. On attempts to manually rupture the cystic structure, follicular cysts burst or rupture under minimal pressure while luteal cysts cannot be ruptured with reasonable force. Both types of cysts respond to LH or gonadotropin releasing hormone (GnRH) therapy, but $PGF_{2\alpha}$ will lyse some luteal cysts and all diestrual CL structures. When applicable, the prostaglandin treatment is preferable to the human chorionic gonadotropin (HCG) or GnRH products due to its much shorter time from administration to estrus and its lower cost.

Treatment and Control: The treatment of choice is luteolytic doses of $PGF_{2\alpha}$. A normal estrus is expected in 3-5 days. The major limitation of this treatment is the difficulty in accurately estimating the amount of luteal tissue present. If the structure being diagnosed as a luteal cyst is really a developing CL (as discussed above, sometimes called a cystic CL), it may not respond because dairy cows do not become highly responsive to the luteolytic action of $PGF_{2\alpha}$ until day 8 after estrus. Luteal cysts also respond to HCG and GnRH therapy effective in the treatment of follicular cysts, but the next estrus could occur 5-21 days after treatment. Manual rupture of luteal cysts is not recommended.

Preventive measures are the same as for follicular cystic ovary disease (*see* above).

EQUINE COITAL EXANTHEMA

(Genital horsepox, Equine venereal balanitis in stallions)

Etiology and Epidemiology: Equine coital exanthema is a benign venereal disease of horses that probably occurs worldwide. It affects both sexes and is caused by equine herpesvirus type 3 (EHV-3). This virus has a single antigenic type but also has small and large plaque variants in tissue culture, indicating that variation may occur in the severity of field outbreaks. Although the primary route of transmission is venereal, outbreaks have been documented in which transmission occurred via contaminated supplies and instruments or by the use of a single glove for rectal examination of many mares. It is probably for this reason that EHV-3 has also been isolated from animals that have not been bred.

Equine coital exanthema is probably transmitted only in the acute phase of the disease; after the lesions have healed, horses do not appear to shed the virus. However, the existence of a carrier state is unclear: the scars that persist after healing may identify potential carriers, but such asymptomatic carriers have not been identified. Immunity is short-lived, but evidence from stallions shows that recurrence is not likely within a single breeding season.

Clinical Findings: Clinical signs in mares develop 4-8 days after sexual contact or veterinary examination and are manifest by the appearance of multiple, circular, red nodules up to 2 mm in diameter on the vulvar and vaginal mucosa, the clitoral sinus, and perineal skin. These lesions develop into vesicles and then pustules and eventually rupture, leaving shallow, painful, ulcerated areas that may coalesce into larger lesions. Edema can develop in the perineum and may extend to between the thighs. Occasionally, ulcers will be found on the teats, lips, and nasal mucosa. Secondary bacterial infection of the ulcers by *Streptococcus* spp is common, causing the ulcers to enlarge and exude a mucopurulent discharge. In such cases, the horse may become febrile. Unless secondary bacterial infection occurs, skin healing is complete within 3 wk, but clitoral and vaginal ulcers heal more slowly. Skin lesions persist for long periods as unpigmented scars. However, pregnancy rates are not reduced.

Lesions in stallions are similar to those in mares and are found on both the penis and prepuce. As a result, intromission is painful, and the stallion may be reluctant to copulate. If copulation does occur during the ulcerative stage, the ulcers may hemorrhage into the ejaculate, reducing sperm viability.

Diagnosis: A tentative diagnosis is based on clinical signs and confirmed by identifying (using electron microscopy) the virus in cells from the margin of ulcers. Typical intranuclear herpesvirus inclusion bodies can also be seen in cytologic or histologic preparations. Acute and convalescent samples for serum neutralization or complement fixation tests can also be diagnostic, but these tests must be interpreted carefully because both EHV-1 and EHV-4 have also been isolated from genital lesions.

Treatment and Prevention: Sexual rest is essential to allow ulcers to heal and prevent the spread of the disease. The use of antibiotic ointments to prevent secondary infections is also advisable. Affected horses should be isolated until all lesions have healed, and disposable equipment should be used for examinations. During the acute phase of the disease mares should be bred only by artificial insemination. No vaccine is available. All animals should be examined carefully before they are allowed to breed, keeping in mind that the incubation period is up to 10 days.

MASTITIS IN LARGE ANIMALS

Mastitis—inflammation of the mammary gland—is almost always due to the effects of infection by bacterial or mycotic pathogens. Pathologic changes to milk-secreting epithelial cells from the inflammatory process often bring about a decrease in functional capacity. Depending on the pathogen, functional losses may continue into further lactations, which impairs productivity and potential weight gain for offspring. Although most infections result in relatively mild clinical or subclinical local inflammation, more severe cases can lead to agalactia or even profound systemic involvement resulting in death. Mastitis has been reported in almost all domestic mammals, as well as humans, and has a worldwide geographic distribution. Climatic conditions, seasonal variation, density and housing of livestock populations, and husbandry practices may affect the incidence and etiology. However, it is of greatest frequency and economic importance in species that primarily function as producers of milk for dairy products, particularly dairy cattle. *See also* UDDER DISEASES, p 1144.

MASTITIS IN CATTLE

Almost any bacterial or mycotic organism that can opportunistically invade tissue and cause infection can cause mastitis. However, most infections are caused by various species of streptococci, staphylococci, and gram-negative rods, especially lactose-fermenting organisms of enteric origin, commonly termed coliforms. From an epidemiologic standpoint, the source of infection may be regarded as contagious or environmental. Except for *Mycoplasma* spp, which may spread from cow to cow through aerosol transmission and invade the udder subsequent to bacteremia, contagious pathogens are spread during milking by milkers' hands or the liners of the milking unit. Species that utilize this mode of transmission include *Staphylococcus aureus*, *Streptococcus agalactiae*, and *Corynebacterium bovis*. Most other species are opportunistic invaders from the cow's environment, although some other streptococci and staphylococci may also have a contagious component. The bedding used for housing cattle is the primary source of environmental pathogens, but contaminated teat dips, intramammary infusions, water hoses used for udder preparation during milking, water ponds or mud holes, skin lesions, teat trauma, and flies have all been incriminated as sources of infection.

Intramammary infections are often described as subclinical or clinical mastitis. **Subclinical mastitis** is the presence of an infection without apparent signs of local inflammation or systemic involvement. Although transient episodes of abnormal milk or udder inflammation may appear, these infections are for the most part asymptomatic and, if the infection persists for at least 2 mo, are termed chronic. Once established, many of these infections persist for entire lactations or the life of the cow. Detection is best done by examination of milk for somatic cell counts (predominantly neutrophils) using either the California Mastitis Test or automated methods provided by dairy herd improvement organizations. Somatic cell counts are positively correlated with the presence of infection. Although variable (especially if determined on a single analysis), cows with a somatic cell count of ≥280,000 cells/mL (≥ a linear score of 5) have a >80% chance of being infected. Likewise, the higher the somatic cell count in a herd bulk tank, the higher the prevalence of infection in the herd. Causative agents must be identified by bacterial culture of milk.

Clinical mastitis is an inflammatory response to infection causing visibly abnormal milk (eg, color, fibrin clots). As the extent of the inflammation increases, changes in the udder (swelling, heat, pain, redness) may also be apparent. Clinical cases that include local signs only are referred to as mild or moderate. If the inflammatory response includes systemic involvement (fever, anorexia, shock), the case is termed severe. If the onset is very rapid, as often occurs with severe clinical cases, it is termed an acute case of severe mastitis. More severely affected cows tend to have more serous secretions in the affected quarter. Although any number of quarters can be infected simultaneously in subclinical mastitis, typically only one quarter at a time will display clinical mastitis. However, it is not uncommon for clinical episodes caused by *Mycoplasma* to affect multiple quarters. Gangrenous mastitis can also occur, particularly when subclinical, chronic infections of *S aureus* become severe at times of immunosuppression (eg, at parturition). As with subclinical mastitis, culture of milk samples collected from affected quarters is the only reliable method to determine the etiology of clinical cases.

Subclinical Mastitis

Epidemiology: All dairy herds have cows with subclinical mastitis; however, the prevalence of infected cows varies from 15-75%, and quarters from 5-40%. Many different pathogens can establish a chronic infection that will only on occasion manifest clinical signs of mastitis. The primary focus of most subclinical mastitis programs is to reduce the prevalence of *Streptococcus agalactiae, Staphylococcus aureus*, and other gram-positive cocci, most notably *Streptococcus dysgalactiae* (which may also be contagious or an environmental pathogen), *Streptococcus uberis*, enterococci, and numerous other coagulase-negative staphylococci, including *S hyicus, S epidermidis, S xylosus* and *S intermedius*. Adult lactating cattle are most at risk for infection, either while lactating or during the dry period. The primary reservoir of infection is the mammary gland; transmission occurs at milking with either milkers' hands or milking equipment acting as fomites. Primiparous heifers have been reported to be infected with staphylococci and streptococci prior to calving, although the prevalence varies greatly among herds and geographic regions. Teat-end dermatitis caused by the horn fly, *Haematobia irritans*, which can harbor *S aureus*, has been associated with increased risk of infection in heifers, especially in warmer climates.

For the contagious pathogens and coagulase-negative staphylococci, there is little or no seasonal variation in incidence of infection.

Treatment: Therapy is given on the premise that treatment costs will be outweighed by production gains following elimination of infection. In the case of contagious pathogens, elimination may also result in a decrease of the reservoir of infection for previously noninfected cows. No significant economic losses will occur as a result of delaying therapy until bacterial culture can be completed. However, many subclinical cases selected as potential therapy candidates have chronic infections; particularly in the case of *S aureus*, prediction of therapeutic outcome by in vitro testing is unreliable. Drug distribution following intramammary administration may not be adequate due to extensive fibrosis and microabscess formation in the gland; it is critical to assess the cow's immune status from a perspective of duration of infection, number of quarters infected, and other variables.

Prevalence of *S agalactiae* infection can be rapidly reduced by treating an entire herd—or more economically, all the infected cows in a herd—with antibacterials. All 4 quarters of infected cows should be treated to ensure elimination of the pathogen and to prevent possible cross-infection of a noninfected quarter. Cure rates can often be 70-90%. Labeled use of commercial intramammary products that contain amoxicillin, penicillin, and erythromycin are as efficacious as procaine penicillin G infusions derived from multiple dose vials. Consequently, commercial intramammary infusions are preferred because of higher quality control for sterility and better reliability for predicting withholding periods for milk and meat after treatment. Treated herds must be monitored by somatic cell counts and bacteriology to further identify and treat cows that were not identified or cured during the initial therapy. Usually, 30-day monitoring intervals are successful. A small percentage of cows will not respond to therapy and are best segregated or culled. In addition, failure to use post-milking teat dipping and total dry cow treatment to prevent new infections during the treatment period will ultimately result in reinfection of the herd. Parenteral therapy is not likely to offer any benefit over intramammary therapy.

Most other streptococci also display in vitro susceptibility to numerous antibacterials, especially β-lactam drugs. Despite this apparent susceptibility, many streptococcal infections are not as easily cured as those caused by *S agalactiae*. Generally, subclinical infections caused by *S uberis* and *S dysgalactiae* should be preferentially treated at the end of lactation with intramammary infusions of commercial dry cow products. Cure rates at this time may exceed 75%.

Staphylococcus aureus intramammary infections often result in deep-seated abscesses. Therapy is difficult, as resistance to antibacterials (particularly β-lactams) is more common compared with streptococcal infections, and *S aureus* may survive intracellularly following phagocytosis when antibacterial concentrations are reduced. Intramammary infusions may cure only 35-40% of infections; however, this number will be substantially lower for chronic infections.

The success rate of therapy for chronic subclinical intramammary infections caused by *S aureus* may be increased by using both parenteral and intramammary therapy. However, systemic therapy involves extra-label drug use, and milk and meat withholding periods must be determined judiciously. Therapy should be administered for periods long enough (5-10 days) to allow effective killing of the pathogen. It is most economical and least likely to result in residues in milk if this therapy is applied to dry cows. Depending on susceptibility testing, lipophilic antibacterial drugs that distribute well into mammary tissue, such as oxytetracycline (11 mg/kg, SID) are the best candidates for systemic administration although several studies have found oxytetracycline to be ineffective. Cure rates may not be much better than those attained from spontaneous cure, and cure must be defined critically. Affected quarters should be monitored bacteriologically for ≥30 days to encompass the refractory period when bacteria may not be isolated.

Occasionally, premature agalactia will occur in chronically infected quarters, particularly quarters infected with resistant pathogens. Culling may be a practical option for these cows. Alternatively, it is common to dry off the infected quarter and continue to milk the cow. This may have some benefit for genetically superior animals within a herd or for cows that are to be maintained until calving. Anecdotally, the milk production from such cows may remain the same. The goal is to eliminate the infection by causing fibrosis of the affected quarter, thus reducing the risk of further pathogenic change or systemic effects on the cow, as well as reducing risk of infection for other cows. Infusion of 60 mL of 2% chlorhexidine into affected quarters twice at 24-hr intervals has been recommended. The quarter should be stripped out before the second infusion. Milk from noninfected quarters must not be sent to market before prior testing for inhibitors. Other methods of stopping a quarter from milking are simply to stop milking the quarter or to excise the teat through banding. This regimen is not recommended for most chronically infected animals.

Dry Cows: The dry period of the lactation cycle is a critical time for the udder health of dairy animals. The mammary gland undergoes marked biochemical, cellular, and immunologic changes. Involution of the mammary parenchyma begins 1-2 days after the end of lactation and continues for 10-14 days. During this time, the gland is particularly vulnerable to new intramammary infections. However, the involuted mammary gland offers the most hostile immune environment for bacterial pathogens. Consequently, the dry period is an ideal time to attain synergy between antibacterial therapy and immune function, without incurring the extensive costs typical of lactating cow therapy. Intramammary administration of antibacterials at the end of lactation has been a standard of dairy mastitis management for 30 yr. Numerous commercial products are available; the majority contain penicillin, cloxacillin, cephapirin, or a macrolide such as erythromycin or novobiocin. One tube per quarter is sufficient and should be administered immediately after the last milking of lactation. Therapy should not be repeated by intramammary infusion; if there is a need to extend therapy, systemic administration should be used as an adjunct to the intramammary infusion. In addition to eliminating existing subclinical infections, one of the most critical roles of dry cow therapy is the prevention of new infections. However, most commercial dry cow products have little or no activity against gram-negative pathogens, and their administration at the start of the dry period will not be effective against new infections that begin during the periparturient period.

Heifers: Heifers were previously considered to be essentially free of intramammary infections before calving, but recent studies have challenged this assumption. Many infections in calving heifers are caused by staphylococcal species other than *S aureus*, which have a high rate of spontaneous cure. However, under some herd conditions, a substantial portion of heifers are infected at calving; some of these infections are caused by pathogens such as *S aureus*. Potential sources include milk (fed to calves) and body sites such as tonsils and skin. There is also a geographic risk factor: fly bite dermatitis of the teat end, which compromises this important physical barrier to infection, may play a role in the pathogenesis. Intramammary infusions of β-lactam antibacterial drugs 7-14 days before expected calving dates reduce the rate of intramammary infections at calving. However, as with cows, strict teat-end antisepsis should be followed before infusion to prevent contamination; labor to handle animals for treatment can be extensive. This is not a recommended management program for many dairies.

However, if herd records indicate that an undesirable proportion of first lactation animals are infected at calving, particularly with staphylococci, this regimen may reduce losses.

Prevention: New infections caused by *S agalactiae* and *S aureus* can be prevented by focusing management efforts on milking technique and hygiene. Clean and dry bedding, clean and dry udders at the time of milking, and lack of teat-end lesions all have a positive effect on control. The single most important management practice to prevent transmission of new infections is the use of an effective germicide (eg, 1% iodophor or 4% hypochlorite) as a postmilking teat dip. These products should be applied as a dip (rather than a spray) immediately after milking. Other practices that may augment teat dipping include use of individual towels for drying teats, gloves for milkers' hands, use of a premilking germicide (spray or dip), cleaning milking units after an infected cow has been milked, or segregation of infected cows into a separate milk group. This last option may be difficult for cattle in free housing that are normally segregated for nutritional or reproductive reasons. Routine milking equipment evaluations should be conducted to ensure that the teat-end vacuum is operating at a proper level and remains stable during milking. Proper pulsator function should be maintained and liners and rubber air hoses should be replaced as needed.

Proper milking hygiene also reduces the new infection rate of noncontagious pathogens, but not to the same extent as for contagious pathogens. More importantly for environmental pathogens, cows should be provided dry, clean housing. Emphasis should be placed on bedding and any other practices that reduce the exposure of the teat end to bacteria. Inorganic bedding supports less bacterial growth than cellulose-based material; thus, sand is preferred over sawdust, straw, recycled paper, or manure. In particular, higher incidence of infections caused by *Klebsiella* has been associated with sawdust bedding. Similarly, a higher incidence of infections caused by environmental streptococci has been associated with straw bedding. Removing udder hair, preventing teat trauma, reducing udder edema in periparturient cows by nutritional management of potassium and sodium intake, and preventing frostbite and fly exposure all have a positive impact on environmental mastitis control.

Clinical Mastitis

When the balance between host defenses and invading pathogens attracts a marked inflammatory response, clinical signs become apparent. Infections from any pathogen can be clinical or subclinical, depending on the duration of infection, host immune status, and pathogen virulence. The control of clinical mastitis usually focuses on the prevention and elimination of pathogens that arise from an environmental reservoir. Thus, the epidemiology and prevention of clinical mastitis is similar to previously discussed concepts regarding the control of subclinical mastitis.

Epidemiology: Except for outbreaks of *Mycoplasma*, clinical mastitis in most dairy herds is caused by environmental pathogens. In addition, many clinical mastitis cases are transient, especially those that are initial episodes for a cow and quarter. Thus, from an epidemiologic perspective, assessment of clinical mastitis is based on incidence and not prevalence. The standard methods of monitoring subclinical mastitis, routine somatic cell counts (SCC) and culture of cows with elevated SCC, are poor indicators of clinical mastitis. Cows with high SCC caused by chronic infections may occasionally display clinical mastitis, although it is usually mild. However, cows with low SCC are also prone to develop clinical mastitis, especially those cases with an acute onset. Herds with low SCC may actually have a higher incidence of clinical cases caused by environmental organisms (30-50 cases/100 cows/yr) than herds with higher SCC. Similarly, routine culture of milk samples from a cow with low SCC is a poor indicator of the probability of developing clinical mastitis, especially if the culture yielded no organisms. Thus, records that indicate the incidence of clinical cases, and data from each case that may determine risk factors (eg, season, age, stage of lactation, and previous episodes) should be recorded as part of a mastitis control program. Milk samples should be collected from affected quarters and, when feasible, antibacterial susceptibility testing performed. For well managed herds in which mastitis caused by contagious pathogens has been controlled, a goal for the incidence of clinical mastitis should be 2 cases/100 cows milking/mo. Severe mastitis cases should be in the range of 1-2 cases/100 cows milking/yr. Typically, 10-40% of milk samples collected from clinical mastitis cases yield no organisms on culture. However, of the samples that do yield organisms, 90-95% of the isolated bacteria include a wide variety of streptococci, staphylococci, or coliforms. If this is not the case, especially if a single pathogen such as a noncoliform gram-negative rod or a fungus predominates, a point source of infection should be considered.

Severe Clinical Mastitis: Coliforms (lactose-fermenting gram-negative rods of the family Enterobacteriaceae) are the most common cause of this form of mastitis. Following infection, coliform numbers in milk increase rapidly, often attaining peak bacterial concentrations within a few hours. A subsequent decline (rapid in most cases but may take several days in truly severe mastitis) in bacterial concentration follows neutrophil migration into the gland. The majority of coliform infections are cleared from the gland with few or mild clinical signs. However, if bacterial concentrations are elevated enough to elicit an acute inflammatory response, systemic involvement is a frequent consequence. Coliform-related mastitis results in a higher incidence of cow death or agalactia-related culling (30-40%) than mastitis caused by other pathogens (2%). Prognosis for cases of *Klebsiella* infection should be particularly guarded, as cows are twice as likely to be culled or die than those infected by other coliforms. Thus, primary therapy for severe clinical mastitis should be directed against coliform organisms, although secondary consideration must be given for causative agents. Supportive care, including fluids, is usually indicated, and in the case of coliform mastitis, may be the most beneficial component of the therapeutic regimen. Antibacterial therapy is ideally based on identification of the causative pathogen; however, this is not attainable for some hours after initial case recognition. In addition, most antibacterial therapeutic regimens currently used for severe clinical mastitis in the USA are not approved by the FDA.

Many inflammatory and systemic changes seen in severe coliform mastitis result from the effects of release of lipopolysaccharide (LPS) endotoxin from the bacteria. By the time therapy is initiated, maximal release of LPS has likely occurred. Thus, the primary therapeutic concern is the treatment of endotoxin-induced shock with fluids, electrolytes, and anti-inflammatory drugs. IV fluids are preferred as the initial method of administration. If isotonic saline is administered, 30-40 L are necessary over a 4-hr period, which can be difficult under farm conditions. A practical alternative is 2 L of 7% NaCl (hypersaline) administered IV. This allows rapid fluid uptake from the body compartment into the circulation. Cows should then be offered free choice water to drink, and if at least 10 gal. is not consumed, 5-7 gal. should be pumped into the rumen. Many cows with endotoxic shock are marginally hypocalcemic, thus 500 mL calcium borogluconate should be administered SC (to avoid potential complications that could arise from IV administration). Alternatively, rapid absorption calcium gels, designed for periparturient hypocalcemia, can be given. If the cow remains in shock, continued fluid therapy should be administered PO or IV as isotonic, not hypertonic, fluids.

Glucocorticoids are particularly helpful in cases of mastitis caused by endotoxin-producing coliforms. They should be administered early in the course of disease for maximal efficacy. Administration of dexamethasone (30 mg, IM) to dairy cows immediately following introduction of *E coli* into the mammary gland has been reported to reduce mammary gland swelling and inhibition of rumen motility. Isoflupredone (10-20 mg, IM) has also been shown to reduce local mammary swelling. Cattle are sensitive to glucocorticoid-induced immune suppression; however, it is unlikely that one-time administration of a glucocorticoid will adversely affect cows with endotoxin-induced severe clinical mastitis. Temporary suppression of inflammation as manifested by reduced neutrophil migration may well be beneficial. Care should be exercised in administering these drugs to pregnant animals; however, severe clinical mastitis in and of itself may cause pregnancy loss in cattle.

There is little published research on the use of glucocorticoids for mastitis caused by gram-positive bacteria. It is reasonable to expect that gram-positive infections would be less likely to benefit from the anti-inflammatory activities of glucocorticoids and may even be adversely affected. Intramammary glucocorticoid administration to reduce local inflammation, without affecting the migration of neutrophils into the gland, is an attractive therapeutic option. Although products that combine antibacterial and glucocorticoid drugs for intramammary administration exist in Europe, it is not clear whether clinical benefit is gained when compared with antibacterial therapy alone. As a general guideline, glucocorticoid treatment should be reserved for severe cases of gram-negative mastitis, with a single dose administered early in the disease course.

NSAID are widely used for the treatment of acute mastitis. Aspirin, flunixin meglumine, flurbiprofen, carprofen, ibuprofen, and ketoprofen have been studied as treatments for experimental coliform mastitis or endotoxin-induced mastitis. Orally administered aspirin should be used with caution in acute coliform mastitis because it may lead to severe rumen atony. If used, the Food Animal Residue Avoidance Databank (FARAD) recommends a milk and slaughter withdrawal interval of 24 hr to reduce the risk of Reye's syndrome in children. Dipyrone has been studied and widely used as a treatment for acute mastitis. However, the use of dipyrone in food animals is specifically prohibited by the FDA and it is no longer available in the USA. Phenylbutazone has also been studied and widely used as a treatment for acute mastitis. However, the FDA and FARAD strongly discourage its use in food animals. The tolerance level for phenylbutazone is zero and detection of any concentration is an illegal residue. In addition, extended withdrawal intervals make phenylbutazone a poor economic choice.

Treatment with ketoprofen improved recovery of cows with acute clinical mastitis in a blinded, placebo-controlled study. Although ketoprofen is available as a veterinary product for use in horses, has a high therapeutic index, has favorable pharmacokinetics for use in lactating dairy cattle, and is approved for use in cattle in France, it is not currently labeled for food animal use in the USA. FARAD recommends withdrawal intervals of 7 days for slaughter and 24 hr for milk, with IV or IM administration, for dosages up to 3.3 mg/kg, SID, for up to 3 days.

Flunixin meglumine is labeled for beef and nonlactating dairy cattle with bovine respiratory disease. It is the only NSAID labeled for use in cattle in the USA and is therefore the most logical choice for treating clinical mastitis. In field studies, increased survival and improved milk production have not been demonstrated following treatment of clinical acute mastitis with flunixin meglumine at a dosage of 1.1 mg/kg. However, in studies of experimental mastitis, this drug reduced the severity of clinical signs such as fever, depression, heart and respiratory rates, and udder pain. FARAD recommends withdrawal intervals of 4 days for slaughter and 72 hr for milk when used as specified. As with the glucocorticoids, NSAID may provide symptomatic relief and promote well-being. Administration early in the course of the infection is likely to increase clinical benefit.

Antibacterial therapy may be of secondary importance relative to immediate supportive treatment of endotoxic shock, but it remains an integral part of a therapeutic regimen. Occasionally, coliform infections do result in chronic mastitis. Research suggests that bacteremia may occur in >40% of severe coliform cases. In addition, numerous other pathogens including gram-positive cocci cause severe clinical mastitis, which can be difficult to distinguish from cases caused by coliforms at initial presentation.

Selection of an appropriate antibacterial for severe coliform mastitis depends primarily on the susceptibility of the organism to the selected drug and the ability to maintain effective concentrations at the primary pharmacologic target (which, in the case of coliform mastitis, is the plasma compartment of the cow).

In one study, IM gentamicin was not more effective in preventing agalactia or death resulting from severe coliform mastitis, or in improving other clinical outcomes, than IM erythromycin or no systemic antibacterials. Cows experimentally challenged with *E coli* and given 500 mg of intramammary gentamicin BID did not have lower peak bacterial concentrations in milk, duration of infection, convalescent SCC or serum albumin concentrations in milk, or rectal temperatures as compared with untreated challenged cows. In additional, gentamicin readily diffused through the milk-blood barrier, resulting in drug residues in the kidney for >6 mo. With increased interest and sophistication of drug residue testing among regulatory agencies, practitioners should carefully consider the 30-45 day half-life for clearance in bovine kidneys and extended milk withdrawal periods following use of aminoglycosides.

Oxytetracycline (11 mg/kg, IV, SID) improved outcome of cows with clinical coliform mastitis (not necessarily severe) as compared with cows that did not receive systemic antibacterials. Ceftiofur sodium (2.2 mg/kg, IM, SID) decreased the mortality and cull rates of cows with severe coliform mastitis. This drug distributes poorly to the mammary gland, supporting the emphasis on treating the cow rather than the mammary gland because of the risk of septicemia.

Intramammary infusion of commercial products that have good activity against gram-positive organisms should be administered to any cow with severe clinical mastitis. This treatment is not likely to affect the outcome of a case caused by coliforms, but may provide some benefit for cases caused by gram-positive cocci. The need for antibacterial therapy in cows with grossly abnormal milk, but with improved appetite, attitude, and milk production should be evaluated critically. Unnecessary extension of therapy in these instances results in increased discarded milk expense for the dairy producer and risk of antibacterials in marketed milk.

Mild Clinical Mastitis: No microorganisms are isolated from 10-40% of bacteriologic cultures of milk samples collected from cows with clinical mastitis. Many mild mastitis cases (nearly 80%) are coliform intramammary infections that resolve before treatment is necessary. In addition, numerous mild clinical mastitis cases are temporary setbacks in the balance between pathogen and host defenses that occurs in more chronic intramammary infections. A "no antibiotic" approach to mild clinical mastitis cases avoids costs of discarded milk and residue risks that are inherent in antibacterial therapy. Although therapeutic and spontaneous cure rates for mild clinical mastitis cases caused by coliforms are similar, information on the efficacy of treatment for mild clinical mastitis cases caused by other pathogens is not extensive. Use of antibacterials for the treatment of clinical cases caused by streptococci has been reported to achieve bacterial cures in 60-65% of cases. However, a comparison of cure rate in treated vs. untreated cows was not reported in many studies. In a study of 3 California dairies, bacteriologic cure assessed at 4 and 20 days after treatment with amoxicillin, cephapirin, or oxytocin (no antibacterial) did not differ for mild clinical mastitis cases caused by streptococci and coliforms. Although milk production and survival did not differ, the rates of both relapses and recurring cases were higher in untreated cows, especially among streptococcal cases. A Colorado dairy study reported similar results, along with an increase in the incidence of clinical mastitis, prevalence of intramammary infections, and herd SCC associated with streptococcal infections following adoption of a no-antibiotic approach to clinical mastitis.

Common sense and individual herd history should determine the course of therapy for mild clinical mastitis cases in dairy herds. For initial occurrences of clinical episodes in any affected quarter, especially those caused by streptococci, use of approved commercial intramammary infusions is likely to be the best option. Assessment of success should be based on bacteriologic cure, but therapeutic success can be monitored more practically by improvement in days of marketed milk. If mastitis recurs regularly in affected quarters in the absence of systemic signs, repeated treatment of what now has become chronic intramammary infection is not warranted. Any moderate increase in cure rates gained by extensive parenteral therapy will not likely overcome the expense of discarded milk and other related treatment costs. If standard regimens achieve less than desired results, it would be better to extend therapy for a prolonged period, rather than to change to other antibacterial drugs or increase the amount of each dose. Alternatively, therapy of mild cases can be withheld until initial bacteriology is performed. If initial culture yields no organisms or coliforms, therapy is not initiated, whereas if gram-positive cocci are isolated, therapy is administered.

Unusual Pathogens: *Pseudomonas aeruginosa* may cause outbreaks of clinical mastitis. Generally, a persistent infection occurs, which may be characterized by intermittent acute or subacute exacerbations. The organism is found in soil-water environments common to dairy farms. Herd infections have been reported after extensive exposure to contaminated wash water (particularly wash hoses), teat cup liners, or intramammary treatments administered by milkers. Failure to use aseptic techniques for udder therapy or use of contaminated milking equipment may lead to establishment of *P aeruginosa* infections within the mammary glands. Severe peracute mastitis with toxemia and high mortality may follow immediately in some cows, while subclinical infections may occur in others. The organism has persisted in a gland for as long as 5 lactations, but spontaneous recovery may occur. Other than supportive care for severe episodes, therapy is of little value. Culling is recommended for cows.

Arcanobacterium (Actinomyces) pyogenes is common in suppurative processes of cattle and pigs and produces a characteristic mastitis in heifers and dry cows. It is occasionally seen in mastitis of lactating udders after teat injury, and it may be a secondary invader. The inflammation is typified by the formation of profuse, foul-smelling, purulent exudate. Mastitis due to *A pyogenes* is common among dry cows and heifers that are pastured during the summer months on fields and that have access to ponds or wet areas. The vector for animal-to-animal spread is the fly *Hydrotaea irritans*. Control of infections is by limiting the ability to stand udder-deep in water and by controlling flies. Preventive treatment of heifers and dry cows in susceptible areas with long-acting penicillin preparations has been effective in reducing infections. Therapy is rarely successful, and the infected quarter is usually lost to production. Infected cows may be systemically ill, and cows with abscesses usually should be slaughtered. (*See also* ACTINOMYCOSIS, p 477.)

Mycoplasma spp can cause a severe form of mastitis that may spread rapidly through a herd with serious consequences. *M bovis* is the most common cause. Other significant species include *M californicum, M canadense,* and *M bovigenitalium*. Onset is rapid, and the source of infection is believed to be endogenous after outbreaks of respiratory disease in heifers or cows. The disease is often seen in herds undergoing expansion in which animals from outside sources have been added. Some or all quarters become involved. Loss of production is often dramatic, and the secretion is soon replaced by a serous or purulent exudate. Initially, a characteristic fine granular or flaky sediment may be seen in the material removed from infected glands. Despite the severe local effects on udder tissue, cows usually do not manifest signs of systemic involvement. The infection may persist through the dry period. Because there is no satisfactory treatment, affected cows should be segregated at least for that lactation, or for their lifetimes. Identification of infected cows can be difficult because of the frequent propensity of infected cows to become asymptomatic carriers. Routine screening of the bulk tank and milk strings may help identify the presence of infected cows. However, culture of the mammary secretion of cows with clinical mastitis is the most reliable surveillance method. If cows continue to display clinical mastitis or systemic signs, they should be culled. Sanitary measures should be strictly enforced, especially at milking or during treatment. Milk from *Mycoplasma*-infected cows should not be fed to calves as this may result in respiratory and inner ear infections. Milk replacer, rather than discarded milk from mastitis cows, should be fed to calves in herds with *Mycoplasma*.

Nocardia asteroides causes a destructive mastitis characterized by acute onset, high temperature, anorexia, rapid wasting, and marked swelling of the udder. Response in the udder is typical of a granulomatous inflammation and leads to extensive fibrosis and formation of palpable nodules. Herd histories suggest that infection of the udder may be associated with failure to ensure asepsis in intramammary treatment of the common forms of mastitis. Slaughter is recommended for infected cows.

Serratia mastitis may arise from contamination of milk hoses, teat dips, water supply, or other equipment used in the milking process. The organism is resistant to disinfectants. Cows with this form of mastitis that continue to display clinical signs should be culled.

Mastitis due to various yeasts has appeared in dairy herds, especially after the use of penicillin in association with prolonged repetitive use of antibiotic infusions in individual cows. Yeasts grow well in the presence of penicillin and some other antibiotics; they may be introduced during udder infusions of antibiotics, multiply, and cause mastitis. Yet, heifers that have never received intramammary infusions may develop yeast mastitis. Signs may be severe, with a fever followed either by spontaneous recovery in ~2 wk or, more rarely, by a chronic destructive mastitis. Other yeast infections cause minimal inflammation and are self-limiting. If mastitis due to yeast is suspected, antibiotic therapy should be stopped immediately. Yeast or other mastitis infections can be reduced if the tip of the plastic infusion tube is only partially (rather than completely) inserted through the teat canal during intramammary therapy.

A chronic, indurative mastitis similar to that caused by the tubercle bacillus has been reported to be caused by acid-fast *Mycobacterium* spp derived from the soil, such as *M fortuitum*, *M smegmatis*, *M vaccae*, and *M phlei*, when such organisms are introduced into the gland along with antibiotics (especially penicillin) in oil or ointment vehicles. The oil apparently enhances the invasiveness of these organisms, and such therapy is contraindicated. These organisms otherwise tend to be saprophytic and to disappear from infected quarters, at least by the next lactation. In the meantime, mastitis is usually moderate. Distinct outbreaks do occur and several have been reported, especially with *M fortuitum* and *M smegmatis*.

Prevention: Bacterins that utilize core-antigen technology based on J5 mutant *Escherichia coli* can be helpful in reducing the incidence and severity of clinical mastitis caused by coliforms. Vaccination programs using these bacterins should minimally include multiple administration during the dry period to reduce the incidence of clinical coliform mastitis that is frequently associated with early lactation.

MASTITIS IN GOATS

The organisms infecting the udder of goats are similar to those in cows. Coagulase-negative staphylococci are generally the most prevalent and can cause persistent infections that result in increased cell counts and low-grade mastitis with some recurring clinical episodes. The level of infection and incidence of mastitis due to *Staphylococcus aureus* tends to be low (<5%), but can result in persistent infections that do not generally respond to therapy. Streptococcal intramammary infections can occur in both subclinical and clinical cases, but are usually much less frequent than in cattle. *Streptococcus agalactiae* is not a common pathogen of mastitis in does.

Mycoplasma infections, primarily *M mycoides* (large colony type) and *M putrefaciens*, sometimes cause serious outbreaks of mastitis in goats (*see also* p 1114). The latter also causes septicemia, polyarthritis, pneumonia, and encephalitis, together with serious disease and mortality in suckling kids. *M capricolum* has also been reported to cause severe mastitis in goats and infection in kids. Does usually recover in ~4 wk.

As with cows, gram-negative organisms cause intermittent infections that may be severe but are usually self-limiting. *Arcanobacterium (Actinomyces) pyogenes* sometimes produces multiple, nodular abscesses.

Does can also exhibit signs of mastitis from caprine arthritis and encephalitis (p 598) and ovine progressive pneumonia (p 1233) secondary to systemic infection. Agalactia is common, as is a hardening of the udder from fibrosis.

Programs for diagnosis, control, and treatment of bacterial mastitis in goats are similar to those in cows. However, monitoring subclinical mastitis with SCC in does is difficult due to poor discrimination between infected and noninfected animals, especially in the later stages of lactation. This is partially because a higher proportion of cells in goat milk are epithelial in origin as compared with cow milk. As lactation progresses, shedding of epithelial cells into milk increases, thus SCC >1,000,000 cells/mL are common in uninfected does in late lactation. Proper milking procedures and good environmental sanitation are needed to reduce the prevalence and spread of infection. Chronically infected goats should be culled, as should goats with *M mycoides* infections and those that do not recover from *M putrefaciens* or *M capricolum* infections.

MASTITIS IN EWES

Mastitis can be an important disease in sheep, with an incidence >2%. In addition to deaths from severe infections, the disease can be a cause of lamb mortality from starvation or of depressed weaning weights of lambs. Peracute, gangrenous (usually due to *Staphylococcus aureus*), acute, subacute, and probably subclinical types occur. The organisms most commonly involved are *S aureus*, coagulase-negative staphylococci, streptococci, *Escherichia coli*, *Mannheimia haemolytica*, and *Arcanobacterium (Actinomyces) pyogenes*.

The principles of diagnosis and treatment used in bovine mastitis can be applied to ewes. Little is known about the control of ovine mastitis, but careful inspection of the mammary glands of ewes before mating to detect and eliminate those with chronic mastitis should be beneficial.

MASTITIS IN MARES

Acute mastitis occurs occasionally in lactating mares, most commonly in the drying-off period, in one or both glands. *Streptococcus zooepidemicus* is the most frequent pathogen, but *S equi, S equisimilis, S agalactiae,* and *S viridans* are also found. A variety of gram-negative bacteria has also been reported. Marked painful swelling of the affected gland and adjacent tissues develops, and the secretion is often seroflocculent. Fever and depression may be present. The mare may walk stiffly or stand with hindlegs apart due to the discomfort.

Treatment is similar to that in cows, but when intramammary infusions are used, they should be inserted separately into both orifices of the teat. Systemic therapy has been suggested to include trimethoprim-sulfonamide (based on 5 mg/kg of trimethoprim, PO, BID) or a combination of penicillin (20,000 IU/kg, IM, BID) and gentamicin sulfate (2 mg/kg, IV, TID). Therapy should be continued on the basis of culture and antibacterial sensitivity testing. Without prompt treatment, abscessation or induration of the gland can occur. Little is known about the frequency and persistence of subclinical intramammary infections in mares.

MASTITIS IN SOWS

Mastitis can be important in swine-raising units. Peracute mastitis can affect sows and gilts and is most commonly associated with coliform (*Escherichia coli, Enterobacter aerogenes,* and *Klebsiella*) infections. It is most common at or just after parturition, and affected sows have a moderate to severe toxemia. The sow's temperature may increase to 107°F (42°C) or may be subnormal. The affected glands are swollen, purple, and have a watery secretion. Sow mortality is high, and the piglets will die unless fostered or fed artificially. Milk production of recovered sows may be impaired in the next lactation. The treatment of peracute coliform mastitis in sows is similar to that in cows. Ampicillin, dihydrostreptomycin, or oxytetracycline administered systemically have been used.

Subacute mastitis may occur in older sows and lead to induration of one or more glands, impairing the sow's ability to nurse a large litter. This form of mastitis is more likely to be associated with infection by streptococci or staphylococci. Granulomatous lesions in the mammae of sows have been associated with *Actinobacillus lignieresii, Actinomyces bovis,* and *Staphylococcus aureus* infections. *Fusobacterium necrophorum* and *Arcanobacterium (Actinomyces) pyogenes* also have been incriminated in sow mastitis. A thorough examination and culture of the mammary glands of the sow are important to diagnose any of the above peracute and subacute types of mastitis. (*See also* POSTPARTUM DYSGALACTIA SYNDROME, p 1134.)

The control of mastitis in sows has not been extensively investigated, but isolating sows in adequately disinfected pens before, during, and for an adequate period after farrowing should help prevent the severe losses associated with coliform mastitis.

METRITIS IN LARGE ANIMALS

ACUTE PUERPERAL METRITIS

In all species, acute puerperal metritis occurs within the first postpartum week. It results from contamination of the reproductive tract at parturition and often, but not invariably, follows complicated parturition. The causative organisms in cattle are most frequently *Arcanobacterium (Actinomyces) pyogenes* in association with gram-negative anaerobic bacteria such as *Fusobacterium necrophorum.* The condition is acute in onset.

Affected cows, mares, ewes, does, or sows are depressed, febrile, and inappetent. A fetid, watery uterine discharge is characteristic of the condition in cows but may not be conspicuous in other species. Milk production is diminished, and nursing young may show signs of food deprivation.

Acute puerperal metritis responds well to systemic antimicrobial therapy combined, if necessary, with NSAID and other supportive measures such as fluid therapy. Penicillin is considered an appropriate drug for systemic treatment of cows with endometritis because it is active against most common pathogens, reaches therapeutic levels in endometrial tissues, and may help prevent some of the potential sequelae of metritis and endometritis, such as endocarditis or renal disease. In cows, daily injections of procaine penicillin G at 20,000-25,000 IU/kg, IM, SID, results in adequate and sustained uterine levels; the same dose of sodium penicillin G requires BID administration. In the early postpartum period, the uterine flora is usually mixed, and some organisms are likely to produce β-lactamase. The use of β-lactamase-resistant penicillins or cephalosporins in such cases may be useful but has not been evaluated. Oxytetracycline requires administration at high levels (11 mg/kg, BID) to maintain uterine tissue concentrations of 5 µg/g, which is below the minimal inhibitory concentration (MIC) for many strains of pathogenic *A pyogenes*. Drainage of the uterine content may be advantageous but should be attempted only after initiation of antimicrobial therapy; it should be done very carefully because the inflamed uterus may be friable, and manipulation of the uterus may result in bacteremia.

METRITIS AND ENDOMETRITIS

Cows: Several specific diseases are associated with metritis or endometritis. These include brucellosis (p 1110), leptospirosis (p 525), campylobacteriosis (p 1108), and trichomoniasis (p 1142). More often, endometritis is the result of nonspecific infections.

The normal uterus is a sterile environment, in contrast to the vagina, which hosts numerous microorganisms. Opportunistic pathogens from the normal vaginal flora or from the environment may invade the uterus from time to time. A healthy uterus is able to rid itself of these transient infections very efficiently; however, in the immediate postpartum period, the uterus of cows is usually contaminated with a variety of organisms. Within days or weeks postpartum, the sterile uterine environment is reestablished in most animals. In those in which infection persists, chronic or subacute endometritis develops and has a detrimental effect on fertility. The prevalence of subclinical endometrial inflammation in dairy cows seems to exceed the prevalence of uterine infection. The pathogenesis of this form of endometritis is not yet understood.

In cows, the causative organisms are most often *Arcanobacterium (Actinomyces) pyogenes*, alone or in association with *Fusobacterium necrophorum* or other gram-negative anaerobic organisms. Signs of infection vary from obvious and persistent purulent exudate from the uterus and vagina to flakes of exudate in otherwise clear estrous mucus. Changes in uterine consistency may occur, but transrectal palpation alone is an insensitive means of diagnosis. Both sensitivity and specificity of diagnosis are improved by speculum examination and may be further improved by such measures as endometrial cytology. Affected cows rarely exhibit any systemic signs of illness, and appetite and milk production are usually unimpaired.

For decades, endometritis in cows has been treated with the intrauterine infusion of a bewildering array of substances. This is now receiving closer scrutiny. Although infusion of antimicrobials may rid the uterus of bacteria, there is little evidence that it eliminates the endometrial inflammation or restores fertility. Intrauterine infusion of cephapirin has enhanced fertility in dairy cows with endometritis. However, many preparations routinely administered into the bovine uterus are detrimental to uterine tissue. Increased concern about milk and carcass residues, along with poor or uncertain results, should discourage intrauterine therapy as a routine approach to management of bovine endometritis. In the rare cases in which systemic signs of illness are seen, systemic administration of antimicrobials is indicated.

Cows are more resistant to uterine infection during estrus, and as cows undergo more estrous cycles after parturition, the prevalence of endometritis diminishes. This has led to increased use of prostaglandin (PG) $F_{2\alpha}$ or its analogs, at usual luteolytic doses, for the management of endometritis. Another potential advantage of the use of $PGF_{2\alpha}$ or its analogs is stimulation of uterine contraction and expulsion of uterine exudate.

Mares: Although profound endometritis accompanies contagious equine metritis (*see* below) in mares, most breeding problems are related to endometritis caused by nonspecific infections. In mares, the most common etiologic agent of endometritis is *Streptococcus zooepidemicus*, but several other organisms may be involved, including *Escherichia coli, Pseudomonas aeruginosa,* and *Klebsiella pneumoniae.* Yeasts and fungi are incriminated in some cases, particularly in mares with reduced resistance, or as a sequela of exuberant antimicrobial therapy. Visible exudate is rarely a feature of endometritis in mares. (Contagious equine metritis is a notable exception.) Endometrial inflammation is best confirmed by examination of endometrial cytology or biopsy samples. Additional support of the diagnosis is provided by ultrasonographic demonstration of intraluminal free fluid, especially during diestrus, or by isolation of potentially pathogenic bacteria from appropriately guarded swabs of the endometrium. Because most causative organisms are common commensals, isolation of bacteria alone is not sufficient evidence for diagnosis.

Intrauterine therapy is still commonly used in mares. Many antimicrobial drugs have been used, and effective doses determined mainly empirically. Some examples include penicillin (5 million U; effective mainly against *S zooepidemicus*), ticarcillin (6 g; broad spectrum), ampicillin (3 g of soluble preparation), gentamicin (2 g, buffered with bicarbonate; effective especially against gram-negative agents), and kanamycin (2 g; effective against gram-negative bacteria). For fungal or yeast infections, 100 mg of amphotericin B or 500 mg of clotrimazole have been effective. Treatment should be continued for several consecutive days, preferably during estrus. Most of the above treatments constitute extralabel drug use in the USA.

Sows: A form of endometritis characterized by profuse vaginal discharge at the onset of estrus has been described in Europe and other regions. The causative agent is usually *Staphylococcus hyicus* or *E coli*, and the disease seems to be transmitted at mating or artificial insemination; signs are seen 15-25 days later during the subsequent proestrus or estrus. Infection may be of long duration with signs recurring at each estrus. Some sows recover spontaneously, but there does not seem to be any effective treatment for those that do not. At necropsy, copious quantities of purulent exudate may be found in the uterus, making this condition more akin to pyometra (*see* below).

Other Species: Endometritis has been seen in sheep, goats, and camelids. In commercial sheep and goat flocks, diagnosis is seldom made antemortem, and treatment is generally impractical. In animals with a persistent uterine discharge, remnants of a macerated fetus should be considered as a nidus of chronic infection. Endometritis in camelids is usually treated empirically based on treatments for cattle and horses.

PYOMETRA

Pyometra is characterized by the accumulation of purulent or mucopurulent exudate in the uterus. In cows, it is invariably accompanied by the persistence of an active corpus luteum and interruption of the estrous cycle. In affected mares, the cervix is often fibrotic, inelastic, affected with transluminal adhesions, or otherwise impaired. Mares may continue to cycle normally, or the cycle may be interrupted. Discharge from the genital tract may be absent or intermittent and corresponding to periods of estrus. As a rule, affected animals do not exhibit any systemic signs of illness, but affected mares may be in poor condition. In both cows and mares, pyometra must be distinguished carefully from pregnancy before treatment is undertaken.

The treatment of choice in cows is administration of $PGF_{2\alpha}$ or its analogs at normal luteolytic doses. Expulsion of exudate and bacteriologic clearance of the uterus follows in 90-100% of treated cases. Although first-service conception rate after treatment may be low, up to 80% of cows may be expected to conceive within 3-4 inseminations. In a small proportion of cows, the treatment may need to be repeated. No intrauterine treatment is recommended in conjunction with the prostaglandin.

In the face of cervical changes, drainage of the affected equine uterus may be virtually impossible. Lavage of the uterus using large volumes of fluid is recommended, but the condition frequently recurs, and permanent cure in these cases requires hysterectomy.

Pyometra occurs in small ruminants, swine, and other species; diagnosis is rendered more difficult by their size and management practices. If pyometra is diagnosed, evacuation of the uterus is recommended.

CONTAGIOUS EQUINE METRITIS

Contagious equine metritis (CEM) is an acute, highly contagious venereal disease of horses (and experimentally of donkeys) characterized by a profuse, mucopurulent vaginal discharge and early return to estrus in most affected mares. Infected stallions and chronically infected mares show no clinical signs. The disease occurs primarily in Europe, but technical challenges in propagation of the causative organism prevent accurate determination of the precise distribution of the disease.

Etiology and Transmission: CEM is caused by the gram-negative, microaerophilic coccobacillus *Taylorella equigenitalis*, also known as the contagious equine metritis organism (CEMO). Important strain differences exist; some strains are resistant to streptomycin (a fact that helps isolate this fastidious, slow-growing organism from contaminants), while others are streptomycin-sensitive. It is best cultured on chocolate Eugon agar at 37°C in an atmosphere of 5-10% CO_2 in air. *T equigenitalis* is asaccharolytic but is positive for catalase, cytochrome oxidase, and phosphatase and unreactive to other conventional biochemical tests.

CEM is transmitted primarily at mating, but infected fomites (instruments and equipment) also play a role. Undetected infected mares and stallions are the source of new outbreaks. Infected stallions show no signs and harbor the organism in the smegma of the prepuce and the surface of the penis, especially in the urethral fossa. The transmission rate is exceptionally high; virtually every mare mated by an infected stallion becomes infected.

Clinical Findings: In mares, a copious, mucopurulent vaginal discharge is seen 10-14 days after infected matings. Mares may return to estrus after a shortened estrous cycle. Although the discharge subsides after a few days, mares may remain infected for several months. Chronically infected mares show no signs. Most mares do not conceive at the time of infected mating. If they do, they may infect the foal at or shortly after birth. Foals so infected may become carriers of CEMO when they reach sexual maturity.

Lesions: Lesions consist of edema and hyperemia of the endometrium, the endocervix, and the vaginal mucosa. The microscopic lesions include invasion of the affected tissues by neutrophils during the acute stage, and by lymphocytes, macrophages, and plasma cells later in the course of the infection.

Diagnosis: Diagnosis depends on isolation of the causative organism. Although other bacterial infections of the genital tract of mares may produce a conspicuous vaginal discharge, this is uncommon, and no other venereal pathogen of the equine reproductive tract is as contagious. In mares, swabs for culture should be taken from the endometrium (preferably during estrus) and from the clitoral fossa and sinuses. Swabs from suspected stallions should be taken from the urethral fossa, the urethra, the preputial cavity, the shaft of the penis and, if possible, the pre-ejaculatory fluid or ejaculate. Stallions should be sampled at least 3 times before being declared free of CEMO. Test-mating suspect stallions to susceptible mares that are then screened bacteriologically constitutes a satisfactory means of determining CEM status. All swabs should be placed in a transport medium (preferably Amies with charcoal), kept on ice or at 4°C, and delivered to a qualified laboratory within 24 hr (or frozen if transport will take longer). A variety of serologic tests has been developed, but none is yet capable of reliably detecting the carrier status.

Treatment and Control: Stallions can be treated by thoroughly cleaning the extended penis with chlorhexidine surgical scrub and then applying nitrofurazone ointment. This should be repeated daily for 5 days, and the stallion retested at least 10 days after treatment. Most mares rid themselves of uterine infection after a few weeks. Those that become chronically infected harbor the CEMO in the clitoral fossa or sinuses. They can be treated by thoroughly cleaning the clitoral area with chlorhexidine surgical scrub and then applying nitrofurazone ointment as for the stallion. In some mares, surgical excision of the clitoral sinuses may be required to rid them of infection.

Control of CEM depends on identification of infected carrier animals and on their treatment or elimination from breeding programs. Strict import regulations exist in many countries to avoid the introduction of CEM, and current prevalence of the disease appears to be low.

POSTPARTUM DYSGALACTIA SYNDROME AND MASTITIS IN SOWS

Numerous etiologies or pathophysiologies can be involved in these syndromes, which is reflected by the use of several different names—mastitis-metritis-agalactia (MMA) complex, agalactia syndrome, dysgalactia syndrome, mammary edema, periparturient hypogalactia syndrome, agalactia toxemia, and puerperal mastitis. However, these names are not synonymous and have often been misused. This syndrome is currently classified according to the number of mammary glands affected, ie, uniglandular or multiglandular mastitis (including postpartum dysgalactia syndrome [PPDS], MMA complex). (*See also* MASTITIS IN LARGE ANIMALS, p 1120.)

Acute or chronic mastitis of only 1 or 2 mammary glands (acute or chronic uniglandular mastitis) in sows is present in nearly all herds. When all mammary glands are acutely affected, it can be a primary or a secondary mastitis (acute multiglandular mastitis) or also a mammary edema (hard udder syndrome), which is very common in primiparous sows. Acute multiglandular mastitis is usually accompanied by systemic signs and agalactia, while hard udder syndrome is not. Both conditions occur within the first 3 days after farrowing and rapidly lead to piglet starvation. Although the problem can be sporadic and limited to a few sows, sometimes it can occur in a greater number of sows and become nearly epidemic.

PPDS is characterized by transitory hypogalactia. It can lead to acute multiglandular mastitis and should be considered as the general cause of lactation failure in the sow. The name MMA complex is a misnomer. Although the mammary glands are swollen and frequently warmer than normal, grossly detectable primary mastitis is uncommon. Likewise, metritis (more commonly endometritis) is only an occasional finding in some herds. Finally, only rarely is there complete agalactia; most sows continue to produce milk but at a greatly reduced rate (hypogalactia or more correctly dysgalactia). In reality, MMA complex is only part of the more general PPDS. The primary clinical signs of the sow's inability to produce a sufficient amount of milk to meet the needs of the piglets are growth retardation and increased mortality in piglets.

Mammary glands of sows are anatomically different from those of cows. In sows, there are no well-identified gland cisterns (gland sinus) in the mammary glands. There are usually 2 complete gland systems and 2 teat orifices per teat. When 3 orifices are present, 1 sinus ends blindly at the base of the teat and does not have glandular tissue. There is no muscular sphincter around the teat orifice. Therefore, intramammary treatment by way of the teat opening is impossible. Mammogenesis occurs almost exclusively during the last half of gestation and repeatedly from one cycle to the next. Because of this, new glandular tissues are produced during each gestation. Therefore, infection of a mammary gland during one lactation has no consequences for the next. However, chronic lesions of the teat canal may be present from one lactation to the next.

ACUTE MULTIGLANDULAR MASTITIS

This syndrome is seen in all types of herds, including those with excellent hygiene and adequate disinfection practices. It occurs mainly during the first 3 days after farrowing and has major consequences for the piglets. Acute multiglandular mastitis can also follow a specific systemic disease of the sow (eg, septicemia, pseudorabies [p 1065], porcine reproductive and respiratory syndrome [p 581]).

Etiology and Pathogenesis: The etiology is multifactorial. Infections of the mammary gland are more often secondary, and many microorganisms have been identified, including *Escherichia coli, Klebsiella* spp, *Enterobacter* spp, *Citrobacter* spp, *Staphylococcus* spp (eg, *S epidermidis*), and *Pseudomonas aeruginosa*. All these microorganisms are common in the environment of sows.

Although many sows in a herd may be severely affected, this type of mastitis is not contagious. After farrowing, the mammary gland is infected by an environmental opportunist. Very few bacteria (often <100) are enough to colonize the mammary gland.

Major herd risk factors are the sow (*see* PPDS, p 1136), the piglets (uncommon primary form), or the environment (eg, some beddings such as wood shavings can be contaminated by *Klebsiella pneumoniae*).

Clinical Findings: Systemic signs such as anorexia, constipation, fever, and depression are common. Local signs include acute induration of the mammary glands as well as severe edema and skin congestion of the mammary region. However, many sows (especially primiparous sows) develop mammary edema without any signs of acute mastitis. Circumstantial evidence suggests that this is usually associated with increasing milk production (often the milk drips during and right after farrowing) to such an extent that piglets are unable to consume all the available milk.

Once acute multiglandular mastitis is established, the secretion (with oxytocin) of milk is no longer possible. Affected sows deny piglets access to the teats by lying on their mammary glands. General signs result from bacterial multiplication and resorption of toxins. Common consequences for the litter include an increase of stillborn piglets, weak piglets, neonatal diarrhea, starvation, hypoglycemia-induced weakness, an increased incidence of crushing by the sow, and increased susceptibility to other diseases and other problems (eg, runt pigs, etc).

Diagnosis: Early diagnosis is not always easy. Most problem litters are thought to be due to early lactation problems. The primary differential diagnoses are peripartum mammary edema, which is often seen in primiparous sows without any systemic signs, and PPDS, which is less spectacular but affects a greater number of sows. A thorough physical examination, including careful palpation of the mammary glands, should be performed. However, it is necessary to be cautious in the interpretation—hard mammary glands without systemic signs do not always indicate acute mastitis. Although frequently seen, peripartum mammary edema is poorly documented. The sows often appear to be in discomfort and lay down, as do sows with mastitis. However, peripartum mammary edema can certainly lead to an acute multiglandular mastitis. In contrast to the situation in cows, interpretation of cellular modifications in the milk is very difficult in sows.

Treatment and Control: Systemic antibiotic therapy should be started as soon as possible (*see* PPDS, p 1136). Longterm control of a herd problem also requires identification and correction of risk factors. General antibiotic therapy as well as corticosteroids are useful to reduce the intensity of the inflammatory reaction. Management techniques to improve hygiene should be implemented as soon as possible. Cross-fostering is often the only effective way to save a litter.

ACUTE UNIGLANDULAR MASTITIS

In lactating or weaned sows, inflammation of only 1 mammary gland is common. Such uniglandular inflammations are more often noticed in old sows.

Etiology and Pathogenesis: The microorganisms involved are the same as those in acute multiglandular mastitis. Sometimes only 1 or 2 mammary glands are affected; the cause should be identified. Traumatic lesions or inaccessibility of teats to piglets are common. Piglets suckling inguinal mammary glands of old sows are often unable to reach the teat during the phase of milk ejection. Usually, piglets have selected a specific gland by 24 hr after birth. A piglet suckling a teat affected by acute uniglandular mastitis will show growth retardation, while littermates remain normal. Milk secretion may be restricted by acquired problems of mammary conformation (as in old sows), traumatic lesions, and other teat abnormalities. Teat lesions may have developed during the previous lactation, the previous weaning-to-estrus interval, or the previous gestation.

Diagnosis: The integrity of the mammary gland should be checked before each farrowing. Except for cases associated with inaccessible teats, risk factors involved in the development of blind teats should be identified. Traumatic teat lesions can be the consequence of injuries induced by piglets or other sows, or by slipping on slatted floors, etc. Unfortunately, these primary lesions often go unnoticed until several weeks or months have passed.

Treatment and Control: The affected gland is lost for the current lactation and sometimes for the next lactation. During subsequent lactations, the number of nursing piglets should be limited, or the sow should be culled.

CHRONIC OR DRY-SOW MASTITIS

Postweaning or dry-sow mastitis is a particular type of uniglandular mastitis. In contrast to cows, it is uncommon in sows. Abscesses are often associated with chronic mastitis. They are most common during fights after weaning, when several weaned sows are grouped in the same pen. Aggressive behavior after piglets are weaned often leads to injuries in the mammary region.

POSTPARTUM DYSGALACTIA SYNDROME

PPDS is a primary cause of neonatal problems (eg, diarrhea, crushing, runting, inanition, poor growth) but is difficult to characterize because of its multiple manifestations and the difficulty in making an etiologic diagnosis. In a given herd, PPDS affects ~15-20% of the sows; a higher percentage is uncommon.

Etiology and Pathogenesis: There are numerous multifactorial etiologies, which complicate the diagnosis and clinical evaluation. Classically perceived as a part of the MMA complex, PPDS should instead be considered a broader pathology. Thus, the MMA complex is essentially a subtype of PPDS, probably the most severe clinically but also the least common.

Evidence suggests that lipopolysaccharide (LPS) endotoxins, a portion of the cell wall of all gram-negative bacteria, play a role in some cases. Bacterial endotoxins can be absorbed from the uterus (eg, endometritis or metritis), mammary glands (eg, acute multiglandular mastitis), or gut (eg, constipation as a consequence of feeding finely ground feed to sows can result in bacterial overgrowth and subsequent absorption of endotoxins from the intestines) and lead to endotoxemia. Identifying the source of the bacterial endotoxins is important to determine the best preventive approach for the particular herd.

The secretion of colostrum is determined by a complex hormonal balance. LPS endotoxins suppress release of prolactin (the main hormone involved in the initiation of lactation) by the anterior pituitary, decrease circulating thyroid hormone, and increase cortisol concentrations. These changes adversely affect production and secretion of colostrum and milk. In addition, the colostrum is as important for its energy content as it is for its immunoglobulin content. Any decrease in the amount of ingested colostrum will result in consequences for the piglets such as diarrhea, inanition, and poor growth.

Other causes of general hypogalactia that should be considered include acute multiglandular mastitis, udder and teat abnormalities, hypocalcemia (uncommon in sows), and acute (agalactia) or chronic (hypogalactia) ergotism (uncommon in practice). Indeed, ergot derivatives suppress prolactin release.

Risk factors are those associated with stress of the sow and with conditions that lead to bacterial multiplication and subsequent endotoxemia. Such factors are numerous and are linked with different entities (eg, cystitis, metritis, vaginitis, constipation, mastitis, etc).

Clinical Findings: PPDS is seen almost exclusively within the first 3 days after farrowing. Associated signs are numerous and vary from herd to herd, as well as within herds. PPDS is commonly associated with fat sow syndrome, prolonged farrowings, and a high postpartum fever. Management practices reported in herds with a high incidence of PPDS include too much manual intervention during parturition or too many parenteral injections to sows (antibiotics, oxytocin, prostaglandins) or piglets (mainly antibiotics). Piglet losses are due to emaciation or diarrhea (or both), as a consequence of poor nutrition during the first few days postpartum.

Diagnosis: Diagnosis is difficult and based on clinical signs. Clinical examination is best performed while piglets are nursing; milk ejection in affected sows is either absent or of brief duration, which causes the piglets to actively nurse for an extended time. During the initial stages, piglets repeatedly attempt to nurse at frequent intervals and do not settle after nursing. As a result of vigorous nursing efforts, the teats may be traumatized. As the energy reserves of the piglets are depleted, their attempts to nurse decrease, and they often migrate to the warmest portions of the farrowing crate. Crushing by the sow is common. Mammary tenderness, swelling, and teat damage are consistent with a diagnosis of lactational insufficiency. The mammary glands vary from grossly normal to swollen, firm, and warm to the touch, sometimes with blotched purple skin. Pure bacterial cultures may be isolated from milk samples. Rectal temperature of the sow varies from normal to markedly increased (>40.5°C). The concept that postpartum rectal temperatures >39.5°C predict early lactation problems must be questioned. Physiologic hyperthermia observed in lactating sows should not be confused with fever. Reduced appetite or anorexia, constipation, and depression may also be seen. Abnormal and copious vaginal discharges may be seen in some sows (eg, endometritis). Cystitis, metritis, vaginitis, constipation, or mastitis in the sow and diarrhea in neonatal piglets should be considered as a general syndrome (requiring an overall diagnosis) rather than as individual problems.

Treatment and Control: Systemic or local therapeutic intervention can sometimes be helpful but only on a short-term basis (antibiotics, NSAID, and sometimes flunixin meglumine to counteract the effects of endotoxins). However, if used longterm, a dependence on antibiotics for puerperal fevers, acute mastitis, vaginitis, endometritis, or neonatal diarrhea can develop rapidly. Oxytocin or prostaglandins (or both) can be useful in cases of prolonged farrowing or postpartum endometritis. By far the most effective method is to cross-foster the piglets from affected to normal sows. Oxytocin (5-10 U/sow) is occasionally effective in reestablishing lactation if used 4-5 times at 2- to 3-hr intervals. In herds in which PPDS is a significant problem, incidence may be reduced by inducing parturition with prostaglandin $F_{2\alpha}$; this results in rapid induction of labor and dilatation of the teats for a shorter period of time. As many risk factors as possible should be identified and corrected or minimized. Systematic manual interventions during farrowing or uterine washings should be limited to only those that are necessary. There is no clear evidence that vaccines have a beneficial effect. Good sanitation tends to decrease the incidence of mastitis in the sow and diarrhea in the piglets, but PPDS is also common in herds in overall good health and with a high level of hygiene.

PROLONGED GESTATION IN CATTLE AND SHEEP

Parturition is induced by the fetus in both cattle and sheep. It is initiated by rising cortisol levels in the fetus that provoke a cascade of endocrine activity in the mother. Fetal cortisol increases as a result of increased adrenocorticotropic hormone (ACTH) production by the maturing fetal pituitary caused by fetal stressors such as hypoxia and hypercapnia. Gestation length is unique to each fetus, but approximate gestation lengths can be ascribed to each species (*see* TABLE 1, p 1087).

In cattle, gestation length is influenced by factors such as the breed of the cow and bull, calf gender, single vs multiple birth, the parity of the cow, and the fetal genotype. Environmental factors including nutrition, ambient temperature, and the season of the year have a smaller influence. The breed of cattle has the greatest influence on gestation length. In European cattle of the *Bos taurus* species, considerable breed variation is recognized (eg, 279 days mean gestation in Holstein-Friesian to 287 days in Charolais). In breeds of the *Bos indicus* species, a slightly longer gestation length is often seen (eg, Zebu cattle have a mean gestation length of 296 days). Within breeds, individual bulls may sire calves with longer gestation length than normal, leading to a higher incidence of dystocia. In sheep, the normal gestation length is 144-150 days.

PROLONGED GESTATION

In dairy cattle, service dates are normally known; hence the date of anticipated parturition is calculated and recorded once pregnancy is confirmed. In beef cattle, in which cows often run with a bull, exact calving dates are not known but individual pregnant cows are expected to calve within a recognized calving season. Individual animals that have not calved at the anticipated time are checked to confirm that they are still pregnant and that their pregnancy appears to be normal.

In sheep, the exact lambing date is seldom known unless ewes were served in hand or by artificial insemination. In most flocks the ewes run with rams and, when served, receive a raddle crayon mark on their rumps to indicate that service has occurred. Crayon color is changed at 14- to 17-day intervals, and following later pregnancy diagnosis, a lambing date within a 14- to 17-day period is calculated. Individual ewes that fail to lamb are culled or further evaluated for pregnancy.

In many cases, prolonged gestation is incorrectly diagnosed because of human error. Miscalculation of the prospective calving or lambing date, failure to record a subsequent service, faulty pregnancy diagnosis, and incorrect identification of animals may lead to a diagnosis of prolonged gestation in an animal that has a normal pregnancy. True prolonged gestation is relatively uncommon; the common denominator is a defective hypothalamic-pituitary-adrenal axis. Suspected cases should be investigated and examined with care. In some cases, the fetus is dead or severely deformed and is of little economic value. The life of the dam may be at risk if prolonged gestation is allowed to continue, and termination of the abnormal pregnancy is recommended.

Prolonged Gestation Associated with Fetal Death

Fetal death may be followed by abortion, fetal maceration, or fetal mummification. In cases of abortion and fetal maceration, the hormonal support of pregnancy is lost. The animal normally shows signs that pregnancy has terminated. An aborted fetus may be found, the dam may show an abnormal vaginal discharge, and she may return to estrus. Fetal bones may be trapped in the uterus.

In cases of fetal mummification, fetal death is often not immediately apparent. In such cases, the corpus luteum persists in the ovary and there is no vaginal discharge. The abnormal pregnancy in such animals continues indefinitely. Affected animals are normally identified when owners notice that external signs of late pregnancy including abdominal enlargement are less obvious than in other members of a group. Clinical examination reveals that the fetus is dead although the dam is pregnant. Rectal examination reveals an irregularly shaped, contracted uterus with a fetal mass but no fetal fluid within it. There is no fremitus in the uterine artery. Ultrasonographic examination of accessible parts of the uterus per rectum confirms the diagnosis. The abnormal pregnancy can be terminated by a single IM injection of prostaglandin $F_{2\alpha}$. The fetus is expelled from the uterus and can be manually removed from the vagina 48 hr later.

In sheep, fetal mummification may be diagnosed by abdominal palpation supported by a transabdominal ultrasonographic scan. Affected animals are normally culled on economic grounds.

Prolonged Gestation Associated with Fetal Deformity

These cases usually occur as the result of some compromise of the pituitary-adrenal axis of the fetus, which is no longer able to initiate parturition. The affected fetus may either die and be aborted or live on indefinitely in the uterus. Genetic, infectious, toxic, and unknown causes have been associated with this problem.

Genetic Abnormalities: In Holstein-Freisian cows, genetically determined prolonged gestation is caused by an autosomal recessive gene of the fetus. The fetal adrenal glands fail to produce corticosteroids at term, in response to fetal ACTH. As a result, the fetus continues to grow until it outgrows its blood supply. Induction with dexamethasone does not induce normal labor and parturition due to insufficient preparation of the birth canal. A cesarean section will save the dam, but the fetus invariably dies due to adrenal insufficiency.

Three genetic abnormalities associated with prolonged gestation in various breeds of cattle involve fetal pituitary abnormalities. In one condition, severe fetal oversize (fetal giantism) is present; in the second, however, the calf has severe craniofacial defects and is much smaller than normal. In the third condition, multiple skeletal abnormalities are present.

Prolonged gestation and fetal giantism has been reported in Holstein, Ayrshire, and Swedish breeds of cattle. Gestation is prolonged by 21-150 days. Pronounced abdominal enlargement is seen in some cases. There is no attempted parturition unless the fetus dies first after having outgrown its blood supply. Cervical relaxation is poor and dystocia invariably results. The calf weighs 48-80 kg at birth and shows signs of postmaturity. The coat and hooves are longer than normal and prominent loose teeth are present in the gums. Breathing is difficult as a result of failure of surfactant release, and the calf may die from hypoglycemia. At necropsy, hypoplasia of the anterior pituitary and adrenal glands is seen.

Prolonged gestation with craniofacial defects in the fetus has been reported in Ayrshire, Guernsey, and Jersey breeds of cattle and is thought to be caused by a recessive gene. Affected fetuses cease to grow at 7 mo gestation. There is no spontaneous parturition in affected Guernsey cattle due to the nonfunctional pituitary gland in the fetus. Calves are usually dead when delivered. Some may show evidence of severe abnormalities of the cranium and face.

Prolonged gestation associated with multiple skeletal abnormalities has been reported in Hereford cattle. Affected calves show evidence of pituitary aplasia or hypoplasia. Arthrogryposis, torticollis, kyphosis, and scoliosis are present, and some calves have cleft palates.

Infectious Causes: Although bovine viral diarrhea virus can cause abortion in cattle, it can also produce congenital defects in the fetus. These include cerebellar hypoplasia, anencephaly, and hydrocephaly. Affected calves may be born with severe defects of the CNS, but prolonged gestation occasionally occurs if pituitary function is compromised. The related pestivirus Border disease virus can produce severe brain and coat abnormalities in fetal lambs. Pituitary compromise in such lambs can lead to prolonged gestation.

Akabane virus, which is found in Africa, Australia, the Middle East, and the Far East, can be transmitted by insects to both pregnant cattle and sheep. Bovine fetuses exposed to the virus at 76-104 days gestation may develop hydranencephaly (fluid-filled cavitation of the brain). Exposure to the virus at 105-174 days of pregnancy may cause both hydranencephaly and arthrogryposis. Affected fetuses may have severe brain damage. The cerebral cortex may be absent and the cranial cavity filled with fluid. Cerebellar hypoplasia may be present, and the brain stem is smaller than normal. Compromise of pituitary function in the affected fetus can lead to prolonged gestation.

Bluetongue virus (p 590), which is found in Africa, Australia, North and South America, and less commonly in parts of Europe, is also transmitted by insects; infection can occasionally cause prolonged gestation. The fetuses of cows exposed to the virus at 60-120 days of pregnancy developed hydranencephaly, while fetuses exposed later in pregnancy developed less severe CNS defects.

Gestation lengths >200 days have been recorded in ewes vaccinated during pregnancy with Rift Valley fever attenuated viral vaccine. Affected lambs developed severe brain defects and skeletal abnormalities. Some ewes developed hydrops amnion by the fourth month of gestation. Ewes in which pregnancy was not terminated developed ketosis.

Toxic Causes: Several plant toxins cause fetal deformity and prolonged gestation when eaten accidentally or fed experimentally. When fed to sheep in early pregnancy, *Veratrum californicum* (skunk cabbage) produces fetal deformities, giantism, and prolonged gestation. Cranial defects and brain and eye abnormalities were seen in fetuses of ewes fed this plant at 14 days of gestation; pregnancy length in some cases was >230 days. The plant contains the amine cyclopamine, which is believed to be responsible for the fetal abnormalities. This plant also contains a number of toxic alkaloids that cause GI disturbance, dyspnea, and convulsions in sheep. *Veratrum album* has similarly caused prolonged gestation and fetal abnormalities in Holstein-Friesian cows in Japan.

An unidentified toxin in the plant *Salsola tuberculatiformis* (cauliflower saltwort) is thought to cause prolonged gestation in sheep. Pregnancy extended >220 days, and affected lambs showed atrophy of the pituitary, adrenal, and thyroid glands. Fetuses appear to be most susceptible to the toxin in the first and third trimesters of pregnancy. Amniotic fluid continues to increase in volume in cases of prolonged gestation associated with this plant. Physical abnormalities such as cleft palate prevent normal swallowing of amniotic fluid in affected fetuses. Excessive fetal weight and the weight of accumulated fetal fluids may lead to rupture of the prepubic tendon in ewes.

Diagnosis: When a number of cases of prolonged gestation occur in a herd or flock, a full investigation should be mounted in an attempt to identify the cause and possibly a preventive program. A genetic abnormality may be determined by a study of pedigrees or by finding an abnormal karyotype in affected fetuses. Possible exposure to toxic plants and viral infection should be investigated. Tests for evidence of pathogenic viruses or serologic evidence of exposure to them may lead to clear evidence of virus involvement. In some cases, the cause of prolonged gestation remains unknown. Evidence of pituitary hypoplasia or compromise may be found, but the underlying cause remains elusive.

Treatment: In a case of suspected prolonged gestation, the patient's breeding records, if available, should be checked to ensure that parturition really is overdue. Treatment of a case in which gestation is not genuinely prolonged may result in the delivery of a premature fetus that is unlikely to survive. Once the true length of gestation is established, a full clinical examination of the dam should be conducted. In cattle, rectal examination of the uterus and its contents is an important diagnostic aid. Fetal parts may be palpable and in some cases it is possible to detect an abnormal cranium. An ultrasonographic scan may confirm the presence of fetal abnormalities including a thin-walled, fluid-filled cranium. The weight of an overdue fetus may cause it to pass under the rumen while still within the uterus, so that it cannot be palpated. In some animals, prolonged gestation is accompanied by the development of excessive amounts of fetal fluid. The origin of excessive fetal fluid can be assessed by analysis of sodium and chloride levels in an aspirated sample. Amniotic fluid contains approximately 120 mmol/L of sodium and 20 mmol/L of chloride. Allantoic fluid contains 50 mmol/L of sodium and 20 mmol/L of chloride. The correlation between hydrops amnii and hydrops allantois and prolonged gestation is tenuous, however. Most fetal giants suffer from oligoamnios.

In true prolonged gestation, the fetus is unlikely to be of any economic value. Treatment should be aimed at fetal delivery with minimal damage to the dam. In cases of fetal giantism, the dam may be distressed by the weight of her fetus and its associated fluids. Painful edema in front of the udder may indicate rupture or impending rupture of the prepubic tendon. A canvas sling support can be placed around the abdomen to prevent further damage until the pregnancy is terminated. General health of the dam should be assessed and economic considerations discussed with the owner before treatment is attempted.

Successful induction of parturition requires an intact hypothalamic-pituitary-adrenal axis. Pregnancy is maintained in cases of prolonged gestation chiefly by continued production of progesterone by the corpus luteum. Spontaneous induction of birth in cases of prolonged gestation fails as a result of insufficient production of fetal cortisol and the failure of luteolysis to occur. Birth in both cows and sheep can be successfully induced by administering both prostaglandin $F_{2\alpha}$ (or its synthetic analog cloprostenol) and the corticosteroid dexamethasone by IM injection. Luteolysis is induced by the prostaglandin, and the maternal hormone cascade that precedes parturition is initiated by the corticosteroid. In cows, 500 μg cloprostenol and 20 mg dexamethasone are given; in sheep 125 μg cloprostenol and 16 mg dexamethasone are recommended. A single dose of these 2 drugs is normally effective. Parturition should begin in 24-72 hr.

Induced parturition should be monitored carefully. Assistance may be required if there is evidence of uterine inertia or damage to the abdominal wall, either of which might make expulsive efforts ineffective. Fetal malposition requiring obstetric assistance may occur once birth commences. If the fetus is very large, dystocia due to fetal-pelvic disproportion may occur, and assisted delivery by careful traction may be attempted. If this is not possible, cesarean section may be required. If the dam is seriously ill, an elective cesarean without an attempt at vaginal delivery may be considered if the patient is considered well enough to withstand surgery.

After fetal delivery, uterine involution may be encouraged by administration of oxytocin. Retention of fetal membranes is managed in the usual way (p 1141). Fluid therapy, antibiotics, and treatment with NSAID such as flunixin meglumine may aid recovery.

RETAINED FETAL MEMBRANES IN LARGE ANIMALS

(Retained placenta)

Cows: Retention of fetal membranes, or retained placenta, usually is defined as failure to expel fetal membranes within 24 hr after parturition. Normally, expulsion occurs within 3-8 hr after calf delivery. The incidence in healthy dairy cows is 5-15%, while the incidence in beef cows is lower. The incidence during lactation is increased by abortion, dystocia, hypocalcemia, twin birth, high environmental temperature, advancing age of the cow, premature birth or induction of parturition, placentitis, and nutritional disturbances.

The precise pathogenesis of retained fetal membranes is poorly understood, but normal maturation and loosening of the placenta begin during late pregnancy and are marked by alterations in the collagen of the placentome. During parturition, changes in uterine pressure, reduction in blood flow, and physical flattening of the placentome during uterine contractions contribute to final loosening and expulsion of the fetal membranes.

Diagnosis is usually straightforward as degenerating, discolored, ultimately fetid membranes are seen hanging from the vulva >24 hr after parturition. Occasionally, the retained membranes may remain within the uterus and not be readily apparent, in which case their presence may be signalled by a foul-smelling discharge. In most cases, there are no signs of systemic illness. When systemic signs are observed, they are related to toxemia. Uncomplicated retention of fetal membranes is unsightly and inconvenient for animal handlers and milkers but generally not directly harmful to the cow. However, cows with retained fetal membranes are at increased risk of developing metritis, ketosis, mastitis, and even abortion in a subsequent pregnancy. Cows that have once had retained fetal membranes are at increased risk of recurrence at a subsequent parturition.

Manual removal of the retained membranes is no longer recommended and is potentially harmful. Trimming of excess tissue that is objectionable to animal handlers and contributes to gross contamination of the genital tract is permissible. Untreated cows expel the membranes in 2-11 days. Routine use of intrauterine antimicrobials has not been found to be beneficial and may be detrimental. Although advocated at various times, oxytocin, estradiol, prostaglandin $F_{2\alpha}$, and oral calcium preparations have not been shown to hasten expulsion of retained membranes. When systemic signs of illness are present, systemic treatment with antimicrobials and NSAID is indicated. In herds in which incidence of retained fetal membranes is unacceptably high, predisposing causes should be sought and eliminated.

Mares: Equine fetal membranes are normally expelled within 3 hr after parturition, but expulsion may be delayed for 8-12 hr or even longer without signs of illness. The cause of retention of fetal membranes often is not known, but the condition is associated with infection, abortion, short or prolonged gestation, and uterine atony. Retention of just a portion of the fetal membranes entirely within the uterus (usually at the tip of the previously nongravid uterine horn) is less conspicuous but equally likely to result in complications. For this reason, the chorionic surface of the expelled membranes should be examined to ensure that they have been completely expelled.

Retention of fetal membranes may mediate development of metritis or even peritonitis. Laminitis is a potential sequela. For these reasons, it is common practice to administer oxytocin, (20 U, IM, every 2-3 hr) beginning 3-4 hr after parturition if the membranes have not yet been expelled. Manual removal of retained membranes carries the risk of uterine damage or prolapse and is not recommended beyond gentle tugging to displace already loosened membranes. In cases of prolonged retention of fetal membranes, antimicrobials should be administered prophylactically, along with NSAID and other therapeutic strategies aimed at preventing laminitis (p 906). Mares that have recovered from retention of fetal membranes do not generally have lower fertility.

Other species: In does and ewes, the incidence of retained fetal membranes increases with larger litter sizes and with assisted parturition. Systemic treatment to guard against infection and gentle traction on exposed membranes may be used. In sows, retained placentae are contained within the uterus and are not visible at the vulva. In this species, entire fetuses may be retained. Usually, the fetus or membranes decompose in situ. This may be accompanied by signs of systemic illness and a purulent vaginal discharge. Although serious or fatal sequelae occasionally occur, the prognosis for recovery and future fertility is surprisingly good. Oxytocin and antimicrobial treatment are indicated.

TRICHOMONIASIS

Trichomoniasis is a venereal disease of cattle characterized primarily by early fetal death and infertility, resulting in extended calving intervals. Distribution is probably worldwide.

Etiology and Epidemiology: The causative protozoan, *Tritrichomonas (Trichomonas) foetus*, is pyriform and ordinarily 10-15 × 5-10 μm, but there is considerable pleomorphism. It may become spherical when cultured in artificial media. At its anterior end, there are 3 flagella about the same length as the body of the parasite. An undulating membrane extends the length of the body and is bordered by a marginal filament that continues beyond the membrane as a posterior flagellum. Although *T foetus* can survive the process used for freezing semen, it is killed by drying or high temperatures.

T foetus is found in the genital tracts of cattle. When cows are bred naturally by an infected bull, 30-90% become infected, suggesting that strain differences exist. Variation in breed susceptibility to trichomoniasis may also exist. Bulls of all ages can remain infected indefinitely but this is less likely in younger males. By contrast, most cows are free of infection within 3 mo after breeding. However, immunity is not longlasting and reinfection does occur. Transmission can also occur when the semen from infected bulls is used for artificial insemination.

Clinical Findings: The most common sign is infertility caused by embryonic death. This results in repeat breeding, and attending stock persons often note cows in heat when they should be pregnant. This, along with poor pregnancy test results, like too many open and late cows, is usually the presenting complaint.

Fetal death and abortions can also occur, but are not as common as losses earlier in gestation. *T foetus* has been found in vaginal cultures taken as late as 8 mo of gestation and, apparently, live calves can be born to infected dams. Pyometra occasionally develops after breeding.

Diagnosis: History and clinical signs are useful but are essentially the same as those of campylobacteriosis (p 1108). Confirmation depends on isolation of *T foetus*, which may be difficult to differentiate from other trichomonads resident in the digestive tract. Diagnostic efforts are directed at bulls because they are the most likely carriers. Suction is applied to a pipette while it is used to vigorously scrape the epithelium in the preputial fornix. Alternatively, douching with saline or lactated Ringer's solution (without preservatives) can be used. Aspirates or douches, concentrated by centrifugation, are examined using darkfield contrast microscopy. This material is also transferred immediately to the surface of a liquid culture medium such as Diamond's medium. Veterinarians have reported better success culturing the organism when using commercially available media-filled pouches. In addition, incubating the media beyond the standard 48 hr may also enhance the accuracy of the diagnosis. Sampling every 48 hr for 10 days from the bottom of the tube and examining at 100-400× may reveal the rolling jerky movements of *T foetus*. Recent studies have examined the possibility of using PCR assays to identify *T foetus* in reproductive samples. Thus far, these tests are primarily in the developmental stage, although some laboratories may be using them for diagnostic support.

Studies suggest that 90-95% of infected bulls will be positive on culture, and that 3 successive cultures at weekly intervals will detect ~99.5% of infected bulls. A vaginal discharge (after treatment of pyometra) or vaginal mucus (obtained toward the end of a luteal phase) may also be of diagnostic value.

The number of times the bull battery should be sampled and cultured to ensure they are negative depends on the prevalence of fetal wastage in the cow herd. With more open and late cows, the frequency of testing should increase to improve the probability that bulls are negative for the protozoan.

Treatment and Control: Various imidazoles have been used to treat bulls, but none is both safe and effective. Ipronidazole is probably most effective but, due to its low pH, frequently causes sterile abscesses at injection sites. In addition, bulls are probably susceptible to reinfection after successful treatment. Resistance to ipronidazole may also be a concern. The biggest problem, however, is that the success of treatment is measured by repeated sampling, which may mean the individual bull can never be definitively called negative. Therefore an unqualified recommendation for his use may not be given.

Control consists of eliminating the infection from the bull battery by culling all bulls and replacing them with virgin bulls or by testing and culling positive bulls. Repeated testing in older bulls may be unsatisfactory, and it may be prudent to cull them all. Reinfection is prevented by exposing only the uninfected (clean) bulls to uninfected (clean) cows. Clean cows are assumed to be those with calves at foot (even though some infected cows may produce a live calf) and virgin heifers. In situations in which several herds are commingled on the same range, caution must be exercised to ensure that cows and heifers are not exposed to potentially infected bulls at the home ranch before they are turned out on the common grazing pasture.

T foetus can be safely eliminated from semen with dimetridazole. Vaccines have been developed for use in cows but none is highly effective, especially in the absence of other control measures.

UDDER DISEASES

See also MASTITIS IN LARGE ANIMALS, p 1120, and PSEUDOCOWPOX, p 699.

DISEASES OF BOVINE TEATS AND SKIN

Bovine Ulcerative Mammillitis (Bovine Herpesvirus II, Bovine Herpes Mammillitis): Bovine herpesvirus II (BHV-II) causes a severe, ulcerative condition of teat and udder skin of dairy cows that is often referred to as bovine ulcerative mammillitis. BHV-II can occur sporadically or in outbreaks and often results in marked loss of milk production as well as high incidence of secondary mastitis.

Early signs may vary, but the lesions often begin as one or more thickened, edematous plaques of varying size on the skin of one or more teats. Vesicles develop and may rapidly rupture, leaving a raw, ulcerated area that becomes covered with a dark-colored scab. The scabs tend to crack and bleed, especially if milking is attempted. The lesions are of variable size and can include much of the teat wall and orifice. Teats are generally painful and affected cows often resist milking, leading to development of mastitis. The highest incidence is often seen in first-lactation cows, but previously unexposed cows of any age are susceptible. Severe lesions may take several weeks to heal.

Diagnosis is based on clinical signs and confirmed by histopathology or by virus isolation from early lesions. Treatment is directed toward supportive care, as there is no effective therapy for this virus. The use of iodophore-containing teat dips with added emollients may help to inactivate the virus. It is important to isolate affected cows and to use separate milking equipment. Furthermore, separate paper towels and clean gloves for milking personnel help to prevent spread of the agent to susceptible animals.

Pseudocowpox: Pseudocowpox is a common condition of teat skin caused by a poxvirus (*see* PSEUDOCOWPOX, p 699).

Bovine Warts (Bovine Papillomavirus, BPV1, BPV5, BPV6): Several strains of bovine papillomavirus cause the development of papillomas or fibropapillomas on teats. In some herds, pale, smooth, raised lesions develop frequently on teat skin and may persist indefinitely without causing problems. In other instances, filamentous or frond-like lesions develop at the teat orifice and interfere with milking. Bovine warts are spread by direct or indirect contact. Diagnosis is usually made presumptively based on examination of the lesion and exclusion of other causes. In many instances, treatment of warts is not necessary, but frond-like lesions that interfere with milking may require excision. The use of autogenous vaccines and virucidal teat dips may be recommended in herd outbreaks.

Teat-end Hyperkeratosis: The development of raised smooth or rough rings at the teat ends of lactating cows is a common occurrence. Teat ends that are affected with hyperkeratosis may progress from smooth, doughnut-shaped lesions that do not affect milking to severely hyperkeratotic rings with radial cracks. The risk of mastitis is increased in severely affected teats because the teat sphincter cannot function properly and proper premilking teat-end disinfection is difficult. Diagnosis is usually made by clinical examination of affected teats. The cause of hyperkeratosis is multifactorial; thus, prevention is directed toward a number of potential risk factors. Hyperkeratosis is often associated with cold weather, probably because of changes in peripheral circulation. Risk factors for the development of hyperkeratosis include incorrect use of teat chemicals, exposure of wet teats to cold weather, improper milking machine settings leading to overmilking, and inadequate premilking cow preparation for milk letdown. After underlying risk factors are addressed, affected teats generally recover over a period of several weeks or over a dry period.

Dermatitis: Dermatitis of the udder has a number of causes including chemical irritants, sunburn, and bacterial infection. Exposure to chemical irritants can occur from bedding additives (eg, some types of limestone) or chemicals used during milking. The irritation usually resolves after removal of the offending substance, but gentle udder washes and the use of emollient products can accelerate healing. Udder impetigo (udder acne) is a bacterial dermatitis characterized by the development of small pustules on the skin of the udder and teats. Staphylococci usually can be isolated from the pustules. Treatment of udder impetigo consists of clipping hair from the affected area and washing the skin thoroughly each day until the condition resolves.

Frostbite: Teat skin can chap and crack when wet teats are exposed to cold winds or frozen bedding areas. Exposure of wet skin to subfreezing temperatures may result in frostbite. Skin affected by frostbite becomes swollen and discolored and ultimately develops a leathery texture. Frostbite is best prevented by ensuring that teat skin is dry before allowing cows access to housing areas or pastures during periods of temperatures <0°F. Care should be taken to ensure that all bedding areas that contact teat and udder skin are thoroughly dry. Teat disinfectact products (eg, powder teat dips and other cold weather formulations) specifically designed for extremely cold weather have been developed and are relatively successful at preventing frostbite after dipping.

Udder Sores (Necrotic Dermatitis): Moist, foul-smelling, necrotic lesions may be observed in areas of tightly adjacent skin of some animals. In heifers, the lateral aspect of the udder and medial aspect of the thigh are often involved. In this area, the udder is pressed tightly against the leg, resulting in chafing, dermatitis, and necrosis. Udder edema is a risk factor for the development of this condition and must be treated concurrently. The necrotic skin should be cleaned daily with an antiseptic solution and thoroughly dried. Mild astringents should be applied. In multiparous cows, a similar condition, which may be associated with mite infestation, is seen at the anterior portion of the udder between the 2 forequarters. The swollen, necrotic area may be treated topically with an approved miticide; however, appropriate milk withholding periods must be observed.

PHYSIOLOGIC DISORDERS

Udder Edema: Udder edema is common in high-producing dairy cattle (especially heifers) before and after parturition. Predisposing causes include genetics, nutritional management, obesity, and lack of exercise during the precalving period. Physiologic edema is not usually painful and occurs when pitting edema develops symmetrically in the udder prior to parturition. Udder edema can become a chronic condition and persist throughout lactation. Treatment should be initiated if swelling threatens the udder support apparatus, or if the edema interferes with the ability to milk the cow. Edema can be treated by milking cows before parturition but this may predispose older cows to parturient paresis (p 806). Massage, repeated as often as possible, and hot compresses stimulate circulation and promote edema reduction. Diuretics have proved highly beneficial in reducing udder edema and corticosteroids may be helpful. Products that combine diuretics and corticosteroids are available for treatment of udder edema.

Precocious Mammary Development: Initiation of milk secretion in heifers prior to calving is occasionally noted. Precocious mammary development in a single gland sometimes results from suckling by herdmates. Symmetric mammary development has been associated with exposure to feedstuffs containing estrogen or contaminated by mycotoxins. Removal of contaminated feedstuffs generally results in resolution of the problem.

Failure of Milk Ejection (Milk Letdown): In rare instances, newly calved heifers may experience problems with milk ejection. Fear of handling or unfamiliarity with the milking process is the usual cause. Care should be taken to ensure that animals are handled calmly and gently and that the milking routine provides for adequate stimulation (>20 sec) before attaching the milking unit. Administration of oxytocin (20 IU, IM) may be necessary in some instances.

Agalactia: Agalactia is seen occasionally in heifers and can be a primary endocrine problem or a localized problem of the mammary gland. In recently fresh cows, agalactia is occasionally caused by a severe systemic disease or by mastitis caused by *Mycoplasma* *bovis*. Agalactia has also been associated with cows grazing or eating endophyte-infested fescue.

"Blind" or Nonfunctional Quarters: These are usually the result of a severe infection, which may occur in dry or lactating cows or in heifers due to sucking by other heifers or calves. On the rare occasion that fibrosis is not extensive, treatment of the affected quarter might clear the infection. Some of these quarters will milk fairly satisfactorily during the next lactation. Rarely, blind or nonfunctional quarters may be congenital.

Congenital Disorders: Congenital aberrations include many structural defects, but the most significant disorder is **supernumerary teats**. These may be located on the udder behind the posterior teats, between the front and hind teats, or attached to either the front or hind teats. Removal of supernumerary teats from dairy heifers is desirable to improve appearance of the udder, to eliminate the possibility of mastitis in the gland above the extra teats, and to facilitate milking. Most are easily removed surgically when the heifer is from 1 wk to 1 yr old (best done at 3-8 mo of age). Supernumerary teats may be surgically removed from preparturient heifers before lactation begins. The incision should be sutured or stapled after teat removal.

TRAUMATIC AND STRUCTURAL DISORDERS

Trauma and Laceration: **Superficial wounds** to the udder and teats may be cleaned with suitable antiseptic solutions and treated as open wounds with frequent application of antiseptic powders or sprays. If the teats are involved, adhesive tape may hasten healing. Wounds involving the teat orifice should be dressed with antiseptic creams and bandaged after milking. Prophylactic treatment with intramammary antibiotics is usually recommended to prevent the development of mastitis.

Lacerations of the large milk vein should be considered an emergency because of the potential for severe hemorrhage; prompt compression and ligation of these lacerations is recommended.

Deeper wounds of the udder and teats should be promptly (within 6 hr) cleansed and sutured or stapled under local anesthesia with appropriate sedation and restraint. When the wound involves the teat cistern, it may be necessary to insert a self-retaining teat cannula with removable cap into the teat for the first 24 hr to prevent milk seeping through the wound (which would delay or prevent healing) and to aid in milking. The affected quarter should be infused with antibiotic preparations.

Teat Obstructions: Acquired teat obstructions are usually the result of proliferation of granulation tissue after the occurrence of an observed or unobserved teat injury. Teat obstructions are usually recognized when they interfere with milk flow. They can range from diffuse, tightly adherent lesions to highly mobile discrete lesions that float throughout the gland cistern. Some "floaters" are caused by formation of small masses from butterfat, minerals, and tissue in mammary ducts during the dry period. These can be recognized by intermittent disruptions in milk flow. They may be removed by forced pressure downward on the teat cistern or by use of specialized instruments inserted through the teat canal. Membranous obstructions in the area of the annular fold at the base of the gland cistern are sometimes observed in heifers. Treatment of these obstructions is generally frustrating.

Complete teat obstruction may result when adhesions fill the teat cistern after severe trauma. Treatment is similar to that for stenosis (*see* below), but the prognosis usually is more guarded. In instances of severe injury, milking of the quarter should be permanently discontinued.

Teat stenosis is characterized by a marked narrowing of the teat orifice or streak canal, which makes milking difficult. It usually results from a contusion or wound that produces swelling or formation of a blood clot or scab or from mastitis infections, (especially in prelactating heifers). Teat obstructions can be diagnosed initially by careful palpation of the affected gland. Complex teat obstructions or obstructions in valuable animals may require diagnostic imaging such as ultrasonography, contrast radiography, or theloscopy. Treatment varies depending on severity. Conservative treatment includes the use of teat cannulas and external pressure to remove obstructions, while serious cases may require surgery. All injuries to, or surgical procedures on, the teat should be handled carefully to prevent infection. Prophylactic antibiotic infusions of the quarter are indicated when the teat or teat orifice is involved. Permanent fistulas into the teat or gland cisterns are best repaired surgically during the dry period.

Breakdown of Udder Support Apparatus: Rupture of the suspensory ligaments of the udder (usually medial ligaments) occurs gradually in some older cows and leads to a dropping of the udder floor resulting in lateral deviation of the teats. Occasionally, acute rupture can occur at or just after parturition. Animals with this condition are at high risk for developing mastitis. There is no successful treatment; supportive trusses generally are not satisfactory. The condition is suspected to have a genetic basis.

Hematomas: Trauma (often related to inadequate housing) can result in contusions and hematomas of the udder. Hematomas usually appear as soft-tissue swellings located anterior to the foreudder or caudodorsal to the rear udder. They may be difficult to differentiate from abscesses. Severe hematomas can result in anemia if not treated. In most instances, hematomas resolve following conservative treatment consisting of pressure wraps and rest. Hematomas should not be incised or drained unless they become infected. Milking should be performed cautiously during the convalescent period. Hematomas that continue to enlarge should be considered an emergency because of the possibility of excessive blood loss and shock.

Abscesses: Subcutaneous abscesses of the udder (not involving the milk-producing tissue) can develop between the skin and the supporting connective tissue of the udder. Diagnosis is by needle aspiration. Abscesses usually develop secondary to wounds, advanced mastitis, infected hematomas, or severe contusions. They should be incised and drained when they are chronic and near the surface of the udder. The wound should be flushed daily with an antiseptic solution or water under pressure until healing is complete.

Bloody Milk: The occurrence of pink- or red-tinged milk is common after calving and can be attributed to the rupture of tiny mammary blood vessels. Udder swelling from edema or trauma is a potential underlying cause. Bloody milk is not fit for consumption. In most cases it resolves without treatment in 4-14 days, providing the gland is milked out regularly. The occurrence of frank blood in a single quarter is likely the result of severe, acute mastitis (p 1120) or trauma, and milking should be discontinued until hemorrhage is controlled. Intramammary antibiotics should be administered if mastitis is suspected.

Teat Sphincter Inadequacy ("Leakers"): High levels of intramammary pressure in high-producing dairy cows may result in milk dripping from teats in cows that are waiting to be milked. Shorter intervals or more frequent milking may be recommended when a large proportion of the herd is affected. Occasionally, cows are observed to leak milk continuously. These cows usually have sustained a severe teat injury or have an abnormal streak canal. In general, little can be done to correct this condition, and most of these cows will develop mastitis; it is recommended that persistent leakers be designated for removal from the herd.

ULCERATIVE POSTHITIS AND VULVITIS

(Sheath rot, Pizzle rot, Enzootic balanoposthitis)

Ulcerative posthitis is principally a disease of sheep but occasionally is seen in goats and cattle (usually in castrated males). Females are less commonly and usually less severely affected.

Etiology and Epidemiology: This moderately contagious disease is caused by *Corynebacterium renale*, a gram-positive, diphtheroid bacterium capable of hydrolyzing urea. When protein intake is high, urinary urea concentration increases. Hydrolysis of urea by *C renale* results in local production of large quantities of ammonia, which is believed to irritate the penis, lamina interna of the prepuce, and skin surrounding the preputial orifice. The condition is more common in male castrates, probably because of the hypoplastic nature of the penis, exacerbated in some cases by failure of penile-preputial separation that leads to pooling of urine in the prepuce. If preputial hair is cut too short or becomes caked with mud or organic matter, drainage of urine away from the preputial orifice (normally facilitated by this hair) is impaired, and ulcerative lesions may develop.

The incidence of ulcerative posthitis is highest in Merino and Angora wethers, which is attributed to the long hair or wool surrounding the prepuce in these animals, allowing urine to soak the area, which in turn is conducive to bacterial growth and activity. The condition can be transmitted experimentally by infective material from a preputial or vulvar ulcer. Ulcerative posthitis or vulvitis has a seasonal occurrence that varies with local animal husbandry methods. Peak incidence corresponds to the time when animals graze lush green pasture (eg, spring and early summer in New Zealand or autumn and winter in southern Brazil) or are fed or have access to high-protein feedstuffs.

Clinical Findings: In mild cases, signs are limited to swelling of the prepuce. In severe cases, swelling and inflammation interfere with urination and result in straining, which needs to be differentiated from urolithiasis (p 1259). Histologic characteristics are acanthosis, parakeratosis, and hyperkeratosis, followed by leukocyte invasion and ulceration. Ulcers and scabs may be found around the preputial orifice, on the lamina interna of the prepuce, and on the shaft of the penis. Urine and exudate may accumulate in the prepuce. The condition may cause severe discomfort. If the preputial orifice or urethra is occluded, affected animals may die. Ulcerative vulvitis begins with signs of vulvar inflammation, including swelling and redness, and progresses to development of a yellow exudate with ulceration and scab formation around the vulva, vestibule, and caudal vagina. The glans clitoridis may be swollen, red, and ulcerated.

Lesions of ulcerative posthitis or vulvitis should be distinguished from those of granular posthitis or vulvitis (associated with *Mycoplasma* spp or *Ureaplasma* spp, p 1150), herpesviral balanoposthitis or vulvovaginitis (p 1193), ulcerative dermatosis (p 703 [sheep only]), or contagious ecthyma (orf, p 697 [goats only]). Removal of the scabs of ulcerative posthitis or vulvitis characteristically results in little or no hemorrhage.

Treatment and Control: If possible, affected animals should be isolated from the rest of the herd and not fed a high-protein diet. Lesions should be examined to ensure that they do not interfere with urethral patency. Clipping and cleaning hair around the prepuce may be beneficial. *C renale* is usually sensitive to penicillins and cephalosporins, which may be beneficial if practical. Ulcerative posthitis is controlled principally by limiting dietary protein to a level consistent with requirements. Implantation of wethers with 70-100 mg of testosterone every 3 mo is effective in preventing ulcerative posthitis. Castration by the "short scrotum" technique to produce induced cryptorchidism results in sterile animals that have higher concentrations of circulating testosterone and a much lower incidence of posthitis than animals castrated by conventional procedures.

UTERINE PROLAPSE AND EVERSION

Prolapse of the uterus may occur in any species; however, it is most common in dairy and beef cows and ewes and less frequent in sows. (It is rare in mares, bitches, queens, and rabbits.) The etiology is unclear and occurrence is sporadic. Recumbency with the hindquarters lower than the forequarters, invagination of the tip of the uterus, excessive traction to relieve dystocia or retained fetal membranes, uterine atony, hypocalcemia, and lack of exercise have all been incriminated as contributory causes. Prolapse of the uterus invariably occurs immediately after or within several hours of parturition, when the cervix is open and the uterus lacks tone. Prolapse of the postgravid uterine horn usually is complete in cows, and the mass of uterus usually hangs below the hocks. The invagination of the contralateral horn can be located by careful examination of the surface of the prolapsed organ. In sows, one horn may become everted while unborn piglets in the other prevent further prolapse. In small animals, complete prolapse of both uterine horns is usual.

In cows, treatment involves removing the placenta (if still attached), thoroughly cleaning the endometrial surface, and repairing any lacerations. Rubbing the surface of the uterus with glycerol helps reduce edema and provides lubrication. The uterus is then returned to its normal position. An epidural anesthetic should be administered first. If the cow is standing, the cleansed uterus should be elevated to the level of the vulva on a tray or hammock supported by assistants, and then replaced by applying steady pressure beginning at the cervical portion (or at the level of the invagination of the nonprolapsed uterine horn) and gradually working toward the apex. Once the uterus is replaced, a hand should be inserted to the tip of both uterine horns to be sure that there is no remaining invagination that could incite abdominal straining and another prolapse. Installation of warm, sterile saline solution is useful for ensuring complete replacement of the tip of the uterine horn without trauma. If recumbent, the cow should be positioned with the hindquarters elevated by placing her in sternal recumbency with the hindlegs extended backward. Replacement of the prolapsed uterus in mares is done in a similar way, usually with the mare sedated but standing, taking care not to perforate the uterus.

In sows and small animals, the uterus may be repositioned by simultaneously manipulating it from outside with one hand and through an abdominal incision with the other. Resection of the uterus is indicated in longstanding cases in which tissue necrosis has occurred. Once the uterus is in its normal position, oxytocin (20 IU, IV, or 40 IU, IM) is administered to increase uterine tone. Administration IV of calcium-containing solutions is indicated in most cases, also as a means of increasing uterine tone. Caslick sutures or other forms of vulvar closure are not useful because the uterine prolapse begins at the apex of the uterine horn, and prevention of recurrence depends on complete and correct replacement of the uterus.

The prognosis depends on the amount of injury and contamination of the uterus. The prognosis is favorable when a clean, minimally traumatized uterus is promptly replaced. There is no tendency for the condition to recur at subsequent parturitions. Complications tend to develop when laceration, necrosis, and infection occur, or when treatment is delayed. Shock, hemorrhage, and thromboembolism are potential sequelae of a prolonged prolapse. In some instances, the bladder and intestines may prolapse into the everted uterus. These require careful replacement before the uterus is replaced. The bladder may be drained with a catheter or needle passed through the uterine wall. Elevation of the hindquarters and pressure on the uterus aid in replacement of bladder and intestines. It may be necessary to incise the uterus carefully (in a longitudinal direction) to replace these organs. In cows, amputation of a severely traumatized or necrotic uterus may be the only means of saving the animal. Supportive treatment and antibiotic therapy are indicated.

VAGINAL AND CERVICAL PROLAPSE

Eversion and prolapse of the vagina, with or without prolapse of the cervix, occurs most commonly in cattle and sheep. A form of vaginal prolapse, different in pathogenesis, also occurs in dogs (see VAGINAL HYPERPLASIA, p 1156). In cattle and sheep, the condition is usually seen in mature females in the last trimester of pregnancy. Predisposing factors include increased intra-abdominal pressure associated with increased size of the pregnant uterus, intra-abdominal fat, or rumen distention superimposed upon relaxation and softening of the pelvic girdle and associated soft-tissue structures in the pelvic canal and perineum mediated by increased circulating concentrations of estrogens and relaxin during late pregnancy. Intra-abdominal pressure is increased in recumbent animals. Added to this, sheep tend to face uphill when lying down, so that gravity assists vaginal eversion and prolapse.

The prolapse begins as an intussusception-like folding of the vaginal floor just cranial to the vestibulovaginal junction. Discomfort caused by this eversion, coupled with irritation and swelling of the exposed mucosa, results in straining and more extensive prolapse. Eventually the entire vagina may be prolapsed, with the cervix conspicuous at the most caudal part of the prolapsus. The bladder or loops of intestine may be contained within the prolapsed vagina. As the bladder moves into the prolapsed vagina, the urethra may be occluded. The bladder then fills and enlarges, which hinders replacement of the prolapsed vagina unless the bladder is first drained. The bladder may even rupture with potentially fatal consequences.

Although most common in mature animals in late pregnancy, vaginal prolapse occurs in young, nonpregnant ewes and heifers, especially in fat animals. Predisposing factors include grazing estrogenic plants (especially *Trifolium subterraneum*) or exogenous administration of estrogenic compounds (usually in the form of growth-promotant implants). Cervicovaginal prolapse is more common in stabled than in pastured animals, suggesting that lack of exercise may be a contributing factor. Vaginal prolapse may also be a problem in cows subjected to repeated superovulation for embryo recovery. A genetic component in the pathogenesis of cervicovaginal prolapse is likely because a breed predisposition exists in both cattle (Brahman, Brahman crossbreds, Hereford) and sheep (Kerry Hill, Romney Marsh). In pigs, vaginal prolapse is often associated with estrogenic activity of mycotoxins.

For replacement of the prolapsed vagina, an epidural anesthetic is first administered. The organ is washed and rinsed, and the bladder is emptied if necessary. Usually, this can be achieved by elevating the prolapsus to allow straightening of the urethra; occasionally, needle puncture through the vaginal wall may be necessary. The vagina is well lubricated (glycerol provides lubrication and reduces congestion and edema by osmotic action) and replaced and then held in position until it feels warm again. Retention is achieved by insertion of a Buhner suture—a deeply buried, circumferential suture placed around the vestibulum to provide support at the point at which the initial eversion of the vaginal wall occurs. The Buhner suture has largely superseded earlier attempts to prevent prolapse by various patterns of sutures in the vulvar lips (which do not prevent the initial eversion of the vagina into the vestibulum) or by methods that relied on placement of a retention device within the vagina (which tend to cause discomfort and further straining). Buhner sutures should generally be removed before parturition to prevent extensive laceration. Although the cervical os may be edematous and inflamed, cervicovaginal prolapse seldom interrupts pregnancy and does not specifically predispose to dystocia or postpartum uterine prolapse, which has a different etiology. Vaginal prolapse in sheep may occur simultaneously in many ewes as a herd problem, making surgery impractical. In these cases, use of a commercially available vaginal retention device (a bearing retainer) may be useful. Sheep may lamb without mishap with these devices in place. Permanent fixation techniques (cervicopexy or vaginopexy) have been described in which the cervix or vaginal wall is anchored to other pelvic structures. They may be useful in individual cases of chronic or recurrent prolapse.

VULVITIS AND VAGINITIS IN LARGE ANIMALS

Contusion and hematoma of the vagina are noted infrequently after parturition in all species but particularly in mares and sows. Occasionally, vaginal hematomas in sows may rupture and cause serious (or fatal) hemorrhage that can be controlled by ligation of the labial branch of the internal pudendal artery. Necrotic vaginitis, vestibulitis, and vulvitis may follow dystocia in all species. Onset of signs, consisting of arched back, elevated tail, anorexia, dysuria, straining, vulvar and perivulvar swelling, and possibly a fetid, serous discharge, begins within 1-4 days of parturition and may persist for 2-4 wk. In most cases, only gentle and conservative treatment is needed. Prophylactic antibiotic treatment is wise because clostridial or other organisms may proliferate in the damaged tissue and cause tetanus (p 495), blackleg (p 488), or other forms of clostridial myositis. Possible consequences of necrotic vaginitis include permanent stricture of the vagina or perivaginal abscessation.

Vestibular lymphocytic follicles, also called granular venereal disease, granular vulvitis, or granular vulvovaginitis, are seen in cows and are characterized by vestibular hyperemia and hyperplasia of the lymphoid nodules of the vestibular mucosa. These lesions do not constitute a specific disease but reflect irritation of the vestibular mucosa. They can be reproduced experimentally by topical application of *Ureaplasma ureolyticum* or *Mycoplasma* spp in goats and cattle.

Infectious pustular vulvovaginitis of cows is caused by bovine herpesvirus 1 (p 1193) and is transmitted by natural service or by nasogenital contact. It is characterized by vaginal lesions. Affected cows show signs of vaginal discomfort (raised tail, frequent urination) and have numerous, round, white, raised lesions of the vestibular mucosa. Within a short time, these lesions progress to pustules and erosions or ulcers. The histologic lesion consists of necrosis of vestibular and vaginal epithelium, with intranuclear inclusion bodies typical of herpesvirus infection. The virus may be secreted in the semen of infected bulls (which have similar lesions of the penis and prepuce). Intrauterine inoculation of the virus produces necrotizing endometritis and cervicitis.

A severe disease characterized by vaginitis in cows and epididymitis in bulls occurs sporadically in eastern and southern Africa, where it is referred to as epivag. The disease is spread by natural mating. In the early stages of infection, cows have intense vaginitis characterized by reddened mucosae without ulcers, erosions, or vesicular lesions. A thick, creamy, white to yellow discharge develops. The infection spreads to the uterus and uterine tubes, and salpingitis and fimbrial adhesions frequently result in permanent infertility. Although epivag has been transmitted experimentally by transferring exudate, the cause is unknown.

Catarrhal bovine vaginitis has been reported from many countries. Although enteroviruses have been associated with this condition, the cause remains unknown. In areas of the world where bovine tuberculosis (p 549) is still endemic, vaginal lesions may be either a primary lesion after service by a bull with genital infection or evidence of uterine disease.

One cause of vulvitis in sheep is ulcerative dermatosis (p 703), which is characterized by crusted ulcers of the vulvar skin, penis, prepuce, and facial skin. Posthitis and vulvitis are also caused by the interaction of a high-protein diet and infection with urease-producing organisms, usually *Corynebacterium renale*. *Demodex* mites have been seen in the vulvar skin of sheep; they usually are not associated with lesions but may produce granulomas.

Equine coital exanthema (p 1119) is caused by equine herpesvirus 3. It is an acute disease without systemic signs. Red papules appear in the vaginal and vestibular mucosae 2-10 days after infection, which occurs as a result of mating with an infected stallion. Lesions extend to the perivulvar skin. The lesions progress rapidly to pustules, then ulcerate, and finally heal, leaving depigmented scars. Stallions show similar lesions on the penis and prepuce. The disease causes discomfort and may prevent mating but does not specifically inhibit fertility.

Dourine (p 34) is a venereal disease of horses. Early signs are characterized by edematous swelling of the vulva and secondary vulvovaginitis of the swollen, irritable tissue.

Coital injuries of cows and mares may be attributable to the relatively large size of the penis in these species compared with the vagina. Injuries of the vulva and vagina may be caused by horned cattle. Vaginal injuries in a variety of species have also been inflicted maliciously.

REPRODUCTIVE DISEASES OF THE FEMALE SMALL ANIMAL

See also MANAGEMENT OF REPRODUCTION: SMALL ANIMALS, p 1786.

DYSTOCIA

Dystocia refers to abnormal or difficult birth. Causes include maternal factors (uterine inertia, inadequate size of birth canal) and/or fetal factors (oversized fetus, abnormal orientation as the fetus enters the birth canal).

Dystocia should be considered in any of the following situations: 1) animals with a history of previous dystocia or reproductive tract obstruction, 2) parturition that does not occur within 24 hr after a drop in rectal temperature to <100°F (37.7°C), 3) strong abdominal contractions lasting for 1-2 hr without passage of a puppy or kitten, 4) active labor lasting for 1-2 hr without delivery of subsequent puppies or kittens, 5) a resting period during active labor >4-6 hr, 6) a bitch or queen in obvious pain (eg, crying, licking, or biting the vulva), 7) abnormal vulvar discharge (eg, frank blood, dark green discharge before any neonates are born [indicates placental separation]).

To determine the appropriate therapy, the cause of dystocia (obstructive vs nonobstructive) must be determined and the condition of the animal assessed. A thorough history regarding breeding dates, previous parturitions, pelvic trauma, etc is desirable. The animal should be examined for signs of systemic illness that, if present, may necessitate immediate cesarean section. The normal vaginal discharge at parturition is a dark green color; abnormal color or character warrants immediate attention. A sterile digital vaginal examination should be performed to evaluate patency of the birth canal and the position and presentation of the fetus(es). Radiography or ultrasonography can determine the presence and number of fetuses, as well as their size, position, and viability.

Medical management may be considered when the condition of the dam and fetuses is stable, when there is proper fetal position and presentation, and when there is no obstruction. Oxytocin (3-20 U in bitches, 2-5 U in queens) given IM up to 3 times at 30-min intervals, with or without 10% calcium gluconate (3-5 mL, IV slowly) may be given in an attempt to promote uterine contractions. If no response follows, a cesarean section should be performed.

Surgery is indicated for obstructive dystocia, dystocia accompanied by shock or systemic illness, primary uterine inertia, prolonged active labor, or if medical management has failed.

FALSE PREGNANCY
(Pseudopregnancy, Pseudocyesis)

False pregnancy is common in bitches and uncommon in queens. It occurs at the end of diestrus and is characterized by hyperplasia of the mammary glands, lactation, and behavioral changes. Some bitches behave as if parturition has occurred, "mothering" by nesting inanimate objects and refusing to eat. The possibility of a true pregnancy should be eliminated by the history, abdominal palpation, and abdominal radiographs and ultrasonography.

The falling progesterone and increasing prolactin concentrations associated with late diestrus are believed to be responsible for the clinical signs. No treatment is recommended because the condition resolves spontaneously in 1-3 wk. In bitches with discomfort secondary to mammary gland enlargement, alternating cold and warm compresses on the engorged mammae or wrapping the abdomen with an elastic bandage may give relief. The owners must be cautioned not to milk out the mammary glands, because that will only stimulate lactogenesis. Tranquilizers (eg, diazepam, PO, up to 4 days) may be considered for bitches with significant behavioral changes. Estrogens should not be used because of the potential for bone marrow suppression. Megestrol acetate, a progestin (2.5 mg/kg, PO, SID for 8 days), is the only drug currently approved for treatment of false pregnancy in bitches in the USA. Prolonged or repeated use of megestrol acetate may cause pyometra. Androgens (eg, mibolerone, 16 μg/kg, PO, SID for 5 days) may decrease clinical signs of false pregnancy in bitches. Mibolerone is not approved for treatment of false pregnancy in bitches in the USA. If owners are distressed by repeated bouts of pseudopregnancy, the bitch should either be bred or undergo ovariohysterectomy.

FOLLICULAR CYSTS

These fluid-filled structures develop within the ovary and result in prolonged secretion of estrogen, continued signs of proestrus or estrus, and attractiveness to males. Ovulation may not occur during this abnormal estrous cycle. Follicular cysts should be suspected in any bitch showing clinical manifestations of estrus for >21 days, or when proestrus plus estrus have lasted for >40 days. Estrous cycles due to follicular cysts in queens may be difficult to differentiate from normal, frequent cycles.

The primary differential diagnosis is functional ovarian granulosa cell tumor. Assessment of vaginal cytology with presence of cornified cells is indicative of elevated serum estrogens.

The treatment of choice is ovariohysterectomy. If the animal is to be bred, induction of luteinization of the cystic follicles may be accomplished by using gonadotropin-releasing hormone (25 μg, IM) or human chorionic gonadotropin (220 IU/kg, IV, or 1,000 IU, half IV, half IM).

MAMMARY HYPERTROPHY IN CATS

(Feline mammary hypertrophy, Mammary dysplasia, Fibroadenoma complex, Mammary fibroadenomatosis, Glandular mammary hypertrophy)

This benign condition is characterized by rapid abnormal growth of one or more mammary glands. There are 2 basic types of hyperplasia of the feline mammary gland—lobular hyperplasia and fibroepithelial hyperplasia. Lobular hyperplasia is seen as palpable masses in one or more mammary glands in intact cats 1-14 yr old. Fibroepithelial hyperplasia occurs in young, cycling, or pregnant cats; in old, intact females and males; and in neutered males after treatment with progestins.

Feline mammary hypertrophy is considered to be a hormone-dependent dysplastic change in the mammary gland. Hyperplasia occurs within 1-2 wk after estrus or 2-6 wk after progestin treatment. The tremendously enlarged glands may appear erythematous, and some of the skin may be necrotic. Edema of the skin and both hindlegs is common, and the condition can easily be confused with acute mastitis.

Ovariohysterectomy or mastectomy is curative, although spontaneous remissions occur. Ovariohysterectomy is followed by regression of the glands and prevents recurrence.

MASTITIS

Mastitis is inflammation of the mammary gland(s), associated with bacterial infection. It occurs in postpartum bitches and less commonly in postpartum queens. Rarely, mastitis is observed in lactating pseudopregnant bitches. Risk factors for developing mastitis include poor sanitary conditions, trauma inflicted by offspring, and systemic infection. Mastitis may be acute or chronic.

Mastitis may be localized (eg, involving a single gland sinus), diffuse in a single gland, or diffuse within multiple glands. The animal may be asymptomatic or critically compromised. Milk from mastitic glands may appear normal grossly or may be abnormal in color or consistency. In acute mastitis, the affected glands are hot and painful. If acute mastitis progresses to septic mastitis, signs of systemic illness such as fever, depression, anorexia, and lethargy may be seen, and the dam may neglect the neonates. In chronic or subclinical mastitis, the main complaint may be failure of offspring to thrive.

Diagnosis is usually evident from the history and physical examination. Microscopic examination of milk may reveal inflammatory cells. Milk from each gland should be evaluated in any postpartum bitch or queen with signs of systemic illness. Before beginning therapy, a milk sample should be collected (or obtained by fine-needle aspiration) for bacterial culture and sensitivity. Culture of milk or fluid expressed from the affected glands yields moderate to heavy growth of *Escherichia coli* or staphylococci.

Broad-spectrum, bactericidal antibiotics should be chosen based on sensitivity tests and with the realization that they will be passed in the milk to the young. Antibiotics such as tetracycline, chloramphenicol, or aminoglycosides should be avoided during lactation unless the neonates are weaned. Cephalexin (5-15 mg/kg, PO, TID) and amoxicillin/ clavulanate (14 mg/kg, PO, BID-TID) are recommended as initial therapeutic agents pending culture results. Hot-packing the affected gland encourages drainage and seems to relieve discomfort. Fluid therapy is indicated in animals with septic mastitis that are dehydrated or in shock. An abscessed mammary gland should be lanced, drained, flushed, and treated as an open wound.

Nonseptic mastitis is seen most commonly at weaning. The affected glands are warm, swollen, and painful to the touch, but the animal is alert and healthy. Warm compresses should be applied to the affected glands 4-6 times daily, and the young should be encouraged to nurse from these glands. When galactostasis occurs at weaning, lactation can be diminished by reducing food and water intake of the dam. The mammary glands should not be stimulated during this time. Appropriate food and water must be provided for the young.

METRITIS

Metritis is infection of the uterus that occurs postpartum. Predisposing causes include prolonged delivery, dystocia, and retained fetuses or placentas. *Escherichia coli* is the most common bacterium isolated from the infected uterus; streptococci, staphylococci, *Proteus* spp, and others are isolated less frequently.

The primary clinical sign is purulent vulvar discharge. Bitches or queens with metritis are usually depressed, with signs of fever, lethargy, and inappetence and may neglect their offspring. Pups may become restless and cry incessantly. Metritis should be considered in any postpartum animal with signs of systemic illness or an abnormal vaginal discharge. A large, flaccid uterus may be palpable. Radiographs should be taken to determine if fetuses or placentas are retained. The hemogram may show leukocytosis with a left shift.

Treatment includes stabilization with IV fluids, supportive care, and antibiotic therapy based on culture and sensitivity testing of the vulvar discharge. Prostaglandin $F_{2\alpha}$ (0.1-0.25 mg/kg, SC, for 2-3 days) or oxytocin (5-20 U in bitches, 2-5 U in queens, IM) may help evacuate the uterine contents. Ovariohysterectomy is recommended after initial stabilization if the animal is extremely ill or if future reproduction is unimportant. Otherwise, it should be considered an elective procedure to be performed when lactation has ceased.

OVARIAN REMNANT SYNDROME

Ovarian remnant syndrome refers to clinical signs indicating presence of functional ovarian tissue in a previously ovariohysterectomized bitch or queen. It is not a pathologic condition but a complication of ovariohysterectomy. It occurs when a retained piece of ovarian tissue revascularizes and becomes functional. The most common presentation is recurrent estrus (eg, vulvar swelling, flagging, standing to be mounted) after ovariohysterectomy.

Differential diagnoses include vaginitis, uterine stump pyometra, and exogenous estrogen therapy. Presumptive diagnosis of ovarian remnant syndrome requires demonstration of a cornified vaginal epithelium in a spayed female. Exploratory laparotomy to find and remove the ovarian remnant is the treatment of choice.

PYOMETRA

Pyometra is a hormonally mediated diestrual disorder characterized by cystic endometrial hyperplasia with secondary bacterial infection. Pyometra is reported primarily in older bitches (>5 yr old), 4-6 wks after estrus.

Etiology: Factors associated with occurrence of pyometra include administration of longlasting progestational compounds to delay or suppress estrus, administration of estrogens to mismated bitches, and postinsemination or postcopulation infections. Progesterone promotes endometrial growth and glandular secretion while decreasing myometrial activity. Cystic endometrial hyperplasia and accumulation of uterine secretions ultimately develop and provide an excellent environment for bacterial growth. Progesterone may also inhibit the WBC response to bacterial infection. Bacteria from the normal vaginal flora or subclinical urinary tract infections are the most likely sources of uterine contamination. *Escherichia coli* is the most common bacterium isolated in cases of pyometra, although *Staphylococcus, Streptococcus, Pseudomonas,* and *Proteus* spp, and other bacteria also have been recovered. Because queens require copulatory stimulation to ovulate and produce progesterone from corpora lutea, pyometra is less common in queens than in bitches. Administration of medroxyprogesterone and other progestational compounds has been associated with development of pyometra in bitches and queens. Pyometra can develop in uterine tissue left after ovariohysterectomy (stump pyometra). It can also occur secondary to postpartum metritis.

By itself, estrogen does not contribute to the development of cystic endometrial hyperplasia or pyometra. However, it does increase the stimulatory effects of progesterone on the uterus. Administration of exogenous estrogens to prevent pregnancy (ie, "mismate shots") during diestrus greatly increases the risk of developing pyometra and should be discouraged.

Clinical and Laboratory Findings: Clinical signs are seen during diestrus (usually 4-8 wk after estrus) or after administration of exogenous progestins. The signs are variable and include lethargy, anorexia, polyuria, polydipsia, and vomiting. When the cervix is open, a purulent vulvar discharge, often containing blood, is present. When the cervix is closed, there is no discharge and the large uterus may cause abdominal distention. Signs can progress rapidly to shock and death.

Physical examination reveals lethargy, dehydration, uterine enlargement, and if the cervix is patent, a sanguineous to mucopurulent vaginal discharge. Only 20% of affected animals have a fever. Shock may be present.

The leukogram of animals with pyometra is variable and may be normal; however, leukocytosis characterized by a neutrophilia with a left shift is usual. Leukopenia may be found in animals with sepsis. A mild, normocytic, normochromic, nonregenerative anemia (PCV of 28-35%) may also develop. Hyperproteinemia due to hyperglobulinemia may be found. Results of urinalysis are variable. With *E coli* uterine infection, isosthenuria due to endotoxin-induced impairment of renal tubular function or to insensitivity to antidiuretic hormone (or both) may develop. A glomerulonephropathy caused by immune-complex deposition may result in proteinuria. These renal lesions are potentially reversible once the pyometra is resolved.

Diagnosis: Pyometra should be suspected in any ill, diestrual bitch or queen, especially if polydipsia, polyuria, or vomiting is present. The diagnosis can be established from the history, physical examination, abdominal radiography, and ultrasonography. Vaginal cytology is often helpful in determining the nature of the vulvar discharge. A CBC, biochemical profile, and urinalysis help exclude other causes of polydipsia, polyuria, and vomiting; they also evaluate renal function, acid-base status, and septicemia. The uterine exudate should be cultured and sensitivity tests performed. Differential diagnoses include pregnancy and other causes of vulvar discharge, polyuria and polydipsia, and vomiting.

Treatment and Prognosis: Ovariohysterectomy is the treatment of choice. Medical management could be considered if salvaging the reproductive potential of the bitch or queen is desired. Fluids (IV) and broad-spectrum, bactericidal antibiotics should be administered. Fluid, electrolyte, and acid-base imbalances should be corrected as quickly as possible, before ovariohysterectomy is performed. The bacterial infection is responsible for the illness and will not resolve until the uterine exudate is removed. Oral antibiotics (based on the results of the culture and sensitivity) should be continued for 7-10 days after surgery.

Medical therapy with prostaglandin $F_{2\alpha}$ ($PGF_{2\alpha}$) can be used for animals to be bred in the future, although prostaglandins are not approved in the USA for use in cats or dogs. $PGF_{2\alpha}$ causes luteolysis, contraction of the myometrium, relaxation of the cervix, and expulsion of the uterine exudate. They should probably not be used in animals >8 yr old or in those not intended for breeding. The delay before clinical improvement and the many side effects of $PGF_{2\alpha}$ preclude its use in a severely ill animal. $PGF_{2\alpha}$ also should be used with caution in bitches or queens with a closed-cervix pyometra because of increased risk of uterine rupture. Pregnancy must be ruled out, as prostaglandins can induce abortion.

Only naturally occurring $PGF_{2\alpha}$ (0.25 mg/kg, SC, SID for 5 days) should be used. Synthetic analogs (eg, cloprostenol, fluprostenol, and prostalene) are much more potent than natural $PGF_{2\alpha}$ but have not been evaluated for use in dogs or cats. Broad-spectrum, bactericidal antibiotics, chosen on the basis of culture and sensitivity tests, should be given for ≥2 wk.

The side effects of $PGF_{2\alpha}$ include restlessness, anxiety, panting, hypersalivation, pacing, tachycardia, vomiting, urination, and defecation. In cats, vocalization and intense grooming behavior also may be seen. These reactions disappear within 2 hr of the injection. The LD_{50} of $PGF_{2\alpha}$ in dogs is 5.13 mg/kg. Severe ataxia, respiratory distress, and muscle tremors may be seen in queens given 5 mg/kg. If severe side effects occur, IV fluids at rates appropriate for treatment of shock are indicated. Uterine evacuation after an injection is variable.

Animals should be reexamined 2 wk after completion of medical therapy. If a sanguineous or mucopurulent vulvar discharge or uterine enlargement is still present, $PGF_{2\alpha}$ therapy, using the same protocol, may be repeated; however, the prognosis for recovery is much worse. After medical therapy, the prognosis for initial resolution of the pyometra is good if the cervix is open, but guarded to poor if closed. Of those animals that respond, as many as 90% of bitches and 70% of queens with open-cervix pyometra may be fertile. Recurrence is likely; of bitches treated medically for pyometra, 70% had recurrence within 2 yr. Therefore, the animal should be bred on the next and each subsequent cycle until the desired number of puppies or kittens has been produced, and then spayed.

SUBINVOLUTION OF PLACENTAL SITES (SIPS)

SIPS is abnormal repair of the endometrial placental sites. This disorder is most common in young bitches (<3 yr old) after whelping a first litter. Bitches with SIPS are normal except for hemorrhagic uterine discharge passing from the vulva for several weeks postpartum. Diagnosis is by exclusion; differentials include metritis, vaginitis, and cystitis. Treatment is supportive. Ovariohysterectomy is recommended for bitches that become anemic enough to require transfusion and for bitches not intended for future breeding.

VAGINAL HYPERPLASIA
(Vaginal fold prolapse, Vaginal hypertrophy, Vaginal prolapse)

In vaginal hyperplasia, a proliferation of the vaginal mucosa, usually originating from the floor of the vagina anterior to the urethral orifice, occurs during proestrus and estrus as a result of estrogenic stimulation. Occasionally, the prolapse continues throughout pregnancy or recurs at parturition. The most common sign is a mass protruding from the vulva. Initially, the surface is smooth and glistening, but with prolonged exposure it becomes dry and fissures develop. A slight vaginal discharge may be present. Although the hyperplastic tissue originates near the urethral orifice, dysuria is uncommon. Vaginal hyperplasia interferes with copulation. Reluctance to breed or failure of intromission may be the only clinical sign if the hyperplastic tissue is contained within the vaginal vault. Vaginal hyperplasia resolves spontaneously as soon as estrogen declines.

The diagnosis is made by the history (stage of the estrous cycle) and examination of the vagina. Estrogenic stimulation could be confirmed by cornification of the vaginal epithelial cells, the presence of the characteristic serosanguineous estrous discharge, and the presence of estrous behavior. The differential diagnosis is vaginal neoplasia, which can be excluded by biopsy of the protruding tissue.

If the hyperplastic tissue is not causing problems, therapy is not indicated. However, if it protrudes from the vulva, it should be kept clean and moist and an antibiotic ointment applied. An Elizabethan collar may be necessary to prevent self-trauma. These animals may be bred by artificial insemination. The hyperplasia regresses as soon as the follicular phase of the estrous cycle has passed. Submucosal resection may be necessary if the mass is extremely large or if mucosal damage is extensive. Recurrence is common even after surgical resection. Vaginal hyperplasia resolves within days of removal of estrogen. Rarely, the hyperplasia recurs at parturition, presumably associated with a burst of estrogen. Ovariohysterectomy, the treatment of choice, permanently corrects this condition by removing the gonadal source of estrogen, thus preventing recurrence.

VAGINITIS

Inflammation of the vagina may occur in prepubertal or mature (intact or spayed) bitches. It is rare in queens. Vaginitis usually is due to bacterial infection, which may be secondary to conformational abnormalities such as vestibulovaginal strictures. Viral infection (eg, herpes), vaginal foreign bodies, neoplasia, hyperplasia of the vagina, androgenic steroids (eg, mibolerone), or intersex conditions also may cause vaginitis.

The most common clinical sign is a vulvar discharge. Licking of the vulva, attraction of males, and frequent micturition also may be seen. Signs of systemic illness are not present, and the hemogram and biochemical profile are normal. The absence of these abnormalities helps differentiate vaginitis from open-cervix pyometra, the most important differential diagnosis. The diagnostic evaluation should include a digital examination of the vagina, vaginoscopy, cytology and if necessary culture of the exudate, and abdominal radiographs or ultrasonography to evaluate the uterus. An anterior vaginal culture may be obtained using a guarded sterile culture swab. The vagina contains normal bacterial flora; therefore, culture results must be interpreted cautiously. A heavy growth, especially of one organism, is probably more significant than a light growth of several organisms.

Predisposing factors such as foreign material or anatomic abnormalities should be corrected. Bacterial infection may respond to local treatment (ie, vaginal douches). Systemic, broad-spectrum, bactericidal antibiotics may be needed for persistent infections. Prepubertal animals often do not require treatment because the vaginitis nearly always resolves with the first estrus. Therefore, it may be wise to delay elective ovariohysterectomy in affected animals until after their first estrous cycle.

REPRODUCTIVE DISEASES OF THE MALE SMALL ANIMAL

See also MANAGEMENT OF REPRODUCTION: SMALL ANIMALS, p 1786, PROSTATIC DISEASES, p 1162, CONGENITAL AND INHERITED ANOMALIES OF THE REPRODUCTIVE SYSTEM, p 1094, and INFERTILITY, p 1796.

ORCHITIS AND EPIDIDYMITIS

Acute inflammation of the testis or epididymis may be caused by trauma, infection (fungal, bacterial, or viral), or testicular torsion. Clinical signs are pain and swelling of the testes, epididymides, and/or scrotum. There may be wounds or other lesions in the scrotal skin. Orchitis and epididymitis are rare in cats.

The scrotal contents should be carefully palpated to identify which structures are involved, including the vas deferens and pampiniform vessels. Ultrasonography is helpful to further evaluate the affected structures and to confirm the presence of testicular torsion and focal lesions in the testis or epididymis. It will also identify less common causes of scrotal enlargement such as scrotal hernia.

Diagnostic tests should always include a rapid slide agglutination test for *Brucella canis*. (*See also* BRUCELLOSIS IN DOGS, p 1159.) Cytologic examination of semen with bacterial and mycoplasmal culture are also helpful, but semen collection from animals that are ill or in pain may be difficult. Testicular specimens for cytology and culture may be obtained by fine-needle aspiration. Testicular biopsy for histopathology and bacterial culture may be performed, if needed, after less invasive diagnostic tests have been completed. Because of the greater risk of granuloma formation, epididymal aspiration and biopsy are rarely done. If future reproduction is not of importance, specimens can easily be obtained at the time of castration.

Treatment is difficult unless the underlying cause can be identified. The prognosis for maintaining fertility is guarded despite aggressive therapy because of the potential for irreversible damage to the germinal epithelium, tubular degeneration, development of immune-mediated orchitis, or obstruction of the duct system. These sequelae may take months to occur. Application of cool water packs may decrease testicular damage caused by local swelling and hyperthermia. In the case of unilateral involvement, the unaffected testis/epididymis must be protected from damage by heat, pressure, and direct extension of the disease process. Hemicastration may be prudent. If bacterial cultures are positive, appropriate systemic antibiotics should be administered for ≥3 wk. There is no successful treatment for *B canis* infection. All antifungal agents interfere with spermatogenesis, either directly or indirectly.

If histopathology is suggestive of an immune-mediated process (eg, lymphocytic-plasmacytic infiltration), treatment with immunosuppressive drugs (eg, prednisone, 1 mg/kg, BID) may be considered. However, lymphocytic-plasmacytic inflammation is also caused by chronic *B canis* infection. Furthermore, as a result of inhibitory effects on the hypothalamic-pituitary-gonadal axis, glucocorticoids can cause testicular atrophy and infertility. The ischemic damage caused by testicular torsion becomes irreversible within hours. When maintaining fertility is not important, castration is the treatment of choice for orchitis and epididymitis due to any cause. Simultaneously, broad-spectrum, bactericidal antibiotics should be administered for 7-10 days if bacterial infection is suspected. Lesions of the scrotal skin are treated the same as other skin lesions.

Chronic orchiepididymitis may develop as a sequela of the acute syndrome, or there may be no previous history of testicular inflammation. Possible causes include those of acute orchiepididymitis, immune-mediated orchitis and epididymitis, neoplasia, and spermatocele or granuloma formation. Most animals are asymptomatic except for infertility. Physical examination often reveals testicular atrophy. Tumors may be palpable. Palpation of the epididymis may reveal induration or enlargement, which may erroneously be interpreted as dramatic relative to the atrophic testis. Epididymal atrophy is uncommon. Other noninflammatory causes of testicular atrophy include previous exposure to excessive pressure, heat, cold, and cytotoxic agents. Hormonal causes (eg, glucocorticoids, estrogen from contralateral Sertoli cell tumor) are also possible. The prognosis for return of normal fertility in cases of chronic orchitis/epididymitis is grave. If warranted by the dog's value as a stud, the diagnostic and therapeutic plan is as described above for the acute condition.

BALANOPOSTHITIS

Inflammation of the penile or preputial mucosa is common in dogs. The normal preputial secretions usually do not result in overt clinical signs. Mild balanoposthitis, resulting in a slight mucopurulent preputial discharge, is present in many sexually mature dogs, resolves spontaneously, and is of little clinical significance. Diagnostic tests and treatment are not necessary, except as needed for reasonable hygiene. Trauma, lacerations, neoplasia, foreign bodies, infection, or phimosis may result in development of more severe balanoposthitis. A mucopurulent preputial discharge is the most common clinical sign. Swelling of the prepuce and pain are rarely present except in cases of trauma or foreign bodies. If signs of systemic illness are present, the possibility of a more serious concomitant disorder should be considered. Balanoposthitis is rare in cats.

The penis and prepuce should be thoroughly examined, to the level of the fornix, for underlying predisposing factors. Sedation or general anesthesia may be needed. Preputial cytology may be helpful. Bacterial cultures of the preputial cavity, although sometimes difficult to interpret due to the presence of normal preputial flora, may be helpful in identifying unusual organisms and determining antibiotic sensitivities for refractory cases.

Treatment includes correcting any predisposing factors, clipping long hair away from the preputial orifice, and thorough flushing of the preputial cavity with a mild antiseptic (eg, dilute povidone-iodine or chlorhexidine) or sterile saline solution. If bacterial infection is suspected, an antibiotic ointment may be infused into the preputial cavity for 7-10 days. Recurrence of mild balanoposthitis is common irrespective of therapy. Castration may diminish genital secretions.

PARAPHIMOSIS

The inability to completely retract the penis into the preputial cavity usually occurs after erection. It is seen most often after semen collection or coitus. The skin at the preputial orifice becomes inverted, trapping the extruded penis and impairing venous drainage. Other causes of paraphimosis include mild phimosis, foreign objects around the penis, a constricting band of hair at the preputial orifice, or trauma. Paraphimosis is easily differentiated from priapism, congenitally shortened prepuce, congenital deformity of the os penis, or paralysis of the retractor penis muscles on the basis of physical examination and palpation.

Paraphimosis is a medical emergency. The exposed penis quickly becomes edematous because its venous drainage is compromised. With continued exposure, it becomes dry and painful. If untreated, ulceration, ischemic necrosis, or gangrene may develop. If recognized early, before severe edema and pain develop, paraphimosis is easily treated. Treatment consists of gentle cleansing and lubrication of the exposed penis. The penis is replaced inside the prepuce by sliding the prepuce first in a posterior direction, extruding the penis further. This everts the skin at the preputial orifice; usually the prepuce then slides easily over the penis. The edema resolves promptly once circulation is restored.

If the everted prepuce does not slide over the edematous, exposed penis, a cold compress may be applied with gentle digital pressure to act as a pressure bandage. Application of hypertonic solutions may also help reduce swelling. With paraphimosis due to other causes, or of longer duration, sedation or general anesthesia is required. It may be necessary to incise the preputial skin to thoroughly examine the preputial cavity, remove restricting material, and relieve venous obstruction. The penis is then replaced in the preputial cavity, and the incision is closed. If the urethra has been damaged, an indwelling urinary catheter may be needed to prevent stricture formation. If necrosis or gangrene is severe, amputation of the penis and prepuce and castration may be necessary.

PHIMOSIS

An abnormally small preputial orifice, resulting in inability to extrude the penis, may be congenital or acquired as a result of neoplasia, edema, or fibrosis following trauma, inflammation, or infection. Clinical signs are variable. Usually, the problem is unnoticed until the dog attempts to mate and is unable to copulate. Diagnosis is established by physical examination of the prepuce and penis. Treatment depends on severity of the stenosis and intended use of the dog. If the dog is not used for breeding, therapy probably is not needed, although castration should be considered to prevent arousal. Surgical enlargement of the preputial orifice is indicated if the animal is to be used for breeding, if the phimosis contributes to balanoposthitis, or in the unlikely event that phimosis interferes with normal micturition.

BRUCELLOSIS IN DOGS

Although dogs occasionally become infected with *Brucella abortus, B suis,* or *B melitensis,* these sporadic occurrences are usually closely associated with infected domestic livestock (*see also* p 1110).

B canis is a cause of abortion in kenneled dogs. Dogs are the definitive host of this organism, and natural infections in other animals are rare. Infection has caused a reduction of 75% in the number of pups weaned in some breeding kennels. The disease disseminates rapidly among closely confined dogs, especially at time of breeding or when abortions occur. Transmission occurs via ingestion of contaminated materials or venereal routes. Both sexes appear to be equally susceptible. Transmission of brucellosis from dogs to humans occurs but appears to be very rare.

Primary signs are abortion during the last trimester of pregnancy without premonitory signs, stillbirths, and conception failures. Prolonged vaginal discharge usually follows abortion. Abortions may occur during subsequent pregnancies. Infected dogs may develop generalized lymphadenitis and frequently epididymitis, periorchitis, and prostatitis. Spondylitis and uveitis are occasional complications. Bacteremia is frequent and persists for ~18 mo after exposure. Fever is not characteristic.

Diagnosis is based on isolation and identification of the causative agent or by serology. The organisms can usually be readily isolated from vaginal exudate, aborted pups, blood, milk, or semen of infected dogs. The most widely used serologic test is an agglutination test by a tube or slide method. Nonspecific agglutination reactions occur in some dogs from which *Brucella* has not been isolated. To eliminate nonspecific antibodies, the serum is treated with 2-mercaptoethanol and retested. An agar gel immunodiffusion test performed in some laboratories is quite specific.

Attempts at immunization have not been successful. Control is based on elimination or isolation of infected dogs identified by positive cultural or serologic tests. Incidence of infection is much lower in kennels where dogs are caged individually. Longterm therapy, eg, with a combination of streptomycin or gentamicin and tetracycline, has been successful in many cases. Neutering of infected dogs is sometimes an alternative to euthanasia.

MAMMARY TUMORS

The frequency of mammary neoplasia in different species varies tremendously. The dog is by far the most frequently affected domestic species, with a prevalence ~3 times that in women; ~50% of all tumors in the bitch are mammary tumors. Mammary tumors are rare in cows, mares, goats, ewes, and sows. There are differences in both biologic behavior and histology of mammary tumors in dogs and cats. About 45% of mammary tumors are malignant in dogs, whereas ~90% are malignant in cats, and dogs have a much higher number of complex and mixed tumors than do cats.

Etiology: The cause of mammary tumors is unknown in any species except mice, in which an oncornavirus is causative in certain inbred strains. Hormones play an important role in the hyperplasia and neoplasia of mammary tissue, but the exact mechanism is unknown. Estrogen or progesterone receptors (or both) have been reported on mammary tumor cells in animals; these may influence the pathogenesis of hormone-induced mammary neoplasia as well as the response to hormone therapy.

Genetic and nutritional effects on mammary neoplasia have been identified in mice and some people but are not as well understood in dogs or cats. It has been demonstrated that the consumption of red meat, obesity at 1 yr of age, and obesity a year prior to diagnosis are associated with an increased risk of mammary gland tumors in intact or ovariohysterectomized dogs. To date, investigations of oncogenes and tumor suppressor genes have not proved helpful at the clinical level. From a practical view, all mammary tumors should be regarded as potentially malignant regardless of the size or number of glands involved. Spread of mammary carcinomas in both dogs and cats is primarily to regional lymph nodes and lungs. In dogs, 5-10% of mammary carcinomas may produce skeletal metastases, primarily in the axial skeleton, but also in long bones.

Canine Mammary Tumors: Mammary tumors in dogs are most frequent in intact bitches; they are extremely rare in male dogs. Ovariectomy before the first estrus reduces the risk of mammary neoplasia to 0.5% of the risk in intact bitches; ovariectomy after 1 estrus reduces the risk to 8% of that in intact bitches. Bitches neutered after maturity have generally been considered to have the same risk as intact bitches. However, questions remain regarding the impact of ovariohysterectomy at the time of tumor excision. Questions also remain about the timing of such surgery relative to survival. In one study, dogs spayed <2 yr prior to tumor excision lived 45% longer than either intact dogs or those spayed >2 yr prior to tumor excision. The 2 posterior mammary glands are involved more often than the 3 anterior glands. Grossly, tumors appear as single or multiple nodules (1-25 cm) in 1 or more glands. The cut surface is usually lobulated, gray-tan, and firm, often with fluid-filled cysts. Mixed mammary tumors may contain grossly recognizable bone or cartilage on the cut surface.

More than 50% of canine mammary tumors are benign mixed tumors; a smaller percentage of malignant mixed tumors are seen. In the latter, epithelial or mesenchymal components, either singly or in combination, may produce metastases. Histologically, canine mammary gland tumors have been classified by the World Health Organization as carcinomas (with 6 types and additional subtypes), sarcomas (4 types), carcinosarcomas (mixed mammary tumors), or benign adenomas. This classification scheme is based on the extent of the tumor, involvement of lymph nodes, and presence of metastatic lesions (TNM system); it includes unclassified tumors and apparently benign dysplasias.

Feline Mammary Tumors: Mammary tumors in cats are most common in older (average 11 yr) intact females. Spaying at an early age, especially before the first estrus, has a sparing effect and reduces the risk, but the degree of protection is less precisely documented than that for dogs. The 2 anterior or thoracic glands are more frequently involved than the posterior glands.

Histologically, most feline mammary tumors are adenocarcinomas, with tubular or papillary types more common than solid or mucoid types. Mixed mammary tumors and sarcomas are less commonly diagnosed than carcinomas. Benign tumors of the feline mammary gland are relatively infrequent and account for only ~10% of these tumors. The TNM clinical staging system is used for mammary tumors in cats as well as in dogs.

A distinct entity called feline mammary hypertrophy or fibroadenomatous hyperplasia has been noted in cats (see p 1153). It affects primarily young, actively cycling, or pregnant cats. It also has been seen in neutered cats, including older males given exogenous progestational drugs (megestrol acetate). The disorder is marked clinically by the rapid growth of one or more mammary glands.

Diagnostic Methods: A mammary tumor is usually suspected on detection of a mass during physical examination. The length of time the mass has been present is usually unknown, but the rate of growth may be helpful in determining prognosis. Palpation of the regional lymph nodes can help determine the extent of spread. Thoracic radiographs, preferably 3 views (a ventral-dorsal and 2 laterals), should be taken to detect pulmonary metastases. Fine-needle aspirates may differentiate between inflammatory and neoplastic lesions but may lead to erroneous conclusions and delay of surgery. The diagnosis is determined by histopathology and is important in defining treatment and prognosis.

Treatment and Prognosis: Mammary tumors are treated surgically, although there is no consensus as to the best procedure. Removal of the tumor alone (lumpectomy), simple mastectomy (removal of the affected gland only), modified radical mastectomy (removal of the affected gland and those that share lymphatic drainage and associated lymph nodes), and radical mastectomy (removal of the entire mammary chain and associated lymph nodes) all have their proponents. In dogs, the more involved procedures have not prolonged survival compared with the others, and the advantages of the simpler procedures are obvious. In cats, radical mastectomy has increased the disease-free interval but not survival time.

In theory, the use of anticancer drugs to combat micrometastatic disease (adjuvant chemotherapy) is a reasonable consideration. However, chemotherapy has not been proved an effective treatment for mammary tumors in dogs. Part of the difficulty of evaluating the response to adjuvant chemotherapy relates to the fact that only about half of the canine mammary tumors diagnosed as malignant on histopathologic examination actually behave that way. A combination of doxorubicin and cyclophosphamide has been used with limited efficacy in cats. Neither radiation therapy nor antiestrogenic compounds have been effective.

The prognosis is based on multiple factors. Most mammary tumors in dogs that are going to cause death do so within 1 yr. Sarcomas are associated with shorter survival times than carcinomas. Other factors, including size of tumor, lymph node involvement, and nuclear differentiation, also affect the prognosis. In cats, tumor size is important; cats with tumors >3 cm in diameter have a median survival time of 6 mo, but cats with tumors <2 cm in diameter have a median survival time of >4 yr.

PROSTATIC DISEASES

Diseases of the prostate gland are relatively common in dogs but less common in other species. Benign prostatic hyperplasia, bacterial prostatitis, prostatic abscesses, prostatic and paraprostatic cysts, and prostatic adenocarcinoma are the most common prostatic disorders in dogs. These disorders all cause enlargement or inflammation of the prostate gland and, therefore, have similar clinical signs that include tenesmus during defecation, intermittent hematuria, recurrent urinary tract infections, and caudal abdominal discomfort. Additional nonspecific signs, such as fever, malaise, anorexia, severe stiffness, and caudal abdominal pain, are often present with bacterial infections and neoplasia. Prostatic adenocarcinoma with bony involvement of the pelvis and lumbar vertebrae may cause hindlimb gait abnormalities. Prostatic enlargement may mechanically interfere with other abdominal organs. Less commonly, prostatic diseases may cause infertility or urinary incontinence. Prostatic adenocarcinoma may cause complete urethral obstruction.

Physical examination of the prostate gland should include abdominal and rectal palpation. An enlarged prostate typically is located further cranial than usual and can be found in the caudal abdomen, rather than within the pelvic canal. Size, shape, symmetry, consistency, mobility, and the presence or absence of pain are assessed by palpation. The normal dorsal sulcus (depression) helps in assessment of shape and symmetry. The historical and physical findings are usually sufficient to localize a disease process to the prostate gland but not to differentiate among the various conditions.

Abdominal radiographs may further define the size, shape, and position of the prostate gland. The sublumbar lymph nodes, lumbar vertebrae, and bony pelvis should be evaluated radiographically for evidence of periosteal new bone and bony metastases. A positive-contrast retrograde urethrogram can be done when an abnormal prostate or paraprostatic cyst is difficult to differentiate from the bladder. Ultrasonography may provide additional information concerning echogenicity of the prostatic parenchyma and may identify focal prostatic lesions that cannot be palpated. Mass lesions within the prostatic urethra and discontinuity of the prostatic urethral wall are both highly suggestive of prostatic neoplasia.

Material for cytologic and microbiologic examination can be obtained by a combination of prostatic massage and urethral catheterization. Material is aspirated from the prostatic urethral lumen using a rubber or plastic urinary catheter. It is usually helpful to have a finger in the dog's rectum during the procedure, so that the position of the tip of the catheter is known. Alternatively, the prostatic fraction of the ejaculate can be collected. Transcutaneous fine-needle aspiration of prostatic parenchyma and biopsy of the prostate gland are also excellent methods. Prostatic massage is easily performed; however, samples are routinely contaminated with urine from the bladder.

Because prostatic fluid normally refluxes into the bladder, urinary tract infection is usually present with bacterial prostatitis. Microbiologic examination of the prostatic (third) fraction of the ejaculate is more accurate for assessment of prostatic infection than is examination of prostatic massage specimens when urinary tract infection is present. Neoplastic cells are often not recovered in specimens obtained by ejaculation or prostatic massage. Fine-needle aspiration of the prostate gland can be performed transrectally or percutaneously, with or without ultrasonographic guidance; while generally safe and simple, this is not without some risk of penetration of surrounding structures. Biopsy is the most definitive, but also the most invasive, diagnostic procedure for differentiating prostatic diseases. Prostatic biopsy is probably best performed via celiotomy, although a skilled ultrasound radiologist may be able to safely obtain satisfactory biopsies.

BENIGN PROSTATIC HYPERPLASIA

Benign prostatic hyperplasia is the most common prostatic disorder and is found in most intact male dogs >6 yr old. It is a result of androgenic stimulation or altered androgen/ estrogen ratio, but why some males are affected and others are not is unknown. In some dogs, hyperplasia may begin as early as 2.5 yr of age and, after 4 yr of age, cystic hyperplasia tends to develop. There may be no clinical signs, or tenesmus, persistent or intermittent hematuria, and bleeding may occur. The diagnosis is suggested by physical and historical findings and by a nonpainful, symmetrically enlarged prostate. Radiology can confirm prostatomegaly. Ultrasonography should show diffuse, relatively symmetric involvement with multiple, diffuse, cystic structures. Cytologic examination of massage or ejaculate specimens reveals hemorrhage with mild inflammation without evidence of sepsis or neoplasia. Definitive diagnosis is only possible by biopsy. Castration is the treatment of choice; prostatic involution is usually evident within a few weeks and is often complete in several months.

For males intended for use in breeding, medical therapy may be feasible. Estrogens have been used to reduce prostatic hyperplasia but cannot be recommended because of potential side effects. Whenever estrogenic stimulation is present (eg, exogenous administration or endogenous production by Sertoli cell tumor), squamous metaplasia of the prostate can develop. Squamous metaplasia can cause prostatic enlargement and worsen the clinical signs. It may also enhance the risk of cystic changes and infection within the prostate. In addition, estrogens can cause negative feedback to the hypothalamus and pituitary (thereby diminishing spermatogenesis) and are potentially toxic to the bone marrow with resultant anemia, thrombocytopenia, and leukopenia. Medroxyprogesterone acetate has been used to treat prostatic hypertrophy in dogs, but testosterone concentration decreased, testicular degeneration occurred, and only 53% of dogs had a detectable decrease in prostatic size.

Perhaps the most effective medical agent for treatment of benign prostatic hypertrophy in dogs is finasteride, which blocks the action of 5 α-testosterone reductase, an enzyme that converts testosterone to dihydrotestosterone. Dihydrotestosterone is considered to be the key hormone for promoting prostatic hypertrophy in both humans and dogs. Giving 1 mg/kg of finasteride, PO, SID for 16-21 wk, to laboratory beagles resulted in a 50-70% reduction in prostatic hypertrophy with no negative effect on semen quality. Lower doses of finasteride (0.1 mg/kg, PO, SID for 16 wk) reduced hypertrophied prostate volume by 43%, resolved clinical signs, reduced dihydrotestosterone concentration by 58%, maintained normal testosterone levels, and had no deleterious effect on semen quality, fertility, or libido in a group of 9 dogs with prostatic hypertrophy. However, prostatic hypertrophy returns if finasteride administration is discontinued. The low dose (0.1-0.5 mg/kg) of finasteride correlates to convenient dosing of one 5-mg capsule of finasteride SID, for dogs weighing 10-50 kg.

PROSTATITIS

Inflammation of the prostate gland usually is suppurative and may result in abscesses. It may be associated with prostatic hyperplasia (*see* p 1163). Various organisms, including *Escherichia coli, Staphylococcus, Streptococcus,* and *Mycoplasma* spp, have been incriminated. Infection may be hematogenous or ascending from the urethra. Because prostatic fluid normally refluxes into the bladder, urinary tract infection often accompanies prostatic infection.

The signs resemble those of prostatic hyperplasia. In addition, malaise, pain, and fever are common. Dehydration, septicemia, and shock may occur in severe cases of acute bacterial prostatitis or prostatic abscess.

The historical, physical, and radiographic findings are suggestive of acute bacterial prostatitis and abscesses. Neutrophilia with a left shift, monocytosis, and/or toxic WBC may be seen. Ultrasonography shows hypoechoic areas consistent with pockets of fluid. Ideally, prostatic material is obtained by prostatic massage, ejaculation, or fine-needle aspiration for cytologic examination and for culture and sensitivity testing. Massage of an acutely infected prostate may liberate organisms into the blood and cause septicemia. For this reason, other methods are preferred. However, dogs with acute bacterial prostatitis or abscesses may be reluctant to ejaculate, and fine-needle aspiration may release organisms into the peritoneal cavity. Urinalysis shows hematuria, pyuria, and bacteriuria. The urine should be submitted for culture and sensitivity testing. Often, the urine and prostatic material yield the same organisms.

Chronic bacterial prostatitis may cause no clinical signs except recurrent urinary tract infection. Physical abnormalities may be limited to the urinary tract. Rarely, prostatic size and shape may be normal. Dogs with chronic bacterial prostatitis are usually willing to ejaculate. Prostatic massage or fine-needle aspiration could also be used to obtain specimens. Prostatic fluid and urine should be submitted for cytologic and microbiologic examination.

Fluid therapy is indicated when acute prostatitis is associated with dehydration or shock. Antibiotics should be selected on the basis of sensitivity testing and given for 1-4 wk. Large prostatic abscesses are best treated by surgical drainage. After the infection is controlled, castration should be considered. Urine or prostatic fluid (or both) should be cultured again after antibiotic therapy and 2-4 wk later to be certain that the infection has resolved.

Chronic bacterial prostatitis may be difficult to resolve. Antibiotic therapy should continue for ≥4 wk. Cultures should be repeated during, and for several months after, antibiotic therapy to ascertain whether resistance or persistent infection has developed. The benefits of castration for treatment of chronic bacterial prostatitis are uncertain; however, it seems reasonable that the prostatic involution after castration would at least help prevent recurrence of infection.

PROSTATIC AND PARAPROSTATIC CYSTS

Large cysts are occasionally found within or associated with the prostate gland. The signs are similar to those seen with other types of prostatic enlargement and usually become apparent only when the cyst reaches a size sufficient to cause pressure on adjacent organs. Large cysts may result in abdominal distention and must be differentiated from the bladder and from prostatic abscesses.

Medical treatment is ineffective, and estrogen therapy is contraindicated. Castration alone is unlikely to be of benefit but may be indicated after the cyst has been removed. Total excision of the prostatic cyst is the treatment of choice. If complete excision of the cyst is not possible, the remaining portion of the cyst may be filled with a leaf of omentum secured with sutures. This "omentalization" of the cyst will provide internal drainage and lead to resolution. Surgical excision is preferable to marsupialization because chronic management of the marsupialization fistula is often problematic.

NEOPLASMS

Adenocarcinoma is the most common neoplasm of the prostate. Transitional cell carcinoma arising from the bladder occasionally invades the prostate. Castration does not protect against future development of prostatic neoplasia in dogs.

The clinical signs of prostatic neoplasia are similar to those of other prostatic diseases. Pain and fever may be present. If the neoplasm infiltrates the urethra, dysuria or urethral obstruction is likely. Gross metastases are present at the time of diagnosis in >80% of dogs with prostatic adenocarcinoma. The most common sites of metastases are the regional lymph nodes, lumbar vertebrae, and bony pelvis. Spread to distant sites (such as the lungs) is uncommon until late in the course of disease. Urethral obstruction caused by prostatic disease in dogs is highly suggestive of neoplasia, as is prostatomegaly in a previously castrated dog. Diagnosis is made by biopsy.

There is no effective curative treatment. Consultation with a veterinary oncologist is recommended. Because of the high incidence of metastases at the time of diagnosis, and the high incidence of urinary incontinence after prostatectomy in dogs, total prostatectomy is not recommended as a treatment. Radiation therapy for prostatic cancer often results in incontinence due to radiation-induced fibrosis of the urinary bladder. Alternative means of ablating prostatic tissue such as transrectal high-intensity focused ultrasound, transurethral intraprostatic absolute ethanol injections, transurethral laser vaporization, or transurethral electrocoagulation have been successful in experimental studies, but have not been performed on dogs with prostatic adenocarcinoma.

CALCULI

When prostatic calculi occur (rarely), there is usually some other prostatic disease as well. Rarely, radiopaque prostatic calculi are incidental findings on abdominal radiographs.

CANINE TRANSMISSIBLE VENEREAL TUMOR

Canine transmissible venereal tumors (TVT) are cauliflower-like, pedunculated, and nodular, papillary, or multilobulated in appearance. They range in size from a small nodule (5 mm) to a large mass (>10 cm) that is firm, though friable. The surface is often ulcerated and inflamed and bleeds easily. TVT may be solitary or multiple and are almost always located on the genitalia. They may be transplanted to adjacent skin and oral, nasal, or conjunctival mucosae. The tumor may arise deep within the prepuce or vagina and be difficult to see during cursory examination. This may lead to misdiagnosis if genital bleeding is incorrectly assumed to be hematuria. The tumor is transplanted from site to site and dog to dog by direct contact with the mass. Initially, TVT grow rapidly. Metastasis is uncommon (5%). When metastasis occurs, it is usually to the regional lymph nodes, but kidney, spleen, eye, brain, pituitary, skin and subcutis, mesenteric lymph nodes, and peritoneum may also be sites.

Because of their homogenous populations of large, round cells with distinctive centrally located nucleoli, TVT are usually easily diagnosed by cytologic examination of fine-needle aspirates or impression smears or by histopathologic evaluation of biopsies. TVT may be difficult to distinguish from other round cell tumors, particularly lymphosarcomas, when they occur in extragenital locations. Prevalence varies from relatively high in some geographic regions to rare in others.

Although spontaneous regression can occur, TVT are usually progressive and are treated accordingly. Complete surgical excision, radiation therapy, and chemotherapy are effective treatments; however, chemotherapy is considered the treatment of choice. Vincristine sulfate (0.5 mg/m^2, IV, once weekly for 3-6 wk) is reported to be effective, except when the tumor is in the CNS or eye. Usually, total remission can be expected by the sixth treatment. Adriamycin (30 mg/m^2, IV, once every 3 wk) also has been effective for those animals that do not respond to vincristine. The prognosis for total remission with chemotherapy or radiation therapy is good, unless there is metastatic involvement of organs other than skin. Complete surgical excision often cannot be achieved because of the anatomic location of many of these tumors. Recurrence is likely in such cases unless adjunct radiation or chemotherapy is used.

■ ■ ■

RESPIRATORY SYSTEM

RESPIRATORY SYSTEM
INTRODUCTION

The respiratory system performs several functions. Most importantly, it delivers oxygen to the cardiovascular system for distribution to the body and it removes carbon dioxide. Gas transfer occurs in the alveoli of the lungs, where the air-blood barrier is a thin, permeable membrane. Failure or major dysfunction of gas transfer due to disease processes that compromise this membrane or its air or blood supply have serious effects. In addition to gas exchange, the respiratory system performs numerous other functions, including maintaining acid-base balance, acting as a blood reservoir, filtering and probably destroying emboli, metabolizing some bioactive substances (eg, serotonin, prostaglandins, corticosteroids, and leukotrienes), and activating some substances (eg, angiotensin). The respiratory system also protects its own delicate airways by warming and humidifying inhaled air and by filtering out particulate material. The upper airways also provide for the sense of smell (olfaction) and play a role in temperature regulation in panting animals.

Large airborne particles are usually deposited on the mucous lining of the nasal passages, larynx, trachea, and bronchi, after which they are carried by the mucociliary "blanket" to the pharynx to be swallowed or expectorated. Small particles may be deposited as deep as the alveoli, where they are phagocytized by macrophages. Defense against invasion by microorganisms and other foreign particles is provided by anatomic structures and by both nonspecific and immunologic mechanisms (both cellular and humoral). These are the factors that determine species and individual susceptibility to disease and that may be manipulated by using various management techniques, vaccines, antimicrobials, and other agents such as interferons and lymphokines. Other factors include the tortuosity of nasal passages; presence of hairs, cilia, and mucus; the cough reflex; and bronchoconstriction. Cellular defenses include the macrophage, which phagocytizes invaders and presents them (or at least their important antigens) to lymphocytes for stimulation of an immune response, and the neutrophil, which often dies in its fight against invaders and must be removed along with its potentially damaging enzymes. Secretory defenses include interferon for antiviral defense, complement for lysis of invaders, surfactant lining the alveoli to prevent their collapse and to facilitate macrophage function, fibronectin to block bacterial attachment, antibodies, and mucus.

The respiratory system must perform many functions, preferably while expending minimal energy. The required effort is increased by processes that oppose expansion of the lung (eg, fibrosis or hydro-, chylo-, pneumo-, or hemothorax), impede the flow of air (eg, nasal tumors, bronchiolitis, bronchoconstriction, laryngeal paralysis, or pulmonary edema), or thicken the air-blood interface (eg, interstitial pneumonia due to viruses or toxins, pulmonary edema).

The anatomy of the respiratory tract differs markedly among species in the following features: 1) shape of both the upper and lower respiratory tract; 2) extent, shape, and pattern of the turbinate bones; 3) branching patterns of bronchi; 4) anatomy of terminal bronchioles, including collateral ventilation; 5) lobation and lobulation; 6) thickness of pleura; 7) completeness of the mediastinum; 8) relationship of pulmonary arteries to bronchial arteries and bronchioles; 9) presence of vascular shunts; 10) distribution of mast cells; and 11) blood supply to the pleura. Each variation in anatomic structure implies variation in function, which can influence the pathogenesis of respiratory disease in a particular species. The 3 main groups of species that have anatomically similar respiratory tracts are 1) cattle, sheep, and pigs; 2) dogs, cats, monkeys, rats, rabbits, and guinea pigs; and 3) horses and humans.

Marked physiologic variations also exist between different species. For example, cattle are prone to retrograde drainage from the pharynx, are predisposed to pulmonary hypertension and reduced ventilation in a cold environment, have relatively small lungs with low tidal volume and functional residual capacity, and are more sensitive to changes in environmental temperatures than are most other species. These anatomic and physiologic differences largely determine why some pathogens affect only some species (eg, *Mannheimia (Pasteurella) haemolytica* affects cattle but not pigs) and why pneumonia is very important in some species (cattle, pigs) but less so in others (dogs, cats).

Hypoxia (lowered oxygenation, often termed anoxia) causes clinical signs of respiratory disease. It can result from the following: 1) reduced oxygen-carrying capacity of the blood (anemic anoxia, as in carbon monoxide or nitrite poisoning, or true anemia due to various causes), 2) reduced blood flow (stagnant anoxia, as in congestive heart failure or shock), 3) insufficient alveolar ventilation or diffusion impairment (anoxic anoxia, as in pneumonia, pulmonary edema, chronic congestion, pneumothorax, or paralysis of respiratory muscles), or 4) inability of tissues to use available oxygen (eg, histotoxic anoxia, as in cyanide poisoning).

Compensatory mechanisms for hypoxia include increased depth and rate of breathing, which is mediated by chemoreceptors located in the carotid and aortic bodies; contraction of the spleen, which forces more RBC into the circulation; and increased cardiac stroke volume and heart rate. If cerebral hypoxia develops, respiratory function may be reduced even further due to depression of neuronal activity. Erythropoiesis is also stimulated with hypoxia, although the degree of polycythemia is species dependent. In addition, myocardial, renal, and hepatic functions may be reduced, as may motility and secretions of the intestine. If compensatory mechanisms are inadequate, a vicious cycle may begin in which all body tissues function less efficiently.

Clinical Signs of Respiratory Malfunction

Nasal discharge may be serous, catarrhal, purulent, or hemorrhagic, depending on the degree of mucosal damage. It indicates increased production of normal secretions, sometimes supplemented by neutrophils (purulent) or blood (hemorrhage). It probably also indicates decreased "grooming" of the nostrils with the tongue when animals are ill. **Epistaxis** (hemorrhage from the nose) is often caused by vascular rupture, such as in mycotic infection of the guttural pouch or exercise-induced pulmonary hemorrhage in horses, or by intranasal fungal infection or neoplasia, systemic coagulopathy, vasculitis, thrombocytopenia (immune-mediated or result of rickettsial infection), hyperviscosity syndrome, or nasal trauma. **Hemoptysis** (the coughing up of blood) occurs after rupture of pulmonary aneurysms in the lungs of cattle with chronic lung abscesses. Bleeding may also result from polyps, neoplasms, granulomas, trauma, thrombocytopenia, and bracken fern or sweet clover toxicity.

Hyperpnea (an increase in rate and depth of pulmonary ventilation) becomes **dyspnea** when the breathing appears to be labored and causing distress. Hyperpnea, however, is not always a symptom of disease (eg, labored breathing following vigorous exercise in an otherwise healthy animal). Infectious respiratory diseases that cause toxemia may further compromise the host, eg, bovine pneumonia due to *M haemolytica*. Dyspnea can be caused by disease of the respiratory tract itself (eg, airway obstruction, pneumonia, bronchitis, or alveolitis) or by other problems (eg, heart failure, acid-base imbalances, thoracic effusions, abnormal oxygen-carrying capacity of the blood, or disorders of neuromuscular function). Labored inhalation seen with obstructive diseases above the thoracic inlet (eg, laryngeal paralysis, cervical tracheal collapse) or with pleural effusions is termed inspiratory dyspnea; labored expiration seen with obstructive diseases below the thoracic inlet (eg, diffuse bronchitis or pulmonary edema) is termed expiratory dyspnea. Other responses include coughing, clear exudates, and shallow breathing with grunting, often associated with the pain of pleuritis. Fixed airway obstructions (eg, tracheal neoplasia, foreign body, or stenosis) or a combination of upper and lower obstructive airway diseases (eg, pleural effusion with congestive heart failure) will result in both inspiratory and expiratory dyspnea.

Causes of Respiratory Malfunction

Anomalies of the respiratory tract are rare but do occur. Examples include cysts in the sinuses and turbinates, tracheal hypoplasia, and accessory lungs. The most common cause of upper respiratory tract malfunction is **rhinitis** (which results in exudation of neutrophils, macrophages, and fluids), or erosion and ulceration (or both) of the nasal mucosa. It may be caused by viral, bacterial, fungal, or parasitic agents, as well as by hypersensitivity reactions, such as localized allergies and anaphylaxis (*see* THE IMMUNE SYSTEM, p 645 et seq). Atrophy of the turbinates (eg, in atrophic rhinitis of pigs) removes a major filtration function and exposes the lungs to much heavier loads of dust and microorganisms. The nasal cavity may be obstructed by tumors, granulomas, abscesses, or foreign bodies. Sinusitis can be a complication of upper respiratory infections or dehorning.

Laryngitis, **tracheitis**, and **bronchitis** result in coughing and possibly inspiratory or expiratory dyspnea. Coughing may be nonproductive if the irritation is caused by mucosal erosion, or productive if due to copious exudate in the major airways. Severe pulmonary edema and emphysema cause extreme respiratory insufficiency.

The most common respiratory disease is **pneumonia**, which is defined as inflammation of the lungs. There are many systems for classifying the various types of pneumonia. One useful method is to classify according to the distribution of lesions in the lungs. **Focal pneumonia** has one or more discrete foci in a random pattern, eg, abscessation due to emboli from other sites, tuberculosis, or actinomycosis. **Lobular pneumonia** accentuates the anatomic pattern of lobules, as in bronchopneumonia caused by *Pasteurella multocida*. **Lobar pneumonia** covers large areas of lobes and is often severe (eg, fibrinous pneumonic pasteurellosis of cattle). **Diffuse** or **interstitial pneumonia** often involves the entire lung, as in maedi of sheep or in hypersensitivity reactions. The appearance or etiology of a particular pneumonia can be described further, eg, gangrenous, parasitic (verminous), aspiration, etc. The initial problem in many pneumonias is thought to be a sudden alteration in the normal nasal bacterial flora, which results in a sudden dramatic increase in one or more species of bacteria. These bacteria are breathed into the lung in large numbers and may overwhelm the normal defense mechanisms, localize, multiply, and initiate inflammation. In addition, stress is often a precursor of viral respiratory infections, particularly in groups of animals that have recently been congregated and stressed by travel, handling, and mixing. Some respiratory viral infections can cause temporary dysfunction of phagocytic mechanisms of the alveolar macrophages. This usually occurs several days after viral exposure. Inhaled bacteria proliferate and pneumonia ensues, often with an overwhelming infection and massive exudation into the alveoli.

Pneumonia also can be caused by direct infection with viruses, bacteria, and fungi, as well as by toxins arriving hematogenously, by inhalation, or by aspiration of food or gastric contents.

Through natural processes, possibly aided by appropriate therapy, the exudate may be removed from the lungs, and the mucosal lesions of the air passages may heal. However, serious sequelae can persist. **Bronchiectasis** is a chronic lesion of the bronchi and parenchyma characterized by irreversible cylindrical or saccular dilatation, secondary infection, and atelectasis. Ulceration of bronchioles caused by viral agents may lead to organized plugs of connective tissue in small bronchioles, a lesion called **bronchiolitis obliterans**, which may cause permanent obstruction, atelectasis, and severe respiratory insufficiency. Constriction of bronchioles in chronic allergic bronchitis and bronchiolitis results in similar clinical signs. Some chronic pneumonias (eg, maedi in sheep) are characterized by firm diffuse lesions due to hyperplasia of lymphoid follicles, hyperplasia of smooth muscle around bronchioles, diffuse fibrosis, and diffuse lymphocytic infiltration. Aspiration pneumonia often leads to gangrene with severe toxemia accompanying the acute inflammatory reaction.

Most infectious pneumonias occur in the anteroventral portions of the lungs. However, infectious agents, as well as neoplasms, can invade the lungs via the blood, which may extensively impair pulmonary function, as can pulmonary edema from chronic heart failure. Pleuritis, empyema, hydrothorax, chylothorax, atelectasis, diaphragmatic hernia, or pneumothorax can also seriously impair respiratory function. Pulmonary thrombosis leads to acute, often fulminant, respiratory failure as a result of a lack of pulmonary arterial blood flow to ventilated regions of the lung. Infarction of the lung can reduce respiratory function but is rare because of the dual blood supply of the organ. Toxic injury, such as in 3-methylindole toxicity in cattle, causes edema, emphysema, and necrosis of alveolar epithelium followed by compensatory hyperplasia of these cells; the effects on gas exchange result in severe hypoxia and dyspnea.

Although pneumonia is most important, several other conditions that occur in the thorax can cause respiratory dysfunction. **Pulmonary edema**, the abnormal accumulation of fluid in the interstitial tissue, airways, or alveoli of the lungs, may occur in conjunction with circulatory disorders, particularly left ventricular failure or increased capillary permeability, occasionally in anaphylactic and allergic reactions, and in some infectious diseases. Head trauma can cause pulmonary edema in dogs. Dyspnea and open-mouth breathing may occur. Animals stand in preference to lying down, lie only in sternal recumbency, or may assume a sitting position. Auscultation of the chest may reveal wheezing and fluid sounds.

Pleuritis (pleurisy) may be caused by any pathogen that gains entrance to the pleural cavity, but it is often an extension of pneumonia. Rapid shallow breathing, fever, and thoracic pain are suggestive of pleuritis. Auscultation of the chest may reveal friction sounds.

Empyema (purulent exudate in the pleural cavity) is caused by pyogenic bacteria or fungi reaching the thoracic cavity via the blood or by extension of a pneumonia, traumatic reticulitis, or penetrating wound of the chest. Cough, fever, pain, and dyspnea may be present.

Hemothorax (the accumulation of blood in the pleural cavity) is usually caused by trauma to the thorax, systemic coagulopathy, or thoracic neoplasia. **Hydrothorax** (the accumulation of transudate in the pleural cavity) is usually due to interference with venous blood flow or lymph drainage. **Chylothorax** (the accumulation of chyle in the pleural cavity) is relatively rare and is seen most often in cats. It may be caused by rupture of the thoracic duct but often is idiopathic. The signs of all 3 conditions include respiratory embarrassment (eg, rapid shallow breathing with inspiratory dyspnea) and weakness.

Pneumothorax (air in the pleural cavity, *see* p 1397) may be of traumatic or spontaneous origin. Air can enter the pleural cavity through penetrating wounds of the thoracic wall or by extension from pulmonary emphysema or ruptured bullae. The lung collapses if a large volume of air enters the pleural cavity. Bilateral pneumothorax may develop if the mediastinum is weak or incomplete. Inspiratory dyspnea or rapid, shallow breathing is evident.

Diagnostic Techniques

Clinical history and physical examination should aid in determining the possible cause and site of respiratory disease. Lateral cervical and thoracic radiographs may be helpful when obstructive upper airway disease or fixed airway obstruction is suspected (eg, tracheal foreign body, masses, foreign bodies, or stenosis). Thoracic radiographs are essential in any patient exhibiting lower respiratory signs (eg, cough, rapid shallow breathing, dyspnea). Blood gas analysis or pulse oximetry may help assess the need for oxygen therapy in a patient with severe dyspnea.

When obstructive upper airway disease is suspected, diagnostic procedures include nasopharyngoscopy, pharyngoscopy, laryngoscopy, and tracheobronchoscopy. Laryngeal function should be assessed, and the presence of obstructive lesions within the nasopharynx, oropharynx, larynx, trachea, or principal bronchi identified.

With diffuse or lobar lung disease, diagnostic procedures include transtracheal wash, bronchoscopy with bronchoalveolar lavage, and transthoracic fine needle aspirates of lung. When bacterial pneumonia is suspected, bacterial culture of transtracheal wash or bronchoalveolar lavage fluid is recommended. Cytologic evaluation of transtracheal or bronchoalveolar lavage fluid may aid in the diagnosis of fungal, parasitic, or allergic lung diseases. Transthoracic fine needle aspirates of lung often are useful in the diagnosis of fungal pneumonia, but have lower yields in the definitive diagnosis of solitary pulmonary lesions. Solitary pulmonary masses often require surgical excision for definitive diagnosis.

In dogs or cats with pleural effusions, thoracocentesis should be performed for cytologic and potentially microbiologic evaluation of fluid. In cats, pleural effusions often occur with cardiac disease and echocardiography should be performed. In animals suspected to have a chylous effusion, serum and fluid triglyceride levels should be determined. Chylous effusions are associated with fluid triglyceride levels greater than that in serum.

Acute nasal discarge, sneezing, or both may suggest the presence of infection (viral or bacterial) or a nasal foreign body. Chronic nasal discharge warrants further investigation via radiography (nose, guttural pouch), nasal computed tomography, rhinoscopy, nasopharyngoscopy, or nasal biopsy. Rhinoscopy may be of limited value if copious thick discharge or hemorrhage is present. Bacterial cultures of nasal tissue may be of value if bacterial rhinitis is suspected; however, in some species (eg, dog and cat) primary bacterial rhinitis is rare and typically occurs secondary to other nasal conditions. Cytologic evaluation of nasal tissue may help diagnose nasal fungal infections. Serologic testing for fungal respiratory infections may be considered, but these findings should correlate with the patient's clinical signs and documentation of the presence of fungal organisms as false-positive and false-negative tests do occur.

Control of Respiratory Disease

Sudden dietary changes, weaning, cold, drafts, dampness, dust, high levels of ammonia, poor ventilation in general, and the mixing of widely divergent age groups all play a role in respiratory disease in groups of animals. Stress and mixing of animals from several sources should be avoided or minimized. Establishing individual animal identification, making accurate clinical and postmortem diagnoses, and maintaining a record system of diagnosis and treatment are important to minimize or control outbreaks of pneumonia.

Immunization can help control respiratory infection. However, control may be compromised by improper timing, use of ineffective or inappropriate vaccines, or overwhelmingly negative management practices. In most cases, severe insults to the natural defenses cannot be reversed later by therapeutic agents and biologicals.

The mucosal surfaces of the respiratory tract contain lymphoid follicles that exchange cells with other parts of the body. However, most of the lymphocytes in the respiratory lining produce only IgA, whereas the cells in the lymph nodes of the respiratory tract produce IgM and IgG. Depending on the agent involved, various cell- and antibody-mediated immune responses occur in the respiratory tract and include opsonization, agglutination, immobilization, neutralization of toxins and viruses, blockage of adherence to cells, lysis, and chemotaxis. Variation in the type of immune response occurs because of age, species, and the means to respond to specific virulence mechanisms of the pathogens involved. Species vary in the type of immune response available at different sites in the respiratory tract. Large antigen droplets may immunize the upper tract with IgA, but small replicating particles may be necessary to immunize the lower tract. To develop adequate antibody levels to protect the lungs, repeated doses of antigen plus adjuvant, or a replicating antigen, are often necessary. These results are seldom achieved under field conditions (eg, many field trials using respiratory vaccines in cattle have not demonstrated statistically significant efficacy).

PRINCIPLES OF THERAPY

See also SYSTEMIC PHARMACOTHERAPEUTICS OF THE RESPIRATORY SYSTEM, p 2033.

Respiratory disease is often characterized by abnormal production of secretions and exudates and by a reduced ability to remove them. The primary goal is to reduce the volume and viscosity of the secretions and to facilitate their removal. This can be accomplished by controlling infection, modifying the secretions, and when possible, improving postural drainage and mechanically removing the material. Therapeutic methods include altering the inspired air and administering expectorants, antitussives, bronchodilators, antimicrobials, diuretics, and other drugs.

Hydration should be maintained. Inhalation of humidified air may facilitate removal of airway secretions. Expectorants are sometimes used with the intention of liquefying these secretions. However, they should be used in conjunction with ancillary respiratory therapy such as improved postural drainage, mild exercise, and thoracic percussion, which (in addition to coughing) encourages expectoration and removal of secretions. Expectorants at traditional dosages are of questionable value. Mechanical removal of tenacious and viscid secretions by aspiration may be necessary in severe airway obstruction.

Antitussive agents are indicated to relieve the discomfort associated with nonproductive coughing but are contraindicated when secretion of airway mucus is excessive. Products that contain atropine also are contraindicated, at least in theory, because atropine increases the viscosity of airway secretions.

Increased airway resistance caused by bronchial smooth muscle contraction can be alleviated with bronchodilators, which may be indicated in animals with asthma-like conditions and chronic respiratory disease. Methylxanthines, such as theophylline and aminophylline, are effective bronchodilators in species other than cattle (and possibly dogs). Isoproterenol, clenbuterol, and epinephrine are also generally effective, and sodium cromoglycate is used in horses for treating small airway disease (eg, heaves). Corticosteroid use is justified in allergic conditions. Antihistamines can be used to alleviate the bronchoconstriction caused by histamine release. Bronchospasm also can be reduced significantly by removing irritating factors, using mild sedatives, or reducing periods of excitement.

In bacterial infection, antimicrobial therapy should be instituted. The goal is to select either the most effective agent against a specific organism or the least toxic agent of several alternatives. Culture and sensitivity testing of airway secretions provide a worthwhile, although not infallible, guide to determining the appropriate antibiotic. Knowledge of tissue penetration and pharmacokinetic characteristics of the antimicrobial agents is important as well. The following agents have proved effective in the listed species: cattle—oxytetracycline, erythromycin, penicillins, and sulfonamides; sheep and goats—oxytetracycline, penicillins, and sulfonamides; pigs—lincomycin, spectinomycin, penicillins, and sulfonamides; dogs and cats—cephalosporins, chloramphenicol, amoxicillin-clavulanic acid, aminoglycosides, trimethoprim-sulfamethoxazole, fluoroquinolones, and tetracyclines; horses—penicillins, sulfonamides, and tetracyclines, the latter with caution due to an occasional side effect of severe diarrhea. Aminoglycosides are useful but can be nephrotoxic. Trimethoprim, usually in combination with a sulfonamide, is useful for respiratory therapy in most species but is not licensed for food-producing animals in the USA. Drugs such as enrofloxacin (approved for small but not large animals in the USA) and ceftiofur may prove efficacious. Broad-spectrum antibiotics should be used if specific bacteria cannot be identified, and once begun, a full course of therapy should be completed. Multiple antimicrobial agents should be used only with full knowledge of the potential drug interactions. Because of residues in food-producing animals, veterinarians must use these products appropriately and provide sound advice to producers.

The hypoxemia caused by most lung disorders usually can be corrected by administering oxygen. However, continuous administration of high concentrations increases the tendency for regional resorption atelectasis, thus worsening the hypoxemia, and can cause pneumonitis on its own. Hypoxemia is often accompanied by variable degrees of hypercapnia and acidemia. Endotracheal intubation and mechanical ventilation may be necessary in animals with acute respiratory failure or in animals that are comatose or apneic. Arterial blood gas and pH determinations, when practicable, are extremely valuable in monitoring treatment.

Diuretics are indicated in pulmonary edema. The osmotic diuretics have a minimal action on diuresis. Carbonic anhydrase inhibitors (eg, acetazolamide) have a moderate action on diuresis, and loop diuretics (eg, furosemide) have a profound effect.

ASPIRATION PNEUMONIA

(Foreign-body pneumonia, Inhalation pneumonia, Gangrenous pneumonia)

Aspiration pneumonia is a pulmonary infection characterized by inflammation and necrosis caused by inhalation of foreign material. The severity of the inflammatory response depends on the material aspirated, the type of bacteria aspirated, and the distribution of aspirated material in the lungs.

Etiology: Faulty administration of medicines is a common cause of aspiration pneumonia. Liquids administered by drench or dose syringe should not be given faster than the animal can swallow. Drenching is particularly dangerous when the animal's tongue is drawn out, when the head is held high, or when the animal is coughing or bellowing. Administration of liquids by nasal intubation is not without risk, and careful technique is especially necessary in debilitated animals.

Inhalation of irritant gases or smoke is an infrequent cause. Aspiration of vomitus or attempts by animals to eat or drink while partially choked can result in aspiration pneumonia as well. Disturbances of deglutition, as in anesthetized or comatose animals (eg, mature cattle under general anesthesia or cows in lateral recumbency), vagal paralysis, acute pharyngitis, abscesses or tumors of the pharyngeal region, esophageal diverticula, cleft palate, megaesophagus, or encephalitis, are frequent predisposing causes.

Cats are particularly susceptible to pneumonia caused by aspiration of tasteless products such as mineral oil. In sheep, poor dipping technique may cause aspiration of fluid. Calves and lambs may inhale inflammatory debris if affected with diphtheritic laryngitis. Inhalation of milk by pail-fed calves can cause an acute necrotizing pneumonia due to the diffuse distribution of foreign material. The muscles of deglutition may be affected in lambs with nutritional myopathy. Pigs fed fine particulate food in dry environments may inhale feed granules. Aspiration pneumonia in cattle following delayed treatment for milk fever is highly fatal. In dogs with myasthenia gravis, aspiration pneumonia is the leading cause of death.

Clinical Findings: A clinical history suggesting recent foreign-body aspiration is of greatest diagnostic value. Horses may develop fevers of 104-105°F (40-40.5°C), which can drop back into the normal range in a few days. Pyrexia is also seen in cats, dogs, and less commonly in cattle. The patient presents with acute dyspnea, tachypnea, and tachycardia. Associated findings are cyanosis and bronchospasm. A sweetish, fetid breath characteristic of gangrene may be detected, the intensity of which increases with disease progression. This is often associated with a purulent nasal discharge that sometimes is tinged reddish brown or green. Occasionally, evidence of aspirated material (eg, oil droplets) can be seen in the nasal discharge or expectorated material. On auscultation, wheezing sounds, pleuritic friction rubs, and crackling sounds of subcutaneous emphysema may be heard. In cows that aspirate ruminal contents, toxemia is usually fatal within 1-2 days. Cattle and pigs recover more frequently than horses, but mortality is high in all species. Recovered animals often develop pulmonary abscesses. In outbreaks after dipping of sheep, losses occur from day 2 to day 7 and then decrease gradually.

Lesions: The pneumonia is usually in the anteroventral parts of the lung; it may be unilateral or bilateral and centers on airways. In early stages, the lungs are markedly congested with areas of interlobular edema. Bronchi are hyperemic and full of froth. The pneumonic areas tend to be cone-shaped with the base toward the pleura. Suppuration and necrosis follow, the foci becoming soft or liquefied, reddish brown, and foul smelling. There usually is an acute fibrinous pleuritis, often with pleural exudate.

Prevention and Treatment: Atropine sulfate helps to control salivation stimulated by general anesthetics (eg, thiobarbiturates). Use of an endotracheal tube with an inflatable cuff prevents fluid aspiration during surgery.

The animal should be kept quiet. A productive cough should not be suppressed. Broad-spectrum antibiotics should be used in animals known to have inhaled a foreign substance, whether it be a liquid or an irritant vapor, without waiting for signs of pneumonia to appear. Care and supportive treatment are the same as for infectious pneumonias. In small animals, oxygen therapy may be beneficial. Despite all treatments, prognosis is poor, and efforts must be directed at prevention.

CHLAMYDIAL PNEUMONIA

Chlamydiae have been identified in various parts of the world as a cause of enzootic pneumonia in cats, calves, mice, sheep, piglets, foals, and goats. In cats, pneumonia may occur as a rare sequela of the more common chlamydial conjunctivitis and rhinitis. The main clinical sign of zoonotic chlamydiosis in humans is pneumonia, generally contracted from pet birds.

Etiology and Epidemiology: The causative agent is *Chlamydophila (Chlamydia) psittaci*. Some respiratory isolates from calves have properties of immunotypes 1 and 6 and are similar to strains recovered from intestinal infections (p 155) and abortions of cattle and sheep (p 1097). Immunotype 6 has been recovered from pneumonic lungs of calves and pigs. Thus, the GI tract of carrier animals should be considered as an important site in the pathogenesis of chlamydial infections and as a potential source of the organisms. Infection most commonly occurs via inhalation of organisms from fecal carriers or other respiratory cases. Chlamydial pneumonia has affected calves under range conditions as well as on dairy farms. The disease in sheep is most frequently seen in feeder lambs assembled from different sources in feedlots or on irrigated pastures. Stressed lambs under these conditions are frequently subject to various secondary bacterial infections, which can result in higher mortality and morbidity rates than are seen in uncomplicated chlamydial respiratory infections.

Clinical Findings: Calves, lambs, and goats with chlamydial pneumonia are usually febrile, lethargic, and dyspneic. They develop a serous and later mucopurulent nasal discharge with a dry hacking cough. Calves of weaning age are affected most frequently, but older cattle may also show signs.

Lesions: The acute pulmonary lesion is bronchointerstitial pneumonia. The anteroventral parts of the lungs are affected but, in severe cases, entire lobes can be involved. The dry cough is attributed to tracheitis. Microscopic changes in the lungs include suppurative bronchitis and alveolitis progressing to type II pneumocyte hyperplasia and interstitial thickening due to an ingress of mixed inflammatory cells. Lymphocytic aggregates are frequently seen around airways and pulmonary vessels.

Diagnosis: Neither clinical signs nor lesions allow a definitive diagnosis of chlamydial pneumonia because they are not sufficiently different from those seen in the bovine or ovine respiratory disease complex. Diagnosis requires isolation of chlamydiae from affected tissues in tissue culture or chick embryo. Chlamydial inclusion bodies may be detected in affected tissues. Diagnosis may be supported by fluorescent antibody tests and serologic assays performed on acute and convalescent samples. Predominantly, IgG_2 antibodies are induced by chlamydial infections in cattle. Subclinical chlamydial infections occur as well.

Prevention and Treatment: Vaccines are not available. Several antimicrobials (eg, penicillin, erythromycin, tylosin, and tetracyclines) can interfere with chlamydial replication, but tetracycline is generally the drug of choice. Treatment must start as early as possible and continue for at least 5-7 days.

DIAPHRAGMATIC HERNIA

A break in the continuity of the diaphragm allows protrusion of abdominal viscera into the thorax.

Etiology: In small animals, automobile-related trauma is a common cause of diaphragmatic hernia, although congenital defects of the diaphragm may also result in herniation (eg, peritoneopericardial hernia). In horses, diaphragmatic hernia may occur less commonly after trauma, dystocia, or recent strenuous activity. In cattle, there is rarely a history of trauma, and hernias are reportedly associated with traumatic reticulitis.

Clinical Findings: The signs vary, depending on the duration and species affected. Dogs and cats are characteristically dyspneic in the acute case. The degree of dyspnea may vary from subclinical to incompatible with life, depending on the amount of herniated viscera. If the stomach is herniated, it may bloat and the animal may deteriorate rapidly. In chronic cases, systemic signs such as weight loss may be more prominent than respiratory signs. Physical examination findings may include the absence of lung sounds and/or the presence of GI sounds on auscultation of the thorax. Congenital peritoneopericardial hernia is most frequently an incidental finding, although findings may be related to the respiratory or GI systems or due to compromised venous return to the heart. In horses, acute, severe colic secondary to the displaced intestines is most frequently seen; respiratory signs occur less frequently. In cattle, diaphragmatic hernias are most frequently associated with traumatic reticulitis and herniation of the reticulum.

Diagnosis: Careful physical examination, including auscultation and percussion, usually suggests the presence of thoracic disease. The definitive diagnosis is most frequently made from radiographs. Loss of diaphragmatic contour, abdominal viscera in the thorax, and displacement of viscera from the abdomen may be apparent. Radiographic contrast studies may be necessary to make the diagnosis. Barium may be given by mouth (GI series), or water-soluble contrast may be injected intraperitoneally (celiogram). Radiographs may be difficult to obtain in horses and cows; ultrasound is useful. Samples from abdominocentesis and thoracocentesis, electrocardiographs, and blood work may be obtained, and surgical exploration of the abdominal cavity may be necessary for definitive diagnosis in these species.

Treatment: Surgical repair of the hernia is the only treatment. Other areas of trauma may be present. Optimally, the animal should be stabilized before surgery.

HYPOSTATIC PNEUMONIA

Hypostatic pneumonia is caused by passive or dependent congestion of the lungs, a condition most commonly seen in older or debilitated animals. Recumbent animals, such as those recovering from anesthesia, can develop hypostatic pneumonia if not repositioned regularly.

Blood is unable to pass readily through the vasculature of the lung, which can lead to a shift in fluid from the circulatory to the pulmonary spaces. It often occurs secondary to some other disease process causing chest pain (eg, congestive heart failure). Shallow respiration can lead to improper ventilation of the dependent lung, loss of surfactant activity, and accumulation of respiratory secretions and inflammatory exudate in lower airways. Compression of the abdominal contents in recumbent patients restricts the downward movement of the diaphragm, reducing tidal volume and ventilation of alveoli.

Coughing is not always a prominent clinical sign, but as the condition progresses, dyspnea and cyanosis become apparent. Secondary bacterial infection is common. Radiographs reveal increased pulmonary density, and the mediastinal space may show atelectasis.

The animal's position must be changed hourly. Exercise should be encouraged insofar as it is compatible with the animal's condition. If a primary cause can be determined, specific therapy should be instituted. Use of narcotics and sedatives should be minimal to encourage movement and to avoid suppression of the cough reflex. Proper hydration is important, but overhydration may increase congestion and should be avoided.

LARYNGEAL DISORDERS

See also LARYNGEAL HEMIPLEGIA, p 1216.

Laryngitis, an inflammation of the mucosa or cartilages of the larynx, may result from upper respiratory tract infection or by direct irritation from inhalation of dust, smoke, or irritating gas; foreign bodies; or the trauma of intubation, excess vocalization, or in livestock, by injury from roping or restraint devices. Laryngitis may accompany infectious tracheobronchitis and distemper in dogs; infectious rhinotracheitis and calicivirus infection in cats; infectious rhinotracheitis and calf diphtheria in cattle; strangles, herpesvirus 1 infection, viral arteritis, and infectious bronchitis in horses; *Fusobacterium necrophorum* or *Corynebacterium pyogenes* infections in sheep; and influenza in pigs.

Edema of the mucosa and submucosa is often an integral part of laryngitis and, if severe, the rima glottidis may be obstructed. Edema may also result from allergy, inhalation of irritants, or surgery in the area. Intubation for anesthesia, especially when attempted with inadequate induction or poor technique, is likely to provoke laryngeal edema. Brachycephalic and obese dogs, and dogs with laryngeal paralysis (*see* below) develop laryngeal edema and laryngitis through severe panting or respiratory effort during excitement or hyperthermia. In cattle, laryngeal edema has been seen in blackleg, urticaria, serum sickness, and anaphylaxis. In pigs, it may occur as a part of edema disease. In horses, cattle, and sheep, laryngeal edema may lead to arytenoid chondropathy.

Laryngeal chondropathy is a suppurative condition of the cartilage matrix that principally affects the arytenoid cartilages; it is believed to result from microbial infection, often as a sequela of inhalation of irritants. It is characterized by necrosis and ulceration of the laryngeal mucosa, over or just caudal to the vocal cords, and abscessation within the arytenoid cartilage. Initially, there is often acute laryngeal inflammation. Later, there is progressive enlargement of the cartilages that commonly results in a fixed upper airway obstruction with stertorous breathing and reduced exercise tolerance. Laryngeal chondropathy occurs in horses, sheep, and cattle, most often young males. There is a distinct breed predisposition in Thoroughbred horses in race training, Texel and Southdown sheep, and Belgian Blue cattle. Laryngeal contact ulcers are common in young feedlot cattle and often result in necrotic laryngitis and chondropathy.

Clinical Findings: A cough is the principal sign of laryngitis when edema is slight and the deeper tissues of the larynx are not involved. It is harsh, dry, and short at first, but becomes soft and moist later and may be very painful. It can be induced by pressure on the larynx, exposure to cold or dusty air, swallowing coarse food or cold water, or attempts to administer medicines. Vocal changes may be evident, especially in small animals. Stridor may result from swelling and reduced motion of the arytenoid cartilages in laryngeal chondropathy. Halitosis and difficult, noisy breathing may be evident, and the animal may stand with its head lowered and mouth open. Swallowing is difficult and painful. Systemic signs are usually attributable to the primary disease, as in calf diphtheria, in which temperatures of 105°F (40.5°C) may occur. Death due to asphyxiation may occur, especially if the animal is exerted.

Edema of the larynx may develop within hours. It is characterized by increased inspiratory effort and stridor arising from the larynx. Respiratory rate may slow as the effort of breathing becomes exaggerated. Visible mucous membranes are cyanotic, the pulse rate is increased, and body temperature rises. Horses may sweat profusely. Dogs with obstructions of the conducting airways may show extreme disturbance of thermoregulation in hot weather; marked hyperthermia is not uncommon. Untreated animals with marked obstruction eventually collapse and often have signs of pulmonary edema.

Diagnosis: A tentative diagnosis is based on the clinical signs, auscultation of the laryngeal region, and exacerbation of stridor by palpation of the larynx. Definitive diagnosis requires laryngoscopy. In conscious horses and cattle, this can be achieved with a flexible endoscope passed per nasum; in dogs and cats, usually anesthesia or analgesia is required. The history and signs usually permit rapid identification of the primary disease and the associated laryngeal involvement. Bilateral laryngeal paralysis, laryngeal abscess, pharyngeal trauma and cellulitis, and retropharyngeal abscesses or masses can cause similar signs.

Treatment: In laryngeal obstruction, a tracheotomy tube should be placed immediately; if a tracheotomy is not possible, airway patency may be established by passage of a pliable tube through the glottis. Corticosteroids should be administered to reduce the obstructive effect of the inflammatory swellings. Concurrent administration of NSAID and systemic antibiotics is also necessary. Administration of diuretic drugs, eg, furosemide, may be indicated for resolution of laryngeal edema and, if present, pulmonary edema. Identification and treatment of the primary disease is essential. Palliative procedures to speed recovery and give comfort to the animal include inhalation of humidified air; confinement in a warm, clean environment; feeding of soft or liquid foods; and avoidance of dust. The cough may be suppressed with antitussive preparations, and bacterial infections controlled with antibiotics or sulfonamides. Control of pain with judicious use of an analgesic, especially in cats, allows the animal to eat, and thus speeds recovery. Subtotal arytenoidectomy is an effective remedy for laryngeal chondropathy of horses, although a return to full athletic capacity in competitive horses is uncertain. Tracheolaryngostomies and permanent tracheostomies have been used successfully to salvage cattle and sheep with laryngeal chondropathy, but carry significant anesthetic risk. A medical alternative for ruminants is prolonged antibiotic therapy, 14-21 days of parenteral lincomycin (5-10 mg/kg), plus initial short-acting corticosteroids.

LARYNGEAL PARALYSIS

This disease of the upper airway is common in dogs and rare in cats. Signs include a dry cough, voice changes, noisy breathing that progresses to marked difficulty in breathing with stress and exertion, stridor, and collapse. Regurgitation and vomiting may occur. Progression of clinical signs is slow, usually taking months to years before respiratory distress is evident. It is a common acquired problem in middle-aged to older, large and giant breeds of dogs, eg, Labrador Retrievers, Irish Setters, and Great Danes. It is seen less often as a hereditary, congenital disease in Bouvier des Flandres, Leonbergers, Siberian Huskies, Bulldogs, and racing sled dogs.

Diagnosis is based on clinical signs; laryngoscopy under light anesthesia is needed for confirmation. Laryngeal movements are absent or paradoxical with respiration. Electromyography shows positive sharp waves, denervation potentials, and sometimes myotonia. Radiographs are not diagnostic. Denervation atrophy is seen on histologic sections of laryngeal muscles.

Differential diagnoses include myositis, recurrent laryngeal or vagal nerve tumor, inflammation, myasthenia gravis, severe hypothyroidism, trauma, and more widespread generalized neurologic degeneration. Therapy is directed at relieving signs of airway obstruction. Tranquilization and corticosteroids are effective temporarily in mild cases. Severe obstruction may require tracheotomy. Definitive therapy is surgical and is directed at enlarging the glottic opening. Currently recommended techniques include arytenoid cartilage lateralization, ventriculocordectomy and partial arytenoidectomy, castellated laryngofissure, or permanent tracheostomy.

LUNGWORM INFECTION

(Verminous bronchitis, Verminous pneumonia)

An infection of the lower respiratory tract, usually resulting in bronchitis or pneumonia, can be caused by any of several parasitic nematodes, including *Dictyocaulus viviparus* in cattle and deer; *D arnfieldi* in donkeys and horses; *D filaria, Protostrongylus rufescens,* and *Muellerius capillaris* in sheep and goats; *Metastrongylus apri* in pigs; *Oslerus (Filaroides) osleri* in dogs; and *Aelurostrongylus abstrusus* and *Capillaria aerophila* in cats. Other lungworm infections occur but are less common.

The first 3 lungworms listed above belong to the superfamily Trichostrongyloidea and have direct life cycles; the others belong to the Metastrongyloidea and, except for *O osleri* and *C aerophila,* have indirect life cycles.

Some nematodes that inhabit the right ventricle and pulmonary circulation, eg, *Angiostrongylus vasorum* and *Dirofilaria immitis,* both found in dogs in certain areas of the world, may be associated with pulmonary disease. Clinical signs relating to a cardiac or a pulmonary syndrome or to a combination of both may occur.

Diseases caused by the 3 *Dictyocaulus* spp are of most economic importance. The cattle lungworm *D viviparus* is common in northwest Europe and is the cause of severe outbreaks of "husk" or "hoose" in young (and more recently, older) grazing cattle. The lungworm of goats and sheep, *D filaria,* is comparatively less pathogenic but does cause losses, especially in Mediterranean countries, although it is also recognized as a pathogen in Australia, Europe, and North America. *D arnfieldi* can cause severe coughing in horses and, because patency is unusual in horses (but not in donkeys), differential diagnosis with disease due to other respiratory diseases can be difficult. *M capillaris* is prevalent worldwide and, while usually nonpathogenic in sheep, can cause severe signs in goats. Other lungworm infections cause occasional sporadic infections in many animal species in many countries.

Epidemiology: *Dictyocaulus* **spp**—Adult females in the bronchi lay larvated eggs that hatch either in the bronchi (*D viviparus*), or in host feces (*D arnfieldi*) after being coughed up and swallowed. The larvae can become infective in feces on pasture after a minimum of 1 wk in warm, moist conditions, but typically in summer in temperate northern climates will require 2-3 wk. Once infective, the larvae can be further dispersed from fecal pats mechanically or by the sporangia of the fungus *Pilobolus.* A proportion of infective larvae will survive on pasture throughout the winter until the following year but, in very cold conditions, most will become nonviable. The principal source of new infections each year is from infected carrier animals, with overwintered larvae providing a secondary but not unimportant contribution in some countries. In the case of *D arnfieldi,* donkeys are the prime source of pasture contamination for horses. Because *D viviparus* infection in cattle is the most economically important, it has been most investigated and many of the observations from it are applicable to the other species. Clinical disease usually develops on first exposure to sufficient infective larvae; the severity of disease and stimulation of an immune response is related to the number of larvae ingested. In cattle and sheep, this usually occurs during their first season at pasture; however, an increase in the number of older cattle affected has been reported and is attributed to the efficiency of some prophylactic anthelmintic regimens, which prevent exposure at an earlier age. Because transmission of infection to horses requires infected donkeys, first infections can occur at any age in that species. Once infected, adults generally become immune to further disease, but a proportion will contract subclinical infections during which they act as a source of further larval contamination. Occasionally, when previously infected adults or groups that have not been exposed to reinfection for >1 yr, and in which immunity may have waned, are exposed to an overwhelming level of infection, clinical disease may recur. In areas in which cattle are housed during winter and first grazing season calves turned out in late April or May, the first infections can be seen between mid June and late July, but most severe infections develop in previously unexposed calves after multiplication of a second generation of infective larvae on pasture between August and early October.

Other Species—Because other lungworm species either require an intermediate host or are found in nonherd animals, disease caused by them is more sporadic. *Metastrongylus apri* in pigs requires an earthworm as intermediate host; thus, infection is confined to pigs with access to pasture and may become more common as a result of organic farming methods. *Muellerius capillaris* and *Protostrongylus rufescens* in sheep and goats require slugs or snails as intermediate hosts, which must be eaten for infection to occur. *Aelurostrongylus abstrusus* is normally transferred to cats after ingestion of a paratenic host such as a bird or rodent that has previously eaten the slug or snail. Adults of *Oslerus osleri* live in nodules in the trachea of dogs, and larvated eggs laid by adults hatch there. Pups become infected from saliva or feces of an infected dog, in the former case by being licked by their dams. *Capillaria aerophila* in cats has a direct cycle, with infective eggs being ingested with food or water.

Pathogenesis: The pathogenic effect of lungworms depends on their location within the respiratory tract, the number of infective larvae ingested, and the animal's immune state. During the prepatent phase of *Dictyocaulus viviparus* infection, the main lesion is blockage of bronchioles by an infiltrate of eosinophils in response to the developing larvae; this results in obstruction of the airways and collapse of alveoli distal to the block. Clinical signs are moderate unless large numbers of larvae are present, in which case the animal may die in the prepatent phase with severe interstitial emphysema. In the patent phase, the adults in the segmental and lobar bronchi cause a bronchitis, with eosinophils, plasma cells, and lymphocytes in the bronchial wall; a cellular exudate, frothy mucus, and adult nematodes are found in the lumen. The bronchial irritation causes marked coughing, and the entire reaction leads to increased airway resistance. A major component of the patent stage is development of a chronic, nonsuppurative, eosinophilic, granulomatous pneumonia in response to eggs and first-stage larvae aspirated into alveoli and bronchioles. This is usually in the caudal lobes of the lungs and is severe when widespread; in combination with the bronchitis, death may result. Interstitial emphysema, pulmonary edema, and secondary bacterial infection are complications that increase the likelihood of death. Survivors may suffer considerable weight loss. If the animal survives until the end of patency (2-3 mo for *D viviparus*), most or even all of the adult worms are expelled, and the cellular exudate resolves over the ensuing 4 wk. Most recover unless secondary infection develops in the damaged lungs during the postpatent phase. In a few animals, clinical signs are exacerbated in the postpatent phase due to development of a diffuse, proliferative alveolitis characterized by hyperplasia of the type II alveolar epithelial cells. The cause is unknown, but it is observed much less in cattle treated with anthelmintics with a persistent action against *D viviparus* such as the macrocyclic lactones ivermectin, doramectin, eprinomectin, and moxidectin.

D filaria is similar to *D viviparus*, but interstitial emphysema is not a common complication. Bronchial lesions predominate in *D arnfieldi* infections; when an alveolar reaction occurs, as in donkeys or foals, there are lobular areas of overinflation due to intermittent obstruction of small bronchi.

The pathogenic effect of the other lungworms has a similar basis, but frequently such severe clinical signs are not produced, perhaps due to a more restricted localization in the lungs and less severe infections. The patent phase and the associated lesions last >4 mo for some lungworms (*M apri* and *A abstrusus*) but can be >2 yr (*M capillaris*). The lesions in pigs with *M apri* are a combination of localized bronchitis and bronchiolitis with overinflation of related alveoli, usually at the edges of the caudal lobes. In pigs, hypertrophy and hyperplasia of bronchiolar and alveolar duct smooth muscle with marked mucous cell hyperplasia are striking features. Near the end of the patent period (as adult worms are killed), gray-green lymphoid nodules (2-4 mm) are formed; fragments of dead worms may be found microscopically in these nodules composed of lymphocytes and plasma cells surrounding a central zone of eosinophils.

In *M capillaris* and *P rufescens* infections, chronic, eosinophilic, granulomatous pneumonia seems to predominate; the reaction is in the bronchioles and alveoli that contain the parasites, their eggs, or larvae. They are surrounded by macrophages, giant cells, eosinophils, and other immunoinflammatory cells, which produce gray or beige plaques (1-2 cm) subpleurally in the dorsal border of the caudal lung lobes. Small (1-2 mm), greenish, nodular lesions may also develop. The effect of these lesions in sheep is minor, perhaps because of the predominantly subpleural location. This infection represents the lower end of the pathogenic spectrum for lungworms.

In cats, *A abstrusus* produces nodular areas of granulomatous pneumonia in the caudal lobes that, if sufficiently generalized, can be clinically significant and occasionally fatal; a notable feature is the hypertrophy and hyperplasia of the smooth muscle in the media of pulmonary arteries and arterioles. The nodules of *O osleri*, found in the mucous membrane of the trachea and large bronchi, can produce extreme airway irritation and persistent coughing. *Capillaria aerophila* infection causes chronic tracheitis and bronchitis.

In adult animals not previously exposed to infection, the lesions and pathogenesis are the same as in young animals. However, in adults with some degree of immunity, reexposure to the parasite (eg, husk in adult cattle) can result in different lesions. Despite the immune response, many larvae reach the lungs before they are killed in the terminal bronchioles and alveoli. Larvae that are not killed in the terminal bronchioles may reach the bronchi and cause a bronchitis characterized by marked eosinophilic infiltration of the bronchial walls and greenish yellow exudate in the lumen comprising eosinophils, other inflammatory cells, and parasitic debris. The reaction associated with this process can lead to severe clinical signs if the nodules are numerous and the eosinophilic bronchitis extensive; this is responsible for the reinfection phenomenon.

Clinical Findings: Signs of lungworm infection range from moderate coughing with slightly increased respiratory rates to severe persistent coughing and respiratory distress and even failure. Reduced weight gains, reduced milk yields, and weight loss accompany many infections in cattle, sheep, and goats. Patent subclinical infections can occur in all species.

The most consistent signs in cattle are tachypnea and coughing. Initially, rapid, shallow breathing is accompanied by a cough that is exacerbated by exercise. Respiratory difficulty may ensue, and heavily infected animals stand with their heads stretched forward and mouths open, and drool. The animals become anorectic and rapidly lose condition. Lung sounds are particularly prominent at the bronchial bifurcation. In adult dairy cattle, milk yield drops severely, and abnormal lung sounds are heard over the caudal lobes. The reinfection phenomenon in adult dairy cattle is usually seen in the fall; although less severe than in initial infections, the signs are widespread coughing and tachypnea and a marked drop in milk yield.

The signs in sheep and goats infected with *D filaria* are similar to those in cattle. Pulmonary signs usually are not associated with *M capillaris* or *P rufescens* in sheep, but the former can affect goats similarly to *D filaria*. *D arnfieldi* is associated with coughing, tachypnea, and unthriftiness in older horses, but few if any signs in foals or donkeys.

The main clinical sign of *M apri* in pigs is a persistent cough that may become paroxysmal. Coughing and dyspnea occur in cats and dogs with *A abstrusus* and *O osleri* infections, respectively. Fatalities are relatively uncommon with these lungworms, although they do occur in kittens.

Diagnosis: Diagnosis is based on clinical signs, epidemiology, presence of first-stage larvae in feces, and necropsy of animals in the same herd or flock. Bronchoscopy and radiography may be helpful. Larvae are not found in the feces of animals in the prepatent or postpatent phases and usually not in the reinfection phenomenon. ELISA tests are available in some laboratories, but because the antigens used are derived from adult worms, the test is mainly of use in detecting cattle that have not been exposed rather than as a differential diagnosis tool in acute respiratory disease. In the early stages of an outbreak, larvae may be few in number. First-stage larvae or larvated eggs can be recovered using most fecal flotation techniques with the appropriate salt solutions. Bronchial lavage can reveal *D arnfieldi* infections in horses. A convenient method for recovering larvae is a modification of the Baermann technique in which large fecal samples (25-30 g) are wrapped in tissue paper or cheese cloth and suspended or placed in water contained in a beaker. The water at the bottom of the beaker is examined for larvae after 4 hr; in heavy infections, larvae may be present within 30 min.

In domestic pets and horses, because of the relative infrequency of infection, diagnosis may be made only after failure of antibiotic therapy to ameliorate the condition. Adults of *Dictyocaulus* spp and *M apri* are readily visible in the bronchi during the patent phases of infection. However, examination of smears from bronchial mucus or histologic sections from lesions may be necessary to confirm the diagnosis during other stages of lungworm infection (and also for other lungworms).

Bronchoscopy can be used to detect nodules of *O osleri* or to collect tracheal washings (dogs and horses) to examine for eggs, larvae, and eosinophils.

Necropsy should include examination of the trachea, particularly at the bifurcation, for *O osleri* and the lesions they induce.

Treatment: Several drugs are useful (*see* TABLE 1). The benzimidazoles (fenbendazole, oxfendazole, and albendazole), and macrocyclic lactones (ivermectin, doramectin, eprinomectin, and moxidectin) are frequently used in cattle and are effective against all stages of *D viviparus*. These drugs are also effective against lungworms in sheep, horses, and pigs. Levamisole is used in cattle, sheep, and goats but treatment may need to be repeated 2 wk later as it is less effective against larvae during the early stages. Fenbendazole has been used successfully in cats for *A abstrusus*. *O osleri* in dogs is a problem, but there is evidence that fenbendazole and albendazole are effective if treatment is prolonged. *C aerophila* in cats is similarly difficult, but three 5-day cycles of levamisole at 9-day intervals has been reported to be successful.

TABLE 1. Recommended Treatments for Lungworms[*]

Parasite	Host	Treatment
Dictyocaulus viviparus	Cattle	Ivermectin, doramectin, moxidectin, eprinomectin, fenbendazole, albendazole, levamisole
D filaria	Sheep, goat	Ivermectin, doramectin, moxidectin, eprinomectin, fenbendazole, albendazole, levamisole
D arnfieldi	Horse, donkey	Ivermectin, moxidectin
Metastrongylus apri	Pig	Ivermectin, moxidectin, doramectin
Aelurostrongylus abstrusus	Cat	Fenbendazole, selamectin[†]
Oslerus osleri	Dog	Fenbendazole, albendazole
Capillaria aerophila	Cat	Levamisole, selamectin[†]

[*]In severe cases NSAID may also be helpful.
[†]Anecdotal evidence for efficacy but no published evidence or label recommendations.

Animals at pasture should be moved inside for treatment, and supportive therapy may be needed for complications that can arise in all species.

Control: Lungworm infections in herds or flocks are controlled primarily by vaccination or anthelmintics. Oral vaccines are available in Europe for *D viviparus* (northeastern areas) and *D filaria* (southeast). Two doses of irradiated infective larvae are given 4 wk apart at least 2 wk before the start of grazing or exposure to probable infection. Used properly, they prevent clinical disease, but some vaccinated animals may become mildly infected to the extent that larvae are excreted to perpetuate further infection.

Anthelmintic prophylaxis has become feasible with the advent of anthelmintics with prolonged activity (eg, ivermectin, doramectin, moxidectin, eprinomectin) and sustained-release intraruminal boluses containing oxfendazole or fenbendazole. With persistent anthelmintics, 2 or 3 treatments during the grazing season, the timing of which depends on local grazing practice and epidemiology, are effective and may, by disrupting developing infections, stimulate immunity to the parasite. Boluses provide continuous anthelmintic protection but, as with the use of multiple treatments, they delay exposure to *D viviparus* until the animal is adult, when infection (albeit usually less severe) can occur. However, these methods have become popular in that GI parasites are controlled simultaneously.

Other more sporadic infections can be controlled more easily by management, eg, avoidance of grazing horses with donkeys, indoor husbandry of pigs, and by not mixing sheep and goats on the same grazing.

MYCOTIC PNEUMONIA

Fungal infection of the lung results in an acute to chronic active, pyogranulomatous pneumonia.

Etiology: *Cryptococcus neoformans, Histoplasma capsulatum, Coccidioides immitis, Blastomyces dermatiditis, Pneumocystis carinii, Aspergillus* spp, *Candida* spp, and other less common fungi have been identified as causative agents of mycotic pneumonia in domestic animals (*see also* FUNGAL INFECTIONS, p 510). Often these agents are found in immunocompromised hosts, but can cause disease in healthy individuals as well. Infection is typically caused by inhalation of spores, which can lead to hemolymphatic dissemination. Pulmonary tissues and secretions are an excellent environment for these organisms. The source of most fungal infections is believed to be soil-related rather than horizontal transmission. Considering the high rate of exposure to these pathogens in certain environments, there are unresolved questions on the epidemiology of the condition, including individual susceptibility, pathogenicity of organisms, the immune response of the host, and concurrent disease. *Blastomyces* and *Histoplasma* are prevalent in the Mississippi and Ohio River valleys, whereas *Coccidioides* is found in the southwestern USA and northwestern Mexico. *Cryptococcus* is often associated with accumulation of pigeon excreta.

Clinical Findings : Mycotic pneumonia is more commonly seen in small animals. *Blastomyces* infections typically occur in young, male, large-breed dogs. In cats, *Cryptococcus* has a predilection for the nasal cavity where it causes a granulomatous rhinitis and sinusitis. Acute, fulminant clinical presentations do occur but are rare, and the most common course of disease is chronic. A short, moist cough is characteristic. A thick, mucoid nasal discharge may be present. As the disease progresses, dyspnea, emaciation, and generalized weakness become increasingly evident. Respiration may become abdominal, resembling that of a diaphragmatic hernia (p 1178). On auscultation, harsh respiratory sounds are heard. In advanced cases, breath sounds are decreased or almost inaudible. Tracheobronchial lymphadenopathy can cause extrinsic airway compression. Neutrophilic leukocytosis or neutropenia with a left shift, nonregenerative anemia, and periodic fever can occur, possibly concurrent with bacterial infections. Radiography will show enlargement of tracheobronchial lymph nodes and variable, nodular to linear, interstitial infiltrates.

Lesions: Multifocal to coalescing lesions of granulomatous to pyogranulomatous inflammation are present in the lungs. Abscess formation and cavitation may be seen in conjunction with yellow or gray areas of necrosis. Causative organisms are present within macrophages or areas of intense inflammation. Dissemination to multiple organ systems (eg, skin, eyes, peripheral lymph nodes, bones, CNS, male genitalia, oral cavity, nasal cavity) may occur.

Diagnosis: A tentative diagnosis of mycotic pneumonia can be made if an animal with chronic respiratory disease exhibits the clinical signs described and does not respond to antibiotic therapy. Definitive diagnosis requires laboratory confirmation. Radiography may be useful. Serology can provide a presumptive diagnosis. Some antigens (eg, histoplasmin, blastomycin) have been developed and are an aid in diagnosis. Cytologic examinations of the sputum or exudates from sites of extrapulmonary inflammation may reveal the infective organism. The clinical diagnosis can be confirmed at necropsy by appropriate microbiology and histopathology. Special stains can be used to highlight the organisms.

Treatment: There is no entirely satisfactory method of treating systemic mycotic infections. Amphotericin may be helpful but is undesirably nephrotoxic. Ketoconazole, and several newer antifungal agents such as itraconazole and fluconazole, show better, but variable, results against fungal pathogens in companion animals. Protracted therapy, at least 2 mo beyond clinical resolution, is usually necessary for resoluton of the infection.

NECROBACILLOSIS

The term necrobacillosis is used to describe any disease or lesion with which *Fusobacterium necrophorum* is associated. It includes necrotic laryngitis (*see* below), necrotic stomatitis of calves, necrotic rhinitis of pigs (p 1226), footrot of cattle (p 882), foot abscess of sheep (p 943), postparturient necrosis of the vagina and uterus, focal necrosis of the liver of cattle and sheep, quittor of horses (p 911), and numerous other necrotic lesions in ruminants and, less commonly, in pigs, horses, fowl, and rabbits. *F necrophorum* is probably a secondary invader rather than a primary etiologic agent and is usually present as part of a mixed infection. However, its necrotizing exotoxin undoubtedly plays a role in the production of characteristic lesions. It is part of the normal flora of the mouth, intestine, and genital tract of many herbivores and omnivores and is widespread in the environment. It is thought to gain entry to the body through wounds in the skin or mucous membranes.

NECROTIC LARYNGITIS
(Calf diphtheria, Laryngeal necrobacillosis)

Necrotic laryngitis is a disease of young cattle characterized by fever, toxemia, inspiratory dyspnea, and stridor. Inflammation of the pharynx, or the laryngeal mucosa and its cartilage, caused by invasion of *F necrophorum* into existing lesions is responsible for the clinical signs. Necrotic laryngitis primarily affects feedlot cattle 3-18 mo of age; however, cases in calves as young as 5 wk and in cattle as old as 24 mo have been documented. It has a worldwide distribution.

Etiology: The primary etiologic agent is uncertain because *F necrophorum*, which is commonly isolated from lesions of affected cattle, is unable to penetrate intact mucous membranes. Contact ulcers on the mucous membranes of the vocal processes and medial angles of the arytenoid cartilages are thought to be the initial lesions; concurrent disease, inhaled irritants, vitamin A deficiency, and poor hygiene in confined animals have all been incriminated as predisposing factors.

Transmission, Epidemiology, and Pathogenesis: Necrotic laryngitis is most common where cattle are closely confined under unsanitary conditions or in feedlots. The prevalence in feedlot calves is estimated to be 1-2%. Most cases are sporadic and occur year round, but disease peaks in the fall and winter. Mixed upper respiratory infections (viruses such as infectious bovine rhinotracheitis and parainfluenza-3; *Mycoplasma* spp; and bacteria, including *Pasteurella* and *Haemophilus*), and the coughing and swallowing associated with these infections, may predispose feedlot cattle to develop erosions involving the vocal processes and medial angles of arytenoid cartilages. These ulcerative laryngeal lesions then provide a portal of entry for *F necrophorum*.

Once it has invaded the mucosa of the pharynx and larynx, *F necrophorum* causes inflammation and necrosis. Edema of the laryngeal mucosa results in variable narrowing of the rima glottidis accompanied by inspiratory dyspnea and stridor. If infection extends into the laryngeal cartilage, laryngeal chondritis develops, which delays healing and inhibits recovery. Pharyngeal lesions cause discomfort and result in painful swallowing motions. The exotoxin produced by *F necrophorum* also causes systemic signs of illness.

Clinical Findings: Initially, a moist, painful cough is noticed. Severe inspiratory dyspnea, characterized by open-mouth breathing with the head and neck extended and loud inspiratory stridor are common findings. Ptyalism; frequent, painful swallowing motions; bilateral, purulent nasal discharge; and a fetid odor to the breath may also be present. Systemic signs may include fever (106°F [41.1°C]), anorexia, depression, and hyperemia of the mucous membranes. Untreated calves die in 2-7 days from toxemia and upper airway obstruction. Longterm sequelae include aspiration pneumonia and permanent distortion of the larynx.

Lesions: Lesions are typically located over the vocal processes and medial angles of arytenoid cartilages. Acute lesions are characterized by edema and hyperemia surrounding a necrotic ulcer in the laryngeal mucosa; lesions may spread along the vocal folds and processes to involve the cricoarytenoideus dorsalis muscle. In chronic cases, lesions consist of necrotic cartilage associated with a draining tract surrounded by granulation tissue.

Diagnosis: Clinical signs are usually sufficient to establish a diagnosis. However, because numerous other conditions can cause signs of upper airway obstruction, the larynx should be visually inspected to confirm a diagnosis. This can be accomplished by means of an orally inserted speculum, laryngoscopy, endoscopy, or radiography, but care must be exercised to avoid further respiratory embarrassment. A tracheostomy should be performed before laryngoscopic or endoscopic examination in cattle with severe inspiratory dyspnea. Differential diagnoses include pharyngeal trauma; severe viral laryngitis (eg, infectious bovine rhinotracheitis); actinobacillosis; and laryngeal edema, abscesses, trauma, paralysis, or tumors.

Treatment and Control: Sulfonamides (an initial dose of 140 mg/kg, IV, followed by 70 mg/kg, IV, SID) or procaine penicillin (22,000 U/kg, IM, BID) are the drugs of choice. NSAID (aspirin, 100 mg/kg, PO, BID, or ketoprofen, 3 mg/kg, IM or IV, SID for up to 3 days) can be used to decrease the degree of laryngeal inflammation and edema. A tracheostomy is indicated in cattle with severe inspiratory dyspnea. The prognosis is good for early cases that are treated aggressively; chronic cases will require surgery under general anesthesia to remove necrotic or granulation tissue and to drain laryngeal abscesses. A 60% success rate has been reported for surgical intervention in advanced cases.

There are no specific control measures for necrotic laryngitis; however, the proposed pathogenesis suggests that control measures for common respiratory pathogens may be beneficial.

PHARYNGITIS

Pharyngitis is an inflammation of the walls of the pharynx. It may accompany most upper airway viral and bacterial respiratory infections, eg, strangles in horses and distemper in dogs.

Functionally, the pharynx is divided into 2 components—the nasopharynx and the oropharynx. In most species, there is a common pharynx that is present at times other than deglutition. The unique caudal pharyngeal-laryngeal anatomy of horses shows complete separation of the pharynx into 2 components. (*See also* PHARYNGEAL LYMPHOID HYPERPLASIA, p 1217.)

Clinical Findings: In general, animals with pharyngitis have a normal desire to eat and drink but may have difficulty swallowing. As a result of secondary peripharyngeal cellulitis and abscessation, some animals may present in an emergency situation (eg, a young foal with gross suppurative pharyngitis from strangles that is obstructing the pharynx and causing asphyxiation). The diagnosis in such cases is based on complete physical examination and radiographic and endoscopic evaluation of the throat, together with cultures of appropriate draining fluids and sites. In small animals, oral pain and resistance to having the mouth opened may indicate retropharyngeal abscessation and the presence of a penetrating foreign body or neoplasia of the mouth or tonsils.

Treatment: The primary treatment is to identify and control or eliminate the predisposing factors. If pharyngitis has been caused by foreign bodies, removal of the offending object and effective surgical drainage accompanied by excision of necrotic tissue should be done under general anesthesia. In race training of horses, multiple therapies for pharyngeal lymphoid hyperplasia are used. Such therapies involve the use of intranasal sprays via catheters that may include a mixture of components (eg, fluorescein, dimethyl sulfoxide [DMSO], and local anesthetic and antimicrobial agents).

Calicivirus infections in cats may cause marked ulceration of the oropharyngeal mucosa, which is difficult to treat without a primary therapy for the virus. Supportive therapy may control secondary bacterial infection. It is important to maintain normal hydration and provide adequate nutrition, which may be accomplished by IV fluid therapy, feeding by pharyngostomy, or both.

Pharyngeal Trauma

The pharynx of large animals may be traumatized iatrogenically from the use of balling guns or attempts to pass probangs *per os* in cattle. In small animals, oropharyngeal foreign bodies are quite common in dogs but less so in cats. Penetrating foreign bodies include pins, needles, and pieces of stick or bone fragments.

PULMONARY EMPHYSEMA

Two major forms of pulmonary emphysema are generally recognized. **Alveolar emphysema** is abnormal permanent enlargement of air spaces distal to the terminal bronchiole and destruction of alveolar septal walls without apparent fibrosis. **Interstitial emphysema** is the presence of air within the supporting connective tissue stroma of the lung (interlobular, subpleural, mediastinal, subcutaneous). Emphysema should be distinguished from alveolar hyperinflation, a common and temporary postmortem finding that occurs secondary to obstruction of air outflow. While the pathogenesis is not fully understood, at least 2 possibilities have been suggested: 1) there appears to be degradation and weakening of alveolar walls and interstitium by inflammatory cell protease activity, particularly neutrophil elastase, in patients with low antiprotease production; and 2) the condition develops secondary to chronic bronchitis or bronchiolitis (bronchiolitis fibrosa obliterans) causing obstruction of airways on expiration. This creates a "check valve" lesion, in which air is able to enter alveoli on inspiration or through communicating pores in alveolar walls, but is unable to leave freely.

Emphysema is an important disease in humans; in other animals it typically occurs secondary to another pulmonary disease process. Chronic obstructive pulmonary disease (COPD) or "heaves" in horses (p 1213) can cause enlargement and destruction of airspaces secondary to chronic generalized bronchiolitis, which is characterized by epithelial hyperplasia, goblet cell metaplasia, peribronchiolar fibrosis, and lymphoplasmacytic inflammation. The association of high numbers of eosinophils with COPD suggests allergic, infectious, and/or toxicologic etiologies for the condition. Congenital lobar emphysema of dogs (as seen in the Pekingese breed) occurs secondary to aplasia or hypoplasia of bronchiolar cartilage. Due to well-developed interlobular septa and lack of collateral ventilation, sheep, pigs, and particularly cattle are susceptible to interstitial emphysema. Any pathologic process that results in forced expiration can cause air to be forced into interlobular septa. The condition may occur as a sequela of acute interstitial pneumonia in cattle. Severe interstitial emphysema can cause subcutaneous emphysema as air dissects along fascial planes from the lungs through the mediastinum and thoracic inlet to the subcutis of the back.

Minor degrees of emphysema may precede death if there was a prolonged struggle or exaggerated respiration. These agonal changes should be differentiated from antemortem lesions.

RESPIRATORY DISEASES OF CATTLE

Respiratory disease is among the most economically important diseases of cattle in production on a worldwide basis. (*See also* CALF DIPHTHERIA, p 1186.)

ALLERGIC RHINITIS AND ENZOOTIC NASAL GRANULOMA

Allergic rhinitis is an uncommon disease of cattle that, when chronic, may lead to granuloma formation. The etiology is an allergic reaction to pollen or fungal spores. Signs are seasonal and occur under warm, moist conditions; they include rhinorrhea, sneezing, and a sudden onset of dyspnea. In the chronic stage, multiple granulomas may form on the mucosal surface of the nasal cavity. Cytologic examination of nasal discharges may reveal eosinophils. Treatment should focus on removing the allergen or removing the animal from the allergen. Treatment with corticosteroids to block the hypersensitivity reaction is a consideration.

SINUSITIS

Etiology: Sinusitis in cattle typically involves the frontal or maxillary sinus. Frontal sinusitis is usually associated with dehorning and maxillary sinusitis with infected teeth. Numerous bacteria have been isolated from sinusitis infections in cattle.

Clinical Findings: Frontal sinusitis may occur immediately after dehorning while the site is still open or months later after the dehorning site has healed. The condition is most often unilateral. Signs may include anorexia, pyrexia, unilateral or bilateral nasal discharge, changes in air flow through the nasal passages, and foul breath. Head carriage may be abnormal. In longstanding cases of frontal sinusitis, there may be distortion of the frontal bone, exophthalmos, and neurologic signs.

Diagnosis: Diagnosis can usually be made on the basis of clinical signs. Percussion may reveal a dull sound over the affected sinus. Radiographs may reveal fluid in the sinus, the presence of dental disease, or bone lysis. Cytology of aspirated material from the affected sinus may reveal purulent material.

Treatment: Sinusitis is treated by draining the affected sinus. Trephine sites should be reviewed for appropriate anatomic landmarks. If an infected tooth is the cause of maxillary sinusitis, the tooth can be repelled through a sinusotomy site created with a trephine. Once drainage has been established, the sinus can be lavaged daily with antiseptic solutions. Treatment with parenteral antibiotics is indicated if systemic signs are present. NSAID can be given for pain relief, if needed. The prognosis is guarded.

Control: The best control method is to dehorn calves at a young age using a closed dehorning technique. If this is not possible, close attention should be paid to disinfection of surgical instruments between animals, dust control, and fly control.

TRACHEAL EDEMA SYNDROME OF FEEDER CATTLE

Tracheal edema syndrome is characterized by extensive edema of the mucosa and submucosa in the dorsal membrane of the lower trachea. The etiology is unknown. Proposed causes include respiratory viruses and bacteria, trauma to the trachea from feed bunks, passive congestion and edema from excessive fat accumulation in the thoracic inlet, hypersensitivity reactions, and mycotoxins.

The condition occurs in heavy feeder cattle in the later two-thirds of the feeding period throughout North America but may be most severe in the summer in southern plains (USA) feedlots. Onset is sudden and appears to be associated with an increase in respirations stimulated by hot weather or exercise. The initial signs are a loud inspiratory noise (stridor) and the onset of dyspnea. Forced movement causes the respiratory distress to worsen. The cattle become cyanotic and typically collapse and die of asphyxiation in <24 hr. Usually, only 1 or 2 animals per pen are affected.

In the acute form, necropsy lesions include edematous and/or hemorrhagic thickening of the submucosa and mucosa of the dorsal trachea extending from the midcervical area to the thoracic inlet. There is extensive hemorrhage in the trachea but no lung lesions. In the chronic form, lesions consist of hyperemia of the caudal third of the trachea with mucopurulent exudate in the trachea. In fatal cases, the lesion becomes completely obstructive.

Movement and handling of affected cattle should be limited. Antibiotics and corticosteroids are recommended for the acute form. Tracheostomy may be required in severe cases. Providing shade and cooling with fans or water sprays is recommended. Animals that recover are prone to relapse and should be sent to slaughter.

BOVINE RESPIRATORY DISEASE COMPLEX

Bovine respiratory disease (BRD) has a multifactorial etiology and develops as a result of complex interactions between environmental factors, host factors, and pathogens. Environmental factors (eg, weaning, transport, commingling, crowding, and inadequate ventilation) serve as stressors that adversely affect the immune and nonimmune defense mechanisms of the host. In addition, certain environmental factors (eg, crowding and inadequate ventilation) can enhance the transmission of infectious agents among animals. Many infectious agents have been associated with BRD. An initial pathogen (eg, a virus) may alter the animal's defense mechanisms, allowing colonization of the lower respiratory tract by bacteria.

ENZOOTIC PNEUMONIA OF CALVES AND SHIPPING FEVER PNEUMONIA

Enzootic pneumonia and shipping fever pneumonia share many similarities in their respective etiologies and pathogeneses and general measures for control and prevention.

Enzootic Pneumonia of Calves

Enzootic pneumonia of calves refers to infectious respiratory disease in calves. The term "viral pneumonia of calves" is sometimes used but is not preferred based on the current understanding of etiology and pathogenesis. Enzootic pneumonia is primarily a problem in calves <6 mo old with peak occurrence from 2-10 wk, but may be seen in calves up to 1 yr of age. It is more common in dairy than in beef calves and is a common problem in veal calves. It is also more common in housed calves than those raised outside. Peak incidence of disease may coincide with decline of passively acquired immunity. Morbidity rates may approach 100%; case fatality rates vary but can reach 20%.

Etiology: The etiology is similar to that for BRD complex in general (*see* p 1190). The pathogenesis involves stress and possibly an initial respiratory viral infection followed by a secondary bacterial infection of the lower respiratory tract. Stress results from environmental and management factors, including inadequate ventilation, continually adding calves to an established group, crowding, and nutritional factors such as poor-quality milk replacers. Partial or complete failure of passive transfer of maternal antibodies is an important host factor related to development of disease. Any of several viruses may be involved, and a variety of bacteria may be recovered from affected calves. Mycoplasmal and bacterial agents including *Pasteurella multocida, Mannheimia haemolytica,* and *Mycoplasma bovis* represent the most frequently isolated pathogenic organisms. The individual viral and bacterial etiologies, clinical signs, lesions, and treatment are discussed under VIRAL RESPIRATORY TRACT INFECTIONS (p 1192) and BACTERIAL PNEUMONIA (p 1195).

Control and Prevention: When calves of varying ages are placed in communal pens, control of enzootic pneumonia is difficult. The severity of the pneumonia may be decreased by improved husbandry, proper housing, adequate ventilation, and good nursing care. Prevention begins with vaccinating the cows against specific respiratory viruses and bacteria 3-4 wk prepartum to improve the quality of colostral antibodies. Calves should receive good quality colostrum at 8-10% of body wt in the first 12 hr after birth. Newborn dairy calves should be housed individually in hutches or stalls and fed whole milk or a high-quality milk replacer with a fiber content of <0.25% until 8-12 wk old. Calves should be vaccinated against respiratory viruses 3-4 wk before the first grouping, although in some situations, the presence of passive immunity may interfere with an active immune response. Calves should be of similar age when assembled into groups and the group should be limited to ≤10. As calves mature, groups can become larger as the size of the herd, facilities, and available labor dictate. An "all in/all out" management style should be practiced when establishing and terminating a group. At minimum, newly purchased calves should be isolated before introduction to an existing group. Newborn beef calves and their dams should be moved from concentrated calving areas as soon as the calf is nursing well and is strong enough to travel.

Shipping Fever Pneumonia

Shipping fever pneumonia is a respiratory disease of cattle of multifactorial etiology with *Mannheimia haemolytica* and, less commonly, *Pasteurella multocida* or *Histophilus somni* (p 606), being the important infectious agents involved. Shipping fever pneumonia is associated with the assembly into feedlots of large groups of calves from diverse geographic, nutritional, and genetic backgrounds. Disease is typically seen in feeder calves 7-10 days after assembly in a feedlot. Morbidity can approach 35%; mortality is 5-10%.

Etiology: The pathogenesis of shipping fever pneumonia involves stress factors, with or without viral infection, interacting to suppress host defense mechanisms, which allows the proliferation of commensal bacteria in the upper respiratory tract. Subsequently, these bacteria colonize the lower respiratory tract and cause a bronchopneumonia with a cranioventral distribution in the lung. Multiple stress factors are believed to contribute to the suppression of host defense mechanisms. Transportation over long distances serves as a stressor; it may be associated with exhaustion, starvation, dehydration, chilling and overheating depending on weather conditions, and exposure to vehicle exhaust fumes. Additional stressors include passage through auction markets; commingling, processing, and surgical procedures on arrival at the feedlot; dusty environmental conditions; and nutritional stress associated with a change to high-energy rations in the feedlot. The individual viral and bacterial etiologies, clinical signs, lesions, and treatment are discussed under VIRAL RESPIRATORY TRACT INFECTIONS (p 1192) and BACTERIAL PNEUMONIA (p 1195).

Control and Prevention: Prevention of shipping fever pneumonia should focus on reduction of the stressors that contribute to development of the disease. Cattle should be assembled rapidly into groups, and new animals should not be introduced to established groups. Auction markets and mixing of cattle from different sources should be avoided if possible. Transport time should be minimized, and rest periods, with access to feed and water, should be provided during prolonged transport. Calves should be weaned 2-3 wk before shipment, and surgical procedures should be performed in advance of transport. Cattle should be processed within 48 hr after arrival at the feedlot. A rest period of 6-12 hr after transport may allow for rehydration and return of cortisol to levels that will have less impact on the immune response to vaccination. Adaptation to high-energy rations should be gradual as acidosis, indigestion, and anorexia may inhibit the immune response. Vitamin and mineral deficiencies should be corrected. Dust control measures should be used. Metaphylaxis with long-acting antibiotics given "on arrival" for cattle at high risk for developing shipping fever pneumonia has been shown to significantly reduce morbidity and improve rate of gain.

The administration of viral respiratory vaccines on entry to the feedlot has been historically controversial, especially with modified live vaccines. These vaccines have been reported to increase the mortality associated with shipping fever pneumonia. Continuous improvements in modified live vaccine production, and the fact that these vaccines do not require a booster, have made them preferred over killed vaccines for on-arrival processing. When possible, vaccinations for the viral and bacterial components of shipping fever pneumonia should be given 2-3 wk before transport and can be repeated on entry to the feedlot.

VIRAL RESPIRATORY TRACT INFECTIONS

Parainfluenza-3 Virus

Etiology: Parainfluenza-3 virus (PI-3) is an RNA virus classified in the paramyxovirus family. Infections caused by PI-3 are common in cattle. Although PI-3 is capable of causing disease, it is usually associated with mild to subclinical infections. The most important role of PI-3 is to serve as an initiator that can lead to the development of secondary bacterial pneumonia.

Clinical Findings and Lesions: Clinical signs include pyrexia, cough, serous nasal and lacrimal discharge, increased respiratory rate, and increased breath sounds. The severity of signs worsens with the onset of bacterial pneumonia. Fatalities from uncomplicated PI-3 pneumonia are rare. Lesions include cranioventral lung consolidation, bronchiolitis, and alveolitis with marked congestion and hemorrhage. Inclusion bodies may be identified. Most fatal cases have a concurrent bacterial bronchopneumonia.

Diagnosis: Diagnostic procedures for PI-3 are similar to those for BOVINE RESPIRATORY SYNCYTIAL VIRUS (p 1192).

Treatment and Prevention: Treatment focuses on the antimicrobial therapy directed toward bacterial pneumonia (p 1195). NSAID are also a therapeutic consideration.

PI-3 vaccines are available and are almost always combined with bovine herpesvirus 1 (infectious bovine rhinotracheitis). Modified live and inactivated vaccines are available for IM administration. Vaccines containing temperature-sensitive mutants for intranasal administration are also available.

Bovine Respiratory Syncytial Virus

Etiology: Bovine respiratory syncytial virus (BRSV) is an RNA virus classified as a pneumovirus in the paramyxovirus family. This virus was named for its characteristic cytopathic effect—the formation of syncytial cells. In additional to cattle, sheep and goats can also be infected by respiratory syncytial viruses. Human respiratory syncytial virus (HRSV) is an important respiratory pathogen in infants and young children. Antigenic subtypes are known to exist for HRSV, and preliminary evidence suggests that there may be antigenic subtypes of BRSV. BRSV is distributed worldwide, and the virus is indigenous in the cattle population.

BRSV infections associated with respiratory disease occur predominantly in young beef and dairy cattle. Passively derived immunity does not appear to prevent BRSV infections but will reduce the severity of disease. Initial exposures to the virus are associated with severe respiratory disease; subsequent exposures result in mild to subclinical disease. BRSV is an important virus in the bovine respiratory disease complex because of its frequency of occurrence, predilection for the lower respiratory tract, and ability to predispose the respiratory tract to secondary bacterial infection. In outbreaks, morbidity tends to be high, and the case fatality rate can be 0-20%.

Clinical Findings and Lesions: Fever (104-108°F [40-42°C]), depression, decreased feed intake, increased respiratory rate, cough, and nasal and lacrimal discharge are common.

Dyspnea, possibly with open-mouthed breathing, may become pronounced in the later stages of the disease. Subcutaneous emphysema may occur. Secondary bacterial pneumonia is a frequent occurrence. A biphasic disease pattern has been described but is not consistent. Gross lesions include a diffuse interstitial pneumonia with subpleural and interstitial emphysema along with interstitial edema. These lesions are similar to and must be differentiated from other causes of interstitial pneumonia. *See also* INTERSTITIAL PNEUMONIA, p 1198. Bronchopneumonia of bacterial origin is usually present. Histologic examination reveals syncytial cells in bronchiolar epithelium and lung parenchyma, intracytoplasmic inclusion bodies, proliferation and/or degeneration of bronchiolar epithelium, alveolar epithelialization, edema, and hyaline membrane formation.

Diagnosis: A diagnosis of BRSV requires laboratory confirmation. BRSV is a difficult virus to detect, although chances of isolation may improve when sampling animals that are in the incubation or acute phases of infection. An antigen detection enzyme immunoassay is useful in detecting BRSV antigen and establishing a diagnosis. Other procedures that have proved useful in detection of BRSV antigen are fluorescent antibody and immunoperoxidase staining.

Paired serum samples can be used to establish a diagnosis. However, the antibody titer of animals with well-developed clinical disease may be higher in the acute sample than in the sample taken 2-3 wk later because the antibody response often develops rapidly, and clinical signs follow virus infection by up to 7-10 days. Single serum samples with high antibody titers from a number of animals in a respiratory outbreak may be useful in making a diagnosis if coupled with clinical signs. Calves that become infected with BRSV in the presence of passively derived antibody may not seroconvert.

Treatment and Prevention: Treatment focuses on antimicrobial therapy to control secondary bacterial pneumonia (p 1195). There is no specific treatment for the viral interstitial pneumonia. Supportive therapy and correction of dehydration may be necessary. There are anecdotal reports of treatment with antihistamines and/or corticosteroids being of benefit. Most cases will recover in several days without treatment.

General control and prevention are discussed under ENZOOTIC PNEUMONIA OF CALVES AND SHIPPING FEVER PNEUMONIA (p 1190). Inactivated and modified live vaccines are available and may serve to reduce losses associated with BRSV.

Bovine Herpesvirus I
(Infectious bovine rhinotracheitis virus, Infectious pustular vulvovaginitis, and associated diseases)

Etiology and Epidemiology: Bovine herpesvirus 1 (BHV-1) is associated with several diseases in cattle: infectious bovine rhinotracheitis (IBR), infectious pustular vulvovaginitis (IPV), balanoposthitis, conjunctivitis, abortion, encephalomyelitis, and mastitis. Only a single serotype of BHV-1 is recognized; however, three subtypes of BHV-1 have been described on the basis of endonuclease cleavage patterns of viral DNA—BHV-1.1 (respiratory subtype), BHV-1.2 (genital subtype), and BHV-1.3 (encephalitic subtype). BHV-1.3 has been reclassified as a distinct herpesvirus designated BHV-5.

BHV-1 infections are widespread in the cattle population. In feedlot cattle, the respiratory form is most common. The viral infection alone is not life-threatening but predisposes to secondary bacterial pneumonia, which may result in death. In breeding cattle, abortion or genital infections are more common. Genital infections can occur in bulls (infectious pustular balanoposthitis) and cows (IPV) within 1-3 days of mating or close contact with an infected animal. Transmission can occur in the absence of visible lesions and through artificial insemination with semen from subclinically infected bulls. Cattle with latent BHV-1 infections generally show no clinical signs when the virus is reactivated, but they serve as a source of infection for other susceptible animals.

Clinical Findings: The incubation period for the respiratory and genital forms is 2-6 days. In the respiratory form, clinical signs range from mild to severe, depending on the presence of secondary bacterial pneumonia. Clinical signs include high fever, anorexia, coughing, excessive salivation, nasal discharge that progresses from serous to mucopurulent, conjunctivitis with lacrimal discharge, inflamed nares (hence the common name "red nose"), and dyspnea if the larynx becomes occluded with purulent material. Nasal lesions consist of numerous clusters of grayish necrotic foci on the mucous membrane of the septal mucosa, just visible inside the external nares. They may later be accompanied by pseudodiphtheritic yellowish plaques. Conjunctivitis with corneal opacity may occur as the only manifestation of BHV-1 infection. In the absence of bacterial pneumonia, recovery generally occurs 4-5 days after the onset of signs.

Abortions may occur concurrently with respiratory disease but may be seen up to 100 days after infection. They can occur regardless of the severity of disease in the dam. Abortions generally occur during the second half of pregnancy, but early embryonic death is possible.

In genital infections, the first signs are frequent urination, elevation of the tailhead, and a mild vaginal discharge. The vulva is swollen, and small papules, then erosions and ulcers, are present on the mucosal surface. If secondary bacterial infections do not occur, animals recover in 10-14 days. With bacterial infection, there may be inflammation of the uterus and transient infertility, with purulent vaginal discharge for several weeks. In bulls, similar lesions occur on the penis and prepuce. (*See also* p 1150.)

BHV-1 infection can be severe in young calves and cause a generalized disease. Pyrexia, ocular and nasal discharges, respiratory distress, diarrhea, incoordination, and eventually convulsions and death may occur in a short period after generalized viral infection.

Lesions: In uncomplicated IBR infections, most lesions are restricted to the upper respiratory tract and trachea. Petechial to ecchymotic hemorrhages may be found in the mucous membranes of the nasal cavity and the paranasal sinuses. Focal areas of necrosis develop in the nose, pharynx, larynx, and trachea. The lesions may coalesce to form plaques.

The sinuses are often filled with a serous or serofibrinous exudate. As the disease progresses, the pharynx becomes covered with a serofibrinous exudate, and blood-tinged fluid may be found in the trachea. The pharyngeal and pulmonary lymph nodes may be acutely swollen and hemorrhagic. The tracheitis may extend into the bronchi and bronchioles; when this occurs, epithelium is sloughed in the airways. The viral lesions are often masked by secondary bacterial infections. In young animals with generalized BHV-1 infection, erosions and ulcers overlaid with debris may be found in the nose, esophagus, and forestomachs. In addition, white foci may be found in the liver, kidney, spleen, and lymph nodes. Aborted fetuses may have pale, focal, necrotic lesions in all tissues, which are especially visible in the liver.

Diagnosis: Uncomplicated BHV-1 infections can be diagnosed based on the characteristic signs and lesions. However, because the severity of disease can vary, it is best to differentiate BHV-1 from other viral infections by viral isolation. Samples should be taken early in the disease, and a diagnosis should be possible in 2-3 days. A rise in serum antibody titer also can be used to confirm a diagnosis. It is not possible to detect a rising antibody titer in abortions, because infection generally occurs a considerable length of time before the abortion, and titers are already maximal. BHV-1 abortion can be diagnosed by identifying characteristic lesions and demonstrating the virus in fetal tissues by virus isolation, immunoperoxidase, or fluorescent antibody staining. Gross and microscopic lesions detected shortly after death may help to establish a diagnosis.

Treatment and Control: Antimicrobial therapy is indicated to prevent or treat secondary bacterial pneumonia. General recommendations for control are discussed under SHIPPING FEVER PNEUMONIA (p 1190). Immunization with modified live or inactivated virus vaccines generally provides adequate protection against clinical disease. Both IM and intranasal modified live vaccines are available, but the IM types may cause abortion in pregnant cattle. The intranasal vaccines can be used in pregnant cattle. The IM vaccines are easier to use and often are the vaccines of choice in feedlots. Breeding and replacement heifers and bulls should be immunized when 6-8 mo old, before breeding, and yearly thereafter. Some recommend that young bulls not be vaccinated because they may be discriminated against when sold for breeding if they have antibody titers. Feeder calves should be immunized 2-3 wk before entry into the feedlot. Eradication of the virus is possible by serologic testing and either culling reactors or running a strict 2-herd system. To aid in eradication, deletion mutant vaccines have been developed that permit discrimination between antibody produced in response to the vaccine and antibody produced in response to natural exposure.

Bovine Viral Diarrhea Virus

Bovine viral diarrhea virus (BVDV) is an RNA virus classified as a Pestivirus in the family Flaviviridae (p 220). The role of BVDV in BRD has been controversial, but appears to be that of a virus capable of inducing immunosuppression, which allows for the development of secondary bacterial pneumonia. Seroconversion to BVDV has been reported to be predictive of the occurrence of respiratory disease in feedlot calves, and BVDV has been reported to be the virus most frequently associated with multiple viral infections of the respiratory tract of calves.

Treatment for BVDV infection is supportive and includes antimicrobials to prevent or treat bacterial pneumonia. General principles of control are discussed under ENZOOTIC PNEUMONIA OF CALVES AND SHIPPING FEVER PNEUMONIA (p 1190). Inactivated and modified live vaccines are available for IM administration. Recently, vaccines containing both the type I and type II genotypes have become available. Modified live vaccines can induce immunosuppression and should be used with caution in highly stressed cattle. Modified live BVDV vaccines are not approved for use in pregnant cattle.

Other Bovine Respiratory Viruses

Several other viruses may potentially be involved in BRD. Bovine herpesvirus-4 has been implicated in several diseases, including BRD. Bovine adenovirus has been associated with a wide spectrum of diseases, with bovine adenovirus type 3 being the serotype most often associated with BRD. Two serotypes of bovine rhinovirus have been recognized to cause respiratory tract infections in cattle. Other viruses reported to be associated with BRD include bovine reovirus, enterovirus, and coronavirus. There is growing evidence that bovine coronavirus may have a more important role in BRD than previously recognized.

These viruses have a role similar to the other viruses previously discussed in that, in combination with other stressors, they can serve as initiators of bacterial pneumonia. Vaccines are not available for prevention of these viral respiratory diseases.

BACTERIAL PNEUMONIA

Pneumonic Pasteurellosis

Etiology: *Mannheimia haemolytica*, serotype 1 is the bacterium most frequently isolated from the lungs of cattle with BRD. Although less frequently cultured, *Pasteurella multocida* is also an important cuase of bacterial pneumonia. *Histophilus somni* is being increasingly recognized as an important pathogen in BRD; these bacteria are normal inhabitants of the nasopharynx of cattle (p 606). When pulmonary abscessation occurs, generally in association with chronic pneumonia, *Arcanobacterium pyogenes* is frequently isolated.

Under normal conditions, *M haemolytica* remains confined to the upper respiratory tract, in particular the tonsillar crypts, and is difficult to culture from healthy cattle. After stress or viral infection, the replication rate of *M haemolytica* in the upper respiratory tract increases rapidly, as does the likelihood of culturing the bacterium. The increased bacterial growth rate in the upper respiratory tract followed by inhalation and colonization of the lungs may occur due to suppression of the host's defense mechanism related to environmental stressors or viral infections. It is during this log phase of growth of the organism in the lungs that virulence factors are elaborated by *M haemolytica*, such as an exotoxin that has been referred to as leukotoxin. The interaction between the virulence factors of the bacteria and host defenses results in tissue damage with characteristic necrosis, thrombosis, and exudation and the development of pneumonia. The pathogenesis of pneumonia caused by *P multocida* is poorly understood. This organism may opportunistically colonize lungs with chronically damaged respiratory defenses, such as occurs with enzootic calf pneumonia or existing lung lesions of feedlot cattle, and cause a purulent bronchopneumonia. *H somni* may invade the lung and cause pneumonia following damage to the respiratory defenses. This organism is capable of systemic spread from the lung to the brain, myocardium, synovium, and pleural and pericardial surfaces; often death can occur later in the feeding period from involvement of these additional organ systems.

Clinical Findings: Clinical signs of bacterial pneumonia are often preceded by signs of viral infection of the respiratory tract. With the onset of bacterial pneumonia, clinical signs increase in severity and are characterized by depression and toxemia. Fever (104-106°F [40-41°C]); serous to mucopurulent nasal discharge; moist cough; and a rapid, shallow respiratory rate may be noted. Auscultation of the cranioventral lung field reveals increased bronchial sounds, crackles, and wheezes. In severe cases, pleurisy may develop, characterized by an irregular breathing pattern and grunting on expiration. The animal will become unthrifty in appearance if the pneumonia becomes chronic, which is usually associated with the formation of pulmonary abscesses.

Lesions: *M haemolytica* causes a severe, acute, hemorrhagic fibrinonecrotic pneumonia. The pneumonia has a bronchopneumonic pattern. Grossly, there are extensive reddish black to grayish brown cranioventral regions of consolidation with gelatinous thickening of interlobular septa and fibrinous pleuritis. There are extensive thromboses, foci of lung necrosis, and limited evidence of bronchitis and bronchiolitis.

P multocida is associated with a less fulminating fibrinous to fibrinopurulent bronchopneumonia. In contrast to *M haemolytica*, *P multocida* is associated with only small amounts of fibrin exudation, some thromboses, limited lung necrosis, and suppurative bronchitis and bronchiolitis.

H somnus infection of the lungs results in purulent bronchopneumonia that may be followed by septicemia and infection of multiple organs. Occasionally, *H somni* is associated with extensive pleuritis.

Pulmonary abscessation can occur as the pneumonia becomes chronic. Abscesses develop in ~3 wk but do not become encapsulated until 4 wk. *Arcanobacterium pyogenes* is frequently cultured from these abscesses.

Diagnosis: Generally, neither serologic testing nor direct bacterial detection are performed, and diagnosis relies on bacterial culture. Because the bacteria involved are normal inhabitants of the upper respiratory tract, the specificity of culture can be increased by collecting antemortem specimens from the lower respiratory tract by tracheal swab, transtracheal wash, or bronchoalveolar lavage. Lung specimens can be collected for culture at postmortem. If possible, specimens for culture should be collected from animals that have not been treated with antibiotics to permit determination of antimicrobial sensitivity patterns.

Treatment: Early recognition by trained personnel skilled at detecting the early symptoms of disease and treatment with antibiotics are essential for successful therapy. Antibiotics effective against the 3 gram-negative bacteria most often involved in BRD should be selected. Responses to treatment should be monitored and periodic culture and sensitivity should be performed to aid in the selection of antibiotics. Long-acting antibiotics have been specifically developed for treating bacterial pneumonia in cattle. It is important that antibiotic therapy extend beyond apparent recovery to avoid relapses. Mass medication in feed or water is of limited value because sick animals do not eat or drink enough to achieve inhibitory blood levels of the antibiotic, and many of these oral antibiotics are poorly absorbed in ruminants. NSAID have been shown to be a beneficial ancillary therapy in treating bacterial pneumonia. If pulmonary abscessation has occurred, it is difficult to achieve resolution with antimicrobials and culling of the animal should be considered.

Control: General principles of control are discussed under ENZOOTIC PNEUMONIA OF CALVES AND SHIPPING FEVER PNEUMONIA (p 1190). The value of *M haemolytica* and *P multo-*

cida bacterins is questionable, and some reports indicate they may even exacerbate the disease. Newer vaccines, which include live culture and subunit vaccines (leukotoxin), show much more promise for disease prevention. Vaccination should be done 3 wk before transport to the feedlot and can be repeated on arrival. In dairy calves, vaccination of the dam may be of benefit by providing passive immunity to the calf. *H somni* bacterins are available, and there is some evidence that they are effective in control of BRD.

Mycoplasmal Pneumonia

The exact role of mycoplasmas and ureaplasmas in BRD requires better definition. Mycoplasmas can be recovered from the respiratory tract of nonpneumonic calves, but the frequency of isolation is greater in those with respiratory tract disease. Mycoplasmas commonly recovered from the lungs of pneumonic calves include *Mycoplasma dispar*, *M bovis*, and *Ureaplasma* spp. *M bovis* has been associated with otitis media in young calves and polyarthritis in feedlot cattle. Experimental infections usually result in inapparent to mild signs of respiratory disease. This does not preclude a synergistic role for mycoplasmas in conjunction with viruses and bacteria in BRD. Lesions include focal pulmonary abscessation and necrosis with histologic lesions of peribronchial and peribronchiolar lymphoid cuffing and alveolitis. Culture of these organisms requires special media and conditions; growth of the organisms may take up to a week. Mycoplasmas are sensitive to several antibiotics, including the tetracyclines and macrolides.

Chlamydial Pneumonia

Chlamydial agents have been implicated in a number of diseases of cattle, including pneumonia. Only mild clinical signs and lesions of bronchopneumonia have been produced by experimental infections. A synergism between *Chlamydia* and *Mannheimia haemolytica* has been demonstrated experimentally. Because this pathogen is infrequently tested for, its overall importance remains undetermined. The organism can be tested for by staining sections of lung lesions with Gimenez stain or by fluorescent antibody. Isolation requires inoculation of yolk sacs of embryonating chicks. Chlamydial agents are sensitive to tetracyclines. (*See also* p 1177.)

CONTAGIOUS BOVINE PLEUROPNEUMONIA

This highly contagious pneumonia is generally accompanied by pleurisy. It is present in Africa, the Iberian peninsula, and parts of India and China; minor outbreaks occur in the Middle East. The USA has been free of the disease since 1892, the UK since 1898, and Australia since 1973.

Etiology: The causal organism is *Mycoplasma mycoides mycoides* small colony type. (*See also* CONTAGIOUS CAPRINE PLEUROPNEUMONIA, p 1231.) Susceptible cattle become infected by inhaling droplets disseminated by coughing in affected cattle. Goats and sheep are not important in the epidemiology. Septicemia produces lesions in the kidneys and placenta, which can be sources of infection. Transplacental infection of the fetus can occur. Viability of the organism in the environment is poor. The incubation period varies, but most cases occur 3-8 wk after exposure. In some localities, susceptible herds may show up to 100% morbidity, but much lower infection rates (~10%) associated with clinical signs are more common. Mortality is likely to be ~50%. Of recovered animals, 25% may become carriers with chronic lung lesions in the form of sequestra of variable size. Because carriers may not be detectable clinically or serologically, they constitute a serious problem in control programs. Breed susceptibility, management systems, and general health of the animal are important factors that influence the infection.

Clinical Findings: In acute cases, signs include fever up to 107°F (41.5°C), anorexia, and painful, difficult breathing. In hot climates, the animal often stands by itself in the shade, its head lowered and extended, its back slightly arched, and its elbows turned out. Percussion of the chest is painful; respiration is rapid, shallow, and abdominal. If the animal is forced to move quickly, the breathing becomes more distressed and a soft, moist cough may result. The disease progresses rapidly, animals lose condition, and breathing becomes very labored, with a grunt at expiration. The animal becomes recumbent and dies after 1-3 wk. Chronically affected cattle usually exhibit signs of varying intensity for 3-4 wk, after which the lesions gradually resolve and the animals appear to recover. Subclinical cases occur and may be important as carriers.

Lesions: The thoracic cavity may contain up to 10 L of clear yellow or turbid fluid mixed with fibrin flakes, and the organs in the thorax are often covered by thick deposits of fibrin. Varying amounts of one or both lungs may be involved, the affected portion being enlarged and solid. On section of the lung, the typical marbled appearance of pleuropneumonia is evident due to the widened interlobular septa and subpleural tissue that encloses gray, yellow, or red consolidated lung lobules. Microscopically, this is a severe, acute, fibrinous pneumonia with fibrinous pleurisy, thrombosis of pulmonary blood vessels, and areas of necrosis of lung tissue; the interstitial tissue is markedly thickened by edema fluid containing much fibrin. In chronic cases, the lesion has a necrotic center sequestered in a thick, fibrous capsule, and there may be fibrous pleural adhesions. Organisms may survive in these sequestra, and the animals become carriers.

Diagnosis: Diagnosis is based on clinical signs, complement fixation test, and necropsy. Confirmation is by histopathology, detection of organisms in pleural fluid using darkfield microscopy, isolation of the organism from lung or pleural fluid, or demonstration of specific antigens in lung tissue by immunodiffusion or immunofluorescence and hyperimmune antigalactan serum. Subclinical disease is detected by complement fixation test. As soon as an outbreak is suspected, slaughter and necropsy of presumptively infected cattle is advisable.

Control: The disease is reportable by law in many countries from which it has been eradicated by slaughter of all infected and exposed animals. In countries where cattle movement can readily be restricted, the disease can be eradicated by quarantine, blood testing, and immunization with attenuated vaccine (eg, T1/44 strain). Where cattle cannot be confined, the spread of infection can be limited by vaccination. Tracing the source of infected cattle detected at abattoirs, blood testing, and imposition of strict rules for cattle movement also can aid in control of the disease in such areas.

Treatment is recommended only in endemic areas because the organisms may not be eliminated, and carriers may develop. Tylosin (10 mg/kg, IM, BID for 6 injections) is reported to be effective.

INTERSTITIAL PNEUMONIA

This classification represents a group of respiratory diseases that are characterized by an acute onset of respiratory distress and a combination of lung lesions that include pulmonary edema and congestion, interstitial emphysema, alveolar epithelialization, and hyaline membrane formation.

Lungworm infection in cattle can also result in an atypical interstitial pneumonia (p 1181).

ACUTE BOVINE PULMONARY EMPHYSEMA AND EDEMA
(Fog fever, Bovine atypical interstitial pneumonia)

Acute bovine pulmonary emphysema and edema (ABPEE) is one of the more common causes of acute respiratory distress in cattle, particularly adult beef cattle, and is characterized by sudden onset, minimal coughing, and a course that ends fatally or improves dramatically within a few days. It is a disease involving groups of cattle; morbidity may be >50%, although usually only a small minority develops severe respiratory distress. Typically, ABPEE occurs in fall, 5-10 days after change to a better, often lush, pasture. A similar condition has been reported on a wide variety of grasses, alfalfa, rape, kale, and turnip tops.

Etiology: Metabolites of the naturally occurring amino acid L-tryptophan probably are responsible for many outbreaks. In the rumen, L-tryptophan is degraded to indoleacetic acid, which can be converted to 3-methylindole by some ruminal microorganisms.

3-methylindole is absorbed into the bloodstream and is the source of the pneumotoxicity after metabolism by the mixed function oxidase system, which is very active in the lungs. Apparently, the level of L-tryptophan in crops is most likely to be high in lush, rapidly growing pastures, particularly (but not exclusively) in the fall.

Clinical Findings: ABPEE is most common in heavy beef cows but may occur in either sex and in dairy or beef cattle under similar management conditions. Nursing calves are unaffected. Outbreaks usually develop within 5-10 days of a change to better grazing and rarely occur in animals that have been on a field >3 wk.

Mild cases may go unnoticed. Cattle are subdued but still alert; there is tachypnea and hyperpnea, but auscultation is usually unrewarding. Such cattle usually recover spontaneously within days. Severely affected cattle show extensive respiratory distress with mouth breathing, extension of the tongue, and drooling. A loud expiratory grunt is common, but coughing is unusual. In the early stages, auscultation reveals surprisingly soft respiratory sounds. Mild exercise increases dyspnea and may precipitate death. If death does not occur, the animals improve dramatically and resume eating by the third day. At this stage, auscultation reveals harsh respiratory sounds and, in some animals, dorsal (emphysematous) crackles. Some cattle have subcutaneous emphysema extending along the back from the withers. Full clinical recovery may require 3 wk.

Lesions: In affected cattle that have died or been slaughtered in extremis, the lungs are heavy and do not collapse normally. They are widely affected with various degrees of firmness; there is extensive edema and emphysema, often with the formation of large air-filled bullae in interlobular and subpleural regions. Submucosal hemorrhages are often present on the larynx and in the trachea and larger bronchi. Histologically, the lesion is characterized by congestion, alveolar edema, hyaline membrane formation, and areas of early alveolar epithelial hyperplasia of type II pneumocytes; occasionally, areas of bronchiolar necrosis may be found. The emphysema is often dramatic and is limited to interstitial fascia where it is accompanied by edema.

In animals that are slaughtered after 3 days of illness, the lungs are still heavy and do not collapse normally. They are pinkish gray and of increased firmness; edema and emphysema are inconspicuous or absent. Histologically, widespread alveolar epithelial hyperplasia characteristic of a diffuse, acute, proliferative alveolitis is seen.

Diagnosis: Diagnosis is based on history, signs, and lesions. Because the syndrome is not specific with regard to cause, evidence must be obtained from management factors such as change in pasture.

Treatment: Severely affected animals have so little pulmonary reserve that any driving or handling must be done with caution to prevent immediate deaths. Removal of cattle from the offending pastures may not prevent the development of new cases for the next 4-7 days. No treatment has been identified that will reverse the fully developed lesions of ABPEE.

Control: One approach to control is dietary management, including the following options: 1) avoiding pastures likely to induce ABPEE, 2) feeding hay before turn out on pasture and limiting exposure time on suspect pastures, 3) limiting grazing time and gradually increasing exposure to the pasture over time, 4) using pastures before they become lush, 5) delaying use of lush pastures until after a hard frost, 6) initially grazing pastures with less susceptible stock (cattle <15 mo of age or sheep), or 7) using strip grazing.

A medical approach to control involves feeding monensin or lasalocid, which inhibit the bacteria that convert L-tryptophan to 3-methylindole. Treatment with monensin can be started 1 day before introduction to pasture, whereas lasalocid requires a 6-day pretreatment period. These drugs are of no benefit after onset of clinical signs.

ANAPHYLAXIS

Anaphylaxis or Type I hypersensitivity reactions in cattle can result in an atypical interstitial pneumonia. The lung is a major target organ in cattle for Type I hypersensitivity. Clinical signs are those of acute respiratory distress. Cattle that die of anaphylaxis may have lesions consistent with those described for atypical interstitial pneumonia. Treatment is the administration of epinephrine; supportive treatment includes anti-inflammatory therapy with corticosteroids or NSAID. If pharyngeal or laryngeal edema is present, a tracheostomy may be indicated.

HYPERSENSITIVITY PNEUMONITIS
(Extrinsic allergic alveolitis, Farmer's lung disease)

A condition that appears to be similar to farmer's lung disease in humans occurs in both acute and chronic forms in adult cattle. The human and bovine forms of the disease may coexist on problem farms due to common exposure to dust from moldy hay.

Etiology: The disease occurs when sensitized individuals inhale antigens from thermophilic actinomycetes, commonly the spores of *Micropolyspora faeni*. The actinomycetes proliferate in vast numbers in hay, grain, or other vegetable material that has overheated to ~150°F (65°C) after damp storage (30-40% moisture content). Dust that contains large numbers of spores is released when this moldy hay is shaken. The small size (1 μm) of the spores allows them to reach the smallest airways and alveoli to provoke a reaction that has been termed a "hypersensitivity pneumonitis"; this is considered to be predominantly a Type III hypersensitivity reaction, although a Type IV hypersensitivity component is suspected (*see* IMMUNOPATHOLOGIC DISEASES, p 648 et seq).

Affected herds exist in areas where significant rainfall usually occurs during the haymaking season, suggesting that a clinical problem may arise only after repeated sensitization and challenge from the spores. Clinical disease tends to arise during the latter half of the winter feeding period and usually only when moldy hay is fed indoors. Under such circumstances, serum antibodies (usually detected by immunodiffusion) to *M faeni* are widespread among adult cattle by the end of each winter feeding period, and many apparently normal cattle are seropositive. By contrast, few adult cattle are seropositive on other farms on which "good" hay or grass silage is fed.

Clinical Findings: Cattle may succumb to the acute form of the disease over a period of weeks. Usually, only severe acute cases are noticed. There is respiratory distress, anorexia, and agalactia in animals ≥5 yr old; coughing and pyrexia also occur, and adventitious sounds are occasionally heard on auscultation. Death is rare.

The chronic disease usually has a higher morbidity; in most instances, the signs are weight loss, poor production, and persistent coughing. Affected cattle are fairly bright and eat reasonably well, but tachypnea, hyperpnea, and coughing are widespread. Auscultation may reveal cranioventral crackles and sometimes, in more severe cases, scattered rhonchi. Exercise intolerance may be seen, and congestive cardiac failure can develop if pulmonary fibrosis is widespread.

Lesions: The macroscopic lesions are often unremarkable; usually, there is mild peripheral lobular overinflation with diffusely scattered, small, gray, subpleural spots. Although transient pulmonary edema may be a feature of severe acute cases, the histologic lesions that are consistently found are interalveolar cellular infiltration, epithelioid granulomata, and bronchiolitis obliterans. In some chronic cases, small foci of alveolar epithelial hyperplasia and metaplasia with interstitial fibrosis are found. These areas may extend to include most, if not all, of the lung substance to produce cases clinically indistinguishable from diffuse fibrosing alveolitis (*see* below). Circumstantial evidence suggests that some cases of diffuse fibrosing alveolitis are the end stage of hypersensitivity pneumonitis.

Treatment and Control: Because it is often impossible to completely shield cattle from further challenge, most recover only partially after dexamethasone treatment (1 mg/5-10 kg body wt). However, improvement is usually marked when cattle are turned out in the spring. Prevention is difficult in areas where hay is likely to be wet during the curing process and it is not possible to alter the feeding regimen.

DIFFUSE FIBROSING ALVEOLITIS
Diffuse fibrosing alveolitis is a chronic, progressive respiratory disease of undetermined cause and possibly of multiple etiologies. A proportion of affected cattle are seropositive for

precipitating antibodies to *Micropolyspora faeni*, and this condition may represent the end stage of hypersensitivity pneumonitis. Other than the respiratory signs, the animals appear alert and maintain a good appetite until the onset of heart failure in the terminal stages. Signs include coughing, increased respiratory rate, dyspnea, and weight loss. Necropsy findings include right ventricular hypertrophy, interalveolar fibrosis, obliteration of the alveolar spaces, alveolar hyperplasia, bronchitis, and bronchiolitis. There is no treatment.

ACUTE RESPIRATORY DISTRESS SYNDROME OF FEEDLOT CATTLE

An acute respiratory distress syndrome has been described in feedlot cattle with clinical signs and pathologic findings of an atypical interstitial pneumonia. The syndrome occurs sporadically and the etiology remains undefined. Bovine respiratory syncytial virus, abnormal production of 3-methylindole in the rumen, dusty conditions, and pre-existing lesions of chronic cranioventral bacterial pneumonia have been suggested as causes or contributing factors. Clinical signs include respiratory distress characterized by tachypnea and dyspnea, and affected cattle may be found dead if clinical signs are unobserved. Lesions are those of atypical interstitial pneumonia with prominent emphysema and edema in the lungs. Treatment protocols have not been defined, and thus would be symptomatic and supportive. Management strategies suggested include vaccinating for bovine respiratory syncytial virus, controlling dust in the feedlot, and avoiding abrupt dietary changes.

4-IPOMEANOL TOXICITY (MOLDY SWEET POTATO) AND PERILLA KETONE TOXICITY (PURPLE MINT TOXICITY)

Clinicopathologic syndromes indistinguishable from acute bovine pulmonary emphysema and edema (ABPEE, p 1198) occur after ingestion of either moldy sweet potatoes infested with *Fusarium solani*, or the wild mint *Perilla frutescens*. Moldy sweet potato toxicity is caused by the ingestion of a furanoterpenoid toxin produced by sweet potatoes (*Ipomoea batatus*) in response to infestation with the fungus *F solani*; the end result is production of the pneumotoxin 4-ipomeanol. Perilla ketone toxicity is caused by ingestion of the leaves and seeds of the plant *P frutescens* (purple mint), which contains a pneumotoxin and is found in the southeastern USA. The pathogeneses of both these conditions are similar to that of ABPEE, as is approach to treatment.

TOXIC GASES

Nitrogen dioxide is a major component of silo gas; in humans, the disease associated with exposure to NO_2 is termed silo filler's disease. Exposure of cattle results in respiratory distress and necropsy findings of atypical interstitial pneumonia. Treatment is empirical and includes diuretics, corticosteroids, and antibiotics to prevent pneumonia.

Zinc oxide is produced during oxyacetylene cutting or arc welding of galvanized pipes. These activities in closed facilities in which cattle are housed may result in toxicity characterized by respiratory distress. Lesions are similar to those described for atypical interstitial pneumonia. Treatment is as described for nitrogen dioxide toxicity.

VENA CAVAL THROMBOSIS AND METASTATIC PNEUMONIA

Etiology: Vena caval thrombosis and metastatic pneumonia is associated with multifocal abscesses in the lung as the result of septic embolism of the pulmonary arterial vascular system arising from septic thrombi in the caudal vena cava. The most common etiology of vena caval thrombosis is ruminal acidosis leading to rumenitis and subsequent liver abscessation, which may result in a thrombus in the candal vena cava if the vessel wall is infiltrated by the abscess. Bacteria most frequently involved include *Fusobacterium necrophorum*, *Arcanobacterium pyogenes*, staphylococci, streptococci, and *Escherichia coli*.

Clinical Findings: The condition usually occurs in adult cattle. Presenting signs can be acute, manifested by respiratory distress, or chronic, manifested by weight loss and chronic coughing. A common presentation is tachypnea, tachycardia, hemic murmurs, coughing, pale mucous membranes, increased lung sounds, hemoptysis, and epistaxis. Pyrexia and melena may also be present. The case fatality rate is essentially 100%.

Lesions: A thrombus will be present in the vena cava and hepatic abscesses may also be noted. Areas of suppurative pneumonia, pulmonary abscesses, aneurysms, and blood clots from ruptured aneurysms may be present in the lung.

Treatment and Control: Because of the poor prognosis, treatment is not indicated. If treatment is attempted, it includes antibiotics and supportive therapy. Control efforts should focus on reduction of the incidence of ruminal acidosis, which can result in rumenitis and subsequent formation of liver abscesses.

RESPIRATORY DISEASES OF HORSES

Viral respiratory infections are common in horses, and the most notable viral pathogens are equine herpesvirus type 4 (EHV-4, rhinopneumonitis), equine influenza, and equine viral arteritis. The clinical manifestations are similar and include pyrexia, serous nasal discharge, submandibular lymphadenopathy, anorexia, and cough. In addition to respiratory disease, equine herpesvirus type 1 (EHV-1) can cause abortion and neurologic disease. Equine viral arteritis produces respiratory disease, vasculitis, and abortion. Equine herpesvirus type 2, equine rhinitis virus, and reovirus are ubiquitous viral respiratory pathogens, and infection results in minimal clinical disease. Adenovirus pneumonia is most often observed in association with severe combined immunodeficiency in Arabian foals. Hendra virus (p 564) is a newly recognized, zoonotic disease of horses identified in Australia. The disease is rapidly fatal in horses, and close contact is necessary for disease transmission.

Secondary bacterial respiratory infections (with the exception of strangles) are primarily initiated by viral disease, because viral respiratory infections impair and/or destroy respiratory defense mechanisms (ie, influenza destroys the mucociliary apparatus, EHV destroys bronchial-associated lymphoid tissue). The most common organisms associated with pneumonia in horses are opportunistic bacteria originating from the resident microflora of the upper respiratory tract. Clinical evidence of a secondary bacterial infection includes mucopurulent nasal discharge, depression, persistent fever, abnormal lung sounds, hyperfibrinogenemia, and leukocytosis. Secondary bacterial disease may result in mucosal bacterial infections (rhinitis and tracheitis), or may produce more serious invasive disease such as pneumonia and pleuropneumonia. *Streptococcus equi zooepidemicus* is the most common opportunistic pathogen of the equine lung, although *Actinobacillus equuli, Bordetella bronchiseptica, Escherichia coli, Pasteurella* spp, and *Pseudomonas aeruginosa* are frequently isolated. *S equi equi*, the causative agent of strangles (p 1212), is a primary bacterial pathogen of the upper respiratory tract and is capable of mucosal invasion without predisposing factors. *Rhodococcus equi* is a primary pathogen of the lower respiratory tract of foals <5 mo of age, which produces pulmonary consolidation and abscessation. *R equi* pneumonia is not reported in adult horses with a functional immune system.

Noninfectious respiratory disease is a common, performance-limiting condition that affects adult horses of various ages. **Inflammatory airway disease** is characterized by excessive tracheal mucus, airway hyperreactivity, and poor exercise performance in young horses. The etiology is unclear, but viral respiratory infection, allergy, and environmental factors may play a role in the pathophysiology. **Reactive airway disease (heaves)** is triggered by exposure to organic dusts in older horses with a genetic predisposition to allergic airway disease. Small airways are obstructed by bronchoconstriction and excessive mucus production. The severity of clinical signs ranges from exercise intolerance to dyspnea at rest.

The respiratory system is one of the most accessible body systems for diagnostic testing. Endoscopic examination allows direct visualization of the upper respiratory tract, guttural pouches, trachea, and mainstem bronchi. Indications for endoscopic examination include upper airway noise, inspiratory difficulty, poor exercise performance, and unilateral or bilateral nasal discharge. Radiographs of the skull are indicated to investigate facial deformity, abnormalities of the sinus (sinusitis, dental abnormalities, and sinus cyst), guttural pouch (empyema, tympany), and soft tissue structures (epiglottis, soft palate). The most important techniques for evaluation of lower respiratory tract secretions are transtracheal wash and bronchoalveolar lavage. Transtracheal wash is indicated to obtain secretions for bacterial and fungal culture of the lower respiratory tract. Bronchoalveolar lavage is indicated for cytologic evaluation of the lower respiratory tract in animals with diffuse, noninfectious pulmonary disease. Nasal swab culture or testing for influenza by culture or ELISA is inappropriate for investigation of pulmonary infectious disease, but is indicated for horses with suspected strangles infection. Thoracic radiography and ultrasound are useful to assess the lower respiratory tract. Thoracic radiography is used to identify abnormalities of the pulmonary parenchyma, mediastinum, and diaphragm. Pulmonary consolidation (pneumonia), peribronchial disease, pulmonary abscessation, interstitial disease, and mediastinal masses (neoplasia, abscess, granuloma) are most easily identified via thoracic radiography. Thoracic ultrasound is the most appropriate technique to evaluate fluid in the pleural space, peripheral pulmonary consolidation, and peripheral pulmonary abscessation. Ultrasonographic examination can identify the volume, location, and character of pleural fluid or air within the pleural space (pneumothorax). Additionally, ultrasound can identify fibrin tags, gas echoes (anaerobic infection), masses, and loculated fluid pockets and allows the clinician to determine the most appropriate site for centesis and to formulate a prognosis. Pleurocentesis is performed in animals with accumulation of fluid in the pleural space and should be conducted with ultrasound guidance. Lung biopsy and fine needle aspirate are invasive procedures and are performed only after other diagnostic procedures have been exhausted. Pulmonary neoplasia, pulmonary fibrosis, and interstitial diseases may require lung biopsy to obtain a definitive diagnosis.

Vaccination does not always prevent respiratory infections in horses, but duration and severity is usually lessened in horses with regular vaccination depending on factors such as the disease and specific vaccine. Vaccines of variable or unknown effectiveness are available for equine influenza, viral rhinopneumonitis, equine viral arteritis, and strangles. The cost and hazards of each vaccination must be weighed against the probability of exposure and potential disease. Vaccination recommendations and schedules will vary according to the use of the horse and its potential for exposure to contagious animals.

Regardless of the type of respiratory disease, environmental factors and supportive care are important to aid recovery. A dust- and ammonia-free stable environment prevents further damage to the mucociliary apparatus. Highly palatable feeds are indicated to prevent weight loss and debilitation during the treatment and recovery period. Adequate hydration will decrease the viscosity of respiratory secretions, facilitating their removal from the lower respiratory tract. A comfortable, dry, temperature-appropriate environment will allow the horse to rest and will minimize the role of the respiratory tract in thermoregulation.

EQUINE HERPESVIRUS INFECTION
(Equine viral rhinopneumonitis, Equine abortion virus)

Etiology and Epidemiology: Equine herpesvirus 1 (EHV-1) and EHV-4 comprise 2 antigenically distinct groups of viruses previously referred to as subtypes 1 and 2 of EHV-1. Both viruses are ubiquitous in horse populations worldwide and produce an acute febrile respiratory disease upon primary infection, characterized by rhinopharyngitis and tracheobronchitis. Outbreaks of respiratory disease occur annually among foals in areas with concentrated horse populations. Most of these outbreaks in weanlings are caused by strains of EHV-4. The age, seasonal, and geographic distributions vary and are determined by immune status and horse population. In individual horses, the outcome of exposure is determined by viral strain, immune status, pregnancy status, and possibly age. Infection of pregnant mares with EHV-4 rarely results in abortion.

Mares may abort several wk to mo after clinical or subclinical infection with EHV-1. An infrequent clinical sequela of EHV-1 infection is development of neurologic disease. The natural reservoir of both EHV-1 and EHV-4 is the horse. Latent infections and carrier states occur with both virus types. Transmission occurs by direct or indirect contact with infectious nasal secretions, aborted fetuses, placentas, or placental fluids.

Clinical Findings: The incubation period of EHV is 2-10 days. Susceptible horses develop fever of 102-107°F (38.9-41.7°C), neutropenia and lymphopenia, serous nasal discharge, malaise, pharyngitis, cough, inappetence, and/or submandibular or retropharyngeal lymphadenopathy. Horses infected with EHV-1 strains often develop a diphasic fever, with cell-associated viremia coinciding with the second temperature peak. Secondary bacterial infections are common and manifest with mucopurulent nasal exudate and pulmonary disease. The infection is mild or inapparent in horses immunologically sensitized to the virus.

Mares that abort after EHV-1 infection seldom display premonitory signs. Abortions occur 2-12 wk after infection, usually between mo 7 and 11 of gestation. Aborted fetuses are fresh or minimally autolyzed, and the placenta is expelled shortly after abortion. There is no evidence of damage to the mare's reproductive tract, and subsequent conception is unimpaired. Mares exposed late in gestation may not abort, but give birth to live foals with fulminating viral pneumonitis. Such foals are susceptible to secondary bacterial infections and usually die within hours or days.

Outbreaks with specific strains of EHV-1 infection result in neurologic disease (see DISEASES OF THE SPINAL COLUMN AND CORD, p 1017). Clinical signs vary from mild incoordination and posterior paresis to severe posterior paralysis with recumbency, loss of bladder and tail function, and loss of sensation to the skin in the perineal and inguinal areas. In exceptional cases, the paralysis may progress to quadriplegia and death. Prognosis depends on severity of signs and the period of recumbency. Neurologic disease associated with EHV-1 is thought to occur more commonly in mares after abortion storms, but it has been reported in barren mares, stallions, geldings, and foals after an outbreak of EHV-1 respiratory infection.

Lesions: The pathogenetic mechanisms of EHV-1 and EHV-4 differ significantly. EHV-4 infection is restricted to respiratory tract epithelium and associated lymph nodes; EHV-1 strains have a predilection for vascular endothelium, especially the nasal mucosa, lungs, adrenal, thyroid, and CNS. EHV-1 gains access to peripheral tissues via cell-associated viremia, which may manifest as abortion or neurologic disease.

Gross lesions of viral rhinopneumonitis are hyperemia and ulceration of the respiratory epithelium, and multiple, tiny, plum-colored foci in the lungs. Histologically, there is evidence of inflammation, necrosis, and intranuclear inclusions in the respiratory epithelium and germinal centers of the associated lymph nodes. Lung lesions are characterized by neutrophilic infiltration of the terminal bronchioles, peribronchiolar and perivascular mononuclear cell infiltration, and serofibrinous exudate in the alveoli.

Typical lesions in EHV-1 abortion include interlobular lung edema and pleural fluid; multifocal areas of hepatic necrosis; petechiation of the myocardium, adrenal gland, and spleen; and thymic necrosis. Intranuclear inclusions are found in lung, liver, adrenal, and lymphoreticular tissues.

Horses with EHV-1-associated neurologic disease may have no gross lesions, or only minimal evidence of hemorrhage in the meninges, brain, and spinal cord parenchyma. Histologically, lesions are discrete and comprise vasculitis with endothelial cell damage and perivascular cuffing, thrombus formation and hemorrhage, and in advanced cases, areas of malacia. Lesions may occur at any level of the brain or spinal cord.

Diagnosis: Equine viral rhinopneumonitis cannot be clinically differentiated from equine influenza (p 1206), equine viral arteritis (p 560), or other equine respiratory infections solely on the basis of clinical signs. Definitive diagnosis is determined by virus isolation from samples obtained via nasopharyngeal swab and citrated blood sample (buffy coat) early in the course of the infection and by serologic testing of acute and convalescent sera.

In cases of suspected EHV-1 abortion, a diagnosis is based on characteristic gross and microscopic lesions in the aborted fetus, virus isolation, and demonstration of viral antigen in fetal tissues. Lung, liver, adrenal, and lymphoreticular tissues are productive sources of virus. Serologic testing of mares after abortion has little diagnostic value. Diagnosis of herpesvirus myeloencephalopathy depends on demonstration of characteristic vascular lesions in sections of CNS tissue of horses that die or are destroyed. Otherwise, the diagnosis is presumptively based on clinical signs and CSF analysis (xanthochromia, albuminocytologic dissociation).

Treatment: There is no specific treatment for EHV infection. Rest and nursing care are indicated to minimize secondary bacterial complications. Antipyretics are recommended for horses with a fever >104°F (40°C). Antibiotic therapy is instituted upon suspicion of secondary bacterial infection evidenced by purulent nasal discharge or pulmonary disease. Most foals infected prenatally with EHV-1 succumb shortly after birth despite intensive nursing and antimicrobial medication. If horses with EHV-1-associated neurologic disease remain ambulatory, or are recumbent for only 2-3 days, the prognosis is usually favorable. Intensive nursing care is necessary to avoid pulmonary congestion, pneumonia, ruptured bladder, or bowel atony. Recovery may be complete, but a small percentage of cases have neurologic sequelae.

Control: Immunity after natural infection with either EHV-1 or EHV-4 involves a combination of humoral and cellular immunity. While little cross-protection occurs between virus types after primary infection of immunologically naive foals, significant cross-protection develops in horses after repeated infections with a particular virus type. Most horses are latently infected with EHV-1 and EHV-4. The infection remains dormant for most of the horse's life, although stress or immunosuppression may result in recrudescence of disease and shedding of infectious virus. Immunity to reinfection of the respiratory tract may persist for up to 3 mo, but multiple infections result in a level of immunity that prevents clinical signs of respiratory disease. Diminished resistance in pregnant mares allows cell-associated viremia, which may result in transplacental infection of the fetus.

For prevention and control of EHV-4- and EHV-1-related diseases, management practices that reduce viral spread are recommended. New horses (or those returning from other premises) should be isolated for 3-4 wk before commingling with resident horses, especially pregnant mares. Management-related stress-inducing circumstances should be avoided to prevent recrudescence of latent virus. Pregnant mares should be maintained in a group away from the weanlings, yearlings, and horses out of training. In an outbreak of respiratory disease or abortion, affected horses should be isolated and appropriate measures taken for disinfection of contaminated premises. No horse should leave the premises for 3 wk after recovery of the last clinical case.

Parenterally administered modified live vaccines are licensed in some countries but banned in others. An inactivated vaccine is the only product currently recommended by the manufacturer as an aid in prevention of EHV-1 abortion. Vaccine should be administered during mo 3, 5, 7, and 9 of pregnancy. Humoral immunity induced by vaccination against EHV-1 and EHV-4 generally persists for only 2-4 mo. Antigenic variation within each virus type means that available vaccines do not cover all strains to which horses can be exposed. Vaccination should begin when foals are 3-4 mo old and, depending on the vaccine used, a second dose given 4-8 wk later. Booster vaccinations may be indicated as often as every 3-6 mo through maturity. Vaccination programs against EHV-1 should include all horses on the premises.

Infection by other Herpesviruses: Equine herpesvirus 2 (EHV-2) is ubiquitous in respiratory mucosa, conjunctiva, and WBC of normal horses of all ages. The pathogenic significance remains obscure. It has been suggested that EHV-2 is the cause of herpetic keratoconjunctivitis. Equine herpesvirus 3 (EHV-3) is the cause of equine coital exanthema (p 1119), a benign, progenital exanthematous disease.

EQUINE INFLUENZA

Etiology and Epidemiology: Equine influenza is highly contagious and spreads rapidly among susceptible horses. Two immunologically distinct influenza viruses have been found in horse populations worldwide except in Australia and New Zealand. Orthomyxovirus A/Equi-1 has not been isolated since 1980. Orthomyxovirus A/Equi-2 was first recognized in 1963 as a cause of widespread epidemics and has subsequently become endemic in many countries. Endemicity is maintained by sporadic clinical cases and by inapparent infection in susceptible horses that are introduced into the population by birth, through waning immunity, or after movement from other areas or countries. A carrier state is not recognized for equine influenza. The clinical outcome after viral exposure largely depends on immune status; clinical disease varies from a mild, inapparent infection to severe disease in susceptible animals. Influenza is rarely fatal except in donkeys, zebras, and debilitated horses. Transmission occurs by inhalation of respiratory secretions. Epidemics arise when one or more acutely infected horses are introduced into a susceptible group. The epidemiologic outcome depends on the antigenic characteristics of the circulating virus and the immune status of a given population of horses at time of exposure. Frequent natural exposure or regular vaccination may contribute to the degree of antigenic drift observed with specific strains of A/Equi-2 virus in some parts of the world.

Clinical Findings and Lesions: The incubation period of influenza is ~1-3 days. Clinical signs begin abruptly and include high fever (up to 106°F [41.1°C]), serous nasal discharge, submandibular lymphadenopathy, and coughing that is dry, harsh, and nonproductive. Depression, anorexia, and weakness are frequently observed. Clinical signs usually last <3 days in uncomplicated cases. Influenza virus replicates within respiratory epithelial cells, resulting in destruction of tracheal and bronchial epithelium and cilia. Cough develops early in the course of infection and may persist for several weeks. Nasal discharge, although scant and serous initially, may become mucopurulent due to secondary bacterial infection. Mildly affected horses recover uneventfully in 2-3 wk; severely affected horses may convalesce for up to 6 mo. Recovery may be hastened by complete restriction of strenuous physical activity. Respiratory tract epithelium takes ~21 days to regenerate; during this time, horses are susceptible to development of secondary bacterial complications such as pneumonia, pleuropneumonia, and chronic bronchitis. Complications are minimized by restricting exercise, controlling dust, providing superior ventilation, and practicing good stable hygiene. Primary complications of vasculitis, myositis, and myocarditis are observed infrequently.

Diagnosis: The presence of a rapidly spread respiratory infection in a group of horses characterized by rapid onset, high fever, depression, and cough is presumptive evidence of equine influenza. Definitive diagnosis can be determined by virus isolation, influenza A antigen detection, or paired serology (hemagglutination inhibition). Nasopharyngeal swabs are obtained for virus isolation and antigen detection. These samples should be obtained as soon as possible after the onset of illness. Virus isolation in chick embryos is highly specific, but less sensitive for detection of influenza due to bacterial contamination of the sample. Antigen detection is performed using a human influenza A kit, which provides immediate results that are not affected by bacterial contamination.

Treatment and Prevention: Horses that do not develop complications require rest and supportive care. Horses should be rested 1 wk for every day of fever with a minimum of 3 wk rest (to allow regeneration of the mucociliary apparatus). NSAID are recommended for horses with a fever of >104°F (40°C). Antibiotics are indicated when fever persists beyond 3-4 days or when purulent nasal discharge or pneumonia are present.

Prevention of influenza requires hygienic management practices and vaccination. Exposure can be reduced by isolation of newly introduced horses for 2 wk. Numerous vaccines are commercially available for prevention of equine influenza. An intranasal modified live influenza vaccine, designed to induce mucosal (local) antibody protection, has demonstrated protection against natural challenge. This vaccine is temperature sensitive and is not capable of replicating beyond the nasal passages. The majority of commercially available influenza vaccines are inactivated, adjuvanted vaccines recommended primarily for IM administration. Because the duration of protection provided by current vaccines is limited, booster injections probably should be administered often, eg, every 3-6 mo. Vaccine manufacturers monitor continuously to ensure influenza strain content reflects, as closely as possible, the antigenicity of current strains of field virus.

EQUINE VIRAL ARTERITIS

Equine viral arteritis (EVA) is caused by an RNA togavirus, and produces clinical signs of respiratory disease, vasculitis, and abortion. Horses with EVA infection present with fever, anorexia, and depression. The clinical signs of respiratory infection due to EVA are serous nasal discharge, cough, conjunctivitis, lacrimation, and palpebral and periorbital edema. Clinical signs of disease persist for 2-9 days. Treatment consists of supportive care (support bandages), and NSAID for fever and inflammation. Antimicrobial therapy is usually unnecessary. A carrier state occurs in some stallions following natural infection and is primarily responsible for persistence of the virus in the horse population. (*See* EQUINE VIRAL ARTERITIS, p 560.)

HENDRA VIRUS INFECTION
(Equine morbillivirus)

Hendra virus (HeV) is the prototype species of a new genus *Henipavirus* within the subfamily Paramyxovirinae. The viral agent is endemic in specific species of fruit bats (also called flying foxes), and close contact with these bats is suspected to have facilitated transfer of the HeV to horses. Horses are infected by oronasal routes and excrete HeV in urine, saliva, and respiratory secretions.

Epidemiology: There have been 3 reported incidents of equine disease. In one outbreak, 14 of 21 horses died. During this outbreak, 2 human caregivers developed influenza-like signs; one did not survive. A morbillivirus cultured from his kidney was identical to the virus isolated from lungs of 5 affected horses. All human cases have been reported in association with equine cases. Very close contact is required to transmit the virus among horses and from horses to humans, and the virus is not considered highly contagious. There was no serologic evidence of infection in 157 humans who had casual contact with infected humans and horses. Gray-headed fruit bats seroconvert and develop subclinical disease when inoculated with HeV; however, widespread subclinical disease or seroconversion is not recognized in horses. Infected horses develop severe and often fatal respiratory disease, characterized by dyspnea, vascular endothelial damage, and pulmonary edema. Depression, anorexia, fever, respiratory difficulty, ataxia, tachycardia, and frothy, nasal discharge are common clinical signs. *See* HENDRA VIRUS INFECTION, p 564.

PLEUROPNEUMONIA
(Pleuritis, Pleurisy)

Pleuropneumonia is defined as infection of the lungs and pleural space. In most instances, it develops secondary to bacterial pneumonia or penetrating thoracic wounds. Spontaneous pleuritis (without accompanying pneumonia) is uncommon in horses. In the USA, ~70% of horses with pleural effusion have pleuropneumonia. The primary differential diagnoses for pleural effusion are neoplastic effusions, heart failure, and hydatidosis.

Etiology and Pathogenesis: Viral respiratory infection, long-distance transportation, general anesthesia, and strenuous exercise are common predisposing factors that impair pulmonary defense mechanisms allowing secondary bacterial invasion. Race and sport horses are particularly at risk. The majority of horses with pleuropneumonia are athletic horses <5 yr of age. Exercise-induced pulmonary hemorrhage may contribute to development of respiratory infection by providing a favorable environment for bacterial replication.

Polymicrobial and mixed anaerobic-aerobic infections are common in horses with pleuropneumonia. The majority of horses with pleuropneumonia have more than one organism isolated from transtracheal aspirates. The most common aerobic organisms are *Streptococcus equizooepidemicus*, *Escherichia coli*, *Actinobacillus* spp, *Klebsiella* spp, *Enterobacter* spp, *Staphylococcus aureus*, and *Pasteurella* spp. Anaerobic bacteria are isolated from 40-70% of horses with pleuropneumonia, and *Bacteroides* spp, *Clostridium* spp, *Peptostreptococcus* spp, and *Fusobacterium* spp are the most common. The etiology of pleural infection in horses is usually bacterial, although *Mycoplasma felis* and nocardial agents have been isolated from pleural effusion.

Clinical Findings and Lesions: Horses with pleuropneumonia present with fever, depression, lethargy, and inappetence. Clinical signs specific to pleuropneumonia include pleural pain (pleurodynia) evident as short strides, guarding, and flinching on percussion of the chest; shallow respiration; and endotoxemia. Horses with pleural pain have an anxious facial expression, stand with their elbows abducted, and are reluctant to move, cough, or lie down. Gait may be stiff or stilted, and some horses will grunt in response to thoracic pressure, auscultation, or percussion. Nasal discharge is a variable sign. Putrid breath or fetid nasal discharge indicates anaerobic bacterial infection. In most cases, the respiratory pattern is characterized by rapid, shallow respiration due to pleural pain and restricted pulmonary expansion from pleural effusion. A plaque of sternal edema is observed in horses with a large volume of pleural effusion. Horses with toxemia have injected mucous membranes, delayed capillary refill time (>2 sec), and tachycardia. Auscultation reveals a lack of breath sounds in the ventral lung fields, and abnormal lung sounds (often crackles) in dorsal lung fields. Cardiac sounds may be muffled or absent, or may radiate over a wider area. Although uncommon, pleural friction rubs are most prominent at end-inspiration and early expiration, and are detected in horses with peracute disease (prior to development of effusion) or after thoracic drainage.

Diagnosis: In horses with peracute pleuropneumonia, laboratory findings reflect bacterial sepsis or toxemia, and include abnormalities such as leukopenia, neutropenia, left shift, hemoconcentration, and azotemia. Horses with more stable disease have leukocytosis, mature neutrophilia, hyperfibrinogenemia, hyperglobulinemia (chronic antigenic stimulation), hypoalbuminemia (loss in pleural space), and anemia of chronic disease.

Thoracic ultrasound is ideal for investigation of pleural effusion, and is indicated in horses with regions of poor to absent breath sound, thoracic pain, and/or dull thoracic percussion. Transudative pleural fluid (neoplastic effusion) appears anechoic, whereas more cellular exudate appears echogenic. Gas echoes represent small air bubbles within pleural fluid, which may indicate an anaerobic pleural infection, a bronchopleural fistula, or iatrogenic introduction of air. Pulmonary atelectasis, consolidation, and abscessation can be identified if the lesions are located in peripheral lung fields. Ultrasonographic evidence of a large area of pulmonary consolidation, in conjunction with serosanguineous suppurative pleural effusion, is consistent with pulmonary infarction and necrotizing pneumonia. Adhesions of the visceral to perietal pleura can be visualized using thoracic ultrasound, and these regions should be avoided during thoracocentesis.

Ultrasound examination should be performed prior to pleurocentesis to determine the best site for maximum drainage and to avoid cardiac or diaphragmatic puncture. Thoracocentesis is performed for diagnostic and therapeutic purposes in horses with pleuropneumonia. Pleural fluid should be drained relatively slowly to avoid hypotension. The hemithorax that appears to contain the most fluid is drained first. Bilateral thoracocentesis is usually necessary. The chest tube may be removed immediately after drainage of the thoracic cavity, or may be secured in place to allow continual drainage. Thoracic radiography is indicated after pleurocentesis to evaluate pulmonary parenchymal lesions, mediastinal structures, and the presence/severity of pneumothorax.

Gross examination of pleural fluid includes evaluation of color, odor, volume, and turbidity. Malodorous pleural fluid is associated with necrotic tissue and anaerobic infection, and indicates a guarded prognosis. Cytologic evaluation of septic pleural fluid reveals purulent exudate (>90% neutrophils) with increased cellularity (25,000-200,000 cells/μL) and increased total protein (>3.0 g/dL). Intracellular and extracellular bacteria may be observed, and Gram's stain examination is used to direct initial antimicrobial therapy. Bacterial culture and sensitivity should also be performed on transtracheal aspirate samples, which yield positive bacterial cultures more frequently than pleural fluid samples.

Treatment: Management of horses with pleuropneumonia includes daily ultrasound examination to monitor fluid production, evaluate effective drainage, identify isolated fluid pockets, and assess peripheral pulmonary disease. The volume and character of pleural fluid will determine whether single, intermittent, or continual drainage is indicated. Continual drainage is preferable in cases with fibrinous, cellular, malodorous, and/or large volume of effusion. A one-way (Heimlich) valve allows constant drainage of pleural fluid with minimal risk of development of pneumothorax. An indwelling chest tube should remain in place as long as drainage is productive. Medical therapy includes broad-spectrum antibiotics, NSAID, analgesics, and supportive care. Broad-spectrum antimicrobial therapy targeting common aerobic and anaerobic bacteria (eg, penicillin, gentamicin, metronidazole) should be instituted pending results of culture and sensitivity. Some horses do not clear the pleural infection over the course of weeks to months of antimicrobial therapy and drainage via indwelling chest tubes. Thoracostomy allows manual removal of organized fibrinous material and necrotic lung; however, this technique should be limited to horses with chronic, stable, unilateral disease with resolving infection in the contralateral hemithorax.

Complications associated with pleuropneumonia include thrombophlebitis, laminitis, bronchopleural fistula, pulmonary abscess, and cranial thoracic mass.

The prognosis for horses with pleuropneumonia has greatly improved over the past 20 yr due to early recognition, advancements in diagnostic testing, and aggressive therapy. The survival rate is reported to be as high as 90% by some investigators with a 60% chance to return to athletic performance. The duration of hospitalization is not indicative of outcome; however, a delay in initiation of appropriate therapy by more than 48 hr promotes development of anaerobic infection and, ultimately, poor response to treatment. Placement of an indwelling chest tube does not limit the prognosis for return to athletic function. Horses with hemorrhagic necrotizing pneumonia respond poorly to conventional therapy and have a low survival rate.

RHODOCOCCUS EQUI PNEUMONIA

Rhodococcus equi is the most serious cause of pneumonia in foals 1-5 mo of age. It is not the most common cause of pneumonia in this age group; however, it has significant economic consequences due to mortality, prolonged treatment, surveillance programs for early detection, and relatively expensive prophylactic strategies. Clinical disease is rare in horses >8 mo of age. Compelling epidemiologic data indicate pulmonary infection probably originates within the first 2 wk of life.

Etiology and Pathogenesis: *R equi* is a gram-positive, facultative intracellular pathogen that is nearly ubiquitous in soil. Only certain types (Vap A, B, C) are pathogenic. The organism is likely present on all premises to some degree; however, disease incidence may be enzootic, sporadic, or nonexistent for specific farms. High ambient summer temperatures, sandy soil, and dusty conditions favor multiplication and dissemination of the organism in the environment. Inhalation of dust particles laden with virulent *R equi* is the major route of pneumonic infection. The organism readily multiplies within the intestine of foals ≤3 mo of age. Foals with pulmonary infections swallow sputum laden with *R equi*, which replicates in their intestinal tract. Manure from pneumonic foals is a major source of virulent bacteria contaminating the environment. The pathogenicity is linked to the ability of *R equi* to survive intracellularly, which hinges on failure of phagosome-lysosomal fusion in infected macrophages and failure of functional respiratory burst upon phagocytosis of *R equi*.

Clinical Findings and Lesions: *R equi* infection is slowly progressive with acute to subacute clinical manifestations. Clinical signs of disease are difficult to detect until pulmonary lesions reach a critical mass resulting in decompensation of the foal. Pulmonary lesions are relatively consistent and include subacute to chronic suppurative bronchopneumonia, pulmonary abscessation, and suppurative lymphadenitis. At the onset of clinical signs, most foals are lethargic, febrile, and tachypneic. Cough is a variable clinical sign; purulent nasal discharge is less common. Thoracic auscultation reveals crackles and wheezes with asymmetric/regional distribution. Pulmonary regions with marked consolidation lack breath sounds and exhibit dull resonance on thoracic percussion. Diarrhea is observed in many foals due to colonic microabscessation.

Intestinal and mesenteric abscesses are the most common extrapulmonary sites of infection. Foals with abdominal involvement often present with fever, depression, anorexia, weight loss, colic, and diarrhea. Intestinal lesion are characterized by multifocal, ulcerative enterocolitis and typhlitis involving Peyer's patches with granulomatous or suppurative inflammation of the mesenteric and/or colonic lymph nodes. The prognosis for foals with abdominal forms of *R equi* is less favorable than for those with pulmonary disease. Septic physitis and osteomyelitis are less common extrapulmonary sites of infection. Vertebral osteomyelitis may result in pathologic vertebral fracture and spinal cord compression, and is a devastating manifestation of *R equi* osteomyelitis. Panophthalmitis, guttural pouch empyema, sinusitis, pericarditis, nephritis, nonseptic uveitis and synovitis, and hepatic and renal abscessation with *R equi* have been reported.

Diagnosis: Routine laboratory evaluation of CBC and serum chemistry reveals nonspecific abnormalities consistent with infection and inflammation. Neutrophilic leukocytosis and hyperfibrinogenemia are common, and the severity of these findings relates to prognosis. Thoracic radiographic evaluation may reveal a pattern of perihilar alveolization, consolidation, and abscessation. The presence of nodular lung lesions and mediastinal lymphadenopathy in foals 1-5 mo of age is highly suggestive of *R equi*. Bacterial culture of transtracheal wash samples is required for definitive diagnosis. Cytologic evaluation of transtracheal wash samples reveals intracellular coccobacilli, identification of which indicates initiation of appropriate antimicrobial therapy pending culture results.

Treatment and Prognosis: The combination of erythromycin (25 mg/kg, PO, QID; esters or salts) and rifampin (5 mg/kg, BID, or 10 mg/kg, SID) is the treatment of choice. These antimicrobials may be bacteriostatic, but their activity is synergistic, and the combination has markedly improved survival of foals. Idiosyncratic hyperthermia and tachypnea can occur with erythromycin administration during periods of warm environmental conditions, and anorexia, bruxism, and salivation may be observed. Life-threatening, antibiotic-induced enterocolitis, due to *Clostridium difficile*, has been observed in the dams of nursing foals treated with erythromycin. Azithromycin is a newer generation macrolide with greater bioavailability than erythromycin. Azithromycin is administered orally (10 mg/kg, SID) with rifampin until clinical signs stabilize, then every other day until resolution of disease. The duration of antimicrobial therapy typically ranges from 4-9 wk.

Supportive therapy includes provision of a clean, comfortable environment and highly palatable, dust-free feeds. Judicial IV fluid therapy and saline nebulization facilitates expectoration of pulmonary exudates. NSAID should be administered as needed to maintain rectal temperature <103.5°F (39.7°C). Nasal insufflation with oxygen is necessary in foals with severe respiratory compromise. Bronchodilator therapy may or may not improve arterial oxygenation. Prophylactic antiulcer medication is indicated in foals that are stressed by respiratory difficulty, pain, frequent handling, hospitalization, and transportation.

The survival rate of *R equi* pneumonia is approximately 70-90% with appropriate therapy. The case fatality rate without therapy (or with inappropriate antimicrobial therapy) is ~80%. Parameters for discontinuation of medical therapy include clinical signs, serum fibrinogen concentration, and radiographic resolution of pulmonary consolidation and abscessation.

Prevention: There are 3 basic strategies to decrease the incidence of *R equi* pneumonia on endemic farms: decreased exposure to the organism, early detection of clinical cases, and enhanced passive immunity for neonatal foals. Foals should be maintained in well-ventilated, dust-free areas, avoiding dirt paddocks and overcrowding. Pneumonic foals should be isolated and their manure composted. Herd surveillance programs for early detection of pneumonic foals on endemic farms include twice weekly physical examination and auscultation, and monthly CBC and fibrinogen concentration. Foals with WBC count >14,000 cells/μL should be further evaluated for *R equi*. Administration of hyperimmune plasma might reduce the incidence and severity of *R equi* within the herd, but it is not completely effective in preventing disease. Hyperimmune plasma (1 L) is administered IV within the first week of life, followed by a second liter at approximately 25 days of age.

ACUTE BRONCHOINTERSTITIAL PNEUMONIA IN FOALS

Acute bronchointerstitial pneumonia is a sporadic, rapidly progressive disease of foals characterized by acute respiratory distress and high mortality.

Etiology, Epidemiology, and Pathogenesis: This relatively new disease has been reported in North America, Australia, and parts of Europe. The etiology is not clear. It is likely that a number of different insults, rather than a single factor, initiate a cascade of events resulting in a final common response of severe pulmonary damage and acute respiratory distress. Warm weather (>85°F [29.4°C]) is a common epidemiologic factor. Many foals have a history of antimicrobial therapy (particularly erythromycin) at the time clinical signs developed. No virus is consistently isolated, and no bacterial agent has been consistently identified. Enteric gram-negative organisms, *Rhodococcus equi*, *Pseudomonas aeruginosa*, and *Pneumocystis carinii* have been cultured from the lungs of affected foals.

Clinical Findings and Lesions: The age of affected foals ranges from 1 wk to 8 mo. Acute bronchointerstitial pneumonia has an acute or peracute onset and is accompanied by high fever. The disease is rapidly progressive, and may result in sudden death due to fulminant respiratory failure. Foals are unable or reluctant to move and are usually cyanotic. Severe respiratory distress is the most striking clinical sign. Clinicopathologic evaluation of foals with acute respiratory distress should include arterial blood gas, CBC, serum chemistry analysis, and thoracic radiographs. Hypoxemia, hypercapnea, and respiratory acidosis are consistent findings. These arterial blood gas findings quantify the severity of respiratory impairment and are used to monitor response to therapy. The hypoxemia of bronchointerstitial pneumonia is relatively resistant to supplemental oxygen therapy. Bronchointerstitial pneumonia is similar to bacterial pneumonia in that hyperfibrinogenemia and neutrophilic leukocytosis are observed in the majority of foals.

Diagnosis: Physical examination and clinicopathologic findings may appear similar to those of foals with severe *R equi* pneumonia (*see* above), and thoracic radiographic examination may be the most valuable diagnostic test to differentiate *R equi* pneumonia from bronchointerstitial pneumonia. Interstitial pneumonia appears as diffuse to caudodorsally distributed interstitial and bronchointerstitial pulmonary opacities. With advanced disease, the radiographic pattern progresses to include patches of a coalescing alveolar nodular pattern with air bronchograms. Transtracheal aspiration may be prohibitively dangerous to perform on a dyspneic foal, but should be done when the patient becomes more stable to obtain samples for bacterial culture/sensitivity, cytologic evaluation, and virus isolation. Cytologic evaluation of tracheal aspirates reveals acute neutrophilic inflammation with or without evidence of sepsis. Bacterial organisms are often recovered from transtracheal aspiration samples or necropsy of foals with bronchointerstitial pneumonia; however, no single organism is consistently recovered.

Necropsy examination reveals diffusely enlarged lungs that fail to deflate upon opening of the thoracic cavity with rib impressions on the visceral pleural suface. The cut surface of lung is mottled with dark red lung interspersed with more normal-appearing lung tissue, and edematous separation of lobules. The most prominent histopathologic findings are severe, diffuse, necrotizing bronchiolitis, alveolar septal necrosis, and neutrophilic alveolitis. Surviving foals develop a proliferative epithelial and interstitial response including bronchiolar and alveolar epithelial hyperplasia, type II cell hyperplasia, and hyaline membrane formation.

Treatment: Because the etiology of bronchointerstitial pneumonia is unknown, therapy is symptomatic. Treatment includes anti-inflammatory therapy, broad-spectrum antibiotics, thermoregulatory control, bronchodilation, supplemental oxygen, and supportive care. Anti-inflammatory therapy with corticosteroids (ie, dexamethasone 0.1 mg/kg, IV, SID) appears to improve survival. An alcohol bath, an air-conditioned stall, and/or a fan are used in conjunction with NSAID to maintain rectal temperature <103.5°F (39.7°C). The suitability of an antibiotic regimen appears to have little bearing on the outcome of bronchointerstitial pneumonia. Nonetheless, broad-spectrum antibiotic therapy should be instituted to treat existing or impending secondary bacterial infections. Additional supportive therapy includes provision of a clean, comfortable environment; highly palatable, dust-free feeds; and ulcer prophylaxis.

Prognosis: Although mortality is high, affected foals that receive aggressive medical care have a reasonably favorable prognosis for survival (70%). The longterm pulmonary consequences after recovery from bronchointerstitial pneumonia are variable, ranging from undetectable to persistent exercise intolerance.

STRANGLES
(Distemper)

Strangles is an infectious, contagious disease of Equidae characterized by abscessation of the lymphoid tissue of the upper respiratory tract. The causative organism, *Streptococcus equi equi*, is highly host-adapted and produces clinical disease only in horses, donkeys, and mules. It is a gram-positive, capsulated β-hemolytic Lancefield group C coccus, which is an obligate parasite and a primary pathogen.

Etiology and Pathogenesis: *S equi equi* is highly contagious, and produces high morbidity and low mortality in susceptible populations. Transmission occurs via fomites and direct contact with infectious exudates. Carrier animals are important for maintenance of the bacteria between epizootics and initiation of outbreaks on premises previously free of disease. Survival of the organism in the environment is dependent on temperature and humidity; it is susceptible to desiccation, extreme heat, and exposure to sunlight, and must be protected within mucoid secretions to survive. Under ideal environmental circumstances, the organism can survive 7-9 wk outside the host. Paddocks and barn facilities used by infected horses should be regarded as contaminated for ~2 mo after resolution of an outbreak.

Clinical Findings: The incubation period of strangles is 3-14 days and the first sign of infection is fever (103-106°F [39.4-41.1°C]). Within 24-48 hr of the initial fever spike, the horse will exhibit signs typical of strangles, including mucoid to mucopurulent nasal discharge, depression, and submandibular lymphadenopathy. Horses with retropharyngeal lymph node involvement will have difficulty swallowing, inspiratory respiratory noise (compression of the dorsal pharyngeal wall), and extended head and neck. Older animals with residual immunity may develop an atypical or catarrhal form of the disease with mucoid nasal discharge, cough, and mild fever. Metastatic strangles ("bastard strangles") is characterized by abscessation in other lymph nodes of the body, particularly the lymph nodes in the abdomen and, less frequently, the thorax.

Diagnosis: Diagnosis is confirmed by bacterial culture of exudate from abscesses or nasal swab samples. CBC reveals neutrophilic leukocytosis and hyperfibrinogenemia. Serum biochemical analysis is typically unremarkable. Complicated cases may require endoscopic examination of the upper respiratory tract (including the guttural pouches), ultrasonographic examination of the retropharyngeal area, or radiographic examination of the skull to identify the location and extent of retropharyngeal abscesses.

Treatment: The environment for clinically ill horses should be warm, dry, and dust-free. Warm compresses are applied to sites of lymphadenopathy to facilitate maturation of abscesses. Facilitated drainage of mature abscesses will speed recovery. Ruptured abscesses should be flushed with dilute (3-5%) povidone-iodine solution for several days until discharge ceases. NSAID can be administered judiciously to reduce pain and fever and improve appetite in horses with fulminant clinical disease.

Antimicrobial therapy is controversial. Most authors agree that initiation of antibiotic therapy after abscess formation may provide temporary clinical improvement in fever and depression, but ultimately prolongs the course of disease by delaying maturation of abscesses. Antibiotic therapy is indicated in cases with dyspnea, dysphagia, prolonged high fever, and severe lethargy/anorexia. Administration of penicillin during the early stage of infection (≤24 hr of onset of fever) will usually abort abscess formation. The disadvantage of early antimicrobial treatment is failure to mount a protective immune response, rendering horses highly susceptible to infection after cessation of therapy. If antimicrobial therapy is indicated, procaine penicillin (22,000 IU/kg, IM, BID) is the antibiotic of choice.

Prevention: Postexposure immunity is prolonged after natural disease in most horses, and protection is associated with local (nasal mucosa) production of antibody against the antiphagocytic M protein. The clinical attack rate of strangles is reduced by 50% in horses vaccinated with IM products that do not induce mucosal immunity. Local (mucosal) production of antibody requires mucosal antigen stimulation. An intranasal vaccine containing a live attenuated strain of *S equi equi* was designed to elicit a mucosal immunologic response. This attenuated strain is not temperature sensitive (inactivated by core body temperature), like the intranasal influenza vaccine. Reported complications include *S equi equi* abscesses at subsequent IM injection sites (live culture), submandibular lymphadenophathy, serous nasal discharge, and purpura hemorrhagica.

Control: Clinically affected horses should be physically separated from the herd and cared for by separate caregivers. The rectal temperature of all horses exposed to strangles should be obtained twice daily, and horses developing fever should be isolated (and potentially treated with penicillin). Contaminated equipment should be cleaned with detergent and disinfected using chlorhexidine gluconate or glutaraldehyde. Flies can transmit infection mechanically; therefore, efforts should be made to control the fly population during an outbreak. Farriers, trainers, and veterinarians should wear protective clothing or change clothes prior to traveling to the next equine facility. Additions to the herd should be carefully scrutinized for evidence of disease or shedding (nasopharyngeal culture) and quarantined for 14-21 days. Two negative nasal swab cultures should be obtained during the quarantine period.

Most horses continue to shed *S equi* for ~1 mo following recovery. Three negative nasopharyngeal swabs, at 4-7 days intervals, should be obtained prior to release from quarantine, and the minimum isolation period should be 1 mo. Prolonged bacterial shedding (up to 18 mo) has been identified in a small number of horses. Guttural pouch empyema is the source of infection in most prolonged carrier states. Bacterial culture of nasopharyngeal swab and/or guttural pouch lavage is used to identify persistent carriers.

RECURRENT AIRWAY OBSTRUCTION
(Heaves, Chronic obstructive pulmonary disease)

Recurrent airway obstruction (RAO) is a common, performance-limiting, allergic respiratory disease of horses characterized by chronic cough, nasal discharge, and respiratory difficulty. Episodes of airway obstruction are observed when susceptible horses are stabled, bedded on straw, and fed hay, whereas elimination of these inciting factors results in remission or attenuation of clinical signs. The pathophysiology involves small airway inflammation (neutrophilic), mucus production, and bronchoconstriction in response to allergen exposure.

Etiology: The average age at onset is 9 yr. Approximately 12% of mature horses have some degree of allergen-induced lower airway inflammation. There is no breed or gender predilection; however, there does appear to be a heritable component to susceptibility.

Clinical Findings: Horses present with flared nostrils, tachypnea, cough, and a heave line. The typical breathing pattern is characterized by a prolonged, labored expiratory phase of respiration. Cough may be productive and often occurs during feeding or exercise. The abdominal muscles respond by assisting with expiration, and hypertrophy of these muscles produces the classic heave line. Characteristic auscultatory findings include a prolonged expiratory phase of respiration, wheezes, tracheal rattle, and overexpanded lung fields. Wheezes are generated by airflow through narrowed airways, and are most pronounced during expiration. Crackles may be present and are associated with excessive mucus production. Mild to moderately affected horses may present with minimal clinical signs at rest, but coughing and exercise intolerance are noted during performance. Horses with RAO are not typically febrile unless secondary bacterial pneumonia has developed.

Horses from the southeastern USA may demonstrate clinical signs on late-summer pasture, which likely reflects sensitivity to molds or grass pollens. This is referred to as **summer pasture-associated obstructive pulmonary disease**. The management is similar to that of a horse with heaves, with the addition of pasture avoidance.

Diagnosis: The diagnosis of RAO is determined in most horses on the basis of history and characteristic physical examination findings. Hematology and serum chemistry results are unremarkable. Radiographic findings in horses with RAO are peribronchial infiltration and overexpanded pulmonary fields (flattening of the diaphragm). Thoracic radiographs are of little benefit in confirming the diagnosis of RAO and may not be necessary in horses with characteristic clinical signs, unless there is no response to standard treatment after 14 days of therapy. However, they may be helpful in identifying the most important differential diagnoses, including interstitial pneumonia, pulmonary fibrosis, or bacterial pneumonia.

Bronchoalveolar lavage is rarely required for diagnosis of fulminant RAO, and is not innocuous in horses that are dyspneic at rest. It is indicated in horses with mild to moderate disease with poor performance and coughing during exercise. Neutrophilic inflammation (20-90% of total cell count) confirms the presence of lower airway inflammation and differentiates horses with eosinophilic pneumonitis, fungal pneumonia, or lungworm infestation from horses with heaves. Curschmann's spirals may be observed on cytologic evaluation and represent inspissated mucus/cellular casts from obstructed small airways.

Treatment: The single most important treatment is environmental management to reduce allergen exposure. Medication will alleviate clinical signs of disease; however, respiratory disease will return after medication is discontinued if the horse remains in the allergen-challenged environment. The most common culprits are organic dusts present in hay, which need not appear overtly musty to precipitate an episode in a sensitive horse. Horses should be maintained at pasture with fresh grass as the source of roughage, supplemented with pelleted feed. Round bale hay is particularly allergenic and a common cause of treatment failure for horses on pasture. Horses that remain stalled should be maintained in a clean, controlled environment. Complete commerial feeds eliminate the need for roughage. Hay cubes and hay silage are acceptable, low-allergen alternative sources of roughage and may be preferred by horses over the complete feeds. Soaking hay with water prior to feeding may control clinical signs in mildly affected horses but is unacceptable for highly sensitive horses. Horses maintained in a stall should not be housed in the same building as an indoor arena, hay should not be stored overhead, and straw bedding should be avoided. Horses with summer pasture-associated obstructive pulmonary disease should be maintained in a dust-free, stable environment.

Medical treatment consists of a combination of bronchodilating agents (to provide relief of airway obstruction) and corticosteroid preparations (to reduce pulmonary inflammation). Bronchodilator therapy will provide immediate relief of airway obstruction until clincal signs of disease are controlled by corticosteroids. Severely affected horses are ideally controlled with aerosolized bronchodilators and systemic corticosteroids. Horses with mild to moderate airway inflammation can be treated with aerosolized corticosteroids and bronchodilators. It is inappropriate to treat RAO with bronchodilators as the sole therapy. NSAID, antihistamines, and leukotriene-receptor antagonists have failed to demonstrate therapeutic benefit.

INFLAMMATORY AIRWAY DISEASE
(Lower respiratory tract inflammation, Small airway inflammatory disease)

Inflammatory airway disease (IAD) describes a heterogeneous group of inflammatory conditions of the lower respiratory tract that appear to be primarily noninfectious. IAD occurs in 22-50% of athletic horses, and is a common cause of impaired performance and interruption of training.

Etiology and Pathophysiology: Proposed etiologies of IAD include allergic airway disease, recurrent pulmonary stress, deep inhalation of dust, atmospheric pollutants, and/or persistent respiratory viral infections. IAD often develops following an overt viral respiratory infection, and may result from inability of the immune system to fully eliminate viruses or bacteria from small airways. *Streptococcus pneumoniae* has been isolated from horses with IAD; however, its role in the pathophysiology is unclear, as this population of horses is largely unresponsive (or transiently responsive) to antibiotic therapy.

Clinical Findings: The most common clinical signs are chronic cough and mucoid to mucopurulent nasal discharge. Fever and auscultable pulmonary abnormalities are rarely observed. Horses with IAD demonstrate poor exercise tolerance at maximal speed. Endoscopic examination reveals mucopurulent exudate in the pharynx, trachea, and bronchi.

Diagnosis: Diagnosis of IAD is based on poor race performance and clinical signs. Bronchoalveolar lavage is performed to characterize the type of pulmonary inflammation. Cytologic evaluation of bronchoalveolar fluid will reveal one of the following inflammatory profiles: 1) mixed inflammation with high total nucleated cells, mild neutrophilia (15% of total cells), lymphocytosis, and monocytosis; 2) increased metachromatic cells (mast cells >2% of total cells); or 3) eosinophilic inflammation (5-40% of total cells). The mixed inflammatory profile likely results from environmental irritation or the consequences of a previous infectious disease.

Treatment: The type of inflammation in bronchoalveolar fluid will dictate the therapeutic plan. Regardless of the cytologic profile, all horses with IAD should receive aerosolized bronchodilator therapy prior to exercise to avert exercise- or irritant-induced bronchoconstriction. In horses with a mixed inflammatory cytologic profile, administration of low-dose, interferon-a is recommended for immunomodulation and antiviral activity. Interferon-α reduces tracheal exudate and improves cytologic profiles in horses with mixed inflammatory IAD. Eosinophilic bronchoalveolar fluid likely represents a Type I hypersensitivity reaction. In addition to tracheal exudates, peripheral eosinophilia, miliary pulmonary opacities, and eosinophilic pulmonary granulomas may be seen in affected horses. If such fluid is identified, the clinician should consider parasitic pulmonary disease in addition to hypersensitivity pneumonitis. Systemic corticosteroid therapy is recommended to reduce pulmonary inflammation in horses with eosinophilic IAD. Mast cell inflammation likely represents a local pulmonary hypersensitivity response and may represent an early form of recurrent airway obstruction (*see* p 1213). In IAD-affected horses with elevated mast cells in bronchoalveolar fluid, aerosol administration of nedocromil sodium (a mast cell-stabilizing drug) improves the clinical signs of respiratory disease and prevents histamine release.

EXERCISE-INDUCED PULMONARY HEMORRHAGE
(Epistaxis, "Bleeder")

Exercise-induced pulmonary hemorrhage (EIPH) occurs in the majority of racehorses and is observed in many other equine sports (eg, polo, barrel racing, 3-day events) that require strenuous exercise for short periods of time. Epistaxis is observed in a small proportion (~5%) of horses with EIPH. Blood in the tracheobronchial tree is identified in 44-75% of racehorses via endoscopic examination, and hemorrhage is detected by cytologic examination of bronchoalveolar lavage in 93% of racehorses.

Etiology: Proposed pathophysiologic mechanisms for pulmonary hemorrhage include high pulmonary vascular pressures during maximal exercise, neovascularization secondary to pulmonary inflammation, coagulation dysfunction, and intrathoracic shear forces generated during exercise. Some research suggests EIPH results from failure of the pulmonary system to accommodate a massive increase in cardiac output to meet the demands of high intensity exercise.

Diagnosis: Endoscopic observation of blood in the airways 30-90 min after exercise provides definitive evidence of EIPH. Other sources of hemorrhage in the upper airway, particularly guttural pouch mycosis (p 1222) and ethmoid hematoma (p 1221), must be excluded during endoscopic examination. If EIPH is suspected and the horse cannot be examined after exercise, cytologic examination of bronchoalveolar lavage fluid for semiquantitative assessment of hemosiderophages is diagnostic. Stains that highlight iron-containing pigments (Prussian blue) facilitate recognition of these cells. Thoracic radiography demonstrates alveolar or mixed alveolar-interstitial opacities in the caudodorsal lung fields; however, radiographic examination of the thorax has little impact on the diagnosis or management of EIPH.

Treatment and Control: Furosemide does not appear to prevent pulmonary hemorrhage, but it does reduce the severity by 70% and improve race performance. Horses with and without EIPH demonstrate equal improvements in race performance after administration, indicating that furosemide may enhance performance via mechanisms unrelated to EIPH. Application of nasal dilator bands reduces RBC counts in bronchoalveolar fluid from affected horses running on a treadmill by 33%. Alternative treatments, including procoagulant agents (eg, vitamin K, conjugated estrogens, aminocaproic acid), antihypertensive drugs, rheologic agents (pentoxyphylline), bronchodilators, prolonged rest, dietary supplements (hepseridin-citrus bioflavinoids), and anti-inflammatory drugs, have not demonstrated therapeutic benefit.

LARYNGEAL HEMIPLEGIA
(Roaring, Left laryngeal hemiplegia)

Left recurrent laryngeal hemiplegia is characterized by paresis or paralysis of the left arytenoid cartilage and vocal fold. It manifests clinically as exercise intolerance and inspiratory respiratory noise ("roaring") during exercise. Right-sided hemiplegia and bilateral (paraplegia) arytenoid dysfunction are uncommon.

Etiology and Pathogenesis: Progressive loss of the large myelinated fibers in the distal portion of the recurrent laryngeal nerves results in neurogenic atrophy of the intrinsic laryngeal musculature, the most crucial of which is the cricoarytenoideus dorsalis muscle. Axonal dystrophy of the left recurrent nerve occurs more commonly than the right, perhaps due to its extended length around the base of the heart. Left laryngeal hemiplegia is likely heritable. Less common causes include direct trauma to the recurrent laryngeal nerve, accidental perivascular injection of irritating substances, and plant (eg, *Cicer arietinum* [chick peas] and *Lathyrus* spp) and chemical intoxications. Lead toxicity should be suspected in horses with bilateral laryngeal paralysis. The peroneal nerve (similar length to the left recurrent laryngeal) may be affected with toxic insults, and axonal dystrophy of the peroneal nerve may manifest as stringhalt (p 925). Although all breeds are affected, there is a higher prevalence in males and long-necked/larger breeds. The prevalence in young Thoroughbreds presented for sale is estimated to be ~3-5%.

Loss of neuromuscular control of the abductor muscle results in collapse of the arytenoid cartilage and vocal fold, which reduces the glottal cross-sectional area. The resistance to airflow necessitates greater respiratory effort. Because of the pliable nature of the glottis, the exaggerated subatmospheric pressure in the airway results in further collapse of the arytenoid cartilage and exacerbation of the impedance to airflow. Upon inspiration during strenuous exercise, the affected side is drawn across the midline (by negative pressure in the airway) until it abuts the abducted normal arytenoid, effectively occluding the airway (dynamic collapse). The characteristic inspiratory whistle results from resonance within the open ventricle on the affected side. The harsher stridor, or roar, is produced by vortex shedding from the edges of the arytenoid cartilage and vocal fold.

Clinical Findings and Diagnosis: The principal clinical signs are inspiratory noise during exercise and exercise intolerance. Affected horses are asymptomatic at rest but have an unusual whinny. Diagnosis is confirmed by endoscopic observation of reduced or absent mobility of the arytenoid cartilage and vocal fold. With laryngeal hemiplegia, the arytenoid cartilage and vocal fold are located in a median position within the laryngeal lumen and are immobile. Asynchronous movements of the laryngeal cartilages occur commonly, with variable clinical relevance. Horses with laryngeal asynchrony, exercise intolerance, and respiratory noise during exercise should have their laryngeal function evaluated endoscopically during treadmill exercise to confirm laryngeal dysfunction.

Differential diagnoses include other pharyngeal conditions producing upper airway obstruction and exercise intolerance. The majority of these conditions are easily differentiated from laryngeal hemiplegia during endoscopic examination. Although arytenoid chondritis may be confused with laryngeal hemiplegia, misdiagnosis can be avoided by observation of the shape and size of the arytenoid cartilages. In arytenoid chondritis, the arytenoids thicken transversely and lose their characteristic "bean" shape. Abduction and adduction are usually limited. The axial (medial) surface of the arytenoid cartilage may be distorted with granulation tissue protruding through the mucosa, and a contact (kissing) lesion may be present on the contralateral arytenoid cartilage. Arytenoid chondritis should always be considered if motility of the right arytenoid is reduced. Radiographic examination of the pharynx may reveal mineralization within the arytenoid cartilages in cases of chondritis.

Treatment: Prosthetic laryngoplasty can stabilize the affected side of the larynx during inspiration and prevent dynamic collapse of the airway during exercise. Laryngeal ventriculectomy may improve airflow and reduce the "roaring" sound during exercise. Prosthetic laryngoplasty is commonly done in racing horses and is the only technique that satisfactorily reduces the impedance to inspiratory flow. Postoperative complications include chronic cough, chronic aspiration of feed, implant failure, and implant infection. Athletic performance will improve after surgery; however, horses are unlikely to develop their predicted performance potential.

PHARYNGEAL LYMPHOID HYPERPLASIA
(Pharyngitis)

Pharyngeal lymphoid hyperplasia (PLH) is a common condition of the dorsal pharyngeal wall observed in young horses (1-3 yr old). Horses do not have discrete masses of lymphoid tonsillar tissue; rather, they have many small foci or follicles of lymphoid tissue spread diffusely over the roof and lateral walls of the pharynx. In mature horses, these follicles blend with mucosal tissue and are unnoticeable. In young, maturing horses, lymphoid follicles appear as prominent, raised nodules on the surface of the pharyngeal roof and extend down the lateral walls of the pharynx and cranially into the nasopharynx. While PLH was once believed to be an important cause of poor performance in racehorses, its clincal significance is now questionable. Virtually all young horses undergo hyperplasia of pharyngeal lymphoid follicles; in most cases, this represents a normal immunologic event.

Occasionally, follicles may enlarge and coalesce with surrounding follicles. In these situations, follicles may appear hyperemic or inflamed and may exude mucoid or mucopurulent material. These cases likely represent a mild or subclinical viral infection and may be associated with impaired performance. Signs of pharyngeal pain include reduced appetite and frequent swallowing. Treatment is not necessary in the vast majority of cases; however, rest and NSAID administration are warranted in horses demonstrating pharyngeal pain.

DORSAL DISPLACEMENT OF THE SOFT PALATE

Dorsal displacement of the soft palate (DDSP) is a performance-limiting condition of the upper respiratory tract, and is a relatively common cause of upper respiratory noise during exercise. During DDSP, the caudal free margin of the soft palate moves dorsal to the epiglottis, creating a functional obstruction within the airway. The cross-sectional area of the pharynx is reduced, and airflow resistance and turbulence are increased.

Etiology and Pathogenesis: DDSP may result from several pathophysiologic mechanisms. Inflammation of the upper respiratory tract due to infection may cause neuropathy of the pharyngeal branch of the vagus nerve as it traverses the floor of the medial compartment of the guttural pouch, resulting in neuromuscular dysfunction of the pharyngeal muscles that control the soft palate. The retropharyngeal lymph nodes are in direct contact with the pharyngeal branch of the vagus nerve, and retropharyngeal lymphadenopathy may result in compression and irritation. Clinical signs can be induced by local anesthesia of this nerve. Congenital hypoplasia of the epiglottis may contribute to DDSP, due to insufficient epiglottal tissue to maintain the position of the caudal border of the soft palate ventral to the epiglottis.

Clinical Findings: DDSP creates a characteristic gurgling respiratory noise, primarily during expiration, due to vibration of the soft palate. Horses may make no noise at the onset of exercise but displace their palate during high-speed exercise, causing them to "choke down." Head position (flexed) may contribute to displacement.

Treatment: The most effective treatment for DDSP in young horses (2 yr olds) and horses with evidence of upper respiratory tract infection is rest and anti-inflammatory therapy. Caudal retraction of the tongue elevates the soft palate and pushes the larynx caudally, both of which may predispose a horse to DDSP. Placing a tongue tie during exercise reduces caudal retraction of the tongue. Sternothyrohyoideus myectomy performed in horses prone to DDSP to alter the anatomy of the upper respiratory tract is successful in ~50% of horses. Soft palate resection (staphylectomy) is frequently performed in horses with DDSP and also has a success rate of ~50%; however, the mechanism of improvement after surgery is unclear. Success has been attributed to reduction in the mass of soft palate obstructing the airway, easier replacement of the shorter soft palate to the subepiglottic position, and firming of the caudal edge of the soft palate to keep it ventral to the epiglottis.

EPIGLOTTIC ENTRAPMENT

Epiglottic entrapment is a less common cause of respiratory noise and exercise intolerance. In this condition, the aryepiglottic fold completely envelops the apex and lateral margins of the epiglottis. The general shape of the epiglottis is visible, and the position (dorsal to the soft palate) is appropriate. However, the distinct serrated margins of the epiglottis and the dorsal epiglottic vascular pattern are obscured by a fold of aryepiglottic mucosa. Clinical signs of epiglottic entrapment include inspiratory and expiratory respiratory noise during exercise and poor exercise performance. Less common signs include cough, nasal discharge, and headshaking. Diagnosis is determined by endoscopic examination. Surgical correction of epiglottic entrapment is axial division of the aryepiglottic fold to free the epiglottis. Axial transection of the aryepiglottic fold may be performed by transendoscopic contact Nd:YAG laser, transnasal or transoral transection via curved bistoury, or direct excision through a laryngotomy or pharyngotomy. Surgical transection is generally curative with a relapse rate of 5%. Some affected horses can race successfully with the condition.

SUBEPIGLOTTIC CYST

Subepiglottic cysts are an uncommon cause of respiratory noise in young horses. They are likely present from birth, but remain undetected until the horse begins exercise training. These cysts are suspected to arise from remnants of the thyroglossal duct. Clinical signs include respiratory noise and exercise intolerance. Large cysts may produce coughing, dysphagia, and aspiration in foals. Diagnosis is determined by endoscopic examination of the upper respiratory tract. The cyst appears as a smooth-walled, fluctuant mass that contains thick yellow mucoid material. Occasionally, the mass is not visible in the nasopharynx, and oral examination under general anesthesia may be required to identify it.

Histologically, subepiglottic cysts are lined with a combination of stratified squamous and pseudostratified columnar epithelium. Treatment involves complete removal of the secretory lining of the cyst. Rupture of the cyst will result in immediate decompression, but recurrence is common. The most common approach is ventral laryngotomy, although transendoscopic Nd:YAG laser surgery has been used for complete excision.

FOURTH BRANCHIAL ARCH DEFECT

The extrinsic structures of the larynx, such as the wing of the thyroid cartilage, cricothyroid muscle, and upper esophageal sphincter, develop from the fourth branchial arches. Aplasia or hypoplasia of one or more of these structures may occur unilaterally or bilaterally. Right-sided defects are more common than bilateral or left-sided defects. The severity of clinical manifestation ranges broadly and is based on the degree of the defect. The most common clinical sign is respiratory noise, although mild dysphagia, eructation, and cough have been reported. Palpation of the larynx will reveal absence of one or both wings of the thyroid cartilage, resulting in failure of the cricothyroid articulation and a palpable space between the cricoid and thyroid cartilages. Radiographic evidence of a fourth branchial arch defect includes dilation of the cricopharynx with a continuous column of air from the pharynx to the cervical esophagus. Rostral displacement of the palatopharyngeal arch may or may not be detected during endoscopic examination. Endoscopic examination during treadmill exercise may reveal dynamic collapse of the vocal folds. Affected horses are unlikely to become effective athletes.

DISEASES OF THE NASAL PASSAGES

Diseases of the Nasal Septum

Diseases of the nasal septum are rare. Most nasal septal disorders are congenital abnormalities that remain undetected until the horse is exercised. Traumatic injury to the bridge of the nose as a juvenile can produce nasal septal deviation and thickening. Other less common diseases of the nasal septum include amyloidosis, fungal infection, and squamous cell carcinoma.

Thickening or deviation of the nasal septum causes low-pitched stertorous breathing during exercise. Facial deformity may be observed. Septal abnormalities may be detected by palpation, visual inspection, and endoscopic examination. Dimensions of the nasal cavity are difficult to appreciate via endoscopic examination; however, abnormalities of the mucosa are easily identified. Precise dorsoventral radiographs of the skull provide definitive evidence of septal deformity, deviation, and thickening. Histologic examination of any nodules or discrete lesions on the septum will identify tumors, amyloidosis, or fungal infections.

Surgical resection of the nasal septum is the only treatment option in most cases. The entire diseased portion of the septum can be excised using obstetrical wire by transecting the septum on the dorsal, ventral, and caudal border. Hemorrhage is substantial during this procedure (4-8 L), and the nasal passages are packed with sterile gauze soaked in saline or in 1:100,000 epinephrine solution to minimize blood loss. Before the horse recovers from anesthesia, a tracheotomy is performed.

Postoperative care includes parenteral antibiotics and NSAID. The packing and tracheotomy tube should be removed 48-72 hr after surgery. All incisions heal by second intention within 3 wk. Horses should be rested for ~2 mo before returning to normal activity. After surgery, most horses make a respiratory noise during work, although less than before surgery, and exercise tolerance is improved. Shortening of the upper jaw, incisor malalignment, or nostril collapse can develop if the procedure is performed in immature horses. Ideally, the surgery should be delayed until maturity.

Nasal Polyps

Nasal polyps are pedunculated growths that arise from the mucosa of the nasal cavity, nasal septum, or tooth alveolus. Polyps are usually unilateral and single but can be bilateral and multiple. They form in response to chronic inflammation by hypertrophy of the mucous membrane or exuberant proliferation of fibrous connective tissue. There is no age, breed, or gender predilection.

Clinical signs are poor airflow through the affected nasal passage; inspiratory dyspnea; unilateral, malodorous, mucopurulent nasal discharge; and low-volume epistaxis. The mass may extend rostrally until it protrudes beyond the nostrils. Polyps are detected via endoscopic and radiographic examination, and histopathologic evaluation of biopsy samples provide a definitive diagnosis. Surgical excision is performed via an incision in the false nostril, a trephine opening, or a bone flap.

Choanal Atresia

Choanal atresia is caused by persistence of the bucconasal membrane that separates the primitive buccal or oral cavity from the nasal pits during embryonic development. Bilateral and unilateral cases have been described in horses. Clinical signs are evident immediately after birth in foals with bilateral disease, because dyspnea is severe and air cannot be detected passing through the nostrils. An endoscope or stomach tube passed through the ventral meatus will be obstructed at the level of the medial canthus of the eye.

Bilateral complete choanal atresia is a life-threatening condition, and a tracheotomy must be performed immediately after birth. It may be possible to perforate a thin membrane by electrocoagulation or laser or by excision through bilateral flaps centered along the midline. Indwelling tube stents should be inserted through both choanae and left in place for 6 wk.

DISEASES OF THE PARANASAL SINUSES

The maxillary sinus is the largest paranasal sinus and is divided by a thin septum into caudal and rostral parts. The frontal sinus has a large communication with the dorsal conchal sinus at its rostral end, thereby forming the conchofrontal sinus. The conchae or turbinates are delicate scrolls of bone that are attached laterally in the nasal passage and contain the conchal sinuses. The caudal and rostral maxillary sinuses have separate openings into the middle nasal meatus, and the caudal maxillary sinus communicates with the frontal sinus through the large frontomaxillary opening. Diseases that originate in one sinus cavity may extend to and involve others.

Most diseases of the paranasal sinuses cause mucopurulent or bloody nasal discharge. Drainage is unilateral, in contrast to disease of the lungs, pharynx, and guttural pouches, because the source of discharge is rostral to the caudal border of the nasal septum. Unilateral facial swelling, epiphora, dull percussion of the sinuses, and inspiratory noise are common manifestations of disorders of the sinuses.

On endoscopy, purulent material, a mass, or blood can be seen in the nasal passage originating from the nasomaxillary opening. Lateral and dorsoventral radiographs of the skull may reveal fluid lines, sinus cysts, solid masses, or lytic/proliferative changes associated with dental disease and neoplasia. Oblique projections in a dorsal to ventral direction may be required to improve views of the tooth roots. Computed tomography is useful, particularly for ventral conchal sinus disease. Centesis of the maxillary or frontal sinuses is performed to obtain fluid for bacterial culture, sensitivity testing, and cytologic examination. With sedation and local anesthesia, the sinuses can be examined in the standing horse by insertion of an arthroscope (4.0 mm). A second portal could be used to insert an instrument into the sinus to obtain specimens, debride tissue, and lavage the sinus cavity.

Sinusitis

Primary sinusitis occurs subsequent to an upper respiratory tract infection that has involved the paranasal sinuses. It usually involves all sinus cavities but can be confined to the ventral conchal sinus. This cavity is difficult to detect radiographically and access surgically. Secondary sinusitis can result from tooth root infection, fracture, or sinus cyst. The first molar, fourth premolar, and third premolar (in decreasing frequency) are the most likely to develop tooth root abscesses. Clinical signs of secondary sinusitis closely resemble those of primary sinusitis including unilateral mucopurulent nasal discharge and facial deformity. Tooth root abscesses typically produce a fetid nasal discharge. Treatment of primary sinusitis involves lavage of the sinus cavity and systemic antimicrobial therapy based on culture and sensitivity results. Secondary sinusitis requires removal of affected cheek teeth or cystic material via sinusotomy.

Ethmoid Hematoma

Progressive ethmoid hematoma is a locally destructive mass of nasal passages and paranasal sinuses of uncertain etiology. The mass resembles a tumor in appearance and development but is not neoplastic. Large hematomas usually arise from the ethmoid labyrinth, and smaller masses arise from the floor of the sinuses. Masses originating in the sinus extend into the nasal passage. An expanding hematoma can cause pressure necrosis of surrounding bone but rarely causes facial distortion; it is primarily observed in horses >6 yr old. Low-grade, spontaneous, intermittent, unilateral epistaxis is the most common clinical sign. Horse with extensive masses may have reduced airflow through the affected nasal passage and fetid breath. In longstanding cases, the mass may protrude from the nares. In most instances, the lesion can be seen extending into the nasal passages on endoscopic examination, and the extent of the mass can be determined radiographically. Conservative management includes intralesional injection of the mass with 4% formaldehyde. Formalin is injected into the mass using a guarded endoscopic needle. The mass typically regresses rapidly, but recurrence is common. Surgical excision is achieved via frontonasal bone flap.

Sinus Cysts

Sinus cysts are single or loculated fluid-filled cavities with an epithelial lining. They develop in the maxillary sinuses and ventral conchae and can extend into the frontal sinus. A congenital form has been described. Sinus cysts are typically found in horses <1 yr old, but can also be seen in those >9 yr old. The primary clinical signs are facial deformity, nasal discharge, and partial airway obstruction. Radiographs are more likely to identify a sinus cyst than endoscopic examination. Multiloculated densities and fluid lines in the sinuses are observed radiographically; occasionally, dental distortion, flattening of tooth roots, soft-tissue mineralization, and deviation of the nasal septum are seen. Treatment involves radical surgical removal of the cyst and associated conchal lining. Prognosis for complete recovery is good, and the recurrence is low. Some horses may have a permanent, mild mucoid discharge after surgery.

GUTTURAL POUCH DISEASE

Empyema

Guttural pouch empyema is defined as the accumulation of purulent, septic exudate in the guttural pouch. The infection usually develops subsequent to a bacterial (primarily *Streptococcus* spp) infection of the upper respiratory tract. Clinical signs include intermittent purulent nasal discharge, painful swelling in the parotid area, and in severe cases, stiff head carriage and stertorous breathing. Fever, depression, and anorexia may or may not be observed. Diagnosis is determined by endoscopic examination of the guttural pouch. Radiographs of the pharynx will demonstrate a fluid line in the guttural pouch and may allow the clinician to identify an associated retropharyngeal mass.

Systemic antimicrobial therapy alone will not resolve the infection; guttural pouch lavage is necessary. Retropharyngeal abscesses can be resolved by rupturing the abscess into the guttural pouch using an endoscopic blade. If endoscopic rupture into the guttural pouch is unsuccessful, surgical drainage is necessary for retropharyngeal abscessation. Guttural pouch empyema may compress the dorsal pharynx and produce upper airway obstruction. Tracheotomy may be necessary to provide a temporary alternative airway in these cases. If guttural pouch empyema is not treated, chondroid material may form in the guttural pouch and will serve as a chronic source of infectious exudate. A small number of chondroids can be removed endoscopically, but accumulations of exudate, chondroid material, or unresolved retropharyngeal abscesses require surgical drainage.

Guttural Pouch Mycosis

Mycotic plaques in the guttural pouch are typically located on the caudodorsal aspect of the medial guttural pouch, over the internal carotid artery. In some instances, fungal plaques may be multiple or diffuse. The most common fungal organism associated with guttural pouch mycosis is *Aspergillus* spp (*see also* p 511). Clincal signs arise from damage to the cranial nerves and the arteries within the mucosal lining of the guttural pouch. The most common sign is epistaxis, due to fungal erosion of the wall of either the internal carotid artery (most cases) or branches of the external carotid artery. Hemorrhage is spontaneous and severe, and repeated bouts may precede a fatal hemorrhagic episode. Dysphagia, Horner's syndrome, and dorsal displacement of the soft palate may develop in response to fungal damage to cranial nerves and the sympathetic nerve that superficially traverse the guttural pouch. Dysphagia is a poor prognostic indicator. Diagnosis is determined by endoscopic examination of the guttural pouch. Treatment consists of topical and systemic antifungal therapy, based on sensitivity testing. Topical antifungal therapy is administered directly on the lesion via infusion through the biopsy channel of an endoscope. A fatal hemorrhagic event can be prevented by occluding the affected arteries along their course through the guttural pouch by means of a balloon-tipped catheter or a coil embolus. It is necessary to occlude the arteries proximal and distal to the lesion to prevent retrograde bleeding from the circle of Willis.

Guttural Pouch Tympany

Guttural pouch tympany is observed in horses ranging from birth to 1 yr of age and is more common in fillies than in colts. The affected guttural pouch is distended with air and forms a characteristic nonpainful swelling in the parotid region. Breathing may become stertorous in severely affected animals. Tympany may result from inflammation or malformation of the pharyngeal orifice of the eustachian tube, which then acts as a one-way valve by allowing air to enter the pouch but preventing its return into the pharynx. Diagnosis is based on clinical signs and radiographic examination of the skull. Severely affected animals may develop a secondary empyema. Tympany is usually unilateral, but bilateral cases have been reported. Medical management with NSAID and antimicrobial therapy resolves the majority of cases due to upper respiratory tract inflammation. Surgical intervention is warranted in patients with malformation of the guttural pouch opening and involves fenestration of the membrane that separates the affected guttural pouch from the normal one. This provides a route for air in the abnormal guttural pouch to pass to the normal side and be expelled into the pharynx. The postoperative prognosis is good.

Rupture of the Longus Capitis Muscle

Traumatic rupture of the longus capitis is the second most common cause (after mycosis) of severe hemorrhage from the guttural pouch. The longus capitis muscle is one of the ventral straight muscles of the head. It inserts on the basisphenoid bone at the base of the skull. The point of rupture occurs at the insertion of the muscle dorsal to the guttural pouch. Rupture results from traumatic poll injury (rearing over backward) and produces profuse hemorrhage. Hemorrhage into the retropharyngeal space can cause asphyxia and death. On endoscopic examination, swelling and hemorrhage can be seen in the most rostral and medial aspects of the guttural pouch by retroflexion of the endoscope. On lateral radiographic examination, an avulsion fracture of the basisphenoid bone may be seen overlying the guttural pouch region. Significant neurologic deficits are often observed with this fracture. Treatment involves stall rest for 4-6 wk; broad-spectrum antibiotics are given for 5-7 days for any infection at the site of muscle rupture. Prognosis for full recovery is good, but persistent neurologic signs or recurrent hemorrhage worsens the prognosis.

RESPIRATORY DISEASES OF PIGS

Respiratory diseases of pigs can be classified into 2 broad categories based on the extent and duration of overt disease: those that affect large numbers of pigs and may be serious but of limited duration, and those that persist in a large number of pigs for indefinite periods. Diseases in the first category can be costly, but the losses are limited rather than ongoing. They include swine influenza (p 1228), classical swine fever (p 570), the pneumonic forms of pseudorabies (p 1065), and porcine reproductive and respiratory syndrome (p 581). The causal viruses may persist in a herd, but outbreaks of overt disease tend to be self-limiting.

The most important syndromes in the second category are atrophic rhinitis, mycoplasmal pneumonia, and pleuropneumonia (see below). Salmonellosis and Haemophilus parasuis infections may be significant problems in some herds. Moderate levels of atrophic rhinitis caused by Bordetella bronchiseptica alone may not be too significant but, when coupled with toxigenic strains of Pasteurella, are an important cause of economic loss due to decreased rate of growth and reduced feed conversion in young pigs. Enzootic pneumonia, when caused by mycoplasma alone, is of little consequence; however, when it is combined with secondary infection, eg, Pasteurella multocida, the resulting condition may be severe. Actinobacillus pleuropneumoniae may be associated with considerable losses in some herds. Migrating worm larvae or the infections listed in the first category often lead to severe problems when they occur with the infections in the second category.

The severity and economic importance of diseases in the second category also are related to population density and to the type and size of herd. They may be of little importance in weanling pig operations but become of major importance in high-density feeder-pig units. Although mortality usually is low, economic damage results from an adverse and uneven effect on growth rate, decreased feed efficiency, and additional costs of drugs, particularly medicated feed. However, when stress can be avoided by proper management, such diseases may result in only minimal losses.

It is possible to set up herds free of diseases in the second category by techniques such as SPF repopulation or medicated early weaning, or by buying pigs from a pneumonia-free herd. The latter method is the least expensive, but because the etiology of diseases in the second category is complex, all the pigs should be purchased from one source. This is also true when purchasing weaned pigs for feeder-pig units.

It is difficult to keep herds free of respiratory diseases. Aerosols have been suspected as sources of pathogen entry into naive farms. Organisms such as Mycoplasma hyopneumoniae have been postulated to be transmitted over distances ≥2 miles, depending on climate, terrain, and density of pigs in the locality; however, this assumption is based on speculation and the use of mathematical models rather than experimental data.

Closed herds, ie, buying in no live animals (using artificial insemination or embryo transfer to bring in new genetic material), help establish immunity to present organisms and avoid introduction of new infections, strains, or serotypes. Multiple site production or an "all-in/all-out" policy, in which the entire barn or air space is emptied before refilling, can be very effective in minimizing the potential effect of chronic pneumonia.

Respiratory disease is endemic in many herds. The main control factors are stress management, stocking density, ventilation, temperature control, and freedom from mixing and moving. Multiple site production or "all-in/all-out" and closed-herd management practices greatly decrease the need for preventive and therapeutic medication.

ATROPHIC RHINITIS

Atrophic rhinitis is characterized by sneezing, followed by atrophy of the turbinate bones, which may be accompanied by distortion of the nasal septum and shortening or twisting of the upper jaw.

Etiology: The etiology is complex and involves at least 2 organisms. Various infections (eg, inclusion body rhinitis and pseudorabies) and noninfectious agents (eg, dust or high ammonia levels) cause sneezing and tear-staining, usually without leading to atrophic rhinitis. *Bordetella bronchiseptica* has long been implicated as a major cause. This bacterium is not host-specific, although strains that cause atrophic rhinitis are generally isolated only from pigs. Dogs, cats, rodents, and other species may harbor *B bronchiseptica* for long periods, but their role in the spread of atrophic rhinitis in pigs is uncertain. Certain toxigenic strains of *Pasteurella multocida* (types A and D), often acting with *B bronchiseptica*, cause permanent turbinate atrophy and nasal distortion. Both organisms can cause clinical atrophic rhinitis. The disease has been divided into 2 forms: **nonprogressive** atrophic rhinitis, due to *B bronchiseptica*, is mild and transient and probably does not greatly affect the animal's growth and performance; **progressive** atrophic rhinitis, due to toxigenic *P multocida*, is severe, permanent, and usually accompanied by poor growth.

Outbreaks of disease usually follow either the introduction of infected pigs or mixing of pigs from different sources. Piglets may be affected at any age, especially with *P multocida*, which also may infect mature animals. Crowding, inadequate ventilation, mixing and moving, and other concurrent diseases are important contributory factors in intensification of the disease.

Clinical Findings: Acute signs, which usually appear at 3-8 wk of age, include sneezing, coughing, and inflammation of the lacrimal duct. In more severe cases, nasal hemorrhage may occur. The lacrimal ducts may become occluded, and tear stains then appear below the medial canthi of the eyes. Some severely affected pigs may develop lateral deviation or shortening of the upper jaw, while others may suffer some degree of turbinate atrophy with no apparent outward distortion. The degree of distortion can be judged from the relationship of the upper and lower incisors if breed variations are considered. In addition to the above clinical signs, outbreaks frequently impair growth rate and feed conversion.

The severity of atrophic rhinitis in a herd depends largely on the presence of toxigenic strains of *P multocida*, the level of management, and the immune status of the herd. The latter is related to both vaccination status and the parity distribution of the sow herd, because younger sows tend to shed more organisms and produce less lactogenic immunity for their nursing piglets than do older multiparous sows.

Lesions: The degree of atrophy and distortion is best assessed by examining a transverse section at the level of the second premolar tooth (the first cheek tooth, up to 7-9 mo of age); some recommend additional parallel sections. In the active stages of inflammation, the mucosa has a blanched appearance, and purulent material may be present on the surface. In later stages, the nasal cavities may be clear, but there may be variable degrees of softening, atrophy, or grooving of the turbinates; deviation of the nasal septum; and asymmetric distortion of the surrounding bone structure.

Diagnosis: The signs and lesions are commonly the basis for diagnosis; however, the presence of toxigenic strains of *P multocida* should be confirmed. Routine monitoring is done in some breeding herds by measuring the degree of turbinate atrophy and giving the herd an atrophy score. Atrophic rhinitis must be differentiated from necrotic rhinitis (p 1226).

Control: It is rarely possible to keep herds entirely free from mild outbreaks of sneezing, and a low level of aberrant turbinates and nasal bones at necropsy is common, even in herds that show no clinical signs of rhinitis. When atrophic rhinitis rises to an unacceptable level in a herd, control measures are usually strategic—chemoprophylaxis, vaccination, temporary closure of the herd to introduction of new pigs, and improved management (eg, better ventilation and hygiene, less dusty feed). Chemoprophylaxis usually includes administration of antibacterial drugs to all sows, particularly prefarrowing, as well as programs of repeated medications for newborn piglets and sometimes for newly weaned pigs. Medication of weaner and grower rations, and sometimes sow rations, is often helpful. Drugs commonly used are ceftiofur, sulfonamides, tylosin, and tetracyclines.

Bacterins against toxigenic *P multocida* and *B bronchiseptica* have been developed. Both toxoid vaccines and bacterin-toxoid mixtures are available against *P multocida*; while both give satisfactory results in most herds, infection can be best prevented with bacterin-toxoid mixtures. Typically, sows are vaccinated 4 and 2 wk before farrowing, and the young pigs at 1 and 4 wk of age. However, vaccination schedules recommended by the manufacturer should be followed. A high level of colostral immunity is acquired by piglets nursing vaccinated sows. An intranasal vaccine using modified live strains of *B bronchiseptica* is also available for young pigs.

MYCOPLASMAL PNEUMONIA
(Enzootic pneumonia)

Mycoplasmal pneumonia is a chronic, clinically mild, infectious pneumonia of pigs, characterized by its ability to become endemic in a herd and to produce a persistent dry cough, retarded growth rate, sporadic "flare-ups" of overt respiratory distress, and a high incidence of lung lesions in slaughter pigs. It occurs worldwide.

Clinical outbreaks of mycoplasmal pneumonia may impair growth rate and feed conversion. This effect is enhanced when large numbers of pigs are closely confined in poorly ventilated buildings under poor husbandry conditions. The effects of the disease are uneven and unpredictable and place limits on the efficiency and flexibility of large production units. However, in swine units with good disease control measures, mycoplasmal pneumonia may remain largely subclinical and is of little economic importance.

Etiology and Epidemiology: The terms "viral pneumonia" and "enzootic pneumonia" are frequently used to describe a characteristic disease syndrome now known to be caused primarily by *Mycoplasma hyopneumoniae*. The pleomorphic organism is fastidious, smaller than most bacteria, and difficult to see clearly under ordinary light microscopes. It can be cultured in specially prepared media, but isolation from field cases is difficult. It is rapidly inactivated in the environment and by disinfectants, but it may survive longer in cold weather. It appears to be host-specific.

Mycoplasmal pneumonia is also frequently complicated by other mycoplasmas, bacteria, and viruses, which affect the severity of the disease. Certain strains of *M hyorhinis*, and perhaps some viruses, may themselves act as primary agents to produce a syndrome resembling the pneumonia caused by *M hyopneumoniae*.

In most countries that use modern pig-farming methods, the lungs of 30-80% of the pigs slaughtered show pneumonic lesions of the type associated with mycoplasmal infection. Pigs of all ages are susceptible, but within a herd, pigs become infected in the first few weeks of life either by their dam or by other young pigs after mixing. Transmission to lactating piglets can occur from sows of all parities. The incidence of lung lesions is highest in pigs 3-5 mo old. Immunity develops slowly, followed by regression of the lung lesions. Older growing and mature pigs may recover completely.

Clinical Findings: In herds in which the disease is endemic, morbidity is high, but clinical signs may be minimal and mortality is low. Coughing is the most common sign and is most obvious when pigs are roused. Individual pigs or groups sporadically develop severe pneumonia. A common predisposing factor is a change of weather, but other stresses (eg, transient viral infections, parasitic migration, and mixing pigs) may also cause outbreaks. The disease is usually more severe when it first enters a herd.

Lesions: Affected lungs are gray or purple, most commonly in the apical and cardiac lobes. Old lesions become clearly demarcated. The associated lymph nodes may be enlarged. Histologically, inflammatory cells are present in the bronchioles; there is perivascular and peribronchiolar cuffing and extensive lymphoid hyperplasia.

Diagnosis: Clinical, pathologic, and epidemiologic findings are usually adequate for diagnosis. *M hyopneumoniae* can be demonstrated in impression smears of the cut surface of the affected lung, identified by fluorescent antibody technique, and sometimes isolated and identified in culture. Serologic tests, principally the complement fixation test, and ELISA are occasionally used on a herd basis, but results may be difficult to interpret. Recently, a PCR test for the detection of *M hyopneumoniae* from nasal swabs has been developed and appears to be very sensitive and specific.

Control: When the disease first enters a herd, mass treatment with antibiotics (eg, tylosin, lincomycin, tiamulin, or a tetracycline) helps to control the severity of signs.

When disease increases in endemic herds, treatment of individual pigs with antibiotics usually results in remission, presumably by controlling secondary bacteria.

Inactivated mycoplasmal cultures have been developed as bacterins and consist of whole cell preparations as well as new subunit bacterins. These induce excellent protection against the development of gross lesions, and significantly reduce clinical signs (coughing) in growing pigs. Recent data indicate that prefarrowing vaccination of sows with *M hyopneumoniae* vaccines significantly reduces colonization of suckling piglets.

The economic effects of the disease can be reduced, and sometimes eliminated, by improvements in housing and husbandry, particularly ventilation and overcrowding, along with medication and vaccination. "All-in/all-out" management of pigs from birth to market is extremely effective at reducing negative effects of disease; following this practice improves growth performance and reduces lung lesions.

In large intensive units, starting with foundation stock free of mycoplasmal pneumonia and adopting strict precautions against direct and indirect contact with pigs from other herds is advisable. Unfortunately, many herds set up in this way do not remain free of mycoplasmas for very long, particularly in areas with a high density of pigs. Field observations suggest that infection can be windborne for at least a mile between large herds in cold, wet weather.

In the USA and parts of Europe, most herds free of mycoplasmal pneumonia were established by the pig repopulation technique. More recently, some have been established by segregated early weaning. The biggest problems with these herd programs are the breakdown rate and the difficulty of monitoring herds that claim to be free of mycoplasmal pneumonia. Current hypotheses for these outbreaks suggest that certain herds may never have successfully eliminated the organism; rather, it coexisted within the population at an undetectable level for extended periods. Use of nasal swab PCR technology has demonstrated the presence of the organism in pigs free of clinical signs, lesions, and antibodies. Analysis of tracheal sections from these pigs by electron microscopy has indicated the presence of the organism on the cilia.

NECROTIC RHINITIS
(Bullnose)

Necrotic rhinitis is an uncommon, sporadic disease of young pigs characterized by suppuration and necrosis of the snout, arising from wounds of the oral or nasal mucosa. Confusion exists in the literature because of the use of the misnomer "bullnose" to also describe atrophic rhinitis (p 1223).

Etiology: *Fusobacterium necrophorum* is commonly isolated from the lesion and undoubtedly contributes to the disease, but other types of organisms are frequently present. They gain entry through damage to the roof of the mouth, often as a result of clipping the needle teeth too short or using blunt clippers.

Clinical Findings and Lesions: Signs include swelling and deformity of the face, occasionally hemorrhage, snuffling, sneezing, foul-smelling nasal discharge, sometimes involvement of the eyes with lacrimation and purulent discharge, loss of appetite, and emaciation. Generally, only 1-2 pigs in the herd are affected.

The facial swelling usually is hard, but incision reveals a mass of pinkish gray, foul-smelling, necrotic tissue, or greenish gray tissue debris, depending on the age of the lesion. The nasal and facial bones become involved, and facial deformity may be marked.

Diagnosis: Necrotic rhinitis is readily differentiated from atrophic rhinitis by the bulging type of facial distortion seen in the former. The character of the exudate and its location within the tissue of the snout or face are also distinctive of necrotic rhinitis.

Prevention and Treatment: Prevention is directed toward avoiding injuries to the mouth and snout, improving pig processing techniques, and improving sanitation. When the disease occurs repeatedly, needle teeth should be clipped carefully.

If the condition is advanced, treatment may not be advisable. Early surgical intervention and packing the cavity with sulfonamide or tincture of iodine may be useful. In young pigs, sulfamethazine given PO is of value.

PASTEURELLOSIS

Pasteurellosis is most commonly seen in pigs as a complication of mycoplasmal pneumonia (p 1197), although swine influenza, Aujeszky's disease, *Bordetella bronchiseptica*, or *Haemophilus parahaemolyticus* may also cause changes in the lungs that lead to disease caused by *Pasteurella* spp. The causative organism usually is *P multocida*. It produces an exudative bronchopneumonia, sometimes with pericarditis and pleuritis. Primary, sporadic, fibrinous pneumonia due to pasteurellae, with no epidemiologic connection with mycoplasmal or other pneumonia, may also occur in pigs. In both primary and secondary forms, chronic thoracic lesions and polyarthritis tend to develop. Diagnosis is based on necropsy findings and recovery of pasteurellae from the lesions. Nontoxigenic strains of capsular type A are the predominant isolates from cases of pneumonia. Toxigenic strains of *P multocida*, in the presence of *B bronchiseptica*, are now associated with atrophic rhinitis (p 1223).

Septicemic pasteurellosis and meningitis occasionally occur in piglets. *Mannheimia haemolytica* has been recovered from aborted fetuses, and septicemia may also occur in adult pigs. There are no distinctive lesions, and the pathogenesis is obscure. Porcine strains of *M haemolytica* are often untypeable and do not belong to the common ovine and bovine serotypes. However, some outbreaks in the UK have been associated with close contact with sheep.

Control of the secondary, pneumonic form of the disease is generally based on prevention or control of mycoplasmal pneumonia. Early and vigorous therapy with antibiotics, or in combination with sulfonamides, is indicated to prevent chronic sequelae for all forms of the disease. An increasing resistance to some antibiotics has been noted among the pasteurellae.

PLEUROPNEUMONIA

Pleuropneumonia is a severe and contagious respiratory disease, primarily of young pigs (≤6 mo of age), although in an initial outbreak, adults also may be affected. It has a sudden onset, short course, and high morbidity and mortality. It occurs worldwide and appears to be increasing in incidence, although some reports suggest that severity is declining in countries where it has been long established.

Etiology: The causal organism is *Actinobacillus pleuropneumoniae*. Transmission is mainly by nose-to-nose contact, and many recovered pigs are carriers. Clinical signs develop within 4-12 hr in experimental infections. Aerosol transmission is limited.

Clinical Findings: Onset is sudden, and in herds that have not been infected previously, spread is rapid. Some pigs may be found dead without having shown clinical signs. Respiratory distress is severe; there are "thumps," and sometimes open-mouth breathing with a blood-stained, frothy nasal and oral discharge. Fever up to 107°F (41.5°C), anorexia, and reluctance to move are typical signs.

Although primarily a disease of growing pigs, adults may abort or develop fatal infections. The course of the disease varies from peracute to chronic. Morbidity may reach 50%, and in untreated cases, mortality is high. Survivors generally show reduced growth rates and persistent cough.

Once established in a herd, the disease may be evident only as a cause of reduced growth rate and pleurisy at the abattoir, although acute disease exacerbations may occur. However, severe lesions may not always be accompanied by equally severe clinical signs. Deaths in transit and carcass condemnation may result. Concurrent infection with mycoplasma, pasteurellae, porcine reproductive and respiratory syndrome, or swine influenza virus is common.

Lesions: The pneumonia is usually bilateral. The characteristic lesion is a severe fibrinonecrotic and hemorrhagic pneumonia with accompanying fibrinous pleuritis. Fibrinous pleuritis and pericarditis may be severe. In acute cases, the lungs are dark and swollen and ooze bloody fluid from the cut surface; hemorrhagic, even necrotic, bullae of various sizes may be present. The trachea may contain bloodstained froth. In chronic cases, the lesions are more organized and localized. Extrathoracic lesions are uncommon.

Diagnosis: An explosive disease onset is suggestive and, when combined with clinical signs and gross lesions, often justifies a tentative diagnosis. Concurrent infections, eg, with pasteurellae, may complicate diagnosis. In herds that have been exposed and developed at least a degree of immunity, the pattern may be less distinctive. Many serologic tests, including complement fixation and ELISA, have been used to confirm a herd diagnosis or detect carriers, but results are not always straightforward. A definitive diagnosis depends on isolation and identification of *A pleuropneumoniae*, a gram-negative coccobacillus that requires V factor (NAD) supplementation for growth. A *Staphylococcus aureus* nurse colony can provide the necessary factor.

Treatment and Control: Rapidity of onset and persistence in infected herds makes treatment difficult. Ceftiofur, tetracyclines, synthetic penicillins, tylosin, and sulfonamides have been used. The first treatment should be parenteral, followed by medication given in water or feed, which also may protect contact pigs.

Because survivors frequently remain carriers, control is difficult, although good results are being claimed for some vaccines. Segregated early weaning, "all-in/all-out" management, reduced stocking rates when possible, and improved ventilation are recommended. In herds free of the disease, replacements should be purchased from herds free of *A pleuropneumoniae*; if the disease proves difficult to control, herd depopulation and repopulation should be considered. Serologic testing is an effective means of detecting previously infected herds but may not identify carrier animals.

SWINE INFLUENZA
(Hog flu, Pig flu)

Swine influenza is an acute, highly contagious, respiratory disease that results from infection with type A influenza virus. Field isolates of variable virulence exist, and clinical manifestation may be determined by secondary organisms. Pigs are the principal hosts of classic swine influenza virus. (Human infections have been reported, but porcine strains of influenza A do not appear to easily spread in the human population. However, deaths have occurred in immunocompromised people.) The disease in swine occurs commonly in the midwestern USA (and occasionally in other states), Mexico, Canada, South America, Europe (including the UK, Sweden, and Italy), Kenya, China, Japan, Taiwan, and other parts of eastern Asia.

Etiology: Swine influenza virus (SIV) is an orthomyxovirus of the influenza A group with hemagglutinating antigen H1 and neuraminidase antigen N1 (ie, H1N1). Recently, new subtypes of SIV have been reported (H3N2, H1N2). Influenza B and C viruses have been isolated from pigs but have not caused the classic disease. The classic type A infection with isolates of mild virulence may favor replication of pseudorabies virus (p 1065), *Haemophilus parasuis* (*see* GLÄSSER'S DISEASE, p 576), *Actinobacillus pleuropneumoniae* (p 1197), and *Mycoplasma hyopneumoniae* (p 1197), any of which may complicate outbreaks. The mixing of carrier and nonimmune pigs is an important predisposing factor. The virus is unlikely to survive outside living cells for >2 wk except in cold conditions. It is readily inactivated by disinfectants.

Transmission and Epidemiology: In North America, outbreaks are most common in fall or winter, often at the onset of particularly cold weather. In warmer areas of the world, infection may occur at any time. Usually, an outbreak is preceded by one or two individual cases and then spreads rapidly within a herd, mainly by aerosolization and pig-to-pig contact. The virus survives in carrier pigs for up to 3 mo and can be recovered from clinically normal animals between outbreaks. In antibody-positive herds, outbreaks of infection recur as immunity wanes. Up to 40% of herds may contain antibody-positive pigs. Carrier pigs are usually responsible for the introduction of SIV into previously uninfected herds and countries.

Pathogenesis: The spectrum of infection ranges from subclinical to acute. In the classic acute form, the virus multiplies in bronchial epithelium within 16 hr of infection and causes focal necrosis of the bronchial epithelium, focal atelectasis, and gross hyperemia of the lungs. Bronchial exudates and widespread atelectasis, seen grossly as plum-colored lesions affecting individual lobules of apical and intermediate lobes occur after 24 hr. The lesions continue to develop until 72 hr after infection, after which the virus becomes more difficult to demonstrate. Losses in reproduction associated with primary outbreaks appear to be secondary because virus has been recovered only rarely from the fetus.

Clinical Findings: A classic acute outbreak is characterized by sudden onset and rapid spread through the entire herd, often within 1-3 days. The main signs are depression, fever (to 108°F [42°C]), anorexia, coughing, dyspnea, weakness, prostration, and a mucous discharge from the eyes and nose. Mortality is generally 1-4%. The overt course of the disease is usually 3-7 days in uncomplicated infections, with clinical recovery of the herd almost as sudden as the onset. However, virus may continue to cycle among pigs when clinical signs are suppressed by immune responses. Some pigs may become chronically affected. In herds that are in good condition, the principal economic loss is from stunting and delay in reaching market weight. Some increase in piglet mortality has been reported, and effects on herd fertility, including abortions in late pregnancy, may follow outbreaks in nonimmune herds.

Lesions: In uncomplicated infections, the lesions usually are confined to the chest cavity. The pneumonic areas are clearly demarcated, collapsed, and purplish red. They may be distributed throughout the lungs but tend to be more extensive and confluent ventrally. Nonpneumonic areas are pale and emphysematous. The airways contain a copious mucopurulent exudate, and the bronchial and mediastinal lymph nodes are edematous but rarely congested. There may be severe pulmonary edema, especially of interlobular septae, or a serous or serofibrinous pleuritis. Histologically, the lesions, when fully developed, are primarily those of an exudative bronchiolitis with some interstitial pneumonia.

Diagnosis: A presumptive diagnosis can be made on clinical and pathologic findings, but confirmation depends on isolation of the virus or demonstration of virus-specific antibody. Virus can be isolated from nasal secretions in the febrile phase or from affected lung tissue in the early acute stage. A retrospective diagnosis can be made by demonstrating a rise in virus-specific antibodies in acute and convalescent serum samples, using the hemagglutination inhibition test. Both H3 and H1 subtype antigens should be included. This test is also used for herd surveys. To diagnose uncomplicated influenza infection, conditions such as pasteurellosis, pseudorabies, porcine reproductive and respiratory syndrome, and chlamydial and *Haemophilus* infections must be eliminated.

Treatment and Control: There is no effective treatment, although antimicrobials may reduce secondary bacterial infections. Expectorants may help relieve signs in severely affected herds. Vaccination and strict import controls are the only specific preventive measures. Good management practices and freedom from stress, particularly due to crowding and dust, help reduce losses. Commercially available killed vaccines that contain both H1N2 and H3N2 subtypes appear to induce a strong protective immune response.

RESPIRATORY DISEASES OF SHEEP AND GOATS

The importance of respiratory diseases in sheep and goats depends on their prevalence, their effect on productivity, the value of the animal (commercial stock versus purebred animals or pets), and for some diseases, their international spread (the effects on the import/export market).

Upper Respiratory Tract: Diseases of the upper respiratory tract of sheep and goats include sinusitis caused by the larvae of *Oestrus ovis*, nasal foreign bodies, and nasal tumors. Clinical signs associated with sinusitis may include some or all of the following: unilateral or bilateral, serous to mucopurulent nasal discharge; decreased or absence of airflow through one or both nostrils; coughing; sneezing; and mild to severe respiratory distress. Although tumors in general are rare in sheep and goats, the nasal cavity is one of the more common sites for their occurrence. The types of nasal neoplasms that have been reported include adenopapillomas (nasal polyps), adenomas, adenocarcinomas, lymphosarcomas (goats), and squamous cell carcinomas (sheep). An enzootic adenoma/ adenocarcinoma has been described in goats and sheep. The tumor histologically appears to be benign or of low malignancy and is caused by a retrovirus. A closely related retrovirus induces tumor formation in the lungs of sheep and goats (see PULMONARY ADENOMATOSIS, p 1234). Surgical exploration of the nasal cavity with removal of the tumor mass has been described. Outcome depends on the tumor type, condition of the animal, and extent of the lesion. Surgical removal of a noninvasive tumor in an otherwise healthy animal can be rewarding.

The most common problems associated with the pharynx and larynx are trauma and abscessation. Pharyngeal trauma usually results from overly aggressive use of equipment used to administer oral medication (eg, balling guns, dose syringes, oral speculums, and stomach tubes). Injuries may result in the formation of discrete abscesses or extensive and diffuse cellulitis, both of which can interfere with swallowing and possibly lead to respiratory difficulty or distress. Bacteria commonly isolated after an incident of pharyngeal trauma include *Arcanobacterium (Actinomyces), Pasteurella multocida, Mannheimia (Pasteurella) haemolytica,* and *Fusobacterium.*

Corynebacterium pseudotuberculosis, the causative agent of caseous lymphadenitis (p 52) in sheep and goats may localize in the regional lymph nodes of the head, especially the pharyngeal lymph nodes. Lymph node enlargement may cause clinical signs similar to those described for traumatic pharyngitis.

Lower Respiratory Tract: The most common problem associated with the lower respiratory tract is pneumonia. Pneumonias can be caused by viruses, bacteria, or parasites. They can be acute, chronic, or progressive.

Viruses associated with acute pneumonia include parainfluenza-type 3 (PI-3), adenovirus, and respiratory syncytial virus. These viral pneumonias most often affect lambs and kids. Chronic, progressive viral pneumonia is most common in adults and includes progressive interstitial retroviral pneumonia (in sheep, ovine progressive pneumonia or maedi [p 1233]; in goats, pneumonia induced by arthritis encephalitis virus [p 598]) and pulmonary adenomatosis (p 1234), also known as jaagsiekte or the contagious lung tumor of sheep and, infrequently, of goats.

Chronic, progressive, proliferative changes in the lungs are usually associated with the lentiviruses (family Retroviridae), or so-called slow-virus infections. In both progressive pneumonia and pulmonary adenomatosis, the entire lung can change in a gradual process of cellular proliferation, which results in progressive weight loss and dyspnea.

M haemolytica, P multocida, Mycoplasma spp, *Chlamydia* spp, *Haemophilus* spp, and *Salmonella* spp are associated with either primary or secondary bronchopneumonia in sheep and goats. Both *P multocida* and *M haemolytica* can be cultured from the upper respiratory tract of normal sheep and goats. Not all factors predisposing to acute respiratory diseases are known, but acute viral infections in a susceptible population of sheep can alter the protective mechanisms in the respiratory tract so that certain bacteria may invade lung tissue, multiply, and cause serious disease. A confirmed synergism is an initial infection with PI-3 virus or adenovirus followed by invasion of *M haemolytica,* biotype A. Also, *Mycoplasma ovipneumoniae* alone can cause a mild bronchopneumonia and is often isolated along with *M haemolytica* from sheep and goats with severe pneumonia, suggesting that the *Mycoplasma* may predispose the lung to invasion by this organism. Additionally, introduction of new animals, high-density stocking, poor ventilation, and a low plane of nutrition can act as stress factors that predispose to development of pneumonia.

Caseous lymphadenitis (p 52) caused by *Corynebacterium pseudotuberculosis* may result in abscessation of the lungs and mediastinal lymph nodes. This can result in a progressive debilitation in sheep and goats with or without obvious clinical signs of respiratory disease.

Parasitic or verminous pneumonias of sheep and goats most commonly are caused by infection with *Dictyocaulus filaria, Muellerius capillaris,* or *Protostrongylus rufescens. (See also* LUNGWORM INFECTION, p 1181). In contrast to the acute viral and bacterial pneumonias, which result in a bronchopneumonia affecting the anterior ventral portion of the lungs, verminous pneumonia affects the diaphragmatic lung lobes. *Dictyocaulus* has a direct life cycle, whereas *Protostrongylus* and *Muellerius* have indirect life cycles and rely on a variety of snails and slugs to serve as intermediate hosts. Adult forms of *Dictyocaulus* and *Protostrongylus* live in bronchi and produce clinical signs of coughing, mild to moderate dyspnea, anorexia, depressed milk production, and loss of condition. Adult *Muellerius* live in alveoli and lung parenchymal tissue and are considered the least pathogenic of the 3 lungworms. *Muellerius* appears to cause more problems for goats than for sheep.

Diagnosis of lungworm infection requires Baermann examination of fecal material. *Dictyocaulus* and *Protostrongylus* can be treated effectively with levamisole (8 mg/kg, SC or PO), ivermectin (0.2 mg/kg, SC or PO), fenbendazole (5-10 mg/kg, PO), moxidectin (0.2 mg/kg, PO or SC), or febantel (5 mg/kg, PO). Ivermectin (0.3 mg/kg, SC or PO), fenbendazole (15 mg/kg, PO, administered twice, 3 wk apart), and albendazole (10 mg/kg, PO) have been reported to be effective in treatment of *Muellerius*.

SHEEP NOSE BOT

The sheep nose botfly, *Oestrus ovis*, is a cosmopolitan parasite that, in its larval stages, inhabits the nasal passages and sinuses of sheep and goats. It also has been seen in bighorn sheep (*Ovis canadensis*) and European ibex (*Capra ibex*) and in uncharacteristic hosts such as humans and dogs. While its incidence in some northern European countries has decreased in recent years, it continues to be one of the most widely distributed sheep parasites in South Africa, Brazil, and countries in the Mediterranean basin.

The adult fly is grayish brown and ~12 mm long. The female deposits larvae in and about the nostrils of sheep without alighting. These small, clear-white larvae (initially <2 mm long) migrate into the nasal cavity; many spend at least some time in the paranasal sinuses. As the larvae (bots) mature, they become cream-colored, then darken, and finally show a dark or black band on the dorsal surface of each segment. The larval period, which is usually shortest in young animals, varies from 1-10 mo. When mature, the larvae leave the nasal passages, drop to the ground, burrow down a few inches, and pupate. The pupal period lasts 3-9 wk, depending on the environmental conditions, after which the fly emerges from the pupal case and pushes its way to the surface. Mating soon occurs, and the female begins to deposit larvae.

Clinical Findings: Once the larvae begin to move about in the nasal passages, a profuse discharge occurs, at first clear and mucoid, but later mucopurulent and frequently tinged with fine streaks of blood emanating from minute hemorrhages produced by the hooks and spines of the larvae. Continuing activity of the larvae, particularly if they are numerous, causes a thickening of the nasal mucosa that, together with the mucopurulent discharge, impairs respiration. Paroxysms of sneezing accompany migrations of the larger larvae. Larvae present in the sinuses are sometimes unable to escape; they die and may gradually become calcified or lead to a septic sinusitis. The purulent inflammation produced in the sinuses occasionally may spread to the brain with fatal results. However, the principal effects are annoyance, with a resulting reduction in grazing time, and loss of condition. Usually only 4-15 larvae are found, although ≥80 may be present.

To avoid the fly's attempts at larval deposition, a sheep may run from place to place, keeping its nose close to the ground, and sneeze and stamp its feet or shake its head. Commonly, especially during the warmer hours of the day when the flies are most active, small groups of sheep gather and face the center of a circle, heads down and close together.

Treatment: Ivermectin at 200 µg/kg, PO or SC, is highly effective against all stages of the larvae.

CONTAGIOUS CAPRINE PLEUROPNEUMONIA

Contagious caprine pleuropneumonia is a highly fatal disease that occurs in goats in eastern Europe, the Middle East, Africa, and Asia.

Etiology: *Mycoplasma* biotype F38 causes a highly contagious, lethal disease in goats that most resembles the earlier descriptions of classic contagious caprine pleuropneumonia.

It appears to be transmitted by infective aerosol. Morbidity can be 100%, and mortality 60-100%. Gathering or housing animals together facilitates spread of the disease.

Pneumonia and pleuropneumonia can be caused by the other mycoplasmas, including *M mycoides capri*, and *M mycoides mycoides* large colony type. Morbidity and mortality rates are similar to those for the above-mentioned organism.

Clinical Findings : Weakness, anorexia, cough, hyperpnea, and nasal discharge accompanied by fever (106°F [41°C]) are often found. Exercise intolerance and eventually respiratory distress develop. A septicemic form of the disease without specific respiratory tract involvement has been described.

Lesions: Typically, the thorax contains an excess of straw-colored fluid, and there is acute fibrinous pneumonia with overlying fibrinous pleurisy. Consolidation is sometimes confined to one lung. The degree of distention of interlobular septa by serofibrinous fluid varies. The tendency to form necrotic sequestra is less than in contagious bovine pleuropneumonia, and lesions may resolve slowly in surviving animals. Fibrinous pericarditis, fibrinopurulent arthritis, and meningitis also occur with some infections.

Diagnosis: The clinical signs, epidemiology, and necropsy findings are used to establish a diagnosis. The causative organism should be isolated and identified, but isolation may be difficult and special media is required for culture. The filamentous forms of the mycoplasma can often be detected on darkfield microscopic examination of the pleural fluid from acute cases. Serologic tests are complement fixation, passive hemagglutination, ELISA, and latex slide agglutination. Serologic cross-reactions may occur.

Control: Quarantine of affected flocks is desirable. Vaccines are available in some countries, and good to excellent protection has been reported. Treatment with tylosin at 10 mg/kg, IM, SID for 3 days, has been effective, as has oxytetracycline (15 mg/kg).

PASTEURELLA AND MANNHEIMIA PNEUMONIAS

Bronchopneumonia caused by *Pasteurella multocida* or *Mannheimia haemolytica* has a cranioventral lung distribution and affects sheep and goats of all ages worldwide. It can be particularly devastating in young animals. It is a common cause of morbidity and mortality in lambs and kids, especially in those that have not received adequate colostrum or in which passive colostral immunity is waning. The disease appears to occur most often in animals that have undergone recent stress such as transportation, weaning, or commingling with animals from unrelated farms. (*See also* PASTEURELLOSIS OF SHEEP AND GOATS, p 615.)

Etiology: *P multocida* and *M haemolytica* are gram-negative rods that can cause pneumonia either alone or in conjunction with other organisms. Primary infections with respiratory viruses such as parainfluenza-type 3, adenovirus, and respiratory syncytial virus, or *Mycoplasma* spp appear to predispose to secondary infection with *Pasteurella* and *Mannheimia*. Both organisms are normal inhabitants of the upper respiratory tract of sheep and goats. *M haemolytica* causes most respiratory tract infections. In adult sheep, biotype A, which causes pneumonia, and biotype T, which causes acute septicemia, have been identified. Also, at least 12 serotypes of *M haemolytica* are recognized in sheep.

Pathogenesis: Stress appears to be an important factor in the breakdown of respiratory tract defense mechanisms, allowing *Pasteurella*, *Mannheimia*, *Mycoplasma* spp, other bacteria, and viruses to invade lung tissue and cause pneumonia. In some laboratory animal species and calves, alveolar macrophage function is impaired after viral pneumonia. This results in decreased clearance of inhaled bacterial pathogens, allowing them to become established. Pathogen-host interactions result in tissue damage, especially because of massive influx of neutrophils. As these neutrophils are lysed, enzymes are released that cause more lung tissue damage. This mechanism may be similar to that of *Pasteurella* and *Mannheimia* pneumonias in sheep and goats.

Clinical Findings: Outbreaks in groups of sheep and goats usually occur 10-14 days after a stress. In a feedlot situation, outbreaks are expected ~2 wk after arrival in the feedlot. Early clinical signs may be observation of sudden death in a few animals or a decline in feed consumption within a group. Fever of 104-106°F (40-41.1°C), serous (early) to mucopurulent (later) ocular and nasal discharges, anorexia, coughing, dyspnea, and lethargy are common. Harsh lung sounds, especially in the cranioventral portions of the lung field, may be auscultated. Morbidity and mortality rates are variable.

Lesions: Lesions are usually confined to the cranioventral lung lobes on both sides. These areas may appear red to purple and feel firm from consolidation. The pleural cavity may contain variable amounts of straw-colored fluid, and yellow fibrin may cover the pleural surface of affected lung lobes from pleuritis. Chronic cases may have extensive pleural adhesions and multiple abscesses of variable size.

Diagnosis: In acute cases, cultures obtained from tracheal swabs or washes or from lung lesions will be diagnostic. Histopathologic examination is useful, especially if other types of pneumonia (eg, retrovirus interstitial pneumonia in adult sheep and goats) are also suspected. In chronic cases, bacterial cultures may be less rewarding; *Pasteurella* or *Mannheimia* may have been the initial problem, but results of cultures taken later may reveal *Arcanobacterium pyogenes*, a common causative agent of lung abscesses.

Treatment and Control: Whenever possible, treatment should be based on bacterial culture and sensitivity, especially in herd or flock outbreaks, when valuable animals are involved, or in acute or chronic cases when initial therapeutic attempts have failed. Commonly recommended antibiotics include ceftiofur (1.1-2.2 mg/kg), oxytetracycline (10 mg/kg, SID, of non-long-acting product, or 20 mg/kg once of the long-acting product), ampicillin (20 mg/kg, BID), and tylosin (10-20 mg/kg, SID or BID). Therapy should continue for at least 24-48 hr after body temperature has returned to normal. Duration of treatment usually is 4-5 days. Acute cases may also benefit from the use of NSAID (eg, aspirin, flunixin meglumine, or ketoprofen) in conjunction with antibiotic therapy. Treatment with NSAID should be of short duration because prolonged use may result in gastric ulceration or renal complications. Use of some of the above antibiotics and NSAID is extralabel, and appropriate withdrawal times to slaughter should be followed.

Inadequate ventilation, crowding, commingling of animals from various farms (feedlot or salebarn situations), poor nutrition, failure of passive transfer of antibodies, transportation, and other stresses have all been associated with pneumonia outbreaks. Control and prevention lies with correction of the predisposing factors whenever practical. At present, there are no bacterins that have proved effective for control of these pneumonias.

PROGRESSIVE PNEUMONIA
(Maedi, Zwoegersiekte, La bouhite, Graaff-Reinet disease, Marsh's progressive pneumonia, Ovine progressive pneumonia)

Ovine progressive pneumonia and maedi-visna are chronic diseases of sheep caused by lentiviruses (family Retroviridae) that are structurally and antigenically similar. Progressive pneumonia virus and maedi (meaning "dyspnea") virus induce chronic progressive pneumonias that present with similar clinical signs. Visna (meaning "wasting") is the term used in many parts of the world to refer to the neurologic form of the disease in sheep, resulting in paresis and paralysis. A closely related lentivirus-induced disease in goats, caprine arthritis-encephalitis (CAE, p 598), affects the nervous system and joints. There appears to be a wide variation in reported seroprevalence for lentiviral infection in sheep, ranging from 49% in the western USA to 9% in the north Atlantic region. This variation has been reported in other countries as well and may result from varied climatic conditions (arid vs more lush climates) and management (range conditions vs close confinement). Finnish breeds may have a greater tendency to become infected than other sheep breeds.

Etiology: The causal lentivirus, which persists in lymphocytes, monocytes, and macrophages of infected sheep in the presence of a humoral and cell-mediated immune response, can be detected by several serologic tests. Seropositive sheep and goats must be considered infected and capable of transmitting the virus. Transmission occurs most commonly via the oral route, usually by ingestion of colostrum or milk that contains virus, or by inhalation of infected aerosol droplets. Intrauterine infection is thought to occur infrequently. All breeds of sheep and goats appear susceptible; however, some resistance to lentivirus infection may exist within breeds. Management practices can influence morbidity rates.

Clinical Findings: Signs rarely occur in sheep <2 yr old and are most common in sheep >4 yr old. The disease progresses slowly, with wasting and increasing respiratory distress as the main signs. Coughing, bronchial exudate, depression, and fever are seldom evident unless secondary bacterial infection occurs. A noninflammatory, indurative mastitis (hardbag) may occur. In the encephalitic form (visna), ataxia, muscle tremors, or circling progresses to paresis and eventually to complete paralysis.

Lesions: Macroscopic lesions of progressive pneumonia are confined to the lungs and associated lymph nodes. The lungs do not collapse when the thorax is opened and are abnormally firm and heavy (2-4 times normal weight). Early lung changes may be difficult to detect, but later in the disease, lungs are mottled by gray and brown areas of consolidation. The mediastinal and tracheobronchial lymph nodes are enlarged and edematous. Interstitial pneumonia, perivascular and peribronchial lymphoid hyperplasia, and hypertrophy of smooth muscle are seen throughout the entire lung. CNS lesions, when they occur, are those of meningoleukoencephalitis with secondary demyelination. All lesions are progressive and result from the cellular immune response of the host, and not directly from viral damage.

Diagnosis: Differential diagnoses of progressive pneumonia include pulmonary adenomatosis (jaagsiekte), verminous pneumonia, and pulmonary caseous lymphadenitis. Necropsy with histopathologic examination of affected lung tissue is very useful in differentiating these various types of pneumonias. Listeriosis, scrapie, louping ill, rabies, cerebrospinal nematodiasis, and space-occupying lesions should be considered when the neurologic form (visna) of the disease is seen.

In the live animal, agar gel immunodiffusion and ELISA tests are available. Both tests provide a specificity that approaches 100%. The sensitivities of the tests are reported to range from 10% to almost 100% depending on the laboratory and testing methods used. Despite this wide range, serologic testing is considered a useful tool in detecting infected sheep, especially if the disease has been confirmed in the flock by histopathologic examination or virus isolation. PCR is a very sensitive and specific technique for detecting the presence of virus. However, because of the cost, PCR is not widely used.

Control: Currently, there is no practical, effective treatment and no vaccines are available. Therefore, the only means for control and prevention is serologic testing and removal of positive animals. Because of the long incubation period and time to seroconversion, retesting animals once a year, or even twice a year, is recommended. In addition to the test and cull approach, consideration should be given to raising neonates in isolation from their dams, especially if the dam is seropositive. Lambs should be fed colostrum from seronegative sheep, or heat-treated sheep colostrum, and raised on milk replacer, milk from seronegative ewes, or heat-treated sheep milk.

PULMONARY ADENOMATOSIS
(Jaagsiekte)

Pulmonary adenomatosis is a contagious, viral, neoplastic disease of the lungs of sheep and more rarely of goats. It has been reported from Europe, Asia, Africa, and South and North America.

Etiology: Respiratory exudates from affected sheep are infectious. The causal agent is a type D retrovirus, jaagsiekte sheep retrovirus (JSRV). A closely related retrovirus, enzootic nasal tumor virus induces nasal epithelial neoplasia in sheep and goats (*see* ENZOOTIC ADENOMA /ADENOCARCINOMA, under UPPER RESPIRATORY TRACT, p 1229). Natural transmission seems to occur generally by the respiratory route. Close contact (eg, at feeding troughs) may spread the virus.

Clinical Findings: The period of incubation after natural infection extends over months so that clinical signs generally become evident when sheep are 3-4 yr old.

The tumors produce clinical signs when they become sufficiently large or numerous enough to interfere with respiration. Affected sheep lose weight and show increasing respiratory embarrassment. Moist rales may be heard even without a stethoscope. Coughing is not prominent, and infected animals are usually afebrile unless secondary infection occurs. Forced lowering of the head often causes frothy mucus to run from the nostrils. Clinical disease ends in death after days or weeks, sometimes due to secondary bacterial pneumonia.

Lesions: Tumors are confined to the lungs and, rarely, the associated lymph nodes. They vary from small nodules to extensive solid areas that involve the ventral parts of one or more lobes and that are firm, gray, flat, and sharply demarcated. Copious amounts of white, frothy fluid are present in the air passages. Histologic changes are caused by uncontrolled proliferation of columnar-shaped type II pneumonocytes and similar cells in the bronchioles (Clara cells).

Diagnosis: Chronic weight loss, dyspnea, moist rales, and copious amounts of serous nasal discharge from accumulated lung fluid in an adult sheep that is afebrile are highly suggestive clinical signs of pulmonary adenomatosis. Within a flock, many sheep may be infected, however, only 1 or 2 may show clinical evidence of disease. Currently, histologic examination of affected lung is still the standard used to confirm the disease. Recent advances in the use of PCR show promise in detecting JSRV in blood mononuclear cells in infected sheep before they show clinical signs of disease.

Control: There is no specific treatment or vaccine available. At this time, the best that can be recommended once a diagnosis is confirmed is removal of all animals showing signs suggestive of pulmonary adenomatosis. However, subclinically infected sheep will serve as a reservoir for the virus.

RESPIRATORY DISEASES OF SMALL ANIMALS

Respiratory diseases are common in dogs and cats. Although clinical signs such as coughing and dyspnea are commonly referable to primary problems of the respiratory tract, they may also occur secondary to disorders of other organ systems (eg, congestive heart failure).

Both young and aged animals are at increased risk of developing respiratory disease. At birth, the respiratory and immune systems are incompletely developed; this facilitates the introduction and spread of pathogens within the lungs, and alveolar flooding may occur. In aged animals, chronic degenerative changes that disrupt normal mucociliary clearance and immunologic anergy may render the lungs more vulnerable to airborne pathogens and toxic particulates.

A varying flora of indigenous commensal organisms (including *Pasteurella multocida*, *Bordetella bronchiseptica*, streptococci, staphylococci, pseudomonads, and coliform bacteria) normally reside in the canine and feline nasal passages, nasopharynx, and upper trachea, and at least intermittently in the lungs, without causing clinical signs. Opportunistic infections by these bacteria may occur when respiratory defense mechanisms are compromised by infection with a primary pathogen (eg, distemper, parainfluenza virus, or canine type 2 adenovirus in dogs, and rhinotracheitis virus or calicivirus in cats), other insults (eg, inhalation of smoke or noxious gases), or diseases such as congestive heart failure and pulmonary neoplasia. Secondary bacterial infections complicate the management of viral respiratory infections of both dogs and cats. Pathogens may continue to reside in the respiratory tract of convalescent animals. When stressed, these animals may relapse; they can also act as a source of infection for others. Poor management practices (eg, overcrowding) are often associated with poor hygienic and environmental conditions, and the resultant stress increases both the incidence and severity of infections. Conditions that favor the spread of infections often occur in catteries, kennels, pet shops, boarding facilities, and humane shelters.

Congenital abnormalities, such as stenotic nares, elongation of the soft palate, and tracheal stenosis, can cause respiratory dysfunction. Neoplastic masses, degenerative changes of the airways, and tracheal collapse can result in dyspnea and other clinical manifestations of respiratory disease.

Tracheal collapse is most common in toy and miniature breeds of dogs and rare in cats. The etiology is unknown. Affected animals have a nonproductive, honking, chronic cough, and inspiratory or expiratory dyspnea. Frequently they are obese and may have concurrent cardiovascular or other pulmonary disease (especially chronic bronchitis). Weight loss (if obese) is critical in management. Other measures include exercise restriction, reduction of excitement and stress, and medical therapy, eg, antitussives, antibiotics, bronchodilators, and corticosteroids.

ALLERGIC PNEUMONITIS

Allergic pneumonitis is an acute or chronic hypersensitivity reaction of the lungs and small airways.

Etiology: An underlying etiology is rarely determined in pulmonary hypersensitivity reactions in dogs and cats. Type I or immediate hypersensitivity is probably the most common mechanism, although Type III and IV mechanisms may also be involved (*see* IMMUNOPATHOLOGIC DISEASES, p 648 et seq). The cellular infiltrate is typically eosinophilic; however, mixed inflammatory infiltrates consisting of mononuclear cells, eosinophils, and neutrophils, or predominantly lymphocytic infiltrates can be seen. **Pulmonary infiltration with eosinophilia** (PIE, p 649) is a group of diseases associated with both pulmonary-associated and peripheral eosinophilia. Not all types of allergic pneumonitis, however, are associated with PIE. Causes of PIE include migrating parasites, reaction to microfilariae of heartworms, lungworms, chronic bacterial or fungal infections (eg, histoplasmosis, aspergillosis), viruses, external antigens, and unknown precipitating factors. Canine heartworm (p 100) pneumonitis occurs when dogs become sensitized to microfilariae. A similar reaction may be seen in cats with heartworms. Migrating intestinal parasites and primary lung parasites may induce either subclinical or mild signs of allergic pneumonitis. **Pulmonary nodular eosinophilic granulomatous syndrome** is a rare, severe PIE-like syndrome occurring in dogs and most often associated with heartworm infection. In this condition, a severe granulomatous hypersensitivity reaction to microfilariae (or other antigen) results in mixed alveolar and interstitial pulmonary infiltrates plus variably sized, multiple pulmonary nodules scattered throughout the lung fields. Associated pathology may include eosinophilic granulomatous lymphadenitis, tracheitis, tonsillitis, splenitis, enteritis, gastritis, and pericholangitis. Pulmonary hypersensitivity also may be caused by drugs and reactions to inhaled allergens; however, this is poorly documented in small animals.

Clinical Findings: Chronic cough is the most common sign. It may be mild or severe, productive or nonproductive, and progressive or nonprogressive. Weight loss, tachypnea, dyspnea, wheezing, exercise intolerance, and occasionally hemoptysis may be seen. Severely affected animals may exhibit moderate to severe dyspnea and cyanosis at rest. Auscultation varies from unremarkable to increased breath sounds, crackles, or wheezes. Fever is usually absent. The degree of dyspnea and coughing is related to the severity of inflammation within the airways and alveoli.

Diagnosis: This is based largely on history and on radiographic and clinicopathologic findings. Thoracic radiographs frequently show irregular patchy alveolar infiltrates and increased bronchial and interstitial markings. Radiographic evidence of heartworm disease or parasitic pulmonary disease may suggest an underlying etiology. Typical hematologic changes are mild leukocytosis, variable peripheral eosinophilia (4-50%), and occasionally basophilia. Fecal analysis and an occult heartworm test are indicated when lung parasitism or heartworm disease is suspected. Bronchoalveolar lavage for cytologic analysis, culture, and detection of larval forms is often helpful. In allergic pneumonitis, bronchoalveolar lavage cytology generally reveals a predominance of eosinophils. Bacterial cultures of aseptically collected lavage specimens are commonly negative.

Treatment: When an underlying cause can be found, elimination of the offending agent and a short-term course of glucocorticoids resolves the problem. Prednisolone beginning at 1-2 mg/kg body wt, PO, and tapered over 10-14 days is often sufficient. When PIE is secondary to heartworm disease or pulmonary parasites, treatment with prednisolone before or during treatment for the parasite controls the pulmonary signs. When an underlying etiology cannot be determined, prolonged therapy with prednisolone for 3 wk to 3 mo is often required. When severe bronchoconstriction is suspected, bronchodilators or β_2-agonists may be helpful. Severely dyspneic animals may require short-term oxygen therapy.

CANINE NASAL MITES

The canine nasal mite, *Pneumonyssoides caninum*, has been reported worldwide including the USA, Canada, Japan, Australia, South Africa, Italy, France, Spain, Norway, Sweden, Finland, Denmark, and Iran.

Etiology and Epidemiology: *P caninum* is known as the canine nasal mite, and has also been reported in a silver fox. There does not seem to be a breed, age, or sex predilection, although one report suggested that dogs >3 yr of age were affected more often and that large breed dogs had a higher incidence than small breed dogs.

The mites live in the nasal passages and paranasal sinuses. The complete life cycle of the *P caninum* is not known or understood. Transmission is thought to be via direct and indirect contact between dogs. There is no evidence to suggest that this organism presents a zoonotic risk.

Clinical Findings: The most common clinical signs associated with nasal mite infestation include epistaxis, sneezing, reverse sneezing, impaired scenting ability, facial pruritus, and nasal discharge, dyspnea, collapse, head shaking, and stridor. Other clinical signs include coughing, restlessness, and collapse. These signs are not specific for nasal mite infection and may indicate many types of upper respiratory disease.

Diagnosis: Differential diagnoses based on the clinical signs include many upper respiratory diseases such as rhinitis (idiopathic, secondary bacterial, or fungal), oral/nasal neoplasia, dental disease (oral nasal fistula), nasal foreign body, or laryngeal paralysis. To rule out concurrent systemic disease, a CBC, serum chemistry profile, and urinalysis should be performed. If epistaxis is present, a one-stage prothrombin time (OSPT), partial thromboplastin time (PTT), and buccal mucosal bleeding time should be considered. An alternative to the OSPT and PTT is the activated clotting time.

Imaging of the nasal chambers via nasal/dental radiographs should be considered. A laryngeal examination may also be indicated if clinical signs are suggestive of disease of the larynx. Alternative imaging modalities such as computed tomography provide excellent images of the nasal cavity and paranasal sinuses. More invasive diagnostic procedures such as rhinoscopy, nasal flushing, and nasal biopsy must be delayed until after imaging, as iatrogenic changes may be hard to distinguish from primary disease.

Rhinoscopy and nasal flushing are the most useful diagnostic tools. Flexible rhinoscopes allow observation of the nasal choanae. This area is best visualized by putting a u-bend in the rhinoscope (retroflexed view) and advancing it into the oral cavity until it can be hooked under the soft palate. Gentle traction is applied, and the endoscopist can view the nasal choanae or the caudal nasal passages as they enter the nasopharynx. Some authors have described flooding the nasal chambers with anesthetic gas or oxygen to encourage the mites to migrate toward the nasopharynx and the endoscope.

Nasal flushing may also be beneficial in identifying *P caninum*. This is generally performed with the patient under general anesthesia with a cuffed endotracheal tube in place. It can be accomplished by packing the oropharynx with gauze and flushing saline through the external nares with a Foley catheter or a tight-fitting syringe and collecting fluid from the oropharynx. Retrograde flushing can be done by placing a modified catheter behind the soft palate, occluding the nasal pharynx, and flushing with saline. This allows fluid to be collected via the external nares. In both cases, the fluid should be evaluated using an illuminated magnifying lens to look for mites.

The definitive diagnosis of nasal ascariasis can be made via endoscopy or nasal flushing if the mites are identified. This does not, however, determine whether the disease is primary or secondary.

Treatment: There are currently no drugs approved for the treatment of *P caninum*; however, both ivermectin (200-400 µg/kg, SC or PO) and milbemycin oxime (1 mg/kg, PO, 3 times at 10-days intervals) have been suggested. The optimal treatment regimen has yet to be determined. Treatment has been reported to be effective in >85% of cases and the prognosis is excellent. Treatment may not completely eliminate clinical signs, however (particularly if infection is suspected rather than demonstrated). In these cases, it is probable that the signs are the result of a concurrent upper airway disease. Most cases are treated based on definitive diagnosis, but empirical therapy has also been performed based on a high index of suspicion.

FELINE RESPIRATORY DISEASE COMPLEX

Feline respiratory disease complex includes those illnesses typified by rhinosinusitis, conjunctivitis, lacrimation, salivation, and oral ulcerations. The principal diseases, feline viral rhinotracheitis (FVR) and feline calicivirus (FCV) infections, affect exotic as well as domestic species. Feline pneumonitis (*Chlamydophila [Chlamydia] psittaci*) and mycoplasmal infections appear to be of lesser importance. Feline infectious peritonitis and pleuritis (p 628) typically causes a more generalized condition but may cause signs of mild upper respiratory tract infection.

FVR and caliciviruses are host-specific and pose no known human risk. Human conjunctivitis caused by the feline chlamydial agent has been reported.

Etiology: Probably 45-50% of feline upper respiratory infections are caused by FVR virus, which is a herpesvirus; incidence of FCV is similar. Dual infections with these viruses are common. Other organisms such as *C psittaci, Mycoplasma* spp, and reoviruses are believed to account for most of the remaining infections.

Natural transmission of these agents occurs via aerosol droplets and fomites, which can be carried to a susceptible cat by a handler. Convalescent cats may harbor virus for many months. Calicivirus is shed continuously, while infectious FVR virus is released intermittently. Stress may precipitate a secondary course of illness. The incubation period is 2-6 days for FVR and FCV, and 5-10 days for pneumonitis.

Clinical Findings: The onset of FVR is marked by fever, frequent sneezing, conjunctivitis, rhinitis, and often salivation. Excitement or movement may induce sneezing. The fever may reach 105°F (40.5°C) but subsides and tends to fluctuate from normal to 103°F (39°C). Initially, a serous nasal and ocular discharge occurs; it soon becomes mucopurulent and copious, at which time depression and anorexia are evident. Severely debilitated cats may develop ulcerative stomatitis, and ulcerative keratitis occurs in some. Signs may persist for 5-10 days in milder cases and up to 6 wk in severe cases. Generally, the mortality is low and prognosis good except for young kittens and aged cats. The illness often is prolonged, and weight loss may be marked. FVR often is complicated by secondary bacterial infections; abortions and generalized infections also have been associated with it.

There are many serologically related strains of feline caliciviruses. They appear to have a predilection for the epithelium of the oral cavity and the deep tissues of the lungs. Some caliciviruses are nonpathogenic. Some induce little more than salivation and ulceration of the tongue, hard palate, or nostrils; others produce pulmonary edema and interstitial pneumonia. Clinically, it is often impossible to differentiate FVR from FCV infection. Two strains may produce a transient "limping syndrome" without signs of oral ulceration or pneumonia. These strains produce a transient fever, alternating leg lameness, and pain on palpation of affected joints. Signs occur most often in 8- to 12-wk-old kittens and usually resolve without treatment. The syndrome may occur in kittens vaccinated against FCV because no vaccine protects against both of the strains that produce the "limping syndrome."

Calicivirus has also been found in cats with lymphocytic-plasmacytic gingivitis and stomatitis (p 308). The superficial lesions heal rapidly, and the infected cat regains appetite 2-3 days after onset. The clinical course usually is 7-10 days. An acute febrile response, inappetence, and depression are common signs. Serous rhinitis and conjunctivitis also can occur.

C psittaci infections characteristically produce conjunctivitis (p 406); infected cats sneeze occasionally. Fever may occur as the disease progresses beyond serous lacrimal discharge to mucopurulent conjunctivitis, lymphoid infiltration, and epithelial hyperplasia. Convalescent cats may undergo relapses.

Mycoplasma may infect the eyes and upper respiratory passages, characteristically producing severe edema of the conjunctiva and a less severe rhinitis.

The occurrence of severe viral upper respiratory disease is rare in adult, properly vaccinated cats. These cats should be tested for other upper respiratory diseases and, less commonly, concurrent immunodeficiency diseases, including feline leukemia virus and feline immunodeficiency virus.

Lesions: Lesions generally are confined to the respiratory tract, conjunctivae, and oral cavity. In FVR, the conjunctivae and nasal mucous membranes are reddened, swollen, and covered with a serous to purulent exudate. In severe cases, focal necrosis of these membranes may occur. The larynx and trachea may be mildly inflamed. The lungs may be congested, with small areas of consolidation; however, pulmonary changes are rarely remarkable in FVR except possibly in stressed, young kittens. The characteristic histologic lesion of FVR is the acidophilic intranuclear inclusion body. During the early stage of the illness, inclusions may be present in sites of epithelial necrosis on the tongue, nasal membranes, tonsils, epiglottis, trachea, and nictitating membranes. Inclusion bodies are transitory. Inclusions are not seen in calicivirus infections.

The characteristic lesion caused by FCV is ulceration of the oral mucosa. Lesions on the tongue or hard palate initially may appear as vesicles, which subsequently rupture. Ulcerations are occasionally found on the epithelium covering the median nasal septum. The more virulent caliciviruses destroy epithelial cells of the bronchioles and alveoli, which causes acute pulmonary edema that progresses through seropurulent bronchiolar hyperplasia and interstitial pneumonia.

Early in the clinical course of feline pneumonitis, the causative organism may be identified in Giemsa-stained conjunctival smears or scrapings. The elementary bodies are intracytoplasmic. Mycoplasmas occur as extracellular coccoid bodies often seen on the surface of conjunctival epithelial cells.

Diagnosis: The presumptive diagnosis is based on such typical signs as sneezing, conjunctivitis, rhinitis, lacrimation, salivation, oral ulcers, and dyspnea. FVR tends to affect the conjunctivae and nasal passages, caliciviruses the oral mucosa and lower respiratory tract. Chlamydial infections result in chronic, low-grade conjunctivitis. These characteristics may be obscured in mixed infections. Cytologic examination of Giemsa-stained conjunctival scrapings is of value for the identification of chlamydiae and mycoplasmas. A definitive diagnosis is based on isolation and identification of the agent. The oropharyngeal mucosa, external nares, and conjunctival sacs are the preferred sampling sites. However, diagnosis of FVR may be difficult due to intermittant shedding of virus and to similar seroprevalence and virus isolation rates in ill and clinically normal cats.

Treatment: Treatment is largely symptomatic and supportive, but broad-spectrum antibiotics are useful against secondary bacterial invaders (eg, amoxicillin with clavulanic acid, cephalosporins, trimethoprim/sulfa, fluoroquinolones, chloramphenicol) as well as directly against *C psittaci*. Tetracyclines are the most effective against *C psittaci*. Nasal and ocular discharges should be removed frequently for the comfort of the cat. Nebulization or saline nose drops may aid in the removal of tenacious secretions. Nose drops containing a vasoconstrictor (eg, 2 drops of ephedrine sulfate [0.25% solution] in each nostril, BID) and antibiotics may be helpful in reducing the amount of nasal exudate. Prolonged use of nasal decongestants, however, may result in rebound nasal congestion and worsening of clinical signs. A bland ophthalmic ointment containing antibiotics (tetracyclines in *C psittaci* infections) is indicated 5-6 times daily to prevent corneal irritation produced by dried exudate. If corneal ulcers occur in FVR infections (herpetic keratitis), ophthalmic preparations containing idoxuridine or acyclovir are indicated in addition to other antibiotic ophthalmic preparations. Lysine (250 mg, PO, BID-TID) interferes with herpetic viral replication and may reduce the severity of FVR infection. If dyspnea is severe, the cat can be placed in an oxygen tent. Fluids may be indicated to correct dehydration, and force-feeding may be necessary. Esophagostomy and gavage may be appropriate for alimentation of severely debilitated cats. Antihistamines (eg, chlorpheniramine maleate, PO, BID [8 mg for adults, 4 mg for kittens]) may be beneficial early in the course of the disease.

Prevention: Two types of modified live virus FVR-FCV vaccines are available. The first type is intended for parenteral administration; cats >9 wk old should be vaccinated twice, with a 3-wk interval. Kittens should be vaccinated at intervals of 3-4 wk until they are ≥12 wk old. In adult cats, revaccination with a single dose every 1-3 yr is indicated.

The second type of vaccine is administered to healthy cats by instillation into the conjunctival cul-de-sacs and nasal passages. Owners should be advised that cats inoculated oronasally may sneeze frequently at 4-7 days after vaccination. Kittens vaccinated when <12 wk old should be revaccinated on reaching this age. Annual revaccination with a single dose is recommended.

Modified live virus FVR-FCV vaccines intended for parenteral administration are available in combination with either chemically inactivated or modified live virus feline panleukopenia vaccines. A parenterally administered vaccine composed entirely of inactivated viruses also is available.

Vaccines containing either chick-embryo- or cell-line-origin *C psittaci* are administered parenterally. A single dose is recommended for cats >12 wk old; younger kittens should be revaccinated when they reach 16 wk. All should be revaccinated annually. These vaccines are indicated in catteries or on premises where *C psittaci* infection has been confirmed. The chlamydial vaccines are available in combination with FVR-FCV and panleukopenia vaccines. Systematic vaccination and control of environmental factors (such as exposure to sick cats, overcrowding, and stress) provide good protection against upper respiratory disease.

LUNG FLUKES

Paragonimus kellicotti and *P westermani* usually are found in cysts, primarily in the lungs of dogs, cats, and several other domestic and wild animals. They also have been found rarely in other viscera or the brain. Infection is most common in China, southeast Asia, and North America. *P westermani* is a parasite of humans and other animals in China and other countries in the Far East.

The adults are fleshy, reddish brown, oval, and ~14 × 7 mm. The eggs are golden brown, oval, distinctly operculated, and ~100 × 60 μm. The eggs pass through the cyst wall, are coughed up, swallowed, and passed in the feces. The life cycle includes several snails as the first intermediate host and crayfish or crabs as the second. Dogs and cats become infected by eating raw crayfish or crabs that contain the encysted cercariae. After penetrating the intestinal wall and wandering in the peritoneal cavity, the young flukes pass through the diaphragm to the lungs where they become established.

Infected animals may have a chronic, deep, intermittent cough and eventually become weak and lethargic, although many infections pass unnoticed. Finding the characteristic eggs in feces or sputum is diagnostic. The location in the lungs is ascertained by radiography. Aberrant infections can be identified serologically.

Daily administration of bithional for 1 wk or every other day for 1 mo is an effective treatment. Fenbendazole (25-50 mg/kg, PO, BID for 14 days) or albendazole (25 mg/kg, PO, BID for 21 days) also are valuable treatments for reducing the number of eggs deposited and eventually killing the parasites. Praziquantel (25 mg/kg, PO, TID for 3 days) may also be effective in eliminating lung flukes in dogs.

LUNG NEMATODES
See also LUNGWORM INFECTION, p 1181.

Aelurostrongylus abstrusus

Aelurostrongylus abstrusus, the most common lungworm of cats, is found in many parts of the world, including the USA, Europe, and Australia. They are small parasites (males 7 mm, females 10 mm), deeply embedded in the lung tissues. The eggs are forced into alveolar ducts and adjacent alveoli where they form small nodules and hatch. Once the larvae escape, they are coughed up, swallowed, and passed in the feces. The larvae seen in the feces of infected animals are tightly coiled, have an undulating tail with a spine, and are <400 µm long. The life cycle includes snails or slugs as first intermediate hosts, and frogs, lizards, birds, or rodents as transport hosts of encysted larvae. When one of these transport hosts is eaten, the larvae migrate from the stomach to the lungs via the peritoneal and thoracic cavities. They reach the lungs within 24 hr and are seen in the feces in ~1 mo.

Although prevalence can be high, clinical and diagnostic signs are often lacking. Chronic wasting, cough, dyspnea, and pulmonary wheezes may be seen. The lungs usually have solidified, gray, raised nodules 1-10 mm in diameter; generalized alveolar disease has been seen in chronic cases. Treatment is difficult and not often necessary, but fenbendazole (50 mg/kg, PO, BID for 10-14 days) or ivermectin (400 µg/kg, SC, once) may be effective.

Capillaria aerophila

Although usually parasites of the frontal sinuses, trachea, bronchi, and rarely nasal cavities of foxes, *Capillaria aerophila* are found in dogs and other carnivores. They are 25-35 mm long. The females produce eggs with bipolar plugs that resemble those of whipworms; however, their shells are colorless to greenish and pitted. The eggs are laid in the lungs, coughed up and swallowed, and passed in the feces. The eggs can be identified from either tracheal washes and bronchoalveolar lavage or fecal flotation. The life cycle is direct; dogs become infected through consumption of feed or water contaminated with larvated eggs. After hatching in the intestine, the larvae reach the lungs and bronchi via the circulatory system. They mature ~40 days after infection. Clinical signs include coughing, sneezing, and nasal discharge. Treatment may be attempted through extended administration of fenbendazole (50 mg/kg, PO, BID for 10-14 days) or with ivermectin (300-400 µg/kg, SC, once).

Filarids

Oslerus (Filaroides) osleri are tracheal worms of dogs, usually found in thin-walled nodules around the bronchial bifurcation. They have been found in the USA, South Africa, New Zealand, India, Great Britain, France, and Australia. The males are ~5 mm long, and the females 10-15 mm. The life cycle is direct, and an infected bitch can transfer larvae in her saliva to her pups while licking and cleaning them. On ingestion, the larvae pass to the blood and are carried to the lungs and bronchi.

A persistent, dry cough is the most common clinical sign. Coughing may later become severe with respiratory distress. Finding larvae in the feces is diagnostic, but because these larvae are lethargic and few in number, bronchoscopy is a better method. Surgical excision of the nodules, combined with administration of fenbendazole, levamisole, or thiabendazole has been effective in treating infected dogs. Chemotherapy alone can be successful but does not always give a complete cure.

Filaroides hirthi is similar to *O osleri* but is found in the lung parenchyma. The females are oviparous. Adults are found in nests in the lung parenchyma, where a focal granulomatous reaction occurs. Diagnosis of low-grade infection can be difficult. Zinc sulfate flotation is usually more successful than using a Baermann apparatus. Treatment with fenbendazole (50 mg/kg, PO, SID for 14 days) or albendazole (50 mg/kg, PO, BID for 5 days and repeated in 21 days) has been reported to be effective.

NEOPLASIA OF THE RESPIRATORY SYSTEM

Tumors of the Nose and Paranasal Sinuses

Tumors of the nose and paranasal sinuses account for 1-2% of all canine or feline tumors. The incidence in dogs is twice that in cats; incidence is also higher in males of both species than in females. The mean age at time of diagnosis is 10.5 yr for dogs and 12 yr for cats. In dogs, 80% of these tumors are malignant, and 60-70% are carcinomas, of which adenocarcinoma is the most common. In dogs, the ethmoturbinates tend to be the site of predilection. Dolichocephalic and mesocephalic breeds appear to be at higher risk than brachycephalic breeds. In cats, 90% of nasal tumors are malignant, the most common being carcinomas and lymphomas. Tumors of the nose and paranasal sinuses typically are very invasive locally and metastasize infrequently; metastasis is more likely in carcinomas and usually occurs late in the disease. Common sites of metastasis are regional lymph nodes, lungs, and brain. Invasion of the paranasal sinuses tends to be greater in dogs than in cats. In general, if untreated, survival is 3-5 mo after diagnosis.

Chronic nasal discharge is the most common clinical finding; it may be mucoid, mucopurulent, or serosanguinous. Initially, discharge is unilateral but often becomes bilateral. Periodic sneezing, epistaxis, and respiratory stertor may occur. Facial and oral deformities result from destruction of bony or soft-tissue sinonasal structures. Retrobulbar extension of these tumors results in exophthalmos and exposure keratitis. Secondary epiphora may occur if the nasolacrimal duct is blocked. Late in the disease, CNS signs (eg, disorientation, blindness, seizures, stupor, and coma) may develop if the tumor extends into the cranial vault.

Diagnosis is based on history and clinical findings and elimination of other causes of nasal discharge, sneezing, or facial deformation. Nasal radiographs or computed tomography typically show increased density of the nasal cavity and frontal sinuses as well as evidence of bone destruction. Computed tomography is vastly superior to plain radiography in diagnosis of chronic nasal diseases. Definitive diagnosis is based on biopsy of tumor tissue.

Treatment largely depends on tumor type and extent of disease. The treatment of choice for canine nasal adenocarcinoma is radiation therapy. Aggressive surgical excision, chemotherapy, radiation therapy, or combinations for other tumor types afford a more favorable prognosis when diagnosis is made early.

Tumors of the Larynx and Trachea

Tumors of the larynx and trachea are rare in dogs and cats. Tumors of the larynx most frequently reported in dogs are oncocytoma, squamous cell carcinoma, mast cell tumor, melanoma, and osteosarcoma; in cats, they are squamous cell carcinoma, lymphosarcoma, and adenocarcinoma. Benign inflammatory polyps of the larynx also occur in dogs and cats. Tumors of the trachea are particularly rare. Osteochondral dysplasia of the trachea (osteochondroma) is a benign tumor of the trachea primarily seen in dogs <1 yr old. Other benign mesenchymal tumors, carcinomas, and sarcomas are occasionally seen.

The most common signs of tumors of the larynx include inspiratory dyspnea, stridor, voice change (hoarse bark or loss of voice), coughing, and exertional dyspnea. Findings typically associated with tumors of the trachea are coughing, dyspnea, stridor, and rarely hemoptysis. Both laryngeal and tracheal tumors may be associated with signs of fixed upper airway obstruction (inspiratory and expiratory dyspnea). The degree of dyspnea often relates to the degree of luminal obstruction.

Diagnosis is made from the history and clinical findings and by eliminating other causes of upper airway obstruction or coughing. The tumor mass may be seen on laryngoscopy or tracheoscopy. Definitive diagnosis is made on biopsy.

Surgical excision and resection is the treatment of choice. Radiation therapy may be palliative for radiosensitive tumors such as squamous cell carcinoma, mast cell tumor, and lymphoma. Surgical resection of tracheal osteochondral dysplasia in dogs is curative.

Primary Lung Tumors

Primary lung tumors are rare in dogs and cats; however, the reported incidence of lung carcinomas has increased at least 100% during the last 20 yr. This is attributed to an increased average life span, better detection and awareness, or, possibly, increasing exposure to environmental carcinogens. Most primary lung tumors are diagnosed at a mean age of 10-12 yr in dogs and 12 yr in cats. There is no consistent breed or sex predilection in either species. Primary lung tumors usually originate from the terminal bronchioles and alveoli; they occasionally occur as a second coincidental tumor, which may make the differentiation between primary and metastatic disease difficult. Of the primary lung tumors in dogs and cats, ≥80% are malignant. Adenocarcinoma and anaplastic carcinoma are the most common types in dogs and cats. Primary lung sarcomas and adenomas are rare in both species. Metastatic spread of primary lung tumors is generally to other areas of the lungs, tracheobronchial lymph nodes, bone, and brain. Intrapulmonary spread via the airways occurs in ~50% of dogs with adenocarcinoma. Metastatic spread to the pleurae, pericardium, heart, and diaphragm may occur; miscellaneous extrathoracic sites include liver, spleen, and kidney. Dogs with papillary (bronchoalveolar) adenocarcinoma have a better prognosis than those with other lung tumors; however, histologic grade and detection of clinical signs are the most important determinants of prognosis and survival. Both recurrence and metastasis tend to occur earlier and with greater frequency in dogs with moderately or poorly differentiated tumors.

Clinical Findings: Primary lung tumors have variable manifestations, which depend on the location of tumor, rapidity of tumor growth, presence of previous or concurrent pulmonary disease, and awareness of the owner. Common signs include cough, inappetence, weight loss, reduced exercise tolerance, lethargy, tachypnea, dyspnea, wheezing, vomiting or regurgitation, pyrexia, and lameness. The most common clinical finding in dogs is a chronic, nonproductive cough. Coughing is uncommon in cats; nonspecific signs, such as inappetence, weight loss, and tachypnea and dyspnea, are more common. In either species, tachypnea or dyspnea indicates massive tumor burden or pleural effusion. Pleural effusion is particularly common in cats with primary lung tumors. Lameness may be due to hypertrophic osteopathy (unusual in cats) or to metastasis to bone or skeletal muscle. Thoracic auscultation may be normal, reflect increased breath sounds compatible with pulmonary airway disease, or be muffled due to pulmonary consolidation or pleural effusion.

Diagnosis: One-third or more of primary lung tumors are recognized incidentally during radiography for other problems, or at necropsy. Thoracic radiographs are essential for a tentative diagnosis in those animals exhibiting compatible clinical signs. Primary lung tumors in dogs may occur as single or multiple circumscribed mass lesions, as a diffuse lung pattern, or as a lobar consolidation. In cats, single circumscribed mass lesions are less common, whereas a diffuse lung pattern or lobar consolidation is more frequent. Pleural fluid accumulation is common in cats and less frequent in dogs. In either species, chest wall involvement and hilar lymphadenopathy may be seen. Tentative diagnosis can be made by ruling out other causes of pulmonary disease with similar radiographic lung patterns. Definitive diagnosis requires biopsy.

Treatment: Surgical resection of tumor via lobectomy of diseased lung lobes is the treatment of choice. Inoperable lesions or metastatic disease may be controlled with chemotherapy. Mean survival time for operable solitary, well-differentiated, primary lung tumors without node involvement in dogs is 15-26 mo; if the lymph nodes are involved or multiple tumors are found at the time of diagnosis, survival time is shortened. Recurrence or metastasis of tumor is a common cause of death.

Metastatic Tumors of the Lungs

A localized tumor may extend to the lungs by dissemination through hematogenous or lymphatic routes or by direct extension of tumor cells. Certain primary tumors, such as mammary adenocarcinoma, osteosarcoma, hemangiosarcoma, and oral melanoma, most commonly metastasize to the lungs. The lungs may be the only site of metastasis, or there may be concurrent metastasis in other organs; in the former, the diagnostic approach is to identify an occult primary tumor or to carefully review the medical history for disclosure of previous tumor removal. Because pulmonary metastasis occurs late in the clinical course of a malignant tumor, prognosis is poor.

The signs of metastatic pulmonary disease are similar to those of primary lung tumors except that coughing is less common. Severity of signs depends on the anatomic location of the tumor and whether the lesions are solitary or multiple.

The diagnosis is similar to that for primary lung tumors. Because of the limitations of routine radiography, small lesions (≤3 mm in diameter), which are present in ≥40% of cases with pulmonary metastasis, may not be seen.

Radiography of the chest should precede removal of tumors with a known high incidence of metastatic spread to the lungs. The major goal of cancer therapy is prevention of metastasis rather than its eradication. Slow-growing or solitary metastatic lesions are best treated by surgical excision. Chemotherapy or radiation therapy may be useful with certain tumor types not amenable to surgical resection. Overall, the prognosis for animals with pulmonary metastasis is poor.

PNEUMONIA

Pneumonia is an acute or chronic inflammation of the lungs and bronchi characterized by disturbance in respiration and hypoxemia and complicated by the systemic effects of associated toxins. The usual cause is primary viral infection of the lower respiratory tract.

Canine distemper virus, adenovirus types 1 and 2, parainfluenza virus, and feline calicivirus cause lesions in the distal airways and predispose to secondary bacterial invasion of the lungs. Parasitic invasion of the bronchi, as by *Filaroides*, *Aelurostrongylus*, or *Paragonimus* spp may result in pneumonia. Protozoan involvement, eg, by *Toxoplasma gondii* (p 547), is rarely seen. Tuberculous pneumonia, although uncommon, is seen more often in dogs than in cats. The incidence of mycotic granulomatous pneumonias is also higher in dogs than in cats. Cryptococcal pneumonia has been described in cats. Injury to the bronchial mucosa and inhalation or aspiration of irritants may cause pneumonia directly and predispose to secondary bacterial invasion. Aspiration pneumonia (p 1176) may result from persistent vomiting, abnormal esophageal motility, or improperly administered medications (eg, oil or barium) or food (forced feeding); it may also follow suckling in a neonate with a cleft palate.

Clinical Findings: The initial signs are usually those of the primary disease. Lethargy and anorexia are common. A deep cough is noted. Progressive dyspnea, "blowing" of the lips, and cyanosis may be evident, especially on exercise. Body temperature is increased moderately, and there may be leukocytosis. Auscultation usually reveals consolidation, which may be patchy but more commonly is diffuse. In the later stages of pneumonia, the increased lung density and peribronchial consolidation caused by the inflammatory process can be visualized radiographically. Complications such as pleuritis, mediastinitis, or invasion by opportunistic organisms may occur.

Diagnosis: Analysis of bronchoalveolar lavage fluid is valuable for the diagnosis of bacterial infections. Cytologic examination can demonstrate the animal's immune response and indicate the intracellular or extracellular location of bacteria. Bacterial culture and sensitivity testing is required and may include anaerobe and mycoplasma culture, especially in refractory cases. A viral etiology generally results in an initial body temperature of 104-106°F (40-41°C). Leukopenia, often expected, may not be seen in many viral respiratory infections (eg, canine infectious tracheobronchitis, feline calicivirus pneumonia, feline infectious peritonitis pneumonia). A history of recent anesthesia or severe vomiting indicates the possibility of aspiration pneumonia. Acutely affected animals may die within 24-48 hr of onset. Mycotic pneumonias are usually chronic in nature. Miliary nodules seen at necropsy may suggest protozoal pneumonia.

Treatment: The animal should be placed in a warm, dry environment. Anemia, if present, should be corrected. If cyanosis is severe, oxygen therapy may be used, administered by means of an oxygen cage, with a concentration of 30-50%. Empirical antimicrobial chemotherapy should be initiated and changed if needed based on results of culture of bronchoalveolar lavage fluid. Supportive therapy should be instituted as needed and may include oxygen supplementation, pulmonary physiotherapy (nebulization and coupage), and bronchodilators. If no response is seen after 48-72 hr of therapy, the treatment plan should be reassessed. Antimicrobial chemotherapy should be continued 1 wk after clinical and radiographic signs resolve.

Animals should be reexamined frequently. Chest radiographs should be repeated at regular intervals to monitor recurrence or note a primary underlying disease process and to detect complications such as lung consolidation, atelectasis, or abscessation.

RHINITIS AND SINUSITIS

Inflammation of the mucous membranes of the nose and sinuses may be acute or chronic.

Etiology: Viral infection is the most common cause of acute rhinitis or sinusitis in dogs and cats. Feline viral rhinotracheitis (FVR), feline calicivirus (FCV), canine distemper, canine adenovirus types 1 and 2, and canine parainfluenza are most frequently incriminated. Chronic states exist for FVR and FCV, with intermittent shedding associated with stress. Bacterial rhinitis or sinusitis frequently is a secondary complication. Primary bacterial rhinitis is extremely rare in dogs and cats. It may result from infection with *Bordetella bronchiseptica* in dogs. Allergic rhinitis or sinusitis is a poorly defined atopy that occurs seasonally in association with pollen production, and perennially, probably in association with house dusts and molds. Smoke aspiration, inhalation of irritant gases, or foreign bodies lodged in the nasal passages also may cause acute rhinitis.

Chronic rhinitis is commonly complicated by secondary bacterial infection because the primary nasal disease results in increased mucus production and altered mucociliary clearance of debris within the nose. Underlying causes of chronic rhinitis include chronic inflammatory disease (lymphoplasmacytic rhinitis), trauma, parasites (*Cuterebra*), foreign bodies, neoplasia, or mycotic infection. In cats, chronic rhinosinusitis is a frequent sequela of acute viral infections of the nasal and sinus mucosa that result in hyperplastic glandular and epithelial changes. Rhinitis or sinusitis may result when an apical tooth root abscess extends into the maxillary recess. Mycotic rhinosinusitis may be caused by *Cryptococcus neoformans*, *Aspergillus* spp, and *Penicillium* spp. Cats are more often affected with *Cryptococcus* spp than dogs, whereas aspergillosis is frequent in dogs but rare in cats.

Clinical Findings: Acute rhinitis is characterized by nasal discharge, sneezing, pawing at the face, respiratory stertor, open-mouth breathing, and/or inspiratory dyspnea. Lacrimation and conjunctivitis often accompany inflammation of the upper respiratory passages. Affected tissues are often hyperemic and edematous. The nasal discharge is serous but becomes mucoid as a result of secondary bacterial infection. If inflammatory cells infiltrate the mucosa, the discharge may become mucopurulent. Sneezing, in an attempt to clear the upper airways of discharge or exudate, is seen most frequently in acute rhinitis and tends to be intermittent in chronic rhinitis. Aspiration reflex ("reverse sneeze"), a short paroxysmal episode of inspiratory effort in an attempt to clear the nasopharynx of obstructing material, may also be seen. Respiratory stertor, open-mouth breathing, and inspiratory dyspnea occur when the nasal passages are narrowed from inflamed mucosa, glandular elements, and secretions. An acute unilateral nasal discharge, possibly accompanied by pawing at the face, suggests a foreign body. Neoplastic or mycotic disease is suggested by a chronic nasal discharge that was initially unilateral but becomes bilateral or that changes in character from mucopurulent to serosanguineous or hemorrhagic.

Diagnosis: Diagnosis is based on history, physical examination, radiographic findings, (especially computed tomography), rhinoscopy, nasal biopsy, and elimination of other causes of nasal discharge and sneezing.

Treatment: In mild or acute cases, supportive treatment may be effective. Severe cases of rhinosinusitis in kittens or adult cats may require parenteral fluids to prevent dehydration, and nutritional support via a nasogastric tube to maintain weight. Chronic secondary bacterial rhinosinusitis may be treated with antimicrobial chemotherapy for 3-6 wk. Intranasal feline herpesvirus vaccine may help shorten and minimize recurrence of clinical signs. Intermittent use of vasoconstrictive nasal decongestants usually provides only temporary relief of congestion. Mycotic rhinosinusitis requires antifungal therapy based on identification of a fungal etiologic agent. Animals that do not respond to medical therapy may require surgery consisting of sinusotomy or rhinotomy, lavage, and biopsy. Cobalt radiation therapy is the most viable treatment for intranasal neoplasia.

TONSILLITIS

Etiology: Tonsillitis is common in dogs but rare in cats. In dogs, it seldom occurs as a primary disease, but when present it is most frequently seen in small breeds. It usually is secondary to nasal, oral, or pharyngeal disorders (eg, cleft palate); chronic vomiting or regurgitation (eg, from megaesophagus); or chronic coughing (eg, with bronchitis). Chronic tonsillitis may occur in brachycephalic dogs in association with pharyngitis accompanying soft palate elongation and redundant pharyngeal mucosa. Chronic tonsillitis in young dogs is thought to represent maturation of pharyngeal defense mechanisms.

Escherichia coli, Staphylococcus aureus, and hemolytic streptococci are the pathogenic bacteria most often cultured from diseased tonsils. Plant fibers or other foreign bodies that lodge in the tonsillar fossa may produce a localized unilateral inflammation or a peritonsillar abscess. Other physical and chemical agents may cause irritation of the oropharynx and one or both tonsils. Tonsillitis may also accompany neoplastic tonsillar masses because of physical trauma or secondary bacterial infection.

Clinical Findings and Diagnosis: Tonsillitis is not always accompanied by obvious clinical signs. Fever and malaise are uncommon unless consequent to systemic infection. Gagging, followed by retching or a short, soft cough, may result in expulsion of small amounts of mucus. Inappetence, listlessness, salivation, and dysphagia are seen in severe tonsillitis.

Tonsillar enlargement may range from protrusion just out of the crypts to a mass of sufficient size to cause dysphagia or inspiratory stridor. A septic, suppurative exudate may surround the tonsil, which may be reddened with small necrotic foci or plaques. Tonsillitis usually is a sign of generalized or regional inflammatory disease; therefore, primary tonsillitis should be diagnosed only after underlying diseases have been ruled out. Squamous cell carcinoma, malignant melanoma, and lymphosarcoma commonly occur in canine tonsils and should be distinguished from tonsillitis. Tonsillar lymphosarcoma generally results in bilateral symmetric enlargement, whereas nonlymphoid neoplasia is usually unilateral.

Treatment: Prompt systemic administration of antibiotics is indicated for bacterial tonsillitis. Penicillins are often effective, but in refractory cases, culture and sensitivity testing may be needed. Mild analgesics are appropriate for severe pharyngeal irritation, and a soft palatable diet is recommended for a few days until the dysphagia resolves. Parenteral administration of fluids is required for those animals that are unable to take food by mouth.

Tonsillectomy is rarely required for chronic primary tonsillitis but provides permanent relief. Other indications for tonsillectomy include tonsillar neoplasia and tonsillar enlargement that interferes with airflow (eg, in brachycephalic breeds).

TRACHEOBRONCHITIS

Tracheobronchitis is an acute or chronic inflammation of the trachea and bronchial airways; it may be primary or secondary depending on the etiologic agent. Bronchitis may extend from the bronchioles to the lung parenchyma.

Etiology: Canine infectious tracheobronchitis (kennel cough, *see* below) is often secondary to viral infection of the respiratory system. Other causes of tracheobronchitis in dogs include parasites, eg, *Aelurostrongylus abstrusus* (also in cats), *Capillaria aerophila, Crenosoma vulpis,* and *Oslerus osleri.*

Tracheitis may be secondary either to diseases of the oropharynx or to chronic coughing related to heart disease or noncardiac pulmonary disease. Other causes include smoke aspiration and exposure to noxious chemical fumes. Exacerbation of a chronic bronchitis affecting middle-aged and older dogs may follow sudden changes in the weather or other environmental stresses. Bronchial asthma (allergic bronchitis) is a syndrome in cats with similarities to asthma in humans. Young cats and Siamese and

Himalayan breeds are most affected. Foreign bodies in the airway and developmental abnormalities such as laryngeal deformities may predispose to bronchitis. Chronic bronchitis most often affects small breeds of dogs, although it is also seen in large breeds. It is characterized by persistent cough for at least 2 mo in the absence of specific pulmonary disease. Bronchiectasis may occur as the end stage of chronic bronchitis in dogs. Recognition of tracheobronchitis as an often secondary disease syndrome underlies the importance of diagnosis and control of an associated primary disease.

Clinical Findings: Spasms of coughing are the outstanding sign. These are most severe after rest or a change of environment or at the beginning of exercise. On auscultation, respiratory sounds may be essentially normal. In advanced cases, inspiratory crackles and expiratory wheezes are heard. The temperature may be slightly increased. The acute stage of bronchitis passes in 2-3 days; the cough, however, may persist for 2-3 wk. Severe bronchitis and pneumonia are difficult to differentiate; the former often extends into the lung parenchyma and results in pneumonia. Feline bronchial asthma may result in cyanosis and dyspnea and may be accompanied by eosinophilia.

Lesions: During the acute and subacute inflammatory stages, the air passages are filled with frothy, serous, or mucopurulent exudate. In chronic bronchitis, they contain excessive viscid mucus. The epithelial linings are roughened and opaque, a result of diffuse fibrosis, edema, and mononuclear cell infiltration. There is hypertrophy and hyperplasia of the tracheobronchial mucous glands and goblet cells. The act of coughing is an attempt to remove the accumulations of mucus and exudate from the respiratory passages.

Diagnosis: The diagnosis is made from the history and clinical signs and by elimination of other causes of coughing. In chronic bronchitis, chest radiographs may show an increase in linear and peribronchial markings. Bronchoscopy reveals inflamed epithelium and often mucopurulent mucus in the bronchi. In addition, the procedure allows collection of biopsy and swab samples for in vitro assay. Bronchial washing is an additional diagnostic aid that may demonstrate causative agents or significant cellular responses (eg, eosinophils).

Treatment: In mild or acute cases, supportive therapy may be effective, but treatment of concurrent disease is also indicated. Rest, warmth, and proper hygiene are important. Broad-spectrum antimicrobial chemotherapy is indicated for treatment of cough. Persistent, nonproductive coughing is best controlled by antitussives that contain codeine. If conservative medical management is unsuccessful, radiographs should be taken of the thorax and cervical trachea, and laboratory tests evaluated to eliminate other differential diagnoses. Bronchoalveolar lavage or transtracheal wash for cytology and culture sensitivity may be indicated to identify an etiologic agent and to determine appropriate antimicrobial chemotherapy. Pulmonary physiotherapy consisting of sodium chloride nebulization and gentle coupage may loosen secretions and stimulate expectoration. A bathroom environment with steam from a hot shower may be substituted for nebulization.

Infectious Tracheobronchitis of Dogs
(Kennel cough)

Infectious tracheobronchitis results from inflammation of the upper airways. It is a mild, self-limiting disease but may progress to fatal bronchopneumonia in puppies or to chronic bronchitis in debilitated adult or aged dogs. The illness spreads rapidly among susceptible dogs housed in close confinement (eg, veterinary hospitals or kennels).

Etiology: Canine parainfluenza virus, canine adenovirus 2 (CAV-2), or canine distemper virus can be the primary or sole pathogen involved. Canine reoviruses (types 1, 2, and 3), canine herpesvirus, and canine adenovirus 1 (CAV-1) are of questionable significance in this syndrome. *Bordetella bronchiseptica* may act as a primary pathogen, especially in dogs <6 mo old; however, it and other bacteria (usually gram-negative organisms such as *Pseudomonas* sp, *Escherichia coli*, and *Klebsiella pneumoniae*) may cause secondary infections after viral injury to the respiratory tract. Concurrent infections with several of these agents are common. The role of *Mycoplasma* sp has not been clearly established. Stress and extremes of ventilation, temperature, and humidity apparently increase susceptibility to, and severity of, the disease.

Clinical Findings: The prominent clinical sign is paroxysms of harsh, dry coughing, which may be followed by retching and gagging. The cough is easily induced by gentle palpation of the larynx or trachea. Affected dogs demonstrate few if any additional clinical signs except for partial anorexia. Body temperature and WBC counts usually remain normal. Development of more severe signs, including fever, purulent nasal discharge, depression, anorexia, and a productive cough, especially in puppies, indicates a complicating systemic infection such as distemper or bronchopneumonia. Stress, particularly due to adverse environmental conditions and improper nutrition, may contribute to a relapse during convalescence.

Diagnosis: Tracheobronchitis should be suspected whenever the characteristic cough suddenly develops 5-10 days after exposure to other susceptible or affected dogs. Severity usually diminishes during the first 5 days, but the disease persists for 10-20 days. Tracheal trauma secondary to intubation may produce a similar but generally less severe syndrome.

Treatment: Preferably, affected dogs should not be hospitalized because the disease is usually highly contagious (and also self-limiting). Appropriate management practices, including good nutrition, hygiene, and nursing care, as well as correction of predisposing environmental factors, hasten recovery. Cough suppressants containing codeine derivatives, such as hydrocodone (0.25 mg/kg, PO, BID-QID) or butorphanol (0.05-0.1 mg/kg, PO or SC, BID-QID), should be used only as needed to control persistent nonproductive coughing. Antibiotics are usually not needed except in severe chronic cases; cephalosporins, quinolones, chloramphenicol, and tetracycline are preferable because they reach effective concentrations in the tracheobronchial mucosa. When needed, the antibiotic should be selected by culture and sensitivity tests of specimens collected by transtracheal aspiration or bronchoscopy. Antibiotics given PO or IM may not significantly reduce the numbers of *B bronchiseptica* in the distal trachea or major bronchi. Thus, in severely affected dogs that are not responsive to parenteral antibiotics, kanamycin sulfate (250 mg) or gentamicin sulfate (50 mg) diluted in 3 mL of saline may be administered by aerosolization BID for 3 days. Aerosolization treatment should be preceded by administration of bronchodilators. Endotracheal injection of antibiotics (eg, gentamicin) is a possible alternative to aerosolization. Corticosteroids may help alleviate clinical signs but should be used concurrently with an antibacterial agent; they are contraindicated in severely ill, coughing dogs.

Prevention: Dogs should be immunized with modified live virus vaccines against distemper, parainfluenza, and CAV-2, which also provides protection against CAV-1. Commercial products frequently combine these agents and may include modified live parvovirus and leptospiral antigens. An initial vaccination should be given at 6-8 wk and repeated twice at 3- to 4-wk intervals until the dog is 14-16 wk old. Revaccination should be performed annually. When the risk of *B bronchiseptica* infection is significant, use of a live, avirulent, intranasal vaccine is preferable to parenteral products containing inactivated bacteria or bacterial extracts. A combination of an avirulent *B bronchiseptica* and a modified live parainfluenza vaccine is available for intranasal use. One inoculation is administered to puppies >3 wk old.

■ ■ ■

URINARY SYSTEM

URINARY SYSTEM
INTRODUCTION

Primary functions of the urinary system include: 1) excretion of waste products of metabolism; 2) maintenance of a constant extracellular environment through conservation and excretion of water and electrolytes; 3) production of the hormones erythropoietin and renin, which regulate hematopoiesis, blood pressure, and sodium reabsorption; and 4) metabolism of vitamin D to its active form (1,25-dihydroxycholecalciferol). Many abnormalities of the urinary system can be diagnosed from the signalment of the patient, history and physical examination findings, serum chemistry profile, urinalysis, and aerobic bacterial urine culture. The history should include information regarding changes in water consumption, frequency of urination, volume of urine produced, appearance of urine, and behavior of the patient. It is also important to obtain information about historical and current drug administration, appetite, diet, changes in body weight, and previous illnesses or injuries. The physical examination should include palpation of the bladder and examination of external genitalia. In dogs, rectal examination should be performed to evaluate the urethra in both sexes and for evaluation of the prostate in male dogs. Rectal examination in cats may not be feasible due to their small size; however, the kidneys are generally easier to palpate in cats than in dogs. A full neurologic examination should be performed on all animals with micturition disorders. Additional diagnostic tests, such as CBC, blood gas analysis for acid-base status, blood pressure, urine protein:creatinine ratio, iohexol clearance test, survey abdominal radiography, abdominal ultrasonography, contrast studies of the upper and lower urinary tract, cystoscopic examination of the urinary bladder, and renal biopsy may also provide valuable information.

Urinalysis: One of the most important diagnostic tests for evaluation of urinary tract disorders is a urinalysis. (*See also* p 1358.) Urine may be collected by one of 4 methods: spontaneous micturition, manual compression of the urinary bladder, catheterization, and cystocentesis. Each method has advantages and disadvantages (*see* TABLE 1). A urinalysis should include method of collection, urine specific gravity, color, turbidity, pH, glucose, ketones, bilirubin ictotest, occult blood, protein, and leukocytes (urine dipstick leukocyte tests are unreliable in cats). Microscopic examination of urine sediment should include RBC, WBC, epithelial cells, renal casts, bacteria, yeast, parasitic ova, fat, sperm, and crystals. Delay in analyzing urine samples can result in artifacts (eg, changes in urine pH, formation of crystals, etc), so it is important to note the time when the sample was collected and the time when it was analyzed. If a sample will not be analyzed immediately, it should be refrigerated.

TABLE 1. Advantages and Disadvantages of Urine Collection Methods

Method of Collection	Advantages	Disadvantages
Spontaneous micturition	No risk (eg, trauma, bacterial infection) to animal. Avoids iatrogenic hematuria.	May contain debris (eg, bacteria, exudate) from lower urinary and genital tract. If bacterial growth appears on urine culture, must differentiate between urethral contamination and urinary tract infection. Quantitative urine culture required.
Manual compression of urinary bladder	Provides method for obtaining urine sample when voluntary micturition has not occurred.	May induce trauma to urinary tract, resulting in hematuria. May be stressful for animal, especially if bladder is painful. If bacterial growth appears on urine culture, must differentiate between urethral contamination and urinary tract infection. Quantitative urine culture required.
Catheterization	Provides method for obtaining urine sample when other methods of collection have failed.	Potential for trauma to urinary tract, especially bladder. More invasive than other methods; sedation may be required. Risk of introducing bladder infection. If bacterial growth appears on urine culture, must differentiate between urethral contamination and urinary tract infection. Quantitative urine culture required. Least desirable method of urine collection.
Cystocentesis	Preferred method of collection for urine culture. Avoids contamination of sample from lower urinary tract.	Potential risk of trauma if performed incorrectly or patient moves during procedure. More invasive than spontaneous micturition. Potential for contamination of sample if needle penetrates colon during procedure.

Protein in urine should be evaluated in light of the urine specific gravity. Protein in a concentrated urine sample may not be significant, whereas the same amount in a dilute sample may be significant. Urine dipsticks provide a semiquantitative assessment of protein and can be influenced by urine pH. Therefore, they should be used only as a screening test for protein, not as a definitive diagnosis of proteinuria. A urine protein:creatinine ratio from a single urine sample or from a 24-hr urine sample is required to quantitate the amount of protein in urine. In dogs, the following guidelines should be used for interpretation of urine protein:creatinine ratios: 0.0-0.3 = normal; 0.3-1.0 = questionable; and >1.0 = abnormal. In cats, a urine protein:creatinine ratio <0.7 is considered normal. Urine protein:creatinine ratios must be interpreted in the context of other information from the urinalysis. Inflammation and hematuria can falsely elevate urine protein:creatinine ratios.

Bacterial Culture of Urine: A urinalysis is unreliable for ruling out a urinary tract infection (UTI). Not all UTI are associated with an inflammatory response. In addition, >10,000 bacterial rods/mL and >100,000 bacterial cocci/mL of urine are required to consistently find bacteria in a urine sample using light microscopy. About 25-30% of all dogs with UTI have urine bacterial counts below these figures at the time of specimen collection, so urine culture is important to rule out a UTI.

Urine samples for bacterial culture may be obtained by the same methods used for obtaining samples for urinalysis; however, the preferred method is cystocentesis. Urine obtained by cystocentesis should be sterile. If urine samples are collected by methods other than cystocentesis, a quantitative urine culture should be requested. If the sample is collected by spontaneous micturition or manual compression, significant numbers of bacteria are present if ≥100,000 colony forming units (CFU)/mL of urine in dogs or ≥10,000 CFU/mL of urine in cats are detected. Samples with >10,000-90,000 CFU/mL in dogs and >1,000-10,000 CFU/mL in cats are suspicious for a UTI. If the sample is collected by catheterization, ≥10,000 CFU/mL in dogs and ≥1,000 CFU/mL in cats is significant, while samples containing 1,000-10,000 CFU/mL in dogs and 100-1,000 CFU/mL in cats are suspicious for a UTI.

Serum Chemistry Profile: Evaluation of serum chemistries, including BUN, creatinine, calcium, phosphorus, and serum electrolytes, is useful in many urinary tract disorders and can provide a crude indication of glomerular filtration rate (GFR). Although elevations in BUN and creatinine are supportive of renal dysfunction, these tests are influenced by nonrenal factors as well. For example, dehydration can cause increases in BUN and serum creatinine not associated with renal failure. BUN can also be influenced by diet and GI bleeding and is considered inferior to creatinine for evaluating GFR. Serum creatinine levels can be falsely lowered in patients with severe muscle wasting and falsely elevated in patients with severe muscle damage. Although BUN and serum creatinine increase as GFR declines, this relationship is not linear. Large changes in GFR early in renal disease cause only small increases in BUN and serum creatinine, while small changes in GFR in advanced renal disease may be associated with large changes in BUN and serum creatinine.

Additional Diagnostic Tests: More sensitive methods for detecting renal dysfunction include plasma clearance tests (eg, inulin clearance), radionuclide techniques, endogenous creatinine clearance, and exogenous creatinine clearance. However, these tests are impractical to perform routinely in clinical practice. The iohexol clearance test is a recently developed alternative for detecting renal dysfunction. It entails recording an accurate body weight, administering a precise amount of iohexol IV, and accurately timing collection of blood samples as directed following administration. This test does not require timed collection of urine samples or special equipment.

Depending on the cause of the urinary tract disorder, radiographic procedures, sonographic examination, and cystoscopic examination of the bladder may provide additional valuable information. The kidneys have a limited range of responses to disease; therefore, renal biopsies are rarely useful when evaluating renal dysfunction. An exception to this is in animals with significant proteinuria.

Blood gas analysis or serum bicarbonate levels provide useful information on acid-base status, especially in animals with renal dysfunction. Metabolic acidosis is a common problem in chronic renal failure and can result in protein catabolism.

PRINCIPLES OF THERAPY

Diseases of the urinary system can result from a variety of pathologic processes, and appropriate therapy (as discussed in the following chapters) depends on the location, severity, and etiology of the problem. See also SYSTEMIC PHARMACOTHERAPEUTICS OF THE

URINARY SYSTEM, p 2040. If the condition is not life threatening, appropriate diagnostic samples should be collected before initiating therapy. It is important to remember that some diagnostic tests and treatments have the potential to cause significant harm. If the specific cause cannot be determined, nonspecific and supportive therapy (eg, monitoring fluids, treating acidosis) should be instituted.

CONGENITAL AND INHERITED ANOMALIES OF THE URINARY SYSTEM

Congenital and inherited anomalies of the urinary system comprise a group of anatomic defects that may have functional consequences. They are uncommon but remain important components of basic medical knowledge for veterinarians.

RENAL ANOMALIES

Renal Dysplasia and Hypoplasia: These defects are most common in dogs and have been reported in many breeds, including Alaskan Malamutes, Bedlington Terriers, Chow Chows, Cocker Spaniels, Doberman Pinschers, Keeshonden, Lhasa Apsos, Miniature Schnauzers, Norwegian Elkhounds, Samoyeds, Shih Tzus, Soft-coated Wheaten Terriers, and Standard Poodles. Renal dysplasia may be unilateral or bilateral. The kidneys are usually small, firm, and pale; they may have a uniformly diminished renal cortex. Histologic examination reveals immature glomeruli, primitive tubules, and secondary inflammatory lesions, especially interstitial fibrous connective tissue.

Affected animals usually have polydipsia and polyuria that precede signs of uremia. Dwarfing may be noticed if the onset of renal failure occurs within the first few months of life. Urinalysis, hemogram, and blood chemistry changes are the same as in other chronic, progressive renal diseases. Uremia is usually identified between 6 mo and 2 yr of age. The diagnosis is suspected based on the breed and age of disease onset and is confirmed by renal biopsy. Treatment is aimed at managing the associated chronic renal failure.

Renal Agenesis: Renal agenesis is always accompanied by ureteral aplasia and may be associated with aplastic reproductive tissues on the same side. The condition is typically an incidental finding so long as the other kidney is functioning normally. Bilateral agenesis results in early perinatal death.

Polycystic Kidneys: Multiple cysts form within the renal parenchyma, and such kidneys are usually grossly enlarged on palpation. This condition may be associated with hepatic biliary cysts. Polycystic kidneys may cause no clinical signs or may lead to progressive renal failure. This condition is familial in Beagles, Cairn Terriers, Persian cats, and domestic long-haired cats. Diagnosis is based on physical and radiographic findings, ultrasonic examination, or exploratory laparotomy. Pyelonephritis may be seen concurrently and precipitate renal insufficiency.

Simple Renal Cysts: These solitary, unilocular cysts generally do not communicate with the renal collecting system; the rest of the kidney is normal. The origin of these cysts is uncertain. They are usually an incidental finding.

Perirenal Pseudocysts: Perirenal pseudocysts are accumulations of fluid that develop external to the renal parenchyma; they have been identified in cats. Their origin is unknown. The accumulated fluid may be located between the renal parenchyma and the renal capsule or between the renal capsule and a thin-walled fibrous sac attached to the capsule. They are termed pseudocysts rather than cysts because they are not lined by epithelium. Because only a limited number have been examined histologically, it is unknown whether all perirenal fluid-filled structures are pseudocysts. The fluid contained within these structures is not urine or lymph but is described as a transudate. Clinical signs are characterized by progressive abdominal enlargement. Abdominal palpation reveals a large, firm, nonpainful mass located in the area of the kidneys. Renal function tests and urinalysis are typically normal; however, a mild azotemia may occur. Diagnosis is made by excretory urography or ultrasonography. Treatment involves exploratory surgery to confirm the diagnosis, drainage of the pseudocyst fluid, and resection of as much of the pseudocyst wall as possible. The prognosis appears to be good; however, only a limited number of cases have been evaluated.

Miscellaneous Renal Anomalies: Double or multiple renal arteries are seen in ~5% of dogs. Other congenital defects include renal malpositioning, renal fusion, and nephroblastoma. Nephroblastoma is an embryonal tumor and is rare in domestic animals except pigs. It may cause no problems but may be very large and cause abdominal distention.

URETERAL ANOMALIES

Ectopic Ureter: This defect is most commonly reported in 3- to 6-mo-old dogs, with females affected 8 times more frequently than males. Other anomalies frequently associated with ectopic ureter include hydroureter, hydronephrosis, renal hypoplasia, bladder hypoplasia, and urethral sphincter incompetence. Continual dripping of urine is the classic sign, although animals with unilateral ectopic ureter may void normally; the inability to void normally suggests bilateral ectopic ureters. A low-grade vaginitis or vulvitis may also be present due to urine scalding. Involved ureters may open into the urethra, the uterus, or the vagina. Unilateral ectopic ureter is seen with equal frequency on right and left sides, and involvement is bilateral in ~25% of cases. Ectopic ureters generally result from disruption of development of the mesonephric and metanephric duct systems. A genetic component is suspected on the basis of identifying high-risk breeds (West Highland White Terriers, Fox Terriers, and Miniature and Toy Poodles) and a familial occurrence in Siberian Huskies and Labrador Retrievers. Diagnosis is confirmed by IV urography that traces the course of the ureter. Successful surgical treatments usually involve transplantation of affected ureters into the bladder, or ureteronephrectomy. Indications for ureteronephrectomy may include severe ipsilateral renal disease such as hypoplasia, hydronephrosis, or pyelonephritis in the presence of a normally functioning contralateral kidney. Important postoperative complications are persistent incontinence, hydronephrosis, and dysuria. Incontinence occurs most often in cases of bilateral ectopic ureters and may be due to abnormal development of the bladder neck and urethra. An adrenergic agent such as phenylpropanolamine (0.5-1.5 mg/kg, PO, every 8-12 hr) may help minimize the incontinence.

Miscellaneous Ureteral Anomalies: Less frequently recognized ureteral anomalies include aplasia, duplication, and ureterocele. Ureteroceles are characterized by dilation of the submucosal ureter segment within the bladder. Diagnosis is by excretory urography. Appropriate therapy is ureteronephrectomy if the lesion is unilateral with secondary hydronephrosis and hydroureter. If the proximal ureter and kidney are normal, excision or incision of the ureterocele, in addition to ligation of any ectopic distal channel, has been successful.

BLADDER ANOMALIES

Urachal Remnants: Congenital anomalies resulting from incomplete urachal closure include patent urachus, urachal diverticulum, umbilical urachal sinus, and intra-abdominal urachal cyst. Clinical signs and appropriate therapy depend on the type of anomaly. Patent urachus is typically associated with continuous urinary incontinence, urine scalding of the ventral abdomen, and development of bacterial urinary tract infections. Urachal diverticula also predispose to urinary tract infection by serving as a nidus for bacteria. Definitive diagnosis of both disorders is by positive contrast cystography. Treatment consists of surgical resection and 2-4 wk of appropriate antibiotic therapy when indicated. Surgical resection is the standard treatment for umbilical urachal sinuses and intra-abdominal urachal cysts.

Miscellaneous Bladder Anomalies: Bladder duplication, dysplasia, hypoplasia, agenesis, and exstrophy have been reported and are often associated with other urinary tract defects. Diagnosis is by physical examination, observation of micturition, and contrast radiography. Clinical signs and therapy depend on the type of anomaly.

URETHRAL ANOMALIES

Congenital or hereditary urethral anomalies are uncommon; they include urethral agenesis, imperforate urethra, hypospadias, epispadias in combination with bladder exstrophy, urethral duplication, urethral diverticula, urethrorectal fistula, and urethral stenosis.

Hypospadias: This developmental defect results from failure of the urethral grooves to fuse during phallus elongation. The urethral opening is ventral and caudal to the tip of the penis and is classified on the basis of anatomic localization as glandular, penile, scrotal, perineal, or anal. The penis or scrotum may be underdeveloped as well. Clinical signs depend on the site of the urethral meatus and include urine scalding and complications of increased susceptibility to urinary tract infection. Although surgical correction also depends on the site of the urethral meatus, a modification of the prescrotal urethrostomy is generally useful.

Urethrorectal Fistulas: These appear to be more prevalent in English Bulldogs, possibly as a congenital defect due to abnormal separation of the embryonal cloaca into the urethra and rectum. Clinical signs include hematuria and dysuria secondary to urinary tract infection. Simultaneous passage of urine from the anus and urethra during micturition may be noted. Appropriate therapy consists of surgical correction and concurrent management of urinary tract infection.

INFECTIOUS DISEASES OF THE URINARY SYSTEM IN LARGE ANIMALS

BOVINE CYSTITIS AND PYELONEPHRITIS
(Contagious bovine pyelonephritis)

Bovine cystitis is an inflammation of the urinary bladder of cattle that may ascend the ureters to cause infection of the kidneys (pyelonephritis). A similar condition is seen in sheep. The condition is sporadic and worldwide in distribution. It is most often seen after parturition (in one study, the average days to onset after parturition was 83), with multiparous cows being at highest risk. In locations where the disease has been studied, the prevalence is low (1-2%).

Etiology and Pathogenesis: The most common causative agents are the *Corynebacterium renale* group of bacteria, including *C renale*, *C cystitidis*, and *C pilosum*, as well as *Escherichia coli*. The latter is most often seen in chronic cases and may be an opportunist following the corynebacterial infection. Other organisms that may be involved include, but are not limited to, staphylococci and streptococci.

The most common causative agents, *Corynebacterium* spp and *E coli*, are ubiquitous in the environment and are common inhabitants of the vagina and prepuce. Pyelonephritis develops from an ascending infection from the bladder. Cystitis may be present without involving the ureters or ascending to the kidney until some event occurs that compromises the defense mechanism of the ureteral mucosa. The organisms attack or colonize the mucosal lining of the bladder and ureters usually after some traumatic insult (such as parturition or abnormal deformity of the vaginal tract). The stresses of parturition, peak lactation, and a high-protein diet (which increases the pH of the urine and is therefore conducive to colonization of the attacking organisms) are all contributing factors.

Clinical Findings and Lesions: The first sign observed may be the passage of blood-stained urine in an otherwise normal cow. As the infection proceeds up the ureters, causing inflammation and subsequent involvement of the kidney, the animal exhibits discomfort manifest by frequent attempts to urinate, anorexia, a slight fever, loss of production, colic with restlessness, tail switching, polyuria, hematuria, or pyuria. In chronic cases, the animal may show colic, diarrhea, polyuria, polydipsia, stranguria, and anemia. As the disease progresses, the bladder becomes thickened and inflamed. The ureters become thickened and dilated with a purulent exudate. The involved kidneys develop multiple small abscesses on the surface that may extend into the cortex and medulla.

Diagnosis: This is based on clinical signs; hematuria; a history of recent parturition; palpation of the left kidney for enlargement, loss of lobulation, and pain; endoscopic vaginal inspection for detection of inflamed and enlarged ureters; microscopic examination of the urine for WBC and bacteria; dipstick screening for proteinuria and hematuria; and urine culture to identify the organism. In early acute cases, enlarged ureters and involvement of the kidney may not be detectable on rectal palpation.

Treatment: Early diagnosis and prompt, sustained treatment are needed for a successful recovery. A catheterized urine sample should be taken for culture and antibiotic sensitivity. The treatment of choice for pyelonephritis due to the *C renale* group is penicillin (22,000 IU/kg, IM, BID) or trimethoprim-sulfadoxine (16 mg combined/kg, IM, BID) for ≥ 3 wk. The dosage, frequency, and length of administration for both of these drugs is extra-label, and adequate precautions must be taken to prevent antibiotic residues from entering the human food chain. *E coli* infections require a broad-spectrum antibiotic. Gentamicin (2.2 mg/kg, IM, BID) for 4 wk has been used successfully in some cases. Due to the extremely long tissue-depletion time, the aminoglycosides may not be indicated in food-producing animals.

Even though the organisms are ubiquitous in the environment, affected animals should be isolated from the herd to restrict buildup of organisms.

PORCINE CYSTITIS-PYELONEPHRITIS COMPLEX

Porcine cystitis-pyelonephritis complex, a leading cause of mortality in sows, has been reported throughout the world. Increased incidence appears to be correlated with changes in management, particularly the adoption of confinement housing for gestating sows. Distinguishing features of endemic cystitis and pyelonephritis within a herd include lack of a temporal relationship between the vulvar discharge and the estrous cycle, minimal effect on herd fertility, low morbidity, high mortality, and an increased frequency in advanced-parity (6+) sows.

Etiology and Pathogenesis: A wide variety of bacteria have been isolated from cases of porcine cystitis and pyelonephritis, including *Escherichia coli*, *Arcanobacterium* (*Actinomyces*) *pyogenes*, *Streptococcus* spp and *Staphylococcus* spp. These endogenous and opportunistic organisms typically inhabit the lower urinary tract and are often referred to as being responsible for nonspecific urinary tract infections. *Actinobaculum suis*, a specific urinary pathogen, is an important cause of ascending infection in swine. Formerly classified in the genera *Eubacterium* and *Actinomyces*, *A suis* is a gram-positive rod-shaped bacterium that grows well under anaerobic conditions and is a commensal organism of the porcine urogenital tract. *A suis* is fimbriated, and the short, wide urethra of the sow enhances accessibility to the bladder. Once within the bladder lumen, the alkalinity of the environment increases due to the cleavage of urea into ammonia via the urease enzyme. The elevated pH enhances bacterial proliferation and causes an inflammatory reaction of the mucosal surface. The alkaline environment also inhibits the growth of competitive microflora and promotes the precipitation of urinary salts and crystals, particularly struvite. Such precipitates not only further increase inflammatory changes in the bladder mucosa but also provide a nidus for bacterial growth and protection from antibiotics and host defense mechanisms. While the primary means for accessibility to the kidneys is not yet completely understood, it is hypothesized that damage to the ureteric valves secondary to bacterial products (possibly originating from *E coli*) may predispose affected animals to pyelonephritis.

Epidemiology: Problems frequently encountered in confinement facilities that hasten the development of porcine cystitis are the reduced availability of water, increased fecal contamination of the perineal area, excessive weight gain, and leg injuries, all of which result in a reduction in the frequency of urination and enhanced bacterial survival in the urogenital tract. *A suis* has been isolated from the preputial cavity of boars at slaughter, the vaginal tract of neonatal piglets sampled immediately following parturition, and the vaginal tract of sows sampled throughout all stages of production. It may also be isolated from voided urine, contaminated parturition sleeves of farrowing attendants, pen floors of farrowing and nursery rooms, and the boots of stockpersons working in the breeding area. The sole route of transmission was believed to be copulation, but it is now understood that the organism is ubiquitous, and the vaginal tract can become colonized anytime in the life of the pig.

Clinical Findings: Clinical signs vary according to the severity and the phase of the disease. In acute and severe cases, affected animals may be found dead, probably from acute renal failure. Symptomatic animals are usually afebrile and may show anorexia, hematuria, and pyuria. The urine is typically reddish brown with a strong odor of ammonia. Urinary pH may increase from normal values of 5.5-7.5 up to 8-9. Animals that survive the initial infection frequently experience weight loss and reduced productivity secondary to end-stage renal disease, resulting in premature removal from the breeding herd. Inflammatory reaction on the mucosal surface of the bladder may be catarrhal, hemorrhagic, purulent, or necrotic, and the bladder wall may be thickened. Struvites can also be found in the lumen. The ureters, often filled with exudate, may increase to as much as 2.5 cm in diameter. Unilateral or bilateral pyelonephritis or pyelitis is the primary lesion in the kidneys. The pelvic region of the kidney, which is frequently distended with blood, pus, and foul-smelling urine, often shows irregular ulceration and necrosis of the papillae. In longstanding cases of pyelonephritis, fibrosis ultimately replaces inflammation.

Diagnosis: Cystitis and pyelonephritis in live animals can best be presumptively diagnosed when frequent micturition of bloodstained and cloudy urine can be observed. Examination of the urine sediments may reveal the presence of inflammatory cells, RBC, granular renal casts, bacteria, and crystals. Due to the striking gross lesions, confirmation of the diagnosis is usually not difficult. In some cases, determination of urea concentration in ocular fluids is a useful aid to postmortem diagnosis of pyelonephritis, especially if it is difficult to ascertain whether the lesions found in the urinary tract are responsible for the death of the animal. To properly isolate the causative organism, care must be taken during sample collection to minimize exposure to oxygen. In the field, the bladder should remain unopened, and the neck of the bladder should be sealed with umbilical tape. Similar care should be taken with renal tissue. Lesions of pyelonephritis can be demonstrated by examination of one kidney; the other should remain unopened with the ureter sealed as previously described. On arrival at the laboratory, a small incision should be made over a portion of the serosal surface of the bladder and kidney, previously seared with a hot iron to reduce surface contamination. A cotton swab should be inserted into the bladder lumen and streaked for isolation on colistin nalidixic acid agar and then incubated at 37°C under anaerobic conditions for 5-7 days. If the culture is to be done at a distant location, swabs can be placed into Kary Blair anaerobic transport media for shipment.

Treatment and Prevention: Treatment of urinary tract infections may be successful if the correct antibiotic is administered early in the disease course. Penicillin and ampicillin are often the drugs of choice, due to their effectiveness in alkaline conditions and their propensity for excretion through the urinary tract. Dosages of 2.2 mg/kg are typically administered IM for 3 days. Oral administration of penicillin and ampicillin is also possible; however, feed-grade products are of little value due to the high degree of anorexia in acutely infected sows and a reduced bioavailability secondary to destruction by gastric enzymes, low pH, and colonic bacteria. Water-soluble ampicillin can be administered at 2.3 mg/kg for 5 days, although bioavailability is questionable and cost may become an issue. Acidification of the urine through oral administration of feed-grade citric acid has been reported. Results showed a reduced incidence of clinical urinary tract disease, as well as highly significant (p <0.0001) differences in urinary pH and bacterial concentration/mL of urine in medicated versus nonmedicated groups. A level of 70 mg of citric acid was administered daily for 14 days with no palatability problems.

Maintaining excellent hygiene during breeding and parturition, as well as throughout the gestation period, is critical for prevention of urinary tract disease. Facilities must be properly designed to reduce the spread of pathogens within the breeding herd and allow for efficient removal of feces from the environment. Free-choice water should be available at all times, as restricting water availability through the use of intermittent delivery systems or poor husbandry results in an increase in abnormal urine parameters in gestating sows, including reduced urine output, elevated specific gravity (>1.026), and increased creatinine concentration. Sows in crates are reluctant to stand except at feeding times and do not drink except at these times. Providing water at correct flow rates is essential to prevent ascending infection by regular urination. Finally, because a higher degree of urinary tract disease can be seen in older sows, proper culling procedures are important to ensure that an optimal parity distribution is maintained within breeding herds.

SWINE KIDNEY WORM INFECTION

Etiology: *Stephanurus dentatus* are stout-bodied worms (2-4.5 cm long) found encysted in pairs along the ureters from the kidney to the bladder. The kidney worm is found worldwide, particularly in tropical and subtropical areas. It is primarily a parasite of swine raised outdoors in the southeastern and southcentral USA. The eggs hatch shortly after being passed in the urine and reach the infective stage in 3-5 days. The larvae are susceptible to temperature extremes, desiccation, and sunlight. Infection is by skin penetration or ingestion of the infective larvae (earthworms may serve as paratenic hosts). The larvae migrate to the liver, where they migrate extensively for 3-9 mo. Larvae then penetrate the capsule and migrate through the peritoneal cavity to the perirenal area. Occasionally, some larvae errantly migrate to other tissues and organs and to developing fetuses. Infections usually become patent in 9-16 mo but may be found as early as 6 mo.

Clinical Findings and Diagnosis: When present in large numbers, kidney worms may adversely affect growth. The principal economic loss results from condemnation of organs and tissues affected by migrating larvae. The most severe lesions are usually in the liver, which shows cirrhosis, scar formation, extensive thrombosis of the portal vessels, and a variable amount of necrosis. Kidney and lung damage are also possible.

When worms are in the kidney or in cysts that open into the ureter, eggs may be recovered in the urine. Prepatent infections are difficult to diagnose, and a definitive diagnosis depends on demonstration of the worms or lesions at necropsy.

Control: Good control practices are indicated in areas where the worm is known to occur. Because of the long prepatent period, control may be achieved with a "gilts only" breeding program, which prevents patent infection from developing. Older boars are replaced with young boars from clean herds, and only gilts are bred and then sold after weaning. Eradication is possible within 2 yr. More commonly, anthelmintics and sanitation (rearing on concrete or in confinement) are used to control kidney worm.

Ivermectin (in-feed for 7 days at 1.8 g/ton) and fenbendazole (in-feed for 3-12 days at 9 mg/kg/day) are effective against *Stephanurus* sp. Levamisole (in-feed at 0.36 g/ton) is also approved for use against this worm.

NONINFECTIOUS DISEASES OF THE URINARY SYSTEM IN LARGE ANIMALS

UROLITHIASIS

For a more general introduction to urolithiasis, *see* p 1279.

Urolithiasis in Ruminants

Uroliths in cattle, sheep, and goats are common. Although uroliths can be found anywhere within the urinary tract, urethroliths are responsible for most clinical problems. Obstruction induced by urethroliths causes urine retention and leads to bladder distention, abdominal pain, and eventual urethral perforation or bladder rupture, with death from uremia or septicemia. It is an important disease of feeder animals but is also seen in mature breeding animals. Urolithiasis is seen most often during winter in steers and wethers on full feed, or on range during severe weather conditions with limited water intake, especially when the water has a high mineral content. Urolithiasis has no specific geographic distribution, and the different urolith types reflect the mineral distribution of the feed. Uroliths occur in either sex, but obstructive urolithiasis develops primarily in males because of anatomic differences.

Etiology and Pathogenesis: Ruminant urolithiasis is considered primarily a nutritional disease. The prevalence of urolithiasis in the USA is highest in calves, lambs, and kids castrated at an early age and fed high-grain diets with roughly a 1:1 calcium to phosphorus ratio or a diet high in magnesium. Ruminants fed high-grain diets with a low calcium to phosphorus ratio are at increased risk of developing struvite uroliths, while ruminants grazing on silica-rich soil are predisposed to form silica uroliths. Diets high in calcium (eg, subterranean clover) may result in calcium carbonate uroliths, while plants such as halogeton or tops from the common sugar beet may be a factor in calcium oxalate formation. The mineral composition of water, in concert with dietary mineral imbalances, probably contributes more to initiating urolith formation than does the lack of water itself. A definitive diagnosis of urolithiasis in a single animal suggests that all males in the population are at risk for the disease.

The distal aspect of the sigmoid flexure of cattle and the sigmoid flexure and urethral process of sheep and goats are the most common sites for uroliths to lodge. Irritation at the site of lodging causes inflammation and swelling that contributes to urethral occlusion. Castration of young males also predisposes to urolith-induced urethral obstruction by removing hormonal influences necessary for mature development of the penis and urethra.

Clinical Findings: Clinical signs may be associated with partial or complete urethral occlusion. Animals with partial obstruction dribble blood-tinged urine after prolonged, painful (stranguria) attempts at urination; before complete occlusion occurs, urine may dry on the preputial hairs and leave detectable mineral deposits. Animals with complete urethral obstruction exhibit tenesmus, tail twitching, weight shifting, and signs consistent with colic. Inappetence, bloat, depression, and rectal prolapse may also be seen. Affected steers may elevate the tail and show urethral pulsations just ventral to the rectum. Goats may vocalize.

Common sequelae of complete urethral obstruction include urethral perforation or urinary bladder rupture. Bladder rupture often results in death from uremia. The disease course may be 5-7 days. Although urethral perforation may also cause uremia and death, it is not uncommon for the ventral abdominal skin to necrose and slough, allowing the development of a pseudourethra.

Diagnosis: Diagnosis based on the history, clinical signs, and physical examination is usually straightforward. Hypersensitivity in the region of the sigmoid flexure may be evident. Palpation may identify abnormal pulsations of the urethra and tissue swelling associated with the obstruction. Rectal palpation may reveal an enlarged, distended bladder, or the bladder may be nonpalpable, consistent with bladder rupture. Examination of the urethral process in sheep and goats may reveal the occluding urolith. If early clinical signs of obstructive uropathy are missed, the animal may show only inappetence, depression, subcutaneous swelling along the penis, or uroperitoneum; abdominal distention due to uroperitoneum must be differentiated from ruminal tympany, peritonitis, peritoneal tumors, and GI tract obstructions. Ballottement allows detection of the fluid, and when viewing the animal from behind, the abdomen appears symmetrically enlarged and pear-shaped. Ultrasound examination of the abdomen reveals a large amount of hypoechoic fluid. Confirmation is obtained by examining fluid collected by abdominocentesis and finding that the creatinine in peritoneal fluid is 2 times or more that in plasma. Subcutaneous swellings along the prepuce and ventral abdomen due to a perforated urethra must be differentiated from traumatic injury, subcutaneous abscesses, and umbilical or ventral hernias. In breeding animals, preputial lacerations with prolapse and sheath infection, and hematoma of the penis must also be differentiated. In animals with clinical signs of acute colic, other causes of abdominal pain must be eliminated; these diseases include indigestion, stasis or obstruction of the GI tract, primary enteritis, abomasal ulcers, and coccidiosis.

Treatment and Control: Treatment of obstructive urolithiasis generally involves establishing a patent urethra and correcting fluid and electrolyte imbalances. In many instances, surgical management of the obstruction is all that is necessary; however, severely uremic and depressed animals require rehydration and correction of acid-base and electrolyte abnormalities. If a rupture of the urinary tract has occurred, hyponatremia, hypochloremia, hyperphosphatemia, and metabolic alkalosis with variable potassium concentrations are found. Treatment with IV normal saline is indicated. The volume of fluid administered should be calculated to correct clinical dehydration. Once the animal is rehydrated, fluid therapy may be continued to encourage diuresis.

Animals with an intact urethra and bladder, with early clinical signs of obstructive urethral disease, may benefit from conservative therapy using antispasmodics and tranquilizers. This is believed to relax the retractor penis muscles with straightening of the sigmoid flexure. However, conservative therapy is only rarely beneficial in small ruminants, and is warranted only in cases of acute or partial obstruction without evidence of urethral or bladder damage; it should not be used in complicated or advanced cases. Uroliths trapped within the urethral process of sheep and goats may be removed by gentle manipulation or by amputation of the urethral process. Proper restraint, tranquilization, and a regional anesthetic are necessary. The techniques may vary, but the typical procedure requires exteriorization of the penis. Although amputation may be effective, relief is typically temporary (<2 days) in most animals, in which obstruction recurs due to the presence of multiple uroliths.

Perineal urethrostomy has also been recommended as an effective surgical technique in castrated males. Short-term complications associated with perineal urethrostomy may include postoperative hemorrhage, surgical wound dehiscence, and subcutaneous urine accumulation. Urethral stricture is a common longterm complication. In addition, perineal urethrostomy is associated with loss of breeding ability in intact males. In more complicated cases, such as those with urethral perforation, amputation of the penis proximal to the sigmoid flexure or near the perineal area may be necessary as a salvage procedure. Animals that develop urethral perforation also require drainage of accumulated subcutaneous urine; this is accomplished by lancing the skin overlying the area of accumulated urine. Topical antiseptics and fly repellents may be applied to these ventral lacerations, and parenteral antibiotics are recommended to prevent infection.

Cystotomy followed by dietary management is believed to be a more effective longterm solution to urolithiasis in sheep and goats than is perineal urethrostomy. Cystotomy allows removal of multiple urocystoliths, permits bidirectional urethral flushing, and poses less risk for urethral stricture. Tube cystotomy is generally considered the treatment of choice, allowing time for the calculi to be expelled spontaneously.

If the bladder is ruptured, the ability to urinate must be restored and uremia corrected. In animals with substantial uroperitoneum, the peritoneal cavity should be slowly drained using a teat tube or trocar. Urine removal may also reduce the severity of peritonitis and make the animal more comfortable. Fluid, electrolyte, and acid-base homeostasis normally returns within 24 hr after restoration of a patent urinary system. Persistent uremia indicates the possibility of hydronephrosis or ascending pyelonephritis, or both. A urethrostomy should be performed to provide unobstructed passage of urine. Attempts to surgically repair the ruptured bladder have been largely unsuccessful due to the chronic distention prior to rupture. The bladder may heal spontaneously after urethrostomy and removal of abdominal fluid; however, these animals are best salvaged within 3-4 mo to avoid further complications. Despite treatment, some animals fail to pass urine effectively and the uroperitoneum recurs. These animals may be treated by performing tube cystotomy, followed by appropriate antibiotic and fluid therapy.

Several measures to prevent the formation of urethral calculi have been recommended. The most important is to provide a calcium:phosphorus ratio of 2:1 in the complete ration. Intensive concentrate feeding, such as in many finishing programs, frequently leads to urolith formation and urethral obstruction. Thus, any feeding program incorporating concentrate feeding must include appropriate calcium supplementation. Adjunct measures to minimize the formation of urethral calculi include adding sodium chloride up to 4% of the total ration. This promotes increased sodium and chloride concentration in the urine, water intake, and urine dilution, which increases the mineral solubility. Ammonium chloride can be used as a urinary acidifying agent (7-10 g/head/day for a 30-kg lamb or kid; 50-80 g/head/day for a 240-kg steer). Urine acidification antagonizes magnesium-ammonium-phosphate crystal formation and has been shown empirically to be a useful preventive measure. These adjunct measures should not be used in lieu of a properly balanced ration. In operations with a significant problem of urolith formation, evaluation of the ration is the most important measure that can be taken to reduce the incidence.

Urolithiasis in Horses

Urolithiasis is a less common condition in horses than in small ruminants or steers. The disease can affect immature horses but is seen most frequently in adults. There is no breed predilection. Urolithiasis is seen more frequently in males than females, which has been attributed to anatomic differences between the male and female urethra.

Equine uroliths have a diameter of 0.5-21 cm, weigh as much as 6.5 kg, and are found most often within the bladder. Most equine uroliths are composed of calcium carbonate, in various hydrated forms, with struvite uroliths occasionally noted. Calcium carbonate uroliths have 2 separate clinical forms. The first form is a concretion of salts and mucoproteins that varies in consistency from friable to firm. These uroliths are usually yellow and oval or irregularly shaped; they frequently have a rough or spiculated surface and are generally soft enough to be fragmented during surgery. The second calcium carbonate form is a firm concretion that is hard and resistant to fragmentation and is typically smooth and white. There appears to be no difference in chemical composition between these forms.

Etiology: The mechanism of urolith formation in horses is unknown, although the alkaline pH and high mineral content of normal equine urine may favor crystal formation and precipitation. Normal equine urine also contains large amounts of mucoproteins, which may serve as a cementing substance to adhere crystals. Consumption of feed and water high in mineral content may increase urinary solute concentrations and thereby promote crystallization and precipitation. Multiple nephroliths may develop in horses with renal papillary necrosis (associated with NSAID administration while dehydrated) and mineralization of the papillae.

Clinical Findings: Clinical signs depend on the urolith location. Most uroliths are located in the bladder and cause dysuria, pollakiuria, and hematuria. Hematuria is most evident after exercise and toward the end of a voided urine stream. Affected horses frequently stretch out to urinate and may maintain this posture for variable periods before and after micturition. Additional signs may include scalding of the perineum in females or of the medial aspect of the hindlimbs in males. Geldings and stallions may protrude the penis flaccidly for prolonged periods while intermittently dribbling urine. Affected horses may occasionally exhibit recurrent bouts of colic or an altered hindlimb gait. Urethral obstruction may also develop as the result of a trapped urolith and is typically accompanied by restlessness, sweating, varying degrees of colic, and frequent attempts to urinate. The bladder is distended on rectal examination. In most fatal cases, a single large urolith, occasionally accompanied by smaller ones, is found in the bladder; less frequently, the urolith may be found lodged at the bladder neck or the ischial arch. Nephroliths are occasionally found via ultrasonography in horses with cystic calculi; owners of such horses should be informed that obstruction may recur.

Bilateral nephroliths are not uncommon in adult horses that have been used for performance. Intermittent chronic obstruction of ureters will eventually cause renal failure, resulting in weight loss and anorexia.

Diagnosis: Tentative diagnosis of urolithiasis is usually based on the history and clinical signs and confirmed most easily by rectal palpation of a firm, ovoid, intravesicular mass at or near the neck of the bladder. In most cases, urolith palpation is not difficult because clinical signs are rarely evident until the stone is several centimeters in diameter. Transrectal ultrasonography with a 7.5 mHz linear probe allows visualization of the stone. If ultrasound examination cannot be performed, the distended bladder should be catheterized to facilitate palpation and eliminate the possibility of urethroliths, urethral stricture, or smegma impaction of the urethral sinus. Urinalysis frequently reveals RBC, neutrophils, calcium carbonate crystals, and proteinuria. Cystoscopy, ultrasonography, and radiology are not essential for detection of urocystoliths in horses but may provide additional diagnostic or prognostic information. Ultrasonography is necessary to identify nephroliths.

Treatment: Several surgical procedures have been described for urocystolith removal. The surgical options include midline or paramedian laparotomy and cystotomy, pararectal cystotomy, subischial urethrostomy, urethral sphincterotomy, and laser lithotripsy. The selection of a procedure is dictated by the size, location, and number of uroliths; the sex and physiologic status of the horse; and the availability of surgical facilities.

UROPERITONEUM IN FOALS

Uroperitoneum is defined as urine leakage into the peritoneal space. In foals, this most commonly results from tearing of the bladder during parturition or rupture of the urachus secondary to umbilical abscessation. Ureteral or urethral tears are rare. Some studies indicate a higher incidence of bladder rupture in males than in females, possibly because the narrower pelvis and the longer, narrower urethra of colts is a predisposing factor. Urachal rupture occurs in both males and females. Traumatic bladder rupture is thought to be caused by uterine contractions on a full bladder as the foal passes through the birth canal. Although most ruptured bladders at birth are thought to be traumatic, the presence of smooth edges and absence of hemorrhage around the tear in some foals suggest a congenital origin (developmental defect of the bladder wall). Most bladder tears are located on the dorsum of the bladder. In the case of a ruptured urachus, infection in the umbilical stump can weaken the urachal wall and result in leakage of urine into the abdomen. Prematurity, cystitis, ascending infection, abdominal trauma, failure of passive transfer, and sepsis may predispose the foal to bladder rupture.

Clinical Findings: Foals generally appear normal at birth but progressively become lethargic, tachycardic, and tachypneic over 24-48 hr. Signs may not appear for a longer period in foals with a ruptured urachus. As the condition progresses, the abdomen becomes noticeably distended, and ballottement may produce a fluid wave. Most foals attempt to urinate often, with small amounts of urine being produced. This stranguria is often misinterpreted as straining to defecate. Other foals may be anuric or urinate normally.

Diagnosis: Blood and peritoneal fluid analysis can be helpful in diagnosis. Foals usually have a neutrophilic leukocytosis. Serum hyperkalemia combined with hyponatremia and hypochloremia are seen due to the high concentration of potassium and low levels of sodium and chloride in the urine, which rapidly equilibrate across the peritoneum. An ECG may show broad QRS complexes and very tall T waves due to hyperkalemia. The increased serum potassium predisposes the foal to bradycardia and cardiac arrhythmias (AV block, atrial standstill, and cardiac arrest) if not corrected. Serum BUN and creatinine values can be normal or increased. Blood gas analysis may also be normal or reveal a metabolic acidosis. Abdominal fluid is pale yellow and copious and can be easily detected on ultrasonographic evaluation. The creatinine level in the peritoneal fluid is at least double that in the serum. This test is the most accurate in diagnosing the problem. If laboratory testing is not available, then 10 mL of methylene blue can be injected into the bladder via a urinary catheter. If the bladder is patent to the peritoneal space, then dye should be seen in the peritoneal fluid within 15 min.

The clinical signs of progressive depression and stranguria can confuse the diagnosis. Differential diagnoses include septicemia (p 567), hypoxic ischemic encephalopathy (p 1039), persistent meconium impaction, or colic for other reasons.

In the case of a urachal rupture, abdominal ultrasonography may be helpful to establish an etiologic diagnosis. Ultrasonography of the umbilical remnants may suggest the presence of infection or abscessation. A large amount of fluid in the abdomen is also seen.

Treatment: Surgery is necessary to correct the defect and, in uncomplicated cases, is very successful. The foal should be stabilized before surgery. Potassium >5 mEq/L should be lowered preoperatively by administration of insulin at 0.1 mg/kg, IV, in 500 mL of normal saline plus 5% dextrose, over 30-40 min. Sodium bicarbonate administration is also helpful in driving potassium into cells. Peritoneal dialysis can be considered if the above treatment is unsuccessful.

The bladder should be repaired using absorbable sutures. Because surgical staples have migrated into the bladder and become the nidus for stone formation at a later date, they should not be used. If the umbilical structures are enlarged (indicating infection), they should be removed at the time of surgery and cultured. After surgical correction of the bladder, an indwelling urinary catheter may be placed for 48 hr to decrease bladder distention and leakage of urine at the repair site.

If a bladder rupture is recognized early in an otherwise healthy foal and the foal is stabilized appropriately prior to surgery, the prognosis for recovery is good to excellent, with success rates as high as 95%. In septic or premature foals, in which complications such as peritonitis, incisional complications, adhesions, and anesthetic death are encountered more frequently, the prognosis is fair.

INFECTIOUS DISEASES OF THE URINARY SYSTEM IN SMALL ANIMALS

Most infectious diseases of the urinary system in small animals are bacterial infections. Common organisms include *Escherichia coli* and *Staphylococcus*, *Klebsiella*, *Proteus*, *Streptococcus*, and *Enterobacter* spp. Bacterial infections of the urinary tract typically ascend from the urethra into the bladder and in some cases into the kidneys. Predisposing factors include abnormalities of urine flow (eg, urine retention), decreased urothelial defense mechanisms, decreased systemic immune defense mechanisms, inadequate urine concentration, or glucosuria. Female dogs are more susceptible to urinary tract infections than male dogs, except for bacterial prostatitis in older uncastrated male dogs. Dogs with concurrent diseases (eg, diabetes mellitus or hyperadrenocorticism) are at greater risk. Adult cats are relatively resistant to bacterial cystitis. Geriatric cats, immunosuppressed cats, or those with systemic diseases (eg, diabetes mellitus, hyperthyroidism, chronic renal failure) are more prone to both cystitis and pyelonephritis. Urinary tract pathogens, except for *Leptospira interrogans*, are not considered zoonotic. However, the potential for multiple drug-resistant pathogens to localize in the urinary system is a concern for both animal and human health. Subtherapeutic treatment regimens and inappropriate antibiotic selection are contributing factors. Animals that receive chronic antibiotic treatment or are immunocompromised may (rarely) become infected with *Candida* spp. Systemic fungal infections such as blastomycosis or apergillosis can involve the urinary system; the kidneys and prostate are the most likely sites.

BACTERIAL CYSTITIS

Bacterial cystitis is infection and inflammation of the urinary bladder. Clinical signs are pollakiuria, hematuria, dysuria, and urinating in inappropriate places. Hematuria may be more noticeable at the end of the urine stream. An animal may exhibit pain on palpation of the caudal abdomen, and the bladder may feel thickened or irregular. Bacterial cystitis is occasionally diagnosed in an asymptomatic animal when a routine urinalysis is performed. Chronic glucocorticoid administration or hyperadrenocorticism are sometimes associated with asymptomatic urinary tract infections.

Urinalysis often shows increased protein and hemoglobin on the dipstick. The WBC part of the dipstick (ie, nitrate) is inaccurate in dogs and cats and should not be used. The urine pH may be alkaline (7.5-9.0) if the bacteria are urease positive (eg, *Staphylococcus* or *Proteus*). An alkaline urine pH by itself is not abnormal, however, as diet and other factors can affect urine pH. Urine sediment should be examined microscopically. Increased numbers of WBC, RBC, and/or bacteria are consistent with cystitis. Bacteria can be confused with stain precipitate; filtering the stain or evaluating the sediment without staining is advised. Lack of visible bacteria in the sediment does not rule out urinary tract infection.

If clinical signs and/or urinalysis are suggestive of infection, a urine culture and antimicrobial susceptibility should be performed. Cystocentesis is the preferred method for sample collection, followed by sterile urethral catheterization or a midstream free catch into a sterile collection cup. A quantitative culture is necessary to interpret the result, especially with samples not collected by cystocentesis. Ideally, the culture should be set up within 2 hr of collection. If the laboratory is off-site, the sample should be refrigerated and processed by the laboratory within 24 hr. If the specimen cannot be refrigerated, commercial collection kits that contain preservatives can be used to maintain a stable bacterial population at room temperature for 24 hr. Laboratories that can provide both quantitative culturing and a minimum inhibitory concentration-based method for antimicrobial susceptibility testing are preferred.

Simple bacterial cystitis is treated for 2 wk with a broad-spectrum antibiotic that achieves a high concentration in the urine. Appropriate initial choices include amoxicillin (10-20 mg/kg, PO, BID-TID), cefadroxil (22-30 mg/kg, PO, BID), or ometoprim-sulfadimethoxine (27 mg/kg, PO, day one, then 13.5 mg/kg, PO, SID). A repeat urine culture 3-5 days following therapy is recommended. If positive, another antibiotic based on the new susceptibility results is given for a longer treatment period (eg, 3-4 wk). Very resistant or recurrent infections should be treated for 4-6 wk. Every course of treatment should be followed by a urine culture, even if the signs have resolved. In animals that have a history of chronic or recurrent infections, a urine culture should be done every month for 3 mo following therapy. If all of these cultures are negative, then a urine culture every 2-4 mo for the next year is advisable. Because resistance to antibiotics can develop during therapy, antimicrobial susceptibility testing should be performed on every positive urine culture.

Animals with resistant or recurrent bacterial cystitis should be evaluated for an underlying cause. The history may reveal chronic glucocorticoid use. Survey abdominal radiographs are frequently diagnostic for cystic calculi. Negative survey films should be followed by double contrast cystourethrography, ultrasonography, and/or cystoscopy to rule out radiolucent urocystoliths, anatomic defects, and neoplasia. A serum biochemical profile and CBC are important to rule out predisposing systemic diseases. Other diagnostic considerations include feline immunodeficiency virus, feline leukemia virus, and hyperthyroidism in cats and hyperadrenocorticism in dogs.

In cases that respond to therapy but continue to have frequent bouts of cystitis without an identifiable cause, low-dose prophylactic antibiotics can be used to prevent ascending bacteria from establishing an infection according to the following protocol: 1) a therapeutic course of an antibiotic for the current infection is completed, 2) no antibiotics are given for 3 days, to allow collection of urine for a post-treatment culture, and 3) the prophylactic protocol is immediately started. Prophylaxis consists of using a broad-spectrum antibiotic (eg, amoxicillin, cefadroxil) at $1/3$ of the total daily dose, given at bedtime, indefinitely. Every 6-8 wk, the antibiotic should be stopped for 3-5 days to obtain a sample for repeat urinalysis and culture. Every new infection should be treated with a therapeutic course of an antibiotic based on culture and susceptibility results. The treatment antibiotic will likely be different than the prophylactic antibiotic. The most valuable therapeutic antibiotics (eg, fluoroquinolones, second-generation cephalosporins) should be reserved for resistant infections. If the recurrent infection is resistant to the prophylactic antibiotic, this antibiotic can still be used for future prophylaxis after the infection is eradicated. Encouraging frequent voiding during the daytime is helpful in preventing recurrent infections.

PYELONEPHRITIS

Kidney infection (pyelonephritis) is usually due to ascending bacteria, although hematogenous spread is possible. The organisms and predisposing causes are similar to those of bacterial cystitis. Renoliths and ureteroliths, which impede the normal flow of urine out of the renal pelvis, are a common cause. In young dogs or cats, congenital malformations (eg, ectopic ureters) are a predisposing cause. Animals at risk for pyelonephritis are the very young, the very old, the immunosuppressed, or those with inadequate urine-concentrating ability. In many instances, an underlying cause is not identified.

Animals with acute pyelonephritis exhibit kidney or flank pain, fever, malaise, and sometimes vomiting, polyuria, and polydipsia. Urinalysis shows proteinuria, pyuria, bacteriuria, and/or hematuria. WBC casts are often present in fresh urine sediment. The urine culture is usually positive; the CBC may show leukocytosis with a left shift. The biochemical profile may be normal or show azotemia (prerenal or renal) and/or hyperglobulinemia. The animal may be in renal failure. Chronic pyelonephritis is more difficult to recognize because clinical signs may be subtle or absent. Polyuria and polydipsia are frequent. In many cases, the disease goes unrecognized until renal failure occurs. Although abnormalities in the urinalysis are present, they are often less dramatic than with acute kidney infection. A single urine culture can be negative if bacterial numbers are low. Other useful diagnostic tests include renal ultrasonography and IV pyelograms. Both studies may show dilation of one or both renal pelvises secondary to inflammation and partial obstruction. Asymmetric renal size and architectural changes with renal pelvic dilatation is highly suggestive of chronic pyelonephritis. In some cases, nephropyelocentesis via ultrasonographic guidance is useful to obtain a sample of urine from the dilated renal pelvis for analysis and culture.

Pyelonephritis should be treated aggressively with broad-spectrum antibiotics, based on urine culture and antimicrobial susceptibility testing, for 4-6 wk. The infection may respond to the same antibiotics recommended for cystitis, but more frequent administration (eg, amoxicillin TID rather than BID) and/or higher dosages are indicated. A fluoroquinolone or a combination of a fluoroquinolone with a β-lactam antibiotic is often effective. Dosages should be the same as for other soft-tissue infections. Animals that are febrile, anorectic, dehydrated, or azotemic should be hospitalized for IV antibiotics and fluid therapy. Fluid therapy may prevent acute pyelonephritis from progressing to acute renal failure and will improve renal perfusion and uremic signs in animals already in renal failure. Animals with acute pyelonephritis may recover normal renal function, depending on the amount of damage that occurred prior to treatment. In selected cases of chronic pyelonephritis with a severely hydronephrotic, nonfunctional kidney, a nephrectomy may be the treatment of choice once the animal has been stabilized. This will remove the source of infection and hopefully save the opposite kidney. IV pyelography and/or renal scintigraphy are useful to assess the relative function of each kidney. If both kidneys are severely affected, medical management alone is the only alternative. Recovery to chronic, stable renal failure is possible in many cases.

The urine should be cultured after the first 5-7 days of therapy to assess antibiotic efficacy. A urinalysis and culture should be repeated 3-5 days following therapy, and then monthly for 3 consecutive months. If all of these cultures are negative, the interval between urine cultures may be gradually lengthened. Animals with pyelonephritis are at high risk for persistence or recurrence of kidney infection.

INTERSTITIAL NEPHRITIS

Acute interstitial nephritis in dogs is caused most often by *Leptospira interrogans* (p 527). Cats can develop leptospirosis, although signs are less severe than in dogs. Other infectious causes of interstitial nephritis in dogs include *Leishmania donovani* and *Borrelia burgdorferi*. Glomerulonephritis is the predominant renal pathology, so these diseases are considered immune complex diseases rather than true infections. Infectious diseases that cause vasculitis in dogs or cats (eg, feline infectious peritonitis, Rocky Mountain spotted fever, ehrlichiosis) may also cause renal failure.

CAPILLARIA PLICA INFECTION

Capillaria plica may infect the urinary bladder, and occasionally the ureters and renal pelvises, of dogs and cats. Distribution is worldwide, and wild animals appear to be the primary hosts. A similar but less common organism, *C felis cati*, is also found in cats. Dogs and cats become infected with *C plica* by eating earthworms that contain the first-stage larvae. The worms are threadlike, yellowish, and 13-60 mm long. The eggs are colorless, operculated, have a slightly pitted shell, and are 63-68 × 24-27 μm in size. Most dogs and cats are asymptomatic. Some animals show signs of pollakiuria, urinary incontinence, and urinating in abnormal places. The eggs are shed in the urine and may be found in the urine sediment. Microscopic hematuria and increased numbers of epithelial cells may also be present. Reported treatments include levamisole, fenbendazole, albendazole, and ivermectin. The treatment of choice is unknown, but a single dose of ivermectin at 0.2 mg/kg, SC, is likely to be effective. It is not FDA approved for this use and is contraindicated in Collie breeds. The parasite may be self-limiting in the absence of reinfection.

GIANT KIDNEY WORM INFECTION IN MINK AND DOGS

Mink are the most common definitive host for *Dioctophyma renale*, the largest known nematode, which has a worldwide distribution. Many other species, including dogs and humans, can become infected. The definitive host contracts the parasite by ingesting encysted larvae in raw fish (eg, pike, bullhead) or frogs, or by ingesting an infected annelid worm. The larvae penetrate the bowel wall and migrate first to the liver and later to the kidneys. In dogs, the parasite often fails to reach the kidneys and may be found free in the abdominal cavity. Kidney worms grow larger in dogs than in mink, reaching up to 103 cm. Female worms are larger than male worms, and both are blood red. Both male and female worms must be present in the same kidney to complete the life cycle. Barrel-shaped, yellow-brown eggs with a thick pitted shell measuring 71-84 × 45-52 μm are shed into the urine.

In the kidneys, the worm(s) cause obstruction, hydronephrosis, and destruction of the renal parenchyma. The right kidney is most commonly affected in both mink and dogs. Kidney failure can result if both kidneys are parasitized. Chronic peritonitis, adhesions, and liver disease are also possible, especially in dogs. Clinical signs are hematuria, pollakiuria, weight loss, and renal or abdominal pain. Urinalysis may reveal proteinuria, hematuria, and pyuria. IV pyelography or ultrasonography shows the enlarged hydronephrotic kidney. The diagnosis is made by finding the eggs in the urine sediment if both sexes of the nematode are present in the kidney and the ureter is patent. Alternatively, exploratory laparotomy may reveal the diagnosis. Worms may be found in the peritoneal cavity, between the lobes of the liver, or within the affected kidney(s) via nephrotomy.

Unilateral nephrectomy is the treatment of choice if the opposite kidney is unaffected. Preventing ingestion of raw fish or other aquatic organisms is recommended, especially in areas where the parasite is known to infect wild animals.

NONINFECTIOUS DISEASES OF THE URINARY SYSTEM IN SMALL ANIMALS

RENAL DYSFUNCTION

Failure of the filtration function of the kidneys leads to the development of azotemia (an excess of nitrogenous compounds in the blood), which may be classified as prerenal, renal, postrenal, or of mixed origin. Prerenal azotemia develops whenever mean systemic arterial blood pressure declines to values <60 mm Hg and/or when dehydration causes plasma protein concentration to increase. Conditions that may lead to the development of prerenal azotemia include dehydration, congestive heart failure, and shock. Prerenal azotemia generally resolves with appropriate treatment, because kidney structure has not been altered, which allows normal function to resume once renal perfusion has been restored. Renal azotemia refers to a reduction in glomerular filtration rate (GFR) of ~75% during acute or chronic primary renal (or intrarenal) diseases. Postrenal azotemia develops when the integrity of the urinary tract is disrupted (eg, bladder rupture) or urine outflow is obstructed (eg, urethral or bilateral ureteral obstruction). Once adequate urine flow is restored, postrenal azotemia will resolve.

Chronic Kidney Disease

This disease process involves a loss of functional renal tissue due to a prolonged (≥3 mo), usually progressive process. Dramatic changes in renal structure may be seen, although structural and functional changes in the kidney are only loosely correlated. Chronic kidney disease often smolders for many months or years before it becomes clinically apparent, and is invariably irreversible and progressive. Although congenital disease results in a transient increase in prevalence in animals <3 yr old, the prevalence increases with advancing age from 5-6 yr. In geriatric populations at referral institutions, chronic kidney disease affects up to 10% of dogs and 35% of cats. The prevalence in the general small animal population is likely to be lower. Several breeds of dogs and cats are afflicted with heritable chronic kidney disease (see CONGENITAL AND INHERITED ANOMALIES OF THE URINARY SYSTEM, p 1253). There is no apparent breed or sex predisposition for nonheritable chronic kidney disease in dogs or cats.

Chronic kidney disease is generally classified into various stages (TABLE 2) based on laboratory tests and clinical signs. In Stage I, a process is damaging the kidneys but azotemia and clinical signs have not developed. Unfortunately, renal disease is uncommonly detected at this stage. In Stage II, the disease has progressed, GFR has fallen to <25% of normal, and azotemia is present, but clinical signs are not yet observed. However, this stage may be associated with impaired urine-concentrating ability and increased urine volume. Stage III occurs when GFR has declined further and both azotemia and clinical signs are often present. Stage IV reflects further progression and severe azotemia, with clinical signs present. This staging system applies to both chronic and acute kidney disease.

Etiology: Attempting to identify the primary process causing the kidney disease, especially in Stages I and II, is important to form a prognosis and treatment plan. Known causes of chronic kidney disease include diseases of the macrovascular compartment (eg, systemic hypertension, coagulopathies, chronic hypoperfusion), microvascular compartment (eg, systemic and glomerular hypertension, glomerulonephritis, developmental disorders, congenital collagen defects, amyloidosis), interstitial compartment

TABLE 2. International Renal Interest Society Classification of Stages of Kidney Disease

Stage	I	II	III	IV
	Nonazotemic Kidney Disease	Mild Renal Azotemia	Moderate Renal Azotemia	Severe Renal Azotemia
Creatinine (mg/dL)				
Dogs	<1.4	1.4-2.0	2.1-5.0	>5.0
Cats	<1.6	1.6-2.8	2.9-5.0	>5.0

(eg, pyelonephritis, neoplasia, obstructive uropathy, allergic and immune-mediated nephritis), and tubular compartment (eg, tubular reabsorptive defects, chronic low-grade nephrotoxicity, obstructive uropathy). Many causes of chronic, generalized renal disease are associated with progressive interstitial fibrosis. The severity of interstitial fibrosis is positively correlated to the magnitude of decline of GFR and negatively correlated with the prognosis. The glomerular, tubulointerstitial, and vascular lesions found in animals with generalized, chronic renal disease are often similar, regardless of the initiating cause. At this point, renal histology may show only marked interstitial fibrosis, which may be called chronic interstitial nephritis. This term describes the morphologic appearance of kidneys with end-stage chronic disease of any cause. Because acute kidney disease may progress to a chronic condition, any cause of acute kidney disease is also a possible cause of chronic kidney disease.

Clinical Findings: Generally, no clinical signs are observed as a direct result of disease until ≥75% of nephron function has been impaired (Stages III and IV). Exceptions are chronic kidney diseases that develop as part of a systemic disease with clinical signs referable to involvement of other body tissues (eg, systemic lupus erythematosus, systemic hypertension) or those associated with marked renal inflammation and capsular swelling leading to flank pain and occasionally to vomiting. Clinical evaluation may identify systemic hypertension and proteinuria with the nephrotic syndrome in any stage. Usually, the earliest clinical signs commonly attributable to renal dysfunction are polydipsia and polyuria, which are not observed until the function of approximately two-thirds of the nephrons has been impaired (late Stage II or early Stage III). Further destruction of renal tissue leads to azotemia without new clinical signs in Stage II, and finally to the clinically apparent uremic syndrome in Stage IV. Initially, uremia is associated with occasional vomiting and lethargy. As disease progresses within Stages III and IV over months (dogs) to years (cats), anorexia, weight loss, dehydration, oral ulceration, vomiting, and diarrhea become fully manifest. Loose teeth, deformable maxilla and mandible, or pathologic fractures may be seen with renal secondary osteodystrophy (p 858), but these are uncommon and generally observed only in young dogs with end-stage congenital renal disease. Physical examination and imaging studies of animals in Stages III and IV usually reveal small, irregular kidneys, although normal to large kidneys can be observed in animals with neoplasms, hydronephrosis, or glomerulonephritis. Mucous membranes are pale in late Stage III and Stage IV, due to the presence of a nonregenerative, normocytic, normochromic anemia.

Diagnosis: In Stages I and II, diagnosis is often missed or made incidentally during imaging studies or urinalyses conducted for other purposes. In Stages III and IV, the BUN, serum creatinine, and inorganic phosphorus concentrations are increased. Potassium depletion, due to renal potassium wasting combined with inadequate intake and the kaliuretic effects of acidosis, is frequently seen in cats and occasionally seen in dogs. Hyperkalemia associated with oliguria and anuria may be noted in terminal Stage IV or whenever marked prerenal azotemia is superimposed on chronic kidney disease. Systemic hypertension and associated complications develop in ~20% of affected cats and dogs and can occur at any stage. Osteoporosis may be seen radiographically, although this late finding is generally not helpful for diagnosis. In healthy dogs and cats, urine specific gravity generally ranges from 1.001-1.070, depending on body needs for water homeostasis; the normal range overlaps the abnormal or inappropriate range. In dogs and cats with dehydration and normal renal function, urine specific gravity should be >1.035. The inability to produce concentrated urine when challenged by dehydration is an early sign of chronic kidney disease; however, dogs with primary glomerular disease, and some cats, may become azotemic while retaining the ability to concentrate urine to a specific gravity >1.035. Even so, concentrated urine is rarely observed when the serum creatinine is >4 mg/dL in an animal with azotemia of renal origin.

The polydipsia and polyuria of chronic kidney disease must be differentiated from diseases that cause primary polydipsia (eg, psychogenic polydipsia, hyperthyroidism) or interfere directly with the urine-concentrating mechanism. This includes conditions that lead to retention of solute in tubular fluid (eg, diuretic administration, diabetes mellitus), central diabetes insipidus, and nephrogenic diabetes insipidus (eg, hyperadrenocorticism, hypercalcemia, pyometra, diseases causing septicemia). Adrenal insufficiency leads to a urine-concentrating defect and may thus be confused with Stage II and III oliguric renal disease because prerenal azotemia may be caused by the vomiting, diarrhea, and polydipsia associated with hypoadrenocorticism. Hyperkalemia, hyponatremia, and/or reduced plasma Na^+/K^+ ratio is most helpful in establishing a tentative diagnosis of adrenal insufficiency, which must be confirmed by hormonal assay(s). Also, animals with hypoadrenocorticism improve rapidly in response to proper therapy.

Combinations of survey radiography, abdominal ultrasonography, serial clinical pathology tests including urinalyses and urine cultures, and blood pressure measurements should be performed to evaluate the severity of disease, establish a prognosis, monitor the response to therapy, and identify complicating factors. Specific renal function tests and renal biopsy may be helpful to identify the exact cause in Stages I-III, but the presence of advanced pathologic changes in Stage IV is nonspecific and often precludes identification of an underlying cause by histologic studies. This condition in late Stage IV is often described as end-stage renal failure clinically and as chronic, generalized nephritis pathologically. Chronic kidney disease should be distinguished from the more readily reversible acute disease. Frequently, differentiation may be accomplished with an appropriate history, physical examination, and laboratory findings, although a renal biopsy may be required (see below). However, therapy for chronic renal failure caused by a range of morphologic lesions is similar, so renal biopies may not be warranted.

Treatment: With appropriate therapy, animals can survive for long periods with only a small fraction of functional renal tissue, perhaps 5-8% in dogs and cats. Recommended treatment varies with the stage of the disease. In Stages I and II, animals usually have minimal clinical abnormalities. Efforts to identify and treat the primary cause of the disease should be thorough. The identification and supportive treatment of developing complications (eg, systemic hypertension, potassium homeostasis disorders, metabolic acidosis, bacterial urinary tract infection) should be aggressively pursued. The systemic hypertension seen in ~20% of animals with chronic kidney disease may be observed at any stage and is not effectively controlled by feeding a low-salt diet. The usual antihypertensive medications are a calcium-channel blocker such as amlodipine besylate (0.1-0.25 mg/kg, PO, SID) or an angiotensin-converting enzyme (ACE) inhibitor such as enalapril (0.5 mg/kg, SID-BID). While these may be administered together, a calcium-channel blocker is usually recommended as initial therapy in cats and an ACE inhibitor in dogs. In addition to providing a continual supply of fresh drinking water and encouraging (and documenting) adequate dietary intake, body condition scoring should be used routinely to assess adequacy of intake. Animals in this stage should be fed standard, commercially available maintenance diets, unless they are markedly proteinuric (see below). All affected animals should be reevaluated every 3-6 mo, or sooner if problems develop.

In Stages II and III, the principles for management of complications are the same, except that the animal should be evaluated every 2-3 mo. These evaluations should include hematology, serum biochemistries, and urinalysis. Because dogs and cats with chronic kidney disease are prone to the development of bacterial urinary tract infections, urine culture should be performed twice annually or if urinalysis suggests infection. The progressive nature of this disease produces a vicious cycle of progressive renal destruction. Measures that may slow this progression include dietary phosphorus restriction (dogs and cats), dietary fish oil supplementation (dogs), antihypertensive agents (hypertensive dogs and cats), and administration of ACE inhibitors. Dietary restriction of phosphate and acid load is essential in this stage, and specialized diets for management of kidney disease should be fed. Potassium citrate or sodium bicarbonate, given PO, may be indicated if the animal is severely acidotic (plasma bicarbonate <15 mEq/L) or remains acidotic 2-3 wk after diet change. If dietary restriction of phosphorus is unsuccessful in maintaining a normal level of serum phosphorus within 2-3 mo, phosphate-binding gels containing calcium acetate, calcium carbonate, or aluminum hydroxide should be administered with meals to achieve the desired effect. In dogs only, there is a clear rationale for the inclusion of dietary n-3 polyunsaturated fatty acids in these stages.

In late Stage III and Stage IV, all of the principles of managing the preceding stages apply, except that the animal should be evaluated every 1-2 mo. Dietary restriction of protein may relieve some of the signs of uremia. High-quality protein (eg, egg protein) should be fed at a level of 2.0-2.8 g/kg/day for dogs and 2.8-3.8 g/kg/day for cats. Commercial diets formulated for cats and dogs with chronic kidney disease generally meet this recommendation. Administration of an H_2-receptor antagonist such as famotidine (5 mg/kg, PO, TID-QID) decreases gastric acidity and vomiting. Anabolic steroids, such as oxymethalone or nandrolone, have been administered to stimulate RBC production in anemic animals, but this is not effective. Recombinant erythropoietin is effective in stimulating RBC production, but antierythropoietin antibodies develop in ~50% of animals and may result in refractory anemia; until species-specific products become generally available, erythropoietin administration is now recommended only for animals showing clinically apparent signs of anemia (eg, weakness, marked lethargy not attributable to other factors), which generally occurs at a hematocrit <20%. Fluid therapy with polyionic solutions, given IV or SC in the hospital or SC by owners at home, is often beneficial in animals with intermittent signs of uremia. Although controversial, oral vitamin D administration may reduce uremic signs. However, vitamin D administration requires prior resolution of hyperphosphatemia and it may induce hypercalcemia. Feeding tubes may help manage chronic anorexia. Euthanasia or renal replacement therapy (renal transplantation and/or dialysis) should be carefully considered if therapy does not improve renal function and alleviate signs of uremia.

Acute Kidney Disease

Acute kidney disease is seen when a sudden, major insult damages the kidneys. The principal causes are toxins (eg, ethylene glycol, aminoglycoside antibiotics, hypercalcemia, hemoglobinuria) and ischemia (eg, embolic showers from disseminated intravascular coagulation or severe prolonged hypoperfusion).

Clinical Findings: Mild, acute kidney disease often goes unrecognized; severe initial or repeated bouts may lead to chronic kidney disease. The stages of acute and chronic kidney disease are the same (*see* above). Most often, acute kidney disease is recognized in Stage IV and is characterized clinically by anorexia, depression, dehydration, oral ulceration, vomiting and/or diarrhea, or oliguria. Physical examination findings often reveal dehydration but otherwise are usually not remarkable, although pain is occasionally elicited on palpation of the kidneys, which may be normal-sized to slightly enlarged.

Diagnosis: A history of hypotension, shock, or recent exposure to known nephrotoxins in an animal with sudden-onset uremia (Stage IV) is the typical clinical picture of an animal with acute kidney disease. The presence of inappropriately concentrated urine (specific gravity 1.007-1.035) in the face of dehydration and/or azotemia suggests renal dysfunction. Differentiating between chronic and acute kidney disease (and establishing a specific cause in acute kidney disease) is important, as the prognosis and specific therapy may differ. Animals with acute kidney disease usually have a compatible history and other urinalysis abnormalities; marked cylindruria is a frequent and definitive finding. Other urinalysis findings may include the presence of a large number of renal epithelial cells and leukocytes in the urine sediment, glucosuria, crystalluria, and/or myoglobinuria/hemoglobinuria. Animals with Stage III or IV acute kidney disease have increased serum urea nitrogen, creatinine, and inorganic phosphorus concentrations and metabolic acidosis. Oliguria or anuria following rehydration, which is often associated with hyperkalemia, is a poor prognostic sign; in contrast, polyuric animals have a better prognosis, although they may become hypokalemic. Anemia is often, but not always, absent—a finding that may be helpful in differentiating acute from chronic kidney disease.

Following injury, the kidney has considerable potential for functional regeneration through the process of compensatory hypertrophy and adaptive hyperfunction. In animals with chronic kidney disease, it is likely that much of these processes has occurred prior to the initial diagnosis. In contrast, animals with acute kidney disease have considerably more potential for improvement of renal function, if they can be sustained through a uremic episode. The duration of the uremic episode may be substantial with some nephrotoxins (eg, 1-3 wk with aminoglycoside antibiotics and 4-8 wk with ethylene glycol). A renal biopsy may be of value in assessment of the severity, extent, cause, and potential reversibility of the disease.

Treatment: If the cause is known, specific therapy should be instituted, eg, 4-methylpyrazole or ethanol for ethylene glycol toxicity in dogs (p 2357). Fluid therapy is indicated for all dehydrated and inappetant animals. A polyionic fluid such as lactated Ringer's solution is satisfactory unless hyperkalemia is present, in which case normal saline is recommended. Sodium bicarbonate may be cautiously added to the fluids to correct acidosis.

In oliguric or anuric animals, therapy to promote increased urine volume is often recommended if the animal is well hydrated and urine production is <0.5 mL/kg/hr. This approach has been questioned because urine flow may increase without corresponding increases in renal blood flow and GFR. Administration of excess fluid to an animal in the maintenance phase of oliguric renal failure may result in life-threatening pulmonary and cerebral edema. Nonetheless, efforts to increase renal blood flow and GFR may enhance urine production and do have a role in the management of these animals. For this therapy, urine production must be quantitatively monitored closely via an indwelling urethral catheter. Monitoring central venous pressure is advised to prevent overhydration. A sequential approach generally includes an initial slight overhydration by administration of a test dosage of 50 mL/kg of polyionic solution IV. If this fails to yield adequate urine flow within 3 hr, further measures include osmotic diuresis (10% or 20% mannitol or dextrose, 0.5-1 g/kg, IV, as a slow bolus over 15-30 min, alternated with infusion of lactated Ringer's solution, 30 mL/kg, IV, over 30 min). Subsequent measures generally include furosemide (2 mg/kg, IV, which can be doubled and then tripled at 2-hr intervals if urine production does not increase above the target of 0.5 mL/kg/hr). However, furosemide may worsen the severity of acute renal failure caused by aminoglycosides. Finally, renal vasodilators (dopamine diluted in 5% dextrose, IV, to provide 1-5 µg/kg/min) plus furosemide (2 mg/kg, IV) may be tried for 2 hr. Dopamine may lead to ventricular arrhythmias and its use as a renal vasodilator has been questioned, particularly in cats. High doses of dopamine may cause renal vasoconstriction. If attempts to restore urine flow fail, aggressive measures should be discontinued to avoid overhydration. Daily fluid therapy based on maintenance and rehydration needs is continued until renal function and clinical condition improve. Feeding tube placement greatly facilitates patient management at this stage and should be implemented for any animal with marked renal azotemia (serum creatinine >10 mg/dL after rehydration).

A second therapeutic option, rather than the aggressive measures discussed above, is to proceed directly to fluid therapy with polyionic solutions while waiting for renal regeneration. Again, feeding tube placement for parenteral nutrition should be implemented in anorectic animals with marked azotemia. Peritoneal dialysis, hemodialysis, or euthanasia may be necessary if none of the above measures restores urine production.

GLOMERULAR DISEASE

Glomerular disease is a well-recognized cause of chronic (but not acute) kidney disease in dogs, and is also occasionally observed in cats. Animals with primary glomerular disease as a cause of chronic kidney disease may have somewhat different clinical and laboratory abnormalities than those with primary tubulointerstitial disease. Damage to the glomerular basement membrane results in albuminuria, which may lead to hypoalbuminemia. Animals may then exhibit signs related to hypoalbuminemia (eg, peripheral edema, hypercoagulability with thrombosis, hypercholesterolemia) instead of or in addition to uremia.

Secondary glomerulopathies, observed as sequelae of systemic or glomerular hypertension in animals with Stage III or IV chronic kidney disease, are common. Although the overall prevalence of a primary glomerulopathy as an inciting cause is not known, it is apparently more common in dogs than cats.

Immune-mediated glomerulonephropathy is characterized by deposition or in situ formation of immune complexes in the glomerular capillary wall, which then incite inflammatory changes (see also p 654). In one study of dogs, the mean age of presentation for glomerulonephritis was 4-8 yr; 55% were males, and there was no breed predilection. Immune-mediated glomerulonephritis has been associated with neoplasia, rickettsial diseases, systemic lupus erythematosus (SLE), heartworm disease, pyometra, chronic septicemia, and adenovirus infection, but it is usually idiopathic. Though multifactorial in origin, the glomerular disease associated with hyperadrenocorticism and diabetes mellitus in dogs is rarely attributable to immune complex formation. In one study of cats with glomerulonephritis, the mean age at presentation was 3-4 yr; 75% were males, and there was no breed predisposition. Primary glomerular disease in cats is most frequently associated with chronic infection by feline leukemia virus (FeLV), feline immunodeficiency virus (FIV), or feline infectious peritonitis (FIP) virus but has also been reported in association with neoplasia and systemic inflammatory diseases. The relatively young age and predilection for males reflects the high prevalence of FeLV infection as a cause in reported feline cases.

Familial glomerulopathies as a primary cause of chronic kidney disease have been reported in several breeds of dogs, including Bernese Mountain Dogs, English Cocker Spaniels, Doberman Pinschers, Greyhounds, Lhasa Apsos, Poodles, Rottweilers, Samoyeds, Shih Tzus, and Soft-coated Wheaten Terriers. These are not immune complex diseases, although some are characterized by proteinuria and associated clinical abnormalities that resemble those caused by immune-mediated glomerulonephropathy.

Amyloid is the name given to any of several chemically inert fibrillar protein subunits that can be deposited in tissue and interfere with normal organ function. (See also AMYLOIDOSIS, p 478.) All of these proteins are deposited in a β-pleated sheet conformation, which results in the unique appearance and chemical properties of amyloid. Most cases of amyloidosis in dogs and cats, including familial amyloidosis in Shar-Peis and Abyssinian cats, are reactive, or secondary, amyloidosis. In this form of the disease, amyloid A protein is deposited in various tissues after serum levels increase as a result of chronic inflammation. When the kidneys are affected, amyloid deposition in the nonfamilial forms in dogs usually occurs in the glomerulus. However, in Shar-Peis, at least 25% of Abyssinian cats, and in many domestic cats with the nonfamilial form of this disease, amyloid is found primarily in the medullary interstitium where it interferes with the renal concentrating mechanism and is more likely to produce nonproteinuric chronic kidney disease than protein-losing glomerular amyloid deposition. Glomerular amyloidosis usually leads to marked proteinuria. The nonfamilial form of amyloidosis usually affects middle-aged to older dogs and cats. Beagles, Collies, and Walker Hounds are reported to be at increased risk. Animals with the familial form of the disease are usually diagnosed at a younger age.

Clinical Findings: Glomerulopathy often leads to proteinuria (primarily albuminuria) and can produce hypoproteinemia, ascites, dyspnea (due to pleural effusion or pulmonary edema), and/or peripheral edema, which may be referred to as the nephrotic syndrome. Protein wasting can produce preferential loss of lean body mass that may be apparent on careful physical examination. Severe or chronic glomerular disease is a cause of chronic kidney disease; most dogs and many cats with glomerular disease eventually develop Stage III or Stage IV disease. Systemic hypertension may be more prevalent in proteinuric chronic kidney disease and may observed at any stage.

Proteinuria may result in loss of antithrombin III through the glomerular basement membrane, leading to a hypercoagulable state in dogs. Proteinuria also contributes to mild thrombocytosis and platelet hypersensitivity, which contribute to coagulation abnormalities in affected dogs, generally when plasma albumin levels are ≤1.0 g/dL. Severe dyspnea secondary to pulmonary thromboembolism or other sequelae of thrombotic disease may be seen in dogs with glomerulonephritis or amyloidosis. It is unclear whether a hypercoagulable state also exists in proteinuric cats, because clinical signs from hypercoagulability have not been reported in cats.

Diagnosis: The serum urea nitrogen, creatinine, and phosphorus concentrations are usually increased, although the degree varies with the stage of chronic kidney disease at the time of diagnosis. Marked proteinuria with edema may be observed in the presence or absence of azotemia. Physical findings are usually nonspecific except that ascites, pleural effusion, and/or peripheral, pitting, nonpainful, subcutaneous edema, are evident in some animals (75% of cats and 15% of dogs). Although uncommon, urine specific gravity may be inappropriately high for the degree of renal dysfunction. Proteinuria is associated with all forms of glomerular disease, but it must be quantitated to determine whether the protein loss is significant. The urine protein to creatinine ratio is determined in a random urine sample to quantify urinary protein loss; a value >0.5 indicates proteinuria but does not define its origin (glomerular, tubular, or lower tract origin). If the sediment examination eliminates inflammatory urinary tract disease and hemorrhage as the source of proteinuria, then the degree of increase may help distinguish tubular proteinuria (typical ratio value of 0.5-2.5), glomerulonephritis (typical ratio value of 0.5-15), and glomerular amyloidosis (typical ratio value of 0.5-40). However, substantial overlap exists in these ranges, and the ratio will tend to be low in the initial stages of a glomerulopathy, increase in severity as the disease progresses, and then decline terminally as GFR falls to very low levels in late Stage IV disease.

Renal biopsy is often required to determine the type of glomerular disease. Membranous glomerulonephritis is reported most frequently in cats; there is a roughly equal distribution of histologic findings in dogs, with glomerular amyloidosis and membranous, proliferative, and membranoproliferative glomerulonephritis all represented. The degree of proteinuria does not always correlate with the severity of the histologic lesions or the degree of azotemia. Systemic hypertension develops in an unusually large proportion of animals with protein-losing glomerulonephritis; therefore, blood pressure should be determined in all animals with evidence of glomerular disease.

A careful search should be made for an inciting disease process. Abdominal and thoracic radiographs, ultrasonography, and specialized serologic tests can rule out various inflammatory, infectious, and neoplastic diseases. In dogs with glomerulonephritis, this includes tests for SLE (eg, antinuclear antibody titer and LE prep) and appropriate antigen or antibody screening tests for other infectious agents and heartworm disease; in cats, tests for infection with FeLV, FIV, FIP, SLE, and heartworm disease should be included.

Treatment: There are 6 basic principles to therapy in glomerulonephropathies: 1) If a cause of immune-complex disease can be identified, it should be treated. 2) Manifestations of the nephrotic syndrome, if present, should be managed with dietary salt restriction and judicious use of diuretics. 3) Antithrombotics (eg, aspirin) should be considered for hypoalbuminemic (plasma albumin <1.0 g/dL) animals as well as those with low serum levels of antithrombin III (<30% of normal). In dogs with marked proteinuria and serum albumin <2 g/dL, low-dose aspirin therapy is appropriate, unless melena is present or gastric ulceration is suspected. However, aspirin is bound to plasma proteins and is eliminated via the kidneys, so the dosage may need to be adjusted. 4) Because proteinuria may promote interstitial fibrosis, treatment to limit glomerular loss of protein is warranted and may include dietary protein restriction and administration of an ACE inhibitor. 5) Efforts to reduce the magnitude and consequences of glomerular immune complex deposition should be considered, especially in animals with biopsy-confirmed glomerular inflammation and no known primary antigenic stimulus. Immunosuppressive drugs (eg, azathioprine, cyclophosphamide, cyclosporine) can be used in dogs with glomerulonephritis, although results are variable. For amyloidosis, dimethylsulfoxide and colchicine have been tried, but without consistent results. These anti-inflammatory drugs should be administered only on a trial basis with owner consent. Corticosteroids seem to be beneficial only in mild glomerulopathy; they may worsen proteinuria in other glomerulopathies and should be avoided in animals with amyloidosis, as they are reported to enhance amyloid deposition. 6) Manifestations of chronic kidney disease will be observed in accordance with the stage of disease. Appropriate therapy has been discussed elsewhere (see above).

Prognosis: Although one study found that mean survival time of dogs with glomerulonephritis was 87 days, the prognosis with early diagnosis and appropriate therapy is much better. In a recent study of dogs with glomerulonephritis, those receiving a placebo medication survived beyond the entire 6-mo duration of the study. The prognosis for animals with amyloidosis is guarded but variable, with reported mean survival times ranging from 49 days to 20 mo.

RENAL TUBULAR DEFECTS

Renal Tubular Acidosis

The form of metabolic acidosis that occurs in Stages II-IV of acute and chronic kidney disease, referred to as uremic acidosis, is due to reduced urine-acidifying ability of diseased kidneys. In uremic acidosis, although the ability of some individual tubular cells to reabsorb bicarbonate and/or secrete hydrogen ions may be normal, there is generally far less total cell mass present. Acid accumulates if the animal is under metabolic or dietary acid pressure, which is common in carnivores and is particularly problematic in cats, which are often fed acidifying maintenance diets.

Rare renal tubular defects in dogs and cats may result in hyperchloremic metabolic acidosis, referred to as renal tubular acidosis. Two types of renal tubular acidosis have been described in dogs and one in cats. In Type I (distal), the ability of the distal tubule to secrete hydrogen ions against a concentration gradient is defective; in Type II (proximal), the ability to reabsorb bicarbonate in the proximal tubule is reduced. Type I has been reported in both species; Type II has also been described in dogs in conjunction with other proximal tubular defects in acquired (gentamicin nephrotoxicosis and an idiopathic form) and heritable (Fanconi syndrome, see below) forms.

Type I renal tubular acidosis has been associated with demineralization of the skeleton (due to buffering of excess hydrogen ions) and nephrolithiasis (due to hypercalciuria from bone resorption) in dogs. Diagnosis is based on the presence of hyperchloremic metabolic acidosis with a urinary pH that is inappropriately high for the degree of systemic acidosis in the absence of bacterial urease modification of urine. Failure to produce acid urine after oral ammonium chloride loading is diagnostic; however, this test is contraindicated in animals that are already severely acidotic. Type II renal tubular acidosis is diagnosed by demonstrating increased urinary fractional excretion of bicarbonate when plasma bicarbonate levels are normal or decreased; this test is not practicable in the clinical setting and diagnosis is presumptively based on history, signalment, and clinical pathology findings.

Therapy consists of oral administration of an alkalinizing agent sufficient to maintain normal blood pH (1 mEq bicarbonate equivalent/kg/day for Type I and 1-6 mEq bicarbonate equivalent/kg/day for Type II, PO). Therapy is more problematic in dogs with Type II renal tubular acidosis, because supplemental bicarbonate is readily lost in the urine.

Fanconi Syndrome

Fanconi syndrome is a generalized proximal tubular reabsorptive defect resulting in excessive loss of many solutes in the urine. It has been reported as an acquired condition in dogs (gentamicin nephrotoxicosis and an idiopathic form) and in a heritable form in a variety of breeds (most notably Basenjis), in which it develops gradually in adults of both sexes. There is excessive urinary loss of glucose, sodium, potassium, phosphorus, uric acid, bicarbonate, and amino acids. Blood glucose concentrations are normal. Serum electrolytes are normal early in the disease, but hypophosphatemia, hypokalemia, and metabolic acidosis are seen in the later stages.

Clinical signs include polydipsia, polyuria, and weight loss. Signs of uremia may be present if the animal is in Stage III chronic kidney disease. Diagnosis is based on documentation of increased urinary fractional excretion of glucose, sodium, potassium, phosphorus, and bicarbonate in the presence of normal plasma concentrations. Differential diagnoses include simple renal glucosuria and chronic kidney disease from other causes. The microscopic renal changes in the heritable form are not remarkable in the early stages but progress to nonspecific findings characteristic of chronic kidney disease. A genetic marker has been developed. A treatment regimen to reverse the tubular defect has not been described. The histologic appearance of the acquired forms of Fanconi syndrome vary, depending on the cause.

Oral supplementation of sodium chloride, potassium, phosphate, and bicarbonate is indicated if the corresponding serum concentration is low. Dogs with acute or chronic kidney disease should be treated symptomatically as appropriate. The heritable disease is slowly progressive despite therapy and usually results in death from uremia.

Renal Glucosuria

This is usually a congenital defect in proximal tubular handling of glucose that results in glucosuria despite normal blood glucose concentration. Affected animals may be asymptomatic, have polydipsia and polyuria, or have recurrent urinary tract infections due to bacterial colonization in the presence of glucose. Diagnosis is made by demonstrating persistent glucosuria despite a normal blood glucose concentration and by identifying no other renal reabsorptive abnormalities. This disease is so uncommonly recognized that little is known about its biologic behavior. The general consensus is that it is not progressive and does not require treatment.

OBSTRUCTIVE UROPATHY

Even though the kidneys would otherwise be able to function normally, obstruction of urine flow at any point below the level of the kidneys leads to accumulation of metabolic wastes and postrenal azotemia/uremia. Obstruction of the urethra by uroliths in dogs and by matrix-crystalline plugs in cats are the most common causes, although uroliths, tumors, or blood clots may obstruct the ureters (or urethra) in either species.

Hydronephrosis is characterized by dilatation of the renal pelvis as the result of partial or complete obstruction of outflow of urine from one or both kidneys. When the obstruction is acute, complete, and bilateral, morphologic changes in the kidneys are less extensive because the period of survival is short. In unilateral or partial obstruction, the animal often survives long enough for severe pressure atrophy of the renal parenchyma and cystic enlargement of the affected kidney to develop. Hydroureter commonly develops when the obstruction is located lower in the tract. Increased hydrostatic pressure results in atrophy of functional renal parenchyma. The pseudodiverticula of the renal pelvis disappear first; later, even the cortex may atrophy. The affected kidneys eventually become grossly enlarged, functionless sacs, filled with urine or serous fluid that may harbor bacteria.

Clinical Findings: Animals with urethral obstruction exhibit pollakiuria, stranguria, and frequently hematuria; abdominal pain may be marked. Signs of uremia develop rapidly and include vomiting, dehydration, hypothermia, and severe depression. The bladder is distended and painful on palpation, and a urethral catheter cannot be readily passed. Bradycardia or cardiac arrhythmias due to hyperkalemia may be present, particularly if plasma potassium is >7 mEq/L. Because compensatory hypertrophy of the non-affected kidney results in a nonazotemic state, unilateral ureteral obstruction commonly is undiagnosed unless the animal has accompanying renal disease or the enlarged, hydronephrotic kidney is palpated or observed during physical examination and/or radiologic or ultrasonographic imaging studies.

Diagnosis: The history, clinical signs, and physical examination usually provide a straightforward diagnosis. Excretory urography or abdominal ultrasonography is necessary in animals with bilateral or unilateral ureteral obstruction. Serum potassium levels should be determined immediately in animals with cardiac arrhythmias. An ECG can provide presumptive evidence of hyperkalemia (bradycardia; tall, peaked T waves; increased PR interval; widened QRS complex; atrial standstill) if laboratory results are delayed.

Treatment: The urethral obstruction should be relieved (*see also* UROLITHIASIS, p 1279). Fluids given IV improve renal function and correct electrolyte and acid-base abnormalities. Normal saline is preferred but not required in hyperkalemic animals. Unless the animal is markedly hyperkalemic (serum potassium >7 mEq/L), has cardiac arrhythmias, or is known to have preexisting kidney disease, it is often best to avoid overcorrection by allowing plasma potassium and acid-base balance to return toward normal via restoration of renal excretory function for 12 hr before administering therapy specifically designed to correct these abnormalities. In animals with severe hyperkalemia and cardiac arrhythmias, bicarbonate (0.5 mEq/kg, given slowly IV over 5 min) or regular insulin and dextrose infusions can be given to drive potassium intracellularly. Because of a postobstructive diuresis that lasts for 1-5 days, hypokalemia and/or dehydration are often observed within 24-48 hr following correction of urethral obstruction. Plasma electrolytes, body weight, urine output, hematocrit, and plasma total solids should be monitored daily, and the type and quantity of fluid administered adjusted appropriately.

Surgery is often necessary to correct complete ureteral obstruction. When possible, the obstruction should be removed to reestablish urine flow. In some cases, ureteroliths will pass through the ureters, eliminating the need for surgery. This may require partial ureteral resection and reimplantation, particularly in cats, which possess a very small and friable ureter. In some cases unilateral nephrectomy may be required, but a kidney should not be removed without clear evidence that the contralateral kidney is capable of sustaining life. Preferred evidence includes the estimation of GFR in the contralateral kidney but could alternatively be based on all of the following criteria: normal renal size, shape, and consistency on ultrasonography; presence of normal vascular and excretory phases on excretory urography; normal renal ultrasonographic examination; and normal renal biopsy.

NEOPLASIA

Neoplasms of the Kidney

Neoplasms of the kidney are uncommon and represent ~0.5-1.7% of all neoplasms in dogs. Benign neoplasms are uncommon, usually incidental findings at necropsy, and generally of little clinical significance. Adenomas, lipomas, fibromas, and papillomas have been reported.

Primary malignant renal neoplasms (except nephroblastomas) are most common in middle-aged to older animals. No breed predilection has been found, except for heritable predilection for the development of bilateral, multifocal cystoadenocarcinomas in German Shepherds, generally between 5-11 yr of age. The most common primary malignant renal neoplasm is carcinoma, which originates from the renal tubular epithelium.

Usually, it is unilateral, located at one pole of the kidney, and well demarcated. Size varies from microscopic to several times that of the normal kidney, and color may be yellow, white, or gray. Renal carcinomas metastasize early to various organs; the opposite kidney, lungs, liver, and adrenals are involved most commonly.

Nephroblastomas (embryonal nephroma, Wilms' tumor) arise from vestigial embryonic tissue. They are seen in young animals and, in dogs, are most commonly diagnosed at <1 yr of age. There is no breed predilection. Males are affected twice as commonly as females. Nephroblastomas are usually unilateral but are occasionally bilateral. They can grow to immense proportions; it is not uncommon to have virtually the entire abdomen occupied by tumor. Metastasis occurs to regional lymph nodes, liver, and lungs.

Transitional cell carcinomas arise from transitional epithelium of the renal pelvis, ureter, bladder, or urethra (see NEOPLASMS OF THE LOWER URINARY TRACT, below). Other primary malignant renal neoplasms are uncommon and include hemangiosarcomas, fibrosarcomas, leiomyosarcomas, and squamous cell carcinomas.

The kidneys are a common site of metastatic or multicentric neoplasms. Metastatic lesions may be unilateral or bilateral. Lymphosarcoma is the most common multicentric tumor involving the kidneys. Up to 50% of dogs and cats with lymphosarcoma have renal lesions and, in some cases, only the kidneys or kidneys and brain are affected. Renal involvement is usually multifocal or diffuse, interstitial, and bilateral, and results in large, irregular kidneys. Lymphosarcoma in cats frequently is associated with infection by feline leukemia virus.

Clinical Findings: Signs are nonspecific and may include weight loss, anorexia, depression, and fever. Bilateral neoplasms may uncommonly destroy sufficient renal tissue to cause chronic kidney disease and associated signs of uremia. Astute owners may notice "lumps" in their animal's abdomen or abdominal enlargement. Persistent hematuria, usually microscopic, may occur. Rarely, renal tumors may produce excessive erythropoietin, which results in erythrocythemia (p 56).

Diagnosis: History and clinical signs may indicate a mass in the area of the kidneys or renomegaly, which can be confirmed by ultrasonography or radiography, although an excretory urogram or renal arteriogram may be required. Radiographs of the thorax may reveal metastatic disease. Neoplastic cells occasionally can be found in the urine sediment. Percutaneous needle aspiration and cytologic examination may be sufficient for the diagnosis of lymphosarcoma in cats and dogs, particularly when there is diffuse involvement or with ultrasonographic guidance when multifocal disease occurs. Histologic examination of tissue obtained by needle biopsy or surgical wedge biopsy is often necessary to determine the type of tumor.

Treatment: Treatment of all renal neoplasms except lymphosarcoma involves surgical removal; unilateral nephrectomy is usually required. Lymphosarcoma is best managed by combination chemotherapy (see CANINE MALIGNANT LYMPHOMA, p 35). Chemotherapy is generally ineffective against renal tumors other than lymphosarcoma.

Neoplasms of the Lower Urinary Tract

Neoplasms of the ureters, bladder, and urethra are uncommon in dogs and rare in cats. The low incidence in cats may be due to a difference in tryptophan metabolism that results in low urinary concentrations of carcinogenic tryptophan metabolites. The mean age of affected dogs and cats is 9 yr.

In the lower urinary tract, primary neoplasms are more likely to be malignant than benign. Papillomas, leiomyomas, fibromas, neurofibromas, hemangiomas, rhabdomyomas, and myxomas are found infrequently.

Among primary malignant neoplasms of the lower urinary tract, transitional cell carcinomas are diagnosed most frequently in both species. Squamous cell carcinomas, adenocarcinomas, fibrosarcomas, leiomyosarcomas, rhabdomyosarcomas, hemangiosarcomas, and osteosarcomas also are found. Transitional cell carcinomas may be solitary or multiple papillary-like projections from the mucosa or may develop as a diffuse infiltration of the ureter, bladder, prostate, and/or urethra. They are highly invasive and metastasize frequently, most commonly to the regional lymph nodes and lungs. Ureteral and bladder neoplasms can cause chronic obstruction to urine flow with secondary hydronephrosis. Urethral tumors are more likely to cause acute obstructive uropathy. Intractable secondary bacterial urinary tract infections are commonly associated with neoplasms of the bladder and urethra.

Clinical Findings: Hematuria, dysuria, stranguria, and pollakiuria are the most common signs. Animals with ureteral obstruction and unilateral hydronephrosis may show signs of abdominal pain and have a palpable, enlarged kidney. Signs of uremia may be apparent in animals with bilateral ureteral obstruction and hydronephrosis or with urethral obstruction. The bladder wall may be thickened, and a cord-like urethra or urethral mass(es) may be palpable rectally.

Diagnosis: History and clinical signs are highly suggestive of lower urinary tract disease in animals with tumors of the bladder or urethra. Urinalysis frequently reveals hematuria, and there may be evidence of secondary infection. Chronic, uncomplicated urinary tract infections must be differentiated from those associated with neoplasms. Neoplastic cells may be found in the sediment, particularly with transitional cell carcinomas. A cystourethrogram, retrograde urethrogram, or ultrasonography is generally necessary to determine the location and extent of the tumor. Biopsy of the tumor is required for definitive diagnosis.

Treatment: Excision of the tumor, if possible, is the most beneficial therapy. Transitional cell carcinomas are frequently located at the trigone of the bladder or in the urethra and may necessitate radical reconstructive surgery of the lower urinary tract. Prognosis is poor for these animals, even with surgery, because recurrence and metastasis occur rapidly. Chemotherapy with cisplatin or piroxicam may prolong the life of affected animals.

DISORDERS OF MICTURITION

Disorders of micturition result from a dysfunction in the storage or voiding of urine and may be neurogenic or non-neurogenic in origin. Urinary incontinence is the failure of voluntarily control micturition, with constant or intermittent unconscious passage of urine. Incontinent animals may leave a pool of urine where they have been lying or may dribble urine while walking. The coat around the vulva or prepuce may be wet, and perivulvar or peripreputial dermatitis can result from urine scalding.

Failure of urine storage is characterized by inappropriate leakage of urine due to failure of bladder relaxation, urethral incompetence, anatomic defects, or overflow of stored urine. Urge incontinence is seen with detrusor irritability, usually associated with cystitis. The most common non-neurogenic incontinence is attributed to deficiency of sex hormones in neutered animals, particularly female dogs, and is referred to as hormonal-responsive urethral incompetence. Idiopathic urethral sphincter incompetence also is seen. Urinary incontinence associated with anatomic defects may be detected in animals at an early age. For example, an animal with a unilateral congenital ectopic ureter may void normally but "dribble" urine intermittently, whereas animals with bilateral ectopic ureters are less likely to void normally. Paradoxical urinary incontinence may develop when there is a partial obstruction of the urethra leading to bladder distention and overflow incontinence.

Failure of normal voiding is characterized by frequent attempts to urinate with stranguria, and passage of only small amounts of urine. Inability to urinate can be due to mechanical obstruction of the urethra by calculi, neoplasms, or strictures; detrusor atony from overdistention of the bladder; or neurologic disease. Animals with abnormalities of the voiding phase may develop overflow incontinence due to dribbling of urine associated with bladder overdistention.

Neurologic causes of micturition disorders can be categorized as upper (UMN) or lower motor neuron (LMN) lesions. Lesions in the sacral spinal cord, pelvic nerve, and detrusor atony lead to LMN signs, which are often characterized by a distended, easily expressed bladder. Dysautonomia in cats is a multisystemic disease characterized by widespread disruption of autonomic system functions, including urinary incontinence of

LMN origin. Damage to the thoracolumbar spinal cord or disease of the cerebrum, cerebellum, or brain stem can lead to UMN signs, which are characterized by a distended bladder that is difficult to express. Another neurologic cause of inability to urinate is functional obstruction (detrusor-sphincter reflex dyssynergia), which occurs when there is incoordination of the normal micturition reflex; this is believed to result from overdischarge of sympathetic nerve impulses to the urethral sphincter, resulting in a failure of urethral relaxation during detrusor contraction. Animals with neurogenic incontinence may leak urine (LMN) and/or develop overflow incontinence due to dribbling of urine associated with bladder overdistension (any neurogenic cause).

Diagnosis: Clinical signs are usually suggestive of a micturition disorder. The history should include age of onset, sexual status of the animal, age at neutering, current medication, and history of previous urinary tract disorders. A thorough physical and neurologic examination is indicated, and the act of voiding should be observed, including estimation of initial and final bladder volume.

Animals with LMN lesions or an atonic bladder have a large, distended bladder that can be expressed with minimal pressure. Animals with mechanical or functional obstruction or with spinal lesions causing UMN also have a large distended bladder, but urine cannot be readily expressed. Caution must be exercised when attempting to express urine from these animals to avoid rupturing the bladder. Plain or contrast radiography, cystoscopy, or ultrasonography are necessary to determine the type and location of mechanical obstruction.

Animals with functional obstruction (reflex dyssynergia) generally exhibit pollakiuria with interrupted urine stream, distended urinary bladder, no identifiable structural cause of obstruction, and overflow incontinence, and generally have an abnormal neurologic examination. A catheter can easily be passed into the bladder in animals with functional obstruction but will not pass in animals with mechanical obstruction.

Treatment: Accurate diagnosis or localization of the lesion is essential for appropriate pharmacologic management. Animals with hormonal incontinence were formerly treated with the appropriate sex hormone—diethylstilbestrol in females and testosterone in males. The dose should be adjusted to the minimum required to maintain continence. Diethylstilbestrol may be unavailable or difficult to obtain. Alternatively, an α-adrenergic agonist drug (eg, phenylpropanolamine, 2-4 mg/kg/day in divided doses) can be given to animals with urethral incompetence. Urge incontinence (detrusor instability) is treated with anticholinergic drugs such as oxybutin chloride (0.5 mg/kg, PO, SID) or propantheline (dogs <20 kg, 7.5 mg/day; dogs >20 kg, 15 mg/day; cats, 7.5 mg every 72 hr). Cholinergic drugs such as bethanechol are used in animals with detrusor atony. Functional obstruction is treated with sympatholytic drugs (eg, phenoxybenzamine, 2.5-10 mg, SID-TID); cholinergic drugs may also be necessary.

Complete mechanical obstruction of the urethra is a medical emergency and should be relieved by catheterization and retropulsion of the obstructing material into the bladder or by surgery. Animals with detrusor atony from overdistention but without neurologic lesions benefit from decompression of the bladder by placement of an indwelling urinary catheter for 3-7 days. This may be done continuously or intermittently. Those with neurogenic atony, which usually does not respond to medical management, may require manual expression of the bladder or catheterization several times daily.

UROLITHIASIS

Some mineral solutes precipitate to form crystals in urine; these crystals may aggregate and grow to macroscopic size, at which time they are known as **uroliths** (calculi or stones). Uroliths generally contain an organic matrix that is believed to vary minimally among uroliths and that constitutes ~2-10% of the stone's chemical composition. The remaining 90-98% of the urolith is composed of minerals that vary depending on the type of urolith. **Urolithiasis** is a general term referring to stones located anywhere within the urinary tract. Uroliths can develop in the kidney, ureter, bladder, or urethra and are referred to as nephroliths, ureteroliths, urocystoliths, and urethroliths, respectively.

Uroliths in all animal species are composed of ~10 different minerals. Identification of the minerals in uroliths by quantitative analysis is unreliable. The type of minerals in uroliths can be readily identified by optical crystallography, infrared spectroscopy, and/or x-ray diffraction. Minerals found in uroliths have a chemical name and often a mineral or crystal name (TABLE 3). Variation in urine characteristics over time can result in more than one crystal type within a single urolith. In such instances, the urolith core corresponds to conditions that were present when the urolith initially formed, and the outer layers correspond to more recent conditions that favored continued growth.

Mechanisms involved in stone formation have not been completely defined. However, three main contributing factors are: 1) matrix—the inorganic protein core may facilitate initial urolith formation, 2) crystallization inhibitors—organic and inorganic crystallization inhibitors may be lacking or dysfunctional in animals with uroliths, and 3) precipitation crystallization factors—a complex relationship among urine solutes and other chemical factors in the urine can lead to conditions favoring crystallization. Regardless of the underlying mechanism(s), uroliths are not produced unless sufficiently high urine concentrations of urolith-forming constituents exist, and transit time of crystals within the urinary tract is prolonged. For selected stones (eg, struvite, cystine, urate), other favorable conditions (eg, proper pH) for crystallization must also exist. These criteria can be affected by urinary tract infection, diet, intestinal absorption, urine volume, frequency of urination, therapeutic agents, and genetics.

Clinical signs associated with urolithiasis are seldom caused by microscopic crystals. However, formation of macroscopic uroliths in the lower urinary tract that interfere with the flow of urine and/or irritate the mucosal surface often results in dysuria, hematuria, and stranguria. Nephroliths often are asymptomatic unless pyelonephritis exists concurrently or they pass into the ureter. Ureteral obstruction may produce signs of vomiting, lethargy, and/or flank and renal pain, particularly if there is acute total obstruction with distention of the renal capsule. The only clinical sign associated with unilateral urethroliths may be pain, which can be difficult to detect in dogs and cats. If these initial signs of ureteral obstruction do not lead to a diagnosis, unilateral ureteral obstruction may result in hydronephrosis with loss of function of the ipsilateral kidney. Ureteroliths may also precipitate a uremic crisis in cats with previously compensated chronic renal failure. Because clinical signs of renal dysfunction are generally not apparent until two-thirds or more of total functional renal parenchyma is lost, clinical signs may not be observed unless both ureters are obstructed, there is contralateral chronic kidney disease, or a renal infection develops. Unilateral ureteroliths may be identified serendipitously during abdominal imaging studies or surgery.

TABLE 3. Urolith Names

Mineral Name	Chemical Formula	Chemical Name
Struvite	$MgNH_4PO_4 \bullet 6H_2O$	Magnesium ammonium phosphate hexahydrate
Whewellite	$CaC_2O_4 \bullet H_2O$	Calcium oxalate monohydrate
Weddellite	$CaC_2O_4 \bullet 2H_2O$	Calcium oxalate dihydrate
Hydroxyapatite	$Ca_{10}(PO_4)_6(OH)_2$	Calcium phosphate (hydroxyl form)
Urate	$C_5H_4N_4O_3$	Urate
Ammonium urate	$NH_4 \bullet C_5H_4N_4O_3$	Ammonium urate
Sodium urate	$Na \bullet C_5H_4N_4O_3 \times H_2O$	Sodium urate monohydrate
Cystine	$(SCH_2CHNH_2COOH)_2$	Cystine
Silica	SiO_2	Silica
Xanthine	$C_5H_4N_4O_2$	Xanthine

Abdominal palpation is helpful in detecting urocystoliths; the bladder wall may be thickened and a grating sensation may be felt when the bladder is palpated. Although palpation may reveal a single large urolith or multiple uroliths by their crepitation, it cannot dependably identify all animals with uroliths; urethral calculi may be detected by rectal palpation or located by passing a catheter. Because multiple uroliths may be present throughout the urinary tract, a complete radiographic examination of the tract is indicated; radiodense calculi >3 mm in diameter are usually visible on radiographs. Urate, and occasionally cystine, uroliths may be radiolucent, requiring contrast radiography or ultrasonography to confirm their presence. Urinalysis, including identification of crystals on microscopic examination of fresh, warm urine and bacterial culture and sensitivity testing, is a critical part of the evaluation and may be helpful in determining the type of urolith present. Ultrasonography and cystoscopy may also be useful.

Urethral Obstruction: Urethral obstruction is common in male dogs and cats. It may occur suddenly or may develop over days or weeks. Initially, the animal may exhibit frequent attempts to urinate and produce only a fine stream, a few drops, or nothing. Animals may also exhibit extreme pain manifested by crying out when attempting to urinate. Complete obstruction causes uremia within 36-48 hr, which leads to depression, anorexia, vomiting, diarrhea, dehydration, coma, and death within ~72 hr. Urethral obstruction is an emergency condition, and treatment should begin immediately.

If the bladder is intact, it is distended, hard, and painful; care should be used when palpating the bladder to avoid iatrogenic rupture. If the bladder has ruptured, it cannot be palpated and urine can sometimes, but not always, be obtained from the abdominal cavity by paracentesis. Animals with spontaneous bladder rupture may appear temporarily improved because the pain associated with bladder distention has been relieved; however, peritonitis and absorption of uremic toxins and potassium occur rapidly and lead to depression, abdominal distention, cardiac arrhythmias, and death.

Hyperkalemia and metabolic acidosis are life-threatening complications of urethral obstruction. An ECG (to record cardiac rhythm and rate) and a serum potassium are indicated. Initial emergency care involves immediate relief of obstruction by catheterization and fluid therapy with normal saline. Occasionally, an obstruction at the external urethral orifice can be dislodged by gentle massage. Sometimes, when a portion of the urethra is dilated with fluid under pressure and then suddenly released, urethral calculi can be flushed out. The urolith nearly always can be flushed back into the bladder by using the largest catheter that can be easily passed to the calculus, occluding the distal end of the urethral lumen around the catheter, and infusing a sterile mixture of equal parts of isotonic saline solution and an aqueous lubricant. If the urethrolith cannot be flushed back into the bladder, a urethrotomy should be performed to remove the obstructing stone(s). Depending on the clinical circumstances, the urethrotomy site may be sutured or a permanent urethrostomy created. Calculi that are flushed back into the bladder should be removed by cystotomy to prevent recurrence, although in some cases they can be dissolved. The stone should be sent for quantitative analysis, and the animal managed medically to prevent stone recurrence based on the results.

Canine Urolithiasis

The most common canine uroliths are magnesium ammonium phosphate, calcium oxalate, or urate; less common uroliths include cystine, silica, calcium phosphate, and xanthine.

Struvite Stones: The most common urinary stones in dogs are composed of struvite. The mineral composition is mostly struvite ($MgNH_4PO_4 \cdot 6H_2O$), but frequently, small amounts of carbonate-apatite and ammonium urate are present. In most cases, struvite uroliths form in association with urinary tract infections with urease-producing *Staphylococcus* or *Proteus* spp. Unlike in cats, in which they are frequent, sterile struvite uroliths rarely form in dogs. They have been detected in a family of English Cocker Spaniels, suggesting a genetic predisposition.

Medical management involves dissolution and prevention of stone formation. In both instances, the aim of treatment is to reduce the concentrations of NH_4^+, Mg^{2+}, and PO_4^{-3} in urine. For dissolution, urine should be extremely undersaturated for struvite; for prevention, the degree of struvite saturation should be sufficiently low to make crystallization unlikely. The choice between surgery, lithotripsy, and medical treatment may not be easy. Owner compliance, the animal's acceptance of the diet, availability of lithotripsy, practice philosophy, and knowledge of the indications and contraindications are necessary to make a decision. If stone dissolution is prolonged or fails, it may be more costly than surgical treatment. Surgical removal of uroliths is often incomplete, with small, hidden uroliths often inadvertently left in the urinary tract serving as a nidus for recurrence.

Before beginning stone dissolution by medical therapy, a physical examination, CBC, serum chemistry profile, urinalysis, urine culture and sensitivity, abdominal radiographs to document stone size, and blood pressure measurement (if possible) should be performed. Contraindications to stone dissolution include heart failure, edema, ascites, pleural effusion, hypertension, hepatic failure, renal failure, and hypoalbuminemia. Renal failure is not always a contraindication for dissolution of struvite nephroliths, however.

Dissolution Protocol: While the use of urinary acidification to reduce urine pH <6 and other individualized dietary maneuvers may prove effective, a few commercially available diets that are generally nutritionally balanced promote struvite stone dissolution. Dogs fed these rations generally have reduced intake of protein, phosphate, and magnesium and a high intake of sodium. This results in osmotic diuresis, reduced daily urea output, and enhanced urine volume. The low urinary urea concentration is one of the most important features of such diets and also reduces ammonia production by the action of urease-producing bacteria. No other food, including treats, should be fed, and adequate fresh water should be available at all times.

Urease-producing urinary tract infections must be treated. The choice of antibacterial should be based on sensitivity testing when possible. Most *Staphylococcus* and *Proteus* infections are sensitive to levels of amoxicillin or ampicillin achieved in the urine of normal dogs. A urease inhibitor can be given but is not usually necessary. Concurrent treatment with a urease inhibitor such as acetohydroxamic acid enhances the rate of struvite stone dissolution, particularly when antibiotic resistance precludes effective antibacterial sterilization of the urine. A reasonably safe dose of acetohydroxamic acid appears to be 12.5 mg/kg, PO, BID. A reversible, mild hemolytic anemia has been seen in dogs given higher doses.

After ~4 wk of treatment, a physical examination, serum chemistry profile, urinalysis, and abdominal radiographs or ultrasonography should be repeated. The stone dissolution protocol should be discontinued if severe side effects develop, although a mild degree of hypoalbuminemia is to be expected and can be tolerated. With good compliance, the following results can be anticipated: urine pH <6.5; urine specific gravity <1.025; serum urea <10 mg/dL. The radiographic stone size should be compared with the size on previous radiographs. Routine testing should be repeated every 4 wk until 4 wk after the stone is no longer visible radiographically; this generally takes 8-12 wk but may take up to 20 wk. Stones that fail to reduce in size after 8 wk of treatment are probably not composed of struvite and should be treated another way, although failure could also result from poor treatment compliance. Renal stones tend to dissolve more slowly than bladder stones.

The recurrence rate after surgical treatment of struvite uroliths has been reported to be ~20-25%, with most recurrences within 1 yr. When surgery is performed to remove multiple small struvite calculi, removing all stone material is often difficult. In such cases, a 4-wk dissolution protocol starting at the time of suture removal aids in preventing recurrence due to residual crystalline material. Once the urinary tract is free of stones, prevention strategies are much more likely to be successful.

Prevention Protocol: The key to prevention of recurrence in animals with a struvite stone associated with infection is achieving and maintaining sterile urine. Routine testing of urine pH by the owner is important. If fresh urine is alkaline, a urinalysis and culture should be done, and the dog treated appropriately if an infection is present.

Once stone dissolution is completed, a prevention program can be considered. The aim is to prevent urinary tract infections with urease-producing microbes. The concentration of major struvite solutes in urine should also be reduced. A commercially available diet may be fed to lower urinary phosphate and magnesium and to maintain an acidic urine. Urease-producing infections should be eliminated, after which owners should regularly check the pH of the first voided urine in the morning after an overnight fast; in most dogs on a normal diet, the urine will be acidic. Checking urine pH weekly is sufficient.

Calcium Oxalate Stones: Calcium oxalate uroliths have been increasing in frequency in dogs. While they may develop in any breed, Miniature Schnauzers, Lhasa Apsos, Yorkshire Terriers, Bichon Frise, Shih Tzus, and Miniature Poodles may be predisposed. Most affected dogs are 2-10 yr old. Hypercalciuria leading to calcium oxalate stone formation can result from increased renal clearance of calcium due to excessive intestinal absorption of calcium (absorptive hypercalciuria), to impaired renal conservation of calcium (renal leak hypercalciuria), or to excessive skeletal mobilization of calcium (resorptive hypercalciuria).

Absorptive hypercalciuria is characterized by increased urine calcium excretion, normal serum calcium concentration, and normal or low serum parathormone concentration. Because absorptive hypercalciuria depends on dietary calcium, the amount of calcium excreted in the urine during fasting is normal or significantly reduced when compared with nonfasting levels. Renal leak hypercalciuria has been recognized in dogs less frequently than absorptive hypercalciuria. In dogs, renal leak hypercalciuria is characterized by normal serum calcium concentration, increased urine calcium excretion, and increased serum parathormone concentration. During fasting, these dogs do not show a decline in urinary calcium loss. The underlying cause of renal leak hypercalciuria in dogs is not known. Resorptive hypercalciuria is characterized by excessive filtration and excretion of calcium in urine as a result of hypercalcemia. Hypercalcemic disorders have been associated only infrequently with calcium oxalate uroliths in dogs.

Routine laboratory determinations should include serum calcium, phosphate, total CO_2, and chloride to eliminate the possibility of hyperparathyroidism and renal tubular acidosis. Dissolution of calcium oxalate stones by medical means has not been established at present. Treatment requires surgical removal or lithotripsy followed by preventive strategies.

Prevention Protocol: Recurrence is a major problem with calcium oxalate uroliths. An "ideal" diet is considered to be low oxalate, low protein, and low sodium, and would maintain urine pH at 6.5-7.5 and urine specific gravity <1.020. A few commercially available canned foods achieve these goals and may minimize the risk of recurrence. Potassium citrate may be added as needed to assure the urine pH is within the desired range; water may be used to provide appropriate reduction in urine concentration. If these urine conditions are achieved and calcium oxalate crystals are still observed in warm, fresh urine, then vitamin B_6 and/or thiazide diuretics can be considered (although of unproven efficacy). Effectiveness of therapy should be reevaluated at 1- to 4-mo intervals by urinalysis. Chlorothiazide diuretics may also be of value.

Urate Stones: Ammonium urate stones are most common in Dalmatians and in dogs with congenital portosystemic vascular shunts. The formation of ammonium urate calculi depends on the urine concentrations of urate and ammonium and on other poorly understood factors. Dalmatians fail to convert most of their metabolic urate to allantoin and thus excrete the bulk of nucleic acid metabolites as relatively insoluble urate. The biologic mechanism responsible for decreased hepatic conversion of urate to allantoin lies not in reduced uricase activity, but in reduced hepatic transport of urate; the rate of urate hepatic transport is about 3 times faster in breeds other than Dalmatians. The net result is only 30-40% of urate is converted to allantoin in Dalmatians compared with ~90% in other breeds.

Dalmatians fed a diet high in animal protein excrete a net acid load in the urine, and urinary ammonium output is subsequently increased. The combined high concentration of ammonium and urate in urine increases the risk of formation of ammonium urate stones. The excretion of acidic metabolites of an animal protein diet is believed to be important in this process because urinary ammonium excretion is enhanced and ammonium urate is insoluble. Urate output has been reported to be the same in Dalmatians that form stones and in those that do not, although in some studies the methods used to determine urine uric acid concentrations were unreliable; ammonium output has not been determined. In dogs with a portosystemic vascular anastomosis, increased urinary ammonium output may partially be due to the increased filtered load of ammonia, because plasma levels of ammonia tend to be increased.

Dissolution Protocol: Urine alkalinization minimizes renal ammonia production; the goal is to achieve a urine pH >7. If required, urine alkalinization can be achieved by administering NaHCO$_3$, 1 g ($^1/_4$ tsp)/5 kg, PO, TID, with food. Potassium citrate, administered to effect (25-50 mg/kg/day) is an alternative, more palatable alkalinizing agent.

Urinary urate output should be reduced. This can be accomplished by feeding a low purine, low-protein commercial diet. In addition, the xanthine oxidase inhibitor allopurinol (15 mg/kg, PO, BID) may be administered to ensure the nucleic acid metabolite load is excreted as a combination of xanthine, hypoxanthine, uric acid, and allantoin, rather than almost entirely as urate. However, the effectiveness of allopurinol in reducing urinary urate output is variable, and urinary urate levels should be measured (although this may be difficult). Allopurinol must be used cautiously in dogs with hepatic disease or primary renal failure because it is metabolized to its active form in the liver and is excreted via the kidneys. It is important that diets high in purines not be fed to dogs receiving allopurinol because xanthine uroliths may result.

Urine volume should be increased to reduce the concentration of all dissolved solutes in urine. This can be achieved by feeding canned diets restricted in protein. By reducing formation of urea, renal medullary urea concentration declines, interfering with the countercurrent system of urine concentration. Adding salt, 1 g ($^1/_4$ tsp)/5 kg, daily to the diet, or mixing water with the food are additional methods. Salt should not be given to animals with hypertension but otherwise poses little risk in normotensive dogs without chronic kidney disease, proteinuria, or hypoalbuminemia.

Prevention Protocol: Prevention strategies aim to reduce the concentration of ammonium and urate in urine to levels unlikely to induce flocculation.

A low-protein, low-purine diet should be fed to reduce urinary urate output. Alkalinization should be used as needed to ensure alkalinuria. Treatment with allopurinol (10 mg/kg, PO, SID) can be considered. Ideally, allopurinol is not needed as a supplement to dietary management; however, if urate crystals persist, a low maintenance dose of allopurinol is appropriate.

These dissolution and prevention strategies were developed for use in Dalmatians in which hepatic conversion of urate to allantoin is reduced, but the liver is otherwise normal. They may not be safe for use in dogs with portosystemic vascular shunts. Such dogs tend to develop hypoalbuminemia, edema, and ascites when fed a low-protein diet. The safety of allopurinol in these dogs has not been established. In addition, alkalinization can predispose to hepatic encephalopathy because of increased GI absorption of dietary protein metabolites.

Cystine Stones: Stones composed almost entirely of cystine form in dogs that have a renal tubular amino acid reabsorption defect known as cystinuria. Healthy dogs demonstrate 97% fractional reabsorption of cystine, while affected dogs excrete a much greater proportion of the filtered cystine load and may even exhibit net cystine secretion. Cystine is a relatively insoluble amino acid; therefore, in high concentration it may precipitate and form stones. Despite excessive urinary loss of cystine in cystinuric dogs, plasma cystine levels remain the same as in healthy dogs; in fact, the only morbidity or mortality associated with the inherited defect of cystine reabsorption is the sequela of urolith formation. Identification of cystine crystals by urinalysis indicates the dog is at risk of forming cystine uroliths. For poorly understood reasons, not all cystinuric dogs develop uroliths. However, the absence of uroliths does not preclude their future development, and preventive measures are indicated.

Cystinuria is thought to be inherited as a sex-linked trait. However, in Newfoundlands it is transmitted as a simple autosomal recessive trait. The defect has also been reported in Dachshunds, Basset Hounds, English Bulldogs, Chihuahuas, Yorkshire Terriers, Irish Terriers, and mixed-breed dogs. Except for Newfoundlands, cystinuria has been recognized almost exclusively in male dogs. A urine cystine concentration of >75 mg/g creatinine in nonfasted dogs is predictive of susceptibility to cystine urolithiasis.

Cystine solubility depends on urine pH, with solubility increasing rapidly when urinary pH is >7.5. Dogs fed meat-based diets tend to excrete acidic urine, which leads to urine cystine supersaturation.

Cystinuria is a lifelong defect of tubular reabsorption and cannot be cured. Cystine stones tend to recur within 1 yr without management to prevent recurrence, and they often recur despite attempts at prevention.

Dissolution and Prevention Protocols: Urinary cystine output should be reduced. Protein-restricted alkalinizing diets have been associated with reducing the size of cystine urocystoliths. Urinary cystine concentration can also be reduced by administering N-(2-mercaptoproprionyl)-glycine (2-MPG, tiopronin) or penicillamine. 2-MPG should be given at 15-20 mg/kg, PO, BID, for dissolution, and at 10-15 mg/kg, PO, BID, for prevention. Penicillamine (15 mg/kg, PO, BID) can be substituted for 2-MPG; unfortunately, ~40% of dogs treated with penicillamine exhibit anorexia and vomiting. The vomiting may be partially resolved by giving the medication with meals; however, a severe reduction in dosage or complete withdrawal is often necessary.

The urine should be alkalinized to a pH >7.5. Sodium bicarbonate added to the diet at 1 g ($^1/_4$ tsp)/5 kg, TID, readily accomplishes this, but because sodium supplementation may enhance cystinuria, potassium citrate (20-75 mg/kg, PO, BID) is preferred.

Urine volume can be increased by mixing water with the food. Salt should not be added to the diet because increased sodium excretion may cause increased cystine excretion. Provided urine volume is adequate and the urine pH is maintained above 7.5, most cystinuric dogs will pass urine that is only slightly supersaturated or undersaturated for cystine. Under such conditions, only relatively small doses of 2-MPG or penicillamine may be necessary to achieve 24-hr undersaturation.

Silica Stones: Early reports indicated a predominance of silica stones in German Shepherds, but many breeds have now been implicated. Urethral obstruction in males is the most common presenting problem, but signs similar to those associated with other types of uroliths also may be noted. The mean age at occurrence is ~6 yr. The stones are usually multiple and develop in the bladder and urethra. Silica uroliths are radio-opaque. They frequently, but not always, have a characteristic "jack-stone" appearance. Identification requires spectrographic analysis and cannot be made with kits for qualitative stone analysis.

The role of diet in spontaneously occurring silica urolithiasis has not been determined, although plants are often an abundant source of silica. If the diet of an affected dog is known to be high in silica, or if silica urolithiasis has been recurrent, a dietary change should be recommended. Only general management principles can be suggested for silicate urolithiasis. Additional salt and/or water should be added to the diet to induce diuresis and to lower the urine solute concentration. When present, urinary tract infections should be eliminated. Diets high in plant proteins should be avoided.

Feline Urolithiasis and Feline Lower Urinary Tract Disease (FLUTD)
(Feline urologic syndrome)

Hematuria, pollakiuria, and stranguria are the characteristic clinical signs of FLUTD in cats. Although the specific underlying etiology of this common disease may not be identified, 2 major disease categories have been suggested based on the presence or absence of mineral precipitates; this discussion is limited to feline urolithiasis.

Feline urolithiasis is a common disease that is seen with equal frequency in both sexes. Until recently, it was thought that most uroliths in cats were small and resembled sand or were gelatinous plugs that differed from typical uroliths in that they contained a greater amount of organic matrix, giving them a toothpaste-like consistency. Matrix-crystalline plugs are most commonly found within the urethra near the urethral orifice and are primarily responsible for urethral obstruction. Recently, prevalence of urolithiasis with grossly observable stones composed primarily of calcium oxalate has increased in cats. The most common feline uroliths are calcium oxalate, magnesium ammonium phosphate, and urate.

Urolithiasis is usually suspected based on clinical signs of hematuria, dysuria, or urethral obstruction. Urinalysis, urine culture, radiography, and ultrasonography may be required to differentiate uroliths from urinary tract infection or neoplasia. Radiography, cystoscopy, or ultrasonography are critically important to detect uroliths because only ~10% of feline urocystoliths can be detected by abdominal palpation. Uroliths with a diameter >3 mm are usually radiodense; however, because smaller uroliths are common, double contrast radiography may be required for detection. Radiographic evidence of uroliths is seen in ~20% of cats with hematuria or dysuria. The usual clinical approach to grossly observable urocystoliths is surgical removal or lithotripsy where available, followed by dietary therapy instituted as a preventive measure. For sterile struvite uroliths, medical dissolution is the preferred treatment.

Calcium Oxalate Stones: Calcium oxalate uroliths are the most common feline uroliths and the most common nephrolith, although their underlying cause is unknown. Common management schemes that involve feeding urine-acidifying diets with reduced magnesium, have reduced the incidence of feline struvite urolithiasis. Magnesium has been reported to be an inhibitor of calcium oxalate formation in rats and humans; thus, the reduced magnesium concentration in feline urine may partially explain the increase in calcium oxalate stones in cats.

Medical protocols that promote calcium oxalate dissolution are not known; therefore, surgery and lithotripsy are the primary means for removal (small bladder stones may be eliminated by voiding urohydropulsion). However, some calcium oxalate uroliths, especially those in the kidneys, may not cause clinical signs for months to years. Because of the unavoidable destruction of nephrons during nephrotomy, this procedure is not recommended unless it can be established that the stones are a cause of clinically significant disease. Recurrence remains problematic. A variety of diets has been formulated to restrict the formation of calcium oxalate uroliths and should be considered appropriate for maintenance in cats with nephroliths and following the removal of urocystoliths. Eliminating any associated urinary tract infections, avoiding mineral and vitamin C and D supplementation, and encouraging water consumption are critical.

Struvite Stones: Three distinct types of struvite uroliths are recognized in cats: amorphous urethral plugs with a large quantity of matrix, sterile struvite uroliths (which form perhaps as a result of certain dietary ingredients), and struvite uroliths that form as a sequela of urinary tract infection with urease-producing bacteria. Struvite uroliths induced by infection are less common than sterile struvite uroliths. An additional type of struvite urolith in cats consists of a sterile struvite nidus that predisposes to urinary tract infection with urease-producing bacteria and subsequent formation of infected struvite laminations around the sterile nidus.

Treatment of sterile struvite urolithiasis focuses on reducing the urine pH to ≤6.0 and on reducing the urine magnesium concentration by feeding magnesium-restricted diets. Reducing urine pH and magnesium concentration is best accomplished by feeding a commercially available prescription diet formulated for this purpose. Generally, neither sodium chloride nor urine acidifiers should be given concurrently with these diets because they are already supplemented with sodium chloride and formulated to produce aciduria. In addition, these diets should not be fed to cats that are acidemic, have azotemia of any cause, or have cardiac dysfunction or hypertension. Urolith size and crystalluria should be monitored every 4 wk by radiographs or ultrasonography and urinalysis, respectively. Struvite crystals should not form if therapy has been effective in producing urine that is undersaturated with magnesium, ammonium, and phosphate. Because small uroliths may not be detected radiographically, the calculolytic diet should be continued for ≥4 wk after radiographic documentation of urolith dissolution. If treatment does not induce complete dissolution of uroliths, it is likely that either the wrong mineral component was identified, the nucleus of the urolith is composed of a different mineral than the outer portion of the urolith, or the owner is not complying with therapeutic recommendations.

Other Feline Stones: Ammonium urate, uric acid, calcium phosphate, and cystine uroliths are less common in cats, but ammonium urate and uric acid account for ~6% of feline uroliths. Although a renal tubular reabsorptive defect and portovascular anomalies have been incriminated as causes in a few cases, the cause of most urate uroliths in cats has not been established. Nonetheless, formation of highly acidic and concentrated urine associated with consumption of diets high in purine precursors (especially liver) appears to be a risk factor.

Medical protocols that consistently promote dissolution of ammonium urate uroliths in cats have not been developed, and surgery remains the most common method of removal. For small stones, voiding urohydropulsion may be effective. Prevention should include feeding a diet low in purine precursors and promoting formation of less acidic urine that is not highly concentrated. Although allopurinol may reduce the formation of urate in cats, studies of the efficacy and potential toxicity of allopurinol in cats are required before meaningful guidelines can be established.

■ ■ ■

BEHAVIOR

BEHAVIORAL MEDICINE INTRODUCTION

An animal's "behavior" is the product of its genetic composition, the environment in which the animal functions, and the animal's experience (ie, what it has learned given its previous genetic × environment interaction). While this section focuses primarily on abnormal behavior of domestic animals, the extent to which an animal's behavior is abnormal is defined by its deviation from "normal." For each group of domestic animals, normal social and group behavior is outlined and followed by a listing of the common behavioral disorders and treatment approaches.

In behavioral medicine, diagnoses are not diseases; correlation is not causality. Behavioral conditions for which there is putative etiologic and pathophysiologic heterogeneity (multifactorial disorders) are complex (TABLE 1).

Phenotypic (functional, phenomenologic) diagnoses are open to various mechanistic bases of all subsequent levels. Some of these more reductionistic levels can be tested using treatment (eg, specific pharmacologic agents), but few phenotypic diagnoses can be specifically tested using behavior modification. Most of the behavioral diagnoses for farm animals are descriptive and relatively nonspecific. Behavioral diagnoses for dogs and cats have been more fully developed and are discussed in the context of the "necessary and sufficient" conditions (or criteria) for diagnosis. The use of "necessary and sufficient" conditions, using the terms as they are used in logical and mathematical applications, is a refinement over descriptive definitions. These conditions act as qualitative, and potentially quantitative, exclusion criteria, allowing for uniform and unambiguous assessment of aberrant, abnormal, and undesirable behaviors.

TABLE 1.   Levels of "Causality" to Consider in Behavioral Diagnosis

Mechanism	Factors
Phenotype	Underlying broad genotype × environment interactions
	Phenomenologic diagnoses
Neuroanatomy	Localization of activity
	Neuroanatomic diagnoses
Neurophysiology and neurochemistry	Chemical or substrate interaction
	Most mechanistic pathophysiologic diagnoses
Molecular	Gene regulation and interaction with substrate
	Most etiologic diagnostic refinements
Genotype	Heritability

A **necessary condition** is one that must be present for the listed diagnosis to be made. A **sufficient condition** is one that can stand alone to singularly identify the condition. Sufficiency is an outcome of knowledge: as more becomes known about the genetics, molecular response, neurochemistry, and neuroanatomy of any condition and its behavioral correlates, a sufficient condition can be defined succinctly and accurately. Definition of necessary and sufficient conditions is not synonymous with a compendium of signs associated with the behavior. The number of signs present and their intensity may be a gauge for the severity of the condition, or act as a flag when there can be variable, nonoverlapping presentations of the same condition.

PRINCIPLES OF BEHAVIORAL DIAGNOSIS AND TREATMENT

Many "health" problems faced by pet dogs and cats are associated with behavioral pathologies or unmet behavioral expectations. A good behavioral history is required before making any behavioral diagnosis. History taking should include the following items: 1) sex, breed, and age of animal (breed predispositions); 2) age at onset of condition or complaint; 3) duration of condition or complaint; 4) description of actual behavior; 5) frequency of condition or behavior (hourly, daily, weekly, monthly); 6) duration of average bout (seconds, minutes, hours); 7) range of duration of bouts; 8) any changes in pattern, frequency, intensity, and duration of bouts; 9) any corrective measures tried and the response (possibly none); 10) any activities that stop the behavior (eg, animal collapses); 11) 24-hr schedule of animal and owner, as well as any day-to-day variability; 12) animal's familial history; 13) anything else that the owner thinks is relevant.

Modern veterinary care should include routine screening questions about specific behavioral complaints (eg, "Any inappropriate or undesirable chewing, any growling, any odd behaviors?") in addition to routine questions that alert veterinarians to potential somatic medical problems. This accomplishes two goals. First, it initiates a dialog with the clients about behavior and lets clients know that behavior is central to good veterinary care. Clients will then feel comfortable asking their veterinarian about behavioral issues. Such dialog represents the best chance for learning of a client's behavioral concerns before these concerns threaten the pet's life. Second, it establishes a baseline of the pet's behaviors. Such a behavioral profile will identify "normal" for that pet and provide a context in which to evaluate behavioral change or client complaints about behavior. This is exactly what is done by recommending routine laboratory evaluation for healthy pets. Length of dysfunction—whether the dysfunction involves a "medical" or a "behavioral" complaint—can affect prognosis, and the extent to which this is true in behavioral medicine is profound.

Basic questionnaires on canine behavior can be easily completed at each visit to encourage routine assessment. Questionnaires should be standardized so that no topic is left uncovered for any patient, and should provide the veterinarian with background data about the dog's history and husbandry. Such data are particularly important if the dog has a behavioral condition that may be genetic in origin or if the veterinarian has not had the dog as a patient since puppyhood. Additional questionnaires can focus on specific behaviors (eg, problems with elimination, interactions with humans or other animals, etc). These questionnaires give clients the vocabulary and opportunity to discuss their pet's behaviors with their veterinarian in an efficient, consistent, and meaningful way. If the veterinarian suspects a problem, but feels that more data are needed, the clients can complete the questionnaires about specific behaviors again in a month or two. When the answers are compared, any trends will become clear and early intervention is then possible. For veterinarians who do not wish to formulate their own questionnaires, there are many published examples that can be incorporated into daily practice. When used continuously from the outset of the relationship with a particular pet, these tools will allow the veterinarian to intervene before many behavior problems become complex.

Veterinarians should also assess how the clients have "trained' their dog and how they have tried to alter the dog's behaviors. The answers may indicate either deliberate or inadvertent abuse. In the USA, the Association of Pet Dog Trainers and American Humane have published guidelines for appropriate and humane training and behavior modification. Without questioning the client about their training experiences, the veterinarian cannot discuss less desirable techniques and explain why replacing them with modern and humane techniques is so important. For clients who are stuck in an abuse cycle, the veterinarian may be able to direct them to help that they otherwise would not have received had the vet not known how the dog was "disciplined."

Because behavioral diagnoses cannot be made on the basis of a one-time event, having the client complete a questionnaire at each visit can clarify the pattern of the animal's behavior. The veterinarian can then ask if the pattern of nonspecific signs (eg, barking, growling, lunging, etc) meets specified diagnostic criteria (eg, fear aggression, protective aggression, etc). The veterinarian and the client must use the same definitions for the same nonspecific signs, and they both must accurately recognize and describe individual behaviors and behavioral sequences that are a concern. Videotapes of patient behaviors can ensure that such communication occurs. Questionnaires rely on client reports and because of this are more subjective. However, when combined with videotapes, the veterinarian can use questionnaires to assess whether the behaviors meet certain diagnostic criteria and how accurately the client can recognize the affiliated patterns. Client understanding and compliance are critical if patients with behavioral disorders are to improve. Only when clients can recognize the behaviors leading to or associated with the problematic ones can they avoid or prevent the provocative situation. By showing the client the problematic behavior on videotape and then working with him or her to substitute a more desirable response, the veterinarian is able to preserve the human-animal bond and help treat the condition.

A brief glossary of terms that are commonly used when discussing behavior follows:

Abnormal Behavior: These activities show dysfunction in action and behavior.

Aggression: Aggression can be defined in a narrow sense (attack) or in a broader sense as a specific example of agonistic behavior. In the latter case, aggression is an appropriate or inappropriate, in-context or out-of-context, inter- or intra-specific threat, challenge, or contest that results in deference or in combat and resolution.

Anxiety: Anxiety is the apprehensive anticipation of future danger or misfortune accompanied by a feeling of dysphoria (in humans) or by somatic signs of tension (vigilance and scanning, autonomic hyperactivity, increased motor activity and tension). The focus of the anxiety can be internal or external.

Conflict: In this motivational state, tendencies to perform more than one type of activity are simultaneously present. Motivational states, except extreme ones associated with survival functions (eg, eating, mating) are extraordinarily hard to identify in animals. Terms describing motivational states (eg, "conflicted," "frustrated," etc) are often used but seldom defined in terms that would allow measurement of the behavior. Accordingly, they do more to blur our understanding than to clarify it. Caution is urged in the use of such nonspecific descriptors. "Conflict" may be best restricted to when there are clear choices and the execution of one causes disharmony in or with respect to the other. The disharmony caused should be easily identifiable and measurable.

Displacement Activity: This type of activity is performed out-of-context, or is "displaced," because the animal is unable—physically or behaviorally—to execute another activity or otherwise occupy itself. This is considerably less specific than redirected activity (*see* below), which implies a substitution of behavior "in kind" but toward another target. When displacement activity occurs, the activity may not be "in kind."

Dominance: Dominance is a concept that has been frequently misapplied. The ethological concept of dominance refers to competitive control over a resource in a limited circumstance and to the ability of a higher-ranking animal to displace a lower-ranking one from that resource. Rank is usually defined by an ability to control the resource (hence the problematic teleology in the argument), or by access and ability to restrict matings (eg, the alpha wolf pair generally is thought to do all the mating); however, extra-pair copulation is almost always more common when assessed by DNA analysis than it was believed to be on the basis of behavioral observations. Dominance is not interchangeable with a hierarchical rank. Dominance ranks, particularly those that are linear and in which a "dominant" animal is identified, are largely artifacts of experimental or manipulated situations. A "dominant" animal is *not* the one engaged in the most fighting and combat. Most high-ranking animals seldom have to contest their right of access to a resource. Instead, high-ranking animals are usually better identified by the character and frequency of deferential behaviors exhibited by others in their social group, and their ability to respond appropriately to a variety of social and environmental circumstances.

Fear: This feeling of apprehension associated with the presence or proximity of an object, individual, or social situation is part of normal behavior and can be an adaptive response. The determination of whether the fear or fearful response is abnormal or inappropriate must be determined by context. For example, fire is a useful tool, but fear of being consumed by it, if the house is on fire, is an adaptive response. If the house is not on fire, such fear would be irrational and, if it were constant or recurrent, probably maladaptive. Normal and abnormal fears usually occur as graded responses, with the intensity of the response proportional to the proximity (or the perception of the proximity) of the stimulus. A sudden, all-or-nothing, profound, abnormal response that results in extremely fearful behaviors (catatonia, panic) is usually called a phobia.

Frustration: This motivational state arises when an animal is engaged in a sequence of behaviors that it is unable to complete because of physical or psychological obstacles in the environment. This term, like "dominance," is overused and usually undefined. Its use often prohibits a true evaluation of what is occurring behaviorally.

Phobia: Most fearful reactions are learned and can be unlearned with gradual exposure. Phobias are defined as profound and quickly developed fearful reactions that do not diminish either with gradual exposure to the object or without exposure (as fears will) over time. Phobias involve sudden, all-or-nothing, profound, abnormal responses that result in extremely fearful behaviors (catatonia, panic). An immediate, excessive anxiety response is characteristic of phobias. Phobias develop quickly, with little change in their presentation between bouts. Fears may develop more gradually and, within a bout of fearful behavior, there may be more variation in response than would be seen in a phobic event. It has been postulated that once a phobic event has been experienced, any event associated with it or the memory of it is sufficient to generate the response. In fact, without reinforcement (eg, exposure of dogs to a shock collar), these phobias can remain at or exceed their former high level for years. In dogs, the genesis for such events is usually either extremely scary and traumatic, or the dog itself has profound internal problems with fear, and the fear itself acts as a reinforcer (unconditioned stimulus). Phobic situations are either avoided at all costs or, if unavoidable, are endured with intense anxiety or distress. There also appears to be a genetic basis for these responses in some canine breeds.

Redirected Activity: These activities are directed away from the principal target and toward another, less appropriate target. This is usually best identified when the recognized activity is interrupted by the less appropriate target or by a third party. In contrast to displacement activity (*see* above), redirected activity appears to be a substitution "in kind" of the interrupted behavior.

Stereotypic Behaviors: These behaviors involve a repetitive, relatively unvaried sequence of movements that has no obvious purpose or function but is usually derived from contextually normal maintenance behaviors (eg, grooming, eating, walking). Inherent in the classification of dysfunction is that the behavior interferes with normal functioning. Not all stereotypic behaviors meet the diagnostic criteria for obsessive-compulsive disorder (OCD), while most OCD involves stereotypic behaviors. A stereotypy is a nonspecific sign and a description—not a diagnosis.

Vacuum Activity: Such activity involves an instinctive or unconscious response in the absence of the stimulus that would normally elicit that behavior. The activity seemingly has no apparent, contextual, useful purpose.

PRINCIPLES OF BEHAVIOR MODIFICATION AND TREATMENT

The most commonly used behavioral techniques include habituation, extinction, desensitization, counterconditioning, and shaping. Flooding is often talked about but seldom used because it has the potential to make most animals worse. While it is claimed that punishment is frequently used, with varying degrees of success, few people correctly employ punishment. For punishment to occur, the aversive stimulus (eg, screaming at the dog, startling the cat with a loud noise, etc) must occur sufficiently close to the onset of the behavior that the probability of the behavior occurring in the future is lessened. Most aversive stimuli are inappropriate in context, duration, or time of application and are more about the client's anger than about changing the behavior.

Most of the humane, passive, or positive techniques involved in behavior modification are not hard to learn and are equally successfully employed as preventive techniques. The following is a short review of the basic principles involved in the techniques and their associated strategies.

Habituation: Habituation is an elementary form of learning that involves no rewards. It is merely the cessation or decrease in a response to a stimulus that results from repeated or prolonged exposure to that stimulus. The stimulus can be positive, neutral, or negative. For example, horses placed in a pasture bordering a road may at first run away when traffic passes, but eventually learn to ignore it. As would be expected, stimuli associated with potentially adverse consequences are more difficult to extinguish with habituation than other stimuli. In prey species, responses to sounds associated with predators should be difficult to habituate because they have been selected for and generally are adaptive; the predator does not have to be present very often for the response to be rewarded. Furthermore, if such responses are even occasionally rewarded, the habituation response will be inhibited. In such circumstances, prolonged exposure to the stimulus may be associated with hypervigilance, exhaustion, and increased anxiety. In fact, this is one explanation for the feedback between anxiety and environmental events, even in situations when the anxiety is pathologic and potentially maladaptive.

Spontaneous Recovery: This phenomenon is associated with habituation. If there is an extended interval between the time the animal last experienced a stimulus to which it had habituated and re-exposure to the stimulus, the animal may again react. Habituation usually occurs more rapidly following spontaneous recovery if no overt fearful associations are involved.

Dishabituation: Dishabituation is the reinstatement of a habituated response as a result of exposure to a stimulus that provokes a response similar to the original. The classic examples of this involve mildly fearful responses—if habituation had just occurred to a certain hand gesture, and another movement occurred that was also worrisome for the animal, the animal could dishabituate to the hand gesture. Rehabituation is the rule unless the event is compounded and made more fearful, or the animal's reaction is extreme (suggesting something innate about the animal's response, not the event itself).

Conditioning: Conditioning refers to associations between stimuli and responses. **Classical conditioning** does not require a reward structure to make these associations, while **operant or instrumental conditioning** uses a reward structure. In operant conditioning, learning is fastest if the positive reinforcer occurs immediately (within 0.5 sec). Delayed and intermittent reinforcements slow the acquisition of the response but work well to reinforce its maintenance. In addition to timing (quantity), value (quality) is also important—the more an animal values a reinforcer, the more quickly and reliably it will acquire the response. Hence, a food treat that dogs do not usually get (eg, cheese, boiled chicken, etc) will be better than their standard kibble in teaching them a new behavior. It is important to realize that not all dogs value food above all else—some prefer interactive play or petting.

Reinforcement: Reinforcement is the application of a stimulus or an event that increases the probability that a certain behavior or class of behaviors will be repeated. A positive reinforcer is a stimulus or an event that occurs after a response that leads to an increase in the response in the future. A negative reinforcer is an aversive event or stimulus that increases the frequency of a behavior, but does so through escape or avoidance. Because people tend to use negative reinforcers in a way consistent with the potential for abuse, they should be avoided by those who feel less than absolutely confident in their timing and control.

Negative reinforcement is *not* to be confused with punishment. Punishment is the application of an aversive or negative stimulus after a response, which leads to a decrease in the frequency of the response. Negative reinforcement is the removal of an aversive stimulus that then leads to an increase in a response.

Second-order reinforcers are signals that can be used at a distance to convey that the reward or the valuable stimulus is coming. Commonly used second-order reinforcers are words ("Good girl!"), hand signals, and clickers or whistles. By carefully pairing these with the reward with which the response to the command has already been paired, second-order reinforcers can elicit the same response as the reward would (at least temporarily—suddenly switching from a first-order reward to only a second-order one should not be done without at least intermittent pairing of the first- and second-order rewards).

"Positive" training and "clicker" training have recently become fashionable. It is possible to do an excellent job at positive training without using any secondary reinforcers. Clicker training requires frequent practice and excellent timing. In situations involving problem behaviors, the animal must be confused as seldom as possible. The incorrect use of clickers may hinder, rather than expedite, a behavior modification program. However, the correct use of clickers is an excellent way to immediately "mark" desirable responses or to associate a positive emotional response with the stimulus. A competent trainer and clear and accurate instructions are therefore needed.

Stimulus and Response Generalization: This occurs when an operantly or classically conditioned response is provoked not only by the object or event that originally provoked it, but by similar stimulus or events. A common example of stimulus response generalization in dogs is to people in uniforms: if a delivery person or meter-reader initially scared the dog or provoked a protective response, this response may then be generalized to others in uniform although the circumstances might not be the same. The more similar the original and subsequent stimuli are, the more similar the responses will be. Stimulus and response generalization may be associated with the development of profoundly anxious or fearful and phobic responses, and understanding this may be key to diminishing the worrisome behavior.

Extinction: A response that ceases when reinforcement/reward is stopped is called extinction. A classic example of extinction of a response involves the dog that jumps up on people for attention. If people pet the dog, the behavior continues; if they stop at once and forever, the dog will eventually extinguish its response because the reward is no longer there. However, any form of intermittent reinforcement—even occasional petting of the dog in response to its jumping—will enhance the continuation of the response. The more valuable the original reinforcer, the longer the reinforcement has been continuing, and the more uncertainty there is about whether the response has been truly removed (ie, presence or absence of intermittent reinforcement), the greater the resistance to extinction.

Resistance to extinction can also occur even without reinforcement, if the reward was good enough and it is tightly coupled with the behavior. Because there is often an association between eliciting the reward and the intensity or rapidity of the performance of the behavior, the intensity or frequency of the behavior one is attempting to extinguish usually increases at the beginning of an extinction process. It is critical that clients *not* give in. Giving in will only make extinction more difficult because the animal has learned that although the client's threshold has increased, the animal can override it.

Overlearning: Overlearning is the repeated evocation and expression of an already learned response. It is a phenomenon that is frequently employed in training for specific events, but may be underused in preventing fearful responses in dogs. Overlearning accomplishes 3 things: it delays forgetting, it increases the resistance to extinction, and it increases the probability that the response will become a "knee-jerk" one, or response of first choice, when the circumstances are similar. This last aspect can be extremely useful in teaching an animal to overcome a fear or anxiety.

Shaping: This learning technique works well for animals that do not know what response is desired by the trainer. Shaping works through gradual approximations and allows the animal to be rewarded initially for any behavior that resembles the desired behavior. For instance, when teaching a puppy to sit, following a slight squat with a food reward will enhance the probability that squatting will be repeated. This squatting behavior is then rewarded only when it becomes more exaggerated, and finally, when it becomes a true sit.

Avoidance: Avoidance is essential until clients can seek qualified help, particularly in the case of aggression. With treatment it may be possible to desensitize the dog to circumstances in which aggressive behavior is exhibited, but avoidance is key in minimizing danger. Clients may be concerned that avoidance means that the dog will now have control, ie, that they are giving in to the dog. This is not what is happening; rather, the dog is not being given the chance to exert control in the manner to which it is accustomed. Every time a dog becomes aggressive, it learns that aggression may help it cope with the situation, thus reinforcing the problem. Even if the event is eventually aborted by an outside force, they learn the experience of exhibiting aggression.

Desensitization: Desensitization is a decrement in response that is produced by gradual exposure to a stimulus that elicits the response. For example, if a puppy has become fearful of or stimulated by the doorbell, use of a tape recording of the doorbell could help stop the undesired response. If the tape is played very softly at first and then only gradually increased in volume at increments designed to elicit no response, the puppy may become desensitized to the doorbell.

In **counterconditioning**, negative or undesirable behavior is extinguished or controlled by teaching the animal to do another behavior (preferably favorable and fun) that competitively interferes with the execution of the undesirable behavior. This is best coupled with desensitization. In the doorbell example, the puppy will learn faster if it is first taught to sit, stay, and relax in exchange for a treat. The puppy must be absolutely quiet and calm, and convey by the look in its eyes, body posture, and facial expressions that it would do anything for its owner. Once this behavior is learned, the desensitization component is added by playing the tape recording at gradually increasing volume. Performing the adoration act for a food reward is incompatible with or competitively exclusive of barking. If at any point the puppy starts to act anxious or to not attend to the client, the tape recording should be lowered in volume until it can relax again. Relaxing is the key— the sitting and staying is merely a facilitator for the relaxation. There is no point in having the dog sit and stay if it is clearly distressed. Relaxation is the first step to changing the behavior.

Counterconditioning coupled with desensitization is an extremely time-consuming technique. The exercises must be constantly repeated so that the response lessens until there is none, and all the patient's communicatory signals must be considered. Clients who are least successful with this technique want both quicker fixes and less work. However, moving too quickly provokes anxiety and sabotages any behavior modification program.

Flooding: Flooding involves prolonged exposure at a level that provokes the response so that the animal eventually gives up. This is exactly the opposite of the approach taken in desensitization. It is far more stressful than any of the other therapy strategies and, used inappropriately, could damage the animal. The most common side effect is enhanced fear. This technique should be used only by those with extensive experience and as a last resort.

Aversive Conditioning/Punishment: This strategy involves the presentation of an aversive stimulus in response to an inappropriate or undesirable behavior; the stimulus is intended to abort the behavior and to decrease the probability of it occurring in the future (the correct definition of punishment). To be most successful, the stimulus designed to abort the behavior must occur as early as possible but certainly within the first 30-60 sec of the onset of the behavioral sequence, and it must be consistent and appropriate. The critical factors in punishment include timing, consistency, appropriate intensity, and the presence of a conditioned response (ie, when the undesirable behavior ends there must be some favorable stimulus or reward, even if it is just praise or a pat). This is the most frequently ignored part of therapy for people whose pets have behavioral problems. People often resort to physical punishment as the correction method of choice, but punishment does not need to be physical. Furthermore, "good" punishment is just as hard work as appropriately executed counterconditioning and desensitization. Punishment is never an "easy out" and has a high probability of failure unless the client understands that its focus is to decrease the probability of future inappropriate events.

PRINCIPLES OF PHARMACOLOGIC TREATMENT

Facile drug use, particularly in the absence of a diagnosis, is not a component of rational treatment and should be avoided. Drug treatment for almost any behavioral condition is most useful when combined with behavior modification.

Prior to incorporating behavioral pharmacology into any treatment program, practitioners should have a reasonable diagnosis or list of diagnoses, an appreciation for the putative mechanism of action of the available drugs, and a clear understanding of potential side effects. In addition, they should have some idea of how the drug will specifically alter the behavior in question. This is critical because it will not only help clients to watch for adverse effects and improvements, but can also help confirm or reject the original diagnosis. Without these guidelines, behavioral drugs may not be given long enough or at a sufficient dosage to attain the desired effect, clients will be unable to participate in the evaluation process, and there will be no objective behavioral criteria with which to assess improvement.

It is important to teach clients to be observant and recognize specific signs of potential adverse reactions. Such reactions can be minimized by performing a premedication CBC, urinalysis, and serum biochemistry profile and by taking a complete behavioral and medical history. Baseline ECGs are recommended for patients with a history of arrhythmia, heart disease, or prior drug reactions; that are on more than one medication; or that may undergo anesthesia or sedation. Liver dyscrasias and cardiac arrhythmias may not rule out the use of a drug, but knowing that they exist can serve as a guide to dosage and antici-

TABLE 2.   Drugs that May Be Useful in the Treatment of Canine Behavioral Diagnoses*

Drug	Formulation	Size	Dosage
Alprazolam	Tablet	0.25, 0.5, 1, 2 mg[†]	0.01-0.1 mg/kg, PO, as needed for phobic or panic attacks[‡]; start with 1-2 mg for a 25 kg dog
Amitriptyline	Tablet	10, 25, 50, 75, 100, 150 mg	1-2 mg/kg, PO, BID to start
Buspirone	Tablet	5, 10 mg	1 mg/kg, PO, SID-TID (mild anxiety); 2.5-10 mg/dog, PO, SID-TID (mild anxiety); 10-15 mg/dog, PO, BID-TID (severe anxiety)[§]
Carbemazepine	Scored tablet Scored chewable tablet	200 mg 100 mg	4-8 mg/kg, PO, BID; 0.5-1.25 mg/kg, PO, TID; 4-10 mg/kg/day, divided TID
Chlordiazepoxide	Tablet[¶]	5, 10, 25 mg	2.2-6.6 mg/kg, PO, as needed
Clomipramine[#]	Scored tablet Capsule (human formulation)	20, 40, 80 mg[**] 25, 50, 75 mg	1-2 mg/kg, PO, BID; increase to 3 mg/kg, BID if necessary[††]
Clonazepam	Tablet	0.125, 0.25, 0.5, 1.0, 2.0 mg	0.125-1.0 mg/kg, PO, BID; range 0.01-1.0 mg/kg, PO, as needed for phobic or panic attacks[‡‡]
Clorazepate	Tablet Capsule	3.75, 7.5, 11.25, 15, 22.5 mg 3.75, 7.5, 15 mg	0.5-2.2 mg/kg, PO, at least 1 hr before provocative stimulus; repeat every 4-6 hr as needed; 11.25-22.5 mg/large dog; ~11.25 mg/medium dog; ~5.6 mg/small dog
Diazepam	Tablet Solution	1, 2, 5, 10 mg 5 mg/mL	0.5-2.2 mg/kg, PO, at least 1 hr before provocative stimulus; repeat every 4-6 hr as needed
Doxepin	Capsule Solution	10, 25, 50, 75, 100, 150 mg 10 mg/mL	3-5 mg/kg, PO, BID-TID
Fluoxetine	Capsule Solution	10, 20 mg 5 mg/mL	1 mg/kg, PO, SID-BID

TABLE 2. (continued)

Drug	Formulation	Size	Dosage
Fluvoxamine	Tablet	25, 50, 100 mg	1 mg/kg, PO, SID-BID
Imipramine	Tablet Capsule	10, 25, 50 mg 75, 100, 125, 150 mg	2.2-4.4 mg/kg, PO, SID-BID; 1-2 or 2-4 mg/kg, PO, SID-BID (start low)
Nortriptyline	Capsule Solution	10, 25, 50, 75 mg 10 mg/5 mL	1-2 mg/kg, PO, BID
Oxazepam	Tablet Capsule	15 mg 10, 15, 30 mg	0.2-1.0 mg/kg, PO, SID-BID
Paroxetine	Tablet Suspension	10, 20, 30, 40 mg 10 mg/5 mL	1 mg/kg, PO, SID
Protriptyline	Tablet	5, 10 mg	5-10 mg/dog, PO, SID-BID (narcolepsy)
Selegiline[#**]	Tablet	5, 10, 15, 30 mg	0.5-1.0 mg/kg, PO, SID
Sertraline	Tablet	25, 50, 100 mg	1 mg/kg, PO, SID
Triazolam	Tablet	0.125, 0.5 mg	0.01-0.1 mg/kg, PO, BID

[*]Most of these are unapproved uses, and caution is indicated.
[†]1- and 2-mg tablets scored
[‡]Not to exceed 4 mg/dog/day. Profound lethargy may occur at 0.75-4.0 mg/dog/day. Dosage may increase slowly over 4 mg/dog/day if obtaining some effect at a lower dosage. Small doses given every 2 hr minimize side effects.
[§]Use high dose for thunderstorm phobia
[¶]Also available as a powder for injection
[#]Veterinary label for some conditions, depending on country
[**]5-mg scored tablet available in Australia and Europe
[††]Constant treatment is associated with slight increase in GI side effects; SID dosing is insufficient for the majority of animals, particularly those with multiple signs, early age onset, or long-standing signs.
[‡‡]Profound lethargy and incoordination may result at dosages >4 mg/day, but higher dosages may be used incrementally if there has been some effect at a lower dosage. Start with 1-2 mg for a 25-kg dog.

pated side effects. Because clients may be distressed after a behavioral consultation, a written reminder of situations for which they should be alert may be helpful. It should also be kept in mind that with few exceptions (eg, clomipramine for separation anxiety in dogs, selegiline for cognitive dysfunction in dogs), the use of the majority of medications prescribed for behavioral problems in pets is extra-label.

Most medications used to treat behavioral problems are tricyclic antidepressants or selective serotonin reuptake inhibitors. Prolonged treatment may be necessary for some pets to prevent relapse, but with good physical and laboratory monitoring there are few associated risks. *See* TABLE 2 and TABLE 3 for recommended dosages for canine and feline behavioral drugs. There have been few well-designed, prospective clinical trials of medication use for behavioral problems in animals, so it should be kept in mind that many of these dosages are based on extrapolation from human use and clinical experience with pets.

TABLE 3. Drugs that May Be Useful in the Treatment of Feline Behavioral Diagnoses[*]

Drug	Formulation	Size	Dosage
Alprazolam	Tablet	0.25, 0.5, 1, 2 mg[†]	0.0125-0.025 mg/kg, PO, BID
Amitriptyline	Tablet	10, 25, 50, 75, 100, 150 mg	0.5-1.0 mg/kg, PO, SID-BID; start at 0.5 mg/kg, BID
Buspirone	Tablet	5, 10 mg	0.5-2.0 mg/kg, PO, SID-TID
Clomi-pramine[‡]	Scored tablet Capsule (human formulation)	20, 40, 80 mg[§] 25, 50, 75 mg	0.5 mg/kg, PO, SID
Clonazepam	Tablet	0.125, 0.25, 0.5, 1.0, 2.0 mg	0.1-0.2 mg/kg, PO, SID-BID
Clorazepate	Tablet Capsule	3.75, 7.5, 11.25, 15, 22.5 mg 3.75, 7.5, 15 mg	0.5-2.2 mg/kg, PO, as needed for profound distress; 0.2-0.4 mg/kg, PO, SID-BID
Diazepam	Tablet Solution	1, 2, 5, 10 mg 5 mg/mL	0.2-0.4 mg/kg, PO, SID-BID; start at 0.2 mg/kg, PO, BID
Doxepin	Capsule Solution	10, 25, 50, 75, 100, 150 mg 10 mg/mL	0.5-1.0 mg/kg, PO, SID-BID; start low
Fluoxetine	Capsule Solution	10, 20 mg 5 mg/mL	0.5-1.0 mg/kg, PO, SID
Fluvoxamine	Capsule	10, 20 mg	0.25-0.5 mg/kg, PO, SID
Imipramine	Tablet Capsule	10, 25, 50 mg 75, 100, 125, 150 mg	0.5-1.0 mg/kg, PO, SID-BID; start at 0.5 mg/kg, PO, BID
Nortriptyline	Capsule	10, 25, 50, 75 mg	0.5-2.0mg/kg, PO, SID-BID
Oxazepam	Tablet Capsule	15 mg 10, 15, 30 mg	0.2-0.5 mg/kg, PO, SID-BID; high dose 1.0-2.5 mg/kg, PO, SID-BID; 3 mg/kg, PO bolus for appetite stimulation
Paroxetine	Tablet Suspension	10, 20, 30, 40 mg 10 mg/5 mL	0.5 mg/kg, PO, SID
Protriptyline	Tablet	5, 10 mg	0.5-1.0 mg/kg, PO, SID-BID; start at 0.5 mg/kg, PO, BID

TABLE 3. (*continued*)

Drug	Formulation	Size	Dosage
Selegiline[‡]	Tablet	5, 10, 15, 30 mg	0.25-1.0 mg/kg, PO, SID-BID; start low
Sertraline	Tablet	25, 50, 100 mg	0.5 mg/kg, PO, SID
Triazolam	Tablet	0.125, 0.25 mg	2.5-5.0 mg/cat, PO, TID

[*]Most of these are unapproved uses, and caution is indicated
[†]1- and 2-mg tablets scored
[‡]Veterinary label for some conditions, depending on country
[§]5-mg scored tablet available in Australia and Europe

NORMAL SOCIAL BEHAVIOR AND BEHAVIORAL PROBLEMS OF DOMESTIC ANIMALS

HORSES

SOCIAL BEHAVIOR

Domestic horses are social animals. In feral situations, they live in a harem group or band with one to several stallions, multiple mares, and those mares' offspring.

One stallion (the highest-ranking or "dominant" animal) is primarily responsible for most of the breeding. In many species, rank is associated with age or some ability to survive and thrive in challenged environments. Old age can be a gauge of the latter. High-ranking males are the first to secure access to a receptive female and the first to displace a female from another band. In the absence of conception, horses cycle every 21 days, except when seasonally anovulatory (fall and winter). Within a harem group, the highest-ranking individual is usually, but not always, a stallion. This high-ranking stallion will force foals to leave the group once they are ~2 yr old, as they begin to become sexually and socially mature.

Snapping (tooth clapping or champing) is a facial expression given by young horses to adults, particularly stallions. It peaks in frequency at 2 mo of age, after which it decreases; it may function to decrease aggression from adults, but is also compatible with displaced nursing behavior. This is not the same behavior as smacking, which is an aggressive threat in which the ears are laid back and the mouth is open with lips smacking, but the lips are not retracted.

Social maturity is not attained until 5 yr of age. Most fillies and all colts leave the natal herd at about this age. Fillies that remain in their natal group may have decreased reproductive success. Young stallions form bachelor herds, and the highest-ranking stallion within this group is usually the next one to acquire a mate. Fillies can join a bachelor herd but are often incorporated into other bands. Stallions are rarely solitary; when this occurs, the stallions appear to be old or infirm.

While hierarchical rank in males is evaluated primarily on the basis of access to females, hierarchical rank in females is determined by effect on group behavior and activity (ie, seeking out resources such as water holes). Horse groups are largely structured by females, and females make the decision about whether to leave or to stay within a harem. Such decisions are usually based not on specific stallions or their characteristics, but on the female's assessment of food resources. High-ranking females can successfully interfere with the nursing of foals by lower-ranking females. Mares have preferred associates, are preferentially groomed, and will groom certain individuals. This pattern is typical of many social animals in that rank is conferred largely by the deference of other animals—not by the results of outright combat.

Hierarchical relationships within groups also depend on the age and sex distribution of the group. The more members of the herd, and the more within each age and sex group, the less likely it is for a linear dominance hierarchy to exist. Relationships within most horse bands are triangular and complex. Hierarchical rank depends on multiple factors and probably their interaction, eg, age or length of residence in the social group, sex (although probably less important than age), size, and inheritance (rank of the mother). These factors are important to consider when addressing problems that may arise in stabled horses.

Hierarchical social effects also exist between herds. Multi-stallion herds are dominant over single-stallion bands, possibly because lower-ranking stallions within a herd conduct most of the fighting that occurs between groups. Herds that are currently occupying an area or using a resource (eg, a water hole) tend to retain it. Groups, as well as individuals within them, follow specific patterns of fecal marking.

Many behavioral problems are associated with confinement. Under free-ranging circumstances, horses will wander and spend >60% of their day foraging. The remainder of their time is spent standing, lying down, or engaging in another activity. This same pattern is the preferred one under barn conditions; even with free choice of grain, horses will choose to eat many small meals a day.

Horses also use free-ranging locomotion as part of their play development. Until ~3 mo of age, most play is solitary. Interactive play peaks at 3-4 mo of age. There are sex differences in play; colts play more than fillies and play different games than do fillies. Colt games focus more on fighting and mounting, while filly games focus more on running and mutual grooming. Fillies will groom both colts and fillies; colts tend to groom only fillies, which has been interpreted as practice for later courtship behavior.

Recent data on the role of play in carnivores suggests such behaviors may be best interpreted as learning how to make and recover from social mistakes. The ability to make a mistake successfully may be more important than previously appreciated. The social experience of play is important for normal social interaction in adult life.

BEHAVIORAL PROBLEMS

Aggression to People or Savagery: The most common correlates of aggression to people are sexual behavior, dominance-associated/impulse dyscontrol aggression (abnormal and out-of-context [see BEHAVIORAL PROBLEMS ASSOCIATED WITH CANINE AGGRESSION, p 1314]), and fear. Understanding which of these is occurring will greatly aid in treatment. Fear can be induced by the behavioral environment (eg, physical abuse or harsh treatment) or by the physical environment (eg, night blindness associated with confinement in a dark stall followed by introduction to pasture with other horses). Savage horses that are exhibiting dominance-associated/impulse dyscontrol aggression behavior toward people have been considered too dangerous to keep. There have been cases of horses killing people in such circumstances. The extent to which early intervention can help modulate these behaviors is unknown.

Treatment involves counterconditioning and desensitization, using rewards for non-aggressive approaches. Rewards could be frequent feedings of highly desirable foods (eg, molasses, apples, vanilla, watermelon), attention, caretaking (epimeletic) behaviors such as grooming, or exercise. The purpose of the frequent feedings is to mimic the natural grazing situation and to associate that and the food reward with the person's presence. All aggressive animals should probably be neutered because there appears to be a genetic basis (albeit poorly understood) for most aggressions, and removal of hormones is associated with less reactive behaviors. Progestins have been recommended as a substitute for castration or ovariohysterectomy but have many side effects that involve multiple organ systems and render the reproductive option moot.

More forceful interventions include techniques designed to increase the equine perception of vulnerability and may include hobbling, the use of paralytic agents (succinylcholine), and controlling access and frequency of light. Because of the danger involved, people have been less willing to try neuropharmacologic intervention, instead resorting to euthanasia. If recognized early, treatment with selective serotonin reuptake inhibitors (eg, fluoxetine) may be successful when combined with behavior modification.

Horses like to turn on lights and can be rewarded with the ability to do so. Horses are prey species and are wary of dogs and other predators; learning to associate light with people, especially if coupled with positive reinforcement, may help.

Aggression to Horses: Aggression to other horses is usually associated with sex, secondary to a fear as described above, or idiosyncratic. Horses have preferred grooming and grazing partners; the extent to which these preferences may be a factor in aggression to other horses is unknown. Treatment can include castration, the use of progestins, and desensitization and counterconditioning that require that the horses are fed by the handler only when in each others' presence. This can be done gradually by introducing horses across one or two fences so that they do not injure each other. Two fences are optimal because they reduce the possibility that the horses could strike each other with their feet. Shock has also been used to treat aggression to horses, based on the principle that fleeing will be rendered undesirable, while concomitantly rendering attack punitive. In cases of profound fear or anxiety, shock will usually either worsen the aggression or render other aspects of the horse's behavior undesirable. Horses are a prey species and have a heightened avoidance system. Accordingly, shock may produce a cessation of the undesirable behavior but also render the horse less interactive, more wary, and more fearful in general. Animal welfare concerns should be a rational component of any cogent behavioral treatment.

Wood-chewing: Wood-chewing may be a residual behavior associated with the equid pattern of browsing. Under free-ranging circumstances, horses will graze 12-14 hr/day. Most wood-chewing occurs in the winter, and it appears to be seen more often in horses that are fed pelleted diets. If horses receive <1 kg of hay/100 kg body wt, wood-chewing can become extreme. It is important to address the primary problem (ie, learn why the horse is engaging in this behavior), rather than merely trying to prevent it, which can make the horse even more secretive. Treatment involves increasing both roughage (hay, sawdust, etc) and exercise through work or increased pasture time. Because of the social factors involved in grazing under free-ranging conditions, animals who chew wood may have less easily recognized, but still extant, social needs that are unmet.

Coprophagia: Coprophagia is a normal behavior in foals that may play a role in B-vitamin supplementation and influence the intestinal flora. It is most common in the first month of life, after which it usually declines. When it is seen in adults, it is usually associated with low roughage, low protein, or a dietary deficiency. In these cases, the primary dietary problem must be addressed; treatment always involves increasing the amount of roughage in the diet and may involve increasing the amount of protein.

Pica: In horses, pica is usually manifest by ingestion of sand or gravel and can result in colonic impaction. In profound circumstances, this may be a ritualistic behavior. Early intervention is important and involves providing the horse with alternative substances that are acceptable (eg, increasing hay). Texture may be important, and the addition of roughage and salt blocks may have a role. In small animals, such behaviors appear to have familial associations, but comparable data are lacking for horses.

Anorexia: Horses form close affiliative attachments with other horses, and anorexia can be associated with changes in these relationships. The most common situation involves separation anxiety in the absence of a preferred equine companion. Addressing the underlying social problem through social facilitation is critical, and treatment with anxiolytic drugs that may also stimulate appetite (eg, benzodiazepines such as diazepam) can help.

Foals usually feed when the mare feeds. During the first month, foals graze only 5 min/hr, but this increases to 45 min/hr by 6 mo of age. Accordingly, weaning methods may be important to prevent anorexia in young horses. Aggressive mares may attack foals that try to share food. Barriers should be erected that safely permit normal development and feeding patterns. Foals may not eat the same plant or same plant part as the mare, and the parts they choose may be based on the height of the plant. Management should address this problem. Creep feeders should be placed near the mare so that the foal does not have to choose between food and contact with its dam. Foals on pasture and those that are nursing do not drink water, but the mares need access to good, clean water.

Obesity: Obesity can be the result of decreased exercise, increased palatable food, and under-stimulation (horses that eat in the absence of other activities). To avoid hyperlipemia, food should not be abruptly removed from obese horses. Reducing intake (by feeding the horse decreased amounts) while increasing exercise is preferable. Horses fed rations that are calorically diluted will compensate by eating more if fed ad lib.

Stall Walking or Circling: Confined, stabled horses can spend >25% of their time in nondirected motor activity within their stall. They may become exhausted or tangled in their bedding; in warm climates, they may become overheated. Classic stall walking or circling is usually in response to separation from another horse or to claustrophobia; it is usually rapid and accompanied by vocalization. Clients should watch for nonspecific signs of anxiety (eg, pacing, startling, changes in typical ingestive and elimination behaviors, changes in vocalization, etc) when stablemates or housing conditions change. The less appreciated form of stall walking involves stereotypic behavior. In this case, the motor activity itself becomes a manifestation of an obsessive-compulsive disorder; it is not accompanied by vocalization. Treatment should address the primary problem, including increasing exercise; providing social company (which need not be a horse); allowing the horse to see other horses; providing thick, clean bedding; feeding frequently (or at least twice per day); providing more open stalls and better access to outside views; and antianxiety or anti-obsessive-compulsive medication. Stall toys are unlikely to fix the problem unless the horse is young and frisky and played with the toys before the problem became apparent.

Weaving: Weaving occurs when a horse that stall walks is tied or prohibited from walking because of restricted space. Horses prohibited from performing other locomotor movements weave. Treatment includes untying the horse, providing a larger stall, turning the horse out onto pasture, and the other treatments recommended for stall walking (*see* above).

Pawing: Pawing is a potentially injurious behavior because it can change the surface of the floor and can cause wear to the horses' hooves. It is a normal, anticipatory behavior and can occur when horses on winter pasture are forced to dig for feed. When horses are confined and fed highly palatable foods, pawing can occur more frequently and more intensely than it would otherwise. Pawing also may be associated with signaling that accompanies escape behavior. The underlying problem should be identified to determine treatment, which should not be directed solely at the nonspecific behavior of pawing. Specific treatments are as for stall walking (*see* above). The pawing should not be rewarded, which is what inadvertently happens when horses paw in anticipation of feeding. The food should be presented to the horse only when the horse is not pawing, or the horse should be brought to the food.

Kicking: Kicking damages horses' legs and stalls. It is often an aggressive behavior that appears when another horse is nearby or when the horse perceives that another horse is nearby. Kicking can also occur in anticipation of food or environmental stimulation (as does pawing). It may occur when the horse cannot achieve its goals (eg, exercise, mating opportunities, monitoring the outside world, etc). All nonspecific kicking is not the same; the underlying basis for the kicking should be determined and treated. Treatment is as for stall walking (*see* above). If aggression is involved, it may require rearranging the social grouping in the barn. Horses can find their own compatible neighbors and can be permitted to choose their own stalls. Hand-feeding the horse can be one way to implement counterconditioning, ie, the horse is fed only when calm and quiet.

Cribbing: Cribbing (windsucking, crib biting) is a distinct behavior, different from wood-chewing, that involves grasping a horizontal surface with the incisors and flexing the neck without swallowing air. In extreme cases, the horse may do this 3,000 times/day. The activity makes a strange, nonflatulent sound. Cribbing is most easily diagnosed by noting the missing U-shaped pieces from the available fencing. Horses that crib have worn teeth and develop thick neck muscles. Cribbers tend to have lower levels of endogenous opiates, and cribbing is postulated to stimulate opiate release. Accordingly, treatment with exogenous opiate blockers (eg, naloxone, nalmefene) may help because it blocks a self-perpetuating loop. Some sweet (and palatable) feeds may also release endogenous opiates and worsen cribbing through positive feedback. Therefore, treatment may involve increasing roughage in the diet, changing companions, and providing greater access to more varied environments (eg, pasture). Unless the horse is very thin or afflicted by flatulent colic, it may be easiest to do nothing.

The assertion that horses learn to crib from other horses has never been substantiated. Cribbing may be more closely related to the group conditions and any resultant anxiety. Cribbing straps prevent the behavior (in theory) by placing pressure on the horse, causing pain when the neck is flexed. Highly motivated horses will crib despite the straps; in such cases, the cribbing may be more a manifestation of an obsessive-compulsive disorder, and treatment with an antiobsessive-compulsive drug may be useful. Experimentally, treatment with narcotic antagonists has reduced cribbing, but these may not be practical for longterm use. Surgical treatments that have been recommended but are often unsuccessful include ventral accessory neurectomy and myotomy. It may be preferable to address the social, physical (eg, duration and form of exercise), and welfare needs of the horse prior to resorting to surgery. If the horse is harming itself when cribbing, a cribbing muzzle may be useful.

Self-mutilation: This may be due to an underlying medical problem (eg, a dermatologic or GI condition involving colic and parasitemia). The progression of the problem should help differentiate a medical problem from one that is primarily behavioral. In horses, most self-mutilation involves biting of the limbs, chest, or flanks. Self-mutilation can appear in sexually frustrated (usually male) or socially incompatible horses, or as a manifestation of an obsessive-compulsive disorder. Treatment should involve correction of the underlying condition. Self-mutilation associated with sexual frustration can be addressed by castration, pasturing with a mare, removing all mares (or horses that induce the behavior, if the problem is primarily social) from the environment, increasing exercise, increasing roughage and decreasing grain, and treatment with progestins or opiate blockers. In the case of an obsessive-compulsive disorder, treatment should involve behavioral and environmental modification and antianxiety or anti-obsessive-compulsive medication.

Foal Rejection: Foal rejection is seen in 3 main forms: mares that will accept the foal but will not let it suckle, mares that are fearful of the foal and run away, and mares that exhibit stallion-like behavior and attempt to kick and bite the foal. Mares may paw at foals to stimulate them to rise from recumbency. This behavior must be differentiated from rejection. Mares can kill their foals if they are experiencing a nutritional stress, and this can be a normal, although uncommon behavior.

The first step in treatment is to protect the foal. If the mare will accept the foal but not let it suckle, the mare should be helped for several nursings until she learns that suckling is pleasurable. Holding her in such a way that she cannot injure the foal may involve either cross-ties or partial barriers through which she can see and smell the foal but that prohibit her from reaching for it. The mare should be examined for mastitis in case she is refusing to suckle because of a painful udder. Pressure resulting from infrequent nursings can be treated using warm water baths and soaks, light massage using a hose, and milking the mare. Foals can suckle up to every 5 min for the first few days of their life, so access to the nipple is important. This nursing and contact form the basis for an ongoing maternal-foal bond. Mares that are afraid of their foals should be treated in the same manner, but the addition of relaxation cues (including darker, quieter stalls and food treats) and mild tranquilizers may help. Dogs have been used to evoke maternal "herding" behavior by stimulating the mare to protect the foal from a potential threat. Mares that attempt to injure their foals must be restrained using stocks or bars. At the same time, the mare can be counterconditioned (preferably prior to foaling) using a stanchion and positive reward. Olfactory and hormonal cues may be important. Noses of mares and foals can be rubbed with fetal membranes, or immediate postpartum cervical stimulation can be practiced. Both of these may stimulate mares to lick, which is important in the first phase of attachment. Mares that lick exuberantly in the first hour may be willing to adopt an orphaned foal. After the first hour postpartum, licking behavior decreases and is replaced by nickering between the foal and mare. These are characteristic behaviors that can be monitored in the course of normal development of the mare-foal bond. Tranquilization can be helpful, if relatively mild uncertainty and anxiety are involved.

Poor Libido: Stallions experience poor libido if they are overused for breeding, have experienced inhibition through the use of antimasturbation devices, are used out of season, or are injured while breeding. Experience is paramount with stallions, and all of these etiologies support the role of bad experiences; owners who want to restrict show or performance horses from masturbating should be so informed. Masturbation is a normal equine behavior and there is no truth to the myth that masturbation depletes semen value—horses that masturbate rarely ejaculate. Although measurement of testosterone levels may be worthwhile, it is usually uninformative because few horses are truly testosterone-deficient. Stallions that have poor libido should be rested if overused. Letting such stallions watch other stallions mate may have a beneficial effect on their libido. Providing them with a variety of teaser mares, mating partners (the Coolidge effect, ie, an increase in mating attempts following introduction of a new partner), and other stallions can also stimulate their interest. Pasturing with a mare in estrus may help. Using an artificial vagina to desensitize a stallion that has been injured can be useful. Treatment with diazepam (to address anxiety) and oxytocin, testosterone, or gonadotropin-releasing hormone (to address the hormonal basis of erection, intromission, and ejaculation) can help. Stallions that will intromit, but not ejaculate, may benefit from hormone-based treatments.

Aggression when Breeding: Stallions that are aggressive when used for breeding are often overused or used out of season. These stallions can benefit from the use of an artificial vagina out of season so that they learn that the experience is pleasurable. Stallions can develop preferences for mating and may not be compatible with the chosen mare; changing the mare may help. If stallions were stabled with mares when they were colts, they may have some social inhibition for mating, and forced mating can result in aggression. The social role is also emphasized by the finding that there is more breeding/hr if bachelor stallions are present. Physical devices (eg, hobbles) or pharmacologic intervention (eg, succinylcholine) have been used to control stallions and to induce learned helplessness. Treating the primary aggression is preferred.

Nymphomania: Nymphomaniac mares "wink" (show clitoris), squat, and urinate frequently. Urine scalding is a real, secondary problem. Mating behaviors and those involved in solicitation are not considered abnormal if they occur every 21 days when the mares cycle. Treatments usually focus on the underlying physiologic correlates of the behaviors. Nymphomaniac mares should be checked for granulosa cell tumors. Treatment has involved the use of progestins and ovariohysterectomy. If behavior problems persist after ovariohysterectomy, the use of dexamethasone will suppress adrenal androgens.

Psychic Estrus: Mares with psychic estrus show estrous behavior without any of the physiologic correlates of heat. Treatment is as for nymphomania (*see* above).

Silent Estrus: Mares exhibiting silent estrus show all of the physiologic correlates of heat without any of the behavioral signs. Tape-recorded sounds of a stallion soliciting mares and breeding them can help, as can the presence of stallion odor. The presence of a known stallion with whom the mare has a good social relationship can help. It may be necessary to permanently or temporarily wean the last foal.

Intraspecific Mounting: Intraspecific mounting is usually mare-mare. Males seldom mount other males unless they bite them, in which case aggression is the primary problem. Mares that mount other mares should be checked for granulosa cell tumors. This can be a normal behavior in some estrous or pregnant mares.

Geldings that Act Like Stallions: Geldings that act like stallions will mount mares, attack foals, fight with other males, and self-mutilate. Some of these geldings are "proud cut" and have residual epididymis. Retained testes may also be implicated. Geldings that still have testosterone may have larger manes, tails, and forelocks than other geldings in their cohort. These geldings can destabilize other social relationships. The behavior of the geldings can encompass the entire range of mating-associated behaviors, including herding, courting (piaf), and flehmen responses. Treatment involves protecting the rest of the group (ie, removing the mares and foals) and using progestins or cyproheptadine, which may block release of adrenocorticotropic hormone from the pituitary gland, or the newer selective serotonin reuptake inhibitors, which address the increased reactivity at a central level.

Problems with Trailering: Problems with trailering include refusing to enter (load) or leave the trailer and scrambling. All of these can be potentially injurious to the horse and are best addressed early. Often, treatment can be as simple as backing the horse into the trailer (using a platform rather than a ramp), walking the horse slowly around and then into the trailer, using an equine or other companion animal that trailers well, and counterconditioning and desensitization using treats. In the latter case, the horse can be fed preferred food in proximity to and then in the trailer. Sedatives may help. Trailers can also be designed to allow bidirectional entry and exit, a turning radius, and a walk-through option. Walk-through trailers may help because the horse is not walking into a dark, uncertain area. Once the horse is calm, the gate can be raised.

CATTLE

SOCIAL BEHAVIOR

There are no free-ranging feral cattle (*Bos*) with which to compare domesticated herds, but wild cattle do exist (Guar, Butang). Cattle live in social groups that are hierarchically structured by age, weight (especially true for polled cattle), the presence and size of horns, sex, and breed. Although the basis of the social group is the female and her calf or calves, males are dominant over females in feral cattle. Small female herds contain one breeding bull; remaining younger or smaller bulls comprise smaller, unstable herds.

In dairy cattle, Holsteins and Ayrshires may be "dominant" over Jerseys; this effect is confounded by the one attributable to weight. In beef cattle, the trend is reversed; lighter breeds appear "dominant" to heavier ones (Angus are more dominant than Shorthorn, which are more dominant than Herefords). In such cases, relative social rank may lead to differential control of grazing and watering areas and shelter. Under free-ranging situations, there does not seem to be a correlation between feeding first or milk production and social rank. Infant cows will hide and lie still for the first few days of life and then form kindergartens with other calves and 1 or 2 cows. Stable social groups usually experience their first agonistic interactions at puberty (if reached). Groups of prepubertal cattle (4-6 mo of age) will form an unstable hierarchy if grouped (eg, feedlot situations). Social status increases with age, and social relationships are not stable until at least 1 yr of age. The peak of social status and control over it occurs at 9 yr of age, after which it declines.

High-ranking animals will approach others with perpendicular postures, whereas lower-ranking animals use parallel approaches. Horning behavior—digging the horns in and pawing the ground—is a threat, regardless.

Bulls will guard cows that are in proestrus and estrus and will frequently smell and lick their vulva. They are stimulated by visual cues that look like the vulva (an inverted U). Flehmen responses are important in cattle, and the vomeronasal organ opens directly into the mouth. Bulls find urine more interesting than mucus. Twin bulls are similar in their behaviors.

BEHAVIORAL PROBLEMS

Most behavioral problems in cattle focus on mating behavior and on the effects of confinement. There may be ontogenic and genetic contributions to temperament and ease with which the animal can be handled. Cattle with off-center or multiple facial hair whorls react differently to chutes and handling than do those with single, central whorls. Given the roles of neuroectodermal induction in early ontogeny, further research into such associations with temperament is warranted.

Reproductive performance is tested in beef bulls (used in natural service). The most common test used is the Blockley test, in which several bulls are tested with several stanchioned cows. Both the number of mounts and the number of completed breedings are noted. There is a heritable basis for the ability to complete service. Fertility is associated with scrotal circumference, which may also be heritable.

Poor Libido: Poor libido is the most common problem in bulls used for artificial insemination. These bulls are kept in an all-male environment. Treatment involves correction of any physical problems coupled with the use of multiple teaser females. Food lures or rewards (molasses) may also stimulate interest.

Buller Steers: Buller steers are those that are mounted by other steers in the group. This causes a secondary problem of weight loss or decreased weight gain because of the resultant physiologic and social turmoil. It is not an uncommon occurrence when steers are first mixed (eg, in feedlots) and may affect 1-4% of the population. It is associated more with social contest than with sexual stimuli (mounting is usually a social display and not just a sexual one). Removing the buller may fix the problem. Overhead electric grills can prohibit other steers from mounting the buller. Most steers in the USA have estrogen implants, which worsen this condition (see p 2169). Avoidance of these implants greatly diminishes the problem.

Masturbation: Masturbation can be a normal behavior in bulls, which usually masturbate twice a day, in the early morning and afternoon. Bulls ejaculate when they masturbate. Unless the masturbation is a manifestation of an obsessive-compulsive disorder (uncommon in bulls), it rarely becomes a breeding problem.

Stereotypic and Obsessive-compulsive Disorders: Cattle have prehensile tongues. Veal cattle that are severely confined have an increased incidence of tongue rolling, which has been correlated with a decreased frequency of abomasal ulcers, leading to the erroneous but often cited conclusion that stereotypic behaviors can be self-medicating. Both tongue-rolling and abomasal ulcers are stress responses induced by confinement. Confined dairy bulls and heifers will also tongue roll. Calves that are early weaned, confined, and milk fed will suck and suckle on any dependent appendage of their other calf companions. Such sucking (or intersucking) results in injury to tails, ears, and prepuces. Hair eating also occurs in these circumstances. Increasing roughage, providing more space, and providing more visual stimuli help reduce both the tongue rolling (and abomasal ulcers) and intersucking.

Balking at Entering Milking Parlors: Dairy cows can become reluctant to enter milking parlors, sometimes as a result of a scary, painful, or otherwise untoward event (eg, abuse, mastitis and pain, unintentional electric shock due to stray voltage problems). In the absence of an untoward event, there are 2 main correlates of this recalcitrant behavior: insufficient reward and a normal social response to a hierarchical social grouping. Cows can be fed during milking or placed in an entry pattern that mimics the social structure of the herd. This problem is usually related to management. Because some cows exhibit handedness or a preference for which side they enter the parlor or are handled/milked, stress can be decreased (and productivity increased) by meeting the cows' needs. Cows may also have preferred bovine parlor-mates.

Heat Detection: While not technically a behavioral problem, detection of heat in dairy cows is a problem for which the solution can be largely behavioral. Dairy cows are in heat for only 4 hr, during which they walk more and eat less. One-fourth of heifers experience a silent heat. Treatment involves learning to recognize the behavioral or olfactory cues of estrus. Dogs and rats can be trained to detect olfactory cues of cows in estrus. Cows can be fitted with computerized pedometers that monitor their walking and eating patterns for heat detection. Heat detectors (dye, etc) can be fitted to the cow's back so that mounting by any other cow is noticed.

Cross-fostering Calves: Orphaned or abandoned calves will steal milk from cows other than their mother. The calf that is stealing the milk will approach the cow from behind, whereas the calf that is born to the cow will approach from the front. Calves will suckle with each other and with other females, if permitted. A cow can be encouraged to accept a calf other than its own by rubbing the calf with the placenta and amniotic fluid of the cow's own calf.

SWINE

SOCIAL BEHAVIOR

Pigs are social animals and form hierarchies at social maturity. Unlike most other social mammals, however, they also form a social hierarchy at birth. This is at least partly the result of teat order—the first pair of teats is often preferred and may produce more milk. Piglets that suckle on the first pair of teats gain more weight than do other piglets. Teat order is formed within the first 48 hr, after which changes are rare. Teat order is stable by 7 days of age. Piglets reinforce the established order early in life and will slash their companions with their teeth, which therefore are usually cut to protect other piglets and the mother. Heavy piglets (ie, the ones that suckled the first pair of teats) continue to reinforce their status through contest. The winner in piglet contests is invariably the heavier pig, which continues to have an advantage later in life. The piglet hierarchy can persist after weaning if the cohort is left together. If the piglets are separated, other factors influence the development of social hierarchies.

Weaning occurs naturally at 14-17 wk but can occur in production or pen situations as early as 6-9 wk. Unfortunately, this period coincides with the period of 11-18 wk during which unpleasant experiences can delay a first pregnancy in gilts and a first successful mating in boars. Boars may be higher ranking, but the same is not true for barrows.

As in cattle, breed is important, and Yorkshires and Large Whites are more aggressive than Hampshires, which are more aggressive than Durocs. The standard porcine social grouping focuses on sows, piglets, and juveniles; males emigrate at ~1-2 yr of age. Pigs have labile social structures, and the extent to which the home ranges of males overlap those of females depends on season and reproduction. Sows within a social group experience synchronous estrus. If allowed to do so, sows will combine their litters so that one sow remains with all of the piglets while the other sows forage. Upon return from foraging, the sows suckle only their own young. Piglets otherwise do not generally mingle with piglets from other litters for the first month.

Communal nesting behavior will occur at night, if allowed. Vegetation and stick nests are usually communally constructed in a protected area (behind a tree or barrier) or at a high point. Undoubtedly, these behaviors are adaptations to avoid predation. Piglets leave the nest permanently at ~9 days of age. Farrowing occurs year round and is more regular under warmer conditions. There are usually 2 farrowing peaks per year.

Overheating is a major problem in pigs, and wallowing in mud is a thermoregulatory behavior. Conditions that decrease expenditure of energy are preferred. This behavior does not represent a desire to be filthy or unclean. Pigs exhibit selective dunging behavior, ie, they choose a location to deposit their feces and faithfully return to it. Given the choice, pigs choose clean conditions in which they can also thermoregulate.

Postweaning sows and prepubertal gilts should be kept in the sight and smell of a boar to induce synchronous estrus (the Whitten effect). They also experience a dormitory effect (the McClintock or Fraser-Darling effect) with regard to synchrony due to the presence of other females. Sexual behavior in pigs is almost universally associated with the "chant de coeur" or song of the heart. Courting pigs are vocal. Boars have a gape response (flehmen), and some boars can detect estrous females through olfactory means. Boars will nuzzle the head, shoulders, flank, and anogenital area of sows during courtship. If the pheromonal cues are present, boars progress to pushing on a sow to see if she will move. If she stands, she is willing to mate. Boars exhibit a unique, pheromonally based solicitation behavior toward females: they "champ"—chewing and gnashing their teeth, producing frothy saliva that is rich in the pheromone androstenol. Androstenol is also present in preputial fluids. Courting boars mark trees with urine and saliva produced by champing. Boars are naturally slow to ejaculate (up to 30 min), which may be a correlate of their long courtship, but mate best if raised in a rich social environment. Boars raised in isolation have decreased sexual performance later in life.

Rooting is a normal foraging behavior in pigs. The nose of a pig is a sensitive sensory organ, and striking a pig on the nose is discouraged. Nose rings may prevent rooting, but no studies have examined the effects that such rings may have on more subtle social and interactive behaviors. All such effects will be magnified by genetic effects on temperament. Pigs bred to have a lower fat content are more reactive and aggressive when handled, leading to earlier slaughter. Handling differences are also known for different breeds of pigs.

BEHAVIORAL PROBLEMS

Cannibalism of Piglets: Piglets may be cannibalized if the sow has a calcium deficiency. Addressing the deficiency resolves the problem. Sows that are not calcium-deficient that cannibalize their piglets are usually primiparous and can be treated with tranquilization and counterconditioning.

Refusal to Nurse: Piglets are seldom anorectic, but if the sow has dysgalactia syndrome (p 1134), she may deny the piglets access to the teats by lying sternally. (Normally, sows allow access by lying in lateral recumbency.) Piglets prefer warm, soft, and fuzzy hairlines. Under normal conditions, grunting in crescendo by the sow stimulates oxytocin and milk letdown, while simultaneously signaling this occurrence to piglets. For sows to continue with milk letdown and to feed piglets, the piglets must exhibit tight tails and put their ears back. Intake of solid food can be stimulated by incorporating some of the sow's milk, sweetening the feed, and creep feeding.

Aggression: Aggression is most common when strange pigs are mixed. However, this is a nonspecific description, and treatment will be more successful if a more specific diagnosis can be made. In general, the social environment can be altered by lowering the lights, providing hides into which the pigs can stick their heads (lower-ranking pigs will hide more), and covering heads with hoods (which affects individual recognitions and social interaction). In addition, the use of the boar pheromone androstenol can augment hierarchies in boars. Tranquilizers (eg, the dopamine blocker azaperone) can help, and some antipsychotic medications (eg, lithium) have been used successfully.

Tail Chewing and Biting: Tail biting occurs if piglets are affected with iron-deficiency anemia (p 13). It is more common in piglets kept on concrete because they cannot engage in normal rooting behaviors. It can also result from escalation of predatory behavior that occurs in the presence of blood. Once piglets taste blood, true aggression ensues. Lack of environmental stimulation coupled with environmental stress may also play a role. Providing the piglets with material in which they can root (eg, peat bark) and with objects to chew can help. Iron supplementation should be the first treatment consideration.

Breeding Problems: The most common problem associated with breeding involves mate choice. Behavioral parameters of estrus as discussed above are critical for successful mating. Sows that are in physiologic, but not behavioral, estrus will not permit breeding, and boars cannot proceed with their mating display. Sows develop preferences for individual boars, and these should be addressed. Sows also may respond to replaying of tape-recorded versions of the "chant de coeur" when accompanied by the olfactory stimulus of androstenol, which is commercially available.

Piglet Crushing: Under free-ranging circumstances, sows give birth in nests that provide hiding areas for the piglets. Hiding areas are not available in farrowing crates, although some crates have bars under which piglets can crawl. Smaller, weaker, and anoxic piglets (those that cannot crawl to safety) are crushed more frequently than other piglets. Crushing is not merely a management-related condition, it is a derivation of other behaviors that have been influenced through artificial selection. Sows are good and protective mothers. Such behaviors interfere with human access to piglets, so less devoted maternal behavior has been selected for to make handling of piglets easier under production conditions.

Good farrowing crates will help prevent crushing. Sloping pens that permit the piglets to roll away can help. Heat lamps placed a distance from the sow provide a thermal gradient that the piglets can exploit while concomitantly rendering the sow only a secondary (and not the only) heat source. Buzzer or alarm systems also can be built into management systems, and sows taught to rise if an alarm sounds.

Stereotypic and Obsessive-compulsive Disorders: The most common stereotypic behaviors include bar biting, tail chewing and biting (in some cases), chain chewing, anal massage, tether manipulation, and polydipsia. Early intervention is most easily accomplished through environmental enrichment. Piglets and pigs can be fed more, encouraged to work for their food by having to root through their bedding for treats, and provided environmental toys (eg, relatively indestructible hard plastic balls, food dispensing toys, logs, clean old tires, etc).

SHEEP

SOCIAL BEHAVIOR

Sheep are extremely social and choose to associate with other sheep. Flocks include multiple females, offspring, and one or more males. Ewes tend to stay in their maternal groups for life, whereas rams can form unstable and easily disbanded bachelor herds. If most rams in a group die, those remaining join another group. Under standard grazing situations, social hierarchies are not as apparent as they are for cattle.

Males in rut will fight with each other. Social rank depends on the presence and size of horns, body mass, and height at the withers and hocks. Age may also play a role because the mortality of lambs from yearling ewes is extremely high. Higher-ranking males concentrate on courting females when in rut and do not graze to the extent that lower-ranking rams do. Groups of 40-50 ewes/adult ram and 25-30 ewes/juvenile ram are common management choices. Mortality in rams is 5 times that in ewes. Unless lower-ranking animals outnumber the higher-ranking male and serve to distract or otherwise occupy him (this need not be cooperative), subordinates are excluded from breeding. While the higher-ranking male usually has larger horns, the role of the demographic environment (ie, the number of lower-ranking males in the group) prevents an extreme selection response for these secondary sex characteristics.

In large groups of sheep or in sheep on large pastures, more subordinates are likely to mate. In tightly confined, relatively small groups, the role that the social order plays in mating is critical, and owners should understand that lower-ranking rams may not mate under such conditions.

Sheep are seasonally polyestrous and reach puberty at 7-12 mo. Mating behavior includes nudging, kicking, or pawing with the front legs, low stretching, and pushing. These same behaviors and head-to-head banging with horn clashing occur in conflicts between males.

Isolation in sheep can cause severe problems associated with stress. Mirrors should be used in the absence of other sheep. Sheep have 3 types of central face recognition cells. Those responsible for the recognition of known versus unknown sheep fire the most frequently. Horn cells fire more frequently with increasing size. The third type of cells fires when a predator (eg, dog, human) appears.

Artificial weaning occurs at 10 wk of age, but these lambs recognize and will return to the ewes after a 2-mo separation. Sheep are naturally weaned at 6 mo of age, usually when their mother again comes into heat. Ewe lambs continue to follow the dam, but ram lambs do not.

BEHAVIORAL PROBLEMS

Homosexuality: Homosexuality is a normal behavior in sheep and is seen in up to 30% of all rams. Incidence of homosexuality is decreased in rams raised in heterosexual groups and in rams that have experience with ewes, but it still persists. It is unclear to what extent such behaviors are facilitated by a sex ratio that has been skewed for mating purposes.

Lamb Stealing: Ewes can steal the lambs of others before their own parturition and then reject their own lamb when it is born. Lambs seek out soft, warm, hairless areas (regardless of where they are), which can help with raising orphaned lambs but render stealing easier. Individual pens or partial barriers can usually prevent theft. Ewes will sequester the lambs at first, and providing them a shelter where this can be done will help. The smell of the wool is important to the ewe for individual lamb recognition, as is the shape and color of the lamb's head. Ewes are more likely to accept lambs that have familiar head coloration.

Lamb Rejection: This can be associated with the social hierarchy or due to behavioral, physiologic, or environmental stresses (eg, rain) at delivery. The smell of the wool is important to the ewe, and lambs that smell unfamiliar are more likely to be rejected. Experimental results show that lambs whose heads have been altered are at risk for rejection. Alteration of the tail does not have the same effect. If the rejection is noted sufficiently early, using a stanchion to confine the ewe with the lamb can address the problem. Tranquilization may be needed.

Cross-fostering: Cross-fostering can be an acceptable solution for abandoned, rejected, or orphaned lambs. Cross-fostering is best addressed by fooling the ewe, using cervical stimulation (using balloons that stimulate oxytocin release and maternal behavior). Covering the lamb to be fostered with a t-shirt that the ewe's own lamb has worn can provide an appropriate olfactory cue, as can the skin of the ewe's own dead lamb.

Stereotypic and Obsessive-compulsive Disorders: In sheep, these include wool-sucking, intersucking, and self-sucking (tails or udder).

GOATS

SOCIAL BEHAVIOR

Social behavior in goats is similar to that in sheep, and horns also play a major factor in their social rankings. Goats also hide early in life but, unlike cows, spend more time away from the nannies for the first 6 wk than for the next 6 wk. The nanny initiates early approaches, and the kid initiates the later ones. Sexual behavior of goats differs slightly from that of sheep. Billy goats throw their head up in the air and ventroflex their neck when they ejaculate. They also frequently urinate on their front legs, which they then rub on the female as part of their courtship ritual. The scent of female urine is important and is transported into the vomeronasal organ during flehmen.

BEHAVIORAL PROBLEMS

Behavioral problems are not commonly reported in goats, perhaps because adult males are expected to charge people if their turf is traversed. Behavioral problems may actually be more rare (as opposed to less frequently reported) in this group because their maintenance conditions more closely mimic those in a free-ranging situation. Domestication may have had less of an impact on the social patterns of goats than is true for other species.

Self-suckling: Goats that abort late in pregnancy or those that have a second pregnancy subsequent to nursing can self-suckle. The latter situation may be illuminating because the behavior did not occur when the nanny was nursing. Treatment involves behavioral and environmental enrichment, social companionship that is stable before pregnancy, and possibly some antianxiety medications.

Stereotypic and Obsessive-compulsive Disorders: These behaviors in goats are similar to those in sheep (*see* above). Goats separated from a group may develop competitive "rearing" or elevation.

CHICKENS

SOCIAL BEHAVIOR

Chickens are social animals, and the focus of the group is the hen and chicks. Roosters practice mate guarding. Most chickens are sent to slaughter before physical maturity. Social maturity does not occur until >1 yr of age. Social rank depends on size, feathers, color, and the demographic environment. Free-range chickens experience more agonistic situations and demonstrate more aggression than do battery chickens. The free-range situation is representative of normal behavior. Battery conditions (eg, housing chickens individually or in small groups in darkened cages with space insufficient to nest and brood) contribute to decreased aggression because of the concomitant debeaking, restrictive caging conditions, and darkness. Tryptophan added to the feed has been correlated with a decrease in aggression. Food intake is heritable in chickens, and most domestic chickens have been selected for high intake. Chickens use nesting material if they have access to it, and adult chickens that have never seen a nesting box will use one if provided. Chickens make fewer trips to nesting boxes if they have to squeeze to enter them.

BEHAVIORAL PROBLEMS

The two most common behavioral problems in chickens—**aggression** and **feather pecking or plucking**—may be associated. Aggression can be manifest as pecking at the head and face or as pecking at and pulling feathers. Dust baths are an essential part of feather hygiene, and some grooming can be social. Feather pecking or plucking occurs in situations of social or physical stress. Treatment for conditions involving outright aggression and self-mutilation involves addressing the underlying problem. Altering social groups and providing environmental enrichment should be included in any treatment program. *See also* CANNIBALISM, p 2271.

DOGS

SOCIAL BEHAVIOR

Dogs, under free-ranging conditions, live in mixed-sex, mixed-age social groups. Relative social ranking is primarily determined by age, although sex may play a role. Females appear to be responsible for guiding most group activities. Social hierarchies are maintained primarily by deference, not—as commonly believed—by agonistic interaction.

Sexual maturity in domestic dogs occurs between 6-9 mo of age (later for giant breeds), while social maturity begins to develop at ~12-36 (mean ~24) mo of age. At social maturity, a relative and fluid hierarchy dependent on age, sex, size, and temperament may develop. In free-ranging groups, dogs that challenge the established social hierarchy may leave and form their own groups if they do not succeed in altering the extant social order. This situation may be analogous to one form of inter-dog aggression that occurs in multiple-dog households. Social maturity is also the time during which problem aggressions and anxieties develop. Roaming, mounting, urine marking, and intra-sexual fighting are facilitated by sex hormones, particularly testosterone. These problems are often prevented or greatly reduced by neutering, especially in males.

Between 3-8 wk of age, dogs tend to focus on other dogs (if available) for their social stimuli, and between 5-12 wk of age on people (if available). Dogs are most receptive to learning about how to deal with novel environments and stimuli until about 16-20 wk of age. After this age dogs do not stop learning from exposure—they just do so at a slower rate, and perhaps in a different way. It is not critical to switch the focus of exposure at one specific period; given adequate opportunity, puppies will learn about the social and physical environments when they are ready. Overtly fearful stimuli should be avoided. Dogs kept exclusively kenneled or not exposed to people by 14 wk of age may have severely undeveloped social skills.

Dogs develop a substrate preference for elimination at ~8½ wk of age, and this may be, overall, the best time to adopt a puppy. Unless there is no other choice, puppies should not be adopted until at least 7½ wk of age. Interstate commerce laws prohibit shipment of dogs before 7 wk of age.

Most domestic dogs, except for Basenjis, have 2 heat cycles per year. Care of the young can be communal, and all members of the group may assist in care if there are no competing nutritional or social stresses. In multi-dog groups, the highest-ranking animals may be the only ones to breed. This is enforced by them and by their interference with the mating of other, lower-ranking animals. There may be pheromonal and hormonal components to these behaviors.

BEHAVIORAL PROBLEMS

The most common behavioral problems in dogs are those associated with aggression, primarily dominance/impulse control aggression, fear aggression, and those associated with fears and anxieties. Most aggressions may be anxiety disorders.

Behavioral Problems Associated with Canine Aggression

An attempt has been made to specify definitional criteria for behavioral diagnoses. The advantage to these is that they do not rely on nonspecific signs, so conditions that share signs are not confused, and conditions that show an atypical form are not ruled out because a nonspecific sign appears discordant. Clusters of nonspecific signs within a diagnosis or those shared in comorbid diagnoses may help to identify treatment and pathological groups. While this system is frequently used, it is not universal. It may be helpful to view these diagnostic categories as guidelines that will continue to be redefined, given that behavioral medicine is a quickly growing and evolving field.

Some of these problems, in feline-specific form, also occur in cats; these include fear aggression, idiopathic aggression, interanimal aggression, pain aggression, play aggression, predatory aggression, redirected aggression, and territorial aggression.

Dominance/impulse control aggression has the following necessary condition: abnormal, inappropriate, out-of-context aggression (threat, challenge, or attack) consistently exhibited by dogs toward people under any circumstance involving passive or active control of the dog's behavior or the dog's access to the behavior. The following condition is sufficient (eg, if it is met there is little doubt that the diagnosis is valid): intensification of any aggressive response from the dog upon any passive or active correction or interruption of the dog's behavior or the dog's access to the behavior. The key is assessment of the dog's need to control for the sake of maintaining control. The behaviors exhibited by dogs with this diagnosis are actually a rule structure that allows the dogs to learn how to act in situations that are potentially unclear, uncertain, and anxiety-provoking to them.

This definition of dominance/impulse control aggression is discrete and does not couple the challenge to food (food-related aggression), toys (possessive aggression), or space (territorial aggression). These aggressions can all be correlates of dominance/impulse control aggression and, when associated with it, may be indicative of a more severe situation. Control and access are key—most of the problems with diagnoses arise from human misunderstanding of canine social systems, canine signaling, and canine anxieties associated with endogenous uncertainty about contextually appropriate responses. Diagnosis cannot be made on the basis of a single event. The behavior, once it begins, will become more visible and consistent, but data on early signs, patterns of change with experience, and changes in intensity are lacking.

The necessary and sufficient conditions are different from the common descriptions of dominance/impulse control aggression that specify that the dog will often react to being pushed on, to being corrected with a leash, or to being pushed from a sofa by a person. The number of situations in which the dog reacts inappropriately, or the intensity with which he or she reacts, do not affect the necessary and sufficient conditions, although these factors may affect the ability to treat the condition, the prognosis, and the risk to people. These dogs are *not* fearful, and they exhibit none of the behavioral or physiologic signs associated with fear. All canine aggressions are likely based to some degree in anxiety, and the uncertainty associated with anxiety is not equivalent to fear.

Fear aggression has the following necessary condition: aggression that consistently occurs concomitant with behavioral and physiologic signs of fear as identified by withdrawal, passive, and avoidance behaviors associated with the sympathetic nervous system. The following condition is sufficient: as above and the aggression is accompanied by urination or defecation, or when the aggression is only active (beyond just posturing) when the target of the aggression is not interacting with the subject.

The actual behaviors associated with fear, fear aggression, and any other aggression that is primarily driven by anxiety are poorly qualified and quantified. However, in contrast to dominance/impulse control aggression, the dog relinquishes control and withdraws. Only when the dog can no longer avoid or withdraw does frank aggression occur. Also, unlike dominance/impulse control aggression, these dogs never deliberately provoke a situation or initially and voluntarily contribute to its escalation.

In extreme cases, the sufficient conditions are clear; in less clear situations, which could be due to uncertainty on the animal's part, caution is urged in ruling out all other aggressions. The most likely diagnosis is the one that is most consistent with all signs and criteria. Fear aggression does not have to occur consistently, although identification of the fearful stimuli will permit assessment of the extent to which the behaviors are consistent and pose a predictable risk. Fear aggression is also seen in cats, in which it is one of the most common types of aggression, both toward other cats and people.

Food-related aggression has the following necessary condition: consistent aggression that is exhibited in the presence, and only in the presence, of pet food, bones, rawhides, biscuits, blood, or human food in the absence of abuse or starvation. The following condition is sufficient: as above with the aggression occurring *only* in the presence of a range or subset of the items listed. This is a restrictive and specific diagnosis. Number or range of items involved, while possibly reflecting danger and risk, do not affect the diagnosis. It is possible that aggressions stimulated by different classes of food indicate varying neurochemical modalities, and these differences may represent subclasses of this diagnosis. This diagnosis serves to highlight that food is not a possession, but rather something very different from a possession. This difference has been noted in neuroanatomic and neurochemical studies of aggression and is probably real. Certainly, a good evolutionary case could be made for aggression related to food being potentially important. While this aggression may be associated with dominance/impulse control aggression (ie, an animal can have both diagnoses, but development of food-related aggression usually precedes development of dominance aggression), it is absolutely, categorically different, based on the necessary and sufficient criteria listed for each. Food-related aggression can be a singular diagnosis, unrelated to any dominance aggression.

Furthermore, if an event related to impulse control aggression only incidentally involved food, or food was the vehicle for the aggression only once (ie, there is no pattern of other food-related responses), and the owner has been able to take or interfere with the food item at other times, the issue is one of control (ie, impulse control aggression), not food.

Idiopathic aggression has the following necessary and sufficient condition: aggression that occurs in an unpredictable, toggle-switch manner in contexts not associated with stimuli noted for any other behavioral aggression diagnosis or with any underlying causal physical or physiologic condition. This diagnosis must be distinguished from any neurologic condition. Intensive characterization of attendant behaviors is necessary to differentiate this from the most common condition with which it is confused—undiagnosed or subtle dominance/impulse control aggression. Explosive, unpredictable aggression can be associated with "rage," a term that should not be used because of the inability to adequately define the analogous emotional conditions in pets that are experienced and described by people. Unpredictability is a function of the quality of observational skills and knowledge. Although idiopathic aggression may be considered a common problem by clients, once a detailed history is collected it becomes clear that this is a rare diagnosis. This form of aggression is also reported to occur in cats. This diagnosis may simply be a misidentified variant of impulse control aggression.

Interanimal or interdog aggression has the following necessary condition: consistent, volitional, proactive aggression that is not contextual given the social signals, threat circumstances, or response received. The following condition is sufficient: as above in the absence of any signal or interaction from the animal that is attacked. It is emphasized that, at some level, the behaviors involved with aggression are normal behaviors. This diagnostic category, while usually associated with changes in social hierarchy that are often related to the development of social maturity in one of the involved animals, does not depend on either hierarchy or social maturity; it depends on the contextual response. This subtle but important distinction supports the contention that social shifts and occasional threats can be normal. A change in behavior is not necessary, although it may be usual, because if this is truly a diagnosis of an abnormal behavior, some animals will respond with aggression regardless of circumstances. More specific categories would be interdog and intercat aggression associated with hierarchical disputes. Interanimal aggression is also seen in cats.

Anthropomorphic terms like sibling rivalry should be avoided. Not only are they likely to be incorrect, they also obscure the difference between truly pathologic aggression and what may be a normal canine redress of mild social conflicts. Caution in generalized and anthropocentric views and terms is urged.

Maternal aggression has the following necessary condition: consistent aggression (threat, challenge, or contest) directed toward puppies in the absence of pain, challenges, or threats to the mother by the puppies. The following condition is sufficient: unprovoked, age-inappropriate attacks on puppies by the mother. When maternal aggression is profound, it is extremely easy to recognize, even though puppies are not necessarily injured or killed. The extent to which discrete aggressive behaviors can be a component of normal maternal behavior has not been well quantified.

Inherited forms of maternal aggression are seen in both cats and dogs. Treatment is important when the condition is familial. The ethics of continued breeding in such circumstances should be considered.

Pain aggression has the following necessary condition: consistent aggressive behavior, in excess of that required to indicate concern and to effect restraint, demonstrated only in a context known or potentially associated with pain but that may not be painful itself. The following condition is sufficient: as above in the absence of any behavioral and physiologic signs of fear as identified by withdrawal, passive, and avoidance behaviors associated with the sympathetic nervous system. Evaluation of pain in animals is very difficult and even more subjective than in humans (*see* PAIN MANAGEMENT, p 1691). This is a diagnosis of degree and correlation: conditions that are known to cause pain (eg, fractured legs) could render the animal resistant to manipulation. Domestic animals do not have opposable thumbs and so may use their mouths to grasp and restrain.

For this diagnosis to be made, fear must not be primary (although anticipation of pain and the attendant anxiety may be involved), and the behaviors must be in excess of those required to indicate the animal's concern. Pain aggression is also seen in cats. Newer protocols for controlling perceived or anticipated pain should decrease the incidence of this condition.

Play aggression has the following necessary condition: consistent aggression that occurs in contexts in which play behaviors (eg, play bows, yips, shoulder blocks [dogs]; chases, charges, pounces [cats]) would normally occur. The following condition is sufficient: out-of-context, consistent aggression in circumstances in which play is relevant, or in-context aggression consistent with the solicitation of play but that involves actions that would discourage play (eg, biting, pain). The normal, accepted, or in-context range of social play behaviors are relatively well defined when compared with abnormal, unacceptable, or out-of-context behaviors. The difficulty is to distinguish rough play (learned in interactions from other animals or people) from truly abnormal behavior. Analysis of discrete behaviors should also distinguish this from attention-seeking behavior. Play aggression is also seen in cats.

In contrast to previously held beliefs, new research has shown that energetic play by humans with dogs (eg, tug-of-war) does not necessarily produce play aggressions. Humans who play energetically and forcefully with their dogs do so best by understanding and using signals that are like those dogs use themselves. The same pattern is likely to be true for cats, especially if appropriate inhibition of damaging play is discouraged through quick signaling and withdrawal of attention.

Possessive aggression has the following necessary condition: aggression that is consistently directed toward another individual that approaches or attempts to obtain a nonfood object or toy that the aggressor possesses or to which the aggressor controls access. The following condition is sufficient: as above, and, in the absence of the object associated with the contentious behavior, aggression does not occur. This diagnosis includes only nonfood items, although there may be some overlap with food-related aggression (eg, rawhide chew toys). The stimuli and neurochemical changes associated with aggression toward objects and toward food are likely very different. While this aggression may be correlated with the occurrence of canine dominance/impulse control aggression (p 1314) or feline status-related aggression (p 1325), the latter behaviors are about control of activity or access—not about control of objects—and the diagnosis of impulse control or status-related aggression should not be made on the basis of a response to an object. For a diagnosis of possessive aggression to be made, the response to the object must be consistent, restrictive, and repeatable. If the animal also fulfills the criteria for dominance or status-related aggression, those diagnoses should be made in addition to, not instead of, the diagnosis of possessive aggression.

Predatory aggression has the following necessary condition: quiet aggression, or behaviors congruent with subsequent predatory behavior (staring, salivating, stalking, body lowering, tail twitching, etc) consistently exhibited in either circumstances associated with predation or toward victims such as human infants or young or ill animals; death is not a necessary sequela, nor is ingestion should death ensue. The following condition is sufficient: quiet, unheralded attacks, generally involving at least one fierce bite and shake, that include staring, salivating, stalking, body lowering, and tail twitching, consistently exhibited toward species-contextual prey items (eg, cats and birds), or toward individuals that exhibit uncoordinated movements and sudden sleep and wake cycles (eg, human infants, young or ill animals, geriatric people); death is not a necessary sequela, nor is ingestion should death ensue. Discrete analyses of the behaviors involved should elucidate different forms of this behavior and the role that the behavior of the victims plays in determining the form that the aggression will take. The latter is important because predatory aggression can also be used to describe aggression to joggers and bicyclists. In the latter case, territorial aggression must be considered, but when predatory aggression involves sentient adult people, it is likely to be categorically different from that described above. Normal, species-typical predatory behavior in the appropriate context is not to be confused with predatory aggression. Predatory aggression also occurs in cats.

Protective aggression has the following necessary condition: aggression that is consistently demonstrated when an individual or class of individuals is approached by a third party, in the absence of an actual, contextual threat from that third party. The following condition is sufficient: as above when the aggression intensifies with decreasing distance, or with vocal or physical cues that could indicate excitement or threat, despite attempts at intervention, correction, or the desire to interact on the part of the individual being "protected." Protective and territorial aggression are often lumped, making it unlikely that the impetus will exist to learn if they are behaviorally discrete. It is important to acknowledge that some degree of in-context, innate protectiveness is desired in most pet dogs. Diagnosis of protective aggression must be made only after the relevance of the context in which it occurs has been evaluated. Many dogs appear to react aggressively when confined to cars. If this is the only circumstance in which the dog is aggressive, the behavior should be considered a variant of normal.

Redirected aggression has the following necessary condition: aggression that is consistently directed toward a third party when the dog is thwarted or interrupted from exhibiting aggressive behaviors to its primary target. The following condition is sufficient: aggression that is instantly and consistently directed toward a third party when the dog is thwarted or interrupted from exhibiting aggressive behaviors to its primary target; the aggression is not accidental, and the dog will actively pursue the third party, particularly if they were associated directly with the interruption of the animal's previous behaviors. Redirected aggression must be differentiated from displacement activity in which both target and behavior have been altered as a result of a thwarted, interrupted, or corrected behavior. This diagnosis is specific and unassailable when identified by discrete behavioral descriptions. The most common diagnostic error is calling a behavior redirected aggression when the aggression was actually accidental and the result of direct intervention in the absence of sufficient time for the aggressors to stop their activity (eg, reaching between 2 fighting animals and being bitten because one animal was already in the process of biting the other and could not stop). Redirected aggression is also seen in cats.

Territorial aggression has the following necessary condition: aggression that is consistently demonstrated in the vicinity of a mobile (eg, car) or stationary (eg, yard) circumscribed area when that area is approached by another individual in the absence of an actual, contextual threat from that individual. The following condition is sufficient: as above in which the aggression intensifies with decreasing distance despite attempts at intervention, correction, or the desire to interact on the part of the approaching individual. If the only context in which the dog protects a territory is when confined in a vehicle, this can be considered a variant of normal behavior. Territorial aggression is also seen in cats, although new research has shown that most aggression exhibited by cats to other cats is about social relationships and not space.

Other Causes of Aggression: In addition to sensory system impairment and changes in an animal's physical and mental ability to negotiate their environment, sudden aggression can also be the result of infection, toxicity, or an atypical drug response. Sudden atypical aggression has been reported for dogs treated with acepromazine, and for dogs and cats treated with diazepam. While the benzodiazepine events are truly paradoxical, those associated with dissociative neuroleptics may not be. Because of their ability to alter perception while rendering the animal relatively immobile, such agents may worsen anxiety-based conditions, not improve them. This is one rationale for advising against the use of acepromazine for the treatment of noise phobias.

Treatment of Behavioral Problems Associated with Canine Aggression: The treatment of aggression can be complex and may best be performed by a specialist. The first step in treating any aggression is to obtain an accurate diagnosis. Then, any provocative circumstances must be avoided—repetition of aggression teaches the dog to be better at executing it and reinforces the association between context and behavior. Most behavior modification focuses on counterconditioning and desensitization using food treats or rewards. Owners must understand the difference between treats and bribes; the latter will guarantee treatment failure. The dog should be taught to defer to the owner for everything it wants. The goal is not to make the dog "submissive," but rather to teach the dog to attend to the owner for cues as to the appropriateness of its behavior. Dogs defer to other dogs by sitting or lying down and waiting for cues that tell them when they can proceed with their next behavior. Sitting or lying down acts as a "stop" command and allows owners to regain control of the situation. These dogs must earn all of their attention—even maintenance attention (eg, feeding, walking). Head collars (head halters, eg, Gentle Leader® or Halti®) can be a great help in treating or preventing problem canine behaviors involving aggression and can render any aggressive dog safer. Almost without exception, physical punishment, including the use of prong collars and electric shock collars, alpha rolls, and dominance downs can make an already aggressive dog worse. Owners should be discouraged from using these techniques, especially in the absence of supervision. Antidepressants (eg, amitriptyline, clomipramine, fluoxetine) have been helpful in treating anxiety associated with the aggression and in facilitating behavior modification. Currently, all behavioral treatment with psychotropic agents is extra-label, requires informed consent, and should be performed only after a thorough physical examination and laboratory evaluation (CBC and serum biochemistry profile).

Behavioral Problems Associated with Canine Elimination

Some of these problems, given attendant species-specific manifestations, also occur in cats, including marking behavior and substrate preference.

Excitement urination has the following necessary condition: urination that occurs only when the dog is engaged in active behavior and is concomitantly demonstrating physical and physiologic signs of excitement (rapid motor activity; high-pitched greeting; panting and salivation associated with open-mouthed, relaxed, greeting face, etc) rather than fear. The following condition is sufficient: urination as above that occurs when the animal is not sitting or lying down (or approaching sitting or lying down) and of which the animal may exhibit no awareness.

Incomplete housetraining has the following necessary condition: consistent and age-inappropriate elimination in undesirable locations or at undesirable times that is not associated with any lack of access or opportunity, other behavioral conditions, or any physical or physiologic condition. The following condition is sufficient: the above in an animal for which this has always been true, ie, there has been no change in behavior. This diagnosis can be made only through exhaustive history and analysis of actual behaviors. Diagnosis is confirmed by a response and adherence to a rigorous housetraining paradigm (eg, leash walking the dog too frequently for "accidents" to occur, praising the dog for use of appropriate substrates and locations). Clients should be advised of canine developmental periods for substrate preferences (~8½ wk). This is one diagnosis that is most easily treated by prevention.

Marking behavior has the following necessary condition: urination or defecation that occurs in frequencies or locations inconsistent solely with evacuation of bladder and bowel but consistent with social and olfactory stimuli. The following condition is sufficient: repeated urination or defecation, associated with species-typical postures distinct from those used in simple elimination, that occurs in frequencies or locations inconsistent solely with evacuation of bladder and bowel but consistent with limited and identifiable social and olfactory stimuli. Marking behavior involving either feces or urine that is voided when squatting is also seen in cats.

Submissive urination has the following necessary condition: urination that occurs in an otherwise housetrained animal only when the animal is exhibiting species-specific postures associated with extreme deferential behavior. The following condition is sufficient: urination that occurs in an otherwise housetrained animal only when the animal is exhibiting species-specific postures associated with extreme deferential behavior and that is worsened by approaches that solicit such deferential behaviors (eg, reaching over, rolling over) in an animal that is showing no signs of fear or aggression.

Substrate preference for elimination has the following necessary and sufficient condition: consistent elimination in an area(s) that is linked by some common sensory aspect, and avoidance or rejection of alternate materials or conditions. Substrate preference for elimination is seen in both dogs and cats, and it is important to note that this is the normal condition for dogs that are well housetrained and for cats that use their litter boxes consistently; however, in those situations, the substrate they prefer is also one that is acceptable to the owners. This becomes a diagnosis only when there is a mismatch in owner-pet preference. When preferences are extremely restrictive, there may be other anxiety-related problems.

Treatment of Behavioral Problems Associated with Canine Elimination: There are 2 main aspects of housetraining: 1) encouraging a preference for substrate and location, and 2) encouraging inhibition of elimination until the appropriate substrate and location are accessible. The latter is largely dependent on cognitive and neuromuscular maturation of the dog. The first age at which the dog is able to voluntarily inhibit elimination and make the cognitive association to do so is ~8½ wk. Appropriate housetraining in dogs involves exposure to the preferred substrate for elimination starting at that age, absence of physical punishment, emphasis on positive reinforcement, frequent trips to the desired area (as often as every 30 min-1 hr for small puppies; smaller breeds have smaller bladders and higher metabolic rates), use of good odor eliminators, and startling the dog for correction only when the dog is caught in the act of eliminating in an inappropriate place. Punishment is not helpful and may be counterproductive. Dogs with submissive urination should never be startled. These are already anxious, uncertain dogs, and any aversive response will reinforce the inappropriate behavior.

Exercising dogs within 15-30 min of eating and immediately after play, awakening, or if they slow down, can help speed the housetraining process. Housetraining an older dog is more a matter of reshaping the animal's behavior and encouraging it to select a more appropriate substrate. For young puppies of small breeds, "litter boxes" may be an appropriate adjuvant. Behaviors that are correlated with the elimination must be avoided (eg, enthusiastic greeting for a puppy with excitement urination). The presence of an older dog (observational learning and scent) can help in housetraining a puppy. Inhibition can be encouraged through the humane use of a crate or restricted area. Prevention is paramount, and owners should know that puppies obtained from pet stores are usually much more difficult to housetrain than those obtained from preferred sources, because they have never had to inhibit elimination and may have learned to play with or eat feces.

Other Canine Behavioral Problems

Some of these problems also occur in cats, in a form specific to that species.

Abnormal ingestive behavior has the following necessary condition: consistent ingestion of abnormal amounts or types of food or nonfood material in a manner or frequency not consistent with previous behavior. The following condition is sufficient: incessant consumption of food or nonfood material, or incessant avoidance of food, in a manner that interferes with normal social functioning. Abnormal ingestive behavior includes pica (consistent ingestion of nonfood material), coprophagia (ingestion of feces that is neither accidental nor incidental), polyphagia, aerophagia, psychogenic water drinking (consumption of water in excess of that necessary to meet daily fluid balance needs or to thermoregulate or lubricate food for ingestion), anorexia, and gorging. Except for pica and aerophagia—which truly seem different from ingestion or lack of ingestion involving food—it is very difficult, although not impossible, to rule out all physiologic causal associations. It is logical that abnormal ingestion of food and abnormal ingestion of water should be classified separately because they are controlled by different, although related, physiologic systems. (The term "psychogenic" does not imply any understanding of the mechanism of the condition and is equivalent to "behaviorally idiopathic.") The sufficient conditions for aerophagia include mechanically forced, volitional swallowing of air that is uncoupled with eating or drinking; behavior may be sufficiently frequent to interfere with normal activities, which can usually be confirmed by owners if questioned. In the extreme, pica, aerophagia, and coprophagia can be signs of obsessive-compulsive disorders.

Attention-seeking behavior has the following necessary condition: the dog uses vocal or physical behaviors to obtain passive or active attention from people when the people are doing something not directly involving the dog. The following condition is sufficient: whenever a person is not directly engaged in passive or active interaction with the animal, the animal uses active or passive behaviors to direct some of the person's attentions to itself and will interrupt human activity to do so. This may be an undesirable behavior, but it is common and may be a variant of normal; it is certainly a behavior that people unconsciously reinforce in their pets. In the extreme form, the dog must solicit the behavior and, if prohibited from doing so, exhibits physical and physiologic signs of anxiety. In this latter case, the attention-seeking behavior is not only abnormal but also is probably a correlate, sign, or subclass of one of the anxieties. Attention-seeking behavior is also seen in cats, typically in the form of vocalizing.

Cognitive dysfunction or senility has the following necessary and sufficient condition: change in interactive, elimination, or navigational behaviors attendant with aging that are explicitly not due to primary failure of any organ system. This is a potential animal model for the age-dependent cognitive changes that occur in humans. The affiliated behaviors may be associated with Alzheimer's-like (senile dementia of the Alzheimer type) lesions. The syndrome occurs in both dogs and cats. It is important to differentiate early cognitive dysfunction from old-age onset separation anxiety. Cognitive dysfunction sometimes involves age-dependent changes in dopaminergic function and microembolic events and is associated with deposition of amyloid plaques; however, the presence of such plaques is not sufficient to diagnose the condition. Many dogs and people with extensive plaque formation experience no decrements in cognitive function.

The following clinical signs may be associated with cognitive dysfunction: 1) Disorientation—the dog or cat seems to get lost in the house or confused when outside. The pet may become increasingly distressed within each episode of disorientation early on in the progression of the cognitive changes, and less so as the changes become more pronounced. 2) Alterations in social and environmental interactions—as cognitive decline progresses, affected dogs and cats interact less with their canine and feline housemates, play less, ignore favored toys, and withdraw from clients, often refusing interaction with them. If forced to interact, the animal can become completely withdrawn, or agitated and more distressed, possibly to the extent of becoming aggressive as a means to decrease interaction. When greeted, affected pets appear not to recognize clients. This profound alteration in client interaction and affect is the change that most distresses clients. 3) Changes in sleep-wake cycle—affected dogs and cats may no longer exhibit standard sleep-wake cycles and instead may pace and/or vocalize during the night. Because cats sleep often during the day as a normal behavior, these changes may be most noticeable in dogs, who will sleep during the day when clients are available to interact with them. Increased vocalization that is repetitive and monotonic is the most common complaint of clients with aging cats. The most distressing aspect of changes in sleep patterns for the clients is that they cannot comfort their pets when they pace and vocalize. Early in the progression of the condition, changes may be manifest only as increased time spent sleeping, which may be considered a normal aging change. Unfortunately, we do not know the extent to which this assumption is true, and such knowledge would allow earlier recognition and intervention for cognitive changes. 4) Changes in elimination behaviors—clients often describe cognitive changes associated with eliminative behaviors as a loss of housetraining. It is likely that there are changes in memory and learning associated with true housetraining (eg, the ability to inhibit elimination unless provided with an appropriate substrate) that are affected as a result of cognitive changes, but in general these dogs are not incontinent. The pets either appear to forget to eliminate when taken to their normal locations and substrates, and then eliminate anywhere when the need is urgent, or they have reduced inhibition and will eliminate wherever they are once they reach a certain threshold stimulus. The extent to which cognition is involved in inhibition of volitional behaviors is largely unexplored in dogs and cats but appears to be important in humans.

There are numerous drugs—and the list is always growing for humans—that may be effective in the treatment of cognitive decline. However, there is only one drug, selegiline, that is approved for canine cognitive dysfunction in the USA. All other use is extra-label, and for some of the medications, canine and feline dosages have not been investigated. Treatment with any cognitive enhancer is likely to be lifelong. Because most of these medications are metabolized through renal and hepatic cycles, pre- and postmedication biochemical evaluation is warranted.

In addition to medications, cognitive enrichment and a prescription diet (Hill's b/d®) have been shown to improve learning and reduce signs of cognitive dysfunction in aged dogs. In the UK, a dietary supplement is available that diminishes signs of cognitive dysfunction. The earlier behavioral, pharmacologic, and dietary intervention are accomplished, the more likely that the dog or cat will improve. However, at present the course of this condition can only be slowed, not aborted.

Compulsive licking has the following necessary condition: licking in excess of that required for standard grooming or exploration. The following condition is sufficient: licking in excess of that required for grooming or exploration that represents a change in the animal's typical behavior and interferes with other activities or functions (eg, eating, drinking, playing, interacting with people) and cannot easily be interrupted. The sufficient condition describes the characteristic manifestations of all obsessive-compulsive disorders (OCD): repetitive, out-of-context behaviors that are not interrupted by conventional stimuli (social or gustatory) for more than a short period, and that consistently interfere with the animal's ability to engage in what were formerly normal behaviors for that age and species. This form of licking can be directed at self (grooming) or toward floors, shiny objects, etc (exploratory). More extreme behaviors are associated with compulsive licking than with excessive licking, which may be just a subset of OCD (*see* below). It is not clear if the forms of the OCD are indicative of varying neuroanatomic or neurophysiologic pathogeneses. It is also possible that compulsive licking and excessive licking are merely 2 recognizable points on a continuum. Diagnosis of OCD is usually made only when the condition is fully developed—early stages are understudied. Compulsive and excessive licking are also seen in cats.

Fearful behavior or fear has the following necessary and sufficient condition: behavior that occurs concomitant with behavioral and physiologic signs such as withdrawal, passive, and avoidance behaviors associated with the sympathetic nervous system, with the absence of any aggression. Fear and anxiety have signs that overlap. Some nonspecific signs, eg, avoidance, shaking, and trembling, can be characteristic of both. The physiologic signs probably differ at some level, and the neurochemistry of each also probably differs. Cats also exhibit fearful behavior.

Generalized anxiety has the following necessary conditions: consistent display of autonomic hyperreactivity, increased motor activity, and increased vigilance and scanning that interferes with a normal range of social interaction. The following condition is sufficient: as above in the absolute absence of any provocative stimuli. This diagnosis is specific and could easily be incorrectly made based on an incomplete history or lack of critical thought. Generalized anxiety should be a diagnosis of last resort, and all of the signs should be concomitantly present under conditions in which any of these signs would have subsided in a normal or asymptomatic animal. Cats also exhibit generalized anxiety.

Hyperactivity has the following necessary condition: motor activity in excess of that warranted by the animal's age and stimulation level that occurs in a consistent, often stereotypical, manner and does not respond to correction, redirection, or restraint. The following condition is sufficient: as above along with sympathetic signs (eg, increased heart rate, increased respiratory rate, vasodilation), even when at rest, in the absence of other signs or significant laboratory data associated with thyroid disease; these dogs respond to treatment with amphetamine or methylphenidate with a paradoxical decrease in motor activity. Most dogs that owners perceive as hyperactive (a diagnosis that does *not* depend on the dog's exercise level compared with its needs) are actually overactive (a diagnosis that *does* depend on the dog's exercise level compared with its needs [*see* below]). True hyperactivity is a specific diagnosis for which specific behavioral signs have been poorly elucidated and is a rare condition.

Inappropriate play behavior has the following necessary and sufficient conditions: play behaviors (eg, play bows, yips, shoulder blocks in dogs; swatting, pouncing, biting in cats) that occur in circumstances that are out-of-context. Such conditions include circumstances in which the behaviors are directed toward inanimate objects, social circumstances in which play is not relevant (challenge), or behaviors that occur in contexts consistent with the solicitation of play but that involve actions that would discourage play (eg, biting, pain).

Neophobia has the following necessary and sufficient condition: consistent, sustained, sudden, profound nongraded response to unfamiliar objects and circumstances manifest as intense active avoidance, escape, or anxiety behaviors associated with the activities of the sympathetic nervous system. Behaviors can include immobility or extremely high activity, along with decreased sensitivity to pain or social stimuli; repeated exposure results in an invariant pattern of response. The stage at which a fear becomes a phobia is unknown but epistemologically important. Deleting patterns related to the development of fears and phobias involves evaluation of the frequency, intensity, and characterization of actual behaviors. Risks for the development of related behaviors are unknown for animals already exhibiting fear or anxiety. A phobic response is difficult to miss but, because of that, is doubtless more complex than is commonly appreciated. This condition may be augmented by extreme deprivation during the relevant sensitive periods (3-20 wk of age in dogs; 2-12 wk of age in cats). Regardless, there is likely to be a strong genetic component. Neophobia is also seen in cats.

Noise phobia has the following necessary and sufficient condition: sudden and profound, nongraded, extreme response to noise manifest as intense active avoidance, escape, or anxiety behaviors associated with the activities of the sympathetic nervous system. The same responses can occur in an animal exposed to any aspect of thunderstorms (eg, noise, dark, changes in barometric pressure or ozone levels). Behaviors, patterns related to the development of fears and phobias, and risks for development are discussed under neophobia (*see* above).

Obsessive-compulsive disorders have the following necessary condition: repetitive, stereotypic motor, locomotory, grooming, ingestive, or hallucinogenic behaviors that occur out-of-context to their normal occurrence, or in a frequency or duration in excess of that required to accomplish the ostensible goal. The following condition is sufficient: as above, in a manner that interferes with the dog's ability to otherwise normally function in its social environment. Although it can be debated whether animals can obsess, it appears that they perceive and experience concern; therefore, it is likely that they can obsess. A separate issue is that of relative intensity, ie, whether a behavior is excessive, or whether a manifestation of an OCD may be a determination of degree. Careful description and recording of behaviors and their durations could provide data that would permit evaluation of the extent to which such behaviors may lie on a continuum. Good histories and observation are important because in some peculiar forms, OCD could resemble seizure-like activity. By definition, some epileptic or seizure-like activity is stereotypic, which is one reason why this explicit and specific diagnosis category is preferable to that of stereotypic behavior. Cats also exhibit OCD. In both cats and dogs, OCD runs in families and, therefore, breed lines. In dogs, the form of OCD exhibited appears to be affected by the jobs/tasks for which the breed was selected (eg, herding breeds often chase their tails).

Overactivity has the following necessary condition: motor activity that is in excess of that exhibited when the animal experiences a regular exercise and interaction schedule. The following condition is sufficient: as above, in the absence of any signs of organic disease or true hyperactivity, and that resolves with increased aerobic activity. The diagnosis of overactivity is contingent on context that includes the age, breed, and social and physical environment of the dog, as well as the owner's perception. It is more often a management-related concern than an abnormality. It must be distinguished from attention-seeking behavior and hyperactivity (*see* above). Overactivity is also seen in cats, in which hyperthyroidism may be the cause.

Pseudocyesis (false pregnancy) has the following necessary condition: maternal behavior exhibited in the absence of pregnancy. The following condition is sufficient: maternal or nesting behaviors exhibited in the absence of pregnancy that develop within 60 days of estrus. Neutering (spaying) the animal after pseudocyesis prevents further occurrences that would otherwise be likely. There may be a greater risk of mammary neoplasia in animals who repetitively experience pseudocyesis.

Roaming has the following necessary and sufficient condition: locomotory activity involving extended absences and greater distances than those needed for the animal to relieve itself. Trajectory of movement may be determined by the presence and estrous cycles of other animals, or by behaviors related to patrol. Roaming is almost always a variant of normal behavior. It is of concern because it can pose a risk to the pet's health and safety. Owners that allow pets to roam may also be in violation of leash or animal control laws. Cats also roam.

Separation anxiety has the following necessary condition: physical or behavioral signs of distress exhibited by the animal only in the absence of or lack of access to the owner. The following condition is sufficient: consistent, intensive destruction, elimination, vocalization, or salivation exhibited only in the virtual or actual absence of the owner (eg, when denied access through a door or when left alone). Behaviors are often most severe within the first 15-20 min of separation, and many anxiety-related behaviors (autonomic hyperreactivity, increased motor activity, and increased vigilance and scanning) may become apparent as the owner prepares to leave. It is important to rule out other situations that could be associated with the common signs of separation anxiety (eg, incomplete housetraining, teething, play, and a response to a truly scary, unique event (such as a robbery).

The extent to which animals with separation anxiety have other anxious behaviors or experience self-mutilation, phobias, or fears is unknown. There is now a well-established comorbid association between separation anxiety and noise and thunderstorm phobias, so any dog exhibiting signs of one condition should be screened for the others. Both sets of conditions should be treated, although treatment schedules and drugs of choice will differ (eg, noise/thunderstorm phobias require that benzodiazepines, preferably alprazolam, be given as needed, and separation anxiety should be treated with tricyclic antidepressants or selective serotonin reuptake inhibitors daily. Contrary to common myth, studies have disproved that this condition is more common in animals that have very attentive owners than in animals with less attentive owners. Regardless, there is a population of dogs with separation anxiety that are hyperattached and must be in sight or touch of their family at all times. This severe variant requires intensive treatment, including extensive behavior modification to teach the dog (and possibly the client) to be less dependent.

Treatment of other Canine Behavioral Problems: Most behavior modification focuses on desensitization and counterconditioning. This is most important in the early treatment of fears, phobias, and anxieties. The earlier the treatment is started, the better the prognosis. Early intervention with antianxiety medication may be preferred for most anxieties, OCD, and phobias (TABLE 2). Noise phobias often respond to diazepam, chlorazepate, or alprazolam (the drug of choice for many of these patients) if administered 1-2 hr before the onset of the expected stimulus. Treatment can then be repeated just before or at the onset of the event and every 4-6 hr as needed. Longterm or maintenance treatment for comorbid anxiety should be instituted using a specific serotonin reuptake inhibitor (eg, fluoxetine, sertraline) or a newer tricyclic antidepressant (eg, clomipramine). Recurrence rates are high, especially if medication is prematurely withdrawn. Pharmacologic treatment will need to be given for at least 4-6 mo and may be lifelong. Because these medications have relatively few side effects, longterm treatment is not problematic if the client complies with recommendations for routine evaluation (eg, physical exam, urinalysis, CBC, serum biochemistry panel, and possibly ECG). In the USA, none of these medications is directly approved for treating behavioral problems in pets aside from clomipramine for separation anxiety in dogs and selegiline for cognitive dysfunction in dogs. In all cases, results are best when medication is combined with a behavioral modification program.

CATS

SOCIAL BEHAVIOR

It is a common myth that cats are asocial. Cats are social, but their social system differs from that of dogs. Cats have neither been exposed to the same extent or direction of artificial selection that dogs have, nor have they been developed in a breed-specific sense to execute specific tasks.

The basic feline social unit is the queen and her kittens. Weaning occurs between 5 and 8 wk, although given the chance, some kittens will occasionally suckle much later. This is probably related more to social behavior than to nutrition. Under free-ranging situations, kittens will remain either with the queen or as part of her extended social group for the first 12-18 mo of life. Male kittens more commonly leave the group before social maturity (2-4 yr) than do females, although all combinations of groupings have been reported for cats. Multiple generations of related females can be found in free-ranging situations, and they may provide some degree of communal care for the young.

Density of free-ranging domestic cats appears directly dependent on food resources. Most domestic cats are solitary hunters. Prey species include those considered by humans to be vermin, which may explain why cats are found worldwide. The small body size of the cat may be another reason that cats have been allowed to coexist with people in the absence of much artificial selection for specific behaviors. Kittens will learn to prefer and to best hunt the prey species that their mother preferentially hunted. Pet cats learn to prefer a certain texture of food.

While sexual maturity is early (6 mo of age), breeding may be inhibited in larger social groups, either directly through male interference with copulation or indirectly by a social hierarchy. Cats are induced ovulators, and high-ranking adult males entering and taking over a group have occasionally been reported to kill nursing young. Such infanticide stimulates ovulation through hormonal effects, and it has been reported that this is a mechanism for guaranteeing the tom's paternity of and genetic investment in the new offspring. This model has been fully developed only for African lions.

Paternity appears to be an important determinant of personality in cats. Toms that are adventurous, outgoing, and friendly appear to produce kittens of similar personality. There appear to be genetically "unfriendly," "timid," or "shy" cats for which no amount of handling can make a difference; the genetic mechanism for this is poorly understood. The role of early experience and exposure for kittens cannot be overemphasized. Kittens between 2 and 7 wk of age that are handled by people are friendlier toward people and more outgoing and may have fewer problems with some forms of aggression, although the latter is poorly quantified. The effect of early handling can augment the paternal effect toward a willingness to explore. Between 12 and 14 wk of age, kittens switch from social play to social fighting and a more predatory play. Early weaning will hasten this change. Kittens that experience extremely restricted nutrition in utero never behave normally. The exact neuroanatomic basis of these changes has not been fully elucidated.

Ancestrally, cats have used open, well-drained, substrates (eg, sand) for elimination. This may reflect their northern African origins. Cats may scratch before, after, or not at all when eliminating, and they may or may not dig to cover their urine or feces. All of these elimination behaviors are variants of normal. Spraying (placement of urine on a vertical surface through projection of a diffuse urine stream that is usually accompanied by elevation and quivering of the tail and possibly treading of the feet) can be a normal elimination behavior in cats; it is a common form of feline marking behavior (as can be the deposition of fecal mounds). Urine marking, roaming, and fighting with other cats are all affected by hormones, and neutering (particularly castration) appears to reduce or prevent their occurrence. Cats are markedly influenced by the role of scent in their environment and mark with urine, feces, and sebaceous secretions. The most common feline behavioral problems are, accordingly, associated with elimination, and anxiety may play a role in their development. The second most common feline behavioral problems involve aggression. Much aggression in cats is subtle and passive, so its real frequency may be seriously underestimated.

BEHAVIORAL PROBLEMS

Many behavioral problems in cats also occur in dogs, including those dealing with some types of aggression and elimination behaviors. For discussion of these behaviors, see BEHAVIORAL PROBLEMS OF DOGS, p 1314. Additional behavioral problems in cats are discussed below.

Behavioral Problems Associated with Feline Aggression

Aggression due to lack of early experience has the following necessary condition: consistently displayed, abnormal, out-of-context threats, contest, or attack demonstrated by cats toward people in any circumstances in which people approach or attempt to care for the cat. The following condition is sufficient: as above, and exhibited in cats known to be unexposed to people until at least 14 wk old. Experimental evidence indicates that early exposure to people is essential for cats if they are not to avoid people; however, confounding factors include the genetic effects of less versus more friendly cats and early traumatic and potentially fear-provoking circumstances. This diagnosis should be used only for cats that have an entire range of abnormal social responses, even given later extensive exposure to people. These cats can behave normally with other cats but always seem to view people warily. Although they can learn to interact with some people relatively normally, these responses do not tend to generalize to other people.

Status-related aggression has the following necessary condition: abnormal, inappropriate, out-of-context aggression (threat, challenge, or attack) consistently exhibited by cats toward people under any circumstance involving passive or active control of the cat's behavior or the cat's access to the behavior. The following condition is sufficient: intensification of any aggressive response from the cat upon any passive or active correction or interruption of the cat's behavior or the cat's access to the behavior. This is a discrete definition of what has been called the "leave-me-alone bite." It is truly the analog (not homolog—canine and feline social systems are not homologous) of the canine condition and is defined in terms that are relevant to feline social systems. Unlike the analogous situation in dogs, this diagnosis in cats is not often comorbid with other aggressions associated with resources such as food (food-related aggression), toys (possessive aggression), or space (territorial aggression). The keys are control and access—most of the problems with diagnoses arise from our misunderstanding of feline social systems, feline signaling, and feline anxieties.

Treatment of Behavioral Problems Associated with Feline Aggression: Treatment of feline aggression is similar in principle and practice to that of canine aggression (p 1314). Cats, too, will work for food rewards in counterconditioning programs. Avoidance (physical, visual, and preferably, olfactory separation of cats who are fighting) is paramount, and early intervention is best. Cats will share time and space and can be encouraged to do so sequentially as part of a comprehensive behavior modification program.

Because feline aggression can be covert, clients and veterinarians may underappreciate the importance of unwitnessed threats that may occur multiple times a day. The cat behaving most appropriately should have free access to the home while the aggressor is humanely confined to a less desirable, protected area and provided with water, food, and litter. If this is not possible, access can be rotated between cats. All cats should still have regular individual interaction with clients. Treatment with tricyclic antidepressants and some newer anxiolytic medications can help tremendously, but concerns regarding extra-label drug use must be communicated to clients (TABLE 3).

Behavioral Problems Associated with Feline Elimination

Elimination aversion for substrate or location has the following necessary condition: consistent avoidance of locations or substrates formerly used for elimination. The following condition is sufficient: consistent avoidance of locations or substrates formerly used for elimination, accompanied by behaviors that are concurrent with active or passive avoidance or distaste that is amplified if the cat is forced to eliminate in the area or on the substrate that the cat finds aversive.

Location preference has the following necessary and sufficient conditions: consistent elimination in an area or a few areas that are restricted to one location and are not linked by some common sensory aspect.

Spraying has the following necessary condition: elimination of urine through species-specific postures, including vertical stance, elevation and quivering of the tail, and treading of the feet, that propel urine against a vertical surface if one is available. The following condition is sufficient: the detection of urine at a height that is equal to that of the cat; dripping could contribute to a secondary puddle on a lower, horizontal surface. Spraying can be a variant of normal feline elimination behaviors and can be performed by both males and females. Cats also spray when they are distressed or anxious.

Substrate preference has the following necessary and sufficient conditions: consistent elimination on a particular surface or substrate (eg, carpet, ceramic tile). The behavior may occur in a single or multiple locations.

Treatment of Behavioral Problems Associated with Feline Elimination: Treatments for feline elimination disorders include addressing any underlying anxieties and their associated active or passive aggressions, observing meticulous litter hygiene, and determining what combination of litter, box, and location is preferred by the cat. The first involves making a competent diagnosis; appropriate social intervention and manipulation (eg, separating the cats); and potentially the use of synthetic pheromones or tricyclic antidepressants, benzodiazepines, or some of the newer selective serotonin reuptake inhibitors (*see* TABLE 3). The second involves regular daily cleaning/sifting of the litter, weekly changing and washing of the litter box, and the use of good odor eliminators after cleaning soiled areas with copious amounts of water and mild soaps. The third involves use of litter substrates that more closely resemble the ancestral substrate (sands, clumpable litters) and alteration of the overall litter environment (changing box shape, size, number, location and type [eg, covered vs open]).

Other Feline Behavioral Problems

Hyperesthesia has the following necessary condition: tactile response in excess of that warranted by external stimuli. The following condition is sufficient: repetitive, uninterruptable tactile response in excess of that warranted by external stimuli, or that may occur in the absence of external stimuli and may be accompanied by locomotor activity and vocalization. Most of the diagnoses pertaining to this condition originate in the dermatologic literature and are purely descriptive of the behaviors (eg, twitchy cat syndrome). It is likely that in the extreme case, this is a subset of OCD, but there is also a considerable range in both normal and abnormal tactile responses.

The most common feline **stereotypic behaviors** are normal ones—stalking, chasing imaginary individuals, grooming, etc. When these occur out of context or in a frequency or duration in excess of that needed to accomplish an actual task, a diagnosis of OCD must be considered. The most common feline OCD involves self-mutilation, excessive grooming, and/or self-directed aggression. These signs, together, have carelessly been called feline hyperesthesia syndrome. Sucking, chewing, and/or ingestion of fabrics or plastic are forms of pica—the ingestion of non-nutritive substances—and involve OCD. Oriental breeds seem to exhibit pica more frequently than other cats. It has been noted that cats that chew do not suck, cats that suck do not ingest, and so forth, suggesting that each of these forms of pica may be different types of OCD neurochemically. Unlike dogs, most cats begin to exhibit OCD following stressors such as a change in feline or human relationships. With pica, there also appears to be a strong familial component, indicating that the genetic potential for the behavior may require provocation from the social environment before the OCD is fully developed. Fortunately, like dogs, cats respond to medications that augment the amount of brain serotonin and that affect neurochemical receptor development through stimulation of 5-HT(1A) receptors.

HUMAN-ANIMAL BOND

Companion animals are now considered to be family members, no longer the outdoor dogs and cats on farms that were typical for many families a few decades ago. The human-animal bond has become a household term, reflecting the entry of dogs, cats, and other pets into our everyday lives. Cats are sharply increasing in popularity and numbers, including households with multiple cats, leading to the emergence of veterinary practices serving only cats. Yet a strong majority of Americans (73%) feel that dogs rather than cats are the better pet, as reported in a 2001 Gallup Poll. A 2002 AVMA study of household pets reported that dogs received 1.9 veterinary visits per animal in 2001, as compared with 1.0 visits per cat. Dogs had a total of 117 million veterinary visits, contrasting with 71 million for cats, but revealing the economic significance of both.

In addition to the growing awareness of the human-animal bond, the roles of animals have expanded into new applications. At the same time, the public is focused on ensuring that animals receive adequate consideration and care. Albert Schweitzer's concept of "reverence for life" has become a standard for decision-making concerning animals. Acknowledgment of the human-animal bond is fast becoming a cornerstone of veterinary practice.

VETERINARY FAMILY PRACTICE, OR BOND-CENTERED PRACTICE

The primacy of pets in clients' lives today resembles their importance in the lives of veterinarians who entered the profession due to their involvement with animals. Clients become deeply attached to and care about the health and well-being of their companions. Their expectations for veterinary care are becoming more similar to that ideally provided in human medicine—clients anticipate superb care for both the animal and themselves. As high-tech medicine expands within veterinary specialties, a more sophisticated level of family support is required and expected by many clients. The current elevated importance of animals, often regarded as part of the family, revolutionizes the nature of veterinary practice to include the entire family. Because veterinarians now deal with the family plus the animal, and no longer just treat the animal, the style and emphasis of companion animal practices have shifted, as reflected in the terms "veterinary family practice" or "bond-centered practice."

Such practices build lifelong relationships with families and their animals. A new animal brought into the family is the occasion to discuss the animal's life cycle with the family and provide an overview that can optimize the likelihood of a positive relationship with few behavioral problems. Emotional needs of the family are addressed along with the medical needs of the animal. Upper-socioeconomic clients are especially likely to view their pets as companions. Many clients with companion animals are families with young children. The animals are acknowledged to play a central and formative role in children's lives. Some studies have reported that pet-owning pre-adolescents score higher on measures of self-esteem and autonomy. Practitioners may consider giving special thought to incorporating children into their communications with the family, making it easy for families with children to be comfortable during consultation (eg, provision of play areas and planning for children to be present in or visibly near the examination room). Hospitals providing extended diagnoses and treatments to animals sometimes find entire families coming in to offer support to the animal, perhaps spending hours to be on hand when the animal is available; these hospitals may want to plan accommodation near at hand for such families.

Providing areas for relaxation, softer light in public areas, and comfortable seating in exam rooms without barriers from the medical staff are some features that improve customer satisfaction. Impeccable cleanliness also matters. In veterinary practices with these values, everyone understands that every medical intervention carries emotional consequences and that medical competence and providing emotional support go hand-in-hand. Various resources provide models for veterinary staffs based on skilled communication.

The key role of communication was revealed in a study of the medical profession showing that physicians who had never been sued laughed more with their patients, asked them more questions, and spent 3 min longer on average with patients than their colleagues who had been sued. A recent study of successful veterinarians reported that nontechnical competencies were essential, including interpersonal relationship-building skills. Using such skills, veterinarians and their staffs facilitate clients' understanding of medical situations and preventive medicine. They can encourage clients to attend puppy socialization classes to improve retention of dogs, assist in behavioral assessments, and prepare clients for providing palliative care or dealing with end-of-life issues. Client adherence is generally lower than believed by veterinarians, but followup communication improves the level of adherence.

Despite optimal communication skills, research has shown that veterinarians inevitably encounter clients who are inattentive, neglectful, over-involved, or cost-focused, and patients who are uncontrolled, dangerous, or dirty, adding to medical and emotional problems. Almost all veterinarians feel they were not prepared by their education and training for dealing with such nonmedical issues. Making plans in advance, with specific protocols for interventions, can prepare the veterinary staff with strategies for these occasions.

HEALTH BENEFITS OF PETS FOR PEOPLE

The companionship of pets relaxes and entertains people. In coming to know their clients, veterinarians can assess the importance of the pet to a family and the extent to which the family members benefit from the potential psychosocial effects of living with an animal. During stressful periods in people's lives, many studies have reported that pets offer meaningful comfort that is protective against depression and loneliness. Elderly women living alone score more favorably on measures of mental health; even college-aged women report less loneliness if living with companion animals rather than alone. Similar comforting effects of animal companions, whether cats or dogs, in warding off depression were reported for patients with Alzheimer's disease who had a companion animal and were cared for at home and for men with AIDS whose social lives were shrinking. Elderly people experiencing typical life stresses are less affected (as measured by number of medical visits) when they have a companion dog, suggesting that a dog can be a stress buffer that softens the effects of adverse events on the person. The interactive caregiving exchanged with the animal allows the person to nurture and feel needed, while also feeling nurtured. The animal's constancy bolsters courage during setbacks, as the animal's affection is unaffected by factors such as the person's physical capabilities or mood.

Companion animals also facilitate social interactions with other people and positive social involvement. The socializing effects of dogs have been documented in public settings and also among people with a variety of disabilities. A companion animal provides a person who has few friends with an ally in making new human acquaintances, while also creating a richer family environment with enhanced companionship. Even one person with an animal lives in a family unit, and has someone who offers a greeting or recognition when the person comes home.

The motivating role of animals is a further antidote to depression. Many people are inspired to walk their dogs, volunteer to take animals into nursing homes for visits, or just actively nurture an animal, whereas without the animal they would be less involved and engaged in living or even depressed. Walking the dog and being outdoors where other social contact arises are two healthful effects of living with a canine companion.

The daily comfort, socialization, and motivation offered by an animal also are associated with cardiovascular benefits. Blood pressure decreases transiently when a person relaxes with, talks to, or just watches an animal. When patients with elevated blood pressure were given medication, and random assignment of pets was made to some patients, those with pets performed better on stressful tasks but did not differ in blood pressure scores, indicating a lower response to stress among pet owners. Several studies show longterm health correlates with animal companionship, although the animals were not randomly assigned to the people, but rather were chosen by them or their families. Cardiovascular measures were better among pet owners than nonowners in a large Australian study. Two studies reported that pet ownership was related to decreased mortality. Recently, survival for 1 yr following heart attack was found to be more likely among people with companion dogs and human social support.

ANIMAL-ASSISTED THERAPY AND ACTIVITIES

The field called animal-assisted therapy originated when the lay public began to take animals into nursing homes and other facilities to share them with residents. This practice has become more formalized. Unless medically supervised, these programs are now termed "animal-assisted activities," whereas those directed as part of medical treatment are termed "animal-assisted therapy." Procedures for screening animals and providing training for the people involved are offered and have been standardized by the Delta Society. However, these are neither legislatively required as part of a certification process, nor is there a conventional educational process for individuals wanting to work in this area. Some individuals within human health professions, such as clinical psychology, social work, occupational therapy, physical therapy, or nursing, have incorporated animal-assisted activities and therapy into their professional practice. Animal-assisted activities and therapy can be observed in some mental health settings where they are a part of treatment.

A much larger number of people continue to volunteer to bring their animals into facilities, often with some screening process and training organized by local groups. Such groups often benefit from veterinary assistance and leadership in developing appropriate screening methods for selection and preparation of both animals and people participating in these programs.

If periodic exposure to an animal via animal-assisted activities or animal-assisted therapy is healthful for someone with special needs, constant exposure may offer even greater benefits. Service dogs provide an example of a full-time animal therapist for the person. An emerging role of service dogs is as psychiatric service dogs, assisting persons with mental illness such as schizophrenia, bipolar disorder, agoraphobia, or anxiety. Like all service dogs, these dogs are trained to perform specific tasks, such as employing tactile stimulation to facilitate recovery from episodes and creating a safe personal space for the owner. It has also been suggested that the relationship between the dog and owner is intrinsically therapeutic.

SERVICE AND OTHER WORKING DOGS

Dogs have been trained to perform specific tasks in partnership with people. Some assist people with disabilities. Others assist in law enforcement, agricultural or bomb sniffing, search and rescue, or war tasks. Significant investments of money and time are required for the specialized training and development of working partnerships with these dogs. As they forge working partnerships with their dogs, the handlers inevitably become emotionally bonded. Details of these working relationships vary. Service dogs, after having several handlers in their early lives, typically spend all their waking hours with a single handler. Some working dogs may be kenneled in a facility when not working, whereas many police dogs live with the families of their handlers.

While every situation involving working dogs is somewhat unique, the dogs are extremely precious and valuable to the handlers. When a medical crisis arises with such a dog, the veterinarian will often be the closest professional at hand and may need to provide support to the handler as well as the animal. Treatments that adversely affect performance, especially for an extended period of time, disrupt functioning. If the client has a disability, special accommodation may be required for communicating with and providing instructions to the client. Attentive listening and respect, while essential for all clients, assumes particular importance in these relationships.

ANIMAL WELFARE

Reducing or preventing the incidence of animal pain or distress and promoting animal well-being (and even pleasure) are overall goals of animal welfare. These goals pertain to animals on farms or in laboratories as well as companion animals. Aversive handling, even if infrequent, has stressful consequences for pigs and other farm animals, with resulting adverse effects on reproduction and development. Aversive handling has similar effects on animals in other settings. Veterinarians are often the first contacts when someone seeks help for animals being badly treated or receiving inadequate care.

Intentional, deliberate abuse of animals is an extreme marker of a likely pattern of abuse elsewhere within a family. Veterinarians who report suspected animal abuse sometimes can avert similar abuse of other vulnerable family members, especially children or the elderly. Two studies reported that >90% of veterinarians would report cases of suspected animal abuse to authorities. A majority agreed that animal abuse in families would tend to be linked with child or elder abuse.

Although sometimes seen by veterinarians, abuse appears less common than the neglect, poor husbandry, or lack of essential medical care of animals, some of which may be inadvertent. A more serious problem occurs with animal hoarders who may be mentally ill. Some communities routinely combine efforts of animal control and mental health agencies when dealing with such cases. The person, perhaps without awareness, acquires more animals than they can care for properly.

A major, widespread societal problem of animal welfare is the abandoning and killing of companion animals. While the incidence of animal relinquishment has decreased somewhat, the problem is still widespread. Behavioral problems of animals and owners' lack of knowledge increase the likelihood of relinquishment. Veterinary teams can provide leadership and education about more realistic expectations of companion animals, and can encourage earlier intervention if problems arise.

EUTHANASIA, PET LOSS, AND GRIEF FOR CLIENTS AND VETERINARIANS

As in any intimate relationship, when an animal companion dies or is ill, people are likely to feel stress, sorrow, and grief. This may include the animal's family and neighbors in the community, as well as the veterinary team that has provided care. The significance of pets dying and the consequent emotional impact on clients is now clearly profiled within the veterinary profession, with educational materials and support groups, hotlines, and counseling available. The relatively short lifespan of dogs and cats means that clients face losing several animals during a lifetime. Most veterinarians themselves have painful memories of losing a particular animal and understand only too well the pain their clients feel. (*See also* EUTHANASIA, p 1379.)

An extra burden comes in assuming responsibility for the moment of death by euthanasia. The philosophical dilemma is the same as that posed by human euthanasia. One must weigh the value of mercy or the Golden Rule to relieve pain and suffering with the wrongness of killing or a religious argument for reverence for life. The difficulty of this decision overlays the loss with feelings of overwhelming guilt and the thought that there must have been some other step that could have been taken. Even with family support, these feelings are not assuaged. Among married couples in one study, about half of the wives and more than a quarter of husbands reported they were quite or extremely disturbed by the death of the family pet.

As an alternative to euthanasia, it is important to offer instruction in providing palliative care for clients who are prepared to offer it. Procedures developed in hospice care can assure high quality, end-of-life care. As in human medicine, families can combine good medical care with pain relief for the animal. The technical aspects of treatment no longer override the compassionate care, as a specific approach is offered for dealing with the family's and animal's distress.

Notwithstanding the anguish that veterinary clients experience, the process of animals dying, especially the act of performing euthanasia, poses a time-consuming and emotionally wearing duty for veterinarians, accounting for 2-4% of encounters. In a recent study, almost all veterinarians felt they were untrained in making explanations to clients at such times. Almost half had regretted a euthanasia, and a majority of private practice veterinarians had felt guilty after performing a euthanasia. After euthanizing their own pets, a majority felt depressed and 30% felt guilty. All of these figures were elevated among women veterinarians, suggesting that their impact may have risen in the intervening years with the gender shift of the profession.

Compassionate veterinarians include themselves in the circle of remembrance of their clients' animals and respect the families' regard for the animal throughout the relationship. A veterinarian can assume that many grieving clients will need a year of recovery to pass through the holidays and family traditions before somewhat accepting a loss and may consider sending a remembrance card to the family after 1 yr.

■ ■ ■

CLINICAL PATHOLOGY AND PROCEDURES

COLLECTION AND SUBMISSION OF LABORATORY SAMPLES

Each veterinary diagnostic laboratory offers a unique set of diagnostic tests that is subject to frequent changes as better tests become available. The protocols for sample collection and submission are also subject to change. The practitioner and diagnostic laboratory staff must maintain good communication in order to complete their diagnostic efforts efficiently and provide optimal service to the animal owner. Practitioners must be specific and clear in their test requests. The laboratory staff can provide guidance when there are questions regarding sample collection and handling, as well as offering assistance in interpretation of test results. Most diagnostic laboratories publish user guidelines with preferred protocols for sample collection and submission, but the following broad recommendations are fairly standard.

Regardless of the type of submission, a detailed case history should be included with the samples to assist laboratory personnel in determining a diagnosis. The information should include: owner, species, breed, sex, age, animal identification, clinical signs, gross appearance (including size and location) of the lesion(s), previous treatment (if any), time of recurrence from any previous treatment, and morbidity/mortality in the group. If a zoonotic disease is suspected, this should also be clearly indicated on the submission sheet to alert lab personnel. The submission form should be placed in a waterproof bag to protect it from any fluids that might be present in the packaged materials. Waterproof markers should be used when labeling specimen bags and containers.

Histology: Microscopic examination of adequately prepared tissue sections is a valuable aid to diagnosis. Cellular changes in diseased tissues are often characteristic of a specific disease or group of diseases. Use of this relatively rapid and inexpensive diagnostic technique can often result in substantial savings in time, money, and animal life. The increasing number of immunohistochemical tests that can be applied to formalin-fixed tissue has further reinforced the utility of this diagnostic technique.

Autolyzed tissues are generally useless for histopathologic examination; prompt necropsy examination and organ sampling are critical. Tissues collected for histologic examination should be representative of any lesions present and, if possible, should include some of the apparently normal surrounding tissue. Tissue should not be frozen before fixation. Samples of the various organs should be cut <1 cm thick (preferably 7 mm) and placed immediately into ≥10 times their volume of phosphate-buffered 10% formalin for fixation. Thin slices or cubes ensure adequate penetration of the fixative. Because the GI mucosa decomposes rapidly, short sections of gut must be opened lengthwise to allow adequate fixation. The tissues should remain in fixative for ≥24 hr; after this initial fixation, the samples may be placed in a smaller volume of fresh formalin for shipment. Samples should be shipped in unbreakable containers and packed in a manner that prevents spillage during shipment. Fixed tissues should be protected from freezing.

If the animal exhibited CNS signs, the brain and portions of the spinal cord should be submitted. When the whole brain may be required, it should be placed in concentrated formalin (40% formaldehyde), to which water is added slowly and mixed until the brain sinks to just below the surface but not to the bottom. The brain should remain in this solution for ≥24 hr, after which it may be removed and placed in a solid container in 10% formalin and either mailed (suitably packed) or held until processing is desired. Often, the brain is halved longitudinally and one-half sent unfixed (fresh), properly refrigerated, for microbiologic tests.

Biopsy samples should be fixed in the same manner as necropsy tissues. Small tumors (<1 cm) should be cut in half, and larger tumors into small pieces or several representative samples.

Microbiology: Laboratory techniques and capabilities for microbiologic examination vary; available tests include bacteriologic culture, virus isolation, in-situ hybridization, PCR, fluorescent antibody tests, latex agglutination tests, and ELISA. Therefore, it is critical to obtain specific instructions from the diagnostic laboratory on sample collection and handling. Usually, unfixed specimens are submitted and should be collected aseptically, as soon as possible after death. If PCR testing is to be performed, it is particularly important to avoid cross-contamination between multiple animals in a submission; this applies to tissues, fluids, and even dissection instruments. Tissues for most microbiologic assays may be frozen before shipment, but freezing is undesirable if samples can be chilled and delivered directly to the laboratory in a short period. Adequate refrigerant should be provided so that samples will remain chilled until they reach the laboratory.

Toxicology: If a known toxin is suspected, a specific analysis should always be requested—laboratories cannot just "check for poisoning." A complete description of clinical and epidemiologic findings may help differentiate poisoning from infectious diseases that can simulate poisoning. Appropriate samples for many of the more common toxicities are listed in TABLE 1. If there is doubt about sample submission procedures, the laboratory should be contacted.

Tissues or fluids for chemical analysis should be as fresh as possible and kept in a refrigerator or preserved chemically; packing with ice is preferred. A polystyrene refrigerator box, metal can, or stout cardboard box may be used for shipment. Packing must withstand breakage if the ice melts. Samples can be preserved for 72 hr if packed in a styrofoam box with dry ice. Packages containing dry ice must be so labeled on the outside and suitably vented to prevent pressure buildup. Adequate refrigeration is of special importance when submitting clean body fluids (such as those obtained from an eye) and material for nitrate or nitrite analysis; these salts are rapidly metabolized by microorganisms.

The containers for packing and transporting specimens should be free of chemicals. Plastic containers, both bags and jars, are ideal; jars with metal screw caps should be avoided. Samples should be packed individually. Containers must be labeled with all information necessary to identify the sample and, if mailed, must conform to postal regulations.

If legal action is a possibility, all containers for shipment should be either sealed so that tampering can be detected or hand-carried to the laboratory and a receipt obtained. The chain of custody must be accurately documented.

If feed or water is suspected as the source of poisoning, samples of these and any descriptive feed tag should accompany the tissue samples. If at all possible, a representative composite sample of the feed should be submitted from the suspect lot or shipment. In some instances, if an adequate amount of involved feed is available, some of it may be fed to experimental animals in an effort to reproduce the signs and lesions seen in the field cases.

Hematology: Routine studies require anticoagulated whole blood and several blood smears. Blood smears should be prepared immediately after the sample has been collected to minimize cell deterioration. Anticoagulated blood should be kept refrigerated; blood smears should not. Ethylenediamine tetra-acetic acid (EDTA) is the anticoagulant of choice for a CBC because it best preserves the cellular components of the blood and prevents platelet aggregation. Blood for coagulation testing should be collected into a blue top tube, which contains sodium citrate. After mixing, the sample should be centrifuged for 5 min, and then plasma should be removed and transferred to a clean tube without anticoagulant. The plasma should be kept frozen until the time of analysis. Whole blood should not be frozen because this causes cell lysis and gross hemolysis, which interfere with testing.

Clinical Chemistry: Most clinical chemistry tests require serum, but an occasional test may require plasma. Anticoagulants present in plasma may interfere with tests; therefore, serum should always be submitted unless plasma is specifically requested. Because lipemia can interfere with a number of chemistry tests, dogs and cats should be fasted for 12 hr before samples are collected. For serum samples, the blood should be drawn into a red top tube or a separator tube. The sample should be held at room temperature for 20-30 min to allow complete clot formation and retraction. Incomplete clot formation may cause the serum to gel due to latent fibrin formation. The clot should be separated from the glass by gently running an applicator stick around the tube walls ("rimming"). The sample should then be centrifuged at high speed (~1,000 g; 2,200 rpm) for 10 min. Rough handling of the sample or incomplete separation of erythrocytes from serum may promote hemolysis, which can interfere with certain tests. If the sample has been collected into a serum separator tube, centrifugation will cause a layer of silicon gel to lodge between the packed cells and the serum. The gel layer should be inspected to ensure the integrity of the barrier, and recentrifugation is recommended if there is a visible crack in this layer. If a red top tube has been used, the serum should be removed and transferred to a clean tube. Serum should be refrigerated or frozen until analyzed.

Many commercial laboratories provide sample containers and mailers.

TABLE 1. Guidelines for Submitting Samples for Toxicologic Examination

Suspected Poison or Analysis	Specimen Required	Comments
Ammonia	Whole blood or serum Urine Rumen contents	Frozen Frozen Frozen (or may add 1-2 drops saturated $HgCl_3$)
Arsenic	Liver Kidney Urine Ingesta Feed	
Arsenical feed additives	Liver Kidney Sciatic nerve	Fixed in formalin
Carbon monoxide	Whole blood	
Chlorates	Stomach contents Urine Feed	Frozen, in airtight container
Chlorinated hydrocarbons	Cerebrum Ingesta Body fat Liver Kidney	Use only glass containers Avoid contamination Refrigerated or frozen
Cholinesterase	Serum Cerebrum	Frozen
Copper (and Ni, Fe, Co, Cr, and Tl)	Kidney Liver Serum Feed Whole blood Feces	
Cyanide	Forage Whole blood Liver	Rush to laboratory or ship promptly, frozen in airtight container
Dicumarol	Forage Liver	
Ethylene glycol	Serum Urine Kidneys	Fixed in formalin
Fluorides	Bone Water Forage Urine	Best to send affected bone(s)
Herbicides (many)	Treated weeds Urine Ingesta Liver or kidney	

TABLE I. (continued)

Suspected Poison or Analysis	Specimen Required	Comments
Lead (also Hg, Mo, Ni, and Tl)	Kidney Whole blood Liver Urine	Heparinized blood preferred
Mercury and molybdenum	Kidney Whole blood Liver Feed	See lead, above
Mycotoxins	Grain, forages Liver, kidney	Consult with laboratory personnel on specific tests
Monensin	Feed Rumen contents Heart Skeletal muscle	Fixed in formalin Fixed in formalin
Nitrate	Forage Water Body fluids (eg, aqueous humor)	Refrigerated
Organophosphates (and carbamates)	Feed Ingesta Urine	Also send urine, blood, and stomach contents from clinically normal animals
Oxalates	Fresh forage Kidney	Do not macerate; freeze Fixed in formalin
Phenols	Gastric or rumen contents	In airtight container
Polychlorinated (and polybrominated) biphenyls	Liver Feed	
Rumen pH	Ingesta	Frozen
Selenium	Whole blood Feed Liver Hair clippings	Heparinized
Sodium (NaCl)	Brain Serum CSF Feed	Other half fixed in formalin
Sodium fluoroacetate (1080)	Stomach contents Liver	Frozen
Strychnine	Liver Kidney Stomach contents	
Sulfates	Water Brain	See TDS, below Fixed in formalin

(continued)

TABLE I. Guidelines for Submitting Samples for Toxicologic Examination *(continued)*

Suspected Poison or Analysis	Specimen Required	Comments
TDS (total dissolved solids)	Water	
Triaryl-PO_4	Ingesta Feed	
Urea	Feed	*See* ammonia, above
Vitamin A (also D and E)	Liver Serum	Frozen
Warfarin (also other anticoagulants)	Whole blood Liver Feed Stomach contents	Heparin or EDTA Refrigerated
Zinc	Liver Kidney Serum	Use "trace minerals" tubes
Zinc phosphide	Liver Gastric contents	

Serology: Serology generally requires serum, but plasma is often satisfactory. Samples should be collected as described for clinical chemistry tests and should always be free of hemolysis. In some instances, paired samples may be required for an adequate diagnosis. The acute sample should be collected early in the course of the disease and frozen. The convalescent sample should be collected 10-14 days later, and both samples should be forwarded to the laboratory at the same time.

Cytology: Air-dried smears are usually acceptable. Rapid air drying of smears minimizes cell distortion, thereby enhancing diagnostic quality. However, depending on the method of staining used, some laboratories prefer alcohol-fixed smears. Samples can be obtained by fine-needle aspiration or by scraping. Imprints (touch preparations) of external lesions can also be used, although these tend to have a greater degree of contamination. Aspirated material should always be smeared before air drying. Smears of fluid can be prepared using a traditional blood smearing technique. Highly cellular fluids may be smeared directly; fluids of low cellularity should be centrifuged to concentrate the cells. Thick material or viscous fluid is more readily smeared using a squash technique in which a second glass slide is placed over the aspirated material and then slid rapidly and smoothly down the length of the lower slide. Blood or cytologic smears should never be mailed to the laboratory in the same package with formalin-fixed tissues because formalin vapors will produce artifacts in the specimen.

Fluid Analysis: Body cavity effusions should be analyzed. Fluid analysis usually includes determination of protein content and total cell count and cytologic examination. Other tests may be performed depending on the source (eg, synovial fluid) or appearance (eg, chylous fluid) of the effusion. A sample of effusion should be collected into an EDTA (purple top) tube for routine analysis. A second sample should be collected into a serum (red top) tube if any biochemical analyses (eg, triglyceride, cholesterol, lipase) are to be performed or if a bacterial culture is desired. Smears for cytologic examination should be prepared immediately after the sample has been collected to minimize cell deterioration and other in vitro artifacts.

DIAGNOSTIC PROCEDURES FOR THE PRIVATE PRACTICE LABORATORY

Numerous laboratory tests can be done in a private practice laboratory. Use of a commercial laboratory versus in-house testing should be evaluated to determine whether in-house testing is practical and economical. Because the availability of diagnostic laboratories and their reporting intervals may be problematic (eg, nights and holidays), performing some diagnostic screening tests in-house is often desirable. However, because the people performing these tests often have minimal technical training, quality control procedures must be rigorous. The time and care that must be devoted to quality control issues may preclude in-house testing in many practices. Errors may occur not only in testing procedures but also in sample collection and handling and in recording results.

Tests can be done using either manual or automated methods. Manual methods tend to be time consuming and are more subject to human error. Automated and semiautomated systems are available but are considerably more expensive. Factors to be considered include instrument and reagent costs (including materials for calibration and quality control), availability of personnel training, technical support, and instrument maintenance and service. Although service contracts can cost up to 10% of the purchase price of an instrument, they are often cost-effective due to the expense of instrument repair.

CLINICAL BIOCHEMISTRY

Clinical biochemistry refers to the analysis of the blood plasma (or serum) for a wide variety of substances—substrates, enzymes, hormones, etc—and their use in the diagnosis and monitoring of disease. Analysis of other body fluids (eg, urine, ascitic fluids, CSF, etc) is also included. One test is very seldom specific to one clinical condition, and basic checklists of factors affecting the most commonly-requested analytes are given below. Thus, rather than 6 tests that merely confirm or deny 6 possibilities, a well-chosen group of 6 tests can provide information pointing to a wide variety of different conditions by a process of pattern recognition. Biochemistry tests should be accompanied by full hematology, as evaluation of both together is essential for optimal recognition of many of the most characteristic disease patterns (see HEMATOLOGY, p 1353).

Basic Test Panel: Most veterinary laboratories offer a basic panel of tests, which represents a minimal investigation applicable to most general situations. For small animals, a typical panel includes total protein, albumin, globulin (calculated as the difference between the first 2 analytes), urea, creatinine, ALT, and alkaline phosphatase (ALP). In addition, a yellow color seen in the plasma should be considered an indication for measuring bilirubin. This panel may be modified as appropriate for other species, eg, glutamate dehydrogenase (GDH) and/or γ glutamyl transferase (γGT) are more appropriate "liver enzymes" for horses and farm animals, or it may be more appropriate to concentrate primarily on muscle enzymes (CK and AST) in athletic animals.

Total protein increases due to dehydration, chronic inflammation, and paraproteinemia. It decreases due to overhydration, severe congestive heart failure (with edema), protein-losing nephropathy, protein-losing enteropathy, hemorrhage, burns, dietary protein deficiency, malabsorption, and some viral conditions (especially in horses). **Albumin** increases due to dehydration. It decreases due to the same factors as total protein, plus liver failure. **Urea** increases due to excess dietary protein, poor quality dietary protein, carbohydrate deficiency, catabolic states, dehydration, congestive heart failure, renal failure, blocked urethra, and ruptured bladder. It decreases due to low dietary protein, gross sepsis, anabolic hormonal effects, liver failure, portosystemic shunts (congenital or acquired), and inborn errors of urea cycle metabolism. **Creatinine** increases due to renal dysfunction, blocked urethra, and ruptured bladder. It decreases due to sample deterioration. Patients with a high muscle mass have high-normal creatinine concentrations, while patients with a low muscle mass have low-normal creatinine concentrations.

ALT increases due to hepatocellular damage, muscle damage, and hyperthyroidism. **ALP** increases due to increased bone deposition, liver damage, hyperthyroidism, biliary tract disease, intestinal damage, Cushing's disease, corticosteroid administration, barbiturate administration, and generalized tissue damage (including neoplasia). **GDH** increases in hepatocellular damage, particularly hepatic necrosis in horses and ruminants. γ**GT** increases in longer-term liver damage; it is particularly useful in horses and ruminants. **CK**, the classic "muscle enzyme," increases markedly in rhabdomyolysis and aortic thromboembolism. Slight increases are reported in hypothyroidism. **AST** increases in both muscle and liver damage and is also reported to increase in hypothyroidism.

In general, plasma enzymes decrease due to sample deterioration. Uncommonly, atrophy or fibrosis of an organ may result in unusually low plasma activities of the relevant enzymes.

Additional Tests: Further tests may be added to the basic panel, according to the principal presenting signs, in order to create panels for polydipsic patients, collapsing patients, etc. These panels are structured so that the patterns of abnormalities typical of all the likely differential diagnoses applicable to the situation can be discerned. For example, a polydipsia panel may add calcium, glucose, and cholesterol. Calcium allows recognition of hyperparathyroidism and other causes of hypercalcemia (which causes polydipsia and renal insufficiency), glucose picks up diabetes mellitus and contributes to the pattern characteristic of Cushing's disease, and cholesterol also adds to the appreciation of the "Cushing's pattern." Renal failure is covered by the tests already contained in the basic panel. In contrast, a "collapsing animal" panel may add calcium and glucose to screen for hypocalcemia or hypoglycemia. Sodium and potassium are included to screen for Addison's disease or hypokalemia. Analytes that might be considered for incorporation in such expanded profiles are described below.

Sodium increases due to Conn's syndrome, restricted water intake, vomiting, and dehydration due to most causes. It decreases due to Addison's disease, loss of any high-sodium fluid such as some forms of renal disease, and insufficient sodium provision during IV fluid therapy. **Potassium** increases due to Addison's disease and severe renal failure (especially terminal cases). It decreases due to Conn's syndrome, chronic renal dysfunction, vomiting, diarrhea, and insufficient potassium provision during intravenous fluid therapy. Congenital hypokalemia occurs in Burmese cats. **Chloride** increases in acidosis, and in parallel with increases in sodium concentration. It decreases in alkalosis, vomiting (especially after eating), and in association with hyponatremia. **Total CO$_2$ (bicarbonate)** increases in metabolic alkalosis and decreases in metabolic acidosis. It is less useful in assessing respiratory acid/base disturbances. **Calcium** increases due to dehydration (which is also associated with increased albumin), primary hyperparathyroidism (neoplasia of parathyroid gland), primary pseudohyperparathyroidism (neoplasms producing parathormone-related peptide or PRP, usually perianal adenocarcinoma or some form of lymphosarcoma), bone invasion of malignant neoplasms, thyrotoxicosis (uncommon), and overtreatment of parturient paresis. It decreases due to hypoalbuminemia, parturient paresis, oxalate poisoning, chronic renal failure (secondary renal hyperparathyroidism), acute pancreatitis (occasionally), surgical interference with parathyroid glands, and idiopathic (autoimmune) hypoparathyroidism. **Phosphate** increases due to renal failure (secondary renal hyperparathyroidism). Decreases are seen in some downer cows and as part of the stress pattern in horses and small animals. **Magnesium** increases are rarely seen, including during acute renal failure. It decreases in ruminants due to dietary deficiency, either acute (grass staggers) or chronic, and diarrhea (uncommon). **Glucose** increases due to high-carbohydrate meals, sprint exercise, stress or excitement (including handling and sampling stress), glucocorticoid therapy, Cushing's disease, overinfusion with glucose/dextrose-containing IV fluids, and diabetes mellitus. It decreases due to insulin overdose, insulinoma, islet cell hyperplasia (uncommon), acetonemia/pregnancy toxemia, acute febrile illness, and idiopathically (in certain dog breeds). **β-Hydroxybutyrate** increases in diabetic ketoacidosis, acetonemia/pregnancy toxemia, and extreme starvation.

Bilirubin increases due to fasting (benign effect in horses and squirrel monkeys, may lead to hepatic lipidosis in cats), hemolytic disease (usually mild increase), liver dysfunction, and biliary obstruction (intra- or extrahepatic). Theoretically, hemolysis is characterized by an increase in unconjugated (indirect) bilirubin, while hepatic and post-hepatic disorders are characterized by an increase in conjugated (direct) bilirubin; however, in practice this differentiation is unsatisfactory. Better appreciation of the source of the jaundice is gained from bile acid measurements. **Bile acids** increase when hepatic anion transport is impaired, usually during liver dysfunction (bile acids are more sensitive than bilirubin to hepatic impairment), and in the presence of a portosystemic shunt (congenital or acquired). The latter condition is characterized by a marked increase in bile acid concentration after feeding, from a fasting concentration that may be normal. It also increases in bile duct obstruction; very little increase is seen in feline infectious peritonitis or mild cases of hepatic lipidosis. **Cholesterol** increases due to fatty meals, hepatic or biliary disease, protein-losing nephropathy (and other protein-losing syndromes to some extent), diabetes mellitus, Cushing's disease, and hypothyroidism. It decreases in some cases of severe liver dysfunction, and occasionally in hyperthyroidism. **Lactate dehydrogenase** is a ubiquitous enzyme with a number of isoenzymes; electrophoretic separation of isoenzymes is necessary to locate the source of increased activity. **Sorbitol dehydrogenase** increases in acute hepatocellular damage in horses but is a very labile analyte. **α-Amylase** increases in acute pancreatitis in dogs and in chronic renal dysfunction. Amylase is not a useful indicator of pancreatitis in cats. **Lipase** increases in acute pancreatitis in dogs (longer half-life than amylase) and also occasionally in chronic renal dysfunction. Lipase is not a useful indicator of pancreatitis in cats. **Immunoreactive trypsin (trypsin-like immunoreactivity)** decreases in exocrine pancreatic insufficiency in dogs. It will also increase (irregularly) in pancreatitis. (*See* TESTS FOR PANCREATIC DISEASE, p 1343.)

Pattern Recognition: The essence of pattern recognition is the identification of a single condition that will explain the totality of the findings— not only biochemical, but clinical and hematologic as well. Further specific investigations are then carried out to confirm or deny this hypothesis. If more than a single condition will explain all the findings, then these must be differentiated by further investigation. While the "textbook" case of any condition is seldom encountered, a "best-fit" approach is usually productive in identifying the most promising avenues of exploration. The postulation of 2 or more simultaneous diagnoses to account for all the abnormalities seen is usually counterproductive.

Handling of Samples: Most biochemistry tests can be performed on either serum or heparinized plasma. A few (principally bile acids) require serum, while potassium is best measured on heparin plasma separated immediately after collection. Glucose measurement requires fluoride/oxalate plasma. Suitable collection tubes with and without anticoagulant are available commercially. Plastic tubes are satisfactory for blood in anticoagulant, but clotted blood must be collected either into glass tubes or plastic tubes specially coated to discourage the clot from adhering to the vessel walls.

Samples for biochemical analysis should be separated as soon as possible after collection to minimize artifacts caused by hemolysis and leakage of intracellular fluid components (eg, potassium) out of the cells. Samples in anticoagulant may be centrifuged immediately, but clotted samples need at least 30 min to allow the clot to form. Fluoride/oxalate samples hemolyze very readily because the cells can no longer respire, so timely separation is especially important. Proprietary gels or plastic beads assist with separation, and these may be incorporated into the collection tube or added before centrifugation.

Larger bucket-type centrifuges will accept almost any type or size of tube, but the rotors require careful balancing. They should be spun at 3,000 rpm for 10 min. Dual-purpose, high-speed microhematocrit centrifuges are favored for in-practice use, as they separate samples more quickly and the same machine can be used for measuring PCV. However, they can handle only a limited range of small-volume tubes.

Some "gel-tube" products may provide a permanent separation of serum or plasma, otherwise this must be separated into a fresh tube. The new tube must be adequately labeled. Samples may then be sent to a professional laboratory or analyzed in the practice.

In-practice Analysis: A number of biochemical analytes may be estimated in the practice without the need for large analytical instruments. **Total protein** is measured by refractometry, using the same instrument as is used to measure urine specific gravity, provided that an instrument with a total protein scale is purchased. It is also valid for protein measurement of ascitic and pleural fluids. The readout may be in g/dL, in which case multiplying the result by 10 will yield the SI unit of g/L. **Urea** may be estimated by chromatographic reaction strips, which correlate well with standard laboratory methods. A rapid whole-blood color comparison strip is also available, but these only read up to ~20 mmol/L and are thus of limited use. A dedicated reflectance meter for urea estimation is not available. **Glucose** meters for use on whole blood are widely available for home use by human diabetic patients. These yield acceptably accurate results on animal blood, although an unexpected hypoglycemia should be confirmed by a professional laboratory. Fresh whole blood may be used, but fluoride blood or plasma is the preferred sample if analysis is not immediate. **Ketones** may be estimated on either urine (preferred sample) or plasma/serum, using the ketone patch of a urine dipstick. The result is qualitative, not quantitative. **Triglycerides** may be visualized in a plasma or serum sample as lipemia. If the milkiness rises to the top of the tube on storage, chylomicrons are present. Otherwise, it is triglycerides. This is a qualitative judgment but is nevertheless useful, especially in equine patients. **Bilirubin** may also be appreciated by eye in most species. Equine and bovine plasma is normally yellow, which makes determination problematic, but in other species, any yellow color is abnormal and indicates an increased bilirubin. Visual assessment of the depth and shade of color may provide additional information.

For emergency in-clinic use, the most important analytes beyond these simple basics are sodium and potassium. A dedicated ion-specific electrode meter is the best way to measure these. Instruments are available that can analyze whole blood, although great care must be taken to avoid artifacts due to unappreciated hemolysis. Critical care meters are also available that can estimate a variety of analytes including glucose, urea, and electrolytes; however, these have not been extensively validated on nonhuman blood, and results should be interpreted with caution.

Extending in-practice analysis beyond these emergency basics requires a dedicated instrument capable of measuring multiple analytes. Two types are available—those based on transmission/absorbance photometry (wet chemistry), and those based on reflectance photometry (dry-reagent chemistry). Transmission/absorbance photometry is the reference method on which all reference values and interpretive guidelines are based. Reflectance photometry methods do not always compare well with the reference method, and are best confined to simpler tests such as glucose and urea. For wider applications, such as enzyme analysis, wet chemistry instruments are preferred.

In-clinic analysis is inevitably more expensive than the same investigations carried out by a professional laboratory, and the range of analytes available is more restricted. Additionally, the level of accuracy or reliability is likely to be lower. Therefore, it is still best practice to regard in-practice analysis as an interim emergency investigation, with the results to be confirmed as appropriate by a professional laboratory. Detailed case work-up of non-emergency patients is best referred to a professional laboratory from the outset, for reasons of cost, accuracy, range of analytes available, and the additional assistance of the clinical pathologist in the interpretation of the results.

If in-clinic analysis is to be relied on for general case work-up, meticulous attention must be paid to quality assurance. Samples of known composition must be run at least daily for each analyte, in both normal and pathologic ranges, and no patient results accepted unless these are within the tolerance limits. Participation in an external quality assessment program is also strongly recommended. Employing a trained technician will address some of these issues but has implications for availability of results out-of-hours and during holidays. The veterinarian in charge of the laboratory is responsible for all the results issued and incurs a legal liability to prove accuracy and reliability. If these cannot be guaranteed to the same standard as a referral laboratory, then results should not be relied on without external confirmation.

Tests For Pancreatic Disease

Pancreatitis: **Serum amylase and lipase activities** have been used for several decades to diagnose pancreatitis in both humans and dogs. Unfortunately, neither of these diagnostic tests is both sensitive and specific for pancreatitis. After total pancreatectomy, significant serum amylase and lipase activities remain, indicating that there are sources other than the exocrine pancreas. Clinical data also suggest a specificity for pancreatitis of only ~50% for both of these markers. Many nonpancreatic diseases, such as renal, hepatic, intestinal, and neoplastic diseases, can lead to increases in serum amylase and lipase activities. Steroid administration can also increase serum lipase activity and cause variable responses in serum amylase activity. Thus, in dogs, measurement of serum amylase and lipase activities are of limited clinical usefulness for the diagnosis of pancreatitis and should only be used until a more definitive diagnostic test, such as abdominal ultrasound, serum canine pancreatic lipase immunoreactivity concentration, or exploratory laparotomy, can be performed. Serum amylase and/or lipase activities that are 3-5 times the upper limit of the reference range, in patients with clinical signs that are consistent with pancreatitis, are suggestive of such a diagnosis. However, it is important to note that ~50% of dogs in this group do not have pancreatitis. In cats, serum amylase and lipase activities are of no clinical value for the diagnosis of pancreatitis. While cats with experimental pancreatitis show an increase in serum lipase activity and a decrease in serum amylase activity, these changes are not seen in cats with spontaneous disease.

Serum trypsin-like immunoreactivity (TLI) concentration measures mainly trypsinogen, the only form of trypsin that should be circulating in healthy individuals. However, trypsin, if present in the serum, is also detected by the assay. In healthy animals, serum TLI is low; during pancreatitis, however, an increased amount of trypsinogen leaks into the vascular space, which leads to an increase in serum TLI. Trypsin that has been prematurely activated may also contribute to this increase. However, both trypsinogen and trypsin are quickly cleared by the kidney. In addition, any prematurely activated trypsin is quickly removed by proteinase inhibitors, such as α_1-proteinase inhibitor and α_2-macroglobulin. In turn, α_2-macroglobulin-trypsin complexes are removed by the reticuloendothelial system. Thus, serum half-life for TLI is short, and a significant degree of active inflammation is required to increase serum TLI. In dogs, serum TLI is of limited usefulness for the diagnosis of pancreatitis. While it is more specific than serum amylase and lipase activity, its sensitivity is lower. For most veterinarians, the longer turnaround time for this test makes the measurement of serum TLI less desirable as a diagnostic test. Assays for the measurement of pancreatic lipase immunoreactivity (PLI) in canine and feline serum have recently been developed and validated. Serum PLI is highly specific for exocrine pancreatic function. Also, serum PLI is far more sensitive for the diagnosis of pancreatitis than any other diagnostic test currently available.

Pancreatic lipase immunoreactivity concentration specifically measures the mass of classical pancreatic lipase in the serum, rather than its kinetic (enzymatic) activity. At the moment, measurement of serum PLI concentration is only available through the Gastrointestinal Laboratory at Texas A&M University. Serum PLI concentration can be used to diagnose pancreatitis in dogs with renal failure, underscoring the high specificity of this new diagnostic test.

Other tests for the diagnosis of pancreatitis in dogs and cats have been evaluated. However, plasma trypsinogen activation peptide (TAP) concentration, urine TAP concentration, urine TAP:creatinine ratio, serum α_1-proteinase inhibitor trypsin complex concentration, and serum α_2-macroglobulin concentration have all been shown to be of little clinical usefulness for the diagnosis of spontaneous pancreatitis in dogs or cats.

Exocrine Pancreatic Insufficiency: In the past, several fecal tests were used to diagnose exocrine pancreatic insufficiency (EPI). Microscopic fecal examination for fat and/or undigested starch or muscle fibers are at best useful to suggest maldigestion. However, in light of wide availability of tests for diagnosing EPI, microscopic fecal examination can no longer be clinically justified. Fecal proteolytic activity had been used for several decades to diagnose EPI in small animals. Most of these methods, particularly the radiographic film clearance test, are unreliable. One method, which uses pre-made tablets to pour a gelatin agar, is the most useful. However, false positive as well as false negative results have been reported; the clinical use of fecal proteolytic activity is limited to species for which more specific assays to estimate pancreatic function are not available.

Serum TLI concentration is the diagnostic test of choice for EPI in both dogs and cats. Assays for TLI measure trypsinogen circulating in the vascular space. In healthy individuals, only a small amount of trypsinogen is present in serum. However, in dogs and cats with EPI, serum TLI decreases significantly and may even be undetectable. The reference range for canine TLI is 5-35 µg/L with a cut-off value of ≤2.5 µg/L considered diagnostic for EPI. Similarly, the reference range for feline serum TLI is 12-82 µg/L, with a cut-off value of ≤8 µg/L diagnostic for feline EPI. Rarely, animals with serum TLI concentrations below the cut-off value do not have clinical signs of EPI. This is probably due to the functional redundancy of the GI tract. At the same time, many dogs and cats with chronic diarrhea and weight loss have mild decreases in serum TLI (2.5-5.0 µg/L). Most of these animals have chronic small-intestinal disease and should be investigated accordingly. However, a small number of these dogs and cats may have EPI. If chronic small-intestinal disease is not diagnosed, serum TLI should be reevaluated in 2-3 mo.

PLI is also highly specific for exocrine pancreatic function and could be used to diagnose EPI. However, there is a small degree of overlap in serum PLI concentrations between normal dogs and dogs with EPI, making the measurement of PLI slightly inferior to TLI for accurate diagnosis.

Recently, an assay for measurement of canine fecal elastase has been developed and validated. This assay is inferior to serum TLI measurement and leads to many false-positive results. It is also more cumbersome and more expensive. It might be useful for the diagnosis of EPI due to obstruction of the pancreatic duct; however, this condition has never been described in dogs or cats.

CLINICAL MICROBIOLOGY

In-house microbiology can be a valuable asset to practitioners, providing quick results with minimal investment. Expensive equipment and materials are not usually necessary for the recovery of common aerobic or facultatively anaerobic bacterial pathogens, such as *Staphylococcus* spp, *Streptococcus* spp, and coliforms. While microbiologic media is not difficult to prepare, it may be more convenient to purchase from a scientific supply house. Most bacteria will grow readily on standard media (blood agar and MacConkey agar plates) when incubated aerobically. Basic equipment should include an incubator, refrigerator, Bunsen burner or portable gas torch, and microscope with low, high, and oil immersion objective lenses. Materials should consist of inoculating loops, prepared microbiologic media, microscope slides, Gram-stain reagents, 3% hydrogen peroxide, oxidase reagent, microbial identification systems, and a current veterinary microbiology textbook.

Specimen Selection and Collection: Although it is not always easy to obtain optimal specimens when working with animals, certain practices can ensure the best possible specimen under the circumstances. Application of the following principles should result in acceptable specimens that produce high-quality microbiology results: 1) Specimens must be obtained aseptically from a site that is representative of the disease process. 2) Swabs are the most common specimen collected, but they are generally not the specimens of choice, as they may become contaminated with commensals during the collection process, and they provide a small sample volume. Swabs are most useful for obtaining specimens from skin pustules, ears, conjunctiva, deep within draining tracts or wounds, soft tissue infections, or the reproductive tract. 3) A sufficient quantity of material should be collected to permit adequate examination. 4) Specimens must be collected at the proper time in the disease process and prior to the initiation of antimicrobial therapy to maximize pathogen recovery. 5) If cultures are not immediately initiated after collection, specimens should be refrigerated.

Specimen Processing: Microbiologic testing should include both direct, microscopic examination and culture of the specimen. Gram-stained smears should be examined using oil immersion in order to determine the correct reaction. Generally, both solid (agar) and liquid (broth) media should be inoculated. Solid media permit colony isolation, rough bacterial quantitation, and selection or differentiation of normal flora from potential pathogens, while broth media allow for the recovery of small numbers of organisms.

Clinical specimens should be inoculated onto both general purpose and selective media to maximize bacterial recovery. Plates containing trypticase/tryptic soy agar with 5% sheep blood are the most widely used types of general-purpose media. Selective and/or differential media include MacConkey agar (gram-negative bacteria), mannitol salt agar (staphylococci), and phenylethyl alcohol agar (gram-positive bacteria). Microbiologic media should be stored in the refrigerator, but allowed to warm to room temperature prior to inoculation.

Transfer of specimens to plated media depends on the type of specimen. Liquid specimens are inoculated by use of a sterile syringe or pipette. Swabs are generally plated directly by rolling the swab over an area ~2 cm in diameter. Feces are inoculated by dipping a swab into the specimen. Surgical biopsy specimens may be touched directly to the agar surface.

Bacterial identification methods depend on obtaining isolated colonies. The most common technique to achieve isolation is to streak plates using a wire loop. After the specimen has been inoculated onto a plate, a wire loop is flamed, cooled, and passed at a 90° angle several times through the initial area of inoculation. The plate is rotated 90°, the loop is flamed and cooled, and the process is repeated 3 more times. This results in 4 quadrants on the plate, which enable quantitation of the relative numbers of bacteria present in a given sample after colonies appear.

After inoculation, plates and tubes should be labeled and placed in an incubator set at 35-37°C. Plates are incubated with their lids down to prevent condensed water from dropping down from the lid onto the agar surface, which can result in confluent bacterial growth.

Bacterial Identification: The first step in culture evaluation is the visual examination of plated media. Most bacteria produce visible colonies in 24 hr, although some require 48-72 hr. Inspection includes examination of colonial morphology, noting both the types and numbers of colonies and any hemolytic reactions on blood-based agar. Further classification is based on the presence or absence of growth on differential or selective media.

After the evaluation of plated media, examination of Gram stains made from each different colony type is performed. Those reactions, combined with colonial morphology, may allow for the presumptive identification of organisms. If >1 colony type is present, subcultures of each are made. A single colony is streaked to a plate of nonselective medium. This will ensure a pure culture of the unknown organism, which is required for biochemical characterization and identification.

Several microbial identification systems are commercially available. Systems may be manual or automated. Each usually contains a complete package for the identification of a particular group of organisms. There are specific systems for staphylococci, streptococci, corynebacteria, nonfermenting gram-negative rods, and Enterobacteriaceae. All are useful for conducting a wide variety of biochemical tests simultaneously. Most manual systems consist of plates or strips made up of a series of wells or cups that contain test substrates. A pure culture of the unknown organism in suspension is added to the test wells. The strips are incubated aerobically at 37°C for 24-48 hr. The wells are viewed for colorimetric changes and a biocode is generated from scoring the test results. This numeric code is compared to those in the system database to obtain an identity for the test organism.

Antimicrobial Susceptibility Testing: There are 2 common procedures for determining the antimicrobial susceptibility of bacteria that are able to grow aerobically within 24 hr. Both procedures have been accepted by the National Committee for Clinical

Laboratory Standards (NCCLS). The first procedure is qualitative and is based on the agar disk diffusion method of Bauer and Kirby. The second procedure is quantitative and involves dilutions of antimicrobial agents, which are tested either in liquid or solid agar media. The latter is referred to as the minimal inhibitory concentration test.

The agar disk diffusion method is more widely used for testing the common, rapidly growing aerobic to facultatively anaerobic pathogenic bacteria. The determination of antimicrobial susceptibility of many fastidious bacteria, such as *Haemophilus parasuis* or *Pasteurella* spp, remains to be standardized. The Bauer-Kirby method is based on the diffusion of an antimicrobial agent impregnated within a paper disk through an agar medium. Briefly, a suspension of actively growing test organism is standardized to a turbidity equivalent to 0.5 on the McFarland scale. Within 15 min of standardization, a sterile swab is dipped into the bacterial suspension and a dry Müller-Hinton agar plate is inoculated by streaking the swab over the entire surface 3 times. To ensure an even distribution of the inoculum, the plate is rotated ~60° each time. Antimicrobial disks are placed on the plate and are gently pressed down to ensure their close contact with the agar surface. Inverted plates are placed in an incubator at 35°C. Plates are examined after 18 hr of incubation. Zones of complete inhibition are measured in millimeters using a ruler. The zone sizes are compared to those published by the NCCLS in order to make an interpretation of susceptible, intermediate, or resistant for each agent tested.

Reliable antimicrobial susceptibility testing results can only be obtained by following standardized procedures. Any procedural deviation may lead to erroneous results. It is imperative to properly store antimicrobial susceptibility test disks and test media and to ensure quality control for each test. Any clinic that does not regularly perform testing on a weekly basis may wish to use a veterinary diagnostic laboratory for this procedure instead.

CYTOLOGY

Cytology is a useful clinical tool for the investigation of disease processes and was originally developed mainly for use in the practice environment. It should be considered as a guide only and rarely provides a diagnosis. It should not be used as a substitute for more accurate diagnostic methods such as histopathology. Most of this section refers to small animals; however, the basic principles apply to all species.

Sample Collection

Fine-needle Aspiration: Using a 21- to 25-gauge needle attached to a 5- or 10-mL syringe, the needle should be inserted into the area to be sampled and repeatedly redirected within the lesion while gentle suction is applied. The resulting sample is often very small and may only be present within the needle, not the syringe. The syringe should be detached, filled with air, re-attached, and gently depressed to express the sample onto a clean, dry, glass slide. The force applied should be minimal in order to avoid rupture of the cells. Another slide is placed on the top of the sample and pulled lengthwise to spread the sample to a single layer if possible.

If blood is collected in the syringe during aspiration, this can be centrifuged and the buffy coat examined for nonblood cells. If the sample is directly smeared onto a slide, a feathered edge should be obtained because this is where the heavier cells will congregate. Blood contamination can be minimized by use of a very fine (25-gauge) needle; this increases the chance of collecting diagnostic cells.

Lymphocytes are particularly fragile, and aspirates of lymph nodes should be made using a needle only with no attached syringe and no suction. The needle should be repeatedly redirected to pack the lumen of the needle with cells; a syringe is then attached in order to carefully express the sample material.

The sample should be air dried as quickly as possible to reduce the effects of shrinkage but should never be heated.

Impression Smears: These are often used for ulcerated surface lesions. They usually only sample the surface inflammatory exudate, rather than deeper tissues, and are of limited value. This technique can also be used on biopsies to give an immediate indication of the type of lesion before sending the sample for histopathologic interpretation. The cut surface of the sample is blotted to remove surface blood and serum, then the dried surface is applied to a clean, dry slide with gentle pressure. Several areas can be prepared on a single slide. The preparations are quickly air dried and then stained as for a fluid sample.

Fluids: When a fluid sample is obtained, centrifugation of the preparation and sampling of the centrifuged sediment is the usual method of cell concentration. Once the slide has been prepared, rapid air drying before staining is necessary.

If the fluid will be sent to a laboratory, adding a few drops of formalin to the sample will preserve cells and prevent bacterial overgrowth during transit. This is particularly useful for bronchoalveolar lavage fluid and urine because these often contain infectious agents and are prone to bacterial contamination at sampling. The laboratory must, however, be told of the presence of formalin because the usual Romanowsky stains cannot then be used. Calcium disodium adetate is often recommended to help preserve cytology samples but its effects are limited.

Staining

The traditional stains for cytology preparations are modified Wright's stain (Wright-Giemsa) and May-Grunwald Giemsa. Over the past few years, however, very good quality, rapid Romanowsky stains have been developed for cytology and hematology use, and these are now often used by professional veterinary diagnostic laboratories. Many different brands of rapid stain are available; more than one should be tried in order to see which is best suited to a particular practice. All are equally rapid but some are easier to complete in a practice environment. Many can be adjusted by returning a finished slide to the stain for deeper color reaction, or if overstained, color can be removed by placing the slide in alcohol. Formalin-fixed material must be stained with either H&E or Papanicolaou stain.

Sample Interpretation

Full sample interpretation may require a professional laboratory, but much information can be obtained in the practice. It is axiomatic that full interpretation requires a good-quality sample. Many samples taken in practice environments are unsuitable for full interpretation. Techniques that appear to be simple may require considerable practice to yield consistent quality. A high quality microscope with a range of objective lenses, including oil immersion, is required to examine smears.

Inflammation: Clinicians must be able to recognize the basic inflammatory cells—neutrophils, eosinophils, lymphocytes, macrophages, and plasma cells. Some tumors contain a large number of inflammatory cells, but these are very uncommon. If inflammatory cells are exclusively present in a sample, it is almost certainly a primary inflammatory lesion.

A large number of **neutrophils** in a cytology preparation indicates acute inflammation and is usually accompanied by smaller numbers of lymphocytes and macrophages. This is most often caused by an infection or foreign body reaction, including furunculotic reactions directed against hair and keratin embedded in the soft tissue. The cytoplasm of neutrophils may contain causative organisms.

Macrophages are medium-sized round cells with oval, sometimes indented, nuclei and moderate amounts of usually vacuolated, foamy cytoplasm. These cells phagocytize organisms, other cells, and debris. They are associated with any tissue damage but especially with chronic inflammation. Chronic inflammation leads to a very mixed cell population, including neutrophils, but there is a much higher proportion of macrophages, plasma cells, and lymphocytes. Spindle-shaped fibroblasts are often also present. Macrophages are also seen within the contents of cysts.

Eosinophils can often be seen in association with mast cells. They are associated with allergies and also are prominent in parasitic diseases, superficial cutaneous viral infection in cats, and fungal infections. They are the predominant cell type in specific eosinophilic conditions, eg, eosinophilic granuloma in cats (rarely dogs) and eosinophilic collagenolytic granuloma in horses. Some canine cutaneous mast cell tumors have a very high proportion of eosinophils and very few mast cells. Eosinophils can be a less specific part of the inflammatory response in certain species (eg, rabbits). Heterophils in birds and reptiles are similar morphologically to eosinophils.

Lymphocytes are part of the chronic inflammatory response and are not specific for a particular stimulus. Most are small, with nuclei approximately the same size as RBC. If mostly medium to large lymphocytes are present, lymphoma should be considered.

Histiocytes are part of the macrophage cell family but appear less activated than macrophages and have many fewer cytoplasmic vacuoles. They are found in cutaneous histiocytoses in dogs and granulomas in all species.

Multinucleated cells are usually seen in small numbers along with other inflammatory cells as part of a granulomatous reaction. They are particularly common in fungal infections and reaction to foreign material, although this association is much less specific in birds and reptiles.

Fibroblasts proliferate as part of the repair reaction associated with tissue damage. When fibroblasts are aspirated from tissue, the cells usually lose their spindle shape and become round, but a few will retain their elongated shape. They have round or oval nuclei, indistinct nucleoli, and moderate amounts of uniform, pale blue-staining cytoplasm. The cytoplasmic boundaries are indistinct with a "wispy" appearance. Fibroblasts may look the same as low-grade spindle cell tumors, and these cannot be definitively distinguished cytologically. If found with inflammatory cells, the spindle cells are most often reactive, but neoplasia cannot be ruled out.

Neoplasia: Ideally, the first stage in the cytologic interpretation of neoplasia is determination of the cells' tissue type. Occasionally, however, this is not possible. The next stage would then be determination of the likely behavior of the cells, which can be done without specifically identifying the cell type. There are 3 basic cell types: epithelial, mesenchymal (ie, supporting or connective), and round. **Epithelial cells** are round, cuboidal, or polygonal and tend to adhere tightly to each other and exfoliate in clusters or sheets. They have a sharp cytoplasmic outline and exfoliate in moderate numbers. **Mesenchymal cells** are tightly adherent and usually exfoliate in very low numbers as single cells or very small, loose aggregates. They are classically spindle shaped but usually become round and plump when removed from the body. **Round cells** have little or no adherence in the body and therefore usually exfoliate in large numbers and lie individually in the smear with no clumping. Cells of this category include mast cells, lymphocytes, histiocytes, plasma cells, and cells of transmissible venereal tumors.

Classification of the cell type and likely behavior may require tissue biopsy; with very few exceptions, histology will be necessary for a definitive diagnosis. However, it may be possible to obtain further information from a cytology sample.

Tumor Behavior

To distinguish benign from malignant tumors, the variation in certain characteristics is assessed within the cell population. As a general rule, the more malignant the cell, the less differentiated it becomes and the more variation there is within the cell population. Benign tumors have cells that are often uniform in size, with a uniform nucleus:cytoplasm ratio, and strongly resemble the cell of origin. Nuclear criteria are the major indicators of malignancy. Criteria for malignancy include variation in cell size and shape, increased cell exfoliation, increased nuclear size, increased nucleus:cytoplasm ratio, variation in nuclear size and an increase in multinucleated cells, increased mitosis with abnormal mitotic figures, a coarse and often clumped chromatin pattern, altered shape of the nucleus due to close approximation of a nucleus from an adjacent cell (nuclear molding), and large (often multiple) nucleoli of irregular and abnormal shape. There are several exceptions, however. Thyroid carcinomas usually have fairly uniform, well differentiated cells. A diagnosis of thyroid carcinoma is usually made on size and capsular and soft tissue invasion, features that are only identifiable histologically. Other tissues in which it may be impossible to differentiate benign from malignant cells include apocrine gland carcinomas, basal cell tumors, melanomas, and proliferative hepatic lesions. Some normal structures, such as hepatoid glands, have more than one cell type (ie, reserve and terminal cells) and can exhibit variation in size or morphology even when benign. Many mammary tumors show marked variation in cell morphology but histologically are classed as benign. These exceptions often make cytologic interpretation unreliable, particularly for the tissues listed.

Lymphoma is most commonly characterized by a uniform population of larger than normal lymphoid cells. Variation in morphology, therefore, is not necessary for a diagnosis of malignancy with this tissue type. Most spindle cell tumors do not metastasize but are locally aggressive and often difficult to remove. The criteria for malignancy are often less important with respect to the behavior of these tumors than for epithelial tumors.

Common Cytology Results

Some specific features of cytology preparations can provide a more accurate interpretation of the sample. Listed below are some common results and their interpretation.

Mature Fat Cells: These are seen in benign lipoma and mature body fat, which cannot be differentiated cytologically. Because fat cells are mesenchymal cells, they tend not to exfoliate well and are usually present in low numbers.

Spindle Cells: It is usually not possible to differentiate reactive spindle cells from those of spindle cell neoplasia. Absence of a reactive stimulus (eg, inflammation or hemorrhage) and a higher cell population with more and larger clumps of cells may indicate neoplasia. Greater variation in the neoplastic criteria indicates more aggressive behavior.

Keratin: Keratin includes nucleated and terminally differentiated non-nucleated squamous epithelial cells. It can be a contaminant from the surface of the animal's skin or the skin of any handlers of the sample and is a common artifact. It can also be sampled from cutaneous keratin-filled cysts, which are always benign and very common, particularly in dogs. Large, densely packed clumps of keratin in restricted areas in the center of the slide suggest that keratin is part of the lesion rather than an artifact.

Blood: This is a common artifact of fine-needle aspiration but can also come from blood-filled spaces in the tissue, which can be non-neoplastic, such as hematomas or severe bruising, or neoplastic lesions, such as hemangiomas and hemangiosarcomas. The presence of spindle cells does not adequately differentiate neoplastic from non-neoplastic causes of hemorrhage (*see* SPINDLE CELLS, above). Use of a very fine needle (25 gauge) can help decrease blood contamination.

Lack of Cells: This is a common problem with cytology samples. If proper technique has been used, absence of cells may indicate mesenchymal cell proliferation (including lipomas), as these tightly adherent cells do not exfoliate well.

Cells with Cytoplasmic Granules: The most important of these is the **mast cell**, because mast cell tumors are common in dogs. These are medium-sized cells with round nuclei. With Romanowsky stains, the granules are dark blue or purple, small (similar to bacteria), and usually found in large numbers in the cytoplasm. Less differentiated mast cells have fewer granules, but cytology is a very poor method of grading these tumors. The cells are fragile; large numbers of granules are released from damaged cells. In dogs in particular, eosinophils are often present and occasionally may be the dominant cell type. Eosinophils are less commonly seen in other species. Mast cell tumors in horses have similar cytology to those in dogs, but mast cell tumors in cats often have cells that are smaller and more uniform, with less distinct granulation.

Thyroid cells can also have dark granules, usually blue or black, called tyrosine granules. These are relatively small, low in number, and can be difficult to see. Black granules are associated with melanocytes and are seen in **melanomas**. Cytology cannot differentiate benign from malignant melanomas but, in dogs, melanomas on haired skin are usually benign and those on nonhaired areas, such as the lips, feet, and mouth, are usually malignant. However, basal cell tumors also often contain cells with melanin. These tumors are usually benign and cytologically can sometimes be difficult to distinguish from melanomas. Melanin can also be seen in macrophages, sometimes in large amounts, but it is usually in much larger clumps within the cytoplasm rather than fine granules that are found in melanocytes. Very fine magenta granules can be seen in **osteoblastic cells** from osteosarcoma. Golden, granular material accumulates in the cytoplasm of macrophages following hemorrhage into soft tissues.

Cells with Cytoplasmic Vacuoles: A large, single vacuole is seen in fat cells. In normal or benign cells, the nuclei are small and often indistinct; the cells are often folded like a collapsed ball. Smaller cells with larger, more prominent nuclei and some cytoplasm in addition to clear vacuoles are more suggestive of malignancy. Cells with multiple, small vacuoles with a foamy appearance include macrophages, sebaceous glandular cells, and salivary cells. These can be very difficult to differentiate. Biopsy site and other clinical features can be a deciding factor in interpretation.

Differentiation of Round Cell Tumors: These cells include mast cells, plasma cells, lymphocytes, histiocytes, and cells of transmissible venereal tumors. Mast cells have very distinctive cytoplasmic granules and are usually easily distinguished except in the small number of cases that have few or no cytoplasmic granules.

Lymphoid cells classically have a very high nucleus:cytoplasm ratio, which is found in few other cells. When neoplastic, **lymphoma** cells are medium to large in size, with a nucleus at least $1^1/_2$ times the size of RBC. Nucleoli are often multiple and may be prominent.

Cells of a **histiocytoma** are not especially histiocytic cytologically. They are round cells with a moderate amount of pale-staining cytoplasm. They are fairly uniform and have nuclei that are eccentric within the cell. Nucleoli are not prominent. Histiocytic cells are slightly more problematic. They are part of the cell line that includes macrophages and inflammatory and reactive cells, as well as highly malignant round cell tumors. Histiocytic cells tend to be larger than other round cells and may be vacuolated, with more cytoplasm and nuclei that are oval or indented. Infiltrates of histiocytic cells are often problematic, even with full tissue biopsy examination, and always require histologic examination to determine malignancy.

Neoplastic plasma cells include **myeloma** cells. These are usually very well differentiated and have most of the characteristics of normal plasma cells but, when neoplastic, are present in very large numbers, along with few other cell types. Benign nodular proliferations of plasma cells—**plasmacytomas**—show more marked pleomorphism and often differ markedly from normal plasma cells. Many have a slightly histiocytic appearance and can be difficult to distinguish cytologically.

Even histologically, it can be very difficult to distinguish cells of transmissible venereal tumors. They tend to have a moderate amount of cytoplasm (more than lymphoblasts), often with small vacuoles. Nuclear chromatin is coarse with 1 or 2 fairly prominent nucleoli. Mitotic figures are often numerous, unlike most cytology preparations of neoplastic lesions, and they tend to show moderate variation in the nucleus:cytoplasm ratio.

Cytology of Specific Sites

Lymph Nodes: Uniform cell populations indicate neoplasia. Size in comparison with RBC is useful. Normal mature lymphocytes or small neoplastic lymphocytes (rare) have nuclei of the same size as RBC. Blast cells, however, have nuclei $\geq 1^1/_2$ times the diameter of RBC. Samples with large numbers of medium blast cells and a moderate number of small lymphocytes are difficult to interpret, and cytologists may not agree on the percentage of blasts that are necessary for a diagnosis of lymphoma.

Submandibular lymph nodes are often difficult to assess. They drain the buccal and nasal areas and are therefore subject to strong antigenic stimuli. They frequently undergo hyperplasia, often histologically atypical, especially in cats. Cats also develop unusual neoplastic conditions affecting this node, such as the T-cell rich B-cell lymphoma and Hodgkin's-like lymphoma. For these reasons, great care must be taken in the inter-

TABLE 2. **Characteristics of Transudates and Exudate**

	Total Protein (g/dL)	Cell Count (cells/μL)
Transudate	<2.5	<1,500
Modified transudate	2.5-7.5	1,000-7,000
Exudate	>3.0	>7,000

pretation of lesions involving the submandibular lymph nodes to avoid false negative or false positive diagnoses of neoplasia. Aspirates from enlarged submandibular lymph nodes often yield only large foamy cells. These cells are of salivary gland origin and may be obtained due to sampling error or hypertrophy of the salivary gland (in cases of sialoadenosis), which may be mistaken for lymph node enlargement.

Body Cavity Fluids: Meaningful analysis of fluid from body cavities requires total protein (measured with a handheld refractometer), total cell count, and a differential of cell types present (TABLE 2). Pure transudates are rare because they rapidly become modified by leakage of fluid from lymphatics or blood vessels and attraction of mixed inflammatory cells. Transudates attract activated macrophages and variable numbers of nondegenerate neutrophils. The lymphocytes that may also be present are classified as small, but most are usually just slightly larger than circulating lymphocytes and are part of the reactive process of the fluid in the body cavity. In addition, when fluid accumulates in the body cavity, the lining mesothelial cells proliferate and are shed into the fluid. These cells are large, often multinucleated, vary in appearance, and often are seen in groups with very large nucleoli. All of these features are usually seen with malignancy but, in this case, the cells are simply reactive and not neoplastic. Care must be taken to differentiate these mesothelial cells from neoplastic cells within the body fluid. Usually, a small number of these cells have a corona around the cytoplasmic envelope, giving a fuzzy outline, which is a distinguishing factor for mesothelial cells.

Mesothelial cells can be present in very large numbers, especially in pericardial fluid. Malignant mesotheliomas are rare in domestic species, but it is not possible to differentiate neoplastic from reactive mesothelial cells on cytologic examination. The degree of polyploidy is not a distinguishing feature.

Mixed inflammatory cells are increased in number as a transudate becomes modified and are present in large numbers in an exudate. Cells that do not fall into these categories may be neoplastic and must therefore be examined using the general criteria outlined above.

Tracheal or Bronchoalveolar Lavage (BAL): Epithelial cells are seen in BAL from normal and diseased animals. The epithelial cells may retain their original structure, with a ciliated surface, but often appear round with indistinct cilia. **Macrophages** come from deep in the alveoli and are part of the normal defense mechanisms. They greatly increase with fluid accumulation in the lung (eg, cardiovascular insufficiency) and in inflammatory conditions, where they are accompanied by other inflammatory cells. Debris, foreign material, hemosiderin, RBC, and microorganisms can sometimes be seen in the cytoplasm of these cells.

Neutrophils are nonspecific inflammatory cells in the respiratory system. They can dominate an inflammatory reaction, even in cases of allergy, but are probably most commonly associated with infection. In bacterial infections, microorganisms can often be seen in the cytoplasm of neutrophils and in extracellular parts of the smear. Great care must be taken to differentiate **eosinophils** from neutrophils in BAL preparations because the granules are often faint and difficult to identify. Eosinophils are ≤5% of cells in BAL from normal dogs but may reach 10% in normal cats. Eosinophils that comprise >10% of cells indicate hypersensitivity. This is most commonly associated with an allergic respiratory disease, although lungworms and heartworms can also cause this reaction. Larvae are sometimes present in lungworm infection, usually in young animals. Nucleated and non-nucleated **squamous cells** are commonly seen in BAL preparations and are often associated with bacteria on the cell surface. This indicates contamination from the pharynx. Bacteria are normal inhabitants of the pharynx, in particular *Simonsiella*, which are very large, ladder-like organisms; their presence confirms contamination from the pharynx. If bacteria are present along with squamous epithelial cells, it may not be possible to conclude whether the bacteria are from the respiratory tree or the pharynx.

Synovial Fluid: Full examination of synovial fluid includes evaluation of protein content, mucin clot formation, and other factors. It is usually not feasible to perform these tests in a practice environment, but cytology is often all that is necessary for an interpretation, particularly when also evaluating the clinical condition of the animal. Normal synovial fluid contains small numbers of joint macrophages or synoviocytes. Cell counts in normal animals vary greatly (eg, 0-400/μL in dogs). Counts >500/μL in dogs are generally considered clinically significant.

Macrophages increase with any damage to a joint, especially in cases of degenerative joint disease. Vacuolation of the cytoplasm, and especially the presence of phagocytosis of debris or RBC, indicate macrophage activation, a feature not seen in normal joint mononuclear cells. In degenerative joint disease, synovial fluid often contains only macrophages.

Hemorrhage is common in synovial preparations but is frequently an artifact. It may also indicate hemarthrosis. Although not always the case in hemarthrosis, RBC may be seen in the cytoplasm of macrophages.

Neutrophils are seen in both septic arthritis and autoimmune joint disease. These 2 conditions can usually be differentiated by the clinical history. In septic arthritis, bacteria may be present within the cytoplasm of phagocytic cells.

Vaginal Cytology: This can be used to identify the various stages of the canine estrous cycle, but results must be interpreted in conjunction with the animal's behavior. A sample of exfoliated cells is obtained from the vaginal vault cranial to the urethral orifice with a cotton-tipped swab or glass rod. Cells are gently rolled onto a glass slide, air dried, and stained. Features to be identified include neutrophils, bacteria, and RBC, along with the types of epithelial cells present. The epithelial cells (in increasing order of differentiation) are parabasal, small and large intermediate cells, and superficial cells. Parabasal cells are small, with central round nuclei, indistinct nucleoli with a relatively narrow band of cytoplasm, and a nucleus:cytoplasm ratio of ~1:1. Small intermediate cells have a similar nucleus but a much larger amount of cytoplasm. Large intermediate cells have a similar nucleus with very large amounts of cytoplasm and an angular, irregular outline. Superficial cells also have large amounts of cytoplasm, but their nuclei are pyknotic (small and contracted) or absent.

Stages of the estrous cycle change gradually. If a preparation does not conform exactly to a specific part of the cycle, judgment must be made regarding what stages are present. In **proestrus**, mixed epithelial cells, including parabasal, small and large intermediate cells, superficial cells, and neutrophils are present. Bacteria are often present in large numbers. In **estrus**, 90% of epithelial cells are superficial cells. There are large numbers of bacteria but no neutrophils. In **diestrus**, parabasal and intermediate cells are more prominent and may total >10% of the total epithelial cells. The number of neutrophils varies. In **anestrus**, parabasal and intermediate cells predominate. Neutrophils and bacteria are few in number. RBC are not helpful in differentiating the stages of estrus.

Nasal Cavity: The cytology of nasal flush preparations is similar to that seen with BAL preparations. A small number of respiratory epithelial cells are usually flushed out along with exudate. A predominance of eosinophils may indicate inhaled allergens, parasites, or fungi and may occasionally indicate bacteria or neoplasia. Eosinophils in the nasal cavity are therefore less indicative of a specific disease than in other sites, eg, the trachea or bronchi.

Neutrophils are the most common exudative cell but, as with BAL, often indicate secondary infection. In the case of intranasal neoplasia, cells with neoplastic characteristics (*see* p 1350) may be present, but absence of these cells does not rule out neoplasia. Only a minority of neoplastic processes actually erode the overlying respiratory epithelium, allowing for exfoliation of neoplastic cells. Similarly, absence of fungal hyphae within the preparation does not rule out fungal infection. Viral inclusions are rarely seen.

Cerebrospinal Fluid: For good interpretation of CSF, cytospin preparations are essential. Even in disease states, the number of cells present in CSF can be very low. CSF cytology examinations show an extremely wide range of normal values. The presence of >1-2 nucleated inflammatory cells in a CSF cytospin preparation or plain smear should be considered potentially significant.

Urine Cytology: Urine can be examined as a wet preparation or as a dried cytology smear. Because of the absence of staining in a wet preparation, these are better limited to examination for crystals and RBC. Although nucleated cells may be seen, in most practice environments they cannot be identified and are better examined using a dried cytology smear.

There are at least 10 common forms of urinary crystals. Identification is not discussed here, but may be readily accomplished by use of good reference illustrations. (*See also* UROLITHIASIS, p 1279.)

Because cells in urine rapidly degenerate, particularly if bacteria are present, centrifuged preparations of urine samples should be examined rapidly after sampling. If this is not possible, boric acid is often added to urine to prevent degeneration and bacterial overgrowth. A better preservation method is the addition of a few drops of formalin; however, Romanowsky stains cannot then be used.

Normal urine usually has no or very few cells. Single urothelial cells are occasionally present. Squamous epithelial cells are also commonly seen in urine and come from the terminal urethra, vagina, vulva, and preputial epithelium. Squamous metaplasia of bladder epithelium following chronic inflammation is rare.

Neoplastic cells in urine are almost always epithelial. They are therefore rounded polygonal cells, often clumped, with marked variation in morphology. Uniform cells are more likely to be normal or may be associated with hyperplasia (eg, some cases of polypoid cystitis).

RBC are commonly seen with neoplastic and inflammatory diseases of the bladder but are also often seen without indication of other pathology. RBC may be artifacts of sample collection but are also common in cases of interstitial cystitis. In cats, this term is often used synonymously with feline urologic syndrome, but interstitial cystitis also is seen in dogs and humans, suggesting other unknown pathogenic factors that can cause this condition. Persistent hematuria, therefore, without cytologic evidence of neoplasia or inflammation, may indicate interstitial cystitis.

See also URINALYSIS, p 1358.

CLINICAL HEMATOLOGY

Hematology refers to the study of the numbers and morphology of the cellular elements of the blood—the red cells (erythrocytes), white cells (leukocytes), and platelets (thrombocytes) and the use of these results in the diagnosis and monitoring of disease. (*See also* HEMATOPOIETIC SYSTEM INTRODUCTION, p 4.)

Red Blood Cells

Three RBC measurements are routinely carried out: packed cell volume (PCV), the proportion of whole blood volume occupied by RBC; hemoglobin (Hgb) concentration of whole lysed blood; and RBC count, the number of RBC per unit volume of whole blood. Although these are separate estimations, they are in effect 3 ways of measuring the same thing, and it is incorrect to attempt to interpret them as separate variables. Inasmuch as they do vary in relation to each other, they allow calculation of 2 further meaningful parameters, mean corpuscular volume (MCV) and mean corpuscular hemoglobin concentration (MCHC), as follows:

$$MCV \ (fL) \ = \ \frac{PCV(\%) \times 10}{RBC(\times 10^{12}/L)}$$

$$MCHC \ (g/dL) \ = \ \frac{Whole \ blood \ hemoglobin \ concentration \ (g/dL)}{PCV(decimal \ fraction)}$$

MCV varies widely between mammalian species, from ~15 fL in goats to ~90 fL in humans. Avian and reptilian red cells are even larger, up to 300 fL. Nevertheless, MCHC varies little with species (or erythrocyte size), at ~33 g/dL.

Several artifacts can cause significant and potentially misleading alterations to measured erythrocyte parameters: 1) old samples cause RBC to swell, thus increasing PCV and MCV and decreasing MCHC; 2) lipemia causes a falsely high Hgb reading, and hence a falsely high MCHC; 3) hemolysis causes PCV to decrease while Hgb remains unchanged, again leading to a falsely high MCHC; 4) underfilling of the tube causes RBC to shrink, causing PCV and MCV to decrease and MCHC to increase; 5) autoagglutination causes a falsely low RBC count, and hence a falsely high MCV.

Visual description of RBC morphology on a Romanowsky stain also provides useful diagnostic information. The most common terms employed include: 1) Normocytic—cells are of normal size. 2) Macrocyte—abnormally large cell, usually polychromatophilic (see below). 3) Microcyte—abnormally small cell, usually caused by a lack of hemoglobin precursors. 4) Anisocytosis—variation in size of cells, due to macrocytes, microcytes, or both. 5) Normochromic—cells are of normal color. 6) Polychromasia—variation in color of the cells. This usually describes the appearance of large, juvenile, bluish-staining polychromatophilic macrocytes. These broadly correspond to the "reticulocyte" seen with new methylene blue staining, in which the reticulum represents the remnants of the nucleus. 7) Hypochromasia—decrease in staining density of the cells, usually due to a lack of hemoglobin precursors, especially iron. 8) Annulocyte—extreme form of hypochromic cell with only a thin rim of hemoglobin.

PCV is the variable normally used to assess the basic status of the erythron—increased in polycythemia, decreased in anemia—although if a sample is too hemolyzed to allow measurement of PCV, a meaningful Hgb measurement may still be obtained. RBC count as such should not be interpreted clinically.

An abnormally high PCV (polycythemia) may be relative, due to a change in the proportion of circulating RBC to blood plasma without any alteration in the size of the erythron, or absolute, due to a real increase in erythron size. Absolute polycythemia may be primary (eg, polycythemia vera or, rarely, erythropoietin-producing tumors) or secondary (a consequence of disease in another organ system). (See also POLYCYTHEMIA, p 56.)

Polycythemia vera and erythropoietin-producing tumors should only be suspected when PCV is very high, normally >0.70. The former is characterized by normal adult erythrocytes and a normal (or low) erythropoietin concentration, while the latter may show a regenerative RBC picture with high erythropoietin concentration. Relative polycythemia may also be associated with very high PCV values, and normal adult RBC. Secondary polycythemia generally shows a more modest increase in PCV, often with evidence of regeneration (more so when the cause is pulmonary or cardiac, less so when the cause is hormonal). It is often possible to make the differential diagnosis of polycythemia on clinical grounds.

Abnormally low PCV (anemia) may be caused by loss of blood (hemorrhage), breakdown of erythrocytes in circulation (hemolysis), or lack of production of erythrocytes by the bone marrow (hypoplasia or aplasia). Presentation varies according to whether the condition is acute or chronic. Aplastic anemia is always chronic in onset because anemia occurs gradually as existing cells reach the end of their lifespan. (*See also* ANEMIA, p 8.)

In acute hemorrhagic anemia, external blood loss is easily appreciated clinically, but blood loss into a body cavity may only be determined on paracentesis. Initially, all hematologic parameters may be normal, as it may take 12 hr for fluid shifts to produce a decrease in the PCV. Within a few days, RBC become regenerative, with juvenile forms appearing in circulation (except in horses, where circulating evidence of regeneration is not readily appreciable). These consist of polychromatophilic macrocytes and normoblasts (nucleated RBC). Late normoblasts have a small, nonviable nucleus and a moderate amount of cytoplasm colored similarly to that of the polychromatophilic macrocytes, while early normoblasts have a larger, viable nucleus and scanty cytoplasm. These are most easily distinguished from lymphocytes by their more densely-staining nucleus. If substantial amounts of blood have been lost from the body, the RBC picture may become hypochromic. Thus, this type of anemia shows an increase in MCV and a decrease in MCHC. If bleeding is into a body cavity, hypochromasia may not be evident because hemoglobin precursors will be recycled. However, slight jaundice may be seen as the sequestered cells are broken down. Some sequestered cells may also be returned to the circulation intact, if somewhat misshapen.

In acute hemolytic anemia, PCV will decrease immediately, and in the early stages some jaundice will be evident. In the very early stages, even a sample collected with extreme care may be markedly hemolyzed. As with hemorrhagic anemia, the RBC will become regenerative within a few days, with polychromatophilic macrocytes and nucleated RBC evident. However, as hemoglobin precursors are not lost from the body, true hypochromasia is not seen.

Chronic hemorrhagic anemia may be difficult to appreciate if blood is lost in the feces or urine, or due to bloodsucking ectoparasites. Anemia may be severe, and the RBC picture will be regenerative on presentation. Hypochromasia is usually very marked. In very longstanding conditions, depletion of iron and other hemoglobin precursors can become so marked that most of the cells are microcytic, and MCV may paradoxically decrease. Intermittent intra-abdominal hemorrhage leads to a somewhat different picture, as blood shed into the peritoneal cavity can be returned to the circulation. PCV may therefore recover quickly, until the next episode, and signs of depletion of hemoglobin constituents do not emerge.

In chronic hemolytic anemia, RBC are regenerative on presentation, except that some cases of autoimmune hemolytic anemia (AIHA) paradoxically show little or no regeneration until treatment has been initiated. Hypochromasia is less marked than in hemorrhagic conditions, and misshapen erythrocytes (including target cells and folded cells) are more common. The spherocyte, in which the erythrocyte loses its classic biconcave shape, is essentially pathognomonic for AIHA. Jaundice may be absent, because the products of the destruction of the erythrocytes may be cleared by the reticuloendothelial system and the liver as quickly as they are formed.

Hypoplastic and aplastic anemia may be mild if RBC production is merely depressed secondary to some other disease. Protein, mineral, or vitamin deficiencies may cause hypoplastic anemia, but these are more likely to be secondary to another disease (eg, chronic hemorrhage or malabsorption) than simple dietary deficiency. Other diseases may cause depression of erythropoietin production, eg, renal failure, deficiencies of hormones that usually stimulate erythropoietin production (eg, hypothyroidism, Addison's disease), and chronic, debilitating conditions such as chronic infections, chronic parasitism, and neoplasia. RBC morphology is nonregenerative and may be hypochromic if a deficiency state is involved. Paradoxically, vitamin B_{12} and/or folic acid deficiency produces a macrocytic RBC picture due to early maturation arrest of the erythrocytes. Neoplasia of the bone marrow may cause severe anemia as erythropoietic elements are crowded out, but some regeneration may be observed as the remaining bone marrow attempts to compensate. In this case, other bone marrow cell lines will also be affected.

True aplastic anemia refers to a failure of the entire bone marrow. The shorter-lived granulocytes and platelets decrease first, followed by a progressively severe anemia that is normocytic and normochromic.

White Blood Cells

The white blood cells consist of the granulocytes (neutrophils in most mammals, heterophils in rabbits, reptiles, and birds; eosinophils; and basophils) and the agranulocytes (lymphocytes and monocytes). Although they are traditionally counted by determining each as a percentage of the total WBC population, meaningful interpretation requires that the absolute number of each type be calculated by multiplying the total white cell count by the fraction attributable to the individual cell type. An increased percentage that is due to an absolute decrease in another cell type is not an increase at all.

Mature **neutrophils** have a lobulated nucleus, but when demand is high immature cells with an unlobulated band nucleus may be released into circulation. They function as phagocytes and are important in infectious conditions and in inflammation. Increased neutrophil counts (neutrophilia) are caused by inflammation, bacterial infection, acute stress, steroid effects, and neoplasia of the granulocytic cell line (granulocytic leukemia can be difficult to differentiate from a simple neutrophilia without special stains or bone marrow biopsy). Decreased neutrophil counts (neutropenia) are caused by viral infections, toxin exposure (including foodborne toxins), certain drugs (eg, carbimazole and methimazole), autoimmune destruction of neutrophils, bone marrow neoplasia not involving the granulocytes, and bone marrow aplasia.

Eosinophils are characterized by prominent pink-staining granules on a Romanowsky stain. They inactivate histamine and inhibit edema formation. Increased eosinophil counts (eosinophilia) are caused by allergic/hypersensitivity reactions, parasitism, tissue injury, mast cell tumors, estrus, and pregnancy or parturition in the bitch. Some large continental dog breeds (eg, German and Belgian Shepherds, Rottweilers) normally have a relatively high eosinophil count. Extremely high eosinophil counts (hypereosinophilic syndrome), possibly due to an out-of-control hypersensitivity reaction, and eosinophil leukemia (a form of chronic myeloid leukemia) are also described. Decreased eosinophil count (eosinopenia) is almost always caused by the action of glucocorticoids, either endogenous or therapeutic.

Basophils are rare in most species and are characterized by blue-staining granules on a Romanowsky stain. They are closely related to mast cells and, like them, initiate the inflammatory response by releasing histamine. An increased basophil count (basophilia) accompanies eosinophilia in some species as part of the hypersensitivity reaction.

Monocytes are large cells with blue-gray cytoplasm, which may be vacuolated, and a kidney bean-shaped or lobulated nucleus. Their main function is phagocytosis, and they are essentially identical to tissue macrophages. An increased monocyte count (monocytosis) may occur in any chronic disease, especially chronic inflammation, and may be very marked in neoplasia. Monocytes also increase as part of the steroid response in dogs.

Lymphocytes mainly develop outside the bone marrow in the lymph nodes, spleen, and gut-associated lymphoid tissue. They are the smallest of the white cells, with a round, evenly staining nucleus and sparse cytoplasm. Their primary function is immunologic, including both antibody production and cell-mediated immune responses. Some survive only a few days, but many are long-lived. The number in circulation is a balance between populations in the blood, lymph, lymph nodes, and splenic follicles and does not necessarily reflect changes in lymphopoiesis. An increased lymphocyte count (lymphocytosis) may occur for physiologic reasons, especially in cats, but significant increases usually indicate leukemia. Immature or bizarre cells may also be recognized. Decreased lymphocyte counts (lymphopenia) are usually due to an effect of corticosteroids, either endogenous (stress or Cushing's disease) or therapeutic and may also accompany neutropenia in some viral infections, especially the parvoviruses. Lymphopenia may also be a feature of solid-organ lymphosarcomas, when leukemia is absent.

Platelets

Mammalian platelets are pale blue granular fragments (much smaller than RBC) that are shed from multinucleate megakaryocytes in the bone marrow; avian and reptilian platelets are true cells with nuclei. They maintain the integrity of the endothelium and act as part of the clotting process to repair damaged endothelium, where they ensure mechanical strength of the clot. Increased platelet counts (thrombocytosis) occur as a reaction to consumption following injury, when large juvenile platelets may also appear; after splenectomy, as splenic stores are liberated to the circulation; after vincristine treatment, which increases platelet shedding from megakaryocytes; and in megakaryocytic leukemia. Decreased platelet counts (thrombocytopenia) are caused by autoimmune reactions, thrombotic/thrombocytopenic purpura, bone marrow suppression and aplasia, bone marrow neoplasia, and equine infectious anemia. Signs are petechiation and ecchymosis more than frank hemorrhage, and little may be seen until the platelet count is $<20 \times 10^9/L$. Platelet functional abnormalities present similarly, but platelet numbers and morphology are normal.

Blood Sample Preparation and Evaluation

In-house hematologic investigations, with a minimum of specialist equipment, can provide almost as much information as a full laboratory analysis, although some estimations are qualitative rather than quantitative.

Blood for hematology should be collected into EDTA anticoagulant and immediately mixed well to avoid clotting. Larger (2.5 mL) tubes yield better results than the smaller (1 mL) pediatric tubes and are less likely to clot. Nevertheless, it is essential to fill the tube exactly to the mark, so smaller tubes may be unavoidable for small patients. White cell morphology deteriorates most quickly, especially in equine blood, so if the sample cannot be analyzed immediately, a thin blood smear should be submitted to the laboratory with the blood sample.

PCV is measured by microhematocrit, which is the reference method. A capillary tube is filled $^3/_4$ full with well-mixed blood and sealed at one end—heat-sealing is best if a bunsen burner is available, otherwise a proprietary clay pad is used. The tube is spun in a high-speed microhematocrit centrifuge for 6 min and the PCV is read using a microhematocrit reader with a sliding cursor. The appearance of the plasma (eg, normal, icteric, hemolyzed, lipemic) and the thickness of the buffy coat, which gives a very rough guide to total WBC count, should be noted.

Further information is obtained from a blood film. This is made by using one slide, with a corner broken off as a spreader, to pull a small drop of blood across a clean slide into a thin film. A suitable film is thin (1 erythrocyte thick) and tapers to a feathered edge before the far end of the slide. The broken corner of the spreader slide ensures 2 straight edges parallel to the long edges of the slide. Immediately after the film is spread, it is dried quickly by fanning the slide in the air. Air-dried smears can be sent to the laboratory in a slide mailer or stained and examined in the practice. Commercial rapid Romanowsky-type stains merely require the slide to be dipped in 3 colored solutions in succession. Cell morphology is clear and comparable to more permanent stains such as Leishman's or May-Gruenwald-Giemsa, although quality deteriorates after a few days. The slide should be allowed to dry naturally or dried with a hair-dryer (do not wipe dry), and examined under oil immersion.

Clinically useful information may be easily achieved in-house for all hematologic variables. The main deficiency is the absence of a numerical WBC count, and hence of numerical values for the differential WBC count. This may be acceptable for an interim emergency investigation, and a WBC count using a hemocytometer slide may be attempted. A mirrored slide with an Improved Neubauer ruling may be used, with a cover slip fitted so that Newton's rings are visible on both sides. The blood sample is diluted 1:20 with Turck's fluid or a similar diluent. An automatic pipette capable of dispensing 0.95 mL and 0.05 mL (50 μL) should be used to ensure an accurate dilution. The sample should be mixed well and allowed to stand for 10 min while the stain is taken up by the cells. The chamber of the hemocytometer is then filled by using a capillary (PCV) tube.

The number of cells in each of the 4 large corner squares of the grid are counted and the total divided by 20 to calculate the total WBC count $\times 10^9$/L.

Several hematologic instruments are available for in-practice use. Those based on centrifugation, where WBC measurements are made by spreading a stained buffy coat, are not true hematology analyzers, but give approximate counts. Although a numerical estimate of total WBC count is provided, the differential WBC count cannot distinguish between lymphocytes and monocytes, and results do not always correlate well with standard methods. This method is only appropriate as an emergency approximation, and a blood film must always be examined in addition. It is also wise to check the PCV by microhematocrit.

Impedance counters (Coulter principle) are used by professional laboratories and perform well in experienced hands. However it is difficult to achieve optimal performance without trained technical staff. Non-Coulter-principle instruments should be avoided for veterinary use, as their results do not necessarily compare well on nonhuman samples. Instruments providing automated differential counts perform less well on nonhuman blood compared to human, and results must never be accepted without also checking a blood film. No hematology laboratory should be without the facility for examining blood films, and a blood film should be examined for every patient sample. Quality assurance issues are the same as for biochemistry laboratories (see p 1339). If accuracy and reliability cannot be guaranteed to the same standard as the referral laboratory, then results should not be relied on without external confirmation.

Red Blood Cells: The size, uniformity of size, and presence of microcytes, macrocytes, and abnormally shaped cells should be noted, along with cell color, uniformity of color, and the presence of hypochromasia, polychromasia, and nucleated RBC. An overall descriptive assessment of the RBC picture should be made, including the degree of regeneration or hypochromasia, if any.

White Blood Cells: A qualitative estimate of numbers should be made (ie, very low, low, normal, raised, high, very high). This can be remarkably consistent with practice. The proportions of each cell type can be estimated, or preferably, a formal differential count of 100 or 200 cells performed. Unusual or abnormal white cell forms (eg, band or toxic neutrophils), or pathologic cells (eg, prolymphocytes, lymphoblasts, or mast cells) should be noted.

Platelets: A qualitative estimate of platelet numbers, based on how many can be seen in a typical high-power field ($\times 1,000$, oil immersion) should be made. Several fields should be examined, more if numbers appear low. Results can be ranked as none seen (on entire slide), rare (very few on entire slide), low in number (<5 per high-power field), adequate (5-20 per high-power field), or abundant (>20 per high-power field). Normal platelet numbers in the horse are about half those of other species. In a sample more than a few hours old, platelets may clump into rafts, leaving areas of the slide apparently devoid of platelets. Slides should be scanned for rafts before reporting platelet numbers as low. Enlarged or macroplatelets should also be noted.

URINALYSIS

Urinalysis is an important laboratory test that can be readily performed in veterinary practice, and is considered part of a minimum database. It is useful in documenting various types of urinary tract diseases and may provide information about other systemic diseases, such as liver failure and hemolysis. Urine may be collected by cystocentesis, urethral catheterization, or voiding and should be evaluated within 30 min. If this is not possible, then it may be refrigerated for up to 24 hr; however, this may alter results of some tests, such as pH, protein, and sediment examination (crystals, casts, and cells).

Urine Appearance

Color: Normal urine is typically transparent and yellow or amber on visual inspection. The intensity of color is in part related to the volume of urine collected and concentration of urine produced; therefore, it should be interpreted in context of urine specific gravity (USG). Significant disease may exist when urine is normal in color. Abnormal urine color may be caused by presence of endogenous or exogenous pigments, but it does not provide specific information. Interpretation of semiquantitative reagent strips, which are colorimetric tests, requires knowledge of urine color because discolored urine may result in a false-positive result. Equine urine may turn brown after a period of time.

Turbidity: Urine is typically clear but may become less transparent with pigmenturia, crystalluria, hematuria, pyuria, lipiduria, or when other compounds such as mucus are present. Depending on the cause, increased turbidity may disappear with centrifugation of the sample.

Odor: Normal urine has a slight odor of ammonia; however, the odor is dependent on urine concentration. Some species, such as cats and goats, have pungent urine odor because of urine composition. Bacterial infection may result in a strong odor due to pyuria; a strong ammonia odor may occur if the bacteria produce urease.

Urine Chemistries

Urine must be at room temperature for accurate measurement of USG and for chemical analysis. These tests are usually done prior to centrifugation; however, if urine is discolored or turbid, it may be beneficial to perform these tests on supernatant (*see* URINE SEDIMENT, below).

Specific Gravity: The USG is determined using a refractometer designed for veterinary samples, which includes a scale calibrated specifically for cat urine. USG for species other than cats should be determined using the scale for dogs. In healthy animals, USG is highly variable, depending on fluid and electrolyte balance of the body. Interpretation of USG, therefore, depends on the clinical presentation and serum chemistry findings (*see also* URINARY SYSTEM INTRODUCTION, p 1250). An animal that is dehydrated or has other causes of prerenal azotemia will have hypersthenuric urine with a USG >1.025-1.040 (depending on species). Dilute urine in a dehydrated or azotemic animal is abnormal and could be caused by renal failure, hypo- or hyperadrenocorticism, hypercalcemia, diabetes mellitus, hyperthyroidism, diuretic therapy, or diabetes insipidus. Glucosuria increases the refractive index of urine, resulting in an increased USG despite increased urine volume.

Semiquantitative, Colorimetric Reagent Strips: Reagent strips such as Multistix® or Chemstrip® can be used to perform several semiquantitative chemical evaluations simultaneously. They are used routinely to determine urine pH, protein, glucose, ketones, bilirubin/urobilinogen, and occult blood. Some reagent strips include test pads for leukocyte esterase (for detection of WBC), nitrite (for detection of bacteria), and USG; these are not valid in animals and should not be used. Reagent strips are adversely affected by moisture and have a limited shelf life. Bottles should be kept tightly capped, and unused strips should be discarded after their expiration date.

Urine pH: Urine pH is typically acidic in dogs and cats and alkaline in horses and ruminants, but varies depending on diet, medications, or presence of disease. Reagent strip colorimetric test pads for pH determination are accurate to within ~0.5 pH units. For example, a reading of 6.5 means the actual pH is likely to be between 6.0 and 7.0. A bacterial urinary tract infection with a urease-producing microbe will result in alkaluria. Urine pH will affect crystalluria because some crystals, such as struvite, form in alkaline urine, while other crystals, such as cystine, form in acidic urine.

Protein: The protein test pad detects primarily albumin in urine. Proteinuria can be seen with inflammation, hemorrhage, or glomerular disease. A positive reaction must be interpreted in light of USG, pH, and urine sediment examination. For example, a trace amount of protein in concentrated urine is less significant than a trace amount of protein in dilute urine. Alkaluria will give a false positive reaction. Likewise, presence of other proteins, such as Bence-Jones proteins, will give false negative results. Proteinuria can be measured using sulfosalicylic acid precipitation, which detects albumin and globulins. If proteinuria is present with an inactive urine sediment, its significance can be verified and quantitated by dividing the urine protein concentration by the urine creatinine concentration (urine protein to urine creatinine ratio; UP:UC). Interpretation of a UP:UC is as follows: <0.5:1 is normal, 0.5-1.0:1.0 is questionable, and >1.0:1.0 is abnormal. It is important to ensure that hematuria, pyuria, and infection are not present before determining a UP:UC because inflammation and hemorrhage result in significant proteinuria.

Glucose: Glucosuria is not present normally because the renal threshold for glucose is >180 mg/dL in most species and >240 mg/dL in cats. With euglycemia, the amount of filtered glucose is less than the renal threshold and all of the filtered glucose is reabsorbed in the proximal renal tubules. Glucosuria can result from hyperglycemia (due to diabetes mellitus, excessive endogenous or exogenous glucocorticoids, or stress) or from a proximal renal tubular defect (such as primary renal glucosuria or Fanconi syndrome). If glucosuria is present, blood glucose concentration should be determined.

Ketones: The ketone test pad detects acetate and acetoacetate, but not β-hydroxybutyrate. Ketonuria is associated with primary ketosis (ruminants), ketosis secondary to diabetes mellitus (small animals), and occasionally with prolonged fasting or starvation. A false positive reaction can occur with presence of reducing substances in urine.

Bilirubin/Urobilinogen: Presence of conjugated bilirubin in urine will result in a positive reaction. A tablet test, Ictotest®, can be used to detect bilirubin as well. Bilirubinuria occurs when conjugated bilirubin exceeds the renal threshold as with liver disease or hemolysis. In dogs with concentrated urine, a small amount of bilirubin can be normal. Pigmenturia may result in a false positive reaction. Urobilinogen, formed from bilirubin by intestinal microflora, is absorbed into the portal circulation and is excreted renally. A small amount of urinary urobilinogen is normal. Increased urinary urobilinogen occurs with hyperbilirubinemia; a negative test may be observed with biliary obstruction. However, the test is not specific enough to be clinically useful.

Occult Blood: The occult blood test pad uses a "pseudoperoxidase" method to detect intact RBC, hemoglobin, and myoglobin. A positive reaction can be due to hemorrhage (hematuria), intravascular hemolysis (hemoglobinuria), or myoglobinuria. The latter 2 processes can be distinguished by examination of plasma—plasma will appear pink to red after intravascular hemolysis, while myoglobin is rapidly cleared from plasma, resulting in clear plasma. As with other colorimetric test pads, discolored urine may yield false positive results. A positive result should be interpreted with microscopic examination of urine sediment.

Urine Sediment

Microscopic examination of urine sediment should be part of a routine urinalysis. For centrifugation, 3-5 mL of urine is transferred to a conical centrifuge tube. Urine is centrifuged at 1,500-2,000 rpm for ~5 min. The supernatant is decanted, leaving ~0.5 mL of urine and sediment in the tip of the conical tube. The sediment is resuspended by tapping the tip of the conical tube against the table several times. A few drops of the sediment are transferred to a glass slide, and a cover slip is applied. Examination of unstained urine is recommended for routine samples. Microscopic examination is performed at 100× (for crystals, casts, and cells) and 400× (for cells and bacteria) magnifications. Contrast of the sample is enhanced by closing the iris diaphragm and lowering the condenser of the microscope. Stains such as Sedistain® and new methylene blue can be used to aid in cell identification but tend to dilute the specimen and introduce artifacts such as stain precipitate and crystals.

Red Blood Cells: In an unstained preparation, RBC are small and round and have a slight orange tint and a smooth appearance. Normal urine should contain <5 RBC/field at 400× magnification. Increased RBC in urine (hematuria) indicates hemorrhage somewhere in the urogenital system; however, sample collection by cystocentesis or catheterization may cause hemorrhage.

White Blood Cells: WBC are slightly larger than RBC and have a grainy cytoplasm. Normal urine should contain <5 WBC/field at 400× magnification. Increased WBC (pyuria) can occur due to inflammation, infection, trauma, or neoplasia. Catheterization or collection of voided urine may introduce a few WBC from the urogenital tract.

Epithelial Cells: Transitional epithelial cells, a common urine contaminant derived from the bladder and proximal urethra, resemble WBC but are larger. They have a greater amount of grainy cytoplasm and a round, centrally located nucleus. In a voided urine sample, squamous epithelial cells may be observed. They are large, oval to cuboidal in shape, and may or may not contain a nucleus. Occasionally, neoplastic transitional cells may be observed in an animal with a transitional cell carcinoma. Neoplastic squamous cells may be observed in an animal with a squamous cell carcinoma.

Cylindruria (Casts): Casts are elongated, cylindrical structures formed by mucoprotein congealing within renal tubules and may contain cells. Hyaline casts have parallel sides and rounded ends and are composed of mucoprotein. They may occur with fever, exercise, and renal disease. Epithelial cellular casts form from entrapment of sloughed tubular epithelial cells in the mucoprotein; they may be observed with renal disease. Granular casts are thought to represent degenerated epithelial cellular casts. Waxy casts have a granular appearance, and are thought to arise from longstanding granular casts. They typically have sharp borders with broken ends. Other cellular casts include erythrocyte casts and WBC casts. Erythrocyte casts form because of renal hemorrhage. WBC casts occur because of renal inflammation, as with pyelonephritis. Fatty casts are not common, but can be observed with disorders of lipid metabolism, such as diabetes mellitus. A few hyaline or granular casts are considered normal. However, presence of cellular casts or other casts in high numbers indicates renal damage, and may be one of the earliest laboratory abnormalities noted with toxic damage to renal epithelial cells (eg, gentamicin, amphotericin B).

Infectious Organisms: The presence of bacteria in urine collected by cystocentesis indicates infection. Small numbers of bacteria from the lower urogenital tract may contaminate voided samples or samples collected by catheterization and do not indicate infection. Bacterial rods are most easily identified in urine sediment. Particles of debris may be mistaken for bacteria. Suspected bacteria can be confirmed by staining urine sediment with Gram's stain; however, aerobic culture is best to confirm a bacterial urinary tract infection. Rarely, yeast and fungal hyphae and parasitic ova may be observed in urine sediment. Their presence is not always associated with clinical disease. Parasitic ova observed include *Stephanus dentatus*, *Capillaria plica*, *C felis*, and *Dioctophyma renale*. Additionally, microfilariae of *Dirofilaria immitis* may be observed in urine sediment.

Crystals: Many urine sediments contain crystals. The type of crystal present depends on urine pH, concentration of crystallogenic materials, urine temperature, and length of time between urine collection and examination. Crystalluria is not synonymous with urolithiasis and is not necessarily pathologic. Furthermore, uroliths may form without observed crystalluria. Struvite crystals are commonly observed in canine and feline urine. Struvite crystalluria in dogs is not a problem unless there is a concurrent bacterial urinary tract infection with a urease-producing microbe. Without an infection, struvite crystals in dogs will not be associated with struvite urolith formation. However, some animals (eg, cats) do form struvite uroliths without a bacterial urinary tract infection. In these animals, struvite crystalluria may be pathologic. Struvite crystals appear typically as "coffin-lids" or "prisms"; however, they may be amorphous. Calcium oxalate crystalluria occurs less commonly in dogs and cats; if persistent, it may indicate an increased risk for calcium oxalate urolith formation. (*See also* UROLITHIASIS, p 1259 and p 1279.) However, calcium oxalate and calcium carbonate crystalluria is common in healthy horses and cattle. Calcium oxalate dihydrate crystals appear as squares with an "X" in the middle or "envelope-shaped." Calcium oxalate monohydrate crystals are "dumb-bell" shaped. An unusual form of calcium oxalate crystals is typically seen in association with ethylene glycol toxicity (p 2357). These crystals occur in neutral to acidic urine. They are small, flat, and colorless, and are shaped like "picket fence posts." Ammonium acid urate crystals suggest liver disease (eg, portosystemic shunt). These crystals occur in acidic urine and are yellow-brown spheres with irregular, spiny projections; however, they may also be amorphous. Certain species, such as birds and reptiles, and certain breeds of dogs, specifically Dalmatians, can normally have ammonium acid urate crystalluria. Cystine crystals are 6-sided and of variable size. They occur in acidic urine. Presence of cystine crystals represents a proximal tubular defect in amino acid reabsorption. Cystinuria has been reported to occur in many breeds of dogs and rarely in cats. Dachshunds, Newfoundlands, English Bulldogs, and Scottish Terriers have a high incidence of cystine urolithiasis. Bilirubin crystals occur with bilirubinuria; however, they may be normal in small numbers in dogs.

Lipids: Fat droplets are commonly present in urine from dogs and cats and may be mistaken for RBC. However, they often vary in size and tend to float on a different plane of focus than the remainder of the sediment. They are not considered to be pathologic.

Spermatozoa: Spermatozoa may be observed normally in urine collected from male dogs.

Plant Material: Occasionally, plant material may be observed in urine samples collected by voiding. When present, they indicate contamination of the urine sample and are not pathologic.

PARASITOLOGY

Internal Parasite Diagnosis in Small Animals

Diagnosis of internal parasites in small animals is typically done by examination of feces for parasite eggs. Fecal samples should be fresh, preferably collected from the rectum using a fecal loop. Specimens submitted to a diagnostic laboratory should be fixed in 10% formaldehyde solution or sent chilled. Other preservative solutions (eg, sodium acetate formalin, polyvinyl alcohol, available in commercial mailer kits) better preserve protozoa and facilitate special staining (eg, trichrome, iron hematoxylin).

Routine examinations should be done by both direct fecal smear and fecal flotation. Direct smears are prepared by mixing feces (an amount of feces fitting on one-half the tip of an applicator stick) with 1 drop each of saline (for motile organisms), and Lugol's iodine stain (to see internal structures, eg, *Giardia*), covering with separate coverslips on the same slide. Flotation methods concentrate diagnostic stages and provide a cleaner final preparation, using about 2 g feces. Sugar (specific gravity [sg] 1.27) and sodium nitrate (sg 1.39) are commonly used flotation media. Zinc sulfate flotation (sg 1.18), repeated on 3 consecutive days, is the method of choice for concentrating *Giardia* cysts, which are intermittently shed, and larvae that crenate in media of higher specific gravity. Motile larvae may be collected and concentrated by Baermann sedimentation; a convenient method for small animals is to place feces on a sheet of gauze in a tea strainer in the opening of a conical glass filled with warm tap water or saline for 1 hr before sediment examination. Special procedures, such as formalin-ethyl acetate sedimentation may be used for parasitic larval stages that do not float well. Sheather's sugar (sg 1.30) can be used to detect small oocysts of *Cryptosporidium* (4-6 μ) or *Toxoplasma* (12 μ) by focusing just under the coverslip on oocysts allowed to "float up twice" in the media film on slides placed on a counter for 10 min before examination.

A direct smear using 1 drop of blood is an effective screening procedure for detection of motile microfilariae of *Dirofilaria*. More accurate examination of blood may be done by a Knotts' test. For the latter, 1 mL blood is added to 9 mL of 2% formalin solution in a 15 mL tube and centrifuged at 1,500 rpm. The supernatant is discarded and a drop of new methylene blue stain is mixed with the sediment "button," which is pipetted onto a microscope slide, covered with a coverslip, and examined to differentiate *Dirofilaria* from nonpathogenic *Dipetalonema* infections. Commercial filtration and staining procedures are effective alternatives to the Knotts' test. Animals on heartworm preventive become amicrofilaremic, and an occult heartworm test for circulating uterine antigen of adult female *Dirofilaria* is the method of choice for treated dogs. Feline dirofilariasis cannot be reliably diagnosed by microfilaremia or antigenemia tests because heartworm numbers are typically too low; antibody titers to *Dirofilaria* are used to detect prior exposure and possible current infection in cats.

Internal Parasite Diagnosis in Livestock

Fresh fecal samples should be collected from livestock from pasture or, preferably, per rectum using plastic gloves (which may be inverted to act as a receptacle after sample collection). A representative number of herd samples should be collected from a minimum of 10 animals to account for the typical high individual variation in numbers of eggs shed. Samples can be combined after thorough mixing to enable examination of a single herd composite sample.

Quantitative fecal egg counts by the Wisconsin centrifugal flotation procedure or similar methods can be used to estimate relative infection burden for nematodes of the "GI parasite complex," while also detecting coccidia and other parasites such as lungworm larvae and tapeworms. Three g of feces are placed in a container, suspended in ~15 mL water, strained through a gauze square into a 15 mL tube, and centrifuged (1,500 rpm for 3 min). The supernatant is decanted and the sediment mixed with saturated sugar solution, filling the tube enough to form a positive meniscus before placing a 22 × 22 mm coverslip on the lip of the tube orifice. The tube is centrifuged again at low speed (1,500 rpm for 5 min). The coverslip, with the surface film containing eggs, is removed and transferred to a microscope slide for counting of trichostrongyle- and strongyle-type eggs. The total is divided by 3 to derive eggs/g (EPG). Other parasites are noted, if present, with a general abundance designation of +1 (few), +2 (small number), +3 (large number), or +4 (too numerous to count).

A saturated solution of table salt (sg 1.20) is a cheap alternative medium for diagnosis of livestock parasites. Magnesium sulfate (sg 1.20) is the preferred medium for swine. Special slides containing chambers with etched areas of known volume are also used for estimating EPG, especially for small ruminants. Feces in a strained solution (usually saturated salt) are introduced into each chamber with a Pasteur pipette, and the eggs are counted under low-power magnification. A commonly used counting slide is the McMaster slide, which has 2 chambers, each with a volume of 0.15 mL under the etched area. For example, if 3 g of feces are mixed with 42 mL of concentrate solution, then each egg counted is multiplied by 50 to yield the number of EPG in the fecal sample. Acceptable correlation between the EPG and the relative worm burden is often possible in young animals, although low (<5 EPG) or negative counts are typically found in adult animals. In young cattle, which generally have EPG counts 10 times that of adult animals, EPG counts >50 reflect a moderate infection, and EPG counts >500 indicate a heavy burden and a need for treatment.

Because fluke eggs do not float readily, quantitative fecal sedimentation procedures are usually used. Two grams of feces are mixed with 35 mL soapy solution (2% liquid detergent) and strained through gauze into a 50-mL centrifuge tube. The tube is filled with soapy water and allowed to stand for 3 min, after which $^1/_2$ of the supernatant is discarded. This is repeated 2-3 times until the supernatant is clean. All but 15 mL is poured off, 2 drops of new methylene blue are added, and the eggs counted with a dissecting microscope in a gridded Petri dish or by examining several coverslipped microscope slides. The liver fluke, *Fasciola*, can be differentiated from *Paramphistomum*, the rumen fluke, by the golden color, more barreled shape, and slightly larger size of *Fasciola* versus the gray color, more pointed end, and smaller size of the usually nonpathogenic rumen fluke. Commercial sieve-sediment kits can reduce sample preparation time by 50%. In cattle, *Fasciola* EPG counts >3 suggest economic losses; EPG >10 may be associated with clinical signs.

Examination for Ectoparasites

Animals with dermatoses should be evaluated by examining for ectoparasites or evidence of their presence. For example, fleas may not be seen on a cat or dog, but small black flecks of excrement that produce a reddish stain when placed on a wet paper towel may be noted. Skin must sometimes be scraped to diagnose parasites. A scalpel blade is used for the deep scrapings (until blood oozes) needed to demonstrate parasites (eg, *Sarcoptes, Demodex* spp) that live in burrows or hair follicles. The scraped material is placed in a drop of mineral oil on a slide, and the entire area under the coverglass is scanned under low-power magnification. A few drops of 10% potassium hydroxide solution may be added to clear debris and allow better visualization.

SEROLOGY

In-house serologic test kits have continued to improve in reliability, ease of use, and types available. They include tests for infectious disease antigens and antibodies, hormones, and immunoglobulin levels. Many of these tests are ELISA that may be microwell or membrane-based, but other types including immunomigration and agglutination tests are also available. Sample requirements may be plasma, serum, whole blood, feces, or saliva, depending on the test format.

Feline Leukemia Virus (FeLV): Serologic testing for FeLV is important in order to identify infected cats and prevent transmission of the virus (*see* p 631). Testing is also recommended prior to vaccination against FeLV because vaccination of infected cats will not limit development or transmission of disease. Most currently available in-house diagnostic kits are designed to detect soluble FeLV-specific *gag* protein p27, which is produced in large amounts during viremia. The time between infection and the presence of detectable antigen varies, but is likely to be within 28 days. Vaccination against FeLV will not yield a positive test result when antigen tests are used, nor will the presence of maternally-derived antibodies in kittens. Testing serum or plasma is considered more reliable than testing whole blood, saliva, or tears. Most test kits have positive and negative controls incorporated into the kit, so technical problems with running the test may be detected. There is a relatively high rate of false positive results with these tests of soluble antigen, especially in a population of cats with a low incidence of disease. A true positive result may reflect either transient or persistent viremia, so clinical decisions should not be based on a single test result. Confirmation of positive results, especially in asymptomatic cats, should be pursued by testing for cell-associated antigen, eg, with an immunofluorescent antibody assay.

Feline Immunodeficiency Virus (FIV): Because the concentration of FIV antigen in the blood of infected cats is often very low, in-house diagnostic tests are designed to detect anti-FIV antibodies rather than antigen. Test kits yield a positive or negative result for antibody rather than a quantitative result. Antibodies usually develop within 60 days of infection, but this time period is quite variable and a few infected cats fail to develop detectable antibody levels. Once present, antibodies appear to be present for life, except for those transiently detectable in kittens that have maternally-derived antibodies. A kitten <6 mo of age that tests positive should be retested after 6 mo of age for this reason. If the test is still positive, the kitten is most likely infected.

With ELISA tests, the incidence of false positives is relatively high. Positive results, especially in asymptomatic cats, should be confirmed by another test such as Western blot. Currently, antibodies produced in response to vaccination with FIV vaccine cannot be reliably distinguished from those produced by natural infection, so results must be interpreted with knowledge of a cat's vaccination history. In addition, kittens born to vaccinated queens are antibody-positive for a variable length of time. PCR testing may be able to distinguish naturally-infected cats from vaccinated cats, but this method is unlikely to become practical for in-clinic laboratories.

Canine Parvovirus (CPV): Both ELISA and immunomigration test kits are available for detection of CPV antigen in feces. These tests are fairly specific for the virus, but sensitivity is somewhat lower for several reasons. Fecal shedding only occurs for ~7-10 days, beginning on day 3-5 following exposure, so virus is not always detectable in dogs with clinical signs. Blood in the stool as well as the formation of antigen-antibody complexes may be associated with false negative results.

Because of interest in measuring serum antibodies to CPV to evaluate the need for revaccination and the presence of possibly interfering maternal antibodies, in-house tests for assay of anti-CPV antibody have become available. These tests are not intended to diagnose parvovirus infection and do not distinguish between natural exposure and vaccine-induced antibodies. Currently available test kits are ELISA for detection of IgG antibody in serum or plasma. They are semiquantitative and use color changes in positive control wells compared to color changes in samples to determine relative antibody levels. The level of anti-CPV antibody that is protective against infection is not known, but results are interpreted based on protective titers measured by other methods.

Canine Distemper Virus: In-house test kits for determination of antibodies to canine distemper virus are available in combination with CPV antibody testing. As with the CPV kits, these tests are semiquantitative ELISA for anti-canine distemper IgG in serum or plasma. They may be used to evaluate the need for revaccination and to determine the level of maternal antibody present in puppies.

Borrelia burgdorferi: Lyme disease (p 485) is caused by the tickborne spirochete *B burgdorferi*. In general, diagnostic tests for this infection have several potential problems, including relatively high levels of false positive results that may be difficult to distinguish from subclinical infections, persistence of antibodies following apparent resolution of clinical disease, interpretation of antibody titers in vaccinated dogs, and the fact that detectable antibody may not be present until 4-6 wk after exposure. There are several in-clinic ELISA test kits for detection of anti-*B burgdorferi* antibodies in serum or plasma. One of these tests uses a synthetic peptide derived from a *B burgdorferi*-specific protein that is important in inducing a humoral immune response by 4-5 wk following infection in dogs. In addition to reducing the level of cross-reaction with other infectious agents because of its specificity, this test does not give a positive result to vaccine antigens and thus appears to distinguish vaccine-induced antibodies from those produced in response to natural infections. Current in-house tests are not quantitative; they give only a positive or negative result and are not suitable for monitoring response to treatment.

Ehrlichia canis: Canine ehrlichiosis (p 638) is a tickborne disease caused by a rickettsial organism. It can be associated with thrombocytopenia, anemia, and neutropenia as well as other nonspecific clinical signs. While identification of *Ehrlichia* morulae in leukocytes can be diagnostic for this infection, serologic assay for detection of antibodies is more common and has better sensitivity. In-house tests for ehrlichiosis are either qualitative (giving only a positive or negative result) or semiquantitative; those currently available are ELISA to be performed on serum, plasma, or whole blood. Newer tests that use recombinant analogs of major outer membrane proteins of *E canis* are more reliable than those using whole *E canis* proteins as the antigen. Because anti-*E canis* antibodies may be very long-lived and may be present in subclinical infections, detection of these antibodies does not distinguish between exposure and *Ehrlichia*-induced illness and cannot reliably indicate success of response to therapy.

Brucella canis: Infection with *B canis* may be subclinical, or it may cause a variety of clinical signs including abortion, infertility, and diskospondylitis (*see* p 1159). Infection most often occurs during mating; thus, testing of breeding animals is important in disease prevention. An in-house test for anti-*B canis* antibody is a rapid slide agglutination test that includes a 2-mercaptoethanol (2-ME) step to reduce false-positive reactions by eliminating nonspecific IgM reactions. This assay detects serum antibody to surface antigens of the bacteria. If the first step (with no 2-ME) shows agglutination, the second step (with 2-ME) is performed to rule out a nonspecific reaction. Although this test is very convenient as a rapid screening test, some newer ELISA techniques performed in reference laboratories have higher specificity and sensitivity, especially in the early stages of infection.

Heartworm Antigen—Dogs: Serologic testing for heartworm antigen in dogs is more sensitive than screening for microfilaremia and, in addition, can detect occult infections. Heartworm antigen is first detectable at ~5 mo postinfection and will usually precede microfilaremia by a few weeks. There are several different antigen test formats available including ELISA with microwells, membrane ELISA, agglutination, and lateral flow membrane immunomigration. Serum or plasma may be used in all kits, and some may be run using whole blood. Some test kits can be stored at room temperature, while others must be stored refrigerated and brought to room temperature before use. Batch testing and single sample testing are both available. All of the test kits have very high specificity. False-positive results are most often due to technical problems such as inadequate washing or failure to read the results at the optimal time. The manufacturer's instructions should be closely followed with any of the test formats.

Sensitivity varies from one test to another and is affected by worm load, worm gender (a female antigen is detected, thus male-only infections will not be detected), and maturity of female worms. None of these tests has 100% sensitivity. When unexpected false results are obtained on an antigen test, additional testing, using a different format, is recommended.

Following adulticide treatment, antigenemia should become undetectable within 4-5 mo. It can take more than a month for some adult heartworms to die, however, so a positive antigen test at 4-5 mo post-treatment does not necessarily indicate treatment failure and the test should be repeated 2-3 mo later.

Heartworm Antibody and Antigen—Cats: Heartworm disease in cats is substantially different from the disease in dogs, and recommendations for serologic testing are consequently different. Cats tend to have a much lower worm burden—often only 1 or 2 worms. Cats also have single-sex infections more frequently than do dogs. Circulating microfilaremia is rare in cats, and microfilariae have a shorter life span. These differences are often attributed to a more effective feline immune response to heartworm infection. Heartworms can, however, cause serious disease in cats.

Heartworm antigen tests are less sensitive for detection of infection in cats than they are in dogs. Antibody testing may be preferred because antibodies are produced to both male and female worms, and they are produced as early as 2 mo after infection, which is much earlier than antigen may be detected. The presence of antibody does not confirm feline heartworm disease, because transient exposure to larvae will stimulate production of antibody. Many early infections are cleared spontaneously, and adult heartworms never develop. A combination of testing for heartworm antigen and anti-heartworm antibody is warranted in cats with clinical signs of heartworm disease when results of a single test are not conclusive.

Test kits for detection of anti-heartworm antibody in cats are marketed in several different formats. These can be run using either plasma or serum and are qualitative rather than quantitative. There are currently test kits specific for heartworm antigenemia in cats as well as those that can be used to test either canine or feline samples.

Canine Pregnancy Diagnosis—Relaxin: The only known pregnancy-specific hormone in the bitch is relaxin, which is produced by the placenta when a fertilized egg is implanted. Relaxin is first detectable in the plasma around day 22-25 following fertilization. It is not present in pseudopregnant or nonpregnant bitches. Relaxin levels peak by about day 40-50 of gestation and drop at parturition, but they may remain detectable for up to 50 days during lactation. In-clinic test kits to measure relaxin include microwell ELISA and immunomigration qualitative tests requiring serum, plasma, or whole blood. The assays appear to have very good specificity; that is, a detectable level of relaxin is not found in nonpregnant bitches. False negatives have been reported in some bitches carrying very small litters or in those with 1 or more nonviable puppies.

Canine Ovulation and Whelping Timing—Luteinizing Hormone: In the bitch, serum luteinizing hormone (LH) is normally present in very low levels except for a dramatic rise just prior to ovulation. Ovulation occurs 2 days after this LH surge, and the LH level returns to baseline within 24-40 hr of peaking. Serum progesterone levels begin to rise at the time of the LH surge. A bitch will be fertile between days 4-7 following the LH surge with the most fertile period on days 5 and 6. In addition, the LH surge determines the gestation period, with parturition occurring between day 64 and 66 following the surge. The LH surge may occur anywhere from 3 days before to 5 days after the onset of estrus behavior, so it cannot be reliably predicted by behavior.

Ovulation timing by measurement of LH requires daily testing, which usually begins when >50% of vaginal epithelial cells are cornified, based on vaginal cytology. There is occasionally a false LH peak that is not followed by ovulation, but it will also not be followed by an increase in progesterone. For that reason, assay of both LH and progesterone are recommended for most accurate ovulation detection. An elevated LH concentration that is not followed by increased progesterone levels is considered a proestrus fluctuation and testing for ovulation should continue.

In-clinic kits to measure LH concentrations in serum are essentially qualitative, with a serum level of <1 ng/mL being read as negative and a positive test indicating LH concentration of >1 ng/mL. Current test kits have a short shelf life.

Canine Ovulation Timing—Progesterone: Serum progesterone begins to increase following the LH surge with a concentration of 2.0-3.9 ng/mL on the day before ovulation and 4.0-10.0 ng/mL on the day of ovulation. Progesterone continues to increase and stays elevated throughout pregnancy or diestrus. As the rise in progesterone is more constant, compared to LH, daily testing is not necessary. It is recommended that testing begin in late proestrus and continue every 2-3 days until a high range is reached, indicating ovulation.

The test kits for in-clinic progesterone testing are semiquantitative ELISA with levels of <1 ng/mL, <2 ng/mL, or <4 ng/mL designated as pre-ovulatory, depending on the kit. Some kits are designed to give 2 additional progesterone ranges (intermediate and high), while others will indicate only pre-ovulatory and "ovulatory day or later" levels. In comparison with other test methods, the in-house test kits are less accurate, particularly in the range of roughly 1.5-10 ng/mL, which is the range of interest for earliest detection of ovulation. Accuracy is greater at higher progesterone levels. As mentioned above, measurement of both LH and progesterone is recommended for most accurate breeding management.

Thyroxine: Assay of total serum thyroxine (T_4) may be used as a screening test for canine hypothyroidism or as a diagnostic test for feline hyperthyroidism. (*See also* THE THYROID GLAND, p 460.) In addition, T_4 concentrations are measured when monitoring therapy for hypo- or hyperthyroidism. An in-house ELISA test kit, which uses an additional instrument to read results, provides semiquantitative information about T_4 concentration in canine and feline sera. The assay is run at 1 of 2 "dynamic ranges" depending on the predicted range of results. Although there are currently few published studies comparing this assay with other test methods for T_4, one comparison of this kit with a radioimmunoassay reported a fairly low correlation in comparing results using the 2 methods.

Foal Immunoglobulin (IgG): Measurement of foal serum IgG concentration within the first 24 hr after birth can be useful in preventing disease related to failure of passive transfer of IgG from mare to foal in colostrum. Use of foal-side testing procedures can facilitate prompt diagnosis and treatment. A foal serum IgG level of >800 mg/dL is generally considered optimal, with <200 mg/dL indicating failure of passive transfer. Concentrations of 200-800 mg/dL are considered evidence of partial transfer.

Although radial immunodiffusion (RID) is considered the most accurate test for IgG concentration, it takes much longer (5-24 hr) than many of the other test methods and thus is not as useful as an indicator of the need for therapeutic intervention. More rapid screening tests include the zinc sulfate turbidity test, glutaraldehyde clot test, and ELISA test kits. The zinc sulfate test estimates IgG in serum based on its precipitation when added to a zinc-containing solution. Turbidity generally becomes visible when there are 400-500 mg/dL IgG. This test takes ~1hr and may be performed with zinc sulfate solutions made in the clinic, or reagents for the test may be purchased as a test kit. The glutaraldehyde clot test requires the addition of 1 volume of serum to 10 volumes of 10% glutaraldehyde and examination of the tubes at timed intervals up to 60 min. The presence of IgG in the serum causes formation of a solid clot in the tube. Clot formation in <10 min generally correlates to an IgG concentration of >800 mg/dL, while a positive reaction within 60 min is interpreted as >400 mg/dL of IgG. Both of these test methods use serum, rather than plasma, so time for the blood to clot and separation of serum must be added to the time needed to perform the test. ELISA test kits for in-house or foal-side testing can use either serum or whole blood as the sample and take ~10 min. They are semiquantitative with color changes corresponding to IgG concentrations of <400 mg/dL, 400-800 mg/dL, or >800 mg/dL. Results, especially at high and low IgG levels, have been shown to correlate well with RID results.

Calf Immunoglobulin: Measurement of IgG concentration in neonatal calf serum is important for the same reasons described for foals. IgG levels are, however, different from those in foals, with >1,000 mg/dL considered evidence of adequate passive transfer and <1,000 mg/dL indicating failure of passive transfer. As with foals, RID is the gold standard for accurate measurement of serum IgG, but the length of time required to complete this assay makes it less useful than other methods. Other methods that have been used include zinc sulfate and sodium sulfite turbidity tests, glutaraldehyde coagulation test, measurement of total serum solids by refractometry, and a lateral flowthrough ELISA test kit.

The sodium sulfite and zinc sulfate turbidity tests are both based on the precipitation of high molecular weight proteins in these solutions. Serum is used as the sample and tests are read after 15-30 min of incubation. Results of these tests vary in sensitivity and specificity depending on the endpoint chosen, and there are some technical difficulties with reagents that can decrease test performance. The glutaraldehyde clot test is performed as in foals, with no clot formation at 60 min indicating failure of passive transfer.

Measurement of serum total protein by refractometer is a fairly reliable indicator of adequate passive transfer in healthy, well-hydrated calves. A level of 5.2 g/dL is roughly equivalent to an IgG concentration of 1,000 mg/dL.

A commercially-available ELISA test kit uses serum as the sample and takes ~20 min. The assay is qualitative in that it indicates an IgG concentration of >1,000 mg/dL or <1,000 mg/dL. Sensitivity and specificity are reasonably good and this test is less influenced by factors such as calf dehydration or reagent instability than some other methods. Manufacturer recommendations for storing and using the kits must be followed.

DIAGNOSTIC IMAGING

RADIOGRAPHY

Radiography is one of the most commonly used diagnostic tools in veterinary practice. It provides a large amount of information to the veterinarian by noninvasive and economical means. It does not alter the disease process or cause unacceptable discomfort to the animal. Although radiography is painless, sedation is often desirable in order to reduce anxiety and stress associated with the procedure.

Equipment: Radiographs are made using a specialized type of vacuum tube that produces x-rays. The tube current, measured in milliamperes (mA), and voltage, measured in kilovolts (kV), determine the strength and number of x-rays produced and are 2 of the 3 exposure factors which can be set on most x-ray machines. Kilovoltage potential (kVp) is the highest potential voltage achieved at a certain kV setting.

Higher kV settings produce more penetrating beams in which a higher percentage of the x-rays produced penetrate the subject being radiographed. There is also a decrease in the percentage difference in absorption between tissue types. This results in a decrease in contrast (long-scale contrast) on the final film. High kVp techniques are most useful for studies of body regions with many different tissue densities (eg, thorax). Higher kVp techniques are appropriate for larger and thicker animals. Increasing kV is not a linear function, and small increases in kVp settings may substantially increase the number of x-rays penetrating the animal. However, this effect is much less dramatic above 85 kVp.

Increasing the mA setting on the machine increases the number of x-rays produced. The energy spectrum of the x-ray beam is essentially unchanged, as is the relative numbers of x-ray photons penetrating tissues of different densities such as bone, soft tissue, and fat. However, the amount of darkening on the film is related to the total number of photons reaching it. Therefore, increasing mA increases film contrast. Changes in mA settings are relatively linear. Increased contrast is desirable where tissue densities are similar (eg, musculoskeletal system).

The third major parameter in the making of a radiographic exposure is exposure time. Increasing the exposure time increases the number of photons produced and hence the darkness of the film. For exposure in the general diagnostic range, this a linear function.

All 3 of the above parameters are interdependent. Exposure time and mA are so much so that the term milliampere-seconds (mAs) is usually used to indicate the product of these 2 factors. Increasing the mA and decreasing the exposure time by a proportionate amount results in a radiograph that is less likely to be degraded by motion. As a rule, it is best to minimize the exposure time but maintain an appropriate mAs and scale of contrast. Increasing kVp increases the number of photons penetrating the patient and also darkens the film. This effect can be used within limits to correct an underexposure. The converse is likewise true.

When correcting a previously unsatisfactory film, underexposure or overexposure should be corrected by adjusting the mAs when examining areas of high contrast (skeleton) or by adjusting the kVp when examining areas of low contrast (thorax). This will maintain the same relative contrast for that anatomic area while adjusting the film darkness.

Establishing a technique chart for making radiographs makes it easy for the operator to arrive at a technique by simply correcting a standardized protocol for the size of the animal being examined and the anatomic area under consideration. It also ensures that radiographs of the same anatomic region will have a consistent appearance from animal to animal. A technique chart must be made for each machine. Some generalizations can be made, however. Exposure factors for the thorax should have mAs values ≤5 unless the animal is very large. Values of 10 for the abdomen and 15-20 for skeletal studies are appropriate. In many modern x-ray machines, the technique chart is built into the machine. The operator need only enter the body part and thickness and the machine automatically sets the technique. This is convenient and reduces mistakes in technique, but the settings may need to be altered to suit the specific equipment, film-screen speed, and the viewer's preferences (eg, contrast level).

Automatic exposure control (AEC) is a system in which the operator sets the kVp and mA and the machine terminates the exposure at the appropriate time. If used properly, this system results in nearly identical film exposures between animals. However, appropriate kV settings are needed, and animal positioning is critical. Identical positioning between animals is required to achieve identical films. Placing the heart or lungs over the AEC sensor results in radically different appearing radiographs. AEC is probably most effective when large numbers of films are being done of the same anatomic area by the same personnel.

X-ray machines today are equipped with collimators that allow adjustment of the size of the beam to the size of the area being radiographed. This reduces the amount of scatter radiation generated, thus improving image contrast and detail. Scatter radiation is also the major source of radiation exposure to operators, so proper collimation is important in reducing this risk.

When a radiograph is taken, some of the x-rays are scattered. When the object being radiographed is ≥10 cm thick, scattering becomes a problem by causing unwanted exposure of the x-ray film. A grid, which is a thin plate made up of alternating thin strips of lead and plastic, can be placed between the animal and the film to reduce the scattered x-rays from exposing the film. The ability of a grid to remove scattered radiation is measured by the grid ratio. The grid ratio is determined by the height of the lead strips divided by the distance between them. A grid with an 8:1 ratio will eliminate more scattered radiation from exposing the film than will a grid with a 6:1 ratio.

Recording of the radiographic image has traditionally been done on specially optimized film. However, even the best silver halide film is relatively insensitive to x-rays. For that reason, the film is usually placed between specially designed phosphorescent screens—panels composed of microscopic phosphorescent crystals embedded in a plastic matrix that directs the spread of the phosphorescent light toward the film. These screens are much more sensitive to x-rays than film. When the x-ray strikes a crystal, it phosphoresces and the light exposes the film secondarily. This process of recording the x-ray image is much more efficient than using film alone and markedly reduces radiation exposure to the patient (sometimes by a factor of 100 or more) and the operator. It also reduces the amount of scatter radiation recorded on the image. The screens and film are contained in a lightproof cassette, which is transparent to x-rays.

Screens and film must be matched for spectral emission and sensitivity. Films produced by one company are generally not optimally sensitive to screens made by another, and it is inadvisable to mix screen and film brands. Screen and film combinations come in different speeds. The larger the crystals in a screen are, the more likely it is to interact with an x-ray and the greater the amount of light produced. Unfortunately, larger crystals also produce larger areas of light, which tend to decrease the detail of the film. Likewise, film with larger silver halide grains is more sensitive to the light creating the exposure but also reduces the detail or resolution of the final image. Therefore, fine grain films are matched to fine crystal screens, resulting in very detailed images that take more radiation to produce. The converse is true for large grain film and large crystal screens. The speed of these combinations is designated by a rating of 100-1,600, with 100 being relatively slow but with very good detail and 1,600 being very fast but with limited detail. Film-screen combinations with speeds of 200-800 are generally used in veterinary medicine. 200-speed systems are used for small body parts and skeletal imaging, while 800-speed systems are used for large abdomens in small animals and thoracic radiography in large animals. Choice of the proper speed system for a specific use is based not only on the area being radiographed but also on the capabilities of the machine. Small portable x-ray machines can be used for larger body parts with fast film-screen combinations, substantially improving the utility of these machines.

Darkroom: Once the film is exposed, it must be processed in a darkroom to make the latent image recorded on the film visible and fix it so that the image remains unchanged once the film is brought into the light. Care should be taken to make sure that no exterior light enters the darkroom. Even very small amounts of white light will markedly fog a film and decrease its diagnostic quality. Safelights used to illuminate darkrooms include filters that remove the frequencies of the light to which the film is sensitive, so that the film will not be exposed. Films vary in their spectral sensitivity; when replacing a safelight filter, the spectral requirements of the filter must be specified.

Developing was traditionally done in hand tanks by placing the film on a rack and immersing it in tanks full of the processing chemicals. However, automatic processors are now readily available and economically feasible. Automatic processing systems improve processing quality and consistency and reduce the processing time. Relatively few films processed per week will justify the purchase of an automated processing system. In any case, film processing must be done in strict accordance with the specified time and temperature requirements of the film being used. These requirements have been standardized for many years, and automated systems are designed to meet them.

Whether processing is manual or automated, the chemicals must be handled with care. Contamination of the darkroom with chemicals can ruin film, screens, and clothes. Fumes from the chemicals may be harmful, and some people may be more sensitive than others, especially to the fixer solution. Cross contamination of the developer solution with fixer will inactivate it and require replacement of the developer. Improper handling of chemicals will result in many artifacts on films as well as potential health hazards to the operators.

Filmless Radiography: Image recording systems developed recently do not require the use of film, screens, or processing chemicals. They have several advantages over conventional radiography: 1) radiographs cannot be lost; 2) there is no need for film storage; 3) the process allows for post-processing manipulation; and 4) images can be transmitted to a remote location for interpretation. These systems fall into 2 categories: 1) computed radiography (CR), in which a semiconductor plate contained in a cassette is exposed in the usual fashion and then read electronically; and 2) direct digital radiography (DR) in which a large array of photoelectric crystals is exposed in the usual fashion and then read in place electronically. In both systems, the radiographs are read and processed electronically by computer, which generates the image on a monitor. The digital images can then be stored electronically and made available to any computer with access to the image archive. The difference between the 2 systems lies in the intermediate step of exposing a plate in CR, which is then placed in a reader. These plates must be replaced periodically due to wear created during the reading process. There is also the issue of whether or not the latent image recorded by the reader is an accurate representation of the true image. The portability of the cassettes is an important benefit in large animal and equine radiography.

Direct digital systems expose the image recording device, which is then directly read by the computer. This is done by embedding millions of photodiodes or similar devices in the surface of the recording plates. Each element (referred to as a pixel) is connected to an electronic recording system that reads the exposure of each pixel and transmits that information to a computer. The computer then reconstructs the image based on the amount of exposure received by each of the photosensitive elements. The image is displayed rapidly and can be viewed before the animal is moved or repositioned. DR systems are very complex electronically and subject to the same insults as any complex computer system. However, when properly cared for, DR systems are durable and reliable. They do not require handling of the image recording plate, which reduces wear and tear on the system. Their main advantages over CR are image display speed and improved spatial and contrast resolution. The flexibility and reliability of these systems is rapidly improving and has reached the point of being introduced to clinical settings. As DR systems grow in capability and acceptance and decrease in cost, it is expected they will eventually replace both CR and traditional film systems in the majority of medical practice.

Animal Restraint: Animals must be adequately restrained and positioned to obtain quality radiographic images. Many animals may be manually restrained by people dressed in appropriate protective apparel; however, manual restraint should be kept to a minimum. In some states, a manual restraint is not allowed except under explicitly defined circumstances. Sedation or short-acting anesthesia is often necessary. Chemical restraint lessens the need for manual restraint, which leads to fewer poor or unacceptable radiographs and usually shortens the amount of time required to complete the examination. In many instances, animals can be restrained using sandbags, tape, and foam pads. With some practice it is often possible to complete the radiographic examination in essentially the same time that it could have been performed using manual restraint, with the added benefit that the animal is less likely to injure personnel.

Animal motion may also be minimized by decreasing exposure time and maximizing mA to achieve the required mAs for the body region examined. Other technical adjustments, such as increasing the kVp or shortening the film focus distance, may be made in some cases. However, major changes in film focus distance will likely cause serious degradation of the image. In most instances it is preferable to chemically immobilize the animal as long as there is not a medical contraindication.

Radiation Safety: Radiographic examinations must be performed with proper respect for radiation safety procedures. Diagnostic x-ray machines are potent sources of radiation and can, if improperly used, result in injurious exposure to personnel over time. The exposure factors used in modern x-ray systems are substantially lower than those used in the past but can still result in injury. It is never acceptable to hold animals without the use of lead-impregnated aprons and gloves to decrease exposure to personnel. Leaded gloves should not be used within the primary beam of the x-ray machine. These gloves and aprons reduce exposure from scatter radiation by a factor of ~1,000 but only reduce exposure from the primary beam by a factor of ~10. Thyroid shields and eye shields are also recommended, especially when radiographing large animals, as the techniques used there are sometimes quite high. Upper limb and skull studies in horses are particularly likely to result in substantial exposure to anyone holding the film or the horse.

Pregnant women and any personnel <18 yr of age should refrain from direct involvement in the making of radiographs whenever possible. If a pregnant woman is directly involved in the making of radiographs, she should wear an apron that completely encircles her abdomen. Individuals involved in the making of radiographic images should be monitored for radiation exposure. This is essential to identify and correct conditions that can result in excessive radiation exposure to personnel. Monitoring of exposure also provides evidence of proper adherence to radiation safety standards if questions arise as to whether an employee's medical condition could be related to radiation exposure.

Interpretation of Images: Radiographic images are complex 2-dimensional representations of 3-dimensional subjects that are generated in a format unfamiliar to the average individual. Interpretation of radiographic images is difficult for the novice. Substantial experience and attention to detail is required to become proficient. The cornerstone of radiographic interpretation is a properly positioned and exposed study. Studies that are poorly or inconsistently positioned are difficult to interpret, and improper technique further decrease the amount of information obtained from the radiograph.

Although interpretation is aided by experience, conscious use of a systematic approach to evaluation of the film will improve the reading skill of even very experienced individuals and will ensure that lesions in areas not of primary interest or near the edge of the film are not missed. Once all of the lesions on the study are identified, a rational cause for those lesions can be formulated. The maximum amount of information is derived from the radiographic study when interpretation is done in light of the clinical and clinicopathologic information available. In this way, the most likely cause for the animal's condition can be determined.

Contrast Procedures: Shortly after radiography developed as a diagnostic specialty, it became evident that radiographic exposure of film alone lacked sufficient contrast to evaluate many structures. Contrast procedures were developed to increase the native contrast of organs, in order to separate them from surrounding tissues. Contrast agents are iodine-based compounds that are radiopaque. IV and intra-arterial contrast agents increase the opacity of the blood and make vascular structures visible. Iodinated contrast agents are cleared primarily by the kidneys, making the collecting system of the urinary tract visible. Orally administered agents, primarily barium sulfate-based compounds, outline the mucosa and lumen of the GI tract. Intrathecal contrast agents allow evaluation of the spinal cord and meninges. These contrast procedures have been largely supplanted by modern imaging procedures, but many of them are still the best way of imaging the structures they are designed to evaluate. Many contrast procedures do not require special equipment and can be performed in the average veterinary practice, but interpretation is best performed by someone with experience.

ULTRASONOGRAPHY

Ultrasonography is the second most commonly used imaging format in veterinary practice. It uses ultrasonic sound waves in the frequency range of 1.5-15 megahertz (MHz) to create images of body structures based on the pattern of echoes reflected from the tissues and organs. Several different types of image formats can be displayed. The most familiar one (and the one that creates the actual image of anatomy) is B-mode, or grayscale scanning. The sound beam is produced by a transducer placed in contact with the animal. An ultrashort pulse of sound is directed into the animal, after which the transducer switches to the receive mode. Echoes occur as the sound beam changes velocity while passing through tissues of varying density. The greater the change in velocity, the greater the strength of the echo. The transducer then reconverts the echoes to electrical impulses recorded by the computer in the ultrasound machine. The strength of the echo, the time required for the echo to return after the pulse, and the direction the sound beam was sent is recorded. Using the information from multiple echoes, the machine creates an image that represents the appearance of the tissues when cut in that same plane on an anatomic specimen. In modern scanning systems, the sound beam is swept through the body many times per second, producing a dynamic, real time image that changes as the transducer is moved across the body. This real-time image is easier to interpret and allows the examiner to scan continuously until a satisfactory image is obtained.

Ultrasonography cannot be used to scan gas-filled or bony tissues. The sound beam is totally reflected at soft tissue/gas interfaces and absorbed at soft tissue/bone interfaces. Gas and bone also "shadow" any other organs beyond them. Bowel gas can inhibit imaging of adjacent abdominal organs, and the heart must be imaged from locations that do not require the sound beam to pass through the lungs.

Sonographic imaging is also limited in regard to the depth of tissue that can be examined. Most scanners will display tissues to a depth of ~24 cm, but the image is often quite noisy at that depth. This is because most tissue echoes do not return directly to the transducer but are reflected in some other direction. By a depth of 24 cm, the loss of energy from the sound beam results in echoes so weak that the scanner cannot separate the returning echoes from the background electronic noise. In addition, some echoes that are not directly reflected may return to the transducer by reflection from a tissue outside the beam path. Such echoes require longer to return to the transducer and are depicted at a spurious location, adding noise to the image. Low-frequency transducers can scan deeper than high-frequency transducers. There is less loss of beam intensity in fluid media, so if the beam passes through a fluid media such as blood in the heart or urine in the bladder, the maximum scanning depth may be increased.

Although ultrasound can be used to evaluate most soft tissues, the heart and abdominal organs still constitute the majority of the examinations performed. In scanning of the abdomen, a systematic evaluation of the abdominal structures is made. Each sonographer develops his or her own system of completely evaluating the abdomen. Systematic evaluation ensures that all structures are scanned. In the past, organs such as the adrenal glands and pancreas were only seen if diseased and enlarged, but modern ultrasound machines operated by an experienced sonographer produce images of such quality that the normal adrenal glands and pancreas can be imaged.

Changes in the size and shape of organs are evident in most cases, but evaluation of the echo pattern is based on comparison with that of other organs and tissues that the examiner has scanned in other patients. The person evaluating the scan must have a firm idea, developed from experience and comparison with known normals, of the normal echo pattern for each organ. The echogenicity of several tissues must be compared, as any organ may have increases or decreases in the echogenicity of its parenchyma. Diseased organs may be either uniformly altered in echogenicity or exhibit focal or multifocal changes. Focal changes are usually easier to detect than uniform changes. Sonographic lesions are sometimes quite characteristic of a given disease process, but more often the changes are nonspecific. While ultrasonography can be quite sensitive to detection of disease, the changes are not specific for a given disease in most cases.

Ultrasonography can also be used to direct biopsy instruments to acquire tissue for a specific pathologic diagnosis. This obviates the need for an open surgical exploration in many cases. Lesions buried within large organs such as the liver and kidneys that might not be detectable at laparotomy may be detected and biopsied with ultrasonographic guidance. Presurgical diagnosis permits more thorough and specific planning of surgical procedures and presurgical treatment of lesions. These procedures can frequently be safely performed under heavy sedation. Ultrasound-guided biopsy and aspiration of lesions can also be performed in large animals without the need for general anesthesia.

Echocardiography: Ultrasonic evaluation of the heart is termed echocardiography. In the past, this was done using the M-mode format of displaying ultrasound information. A narrow beam of sound is projected into the heart, and the echo pattern and strength are displayed onto a persistence screen with the x-axis of the display representing time (y-axis is depth), similar to the familiar format of an electrocardiogram. The pattern and amplitude of movement of the walls of the chambers of the heart and valves could be evaluated, as well as the size of the respective structures along the path of the sound beam. Considerable experience is required to obtain and interpret diagnostic studies. In recent years, the M-mode examination has been coupled with real-time B-mode studies to improve the accuracy of beam placement and add additional information, such as shape of the chamber.

Ultrasonographic images are also used to acquire quantitative information about cardiac function. Measurement of specified parameters may be made on either the M-mode scan or on the 2-dimensional B-mode image. Mathematical formulas are then applied to determine values for cardiac output, ventricular contractility, ejection fraction, ventricular wall stiffness, and other cardiac functions.

Doppler ultrasound makes use of the familiar phenomenon that sound emitted from a moving object such as a train has a different apparent frequency to someone standing still relative to the moving object. If the object is moving away from the observer the frequency of the sound is lower; conversely, if the emitter is moving toward the observer the frequency of the sound is higher. The same is true of ultrasound. Echoes from moving RBC change the frequency of the sound reflected back to the transducer. The amount by which the frequency is shifted is proportional to the velocity of the RBC; whether it is a positive or negative frequency shift is used to determine blood flow direction. This is used to identify valvular regurgitation (insufficiency), increased flow velocity (as in a stenosis), or abnormal movement of the blood in the heart or vessels elsewhere in the body. Doppler signals may be displayed in 2 formats. In the first, spectral Doppler, a sound beam is used to evaluate a specific small volume within the vessel of interest. This display resembles the M-mode display except that the frequency shift, or velocity, is substituted on the y-axis. The second way to display Doppler frequency shifts is to select a larger area of the scan and a real time B-mode image, encoding the velocities and direction as a color spectrum. The color (usually red or blue) depicts blood flow direction and the hue depicts mean flow velocity. This allows evaluation of larger areas, but at the price of lower temporal resolution. For this reason color-encoded B-mode flow studies are used to guide placement of spectral sample volumes to acquire more accurate and complete information. Thus, Doppler studies complement and improve the accuracy and specificity of echocardiograms. Quantitative evaluation of spectral Doppler studies also allows the examiner to determine values such as pressure gradients across valves and stenotic areas or resistance to flow of blood entering an organ.

Ultrasound contrast agents increase the reflectivity of blood and any tissue through which blood flows. Enhancement of blood reflectivity is usually accomplished by the formation of transient microscopic bubbles in the plasma. The increase in echogenicity is related to the amount of blood flowing through the tissue. The bubbles are quickly absorbed into the plasma and therefore do not constitute an embolism hazard. The ability to evaluate the vascularity of a tissue provides additional information about the type of lesion present. For instance, granulomas generally have poorer blood flow than normal tissue and do not enhance as much as the surrounding tissue, while tumors may enhance more and retain the contrast for a longer time than the surrounding tissue. Contrast agents hold great promise for improving both the sensitivity and specificity of ultrasonographic examinations.

COMPUTED TOMOGRAPHY

In computed tomography (CT), an x-ray tube moves around the body and continuously projects a thin fan of x-rays through the body. Electronic detectors opposite the x-ray tube continuously monitor the number of x-rays passing through the body and the angle at which the beam is being projected. The number of x-rays reaching the detector changes as the beam passes through different tissues because of the tube movement. A computer mathematically evaluates the data and determines the most probable density of any point within the volume of tissue scanned. This density is then displayed on a monitor. Together, all of the densities make an image of the cross-section of the body through which the beam passed, referred to as a slice. The animal is then moved a few millimeters and the process repeated. By sequentially scanning a body area, the entire volume of interest can be imaged without any superimposition of structures. CT also has much better contrast discrimination than standard radiographs, so structures such as individual parts of the brain or individual muscle bellies are seen as separate and distinct on the CT scan. X-ray contrast media is frequently used to further enhance the contrast between structures and help characterize lesions.

The first scanners were slow and cumbersome with limited resolution. However, modern multi-slice CT scanners with supercomputer capabilities can acquire up to 16 cross-sectional images per rotation; each rotation may be <1 sec. These systems are capable of continuous rotation (helical or spiral scanning) and can perform a complete scan of the abdomen or thorax in a human on a single breath hold (≤17 sec). The image reconstruction time is correspondingly short, and the entire study can be completed in less time than was originally required to acquire a single image. Even with such extraordinarily fast systems, veterinary patients must still be anesthetized and immobilized to perform the studies, but the period of anesthesia is short and the value of the information derived is great. Modern reconstruction algorithms also allow 3-dimensional reconstruction of structures with a given density. Bones can be depicted without the overlying soft tissues and vascular structures that have been contrast enhanced can be depicted without any overlying tissues. The newest scanners can produce images of vessels that rival those obtained by conventional contrast angiography.

CT scans can be used to detect structural changes deep within the body, including tumors, abscesses, vascular abnormalities, occult fractures, and hematomas. The radiologist must have a firm knowledge of anatomy and be able to ascertain the identity of structures in any plane through the body. Knowledge of physiology and artifacts are also paramount in evaluating CT scans. Extensive experience and training are required to become adept at the interpretation of these images. Because of the expense and size of the equipment, the need for specialized experience, and the number of animals for which it is indicated, CT scanners are typically limited to specialty and academic practices.

MAGNETIC RESONANCE IMAGING

Magnetic resonance imaging (MRI) is the newest form of imaging in general use today. In this imaging modality a powerful magnet, up to 40,000 times as strong as the magnetic field of the earth, is used to transiently align the hydrogen atoms in the body with the magnetic field. All atoms with odd atomic numbers are affected, but the effect on hydrogen overshadows the effect on other natural elements within the body. If the field is abruptly turned off or reversed, the hydrogen atoms lose their alignment or realign in the opposite direction. The rate at which they do this is restricted by the molecule of which they are a part. During this relaxation or realignment phase, the hydrogen atoms emit radio waves that can be detected by highly sensitive equipment. The frequency of these waves depends on the strength of the magnetic field. By constructing the magnetic field of the scanner in such a way that each small discrete volume (referred to as a voxel) has a different field strength, each of these volumes can be represented by a frequency. Then, by evaluating the signal strength and duration for each frequency, the chemical composition of each voxel can be estimated. In practice this is done by representing the signal strengths for each volume on a monitor, much as is done with CT. The signal strength from each volume element is very small, so many repetitions or pulses of the magnet field application and relaxation are required to provide a statistically significant determination of the relative signal strength from the volume elements. Thus, each scanning sequence may require several minutes to perform. Sequential examination of slices through the body is done in the same way that CT examinations are performed. MRI differs from CT in that the data for all the slices in the volume being imaged are acquired simultaneously; however, only 1 set of planes is acquired at a time. Scans are typically acquired in more than 1 of the 3 orthogonal planes, with different magnet pulsing sequences to highlight different types of tissue. Also, unlike CT, MRI scans are seldom reformatted to project oblique planes, although 3-dimensional rendering is occasionally done.

MRI interpretation requires a firm knowledge of sectional anatomy as well as knowledge of the physics of the imaging system. Because this type of imaging is based on chemical composition of the body rather than density, it provides exquisite detail and contrast of body structures. However, the duration of data acquisition limits its use in areas of substantial movement, such as the chest. MRI does not image cortical bone well, and therefore is of limited use in the evaluation of bony lesions, although it is quite applicable to imaging of bone marrow and cartilage. Like CT, MRI was initially used primarily for neuroimaging and is still the mainstay of imaging in that area. MRI is also now being used frequently for joint and muscle imaging.

Most MRI systems are large and expensive to purchase, install, and maintain. The length of time required dicates that studies be performed under general anesthesia. Because powerful magnets are used, ferromagnetic material may not be brought into the room due to safety considerations. For veterinary patients, this means that injectable anesthesia is typically used unless special anesthesia machines are available. These factors, combined with the specialized knowledge required to perform studies and interpret the images, generally limits these instruments to large private and academic referral specialty practices.

NUCLEAR MEDICINE IMAGING
(Nuclear scintigraphy)

Nuclear medicine imaging involves dosing the patient with a very small amount of a gamma ray-emitting radioisotope. The material is then detected within the body with a gamma camera. The isotope may be injected, ingested, or inhaled as appropriate for the study being performed. The radioisotope is usually part of a larger molecule that has a specific affinity for the tissue or organ of interest. For instance, some organic phosphonates have an affinity for bone, and isotopes bound to sulfur colloids will localize in the liver and spleen. Very few radioisotopes have direct affinity for a given tissue; iodine is the notable exception and localizes very strongly in the thyroid. Inhaled gases or aerosols localize in the airways and lungs. In veterinary medicine, the most commonly used isotope is metastable technetium 99 (^{99m}Tc), although radioactive iodine, indium, and thallium are also used in specific instances.

The image data is collected by a device called a gamma camera, which detects the gamma rays emitted by the radioisotope. The data collected can be displayed directly on a monitor or projected onto a film as a permanent record. Most systems also send the data to a computer system for analysis, which allows enhancement of count differences and determination of organ margins. The operator can select regions of interest to be analyzed for count content and for counts over time. When the study uses a radiopharmaceutical that is metabolized or has a limited residence time in an organ, organ function can be determined. These dynamic studies can be used to evaluate the function of organs such as the lungs, kidneys, and heart. Such studies may reveal abnormalities that static forms of anatomic imaging cannot detect. Functional imaging is the great strength of nuclear medicine studies and allows disease detection earlier and more readily compared with anatomic imaging systems. Only advanced MRI studies can emulate this functional aspect of scintigraphic imaging, but those systems are much more limited in scope and availability.

Single photon emission computed tomography and positron emission tomography (PET) are advanced scintigraphic imaging techniques that are widely used in human medicine for detection and evaluation of many diseases. Both of these techniques yield a CT-like cross-sectional image based on the deposition of radionuclides within the body. Such images have greater sensitivity than planar images and improved specificity as well. PET imaging in particular has seen tremendous growth in the last decade and is now routinely used in the staging and evaluation of many diseases, especially cancer. This technology, which is based on the use of positron-emitting isotopes of lighter elements such as oxygen, nitrogen, carbon, and fluorine, can evaluate the metabolism and localization of these elements with great sensitivity. Unfortunately, the cost of the instruments and radiopharmaceuticals and the lack of expertise in veterinary medicine to interpret the studies currently limits their use to research and rare clinical cases in teaching institutions.

RADIATION THERAPY

Although not an imaging modality, radiation therapy has long been the province of radiologists because it also uses ionizing radiation. Radiation therapy has seen dramatic increases in demand and sophistication in recent years, which has led to creation of a board specialty in radiation oncology, granted by the American College of Veterinary Radiology, that is specifically limited to certification in radiation oncology. Radiation therapy has advanced to the point that only a few radiologists now actively practice in both the fields of imaging and therapy.

Radiation therapy practices generally use linear accelerators as the source of the ionizing radiation used to treat neoplasia. These machines produce powerful x-rays and electron beams with energies of 4-12 million electron volts. The x-rays are used to treat deep-seated tumors, whereas electron beams are generally used to treat tumors of the skin and subcutis. Linear accelerators are complex machines that require the support of a medical physicist to maintain safe and effective use. This increased support load is offset by the machine's flexibility and speed, which is necessary as treatment techniques become more sophisticated and complex. Another significant advantage is the lack of need for long-lived radioactive materials, such as 137-cesium and 60-cobalt, which were used in older radiation therapy machines and had to be periodically replaced and disposed of by highly trained specialists. Care and use of these isotopes also requires many safety inspections as mandated by law.

Computerized treatment planning systems are used to improve the localization and distribution of the therapeutic beam within the patient. This limits the dose to normal tissues and also increases the dose to the neoplastic tissue being treated, increasing cure or control rates and reducing the severity of normal tissue complications. These programs are best used in conjunction with CT or MRI images, which determine the position and extent of the tumor within the body and its relative position to normal structures. Many hours of planning may be required to generate a treatment plan for a large, complex tumor.

Whenever possible, elimination of a tumor by surgery is preferred. However, in many instances large neoplasms, or those in critical areas such as the brain, are not amenable to complete or even partial surgical removal. Even when a tumor is grossly removed, microscopic foci of neoplastic cells may extend beyond the limits of the surgical field. In all of these instances radiation therapy, often in combination with chemotherapy, is useful in treating the remaining cancer. Radiation therapy is often the treatment of choice for brain tumors, nasal tumors, and other neoplasms of the head and neck. It may be the only treatment option for cancer of the vertebral column and pelvic canal. Radiotherapy is also used to treat tumors in the mediastinum and soft tissues of the skin and subcutis either before or after surgery. It is seldom used in the treatment of lung neoplasia or in the treatment of neoplastic disease of the abdominal cavity, due to the mobility of tumors in these areas. As the sophistication of radiotherapy techniques increases, more and more types of neoplasia are being treated at least in part by radiation therapy.

Brachytherapy is the implantation of radioactive sources into the tumor to achieve radiation therapy. It is seldom used for treatment of cancers in animals due to the difficulties associated with maintenance of the sources and keeping the sources in place within the tumor. The notable exception to this is the use of radioiodine to treat thyroid adenomas in cats. Implantable radiation sources that are so small that they are permanently implanted within the body blur the margins between radiation therapy and nuclear medicine. Such techniques may well increase the interest in and availability of brachytherapy procedures in the future. Due to the risk of excessive radiation exposure and contamination of the patient or hospital, these procedures should only be performed by people with appropriate training.

DISPOSAL OF CARCASSES AND DISINFECTION OF PREMISES

When animals die or are slaughtered on farms, carcasses and parts that are unfit for use as food should be disposed of and the premises cleaned promptly in a manner that prevents any infectious or toxic health hazard to domestic or wild animals or humans. Information on the safe and lawful disposal of carcasses can be obtained from local environmental protection agencies. When the circumstances under which death has occurred suggest a transmissible disease or toxic hazard, the nearest animal health official should be notified immediately.

As general precautions, persons handling carcasses and disinfectants should wear protective clothing and be properly equipped to complete the tasks of disposition and disinfection. The method of disposal should preclude contamination of soil, air, and water. Hides and other parts of animals that have succumbed to infectious diseases or toxins should be safely disposed of and not retained for use.

Sheep or cattle diagnosed with or suspected of being affected by **scrapie** (p 1071) or **bovine spongiform encephalopathy** (p 991), respectively, must not be rendered. The preferred means of disposal for these animals is incineration, although they may also be buried (*see* below).

Rendering: Ordinarily, rendering is a safe, rapid, and economical method of disposal of carcasses. Renderers are required to use equipment and methods that prevent health hazards. Local regulations specify requirements for transportation of carcasses to rendering plants.

Burial: When a site acceptable to the local environmental protection agency is available, burial is usually the preferred method of disposal. In selecting a burial site, it is necessary to consider the adequacy of soil depth and to avoid underground electrical cables, water pipes, gas pipes, septic tanks, and water wells. The burial pit or trench should be at least 2.3 m wide and 3 m deep (7×9 ft). The pit is a cave-in hazard and must not be entered without proper shoring, and any other appropriate precautions should be taken. At this depth, 1.3 m^2 (15 ft^2) of floor space will accommodate a mature bovine or equine carcass, 5 mature pigs or sheep, 100 mature chickens, or 40 mature turkeys. For each additional meter (3 ft) in depth, the number of animals per 1.3 m^2 of floor space may be doubled. Contaminated litter, soil, manure, feed, milk, or other material should be placed in the pit with the carcasses and covered with at least 2 m (6 ft) of soil. The covering soil should not be compacted. Decomposition and gas formation cause cracking, bubbling, and leaking of fluids from a compacted burial site. The soil should be mounded and neatly graded.

Burning: Burning in an incinerator that is operated in compliance with local laws and ordinances is an excellent means for disposing of one or a few carcasses and is the preferred means for sheep with scrapie and cattle with bovine spongiform encephalopathy.

Burning carcasses in an open site should be done only when legally permitted. Burning poultry carcasses should be considered only when burial is not feasible. The burn site should be away from public view and on flat, open ground that is clear of buildings, hay or straw stacks, overhead cables, and shallow underground pipes or cables. Locations upwind from houses, farm buildings, roads, or populated areas, and those from which precipitation runoff may contaminate the environment, should be avoided. Carcasses must be placed on a quantity of combustible supporting materials sufficient to reduce them completely to ashes. The material must also be arranged in a manner to permit an adequate flow of air to the fire. Gasoline or other highly volatile combustible liquids should not be used.

To prepare the fire bed, an area of ground should be staked out to accommodate the number of carcasses to be burned: 8×3 ft for each mature cow or horse, 5 mature pigs or sheep, 100 mature chickens, or 40 mature turkeys. The fire bed burns best if at a right angle to the prevailing wind.

Under favorable conditions, burning should be complete in 48 hr. Additional fuel should be added as needed. When the fire has died out, the ashes should be buried and the area cleaned, graded or plowed, and prepared for seeding.

Other Disposal Methods: Composting, fermentation, and dry extrusion methods have been developed to process certain dead animals and animal waste, destroy pathogenic organisms, reduce volume, and produce feedstuffs. Local environmental protection agencies and state agriculture departments should be consulted concerning the acceptability of these and other possible alternative disposal methods.

Disinfection of Premises: Removal and safe disposal of manure, feed, and debris by burial or burning, followed by thorough scraping and cleaning of all buildings and equipment, must precede the application of chemical disinfectant. Except for steam cleaning, cleaning with aqueous solutions is practical only at temperatures above freezing. A cleaning agent such as trisodium phosphate or sodium carbonate dissolved in hot water will facilitate cleaning. All traces of the cleaning agent must be rinsed away with clear water before disinfectant is applied. Provision must be made to contain and safely dispose of cleaning solutions, rinse water, and disinfectant.

Disinfectants recommended for general use on surfaces free of organic matter are sodium or calcium hypochlorite (1,200 ppm available chlorine), iodine, phenol, and quaternary ammonium compounds. Newer disinfectants use a combination of products (eg, quaternary ammonia and glutaraldehyde) to enhance efficacy. Information on disinfectants for specific animal disease agents can be obtained from state or federal animal health agencies. Disinfectants should bear the approval statement of the Environmental Protection Agency in the USA, or of a similar agency in other countries. Label instructions for application must be followed.

EUTHANASIA

Euthanasia is defined as an easy, painless death. In regard to animals, euthanasia is the act of killing an animal in a humane manner. The primary objectives of animal euthanasia are: 1) relieving pain and suffering of the animal(s) to be euthanized, 2) minimizing the pain, anxiety, distress, and fear the animal experiences before consciousness is lost, and 3) inducing a painless and distress-free death.

Observing the behavioral and physiologic responses of animals is beneficial in assessing whether the objectives of euthanasia are being met. A variety of behaviors and physiologic responses may be demonstrated by animals experiencing pain and/or fear, including (but not limited to) distress vocalizations, struggling, escape attempts, agitation, freezing, aggression, fearful postures or facial expressions, trembling, salivating, urinating, defecating, evacuation of anal sacs, pupillary dilation, panting, tachycardia, and sweating. Response to euthanasia procedures (handling, restraint, confinement, venipuncture, gas odors, etc) varies among species and among individuals, necessitating careful monitoring of every euthanasia.

Loss of physiologic function during euthanasia should occur in the following order to help prevent fear and distress: 1) rapid loss of consciousness, 2) loss of motor function, 3) arrest of respiratory and cardiac function, and finally, 4) permanent loss of brain function. If loss of motor or respiratory and cardiac function precedes loss of consciousness, animals become fearful and experience distress. In some species, particularly rabbits and chickens, tonic immobility may be induced by fear, and care must be taken to not confuse this behavioral response with loss of consciousness.

Before the carcass is disposed of, death must be verified by a means appropriate to the species and the method of euthanasia. Care must be taken not to confuse narcosis with death. Determination of death in ectothermic animals may be more difficult due to differences in their physiology.

Euthanasia frequently results in chemical tissue residues, necessitating proper disposal to prevent contamination of the environment or other animals (eg, scavengers, predators).

The methods used for euthanasia of animals intended for consumption by humans or other animals in the USA must meet the requirements of the USDA; chemical agents that result in chemical tissue residues cannot be used unless approved by the FDA.

Other factors that must be taken into account in animal euthanasias include the safety of operators, observers, and other animals; human psychological responses to euthanasia, eg, sadness and grief; and fear and anxiety of other animals exposed to the behaviors, vocalizations, and pheromones of animals being euthanized. Counseling services and pet loss support hotlines are available for grieving pet owners in some communities and veterinary colleges. Personnel involved in euthanasias or animal slaughter may also experience negative psychological consequences. Workplace support programs and accessibility to counseling may help alleviate the stress felt by euthanasia personnel.

The operator must be knowledgeable regarding the agent, method, equipment, and behavior and physiology of the species and individual animal(s) to be euthanized; be trained in the technique; and have demonstrated skill in the euthanasia operation to be performed.

Selection of an appropriate method and agent of euthanasia is paramount in assuring a humane death. Selection is based on the behavior, physiology, and metabolism of the species, as well as any particular characteristics of the individual animal(s) that would influence the ability to use a particular method. The setting, the available means of animal restraint, the skill and knowledge of the operator, the number of animals to be euthanized, and the purpose for which the animal(s) is to be used are also determining factors in selection of the methods and the agent. Euthanasia in circumstances other than the clinical veterinary setting, eg, wildlife in the field, may limit the euthanasia options. However, in all circumstances, humaneness to the animal should be a prevailing concern. Slaughter of animals for food, fur, or fiber, and euthanasia of wildlife and feral animals should all adhere to the same humane standards for euthanasia.

Acceptable methods and agents for euthanasia of different species of animals are listed in TABLE 3. It is the obligation of the operator to know the physiology and behavior of the species to be euthanized, and the specific technical information and safety precautions for the method and agent selected. The 2000 report of the American Veterinary Medical Association panel on euthanasia provides additional details, as well as references for specific technical and safety information.

Inhalant agents should not be used alone in animals <16 wk old because neonatal animals are more resistant to hypoxia and it takes longer for them to die. Reptiles, amphibians, diving birds, and diving and burrowing mammals may have a prolonged time to loss of consciousness with inhalant gases. **Inhalant anesthetics** are useful for small animals (<7 kg) in which injections are difficult. The order of preference of inhalant

---

TABLE 3. Agents and Methods of Euthanasia by Species

Species	Acceptable*	Conditionally Acceptable†
Amphibians	Barbiturates, inhalant anesthetics (in appropriate species), CO_2, CO, tricaine methane sulfonate (MS-222), benzocaine hydrochloride, double pithing	Penetrating captive bolt, gunshot, stunning and decapitation, decapitation and pithing
Birds	Barbiturates, inhalant anesthetics, CO_2, CO, gunshot (free-ranging only)	N_2, argon, cervical dislocation, decapitation, thoracic compression (small, free-ranging only)
Cats	Barbiturates, inhalant anesthetics, CO_2, CO, potassium chloride in conjunction with general anesthesia	N_2, argon
Dogs	Barbiturates, inhalant anesthetics, CO_2, CO, potassium chloride in conjunction with general anesthesia	N_2, argon, penetrating captive bolt, electrocution
Fish	Barbiturates, inhalant anesthetics, CO_2, tricaine methane sulfonate, benzocaine hydrochloride, 2-phenoxyethanol	Decapitation and pithing, stunning and decapitation/pithing

TABLE 3. *(continued)*

Species	Acceptable[*]	Conditionally Acceptable[†]
Horses	Barbiturates, potassium chloride in conjunction with general anesthesia, penetrating captive bolt	Chloral hydrate (IV, after sedation), gunshot, electrocution
Marine mammals	Barbiturates, etorphine hydrochloride	Gunshot (cetaceans <4 m long)
Mink, fox, and other mammals produced for fur	Barbiturates, inhalant anesthetics, CO_2 (mink require high concentrations for euthanasia without supplemental agents), CO, potassium chloride in conjunction with general anesthesia	N_2, argon, electrocution followed by cervical dislocation
Nonhuman primates	Barbiturates	Inhalant anesthetics, CO_2, CO, N_2, argon
Rabbits	Barbiturates, inhalant anesthetics, CO_2, CO, potassium chloride in conjunction with general anesthesia	N_2, argon, cervical dislocation (<1 kg), decapitation, penetrating captive bolt
Reptiles	Barbiturates, inhalant anesthetics (in appropriate species), CO_2 (in appropriate species)	Penetrating captive bolt, gunshot, decapitation and pithing, stunning and decapitation
Rodents and other small mammals	Barbiturates, inhalant anesthetics, CO_2, CO, potassium chloride in conjunction with general anesthesia, microwave irradiation	Methoxyflurane, ether, N_2, argon, cervical dislocation (rats <200 g), decapitation
Ruminants	Barbiturates, potassium chloride in conjunction with general anesthesia, penetrating captive bolt	Chloral hydrate (IV, after sedation), gunshot, electrocution
Swine	Barbiturates, CO_2, potassium chloride in conjunction with general anesthesia, penetrating captive bolt	Inhalant anesthetics, CO, chloral hydrate (IV, after sedation), gunshot, electrocution, blow to the head (<3 wk of age)
Zoo animals	Barbiturates, inhalant anesthetics, CO_2, CO, potassium chloride in conjunction with general anesthesia	N_2, argon, penetrating captive bolt, gunshot
Free-ranging wildlife	Barbiturates IV or IP, inhalant anesthetics, potassium chloride in conjunction with general anesthesia	CO_2, CO, N_2, argon, penetrating captive bolt, gunshot, kill traps (scientifically tested)

[*]Acceptable methods are the preferred means of euthanizing animals of a given species. Those listed are in addition to anesthetic overdose and euthanasia formulations (*see* text above).

[†]Conditionally acceptable methods are those that may be used if conditions prevent the use of any acceptable method for that species (eg, in slaughtering animals for food). All factors in any situation must be carefully considered to select the best alternative method that assures humaneness in handling and killing the animal and safety for the operator performing the procedure.

Adapted, with permission, from the *2000 Report of the AVMA Panel on Euthanasia* and the *1997 Report of the Working Party for the European Commission on the Recommendations for Euthanasia of Experimental Animals.* For complete information, including methods of euthanasia not described here, please refer to the full reports.

anesthetics for euthanasia is halothane, enflurane, isoflurane, sevoflurane, methoxyflurane, and desflurane, with or without nitrous oxide.

Injectable agents are the most rapid and reliable and are preferred when venipuncture can be accomplished without causing fear to the animal or unnecessary risk to the operator. All barbituric acid derivatives are acceptable IV euthanasia agents. Certain injectable agents (eg, strychnine, nicotine, caffeine, magnesium sulfate, cleaning agents, solvents, disinfectants, other toxins or salts, potassium chloride as a sole agent, and all neuromuscular blocking agents) are absolutely not acceptable and are condemned as agents of euthanasia.

Physical methods of euthanasia, including captive bolt, gunshot, cervical dislocation, decapitation, microwave irradiation, and thoracic compression can be humane methods of euthanasia when used properly by skilled operators with well-maintained equipment and when other means of euthanasia are impractical or contraindicated by the intended use of the animal. Exsanguination, stunning, and pithing should not be used as sole methods of euthanasia but as adjuncts to other methods.

MEAT INSPECTION

Inspection of meat by qualified individuals to eliminate from the food supply unwholesome, adulterated, or mislabeled meat or meat products helps to protect consumers from the infectious, toxic, and physical hazards that may originate in food animals, the environment, or humans. The standard procedures do not cover every possibility concerning the acceptability of carcasses, organs, or other animal parts; personal judgment is also required to ensure that only wholesome, unadulterated product is approved for food. (*See also* CHEMICAL RESIDUES IN FOOD AND FIBER, p 1962.)

Inspection activities are divided into antemortem, postmortem, and processing inspection.

Premortem Inspection

Premortem inspection is conducted at the abattoir on the day of slaughter to detect and condemn animals that are unfit for slaughter and to note signs or lesions of diseases that may not be apparent after slaughter (eg, rabies, listeriosis, and heavy metal poisoning). During inspection, animals should be confined in a lighted enclosure so that they can be clearly observed at rest and in motion. The animals must not be allowed to enter into any area of the facility where slaughtering, dressing, or handling of edible products is performed until they have been inspected and found to be acceptable candidates for human consumption. Gates, chutes, and equipment must be available to segregate abnormal animals for closer examination and proper identification.

Seriously crippled animals, animals commonly termed "downers," and disabled or moribund animals are not acceptable candidates for slaughter as food. Rectal temperatures should be verified on any animal suspected of being febrile. Body temperature should be ≤106°F (41°C) for pigs and 105°F (40.5°C) for cattle, sheep, goats, horses, and mules. Animals with signs or lesions that do not warrant immediate condemnation can be identified as "suspects" so that their carcasses and viscera can be inspected separately. Certain animals may be retained to allow recovery from minor diseases or to permit depletion of residues of chemical and biologic substances. Animals that may have been treated with or exposed to substances that may make the edible tissues unfit for human food should not be slaughtered for such.

Animals that have reacted to a test for leptospirosis, anaplasmosis, or tuberculosis, and goats that have reacted to a test for brucellosis, are unacceptable as food. The temperature of bovine tuberculosis reactors should be taken on antemortem inspection.

Animals suspected of having a foreign disease or parasite should be held and reported immediately to the nearest state or federal animal health official.

Animal welfare and humane slaughter concerns are becoming increasingly important to the livestock industry. Slaughtering plants in the USA are now routinely observed to ensure full compliance with the provisions of the Humane Methods of Slaughter Act of 1978 and related regulations. Humane handling of livestock prior to slaughter is necessary and includes methods of stimulation, nonabuse by plant workers, provision of feed and water, safe pen construction, nonslip floors, and protection from adverse weather conditions.

Most large meat purchasers require that meat-producing animals be killed in compliance with humane slaughter regulations. Therefore, these animals must be rendered insensible to pain by a single blow, gunshot, or an electrical, chemical, or other method that is rapid and effective before shackling, hoisting, or cutting.

Recognized ritual slaughter, such as kosher and halal (Muslim), are exempted from these requirements.

Postmortem Inspection

Animals should be inspected immediately after slaughter and evisceration for possible changes and lesions that indicate unsuitability of the meat for food. Postmortem examination requires observation of all parts of the carcass, dressing procedures, equipment, and facilities to prevent contamination of edible parts. The inspector must ensure that condemned carcasses and parts are disposed of safely. The following are unacceptable for human food: the lungs, thyroid glands, laryngeal muscles, and lactating mammary glands; brains, cheek meat, and head trimmings from animals that were stunned by lead, sponge iron, or frangible bullets; and carcasses suspected of containing sulfonamides, antibiotics, or other residues. Spinal cords and CNS tissue must be discarded to eliminate threat of bovine spongiform encephalopathy in the food supply.

A routine postmortem inspection should include the following procedures:

Cattle—*Head:* Incise and visually examine the left and right mandibular, parotid, atlantal, and suprapharyngeal lymph nodes. Examine 2 incised layers of both masseter muscles. Examine and palpate tongue. *Viscera:* Examine mesenteric lymph nodes and abdominal viscera. Examine and palpate ruminoreticular junction. Examine esophagus and spleen. Incise and examine anterior, middle, and posterior mediastinal lymph nodes and right and left bronchial lymph nodes. Examine and palpate costal and ventral surfaces of the lungs. Incise heart from base to apex through interventricular septum and examine and cut inner and outer surfaces. Incise and examine hepatic (portal) lymph nodes. Incise bile duct in both directions and examine contents. Examine and palpate ventral and dorsal surfaces and renal impression of liver. *Carcass:* Examine internal and external surfaces. Palpate superficial inguinal or supramammary and internal iliac lymph nodes. Examine and palpate kidneys and diaphragm.

Calves and Veal—*Head:* Incise and examine suprapharyngeal lymph nodes. *Viscera:* Examine and palpate lungs, bronchial and mediastinal lymph nodes, and heart. Examine spleen. Examine and palpate dorsal and ventral surfaces of the liver and palpate portal lymph nodes. Examine abdominal viscera. *Carcass:* Examine exposed inner and outer surfaces. Palpate internal iliac lymph nodes and kidneys.

Sheep and Goats—*Head and Carcass:* Examine outer surfaces and body cavities. Palpate back and sides of carcass. Examine neck, shoulders, and head. Palpate prescapular lymph nodes. Examine and palpate kidneys. Palpate femoral, superficial inguinal or supramammary, and popliteal lymph nodes. Incise lymph nodes when necessary to rule out caseous lymphadenitis. *Viscera:* Examine abdominal viscera, esophagus, mesenteric lymph nodes, omental fat, and spleen. Examine bile duct and gallbladder and their contents. Examine and palpate liver and costal and ventral surfaces of lungs. Palpate bronchial and mediastinal lymph nodes. Examine and palpate heart.

Pigs—*Head:* Examine head and cervical muscles. Incise mandibular lymph nodes. *Viscera:* Examine and palpate spleen and mesenteric lymph nodes. Palpate portal lymph nodes. Examine dorsal and ventral surfaces of the liver. Palpate right and left bronchial and mediastinal lymph nodes. Examine and palpate dorsal and ventral surfaces of the lungs. Examine and palpate heart. *Carcass:* Examine internal and external surfaces and incise any suspected abnormalities. Examine and palpate kidneys.

Horses—*Head:* Examine surfaces. Palpate, incise, and examine mandibular, pharyngeal, and parotid lymph nodes; guttural pouches; and tongue. *Viscera:* Examine and palpate lungs and bronchial and mediastinal lymph nodes, and incise any suspected abnormalities.

Examine and palpate spleen, liver, and portal lymph nodes. Incise hepatic duct. Examine remaining viscera. *Carcass:* Examine internal and external surfaces. Palpate superficial inguinal or supramammary and internal iliac lymph nodes. Examine and palpate kidneys and diaphragm. Examine and incise the internal abdominal walls for possible parasitic cysts. Examine spinous processes of thoracic vertebrae, supraspinous bursa, and first 2 cervical vertebrae for fistulous conditions. Examine axillary and subscapular tissues of white and gray horses for melanosis.

Poultry—Examine external surfaces for dressing defects, bruises, and disease lesions. Palpate tibias for bone diseases. Examine internal surfaces, lungs, and kidneys in place. Examine viscera and palpate liver, heart, and spleen.

General Condemnations

Livestock clearly showing at premortem inspection any irreversible disease or condition that justifies condemnation as unfit for use as food should be humanely destroyed and disposed of (*see* DISPOSAL OF CARCASSES AND DISINFECTION OF PREMISES, p 1377).

Carcasses contaminated by infectious, toxic, or hazardous physical agents should not be approved for use as food. Carcasses with generalized conditions or diseases, including malignant tumors, that have so altered the normal characteristics of the meat as to cause it to be inedible or sufficiently abnormal to be reasonably considered unfit for food should not be approved. Localized conditions that do not affect the wholesomeness of the entire carcass should be removed by trimming so that the remainder of the carcass can be used for food.

Special Considerations for Tuberculosis: The entire carcass should be condemned when there is evidence of tuberculosis, including the following: 1) An active lesion is present. 2) The animal is cachectic. 3) A lesion is present in muscle, intermuscular tissue, bone, joint, abdominal organs other than the GI tract, or in a lymph node associated with these parts. 4) Extensive lesions are present in the thoracic or abdominal cavity. 5) Lesions are multiple, acute, and actively progressive. 6) The nature or extent of lesions does not indicate localization.

An organ or part should be condemned when it or its corresponding lymph nodes contain lesions. When lesions in pigs are localized and are found at only 1 primary site of infection, such as the cervical lymph nodes, the unaffected parts are acceptable for food after condemnation of the affected organ or part. Even though certain carcasses minimally affected with tuberculosis may be considered safe after commercial cooking, this procedure is not recommended for carcasses that are not inspected in facilities inspected by federal or state officials.

Detection of Unwholesome Meat

Meat for human consumption should be prepared from animals that were healthy and have been exsanguinated. Animals having infectious, toxic, or physical agents that may be hazardous to human health or that are otherwise unwholesome in their tissues should not be used for food. Fitness for food can be determined by a comprehensive evaluation that may include organoleptic, histologic, microbiologic, chemical, and toxicologic examinations.

Meat should be examined under light of adequate intensity. Foreign objects on the surface or visible within the tissue should be collected for further examination. Items such as feathers, hair, fibers, parasites, or insect larvae may provide valuable data on the species, origin, and handling of the meat. Texture, color, and odor should be noted. Meat should be firm, and cut surfaces should be glossy. Gray or green discoloration may indicate bacterial action. Dark-red meat may result from postmortem retention of blood in animals that were not exsanguinated. A stable, bright-red color may indicate the unwholesome addition of sulfite. Ultraviolet light may be used to visualize rodent urine and fluorescent substances produced by certain spoilage bacteria. Areas of bruising, hemorrhage, or inflammation should be readily recognized. Odors from contaminating chemicals, urine, fish, or other sources are unacceptable. When there is uncertainty about odors, a possible unwholesome odor can be enhanced by boiling or frying the meat.

Histologic examination may be used to evaluate abnormalities caused by infectious, toxic, or physical agents. Similarly, microbiologic examination may be used to evaluate spoilage and determine the presence of infectious organisms capable of causing illness in consumers. Chemical and toxicologic examinations should be done when the presence of adulterative or toxic substances is suspected. It may be necessary to increase random microbial testing of meat products to ensure their freedom from bacterial contamination.

Abattoir Sanitation

Abattoir buildings, equipment, personnel, and operating procedures should assure the continued wholesomeness and freedom from adulteration of carcasses and meat. Floors, walls, and ceilings should be constructed of materials and in a manner that allows sanitary operation and thorough cleaning. An ample supply of hot and cold water and cleaning materials should be conveniently available for slaughtering, cleaning, and personal hygiene. Water of at least 180°F (82°C) should be available for sanitizing tools and equipment after cleaning. Equipment, knives, and utensils that have contacted diseased carcasses should be cleaned and sterilized before being used again. Waste-water drainage, with proper trapping and sewage disposal, should be adequate to maintain the abattoir in a sanitary condition. Ventilation should be sufficient to assure that edible product areas are free of noxious odors. Access of flies, rodents, and other vermin should be prevented. Lighting should be maintained at an intensity adequate for cleaning and inspection. Equipment should be of such material and so constructed as to be readily and thoroughly cleaned and should be properly maintained. Separate, clean containers for edible and inedible materials should be provided at convenient locations. Tables or racks should be provided for heads. Personnel should wear clean garments and follow all sanitation and hygiene procedures.

PREPURCHASE EXAMINATION OF HORSES

See also THE LAMENESS EXAMINATION, p 898.

Prepurchase examinations are often requested by a potential buyer of a horse. The objective is to reduce the buyer's risks in relationship to the general health and athletic soundness of the horse for sale. The examination is not meant to guarantee soundness of the horse, but is an attempt, on the part of the veterinarian, to ascertain any preexisting problem or any potential problem that may affect future soundness (eg, degenerative joint disease).

The examining veterinarian should have experience with the specific breed, as well as knowledge of the purpose for which the horse is being purchased. Ideally, the examiner should also be aware of any related organizational regulations that may influence the prepurchase examination. All notes generated during the examination should be kept in the buyer's file and a report should be generated for the buyer. The examination should be conducted in a thorough and organized manner, as prepurchase examinations are a common cause for litigation from dissatisfied buyers. The major problems related to litigation are lack of understanding of the prepurchase examination process and the client's excessive expectation of a secure investment.

At the onset, the roles of all the parties involved (eg, buyer, trainer, legal agent) in the purchase of the particular horse should be defined. Trainers may or may not have legal agent status. The trainer does have the potential to be responsible for assessing buyer's expectations for the horse's athletic future and also whether the horse is suitable for the buyer. If an agent is representing the buyer, the examining veterinarian should encourage all information gathered to be communicated to the buyer, along with the report. Buyers of horses have different levels of experience and practical expectations. The veterinarian should ascertain the particular buyer's expectations and define the limitations of the examination, emphasizing that the examination does not eliminate risks.

The buyer is the owner of the information, but needs to maintain a level of confidentiality so that the reputation of the horse is not potentially altered due to inappropriate dissemination of medical information. Through requests by the buyer or the buyer's agent, the seller and/or their veterinarian may agree to provide the horse's medical history to the examining veterinarian. These medical records are returned at the end of the examination. Trial periods are often acceptable and encouraged, especially if the seller can be assured of the horse's safety. One option is to house the horse in a mutually known, professionally managed barn. The seller may request that the horse be insured.

The simplest way for the veterinarian to accumulate history prior to the examination is to have the seller fill out and sign a history form. This helps to legally bind the seller in the transaction and gives information that may or may not have been known to the buyer, their agent, or the examining veterinarian. A similar questionnaire can be devised for the buyer as to their expectations, potential use, and previous experience with the horse in question. Examples of such forms are readily available on the Internet and may be modified as needed.

Traditionally, it is recommended that the examining veterinarian have had no contact with the horse or seller in a previous medical or personal role. However, this is often not possible when the horse is being sold within a small community or within the same boarding barn. In such situations, the relationship of the veterinarian to all parties involved should be clearly stated. The opposite situation can occur when the horse is being purchased out of town and the examining veterinarian is not the routine veterinarian for the buyer. The examining veterinarian may want to have the buyer's routine veterinarian review the examination report and any ancillary information, such as radiographs, laboratory tests, etc. Also, if any particular question arises during the examination, an opinion from a board-certified veterinary specialist might be indicated.

If the veterinarian has working knowledge of competition rules related to the discipline in which the horse is being purchased (eg, height requirements), he or she should explain how these rules may apply to the prepurchase examination. The veterinarian should counsel the buyer to learn the specific rules and verify "cards" that belong to the pony or horse. Having the buyer verify any rule requirements may help reduce future problems.

State and international disease testing and other requirements should be reviewed with the buyer and complied with by the examining veterinarian. Drug testing should be offered to the buyer and its limitations discussed. If the horse is purchased at a competition, or the seller is not known to the buyer, drug testing should be strongly recommended. Even when a buyer does not wish to have drug testing, examiners often collect blood at the time of the exam and store the serum or plasma frozen. It would then be available if any questions arose after the purchase.

Prepurchase examinations of performance horses often are conducted under several different conditions of training. The ideal situation is that the horse is currently active in the particular level of competition for which it is being purchased. However, prepurchase examinations can involve some inherent predictability even though they are not classically meant for prediction of a horse's health. The following are examples of conditions an examiner may face. Any of these or other modifying conditions should be noted as part of the examination notes: 1) A horse is currently in early training for a specific athletic endeavor and the buyer is ultimately looking to have the horse compete at a higher level. 2) A horse is coming off a lay-off period and has only been back in work for a brief period of time. 3) An older horse that has some infirmities and is being purchased as a schoolmaster by a less experienced rider, in which case the physical demands will potentially decrease with the new buyer. 4) A horse is being purchased for a financial investment. 5) A horse is being purchased as a pleasure or trail horse where the workload is not high but the horse's attitude is extremely important. In each of these conditions, different approaches are needed, and different questions should be asked and understood by the examiner.

Examinations of pretraining and brood stock present different issues to the examining veterinarian. The examiner must be alert to potential limiting conditions of the suckling, weanling, or yearling that would diminish its ability to perform its potential future work. In examining mares and stallions, experience with reproductive examination procedures is needed. (*See also* BREEDING SOUNDNESS EXAMINATION OF THE MARE, p 1761, and BREEDING SOUNDNESS EXAMINATION OF THE MALE, p 1770.) In all situations, thorough knowledge of the rules of the specific breed and any governmental disease regulations is critical.

The examination for a performing horse can be divided into 4 sections. The first part is observing the horse in the stall. The second includes observing the horse on a lead strap at a walk and a trot on a straight line, doing flexion tests, and in a circle with a longe line. The third part of the examination involves observation of the horse while it is being ridden. The fourth part includes diagnostic procedures such as radiography and ultrasound.

During the first part of the examination, a thorough identification of the horse should be recorded. This can be a written description of its color and age verification with inspection of the teeth. Notations of markings and any other permanent peculiarities to the horse's body are also beneficial. The most common markings include a star, stripe, blaze, or snip on the face of the horse. Any white markings on the legs should also be described. Other markings that are valuable to record include whorls on the face and neck, brands, and tattoos. The presence of any scars, splints, or joint effusion should be noted. In some cases, brands or tattoos can give information, such as age (eg, American Jockey Club tattoos have an alphabet letter before the number; "A" represents the years 1971 and 1997). The date, time, and place of the examination should also be recorded. An ophthalmologic examination should be done, as well as auscultation of the heart and lungs, temperature and pulse recordings, and oral examinations. It is also worth looking in the stall for the character of the manure and feed and/or oral medication remaining in the feed bucket.

The second phase of the examination outside the stall can begin with general body and skin condition. The body condition score (1-9) can be assigned a number from thinness (1) to obesity (9). Scores of 4, 5, or 6 are considered normal. Next, visual observation and palpation of the limbs, hoof examination (including hoof testers), passive and active flexion tests, and watching the horse move on different surfaces on a straight line and in a circle should be done. It is also valuable to complete a basic neurologic examination.

Many examiners feel that it is helpful to watch the horse being ridden to rule out any subtle unsoundness. It also gives the examiner some observations and insight into the potential of the rider, if it is the buyer. These observations are worth noting, even though it is the trainer's and buyer's responsibility to determine the suitability of the horse.

The fourth part of the examination should include any diagnostic procedures that may be necessary to determine soundness, including radiographs (particularly of the feet, hocks, and stifles), ultrasonography, and nuclear scans. (*See also* THE LAMENESS EXAMINATION, p 898.) Radiography is the most common diagnostic procedure performed. A recent retrospective analysis of radiography in equine prepurchase examinations suggests that higher radiographic grades (eg, 2-3) in the navicular bone and distal phalanx are associated with lameness, whereas similar grades in the tarsus were less likely to be associated with lameness.

A summary report should be prepared and given to the buyer. There are many published samples of these reports, available in letter or check-off list form. The report should describe any abnormal or undesirable findings and include an opinion as to the functional effect of these findings. The American Association of Equine Practitioners publishes an annual Resource Guide in their membership directory that provides guidelines for reproduction, medications, sale issues such as cryptorchidism, dental malocclusions, postsale examination of the upper respiratory tract of horses intended for racing, radiograph custody, and sale disclosure. Specific guidelines for reporting prepurchase examinations are also included.

PREPURCHASE EXAMINATION OF RUMINANTS AND SWINE

See also BIOSECURITY, p 1679.

The health of animals that are to be sold or moved to other premises is highly important. Both the purchaser and regulatory officials want assurance that the animals are healthy and will not introduce disease into the new herd or new area.

Many countries also have health regulations for exportation of animals. These regulations have been developed to protect foreign markets by assuring foreign animal disease regulatory officials and animal purchasers that the animals are healthy and can be added to their herds with confidence.

Animal health requirements vary with the country, species, age, sex, intended use of the animal, and specific demands of the purchaser. Local animal disease regulatory officials should be contacted for regulations that apply to the specific situation. The following describes general requirements for animal movement in the USA.

When breeding cattle are sold, they must be certified to be free of brucellosis and tuberculosis and, in some states, bluetongue. The certificate, which must be signed by the seller and an accredited veterinarian, certifies that the veterinarian has inspected the animals and that they are not showing signs of infectious or communicable disease. When the herd or geographic area of the seller has been declared free of specific diseases by animal disease regulatory agencies, testing the sale animals for those diseases is usually not required. Pregnancy status of breeding-age females is usually determined, and semen is usually evaluated when breeding-age bulls are sold. When breeding swine are sold, they must be tested for (and found free of) brucellosis and pseudorabies. A detailed examination often is demanded by the purchaser of valuable breeding or performance animals; in the latter, determination of soundness is of prime importance. The prospective purchaser may also select a second veterinarian to perform an additional inspection.

In the examination of any animal before sale, several points should be emphasized: 1) The veterinarian is working for the person paying the fee and reports only to that person. The person responsible for compensating the veterinarian should be informed of the cost before the inspection. 2) The purpose for which the animal is to be used should be clearly established before the examination. 3) The examining veterinarian must be knowledgeable not only in the care and treatment of animals but also must be aware of the purpose for which they will be used.

Because legal action against the examining veterinarian is a possibility, a veterinarian may refuse to provide a written report for prepurchase examinations. However, a written record of findings should be made because it may be needed at a future date. The responsibility of the veterinarian is to supply information and identify abnormalities; the prospective purchaser must make the decision whether to purchase.

The examination is divided into 3 parts: history, clinical examination, and special examinations or diagnostic procedures.

History: A complete history should be obtained by questioning the seller, examining the seller's records, and observing the remainder of the herd and the management conditions. The animal's breed, sex, age, color, markings, tattoos, ear tags, brands, and other identification aids should be noted. Its registration papers should be checked, and its identity definitively established. For a breeding animal, the records of its sire and dam also should be considered, including their breeding ability, the possibility of heritable defects in the line to which each belongs, and, if dead, the cause of death. Also, breeding records of the animal itself should be reviewed to determine its fertility. Breeding records of the herd of origin of the animal should be examined for evidence of disorders that may affect reproduction. If the animal is an adult female, the breeding dates and stage of pregnancy, if applicable, should be noted.

Records should be examined to determine whether the animal has had any previous diseases, injuries (and their severity), or surgical procedures. Previous vaccinations, their type, and date of administration should be noted. The health of the herd of origin and possible contacts with other animals before the sale should be determined because animals so exposed could be in the incubation period of disease. It should also be established whether the animal received any drugs or medication that could alter its normal state. If this cannot be established in the history, it may be prudent to perform assays for suspected medication.

Clinical Examination: All areas of the body and its functions should be examined. The clinical examination should establish the current state of the animal's health and condition of each body system.

Special Examinations and Diagnostic Tests: Some diagnostic tests are routinely performed at the time of sale. Additional diagnostic tests and special examinations may be required by the regulatory officials in the purchaser's locale, demanded by the buyer, or indicated by the findings of the clinical examination. When certain diseases are not present in the seller's locale but are endemic in the purchaser's locale, vaccination (if available) for those diseases is frequently required before movement. Therefore, the regulations of the state or country to which the animal is to be sent must be thoroughly understood and followed, or the sale may be declared void.

If a male is to be purchased for breeding purposes, a complete breeding soundness examination (p 1757) should be conducted.

■　■　■

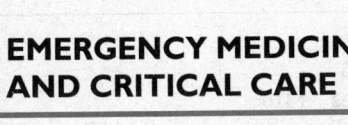

EMERGENCY MEDICINE AND CRITICAL CARE

EMERGENCY MEDICINE
INTRODUCTION

Emergency patients present special challenges because underlying problems may not be evident for 24-48 hr after initial presentation. Problems can arise from an acute illness, from a chronic illness that has decompensated, or from an unexpected complication of another illness. All postoperative patients are considered critical care patients until life-threatening anesthetic or surgical complications are ruled out. The golden rule of emergency medicine is to treat the most life-threatening problems first.

Variables that contribute to the overall success of emergency treatment include the severity of the primary illness or injury, the amount of fluid or blood lost, age of the animal, previous health problems, the number and extent of associated conditions, time delay in instituting therapy, the volume and rate of fluid administration, and the choice of fluids (eg, crystalloid, blood components, or synthetic colloids). Therapy must be done at the right time, in the right amount, and in the right order. Therapeutic failures are generally a result of failing to act expeditiously at a crucial moment.

Specialized care often begins with the owner's initial telephone call. Instructing the owner on first aid and transport procedures can be life-saving for the animal. The clinic and staff must be in readiness, especially if more than one animal in critical condition arrives at the same time. The primary survey, or **triage** (*see* p 1394), requires a quick and accurate assessment and decision regarding the stability of the animal. As life-threatening airway, breathing, and circulation problems are identified, immediate treatment is initiated. Once the animal has been stabilized, a more systematic and organized approach to the history and physical examination (secondary survey) and more specific diagnostic and therapeutic procedures aimed at the underlying etiology can be done.

First Aid and Transport: Owners can provide significant medical assistance at the scene of the injury. At the time of the initial telephone call, the owner should be questioned about the level of consciousness, breathing pattern, and perfusion of the animal. The first concern is for the safety of the owner. Placing a light cloak or cloth over the head of the animal can lessen external stimuli that may cause fearful and aggressive reactions. Cats can be placed in dark boxes to minimize stress during transport; the box should have holes large enough so that the cat can be observed.

When moving the animal, motion of the head, neck, and spine should be minimized. A flat, firm board of wood, cardboard, or thick fabric can be used to provide support. Radiographs can also be taken through these materials without having to move the animal.

Mouth-to-nose resuscitation and chest compressions may provide enough respiratory and circulatory support to maintain life during transport. If the animal is unconscious and not breathing, the owner should be instructed to close the animal's mouth, place their lips over the animal's nostrils, and initially give 3-4 strong breaths. If the animal's breathing does not become spontaneous, the owner should breathe for the animal 10-12 times/min. The owners can also be instructed to compress the esophagus behind the trachea so that most of the air will go down the airway instead of into the stomach. If a heart beat cannot be detected, chest compressions and ventilations at a 5:1 ratio can be performed. Of course, someone else will have to drive during transport.

Owners should be asked if hemorrhage is ongoing or if bleeding was seen at the site of injury. Pulsating arterial bleeding should be controlled by direct digital pressure and then by a pressure bandage. Any long pieces of fabric or gauze can be used. Often washcloths and hand towels are adequate when applied with mild pressure. Additional material can be placed over the original bandage if it becomes soaked with blood.

Penetrating foreign objects should be left in place, but the owner should guard against further penetration or movement of the object. When an arrow has penetrated the abdominal cavity, the shaft of the arrow should not be allowed to move during transport so that bowel segments are not lacerated by the blades. It is often necessary to stabilize the shaft of the arrow just outside the body and, holding it firmly, cut the shaft off.

In dogs with fractures below the elbow or hock with significant displacement, support should be provided. The owner can make a support splint from a rolled newspaper or magazine, which is then secured in place by long pieces of fabric.

Animals with altered mentation after trauma should be transported with the head level or elevated 20°. There should not be any jerking or thrashing motions and no compression of the neck or jugular veins.

Ready Area: A central area of the clinic should be designated as the "ready area," where therapeutics and equipment are organized and available for immediate use. An emergency treatment or crash cart should contain endotracheal tubes of various sizes, a laryngoscope, syringes with needles of different sizes, and drugs for cardiac resuscitation. Oxygen and a small and large ambu bag should be immediately available. Other necessary materials include hair clippers, tape, intravenous and intraosseous catheters with flushing solutions, intravenous isotonic crystalloids, synthetic colloids, bandage material, and trauma transport materials. Additional equipment that would be beneficial include a defibrillator, an ECG machine, a suction unit with various tips, and an indirect blood pressure measurement unit.

EVALUATION AND INITIAL TREATMENT OF THE EMERGENCY PATIENT

PRIMARY SURVEY OR TRIAGE

Triage is the art of assigning priority to emergency patients and their problems based on rapid assessment of historical and physical parameters (*see* TABLE 1). Several historical or observed problems warrant transfer of the animal to the treatment area regardless of physical findings. These problems include trauma, poisonings, profuse diarrhea, urethral obstruction, labored breathing, seizures, loss of consciousness, excessive bleeding, prolapsed organs, potential snake bite, heat prostration, open wounds exposing extensive soft tissue or bone, shock, anemia, burns, and dystocia.

Airway, breathing, and circulation are evaluated sequentially, followed by examination for sources of hemorrhage and determination of the level of consciousness. The most common reasons for an animal "dying before your eyes" include: 1) airway—airway obstruction or disruption; 2) breathing—tension pneumothorax, alveolar flooding (edema fluid or blood), severe bronchoconstriction with air trapping or brain-stem pathology affecting ventilation; and 3) circulation—cardiopulmonary arrest, extreme bradyarrhythmias or tachyarrhythmias, cardiac tamponade, or ongoing internal or external hemorrhage.

AIRWAY

Life-threatening airway pathology (catastrophic or severe) includes complete large airway obstruction and partial obstruction of the large and small airways.

Diagnosis: Animals with complete large airway obstruction are unconscious and apneic. Partial large airway obstruction causes noisy breathing, heard without the aid of a stethoscope. Cyanosis and anxiety are present with loud, low-pitched referred airway sounds heard throughout the thorax on auscultation. Compromise of the extrathoracic airway (nasal passages, pharynx, larynx, or cervical trachea) causes inspiratory stridor; compromise of the intrathoracic trachea or bronchi causes expiratory stridor. Possible causes of large airway pathology include foreign bodies, edema, paralysis of the larynx, tracheal collapse, elongated soft palate, and aspiration of stomach contents. Animals with severe small airway obstruction have labored breathing with an expiratory push of the diaphragm, cyanosis, and anxiety. Auscultation reveals high-pitched wheezes throughout the lung field. In severe life-threatening situations, the animal is cyanotic,

TABLE 1.   Parameters to Evaluate During Triage

Parameter	Evaluation	Significance
Mucous membrane color	Pink	Normal PCV and adequate perfusion
	Pale or white	Anemia or shock
	Cyanotic	Severe hypoxemia
	Yellow	Increased serum bilirubin due to hepatic disease or hemolysis
Capillary refill time	1-2 sec	Normal perfusion and rapidity with which capillaries refill with blood
	>2 sec	Poor perfusion or peripheral vasoconstriction
	<1 sec	Hyperdynamic states; could be associated with fever, heat stroke, distributive shock, or early compensatory stage of hypovolemic shock
Heart rate	70-120 bpm (small dogs) 60-120 bpm (large dogs) 120-200 bpm (cats)	Normal heart rates, indicate that at least one component of cardiac output is normal
	Bradycardia	Decreased cardiac output and subsequent poor perfusion; cats in particular will develop bradycardia (<120 bpm) in shock; an irregular, slow heart beat can be associated with imminent cardiac arrest or conditions such as sick sinus syndrome
	Tachycardia (dogs >180 bpm, cats >220 bpm)	Compromised diastolic filling; sinus tachycardia often results from hypovolemic shock or pain; tachycardia that is irregular or associated with pulse deficits usually indicates an arrhythmia, and an ECG is indicated
Pulse rate and quality	Strong and synchronous with each heart beat	Normal; both femoral and digital pulses should be palpated
	Irregular	Usually indicative of a cardiac arrhythmia
	Bounding	Hyperdynamic state
	Weak	Decreased cardiac output, peripheral vasoconstriction, or decreased pulse pressure
Level of consciousness	Alert and responsive to surroundings	Normal overall neurologic and metabolic state
	Depressed (less responsive to visual and tactile stimuli, sleepy appearance but still arousable)	Can be caused by any illness
	Stupor (arousable only with painful stimuli)	Severe neurologic or metabolic derangements
	Comatose (unarousable with any stimuli) or seizures (usually associated with whole body convulsions, salivation, facial tremors, possibly involuntary urination and defecation)	Abnormal cerebral electrical activity from primary neurologic disease or secondary to metabolic derangements seen in diseases such as diabetes, hepatic encephalopathy, or toxin exposure; accurate history or prior health problems, current medications, and possible toxin exposure important

open-mouth breathing, collapsed, and asphyxiating. Common etiologies include anaphylactic reactions; asthma (cats); and bronchial obstruction from edema, mucus, exudates, or foreign material.

Treatment: Unconscious, apneic animals require immediate tracheal intubation. If the upper airway is obstructed, oxygen can be supplemented by a transtracheal catheter inserted below the obstruction until a tracheotomy is quickly performed. Once an airway is established, ventilation is initiated with 100% oxygen via an ambu bag. Should auscultation during ventilation detect absent or muffled lung sounds indicative of pleural fluid or air, immediate thoracocentesis is warranted. Heart sounds and pulses are checked and when absent, cardiopulmonary-cerebral resuscitation (p 1401) is initiated.

With partial large airway obstruction, flow-by oxygen is delivered through oxygen tubing at a high flow rate aimed at the open, panting mouth until an airway is secured. Heavy sedation using a narcotic/tranquilizer combination may be used to relieve anxiety and struggling, to allow a cursory examination of the pharynx and larynx, and to remove pharyngeal foreign bodies. When tracheal intubation is necessary, general anesthesia (eg, etomidate, ketamine/diazepam, propofol) should be induced rapidly. The ability of the laryngeal folds to move should be assessed during intubation. A tracheotomy is necessary when pharyngeal, laryngeal, or tracheal pathology prevents orotracheal intubation. A transtracheal catheter can be used to provide oxygen support during stabilization. When the airway pathology lies within the thoracic cavity, airway patency must be established down to the bifurcation of the trachea.

Cyanosis from small airway obstructive disease is treated by providing oxygen by flow-by, hood, or nasal cannula and sedation with a narcotic/tranquilizer combination. Epinephrine is given for its bronchodilatory effects both in anaphylaxis (0.01-0.02 mg/kg, IV) and in life-threatening asthma (0.02 mg/kg, IM). Corticosteroids (prednisone sodium succinate, 15 mg/kg, IV, or dexamethasone, 2-4 mg/kg, IM or IV) are given for allergic bronchitis or asthma. Other bronchodilators, such as aminophylline or terbutaline, are given IM or nebulized in the case of an animal in crisis.

BREATHING

Diagnosis: Compromised breathing in both dogs and cats manifests with an increased respiratory rate and effort, immediately followed by a change in the respiratory pattern. Postural changes follow; dogs stand with the elbows abducted and the back arched, while cats may sit crouched on all 4 limbs with the sternum slightly elevated or high on the rear haunches with the head and neck extended. Obvious labored, open-mouth breathing and cyanosis develop last and indicate significant loss of pulmonary function.

The location of the pathology—pleural space or parenchymal disease—is determined at presentation by careful observation of the breathing pattern and auscultation of the thorax. This will direct resuscitative efforts. Taking radiographs or performing stressful diagnostic procedures before the animal has been stabilized can lead to rapid decompensation.

Pleural space disease causes dysynchronous breathing. The chest expands on inspiration as the abdomen is pulled inward, then the chest moves inward on expiration as the abdomen expands. In cats, breathing is slower and more deliberate than in dogs. The respiratory pattern is the same whether air, fluid, or abdominal contents are in the pleural space. Thoracic auscultation reveals muffled lung sounds over the affected regions.

Lung parenchymal disease causes quiet, smooth breathing, with the chest and abdominal wall moving in the same direction. Inspiration and expiration are equally labored unless concurrent small airway edema or constriction adds an expiratory push. Cats demonstrate rapid, shallow synchronous breathing with active movement of the cupula. Thoracic auscultation reveals louder than normal lung sounds in early phases. As disease progresses, harsh lung sounds with moist crackles and rales are heard over the affected lungs. The most common cause of lung parenchymal disease is pulmonary edema. Other abnormalities to exclude include CNS disease, pneumonia, aspiration, pulmonary contusions, or hemoglobin abnormalities. Rapid evaluation of the heart for a murmur, gallop, or arrhythmia aids in identifying cardiogenic versus noncardiogenic causes of the parenchymal pathology.

Treatment: Oxygen is administered immediately via flow-by, mask, hood, or plastic bag techniques. Sedation with a narcotic/tranquilizer combination can relieve struggling and anxiety. Longterm continuous supplemental oxygen is best provided by nasal oxygen catheter. The intranasal oxygen catheter is placed after topical anesthetic has been instilled into the nostril where the tube is to be inserted. Nasal oxygen flow rates of 50-100 mL/kg/min deliver 40-60% inspired oxygen while allowing the animal to be examined and treated. If cyanosis and decompensation persist, intubation and positive-pressure ventilation with 100% oxygen is necessary.

Catastrophic pleural space disease with rapid cardiovascular decompensation, absent lung sounds throughout the thorax, and a barrel-shaped chest suggests tension pneumothorax. Lidocaine is injected for local anesthesia and a small skin incision is made between ribs (at the seventh to eighth intercostal space). Hemostats are used to enter the pleural space, relieving the tension within the thorax. This allows cardiovascular filling and lung re-expansion. The open pneumothorax is then managed by placing a chest tube and surgically closing the intercostal incision.

When breathing is severely compromised by pleural air or fluid without tension pneumothorax, the pleural space should be drained by thoracocentesis. The intended site is clipped and aseptically prepared (when time permits). If fluid is expected, the needle is inserted ventrally between the sternum and the costochondral junction. When air is to be recovered, the needle is inserted into the dorsal half of the thorax, above the costochondral junction. A local anesthetic is placed into the skin, subcutaneous tissue, and intercostal muscle at the site to be tapped. After the needle is inserted just through the skin, a drop of saline is placed in the hub of the needle. The needle is then gradually inserted straight into the thorax (with the needle perpendicular to the chest wall) until the saline in the needle hub moves. The movement of the saline in the hub indicates that the pleural space has been entered. The needle is immediately directed so that it lies against the parietal pleura. This prevents laceration of the lung by the needle as the lung re-expands. As soon as the pleural space is entered, the evacuation apparatus (usually an IV extension set, 3-way stopcock, and syringe) is attached and aspiration begins. In animals in which the pleural space cannot be emptied (eg, tension pneumothorax, ongoing hemorrhage) or when repeated chest taps are required within minutes to hours, an indwelling chest tube should be placed for continuous closed suction.

Lung parenchymal disease is primarily treated using oxygen supplementation, diuretics (furosemide, 1-7 mg/kg, IV), and sedation to relieve anxiety. Cardiogenic edema is usually associated with a gallop, murmur, or arrhythmia and is treated with nitroglycerin ointment ($^1/_4$ in. in cats and $^1/_2$ in. in larger dogs) applied topically to a shaved area of the abdomen. After initial stabilization, further diagnostic procedures (eg, thoracic radiography and echocardiography) aid in determining the cause and specific therapy.

CIRCULATION

Diagnosis: Animals with circulatory compromise have alterations in their perfusion parameters (ie, heart rate, mucous membrane color, capillary refill time [CRT], and pulse intensity). Careful auscultation of the heart for a murmur, gallop, or arrhythmia and the lungs for evidence of fluid is important to help identify heart failure as a cause of cardiogenic shock.

In the early compensatory stages of hypovolemic shock in dogs, there is a rapid heart rate, pink to red mucous membranes, rapid CRT, and bounding pulses. This stage is rarely seen in cats unless there is significant pain. As the pathology progresses, dogs begin to have pale mucous membranes, prolonged CRT, weak pulses, and tachycardia—the classic signs of the middle stage of early decompensatory shock. Cats have gray mucous membranes, slow CRT, weak or absent pulses, hypothermia, and a normal or low heart rate. As shock approaches the terminal stages, the heart rate slows in both dogs and cats, and animals begin to lose consciousness. Clinical signs in this terminal stage include heart failure, pulmonary edema, severe hypotension, oliguria, and abnormal respiratory patterns. Cardiopulmonary arrest is a common sequela.

Treatment: The therapeutic goal is to deliver oxygen and substrate to the tissues. This requires a heart that effectively pumps blood, adequate hemoglobin and intravascular volume, vascular tone and patency, and sufficient oxygen and substrate. General guidelines for treatment of hypovolemic and distributive shock are described below, but modifications may be needed for specific animals.

Oxygen Supplementation: Oxygen (at least 40-60% concentration) should be administered by flow-by technique, mask, bag, nasal cannula, endotracheal tube, or transtracheal catheter.

Hemostasis: Control of ongoing hemorrhage is essential for stabilization and often required before restoration of circulation. The animal must be carefully examined on both sides for any evidence of bleeding. Direct pressure should be immediately placed over the bleeding skin site, and bleeding arteries clamped. When blood slowly oozes from a skin wound, a compression bandage should be placed. If more aggressive hemostasis is required, a pneumatic cuff can be placed above the bleeding site and inflated until hemorrhage stops.

Intrathoracic or abdominal hemorrhage may not become evident until blood pressure and circulation are restored. Ongoing abdominal hemorrhage is initially managed by small volume fluid therapy and abdominal counterpressure. Ongoing intrathoracic hemorrhage should be managed by a chest tube to evacuate the blood and to allow measurement of the volume lost. Exploration of these body cavities is often required for assessment and definitive hemostasis.

Intravascular Volume Replacement: Intravenous or intraosseous catheters are used, with multiple catheters placed for rapid, large volume infusion in dogs >30 kg body wt. Isotonic crystalloids can be administered by repeated low volume boluses (10-15 mL/kg) until desired endpoints of resuscitation are reached. However, the interstitium is at risk for fluid overload with crystalloids alone. The concurrent use of colloids and crystalloids can reduce the amount of crystalloid required, rapidly expand the intravascular space with a smaller volume of fluid infused, and reduce the amount of fluid extravasating into the interstitial spaces of vital organs (eg, lung, brain). Isotonic crystalloids are given with hetastarch or stroma-free hemoglobin. Whole blood, stroma-free hemoglobin, or packed red cells are necessary during initial volume resuscitation when hemorrhage has been significant.

Small volume resuscitation is used to avoid volume overload or hypertension and is ideal for animals with head injury, pulmonary edema or contusions, abdominal or intrathoracic hemorrhage, heart disease, and all cats in hypovolemic shock. Isotonic crystalloids are given (10-15 mL/kg, IV) followed by hetastarch or stroma-free hemoglobin (dogs 5 mL/kg, IV; cats 1-5 mL/kg, IV slowly) repeated to effect. The least amount of crystalloids and colloids possible are used to obtain and maintain a systolic blood pressure of 90 mm Hg. *See* FLUID THERAPY (p 1409) for an in-depth explanation.

Pain Control: Analgesia is provided during initial fluid resuscitation for optimal cardiovascular response and relief of anxiety. Narcotics are administered systemically, and local anesthetics can be infiltrated into the affected area.

Warming: Animals in shock should be warmed during fluid resuscitation until rectal temperatures are >98°F.

Corticosteroids: Corticosteroids are administered when a deficiency is suspected (ie, Addisonian crisis, adrenal depletion). High-dose steroid administration has not been proved to improve mortality in hypovolemic, septic, or cardiogenic shock and has been associated with increased morbidity.

Cardiovascular Support: Pharmacologic agents (positive inotropes, systemic vasodilators, and vasopressors) can be used when fluid infusion has adequately replaced intravascular volume (ie, central venous pressure >5 cm H_2O) but fails to restore blood pressure and perfusion, or when poor cardiac contractility is thought to contribute to hypotension. A positive inotropic agent can be administered (eg, dobutamine, initially at 2-5 µg/kg/min, and the dosage titrated for optimal cardiac output). Stroma-free hemoglobin (dogs 5 mL/kg; cats 1-3 mL per cat, slowly) can be administered for its colloid effect as well as its mild pressor effect. The initial dose may be followed by a slow constant rate of infusion (dogs 10-15 mL/kg/day; cats 1-3 mL/hr up to 5 mL/kg/day) to maintain perfusion if the initial dose was successful and further support is anticipated.

Dopamine (5-20 mg/kg/min, IV, constant rate infusion) can be infused for vasopressor effects and delivered, in the smallest dosage, needed to maintain mean arterial pressure >80 mm Hg, as another option. The blood flow to the kidneys and GI tract, as well as other organs, may have been significantly impaired during shock. Urine output, heart rate, potential arrhythmias, pulse intensity, and mucous membrane color should be closely monitored as further vasoconstriction can worsen function. If organ function declines or if arrythmias become a problem, the IV drip should be stopped; the effects of dopamine should reverse within 5-10 min.

Rear Limb and Abdominal Binding: When ongoing abdominal hemorrhage is suspected from trauma, binding the rear limbs and abdomen can improve perfusion. This procedure compresses the arteries and arterioles within the bound regions, increasing regional vascular resistance. Bleeding from vessels within the region is slowed or arrested while blood is redirected from the periphery to the more central (core) circulation. Binding can be accomplished by applying towels and stretch bandage wrap, using techniques similar to placing a large padded bandage. Beginning at the toes, the rear limbs are bound upward with the abdomen bound last. Prior to binding the abdomen, a small cloth roll should be placed along the midline from sternum to pelvis for padding. This prevents the wrap from impairing ventilation or fracturing the spleen or liver. Abdominal binding should be avoided in cases of intrathoracic or intracranial hemorrhage. Once perfusion has stabilized, the wrap is removed slowly by sections, from the abdomen moving caudally. Any signs of decompensation warrant rapid rebinding of the region last unwrapped.

SECONDARY SURVEY

The secondary survey of emergency patients is the process of obtaining significant historical information, performing a complete physical examination, and collecting general diagnostic information. These data are used to identify specific historical or physical problems and to direct the formulation of a specific diagnostic, therapeutic, and monitoring plan.

The **history** should be recorded in a concise format. The presenting complaint is obtained from the owner, who can provide information such as when the animal was last completely normal. A chronology of the daily progression of abnormalities since the onset of signs can be useful. Background information includes past medical problems, medications, drug and food sensitivities, blood transfusions, and the date of last vaccinations. Other organ systems not seemingly involved should also be evaluated.

A complete **physical examination** should be performed, working from head to tail. Particular attention should be given to heart and lung auscultation for abnormalities, and to abdominal, rectal, and joint palpation for pain or enlargements. Acute abdominal pain requires localization of the pain and auscultation of the abdomen for bowel sounds to localize the problem to the reticuloendothelial, reproductive, urinary, or GI systems; the peritoneal space; or the muscle, skin, nerves, or fat around the abdominal wall. Fever of unknown origin directs examination to the peritoneal cavity and to the reproductive, urinary, pulmonary, and cardiovascular systems.

An initial **minimum database** should consist of a PCV, total solids, glucose, BUN, urinalysis (before fluid administration), and sodium and potassium levels. When coagulation disorders are suspected or surgery is anticipated, blood smears to estimate platelet number, buccal bleeding time to evaluate platelet number and function, and activated clotting times to test the intrinsic clotting cascade should be done as soon as possible.

SPECIFIC DIAGNOSTICS AND THERAPY

TRAUMA

The nature of the trauma can direct diagnostic and therapeutic efforts. Blunt trauma is commonly associated with thoracic and abdominal bleeding, organ rupture, fractures, and neurologic injuries. Penetrating trauma is typically localized to the path of the penetrating object. Falling from a height causes long bone and facial bone fractures as well as thoracic injuries. A dog bitten by another larger dog can have deep penetrating bite wounds and frequently spinal injuries and tracheal rupture from the thrashing motions experienced during the attack. Resuscitation of the airway, breathing, and circulation; control of hemorrhage; and pain relief are followed by a careful evaluation of the nervous system, chest, abdomen, and skeletal system.

The traumatized animal should be approached as if multiple injuries are present. The neck and spine should be immobilized until a thorough examination for spinal fractures or luxations is made. Thoracic auscultation for cardiac arrhythmias and lung sounds should be done to determine the presence of chest injuries. The abdomen should be palpated for pain, fluid, or hernias. Extremity fractures should be supported by bandages or splinted to prevent further injury if there is significant swelling or displacement of bone. Because many problems are not apparent for 12-24 hr after trauma occurs, careful monitoring allows early detection of potentially life-threatening complications.

Initial diagnostic work should include the minimum database before fluids are administered. This baseline information is used to determine the response to therapy. Survey lateral radiographs of the chest and abdomen can demonstrate changes resulting from thoracic and abdominal trauma.

Thoracic Trauma

Pulmonary contusions, pneumothorax, cardiac arrhythmias, pleural hemorrhage, pericardial hemorrhage, rib fractures, flail chest, and diaphragmatic hernia are but a few of the potentially life-threatening complications that must be considered in thoracic trauma. Oxygen supplementation and analgesics allow careful physical examination. An ECG, thoracic radiographs, blood gas analysis, and diagnostic or therapeutic centesis aid in determining the extent and severity of the problems.

Severe pulmonary contusions cause hypoxemia, labored breathing in a pattern consistent with parenchymal disease, and crackles and rales on pulmonary auscultation. If the animal does not improve with supplemental oxygen, rapid sedation, intubation, and positive-pressure ventilation with 100% oxygen are indicated. The airway should be suctioned to evacuate blood and debris that is obstructing the flow of air.

Labored breathing with a choppy pattern consistent with pleural air or fluid warrants thoracocentesis. When a negative pressure cannot be achieved, repeated thoracocentesis or continuous drainage of the pleural space by chest tube is required. Large quantities of whole blood removed on thoracocentesis or ongoing leakage of air after 72 hr of pleural drainage are indications for surgical exploration of the chest.

The chest cavity should be palpated for rib fractures with displaced bone, flail segments, avulsion of ribs, torn intercostal muscles, and herniations. When flail segments impair ventilation, the segment is stabilized by securing it to an external frame of metal rods or cast material formed to the shape of the chest. Penetrating bite wounds over the chest should be explored under anesthesia for debridement and drain placement; the thorax will need to be entered if the wound is penetrating.

The heart should be auscultated, and an ECG evaluated for arrhythmias. The most common arrhythmias seen with thoracic trauma are sinus tachycardia, ventricular premature contractions, and ventricular tachycardia. Treatment with lidocaine is warranted if the arrhythmias impair perfusion, if the rate is rapid, if ventricular premature contractions are multiform, or if there are prefibrillatory rhythms (R on T phenomenon, torsades de pointes, ventricular flutter).

Abdominal Trauma

The extent and severity of abdominal injuries are not initially obvious unless there is visceral dehiscence. The abdomen should be examined closely for evidence of bruising, road burns, lacerations, protrusions, localized swelling, distention, and pain. Animals with evidence of abdominal pain and in shock should be considered to have intra-abdominal hemorrhage until proved otherwise. Rupture or laceration of the spleen or liver are the most likely sources. Retroperitoneal hemorrhage from damaged muscle or avulsion of the kidneys or a mesenteric vessel are other common sources. However, all abdominal organs have blood vessels that are susceptible to the shearing forces from blunt trauma and are possible sites of significant bleeding. Small volume fluid resuscitation to achieve low normal blood pressure is indicated to avoid increases in arterial or venous pressures that can disrupt a blood clot. Abdominal distention from hemorrhage is generally not apparent until fluid therapy has been ongoing and intravascular blood pressures have increased enough to cause continuous hemorrhage. Rear limb and abdominal binding (p 1399) are indicated early to reduce the amount of hemorrhage.

After injury of any abdominal organ, clinical signs of organ dysfunction or hollow viscus rupture typically develop over a period of hours. Acute abdominal pain is a key physical finding. Survey abdominal radiographs can demonstrate organ displacement, distention, rotation, or free abdominal fluid. Fluid can be recovered by abdominocentesis from a tap of each abdominal quadrant or an ultrasound-guided tap. When free fluid is not readily identified, a diagnostic peritoneal lavage is done. A fenestrated catheter is placed into the peritoneal space, and warm isotonic saline (20 mL/kg) infused into the abdomen. The fluid is allowed to dwell for several minutes and distribute throughout the abdomen; it is then drained and evaluated.

Clear fluid indicates that the possibility of significant abdominal hemorrhage is minimal. Fluid with a 1% PCV indicates mild abdominal hemorrhage, while fluid with a PCV >5% indicates significant abdominal hemorrhage that warrants careful monitoring. The fluid should be examined cytologically for evidence of WBC, plant or meat fibers, free bacteria, or bacteria within WBC. Biochemical evaluation for creatinine and potassium, bilirubin, amylase, and phosphorus help identify urinary bladder rupture, gallbladder rupture, pancreatic injury, or ischemic bowel, respectively. The abdominocentesis or peritoneal lavage can be repeated in several hours if fluid from the first tap did not indicate a significant problem but the clinical signs continue or progress.

Criteria for emergency exploratory laparotomy include ongoing hemorrhage; inability to stabilize shock; evidence of organ rupture, rotation, or laceration; diaphragmatic hernia with labored breathing or the stomach in the chest; or peritonitis after abdominal trauma. Retroperitoneal or severe fascial compartment hemorrhage (associated with pelvic fractures) is suspected in those acutely traumatized animals that still have signs of a declining PCV, nonresponsive hemorrhagic shock, and no significant findings on peritoneal lavage. Radiographs typically show expansion and loss of detail in the retroperitoneal space. An IV pyelogram should be done to help delineate disruption in the renal vascular supply or in the retroperitoneal portion of the ureter before proceeding with exploratory surgery in this situation.

CARDIOPULMONARY-CEREBRAL RESUSCITATION

The success of cardiopulmonary-cerebral resuscitation (CPCR) efforts depends on the underlying cause of the arrest and on the timeliness and effectiveness of the intervention. The basic initial steps of CPCR promote oxygenation, ventilation, and circulation. CPCR progresses with advanced life support, using electrocardiographic evaluation of cardiac rhythms, administration of drugs, and defibrillation when necessary. Often, basic life support takes on an advanced form when circulation must be promoted by surgical intervention.

Basic Life Support

Mouth-to-nose resuscitation should be performed until endotracheal intubation and positive-pressure ventilation with 100% oxygen can be accomplished. Two quick breaths are given while the chest is auscultated to assess endotracheal tube placement. Ventilations should be provided at 20-60 breaths/min.

Circulation should be promoted by compressing the chest externally over the area of the heart, generally the fourth and fifth intercostal space, while the animal is in lateral recumbency. Dogs weighing >15 kg can be placed in dorsal recumbency, and chest compressions applied over the caudal one-third of the sternum. The compression rate should be 60-120/min. Each compression should be delivered quickly in a cough-like fashion and should compress the chest wall ~30%. In dogs weighing <15 kg, the direct compression of the heart may contribute to forward blood flow, but the change in pressure that occurs in the thorax as a whole is considered to be the more important mechanism for generating forward flow.

Perfusion should be quickly assessed to determine the effectiveness of basic life support procedures. If perfusion is inadequate, procedures should be modified as necessary. Abdominal counterpressure can be initiated if there is no intra-abdominal pathology. Abdominal counterpressure is performed by placing both hands on the ventral surface of the abdomen and thrusting quickly in a dorsal direction, timing the abdominal compression to occur between chest compressions. The goal is to improve venous return to the heart during the diastolic phase of the compression cycle.

Many clinicians think that immediate defibrillation of an animal with a witnessed arrest offers the best prognosis for recovery. One of the most treatable arrest arrhythmias is ventricular fibrillation, and defibrillation is the treatment of choice. If the arrhythmia is something other than ventricular fibrillation, it is thought that one-time defibrillation does minimal, if no, harm.

Advanced Life Support

In advanced life support, an ECG is obtained to characterize arrhythmias, followed by drug administration or defibrillation as indicated. The purpose is to reestablish electrical and myocardial activity of the heart. Five major arrhythmias are frequently associated with cardiac arrest: ventricular flutter, ventricular fibrillation, asystole, pulseless idioventricular rhythm, and electromechanical dissociation. Drugs are selected based on the arrhythmia and can be administered by intravenous, intraosseous, intratracheal, intracardiac, or sublingual routes (TABLE 2).

Isotonic balanced electrolyte crystalloid solutions should be rapidly infused to restore volume and promote perfusion. Synthetic colloids such as hetastarch or dextran 70 or stroma-free hemoglobin rapidly expand the intravascular volume with a much smaller volume required. Overzealous fluid administration can result in fulminant pulmonary edema due to poor myocardial contractility or arrhythmias.

If the basic life support is unsuccessful (determined by failure of spontaneous respiration or inability to generate detectable forward blood flow) after 5-10 min, open-chest

TABLE 2. Drugs Used in Cardiopulmonary-cerebral Resuscitation, Dosages, and Indications

Drug	Dosage*	Indications
Epinephrine	1 mL/5-10 lb (1:10,000 concentration)	Asystole, ventricular fibrillation
Atropine	0.1 mL/5 lb (0.5 mg/mL solution)	Sinus bradycardia, asystole
Sodium bicarbonate	0.2-2.0 mL/kg (1 mEq/mL solution)	Severe metabolic acidemia associated with prolonged cardiopulmonary resuscitation efforts (must adequately ventilate to be effective)
Calcium gluconate	1 mL/5-10 kg (2% solution without epinephrine)	Electromechanical dissociation, pulseless idioventricular rhythm
Prednisolone or methylprednisolone sodium succinate	5-15 mg/kg	Electromechanical dissociation
Dexamethasone sodium succinate	1 mL/kg (4 mg/mL solution)	Electromechanical dissociation
Lidocaine	2-4 mg/kg	Ventricular flutter, ventricular fine fibrillation

*Dosage should be doubled if given via intratracheal or sublingual route.

cardiopulmonary resuscitation (CPR, *see* below) is indicated. There are instances when open-chest CPR is indicated during initial basic life support, such as severe trauma with blood loss or in a large dog in which external compressions are unlikely to generate an adequate forward blood flow.

Arrhythmias of Cardiac Arrest

Asystole: Asystole appears as a flat line on the ECG and suggests complete absence of electrical activity. Animals in asystole can be assumed to have hyperkalemia until proved otherwise. Regular insulin at 0.2 U/kg, followed by glucose at 2 g/U of insulin often starts the heart beating again. If it does not, the prognosis is grave. Atropine and epinephrine can be administered in an attempt to generate impulses. Many arrhythmias that appear to be asystole are, in fact, fine ventricular fibrillation. For this reason, open-chest heart massage and direct observation of myocardial activity are warranted early with this arrhythmia. Administration of epinephrine and defibrillation may be indicated.

Ventricular Flutter: This rhythm is more chaotic than ventricular tachycardia and is prefibrillatory. Lidocaine is the drug of choice to block the excited focus. If lidocaine is ineffective after 2 boluses and perfusion is absent, defibrillation may be required.

Ventricular Fibrillation: This rhythm implies that multiple foci within the ventricles are firing rapidly and independently, resulting in no coordinated mechanical activity. There are no ventricular contractions and no cardiac output. The goal is to abruptly stop the electrical activity and allow one strong focus to take over. Defibrillation is more successful when there are few, strong foci (coarse fibrillation) than when there are multiple, weak foci (fine fibrillation). When the fibrillation is fine, an attempt is made to convert it to coarse by use of epinephrine (if no effect, then lidocaine) before defibrillation.

Electromechanical Dissociation (EMD): The ECG tracing can be normal or show an arrhythmia, but the heart has no muscular activity, ie, no contractions and no cardiac output. In this arrhythmia, it is vital that thoracic auscultation be performed in tandem with ECG evaluation. There are no heart sounds or pulse activity. However, severe hypovolemia, pericardial effusion, and significant accumulation of fluid or air in the pleural cavity can prevent detection of heart sounds in a beating heart. The ECG associated with these conditions demonstrates tachyarrhythmias, in contrast to the usually normal or slow rate of EMD. EMD has a grave prognosis. Epinephrine and glucocorticoids may be given in an attempt to correct this arrhythmia.

Pulseless Idioventricular Rhythm: This electrical activity originates from an ectopic ventricular focus that produces insufficient pressure to generate a peripheral pulse. Generally, this is a slow ventricular rhythm. Lidocaine should not be given because it can eliminate the single focus. Dexamethasone, vasopressors, or positive inotropes may help. Epinephrine may be given, one dose IV, followed by a constant rate infusion administered in the fluids.

Open-chest Cardiopulmonary Resuscitation
(Emergency thoracotomy)

If possible, a quick clip of the hair along the intended incision site is helpful. Usually, there is no time for a full aseptic preparation of the area. A scalpel blade is used to incise the skin and subcutaneous tissues along the cranial border of the fourth or fifth rib from the spine to sternum. A Carmalt forceps is used to bluntly dissect through the underlying muscle tissues and push through the pleura. After the pleura is entered at the ventral aspect of the incision, Mayo scissors are used to incise the muscles dorsally along the entire length of the intercostal space. After the chest cavity is open, the pericardiodiaphragmatic ligament is elevated and incised with scissors, extending the incision dorsally to just ventral to the phrenic nerve. The heart is then lifted out of the pericardial sac and observed for any coordinated spontaneous contractions. If no cardiac contractions are noted, the heart is grasped with one or both hands and compressed progressively from the apex to the base. The compression is then released to allow the cardiac chambers to refill with blood. The descending aorta can be isolated and temporarily cross-clamped to direct blood flow to the brain. Aortic cross-clamping can be performed with atraumatic vascular clamps, rubber shod clamps, Forrester sponge forceps, or by passing a rubber tube or umbilical tape around the aorta and tightening by sliding a hemostat down just above the aorta. Aortic cross-clamping can be performed for 10 min without serious complications.

An ECG is evaluated and drugs given as indicated during advanced life support procedures. Return of spontaneous circulation allows lavage of the thorax with large quantities of sterile, warm, isotonic saline; placement of a chest tube; and surgical closure of the thorax. Cardiovascular support (see p 1398) is frequently required to maintain circulation while the underlying cause of the arrest is treated.

FLUID THERAPY

Cardiac function; intravascular volume; and vascular tone, integrity, and patency are critical to normal circulation. An abnormality in one or more of these components of circulation leads to compensatory changes to maintain perfusion. The hemodynamic and cellular changes that develop as a result of these abnormalities are called shock. As shock progresses, oxygen and substrate delivery to the tissues becomes insufficient to meet energy requirements for cellular maintenance and repair. If shock progresses and cellular energy demands cannot be met, the ensuing organ failure leads to death. Early recognition of the type and stage of shock is vital to establishing a successful fluid therapy plan.

Shock is typically classified into 3 categories: hypovolemic, cardiogenic, and distributive. Hypovolemic shock develops when there is a blood volume deficit ≥15%. Cardiogenic shock results when the heart fails as a pump. Common etiologies include pulmonary emboli, cardiac tamponade, valvular insufficiency, cardiomyopathy, and cardiac arrhythmias. Distributive shock is caused by maldistribution of blood flow away from the central circulation as a result of peripheral vasodilation. The different types of shock may have different hemodynamic profiles during the early and middle stages. Frequently, more than one type of shock is present.

FLUID THERAPY PLAN

Fluid therapy is used to replace intravascular volume (perfusion) or interstitial fluid volume (dehydration), or to correct electrolyte abnormalities (hypercalcemia, hypokalemia, hyper- or hyponatremia). More accuracy is required in formulating the fluid therapy plan for the critically ill than in the usual hospital patient, because the kidneys and cardiovascular system, which can correct most fluid therapy miscalculations, may be compromised. It is important to understand the dynamics between the fluid compartments and the specific components of each fluid to select the best fluid for the individual situation. The volume and rate of administration are guided by pathologic conditions such as cardiac disease, systemic inflammatory response syndrome diseases, fluid loss into the third body fluid space, blood pressure, and pulmonary and cerebral edema.

Fluid Compartment Dynamics

Water comprises 60% of body weight. Of this water, $2/3$ is intracellular, and $1/3$ is extracellular. Of the body water that is extracellular, $1/4$ is intravascular, and $3/4$ is interstitial. The membranes separating these compartments are freely permeable to water, which moves under the force of osmotic pressure until the osmolality of each compartment is equal. When "free water" (no osmotically active particles) is added to one body compartment, it is distributed evenly throughout all body water compartments. The replacement of 3 L of free water in the intravascular space results in a net increase of only 250 mL in the intravascular volume after equilibration.

When a solution isotonic with plasma is infused, the fluid distribution is different. With no difference in osmolality, there is no osmotic pressure to cause the water to move into the intracellular space. The membrane separating the intravascular and interstitial compartments is freely permeable to water and small ions, while the membrane surrounding the intracellular space is not. But only $1/4$ of the volume of isotonic fluids infused remains in the intravascular space after 30 min due to the influences of osmotic and hydrostatic forces.

The intravascular and interstitial fluid compartments are separated by a semipermeable membrane. In solution in the intravascular compartment are large molecular weight molecules, called colloids, that cannot easily cross the membrane because of the minute size of the membrane pore. The force exerted on the membrane caused by the osmotic gradient created by these colloids is called the colloidal oncotic pressure (COP). The natural particles in blood that create COP are proteins—globulins, fibrinogen, and albumin. Albumin is the smallest (~69,000 daltons) and most numerous. Whether or not fluid remains in the intravascular space or moves into the interstitium is the result of the differences between the COP and hydrostatic pressure in the 2 compartments. Fluid moves into the interstitial space when intravascular hydrostatic pressure is increased over COP, membrane pore size increases, or intravascular COP becomes lower than interstitial COP. When this is replenishing an interstitial volume deficit, the result is rehydration. An excessive volume causes edema.

The usual pressure pushing the fluid across the semipermeable membrane is 17 mm Hg. A total protein of 5.2-5.4 g/dL usually creates a COP of 17 mm Hg. A total protein below this range indicates that colloids should be included in fluid therapy; continued administration of crystalloids increases the intravascular hydrostatic pressure, further dilutes total protein, and accelerates fluid flow across the membrane.

Fluid Compartment Deficits

Fluid deficit in the intravascular space results in poor perfusion and inadequate tissue oxygenation. This volume deficit results in a lower vessel wall tension and stimulation of the baroreceptors. Physical parameters that reflect perfusion status include heart rate, pulse intensity, capillary refill time, mucous membrane color, and rectal temperature. Fluids administered must remain in the intravascular space, increase the vessel wall tension, and obliterate the need for the baroreceptor compensatory response. Most animals with an intravascular deficit (poor perfusion) also have concurrent extravascular deficits. This warrants the simultaneous administration of crystalloid solutions when colloids are used for correction of the intravascular deficit.

Fluid deficit in the extravascular space (interstitial and intracellular) causes dehydration. This results in tenting of the skin, dry mucous membranes, sunken eyes, and dullness of the cornea. Perfusion parameters should be evaluated simultaneously to determine whether poor perfusion is compounding the dehydration. To replenish the extravascular spaces, crystalloid fluids that are the same tonicity as plasma are used. Crystalloids are water-based solutions with low molecular weight molecules that are freely permeable across the capillary membrane. The concentration of these molecules in relation to normal plasma indicates the tonicity of the fluid. If the concentration is similar to normal plasma, the solution is called isotonic.

Physical and laboratory parameters are used to quantify the degree of dehydration. Semidry oral mucous membranes, normal skin turgor, and eyes maintaining normal moisture indicate 4-5% dehydration. Dry oral mucous membranes, mild loss of skin turgor, and eyes still moist indicate 6-7%. Dry mucous membranes, considerable loss of skin turgor, and eyes retracted indicate 8-10%. Very dry oral mucous membranes, complete loss of skin turgor, severe retraction of the eyes, dull eyes, and possible alteration of consciousness indicate 12%.

The physical guidelines for estimating dehydration are misleading in 2 common clinical situations. Chronically emaciated animals may have metabolized the fat from around the eyes and the collagen in the skin, resulting in poor skin turgor and sunken eyes despite normal hydration. Animals with rapid fluid loss into a third body fluid space (a space within the body cavity where fluid from the local interstitial and intravascular spaces leak) have rapid fluid shifts from the intravascular compartments into these spaces before clinical evidence of interstitial fluid loss is seen. Both situations require evaluation of mucous membrane and eye moisture, PCV, and total solids before dehydration can be estimated.

The intravascular space can be replenished using crystalloid solutions alone. However, large quantities of crystalloids may be required to provide volumes sufficient to blunt the baroreceptor response after 1 hr of infusion. The extra interstitial volume for a short period does not cause a problem in most animals, and if renal function is normal, the additional volume is eventually excreted. However, the brain and heart do not have "forgiving" interstitial spaces in disease, and additional interstitial fluid can cause organ failure.

Many conditions can increase capillary permeability and cause systemic inflammation (eg, parvoviral diarrhea, pancreatitis, septic shock, massive trauma, heat stroke, cold exposure, burns, snake bite, and systemic neoplasia). Increased vessel permeability is an additional factor that favors movement of crystalloid fluid from the intravascular space into the interstitial space and complicates maintenance of intravascular volume. A combination of a large molecular weight colloid (to hold the water in the vessels) and crystalloids (to replenish the interstitial spaces) is recommended. In addition, many of these animals have a third body fluid space, most likely due to significant regional inflammation. The end result is massive fluid requirements, which make maintaining fluid balance (especially intravascularly) difficult. It is almost impossible to predict how much fluid will be required to maintain perfusion and hydration in these critical patients. Fluid selection becomes critical, with the rate and volume titrated until the goals of resuscitation have been met (ie, normal heart rate, blood pressure, perfusion parameters).

FLUID SELECTION

Proper fluid selection begins by determining the site(s) of the deficit and the type of fluid to administer—colloid, crystalloid, or a combination of both.

Colloids

When colloids are to be administered, it must be decided whether natural colloids (eg, plasma or whole blood) or a synthetic colloid (TABLE 3) is to be used. When the animal requires RBC, clotting factors, antithrombin III, or albumin, blood products are the colloids of choice.

During maintenance therapy, when the albumin is <2 g/dL, fresh frozen plasma is used. The goal is to give plasma until the albumin is >2 g/dL; synthetic colloids can then be used to add the remaining volume in larger animals.

When the initial goal is to rapidly improve perfusion in an animal without obvious significant blood loss, a synthetic colloid can achieve the desired volume expansion rapidly. Choices of synthetic colloids include dextran, hydroxyethyl starch (HES), and stroma-free hemoglobin.

Dextrans are polysaccharides composed of linear glucose residues. They are produced by the enzyme dextran sucrase during growth of various strains of *Leuconostoc* bacteria in media containing sucrose. Dextrans are isotonic and can be stored at room

TABLE 3. Synthetic Colloids			
Colloid	Average Molecular Weight (daltons)	Molecular Weight Range (daltons)	Half-life (hr)
Dextran 70	70,000	10,000-80,000	25
Hetastarch	450,000	10,000-3.4 million	25
Stroma-free hemoglobin (Oxyglobin®)	65,000-130,000	Up to 500,000	30-40

temperature. Dextran is broken down completely to CO_2 and H_2O by dextranase present in spleen, liver, lung, kidney, brain, and muscle at a rate approaching 70 mg/kg every 24 hr. In normal dogs, dextran 70 increases plasma volume 1.38 times (138%) the volume infused.

Hemostatic changes in healthy experimental dogs given dextran 70 include an increase in the buccal mucosal bleeding time and partial thromboplastin time and a decrease in Von Willebrand's factor antigen and factor VIII coagulant activity, without clinical bleeding. Fibrinogen concentration decreases in excess of that which can be explained by dilution in dogs. Dextran copolymerizes with the fibrin monomer, destabilizing clot formation. Blood glucose levels may be elevated during dextran metabolism. Dextran 70 may cause a change in the total solids value that does not reflect actual protein content and may interfere with blood crossmatching. Moderate to life-threatening reactions in dogs have been rare.

Hydroxyethyl starch (HES) is the parent name of a polymeric molecule made from a waxy species of either maize or sorghum and is composed primarily of amylopectin (98%). The disappearance of HES molecules from the body depends on their rate of absorption by tissues (liver, spleen, kidney, and heart), gradual return to circulation, uptake by the reticuloendothelial system, enzymatic degradation to smaller particles by amylase, and clearance through urine and bile. Blood α-amylase-mediated hydrolysis reduces the molecular weight to <72,000 daltons. Metabolism of HES retained in tissue is probably performed by cytoplasmic lysosomes. A rise in serum amylase is to be expected without alteration in pancreatic function.

The degree of substitution, rather than molecular weight, is the major determinant of how long the different types of HES survive in the blood. When hetastarch (the most common HES) is infused at 25 mL/kg in healthy dogs, the initial increase in plasma volume is 1.37 times (137%) the volume infused. Intravascular persistence is significantly greater than that of dextran 70, with 38% of hetastarch remaining compared with 19% of dextran 24 hr after infusion. Administration by constant rate infusion may provide a constant supply of larger molecular weight particles, perhaps maintaining and augmenting plasma COP in animals with albumin loss.

Hetastarch favors retention of intravascular fluid and prevents washout of interstitial proteins. In hypo-oncotic situations, hetastarch infusion has a great advantage over other colloids because the larger molecules remain intravascular, limiting pulmonary fluid flux. It is nontoxic and nonallergenic in dosages up to 100 mL/kg in dogs. Many cats have a moderate reaction—nausea and occasional vomiting—with rapid infusion. However, when hetastarch is given slowly (over 5-15 min), this side effect is eliminated.

Hetastarch is associated with minor alterations in laboratory coagulation measurements but not with clinical bleeding unless daily maximum dosages (40 mL/kg/day) are exceeded. Dilutional effects on coagulation, cells, and proteins are produced in response to the volume expansion of the plasma.

Stroma-free hemoglobin (Oxyglobin®) is a polymerized bovine hemoglobin-based solution that increases plasma and total hemoglobin concentration. This solution is indicated for the treatment of anemia and hypovolemia with tissue hypoxia. It has colloidal properties similar to those of hetastarch and exerts mild vasopressor activity. The dark hue of the solution causes discoloration of the serum that can interfere with some serum chemistry tests, depending on the type of analyzer and reagents used.

◀ TABLE 3. (continued)		
Colloid Oncotic Pressure (mm Hg)	**Concentration (%)**	**Maximum Water Binding (mL water/g colloid)**
—	6	29
30	10	20
—	13	—

Bilirubinuria will be present. Dosages ≤30 mL/kg/day have been approved for dogs, with the rate of infusion <10 mL/kg/hr. When given to an animal that has a normal blood volume, administration must be slow and carefully monitored to avoid volume overload resulting from the colloidal and pressor properties of the solution.

Crystalloids

The particular crystalloid to administer is determined by the measured or estimated sodium and potassium concentrations and by the osmolality of both the animal's serum and the fluid to be administered (TABLE 4). When blood parameters are unknown, it is best to initially select a fluid with electrolyte content, pH, and osmolality most like serum (eg, lactated Ringer's, Plasmalyte-A®, Normosol-R®).

Sodium Content: When serum sodium estimations are normal, a balanced isotonic electrolyte solution can be used for volume replacement. In animals with decreased serum sodium content, volume replacement should be with isotonic saline (0.9%). If the serum sodium is measured at <115 mEq/L (resulting in neurologic abnormalities), care must be taken not to increase the sodium concentration too quickly.

Increased serum sodium values most commonly reflect a loss of solute-free water. The animal should be reperfused and rehydrated using an isotonic fluid. The free water can then be replaced using 2.5% dextrose in half-strength lactated Ringer's, 2.5% dextrose in half-strength saline, 0.45% saline, or 5% dextrose in water. This must be done carefully, and the sodium concentration lowered slowly.

Potassium Content: When serum potassium estimations are normal, a balanced electrolyte solution can be used. Hypokalemia can be difficult to recognize clinically. Few clinical situations warrant potassium supplementation beyond the content of lactated Ringer's or Plasmalyte-A® during initial volume replacement. Once the animal has been stabilized, potassium chloride should be added to the fluids, administered at a rate ≤0.5 mEq/kg body wt/hr. Typically, 20 mEq is added to a liter of balanced isotonic crystalloids used as maintenance fluids. Serum potassium values should be obtained before supplementation when possible.

In animals with hyperkalemia, fluids should be selected carefully. When oliguric renal failure is suspected as the cause of the hyperkalemia, potassium-free solutions, such as 0.9% saline, are used for volume replacement. Clinical conditions requiring potassium-free solutions include oliguric renal failure, heat stroke, adrenal insufficiency, and

TABLE 4.   Crystalloids

Crystalloid	Tonicity	Sodium (mEq/L)	Potassium (mEq/L)	Calcium (mEq/L)	Osmolality (mOsm/L)
Lactated Ringer's solution	Isotonic	130	4	2.7	273 (pH 6.7)
Plasmalyte-A®	Isotonic	140	5	—	294 (pH 7.4)
Normosol-R®	Isotonic	140	5	—	295 (pH 7.4)
Normal saline (0.9%)	Isotonic	154	—	—	308 (pH 5.7)
Dextrose (2.5% in 0.45% saline)	Isotonic	77	—	—	280 (pH 4.5)
Dextrose (5%) in water	Hypotonic	—	—	—	253 (pH 5.0)
Saline (7.5%)	Hypertonic	1,232	—	—	2,464 (pH 5.2)
Normosol-M® with 5% dextrose	Hypertonic	40	13	—	363 (pH 5.2)

massive muscle breakdown. When it is determined that the hyperkalemia will resolve after volume replacement and fluid diuresis (such as in feline urethral obstruction), a balanced electrolyte solution should be used. These solutions have a normal pH and promote potassium excretion.

Osmolality: Osmolality is defined as the number of solute particles per unit of solvent. Four main serum components are responsible for normal serum osmolality: sodium, potassium, BUN, and glucose. Normal serum osmolality is 290-310 mOsm/L.

Animals with increased serum glucose or sodium or markedly increased BUN values have hyperosmolar serum. Fluids that do not contribute significantly to serum osmolality should be used for volume replacement.

Hyperosmolar solutions include hypertonic saline and Normosol-M® with 5% dextrose, or any isotonic fluid that has glucose added. Except for hypertonic saline, the hyperosmolar glucose-containing solutions are meant to be maintenance solutions used in animals in which fluids are not shifting rapidly from the vascular compartment to a third body fluid space. They are usually not used as volume replacement solutions.

Hypertonic saline provides a supranormal concentration of sodium and is generally given in a 3%, 7%, or 7.5% IV solution. The effect is to rapidly draw water from the interstitial space into the intravascular space and to rapidly expand the intravascular volume. However, adequate interstitial fluid is required to obtain the desired effect. In addition, because these solutions are crystalloids, the fluid will extravasate into the interstitium within 1 hr in a healthy animal, and possibly sooner in a diseased animal. It is common practice to administer hypertonic saline with a colloid, so that the water brought into the intravascular space can be at least partially retained there by the colloid. Hypertonic saline administration is rarely indicated.

RATE AND VOLUME OF ADMINISTRATION

The initial condition of the animal must be accurately assessed through historical, physical, and laboratory findings. Inciting causes, duration of signs, and observed loss of body fluids aid in determining fluid rate and volume. Perfusion and hydration must be determined.

Poor perfusion and low blood pressure due to hypovolemia mandate rapid volume replacement. Capillary leakage leading to volume deficits warrants fluid therapy using a colloid and crystalloid combination. Hypotension associated with heart failure requires carefully monitored conservative volume replacement. In heart failure, rates above maintenance are rarely required.

When crystalloids alone are used for replacing intravascular volume causing perfusion deficits, the volume administered is determined by titrating to effect. A pretreatment blood pressure is obtained. Increments of isotonic crystalloids (10-15 mL/kg) are infused IV. The animal's perfusion parameters are assessed between boluses to determine the effect of the therapy. If the desired endpoints of resuscitation have not been met, another bolus is given (up to 90 mL/kg/hr in dogs, 40-55 mL/kg/hr in cats). Careful monitoring is required to avoid interstitial volume overload.

A balanced approach to correcting perfusion deficits due to hypovolemia incorporates the administration of both large molecular weight colloids and crystalloids. A pretreatment blood pressure and heart rate are obtained. Isotonic crystalloids (10-15 mL/kg) are given IV, followed by hetastarch at 5 mL/kg IV, given rapidly in dogs and over 2-5 min in cats. Perfusion parameters, including blood pressure, are reevaluated. If the blood pressure has not reached the desired endpoint (systolic blood pressure >90 mm Hg in dogs and >40 mm Hg in cats), another bolus (5 mL/kg) of hetastarch is administered.

Once the blood pressure is >40 mm Hg in cats with rectal temperatures <98°F (36.7°C), aggressive warming procedures are initiated until the rectal temperature is >98°F (within 30 min). Often, warming a cat after the initial fluid infusion increases blood pressure to >90 mm Hg without additional fluid administration. Should the temperature rise above 98°F and the blood pressure remain <70 mm Hg, repeated doses of hetastarch can be given until the central volume has been restored.

When systemic inflammatory response syndrome diseases cause increased capillary permeability, hetastarch (dog: 20 mL/kg/day; cat: 5-10 mL/kg/day) is given by constant rate infusion after the initial resuscitation boluses to maintain the colloidal oncotic pressure.

Stroma-free hemoglobin (dog: 5-10 mL/kg, IV; cat: 0.25-1.0 mL/kg, slow IV infusion) can be titrated in place of hetastarch when blood loss is suspected, severe anemia is present from any cause, organ or tissue hypoxia or ischemia is anticipated, or conditions require rapid, small volume resuscitation.

When water and electrolyte loss into a third body fluid space has been substantial or ongoing fluid loss is anticipated (eg, parvoviral diarrhea, pyometra, heat stroke), rapid infusion of additional crystalloids is required during the resuscitation phase to replace losses. If adequate perfusion is not restored by replacing intravascular volume, then other pharmacologic means of cardiovascular support are used (*see* p 1398). Once perfusion has been restored, dehydration is estimated and corrected using isotonic crystalloids. Peracute dehydration should be corrected over 1-2 hr, acute over 1-4 hr, and more chronic problems over 4-12 hr. Dehydration is calculated as follows: % estimated dehydration × kg body wt = mL of fluid deficit. The hourly maintenance fluid rate is added to the hourly rate for rehydration to determine the total hourly fluid infusion rate. Hydration status should be closely monitored to determine if the rate or volume requires adjustment.

Maintenance fluid therapy is meant to replace both ongoing and insensible losses. When there is no vomiting, diarrhea, fever, or loss into the third body fluid space, the average maintenance rate is 40-60 mL/kg/day. During fever, the maintenance rate increases an extra 15-20 mL/kg/day. Fluid losses through vomiting, diarrhea, the third body fluid space, and polyuria must also be estimated and replaced.

MONITORING PROCEDURES FOR THE CRITICALLY ILL ANIMAL

The key to successful management of critically ill small animals is anticipation, not reaction. Animals must be aggressively treated and actively monitored to detect organ compromise before organ failure occurs. Resuscitation, support, and stabilization of the animal for extended periods are often necessary before or throughout the course of definitive therapy.

Tissue hypoxia and organ compromise or failure can be a direct result of the primary disease or can be secondary to the disease or its therapy. Organs frequently affected include the heart and blood vessels, kidneys, lungs, GI tract, and liver. When the disease process is multisystemic, problems such as malnutrition and coagulopathies must be anticipated. Optimal care requires a thorough and methodical approach to diagnostic procedures, monitoring, specific therapeutics, and supportive care.

The Rule of Twenty

The Rule of Twenty is a list of 20 critical parameters that should be evaluated at least daily in all critical animals. It can be used as a guide to assess the status and therapeutic strategy for each case.

Fluid Balance: The goal of fluid therapy (p 1404) is to provide adequate intravascular volume (as gauged by blood pressure and central venous pressure) and hydration (as gauged by clinical assessment of mucous membrane moistness, skin turgor, and urine output) without overloading the interstitial space. Animals with systemic inflammatory response syndrome (SIRS) diseases may require much more fluid than expected because of massive losses into the third body fluid space or into the interstitium due to loss of endothelial integrity.

Oncotic Pull: Normally, albumin provides the major intravascular oncotic pull. In conditions in which there has been massive blood loss or leakage of plasma protein due to an exudative process, albumin is lost from the intravascular space. This loss of intravascular oncotic pressure combined with increased capillary permeability associated with many SIRS diseases requires treatment using artificial colloids that have a higher molecular weight than that of albumin.

Glucose: The goal is to maintain glucose between 100 and 150 mg/dL. Septic animals are at an increased risk of hypoglycemia that can be severe enough to cause neurologic dysfunction ranging from weakness to stupor or seizures. Acutely traumatized animals are also prone to insulin resistance due to large amounts of circulating stress hormones and may develop hyperglycemia severe enough to require treatment with insulin.

Electrolytes and Acid-Base Balance: Critically ill animals are commonly anorectic, or their oral intake is less than their caloric requirements. Under these circumstances, most animals require potassium supplementation in the IV fluids. Hypokalemia can be a contributing factor in weakness and ileus. Hyperkalemia can be a life-threatening complication of reperfusion injury or renal failure. Other important electrolytes to monitor include sodium, ionized calcium, phosphorus, and magnesium.

Most metabolic acidosis seen in critically ill animals is due to poor perfusion and the production of lactic acid. Treatment involves maximizing cardiac function and intravascular volume as required to improve blood flow and oxygen delivery. Rarely is the administration of sodium bicarbonate ($NaHCO_3$) warranted for perfusion-related acidosis. Acidosis is associated with underlying diseases that produce acids as part of their specific pathology, such as oliguric renal failure (eg, primary renal failure, ethylene glycol toxicity) or diabetic ketoacidosis. Once perfusion and hydration are corrected, the acid-base status is reassessed. If severe metabolic acidosis persists, slow supplementation of the fluids with $NaHCO_3$ to a serum value of 13-15 mEq/L is warranted. The dosage of $NaHCO_3$ is calculated as follows:

$$mEq\ NaHCO_3 = 0.3 \times (15 - measured\ NaHCO_3) \times kg\ body\ wt$$

Serum bicarbonate levels are carefully monitored to meet patient requirements.

Oxygenation and Ventilation: Arterial blood gases are used to detect hypoxemia or hypercarbia. Serial monitoring helps to determine if the lungs are exchanging gas effectively and is recommended in the initial management of animals with respiratory compromise to determine the adequacy of oxygen supplementation and whether mechanical ventilation is necessary. If hypoxemia is unresponsive to oxygen supplementation or hypercarbia is present, mechanical ventilation is necessary. During ventilation, serial arterial blood gas measurements should be performed to gauge the adequacy of mechanical ventilation and to adjust the ventilator settings.

Level of Consciousness: A decline in an animal's level of consciousness warrants investigation to exclude metabolic causes, such as hypoglycemia, hepatic encephalopathy, acidosis, electrolyte or osmotic derangements, or sudden development of shock.

Blood Pressure: Blood pressure should be monitored via direct or indirect methods. The goal is to maintain mean arterial blood pressure >60 mm Hg (systolic >90 mm Hg). In hypotensive animals, treatment consists of volume infusion to increase intravascular volume, oxygen administration, and pain control. The need for positive inotropes should be assessed. If intravascular volume (central venous pressure >8 cm H_2O) and cardiac function are adequate, then vasopressor therapy with a constant rate infusion of dopamine at 5-15 µg/kg/min, beginning at the lower end of the dosage range and increasing by 2-µg increments is recommended. Stroma-free hemoglobin can also be used for its pressor effects.

Heart Rate, Rhythm, and Contractility: Specific antiarrhythmic therapy should be instituted when perfusion is compromised by the arrhythmia and when oxygen supplementation and analgesics have been unsuccessful in controlling the arrhythmia. An echocardiogram can be performed to evaluate cardiac contractility in SIRS diseases and to detect underlying cardiac diseases. If cardiac contractility is decreased, dobutamine at 5-10 µg/kg/min (dogs) or 2.5-5.0 µg/kg/min (cats) should be given.

Albumin: Part of the oncotic activity normally provided by albumin can be provided by synthetic colloids, but only albumin can perform other functions such as cation and hormone transport. Plasma transfusion is indicated when the albumin level is <2 g/dL. The interstitial albumin stores are replenished first, so multiple units of plasma may be necessary to increase serum albumin levels. Conversely, in cases of albumin depletion, the interstitial stores are drawn upon to replace the serum albumin, so a low serum albumin reflects a total body deficit of albumin.

Coagulation: Disseminated intravascular coagulation (DIC) can develop in any animal that has undergone a period of relative vascular stasis as occurs during shock, severe tissue damage, or capillary damage. In the early stages of DIC, there may be no clinical signs. However, as DIC progresses, its effects are obvious and catastrophic. The goal is to detect DIC in the early stages and to prevent its progression.

Early DIC is characterized by a hypercoagulable stage in which serum antithrombin III levels are decreased and the coagulation cascade is activated by any of the precipitating causes. Activation of the coagulation cascade throughout the body depletes the clotting factors and decreases the peripheral platelet count as platelets are incorporated into the clots that form. At this stage, the prothrombin time and partial thromboplastin time are decreased. However, this stage rapidly progresses to a hypocoagulable stage as the coagulation factors are consumed. In this late stage, the prothrombin time, partial thromboplastin time, and fibrinogen degradation products are increased.

Treatment of DIC focuses on treating the underlying disease and removing the stimulus for continued activation of the coagulation cascade. In the early hypercoagulable stages, treatment focuses on maximizing the function of antithrombin III, which is the most abundant natural inhibitor of the serine proteases of the coagulation cascade. When antithrombin III levels are adequate, heparin can be administered SC at low dosages (50-100 U/kg, TID). If antithrombin III levels are <60% of normal, then fresh frozen plasma transfusions should also be given to increase the level to ≥80%. In animals with diseases known to predispose to DIC, coagulation parameters (at minimum, an activated clotting time and platelet estimate) should be monitored daily.

Red Blood Cell and Hemoglobin Concentration: Because Hgb carries most of the oxygen in the blood, maintaining adequate Hgb levels is essential to maintaining adequate oxygen delivery. In an animal that is acutely anemic or suffering from SIRS diseases, the PCV should be maintained at >20%. In some cases of hemolytic or chronic anemia, the PCV may be allowed to become much lower before transfusion. In animals with a PCV >55% (other than sight hounds and high altitudes), treatment with IV fluids, and phlebotomy in cases of absolute polycythemia, should be performed to prevent microvascular sludging and hypertension that can develop as a result of the increased blood viscosity.

Renal Function: In animals that have had a hypotensive episode or are receiving potentially nephrotoxic medications, renal function should be evaluated daily. Urine output should be at least 1 mL/kg/hr. Serial urinalyses to detect glucosuria, proteinuria, or cylinduria are useful for evaluating acute tubular injury before the damage progresses to overt renal failure and azotemia.

Immune Status, Antibiotic Dosage and Selection, and WBC Count: Strict aseptic technique should be observed when examining or treating animals that are neutropenic or receiving immunosuppressive drugs. These animals should be isolated from other animals and handled by a single person who washes his or her hands and dons gloves before handling the animal. Antibiotics are selected based on the site of infection and the most likely types of bacterial infection. Ultimately, antibiotic selection should be based on the results of culture and sensitivity, but empiric treatment is necessary pending these results.

In animals that have sustained a hypotensive episode or have a GI disease that would allow bacterial translocation, broad-spectrum bacterial coverage should be provided until the results of culture are available or until the risk of systemic infection has passed. However, the numbers of antibiotics administered empirically on a routine basis should be minimized to minimize the development of resistant organisms in the hospital environment. A first-generation cephalosporin is useful for gram-positive and gram-negative infections. Cefazolin can be administered at 40 mg/kg, initially, followed by 20 mg/kg, TID-QID. If a resistant bacteria is suspected, gentamicin can be given at 3-5 mg/kg, IV, SID, to more specifically target gram-negative organisms after hydration and perfusion have normalized. The once-daily dosage is less likely to cause renal toxicity and has the same antibacterial effect as a divided dosage schedule. Metronidazole at 5-7.5 mg/kg, given slowly IV over 20 min every 6-8 hr, is used for suspected anaerobic infections.

GI Motility and Mucosal Integrity: Critically ill animals, even those without a primary GI disease, are prone to gastric atony, ileus, and stress-induced gastric ulceration. Auscultation for bowel sounds should be performed 3 times a day. Metoclopramide (1-2 mg/kg/day as a constant rate infusion) is useful because of its central antiemetic effects and its ability to increase progressive gastric and intestinal motility. Other motility modifiers to consider include cisapride, ranitidine, and erythromycin. Placement of a nasogastric tube to allow removal of accumulated gas and fluid reduces the possibility of aspiration of refluxed gastric contents and allows continuous decompression. The nasogastric tube also can be used to introduce small amounts of a liquid diet to provide nutrition to the enterocytes, which will help prevent gastric ulceration and intestinal mucosal compromise with secondary bacterial translocation. Antiemetics are used in animals that continue to vomit frequently despite placement of a nasogastric tube (and that have no obstructive intestinal lesion) to improve patient comfort and reduce the incidence of aspiration, vagal-induced collapse, and bradycardia that can accompany the vomiting reflex. Metoclopramide blocks the dopaminergic receptors in the chemoreceptor trigger zone (CRTZ) and central vomiting center, and acts peripherally by promoting gastric emptying. Ondansetron blocks serotonin and acts at the CRTZ and the central vomiting center. Vomiting refractory to all other treatments in an otherwise stable animal with normal blood pressure can be treated with chlorpromazine (dogs: 0.05-1 mg/kg, IV, every 4-8 hr; cats: 0.01-0.025 mg/kg, IV, every 4-8 hr). A combination of antiemetics that have different mechanisms of action is often required to arrest refractory emesis.

Drug Dosages and Metabolism: If renal or hepatic function is compromised, some drug dosages should be decreased to account for decreased elimination. Also, drug treatments should be reviewed daily to ensure that the dose has been calculated correctly and that it is appropriate for the animal's current weight.

Nutrition: Enteral feeding is always preferred if the GI tract can tolerate it. Microenteral nutrition can be performed in all animals, even those with GI disease. If nutritional needs cannot be met enterally, then nutrition should be provided parenterally. Partial parenteral nutrition, using amino acid solutions, can be given in a peripheral vein and provide part of the animal's caloric requirements in a form that can be readily metabolized. The amino acids are used in gluconeogenic pathways to provide energy and thus prevent catabolism of visceral and muscle proteins. The acutely ill animal, unlike the chronically malnourished animal, uses protein preferentially as a fuel source.

In animals that remain anorectic and for which there is no medical contraindication for full enteral feeding, attempts to gradually provide maintenance caloric requirements should be made first by syringe feeding if well tolerated. Feeding liquid diets through a nasogastric tube is also well tolerated. For longterm feeding, an esophagostomy, gastrotomy, nasojejunostomy, or jejunostomy tube can be placed.

Feeding is instituted by starting with small volumes of a dilute liquid diet solution (eg, CliniCare®). For the first 12-24 hr, the amount of diet calculated to provide one-third of the daily caloric requirement is diluted 1 part liquid diet to 2 parts water. This volume is then delivered by constant rate infusion over 12-24 hr or divided into small boluses every 2-4 hr. Each time a bolus feeding is administered and every 6 hr during a constant infusion, the feeding tube should be suctioned to determine if any residual volume is present that would necessitate decreasing the volume infused or adding prokinetic agents. After suctioning, the tube should be flushed with saline. If this initial feeding of dilute diet is tolerated, the concentration is increased to 2 parts liquid diet mixed with 1 part water during the next 12-24 hr. If this is tolerated, then the undiluted diet can be delivered to provide the full caloric requirements. As the animal recovers, bolus feeding can be introduced by gradually decreasing feeding frequency and increasing volumes.

Pain Control: Pain activates the stress hormone systems of the body and contributes to morbidity and mortality. Signs of pain, such as increased heart rate and pale mucous membranes, can mimic signs of shock. (*See also* SYSTEMIC PHARMACOTHERAPEUTICS OF THE NERVOUS SYSTEM, p 2014, and PAIN MANAGEMENT, p 1691.)

Analgesia in critical animals can safely be provided by opioids titrated to effect. Preemptive administration of analgesics is recommended when possible. Animals that may not show obvious signs of pain but are known to have a painful condition should receive analgesics as part of their treatment (TABLE 5). Opioids have minimal cardiovascular side effects, and their effects are reversible with antagonists (eg, naloxone). Regardless, long-acting opioids are best avoided in unstable animals. Morphine is a potent, inexpensive analgesic that can be given IV as a slow bolus, followed by a constant rate infusion or intermittent IM injections. Reports of IV morphine causing hypotension due to histamine release do not seem to be clinically significant if the bolus is given over 5-10 min. A constant

TABLE 5. Analgesics Used in Emergency Practice

Drug	Dosage	Comments
Morphine	Dogs: 0.05-0.4 mg/kg, IV, every 1-4 hr; 0.2-1.0 mg/kg, IM or SC, every 2-6 hr; 0.1 mg/kg diluted with 0.9% saline administered epidurally at 0.23 mL/kg, every 8-24 hr Cats: 0.05-0.2 mg/kg, IM or SC, every 2-6 hr	Incremental IV bolus technique: dogs—increments of 0.1 mg/kg until analgesia appears adequate; cats—increments of 0.02 mg/kg. In dogs, this can be followed by a constant rate infusion at 0.1 mg/kg/hr that can be increased incrementally if needed.
Oxymorphone	Dogs: 0.02-0.1 mg/kg, IV, every 2-4 hr; 0.05-0.2 mg/kg, IM or SC, every 2-6 hr Cats: 0.02-0.05 mg/kg, IV, every 2-4 hr; 0.05-0.1 mg/kg, IM or SC, every 2-6 hr	
Fentanyl	Dogs: 0.003-0.1 mg/kg, IV, every 30-60 min; 0.01 mg/kg/hr, IV as a constant rate infusion	
Fentanyl transdermal patch	Patch size µg/hr: 1/2 of 25 for animals <2.5 kg body wt; 25 for animals 2.5-10 kg body wt; 50 for animals 10-20 kg body wt; 75 for animals 20-30 kg body wt; 100 for animals >30 kg body wt	One-half patch applied by removing adhesive backing from half of the patch. The patches cannot be cut because the fentanyl will leak out of the reservoir.
Butorphanol	Dogs: 0.2-0.8 mg/kg, IM, IV, or SC, every 1-3 hr Cats: 0.1-0.4 mg/kg, IM, IV, or SC, every 1-3 hr	
Buprenorphine	Dogs 0.005-0.02 mg/kg, IM or IV, every 1-6 hr Cats: 0.005-0.01 mg/kg, IM or IV, every 4-8 hr	

rate infusion provides constant analgesia and is often more convenient and less painful than intermittent IM or SC injections.

For longterm control of pain, intermittent IV boluses of injectable opioids or constant rate infusions can be used. Transdermal fentanyl patches are being used more commonly but require up to 12 hr to reach therapeutic blood levels; analgesia must be provided by injection until adequate blood levels have been reached.

Nursing Care: Providing nursing care to critically ill animals requires a skilled, knowledgeable, attentive, and highly trained nurse. Recumbent animals should be turned from one side to the other every 4 hr or maintained in variations of sternal recumbency to prevent decubital ulcers and atelectasis. Physical therapy 3-4 times a day is important for maintaining range of motion and muscle tone and blood flow. The catheter sites should be inspected daily for signs of infection or displacement. Catheters should be labeled and marked with the date of placement. When catheters are removed, the tips should be saved for possible culture if there is evidence of inflammation at the catheter site.

Wound Care and Bandage Changes: Bandages should be changed anytime they become soiled or wet. Distal limb edema can be improved by placing light compression wraps that are changed every day. (*See also* WOUND MANAGEMENT, p 1419.)

Tender Loving Care: Owner visits should be encouraged. Animals should be handled and spoken to kindly to minimize stress and anxiety that could dislodge a catheter or result in a cardiac arrhythmia. Consolidating several treatments at one time and turning down the lights at night, when the animal's condition permits, allows the animal some time to rest and sleep undisturbed.

OPHTHALMIC EMERGENCIES

Ophthalmic emergencies require rapid diagnosis and appropriate and often aggressive therapy for maintenance of vision.

TRAUMATIC PROPTOSIS

Traumatic proptosis may follow blunt trauma (eg, being hit by a car, fight with another animal). During trauma, the globe is luxated from the orbit, and eyelid spasms prevent its retraction. Secondary orbital hemorrhage and swelling displace the globe further from the orbit. Corneoconjunctival drying and malacia follow. Prognosis depends on pupil size and reflexes, duration of exposure, other globe or orbital damage, breed (brachycephalics are predisposed), and other systemic trauma. About 40-60% of dogs, but very few cats, recover vision. Treatment begins by providing moisture to lubricate the exposed corneoconjunctiva. General anesthesia followed by a lateral canthotomy, and complete temporary tarsorrhaphy with usually 2 or 3 interrupted horizontal mattress sutures (placed at one-half thickness of the eyelids) and stents should be followed by systemic antibiotics and corticosteroids, as well as topical antibiotics and mydriatics (if miosis is present). Sutures and stents are removed when a brisk blink reflex returns (usually 7-21 days). Complications include corneal ulceration, enophthalmia, optic nerve degeneration, keratoconjunctivitis sicca, and medial rectus muscle injury.

TRAUMATIC RETROBULBAR HEMORRHAGE

Retrobulbar hemorrhage follows trauma sufficient to damage the orbital vasculature and cause exophthalmos, iridocyclitis, and lagophthalmos. The lagophthalmos is associated with an impaired blink reflex and acute exposure keratitis. Subconjunctival and intraocular hemorrhage may also be present, and the latter can prevent intraocular examination. Corneal and scleral lacerations should be excluded by ophthalmic examination, and b-scan ultrasonography to detect retinal detachment is recommended in eyes with intraocular hemorrhage.

Medical and surgical therapy consists of topical and systemic antibiotics and corticosteroids, mydriatics if pupillary dilation is necessary, and a complete temporary tarsorrhaphy to protect the cornea until a brisk blink reflex returns. Prognosis is guarded, as secondary glaucoma and phthisis bulbus are not infrequent. Intraocular hemorrhage is usually allowed to reabsorb.

CORNEAL FOREIGN BODIES

Corneal foreign bodies are seen most frequently in dogs, cats, and horses. They are usually organic material, but sand, metal, and glass foreign bodies are also seen. Presenting signs include variable blepharospasm, tearing, and a variable secondary iridocyclitis (aqueous flare, miosis, iridal swelling, ocular hypotony, and possible hypopyon). Ophthalmic examination reveals a foreign body on the conjunctival surface, in the posterior third eyelid fornix, or on or in the cornea. Foreign bodies that adhere to the ocular surfaces are usually removed under topical anesthesia with either vigorous irrigation or small serrated ophthalmic forceps. If the foreign body has embedded within the deeper corneal layers or has penetrated into the anterior chamber, general anesthesia is required for careful removal from either the anterior corneal surface or the anterior chamber. The corneal wound is apposed with simple interrupted 6-0 to 8-0 absorbable sutures. Postoperative therapy includes topical and systemic broad-spectrum antibiotics, mydriatics, systemic NSAID, and if necessary, drugs to reduce intraocular pressure. Prognosis for vision is usually good. Infrequent complications include variable corneal scar formation, septic endophthalmitis, cataract formation, and secondary glaucoma.

PENETRATING INTRAOCULAR INJURIES

Penetrating intraocular injuries with retained foreign bodies are seen most frequently in dogs and cats. They are often associated with lead pellets and bullets that partially or totally traverse the ocular tunics, but splinters or spines (eg, cactus) can also cause a penetrating injury. Pellets or bullets usually cause self-sealing, slightly tan corneal defects, may cause intraocular hemorrhage, and may traverse the lens and posterior segment wall. Perforation of the lens leads to rapid cataract formation. Vitreal and retinal hemorrhage and retinal detachments are likely. Ophthalmic ultrasonography and orbital radiology are most helpful is assessing pellet location and the integrity of the intraocular and orbital tissues. Lens rupture is also a common sequela of cat claw injuries.

Penetration of the lens requires lens removal as soon as possible, as escape of lens material causes gradually intensifying lens-induced uveitis that often progresses to secondary glaucoma and phthisis bulbus. The posterior segment changes usually resolve provided the retina eventually re-attaches. Focal retinal degeneration in the area of retinal detachment is common. Prognosis is guarded and based, in part, on the response to therapy and gradual clearing of the intraocular media.

Therapy is directed at controlling the post-traumatic inflammation and maintaining normal levels of intraocular pressure. Mydriatics and topical and systemic antibiotics and corticosteroids are administered to control the uveitis. Intraocular hemorrhage is allowed to resolve with anterior chamber hemorrhage usually disappearing in ~1-2 wk and the vitreal hemorrhage resolving in 3-6 mo.

DEEP STROMAL CORNEAL ULCERS, DESCEMETOCELE, AND IRIS PROLAPSE

Deep corneal ulcers, descemetocele, and iris prolapse are seen with some frequency in dogs, cats, and horses. These conditions require immediate surgical support of the weakened cornea as they can threaten or seriously compromise corneal integrity. In dogs, the brachycephalic breeds and dogs with keratoconjunctivitis sicca are most vulnerable. These corneal defects often develop in the center of the cornea and can markedly impair vision. Important diagnostic aids are the Schirmer tear test to measure aqueous tear production and topical fluorescein to examine the corneal ulcer. Corneal culture and cytology can assist in choosing topical and systemic antibiotics. Secondary anterior uveitis with aqueous flare, miosis, ocular hypotony, and hypopyon is common.

Corneal ulcer depth must be accurately estimated using magnification, focal illumination, and topical fluorescein. Central corneal ulcers are more vulnerable because they require more time for the healing response and vascularization. Adequate ulcer debridement is essential for successful adherence of a conjunctival graft. The corneal ulceration (stromal, descemetocele, or iris prolapse) is covered with the bulbar conjunctival graft (360°, 180°, bridge, or pedicle) that appears most appropriate. For full-thickness corneal ulcers with iris prolapse, conjunctival grafts are also used, but the postoperative corneal opacity is usually larger and more dense. Postoperative therapy includes topical and systemic broad-spectrum antibiotics, systemic NSAID or corticosteroids, and mydriatics. Treatments are gradually tapered and administered for 4-8 wk. Postoperative complications include variable corneal scar and pigmentation, secondary cataract formation, and rarely, bacterial endophthalmitis.

CORNEAL LACERATIONS

Corneal lacerations are seen most frequently in dogs and horses and infrequently in cats. Bites, self-inflicted trauma, and other accidents can partially or totally penetrate the cornea. Partial-thickness corneal lacerations are usually highly painful and require apposition with simple interrupted absorbable sutures to the healthy cornea. Excision of the lacerated section is not recommended.

For full-thickness corneal lacerations, signs usually include pain, blepharospasm, tearing, a corneal defect, and variable iris prolapse. Marked aqueous flare, hyphema, miosis, and distortion of the pupil are common. Often, the size of the iris prolapse is much larger than the underlying corneal laceration. Prognosis depends on size and position of the corneal laceration, other ocular tissue involvement, age of the animal, duration of the injury, and other systemic injuries. If the entire eye cannot be examined directly, b-scan ultrasonography is used.

The corneal laceration is apposed with simple interrupted 6-0 to 8-0 absorbable sutures. To provide additional protection and support, the sutured laceration may be covered with a third eyelid flap, bulbar conjunctival graft, or partial temporary tarsorrhaphy. Postoperative therapy to control the secondary iridocyclitis consists of topical and systemic antibiotics, systemic NSAID, and mydriatics. Postoperative complications include variable and often dense corneal scarring, cataract formation with posterior synechiae, secondary glaucoma, phthisis bulbus, and bacterial endophthalmitis.

GLAUCOMA

Animals are usually presented with high-pressure glaucoma because intraocular pressure (IOP) >30-50 mm Hg results in clinical signs of buphthalmia, mydriasis, corneal edema, episcleral venous congestion, and variable ocular pain. The underlying glaucoma may be either open or narrow-closed angle, and either acute or chronic. Dog breeds most often affected with primary glaucoma include the American Cocker Spaniel, Basset Hound, Chow Chow, Akita, Chinese Shar-Pei, Norwegian Elkhound, and Samoyed. Diagnosis depends on accurate tonometry. The Tono-Pen™ applanation tonometer is the most versatile. Gonioscopy and other diagnostic methods are used to evaluate the anterior chamber angle and the posterior segment including the optic nerve head.

The goals of therapy are to rapidly lower IOP and to preserve as much vision as possible. Short-term treatment includes mannitol (1-2 g/kg, IV), topical β-blockers and carbonic anhydrase inhibitors, systemic carbonic anhydrase inhibitors, and either miotics (pilocarpine or demecarium) or prostaglandin analogs. The beneficial effects of the topical medications are not usually apparent until IOP is ≤30 mm Hg. If mannitol treatment does not lower IOP within 2-4 hr, anterior chamber paracentesis under general anesthesia may be attempted. Longterm therapy usually includes topical and systemic ocular hypotensive medications, laser cyclophotocoagulation, cyclocryotherapy, intraocular implant insertion, and anterior chamber shunts.

ANTERIOR LENS LUXATION

Anterior lens luxation usually affects middle-aged dogs of the terrier breeds and is seen most frequently in Smooth and Wire Haired Fox Terriers and Jack Russell Terriers.

It is associated with zonular defects, and appears as acute corneal edema, elevated IOP, blepharospasm, tearing, and ciliary flush. The lens is in front of the pupil and often totally within the anterior chamber. Pupillary blockage with vitreous adherent to the posterior lens capsule is common and can markedly elevate IOP within the posterior segment. Applanation tonometry from the central cornea may yield erroneous low IOP levels. Direct examination of the posterior segment is not usually possible, and b-scan ultrasonography may be used to evaluate the vitreous and retina.

Treatment consists of lowering IOP to normal levels (usually with mannitol, 1-2 g/kg IV); transpupillary aqueous humor flow may be reestablished with moderate dilation with 10% phenylephrine. Lens removal by intracapsular extraction or phacoemulsification is performed as soon as possible. Postoperative treatment consists of topical and systemic antibiotics and corticosteroids, and maintenance of a moderate but moving pupil. IOP is closely monitored and any increases treated with topical β-blockers, topical and systemic carbonic anhydrase inhibitors, and prostaglandin analogs. Longterm postoperative complications include anterior uveitis, secondary glaucoma, and retinal detachment.

ACUTE VISION LOSS

Acute loss of vision may occur with many ophthalmic and CNS diseases, usually with abrupt onset of blindness, anisocoria, mydriasis, and loss of both direct and indirect pupillary light reflexes. Bilateral loss of vision is more common, but unilateral vision loss can occur particularly when the other eye is blind. For acute vision loss, large amounts of the retina must be involved; lesions of the optic nerve can cause blindness as the disease process can be quite localized. The evaluation includes thorough ophthalmic and general physical examinations, as many systemic diseases may cause blindness. Because visual field evaluation cannot be performed in animals, subjective tests for vision are necessary and include the menace test, dazzle reflex, maze test in both light and dark illumination, and electroretinography.

OPTIC NEURITIS

Optic neuritis may be divided into papillitis (an inflamed optic nerve head visible with an ophthalmoscope) and retrobulbar optic neuritis, which includes mydriasis, absence of pupillary reflexes, and blindness without any ophthalmoscopic abnormalities. Flash electroretinography, combined with vision evoked potentials and fluorescein angiography may be used to confirm optic neuritis. A CBC, blood chemistry profile, neurologic examination, radiology, and vitreous and CSF analyses may be indicated.

Papillitis is common in granulomatous meningoencephalitis in dogs; systemic viral, bacterial, and fungal infections in dogs, cats, horses, and cattle; and trauma. It appears as a swollen optic nerve head with blurred margins, variable hemorrhages, and exudates. Peripapillary retinitis is often present and appears as a translucent to opaque retina adjacent to the optic disk. Therapy is directed at the underlying systemic disease. Systemic corticosteroids may be used for the optic neuritis. A positive response includes return of the pupillary reflexes and normal pupil size in several days, followed by vision a few days later.

SUDDEN ACQUIRED RETINAL DEGENERATION (SARD)

SARD is seen in dogs. Clinical findings include acute loss of vision (often occurring over several days), widely dilated and poorly responsive to nonresponsive pupils, and a normal-appearing ocular fundus. Dogs affected most often are middle-aged and sometimes have liver disease and hyperadrenocorticism with clinical signs of weight gain, polyuria, polydipsia, and polyphagia. Electroretinography indicates loss of outer retinal function; complete retinal and optic nerve degeneration becomes apparent over several weeks. There is no effective treatment.

RETINAL DETACHMENT

Retinal detachment is being diagnosed more commonly and is an important cause of vision loss (either unilateral or bilateral). It is an important postoperative complication of cataract and lens surgery. Once retinal detachment is detected, immediate medical and/or surgical treatment can reduce the resultant retinal degeneration and facilitate restoration of vision. Contributing factors include breed (eg, Shih Tzu with vitreal syneresis), previous cataract or lens removal, trauma, systemic hypertension (cats and dogs), and systemic mycoses (dogs and cats). History, complete ophthalmic and systemic examination, CBC, blood chemistry profile, and other diagnostic tests are important to determine the underlying cause. Ophthalmoscopy, b-scan ultrasonography, electroretinography, and blood pressure measurement are important diagnostic tests for retinal detachment.

Exudative nonrhegmatogenous retinal detachments may resolve with resolution of the inflammatory or hemorrhagic intra- and subretinal exudates. Some retinal degeneration usually occurs, but vision may return. Retinal detachments secondary to Collie eye anomaly (p 402) may be treated successfully by diode laser photocoagulation of the surrounding retina. Repair of rhegmatogenous retinal detachments, characterized by retinal breaks (holes and tears), may be attempted using vitreoretinal techniques that are routine in humans, including intraocular gases, silicone oil, scleral buckling, and laser or cryoretinopexy.

WOUND MANAGEMENT

Wound healing is the restoration of the normal anatomic continuity to a disrupted area of tissue. An understanding of the normal process of wound healing is essential to make well-founded decisions in the management of wounds. Correctly using the principles of wound management help avoid premature wound closure and its potential complications.

Wounds may be classified as clean, contaminated, or infected. Clean wounds are those created under aseptic conditions, eg, surgical incisions. The number of bacteria present can determine the difference between contaminated and infected wounds. As a guideline, $>10^5$ bacteria per gram of tissue is considered adequate to cause infection. The level of contamination, blood supply, and the cause of the wound all contribute to the development of the necessary conditions for infection, and each case must be assessed independently.

GENERAL PRINCIPLES OF WOUND HEALING

Although there are many types of wounds, most undergo similar stages in healing that are mediated by cytokines and other chemotactic factors within the tissue. The duration of each state varies with the wound type, management, microbiologic, and other physiologic factors. There are 4 major stages of wound healing after a full-thickness skin wound.

Inflammation is the first stage of wound healing. It can be divided into 2 phases. During the initial phase, vasoconstriction occurs immediately to control hemorrhage, followed within minutes by vasodilation. During the second phase, cells adhere to the vascular endothelium. Within 30 min, leukocytes migrate through the vascular basement membrane into the newly created wound. Initially, neutrophils predominate (as in the peripheral blood); later, the neutrophils die off and monocytes become the predominant cell type in the wound.

Debridement is the second stage of wound healing. Although neutrophils phagocytose bacteria, monocytes, rather than neutrophils, are considered essential for wound healing. After migration out of the blood vessels, monocytes are considered macrophages, which then phagocytose necrotic debris. Macrophages also attract mesenchymal cells by an undefined mechanism. Finally, mononuclear cells coalesce to form multinucleated giant cells in chronic inflammation. Lymphocytes may also be present in the wound and contribute to the immunologic response to foreign debris.

Repair is the third stage of wound healing. It consists of fibroblast, capillary, and epithelial proliferation phases. During the repair stage, mesenchymal cells transform into fibroblasts, which lay fibrin strands to act as a framework for cellular migration. In a healthy wound, fibroblasts begin to appear ~3 days after the initial injury. These fibroblasts initially secrete ground substance and later collagen. The early collagen secretion results in an initial rapid increase in wound strength, which continues to increase more slowly as the collagen fibers reorganize according to the stress on the wound.

Migrating capillaries deliver a blood supply to the wound. The center of the wound is an area of low oxygen tension that attracts capillaries following the oxygen gradient. Because of the need for oxygen, fibroblast activity depends on the rate of capillary development. As capillaries and fibroblasts proliferate, granulation tissue is produced. Because of the extensive capillary invasion, granulation tissue is both very friable and resistant to infection.

Epithelial cell migration begins within hours of the initial wound. Basal epithelial cells flatten and migrate across the open wound. The epithelial cells may slide across the defect in small groups, or "leapfrog" across one another to cover the defect. Migrating epithelial cells secrete mediators, such as transforming growth factors α and β, which enhance wound closure. Although epithelial cells migrate in random directions, migration stops when contact is made with other epithelial cells on all sides (ie, contact inhibition). Epithelial cells migrate across the open wound and can cover a properly closed surgical incision within 48 hr. In an open wound, epithelial cells must have a healthy bed of granulation tissue to cross. Epithelialization is retarded in a desiccated wound.

Maturation is the final stage of wound healing. During this period, the newly laid collagen fibers and fibroblasts reorganize along lines of tension. Fibers in a nonfunctional orientation are replaced by functional fibers. This process allows wound strength to increase slowly over a long period (up to 2 yr). Most wounds remain 15-20% weaker than the original tissue.

INITIAL WOUND MANAGEMENT

The first step in wound management is assessment of the overall stability of the animal. Obvious open wounds can detract attention from more subtle but potentially life-threatening problems. After initial assessment, the animal should be stabilized. First aid for the wound should be performed as soon as safely possible. Active bleeding can be controlled with direct pressure. A pneumatic cuff, instead of a tourniquet, should be used in cases of severe arterial bleeding; the cuff should be inflated until the hemorrhage is controlled. Use of a cuff avoids neurovascular complications that can be associated with narrow tourniquets.

The wound must be protected from further contamination or trauma by covering it with a sterile, lint-free dressing. The delay between examination and definitive debridement should be minimized to decrease bacterial contamination. If the wound is infected, a sample should be collected for culture and sensitivity testing. Antibiotic therapy should be instituted in all cases of dirty, infected, or puncture wounds. A broad-spectrum bactericidal antibiotic, eg, a first-generation cephalosporin, is generally recommended pending culture results. Analgesia is also indicated for pain relief.

Wound Lavage: Irrigation of the wound washes away both visible and microscopic debris. This reduces the bacterial load in the tissue, which helps decrease wound complications. Assuming the solution is nontoxic, the most important factor in wound lavage is use of large volumes to facilitate the removal of debris. The recommended lavage is a moderate pressure system using a 35-mL syringe and a 19-gauge needle that delivers lavage fluid at 8 lb/sq in. The use of antibiotics in the lavage fluid is controversial.

The ideal lavage fluid would be antiseptic and nontoxic to the healing tissues. Although isotonic saline is not antiseptic, it is the least toxic to healing tissue. Surgical scrub agents should not be used because the detergent component is damaging to tissue. Dilute antiseptics can be used safely. Chlorhexidine diacetate 0.05% has sustained residual activity against a broad spectrum of bacteria, while causing minimal tissue inflammation. However, gram-negative bacteria may become resistant to chlorhexidine. Stronger solutions of chlorhexidine are toxic to healing tissue. Povidone-iodine

1% is an effective antiseptic, but it has minimal residual activity and may be inactivated by purulent debris.

Debridement: After wound preparation and hair removal, debridement can be performed. Skin and local tissue viability should be assessed. Blue-black, leathery, thin, or white skin are signs associated with nonviability. Necrotic tissue should be sharply excised. The debridement may be done in layers or as one complete section of tissue. Tissues that have questionable viability or are associated with essential structures such as neurovascular bundles should be treated conservatively. Staged debridement may be indicated.

After initial inspection, lavage, and debridement, a decision must be made whether to close the wound or to manage it as an open wound. Considerations include the availability of skin for closure and the level of contamination or infection. If the wound is left open, it should be managed for optimal healing.

Wound Closure: Although **primary closure** is the simplest method of wound management, it should be used only in ideal situations to avoid wound complications. Wounds may be closed with suture, staples, or cyanoacrylate. Clean wounds that are properly debrided usually heal without complication. With a primary closure, the layers should be individually closed to minimize "dead space" that might contribute to seroma formation. The types of suture and suture patterns used depend on the size and location of the wound and on the size of the animal.

Primary closure may not be appropriate for a grossly contaminated or infected wound. If closure is a suitable goal, it may be delayed until the contamination or infection is controlled. The wound can be managed short-term as an open wound until it appears healthy. At that time, the wound can be safely closed with minimal risk of complications. The time between initial debridement and final closure vary according to the degree of contamination or infection. Minimally contaminated wounds may be closed after 24-72 hr. Longer periods may be required for heavily infected wounds.

Wounds that are closed >5 days after the initial wounding are considered to be a **secondary closure**. This implies that granulation tissue has begun to form in the wound before closure.

Open Wound Management: When a wound cannot or should not be closed, open wound management (ie, second-intention healing) may be appropriate. Such wounds include those in which there has been a loss of skin that makes closure impossible or those that are too grossly infected to close. Longitudinal degloving injuries of the extremities are especially amenable to open wound management. Open wound management enables progressive debridement procedures and does not require specialized equipment (such as may be needed with skin grafting). However, it increases cost, prolongs time for healing, and may create complications from wound contracture.

Open wound management is based on repeated bandaging and debridement as needed until the wound heals. Initially, wet-to-dry dressings are used. These dressings help with mechanical debridement at every bandage change. Until a granulation bed forms, the bandage should be changed at least once daily. In the early stages of healing, the bandage may need to be changed as often as twice daily. After granulation tissue develops, the bandage should be changed to a dry, nonstick dressing so the granulation bed is not disrupted. Both the granulation bed and the early epithelium are easily damaged, and disruption of the granulation bed delays wound healing.

DRAINS

Drains are used to direct fluid out of a wound or body cavity. Passive drainage techniques require gravity or capillary action to draw fluid from the wound or cavity. Penrose drains are soft, flat, commonly used passive drains made from latex. These drains must be placed in gravity-dependent locations to ensure proper function. A firmer drain can be constructed from a red rubber or silicone tube. A double lumen or sump drain allows fluid to drain through the outer lumen and air to enter from the inner lumen. Active drains require some type of negative pressure to pull fluid from the wound. Red rubber or silicone drains can be used with a closed system and low-pressure suction maintained with the intermittent use of low-pressure pumps or handheld rechargeable devices. The use of active, closed-drain systems decreases the likelihood of ascending infection that can be associated with passive drains. Drains should be left in place until the draining fluid decreases in quantity and no longer appears purulent. The fluid can be evaluated by cytologic examination.

BANDAGES

The goals of bandaging include limiting hemorrhage, immobilizing the area, preventing further trauma or contamination of the wound, preventing wound desiccation, absorbing exudate, and aiding in mechanical debridement of the wound. When constructing bandages, several principles must be followed to avoid complications. The bandages should be sufficiently padded, applied evenly and snugly, composed of 3 layers (primary, secondary, and tertiary), and placed to avoid traumatizing the newly formed granulation tissue or epithelium.

The first or primary layer directly contacts the wound to allow tissue fluid to pass through to the secondary layer. The first layer may be adherent or nonadherent. A nonadherent bandage is usually a fine mesh, nonstick material and is indicated when a healthy granulation bed has developed. This layer prevents tissue desiccation and causes minimal trauma. An adherent bandage uses a wide mesh material allowing tissue to become incorporated into the bandage. This tissue is then removed with the bandage change. Adherent bandages are classified as dry to dry, wet to dry, or wet to wet based on the composition of the primary layer. Dry-to-dry bandages consist of dry gauze applied to the wound. The bandages are painful to remove but enable excellent tissue debridement. Wet-to-dry bandages are made with saline-moistened gauze placed directly on the wound. They are also painful to remove but result in less tissue desiccation than dry-to-dry bandages. Wet-to-wet bandages tend to damage the tissue bed by keeping it too moist.

The secondary layer of a bandage absorbs tissue fluid, pads the wound, and supports or immobilizes the limb. This layer is frequently composed of cast padding or roll cotton. The tertiary layer functions to hold the primary and secondary layers in place, provide pressure, and keep the inner layers protected from the environment. This layer is composed of adhesive tape or elastic wraps.

SURGICAL TECHNIQUES

Advancement flaps can be used to move skin and relieve tension. The simplest type of advancement flap involves sliding skin to cover an adjacent defect. These flaps are elevated without regard to their vascular supply. Flap survival depends on the subdermal vascular plexus from the flap base and revascularization from the recipient bed. With subdermal plexus flaps, the vascular supply is affected by the width of the flap base. A high length/width ratio decreases the likelihood of survival as blood supply will not reach the distal end of the flap. Any flap placed in tension carries a high risk of failure.

The basic advancement flap technique is known as the **single pedicle advancement flap**. Two slightly divergent incisions are made perpendicular to the defect. The tissue is undermined, advanced, and sutured to close the original defect. For larger wounds, two single pedicle flaps are safer than one large flap. Two advancement flaps are combined to form the "H" plasty. There are several other well described flap techniques, including the bipedicle advancement flap and the "V-Y" advancement flap. In each of these techniques, the coverage depends on stretching the skin over the defect. For this reason, the use of these techniques may be limited by the regional anatomy, such as the region around the eyelids.

Flaps designed to incorporate a direct cutaneous artery are known as **axial pattern flaps** (arterial pedicle graft). The flaps can be used to cover a large area of tissue and carry along a new blood supply to ensure flap survival. Muscle-based pattern flaps can also be used to reconstruct a body wall defect in addition to covering a loss of skin. The surviving area of axial pattern flaps is 50% greater than a corresponding subdermal plexus flap and therefore allows coverage of a larger area. Because axial pattern flaps are based on arteries, they must have consistent landmarks and do not cover all regions of the body. The best described of the axial pattern flaps is based on the caudal superficial epigastric artery. Based in the caudal aspect of the abdominal wall, this flap can extend cranially to include mammary glands 2-5.

Free skin grafts are used for cases with massive tissue loss such as large burns or degloving injuries. The grafts are best used as a split mesh. This allows drainage and helps prevent seroma formation. Skin grafts will not remain viable if laid over squamous epithelium, denuded bone, cartilage, or tendon. The grafts must have a healthy, vascularized bed. Initially, nutrition for the flap is maintained as capillary action pulls serum into the dilated capillaries of the skin graft, creating graft edema. Anastomosis with recipient bed vessels (inosculation) begins within 48-72 hr of surgery. The edema may worsen immediately following inosculation, as venous return is not adequate initially. The edema should resolve as normal blood flow returns to the flap by day 4-6 following surgery.

All skin flaps and grafts require a clean, healthy recipient bed for survival. This is especially important for subdermal plexus flaps and free tissue transfers because they do not contain a direct cutaneous arterial supply. The recipient bed must be free of debris, infection, and necrotic tissue.

While flaps may have well described anatomic markers, determining their viability may not be as easy. The simplest, but least accurate, methods for the assessment of a flap's viability are subjective measures including the assessment of color, warmth, sensation, and bleeding. Purple color cannot be used as a predictor of viability. Contused, purple skin is often viable. Progression from deep purple to black indicates necrosis. Skin temperature may be affected by the state of vasodilation and is therefore not an accurate method of assessing viability. Bleeding from a cut surface may occur in viable flaps as well as nonviable flaps that still have some arterial function but poor or no venous return. After movement of a flap, a flap may develop edema for the first few days until venous vascularization is completed.

FACTORS THAT INTERFERE WITH WOUND HEALING

Factors that interfere with wound healing may be divided by source into physical, endogenous, and exogenous categories. **Physical factors** are environmental issues. Temperature affects the tensile strength of wounds. Ideal conditions allow wound healing to occur at 30°C. Decreasing the temperature to 12°C results in a 20% loss of tensile wound strength. Adequate oxygen levels are also required for appropriate wound healing. Because of vessel disruption, wounds contain lower oxygen levels than surrounding healthy tissue. Low levels of oxygen interfere with protein synthesis and fibroblast activity, causing a delay in wound healing. Oxygen levels may be compromised for many reasons, including hypovolemia, the presence of devitalized tissue, and excessively tight bandages.

Endogenous factors (previously known as systemic factors) typically reflect the overall condition of the animal. Anemia may interfere with wound healing by creating low tissue oxygen levels. Hypoproteinemia delays wound healing only when the total serum protein content is <2.0 g/dL. Because wound healing is a function of protein synthesis, malnutrition may alter the healing process. The addition of DL-methionine or cysteine (an important amino acid in wound repair) prevents delayed wound healing. Uremia can interfere with wound healing by slowing granulation tissue formation and inducing the synthesis of poor quality collagen. Although diabetes is a known problem with wound healing in humans, it has not been demonstrated to cause a problem in animals. Obesity contributes to poor wound healing primarily as a consequence of poor suture holding in the subcutaneous fat layers.

Exogenous factors include any external chemical that alters wound healing. Cortisone is commonly implicated in wound complications. Corticosteroids markedly inhibit capillary budding, fibroblast proliferation, and the rate of epithelialization. Similar to cortisone, vitamin E adversely affects wound healing by slowing collagen production. This effect may be reversed with vitamin A. Additional vitamin A will not improve wound healing in the absence of vitamin E or cortisone. Vitamin C is required for the hydroxylation of proline and lysine. Zinc is required for epithelial and fibroblastic proliferation;

however, excessive zinc delays wound healing by inhibiting macrophage function. Radiation is detrimental to wound healing. Given 7 days prior to wound creation, healing is impaired. Administered 7 days following wound creation, it has no effect on wound strength. Cytotoxic drugs may also delay wound healing. Alkylating agents (eg, cyclophosphamide, melphalan) slow wound healing by blocking DNA synthesis.

MANAGEMENT OF SPECIFIC WOUNDS

Lacerations: Uncomplicated simple lacerations are usually managed by complete closure if they are not grossly contaminated. The wound should be thoroughly lavaged and debrided as necessary before closure. If tension is present on the wound edges, it should be relieved by tension-relieving suture techniques, sliding tissue flaps, or grafts. Deep lacerations may be treated according to the same principles, depending on the extent of the injury. Damage to underlying structures (eg, muscles, tendons, and blood vessels) must be resolved before closure. If a laceration is grossly contaminated with debris, primary closure of the wound may not be indicated. Contaminated wounds may be closed with drains or treated as an open wound.

Bite Wounds: Bite wounds are a major cause of injuries, especially in free-ranging animals. Cat bites tend to be small, penetrating wounds that frequently become infected and must be treated as an abscess with culture, debridement, antibiotics, and drainage. Dog bites have a more varied presentation. Because of the slashing nature of dog bite injuries, the major tissue damage is usually found beneath the surface of the wound. While only small puncture marks or bruising may be evident on the surface, ribs may be broken or internal organs seriously damaged. The animal should be thoroughly examined and stabilized before definitive wound care is begun. The wound should be surgically extended as far as necessary to allow a thorough examination and determination of its extent before a decision on the repair can be made. After a proper assessment, debridement can be performed. Unless en bloc debridement is performed, complete wound closure is usually not recommended because the sites are usually contaminated. Closure can be accomplished with drains, as a delayed closure, or by second intention depending on the extent of the injury.

Degloving Injuries: Degloving injuries result in an extensive loss of skin and a varied amount of deeper tissues. These injuries are a result of a shear force on the skin. Sources include fan belt injuries and loss of tissue during a collision with a motor vehicle. With a physiologic degloving injury, the skin is still present but completely freed from the underlying fascia. If the injury results in a loss of blood supply to the skin, necrosis may develop later. In an anatomic degloving injury, the skin is torn off the body. Anatomic degloving injuries frequently require marked and repeated debridement. Differentiating viable and nonviable tissue may be a problem in the early wound debridement process. An attempt should be made to salvage tissue in which viability is questionable. Subsequent debridement can be used to remove any necrotic tissue. In orthopedic injuries that typically accompany degloving injuries, final stabilization may be delayed until local infection is under control.

Gunshot Injuries: In gunshot injuries, most of the damage is not visible. As the projectile penetrates, it drags skin, hair, and dirt through the wound. If the projectile exits the body, the exit wound is larger than the entrance wound. The amount of damage caused by the projectile is a function of its shape, aerodynamic stability, mass, and velocity. High-velocity projectiles tend to produce more damage as a result of impact-induced shock waves that move through the tissue. The shock waves create blunt force trauma resulting in tissue and vascular damage.

Gunshot wounds are always considered to be contaminated, and primary closure is generally not recommended. These wounds should be managed as open wounds or by delayed primary closure. After initial assessment and stabilization of the animal, the wound may be explored to evaluate the extent of damage and to determine a plan for repair. If the projectile caused a fracture, the method of repair depends on the location and type of fracture. External fixation or bone plates are common choices for rigid stabilization of the fracture so that the soft tissues may be appropriately managed. Gunshot wounds to the abdomen are an indication for an exploratory celiotomy. Gunshot wounds to the thorax may require a thoracotomy if hemorrhage or pneumothorax cannot be conservatively managed.

Pressure Wounds: Pressure wounds or decubital ulcers develop as a result of pressure-induced necrosis. Pressure wounds can be extremely difficult to treat and are best prevented. Preventive measures include changing the position of the animal frequently, maintaining adequate nutrition and cleanliness, and providing a sufficiently padded bed. Factors that predispose to pressure wounds include paraplegia, tetraplegia, improper coaptation, and immobility. Mild ulcers may be managed with debridement and bandaging to prevent further trauma to the affected site. More severe wounds require extensive surgical management. After debridement and development of a granulation bed, an advancement flap or pedicle graft may be required for closure.

EQUINE EMERGENCY MEDICINE

Equine emergencies can be challenging for veterinary practitioners and emotionally charged for owners. Problems can be reduced by educating owners about emergency preparedness and first aid procedures. The most common types of equine emergencies are abdominal pain (colic), trauma and lacerations, and acutely ill foals.

EQUINE EMERGENCY PROCEDURES

Emergency Fluid Therapy

Injuries with blood loss, exhaustion, acute rhabdomyolysis, and overheating are conditions that require emergency fluid replacement. Fluids can be administered for maintenance purposes, when fluid intake is physically not possible, or for replacement purposes when excessive losses have been incurred or ongoing losses are anticipated.

In athletic horses, replacement therapy is the mainstay of fluid therapy. Designing a replacement fluid therapy regimen requires consideration of the volume and type of fluids required as well as the route and rate of administration. The volume of fluid to give on a daily basis can be calculated using the following: volume to administer (L) = maintenance (60 mL/kg/day) + immediate losses (body wt [kg] × estimate of dehydration) + ongoing losses. Ongoing losses can be difficult to determine. Maintenance volumes are ~1L/hr for adult horses. Dehydration can be estimated by using clinical and laboratory parameters (TABLE 6). These numbers should be considered in relation to the horse's clinical condition. For example, a nervous horse may have a transiently high heart rate in response to excitement and a high PCV because of splenic contraction.

Ongoing losses can be difficult to estimate, as losses through the GI tract are hard to measure. The equine GI tract secretes and reabsorbs the equivalent of the extracellular volume (~30% of body wt) on a daily basis. If ileus is present, the amount of reflux can be

TABLE 6. Physical and Laboratory Parameters for Estimation of Dehydration in Horses

% Dehydration	Heart Rate (bpm)	Capillary Refill Time (sec)	PCV (%/L)	Total Protein (g/L)	Creatinine (mg/dL)
6%	40-60	2	40	7	1.5-2
8%	61-80	3	45	7.5	2-3
10%	81-100	4	50	8	3-4
12%	>100	>4	>50	>8	>4

quantitated. If the large colon is not reabsorbing water (eg, diarrhea), losses can be significant. With severe diarrhea, ~50% of extracellular fluids can be lost on a daily basis.

This calculation provides only a crude estimate; volumes should be adjusted based on objective responses to fluid administration such as heart rate, pulse quality, capillary refill time, urine production, PCV, total protein, and creatinine. These parameters should be monitored as often as dictated by the horse's clinical condition. In a horse in severe shock, cardiovascular parameters may need to be monitored continuously, or at least every 15 min until an improvement is noted. In a horse with severe ongoing fluid losses, cardiovascular parameters should be monitored at least every 4 hr, and laboratory parameters as frequently as 4 times a day until stabilized. Following these evaluations, the estimate of fluid requirements can be adjusted.

Fluids available for administration in horses include **crystalloids** (fluids containing substances that freely cross the capillary membrane, including balanced electrolyte, saline, and dextrose solutions) and **colloids** (fluids that are retained in the vascular space for a certain number of hours because of their larger molecular size). Colloids include plasma, albumin solutions, dextrans, and hydroxyethylstarch. Crystalloids are most commonly used for replacement fluid therapy in athletic horses, whereas colloids are mostly reserved for resuscitation purposes.

Two basic types of crystalloids are available for horses: **balanced electrolyte solutions** (BES), which are solutions that contain electrolyte in concentrations similar to those in plasma, and **saline solutions**, which contain only sodium chloride. Although considered a crystalloid, dextrose solutions are rarely used alone. The decision to choose BES or saline is based, if available, on a serum chemistry profile. Saline is chosen if the sodium concentration is <125 mEq/L and there is no edema, there is a metabolic alkalosis, or the potassium is >5.9 mEq/L. Otherwise, a BES is used. If serum chemistries are unavailable, a BES is safe, unless hyperkalemic periodic paralysis is suspected, in which case saline, dextrose, and/or sodium bicarbonate should be used.

The addition of colloids to a fluid therapy regimen serves 2 purposes—preventing edema formation in hypoproteinemic states and sustaining the intravascular fluid volume. Products containing antibodies are also available for the treatment or prevention of endotoxemia, *Rhodococcus equi* pneumonia, West Nile virus infection, and clostridial diseases. Colloidal solutions are available in natural or synthetic forms. Natural colloids are plasma, serum products, or albumin. In general, plasma is selected when an increase in oncotic pressure is needed and coagulation factors or specific anticoagulants such as antithrombin III are required. Albumin solutions are not commonly used, as the intravascular half-life of albumin in states of compromised vascular permeability is short, and they do not have the added benefits of whole plasma. The synthetic colloid most commonly used in horses is hydroxyethylstarch. It is used to increase plasma oncotic pressure, and its effect is best evaluated either by clinical response (decreased edema) or increased oncotic pressure (measured by colloid osmometry). A refractometer cannot be used to monitor the effect of synthetic colloid administration.

The goal of fluid therapy in shock states is to rapidly expand circulating blood volume to improve perfusion and oxygen delivery. Isotonic crystalloids must be administered at a rapid rate of up to 60-80 mL/kg in the first hour (~1 blood volume) for maximal beneficial effects. Hypertonic saline can rapidly expand circulating volume by redistributing extravascular fluids into the vascular space. Because of redistribution, hypertonic solutions in horses have a short duration of effect (~45 min). Colloid solutions can be used to sustain the effect of hypertonic crystalloid solutions to several hours. For resuscitation, a combination of hypertonic saline (4 mL/kg) and hetastarch (4 mL/kg) has the most beneficial and sustained effects.

The flow rate of fluids through an administration system is directly proportional to the diameter of the line and inversely proportional to the viscosity of the fluid and the length of the line. Teflon® or polyurethane 14-gauge catheters are used routinely in adult horses. When gravity flow is used, a rate of 2-3 L/hr can be achieved when fluids are ~10 ft higher than the jugular vein. For more rapid flow, 10- or 12-gauge catheters with large-bore connecting sets can be used, but 10-gauge catheters are more thrombogenic. Finally, both jugular veins can be cannulated for increased fluid administration, and a pressure bag system or a pump used to increase the flow rate. Peristaltic pumps can cause endothelial damage and increase the risk of thrombosis.

Nasogastric Intubation

Nasogastric intubation is an essential and possibly life-saving procedure performed in cases of equine colic. The tube is passed in the ventral meatus, using the thumb to keep it directed correctly. If a hard structure (the ethmoidal area) is encountered, the tube should be redirected more ventrally. Once the pharynx is reached, a soft resistance is felt. The tube can be turned 180° to direct the curvature dorsally toward the esophagus. The horse is stimulated to swallow, and the tube is then pushed in the esophagus. Blowing into the tube to dilate the esophagus helps facilitate insertion. If the horse coughs, the tube should be withdrawn and the procedure repeated until it is correctly positioned. The tube is advanced into the stomach (14th rib). If difficulty is encountered in passing the cardia, 60 mL of mepivacaine can be injected into the tube. Once the tube is in place, if there is no spontaneous reflux, the stomach should be lavaged (ie, it should not be assumed that any reflux will come out spontaneously). Medication should never be administered by nasogastric tube to a horse with colic without checking first for reflux. To do so, the tube is filled with water using a pump, and the end of the tube is directed downward to verify the presence of gastric contents. Subtracting the amount pumped in from the amount obtained determines "net" reflux.

Nasogastric reflux is not normal. Occasionally a small amount of reflux (≤1 L) is obtained if a horse has had a tube in place for a long time. When reflux is obtained, the amount, character, and timing in relationship to the onset of colic is noted. In addition, the response to gastric decompression should be noted.

Typically, reflux accompanies small-intestinal ileus, either functional or mechanical. Lesions of the proximal small intestine produce large amounts of reflux early in relationship to the onset of the colic. With lesions of the distal small intestine (ileum), there is initially no reflux, but it usually is found several hours after the onset of colic. Occasionally, large colon disease can be associated with reflux, if the colonic distention exerts pressure on the duodenum as it curves over the base of the cecum.

Foul-smelling, fermented, or copious bloody reflux is associated with anterior enteritis. With intestinal obstruction, the reflux is usually composed of fresh feed material and intestinal secretions. Reflux originating from the small intestine is alkaline, whereas reflux composed of gastric secretions is acidic. Because gastric outflow obstruction is rare in horses, pH is usually not measured. Response to gastric decompression should be noted. Horses with functional ileus show relief of pain, and the heart rate decreases in response to decompression. Horses with a mechanical obstruction usually remain painful, although some horses respond. The rest of the examination should focus on determining whether functional or mechanical ileus is present. The amount of reflux obtained should be noted, and the volume of fluids given IV should be adjusted accordingly. Horses with functional ileus generally need gastric decompression every 4 hr, although if severe, every 2 hr may be required. The nasogastric tube should be left in place only as long as required, as it will cause pharyngeal and laryngeal irritation in some horses.

Abdominocentesis

Abdominocentesis is important in the evaluation of abdominal disease (eg, colic, weight loss, or postoperative problems). Ultrasonography can be used to determine the best location for obtaining a fluid sample, which can be collected using an 18-gauge needle, a catheter, or a cannula. The fluid is collected using sterile technique and placed in an anticoagulant or culture tube.

Normal values for abdominocentesis include a total protein <2.5 g/dL and WBC <5,000 cells/μL. On cytology, neutrophils comprise ~40% of cells; the remainder are lymphocytes, macrophages, and peritoneal cells. With intestinal strangulation, protein increases in the first 1-2 hr. After 3-4 hr of strangulation, RBC are present, and after 6 hr or more, WBC increase gradually, as intestinal necrosis progresses.

Enterocentesis sometimes is seen and should be differentiated from intestinal rupture. With enterocentesis, cytology reveals plant material, bacteria, and debris, but no cells. The horse's clinical condition is not consistent with rupture, although in early rupture (2-4 hr), clinical signs may not be seen. Cytology of abdominal fluid with intestinal rupture shows neutrophils, bacteria, and bacteria that have been phagocytized by neutrophils.

Blood contamination that occurs during the procedure should be differentiated from internal hemorrhage or severely devitalized bowel. Blood from skin vessels usually swirls in the sample and spins down when centrifuged, leaving the sample clear. If an abdominal vessel is punctured, blood will also spin down. All fresh blood contamination shows platelets, which are not present with blood >12 hr old. If the spleen is accidentally punctured, centrifugation reveals a PCV higher than the peripheral PCV. In internal hemorrhage, blood is hemolyzed (leading to a reddish supernatant after centrifugation), there are no platelets, and erythrophagocytosis may be seen. Ultrasonography also reveals fluid swirling in the abdomen. Because Ca edetate in the sample will falsely elevate the total protein, it is useful to shake it out of the tube.

Abdominal surgery increases the total protein (TP) for 3-4 wk and WBC for up to 2 wk. Neutrophils appear nondegenerate. After an enterotomy or an anastomosis, degenerate neutrophils and occasional bacteria may be seen in the first 12-24 hr. The WBC count remains elevated for 2 wk, but the neutrophils appear nondegenerate on cytology, and there are no bacteria. The TP remains elevated for 1 mo after surgery. If septic peritonitis is present, clinical signs will be consistent with bacterial infection (eg, fever, depression, anorexia, ileus, pain, endotoxemia). The WBC and TP are markedly elevated. On cytology, >90% of cells are neutrophils, and they appear degenerate. Free and phagocytized bacteria are seen.

Trocarization

Trocarization is useful to decompress the abdomen when abdominal compartment syndrome is present (severe distention associated with pain and dyspnea). Trocarization should be performed only for large colon distention, never to decompress the small intestine. Thus, it is important to identify the segment of intestine that is involved prior to the procedure. In adult horses, this can be done by rectal palpation. In foals or small horses, radiographs and/or ultrasonography can be used. The distended segment of large colon must also be close to the body wall so it can be safely reached. The most common site for trocarization is the right upper flank area, just cranial to the greater trochanter at the location of the cecal base. After decompression, the trocar is removed, and an antibiotic (usually gentamicin) is infused as the catheter is withdrawn.

Peritonitis and local abscessation are the 2 most common problems encountered after trocarization. The horse is observed for 24 hr for signs of peritonitis. Peritonitis is confirmed with abdominocentesis, and systemic broad-spectrum antibiotics are administered until it is resolved. A local abscess can be drained externally.

Tracheostomy

If possible, the planned incision site for a tracheostomy should be clipped, prepped, and infiltrated with a local anesthetic. In acute respiratory distress, this may not be possible, and the procedure is done without preparation.

An 8- to 10-cm longitudinal incision is made at the junction of the proximal and middle third of the neck, just above the "V" made by the junction of the sternothyrohyoideus muscles. Care must be taken to stay on midline, to favor drainage. The sternothyrohyoid muscles are separated on the midline, and the trachea is exposed. A transverse incision is made between 2 tracheal rings, taking care to avoid damaging the tracheal cartilages. If the horse's head is elevated during the procedure, the tracheal incision should be made distal in relationship to the skin incision, to avoid covering the incision when the head is lowered. In emergency situations, a J-type tracheostomy tube is used because of ease of insertion. When the horse is calm or if the situation is not critical, a self-retaining tube is preferred for maintenance, as J-tubes tend to fall out. If the animal is to be ventilated, a silicone-cuffed tube allows for closed-system ventilation.

The tracheostomy tube should be cleaned daily and changed as needed. Petroleum gel applied around the incision helps to avoid skin scalding. In general, but particularly in foals, tracheostomy tubes should be removed as early as possible to avoid permanent tracheal deformity. To help determine when the tube can be removed, it can be temporarily occluded to see if the horse can breathe without it. Once the tube has been removed, the site is cleaned of exudate twice daily and allowed to heal by second intention. It will generally close in 10-14 days and heal in 3 wk.

EQUINE TRAUMA AND FIRST AID

Common emergencies involving the musculoskeletal system include fractures, luxations, lacerations, puncture wounds, infections, and exertional rhabdomyolysis. Although many of these conditions cannot be treated in the field, accurate identification and provision of appropriate emergency treatment are essential for a successful outcome.

Fractures and Luxations

A thorough physical examination is warranted, but completion can be complicated by the severity of the injury and other factors (eg, anxiety, exhaustion, dehydration, owner/trainer anxiety). The goals of initial coaptation of fractures are to relieve anxiety, prevent further injury, and allow safe transportation for additional evaluation. Emergency coaptation of unstable limbs should be performed before radiographic evaluation or transportation to a surgical facility.

Initial Assessment: Fractures or luxations should be suspected if a loud crack is heard, there is acute non-weightbearing lameness, or the limb is misaligned or visibly unstable. Physical examination should be completed in the best possible setting to avoid further injury to the horse or bystanders. If the horse is recumbent, examination should be completed before attempting to stand the horse. If the horse is standing, examination should be completed before attempting to move the horse. Sedation and a twitch can be used to aid restraint. For sedation, an α_2 agonist such as xylazine, or xylazine and acepromazine, can be used. If sedation is needed immediately after maximal exercise, up to double the standard dosage regimen may be required to achieve effective sedation. Butorphanol or detomidine should be reserved for horses that are not controlled with xylazine. Because α_2 agonists often cause the horse to lean forward, which may increase the weight on an injured forelimb and decrease the ability to manipulate the limb, the minimal effective dose should be used. If the horse is recumbent and a serious injury is suspected, general anesthesia can be safely induced following maximal exercise using sedation with a combination of xylazine and acepromazine, followed by induction of anesthesia with ketamine and diazepam or tiletamine-zolazepam. The combination of guaifenesin and thiopenthal results in more hypotension and is less desirable. Circulatory status should be briefly assessed by evaluating heart rate, mucous membrane color, capillary refill time, and pulse quality. A heart rate >80 bpm accompanied by a delayed capillary refill time and poor peripheral pulse quality indicates the need for IV fluid support.

Once the general status of the horse has been assessed, location and assessment of the injury follows. It is useful to divide the limbs into 4 levels, which help define the method of coaptation. Level 1 injuries involve the limbs from the fetlock down and include extensor and flexor tendon injuries located at the level of the metacarpus/metatarsus. Level 2 injuries involve the limbs from the fetlock to the carpus or hock. Level 3 injuries involve the forelimbs from the carpus to the elbow or the hindlimb from the hock to the stifle. Level 4 injuries involve the forelimb above the elbow or the hindlimb above the stifle.

The presence of a fracture can be determined by instability, crepitus, or abnormal motion. Luxations should be suspected when there is abnormal lateral to medial motion at the level of a joint. Radiographs are indicated to confirm the presence of a fracture or luxation. If radiographic equipment is unavailable on site, external coaptation should be applied as if a fracture or luxation exists and the horse transported to a referral facility for further examination. Incomplete (hairline) fractures of the radius, tibia, and other bones can be difficult to demonstrate radiographically, particularly in field conditions. Therefore, in the presence of severe lameness with pain localized to a long bone, external coaptation should be completed before transportation to avoid catastrophic displacement of a fracture. Laboratory determinations of biochemistry profile indices are becoming more commonly available, even in field situations. If available, parameters of hydration and electrolyte balance are useful to dictate fluid volume and type.

Emergency Treatment: Therapeutic aims of the initial management of traumatic injuries are to relieve anxiety, immobilize the fracture or luxation for transportation, prevent further damage, and provide safe transportation. The principles of emergency coaptation of traumatic injuries in horses include appropriate wound care before application of external coaptation, provision of adequate padding to prevent skin abrasions, immobilization of the joint below and above the area of injury, prevention of lateromedial and craniocaudal motion, and never ending a splint in the middle of a long bone segment or at the end of a fracture line.

Wounds should be carefully cleaned and debrided. An antiseptic ointment can be applied and held in place with conforming gauze. Cotton padding is applied to the entire length of the segment to be immobilized and held in place with gauze, followed by nonstretch bandage material. The bandage should be snug, to avoid loosening with packing of the cotton material. Splints are then applied and held in place, ideally with fiberglass casting tape. This is particularly useful in stabilizing a luxation. If unavailable, heavy tape can be used. The splints must be well padded to avoid the development of sores.

Immobilization of Level 1 Injuries: Level 1 injuries include phalangeal fractures; fetlock, pastern, or coffin joint luxations; and severance of one or more flexor tendons. Although technically Level 1 injuries, extensor tendon lacerations require a different mode of splint application and are discussed separately. Forelimb and hindlimb immobilization differ slightly, because of the presence of the reciprocal apparatus in the hindlimb.

In forelimb injuries, immobilization is best accomplished by aligning the cannon bone with the phalanges to establish a straight column. The horse will bear weight on its toe. The forelimb is held above the carpus and bandaged, and the splint applied on the cranial aspect of the distal limb, extending from the toe to the carpus. If there is lateromedial instability, a lateral splint can also be applied.

In the hindlimb, the reciprocal apparatus prevents extension of the distal limb if the animal is non-weightbearing. Therefore, the limb is best immobilized by applying the splint on the caudal aspect of the limb, from the toe to the point of the hock. If there is lateromedial instability, a lateral splint should also be placed.

A commercially available splint may be used for Level 1 injuries other than fetlock or pastern luxations; however, it does not provide enough lateral-to-medial stability for luxations. The splint is readily available, easy to apply, and effective in achieving immobilization. Two configurations are available—one with a slightly forward-angled bar (for the forelimb) and one with a backward angle with a curve at the level of the fetlock (for the hindlimb). The forward angle configuration is more effective for either fore- or hindlimb injuries. The hindlimb splint has a heel piece to facilitate weightbearing. Alternatively, a heel piece can be welded onto the splint to increase the weightbearing surface area. Nonslip tape should be placed on the foot plate to make it less slippery, particularly on cement floors.

When both extensor tendons of the forelimb or hindlimb are completely severed, the horse will knuckle over, which can injure the dorsal aspect of the fetlock and further disrupt the wound. In this instance, external coaptation is needed to prevent knuckling over at the fetlock. A splint is applied to the cranial aspect of the fore- or hindlimb, with the hoof flat on the ground.

Immobilization of Level 2 Injuries: Examples of level 2 injuries include cannon bone fractures, wounds of the carpus or hock, olecranon fractures, and radial nerve paralysis. In level 2 injuries of the forelimb, 2 splints are needed, applied at a 90° angle, with one lateral and one caudal. The splints should extend from the hoof to the elbow. For olecranon fractures and radial nerve paralysis, the goal of immobilization is to prevent tendon contracture and injury to the dorsal aspect of the limb. Only a caudal splint is needed for these injuries. In hindlimb injuries, as in the forelimb, 2 splints are needed (applied laterally and caudally, from the hoof to the stifle). The angle of the hock makes it difficult to apply a caudal splint. Therefore, the caudal splint can end at the point of the hock, rather than at the stifle. Alternatively, a splint can be molded and applied to the hock.

Immobilization of Level 3 Injuries: Level 3 injuries include fractures of the radius or tibia. With fracture, the flexor muscles become abductors, resulting in displacement and comminution of the medial aspect of the limb. The medial aspect of both the radius and ulna does not include a muscle mass to help prevent penetration of the skin by fractured bone. The goal of external coaptation is to prevent abduction of the limb. On the forelimb, the splint is applied to the lateral aspect of the limb and must extend from the hoof to the withers. The tip of the splint can be taped around the chest for further stability. On the hindlimb, the splint is applied to the lateral aspect of the limb, extending from the hoof to the hip.

Immobilization of Level 4 Injuries: Level 4 injuries include fractures of the scapula, humerus, femur, and pelvis. External coaptation is not recommended for these injuries, as these areas are not amenable to bandaging. Hematomas and swelling around the injury may provide functional immobilization. A bandage should not be applied to the distal limb, as it will make it more awkward to move and may increase motion at the fracture site. If the pelvis is fractured, the need for transportation should be discussed, as moving of the fracture segments may lacerate major blood vessels. General anesthesia for pelvic fracture should be delayed for 3-4 wk to avoid fatal hemorrhage.

Guidelines for Safe Transportation

Before loading an injured horse, proper functioning of the vehicle should be assured, the horse stabilized, and the injury immobilized as much as possible. A low ramp facilitates loading and unloading of an injured horse. While in the trailer, the horse may lean on the wall and partitions to help reduce the load on the injured leg. It will be easier for the horse to travel with partitions in place rather than loose in a makeshift stall. A sling can be placed under the abdomen to help the horse take weight off the injured limb. Many trailers have standing stalls at 45° angles (slant load trailers), which help horses balance during transport. If a regular straight-load trailer is used, the horse should face backward for a forelimb injury, and forward for a hindlimb injury, to help cushion sudden stops. Providing hay helps relieve anxiety, and frequent stops should be made to check on the status of the horse and provide drinking water. If significant cardiovascular compromise exists, IV fluids can be administered while in transit.

If the horse is severely injured and needs to remain recumbent, it can be pulled onto the trailer using a large tarp or blanket. The horse should be kept sedated during transport, to avoid injuries. A head protector or bandage can be used to protect the eyes and head from self-induced trauma. Bandages should be applied to the lower limbs to avoid trauma caused by paddling.

Wounds and Lacerations

Wounds and lacerations are common in horses. The steps involved in the management of these injuries include identification of all involved structures, control of hemorrhage, and evaluation of the need for referral. Referral to a surgical facility is recommended if there are tendon injuries, penetration of a synovial structure, extensive degloving injury, or severe blood loss. In addition to wound management, tetanus prophylaxis, analgesia, and appropriate antibiotic therapy are indicated. If severe blood loss has occurred, cardiovascular support should be provided before or during transportation, or both.

Assessment: A brief physical examination should be completed before addressing the primary problem. If the wound is located on a limb, the presence and degree of lameness should be noted as indicators of a potentially more serious injury. The following characteristics are then evaluated: location, hemorrhage, configuration, penetration of a body cavity, and involvement of synovial structures or tendons. Wounds over joints, tendon sheaths, or tendons (particularly flexor tendons) and those that expose or penetrate to bone should be explored thoroughly for injury to important underlying structures. Severe hemorrhage may need to be controlled before further wound assessment is possible. A pressure bandage is applied directly over the bleeding area. Attempts to find the bleeding vessels are usually not successful. Certain wound configurations may lead to significant damage to the blood supply to the skin and subcutaneous tissues and result in sloughing (eg, an inverted "V" configuration or significant bruising or trauma to adjacent tissue). Wounds over the chest or abdomen may penetrate important organs. In the case of thoracic wounds, development of an open or closed pneumothorax can lead to severe respiratory distress. Any horse with chest trauma and respiratory distress should be evaluated for the presence of pneumothorax.

The potential involvement of a synovial structure should be immediately determined. The horse should be restrained and sedated as needed for this procedure. A site of entry of the joint or tendon sheath remote from the wound is chosen, clipped, and prepared aseptically. Using sterile technique, saline or a balanced electrolyte solution is injected into the synovial structure. The amount needed to achieve distention can vary from a few mL in the case of a distal tarsal joint injury to ≥100 mL for the femoropatellar joint. All possible joint compartments should be assessed. The wound is observed for leakage of the injected solution.

Extensor tendon injury of the distal limbs results in inability to appropriately place the hoof on the ground, resulting in the horse knuckling over. This suggests involvement of both tendons in proximal metacarpal or metatarsal injuries. Flexor tendon injuries result in hyperextension of the fetlock (superficial digital flexor), lifting up of the toe (deep digital flexor), or complete dropping of the fetlock to the ground (severance of the suspensory ligament). For this to be observed, the horse must bear weight on the limb at least transiently. In the case of complete suspensory breakdown, severe stretching of digital vessels can lead to thrombosis and avascular injury to the hoof. In complete breakdown injury, it is critical to support the fetlock and not allow weightbearing until further stabilization is performed. The goals of initial wound care are to decontaminate the wound as much as possible and prevent further contamination during transportation. This is done by lavage with saline and sharp debridement of gross contaminants. Local antiseptics or antibiotics can then be packed in the wound for further decontamination. Immobilization of the limb (*see* above) is needed if there is injury to a supporting structure (bone tendon) or significant instability (luxation).

Pneumothorax: An open chest wound can result in the development of pneumothorax and lead to respiratory distress manifested by a restrictive pattern of breathing. On auscultation, there is no sound in the dorsal lung fields. Because of the incomplete mediastinum in horses, a unilateral chest wound can lead to bilateral pneumothorax. An open pneumothorax is managed by providing a temporary seal over the chest wound. The wound is bandaged and an airtight layer of material (eg, conforming plastic sheets) is applied. The chest is then evacuated by inserting a 14-gauge catheter, using aseptic technique, in the dorsal aspect of the 12th intercostal space and aspirating the air out of the chest. Use of a 3-way stopcock facilitates this procedure.

Penetrating Abdominal Wounds: Penetrating abdominal wounds are serious and potentially fatal injuries that can lead to penetration of a viscus or development of peritonitis. If a penetrating wound is suspected, it should be cleaned, explored for the presence of a foreign body, and debrided. Abdominocentesis can be performed to detect fecal contamination, indicating a ruptured viscus. However, abdominocentesis may not be diagnostic in the early stages of peritoneal contamination, as indicators of peritonitis take several hours to develop. The wound can be bandaged, and broad-spectrum systemic antibiotics initiated. In the presence of a large wound, or if abdominal musculature is involved, the abdomen can be supported.

Head Injuries

Head injuries can result in severe CNS damage. Injury can be primary (ie, contusion, lacerations, or hemorrhage causing acute damage) or secondary (ie, subsequent edema, reperfusion injury, and necrosis). Head injury therapy is designed to minimize secondary CNS damage. Causes of head injury in athletic horses include direct trauma from a fall, blows to the head, and falling over backward onto the poll region. The associated injuries include basisphenoid fractures and avulsion of ventral straight muscles of the head. Basisphenoid fractures can result in acute optic nerve damage and cerebral signs. Temporary or permanent blindness may result. The diagnosis is made by radiography; treatment is supportive care and is focused on minimizing secondary brain damage. Rectus and longus capitis muscle rupture occurs most commonly from falling over backward. The muscles attach to the base of the cranium; with injury, hematoma and even avulsion fractures of the muscular insertion may result. Because of the location of these muscles within the guttural pouch septum, hematomas may rupture into one of the guttural pouches, resulting in epistaxis that may require blood transfusion. When epistaxis of guttural pouch origin, in conjunction with a large hematoma in the guttural pouch septum, is identified, diagnosis is made by endoscopy. Radiographs are useful to demonstrate an avulsion fracture accompanied by a soft-tissue opacity overlying the guttural pouches.

Treatment: Horses with head injury can be severely ataxic and should be handled and moved with extreme caution. If the horse is down, short-term general anesthesia is best used while moving the horse to a referral facility for further evaluation. If hypoventilation develops, the horse should be intubated and ventilation assisted to prevent hypercapnia. NSAID are used to minimize inflammation. Although controversial, corticosteroids may be indicated if used in the immediate phase of injury. Dimethyl sulfoxide (DMSO) is often used to minimize secondary edema. Magnesium has recently been proposed as another therapeutic agent for acute head injury.

Ocular Injuries

Ocular injuries are usually traumatic in origin, and include periocular lacerations, corneal lacerations or foreign body penetrating injuries, and direct blows to the eye causing retinal detachment. See also OPHTHALMIC EMERGENCIES, p 1415. Evaluation of acute ocular injury includes evaluation of the different structures of the eye, as well as evaluation of cranial nerve function. Eyelids, conjunctiva, cornea, lens, and fundic examinations can be performed to assess the degree of damage. Vision can be assessed by the menace response, supplemented with obstacle course testing. Oculomotor, trochlear, and abducent nerve function are assessed by the position of the eye and pupillary light responses. Facial nerve and sympathetic innervation to the eye are assessed by eyelid tone and position of the eyelashes.

Treatment of acute ocular injuries includes minimizing pain and inflammation, preventing infection, and preventing further injuries. If penetration by a foreign body is suspected, rapid surgical intervention is indicated to prevent further injury. Anti-inflammatory drugs that are used to minimize pain and inflammation associated with ocular injuries include NSAID, DMSO, and topical osmotic agents. Pain from pupillary spasm can be minimized by dilating the pupil with atropine. Direct sunlight should be minimized by protecting the eye. Acute injuries can be associated with ulceration and secondary bacterial invasion. Use of a broad-spectrum topical antibiotic may prevent secondary infection of an ulcer. Horses that are acutely blind cannot move around their environment well. Further injury should be prevented by protecting the blind eye and by carefully handling the horse.

OTHER COMMON CONDITIONS REQUIRING EMERGENCY TREATMENT

Esophageal Obstruction
(Choke)

See also ESOPHAGEAL OBSTRUCTION, p 174.

Intraluminal esophageal obstruction is common in horses and is generally caused by impaction of feed material. The most frequent sites of impaction are the proximal esophagus and just cranial to the thoracic inlet. Predisposing factors include bolting of food, improper chewing of food (poor dentition), recent sedation, poor feed quality, and dehydration.

Diagnosis: Clinical signs of choke include nasal discharge containing saliva and feed material, hypersalivation, coughing, and frequent attempts to swallow. Esophageal obstruction is identified by palpation of the neck, passage of a nasogastric tube, or endoscopy. In refractory cases, radiography and contrast radiography may be used, particularly if a foreign body, stricture, or diverticulum is suspected.

Treatment: Once the presence of an obstruction has been confirmed, the horse should be muzzled to prevent packing of feed at the obstruction site. Many obstructions resolve with sedation and consequent relaxation of the esophageal musculature. An α_2 agonist such as xylazine or detomidine provides good relaxation. Recently, oxytocin (0.11 mg/kg, IV) has been demonstrated to provide good esophageal relaxation and has been used successfully to resolve esophageal obstructions. Once an esophageal relaxant has been given, the obstruction often resolves within ~1 hr. If the horse is dehydrated, IV fluids may also help resolve the obstruction.

If the obstruction has not resolved after ~1 hr, a nasogastric tube is passed, and after adequate sedation (to lower the head), gentle lavage with water or 0.9% saline is used to flush the esophagus. Mineral oil should never be used due to the risks associated with aspiration. An esophageal lavage tube—essentially a nasogastric tube with a cuff—is useful to help resolve the obstruction. Alternatively, an endotracheal tube can be passed through the nasal passages and into the esophagus, and a smaller nasogastric tube is used for lavage. These procedures can be repeated intermittently and are facilitated by general anesthesia. However, if unsuccessful after a few hours, further tests may be required to exclude the presence of a foreign body.

After the obstruction has been relieved, endoscopy can be used to assess the esophageal mucosa. Circumferential ulceration can lead to stricture formation with recurrence of the obstruction. Horses that have choked are at risk for recurrence in the 2-4 wk after the initial event even without visible esophageal damage. Feeding a slurried, pelleted diet or grass can prevent recurrence. When the esophagus has been damaged, narrowing maximizes at 30 days. Before attempts are made to resolve a potential stricture, the horse should be managed medically with dietary modification for 60 days. Broad-spectrum antibiotics are administered to prevent or treat aspiration pneumonia, along with anti-inflammatory drugs. Sucralfate has been advocated to facilitate healing of ulcers.

Rectal Tears

See also RECTAL TEARS, p 152.

Rectal tears are serious injuries in horses. Prevention is key, but if a rectal tear should occur, appropriate and timely referral can result in a successful outcome. Rectal tears are classified into 4 grades based on the number of layers involved and their craniocaudal location. Grade I involves the mucosa and submucosa only; grade II involves the muscularis, with a mucosal-submucosal hernia; and grade III involves the mucosa, submucosa, and muscularis, leaving the serosal layer intact. In the case of a grade III tear located in the retroperitoneal area, there is no serosa, so the tear is complete and extends perirectally. Grade IIIa tears leave the visceral peritoneum intact; grade IIIb tears are located in the mesorectum. Grade IV involves the mucosa, submucosa, muscularis, and serosa. There is potential for fecal contamination of the abdomen. Most tears resulting from rectal palpation are located dorsally within the peritoneal cavity and extend into the mesocolon.

Diagnosis: A rectal tear is suspected when there is sudden loss of resistance during palpation, and when a copious amount of fresh blood is present on the rectal sleeve. Blood-tinged mucus usually indicates mucosal irritation only. If a tear is suspected, the severity should be immediately assessed and measures taken to initiate treatment or referral.

The horse should be sedated during assessment and an epidural performed if there is any straining. Propantheline bromide can be given to decrease peristalsis. A speculum should not be used, as it can worsen the tear. Digital palpation (preferably bare handed) is carefully performed. A thin flap of tissue indicates a tear through only the mucosa. If a large cavity with a thin membrane is noted, then a grade III tear is present. If intestine can be palpated, the tear is a grade IV.

Treatment: Grade I and II tears can be managed medically with antibiotics and a laxative diet (oil, grass) and analgesics (flunixin meglumine) to facilitate defecation. Grade III and IV tears should be referred to a surgical facility. However, it is essential to prevent fecal contamination during transportation. Rectal packing is highly recommended to achieve this goal. The horse is sedated, and an epidural is performed, using a combination of xylazine and mepivacaine. A tampon composed of a 6.5-cm stockinet filled with cotton is inserted until located at least 10 cm cranial to the tear, and the anus is occluded with a purse-string suture or towel clamp. It is important to insert the stockinet before filling it completely, to avoid further enlargement of the tear. The horse should be given systemic broad-spectrum antibiotics, flunixin meglumine, and appropriate tetanus prophylaxis. Prevention of fecal contamination of grade III and IV tears during referral can determine whether the outcome will be successful.

At the referral facility, the tear is reassessed to check for additional damage during transportation. An abdominocentesis is performed to check for peritonitis. Following assessment, several treatment options are available. For grade II tears with no fecal contamination, primary repair by a rectal approach can be attempted using 1-handed ties. The horse should be monitored carefully for development of a perirectal abscess. For grade III retroperitoneal tears with fecal contamination, the tear can be packed with iodine-soaked gauze and the cavity cleaned out daily. In mares, the cavity may be drained into the vagina and the tear closed primarily. A laxative diet is provided, with additional laxatives such as mineral oil. These horses are often painful when defecating, so analgesics are provided as needed. The most serious complication of retroperitoneal tears is development of an abscess that migrates forward into the abdominal cavity (point of least resistance). This is prevented by ensuring appropriate drainage into the rectum or vagina. For grade III and IV peritoneal tears in a caudal location, primary repair through a rectal approach can be attempted. A successful primary repair of a grade IV tear using a linear stapling device has been reported. This approach requires that the abdomen has not been contaminated or that the contamination is minimal. Alternatively, these tears can be treated through a ventral midline approach, followed by an antimesenteric incision in the caudal small colon and repair through the lumen. The abdominal approach is very caudal and involves separation of the udder in mares or a preputial reflection in males. This approach has the advantage of allowing the large colon to empty, thus reducing fecal load.

Grade III and IV tears can also be treated by insertion of a rectal liner. Rectal liners are made from a plastic ring glued to a rectal sleeve. The liner is sutured to the small colon mucosa, via an enterotomy, and the sleeve protects the tear during healing. The ring is sloughed in ~10 days with normal mucosal turnover. In other cases, a loop colostomy can be performed to maintain patency of the distal segment. The colostomy is performed as the first step; after healing of the tear, colonic continuity is reestablished. In all fecal diversion procedures, an attempt should be made to also close or approximate the tear. If large, it may heal with a fistula.

Postcastration Evisceration

Postcastration evisceration is always a risk following open castrations, but the risk is increased in Standardbreds and Belgians (due to their larger inguinal rings) or after castration of an adult stallion.

Diagnosis: Evisceration of omentum or small intestine is first identified by a structure hanging out of the surgical incision. It is important to instruct the owner to keep the horse quiet and to support the eviscerated structure with a towel to avoid further stretching or damage. Examination quickly reveals what structure(s) is involved so that treatment can be initiated.

Treatment: In cases of omental evisceration, a rectal palpation should be performed to ensure that only omentum is involved. A short-term general anesthetic is given. The omentum and scrotum are cleaned and prepped, and the omental segment is emasculated. The scrotum is packed with gauze and closed, and the horse is given systemic antibiotics. The packing can be removed after 2 days, with antibiotics continued for 24 hr after removal of the pack.

If small intestine is eviscerated, a short-term general anesthetic is given. The intestine is copiously lavaged and examined for damage. Avulsion of mesenteric vessels or strangulation require resection, so the scrotum should be sutured closed and the horse referred to a surgical facility. If the intestine appears healthy, it is replaced in the abdomen, which often requires cutting the internal inguinal ring. Care should be taken to replace the intestine within the peritoneal cavity through the inguinal canal and not through a separate, iatrogenic opening. If the herniation cannot be reduced confidently, the scrotum should be packed and the case referred. If the herniation can be reduced, the inguinal canal and scrotum are packed with sterile gauze, and the scrotum is sutured closed (leaving a short segment of gauze exposed). Systemic broad-spectrum antibiotics are administered, and the horse is monitored closely for development of colic or ileus, which indicate intestinal devitalization. Should that occur, the horse must be referred for an abdominal exploratory surgery. If the horse progresses well, the packing can be removed in 48 hr, and the antibiotics discontinued 24 hr after removal of the packing.

NEONATAL INTENSIVE CARE AND NEONATAL EMERGENCIES

Initial Assessment

Early recognition of abnormalities is of utmost importance for the successful management of critically ill foals (*see also* MANAGEMENT OF THE NEONATE, p 1683). Immediately following birth, the cardiovascular and respiratory systems of the foal must adapt to extrauterine life. These critical events are undermined by factors such as inadequate lung development, surfactant deficiency (primary or secondary), viral or bacterial infection, placental abnormalities, in utero hypoxia, and meconium aspiration.

Spontaneous breathing should begin within 1 min of birth and many foals attempt to breathe as their thorax clears the pelvic canal. During the first hour of life, the respiratory rate of a healthy foal can be as high as 80 breaths/min, but should decrease to 30-40 breaths/min within a few hours. Auscultation of the thorax shortly after birth reveals a cacophony of sounds as airways are opened and fluid is cleared. End-expiratory crackles are consistently heard in the dependent lung during and following lateral recumbency. It is not unusual for a newborn foal to appear slightly cyanotic during this initial adaptation period, but this should resolve within minutes of birth. Similarly, the heart rate of a healthy newborn foal has a regular rhythm and should be at least 60 bpm at the first minute. A continuous murmur can usually be heard over the left side of the heart, although its loudness may vary with position. Variable systolic murmurs, thought to be flow murmurs, may be heard during the first week of life. Murmurs that persist beyond the first week of life in an otherwise healthy foal should be more thoroughly investigated, as should any murmur associated with persistent hypoxia.

Foals are normally nonresponsive while in the birth canal. This lack of responsiveness has lead to presumption of fetal death during dystocia. Other tests should be attempted before determining that a foal has died during birth, eg, detection of pulses in the tongue, neck, or any presented limb; or palpation of the thorax for a heartbeat.

If the foal's nose is accessible, nasotracheal intubation will allow measurement of CO_2 tension in the exhaled gas. Nasotracheal intubation of foals under these circumstances can be quite readily performed with minimal practice. Long endotracheal tubes of several sizes (7-12 mm outer diameter) with an inflatable cuff should be available. The tube can be passed blindly using a finger in one nostril for guidance; position can be checked by palpation of the throat. The cuff is inflated, and manual ventilation with either 100% oxygen or room air is begun. CO_2 tension is measured continuously using a capnograph or single-use disposable end-tidal CO_2 monitor. End-tidal CO_2 varies in foals during birth, depending on cardiac output and ventilation frequency, but it should be consistently >20 mm Hg and is usually closer to 30 mm Hg. Once manual ventilation of a living foal is established, it must be continued until the foal is completely delivered.

The righting reflex is present as the foal exits the birth canal, as is the withdrawal reflex. Cranial nerve responses are intact at birth, but the menace response may take as long as 2 wk to fully develop, and its absence should not be considered diagnostic of visual deficits in a newborn foal. Within an hour of birth, normal foals demonstrate auditory orientation with unilateral pinna control. The normal pupillary angle is ventromedial in newborn foals; this angle gradually becomes dorsomedial over the first month of life. Foals should be able to stand on their own within 2 hr of birth and nurse unaided by 3 hr postpartum. Normal foals may defecate shortly after standing but may not attempt defecation until after successfully suckling from the dam. Urination is more variable, with fillies usually urinating before colts. It is not unusual for colts to fail to "drop" their penis when urinating over the first few days of life.

The gait of newborn foals is hypermetric, with a base-wide stance. Extreme hypermetria of the forelimbs, usually bilateral but occasionally unilateral, has been observed in some foals associated with perinatal hypoxic/ischemic insults, but this gait abnormality usually resolves without specific therapy within a few days. Spinal reflexes tend to be exaggerated. Foals also exhibit an exaggerated response to external stimuli (eg, noise, sudden visual changes, touch) for the fist few weeks of life.

Dystocia and Resuscitation

Most newborn foals make the transition to extrauterine life easily. However, for those in difficulty, it is of utmost importance to recognize the condition immediately and institute appropriate resuscitation. A modified Apgar scoring system has been developed as a guide for initiating resuscitation and determining probable level of fetal compromise. A brief physical examination should be performed prior to initiating resuscitation, as there are humane issues concerning foals with serious problems such as severe limb contracture, microophthalmia, and hydrocephalus, among others.

The initial assessment begins during presentation of the fetus. While the following applies primarily to the birth of a foal from a high-risk pregnancy, quiet and rapid evaluation can be performed during any attended birth. The goal in a normal birth of a healthy foal is to minimally disturb the bonding process. This also applies to high-risk births, although some disruption of normal bonding is inevitable.

The strength and rate of any palpable peripheral pulse should be evaluated. The apical pulse should be evaluated as soon as the chest clears the birth canal. Bradycardia (pulse <40 bpm) is expected during forceful contractions, and the pulse rate should increase rapidly once the chest clears the birth canal. Persistent bradycardia is an indication for rapid intervention.

The fetus is normally hypoxemic when compared with the newborn foal, and this hypoxemia is largely responsible for the maintenance of fetal circulation by generation of pulmonary hypertension. During normal parturition, mild asphyxia occurs and results in fetal responses that lead to a successful transition to extrauterine life. If more than mild transient asphyxia occurs, the fetus is stimulated to breathe in utero; this is known as **primary asphyxia**. If the initial breathing effort resulting from the primary asphyxia is not effective, a second gasping period, the **secondary asphyxia** response, occurs in several minutes. If asphyxia does not improve, the foal enters **secondary apnea**, which is irreversible unless resuscitation is initiated. Therefore, the first priority of neonatal resuscitation is establishing an airway and breathing pattern. Foals that are not spontaneously breathing are assumed to be in secondary apnea. The airway should be cleared of membranes as soon as the nose is presented. If meconium staining is present, the airway should be suctioned before delivery of the foal is completed and before the foal breathes spontaneously. Suction should be continued to the trachea if aspiration of the nasopharynx is productive. Overzealous suctioning worsens bradycardia, as it worsens hypoxia. Suctioning should end once the foal begins breathing spontaneously because hypoxia will worsen with continued suction. If the foal does not breathe or move spontaneously within seconds of birth, tactile stimulation is necessary. If tactile stimulation does not result in spontaneous breathing, the foal should be immediately intubated and manually ventilated. Mouth-to-nose ventilation can be used if nasotracheal tubes or an ambu bag (or equivalent) are not available. Hyperventilation with 100% oxygen is the best choice to reverse fetal circulation. However, recent evidence suggests that there are no apparent clinical disadvantages in using room air rather than 100% oxygen for ventilation of asphyxiated human neonates.

Almost 90% of foals requiring resuscitation respond to hyperventilation alone and require no additional therapy. Nasotracheal intubation can be initiated while the foal is in the birth canal if the foal is not delivered rapidly (eg, dystocia). This "blind" technique may require some practice but can be lifesaving. The nasotracheal tube also provides a convenient site for administration of intratracheal medications, such as epinephrine. Once breathing is spontaneous, humidified oxygen should be provided via nasal insufflation at 8-10 L/min.

Chest compressions should be initiated if the foal remains bradycardic despite ventilation and a nonperfusing rhythm is present. The foal should be placed on a hard surface in right lateral recumbency with the topline against a wall or other support. Approximately 5% of foals are born with fractured ribs, and an assessment for the presence of rib fractures should be done before initiating chest compressions. Many of these fractures can be identified by palpating the ribs. They are usually multiple and consecutive on one side of the thorax, located in a relatively straight line along the part of the rib with the greatest curvature dorsal to the costochondral junction. Unfortunately, ribs 3-5 are frequently involved, and their location over the heart can make chest compression a potentially fatal exercise. Auscultation over the ribs during breathing results in a recognizable "click," identifying rib fractures that may have escaped detection by palpation.

Drug therapy should be started if a nonperfusing rhythm persists for >30-60 sec in the face of chest compression. Epinephrine is the drug of choice, although the best dose and frequency of administration for resuscitation are controversial. Vasopressin is gaining attention as a cardiovascular resuscitation drug, but experience with it is limited. Atropine is not recommended in bradycardic newborn foals, as the bradycardia is usually due to hypoxia and atropine can increase myocardial oxygen debt if the hypoxia is not corrected. Doxapram is not recommended because it does not reverse secondary apnea, the most common apnea in newborns.

Immediately after birth, the foal must adapt to independent thermoregulation. In response to the catecholamine surge associated with birth, uncoupling of oxidative phosphorylation occurs within mitochondria, releasing energy as heat. This nonshivering thermogenesis is impaired in newborns undergoing hypoxia or asphyxiation and in those that are ill at birth. Infants born to mothers sedated by benzodiazepines are similarly affected, a consideration in the choice of sedative and preanesthetic medications in mares with dystocia or undergoing caesarian section. Heat losses by convection, radiation, and evaporation are quite high in most areas where foals are delivered, resuscitated, and managed, and care must be taken to ensure cold stress is minimized in both newborn and critically ill foals. The foal should be dried and placed on dry bedding once resuscitation is complete. Supplementary heat, in the form of radiant heat lamps or warm air circulating blankets, may be required.

Fluid therapy should be used conservatively during postpartum resuscitation. The neonate is not volume depleted unless excessive bleeding has occurred. Some compromised newborn foals are actually hypervolemic. Because the renal function of the equine neonate is substantially different from that of adult horses, fluid therapy cannot be simply scaled down. If IV fluids are required for resuscitation, and blood loss is identified, administration of 20 mL/kg of a nonglucose-containing polyionic isotonic fluid over 20 min (~1 L for a 50-kg foal) can be effective. Indications for this "shock bolus" therapy include poor mentation, poorly palpable peripheral pulses, and the development of cold distal extremities, compatible with hemorrhagic shock. The foal should be reassessed after the initial bolus, and additional boluses administered as necessary. Glucose-containing fluids can be administered after resuscitation at a rate delivering 4-8 mg/kg/min glucose (~240 mL/hr 5% dextrose or 120 mL/hr 10% dextrose to the average 50-kg foal), particularly in the obviously compromised foal. This therapy is indicated to help resolve metabolic acidosis, support cardiac output as myocardial glycogen stores have likely been depleted, and prevent postasphyxial hypoglycemia.

Prematurity, Dysmaturity, and Postmaturity

Traditionally, prematurity is defined as a birth at <320 days gestation in the horse. Because gestation length ranges from 310 days to >370 days in some mares, it is possible for a mare whose usual gestation length is 315 days to have a term foal at 313 days, while a mare whose usual gestation length is 365 days may have a premature foal at 340 days. Foals that are born post-term but small are termed dysmature. A postmature foal is a post-term foal that has a normal axial skeletal size but is thin or emaciated. Dysmature foals may have been classified in the past as "small for gestational age" and are thought to have suffered placental insufficiency; postmature foals are usually normal foals that have been retained too long in utero, perhaps due to an abnormal signaling of readiness for birth, and have outgrown their somewhat aged placenta. Postmature foals become more abnormal the longer they are maintained and may also suffer from placental insufficiency. They are most commonly born to mares ingesting endophyte-infested fescue.

Prematurity, dysmaturity, and postmaturity may be associated with high-risk pregnancy. Iatrogenic causes include early elective induction of labor, based on inaccurate breeding dates or misinterpretation of late-term colic or uterine bleeding as ineffective labor. The majority of causes are idiopathic. Even if undetermined, the cause may continue to affect the foal after birth. All body systems may be affected by prematurity, dysmaturity, and postmaturity, and thorough evaluation is necessary.

Respiratory failure is common in these foals, and is related to immaturity of the respiratory tract, poor control of respiratory vessel tone, and weak respiratory muscles, combined with poorly compliant lungs and a greatly compliant chest wall. It is not usually due to surfactant deficiency. Most foals require oxygen supplementation and positional support for optimal oxygenation and ventilation. Effort must be expended to maintain these "floppy foals" in sternal recumbency. Some may require mechanical ventilation. These foals also require cardiovascular support but are frequently unresponsive to commonly used pressors and inotropes, including dopamine, dobutamine, epinephrine, and vasopressin. Careful use of these drugs and judicious IV fluid therapy are necessary. Renal function, reflected in low urine output, is often initially poor due to a delay in making the transition from fetal to neonatal glomerular filtration rates. The delay can be due to true failure of transition or secondary to hypoxic or ischemic insult. Fluid therapy should be used cautiously in these cases, and initial fluid restriction may be necessary to avoid fluid overload. Many premature, dysmature, or postmature foals have suffered a hypoxic insult and present with all of the disorders associated with perinatal asphyxial syndrome, including hypoxic ischemic encephalopathy. Treatment is similar to that of term foals with these problems. These foals are also predisposed to secondary bacterial infection and must be examined frequently for signs consistent with early sepsis or nosocomial infection.

The GI system of these foals is not usually functionally mature due to a primary lack of maturity or secondary to hypoxia. Dysmotility and varying degrees of necrotizing enterocolitis are common. Both hyperglycemia and hypoglycemia are frequently encountered. Hyperglycemia is generally related to stress, increased levels of circulating catecholamines, and rapid progression to gluconeogenesis, while hypoglycemia is associated with diminished glycogen stores, inability to engage gluconeogenesis, sepsis, and hypoxic damage. Immature endocrine function may be present, particularly regarding the hypo-thalamic-pituitary-adrenal axis, and contributes to metabolic derangements. If possible, enteral feeding should be delayed until metabolic and cardiorespiratory parameters are stable. When enteral feeding is initiated, small volumes should be provided at first and slowly increased over several days.

Musculoskeletal problems are frequent, particularly in premature foals, and include significant flexor laxity and decreased muscle tone. Postmature foals may be affected by flexural contracture deformities, most likely due to decreased intrauterine movement as they increase in size.

Premature foals frequently exhibit flexor laxity and decreased cuboidal bone ossification that predisposes them to crush injury of the carpal and tarsal bones if weightbearing is not strictly controlled. Physical therapy, in the form of standing and exercise, is indicated in the management of these problems; however, care should be taken to ensure that the foal does not become fatigued and stand in abnormal positions. Bandaging of the limbs only increases laxity, although light bandages over the fetlock may be necessary to prevent injury if flexor laxity is severe. These foals are predisposed to angular limb deformity and must be closely monitored for development of this problem as they mature.

The overall prognosis for premature, dysmature, and postmature foals remains good with intensive care and attention to detail. Many foals (up to 80%) survive and become productive athletes. Complications associated with sepsis and musculoskeletal abnormalities are the most significant indicators of poor athletic outcome.

Hypoxic Ischemic Encephalopathy

A wide spectrum of clinical signs is associated with hypoxic ischemic encephalopathy (HIE), ranging from mild depression with loss of the suck reflex to grand mal seizures. Affected foals are typically normal at birth but show signs of CNS abnormalities within a few hours. However, some foals are obviously abnormal at birth, and some do not show signs until 24 hr of age. HIE is commonly associated with adverse peripartum events, including dystocia and premature placental separation, but some foals have no known peripartum period of hypoxia, suggesting that unrecognized in utero hypoxia occurred.

Perinatal brain damage in the mature fetus usually results from severe uterine asphyxia due to an acute reduction of uterine or umbilical circulation. The fetus responds to this challenge by activation of the sympathetic adrenergic nervous system, causing a redistribution of cardiac output that favors the central organs—brain, heart, and adrenal glands. If the hypoxic insult continues, a point is reached beyond which the fetus cannot maintain this centralization of circulation, cardiac output falls, and cerebral circulation diminishes. The loss of oxygen results in neuronal injury and death. Once the anoxic event is over, protein synthesis remains inhibited in specific areas of the brain and returns to normal in less vulnerable areas. Loss of protein synthesis appears to be an early indicator of cell death due to the primary hypoxic/anoxic event. A second wave of neuronal cell death occurs during the reperfusion phase and is thought to be similar to classically described postischemic reperfusion injury, in that damage is due to production and release of oxygen radicals, synthesis of nitric oxide, and inflammatory reactions. Additionally, an imbalance between excitatory and inhibitory neurotransmitters occurs. The secondary cell death that occurs is thought to be due to apoptosis and to the neurotoxicity of glutamate and aspartate resulting from increased intracellular calcium levels. The excitotoxic cascade that evolves during HIE extends over several days from the time of insult and is modifiable. Magnesium (constant rate infusion) can be used during the post-injury period in an attempt to modify the excitotoxic cascade injury by inhibition of receptor activity.

Therapy for the various manifestations of hypoxia and ischemia involves control of seizures; general cerebral support; correction of metabolic abnormalities; maintenance of normal arterial blood gas values, tissue perfusion, and renal function; treatment of GI dysfunction; prevention, recognition, and early treatment of secondary infections; and general supportive care. Seizures must be controlled because they increase cerebral oxygen consumption by 5-fold. Diazepam and midazolam can be used for emergency control of seizures. If seizures are not readily stopped with diazepam, or >2 seizures are recognized, then treatment using a midazolam constant rate infusion can be instituted or phenobarbital therapy initiated.

Sepsis

Sepsis in foals can be quite subtle initially, and the onset of clinical signs is variable, depending on the pathogen involved and the immune status of the foal. Failure of passive transfer of immunity can contribute to the development of sepsis in a foal at risk. The current recommendation is that foals have IgG levels ≥800 mg/dL for passive transfer to be considered adequate. Other risk factors for the development of sepsis include any adverse advents at the time of birth, maternal illness, or any abnormalities in the foal. Although the umbilicus is frequently implicated as a major portal of entry for infectious organisms, the GI tract may be the primary site of entry. Other portals of entry include the respiratory tract and wounds.

Early signs of sepsis include depression, decreased suck reflex, increased recumbency, fever, hypothermia, weakness, dysphagia, failure to gain weight, increased respiratory rate, tachycardia, bradycardia, injected mucous membranes, decreased capillary refill time, shivering, lameness, aural petechiae, and coronitis. The survival rate of foals treated for sepsis has improved. If sepsis is recognized early, foals may have a good outcome, depending on the pathogen involved. Gram-negative sepsis is more commonly diagnosed, but gram-positive septicemia is being recognized more frequently. It is important to isolate the organism involved early in the course of the disease. Blood cultures and, if localizing signs are present, samples should be obtained as appropriate. Until antimicrobial sensitivity patterns for the pathogen involved are obtained, broad-spectrum antimicrobial therapy should be initiated. IV amikacin and penicillin are good first-line choices, but renal function should be monitored closely. Other first-line antimicrobials include high-dose ceftiofur sodium or timentin. Failure of passive transfer should be treated if present. Intranasal oxygen insufflation at 5-10 L/min should be provided, even if hypoxemia is not present, to decrease the work of breathing and provide support for the increased oxygen demands associated with sepsis. Mechanical ventilation may be necessary in cases of severe respiratory involvement seen with acute lung injury or acute respiratory distress syndrome. If the foal is hypotensive, pressor agents or inotropes may be administered by constant rate infusion. Inotrope and pressor therapy is generally restricted to referral centers, where these drugs can be given as constant rate infusions and blood pressure can be closely monitored. NSAID are used by some practitioners, as are corticosteroids in specific circumstances. Use of these drugs should be judicious, as they may have several negative consequences including, but not limited to, renal failure and gastric or duodenal ulceration.

Supportive care is important in the treatment of septic foals. Foals should be kept warm and dry and turned at 2-hr intervals if they are recumbent. Feeding septic foals can be a challenge if GI function is abnormal; total parenteral nutrition may be needed. If at all possible, foals should be weighed daily and blood glucose levels monitored frequently. Some foals become persistently hyperglycemic on low glucose infusion rates. These foals may benefit from constant rate low-dose insulin infusions. Recumbent foals must be examined frequently for decubital ulcers, corneal ulcers, and for heat and swelling associated with joints and physis.

The prognosis for foals in the early stages of sepsis is fair to good. Once the disease has progressed to septic shock, the prognosis becomes less favorable, although short-term survival rates are as good as those seen in human patients. Longterm survival and athletic outcomes are fair. Racing-breed foals that make it to the track perform similarly to their age-matched siblings.

■ ■ ■

AMPHIBIANS

The class Amphibia is composed of 3 orders: Anura (frogs and toads), the largest with over 3,500 species; Caudata (salamanders, newts, and sirens) with about 375 species; and Gymnophiona (caecilians) with about 160 species.

Environmental Considerations

Captive amphibians require proper environmental conditions in order to remain healthy. As ectotherms, amphibians thermoregulate by shuttling back and forth between different temperatures in their environment. The range of temperatures necessary for proper metabolism, called the preferred operating temperature zone (POTZ), varies between species. Metabolism, including the regulation of immune function and digestion, can be adversely affected if the animals are kept at temperatures outside of their POTZ. Infectious diseases and malnutrition are common problems in tropical amphibians kept at suboptimal temperatures.

Amphibians require moisture to prevent desiccation. Aquatic amphibians may be accommodated in aquariums with appropriate areas for swimming. Terrestrial amphibians need a shallow container of water in the enclosure. Moisture may also be provided by incorporating small streams, waterfalls, or ultrasonic humidifiers into enclosures, or by misting frequently with a spray bottle. Because amphibians have a semipermeable skin that readily absorbs potentially harmful substances, the water must be clean and free of toxins such as chlorine, ammonia, nitrite, pesticides, and heavy metals. Chlorine can be removed from tap water by placing the water in a barrel and circulating it through a carbon filter for ≥24 hr prior to use. Some municipal water supplies may include chloramines. The chloramine bond must be split with specific dechlorinizing agents, after which water can be filtered to remove the chlorine. External canister filters or undergravel filters help maintain water quality in tank waterfalls, streams, and ponds.

Substrates that can be used include gravel, soil, sphagnum moss, and mulch. Gravel should be either too large to be swallowed or small enough to be easily passed in the feces. Soils with chemical additives such as fungicides must not be used. Substrates such as sphagnum moss, untreated hardwood mulches, and leaf litter can be used, but cedar and pine mulches have toxic oils and should be avoided. Some amphibians cannot tolerate low pH and may develop skin irritation if they come into contact with peat moss and sphagnum moss. Heating soils to 200°F for 30 min is recommended to kill arthropods, such as trombiculid mites, and helminth parasites. Freezing substrates at <32°F is also effective for removing many infectious organisms.

Adequate ventilation (1-2 fresh air changes/hr) is needed in order to prevent disease in amphibians. Live plants are recommended furnishings for terrestrial amphibians as they purify the air, remove organic wastes in the soil, filter light, generate humidity, and provide hiding and perching places. Aquatic plants oxygenate the water, remove nitrogenous waste, provide hiding places, and are often a source of nutrition for larval amphibians. Full-spectrum lighting using bulbs that emit biologically active ultraviolet-B (280-320 nm) is recommended in order to prevent metabolic bone disease. Bulbs must be changed every 6-8 mo or according to the manufacturer's specification.

Bleach (30 mL/L of water) can be used to disinfect tools and housing materials. A minimum of 30 min of contact time is recommended. Several sets of tools should be kept on hand when working with >1 colony of animals. Humidifiers and spray bottles must be disinfected weekly to remove potentially pathogenic bacteria, including *Pseudomonas* spp and *Aeromonas* spp.

Clinical Techniques

All possible routes of escape from the examination room, such as ventilation ducts and sink drains, should be blocked prior to handling amphibians. Recommended supplies include a mist bottle containing dechlorinated water, which can be used to keep amphibians moist when handled, dip nets, a small air pump with airline and air stone, a water quality test kit, a small room humidifier, tryptic soy broth blood culture vials, the anesthetic tricaine methane sulfonate, and a microliter syringe. Fine-tipped culture swabs, glass slides, coverslips, scalpel blades of various sizes, an assortment of needles and syringes, sterile red-rubber tubes, and sterile saline should also be readily accessible.

The history should include a description of the animal's diet and appetite; environmental parameters of the animal's habitat including humidity, temperature, water quality, and lighting; social structure and reproductive status; the recent introduction or loss of animals; and the use of medications. Problems noted by clients should be described in detail. A review of food and water quality records is useful in identifying important trends. A water sample from the animal's enclosure should be analyzed for ammonia, nitrite, pH, hardness, alkalinity, and copper using a simple test kit readily available from most pet stores. Clients must take air and water temperatures at the time of water collection.

Prior to handling, the animal's body condition, agility, posture, and behavior should be noted. Parasitic or microbial infections, malformation, or nutritional deficiencies may cause asymmetry. Loss of muscle mass commonly occurs as a result of improper nutrition, improper environmental temperatures, or chronic disease (eg, mycobacteriosis, chromomycosis, microsporidiosis). Neurologic impairment may be detected by first watching the animal move about its enclosure and then assessing its response to the introduction of stimuli. Neurologic impairment may also be suspected if an amphibian is unable to maintain equilibrium or exhibits an abnormal swimming pattern. When handled, most amphibians attempt to escape, withdrawing limbs that are grasped. Placed upside down, most species will attempt to right themselves. Touching the eyes typically elicits a blink reflex or withdrawal of the globe.

A cool, bright light and magnification are required when performing a physical examination. The mouth can be opened using the edge of an index card, a plastic card, or a rubber spatula. The color of the mucous membranes should be evaluated and any lesions noted (eg, retrobulbar injury, orogastric intussusception). Ulcerations, erythema, hemorrhage, and pigment loss in the skin are indicative of poor husbandry, trauma, and infections (microbial and parasitic). Improper substrate or sanitation leading to bacterial and fungal infections can cause lesions on the feet. Touch preparations or skin scrapings of affected areas are easily made and can be stained with Wright's-Giemsa and Gram stains for cytologic evaluation. Heart rate can often be determined by watching the skin overlying the xiphoid or using a hand-held 8-MHz transcutaneous Doppler system. Because pulmonic respiration (if present) depends on positive pressure ventilation from buccal pumping, respiratory rate should be assessed by watching the rapid movements of the intermandibular space. The nares should be free of obstruction from mucus, which may be indicative of respiratory disease. *Rhabdias* spp, a nematode that has a direct life cycle, can cause respiratory infections in captive animals. Ova or larvae may sometimes be detected in oropharyngeal mucus. Ocular lesions are often detected and may include conjunctival, corneal, iridal, and lenticular changes. Corneal diseases, including nonspecific keratitis and lipid keratosis, are common. Corneal scrapings are easily collected for cytologic examination. Panophthalmitis and uveitis are associated with systemic or localized infection. A sample of aqueous or vitreous humor can be collected with a small-gauge needle for cytology, as well as for bacterial and fungal culture. Coelomic palpation may detect retained egg masses, bladder stones, foreign bodies, or neoplasms. Hydrocoelom and subcutaneous edema (anasarca and ascites) are commonly seen and may be caused by lymph heart failure, cardiac failure, renal or hepatic disease, microbial infection, parasitism, toxicosis, or other unknown factors. Collection of fluid for biochemical analysis, cytologic evaluation, and culture for bacteria and fungi is recommended. Blood collected from the ventral abdominal vein, lingual vein, femoral vein, coccygeal vein, or by cardiac puncture and placed into lithium heparin can be used for hematologic evaluation. A volume equal to 1% of the body weight of a healthy amphibian and 0.5% of the body weight of a sick amphibian may be taken. Normal values have not been established for most species of amphibians. Urine may be collected for analysis from those anurans that urinate when first restrained. Stool samples uncontaminated by environmental organisms may be collected from species such as dart frogs by feeding the animal just prior to placing it on a clean moist paper towel. Direct and float examinations are useful in identifying protozoa and metazoa.

Anesthesia: Anesthesia may be required for further examination or for diagnostic and surgical procedures. Tricaine methane sulfonate, ketamine hydrochloride, halothane, and isoflurane may be used. Tricaine methane sulfonate is a fine white crystal that is highly soluble in water. It can be prepared and stored as a 10 g/L stock solution, which is diluted just prior to use. Administration is by bath, as most amphibians will absorb tricaine through the skin. The dosage used for many large amphibians is 2-3 g/L for induction. For short procedures, the amphibian should be immediately removed and rinsed with fresh water. For longer procedures, the amphibian may be placed into a maintenance solution of 100-200 mg/L after it has been induced. In smaller amphibians, an induction dosage of 100-200 mg/L is safer. Aeration must be provided in the anesthetic solution in order to avoid hypoxia. Tricaine produces an acidic solution that must be buffered to a pH of about 7 using sodium bicarbonate, sodium hydroxide, or sodium hydrogen phosphate. Isoflurane gas can also be bubbled into an anesthetic bath placed in a sealed container; this will allow both percutaneous and inhalation absorption. Ketamine hydrochloride injected percutaneously or into the dorsal lymph sac at a dosage of 75-125 mg/kg body weight can be used; however, a surgical plane of anesthesia can be difficult to maintain, and recoveries are long.

Infectious and Nutritional Diseases

Bacterial Diseases: "Red-leg" syndrome commonly refers to the hyperemia of the ventral skin that accompanies systemic infection in amphibians. Saprophytic, gram-negative bacteria such as *Aeromonas* spp, *Pseudomonas* spp, *Proteus* spp, and *Citrobacter* spp typically cause red-leg. Viruses, fungi, and other pathogens may cause similar lesions. Ventral hyperemia is a nonspecific sign and may also be seen with toxicosis. Malnourished, newly acquired amphibians that are maintained in poor-quality water or other inappropriate environmental conditions are particularly susceptible. Clinical signs include lethargy; emaciation; ulcerations of the skin, nose, and toes; and characteristic cutaneous pinpoint hemorrhages of the legs and abdomen. Hemorrhages may also occur in the skeletal muscles, tongue, and nictitating membrane. In acute cases, these signs may be absent. Histologic evidence of systemic infection may include inflammatory or necrotic foci in the liver, spleen, and other coelomic organs. Blood or, if present, coelomic fluid, should be cultured prior to beginning therapy. Individuals can be treated initially with enrofloxacin (5-10 mg/kg, PO or IM, SID), oxytetracycline (50 mg/kg, PO, BID), or chloramphenicol (50 mg/kg, PO, BID) prior to receiving culture and sensitivity results. If fungal infection is suspected, a 0.01% itraconazole bath (5 min, SID for 8 days) may be effective.

Mycobacteriosis, caused by acid-fast bacilli including *Mycobacterium fortuitum*, *M marinum*, and *M xenopi*, occurs principally in debilitated amphibians. While often an infection of the integument, ingestion of infectious organisms may also lead to GI disease and systemic infection. Affected amphibians may exhibit gray nodules in the skin, liver, kidneys, spleen, lungs, and other coelomic organs. Infected amphibians may eat well but still lose weight. Acid-fast bacilli may be detected in feces and oropharyngeal mucus. A premortem diagnosis can be made by finding acid-fast bacilli in animals with external lesions. Culture of mycobacteria requires special media such as Lowenstein-Jensen agar but is frequently unsuccessful. Treatment is not recommended for this potentially zoonotic disease.

Chlamydiosis is a serious infection of amphibians. Originally attributed to *Chlamidophila (Chlamydia) psittaci*, the causative agent may be reclassified given recent taxonomic changes in this genus. The disease was originally recognized in a mass mortality of African clawed frogs (*Xenopus laevis*) fed uncooked beef livers. Infected frogs may die peracutely or exhibit lethargy, disequilibrium, cutaneous depigmentation, petechiae, and edema. Histologically, intracytoplasmic basophilic inclusion bodies can be identified in sinusoidal lining cells of the liver and spleen. Secondary bacterial infections are frequently present in affected amphibians and must be treated appropriately. Antibiotic treatment including doxycycline (5-10 mg/kg, PO, SID) or oxytetracycline (50 mg/kg, PO, SID) may be effective against chlamydial infection.

Fungal Diseases: Many of the fungi that infect amphibians are difficult to distinguish grossly as they produce similar clinical effects, including lethargy and skin ulcerations. Some fungi can be identified via the examination of a wet mount prepared from a skin scraping, while others require culture, histology, and special stains. Treatment includes proper hygiene and the use of topical or systemic antifungal agents such as itraconazole, as above. Other antifungal drugs such as fluconazole may also be effective.

Chytridiomycosis is currently the most serious fungal infection in amphibians and has been implicated in the decline of frog populations in many parts of the world. It is caused by *Batrachochytrium dendrobatidis*, a fungus that feeds on keratin found in the outer epidermal layers of the skin. Amphibians are the only known vertebrate host for any of the chytrid fungi. Clinical signs include anorexia, lethargy, excessive shedding of skin, pupillary miosis, and muscle incoordination. Visualizing the spherical, single-celled organisms in skin scrapings stained with Wright's-Giemsa or Gram stains using a light microscope is diagnostic. On histopathology these organisms are associated with hyperkeratosis and underlying dermal infection. Treatment includes the topical administration of itraconazole (0.01% bath for 5 min, SID for 8 days) and making sure that animals are kept well within their normal thermal range. Systemic antifungal drugs appear to be ineffective in treating this infection of the epidermis.

Saprolegniasis refers to disease caused by several genera of opportunistic fungi or "water molds" that infect the gills and/or skin of aquatic and larval amphibians. When in water, newly affected animals appear to have a whitish cotton-like growth on their skin. As the fungal mat ages, it may become greenish due to the presence of algae. Once removed from water, the fungal mat collapses and is difficult to see. Other clinical signs include lethargy, respiratory distress, anorexia, and weight loss. Skin ulcerations may occur as the infection progresses. A diagnosis of saprolegniasis is made by finding hyphae and the thin-walled zoospores in a skin scrape. Treatment with a malachite green dip (67 mg/L for 15 sec, SID for 2-3 days) or copper sulfate (500 mg/L for 2 min, SID for 5 days, then once weekly until healed) may be effective. Secondary bacterial and parasitic infections may be present in animals with dermal ulcers. Poor water quality conditions should be corrected.

Chromomycosis is caused by pigmented or black fungi from several genera (eg, *Cladosporium*, *Fonsecaea*, *Phialophora*, *Ochroconis*, and *Wangiella*). These fungi may be found in organic substrates such as topsoil and decaying plant matter. Clinical signs may include anorexia, weight loss, granulomatous skin lesions or ulcers, coelomic distention, and neurologic disease. Diagnosis is usually made postmortem by finding disseminated granulomas with pigmented fungal cells and hyphae. Culture is frequently unsuccessful; histopathology may be necessary to confirm the diagnosis. Treatment using itraconazole (10 mg/kg, PO, SID for 30 days) may be given, but the prognosis is poor once the infection is disseminated.

Parasitic Diseases: Many of the protozoa and metazoa found in and on amphibians are not associated with disease unless the host amphibian is stressed or immunocompromised. Recently caught or transported amphibians are particularly susceptible to parasitism, as are those kept in poor hygienic conditions and outside their POTZ. Parasites with indirect life cycles tend to die out when wild-caught amphibians are brought into captivity if the intermediate or final host is not present. Conversely, infections by parasites with a direct life cycle may be magnified in a closed environment. Excellent hygiene is essential for parasite control and includes the routine removal of sloughed skin, fecal material, uneaten food, and carcasses from animal enclosures. External parasites may be found by close examination of amphibians using magnification and a bright, cool light. A skin scrape or biopsy may be required to identify parasites causing nodules or epidermal lesions. Internal parasites are often identified through examination of fresh fecal samples. Some small frogs are translucent enough to allow the visualization of nematodes using transillumination. In some cases, metazoan and protozoan parasites are found only at necropsy. Finding flagellates, ciliates, and opalinids in the feces is normal and does not require treatment in healthy amphibians. While many larval nematodes found in the feces are nonpathogenic, treatment is recommended because pathogenic and nonpathogenic species cannot be readily distinguished.

Rhabdiasis, caused by the lungworm *Rhabdias* sp, commonly causes pulmonary damage and secondary infections in captive amphibians. This nematode has a direct life cycle with free-living phases. Adult worms live in the lungs where they deposit larvated eggs that are coughed up, swallowed, and then excreted into the environment. Infective L3 larvae then burrow through the skin of a new host where they mature and migrate to the lungs. Clinically affected animals may appear anorectic, thin, and generally debilitated. A premortem diagnosis may be made by finding ova or worms in oral and nasal secretions. Infection should be suspected when nematode larva and larvated eggs are found in fresh feces from an animal with clinical signs. When rhabdiasis is suspected, treatment using fenbendazole (100 mg/kg, PO, SID for 2 days then repeated 12-14 days later) or ivermectin (200-400 µg/kg, PO, once, repeated 12-14 days later) is recommended. Following the second of each 2-day fenbendazole treatment or each dose of ivermectin, the animals should be moved into a newly established environment to prevent reinfection from free-living life stages.

The capillarid nematode *Pseudocapillaroides xenopi* burrows into the skin and is known to affect colonies of the aquatic African clawed frog. Clinical signs include discoloration, roughening, pitting, and ulceration of the skin. As the infection progresses, lethargy, anorexia, and sloughing of the skin occur. Diagnosis is made by finding small, white nematodes beneath the mucus on the skin; skin scrapings may show larvae and ova. Treatment by adding thiabendazole (0.1 g/L) to the water may be effective. Levamisole and other anthelmintics may also be effective. Frequent water changes with removal of shed skin containing the parasite are required in order to prevent the amplification and spread of infection to cage mates.

Viral Diseases: Renal adenocarcinomas (Lucké tumors) are relatively common in leopard frogs (*Rana pipiens*) wild-caught in the northeastern and north central USA. Few frogs with tumors are seen in the summer because viral replication is temperature-dependent. Virus particles and inclusion bodies are seen when frogs are in hibernation; at 41-50°F (5-10°C). Metastasis of the tumor to liver, lungs, and other organs is common; both the primary and metastatic tumors can become very large. There is no treatment. The neoplasm is a model of herpesvirus-induced cancer.

Iridoviruses have been identified in many wild populations of amphibians across the world. Some of these cause lesions very similar to bacterial dermatosepticemias. The original viral lesions may be overwhelmed by secondary invaders, and many outbreaks of "red-leg" may have had an underlying and undiagnosed viral infection. There is no treatment for iridoviral disease other than supportive care and appropriate treatment for the secondary infections with bacteria or fungi.

Nutritional Diseases: Longterm maintenance of most amphibians requires live food. While most adult terrestrial and aquatic amphibians feed on invertebrates, including earthworms, bloodworms, black worms, white worms, tubifex worms, springtails, fruit flies, fly larvae, mealworms, and crickets, some amphibians feed on vertebrates and require live minnows, guppies, goldfish, or neonatal mice or rats. Vitamin and mineral supplements are necessary to prevent nutritional disease. These are commonly administered by "gut loading" insects using commercially available diets high in calcium or by coating insects with powdered multiple-vitamin preparations that include vitamin D_3 and calcium (also known as "dusting").

Metabolic bone disease is frequently seen in amphibians consuming nonsupplemented invertebrates. With the exception of earthworms, most invertebrates used as food have an inverse calcium:phosphorus ratio. This results in mandibular deformity, long bone fracture, scoliosis, and eventually tetany and bloating. Diagnosis is made radiographically by finding thinning cortices of long bones, mandibular and hyoid bone deformities, pathologic fractures, and in severe cases, GI gas. Treatment includes correcting the diet and administering calcium glubionate 1 mL/kg, PO, SID for 30 days. Full spectrum lighting with biologically active ultraviolet-B light should be provided. Vitamin D_3 can also be administered in severe cases.

Thiamine deficiency is seen in amphibians fed frozen fish containing thiaminase. Clinical signs include tremors, seizures, and opisthotonos. Initial treatment is the administration of thiamine at 25-100 mg/kg IM or intracoelomic, followed by thiamine 25 mg/kg body wt, PO, with each meal. Thiamine deficiency can be prevented by routinely supplementing diets with 250 mg thiamine/kg of fish fed.

Obesity is a disease. Overfeeding is the primary cause of obesity, as many amphibian species will continue to consume prey as long as it is available and without regard for their energy needs. The oversized fat bodies may be palpated within the coelomic cavity; however, in females, ultrasound may be necessary to differentiate enlarged fat bodies from egg masses. Treatment for active species includes enlarging the size of the enclosure to allow increased activity. Maintaining the amphibian at the upper end of its POTZ will accelerate metabolic rate and increase caloric use. Lastly, a reduction in caloric intake may be used to control weight.

Amphibians as Laboratory Animals

Amphibians have long been used as laboratory animals. Species that are captive born and readily available from commercial suppliers include the African clawed frog (*Xenopus laevis, X tropicalis*), the African dwarf frog (*Hymenochirus boettgeri*), the fire-bellied toad (*Bombina orientalis*), the axolotl (*Ambystoma mexicanum*), and the tiger salamander (*A tigrinum*). Wild-caught species collected by researchers or vendors for use in the laboratory include the northern leopard frog (*Rana pipiens*, sometimes called the grass frog), bull frog (*R catesbeiana*), cane toad (*Bufo marinus*, sometimes called the marine toad), and the mud puppy (*Necturus maculosus*). Other North American ranid frogs are sometimes used. When collecting or importing amphibians, it is important to abide by state laws and obtain required permits.

Pelleted diets are available for some aquatic species, like African clawed frogs, bullfrogs, and axolotls, making it easier to feed large groups. These foods must be stored in a cool, dry location to maintain freshness. Uneaten food should be removed after all animals appear satiated to avoid fouling the tank. Handling and research protocols should be developed in order to minimize stress to the animals. Overcrowding must be avoided to maintain sanitation, prevent disease transfer, and reduce social stress.

Most aquatic species used for laboratory studies are kept in large, recirculating systems that have multiple tanks using a common water supply. Water is filtered, sent to individual tanks, and then returned for filtration and disinfection. Proper water quality is maintained using one or more different types of filtration. These include a mechanical filter to remove suspended waste material, a biofilter to convert nitrogenous wastes to less toxic compounds, and a chemical filter to remove dissolved organic compounds. The addition of an ultraviolet sterilizer to inactivate microorganisms is highly recommended. Bulbs must be kept clean and changed every 6-8 mo for the ultraviolet sterilizer to remain effective. Ozone, a potent oxidant, may also be used with caution to remove suspended organic material and potential pathogens from the water.

Ammonia toxicosis is common in systems that have not established a good biofilter. Amphibians exposed to inappropriate levels of ammonia typically produce excess mucus, become dull in color, and attempt to escape. Amphibians should be removed from the contaminated water and rinsed thoroughly with dechlorinated and well oxygenated fresh water. A diagnosis can be confirmed if the source water has ammonia at levels >0.5 ppm, although toxicity can be seen at levels >0.1 ppm for some species. Many tropical fish stores sell test kits that check for ammonia.

CAGED BIRDS

Recent advances in avian medicine have changed the emphasis from infectious diseases and emergency medicine to wellness care. The importance of nutrition and behavior in the health of psittacines has been acknowledged and plays a major role in pet bird wellness programs. Mass importation of wild-caught psittacines was curtailed in the mid-1980s. The current pet bird population is comprised primarily of captive-bred parrots. This has resulted in novel medical concerns and unique behavioral challenges.

MANAGEMENT

The ability to mask clinical signs until the late stages of disease and high metabolic rates in birds can result in oxygen deprivation and death during treatment or diagnostic sampling. Thus, diagnosis and treatment must be performed in a step-wise fashion, with constant reevaluation of the bird's ability to tolerate further procedures. Good client communication will allow the owner to understand the potential severity of the situation and the need for diagnosis and treatment to proceed in a specific sequence.

History: The bird should be brought in its own cage if practical. Some tentative diagnoses (eg, zinc toxicity from galvanized wire or dishes, loose perches, territorial or sexual behavior, and nutritional disorders) can be based on examination of the cage.

Practitioners should be familiar with general behaviors of common avian species. As prey animals, companion birds generally exhibit "masking" behavior to hide signs of illness. Masking behavior may include continuing to vocalize, keeping the feathers smooth (as opposed to fluffed as when sleeping) and exhibiting exaggerated eating behavior. Captive raised birds exhibit masking behavior to varying degrees. Owners are often attuned to seemingly minor behavioral differences in their hand-raised bird, such as not vocalizing in the morning, or not joining the family to interact or eat. These changes should be considered potential signs of illness. Owners with less experience or less interaction with their birds are not as likely to notice these early signs. These owners often present their birds in a more advanced state of decompensation. When birds are not handled regularly, the feathers effectively mask even severe emaciation or abdominal distention.

The length of time that a bird has been in the household is inversely proportional to the probability that illness will be due to a primary infectious disease. Chronic malnutrition and secondary infection are more common in birds without recent exposure to potentially infectious psittacines. Newly acquired birds, or those exposed to other birds outside the household via bird shows or pet store visits, are most likely to be affected by contagious diseases. Malnutrition is a major cause of subclinical disease in birds, which often becomes clinical when a secondary infection occurs.

A thorough history should include the original source of the bird, whether it was raised by its parents or by hand; previous medical conditions or treatments received; current diet (both what is offered and what is actually consumed); and current environment, including caging, changes in diet or caging, other pets in the household and the bird's interaction with them, recent interaction with other birds, temperature and humidity at which the bird is maintained, indoor and outdoor exposure, and photoperiod regulation.

Physical Examination: While taking the history, the clinician should observe the bird and note its behavior prior to restraint. The veterinarian should be seated, in order to decrease a perceived predatory threat and allow the bird to relax. The bird's respiration should be observed. Open-mouthed breathing, panting, marked tail bobbing, increased respiratory effort, or audible respiratory sounds should be noted. Subsequent handling may need to be abbreviated. Birds that are ill may smooth their feathers again briefly upon entrance of the clinician, but soon resume a fluffed and sleepy appearance. While the presence of this classic "sick bird" presentation is significant, its absence is not a guarantee of wellness.

Handling techniques should be designed to minimize stress. Some birds are towel-trained to accept the towel as a refuge, and this can minimize stress during handling. Also, birds may have been trained to allow the owner to groom their nails or wings. The degree to which the owner is allowed to assist in the veterinary office will vary with the practitioner, the owner, and the situation. Regardless of the owner's involvement, attention must be paid to the psychological effect of the veterinary visit on the bird. Certain species, particularly African Gray parrots (*Psittacus erithacus*) are noticeably sensitive and prone to the development of phobias. Luckily, these birds can also be soothed by quiet talking and eye contact during restraint.

Practitioners should be familiar with techniques that can be used in the animal hospital and also with basic behavioral tendencies of different species that may aid owners in their interactions with their birds at home. For instance, Umbrella cockatoos (*Cacatua alba*) of any age will usually allow a complete examination while cuddled to the practitioner's body, and will allow the mouth to be held open sufficiently to do a thorough oral examination. These same birds, however, often do not readily step onto a hand. Conversely, most *Amazona* spp will step onto anyone's hand when at an inferior height, but will generally not allow cuddling or comply with an oral exam.

Restraint of psittacines involves immobilization of the head, generally with a thumb on one side of the mandible and the index or middle finger on the other. The feet and the distal reminges (primary wing feathers) are held by the opposite hand in medium to larger parrots. This leaves the thorax and abdomen free to expand with respiration. If the primary wing feathers have been trimmed, a towel may be useful in preventing the wings from flapping during restraint.

The bird's reactions to the potential stress of handling and examination must be monitored during restraint. If respiration becomes excessively labored, the bird's grip with its feet weakens, or it fails to move its head when manual restraint is lessened, it may not be getting enough oxygen and should be returned to the cage or table. Severely ill birds may not tolerate even minimal handling or repositioning; placement of the entire cage into an oxygen-rich, humidified, heated enclosure may be needed prior to any procedures.

Obtaining an accurate weight is essential for monitoring general health and illness. The general condition of the feathers and skin should be noted, including the symmetry and integrity of the beak and nails. Pectoral muscling can be used as a very rough guide to a bird's general body condition. However, although obese birds may carry some excessive fat over the pectoral muscles, much of it is deposited subcutaneously over the neck, thighs, and in the sterno-pubic area. The wings and legs should be symmetric in their degree of extension, flexion, range of motion, and strength of grip. The joints should likewise be symmetric and nonpainful on palpation. Matted feathers over the cere indicate nasal discharge. More excessive dried debris over the head usually indicates vomition.

Respiration may increase during restraint due to stress, hyperthermia, underlying disease, or obesity. Panting, when it occurs, should abate within ~3 min after release, or underlying cardiopulmonary disease may be present. Auscultation of the lungs can be performed over the dorso-cranial thorax. Arrhythmias may occur, but can be difficult to categorize due to the rapid heart rate of birds. The cloaca should have sufficient tone to provide tight closure.

Routine Grooming Procedures: **Wing clipping** is frequently requested by owners. Communication about wing trims is vital. Owners may assume that a wing trim is required at regular intervals. The fact that a wing trim is a deterrent to flight, not a guarantee, should be emphasized. A bird that can only glide to the ground indoors may be able to fly outdoors on a windy day. The basic types of wing trims are: 1) Removing 4-7 of the distal primary flight feathers from both wings, below the level of the coverts. The number of feathers that must be removed is inversely proportional to the bird's weight. 2) Leaving 1-4 distal primary feathers and removing the remainder of the primaries from both wings. This clip has fallen out of favor, but some owners have used it for many years. If it has worked well for their bird, it may be wise to continue its use. 3) Removing a variable number of primary feathers from just 1 wing. This clip is unnecessarily severe in many cases, but some owners have found it a useful and effective deterrent to flight. Some smaller birds are able to compensate by holding their tails to the side and are still able to fly.

Nail trimming is often requested, usually for the owner's comfort and not due to any true overgrowth of the nails. Owners should be cautioned that nail trimming decreases the bird's stability and increases the chance that it will fall from its perch. Generally, a compromise can be reached by blunting the needle-like tip while still leaving sufficient nail to allow a stable grip.

Various types of equipment can be used for nail trims, depending on the size of the bird. Human fingernail trimmers work well to remove the tips of the nails from very small birds. Cat claw trimmers, White's nail trimmers, and hobby drills with sanding bits are all useful. The sanding tools are also excellent for removal of excess keratin that can accumulate on the lateral surfaces of the beak. Birds with beak deformities often have underlying nutritional deficiencies, disease, or previous trauma. Normal, healthy birds that are provided with adequate environmental abrasive surfaces rarely require beak trims.

Concrete (cement) perches are available in various sizes and textures. These can work well for medium-sized psittacines (~250-700 g) when a suitable size is selected and properly placed in the cage. These perches eliminate the need for both nail trimming and removal of excess keratin from the beak. The perch should be placed where the bird is forced to stand for brief periods (eg, in front of a food bowl or treat cup). To avoid irritation to the plantar surfaces of the feet, the concrete perch should not be the main perch on which the bird sits to preen or sleep.

Many birds are **leg banded**, either for individual identification or to indicate a proper quarantine history. Bands present certain hazards to the bird, but removal also entails some risk if the proper equipment is not available. Open (gap present), rolled, steel rings are the traditional quarantine bands, and are becoming much less prevalent since the

TABLE 1. Blood Collection and Bolus Fluid Administration in Common Avian Species

Bird	Approximate Body Weight (g)	Maximum Recommended Blood Sample Volume (mL)	Initial Amount of IV Fluids for Bolus Administration (mL)
Finch	10	0.10	0.5
Budgerigar	30	0.25	1.0
Cockatiel	85	0.75	2.0
Amazon	400	3.00	8.0
Macaw	950	5.00	12.0

cessation of importation. These steel import bands are extremely strong and require removal by a full-size bolt cutter with sharp edges. Closed aluminum bands (placed by breeders of captive-raised birds while they are still small) should be stabilized to prevent twisting while being cut. These bands require 2 cuts to remove; a sharp, properly designed instrument for removal decreases the danger of leg trauma. Full circle plastic bands can be removed in the same manner. **Microchipping** is replacing or augmenting banding as a means of identification. The standard for placement of these chips in psittacines is in the left pectoral muscles. Adverse reactions or failures in birds have been infrequent.

Clinical Pathology: Hematology and blood chemistry are especially important in birds because physical examination tends to be less revealing than in other animals. The quantity of blood that can be drawn depends on the weight and health of the bird (TABLE 1). Blood is usually collected from the right jugular vein, which is larger than the left. The basilic (wing) vein can also be used, but is prone to hematoma formation. In medium to larger psittacines, seabirds, and poultry, the medial metatarsal vein can also be used. Coating a syringe with an anticoagulant before collection may be helpful in smaller species in which sample collection may take longer.

The normal hematocrit also varies between species. For example, cockatiels normally have higher PCV than most birds, averaging 50-55%. Cockatoos (*Cacatua* spp), however, often have PCV in the low- to mid-40% range. Elevations in various leukocytes can provide an indication of the underlying disease.

Normal ranges of hematology are still being studied for various avian species. RBC are nucleated, so traditional mammalian methods of WBC determination are not adequate. Various diluents (eg, Eosinophil Unopette®, Natt-Herricks® solution) are available to enable accurate WBC determinations. Estimated WBC counts are inherently less accurate, but can be useful when the individual performing the estimate produces blood smears of consistent quality and thickness. Normal total WBC counts vary with species and age. Very young birds often have significantly higher WBC counts than adults. Adult cockatiels often have total WBC counts of $4,000\text{-}7,000 \times 10^3$. Adult macaws are usually at the high end of the normal avian range ($12,000\text{-}15,000 \times 10^3$).

Physiologic differences in birds create variations in normal values for many **biochemical measurements**. Due to the excretion of uric acid rather than urea as the primary product of protein metabolism, uric acid levels are significantly higher in birds than in mammals, while BUN is lower. However, elevations from this low BUN level may be seen with dehydration. Uric acid may be elevated in severe renal disease or with articular gout (*see* MISCELLANEOUS DISEASES, p 1472). No reliable biochemical indicator is currently available to detect early renal impairment. Serum or plasma glucose is normally higher in birds than in mammals, with levels of 150-400 g/dL common, depending on species. Levels that indicate diabetes also vary with species and individuals, but often are 650 to >1,000 g/dL (*see* p 1472). Hepatic enzymes measured commonly include AST and lactic dehydrogenase (LDH), which have normal values several times those of mammals (AST, 10-400 U/L; LDH, 75-450 U/L). Measurement of CPK is often performed concurrently to differentiate increased values of AST due to muscle necrosis from those due to hepatic damage. LDH is a short-lived enzyme of limited usefulness in the detection of hepatic necrosis. ALT levels are very low compared to mammals (5-15 U/L). Birds have low bilirubin reductase levels; therefore, total bilirubin is normally also very low, and elevation with hepatic disease is not consistent (total bilirubin range 0-0.1 mg/dL). Bile acid measurements are useful indicators of hepatic function, with levels <100 mol/L considered normal for most avian species.

Calcium and phosphorus values are similar to those found in mammals. These levels may increase up to 3-fold in the hen in preparation for egg laying (ie, calcium ~30 mg/dL and phosphorus >10 mg/dL), usually with a relatively normal ratio of these minerals. Total solids as measured via refractometer are significantly lower in birds than in mammals, with levels of 3.0-5.5 g/dL normal for most species.

Routine Medical Procedures: **Injections** can be given by a number of routes. SC injections are used for fluid administration and some vaccinations, and they are gaining acceptance for the administration of routine medications such as antibiotics. Preliminary studies show that the SC route may be as effective as IM injections for many medications, without the associated muscle necrosis. To ensure that the medication or fluid being injected is actually deposited subcutaneously, the skin must be clearly visualized; use of alcohol is recommended to aid in visualization. Insulin syringes (50 U or 0.5 mL) with 27-gauge needles are invaluable for accurate dosing when small quantities must be administered. SC fluids are often used in birds. In order to maximize their absorption and minimize the stress produced, fluids should be warmed to 102-106°F and hyaluronidase added at 100-150 U/L. Sites of administration include the back, the inguinal web, and the skin over the breast muscle. The medial aspect of the patagium (wing web) may be used but can cause a temporary wing droop or wing discomfort. Maintenance fluids are estimated at 50 mL/kg divided BID-TID. In dehydrated birds, 30 mL/kg is often administered until hydration is reestablished.

IM injections are given into the pectoral muscles in most pet birds; leg muscles are also used in some species. The muscle fibers of birds are more vascular and tightly packed than those in mammals, making both muscle necrosis and inadvertent IV injection more likely.

IV injections are occasionally indicated in birds. Common medications administered IV include doxycycline, amphotericin B, chemotherapeutics, contrast media, and fluids.

Indwelling catheters can be placed in the jugular, basilic, or media metatarsal veins for constant rate infusions or intermittent fluid administration. Intraosseous catheters can also be inserted, generally in the proximal tibiotarsal bone. A standard hypodermic needle may be used (usually 25-gauge for initial entry, followed by a second 22-gauge needle sutured in place), or a spinal needle with stylet may be used for larger birds. Without a stylet or second needle, a bone plug may obstruct the needle. The intraosseous or IV catheter is intermittently flushed with heparinized saline whenever fluids are not running.

Crop (gavage) feeding may be used to maintain caloric needs in anorectic birds. Many commercial formulas are available and convenient to use. Adequate hydration must be established prior to initiating crop feeding to prevent desiccation of the crop food and stasis of the GI tract. In adult birds, generally 30 mL/kg can be administered TID-QID. Baby birds have a much more distensible crop and will hold about 10% of their body wt per feeding (100 mL/kg). Oral medications may be added to the crop feeding or given directly by mouth. The technique of holding the bird so that the medication is administered into the commissure of the mouth and rolls onto the tongue will minimize stress, loss of medication, and the danger of aspiration. Medications administered in the water are only indicated in special circumstances. Accurate dosing, stability of the medication, and palatability make this route undesirable in most cases.

Sedation is sometimes desirable for diagnostic or treatment procedures. Isoflurane or sevoflurane anesthesia delivered via face mask can safely sedate most stressed or mildly debilitated birds and provide a rapid recovery. Intubation in birds >200 g is relatively easy, as the absence of an epiglottis facilitates visualization of the tracheal opening and arytenoids. Fasting before anesthesia should be of minimal duration; 4 hr fasts are typical. Regardless of the duration of the fast, the crop should be palpated for the presence of food or fluid prior to anesthesia. Delayed crop emptying is common in clinically ill birds. If anesthesia must be administered to a bird with food or water still in the crop, the head should be elevated for the duration of anesthesia, regardless of whether or not the bird is intubated.

Environmental management is very important, and severely ill birds benefit greatly from an increased environmental temperature and humidity (eg, use of commercial incubators with temperature and humidity controls). For at-home emergencies, a warm environment can be created by wrapping clear plastic wrap around 3 sides of the cage and placing an electric heating pad on the remaining side. Inexpensive digital thermometers with remote probes are readily available for accurate monitoring of environmental temperatures. A quiet location, away from the sound of barking dogs and other excessive activity, will decrease stress.

The cage arrangement can be critical for ill birds. If a perch is supplied, the food and water must be elevated so that the bird has ready access without having to climb down from the perch. Often it is best to remove perches from the cages of ill birds so they can more easily access their food, and so they do not expend energy simply trying to maintain their perched position.

PEDIATRIC DISEASES

Pediatric diseases in psittacine chicks can present a diagnostic challenge. Intensive hand-rearing methods often create problems, as do husbandry errors (TABLE 2). Proper nursery management, incubation, and production techniques are fundamental to the prevention of pediatric problems in parrot chicks. Captive breeding has greatly increased the frequency of pediatric diseases. Birds that would have perished due to illness in the wild can often be treated in captivity. Unfortunately, captive breeding has also increased the frequency of diseases related to genetic manipulation (eg, breeding for colors) and developmental problems created with artificial incubation and hand-feeding.

Certain viral diseases, notably polyomavirus and circovirus, are most often seen in pediatric psittacines (*see* VIRAL DISEASES, p 1466).

Foreign Bodies: An ingluviotomy is performed in order to gain access to the mucosal surface and lumen of the crop, proventriculus, or ventriculus. Removal of a foreign body, such as a feeding tube, is the most common indication for this procedure in pediatric birds. In larger or older birds, a rigid endoscope may be necessary to visualize and extract ingluvial (crop) foreign bodies. The endoscope may be used either orally or through an ingluviotomy incision, depending on the accessibility of the foreign body.

Crop Burns: Damage to the crop is most often from thermal burns caused by improperly heated hand-feeding formula. The severity of the burn and the bird's reaction vary greatly. Some birds become ill from the tissue damage and may develop endotoxemia and die despite intensive supportive care. Other birds are totally asymptomatic and are presented by their owners when either food or a hole is noticed in the area of the crop. In the latter case, the crop has already fistulated, creating a demarcation between healthy tissue and necrotic tissue. Surgery should be delayed until the area has begun to granulate, allowing the development of a healthy tissue bed for surgical reconstruction. This decreases the quantity of tissue that must be resected. Supportive care is provided until surgery can be performed.

Hepatic Lipidosis: The liver in neonates is typically larger relative to the total body weight than in adult birds, so some degree of hepatomegaly is normal in chicks. However, neonates with hepatic lipidosis typically have the following characteristics: 1) they are usually still being hand fed, often with a commercial formula to which the owners have added peanut butter, oil, or some other high-fat food, and 2) they are usually heavy for their age and exhibit severe respiratory distress. These birds must be handled gently and minimally. Cool oxygenation is the best first step. They have virtually no lung and air sac capacity and are presented because the stress of feeding and breathing at the same time has exceeded their oxygen reserves. Drastically reducing the quantity of crop food per feeding, adjusting the content of the formula, and adding lactulose to the formula are

TABLE 2. Common Pediatric Disorders in Psittacines

Disorder	Species Commonly Affected	Agents (if known)	Typical Signs
"Sour crop" (crop stasis)	Any	Various	Crop stasis (crop contents not moving)
Crop burns	Any	Microwave heating of feed, water for formula too hot	Pink edematous patch, followed by dark crust, fistula
Vomiting or regurgitation	Any	Common causes include ingested shavings, viral diseases, bacterial or yeast infections, overfeeding, weaning	Formula or fluids vomited
Ventricular obstruction	Any	Ingested shavings, corncobs, feeding tubes, etc	Vomiting, dehydration
Aspiration	Any, usually neonatal chicks	Overfeeding, overhandling, obesity	Acute respiratory distress, death
Pharyngeal puncture	Macaws, others aggressive feeders	Feeding syringe tip	Edema, swelling, and erythema of neck; anorexia; depression; death
Crooked beak (maxillary) or mandibular prognathism	Macaws, cockatoos	Unknown	Upper beak deviates from center, lower beak protrudes
Splayleg	Cockatiels, others	Multifactorial, including substrate, diet, genetic factors	Outward rotation of one or both legs
Weak neck (torticollis)	African Gray parrots, cockatiels, macaws	Unknown	Head lies laterally
Toe necrosis	Any	Possibly incorrect humidity or septicemia, check for fibers	Swelling or blackening of toes, distinct constriction
Neonatal feather dystrophy or loss	Cockatoos, others	Psittacine circovirus, polyomavirus especially in small species	Feather damage or loss, depression, death
Depression, anorexia	Macaws, Amazons, others	Psittacosis, improper husbandry, any illness	Hepatomegaly, splenomegaly, possibly other signs
Hepatomegaly, acute onset dyspnea in well-fleshed baby	Cockatoos	Hepatic lipidosis	Dyspnea, anorexia, abdominal enlargement
Pallor, GI stasis, subcutaneous hemorrhages, death, melena, hematuria	Amazons, macaws, others	Polyomavirus	Dehydration, vomiting, sudden death, hemorrhage in various locations, bursal necrosis

the general nutritional changes required. Parenteral fluid supplementation, when tolerated, should be added to keep the initially hyperthermic bird hydrated and to help detoxify the body, as the liver is generally not functioning adequately. When possible, blood samples should be obtained to check for concurrent infection or other diseases.

Low Body Weight: Young, recently obtained cockatiels often have low body weights for their age (commonly 45-70 g rather than 75-110 g) and a stunted appearance. These birds may have underlying congenital or developmental problems, including decreased hepatic function and decreased immunocompetence. With supportive care, some of these birds will survive, but many will not. Birds that survive may have a fairly normal life or may require repeated hospitalization due to relapses.

"One Week Post-purchase Syndrome": Young cockatiels with this syndrome were often purchased soon after arriving at the pet store. In nature, they would be eating partially on their own but still receiving supplementation from their parents. When such a bird is sold as "weaned" to an uninformed owner, it generally takes about a week for the bird's insufficient food intake to create noticeable debilitation and weakness. The veterinarian is then presented with an emaciated, dehydrated infant that may or may not be beyond medical treatment.

Splay Leg: The etiology of this condition is unknown. Parental "over-sitting," nest box flooring that is too slick, congenital ligamentous abnormalities, and nutritional deficiencies of the parents or diet may all contribute. Various types of external coaptation, designed to get the hips back under the bird, are often successful. Surgical correction has also been described. The younger the bird is at the time of the attempted correction, the shorter the period that will be needed for correction and the greater the success rate.

Mandibular Prognathism: This commonly occurs in clutches. If detected early, many can be manually manipulated to avoid prosthesis application. The prostheses can be cumbersome, painful, and often need to be re-applied. In extreme cases, however, prostheses are necessary and effective.

Constricted Toe Syndrome: This is fairly common in neonates, often affecting >1 digit. An annular band of fibrous tissue forms at a joint of the digit, impeding circulation. The etiology is unknown, although both excessively low and high humidity and septicemia have been proposed. When detected early, debridement of the annular band and application of a moist dressing is often effective. Creating small longitudinal cuts on the medial and lateral surfaces to allow for swelling and circulation, and suturing of the digit over the incised area, followed by a dressing, are sometimes needed. If circulation loss is severe and necrosis is apparent, amputation may be necessary.

Eyelid Atresia: Most common in cockatiels, varying degrees of eyelid atresia usually occur in several members of the same clutch. If some eyelid margin remains and there is a sufficient opening for vision, the bird may lead a close to normal life. Attempts to slit the skin in this area and maintain patency of the margins is rarely successful because of the propensity for the skin margins to heal together. One case of a vent tissue graft was partially successful and may hold promise.

"Lockjaw": This syndrome can appear in clutches, most commonly in cockatiels. *Bordetella* sp has been implicated in the sinusitis and secondary osteomyelitis associated with this disease.

BACTERIAL DISEASES

The gram-negative bacteria of the family Enterobacteriaceae are common avian pathogens, although many are regarded as opportunists. *Escherichia coli, Pseudomonas, Aeromonas, Serratia marcescens, Salmonella, Klebsiella, Enterobacter, Proteus,* and *Citrobacter* spp are frequently isolated.

Salmonellosis is not often reported, but may produce clinical disease in birds that are immunocompromised or stressed.

Pasteurella spp have been reported as possible septicemic agents in birds attacked by pet cats or rats.

Mycoplasma spp have been implicated in the chronic sinusitis often found in cockatiels. This organism is difficult to culture, and the true incidence is unknown.

Avian tuberculosis is a common problem in the gray-cheeked parakeet and other *Brotogeris* spp, in addition to affecting a wide variety of other avian species in collections.

Mycobacterium avium, M intracellulare, and *M genavense* are the 3 species most frequently linked to pet bird mycobacteriosis. The most commonly affected organs in caged birds are the GI tract, liver, and spleen.

Staphylococci and streptococci (especially hemolytic strains) and *Bacillus* spp are thought to be responsible for several dermatologic conditions in psittacines. Staphylococci are often isolated from lesions of pododermatitis (bumblefoot) in many avian species.

Clostridial organisms are common secondary invaders of damaged cloacal tissue in birds with cloacal prolapse or papillomatosis. Several specific syndromes of birds can arise from various other species of Clostridia. A Gram's stain or other direct cytologic examination is necessary to identify these organisms, as aerobic cultures in these cases prove negative or identify bacteria that are not significant.

See TABLE 3 for a partial list of antimicrobials frequently recommended for caged birds.

Chlamydiosis

(Psittacosis, Ornithosis)

Chlamydia psittaci has been reclassified as *Chlamydophila psittaci.* Several parameters of this organism are being reexamined, including incubation, necessary duration of treatment, and degree of zoonotic potential. However, current state and federal regulations governing the testing, reporting, treatment, and quarantine for *Chlamydophila* should be followed pending official changes in the guidelines.

Clinical presentations of *Chlamydophila* in psittacine birds vary. Nonspecific signs may include ocular, nasal, or conjunctival irritation and discharge; anorexia; dyspnea; depression; dehydration; polyuria; biliverdinuria; and diarrhea. Establishing a definitive diagnosis can be challenging. Culture of the organism or finding elementary bodies in tissue specimens are the most definitive methods of diagnosis. Various antibody and antigen tests are available, including PCR. Due to the intracellular nature of this organism, and the reduction in numbers that accompanies antibiotic use, false-negative antigen tests are common. Acutely ill birds may not mount an antibody response, also yielding false-negative results. Lastly, exposed but clinically normal birds may produce appreciable antibody titers. Laboratories should be consulted prior to shipment to identify appropriate samples, shipping methods, and tests to request.

Doxycycline (20 mg/mL formulation, PO or IM) is commonly used for treatment of *Chlamydophila* infection. Formulations of doxycycline in the seed and water and chlortetracycline-impregnated seeds or other foods are available or can be manufactured for treatment of affected flocks. These indirect modes of antibiotic administration depend on ingestion of sufficient quantities of antibiotics to maintain effective blood levels, which may not always occur.

MYCOTIC DISEASES

Candidiasis

Candida albicans is an opportunistic yeast and is not generally considered a primary pathogen. Small numbers of *Candida* are commonly found in the digestive tract of birds and may become pathologic when normal digestive flora are disrupted by immunosuppression. (*See also* CANDIDIASIS, p 2201.)

Candidiasis most commonly affects unweaned chicks. Infection may be totally endogenous, with overgrowth due to the above-mentioned factors. It may also be caused or exacerbated by oral inoculation of large numbers of *Candida*, either by parental feeding or by hand feeding with utensils that are inadequately cleaned.

TABLE 3.   Antimicrobials Used in Caged Birds*

Agent	Dosage	Route and Frequency[†]
Amikacin sulfate	15 mg/kg	IM, BID
Carbenicillin	150 mg/kg	IM, BID
Ceftazidime sodium	75 mg/kg	IM, TID
Chloramphenicol succinate	80 mg/kg	IM, TID
Chloramphenicol palmitate	50 mg/kg	PO, TID
Chlortetracycline premix, 100 g/lb	100 g/20 lb (9 kg) oral mash	Sole food source (for control of psittacosis) for 45 days[‡]
Chlortetracycline seeds	0.5% mg/g of seed (0.05%)	Sole food source for 45 days[‡]
Chlortetracycline pellets	4-10 mg/g (0.4-1%)	Sole food source for 45 days[‡]
Ciprofloxacin (tablets)	25 mg/kg	PO, in suspension, BID
Clavulinic acid/amoxicillin	75-100 mg/kg	PO, TID
Doxycycline suspension	25 mg/kg	PO, BID for 45 days[‡]
Doxycycline injectable, 20 mg/mL	50-100 mg/kg	IM, every 5 days, then weekly for 6 treatments[‡]
Doxycycline hyclate, capsules	1,000 mg/kg of oral mash	Added to beans, corn, rice, oatmeal to make up a mash; sole food source for 45 days[‡]
Enrofloxacin, oral or injectable	15 mg/kg	PO or IM, BID
Enrofloxacin, oral or injectable	200 mg/L	Drinking water
Trimethoprim/sulfamethoxazole, oral	30-75 mg/kg	PO, SID-BID
Trimethoprim/sulfamethoxazole, injectable suspension	50 mg/kg	IM, SID-BID
Tylosin, soluble powder (tylosin tartrate)	1 mL/L	Drinking water
Tylosin, injectable	35 mg/kg	IM, q 12 hr

*Most of these are unapproved uses, and caution is indicated.
[†]May vary with etiology and species treated
[‡]Duration and dosage for treatment of *Chlamydophila*

Clinical Findings: Delayed crop emptying with a thickened crop is the most common finding in hand-fed birds. Regurgitation, weight loss, and depression may follow. *See* TABLE 4 for differential diagnoses for regurgitation in birds. Adult birds may harbor low-grade candidiasis with few overt clinical signs.

Diagnosis: Diagnosis is usually based on cytology. In more severe cases, when tissue invasion has occurred, the budding yeast will produce hyphae that can be seen in scrapings obtained from the crop or pharynx, or from the feces.

Treatment: If a reservoir of exogenous *Candida* is present (eg, poor nest box or feeding tube hygiene), then eliminating the source of the *Candida* is critical. In neonates, the crop must often be emptied and smaller amounts fed until crop stasis has been resolved.

TABLE 4. Differential Diagnoses for Regurgitation in Pet Birds

Problem	Species Commonly Affected	Common Agents (if known)	Typical Signs
Toxicities	Various	Lead, zinc, pesticides, medications	Vomiting, abnormal droppings, lethargy, possible CNS signs
Oral upper GI irritation	Cockatiel, various	Plants (*Pothos, Philodendron*), various medications, other caustic materials	Lethargy, ptyalism, passive regurgitation of water, erythema of tongue and pharynx
Proventricular dilatation syndrome	Macaws, miniature macaws, African Gray parrots, cockatoos, others	Suspected virus	Weight loss, vomiting, seeds in feces, possible CNS signs
Bacterial GI infections	Various	Gram-negative bacteria	Vomiting, watery droppings, lethargy
Candidiasis	Cockatiels, lovebirds, others	*Candida*	Regurgitation, crop distention, oropharyngeal and crop lesions
Trichomoniasis	Budgerigars, cockatiels, doves, others	*Trichomonas*	Regurgitation, mouth and crop lesions (white matter), mucus in crop
Ventricular, proventricular, or crop obstruction	Cockatoos, macaws, *Eclectus* parrots, cockatiels, others	Wood shavings, corncob bedding, other bedding, fibers, foreign bodies, ascarids	Vomiting, depression, weight loss
Proventricular adenocarcinoma	Various	Neoplasm	Vomiting, weight loss, lethargy, severe pain, sudden death
Internal papillomatosis	Amazons, macaws	Unknown, possibly herpesvirus	Vomiting, straining to defecate, secondary cloacal and choanal infections
Abdominal mass	Budgerigars	Renal or gonadal mass—usually neoplasia	Weight loss, lameness, vomiting
Behavioral	Various	Courtship behavior	Regurgitation on mirror, owner, toy, or cagemate

Metoclopramide may aid in crop motility and preventing regurgitation. Nystatin (300,000 U/kg) is the most commonly used medication for candidiasis. Because it is fungistatic and is only effective when it directly contacts infected tissue, it is often administered TID, prior to feeding. Some *Candida* infections are resistant to nystatin, and in some birds immunosuppression precludes clearing of the infection by use of only a fungistatic agent. In these cases, systemic medications such as fluconazole (10 mg/kg, BID) are often used.

Flock treatment has historically been accomplished with the use of chlorhexidine at 10 mL/gal. of drinking water for 1-3 wk. Because chlorhexidine is a disinfectant, its use will also deplete the normal digestive flora. Acidification of the upper GI tract by use of apple cider vinegar has also been reported to resolve *Candida* overgrowth.

See TABLE 5 for some antifungals used in caged birds.

TABLE 5. Antifungals Used in Caged Birds*

Agent	Dosage	Route and Frequency
Amphotericin B	1 mg/kg intratracheal; 0.25-1 mg/mL sterile water for nebulization	Given intratracheally SID; nebulized 10-20 min, BID
Fluconazole (tablets)	5 mg/kg	PO, SID
5-Flucytosine	0.25 mg	PO, BID
F-10[†] (quaternary ammonium disinfectant)	1.5/400 mL distilled water	Nebulization for cutaneous and possibly respiratory fungus
Itraconazole liquid 10 mg/mL	5-10 mg/kg	PO, SID-BID (lower dosage and use cautiously in *Psittacus erithracus*)
Ketoconazole	10-30 mg/kg	—
Terbinafine	10 mg/kg	PO, SID
Nystatin oral suspension (100,000 U/mL)	1 mL/350 g	PO, BID

*Most of these are unapproved uses, and caution is indicated.
[†]Quaternary ammonium and biguanidine compound; nontoxic, ampholytic surfactant

Aspergillosis

Fungal infections in pet birds are generally caused by *Aspergillus fumigatus*. An opportunistic organism, it is often found in the same locations and under the same conditions as many bacterial secondary invaders. Malnutrition, especially vitamin A deficiency, is a common predisposing factor. Poor hygiene and inadequate ventilation, especially in warm, humid climates, can increase the incidence of this disease.

Clinical Findings: Rhinitis caused by *Aspergillus* is similar in appearance to bacterial rhinitis or sinusitis. A Gram's stain or modified Wright's stain of lesions or debris will often demonstrate the fungal hyphae. Infraorbital sinusitis involving aspergillosis often must be surgically debrided prior to effective therapy. Extensive or chronic fungal sinusitis may lead to osseous changes and permanent malformation of the upper respiratory architecture.

Tracheitis due to aspergillosis can occur in immunocompromised birds. *Aspergillus* granulomas often form in the syrinx of both psittacines and raptors and are particularly challenging to treat. Changes in vocalization may occur prior to dyspnea. Often these birds will stretch out their necks in order to attempt to get more oxygen.

Lower respiratory disease, including air sacculitis, often involves invasion by *Aspergillus*. Granulomas of the air sacs or coelomic cavity are also common, usually in the caudal thoracic or abdominal air sacs. These lesions may require surgical resection.

Diagnosis: Antibody titers are of use in some species for aid in diagnosis of this condition. Antigen tests may also be helpful. False negatives and false positives occur with these tests. Serum electrophoresis with elevated β-globulins is consistent with aspergillosis. An absolute monocytosis and heterophilia with a significantly increased total WBC count are usually present. Direct visualization, cytology, and fungal culture may be necessary to confirm the diagnosis. Low fungal viability may yield a negative culture despite confirmation by cytology.

Treatment: There have been significant advances in the treatment of aspergillosis in recent years. Amphotericin B is still used in nebulization, nasal flushes, and intratracheal and IV administration and is the only completely fungicidal agent available. For nebulization, it is used at a concentration of 0.25-1 mg/mL of sterile water. The concentration for nasal and sinus flushes is generally more dilute (0.05 mg/mL of sterile water). Amphotericin should not be diluted with NaCl, because this decreases its potency.

The addition of hyaluronidase to the nasal flush may increase the penetration of the antimicrobial agent by its action on hyaluronic acid in the caseated debris in the sinus. The usual dosage for hyaluronidase is 75-150 IU/10 mL of flush. The appropriate antimicrobial may be added to this flush solution. Several flushes of unmedicated warm isotonic saline or sterile water should be employed prior to a final infusion of the medicated mixture. Organic debris obtained by these preliminary flushes can be used for cytology and culture. Care must be exercised to maintain the bird's head in a downward position to avoid the potential for aspiration of the infected debris into the lower respiratory tract.

Itraconazole (5-10 mg/kg, PO, every 24-48 hr) is the most commonly used azole for systemic *Aspergillus* infections in the USA. African Gray parrots (*Psittacus erithacus*) seem particularly sensitive to regurgitation and anorexia and generally receive a lower dosage—2.5-5 mg/kg, SID. Clotrimazole (10 mg/mL) is being used more frequently for nebulization in birds. Terbinafine (10 mg/kg, PO, SID) is used with increasing frequency in conjunction with or in lieu of itraconazole.

Although treatment protocols have improved, many birds infected with aspergillosis have underlying problems. Chronic vitamin A deficiency and squamous metaplasia, immunocompromise, and the scarring and thickening of air sacs that occur following an infection all provide an environment for reinfection, which is common.

If *Aspergillus* granulomas have formed, surgical removal (with placement of an abdominal breathing tube) can be attempted, as can flushing or aspiration of the granuloma using endoscopic equipment. Recurrence of the granuloma, secondary inflammatory changes, and the production of hyaline membranes subsequent to infection in this area are common.

Avian Gastric Yeast

(Macrorhabdosis)

Previously described as a bacterium, this organism has a worldwide distribution and a wide variation in pathogenicity. Its site of colonization is the GI tract, primarily the proventriculus.

Clinical Findings: The most common presentation of avian gastric yeast is chronic weight loss. Regurgitation is common, and polyphagia followed by decreased food intake often occurs. Stools may contain undigested seeds or pellets. These clinical signs may mimic proventricular dilatation disease. Mortality is high, but recovery may occur. In recovered birds, both relapses and potential shedding of the organism in the stool are likely. This disease is often seen in conjunction with immunosuppression, such as that seen in circovirus infection.

Diagnosis: Wet mount, modified Wright's, or Gram's stain preparations of feces often reveal organisms. The agent responsible for avian gastric yeast infection appears as a large, gram-positive rod, with mottling or stippling throughout its length. Although the size and length may vary, organisms recovered from the stool are generally several magnitudes larger than the normal digestive bacilli found in birds. This organism is difficult to culture.

Treatment: The goals of treatment are to reduce the number of organisms and improve the general health and immunocompetence of the bird. Amphotericin B has been used most often in the treatment of avian gastric yeast. Various azoles may also be effective. Acidification of the proventriculus has been reported to create an environment less conducive to the proliferation of avian gastric yeast.

Malassezia sp

Malassezia sp dermatitis has been reported frequently and is often diagnosed by histopathology rather than culture. The recommended treatment is fluconazole (5-10 mg/kg, PO, BID). Topical therapy with either dilute chlorhexidine spray (0.1%) or clotrimazole has been used.

Miscellaneous Mycoses

Dermatophytosis, including *Trichophyton* and *Microsporum* spp, is occasionally reported in pet birds. Treatment protocols for dogs and cats are used (*see* p 705). *Cryptococc-*

cus has been occasionally reported to cause facial dermatitis in birds. Therapy includes debridement and longterm itraconazole. This organism may cause zoonotic infections. Histoplasmosis and mucormycosis are also occasionally reported in pet birds.

PARASITIC DISEASES

See also POULTRY, p 2185 et seq.

Parasites of the Circulatory System

See also BLOODBORNE ORGANISMS, POULTRY, p 2190.

Protozoa: *Haemoproteus* was previously documented with great frequency in imported *Cacatua* sp. *Leucocytozoon*, *Plasmodium*, and *Atoxoplasma* spp are all seen occasionally in various species, most commonly in raptors, canaries, and Columbiformes, and are currently not of major significance in psittacines. Atoxoplasmosis is still diagnosed in canaries.

Parasites of the Gastrointestinal System

Giardiasis: This intestinal protozoal disease is seen most often in cockatiels. Adult birds may be latent carriers. Transmission is presumably direct (ingestion of infective cysts). Affected cockatiels occasionally exhibit feather pulling in the axillary and inner thigh regions, along with vocalization. A true causal relationship between giardiasis and these clinical signs has not been proved. Droppings of affected cockatiels may be voluminous and aerated (a "popcorn" appearance).

Microscopic examination of a warm saline mount of fresh feces may reveal motile trophozoites. Because the presence of cysts is variable, serial tests are advised. A drop of Lugol's iodine solution added to the preparation aids in detection of the cysts. For postmortem diagnosis, gram-stained impression smears from the proventriculus and duodenum are often useful.

Metronidazole (50 mg/kg, SID for 5-7 days) is the recommended treatment. Treatment of giardiasis in cockatiels with fenbendazole at dosages extrapolated from dogs has been anecdotally reported to cause death and should be avoided.

Trichomoniasis: *Trichomonas gallinae* (called frounce in birds of prey and canker in Columbiformes) is occasionally seen in pet birds, notably budgerigars. Whitish yellow, caseous lesions adherent to the mucosa of the oropharynx, crop, and esophagus may occur in raptors and Columbiformes. Budgerigars generally do not have oral lesions but do have increased salivation and regurgitation. Transmission is by direct (parents feeding young) or indirect (ingestion of contaminated food and water) contact; raptors may become infected by ingesting infected pigeons or doves. Microscopic examination of a warm saline mount of material from the oral cavity may reveal the flagellated organism.

Treatment is generally either carnidazole (20 mg/kg, PO, once), ronidazole (5 mg/kg, SID for 14 days), or metronidazole (40-60 mg/kg, PO, SID for 5 days).

Other Protozoal Diseases: Other protozoan parasites such as **coccidia** are much more common in gallinaceous or Columbiforme birds, although coccidial oocysts have been reported occasionally in psittacines and passerines. **Cryptosporidiosis** has been seen in a variety of psittacine birds and Gouldian finches, but is thought to be a secondary rather than a primary pathogen. **Atoxoplasmosis** is a highly pathogenic protozoal disease that causes hepatomegaly and splenomegaly in canaries, with coccidia-like oocysts shed in the feces.

Roundworms: Various genera and species occur in caged birds, and wild birds may transmit certain nematodes to captive parrots housed outdoors. Transmission is direct, via ingestion of embryonated ova. Clinical findings include loss of condition, weakness, emaciation, and death; intestinal obstruction is common in heavy infections. Diagnosis of intestinal nematode infection is by fecal flotation, although shedding of ova may be intermittent. Pyrantel pamoate (20 mg/kg, PO) or fenbendazole (20 mg/kg, PO) are generally effective. In warm climates where exposure via outdoor aviaries is likely, routine deworming with one of these anthelmintics is often performed.

Cestodes: Cestodes have become uncommon following the shift from imported to domestically bred birds. Cestodiasis is most common in cockatoos, African Gray parrots, and finches. Intermediate hosts are most likely insects and arachnids of various types, earthworms, and slugs. Clinical signs are rarely present, but proglottids are sometimes recognized in the droppings of affected birds.

Praziquantel (8 mg/kg, PO or IM) is the recommended treatment. Recurrence is rare in the majority of cases in which the intermediate host is not indigenous to where the bird is housed.

Filarid Nematodes: Filarid nematodes have also become much less common since importation of psittacines was curtailed. In the past, clinical signs were generally rare, but some imported South American psittacines had subcutaneous filarid granulomas, often on the legs or feet. Treatment by surgical removal or ivermectin injection (200-400 μg/kg) has been recommended.

Parasites of the Integumentary System

Scaly Face (Leg) Mite: *Cnemidocoptes pilae* is common in budgerigars and rare in all other psittacines. In budgerigars, white, porous, proliferative encrustations involving the corners of the mouth, cere, beak, and occasionally the periorbital area or the legs are typical. Even after successful treatment, beak deformity may persist. Passerines can also be parasitized but have different clinical signs. In passerine birds (particularly the canary and the European goldfinch), crusts form on the legs and surfaces of the digits ("tassel foot"). Immunocompromise plays a role in the expression of these mites in both psittacines and passerines; individuals that are immunocompetent are generally not affected.

The mites can be recovered from facial scrapings of budgerigars, although the clinical appearance is generally pathognomonic. In passerines affected with *Cnemidocoptes*, skin scrapings of the legs often result in hemorrhage and are generally not recommended. Ivermectin at 200-400 μg/kg, PO or by injection, is generally effective. The treatment is usually repeated in 2 wk.

Feather Mites: Psittacines are seldom affected by any type of feather mite, although owners commonly believe the opposite. Occasionally, infestation with the red mite (*Dermanyssus gallinae*) may be found in outdoor aviaries, especially in nest boxes. A causative relationship between mites and feather picking is often assumed by owners of feather-picking birds, although this is rarely the case. Behavioral and/or systemic factors are more often related to feather loss (*see* p 1474). Signs of feather mite infestation include restlessness (especially at night), anemia, and death, most notably in young chicks confined to the nest box. Diagnosis is by visual inspection and microscopic examination if needed for confirmation. Covering the cage at night with a white sheet and examining the underside of the cover for mites the following morning aids in mite collection.

Individual birds may be treated with pyrethrin sprays, 5% carbaryl powder, or ivermectin. Nest box treatment includes mixing 5% carbaryl powder into the nest box substrate. Cages should be cleaned thoroughly, and wooden nest boxes may need to be discarded and replaced.

Parasites of the Respiratory System

Air Sac Mites: *Sternostoma tracheacolum* parasitizes the entire respiratory tract, most frequently of canaries and Gouldian finches. All stages of the mite are found within the respiratory tissues. The life cycle is poorly understood.

In mild infections, birds are usually asymptomatic; in heavy infections, audible dyspnea (high-pitched noises and clicking), sneezing, tail bobbing, and open-mouthed breathing are noted. Copious amounts of saliva will be located in the oropharynx, and ptyalism may be present. Signs are exacerbated by handling, exercise, and other stresses. Mortality can be high. Transillumination of the trachea in a darkened room occasionally reveals the mite. Response to treatment can assist in reaching a diagnosis.

When the recovery of an individual bird is paramount, treatment should be administered quickly and with minimal handling. Ivermectin (200-400 µg/kg) may be administered, and the dose repeated in ~2 wk.

Gapeworm: *Syngamus trachea* parasitizes gallinaceous birds and passerines but is extremely rare in caged birds.

Sarcocystosis: Sarcocystosis is a major cause of mortality in parrots housed outdoors in the southern USA. In severely affected areas, even indoor birds can be infected via contaminated food. The oocysts are passed from infected opossum feces by insects (eg, cockroaches) or rats into the feed cups of birds. The feces of these transport hosts are then consumed by the birds, and a rapidly fatal disease can develop. Old World species are immunologically naive to this disease, and a high mortality rate is observed in untreated birds such as cockatoos, African Grays, and *Eclectus* parrots. Although not directly contagious, birds in communal aviaries are often affected simultaneously, and large die-offs have been documented.

Clinical signs generally consist of lethargy, passive regurgitation of water, and anemia. Prolonged treatment with trimethoprim/sulfa (25 mg/kg, SID-BID) and pyrimethamine (0.5 mg/kg, PO, SID) is often effective. No specific diagnostic test is available, although certain plasma electrophoresis results may be indicative, and an antibody test has been developed. Muscle biopsies may be conclusive for the encysted stages but are not commonly performed. Response to treatment is generally monitored by serial PCV sampling.

Gross necropsy signs include increased lung density and hemorrhage and renal pathology. Occasionally, clinical signs will reflect CNS involvement. Histopathology samples should include lung, kidney, muscle, and CNS tissue if neurologic signs were apparent.

VIRAL DISEASES

Avian Polyomavirus
(Papovavirus, Budgerigar fledgling disease, Psittacine polyomavirus)

Avian polyomavirus (AVP) primarily affects young birds. It is a primary infectious cause of nestling psittacine mortality, especially in mixed collections and open aviaries. The typical presentation is a well-fleshed juvenile, just prior to fledgling age, with acute onset of lethargy, crop stasis, and death within 24-48 hr. Subcutaneous hemorrhages are often noted when injections are administered. Asymptomatic adults may be carriers. Prevalence of the virus in adult psittacines, including budgerigars, is thought to be high.

Gross necropsy findings in deceased chicks often include pale skeletal musculature and subcutaneous ecchymotic hemorrhages. The kidneys and liver are enlarged and may be pale, congested, and mottled, or have pinpoint, white foci. Petechial or ecchymotic hemorrhages may also be present on viscera, particularly the heart. The heart is sometimes enlarged and may show hydropericardium. Intranuclear inclusion bodies are often seen in the liver, kidneys, heart, spleen, bone marrow, uropygial gland, skin, feather follicles, etc. DNA probe testing of blood and of choanal and cloacal swabs from live birds are also commonly performed.

Control methods include not housing budgerigars or lovebirds on the premises of psittacine breeding facilities, monitoring standard hygiene procedures closely, preventing access to the nursery by visitors or any returned bird or outside bird, using biosecure shipping containers, not allowing retailers or wholesalers to mix neonates from multiple sources in the same airspace, and using 90-day quarantine procedures for all birds entering the flock. Screening should first be done to ensure that AVP is not already present. This involves collection of cloacal and choanal swabs for PCR testing for viral shedding and blood for virus-neutralizing antibody to identify birds with previous viral exposure.

A vaccine is available, and the first dose may be given as early as 4 wk old to properly complete the vaccination series and allow full immunity to develop.

Psittacine Beak and Feather Disease

Psittacine beak and feather disease (PBFD) is caused by a psittacine circovirus. The name is not representative of the typical clinical presentation, which does not include beak abnormalities and is less likely to have the severe, classic feather abnormalities that were seen in cockatoos when the disease was first documented. PCR screening has greatly decreased the prevalence of the virus in *Cacatua* spp. Disease is still noted, however, in African Gray parrots, *Eclectus*, lovebirds (*Agapornis*), lorikeets, and other species. This debilitating infection may affect any psittacine, although Old World species are most susceptible, and has been reported in wild and domestic birds. The natural infection appears to occur primarily in juvenile birds, with few instances of clinical infection seen in birds >3 yr old.

Typical findings include feather loss, abnormal pin feathers (constricted, clubbed, or stunted), abnormal mature feathers (blood in shaft), and lack of powder down in applicable species. Pigment loss may occur in colored feathers. Immunosuppression is present. Acute infections in chicks also occur, with several days of depression followed by profound changes in the developing feathers and sudden death.

Diagnosis is based on gross appearance, PCR, and biopsies of affected feather follicles showing basophilic intracytoplasmic inclusions. PCR may be able to detect infection in birds that still appear healthy.

The contagious nature of PBFD and its probable terminal outcome in clinically affected birds warrant isolation and eventual euthanasia in most clinical cases. Strict hygiene with attention to dust control, screening protocols including PCR, and lengthy quarantines are highly recommended in cockatoo breeding colonies. The removal of all eggs for cleaning and incubation may also be helpful.

Pacheco's Disease
(Pacheco's herpesvirus)

Pacheco's disease (PD) is a highly contagious, acute disease of psittacines caused by a herpesvirus. It is associated with stress, which can cause clinically healthy carriers to shed virus and initiate infection in susceptible birds. It is spread by direct contact and by aerosol or fecal contamination of food or water. Macaws, Amazon parrots, Monk parakeets, and conures are often involved in outbreaks. Old World species are less likely to be either inapparent carriers or clinically susceptible. Patagonian species and some *Aratinga* sp may be natural hosts in the wild, and some individuals of these species may asymptomatically shed virus when stressed. Other species can also act as carriers.

Terminal signs include acute death in well-fleshed birds and bright yellow urates with scant feces. Due to the acute nature of the disease, no gross histologic lesions may be evident. Most affected birds, however, will have an enlarged liver, splenomegaly, and renomegaly. The liver may be mottled or grossly discolored. Ecchymotic and petechial hemorrhages may be present on the pericardium and within the mesenteric fat. Primary differential diagnoses for PD include acute salmonellosis, polyomavirus, and psittacine reovirus. Acyclovir (80 mg/kg, TID, or 400 mg/kg feed) can be used during an outbreak; however, the risk of increased transmission due to handling is great.

Other clinically significant herpesviruses include the strain responsible for papillomatous foot lesions in *Cacatua* sp and the depigmentation lesions noted on the feet of macaws. The internal papillomatous disease of macaws (most notably green-wing macaws, *Ara chloroptera*) and Amazon parrots is thought to be caused by a herpesvirus related to that causing PD. Amazon tracheitis is also caused by a herpesvirus, although the frequency of occurrence of this infection is low.

Poxvirus Infections

Because of import restrictions, poxvirus in blue-fronted Amazon parrots is no longer seen. In pet bird practice, veterinarians will generally encounter only canary, lovebird, and pigeon poxviruses, which have specific host ranges.

Clinical Findings: Three different clinical presentations have been described: 1) Cutaneous, the most common, with discrete papules, pustules, or crusty scabs (depending on the stage of infection) developing on unfeathered areas, such as the face—notably the periorbital area and commissures of the mouth—and the legs and feet. Mortality is low, and the infection usually is self-limiting. 2) Diphtheritic ("wet" form), which may progress from the cutaneous form or present independently. Blepharitis, chemosis, and conjunctivitis are followed by fibrinonecrotic lesions on mucous membranes of the oropharynx, upper respiratory tract, and esophagus. Mortality is often high. 3) Acute onset of generalized signs, including depression, cyanosis, anorexia, and rapid death.

The virus causes eosinophilic, intracytoplasmic inclusion bodies (Bollinger's bodies), which displace the nucleus of epithelial cells and cause cellular swelling. Scarring of eyelids and small opacifications of the cornea are common sequelae, although permanent damage is relatively minor compared with the original lesions.

Diagnosis: Diagnosis is by virus isolation and typical histologic findings of epidermal hyperplasia with ballooning degeneration, intraepithelial vesicles, and eosinophilic, intracytoplasmic inclusion bodies.

Treatment and Control: Parenteral vitamin A, ophthalmic ointments, heat, humidity, parenteral antibiotics, daily cleansing of the affected areas, and attention to diet is recommended. Transmission is via insect vectors (mosquito bites) or other entry through breaks in the skin. Therefore, mosquito control and indoor housing are vital to prevent outbreaks. Vaccines for canarypox and pigeonpox are available, but are specific for their host species.

Viscerotropic Velogenic Newcastle Disease
(Exotic Newcastle disease)

Viscerotropic velogenic Newcastle disease (VVND, p 2255), caused by a paramyxovirus, is a significant threat to the poultry industry. Transmission is by respiratory aerosols, fecal contamination of food or water, direct contact with infected birds, and fomites.

Birds may be asymptomatic or die acutely. Signs include depression, anorexia, weight loss, sneezing, nasal discharge, dyspnea, conjunctivitis, bright yellow-green diarrhea, ataxia, head bobbing, and opisthotonos. In prolonged cases, unilateral or bilateral wing and leg paralysis, chorea, torticollis, and dilated pupils also may be seen. Primary differential diagnoses include other paramyxoviruses (non-Newcastle), psittacine proventricular dilatation syndrome, and heavy metal toxicosis.

Lesions include hepatomegaly, splenomegaly, petechial or ecchymotic hemorrhages on serosal surfaces of all viscera and air sacs, airsacculitis, and excess straw-colored peritoneal fluid. Diagnosis is by viral isolation.

Only symptomatic treatment is possible and thus not advised. If suspected, VVND must be reported to appropriate authorities. Vaccination is prohibited in birds entering the USA because it does not eliminate the carrier state and hampers viral detection during quarantine.

There are several less pathogenic paramyxovirus strains. Paramyxovirus group 3 is reported most frequently in *Neophema* spp, lovebirds, and Gouldian finches. Clinical signs may be absent, resulting in acute death. In disease of longer duration, respiratory signs, pancreatitis, and torticollis may occur.

Avian Influenza

Avian influenza is caused by orthomyxoviruses. Due to the zoonotic potential of some strains, and the recent discovery of new mutations, this virus may become a more significant pathogen. Both zoonotic potential and economic effects on the poultry industry are causes of concern. (*See also* AVIAN INFLUENZA, p 2297.)

NEOPLASTIC DISEASES

As the average age of pet birds has increased, so has the incidence of neoplasia. Avian neoplasias encountered in practice encompass most of the common locations and categories seen in other companion animals, with variations in distribution and morbidity.

Pseudoneoplastic Skin Conditions

Xanthomas are generally subcutaneous, yellow, fatty masses. The distal wing, keel, and the sternopubic area are common locations, although xanthomas may be found anywhere. Cockatiels and budgerigars are overrepresented, although xanthomas are seen in most psittacine species. The etiology is unknown; however, dietary improvement, including sufficient vitamin A or vitamin A precursors, has been curative in less advanced cases. Xanthomas tend to be very vascular. Surgical excision, if elected, should be undertaken with strict attention to hemostasis.

Lipomas occur most frequently in budgerigars but are rare in psittacines. They are most often located on the keel or in the sternopubic area.

Cutaneous and Subcutaneous Neoplasia

Fibrosarcomas may be lobular, subcutaneous masses without skin involvement or may be seen as erythemic skin lesions. Fibrosarcomas tend to be locally invasive and recurrent. Surgical excision has been followed by both radiation and chemotherapy with some success.

Squamous cell carcinomas are most prevalent at mucocutaneous junctions of the head, on the distal wing, and on the phalanges. These tumors also tend to be locally invasive, and radiation therapy has been attempted with some success. The uropygial (preen) gland may also develop squamous cell carcinoma.

Musculoskeletal neoplasms that have been reported in psittacines include osteosarcoma, chondroma, chondrosarcoma, hemangioma, and leiomyosarcoma. Wide surgical resection is the suggested treatment, although extrapolation from canine and feline oncology may suggest other methods.

Internal carcinomas include **ovarian neoplasias** (various cell origins), **renal carcinomas**, **hepatic adenocarcinoma**, and **hepatobiliary adenocarcinoma** (related to papillomas in Amazon parrots). Both carboplatin and cisplatin have been used successfully in various forms of internal carcinoma. Toxicity studies with cisplatin in cockatoos indicate that psittacine tolerance for this drug may be greater than that of mammals. **Gastric carcinomas**, generally diagnosed at necropsy, are often found at the proventricular-ventricular junction. Death from gastric neoplasia may be due to hemorrhage, gastric perforation and sepsis or endotoxic shock, or inanition and subsequent wasting.

Pituitary adenomas are most prevalent in budgerigars and cockatiels. They may be seen as acute neurologic conditions (eg, seizures, opisthotonos). Affected birds may also show signs related to the pituitary hormone(s) that are affected (eg, polydipsia and polyuria).

Thymoma and thyroid adenocarcinoma have also been reported in several psittacine species. Primary **pancreatic neoplasias** of variable cell origins have been reported.

Lymphoma may result in various clinical signs in pet birds, much as it does in other companion animals. Both chemotherapy and radiation therapy have been successful treatment for lymphoma. No evidence of retroviral activity has been associated with psittacine lymphoma.

Primary respiratory neoplasia is uncommon in psittacines, except for a mixed pulmonary tumor reported in cockatiels. Metastatic pulmonary neoplasia may occur, but it is not noted with the same frequency as in dogs.

NUTRITIONAL DISEASES

Avian nutrition has greatly improved in the past decade. Pellets and even organic formulated diets are now available, and domestically raised psittacine juveniles generally accept these readily. However, the nutritional requirements for individual psittacine species are still largely unknown. Many of the illnesses seen in pet birds have their basis in malnutrition. This includes hepatic disease, renal insufficiency, respiratory impairment, musculoskeletal disease, and reproductive problems. For information on appropriate nutrition in pet birds, *see* p 1845.

Vitamin A Deficiency: This is frequently unrecognized in its subclinical forms in pet birds. White plaques (hyperkeratosis) in and around the mouth, eyes, and sinuses are typical. Blunting or absence of the choanal papilla is common. Chronic epithelial conditions, eg, pododermatitis, sinusitis, and conjunctivitis, that have been refractory or recurrent often have vitamin A deficiency as the primary etiology. Parenteral vitamin A can be given IM at 100,000 U/kg. Vitamin A precursors, such as spirolina, sprinkled daily over the food are a way to supplement birds deficient in vitamin A. The diets of all caged birds should be evaluated for vitamin A content.

Iodine Deficiency: Goiter, or thyroid hyperplasia, was previously a serious problem of pet budgerigars and still occurs in certain areas. The thyroid gland in budgerigars is normally ~3 mm long but can enlarge to ≥1 cm. Classic signs include respiratory stridor, wheezing, or clicking due to the pressure of the thyroid on the syrinx. Regurgitation is seen in some severe cases, and the right jugular vein may be engorged; these signs are caused by mechanical obstruction of the thoracic inlet. Affected birds tolerate stress poorly. Lugol's iodine (1 drop/250 mL of drinking water) can be used until conversion to a pellet or seed is accomplished and clinical signs have subsided.

Calcium, Phosphorus, and Vitamin D$_3$ Imbalance: Seed diets have been well known for their calcium:phosphorus imbalance and amino acid deficiencies. Sunflower seeds, which tend to be selected preferentially by many psittacines, are low in calcium, deficient in essential amino acids, and high in fat. Safflower seeds are actually higher in fat content than sunflower seeds, contrary to popular belief, and also contain inadequate amino acids and calcium.

Acute Hypocalcemia in African Gray Parrots: This syndrome is characterized by weakness, tremors, and seizures. The exact etiology is unknown, although parathyroid hormone abnormalities in this species are being studied. Parenteral calcium may effect immediate improvement. Differential diagnoses include heavy metal toxicosis, trauma, and idiopathic epilepsy.

Vitamin D Toxicosis: Although excess calcium intake is not thought to cause clinical problems in most cases, excess vitamin D$_3$ can cause harmful calcium accumulation in tissues such as the kidneys. Supplements should be used carefully, and excess vitamin D$_3$ should not be administered to susceptible species (eg, macaws).

Additional Nutritional Concerns: In addition to the well documented nutritional deficiencies in the traditional diets designed for psittacines, described above, the following dietary concerns should also be noted: 1) the relative inability of birds to use the vitamin A in raw carrots due to a lack of cellulase; 2) the potential sensitivity of individual birds to dyes and preservatives that are added to some seed and pelleted foods; 3) the high incidence of hepatic lipidosis in sedentary captive birds consuming primarily seed diets; 4) the occurrence of hepatic fibrosis and cirrhosis secondary to aflatoxicosis from improperly stored seed and pet-grade peanuts; 5) the difference between food provided by well-meaning owners for their birds to eat (table foods, formulated pelleted diet, vegetables, etc) and what the birds actually consume (seed); and 6) the low palatability of most vitamin and mineral supplements added to water, which are not only ineffectual, but can lead to decreased water consumption and dehydration.

REPRODUCTIVE DISEASES

Egg Binding: This is a common occurrence in captive hens, most notably in cockatiels, budgerigars, and lovebirds. Usually these birds are chronic egg layers, and calcium deficiency, general depletion of nutritional stores, and potential oviductal inertia may be causes. Supportive care (ie, rehydration, injectable calcium, warmth) before attempting extraction of the egg is critical. A single injection of a short-acting glucocorticoid (for potential renal and cloacal swelling as well as shock) and an antibiotic for potential sepsis may also be given, although glucocorticoids should be used carefully in birds. Oxytocin and the avian equivalent, arginine vasotocin, both cause uterine contractions and can help induce oviposition, as can the prostaglandins F$_{2\alpha}$ and E$_2$. If the egg is adherent to the uterine wall or unable to descend (often due to soft tissue swelling or collection of urates and stool), the administration of these drugs could theoretically lead to uterine rupture, but this has rarely been reported.

If the egg does not pass with medical management, inhalant anesthesia and manual extraction may be used. The decreased stress (due to decreased pain) and increased muscle relaxation warrant the slight anesthetic risk. The head should be held elevated to aid respiration. Barring adherence of the egg to the uterus, steady digital pressure applied between the end of the sternum and the egg will cause the slow descent of the egg. At this point, the uterus will often evert and reveal the white pinhole where the uterine opening is located. This opening will gradually dilate. Very seldom will any additional pressure or manipulation be required. After the egg is delivered, the uterus will normally involute. If any hemorrhage has occurred, antibiotics are indicated to prevent cloacal or uterine infection. Postoperatively, the hen will continue to be depressed, with labored breathing. By the next day, she will appear clinically normal. A second egg may be produced within the next 24 hr, so repeated palpation is indicated.

Egg binding may also be seen in larger psittacines, although excessive previous laying is not usually associated with the condition in these birds. Obesity, general nutritional inadequacy, behavioral, and husbandry conditions may be involved.

Cystic Ovarian Disease: Birds with cystic ovarian disease often present with a history of previous egg production. Egg laying may not have occurred for several years. Owners may have noticed reproductive behavior until the recent onset of illness. Generally, these birds are depressed, inactive, and often dyspneic. Abdominal palpation often reveals distention with ascitic fluid.

The fluid from cystic ovarian disease is usually a transudate, although it should be examined for evidence of secondary infection or egg-yolk peritonitis. Careful aspiration of fluid from the ventral midline may relieve respiratory distress.

Radiographs, when the bird is stable, will often demonstrate hyperostosis of the femurs and other long bones. On the lateral view, the ventriculus will be displaced cranially, and a space-occupying mass will be noted in the renal and gonadal area. Ultrasonography can often detect cystic follicles, in additional to normal follicular development.

Treatment with leuprolide acetate (100-800 µg/kg, IM, every 30-45 days) will cause follicular atresia and a decrease in cystic ovarian size and activity. Surgery may not be needed if there is no concurrent infection or neoplasia.

Cloacal Prolapse: This syndrome is extremely common in adult Umbrella and Moluccan cockatoos. The exact cause has not been proven, but the following characteristics have been associated with most cases: 1) hand-raised, 2) delayed weaning and/or continued begging for food, 3) close attachment to at least one person, 4) signs of either a child/parent or a mate/mate relationship with the owner, who may not be aware of these signs, and 5) a tendency to hold the stool in the vent for prolonged periods (eg, overnight), rather than defecating in the cage. Cockatoos that are independent of humans do not have this medical problem. Although the etiology is unknown, proposed causes include prolonged begging for food, causing straining and dilation of the vent; misplaced sexual attraction to a person, causing vent straining and movement; and retention of stool in the vent for prolonged periods, stretching and dilating the vent. The cause may be a combination of these factors.

If detected and treated early, surgery combined with behavioral modification can correct the problem and prevent secondary infections and other complications. Behavioral modification is often difficult for owners to accomplish because in many ways it involves breaking the close bond that they have with their bird. If the bird still perceives its owner as either a parent or mate, it will continue to strain and the problem will likely recur. Behaviors that should be avoided include stroking the bird, especially on the back (ie, petting); feeding the bird warm foods, or food by hand or mouth; and cuddling the bird close to the body. If an owner is serious about trying to change their bird's behavioral patterns, the aid of a behavioral consultant will likely be necessary.

TOXICITIES

Heavy Metal Toxicosis: Lead and zinc intoxication are the most commonly encountered toxicities in caged birds. Paint, stained-glass lamps or windows, lead curtain weights, lead solder, and other lead metal objects are frequently sampled by pet birds. Galvanized cage wire and other metal objects coated with a shiny metal to prevent rust may be sources of zinc.

Clinical signs of heavy metal poisoning include passive regurgitation of water, polydipsia, depression, biliverdinuria, lethargy, and weakness. Some species, such as *Amazona* and *Eclectus*, may show hemoglobinuria with lead toxicity. Neurologic hyperexcitability or seizures may occur in lead toxicosis.

Diagnosis is usually based on serum levels of lead or zinc. The laboratory should be contacted for proper submission methods. In acute cases, and for tentative diagnosis pending heavy metal serum levels, radiographs often show metal-dense material within the ventriculus. Calcium edetate (30-50 mg/kg, IM, TID until asymptomatic) is indicated in all cases, and response to therapy is usually rapid. D-penicillamine (30-50 mg/kg, BID) and other oral chelation agents may be used once the bird is stable.

Polytetrafluoroethylene Toxicosis: Nonstick bakeware coating may give off lethal acidic gases if pans are overheated. Other aerosols, including some carpet fresheners, plastics melted or burned in a microwave oven, or new heating duct systems may also be irritating or toxic to caged birds.

Iron Storage Disease: Hemochromatosis is the current popular scientific designation of this disease, but the specific histopathologic and physiologic changes that define hemochromatosis may not be the same as those seen in birds. Therefore, it is recommended that this condition be referred to simply as iron storage disease. It is common in pet mynahs and toucans, as well as in certain zoo birds such as the bird of paradise. It has also been occasionally reported in pet psittacine species, particularly lories. Iron storage disease is reported to be associated with excessive intake of dietary iron. However, not all birds become affected when kept on similar diets. Stress or genetic factors may also play a role. Certain foods rich in vitamin C, such as citrus fruits, increase dietary iron uptake. Current recommendations are that the diet for toucans and mynahs contain <50-100 ppm of iron. Once clinical signs appear, low-iron, low-vitamin C diets and periodic phlebotomy have been helpful in control. Recommending low-iron diets routinely for pet mynahs and toucans is prudent (commercial formulas are available).

TRAUMATIC INJURY

When an owner presents a bird with a "bleeding" emergency, it is important to distinguish between frank external hemorrhage (eg, wing, beak, foot) and blood on the cage or on the bird but with no active bleeding. Continued frank hemorrhage requires intervention, whereas hemorrhage that has ceased is best left undisturbed.

Birds in respiratory distress are initially placed in an incubator with oxygen. Unless they are showing signs of overheating (panting, wings held out) or head trauma, the incubator should be warmed. An antibiotic injection and SC fluids are administered as soon as it seems safe to do so. This may be before placement into the incubator or sequentially; antibiotic injections are less stressful than SC fluid administration. Hypovolemic shock, with the respiratory reserve being exceeded, is the initial concern. Septic shock or septicemia is of concern within a short period after stabilization in birds with penetrating or extensive wound trauma.

Minor or external trauma should be treated with the goal of the bird's survival first and treatment of traumatized tissue second. For example, a bird that has been struggling for hours with its leg band caught, and that may possibly have a fractured tibiotarsal bone, is in more danger of dying from stress related to the prolonged struggling than from the fracture. Attention to reestablishing homeostasis, with temporary stabilization of the traumatized tissue, should occur first. When this has been accomplished, the traumatized site can be treated.

MISCELLANEOUS DISEASES

Proventricular dilatation disease (PDD) is characterized by chronic weight loss (often following an initial increase in appetite), the passage of undigested food (most easily recognized when whole seeds are found in the droppings), and regurgitation. A dilated proventriculus may be seen radiographically. Neurologic signs may occur in some species. Outbreaks are sporadic, with a low morbidity and a high mortality.

Typical histologic findings include multifocal lymphocytic, plasmacytic ganglioneuritis of the proventriculus and portions of the GI tract. Histologic and epidemiologic findings suggest a viral etiology, which possibly exerts its effect via neuronal damage. Therefore, the virus may not be detectable in the host at the time of clinical disease. Premortem diagnosis is difficult and is usually based on clinical signs, radiographs demonstrating an enlarged proventriculus, and exclusion of other differential diagnoses such as heavy metal intoxication, foreign body obstruction, internal papillomatosis, internal neoplasia, and GI infectious disease (including bacterial and fungal proventricular infections). Clinical pathologic findings are variable, but increased serum CPK and a mild lymphocytosis, monocytosis, or heterophilia may be seen. Proventricular biopsies in affected birds are prone to dehiscence due to low total protein subsequent to malabsorption. Crop biopsies are a less invasive diagnostic tool and may be useful if the sample taken contains sufficient innervation to be diagnostic; however, a negative crop biopsy does not rule out the presence of PDD.

Treatment for PDD includes providing easily digestible foods and may be aided by the administration of an NSAID. In aviaries with confirmed cases of PDD, increased separation of the birds and ventilation of the aviary is recommended to decrease or eliminate this disease.

Cloacal papillomatosis (internal papillomatosis) is thought to be transmissible, although an infectious agent has never been recovered. This syndrome tends to occur as a flock problem, particularly in breeding colonies of macaws and Amazon parrots. Prolapsed tissue is erythematous and originates from the inside rim of the cloaca. Spread to the mouth and upper GI tract is not uncommon. Surgical removal (surgical resection, electrocautery, cryosurgery, or radiosurgery) or chemical cautery (ie, topical silver nitrate) is indicated but cannot be regarded as a permanent cure. Relapses may occur from year to year, and autogenous vaccines may or may not be helpful. Multiple resections can be performed, but sequelae include stricture and secondary cloacal infections, notably *Escherichia coli* and *Clostridium* spp.

Diabetes mellitus is seen in pet birds and causes fairly typical signs of polyuria, polydipsia, and high glucose levels in blood and urine. Normal glucose levels in birds are significantly greater than those in mammals. Diabetes is often seen in conjunction with obesity or pancreatic or reproductive problems and may be transient in such cases. Depending on the species, a deficiency of insulin or a relative increase in glucagon may be noted. Treatment with insulin often results in extremely short-term correction of blood glucose elevations. Oral hypoglycemic agents administered in the water may be effective and allow birds to self-regulate (ie, as the blood glucose drops back toward normal, the amount of medicated water imbibed decreases).

Gout is the abnormal deposition of uric acid in the body. Articular gout occurs in the joints of birds (most often the metatarsal and phalangeal joints) and tends to be severely painful. If pain control cannot be accomplished, euthanasia should be considered. Diagnosis of articular gout is by the identification of gout tophi—whitish yellow, subcutaneous and intra-articular deposits that demonstrate uric acid crystals upon staining. Surgical removal of these tophi is not practical in most cases because they are extremely vascular and the risk of fatal hemorrhage is high. Additionally, unless the underlying condition can be identified and corrected or controlled, new tophi will appear very rapidly. Allopurinol (10-30 mg/kg, PO, BID) and colchicine (0.04 mg/kg, PO, SID-BID) may be useful in the control of articular gout. Visceral gout is seldom diagnosed premortem. The serosal surface of various organs and the renal tubules are the location of uric acid deposition. Acute death is often the only clinical sign noted. Serum uric acid levels are seldom elevated with visceral gout. The genetic, nutritional, or environmental factors that predispose a bird to gout are not fully understood. However, uric acid levels should be determined in birds with gout, and birds with elevated levels should be placed on a low-protein diet.

Feather cysts are ingrown feathers that result in a granulomatous mass. Initial resection is not a major procedure, but recurrence is common unless the extensive dissection of the feather follicle is accomplished. In birds with multiple affected feathers, such as the genetically predisposed Norwich canary, this is not practical.

Feather Destructive Behavior

The phrase "feather plucking" is commonly used to describe behavior that ranges from mild overpreening to self-mutilation. Management of this condition is frequently challenging. Feather plucking seldom has a single etiology, and it is prudent to thoroughly explore all possible contributing factors, including underlying medical problems. Good communication concerning feather plucking in birds at the onset will help clients realize that the odds are not in favor of a simple (or indeed, any) cure. The goal should be to improve the health of the bird and to reduce or eliminate the plucking behavior if possible.

Possible medical etiologies for feather plucking include: 1) Endoparasites (especially giardiasis in cockatiels) and occasionally tapeworms or roundworms. 2) Ectoparasites (rarely); the red mite (*Dermanyssus gallinae*) is the most common ectoparasite involved in feather plucking. 3) Hepatic disease, with associated pruritus. 4) Coelomic cavity granuloma or mass. 5) Neoplasia, which typically causes localized plucking of the area associated with an underlying mass. 6) Folliculitis or dermatitis. These conditions can be primary, or secondary to excessive plucking and/or mutilation. Bacteria, viruses, fungi, or yeasts may be involved. 7) Allergies. Although difficult to confirm, a change in environment or diet when allergens are suspected may lead to a decrease in plucking and a tentative diagnosis by elimination. 8) Endocrine abnormalities, the most likely being hypothyroidism. Hypothyroidism is overdiagnosed; however, due in part to the lack of established normal values for avian thyroid levels, the low range for baseline T_4 noted in birds, and the absence of a reliable thyroid stimulating hormone response test. Nevertheless, some obese birds that demonstrate a lack of weight loss following a rigid diet, accompanied by poor quality feathers and infrequent molts, may be thyroid deficient. The plucking exhibited by these birds is often an attempt to rid themselves of old, damaged feathers. 9) Heavy metal toxicity, notably zinc. Barbering and feather plucking from zinc ingestion has been reported. Many of these cases will not have radiographic evidence of heavy metal and require a blood zinc analysis for diagnosis.

Malnutrition is likely a more common contributing factor to feather plucking than the medical conditions listed above. Basic seed and table food diets often create multiple nutritional deficiencies. These deficiencies cause abnormal skin and feather development resulting in plucking behavior, as well as a myriad of other medical problems that may occur later in life. The dyes and preservatives added to seeds and most pelleted diets may be detrimental to birds. This seems to be most common in species such as African Gray parrots, *Eclectus* parrots, and some cockatoos. The relatively low humidity in most households also has a drying effect on the skin. Being deprived of natural sunlight, fresh air, humidity, and the normal light/dark cycle has negative physiologic and psychologic effects on birds.

Although treatment of medical and environmental factors may reduce the severity of feather plucking, a strong behavioral component is often involved. Treatment of some of the above-mentioned problems may lead to initial improvement, followed by a relapse. Psychological stressors can lead to feather plucking as a displacement behavior (*see* p 1292). Unfortunately, once the stress has been relieved, the habit may still remain. Feather plucking does not occur in the wild, where birds are occupied with finding food, maintaining their social status in the flock, seeking a mate, avoiding predators, and breeding and raising young. Therefore, often the best-kept birds, which have all their apparent needs met, will pluck their feathers for behavioral reasons. Psychological conditions that may cause feather plucking in birds vary. Overstimulation may cause plucking in a nervous bird. Another bird that was plucking from boredom may feel both stimulated and slightly threatened by increased activity in the home and stop plucking in order to pay attention to the environment and guard itself against potential predators. Birds that reach sexual maturity may begin to pluck as an outlet for their increased energy and agitation. Owners of these birds often report that their birds are showing more cage territoriality, more aggression toward family members, and potentially, sexual behavior toward a perceived human mate or inanimate objects.

A thorough understanding of the bird's environment and the associated behavioral changes that have accompanied the onset of plucking is required in order to make appropriate suggestions for environmental manipulation. When the history suggests a social or sexual cause of plucking, the veterinarian and owner may elect to combine environmental manipulation with either hormonal or psychotropic medications (TABLE 6). Neither of

TABLE 6. Psychotropic Medications Used for Feather Plucking in Caged Birds

Medication	Dosage	Comments
Psychotropic Medications		
Amitriptyline	1-2 mg/kg, PO, SID-BID	Maximal effects may require treatment for several weeks
Clomipramine	1 mg/kg, PO, SID	Effects similar to amitriptyline, but may be effective in some cases where amitriptyline is not
Diazepam	2.5-4.0 mg/kg, PO, as needed	Limited usefulness; most birds require a dosage that causes sedation in order to inhibit plucking
Haloperidol	0.15 mg/kg, PO, SID for larger birds; 0.2 mg/kg, PO, BID for smaller species	Serious side effects, including anorexia, hepatic dysfunction, and CNS signs have been reported; most often used in cockatoos
Fluoxetine	2 mg/kg, PO, BID	Effectiveness reported to vary; maximal effects may require treatment for several weeks
Hormones		
Medroxyprogesterone acetate	—	Decreases sexual behavior; not recommended due to serious side effects including weight gain, polyuria, polydipsia, lethargy, hepatopathy, diabetes mellitus, and death
Gonadotropin-releasing hormone agonist	300-800 µg/kg, IM	Decreases sexual behavior by negative feedback reducing production of sex hormones

*All are extra-label usages.

these categories of drugs tends to produce longterm positive results, and side effects may be seen. In addition to traditional medical therapies, acupuncture has been reported to be helpful in some cases. Dietary supplementation with omega fatty acids has been reported to be helpful. Whether this is due to the antiprostaglandin effect or a true fatty acid deficiency is not certain.

An ideal medical treatment is not likely to be found for feather plucking in captive birds. Environmental manipulation, ensuring quality nutrition, and psychological adaptations suited to the species and temperament of the bird offer the best hope for reducing this syndrome. Referral to a behavioral consultant may be helpful.

FERRETS

The domestic ferret (*Mustela putorius furo*) is in the order Carnivora, family Mustelidae, and has been in captivity for over 2,000 years. They are used as research animals, often in studies of the respiratory system and as models for *Helicobacter* sp infection, and have become popular pets over the last decade in the USA. They are also used as hunting animals in Europe, Australia, and New Zealand.

Management

The male ferret (hob) can weigh up to 2 kg; the female (jill) can weigh up to 1.2 kg. Sexual maturity is reached at 4-8 mo and occurs in the first spring after birth. The vast majority of ferrets are spayed or neutered before 6 wk of age primarily because females are induced ovulators and can develop severe hyperestrogenism if not bred. Ferrets also have less of the musky smell that is characteristic of Mustelids if they are gonadectomized early in life. The anal scent glands are usually removed when they are neutered/spayed. Most physiologic data for ferrets are similar to that of the domestic cat. Ferrets require high levels of fat and protein in the diet and should be fed commercial ferret food or high quality cat or kitten food. Many adult ferrets have a large spleen. This is usually caused by extramedullary hematopoiesis and is nonpathogenic; ultrasonography and aspiration can be used for a definitive diagnosis.

Vaccinations: Current recommendations are to vaccinate annually for rabies and canine distemper. There is one FDA-approved rabies vaccine for ferrets in the USA. It should be given to ferrets >16 wk old and repeated annually. If this vaccine is unavailable, then an inactivated vaccine of murine origin should be substituted. Canine distemper vaccines for ferrets should be of chick embryo or recombinant origin. Vaccines of mink or ferret culture should not be used as they may cause disease. There are currently 2 FDA-approved distemper vaccines in the USA for ferrets. Ferrets should be vaccinated at ~8, 10, and 12 wk of age and then yearly. Vaccine reactions occur frequently in ferrets and it is recommended that vaccinated animals be monitored for 20-30 min following vaccination. Ferrets raised commercially are often vaccinated for *Clostridium botulinum* type C at 6-8 wk old.

Infectious Diseases

Bacterial Diseases: *Helicobacter mustelae* is found in the stomach and duodenum of most, if not all, ferrets after weaning. It can induce chronic, persistent gastritis and ulcer formation similar to the disease in humans. Gastric lymphoma may occur in chronic cases. Clinical signs include inappetence, vomiting, bruxism, diarrhea, melena, and hypersalivation. Lethargy, weight loss, and dehydration can also occur. These animals may be painful on cranial abdominal palpation. Definitive diagnosis requires examination of tissue from surgical or endoscopic biopsy. Silver stains and urease tests should be performed on the biopsy specimens. A molecular assay is available for fecal samples. Treatment is with multidrug regimens including amoxicillin (20 mg/kg, PO, BID), metronidazole (20 mg/kg, PO, BID), and bismuth subsalicylate (1 mg/kg, PO, BID). Clarithromycin (25 mg/kg, PO, SID) and omeprazole (1 mg/kg, PO, SID) can be used for refractory cases. Treatment is usually for 21 days.

Lawsonia intracellularis can cause a proliferative bowel disease, especially in younger ferrets. Signs include diarrhea, weight loss, and rectal prolapse. Treatment is with chloramphenicol (25 mg/kg, PO, BID) for 14-21 days.

Other bacterial infections are similar to those seen in other carnivores. Ferrets are susceptible to *Mycobacterium avium*, *M bovis*, and *M tuberculosis*. Intradermal testing is not reliable.

Viral Diseases: Ferrets are susceptible to **canine distemper virus**. Transmission is by aerosol or exposure to infected secretions. Clinical signs are seen 7-10 days after infection and start as fever and dermatitis on the chin and inguinal area, progressing to anorexia, erythema of mucus membranes, and mucopurulent ocular and nasal discharge. Brown crusts on the face and eyelids and hyperkeratosis of the footpads also occur. Respiratory signs develop and progress rapidly. Diagnosis is by history, clinical signs, and positive immunofluorescent antibody testing or histopathology. Mortality is close to 100% and typically occurs 12-14 days after infection.

Human influenza virus causes fever, lethargy, anorexia, nasal discharge, sneezing, and depression in ferrets. Treatment is supportive and includes antibiotics for secondary infections, antihistamines, and amantadine (6 mg/kg, nasally, BID). Recovery is usually within 7-14 days.

Epizootic catarrhal enteritis is highly transmissible and is often brought into a group of ferrets by an asymptomatic juvenile animal. Although the etiology is not confirmed, a coronavirus is highly suspected. Clinical signs are seen 2-14 days after introduction of the new ferret or exposure through fomites and include anorexia, vomiting, green or mucoid diarrhea, melena, dehydration, lethargy, and weight loss. The disease is most severe in older ferrets, which may take months to fully recover. The virus causes blunting of the intestinal villi and consequent maldigestion and malabsorption. Definitive diagnosis is difficult, although scanning electron microscopy of the feces may identify coronavirus. Elevated ALT and alkaline phosphatase may occur secondarily to hepatic lipidosis. Treatment is supportive and includes fluids, nutritional support, broad spectrum antibiotics, and GI protectants. Prevention is by quarantine of new ferrets, thorough cleaning of new bedding and toys, and washing hands and changing clothes after handling other ferrets.

Aleutian disease is a parvovirus originally seen in mink, but at least 2 distinct ferret strains of the virus have been identified (*see* p 1545). The virus causes immune complex deposition on organs resulting in a variety of nonspecific clinical signs such as progressive weight loss, weakness, ataxia, hepatomegaly, and splenomegaly. A severe hypergammaglobulinemia is the most consistent finding on blood work. A presumptive diagnosis is based on clinical signs and hyperglobulinemia. The 2 most common tests for the virus antibody are counterimmunoelectrophoresis and immunofluorescent antibody tests. Definitive diagnosis is difficult because many apparently normal ferrets have positive titers. No specific treatment exists.

Fungal Diseases: Ferrets are susceptible to *Microsporum canis* and *Trichophyton mentagrophytes*. Transmission is by direct contact or fomites and is often associated with overcrowding and exposure to cats. Infection is more common in kits and young ferrets and is often seasonal and self-limiting. Other fungal diseases in ferrets include cryptococcal meningitis and blastomycosis causing granulomatous meningoencephalitis. Fungal pneumonia is uncommon in ferrets but can be caused by *Blastomyces dermatitidis* and *Coccidioides immitis*.

Parasitic Diseases: Earmites are the most common ectoparasite in ferrets and are caused by *Otodectes cyanotis*. The same organism is found in dogs and cats, and the disease can be passed between species. Diagnosis and treatment are as for dogs and cats (*see* OTITIS EXTERNA, p 421). Fleas are occasionally seen in ferrets, especially in households with multiple pets, and can be transmitted between ferrets and other household pets. Diagnosis is by visualization, and treatment is the same as for cats (*see* FLEAS AND FLEA ALLERGY DERMATITIS, p 710). Many of the long-acting topical treatments, such as fipronil, last longer in ferrets because of the increased sebum in the coat. Mange in ferrets is caused by *Sarcoptes scabei* and can be seen as a generalized dermatitis or can be limited to the feet, toes, and pads in a pedal form unique to ferrets. Ferrets that are housed outside may be infested with *Hypoderma* or *Cuterebra* spp larvae (*see* CUTEREBRA INFESTATION IN SMALL ANIMALS, p 710).

Heartworm, caused by *Dirofilaria immitis*, can be found in ferrets, especially if given outdoor access in endemic areas. Disease can be caused by even a single worm. Clinical signs include lethargy, coughing, dyspnea, and ascites. Echocardiographic identification of the worms in the right ventricle may be difficult because of the relatively small number of worms present. Peripheral microfilaremia is uncommon in ferrets; therefore, antigen testing is more beneficial. Treatment is as in dogs and cats using longterm and antithrombotic drugs and adulticides (*see* HEARTWORM DISEASE, p 100). Coccidiosis can cause disease in young ferrets including diarrhea, lethargy, and rectal prolapse. Diagnosis and treatment are similar to those in dogs. If present, rectal prolapse usually resolves after treating the underlying disease. Topical hemorrhoidal creams may be helpful.

Neoplasia

Cutaneous mast cell tumors are probably the most common skin tumors in ferrets. These tumors can appear anywhere on the body but typically affect the trunk and neck. The tumor appears as a raised, irregular, and often scabbed mass. Systemic signs are rare, but the tumors may bleed when scratched. Treatment is by excision.

Lymphoma is common in ferrets and can affect many organ systems including the lymph nodes, spleen, liver, heart, thymus, and kidneys. Disease of the spine and central nervous system has also been seen. Lymphoma of young ferrets can be rapidly progressive, whereas it is often a chronic disease in adults. Clusters of lymphoma have been seen in related or cohabitating ferrets, and a viral agent is suspected. Diagnostics should include a CBC, chemistry panel, radiographs, ultrasonography, and aspirates of any suspected tissues. Treatment protocols for ferrets have not been standardized but can include removal of the neoplastic tissue, if possible; chemotherapy; and/or radiation therapy. Immunosuppression is a common problem with chemotherapy in the ferret and frequent CBC are imperative with any treatment protocol.

Chordomas and chondrosarcomas have been reported in ferrets. Chordomas typically appear as firm masses on the tail. They may become ulcerated from dragging on the ground, but otherwise they cause few problems. These tumors have also been reported at the cervical region. Surgical removal is suggested when possible. Chondrosarcomas can occur anywhere along the spine, ribs, or sternum and tend to cause spinal cord compression and associated clinical signs. Treatment should include removal, if possible.

Splenomegaly is common in adult ferrets and is usually caused by extramedullary hematopoiesis; however, lymphoma and hemangiosarcoma can occur.

Endocrine Disorders

Insulinomas are very common in ferrets >2-3 yr of age. These functional tumors of the pancreatic β cells cause elevated insulin levels, resulting in hypoglycemia and its associated clinical signs such as weakness, lethargy, posterior paresis, hypersalivation, bruxism, and seizures. Diagnosis is based on demonstration of hypoglycemia and corresponding normal or elevated insulin levels. Other blood work is usually normal. Ultrasonography only occasionally reveals pancreatic masses. Medical and surgical treatments are possible, but there is no cure. Surgical treatment involves removing discrete tumors via nodulectomies or partial pancreatectomy. Micrometastasis within the pancreas is common; therefore, removal of the entire tumor is unlikely. A period of euglycemia occurs following surgery in some cases, but most cases require continued medical treatment. Major benefits of surgery are reducing the severity of signs, easing case management, and moderately increasing survival time. Medical management includes use of prednisone (0.5-2.0 mg/kg, PO, BID) and diazoxide (5-30 mg/kg, PO, BID), alone or together, to counteract the effects of the tumor; however, this does not reduce the tumor directly. Prednisone increases resting blood glucose levels while diazoxide decreases insulin release from the β cells and competes at peripheral insulins receptors. Typically, prednisone is used first until the dosage is >1.5 mg/kg and then diazoxide is added. Medical treatment is lifelong, and glucose levels should be monitored 5-7 days after changing doses and at least every 3 mo afterwards.

Hyperadrenocorticism in ferrets is caused by excessive secretion of the sex hormones progesterone, testosterone, and estrogen by the zona reticularis of the adrenal gland. It can be seen in ferrets as young as 1.5 yr old. The most common clinical sign is hair loss beginning on the tail and rump and progressing up the flank and head. In females a swollen vulva and enlarged mamillae may also be seen, while males may develop aggression and stranguria secondary to prostatic enlargement. Bone marrow suppression with severe hyperestrogenemia may occur. A presumptive diagnosis is made on history and physical examination. The enlarged adrenal glands are often palpable cranial to either kidney. CBC and chemistry panels are typically normal. Radiographs are not useful because the masses do not calcify as commonly as in other species. Ultrasonography can demonstrate enlargement of the gland(s). Definitive diagnosis requires measurement of sex hormones, which can be performed in a panel at the University of Tennessee. Medical and surgical treatments exist. Surgical removal of the adrenal gland(s) is more likely to be curative than medical management, but there is still a recurrence rate of ~50%. The left gland is easier to remove because the right gland is closely associated with the caudal vena cava. If both sides are affected, a subtotal adrenalectomy can be performed. Histology of these glands may reveal hyperplasia, adenoma, or adenocarcinoma. Functionally all 3 grades are similar, and metastasis is unlikely. Hypoadrenocorticism may develop in situations where both adrenal glands are completely or partially removed and can be treated with mineralocorticoid and glucocorticoid supplementation. Medical management is aimed at reducing the clinical signs but does not affect the adrenal gland. Leuprolide acetate is the most common drug used. The mechanism is not completely understood but is probably related to down-regulation of peripheral hormone receptors. Leuprolide is a repositol formulation of a GnRH agonist. Using the 1-mo or 4-mo depot form (IM suspension), dosage is 100 μg once a month or 2 mg/kg every 4 mo. Owners should be advised that this is a lifelong treatment to control the clinical signs of the disease; however, longterm treatment may result in suppression of signs while the tumor continues to enlarge. Ferrets should be closely monitored via ultrasound every 6 mo if longterm leuprolide is used. Melatonin can also be used at 1 mg per ferret, orally, SID, to counteract alopecia. It may help with other signs as well. Other drugs used to control sex hormone levels in humans are beginning to be used in ferrets and show promise in controlling clinical signs.

Other Noninfectious Diseases

Gastric foreign bodies are common in ferrets because of their inquisitive nature. Foreign bodies are usually soft rubber or plastic items, but can also be trichobezoars. Clinical signs include anorexia, bruxism, hypersalivation, cranial abdominal pain, diarrhea, and melena. Vomiting is more common with gastritis than with foreign bodies. Diagnosis is with plain or contrast radiography. Treatment involves surgical or endoscopic removal. Gastritis should be treated following removal of the foreign body.

Dilated cardiomyopathy occurs in ferrets >4 yr old. Clinical signs can be similar to insulinoma, so both should be ruled out when examining a ferret with lethargy, weakness, ascites, increased respiratory effort, or exercise intolerance. Diagnosis is by radiography and echocardiography. Treatment is based on echocardiographic abnormalities.

Renal disease in ferrets is similar to other species. Renal cysts are common in adult ferrets and usually do not cause a problem unless present in large numbers. Uroliths can develop in ferrets fed diets high in plant proteins and are usually composed of struvite.

FISH

See also AQUACULTURE SYSTEMS, p 1702.

Aquatic medicine has emerged as a recognized specialty within the practice of zoological medicine. Fish medicine, an important component of the aquatic specialty, is evolving with distinct subspecialties of aquaculture or production medicine (*see* p 1702), and pet fish medicine that focuses on individual animals. Although reference will be made to aquaculture medicine, the emphasis of this chapter is on pet fish medicine. In addition to aquaculture and pet fish practice, aquatic species are increasingly important as laboratory models for biomedical research and toxicology studies. Maintenance and husbandry of aquatic species is becoming a component of laboratory animal practice.

Many fish sold through the pet trade are raised on farms in south Florida. Live bearers (ie, guppies, platties, and swordtails) are pond raised and harvested by trapping. Most other fish are categorized as egg layers, which are often hatched indoors and then moved into fertilized ponds for grow-out. At the end of the production cycle, which is usually 3-6 mo, ponds are drained, and fish are harvested with a seine net and prepared for shipment.

A large percentage of fish sold through the pet trade is imported. Some of these fish are wild caught, while others are raised on small production facilities, many of which are located in southeast Asia. Virtually all marine fish, except for clown fish (*Amphiprion* spp), are wild caught. The pet trade is a global industry, and fish may be moved through several dealers before reaching a retail outlet.

Koi and fancy goldfish for ornamental garden ponds have grown in popularity. Many are imported from Japan (koi) or China (fancy goldfish). Imported, show quality fish sell for hundreds to thousands of dollars each. Koi are very hardy and quite tolerant of medical and surgical procedures. Owners value individual animals and are often eager to invest in veterinary care for these pets.

Clinical management of individual pet fish, exhibit animals, and valuable broodstock has changed dramatically in recent years. Advances include use of nonlethal methods for diagnosing disease and more sophisticated treatment options. Radiology and ultrasound are particularly well suited for disease diagnosis in aquatic species. Development of blood culture techniques to accurately identify bacterial agents and run sensitivity tests prior to the start of antibiotic therapy has been particularly useful in decreasing the need to euthanize, or surgically biopsy, an animal to achieve an accurate diagnosis. Surgical advances, including use of exploratory laparotomy and swim bladder repairs, have salvaged animals that previously would have been euthanized.

PHYSIOLOGY

Fish are poikilothermic, and all physiologic processes are greatly influenced by water temperature. In freshwater, the internal tissues of fish are hyperosmotic, whereas in saltwater they are hypo-osmotic. Surface injuries to the skin make osmoregulation more difficult and may be of serious consequence due to loss of fluid balance and circulatory collapse.

Fish lack organized lymph nodes and Kuppfer's cells. Phagocytic tissue is located in the hematopoietic tissue of the spleen and kidney and often in the atrium of the 2-chambered heart. The structure of the fish kidney varies with the species; generally it is divided into an anterior "head" kidney and a posterior "caudal" kidney, located retroperitoneally, ventral to the vertebral column. Hematopoietic, renal, and endocrine tissues are found in the kidney. Divalent ions are excreted principally via the kidney, and monovalent ions and nitrogenous excretions via the gills. Accordingly, lesions of the kidney and gills may seriously interfere with respiration, excretion, and fluid balance.

The swim bladder in bony fish, which originates as an appendage of the foregut, regulates body buoyancy and may also be used for sound production. Gas is either secreted by or absorbed into the swim bladder to maintain buoyancy or specific gravity and balance. A sensory lateral line system along the sides of the body and head receives stimuli from the aquatic environment and mediates adaptive responses through the CNS.

A humoral antibody system occurs in all fish but varies considerably between classes. Although antibody production often is temperature dependent, specific serum antibodies can be demonstrated. B lymphocytes, found in the spleen and liver, are responsible for production of immunoglobulins found in the serum and tissue fluids of fish. However, fish lack the potent immunoglobulins similar to IgG of other animals. Fish do increase production of IgM, similar to other vertebrates, when responding immunologically to many infectious agents. Fish depend on increases in environmental temperature for efficient antibody production during infections (or after vaccinations), when most pathogens are replicating at a more rapid rate. The optimal temperature for antibody production varies with the species of fish (warmwater or coldwater). Extreme increases in environmental temperature (above that of the natural habitat) inhibit antibody production. T lymphocytes of fish, like those of other vertebrates, are responsible for cell-mediated immunity. Immunity is not as age dependent in fish as it is in other animals; young fish are usually immunocompetent and can be vaccinated successfully. Antibodies are found in the mucus of the fish skin and GI tract.

While anamnestic immunologic responses have been documented in fish, the duration of acquired immunity appears limited. Immunity lasts longer with individual parenteral administration of antigens than with mass bath methods. Although vaccination of fish against specific diseases has been economically important in preventing losses, there is a need for improved methodology.

NECROPSY AND DIAGNOSTIC TECHNIQUES

While the same principles are used in necropsy of fish as in other animals, greater emphasis is placed on an accurate history, premortem signs, fresh necropsy material, and direct microscopic examination of fresh tissue smears and squash preparations.

Fish decompose quickly, and many saprophytic microorganisms reproduce rapidly in the decaying tissues, which complicates isolation of pathogens unless samples are collected immediately after death. A general fish necropsy may include blood collection (premortem); biopsy of gill, skin, and fin tissues; bacterial or viral culture of internal organs; and histology. A diagnostic facility that is familiar with fish necropsy protocols and aquatic microbiology should be used. Whenever possible, fish should be submitted alive. If the fish has just died, the eyes should be clear and the gills normal in coloration and texture. Freshly dead fish can be wrapped in a moist paper towel and submitted on ice. A water sample should also be submitted with the fish.

Fresh tissue samples of gill filaments, skin mucus, and fins should be collected, prepared as a wet mount, and examined under a light microscope at 100× and 400×. Fresh water should be used to prepare wet mounts of external tissues from freshwater fish, and saltwater should be used to prepare wet mounts from marine fish. If uncertain, use water from the tank or from the submitted water sample. Tissue should be examined for morphology and for the presence of parasites, fungi, or bacteria. Ensuring that the salinity used to prepare mounts is similar to the salinity present in the environment should allow organisms to remain viable long enough to allow identification. Microscopic examination of internal organs is also recommended if the fish has been euthanized. Unstained sections of stomach and intestine should be examined for the presence of parasites. Unstained sections of spleen, kidney, and liver should be examined for the presence of parasites, granulomas, or other anomalies.

Blood can be collected from the caudal vein of fish larger than 25-100 g, depending on species, and hematologic parameters measured. Use of hematology and serum chemistry is limited because normal values are not readily available; however, the information may still be clinically useful. Serology may be diagnostic in certain cases (eg, heavy metal toxicity). Whole blood (1-2 drops) can be incubated in brain heart infusion broth at room temperature on an electric rotator. If cloudiness indicative of bacterial growth develops, a loop of the blood-broth mix can be used to attempt primary isolation of a systemic bacterial pathogen.

If the fish is to be sacrificed, it should be euthanized and opened under sterile conditions. Bacterial cultures should be taken from the posterior kidney and streaked onto blood agar. Although blood agar supplemented with salt is helpful for marine fish, it is not necessary if an enriched blood agar is used. Ordal's or similar cytophage media should be available for isolation of myxobacteria (slime bacteria). Sabouraud's is an excellent all-purpose media for the isolation of fungal agents. Lowenstein's media is recommended for isolation of *Mycobacteria* spp. Mueller-Hinton is the media of choice for sensitivity testing of most common bacteria isolated from fish. If abscesses or other obvious anomalies are visible, those sites should also be cultured. As a general rule, bacterial or fungal cultures taken from fish tissue should be incubated at room temperature (25°C). Some agents of concern will not grow at all at 37°C, the standard temperature for incubation of cultures taken from mammals. An acid-fast stain should be available to rapidly rule out mycobacteriosis when granulomatous or other suspect material is seen. If fish are seen spinning before death, or showing other behavioral indications of neurologic disease, brain cultures are indicated.

With the exception of lymphocystis and carp pox, viral diseases of pet fish have been of minimal concern to clinicians. This is changing as new diseases are being recognized. Most viral diseases of pet fish are identified using electron microscopy (*see* p 1510). Spring viremia of carp, a disease listed as notifiable by the OIE, was reported in koi in the USA for the first time in 2002. The disease should be considered of regulatory concern in the USA. Veterinarians working with coldwater species, particularly salmonids, should be familiar with guidelines of the Fish Health Section of the American Fisheries Society for identifying and reporting viral diseases. Infectious salmon anemia, a viral disease first reported in the USA (Maine) in 2000, is of particular concern.

THERAPEUTIC CONSIDERATIONS

Therapeutic options in fish are limited. FDA-approved drugs commercially available for use in food fish are listed in TABLE 7. In addition, the FDA has listed several compounds as being of "low regulatory concern" (TABLE 8). These compounds, though not fully

TABLE 7. FDA-approved Drugs for Aquaculture Use in the USA (2002) ▶

Drug	Species	Indications
Chorionic gonadotropin	Male and female brood finfish	Aid spawning
Oxytetracycline monoalkyl trimethyl ammonium	Pacific salmon	Mark skeletal tissue
	Salmonids	Control ulcer disease furunculosis, bacterial hemorrhagic septicemia, and *Pseudomonas* infection (*Hemophilus piscium, Aeromonas salmonicida, A liquifaciens, Pseudomonas*)
	Catfish	Control bacterial hemorrhagic septicemia and *Pseudomonas* infection (*A liquefaciens, Pseudomonas*)
	Lobster	Control gaffkemia (*Aerococccus viridans*)
Sulfadimethoxine ormetoprim	Salmonids	Control furunculosis (*Aeromonas salmonicida*)
	Catfish	Control enteric septicemia (*Edwardsiella ictaluri*)
Tricaine methane-sulfonate	Fish (Ictaluridae, Salmonidae, Esocidae, Percidae); other aquatic poikilotherms	Sedation/anesthesia
Formalin (Formalin-F® Natchez Animal Supply Co; Paracide-F®, Argent Laboratories)	Select finfish: salmon, trout, catfish, bluegill, largemouth bass	Control protozoa (*Chilodonella, Costia, Epistylis, Ichthyophthirius, Scyphidia, Trichodina* spp) and monogenean trematodes (*Cleidodiscus, Dactylogyrus, Gyrodactylus* spp)
	Select finfish eggs: salmon, trout, esocids	Control fungi of the family Saprolegniaceae
Formalin (Parasite-S® Western Chemical)	All finfish	Control protozoa (*Chilodonella, Costia, Epistylis, Ichthyophthirius, Scyphidia, Trichodina* spp) and monogenean trematodes (*Cleidodiscus, Dactylogyrus, Gyrodactylus* spp)
	All finfish eggs	Control fungi of the family Saprolegniaceae
	Penaeid shrimp	Control protozoan parasites (*Bodo, Epistylis,* and *Zoothamnium* spp)

◀ **TABLE 7.** *(continued)*

Dosage Regimen	Limitations/Comments
50-510 IU/lb (males) 67-1816 IU/lb (females)	Up to 3 doses; total dose not to exceed 25,000 IU in fish intended for human consumption
250 mg/kg/day for 4 days	Salmon <30 g; in feed as sole ration; 7 day withdrawal time; also hydrochloride form
2.5-3.75 g/100 lb/day for 10 days	In mixed ration; water temperature not <48.2°F; 21-day withdrawal time
2.5-3.75 g/100 lb/day for 10 days	In mixed ration; water temperature not <62°F; 21-day withdrawal time
1 g/lb medicated feed for 5 days	In feed as sole ration; 30-day withdrawal time
50 mg/kg/day for 5 days	In feed; 42-day withdrawal time
50 mg/kg/day for 5 days	In feed; 3-day withdrawal time
15-330 mg/L (fish); 1:1,000 to 1:20,000 (other poikilotherms)	Powder is added to water; concentration depends on desired degree of anesthesia, species, size, water temperature and softness, stage of development; preliminary tests of solution should be made with a few fish; 21-day withdrawal time (fish); laboratory or hatchery use only in other poikilotherms; water temperature >50°F
Tanks and raceways—salmon and trout, >50°F—up to 170 µL/L up to 1 hr; all other finfish—up to 250 µL/L up to 1 hr; earthen ponds—15-25 µL/L indefinitely	Drug must not be subjected to temperature <40°F; do not apply to ponds when water is warmer than 80°F, there is a heavy phytoplankton bloom, or dissolved oxygen is <5 mg/L; ponds may be retreated in 5-10 days if needed; do not treat ponds containing striped bass
1,000-2,000 mg/L	Preliminary bioassay should be conducted to determine species sensitivity
Tanks and raceways—salmon and trout >50°F—up to 170 µL/L up to 1 hr; <50°F—up to 250 µL/L up to 1 hr; all other finfish—up to 250 µL/L up to 1 hr; earthen ponds—15-25 µL/L indefinitely	*See* Formalin F® and Paracide F® in select finfish, above
All finfish eggs—1,000-2,000 mg/L for 15 min; acipenseriformes up to 1,500 mg/L for 15 min	*See* Formalin F® and Paracide F® in select finfish eggs, above
Tanks and raceways—50-100 µL/L up to 4 hr daily; earthen ponds—25 µL/L single treatment	*See* Formalin-F® and Paracide-F® in select finfish, above

TABLE 8. Drugs Designated as Low Regulatory Priority for Aquaculture by the FDA[*]

Drug	Dosage	Indication
Acetic acid	1,000-2,000 mg/L for 1-10 min	Parasiticide
Calcium chloride	Amount necessary to raise calcium concentration to 10-20 mg/L $CaCO_3$; up to 150 mg/L indefinitely	Egg hardening; maintain osmotic balance during handling and transportation
Calcium oxide	Concentration of 2,000 mg/L for 5 sec	Protozoacide
Carbon dioxide gas		Anesthetic
Fuller's earth		Reduce adhesiveness of fish eggs to improve hatchability
Garlic (whole)		Control of helminth and sea lice infestations of marine salmonids
Hydrogen peroxide	250-500 mg/L	Fungicide
Ice		Reduce metabolic rate during transport
Magnesium sulfate	30,000 mg $MgSO_4$/L and 7,000 mg NaCl/L solution for 5-10 min	Monogenean trematode and external crustacean infestations in freshwater species
Onion (whole)		External crustacean and sea lice infestations in salmonids
Papain	0.2% solution	Remove gelatinous matrix of fish egg masses to improve hatchability and prevent disease
Potassium chloride	Dosages necessary to increase chloride ion concentration to 10-2,000 mg/L	Osmoregulation; relieve stress and prevent shock
Povidone iodine	100 mg/L solution for 10 min	Egg surface disinfectant
Sodium bicarbonate	142-642 mg/L for 5 min	Anesthetic
Sodium chloride	0.5-1.0% indefinitely	Osmoregulation; relieve stress and prevent shock
	3% solution for 10-30 min	Parasiticide
Sodium sulfite	15% solution for 5-8 min	Improve egg hatchability
Thiamine hydrochloride	Up to 100 mg/L for up to 4 hr (eggs); up to 1,000 mg/L for up to 1 hr (sac fry)	Prevent or treat thiamine deficiency in salmonids
Urea and tannic acid	15 g urea and 20 g NaCl/5 L water for 6 min, followed by separate solution of 0.75 g tannic acid/5 L of water for 6 additional min (treats ~400,000 eggs)	Denature adhesive component of eggs

[*]FDA states that it is unlikely to object to the use of these substances if they are used for the indications listed, at prescribed levels, and according to good management practices; if they are of an appropriate grade for use in food animals; and there is not likely to be an adverse effect on the environment.

approved, are considered innocuous enough for use in food fish. Of these, salt is the most important. A few compounds, including copper sulfate and potassium permanganate, are not FDA-approved, but are used in aquaculture under the provision of "moderate regulatory concern." Finally, there are several non-FDA approved compounds that are used in pet fish practice under controlled conditions. These have no legal status at present and have no place in food animal practice. In addition to being aware of FDA concerns, fish practitioners should be familiar with state environmental regulations. Federal and state environmental regulations are of greatest concern when treating outdoor ponds.

FDA-approved Drugs: FDA-approved drugs for use in aquaculture in the USA include 2 antibiotics, 1 parasiticide, 1 anesthetic, and 1 spawning hormone. In many cases, therapeutic management of fish other than catfish or salmonids requires extra-label use of drugs.

Oxytetracycline is approved for use in Pacific salmon (for marking bony tissue), salmonids, catfish, and lobsters. It is widely available and has a broad spectrum of activity against gram-negative bacteria. Clinical evidence suggests that it is quite effective against myxobacteria, which do not grow on Müller-Hinton agar, making sensitivity testing difficult. Its main disadvantage is that it is only available in sinking feeds, which may make it difficult to determine whether it has been eaten, especially when treating fish in ponds. Because oxytetracycline has been used extensively for several decades, significant bacterial resistance has developed. Reliance on bacterial sensitivity test results is recommended.

A potentiated sulfonamide is approved for use in salmonids with furunculosis (*Aeromonas salmonicida*) and in channel catfish infected with *Edwardsiella ictaluri*. It should be fed at a dosage of 50 mg/kg for 5 days. The drug binds to the skin, and salmonid products are generally sold with intact skin, so longer withdrawal times (42 days) are required. This drug is available in floating feed, which makes it easier to determine whether it has been eaten. Clinical evidence suggests that it is not always effective against myxobacteria; therefore, it is not recommended as the drug of choice if columnaris is an important component of an epizootic.

Formalin is FDA approved for use in finfish and penaeid (saltwater) shrimp. Parasite-S® is labeled for all finfish and penaeid shrimp; 2 other brands, Formalin-F® and Paracide-F® are labeled for select finfish species (TABLE 7, p 1482). Methanol may be added to formalin products as a preservative. Formalin eliminates protozoan parasites and monogenean trematodes from the external surface of fish. It can be used as a prolonged bath at concentrations of 15-25 mg/L. The lower concentration is recommended for pond use because formalin removes dissolved oxygen from the water. Vigorous aeration during formalin treatment is essential. A concentration of 25 mg/L is equal to 2 drops/gal. (useful for delivering formalin to aquarium fish). When treating at ≤25 mg/L, a water change is not necessary following chemical administration. At this concentration, formalin has minimal impact on biofiltration; however, if ammonia is tested using Nessler's reagent, a very high reading may be observed for several days. This is an artifact caused by the interaction of the 2 compounds. Short-term baths with formalin can be provided at concentrations up to 250 mg/L for 30-60 min. At water temperatures >77°F (25°C), the concentration should be decreased to ~170 mg/L. Fish should never be left unattended during treatment and if adverse reaction to the chemical becomes apparent, the fish should be immediately placed in clean water. If formalin is allowed to chill to <45°F, a white precipitate, paraformaldehyde, will form. Because paraformaldehyde is highly toxic to fish, formalin should never be used if a precipitate or cloudiness is observed. Formalin is carcinogenic and potentially toxic to workers; material safety data sheets should be on hand in businesses where the chemical is used, and employees should be informed of appropriate safety precautions.

Tricaine methanesulfonate (MS-222) is FDA approved for use as a sedative and anesthetic in food fish and is often used to sedate broodstock for handling and injection of hormones for spawning. It is also useful for pet fish and is effective for sedation, surgical anesthesia, and euthanasia. Sedation can generally be achieved with concentrations between 50-100 mg/L, although species-specific sensitivities should be expected. Induction for most species may be near 125 mg/L; however, when working with unfamiliar species it is best to start at a lower concentration (ie, 50 mg/L) and increase the concentration until the desired effect is achieved. Because MS-222 is an acid, the chemical should be buffered (2 parts sodium bicarbonate by weight to 1 part MS-222). Following induction, the concentration may be decreased to 50-100 mg/L to maintain the desired depth of anesthesia. Respiration should be monitored; if opercular movement ceases, fish should be immediately moved to clean water. MS-222 can also be used to euthanize fish at concentrations of 1,000-10,000 mg/L. For small animals, a squirt bottle with a stock solution of 10,000 mg/L can be used to quickly apply a lethal dose of chemical to the gills. The compound will not remain stable for more than a few weeks when used in this manner. As it degrades, the color of the solution will change from clear to brownish. MS-222 is light sensitive and should be kept in a brown bottle when stored as a solution.

Chorionic gonadotropin is FDA approved as a spawning aid for finfish. Veterinarians may work as part of a team for fish hatcheries and may be asked to assist in obtaining spawning hormones.

Salt: Salt can be used for many purposes, including destruction of single-celled protozoans and management of osmoregulation. Seawater is 3% salt, which is 30,000 ppm. By increasing or decreasing the amount of salt to which a freshwater fish or marine fish, respectively, is exposed, osmoregulatory stress can be minimized and many parasites eliminated. For freshwater fish, a 3% dip is an effective ectoparasiticide and is strongly recommended when moving fish. However, tolerance varies by species. Most freshwater fish will tolerate 3% salt for 30 sec up to several minutes, after which they show signs of stress, commonly manifest by rolling on their side. Recovery is rapid if fish are promptly removed from the salt solution. The use of salt is a quick, effective, inexpensive, and readily available means of minimizing the introduction of protozoans into a system with new fish. A solution of 0.5-1.0% salt is recommended for transportation of freshwater fish, and most species will tolerate this concentration for several hours or days. A solution of 0.02-0.2% (200-2,000 ppm) salt can be added to freshwater recirculating systems as a continuous treatment to minimize parasitic protozoa in the system. Salt is less caustic than other parasiticides and seems to optimize healing of epithelial surfaces. Unfortunately, it is not practical for use in ponds (other than for control of nitrite toxicity) because of the massive quantities that would be required to achieve a nominal level of salinity. Addition of salt may be practical in small ornamental ponds of a few thousand gallons. Less information is available on lowering salinity for marine fish, but it is a technique that should not be overlooked.

Non-FDA-approved Compounds: Copper sulfate ($CuSO_4$) is not approved by the FDA; however, a number of compounds containing $CuSO_4$ have been approved by the US Environmental Protection Agency (EPA) as algicides for use in aquatic sites. $CuSO_4$ is currently designated as "of moderate regulatory concern" and is used in food fish practice; however, practitioners must keep themselves informed of possible changes in the status of this chemical. $CuSO_4$ has been used for many years as a parasiticide and is particularly useful in large production ponds because of its relatively low cost. Copper is highly toxic to fish, and safe use depends on its interaction with carbonate salts in water. In freshwater systems, the concentration of $CuSO_4$ applied should be based on the total alkalinity (TA) of the water. If TA is <50 mg/L, copper cannot be used safely without performing a bioassay. If TA is 50-250 mg/L, a safe concentration of $CuSO_4$ can be determined by dividing the TA by 100. For example, if TA = 100 mg/L, a safe concentration of $CuSO_4$ would be 1 mg/L. If TA is >250 mg/L, the concentration of $CuSO_4$ should not exceed 2.5 mg/L. Other concerns when treating a pond with $CuSO_4$ (in addition to its direct toxicity to fish) relate to its algicidal activity. Rapid death of an algal bloom can precipitate a catastrophic oxygen depletion. Use of $CuSO_4$ in ponds not equipped with supplemental aeration is risky. Use of $CuSO_4$ is hazardous if a pond has a heavy algal bloom (secchi disc ≤18 in.) or if the water is already deficient in oxygen due to other factors, (eg, cloudy weather or high water temperature). $CuSO_4$ is efficacious against most protozoal parasites, is economical, and despite these concerns, may be an excellent choice when multiple treatments are required (eg, in an epizootic of *Ichthyophthirius multifiliis*). In saltwater systems, copper is sometimes applied in a chelated form because it stays in concentration longer. Chelated compounds may be difficult to use safely and require careful monitoring. $CuSO_4$ can be used to treat marine fish, but the concentration of active copper must be closely monitored (test kits are available) and should be maintained at 0.2 mg/L for up to 3 wk. Safe and effective use of copper in marine systems requires that Cu^{2+} concentrations be tested at least once a day. Copper is extremely toxic to invertebrates, so these must be removed before the water is treated. Copper is also toxic to plants and should not be used in ornamental ponds that have been stocked with valuable plants. Finally, copper will impact bacteria in biofilters and a transient increase in ammonia should be expected for several days following treatment. Monitoring ammonia until measurable concentrations subside is recommended.

Potassium permanganate ($KMnO_4$) is not approved by the FDA but is also in the group designated "of moderate regulatory concern." $KMnO_4$ is used as an external parasiticide, fungicide, and bactericide. It is a strong oxidizing agent and "burns" organic material off the external surface of the fish. Overuse, particularly multiple uses within a short period of time, will kill fish. Use of $KMnO_4$ no more than once a week seems safe for many fish. The concentration of $KMnO_4$ used varies with the permanganate demand of the water. Permanganate demand is greater in water with a high organic load than in water with little organic matter. To determine the permanganate demand, a bioassay can be performed; the water to be treated is placed in small containers and $KMnO_4$ is added in incremental concentrations of 2 mg/L. The correct concentration for therapeutic use will be the lowest concentration that maintains a pink color for at least 8 hr. A practical method is to apply $KMnO_4$ at 2 mg/L in the morning—if the color changes from pink to brown or clear in <8 hr, the treatment should be repeated. If the concentration of $KMnO_4$ required to maintain a pink color for at least 4 hr is >6 mg/L, then the organic load is excessive, and sanitation practices should be evaluated. In large production ponds, little can be done to decrease the accumulation of organic material in ponds other than draining the pond, drying the bottom, and discing it. This is not done very often, perhaps once in 10-15 yr. In smaller systems (<0.1 acre), mechanisms may be in place to facilitate cleaning and removal of debris. $KMnO_4$ has little impact on biofilters when applied at 2 mg/L or less.

Hydrogen peroxide (H_2O_2, 3%) is currently used to control protozoan parasites in both food and ornamental species as an alternative to $CuSO_4$ and $KMnO_4$. H_2O_2 is categorized as "low regulatory priority" by the FDA and is used in the salmonid and hybrid striped bass industries. Food grade H_2O_2 is 35% active and is the best product for aquaculture use. The primary use of H_2O_2 is the control of sea lice and aquatic fungi on fish or fish eggs. It may also help control bacterial gill disease and columnaris. Dosages are variable and some fish may not tolerate this chemical. It is applied as a short-term bath, often for 15-30 min intervals. A dosage of 250 mg/L would be 2.7 mL of the 35% solution/gal. of water. Practitioners unfamiliar with use of this compound should experiment with it in a bioassay before applying it to a valuable group of fish. Efficacy can be monitored by evaluation of gill and skin biopsy material before and after treatment.

Erythromycin is not FDA approved but has been used in management of bacterial kidney disease of salmonids and streptococcal infections in food and nonfood species. It can be incorporated into fish food at a dosage of 100 mg/kg body wt and fed for 14 days. FDA permission is required for use in food animals.

Another group of compounds have been designated by FDA as "high regulatory priority," ie, their use is likely to result in enforcement action by the FDA. The most important of these compounds are chloramphenicol, the nitrofurans, and malachite green. These compounds should never be used in food animals for any reason, and their use in nonfood species is discouraged.

Pet Fish Practice: Some drugs are used in pet fish practice that are not appropriate for aquaculture use, including both antibiotics and parasiticides. None of these compounds are approved for the uses described, and safety and efficacy data are sparse. Nonetheless, these treatments are considered somewhat routine in the practice of ornamental fish medicine.

Kanamycin has been used with some success to treat bacterial diseases of ornamental fish, including koi. It can be administered orally at 20 mg/kg, by injection at 20 mg/kg, or in a bath at a concentration of 750 mg/L for 2 hr. Anorectic fish can be medicated with a bath treatment or by injection, repeated daily, until fish begin to eat, at which time the drug can be incorporated into the feed to complete the treatment period. Treatment should be continued for 7 days beyond the alleviation of clinical signs. Aminoglycosides are toxic to fish and should be used with caution. Severe kidney lesions have been reported in goldfish treated with gentamicin. Toxicity may be exacerbated by a high ammonia concentration in the water.

Organophosphates have been used in nonfood fish practice for decades to control monogenea, crustaceans, and leeches. Historically, there was an approved compound, Masoten (used at a concentration of 0.25 mg/L active ingredient), for use in ponds stocked with nonfood fish, however the label expired and was not renewed. Use of organophosphates in aquaria is still practiced, and the dosage is often increased slightly in marine systems due to the higher pH. Use of organophosphates in outdoor ponds is not generally recommended because of legal and environmental concerns.

Metronidazole is used to control flagellated protozoans and can be delivered in a medicated food or as a bath when fish are anorectic. A concentration of ~7 mg/L (~250 mg metronidazole dissolved in 10 gal. of water) can be administered daily for 5 days. A daily water change a few hours after treatment is recommended. Metronidazole can be administered at 50 mg/kg PO, for 5 days. Anecdotal information suggests that excessive treatment (10 times the recommended dosage for 30 days) with metronidazole may be associated with reproductive failure in some fish.

Fenbendazole has been used to control intestinal helminths in fish. A dosage of 25 mg/kg, delivered in food for 3-5 days, has been commonly recommended, but this regimen has not been evaluated in controlled trials.

Praziquantel has also been used successfully in fish to control intestinal cestodes as well as monogenean trematodes on the gills and skin. The most common use of praziquantel is as a prolonged bath in large marine aquaria for control of monogenean trematodes, particularly *Neobenedenia* spp. It is applied at a concentration of 2 mg/L, and limited work indicates that the compound remains active for several weeks. Praziquantel can also be administered PO at a dosage of 35-125 mg/kg for up to 3 days or as a short-term bath treatment at a concentration of 10 mg/L for 3 hr.

Chloroquine has been used to control *Amyloodinium* sp in ornamental marine fish. It is applied as a prolonged bath at concentrations of 2 mg/L. Efficacy in recirculating systems seems to be very good; however, there are essentially no data on treatment intervals, effects on biofilters, or other basic husbandry data.

FISH HEALTH MANAGEMENT

When working with fish, disease prevention is always more rewarding than treatment. Once fish are sick, accurately identifying all problems present can be difficult, and treatment must be administered early in the course of an epizootic to be effective. In most cases, a comprehensive program of fish health management should be based on the principles of water quality, nutrition, sanitation, and quarantine. Water quality and nutrition are discussed below. Sanitation includes maintenance of a clean environment with minimal accumulation of organic debris, proper disinfection of nets and equipment, and thorough disinfection of fish-holding units between groups of fish. While these practices are more applicable to hatchery management and intensive, indoor systems than to pond or sea-cage culture, efforts to maintain as clean an environment as possible within the constraints of the operation will help minimize disease outbreaks. New fish should be quarantined for at least 3 wk, with 30-60 days preferred for valuable pets or zoologic specimens. Producers may be constrained by production practices; however, they may be forced to address quarantine concerns as regulations are enforced in an effort to prevent the introduction of viral diseases to aquaculture facilities.

ENVIRONMENTAL DISEASES

Because poor water quality is the most common cause of environmentally induced diseases, some means of assessing water quality is essential. Inexpensive test kits are easy to use and provide information that is reasonably accurate. Professional aquaculturists or advanced tropical fish hobbyists should be encouraged to purchase their own water-testing equipment and use it on a regular basis. Veterinarians practicing fish medicine need a comprehensive understanding of the dynamics and management of water quality.

Basic parameters of water quality can be grouped into 4 major categories: dissolved gases, nitrogenous compounds, carbonate compounds, and salinity (*see also* p 1705). The significance of these parameters varies with the type of system, species, and stocking density; however, low dissolved oxygen and high ammonia are the 2 water quality parameters most likely to kill fish directly.

In addition to water quality problems, aquatic organisms are sensitive to a wide variety of toxicants. One toxicant worthy of special mention is chlorine, a common additive to city water that is also used as a disinfectant on aquaculture facilities. It is highly toxic to fish, with adverse effects seen at concentrations of 0.02 mg/L and deaths occurring at 0.04 mg/L. A simple, colormetric test is available to measure chlorine in aquatic systems. No chlorine should be present at any time live animals are present. Sodium thiosulfate can be used to eliminate chlorine from a system. To use this chemical effectively, the total volume of water to be treated and the concentration of chlorine present must be determined. One mg of chlorine/L is eliminated by each 7.4 mg of sodium thiosulfate/L added to the system.

Some municipalities use chloramine, rather than chlorine, as a disinfectant. Chloramine is a compound in which the chlorine molecule is stabilized by aminating it. The resultant compound releases ammonia when water is dechlorinated with sodium thiosulfate. A properly conditioned biofilter should be able to metabolize the ammonia as it is released, but a new or damaged bacterial bed will not be able to manage the influx of ammonia from deamination of chloramines. Products that remove ammonia and chlorine from city water treated with chloramine are sold in pet stores. These products can be invaluable in an emergency but should not be used as a substitute for proper management and effective filtration.

Dissolved Gases: Of the dissolved gases, oxygen is the most important. In ponds, photosynthesis by algae is the primary source of oxygen. A diurnal cycle is established, which coincides with photosynthetic activity. During daylight hours, when photosynthesis is occurring, oxygen levels rise and carbon dioxide levels fall. At night, respiration is the driving force, resulting in a decrease in dissolved oxygen (DO) and an increase in carbon dioxide. Most finfish thrive when the DO concentration is >5 mg/L. When DO is <5 mg/L, fish become stressed; depending on species, size, and duration of exposure, a fish kill may result. Cardinal signs of a fish kill caused by hypoxia include sudden, significant mortality, usually noticed early in the morning (when oxygen levels are lowest); often, large fish are affected more than small fish. Hybrid striped bass may display a characteristic posture—an arched back, flared gills, and open mouth. Certain species are more sensitive to low DO than others. For example, hybrid striped bass may die at DO levels of 2-4 mg/L, yet channel catfish rarely succumb until DO falls below 1 mg/L. Fish that are hypoxic often school near the surface of the water and may be seen trying to gulp air, a behavior referred to as "piping." Differential diagnoses for piping include low DO, high nitrite, and gill disease.

Although low DO is most common early in the morning, it can occur at any time. The most common causes in ponds are cloudy weather, death of an algal bloom, and pond turnover. Cloudy, overcast skies decrease the amount of light reaching the surface of the pond, which results in decreased photosynthetic activity and poor oxygen production. Algae can die at any time; however, a common cause of algal mortality is chemical treatment. After an algae die-off, pond water changes color, usually from green to brown. Concurrent with the decrease in DO, the total ammonia nitrogen increases and the pH decreases. The bloom will generally return naturally within a week or so; however, the pond should be monitored closely during the transitional period and aerated as necessary. Pond turnover is most common in deep ponds (>6 ft) and involves a phenomenon referred to as stratification. Water at the bottom of the pond cools, and a temperature gradient, called the thermocline, develops between warm surface water and cool bottom water. The thermocline acts as a physical barrier between the surface water (epilimnion) and bottom water (hypolimnion). Because photosynthesis, and hence oxygen production, occurs at the surface, the hypolimnion becomes hypoxic and develops a biologic oxygen demand. When the pond is mixed, or "turns over," the oxygen is removed as the biologic oxygen demand of the hypolimnion is satisfied. This sudden removal of oxygen can result in oxygen depletion and a fish kill. The most common cause of pond turnover in the southern USA is a summer thunderstorm, in which energy released from cold rain coupled with wind and wave action is sufficient to mix the pond. Pond turnover can result in catastrophic oxygen depletion and, once a pond has stratified, turnover can be caused by seining, aeration, or other management practices that result in mixing of the epilimnion and hypolimnion. Pond turnover can be avoided by performing a weekly oxygen profile during periods of greatest risk.

Gas bubble disease is caused by supersaturation of water with dissolved gases. It is more common in coldwater aquaculture, in which cold, inflowing water, already saturated with gas, may be heated without adequate time or aeration for volatilization of excess gas. It also commonly results when water from deep wells, often high in nitrogen gas and carbon dioxide, is brought into an aquaculture facility without proper aeration. The disease can also be caused in small pools or tanks by leaving a garden hose running on the bottom of the tank. Once the hose is submerged, there is no release of excess gas to the atmosphere, resulting in supersaturation of tank water and acute mortality. Gas bubble disease has also been associated with faulty pumps and, although rare in ponds, the presence of heavy algal blooms with afternoon DO levels >25 mg/L. Gas bubble disease is manifest by exophthalmos and the presence of tiny gas emboli in fins or tissue. The presence of gas emboli in gill capillaries is diagnostic. Treatment of gas bubble disease is vigorous aeration to volatilize excess gas.

Carbon dioxide (CO_2) can be toxic to fish when present at concentrations >20 mg/L. Water from affected systems is acidic. A quick field test for excessive CO_2 involves vigorous aeration of a bucket of suspect water for 1 hr. A significant increase in pH (ie, >1 unit) over the hour is indicative of excess CO_2. Hybrid striped bass exposed to toxic levels of CO_2 will hover at the surface with their backs out of the water and will be extremely lethargic. If fish are treated with salt under these conditions, they may try to leave the water and significant mortality can result. Treatment for CO_2 toxicity is vigorous aeration.

Hydrogen sulfide (H_2S) is highly toxic to fish. The 2 most common sources of H_2S in an aquaculture facility are water from a deep well or anoxic organic material from the bottom of a tank or pond. Regardless of source, contamination of water with H_2S results in acute mortality of fish. Although test kits are available to detect H_2S, a presumptive diagnosis can be made from the sulfide smell within the culture facility. H_2S can be eliminated by thoroughly aerating water before it enters the culture facility and by maintaining standards of sanitation that minimize accumulation of organic debris in fish-holding units.

Nitrogenous Compounds: Nitrogenous wastes enter the aquatic system directly from excretion by fish or degradation of fish food. Fish foods are generally very high in protein, often >38%, and can add significant quantities of nitrogen to a system. Nitrogen is eliminated from fish by the passive diffusion of ammonia (NH_3) from gill capillaries. Once NH_3 is released into the water, it enters the nitrogen cycle, a natural process in which bacterial populations change ammonia to nitrite (NO_2) and then to nitrate (NO_3). Nitrate can be anaerobically converted to nitrogen gas (N_2), which is volatile and quickly leaves the system. Plants or algae in the system may use nitrogen products directly.

NH_3 is highly toxic and frequently limits fish production in intensive systems. It is also dynamic, and when it enters the aquatic system, an equilibrium is established between NH_3 and ammonium (NH_4^+). Of the two, NH_3 is far more toxic to fish, and its formation is favored by high pH and water temperature. When pH exceeds ~8.5, any NH_3 present can be dangerous. In general, a normally functioning aquatic system should contain no measurable NH_3 because as soon as it enters the system, it should be removed by bacteria (*Nitrosomonas* spp). Test kits used for aquaculture do not measure NH_3 directly but instead measure the combination of NH_3 and NH_4, referred to as total ammonia nitrogen (TAN). A TAN of 1 mg/L is usually not cause for concern unless the pH is >8.5. However, if the amount of NH_3 is increased, an explanation should be sought. The amount of toxic NH_3 present can be calculated using the TAN, pH, and water temperature. When NH_3 levels exceed 0.05 mg/L, damage to gills becomes apparent; levels of 2.0 mg/L are lethal for many fish.

Overfeeding or malfunction (death) of a biologic filter are common causes of increased NH_3. If possible, a water change (≥50%) should be done as soon as high NH_3 levels are detected. Feeding should be discontinued or significantly reduced until the problem has been corrected. In a production pond, a water change is not feasible; however, stocking density and feeding rate should be assessed, and fresh water run into the pond if possible.

Two conditions encountered in pet fish medicine are characterized by high NH_3 concentrations. The first, referred to as new tank syndrome, is fairly well recognized by hobbyists. NH_3 levels are high in the affected system because the biofilter has not had time to develop. It takes at least 3-6 wk for a new filter to develop a bacterial bed that is adequate to metabolize NH_3 from even a small population of fish. Beginning aquarists are likely to overstock and overfeed new systems, resulting in significant NH_3 spikes and sick or dying fish.

The second condition, called old tank syndrome, is less frequently recognized. It is characterized by extremely high ammonia levels (TAN may be near 40 mg/L in severe cases), extremely low pH (usually <6, may be <5 in severe cases) and a complete absence of alkalinity. The condition is caused by complete exhaustion of buffering capacity within a system, usually precipitated by improper management over a period of months. As the buffering capacity (alkalinity) is exhausted, organic acids that have accumulated drop the pH and the acidic environment kills the biofilter, leading to an accumulation of NH_3. When correcting such a situation it is important to eliminate as much "bad" water as possible and avoid a shift in residual NH_3 to the toxic un-ionized state as pH rises. A simple water change under such circumstances can result in catastrophic mortality, as pH rises above 7 and ammonia shifts to the un-ionized form. Over-the-counter products that chemically remove NH_3 can be helpful in preventing mortality, but the system must be thoroughly cleaned and restarted. It may take several weeks for the system to recover.

The second breakdown product in the nitrogen cycle is NO_2, which is also toxic to fish. NO_2 can enter the bloodstream passively across the gill epithelium. It complexes with hemoglobin to form methemoglobin, resulting in methemoglobinemia or brown blood disease. As in other species, RBC containing methemoglobin are unable to transport oxygen, resulting in a physiologic hypoxia regardless of oxygen content in the water. There are species-specific differences in fishes' susceptibility to NO_2 toxicity (eg, centrarchids [bass, bluegill, etc] are refractory to methemoglobinemia). Marine fish were thought to be protected from NO_2 toxicity by salts in their environment; however, red drum have developed brown blood disease in the presence of NO_2. A tentative diagnosis of brown blood disease can be made by observing the characteristic chocolate brown color of the gills. Blood samples will also be an abnormal color. Methemoglobin concentrations in the blood can be determined, although this is not necessary for clinical management. A water quality test can confirm the presence of NO_2. Fish affected with methemoglobinemia typically show signs of hypoxia, often manifest by piping. The most rapid treatment for NO_2 toxicity is a water change, but this may not be feasible in production ponds. Increasing chloride Cl⁻) concentration in the water creates a competitive inhibition at the gill epithelium between Cl⁻ and NO_2. By increasing the concentration of Cl⁻, so that there are 6 parts Cl⁻ to 1 part NO_2, the percentage of Hgb converted to methemoglobin will decrease dramatically, providing immediate relief to the fish and stopping most further mortality within 24 hr. Salt can be used to increase the concentration of Cl⁻. To determine the amount of salt required, the concentrations of NO_2 and Cl⁻ present must be measured, by commercial test kits. The concentration of Cl⁻ needed (mg/L) = (6 × NO_2) - Cl⁻ present. Once the concentration of Cl⁻ needed is known, the volume of water can be calculated in acre-feet (1 acre foot = 1 surface acre, 1 foot deep), and salt can be added to increase Cl⁻ to the desired concentration (4.5 lb of salt will add Cl⁻ at 1 mg/L to 1 acre-foot of water). In aquariums and garden ponds, a water change and filter maintenance are recommended, although salt may still be used to halt mortality.

Carbonate Compounds: The carbonate cycle is another important concept in water quality management, and its complexity is reflected in the dynamic interactions between CO_2, pH, total alkalinity, and total hardness. In aquatic systems containing algae or plants, CO_2 fluctuates on a diurnal basis, similar but opposite to fluctuations in dissolved oxygen. As CO_2 concentration changes, the pH of the water also changes. As CO_2 concentration decreases during daylight hours, pH rises, reaching its peak late in the afternoon. Conversely, as CO_2 concentration increases during the night, pH falls, reaching its lowest level just before daylight. A diurnal pH change from 6.5 to 9.0 is not unusual in a freshwater fish pond with a healthy algal bloom. Most freshwater fish can tolerate reasonable fluctuation in pH, and the lethal limits for many species are about 4 and 10. Marine fish are much less tolerant of pH fluctuation; the marine environment is much more stable, with a pH of 8.2-8.3.

Although fish kills caused by improper pH are rare, hydrated lime (CaOH) is sometimes added to freshwater ponds by mistake. CaOH will rapidly increase the pH to >10, killing all fish present. Correct liming of ponds is discussed below. Of greater clinical significance is the effect of pH on NH_3 toxicity. The toxicity of NH_3 increases dramatically as pH rises; consequently, it is possible to have fish in a freshwater pond die of acute NH_3 toxicity late in the afternoon when pH is high. A history of sudden deaths late in the day, with fish seen spinning or skittering near the surface before death is typical. The diagnosis is confirmed by testing total ammonia nitrogen (TAN, see above), pH, and water temperature. Calculation of NH_3 levels may reveal toxic concentrations >1.0 mg/L at the time deaths occurred.

CO_2 released into an aquatic system enters the carbonate cycle: $H_2O + CO_2 \leftrightarrow H^+ + HCO_3^- \leftrightarrow 2H^+ + CO_3^{2-}$. The process is driven by the presence of carbonate (CO_3^{2-}) in the system, which is measured using a test referred to as total alkalinity (TA). For most fish, water should ideally be of moderate alkalinity, 100-250 mg/L. When TA is <50 mg/L, water is considered low in alkalinity, and buffering ability will not be adequate to prevent major pH fluctuations. Toxicity of copper sulfate, an algicide and effective parasiticide, is closely associated with TA, and the compound cannot be used safely if the TA is <50 mg/L. To raise alkalinity, dolomite or agricultural limestone may be added to the system. In freshwater ponds, the lime requirement of the pond may be determined from sediment samples submitted to a soil laboratory. If this service is not available, 1-2 tons of agricultural limestone are recommended per surface acre of water. Once limestone has been applied, 2-4 wk are required for maximum effect. This treatment should not have to be repeated for several years unless the pond is drained. In smaller systems, dolomite may be purchased in 50-lb bags and used to effect. Alkalinity should be ≥100 mg/L in freshwater systems and ≥250 mg/L in saltwater systems.

Total hardness (TH) has been confused with TA in the past. Both TH and TA are reported as mg/L of $CaCO_3$. The difference is that the test for TA measures the CO_3^{2-} fraction and the test for TH measures the calcium (Ca^{2+}) fraction. The test for TH is also influenced by the presence of other divalent cations in the system, including magnesium, manganese, iron, and zinc. TH is important in determining the amount of calcium available to young fish. Catfish hatcheries should have a minimum calcium concentration of 20 mg/L. Calcium chloride can be added to water to increase calcium concentration.

Salinity: The salinity of seawater is determined by a complex array of salts. Seawater is 3% salt, or 30,000 ppm. For marine fish, many of the micronutrients present in sea water are essential, so it is necessary to buy or make "sea salts." In freshwater, salinity may be increased to some degree using table salt (NaCl). Salt is often used in freshwater systems to reduce osmoregulatory stress or to eliminate certain ectoparasites. Salinity can be measured with a clinical refractometer or with a hydrometer purchased from a pet store.

NUTRITIONAL DISEASES

Nutritional management of fish is highly variable, depending on species and system. For established foodfish industries, high-quality diets are readily available. For emerging industries and ornamental fish, particularly marine species, nutrition is one of the greatest constraints to development of commercial culture. Fish generally require a high-protein diet, with a significant percentage of protein provided by fish meal. Most fish do not synthesize ascorbic acid; therefore, adequate supplementation is necessary. Ascorbic acid should be provided in a stabilized form, often referred to as "stay C." Proper storage of feeds in a cool, dry place is necessary to minimize nutritional degradation.

Classic ascorbic acid deficiency has been referred to as "broken back disease" by fish farmers because of the collapse of the vertebral column that occurs secondary to inadequate collagen synthesis. Less dramatic signs of deficiency include impaired wound healing and immune function. Of the B vitamins, folic acid deficiency has been associated with poor growth and, in channel catfish, with anemia. Pantothenic acid deficiency has caused gill disease. Acute thiamine deficiency has been associated with neurologic signs, including convulsions and death; chronic deficiency has resulted in loss of equilibrium, edema, and poor growth. Riboflavin deficiency has been associated with vascularization of the cornea, hyperpigmentation, clouding, and hemorrhage of the eyes. Niacin, biotin, and pyridoxine deficiencies have been associated with neurologic abnormalities, including spasms and convulsions. Choline and inositol deficiency have been linked to poor growth. Vitamin A deficiency has been associated with poor growth and retinal atrophy. Vitamin E deficiency has been related to myopathy, including muscular deformities. Skeletal muscle abnormalities have been associated with selenium deficiency and rancid feeds. Rancid feeds have also been linked to steatitis. The nutritional requirements for trout, salmon, catfish, warmwater fishes, and aquarium fishes have been published by the National Academy of Sciences.

Feeding methods and rates vary with species, age, system, and water temperature. A maintenance diet is generally considered to be 1-2% of body wt/day, whereas a diet for growth may be 3-5% of body wt/day. In many systems, feeding behavior is an important indicator of health. Vigorous feeding is desirable, and a sudden decrease in appetite should be cause for alarm. To minimize size variation within a population, feed should be distributed over as broad an area as possible. Smaller, more frequent feedings are preferable to one large feeding, especially for young fish.

PARASITIC DISEASES

All of the major groups of animal parasites are found in fish, and apparently healthy wild fish often carry heavy parasite burdens. Parasites with direct life cycles can be important pathogens of cultured fish; parasites with indirect life cycles frequently use fish as intermediate hosts. Knowledge of specific fish hosts greatly facilitates identification of parasites with marked host and tissue specificity, while others are recognized because of their common occurrence and lack of host specificity. Examination of fresh smears that contain living parasites is often diagnostic.

The most common parasites of fish are protozoa (TABLE 9). These include species found on external surfaces and species found in specific organs. Most protozoa have direct life cycles, but the myxosporidia require an invertebrate intermediate host.

Protozoa Infecting Gills and Skin

Ciliates: Ciliated protozoa are among the most common external parasites of fish. Most ciliates have a simple life cycle and divide by binary fission. Ciliates can be motile, attached, or found within the epithelium. The most well-known organism in the latter group is *Ichthyophthirius multifiliis*, which has a more complex life cycle than the other ciliates.

The infection caused by *I multifiliis* is referred to as "ich" or "white spot disease," although the latter name is misleading because fish can die from an infection without ever developing the classic, white blister-like lesions. This parasite is an obligate pathogen and cannot survive without the presence of living fish. It is readily identified using a light microscope at magnifications of 40× or 100×. It is large (0.50-1 mm), round, and completely covered with cilia. It has a characteristic horseshoe-shaped macronucleus. Its characteristic movement varies from constantly rotating to ameboid-like. The immature stages of the parasite (tomites) must find a host within a specified time, which varies with water temperature from several days (warm water) to weeks (cold water), or they will die. With large, complex systems, removing fish and leaving the system fallow is an acceptable means of preventing reinfection. The tomites penetrate mucus of the epidermis and gills, where they feed on epithelial and blood cells extracted from the superficial capillaries. Once encysted under the epithelium, *I multifiliis* is refractory to chemical treatment. After reaching maturity, it leaves the host and sinks to the bottom sediment, where it divides within a cyst-like structure. While encysted, it is also refractory to chemical treatment, but cysts may be removed by aggressive cleaning and removal of debris from gravel substrates. The organism multiplies within the cyst, producing 500-1,200 tomites from each adult parasite. The speed of the life cycle is determined by water temperature. The life cycle is completed in 4 days at water temperatures of 24-26°C but takes 35-40 days at 7°C. Multiple chemical treatments

TABLE 9. Protozoan Parasites of Fish*

	Parasites	Tissue	Susceptible Species
External ciliates (motile)	*Ichthyophthirius* (FW); *Cryptocaryon* (SW)	Gills, skin, fins	All
	Trichodina (FW, SW); *Chilodonella* (FW); *Brooklynella* (SW)	Gills, skin, fins	All
	Tetrahymena (FW); *Uronema* (SW)	Skin, eye	All ("guppy killer")
External (sessile)	*Ambiphyra*; *Apiosoma*	Gills, skin, fins	Primarily pond fish
External flagellates	*Ichthyobodo, Cryptobia* (*see also* internal)	Gills, skin, fins	All
	Oodinium (FW); *Amyloodinium* (SW)	Gills, skin	Salt water fish more susceptible, especially clown fish and red drum
Internal flagellates	*Spironucleus*; *Hexamita*	Intestine	All cichlids, betas, gouramis, other aquarium fish
	Cryptobia	Stomach	African cichlids
	Trypanosoma	Blood	Plecostomus (blue-eyed)
Coccidia	*Coccidia*	Intestine	Multiple
Myxosporidians (IH)	*Myxosoma cerebralis* (whirling disease)	Head, cartilage, backbone	RBT, salmonids
	Ceratomyxa shasta	Posterior intestine	Salmonids (Pacific NW)
	Aurantiactinomyxon ictaluri (PGD, HGD)	Gill	CCF
	Henneguya	Gill	CCF, other
	Sphaerospora auratus (renal dropsy)	Kidney	Goldfish (pond-reared)
	Proliferative kidney disease	Kidney	RBT, all salmonids
Microsporidians (DH)	*Pleistophora ovariae*	Ovary	Golden shiner
	P hyphessobryconis	Skeletal muscle	Neon tetra (neon tetra disease), AF, other FW aquarium species

*FW, fresh water; SW, salt water; RBT, rainbow trout; CCF, channel catfish; AF, angelfish; IH, intermediate host; DH, direct host; PGD, proliferative gill disease; HGD, hamburger gill disease

Signs	Diagnosis	Treatment
White spot disease; no spots visible if on gills only	Wet mount	FW—formalin, $CuSO_4$, SW—formalin, Cu^{2+}, formalin
High respiration rate, piping, excess mucus, flashing, loss of condition	Wet mount	FW—formalin, $CuSO_4$, SW—formalin, Cu^{2+}, formalin
Mucus, flashing, intraocular lesions, popeye	Wet mount	External as above; improve sanitation Internal: no treatment
Excess mucus, flashing, piping, loss of condition	Wet mount	Formalin, $KMnO_4$; management—decrease crowding, correct sanitation
Blue slime, flashing, piping, excess mucus, loss of condition	Wet mount	Formalin, $CuSO_4$, $KMnO_4$, salt
Mortality, lethargy, piping; "velvet" (if on skin)	Wet mount	Chloroquine (nonfood fish only); freshwater dips for marine food fish
Weight loss (anorexia), mortality of fry and juveniles	Wet mount	Metronidazole (nonfood fish only)
Extreme weight loss, anorexia	Wet mount, histology	None; management—correct sanitation, feeding, stocking density
Anemia, mortality	Wet mount	none
Weight loss, mortality	Histology	Sulfamethazine (efficacy questionable)
Blacktail, skeletal deformity	Histology, isolation of parasite	None; regulatory concern
Weight loss, distended and hemorrhagic vent	Wet mount, histology	None; regulatory concern
Mortality, piping	Wet mount, histology	None
None, severe hypoxia	Wet mount	None
Mortality, severely enlarged and cystic kidney	Histology	None
Lethargy, darkening, fluid accumulation, exophthalmia	Wet mount, histology	None
Sterility	"Marbled" ovarian tissue on wet mount	None; management—annual replacement of female brood stock
Abnormal locomotion	Wet mount, histology	None

(with intervals determined by water temperature) are required for successful treatment of *I multifiliis*. At warm temperatures typical of home aquaria (eg, >26°C), infected fish should be treated every 2-3 days. Copper sulfate is the treatment of choice for pond fish, and either copper sulfate or formalin for fish in tanks. Potassium permanganate is not recommended because it is caustic to the gills, and repeated treatments may result in death of the fish.

Cryptocaryon irritans is a parasite of marine fish that closely resembles *I multifiliis*. *Cryptocaryon* spp infections are usually controlled by maintaining copper concentrations of 0.2 mg/L for 3 wk. Because copper is so toxic and difficult to use, formalin is an alternative for less experienced owners. A protocol similar to that recommended for freshwater fish is appropriate (ie, apply the chemical every third day if the tank is maintained at 24-26°C). If treating with formalin in marine tanks, the total duration of treatment should be extended. A minimum treatment time in marine systems is 3 wk. In a marine system, fish must be separated from valued invertebrates before beginning treatment as either copper or formalin will kill them.

There are two important groups of ciliates that are motile and move on the surface of skin and gills of fish. These can be found in fish from all geographic areas and all types of aquatic systems. They include *Chilodonella* spp (which has a marine counterpart, *Brooklynella* spp) and the trichodinids, which are found on both freshwater and marine fish. Fish with chilodonelliasis typically lose condition, and copious mucous secretions may be noticed in areas where infestation is most severe. If gills are heavily infested, the fish may show signs of respiratory distress, including rapid breathing and coughing. The gills may be visibly swollen and mucoid. If the skin is heavily infested, it may have a cloudy appearance, associated with excessive mucus, and the fish may be irritated as evidenced by flashing (scratching) and decreased appetite. *Chilodonella* can be easily identified from fresh biopsies of infected tissues. They are 0.5-0.7 mm, are somewhat heart-shaped with parallel bands of cilia, and move in a characteristic slow spiral.

Several genera of peritrichous ciliates have been grouped together and are collectively referred to as the trichodinids. These include *Trichodina, Trichodinella, Tripartiella,* and *Vauchomia* spp. Clinical signs associated with trichodinid infestation are similar to those of chilodonelliasis, although secretion of mucus is not usually as noticeable. Trichodinids are easily identified from biopsies of infected gill or skin tissue. They are readily visible using a light microscope at 40-100×. Trichodinids move along the surface of infested tissue and appear as little saucers or, from a lateral view, as little bubbles. The body of the organism may be cylindrical, hemispherical, or discoid. Trichodinids are characterized by an attaching disc with a corona of denticles on the adoral sucker surface.

Tetrahymena corlissi, another ciliate, may be motile and surface-dwelling but is also occasionally found within tissue, including skeletal muscle and ocular fluids. Similar protozoa, *Uronema* spp, are found on marine fish. *Tetrahymena* spp are pear-shaped and 10-20 μm long, with longitudinal rows of cilia and inconspicuous cytostomes. External infestations of *Tetrahymena* spp are not uncommon on moribund fish removed from the bottom of a tank or aquarium and are often associated with an environment rich in organic material. As long as *Tetrahymena* spp are restricted to the external surface of the fish, they are easily eliminated with chemical treatment and sanitation. When they become established internally, they are not treatable and can cause significant mortality. Fish with intraocular infections of *Tetrahymena* spp develop extreme exophthalmos. The parasite is readily identified by examining ocular fluids with a light microscope.

Ambiphyra and *Apiosoma* are a sessile ciliates that can be found on the skin, gills, and fins of fish. These seem to be more common in pond fish than tank-reared fish and have a predilection for organically rich environments. They are not generally found on marine fish. When examined from a lateral view, *Ambiphyra* is the shape of a tin can with a ciliated band around the middle and at the cytostome, which is distal to the attachment site. *Apiosoma* spp are vase-shaped. Neither *Ambiphyra* spp nor *Apiosoma* spp are particularly pathogenic if present in low numbers (no more than 1-2/low-power field); however, when present in high numbers, these parasites can cause significant epithelial damage, predisposing fish to opportunistic pathogens in the environment and compromising respiration and osmoregulation. Infested fish demonstrate flashing, decreased appetite, loss of condition, and hyperplasia of infested epithelial surfaces. Severe infestation of the gills is particularly damaging. The organisms can be controlled with a single treatment of formalin, copper sulfate, potassium permanganate, or a salt dip. Excessive crowding and poor sanitation are frequently associated with heavy infestations and should be corrected.

Heteropolaria spp is a stalked, colonial ciliate that most frequently attaches to bony surfaces of fish, particularly the tips of fin rays and opercula. It is most common in freshwater gamefish, particularly centrarchids, (eg, largemouth bass, bluegill, and sunfish) and is frequently associated with development of "red sore disease." In the earliest stages of infection, bony protuberances appear slightly raised and erythematous; as the colony grows, they appear cottony. Examination of material with a light microscope is required to differentiate *Heteropolaria* spp from fungal hyphae, and mixed infections are common. Further progression of the disease is typified by development of shallow ulcers on the lateral surface of the fish. A wet mount of fresh tissue from the margin of the lesion is required to differentiate between *Heteropolaria* spp, fungal hyphae, and columnaris bacteria. Coinfection with the bacterium *Aeromonas hydrophila* is typical of red sore disease. If deaths occur, a single treatment of potassium permanganate or copper sulfate should be administered. If systemic bacterial infection is a component of the epizootic, antibiotics should be provided in medicated feed, if affected fish will accept a pelleted diet.

Flagellates: *Ichthyobodo (Costia)* spp are some of the most common and smallest (~15 × 5 μm) flagellated protozoan parasites of the skin and gills. They are flattened, pear-shaped organisms with 2 flagellae of unequal lengths. *Ichthyobodo* moves in a jerky, spiral pattern, and free-swimming organisms are fairly easy to identify in direct smear preparations. Once attached, the organism can be difficult to see and is often missed by the novice, but movement typical of a flickering flame is characteristic. Affected skin often has a steel-gray discoloration and gills may appear swollen. Copious mucus production, sometimes referred to as "blue slime," is characteristic of costiasis. Behavioral signs of infestation include lethargy, anorexia, piping, and flashing. In acute cases, fish may appear hypoxic and swim to the surface frequently. In chronic cases, fish are weak, thin, and anorectic. The disease affects aquarium, pond, and marine fish. *Ichthyobodo* is readily controlled with salt, formalin, copper sulfate, or potassium permanganate baths. Because the parasite has a direct life cycle, a single treatment should be adequate. If reinfestation occurs, sanitation and quarantine practices should be evaluated.

One of the most serious health problems of captive marine fish is the parasitic dinoflagellate *Amyloodinium* spp. Its freshwater counterpart, *Oodinium* spp, is less common but can also result in high mortality. These parasites produce a disease that has been called "velvet," "rust," "gold-dust," and "coral disease" because of the brownish gold color they impart to infected fish. The pathogenic stages of the organism are pigmented, photosynthetic, nonflagellated, nonmotile algae that attach to and invade the skin and gills during their parasitic existence. When mature, these parasites give rise to cysts that contain numerous flagellated, small, free-swimming stages that can initiate new infections. Control of *Amyloodinium* is challenging, and the prognosis is guarded. Copper sulfate is the only therapeutic option for food animals in the USA, and repeated treatments are necessary to break the life cycle. In marine systems, chelated copper solutions can be used, but the concentration of free copper ions must be closely monitored and should be maintained at 0.2 mg/L for 3 wk. Copper is highly toxic to invertebrates, which must be removed from the system before treatment. When possible, environmental manipulation may be helpful. Progress of the disease may be delayed by reducing lighting and by lowering temperature and organic load. For nonfood species, chloroquine has been used at 10 mg/L as an indefinite bath; it is apparently effective but is not approved for this use. Formalin and potassium permanganate are not effective in controlling *Amyloodinium* spp or *Oodinium* spp. There is some controversy as to the effect of altered salinity on these organisms, because some species seem to thrive in brackish waters. Therefore, adjustments in salinity (increase for freshwater fish, decrease for marine fish) during an epizootic should be carefully monitored for evidence of efficacy.

Internal Protozoan Parasites

Hexamita and *Spironucleus* spp are common, small (~9 μm), bilaterally symmetric, flagellated (4 pairs) protozoa most frequently found in the intestinal tract and occasionally in skin lesions or degenerating soft tissues of finfish. These genera are similar but differ slightly in the position and shape of their nuclei (2 within 1 organism). Pathogenicity of these organisms is variable and correlated with the number present. If there is a question as to whether treatment is warranted, the number of organisms present can be assessed in a wet mount of intestine. If <5 organisms per low-power field (LPF) are present, treatment is probably not necessary; if 5-15 organisms/LPF are present, treatment should be administered if fish are in poor condition; and if >15 organisms/LPF are present, treatment is strongly recommended. The only treatment available for hexamitiasis is metronidazole (use only in ornamental species), which should be given orally but can be administered as a bath if fish are anorectic. The number of organisms present in infested freshwater angelfish increases dramatically after shipping and handling. Chronic problems have been seen in fish maintained in unsanitary or crowded conditions. Preventive treatment of ornamental cichlids is recommended before shipping, and broodstock should be evaluated periodically. The hatchability of eggs from heavily infested adult angelfish (freshwater) seems to be significantly decreased; resultant fry may be weak with poor longterm survival.

Cryptobia and *Trypanosoma* spp are slender, elongated (6-20 μm), actively motile, biflagellated protozoa that are easily detected in fresh blood and tissue smears of both marine and freshwater finfish. Hematogenous forms are generally described as *Trypanosoma* and have a well-developed undulating membrane. Trypanosomes may be transmitted by leeches and have been associated with anemia in blue-eyed plecostomus imported from South America. *Cryptobia iubilans* has been associated with granulomatous disease in African cichlids and discus. Clinical disease is manifest by severe weight loss and cachexia. Clinically affected fish should be culled. Presumptive diagnosis can be made from microscopic examination of fresh tissue. Typically, granulomas will be found in the stomach, which may be visibly thickened. Acid-fast material will not be found in granulomas caused by *Cryptobia*. Motile flagellates may be visible using magnification of 400× or greater. Transmission electron micrographs are required to confirm the diagnosis of *C iubilans*.

Sporozoans: Coccidiosis, while common in freshwater or marine finfish, is rarely diagnosed in live fish. Many species of finfish are affected. The life cycles of many fish coccidia are unknown, and some involve >1 host to complete their development. In addition to intestinal infection, the internal organs also are commonly affected; sporulated *Eimeria*-like oocysts and sexual and asexual stages are commonly found in direct smears and histologic sections of the internal organs. Sulfamethazine, at 22-24 g/100 kg of fish wt/day in the feed for 50 days at 50°F (10°C), is used to treat food fish (21-day withdrawal time) in some countries. For aquarium fish, 10 ppm in the aquarium water once a week for 2-3 wk has been reported to be preventive, but safety and efficacy data are sparse.

Myxosporidians are common fish parasites. The myxosporidian spore consists of 2 valves, a suture line, and 1-4 polar capsules that contain coiled, extensible filaments and an infective central body called the sporoplasm. Evidence suggests that myxosporidia have indirect life cycles and use other aquatic organisms (eg, annelids) as intermediate hosts. Hence, myxosporidian infections are more common in, and more pathogenic for, wild fish or fish reared intensively in outdoor fish ponds. The organisms tend to be host- and tissue-specific. Accordingly, expression of the disease is related to the specific pathogen and host.

Myxosoma cerebralis, an important pathogen of young salmonids, is responsible for whirling disease, also known as "blacktail." Typically, infected fingerlings show rapid tail-chasing behavior when startled, and the peduncle and tail may darken significantly. As infected fish age, skeletal deformity may result from damage to the cartilaginous structures, particularly the skull and vertebral column. Recovered fish remain carriers, and adults do not show signs, although skeletal deformities do not resolve. The disease can be prevented by purchasing uninfected breeding stock and maintaining them in an environment free of the intermediate hosts. A presumptive diagnosis of whirling disease is made by detection of spores from skulls of infected fish. Samples can be submitted to a fish disease laboratory, or procedures described by the American Fisheries Society can be followed. Diagnosis may be confirmed histologically or serologically. Whirling disease is of regulatory concern in some states.

Salmonid ceratomyxosis is caused by *Ceratomyxa shasta*, a myxosporidian endemic to specific watersheds in the Pacific northwest. The disease occurs in wild fish as well as in fish from hatcheries that use contaminated water. The most typical presentation includes hemorrhage and fibrinous inflammation in the posterior intestine, but other visceral organs and musculature can also be infected. Grossly, fish may appear emaciated, with a distended abdomen and hemorrhagic vent. A presumptive diagnosis can be made by examination of a wet mount of the posterior intestine and visualization of the kidney-bean-shaped trophozoites. The presence of the organism can be confirmed histologically. Some states consider *C shasta* a reportable disease.

Proliferative gill disease of catfish is caused by the myxosporidian *Aurantiactinomyxon ictaluri*. The organism has a complex life cycle, with the oligochete worm *Dero digitata* serving as the intermediate host. Channel catfish may be an aberrant host for *A ictaluri*, and the disease is usually associated with new ponds or previously infected ponds that have been drained and refilled. Although proliferative gill disease can cause catastrophic mortality approaching 100%, losses may be as low as 1%. Disease occurs at water temperatures of 16-26°C, and mortality is exacerbated by poor water quality, particularly low dissolved oxygen or high levels of un-ionized ammonia. Gills of affected fish are severely swollen and bloody, resulting in the colloquial name "hamburger gill disease." A presumptive diagnosis can be made from a wet mount of infected gill tissue, in which filaments appear swollen, clubbed, and broken. Cartilaginous necrosis is strongly supportive of a diagnosis of proliferative gill disease; however, histology is required for confirmation.

Many species of myxosporidians produce nodular or cystic lesions in the skin, gills, muscle, or visceral organs of fish, depending on their host species and tissue preference. *Henneguya* is commonly found in white, cystic skin lesions of cultured channel catfish and aquarium fish; it is easily identified by the forked-tail appendage of the spore seen microscopically. If ponds are dried and limed heavily, infection can be eliminated, apparently by reduction of the intermediate hosts. Aquarium infection can be self-limiting in the absence of intermediate hosts. *Henneguya* may also be seen in wet mounts of gill tissue. Although an occasional cyst may be considered an incidental finding, severe damage has been associated with diffuse distribution of interlamellar cysts.

Renal dropsy in pond-reared goldfish is caused by the myxosporidian *Sphaerospora auratus*. The disease is characterized by renal degeneration and ascites and is usually diagnosed by identification of spores in histologic sections of the kidney. Newly purchased pond-reared goldfish placed in aquaria may show signs of the disease, including death. No practical treatment is available. The carp-dropsy complex is a disease of carp and goldfish characterized by dropsy and exophthalmos. It is associated with *S angulata* infection and may be complicated by viral infections (such as spring viremia of carp), carp swim-bladder disease, or bacterial septicemias. Deaths may be acute or occur over a 6-mo period. The response to drug treatment is generally poor.

Proliferative kidney disease (PKD) is one of the most economically important diseases affecting salmonid industries of North America and Europe. Rainbow trout are particularly sensitive to the disease, although all salmonids seem susceptible. PKD is caused by an unnamed myxosporidian parasite, sometimes referred to as the PKD parasite. PKD has been reported in both captive and free-ranging salmonid populations. It occurs most commonly in the summer when water temperatures are >12°C, and the parasite primarily infects yearling and younger fish. Clinical signs include lethargy, darkening, and fluid accumulation indicated by exophthalmos, ascites, and lateral body swelling. Infected fish are frequently anemic, resulting in gill pallor. Grossly, the posterior kidney appears gray, mottled, and significantly enlarged. Presumptive diagnosis can be based on observation of suspect organisms, 10-20 μm in diameter, in Giemsa-stained wet mounts of kidney tissue. Histologic examination of infected tissue, stained with H&E, is required for confirmation. Avoidance is the best preventive measure, although losses may be minimized by improved husbandry. Bacterial infections, particularly *Aeromonas salmonicida*, are common sequelae of PKD epizootics and, if uncontrolled, can result in substantially increased mortality. There is no treatment; however, fish that recover from the infection are resistant to subsequent outbreaks. Infected stocks in nonendemic areas should be depopulated, the premises sanitized, and disease-free stock obtained for replacement.

Microsporidians are tiny, intracellular, spore-forming organisms with single polar filaments that are common parasites of finfish. They are host- and tissue-specific and can also infect helminth parasites of fish. The spores are extremely resistant.

Pleistophora ovariae infects ovarian tissue of golden shiners (bait fish), resulting in sterility. It is an important disease in the bait-fish industry. The organism has no intermediate host and is transmitted horizontally (through ingestion of infective spores) or vertically (through infected ova). Fertility declines as fish age, eventually resulting in sterility. Grossly, infected ovarian tissue appears marbled. The diagnosis is confirmed by examination of a wet mount of suspect tissue, revealing the presence of microsporidian spores. Although there is no treatment, the problem can be managed by discarding female broodstock when they reach 1 yr of age and replacing them annually. Although the young females remain infected, the disease is not yet sufficiently advanced to have a major impact on fertility.

Neon tetra disease is caused by *Pleistophora hyphessobryconis*, which infects the skeletal musculature of a number of species of aquarium fish, including tetras, angelfish, rasporas, and barbs. Infected fish may exhibit abnormal locomotion caused by muscle damage, and muscle tissue may appear marbled or necrotic at necropsy. The parasitic spores are readily visualized in wet mounts of infected tissue. There is no treatment for the infection, although removal of moribund fish helps prevent transmission by eliminating cannibalism within the population.

Helminthiasis

Helminths are common in both wild and cultured fish (TABLE 10). Fish frequently serve as intermediate or transport hosts for larval parasites of many animals, including humans. Helminths with direct life cycles are most important in dense populations, and heavy parasite burdens are sometimes found. In general, heavy parasite burdens seem to be more common in fish originating from wild sources.

Monogenean trematodes, which have direct life cycles, are common, highly pathogenic, obligatory parasites of the skin and gills. They are ~0.1-0.8 mm long and are best seen microscopically. The worms can be identified by their characteristic hold-fast organ, the haptor, which is armed with large and small hooks. Aquarium and cultured fish are subject to a rapid buildup of parasites by continuous infection and worm transfer to other fish in the tank or pond. Although many species are host-specific, the more common types seen in aquaria are less selective. The 2 most common genera are *Gyrodactylus* and *Dactylogyrus*. *Gyrodactylus* gives birth to live young, which can be seen within the body of the adult worm, and frequently are skin parasites; *Dactylogyrus* lays eggs and is principally a parasite of the gills. *Cleidodiscus* is an important monogene found on the gills of channel catfish. *Neobenedenia* and *Benedenia* are important monogeneans in marine fish. Infected fish show hyperactivity and erratic swimming, often flashing above the water surface or rubbing the sides of their bodies against an object in the aquarium to dislodge the worms. Fish become pale as colors fade. They breathe rapidly and distend their gill covers, exposing swollen, pale gills. Localized skin lesions appear with scattered hemorrhages and ulcerations. Mortality may be high. To prevent the disease, introduction of infected fish should be avoided. Formalin is often the treatment of choice for monogenean infestations. Multiple treatments at weekly intervals are recommended for *Dactylogyrus* because eggs may be resistant to chemical treatment. Organophosphates have been used successfully in nonfood fish but are not approved for this use. Trichlorfon (active ingredient) as a prolonged bath (0.25 mg/L) is effective. Organophosphates break down rapidly as pH and temperature rise, therefore slight increases in concentration may be necessary in marine systems. A bioassay is recommended if practitioners are uncertain how to proceed. Use of organophosphates in ponds may be restricted by federal or state environmental regulations. Monogenes on marine fish can be removed using freshwater dips for 1-5 min, depending on the tolerance of the species; however, eggs will not be damaged or removed. Trichlorfon can be used in marine systems, but some species are highly sensitive to it, particularly elasmobranchs. Increased ammonia levels should be anticipated after chemical application. Praziquantel (2 mg/L) has become the treatment of choice for monogenean infestations of aquarium fish, particularly marine species. The high cost of praziquantel is offset by excellent efficacy and target animal safety reported to date.

Digenean trematodes have complicated life cycles, with several larval stages that infect one or more hosts. With rare exceptions, the first intermediate host is a mollusc, without which the life cycle generally cannot be completed. A diagnosis usually can be established by gross or microscopic examinations that reveal the cercarial, metacercarial, or adult worms in any of the tissues or body cavities of the fish. Fish tend to form pigmented tissue encapsulations that encyst the parasites. Depending on the color of the cysts in the skin, the condition is called black, white, or yellow grub disease. Heavily parasitized fish often are weak, thin, inactive, and feed poorly. Treatment is not recommended.

Pond-reared, juvenile, tropical fish may develop severe gill disease from metacercarial cysts in gill tissue. Although acute death is occasionally seen, infected fish more commonly die during harvest or shipping when they may be exposed to suboptimal dissolved oxygen concentrations. Treatment of infected fish has not been successful; however, prevention of the disease by elimination of the intermediate host, a freshwater snail, has been effective. Snails can be controlled in fish ponds by applying a copper sulfate treatment at night when they are active. A molluscicide, Bayluscid®, is available as a restricted-use pesticide in some areas (eg, Puerto Rico, Florida) for control of aquatic snails. It cannot be applied to ponds containing live fish but is extremely effective in eliminating snails if applied 1-2 wk before stocking.

Bolbophorus confusus is a digenean trematode that has recently been reported to cause mortality in channel catfish fingerlings in production ponds in Mississippi, Louisiana, and Alabama. The definitive host of *B confusus* is the white pelican, and the first intermediate host is the ram's horn snail (*Heliosoma* spp). Cercariae released from snails encyst in fish tissue, forming metacercariae in any tissue, but the majority are found in skin and skeletal muscle of the peduncle of juvenile channel catfish. Severe disease occurs when metacercariae encyst in visceral organs, particularly the posterior kidney and liver. Involvement of these organs can result in a presentation similar to enteric septicemia or channel virus disease, characterized by fluid accumulation in the abdomen and exophthalmia. Skin and muscle lesions typically result in raised bumps that are white to reddish in color. Visceral involvement can result in high mortality (95%) of small fish. Heavy infestation of older fish may result in anorexia, lethargy, and loss of condition. Digenea in skeletal muscle can result in condemnation of affected carcasses by processing plants.

Ponds at greatest risk to *B confusus* are those frequented by white pelicans. Pelicans are federally protected; however, assistance for control of nuisance wildlife is available through Wildlife Services of the USDA. Snail control is an important part of an overall control strategy and requires a mix of chemical, biological and aquatic plant control strategies. Copper sulfate is effective against snails but will not penetrate when they are buried in mud or sealed into their shells. Treatment is likely to be most effective in summer and early fall when snails are actively feeding. Nocturnal application of copper sulfate has been helpful in ornamental fish ponds, but care must be taken not to precipitate an oxygen depletion by killing plants and algae. Bayluscide® may be labeled in some states for control of aquatic snails. Chemical control will not eliminate snails, and efforts should be augmented by control of aquatic weeds. Snails climb emergent vegetation to lay eggs, so eliminating vegetation can decrease reproduction. Finally, biologic control may be attempted using black carp; however, these are an exotic species and stocking is prohibited in many geographic areas. Red-ear sunfish are also known to eat snails, but their potential impact on snail populations has not been tested. Due to the complexity of this problem, and rapid generation of new information, practitioners are urged to consult with extension and other aquaculture specialists.

Both larval and adult tapeworms are common in fish. Larval forms encyst in visceral organs and muscle, while adults usually are found in the intestinal tract. Aquatic Crustacea are the most common intermediate host for fish; accordingly, wild and cultured pond fish may be heavily infected. *Diphyllobothrium latum*, the broad fish tapeworm infection of humans, is acquired by eating larval tapeworms in the flesh of food fish. Aquarium fish may be purchased with heavy cestode infections but have limited exposure once in

TABLE 10. Helminth Parasites of Fish [*]

	Parasites	Tissue	Susceptible species
Monogenes	*Gyrodactylus* (live bearer)	Skin, fins	Goldfish, koi (predisposed)
	Dactylogyrus (egg layer) *Cleidodiscus*	Gills	Goldfish, koi, AF, discus (predisposed), CCF
	Benedenia; Neobenedenia (egg layer)	Cornea, gills, skin	Marine tropicals, other marine species, marine AF (predisposed)
	Polyopisthocotylea	Gill	SB
Digenes (IH usually mollusc)	Heterophyidae	Gill	Redtail shark, black shark, rainbow shark, AF (FW), other pond-reared fish, aquarium fish
	Clinostomum	Skeletal muscle	LMB, centrarchids, HSB
	Bolbophorus confusus	Skeletal muscle, viscera	CCF
	Posthodiplostomum	Viscera, heart, posterior kidney	LMB, bluegill, centrarchids, salmonids, other fish
	Diplostomum	Eye (lens)	Fish are IH (unspecified species)
Cestodes	*Diphyllobothrium latum*	Viscera, musculature	Salmonids, other FW species
	Corallobothrium	Intestine (adult)	CCF
	Proteocephalus ambloplitis	Ovary (larval stage)	LMB
	Bothriocephalus acheilognathi	Intestine (adult)	Carp, aquarium fish
Acanthocephalids	*Acanthocephalus*	Intestine	Wild-caught salmonids, wild-caught marine fish
Nematodes (fish as DH)	*Capillaria*	Intestine	AF, discus, other aquarium fish
	Camillanus	Posterior intestine	LMB, other centrarchids
	Philometra	Posterior intestine	Aquarium fish
Nematodes (fish as IH)	*Eustrongylides*	Encysted in coelom	AF, other aquarium species
		Encysted in viscera	LMB, centrarchids
Leeches	Leech	Skin	FW game fish, aquarium fish

[*]CCF, channel catfish; AF, angelfish; SB; striped bass; LMB largemouth bass; HSB, hybrid striped bass; FW, freshwater; IH, intermediate host; DH, direct host; KMnO₄, Potassium permanganate

TABLE 10. *(continued)*

Signs	Diagnosis	Treatment
Excess mucus, flashing, weight loss	Wet mount	Formalin, $KMnO_4$, praziquantel (aquarium)
Piping, coughing, weight loss, skin lesions	Wet mount	Formalin, $KMnO_4$, praziquantel (aquarium)
Eye lesions, flashing, weight loss, mortality	Wet mount	Praziquantel (aquarium), FW dips (eggs remain in system)
Pale gills, piping, mortality	Wet mount	Formalin, FW dips
Flared gills, hypoxia, piping, do not tolerate shipping and handling	Wet mount	None; management—snail control in production ponds; minimize access of birds to fish ponds
Yellow grub	Direct visualization, wet mount	None; management—snail control in production ponds
None	Direct visualization, wet mount	None
None	Direct visualization, wet mount	None; management—as above is applicable
Cataracts, blindness	Direct visualization, histology	None
Adhesions, sterility (if gonads affected)	Direct visualization, wet mount	None
None	Direct visualization, wet mount	None in food animals
Sterility	Direct visualization, wet mount	None
Weight loss, enteritis, mortality	Direct visualization	Praziquantel (aquarium)
Enteritis, mortality	Direct visualization	None
Weight loss, pot belly	Direct visualization, wet mount	Fenbendazole, levamisole (aquarium)
Visualize worms protruding from anus	Direct visualization	None
Visualize worms protruding from anus	Direct visualization	Fenbendazole, levamisole (aquarium)
Weight loss, pot belly	Direct visualization	None
Often none	Direct visualization	None
Anemia, weight loss	Direct visualization	Organophosphates (aquarium, no effluent)

the aquarium (unless fed infected intermediate hosts). There is no safe, effective treatment for larval tapeworm infections. *Corallobothrium* spp are tapeworms occasionally found in the intestinal tract of channel catfish; however, their clinical significance is minimal. Larval migrations of the bass tapeworm, *Proteocephalus ambloplites*, have been associated with reproductive failure in free-ranging populations of largemouth bass. Although usually an incidental finding, heavy infestations of tapeworms have been associated with mechanical obstruction of the lumen of the gut. The Asian tapeworm, *Bothriocephalus acheilognathus*, is occasionally seen in carp and aquarium fish. It is usually found in the anterior intestine and may be associated with enteritis and degeneration of the intestinal wall. Praziquantel is the drug of choice for treatment of cestodes in fish, but it is not approved for any aquatic use. It can be applied as a bath (2 mg/L for prolonged immersion or 10 mg/L for 3 hr) or in a medicated food (50 mg/kg, 1 time).

Acanthocephala (thorny-headed worms) are common in wild fish as both larval tissue stages and adult intestinal parasites. They are more common in salmonid and marine fish. Arthropods are the first intermediate host. Adult acanthocephala are easily recognized by their protrusible proboscis, armed with many recurrent hooks.

Nematodes are common in wild fish that are exposed to the intermediate hosts. Fish may be definitive hosts for adult nematodes, or they may act as transport or intermediate hosts for larval nematode forms (anisakids, eustrongylids, and others) that infect higher vertebrate predators, including humans. Encysted or free nematodes can be found in almost any tissue or body cavity of fish. Aquarium and cultured pond fish may be heavily infected if crustacean intermediate hosts are present. *Cyclops* and *Daphnia* spp are common intermediate hosts for *Philometra* sp, a nematode that is pathogenic for guppies and other aquarium fish. These blood-red worms can be seen in the swollen abdominal cavity and protruding from the anus of affected fish (red worm disease). *Capillaria* spp are commonly found in aquaria fish, particularly freshwater angelfish. Heavy infections in juvenile angelfish have been associated with poor growth rates and an inability to withstand shipping and handling. Treatment with fenbendazole (25 mg/kg for 3 days) is recommended, but efficacy has not been firmly established. Levamisole (10 mg/L) administered as a bath treatment for 3 days has also been recommended. Ivermectin is highly toxic to aquarium fish, particularly cichlids, and its use is not recommended.

Leeches are parasitic bloodsuckers of fish and also serve as vectors for blood parasites of fish (eg, *Trypanosoma, Cryptobia*, and haemogregarines). They can produce a debilitating anemia due to chronic blood loss and disease. Leech infestations are most common in wild fish, but aquarium and pond infestations can occur by introduction of infested fish, plants, etc. Trichlorfon (0.25-1 ppm in aquarium water, use higher dosages at higher pH) is effective but is not approved for use in food fish, and environmental regulations may restrict its use in outdoor ponds. Multiple treatments may be required because eggs are resilient and juveniles may continue to hatch. Preventive measures include avoiding leeches (ie, effective quarantine) and depopulating infested aquarium fish. Infestations in recreational fishing ponds are often self-limiting.

Copepods

Some copepods, during specific stages of their complicated life cycle, are obligatory parasites of finfish. They lose their copepod form, including their appendages, and become rod- or sac-like structures specifically adapted for piercing, holding, feeding, and reproducing. Grossly, they appear as barb-like attachments to the skin or gills, where they feed on blood and tissue fluids. They can cause hemorrhage, anemia, and tissue destruction, as well as provide a portal of entry for other pathogens. Many different species of these parasites can be found on freshwater and marine fish. The anchor worms, *Laernea* spp, are commonly found in a wide variety of aquarium- and pond-reared fish, including goldfish and other cyprinids. *Ergasilus* spp infest the gills.

Lice (*Branchiuria*) are related to the parasitic copepods and have flattened bodies adapted for rapid movement over the skin surface. By means of hooks and suckers, they periodically attach for feeding by inserting the piercing mouth part (stylet) into the skin.

Sea lice (*Lepeophtheirus salmonis*) are a significant disease problem of pen-reared salmonids which can be treated with hydrogen peroxide. *Argulus* spp are lice commonly found on aquarium, pond-reared, and wild fish. Trichlorfon at 0.25 ppm of aquarium water is the drug of choice for treating infested aquarium fish but is not approved for use in food fish. Infested fish should not be introduced.

BACTERIAL DISEASES

Epidemics of bacterial diseases are common in dense populations of cultured food or aquarium fish. Predisposition to such outbreaks frequently is associated with poor water quality, organic loading of the aquatic environment, handling and transport of fish, marked temperature changes, hypoxia, and related stressful conditions. High concentrations of waterborne bacteria are normally found in ponds and aquaria. Many of these bacteria are opportunistic facultative pathogens, which are activated by an adverse environment, a debilitated host, or a primary pathogen. In sharp contrast, obligatory bacterial pathogens of finfish require the presence of fish for replication and are unable to survive alone for long in the aquatic environment.

Most bacterial pathogens of fish are aerobic gram-negative rods. Diagnosis is by isolating the organism in pure culture from infected tissues and identifying the bacterial agent.

Some of the most common bacterial infections that are associated with stressful conditions in freshwater systems are *Aeromonas hydrophila*, *A sobria*, and *Pseudomonas* spp. These opportunistic organisms frequently cause disease in freshwater fish, usually under warmwater conditions, although all species are susceptible. They produce very similar clinical syndromes, sometimes referred to as **hemorrhagic septicemia**. Nutritional deficiencies, traumatic injuries, parasitism, and sharp seasonal temperature changes appear to be predisposing factors. The acute form is characterized by signs of a septicemic infection with external reddening, and hemorrhages are found in the peritoneum, body wall, and viscera. Control is based on removal of predisposing factors. If antibiotic therapy is warranted, the drug selection should be based on sensitivity testing when possible.

Aeromonas salmonicida is a gram-negative, nonmotile, rod originally described as the cause of a septicemic disease of salmonids (**furunculosis**) and goldfish (**ulcer disease**). It is also a pathogen of many other freshwater and marine fishes and may produce high mortality. *A salmonicida* is a very important disease of koi and fancy goldfish, and is of particular concern in imported specimens. In the acute form, hemorrhages are found in the fins, tail, muscles, gills, and internal organs. In more chronic forms, focal areas of swelling, hemorrhage, and tissue necrosis develop in the muscles. These lesions progress to crateriform abscesses that discharge from the skin surface (furuncles). Liquefactive necrosis occurs in the spleen and kidney. Diagnosis is made by isolating and identifying a pure culture of the organism from infected tissue. Avoidance through use of good quarantine practices, and vaccination when appropriate, is preferable to treatment. Vaccination is available for koi, but information on efficacy is limited. Successful treatment is possible, based on appropriate antibiotic therapy. Blood culture (*see* p 1480) is an effective and nonlethal method for effective identification and sensitivity testing of *A salmonicida* isolates from valuable koi. Prevention and control of *A salmonicida* in fish and eggs is also of concern to the salmonid industry. Fish and fish eggs should be obtained from disease-free sources. Eyed fish eggs can be treated for 10-15 min in a solution containing iodine at 100 mg/L at a pH of 7 and a temperature of 10-15°C, although the drug is not approved for use on food-fish eggs. Eggs should be rinsed immediately after treatment. Antibiotic treatment should be based on results of sensitivity testing. Commercial vaccines are available for prevention of *A salmonicida* in salmonids.

Vibriosis is a potentially serious, common systemic disease of many cultured, aquarium, and wild marine and estuarine fishes; it is less common in freshwater fish. *Vibrio anguillarium* and other *Vibrio* spp are responsible for the disease, which produces systemic manifestations, including hemorrhages and ulcerations of the skin, fin, and tail, and hemorrhagic and degenerative changes of internal organs. Diagnosis requires identification of pure isolates from infected tissues. Isolation of *V cholera* from fish is not uncommon and should not cause alarm as long as the isolate is the non-O type. Preventive measures include minimizing stress and crowding. Coldwater vibriosis (Hitra disease), a serious problem in sea farming of salmonids, is characterized by high mortality, resistance to drug therapy, and stress mediation. The etiologic agent is *V salmonicida*. Because *Vibrio* spp are ubiquitous in marine environments, avoidance is difficult. Preventive vaccination with formalin-killed *Vibrio* is used in the salmonid industry. Antibiotic therapy should be based on results of sensitivity testing.

Yersiniosis (enteric redmouth disease) is a serious acute or chronic bacterial disease of intensively cultured salmonids. The etiologic agent is *Yersinia ruckeri*. Signs are darkening and hemorrhage of the mouth (red mouth), skin, anus, and fins. Chronic signs are associated with inappetence, exophthalmos, and swelling and degenerative changes of internal organs. Mortality rates are variable but are exacerbated by poor water quality and related stressors. Diagnosis is by isolation and identification of pure cultures of the organism obtained from the internal organs of infected fish. Fish that survive remain carriers and may cyclically shed bacteria, particularly when exposed to stressful conditions and water temperatures of 15-18°C. Depopulation of infected fish and avoidance of introduction of infected fish can be recommended, but preventive vaccination is the usual procedure in endemic areas. Yersiniosis can be treated successfully with antibiotics, which should be selected based on a sensitivity test. Therapy should be continued for at least 14 days.

Edwardsiella ictaluri causes **enteric septicemia of catfish**, the most important infectious disease in the channel catfish industry. Infection occurs in the spring and fall when water temperatures are 22-28°C, and mortality may be exacerbated by handling stress, chemical treatment, or poor water quality. The disease occurs in 2 forms—the enteric (or intestinal) form and the meningeal form. In the enteric form, infected fish may develop skin lesions characterized by massive petechial hemorrhage around the mouth, operculum, and eyes, or they may develop measles-like red punctate lesions along the body wall. There is a hemorrhagic enteritis, and the intestine may be hemorrhagic and fluid- or gas-filled. Liver lesions are common and may be evident as multifocal areas of necrosis, abcessation, or hemorrhage. In contrast, in the meningeal form, few external signs may be seen in infected fish. The bacteria enter the CNS through the olfactory system, and affected fish develop severe meningitis. In fingerlings, the inflammation may be severe enough to erode the skull, resulting in the characteristic "hole-in-the-head" lesion. Fish affected with the meningeal form may demonstrate bizarre behavior, including spinning, erratic swimming, and general disorientation. Diagnosis is based on bacterial culture and isolation. Brain culture is indicated whenever *E ictaluri* is suspected. *E ictaluri* will grow on blood agar incubated at 25°C for 48 hr. Antibiotic therapy should be based on results of sensitivity testing. Oral vaccination is available for channel catfish fingerlings.

Edwardsiella tarda causes intestinal disease in a variety of aquatic and terrestrial organisms, including fish, reptiles, and mammals (including humans). In catfish, this bacterium causes a disease referred to as **emphysematous putrefactive disease of catfish**, descriptive of the characteristic malodorous, gaseous lesions. Infection is usually limited to 5-10% of the population, and mortality is chronic. Clinically, affected fish may be unable to swim normally because of abnormal buoyancy created by gas-filled lesions in the skeletal musculature. When lesions burst, they are extremely malodorous. *E tarda* has been reported in freshwater and marine aquaria across a fairly wide temperature range, and in free-ranging largemouth bass. Clinical signs include significant ulceration of skin as well as systemic disease. Overall mortality rates are generally low, usually <5%. The organism is easily isolated using blood agar incubated at 25°C for 24 hr. Antibiotic treatment based on results of sensitivity testing is effective.

The order Cytophogales (Myxobacterales, slime bacteria, fish slime bacteria) includes an important group of opportunistic pathogens of fish that are common inhabitants of soil and water. The gram-negative, rod or filamentous bacteria have a distinctive gliding motion and form palisading masses on infected tissue. Skin or gill lesions have slimy or cotton-like surface exudates, which usually cover surface necrosis, ulcerations, and marginal hemorrhages. *Flavobacterium columnaris*, the member of this group responsible for **columnaris disease** (cottonmouth disease, saddleback), is most common in warm water and warmwater species of fish. A presumptive diagnosis can be made from visualization of typical myxobacteria on wet mounts of infected skin or gill tissue. If the disease is diagnosed early in the course of infection, a treatment with potassium permanganate may be efficacious. If the disease becomes chronic, it may have become systemic, in which case treatment with oxytetracycline for 10 days is recommended. Columnaris disease can be confirmed by isolation of the organism on Ordal's or other cytophage media. Sensitivity tests are difficult to perform because *F columnaria* will not grow on Müller-Hinton media. Columnaris disease can be prevented by reducing organic loading and avoiding traumatic injuries. *Cytophaga psychrophila* causes coldwater (peduncle) disease and fin and tail rot. It most commonly infects coldwater fish but can be found in warmwater fish subjected to low temperatures. The lesions are especially common on the dorsal, posterior surface of the fish under the dorsal fin but may be found on any part of the body. Advanced cases show necrosis and ulceration of the peduncle. Both *Flavobacterium* and *Cytophaga* infections can be controlled by oxytetracycline.

Bacterial gill disease is a disease complex most frequently reported in young cultured salmonids or fish cultured under conditions of high organic loading. It has been seen occasionally in aquarium fish. It may be initiated by crowding and poor water quality, particularly high organic loads, high ammonia levels, and silt. Although bacteria in the genera *Flavobacteria* have been implicated as the cause, the association is still somewhat tentative. Opportunistic bacteria, including *Aeromonas* and *Pseudomonas* spp, may follow as secondary invaders of traumatized gill tissue. Signs of the disease are related to respiratory embarrassment due to impaired gill function. Gills appear swollen and mottled, with patchy areas of bacterial growth that can be confirmed by microscopic examination of direct gill smears. Hyperplasia, adhesions, and deformity of the gill lamellae can be seen. In young fish affected with the disease, mortality is high and morbidity sustained. Prevention efforts include improving water quality and avoiding overstocking. A single treatment with potassium permanganate, followed by addition of salt to the system (0.02-0.5%), depending on species and type of system, may be beneficial in controlling losses, but sanitation is critical for long-term resolution of the problem. Antibiotic therapy may be used as needed to control secondary bacterial problems.

Bacterial kidney disease (corynebacterial kidney disease) is economically important in cultured salmonids. The cause is *Renibacterium salmoninarum*, an obligate intracellular parasite that is one of the few gram-positive organisms that causes disease in fish. Clinically, infected fish appear lethargic and darkened. Typical lesions include grayish, localized, or conglomerate granulomata in the viscera, especially the kidney or body wall; exophthalmos; blindness; and emaciation. A presumptive diagnosis can be based on visualization of small gram-positive rods in kidney imprints. Definitive diagnosis requires isolation and identification of the bacteria by using a selective medium that contains cysteine and incubating at 15°C for 3-6 wk. *R salmoninarum* is transmitted both horizontally and vertically, and fish that survive an epizootic remain carriers. Infected female fish should be injected with erythromycin (11-20 mg/kg, IM) 14-60 days before spawning to prevent vertical transmission. Erythromycin (100 mg/kg for 10-21 days) is efficacious when administered in feed early in the course of an outbreak; however, it is not FDA approved for this use. Obtaining disease-free stock and preventing contamination by infected wild fish are the best preventive measures.

Gram positive bacteria of concern to fish culturists and aquarists include *Streptococcus* and related genera, *Lactococcus*, *Enterococcus*, and *Vagococcus*. Infections caused by these organisms are uncommon but can cause significant mortality (>50%) when they do occur. Chronic infections may continue for weeks, with only a few fish dying each day. Species known to be susceptible include salmonids, assorted marine fish (eg, mullet, sea bass), tilapia, sturgeon, and striped bass. Susceptible aquarium species include rainbow sharks, red-tailed black sharks, rosey barbs, danios, and some tetras and cichlids. In general, all fish should be considered susceptible. A characteristic manifestation of

Streptococcus infection is neurologic disease, often manifest by spinning or spiraling in the water column. Brain and kidney cultures from suspect fish should be incubated on blood agar at 25°C for 24-48 hr. Gram stains of pinpoint bacterial colonies reveal typical chains of gram-positive cocci, which allows a presumptive diagnosis. Confirmation requires definitive identification of the organism. Antibiotic therapy should be based on sensitivity testing. Erythromycin is often the drug of choice but it is not FDA approved for this use. Mortality should cease within 48 hr of treatment with the correct antibiotic if complicating factors are not present. If fish are anorectic, therapy may be difficult because erythromycin does not absorb well when administered as a bath. Sources of infection may be environmental or include live foods, such as tubifex worms, amphibians, or previously infected fish. Future epizootics can be prevented if the source of infection is identified and eliminated.

Streptococcus iniae has been reported to cause disease in fish and mammals, including humans. In aquaculture, it is encountered most frequently in the intensive culture of tilapia and hybrid striped bass. Human cases have been reported rarely; in several cases individuals developed *S iniae* infection after handling raw fish, primarily tilapia, with open wounds on their hands. Most affected individuals had significant predisposing disease. The most common problem reported was cellulitis, and infections resolved following antibiotic therapy. When *Streptococcus* is isolated from aquatic species, a subculture of the organism should be sent to a laboratory that can determine whether or not it is *S iniae*. If confirmed, at-risk personnel should be restricted from handling infected fish.

Mycobacteriosis is a chronic or acute, systemic, granulomatous disease that occurs in aquarium fish and cultured food fish, particularly those reared under intensive conditions. Predisposing environmental factors include low dissolved oxygen, low pH, and high organic load, all of which are found in recirculating aquaculture systems. The causative bacteria can be any number of species of *Mycobacterium*, including *M piscium*, *M marinum*, and *M fortuitum*. These gram-positive, acid-fast, nonmotile bacteria are difficult to grow but can be isolated using Lowenstein-Jensen media following incubation at 25°C for 3-4 wk. Signs are variable and often resemble those of other diseases, including emaciation, ascites, skin ulceration and hemorrhages, exophthalmos, paleness, and skeletal deformities. On necropsy, gross lesions of viscera consist of grayish white, necrotic foci that sometimes coalesce to form tumor-like masses. A presumptive diagnosis is based on visualization of acid-fast rods in granulomatous material from suspect lesions. Definitive diagnosis requires isolating and identifying the bacteria. Because the disease can produce skin lesions and an allergic dermatitis in humans, and because treatment does not eliminate the disease, infected fish are usually destroyed. Aquarists should be informed of potential risks if handling or cleaning contaminated fish or exhibits. An aquarium should be disinfected before other fish are added. Mycobacteria are not always killed by bleach; disinfection with alcohol or phenolic compounds is recommended.

Piscirickettsia salmonis has been described in salmonid species from Chile, Norway, Ireland, and Canada. Rickettsial-like organisms have been reported in tilapia, sea bass, and blue-eyed plecostomus. It is unclear whether organisms reported in different groups of fish are separate species. Of the salmonid species, coho salmon seem to be the most susceptible. These organisms do not appear to be a zoonotic threat as they do not seem able to survive at mammalian body temperatures. Rickettsial disease can result in acute mortality affecting up to 95% of fish with few gross signs. In tilapia, acute mortality events may be triggered by sudden drops in temperature. Chronic disease is manifest by nonspecific external lesions including anorexia, pale gills, and skin lesions. Internally, lesions are more typical, with granulomatous lesions possible throughout the viscera. The most characteristic lesions may be found in liver and kidney tissue, and have been described as gray to yellow mottled areas with ring-shaped foci. Histologically, intracellular organisms may be seen in macrophages and hematopoietic tissue in the liver, spleen, and kidney. Blood or tissue smears stained with Giemsa or acridine orange may reveal the intracellular organisms, often appearing as paired, curved gram-negative rods in macrophages or hepatocytes. Rickettsia-like organisms can be isolated using a variety of cell lines; however, confirmation of a suspect case may also be based on serology. Transmission of rickettsial-like diseases in fish is not understood. In terrestrial species a vector is often required; however, *R salmonis* has been demonstrated to survive for 14 days in sea water, suggesting that horizontal transmission in the absence of vectors may be possible in aquatic species. Antibiotic control of these organisms appeared promising from in vitro work, but in vivo studies have not been as successful. It may be that intracellular organisms are sequestered from antibiotics.

Many other less commonly recognized bacterial diseases have been described in fish. These include pasteurellosis, *Haemophilus piscium* infection (ulcer disease), *Eubacterium* infection (fish meningitis), and others. Diagnosis of these diseases requires isolation and identification of the specific bacterial agent.

MYCOTIC DISEASES

Aquatic fungi often are considered secondary tissue invaders that follow traumatic injuries, infectious agents, or environmental insults such as poor water quality. Because many fungi grow on decaying organic matter, they are especially common in the aquatic environment. Fish egg masses, which usually contain tissue debris and dead ova or embryos, are especially vulnerable. Iodophors of varying iodine concentrations are used to prevent mycotic infections of nonfood-fish eggs, which can be disinfected by a 100 ppm iodine bath for 10-15 min. This solution is toxic for hatched fish, and only eggs should be treated. Formaldehyde, up to 2,000 ppm for 15 min, can be used to treat eggs of food fish (salmonid and esocid) for the control of fungi. Chronic fungal infections of eggs may suggest improper incubation temperature or poor sanitation.

Saprolegnia infections are among the most common fungal infections of fish and fish eggs. Gross signs are grayish white, cotton-like growths on the skin, gills, eyes, or fins that may invade deeper tissues of the body. Microscopically, saprolegniasis can be recognized by making direct smears from the infected tissues and observing the nonseptate hyphal elements and mycelia. The sexual stages of the fungus can be seen only in cultures of the organism and are required for specific identification. Sabaroud's dextrose agar is acceptable for primary isolation of oomycetes, including the genera *Saprolegnia*. Preventive measures include removal of predisposing causes, eg, inadequate sanitation, excessive chemical treatment, or the presence of dead, infected fish and decaying organic material. If the environment is clean and skin pathogens have been eliminated, a single treatment with potassium permanganate is often adequate to control external saprolegniasis.

Ichthyophonus hoferi causes an internal fungal infection. It is occasionally seen in wild fish as well as in aged cultured and aquarium fish. The disease is generally chronic and progressive. It usually is detected on necropsy when the characteristic spherical cyst stages are seen microscopically in the smears of granulomatous lesions of the heart, liver, spleen, kidney, skin, and muscle. Lordosis and scoliosis are occasionally seen in infected rainbow trout. Culture of suspect lesions is recommended, and Sabaroud's dextrose agar is acceptable for primary isolation. Preventive measures include removing infected fish and avoiding feeding raw fish products.

Branchiomycosis is a fungal disease of gill tissue characterized by respiratory distress and gill necrosis. The causative agents are *Branchiomyces sanguinis* and *B demigrans*, which are opportunistic pathogens found in decaying organic materials in the aquatic environment. Branchiomycosis typically occurs in warm ponds (water temperature >20°C) with high organic loads. It seems endemic in eastern Europe, where it is an important problem in food fish industries; it is also occasionally reported in the USA. Affected fish show signs typical of hypoxia. Gross examination of gills reveals necrotic, mottled, and pale tissue. A presumptive diagnosis can be made by observation of characteristic aseptate, branched hyphae in gill lamellae. Branchiomycosis is prevented by avoiding predisposing conditions. Ponds that are at risk should be kept as clean as possible, and stocking rates decreased when water temperatures approach 20°C.

Many other less common mycotic infections have been reported in fish, including infections with *Achyla, Aphanomyces, Dermocystidium, Ichthyosporidium, Basid-*

iobolus, Phoma, Candida, Cladosporium, Fusarium, Penicillium, Ichthyochytrium spp, and others. *Fusarium* is emerging as an important disease of captive marine fish, particularly elasmobranchs. Many of these organisms have questionable status as fungi, and laboratory culture of their complete life cycle is required for accurate diagnosis.

VIRAL DISEASES

Descriptions of viral diseases of fish are rapidly expanding. Viruses are being reported in new species and interpretation of the significance of findings is also changing. The OIE lists 5 viral diseases of fish as notifiable: epizootic hematopoietic necrosis, infectious hematopoietic necrosis, spring viremia of carp, viral hemorrhagic septicemia, and *Oncorhynchus masou* virus. In the USA, these diseases should be reported to the USDA. Infectious salmon anemia is not listed as notifiable by the OIE in the 2002 edition of the International Aquatic Animal Health Code; however, it is considered a reportable disease in the USA. Sources for current information on regulatory requirements for aquatic species include the OIE, USDA, state veterinarian offices, state departments of agriculture, and university extension veterinary aquaculture specialists.

While viruses of homeothermic animals are cultured at uniform temperatures, fish viruses have wider, but specific, temperature tolerances in fish cell cultures at lower temperatures. Because of this relatively defined temperature range, variation in temperature may enable control, although often it merely induces latency. Because many viral diseases of fish are geographically limited, regulatory agencies and fish farms in disease-free areas consider them as exotic diseases and require certification of introduced stocks. Many produce high mortality in young fish and little or no losses in adults, which may become carriers. For these reasons, avoidance of carriers and certification of SPF replacement stocks are frequently required. Specific testing procedures are available. Vaccines are not yet commercially available for viral diseases of fish. Drugs are not effective, although antibiotics and other drugs may be used to control secondary bacterial infections that frequently follow viral diseases. Management techniques that minimize stress and crowding, biosecurity measures, and temperature manipulation hold the greatest promise for control of many piscine viral diseases.

Herpesviruses: Channel catfish virus (CCV) disease is an acute, virulent herpesvirus infection of fry and fingerling channel catfish that can cause mortality of >80% at water temperatures ≥25°C in small fish (≤5 cm). As fish age, mortality decreases, and clinical infection in fish >1 yr old is rare. Acute infection often includes a recent history of a stressful event such as handling or transport, low dissolved oxygen, or chemical treatment. Infected fish show signs of ascites, exophthalmos, and hemorrhages in fins. The cell line of choice for virus isolation is channel catfish ovary, followed by serum neutralization to confirm identification. Typical cytopathic effects include cell fusion, syncytia formation, and intranuclear inclusions. There is evidence for vertical transmission of CCV; consequently, survivors of an epizootic should not be used for broodstock. Although CCV can cause severe mortality when an outbreak is in progress, the annual number of cases of CCV in the catfish industry is relatively low.

Herpesvirus disease of salmonids has been subdivided into 2 types, HPV-1 and HPV-2, based on serology and DNA homology. HPV-1 has been isolated from salmonids in the western USA only, from ovarian fluid of moribund rainbow trout, from steelhead trout dying of other causes, and experimentally from chinook salmon. Signs of HPV-1 in prespawning rainbow trout included darkening and fluid accumulation, as evidenced by exophthalmos, ascites, and edema of visceral organs and skeletal muscle. A presumptive diagnosis is based on observation of the typical herpesvirus cytopathic effect, including giant cell formation and Cowdry Type A inclusion bodies, in salmonid cell lines. Confirmation requires serum neutralization. HPV-2, previously referred to as *Oncorhynchus masou* virus, refers to a group of salmonid herpesviruses from Japan, all of which are oncogenic except for one strain, NeTVA. These viruses are on the list of 5 fish diseases categorized as notifiable by the OIE. HPV-2 has been isolated from masou, kokanee, coho, and chum salmon, and experimentally from rainbow trout. The virus was initially isolated in 1978 from ovarian fluid of clinically normal masou salmon that were producing fry with poor survival rates. Fish with clinical disease may be lethargic and anorectic. Darkening and petechiation of the body wall may be evident. Tumorigenic strains result in development of epitheliomas on fins or mandibles of survivors. A presumptive diagnosis is made from observation of the typical herpesvirus cytopathic effect on salmonid cell lines. Confirmation requires serum neutralization.

Herpesvirus disease of turbot is a disease of wild and cultured turbot that causes massive hypertrophy and fusion of epithelial cells of the skin and gills of young fish. Mortality is associated with heavy gill infections and poor water quality. High levels of oxygenation are essential for fish with respiratory distress. Diagnosis is by examination of skin scrapings or histologic sections for the characteristic fusion of giant cells.

A recently described herpesvirus has been blamed for serious disease in koi, with mortality rates reported to reach 100%. The disease is characterized by severe necrosis of gill epithelium. Affected fish are lethargic and show signs of respiratory distress, eg, piping and laying near inflows of oxygenated water. Grossly, copious mucus secretion may be noted on the gills and skin, and gross necrosis of gill tissue may be evident. Presumptive diagnosis of koi herpesvirus may be based on histologic evidence of epithelial necrosis of gill tissue and possible intranuclear inclusions. Transmission electron microscopy should demonstrate herpesvirus particles within inclusions. Laboratory tests to confirm the diagnosis are not currently available. Currently, koi affected with systemic herpesvirus infection should be destroyed and contaminated facilities disinfected.

Carp pox is one of the oldest recognized fish diseases. It is caused by cyprinid herpesvirus-1. Pox lesions may occur on other species of fish, and are sometimes referred to as fish pox. Lesions typically are smooth and raised and may have a milky appearance. They are benign, non-necrotizing areas of epidermal hyperplasia. Severe cases may result in development of papillomatous growths, and these may be a site of complicating bacterial infection. Generally, lesions are self-limiting and of minimal clinical significance. Carp pox can be a significant problem with koi because the aesthetic quality, and hence the market value, of the animal is severely compromised. For the serious koi enthusiast, carp pox-affected fish should be culled, preferably during quarantine. Surgical removal of pox lesions has not been rewarding.

Rhabdoviruses: Infectious hematopoietic necrosis is caused by a rhabdovirus and is endemic in salmonid (*Oncorhynchus* spp) populations in the Pacific Northwest and Alaska. The disease is listed as notifiable by the OIE. Disease has been reported in Atlantic, chum, chinook, sockeye, and kokanee salmon and in cutthroat, steelhead, and rainbow trout. Lake trout and Arctic char, members of the genus *Salvelinus*, appear resistant. Experimental infection of nonsalmonid fish demonstrated mortality of 43% and 87%, respectively, in sea bream and turbot. Infectious hematopoietic necrosis has also been isolated from leeches, parasitic copepods, and mayflies. Sporadic epizootics have been reported in several states in the USA and in Japan, Italy, France, Taiwan, Belgium, and Korea. Most epizootics have been attributed to importation of infected eggs or fry. Acute disease in fry <2 mo may result in high mortality (>90%) with few external signs. Disease usually occurs at water temperatures of 10-12°C, although outbreaks occasionally occur at temperatures >15°C. Typical signs include lethargy with sporadic hyperexcitability, including whirling. Sick fish may be darkened with distended abdomens, exophthalmia, pale gills, and mucoid fecal casts. Important differential diagnoses include infectious pancreatic necrosis and viral hemorrhagic septicemia. Hematopoietic tissue in the kidney and spleen are most severely affected by necrosis. Risk factors include age (fish <2 mo are most susceptible), density, and water temperature. Hauling young fish around dams in trucks may be a significant risk factor because of crowding during transit. Although most disease outbreaks have been reported in freshwater, active disease has occurred in Atlantic salmon housed in sea cages. Diagnosis is by viral isolation (from kidney and spleen of young fish and ovarian fluid of broodstock), with confirmation by serum neutralization. Rapid serologic tests have been developed and are becoming more available. A nonlethal test involving viral isolation from mucus has been reported. The disease is transmitted horizontally through the water, and vertical transmission seems likely. There is some controversy as to whether the virus is present on the outside of the egg or within the egg, as disinfection with iodophors (100 mg/L) seems to stop >99% of vertical transmission. Asymptomatic carrier fish serve as reservoirs of infection.

Viral hemorrhagic septicemia, the most important viral disease affecting cultured rainbow trout in Europe, is caused by a rhabdovirus in the family rhabdoviridae. The disease is believed to have spread to Europe >100 years ago when rainbow trout were first imported from the USA. The disease causes marked necrosis of hematopoietic tissue in the kidney, particularly the anterior kidney, but largely spares excretory tubules in the posterior kidney. In addition to rainbow trout, brook and lake trout (genus *Salvelinus*), and Atlantic salmon and brown and golden trout (genus *Salmo*) are susceptible. The virus also causes disease in a variety of freshwater and marine coldwater fish including pike, turbot, white fish, and sea bass. New information indicates that viral hemorrhagic septicemia is found in free-ranging marine fish in the Pacific Northwest including anadromous salmon (coho and chinook) as well as haddock and cod in the North Sea. The disease occurs in 3 forms—acute, chronic, and nervous. Acute mortalities occur in rainbow trout fry <3 g and <30 days old. In these fish, the kidney is swollen and the anterior segment is necrotic and pale. The liver may be pale with hemorrhagic mottling, and systemic hemorrhage may be visible in the eyes, skin, skeletal muscle, and viscera. The most notable lesion is widespread hemorrhage in the liver, adipose tissue, and within skeletal muscle. Moribund fish lie on the bottom of the tank and may exhibit sporadic flashing and corkscrew swimming behavior. As fish age, mortalities drop from 80-100% to 10-50%. The chronic form is a persistent infection characterized by the ability to isolate virus from all tissues and low red and white blood cell counts. Chronically infected fish may exhibit few visible external signs. The nervous form of the disease has been reported primarily in cultured freshwater fish but was recently reported in marine fish. The optimal temperature for active infection is 9-12°C; the virus is unable to replicate at temperatures >15°C. The cell line of choice for virus isolation is bluegill fry (BF-2). Viral identification is confirmed by serum neutralization. Newer diagnostic tests include immunofluorescence, ELISA, and PCR. Viral hemorrhagic septicemia is a heavily regulated disease with disease-free geographic regions defined in Europe. No vaccine is commercially available.

Spring viremia of carp (SVC) is an acute, virulent, usually hemorrhagic disease of cultured carp caused by Rhabdovirus carpio. The disease is listed as notifiable by the OIE. Historically, it was reported in Europe and the former USSR; however, an outbreak in the USA was confirmed in the spring of 2002. SVC causes disease in common carp, including koi, as well as grass, bighead, silver, and crucian carp. Limited experience suggests that common goldfish may be susceptible. Clinical signs are nonspecific and may include darkening of the skin, exophthalmia, ascites, pale gills, hemorrhage, and a protruding vent with thick mucoid fecal casts. Pinpoint hemorrhage in the swim bladder is indicative of SVC, if present. Coinfection with *Aeromonas* or other systemic bacteria may obscure the presence of the virus and is referred to as carp-dropsy complex. The bacterial component of the infection can be controlled with antibiotics. The disease causes death in both adult and young fish. Affected fish may lie on their sides on the bottom of the tank, lose motor control, have ascites, and show petechiation of the skin, gills, and visceral mass. Clinical disease may be controlled by raising water temperature >22°C; maximum mortality can be expected at temperatures <18°C. The virus is readily isolated in common fish cell lines and identified by serum neutralization and fluorescent antibody tests.

Pike fry rhabdovirus disease is an acute hemorrhagic infection of young northern pike, thus far known only in Europe. Affected fry have pale gills, exophthalmos, and hydrocephalus. Kidney tubules show degeneration and necrosis. The causal agent is readily isolated in a variety of cell cultures. Identification is by serum neutralization.

Infectious pancreatic necrosis is an acute, systemic, contagious disease of salmonid fry and fingerlings cause by a birnavirus. The virus is the archetype of the aquatic birnaviruses, which are further subdivided into 2 serotypes, A and B, that do not crossreact using serum neutralization. The Serotype B group currently consists of only 10 isolates, all European in origin. In contrast, the A serotype contains >200 isolates that have been further subdivided into 9 serotypes, A_1-A_9. Morbidity and mortality occur only in young animals, usually <3 g; however, virus can be isolated from survivors for the duration of their lives resulting in a persistent carrier state. Recrudescence of disease in survivors has not been reported. The virus is vertically and horizontally transmitted, widespread, and reported worldwide, except in Iceland and Australia. Rainbow trout are highly susceptible to disease. In the USA, striped bass and their hybrids are recognized as potential carriers. Other species affected include freshwater eels (*Anguilla* spp), yellowtail, turbot, sea bass, and menhaden, as well as aquatic invertebrates including molluscs and crustaceans. Brook trout are believed to be reservoirs of infection in the USA. Clinical infection is nonspecific. Diseased fish may be anorectic, ataxic, and display a corkscrew swimming pattern. Externally, fish are darkened; exophthalmia and external petechiation may be evident. Internally, petechiae may be visible on viscera; the gut is typically empty and may contain a yellow exudate. Fecal pseudocysts may be evident in the water column. Histologically, focal areas of coagulative necrosis involve acinar and islet cells of the pancreas and hematopoietic cells of the kidney. Intracytoplasmic viral inclusions may be visible in pancreatic acinar cells. Infection should be confirmed with viral isolation followed by serum neutralization. Most fish cell lines are susceptible. The virus can also be identified using fluorescent antibody, complement fixation, and ELISA techniques. There is no treatment for infected fish, but avoidance can be accomplished by purchase of SPF stocks, quarantine, and disinfection of eggs with iodophores (20-50 mg/L). Infectious pancreatic necrosis is not regulated by the USDA, but state regulations do exist in various parts of the country.

Iridoviruses: Lymphocystis disease is a unique, typically chronic, viral infection of wild or captive marine and freshwater fish. The causal agent is an icosahedral DNA virus ~300 nm in diameter, of the Iridoviridae family. Infection may be manifest by benign cauliflower-like lesions typically located on fins. The disease affects a wide range of fish and is generally considered global. Within the aquarium trade, painted glass fish are commonly infected. Presumptive diagnosis is based on the presence of enlarged fibroblasts (up to 1 mm), which are easily visualized with a light microscope. Microscopic examination typically reveals the appearance of grape-like clusters of virus-laden cells. Diagnosis is confirmed histologically. Feulgen-positive cytoplasmic inclusions and a hypertrophied nucleus are pathognomonic. The disease is usually self-limiting but is of aesthetic concern.

Viral erythrocytic necrosis is an OIE-notifiable disease. It has been reported in >20 species of marine and anadromous fish (both cultured and free ranging) and is characterized by erythrocytic degeneration. Affected species include Pacific herring, Atlantic cod, and Pacific salmonids (chum, pink, coho, and chinook), steelhead trout, and cultured eels in Taiwan. The disease is chronic, and external signs may be subtle or nonexistent. Sick fish are anemic, which may result in pale gills and internal organs. Severity of the disease is related to age and species of fish, with juveniles <1 g most severely affected. The characteristic lesion is a single eosinophilic cytoplasmic inclusion body in the circulating erythrocytes of anemic fish. The inclusions are best visualized from Giemsa-stained fresh blood smears. Transmission electron microscopy has demonstrated hexagonal virus particles, presumptively classified as an iridovirus, in the cytoplasm of cells containing inclusions. To date, the agent has not been successfully isolated. Histologically, increased hematopoietic activity may be evident in the kidney, and round cytoplasmic inclusions (0.8-4 μm) are found in circulating RBC. Inclusions stain pink or magenta with Giemsa. Other degenerative changes may be evident in RBC, including cytoplasmic vacuolation and margination of nuclear chromatin. Hemolytic anemia with concurrent hemosiderosis and erythroblastosis has been reported in moribund Pacific herring. Multinucleated giant erythroblasts may occasionally be seen in peripheral blood, and macrophages may phagocytize abnormal erythroblasts. A presumptive diagnosis is based on the presence of typical cytoplasmic inclusions in circulating erythrocytes of anemic fish. Confirmation requires visualization of hexagonal virus particles in cytoplasm of affected erythrocytes using transmission electron microscopy. A marine reservoir is suspected but has not been identified. Vertical transmission is suspected due to the high prevalence of infection in fry from infected broodstock.

The ranaviruses are an important group within the family Iridoviridae that affect fish. One of these, epizootic erythropoietic necrosis (EHN) is listed as a notifiable disease by OIE. It was first reported in redfin perch in Australia in the spring of 1984, but has also been shown to cause disease, albeit less severe, in rainbow trout. Similar viruses have been reported in sheatfish in Germany and black bullhead catfish in France and Italy. EHN is endotheliotropic, producing necrotic lesions in the endothelium of blood vessels and some visceral lesions. Behavioral signs include lethargy, darkening, and erratic swimming. Mortality occurs after 4-5 days. The most consistent lesion associated with EHN is focal necrosis of hematopoietic tissue in the anterior kidney and liver. Necrotic hematopoietic cells may be visible within blood vessels. Presumptive diagnosis is based on clinical signs and isolation of the suspect agent in cell culture. Bluegill fry (BF-2) is the cell line of choice. Detection may also be accomplished using ELISA, immunofluorescence, or electron microscopy. Epizootics of EHN in redfin perch are most common in the spring and summer and almost exclusively involve juvenile fish. Survivors seem to be resistant to future infection. There is no evidence of vertical transmission of EHN, and redfin perch carriers have not been detected. An unidentified reservoir and carrier host is suspected. Fomite transmission of EHN has been demonstrated, and birds have also been shown to carry infected material.

Largemouth bass virus is a ranavirus that was isolated from moribund largemouth bass in South Carolina in 1995. It was previously isolated from largemouth bass in several Florida lakes but had not been directly associated with disease. In recent years it has been found in largemouth bass in most southeastern and many midwestern states. The disease is not well understood because the virus is commonly isolated from tissues of clinically normal fish. In the 1995 fish kill, ~1,000 fish died over a 2-3 mo period in an area that encompasses >66,000 hectares. Lesions were nonspecific and are still poorly described. Fat-head minnow (FHM) is the cell line of choice for isolation of virus.

Several other iridoviruses have been described in ornamental fish. Two of these were initially reported as being closely related to largemouth bass virus, but more recent work indicates that the isolates from guppy and doctor fish are not as closely related as originally thought. An iridovirus has been described in freshwater angelfish (*Pterophyllum scalare*) showing signs of systemic disease, but the agent has not been isolated. An iridovirus has been isolated from gouramis in the genus *Trichogaster* using a tilapia heart cell line. This virus does not grow on FHM cells or other common cell lines used for isolation of fish viruses. The gourami virus has been associated with systemic disease and mortality of *Trichogaster* spp gouramis. Efforts to fulfill River's postulates were supportive though not conclusive. Clinical disease with largemouth bass virus and the gourami iridovirus seems more severe at water temperatures ≥30°C, based on very limited information.

Infectious salmon anemia is an emerging disease in USA aquaculture. It is classified as a significant disease by OIE, but the USDA has listed it as a federally notifiable disease in the USA. The first report was from farmed Atlantic salmon on the west coast of Norway in 1984. Affected fish were lethargic and severely anemic (PCV <5% in moribund fish). The causative agent is an orthomyxovirus. Acute outbreaks result in high mortality. Initial signs include lethargic fish hanging around the edges of the cage. As the disease progresses, moribund animals lie on the bottom. The most obvious external lesions are pale gills and hemorrhage in the anterior chamber of the eye. Internally, the liver appears dark and hemorrhagic, an important indication of infectious salmon anemia. Other lesions may include a fibrinous capsule around the liver, a distended stomach filled with viscous mucus, and sometimes hemorrhagic areas on the mucosa. Infected fish often have obvious ascites, and hemorrhage may be present in skeletal muscle. Histologically, the most important lesion is multifocal, hemorrhagic hepatic necrosis, which may appear zonal; hepatocytes may be dark and swollen and necrotic areas are eosinophilic. Circulating RBC are small, and evidence of cytoplasmic vacuolation, nuclear degeneration, and cell fragmentation may be seen. Affected fish may develop lymphocytopenia and thrombocytopenia and an apparent increase in immature RBC in the peripheral circulation. Signs of chronic infection are more subtle but may include hemorrhage in the swim bladder and skin. Diagnosis is based on clinical signs, with emphasis on anemia (PCV <10%), the gross appearance of a dark liver, and hepatic necrosis. Confirmation can be by viral isolation using the SHK-1 cell line. Virus may be visualized in endothelial cells of cardiac blood vessels using transmission electron microscopy. The agent is enveloped, slightly pleomorphic, and ~100 nm in size. Suspected cases can also be verified using an immunofluorescent antibody technique on frozen tissue. Transmission is horizontal and virus is shed in skin, mucus, feces, and urine. Sea lice (*Lepeophtheirus salmonis*) may be a vector; disease outbreaks seem worse when sea lice are present. Currently there is no evidence of vertical transmission. Sea trout have been proposed as a possible reservoir of infection. Protective immunity has been demonstrated in salmon that survive an outbreak. The disease is heavily regulated in Norway and now in the USA, where the USDA should be notified immediately of any suspected cases.

MISCELLANEOUS NONINFECTIOUS DISEASES

Wild fish populations are monitored for detection of toxic pollutants. Many sources indicate that the industrial and domestic production of sulfur dioxide fumes from the combustion of fossil fuels has been responsible for acid rain and the resultant high mortalities in fish in natural bodies of water. The formation of toxic aluminum compounds in acid waters also has been incriminated as a cause of fish morbidity and mortality. The discharge of toxic substances into natural waters has resulted in fish kills; some pollutants are being investigated as carcinogens because of a high incidence of tumors in fish in defined bodies of water, both marine and freshwater. Higher incidences of tumors have been found in bottom-dwelling species and are thought to be related to carcinogens in the sediment. Ulcerative dermatitis and fin and tail rot have been described in marine fish such as flounder, salmon, sea trout, and others. Although aquatic pollutants have been incriminated, the etiology of these conditions remains obscure.

Cultured, pond-reared food fish are subject to environmental pollutants such as industrial pollutants, fertilizers, pesticides, road salt, and other runoff from surface drainage into fish ponds. Aquarium fish also have environmental problems due to accidental or intentional introduction of toxic substances, including drugs for medication, disinfectants, soaps, and aerosol sprays.

Feed intoxications of fish are commonly due to spoilage and rancidity. A dramatic food intoxication is aflatoxicosis, which results from ingestion of fish feeds contaminated with aflatoxin produced by *Aspergillus flavus*. Rainbow trout and other salmonids are particularly susceptible to aflatoxicosis, which results in the induction of rapidly growing hepatomas and high mortality. Other toxin-producing molds can produce similar intoxication.

Pansteatitis and swim-bladder thickening due to toxic cottonseed in fish meals incorporated in a diet low in vitamin E are reportedly associated with high mortality in cultured fish. Contaminated binders, used in making pelleted fish feeds, and salt contamination have been reported. The latter may result from errors in feed formulation or from contamination with seawater during storage. Heavy metals, plastics, oil, phenolic compounds, and other organic substances have been reported to be toxic for fish, which have become standard laboratory animals for bioassays of such toxic substances.

Neoplastic diseases similar to those found in other animals are found in fish. Their incidence frequently is higher in some geographic areas and in certain species. Some tumors are genetically mediated, such as the malignant melanoma of the gypsy-swordtail cross, and possibly the pseudobranch tumor of cod, thyroid tumors, malignant lymphosarcoma of northern pike, and fibromas or sarcomas of goldfish. The reported incidence of tumors in sharks, skates, and rays is low.

Gonadal tumors are important neoplastic disorders of koi. Typically fish present with a swollen abdomen, and depending on the severity of disease, there may be significant loss of condition. The presence of a mass can be confirmed with ultrasound. Biopsy of tissue may not offer a clear diagnosis. Laparotomy of affected fish often reveals a circumscribed mass of gonadal tissue. Fish that are not excessively debilitated are excellent surgical candidates for removal of the mass.

Coloration anomalies and yolk-sac anomalies or deformities are common in cultured fish and may be of genetic or environmental origin. For example, blue-sac disease, a condition of larval rainbow trout, is believed to be associated with unsuitable hatchery water, and pseudoalbinism in cultured flatfish is associated with excess light levels shortly after hatching.

Sunburn can occur in surface swimming fish or can be induced (even in bottom-dwelling species) by feeding photodynamic drugs such as phenothiazine, although ultra-violet light penetrates water poorly.

Nephrocalcinosis and visceral granuloma are found particularly in salmonid culture, induced supposedly by a high level of carbon dioxide in the water; this produces a metabolic acidosis and urinary and tissue precipitation of calcium, around which extensive granulomata develop.

FOXES

MANAGEMENT

Cleanliness is of extreme importance in raising foxes (*Vulpes* spp). Usually, foxes are kept in individual pens with an attached kennel. Pens with raised, woven-wire bottoms, which disrupt the life cycle of many parasites, should be used.

The ration for ranch-raised foxes is roughly the same as that for mink and consists of a commercial cooked cereal with chicken, beef byproducts, and fish (p 1544). Commercially available fox pellets have also given satisfactory performance.

The gestation period of foxes is ~52 days, and foxes have one litter per year. Blue foxes should average 6-7 pups per litter, silver foxes 3-5 pups. The vixen usually shows signs of estrus in late January and February. Most females are in standing heat for 2-3 days and are bred 2 or 3 times during this period. Many ranchers use vaginal cytology or electronic "rut gauges" to determine the proper time for best mating. Most often, a polygamous mating system is used, and the female is taken to the pen of the male. Artificial insemination is becoming widely used on larger ranches.

Pelts are usually collected in November or December.

DISEASES

Distemper: Foxes are susceptible to canine distemper virus (p 625), which is easily transmitted between dogs, mink, ferrets, raccoons, and other susceptible species. Because of the high population density in confinement and the high transmissibility of the virus, mortality on unvaccinated farms may be 50% in breeding stock and 75% in pups. The diagnosis is based on clinical signs, histologic lesions (including the presence of inclusion bodies), ELISA, immunohistochemistry, and fluorescent antibody procedures. The most effective control procedure during an outbreak is to immediately destroy all foxes showing signs of disease and to vaccinate all others. All dead animals should be incinerated, and all equipment thoroughly disinfected. Because there are no licensed distemper vaccines for foxes, mink vaccine has been used. Vaccination of weaned pups at 12-13 wk of age is suggested. Annual vaccination of breeder foxes is recommended.

Fox Encephalitis: This disease, caused by the same virus that causes infectious canine hepatitis (p 637), may cause serious losses when unvaccinated foxes are raised intensively. Mortality may be 2-40% on affected ranches. Fox encephalitis has a rapid course. The virus invades cells in the liver and kidneys and the endothelial lining of small blood vessels. Signs include anorexia, bloody diarrhea, depression, and often nervous signs such as convulsions and paralysis. Death occurs in a few hours to a few days. Signs and death are due to hemorrhage of small vessels throughout the body, including the brain. Diagnosis is confirmed by demonstrating typical intranuclear inclusion bodies in liver, kidney, and endothelial cells; virus isolation; or fluorescent antibody techniques. An inactivated vaccine is available. Pups from unvaccinated vixens are vaccinated at weaning, and others when 10-12 wk old. Breeders should be given booster vaccinations in December or January.

Salmon Poisoning: *Neorickettsia helminthoeca* is the cause of salmon poisoning disease (p 642), which is the result of eating salmon or trout that harbor the vector fluke,

Nanophyetus salmincola. Signs include fever, inappetence, vomiting, lethargy, and diarrhea. Treatment is the same as for dogs. Untreated foxes usually die.

Botulism: Improper handling and storage of food is the usual source of botulism in foxes as well as in mink. Storage of meat byproducts in metal drums, in which anaerobic conditions prevail, is an excellent medium for production of botulism toxin. In almost all instances, type C toxin has been incriminated. Signs include flaccid paralysis and abdominal breathing, usually followed by death. Because vaccines approved for foxes are not available, those approved for mink are used. (*See also* BOTULISM, p 490.)

Canine Parvovirus: While canids in zoological parks have succumbed to canine parvoviral infection, there have been no reported outbreaks of canine parvovirus (p 319) on commercial fox farms; however, the prospect of an outbreak should be kept in mind. Vaccination of silver foxes with inactivated canine parvovirus vaccines should be considered, whereas blue foxes might be better protected with mink virus enteritis vaccines.

Parasites: Internal and external parasites are controlled by means essentially the same as those recommended for dogs.

Fleas (*Ctenocephalides canis*) cause skin irritation and sometimes severe anemia and are particularly harmful in pups. Ear mites (*Otodectes cynotis*) are common in ranch-raised foxes. Infected foxes shake their heads and dig at the base of the ears with their front paws. Secondary bacterial or mycotic otitis may result. Some foxes hold their heads to one side. (*See also* FLEAS, p 710, and OTITIS EXTERNA, p 421.)

Sarcoptic mange (*Sarcoptes scabiei*) may cause serious economic loss in ranch-raised foxes. Clinical signs are similar to those seen in dogs. Ivermectin at 200 µg/kg, SC, has been used successfully to treat outbreaks; however, idiosyncratic reactions have been reported in some dogs at this dosage, and caution is suggested. (*See also* p 746.)

Hookworms (*Uncinaria stenocephala*) in commercially raised foxes can cause deaths in pups. Fox pups are infected by larvae in the vixen's milk. Anemia may be profound, and pups may die beginning at 12 days of age. Fecal samples from these pups often are negative for eggs, and death may occur before the infection becomes patent. Pups with milder infection may grow poorly, appear emaciated, and have a marginal anemia. Treatment involves worming pups at 10 and 21 days with pyrantel pamoate. The vixen also should be wormed when the pups are 21 days old.

Foxes are commonly infected with ascarids (*Toxocara canis*), which may cause vomiting, diarrhea, abdominal distention, lethargy, and occasionally intestinal obstruction. Migration of ascarid larvae may cause parasitic pneumonia. Fox pups may be infected in utero or after whelping by ingesting eggs. Treatment involves worming pups at 10 and 21 days of age with pyrantel pamoate or piperazine.

Two lungworms, *Capillaria aerophila* and *Crenosoma vulpis*, infect foxes. Lungworm infection and the consequent chronic bronchitis or pneumonia may cause death in ranch-raised foxes. (*See also* p 1181.)

Foxes may be infected with coccidia, the most common being *Isospora bigemina*. The signs are mild to bloody diarrhea, anorexia, and death. Treatment is the same as for dogs. (*See also* p 2201.)

Dermatomycosis: Although dermatomycosis appears to be rare in the USA, *Trichophyton mentagrophytes* has been incriminated in an outbreak. It is reported to be common in foxes in the former USSR. (*See also* p 704.)

Nutritional Diseases: Rickets may occur in young foxes shortly after weaning. Affected pups appear bowlegged due to curvature of the long bones and joint enlargement. Sometimes the facial bones are distorted and the costochondral junctions enlarged. Rickets is treated by correcting the ratio of calcium to phosphorus in the diet and supplementing with vitamin D. (*See also* p 853.)

Chastek paralysis (p 1547) is a vitamin B_1 deficiency induced by feeding certain types of raw fish that contain the enzyme thiaminase. Early in the course of the disease, a few foxes may have an abnormal gait as though their legs were stiff; within 12-36 hr, they have extensive spastic paralysis and are unable to rise. Convulsions often occur shortly before death.

Raw fish should be removed from the diet, and daily injections of 100 U of thiamine given. Cooking of fish that contain thiaminase before mixing prevents the deficiency.

Biotin deficiency occurs when high levels of uncooked eggs (particularly turkey eggs) are fed, causing gray underfur and loss of guard hairs. Preventive measures are described for the disease in mink (p 1547).

Cardiac myopathy has been seen only when fox pups are fed certain commercial pellets. Some factor(s) is deficient in the pup's early growth phase, which results in an enlarged right ventricle. Supplementing the ration with liver or meat is preventive.

LABORATORY ANIMALS

Management

Consistently delivered quality programs of husbandry and veterinary care provide the foundation enabling valid scientific research. For proper management of research animals, the animal care and research staff must be responsible, sensitive to the animals' health and well-being, well trained in the humane care and use of laboratory animals, highly motivated, experienced, and diligent in performing their duties and responsibilities. Standard operating procedures must be established, and training and supervision provided to assure a consistently applied and uniformly high level of animal care. Within research facilities, environmental conditions must be carefully controlled so that, along with conscientiously applied programs of animal care and use, the best possible conditions for conducting research are provided. *The Guide for the Care and Use of Laboratory Animals* (1996, National Academies Press, available online) is a primary reference for information on basic principles and standards for laboratory animal management.

Laboratory rodents that are disease- and pathogen-free and that do not possess antibodies indicative of past infection are readily available from commercial vendors. Procuring such animals from high-quality sources, transporting them in filtered shipping containers, and maintaining them in facilities with both physical and procedural barriers to the introduction of infectious agents are effective measures to prevent disease within a colony.

However, although there are colonies of some species of primates that are free of most agents that cause infectious disease in these species, many primates used are of feral origin. For this reason, appropriate quarantine, isolation, and conditioning programs should be implemented in addition to the program followed in the importers' facilities.

Housing: Cages, pens, or runs should provide adequate space to allow for normal physiologic needs, permit postural adjustments, and meet requisites for species-specific behavior. When possible, compatible groups of social animals should be housed together. Primary enclosures should be constructed of durable materials, easily cleaned and sanitized, and designed for comfort and safety. Static microisolation (filter top) cages and, recently, more advanced individually ventilated caging systems have been used widely for rodent housing to impede cage-to-cage transmission of infectious agents. Additionally, individual ventilation of cages serves to delay deterioration of the environment within the cage and maintain a more consistent and wholesome microenvironment. A potential drawback that must be considered in the use and management of ventilated cages is that hairless genotypes and neonates may be prone to chilling. This risk can be reduced by providing nesting material.

Federal law in the USA requires that laboratory dogs have an opportunity to exercise regularly and have sensory contact with other dogs unless restricted by experimental or behavioral considerations. Housing for nonhuman primates must provide social and environmental enrichment to promote their psychological well-being compatible with the experimental and practical constraints of the housing situation. Successful enrichment strategies for nonhuman primates have included pair or group housing; variation in the dietary content and method of presentation; diversification of the internal cage environment with ancillary apparatus (eg, perches, swings, or ladders); provision of devices to enhance visual, auditory, or tactile stimulation; and participation in challenging, nonaversive behavioral laboratory studies. Efforts to extend and adapt environmental enrichment practices to other laboratory animal species warrant consideration and have been implemented in some institutions.

Temperature, relative humidity, ventilation rates, lighting conditions (spectrum, intensity, and photoperiod), gaseous pollutants (eg, ammonia), and noise should be carefully controlled at all times and monitored as appropriate. Unstable environmental conditions can have a profound effect on the comfort, well-being, and metabolism of animals and therefore on the quality of experimental data derived. In general, temperature should be maintained at 64-79°F (18-26°C) for most rodents, 61-72°F (16-22°C) for rabbits, 59-64°F (15-18°C) for ferrets, and 64-84°F (18-29°C) for primates. Within these ranges, optimal systems should maintain temperatures within ±1°F of the set point. Relative humidity should be maintained at 30-70% for most species and preferably within 10% of the set point. Ventilation rates should be 10-15 fresh air changes/hr. Air should not be recirculated unless it has been treated to remove particulate and gaseous contaminants. Lighting should be distributed evenly and sufficiently intense to promote animal well-being and to allow personnel to observe the animals and to perform all husbandry and sanitation duties safely and effectively. Diurnal or day-night cycles, as determined by species' requirements, should be controlled by automatic timers to maintain circadian and neuroendocrine regulation. The microenvironment within certain types of caging may be very different from that of the macroenvironment of the room. Carefully conducted research is needed to define the optimal environmental conditions for each species or group of species at the cage level.

Bedding: Bedding materials should be nonirritating, absorbent, free of chemical contamination and pathogens, and unpalatable. Adequate quantities should be used to keep animals dry and clean between changes of bedding or caging. Hardwood bedding products and others not made with softwoods are recommended because softwood products contain volatile oils that may alter hepatic enzyme systems and affect certain kinds of research.

Feeding: Feed should be of adequate quantity, palatable, free of contaminants, and nutritionally adequate, according to specific species requirements. Feeds specifically manufactured for research animal use are preferred because they are more likely to be uniformly constituted, free of contaminants, and mill dated. Feed should be manufactured, transported, stored, and used in ways that minimize its deterioration, contamination, or infestation. Most small animals are fed ad lib; rabbits, laboratory carnivores, swine, aquatic amphibians, and primates may be restricted to measured quantities of feed each day. In addition to commercially prepared and usually pelleted diets, semisynthetic or completely synthetic diets can be prepared for use in certain kinds of research. Autoclavable or irradiated diets are available for rodents and can be used when sterilization of feed is desired.

Water: Potable, uncontaminated water should be provided in adequate quantities to meet specific species requirements. Quality assurance programs that measure pH, hardness, chemical content, and microbial load are recommended. Highly purified, deionized, acidified, chlorinated, or sterile water may be required under certain experimental or husbandry conditions. Water is usually provided ad lib in manually filled or automatic watering devices.

Water quality is the most important environmental variable for amphibians and a key determinant of health. Inadequate water quality or fluctuations of water temperature are physiologic stressors that impact the intake, digestion, and use of food; alter the immune system; and predispose to opportunistic infection. Water for aquatic amphibians should be free of nitrite, ammonia, chlorine, and with total coliform counts not exceeding 200/mL. The pH should be 6.5-8.5. While aquatic amphibians may be maintained in small containers of standing water, water recirculation with biologic filtration and periodic partial replenishment with fresh water are helpful in suppressing bacterial counts and preventing the build-up of toxic chemicals. The ideal water temperature range for most aquatic amphibians is 64-72°F (18-22°C). (*See also* AMPHIBIANS, p 1445.)

TABLE 11. Selected Physiologic Data of Laboratory Animals *   ▶

Species	Gestation Period (days)	Litter Size	Age and Body Weight at Sexual Maturity
Mice	19-21	6-10	6 wk (20-30 g)
Rats	21-23	6-14	3 mo (0.2-0.3 kg)
Guinea pigs	59-72	1-4	3-4 mo (0.4-0.5 kg)
Hamsters, golden	15-18	4-10	2 mo (85-110 g)
Gerbils	25	2-9	3 mo (60-100 g)
Rabbits	30	4-12	5-6 mo (3-4 kg)
Squirrel monkeys	150	1	3-5 yr (0.6-1.1 kg)
Rhesus monkeys	164	1-2	3-4 yr (5-11 kg)
Chimpanzees	227-235	1	7-10 yr (40-50 kg)
Baboons	164-186	1	3-5 yr (11-30 kg)

*See also FEATURES OF THE REPRODUCTIVE CYCLE, p 1088.

Sanitation: A uniformly high level of sanitation is mandatory. Housing rooms and ancillary support space should be cleaned and sanitized as often as necessary to keep them free of dirt, debris, and potentially harmful contamination. Primary enclosures also should be cleaned and sanitized as often as necessary to keep animals clean and dry. For rodents in solid-bottom cages, usually 1-3 changes per week will suffice; for rodents, rabbits, and nonhuman primates in suspended cages over excreta pans, cage changes every other week should be adequate. For larger animals, excreta and soiled bedding should be removed daily, and primary enclosures cleaned and sanitized daily to at least every other week. Water bottles and other watering or feeding devices should be cleaned and sanitized at least weekly. Automatic watering devices on cages, racks, or in rooms should be drained, rinsed, and sanitized at regular, frequent intervals. Heating cages and other equipment to 180°F (82.2°C) or using appropriate chemical disinfection (eg, hypochlorite solutions) kills nonsporeforming pathogenic bacteria and viruses. All caging and other equipment should be rinsed thoroughly after treatment with detergents or disinfectants.

Vermin Control: Professionally directed programs to prevent, identify, and eradicate or control insects or escaped or feral rodents must be instituted. The use of pesticides should generally be confined to areas not used for animals or for storage of feed or bedding. Relatively inert substances, such as silica aerogel or boric acid powder, are recommended and are useful in control of crawling insects, eg, cockroaches.

Colony Monitoring

While most commercially reared rodents, some rabbits, and relatively fewer dogs, cats, and primates can be obtained as SPF animals, resident animal colonies must be monitored for naturally occurring disease as a measure of the effectiveness of the prevention and control program. Investigators should be informed regularly as to the health status of their research animals. In addition to monitoring for infectious disease, a quality assurance program should monitor for genetic integrity, especially for inbred mouse strains that are bred and maintained in the research facility, as well as for environmental factors (quality of feed, water, and bedding; efficacy of sanitation programs; air handling and quality; lighting; noise; etc) that can affect colony health.

Colony health monitoring consists of a defined program of regular physical and laboratory evaluations of animals within a unit, as well as a morbidity and mortality reporting system that enables timely identification of potential problems. Thorough investigations of illnesses and deaths in a colony are essential components of such a program. For selected physiologic data of some laboratory animals, *see* TABLE 11.

Total RBC ($\times 10^{12}$/L)	Total WBC ($\times 10^9$/L)	Average Body Temperature (°C)	Water Consumption (per day)[†]
7-11	4-12	37	4-7 mL
7-10	5-15	38	30 mL
5-7	7-14	38	150 mL
6-7	7-10	38	30 mL
7-8	8-11	39	4 mL
5-7	6-12	39	300-700 mL
5-8	5-11	39	70-110 mL
5-7	4-16	38	0.2-1.0 L
5-6	6-14	37	2.2-2.7 L
4-6	4-15	39	1.0-1.5 L

TABLE 11. *(continued)*

[†]Varies with number of animals per cage, moisture in feed, temperature, etc

While certain general principles apply, a health monitoring program must be specifically developed for each species maintained in a facility. For example, generally all primates are quarantined and isolated on arrival. Physical examinations, tuberculin testing, and baseline hematologic and other clinical pathologic tests should be performed. In addition, serologic evaluation for *Cercopithecine herpesvirus* type 1 (*Herpesvirus simiae*, B virus), simian retroviruses, and other specific agents may be done, depending on the species of primate. Primates should be released from quarantine only when both the health status and suitability for use are determined. Furthermore, primates should have quarterly, semiannual, and annual health surveillance screens, each consisting of defined elements. (*See also* NONHUMAN PRIMATES, p 1549.)

For colony-bred rats and mice, programs for disease monitoring can consist of any or all of the following: 1) vendor surveillance, 2) quarantine and isolation evaluation, 3) ongoing clinical and postmortem evaluation during the course of studies, 4) sentinel animal programs, and 5) evaluation at termination of the study. In addition, all transplantable tumors, cells, or other biologic products destined for animal passage should be screened for murine and zoonotic pathogens. Of particular concern to colony health is the occasional and justifiable need to obtain animals from less well-defined sources, such as an investigator's colony or other nonapproved source. The presence of infectious agents either in transplantable tumors or noncommercial animal sources can pose a substantial threat to resident colonies and personnel.

LLAMAS AND ALPACAS

The 4 members of the South American camelids are the llama, alpaca, guanaco, and vicuña. The species evolved in the Andes, with the guanaco and vicuña probably serving as the foundation stock for the llama and alpaca.

Mature alpacas weigh ~60-80 kg and stand 76-97 cm at the withers. Alpacas are primarily used as fiber-producing animals. The fiber grows rapidly and requires shearing every 12-24 mo. Mature llamas are significantly larger animals, weighing 120-200 kg and standing 102-127 cm at the withers. Llamas were primarily developed as pack animals and can carry loads of 25-40 kg. Males and females of both species have approximately similar mature weights. Guanacos are not easily tamed, although a significant number have been exported from South America. Guanacos are similar in size to llamas but weigh somewhat less.

Unlike llamas and alpacas, in which coloration patterns vary, guanacos have a consistent light brown or tan coat over the neck, back, and outside of the legs, with white on the under-belly and medial surface of the legs. Vicuñas are nondomesticated and slightly taller than alpacas, with a longer neck, much shorter fiber, and a characteristic "bib" of long fibers in the chest region. Vicuñas have extremely fine fiber and are considered an endangered species.

All South American camelids have 74 chromosomes and are cross-fertile, producing fertile F-1 progeny. The most common cross is a llama × alpaca mating, producing a "hua-rizo" that is intermediate in size, body characteristics, and fiber quality. None of the other crosses are common, although the structural similarities between llamas and guanacos make identification of hybrids particularly difficult. Intact male llamas and alpacas are called males, or less frequently machos, while castrated males are referred to as geld-ings. Females are called females, or occasionally hembras. The neonates and young up to ~6 mo of age are called crias.

There are no distinct llama breeds. All llamas have characteristic "banana-shaped" ears, a level back, and a high tail set. In contrast, there are 2 morphologically distinct types of alpacas—the Huacaya and Suri. The more common Huacayas have a lofted fiber coat with coverage down the legs and around the face. Suri have a flat-lying corded fiber structure with less coverage on the head. A suri-style llama has recently been introduced into the North American market. Alpacas have shorter "spear-shaped" ears, a lower tail set, slightly more humping to the back, and a sloping rear end. Llamas and alpacas can-not necessarily be differentiated from one another based on fiber coverage.

South American camelids are most closely related to the old world camelids (Bac-trian and dromedary), having the same number of chromosomes, similar anatomy and physiology, and general patterns of disease susceptibility. Although cows, sheep, and goats are frequently used as reference points for drug dosage extrapolation, disease sus-ceptibility, and management decisions, it is important to remember that South American camelids and common domestic ruminants are only distantly related.

MANAGEMENT

Llamas and alpacas are adaptable to a wide climatic range and have been success-fully raised in regions with winter temperatures as low as -20°C if reasonable wind shel-ter is provided. Heat stress is a significant problem if animals have moderate to heavy fiber coats and are subjected to high temperature and humidity. Shearing, leaving re-maining fiber at least 2 cm long to prevent sunburns, and providing access to shade and sufficient water will usually allow South American camelids to handle moderately high temperature and humidity. Air conditioning, misters, and damp sand pits are helpful to maintain heavy fiber coats in warm, humid climates. Llamas and alpacas can adapt well to damp climates as long as the temperature does not get too high, and few problems of either footrot or "rain rot" are encountered.

Llamas and alpacas can be housed with other species, including goats and sheep. Indi-vidual llamas can also be successfully housed with sheep flocks and can be effectively used as guard animals. These camelids are herd animals and do poorly if isolated from cohorts or other animals; ill animals should be housed with herdmates if appropriate. If sufficient space is available, large groups of males (or females) can be pastured together. In the presence of nonpregnant females, however, intact males and recently castrated geld-ings will commonly spend much of their time fighting, typically biting at the ears, neck, and scrotum. Llamas and alpacas generally do not destroy fences and can usually be confined behind a 1.5-m or 1.2-m fence, respectively. Barbed wire is not needed for containment.

A somewhat unique behavioral characteristic of South American camelids is the use of communal dung piles. Animals urinate and defecate on the same pile, with favorite sites being entryways to barns and other inconvenient locations. Normal feces are pel-leted and firm. Unless forage becomes very limited, animals will not graze in areas around or downstream from dung piles. The urethral diameter in both males and females is small, and the process of urination takes much longer than in other species of comparable size.

Handling: Llamas and alpacas are highly trainable and most animals can be easily taught to come into a barn or corral for food. Many animals can be restrained by an arm around the base of the neck and another arm holding the tail or flank region on the opposite side. Most domesticated South American camelids are halter trained and can be easily led into a smaller area for examination and treatment. Specially designed llama chutes should be used for reproductive examinations and other potentially uncomfortable procedures. In contrast, alpacas respond better to most procedures if assistants, and not restraint chutes, are used to hold the animals. With both llamas and alpacas, it is particularly important to maintain control of the animal's head. The neck is very muscular and can move with amazing speed. Sedation is not needed for most procedures.

Feeding and Nutrition: Most mature males, and females during midgestation, will maintain appropriate body condition on 10-14% crude protein grass hay with total digestible nutrients (TDN) of 50-60%. Late gestation and heavily lactating females require a slightly higher percentage of crude protein and TDN of 65-70%. Under basal conditions, most camelids eat 1.4-1.8% of body wt/day on a dry-matter basis. Legumes are usually not needed and may result in obesity. Body condition can best be assessed by palpating the amount of tissue over the lumbar vertebrae.

Seasonal hypovitaminosis D, characterized by diminished growth, angular limb deformities, kyphosis, and a reluctance to move, can be a problem in heavily fibered animals raised in regions with poor sun exposure during winter months. The problem is most severe in rapidly growing, fall-born crias. Serum phosphorus of <3.0 mg/dL, a calcium:phosphorus ratio of >3:1, and vitamin D concentrations of <15 nmol/L in crias <6 mo old are diagnostic. Normal phosphorus and vitamin D concentrations in this age group are 6.5-9.0 mg/dL and >50 nMol/L, respectively.

Anesthesia: Xylazine (0.1-0.2 mg/kg, IV) can be used for sedation without recumbency; higher dosages (0.3-0.4 mg/kg, IV) will result in recumbency and provide a light plane of anesthesia for 20-30 min. Xylazine (0.25 mg/kg, IV, or 0.35 mg/kg, IM) followed by ketamine (3-5 mg/kg, IV, or 5-8 mg/kg, IM) 15 min later will provide 30-60 min of restraint. Simultaneous administration of xylazine (0.4 mg/kg, IM) and ketamine (4.0 mg/kg, IM) will usually provide 15-20 min of restraint. Butorphanol (0.1-0.2 mg/kg, IM) can provide sedation of short duration.

Llamas and alpacas tolerate general anesthesia well and usually do not require tranquilization before induction. Premedication with atropine (0.02 mg/kg, IV, or 0.04 mg/kg, IM) will prevent bradyarrhythmias and decrease salivary secretions. Induction and maintenance of anesthesia are similar to that in other domestic species.

Clinical Pathology: Hematology and clinical chemistries are similar to those in other species with a few significant differences. Camelid RBC are relatively small and may produce anomalous results when evaluated using an automated cell counter. Therefore, instrument adjustment or manual determination is needed for accurate estimations of RBC numbers and the RBC indices. Normal PCV is 27-45%, and normal RBC numbers are 10.1-$17.3 \times 10^6/\mu L$. Normal WBC counts are 8,000-21,400/μL.

Basal glucose concentrations in llamas and alpacas are more typical of monogastric species than ruminants. Basal levels are 82-160 mg/dL, but glucose levels >300 mg/dL are common after stressful events. For additional hematologic and serum biochemical reference ranges, *see* p 2584 and p 2586.

Antibiotic Use: No drugs are currently approved for use in llamas and alpacas. However, the following antibiotics are used for treatment of sensitive bacteria: ceftiofur (2.2 mg/kg, IM or IV, BID), trimethoprim/sulfamethoxazole (3/15 mg/kg, IV, BID), ampicillin sodium (6 mg /kg, IM or IV, BID), enrofloxacin (5 mg/kg, IV, BID), gentamicin (0.75 mg/kg, IV, TID or 4-5 mg/kg, IV, SID), tobramycin (4 mg/kg, IV, SID), amikacin (12 mg/kg, IV, SID). Administration of ampicillin trihydrate IM does not result in clinically useful serum concentrations.

REPRODUCTION

Reproductive Physiology

Females: Relative to body size, the nonpregnant reproductive tract of South American camelids is relatively small. The uterine morphology is similar to that of a cow with relatively long horns and a short uterine body. The cervix can be felt on rectal palpation and has 2 or 3 rings. The urethra opens into the floor of the vagina. A suburethral diverticulum is present.

Ovarian activity typically begins at ~6-8 mo of age. Due to the small size of females and the higher rate of dystocia associated with early matings, females are usually not bred until they are 18 mo old and weigh 40 kg (alpaca) or 90 kg (llama). If a female is receptive, she will usually assume a position of sternal recumbency (cush) within seconds to a few minutes after introduction of a male and allow the male to breed. Once intromission has occurred, the male will typically begin a vocalization described as "orgling." The volume of the ejaculate is relatively small (2-5 mL) and is deposited directly into the body of the uterus. Ejaculation occurs over an extended period of time. The cervical stimulation and perhaps components in the semen stimulate reflex ovulation ~24 hr after mating. The fertilized oocyte is usually found in the uterus by day 7 after mating, with implantation occurring by ~30 days of gestation. The type of placentation is diffuse epitheliochorial, and the placenta fills both horns. While ovulation occurs bilaterally, ~95% or more of the pregnancies are carried in the left horn. Live births of twins are extremely uncommon, with most twins being aborted by 5-7 mo of gestation.

If the female has a functional corpus luteum (CL), she will aggressively refuse the male's efforts to mount. An indication of pregnancy is the female's rejection of the male if he is reintroduced >15 days after the initial breeding. Progesterone concentrations of >1.0 ng/mL are typical in females with a functional CL and can be used for confirmation of both ovulation at 6-9 days after mating and pregnancy at >21 days after mating. Persistent CL are periodically seen and account for most of the 2-5% false-positive results when using serum progesterone for pregnancy confirmation. Rectal palpation is practical in llamas at >30 days of gestation. It is usually not possible to safely perform rectal palpation in alpacas. Pregnancy can be diagnosed by rectal ultrasound from >28 days of gestation and by transabdominal ultrasonography from >90 days.

Gestation in llamas and alpacas is ~342 ± 10 days. Most births (>70%) occur between midmorning and mid- to late afternoon. Owners are often concerned about prolonged gestation, which is most frequently the result of inaccurate breeding dates. Dystocias due to excessively large crias are rare.

There are few reliable indications of pending delivery. Stage I labor typically lasts 1-6 hr and may be accompanied by increased frequency of urination, increased "humming," and separation from the herd. Stage II labor is rapid (typically <30 min), with delivery of a cria weighing 5.5-8.0 kg (alpaca) or 11-16 kg (llama). Stage III labor lasts 4-6 hr. Retained placentas are rare. Uterine involution begins shortly after birth, and most females can conceive 14-28 days after delivery. Females have 4 teats and do not exhibit significant mammary enlargement during the postpartum period. Mastitis is rare.

Males: Both testicles should be fully descended at birth. Testes should be at least ~2 × 4 cm and 3 × 6 cm in mature alpacas and llamas, respectively. Relative to body size, testes of South American camelids are smaller than those of many other domestic livestock species and are held close to the body wall. The urethra is relatively small and contains a urethral diverticulum at the level of the ischial arch. The penis is fibrous, with a sigmoid flexure just before its distal tip. A cartilaginous process is present at the tip of the penis, and the urethra opens 1-2 cm back from the tip. Urinary calculi are relatively common and have a poor prognosis due to the small urethral diameter (3.5-5 French).

Although androgen production begins at <8 mo of age, and sperm can be collected by electroejaculation as early as 14 mo of age, preputial adhesions prevent full penile extension and copulation until 18-24 mo of age or older. Most males enter breeding programs when 18-24 mo old, and most animals are fertile by 30 mo of age. Sexual maturity may be later in alpacas than in llamas.

Semen evaluation is difficult in camelids due to the small total volume of semen and the dribble ejaculation. While males can be trained to mount a phantom or dummy, semen collection usually requires heavy sedation or anesthesia and electroejaculation. Semen collection, even from males of known fertility, is inconsistent. Likewise, uterine collection of semen samples after copulation is also unreliable.

Management of Reproductive Problems

Fertility problems are relatively common in llamas and alpacas. Although most problems primarily involve females, problems with males include hypoplastic testes and heat stress. The latter is characterized by scrotal edema, decreased activity, and reluctance to breed. Shearing, adequate shade, and sufficient water usually resolve the problem, although fertility may not return to normal for up to 6 wk. If other males are present in the same or adjacent pastures, conception rates may decline because they spend progressively more of their time fighting with other males. When working with inexperienced males, vaginal intromission should be visually confirmed.

Due to the relatively high incidence of congenital anomalies, anatomic problems (eg, uterus unicornis, hypoplastic ovaries, double cervixes, and segmental aplasia of the vagina or uterus) must be considered as causes of infertility in primiparous animals. In multiparous animals, vaginal strictures, uterine infections, and cervical damage are also relatively common. Significant to complete uterine strictures are a common sequelae of dystocias. The diagnostic approach to all these conditions is similar to that used in mares, except that rectal palpation cannot usually be safely done in alpacas. If uterine biopsies or cultures are appropriate, the cervix can be dilated in ~24 hr by administration of estradiol cypionate, 2-3 mg, IM.

Rupture of a mature follicle (>7 mm) can reliably be induced with human chorionic gonadotropin (hCG) at 5,000 IU or GnRH at 1.0 μg/kg, IM. Increased progesterone concentration (>1.0 ng/mL) 7 days after copulation or treatment with hCG or GnRH is indicative of CL formation. Although persistent CL have been identified, they are relatively rare. Two doses of cloprostenol (250 mg, IM) at 24-hr intervals will result in regression of a persistent CL and abortion in llamas in early to midgestation. Induction of parturition with prostaglandins or glucocorticoids is not recommended.

HERD HEALTH

Neonatal Care: Crias should be on their feet and attempting to nurse within 2 hr after birth and every 1-2 hr thereafter for the first few days. While weight gain for the first 24 hr postpartum may be minimal, thereafter llamas should gain 250-500 g/day and alpacas 100-250 g/day. Healthy crias should approximately double their birth weight by 1 mo of age.

Routine cria care should include weighing and dipping the navel in 7% tincture of iodine or 0.5% chlorhexidine 3 times during the first 24 hr after birth. Supplemental selenium should be provided by injection (0.5 mg for alpacas, 1.0 mg for llamas) if appropriate for the area.

Parasite Control: Parasite control programs vary according to climatic conditions, population density, and parasite load, and should be developed according to local conditions. As a general rule, 2-4 treatments/yr usually provide sufficient control.

No drugs have been approved for use in South American camelids. However, anthelmintics that are generally recognized as safe and efficacious include ivermectin (0.2 mg/kg), pyrantel pamoate (18 mg/kg), and fenbendazole (5-10 mg/kg). Although not critically evaluated, the topical formulation of ivermectin appears to be efficacious when applied to the skin, not the fiber. Liver flukes can be a significant problem. Control with clorsulon (7-14 mg/kg) or albendazole (10 mg/kg) is usually effective, although repeated clorsulon treatment after 6-8 wk may be necessary.

Vaccinations: Most vaccination protocols for llamas and alpacas have been empirically derived. All animals should receive *Clostridium perfringens* type C and D vaccinations and tetanus toxoid. In regions where liver fluke (*Fasciola hepatica*) infections are a problem, use of polyvalent *Clostridium* vaccines against *C novyi*, *C septicum*, *C sordellii*, and *C chauvoei* are warranted. One successful approach has been to give an initial vaccination at 3 mo of age, a booster 30 days later, and annual boosters thereafter.

Abortions secondary to *Leptospira* spp infections are intermittently a problem and can usually be prevented using a similar vaccination schedule, although some practitioners administer boosters twice a year. Killed rabies vaccines have been used with unknown efficacy in endemic areas. Vaccinations for equine herpesvirus 1 are probably not warranted in most situations.

Dental Development and Care: The deciduous dental formula in the llama and alpaca is 2 $(I\frac{1-2}{3} \ C\frac{1}{1} \ P\frac{2-3}{1-2})$ with the upper I1 and I2 missing in both juveniles and adults. The upper second incisors may be radiographically apparent but do not erupt. The dental pad is similar to that of a cow. At birth, the first 2 pairs of lower incisors are normally through the gum line with lack of eruption of I1 and I2 being one indication of prematurity. The adult dental formula is 2 $(I\frac{1}{3} \ C\frac{1}{1} \ P\frac{1-2}{1-2} \ M\frac{3}{3})$. The mandibular deciduous incisors I1-I3 are replaced at ~2-2$\frac{1}{2}$, 3-3$\frac{1}{2}$, and 3-6 yr, respectively, although determining age by the teeth is notoriously inaccurate in these species.

A unique feature of South American camelids is the development of the upper I3 and upper and lower canine teeth on both sides into "fighting" teeth that grow to >3 cm long. The teeth can cause serious damage to other males during fights and usually need to be cut flush to the gum with obstetrical wire, beginning at ~3 yr of age and every 2-4 yr thereafter. Fighting teeth in females rarely penetrate the gumline and seldom, if ever, need to be cut. Growth of fighting teeth usually stops after castration. Tooth extraction to avoid periodic trimming is impractical due to very deep, curved roots.

The incisors are open-rooted in alpacas and continue to grow throughout life. Poor occlusion of the incisors and dental pad necessitate periodic tooth trimming and appears to be more of a problem in alpacas than in llamas. Cheek teeth are rooted and do not require regular floating, although premolar and molar occlusion should be checked and problems corrected in older animals exhibiting difficulty in chewing or weight loss.

Abscesses of the lower second premolar and first and second molars are frequently seen as a hard, well-developed swelling on the lateral surface of the mandible over the affected teeth. A draining track may or may not be present. The area is usually not painful on palpation, and most animals maintain body condition. No bacterial agent has been consistently isolated from the abscesses. Antibiotic therapy is sometimes palliative, although rarely curative. Due to inadequate exposure, tooth extraction usually requires making a lateral incision over the affected teeth, splitting the tooth due to the divergent roots, and repelling the tooth into the oral cavity. Care should be taken during extraction to avoid fracturing the mandible. Problems with other teeth are rare.

Nail Trimming: Nail growth varies significantly from animal to animal. Some individuals rarely need foot care, while others require nail trimming every 2-3 mo. The nails should be trimmed flush with the bottom of the pad.

DISEASES

Congenital and Inherited Anomalies

While few congenital anomalies have conclusively been shown to be inherited, it is assumed that defects inherited in other species, eg, umbilical hernias, are probably inherited in South American camelids as well. Accordingly, breeding decisions should take this into consideration.

Choanal atresia, a condition caused by failure of the caudal nares (choanae) to open during embryologic development, is probably the most widespread congenital defect in South American camelids. The defect can be unilateral or bilateral and may result in complete or partial blockage. Accordingly, the primary clinical presentation is a variable degree of respiratory distress in the neonate. The cheeks may flare noticeably during inspiration. (Flaring of the nostrils occurs in the presence or absence of choanal atresia.) Distress becomes more apparent during nursing, and crias commonly gasp as milk is inhaled. Surgical correction is not recommended.

Wry face is characterized by a slight (<5°) to severe (>60°) lateral deviation of the maxilla. The mandible may or may not have a similar deviation. The occlusion of the nares and lack of apposition of the incisors and dental pad usually necessitate euthanasia of the cria. The relationship of this defect, if any, to choanal atresia is unclear.

Eye and ear defects, such as juvenile cataracts, are seen occasionally. There may be an association between blue eyes and deafness in some lines of white animals. Fused (tip or base) and short ("gopher") ears are recognized heritable defects.

Cardiac defects are relatively common, and ventricular septal defects are more common than patent ductus arteriosus and various transpositions of the great vessels.

Numerous **musculoskeletal defects** have been identified, including syndactyly and polydactyly. Arthrogryposis, rotated talus(es), angular limb deformities of the front limbs, and tendon laxity are occasionally also observed in South American camelids.

Other congenital anomalies identified in llamas and alpacas include **atresia ani, umbilical hernias**, and several different types of **tail defects**, including a pronounced lateral deviation of the tail at the base.

Urogenital defects are much more common in South American camelids than in many other species. Significant defects include uterus unicornis, hypoplastic ovaries, double cervices, segmental aplasia of the vagina or uterus, hypoplastic testes, and clitoral hypertrophy. Unilateral absence of a kidney is periodically seen, commonly in association with choanal atresia. Total absence of kidneys has also been seen.

Bacterial Diseases

Brucellosis, tuberculosis, and Johne's disease (paratuberculosis) have been identified in South American camelids, although the naturally occurring incidence of these infections is low. *Clostridium perfringens* type A is a very important pathogen under some circumstances, especially in South America, and results in a high death rate in crias <4 wk old. Enterotoxigenic strains of *C perfringens* type A are believed to be particularly lethal. Clinical signs are similar to type A infections in other species with a rapid onset of neurologic changes, followed shortly by death.

Viral Diseases

Most camelids are seropositive for a presumptively nonpathogenic adenovirus that is specific to llamas. Occasionally, an animal will develop a titer to bovine viral diarrhea virus, and a few animals have developed a mild diarrhea or respiratory disease, presumably in response to the virus. Equine herpesvirus 1 infections with associated neurologic signs and blindness have been seen in a small number of alpacas. Although an occasional animal will develop a serologic response to bluetongue virus, all seropositive animals have been asymptomatic. South American camelids can also contract foot and mouth disease, although clinical disease is usually relatively mild; the carrier status of infected animals is unknown.

Gastrointestinal Diseases

The oral cavity and esophagus of South American camelids are unremarkable. The stomach has 3 distinct compartments (C-1, 2, and 3) that do not correlate directly with the 4 chambers of the ruminant stomach. The remarkable features of the small and large intestines are the short mesentery of the small intestine, which results in a convoluted appearance, and the freely moveable spiral colon. The spiral colon is generally a flat single spiral, although variations include a double spiral or corkscrew appearance. Torsions at the base of the spiral colon occasionally occur.

Megaesophagus: Moderate to severe dilatation of the esophagus is relatively common in llamas and alpacas. Signs include chronic weight loss frequently associated with postprandial regurgitation or "frothing" of food. If the cervical esophagus is dilated, it is also sometimes possible to watch boluses of food move up and down the esophagus. There is no identified age or sex predilection, and no etiology has been established. A suspected case of megaesophagus should be confirmed with barium contrast radiography. No treatments (surgical or changes in feeding practices) have been successful. The longterm prognosis is fair to poor, with some animals maintaining condition for an extended period and others continuing to lose weight.

Stomach Atony: Atony of the stomach (C-1 and C-2) is an occasional problem of unknown etiology. Signs can include decreased or complete cessation of food consumption, loss of body condition, and depression. Other GI problems, eg, diarrhea, may be present. Although no etiology has been identified, supportive therapy including fluids is frequently helpful. Lack of food for 3-5 days will also usually cause the death of bacteria and protozoa in C-1 and C-2. Transfaunation (0.5-1.0 L) of camelid C-1 or strained rumen contents (sheep or cow), administered by gavage, frequently results in a dramatic improvement in appetite and reestablishment of the appropriate flora.

Ulcers: Partial and complete thickness erosions of the acid-secreting distal portion of C-3 and the most proximal portion of the duodenum are relatively common. Signs may include decreased food consumption, intermittent to severe colic, and depression. However, a few animals with perforated ulcers and severe peritonitis have, surprisingly, been asymptomatic. While the etiology has not been clearly established, stress appears to be a significant component, with problems often developing 3-5 days after serious injuries, fractures, traumas, etc. The role of exogenous glucocorticoids in the development of these ulcers is unknown.

No reliable premortem diagnostic procedures are available; treatment is usually based on history and clinical signs. Sucralfate (20-40 mg/kg, QID) can be tried; although its efficacy is unknown, it does not appear to cause any adverse reactions. H_2-blockers (eg, cimetidine, ranitidine) are metabolized extremely rapidly and are of uncertain value. Parenteral administration of omeprazole (0.4 mg/kg, BID) is effective in reducing acid production. Stress reduction, including housing with a cohort animal, and supportive therapy are helpful.

Pancreatitis: Exocrine pancreatic problems are occasionally seen. Signs include decreased food consumption, depression, and nonspecific ill health. Increased amylase (normal, 650-1,850 IU/L) and lipase (normal, 19-159 IU/L) concentrations are consistent with a diagnosis of pancreatitis. Peritoneal amylase and lipase concentrations are usually higher than temporally matched serum samples in animals with active pancreatitis. Protein and WBC counts of peritoneal fluid are usually increased. Therapy is nonspecific and supportive, including antibiotics and total parenteral nutrition if indicated.

Hepatic Disease: The visceral surface of the liver normally has multiple fissures, while the parietal surface is smooth and lobation is indistinct. South American camelids appear to be particularly susceptible to *Fasciola hepatica*, with fecal shedding beginning 10-12 wk after infection. Clinical signs can include ill thrift, diminished growth, and acute death. Icterus is rarely seen. Increased serum bile acids (>25 μmol/L) and enzyme concentrations (normal, alkaline phosphatase 15-121 IU/L and AST 66-235 IU/L) are also diagnostically useful.

Hepatic Lipidosis: Hepatic lipidosis is a relatively common problem in South American camelids. Clinical signs associated with liver failure in other species are frequently observed, although acute death without prior indication of pending problems has also been reported. The etiology has not been clearly established, but stress and/or abrupt decrease in food consumption appear to play a role. Treatment is symptomatic. Mortality in untreated animals is frequently high.

Small- and Large-intestinal Diseases: Diarrhea is relatively uncommon in llamas and alpacas. The primary recognized cause of diarrhea in the neonate is *Eimeria* spp infection. Some crias will also experience a transitory diarrhea 2-3 wk after birth. Identified causes of diarrhea in older animals include *Salmonella* spp, *Giardia* spp, *Cryptosporidium parvum*, and *Mycobacterium paratuberculosis*. Treatment options are the same as for other species. In *M paratuberculosis* infections, there is usually chronic weight loss, with diarrhea seen only infrequently in the terminal phase of the disease. The question of differential age susceptibility to *M paratuberculosis* infection has not been resolved. Lymphosarcoma is the only neoplasia found with significant frequency in South American camelids and has gross pathologic lesions similar to that of

Johne's disease, specifically a marked thickening of the intestinal wall and dramatic enlargement of the mesenteric lymph nodes.

Respiratory Diseases

Auscultation of llamas and alpacas is difficult and frequently unrewarding. Little air movement is heard under most conditions, and identification of areas of infection or consolidation is usually not possible. Lateral radiographs are usually required for the diagnosis of pneumonia. Bacterial infections of the lung are relatively rare, with *Streptococcus* and *Corynebacterium* spp being the most common isolates.

MARINE MAMMALS

Marine mammals are a diverse group of species that include cetaceans, pinnipeds, sirenians, sea otters, and polar bears. The cetaceans consist of 2 major groups with different physiology and anatomy—toothed whales (Odontocetes) and baleen whales (Mysticetes). The pinnipeds consist of 3 major groups—true seals (Phocidae), eared seals (Otariidae), and walruses (Odobenidae). Sirenians (Sirenidae) are of a single family that includes manatees and dugongs. The sea otter (*Enhydra lutris*) is a marine member of the Mustelidae, and the polar bear (*Ursus maritimus*) is the only member of the Ursidae that is considered marine.

Few pharmaceuticals or vaccines are approved for use in marine mammals. Many recommendations can be made based on personal experience or published reports, but clinicians should be cautious in their application.

MANAGEMENT

The general rule in maintaining marine mammals in captivity is to duplicate their natural environment as closely as possible. Most live in marine habitats, although some species migrate into freshwater; Baikal seals (*Phoca sibirica*) and 5 species of river dolphins have adapted completely to freshwater habitats. Manatee subspecies vary in the time they spend in freshwater, but the dugong (*Dugong dugong*) is completely marine.

Marine cetaceans should be kept in water with a salinity of 25-35 g/L, preferably using balanced sea salts. Water for captive marine cetaceans should be maintained as close to the pH of mid-ocean waters (8-8.3) as possible. Freshwater cetaceans and seals require water similar to that of their natural habitat. In the USA, the Marine Mammal Protection Act of 1972 specifies that coliform bacterial counts of water for captive marine mammals must be ≤1,000 MPN (most probable number per 100 mL).

Marine mammals kept in the extremes of their temperature tolerance range are more susceptible to environmental and infectious disease. In general, cetaceans and pinnipeds are better adapted to cold than to heat but species-specific tolerances differ. Inappropriately combining different species for display purposes can result in compromises that jeopardize the well-being of some species.

Good air quality, especially in indoor facilities (10-20 air changes/hr) is as important as good water quality. Photoperiods, light spectral and intensity requirements, sound tolerances, and flight distance requirements are not well established for any cetacean. Extremes in any of these factors should be considered detrimental in the absence of specific data for the species in question.

Environmental requirements of pinnipeds are similar to those of cetaceans except that pinnipeds can "haul out" on land. Although captive pinnipeds can be kept in freshwater if given additional salt in their diet, saltwater pools that meet the specifications listed above for cetaceans are preferred. Most pinnipeds obtain their metabolic water requirements in food and do not require access to freshwater if provided fish with a high-fat content. However, it is common practice to allow pinnipeds access to potable water.

Pools for captive pinnipeds should provide shelter from wind and some shade. Haul out requirements are different for each species, and some pinnipeds (eg, the Northern fur seal [*Callorhinus ursinus*]) require very specific timing of access to land (eg, only at the pupping season).

Sirenians are warm-water species with water requirements similar to those of cetaceans, although the most common sirenian in the USA, the Florida manatee (*Trichechus manatus latirostris*), migrates between marine and freshwater environments seasonally. Manatees do better in captivity if salinity is changed seasonally to match migration in the wild.

In captivity, the sea otter thrives best in a cold marine water system. Because the fur of the sea otter is its major protection against hypothermia, the water must be kept completely free of oils and organic material that could mat or damage the coat.

The polar bear naturally lives on arctic and subarctic ice. It has successfully adapted to subtropical climates in captivity but is more susceptible to disease in warm climates. Polar bears traditionally have been provided with freshwater in captivity. Proper attention to filtration and water quality is beneficial.

Restraint

Marine mammals must be restrained for thorough examinations. Trained cetaceans and pinnipeds can be taught behaviors that facilitate examination and collection of diagnostic samples. For these animals, the presence of familiar attendants is important.

For complex procedures or untrained animals, the safest approach to restraining a cetacean is to remove it from the water. Captive enclosures should allow water drainage so that cetaceans can be stranded without the use of nets. As the animal begins to lose buoyancy in the draining water, it should be positioned over thick foam pads to minimize struggling and injury. Nets are an alternative for corralling or catching small cetaceans kept in sea pens or encountered in the wild; however, experienced personnel are required to minimize the risk of drowning or injury to the animal or staff. Netted cetaceans are placed on foam or specially designed stretchers that can be suspended above water level to support and restrain the animal.

Small cetaceans (dolphins) can often be restrained by the weight of 3 or 4 attendants—1 person controls the peduncle of the tail fluke and the others apply weight to the animal's body. The pectoral fins should be placed alongside the animal in a natural position to avoid permanent damage. In larger cetaceans (whales), the powerful tail fluke may need to be secured with a rope loop around the tail stock, taking care to prevent abrasions or lacerations with the restraint loop.

Capturing pinnipeds is generally easier on dry ground, although small ones can be captured in the water with end-release hoop nets. Larger animals should not be netted in water but should be coaxed or driven from the water or have the water drained from their pool. On land, hoop nets can be used on larger animals, but cargo nets, baffle boards, and "come-along" poles also can be helpful. Once captured, small seals can be restrained for some procedures by an experienced handler sitting on the seal's back and holding the head. Larger pinnipeds or more complex procedures require an appropriately designed squeeze cage.

Sirenians are relatively docile; problems in restraint are generally due to their bulk and weight, and caution is recommended because they tend to roll. They can be handled in much the same way as cetaceans. Sea otters can be restrained like most other large mustelids. Hoop nets can be used to remove them from pools. Once they are out of the water, restraint bags, squeeze boxes, or other restraint devices for small wild carnivores can be used. Polar bears are large and dangerous, and manual restraint is not advised.

Anesthesia

Physiologic adaptations to diving and marine environments make general anesthesia of cetaceans and pinnipeds difficult. Anesthetic drugs commonly used in other animals often have narrow margins of safety or cause unexpected reactions in marine mammals. Tranquilizers, sedatives, and anesthetics should be administered to marine mammals only by personnel experienced in their use. Specialized anesthetic machines and respirators are required for cetaceans. Sirenians rarely require general anesthesia or tranquilization for treatment. Sea otters can be sedated with diazepam (0.2 mg/kg body wt) or tiletamine-zolazepam (1 mg/kg). Surgical anesthesia can be obtained with higher dosages of tiletamine-zolazepam (2 mg/kg) or with halothane, isoflurane, or sevoflurane, with or without nitrous oxide. Polar bears are routinely immobilized with etorphine, tiletamine-zolazepam with or without medetomidine, ketamine with xylazine, or a variety of other agents used IM. The required dose is highly dependent on the individual animal and environment.

ENVIRONMENTAL DISEASES

Corneal Edema: Corneal opacity is frequent in captive pinnipeds kept in either freshwater or saltwater; it is also seen in captive cetaceans but is rare in wild animals. It can be due to various environmental problems. Transient cases can be caused by simply moving an animal to freshwater from saltwater, or vice versa. Lack of shade and excessive bright light have been implicated. Unsanitary water conditions (eg, high bacterial loads or overuse of oxidative disinfectants in the water) also have been associated with the disease. Nutritional deficiencies have been suggested as causes, but response to supplementation with vitamin C or A has not been dramatic. The condition is usually self-limiting if the underlying insult to the cornea is removed.

Corneal Ulcers: These occur frequently in captive pinnipeds and cetaceans. They can be the result of direct trauma or the sequelae of unresolved or untreated cases of corneal edema. Diagnosis is by observation of epithelial defects on corneas stained with fluorescein. In trained animals, small lesions can be treated topically. In untrained animals, subconjunctival injections of antibiotics and steroid are required. Extensive lesions benefit from protection by suturing the eyelids. Deep ulcers or lacerations in danger of eroding Descemet's membrane should be stabilized with a thin methylacrylate patch. As in corneal edema, successful resolution and prevention of recurrence depend on removal of the underlying cause.

Foreign Bodies: Many captive marine mammals develop the habit of swallowing objects dropped into their pools. In cetaceans, the opening to the second compartment of the stomach is small, and foreign objects remain in the first compartment. In pinnipeds, the small pylorus prevents passage of most foreign bodies. Frequently, no clinical signs are evident. On occasion, anorexia, regurgitation, or lethargy may be seen. Diagnosis is often made by observing the animal swallow an object. Smaller animals can be radiographed; in small cetaceans, the esophagus can be palpated to establish the presence of foreign bodies. Animals occasionally regurgitate foreign bodies; however, assisted removal is usually indicated. Removal is usually best performed by gastroscopy, which is also used as a method of diagnostic confirmation. All efforts should be made to prevent ingestion of foreign bodies. Training animals to retrieve for reward as a displacement to swallowing foreign objects is thought to be beneficial.

Gastrointestinal Ulcers: GI ulcers are a significant problem in captive marine mammals. Ulcers of the first compartment of the cetacean stomach are a common necropsy finding and pose less severe clinical problems than do ulcers of the pyloric region or proximal duodenum. Gastric ulcers in pinnipeds frequently progress to perforation, which results in peritonitis and subsequent death. Gastric ulcers also occur in sirenians. Although ulcers in cetaceans perforate less frequently than in pinnipeds, they should be treated as a serious clinical problem. Various etiologies, including parasitic damage and increased histamine content of spoiled fish, have been suggested, but the disease must be considered primarily an environmental or stress-related condition. Dramatic environmental changes, including changes of personnel or companion animals, can precipitate serious GI ulceration in cetaceans or pinnipeds.

Clinical signs include lethargy, partial anorexia, abdominal splinting, pallor, and occasionally regurgitation. Animals with bleeding ulcers show anemia and possibly leukocytosis. Diagnosis generally is based on identification of mammalian RBC in gastric washes; confirmation is by endoscopic visualization of the lesions. Palliative treatment of nonperforating ulcers consists of administration of cimetidine (4.5 mg/kg, BID) and alumina-gel-based antacids with or without simethicone, along with frequent small meals. The underlying cause must be identified and corrected for successful resolution. Management of perforating ulcers with resulting peritonitis must include intensive broad-spectrum antibiotic and fluid therapy. As in humans, stress-induced GI ulcers are more likely to develop in marine mammals that have previously had an ulcer.

Trauma: Traumatic lesions (eg, cuts, wounds from gunshots or propeller blades) are common in marine mammals. Propeller injuries are a major problem in manatees, which commonly enter heavily navigated recreational waters in Florida. Traumatic wounds should be cleaned, debrided, and generally allowed to heal as open wounds unless body cavities are breached. Antibiotics should be administered during convalescence to prevent gross infection. Maintenance of good water quality and a high plane of nutrition is beneficial to the healing process. Large wounds frequently heal uneventfully.

Oil Exposure: Exposure of marine mammals to spills of petroleum hydrocarbons is a major concern. Sea otters are particularly susceptible to the impact of oil spills because of their natural grooming habits and their lack of an insulating blubber layer. Hepatotoxicity, renal toxicity, GI damage, and loss of homeothermic ability are important effects of exposure to petroleum hydrocarbons; however, the most devastating effects are due to direct pulmonary damage from inhalation of volatile hydrocarbons.

Experimental evidence suggests cetaceans and pinnipeds will avoid petroleum spills if possible (unlike sea otters) and are relatively resistant to toxicities from direct skin contact. Ingestion of large quantities of oil by these species is unlikely and although baleen fouling occurs in mysticete whales, it is usually resolved with 24-36 hr. Pinnipeds and cetaceans are susceptible to severe pulmonary damage due to inhalation of volatile hydrocarbons as are other mammals, including humans. Efforts to reduce human exposure to hydrocarbons when dealing with oil-contaminated animals must be a top priority. Treatment of exposed animals includes removal of oil from both the skin, using mild detergents (eg, 2% New Dawn), and the GI system (activated carbon gavage), along with physiologic supportive therapy. It is critical to recognize that capture, transport, and holding stresses appear to lower the threshold of hydrocarbon toxicity in these animals.

NUTRITION AND NUTRITIONAL DISEASES

Generally, captive animals fed a diet that is solely or primarily fish are provided dead fish that have been frozen. The logistics and difficulty in providing this fish can lead to some special nutritional concerns. All fish are not of equal nutritional value; diets consisting of a single species of fish are unlikely to provide balanced nutrition for any animal. Similarly, one diet will not serve all piscivores equally. Only fish suitable for human consumption should be fed. (*See also* NUTRITION: EXOTIC AND ZOO ANIMALS, p 1843.)

Storage and thawing of frozen fish must be monitored carefully. Feed fish should be held at -19°F (-28°C) to reduce deterioration of their nutritional value through oxidation of amino acids and unsaturated lipids. Dehydration of frozen fish can also be a problem for animals that obtain their water from their food. Fatty fish should not be stored >6 mo. Few fish, with the possible exception of capelin, should be stored >1 yr. To retain optimal vitamin content and reduce moisture loss, frozen fish should be thawed in air under refrigeration. Thawing in water leaches away water-soluble vitamins. Thawing at room temperature encourages bacterial growth and spoilage.

The energy requirements of marine mammals vary with age, environmental temperatures, and condition. Young growing dolphins and smaller pinnipeds generally require 9-15% of their body weight in high-quality fish per day. Older animals may need only 4-9% of their body wt for maintenance. Larger species (whales, elephant seals) generally require less food (2-5% of body wt) as adults.

Sirenians thrive on a diet of hydroponic grass and various lettuces and vegetables, supplemented with high-protein monkey chow, carrots, bananas, and multivitamin-mineral supplements used particularly to balance calcium/phosphorus ratios. It is thought that sirenians ingest considerable animal protein incidentally during grazing in the wild. Intake requirements have been estimated at 7-9% of body wt daily. Sirenians are generally fed several times a day to accommodate their grazing feeding pattern.

Sea otters are usually fed diets consisting of various invertebrates (echinoderms, molluscs, occasional crustaceans) and fish. Adult animals require ~25-30% of their body wt in food each day.

Polar bears in the wild have high-lipid diets, particularly in winter when they subsist heavily on seals. They are considered to have an exceptional dietary requirement for vitamin A, and some dermatologic conditions respond to daily supplementation of 20,000-1,000,000 IU in the diet. Polar bears are commonly fed large amounts of fish in captivity.

Neonatal Nutrition: Young unweaned marine mammals are frequently encountered in strandings and must be fed a diet resembling their dam's milk. In captivity, neonates may be abandoned by their parents and require artificial rearing. The milk of marine mammals has a high lipid content. Most species are carbohydrate intolerant, and neonates fed formulas with carbohydrates develop severe, life-threatening, bacterial gastroenteritis. Most neonatal marine mammals also require immense caloric density in replacement milks. In the past few years, milk replacement formulas based on commercial component-based milk replacers, eg, Zoologic® Milk Matrix have begun to supplant some of the very complex scratch-made formulas used in the past. When confronted with a marine mammal neonate to raise, contacting one of the major marine mammal rescue centers for advice is recommended.

Phocid and otarid seals can be reared on the same milk replacer-based formulas. Pinniped pups should be fed every 4 hr in their first week of life; gradually, the amount of formula fed should be increased and the feedings dropped to 5/day. Harbor seal (*Phoca vitulina*) pups should be tube fed until 2-3 wk old, when they can be weaned to small pieces of fish. Elephant seal pups require tube feeding until they are 4 wk old, when weaning can begin. California sea lion (*Zalophus californianus*) pups can be force fed fish as early as 4 wk of age and be free feeding by 6 wk.

Neonatal walruses (*Odobenus rosmarus*) have been reared on milk replacer-based formulas as well as on whipping-cream base extended with ground molluscs (clams) rather than fish. They also seem to tolerate carbohydrates reasonably well. Walruses have a much longer nursing period than other pinnipeds.

Neonatal cetaceans have longer nursing periods than pinnipeds. Success at bottle rearing has improved with experience, and individuals from species ranging from common dolphins (*Delphinus delphis*) to gray whales (*Escrichtius robustus*) have been reared successfully. The fat content of cetacean milks varies considerably; bottlenose dolphin (*Tursiops* spp) milk is ~17% fat (half that of most pinniped milks); beluga whale (*Delphinatperus leucus*) milk, 27%; harbor porpoise (*Phocoena phocoena*) milk, 46%; and mysticete blue whale (*Baleanoptera musculus*) milk, 42%. Formulas based on commercial component milk replacers supplemented with ground fish and oils have been used successfully in bottlenose dolphins and harbor porpoises using a lamb's nipple or stomach tubing.

Neonatal sirenians begin to nibble sea grasses shortly after birth but may continue to nurse up to 18 mo. They can be reared on artificial milks with early weaning. Neonatal sea otters also have been reared successfully from birth on artificial formulas. Neonatal polar bears are extremely altricial and are a challenge because of an apparently immature immune system. Polar bear milk is high in fat (31%) and contains minimal lactose. Polar bears have been successfully reared on formulas with a whipping cream or oil base.

Thiamine Deficiency: This can be seen in any piscivorous animal. Thiamine in the food is destroyed by the activity of thiaminase enzymes or antithiamine substances in the fish being fed. These active enzymes also destroy supplemental thiamine that is placed in fish if it sits for long periods before feeding. Clinical signs of thiamine deficiency are primarily of CNS disturbances. Affected animals may show anorexia, regurgitation, or ataxia. The condition can progress to seizures, coma, and death.

Animals with clinical signs of thiamine deficiency respond rapidly to IM injection of thiamine hydrochloride (up to 1 mg/kg body wt), followed by oral supplementation. Control usually involves supplemental thiamine at 25 mg/kg food, preferably administered 2 hr before a main feeding.

Vitamin E Deficiency (Steatitis, White Fat Disease): The antioxidant properties of vitamin E are believed to play an important role in maintaining the integrity of cellular membranes. Oxidative processes during the storage of fish destroy vitamin E and other antioxidants. Steatitis has been induced experimentally in phocid seals, and relationships between vitamin E deficiency and hyponatremia are suspected. Captive piscivores commonly are supplemented PO with vitamin E at a rate up to 100 mg/kg of feed, which generally maintains high serum levels of the vitamin. This does not appear necessary if feeder fish are properly stored and thawed.

Hyponatremia (Salt Deficiency, Addison's Disease): Hyponatremia in pinnipeds is closely related to adrenal exhaustion and development of Addison's disease, which links the syndrome to environmental stressors rather than to a simple primary salt deficiency. It is most common in pinnipeds maintained in freshwater exhibits but can be seen in animals kept in saltwater. It is more common in phocid seals but occurs in otarids and other marine mammals. Signs include periodic weakness, anorexia, lethargy, incoordination, tremor, and convulsions. Serum sodium levels can fall to <140 mEq/L. Severely affected animals may collapse in an Addisonian crisis, which can be fatal.

Emergency therapy consists of sodium chloride infusion and replacement corticosteroids. Longterm management of advanced cases requires mineralocorticoid supplementation in conjunction with oral sodium chloride supplements and periodic monitoring of serum sodium levels. Control consists of provision of saltwater pools or supplementation of sodium chloride (3 g/kg food) in the diet of captive pinnipeds maintained in freshwater pools. Animals on salt supplementation should have continuous access to freshwater.

Histamine Toxicity (Scombroid Poisoning, Mackerel Poisoning): Scombroid fish (mackerel, tuna) and other dark-fleshed fish have a short shelf life, even when frozen at low temperatures. A complex of substances, including histamine formed by bacterial decarboxylation of the large amount of histidine found in the flesh of the fish, is responsible for the signs seen in affected marine mammals. The toxicity can also occur with nonscombroid fishes, including poorly handled herring, anchovies, or pilchard. It is most common in pinnipeds but is seen in other marine mammals. Clinical signs include anorexia; lethargy; a red, inflamed mouth or throat; and conjunctivitis and increased lacrimation. Occasionally vomiting, diarrhea, pruritus, urticaria, or postures indicative of abdominal pain are seen. Antihistamines, including cimetidine, may provide symptomatic relief, but the condition is generally self-limiting and the animal begins feeding within 2-3 days. In more severe or acute cases, epinephrine is effective in counteracting the histamine reaction. Cortisone and diphenhydramine hydrochloride can be beneficial in the face of respiratory difficulty. Control consists of avoiding scombroid fish in the diet or careful attention to their quality, storage, and handling when used.

BACTERIAL DISEASES

Actinomycetes: Nocardiosis is commonly reported in debilitated marine mammals. It has been diagnosed in bottlenose dolphins, beluga whales, pilot whales (*Globicephala* spp), harbor porpoises, killer whales (*Orcinus orca*), false killer whales (*Pseudorca crassidens*), spinner dolphins (*Stenella longirostris*), and leopard seals (*Hydrurga leptonyx*). Infections due to *Actinomyces* spp also have been diagnosed in bottlenose dolphins.

Brucellosis: Brucellosis is a relatively recent development in marine mammals, with initial reports of serologic evidence of the disease in 1994. Since that time, a wide range of pinniped and cetacean species have been shown to have antibodies to *Brucella* spp. Several marine *Brucella* species have been cultured, and genetic analyses show these to be different from known terrestrial *Brucella* spp. Strains from dolphins, porpoises, and pinnipeds appear to be distinct from each other, but strains from one type of animal do not seem to vary much from the Atlantic to the Pacific ocean. Diagnosis remains controversial with challenges in both culture techniques and serologic methods. Little is known about the pathophysiology of brucellosis in marine mammals, although some postulate that transitory reproductive dysfunction is a component of the disease. Clinical experience with the disease is not extensive and no therapy or control methods are established. Zoonotic potential has not yet been determined.

Clostridial Myositis: Severe myositis due to infections with *Clostridium* spp has been diagnosed in captive killer whales, pilot whales, bottlenose dolphins, California sea lions, and manatees. All marine mammals are probably susceptible. The disease is characterized by acute swelling, muscle necrosis, and accumulations of gas in affected tissues, accompanied by a severe leukocytosis. Untreated, it can be fatal. Diagnosis is based on detection of gram-positive bacilli in aspirates of the lesions and is confirmed by anaerobic culture and identification of the organism. Treatment includes systemic and local antibiotics, surgical drainage of abscessed areas, and flushing with hydrogen peroxide. Commercially available, inactivated clostridial bacterins are used routinely in some facilities, although efficacy in marine mammals has not been studied. Botulism has been reported in captive California sea lions during an endemic outbreak of the disease in waterfowl. Affected animals stopped eating and appeared unable to swallow several days before dying.

Pneumonia: The chief cause of death in captive marine mammals is believed to be pneumonia. It is not common in polar bears. Most cases of marine mammal pneumonia have significant bacterial involvement, and most organisms cultured from terrestrial species have been identified in marine mammals. Pneumonia often can be considered the result of mismanagement. Marine mammals require good air quality, including high rates of air exchange at the water surface in indoor facilities. Tempered air or acclimation to cold temperatures is also important to prevent lung disease, even in polar species. Animals acclimated to cold temperatures are usually quite hardy; however, sudden transition from warm environments to cold air, even with warmer water, can precipitate fulminating pneumonias, particularly in nutritionally or otherwise compromised animals. Clinical signs include lethargy, anorexia, severe halitosis, dyspnea, pyrexia, and marked leukocytosis. The disease can progress rapidly. Diagnosis is usually based on clinical signs and confirmed by response to therapy. Treatment consists of correction of environmental factors and intensive antibiotic and supportive therapy. The initial antibiotic is usually broad-spectrum, commonly cephalexin (40 mg/kg, TID or QID); adjustments are based on cultures and sensitivities from blowhole or tracheal samples.

Erysipelas (Diamond Skin Disease): Erysipelas can be a serious infectious disease of captive cetaceans and pinnipeds. The organism, *Erysipelothrix rhusiopathiae*, which causes erysipelas in pigs and other domestic species, is a common contaminant of fish. A septicemic form of the disease in marine mammals can be peracute or acute; affected animals die suddenly either with no prodromal signs or with sudden depression, inappetence, or fever. A cutaneous form that causes typical rhomboidal skin lesions is a more chronic form of the disease. Animals with this form usually recover with timely antibiotic treatment.

Necropsy of peracute cases generally fails to reveal grossly discernible lesions other than widespread petechiation. Diagnosis is based on culture of the organism from the blood, spleen, or body cavities. Arthritis has been found in animals that have died with the chronic form.

Treatment of the peracute and acute forms has rarely been attempted because the absence of prodromal signs obscures the diagnosis. Animals with the dermatologic form usually recover with administration of penicillins, tetracyclines, or chloramphenicol and supportive treatment.

Control seems primarily related to the provision of high-quality fish that is properly stored and handled. Vaccination is controversial, and vaccine breaks can occur. Vials of killed erysipelas bacterin should be cultured for surviving organisms before use in marine mammals. Modified live bacterins should be avoided for the initial vaccination. Fatal anaphylaxis can occur on revaccination. For this reason, some vaccination programs have been reduced to one-time administration even though antibody titers fall below the presumed effective level.

If cetaceans are to be revaccinated, sensitivity tests should be performed by injecting a small amount of bacterin submucosally on the lower surface of the tongue. Hypersensitive animals develop swelling and redness at the injection site within 30 min. Because the vaccine is extremely irritating, no more than 3-5 mL should be used at any one site, even in nonsensitive mammals. A long needle (≥2 in. [5 cm]) should be used to assure that the vaccine is deposited in the muscle and not between muscle and blubber, or a sterile abscess can result. Bacterin should be administered in the dorsal musculature anterior and lateral to the dorsal fin. Administration posterior to the dorsal fin can result in a severe tissue reaction, immobilizing the animal for several days. To maintain high antibody titers, a booster after 6 mo and annual revaccination are required.

Leptospirosis: This has been diagnosed in otarid pinnipeds and bears. In seals, the disease is characterized by depression, reluctance to move, polydipsia, and pyrexia. It may also cause abortions and neonatal deaths in California sea lions and Northern fur seals. Lesions include a severe, diffuse, interstitial nephritis, with renal tubules packed with spirochetes. The gallbladder may contain inspissated black bile, but hepatitis may not be apparent grossly. Hyperplasia of Kupffer's cells, erythrophagocytosis, and hemosiderosis are seen histologically. Gastroenteritis can be a feature. Antibodies to various *Leptospira* serovars (*L canicola, L icterohaemorrhagiae, L autumnalis,* and *L pomona*) have been identified in affected animals by fluorescent antibody techniques. Treatment in pinnipeds is similar to that in dogs (p 527). Control in captive animals requires serologic examination of new animals during quarantine. Captive animals can be vaccinated in endemic areas. *Leptospira* is zoonotic, and appropriate precautions should be taken.

Streptothricosis (Dolphin Pseudopox, Cutaneous Dermatophilosis): Streptothricosis (*Dermatophilus congolensis*), a subcutaneous bacterial disease, has been reported in pinnipeds and polar bears. It must be distinguished from sealpox. Simultaneous infections of streptothricosis and pox have been recorded in sea lions. Cutaneous streptothricosis usually manifests as sharply delineated nodules distributed over the entire body and usually progresses to death. Diagnosis is based on demonstration of the organism in biopsies or culture. Treatment with prolonged high dosages of systemic antibiotics can be successful. *Sporothrix schenckii*, the cause of a subcutaneous mycosis, has been reported in Pacific white-sided dolphins (*Laegenorhynchus obliquidens*).

Tuberculosis: Marine mammals are susceptible to various mycobacteria. Unconfirmed tuberculosis has been reported in a stranded, wild bottlenose dolphin in the Mediterranean, and indirect evidence points to *Mycobacterium tuberculosis* being possibly endemic in free-ranging otarids off the coast of Australia. (Originally thought to be *M bovis*, subsequent molecular assessment places the isolates from free-ranging southern hemisphere pinnipeds in a unique cluster in the *M tuberculosis* complex.) Subantarctic fur seals (*Arctocephalus tropicalis*)) are thought to be the common link in the spread of the disease to other pinniped species because they cohabit with the other known affected species, Australian sean lions (*Neophoca cinerea*) and New Zealand fur seals (*Arctocephalus forsteri*). Otherwise, mycobacteriosis has been a disease of captivity. Pinnipeds, cetaceans, and sirenians have developed disease due to *M bovis, M smegmatis, M chitae, M fortuitum, M chelonei,* and *M marinum*. Cutaneous and systemic forms are seen. There are strong indications that immunosuppression may be involved in the development of infections by the atypical mycobacteria. Intradermal testing with high concentrations of bovine or avian purified protein derivative tuberculin can be used to screen exposed animals; however, anergy occurs. In pinnipeds, injections in the webbing of the rear flippers should be read at 48 and 72 hr. ELISA screening has identified antibodies in seals but requires further evaluation before it can be considered a screening test. Diagnosis is made by culture and identification of the organism from lesion biopsies, tracheal washes, or feces. Mycobacteriosis in marine mammals is an emerging disease and is probably of public health significance. (*See also* p 549.)

Miscellaneous Bacterial Diseases: Marine mammals are probably susceptible to the entire range of pathogenic bacteria. *Pasteurella multocida* has caused several outbreaks of hemorrhagic enteritis with depression and abdominal distress leading to acute death in dolphins and pinnipeds. It has also been reported to cause pneumonia in pinnipeds. In dolphins, *Mannheimia (Pasteurella) haemolytica* has been incriminated in hemorrhagic tracheitis that responded to chloramphenicol therapy.

Plesiomonas shigelloides has been responsible for gastroenteritis in harbor seals. *Burkholderia (Pseudomonas) pseudomallei* has caused serious fatal outbreaks of disease in various marine mammals in captivity in the Far East. *Salmonella* spp have caused fatal gastroenteritis in manatees and beluga whales. Staphylococcal septicemia has caused the death of a dolphin with osteomyelitis of the spine (pyogenic spondylitis). Another case of intradiskal osteomyelitis, due to *Staphylococcus aureus*, was treated successfully with a prolonged course of cefazolin sodium and cephalexin. *S aureus* also has been incriminated in a fatal pneumonia in a killer whale. *Vibrio* spp infect slow-healing wounds of cetaceans managed in open sea pens.

MYCOTIC DISEASES

Captive marine mammals seem particularly prone to fungal infections (*see also* p 510). Most appear to be secondary to stress, environmental compromise, or other infectious disease. Some systemic mycoses have distinct geographic distributions. Diagnosis is based on clinical signs and confirmed by identification of the organism in biopsy or, preferably, culture. Wet mounts in lactophenol or cotton blue may render an immediate diagnosis with some of the morphologically distinct fungi. Tissue smears cleared in warm 10% potassium hydroxide can be examined to identify characteristic fruiting bodies or hyphae.

Topical medication of pinnipeds for dermatophytosis is feasible. Smaller cetaceans can be kept out of water in a sling for 2-24 hr, provided areas of the body not being treated are kept moist. Otherwise, systemic therapy is used.

Aspergillosis: Fatal pulmonary aspergillosis has been diagnosed in several species of cetaceans including bottlenose dolphins and killer whales, and in several pinnipeds including Antarctic fur seals (*Arctocephalus gazella*), harbor seals, and California sea lions. Cutaneous aspergillosis has been seen in gray seals (*Halichoerus grypus*) with concomitant mycobacteriosis. The respiratory form has been a postmortem diagnosis. Cutaneous lesions respond to topical povidone-iodine with ketoconazole therapy (10 mg/kg, PO, SID).

Candidiasis: This common mycotic disease in captive cetaceans occurs secondary to stress, unbalanced water disinfection with chlorines, or indiscriminate antibiotic therapy. Candidiasis is also reported in pinnipeds. In cetaceans, the lesions usually are found around body orifices. At necropsy, esophageal ulcers are often found, particularly in the area of the gastroesophageal junction. In phocid pinnipeds, inflammation at the mucocutaneous junctions, particularly at the commissures of the mouth and around the eyes, anus, and vulva, is the common presentation. Diagnosis is based on identification of the yeast in cultures or biopsy. Candidiasis generally responds well to ketoconazole (6 mg/kg, PO, SID) along with correction of any environmental deficits. Supplementation with prednisolone (0.01 mg/kg) may be appropriate to compensate for ketoconazole inhibition of glucocorticoid production. Fluconazole (2 mg/kg, BID) has also been used successfully. One anecdotal report suggests a possible toxic reaction to ketoconazole in a northern elephant seal (*Mirounga angustirostris*). Early detection and treatment is usually successful. Another opportunistic yeast, *Cryptococcus neoformans*, has been diagnosed in fatal advanced pulmonary disease in a bottlenose dolphin.

Dermatophytosis: Mycotic dermatitis due to *Trichophyton* spp or *Microsporum canis* generally responds to topical povidone-iodine or oral griseofulvin (or both).

Lobomycosis: This disfiguring cutaneous disease is caused by infection with *Lacazia loboi*. The disease has only been reported in humans and in Atlantic bottlenose Sotalia (*Sotalia fluviatilis*) dolphins. Culture of the organism has not been possible. Excisional therapy and systemic antifungal drugs have been used with varying success. Zoonotic transmission has not been demonstrated.

Systemic Mycoses: The systemic mycoses of marine mammals are a zoonotic risk, and precautions should be taken to prevent infection when handling dead and diseased animals. Blastomycosis has caused fatal disease in bottlenose dolphins, California sea lions, a Stellar sea lion (*Eumetopias jubatus*), Northern fur seals, and polar bears. Fatal systemic histoplasmosis has been reported in a captive harp seal (*Pagophilus groenlandicus*), a bottlenose dolphin, and a Pacific white-sided dolphin. Coccidioidomycosis has been found in bottlenose dolphins, California sea lions, and sea otters. Blastomycosis has been successfully treated with intensive management including 70 days of itraconazole (3.5 mg/kg, PO, SID) combined with antibiotic and supportive therapy when indicated.

Zygomycetes: Dermatologic conditions caused by various *Fusarium* spp have been reported in pygmy sperm whales (*Kogia breviceps*), Atlantic white-sided dolphins (*Laegenorhynchus acutus*), harbor seals, gray seals, California sea lions, and northern elephant seals. Diagnosis is based on culture or organism identification from biopsy. Cases have responded to ketaconazole (5 mg/kg, SID for 10 days), fluconazole (0.5 mg/kg, BID for 21 days), or itraconazole (1 mg/kg, SID for 120 days). *Mucor* spp and *Entomophthora* spp have caused fatal disease in bottlenose dolphins, harbor porpoises, and harp seals. A wide range of other zygomycetes have been diagnosed as a cause of fatal disseminated disease in various species of marine mammals. These should be considered diseases of debilitated animals; the underlying cause of the low host resistance to these opportunistic infections must be corrected if therapy is to be successful. Amphotericin B is the therapy of choice for zygomycete infections, but newer imidazoles warrant consideration.

PARASITIC DISEASES

Marine mammals are susceptible to all of the major groups of parasites, including various nematodes, trematodes, cestodes, mites, lice, and acanthocephalans. Clinical experience with many of these is limited, while others are commonly seen in recently captured specimens.

Acanthocephalans: Cetaceans are the primary host of *Bolbosoma* spp but can be infested with parasites of the genus *Corynosoma*, which have pinnipeds and sea otters as primary hosts. *Bolbosoma* spp have been reported in pinnipeds. *C enhydra* has only been reported from sea otters. Diagnosis is by detection of eggs in feces, but clinical disease and therapy are not well documented. Three species of *Profilicollis* (also found in birds) are reported to cause peritonitis associated with intestinal perforation in sea otters. Mortality usually occurs before the parasite produces ova. Premortem diagnosis is problematic. No successful treatment has been reported.

Acariasis: Nasal and lung mites are found in phocid and otarid seals. Lung mites cause rattling coughs. Nasal mites cause nasal discharge but apparently little discomfort. Diagnosis is made by identifying the mite in nasal secretions or sputum. The life cycles of these mites are unknown. Infections have been cleared rapidly with 2 injections of ivermectin at 200 μg/kg, 2 wk apart. Treatment of infected animals eliminates the problem in captive enclosures without environmental treatment. Mites have been associated with large, roughened lesions of the laryngeal area of cetaceans, but their overall significance or treatment is unknown.

Demodectic mange has been diagnosed in California sea lions. Nonpruritic, alopecic lesions with hyperkeratosis, scaling, and excoriation occur on the flippers and other body surfaces that contact the substrate. Diagnosis is made by deep skin scrapings and identification of the mite. Secondary bacterial infection that results in pyoderma occurs in chronic cases. Treatment is the same as in dogs (p 746). Predisposing factors in pinnipeds are unknown. The mites are not readily transmitted among contact animals.

Heavy infestations of sucking lice are common in wild pinnipeds and can cause severe anemia. The lice can be seen grossly and are readily transmitted. They are highly sensitive to ivermectin as well as chlorinated hydrocarbon insecticides. Rotenone powder is also effective. The affected animal must be removed from the water, allowed to dry before being dusted, and kept out of the water ≥12 hr. Treatments must be repeated in

10-12 days. Animals in captivity can be freed of parasites, provided no new sources of infestation are introduced.

Lungworm: Lungworms are common in all pinnipeds. Sea lions have *Parafilaroides decorus*, while true seals are usually parasitized by *Otostrongylus circumlitus*. The latter parasite is also found in the hearts of some phocids; however, it does not produce a microfilaremia. Both of these parasites use fish as intermediate hosts. There are at least 4 species of lungworms in various cetacean hosts, including *Halocercus lagenorhynchi*, which has caused prenatal infections in Atlantic bottlenose dolphins.

Lungworm infection can be diagnosed by examination of feces or bronchial mucus. Anorexia, coughing, and sometimes blood-flecked mucus are the first signs of pulmonary parasitism. Treatment of *P decorus* infection consists of mucolytic agents administered intratracheally, antibiotics to treat any concomitant bacterial pneumonia, ivermectin, and concurrent prednisone or dexamethasone. Diagnosis of *O circumlitus* in elephant seals is complicated by mortality occurring after generalized clinical signs of depression, dehydration, and neutrophilia before the parasites become patent and first-stage larvae can be detected in sputum or feces. Some success in treatment has been reported using intratracheal administration of levamisole phosphate (5 mg/kg, SID for 5 days); however, combined therapy with ivermectin and fenbendazole given 3 days after initiation of therapy with dexamethasone, antibiotics, and mucolytic agents may be more effective. Cetacean lungworms probably are also susceptible to levamisole and ivermectin; however, the sudden deaths of 2 beluga whales injected IM with levamisole phosphate suggest this drug administered by that route may be contraindicated. A percentage of pinnipeds also show neurologic reactions to IM injection of levamisole; PO or SC administration has been recommended.

Lungworm infections often remain asymptomatic for long periods with clinical signs appearing only when an animal becomes debilitated for other reasons. In captivity, lungworm infections are usually self-limiting if larvae are not introduced in fresh fish intermediate hosts. Feeding frozen fish prevents reinfection.

Heartworm: Heartworms of the genus *Acanthocheilonema (formerly Dipetalonema)* are a common necropsy finding in pinnipeds but have not been reported in cetaceans, sea otters, or sirenians. Phocid seals are affected by *D spirocauda*, and otarids are infected subcutaneously by *D odendhali*. Transmission of *A spirocauda* is thought to be by the seal louse (*Echinophthirius horridus*). Both groups of pinnipeds can be infected with the canine heartworm *Dirofilaria immitis* in endemic areas; however, phocid seals are abnormal hosts. Dirofilariasis is diagnosed by identifying microfilariae in the blood. Transmission is thought to be by the same mosquitos that bite dogs. A graded regimen of levamisole phosphate progressing to a high dosage (40 mg/kg, SID for 1 wk) has successfully cleared infection in captive pinnipeds, with the advantage of oral administration. Prevention in endemic areas has been successful with oral administration of ivermectin (canine dosages) monthly or diethylcarbamazine (3.3 mg/kg) weekly, in food during the mosquito season (*see also* p 100).

Other Nematodes: The Anasakidae are pathogenic nematodes found in the stomach of marine mammals. Granulomas form at their attachment sites and can lead to blood loss, ulceration, and ultimately perforation and peritonitis. Raw fish is most often incriminated as the source of infection. Infections with *Contracaecum* spp are common in wild cetaceans and pinnipeds. Polar bears in captivity are prone to heavy ascarid infection. Gastric nematodes can be successfully treated with oral dichlorvos (30 mg/kg), fenbendazole (11 mg/kg), or mebendazole (9 mg/kg) given twice, 10 days apart. Ivermectin may be considered.

Hookworms (*Uncinaria* spp) are found in pinnipeds. Severe infections are known only in the fur seals. Newborn pups are infected via colostrum. Disophenol (12.5 mg/kg) or ivermectin (100 µg/kg) injected SC are effective against these parasites.

Many species of a large spirurid nematode (*Crassicauda* spp) infect the cranial sinuses, major vessels, kidneys, and mammary gland ducts of cetaceans. Successful treatments are not documented but are potentially possible with systemic parasiticides.

Cestodiasis: *Diphyllobothrium pacificum* is commonly found in sea lions, and heavy infection is thought to cause intestinal obstruction. Praziquantel (10 mg/kg) or niclosamide (160 mg/kg) are effective treatments. Other cestodes commonly seen include *D lanceolatum* in phocid seals, *Diplogonoporus tetrapterous* in all pinnipeds, and *Tetrabothrium forsteri* and *Strobilocephalus triangularis* in cetaceans. Cetaceans are also commonly infected with subcutaneous tapeworm cysts throughout the blubber. These usually are the larval forms of tapeworms of sharks. Several species of cestodes are reported in sea otters and polar bears, but are not known to have clinical significance.

Trematodiasis: Fluke infections are common in pinnipeds and cetaceans; *Nasitrema* spp are found in the nasal passages and sinuses of cetaceans. Ova of these trematodes have been associated with necrotic foci in the brains of animals showing behavioral aberrations and have been incriminated as a cause of localized pneumonia in cetaceans. Infections are often accompanied by halitosis and brown mucus around the blowhole and occasionally by coughing. Diagnosis is based on demonstration of typical operculated trematode ova in blowhole swabs or feces. Oral praziquantel (10 mg/kg, 2 treatments 1 wk apart) is usually effective. Reinfection can be prevented by not feeding fresh or live fish.

Zalophotrema hepaticum is an important hepatic trematode of California sea lions; it causes biliary hypertrophy and fibrosis of the liver. Signs are usually seen in adults and include icterus, lethargy, and anorexia. Bilirubinemia and increased serum hepatic enzymes are common. Diagnosis is based on identification of trematode ova in the feces. Treatment with praziquantel (10 mg/kg) or with bithional (20 mg/kg) has been successful.

Various other trematodes infect the stomach, intestines, liver, pancreas, and other abdominal organs of marine mammals. Pancreatic fibrosis due to trematodiasis is a common necropsy finding.

Coccidiosis: Coccidia (*Eimeria phocae*) have been found in harbor seals with a fatal, bloody diarrhea. It is thought that clinical disease with this parasite is rare unless the host is stressed through capture, handling, or husbandry changes. A coccidian, *Cystoisospora delphini*, has been reported as the cause of enteritis in bottlenose dolphins; however, other workers consider the parasite to have been a fish coccidia not associated with the disease. *Eimeria trichechi* reported from the Amazonian manatee (*Trichechus inunguis*), and *E nodulosa* reported from the Florida manatee, are also not associated with disease. These coccidia are probably susceptible to anticoccidial drugs used against other species, eg, amprolium. (*See also* p 163.)

Sarcocystis: *Sarcocystis neurona* is found in high prevalence in the California population of sea otters. Infection can be asymptomatic or cause severe encephalitis characterized by generalized neurologic signs. Methods of premortem diagnosis are currently under development. No successful treatment has been reported. *Sarcocystis* spp have been found in the muscles of many cetacean, otarid, and phocid species and do not seem to be associated with any recognized clinical signs.

Toxoplasmosis: *Toxoplasma gondii* is known to infect the California population of sea otters causing disease that ranges from asymptomatic infection to severe encephalitis. Fatal meningoencephalitis due to *T gondii* has also been reported in a Florida manatee. *Toxoplasma* spp encephalitis is also reported in harbor seals and Northern fur seal. Disseminated toxoplasmosis is reported in California sea lions. *T gondii* is reported from Atlantic bottlenose, Risso's (*Grampus griseus*), striped (*Stenella coeruleoalba*), and spinner dolphins. Methods of premortem diagnosis are currently under development. No successful treatment has been reported.

VIRAL DISEASES

Adenovirus: Adenovirus has been isolated from a sei whale (*Balaenoptera borealis*) and bowhead whales (*Balaena mysticetus*) and in livers from 6 young stranded California sea lions with hepatitis. No disease was noted in the cetaceans. Pinnipeds developed weakness, emaciation, photophobia, polydipsia, abdominal splinting, blood-tinged diarrhea, and eventually posterior paresis; a relative lymphopenia and monocytosis were seen. All pinnipeds developed pneumonia and died within 28 days.

The most prominent histologic lesion in all cases was hepatic necrosis. Massive coagulation necrosis without apparent zonal distribution occurred in some animals. Basophilic intranuclear inclusions in hepatocytes or granular amphophilic intranuclear inclusions in Kupffer's cells were seen. No evidence of adenovirus was detected in the lungs. Adenovirus from California sea lions is not known to cause disease in humans.

Caliciviruses (San Miguel Sea Lion Virus): Caliciviruses have been isolated from otarid seals, walrus, Atlantic bottlenose dolphins, and opaleye fish (*Girella nigricans*). The marine caliciviruses appear to be serotypes of vesicular exanthema of swine virus (VESV, p 590). Several species of mysticete cetaceans have antibodies to different serotypes of VESV. By 4 mo of age, most California sea lions have neutralizing antibodies to one or more of the serotypes. Opaleye fish are probably responsible for the endemic status of caliciviruses in marine mammals that inhabit the coastal waters of California. To date, infections have not been diagnosed in marine mammals in the Atlantic Ocean.

The most consistent lesion in marine mammals is skin vesicles. In pinnipeds, the vesicles are most prevalent on the dorsal surfaces of the fore flippers. In dolphins, vesicular lesions have been seen in association with "tattoo" lesions and old scars. Vesicles are 1 mm to 3 cm in diameter. They usually erode and leave shallow, fast-healing ulcers, but occasionally vesicles regress and leave plaque-like lesions. Skin lesions usually resolve without treatment. Infection may cause premature parturition in pinnipeds. Affected pups have interstitial pneumonitis and encephalitis and fail to thrive.

Inoculation of marine caliciviruses into pigs causes vesicular lesions identical to those seen in vesicular exanthema. In humans, heavy exposure to marine caliciviruses can result in neutralizing antibodies. Localized lesions in an accidental laboratory exposure as well as isolation of calicivirus from a clinically ill primate indicates that these viruses should be handled carefully.

Herpesvirus: Herpesviruses have been isolated from neonatal harbor seals, a California sea lion, and a gray seal. Herpesvirus-like particles have been demonstrated in skin lesions from beluga whales and dusky dolphins (*Lagenorhynchus obscurus*). Herpesvirus-like lesions occur in a wide variety of other pinnipeds and cetaceans. Two distinct herpesviruses have been characterized from harbor seals and gray seals. Phocid herpesvirus type-1 (PhHV-1) is an α-herpesvirus similar to canine herpesvirus. Phocid herpesvirus-2 (PhHV-2) is a putative γ-herpesvirus. Other than a postmortem diagnosis of herpesvirus encephalitis in a dead harbor porpoise, reports of herpesviral disease in cetaceans have been limited to skin and mucosal lesions with little clinical significance. A herpes-like virus was found associated with sublingual ulcers in sea otters stressed in oil spill rehabilitation processing.

Young harbor seals from Atlantic waters infected with PhHV-1 develop nasal discharge, inflammation of the oral mucosa, vomiting, diarrhea, and fever, followed by coughing, pneumonia, anorexia, and lethargy that can result in death in 1-6 days. Morbidity can approach 100% in stressed seals in crowded conditions; mortality is ~50%. The incubation period appears to be 10-14 days. Pacific harbor seals with PhHV-1 tend to develop signs related to adrenal and hepatic dysfunction.

PhHV-2 has been associated with recurring circumscribed areas of alopecia ~0.5 cm in diameter in gray seals. Herpetic lesions in beluga whales are generally circular, up to 2 cm in diameter, and may appear slightly depressed with a target appearance or be raised and proliferative. The centers of some lesions are necrotic or may contain verrucous growths. Systemic infections have not been documented in the whales.

Diagnosis is often made at necropsy or by clinical signs and observation of characteristic intranuclear inclusion bodies in biopsies of early skin lesions. In seals, interstitial pneumonia caused by herpesvirus must be distinguished from bronchial pneumonia caused by influenza virus.

In systemic herpesvirus infection, therapy is supportive. In a documented epidemic, oral acyclovir did not eliminate the infection but appeared to significantly shorten clinical signs in primary infections. Vaccination with 1 mL of trivalent poliovirus vaccine to control recrudescence of suspected herpesvirus lesions has been used with some success; although it reduced the severity of recrudescence in seals, there is a potential public health risk because live poliovirus may be shed after vaccination. Stress and immunosuppression are associated with recrudescence of latent infections. There is no evidence that the herpesviruses of pinnipeds or cetaceans are zoonotic.

Influenza Virus: Four different influenza A viruses have been isolated from harbor seals and 2 other subtypes from a stranded pilot whale. Infection is probably common. Only nonspecific clinical signs were reported in the stranded pilot whale, which had difficulty maneuvering, was emaciated, and was sloughing skin. Disease due to influenza virus in seals is better characterized. Even well-fed captive animals become weak, incoordinated, and dyspneic. Swollen necks due to fascial trapping of air escaping through the thoracic inlet is reported. Occasionally, white or bloody nasal discharge will be evident. The incubation period during epidemics in harbor seals is ≤3 days. Many factors probably contribute to the explosive nature of the reported epidemics. High population densities and unseasonably warm temperatures contribute to high mortality.

In harbor seals, influenza pneumonia is characterized by necrotizing bronchitis and bronchiolitis and hemorrhagic alveolitis. In the pilot whale, the lungs were hemorrhagic and a hilar node was greatly enlarged. For differential diagnosis, *see* HERPESVIRUS above.

The virulence of epidemics has precluded attempts at intensive supportive care. Persons whose eyes were contaminated while doing necropsies, or by being sneezed on by affected seals, have developed keratoconjunctivitis within 2-3 days, and identical virus has been recovered. All affected people have recovered completely within 7 days without developing any antibody titers, which suggests that the reaction is local, as occurs with Newcastle disease virus.

Morbillivirus: Phocid seals are susceptible to canine distemper virus (p 625) and to a closely related but distinct morbillivirus (phocine distemper virus [PDV]). Generally, young seals are affected and show depression, anorexia, crusting conjunctivitis, nasal discharge, and dyspnea. Pneumonia develops and mortality can be high in previously unexposed animals. Outbreaks in wild harbor seals have been extensive in the North Sea. Seals vaccinated with canine distemper vaccine have been rendered immune to challenge with the virus (suspension of organ material) obtained from dead wild seals. Deaths of seals in Lake Baikal, Russia, in 1987 were due to canine distemper virus.

A delphinoid distemper virus (cetacean morbillivirus [CMV]), closely related to rinderpest (p 619) and peste des petits ruminants (p 616), has been implicated in the deaths of harbor porpoises and common dolphins off the coast of the UK, striped dolphins in the Mediterranean, and bottlenose dolphins in the western Atlantic and Gulf of Mexico. Pilot whale calves, white-beaked dolphins (*Laegenorhynchus albirostris*), harp seals, hooded seals (*Cystophora cristata*), and Mediterranean monk seals (*Monachus monachus*) have been affected by PDV and/or CMV infections. Harp seals and pilot whales have been incriminated as apparent reservoirs in the wild of PDV and CMV, respectively.

Therapy is supportive. Mortality in naive populations is high, often due to secondary infections facilitated by the immunosuppressive impact of active morbillivirus infection. Vaccination with a subunit vaccine is practiced in European rescue centers and appears to be protective, but this approach has not been applied in North America, in large part due to lack of availability of the appropriate vaccine.

Poxvirus: Poxvirus has been identified morphologically in skin lesions of both captive and free-ranging pinnipeds and cetaceans. Lesions in California sea lions, harbor seals, and gray seals are probably due to parapoxviruses; lesions in South American sea lions (*Otaria byronia*) and Northern fur seals are probably not. An orthopox virus has been isolated from pox-like lesions on a gray seal. An unclassified poxvirus has also been associated with skin lesions in Atlantic bottlenose dolphins and in a stranded Atlantic white-sided dolphin. Cases in killer whales, dusky dolphins, long-beaked common dolphins

(*Delphis capensis*), Hector's dolphins (*Cephalorhynchus hectori*), and Burmeister's porpoises (*Phocoena spinipinnis*) have also been reported.

Outbreaks typically occur in postweanling pinnipeds recently introduced into captivity. The incubation period is 3-5 wk. A break in the epithelial surface may be required to start an infection. Lesions can recur. Small, cutaneous, raised nodules (0.5-1 cm in diameter) occur on the head, neck, and flippers of affected pinnipeds. These may increase to 1.5-3 cm in diameter during the first week and may ulcerate or develop satellite lesions during the second week. After the fourth week, lesions begin to regress, although nodules are reported to persist as long as 15-18 wk. Areas of alopecia and scar tissue may remain after resolution.

Cutaneous poxvirus infections in cetaceans can occur on any part of the body but are most common on the head, pectoral flippers, dorsal fin, and tail fluke. They range from ring or pinhole lesions to black, punctiform, stippled patterns ("tattoo" lesions). Ring or pinhole lesions appear as solitary, 0.5-3 cm, round or elliptical blemishes, which sometimes coalesce. They are usually light gray and may have a dark gray border, although the reverse color pattern is also seen. Lesions may persist for months or years without apparent ill effects to the animal.

Major differentials include cutaneous streptothricosis and calicivirus. Diagnosis is based on the presence of eosinophilic, intracytoplasmic inclusion bodies in lesion biopsies and is confirmed by identification of typical poxvirus particles by electron microscopy.

Poxviruses of marine mammals do not appear to cause systemic infections. Although animals with cutaneous poxvirus lesions have died, other factors were responsible. Therapy to control secondary bacterial infections is indicated only when skin lesions suppurate. The parapoxviruses of pinnipeds can cause isolated lesions on the hands of persons not wearing gloves during contact with infected animals.

Miscellaneous Viral Diseases: A ringed seal (*Phoca hispida*) in Norway was wounded and appeared confused; its overall condition deteriorated over 5 days, and it became aggressive. Rabies was confirmed by immunofluorescent examination of the brain. At the time, there was an epidemic of rabies in foxes in the area. Other rhabdoviruses isolated from cetaceans, which are not recognized by antisera to representatives of the Lyssavirus, Ephemerovirus, or Vesiculovirus genera, may be related to rhabdoviruses of fish.

Papillomavirus infections have been reported in a wide range of cetaceans including narwals (*Monodon monoceros*), and several species of mysticete whale. Lesions are typical of those found in terrestrial species. No therapy is available. Lesions are usually self-limiting.

Hepadnavirus infection with a hepatitis B-like agent has been documented in a Pacific white-sided dolphin with a long history of recurrent illness in captivity. No evidence of zoonotic transmission was identified.

The only retrovirus identified to date in a marine mammal was a spumavirus isolated from recurring skin lesions in a California sea lion that subsequently died of *Pasteurella* pneumonia complicated with herpesvirus.

Immunohistochemical staining consistent with coronavirus infections was found in 2 adult harbor seals that died without clinical signs and a third that died acutely after a brief period of anorexia and behavioral aberration.

An enterovirus of unknown pathogenicity isolated from a rectal swab of a California gray whale has now been reclassified as a calicivirus. Antibodies, unassociated with disease, against human influenza virus (after challenge) and poliomyelitis virus were found in bottlenose dolphins.

Severe enteritis and vomiting that rapidly led to death in a captive beluga whale was suggestive of parvovirus enteritis, but no virus was isolated.

NEOPLASTIC DISEASES

Tumors in marine mammals are infrequent, although a wide variety has been reported. They are of little consequence except for malignant lymphoma in harbor seals, in which horizontal transmission can occur in a closed population.

MINK

MANAGEMENT

Mink (*Mustela vison*) are housed individually in raised wire mesh pens. A nest box with a hole for entry is attached outside or placed within the pen. Wood used for the nest box should not be painted or treated with wood preservatives. Soft, awn-free marsh hay, chopped straw, untreated wood shavings, or fine wood-wool make suitable nest material. Nest boxes should be cleaned and nest material replaced as required, especially before whelping. Sheds are used throughout the year and should admit natural daylight. There should be plenty of air circulation in the warmer months.

Mink feed may be supplied as a wet gruel placed on top of the wire or as a commercially prepared, dry, pelleted ration placed in feed hoppers. During the weaning and postweaning periods, food is supplied on feeding trays placed on the floor of the pen for small kits that cannot reach the top of the pen. Fresh water should always be available. Watering cups fastened to the outside of the pen with a lip protruding inside are commonly used. Automatic watering systems with individual nipples or flotation cups are used in sheds, temperature permitting.

Cold storage facilities are necessary to freeze and store the meat portion of the ration. A day's supply of fish and meat byproducts is thawed, commercial cereal added, and the combined ration mixed with water to a consistency that will remain on the wire of the pen without dropping through. Ready-mixed feeds may be delivered daily, either ready to feed or in frozen blocks that are thawed as required. Dry pelleted diets are used on some ranches for part or all of the year.

Ranchers usually keep 1 male for each 5 female breeders. Mink are seasonal breeders, with sexual activity controlled by increasing periods of daylight. Artificial lights in the sheds must be used with caution because they may adversely affect photoperiod and interfere with the normal reproductive cycle. In the northern hemisphere, the breeding season begins in late February or early March and lasts ~4 wk. Mating should occur within 1 hr after the female is placed in the male's pen. If fighting ensues, they should be separated. Ovulation is induced by coitus. Females mated before mid-March are usually mated again after 7-8 days, often with an additional mating the following day; thus, individual females may be mated 2 or 3 times. Ova from 2 matings have been known to develop in the same litter. Implantation of the fertilized ova is delayed, so the apparent gestation period is 40-75 days.

Mink have one annual litter of 1-12 kits (average 4). Most kits are born during the last week in April and the first 2 wk in May. Kits are blind, hairless, and weigh ~10 g when born but grow rapidly throughout the summer to reach a weight of ~800 g (females) or 1600 g (males) by October. Kits are weaned at ~6-8 wk of age and may be separated shortly thereafter and housed in single pens. Adult mink are extremely agile, strong, and vicious. Handling requires the use of special leather gloves or wire catching cages.

Pelt collection usually is done in November or December. The most humane way to kill mink is with carbon monoxide.

BACTERIAL DISEASES

Botulism: Botulism (p 490) occasionally causes heavy losses in unvaccinated mink that consume feed containing type C toxin. Usually, many mink are found dead within 24 hr of exposure to the toxin, while others show varying degrees of paralysis and dyspnea. Necropsy findings are nonspecific and related to death from respiratory paralysis. Diagnosis is confirmed by inoculation of serum or filtered tissue from affected mink into mice. The immunotype of the botulism toxin is type C in almost all outbreaks.

Toxic feed should be removed, and stored feed or ingredients examined for the toxin. Recovered mink are not immune to further challenge. Annual vaccination of kits and breeders with a combination botulism (type C) toxoid and *Pseudomonas* bacterin is recommended to prevent outbreaks. Kits should be vaccinated after 6 wk of age.

Hemorrhagic Pneumonia: *Pseudomonas aeruginosa* may result in serious losses. Mink of all ages are affected, particularly during the stress of fall molt. Mink are usually found dead with no prodromal signs. A bloody nasal exudate may be seen at the time of death. Gross lesions include a severe hemorrhagic pneumonia with swelling and consolidation of one or more lung lobes. Treatment involves immediate vaccination of the entire herd. *Pseudomonas* bacterins containing subtypes 5, 6, 7, and 8 are available commercially.

Urinary Infections and Urolithiasis: Urinary tract infections, commonly called "plum bladders," cause serious losses in females in late spring (during pregnancy and lactation) and in males in late summer and autumn (during the rapid growth and furring period). Several predisposing factors have been suggested, including contamination of food, cages, or nest boxes by pathogenic bacteria; decreased water intake; or increased ash intake.

Mink may die without showing signs, or they may have difficulty in urinating or dribble urine. Occasionally, hematuria may be seen. Necropsy findings include acute hemorrhagic cystitis or pyelonephritis, usually associated with calculi (magnesium ammonium phosphate) in the bladder or kidneys. Various organisms, including staphylococci, coliforms, and *Proteus* sp, have been isolated.

In severe outbreaks, culture and antibiotic sensitivity tests should be done, and medication added to the feed. Good sanitation to reduce environmental contamination, increasing the water supply, and culling families in which the condition is seen help prevent the condition. When a continual problem exists (with magnesium ammonium phosphate calculi), feed-grade (75%) phosphoric acid may be added to the feed (0.8 lb/100 lb [8 g/kg] of wet mixed feed), from March to early June and from mid-July to October, to reduce the pH of the urine; phosphoric acid should not be used in young mink. Salt (NaCl, 0.5%) may be added to the diet to increase water consumption.

Mastitis: A variety of bacteria, mainly staphylococci, streptococci, and *Escherichia coli*, are involved in mastitis in mink. Staphylococcal mastitis typically results in abscessation of affected glands or subclinical disease evidenced only by mild diarrhea in the kits. *E coli* causes a peracute, necrotizing mastitis similar to that seen in dairy cattle. Predisposing factors include poor nest box and cage sanitation, rough or sharp edges to the entrance of nestboxes, and high bacterial contamination of feed. Treatment and prevention involve improving management and treating individual animals or the herd with appropriate antibiotics based on sensitivity testing.

Miscellaneous Bacterial Diseases: Various diseases or signs of disease, including septicemia, pneumonia, purulent pleuritis, abortions, abscesses, cellulitis, and enteritis occur sporadically; occasionally, they may become herd problems. Many bacteria, including *Proteus*, *Klebsiella*, and *Campylobacter* spp, coliforms, streptococci, staphylococci, and salmonellae, have been isolated.

Treatment should be based on antibacterial sensitivity tests. Drugs may be administered parenterally or in the feed or water. Dosage can be estimated on the basis of body wt—female mink weigh ~$1^3/_4$-2 lb (0.8-1 kg), and males ~4-$4^1/_2$ lb (1.8-2.1 kg). Dosages recommended for cats should be used and adjusted for weight. However, some sulfonamides (eg, sulfaquinoxaline and sulfamethazine) and streptomycin should not be used in mink. Trimethoprim/sulfadiazine causes abortions in pregnant female mink.

The source of infection should be determined and eliminated. Enteritis often is caused by contaminated or spoiled feed. Abscesses are often caused by injury from wire or splintered wood in the pens, awns in hay or straw used for bedding, or spicules of bone in the feed. Outbreaks of tularemia, anthrax, brucellosis, tuberculosis, and clostridial infections have been caused by feed contaminated with tissue of animals that have died or are carriers of these infections. Careful selection of feed ingredients and disinfection of equipment and pens are important in the prevention and control of many infections. Dead stock should not be used as mink feed.

VIRAL DISEASES

Aleutian Disease (Plasmacytosis): This slow virus infection is characterized by poor reproduction, gradual weight loss, oral and GI bleeding, renal failure and uremia, and high mortality. All color phases of mink may be infected, but light color phases genetically derived from the Aleutian color phase are most susceptible. The cause is a parvovirus not related to mink viral enteritis (*see* below). Transmission occurs in utero and by direct or indirect contact with infected mink.

After infection, immunoglobulin levels frequently increase markedly. Immunoglobulins are unable to neutralize the virus; immune complexes form and deposit in various tissues, resulting in immune-complex glomerulonephritis and arteritis. Gross pathologic changes include splenomegaly, renal changes (varying from swelling and petechiation to atrophy and pitting), and enlargement of mesenteric lymph nodes. Histologic lesions include plasma cell infiltration in the kidneys, liver, spleen, lymph nodes, and bone marrow; bile duct proliferation; membranous glomerulonephritis; and fibrinoid arteritis. Kits from dams negative for Aleutian disease virus may die from acute interstitial pneumonia.

The disease is controlled through a test and slaughter program. Positive mink are identified by blood testing for specific antibody by counterimmunoelectrophoresis. All positive mink should be culled. Mink that are to be kept for breeding stock should be tested in late fall (before selection of breeding stock and pelting) and in January or February (before breeding). New introductions to the herd should be tested.

There is no vaccination or effective treatment. The virus is present in the saliva, urine, feces, and blood of infected mink. Pens should be steam cleaned and dipped in or sprayed with 2% sodium hydroxide. Equipment should be disinfected after handling, vaccinating, or testing mink on infected farms. Raccoons and flies may serve as vectors, and their control is essential.

Distemper: Mink of all ages are susceptible to canine distemper virus (p 625). The incubation period is 9-14 days. The virus may be recovered from infected mink 5 days before clinical signs appear. Recovered mink may continue to shed the virus for several weeks. Transmission may be direct (through contact or aerosol) or indirect.

Clinical signs include nasal and ocular discharge; hyperemia, thickening, and crustiness of the skin on the muzzle, feet, and ventral abdominal wall; neurologic signs (convulsions and "screaming fits"); or a combination of these. Histologic ELISA, immunohistochemistry, or fluorescent antibody examination may reveal intracytoplasmic or intranuclear inclusions or distemper antigen in epithelial cells of the bladder, kidneys, bile ducts, intestine, lungs, trachea, and occasionally brain.

In outbreaks, affected mink should be culled, and the balance of the herd vaccinated as soon as possible. Deaths from neurotropic distemper may occur until 12 wk after vaccination. Kits should be vaccinated prophylactically when 12 wk old with a modified live vaccine (parenteral or aerosol route). Ordinarily, adults are vaccinated at the same time, although vaccination of adults in alternate years may be sufficient.

Mink Viral Enteritis: This highly contagious disease is caused by a parvovirus related to, but not identical with, that of feline panleukopenia (p 635). All ages are susceptible, but the disease is most serious in kits. Transmission usually occurs by the fecal/oral route; the incubation period is 4-8 days.

Clinical signs include sudden anorexia; depression; watery, mucoid, blood-tinged diarrhea; dehydration; and death. Characteristic gross lesions include a flaccid, dilated, hyperemic small intestine with liquid fetid contents. Some mink may die suddenly with no gross lesions. Intestinal lesions are characterized by erosion of surface mucosa, blunting and attenuation of villi, and dilation of crypts. Ballooned epithelial cells may contain inclusion bodies similar to those of feline panleukopenia. Splenic and lymph node lesions include lymphoid depletion and necrosis.

Early in an outbreak, all mink showing signs should be culled or isolated, and all clinically normal mink should be vaccinated immediately. Affected mink can be treated PO with a mixture of kaolin, pectin, and neomycin. Mink viral enteritis can be prevented by vaccination. All mink should be vaccinated when they reach 12 wk old with a combination 4-way vaccine containing mink viral enteritis, distemper, botulism, and *Pseudomonas*. Annual vaccination is recommended.

Aujeszky's Disease (Pseudorabies): This occurs occasionally in mink fed pork products contaminated with pseudorabies virus (p 1065). Mortality may be high and clinical signs are referable to the CNS (tonic and clonic convulsions, excitement alternating with depression, and self-mutilation in some cases). Diagnosis is confirmed by virus isolation or serology. Because contaminated pork is the usual source of infection, all pork products should be cooked before being fed to mink.

Transmissible Mink Encephalopathy (Mink Scrapie): This progressive neurologic disease of mink is rare, but mortality may reach 60-90% of the ranch population. The incubation period is 8-12 mo. Mink usually bite compulsively, are incoordinated and somnolent, scatter feces in the pen, and flip their tails up over their backs (like squirrels). Histologic lesions of the brain are spongiform changes of the gray matter, astrocytosis, and neuronal vacuolation. The demonstration of disease-specific prion protein in nervous tissues aids in the diagnosis. While the means of transmission is unknown, "downer" cattle are suspected to be the source of the agent. There are no vaccines or treatment.

Epizootic Catarrhal Gastroenteritis: Millions of mink have been affected by an agent (most likely a virus) that causes an acute catarrhal gastroenteritis. The disease usually occurs in adult dark mink. Outbreaks occur most frequently during times of stress, eg, during early fall molting, spring mating, and whelping seasons. Clinical signs (mucus in the feces and partial anorexia) rarely last longer than 5-6 days. Death may occur if the affected mink are immunosuppressed by the Aleutian disease virus. There are no commercially available vaccines. Treatment is symptomatic and of questionable value. It is important to differentiate this condition from mink viral enteritis.

NUTRITIONAL DISEASES

Steatitis (yellow fat disease, p 968) occurs in young, rapidly growing mink as a result of excessive, rancid unsaturated fatty acids and a deficiency of vitamin E in the diet. Affected mink may be found dead, or they may exhibit slight locomotor disturbances followed by death. Necropsy findings include yellow, edematous internal or subcutaneous fat that contains an acid-fast pigment. Control consists of removal of the source of the rancid fats and proper storage of feed. Stabilized vitamin E may be administered in the feed (15 mg/mink) for 4 wk, and affected kits should be injected parenterally with 10-20 mg vitamin E for several days. The condition can be prevented by feeding a nutritionally sound diet with added vitamin E.

Chastek paralysis (thiamine deficiency) results from feeding certain raw fish that contain the enzyme thiaminase. These include whitefish, freshwater smelt, carp, goldfish, creek chub, fathead minnow, buckeye shiner, sucker, channel catfish, bullhead, minnow, white bass, sauger pike, burbot, and saltwater herring. Affected mink gradually become anorectic, lose weight, and die after terminal convulsions and paralysis. Fish that contain high levels of thiaminase should be thoroughly cooked at 181°F (83°C) for ≥5 min, or fed raw as a portion of the diet only on alternate days. Mink injected with thiamine hydrochloride, 50 mg, SC, recover rapidly. Adequate thiamine (brewer's yeast) should be included in the ration.

Rickets occurs due to the rapid growth rate of kits when rations are deficient in vitamin D, calcium, or phosphorus. Affected kits usually crawl unsteadily in a frog-like posture, have rubbery bones, and are smaller than normal. The diet should be supplemented as required, and severely affected kits may be treated individually. (*See also* p 853.)

Nursing disease is a metabolic disease that affects lactating mink ~40 days after whelping. It is characterized by rapid dehydration, serum electrolyte imbalances, renal shutdown, and death. Treatment can be successful if affected females are identified as soon as they begin refusing feed and rehydrated with IP or SC sterile fluids. The disease is multifactorial; although there appears to be a genetic predisposition in certain light color mutations, it is more severe in females with large litters and during hot weather. Often, affected females have concurrent subclinical mastitis. Adequate water, environmental cooling systems, fostering kits from large litters to make litter size more manageable for the female, and early weaning help prevent this condition.

Cotton underfur usually indicates anemia and may be caused by certain fish (Pacific hake, coalfish, whiting) that interfere with iron metabolism in mink, which affects melanin pigment formation. Thoroughly cooking the offending fish at 181°F (83°C) for ≥5 min or feeding it on alternate days prevents the condition.

Biotin deficiency, which can cause gray underfur and loss of guard hair, occurs when high levels of uncooked eggs, particularly turkey eggs, are fed. Avidin, a factor present in eggs, inactivates biotin, a vitamin required for pigmentation and hair growth. Affected mink may be injected with 1 mg biotin twice weekly for 4 wk, and biotin may be added to the ration. Biotin deficiency can be prevented by cooking eggs at 196°F (91°C) for 5 min.

POISONING

Lead poisoning (p 2404) may occur in mink that have ingested lead-containing paint from wire or other equipment. Affected mink gradually lose weight and die within 1-2 mo with clinical signs consistent with either gastroenteritis or CNS disturbance. Individual mink may be treated with calcium edetate as a chelating agent. All sources of lead should be removed.

Insecticides other than pyrethrum, piperonyl butoxide, and rotenone may be highly toxic to mink. Even these insecticides should not be used on mink <8 wk old, or where such mink can contact them (eg, nest boxes). Other insecticides should be avoided whenever possible. (*See also* p 2393.)

Wood preservatives (chlorinated phenols, cresols) can cause death of kits in the first 3 wk of life and occasionally of older mink. They should not be used where mink can chew on treated wood (pens, nest boxes, or nest litter). Shavings used as nest-box litter should not contain wood preservatives.

Diethylstilbestrol causes reproductive failure and a high incidence of urinary tract infections in mink and should not be included in the ration. Similarly, thyroid and parathyroid glands included in meat trimmings fed to mink may result in reproductive failure if present at high levels.

Chlorinated hydrocarbons and **polychlorinated biphenyls** contained in the ration can cause reproductive failure. Mink appear to be exquisitely sensitive to **polybrominated biphenyls**; 1 ppm in the ration has caused litter size and offspring viability to decrease. (*See also* p 2367.)

Dimethylnitrosamine (DMNA) is hepatotoxic in mink. In the past, addition of sodium nitrate as a preservative to herring meal resulted in formation of DMNA, which causes hepatic degeneration, ascites, and extensive internal hemorrhage.

Sulfaquinoxaline upsets normal blood-clotting mechanisms of mink and causes extensive internal hemorrhage. **Streptomycin** is toxic to mink.

MISCELLANEOUS DISEASES

Fur-clipping and **tail-biting** are common in mink and may be caused by captivity. Fur-clipping decreases the value of the pelt, and tail-biting frequently results in fatal hemorrhage. There is no effective treatment—all mink demonstrating these behaviors should be culled.

Urinary incontinence (wet belly disease) is a nonfatal condition that usually affects obese males in the late summer and autumn. It is characterized by dribbling of urine and staining of the pelt around the urinary orifice. Because affected areas of the pelt must be discarded, the condition is of economic importance. The cause is unknown, but genetic strain, high dietary fat level, and obesity appear to have the greatest influence on incidence. Affected mink should have an ample water supply.

Starvation and **chilling** cause death in mink fed inadequate fat or provided with too little feed during the winter and early spring. Affected mink are thin and may run until they collapse and die, or they may be found dead in their cages. Such deaths usually occur after the environmental temperature decreases suddenly, especially in the early spring when mink are being brought into breeding condition. Necropsy reveals emaciation and an absence of body fat, in some cases accompanied by hepatic lipidosis and gastric ulceration. This results from improper management and must be differentiated from infectious diseases.

Gray diarrhea in mink clinically resembles chronic pancreatic necrosis in dogs and is characterized by a ravenous appetite and the passage of large amounts of gray, fetid feces. Affected mink appear to die of starvation. No pancreatic abnormalities, viruses, bacteria, or parasites have been demonstrated to be causes. Treatment is of questionable value.

Gastric ulcers and **hepatic and renal lipidosis** are common in mink and usually are associated with high levels of dietary fat or with other diseases or stresses that result in several days of inappetence (eg, during late gestation, the period of weaning kits, or the fall period of furring up).

Hereditary diseases such as hydrocephalus, hairlessness, "screw neck," "bobbed tails," Ehlers-Danlos syndrome, hemivertebrae, and tyrosinemia occur occasionally. Culling the sire, dam, and littermates of the affected mink is necessary for control.

Coccidiosis (p 163) occasionally causes losses in young mink. Affected mink have diarrhea, dehydration, and weight loss. Coccidiostats may be used to control outbreaks. Coccidiosis can be prevented through good sanitation and regular manure removal.

Myiasis develops in mink when flies of *Wohlfahrtia* spp lay maggots directly on the skin of kits. The larvae penetrate the skin and produce inflammation and lesions that resemble abscesses. Affected kits become restless, lose condition, and may die. Malathion dust (5%) placed beneath the litter in the nest boxes beginning a few days before the flies appear may help prevent infestation. It should not be used before whelping or until the kits are 1 wk old. Treatment may be repeated once after a 2-wk interval. (*See also* CUTEREBRA INFESTATION IN SMALL ANIMALS, p 710, and INSECTICIDE AND ACARICIDE TOXICITY, p 2393.)

NONHUMAN PRIMATES

The nonhuman primate species most widely used in research are the macaques, *Macaca mulatta* (rhesus monkey), *M fascicularis* (cynomolgus monkey), and *M nemestrina* (pig-tailed monkey); some African species, primarily *Cercopithecus aethiops* (African green monkey, vervet) and *Papio* spp (baboons); and some of South American origin, *Saimiri sciureus* (squirrel monkey), and *Aotus trivirgatus* (owl monkey). *Saguinus* spp (marmosets) and *Callithrix* spp (tamarins, marmosets), also of South American origin, have had more limited use.

Increased restrictions on exportation or availability of nonhuman primates from countries of origin have led to decreased importation and increased domestic production, with an attendant increase in cost. Importation of nonhuman primates into the USA is prohibited except for scientific, educational, and exhibition purposes.

Primates are susceptible to, and may carry, numerous infectious diseases, many of which are anthroponoses and zoonoses. Consequently, they should be quarantined before use for 1-3 mo to permit adequate evaluation of their health status and adaptation to the laboratory environment. The general principle for quarantine is to completely isolate each group of animals and not mix animals from different shipments or sources without restarting the quarantine period. Recently imported animals that die or become severely ill must be necropsied and reported to the Centers for Disease Control and Prevention, Division of Quarantine.

For nonhuman primate therapeutics, *see* TABLE 12.

Bacterial Diseases

Gastrointestinal Diseases: The bacteria most commonly associated with GI disease in primates are *Shigella* and *Campylobacter jejuni*; occasionally, enterotoxigenic

TABLE 12. Nonhuman Primate Therapeutics*

Antibiotics	
Amoxicillin	11 mg/kg, IM or SC, SID 11 mg/kg, PO, BID
Cefazolin	25 mg/kg, IM or IV, BID
Ceftriaxone	25 mg/kg, IM or IV, SID
Enrofloxacin	5 mg/kg, IM, SID
Erythromycin	30-50 mg/kg, IM, BID
Gentamicin	3-5 mg/kg, IM or SC, SID
Penicillin G potassium + penicillin G benzathine	20,000-60,000 U/kg, IM, SID or BID
Trimethoprim-sulfamethoxazole syrup	Trimethoprim at 4 mg/kg, PO, BID; sulfamethoxazole at 20 mg/kg, PO, BID
Parasiticides	
Fenbendazole	50 mg/kg, PO, daily for 3 days, repeated in 2 wk
Ivermectin	200 µg/kg, IM or SC
Mebendazole	22 mg/kg, PO, daily for 3 days, repeated in 2 wk
Metronidazole	30-50 mg/kg, PO, daily for 5 days
Praziquantel	5 mg/kg, IM
Thiabendazole	100 mg/kg, PO, once, repeated in 3 wk
Anesthetics and Analgesics	
Ketamine hydrochloride	10 mg/kg, IM, for restraint only; with diazepam or midazolam at 0.5 mg/kg, IM, for additional muscle relaxation
Inhalant gas (isoflurane, halothane)	1-2%; maintenance of surgical plane of anesthesia
Banamine (analgesic)	1 mg/kg, IV or IM, BID
Buprenorphine	0.01-0.05 mg/kg, IM, SC, BID-TID
Butorphanol tartrate	0.1-0.15 mg/kg, SC, QID
Propofol	1 mg/kg, IV, induction, 0.3-0.5 mg/kg/min constant rate infusion
Tiletamine-zolazepam	3-5 mg/kg, IM, for restraint only

*All are extra-label uses.

Escherichia coli, Pseudomonas aeruginosa, Yersinia spp, *Lawsonia intracellularis, Salmonella,* and *Aerobacter aerogenes (hydrophila)* are implicated. Primates may be intermittent, asymptomatic carriers of any of these organisms. *Helicobacter* spp have been implicated as a cause of gastritis, anorexia, and vomiting.

GI diseases may be major problems in primates. Clinical signs include watery or mucoid blood-tinged feces, rapid dehydration, emaciation, and prostration. Rectal prolapse is an occasional sequela. Helminths or protozoa may be a complicating factor. Mortality can be extremely high in acute outbreaks unless treatment is instituted promptly to restore and maintain normal fluid and electrolyte balance. The most common lesions at necropsy are hemorrhagic enteritis, enterocolitis, colonic ulcers, or simply colitis.

Clinical signs and death are generally due to dehydration, hypokalemia, and metabolic acidosis. Hydration should be maintained with parenteral electrolyte solutions.

Although medications may often be easily administered parenterally, potassium, B vitamins, electrolytes, bismuth subsalicylate, and antibacterial agents can be administered PO or by nasogastric tube in most primates. Culture and identification of the infecting organism along with assessment of antibiotic sensitivity may be needed for effective therapy. Enrofloxacin (5 mg/kg, SID) or the combination of trimethoprim (4 mg/kg body wt) and sulfamethoxazole (20 mg/kg of body wt), administered as a total daily oral dosage for 10 days, are useful in treating active shigellosis. Erythromycin (30-50 mg/kg, IM, BID for 7-14 days) is recommended for treating *Campylobacter*-associated diarrhea.

Pneumonia: Upper respiratory disease and pneumonia of bacterial origin can cause widespread illness and death, particularly in newly imported primates. Causative agents include *Streptococcus pneumoniae, Klebsiella pneumoniae, Bordetella bronchiseptica, Haemophilus influenzae,* and various species of streptococci, staphylococci, and pasteurellae.

Pneumonia may accompany or follow other primary disease (eg, dysentery). Clinical signs may include coughing, sneezing, dyspnea, mucoid or mucopurulent nasal discharge, lethargy, anorexia, and weight loss. The principal lesions seen at necropsy are those of bronchopneumonia or lobar pneumonia. Empiric antibiotic therapy with trimethoprim/sulfamethoxazole, penicillin, or cephalosporin (either of the latter 2 in combination with an aminoglycoside) generally is indicated. Cultures from pharyngeal swabs or transtracheal lavage are useful in isolating the causative agent and determining the specific antibiotic sensitivity. Intensive nursing and other supportive therapy, such as fluid and oxygen administration, may also aid recovery in selected cases.

Tuberculosis: All primates are susceptible to tuberculosis, although major differences exist in the prevalence of cases in different species. Most cases of tuberculosis in nonhuman primates have been reported in Old World primate species such as rhesus monkeys. Reports in New World species such as squirrel monkeys are much less frequent. Tuberculosis occurs at an attack rate of <1% of quarantined Old World primates, but 45% of cases (especially cynomolgus monkeys) may not be diagnosed until after the first 30 days of quarantine. Clinical signs are not a reliable indication of the extent of tuberculosis in monkeys. A monkey that appears healthy may have extensive miliary disease involving thoracic and abdominal organs; signs of debilitation may appear only shortly before death. However, advanced tuberculosis should be suspected in animals that cough; lose appetite or weight; and/or have enlarged or draining lymph nodes, skin wounds that fail to heal, or abdominal masses. A testing program is mandatory; the tuberculin skin test is the primary diagnostic method for routine surveillance. Tuberculin tests should be done on all primates on arrival at the facility and at 2-wk intervals thereafter until at least 3 consecutive negative tests have been recorded for the entire group. The last test should be administered within 14 days of the introduction to a maintenance colony.

The time from initial infection to skin-test conversion is dependent on the route of exposure, the infecting inoculum, and the strain of organism, but normally occurs in 3-4 wk in rhesus monkeys. Late in the disease, anergy can result in a negative skin test. Anergy may also be induced by concurrent viral infection, such as measles, or immunosuppressive disease. After their release from quarantine, all primates should be skin-tested at least semiannually, and quarterly testing is recommended. The test consists of injecting mammalian tuberculin or Old Tuberculin (15 mg or 1500 tuberculin units) intradermally at the margin of the upper eyelid. The animal is examined at 24, 48, and 72 hr. A positive hypersensitivity reaction is marked by edema and induration resulting in some degree of ptosis. Radiographic examination of the chest may aid diagnosis in well-established cases but is unreliable because lesions rarely calcify or cavitate as they do in humans. Additional diagnostic tests, such as culture, PCR, and staining of a gastric lavage or transtracheal wash sample, ELISA, and comparative abdominal skin testing with avian and atypical tuberculins, may aid in diagnosis. Biopsies of positive or suspicious abdominal tests may be useful in identifying true delayed type hypersensitivity reactions. Due to the public health risk, euthanasia is recommended for all positive reactors.

Tuberculosis should then be confirmed by necropsy. When a positive case is identified, the entire group of primates in a maintenance colony should be quarantined. For animals in quarantine, the period should be restarted and testing should be continued. Personnel working in primate facilities should have regular skin tests.

Mycotic Diseases

See also FUNGAL INFECTIONS, p 510.

Microsporum and *Trichophyton* spp rarely infect primates. Topical treatment of ringworm with undecylenic acid ointment or 1% tolnaftate cream, BID for 2-3 wk, or administration of griseofulvin at 25 mg/kg, PO, for 3-4 wk, is recommended. *Candida* spp are common saprophytes of the skin, GI tract, and reproductive tract; they act as facultative pathogens in debilitated primates. Ulcers or white, raised plaques may be seen on the tongue or mouth; the fungus may also attack fingernails. Oral lesions must be differentiated from those of trauma, monkeypox, or herpesvirus infections. A topical cream containing nystatin is effective in superficial infections. Oral nystatin (200,000 U, QID, continued for 48 hr after clinical recovery) is effective for candidiasis of the GI tract. *Dermatophilus congolensis* has been reported in owl monkeys. Papillomatous lesions are seen on the face and extremities. The infection is transmissible to humans. Aspergillosis may occur in various primate species, and the organism usually is a facultative pathogen.

Parasitic Diseases

Newly imported primates harbor numerous parasites. Some are commensal; others can be made self-limiting by strict sanitation and good husbandry. However, some can cause serious diseases or debilitation and should be removed by specific treatment.

Arthropods: Pulmonary acariasis (*Pneumonyssus* spp) is common in wild-caught Asian and African primates, particularly rhesus monkeys and baboons. Infection is rare in laboratory-raised primates. The life cycle of *Pneumonyssus* spp is not well understood. Infestations usually do not produce serious symptomatic disease, although they may cause sneezing and coughing. Lesions include dilation and focal chronic inflammation of terminal bronchioles. The gross lesions may occasionally be confused with tuberculous granulomas. Ivermectin (200 µg/kg body wt, SC) has been used for treatment in closed breeding colonies.

Mange mites (*Psorergates* spp, *Sarcoptes scabiei*) or sucking lice (*Pedicinus obtusus* [*longiceps*]) are seen occasionally, particularly in feral animals, and may produce dermatoses. Systemic treatment with ivermectin (200 µg/kg) repeated every 3 wk or topical treatment with pyrethrin, repeated after 3 days if necessary, is recommended. Use of more toxic parasiticides should be avoided because of the possibility of ingestion during grooming.

Helminths: *Oesophagostomum* may cause characteristic granulomatous nodules in the large bowel associated with development of the worms and with an immune reaction of the host. The nodules may rupture and cause peritonitis. *Strongyloides* and *Trichostrongylus* are invasive—adults may cause enteritis and diarrhea, larvae may cause pulmonary lesions during migration. These helminths, as well as *Trichuris*, can be treated effectively with thiabendazole (100 mg/kg body wt), administered PO at intervals of 2-4 wk or ivermectin (200 µg/kg) SC. The effectiveness of anthelmintic treatment is enhanced by aggressive environmental hygiene practices. *Prosthenorchis* are acanthocephalans, common in Central and South American primates, that burrow into the mucosa of the ileocecal junction and sometimes perforate the bowel or cause obstruction when present in large numbers. Cockroaches are intermediate hosts, and their elimination, along with strict sanitation, is essential for control of infection. *Dipetalonema* and *Tetrapetalonema* are filarid worms found in the peritoneal cavity of New World species; large numbers may be present with very limited host reaction. Lungworms such as *Filaroides* are commonly found in many South American monkeys.

Cestodes: *Bertiella studeri* and other enteric cestodes may be found in animals of feral origin and are treated effectively with praziquantel (5 mg/kg, IM). Somatic larval (cystic) cestodiasis has been reported.

Protozoa: Primates may serve as hosts of various intestinal amebae. *Entamoeba histolytica* is the principal pathogenic form in nonhuman primates (as in humans). It has only rarely been reported as pathogenic in monkeys, mostly in South American spider and woolly monkeys. In a heavy infection, it may cause severe enteritis and diarrhea, and cysts may be demonstrated in the feces in large numbers. *Giardia* inhabit the upper small intestine and may cause diarrhea. Treatment with metronidazole (50 mg/kg, PO, SID for 5-10 days) is recommended.

Blood parasites, such as *Plasmodium*, *Leishmania*, and *Trypanosoma* spp, are also found. Generally, there is an equilibrium between the parasite and the natural host, with infections not causing overt clinical disease. Transmission of simian malarias to humans, although rare, has occurred in areas where the appropriate mosquito vectors are present. Some primate species (eg, owl monkeys) are excellent models for malarial research.

Naturally occurring toxoplasmosis (*Toxoplasma gondii*) has been reported in Central and South American primates. Clinical signs of infection tend to be nonspecific (lethargy, anorexia, diarrhea). Hepatic focal necrosis and fibrinous pneumonia with edema are common histologic findings. *Toxoplasma* can be demonstrated in blood smears in acute cases. (*See also* p 547.)

Viral Diseases

A number of herpesviruses affect primates; many exist as latent or subclinical infections in reservoir hosts but cause severe disease or death when transmitted naturally to other hosts. All macaques are considered to be potential shedders of *Cercopithecine herpesvirus* type 1 (*Herpesvirus simiae*, B virus). The infection is generally subclinical or mild (conjunctivitis or oral vesicles) in *Macaca* spp but usually causes a fatal encephalitis and encephalomyelitis in humans. Transmission may occur via a bite, scratch, or contamination of a superficial wound or mucous membranes (eg, conjunctiva) with infectious saliva, conjunctival secretion, or genitourinary secretions. Human fatalities due to B virus encephalitis illustrate the importance of using appropriate precautions and protective attire to prevent direct or indirect contact with macaque secretions and body fluids.

Saimiriine herpesvirus type 1 (herpesvirus T) causes mild herpetic lingual ulcers and stomatitis in squirrel monkeys, but fatal epizootics have followed natural transmission to owl monkeys and marmosets. The human herpesvirus, herpes simplex virus type 1, causes a mild infection in humans and certain other primates, but owl monkeys, gibbons, and tree shrews (*Tupaia glis*) are highly susceptible and may die; signs may include ulcerations of the mucous membrane or skin, conjunctivitis, meningitis, or encephalitis.

Naturally occurring, clinically silent infections of hepatitis A virus (the virus of infectious hepatitis) have been observed in chimpanzees (*Pan troglodytes*) and monkeys. Increased AST and ALT values are of diagnostic significance in primates. Human infections have been contracted from chimpanzees.

Because vaccines are not available to protect primate colony personnel or the primates against herpes and some viral hepatitis infections, exposure should be prevented. This is best accomplished by carefully training personnel in the handling of primates; using protective clothing, face masks, goggles or shields, and gloves; separating primates in species-specific rooms; and paying strict attention to hygienic standards.

Several other viruses commonly produce clinical disease in newly imported primates. Rubella infection (measles) acquired via human contact can assume epizootic proportions. The virus causes a nonpruritic, exanthematous rash on the chest and lower portions of the body; it may also cause interstitial giant-cell pneumonia, rhinitis, conjunctivitis, and, particularly in New World monkeys, gastroenteritis. There is no specific treatment. Vaccination of infant rhesus monkeys, other macaques, and marmosets with human measles vaccine is recommended. Monkeypox and other poxvirus infections may occur in primate colonies. Monkeypox is a reportable, zoonotic disease characterized by a maculopapular rash and variolous pustules. (*See also* p 2574.) Affected monkeys usually survive; after recovery, they are immune to challenge.

Immunosuppressive disease in nonhuman primates may be caused by a number of retroviruses including type C and D oncornaviruses and several simian immunodeficiency viruses (SIV). The SIV are lentiviruses closely related to human immunodeficiency virus 1 (HIV-1) and HIV-2. Unique isolates have been found in different species of nonhuman primates. SIV are of low pathogenicity in African species and are often clinically silent, but may cause devastating disease similar to AIDS in macaques. They have been demonstrated to infect humans, although the longterm consequences of infection are unknown. Likewise, the 2 type D oncornaviruses (simian retrovirus D1 and D2) may cause an immunodeficiency predisposing to a complex of diseases such as fibromatosis, atypical mycobacteriosis, intestinal cryptosporidiosis, pneumocystic pneumonia, disseminated cytomegalovirus infection, and candidiasis in colonies of macaques, African green monkeys, and sooty mangabeys (*Cercocebus atys*). Type C retrovirus infection results primarily in lymphoproliferative disease in Old World monkeys and apes. There is great host-interspecies variation in clinical signs and susceptibility from virus to virus. Transmission between primates is via direct or indirect contact with infected blood and other body fluids or from dam to offspring.

Hemorrhagic viral zoonoses, such as Ebola, Marburg, and mosquito-borne yellow fever, are risks with wild-caught animals. An important differential diagnosis for these zoonoses is simian hemorrhagic fever. This arterivirus infection is subclinical in African monkeys, but is highly contagious and fatal for Asian species. Hemorrhagic necrosis of the proximal duodenum is a pathognomonic lesion.

Nutritional Diseases

See also NUTRITION: EXOTIC AND ZOO ANIMALS, p 1843.

All laboratory primates are susceptible to vitamin C deficiency. Hypovitaminosis C may cause immunosuppression and increase susceptibility to infectious diseases before clinical signs of the deficiency appear. Commercial monkey diets contain vitamin C that is stable for 3 mo after the diet is milled and packaged, if properly stored. Supplemental sources are green leafy vegetables and citrus fruits. Orally administered pediatric vitamin preparations that contain ascorbic acid are readily accepted. Daily intake of vitamin C at 3-6 mg/kg body wt prevents scurvy. Scurvy should be treated with ascorbic acid at dosages of 25-50 mg/kg daily until clinical signs resolve and dietary consumption of adequate vitamin C is restored. Primates require vitamin D to prevent rickets and osteomalacia. Asian and African primates can use provitamin D_2 (in plant materials); Central and South American primates cannot and require provitamin D_3. Fish-liver oils provide an adequate source of D_3, or as little as 1.25 IU/g of diet can be added to the ration. Exposure of monkeys to sunlight facilitates conversion of vitamin D to active forms. Without adequate D_3, New World primates may develop osteodystrophia fibrosa (p 856).

Miscellaneous Conditions

Acute Gastric Dilatation: Life-threatening bloat occurs sporadically in primate colonies and may be associated with feeding following a prolonged fast or periods of water restriction or accidental overfeeding. Etiologic factors include intragastric fermentation associated with *Clostridium perfringens* and abnormal gastric function. Monkeys become acutely ill with clinical findings similar to those seen in small animals (*see* p 325). Acute gastric dilatation is often fatal unless emergency treatment is given. The stomach must be evacuated and fluids replaced, in like volume, with electrolyte solution given parenterally. Shock and dehydration usually occur and require prompt treatment. Periodic evacuation of the stomach may be necessary for several days until GI function is normal. Metabolic alkalosis may result from continued loss of hydrochloric acid. Adequate sodium, chloride, and potassium must be provided via parenteral fluid therapy.

Trauma: Trauma from cagemate aggression or self-mutilation (biting or hair pulling) may occur occasionally, as may thinning of the hair due to self-induced alopecia. Massive soft tissue injury, such as that which occurs from mob attacks, causes release of intracellular contents (ie, hypercreatinemia, hyperkalemia) leading to renal failure and death. Aggressive, regular fluid therapy is indicated to avert renal shutdown and antibiotics should be given to prevent infection and sepsis. While measures should be taken to enhance the psychologic well-being of primates—such as group housing, exercise pens, shelters, foraging activities, and cage toys—animals in social groups should also be provided facilities for refuge and escape.

Tetanus: Infection with *Clostridium tetani* is a risk with free-ranging and outdoor-housed monkeys, particularly as a consequence of fighting, parturition, frostbite, and other forms of skin trauma. Immunization with tetanus toxoid should be considered for populations at risk. (*See also* TETANUS, p 495.)

OSTRICHES

Ostriches are large, flightless birds belonging to the ratite group. Mature ostriches may stand 2.4-2.8 m tall and weigh 160 kg. Males are black and white, females are brown. There are 3 recognized subspecies of ostriches in the USA: the red neck, the blue neck, and a hybrid African black.

The major anatomic differences between ostriches and other birds include rudimentary wings, a digestive system modified for grazing, and the loss of 3 phalanges as an adaptation for running. Ostrich keels are flattened; the birds have rudimentary pectoral muscles. Ostriches have several anatomic adaptations of the GI tract that allow grazing with other ungulates in their native habitat, including a large sac-like proventriculus with a defined area of secretory glands. The ventriculus (gizzard) is a large bivalved structure found just caudal to the keel bone on the standing bird. Ostriches are hindgut fermenters and rely on microflora, as do other grazing animals, for digestion of their highly fibrous diet. The colon comprises 60% of the length of the intestinal tract (compared with 6% in domestic chickens).

MANAGEMENT

Restraint: If an ostrich cannot see, it will usually stand calmly without tranquilization for physical examination, venipuncture, sample collection for cultures, radiographs, and ultrasound. Ostriches are curious by nature and can frequently be hooded when approached while carrying a feed bucket. A hood is placed on the restrainer's arm. The beak is grasped with the hand wearing the hood, and the head is pulled to chest level as the hood is slipped over the bird's head with the free hand. It is helpful to have someone step behind the bird to lift up on the pelvis if the bird is backing away.

Juvenile birds from 4 mo to yearlings are best handled by slowly and calmly herding them into an enclosed barn. If they cannot see out and are crowded into a corner, they will sit and can then be easily handled. If there is no enclosed area, portable panels can be used to crowd the birds into a small area.

Physical and Laboratory Examination: Before an ostrich is restrained, it should be examined moving in its enclosure for conformation, gait, body condition, respiration rate and character, and behavior-related problems.

The enclosure should be examined for fresh droppings and urine. Orange to red urine is generally from a porphyrin pigment in the diet and is noticed when urine concentration increases. Green urate may indicate muscle or liver disease. The droppings should be examined for tapeworm segments and collected for fecal flotation.

The eyes and sinuses are examined for any discharge or swelling, and the beak and oral cavity for any lesions. The neck is palpated, especially in the area of the thoracic inlet, for any swellings. Overall body condition should be noted, and a body score assigned based on fat percentage. The feathers and skin should be examined for lesions or parasites. The thorax should be auscultated. The abdomen is palpated from the ventriculus, which lies immediately caudal to the breastplate, to the proventriculus, which can be palpated between the legs. The caudal abdomen is palpated and balloted for any evidence of fluid buildup or retained eggs. Finally, a cloacal examination is performed to verify normal anatomy. When indicated, samples for culture can be taken from the trachea and vagina, and blood drawn for a CBC and serum chemistry. (For hematologic and serum biochemical reference ranges, see TABLES 6 and 7, p 2584 and p 2586). Sodium heparin is the preferred anticoagulant. A slide should be prepared immediately for cytologic evaluation. Cellular morphology is extremely important and should be interpreted by an experienced technician.

Good sites for venipuncture and catheterization in ostriches of all ages are the cutaneous ulnar veins on the ventral side of the wings and the medial metatarsal veins. Venipuncture and catheterization of the jugular vein should be avoided if possible because hematomas form easily, and sudden movement by the ostrich can result in lacerations and exsanguination. The right jugular vein is more developed than the left.

Anesthesia: There are many protocols for induction and maintenance of anesthesia in ostriches. For example, anesthesia can be induced in birds <18 kg by 5% isoflurane (8% sevoflurane) administered via mask and maintained on 2% isoflurane (3-4% sevoflurane). Halothane or methoxyflurane can also be used, but the recovery is not as smooth. Birds >18 kg should be premedicated with xylazine at 1 mg/lb, IM. When the ostrich is relaxed (~5-10 min), ie, nictitating membrane up, head down, and wings forward, a combination of ketamine at 8-10 mg/kg, mixed with an equal volume of diazepam or 0.2-0.4 mg/kg, should be administered IV. The ostrich is hooded, and the only support given is lightly lifting up on the pelvis as the ostrich sits down. Induction and recovery are generally smooth with this protocol. The ostrich should be intubated and maintained on 2-5% isoflurane throughout the surgical procedure. Other induction protocols include xylazine as a tranquilizer at 2-4 mg/kg, IM, followed in 5 min by ketamine at 8-10 mg/kg, IV. A combination of xylazine at 1-2 mg/kg and ketamine at 8-10 mg/kg can be given IV. After induction, maintenance on isoflurane, halothane, or methoxyflurane is possible. Tiletamine-zolazepam at 4-6 mg/kg provides a smooth induction. However, a true surgical plane of anesthesia is not reached, and multiple dosing is required to prevent sudden movement. The recovery can be prolonged and difficult, and the bird difficult to maintain in sternal recumbency due to violent thrashing.

Positioning for surgery and recovery is important. If the bird is in lateral recumbency, the "down" leg should be padded to prevent myositis and neuritis. If a temporary paralysis is present on recovery, the foot should be bandaged (figure-of-8) in a normal standing position for 72-96 hr after surgery. If the bird is in dorsal recumbency, it should be well padded, and the legs extended caudally to prevent neuritis and paralysis. In both positions, the head should be elevated above the proventriculus to prevent reflux of fluid.

The bird should be placed in sternal recumbency in a dark, quiet area with its head elevated for recovery. If the bird must recover in a potentially hazardous location, it should be prevented from flipping over backward. This can be accomplished by tying a soft cotton rope from one ankle over the back as far forward as possible (just under the attachment of the wings), to the other ankle. Tying the ankles together under the bird in the sitting position will add further security.

Surgical Procedures: Proventriculotomy is a common surgical procedure in ostriches. It is indicated for removal of foreign material (eg, hardware, rocks, etc) from the proventriculus or for impaction of the proventriculus with forages. In young birds, incisions should be made carefully because the abdominal wall is very thin.

Nutrition: There has been little research on ostrich nutrition. The formulations of commercial diets are based on extrapolations from poultry. Current trends are to feed 21-23% protein from hatching to 3 mo of age, then reducing the protein level to 14-18%. When an ostrich is 3-6 wk old, the microflora of the cecum and large intestine is similar to that of the rumen. Therefore, ostriches have the ability to digest fiber from a young age. Sheep and goat pellets supplemented by grazing are a more economic alternative to commercial ostrich diets. Chicks allowed to hatch in the nest are coprophagic, eating feces from the parents for the first few weeks of life. (*See also* NUTRITION: EXOTIC AND ZOO ANIMALS, p 1843.)

Vaccination: Although the use of clostridial vaccines in ostriches has been advocated, efficacy is unknown. Use of killed vaccines for equine encephalomyelitis virus has also been advocated based on the isolation of the virus from ostriches, but Koch's postulates have not been fulfilled in determining the role of encephalitis viruses in production of disease. When indicated in a specific flock, autogenous bacterins for *Salmonella*, *Escherichia coli*, and clostridial diseases have been used.

REPRODUCTION

Physiology

Ostriches become sexually mature at 18-36 mo of age. Ostrich reproduction depends on the photoperiod and environmental temperature. In the USA, the breeding season varies from north to south. Birds in the northern USA lay eggs from May to September; birds in the southern USA may lay all year.

In males, testosterone production increases with increasing day length. The testes increase in size (200-400%) during the breeding season, and secondary sexual characteristics such as reddening of beak and legs, vocalization (booming), and territorial displays (kanteling) appear. Spermatozoa production starts at the same time. Avian semen is collected by 1 of 3 techniques: electroejaculation, forced massage, or voluntary ejaculation. None of these methods works well with ostriches because of their physical size, demeanor, and lack of sexual imprinting. Ostrich semen that has been collected by a combination of forced massage and voluntary response is heavily contaminated with urine, making assessments of concentration, volume, and pH unreliable.

As sexual maturity approaches in females, gonadotropin stimulation of the ovary results in a hierarchy of follicular development being established. Each maturing follicle is steroidogenically active, as is the postovulatory follicle. This hierarchy of follicles (F1, F2, and F3) and postovulatory follicles must be maintained for ovulation to occur. In other avian species, the administration of exogenous gonadotropins results in a preponderance of F2 follicles, and ovulation is blocked. Ovulation is controlled by luteinizing hormone (LH) as it is in mammals; however, avian species have 3 LH peaks in a 24-hr period rather than 2 in a 21-day cycle. Oviposition occurs late afternoon to early evening, with the time of lay becoming a few minutes later each day. Ostrich hens are indeterminate layers; they lay every other day in the evening during the breeding season. In the wild, an average clutch is 20-22 eggs.

Reproductive Behavior: The scrape (nest) consists of a shallow depression in the ground that is formed and protected by the male. If left to parental care, the male sits on the nest at night and the female during the day. In free-ranging groups, the dominant hen incubates the eggs during the day. The dominant hen recognizes her eggs, and if the nest is overcrowded, she will remove eggs laid by other females. Nondominant hens may lay in several nests and be bred by several males. Both males and females brood the chicks.

Reproductive Failure: Eggs are candled at 7-10 days of incubation to determine fertility and evaluate for early embryonic death. The embryonic disk floats up and can be examined for development; this is best performed during the incubation cycle because early dead embryos will not be seen after 40 days of incubation. Early embryonic death has many causes, including poor nutrition in the hen, toxins, improper egg storage, and improper incubation.

Behavioral problems may result in failure to copulate. Although ostriches are gregarious in nature, with one male breeding several hens, they do have preferences, and incompatibility is common when the birds are not allowed to select their mates. Seasonal infertility is common early in the breeding season when the hen comes into production before the cock has mature spermatozoa. Late in the season, nutritional influences may also play a role. In other avian species, deficiencies of vitamins A, E, and selenium have been linked to infertility. Environmental conditions may result in behavioral infertility. Extreme environmental temperatures may also adversely affect fertility.

Incubation: In South Africa, many producers allow adult ostriches to incubate their eggs in scrapes. In the USA, commercial incubators are used. Incubators should be stainless steel for ease of cleaning, have proper air flow, and maintain a consistent temperature throughout. The incubation period averages 42 days at a temperature between 96-98°F. Most ostrich eggs weigh 1,300-1,600 g (range 800-2,100 g). Larger eggs require lower temperatures and may take 1-2 days longer to hatch.

Humidity in the incubator is set to maintain a 12-15% egg weight loss during the incubation period. In general, this will range from 20-35% relative humidity. Ostrich eggs that lose <12% of their initial weight during incubation often require assistance to hatch, and the chicks are edematous and have poor first week survival. Although eggs that lose >16% of their initial weight may have good hatchability, chick mortality from 2-3 wk of age will be high. Eggs have been successfully stored up to 14 days without a significant decrease in hatchability. Eggs that are stored >7 days should be turned 2-3 times daily. If the producer has a wide range of egg sizes, multiple incubators allowing different relative humidity settings are beneficial. Proper temperature, humidity, and ventilation in the room housing the incubator are essential for its function. Fresh air flow into the incubator is required to supply an adequate amount of oxygen to the embryo and to exhaust carbon dioxide. Air flow within the incubator is important in maintaining uniform temperature, humidity, and oxygen levels. Ostrich eggs should be incubated with the air cell up and turned through a 90° angle, 45° from vertical in two directions, at least 3 times a day. Most commercial incubators turn the eggs every 2 hr.

Eggs should be candled weekly so that infertile and nonviable eggs can be removed from the incubator. A small, bright flashlight can be used to illuminate the eggs from the ventral surface as they sit in the incubator.

Hatching: Proper hatchery management is essential to the success of any ostrich production operation. Egg collection and handling techniques, incubation, hatching, and chick management during the first 24 hr of life should all be evaluated. Eggs should be collected as soon as possible after oviposition. For best results, eggs should be laid in a clean, dry environment, and any wet or muddy eggs should be culled.

Eggs can be stored safely for up to 14 days at 55-60°F with a relative humidity of 60-75%. The benefit of storing eggs comes from allowing batch hatches, which allows time for proper hatcher sanitation between hatches.

Ostrich eggs are transferred from the incubator to the hatcher either at 40 days of incubation or when the chick pips into the air cell. The temperature and humidity setting in the hatcher should be the same as in the incubator. The chicks should be allowed to hatch unassisted and should be removed from the hatcher when they can stand, generally 4-12 hr after hatching.

Reproductive Diseases: Many diseases can result in reproductive failure, either through failure to produce eggs or through production of abnormal or contaminated eggs. Bacterial salpingitis or metritis is common. The etiologic agents vary, as does the severity of the infection. In mild cases, only the uterus or shell gland is affected (metritis), and clinical signs range from abnormal shells to no egg production at all. Infection may result from retrograde bacterial invasion (from breeding or uterine fatigue), extension of airsacculitis, or perforation of the abdominal cavity by a foreign body. Affected hens generally have a history of erratic egg production, malformed or odoriferous eggs, or a sudden stop in production. On physical examination, temperature and respiration are variable, there may be a discharge below the cloaca, and hens may have a fetid odor. Affected hens often have WBC counts ranging from 8,000 to >100,000. Ultrasonography and radiology are useful in assessing the amount and consistency of exudate in the oviduct. Treatment is based on culture and sensitivity. When large amounts of exudate are present in the oviduct, normograde lavaging of the oviduct is indicated; if it is a valuable hen, systemic antibiotics should be administered. Cocks may develop ascending infections of the seminiferous tubules. Gram-negative organisms are generally isolated; treatment should be based on culture and sensitivity. The prognosis is guarded.

Egg binding is a common problem in ostrich hens. It is thought to be genetically predisposed and complicated by poor nutrition, obesity, metritis, or environmental factors. Although some hens may have a history of straining or vaginal prolapse, most exhibit no clinical signs. In thin hens, the egg may be palpable in the caudal abdomen. Radiology or ultrasonography is generally required for diagnosis. Medical treatment consists of injections of vitamins A, D, and E; calcium; and oxytoxin. The decision to treat medically versus surgically is based on age, assurance that no infection is present, history of the individual hen, and economics. Breaking the egg in the uterus is dangerous due to the risk of lacerations from shell fragments, and surgical intervention is generally required.

Prolapsed phalluses are seen in cocks that are debilitated from other diseases, eg, hardware disease, peritoneal hernia, or sand impaction. Cocks may also prolapse near the end of breeding season due to extreme weather fluctuations or fatigue. Frostbite or necrotizing dermatitis is a frequent sequela. The prognosis for return to normal function is good if the damage is not too extensive and the condition is treated promptly by cleaning and replacing the phallus within the vent 3 times a day until the bird can retain it in the cloaca. If this is not successful after 72 hr, a purse-string suture can be placed in the cloaca. Systemic antibiotics and NSAID are indicated. Males should be separated from females during treatment and for 10 days after resolution of the condition.

CHICK MANAGEMENT

The basic principles of animal husbandry and aviary management, including an "all-in/all-out" system of management, biosecurity of the flock and facility, and a stress-free environment, are inherent to successful ostrich production.

Although, the term "fading chick syndrome" has been adopted in the lay literature to describe any chick that is losing weight, this is often just a sign of poor management. Generally, the level of identifiable infectious or contagious disease is low, and most clinical signs are produced by stress factors such as poor ventilation, overcrowding, excessively high ambient temperatures, overuse of antibiotics, improper incubation or hatching procedures, improper nutrition, and other management-related disease. When considering sick chicks, it is also important to evaluate the population at risk and take appropriate steps to prevent other chicks from developing the problem. This often means elimination of clinically ill chicks by appropriate quarantine or euthanasia. If an infectious disease is involved, treating the individual chick in its environment places all the other chicks at risk.

The most successful management systems are those that allow groups of chicks that hatch together (eg, within 1 wk) to be placed in a clean pen and kept in that pen until 3 mo of age with no additions to the group. The pen is then cleaned, disinfected, and left empty for 30 days before more chicks are placed there. Social groups of ~20 are desirable.

Ostrich chicks do well on a wide range of substrates (including sand, grass, alfalfa, or native pasture) if they are introduced to the substrate at hatch, have adequate space, and have enough feeders and waterers available. Ostrich chicks up to 3 mo old grow best and have the fewest management-related diseases (eg, proventricular impaction, leg problems, feather picking) if they have 100-133 sq ft of pen space per bird. Ostrich chicks do not do well on concrete flooring. Adequate exercise is important to promote normal leg growth and digestive function.

Ventilation is the most commonly overlooked management aspect of ostrich production. In the attempt to keep chicks warm, producers may eliminate ventilation in barns and brooder areas. Additionally, keeping ostrich chicks too hot for extended periods of time may interfere with normal development of the immune system (as it does in other avian species). Keeping the barn or brooder 70-72°F with an additional heat source overhead is adequate. Chick behavior can indicate whether they are too hot (wings extended and panting) or too cold (huddling near the heat source). Normal chicks are gregarious, curious, and active.

Traffic flow in chick-rearing areas should also be monitored closely. Traffic movement on any farm should be unidirectional, with personnel moving from the youngest birds to the oldest. A closed flock is essential for disease prevention and control.

INFECTIOUS DISEASES

Infective agents associated with disease in ostrich chicks include bacterial, fungal, viral, and parasitic agents. However, the isolation of disease agents in a sick chick must be considered in conjunction with a review of nutritional, environmental, management, and genetic factors.

Diarrhea is the most common clinical symptom in ostrich chicks. Many chicks will have diarrhea when the yolk sac is absorbed and they start eating well, at 8-12 days of age. If the chicks are alert and active, no treatment is needed. Chicks will also develop diarrhea after a sudden change in diet; they can be treated with bismuth subsalicylate, but chicks should be allowed to acclimate slowly to a new diet. Bacterial causes of diarrhea include *Escherichia, Salmonella, Pseudomonas, Campylobacter jejuni, Klebsiella, Clostridium perfringens, Clostridium colinum, Mycobacterium* (adults), *Streptococcus,* and *Staphylococcus.* The appropriate antibiotic should be determined by culture and sensitivity testing, and the source of the bacteria identified (eg, barn, hatcher, inadequate hygiene, airborne vectors such as flies, etc). Viral agents (suspected pathogens) that may cause diarrhea include paramyxovirus, reovirus, herpesvirus, birna-like virus, enterovirus, adenovirus, and coronavirus. Treatment for viral diarrhea is symptomatic only, and any potential source of the virus (eg, wild birds, infected hens, people) should be eliminated. GI obstruction is another cause of diarrhea; treatment is surgical, and any changes in environment or feed should be made slowly to prevent recurrence. In cases of fungal candidiasis, antibiotic treatment should be stopped, and a dry environment should be maintained. Although the pathogenicity of protozoa in ostrich chicks is unknown, metronidazole can be administered. Enteritis may also be caused by management errors, including overmedication and excess electrolytes in water during hot weather.

The incidence of **yolk sacculitis** generally is low in naturally hatched chicks. However, owners often assist the chick in hatching or tie off the omphalomesenteric vessels, using a variety of techniques, and bandage the abdomen. These practices often result in yolk sacculitis. The yolk sac may also be contaminated through the ostium at the ileal opening when absorption of the yolk material by the vitelline membrane (yolk sac lining) is delayed. Bacteria commonly isolated from the yolk sac are gram-negative; however, yolk sac retention secondary to noninfectious causes also occurs. The temperature of incubation determines the rate of yolk sac absorption.

Poxvirus infections in young chicks produce typical pox lesions on the face, ears, and neck. The disease (transmitted by insects) is self-limiting and mortality is low. Vaccination of a flock with fowlpox vaccine during an outbreak may stop the spread of disease. Staphylococcal dermatitis occurs as a secondary problem in debilitated chicks, especially when external parasites are a problem.

Parasitic Diseases

Protozoa: A number of intestinal protozoa, including *Hexamita, Giardia, Trichomonas, Cryptosporidium,* and *Toxoplasma,* have been isolated from ostrich chicks. Their pathogenicity is unknown, and immunosuppression may be required for disease to develop. Metronidazole at 10 mg/kg, PO, BID is administered. Coccidiosis is common, and although coccidia are not believed to be pathogenic, it can be treated with sulfa drugs.

Cestodes: The tapeworm *Houttuynia struthionis* is common in Africa but is seen only sporadically in the USA. The intermediate host is not known. Diagnosis is made by observing tapeworm segments in the feces. Treatment is fenbendazole, 15 mg/kg, PO, SID for 5 days.

Nematodes: The wireworm *Libostrongylus douglassii* is the most economically significant GI parasite of ostriches. Mature worms and late larval stages live in the crypts of the glandular portion of the stomach. Diagnosis is based on finding trichostrongyloid-type eggs in the feces. Treatment is ivermectin at 0.2 mg/kg, fenbendazole at 15 mg/kg, or levamisole hydrochloride at 30 mg/kg. Another nematode with clinical significance is *Baylisascaris,* which is transmitted from skunks or raccoons through feed. It is a neurotropic parasite that causes CNS lesions and signs. Restricting exposure to raccoon and skunk feces is the best prevention.

Arthropods: Three types of arthropods affect ostriches—lice, ticks, and quill mites. Biting lice, *Struthioliperurus struthionis*, result in skin and feather damage. The mites can be seen on the feather shaft. Treatment is 5% carbaryl dust at 14-day intervals. A number of ticks affect ostriches, their main significance being disease vectors. The feather mites of ostriches live in the vein on the underside of the feather and feed on blood. They can be visualized as small, reddish, dust-like particles in the feather vein. Treatment for ticks and mites is ivermectin at 0.2 mg/kg at 30-day intervals.

DIGESTIVE SYSTEM DISORDERS

Impaction of the proventriculus and ingestion of foreign bodies are management-related problems. Chicks are at high risk of impaction for the first 2 wk after movement to a new environment, with or without a change in substrate or diet. Proventricular impaction is also seen as a sequela of diseases involving ileus of the GI tract. Impactions with sand and concentrated feed can be managed medically with psyllium laxatives and supportive therapy. Impactions with forages or foreign material (eg, hardware) require proventriculotomy.

Cloacal prolapses are common in young chicks. Frequently the chick has diarrhea or an impaction within the GI tract that causes straining and subsequent prolapse of the cloaca. The cloaca is easily replaced, and a purse-string suture is placed for 24-48 hr.

Intestinal torsion or volvulus, primarily involving the colon, occurs in ostriches of all ages. It can be seen as a flock problem when the diet is suddenly changed, especially if the new diet has a high fiber content. Clinical signs include scant to no feces, slight diarrhea, abdominal enlargement, and vomiting. Abdominocentesis and radiography are diagnostic. When diagnosis is made early, surgical intervention is corrective but often not economically feasible.

MUSCULOSKELETAL DISORDERS

Clinical signs of rickets include enlarged joints and epiphyses, lameness, and pathologic fractures. Rickets (p 853) is caused by a lack of calcium and phosphorus, lack of vitamin D_3, or calcium and phosphorus imbalance. Calcium oversupplementation is common and results in a phosphorus deficiency. Rickets can be induced in young chicks if they are housed under inappropriate light for 10 days.

The etiology of tibiotarsal rotation (rotated leg) is multifactorial. Inadequate exercise, floor heating, and improper nutrition (primarily oversupplementation) may also be contributing factors. Soft-tissue injuries that result in unequal weight bearing have been implicated. There is an avascular necrosis of the cartilage core in the tibiotarsus, resulting in rotational deformity in some birds. Several treatments have been tried, but economics usually dictate euthanasia.

Curled toes are common and unlikely to be related to riboflavin deficiency, which produces curly toe paralysis in chickens. In ostriches, curled toes are usually an individual rather than a flock problem. Splinting the toes when the chick is <10 days old corrects most cases.

Slipped tendon is more common in chicks than in adults but occurs in ostriches of all ages. In this condition, the gastrocnemius tendon slips from the caudal aspect of the hock. Slipped tendon often occurs bilaterally, and both legs are generally repaired at the same time. The prognosis is good.

Myositis results from capture, transport, attack by predators, or fighting. Borderline nutritional deficiencies may exacerbate stress-related myositis. Clinically, the ostriches are often unable to stand. Fluid therapy to correct metabolic acidosis and to affect diuresis, combined with anti-inflammatory therapy and antibiotics to prevent clostridial disease, is indicated. The administration of vitamin E at 5.0 mg/kg, with or without selenium at 0.06 mg/kg, is recommended. If nutritional deficiencies are expected, oral vitamin E can be added to the diet or drinking water.

Various treatments, including slinging the bird to exercise the legs and swimming, have been tried for myositis secondary to overexertion or trauma. However, handling the bird in this manner is very stressful; it is preferable to allow the bird to sit until it can stand on its own, which may take up to 90 days. If the bird is alert and has a good appetite, the prognosis for recovery is good.

TOXICITIES

Many toxicities have been documented in ostriches. Exogenous selenium may cause acute selenium toxicity, leading to pulmonary edema and congestion. The feed additives furazolidone and monensin have been associated with myositis and malabsorption syndromes. Gossypol in commercial ostrich feed contaminated with cattle feed caused a malabsorption syndrome. Cantharidin from blister beetles results in hemorrhagic gastritis and enteritis. Nicotine from cigarette butts results in CNS signs. Toxic plants that contain solanine (eg, silverleaf, nightshade) result in vomiting and diarrhea. Plants that contain high levels of nitrates result in dyspnea and CNS signs. Ammonia toxicity is seen in poorly ventilated barns and results in corneal edema, epiphora, and dyspnea.

TRAUMA

Wing luxations and fractures can result from hauling or breeding accidents. Most cases of wing luxation are actually radial paralysis rather than a true joint luxation. Taping the wings up over the back for 1-2 wk generally alleviates the condition. Fractured wings, depending on the location of the fracture, can be repaired with a half-Kirschner apparatus or splints (or both). Occasionally, intramedullary pinning is required.

Neck lacerations involving the trachea and esophagus are common fence injuries. Primary closure of the trachea is required. Primary closure of the esophagus in fresh injuries is successful; if the injury is old, the esophagus will granulate. With severe injuries, an esophagotomy tube, placed in the distal third of the cervical portion of the esophagus, may be required for alimentation.

Lower leg injuries due to cable fencing are also common. Standard principles of wound management (p 1420) should be applied, including debriding and bandaging the wound. If bone is exposed in a lower leg injury, radiography at weekly intervals is recommended because stress fractures can occur. Soft tissues often are healing normally 3 wk after trauma, but the bird may have a fracture of the tarsometatarsus. Phalangeal luxation is common, especially if birds are kept in icy or muddy areas. If the luxation is not treated promptly, casting the foot in a normal flexed position for 5-6 wk generally allows enough soft-tissue fibrosis and repair to hold the luxated joint in place. When casting alone is unsuccessful, joint arthrodesis according to standard equine procedures can be performed.

POTBELLIED PIGS

Potbellied pigs (PBP) have a short to medium wrinkled snout, small erect ears, large jowls in proportion to the head, short neck, pronounced potbelly, swayed back, and straight tail with a switch at the end. The CON and LEA lines of PBP at 1 yr of age should not be >18 in. at the withers (ideal height ≤14 in.) or weigh >95 lb (ideal weight ≤50 lb). The life span of PBP is probably 8-20 yr with ~10-15 yr typical. Very small or obese PBP may have a shortened life span. For hematologic and serum biochemical reference ranges, *see* p 2584 and p 2586.

MANAGEMENT

Environment: PBP are sensitive to extremes of heat and cold and should be provided a clean, dry, draft-free environment. Adults are usually comfortable in a temperature range of 65-75°F (18.3-23.9°C). Because pigs do not sweat, temperatures ≥85°F (29.4°C) are stressful to adult swine. Extended exposure to high temperatures combined with high humidity may be fatal to PBP not acclimated to such an environment. Cooling methods for adult PBP include moving air across the body, wetting the skin for evaporative cooling (more efficient as humidity decreases), providing shade, and resting on cool surfaces.

Newborn pigs are very susceptible to drafts and chilling and require an environmental temperature of ~90°F (32°C). Chilled pigs will pile on each other and shiver, and their hair will stand on end. A poor environment may cause neonates to become moribund and hypoglycemic (p 1686) within 24-36 hr. Heat lamps or pads can be used to provide supplemental warmth, but their use should be monitored closely; pigs that become too hot will spread out and pant.

Housing: PBP may be housed outdoors or indoors (or both) but must be appropriately acclimated to the specific environmental situation.

PBP housed outdoors should have a large pen (≥50 sq ft/pig) with a structure (eg, a large doghouse) within to provide a sleeping, feeding, and watering area. Pigs instinctively eat and sleep in one area, and defecate and urinate in another. They will use dirt for elimination, and daily removal of feces and addition of fresh dirt to cover and absorb urine is required. Hay or straw may be added to partially satisfy the need to root. However, "rooted-up" pen ground should be filled in with fresh dirt from time to time. Fencing should be well secured in the ground to prevent it from being rooted up, but it should also be portable so that the entire pen can be moved periodically, giving access to fresh, clean dirt. The old pen dirt should then be smoothed out even with the soil surface and left unused for several months before being used again. If pens are maintained on solid surfaces (eg, concrete pads), feces and urine should be removed daily, and fresh hay or straw provided as needed. Water dispensers must be secured to keep pigs from spilling the water by rooting or damaging the device by chewing.

PBP housed indoors should have a particular area (eg, a laundry room), with an elimination area in one corner and a sleeping and eating area in another corner. A litter box with the side cut down to accommodate easy entry and exit may be used as an elimination area. Nontoxic material should be used for litter because pigs are curious and tend to chew on everything. A blanket may be provided to allow the pig to burrow under and partially satisfy the need to root while indoors; a box of dirt is another alternative.

Exercise: PBP should be exercised whether kept outside or indoors. They may be trained to walk on a leash or released into exercise areas. Exercise and all other routines should be at about the same time every day. Daily exercise is important not only for physical health but also to relieve boredom that may otherwise manifest as destructive chewing or rooting or as aggressiveness. Even if the PBP does not exercise much when given the opportunity to do so each day, the various stimuli from an outside environment appear to be beneficial to overall temperament.

Vaccinations: Neutered PBP should be vaccinated against erysipelas, *Actinobacillus pleuropneumoniae,* and leptospirosis. Combination vaccines are available for domestic commercial swine but are not specifically approved for PBP. Because bacterins are used, 2 initial vaccinations 3-4 wk apart are followed by boosters every 6 mo. If exposure is limited, pet PBP may receive yearly boosters at the time of annual physical examinations. Breeding PBP should be minimally vaccinated against erysipelas, leptospirosis, and parvovirus. Such PBP should be vaccinated twice, 3-4 wk apart, before breeding and before rebreeding or every 6-12 mo. Bacterins containing all these antigens are also available for domestic commercial swine but not PBP. Other vaccines should be used as exposure risk indicates. For example, tetanus toxoid vaccine may be used in PBP housed outside and in contact with other species (eg, petting zoos). Routine vaccination against various pathogens not only minimizes sickness in PBP but helps prevent zoonotic disease and may satisfy requirements for pet licensure. Safety and efficacy are concerns when using domestic commercial swine vaccines in PBP. Consideration should always be given to how much antigen per body weight is injected via vaccines. Excessive antigen administration may cause adverse reactions. No rabies vaccine is approved for use in PBP (or any swine). Swine are susceptible to rabies, but only 1-3 cases/yr have been confirmed in the USA in recent years.

Parasite Control: External and internal parasites are possible health problems in PBP, and the zoonotic potential of sarcoptic mange and roundworms should be considered when counseling clients. Fecal samples via fecal flotation may be evaluated in PBP after 6 wk of age. Dewormers, such as oral fenbendazole at 3 mg/kg, SID for 3 days; ivermectin at 300 µg/kg, SC; or doramectin at 300 µg/kg, IM, should be used as indicated. Injectable ivermectin and doramectin are highly effective against sarcoptic mange, the most common external parasite in PBP.

Dental Care: The 8 needle teeth (4 deciduous lateral incisors and 4 deciduous canines) of newborn PBP should be trimmed to prevent injury to littermates and laceration of the sow's underline. Four permanent canine teeth erupt at ~5-7 mo of age and are first trimmed at or after 1 yr of age. Elongated permanent canine teeth may cause discomfort, malocclusion, and persistent chewing motion and salivation. In neutered or intact male and female PBP, the canine teeth grow continually and should be cut about once a year using obstetrical wire, mechanical saws, or other instruments. Sedation or anesthesia is required. Teeth should be cut as close as possible to the gum line without cutting the oral mucosa or lips; there should be no exposed root canal after cutting. Tetanus antitoxin (500-1,500 U, depending on PBP size) and antibacterials are usually administered. In PBP properly vaccinated with tetanus toxoid, a tetanus antitoxin injection is unnecessary. Tartar buildup on the incisors, canines, and lateral surfaces of premolars and molars can be removed manually by instrument scraping at the same time the canine teeth are cut. Dental cleaners for small animals may be used with care, positioning the head of the PBP downward during use to prevent water aspiration.

Geriatric PBP may have abscessed and/or exposed tooth roots; sedation (tiletamine-zolazepam 2.2 mg/kg, IM, in ham) and examination of the oral cavity with or without endoscopy is indicated if anorexia and/or bruxism are reported. Radiographs may be necessary to diagnose tooth root abscession. PBP seem to recover well after tooth extraction followed by antibiotics and tetanus prophylaxis.

REPRODUCTION

Females: First estrus occurs as early as 3 mo of age in gilt piglets. The lack of estrus or a distended abdomen in a young gilt may be due to pregnancy if she has been exposed to littermate boars. If the female does not cycle, the abortifacient prostaglandin $F_{2\alpha}$, given as 2 injections (8 mg and 5 mg in a 25-kg pig) 12 hr apart, can be administered when corpora lutea have become susceptible to luteolysis after day 13 after estrus. Estrus should occur 3-7 days later.

Dystocia is another reproductive problem in PBP. Because the birth canal is too small for inspection for unborn pigs via palpation, radiography or ultrasound may be indicated to reveal undelivered piglets. Oxytocin (5-10 U) may be used to aid delivery if the vaginal canal is patent. The decision to perform a cesarean section, if indicated, should be made promptly, before the sow becomes toxic and has friable uterine tissue and vessels. Cesarean section may be performed by several approaches, but the right flank approach has 2 advantages: the piglets nurse away from the incision, and gravity pulls the incision shut, minimizing the chance of dehiscence. However, regardless of surgical approach, surviving piglets will probably require hand-raising.

Ovariohysterectomy ideally should be done in PBP at 4-6 mo of age. Older female PBP generally display irritable behavior for 2-3 days of estrus out of every 21 days of the estrous cycle. Performing an ovariohysterectomy during estrus is a formidable task because of the tremendous vasculature in the broad ligaments of the horns of the uterus, and surgery should be delayed until ~7-10 days after estrus. Early spaying may also reduce the risk of ovarian cysts, uterine tumors, and cystic endometrial hyperplasia. An obviously distended abdomen accompanies large ovarian or uterine masses (≥20-30 lb). Vulvar hemorrhage may be a sign of uterine tumor and can be life-threatening. Although most ovarian or uterine masses can be surgically removed, some are so extensive and invasive that euthanasia is required. A distal midline approach, as if performing a cystotomy, has been routinely used for ovariohysterectomy because it is more difficult to expose the cervical end of the reproductive tract than the ovarian end. Penetration of the cervix by sutures should be avoided when ligating the uterine stump to prevent intermittent post-surgical hemorrhage from the vulva. A right flank approach may be used in extremely obese PBP, in which wound dehiscence could be a complication. Isoflurane anesthesia provides excellent muscle relaxation. Malignant hyperthermia (p 832) has been reported only once in a PBP under isoflurane gas anesthesia, so it is thought to be rare in PBP. Because some PBP may become apneic when placed in prolonged dorsal recumbency, intubation is preferred to masking; however, PBP may be difficult to intubate, and prolonged efforts at intubation may cause laryngeal edema and postsurgical complications.

Males: PBP boars retained for breeding should be kept in secure pens; they should not be kept as pets because of the unpredictable behavior of boars around other animals or people. Neutering is usually performed at 8-12 wk of age, using injectable or isoflurane anesthesia. One protocol for injectable anesthesia is xylazine at 2.2 mg/kg, IM, followed by tiletamine-zolazepam at 6.6 mg/kg, IM, both injections in the hams. Determining whether both testicles are descended before surgery is important because cryptorchidism is seen in PBP. An inguinal hernia is another possible complicating factor. The midline skin incision is made cranial to the scrotum, and structures such as the vas deferens and blood vessels are ligated and excised similar to the procedure in dogs. Both inguinal ring areas should be closed to prevent herniation after surgery. Removal of tunic, cremaster muscle, and extraneous subcutaneous tissue, followed by closure to obliterate empty space, will help prevent seroma formation. At the time of castration, the preputial diverticulum or "scent gland" may be removed by eversion and excision to minimize the pooling and discharge of foul-smelling preputial fluid after castration. Umbilical hernia may complicate removal. Tetanus antitoxin (if no current tetanus toxoid vaccination) and antibacterial injection are given after surgery of the reproductive tract.

FEEDING AND NUTRITION

Fresh water should be available at all times to prevent dehydration and salt toxicity (water deprivation). Balanced diets are essential to provide proper daily nutrients and prevent obesity. Starter, grower, and maintenance rations for PBP are commercially available as crumbles or pellets. The recommended amount per body weight should be fed divided into at least 2 meals/day. Rations for commercial domestic swine, which are available in meal, crumble, or pellets, may also be used with professional veterinary guidance. Green leafy vegetables, alfalfa, and green grasses (but not weeds, because some are toxic) can be added to the ration to satisfy appetite. Fruits such as apples and grapes may be given in limited amounts. High-energy treats should be avoided because PBP tend to become overweight.

Even when calorie intake is restricted, weight loss is difficult because the minimal amount of exercise possible in obese PBP consumes few calories. Lameness is another common factor limiting exercise capacity. Swimming is an alternative form of exercise for obese, lame PBP.

Young weaned PBP thrive best if adequate colostrum was consumed within the first 24 hr of life. PBP deprived of colostrum easily succumb to diarrheal and septicemic disease. For early nutrition, commercial milk replacers are available, but 2-3% pasteurized milk or powdered milk also can be used successfully. About 1 oz every 4-6 hr should be fed from a bottle with a nipple until the pig is trained to drink the milk from a shallow bowl or pan; usually, this can be done in <24 hr. The volume fed should be increased as the pig grows but decreased if diarrhea occurs. Overeating diarrhea may be controlled with kaolin/pectin preparations given every 4 hr. Infectious diarrhea that may be from gram-negative bacteria (eg, *Escherichia coli*) should respond to parenteral or oral gentamicin or oral spectinomycin. The diet can be converted to solid feed by mixing a small amount with milk to make a gruel and gradually increasing the ratio of feed to milk (conversion to all feed in ~14 days). Increasing amounts of fresh water should be provided as the diet is converted.

Urolithiasis from triple phosphate crystalluria may occur in male or female PBP but can be prevented through addition of urinary acidifiers to the ration. One commercial PBP feed contains ammonium chloride, and feed additives containing ammonium chloride or citric acid are available. Owners may feed fruits or vitamin C in an attempt to acidify the urine. A constant source of clean, fresh water is also important to prevent the accumulation of triple phosphate crystals. Adding fruit juice to water may increase water consumption and help acidify the urine. Inadequate water consumption by sedentary PBP in cool weather has been associated with urolithiasis.

DISEASES

Furnishing adequate housing, nutrition, and care will minimize disease in PBP, as in other species. Many diseases of PBP are similar to those of domestic commercial swine, although some are more common in PBP.

Gastrointestinal System

Gastritis and gastric foreign bodies are common in PBP because they are omnivorous and prone to ingest many types of objects. This may be related to normal curiosity, boredom, and/or a seemingly insatiable appetite. Keeping PBP indoors where they are unable to root and restricting calorie intake to prevent obesity probably contribute to this continual search for food. Dividing the daily ration into 2 or more portions and furnishing low-calorie foods (eg, lettuce, cabbage, celery, carrots, or green grasses) may help satisfy appetite. If an ingested foreign body is small or pliable enough, it may pass through the GI tract and cause mild gastritis that is self-limiting or only requires antibiotic therapy. Larger objects may remain in the stomach or partially pass into the duodenum or a more distal part of the small intestine. Clinical signs such as vomiting and colic can be acute but may be more subtle and increase in intensity over several days or weeks. Radiographs may demonstrate obvious foreign material or delayed gastric emptying. CBC may indicate infection but are usually not informative; serum enzyme and electrolyte panels may only reflect dehydration. Surgical correction is indicated but may not be successful if extensive necrosis of GI tissue is present. Fluid replacement and nutritional supplementation plus antibacterial therapy and tetanus prophylaxis are indicated in convalescing PBP.

Lower GI obstruction due to bowel stricture occurs in geriatric PBP. Anorexia, scant fecal production, and a bloated abdomen with massively distended intestines seen radiographically are typical. Sedation and endoscopic examination of the oral cavity, esophagus, and stomach are indicated to rule out other problems. Exploratory laparotomy and anastomosis with or without bowel resection is usually remedial.

Colibacillosis or *E coli* diarrhea is generally an important disease in young PBP. Mortality may be high in piglets that have not ingested adequate colostrum in their first 24 hr of life. Older PBP apparently develop resistance to colibacillosis. Diagnosis is through signalment, history, and fecal culture. Sanitation to minimize infective doses of pathogenic coliforms in the environment of young, nursing PBP is important for prevention. Commercial swine vaccines to prevent colibacillosis are available but must be given to sows before farrowing to stimulate immunity and secretion of IgA into the milk. Treatment is based on in vitro antibacterial sensitivity testing, but antibiotics such as oral or injectable gentamicin or injectable ceftiofur are usually effective.

Enterocolitis from *Salmonella typhimurium* infection can affect PBP of any age, but it usually occurs after weaning. Sources of salmonellae include waste food from overturned garbage cans, exposure to carrier swine (such as the dam), or fecal material from other animal species. Mild to severe diarrhea with mucus and blood can result. Diagnosis is through signalment, history, and fecal culture or PCR. *Salmonella* spp are characteristically resistant to many antibiotics, so in vitro antibacterial sensitivity testing is important. Parenteral gentamicin at 2.2 mg/kg, SID for 3 days, or enrofloxacin at 2.2 mg/kg, BID for 3 days, may be effective in the interim. Untreated PBP may die. Some recovered PBP may develop rectal stricture after enterocolitis, resulting in megacolon and a distended abdomen. Subsequent straining to defecate can cause rectal prolapse. Surgical correction of the rectal prolapse will not correct the underlying problem. Owners should be advised that many *Salmonella* spp, including *S typhimurium*, are zoonotic. Healthy PBP may be tested via fecal culture or PCR to determine their salmonella status. Multiple tests are more accurate predictors than single tests. Vaccines available for commercial swine have not been used much in PBP.

Bacteremia or septicemia after *S choleraesuis* infection may also affect PBP, usually after weaning. Sources of infection are similar to those of *S typhimurium*. Mild to inapparent diarrhea followed by fever, lethargy, anorexia, cyanosis of extremities, recumbency, and death may ensue. Diagnosis, treatment, prevention, and zoonotic potential are similar to those of *S typhimurium*, except zoonosis is mainly a threat in immunocompromised people.

Constipation may be seen in PBP; however, each normal bowel movement of a PBP is typically 1 main cylindrical formation made up of smaller, multiple fecal balls (which give the impression that the PBP is constipated). True constipation may be due to low water intake in sedentary PBP or to an actual disease state. Enemas may be contraindicated if there is pathology such as colitis. Therefore, careful evaluation is warranted before treatment is administered. In simple constipation, mineral oil and other fecal softeners may be used, as may mild laxatives such as sodium sulfate or magnesium sulfate. These should be given with food, if possible, as forced PO administration can result in aspiration pneumonia and death, especially with mineral oil. Encouraging increased water intake by flavoring with fruit juice or liquid gelatin may be helpful. Regular exercise is also beneficial in promoting normal feces.

Rectal prolapse occurs due to straining from bowel irritation from diarrheal disease, rectal stricture after *S typhimurium* enterocolitis or previous rectal prolapse repair, cystitis or urolithiasis, persistent coughing, dystocia, or possibly genetic predisposition. Small, uncomplicated, recent rectal prolapses may be repaired via anesthesia and purse-string closure of the rectum that allows for minimal passage of feces. Larger, complicated prolapses require surgical excision and suturing. Recurrence is less likely after surgery but is possible regardless of method of repair.

Integumentary System

Dry, flaky skin with pruritus that varies from minimal to severe is seen in virtually all PBP. Wiping the skin down with wet towels each week will remove the flakes. Moisturizing lotions (eg, aloe vera) will also temporarily alleviate this problem. Fatty acid supplementation can be used as a more longterm remedy, but caution must be exercised not to promote obesity.

Sarcoptic mange is the most important ectoparasitic disease of PBP. Clinical signs of intense pruritis and dermatitis are the basis for a presumptive diagnosis. In many cases, the owners have pruritic skin lesions on the arms or abdomen. Examination of PBP skin scrapings (deep enough to contain some blood) from several sites usually confirms the diagnosis in advanced cases but may be negative in less advanced cases if very few mites are present. In young PBP, the source of infestation is usually the dam; in older PBP, the source is usually other infested pigs. Young PBP isolated from other pigs and kept as pets may harbor mange mites as a subclinical problem until mite populations increase sufficiently to make the condition obvious. Treatment with ivermectin (300 μg/kg, SC, repeated in 2 wk) or doramectin (300 μg/kg, IM, repeated in 3 wk), is indicated. Recently acquired young PBP may be given a routine preventive injection of either parasiticide when first presented for examination.

Melanomas and hemangiomas are important skin tumors in swine, and tumor removal and evaluation of metastatic potential through histopathology is important for prognosis. Spontaneous regression of melanomas, with subsequent depigmentation of the hair, skin, and iris, is occasionally seen in both PBP and domestic commercial swine; affected swine usually have normal life spans.

Sunburn may develop in PBP exposed to sudden high-intensity sunlight. Skin lesions may or may not be obvious, but affected PBP appear painful and seem to have hindlimb weakness or paresis. A sunburned PBP may be "down in the back legs" and show intense pain with vocalization. A thorough history is important for the diagnosis. Exposure to further sunlight should be prevented. Symptomatic treatment is remedial.

Erysipelas (p 2225), caused by *Erysipelothrix rhusiopathiae*, is a generalized bacterial infection that causes skin erythema and necrosis, arthritis, vegetative valvular endocarditis, and/or death. Clinically normal PBP may carry the organisms in their tonsils and other lymphoid tissue, and stress may result in development of clinical signs. PBP should be routinely vaccinated with an erysipelas bacterin twice, 3-4 wk apart, and then given boosters every 6-12 mo. PBP with erysipelas should be treated aggressively with penicillin (22,000 IU/kg, SID for 3 days) and isolated to minimize risk of zoonotic exposure. If the PBP is allergic to penicillin products, an alternative antibiotic, such as erythromycin, can be used. Recovered PBP may have chronic arthritis or valvular endocarditis.

Musculoskeletal System

Lameness due to lower back, hindlimb, or forelimb weakness is common in PBP. Due to conformation, PBP are susceptible to muscle pulls and ligament damage as well as fractures of the back and all limbs. Because PBP usually struggle against manual restraint (predisposing to injury), sedation or anesthesia is often used for procedures such as prolonged examination, radiography, foot trimming, blood collection, and dental work. Tiletamine-zolazepam at 2.2 mg/kg body weight, IM (in the ham), provides excellent analgesia and chemical restraint for these minor procedures; recovery time, although smooth, is prolonged. Isoflurane is also used and has the advantage of a rapid recovery time. Fasting for 24 hr and withholding water for 4-6 hr before sedation or anesthesia is recommended.

PBP with injuries to the back or limbs are usually treated with anti-inflammatory drugs such as buffered aspirin with antacid, flunixin meglumine, or glucocorticoids (eg, dexamethasone). Polysulfated glycosaminoglycan and/or glucosamine/chondroitin sulfate products may be tried in nonresponsive cases.

Fractures of the distal humerus and elbow area and femur are common. These occur from jumping off furniture (distal humerus), dog bites (elbow area), restraint (elbow area and femur), equine kicks (femur), and other trauma. Repair via pins, screws, plates, and external devices successfully restore some range of motion as long as fractures are immobilized properly and any sepsis is controlled.

Infectious arthritis may affect the very young to the older PBP. Lameness with or without joint swelling in one or more limbs is the usual clinical finding. *Erysipelothrix rhusiopathiae, Streptococcus* spp, *Mycoplasma hyosynoviae, M hyorhinis, Staphylococcus* spp, and *Haemophilus parasuis* are possible causes. Treatment early in the disease course with an effective antimicrobial (eg, lincomycin at 11 mg/kg, BID for 3 days) may be effective. Treatment after chronic changes have already occurred, antimicrobial ineffectiveness against the etiologic agent, or misdiagnosis are reasons for treatment failure and persistence of lameness. In chronic cases for which pain management is part of the treatment strategy, treatment with anti-inflammatory drugs should be considered. Polyarthritis from neonatal infection of the navel may be due to various environmental bacteria, including *Pseudomonas* spp. If degenerative arthritis and joint fusion from chronic inflammation are present after polyarthritis, euthanasia may be warranted. Osteochondrosis may also be considered in shoulder, elbow, hip, and stifle lameness, but this condition is not common in slow-growing, light-muscled animals such as PBP.

Overgrown and/or cracked hooves are a common cause of lameness. Regular exercise on abrasive surfaces (eg, concrete) will wear hoof ends and help keep them the appropriate length. In PBP that have overgrown, elongated hooves, normal hoof length can be maintained by routine hoof trimming under sedation or anesthesia each year. Hoof cracks can be caused by overgrown hooves. PBP with cracked hooves may additionally require antiseptic cleaning with tamed iodine and systemic antimicrobial therapy (ceftiofur at 4.4 mg/kg, SID for 3-10 days, or ampicillin at 11 mg/kg, PO, BID for 7-10 days).

Zygomycosis from *Mucor* spp infection has occurred in the distal hindlimb of a PBP. The large growth that encompassed the entire foot was composed of infected/abscessed tissue that involved bone. Amputation was remedial.

Tetanus may occur after wound contamination from dog bites, skin abrasions, oral cavity abrasions, or surgical procedures. Tetanus toxoid should be considered as part of the routine vaccination schedule of PBP at high risk of exposure. If there is no current tetanus toxoid vaccination, tetanus antitoxin (500-1,500 U, depending on body weight) should be administered IM in the neck after recovery from any surgery or dental procedure (eg, trimming of canine teeth). Treatment for tetanus is by massive doses of tetanus antitoxin and penicillin early in the disease along with tranquilizers, isolation to minimize external stimuli, and supportive therapy.

Nervous System

Systemic bacterial infection can be caused by (in approximate decreasing order of importance) *Streptococcus suis* type 2, other *Streptococcus* spp, *Salmonella choleraesuis*, *Haemophilus parasuis*, *Escherichia coli*, other gram-negative bacteria, and *Listeria monocytogenes*. PBP are most commonly affected from birth through 4-6 mo of age. Treatment with the appropriate antibacterial therapy (such as ceftiofur) in the early stages of infection is most effective; however, death may be the first clinical sign. Because *S suis* type 2 is a zoonotic disease agent, care should be exercised to prevent human infection when performing necropsies on pigs dying from suspected CNS disease.

Overheated PBP may be depressed, inactive, and have a subnormal temperature. The prognosis is grave, but some affected PBP may respond to symptomatic treatment for cooling (*see* ENVIRONMENT, p 1562).

Salt toxicity occurs after water deprivation for ≥36 hr and sudden rehydration or, less commonly, after prolonged consumption of high-salt foods. Owners may not be aware of low water consumption in sedentary PBP, especially when water is provided free-choice. Cool weather may further contribute to reduced water intake. Affected PBP may have seizures, walk aimlessly, or show other CNS signs such as blindness or postural abnormalities. Diagnosis in the affected live animal is confirmed by high levels of serum sodium, usually 160-183 mEq/dL (normal range 142-153 mEq/dL). Gradual rehydration and symptomatic treatment to counteract cerebral edema is indicated, but severely affected PBP may only be stabilized to a vegetative and blind status. Owners usually request euthanasia because of irreversible brain damage in such PBP. The histopathologic finding of eosinophilic infiltration into brain tissue is also diagnostic.

Seizure from unknown cause occurs in PBP. Animals <1 yr old seem most susceptible. Frequency may range from 1-2 seizures per month to several per day. Infrequent seizures may require no preventive medication. Diazepam is used to control more frequent episodes. Phenobarbital in addition to diazepam may be required control the most severe cases. Seizures may cease as the affected PBP ages.

Respiratory System

Atrophic rhinitis (p 1223) is an infectious disease of younger PBP that initially causes sneezing, nasal discharge, tearing, and growth retardation. *Bordetella bronchiseptica*, *Pasteurella multocida* types D and A (that produce types D and A toxins), and cytomegalovirus are common bacterial and viral causes. Transmission is predominately from dam to offspring before weaning but may be pig-to-pig after weaning. The more severe the rhinitis, the more likely that permanent distortion of the snout may occur as the pig ages. There is no remedy for a crooked nose resulting from earlier rhinitis and nasal turbinate inflammation, and snout deviation usually worsens with age. Intermittent nosebleed, with or without a crooked snout, may also be a sign. Early treatment with appropriate antibacterials such as amoxicillin or ampicillin is indicated for acute atrophic rhinitis. Chronic nosebleed may be treated by cooling the nasal area with cold water and keeping the pig calm to reduce air movement across the nasal turbinates. Increasing the humidity of inspired air may be helpful in dry climates. Vaccines are available but must be used in pregnant females before farrowing and in unweaned pigs to be most effective.

Pneumonia can be a very serious disease in PBP because of their relatively small lung capacity. The most common cause of pneumonia is from initial *Mycoplasma hyopneumoniae* infection, which immunocompromises the lungs, followed by *P multocida* infection. Young pigs contract these infectious agents from their dams or from mixing with infected pigs after weaning. Antibiotic treatment may be more effective if directed against *P multocida*, because this bacterium becomes the most important pathogen once coughing is present for several days. Vaccines available for *M hyopneumoniae* in domestic commercial swine have been used in young PBP to prevent mycoplasmal pneumonia and subsequent *Pasteurella* pneumonia. Vaccination in older PBP is probably unnecessary unless risk of exposure warrants continued use.

Actinobacillus pleuropneumoniae may cause a life-threatening pneumonia that may occur after infection from the sow or exposure to carrier animals. Clinical signs range from coughing, fever, and lethargy to sudden death, depending on the serotype of *A pleuropneumoniae.* Prompt antibiotic treatment with penicillin or ceftiofur is indicated. Recovered PBP usually have permanent tissue loss in affected lung areas and may have recurrent respiratory problems. Vaccines available for domestic commercial swine should be used routinely in PBP.

Swine influenza (p 1228) is an important viral pneumonia in PBP that are taken to fairs and exhibitions and, therefore, exposed to other pig populations. It is usually self-limiting after 7-10 days but can be fatal. H1N1, H3N2, and H1N2 are the most common strains in domestic swine. H1N1, bivalent, and trivalent vaccines are now used in domestic swine and could be used in PBP. Swine influenza is a zoonotic disease.

One limited survey for porcine reproductive and respiratory syndrome (PRRS) virus antibody in PBP in Florida showed no evidence of infection. PRRS is also extremely rare in feral swine in the USA.

Urinary System

Cystitis and urolithiasis are common in both male and female PBP. Signs include frequent urination or straining to urinate. Urinalysis, urine culture, CBC, serum chemistry, radiography, and ultrasound are important diagnostic aids. A sterile urine sample for culture can be obtained via cystocentesis. Cystitis without triple phosphate crystalluria should respond to extended antibacterial therapy based on in vitro sensitivity testing. Acidification of the urine may also help minimize recurrence of infection. Nephritis can occur after cystitis as an ascending infection. Leptospirosis may be a primary cause of nephritis. Increased BUN and creatinine values may aid in the diagnosis of nephritis and kidney failure. Routine vaccination for 6 *Leptospira* serovars is recommended because such multivalent bacterins include *L bratislava* and *Leptospira pomona*, the most common types infecting commercial swine. Vaccination may possibly reduce renal shedding of leptospires should PBP become chronically infected and, therefore, minimize transmission of this zoonotic disease.

In a PBP that is straining and unable to urinate, the bladder size should be reduced immediately by cystocentesis after sedation and radiography (plain or contrast) or ultrasonography to evaluate the location of urethral and bladder stones. If the blockage is in the urethra, cystotomy is recommended (both sexes) to identify and remove calculi in all possible locations. Calculi in a male's urethra may be removed by cutting through the sheath to expose the distal penis, catheterizing the urethra, and backflushing into the bladder. Calculi that cannot be removed by this method must be surgically removed by incising the urethra at the location of the blockage. Suturing of the urethra is followed by cystotomy, bladder flushing (cystotomy/flushing minimizes recurrence), and inspection for more calculi. The bladder is then closed, and a Foley catheter is inserted into the bladder, tunneled through the abdominal muscles, and sutured to the skin to accommodate the flow of urine while the urethra heals. Several days later, the Foley catheter is occluded, and the urethra is inspected to determine patency and urine flow; if not patent, the Foley catheter is opened again, and the process is repeated several days later. When the urethra becomes patent, the Foley catheter is removed and the drainage site allowed to granulate closed. Although female urethras are short, blockage can still occur. Because urethral catheterization is difficult without endoscopy, a Foley catheter is inserted into the vagina and inflated, and a purse-string suture is placed at the vulva. Retrograde flushing through the urethral opening in the vaginal floor is attempted. A cystotomy is then performed to remove all possible calculi, followed by routine closure of the bladder. Foley catheter placement into the bladder may not be necessary. Further treatment includes antibiotic therapy and acidification of the urine. Despite these efforts, some affected PBP do not recover and require euthanasia. Perineal urethrostomies are usually only temporarily successful because the surgical site becomes occluded by amorphous material or urethral polyps, and patency cannot be reestablished. However, surgical methods have been described to correct failed perineal urethrostomies in PBP. Rupture of the bladder is a grave complication because normal bladder tone may not return even after stones have been removed and the bladder has been surgically repaired. Laser lithotripsy has been recently used to fracture urethral calculi not removable by flushing.

Routine urinalysis as part of an annual examination may enable early diagnosis and prevention of serious urinary tract disease in PBP.

Psychogenic water consumption should be considered in PBP (especially young PBP) with polydipsia and polyuria. PBP may develop a habit of drinking water and urinating frequently because of possible boredom or unknown causes. Cystitis and crystalluria should be eliminated as differential diagnoses. Measuring urine specific gravity before and after a 12-hr water fast will demonstrate whether the affected PBP is able to concentrate urine. Ability to concentrate urine indicates normal kidney function and helps rule out diabetes insipidus. Estimating the daily water intake and urine output will further aid the diagnosis of psychogenic water intake or establish that water consumption and urination are in fact normal. Relieving boredom may be helpful to change this behavior. Affected young PBP typically outgrow this condition. If water is restricted and offered only with meals, care must be taken to prevent salt toxicity.

RABBITS

The European or Old World rabbit (*Oryctolagus cuniculus*) is the only genus of domestic rabbits. Wild rabbits and hares include cottontail rabbits (*Sylvilagus*) and the "true" hares or jackrabbits (*Lepus*). Rabbits have been bred for fur, meat, wool, exhibition, and for use as laboratory animals.

MANAGEMENT

Management of rabbits for meat, fur, or wool production is quite different from the maintenance of a pet or house rabbit. The American Rabbit Breeders Association provides guidance for both production and pet rabbit care. The House Rabbit Society is another resource regarding pet rabbit care.

Restraint: Proper handling and restraint is important. Rabbits have powerful hind limbs, which can kick out and lead to broken backs. Rabbits should never be held by the ears; they should be scruffed at the neck and the body firmly supported at the rump. If they are not held properly and securely, fractures or luxations of lumbar vertebrae may follow struggling.

Physical Examination and Sample Collection: Most techniques for physical examination suitable for dogs and cats may be applied to rabbits. A thorough oral exam including palpation of the face and bottom of the jaw should be performed to evaluate dental health. An otoscope or a pediatric nasal speculum can assist visualization of the molars. Sex can be determined by depressing the external genitalia to reveal a slit-like vulva in females and penis in males. The testicles descend at 10-12 wk. Normal body temperature is 103.3-104°F. Body temperature <100.4°F or >105°F is cause for concern.

Blood can be collected from the auricular or central ear artery, cephalic vein, lateral saphenous vein, and the jugular vein. The auricular or marginal ear vein provides a site for venous administration or catheterization. Application of a topical anesthetic cream greatly facilitates these procedures.

Clinical Pathology: Rabbit clinical pathology varies from other domestic animals. The normal neutrophil:lymphocyte ratio is 1:1. The rabbit neutrophil is called a "pseudoeosinophil" or heterophil due to red-staining cytoplasmic granules. Both the heterophil and the granules are smaller than the eosinophil and eosinophil red granules. Rabbit calcium metabolism results in higher blood calcium levels and a wider range than other animals, which can lead to erroneous diagnosis of hypercalcemia. Rabbit urine ranges from yellow to brown or reddish. A dipstick can quickly differentiate normal rabbit urinary pigments from hematuria. Traces of glucose and protein are normal in rabbit urine.

Therapeutics: Very few products are licensed for use in rabbits, leading to extra-label use of drug therapies approved for use in other species. Particular caution must be applied to the use of antibiotics that suppress normal GI microflora and result in enteric dysbiosis and/or enterotoxemia. This has been called "antibiotic toxicity." Antibiotics contraindicated in rabbits include clindamycin, lincomycin, erythromycin, ampicillin, amoxicillin/clavulanic acid, and cephalosporins. The flea treatment fipronil is contraindicated in rabbits due to severe toxic reactions in some individuals. Therapeutic treatment may require aggressive nutritional support via syringe feeding, orogastric tube (14 French), nasogastric tube (4-8 French), or pharyngostomy tube (soft esophagostomy tube designed for cats). A gastrotomy tube is less successful than in dogs or cats.

Reproduction: Rabbit breeds of medium size are sexually mature at $4-4^{1}/_{2}$ mo, giant breeds at 6-9 mo, and small breeds (eg, the Polish Dwarf and Dutch) at $3^{1}/_{2}-4$ mo of age. The rabbit is an induced ovulator and, contrary to popular belief, has a cycle of mating receptivity; rabbits are receptive to mating ~14 of every 16 days. The degree of mating receptivity is indicated by the color of the vaginal orifice and by the amount of moisture on the labia. A doe is most receptive when the vagina is red and moist. Does that are not receptive have a whitish pink vaginal color with little or no moisture. Many breeders test mate the doe 10-16 days after breeding, as a means of detecting pregnancy, but this is unreliable. Palpation of the doe's abdomen for "grape-sized" embryos in the uterus is a much better technique for detecting pregnancy. The best time to palpate is 12 days after breeding. Pseudopregnancy is common in rabbits and can follow any induced ovulation, the introduction of a male rabbit in the environment, or other stimuli.

A ratio of 1 buck to 10 does is common practice, but many commercial growers find that 1 buck to 20-25 does is more economical. Bucks can be used daily without decreasing fertility; more frequent use requires periods of rest. The doe should always be taken to the buck's cage for breeding. The breeding program should continue year round. Does that have experienced long periods of rest between litters tend to become obese and difficult to breed. Does that are constantly in gestation and lactation may become underweight, and their receptivity to the buck and fertility decrease dramatically. If breeding is delayed several weeks and the doe is given full feed, weight is quickly regained.

The gestation period is ~31-33 days. Does with a small litter (usually ≤4) seem to have a longer gestation period than does that produce larger litters. If a doe has not kindled by day 32 of gestation, oxytocin (1-2 IU) should be given to induce parturition; otherwise, a dead litter is almost always delivered sometime after day 34. Occasionally, pregnant does abort or resorb the fetuses due to nutritional deficiencies or disease.

Nest boxes should be added to the cages 28-29 days after breeding. If boxes are added too soon, the does foul the nests with urine and feces. A day or two before kindling, the doe pulls fur from her body and builds a nest in the nest box. The young are born naked, blind, and deaf. They begin to show hair on day 2-3 after birth, and their eyes and ears are open by day 10. Neonatal rabbits are unable to thermoregulate until about day 7. Rebreeding can occur any time after parturition. Some commercial growers use accelerated breeding schedules and rebreed 7-21 days after parturition, while most people raising for show or home use rebreed 35-42 days after parturition.

Most medium-sized female rabbits have 8-10 nipples, and many kindle 12-15 young. If a doe is unable to nurse all the kits effectively, kits may be fostered by removing them from the nest box during the first 3 days and giving them to a doe of the same age with a smaller litter. If the fostered kits are mixed with the doe's own kits and covered with hair of the doe, they are generally accepted. Moving the larger kits to the new litter instead of the smaller kits increases the chance of success. Does nurse only 1-2 times daily. Kits nurse <3 min. Kits are weaned around 4-5 wk of age.

Rearing Orphaned Infants: Kits can be hand-reared, but mortality is high. They should be kept warm, dry, and quiet. Kitten milk replacer or a formula of $^{1}/_{2}$ cup evaporated milk, $^{1}/_{2}$ cup water, 1 egg yolk, and 1 tbsp corn syrup can be used. Feedings vary from $^{1}/_{2}$ tsp to 2 tbsp, depending on the age of the kits. Kits start eating greens around day 15-18.

Surgery: Preoperative fasting is not required or recommended. Rabbits cannot vomit. Additionally, rabbit stomachs are never empty, even after prolonged fasting. Premedication with butorphanol or diazepam can reduce stress from preoperative handling. Premedication with atropine may be of little use as many rabbits have an atropinase. Instead, glycopyrrolate may be used to reduce bradycardia and upper airway and salivary secretions (0.01-0.1 mg/kg, IM or SC, or 0.01 mg/kg, IV). Isoflurane is recommended for general anesthesia. The long and narrow pharynx and the large tongue make rabbits difficult to intubate, but it is possible with practice. Laryngospasm can be limited by applications of lidocaine on the epiglottis. A laryngoscope with a Miller 0 blade, rabbit oral specula, and cheek dilators can assist in successful placement of an endotracheal tube (2.0-4.0 mm). Adequate general anesthesia can be achieved with injectable ketamine (35-50 mg/kg) in combination with a tranquilizer such as xylazine (5-10 mg/kg) given IM. It is critical to get rabbits eating postoperatively, and analgesic treatment for 1-2 days will help prevent inappetence. A painful rabbit may exhibit teeth chattering or grinding while sitting in a "hunched" position. Analgesic treatment may include opioid drugs such as buprenorphine (0.01-0.05 mg/kg, SC, IM, or IV, BID-TID) or butorphanol (0.05-0.4 mg/kg, SC or IM, BID-TID) or NSAID such as carprofen (1.5 mg/kg, PO or SC, BID), flunixin (0.5-2 mg/kg, PO, deep IM, or IV, SID for no more than 3 days), or meloxicam (0.1-0.2 mg/kg, SC or PO, SID). Hay and water should be offered as soon as possible following surgery. Alfalfa hay tends to entice a reluctant appetite.

Castration can reduce aggressive behavior and is suggested for house rabbits and group-housed rabbits. It has no advantage for meat-type rabbits. The scrotums are lateral and anterior to the penis, as in marsupials and not as in most other placental mammals. Castration is performed using a closed technique or by an open technique with closure of the large superficial inguinal ring to prevent herniation.

Female pet rabbits should be spayed due to the risk of uterine cancer. Rabbits have 2 uterine horns connected to the vagina by separate cervices. The oviduct loops around and is much longer than in cats or dogs. Older or multiparous rabbits will have a more complicated spay due to the large amount of fat in the mesometrium. Postoperative adhesions are a common complication, which may be reduced by calcium-blocker treatment (verapamil, 200 µg/kg, SC, TID for 3 days).

When gastrotomies are performed to remove a hairball, the stomach is elevated by stay sutures through a cranial celiotomy incision. An incision is made through the greater curvature of the stomach. The hairball is often so firm and well packed that it may be removed in one piece. It is important to remove fur from the pyloric sphincter and to examine the stomach lining for abnormalities. A fine absorbable monofilament suture is preferred over gut suture due to the acidic environment of the rabbit stomach. Sutures should incorporate, but not penetrate, the gastric mucosa. Pre- and postsurgical care should include fluids and antibiotic therapy. Animals remain anorectic and force feeding is typically required.

Rabbits will chew out skin sutures; therefore, skin closure should be performed with a 4-0 absorbable synthetic suture with a cuticular-cuticular pattern. Rabbits tolerate staples. Tissue glue has also been used successfully.

Euthanasia: Rabbits may jump or scream when the traditional overdose of barbiturate is given in the marginal ear vein. Sedation with ketamine (50 mg/kg), alone or in combination with a tranquilizer such as acepromazine or xylazine, is recommended prior to administration of the barbiturate. As a further precaution, euthanasia solution may be diluted 1:1 with saline to prevent a negative reaction.

Other Management Techniques: Toenails on the rear limbs may severely scratch unprotected arms of handlers. Nails should be trimmed every 1-2 mo.

Some breeders tattoo or place ear tags on their rabbits for identification purposes. For show purposes, the right ear is reserved for registration marks applied by registrars of the American Rabbit Breeders Association.

HOUSING

Pet Rabbits: A rabbit hutch placed in the back yard, basement, or garage has been and continues to be traditional housing for rabbits. The hutch should be conveniently accessed for proper care of the rabbit, as diseases of neglect are common in rabbits abandoned in a hutch at the back of the yard. There should be adequate ventilation and protection from dogs or other predators.

House Rabbits: Rabbits can become a more integrated part of the household when they are trained to a litter box and accustomed to periodic confinement housing. Rabbits have a tendency to chew on things and may gnaw furniture, curtains, carpeting, or electrical wiring, which is dangerous for the rabbit and creates a fire hazard. Rabbits should be confined to safe quarters when unsupervised.

Cages and Ancillary Equipment: Rabbits gnaw, and caging should be constructed of materials that will hold up. Cages should be easily sanitized and allow easy manure removal. All-wire cages with a minimum of 12-gauge wire (16-gauge recommended for cage floor to support the weight of the rabbit) are preferred. Cages can be suspended from the ceiling with wire or set on metal frames. The size of the hutch depends on the size of the rabbit. Giant breeds (>12 lb) require a minimum of 30 × 36 in. to 36 × 48 in. Medium breeds (7-12 lb) require 24 × 30 in. to 30 × 36 in. Smaller breeds can be accommodated by 18 × 24 in. The cage should be equipped with a feed hopper and a watering system. Feed hoppers are best constructed of sheet metal with holes or a screen in the bottom for removal of "fines" (small broken feed particles). Rabbits drink more than other animals of similar size and they should be offered ad lib potable water. Rabbits often chew on the watering valve and eventually destroy it unless it is made of stainless steel or has a stainless centerpiece. Water bottles with sipper tubes work well. Crocks and cans are sometimes used in small rabbitries; such containers are easily contaminated and should be washed and disinfected daily. A barren cage is inadequate; the cage environment should be enriched to give the rabbit something to do. Optimally, rabbits should be given run time outside of the cage daily.

Nest boxes should be constructed so that they can be easily placed in the cage and later removed for cleaning and disinfecting between litters. Disinfecting the nest box after cleaning and again just before placing it in the cage helps reduce incidence of disease. The box should be large enough to prevent crowding but small enough to keep the kits warm. A standard size nest box for medium-sized rabbits is 16 × 10 × 8 in. high. Wooden, metal, or plastic nest boxes with nesting material (eg, straw, hardwood shavings, shredded sugarcane) serves well in either warm or cold weather. Shredded paper, hay, leaves, and other materials have been used with less success. Rough edges such as splintering wood should be avoided as they contribute to mastitis when does hop in and out of the nest box.

Pens: Pens should have a nonslip floor and may be bedded with straw or shredded paper covered with straw or hay to increase absorbency. Shavings or sawdust are not the best as the scent is too powerful. Pen sides should be at least 4 ft high.

Group Housing: When setting up group housing, compatibility is a major factor. Personalities should be evaluated for docility and aggressiveness. Strain influences personality. Rabbits that have grown up together are best, although adult males may be so aggressive toward each other that serious fights occur. Neutering may improve compatibility. A general guide is "same sex and same size." A period of adjacent proximity is prudent prior to group housing rabbits. Another factor to consider is stocking density. Floor space recommendations vary from 3.5-10 sq ft/rabbit to allow territory establishment. Others recommend 3.5 hop lengths per rabbit as a rule of thumb. Regardless, group-housed rabbits should be provided escape and hiding places and should be frequently monitored.

Production Housing: Housing requirements for rabbits depend on climate. Minimal housing (an A-frame roof without sides) can be used in moderate climates, while a climate-controlled rabbitry may be necessary in hot or cold climates. Rabbitries should be located on nearly level ground and use well-drained soil or tile-drained pits for manure. Shade should be provided over as much of the rabbitry as possible. Rabbits are prone to heat stress. While they tolerate subzero temperatures when provided proper shelter, the optimal rabbit environment is 61-72°F. Good ventilation at all times is imperative.

Sanitation: Cleaning frequency depends of the type of facility or caging system. Rabbits typically choose a preferred latrine site, such as a corner of the cage. Sanitation is especially important in rabbit production. Poor sanitation leads to disease and deaths; therefore, cleaning and sanitizing must be constant. Nest boxes must be disinfected between uses. Cages, feeders, and watering equipment should be sanitized periodically with an effective and inexpensive sanitizing solution such as diluted household chlorine bleach (1 oz/1 quart water) or other less corrosive disinfectants. Complete cleaning should be performed before housing new stock.

An active rabbitry constantly experiences a loose hair problem. Does pull hair from their bodies to make nests, and some of this hair becomes airborne. It sticks to almost any surface, including cages, ceilings, and lights, and must be removed periodically. The most effective ways to remove hair from cages are washing or using a propane torch or flame. Washing, brushing, sweeping, and vacuuming also are effective in other parts of the rabbitry. Pens or wire-floored cages should be brushed or hosed every 2 wk. An acid wash may be required to descale rabbit urine from solid floor pans.

Frequent manure removal is essential. Excess manure leads to unacceptable levels of ammonia in the air, which predisposes to respiratory disease. The manure can be composted in an efficient pit system.

NUTRITION

Rabbits are small herbivores with specialized feeding and digestive strategies. They are selective eaters and choose nutrient-rich leaves and new plant shoots over mature plant material that is higher in fiber. They have a high metabolic rate and only by selecting the most nutritious plant parts can they meet their requirements. Rabbits are nonruminant herbivores with an enlarged hindgut. The large cecum supports a population of microorganisms that uses nutrients not digested in the small intestine. Separation of digesta on the basis of particle size occurs in the hindgut. Peristaltic action rapidly moves large particles, primarily lignocellulose, through the colon and excretes them as hard fecal pellets. Antiperistaltic action moves small particles and soluble material into the cecum, where they undergo fermentation. At intervals, the cecal contents are expelled as "soft feces" and consumed by the rabbit directly from the anus. This reingested material provides microbial protein, vitamins (including all the B vitamins needed), and small quantities of volatile fatty acids, which are essential in rabbit nutrition. However, because amino acids obtained in this manner make only a minor contribution to the rabbits' protein needs (particularly young, growing rabbits), the diet must supply the additional amino acids, although the requirements for essential amino acids in rabbits have not yet been defined.

Rabbits digest fiber poorly because of the selective separation and rapid excretion of large particles in the hindgut. A generous amount of fiber in the diet (~15% crude fiber) is needed to promote intestinal motility and minimize intestinal disease. Fiber may also absorb bacterial toxins and eliminate them via the hard feces. Diets low in fiber promote an increased incidence of intestinal problems, eg, enterotoxemia. This may be a result of the higher starch content of low-fiber diets. Starch is a substrate for the proliferation of pathogenic bacteria such as *Clostridium spiroforme*, which produce a potent toxin. High-fiber diets (>20% crude fiber) may result in an increased incidence of cecal impaction and mucoid enteritis. Volatile fatty acids produced in the cecum are important metabolites because they aid in the control of pathogenic organisms by helping to maintain a low pH in the cecum.

A dietary supply of vitamins A, D, and E is necessary. Bacteria in the gut synthesize B vitamins and vitamin K in adequate quantities; thus, dietary supplements are unnecessary. Disease and stress may increase the daily vitamin requirements. Feed preparation and storage must be done in a manner that will reduce losses from oxidation, which destroys vitamins A and E more readily than other vitamins. Diets containing ≥30% of alfalfa meal generally provide sufficient vitamin A. Levels of vitamin A in the diet must be >5,000 IU/kg and <75,000 IU/kg. Levels out of this range may cause abortion, resorbed litters, and fetal hydrocephalus. Vitamin E deficiency has been associated with infertility, muscular dystrophy, and fetal and neonatal death.

All the components of the basic diet (ie, protein, fiber, fat, and energy) should be managed in consideration of the life stage (growth, gestation, lactation, maintenance),

TABLE 13. Nutrient Requirements of Rabbits ▶

	Protein (%) Total	Protein (%) Digestible
Maintenance	12	9
Growth and finishing	16	12
Pregnancy	15	11
Lactation (with litter of 7-8)	17	13

breed, condition, and lifestyle of the rabbit. Ratios should meet the nutrient requirements of the National Research Council (TABLE 13). Pelleted rabbit feeds provide good nutrition at reasonable cost. Fresh, clean water should always be available. Rabbits fed hay (alfalfa or clover) and grain (corn, oats, barley) should be provided with a trace mineral salt block. Prolonged intake of typical commercial diets containing alfalfa meal by laboratory or pet rabbits kept for extended periods under maintenance conditions may lead to kidney damage and calcium carbonate deposits in the urinary tract. Reducing the calcium level to 0.4-0.5% of the diet for nonlactating rabbits helps reduce these problems. This can be accomplished by feeding pelleted diets with a timothy hay base. Adult pet rabbits not intended for breeding should be fed a high-fiber pelleted diet, restricted to $^1/_4$ cup/5 lb body wt/day to prevent obesity and maintain GI health. At this level of restriction, ad lib hay is necessary to avoid trichobezoars and general gut stasis.

Rabbits are efficient converters of poorly digestible materials to meat. Therefore, it is easy to overfeed or underfeed does and growing, adolescent rabbits (fryers). The amount to feed depends on the age of the fryers or on the stage of pregnancy or lactation of the does. A general rule in feeding fryers is to feed all that can be consumed in 20 hr, with the feed hopper empty ~4 hr/day. Does are usually fed ad lib once they kindle. The general practice is to bring the doe from restricted to full feed slowly during the first week of lactation. Does that are bred to kindle 5 times during the year generally have their feed restricted between litters; those bred intensively should be on full feed continuously once they begin the first lactation.

BACTERIAL AND MYCOTIC DISEASES

Pasteurellosis

Pasteurellosis is common in domestic rabbits. It is highly contagious, and is transmitted primarily by direct contact, although aerosol transmission may also occur. The etiologic agent is *Pasteurella multocida*, a gram-negative, nonmotile coccobacillus. In conventional colonies, 30-90% of apparently healthy rabbits may be asymptomatic carriers. Several barrier colonies of laboratory rabbits have been established as *Pasteurella*-free.

Clinical Findings: Pasteurellosis presents with a variety of clinical symptoms including rhinitis, pneumonia, abscesses, reproductive tract infections, torticollis, and septicemia.

Rhinitis (snuffles or nasal catarrh) is an acute, subacute, or chronic inflammation of the mucous membranes of the air passages and lungs, induced primarily by *Pasteurella*, but *Pseudomonas*, *Bordetella bronchiseptica*, *Staphylococcus*, and *Streptococcus* have also been isolated. The initial sign is a thin, serous exudate from the nose and eyes that later becomes purulent. The fur on the inside of the front legs just above the paws may be matted and caked with dried exudate or this area may be clean with thinned fur as a result of pawing at the nose. Infected rabbits usually sneeze and cough. In general, snuffles occurs when the resistance of the rabbit is low. Recovered rabbits are likely carriers. Pneumonia can ensue.

Pneumonia is common in domestic rabbits. Frequently, it is a secondary and complicating factor in the enteritis complex. The cause is typically *P multocida* but other bacteria such as *Klebsiella pneumoniae*, *Bordetella bronchiseptica*, *Staphylococcus aureus*, and

TABLE 13.	(Continued)		
Fat (%)	Fiber (%)	Digestible Carbohydrates (NFE, %)*	Total Digestible Nutrients (%)
1.5-2	14-20	40-45	50-60
2-4	14-16	45-50	60-70
2-3	14-16	45-50	55-65
2.5-3.5	12-14	45-50	65-75

*NFE = nitrogen-free extract

pneumococci may be involved. Upper respiratory disease (snuffles, *see* above) is often a precursor of pneumonia. Inadequate ventilation, sanitation, and nesting material are predisposing factors. The number of cases of pneumonia is directly proportional to the level of ammonia in a rabbitry. Rabbits usually succumb within 1 wk after signs appear. Affected rabbits are anorectic, listless, dyspneic, and have a fever. Necropsy reveals bronchopneumonia, pleuritis, pyothorax, or pericardial petechiae. Diagnosis depends on signs, lesions, and culture results. Antibiotic treatment often fails because the pneumonia is advanced before it is detected.

Otitis media or interna ("Wry neck" or head tilt) results from *P multocida* or *Encephalitozoon cuniculi* infection. An accumulation of pus or fluid in the middle or inner ear causes the rabbit to twist its head, eg, "wry neck" or torticollis. However, not all rabbits with middle ear infections show torticollis. Longterm antibiotic treatment is required for drug penetration into the affected area. Antibiotic therapy may only prevent worsening of clinical signs and as the prognosis is guarded, most colony rabbits with this condition are culled.

Mature bucks and young rabbits seem particularly susceptible to **conjunctivitis**, (weepy eye) caused by *P multocida* or *S aureus*; however, the incidence is low. Transmission is by direct contact or fomites. Affected rabbits rub their eyes with their front feet. Ophthalmic ointments containing sulfonamides, antibiotics, or antibiotics and a steroid are satisfactory for treatment, but recurrence is common. Flushing the lacrimal duct with an antibiotic solution is often beneficial in chronically affected show rabbits. Conjunctivitis also accompanies rabbitpox (p 1582) and myxomatosis (p 1581).

Subcutaneous and visceral **abscesses** caused by *Pasteurella* may be clinically silent for long periods and spontaneously rupture. When bucks penned together fight, their wounds frequently develop abscesses. With colony rabbits, it is usually advisable to eliminate rather than to treat the affected rabbit; with pet rabbits, drainage of the abscess accompanied by antibiotic therapy based on culture and sensitivity tests has been successful, although recurrence of signs is common.

Pasteurella often causes **genital infections**, but several other organisms also may be involved. They are manifest by an acute or subacute inflammation of the reproductive tract, and most frequently are found in adults, more often in does than bucks. If both horns of the uterus are affected, the does often become sterile; if only one horn is involved, a normal litter may develop in the other. The only sign of pyometra may be a thick, yellowish gray vaginal discharge. Bucks may discharge pus from the urethra or have an enlarged testicle. Chronic infection of the prostate and seminal vesicles is likely, and because venereal transmission may ensue, it is best to cull the animal in a production rabbitry colony. Surgical removal of the infected reproductive organs in conjunction with antibiotic therapy is indicated for pet rabbits. The contaminated hutch and its equipment should be thoroughly disinfected.

Rabbits may develop *Pasteurella septicemia* and die acutely without any clinical signs. Septicemia necropsy findings may reveal only congestion and petechial hemorrhages in multiple organs.

Diagnosis: Diagnosis of pasteurellosis is based on clinical signs and isolation of *P multocida*. Carriers can be identified by an indirect fluorescent antibody test on nasal swabs. A technique that uses small, saline-moistened, pediatric nasopharyngeal swabs has proved superior to the standard, larger nasal swab. The swab is directed medially through the external nares past the turbinates and onto the dorsal surface of the soft palate. The swab is then retracted and can be used in the fluorescent antibody test or plated onto a culture medium. An ELISA test for detecting antibodies against *P multocida* may also prove beneficial in detecting carriers.

Treatment and Control: Treatment is difficult and may not eradicate the organism. Antibiotics seem to provide only temporary remission, and the next stress (eg, kindling) may cause relapse. Enrofloxacin (200 mg/L of drinking water for 14 days or 5-10 mg/kg parenteral, BID for 14 days) is effective for upper respiratory *P multocida* infections. Tilmicosin (25 mg/kg, SC) has been reported as an effective treatment for pasteurellosis. Procaine penicillin (60,000 IU/kg for 10 days) was recommended for indiviual rabbits, but its use should be cautioned as deaths from enterotoxemia often follow penicillin administration.

An effective vaccine has not been developed; therefore, the best method of control in large rabbitries is strict culling. Two methods to free a production colony of *Pasteurella* have been reported. The first involves culture and culling of positive animals; once the colony is *Pasteurella*-free, it must be maintained in isolation. In the second method, pregnant does past kindling are treated with enrofloxacin. While does remain *Pasteurella*-culture positive the kits remain *Pasteurella*-culture negative. Carriers can be identified by an indirect fluorescent antibody test on nasal swabs.

Listeriosis

Listeriosis, a sporadic septicemic disease characterized by sudden deaths or abortions, is most common in does in advanced pregnancy. Poor husbandry and stress may be important in initiating the disease. Clinical signs are variable and nonspecific and include anorexia, depression, and weight loss. In contrast to the disease in cattle and sheep, listeriosis seldom affects the CNS in rabbits. The causal agent, *Listeria monocytogenes*, spreads via the blood to the liver, spleen, and gravid uterus. At necropsy, the liver consistently contains multiple, pinpoint, gray-white foci. Because diagnosis is rarely made premortem, treatment is seldom attempted. *L monocytogenes* can infect many animals, including humans. It is difficult to isolate with normal methods, and special techniques are often required.

Intestinal Diseases

Intestinal disease is a major cause of death in young rabbits. Although most diarrheal diseases were once lumped together (as the enteritis complex) or simply called mucoid enteritis, specific diseases are being delineated. Diet, antibiotic treatment, and other factors create disturbances of the GI microflora and may predispose rabbits to dysbiosis and intestinal disease. For discussion of hairballs, *see* p 1587.

Enterotoxemia: Enterotoxemia is an explosive diarrheal disease, primarily of rabbits 4-8 wk old. It occasionally affects adults and junior stock. Signs are lethargy, rough coat, a perineal area covered with greenish brown fecal material, and death within 48 hr. Often, a rabbit looks healthy in the evening and is dead the next morning. Necropsy reveals the typical lesions of enterotoxemia, ie, a fluid-distended intestine with hemorrhagic petechiae on the serosal surface. The primary causative agent is *Clostridium spiroforme*, which produces an iota toxin. Little is known about transmission of the organism; it is assumed to be a commensal that is normally present in low numbers. The type of diet seems to be a factor in development of the disease; enterotoxemia is seen less often when high-fiber diets are fed. Because lincomycin, clindamycin, and erythromycin induce *Clostridium*-related (eg, *C difficile*) enterotoxemia due to their selective effect on normal gram-positive bacteria, they are contraindicated in rabbits. Enterotoxemia is a consideration for most antibiotic therapy, and it has been seen after administration of penicillins and cephalosporins. The incidence rate is 40-80% after oral penicillin therapy, which should be considered contraindicated in rabbits. These diarrheas are remarkably similar to those that occur naturally (described above as enterotoxemia). Treatment of colony rabbits is seldom attempted because of the rapidity of death. However, when population size permits, cholestyramine has been used with promising results, both as a preventive and a treatment. Reducing stress of the young rabbits (weaning, etc) and ad lib feeding of hay or straw are helpful in prevention. Adding 250 ppm of copper sulfate to the diet of young rabbits also helps prevent enterotoxemia. Individual animal treatment for enterotoxemia should include supportive fluid therapy. There is little evidence that antibiotics are helpful. Diagnosis depends on history, signs, lesions, and demonstration of *C spiroforme*. Centrifugation of intestinal contents at 20,000 g for 15 min followed by culture of the supernatant-pellet interface will reveal the organism. For a definitive diagnosis, the presence of iota toxin in the supernatant of centrifuged cecal contents can be demonstrated by in vivo or in vitro assays.

Tyzzer's Disease: Tyzzer's disease (p 160), caused by *Clostridium piliforme* (formerly *Bacillus piliformis*), is characterized by profuse watery diarrhea, anorexia, dehydration, lethargy, staining of the hindquarters, and death within 1-3 days in weanling rabbits 6-12 wk old. Acute outbreaks have been associated with >90% mortality. Some rabbits may develop chronic infections that present clinically as a wasting disease. Infection occurs by ingestion and is associated with poor sanitation and stress. The lesions consist of necrotic enteritis along with multifocal necrosis in the liver and heart. Diagnosis is made histologically; special stains (eg, Giemsa or Warthin-Starry silver) show the characteristic intracellular bacterium. Culturing is impractical because the bacterium does not grow on artificial media. Serologic tests are available from laboratory animal diagnostic laboratories. Tyzzer's disease affects a wide spectrum of other species but has not been reported in humans, although titers have been documented in pregnant women. Although antibiotics used in treatment of other animals have not been effective in rabbits, oxytetracycline has been of some value in limiting an outbreak. No vaccine is available. Aggressive disinfection and decontamination of the housing facility to reduce the presence of hardy spores is indicated with either 1% peracetic acid or 3% hypochlorite.

Colibacillosis: *Escherichia coli* as a cause of rabbit diarrhea has been confused by the circumstance that *E coli* often proliferate when rabbits develop diarrhea for any reason. Enteropathogenic strains of *E coli* (serotype O103) commonly express the eae gene, which codes for intimin, an outer membrane protein associated with the attaching and effacing lesions. Serotypes O15:H, O109:H2, O103:H2, O128, and O132 are also important. Normal healthy rabbits do not have *E coli* of any strain associated with their GI tract.

Two types of colibacillosis are seen in rabbits, depending on age. Rabbits 1-2 wk old develop a severe yellowish diarrhea that results in high mortality. It is common for entire litters to succumb to this disease. In weaned rabbits 4-6 wk old, a diarrheal disease very similar to that described for enterotoxemia is seen. The intestines are fluid filled, with petechial hemorrhages on the serosal surface, similar to the pathology described for both Tyzzer's disease and enterotoxemia (*see* above). Death occurs in 5-14 days, or rabbits are left stunted and unthrifty. Diagnosis is made by isolating *E coli* on blood agar and then having the isolate biotyped or serotyped. Electron micrographs of *E coli* attached to the mucosa are also helpful. In severe cases, treatment is not successful; in mild cases, antibiotics are of value. Severely affected rabbits should be culled, and facilities thoroughly sanitized. High-fiber diets appear to help prevent the disease in weaned rabbits.

Proliferative Enteropathy: Proliferative enteropathy caused by *Lawsonia intracellularis* has been reported to cause diarrhea in weanling rabbits. Clinical symptoms include diarrhea, depression, and dehydration, which resolve over 1-2 wk. Disease does not cause death unless associated with a dual infection with another enteropathogenic agent. Diagnosis is based on necropsy findings of a thickened and corrugated ileum and histologic identification of the rod-shaped to curved or spiral silver-staining organism in crypt enterocytes. The organism requires cell-containing media (enterocytes) for culture. Immunohistochemistry and PCR may be useful to identify *L intracellularis*. Isolation of sick animals and symptomatic treatment is advised.

Mucoid Enteropathy: Mucoid enteropathy is a distinct diarrheal disease of rabbits, characterized by minimal inflammation, hypersecretion, and accumulation of mucus in the small and large intestines. While the etiology is unknown, it may occur concurrent with other enteric diseases. Predisposing factors include dietary changes, dietary fiber <6% or >22%, antibiotic treatments, environmental stress, and challenges with other bacteria. Clinical signs are gelatinous or mucus-covered feces, anorexia, lethargy, subnormal temperature, dehydration, rough coat, and often a bloated abdomen due to excess water in the stomach. A firm, impacted cecum may be palpable. The perineal area is often covered with mucus and feces. Diagnosis is based on clinical signs and necropsy findings of gelatinous mucus in the colon. Rabbits may live for ~1 wk. Treatment is unrewarding, but intense fluid therapy, enema removal of mucus mass, antibiotics, and analgesics may be tried. Prevention is the same as for any rabbit enteropathy.

Mastitis
(Blue breasts)

Mastitis is common in commercial rabbitries and is occasionally seen in smaller units. Poor sanitation enhances spread throughout the rabbitry. Mastitis affects lactating does and may progress to a septicemia that rapidly kills the doe. Generally, it is caused by staphylococci, but streptococci and other bacteria have been isolated. Initially, the mammary glands become hot, reddened, and swollen. Later, they may become cyanotic, hence the common name, "blue bag." The doe will not eat but may crave water. Fever ≥105°F (40.5°C) is often noted. If antibiotic treatment is started early (the first day the doe goes off feed), the rabbit may be saved and damage limited to 1-2 mammary glands. If >2 glands are lost, keeping the doe may not be economical. Because penicillin often causes diarrhea in rabbits, does should be treated only after the pelleted ration has been replaced with hay or some other high-fiber diet (*see* ENTEROTOXEMIA, p 1578). Kits should not be fostered to another doe because they will spread the infection to the foster mother. Handrearing of infected young may be attempted but is difficult. The incidence of mastitis can be reduced if nest boxes are maintained without rough edges to the entrance, which can traumatize the teats when the doe jumps in and out of the nest box. It is essential for the nest box to be sanitized both before and after use. Vaccines have not proved to be beneficial in preventing mastitis.

Treponematosis
(Vent disease, Syphilis, Spirochetosis)

Treponematosis, a specific venereal disease of domestic rabbits, is caused by the spirochete *Treponema paraluis cuniculi*. It occurs in both sexes and is transmitted by coitus and from the doe to offspring. Although closely related to the organism (*T pallidum*) that causes human syphilis, *T cuniculi* is not transmissible to other domestic animals or humans. The incubation period is 3-6 wk. Small vesicles or ulcers are formed, which ultimately become covered with a heavy scab. These lesions usually are confined to the genital region, but the lips and eyelids may be involved. Infected rabbits should not be mated. Diagnosis is based on the lesions and observation of the spirochete's corkscrew motility under darkfield microscopy. Serologic tests used to diagnose *T pallidum*, such as the VDRL slide test and the rapid-plasma regain card test are widely available and can be used to diagnose *T cuniculi*. Hutch burn is a differential diagnosis.

Benzathine penicillin G, 42,000 IU/kg, SC, at weekly intervals for 3 wk, is necessary to eradicate treponematosis from a herd. All rabbits must be treated even if no lesions are present. Lesions usually heal within 10-14 days, and recovered rabbits can be bred without danger of transmitting the infection. A potential side effect of penicillin treatment is diarrhea and the possibility of an enteritis outbreak due to proliferation of gram-negative bacteria in the gut. Rabbits treated with penicillin should be switched to hay and treated with antidiarrheals immediately if needed (*see* ENTEROTOXEMIA, p 1578).

Dermatophytosis
(Ringworm)

Clinical dermatophytosis commonly affects individual rabbits, but epizootics can also occur. Ringworm is generally associated with poor husbandry, poor nutrition, and other environmental stressors. The cause is most commonly *Trichophyton mentagrophytes* and occasionally *Microsporum canis*. Transmission is by direct contact. Fomites, such as hair brushes, that evade proper disinfection can play a significant role in spreading infection. Asymptomatic carriers are very common. The lesions usually appear first on the head and may spread to any area of the skin. Affected areas are circular, raised, reddened, and capped with white, bran-like, flaky material. A negative result with a Wood's lamp illumination does not rule out dermatophytosis, as all agents do not fluoresce. Hair plucked from the edge of the lesion may be cultured on special media, such as dermatophyte test media or Sabouraud's agar. A KOH skin scraping taken from the periphery of the lesion that reveals fungal forms confirms the diagnosis. Because rabbits with active infections are infectious for humans and other animals, they should be either isolated and treated or killed. Griseofulvin at an individual dosage of 25 mg/kg body wt, SID for 2 wk or in the feed at 825 mg/kg of feed is effective but not approved for use in rabbits; it should not be used in rabbits intended for human consumption. Griseofulvin may be teratogenic and should not be used in pregnant does. Topical antifungal creams containing itraconazole, clotrimazole, or miconazole may be effective extra-label treatments. For rabbitries, treatment with either 1% copper sulfate as a dip or 8 oz of MECA (metabolized chlorous acid/chlorine dioxide compound, 1:1:10 mix of base:activator:water) sprayed on 6 times in a 26-day period was shown to be effective.

Tularemia

Tularemia is rare in domestic rabbits, but wild rabbits and rodents are highly susceptible and have been involved in most epizootics. Up to 90% of human cases are linked to wild lagomorph exposure. The etiologic agent, *Francisella tularensis*, is an aerobic nonmotile gram-negative, pleomorphic, bipolar coccobacillus that is prevalent in the south central USA. It is highly infectious and passed through the skin, through the respiratory tract via aerosols, by ingestion, and via bloodsucking arthropods. Tularemia causes an acute fatal septicemia. Diagnosis is based on necropsy findings of septicemic bacterial disease with numerous small, bright white hepatic foci, congestion, and enlargement of the liver and spleen. Treatment of the animal is not indicated. Tularemia is a reportable disease.

VIRAL DISEASES

Viruses are not important causes of clinical disease of rabbits in the USA but include the infectious fibromas, papillomatosis, rabbitpox, myxomatosis, and a herpesvirus infection (Virus III). Rotaviral enteritis also has been diagnosed in the USA and seems to contribute to the overall problem of intestinal disease in rabbits. Viral hemorrhagic disease is found in almost every country that raises rabbits except the USA. In April 2000, USDA diagnosed rabbit calicivirus in a backyard facility in Iowa. Rapid response and cooperation between federal and state agencies contained this outbreak and eliminated the source of infection. The USA is currently considered free of rabbit hemorrhagic disease.

Myxomatosis

Myxomatosis is a fatal disease of all breeds of domesticated rabbits caused by myxoma virus, a member of the poxvirus group. Myxomatosis is called "big head" and is characterized by mucinous skin lesions or myxomas. Wild rabbits like the cottontail (*Sylvilagus*) and jackrabbits (*Lepus*) are quite resistant. Myxoma virus-infected *Sylvilagus* develop fibroma-like lesions similar to those caused by rabbit fibroma virus. All other mammals are refractory to the virus. Myxomatosis has a worldwide distribution. In the USA, myxomatosis is restricted largely to the coastal area of California and Oregon, where epidemics occur infrequently but sporadic cases are common. These areas correspond to the geographic distribution of the California brush rabbit (*S bachmani*), the reservoir of the infection. Losses in rabbitries may be 25-90%. Transmission occurs via mosquitos, fleas, biting flies, and direct contact.

The initial sign is conjunctivitis that rapidly becomes more marked and is accompanied by a milky ocular discharge. The rabbit is listless and anorectic, with a fever that frequently reaches 108°F (42°C). In acute outbreaks, some rabbits may die within 48 hr after signs appear. Those that survive become progressively depressed and develop a rough coat. The eyelids, nose, lips, and ears become edematous, which gives a swollen appearance to the head. In females, the vulva becomes inflamed and edematous; in males, the scrotum swells. A characteristic sign at this stage is drooping of the edematous ears. A purulent nasal discharge invariably appears, breathing becomes labored, and the rabbit goes into a coma just before death, which usually occurs within 1-2 wk after clinical signs appear. Occasionally, a rabbit survives for several weeks; in these cases, fibrotic nodules appear on the nose, ears, and forefeet. Rabbits inoculated experimentally with laboratory strains of the virus invariably develop small nodules at the point of injection after several days; similar nodules develop later on other parts of the body, particularly the ears.

Few characteristic gross lesions are found at necropsy in the acute form of the disease. The spleen is occasionally enlarged and is almost always devoid of lymphocytes when examined histologically. In rabbits that survive longer, subcutaneous edema and nodular skin tumors are seen. The seasonal incidence of the disease, clinical signs (especially the swollen genitalia), and high mortality are all of diagnostic significance. Large, eosinophilic, cytoplasmic inclusion bodies in the conjunctival epithelial cells are also helpful in diagnosis.

An attenuated vaccine prepared from a myxomatosis virus has protected rabbits infected under both field and laboratory conditions. This vaccine is not available in the USA, and because there is no effective treatment, euthanasia and burying or burning of affected rabbits is indicated. Preventive measures include protecting rabbits from exposure to arthropod vectors.

Rabbit (Shope) Fibroma Virus

Shope fibromas are found under natural conditions only in cottontails, although domestic rabbits can be infected by inoculation of virus-containing material. Fibromas may be found in domestic rabbits in areas where they are endemic in wild rabbits and where husbandry practices allow contact with arthropod vectors.

A fibroma virus, a member of the poxvirus group, causes this tumor, which is found on the legs, feet, and ears. The earliest lesion is a slight thickening of the subcutaneous tissues, followed by development of a clearly demarcated soft swelling. These tumors may persist for several months before regressing, leaving the rabbit essentially normal. Intracytoplasmic inclusion bodies are seen when sections of the tumor are examined histologically. Because Shope fibromas are of little significance in domestic rabbits, no control measures have been developed.

Rabbitpox

Rabbitpox is an acute, generalized disease of laboratory rabbits (*Oryctolagus*) that apparently has not been recognized in wild rabbits (*Sylvilagus*). A few outbreaks have been reported in the USA since 1930. The causative virus is closely related to vaccinia virus, and some outbreaks may have been caused by a virulent strain of vaccinia. Pox lesions may or may not be present on the skin. Most rabbits develop a fever and nasal discharge. The mortality varies but is always high. The most characteristic lesions seen at necropsy are a skin rash, subcutaneous edema, and edema of the mouth and other body openings. Because of the edematous condition, "poxless" rabbitpox may be confused with myxomatosis. The virus may be isolated or the infection diagnosed serologically by methods appropriate to vaccinia. (*See also* POX DISEASES, p 698.) Spread through a rabbitry is rapid, but rabbits inoculated with smallpox vaccine (vaccinia virus) are immune. Rabbitpox virus does not infect humans.

Papillomatosis

Two types of infectious papillomas occur infrequently in domestic rabbits. The oral papilloma, caused by the rabbit oral papillomavirus, is the most important clinically. The lesions consist of small, grayish white, pedunculated nodules or warts on the undersurface of the tongue or on the floor of the mouth. The second type, caused by the cottontail (Shope) papillomavirus, is characterized by horny warts on the neck, shoulders, ears, or abdomen and is primarily a natural disease of cottontail rabbits. Arthropod vectors transmit the Shope papillomavirus; therefore, arthropod control could be used as means of disease prevention. The oral papillomavirus is distinct from the Shope papillomavirus (which is also distinct from the Shope fibroma virus). Skin tumors caused by the Shope papillomavirus never occur in the mouth. Neither type of papillomatosis is treated, and the condition usually resolves spontaneously over time.

Rotaviral Infection

Rotavirus has been isolated from rabbits with diarrhea in many different countries. In serologic studies of rabbit colonies around the world, almost 100% of the adult rabbits in some rabbitries were positive for rotavirus, demonstrating its widespread nature. Rotavirus is shed in the feces of infected rabbits and, therefore, is probably transmitted by the fecal-oral route. Young rabbits of weaning age are most susceptible. It is probable that rotavirus is only mildly pathogenic, but most rotavirus infections are complicated with pathogenic bacteria such as *Clostridium* spp or *E coli*. The mixed infection results in a much more deadly syndrome. There is no treatment, but the infection appears to be self-limiting if susceptible rabbits are not continually introduced into the population. Experimentally, the virus is shed for only 1 wk after inoculation. Therefore, cessation of breeding for 4-6 wk seems to allow the disease to run its course because seropositive does do not infect their offspring.

Rabbit Calicivirus Disease
(Viral hemorrhagic disease)

Rabbit calicivirus disease was first reported in 1984 in the People's Republic of China, from whence it spread through the domestic and wild rabbit populations in continental Europe. The first report of the virus in the Western hemisphere was in Mexico City in 1988. Mexico successfully eradicated the virus by 1992. Recent outbreaks of rabbit calicivirus disease occurred in Australia (1995), New Zealand (1997), and Cuba (1997). In 1995, as a result of a laboratory accident in southern Australia, the virus escaped and killed 10 million rabbits in 8 wk. Rabbit calicivirus disease was confirmed in a group of 27 rabbits in Iowa in April, 2000, in the USA. The source of infection was not determined. The outbreak was contained, the virus eradicated, and the USA remains disease free.

Rabbit calicivirus disease is highly infectious in European rabbits (*Oryctolagus*), but cottontail rabbits and jackrabbits are not susceptible. Humans and other mammals are not affected. The calicivirus is highly contagious and can be transmitted by direct contact with infected rabbits or indirectly by fomites. Infection results in a peracute febrile disease causing hepatic necrosis, enteritis, and lymphoid necrosis, followed by massive coagulopathy and hemorrhages in multiple organs. Rabbits show few clinical signs and die within 6-24 hr of fever onset. Morbidity is often ~100% and mortality 60-90%. This is a reportable disease.

PARASITIC DISEASES

Coccidiosis

Coccidiosis is a common and worldwide protozoal disease of rabbits. Rabbits that recover frequently become carriers. There are 2 anatomic forms: hepatic, caused by *Eimeria stiedae*, and intestinal, caused by *E magna, E irresidua, E media, E perforans, E flavescens, E intestinalis*, or other *Eimeria* spp. Transmission of both the hepatic and intestinal forms is by ingestion of the sporulated oocysts, usually in contaminated feed or water.

Hepatic Coccidiosis: Severity of disease depends on the number of oocysts ingested. Young rabbits are most susceptible. Affected rabbits may be anorectic and have a rough coat. Hepatic coccidiosis is most often subclinical, but growing rabbits may fail to make normal gains. Infrequently, death may follow a short course. Rabbits usually succumb within 1 mo after a severe experimental exposure. At necropsy, small, yellowish white nodules are found throughout the hepatic parenchyma. In the early stages, they may be sharply demarcated, while in the later stages they coalesce. The early lesions have a milky content; older lesions may have a more cheese-like consistency. Microscopically, the nodules are composed of hypertrophied bile ducts or gallbladder. Diagnosis of this form of coccidiosis is based on the gross and microscopic changes, along with demonstration of the oocysts in the bile ducts. An impression smear of a lesion in the liver examined under light microscopy often reveals oocysts. The oocysts may also be demonstrated by fecal flotation.

Treatment is difficult, and control rather than cure is expected. Sulfaquinoxaline administered continuously in the drinking water (0.04% for 30 days) prevents clinical signs of hepatic coccidiosis in rabbits heavily exposed to *E stiedae*. However, it may not prevent the lesions. Sulfaquinoxaline may also be given in the feed at 0.025% for 20 days, or for 2 days out of every 8 until marketing. Because feed-grade sulfaquinoxaline can be difficult to obtain, liquid sulfaquinoxaline is used more commonly. Withdrawal time is 10 days for rabbits used for food. Other coccidiosis treatments do not have approved withdrawal times for meat rabbits. Other sulfa drug treatments include sulfadimethoxine (0.5-0.7 g/L drinking water) and sulfadimerazine (2 g/L drinking water). Other coccidiostats that may prove to be effective include salinomycine, diclazuril, and toltrazuril. Treatment is best administered for a minimum of 5 days and repeated after 5 days. Rabbits that are treated successfully are immune to subsequent infections.

Treatment will not be successful unless a sanitation program is instituted simultaneously. Elimination of fecal-oral transmission of infective oocysts is achieved by preventing feed hoppers and water crocks from becoming contaminated with feces. Hutches should be kept dry and the accumulated feces removed frequently. Wire cage bottoms should be brushed daily with a wire brush to help break the life cycle of the protozoa. Ammonia (10%) solution is lethal to oocysts and is the best choice to disinfect cages or ancillary equipment exposed to fecal material.

Intestinal Coccidiosis: This form of coccidiosis can occur in rabbits receiving the best of care, as well as in rabbits raised under unsanitary conditions. Typically, infections are mild and often no clinical signs are seen. In early infections, there are few lesions; later, the intestine may be thickened and pale. Good sanitation programs that can eliminate hepatic coccidiosis do not seem to eliminate intestinal coccidiosis. Intestinal coccidiosis is generally diagnosed by fecal flotation and microscopic identification of the oocysts (species). It is important to distinguish coccidian oocysts from the nonpathogenic yeast *Saccharomycopsis (Saccharomyces) guttulatus* that can also be found in large numbers. Treatment is similar to that for hepatic coccidiosis except that sulfaquinoxaline is given for 7 days and repeated after a 7-day interval.

Larval Worm Infection

Although adult tapeworm infections are rare in domestic rabbits, the discovery of larval tapeworm cysts on the serosal peritoneum is common. Rabbits are intermediate hosts for 2 species of canine tapeworm, *Taenia serialis* and *T pisiformis*. Although *T serialis* is rare in domestic rabbits, it is somewhat more common in wild ones. The larval stage of *T pisiformis*, a cysticercus, is found attached to the mesenteries. Before forming these fluid-filled cysts, the young larvae migrate through the liver, where they leave white, tortuous subcapsular tracts. Generally, there are no clinical signs, and diagnosis occurs at necropsy. Treatment is usually not attempted, but control is accomplished by restricting access of dogs (the final host of the tapeworm) to the area in which food and nesting material are stored. Dogs should not be fed infected dead rabbits because this perpetuates the cycle. Mebendazole at 1 g/kg of feed (50 mg/kg) for 14 days is reported to be an effective treatment.

Baylisascaris procyonis has been reported in rabbits. Signs are similar to those induced by *Encephalitozoon cuniculi*. No treatment is available.

Ectoparasites

The ear mite *Psoroptes cuniculi* is a common parasite of rabbits worldwide. Mites irritate the lining of the ear and cause serum and thick brown crusts to accumulate, creating an "ear canker." Infested rabbits scratch at and shake their head and ears. They lose flesh, fail to produce, and suffer secondary infections, which may damage the inner ear, reach the CNS, and result in torticollis. With the rabbit well restrained or under general anesthesia, the brown crumbly exudate should be removed with cotton soaked in dilute hydrogen peroxide. The ear should be treated with any of the miticides approved for use in dogs and cats. Those products containing a cerumenolytic agent are particularly useful in removing the heavy, crusted material. The medication should be applied within the ear and down the side of the head and neck. The incidence is much lower when rabbits are housed in wire cages than in solid cages. The mite is readily transmitted by direct contact. A variety of injectable ivermectin treatment regimes effective against both fur and ear mites have been reported, with the dosage of ivermectin 200-400 µg/kg, SC, 2-3 treatments 10-21 days apart.

Fur mite infestations are common, and 2 genera, *Cheyletiella* and *Listrophorus*, are found worldwide. A number of different species of the genus *Cheyletiella* are found on rabbits. The most common in North America is *C parasitovorax*. The genus *Listrophorus* has but 1 species, *L gibbus*. These mites live on the surface of the skin and do not cause the intense pruritus seen with sarcoptic mange. Fur mite infestations usually are asymptomatic unless the rabbit becomes debilitated. *Cheyletiella* may be noticed as "dandruff." Scraping the dandruff onto a dark paper or background will demonstrate the "walking dandruff" as *Cheyletiella* is called. Transmission is by direct contact. Diagnosis is accomplished by skin scraping and light microscopy. *Cheyletiella* mites may cause a mild dermatitis in humans. Weekly dusting of animals and bedding with permethrin powder can control *Cheyletiella* mites.

Rabbits are rarely infested with either *Sarcoptes scabei*, or *Notoedres cati*. These mites burrow into the skin and lay eggs. The rabbits are extremely pruritic and it is difficult to eliminate the parasites on domestic rabbits. The condition is extremely contagious and can be transmitted to humans.

Fleas of the following species, *Ctenocephalides felis*, *C canis*, and *Pulex irritans*, can affect rabbits and many other animals. Imidacloprid is a flea adulticide that kills on and contact and has been successfully used to treat rabbits infested with fleas. Fipronil is contraindicated for use in rabbits due to potential toxicity.

Encephalitozoonosis
(Nosematosis)

Encephalitozoon (Nosema) cuniculi is a widespread protozoal (microsporidian) infection of rabbits and occasionally of mice, guinea pigs, rats, and dogs. Usually, no clinical signs are seen. The mode of transmission is not definitely known, but the organism is shed in the urine. It seems to be mildly contagious in a rabbitry. At necropsy, the most significant lesion is pitting of the kidneys. Microscopic lesions consist of focal granulomas and pseudocysts in the brain and kidneys. Sometimes a severe, focal, interstitial nephritis is seen. Diagnosis is made by histologically identifying the lesions (pseudocysts) and observing the organisms when stained with Giemsa, Gram's or Goodpasture-carbol fuchsin stains. Several serologic and skin tests are helpful in screening rabbits for antibodies to the organism. Effective treatment has not been established. Prevention entails good sanitation and, possibly, serologic screening of breeding stock with elimination of positive reactors. A differential diagnosis is an aberrant migration of *Baylisascaris* spp into the nervous system. Encephalitozoonosis is an emerging disease of immunodeficient humans.

Pinworms

Passalurus ambiguus, the rabbit pinworm, usually is not clinically significant but often is upsetting to owners. It is common in many rabbitries and is distributed worldwide. Transmission is by ingestion of contaminated food or water. The adult worm lives in the cecum or anterior colon. Diagnosis is made by observing the adults at necropsy or by finding the eggs during examination of the feces. Single treatments are not very effective because the life cycle is direct and reinfection is common. Piperazine citrates in the water (3 g/L) for alternating 2-wk periods or fenbendazole (50 ppm in feed for 5 days) are effective treatments. Rabbit pinworms are not transmissible to humans.

NONINFECTIOUS DISEASES

Broken Back

Fracture or dislocation of lumbar vertebrae with compression or severing of the spinal cord is common in both pet and commercial rabbits. Common signs include posterior paresis or paralysis and urinary and fecal incontinence due to loss of sphincter control. Initial signs of paralysis may resolve within 3-5 days as swelling around the cord diminishes. Supportive therapy includes anti-inflammatory glucocorticoids (eg, dexamethasone) to reduce damage from swelling. Paralysis after 1-2 wk or incontinence indicates a grave prognosis and warrants euthanasia.

Cannibalism

Young does may kill and eat their young for a number of reasons, including nervousness, neglect (failure to nurse), and severe cold. Dogs or predators entering a rabbitry often cause nervous does to kill and eat the young. Cannibalism of the dead young occurs as a natural, nest-cleaning instinct. If all management practices are proper and the doe kills 2 litters in a row, she should be culled.

Dental Malocclusion

The incisors, premolars, and molars of rabbits grow throughout life. The normal length is maintained by the wearing action of opposing teeth. Malocclusion (mandibular prognathism, brachygnathism) probably is the most common inherited disease in rabbits and leads to overgrowth of incisors with resultant difficulty in eating and drinking. Dental trimming is often done with combined anesthesia of diazepam (7-10 mg/kg, IM) followed in 20 min with ketamine (25 mg/kg, IM). Overgrown teeth can be cut with bone or wire cutters, however a grinding tool or dental burr is safer. When trimming with a dental burr, minimal pressure should be applied to keep the burr cool. The pulp, which looks like a pink tinge in the dentin, should not be exposed. If this occurs, the risk of pulp necrosis is avoided by performing a partial pulpectomy. The tooth should be aseptically prepared and the pulp burred out and filled with calcium hydroxide. Hard fillings are contraindicated in the continuously erupting tooth.

Occasionally, the cheek teeth overgrow and cause severe tongue or buccal lesions. Because malocclusion is generally considered to be inherited, rabbits with this condition should not be bred. However, young rabbits can damage their incisor teeth by pulling on the cage wire, which results in misalignment and possibly malocclusion as the teeth grow. This condition is difficult to differentiate from genetic malocclusion, and these rabbits should also be culled. Genetic malocclusion generally can be detected in rabbits 3-8 wk old.

Dental Abscesses

Dental abscesses may develop as a consequence of foreign bodies (eg, plant material embedded between the tooth and gum), pulp exposure following tooth trimming, or other diseases. It may be that rabbit incisors wear differently depending on diet, and a pelleted diet may predispose the rabbit to dental disease. Multiple teeth are commonly affected. A thorough oral exam and diagnostic radiographs are indicated. Dental extractions may be accomplished using a fine-tipped dental elevator worked along the root to free the tooth. Incisors are curved and require use of a specialized rabbit incisor luxator or similar curved instrument for removal. Curettage of the alveolus to destroy the apical germinal tissue is required to prevent regrowth of the tooth. Regrowth is unlikely if the pulp remains in the extracted tooth, but followup radiographs in 2-3 mo will confirm successful extraction. Infected sockets are left open to drain or filled with a doxycycline periceutical gel. Gingival tissues should be sutured as needed. Surgical removal of the lateral wall of the alveolus may be needed to remove an abnormal tooth. Extraction of cheek teeth involves routine elevation and luxation if the dental anatomy is normal. Extraction of multiple cheek teeth carries a very poor prognosis for recovery. Continued monitoring of the occlusal surface and followup adjustment is expected.

Hair Chewing and Hairballs
(Trichobezoars)

Rabbits groom themselves constantly, so the stomach contents often contain hair, which is normally passed through the GI tract and excreted with the fecal pellets. The stomach of a healthy rabbit is never empty and the gastric contents often include a large amount of ingested hair. Hair chewing is generally a result of low fiber in the diet and can be corrected by increasing the fiber or feeding hay along with the pellets. Adding magnesium oxide to the diet at 0.25% also may be helpful. In some cases, hair chewing is a result of boredom. Providing environmental enrichment often halts this abnormal behavior.

The hair becomes a problem only if excess amounts are consumed or if it accumulates in the stomach and blocks the pylorus. If this happens, the rabbit becomes anorectic, loses weight, and dies within 3-4 wk. Premortem diagnosis of pyloric obstruction can be difficult, as palpable hairballs can be an incidental finding and radiography is often nondiagnostic.

GI hypomotility or gut stasis is the primary concern when presented with clinical illness associated with a hairball. Hairballs are more likely a result of anorexia, not its cause. Gas accumulation creates visceral distention and pain. Decreased food intake and GI hypomotility result in elevation of cecal pH and alteration of cecal microflora, creating cecal dysbiosis. Alterations in water and electrolyte balance result in ketoacidosis and hepatic lipidosis. Gastric ulceration and gastric rupture may occur.

The goals of treatment are to remove the obstruction, stimulate motility, restore GI microorganism balance, and relieve dehydration and anorexia. Treatment includes motility stimulants such as metoclopromide (0.5 mg/kg, PO or SC, TID-QID), fluid therapy, pain medication, and antiulcer therapy. Reestablishment of GI microflora may be assisted by probiotic treatment or cecotrophs from healthy rabbits.

Several remedies have been proposed to assist in the break up or passage of a hairball. Pineapple juice contains the digestive enzyme bromelain and has been used to treat early cases of trichobezoars; an adult rabbit is given 10 mL of fresh or frozen juice through a stomach tube or intubation needle, SID-BID for 3 days. Both the fluid and the enzyme help to break up the matrix of the hairball. Canned pineapple juice is not as effective because the canning process destroys the enzyme. Papaya contains the enzyme papain, also called papayazyme. Papain enzymes do not break down the hair itself, but may help break down the mucus that holds the hairball together. Human health food or nutrition stores carry bromelain and papayazyme supplements as aids to digestion. Mineral oil and laxatives are not effective in removing the hair mass. Roughage (hay or straw) should be fed during the treatment to help carry the hair fibers through the GI tract and out with the feces. Surgical treatment is certain but risky.

Prevention is the best option. Providing a high fiber diet, avoiding stress and obesity, environmental enrichment, and daily combing to remove loose hair effectively prevents this condition. Clinical research does not support routine doses of mineral oil, wetting agents, or proteolytic enzymes as effective preventives.

Heat Exhaustion

Rabbits are sensitive to heat. Hot, humid weather, along with poorly ventilated hutches or transport in poorly ventilated vehicles, may lead to death of many rabbits, particularly pregnant does. Affected rabbits stretch out and breathe rapidly. Hutches should be constructed so that they can be sprinkled in hot, humid weather. Free access to cool water should be provided. When the environment can be controlled, optimal conditions are a temperature of 50-70°F (15.5-21°C) and a relative humidity of 40-60%, with 10-20 air changes/hr. Wire cages are preferable to solid hutches. Treatment consists of immersing rabbits in cold water during the heat of the day, especially those that will kindle in the next day or two. Breeding bucks may lose a majority of viable sperm and might not breed successfully for several weeks while new sperm production replaces the sperm killed by thermal stress.

Hutch Burn
(Urine burn)

Hutch burn is often confused with treponematosis and can be truly differentiated only by the absence of spirochetes on darkfield microscopy and by the lack of antibodies to *Treponema cuniculi*. It is caused by wet and dirty hutch floors and affects the anus and external genitalia. Also, rabbits that lack adequate sphincter control of the bladder constantly dribble urine and may be affected. The membranes of the anus and genital region become inflamed and chapped. The area soon becomes secondarily infected with opportunistic pathogenic bacteria. Brownish crusts cover the area and a hemorrhagic, purulent exudate may be present. Keeping hutch floors clean and dry and applying nitrofurazone or an antibiotic ointment to the lesions hastens recovery.

Ketosis
(Pregnancy toxemia)

Ketosis is a rare disorder that may result in death of does at or 1-2 days before kindling. The disease is more common in first-litter does. Predisposing factors include obesity and lack of exercise. The probable cause is starvation. For some reason not well understood, there is anorexia. Other signs are dullness of eyes, sluggishness, respiratory distress, prostration, and death. The most significant lesions are fatty liver and kidneys. The body mobilizes fat and transports it to the liver to be broken down for energy, thus the fatty liver. Diagnosis depends on clinical signs and necropsy lesions. Injection of fluids that contain glucose may be helpful in correcting the disease. Breeding junior does early, before they become too fat, is also helpful. Hairballs in the stomach are often a factor in ketosis.

Moist Dermatitis
(Wet dewlap)

Female rabbits have a heavy fold of skin on the ventral aspect of the neck. As the rabbit drinks, this skin may become wet and soggy ("slobbers"), which leads to inflammation. Contributing factors include dental malocclusion, open water crocks, and damp bedding. The hair may slip, and the area may become infected or flyblown. The area often turns green if infected with *Pseudomonas* sp. Automatic watering systems with drinking valves generally prevent wet dewlaps. If open water receptacles are used, they should have small openings or be elevated. Once the area is infected, the hair should be clipped and antiseptic dusting powder applied. In severe cases, parenteral antibiotics may be necessary.

Ulcerative Pododermatitis
(Sore hocks)

This disease does not involve the hock but the plantar surface of the metatarsals and, less commonly, the volar surface of the metacarpal-phalangeal region. The cause is either pressure on the skin from bearing the body weight on wire-floored cages or trauma to the skin from stamping, with secondary infection of the necrotic skin. Several factors, including accumulation of urine-soaked feces, nervousness, posterior paralysis after a spinal cord injury, and the type of wire used, may influence development. Genetics are also involved. Heavy-breed rabbits such as the Rex, Flemish Giant, and Checkered Giant are more susceptible. Affected rabbits sit in a peculiar position with their weight on their front feet; if all 4 feet are affected, they tiptoe when walking. Various debriding agents can be used to clean the lesion, followed by topical antibiotic treatment along with parenteral antibiotics. Radiographs rule out osteomyelitis with severe lesions. The rabbit must be removed from the cage or given a solid floor (board or mat) on which to sit or rest. Because treatment is difficult and time consuming and the condition often recurs, affected commercial animals should be culled. Because big feet and thick footpads are hereditary, selection of breeding stock for these traits has reduced the incidence of pododermatitis.

Urolithiasis

Urolithiasis is seen routinely in pet rabbits and occasionally in commercial rabbitries. It is generally suspected when hematuria is seen. (A dipstick can quickly rule out normal pigment causes of red urine.) Uroliths are caused by calcium carbonate and triple phosphate crystals precipitating out of normal urine when the pH increases to 8.5-9.5. Normal rabbit urine has an average pH of 8.2. Several factors have been incriminated in urolithiasis, including nutritional imbalance (especially the calcium:phosphorus ratio), genetic predisposition, infection, inadequate water intake, and metabolic disorders. Treatment involves surgically removing the uroliths, acidifying the urine, and reducing dietary calcium. Because alfalfa is high in calcium and one of the main dietary components of rabbit pellets, removal of the pellets and a switch to grass or timothy hay and rolled oats is beneficial in preventing recurrence.

Heritable Diseases

Hydrocephalus: Hydrocephalus, characterized by an enlarged head, is occasionally seen in neonatal rabbits. The top of the skull appears dome-shaped, and the fontanelle is wider than normal. Most affected rabbits are born dead; occasionally, they live for several weeks but generally exhibit neurologic signs. At necropsy, the brain is enlarged; on cut section, the ventricles are greatly enlarged and filled with CSF. The cause can either be genetic or result from dietary deficiency or excess of vitamin A. In the case of a dietary deficiency or hypervitaminosis, poor reproduction (low fertility, small litter size, abortion, etc) also is seen in the breeding herd. A correct assessment of vitamin A becomes critical in treatment, and both serum and liver should be analyzed. In deficiency, the serum level of vitamin A is below normal (2.6-4.2 IU/mL). In toxicity, the serum level can be normal, but the concentration of vitamin A in the liver is very high (>4,000 IU/g). Treatment of the deficiency involves increasing the carotene content of the diet or adding a vitamin A supplement. Treatment of hypervitaminosis A requires reducing vitamin A in the diet. However, reducing the amount of vitamin A stored in the liver is extremely difficult. If the doe's reproduction has been impaired, replacing the doe is probably more cost-effective than trying to decrease the vitamin A level. Because genetic hydrocephalus appears to be inherited recessively, control requires culling both parents.

Buphthalmia (Blue Eye, Moon Eye, Infantile Glaucoma): Buphthalmia is an autosomal trait with incomplete penetrance that results in variable clinical severity. Intraocular pressures begin to rise as early as 3 mo. One or both eyes may be affected. There is no described treatment, but affected animals should not breed.

Splay Leg: Splay leg is presumed to be an inherited disorder presenting with abduction of one or more legs as early as 3-4 wk of age. The right rear limb is most commonly affected, although the condition may be unilateral or bilateral.

Neoplasia

By far, the most common tumor in rabbits is uterine adenocarcinoma. Susceptibility is related to breed. The disease may present as multiple tumors that often metastasize to the liver, lungs, and other organs. This disease is the primary reason to recommend spaying of nonbreeding female rabbits. Monitoring for metastasis should follow surgical removal of uterine adenocarcinoma. Malignant lymphomas (lymphosarcoma) are relatively common and may occur in rabbits <2 yr old. Typically, lymphosarcoma presents with a tetrad of lesions including enlarged kidneys, splenomegaly, hepatomegaly, and lymphadenopathy.

REPTILES

Reptiles can be easily recognized by their horny or scaly integument. The class Reptilia comprises 4 orders: Rhynchocephalia, in which the sole species is the tuatara; Crocodilia, which includes alligators, caimans, crocodiles, and gavials; Chelonia, which contains tortoises and turtles; and Squamata, which contains lizards and snakes.

There are many morphologic and biologic differences between reptiles and other vertebrates. Most reptiles are ectothermal poikilotherms, while most mammals and birds are endothermal homeotherms. Structurally, reptiles other than the crocodilians have an incomplete ventricular septum, yet functionally, the heart acts more like a 4-chambered heart. A renal portal system exists in addition to the hepatic portal system. Fertilization occurs internally, and the embryos develop within amnionic eggs, either externally (oviparity) or internally (viviparity).

MANAGEMENT

Poor management practices are thought to be the underlying cause of most health problems in captive reptiles. In the absence of sound management, captive reptiles commonly develop immune system dysfunction, leaving them susceptible to many infectious diseases. To ensure a high quality of life, reptiles should be kept in an environment as similar to that of their native habitat as possible.

Temperature: Most reptiles are ectotherms; the heat generated from metabolic activity is limited, and control mechanisms, apart from behavior, to retain the heat produced are lacking. To control daily fluctuations in body temperature, many reptiles seek out cool or warm areas. In their natural habitat, they are quite adept at behavioral mechanisms aimed at maintaining their body temperature within a relatively narrow range compared with the ambient temperature. While unable to produce a true fever, when infected with bacterial agents, reptiles move to warmer areas in their environment to create a "behavioral fever." Therefore, the cage or enclosure used to house reptiles should provide a thermal gradient (within the preferred optimal temperature zone for each species) that enhances physiologic and psychologic well-being. Reptiles also use a thermal gradient to facilitate digestion, increase antibody production, and increase the distribution and clearance of certain antibiotics. Sick reptiles should initially be maintained at the upper range of their preferred optimal temperature. Tropical species generally prefer temperatures of 80-100°F (27-38°C) and temperate species, 68-95°F (20-35°C). Semiaquatic turtles prefer a slightly lower range. Lethal temperatures for some species may be within 10°F (5°C) of the upper limits of the preferred range.

Most reptiles prefer basking sources of heat, perhaps being the most similar to their normal environment. Basking lights are preferred for chelonians and lizards; this can be an incandescent bulb, infrared device, mercury vapor lamp, or a ceramic bulb heater. Heat lamps can be used, but overheating is a common problem. These sources should all be protected from reptile contact and placed >18 in. (45 cm) from the substrate. Smaller enclosures with limited ventilation should have a reptile thermostat with a probe attached to the heat source, and all cages should have a thermometer. It is prudent to place thermometers in both the directly heated and unheated regions of the enclosure. Undertank heaters are also useful heat sources primarily for lizards and snakes; when used in conjunction with a basking light, they can provide heat at night as well as day. Undertank heaters should cover no more than 30% of the available cage space and be designed for this application. Two more recent innovations for reptile heating are mercury vapor bulbs and infrared heaters. Mercury vapor lamps are very good basking lights and also provide some ultraviolet light in the wavelengths appropriate for reptile use. Infrared panels are produced in a variety of sizes. They can easily be attached to the roof of the cage so as to radiate heat down toward the substrate. Infrared heaters are unique in that they tend to heat objects in the field of the heat waves, without overheating the enclosure. Neither infrared nor ceramic heaters produce light. As with any basking light or device, the user should always check the substrate temperature. If the heated surface is too warm for maintaining comfortable contact, it is too warm for the reptile as well. "Hot-rocks" are less popular because the heat they provide is inconsistent and thermal burns are commonly linked to their use.

Reptiles become inactive at lower temperatures (torpor). This is a normal seasonal event for temperate species, and hibernation is generally required for optimal reproduction and longterm physiologic well-being. However, hibernation should never be attempted with a compromised reptile because immune status and function is suppressed by both seasonal changes and temperature reduction. Tropical species may decrease their level of activity due to minor temperature fluctuations, but they should not be hibernated. Temperature extremes and rapid fluctuations of temperature in the animal unit should be avoided. Knowledge of the seasonal husbandry requirements of each captive reptile is vital.

Photoperiod: Photoperiod requirements for reptiles are based on circadian and circannual activity requirements. For temperate species, variations in photoperiod are used as environmental cues to synchronize reproductive cyclicity with optimal environmental conditions. For tropical species, variations in photoperiod are less important in synchronizing reproductive cyclicity. However, the single most important factor in stimulating reproductive activity in captive reptiles is temperature change.

Fluctuations in photoperiod of ~10 hr of daylight for winter months to ~14 hr of daylight for summer months are common for many tropical and subtropical areas. Temperate areas experience changes in photoperiod ranging from ~8 hr of daylight during the winter to ~16 hr during the summer.

Lighting Requirements: Feeding behavior, activity, and to a lesser extent, reproduction in reptiles are improved with full-spectrum light. This requires the use of fluorescent tubes with spectral qualities similar to natural sunlight, including ultraviolet (UV). Bulbs that produce UVB wavelengths in the range of 290-320 nm are the most appropriate. Mercury vapor lamps are the only non-fluorescent bulbs available that can also provide UV light, despite the claims of many incandescent bulb manufacturers. The provision of the proper UV spectrum is essential to the conversion of cholesterol byproducts into active vitamin D_3 in reptilian skin. While exposure to unfiltered sunlight is the best form of UV available, sunlight filtered through most glass or plastic is virtually devoid of UV rays. UV-producing bulbs should be placed within range of resting or basking surfaces so that the reptile can obtain adequate UV exposure. Typical UV-producing lights should be within 18 in. of resting or basking areas, while mercury vapor lamps can be several feet away. The practice of using a black light in combination with full spectrum bulbs has been shown to be of merit in promoting reproductive activity in lizards, but does not appreciably increase UVB exposure. As even the best "full-spectrum" bulbs available are a poor substitute for natural sunlight, a species appropriate supplement that contains vitamin D_3 may be necessary. (*See* NUTRITION AND NUTRITIONAL DISEASES, p 1597.)

Water and Humidity: Semiaquatic species require enough water to allow complete immersion. Feeding, reproduction, and social interaction occur aquatically in many species. Water quality should be controlled through filtration and aeration to prevent accumulation of toxic organic wastes and overgrowth of pathogenic organisms. For estuarine species, water salinity should be monitored. Water pH for some species of aquatic turtles may need to be adjusted to that of the natural habitat.

Requirements for water intake are linked to availability in the natural habitat. Aquatic and semiaquatic species tend to be ureotelic (urea excretors), which results in significant water loss. Species from drier environments tend to be uricotelic (uric acid excretors), which conserves water. Loss of water through the skin occurs in many species when deprived of soaking areas; loss in crocodilians may be as high as 20% of body wt. Likewise, transcutaneous absorption of water has also been documented. Many species drink readily from pools or bowls, but a number of small lizards (eg, anoles, true chameleons) drink by lapping water droplets that accumulate through condensation. Misting the environment or creating a drip system provides options for water intake.

The humidity should mimic that of the natural environment of the captive species. Excessively low humidity (<35%) can result in abnormally dry skin and dysecdysis, especially in species that are not adapted to an arid environment. Excessively high humidity (>70%) can result in bacterial or fungal blooms and predispose to cutaneous infections.

Enclosure Design: Many reptiles appear nervous and insecure in captivity. This can be minimized by providing appropriate cage "furniture" and hiding spaces. Arboreal species should be provided with horizontal and vertical tree branches or other appropriate climbing material. Terrestrial species usually require more horizontal space. Many terrestrial and fossorial species require hiding places, eg, boxes, tree trunks, rocks, or other objects. For some species, a solid black border painted on the glass wall 8 in. (20 cm) from the cage bottom provides added security. Community housing of highly social, diurnal species often requires placing several stations for basking, eating, and drinking that are all out of the view of dominant conspecifics and any human observers. Overcrowding must be avoided to reduce stress and competition for food, water, basking sites, mates, etc. Aggressive species may have to be separated during feeding to prevent injury to cagemates. Fighting can be reduced significantly by housing compatible species together.

Substrates: Cage substrates should be disposable, inexpensive, nontoxic, and nonabrasive. They should provide minimal areas for microbial growth and facilitate cage cleaning. Newsprint, sand, peat moss, potting soil, wood shavings, cypress mulch, corncob bedding, walnut bedding, gravel, alfalfa pellets, and artificial turf have all been used successfully for most snakes. The pungent volatile substances in cedar shavings may cause mucosal and respiratory irritation as well as potential neurologic problems. Snakes <18 in. (45 cm) long should not be fed while on "loose" substrates (shavings, corncob, walnut, small gravel, etc) because these substrates accumulate around the mouth (predisposing to stomatitis) and may be swallowed (predisposing to intestinal impaction). Many experienced herpetologists remove the snake from its normal cage and feed it in a separate cage on newspaper. This results in conditioned behavior that is thought by some to decrease feeding frenzy activity in large snakes when approached in their normal, nonfeeding cage.

Ease of cleaning is a legitimate reason to choose a less complicated substrate, as the more elaborate substrates tend to be cleaned less frequently. In dealing with parasites (eg, reptile mites, parasite ova) and overgrowth of bacterial and fungal agents, it is essential to be able to clean thoroughly and frequently. Newspaper is perhaps the substrate of choice for sick reptiles because it is inexpensive, easy to clean, and allows regurgitated material, feces, etc, to be easily observed.

Substrate choice is also determined by the humidity level desired for a particular reptile. Cypress mulch can hold moisture and is resistant to mold. In contrast, corncob bedding is readily available but is expensive and subject to severe molding if wet. Mixtures of sand, peat moss, and soil hold moisture and allow burrowing. Sand or soil can also be used for a drier substrate. Microhabitats within an enclosure can provide increased humidity without creating high humidity levels in the entire cage.

Sand, potting soil, and leaf litter are adequate substrates for many species of lizards, turtles, and tortoises. Alfalfa pellets (common rabbit pellets) are also a useful bedding for turtles and tortoises. It is inexpensive and easy to clean, and the pellets are nutritious if eaten.

Crocodilians and aquatic turtles can be maintained on a combination of sand, gravel, and cement substrates if basking areas are provided. Gravel should be large enough that it cannot be ingested.

Sanitation: Sanitation is essential for successful longterm maintenance of reptiles. Cages should be kept free of excreta, and uneaten food should be removed and disposed of daily. Internal parasites are one of the most common health problems seen in captive reptiles; and many parasites have direct life cycles, which exacerbates infection if fecal waste is not removed. Tools used for scooping wastes should be disinfected with a quaternary ammonium compound before use in each cage to reduce the possibility of disease transmission. All substrates should be completely replaced at least every 3 mo. Aquatic and terrestrial environments should be disassembled and disinfected at least every 3 mo. Water dishes should be thoroughly cleaned at least once every 2 wk. Although turtles appear to tolerate chlorine in treated water reasonably well, its effects are undetermined. While chlorine may result in transient irritation of eyes of aquatic turtles not used to chlorine, it appears to be beneficial in controlling pathogen levels in the water.

Chemical Restraint: There are many circumstances where chemical restraint is indicated to perform a complete and thorough physical examination. If the reptile is likely to injure veterinary personnel or itself during examination, chemical restraint should be used (*see* below). While sedated, as many diagnostic and treatment procedures as possible should be performed at the same time.

Sedation and Anesthesia

Anesthesia in reptiles has been improved by research and clinical experience, resulting in protocols for the use of injectable agents and inhalant gases to provide a wide range of sedation and surgical anesthesia. Several anesthetic techniques are inappropriate for use in reptiles. Hypothermia reduces movement but does not induce analgesia and, therefore, is unacceptable and inhumane. Barbiturates and ether have been used in reptiles but are not recommended; their duration of action is prolonged, metabolic dysfunction may occur, and the depth of anesthesia is difficult to assess and manage.

Before elective surgery, the reptile should be acclimated to a temperature within the upper levels of its preferred range. If a reptile is not properly warmed, uptake, action, transformation, and excretion of sedatives and anesthetics will be dramatically delayed. The use of a warm water circulating pad or heated air blanket on the surgery table will help maintain body temperatures during induction and maintenance of anesthesia. The same temperature considerations are just as important during recovery, as drug transformation and elimination is much slower in reptiles and is exacerbated by low temperatures. More consistent anesthetic results will be achieved with temperature maintenance prior to, during, and after surgery.

Preanesthetic Medications: If possible, reptiles should be fasted for ≥24 hr. A large snake undergoing an elective procedure would be better held off food for several days. It is very rare for a reptile to aspirate, as the glottis is closed at rest. A very large meal can interfere with tidal volume (*see* below), so fasting also improves ventilation.

There are no studies justifying the use of anticholinergics in reptiles. In fact, the use of atropine has been linked to GI atony problems postoperatively. However, if the practitioner feels that an anticholinergic agent is indicated, atropine sulfate at 0.01-0.04 mg/kg IM or glycopyrrolate at 0.01 mg/kg IM or SC may be given at least 30 min prior to induction to decrease oral secretions and avoid profound bradycardia. Most reptile surgeons do not report any problems when omitting these drugs and their main application appears to be reducing viscous secretions hindering intubation.

Tranquilizers may be given prior to other sedatives or anesthetics to decrease the amount of drugs required for induction and maintenance of anesthesia. They may produce a smoother, less violent recovery, but may also increase recovery time. Acepromazine at 0.1-0.5 mg/kg IM and chlorpromazine at 10 mg/kg IM have been reported to smooth induction and reduce maintenance drug levels.

It is unclear whether opiates produce sedation in reptiles. However, many practitioners report that employing this group of drugs as a preanesthetic allows for a quicker induction and less violent recovery. With the current emphasis on pain management it is important to consider analgesia with regard to reptiles. Buprenorphine may produce

TABLE 14. Pain Medications Used in Reptiles

Drug	Species	Dosage and Route	Comments
Banamine	Lizards	1-2 mg/kg, SID for 1-2 doses	Green iguanas post-operatively
Buprenorphine	All	0.005-0.02 mg/kg, IM, every 24-48 hr	Long-lasting analgesia
Butorphanol	Tortoises	0.2 mg/kg, IM or SC	Analgesia, sedation, preanesthetic
	Lizards	0.05 mg/kg, IM, SID for 2-3 days	Green iguanas, postoperatively
	Lizards	1.0-1.5 mg/kg, IM or SC	30 min prior to isoflurane for induction
Carprofen	All	1-4 mg/kg, PO, IM, SC, or IV, SID	NSAID
Ketoprofen	All	1-2 mg/kg, SC or IM, SID	NSAID
Lidocaine (1%)	All	≤10 mg/kg	Local anesthetic, glottis for induction
Meperidine	Snakes	5-10 mg/kg, SID-BID	Analgesia, but no sedation
Morphine	Crocodiles	0.5-4.0 mg/kg, intra-coelomic	Analgesia
Pentazocine	All	2-5 mg/kg, IM, SID-QID	Analgesia
Prednisolone	All	2-5 mg/kg, PO or IM	Anti-inflammatory for chronic pain

analgesia for 24-48 hr, but data is lacking. Dosages are listed in TABLE 14 and should be considered to last for at least several hours. Butorphanol can be given to reptiles in dosages up to 2 mg/kg but the duration of activity is short lived.

Ventilation: Because reptiles breathe so seldom under sedation or anesthesia, assisted ventilation provides for better gas exchange. Tracheas of lizards and snakes are made up of incomplete, C-shaped tracheal rings, whereas tracheas of crocodilians, turtles, and tortoises are composed of complete tracheal rings. Most reptiles have a very long trachea, except turtles which have a short trachea that bifurcates just after entering the cranial coelomic inlet. The glottis of reptiles remains closed between breaths or at rest but opens for respiration. The larynx and glottis are found in the rostral part of the mouth, at the base of the tongue, and intubation is easily accomplished if the reptile is adequately sedated. Turtles and tortoises have very thick, fleshy tongues in a smaller mouth, sometimes making it more difficult to locate the glottis and intubate these reptiles. With the mouth opened and the tongue visualized, slight digital pressure directed upward at the base of the throat often lifts the glottis into view. Like cats, reptiles are easier to intubate if the surface of the glottis has been swabbed with a topical anesthetic, such as 1% lidocaine. Intubation may also be facilitated by using a stylet within the lumen of the endotracheal tube to keep smaller diameter tubes from folding.

In general, reptilian lungs are very simple structures accommodating a larger tidal volume but a smaller surface for gas exchange. The left lung is absent or vestigial in most snakes, with the exception of boids (boas and pythons). The right lung extends caudally in snakes, becoming more of an air sac in the lower third of the body. Most reptiles do not have a functional muscular diaphragm and therefore have a combined pleuroperitoneum or coelomic cavity. The muscles of the abdomen and trunk complement the intercostal muscles to generate negative pressure, causing the lungs to expand. Activity of smooth muscles within the lung wall also helps to move air in and out of the lungs. Turtles have a membranous separation between the lungs and remaining viscera, but do not have intercostal muscles. Turtles breathe by changing the positions of the coelomic viscera and limbs, thereby creating pressure differences within the lungs. Crocodilians have a membranous pseudodiaphragm, which does not function as a mammalian diaphragm does.

The clinically significant difference between mammalian and reptilian respiration is that, at a surgical plane of anesthesia, the skeletal muscles of reptiles will not be able to assist breathing and so assisted ventilation will be required. Further, if the reptile is positioned in dorsal recumbency, viscera will compress the lungs, increasing the need for assisted ventilation. It is important to avoid rupturing the lungs during ventilation. A positive pressure of 4-8 cm H_2O at a rate of 2-5 breaths/min is recommended. Employing the reptile's conscious respiratory rate at rest may provide a better guideline for selecting the ventilation frequency (breaths/min).

Apnea is a common problem with high or repeated doses of induction agents and ventilation is critical in maintaining reptiles until they resume breathing. Many clinicians use specialty ventilators that function according to parameters set prior to anesthesia. Ventilation by simply bagging the reptile is also useful, albeit less precise, and is recommended in the absence of a ventilator.

Monitoring Vital Signs: Reptiles can and should be monitored during anesthesia and surgery. Heart rates can be assessed by blood pressure monitor, esophageal stethoscope, and ECG. However, heart rate alone may not give an adequate picture of a reptile's health, as the heart may continue to beat for minutes to hours after removal from a reptile's body. Trends in heart rate and amplitude of heart sounds should be monitored to help determine whether anesthesia can be continued. A decreasing rate and amplitude suggest that a decrease or cessation of anesthesic agent(s) may be appropriate. Pulse oximeters should also be used when possible to review trends in blood oxygen saturation. In most mammals, breathing is stimulated by decreasing blood levels of oxygen or increasing levels of CO_2. In reptiles, CO_2 levels have less effect on respiration, which is stimulated primarily by dropping oxygen levels and temperature. Reptiles have some pulmonary stretch receptors that are sensitive to CO_2, and as CO_2 increases, so does tidal volume. As the blood level of oxygen decreases, the frequency of respiration increases. In mammals, pulse oximeter readings >90% are preferred; however, in some reptiles respiration is not stimulated until oxygen levels are <20%, so different standards are employed. Pulse oximeters are not calibrated for reptiles, and their values differ greatly from those obtained from use in mammals. While it is impossible to give exact pulse oximeter readings that should be maintained during anesthesia, trends are important. If the heart rate and oximeter readings are unstable and steadily decreasing, then anesthesia may need to be decreased or stopped.

Reptiles that are ventilated every 1-2 min with room air postoperatively start breathing and recover more quickly than those ventilated frequently with 100% oxygen. Frequent ventilation with oxygen does not allow the oxygen level to drop or the CO_2 level to rise to a point where respiration is stimulated.

Anesthetic Death: It is rare for heart rate and pulse oximeter readings to drop to the point where they cannot be accurately measured. When this occurs, all reflexes, respiration, and signs of life are absent. In mammals this would lead to certain death without proper resuscitation. However, death should not be pronounced in a deeply anesthetized reptile until a period of several hours of support and recovery has been provided. If possible the reptile should be ventilated intermittently. A normal body temperature should be maintained as well, because respiration is stimulated by warmer temperatures. In cases of a blocked glottis, lack of ventilation, or refusal to breathe, reptiles likely use other methods of gas exchange, or rely on anaerobic respiration. It is thought that the cloacal and pharyngeal mucosal membranes, and even some cutaneous membranes, allow limited gas exchange. Most reptiles can also switch to anaerobic metabolism, allowing survival for many hours with little or no additional oxygen.

Injectable Anesthetics: Many of the injectable anesthetics used in mammals are also appropriate for reptiles.

Ketamine Hydrochloride: Ketamine is best used as an induction agent prior to the use of a gas inhalant. Tranquilizing effects are seen at lower dosages (5-20 mg/kg), adequate for induction of anesthesia or for minor procedures of short duration. Smaller specimens may require proportionally slightly higher dosages. Due to the slow onset and long recovery period, this drug is not used as frequently as in the past. The amount needed for anesthesia varies considerably by species. Dosages of 20-40 mg/kg produce 2-20 min of anesthesia after an induction period of 10-60 min. Dosages of 40-100 mg/kg produce variable lengths of anesthesia (20 min to literally hours) after an induction period of 10-60 min. The anesthesia induced is seldom adequate for longer or more invasive procedures. Recovery occurs in 24-96 hr, depending on dose and temperature. The reptile should be hospitalized until fully aroused. Dosages >110 mg/kg may cause respiratory arrest and decrease cardiac rate. The mechanism for ketamine elimination is unknown, but since reptiles have a renal portal system which passes blood from the caudal half of the body through the kidneys prior to its reaching the systemic circulation, it would be inappropriate to inject ketamine in the rear half of the body.

Tiletamine-Zolazepam: An excellent drug for induction prior to gas anesthesia, tiletamine-zolazepam is similar to ketamine, but more potent, more predictable, and has shorter induction and recovery times. Tranquilizing effects are seen at 4-10 mg/kg, given IM or SC, with an induction time of 5-30 min and a recovery time of 1-12 hr. Tiletamine-zolazepam is not recommended as a stand-alone anesthetic; dosages of up to 90 mg/kg are required to produce anesthesia. At those levels, the reptiles are anesthetized for up to 16 hr and may take >22 hr to recover. If initial doses fail to create enough sedation to allow intubation, an additional dosage of 2-5 mg/kg may be given IV.

Propofol: Propofol is a good choice for very short sedation or induction for gas anesthesia. Advantages of propofol include a rapid and smooth induction, rapid tissue degradation with rapid recovery, few excitatory side effects, and minimal accumulation with repeated doses. While the preferred method of administration is IV, some practitioners report good results administering propofol by an intraosseous route. An initial IV dosage of 5-10 mg/kg will cause rapid induction (within 1 min) and last for 5-20 min. Recovery from propofol is relatively rapid, often within 20-60 min. Subsequent dosages (2.5 mg/kg) have been shown to increase apnea, so intubation is strongly recommended. Once the reptile is intubated, positive pressure ventilation is recommended so that the gas anesthetic, if being used, will become effective prior to the propofol wearing off. While subsequent IV doses can be administered, it is possible to give this drug via continuous infusion through an indwelling catheter. Propofol can also be given through a cardiac catheter, which is easily placed in snakes, but this route is generally not accessible in turtles and lizards. Arousal and recovery are rapid, and reptiles can be sent home the same day. This drug is of limited use in reptiles in which an IV route cannot be obtained. Perivascular tissue damage has not been seen, but reptiles will often flinch after administration, perhaps due to injection pressure more than the drug itself.

Medetomidine: Medetomidine has been used for sedation, primarily as an induction agent, but also mixed with other sedating drugs. In general, it is unpredictable in reptiles and not a good choice for producing surgical anesthesia. The interest in this drug is primarily due to the reversal potential, using atipamizole, which would help to eliminate problems associated with delayed arousal and prolonged recovery. In a study of gopher tortoises, medetomidine at 75 μg/kg mixed with ketamine at 7.5 mg/kg administered IM allowed for brief sedation and intubation ~20 min after administration. Reversal with atipamizole at 5× the dosage of medetomidine significantly reduced the recovery time, which was about 60 min. In another study, an IV dosage of 25-100 μg of medetomidine mixed with 4-8 mg/kg of ketamine in tortoises induced sedation in 4-16 min, followed by recovery in 5-30 min when reversed with 400 μg of atipamizole IV. The use of medetomidine alone in green iguanas has produced disappointing results.

Gas Anesthesia: Induction with gas inhalants (eg, sevoflurane, isoflurane, halothane) is possible but not always practical. It is not unusual for a reptile placed in a gas induction chamber to hold its breath (*see* above) when exposed to the annoying odor, and adequate induction can take anywhere from several minutes to hours. This is especially true of chelonians and crocodilians. Induction with other agents such as tiletamine-zolazepam (IM, SC, or IV) or propofol (IV), followed by intubation for maintenance of gas administration, is ideal.

Sevoflurane and isoflurane are preferable to halothane due to a quicker induction, safer maintenance, and improved recovery times. The newest anesthetic gas, flurane, is currently limited in use due to price, but provides advantages comparable to isoflurane over halothane. While administration of the gas can be continued with a nose cone, intubation is preferable. The continued use of a nose cone beyond induction will eliminate the possibility of ventilation.

Sedating Debilitated Reptiles: When possible, all underlying diseases and medical issues should be addressed prior to sedation/anesthesia. However, occasionally a debilitated animal will need to be sedated. For fractious or difficult reptiles, propofol at 5 mg/kg IV is the safest drug with the quickest induction and recovery. If giving an IV dose is not practical, then tiletamine-zolazepam at 2-5 mg/kg IM or SC is also a viable drug but has longer induction and recovery times. Both regimens can be followed by intubation and maintenance on sevoflurane or isoflurane. Induction with gas via nose cone or induction chamber can be attempted, but often is prolonged due to the reptile's ability to hold its breath and minimize ventilation. Another option is the use of a local anesthetic. Lidocaine (1%) has been used successfully, but toxicity can result if >10 mg/kg is given. Local anesthetics can also be with injectable induction agents at lower dosages.

Pain Management: As mentioned previously, the use of local anesthetics for minor procedures or in debilitated reptiles is encouraged. As an example, 1% lidocaine can be infiltrated into an abscess that needs to be lanced, and no further sedation may be required. Initially it appeared that reptiles were somewhat refractory to opiates, requiring higher dosages of narcotics than would be expected. However, it is now thought that although opiates do not produce sedation in reptiles, they do provide analgesia. See TABLE 14 for dosages of analgesic drugs. NSAID have recently been adapted for use in reptiles. While studies are lacking, empirical data suggest that they may be useful for controlling pain. Carprofen has been given at dosages ranging from 1-4 mg/kg, PO, IM, SC, and IV every 12-72 hr. Ketoprofen has been given at dosages ranging from 1-2 mg/kg, SC or IM, SID.

Sex Determination

In snakes, sex can be determined by using a cloacal probe of appropriate size. The end of the probe must be smooth and rounded to avoid injury to the delicate cloacal tissues. The lubricated probe is inserted into the cloaca and directed caudally just lateral to the midline. In females, the probe will enter 2-4 subcaudal scales; in males, it will enter 8-12 subcaudal scales (the hemipenal sacs). Some species of lizards show sexual dimorphism; for species that do not, the hemipenis of the male can be extruded from the vent by placing pressure caudal to the vent with the thumb and rolling the thumb cranially. Some species of lizards can be probed in a similar fashion to that used with snakes. Gila monsters, bearded lizards, and some skinks are difficult to sex reliably; ultrasonography or coelioscopy may be required. A more recent technique involves injecting saline in the ventral tail of helodermatids distal to the hemipenes. The saline causes irritation and/or increases pressure, and the hemipenes temporarily evert. A working knowledge of these lizards, and the position of the hemipenes, is required to perform such a procedure. The penis of male crocodilians can be identified by deep digital palpation of the cloaca.

Male turtles have a longer tail than females, and the cloacal opening in males is more toward the tail tip. In semiaquatic species, males are smaller and have longer claws. Males may also have a spur on the hindlegs. Terrestrial turtles and tortoises have distinct differences in the shape of the plastron, which is concave in males and flat in females. Some male tortoises also have an enlarged gular scale pair.

NUTRITION AND NUTRITIONAL DISEASES

The nutritional requirements of reptiles are poorly defined. Research is limited, and most recommendations are empiric. The required levels of macronutrients, protein, carbohydrates, and fat in the diet are thought to be qualitatively similar to those of mammals. (*See also* NUTRITION: EXOTIC AND ZOO ANIMALS, p 1843.)

Feeding behavior, digestion, and assimilation are related to environmental temperature and activation of the associated enzyme systems. Because ectotherms have a reduced metabolic rate, they feed less frequently. Humidity, light source, population density, and food type also affect feeding behavior. In turtles and some herbivorous lizards, the color of the food contributes to food acceptance; red and yellow are often preferred colors. Some reptiles habituate to certain foods and are unwilling to accept alternatives. Providing a variety of foods at each feeding, especially to younger reptiles, may alleviate this problem.

Quality is important when feeding whole-animal foods. Goldfish, mealworms, crickets, wax moth larvae (*Galleria* spp), mice, or rats intended for use as reptile food should be fed a complete and balanced diet so that they provide adequate nutrients. Herbivores and omnivores also require balanced rations. Many vegetable diets are deficient in calories, protein, and calcium. Insects and grubs are deficient in available calcium, and supplementation is required. Two common techniques to supplement insect prey are "gut loading" and using powdered vitamin/mineral supplements. Gut loading refers to allowing the insects to feed on a nutritious mixture of cereals and vegetables immediately before being fed to the reptile. Crickets brought home from a pet store and never fed have little nutrient value. Placing the insects in a bag with vitamin and mineral powders and shaking the bag will coat the insects with the powder. Although some of the powder will fall off, the newer microfine powders adhere remarkably well. Adding calcium and calcium-rich foods to the diet of crickets and wax moth larvae intended as prey increases their calcium:phosphorus ratio to a more acceptable level.

Anorectic reptiles may require force feeding to correct severe deficiencies. Initial feedings should replace fluids and electrolytes. Feeding a malnourished reptile in the face of severe dehydration will create a hyperuricemia often severe enough to induce visceral gout (*see* below). Dehydration is recognized by lateral skin folds, loss of skin turgor, and in severe cases, sunken eyes.

Fluids can be administered by soaking, oral, intracoelomic, intravenous, intraosseous, or subcutaneous routes. The soaking of mildly dehydrated reptiles can lead to per cloaca absorption of fluids and is an easy and practical means of hydrating reptiles. For reptiles that are alert enough, oral fluids are preferred to more invasive forms. Hypo-osmotic fluids are preferred; some practitioners avoid the use of lactated Ringer's solution. In reptiles that are active and mobile, enteric fluids can be delivered via red rubber urethral catheters or ball-tipped feeding needles, depending on the size of the reptile. Quantities of fluids should not exceed 2-3% total body wt in chelonians or 10-20 mL/kg in lizards and snakes. If this method seems too stressful or regurgitation occurs, fluids can be given intracoelomically. Reptiles lack a functional diaphragm, so large volumes of fluid may compromise lung capacity and tidal volume. Injected fluids must be sterile, and quantities are the same as for enteral fluids. Subcutaneous fluids, especially in turtles and lizards, can also be used. Fluid quantities and types are the same as with intracoelomic administration. Intraosseous fluid administration requires the placement of an indwelling needle or catheter, best placed in the tibia or femur depending on the size of the reptile. Fluid quantities and types are the same, but should be strictly administered via a fluid/syringe pump for accuracy.

A malnourished or starving reptile is similar in appearance to a dehydrated reptile. Loss of subcutaneous tissue, prominent bones, and a gaunt, sunken appearance are noted. Initial force feedings are best done with a prepared mixture rather than with whole animals. A good diet for force feeding carnivores is a commercially available product (Canine/Feline a/d[®]) designed for debilitated and cachectic dogs and cats. It contains vital amino acids, minerals, and easily digested nutrients, and the protein content of 8.5% makes it safe to use in animals with borderline to slightly increased uric acid levels. Mixing a/d 1:1 with liquid Ensure[®] provides a good force feeding mixture. In smaller specimens, it is fed through either a soft red urethral tube with an end that has been adapted to a syringe or a ball-tipped feeding needle at a rate of 28 g/kg every 3-7 days. This rate of administration varies with species, temperature, and response to feeding. In chronically dehydrated animals, it can be further diluted with Normosol® solution or a pediatric (human) oral electrolyte maintenance solution. Because a/d has a relatively high purine level, it should not be used for longterm maintenance.

For herbivorous reptiles, a force-feeding mixture is created by moistening 1 cup of commercial rabbit pellets (alfalfa) in water, adding an equal volume of liquid Ensure and 1 small banana, and mixing in a blender. This can be force fed at 28 g/kg every few days as needed. Oral electrolyte solutions can be added in very dehydrated animals. A commercial product (Herbivore Critical Care [Oxbow®]) can be mixed with water and then force fed.

Once initial force feedings have been done, small whole animals can be force fed to snakes and carnivorous lizards. The prey should be lubricated with egg white and then gently advanced into the back of the mouth, after which the reptile is allowed to swallow.

Environmental factors (temperature, light, humidity, etc) should be optimized for all anorectic reptiles. Fluids and nutrients will not be used properly under suboptimal conditions.

Nutrient Requirements

Water is essential for normal hydration. The ability of arid species to conserve water is not indicative of a reduced intake requirement. In several species, reduced water availability has resulted in lowered growth rates without apparent changes in the physiologic status of the animals.

The **protein** content of the diet has traditionally been recommended to be ~18-20% for carnivores and 11-12% for herbivores. Amino acid requirements are identical to those of mammals, with the addition of histidine in reptiles. Inadequate protein levels result in weight loss, muscle wasting, increased susceptibility to secondary infections, failure to reproduce, and slower healing after injury. A nonresponsive infection can be the result of a primary nutritional deficiency. Many newer commercial diets offer protein levels up to 28-32%, which may prompt rapid growth but can have severe longterm consequences (eg, hyperuricemia, see below). Consequently, lower protein levels are currently recommended, particularly for uricotelic reptiles.

Excess protein is common in the diet of carnivorous lizards when excessive meat products are fed rather than whole animals. Feeding excessive amounts of high-protein cat foods has been implicated in cases of excess protein and vitamin D_3. Many nutritionists recommend not feeding cat foods to reptiles. Dog food, especially low-fat varieties, can be used sparingly as part of a complete and balanced diet in both carnivores and omnivores. The overuse of high-protein diets prepared for carnivores has been incriminated in causing disease in tortoises and iguanas.

Feeding excess protein can result in hyperuricemia, in which uric acid is deposited in internal organs; this may lead to primary visceral gout, a debilitating and often fatal condition. Uric acid levels can also be increased by dehydration or renal damage. Hyperuricemia leading to visceral gout from these causes is referred to as secondary visceral gout. (See also p 1615.)

Most protein deficiencies are seen in herbivorous species on "salad-type" diets or in anorectic individuals. Herbivore diets may be supplemented with alfalfa sprouts, bean sprouts, soy beans or meal, invertebrates, or soft-moist or low-fat dog food (used sparingly). Anorectic reptiles may require force feeding, environmental alteration, or sufficient variety in the diet to identify a preferred food item.

Carbohydrates do not appear to be essential to carnivorous species but, in many cases, caloric requirements can be met by adding carbohydrates to the diet or through gluconeogenesis of dietary protein. Crocodilians appear unable to assimilate certain polysaccharides. Blood glucose values are variable for each order and may remain increased for as long as 1 wk after a meal. Blood glucose is increased during breeding seasons, especially in males.

Clinical hypoglycemia has been reported in captive crocodilians. Signs include mydriasis, tremors, opisthotonos, loss of the righting reflex, and death. Overcrowding and stress with the prolonged release of adrenergic compounds is thought to be causative. Hypoglycemia without clinical signs is normally seen in alligators during the winter.

Fiber is required for the normal functioning of the digestive tract. In large land tortoises and other herbivorous species, adding roughage (eg, hay) to the diet has eliminated chronic malodorous diarrhea.

Specific **fatty acid** requirements have not been determined for reptiles, but 0.2% linoleic acid in the diet is recommended. Deficiencies have not been reported, but reduced stores in the visceral fat have been associated with small clutch size during the breeding season. Atherosclerosis has been reported; restriction of cholesterol may be an important longterm dietary consideration in captive reptiles.

Mineral deficiencies are seen frequently in captive reptiles, especially chelonians and lizards. Vitamin and mineral deficiencies are rare in snakes that are fed nutrient-rich whole prey. A vitamin/mineral supplement should be added to the diet of every captive reptile; many products specific for use in reptiles are commercially available.

Calcium is the most important mineral deficiency in reptile nutrition. A calcium:phosphorus ratio of at least 1.2:1 is generally recommended. However, in some situations (eg, females laying large numbers of calcareous eggs, or rapidly growing juveniles), a ratio approaching 2:1 or greater, is more appropriate. With carnivorous diets, skeletal muscle has a calcium:phosphorus ratio of ~1:25; beef heart and liver, ~1:44. Feeding a pure meat diet not only provides excessive protein but also is extremely poor in calcium and rich in phosphorus. Such carnivorous diets should be altered to include whole prey or a low-fat, low-protein dog food. Calcium should be supplemented with products developed for reptiles that ideally contain no phosphorus.

The chitinous exoskeleton of insects is devoid of calcium and, therefore, insectivores must obtain dietary calcium from insects "gut loaded" and powdered with calcium supplements (*see* p 1597).

Herbivores should be encouraged to eat items rich in calcium, including cabbage, kale, okra, sprouts, collard greens, and bok choy. These foods typically are also rich in vitamin A. A calcium supplement with no phosphorus should be routinely given to herbivores, up to twice weekly in normal specimens.

Vitamin D is also required for proper calcium metabolism and balance. Animals housed outside with access to natural, unfiltered sunlight usually have adequate levels of vitamin D_3 because inactive vitamin D precursors in the skin are converted to vitamin D_3 when the skin is exposed to ultraviolet (UV) light. Access to UV light has been recommended in reptiles not exposed to unfiltered sunlight (*see* LIGHTING REQUIREMENTS p 1591). Reptiles fed whole mammalian prey generally consume adequate levels of preformed vitamin D_3. The food items of insectivores should be fortified by gut loading and powdering. Herbivores that have limited exposure to UV light should receive supplemental vitamin D_3. Most reptile supplements that contain calcium also contain limited (but adequate) amounts of vitamin D_3. Excessive levels of oral vitamin D_3 can lead to the excessive absorption and utilization of calcium.

An inappropriate calcium:phosphorus ratio or inadequate levels of vitamin D can result in nutritional secondary hyperparathyroidism, fibrous osteodystrophy, osteomalacia, cystic calculi, cloacal calculi, and rickets. Pathologic fractures, bone deformities, and soft or deformed shells in turtles may occur. Terminal signs may include tetanic seizures. The skeletal maladies that result from abnormal calcium:phosphorus metabolism are referred to as metabolic bone disease.

Treatment consists of correcting the calcium:phosphorus ratio and administering vitamin D_3, if appropriate, either by injection, per os, or by exposure to an appropriate UV source. A dietary history should be obtained and evaluated, and deficiencies corrected. If a calcium supplement is to be provided in the initial stages of treatment, it should not contain phosphorus. An excellent calcium source is calcium glubionate, given PO at 1 mL/kg, as long as is needed. Other sources of dietary calcium include crushed cuttlebone, crushed oyster shell, crushed or pulverized calcium lactate, or commercially available products. In severe cases, a calcium injection can be given before the oral supplementation. Calcium gluconate (10%) can be given at 250 mg/kg, IP, for 1 dose only, and calcium lactate at 5 mg/kg, IM or SC, daily for 1-7 days.

To avoid toxicity, vitamin D should not be injected more than once every 2-4 wk at a dosage of 200 IU/kg, IM. Excessive supplementation of vitamin D combined with plentiful calcium may result in soft-tissue calcification. Green iguanas fed excessive levels of cat food developed calcification of soft tissues thought to be due to hypervitaminosis D. Oversupplementation of vitamin D and calcium is thought to be one of the main causes of renal disease in mature lizards, especially green iguanas and bearded dragons.

Calcitonin has been used at dosages of 50 IU/kg, IM, once a week for 2 treatments in green iguanas with metabolic bone disease caused by nutritional secondary hyperparathyroidism. Calcitonin inhibits bone resorption and acts as an antagonist to parathyroid hormone, but there is debate whether calcitonin accomplishes for reptiles what it does for mammals. Calcium supplements should begin before the calcitonin is used, because the latter can cause severe hypocalcemia.

Iodine deficiency can manifest as lethargy and an abnormal swelling at the thoracic inlet (goiter). Feeding of goitrogenic compounds, including certain green forages, may precipitate the problem. The imbalance is corrected by supplementation with a balanced vitamin-mineral mixture containing iodine, or iodized salt (0.5% of the diet).

Iron and **copper** deficiencies associated with anemia have been reported in turtles.

Vitamin A deficiency is seen frequently in captive turtles. Aquatic turtles rarely are involved because they typically eat whole prey that contain preformed vitamin A. However, some adult aquatic turtles eat a more herbivorous diet, and the first documented case of hypovitaminosis A was in a red-eared slider. Terrestrial turtles are more commonly affected. Herbivorous tortoises fed correctly eat diets high in β-carotene that is converted to vitamin A and rarely exhibit signs. Box turtles, particularly in the USA, appear most at risk usually due to diets (fed in captivity) that contain little vitamin A. Signs of hypovitaminosis A include palpebral edema, chronic respiratory disease, and renal disease. Squamous metaplasia of epithelial structures is characteristic, especially of the lacrimal glands, producing a thickened, sticky discharge in addition to swollen eyelids. The eyes may eventually remain closed, impairing the ability of the turtle to find food. Secondary infections of the eyes, respiratory system, and skin are common. Treatment consists of short daily soaks to allow the turtle to drink and wash its eyes, application of an antibiotic ophthalmic ointment for both moisture and secondary infections, and administration of vitamin A at 200 IU/kg, once every 2 wk for no more than 2 injections. For less severe cases, oral vitamin A can be supplied via cod liver oil at a rate of 1 drop in the food twice a week. Oral supplementation is generally preferred due to the potential toxicity of the injections. Commercially available vitamin products are also available for reptiles. Dietary levels of vitamin A should be increased for up to 6 wk before hibernation in turtles and tortoises. Severe hyperkeratosis and dysecdysis, which in the past have been associated with hypovitaminosis A, are more commonly due to hypervitaminosis A. Vitamin A administered at dosages recommended in the past would induce severe skin irritation and shedding, often within days.

Vitamin B_1 deficiency can result from diets containing fish with high thiaminase levels, and exogenous supplementation is required. Weight loss with adequate food intake is characteristic, but neurologic signs can also occur. Goldfish have low thiaminase activity, while smelt have extremely high levels. Freezing of fish decreases parasite loads but increases thiaminase levels. Posterior paresis progressing to flaccid paralysis and the loss of the righting reflex has been seen in iguanas and garter snakes, respectively, and is associated with a B-complex deficiency. Deficiencies of the water-soluble vitamins often involve more than 1 vitamin and require treatment with a multivitamin preparation.

Biotin deficiency, associated with the feeding of unfertilized, uncooked chicken eggs, has been reported in helodermatids, some varanids, tegus, and larger skinks. Anorexia and weakness are the primary signs. Avidin, an antibiotin substance, is found in ovalbumin. Feeding fertilized eggs reduces the amount of avidin in the egg, and biotin supplementation reduces the frequency of the condition.

Vitamin C is produced endogenously in reptile kidneys. Vitamin C deficiency has been incriminated (but never proved) in cases of infectious stomatitis, and oral or injectable supplementation of vitamin C (from 25 mg to several grams, depending on the size of the reptile, daily or as needed) has been suggested, especially when renal disease is present. While not proved beneficial, vitamin C supplementation at this dosage is safe and will do no harm.

Vitamin-K-responsive coagulopathies characterized by prolonged gingival bleeding after loss of deciduous teeth have been reported in crocodilians. Treatment with vitamin K at 0.5 mg/kg body wt has been suggested.

Steatitis has been reported in crocodilians fed mackerel and tuna and in snakes fed obese rats. Ceroid deposition was seen at necropsy. Vitamin E supplementation at 100 IU/kg has been recommended as a preventive, but it is more important to avoid feeding fish that have been frozen and thawed improperly, stored too long, or left uneaten for ≥1 day.

BACTERIAL DISEASES

Bacterial diseases are common in all reptilian orders. Most infections are caused by opportunistic agents that infect immunosuppressed hosts. A comprehensive approach is required to ensure the success of a therapeutic plan. It is important not only to determine the causative agent but also to correct environmental and nutritional deficiencies. Treatment with antibiotics (*see* TABLE 15) for a specific microbial agent in the absence of proper heat, light, hydration, nutrition, etc, will not be successful.

Culture and sensitivity are essential in determining appropriate therapy. Most bacterial infections involve gram-negative bacteria, many of which are considered to be commensal organisms. These agents can remain dormant until the reptile becomes immunosuppressed. Anaerobic infections are more common than once thought and may be involved in up to 40% of all bacterial infections. If a therapeutic agent was selected based on an aerobic culture and sensitivity and response is poor, then the presence of an additional anaerobic agent should be considered.

Although it has been advocated that all antimicrobial drugs be administered parenterally, orally administered drugs, can be used effectively. The factors involved in oral administration that can alter absorption and use of a drug include GI transit time, temperature, and the presence of food. However, drugs administered orally at a given temperature and in the absence of food appear to have a fairly predictable rate of absorption and use. Oral medications are especially useful in extremely small specimens (eg, the true chameleons and smaller geckos) that lack adequate muscle mass for, and will be adversely affected by, a painful injection. Parenteral injections are preferred in larger specimens or when working around the head and mouth would be dangerous. The normal route of administration (IM or SC) should be used.

Environmental temperatures should be maintained near the upper limit preferred by the species to enhance immune function. Higher metabolic rates of anorectic reptiles may necessitate force-feeding or increased rate of feeding. However, heat and feeding also raise uric acid levels. If a particular drug is potentially nephrotoxic, uric acid levels should be determined before the drug is administered; if the uric acid level is increased, feeding should be delayed (so as not to further increase uric acid levels). Fluid administration should be considered as well.

Because most infected reptiles have some level of immunosuppression, bactericidal drugs are preferable to bacteriostatic ones.

The aminoglycosides are some of the most frequently used antibiotics against the gram-negative organisms of reptiles. However, neomycin, streptomycin, kanamycin, and gentamicin should not be used systemically in reptiles because they have been associated with numerous reports of renal toxicity. Amikacin is the aminoglycoside of choice.

Mixed or resistant infections may require combinations of antibiotics. Amikacin is commonly used in conjunction with penicillin drugs (eg, ampicillin, carbenicillin, or piperacillin) in the treatment of severe gram-negative sepsis such as that caused by *Pseudomonas*. Ceftazidime can be given with amikacin or enrofloxacin to broaden the spectrum as well as to take advantage of the ability of ceftazidime to control anaerobic bacteria. Metronidazole can be given with either amikacin or enrofloxacin for the same reason.

A number of infectious conditions are similar in appearance regardless of species. **Septicemia** is a common cause of death. The systemic disease may be preceded by trauma, local abscessation, parasitism, or environmental stress. *Aeromonas* and *Pseudomonas* spp are frequently isolated; the former may be transmitted by the snake

TABLE 15. Antimicrobial Drugs for Use in Reptiles

Drug	Species	Dosage and Route	Comments	Contraindications
Ampicillin	All but tortoise	3-6 mg/kg, SID-BID	Anaerobic infections or in combination with aminoglycosides	
	Tortoise	50 mg/kg, IM, BID		
Amikacin	Alligator	2.25 mg/kg, IM, every 72 hr	Potentially nephrotoxic	Renal insufficiency, dehydration
	Tortoise	5 mg/kg, IM, every 48 hr		
	Snake	5 mg/kg, IM, first dose, then 2.5 mg/kg every 72 hr		
	Lizard	5 mg/kg, IM, every 24-72 hr		
Carbenicillin	Snake	400 mg/kg, IM, SID	Painful injection	Small muscle mass
	Tortoise	400 mg/kg, IM, every 48 hr		
	Lizard	400 mg/kg, IM, SC, every 48 hr		
Ceftazidime	Snake	20 mg/kg, IM, SC, every 72 hr	Good for *Pseudomonas*	
Cephazolin	All	20 mg/kg, IM, SC, SID		
Chloramphenicol	Snake	50 mg/kg, SC, every 12-72 hr (species dependent)	Bone marrow suppression in water snakes	
Ciprofloxacin	Snake	10 mg/kg, PO, every 48-72 hr	Must be mixed with distilled water	
Doxycycline	Tortoise	50 mg/kg, loading dose, then 25 mg/kg, IM, every 72 hr	Painful injection	
	All	5-10 mg/kg, PO, SID as needed		
Enrofloxacin	All	5-10 mg/kg, PO, every 24-48 hr	Tissue necrosis common at IM injections; skin discoloration and necrosis at SC sites	
	Box turtle	5 mg/kg, IM, every 72 hr	Painful	Small tissue mass may cause necrosis

TABLE 15. Antimicrobial Drugs for Use in Reptiles (continued)

Drug	Species	Dosage and Route	Comments	Contraindications
	Herrmann's tortoise	10 mg/kg, IM, SID	Painful	
	Green iguana	5 mg/kg, PO, IM, every 24-48 hr	Painful	
	Gopher tortoise	5 mg/kg, IM, every 24-48 hr	Painful	
	Star tortoise	5 mg/kg, IM, SID-BID	Painful	
	Monitor	10 mg/kg, IM, every 5 days	Painful	
	Snake	11 mg/kg, IM every 48 hr		
Ketoconazole	Tortoise	15-30 mg/kg, PO, SID	Potentially hepatotoxic	Hepatic disease
Metronidazole	Iguana	20 mg/kg, PO, every 24-48 hr	Use every 24 hr for resistant anaerobes	
	Snake	20 mg/kg, PO, every 48 hr		
Nystatin	Snake	100,000 IU/kg, SID	Yeast enteritis	
Oxytetracycline	Tortoise	5-10 mg/kg, IM, SID	Mycoplasma in tortoises	
	Alligator	10 mg/kg, PO, SID		
	Crocodile	10 mg/kg, IM, every 7 days	Mycoplasmosis	
Piperacillin	All	50-200 mg/kg, IM, every 24-48 hr	Useful to add to aminoglycoside	Fluid support
Tetracycline	All	10 mg/kg, PO, SID	Seldom used	
Ticarcillin	All	50-100 mg/kg, SID		Fluid support
Trimethoprim	All	30 mg/kg, every 48 hr	Need proper hydration	Dehydration
Tylosin	All	5 mg/kg, SID for 10-60 days	Mycoplasmosis	

mite *Ophionyssus natricis*. Death may be peracute or chronic. Common signs are respiratory distress, lethargy, convulsions, and incoordination. Petechiae may be found on the ventral abdomen, and chelonians develop erythema of the plastron. Sanitation and husbandry can be significant factors in reducing outbreaks. Affected reptiles should be isolated, and antibiotic therapy initiated.

Septicemic cutaneous ulcerative disease (SCUD) in turtles is often caused by *Citrobacter freundii*. *Serratia* spp may act synergistically by facilitating entry of *C freundii* into the turtle. The scutes are pitted and may slough with an underlying purulent discharge. Anorexia, lethargy, and petechial hemorrhages on the shell and skin are seen; liver necrosis is common. Systemic antibiotics are recommended. Good sanitation is paramount in prevention.

Another shell disease of turtles is caused by *Beneckea chitinovora*, a common infectious agent of crustaceans. Erythema and pitting of the shell with ulceration is seen. Septicemia is uncommon. Treatment with topical iodine is recommended. The practice of feeding crayfish is often implicated in this condition and should be discouraged.

Ulcerative or **necrotic dermatitis (scale rot)** is seen in snakes and lizard. Humidity and environmental contamination have been considered the main predisposing factors. Moist, contaminated bedding allows bacterial and fungal growth which, when coupled with exposure to fecal degradation products, can predispose to small cutaneous erosions. Secondary infection with *Aeromonas* spp, *Pseudomonas* spp, and a number of other bacteria may result in septicemia and death if untreated. Erythema, necrosis, and ulceration of the dermis, and an exudative discharge are common. While lesions are often a sequelae of skin injuries, they more often develop from within, as is the case with classic necrotic dermatitis in the ball python. The disease can develop even when these animals are maintained under pristine conditions, so it is not simply a matter of excessive moisture and poor hygiene. The condition starts with hemorrhage into scales, followed by pustules that eventually lead to open and ulcerated lesions. Treatment with systemic antibiotics, topical antibiotic ointment, and excellent hygiene and husbandry are essential.

Blister disease has traditionally been considered a separate entity but is simply an early stage of ulcerative (necrotic) dermatitis. The cutaneous involvement is characterized by pustules or blisters that may resolve without development of ulcerative lesions if treatment is started early. A low-grade thermal injury may mimic blister disease due to the potential development of fluid filled vesicles.

Abscesses caused by traumatic injury, bite wounds, or poor environmental quality are seen in all orders of reptiles. Subcutaneous abscesses are seen as nodules or swellings. Differential diagnoses include parasitic nodules, tumors, and hematomas. Isolates of the anaerobic organism *Peptostreptococcus* and of the aerobes *Pseudomonas, Aeromonas, Serratia, Salmonella, Micrococcus, Erysipelothrix, Citrobacter freundii, Morganella morganii, Proteus, Staphylococcus, Streptococcus, Escherichia coli, Klebsiella, Arizona,* and *Dermatophilus* have been recovered from reptilian abscesses, often in combinations. Small localized abscesses should be completely excised to avoid recurrence, which is frequent. Larger abscesses should be incised, followed by aggressive local wound treatment. The lining of the abscess must be aggressively scraped to remove as much material as possible. Appropriate systemic antibiotics may also be indicated. Anaerobic bacteria are common in these lesions, and an appropriate antimicrobial agent (eg, metronidazole, ceftazidime, or a potentiated penicillin product) may need to be used or added to a current regimen.

Visceral abscessation may occur as a result of hematogenous infection. Abscesses of the female reproductive system are common and may result in coelomitis. Surgical intervention is indicated; systemic antibiotics alone are rarely successful.

Subspectacle abscessation is seen in snakes, and conjunctivitis in the other orders. The severity ranges from mild inflammation to panophthalmitis and may occur as a result of ascending infectious stomatitis (*see* below). Topical antibiotic ointments are used in turtles, lizards without spectacles, and crocodilians. In snakes and lizards with spectacles, drainage is achieved by surgically removing a small wedge from the spectacle and flushing the subspectacular space and lacrimal duct with an antibiotic solution (eg, gentamicin). Some affected reptiles, especially turtles, may need supplemental vitamin A.

Star-gazing refers to any neurologic disorder characterized by mental dullness, abnormal posturing, and an inability to move forward in a normal fashion. This is more commonly seen in, but not restricted to, snakes, and is characterized by a severely twisted cervical positioning, creating a "starward gaze." A retrovirus causing a viral meningitis/encephalitis in boids (boas and pythons) is the most commonly diagnosed "star-gazing" syndrome. The virus is not a new; rather, there is increased awareness of an epidemic in the making for over 2 decades. This syndrome is referred to as **inclusion body disease** due to the presence of characteristic inclusion bodies in affected cells (*see* VIRAL DISEASES, p 1611). Among other possible causes of star-gazing protozoa, heat damage, trauma, and bacterial agents are the most common. Bacterial meningitis or encephalitis usually results from hematogenous infection or bacterial emboli from an abscess elsewhere in the body. The prognosis varies with the cause but is generally guarded. Systemic antibiotics that can cross the blood-brain barrier (eg, ceftazidime, metronidazole, penicillins, etc) are indicated in bacterial cases. Prednisolone acetate at a dosage of 1 mg/kg, IM, once has been recommended for inflammation associated with these infections. Because lesions may resolve slowly, an early response to therapy is rarely seen, and good supportive care (eg, fluids and nutrient supplementation) is essential.

Infectious stomatitis is seen in snakes, lizards, and turtles. It is characterized early by petechiae in the oral cavity; caseous material develops along the dental arcade as the condition worsens. In severe cases, infection extends into the bony structures of the mouth. *Aeromonas* and *Pseudomonas* spp, common oral inhabitants, are most frequently isolated, along with a variety of other gram-negative and gram-positive bacteria. Respiratory or GI infection may develop in poorly managed cases. Debridement, irrigation with antiseptics or antibiotics, systemic antibiotics, and supportive therapy are indicated. In severe cases with ulceration or granuloma formation, more aggressive surgery may be indicated. Vitamin supplementation, especially with vitamins A and C, has been advocated but does not always affect the disease course.

Respiratory infections are common; the incidence can be influenced by respiratory or systemic parasitism, unfavorable environmental temperatures, unsanitary conditions, concurrent disease, malnutrition, and hypovitaminosis A. Open-mouth breathing, nasal discharge, and dyspnea are frequent signs. *Aeromonas* and *Pseudomonas* spp are frequently isolated, but many respiratory infections are mixed. Septicemia may develop in severe or prolonged cases. Treatment consists of improving husbandry and initiating systemic antibiotics. Nebulization therapy with antibiotics diluted in saline, in combination with acetylcysteine, has been used together with parenteral antibiotics to treat bacterial pneumonia. Reptiles with respiratory infections should be maintained at the mid to upper end of their preferred optimal temperatures. Increased temperatures are important not only to stimulate the immune system but also to help mobilize respiratory secretions. Turtles often have an underlying vitamin A deficiency, and supplementation at 200 IU/kg, IM, should be given once a week for 2 wk if needed. Many turtles treated for pneumonia fail to improve until after treatment for vitamin A deficiency.

Ear infections occur in turtles, most frequently in box turtles and aquatic turtles. Marked swelling is seen at the tympanic membrane, and caseous material is present. *Proteus* spp, *Pseudomonas* spp, *Citrobacter* spp, *Morganella morganii*, *Enterobacter* spp, and other bacteria have been isolated. Drainage and systemic antibiotics are appropriate. The tympanic membrane must be incised, and aggressive curettage of the area performed. The open area should be flushed with diluted povidone-iodine or a similar product for a few days to prevent premature closure and to keep the area clean. Ear infections may be secondary to hypovitaminosis A; parenteral and dietary supplementation of vitamin A may be beneficial.

Infectious cloacitis is characterized by edema and hemorrhagic discharge. The cause may be traumatic. Cloacal calculi may form in vitamin or mineral imbalances and should be manually removed and followed by dietary correction. In pericloacal abscesses, the infection often migrates cranially by subcutaneous or coelomic tissue pathways. Ascending urinary or genital tract infections are common sequelae. Aggressive therapy, including surgical debridement, local wound treatment, and appropriate systemic antibiotics, is indicated. Fecal examinations should be performed to identify potential parasitic causes.

Mycobacterial infections are often associated with chronic wasting and are seen as granulomatous lesions at necropsy. Chelonians generally exhibit pulmonary involvement, while lizards, snakes, and crocodilians show visceral granulomas. Rifampin and isoniazid are hepatotoxic in reptiles, and the longterm administration required is unlikely to be safe. The species isolated are *Mycobacterium ulcerans*, *M chelonae*, *M hemophilus*, and *M marinum*. All are cultured at reduced temperatures and may require long periods for growth.

Salmonella, *Arizona*, and *Edwardsiella* spp have been isolated from clinically normal turtles. The zoonotic nature of these organisms must be considered when handling or treating turtles. Attempts to eliminate these microorganisms from infected turtles and their eggs have been unsuccessful.

PARASITIC DISEASES

Ectoparasites

A limited number of ectoparasites are seen, except on wild and newly acquired reptiles. Mites are distributed worldwide, and most reptilian species are affected. Reduced vitality and, in heavy infestations, death due to anemia may occur. Skin of affected reptiles appears coarse, and dysecdysis is frequent. The mite is <1.5 mm long and is often found near the eyecaps, gluttal folds, or any other indentation on the reptile. Mites may also be associated with mechanical transmission of *Aeromonas hydrophila*, a variety of other bacteria, and rickettsial agents, and they very likely act as a vector in inclusion body disease of boid snakes.

Mites are visible to the naked eye but are hard to see in small numbers. If mites are suspected, gently rubbing the reptile while it is standing over a piece of white paper will allow the mites to be seen after they have fallen off. Affected reptiles often spend an inordinate amount of time soaking to drown the mites. Examination of the water dish can reveal the drowned remains of many mites. The gluttal folds, involutions around the face, and the space between the eye and its orbit are favored areas and should be inspected carefully.

There are many methods of treatment. In all cases, cages should be cleaned thoroughly, and substrate materials, branches, and disposable cage furniture eliminated. Newspaper bedding should be used until treatment is completed to facilitate frequent cleaning and to eliminate egg-laying sites. In small collections with a few cages, small pieces of dichlorvos strips are placed in containers (eg, jars or vials) in which holes have been made. This prevents the reptile from direct contact with the strip but allows penetration of the dichlorvos vapors. The container should be placed in the cage for 3-4 hr at least 2-3 times a week for at least 3 wk. The cage must be well ventilated, and the water dish should be removed while the container is in the cage.

Toxicity can and will occur if the pest strips are used in nonventilated cages. For large collections with multiple cages, trichlorfon and ivermectin sprays work best, although trichlorfon may be removed from the market in the USA. Trichlorfon, available as an 8% solution, should be diluted to 0.15% by adding 8 mL of the solution to 400 mL of water; this is stable for up to 30 days. The cage and the reptile should be sprayed thoroughly once every 10-14 days as needed. The water dish should be removed while spraying and not returned until the spray has dried. Trichlorfon must not be used in a closed cage; ventilation is essential. Trichlorfon is contraindicated in geckos.

Ivermectin, available as a 1% solution, should be diluted by adding 1 mL (10 mg) to 1 L of water; this is stable for up to 30 days. The cage and reptile should be sprayed thoroughly every 4-5 days for up to 3 wk. The water dish should be removed while spraying and drying. Ivermectin is contraindicated for use in turtles and tortoises, and while a dilute spray is likely safe, the potential for toxicity is real.

Pyrethrins and pyrethroids have been used with conflicting information and accounts of efficacy. Pyrethrins, especially those with residual action, may be used outside the cage to help control mites in the environment. Herpetoculturalists have reported severe or fatal consequences following the application of a pyrethrin spray product on snakes. Apparently, the animals were lightly but thoroughly sprayed with the product and then returned to poorly ventilated shoebox cages. In one reported incident, 20 out of

30 snakes died within 2 hr. It appears that the aerosolized pyrethrin in a poorly ventilated container is quite dangerous. Pyrethroids, or synthetic pyrethrins, are supposed to be more potent but far less toxic. Many veterinarians and hobbyists have successfully used the pyrethroids diluted as a sponge-on application, as long as ventilation is adequate.

The larvae of trombiculid mites (chiggers) are seen occasionally but are not considered to be pathogenic.

Ticks are frequently found on reptiles, and heavy infestations may result in anemia. Argasid ticks may cause paralysis, with muscle degeneration at the site of the bite. The transmission of green-lizard papilloma-associated virus, several hemogregarines, and the filarid worm *Macdonaldius oscheri* has been associated with ticks. Ticks can be removed manually. Systemic antibiotics are often indicated due to systemic infections associated with multiple cutaneous bite wounds and, potentially, with transmission of pathogenic bacteria.

Leeches have been found on the legs, head, neck, and in the oral cavity of a variety of turtles and crocodilians.

Turtles frequently have cutaneous myiasis. Botflies (including *Cuterebra* sp) create a cutaneous wound in which to lay their eggs, which hatch into bots that live in their cyst-like structures until they are mature enough to leave the wound. These lesions are characterized as a lump under the skin; on closer inspection, they have an opening that is often lined by a black, crusted material. Treatment consists of slightly expanding the natural opening and manually removing the bot with a forceps. The wound is then flushed with povidone-iodine, chlorhexidine, etc, and an antibiotic ointment is instilled. Systemic antibiotics are indicated in reptiles that have multiple lesions. Cutaneous myiasis also occurs secondary to existing wounds, and maggots must be manually removed and the underlying lesion treated with topical and systemic antibiotics as needed. During heavy fly season, turtles often are housed indoors or with screens over their enclosures to offer some protection.

Ectoparasite infestations are best prevented by thorough screening and quarantine of all new animals entering a collection.

Endoparasites

The stress of captivity coupled with a closed environment predisposes to a heavy internal parasite burden in reptiles. Many common endoparasites of reptiles have direct life cycles and can multiply to staggering numbers. Every effort must be taken to rid reptiles of parasite burdens, and the environment of intermediate hosts.

Pathogenic trematodes infect the vascular system of turtles, and the oral cavity, respiratory system, renal tubules, and ureters of snakes. Chemotherapeutic agents have not been effective in eliminating these parasites, although praziquantel administered at 5-8 mg/kg, IM or PO, has shown some promise.

Tapeworms are found in all orders of reptiles but are rare in crocodilians. Reptiles may act as the definitive, paratenic, or intermediate hosts for a large number of species. Although most species of tapeworms are generally nonpathogenic in wild reptiles, weight loss and death have been reported. The complex life cycle of cestodes and restricted geographic range of intermediate hosts limit the number of cases in captive reptiles. When present, proglottids may be found around the cloaca, or typical cestode ova may be isolated from feces. Treatment is with praziquantel at 5-8 mg/kg, IM or PO, repeated in 2 wk. Plerocercoids of the genus *Spirometra* may be found as soft swellings in the subcutis. These larval stages may be removed surgically.

Nematodes are found in all orders of reptiles, and several genera are important. *Strongyloides* spp frequently inhabit the intestinal tract of reptiles; larvae are seen in the respiratory tract and respiratory exudate. In snakes, the larvae have been seen within granulomas distributed throughout the body wall, suggesting that the larvae may be able to penetrate the skin. Overwhelming parasitism is common when poor hygiene results in highly contaminated environments. *Rhabdias* and related species have been found in the lungs of a variety of snakes; embryonated ova may be found in the oral cavity and in lung aspirates. Embryonated ova and free larval forms may be seen in the feces. Larvae resembling *Rhabdias* also have been seen in the gingiva of snakes with stomatitis. Infections often are subclinical but may be associated with secondary bacterial pneumonia. In severe cases, death may result.

Stomach worms of the genus *Physaloptera* are seen in lizards. Gastric ulceration may occur in severe infections. Ova are elliptical and may be embryonated. Numerous snakes are infected by *Kalicephalus* spp. This hookworm, capable of transcutaneous infestation, prefers the upper GI tract and causes erosive lesions at sites of attachment. Ova are similar to those of *Physaloptera* spp. Large granulomas caused by the above species have also caused GI obstruction in snakes.

Ascarids frequently infect reptiles. Ova are similar to those of ascarids from mammalian hosts. Severe lesions and death may be seen in infected snakes. Clinically infected snakes frequently regurgitate partially digested food or adult nematodes and are anorectic. The major lesions are large granulomatous masses in the GI tract; they may abscess and perforate the intestinal wall.

Many other nematode species may be found in reptiles. Capillarid, trichurid, and oxyurid ova may be found on fecal examination. The nonpathogenic larval and oval forms of parasites of prey items (eg, *Syphacia obvelata*, the mouse pinworm) may be found when infected prey is consumed. Treatment should be attempted when evidence of parasitism is present.

Some larval forms of nematodes are suspected or confirmed to penetrate the skin (eg, *Strongyloides* and *Kalicephalus*), bypassing the oral reinfection route. The subtle nature of reinfection by this route often goes unnoticed until the reptile is overwhelmed by parasites. Close attention to the immediate removal of excreta and fastidious sanitation help to reduce parasite burdens in captivity.

The drug of choice for treating nematode infections is fenbendazole at 10-25 mg/kg, PO, for 3-5 days. Administration is stopped for 10 days, and then the 3- to 5-day regimen is repeated. Administering fenbendazole on consecutive days is more effective than giving doses once every 7-10 days. If protozoans are to be treated concurrently, dosage may be increased to 50 mg/kg fenbendazole with the aforementioned regimen. When parasites are resistant to fenbendazole or have not been eliminated after 2 oral courses, the reptile can be treated with ivermectin at 0.2 mg/kg, PO, once every 7-10 days for 3 treatments. Fenbendazole has a much broader margin of safety than ivermectin and should be used first. Complications, from mild ataxia to paralysis and death, have been associated with the use of ivermectin, although it has been used safely in snakes and lizards at 0.2-0.4 mg/kg. In turtles, ivermectin toxicity (paresis) has been seen at dosages as low as 0.025 mg/kg; therefore, ivermectin is not recommended for use in turtles. Levamisole at 10-50 mg/kg via intracoelomic, IM, or SC injection, and at 200 mg/kg, PO, has been reported to be effective for *Rhabdias* spp. The margin of safety for levamisole is very narrow, and it should be used with caution.

Dermal lesions caused by the spirurid worm *Dracunculus* spp may be seen. Numerous species of spirurids infect the mesentery, coelomic cavity, and blood vessels. These worms require a mechanical vector, so their incidence is reduced in captive-bred reptiles or in reptiles that have been in captivity longterm. Treatment consists of increasing the environmental temperature to 95-98°F (35-37°C) for 24-48 hr. However, some "cool-adapted" reptiles may not tolerate this treatment.

Pentastomes are found in a wide variety of reptiles, with variable pathogenicity. Pentastomid infections are occasionally associated with pneumonic signs, but these primitive arthropods can inhabit any tissue and symptoms will vary with their migration path and tissues responses. Pentastomes were initially found primarily in tropical poisonous snakes; however, as more necropsies on reptiles were performed, more were found. Necropsy results from 88 bearded dragons showed that 11 were infested with pentastomes. No truly effective treatment has been reported, but praziquantel at dosages >8 mg/kg and ivermectin at 5-10 times normal dosages have been shown to reduce ova numbers being shed, but have not eliminated the worms. The most novel approach has been to endoscopically locate and mechanically remove all the adult pentastomes. Recognization of pentastomal infestations is important because these parasites are thought to present a risk of zoonotic infection. Euthanasia is a valid consideration due to public health concerns.

Protozoal Diseases

Numerous protozoans are found on reptiles; many are harmless commensals. The most serious protozoal pathogen of reptiles is *Entamoeba invadens*. Clinical signs are anorexia, weight loss, vomiting, mucoidal or hemorrhagic diarrhea, and death. Entamebiasis may be epidemic in large snake collections. Herbivores appear less susceptible than carnivores; a number of reptiles that seldom become affected or die can serve as carriers, including garter snakes, northern black racers, and box turtles. While most turtles are resistant, the giant tortoises are susceptible. Other resistant groups include eastern king snakes, crocodiles, and cobras (possibly as an adaptation that allows them to eat snakes). Most boas, colubrids, elapids, vipers, and crotalids are highly susceptible. Transmission is by direct contact with the cyst form. Hepatic abscesses containing numerous *E invadens* trophozoites are common in chronic cases. At necropsy, gross lesions may extend from the stomach to the cloaca. The intestine shows areas of ulceration that tend to coalesce, caseous necrosis, edema, and hemorrhage. Multifocal abscesses in a swollen, friable liver are seen in the hepatic form. Identification of trophozoites or cysts in a wet preparation of fresh feces or tissue impressions, or in histologic sections, is diagnostic. Turtles and snakes should not be housed together.

E invadens is best treated with metronidazole (20 mg/kg, PO, every 48 hr). Iodoquinol (50 mg/kg, PO, SID) has been advocated for a 3-wk course in chelonians. Dimetridazole may be given PO for 10 days at 40 mg/kg. Emetine hydrochloride may be given at 2.5-5 mg/kg, IM or SC, SID for 10 days. Tetracycline and paromomycin have been used but are considered ineffective against the hepatic form. The zoonotic potential for this disease should not be taken lightly, and strict sanitation and hygiene measures should be observed.

Flagellates, especially *Hexamita* spp, have been reported to cause urinary tract disease in chelonians and intestinal disease in snakes. The "giardia" seen in some cases of enteritis in snakes may actually be *Hexamita* or one of the relatively nonpathogenic flagellates that inhabit the intestinal tract of snakes. Differentiation between the species requires expertise, and special preservatives and stains are required to identify most of these organisms. Metronidazole at 25-50 mg/kg, PO, repeated in 3-5 days has been used to treat flagellates. Indigo snakes, king snakes, and uracoan rattlers should be treated at the low end of this dosage range. Fenbendazole at 50 mg/kg, PO for 5 days is more effective at eliminating *Giardia* in mammals than is metronidazole. Early studies with fenbendazole are very encouraging and it would appear to be the drug of choice for treating flagellates.

Several coccidial organisms have been reported: *Klossiella* from the kidney, *Isospora* from the gallbladder and intestine, and *Eimeria* from the gallbladder. The severity of disease varies with the coccidia and affected species. Due to their direct life cycle, these parasites can increase to tremendous numbers, especially in immunosuppressed reptiles. Oocysts are not fragile and can survive for weeks in a dessicated condition. Fastidious, daily cleanings are necessary to remove all feces and feces-contaminated food and water. Insects and other food items must be removed on a daily basis as they are another source of contamination (eg, crickets may eat the oocysts while gathering fluid from the feces). Treatment is sulfadimethoxine at 50 mg/kg, PO, for 3 days and then every 48 hr until infection is resolved. Treatment often takes 2-3 wk and success should be measured by serial fecal samples.

Trimethoprim/sulfa at 30 mg/kg every 48 hr as needed is another drug useful in the treatment of coccidia. Care should be taken when using sulfa in reptiles with dehydration or renal compromise. If in doubt, a balanced electrolyte solution should be administered PO at appropriate dosages. Even under the best conditions, treatment will eliminate coccidia in only 50% of cases. Treatment resulting in a reduction of coccidia is still important and coccidial numbers should be periodically monitored.

Plasmodial (malarial) organisms, as well as other intracellular blood protozoans, have been reported in reptiles. Their significance is unknown, and treatment is not considered necessary.

Cryptosporidiosis is frequently reported in association with postprandial regurgitation, marked weight loss, and chronic debilitation. The organism affects the GI mucosa (in snakes), resulting in marked thickening of the rugae and loss of segmented motility.

A mass in the gastric region is often, but not always, palpable, and contrast radiographs or endoscopic examination reveals rugal thickening. Many lizards, including old world chameleons and savannah monitors, are affected primarily in the intestine. Mucosal thickening develops as a result of invasion by numerous cryptosporidial organisms. Diagnosis can be made using acid-fast stains on fresh feces or on the coating from regurgitated items or endoscopic gastric biopsies, which will identify the tiny oocysts. While several treatments have been suggested, none have been consistently effective. Intensive supportive care will often stabilize and help prolong the life of the affected reptile. Euthanasia is a valid option for the infected reptile. Cryptosporidiosis was previously considered a zoonotic disease; however, it now appears that the strains commonly found in reptiles do not affect mammals.

MYCOTIC DISEASES

Excessively high humidity, low environmental temperature, concurrent disease, malnutrition, and stress from poor husbandry may be factors in the development of mycotic diseases in reptiles. Little is known about the pathogenesis of systemic mycoses, which can develop over a long period, but maintaining good sanitation and husbandry reduces the frequency of infection. *Aspergillus, Metarhizium, Mucor, Paecilomyces*, and *Penicillium* spp are a few of the organisms that have been isolated from reptiles with systemic mycoses. Reports of successful treatment of systemic mycoses in reptiles are few. Suggested treatments for deep fungal respiratory infections include amphotericin B (5 mg/kg body wt, nebulized in 150 mL of saline for 1 hr, BID), and thiabendazole (50 mg/kg) and ketoconazole (35 mg/kg) in combination, administered PO, SID. For superficial or localized mycotic infections, surgical removal of the granuloma with local wound treatment is advised. *Basidiobolus* spp, pathogenic for mammals, are found in feces of normal reptiles.

Dermatophytosis has been described in all orders of reptiles. *Geotrichum, Fusarium*, and *Trichosporon* are the genera most frequently isolated. In most cases, cutaneous injury precedes a secondary fungal infection. Chelonians with fungal infections of the shell can be treated by local debridement and topical application of Lugol's solution or povidone-iodine. Griseofulvin, at 20-40 mg/kg, PO, every 72 hr for 5 treatments, has been recommended for mycotic skin infections. Topical 1% tolnaftate cream has also been effective. Exposure to ultraviolet light also may be beneficial.

Ulceration of GI tissues has been associated with infections by *Mucor* and *Fusarium* spp. Chronic visceral granulomatous disease of liver, kidneys, and spleen has been caused by *Metarhizium* and *Paecilomyces* spp. Few signs other than weight loss are seen before death. Animals may continue to feed until a few days before death.

The most frequent sites of mycotic infection are the skin and respiratory tract. *Metarhizium, Mucor*, and *Paecilomyces* spp are frequent isolates. *Aspergillus* spp has been isolated from pulmonary lesions in the chuckwalla (*Sauromalus obesus*). Most infections involve granuloma or plaque formation with resultant signs of respiratory distress before death.

Candidiasis in large snakes has been treated with nystatin (100,000 U, PO, for 10 days).

VIRAL DISEASES

Few viruses have been clearly proven as etiologic agents of disease in reptiles, but several have been linked strongly enough for them to be considered the causative agent until proven otherwise.

Inclusion Body Disease (IBD) of Boid Snakes: Boa constrictors and several species of pythons are most commonly affected by IBD. Boas are considered to be the normal host for this retrovirus because so many (up to 50% of those tested) are infected and they can harbor the virus for years without symptoms. Early symptoms, possibly precipitated by any factor causing immune suppression, include a history of unthriftiness, anorexia, weight loss, secondary bacterial infections, poor wound healing, dermal necrosis, and regurgitation. In essence, IBD should be considered in every sick boa.

Typical findings in the acute phase of the disease include leukocytosis and a normal chemistry panel. As the disease progresses, white cell counts tend to decline to subnormal levels. Blood chemistry results are variable depending on how debilitated and dehydrated the boa becomes, but organ damage may appear. As the disease becomes chronic, some boas will exhibit neurologic symptoms ranging from mild facial tics and abnormal tongue flicking to failure of the snake to right itself when placed in dorsal recumbency and severe seizures.

Pythons are thought to be an abnormal host to the IBD retrovirus because the course of disease is more acute and neurologic symptoms more profound. In most pythons the acute symptoms that boas exhibit will be missed, and they will be presented with severe neurologic disease. While the active disease can linger for months or more in boas, most pythons die within days or weeks of the onset of clinical signs.

Exposure to this retrovirus appears to be due to a transfer of body fluids. Breeding, fight wounds, and fecal/oral contamination are common ways of transfer. Casual handling of an infected specimen and then a normal specimen does not appear to create enough viral exposure to cause infection. However, any immunocompromised reptile may be susceptible under the right circumstances. The snake mite is assumed to be responsible for the spread of the virus in large, well-maintained collections.

A tentative diagnosis is based on the history and clinical signs. Blood work will vary depending on the stage of the disease, but few diseases in snakes will cause such elevated white cell counts in the early stages. On blood smears, inclusion bodies are frequently found in the cytoplasm of leukocytes. One strain (3 strains have been isolated) of the virus frequently produces inclusion bodies in the cytoplasm of erythrocytes. The inclusion bodies are highly suggestive, but not 100% reliable. A definitive diagnosis is obtained via biopsy of internal tissues in which the characteristic inclusion bodies are found, eg, the liver, kidney, esophageal tonsils, and stomach. An ELISA is being developed.

IBD is not curable, and many clients may choose euthanasia. However, individuals may elect to isolate their snakes and treat with supportive and palliative measures. It is essential to educate clients not to sell infected specimens or their offspring, as this has caused the disease to spread worldwide.

Other Retroviruses: Retroviruses have also been found in Russell's viper, corn snakes, and California kingsnakes in association with malignant tumors. A retrovirus isolated from a sarcoma in a Russell's viper was designated as viper virus. A related virus was isolated in a corn snake from a rhabdomyosarcoma and designated cornsnake retrovirus.

Adenoviruses: Adenoviruses have been implicated in fatal hepatic or GI diseases in snakes (gaboon vipers, ball pythons, boa constrictors, rosy boas, and rat snakes), lizards (Jackson's chameleons, savannah monitors, and bearded dragons) and crocodilians.

In bearded dragons, the route of transmission appears to be fecal/oral contamination. Clinical signs are more commonly noted in juvenile dragons but can affect adults, usually to a lesser extent. Symptoms are vague and include lethargy, weakness, weight loss, diarrhea, and sudden death. The morbidity is high in young bearded dragons, but survival is increased with supportive care. Fluid administration, force-feeding, and antibiotics for secondary infections are useful.

As the signs of disease in bearded dragons are vague and similar to those caused by coccidia and nutritional disorders, it is important to confirm the diagnosis. Characteristic intranuclear inclusion bodies are found in several internal organs, primarily the liver. When working with a large breeding group of lizards, it is practical to sacrifice a failing specimen in order to make a diagnosis. Premortem diagnosis can be accomplished by liver biopsy. Identification of adenovirus from fresh feces may be possible in the near future.

Recovered lizards should be quarantined for at least 3 mo. Duration of viral shedding after recovery is unknown, so clients should be discouraged from selling or trading previously infected animals.

Herpesviruses: Herpesviruses have been isolated from freshwater turtles, tortoises, and green sea turtles. In freshwater turtles, the virus may be associated with hepatic necrosis. In tortoises the virus may cause necrosis of oral mucosa accompanied by anorexia, regurgitation, and oral and ocular discharge. Treatment in tortoises includes isolation, supportive care, and application of 5% acyclovir to oral lesions. Acyclovir given at 80 mg/kg, PO, SID appeared to improve the lesions in a desert tortoise. Herpesvirus is diagnosed by the presence of intranuclear inclusion bodies and electron microscopic demonstration of viral particles.

Herpesvirus infection in green sea turtles is called gray patch disease. Epizootics of small, circular papular skin lesions that coalesce into patches are associated with young turtles maintained in crowded, warmer, stressful situations. Biopsies of the skin reveal basophilic intranuclear inclusion bodies in epidermal cells; viral particles are noted in the cytoplasm by electron microscopy. There is no specific treatment, but reduction of crowding and stress appears to decrease the incidence.

Paramyxovirus: Paramyxovirus infections are more common in viperid snakes, but have been reported in nonvenomous snakes as well. This highly contagious virus causes predominantly respiratory signs; transmission appears to be from respiratory secretions. Secondary bacterial infections are common due to the severe inflammation initiated by the virus, and it is not unusual to note nasal discharge, open-mouth breathing, caseated pus in the oral cavity, and labored breathing. Neurologic involvement, including tremors and opisthotonos, is occasionally noted.

Paramyxovirus should be suspected in any respiratory infection that does not respond to treatment with supportive care, antibiotics, and nebulization. Postmortem samples of lung tissue can be submitted to detect viral particles by histology and electron microscopy. A hemagglutination inhibition test is used to measure antibodies against ophidian paramyxovirus in zoos and private collections; positive titer should be used as a screening tool to aid in eliminating infected animals and preventing carriers from entering noninfected collections.

There is no specific treatment, but supportive care and antibiotics may prove useful. Affected specimens should be isolated and strict hygiene employed. Although a vaccine is under development, it is currently not effective.

Papillomas: Viral particles appear to be transmitted from one European green lizard to another via bite wounds. The resulting papillomas are 2-20 mm in diameter and may be single or multiple. While there are no symptoms in the initial phase, affected lizards may become lethargic, anorectic, and die. Diagnosis involves detection of viral particles by electron microscopy. Treatment consists of surgically removing single masses, although regrowth is common. Isolating affected lizards is perhaps the only means to prevent spread.

A papilloma-type virus also appears to affect Bolivian side-neck turtles and appears as white, oval skin lesions distributed over the head. Ulcerative shell lesions are also seen, primarily on the plastron. Diagnosis is made by identifying viral particles on electron microscopy. Treatment is supportive and palliative, and affected animals should be isolated.

Fibropapillomatosis: Sea turtles, primarily free-roaming green sea turtles, have been found to have fibropapillomatous lesions. The route of transmission is not known. The light gray to black masses range in size up to 10 cm in diameter. The location of the masses seems to dictate the severity of symptoms. Masses occurring on periocular tissue can obscure vision. Growths on the flippers can interfere with swimming and the ability to forage for food. Internal masses also occur, primarily in the lungs, liver, kidneys, and GI tract. Diagnosis is made by characteristic lesions and histologic exam. Treatment consists of surgical removal, with wide margins to help reduce recurrence. Some turtles recover spontaneously, while those with internal lesions usually perish. It is suspected that fibropapillomas are caused by an infective agent, and infected specimens should be isolated from other healthy turtles.

Other Viruses: Many other viruses have been reported, but little information exists regarding their diagnosis, control, and treatment. An iridovirus was found in a Herman's tortoise, which died without prior signs of disease. Progressive anemia in Australian geckos has been linked to an iridovirus. Two nonpathogenic rhabdoviruses were isolated from *Ameiva* sp lizards. In addition to herpesviruses and adenoviruses, parvoviruses and picornaviruses have been found in the intestinal tract of snakes, but their exact role is unknown. A poxvirus-like virus has been isolated from circumscribed cutaneous lesions in a caiman and from dermal lesions in a tegu. A reovirus isolated from 4 Chinese vipers was associated with death without prior signs of illness.

ENVIRONMENTAL DISEASES AND TRAUMATIC INJURIES

Abnormal beak growth, which inhibits feeding, occurs in turtles and tortoises; it is often associated with nutritional secondary hyperparathyroidism leading to hypocalcemia, which may cause distortion of the skull as it develops and thus interfere with normal occlusion and wear. Increased levels of protein from feeding excessive amounts of dog food or monkey chow may contribute to accelerated growth of these tissues. A lack of "chewable" foods in captivity also contributes. Treatment consists of trimming or grinding the mouthparts into a more normal conformation. The condition usually recurs due to primary malocclusion, and longterm maintenance is required.

Aggression at mating and feeding is common in crocodilians, some semiaquatic turtles, some skinks and iguanas, and many other lizards. Injuries to cagemates can be severe and are best avoided by separating animals at feeding and reducing the number of animals allowed in a breeding group. When separated individuals are placed together for breeding, they should be carefully monitored. If reptiles must be kept together, it is vital that the enclosure is large enough to accommodate a perch and/or hiding area for each reptile. Food and water is best placed in multiple locations to prevent dominant cohabitants from intimidating the others.

Fractures due to trauma are seen in all species. Long bones may be repaired with splints or internal fixation devices. A simple way of splinting the legs of lizards is to tape the injured leg to the body (front legs) or the tail (rear legs). These splints are tolerated well and protect the injured limb from further injury.

Injury to the spinal column must be assessed individually; when clear displacement is not evident, radiographic evaluation should be done. Spinal injuries caudal to the vent may be tolerated, but injuries cranial to the vent frequently result in constipation and retention of urates. Many green iguanas suffer spinal injuries just over the pelvis, leaving the lizard paralyzed in the rear. Environmental changes (eg, low branches, shallow water dish, nonabrasive substrates) and teaching the owner how to empty the cloacal content will allow the lizard to live a useful, comfortable life. As these fractures are often secondary to metabolic bone disease, a thorough history of the reptile's husbandry may also reveal the need for nutritional changes.

Burns (associated with the use of incandescent lights or other heat sources) are treated by cleansing the site, applying antibiotic ointment; and placing the reptile in a clean, dry environment. Silvadene cream is the preferred topical dressing as it is water miscible and is effective against yeast and bacteria, including *Pseudomonas* spp. In uninfected burns, sterile skin protectants can be applied to the area to act as a "second skin." These products allow access to the water and help keep contaminants out. In severe burn cases, intracoelomic or SC administration of fluids may be needed to prevent dehydration, and systemic antibiotics may be required to prevent or treat secondary opportunistic bacteria, eg, *Pseudomonas* spp. Pain management and assisted feeding techniques may also be applied.

Crush injuries to turtles may result in fractures to the plastron, the carapace, or both. If very contaminated, the tissues should be gently debrided, flushed, and appropriately bandaged. Holes can be created to allow the legs to remain exposed, if desired. Systemic antibiotics should be initiated. Once stable, the wounds should be cleaned again, and the fractures realigned under general anesthesia and repaired using an epoxy resin. These injuries also can be repaired using a quick-setting epoxy glue layered over fiberglass screen. Dental and orthopedic cements have also been used to stabilize fractured tissues. Healing is slow and may require >1 yr.

Ecdysis (shedding) is the hormonally mediated process by which reptiles shed the outer keratinized skin in response to growth or wear. In snakes and some lizards, the process results in shedding the entire layer of skin as a single piece. Crocodilians and many lizards shed small sections of skin intermittently. Turtles follow this pattern on scaled areas and shed coverings from individual scutes one at a time. Large, moderately abrasive rocks or other articles for reptiles to rub on during ecdysis facilitate a normal shed. Before shedding, snakes become anorectic, and their color becomes mildly translucent and dull, which is especially evident over the eyecaps (opaque). Increased irritability and aggressiveness are frequent. The shed begins around the mouth, and the old skin is everted as it is shed.

Once a reptile becomes opaque, the humidity should be slightly increased to decrease the potential for a retained shed. Lightly misting the cage at least daily and providing a hidebox with moist sphagnum moss or a soaking container are all proven techniques.

Dysecdysis refers to an incomplete or inadequate shed. Low humidity and other stresses, including decreased thyroid function, ectoparasitism, nutritional deficiencies, infectious diseases, and lack of suitable abrasive surfaces, have been incriminated as contributing factors. Often, eyecaps or annular bands on the tail or digits are retained. Eyecaps are best treated by the application of an ophthalmic ointment BID for several days until they either fall off or can be grasped with a pair of fine forceps and removed. Patience is advised—eyecaps should never be forced off because of the possibility of damaging the spectacle.

Recalcitrant, retained sheds are best treated by soaking the reptile in warm (77-82°F [25-28°C]) water for several hours and then pulling gently with a gauze sponge. A humidity chamber also works well and can be as simple as a 10-gal. aquarium with an undertank heater in which wet bath towels are placed. The top can be covered with a light cloth to increase humidity levels, but excessive heat must be avoided and can be relieved by allowing more ventilation if needed. Retained sheds are best prevented rather than treated (see above).

Rodent bites, inflicted by uneaten prey, frequently cause traumatic injuries; secondary infection and abscessation are common sequelae. When possible, rodents that have been freshly sacrificed or frozen and thawed should be offered to prevent injury to the reptile (dead prey should be discarded after 24 hr if left uneaten). The feeding of live prey is illegal in many European countries. Fresh bite wounds may be treated by cleansing and saturating with povidone-iodine (diluted 1:10). Parenteral antibiotics, based on results of culture and sensitivity tests, should be used. Untreated wounds frequently abscess and are seen as a soft or hard swelling. The abscess, including the fibrous capsule, should be removed surgically, and the defect sutured. Open or draining abscesses should be curetted, flushed with a povidone-iodine or Lugol's solution, and parenteral antibiotics administered. Antibiotic ointments with proteolytic enzymes may be helpful. (See also ABSCESSES, p 1605.)

METABOLIC AND ENDOCRINE DISEASES

Gout is seen in all orders of reptiles; visceral and articular forms have been reported. (See also p 1472 and p 2271.) Radiographs often reveal mineralized tophi in affected organs and joints. Primary visceral gout is the accumulation of urate microcrystals in organs secondary to a chronic hyperuricemia and is generally caused by excessive protein in the diet. Secondary visceral gout is due to chronic hyperuricemia due to such causes as dehydration and renal damage. Gout can be very debilitating, causing discomfort to the point that some reptiles refuse to move, eat, or drink.

Primary visceral gout is treated by correcting the diet. Secondary visceral gout is treated by attempting to correct the underlying problem, be it dehydration or renal failure. The prognosis is poor in advanced cases. Allopurinol (20 mg/kg) with colchicine may be beneficial if the diagnosis is made early. Tortoises treated with allopurinol seem to respond better than other reptiles. Drug administration usually must be longterm because signs typically recur if treatment is discontinued. Euthanasia must be considered in reptiles in which movement is painful and appetite becomes suppressed.

Endocrine diseases are not often documented in reptiles. However, diabetes mellitus has been reported in chelonians; glucosuria and hyperglycemia are the primary findings, and polyphagia may or may not be apparent. The etiology is undetermined. Pancreatectomy in lizards may result in hypoglycemia, implying that other hormones, such as glucagon or somatotropin, may play a role in the pathogenesis of diabetes mellitus in reptiles. Hypothyroidism and thyroid hyperplasia have been reported mainly in Galapagos Islands tortoises. It has been speculated that high amounts of dietary iodine in the natural diet may play a significant role. Feeding goitrogenic foods to tortoises has been incriminated in development of this condition. The primary clinical sign is subcutaneous edema.

NEOPLASTIC DISEASES

Neoplasia should always be included in the differential diagnosis of disease in reptiles, as neoplastic masses are much more common in reptiles than previously thought. In addition to spontaneously developing neoplastic diseases, tumors have been associated with parasitism and oncogenic viruses. Tumors in reptiles are usually primitive and easily identified. Cytologic examination of a fine-needle aspirate is a quick and easy way to tentatively identify tumors, but surgical biopsies are generally preferred. Techniques such as radiography, ultrasonography, cytology, histopathology (biopsy), and viral isolation provide improved diagnostic capabilities. Once neoplasia is diagnosed, treatment protocols similar to those used in other animals could be adapted.

RODENTS

CHINCHILLAS

Chinchillas are increasingly popular as companion animals. Individual pets are typically seen for conditions related to age, trauma, or improper care, while infectious diseases are more often reported in colony animals raised for fur production. Viruses are uncommon, most bacterial infections are opportunistic, and tumor reports in chinchillas are very rare despite their 20-yr lifespan.

Management

Physical Examination: The animal's overall appearance and behavior should be noted. Sick chinchillas may show weight loss, hunched posture, abnormal gait, scruffy hair coat, or labored breathing. They may be lethargic or unresponsive to stimulation. Respiratory or GI conditions are most commonly encountered and may be signaled by ocular and nasal discharges or diarrhea. Feet should be examined for sores or broken nails. Teeth may be discolored or overgrown. Ears should be examined for discharges or inflammation and eyes for discharges or conjunctivitis. The submandibular area should be examined for swellings. Labored breathing and abnormal respiratory sounds should be noted. The abdomen should be palpated for masses.

Chinchillas should be handled calmly and gently to minimize stress. Docile, nonpregnant animals can be removed from a cage by grasping and lifting the base of the tail while using the opposite hand to support the body. Otherwise, the animal should be guided into its nesting box or a small enclosure with an open end. Routine restraint can be accomplished by wrapping a towel around the body. For longer periods of examination or treatment, a squeezable restraining device can be used. Small chinchillas may be grasped gently around the thorax, taking care not to restrict breathing. Pregnant females should not be handled unless necessary. Pregnancy is detectable by palpation at 90 days gestation and may also be determined by regular weighing. After 6 wk, weight gain in pregnant chinchillas will increase rapidly.

A protective reaction in chinchillas known as **fur slip** results in the release of a large patch of fur revealing smooth, clean skin underneath. It may also occur with improper handling, fighting, or anything that overexcites chinchillas. The fur can take several months to regrow and frequently results in a different shade. To prevent this phenomenon, chinchillas should be handled gently with minimal stress.

Disease Treatment and Prevention: Sick chinchillas are easily stressed and should be handled minimally. Antibiotics are not well tolerated due to adverse changes in GI flora. For drug or therapeutic administration in chinchillas, PO, SC, IM, IV, and IP routes are used. Oral medications or fluids can be administered with a small syringe or eyedropper, carefully positioned at the diastoma. If the animal is able to eat, medications can be mixed with food or water. A stomach tube passed through a speculum may be necessary to directly deposit medications in the stomach. Some medicines can be administered rectally. The flank and interscapular regions are common sites for SC injections, which can also be given in the inner thigh area to minimize potential pelt damage. The large thigh muscles are preferred sites for IM injections and should be limited to volumes <0.3 mL, using a 23-gauge or smaller needle. Femoral, cephalic, and lateral saphenous veins are the best sites for IV injection and blood collection.

Dehydration is evidenced by dry stools, dark urine, and skin tenting. Fluid therapy should be isotonic and selected according to the animal's condition. Anorectic animals may require force feeding by gavage.

Housing: Many health problems can be avoided by providing proper and consistent diets, clean sources of water, nonabrasive contact bedding materials (soft wood shavings, Fuller's earth, or cat litter), and frequent disinfection and sanitation of housing equipment. The housing environment should be dry, free of drafts, and moderately cool. Indoors, the chinchilla's preferred temperature range is 50-60°F (10-16°C). While chinchillas can gradually adapt to outdoor temperatures <32°F, they are prone to heat stroke at temperatures >80°F. Commercial dust baths, or mixtures of silver sand and Fuller's earth (9:1), 2-4 in. deep, should be offered to chinchillas daily for ~10 min. This satisfies the chinchilla's desire to keep its fur clean and groomed. Such mixtures should not remain in the cage for long periods of time because they will become soiled with feces and food debris.

Nutrition: In the wild, herbivorous chinchillas eat a diet high in fiber. Commercial pelleted diets formulated for chinchillas or guinea pigs provide adequate nutrition alone or may be supplemented by small amounts of high-quality hay. New ingredients in the diet should be introduced gradually to help prevent GI disorders. Chinchillas do not regurgitate and thus cannot quickly expel contaminated or spoiled food. Hay should be stored in a well-ventilated, dry area and fed to chinchillas fresh daily. Inadequate nutrition may result in higher mortality rates or developmental problems in young kits, decreased lactation in nursing females, or disturbances in normal GI flora. Chinchilla feces are typically dry, and coprophagia is normal. Watering systems should be sanitized regularly to prevent contamination by opportunistic bacteria such as *Pseudomonas aeruginosa*.

Respiratory Diseases

Choke: Chinchilla anatomy precludes the ability to vomit; choking may be observed when the entrance to the trachea is occluded by a large piece of food or bedding or in postpartum females that eat their placentas. Aspiration of tiny particles from the foreign body can irritate the lower respiratory tract and precipitate a suffocating, edematous response leading to drooling, retching, coughing, and dyspnea as the chinchilla attempts to dislodge the foreign body. If untreated, choking may lead to asphyxiation and death.

Upper Respiratory Tract Infections: Humid, crowded, and poorly ventilated housing conditions may contribute to an increased incidence of respiratory disease in chinchillas. Bacterial infections of nasal sinuses and mucous membranes are seen more often in young or stressed chinchillas. *Streptococcus* spp, *Pseudomonas aeruginosa*, *Pasteurella* spp, and *Bordetella* spp may act as primary or opportunistic pathogens. Clinical signs include sneezing, nasal discharge, and conjunctivitis. In acute cases, animals die suddenly. Untreated animals may progress to pneumonia (*see* below) or death. Grossly, sinus cavities are necrotic and filled with mucopurulent debris, and infection may extend to the brain. Diagnosis is based on clinical signs and culture and isolation of the organism. Treatment includes appropriate ocular and systemic antibiotics and general supportive therapy, including gently soaking the nose and eyes with warm water compresses and removing any crusts. Prevention includes keeping young chinchillas in a warm and draft-free environment, maintaining good husbandry and sanitation, and separation of affected or carrier animals.

Pneumonia: Pneumonia, with inflammation of the lung parenchyma and airways, is usually associated with bacterial infection. *Bordetella* spp, *Streptococcus* spp, and *Pasteurella* spp have been isolated, sometimes concurrently. Housing in cold, damp environments may lead to lowered resistance. *Histoplasma capsulatum*, a fungus found in contaminated hay, has also been reported in chinchillas. Clinical signs of respiratory distress include mucopurulent nasal discharge, sneezing, and labored breathing. Infection may be accompanied by conjunctivitis, fever, weight loss, lethargy, depression, or anorexia. Auscultation reveals wheezing sounds across the entire lung field. Grossly, lesions may range from a focal bronchopneumonia involving only a small area of 1 lobe to complete consolidation; small amounts of purulent debris can be expressed from the bronchioles on cut surface. Sudden death with sepsis may occur in epizootic outbreaks. Diagnosis is based on clinical signs, pneumonic lesions observed at necropsy, and isolation of the causative organism from nasal or conjunctival washes. Treatment is usually not effective in severe cases with total consolidation of the lungs, but antibiotics may be attempted in focal bronchopneumonia. In addition, supportive therapy includes parenteral fluids; warm, dry housing; and stress reduction. Prevention and control in colonies depend on maintenance of good husbandry and sanitation and separation of affected or carrier animals.

Eye and Ear Diseases

Conjunctivitis: Conjunctivitis is seen occasionally in young chinchillas. Catarrhal or mechanical conjunctivitis may result from an ocular foreign body. Purulent conjunctivitis may signal bacterial infection of the eye secondary to mechanical conjunctivitis or, in nursing animals, result from direct contact from vaginitis in the dam. *Staphylococcus* spp and *P aeruginosa* infections have been reported. Chinchillas may develop conjunctivitis secondary to dust-bath irritation. Clinically, infected eyes exhibit hyperemic conjunctiva, edema, and a serous or purulent ocular discharge. Infections usually resolve with topical antibiotic treatment and dust baths should be removed until the condition has completely resolved. Dust baths should be avoided with periparturient females to prevent neonates from accumulating dust in their eyes or mouth.

Otitis Media: This disease is frequently seen in young chinchillas secondary to respiratory infection or trauma. Scar tissue can enclose the healing ear canal and trap cerumen and debris inside. The tympanic membrane may become thickened and inflamed. Inflammation may progress to the inner ear or meninges, with accompanying neurologic signs of ataxia, torticollis, or circling and rolling. Treatment of otitis media is hampered by tissue proliferation and risk to the large, fragile tympanic bullae. Surgery may be necessary to reopen a closed ear canal. Cautery of the ear canal edges may help prevent reclosure. Regular cleaning, in addition to topical and systemic antibiotics, can help ensure that the ear canal remains patent until healing is complete.

Ear Trauma: The chinchilla's large, delicate ear pinnae are easily traumatized, most often from bite wounds or, if exposed to extreme cold, frostbite. Therapy includes cleaning the traumatized area with antiseptic solution and antibiotic ointment. Suturing large ear lacerations is usually not effective and not recommended. If severe damage is present, ear tissue may require significant debridement or partial surgical removal. If lesions are left open, appropriate systemic antibiotics should be administered to minimize potential for infection. Trauma can result in rapid hematoma development with blood and serum filling the space between skin and cartilage. Hematomas should be lanced and contents gently removed to avoid further damage to the ear. The skin over the hematoma must remain in contact with the underlying cartilage and should be immobilized by sutures if necessary.

Gastrointestinal Diseases

Malocclusion (Slobbers): Tooth abnormalities are common in chinchillas and may be observed by the time they are 6 mo old. Malocclusion caused by a nutritional mineral imbalance may also be noted in primiparous females. Clinically, malocclusion leads to unthriftiness, rough hair coat, anorexia, and weight loss. Frequently, excess salivation results in inflammation and alopecia of the skin on the chin and ventral neck. Uncorrected cases may develop periodontitis, alveolar periostitis, or secondary bacterial infections. Overgrown teeth or roots can penetrate the mandible or hard palate, demonstrated by mucopurulent draining tracts or ocular and nasal discharge. Mastication becomes increasingly difficult and severe malnutrition may lead to hypoglycemia and ultimately seizures, paralysis, coma, and death. The oral cavity should be thoroughly examined by otoscope or small speculum, sedating the animal if necessary. Brown spots on the lingual surfaces are indicative of tooth decay; the normally orange incisors may fade with dental disease. Premolar and molar teeth may be loose, broken, or sharply pointed. Sometimes feed or foreign bodies are impacted between the teeth and the underlying oral mucosa. Radiography is a helpful tool for checking tooth position and overgrowth of the roots, which are normally not embedded in bone. Computed tomography provides even earlier detection of pathologic changes. Malocclusion is a chronic condition requiring monthly prophylactic care. Treatment involves trimming and filing teeth, removing food or foreign body impactions, and cleaning any mucosal ulcerations. Because chinchilla teeth grow constantly, appropriate materials (eg, pumice stones, chew blocks) to gnaw are required. A commercial pelleted diet should provide adequate nutrition. If the diet is marginal, it should be supplemented with Vitamin C, dicalcium phosphate, and trace minerals. Teeth and body weight should be frequently monitored to avoid further problems. While individual chinchillas with malocclusion can be managed by careful observation and dental prophylaxis, they should not be bred.

Diarrhea: Chinchillas with GI disorders often have similar clinical signs that may represent any of several nutritional, bacterial, protozoal, parasitic, or stress-induced etiologies. Clinically, infected animals may die acutely without symptoms or in chronic cases of gastroenteritis, exhibit a range of signs including lethargy, anorexia, rough hair coat, perineal staining, hunched posture, listlessness, dull eyes, dehydration, weight loss, pain on abdominal palpation, flatulence, fever or hypothermia, and diarrhea or constipation. Fecal consistency ranges from hemorrhagic to mucoid, and abdominal straining can lead to rectal prolapse. Treatment of diarrhea is similar for most causes. Dietary roughage should be increased and grains and concentrates decreased. This can be accomplished by providing hay in addition to a commercial pelleted diet. Feeding *Lactobacillus* spp, in the form of yogurt with active cultures, may help reestablish normal bacterial flora within the digestive tract. Supportive care is important, and hydration must be maintained by oral or parenteral fluids. Antibiotics should be used cautiously, because they may further disrupt the bacterial flora of the GI tract and exacerbate the diarrhea. Albendazole and fenbendazole are preferable to metronidazole in treating protozoal infections.

Sudden dietary changes and administration of inappropriate antibiotics (eg, erythromycin, clindamycin, lincomycin, cephalosporins, penicillin, ampicillin, or amoxicillin) can alter a chinchilla's normal gram-positive flora, allowing overgrowth of various gram-negative coliforms and clostridial bacteria. Enterotoxemia is most commonly caused by infection with *Clostridium perfringens*. Clinical signs range from diarrhea to emaciation, lethargy, dehydration, and death. Grossly, both spleen and liver are enlarged. Diagnosis is based on serology and identification of the toxin in gastric contents. Vaccinating with clostridial toxoid may reduce morbidity and mortality in colony outbreaks. Other bacteria reported to cause gastroenteritis and diarrhea in chinchillas through contaminated environment or feed include *Salmonella arizona, S enteritidis, Corynebacterium* spp, *Yersinia pseudotuberculosis, Y enterocolitica, Escherichia coli,* and *Proteus* spp.

Frequently prevalent in otherwise clinically normal chinchillas, protozoa such as *Giardia, Trichomonas,* and *Balantidium* spp may cause enteritis, typhlocolitis, and diarrhea under conditions of stress, poor sanitation, or coincidental bacterial enteritis. Fecal wet mounts demonstrate a marked increase in the number of flagellated or ciliated protozoa. *Giardia* spp can also be detected serologically by an indirect fluorescent antibody test. Other enteric protozoa reported to infect chinchillas include *Cryptosporidium* spp and *Eimeria chinchillae.*

Trematodes, nematodes, and cestodes have been observed on fecal floats, but have not been associated with enteritis or diarrhea except in cases of severe infestation.

Gastroenteritis may result from any rapid changes in the chinchilla's normal diet. Increased intake of cellulose and fiber (fruits and green vegetables) can led to decreased peristalsis and invasion of the intestinal mucosa by opportunistic bacteria. Diets low in fiber and high in carbohydrates, fats, and protein can affect normal cecal fermentation and motility and result in typhlitis. Feed or drinking water can also be contaminated by bacteria, molds, or chemicals. Vitamin A, B complex, or C deficiency may result in gastroenteritis. Young kits often develop diarrhea secondary to agalactia or use of milk replacers.

Constipation: More common than diarrhea, constipation typically results from insufficient dietary fiber and roughage. Dehydration, environmental stress, intestinal obstruction, obesity, lack of exercise, trichobezoars, and uterine compression in gravid females may also result in constipation. Chinchillas may strain to defecate and have decreased fecal output. Fecal pellets are thin, short, hard, malodorous, and sometimes stained with blood. Chronic cases may lead to rectal prolapse, intestinal torsion, cecal impaction, or colonic flexure. To provide relief, dietary fiber should be increased by providing alfalfa cubes, adding mineral oil to the feed, and administering soapy, warm-water enemas. Persistent intestinal blockage may be due to intestinal adhesions, tumors, abscesses, impactions, or foreign bodies. These may be palpated abdominally or identified on radiographs using contrast media. Enterotomy and intestinal anastomosis may be required in such cases.

Gastric Tympany (Bloat): Bloat can result from sudden dietary changes, especially overeating. It has been reported in lactating females 2-3 wk postpartum and may be related to hypocalcemia. Gas production from the bacterial flora in static bowel rapidly accumulates within 2-4 hr. Affected animals are lethargic, dyspneic, and have a painful distended abdomen. They may roll or stretch while attempting to relieve their discomfort. Treatment may require passage of a stomach tube or paracentesis to relieve gas build-up. Lactating females may respond favorably to calcium gluconate administered IV slowly to effect.

Gastric Ulcers: Gastric ulcers are common in young chinchillas and are frequently caused by feeding coarse, fibrous roughage or moldy feeds. Clinically affected animals may be anorectic or asymptomatic. Lesions may only be noted at necropsy, with gastric mucosal ulcers and erosions covered by thick, black fluid. Prevention includes decreasing dietary roughage and feeding a commercial pelleted diet.

Integumentary Diseases

Dermatophytosis (Ringworm): Fungal skin infections in chinchillas are infrequent. The most commonly isolated dermatophyte is *Trichophyton mentagrophytes*; *Microsporum* spp are seen occasionally. Outbreaks of active disease in colonies may accompany the introduction of a new chinchilla. Small patchy areas of alopecia are seen mostly around the ears, nose, and feet, but can be found on any part of the body. Lesions are characterized by irregular or circular-shaped, crusty, flaky skin lesions with reddened margins. Transmission is by direct contact or by fomites, such as cage bedding. Diagnosis is based on lesions, Wood's lamp examination, and by isolation of the causative agent in or on infected hairs. Some animals may be asymptomatic carriers. Effective treatment consists of 5-6 wk of oral griseofulvin or itraconazole. Griseofulvin is teratogenic in other species and should be avoided in pregnant females. Isolated skin lesions may be treated effectively with topical griseofulvin, tolnaftate, or butenafine creams applied daily for 7-10 days. Antifungal powders may be added to the chinchilla's dust bath. Prevention includes decreasing potential for stress, culling affected stock from colonies, quarantine of new additions to colonies, and adequate sanitation. Ringworm is contagious to humans and other animals.

Abscesses: Abscesses in chinchillas may occur secondary to bite wounds or other trauma. *Staphylococcus aureus* and *Streptococcus* spp are the most common bacteria isolated. An abscess may remain hidden under the animal's thick coat and only become evident after it ruptures. Ruptured abscesses should be expressed to empty remaining contents and flushed with antiseptic solution. Appropriate topical antibiotic creams may be applied as needed. Unruptured abscesses can be surgically removed and appropriate parenteral antibiotics administered. Abscesses removed surgically often heal better than those that are lanced, drained, and flushed.

Fur Chewing: Currently thought to be an abnormal behavior, chinchillas chew their own or each other's fur, resulting in a moth-eaten appearance. The phenomenon is reported to occur in 30% of chinchillas. Factors that may be related to the pathogenesis include boredom, stress, malnutrition, warm or drafty environments, or increased thyroid and adrenocortical activity. Fur-chewing mothers tend to pass this disorder to their offspring, and affected chinchillas usually have a nervous disposition. Clinically, hair loss is observed along the shoulders, flanks, sides, and paws. The affected areas appear darker due to the exposed underfur. A variety of approaches to control the behavior has been attempted, including decreasing room humidity and temperature and removing the darker underfur from affected areas and applying povidone-iodine ointment to the skin for disinfection and facilitation of scale removal. Identifiable stressors should be minimized. Papaya cubes or tablets may help prevent trichobezoar formation and potential intestinal blockage.

Multisystemic Diseases

Septicemia: Multisystemic infections may be secondary to untreated bacterial gastroenteritis (*Streptococcus* spp, *Enterococcus* spp, *Pasteurella multocida*, *Klebsiella pneumoniae*, and *Actinomyces necrophorum*), although some nonenteric bacteria have also been isolated. Animals may be asymptomatic and die suddenly or develop nonspecific signs of anorexia, lethargy, rough hair coats, and diarrhea. At necropsy, septicemic organs are diffusely congested and may contain bacterial emboli. Diagnosis is based on isolation of bacteria in blood or affected organs. Treatment includes appropriate antibiotics and general supportive care.

Heat Stress: Chinchillas are highly susceptible to sudden changes in their environment, especially temperatures >80°F. Clinical signs include initial restlessness, shallow rapid respiration, hypersalivation, weakness, hyperthermia, coma, and death. Gross lesions include markedly congested lungs. To treat, the animal should be cooled down slowly and carefully via cool water baths or alcohol sprays and provided with general supportive care such as parenteral fluids and corticosteroids.

***Pseudomonas aeruginosa* Infection:**   Commonly found in drinking water and the cage environment, *P aeruginosa* may cause opportunistic infections secondary to stress. Transmission occurs by aerosol, direct contact, and fecal-oral routes. Neonatal infection may result from nursing an infected dam. Clinical signs include anorexia, depression, diarrhea or constipation, corneal or oral ulcers, intradermal pustules, conjunctivitis, genital swellings, mastitis, abortion, infertility, and acute death. Gross lesions may be seen in multiple organs with abscesses, generalized lymphadenopathy, and multifocal necrosis. Diagnosis is based on isolation and identification of the bacteria; treatment includes appropriate antibiotics. To prevent infection, general animal husbandry and sanitation and disinfection practices should be improved. Vaccines have been developed for colony animals raised for fur.

***Listeria monocytogenes* Infection:**   *L monocytogenes* is often associated with poor sanitation and contaminated feedstuffs or drinking water and occurs mostly in colony animals raised for fur. Transmission is by the fecal-oral route. While this environmental bacterium can infect many species of animals and humans, chinchillas are highly susceptible. Systemic infection may include visceral and encephalitic forms. Clinical signs, if present, include anorexia, depression, weight loss, constipation or diarrhea, and abdominal pain. With CNS involvement, additional signs include droopy ears, torticollis, ataxia, circling, and convulsions progressing to death. Gross lesions include fibrinous peritonitis, interstitial pneumonia, and widespread multifocal miliary necrosis. Any organ may be affected. The classic histologic lesions include monocytic perivascular cuffing in brain sections. Diagnosis is based on bacterial isolation. Treatment of clinically ill chinchillas is not effective. Affected colony animals should be removed and attention given to cleaning the environment, water, and diet. Chinchillas not exhibiting clinical signs can be inoculated with autogenous bacterins or treated with prophylactic antibiotics, such as chloramphenicol or oxytetracycline.

Yersinia spp Infection: Both *Y pseudotuberculosis* and *Y enterocolitica* are gram-negative bacteria frequently isolated from chinchillas. Exposure to asymptomatic wild rodents is the most likely source of contamination. Transmission is both horizontal (fecal-oral) and vertical (transplacental and milkborne). Infections may be asymptomatic or, in epizootics, cause high morbidity and mortality with lethargy, depression, anorexia, weight loss, constipation or diarrhea, and sudden death. With *Y pseudotuberculosis*, granulomatous lesions are found primarily in the liver, spleen, and lungs. *Y enterocolitica* causes similar lesions in the liver, spleen, intestines, lymph nodes, kidneys, and lungs. Diagnosis is based on bacterial isolation. Treatment of clinically ill chinchillas is not effective. Affected colony animals should be removed and attention given to cleaning the environment, water, and diet. Chinchillas not exhibiting clinical signs can be inoculated with autogenous bacterins or treated with prophylactic tetracycline.

Reproduction

Pet owners should be encouraged to maintain chinchillas in single-sex groups to provide companionship but avoid producing large numbers of offspring. Male chinchillas must be grouped before weaning or castrated to prevent fighting. When breeding, potential mates should be introduced before the female enters estrus to reduce fighting and increase compatibility. Males need a refuge box to escape potentially aggressive nonestrous females. Specially fitted muzzles or collars can be applied to the female to prevent her from biting or chasing the male. Repeated female-to-male aggression can lead to a conditioned avoidance response in the male, making him an unsatisfactory breeder. Polygamous and harem mating systems are commonly employed by breeders. As chinchillas approach parturition, they may become less active, anorectic, and aggressive toward previously compatible cagemates. Chinchilla dams do not typically build nests at parturition, although a nesting box may help decrease neonatal mortality caused by drafts or cold stress. Hypothermic kits should be warmed and revived quickly to prevent mortality.

Infertility: Decreased reproductive performance may be due to several causes, including malnutrition, abnormal sperm, hormonal imbalance, infectious disease, lack of experience, lethal genes from inappropriate crosses, or poor conditioning. Infectious and dietary factors are often implicated. Obese females produce smaller litters. Matings between or among chinchillas homozygous for White and Velvet coat color genes should be avoided. Breeders should have access to a fresh commercial pelleted diet and adequate roughage, and colonies should be screened carefully for any heritable physical defects.

Abortion: Pregnancy termination may be caused by improper handling, trauma, inadequate nutrition, septicemia, fever, or interruption of the uterine blood supply. At term, suddenly startled females may spontaneously abort. Frequently the female will immediately ingest the aborted kits. Abortion may take place unnoticed, but should be suspected if a female chinchilla suddenly loses weight. Often, a bloody vaginal discharge and perineal staining are observed. Treatment for post-abortion females includes flushing the reproductive tract gently with an antiseptic solution and administration of appropriate parenteral antibiotics.

Retained or Mummified Fetus: A fetus that dies late in gestation may be delivered normally along with the live young, remain within the uterus, or become mummified. If a dead fetus is retained, the parturient female may neglect her live kits and become increasingly depressed as toxicity develops. A fetus that dies early in gestation is normally resorbed without complication, but loss of fetal fluids may lead to mummification. A mummified fetus can remain within the uterus for extended periods of time and prevent further pregnancies. Causes are thought to be similar to those for infertility (*see* above), with poor conditioning or infectious diseases being the most likely. All female chinchillas should be examined as soon as possible following parturition to determine if there are retained fetuses. Abdominal palpation may not be conclusive and radiography should be used to provide a definitive diagnosis. A female not able to pass a retained fetus may require cesarean section.

Dystocia: Dystocia is very rare in chinchillas, but may be observed with an abnormally large or misplaced fetus or in young females bred too early. Poorly conditioned females may also develop primary uterine inertia or lack sufficient strength to deliver the kits. If labor continues >4 hr, oxytocin (1 U) or 0.5 ml of 20% calcium solution should be administered IM. If dystocia continues, a cesarean section should be performed.

Metritis: A retained placenta or fetus may lead to bacterial contamination and inflammation of the uterus. Chinchillas with metritis may have anorexia, agalactia, abnormal gait, high fever, swollen discolored vulva, and a malodorous, mucopurulent vaginal discharge. Kits are at risk of infection through contact with infected discharge. Early detection and treatment are essential because affected females can develop a severe, fatal septicemia with sudden deterioration and death. Oxytocin induces uterine contractions and expulsion of mucopurulent debris. The reproductive tract can be irrigated with an antiseptic solution, followed by sulfathiazole in mineral oil, using a small rubber catheter to deliver the solution into the uterus. Appropriate systemic antibiotics should be administered and general support provided.

Pyometra: Following an episode of metritis or retained placenta, and occasionally observed in unbred females, bacterial infection may lead to pyometra with accumulation of mucopurulent debris within the uterus. Clinically, chinchillas lose weight and have a rough hair coat and a mucopurulent vaginal discharge staining the perivulvar areas. Often, affected females are no longer capable of successful breeding and should be culled. Medical treatment of pyometra is ineffective and ovariohysterectomy is recommended.

Agalactia: Inadequate milk production in postpartum chinchillas depends on a variety of age, genetic, infectious, and nutritional factors. Kits from agalactic females are vocal, restless, lose weight, and may die. Following parturition, the female's mammary glands should be examined for milk production. If females have not begun to produce adequate milk within 72 hr, oxytocin should be administered to stimulate milk letdown. Cross-fostering with compatible females or guinea pigs may be necessary in unresponsive cases or large litters.

Mastitis: Mammary glands of lactating females should be observed frequently for injuries caused by the sharp teeth of nursing kits. Superficial lesions can be treated with topical antibiotics and warm compresses. More extensive tissue trauma can lead to inflammation and infection. With clinical mastitis, mammary glands are warm, firm, enlarged, and painful. Milk may be thick or bloody and clotted. Appropriate systemic antibiotics are indicated and kits may need to be cross-fostered or hand-raised.

Hair Rings: In male chinchillas, a ring of hair may surround the penis within the prepuce and cause a secondary paraphimosis, urethral constriction, and urinary retention. Affected males may be observed excessively grooming, straining to urinate, and frequently cleaning their penis. Hair rings often develop following copulation. Treatment includes lubricating the penis or mild sedation to facilitate gentle removal of the fur ring.

Nervous System Diseases

Baylisascaris procyonis **Infection (Cerebral Nematodiasis):** *B procyonis*, a roundworm of raccoons, may cause cerebral nematodiasis in infected chinchillas. Transmission occurs following ingestion of feed contaminated with raccoon feces. Infected chinchillas may exhibit a variety of CNS signs, including ataxia, incoordination, head tilt, tumbling, paralysis, recumbency, coma, and death. Histopathology is diagnostic and characterized by meningitis, multifocal necrosis, and sections of ascarid larvae throughout the midbrain, medulla, and cerebellum. Treatment is ineffective. Prevention includes appropriate husbandry and adequate sanitation practices. *B procyonis* is potentially zoonotic and causes a fatal encephalopathy in humans.

Protozoa: *Toxoplasma gondii* and *Frenkelia* spp are protozoa associated with necrotic meningoencephalitis in chinchillas. Infections are rare and clinical signs may include incoordination, lethargy, depression, anorexia, weight loss, dyspnea, cyanosis, and purulent nasal discharge. Gross lesions include hemorrhagic lungs and enlarged spleen and lymph nodes. Microscopically, *Toxoplasma* pseudocysts or bradyzoites may be observed in lungs, liver, intestine, pancreas, myocardium, or brain. Tachyzoites are found in blood and lymphatic fluids. Diagnosis is accomplished by serology or demonstrating cysts with Giemsa- or periodic acid-Schiff-stained tissue sections. Active infections can be treated with sulfonamide antibiotics but these are not effective against the encysted stage of toxoplasmosis.

Herpesvirus 1 Infection: Spontaneous human herpesvirus 1 infection has been reported in chinchillas. Clinical signs include conjunctivitis and various neurologic signs, including seizures, disorientation, recumbency, and apathy, progressing to death. Histologic lesions include nonsuppurative meningitis, polioencephalitis with neuronal necrosis and intranuclear inclusion bodies affecting primarily the brain stem and cerebral cortex, ulcerative keratitis, uveitis, retinitis, retinal degeneration, optical neuritis, and purulent rhinitis. Diagnosis is based on clinical signs and demonstrating the lesions via immunohistochemistry. Treatment is not likely to be effective and affected animals should be removed from breeding colonies. Chinchillas may serve as a temporary reservoir for human infections.

Thiamine Deficiency: Required for normal carbohydrate metabolism and protein synthesis, thiamine or vitamin B_1 deficiency causes reversible damage to peripheral motor nerves. Affected chinchillas may show neurologic signs such as trembling, circling, convulsions, or paralysis. Treatment consists of IM injections of thiamine or B-complex vitamins. Natural thiamine sources are found in leafy vegetables, high-quality hay, and wheatgerm meal, or supplements can be added to the diet (1 mg thiamine/kg feed).

Musculoskeletal Diseases

Tibial Fractures: Transverse or spiral traumatic fractures of the tibia are commonly seen when chinchillas accidentally catch their legs on wire caging. Healing is generally rapid, with callus formation in 7-10 days, and can be facilitated by external coaptation or internal fixation. To prevent potential limb injuries, caging should have solid floors or mesh openings ≤15 × 15 mm.

Calcium:Phosphorous Imbalance: A dietary imbalance in the ratio of calcium to phosphorus or phosphorus deficiency may result in severe muscle spasms in young or pregnant chinchillas. Muscles of the hindlimbs, forelimbs, and face are affected. Treatment with calcium gluconate, given IP or IV to effect, is recommended. Prevention is accomplished by feeding a well-balanced, nutritionally complete diet.

GERBILS

Mongolian gerbils (*Meriones unguichulatus*) are characterized by their nonaggressive nature, monogamous mating behavior, conservation of water and temperature, lack of odor, and relative lack of spontaneous disease. There are several coat color varieties. Normal lifespan is 2-3 yr and adult body weight is 50-90 g, with males being slightly larger than females. Individual pets may often be seen for conditions related to age, trauma, or improper care.

Management

Physical Examination: The animal's overall appearance and behavior, particularly in relation to its cagemates, should be noted. Sick animals are often isolated from others and may demonstrate weight loss, hunched posture, lethargy, rough hair coat, labored breathing, and a loss of exploratory behavior. Early signs of illness involve changes in the color, consistency, odor, and amount of urine and feces. The perineal area should be checked for fecal or urine stains or discharges from the vulva in females. Fecal samples may be taken for parasite detection and bacterial culture. The fur and skin should be examined for alopecia, fight wounds or other trauma, ectoparasites, and elasticity for evidence of dehydration. The oral cavity should be checked for overgrown teeth. Ears should be examined for discharges or inflammation and eyes for discharges or conjunctivitis. Feet should be examined for sores and overgrown or broken nails. The abdomen should be palpated for masses. Normal body temperature is 98-102°F (37-39°C). Respiratory rate or signs of labored breathing should be noted. The thorax can be ausculted with a pediatric stethoscope. Gerbils have a large ventral, abdominal marking gland that is androgen-dependent and larger in males. Females mark their territory following parturition and become more aggressive. Reflecting their desert origins, gerbils excrete little urine and their fecal pellets are normally hard and dry. Gerbil tails are fragile and animals should only be handled by the base of the tail to avoid damage.

Disease Treatment and Prevention: For drug or therapeutic administration in gerbils, PO, SC, IM, IV, and IP routes are used. The gerbil's intestinal flora is not as sensitive to antibiotics as that of hamsters and guinea pigs. Oral medications or fluids can be administered into the oral cavity with an eye dropper or directly into the stomach by gavage with a ball-tipped needle. The flank and interscapular regions are common sites for SC injections ≤1.0 mL. The caudal quadriceps or hamstring muscles are preferred sites for IM injections and should be limited to volumes <0.1 mL or necrosis may result. Intraperitoneal injections ≤4-5 mL are administered on either side of the midline in the inguinal region with the gerbil's head tilted downward to avoid the large cecum. IV injections (≤0.1 mL) and blood collection are very difficult in gerbils, because they have few accessible veins. Those which may be attempted include the lateral tail, anterior cephalic, and lingual veins. Appropriate needle sizes are 27-30 gauge. In critically ill animals, interosseous injections can be made in the tibial crest using a 22-gauge spinal needle under anesthesia. Small amounts of blood can be collected via toenail clip or by puncturing a footpad or ear pinna. Larger amounts of blood may be collected from anesthetized animals intracardially or via the retro-orbital sinus.

Dehydration may occur with diarrhea or other illnesses; fluid therapy should be isotonic and selected according to the animal's condition. Prevention of health problems should be emphasized to pet owners, including proper and consistent diets, clean sources of water and bedding, and frequent disinfection and sanitation of housing equipment. Indoors, gerbils should be maintained between temperatures of 60-70°F (16-21°C) and relative humidity <50%. Sand baths are used to keep hair coats from becoming too oily. Caging should have solid bottoms since gerbils often stand erect on their hindlimbs.

Dental Care: Overgrown incisor teeth in gerbils are not as common as in other rodents. If present, they may result in anorexia, depression, and weight loss. Treatment involves periodic trimming of affected teeth and provision of materials for the gerbil to gnaw and wear teeth down naturally.

Gerbils maintained on standard commercial pelleted feeds will develop severe, progressive periodontal disease starting at 6 mo of age, leading to tooth loss in 2 yr.

Nutrition: Gerbils can be maintained on good quality commercial rodent diet with 18-20% protein but may have deficiency problems when fed primarily homemade diets, sunflower seeds, or table scraps, which lack specific nutrients. Sunflower seeds are high in fat and low in calcium. Pelleted chow (5 g/day) has been recommended to avoid obesity and diabetes. Gerbils hoard food. They are not normally coprophagic, unless diets lack adequate nutrient value. Two-wk-old weanling gerbils are sensitive to food and water deprivation. Food pellets should be soaked in water for easier consumption. Normal water intake for adults is 4 mL/day. Watering systems should be sanitized regularly to prevent contamination by opportunistic bacteria.

Among gerbils fed commercial pelleted diets, 10% may develop obesity, along with lipemia, reduced glucose tolerance, elevated insulin levels, and endocrine pancreatic lesions.

Gastrointestinal Diseases

Tyzzer's Disease (*Clostridium piliforme*): The most commonly reported infectious disease in gerbils is caused by *C piliforme*, a gram-negative, obligately intracellular, sporeforming bacteria with a broad host range. Gerbils are among the most susceptible species to infection, with high morbidity and mortality in colony outbreaks. Transmission is via the fecal-oral route, and clinical disease is reported more often in younger or stressed animals. Infection primarily targets the liver and intestines, and clinical signs include depression, rough hair coat, hunched posture, anorexia, dehydration, watery diarrhea, and death within 5 days of infection. Septicemia may lead to myocardial lesions and encephalitis with additional clinical signs of torticollis, rolling, and sudden death. Gross lesions include dilation and hyperemia of large intestines; foamy, yellow fecal contents; and liver and heart necrosis. Diagnosis is based on signs and demonstration of the gram-negative intracellular organisms with Giemsa or silver stains in histologic sections of the intestine, liver, or heart. Infection can also be diagnosed by PCR. Serologic detection by ELISA is variable. Supportive fluids and treatment with tetracycline or metronidazole are recommended to reduce colony mortality. Affected and exposed animals should be removed to prevent further spread. Because the bacteria form spores, the housing environment should be thoroughly sanitized and disinfected.

Salmonellosis: *Salmonella enteritidis*, *S typhimurium*, and *Salmonella* Group D infections have been reported in gerbils. Morbidity and mortality are reported to be higher in younger animals. Clinical signs include diarrhea, dehydration, weight loss, rough hair coat, depression, abdominal distension, abortion, or sudden death. Testicular enlargement was also observed in an outbreak of Group D salmonellosis. Transmission is associated with food or bedding contaminated by insects and wild rodents. Gross lesions include enlarged liver and spleen, with small, white focal necrosis, patchy pulmonary hemorrhage, peritonitis, and enteritis. Diagnosis is based on isolation of the organism from affected organs, fecal contents, or blood. Treatment is generally not recommended. Affected or exposed animals should be isolated and the environment sanitized and disinfected to eliminate any potential sources of contamination. Salmonellosis is zoonotic and potential exists for an asymptomatic carrier state.

Nematodes: Oxyurid pinworms, including *Syphacia obvelata*, *S muris*, and *Dentostomella translucida* may be seen in gerbils. Transmission is by the fecal-oral route. Mild enteritis may occur with heavy infection in other rodent species, but no clinical signs have been reported in gerbils. Diagnosis includes identifying perianal eggs retrieved from cellophane tape impression smears or fecal flotation. Treatment includes 2 separate 7-day courses of piperazine (10 mg/mL water) or ivermectin (0.2 mg/kg), separated by 5 days to account for the pinworm's life cycle. Fenbendazole mixed in the feed at 0.1% and fed 3-4 wk should also eliminate pinworm infection. Because pinworm eggs are light and may aerosolize, it is important to sanitize and disinfect the housing environment.

Cestodes: Gerbils can be infected by *Rodentolepis nana* (dwarf tapeworm) or *Hymenolepis diminuta*. *R nana* has a direct life cycle and may potentially infect humans if ingested. Both tapeworms can be transmitted indirectly; cockroaches, beetles, or fleas act as intermediate hosts. Although usually asymptomatic, heavy infections may cause dehydration and mucoid diarrhea. Diagnosis is by identification of hexacanth ova in fecal contents or viewing adults in histopathologic sections of small intestine. Recommended treatment is niclosamide fed at 10 mg feed/100 g body wt for two 7-day periods separated by 1 wk. Also effective are thiabendazole (0.33% mixed in the feed for 7-14 days) or praziquantel (5-10 mg/kg, IM, SC, or PO, repeated in 10 days). The animal's environment should be appropriately sanitized and disinfected and potential intermediate hosts eliminated.

Integumentary Diseases

Facial Dermatitis (Nasal Dermatitis, Sore Nose): In juvenile and adult gerbils, environmental stressors such as incompatible cagemates, high humidity, and overcrowding cause release of Harderian gland porphyrin secretions around the external nares and eyes. Accumulation of the reddish-brown porphyrin pigment causes skin irritation and eventually leads to self-trauma, localized alopecia, and moist dermatitis with erythema, scabs, and ulceration. *Staphylococcus saprophyticus, S xylosis,* and *S aureus* may secondarily invade and exacerbate the dermatitis, spreading to the forepaws and ventral thorax and abdomen. Skin lesions are pruritic and frequent scratching may result in bleeding. Infection may also extend to the maxillary sinuses. The condition may be self-limiting with spontaneous recovery or, more often, progressive with bacterial infection. With accumulating effects of disease, affected gerbils develop anorexia and adipsia, lose weight, and may die. Diagnosis is based on clinical signs and isolation of secondary bacteria. Treatment includes carefully cleaning the skin lesions and applying topical antibiotics (chloramphenicol 1% ophthalmic ointment, TID). Prevention requires careful control of environmental temperature and humidity or other sources of stress and providing sand baths or clay bedding.

Alopecia: Patchy facial hair loss may result from constant rubbing on metal cage feeders or excessive burrowing behavior. Alopecia and lesions around the tail and hindquarters may result from cage overcrowding, fight wound trauma, and barbering (hair chewing by cagemates). Improper handling may cause tail fur loss or skin slipping. The underlying exposed tail becomes necrotic and requires amputation with cautery. Prevention includes correcting adverse environmental conditions and separating affected animals. Gerbils should only be handled by the base of the tail to prevent degloving.

Rough Hair Coat: A rough and matted hair coat often indicates excessive environmental humidity (>50%). This condition is often observed in gerbils housed in solid-topped aquariums or cages. It can be prevented by providing adequate air exchange to remove excess environmental moisture.

Acariasis: *Demodex meriones* is occasionally reported in gerbils. Old age and debilitation are important predisposing factors. Dry, scaly dermatitis and alopecia are observed over the back and rump. Treatment is by application of a topical amitraz and water mixture (0.66 mL in 1 pint [473 mL] water) 3-6 times at 2-wk intervals. Bedding should be changed frequently and the environment sanitized and disinfected.

Ventral Scent Gland Tumor: In older gerbils, the ventral scent gland is at risk for developing adenomas or squamous cell carcinomas. Affected glands may ulcerate or develop secondary bacterial infections, but rarely metastasize. Other cutaneous tumors include squamous cell carcinomas and melanomas affecting the ear and feet. Masses may be surgically removed. The prognosis varies with the size, stage, and timing of surgical excision.

Nervous System Diseases

Epilepsy (Seizures): Gerbils may develop spontaneous epileptiform seizures. Precipitating factors include sudden stress, improper handling, or introduction to a novel environment. The incidence is reported to be ~20%. This condition appears to be inherited and related to deficiency of cerebral glutamine synthetase. Clinical onset begins in 2- to 3-mo-old gerbils, with seizure incidence and severity increasing up to 6 mo of age, after which occurrences decrease with age. Seizures last several minutes and range from mild hypnotic episodes with twitching ears and whiskers to severe myoclonic convulsions with extensor rigidity. Mortality is rare and there is no permanent damage. A refractory period of ≤5 days can follow more severe seizures. Seizures can be suppressed in genetically predisposed gerbils if they are frequently stimulated by handling during the first 3 wk of life. Anticonvulsant therapy is unnecessary.

Streptomycin Toxicity: A direct neuromuscular blockade is seen with high doses of streptomycin. This inhibits acetylcholine release and results in an acute toxicity characterized by depression, ascending flaccid paralysis, coma, and death within minutes after administration.

Miscellaneous and Geriatric Diseases

There are several causes of **infertility** in gerbils, including ovarian cysts, incompatibility, sexual immaturity, senescence, overcrowding, ingestion of pesticides or other toxins, nutritional deficiencies, environmental disturbances, low ambient temperatures and systemic disease. Cystic ovaries occur in 20% of older female gerbils and are the major reason for infertility and decreasing litter sizes. Aged females may also develop metritis, dystocia, cystic endometrial hyperplasia, and myometrial mineralization. Older males may develop orchitis, prostatitis, and testicular mineralization.

Gerbils >1 yr old frequently develop **glomerulonephritis**. Clinical signs include polyuria, polydipsia, and progressive weight loss. Grossly, kidneys are shrunken, fibrotic, and pitted. Concurrent neoplasia often occurs. Supportive fluid therapy may be required.

Spontaneous **aural cholesteatomas** occur in 50% of gerbils >2 yr old. Masses displace the tympanum into the middle ear. Compression and secondary infection result in bone necrosis and inner ear destruction. Clinical signs include head tilt.

There is a potential for development of **lead toxicity** in pet gerbils due to their gnawing behavior and the urine-concentrating ability of the kidneys. Chronically, gerbils become emaciated, livers are small and pigmented, and kidneys are small and pitted. Microscopically, acid-fast inclusions are noted in proximal collecting tubules and hepatocytes.

Gerbils >10 mo old may develop **amyloid deposits** in the spleen, liver, lymph nodes, exocrine pancreas, adrenal gland, heart, and intestines. Clinical signs include anorexia, dehydration, weight loss, and death.

Older male gerbil breeders have an increased incidence of **focal myocardial necrosis**, fibrosis, and ischemic lesions.

Aged gerbils may develop a protruding nictitating membrane and bulbar conjunctiva with proptosis.

GUINEA PIGS

Infectious diseases in guinea pigs are more often seen in colony settings, while individual pets may be seen for conditions related to aging, trauma, or improper care. Viruses and internal parasites are uncommon. Tumors are rare in younger animals, but an increased incidence of neoplasia appears after 5 yr.

Management

Physical Examination: Overall appearance and behavior should be noted. Sick guinea pigs may show evidence of weight loss, hunched posture, abnormal gait, drawn in abdomen, scruffy hair coat, or labored breathing. They may be lethargic or unresponsive to stimulation. Respiratory and GI conditions are most commonly encountered, thus ocular or nasal discharges or diarrhea may be present. Feet should be examined for sores or broken nails. Teeth may sometimes overgrow and should be checked. Ears should be examined for discharges or inflammation and eyes for discharges or conjunctivitis. The submandibular area should be examined for swellings.

Disease Treatment and Prevention: Sick guinea pigs are easily stressed and should be handled sparingly. Antibiotics are not well tolerated due to adverse changes in GI flora. Most disease treatments should include vitamin C supplementation. Dehydration may occur with diarrhea or other illnesses and may be assessed by dry stools, dark urine, or skin tenting. Fluid therapy should be isotonic and selected according to the animal's condition. Anorectic animals may require force feeding by gavage. Prevention of health problems should be stressed to pet owners. Proper and consistent diet, clean water, non-abrasive contact bedding materials, frequent disinfection and sanitation of housing equipment, and providing a low-stress environment all help to prevent introduction of infectious or opportunistic pathogens. Guinea pigs are highly susceptible to sudden changes in their environment, especially sudden exposure to temperatures >70°F and should not be housed in direct sunlight to prevent heat stress.

For pet owners, maintaining single-sex groups provides companionship and avoids producing large numbers of offspring. To prevent fighting, males should be grouped together before weaning or castrated. Guinea pigs should not be exposed to other pet species, as they may panic and become stressed; isolation also prevents introduction of contagious pathogens such as *Bordetella bronchiseptica*.

Antibiotic Toxicity: Guinea pigs and hamsters are highly susceptible to the toxic effects of many commonly used antibiotics. Toxicity may result directly from some antibiotics (eg, streptomycin or dihydrostreptomycin). Other gram-positive and broad-spectrum antibiotics (eg, penicillin, ampicillin, lincomycin, clindamycin, gentamicin, vancomycin, erythromycin, tylosin, tetracycline, chlortetracycline) may reduce normal GI anaerobes and gram-positive bacteria and lead to overgrowth of coliforms and clostridial bacteria. Enterocolitis and endotoxemia develop after antibiotic administration, with diarrhea, anorexia, dehydration, hypothermia, and death in 3-7 days. Animals may die suddenly without exhibiting clinical signs. The clinical outcome depends on drug dosage, pathogen presence and strain, and host resistance. A presumptive diagnosis is based on a history of antibiotic administration, clinical signs, and an overabundance of gram-negative bacteria on fecal smears. Treatment is usually ineffective, other than providing general support and discontinuing antibiotic administration. Antibiotics with a primarily gram-positive spectrum should not be used in guinea pigs or hamsters. Broad-spectrum antibiotics, such as chloramphenicol and enrofloxacin, should not be used orally because of their direct effect on the intestinal flora, but can be used parenterally with caution. If ingested, topical antibiotic ointments may also be toxic. Malnutrition and vitamin C deficiency predispose guinea pigs to clostridial enterotoxemia.

Nutritional and Metabolic Diseases

Vitamin C Deficiency (Scurvy, Scorbutus): Like humans and other primates, guinea pigs lack the gene to produce the hepatic enzyme l-gulonolactone oxidase, necessary for the formation of ascorbic acid. Without a sufficient exogenous source, tissue stores of vitamin C are rapidly depleted. The resultant defects in collagen synthesis and blood clotting result in lameness, swollen joints, and hemorrhages throughout subcutaneous tissues, skeletal muscles, subperiosteum, adrenal cortex, and intestines. Clinical signs of vitamin C deficiency include painful locomotion, weakness, lethargy, rough hair coat, anorexia, weight loss or failure to gain weight, anemia, diarrhea, increased susceptibility to opportunistic infections, and sudden death. Diagnosis is based on dietary history and clinical signs, especially hemorrhages and joint defects. Subclinical vitamin C deficiency may be seen secondary to several conditions that preclude adequate nutrition. Treatment includes daily administration of vitamin C (5-10 mg/kg, PO or IM, for 1-2 wk). Multivitamin preparations should be avoided due to potential toxicity of other vitamins. Foods should provide a minimum of 10 mg vitamin C daily (30 mg daily for pregnant sows). Commercial guinea pig diets should be stored properly under cool and dry conditions and used within 90 days of the milling date. Vitamin C may also be supplied daily at levels of 250-500 mg/L in fresh drinking water.

Anorexia: Loss of appetite is a problem observed in many guinea pig diseases, postsurgical recovery, ketosis, exposure to drafts, water deprivation, or malocclusion. Changes in feed or water or the feeders or watering devices may also trigger inappetence. Without supportive care and nutrition, the anorectic animal's condition may rapidly deteriorate, resulting in hepatic lipidosis and eventual death. Irreversible ketosis may develop even in guinea pigs that resume eating. Treatment includes provision of preferred or sweetened foods, high caloric food supplements, yogurt, blended baby food, ground pelleted diet, 50% glucose solution, and vitamin C. Sick guinea pigs that refuse to eat may temporarily require force feeding via nasogastric or orogastric intubation.

Pregnancy Toxemia (Ketosis): Obesity or large litter size leading to uterine ischemia, fasting during the late stages of pregnancy, low energy intake, lack of exercise, environmental stress, and inherited hypoplasia of uterine vessels may contribute to the development of pregnancy toxemia in guinea pigs. This syndrome usually occurs during the final 2-3 wk of gestation or first week postpartum and most commonly affects pregnant sows with their first or second litters. Although its occurrence in pregnant guinea pigs is common, ketosis is also reported in obese males and nonpregnant females. Clinical onset may be asymptomatic with sudden death or progressive with lethargy, anorexia, adipsia, muscle spasms, incoordination, coma, and death within 4-5 days. Abortion may occur. Laboratory findings include aciduria, proteinuria, ketonuria, hyperkalemia, hyperlipemia, anemia, and thrombocytopenia. Gross lesions include fatty livers and uterine and placental hemorrhage or necrosis. Treatment is rarely successful, but oral propylene glycol and parenteral calcium gluconate and corticosteroids have been recommended. With the onset of clinical signs, the prognosis is generally poor. Preventive measures include limiting food intake to avoid obesity, not fasting, avoiding exposure to stress during late pregnancy, and providing a high-quality ration throughout gestation.

Hypocalcemia (Eclampsia): Pregnant sows may develop acute calcium deficiency from the metabolic demands of parturition and lactation. This condition is seen more often in multiparous, obese, and stressed females, 1-2 wk prior to or immediately after parturition. Similar to pregnancy toxemia (*see* above), affected animals may be asymptomatic and die suddenly, or show dehydration, depression, anorexia, muscle spasms, and convulsions. Gross lesions are also similar to pregnancy toxemia, but are usually more severe. Hypocalcemic guinea pigs should be administered calcium gluconate. Prevention includes feeding a high-quality commercial diet formulated for guinea pigs.

Metastatic Calcification: Often asymptomatic, metastatic calcification occurs primarily in male guinea pigs >1 yr old. Clinical signs may include weight loss, muscle and joint stiffness, renal failure, or more often, sudden death. Gross lesions include calcium deposits in the lungs, liver, heart, aorta, stomach, colon, kidneys, joints, and skeletal muscles. The increase in organ mineralization is thought to be related to inappropriate diets high in calcium and phosphorus and low in magnesium and potassium. This condition may be minimized or prevented by feeding diets that contain adequate magnesium (0.3-0.4%), calcium (0.9-1.1%), phosphorus (0.6-0.7%), and potassium (0.4-1.4%), ≤6 IU of vitamin D/g, and with a calcium:phosphorus ratio of 1.5:1.

Vitamin E Deficiency (Nutritional Muscular Dystrophy): Guinea pigs fed diets deficient in vitamin E may develop clinical signs of stiffness, hindlimb weakness, lameness, lethargy, decreased reproductive performance, conjunctivitis, or death 1 wk after onset. Serum CK levels are elevated. Grossly, muscles appear pale due to coagulative necrosis. Treatment may be attempted by administering vitamin E daily. Diets should provide vitamin E at 50 mg/kg and be stored under cool, dry conditions.

Respiratory Diseases

Pneumonia: The most frequent cause of death in guinea pigs is pneumonia, usually associated with bacterial infection. While *Bordetella bronchiseptica* is the most commonly diagnosed agent, other pathogens such as *Streptococcus pneumoniae* or *S zooepidemicus* may be involved. Less frequently, *Klebsiella pneumoniae, Pasteurella pneumotropica, Pseudomonas aeruginosa, Citrobacter freundii, Staphylococcus aureus,* or adenovirus may be implicated. Clinical signs of respiratory distress may include mucopurulent nasal discharge, sneezing, and labored breathing. Infection may be accompanied by conjunctivitis, fever, weight loss, depression, or anorexia. Sudden death with sepsis often occurs during epizootic outbreaks. Diagnosis is based on clinical signs, pneumonic lesions observed at necropsy, and isolation of the causative organism from nasal or conjunctival washes. Radiographs may also show the presence of pulmonary lesions. Treatment is generally supportive and consists of fluid administration, forced feeding if necessary, oxygen therapy, and vitamin C. Antibiotic therapy should be undertaken cautiously because most commonly used antibiotics are toxic for guinea pigs. Parenteral antibiotics considered safe in guinea pigs include chloramphenicol, enrofloxacin, and trimethoprim-sulfa. Nebulization may be a more effective means of administering antibiotics in severe cases. Antibiotics that cause diarrhea should be discontinued. In colonies, prevention and control depends on maintaining good husbandry and sanitation practices and removing affected or carrier animals.

***Bordetella bronchiseptica* Infection:** Asymptomatic guinea pigs may harbor this gram-negative, nonsporeforming rod in the nasal cavity and trachea. Subclinical infections are more common in colonies, but epizootic outbreaks can occur rapidly with high morbidity and mortality. Transmission is by aerosol or, in its genital form, through sexual contact. Genital infection may cause infertility, stillbirths, and abortions. Several other species may be asymptomatic upper respiratory carriers, including dogs, cats, rabbits, rats, and mice. Contact with these potential hosts should be avoided. Necropsy may reveal lung consolidation and mucopurulent exudate in the bronchi, trachea, and middle ear. Vaccination with a nonadjuvant canine bacterin may protect guinea pigs for several months. Although generally considered to be safe, bacterins must not contain aluminum hydroxide because guinea pigs are easily sensitized. Vaccination may cause a localized, mild upper respiratory infection.

***Streptococcus pneumoniae* Infection:** A gram-positive coccus, seen in pair and chain formations, *S pneumoniae* may be asymptomatically carried by guinea pigs. Epidemics may occur due to starvation or stress, with resultant high morbidity and mortality. Transmission is by aerosol or direct contact. Necropsy reveals an acute, fibrinopurulent bronchopneumonia. Other lesions may include pleuritis, pericarditis, otitis media, peritonitis, endometritis, and arthritis. Diagnosis is based on clinical signs, gross lesions, gram stain of tissue smears, and isolation of the organism. Appropriate antibiotics may control a colony outbreak, but will most likely create subclinical carriers.

Adenovirus Infection: Adenovirus is species-specific for guinea pigs and may cause a primary respiratory pneumonia. The asymptomatic carrier state is thought to be common, but prevalence is unknown. Clinical disease, while rare, can be initiated by stress or inhalation anesthesia and occurs more often in immunocompromised, young, or aged animals. Morbidity is low, but animals usually die suddenly without clinical signs. In addition to various bacterial infections, other differential diagnoses include Sendai virus, parainfluenza, cytomegalovirus, and herpesvirus.

Eye and Ear Diseases

Conjunctivitis: Ocular discharge, conjunctival hyperemia, and redness around the eyelid margins are frequently the result of infection with *Chlamydophila (Chlamydia) psittaci*, or other bacteria (*Bordetella bronchiseptica*, *Streptococcus* spp, *Salmonella* spp, *Staphylococcus aureus*, or *Pasteurella multocida*). Chlamydial infection is typically self-limiting and subclinical, most often noted in guinea pigs 4-8 wk old. Full recovery normally takes place within 4 wk. Diagnosis is based on demonstrating antigenic immunofluorescence or intracytoplasmic inclusion bodies in Giemsa- or Macchiovello-stained conjunctival smears. Treatment for chlamydial infection, if necessary, should include sulfonamide systemic or ophthalmic antibiotics.

Otitis Media and Interna: Otitis may be seen with bacterial infections, most commonly *Bordetella bronchiseptica*, *Streptococcus pneumoniae*, *S zooepidemicus*, *Klebsiella pneumoniae*, *Staphylococcus aureus*, and *Pseudomonas aeruginosa*. Opportunistic nasopharyngeal pathogens seen less frequently include *Pasteurella* spp and *Actinobacillus* spp. Otitis media is usually subclinical and may coincide with bacterial infections causing pneumonia. The tympanic membrane is thickened and a purulent discharge may be present. Deafness may occur in severe cases. If infection migrates to the inner ear, additional neurologic signs can develop, including ataxia, head tilt, circling, or rolling. Because it is difficult to navigate the guinea pig's tiny ear canals with an otoscope, the diagnosis is best obtained by radiography. Osteosclerosis and bony lysis of the osseous bullae are radiopaque. Treatment is supportive for the underlying cause, but most cases of otitis are generally unresponsive.

Gastrointestinal Diseases

Diarrhea: A variety of organisms may adversely affect the guinea pig's GI system, causing clinical signs ranging from diarrhea to emaciation, lethargy, dehydration, and death. Potential pathogens include *Clostridium piliforme* (Tyzzer's disease), *Escherichia coli*, *Salmonella* spp, *Citrobacter freundii*, coronavirus-like particle, *Eimeria* *caviae, Balantidium coli, Cryptosporidium wrairi,* and *Paraspidodera uncinata* (cecal worm). Affected animals may die acutely without symptoms or, in chronic cases of gastroenteritis, exhibit a range of signs such as lethargy, anorexia, rough hair coat, perineal staining, loose stools, hunched posture, listlessness, dull eyes, dehydration, weight loss, pain on abdominal palpation, flatulence, and fever or hypothermia. Treatment of diarrhea is similar for most causes. Dietary roughage should be increased and grains and concentrates decreased. This can be accomplished by providing hay in addition to a commercial pelleted diet. Feeding *Lactobacillus* spp, in the form of yogurt with active cultures, may help reestablish normal bacterial flora within the digestive tract. Supportive care is important, and hydration must be maintained through oral or parenteral fluids. Antibiotics can further disrupt the bacterial flora of the GI tract and exacerbate the diarrhea and thus should be used cautiously.

Ptyalism (Slobbers) and Malocclusion: Several diseases are characterized by wet, matted hair around the mouth, chin, and ventral neck. Drooling occurs whenever mastication or deglutition is impaired, usually secondary to dental abnormalities. However, subclinical vitamin C deficiency can also cause ptyalism due to mandibular deformity, as can folate deficiency, excess dietary fluoride, genetic factors, and teeth deviated by periodontal infection or trauma. Like other rodents, guinea pig teeth grow continuously. Malocclusion may result in tooth overgrowth and difficult mastication. When ptyalism is noted, the mouth should be evaluated carefully. Premolar and anterior molar teeth are more commonly affected, but incisors are often noted first. Significant weight loss and oral bleeding may result, and tooth root abscesses may lead to sinus infections. Incisor teeth can be clipped or cheek teeth filed to improve occlusion, but if malocclusion continues, dental prophylaxis at monthly intervals may be necessary. If vitamin C deficiency has resulted in mandibular deformity, the prognosis is poor. Colony animals should be removed to prevent passing the condition to progeny.

Skin Diseases

Dermatophytosis (Ringworm): Fungal skin infections in guinea pigs are caused most often by *Trichophyton mentagrophytes* and less frequently by *Microsporum* spp. Many animals are asymptomatic carriers of fungal pathogens, which are ubiquitous in the environment. Active disease is seen more often in younger or stressed guinea pigs, with patchy alopecia, usually starting at the head and characterized by irregularly shaped, crusty, flaky skin lesions with reddened margins. Facial lesions occur around the eyes, nose, and ears, but the disease can spread over the posterior portions of the back. Transmission is by direct contact or on fomites, such as bedding. Diagnosis is based on lesions, Wood's lamp examination, and by isolation of the causative agent in or on infected hairs. Ringworm usually is self-limiting if good husbandry and sanitation are maintained. Secondary bacterial infections may cause small pustules and skin abscesses. Effective treatment consists of 5-6 wk of oral griseofulvin. Griseofulvin is teratogenic and should not be given to pregnant females. Isolated skin lesions may be treated effectively with topical griseofulvin, tolnaftate, or butenafine creams applied daily for 7-10 days. Prevention includes decreasing any potential for stress, culling affected stock from colonies, good husbandry practices, and adequate sanitation of the environment. Ringworm is highly contagious to humans and other animals.

***Staphylococcus aureus* Infection (Pododermatitis, Bumblefoot):** Chronic inflammation, ulceration, and hyperkeratosis may be observed on one or more footpads. *S aureus* is frequently isolated from lesions, probably entering the skin through abrasions. Predisposing factors include obesity, wire floor caging, poor sanitation, and trauma. Chronic cases may progress to lymphadenopathy, arthritis, tendinitis, and amyloid accumulation in kidney, liver, adrenal glands, spleen, and pancreatic islets. Diagnosis is based on clinical signs and culturing the organism. If detected early, animals should be switched to smooth-bottom flooring, sanitation improved, and bedding changed to softer material. Wounds should be cleaned and hair clipped around the lesions. Overgrown nails should be trimmed. Affected feet should be soaked in warm disinfecting solution such as chlorhexidine or dimethyl sulfoxide combined with appropriate topical antibiotics.

Severe cases may require appropriate parenteral antibiotics (eg, chloramphenicol, trimethoprim-sulfa, enrofloxacin) and dexamethasone. Cases unresponsive to therapy may require amputation at the sacrohumeral joint to prevent amyloidosis.

Alopecia: Several underlying causes may lead to hair loss. Barbering or hair chewing can be a self-inflicted abnormal behavior or result from social status conflicts among adult males or between adults and weanlings. Patchy hair loss is often observed and the underlying skin may or may not have evidence of bite wounds and possible secondary dermatitis. Preventive measures include separating affected animals, decreasing environmental stress, early weaning, and feeding long-stemmed hay. Genetic and metabolic factors are thought to be responsible for thinning hair loss observed in frequently bred female guinea pigs. Hair usually regrows following the cessation of breeding. Weaning animals may also demonstrate thinning hair loss as the hair coat changes to coarser adult fur or when fed protein-deficient diets.

Severe infestation of **fur mites** (*Chirodiscoides caviae*) may result in pruritus and alopecia along the posterior trunk of the body, while underlying skin is relatively unaffected. Subclinical cases may be asymptomatic. *Trixacarus caviae*, a sarcoptid mite common to guinea pigs, burrows into the skin and may produce intense pruritus, alopecia, and dermatitis. Distribution is on the inner thighs, shoulders, and neck. Underlying skin may be dry or oily and thickened or crusty. Severely infected animals may show signs of secondary bacterial infection and stress, including weight loss, lethargy, and running about the cage; untreated cases may progress to convulsions and death. Transmission of either mite is by direct contact or contaminated fomites. Diagnosis is made by examining hair shafts or skin scrapings and identifying the mite. *Chirodiscoides* mites are found only in the fur, are ovoid and elongated, and often found in male-female pairs. *Trixacarus* mites are found by skin scrapings or biopsy. Treatment includes dusting with permethrin or carbamate powders or sprays. Ivermectin may be administered twice at 7- to 10-day intervals, although infections are reported to persist. Prevention includes improving sanitation and decreasing environmental stress.

Lice infestation is usually asymptomatic but in severe cases may lead to pruritus, alopecia, and dermatitis around the neck and ears. Lice may be observed directly on hair shafts with a magnifying glass. *Gyropus ovalis* is seen more commonly and is long and slender compared to *Gliricola porcelli*. Affected guinea pigs should be treated with permethrin or carbamate dusts or sprays or ivermectin. Prevention includes improving sanitary conditions in the animal's environment.

Reproductive Diseases

Mastitis: Acutely inflamed mammary glands are frequently observed during lactation. Trauma or skin lacerations may predispose females to infection with a variety of bacteria, including *Escherichia coli*, and *Pasteurella, Proteus, Klebsiella, Staphylococcus, Streptococcus*, and *Pseudomonas* spp. Clinically, the affected mammary glands are painful and enlarged, warm, firm, and cyanotic. Sepsis may occur and lead to fever, anorexia, depression, dehydration, agalactia, maternal neglect, or death. Milk may be thick or bloody and clotted. Treatment includes appropriate antibiotics, such as chloramphenicol, trimethoprim-sulfa, or enrofloxacin. Prevention includes improving sanitation and animal husbandry practices and removal of potentially abrasive bedding material.

Generalized Diseases

Streptococcal Lymphadenitis (Cervical Lymphadenitis, Lumps): Inflammation and enlargement of the cervical lymph nodes is common in guinea pigs. The causative organism is usually β-hemolytic, gram-positive, encapsulated *Streptococcus zooepidemicus*, although *Streptobacillus moniliformis* or other bacteria may also cause a similar syndrome. Organisms may gain entry to the lymphatics from abrasions of the oral mucosa or from the upper respiratory tract. Clinically, large and sometimes unilateral swellings or abscesses are palpable in the ventral neck. Lymph nodes are variably affected. Systemic involvement may extend to cause otitis media, panophthalmitis, pneumonia, or acute septicemia in younger animals. Other clinical signs depend on the body systems involved and may include head tilt, sinusitis, conjunctivitis, labored breathing, cyanosis, hematuria, hemoglobinuria, abortions, stillbirths, arthritis, peritonitis, pericarditis, hepatitis, or sudden death. Transmission is by aerosol, genital contact, or direct entry through skin lesions or oral cavity abrasions. Gross lesions vary with organ involvement, with chronic suppurative abscesses in cervical lymph nodes, pleura, lungs, liver, uterus, or middle and inner ears. Diagnosis is based on clinical signs, bacterial culture, and identification of chains of gram-positive organisms on direct smears from abscesses. Antibiotic therapy may not be effective in controlling or eliminating the organism, although chloramphenicol, trimethoprim-sulfa, cephalosporin, or enrofloxacin may be used. Abscesses can rupture spontaneously, be surgically incised and drained, or preferably removed, but this may result in septicemia. For prevention, abrasive materials in feed or litter should be avoided. Malocclusions and overgrown teeth should be corrected and upper respiratory infections treated if present. Sanitation should be improved and affected and exposed guinea pigs removed from colonies to prevent further spread.

Salmonellosis: Various serotypes of *Salmonella* (*S typhimurium*, *S enteriditis*, and *S dublin*) may infect guinea pigs. All ages are susceptible, but disease is more often observed in younger or stressed animals. Infection may be subclinical, and diarrhea is rarely present. Clinical signs include conjunctivitis, fever, lethargy, anorexia, rough hair coat, palpable hepatosplenomegaly, cervical lymphadenitis, and abortion in pregnant sows. Mortality is often high in epizootic outbreaks. If animals recover, intermittent shedding of organisms may occur. Transmission is by direct contact with ocular secretions of infected animals or oral-fecal route. Infection may enter a colony through feed, bedding, or water contaminated by wild rodents. Fresh vegetables, such as cabbage or kale, or hay are potential sources of *Salmonella*. Grossly, infected animals have enlarged spleens and lymph nodes, with multifocal necrosis in the liver, spleen, or other organs in chronic cases. Diagnosis is accomplished by isolating the organism from blood, ocular secretions, lymph nodes, or spleen. Due to zoonotic considerations and potential for a carrier state, treatment is not recommended.

Yersinia pseudotuberculosis Infection: Clinical illness due to *Y pseudotuberculosis* may take one of several forms: acute septicemia with sudden death, chronic wasting with diarrhea and death in 3-4 wk, cervical lymphadenopathy, or subclinical infection and carrier state followed by clinical infection. Transmission occurs via ingestion of contaminated feed, bedding, or water; inhalation; or through skin wounds. Diagnosis is confirmed by isolation of the organism from blood or abscesses. Gross lesions include enlarged or abscessed lymph nodes and necrosis of liver and spleen. *Yersinia*-infected colonies should be depopulated, the environment disinfected, and sanitation and husbandry corrected.

Neoplasia

Although skin tumors and leukemia may affect younger guinea pigs, other types of cancer are rarely seen in guinea pigs until they are 4-5 yr old. Thereafter, the incidence may reach 15-30%. Inbred strains are more often affected.

HAMSTERS

Syrian hamsters (*Mesocricetus auratus*, golden hamster) are the species most commonly encountered in companion and laboratory animal medicine, although a number of other close relatives have gained popularity in recent years, including the Chinese hamster (*Cricetulus griseus*), European hamster (*Cricetus cricetus*, black-bellied hamster), Armenian hamster (*Cricetulus migratorius*, migratory gray hamster), Djungarian hamster (*Phodopus sungorus*, Siberian, Russian, or furry-footed hamster), Turkish hamster (*M brandti*, Brandt's hamster), and others. Among Syrian hamsters, there are several hair and coat color varieties. Infectious diseases are uncommon compared to other rodent species, but hamsters are susceptible to a wide range of experimentally induced pathogens and oncogenic tumors. Individual pets may often be seen for conditions related to age, trauma, or improper care.

Syrian hamster adults average ~6 in. in length and 120 g body wt. The normal lifespan is 18-24 mo. Females are typically larger and more dominant and aggressive than males.

Anatomically, hamster cheek pouches are highly distensible components of the lateral buccal walls used primarily to store and transport food. These immunologically privileged sites can easily be evaginated under anesthesia if impaction occurs. Hip or flank glands, more prominent in males, are sebaceous glands with pigmented cells and terminal hairs that produce oily secretions during sexual arousal in both sexes. These secretions are important for territorial marking. Hamsters are nocturnal and should be well secured in their housing environments to prevent escape. While they do not truly hibernate, hamsters can be induced to enter pseudohibernation at temperatures <41°F (5°C).

Aggression may occur with introduction of new hamsters to a group, although same-sex weanlings raised together usually remain compatible. Pregnant females develop a distended abdomen and rapidly gain weight by day 10 of gestation. The relatively immature pups are delivered by day 16 of gestation. Pseudopregnancy may result from infertile matings.

Management

Physical Examination: The animal's overall appearance and behavior, particularly in relation to its cagemates, should be noted. Sick animals are often isolated from others and may show weight loss, hunched posture, lethargy, rough hair coat, labored breathing, and a loss of exploratory behavior. Early signs of illness involve changes in the color, consistency, odor, and volume of urine and feces. The perineal area should be checked for fecal or urine stains or discharges from the vulva in females. Fecal samples may be taken for parasite detection and bacterial culture. The fur and skin should be examined for alopecia, fight wounds or other trauma, ectoparasites, and elasticity for evidence of dehydration. The oral cavity should be checked for overgrown teeth or impacted cheek pouches. Ears should be examined for discharges or inflammation and eyes for discharges or conjunctivitis. Feet should be examined for sores and overgrown or broken nails. The abdomen should be palpated for masses. Body temperature is normally 98-101°F (37-38.5°C). A pediatric stethoscope should be used to auscultate the thorax.

Hamsters are not normally aggressive, but can be provoked if suddenly startled or awakened or roughly handled. It may be easier to scoop hamsters up in a small container rather than pick them up directly. Their highly elastic skin should be grasped sufficiently to prevent the animal from biting.

Disease Treatment and Prevention: For drug or therapeutic administration in hamsters, PO, SC, IM, IV, and IP routes are used. Antibiotics effective against gram-positive bacteria are not well tolerated by hamsters due to adverse changes in GI flora (*see* p 1636). Oral medications or other fluids can be administered into the oral cavity with an eye dropper or directly into the stomach by gavage with a ball-tipped needle. The flank and interscapular regions are common sites for SC injections ≤1.0 mL. The caudal quadriceps or hamstring muscles are preferred sites for IM injections and should be limited to volumes <0.1 mL or necrosis may result. Intraperitoneal injections up to 4-5 mL are administered on either side of the midline in the inguinal region with the hamster's head tilted downward to avoid the large cecum. IV injections (≤0.1 mL) and blood collection are very difficult in hamsters because they have few accessible veins. Those that may be attempted include the lateral tarsal, anterior cephalic, and lingual veins. Appropriate needle sizes are 27-30 gauge. In critically ill animals, interosseous injections can be made in the tibial crest using a 22-gauge spinal needle under anesthesia. Small amounts of blood can be collected via toenail clip or by puncturing a footpad or ear pinna. Larger amounts may be collected from the retro-orbital sinus of anesthetized animals. Dehydration may occur with diarrhea or other illnesses. Fluid therapy should be isotonic and selected according to the animal's condition. Prevention of health problems should be emphasized to pet owners, including complete and balanced diets, clean sources of water and bedding, and frequent disinfection and sanitation of housing equipment. Indoors, hamsters should be maintained at temperatures of 64-79°F (17-26°C).

Dental Care: Overgrown incisors may result in hypersalivation, anorexia, and weight loss. Treatment includes periodically trimming affected teeth and providing materials for the hamster to gnaw and wear teeth down naturally.

Finely ground food is sometimes retained in molar teeth, making hamsters prone to development of dental caries.

Nutrition: In the wild, hamsters are omnivorous. Commercial pelleted diets formulated for rats and mice with 15-20% protein provide adequate nutrition. Although supplements are generally unnecessary, the 25% higher fiber found in commercial rabbit diets may be supplemented to offset the amount of dietary protein consumed. Hamsters tend to hoard food and will hide food pellets in their cheek pouches or around the cage floor. They are normally coprophagic. Watering systems should be sanitized regularly to prevent contamination by opportunistic bacteria.

Vitamin E Deficiency: Vitamin E deficiency may lead to hemorrhagic necrosis of the CNS in fetal hamsters. Clinically, female hamsters may deliver weak or stillborn pups or cannibalize their litters. Grossly, hemorrhage or edema is observed in the calvarium and spinal canal. In adult hamsters, Vitamin E deficiency may lead to nutritional myopathy and paralysis. This condition can be avoided by provision of a balanced diet formulated specifically for hamsters.

Gastrointestinal Diseases

Diarrhea: Diarrhea in hamsters, sometimes collectively referred to as "wet tail" by its clinical appearance, may signal one of several GI diseases.

Proliferative Enteritis (Proliferative Ileitis, Wet Tail): Proliferative enteritis is a frequent cause of diarrhea in hamsters. Recently, the causative agent was determined to be identical to *Lawsonia intracellularis*, a bacteria that causes proliferative enteritis in swine. Precipitating factors include recent transport, overcrowding, surgery, and dietary changes. Clinically, it is more common in younger hamsters with sudden onset, high morbidity and mortality, and signs of watery diarrhea and matting of fur around the tail and ventral abdomen. Affected hamsters may be lethargic, anorectic, and lose weight. Transmission is by the fecal-oral route. Gross pathology may include ileal thickening, enlarged mesenteric lymph nodes, peritonitis, and abdominal adhesions. Definitive diagnosis includes typical signs and lesions and PCR identification of the organism from fresh or frozen intestinal contents. Treatment includes supportive fluids (oral electrolyte solutions or lactated Ringer's solution, SC) for dehydration (5-15% body wt), 1-2 mL bismuth subsalicylate, PO, and appropriate antibiotics such as tetracycline, enrofloxacin, metronidazole, or trimethoprim-sulfa, which can be administered via the drinking water. Some reports indicate the effectiveness of erythromycin (20 mg/kg body wt, PO, or 200 mg/mL drinking water), although it carries a higher risk for antibiotic toxicity. Affected animals should be isolated to prevent further spread and the environment properly sanitized and disinfected.

Tyzzer's Disease (*Clostridium piliforme*): Occasionally reported in hamsters and other rodent species, *C piliforme* may cause clinical signs of enteritis similar to *Lawsonia* spp with anorexia, dehydration, watery diarrhea, and sudden death. Transmission is by the fecal-oral route, and clinical disease is reported more often in younger or stressed animals. Gross lesions include dilation and hyperemia of large intestines; foamy, yellow fecal contents; and hepatic and cardiac necrosis. Diagnosis is based on signs and demonstrating the gram-negative intracellular organisms with Giemsa or silver stains in histologic sections of the intestine, liver, or heart. Infection can also be diagnosed by PCR. Serologic detection by ELISA is variable. Supportive fluids and treatment with tetracycline or metronidazole are recommended to reduce colony mortality. Affected and exposed animals should be isolated to prevent further spread. Because the bacteria is a spore-former, the housing environment should be thoroughly sanitized and disinfected.

Antibiotic-associated Enterocolitis (Clostridial Enteropathy): Administration of antibiotics selective for gram-positive bacteria such as lincomycin, clindamycin, ampicillin, vancomycin, erythromycin, gentamicin, penicillin, and cephalosporins may cause a fatal enterotoxemia with profuse diarrhea and high mortality within 2-10 days. Normal hamster bacterial microflora includes *Lactobacillus* and *Bacteroides* spp. Following inappropriate antibiotic administration, overgrowth with *Clostridium difficile* results, leading to an acute colitis. The cecum is distended with fluid, and intestinal hemorrhages are evident. Diagnosis includes history of antibiotic administration and identification of the causative organism via anaerobic culture. There are also reports of enteropathy associated with *C difficile* overgrowth in hamsters not treated with antibiotics. Prognosis for affected animals is poor. Treatment is generally supportive, with parenteral fluids and kaopectate. Oral gavage of a fecal suspension derived from normal hamsters may help reestablish normal intestinal bacterial flora.

Salmonellosis: *Salmonella enteritidis* and *S typhimurium* infections are uncommon in hamsters. Clinical signs, lesions, and diagnosis are as described in gerbils (p 1624).

***Escherichia coli* Infection:** Although clinically similar to other causes of diarrhea in hamsters, histopathologic changes of *E coli* infections do not include hyperplasia of the intestinal epithelium. Diagnosis is based on isolation of the organism. Treatment and prevention are similar to that for proliferative enteritis.

Protozoa: Normally abundant in hamsters, protozoal organisms such as *Giardia muris mesocricetus, Spironucleus muris,* and *Tritrichomonas muris* may cause opportunistic intestinal infections and diarrhea in young or stressed animals. Fecal smears may show a large number of protozoa. Treatment includes metronidazole in the drinking water for 14 days.

Nematodes: Pinworm infections, including *Syphacia obvelata* and less often, *S muris* and *S mesocricetti,* are rare causes of intestinal diseases in hamsters. Diagnosis and treatment are as described in gerbils (p 1624).

Cestodes: Infection of hamsters with *Rodentolepis nana* (dwarf tapeworm) or *Hymenolepis diminuta* are relatively common when compared to mice and rats, although usually asymptomatic. Heavy infections may cause enteritis, intestinal impaction, and mesenteric lymph node abscesses. Diagnosis and treatment are as described in gerbils (p 1624).

Constipation: Constipation may be associated with tapeworms in the small intestine, ingestion of bedding and subsequent intestinal obstruction, and intestinal intussusception caused by enteritis, pregnancy, poor diet, or insufficient drinking water. Treatment requires correcting the primary cause. Enterotomy and intestinal anastomosis may be necessary.

Actinomycosis: Rare in hamsters, *Actinomyces bovis* can lead to salivary gland abscessation and mucopurulent discharge. Diagnosis is based on isolation of the organism on anaerobic culture. Treatment includes lancing and draining the abscesses and appropriate antibiotics.

Cholangiofibrosis (Cholangiohepatitis, Chronic Hepatitis and Cirrhosis): Chronic hepatitis and cirrhosis are sometimes seen in older hamsters, more often in females. Clinically, serum ALT and bilirubin are significantly elevated. The etiology is unproven, but *Helicobacter cholecysticus* has been isolated from gallbladders of affected hamsters. There is no effective treatment.

Skin Diseases

Cutaneous Abscesses: Skin abscesses may occur secondary to fighting or other trauma. These are frequently located around the head; *Staphylococcus aureus, Streptococcus* spp, *Pasteurella pneumotropica,* and *Actinomyces bovis* are common bacterial isolates. If cervical lymphadenitis is observed, the cheek pouches may also be infected. In male hamsters, hypersecretory flank glands may be infected. Wood shavings in bedding sometimes penetrate the footpad and lead to degeneration and atrophy of digits and necrotic ulcers along the shoulders. Diagnosis is based on isolation of the organism on aerobic and anaerobic cultures. Treatment includes surgical drainage and appropriate antibiotics. Ruptured abscesses should be expressed to empty remaining contents and flushed with antiseptic solution; a topical antibiotic cream may be applied as needed. Unruptured abscesses can be surgically removed and appropriate parenteral antibiotics should be administered. If flank glands are involved, the hair around the lesions should be clipped and cleaned and appropriate topical antibiotics with a corticosteroid applied.

Castration may decrease flank gland secretory activity. Fighting hamsters should be separated and caging checked for sharp edges or protrusions. Bedding with wood shavings should be avoided.

Alopecia: Constant rubbing on feeders or sides of the cage, nutritional protein deficiency, and barbering (hair chewing by cagemates) may lead to patchy areas of hair loss. Mite infestation, adrenal tumors, thyroid deficiency, and chronic renal disease may also cause hair loss.

Dermatophytosis (Ringworm): Fungal skin infections occur infrequently in hamsters. The most commonly isolated dermatophytes are *Trichophyton mentagrophytes* and *Microsporum* spp. Infection may be asymptomatic or result in small, patchy alopecia. Lesions are characterized by irregular to circular, crusty, flaky skin lesions with reddened margins. Transmission is by direct contact or fomites such as cage bedding. Diagnosis is based on lesions, Wood's lamp examination, and isolation of fungus in or on infected hairs. Effective treatment may include topical fungicidal ointments, clipping hair from affected areas, povidone-iodine scrubs, or oral griseofulvin. Ringworm is contagious to humans and other animals.

Acariasis: Two species of demodectic mites, *Demodex criceti* and *D aurati*, are commonly found on hamsters. Increased incidence has been reported in males and older animals or secondary to malnutrition or concurrent disease. Dry, scaly dermatitis and alopecia are often seen over the back and rump. Denuded areas are nonpruritic, dry, and scaly. Other species of mites reported in hamsters include *Sarcoptes scabei*, *Notoedres* spp (ear mite), *Speleorodens clethrionomys* (nasal mite), and *Ornithonyssus bacoti* (tropical rat mite). *Notoedres* may cause dermatitis of the ears, face, feet, and tail. Diagnosis is by identification of the mites in skin scrapings or digestion of hair samples in 10% potassium hydroxide or sodium hydroxide. Treatment for demodicosis includes 1% selenium sulfide shampoo and topical amitraz. Ivermectin is recommended for treating other mite species. Bedding should be changed frequently and the environment sanitized and disinfected.

Respiratory Diseases

Pneumonia: Pneumonia, although uncommon in hamsters, may result from infections of several bacteria individually or in combination with viruses or mycoplasmas. Potential bacterial pathogens include *Streptococcus pneumoniae*, *S agalactiae*, *Pasteurella pneumotropica*, other *Pasteurella* spp, *Staphylococcus aureus*, *Klebsiella pneumoniae*, *Bordetella* spp, *Corynebacterium paulometabulum*, and *Salmonella* spp. Many of these bacteria are normal respiratory or GI flora, but sudden environmental changes, especially temperature, may lead to stress and opportunistic infection. Clinical signs of acute respiratory disease include mucopurulent nasal or ocular discharge, dyspnea, anorexia, and depression. Diagnosis is based on clinical signs, pneumonic lesions observed at necropsy, and isolation of the causative organism from nasal or conjunctival washes. Treatment is generally unrewarding, but appropriate antibiotics (chloramphenicol, trimethoprim-sulfa, or enrofloxacin) may be effective in mild cases. Additional supportive therapy includes parenteral fluids; warm, dry housing; and minimizing stressors. In colonies, prevention and control depends on proper husbandry and sanitation practices and isolating affected animals.

Sendai virus (Parainfluenza 1) is an RNA paramyxovirus occasionally seen in hamsters. A highly contagious virus most often transmitted by aerosol, Sendai may cause nasal discharge, dyspnea, pneumonia, and mortality in newborn hamsters, but is often asymptomatic in adults. Secondary bacterial infections may also develop. Histologic lesions of Sendai virus infection include a mild necrotizing bronchiolitis and focal interstitial pneumonia. Diagnosis is accomplished by ELISA and immunofluorescent antibody tests. Treatment is supportive with subcutaneous fluids, nutritional support, and appropriate antibiotics for secondary bacterial infections. Prevention includes avoiding contact with potentially infected hamsters or other rodents.

Generalized Diseases

Lymphocytic Choriomeningitis Virus (LCMV, Arenavirus) Infection: This RNA arenavirus is occasionally reported in hamsters, although wild mice usually serve as the natural reservoir. Contaminated tumors or cell lines are the usual source of LCMV in laboratory outbreaks. Infection may be transmitted in utero, congenitally, or horizontally via aerosol or direct contact with urine or saliva or animals shedding virus. Generally, the disease is subclinical and many animals clear the infection, but hamsters with persistent infections shed large quantities of virus in the urine and can serve as a source of human infection. Some hamsters develop a chronic wasting disease with convulsions, depression, weight loss, and decreased reproduction in females. Gross lesions may include enlarged liver and spleen, swollen or shrunken and pitted kidneys, or lymphadenopathy. Histologically, there are lymphocytic infiltrates and vasculitis in the liver, spleen, lung, meninges, and brain, and chronic glomerulonephropathy. Diagnosis is based on pathology and serologic detection of antibodies via ELISA or immunofluorescent antibody tests. There is no effective treatment. Affected animals should be euthanized and the environment appropriately sanitized and disinfected. Potential sources of wild rodent contamination should be eliminated. The zoonotic potential is significant; LCMV may cause influenza-like symptoms or viral meningitis or encephalomyelitis in humans.

Amyloidosis: Amyloidosis causes soluble proteins to polymerize as insoluble fibrils and is commonly observed in hamsters >1 yr old and in those with chronic infections. The condition is usually subclinical until renal function is impaired by amyloid deposits. Azotemia then leads to clinical signs of anorexia, rough hair coat, hunched posture, generalized edema, and depression. Disease occurs more often in female hamsters due to sex hormone regulation of amyloid. Clinically, an increase in serum albumin is accompanied by an increase in serum globulins, proteinuria, and hypercholesterolemia. Grossly, kidneys, adrenal glands, and liver are pale and enlarged. Histologic lesions are easily visualized with Congo red stain. Treatment includes general supportive care, but the prognosis is poor.

Polycystic Disease: A common lesion in hamsters >1 yr old, polycystic disease most often affects the liver, creating single or multiple thin-walled, fluid-filled cysts ≤3 cm in diameter. Other tissues affected include epididymis, seminal vesicles, pancreas, endometrium, ovaries, and adrenal glands.

Yersiniosis (Pseudotuberculosis): Infection with *Yersinia pseudotuberculosis* in hamsters usually results from fecal contamination of food or water by wild rodents and birds. Clinically, the infection leads to either an acute septicemia or chronic emaciation and intermittent diarrhea. Grossly, caseous lesions develop in the mesenteric lymph nodes, spleen, liver, lungs, gallbladder, and intestinal walls. Diagnosis is based on serology and isolation of the causative agent. Treatment is not effective nor recommended. Because it is a zoonotic pathogen, colonies should be depopulated, potential sources of infection eliminated, and housing thoroughly sanitized and disinfected.

Tularemia: *Francisella tularensis* is rarely reported in hamsters. It causes acute septicemia with high morbidity and mortality. Transmission is either direct or indirect through arthropod vectors. Clinically, animals may have rough hair coats, and death occurs within 48 hr of onset. Gross lesions include hemorrhagic lungs, enlarged and necrotic liver and spleen, prominent Peyer's patches, and enlarged mesenteric lymph nodes. Treatment is not effective nor recommended. It is a zoonotic pathogen; colonies should be depopulated, potential sources of infection eliminated, and housing thoroughly sanitized and disinfected.

Reproductive Diseases

Infertility and Perinatal Mortality: Decreased reproductive performance may result from old age, malnutrition, abnormal light cycles, normal winter seasonal quiescence, cold environment, breeding pair incompatibility, inadequate nesting material, and anestrous or primiparous females. Pregnant females may abort, abandon, or cannibalize their litters for a variety of reasons, including inadequate nutrition or availability of water, large fetal loads, group housing, excessive handling of mothers or pups, presence of a male in the cage postpartum, inadequate nesting materials, agalactia, mastitis, sick or deformed pups, or noise. Optimal female hamster reproduction occurs between 5 wk and 15 mo of age. Both monogamous pairs and polygamous harem mating systems are commonly employed by breeders. As hamsters approach parturition, they may become restless and active, and vulvar bleeding is evident. At parturition, hamsters should be given nesting material to provide additional security and privacy and prevent hypothermia, abandonment, or cannibalization of newborn litters. Litters should not be disturbed for at least 7 days postpartum, especially in primiparous females. Cross-fostering of pups is rarely successful. Normal litter size averages 6-8 pups and weaning occurs 21-28 days postpartum.

Mastitis:　Acute bacterial mastitis in hamsters has been associated with opportunistic infections of β-hemolytic *Streptococcus* spp. Clinical signs are noted 7-10 days after parturition. Affected mammary glands are swollen and mucopurulent exudate may be present. Females may cannibalize their litters. Diagnosis is based on isolation of the organism; treatment includes appropriate antibiotics.

Cardiovascular Diseases

Atrial Thrombosis:　Atrial thrombosis and congestive heart failure frequently occur in older female hamsters and are often associated with amyloidosis. Thrombi are most commonly found in the left atria. Clinically, disease is recognized by dyspnea, tachycardia, and cyanosis due to congestive heart failure. There is no effective treatment.

Urinary Diseases

Arteriolar Nephrosclerosis (Hamster Nephrosis):　This degenerative renal disease is found most frequently in aged hamsters and is more common in females. Hamsters have weight loss, polyuria, and polydipsia. Etiologies are thought to be secondary to chronic lymphocytic choriomeningitis virus infection, renal vascular hypertension or antigen-antibody complex deposition. Amyloidosis may be concurrent. Grossly, affected kidneys are irregular, granular and pitted. Histologic changes include interstitial fibrosis, basement membrane thickening, and tubular dilation with proteinaceous eosinophilic material and casts.

Ocular Diseases

Conjunctivitis:　Conjunctivitis and facial swelling may occur secondary to trauma, maloccluded or overgrown teeth, or abscessed tooth roots. Conjunctivitis may also be present with bacterial infections, bedding dust, or bite wounds. Warm water can be used to help open closed eyelids. Eyes should be flushed with saline solution and boric acid or appropriate antibiotic ophthalmic ointment applied as needed.

Neoplasia

Spontaneous malignant neoplasms are reported in 4% of Syrian hamsters, with marked variation in individual colonies, reflecting both genetic and environmental influences. The majority of hamster tumors are benign and originate in endocrine or alimentary organs. Adrenocortical adenomas are among the most frequently observed. Cutaneous lymphomas are seen in adult hamsters with clinical signs of lethargy, weight loss, patchy alopecia, and dermatitis. The most common malignant tumor is lymphosarcoma and may involve the thymus, thoracic lymph nodes, mesenteric lymph nodes, spleen, or liver. Other tumors reported include uterine carcinoma, intestinal polyps, glioblastoma, astrocytoma, medulloblastoma, ependymoma, pineocytoma, melanoma, benign tumors of hair follicles or sebaceous glands, keratoacanthomas, squamous papillomas and carcinomas, lymphosarcomas, and basal cell tumors.

PRAIRIE DOGS

Black-tailed prairie dogs (*Cynomys ludovicianus*) are gregarious ground squirrels that are increasingly popular as companion animals, although not without some controversy. Although wild-caught prairie dogs can adapt to captive indoor environments and even bond with humans, they may also be stressed or injured when removed from their natural setting and social hierarchy. Prairie dogs will bite and may harbor zoonoses. In research settings, prairie dogs have proven useful animal models of biliary physiology, gallstone disease, and *Clostridium difficile* cecitis. Several *Cynomys* spp are listed as threatened or endangered by the USA Fish and Wildlife Service, and the black-tailed prairie dog may become subject to provisions of the Endangered Species Act.

Adult prairie dogs are 12-16 in. (30-40 cm) long and weigh 2-4 lbs (1-2 kg), with males slightly larger than females. They have rudimentary cheek pouches and tails covered with fur. The natural lifespan is 8 yr for females and 5 yr for males, although that may be extended in captivity. In nature, prairie dogs live in large and complex social hierarchies referred to as towns, which may cover several acres. Towns are subdivided into colonies or wards that are further subdivided into distinct social family units called coteries. Coteries usually consist of an adult male, 1-4 adult females, and any offspring <2 yr old. Prairie dogs are diurnal and more active during the cooler hours of the day, when they feed and socialize. Female prairie dogs are monoestrous and produce an average litter of 4-5 pups in the spring. The gestation period is 34-35 days and pups are born blind and hairless. After weaning at 7 wk of age, young males soon move away, while females typically spend their entire lives in their original coterie. Female-female aggression increases significantly during pregnancy and lactation.

Physical Examination: The animal's overall appearance and behavior, particularly in relation to its cagemates, should be noted. Early signs of illness involve changes in the color, consistency, odor, and volume of urine and feces. The perineal area should be checked for fecal or urine stains or discharges from the vulva in females. Fecal samples may be taken for parasite detection and bacterial culture. The fur and skin should be examined for alopecia, fight wounds or other trauma, ectoparasites, and elasticity for evidence of dehydration. The oral cavity should be checked for overgrown teeth or impacted cheek pouches. Ears should be examined for discharges or inflammation and eyes for discharges or conjunctivitis. Feet should be examined for sores and overgrown or broken nails. Body temperature is normally 96-102°F (35-39°C). The thorax should be ausculted with a pediatric stethoscope.

Disease Treatment and Prevention: For drug or therapeutic administration in prairie dogs, PO, SC, IM, IV and IP routes are used. Like chinchillas and guinea pigs, the prairie dog's intestinal flora is sensitive to the adverse effects of gram-positive antibiotics on normal GI flora. Overgrowth of gram-negative bacteria can rapidly lead to septicemia and endotoxin production. Supplemental *Lactobacillus* in the diet may help offset prolonged antibiotic therapy. Drugs and dosages described for guinea pigs and chinchillas generally suffice for use in prairie dogs. Oral medications or other fluids can be administered with an eye dropper or directly into the stomach by gavage with a ball-tipped needle. The flank and interscapular regions are potential sites for SC injections. The caudal quadriceps or hamstring muscles are preferred sites for IM injections. Restraint for IM or SC injections can be accomplished by wrapping the animal in a towel. Intraperitoneal injections are administered on either side of the midline in the inguinal region with the prairie dog's head tilted downward to avoid the large cecum. IV injections and blood collection may be attempted via the cephalic or lateral saphenous veins or jugular vein under anesthesia. Smaller amounts of blood can be collected via toenail clip or puncturing a footpad or ear pinna. Dehydration may occur with diarrhea or other illnesses and fluid therapy should be isotonic and selected according to the animal's condition.

Nutrition and Housing: Prairie dogs can be maintained on good quality commercial rodent diet, alfalfa cubes, and ad lib timothy or grass hay. Pelleted diets and alfalfa should be decreased as animals mature to prevent obesity or gallbladder disease. They do not require treats. Prairie dogs have voracious appetites and during summer will normally store up fat reserves for hibernating in winter. Although prairie dogs are not true hibernators, they may enter a dormant state if exposed to ambient temperatures <55°F (13°C). Watering systems should be sanitized regularly to prevent contamination by opportunistic bacteria. Prairie dogs can be trained to use a litter pan for elimination. Their housing should be well-secured because the prairie dogs' natural curiosity and chewing behavior will likely expose them to a number of household dangers such as toxic chemicals or electrical cords. Large plastic rodent cages can be placed inside a larger container to prevent bedding from spreading around during burrowing activities. Animals kept as pets or research animals should be provided adequate space and materials for burrowing. Nest boxes can be used to simulate the natural burrow environment. Prairie dogs should be maintained at temperatures of 69-72°F (20.5-22°C) and relative humidity of 30-70%.

Diseases

Sylvatic Plague: Prairie dogs are highly susceptible to infection with *Yersinia pestis*, a gram-negative, nonsporeforming, pleomorphic bacteria that causes sylvatic plague. Transmission primarily results from flea bites or via aerosolization and direct contact. Currently, sylvatic plague is widespread throughout the western USA. Plague epizootics have very high morbidity and mortality in prairie dog populations, which may limit further spread. Infected animals may be lethargic and anorectic. Gross lesions may be limited due to the animal's rapid death. Subtle lesions that may be present include splenomegaly, hemorrhagic lymphadenitis, and pulmonary edema. Diagnosis is based on history of sudden high mortality, direct fluorescent staining, and isolation of the causative organism. Of all human plague cases reported to the CDC where a source of infection was identified, 31/240 (13%) were attributable to contact with prairie dogs. Preventing transmission of plague infections to humans requires adequate personal protective equipment (eg, goggles, masks, respirators, gowns, gloves, etc), appropriate sanitation and disinfection, wild rodent control, flea removal from all animal species present (carbamate flea dust), avoidance of sick or dead animals, and appropriate antibiotics (tetracyclines, trimethoprim-sulfa).

Tularemia: *Francisella tularensis* is a gram-negative bacteria; infection is rarely reported in prairie dogs. Infection may cause an acute septicemia with high morbidity and mortality. Transmission is either direct or indirect through arthropod vectors. Clinically, animals may have ataxia, dehydration, severe diarrhea, and sudden death. Gross lesions include purulent bronchopneumonia and multifocal necrosis of liver and spleen. Diagnosis is based on direct fluorescent antibody tests and isolation of the causative bacteria from culture of liver and spleen. Treatment is not effective nor recommended. Because tularemia is zoonotic, colonies should be depopulated, potential sources of infection eliminated, and housing thoroughly sanitized and disinfected.

Monkeypox Infection: A recent case documented transmission of monkeypox virus from infected Gambian rats to prairie dogs at an exotic pet distributor in the USA. Clinical signs include profuse nasal discharge, ocular discharge, dyspnea, lymphadenopathy, and mucocutaneous lesions. Both animal-to-animal and animal-to-human transmission have been confirmed. Primary transmission is by direct contact with infected animals or ingestion of inadequately cooked flesh. There is no effective treatment. Because monkeypox virus is zoonotic, infected colonies should be depopulated, potential sources of infection eliminated, and housing thoroughly sanitized and disinfected. Wild animal species of differing origins should be housed separately.

Diarrhea: Several conditions may cause diarrhea in prairie dogs, including overeating, rapid dietary changes, *Eimeria* sp intestinal coccidia, *Salmonella* sp or *Clostridium piliforme* (Tyzzer's disease) bacterial infections (*see* p 1626), or antibiotic-induced changes in intestinal flora. Poor eating habits should be corrected. Supportive therapy includes parenteral fluids and oral bismuth subsalicylate (0.2-0.5 mL/lb, TID). Coccidia may be treated with sulfadimethoxine. In cases of antibiotic-induced toxemia, *Lactobacillus acidophilus* can help reestablish GI microflora.

Respiratory Disease: In wild prairie dogs, respiratory disease with dyspnea or pneumonia may be due to infectious causes such as *Pasteurella multocida* bacteria or *Pneumocoptes penrosei* (pulmonary mites). Diagnosis requires isolation of infectious organisms. Treatment includes general support, appropriate antibiotics, and ivermectin for control of mites. Noninfectious respiratory disease is more commonly seen in captive prairie dogs. Diet and environmental conditions are suspected to be underlying causes. Clinically, prairie dogs have open-mouth breathing, which may be due to nasal discharge, airways blocked by inhalation of foreign bodies (eg, dust, lint) or dental problems. Volatile oils in cedar bedding may lead to both respiratory disease and allergies. Noninfectious rhinitis or other allergic discharges have been reported to respond favorably to oral antihistamines and nasal decongestants.

Preputial Blockage: Intact adult males in captivity that do not mate can develop an accumulation of urine, secretions, and debris in the prepuce. If this material concentrates and hardens, it may lead to discomfort, bacterial infection, and necrosis of the penis. This condition is most commonly observed during or following the annual reproductive season in October-January. Purulent discharge may be seen around the preputial orifice with variable signs of urinary incontinence. Treatment under sedation involves manually removing preputial debris and thoroughly cleansing the prepuce with 10% povidone-iodine solution. If bacterial infection is suspected, isolating the organism through culture and sensitivity are indicated to determine treatment.

Malocclusion: Overgrowth of the incisors and molars may occur. If the condition interferes with eating, prairie dogs will become anorectic and lose weight and condition. They may also hypersalivate, with excess moisture on their muzzles and ventral thorax, along with partially eaten food. If maloccluded teeth continue to grow, adjacent tissues may be traumatized. To treat, the animal should be sedated or anesthetized and overgrown teeth clipped back to normal length using bone forceps or nail trimmers or, in the case of fractured teeth, a high-speed rotary hand tool. Affected animals should be removed from breeding populations if the trait appears to be heritable.

Alopecia: The most frequent causes of hair loss in prairie dogs include self-trauma from rubbing on wire cages, poor nutrition, ectoparasites (fleas, lice, ticks), and dermatophytes (*Microsporum* and *Trichophyton* spp).

Fungal infection may be asymptomatic or cause small, patchy areas of alopecia. Lesions are characterized by irregular or circular, crusty, flaky skin lesions with reddened margins. Transmission is by direct contact or on fomites such as cage bedding. Diagnosis is based on lesions, Wood's lamp examination, and isolation of fungus in or on infected hairs. Effective treatment may include topical fungicidal ointments, clipping hair from affected areas, povidone-iodine scrubs, or oral griseofulvin. Ringworm is contagious to humans and other animals. Ectoparasites can be treated with 0.5% malathion dips or cat flea preventatives and environmental control.

Fractures: Poor nutrition with low levels of calcium or trauma may result in fractured leg bones. Unless the prairie dog is restrained from chewing off bandages, casts, or splints, affected limbs may require amputation. Fractures require ≥3-6 wk to heal. Pelvic fractures are common in adult prairie dogs and may heal on their own if the animal is housed in a way that prevents climbing.

Pododermatitis: Rough cage floors, poor sanitation, or traumatic lesions of the feet may lead to abrasions, ulcers and chronic infection by opportunistic infections of *Staphylococcus aureus*. Diagnosis is based on clinical signs and culture of the organism. If detected early, animals should be switched to smooth-bottom flooring and sanitation should be improved, including more frequent changes of softer bedding material. Nails may require frequent trimming. Wounds should be cleaned and hair clipped around the lesions. Affected feet should be soaked in warm, disinfecting solution such as chlorhexidine or dimethyl sulfoxide combined with appropriate topical antibiotics. Severe cases may require appropriate parenteral antibiotics (eg, chloramphenicol, trimethoprim-sulfa, enrofloxacin) and dexamethasone.

Neoplasia: In prairie dogs, primary hepatocellular carcinoma is a relatively common tumor. Many cases are also associated with chronic active hepatitis. Odontomas are significant causes of upper respiratory signs in prairie dogs and may be related to mechanical trauma of upper incisor teeth. Other reported tumors include renal cortical adenoma, gastric adenocarcinoma, lipoma, and epiglottal fibrosarcoma.

Baylisascaris spp Infection: Following raccoon contamination of captive prairie dog environments, *Baylisascaris* larvae may migrate to the CNS and cause ataxia, incoordination, head tilt, and loss of righting reflexes. Gross lesions may not be apparent, but cross-sections of large ascarid larvae are found on histology of the brain. There is no treatment.

Taenia mustelae Infection: Wild-caught prairie dogs may have fluid-filled cysts in the liver that contain encapsulated larval cestodes (*T mustelae*).

Zoonoses

In general, prairie dogs, should be handled with utmost care and housed and maintained separate from other wild rodent species. There is great potential for crossover of infectious diseases to this very susceptible host.

RATS AND MICE

Rats (*Rattus norvegicus*) and mice (*Mus musculus*) are the most commonly encountered rodent species in companion and laboratory animal medicine. They are social, active, intelligent, and make good pets. Their adaptiveness, small size, rapid reproduction and extensive genetic characterization also greatly enhance their value as laboratory animals. Among laboratory rats and mice, there are >1,000 inbred and outbred strains and thousands more genetic mutants. Pet rodent pedigrees may be hard to determine.

Male rats and mice are typically larger than females. Both rats and mice have Harderian glands that produce a reddish-brown porphyrin pigment frequently observed around the eyes and face of sick or stressed animals. Neither rats nor mice can vomit and rats do not have gallbladders. Albino rodents have degenerative retinas and poor eyesight. Mice and rats are nocturnal and are usually more active during the dark cycle. They may spend hours grooming themselves and their cagemates. Aggression is unusual in domesticated rats or in mice raised together as littermates, although female and male mice of certain strains (C57B1/6 or BALB/c) are prone to fighting. When new groups of animals are housed together, they should be observed carefully for fight trauma and weight loss or abnormal behaviors such as hair chewing or barbering.

Onset of puberty and the estrous cycle are influenced by exposure to pheromones, especially in mice. Females are typically brought to the male's cage for breeding and both monogamous and polygamous breeding schemes are commonly used by breeders. Average gestation is 19-21 days for mice and 21-23 days for rats. Pregnancy is detectable at day 14 in both rats and mice by palpation, weight gain, and evidence of mammary development. Tissue paper can be used by females for nesting material. The average litter size is 10-12 pups for mice and 6-12 pups for rats. Weaning occurs 21-28 days postpartum in mice and 21 days postpartum in rats. The normal lifespan is 1.5-2.5 yr in mice and 2.5-3.5 yr in rats.

Management

Physical Examination: The animal's overall appearance and behavior, particularly in relation to its cagemates, should be noted. Animals that rear up and face an approaching hand are more likely to bite. Mice can be picked up by the base of the tail or removed from their cage in cupped hands. For restraint, mice can be grasped by the loose skin of the neck with the tail held between the palm and little finger. Rats may be grasped gently over the shoulders and lifted up. The head can be restrained by placing the thumb and forefinger just behind the jaws. They can also be steadied by grasping the tail, but only at the base to prevent degloving. Adult body weight is 20-40 g in mice and 250-500 g in rats.

Sick rodents may be isolated from cagemates and potentially show clinical signs, including weight loss, hunched posture, lethargy, rough hair coat, rapid or labored breathing, and closed or squinted eyes. Early signs of illness can involve changes in the color, consistency, odor and volume of urine and feces. The perineal area should be checked for fecal or urine stains or discharges from the vulva in females. Fecal samples may be taken for parasite detection and bacterial culture. Fur and skin should be examined for alopecia, fight wounds or other trauma, ectoparasites and elasticity for evidence of dehydration. Subcutaneous swellings may indicate abscesses or tumors. The oral cavity should be checked for overgrown incisor teeth. Ears should be examined for discharges or inflammation and eyes for discharges or conjunctivitis. Porphyrin pigment around the eyes, face, or forepaws may indicate stress. Feet should be examined for sores and overgrown or broken nails. The abdomen can be palpated for masses. Normal body temperature is 99.5-100.6°F (35.9-37.5°C) in rats and 98-101°F (36.5-38°C) in mice. The thorax can be ausculted with a pediatric stethoscope.

Disease Treatment and Prevention: Drug or therapeutic administration in mice and rats includes PO, SC, IM, IV, and IP routes. Oral medications or fluids can be administered into the oral cavity with a ball-tipped needle (20 gauge for rats, 22 gauge for mice). Maximal volumes for oral medications should be limited to 1.0 mL in rats and 0.1 mL in mice. The flank and interscapular regions are common sites for SC injections up to1.0 mL in mice and 5.0 mL in rats using 23- to 25-gauge needles. The caudal quadriceps or hamstring muscles are preferred sites for IM injections and should be limited to volumes <0.1 mL in mice and <0.2 mL in rats to prevent necrosis. IP injections up to 2.0 mL in mice and 5.0 mL in rats are administered in the lower right quadrant of the abdomen with the animal's head tilted downward to displace and avoid the large cecum. IV injections and blood collection may be attempted using the lateral tail veins with a 25-gauge needle. (Warm water may help dilate the tail veins prior to injection or blood collection.) Small amounts of blood can be collected by nicking the tip of the tail or the lateral saphenous vein along the rear leg. Larger amounts may be collected from the lateral tail veins or retro-orbital sinus of anesthetized animals. In terminal procedures under deep anesthesia, blood may be collected from intracardiac puncture. The total volume of blood collection should be ≤1% of body wt (eg, 0.2 mL for a 20 g mouse, 3.0 mL for a 300 g rat). While antibiotics generally do not cause the severe gram-negative enterotoxemia seen in hamsters and guinea pigs, little is known about drug efficacy in rats and mice. Bacterial infections may respond favorably to antibiotic treatment, but many pathogens persist and relapses may occur. Therapy for common viral infections is generally supportive as there are no specific treatments. Dehydration may require isotonic fluid therapy (0.9% saline or 5% dextrose). Animals not drinking water orally require 40-80 mL fluids/kg/day, administered SC or IP in divided doses 3-4 times per day (eg, 1-2 mL/day for a 25 g mouse or 16-32 mL/day for a 400 g rat). Rats and mice have a limited capacity for thermoregulation and may overheat or develop hypothermia easily. Indoors, mice and rats should be maintained at 64-79°F (18-26°C) and 40-70% relative humidity.

Dental Care: Overgrown incisors may be congenital or caused by trauma. As the condition progresses, it often leads to difficulty in eating, weight loss, dehydration, and secondary oral and facial trauma. Treatment includes periodically trimming affected teeth with a nail clipper or dental bur and providing appropriate materials for rats and mice to gnaw on and wear teeth down naturally.

Infectious Disease Control in Colonies: Control of infectious diseases in laboratory rodent colonies often requires depopulation or rederivation to prevent further transmission or adverse effects on experiments. Control efforts may include cessation of colony breeding for 6-8 wk to limit the introduction of newly susceptible animals, although this method does not work with immunodeficient mice or rats. More reliable methods of eliminating colony infection include depopulation and restocking with uninfected mice or rederivation by cesarean section or embryo transfer. Colony husbandry practices must be modified to prevent reintroduction of the virus from feral or wild rodents, including vendor screening, monitoring potential infection of tumors and cell lines, quarantine, and use of filtered cage tops or microisolator caging.

Heat Stress: Rats and mice have a limited capacity to regulate body temperature. They do not have sweat glands, nor do they pant. Their primary thermoregulatory mechanism occurs through tail vein dilation or constriction. Ambient temperatures >85°F (29.4°C), high humidity levels (>80%), poor ventilation, and overcrowding predispose rodents to heat exhaustion. Affected animals have high mortality, increased respiratory rates, and increased water consumption. Diagnosis includes history of exposure to high temperatures, lack of water, clinical signs, and gross lesions of hyperemic lungs and mesenteric vessels and thymic hemorrhage. Treatment includes cool water baths, oral gavage with water, and administration of SC saline or 5% dextrose.

Nutrition: In the wild, mice and rats are omnivorous. Commercial pelleted diets formulated for maintenance of laboratory and pet rodents contain ~14-20% protein, 4-5% fat, and are hard enough to wear down constantly growing incisor teeth. Feed should be provided free choice, stored in cool and dry conditions, and used prior to its expiration date. Occasional food treats are permissible, but should be used sparingly to avoid dietary problems. Both rats and mice are normally coprophagic. Watering systems should be sanitized regularly to prevent contamination by opportunistic bacteria.

Gastrointestinal Diseases

Transmissible Murine Colonic Hyperplasia: *Citrobacter rodentium* is a gram-negative, enteric bacteria that causes colonic mucosal hyperplasia. Affected mice have rough hair coats, weight loss, lethargy, runting, diarrhea, and prolapsed rectum with high morbidity and variable mortality. Disease may be self-limiting in adult animals, with recovery in 4-6 wk. Transmission is by fecal-oral ingestion. Adults are less susceptible than suckling and recently weaned pups, and higher mortality may occur in inbred strains. Gross lesions include thickening of the descending colon and cecum. Diagnosis is confirmed by isolation and biotyping of the causative organism and gross and histologic pathology. Nonpathogenic *Citrobacter* sp may also be found in mouse intestines. Treatment includes neomycin (2 g/L drinking water), oxytetracycline (500 mg/L drinking water), or 12.5% sulfadimethoxine in drinking water to control symptoms, although antibiotics alone will not completely eliminate the infection. Rectal prolapses can be reduced using a moistened cotton microswab. Infected animals should be removed from colonies to prevent further spread and the environment properly sanitized and disinfected.

Tyzzer's Disease: Occasionally reported in mice and rats, Tyzzer's disease is caused by *Clostridium piliforme*. Nonspecific clinical signs include anorexia, dehydration, watery diarrhea, and sudden death. Transmission is by the fecal-oral route, and clinical disease is reported more often in younger or stressed animals. Gross lesions include dilation and hyperemia of large intestines with foamy, yellow fecal contents and hepatic and cardiac necrosis. Diagnosis is based on signs and demonstrating the gram-negative intracellular organisms using Giemsa or silver stains on histologic sections of the intestine, liver, or heart. Infection can also be diagnosed by PCR or ELISA. Supportive fluids and treatment with oxytetracycline (500 mg/L drinking water) or metronidazole (2.5 mg/mL drinking water with 1% sucrose added for palatability) are recommended to reduce colony mortality. Affected and exposed animals should be isolated to prevent further spread.

***Helicobacter* sp Infection:** *H hepaticus, H bilis, H rodentium,* and *H typhlonicus* are gram-negative, spiral, motile bacteria that can cause enterohepatic disease in mice. Transmission is by the fecal-oral route. Many *Helicobacter* spp are considered commensal intestinal flora in rodents. Rats and hamsters are not reported to develop disease, but may serve as a reservoir of infection for mice. Most mice colonized with *Helicobacter* spp are asymptomatic until 6 mo of age. Infected females from susceptible immunocompetent mouse strains (eg, A/J, BALB/c, C3H) and immunocompromised mice may develop proliferative, inflammatory typhlitis and colitis, often accompanied by a prolapsed rectum. Infected male mice from susceptible immunocompetent strains (eg, A/J) develop chronic active hepatitis, which may progress to hepatic carcinoma. Diagnosis includes isolation of the organism, although culture is difficult and not all pathogenic *Helicobacter* spp cause liver disease. Characteristic bacteria may be visualized in microscopic sections of liver and PCR may be performed on fecal specimens. Treatment with a combination of bismuth subsalicylate, metronidazole, and ampicillin may control signs, but will not eliminate infection. Infected animals should be removed from colonies to prevent further spread and the environment properly sanitized and disinfected.

Mouse Hepatitis Virus (MHV) Infection: MHV is a highly contagious polytropic RNA coronavirus infection of both pet and laboratory mice. Potential routes of transmission include fecal-oral, direct contact, aerosols, and fomites. Clinically, there are 2 main patterns of disease based on the tropism of the viral strain. The enteric pattern infects intestinal mucosa and, to a lesser extent, upper respiratory tract, liver, and brain. The respiratory pattern features viral replication in the nasal cavity and lungs, with subsequent viremia and dissemination to other organs; intestinal involvement is minimal. Disease expression varies with viral strain and host factors including age, genotype, and immune function. In immunocompetent mouse strains, MHV infections are usually subclinical and end in 2-3 wk as antibodies develop. With epizootic infections of virulent MHV, younger mice may develop watery diarrhea with high morbidity and mortality. Infection of immunodeficient mouse strains can lead to a chronic and fatal wasting disease and eventual death. If present, gross lesions include gaseous distention of the intestines in young mice and multifocal hepatic necrosis in older mice. Histopathology may reveal blunt intestinal villi, syncytia within the mucosal epithelium, or focal liver necrosis. Diagnosis is accomplished by characteristic histopathology, ELISA or immunofluorescent antibody (IFA) serology, or PCR of tissue or fecal specimens to detect viral antigen. Other than supportive therapy, there are no effective treatments.

Sialodacryoadentitis Virus and Rat Coronavirus Infection: These coronaviruses infect the upper respiratory tract, Harderian glands, lacrimal glands, and the submandibular and parotid salivary glands in rats. They are highly contagious and transmitted by direct contact, aerosols, and fomites. While morbidity is high, viral infection is usually subclinical and mortality is low. Infected rats may exhibit a 2- to 3-wk course of sneezing, photophobia, and a reddish-brown oculonasal discharge (porphyrin pigment). Infected lacrimal glands cause decreased tear production and can eventually lead to keratoconjunctivitis, corneal ulceration, and cataracts. Gross lesions include rhinitis, enlarged submandibular and parotid salivary glands, edematous cervical lymph nodes, swollen lacrimal glands, corneal ulcers, and cataracts. Diagnosis includes classic pathologic lesions, ELISA and IFA serology, and PCR of Harderian or submandibular salivary glands. Lesions are usually self-limiting, and infected animals recover with immunity.

Mouse Rotavirus Infection (Epizootic Diarrhea of Infant Mice, EDIM): EDIM is caused by an RNA group A rotavirus that replicates in small-intestinal epithelial cells. Transmission occurs via fecal-oral, direct contact, and aerosol routes. Infection is inapparent in adult mice, but carriers can infect susceptible neonatal mice that subsequently develop watery, yellow diarrhea and perianal impactions. Mortality is low and infected mice continue to nurse, a clinical feature that can be used to differentiate rotavirus from MHV, in which young mice often quit nursing. Mice that survive rotavirus infection frequently have stunted growth. Grossly, intestines are distended with gas and mucoid fecal material. Diagnosis includes detection of viral antibody using ELISA or IFA serology, or viral antigen with PCR or ELISA assay of fecal contents. Perianal fecal masses can be removed with warm water soaks. Other treatment is generally supportive.

Nematodes: Oxyurid pinworms are relatively common intestinal parasites in mice and rats. More common pinworms observed in mice include *Syphacia obvelata* and *Aspiculuris tetraptera*, and in rats, *S muris*, although infections may cross over between species. *Syphacia* spp deposit eggs in the perianal region, while *A tetraptera* release eggs into the colon that are passed in fecal pellets. All have direct life cycles and transmission is by the fecal-oral route. Infected mice are usually asymptomatic. Mild enteritis and rectal prolapse may occur with heavy infection or in immunocompromised animals. Diagnosis includes identifying perianal eggs retrieved from cellophane tape impression smears (*Syphacia* spp) or fecal flotation (*A tetraptera*) or visualizing white, hair-like adult nematodes in the cecum or colon. Treatment includes 3 separate 7-day courses of piperazine (4-7 mg/mL drinking water) or ivermectin (0.4 mg/kg, SC or PO) separated by 5 days to account for the pinworm's life cycle. Fenbendazole mixed in the feed at 0.1% and fed 3-4 wk also eliminates pinworm infection. Because *Syphacia* spp eggs are light and may aerosolize, it is important to sanitize and disinfect the housing environment.

Cestodes: Infection of rats and mice with *Rodentolepsis nana* (dwarf tapeworm) or *Hymenolepsis diminuta* (rat tapeworm) is relatively uncommon and usually asymptomatic. *R nana* has direct life cycle and can potentially infect humans if ingested. Both tapeworms are transmitted indirectly; cockroaches, beetles, or fleas are intermediate hosts. Heavy infections can lead to enteritis, diarrhea, and weight loss. Diagnosis is by identifying hexacanth ova in fecal contents or viewing adults in histopathologic sections of small intestine. Recommended treatment is niclosamide mixed in powdered feed at 10 mg feed/100 g body wt for two 7-day periods separated by a week. Also effective are thiabendazole (0.33% mixed in the feed for 7-14 days) or praziquantel (5-10 mg/kg, IM, SC, or PO, repeated in 10 days). The animal's environment should be appropriately sanitized and disinfected and potential intermediate hosts eliminated.

Mice and rats are potential intermediate hosts for the cat tapeworm *Taenia taeniaformis*. The cysticercoid cyst (*Cysticercus fasciolaris*) embeds in the liver, which may become enlarged with numerous cysts. Infection occurs when mice and rats ingest ova in feed or bedding contaminated with cat feces. Treatment is not required, but prevention includes eliminating potential sources of infection.

Protozoa: Occasionally seen in younger or stressed rats and mice, protozoa such as *Giardia muris*, *Spironucleus muris*, and *Tritrichomonas muris* may cause opportunistic intestinal infections leading to abdominal distension, runting, and diarrhea. Transmission is by the fecal-oral route. Fecal smears may show a large number of protozoa. Treatment includes metronidazole (2.5 mg/mL drinking water for 14 days). This may decrease parasite loads, but only rederivation by cesarean section or embryo transfer will successfully eliminate colony infection.

Respiratory Diseases

Murine Respiratory Mycoplasmosis (MRM): *Mycoplasma pulmonis* is a gram-negative, pleomorphic bacteria that colonizes respiratory epithelium and causes both acute and chronic respiratory disease in rats and mice. Transmission includes direct contact, aerosol, and intrauterine routes. Incidence is low in laboratory rodent colonies, but mycoplasmal infection may still be encountered in pets. MRM is often subclinical, although respiratory symptoms can be exacerbated by concurrent bacterial and viral infections or high intracage ammonia levels. Overt disease is characterized by reddish-brown ocular and nasal discharge, head tilt, rough hair coat, hunched posture, anorexia, labored breathing, and coughing. Uterine mycoplasmal infection may decrease litter size. Gross lesions include purulent discharge in nasal mucosa and tympanic bullae, trachea, and bronchi. Pneumonic lungs have a red, brown, and yellow cobblestone appearance. Purulent discharge may also be present with uterine and ovarian infections. Histopathologic lung lesions include peribronchiolar lymphoid hyperplasia. Diagnosis is based on clinical signs, lesions, and isolating the organism, although it is difficult to culture. ELISA and PCR provide the most rapid diagnostic tests. Serum samples should be collected from older animals, because antibody development may take up to 8 wk. Immunocytochemical techniques can also be used to identify the organism on histologic sections of trachea and lungs. While antibiotic treatment with tetracycline (500 mg/L drinking water) or tylosin (500 mg/L drinking water) helps suppress clinical respiratory disease, eliminating infection from a colony requires depopulation and restocking with uninfected rodents or rederivation by embryo transfer. Cesarean section may not be successful due to the potential for uterine infection.

Cilia-associated Respiratory (CAR) Bacillus Infection: CAR bacillus is gram-negative filamentous bacteria found on the cilia of the respiratory tract. It causes a chronic respiratory disease similar to *M pulmonis* infection and is often seen concurrently with mycoplasmas or viruses. Clinical disease is more often seen in rats. If present, respiratory lesions and signs are similar to mycoplasmal infection. The most likely mode of transmission is by direct contact. Because isolation and culture are difficult, diagnostic methods include ELISA serology and PCR assay of nasal swabs. The bacilli can be visualized using Warthin-Starry or immunoperoxidase stains on histologic lung sections. Treatment is not likely to eliminate infection, although ampicillin (500 mg/L drinking water), sulfamerazine (500 mg/L drinking water), and enrofloxacin (165 mg/L drinking water) have been reported to reduce colony mortality. Rats may be asymptomatic carriers and should not be housed with mice.

Streptococcus pneumoniae **Infection:**   Infection of mice and rats with *S pneumoniae* is uncommon. Transmission occurs by direct contact and aerosol. Animals may be asymptomatic or develop mucopurulent nasal discharge, rhinitis, sinusitis, and conjunctivitis. Septicemia produces lesions in reproductive organs and meninges. Young, old, and stressed rodents are at higher risk for infection. Gross lesions include fibrinopurulent pleuritis, pericarditis, pneumonia, and otitis media. Diagnosis is based on isolation of the organism, gross fibrinopurulent lesions, and tissue impression smears demonstrating the characteristic bacteria. Treatment with oxytetracycline (500 mg/L drinking water for 7 days) may decrease morbidity and mortality in epizootics, but does not eliminate the infection.

Corynebacterium kutscheri **Infection (Pseudotuberculosis):**   *C kutscheri* is a gram-positive bacteria that may infect stressed rats and mice. Bacteria are typically harbored in nasal passages and infection is asymptomatic. Transmission occurs by direct contact. Sick animals may have rough hair coats, hunched posture, anorexia, oculonasal discharge, and dyspnea. In rats, gross lesions include large, white caseous foci in the lungs. Mice have granulomatous lung lesions and purulent, necrotic lesions in abdominal organs. Diagnosis is based on identifying the organisms in gram-stained lung sections or impression smears or through bacterial culture. Treatment with oxytetracycline (500 mg/L drinking water for 7 days) may decrease morbidity and mortality in epizootics, but does not eliminate the infection.

Pasteurella pneumotropica **Infection:**   *P pneumotropica* is a gram-negative coccobacillus of low pathogenicity in rats and mice. Most animals are asymptomatic carriers and transmission occurs by aerosols, fecal-oral, and direct contact routes. It is generally an opportunistic pathogen that may proliferate concurrently with other respiratory pathogens. Clinical signs include conjunctivitis, panophthalmitis, oculonasal discharge, dyspnea, and head tilt. In immunodeficient mice, subcutaneous abscesses, mastitis, metritis, and accessory sex gland abscesses are sometimes observed. Infected tissues are characterized by mucopurulent inflammation and necrosis. Diagnosis is by isolation of the organism and ELISA in mice. Treatment with enrofloxacin (165 mg/L drinking water for 2 wk) has been effective in eliminating colonization.

Sendai Virus Infection: Sendai virus is an RNA paramyxovirus of the Parainfluenza family. It is highly contagious in mice and rats and causes an acute respiratory infection with no carrier state in immunocompetent animals. Sendai virus is transmitted by aerosols and direct contact with infected animals. Infection is usually subclinical, although sick animals may show signs of stunted growth and respiratory involvement with secondary bacterial pathogens. Gross lesions may include patchy lung consolidation and mild interstitial pneumonia. Perivascular lymphocytic cuffing is often observed on microscopic lung sections. Diagnosis is by ELISA, IFA, or PCR. Infection is generally self-limiting.

Pneumonia Virus of Mice (PVM) Infection: Caused by an RNA paramyxovirus of the Pneumovirus family, infection and disease in mice is almost identical to that caused by Sendai virus (*see* above). PVM may also infect rats, in which it is usually asymptomatic.

Rat Respiratory Virus (RRV) Infection: A respiratory disease recently identified in laboratory rats worldwide is thought to be of viral origin and has been tentatively named

RRV. It has been passed from infected rat lungs to reproduce disease in naive rats, but its taxonomic classification remains incomplete. RRV is transmitted by direct contact and through fomites. Most infected rats are asymptomatic. Gross lung pathology is different from other causes of rat respiratory disease, with 1-4 mm gray foci randomly distributed throughout all lung lobes. Histopathology of pulmonary lesions shows angiocentric inflammatory cells of variable severity extending to surrounding interstitium. Diagnosis of RRV is currently limited to gross and microscopic pathology, with IFA serology under development. Control measures have not been established because knowledge of the virus is incomplete.

***Pneumocystis carinii* Infection:**   *P carinii* is a latent pathogen of the respiratory tract in humans and virtually all domestic species, including rats and mice. It spreads by aerosol inhalation of infective cysts. Immunocompetent animals are asymptomatic, but infected rodents immunosuppressed by illness or treatment sometimes develop fatal pneumonia. Clinically affected mice show signs of wasting, rough hair coat, scaly skin, hunched posture, tachypnea, cyanosis, and death. Grossly, lungs are rubbery and fail to deflate. Microscopically, interstitial pneumonia includes alveoli filled with eosinophilic foamy material. Periodic acid-Schiff and Giemsa stains are used to visualize trophozoite stages and a silver methanamine stain is used to demonstrate cysts. PCR may also be used to diagnose infection. Antibiotic treatment such as trimethroprim-sulfa in the drinking water may be attempted to alleviate clinical signs. Eliminating infection is difficult due to the organism's ubiquitous presence in the environment, but rederivation through cesarean section or embryo transfer should be effective.

Skin Diseases

***Staphylococcus* spp Infection:**   *S aureus* and *S epidermidis* are gram-positive bacteria commonly found on the skin of most animal species, including mice and rats. In rats, ulcerative dermatitis may be observed on the head and neck, often secondary to skin trauma from fighting or scratches. Cutaneous infection in nude mice may lead to conjunctivitis and facial abscesses. Abscesses occasionally enlarge and form disfiguring subcutaneous lumps around the face and head (furunculosis). Treatment includes topical antibiotic or antibiotic/steroid ointments. Therapy may be prolonged without correcting the irritant stimulus, and immunosuppressed animals do not respond well. Clipping toenails of the hindfoot helps prevent further damage caused by scratching.

***Corynebacterium bovis* Infection:**   *C bovis* causes scaly skin hyperkeratosis in nude mice. With the exception of other hairless strains, most infected immunocompetent mice are asymptomatic. Bacteria can be present on the skin or in the oral cavity, and transmission occurs by direct contact and fomites. Clinically, affected mice have weight loss, pruritus, and transient hyperkeratosis, primarily along the dorsum. Mortality is low. Diagnosis is based on isolation of the causative organism, PCR for bacterial antigen, gross lesions, and histopathology. Treatment with ampicillin or penicillin may help alleviate clinical signs.

Dermatophytosis (Ringworm):   Fungal skin infections occur infrequently in mice and rats. The most commonly isolated dermatophytes are *Trichophyton* and *Microsporum* spp. Infection is often asymptomatic or characterized by small, patchy areas of alopecia with reddened margins, dermatitis, and flaky exfoliation. Transmission occurs by direct contact or on fomites such as cage bedding. Diagnosis is based on lesions, Wood's lamp examination, isolation of fungus in or on infected hairs, and histology of lesions with a silver stain. Effective treatment includes topical fungicidal ointments, clipping hair from affected areas, povidone-iodine scrubs, or oral griseofulvin (25 mg/kg for 30-60 days). Ringworm is contagious to humans and other animals.

Acariasis: Several mites may infest the skin and fur of mice, most often *Myocoptes musculinus* and *Myobia musculi* and less frequently, *Radfordia affinis* and *Psorergates simplex*. The most commonly reported rat fur mite is *R ensifera*. Transmission is by direct contact. Clinically, rodents may be asymptomatic, or with heavy infestation, demonstrate constant scratching leading to self-induced skin trauma, alopecia, and ulcerative dermatitis. Black-haired mice are reported to be more sensitive to infection. Mites spend their entire life cycle on the host. Lesions are often found along the head and neck and between the shoulder blades. Chronic cases sometimes develop secondary bacterial infections. Diagnosis is accomplished by direct observation of mites or eggs from hair and skin of dead or anesthetized mice. As pelts of recently deceased mice cool to room temperature, mites will crawl up to the tips of the hairs, appearing as white specks. Treatment includes application of silica or pyrethrin dusts, ivermectin solutions in drinking water (equine preparation at 8 mg/L drinking water once a week for 3 wk), or 0.1% ivermectin solutions applied topically. Caution should be exercised (eg, testing) before colony treatment because ivermectin may be toxic in certain strains of mice. Repeat treatments should account for the mite's life cycle. Unhatched eggs may lead to reinfection.

Pediculosis: *Polyplax spinulosa* and *P serrata* are blood-sucking lice commonly encountered in wild rats and mice, but rarely seen in laboratory rodents. The lice spend their entire life cycle in the host and transmission occurs by direct contact. Clinical signs with heavy infestation include pruritus, restlessness, debilitation, and anemia. Diagnosis is based on identification of adult lice, nymphs, or eggs on the fur. Treatment and control area similar to mite infection (*see* above).

Fleas: Rodent fleas (*Xenopsylla* and *Nosopsylla* spp) are uncommon in laboratory or pet rats and mice, but can signal contamination by wild rodents. They are also important potential vectors of zoonotic disease such as *Yersinia pestis*, *Rickettsia typhus*, and *Rodentolepis nana* tapeworms. Diagnosis is based on identification of fleas on affected rodents. Treatment includes carbaryl dusts or pyrethrin sprays and preventing wild rodent contamination.

Ringtail: Low environmental humidity, high temperatures, and drafts predispose young rats and mice to develop annular constrictions of the tail and occasionally feet or digits. Localized edema can lead to dry gangrene and tissue sloughing. Diagnosis is based on clinical signs and history. Treatment is supportive, and tail stumps usually heal without complication. Prevention is accomplished by providing environmental humidity of 40-70%, reducing drafts, and maintaining room temperatures at 70-74°F (21-23°C).

Barbering: Barbering is an abnormal behavior frequently observed in groups of male or female mice and occasionally rats. Dominant members of the group chew the hair and whiskers of subordinates. Affected areas around the face or anterior dorsum appear clean shaven, although the underlying skin is normal. Treatment consists of removing the dominant mouse that has not been barbered.

Fight Wounds: Mice and rats, usually males, often fight and cause trauma to the face, back, and genital areas. Clinically, the skin may have focal alopecia and scabs. Affected mice lose weight and sometimes die. Secondary bacterial infection and abscesses may occur. Tail biting can lead to gangrene and sloughing. Treatment includes cleaning the wounds with povidone-iodine solution, lancing and draining abscesses, and appropriate topical antibiotic ointments. Aminoglycosides are toxic and should be avoided. Control is achieved by separating affected mice.

Generalized Diseases

Salmonellosis: *Salmonella enteritidis typhimurium* is uncommon in laboratory or pet rats and mice. Incidence is higher in pregnant and parturient females and infants. Clinical signs may include diarrhea, dehydration, weight loss, rough hair coat, depression, abdominal distension, abortion, or sudden death. Transmission is by the fecal-oral route and often associated with food, water, or bedding contaminated by wild rodents. Gross lesions include enlarged liver and spleen with areas of small, white focal necrosis, patchy pulmonary hemorrhage, and enteritis. Diagnosis is based on colony history of decreased reproduction and isolation of the organism from affected organs, fecal contents, or blood. Treatment is generally not recommended. Affected animals should be isolated and the environment sanitized and disinfected to eliminate any potential sources of contamination. Salmonellosis is zoonotic and the potential exists for an asymptomatic carrier state.

Streptobacillus moniliformis Infection: *S moniliformis* is a gram-negative bacteria of the upper respiratory tract that causes no clinical signs in its natural host, the rat. Infection of mice, however, can lead to an acute septicemia and high mortality. Survivors may develop chronic arthritis and limb deformities. Although the agent is rarely reported in laboratory rodents, infection is important due to its potential to cause rat-bite fever, a flu-like disease in humans. Diagnosis depends on isolation of the causative organism from blood, joint fluid, or affected organs.

Pseudomonas aeruginosa Infection: *P aeruginosa* normally colonizes nasal cavities and intestinal tracts of rats and mice that are not maintained on sterile or treated water. Disease is rare in immunocompetent animals, but opportunistic infection with septicemia and endotoxemia can occur in immunosuppressed animals. Infected animals may die acutely with no signs or develop rough hair coats, hunched posture, anorexia, and torticollis. Gross lesions may be absent acutely, but *Pseudomonas*-infected organ abscesses contain green-tinged purulent material due to pyocyanin and pyoverdin pigments. Exudate may also be found in the middle ear. Systemic disease cannot be easily treated due to the ubiquitous nature of the organism. Efforts should be focused on prevention by supplying acidified or chlorinated drinking water and adequate sanitation of the housing environment and watering equipment.

Mousepox Infection: Mousepox is caused by ectromelia virus, a DNA poxvirus closely related to vaccinia virus. Transmission occurs by the fecal-oral route or contaminated urine; direct contact with abrasions in the skin provide the main route of entry. In laboratory settings, ectromelia can also be transmitted by inoculation with contaminated tumors, cell lines, or serum products. Disease severity is dependent on the strain of mice involved, with A, C3H, DBA/2, and BALB/c being highly susceptible and AKR and C57BL/6 resistant. Overall, disease is rarely reported, but sporadic outbreaks with high morbidity and mortality may be seen if naive mice are exposed. Affected animals have a hunched posture, conjunctivitis, and facial swelling. Mice that survive the acute phase often develop a skin rash and progressive swelling, necrosis, and amputation of extremities. Gross pathology in acute disease includes visceral congestion, splenomegaly and splenic necrosis, hepatic necrosis, and peritoneal exudate. As the disease progresses, other lesions observed include focal pancreatic necrosis, splenic fibrosis, erosive enteritis, and ulcerative vesicles on the skin of extremities. Microscopically, intracytoplasmic inclusion bodies can be observed in epithelial cells from skin ulcers and in sections of small intestine or pancreas. Diagnosis is accomplished by electron microscopy, PCR, ELISA, or IFA. There is no treatment.

Hantavirus Infection: Hantavirus is an RNA bunyavirus of wild rodents with zoonotic implications for humans. In the USA, infection has been reported in deer mice (*Peromyscus* spp) and cotton rats (*Sigmodon hispidus*). Laboratory infection of rats has been reported due to infected transplantable tumors and cell lines. Infection has not yet been reported in pet rodents. In the natural host, infection is persistent, but usually asymptomatic. Hantavirus infection is transmitted by aerosols or bites contaminated by infected urine, feces, or saliva. Diagnosis is made by ELISA, IFA, or PCR. Control should include exclusion of sources of potential wild rodent contamination. Human infections may result in severe infections with renal or pulmonary involvement.

Parvovirus Infection: Multiple variants of single-stranded DNA parvoviruses infect mice and rats. Only Kilham rat virus (KRV) has been reported to cause clinical disease in rats. Other rat parvoviruses (Toolan's H-1 virus, Rat minute virus, and Rat parvovirus) are antigenically distinct from KRV and not associated with naturally occurring disease. Both Mouse parvovirus (MPV) and Minute virus of mice (MVM) are asymptomatic in natural infections of mice. MVM can cause experimental disease and MPV modulates the immune system. All parvoviruses are highly contagious. Transmission is usually from direct contact with infected urine or feces and fomites. Clinical signs in colony epizootics of KRV include decreased fertility, fetal resorption, and runted, small litters. KRV infection of juvenile male rats may result in fatal hemorrhage and necrosis in the brain and gonads. KRV and MPV infections often persist in lymphoid tissue for many weeks. Gross pathology of KRV infection includes cerebellar hypoplasia, scrotal hemorrhage, and occasionally jaundice. Diagnosis includes ELISA and IFA, although cross reactions occur among the parvoviruses in rats and mice. PCR can identify and speciate specific parvoviruses. New ELISA tests based on structural proteins distinguish between MVM and MPV. Parvoviruses survive for weeks in the environment and sanitation with parvovirucidal disinfectants is necessary to prevent reinfection. Cell lines and other biologic material also should be screened for potential infection.

Lymphocytic Choriomeningitis Virus Infection (LCMV, Arenavirus): Lymphocytic choriomeningitis, caused by an RNA arenavirus, is occasionally reported in mice, rats, and hamsters, although wild mice usually serve as the natural reservoir. Contaminated tumors or cell lines are often the source of LCMV in laboratory outbreaks. Infection can be transmitted in utero, congenitally, or horizontally via aerosols or direct contact with urine or saliva of animals shedding virus. Clinical signs depend on the animal's age and immune status, as well as the viral strain, route of transmission, and dose. The disease is usually subclinical, and most animals clear the infection; others may have persistent viruria and viremia and shed large quantities of virus in the urine. Some rodents develop a chronic wasting disease with renal failure, convulsions, depression, weight loss, and decreased reproduction in females. Gross lesions may include enlarged liver and spleen, swollen or shrunken and pitted kidneys, and lymphadenopathy. Histologically, there are lymphocytic infiltrates and vasculitis in the liver, spleen, lung, meninges, brain, and chronic glomerulonephropathy. Large intracytoplasmic inclusions are present in plasma membranes. Diagnosis is based on pathology, ELISA or IFA, and PCR of kidney or brain tissues. There is no effective treatment and rederivation attempts may fail since transovarian and transuterine infection is possible. Affected animals should be euthanized and the environment appropriately sanitized and disinfected. Potential sources of wild rodent contamination should be eliminated. The zoonotic potential of LCMV is significant and may cause influenza-like symptoms, viral meningitis, and encephalomyelitis in humans.

Reproductive Diseases

Decreased reproductive performance in rodents can result from a variety of causes, including age, malnutrition, abnormal light cycles, cold environment, cystic ovaries, neoplasia, inadequate nesting material, anestrus, or primiparous females. Pregnant females may abort, abandon, or cannibalize their offspring. Common causes include inadequate nutrition or availability of water, large fetal loads, group housing and overcrowding, excessive handling of mothers or pups, presence of a male in the cage postpartum, organophosphate or estrogen contamination of feed, inadequate nesting materials, agalactia, mastitis, sick or deformed pups, and excessive noise. Some commensal GI flora such as *Escherichia coli*, *Proteus*, and *Klebsiella* spp have been isolated from abscessed preputial glands and uterine tract infections of mice. At parturition, female rodents should be given nesting material, both to provide additional security and privacy and to prevent hypothermia, abandonment, or cannibalization of newborn litters. Rodent litters should not be disturbed for at least 7 days postpartum, especially in primiparous females.

Urinary Disease

Leptospirosis: *Leptospira interrogans ballum* and *L interrogans icterohemorrhagiae* are gram-negative bacterial infections reported in wild mice and rats, respectively. Animals develop asymptomatic, persistent infections that colonize renal tubules and are shed in the urine. Diagnosis is based on isolating the causative agent or serology. Leptospirosis is significant for its zoonotic potential.

***Trichosomoides crassicauda* Infection:** *T crassicauda* is a rarely reported nematode of rats that infects the urinary bladder. Severe burdens may result in unthriftiness, dysuria, and eosinophilia. Treatment is similar to that for cases of intestinal pinworms (*see* above).

Nervous System Diseases

Mouse Poliovirus Infection (Theiler's Meningoencephalitis Virus, GD VII strain): This virus causes demyelination in the brain and spinal cord of mice. Natural enteric infection is usually asymptomatic, but occasionally mice develop a posterior flaccid paralysis. Gross lesions are not present and there is no treatment. Diagnosis is based on immunohistochemistry of infected brain or spinal cord, ELISA, or PCR. Contaminated transplantable tumors or cell lines may be a source of infection. The nonenveloped virus is resistant to inactivation and requires thorough sanitation.

Geriatric Diseases

Mice: **Amyloidosis** causes soluble proteins to polymerize as insoluble fibrils and is commonly observed in aged C57BL/6 mice. Amyloid deposits are found in intestine, spleen, liver, lung, thyroid, and mesenteric lymph nodes. Clinical signs depend on the organ system involved. Microscopic lesions are easily visualized with Congo red stain. Treatment involves general supportive care.

Dystrophic calcification regularly occurs in the cardiac muscle of some inbred mouse strains (CBA, DBA/2, C3H, and BALB/c). Soft tissue mineralization occurs less often in kidney, liver, stomach, small and large intestines, and gonads. Associated clinical disease is rare.

Atrial thrombosis and congestive heart failure frequently occur in older mice of RFM and other strains. Clinical disease is characterized by dyspnea, tachycardia, and cyanosis. There is no effective treatment.

An autoimmune form of **glomerulonephritis** may cause renal dysfunction and associated morbidity in mice.

Osteoarthrosis is common in aged mice and can lead to difficult locomotion. Treatment is supportive with aspirin or acetaminophen provided in the drinking water.

Retinal degeneration is genetically linked in certain mouse strains or can occur secondary to environmental light exposure, resulting in blindness. Most mice compensate by their keen senses of smell and touch. **Cataracts** may occur in older mice or secondary to decreased tear production and dessication sometimes observed during anesthesia.

Rats: **Progressive glomerulonephrosis** is a common disease of aged rats. The presence and severity of disease is influenced by gender, genotype, and dietary factors such as protein content and total calorie consumption. Affected animals are lethargic and lose weight. Hypertension and secondary renal hyperparathyroidism may be secondary outcomes. In severe cases, rats have proteinuria and affected kidneys are pitted on the surface. Microscopically, lesions include glomerulopathy with thickened glomerular capillaries, dilated tubules with proteinaceous casts, and interstitial fibrosis. Treatment is supportive, but the condition is ultimately fatal.

Commonly seen in 12- to 18-mo old rats, **myocardial degeneration** is more frequently observed in males. Clinically, rats are asymptomatic, but gross lesions of gray foci may be present in the wall of the left ventricle.

Spontaneous **degeneration of the spinal cord and peripheral nerves** may occur in rats >2 yr old. Clinical signs include hindlimb paresis or paralysis. Demyelination is most prominent in the ventral root ganglia and associated motor nerves of the lumbosacral spinal cord and cauda equina.

Polyarteritis nodosa is an inflammatory condition of blood vessels in multiple organs. The etiology is unknown. Clinical disease can be caused by ruptured aneurysms or myocardial infarcts.

Uroliths occur in the renal pelvis and urinary bladder of older rats. Rats are either asymptomatic or have clinical signs including hematuria, cystitis, or anuria and hydronephrosis with obstruction, leading eventually to uremia and death.

Proliferation and fibrosis of portal bile ducts is common in aged rats. Most cases are asymptomatic.

Neoplasia

Mice: Development of neoplasia in mice is dependent on various factors, including strain of mouse, environment, age, and infection by oncogenic viruses.

Mammary adenocarcinomas are commonly observed in mice and can be located anywhere in the subcutaneous region due to extensive distribution of mammary tissue. These tumors can be induced by mouse mammary tumor viruses and transmitted vertically or horizontally through the placenta or milk. Mammary tumors are soft, highly vascularized, and may be necrotic or filled with blood. Mammary tumors can be surgically removed, but unlike benign fibroadenomas in rats, the prognosis is poor due to local tissue invasion and frequent metastasis to the lungs. Spontaneous **lymphosarcomas** are very common in certain strains of mice. Benign **respiratory adenomas** are common in certain strains (A strain) and older mice. Grossly, white nodules are observed on the pleural surface of the lungs.

Rats: The most common tumor of rats is the **benign mammary fibroadenoma**. Because rats have extensive mammary tissue, subcutaneous tumors may be found anywhere on the body. Tumors can occur in either females or males. Clinically, the tumors appear as subcutaneous lumps and can grow quite large, eventually ulcerating or interfering with eating and drinking or locomotion. Benign mammary tumors are usually encapsulated and prognosis improves with surgical removal. Recurrence in another location is frequent, but progression to malignancy is rare.

Pituitary adenomas are very common in rats, especially females, and incidence is increased by ad lib feeding of high-calorie diets. Clinically, rats may have head tilt and depression or die suddenly. Grossly, tumors vary in size. They are soft, have well-defined margins, and hemorrhage may be present. They frequently compress adjacent brain tissue, which may lead to hydrocephalus. Pituitary tumors commonly secrete prolactin.

Spontaneous leukemia with circulating atypical mononuclear cells is common in aged Wistar-Furth and Fischer 344 rat strains. Clinical signs include jaundice, anemia, weight loss, and lethargy. Gross lesions include splenomegaly, hepatomegaly, and lymphadenopathy.

Tumors of the Zymbal's gland occur infrequently. They are observed at the base of the ear in older rats and can be benign or malignant.

Most testicular tumors in rats are benign Leydig cell tumors. They are bilateral and soft, with multiple areas of hemorrhage. The highest incidence is reported in Fischer 344 and ACI/N rats.

Keratocanthomas are benign neoplasms of the skin found on the chest, back, or tail. The tumor's center is sometimes filled by a keratin plug.

SUGAR GLIDERS

Sugar gliders (*Petaurus breviceps*) are small nocturnal marsupials native to Australia and New Guinea that feed on insects and plant exudates, possess gliding membranes for energy-efficient locomotion, and live in colonies that nest in tree hollows. They are generally robust in captivity when proper husbandry practices are followed. They can be susceptible to infection with common bacteria including *Pasteurella*, staphylococci, streptococci, mycobacteria and *Clostridia*. Of zoonotic concern, *Salmonella*, *Giardia*, leptospirosis, and toxoplasmosis are known to occur in sugar gliders. Clinical signs and lesions are similar to those seen in other animals, with depression, loss of appetite, and weight loss being the most readily detected signs. Antibiotic therapy is well tolerated. Sugar gliders possess a well-developed caecum that utilizes bacterial fermentation to break down complex polysaccharides contained in gum. However, they do not appear to suffer adverse effects from antibiotic therapy, perhaps because they are omnivores and captive diets provide ample energy without the need for fermentation. Choice of antibiotic should be determined by signs, diagnostics, and if needed, culture and sensitivity.

Chloramphenicol palmitate and enrofloxacin compounded into liquid formulations are commonly prescribed and easy to administer.

Internal parasites rarely cause disease, but strongyle eggs have been seen on fecal flotation. The recorded internal parasites are nematodes of the genus *Parastrongyloides* and *Paraustrostrongylus* and a liver trematode of the genus *Athesmia*. Wild sugar glider nests generally contain a range of host-specific mites and fleas, but ectoparasites are uncommon in captivity. Dusting with carbaryl powder (50 g/kg) has been effective in controlling fleas and mites. Both the nest and the animal should be treated. Ivermectin (0.2 mg/kg, SC or PO) has also been used to control internal and external parasites.

Pet sugar gliders maintained on a mainly fruit diet are very susceptible to nutritional osteodystrophy. This condition manifests clinically as a posterior paresis progressing to hind limb paralysis. Radiography reveals osteoporosis of the vertebral column, pelvis, and long bones in particular. Treatment involves cage rest, administration of calcium, and correction of the diet. Diets should contain a daily protein source—a commercial extruded protein pellet, mealworms, crickets, or small amounts of cooked skinless chicken—as well as fruits and vegetables. Use of a phosphorus-free calcium with vitamin D_3 and a multivitamin supplement can help prevent nutritional disease.

Another common condition associated with poor nutrition occurs in the eyes of juvenile sugar gliders if the mother has been fed a diet too high in fat. White fatty deposits appear within the young glider's eye and can lead to blindness.

Dental disease is more frequent in sugar gliders fed diets high in soft textured carbohydrates. Feeding insects with hard exoskeletons can help maintain dental health.

Neoplasia, particularly lymphoid neoplasia, is common in oppossum and glider species.

Sugar gliders may be aggressive and may cause severe trauma to each other, particularly during mating and introduction of new adults. These injuries often occur around the face and may include corneal abrasions. In the wild, female young disperse from the colony prior to puberty (7-10 mo) and may be attacked in captivity if not removed soon after weaning.

Behavioral disorders can occur in sugar gliders housed alone, with incompatible mates, or in inappropriate cages. It is essential to provide sugar gliders with a secure

TABLE 16. Selected Physiologic Data for Sugar Gliders

Lifespan	9-12 yr
Adult male body wt	115-160 g
Adult female body wt	95-135 g
Respiratory rate	16-40/min
Heart rate	200-300 bpm
Body temperature	97.3°F (36.3°C)
Thermoneutral zone	80-88°F (27-31°C)
Food consumption	15-20% body wt/day
Dentition	Diprotodont
Dental formula (ICPM)	3 1 3 4
	1 0 3 4
Puberty	7-10 mo
Estrous cycle	29 days
Gestation period	15-17 days
Litter size	2 (81%)
Birth weight	0.2 g
Pouch emergence	70-74 days
Weaning	110-120 days

TABLE 17. Selected Hematologic and Serum Biochemical Values for Sugar Gliders

	Conventional (USA) Units	SI Units
Hematology		
Hemoglobin	13-15 g/dL	130-150 g/L
Hematocrit	45-53%	0.45-0.53 L/L
Red blood cells	5.1-7.2 × 10^6/μL	5.1-7.2 × 10^{12} /L
Mean corpuscular Hgb concentration	30-33 g/dL	300-330 g/L
Mean corpuscular Hgb	18.2-20.6 pg	18.2-20.6 pg
White blood cells	5.0-12.2 × 10^3/μL	5.0-12.2 × 10^9/L
Neutrophils	1.5-3.0 × 10^3/μL	1.5-3.0 × 10^9/L
Lymphocytes	2.8-9.2 × 10^3/μL	2.8-9.2 × 10^9/L
Monocytes	0.06-0.2 × 10^3/μL	0.06-0.2 × 10^9/L
Eosinophils	0.02-0.14 × 10^3/μL	0.02-0.14 × 10^9/L
Basophils	0	0
Plasma proteins	5.6-6.9 g/dL	56-69 g/L
Albumin	3.0-3.5 g/dL	30-35 g/L
Globulin	2.2-3.6 g/dL	22-36 g/L
Biochemistry		
ALT	50-106 U/L	50-106 U/L
AST	46-179 U/L	46-179 U/L
Calcium	6.9-8.4 mg/dL	1.7-2.1 mmol/L
CPK	210-589 U/L	210-589 U/L
Creatinine	0.2-0.5 mg/dL	17.7-44.2 μmol/L
Glucose	130-183 mg/dL	7.2-10.0 mmol/L
Phosphorus	3.8-4.4 mg/dL	1.2-1.4 mmol/L
Potassium	3.3-5.9 mEq/L	3.3-5.9 mmol/L
Sodium	135-145 mEq/L	135-145 mmol/L
Urea	18-24 mg/dL	6.4-8.6 mmol/L

nest box or pouch. Anxiety can manifest as overgrooming with fur loss, particularly at the base of the tail. Self-mutilation, over- or under-eating, polydipsia, coprophagia, cannibalism, and pacing are also associated with stress. Sexually mature male sugar gliders have also suffered from priapism where the penis remained extruded from the cloaca and became traumatized and devitalized, necessitating amputation.

Sugar gliders possess androgen-sensitive frontal (forehead), gular (throat), and paracloacal glands, which they use to mark each other and their furniture. It is normal for fur to be sparse around the frontal gland when active.

For normal physiologic, hematologic, and serum biochemical values in sugar gliders, see TABLE 16 and TABLE 17.

To assist in making clinical diagnoses, blood samples may be obtained from the jugular vein, medial tibial artery, or lateral tail vein of sugar gliders anesthetized with isoflurane administered via mask and T-piece. Blood volumes of up to 1% of the animal's body wt can be collected; typically 0.5 to 1.0 mL is obtained. The jugular vein is difficult to access due to the short neck and loose skin, but if the hair is clipped and a tuberculin syringe is pressed near the thoracic inlet to hold up the vein, it can often be accessed. A

25-gauge needle can be bent at its base to facilitate venipuncture. The medial tibial artery runs very superficially just distal and medial to the stifle joint and can be sampled with a 27- or 25-gauge needle and 0.5-1.0 mL syringe. The size of the lateral tail vein is most suited to skin prick and droplet collection into capillary tubes.

Whole body radiography with both lateral and ventrodorsal views is a useful tool for clinical assessment. It is particularly difficult to detect pneumonia in animals of this size without the use of radiography. Even severely compromised sugar gliders will generally tolerate short anesthesia with isoflurane to allow diagnostic radiographs to be obtained. Limbs should be taped in an extended position to allow a clear view of body cavities.

Fluid therapy is usually limited to SC administration, although the intraosseous route could be considered in critical cases. A 22-gauge $^3/_4$-in. needle can be positioned in the femur using the same technique as for rats, or a smaller gauge catheter can be placed in the proximal tibia. Fluid volume requirements are 20-25 mL/kg daily. Preferred fluids are lactated Ringer's solution, 0.9% NaCl, or 2.5% dextrose in saline.

ZOO ANIMALS

The physical health as well as the social and behavioral well-being of zoo animals depends on enclosure design, nutrition, husbandry, management, group social structure, behavioral enrichment, and good medical and surgical care. Naturalistic enclosures with soil and vegetation are appealing to the public and more stimulating for the animals, but they present challenges for both sanitation and parasite control programs and may complicate restraint procedures. Mixed species exhibits may increase risk of disease transmission between species and can result in interspecific aggression if appropriate choices are not made.

This chapter provides a general discussion of management practices, preventive medicine, clinical care programs, and some of the more commonly encountered disorders in zoo animals. For more specific information, refer to other chapters within this section (eg, AMPHIBIANS, p 1445; MARINE MAMMALS, p 1529; LLAMAS AND ALPACAS, p 1521; OSTRICHES, p 1555; NONHUMAN PRIMATES, p 1549; REPTILES, p 1590; VACCINATION OF EXOTIC MAMMALS, p 1666).

MANAGEMENT PRACTICES

Husbandry: The animal's exhibit should approximate its natural environment and enhance the visual experience for zoo visitors. Many healthy mammals and birds can tolerate a fairly wide temperature range if given access to shade and water in hot weather and to a dry, draft-free shelter with a warm spot and ample food to meet increased energy requirements in cold weather. It is essential to ensure that each animal has access to the protected environment and that one dominant individual does not exclude others from shelter, food, or water; such exclusion can result in frostbite or even death due to exposure. Feed receptacles should be designed to avoid fecal contamination and be easy to clean.

With large numbers of birds or mammals, and especially in mixed species exhibits, several watering and feeding stations should be established at appropriate heights to reduce injuries or deaths resulting from territorial conflicts. The timing of feedings is important. In many species, it is best to feed small amounts throughout the day to stimulate activity; this is beneficial for the animal and results in a better display. Food can also be used to attract an animal to an area where it is more easily and safely examined or treated.

Reproduction: The biology and social behavior of animals must be understood to promote reproduction. Species should be maintained alone, in pairs, or in groups, depending on their established social systems. For example, in mixed species groups of Artiodactyla, it is possible to establish species estrous cycles through a variety of techniques, including monitoring hormone levels in the urine and feces. Monitoring reproductive cycles may be used to determine when to introduce and remove breeding males, with males of other species rotated to coincide with the estrous periods of the females of each species. This may also reduce injuries from interaction between breeding males. At parturition, the males of some species should be removed for several weeks to prevent attacks on the postpartum females or their offspring. In colder climates, males should be introduced at a time that will allow births to occur during warm weather.

Artificial reproductive technologies such as artificial insemination, in vitro fertilization, and embryo transfer have been successfully employed in diverse zoo species. These efforts have made a significant difference in some endangered species breeding programs (eg, black-footed ferret). However, success requires substantial financial, personnel, and resource investments to determine basic parameters of reproductive cycles and responses to pharmacologic manipulation.

An emerging management priority in maintenance of zoologic collections is the need for selective reproduction. Indiscriminate reproduction is unethical and carries with it the potential for overproduction that exceeds the capacity of the exhibit, the zoo, or other zoos to appropriately house the progeny. Overly successful breeding programs carry a risk of limiting resources that could compromise other captive propagation programs. Contraceptive efforts in zoos are multifaceted and include permanent techniques (castration, vasectomy, ovariohysterectomy, tubal ligation), as well as reversible ones such as separation of the sexes, administration of birth control pills, hormonal implants, gonadotropin releasing hormone agonists, and oral or injectable progestins. Reversible contraception can also be used to control timing of reproductive cycles. There is ongoing work with immunocontraception through administration of porcine zona pellucida vaccines.

PREVENTIVE MEDICINE

The foundation of a medical program for zoo animals is preventive medicine, because diagnostic procedures and treatments are less straightforward with zoo animals than domestic species. Preventive medical programs should be continuous and include attention to individual specimens as well as the herd, troop, or flock. Components of the program include quarantine of new arrivals, periodic fecal examinations and treatments for parasites, booster vaccinations, health screening procedures, necropsy examination of deceased specimens, and a comprehensive pest control program. Animals should be evaluated to ensure their health and comply with local, state, and federal health requirements before shipment to other zoos or before release in managed reintroduction programs. Preshipment evaluations can also be used as an opportunity to assess the overall health status of the group in which the animal has been living.

Quarantine: Animals entering a collection must undergo quarantine. Quarantine facilities should be designed to allow handling of animals and proper cleaning and sanitizing of enclosures. Shipping crates should be cleaned and disinfected before they leave the quarantine area, and the crates' contents disposed of appropriately. Quarantine facilities require barriers against ingress of potential vectors and vermin. Separate keepers who are skilled at recognizing signs of stress and disease and who will carefully monitor feed intake and fecal characteristics should care for quarantined animals.

During quarantine, animals should receive appropriate vaccinations and diagnostic testing (eg, tuberculosis, heartworm). They should be examined and treated for ecto- and endoparasites and screened for enteric bacterial pathogens. Before release, animals should receive physical and laboratory examinations, which may include radiographs, serology, hematology, and clinical chemistries. Serum should be frozen for future reference and possible epidemiologic studies. All procedures and results should be recorded in each individual animal's medical record, which is an essential component of the medical program. Each animal should also be identified by some permanent method (eg, tattoo, tag, band, eartag, transponder) to ensure future identification.

When new animals are introduced to enclosures, caution and forethought are necessary to prevent self-induced trauma. Visual barriers, eg, suspending canvasses from fences or enclosure walls or obscuring glass with soap to provide a visual cue, are standard management steps to protect newly introduced specimens from accidents during acclimation to a new exhibit.

Parasite Control: Like domestic animals, zoo animals are vulnerable to a wide variety of ecto- and endoparasites, and similar drugs are used for treatment. Care must be exercised in the choice of medications due to species-specific sensitivities to some drugs. Young animals and those stressed by shipment, disease, or injury are the most likely to be adversely affected by parasites. At these times, commensal parasites (especially protozoa) can cause disease. Acute diarrhea can result from massive infections of *Coccidia, Trichomonas, Giardia,* or *Balantidium* spp. Amebiasis, which is fairly common in primates and reptiles, can be fatal in a compromised animal. Intestinal parasites may be a major, continuous problem in species kept in naturalistic exhibits or on dirt substrate or pasture, especially in young, newly introduced, or stressed individuals. In these situations, incorporating anthelmintics directly into the feed is helpful. As in domestic species, anthelmintic resistance may develop and necessitate a change in medication. Parasites with indirect life cycles are less frequently a problem if the exhibit area is free of intermediate hosts.

Vaccination: Vaccination of zoo carnivores is essential because of their susceptibility to various diseases such as feline panleukopenia, feline rhinotracheitis, feline calicivirus, rabies, canine distemper, and canine parvovirus. (*See also* VACCINATION OF EXOTIC MAMMALS, p 1666). Previously, only killed virus vaccines were recommended, but recent studies have shown that some modified live vaccines are safe for use in select species. Further studies are required because some modified live vaccines (especially canine distemper) produce fatal disease in certain species. A canarypox-vectored recombinant canine distemper vaccine has proven safe for use in those species susceptible to modified live virus vaccine-induced disease. Appropriateness of rabies vaccination depends on the circumstances of each collection. If indicated in rabies-endemic areas for the protection of individual animals, only a killed rabies vaccine should be used. The decision to vaccinate zoo animals for less common diseases for which a vaccine is available should be made on an individual basis.

Necropsy: All dead animals should be necropsied. This should include gross and histopathologic evaluation of tissue and viral, bacterial, or fungal cultures when appropriate. Tissues should also be saved for potential future examinations. A thorough pathology examination allows evaluation of medical, management, and nutritional programs. It is also valuable in identifying problems requiring immediate action to safeguard the health of the collection. Variations in anatomy should be recorded because such observations may aid in future diagnostic procedures or therapy in the species.

Pest Control: A successful control program is continuous and requires a concerted effort by zoo staff to minimize harborage and food for pests, in addition to the use of mechanical and chemical control methods. Choice of agent, method of use, and storage may minimize zoo animals' access to pesticides and the risk of secondary poisoning. Common zoo pests may serve as important disease vectors. For example, cockroaches are intermediate hosts for GI parasites of primates and birds; rodents can harbor and spread *Listeria* spp, *Salmonella* spp, *Francisella tularensis,* and *Leptospira* spp. Wild and feral carnivores such as foxes, raccoons, and domestic dogs and cats can devastate animal collections through predatory attacks and may be important vectors for viral diseases such as rabies, parvovirus, and canine distemper. Raccoons may also transmit *Baylisascaris* parasites, which can cause larval migration resulting in fatal neuropathy in some species. Pigeons and starlings are potential reservoirs for avian diseases; they consume or contaminate animal food and deposit droppings everywhere.

CLINICAL CARE PROGRAMS
The mainstay of the zoo medical program is a qualified and dedicated keeper staff. The keepers know the individuals under their care and observe them daily. They are the

first to recognize abnormalities such as anorexia, inactivity, abnormal feces, or changes in behavior that may reflect early medical problems. Overzealous reporting of observations is preferable to indifference. Because many zoo animals, especially prey species, instinctively conceal overt signs of illness until the disease process is well advanced, it is necessary to make keepers aware of the significance of what may seem to be trivial changes. Past associations with the veterinarian may arouse some animals' responses to the veterinarian's presence, which will mask subtle changes noticeable to keepers.

Once a diagnosis is made, the treatment of zoo animals is similar to that of domestic species except in the method of drug administration and restraint. A comparative medical approach is generally most successful and productive and utilizes application of medical or surgical information about diseases affecting free-ranging animals, related domestic animals, or humans. Frequently, human medical, veterinary, or dental specialists are consulted for advice or assistance with complicated medical or surgical cases. Knowledge of comparative anatomy, physiology, behavior, nutrition, pathology, and taxonomy is useful. Attention must be paid to both individual and population health.

Behavioral Training: An active behavioral training program enables improved health care. Through positive reinforcement, amphibians, reptiles, birds, and mammals in zoo settings have been trained to perform behaviors on command that facilitate accomplishment of various management or medical procedures. Management behaviors include shifting on and off exhibit, onto scales, and into restraint devices or shipping containers. Medical procedures include urine collection, venipuncture, IM injection, tuberculin testing, and rectal or vaginal examination. Often these behaviors are incorporated into behavioral and environmental enrichment programs. Enrichment programs are designed to encourage animals to display more of their normal behavioral repertoire, eg, increasing opportunities for foraging or social interaction, which allows animals to spend their time more as they would in nature.

Physical Restraint: Most zoo animals resent being handled and resist manual restraint. Struggling with an animal to administer treatment may do more harm than can be offset by treatment. Physical restraint is indicated in some species for minor manipulation or close observation. Restraint devices (squeeze cages) or chute systems are frequently used for difficult to handle, larger, or dangerous species. Many procedures can be performed on unanesthetized animals so confined, including limited physical examinations, tuberculin testing, administration of injections or anesthetics, collection of blood samples, trimming malformed claws or overgrown hooves, and application of topical medications.

While the dimensions and construction of these devices vary, some operate by movement of one wall to restrain the animal against the other. Openings are provided to allow safe access to the animal. Many restraint devices for hoofstock are designed with a "V" shape; once the animal enters, the floor is lowered and the animal's body is restrained by the "V" with its feet suspended off the ground. Whenever possible, animals should be trained to enter or be enticed, rather than forced, into the restraint device. Ideally, these facilities should be designed as part of the animal's regular quarters and located in an area where the animal is normally shifted as part of the daily routine. Exhibits should contain nest boxes or restraint pens equipped with doors that operate remotely to confine the animal. From these areas, the animal can be transferred to a restraint device, anesthetic chamber, or shipping container. Weighing facilities are essential.

Small mammals and birds may be caught and restrained in long-handled hoop nets. These nets must be deep enough that the animal can be confined in the blind end, with the upper part of the net twisted to prevent escape.

Personnel participating in capture or restraint procedures must understand their role and be aware of the behavioral characteristics and physical abilities of animals. This is essential to ensure safety of both animals and personnel. Heavy gloves protect handlers from teeth and claws when animals are manually held after capture. Care must be used to avoid excessive pressure on animals, because gloves hinder dexterity and the perception of the pressure being exerted. Gloves are also difficult to clean and can be a fomite for transmitting infectious agents.

Diagnostic Techniques: The fundamental diagnostic technique is a good history and thorough visual and physical examination (often requiring anesthesia). Ease of sample collection for laboratory testing (CBC, biochemical profile, serology, cytology); fecal examination for parasites; urine for urinalysis; and aerobic, anaerobic, fungal, and viral culture is dependent on species anatomic differences compared with other more commonly treated species. Radiography and ultrasonography are commonly employed. Endoscopy, laparoscopy, and minimally invasive surgery are utilized when indicated. Computed tomography and MRI are less commonly utilized but also have a role in specific cases. Virtually any technique used for other species can be modified for use in zoo species.

Drug Administration: Few drugs are approved for use in zoo species, but extra-label drug use laws allow drugs to be legally used in species for which they are not licensed. Providing quality medical care to zoo animals requires that medications be used without documented therapeutic benefit, dosage, treatment schedule, contraindication, and toxicity data in zoo animals. Therefore, extrapolation from what is known about these parameters in other species is necessary. When prescribing, these factors must be kept in mind if therapy is to be beneficial, especially with drugs that have the potential for organ toxicity. The different metabolic rates of various animals, eg, snakes vs birds, must be considered when extrapolating drug dosages. Antibiotic, antifungal, and analgesic treatments, as well as anesthetic dosages, are becoming less empirical due to increasing species-specific knowledge resulting from pharmacokinetics studies in zoo species. When using a drug on a group of animals for the first time, it is often wise to initially administer it to just one or two individuals. If no adverse effects are seen, the rest of the group can then be treated.

In general, zoo animals can be placed in metabolic groups. Dosages should be extrapolated within such groups when data are available. Dosages are generally higher in small animals and lower in large animals in the same metabolic group; an animal 15 times the size (body wt) of a smaller animal may require only half the dosage rate of the smaller animal when both belong to the same energy or metabolic group. If available, pharmacokinetic data for the species being treated should be consulted first.

Drug administration can be challenging. Oral medication has the advantage of minimal disturbance to the animal, but ensuring adequate individual intake may be a problem, especially when animals are housed in a group. Mixing the medication with favorite foods or treats is helpful. Oral antibiotics in hoofstock and other species can disrupt normal bacterial flora and lead to GI problems. Oral sedative or anesthetic administration can result in variable onset, duration, and depth of effect due to inadequate consumption or delayed absorption. IM injections with a hand syringe can be difficult unless a restraint device or other means of physical restraint is used. Remote IM injections may be made by firing a projectile syringe from a dart gun. However, these injections may be painful and may add the trauma of dart impact and injection, especially when delivering large volumes (eg, 10 mL) over long distances (50 m). Problems can be minimized through careful selection of the most appropriate drug and drug concentration, as well as the type of dart gun for the intended use. In addition, practice with projectile darts is mandatory before their use. Marksmanship, as well as familiarity with the weapon, is essential—such weapons in the hands of a novice can be fatal. Other less traumatic methods of IM injection, over shorter distance, include syringe poles or blow guns. Through behavioral training, it is also possible to administer IM injections through voluntary participation of the animal. IV therapy is generally restricted to anesthetized animals or those maintained in restraint devices or small enclosures for the duration of treatment.

Anesthesia: Safe anesthesia of zoo animals is of special concern. Many procedures routinely accomplished on domestic animals with minimal restraint require anesthesia of zoologic species for the welfare and safety of both zoo animals and personnel. Prior to initiation of anesthesia in a zoo animal, the operator should be familiar with the species and choice of anesthetic agent. Anesthesia records for the individual, other specimens of the same species in the collection, or published references for the species should be reviewed. Consultation with someone knowledgeable in the field is advised, as there are great differences in effective drugs and dosages in the diversity of species in a zoologic practice.

Many factors influence an animal's response to anesthetic drugs, including age, sex, stage of reproductive cycle, general nutritional status, and most especially mental state before drug administration. Variations may be marked between species as well as individuals and between different collections of the same species. An excited animal usually requires more drug and, once anesthetized, has a greater tendency to develop capture myopathy secondary to hyperthermia, respiratory depression, and acidosis. Capture myopathy can also occur in manually restrained animals and is more common in ungulates or long-legged birds (*see* p 955). Monitoring of anesthetized animals may include heart and respiratory rates, temperature, ECG, and blood oxygen saturation through pulse oximetry. Attention must be paid at all times to appropriate positioning and padding of anesthetized animals and extremes of environmental conditions to prevent secondary comlications.

The nature of an enclosure in which animals are to be anesthetized should be carefully considered before initiation of an anesthetic episode to minimize complications. For example, prey species that are darted may startle and hit fences or other barriers. In herd situations, the herd members may attack and injure or kill the darted animal as anesthetic induction begins (eg, ataxia).

Xylazine (an α_2-adrenoreceptor agonist) used alone produces adequate sedation in some ungulates, mainly bovids, to allow manipulative procedures. The sedative effects can be antagonized by administration of yohimbine, tolazoline, or atipamezole. Xylazine should not be used as the sole anesthetic agent in dangerous carnivores because they may appear sedated but can respond aggressively when stimulated.

The cyclohexamine ketamine (either alone or in combination with tranquilizers or sedatives such as xylazine or medetomidine) is a common anesthetic for small to medium-sized mammals, especially carnivores, primates, and some ungulates. A concentrated ketamine preparation (200 mg/mL) can be obtained from compounding pharmacies with a resultant decrease in the required injection volume. Combining ketamine with a sedative or tranquilizer speeds induction, minimizes excitement, increases muscle relaxation, and provides a smoother anesthetic induction and recovery than using ketamine alone. The ability to reverse the sedative effects of xylazine or medetomidine with the antagonists yohimbine, tolazaline, or atipamezole enables the use of a lower ketamine dosage and a more complete and rapid reversal upon completion of the procedure.

Tiletamine-zolazepam, a dissociative anesthetic-tranquilizer combination, is relatively safe in most species, has a rapid induction, and can be concentrated to 200 mg/mL to allow a small delivery volume. A disadvantage of this drug is that no complete antagonist exists; therefore, recoveries can be longer than with other drug combinations that can be completely reversed. It is commonly used for anesthesia of carnivores and primates.

The rapid onset and short duration of anesthesia induced by the sedative-hypnotic propofol renders it particularly attractive for use in zoo species. However, due to the necessity for IV administration, its use is limited to species such as reptiles, birds, and small mammals that can safely be manually restrained for drug administration. It is also useful as an adjunct anesthetic agent in large mammals first immobilized with another drug combination.

The potent opioids etorphine and carfentanil, alone or in combination with other agents (eg, acepromazine, xylazine, detomidine), have been used extensively for anesthesia of ungulates, elephants, and rhinoceros. The antagonist of choice for etorphine or carfentanil is naltrexone, a pure narcotic antagonist, which induces complete reversal when given at 100 mg of naltrexone per mg of carfentanil or etorphine. The reversal dosage of naltrexone can be given IV or IM, and in species prone to renarcotization after reversal, additional naltrexone may be administered SC. It can also be given IM 6-8 hr later by remote delivery to prevent renarcotization when the animal is not being observed. Accidental exposure of people to etorphine and carfentanil is quite dangerous. Therefore, they should only be used by trained, experienced personnel, and only after development of accidental-exposure protocols.

Various drug combinations (utilizing ketamine, telazol, medetomidine, detomidine, butorphanol, midazolam, diazepam, or xylazine) have been developed for specific species and purposes. Administration to novel species should be undertaken with care.

Isoflurane has become the inhalation anesthetic of choice for small mammals, birds, and reptiles. It is also used as a supplement to an injectable anesthetic or as an anesthetic maintenance agent to prolong anesthesia in virtually all species. Isoflurane is safe and potent and has minimal side effects, short induction, and quick recovery periods. Sevoflurane, if available, has the advantage of even shorter induction and recovery periods and may be preferred over isoflurane in some species. Small animals can be induced with a face mask or placed in an anesthetic chamber. Injectable anesthesia can be maintained or supplemented using a face mask, nasal cannulae, or intratracheal intubation depending on the species and anesthetic plane.

Regulatory Issues: Collection, transport, and exhibition of wild animals requires compliance with local, state, and federal laws. Permits may be necessary to maintain these species. Institutions in the USA must comply with appropriate rules and regulations such as those of the USDA, United States Fish and Wildlife Service, National Oceanographic and Atmospheric Administration, and National Marine Fisheries Service. Some specific health requirements in the USA include compliance with the USDA's Animal Welfare Act and Permanent Post-entry Quarantine regulations and the Centers for Disease Control and Prevention's regulations governing importation of primates and maintenance of colonies of captive bats.

Zoonoses: Free-ranging and captive wild animals may harbor zoonotic diseases that pose a potential health risk for those who work with these animals. Reptiles are commonly asymptomatic carriers of *Salmonella* spp. Avian species may be infected with *Chlamydophila* spp. Tuberculosis infections in mammals, especially primates and ungulates, can be transmitted from people or harbored and shed by animals to infect zoo staff. Many enteric bacterial or parasitic pathogens of primates can be transmitted to humans. Bats may be a source of *Histoplasma* spp or rabies. Carnivorous species of reptiles, birds, and mammals that consume uncooked meat-based commercial diets or whole prey may develop an asymptomatic *Salmonella* carrier state. Numerous zoo species, as well as feral domestic or native species on zoo grounds, may harbor *Leptospira* spp. Recognition of these zoonotic diseases and institution of procedures to minimize the disease risk to zoo staff and the visiting public are important components of a zoologic practice. Personal protective equipment (eg, disposable gowns, gloves, face shields) should be used as required by zoo personnel. Frequent hand washing is also recommended. (*See also* ZOONOSES, p 2545.)

COMMON DISORDERS AND PROCEDURES

In general, the disease processes and treatments of zoo species are similar to those of domestic pets, agricultural species, laboratory animals, or humans. Commonly encountered medical problems include acute or chronic gastroenteritis, traumatic injuries (bite or gore wounds, lacerations, fractures, luxations), localized (abscess or cellulitis) or generalized (septicemia) bacterial infections, parasitic infestations, obstetrical problems, lameness, arthritis, and GI foreign bodies.

Avian *Aspergillus* infection generally results in chronic respiratory tract disease (*see also* p 1462). Affected birds may exhibit weight loss, markedly elevated WBC counts, and in later stages, dyspnea. Death can also occur peracutely if there is a localized aspergilloma that occludes the trachea or in cases of fungal septicemia. Necropsy generally demonstrates extensive fungal granulomas in the air sac and lungs. Species that are more sensitive to *Aspergillus* infections are penguins, pheasants, and waterfowl. Treatment is generally unrewarding due to the advanced state of infection when diagnosed, but can include oral (flucytosine or itraconazole), IV (amphotericin B), or nebulized (enilconazole) antifungal medications.

Infectious pododermatitis (bumblefoot) is a common disorder of birds. It can be either unilateral or bilateral and is characterized by lameness, inflammation, and swelling of the footpad due to localized bacterial infection. Sequelae of infection can include chronic pododermatitis, septicemia, or amyloidosis. It can occur due to injury, infection, inappropriate substrate, obesity, or unilateral limb problems (trauma, arthritis) that result in excess and abnormal weight bearing on the contralateral foot. Treatment includes correction of the primary problem, local and systemic antibiotic and symptomatic treatment, and in more advanced cases, surgery.

Avian mycobacteriosis is a chronic problem in many bird collections, and control measures are difficult because premortem tests are unreliable (*see also* p 2267). Aggressive sanitation of the infected enclosures and culling of infected and exposed birds may help limit disease dissemination but will not eliminate it. Marsupials and young primates may also develop infection when exposed to infected birds or contaminated environments (such as in a mixed species exhibit). The disease in marsupials can manifest by development of lung or bone lesions and is resistant to most therapies. The disease in primates is often benign but may result in nonspecific tuberculin test responses.

Prevention of flight in birds is accomplished by amputating one wing just distal to the radiocarpal joint (pinion) or less commonly by performing a tenectomy and fusing the radiocarpal joint. Pinioning of young birds soon after hatching is easier and more successful. The appropriateness of performing this procedure on adult birds is controversial. (*See also* p 1453 et seq.)

Bone fractures are repaired with splints, casts, surgical fixation, or a combination of these methods. Because maintaining a splint on a zoo animal can be difficult, rigid internal fixation or an external fixater are preferable. For best results, fixation should be rigid, strong, and require minimal postoperative care. Because casts must be left in place for 6-8 wk, freedom of movement and a minimum of discomfort must be assured. Newer lightweight, strong, waterproof, fiberglass casting material is especially useful.

Mammalian tuberculosis still occasionally occurs in zoo collections, and routine screening of primates, hoofstock, and keeper staff is indicated (*see also* p 549). Interpretation of intradermal tuberculin tests can be problematic in nondomestic species due to the occurrence of nonspecific responses. When a test is suspicious or positive, a complete health evaluation should be performed including additional tests such as radiographs and gastric and bronchial lavage for mycobacterial cytology and culture. Diagnostic immunologic tests are available for zoo bovids and cervids and include lymphocyte stimulation tests and ELISA. Other tests under development include antigen 85 and γ-interferon testing.

Hoof and nail trims are necessary when overgrowth occurs and are most often required in ruminants, equids, elephants, rhinoceros, and larger carnivores. These procedures should be conducted on a regular basis to avoid excessive overgrowth. On occasion, the services of an equine farrier are employed for more complicated cases such as when an equid has foundered. Elephant foot care is especially important to prevent chronic musculoskeletal problems and can usually be accomplished in an awake elephant through training. Many other species require chemical immobilization for foot care.

Mandibular osteomyelitis (lumpy jaw) is a common problem of small ruminants and macropods (wallabies and kangaroos). It can occur secondary to coarse feed, oral trauma, or dental disease. Animals generally present with localized facial swelling and a foul oral odor or discharge. Treatment consists of lancing the abscess, debriding infected bone, removing affected teeth if indicated by radiographs, and treating with systemic antibiotics.

Dentistry in zoo animals presents unique problems. The roots of canine teeth in primates and carnivores are more extensive than the exposed crown. Simple traction and rotation cannot remove such teeth intact; dislodging with a dental elevator is essential. A small electric drill or bone chisel is used to remove a section of alveolar bone around the root. Root canals are indicated when a large canine tooth is fractured and viable pulp exposure occurs. Specialized long dental instruments are required to remove the nerve tissue from these elongated canals. The incisor teeth of rodents, such as beavers, porcupines, and capybaras, grow continually; unless these animals are supplied with coarse feed or logs to gnaw on, their incisors grow excessively and interfere with their ability to feed. Periodontal disease in zoo animals is treated by routine cleaning (under general anesthesia) and by providing adequate chewing substances to supplement the soft, prepared diets fed to many zoo animals.

Due to excellent management, husbandry, nutrition, and veterinary care, many zoo animals live to advanced ages. Care of **geriatric specimens** is becoming increasingly common, including such disorders as diabetes, heart failure, chronic arthritis, and neoplasia. The same diagnostic and therapeutic principles of management of these disorders in humans or domestic animals may be successfully applied to the care of affected zoo animals.

VACCINATION OF EXOTIC MAMMALS

Because a number of diseases of domestic animals also infect certain wild animals, vaccination of captive exotic mammals is desirable when they are at risk of exposure. However, commercial vaccines are approved for use only in domestic species; therefore, recommendations for use in exotic mammals are extra-label and based on limited published data and anecdotal experience (TABLE 18).

In general, inactivated viral or bacterial vaccines are preferable to modified live virus (MLV) vaccines. Although MLV vaccines are avirulent in domestic counterparts, they may be insufficiently attenuated to be nonpathogenic in exotic species. This is especially true for rabies and distemper vaccines. In certain instances, MLV vaccines are recommended in exotic species, based on considerable experience in zoos, with satisfactory safety results and limited serologic data; however, studies evaluating protection against virulent virus challenge typically have not been done.

In general, animals with active clinical illness should not be vaccinated. When using remote delivery systems (eg, darting syringe guns), one must be sure that a full dose has been delivered. Syringe darts may rebound quickly on impact and fail to deliver the dose required to elicit a satisfactory immune response.

Canine Distemper: All members of the families Canidae, Procyonidae, Mustelidae, and some members of Viverridae are considered susceptible. The susceptibility of Hyaenidae and Ursidae is questionable, even controversial. Clinical distemper in exotic carnivores usually resembles that in dogs but often appears primarily as a neurologic disease that results in the affected animal losing its fear of humans; thus, the disease can be confused with rabies. There have been recent reports of clinical canine distemper infection in wild felids such as lions; however, vaccination of feline species in zoos is not deemed necessary.

Caution is advised in vaccinating wild-caught animals because they may be incubating the disease. There is marked variation among species and individuals in their reaction to MLV vaccines, and different MLV vaccines vary considerably in their degree of attenuation. While a killed virus vaccine would be preferred, none are currently available. Several MLV vaccines of chick embryo or avian tissue culture origin have been used in zoos for several years and appear to be the best attenuated and therefore safest, based on limited studies. It is prudent to consult a zoo veterinarian for recommendations of specific products, although there are differences in experiences with specific vaccines. MLV vaccines marketed for use in mink generally are more highly attenuated and are recommended for use in all Mustelidae. However, European mink have developed canine distemper even when such vaccines have been used. Ferret-origin MLV vaccines are poorly attenuated and therefore contraindicated for use in any nondomestic carnivore. Single doses of MLV vaccines are administered SC or IM to young animals after weaning, with monthly booster doses up to 4 mo of age and annual revaccination thereafter. For both the red panda and the giant panda, only specially made killed-virus adjuvanted canine distemper vaccine is used.

Canine Parvovirus and Feline Panleukopenia: Canine parvovirus, raccoon parvovirus, and feline panleukopenia virus are closely related antigenically and pathogenetically. Wild Canidae, Felidae, most Mustelidae, Procyonidae, and Viverridae are considered susceptible to one or more of these parvoviruses. MLV vaccines that are safe for one

TABLE 18. Vaccinations Recommended for Exotic Mammals

Animal Group	Disease or Vaccine	Vaccine Type[*]	Vaccination Frequency
Primates (especially Pongidae): monkey, ape	Poliomyelitis	MLV	Annual
	Measles	MLV	Annual
	Mumps	MLV	Annual
	Rubella	MLV	Annual
	DPT[†] or tetanus	K	Annual
Canidae: fox, wolf, coyote, wild dog	Canine distemper	MLV[‡]	Annual
	Canine adenovirus 2	MLV	Annual
	Canine parvovirus	K	Annual
	Canine parainfluenza	MLV	Annual
	Leptospira bacterin-CI[§]	K	Annual
Felidae: exotic cats	Feline panleukopenia	K/MLV[‡]	Annual
	Feline rhinotracheitis	K/MLV	Annual
	Feline caliciviruses	K/MLV	Annual
Mustelidae/Viverridae/ Procyonidae: raccoon, skunk, ferret, coati, genet, otter, weasel, mink, kinkajou	Canine distemper	K/MLV[‡]	Annual
	Feline panleukopenia	K/MLV	Annual
	Canine adenovirus 2	K/MLV	Annual
	Leptospira bacterin-CI	K	Annual
Ursidae: bear	Canine adenovirus 2	K	Annual
	Leptospira bacterin-CI	K	Annual
Hyaenidae: hyena, aardwolf	Canine distemper[¶]	K/MLV	Annual
	Feline panleukopenia[¶]	K/MLV	Annual
Artiodactyla/Ruminantia: deer, sheep, cattle, goat, antelope, camelids	BVD[#] (in endemic areas)	K	Annual
	8-way *Clostridium* bacterin	K	Annual
	5-way *Leptospira* bacterin	K	Annual or every 6 mo
	Parainfluenza 3	MLV	Annual
Perissodactyla Equidae: ass, zebra	Tetanus	K	Annual
	EEE[**]	K	Annual
	WEE[††]	K	Annual
	Equine rhinopneumonitis	K	every 4 mo
Suidae/Tayassuidae: pigs, peccaries	5-way *Leptospira* bacterin	K	Annual
	Erysipelas bacterin	K	Annual

[*]MLV, Modified live virus; K, killed
[†]DPT, diptheria, pertussis, and tetanus
[‡]Not ferret origin; avian embryo or cell culture origin preferred
[§]Canicola or icterohaemorrhagiae
[¶]Controversial; some believe hyaenids are not susceptible
[#]Bovine viral diarrhea
[**]Eastern equine encephalomyelitis
[††]Western equine encephalomyelitis

species may be insufficiently attenuated for others. Therefore, only inactivated vaccines of tissue or tissue-culture origin should be used in exotic species. Recommendations for dosage and frequency of vaccination have been determined somewhat empirically: for small species, 1 standard small animal dose (1 or 2 mL) is given SC or IM; for larger species, 2 mL/10 lb (4.5 kg) body wt to a maximum of 10 mL is given. A booster dose should be given at 10-14 days, and vaccination repeated at 6- to 12-mo intervals. Combination vaccines containing MLV canine distemper, canine adenovirus 2, canine parainfluenza, and feline panleukopenia or canine parvovirus have been used in wild Canidae without adverse effects, but experience of zoo veterinarians has been variable. Similarly, there are combination MLV feline vaccines that contain feline panleukopenia, feline rhinotracheitis, and feline caliciviruses. Most zoo veterinarians report good results with such vaccines in exotic felids, but a few report conflicting results. Combination killed feline panleukopenia, feline rhinotracheitis, and feline calicivirus vaccines are preferred.

Equine Encephalomyelitis (Eastern, Western, and Venezuelan): Wild Equidae are susceptible to equine encephalomyelitis. Vaccination should follow guidelines recommended for domestic horses in endemic areas. Inactivated trivalent (EEE, WEE, VEE) or bivalent (EEE, WEE) vaccines, or combinations of these with tetanus toxoid, are administered according to manufacturers' instructions, usually intradermally or IM, depending on the product used. Initial immunization consists of 2 doses, 1-2 wk apart. Annual revaccination with intradermal products consists of 2 doses, 1-2 wk apart; combination IM products usually consist of a single injection.

Equine Herpesvirus 1 Infection: This can cause abortion in exotic Equidae. Only killed virus vaccines are recommended because it is not known whether MLV vaccines are adequately attenuated. A single vaccination should be given to foals at 3-4 mo of age and at 4-mo intervals up to 1 yr. Mares should be immunized every 4 mo to maintain adequate protection against abortion because even after recovery from natural infection, protective immunity lasts only ~4 mo.

Erysipelas: *Erysipelothrix rhusiopathiae* is pathogenic for wild Suidae and Tayassuidae (peccaries). Erysipelas bacterin (2 mL) is administered SC at 2-3 mo of age, with a repeat dose in 3-5 wk, and a single annual booster (*see also* p 2225). Cetaceans, especially dolphins, are also susceptible to erysipelas (p 1535).

Feline Caliciviruses: Exotic felids are susceptible to feline caliciviruses. As with feline rhinotracheitis virus, vaccines against this disease are combined with other feline vaccines. Vaccination recommendations are the same as for feline rhinotracheitis.

Feline Herpesvirus Rhinotracheitis: Feline viral rhinotracheitis is a serious disease threat in exotic Felidae. Vaccines currently available are killed or MLV, usually in combination with other agents (eg, canine parvovirus and feline panleukopenia). These are given IM or SC in a single dose at weaning. Doses are then given at monthly intervals to 4 mo and annually thereafter.

Infectious Canine Hepatitis (Canine Adenovirus 1 [CAV-1]): All Canidae are susceptible. In foxes, the disease is called fox encephalitis due to a predominant neurotropism and neurologic signs (p 1516). Recently, evidence has emerged that Ursidae may be susceptible to CAV-1 infection. No killed virus vaccines are commercially available. MLV vaccines that contain combinations of canine distemper and CAV-1 or CAV-2 are used. The CAV-2 MLV is considered less likely to cause adverse postvaccinal reactions (eg, corneal opacity) than the CAV-1 MLV and is preferred for immunization against diseases caused by CAV-1 or CAV-2. These viruses are closely related antigenically and provide cross-protection. Single doses of such combination vaccines are administered SC or IM at weaning and thereafter as for canine distemper.

Leptospirosis: Leptospirosis is occasionally seen in exotic Canidae, Procyonidae, Ursidae, Mustelidae, Suidae, Tayassuidae, and in Cervidae and other ruminants of the families Bovidae, Camelidae, Giraffidae, etc. Bacterins that contain immunogens against *Leptospira interrogans* serovars *canicola* and *icterohaemorrhagiae* are used in the carnivores listed above. Ruminants, pigs, and peccaries are immunized with bacterins that contain serovars *pomona, hardjo, icterohaemorrhagiae, canicola,* and *grippotyphosa.* Carnivores are vaccinated with a 1 or 2 mL dose, IM or SC, at 6-8 wk of age, repeated in 14 days. Boosters are given every 6 mo. Hoofed animals are immunized with 5 mL of pentavalent bacterin IM; annual or, preferably, semiannual boosters are recommended. Vaccination does not necessarily prevent shedding of the causal organism(s).

Measles, Mumps, and Rubella: Pongidae are immunized against measles, mumps, and rubella at 2-3 mo of age with 0.5 mL of MLV human vaccine injected SC. This vaccination is also recommended for monkeys. Annual booster doses are given.

Parainfluenza 3: Wild sheep and goats are susceptible to pneumonia similar to shipping fever pneumonia of domestic sheep. Parainfluenza 3 (PI-3) is recognized as an important primary component, along with stress and *Mannheimia (Pasteurella) haemolytica*. Modified live virus PI-3 vaccines, particularly those administered intranasally, have been useful in reducing incidence of lamb pneumonia. Vaccine is administered at 3-4 mo of age, 1 mL in each nostril, and repeated 3-4 wk before anticipated shipment and annually thereafter.

Poliomyelitis: Primates, particularly the Pongidae (great apes) are susceptible to poliomyelitis. Oral trivalent MLV poliomyelitis vaccine is preferred to parenteral inactivated vaccine due to ease of administration. A single human dose (0.5 mL) is given PO on a sugar cube after 6 mo of age and annually thereafter. Vaccinated animals should be isolated from unvaccinated primates (including humans) for 1 mo after inoculation.

Rabies: All wild mammals are susceptible (*see also* p 1067). In areas where the incidence of rabies in free-living wildlife is high, mammals in zoos or kept as pets may be at high risk of exposure. In such cases, vaccination is recommended. However, the efficacy of parenteral rabies vaccination of wild animals has not been established, and no vaccine is licensed for use in wild animals. When vaccination is considered necessary, only killed virus vaccine should be used. Several inactivated vaccines prepared of nervous tissue (eg, murine, ovine, or caprine) or tissue-culture have been found satisfactory in terms of safety and immunogenicity, the latter based on limited tests that demonstrated adequate antibody responses in some exotic carnivores. The human diploid cell-line origin killed virus vaccines appear to have the best immunogenicity in domestic species. These vaccines should be administered by deep IM injection. Young animals are vaccinated at 3-4 mo of age, and vaccinations must be repeated annually. MLV rabies vaccines licensed for domestic animals should never be used in exotic animals because they are often insufficiently attenuated and may produce clinical rabies and death. Evaluation of vaccines intended to control rabies in wildlife continues in several countries.

Wild-caught animals, especially foxes, raccoons, and skunks, even when very young, may have been exposed to rabies and may be in the incubative phase. Because the incubation period can be quite prolonged (up to 1 yr), a short observation period is inadequate. The National Association of State Public Health Veterinarians recommends that wild-caught animals that will have public contact in zoos should be quarantined for ≥180 days.

Because of the potential for rabies exposure, keeping wild animals as pets, especially wild-caught carnivores, should be discouraged and is illegal in many jurisdictions.

Tetanus: Primates, exotic Equidae, Proboscidae (elephants), Pongidae, Cervidae (deer), camelids, and wild sheep and goats should be immunized against tetanus. Exotic Equidae and elephants are vaccinated on the same schedule as domestic horses; primary immunization at 3-4 mo of age consists of 2 IM injections of tetanus toxoid, 1 mo apart. A single booster dose is given annually.

Pongidae are often vaccinated against tetanus using the diphtheria, tetanus toxoid, and phase 1 pertussis (DPT) vaccines intended for use in human children or monovalent human tetanus toxoid. Primary immunization consists of 0.5 mL vaccine injected IM on 3 occasions at 3-mo intervals, with a booster dose 1 yr after the third injection. Thereafter, booster immunizations of 0.5 mL of diphtheria-tetanus toxoid or tetanus toxoid alone are given every 3-5 yr or after potential exposure due to injury. Monovalent tetanus toxoid is preferred because pertussis and diptheria are not considered health risks for nonhuman primates.

Wild sheep and goats and cervids are sometimes immunized beginning at 10-12 wk of age with multivalent clostridial bacterin-toxoids containing immunogens for *Clostridium tetani*, *C perfringens* (types B, C, D), *C septicum*, *C chauvoei*, *C novyi*, *C sordellii*, and *C haemolyticum* in areas of high exposure risk. The initial dose is 5 mL followed in 6 wk by a 2-mL dose, administered SC. A 2-mL booster dose should be given annually.

Miscellaneous: A number of infectious diseases, eg, bovine viral diarrhea (BVD), bluetongue, malignant catarrhal fever, and epizootic hemorrhagic disease of deer, may appear as serious local problems but are not widespread in zoos. Unfortunately, satisfactory vaccines for many infectious diseases are not available for exotic animals. Inactivated BVD vaccines are recommended in situations in which BVD has been a problem. Annual vaccination with 1 standard bovine dose IM should begin at 3 mo of age.

Satisfactory vaccines for bluetongue, epizootic hemorrhagic disease, and malignant catarrhal fever are not currently available but are needed for exotic ruminants in many regions of the USA.

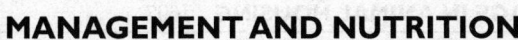

MANAGEMENT AND NUTRITION

GOATS   1866

HORSES   1872

PIGS   1889

RABBITS   1571 (EXL)

SHEEP   1902

MANAGEMENT AND NUTRITION
INTRODUCTION

Proper management and nutrition are essential to the health and well-being of domestic animals, particularly agricultural species that are expected to maintain a high level of production while relying on their managers to meet all their physiologic and behavioral needs. As livestock production becomes more intensified, the need to ensure that management and nutrition do not limit animal health or productivity increases.

Management and nutrition are also central to the prevention and control of many infectious and noninfectious diseases. Although infectious diseases require the presence of a specific infectious organism(s) (eg, a bacterium, virus, parasite), the mere presence of the causal microbe is not usually sufficient to assure that disease will develop. Other environmental and host factors influence whether the infected animal develops clinical disease or has reduced productivity as a result of the infection.

The most effective method of preventing infectious disease is to eradicate and exclude the organism(s) causing the disease. Often, this is impossible or impractical. It becomes necessary to control the infectious disease by minimizing circumstances that favor the spread of the infectious agent, mitigating the environmental circumstances that contribute to development of the disease in the presence of the infectious agent, and minimizing circumstances that increase the host's susceptibility. These circumstances that contribute to the development of a disease are termed risk factors for the disease. They can be grouped into several categories: microbe risk factors, environmental risk factors, and host risk factors. Identifying and mitigating the impact of these risk factors is the goal of a management strategy to prevent specific diseases and maintain productivity.

This multifaceted approach of using management to control and prevent disease is particularly important in dealing with many of the diseases that commonly are seen in food animal production (eg, pneumonia in young animals, GI disease in neonates, bovine respiratory disease complex of feedlot cattle) as well as in companion animals (eg, respiratory disease in catteries, kennel cough in canine boarding facilities). These diseases have either a complex etiology involving the interaction of several microbes or are caused by pathogens for which there are no reliable treatments (eg, viruses, some parasites). Prevention and control of these diseases often depends on implementing management practices to mitigate recognized risk factors for disease and impaired productivity. Often these are general management practices, but effective control of many diseases requires the implementation of management practices to address specific risk factors for individual pathogens.

The need to identify and implement multifaceted management strategies that can maintain health and enhance productivity is likely to increase and will be driven by forces from both within and outside the industry. Recognizing and making these management changes will require the collaborative efforts of all groups working in livestock production including veterinarians, animal scientists, and nutritionists.

Animal agriculture is under pressure from consumers and public interest groups to address concerns arising from current industry practices. These concerns include the potential link between antimicrobial resistance in human pathogens and drug use in animals, the relationship between environmental contamination and disposal of animal waste, the role of agricultural practices in human foodborne illness, and the impact of current management practices on animal welfare. Even if there is no conclusive evidence linking livestock production to these public health issues, livestock production practices will likely change in response to the perceived or potential link. Animal agriculture will need to change current management practices while developing and adopting new approaches to deal with health and production problems. Making these changes will require a substantial investment in research.

Animal agriculture is also under pressure from within the industry to change many current management practices. Recent well-publicized outbreaks of disease such as the epidemic of foot-and-mouth disease in the UK and transmissible spongiform encephalopathies in several species have focused the industry's attention on biosecurity as a disease prevention and control strategy. A biosecurity program is a series of management practices with the objectives of preventing the introduction of infectious or other disease causing agents and preventing the further spread of agents that are introduced or are already present (*see also* BIOSECURITY, p 1679).

Many in animal agriculture also support on-farm food safety initiatives. These programs are often HACCP-based (Hazard Analysis and Critical Control Point) and are developed and implemented by the commodity group involved. They emphasize the central role of management in ensuring the quality and safety of food produced on farms. Developing, implementing, and auditing these management programs is seen as essential to maintaining consumer confidence. These programs require the implementation and documentation of management practices to reduce the risk of physical, chemical, or microbial hazards entering the human food supply through production on farms.

Proper nutritional management is essential to animal health and productivity. Nutrition plays a role in influencing the animal's susceptibility to disease (eg, feline lower urinary tract disease) as well as in managing certain diseases (eg, diabetes, hyperlipidemia). Rations/diets must be formulated to provide for the basic physiologic needs (eg, energy, protein, fats, carbohydrates, vitamins, minerals) of the animal and to ensure optimal growth and productivity. Ration formulation must consider the age, sex, breed, lactation and gestational status, and physical activity of the animal. In agricultural production systems, feed preparation and delivery are often as important in ensuring animal health and productivity as the actual nutritional value of the ration.

Nutritionally related diseases include diseases associated with a nutritional excess (eg, direct toxic effect, digestive upset), nutritional deficiency (either primary or secondary deficiency), or nutritional imbalance. In animal agriculture, health is heavily influenced by feeding management. Inadequacies in nutritional delivery can directly cause disease (eg, ruminal acidosis, laminitis) or increase susceptibility to disease (eg, type D *Clostridium perfringens* enterotoxemia). Nutritionally related diseases in small animals include both diseases of excess (eg, developmental orthopedic disease in dogs related to excess calcium and energy) and diseases of deficiency (eg, blindness in cats related to taurine deficiency). Feeds and feeding management also influence animal health if feeding results in exposure to foodborne physical hazards (eg, sharp objects), chemicals (eg, mycotoxins, toxic plants) or microbes (eg, molds, *Salmonella* spp). Nutritional and waste management practices are also important in preventing and controlling infectious diseases that are spread through fecal-oral transmission (eg, salmonellosis, paratuberculosis in ruminants, toxoplasmosis in cats).

BIOSECURITY

Biosecurity is any practice or system that prevents the spread of pathogens and other harmful agents from infected animals to susceptible animals or that prevents the introduction of infected animals into a herd, region, or country in which the infection has not yet been identified. The harmful effects of these agents may be direct (eg, salmonellosis in humans), or indirect (disruption of the food supply). In addition, naturally produced poisons such as mycotoxins, toxic chemicals, and pesticides have the potential to disrupt beneficial and necessary biologic systems, and can therefore also be considered to threaten biosecurity. The fundamentals of biosecurity have been practiced in veterinary medicine for more than 100 years; however, its importance in protecting animal agriculture and the food supply have received renewed attention because of recent global animal health disasters and the threat of bioterrorism.

The goal of a biosecurity plan is to prevent the transmission of infectious agents among individuals, groups of animals, farms, or geographic regions; biocontainment plans are designed to control the spread of a disease that already exists in a herd or region. There are many possible routes of transmission; some of the more common include direct animal-to-animal contact (via horizontal or vertical transmission) within the herd, contact with wildlife or other species of livestock, contaminated feed or water, mechanical vectors (eg, vehicles and farm implements), animal vectors, airborne transmission, and visitors. From the human health perspective, the ultimate goal of biosecurity is to safeguard the human food chain.

Currently, the challenge to enhance biosecurity is very real. The recent epidemics of bovine spongiform encephalopathy (BSE) and foot-and-mouth disease in cattle have created major concerns about biosecurity. Much could be done at a herd level to improve herd health and productivity by implementing "biosecurity plans" that are designed to prevent the spread of infectious diseases. Regarding zoonotic and foodborne disease, herd level biosecurity to control human pathogens in cattle is likely to be an important first step in any Hazard Analysis and Critical Control Point (HACCP) plan to safeguard human health.

A successful biosecurity plan for an individual herd requires the coordinated efforts of the herd owner and the veterinarian. A major prerequisite is record-keeping of all animal health events, including introductions of animals to the illnesses, individual animal identification, deaths of animals and the results of necropsies, reasons for culling and dispositions of culled animals, details of vaccinations, and vaccines used.

CURRENT BIOSECURITY PRACTICES

A recent evaluation of biosecurity practices in the USA suggested that cow-calf producers commonly engage in management practices that increased the risk of introducing infectious diseases to their herds, such as importing cattle, failing to quarantine imported cattle, and communal grazing. Producers were found to inconsistently adjust for the increased risk of their management practices by increasing the types of vaccines given, increasing the quarantine time or proportion of imported animals quarantined, or increasing testing for various diseases in imported animals.

Similarly, biosecurity practices in dairy cattle herds in Iowa and Wisconsin were evaluated in 1998. In most herds, comprehensive biosecurity programs for incoming cattle were not used. Nearly 60% of herds obtained cattle from sources for which it was difficult to document genetic backgrounds and health testing for incoming cattle, and only ~50% quarantined new cattle on arrival. Despite high rates of vaccination for bovine viral diarrhea, all herd owners and managers indicated that herd biosecurity was compromised as a result of expansion. Herds that added cattle with unknown backgrounds and health status experienced the largest number of diseases.

At least 4 categories of biosecurity in dairy herds exist: 1) replacement cattle are not purchased and animals are not taken to cattle shows or fairs (highest biosecurity), 2) replacement cattle are not purchased but animals are taken to shows and fairs, 3) replacement cattle are purchased but are isolated on arrival, and 4) replacement cattle are purchased but not isolated on arrival (riskiest herds).

BENEFITS OF BIOSECURITY

The benefits of improved biosecurity to the livestock producer include increases in production, productivity, and profit; improved animal welfare; more efficient use of resources; reduced use of medication, such as antibiotics and anthelmintics, with an associated reduction in the risk of resistant pathogens emerging; and enhanced value of the individual herd.

In turn, benefits of improved biosecurity to the food-producing animal industry might include maximizing export markets by the prevention of disease-oriented barriers; decreasing economic losses from some diseases that cannot be treated and controlled using vaccinations or other management strategies (eg, *Mycoplasma bovis* mastitis); negotiating more favorable global trade issues and policies; preventing introduction of foreign diseases; controlling the spread of infections from region to region and farm to farm; preventing zoonoses; and producing wholesome meat and milk free of pathogens.

PRINCIPLES OF BIOSECURITY

The components of biosecurity include management and placement programs, farm layout, decontamination, pest control, and immunization. All these factors directly affect productivity and profitability. For some diseases, preventing the spread of infectious agents from a certain age group to younger age groups is desirable (eg, attempting to control the spread of enzootic pneumonia in calves by raising them in calf hutches).

The introduction of new infections into herds can be prevented or minimized by purchasing animals directly from herds known to be free of a particular disease. The adoption of this principle requires awareness of the possibility of purchasing unknown infected animals and testing animals for the infection before entry into the herd. It may also require keeping the introduced animal in quarantine for several weeks after arrival before it is added to the existing herd. New infections can also be prevented within herds by separating neonates from their dams immediately after birth and rearing them in isolation from infected animals.

Each farm should develop a specific disease control and biosecurity protocol. A closed farming system to prevent the introduction of infectious diseases is technically possible and can be economical. For example, a closed dairy farming system can prevent the introduction of infectious bovine rhinotracheitis virus, bovine viral diarrhea virus, leptospirosis, Johne's disease, tuberculosis, and salmonellosis and can be a good starting point for eradication of these infectious diseases from the herd. Limited field studies have found that closed dairy farms had a higher birth rate per 100 dairy cows, a lower average age at first calving, and lower costs for veterinary services.

Biosecurity measures to prevent the introduction of infectious agents into herds are most advanced in the swine industry, in which workers, visitors, veterinarians, and other service personnel must remove their street clothing, take a shower, and use clothing provided by the swine enterprise before they are allowed to enter the premises. In such high security swine herds, no replacement breeding stock are purchased and all new genetic lines may be introduced through artificial insemination.

ERADICATION AND PREVENTION OF AN INFECTIOUS DISEASE

Some infectious diseases can be eradicated from a herd, geographic area, or country. Eradication means complete elimination of the causative agent from the individual, usually by treatment or by removal or disposal of the infected animal(s) from the herd so that no additional cases are seen unless introduced from the outside. The control of disease by eradication has been a strategy used for many years, even before the specific causes of diseases were known. Diseases can be eradicated in several ways.

Compulsory Destruction and Disposal of Exposed Animals: This method is used by regulatory veterinary authorities for the eradication of exotic or foreign diseases, such as foot-and-mouth disease, in countries that have a policy of being free of the disease. All clinically affected and in-contact susceptible animals are identified, killed, and disposed of by burning or burying. It may include destruction of animals from an adjoining farm that may have had contact with the affected herd through the movement of personnel between farms. All infected farms are quarantined, and movement of animals in a specified area may be prohibited. Following disposal of the herd, standardized cleaning and disinfection procedures and a period of vacancy are mandatory, followed by the use of sentinel animals to ensure that disease does not develop before the farm is repopulated with the original species of livestock.

Identification and Disposal by Slaughter of Infected Animals: Diagnostic tests are used to identify infected animals, which are then removed from the herd and disposed of by slaughter for salvage. Only those animals that test positive for the infection are removed from the herd and, depending on the particular disease, all remaining animals that test negative in the herd are retested at suitable intervals until all animals are negative on one or more tests. Animals found to be positive at each test are removed and sent to slaughter. This method has been used for the eradication of diseases such as tuberculosis, brucellosis in cattle, enzootic bovine leukosis, and Johne's disease. The identification of infected animals depends almost entirely on diagnostic tests, which are not 100% sensitive and specific. Therefore, this method, although highly successful, is not as reliable as the policy of destroying entire herds of animals for the eradication of foreign diseases.

In an individual herd, a disease caused by a specific pathogen can be eradicated by disposal of the entire herd (depopulation), followed by a period of vacancy of the buildings, and then by repopulation with animals from herds certified to be free of the infectious disease. Animals that are imported into a herd or into a country may be quarantined for a period of time and tested for the presence of infection before they are introduced into the herd.

When certain diseases caused by specific pathogens have been eradicated from a herd, the herd can be closed. In this case, no further live animals are introduced, which prevents the entry of unknown infected animals. Genetic improvement in the herd is achieved through artificial insemination, embryo transfer, and selection within the herd.

Elimination of Infection by Treatment: This method involves the treatment of infected animals that have been identified by clinical examination or diagnostic tests. Examples include the use of antibiotics for the treatment of cattle with leptospirosis and cattle with mastitis caused by *Streptococcus agalactiae*. Appropriate withdrawal periods for milk and meat production must be followed to prevent drug residues.

Following eradication of the infection, constant surveillance to prevent the entry of unknown infected animals into the area or the herd is necessary. For notifiable diseases, this requires a regulatory system that certifies that exported and imported animals are free of certain infectious agents. For the individual livestock producer who wants to purchase breeding stock, it requires an effective testing system to certify that the purchased animals are free of the disease and that they originate from a herd that has been free of the disease for a specified period of time.

PREVENTING INTRODUCTION OF INFECTIOUS DISEASES

Central to a biosecurity policy is the strict control of movements into the herd. While it is not appropriate for many herds to be closed, due to management constraints such as co-grazing or a production system based on the rearing of purchased stock, many breeding herds could be managed as "partially closed" units. However, even in essentially closed herds, cattle are occasionally introduced. This requires a rigorous policy to manage the introduction of these animals.

In herds that are not of a particularly high health status, the introduction of animals has inherent risks. The introduced animals may bring with them a pathogen not previously present, leading to disease in the indigenous population (eg, Johne's disease). They may also introduce a different strain of a pathogen (eg, anthelmintic-resistant GI nematodes or virulent infectious bovine rhinotracheitis virus) or may themselves become infected with a disease endemic in the indigenous population. Even if there is no desire to achieve or maintain a high-health-status herd, the risk of introducing more virulent strains of a pathogen or drug-resistant pathogens is very real whenever cattle move between herds.

Prepurchase Testing of Animals: When it is considered essential that only cattle free of certain infections are allowed into a herd, the safest strategy is to purchase animals directly from herds in which a certified testing program has demonstrated that the disease(s) is absent. When such animals are not available, the probability that an animal is infected with a particular disease should be minimized. For example, animals should preferably be purchased directly from a breeder rather than from a dealer or through an auction market. Purchased cattle should then be isolated on arrival and undergo a specific testing regimen before entering the main herd. This testing protocol should be designed to eliminate, or reduce as far as realistically and economically possible, the risk of introducing the target diseases. (*See also* PREPURCHASE EXAMINATION OF RUMINANTS AND SWINE, p 1387.)

Quarantine: Animals being introduced into a herd or a country from another source herd or country may be quarantined in an isolation facility for a specified period of time, during which they are monitored clinically or by laboratory testing for evidence of infectious disease. If there is no evidence of infectious disease after a specified period of time, the restrictions on the quarantined animals are lifted, and they are allowed to mix with the importing herd or the general population. During the period of quarantine, transmission of infectious agents from the quarantined animals to the importing herd must be prevented by ensuring that feed and water supplies and personnel are kept separate from the nonquarantined animals.

Control of Wildlife Vectors: The control of some infectious diseases of food-producing animals, especially cattle, depends on control of disease in wildlife vectors that are reservoirs of infection.

CONTROL OF ENDEMIC INFECTIOUS DISEASES

The inability to completely eradicate many infectious diseases leaves control as the most practical alternative. The ideal objectives of control are to reduce the prevalence of existing infections and the incidence of new infections, and to reduce the morbidity and mortality rates from clinical disease.

One of the most important principles of infectious disease control is to minimize the infection pressure on noninfected susceptible animals and prevent new infections. This is accomplished by maintaining a clean environment so that contamination of the feed and water supplies, bedding, and other materials with infectious agents is minimized. The environment must not be allowed to become heavily contaminated with pathogens shed by carrier animals. High population densities or crowding must be avoided to control the spread of infection among animals. Feed and water supplies must be handled and situated to avoid fecal contamination. However, a controlled infection pressure may be useful. Low levels of contamination below those that result in clinical disease can result in effective immunization, as is seen in coccidiosis.

A second principle is to reduce the environmental and host risk factors that increase susceptibility to disease. Some common environmental risk factors include inadequate housing and ventilation, rapid changes in weather, and sudden exposure to cold and windy weather. Examples of host risk factors include failure of colostral transfer in newborn animals, inadequate nutrition, deficiencies of trace minerals such as selenium and copper, genetic susceptibility, total lack of immunity because of no previous exposure to the antigen (either by natural infection or vaccination), age of animal (the young are more susceptible), stress, food deprivation, immunosuppression, ineffective vaccination practices, concurrent infections, and mixing animals of different ages and from different sources, as is commonly done in commercial feedlots.

Investigation of Epidemics of Infectious Disease

Epidemics of infectious disease are seen even in well-managed herds. The veterinarian should, whenever possible, visit the herd and conduct a thorough epidemiologic investigation of the epidemic, including clinical examination of affected animals. Appropriate laboratory samples should be collected from both affected and normal animals. The aim is to identify risk factors and attempt to eliminate or modify them. The investigation and clinical management of herd epidemics also involves providing recommendations about appropriate treatment, such as antimicrobial therapy, and advice on the withholding of milk from lactating dairy cattle or the slaughter of animals until the withdrawal period is over. Detailed epidemiologic and clinical data must be recorded for the duration of the epidemic. The appropriate analysis and interpretation should be made, followed by a final report to the producer.

Vaccination Programs

Several criteria must be considered in determining whether vaccination is either possible or desirable in controlling a specific disease. The first is the absolute identification of the causal agent. Second, it must be established that an immune response can actually protect against the disease in question. Third, there must be assurance that the risks of vaccination do not exceed those associated with the chance of developing the disease in question. The decision to use vaccines for the control of any disease must be based on considerations not only of the severity of the problem, but also of the prospects for its control by other techniques, such as removing or reducing risk factors.

Producers should record the date on which animals were vaccinated and the brand name and batch number of the vaccine used. Proper implementation of vaccination protocols is necessary to optimize efficacy of vaccines. Periodic reviews of the management practices in a herd are necessary to ensure that the vaccinations are actually done. Label directions should always be followed regarding the use of the vaccine, how it should be stored, whether unused portions can be used at another time, the route of administration, the proper use of needles and syringes, and the hazards of chemical sterilants when using a live vaccine.

PREVENTING SPREAD OF INFECTIOUS AGENTS

Livestock producers and veterinarians must ensure that infections are not spread from one herd or farm to adjacent farms. Culled animals should not be sent to slaughter if they are known to be infected with certain diseases. Disposal of animals that die of an infectious disease must be careful and adequate. (*See* DISPOSAL OF CARCASSES AND DISINFECTION OF PREMISES, p 1377.) All animal attendants should be educated about infectious disease control, and outside contact with animals must be limited.

MANAGEMENT OF THE NEONATE

LARGE ANIMALS

Management is especially important at birth when both dam and fetus are at increased risk of trauma and death. Some conditions and problems are common to all large animal neonates. There is no prepartum transplacental transfer of antibodies from dam to fetus, which renders all large animal neonates susceptible to failure of passive transfer of antibodies if adequate amounts of good quality colostrum are not consumed during the early postpartum period. Dystocia increases the risk of serious injury to the dam while exposing the fetus to potential bouts of life-threatening asphyxia and acidosis. During the early postpartum period, all neonates are susceptible to hypoglycemia, hypothermia, septicemia, peripartum asphyxia, and mismothering. These conditions pose more of a problem in certain species due to differences in the delivery process itself, the type of placentation, the presence of single or multiple neonates, and the innate susceptibility of the neonate to birth stresses. There are usually more financial constraints surrounding the care of calves, lambs, kids, and piglets than of foals. In general, more time and finances are focused on foals due to the fact that a relatively long gestation and sudden delivery results in the birth of only a single neonate.

Parturition

Dams should be vaccinated prepartum to improve colostral quality and enhance neonatal immunoprotection against specific infectious diseases. Ideally, pregnant females should not be moved prior to parturition because their colostrum also contains antibodies against various bacterial and viral pathogens in their environment. To reduce exposure to infectious diseases, the dam should be isolated from new arrivals and any transient animal populations.

Whenever practical, the dam should be provided with separate quarters for delivery that are spacious, well lit, well ventilated, clean, disinfected, and that provide good footing. During parturition, particularly in the case of primiparous animals, an attendant should be available. Birth is a physiologic process that usually occurs without intervention, which, if inappropriate, may permanently injure the reproductive tract or injure or kill the neonate(s). A reasonable period of labor must be permitted for the cervix to dilate and for the vagina and vulva to prepare for passage of the fetus. Veterinary assistance should be secured for more involved cases of fetal malpositioning. Ideally all deliveries in horses should be attended due to the mare's short (<30-40 min) and relatively forceful stage II labor. Dystocias during unattended deliveries in mares often result in death or injury to the fetus and/or dam. Foals surviving difficult births often require resuscitation or oxygen administration and supportive care. In cattle, cesarean sections save many calves that would not survive delivery through a narrow birth canal, particularly in fat or immature dams.

Immediate Postpartum Care

After delivery, the neonate's respiratory tract should be cleared immediately. A portion of the placenta may cover the nostrils, or inhaled amniotic fluid may block air passages. Meconium staining of the fetus or fluids is suggestive of birth stress and peripartum asphyxia. Meconium can physically obstruct the larynx and lower airways if inhaled, and it should be removed. Artificial respiration and elevation of the neonate's hindquarters often assist in initiating respirations. Smaller animals can be held head down and, while carefully supported, swung through a small arc to promote drainage of the respiratory tract. Brisk rubbing with a towel and extension of the limbs also stimulates respiration.

Neonates experiencing postpartum apnea require artificial respiration using mouth-to-nose resuscitation or ventilation via an endotracheal tube. Prompt insertion of a cuffed endotracheal tube into the trachea and application of suction followed by positive-pressure ventilation can save some animals that would otherwise die. Calves and small ruminants can be intubated orally using a laryngoscope and an endotracheal tube with a rigid stylet. Calves can be intubated blindly via palpation of the larynx with the head and neck in an extended position. Foals can be intubated orally or nasally using a long, cuffed nasotracheal tube. Ideally, meconium or excessive amniotic fluid should be removed by suctioning of the nasal passages and nasopharynx, followed by positive-pressure ventilation administered via a handheld resuscitation bag. If spontaneous respirations are abnormally slow or labored and accompanied by bradycardia, oxygen supplementation is indicated. Oxygen can be administered using a face mask equipped with an exhalation valve or via an intranasal cannula placed up one nostril to a level just below the medial canthus of the eye. Oxygen flows of 3-7 L/min are usually adequate. Maintaining the neonate in sternal recumbency allows ventilation of both lung fields and reduces dependent lung atelectasis.

If cardiac arrest accompanies respiratory arrest, then chest compressions should be initiated after ventilation has been started. Larger neonates should be placed on their right side and cardiac compression applied just caudal to the left elbow and just above the costochondral junction. If cardiac arrest persists, IV epinephrine should be given at an initial IV dosage of 0.01-0.02 mg/kg. If there is no response within 3 min, additional epinephrine can be given IV or intratracheally at a dosage of 0.1 mg/kg at 3- to 5-min intervals.

If birth was normal and the umbilical cord was not ruptured in the process, the cord should be left intact for ~5 min; contraction of the uterus forces placental blood into the neonate, thus increasing its chances of survival and reducing the risk of neonatal anemia. After the cord is broken, 2% iodine or chlorhexidine solution should be applied to the stump twice daily until the umbilical remnant is dry. All meconium should be passed within 24 hr of delivery. Foals are often given prophylactic gravity enemas to reduce the risk of meconium impaction. In areas where screw worms are a problem for ruminants, repellent should be applied. Because some dams, especially primiparous ones, may be apprehensive and injure their offspring by butting, striking, kicking, or biting, the attendant should protect the newborn from injury until the dam accepts it or remove it completely from the stall. Mares that attempt to kick or bite their newborn foals can be sedated with acepromazine. Hobbles and a grazing muzzle can be used on the mare to help prevent injury to her foal. Whenever there are signs of mismothering, it is important to reduce unnecessary traffic into and around the birthing stall while ensuring that calm, competent handlers are in attendance to facilitate bonding between dam and offspring.

All large animal neonates are born essentially without circulating γ-globulins due to the lack of in utero transfer of immunoglobulins to the fetus. Ingestion of colostrum that contains adequate amounts of IgG, IgM, and IgA is essential. When absorbed through the gut wall and when in the gut lumen, these immunoglobulins protect the neonate against systemic and enteric diseases. The effectiveness of colostrum in disease prevention and control is determined by the amount ingested, the concentration of specific immunoglobulins, and the absorptive capability of the neonate's gut wall. Colostrum from primiparous animals may be deficient in immunoglobulins. Premature lactation in mares is another common cause of poor colostral quality.

Newborns should receive colostrum as soon after birth as possible, preferably within the first 30-90 min. They should be observed closely and assisted if necessary to make certain that they nurse. If the neonate is too weak to nurse, colostrum should be fed via bottle or stomach tube. When colostrum from the dam is not available, it should be secured from another animal or from a previously frozen supply. Foals should receive a minimum of 1 L, and calves 2 L of colostrum. Following adequate colostrum ingestion, healthy foals and ruminants should have serum IgG concentrations >800 mg/dL and >1,600 mg/dL, respectively. Neonates >24 hr old with failure of passive transfer of colostral antibodies are unable to absorb immunoglobulins received PO due to a decrease in gut wall permeability. These older individuals must receive parenteral antibody supplementation using plasma from the dam or a commercial source. The minimal volume of plasma required is usually 20-40 mL/kg.

Early assessment of the newborn allows timely detection of illness and identification of potentially life-threatening congenital malformations. Early recognition of a hopelessly deformed neonate allows an owner to consider euthanasia versus prolonged care and treatment. Many birth defects are heritable, but it is often difficult to differentiate between those that are and those that are not. Surgical correction of some abnormalities is possible but usually not desirable if the animal will be used for breeding. Examples of potentially life-threatening congenital defects include severe craniofacial malformations, cleft palate, scoliosis, ventral septal defect, severe limb contracture, and atresia coli. Other defects such as umbilical or inguinal hernias are often self-correcting within the first few months of life.

Large animal neonates are precocious and should be able to stand and nurse within 1-3 hr of birth. Newborn foals and calves have a body temperature of 99-102°F (37-38°C) and a pulse of 80-110 bpm. Early signs of neonatal compromise include a weak or absent suckle reflex, inability to stand, depressed or somnolent attitude, and injected mucous membranes and/or sclera. Common periparturient conditions that result in reduced neonatal vigor include hypothermia, hypoglycemia, septicemia, diarrhea, peripartum asphyxia, and prematurity or dysmaturity. If newborn animals become sick, diagnosis and treatment must be prompt because they have little reserve and die quickly. Proper nursing care often determines whether a sick animal will live or die and should not be neglected.

Hypothermia: Although most newborn livestock can withstand very cold temperatures once they are dried (except piglets, *see* below), their extremities may freeze if they are born into a cold environment. In climates where winter temperatures are low, protection should be provided. If economic conditions make this unfeasible, animals should be bred to give birth later in the winter or early spring.

Every effort should be made to maintain body heat during inclement weather. For large animals, it usually is not practical or advisable to heat a large barn to maintain the temperature during extremely cold weather. In such cases, it is advisable to partition small areas that can be more economically heated for severely stressed animals. If used, heat sources should be regulated to meet the needs of the species of animals being managed (eg, piglets require a much warmer environment than calves or foals). A radiant heat lamp placed beyond the animal's reach probably is the most effective method of maintaining body heat in sick neonates.

Neonatal Hypoglycemia: Hypoglycemia develops as a result of decreased caloric intake and/or increased catabolism. Decreased intake can be associated with inability to nurse due to neonatal factors such as weakness, prematurity, peripartum asphyxia, or competition between siblings, or it may be due to maternal factors such as agalactia, mastitis, or maternal rejection. Increased catabolism is often due to septicemia resulting in increased glucose consumption by bacteria and decreased glucose uptake by host cells due to peripheral insulin resistance.

Septicemia with secondary loss of nursing vigor is the most common cause of severe hypoglycemia (glucose <20-40 mg/dL) in newborn foals. Affected foals often exhibit temperature instability and varying degrees of hypovolemic and hemodynamic shock. In addition to parenteral glucose supplementation, septic foals require IV antibiotics, parenteral fluid therapy, and respiratory and nutritional support. Although the intraperitoneal route is used for glucose administration in piglets and small ruminants, it should not be used in foals.

Neonatal hypoglycemia is most common in piglets <1 wk old. It is a contributing factor that leads to death in many diseases and accounts for 15-35% of total piglet mortality. With only partial gluconeogenic ability, limited energy reserves, and essentially no brown fat, newborn piglets rely on glycogen reserves and, most importantly, frequent nursing. Piglets are predisposed to hypoglycemia if the sow has any disease that decreases or inhibits milk production or letdown. Large litter size with an inadequate number of teats precludes proper nursing. In addition, if the lower rail of the farrowing crate impairs access to the udder, inadequate milk intake and hypoglycemia can result.

Piglets have an effective metabolic response to cold and fully functional peripheral vasoconstriction, but their lack of insulating subcutaneous fat (until 1-2 wk old) allows marked heat loss. In drafty or wet environments, on cold floors, or in low ambient temperatures, maintenance of body temperature demands rapid glucose use, which depletes glycogen reserves; if milk intake is impaired, hypoglycemia and death result.

One or more piglets in a litter may be involved. Initially, behavior changes from vigorous sucking or play alternating with sleep to solitary lassitude. Affected piglets wander aimlessly with a faltering gait and cry weakly. The piglets are gaunt with poor muscle tone and pale, cold, clammy skin. They are hypothermic and unresponsive to external stimuli. As incoordination increases, piglets may stand with legs splayed, followed by sternal or lateral recumbency. Terminally, they exhibit convulsions with jaw champing, salivation, opisthotonos, nystagmus, forelimb and hindlimb contraction, coma, and death. Many affected piglets are crushed by the sow.

Blood glucose levels fall from a normal of 90-130 mg/dL to as low as 5-15 mg/dL; piglets usually manifest clinical signs when levels are <50 mg/dL. Any condition that impairs food intake by neonatal pigs can complicate the diagnosis. Generally, however, hypoglycemia can be diagnosed by examination of the sow and environment for predisposing factors and by the piglet's response to glucose therapy.

Piglets should be treated with 15 mL of 5% glucose given IP and placed in a warm environment. A heat lamp can be used. Shivering and more activity should follow within 5-10 min. Severely hypoglycemic and hypothermic piglets may not respond. Sustained energy intake must be provided to avoid relapse. If oxytocin fails to promote milk letdown in the sow, 20 mL of 5% dextrose, cow's colostrum, or evaporated milk diluted one-half with water can be administered intragastrically to each piglet through a small plastic cannula (with care, to avoid damage to the pharyngeal diverticulae), or treatment with glucose IP can be repeated every 4-6 hr. Active piglets learn quickly to drink from a dish. Foster-suckling of piglets is possible in batch farrowing units; most sows accept piglets during the milk letdown period if introduced quietly within the first 24 hr after farrowing. Redistribution of piglets from litters of uneven sizes may reduce mortality from starvation and hypoglycemia. Any primary disease of the sow should be treated, and any faults within the environment corrected. Piglets should be held in a draft-free creep area heated to 95°F (35°C) during the first week of life. Cold-stressed and marginally hypoglycemic piglets are more susceptible to other neonatal diseases.

Septicemia: The most common routes of infection for large animal neonates are the placenta, the GI and respiratory tracts, and the umbilical remnants. Bacterial sepsis is most commonly associated with disseminated gram-negative bacterial infection. During sepsis, the release of bacterial endo- or exotoxins results in overactivation of the host's immune system and uncontrolled release of endogenous mediators. This response precipitates a cascade of metabolic and hemodynamic changes that often culminates in multiple organ system failure. The endpoint is septic shock and is characterized by circulatory failure, perfusion deficits, and an inability of the body to use existing metabolic substrates effectively.

Factors predisposing to the development of septicemia include overcrowding; poor ventilation and sanitation; inappropriate umbilical disinfection; and periparturient stresses including premature delivery, dystocia, cesarean section, peripartum hypoxia, severe maternal illness, and failure of passive antibody transfer. Early signs of neonatal sepsis include lethargy, hypotonia, decreased nursing vigor, loss of suckle reflex, hyperemic mucous membranes with rapid capillary refill time associated with peripheral vasodilation, increased cardiac output, tachycardia, bounding peripheral pulses, extremities that are still warm, tachypnea, and variable body temperature. Increased vascular permeability contributes to the development of petechial hemorrhages on the gums, sclera, coronary bands, and inside the ears. During late sepsis, signs of shock develop. Affected neonates are usually recumbent, dehydrated, and moribund. Clinical signs include severe hypotension; tachycardia; cold extremities; dry, injected mucous membranes with a toxic ring; and prolonged capillary refill time. Gut motility is reduced or absent and is accompanied by gastric reflux, abdominal distention, and diarrhea or constipation. Tachypnea, dyspnea, rib retractions, and expiratory grunting characterize respiratory failure. One of the earliest laboratory signs of sepsis is the development of leukopenia, neutropenia, and a degenerative left shift accompanied by dehydration.

Successful treatment of neonatal sepsis depends on early recognition and aggressive support using systemic, broad-spectrum, bactericidal antibiotics, IV fluids (crystalloids and colloids), plasma, enteral and/or parenteral nutritional support, and oxygen therapy.

Neonatal Diarrhea: Diarrhea is a common problem for all large animal neonates. In ruminants, causes of neonatal diarrhea include rotavirus, cryptosporidia, coronavirus, *Campylobacter* spp, enterotoxigenic *Escherichia coli*, and *Salmonella*. In calves, bovine viral diarrhea virus is another important etiologic agent. Causes of diarrhea in newborn foals include rotavirus, *Salmonella*, *Clostridia* spp, *Strongyloides*, and necrotizing enterocolitis. Therapy for neonatal diarrhea focuses on maintaining hydration and preventing electrolyte imbalances such as metabolic acidosis, hyponatremia, and hypochloremia, while treating the underlying cause.

Peripartum Asphyxia: Asphyxia is the result of impaired oxygen delivery to cells and usually results from a combination of hypoxemia—decreased oxygen concentration in the blood—and ischemia—decreased tissue perfusion. Periparturient asphyxia can result from any event that impairs uteroplacental perfusion prepartum or intrapartum or disrupts normal distribution of blood flow postpartum. Neonatal asphyxia has been associated with normal deliveries, dystocias, induced deliveries, cesarean sections, placentitis, premature placental separation, meconium-stained foals, the birth of multiple fetuses, severe maternal illness, and post-term pregnancies.

Neonates with periparturient asphyxia display a wide spectrum of neurologic signs that include jitteriness, hyperalertness, stupor, somnolence, lethargy, hypotonia, seizures, extensor rigidity, tonic posturing, aimless wandering, head pressing, loss of affinity for the dam, inability to find the udder, abnormal vocalization (barking, high pitched cry), loss of suckle, dysphagia, odontoprisis, central blindness, anisocoria, nystagmus, eye deviation, head tilt, head and neck turn, irregular respiration, apnea, abnormally slow respiratory rate, dysmetric gait, and proprioceptive deficits. Hypoxic neonates may also experience gut stasis and renal ischemia. Therapy includes anticonvulsants to stop seizures (eg, diazepam, phenobarbital), medication to control cerebral edema (eg, IV dimethyl sulfoxide, IV mannitol), antibody administration to prevent secondary sepsis, nutritional support to prevent hypoglycemia, and vigilant nursing care to prevent injury while the neonate is recumbent or disoriented.

Prematurity and Dysmaturity: Possible causes of prematurity or dysmaturity include the following: in utero viral infection, acute or chronic bacterial placentitis, congenital fetal abnormalities, maternal endocrine abnormalities, chronic placental insufficiency, maternal hydrops allantois/amnii, incompetent cervix, severe maternal illness, and prolonged maternal fasting.

Clinical signs include low birth weight; generalized muscle weakness; inability to maintain sternal recumbency or stand unassisted; short, silky hair coat; domed forehead; floppy ears and soft lips; diminished suckle reflex and ineffective swallow; delayed time to nurse; periarticular ligamentous laxity and flexor tendon laxity; delayed time to stand; hypothermia due to poor thermoregulatory control; intolerance to oral feeding due to immature GI function resulting in colic, gastric reflux, abdominal distention, and diarrhea; increased work of breathing; tachypnea and respiratory distress due to lung and chest wall immaturity; and incomplete ossification of cuboidal bones. Premature neonates require good nursing care and excellent nutritional support until they are able to stand and nurse normally. Until that time, premature newborns are at increased risk of respiratory distress and septicemia.

SMALL ANIMALS

Puppies and kittens commonly present for severe illnesses or for rearing as an orphan between birth and 12 wk of age. Illnesses may have been acquired in utero, around the time of birth (0-2 wk of age), or in the postweaning period (6-12 wk of age). Illness during the postweaning period is primarily caused by infectious diseases and/or malnutrition potentiated by weaning stress, exposure to pathogenic organisms in the immediate environment, and diminished local and/or systemic immunity. Most puppy and kitten illnesses result from congenital anomalies, nutritional diseases resulting from improper diets fed to the mother or her young, abnormally low birth weights, traumatic insults during or after birth (dystocia, cannibalism, maternal neglect), neonatal isoerythrolysis, or infectious diseases.

A thorough history (including information on parents and littermates) and physical examination are key components in the assessment of sick neonates. Weight should be compared with that of healthy littermates. Values such as temperature, blood pressure, and many hematologic and biochemical parameters can differ significantly between adults and neonates, so appropriate reference data must be used. A blood sample can be obtained via jugular venipuncture using a 22-gauge needle with a 3-mL syringe. Collection tubes designed for small volumes should be used.

Immediate Postpartum Care
See also MANAGEMENT OF REPRODUCTION: SMALL ANIMALS, p 1795.

Hypoxia or anorexia is a common cause of death in neonates. Immediately following parturition (whether by natural delivery or cesarean section), several procedures should be performed. The airway should be cleared and free of any membranes from the placenta, fluid, and meconium within 1-3 min of birth. The placental membranes should be torn and removed quickly from around the head, especially those covering the openings of the nostrils. Quickly afterward, fluid should be gently suctioned and swabbed from the mouth and opening of the throat. Thereafter, fluid can be expelled from the upper and lower airways by gently swinging the neonate headfirst in a downward path while supporting its head and trunk in a dry, warm towel. If respiration does not begin spontaneously, chest and facial massage with a dry, warm towel may be needed. Effects of narcotics or barbiturates used during cesarean section may be reversed by instilling one to two drops of naloxone or doxapram onto the tongue and roof of the mouth of the neonate. If the neonate is still unresponsive, oxygen is provided through a facemask.

Cardiac arrest or a failing heartbeat generally follow poor respiration that does not respond to treatment. If no heartbeat is detected, the chest is massaged in the area of the heart. If the heart rate is <60 bpm, diluted epinephrine may be placed into the throat or mouth. However, these neonates rarely survive.

Hypothermia develops if external warming is not provided immediately after birth. Neonates should be quickly dried after birth and kept warm. Room temperature should be ~84-86°F (28.9-30°C).

Routine Health Management

Puppies and kittens should be checked for GI parasites at ~3 wk and dewormed at regular intervals—every other week until they reach 2 mo of age, then monthly until they reach 6 mo of age. Heartworm preventive medication should be started at 6-8 wk of age in areas where heartworm disease is endemic. The initial vaccination series for puppies and kittens usually begins at 6 wk of age with boosters given at 9 wk, 12 wk, and sometimes 15 wk. Rabies vaccine should be given as required by law (at 3 mo of age in most states in the USA).

Bacterial Infections

The bacterial invasion of the bloodstream that is regularly seen in puppies and kittens after birth would rarely be of any consequence in healthy adults. Factors predisposing puppies and kittens to septicemic conditions include coexistence of inadequate nutrition and thermoregulation, viral infections, parasitism, and developmental and heritable defects of the immune system.

Etiology: Bloodstream invasion is usually by the more common bacteria, such as *Staphylococcus, Escherichia, Klebsiella, Enterobacter, Streptococcus, Enterococcus, Pseudomonas, Clostridium, Bacteroides, Fusobacterium,* and *Salmonella* spp. Of these, gram-negative bacilli are seen most often. They may enter the bloodstream from the GI tract or from peritoneal, respiratory tract, skin and wound, or urinary tract infection.

Clinical Findings: The clinical manifestations of neonatal illness do not always allow specific identification of the cause. Furthermore, many puppies and kittens have unusual clinical presentations that may not be immediately associated with a specific illness. Death can occur so suddenly that noticeable signs are virtually absent. More typically, puppies and kittens cry often and show signs of restlessness, weakness, hypothermia, diarrhea, altered respiration, hematuria, failure to thrive, and cyanosis; in advanced stages, they may slough parts of their extremities.

Diagnosis: Neonatal illness is usually diagnosed based on the case history and physical examination findings. Ideally, a CBC, plasma chemistry profile, urinalysis, urine and/or blood culture, and culture of suspected sources of infection is obtained. When dealing with neonatal sepsis, conducting a thorough search for the primary source of infection and collecting appropriate bacterial culture samples before initiating antimicrobial therapy is imperative.

The hemograms of septicemic puppies and kittens are usually characterized by a normochromic, normocytic anemia. Thrombocytopenia and mild to moderate neutrophilia with a left shift may be present. Hypoglycemia is consistent with, but not specific for, neonatal sepsis. The remaining laboratory values from the plasma chemistry profile and urinalysis may reflect a specific organ failure.

Treatment: Early prompt care for the ill puppy or kitten is required. Because many neonatal diseases may cause sudden death, puppies and kittens suspected of having a severe illness should be treated immediately. In most instances, rewarming, fluid replacement, and antimicrobial therapy are started empirically. Severely ill puppies and kittens may also require glucose therapy (5% dextrose, IV or intraosseously) if hypoglycemia is present. Animals that are profoundly depressed or seizuring can be given 10-20% dextrose at 1-2 mL/kg.

Many newer antimicrobial agents have either an increased spectrum of activity or a diminished toxicity relative to previously available antimicrobial agents. However, specific pharmacokinetic data have not been obtained either in adults or in puppies and kittens, and therefore, the use of these antimicrobial agents remains somewhat empiric.

Drug distribution, especially in puppies and kittens <5 wk old, differs from that of adults because of differences in body composition, such as lower total body fat, higher percentage of total body water, lower concentrations of albumin, and a poorly developed blood-brain barrier. Because of these differences, a reduction of as much as 30-50% of the adult dose, or changes in dosing frequency, may be necessary when treating septicemic puppies and kittens.

Fluid replacement therapy and antimicrobial agents should be administered IV or intraosseously in severely ill puppies and kittens, as systemic absorption following PO, SC, or IM administration may not be reliable. Most drugs ingested by the lactating bitch or queen appear in her milk. The amount generally is 1-2% of the mother's dose; therefore, severely ill puppies or kittens should never be treated only by treating the lactating mother. β-Lactam antimicrobial agents (eg, penicillins, cephalosporins, combined β-lactam/β-lactamase inhibitors) are the first choice for the treatment of septicemic puppies and kittens.

Malnutrition

Malnutrition develops when basic nutritional requirements for puppies or kittens are not being met and is especially common during the time when they depend entirely on the mother. Several factors can contribute to malnutrition in nursing puppies or kittens, including death of the mother, maternal neglect, a larger litter than can be cared for properly, and partial or complete lactation failure by the mother due to mastitis, metritis, or underdeveloped mammae. In addition, puppies and kittens may be born underdeveloped, be so weak and sick that they cannot suckle, or have a congenital anomaly that precludes adequate milk intake. Failure to provide an adequate growth diet at 3-4 wk of age can also result in malnutrition.

Immediate recognition of a malnourished puppy or kitten is usually based on their smaller, lighter appearance, feeble attempts to feed, and/or inability to attain adequate weight gain for their age. High-pitched, constant crying or inactivity with an accompanying weak sucking reflex are advanced indications that the nursing puppy or kitten is malnourished. Reduced body tone and muscle strength may be evident on handling. Coexisting congenital anomalies that are not immediately life-threatening may be detected on physical examination as well.

Correction of malnutrition in nursing puppies or kittens generally requires that proper nourishment be provided. Complications that are frequently encountered during the management of malnutrition are diarrhea, dehydration, hypoglycemia, and hypothermia. If diarrhea develops during feeding of adequate amounts of commercial milk replacement formula, the amount of solids fed should be reduced to one half of that offered. This can be done by diluting the milk replacement formula 1:1 with water or preferably with a mixture of equal parts of Ringer's solution and 5% dextrose/water solution. As the condition of feces improves, the amount of solids can be gradually increased to the recommended level. Hypoglycemia and dehydration develop quickly when malnourished puppies or kittens are not adequately fed. Milk replacement formula should not be fed to a weak and severely chilled puppy or kitten that possesses a diminished sucking reflex or body temperature <35°C (95°F). Giving an equal mixture of warm Ringer's solution and 5% dextrose/water solution parenterally or administering a warm nutrient-electrolyte solution PO every 15-30 min can help to alleviate or prevent dehydration and mild hypoglycemia.

CARE OF ORPHANED NATIVE BIRDS AND MAMMALS

It is important to determine if an animal is truly orphaned. In many cases, if a bird is returned to its nest or the mammal is left alone and monitored, the parent returns to care for it. Handling of baby birds to return them to their nest does not preclude the parents from accepting them. If an animal or bird is taken for hand-rearing, warmth, hydration, and energy are critical. Because most orphans initially cannot maintain or regulate their body temperature, supplemental heat must be provided with the aid of heating pads, hot water bottles, or incandescent light bulbs. Providing a heat gradient, so that the orphan can select its own comfort zone is ideal. The orphan must be insulated from direct heat to prevent thermal burns. Electric coil heating devices can develop hot spots when worn or damaged. The initial temperature range should be 26-32°C. A hypothermic orphan should not be fed until the body temperature is near normal. During rewarming, hydration and energy can be provided with oral saline and 10-20% dextrose solutions.

Various diets are used to feed altricial birds; they generally contain cooked egg yolk, canned dog food, and baby cereal, which is mixed with water or electrolyte solution in a 1:1 ratio to make a slurry that is fed through a medicine dropper. A few drops of pediatric multivitamins are added to all formulas for orphans. Multivitamin supplements with iron should be avoided, as some birds are prone to iron-storage disease.

Young birds should be stimulated by rustling the nest or tapping them on the upper beak to stimulate gaping. The food is then delivered to the back of the mouth; the bird will stop gaping when it is full. The bird should be fed every 15 min for 1-2 hr and then hourly for 12 hr during the day; its weight and crop emptying should be closely monitored. In some cases, the chick may require feeding around the clock. Crop stasis can develop with overfeeding, formula that is too warm, or secondary yeast infections.

A satisfactory diet for pigeons and doves consists of dry dog food soaked in water (1:1) to form a slurry.

When feeding mammals, once the infant has been stabilized, the formula is introduced gradually using $1/2$ strength for 1-2 days, then $3/4$ strength for 1-2 days, and then full formula. There may be a slight weight loss, but this procedure usually avoids GI upsets.

Handrearing of orphaned skunks, foxes, and raccoons is inadvisable because of the rabies hazard and local regulations. Local fish and game officials and local licensed rehabilitators should be consulted. For raising squirrels and opossum, a commercial milk replacer should be fed every 3 hr for 18 hr/day. Rabbits are very difficult to raise by hand; they can be offered this formula 2-3 times a day. Cow's milk or goat's milk cannot be used universally, as the total solids and casein:whey ratios may not be appropriate for other species.

See also HANDREARING MAMMALS, p 1852.

PAIN MANAGEMENT

Behaviors suggestive of pain are routinely used to diagnose injuries and diseases, guide therapy, and provide prognostic information. Obvious signs of pain alert owners and veterinarians to the fact that something is wrong with the animal. Thus, there is nothing novel about considering pain to be important clinically in the overall evaluation of an animal. What is relatively new is the understanding of the complexity of pain and the recent emphasis on the ethical and medical obligations to treat pain in animals. Although there is some limited survey data and anecdotal evidence to suggest that the management of pain is receiving more attention in veterinary medicine than before, the assessment, prevention, and treatment of pain has yet to become an integral part of every physical examination and treatment plan.

PAIN PERCEPTION

Pain serves a protective role to alert an individual to injury from the environment or from within the individual. Based on what is known to date, all vertebrates, and some invertebrates, experience pain in response to actual or potential tissue damage. Many different types of pain are encountered, with the most common being acute, chronic, cancer, and neuropathic pain. Acute pain is the normal predicted physiologic response to an adverse chemical, thermal, or mechanical stimulus. It may also be the initiation phase of an extensive, persistent nociceptive and behavioral cascade triggered by tissue injury. Acute pain generally improves within the first 3 days following an event such as surgery, but may persist for weeks or months. Chronic pain may be defined as pain that persists for longer than the expected time frame for healing or pain associated with progressive nonmalignant disease (such as osteoarthritis). Cancer pain refers to pain that is the result of primary tumor growth, metastatic disease, or the toxic effects of chemotherapy and radiation. Neuropathic pain refers to a persistent pain syndrome resulting from damage to a peripheral nerve, dorsal root ganglion or dorsal root, or the CNS. Neuropathic pain is recognized in veterinary medicine much less often than in human medicine.

For an animal to experience pain, nociceptive information must be sent to the higher centers in the CNS to be integrated and interpreted into the sensory experience of pain. Noxious stimuli (heat, cold, mechanical, chemical) activate free sensory nerve endings known as nociceptors. A-δ and C-fibers transmit sensory information from the nociceptors to the dorsal horn of the spinal cord, which directs and modulates the input from sensory neurons. Nociceptive information arriving in the dorsal horn of the spinal cord may activate motor neurons responsible for the reflex responses to noxious stimuli (such as withdrawing a limb). Importantly, the nociceptive sensory input may be amplified or inhibited by spinal interneurons. Sensory information is relayed to higher centers in the CNS along a variety of pathways that differ according to species. In general, nociceptive information ascends the spinal cord along superficial and deep pathways to the brain stem with connections to the thalamus, reticular formation (responsible for level of arousal), and limbus (responsible for emotions). From these areas of the brain, nociceptive information is relayed to the cortex where it is recognized as pain. Activity in spinal nociceptive pathways is strongly influenced by descending antinociceptive systems that originate in the brain stem. Endogenous antinociceptive neurotransmitters (eg, endorphin, enkephalin, and dynorphin) inhibit the transmission of nociceptive information in the spinal cord and brain.

The neuroanatomic components of the nociceptive/pain pathways and pain-suppressing systems can change in response to sustained sensory input. Peripheral sensitization of nociceptors and central sensitization of nociceptive neurons and pathways in the spinal cord and brain can develop as a result of extensive tissue trauma or nerve injury. The process of peripheral and central sensitization has been termed "wind-up" and refers to the neuroanatomic changes that result in heightened or exaggerated pain states. Additionally, chronic pain sometimes does not respond to conventional analgesic therapy due to changes in the CNS processing of nociceptive input. Thus, changes in the CNS in response to repeated and sustained nociceptive input (ie, pain) complicate the clinical management of pain.

RECOGNITION AND ASSESSMENT OF PAIN IN ANIMALS

The assessment of pain in animals can be challenging. Recognizing pain in animals is not intuitive, particularly by individuals unfamiliar with normal behavior for a species or individual. In recent years, there has been an increased focus on determining and measuring species-specific pain behaviors, which should improve recognition and treatment of pain in animals. Nevertheless, the assessment of pain in animals remains a subjective and inaccurate undertaking. Numerous factors complicate the evaluation of pain in animals. Any pain scale should consider the following characteristics: species, breed, environment and rearing conditions, age, gender, cause of pain (eg, trauma, surgery, pathology), body region affected (eg, abdominal pain, musculoskeletal pain), character of pain state (eg, acute, chronic), and pain intensity. Any pain scale or methodology employed to assess pain should be able to recognize individual sensitivities. Differences in pain tolerance have been demonstrated experimentally in people and animals, and play an important role in the clinical management of pain.

No "gold standard" exists to measure pain in animals or to compare one type of scale or measurement instrument with another. All of the **pain scales** used in animals rely on the recognition and/or interpretation of some behavior and are subject to some degree of variability among observers. Pain scales that are based on the determination of the presence or absence of species-specific behaviors, and that minimize the interpretation of those behaviors, are likely to be more accurate than generic scales that rely heavily on subjective assessment and interpretation. All current methods used to measure pain in animals are prone to errors of under- or overestimation. Even if the amount of pain is correctly estimated, determining how well the individual animal is coping with the pain may be difficult. This is particularly true if the animal is removed from its normal environment. Finally, all current methods assess the effects of physical pain; none has been designed to evaluate mental or psychological dimensions of pain that an animal may experience.

Physiologic parameters (eg, changes in heart rate, respiratory rate, arterial blood pressure, pupil dilation) may be used to assess responses to an acute noxious (painful) stimulus, particularly during anesthesia, and to assess pain in some clinical situations (eg, horses with acute colic pain). However, physiologic measurements often do not differentiate between animals that have undergone surgery and are experiencing pain and those that did not undergo surgery. Likewise, animals experiencing chronic pain may have normal physiologic parameters. Lack of change in physiologic responses should not be construed to mean there is no pain if other clinical signs suggest otherwise. Physiologic parameters are not specific enough to differentiate pain from other stressors such as anxiety, fear, or physiologic responses to metabolic conditions (eg, anemia).

Unfamiliarity with normal behaviors typical of a particular species or breed makes recognition of pain-induced behaviors difficult or impossible. **Behavioral changes** indicative of pain may be too subtle or take too long to recognize under routine clinical situations in both large and small animals. Sporadic observation of animal behavior may not reveal signs of pain. Except in the most severe circumstances, signs of pain may be "masked" by behavior that is stereotypical of the species being observed. For instance, dogs may wag their tails and greet observers in spite of being in pain. Flock animals, such as sheep, may be startled when an observer approaches and attempt to conceal any signs of pain by staying bunched up with the rest of the flock. Behavioral changes indicating pain may not be what we expect. A cat sitting quietly in the back of the cage after surgery may be painful; however, pain would not be recognized if the caregiver expects to see more active signs of pain such as pacing, agitation, or vocalization.

In general, responses to acute surgical and traumatic pain are likely to be more marked and readily recognizable than clinical signs associated with chronic pain. Clinical criteria used to assess chronic pain, eg, lack of activity, lack of grooming, decreased appetite, weight loss, are not specific signs of pain and point only to an underlying problem in need of further diagnosis. Evaluating the degree of lameness of affected limb(s) is often used to assess chronic orthopedic pain. For socialized animals, observations of owners are essential to detect more subtle signs of chronic pain such as changes in attitude or interaction with family members. Response to therapy, such as increased activity after administering an NSAID, may provide important information regarding the role that pain has played in behavioral changes.

Cancer pain may have components of acute pain (eg, expansion of a tumor or secondary responses to surgical, radiation, or chemotherapy treatment) and components of chronic pain. Thus, assessment of cancer pain requires the caregiver to use methods that can detect behavioral changes associated with both acute and chronic pain.

PAIN ALLEVIATION

Acute perioperative, traumatic, and disease-related (eg, cancer, pancreatitis, pleuritis) pain is generally treated pharmacologically with one or more analgesics. The optimal drug or drug combinations are determined principally by the anticipated severity of pain, health status, and available drugs for the given species. The more extensive the tissue trauma or disease-induced tissue damage is, the greater the need to use analgesics from more than one drug class (multimodal or balanced analgesia). Multimodal analgesia maximizes the beneficial analgesic effects of multiple drugs through additive or synergistic interactions while minimizing adverse drug effects by lowering the dose of any individual drug. A perioperative approach to managing surgically induced pain should be used, beginning with the administration of an analgesic before surgery (preemptive analgesia) and continuing with appropriate analgesia throughout the intraoperative periods. Three days is a useful guideline for the duration of analgesic therapy following acute surgical pain. Depending on multiple factors (eg, procedure performed, species, breed) some animals require a shorter duration of therapy, whereas other animals require analgesia for longer periods. Aggressive prevention and management of acute pain often prevents wind-up of the nociceptive pathways and hastens a return to normal function.

Minimizing stress and ensuring that overall care and husbandry are in accordance with the needs of the animal improve pain management. Proper housing conditions, nutritional support, and interaction with other animals and/or people should be optimal for the given species and breed. For example, separating a sheep from the flock for pain management may be quite stressful, whereas separating a house pet from other animals may not be stressful provided there is sufficient interaction with human caregivers. Managing painful and distressed animals requires a combination of good nursing care, nonpharmacologic methods (eg, bandaging, ice packs or heat, physical therapy), and pharmacologic methods. Pharmacologic methods available for the treatment of pain generally involve opioids, NSAID, corticosteroids, local anesthetics, α_2-agonists, and ketamine.

In the management of acute postoperative and traumatic pain, the following should be considered: 1) Pain is easier to prevent than treat once it is established. Perioperative analgesia should cover the entire operative period, beginning before the start of surgery and continuing for hours to days into the postoperative period. 2) As-needed dosing schedules are less effective than scheduled analgesic dosing to treat pain. As-needed dosing schedules require the animal to demonstrate overt pain behaviors to the extent that they are recognized by the veterinarian and/or owner. 3) Traditional NSAID may be ineffective as the sole agent for treatment of acute postoperative pain, whereas NSAID in combination with other analgesic drugs (ie, multimodal analgesia) may be very effective. 4) The therapeutic and side effects of analgesics are dose-dependent. Combining analgesic drugs allows for reduction in the dose of any one analgesic. 5) Agonist-antagonist opioids (eg, butorphanol) have a "ceiling" effect on analgesia. 6) Many animals benefit from the management of anxiety. Acepromazine is an effective anxiolytic in small animals, but should only be used after appropriate analgesics have been administered. Acepromazine does not have analgesic properties. 7) If in doubt about the role of pain in an animal, treat for pain and observe the results. 8) Appropriate analgesia following surgery or trauma will allows animals to rest. Dogs and cats often sleep, but should be arousable following surgery if their pain is controlled. 9) Aggressive analgesic therapy of several days' duration should be tapered rather than stopped abruptly. 10) Many animals benefit from combined or multimodal therapy (eg, combining an α_2-agonist and an opioid, also administering an NSAID).

ANALGESIC PHARMACOLOGY

Opioids

The opioids are a diverse group of naturally occurring and synthetic drugs used primarily for their analgesic activity. Despite some well-known side effects and disadvantages, opioids are the most effective analgesics available for the systemic treatment of acute pain in many species, particularly dogs and cats. Opioids combine reversibly with specific receptors in the brain, spinal cord, and periphery, altering the transmission and perception of pain. In addition to analgesia, opioids can induce other CNS effects that include sedation, euphoria, dysphoria, and excitement. (*See also* TABLE 14, p 2013.) The clinical effects of opioids vary between the μ opioid receptor agonists (eg, morphine, hydromorphone), partial mu agonists (ie, buprenorphine), and agonist-antagonists (eg, butorphanol). Species and individual differences in the response to opioids are marked, necessitating the adjustment of doses for different species. For example, a 30-kg dog may receive a preoperative dose of morphine (15-30 mg) that is similar to that of a 300-kg horse. The clinical effect of an opioid depends on additional patient factors, including the presence or absence of pain, health status of the animal, concurrent drugs administered (eg, tranquilizers), and individual sensitivity to opioid effects.

Nonsteroidal Anti-inflammatory Drugs and Corticosteroids

NSAID are useful adjuncts in the treatment of postsurgical pain in a variety of species. Decreasing inflammation following surgery or trauma can greatly improve analgesia. A significant advantage of NSAID over other analgesics is that an owner can easily administer them for several days after the animal has been discharged from the hospital. NSAID are also readily available, have a relatively long duration of action, and are generally inexpensive. NSAID have long been used to decrease inflammation and provide analgesia and should be considered as part of the analgesic plan provided the animal does not have pre-existing renal, hepatic, coagulation, or GI problems. NSAID should be administered only to well hydrated animals.

Corticosteroids also reduce inflammation and provide analgesia. Corticosteroids are used less frequently in the postoperative period due to the potential for decreasing immune function and due to other well-known side effects (eg, immune suppression, polyphagia, polydipsia, polyuria) following repeated dosing. Corticosteroids and NSAID should not be administered concurrently.

For pharmacology of NSAID and corticosteroids, *see* ANTI-INFLAMMATORY AGENTS, p 2125.

α₂-Agonists

Xylazine, medetomidine, detomidine, and romifidine are potent analgesics. α₂-Agonists are used in large animals for standing restraint that includes analgesia and sedation, although there is evidence to suggest that the sedation lasts longer than the analgesia. Combination therapy of α₂-agonists and opioids induces profound analgesia and sedation that is additive or synergistic as compared with the effects of either drug alone. α₂-Agonists are used as part of multimodal analgesia in the perioperative period in many species. Notwithstanding the beneficial analgesic properties, many practitioners are uncomfortable with the use of these drugs for maintenance of analgesia following surgery or trauma due to the deep sedation that accompanies analgesic doses of the α₂-agonists in small animals and the potential for excessive sedation and ataxia in large animals. Xylazine and medetomidine may be reversed in small animals following surgery to hasten recovery and minimize cardiopulmonary depression. Once reversed, however, these drugs provide no analgesia. α₂-Receptors play an important role in the modulation of pain by the CNS. They may be used to induce analgesia when administered as anesthetic premedications (preemptive analgesia) and may be used to supplement postoperative analgesia. Postoperatively, much lower doses of α₂-agonists are generally used than would be required preoperatively.

Ketamine

Ketamine has long been known to provide excellent superficial analgesia but rather poor visceral analgesia. Recently, interest in ketamine has increased because of its potential role in preventing wind-up (sensitization) of central nociceptive pathways. Ketamine is an antagonist of the excitatory neurotransmitter glutamate at the N-methyl-D-aspartate (NMDA) receptors in the spinal cord and brain. Inhibition of the NMDA receptors prevents or decreases exaggerated pain states in laboratory animals and people. Thus, ketamine may be incorporated into the anesthetic protocol to prevent the development of exaggerated or chronic pain states.

LOCAL AND REGIONAL ANALGESIC TECHNIQUES

Local and regional anesthetic techniques are extensively used in large animals for a variety of minor and major surgical procedures. Local anesthetics are used in small animals much less frequently and primarily to facilitate suturing of minor lacerations. Due to the relative ease and safety of inducing general anesthesia in small animals, local and regional anesthetic techniques are often overlooked. Nevertheless, local anesthetic techniques provide an excellent alternative to general anesthesia for select cases, and are increasingly being used in conjunction with general anesthesia to improve postoperative analgesia. Local anesthetics used prior to surgery may decrease the requirement for potent injectable and/or inhalant general anesthetics.

Conduction blockade of nerve fibers by local anesthetics is related to the size of the nerve, amount of myelination, and frequency of activity. Small sensory and autonomic fibers tend to be anesthetized before larger motor and proprioceptive fibers. Nerves that are repetitively stimulated are more sensitive to local anesthetics than resting nerves. The most commonly used agents are lidocaine, mepivacaine, and bupivacaine. Bupivacaine is the preferred drug for postoperative analgesia because of a relatively long duration of action (~3-8 hr). Bupivacaine (0.25-0.75%), with or without epinephrine, is administered in a dose not to exceed 3 mg/kg (dogs) for line or ring blocks of an incision, ring blocks prior to declaw in cats (epinephrine-containing solutions should not be used for distal extremity ring blocks), intercostal nerve blocks and intrapleural local anesthesia (diluted to twice the volume) following a thoracotomy, proximal nerve infiltration during limb amputations, tissue infiltration for lateral ear resections, and local blocks of facial nerves (maxillary, infraorbital, mental and mandibular nerves). Bupivacaine is frequently administered into the epidural space at the lumbosacral space for pelvic limb and perianal procedures.

CHRONIC PAIN

The treatment of chronic pain relies on pharmacologic and nonpharmacologic methods. Some chronic pain responds to drugs used to treat acute pain, such as opioids and NSAID; however, other types of chronic pain require the addition of novel drugs such as an anticonvulsant (eg, gabapentin). The nonpharmacologic treatment of chronic pain depends on the underlying cause and the species. Therapy should be tailored to the individual animal.

The nonpharmacologic goals for managing osteoarthritis pain in dogs include increasing mobility, limiting disease progression, and possibly facilitating tissue repair within the joint. Weight control or reduction and mild to moderate amounts of exercise may be beneficial. Excessive and strenuous exercise should be avoided as it may further strain the joints. Providing warmth during cold and damp weather and extra bedding or padding may also improve comfort. Surgically removing loose fragments of bone, joint mice, and osteochondrosis lesions, and restoring joint stability is often necessary to slow the progression of disease and reduce pain. Joint replacement or arthrodesis may be indicated in severe cases. Chondroprotective agents such as glycosaminoglycans, chondroitin sulfates, and glucosamine may help heal cartilage, stimulate cartilage matrix synthesis, and inhibit enzymatic degradation of cartilage. However, the efficacy of these agents may vary with specific product used, route of administration, and underlying musculoskeletal problems. Acupuncture and physical therapy have been used to treat chronic osteoarthritis pain in animals with promising results.

STRAY VOLTAGE IN ANIMAL HOUSING

The term stray voltage has been used to describe a special case of voltage developed on the grounded neutral system of a farm. If this voltage reaches sufficient levels, animals coming into contact with grounded devices may receive a mild electric shock that can cause a behavioral response. At voltage levels that are just perceptible to the animal, behaviors indicative of perception (eg, flinches) may result with little change in normal routines. At higher levels, avoidance may result. The term stray voltage is often applied incorrectly to other electrical phenomena such as electric fields, magnetic fields, and most recently, electric current flowing in the earth.

A great deal of research on the effects of stray voltage on farm animals has been conducted over the past 40 yr. The effects of stray voltage are seen most often in dairy cattle. The most sensitive cows (<1%) begin to react to 60 Hz electrical current of 2 milliamps (measured as the root mean square average or rms) applied from muzzle to hooves or from hoof to hoof. This corresponds to a contact voltage level of ~1 volt (60 Hz, rms). As the voltage and current increase, a larger percentage of cows react with behavioral responses that become more pronounced. Numerous studies have documented avoidance behaviors at levels above the first reaction threshold. The median avoidance threshold for 60 Hz current flowing through a cow is ~8 milliamps (4-8 volts, rms). This response assumes that the cow comes into contact with objects that have different voltages and that this voltage causes sufficient current to flow through the cow. Even when the threshold is exceeded, not all the animals respond behaviorally all the time, nor do they exhibit the same signs; however, as the voltage increases, signs in the herd become more widespread and uniform.

In most situations, cows are less sensitive to current and more sensitive to voltage than are people. While the resistance of cow and human tissues is similar, the contact resistance is generally lower for cows than for humans, particularly in wet environments. The resistance of a cow's body plus the contact resistance with the floor is commonly estimated as 500 ohms for a cow standing on a wet floor. Cows standing on a dry surface typically produce ≥1,000 ohms resistance. Cows standing or lying on dry bedding have a resistance many times higher than this. The resistance of a human can be as low as 1,000 ohms for wet hand-foot contact to >10,000 ohms for dry hand-foot contact. The contact voltage to produce sensation can therefore be higher for humans than for cows, depending on the conditions of the contact points.

The scientific evidence strongly suggests that there is no relationship between behavioral responses to stray voltage and physiologic or hormonal responses. There is no apparent relationship among behavioral modifications, milk production, and animal health. The only studies that have documented adverse effects of voltage and current on cows had both sufficient current applied to cause aversion and forced exposures (ie, animals could not eat or drink without being exposed to voltage and current). It is typical for voltage levels to vary considerably at different locations on a farm. Decreased water and/or feed intake or undesired behaviors result only if current levels are sufficient to produce aversion at locations that are critical to daily animal activity, eg, feeders, waterers, and milking areas. If an aversive current occurs only a few times per day, it is not likely to have an adverse effect on cow behavior. The more often an aversive voltage occurs in areas critical to cows' normal feeding, drinking, or resting, the more likely it is to affect cows.

Recent research has investigated the effects of high frequency or short duration transient voltages on cows. The main sources of these transient voltages on a farm are improperly installed electric fences and switching of electrical devices. The very high frequency switching transient pulses decay quickly and do not travel far from their source. Exceptions to this are electric fences, which produce a powerful electric impulse designed to control animals. Improper installation of these devices can cause these pulses to appear in unintended areas on the farm. As the duration of the pulse gets shorter, more voltage and current is required to perceive an electrical pulse.

Although stray voltage problems can also affect beef cattle, pigs, and poultry, they are less frequent because the electric demand in those operations is lower.

Clinical Findings: No one sign is pathognomonic; a wide variety of signs has been reported in cows exposed to different levels of voltage. Documented signs are behavioral changes and decreased number of drinks of water per day and increased length of time per drink. Amount of water consumed is not affected. Intermittent periods of poor performance, poor milk letdown and incomplete or uneven milk-out, abnormal behavior during milking, increased milking time, refusal of feed or water, increased somatic cell counts in milk, and increased mastitis are signs often attributed by farmers to stray voltage; however, none of these signs were evident in numerous controlled studies. These signs are often caused by other factors, such as abusive cow handling, faulty milking machines, poor milking techniques and hygiene, and nutritional deficiencies. Therefore, animal behavior or other signs cannot be used to diagnose stray voltage problems. The only way to determine if stray voltage is a potential cause of abnormal behaviors or poor performance is to perform electric testing (*see* below). A thorough investigation of the entire production unit should be conducted to determine other sources of problems.

Signs in pigs are similar, although growing pigs are about twice as resistant to stray voltage as are dairy cows. Continuous exposure via feeders or waterers of up to 5 volt AC had no detrimental effect on fattening pigs. Sows show aggressive behavior, reduced appetite and water consumption, and uneven milking (increased starve-out in litters).

The problem in poultry is not well defined. When birds are raised on the ground, exposure to large voltages (>40 volts AC) is required to deliver detrimental currents on feeders or waterers. Voltages in this range fall outside the definition of stray voltage.

Diagnosis: For confirmation, a potential of 2-4 volt (60 Hz, rms) must be measured between 2 points that a cow might contact (point-to-point or cow contact measurement), and some cows should exhibit signs of exposure. This measurement provides the best indication of exposure levels. Voltage levels should be monitored at different times of the day and on different days because the threshold level may be exceeded intermittently. When exposure during milking is suspected, measurements should be made with all electrical milking equipment turned on (both 110 and 220 volt). Although levels of exposure up to 2-4 volts AC are not detrimental, farms on which these levels have been detected should be monitored to ensure that higher levels do not occur intermittently.

Point-to-reference ground measurements can be useful for diagnostic purposes. Cow contact measurements are typically $^1/_2$ to $^1/_3$ of point-to-reference voltage and current levels. A reference ground is established with a 4 ft (1.3 m) copper-clad rod driven into the ground 25 ft (8.5 m) from any grounding rods or electrical equipment. The other contact point is typically the secondary neutral buss in the service entrance panel to the barn or some other part of the grounded neutral system. The voltmeter should have high input impedance with full scale reading of 2-5 volts in 0.1 volt increments. Voltage readings at cow contact points should be made with a 500-1,000 ohm resistor across the 2 measuring leads to the cow contact points in addition to open circuit measurements. Readings without the use of a shunt resistor are meaningless. If >1 volt, 60 Hz rms is detected at the cow contact points, having a qualified electrician and/or the local power supplier evaluate the situation is advisable.

Long, insulated meter leads (6-10 ft [2-3 m]) facilitate measurements on the farm and give a reasonable estimate of 60-Hz electric events, but introduce considerable noise to higher frequency measurements.

The measurement of high frequency events requires proper equipment and careful measurement technique. Details on sensitivity levels and measurement techniques are available through electric power suppliers.

Prevention and Control: Most on-farm sources of stray voltage are due to wiring systems that do not meet wiring codes and standards. Deficiencies may include loose or corroded connections, ground faults (shorts), undersized wiring, or wiring damaged by animals, accidents, or moisture. An electrician should examine the system and repair any defects. Voltage produced by non-faulty 240-volt equipment usually indicates the distribution system as the source and is the responsibility of the utility company to examine and correct.

Cows have been shown to resume normal behaviors within 1 day of removal of adverse voltage and current levels. Conditions produced by abnormal behaviors may take longer to resolve but should improve within 1 mo.

Electric systems should comply with wiring codes and standards at all times to protect both animals and people. Whenever suggestive signs cannot be attributed to other causes, measurements should be taken to determine if a voltage potential exists, and the results recorded for future comparisons. A review of electromagnetic fields and other electrical exposures concluded that there was no evidence to suggest that they are harmful to cows at the typical exposure levels found on farms.

VENTILATION

Ventilation is often associated with respiratory health of animals; the quality of the air that animals breathe directly influences animal health and disease. But ventilation—directly and indirectly—impacts many other aspects of animal health as well. Good ventilation in the lying area of lactating animals helps bedding stay dry, a factor in favor of good mammary health. Good ventilation along alleys helps to keep walking surfaces dry, which contributes to healthy feet. Good ventilation may lead to greater productivity, eg, maintaining air movement in the eating area makes animals more comfortable, which is especially important during hot weather as an aid to maintaining dry matter intake. A comfortable, well-ventilated lying area encourages animals to lie down, an important contribution to many aspects of animal health.

During ventilation, outside air is brought into a barn where it collects moisture, heat, and other contaminants. Air is then exhausted to the outside. To determine ventilation rates, the focus is on the moisture content of the air, measured by relative humidity.

AIR QUALITY

Air quality is not easily defined. It is related to ventilation and the absence (or presence) of contaminants in the air. For animals, good air quality generally implies that the ambient air causes no harmful effects on the animals in the space. Ambient air contains varying amounts of water vapor. Moisture in the air becomes a problem when it exceeds the relative humidity range of 60-75% preferred for animals; above this level, it is considered to be an air contaminant. Other contaminants may include pathogens, harmful gases, dust, and undesirable odors. Concern arises from the concentration of a contaminant above some predetermined level rather than the mere presence of the contaminant itself.

Numerous viral pathogens known to survive in aerosols are apparently spread by the airborne route. Two factors can be significant in the relationship between microbial aerosols and disease incidence: 1) the survival time of the aerosolized pathogen, and 2) the total number of pathogens per volume of air (ie, concentration). Survival is influenced by conditions of the ambient air; conditions of the ambient air and concentration relate to ventilation.

Relative humidity is the most important factor influencing pathogen survival and concentration, but its effects vary greatly between pathogens—some survive best in humid conditions, others survive best in dry air. Maintaining a relative humidity in the range of 60-75% apparently results in the shortest survival time for the greatest number of potential pathogens. Ventilation is used to remove moisture from an animal space with the intention of maintaining relative humidity in this range. Inside air is diluted with outside air, reducing moisture levels. Continuous replacement of contaminated air with fresh, outside air is also the most effective way to reduce the concentration of aerosol pathogens.

Most likely, reducing the concentration of any air contaminant, including gases and dust, is important to reducing its detrimental effect. For example, ammonia is produced by the decay of feces and urine and is probably the most significant air pollutant in cattle barns. Allowed to accumulate, ammonia's irritating effects on the respiratory epithelium appear to directly reduce the number of ciliated cells and thus decrease the efficiency of mucociliary transport.

THE DILUTION EFFECT OF VENTILATION

Dilution reduces heat and concentrations of moisture, as well as concentrations of airborne disease organisms, harmful gases and dust, and undesirable odors. The dilution rate of ventilation is often expressed in air changes per unit time. For example, a ventilation rate of 4 air changes/hr implies that the entire volume of the ventilated space is replaced 4 times every hour. In fact, some of the air may bypass the occupied zone in the barn, depending on geometry of the space, design of diffusers controlling inlet air, etc. Therefore, the effectiveness of ventilation is not 100%, but perhaps approaches 65%. Ventilation effectiveness becomes important to the actual dilution achieved by a particular rate of ventilation (ie, to the ability of ventilating air to reduce the concentrations of contaminants in the animal space). For a ventilation effectiveness of 1.0, one air change would achieve a complete change of air in the space, yielding a 100% reduction in contaminant levels (if the condition of the outside air is considered to be the reference standard). But if ventilation effectiveness is only 0.65, one air change will reduce contaminant levels by only 65%. As ventilation effectiveness diminishes, the ventilation rate required to achieve a certain air change rate increases.

When ventilation is reduced below recommended levels—usually in a misguided effort in cold climates to warm the barn using animal heat—less moisture is removed. Sometimes the consequences of the resulting moisture buildup and lack of proper ventilation (eg, condensation) are masked by 1) insulating the barn, 2) using a greenhouse effect, 3) providing supplemental heat, or 4) dehumidifying the inside air. For example, adding heat to the air reduces relative humidity, without the need for air exchange. It is quite possible to have substantial quantities of moisture added to the air and, if accompanied by heating, keep the relative humidity within an acceptable range. If relative humidity is the only measure of air quality, it may be deemed to be satisfactory. However, even though excess moisture may not be apparent, the reduced dilution does result in increased concentrations of airborne disease organisms, harmful gases and dust, and undesirable odors. If these increases are ignored, animal health problems are inevitable. In addition, heating of barns is rarely economical in cold climates.

COLD WEATHER VENTILATION

A minimal ventilation rate is required in animal housing in cold weather, regardless of outside temperature. This minimal rate is necessary whether the barn is designed to be a warm barn or a cold barn in winter. In addition, the minimal ventilation should be continuous to maintain concentrations of contaminants in the air at minimal levels. The minimal rate depends on outside weather; design conditions; number, type, age, and size of animals; and whether the barn is intended to be cold or warm.

Barn Categories and Winter Temperatures

Barn environments can be categorized according to temperatures maintained in the barn in winter. The particular environment, based on desired indoor temperature, must be established before ventilation system design can begin. In **cold barns**, indoor temperatures are allowed to fluctuate with outdoor temperatures. Ventilation is sufficient to maintain indoor temperatures within 3-6°C of outdoor temperatures. Ventilation is largely unregulated, except to adjust for seasonal changes. In general, a cold barn with natural ventilation has no insulation, open ridge and eaves, and sidewalls and endwalls that open. Providing an open ridge along with open eaves has long been recognized as a means of using a stack effect to cause air exchange, especially for controlling moisture in winter. Indoor temperatures are expected to be a few degrees warmer than outdoor air temperature due to the heat given off by the animals being housed. Current recommendations call for providing a ridge opening of 5 cm per 3 m of barn width and equivalent open area divided between the 2 eaves. Raised ridge caps are to be avoided. Their performance is unpredictable due to local wind patterns, which often channel winds into the structure and increase the entry of snow and rain. The combination of the open ridge and eaves should be viewed as the sole source of ventilation only during the most severe winter weather, ie, during periods when temperatures reach the lowest levels or times when conditions are especially windy or stormy. During all other times in winter, additional ventilation should be provided.

Warm barns are well insulated and, by necessity, have well-controlled ventilation systems. These barns are designed to provide a relatively uniform environment throughout the winter. Tie stall barns for dairy cows (indoor temperatures at least above freezing) and farrowing and nursery barns for swine (indoor temperatures 25-30°C) are examples of this type of housing. Keys to success include ventilating fans and controls chosen to match the needs of the animals being housed, a well-insulated building, supplemental heating (if required), and a ventilation system that is well managed and regulated to compensate for changing outside climatic conditions.

Some barns do not fit into either the warm or cold category. **In-between or modified environment barns** usually have indoor temperatures in winter above freezing. These buildings have some insulation, perhaps only under the roof, and are naturally ventilated (usually with an open ridge, eaves, and sidewalls). Unfortunately, even though a minimal ventilation rate is always necessary, ventilation openings may be closed or blocked during extreme weather to keep manure from freezing and/or for other reasons. This practice can result in inside temperatures rising 10-20°C above the outside temperature, significantly higher than the 3-6°C temperature difference limit considered acceptable for cold barns. This alone can create problems because of excess moisture buildup and a high relative humidity. Even more seriously, openings remain closed or blocked after severe weather conditions have passed. As a consequence, blocked ventilation openings restrict airflow during less severe conditions, resulting in underventilation and poor environmental conditions. A properly designed and managed in-between barn is more like a warm barn, in terms of both design and operation, than a cold barn. Thus, to avoid problems, the design and management of in-between barns should follow the guidelines for a warm barn.

Consequences of Mismanaged Ventilation in Winter

Underventilation in winter is one of the most serious threats to the environment of animals. Both improper design and improper management of the ventilation may compromise animal health. In colder climates, problems are most likely during winter, spring, and fall, especially during rainy weather and warmer days coupled with cold nights.

Reduced Dilution of Ambient Air: Adjusting ventilation for severe winter weather and not readjusting to allow increased ventilation when milder winter weather appears is a major reason for air quality problems in barns in winter. This is especially true for cold barns with manually controlled natural ventilation. For example, ventilation openings are closed in anticipation of a windy, cold, blustery night, but are not opened the next day when, although the temperature may still be cold, the wind subsides and the sun shines. The lack of wind reduces ventilation and thus air exchange and the positive effects of dilution.

Sometimes good ventilation system management does call for openings to be reduced. For example, a slot inlet in a mechanically ventilated tie stall barn may be adjusted, or fabric may be placed over an open sidewall to match the lower ventilation rate in winter. All openings should never be covered, however, because this leaves no means of air exchange for moisture control.

Building Components Affected by Poor Ventilation: In addition to adversely affecting the animal environment, the design and operation of naturally ventilated barns also influence moisture-related deterioration in wood members and metal fasteners. In naturally ventilated dairy free-stall barns in Michigan, where air exchange in winter was defeated by blocking ventilation openings, average wood moisture contents >30% dry basis (capable of supporting wood decay and corrosion in metal fasteners) were found after 2-3 mo of cold weather operation. Moreover, restricted air movement in these barns inhibited drying and allowed wood moisture content to remain elevated even during warm weather. Warm, moist conditions favor growth of mold, bacteria, and decay fungi and accelerate metal corrosion. The presence of insulation under the roofing in these barns fostered the situation. In barns in which design details and management efforts allowed optimal air exchange rates, increases in moisture were minimal. Even if free water from precipitation and condensation caused slightly elevated moisture contents, adequate air exchange, especially during warm weather, promoted drying of wood truss components so that deterioration was not a problem.

WARM WEATHER VENTILATION

In barns with natural ventilation, the combination of the open ridge and eaves is the source of ventilation during the most severe winter weather, ie, during periods when temperatures reach the lowest levels or times when conditions are especially windy or stormy. During all other times in winter, however, additional ventilation must be provided. Typically, doorways are left open, portions of the endwall sections of the gable roof may be left uncovered, or sidewalls away from prevailing winter winds may be left open for this purpose. Then, as temperatures rise into spring and summer, sidewalls and endwalls are fully opened. As a general rule, too much ventilation is preferred over too little.

Hot, muggy summer weather is one of the most critical times for animal health, comfort, and productivity. For barns with natural ventilation, completely open sidewalls and endwalls allow wind to blow through the animal zone for heat stress reduction. However, when winds are calm, providing adequate air movement to avoid heat stress is difficult. Supplemental cooling can be provided in several ways. Fans are commonly used to increase air movement. The increased air velocity over the skin increases the rate at which animals are able to dissipate excess body heat. Two other methods rely on evaporative cooling to either cool the air around the animals or wet the animal's skin and allow body heat to evaporate the water. However, water should be added to the animals' environment only if ample air movement is present.

Barns with mechanical ventilation require staged fans to provide ventilation ranging from the minimal continuous rate, through an intermediate rate for spring and fall, to a high rate for summer. An air exchange rate of 60 air changes/hr is considered the absolute minimum for summer. Often, ventilation rates of 90-120 air changes/hr are provided for hot weather.

AQUACULTURE SYSTEMS

See also FISH, p 1479, for discussion of specific diseases in fish.

The culture of aquatic organisms for food dates back thousands of years, and still exists in many parts of the world, as low-intensity farming requiring little energy input or manipulation of the animal or its environment. A vast amount of production is carp, tilapia, and other locally produced and consumed finfish. This farming is extensive as opposed to intensive and contributes substantial amounts of protein to local diets.

Intensive aquaculture is analogous to a highly productive farrow-to-finish swine operation, while extensive aquaculture can be compared to a low yield (per land area) cattle ranch. Intensive production of aquatic food animals is a relatively recent development and owes many technologic advances to shrimp and catfish farming in warm water, and salmon and trout farming in cold water. Many marine finfish have only recently reached commercial production levels, including halibut, turbot, Atlantic cod, and many other species. Although fish farming husbandry follows similar patterns to agriculture, there are some unique differences. Variations in specific methods for growing aquatic species make it impractical to describe all but generalities. Aquaculture systems for the common species of salmon, trout, and catfish are discussed as examples of the life cycles and husbandry involved in farming fish.

The general principles for the culture of aquatic organisms are similar to those of terrestrial food animals. Good husbandry requires a source of juveniles, an ability to contain the stock, and appropriate nutritional and environmental conditions for growth and health. Some fish species, such as eels, and many of the farmed mollusc (eg, mussels) or crustacean (eg, shrimp) species are still collected in the wild as juveniles and raised to harvest weight. However, genetic improvement and manipulation of the life cycle to optimize productivity is favored by the reproduction of selected brood stock. Historically, the early life stages of salmonids were cultivated by taking eggs from wild brood stock and transporting them around the world to be released as juveniles into local streams. It has been since only about 1970 that the marine growout stages of salmon have been intensified to the level that would be referred to as livestock farming for profit-oriented food production.

Diadromous fish (eg, Atlantic salmon) spawn in freshwater but live their adult stages in seawater. Catadromous fish (eg, American eel) live as adults in freshwater but return to seawater to spawn. Because these 2 environments are radically different, the physiology of fish must change to accommodate the hyperosmotic state when in freshwater and the hypo-osmotic state when in seawater. Fish in freshwater environments must spend energy to concentrate ions (eg, Na^+ and Cl^-) and excrete water, while fish in seawater must excrete ions and concentrate water. Fish that have life stages in each of these environments adapt physiologically by changing their gill chloride cell capacity and renal function. Gill and skin diseases can disrupt the integrity of the osmotic barrier, causing electrolyte and fluid imbalances that overwhelm the ability of the fish to compensate.

Breeding and Hatchery Operations

Fish can have either a single (eg, salmonids) or multiple (eg, the gadid family, which includes cod and haddock) release of eggs. Generally there is a defined spawning season, which may be less intense in species cultured closer to the equator. Fecundity can range from 10,000 eggs per female, exemplified by Atlantic salmon, to millions of eggs, as is seen in cod. Salmon eggs tend to have a large amount of yolk that is rich in nutrients. This is necessary to support the development of the embryo in a cold stream over a period of months. Because the eggs require clean, cool, well-oxygenated water, they are buried in the gravel of a rapidly moving stream at the time of spawning to prevent them from washing downstream. On hatching from the egg membranes, alevins or sac-fry continue to derive their nutrition from the yolk reserves, so they remain buried in the gravel. As the yolk sac is consumed, the fry emerge from the gravel to access the surface to both fill the swim bladder with air and obtain food. Salmonid hatcheries are designed to provide these basic necessities for early life.

All natural spawning of salmonids is in freshwater. Regardless of the aquatic environment for mature brood stock, they will spawn only if provided the proper substrate (ie, gravel bottoms) on which to lay eggs. Because spawning will not occur in tanks or sea cages, commercial production takes advantage of this and maintains brood stock until they can be manually stripped of their eggs and sperm (milt). Salmon eggs are very sensitive to saltwater, and contamination with saltwater must be carefully avoided during collection. Alternatively, brood stock may be transferred to freshwater tanks prior to spawning.

Catfish eggs are adhesive and are deposited in a mass within hollow containers made to mimic spaces under logs or river bottom cavities. The male normally provides a flow of oxygenated water over the eggs using the fanning movement of his fins. In production, the eggs are transported to hatchery troughs for incubation, with flowing water agitated by paddle wheels or air-driven systems to mimic natural incubation conditions. After hatching, sac-fry swim to the bottom of the trough where they absorb the energy from their yolk sacs. Once this is depleted, they swim to the surface and begin to feed on artificial diets. In less intensive systems, the fry may be stocked into ponds that have been fertilized to produce a rich plankton source of food.

Salmonid eggs are quite resistant to handling stresses for the first few days after fertilization, but then become very sensitive to any movement, light, or sudden environmental change. For this reason, all handling and transport must take place immediately after fertilization or, more commonly, wait until after the eggs have developed visible eyes ("eyed eggs") at which time they can tolerate less-optimal conditions. In hatcheries, the conditions for sensitive egg stages can be satisfied with stacked trays or tank inserts using unidirectional flow through a supportive screen mesh on which the eggs lay motionless and in the dark. Cool (10°C), well-oxygenated water and the occasional removal of dead, opaque eggs are the primary requirements at this stage. Rapid water flow can damage eggs or yolk sacs, and high water temperatures can increase the incidence of skeletal deformities and mortality. Nonviable eggs attract saprophytic fungi that are present in most water sources. For this reason, regularly removing dead eggs without disturbing other eggs in the group is important.

As the yolk sac is internalized and reserves are exhausted, the salmonid fry begin feeding on a crumble diet. This stage is referred to as the first-feeding fry stage and these fry leave the low current microenvironment of the tank bottom to access food and air. Feed must be available soon after the yolk sac reserves are depleted, otherwise the fry will be malnourished and more likely to die. Progeny from the same spawning pair reared under the same growing conditions develop at slightly different rates, which results in a period of time during which some fry are feeding and some remain on the tank bottom relying on their yolk reserves for nutrition. During this period, the management of feed and waste is critical, as too much feed contaminates the tank bottom, exposing the nonfeeding fry to higher ammonia levels from the breakdown of feed and feces and to more particulate matter. Reduced water quality challenges their health, particularly of the gills and skin. Tanks are generally designed to make use of water flow to remove uneaten food and excreted waste. At this delicate stage, however, water flow sufficient to remove waste is too extreme for fry with attached yolk sacs.

Grow-out Operations

Once the fry are feeding, they grow rapidly. The variability in the initiation of feeding and different development rates can result in large size variations among fish in a tank. In many aquaculture settings, slow-growing individuals represent an economic inefficiency that will continue until harvest. This problem is best managed by early culling of poor performers. Identification and removal of slowly growing fish prevent greater economic losses in the future. Hierarchies based on size are established within fish groups; if fish sizes continue to diverge, small fish have more nutritional, environmental, and health challenges. This can eventually affect the health of the entire group, eg, the small fish may act as a nidus for infections. In the wild, poor-performing fish are likely to become prey, but in hatcheries it is necessary to sort sizes repeatedly to reduce the impact of diverging growth patterns on productivity.

Many different containment systems are used for finfish grow-out, including earthen ponds (eg, catfish), concrete raceways, concrete or fiberglass tanks, or lake or ocean net pens. Fish can be maintained in small groups if their value is exceptionally high (eg, genetically selected brood stock, ornamental species). Much larger groups (>10,000) are typical, however. Large circular net pens containing >40,000 market-sized salmon can measure 25 m in diameter and 10 m in depth, while standard catfish ponds have surface areas of 6-10 hectares and contain >100,000 fish.

Harvest weight depends on markets and the optimizing of economic efficiency. Typically, Atlantic salmon are harvested at 3-4.5 kg while rainbow trout and catfish harvested for home consumers are 0.5-0.75 kg. Food is withheld 24-72 hr prior to slaughter to evacuate intestinal contents and improve shelf life of the carcass. In recent years, improved attention to the welfare of the fish and reduced preslaughter stress has resulted in less metabolic acidosis, which in turn has led to a greater quality and consistency of saleable product. Fish are crowded or seined, then either transported by net or pumped onto a harvest vehicle where they are either chilled in ice and exsanguinated or stunned by percussion. Catfish and salmon production systems often use live-haul in well-boats to contain the slaughter effluents and reduce disease transmission.

Husbandry Procedures

Size sorting procedures are important tools for fish farmers to separate faster growing fish from their slower growing cohorts, reduce hierarchal disadvantages, and reestablish the optimal growing conditions for all individuals. It is also an opportunity to cull poor performers. Size sorting is accomplished when fish are very small using bar graders. Fish are put into a basket, the bottom of which has parallel bars a standard distance apart. The smaller fish pass through the bars while the larger fish remain behind. The larger fish are then placed into another basket with parallel bars a slightly greater distance apart, and so on. In this way, the size is graded by the greatest width of the fish. Similar methods are used in passive grading, in which a wall of parallel bars is used to make a compartment within the tank, allowing the smaller fish to swim out. Fish can also be graded by passing them down a gradually widening space, in which the small fish fall through first. Size sorting usually is performed at least 3 times during the hatchery stages and once during the grow-out stage, eg, in Atlantic salmon.

Anesthesia is necessary to handle fish for various management procedures such as weight samples, vaccination, and health monitoring (eg, parasite counts). Several anesthetics are available, but few are approved for use in fish. Tricaine methane-sulfonate (TMS or MS-222) is most commonly used. Metomidate and eugenol (a derivative of clove oil) have been used as both sedatives and anesthetics. All anesthetics used in fish farming are typically given as a bath.

Feed and feed delivery management comprise the greatest components of the cost of production in fish farming. It accounts for 40-45% of the cost of production for Atlantic salmon. Prepared feeds—often in pellet form—are most common for salmonids and other intensively farmed fish. Typical feed conversion efficiencies (feed weight:fish weight gain) for salmon are <2:1 and approach 1:1 during certain life stages. For those species with less-defined diets or that are less adapted to prepared feeds, crude mixtures using less valuable fish are used. Many species require live feed (eg, zooplankton), particularly for early juvenile or larval stages. Fish are fed by hand, by automatic distributors on electrical or mechanical spring timers, or by blowers if large amounts of feed must be distributed. Feed wastage must be minimized to reduce both cost and impact on the local aquatic environment.

Optimal **water quality** must be maintained for best productivity and health. Water sources for fish farms vary and include abiotic well water, surface water (streams or lakes), and estuary or marine sources for net pens. Transporting new water to the holding units requires energy, and pumping costs can be prohibitive for many facilities. Well water is often used for young fish because of the need to avoid pathogens before the fish have been immunized.

Water quality is influenced by the source of the water and also by the fish themselves. Consumption of oxygen and production of carbon dioxide and nitrogenous wastes (ammonia) requires that the producer adjust parameters to meet optimal levels, particularly if water is to be recirculated. Water reuse has become very important to fish culture. It allows stricter control of water quality, the reduction or avoidance of exposure to new pathogens, minimization of environmental impacts, and better regulation of water temperature. Although removal of metabolic waste products through mechanical and biologic filtration and replenishment of gases is a constant and costly demand of recirculation systems, it is justified in situations requiring a high health status (eg, juvenile stages), or when the added benefit of heat recovery reduces the costs of warming water and encourages faster growth.

Health Management

See also FISH HEALTH MANAGEMENT, p 1488.

Health assessments may require sampling of fish from tanks, raceways, ponds, or net pens. As holding units can contain >50,000 individuals, collecting a representative sample is important. Crowding fish, or attracting them with feed, and then repeatedly dipping out a number, is not truly random sampling, but it may provide some information about the group. If each fish is being handled individually for a procedure, such as for injectable vaccines, it is possible to systematically select a sample at that time. Accuracy is important when estimating weight for drug dosage calculations, estimating disease prevalence or parasite burdens, or making decisions regarding the timing of harvests.

Counting deaths for inventory records is a constant challenge in aquaculture operations. Accurate starting inventories must be adjusted for dead fish collected near effluent pipes, the sides of ponds, by net pen divers, or by using mortality collection systems (eg, airlifts or mortality socks in nets). Dead fish generally sink and can decompose or be eaten by other fish in the group or by predators. Unaccounted losses can be costly when calculating biomass for feed amounts, drug dosages, or harvest sales.

Due to the direct contact or indirect sharing of water and biologic products with wild fish species, aquatic livestock exchange pathogens with their environment. Disease prevention and management must account for this interaction. Although many infectious agents do not readily cause disease in different fish species, there are sufficient pathogens that can cross-infect and also sufficient wild populations of the same species living near aquaculture establishments that it is almost impossible to prevent some diseases. Closed containment using recirculated water has become a viable strategy to isolate cultured fish from wild.

Vaccination: Vaccination is an important health management tool in fish farming. There are 2 primary routes of vaccination—immersion and injection. Immersion is generally used for small fish and is easier to administer. A 60-sec exposure to a concentrated killed bacterin is the most common method. Although immersion provides limited antigenic stimulation, and usually a shorter duration of response, it is particularly useful for fish that will be exposed to the pathogen early in their life cycle, eg, in salmon with *Aeromonas salmonicida* (furunculosis). Vaccination is not very effective when fish weigh <1 g, but there is a minor response. One or two boosters can be given to provide reasonable protection. Vaccination by intraperitoneal injection stimulates a greater immune response, and the addition of adjuvants provides for a longer duration of response. Due to the amount of vaccine administered, the level of protection, and other factors, injection is generally most cost effective in fish >10 g (for salmon). Mass vaccination by injection, preceded by anesthesia, is routinely done at salmon hatcheries as an effective disease prevention practice.

Treatment Methods: Disease treatments in aquaculture can be accomplished either topically or through injection for individual fish if circumstances permit. Injection is usually reserved for very valuable fish, such as brood stock. Most treatments use immersion or in-feed delivery methods. Immersion is primarily used for surface infections involving gills or skin, while in-feed treatments are reserved for systemic diseases. The issue of chemical release into the environment following immersion treatments must be addressed. Aquaculture in-feed treatments are successful only if the fish are still eating, which means that treatments must be initiated early in any disease outbreak. Fish that are anorectic due to illness will not receive the treatment and may contribute to the progression of disease in the population. Treatment of nontarget organisms is a concern with any of the methods in open aquaculture systems.

Few drugs are available for treating diseases in aquaculture. As with virtually every aspect of fish farming, water temperature has a great impact on the dynamics of disease outbreaks and their treatment. The kinetics of absorption and residue depletion of chemotherapeutics in fish depends on temperature, species, and disease states. Treatments are administered to large groups of fish; therefore, individual fish variation in appetite may alter the actual dose received. Calculating the appropriate dose depends on the accuracy of the weight estimates and the variation of size within the group. The greatest impact on withdrawal periods before the flesh is safe for human consumption, however, remains the half-life of the drug, which is affected by the metabolism of the fish and the temperature of the water.

HEALTH-MANAGEMENT INTERACTION: CATTLE

BEEF CATTLE BREEDING HERDS

Several managerial practices increase productivity within cow-calf herds when they can be implemented practically. These practices are mostly associated with reproduction, as improvements in herd fertility offer more potential for increased profitability in cow-calf operations than production traits. They include a restricted breeding season, identification of the optimal calving season, breeding season evaluation, a good heifer replacement program, proper nutrition, good herd health, prior bull evaluation, cross-breeding, and maintaining good records. Other management practices associated with increased beef herd profitability include partial budgeting, fly control, use of growth promotants and creep feeding in calves, precalving parasite control in cows, and improved calf management.

Reproduction

In most regions of the world, there is an optimal period for females to calve, suckle, and rebreed. This period is mostly related to nutritional opportunity, although other environmental factors such as heat stress and parasite populations may play a role. Producers have traditionally aimed for females to calve at this optimal period because they tend to breed back faster, and their calves are more likely to thrive, than those that calve at less opportune times. Benefits of restricted breeding seasons (<80 days) include enhanced production potential, favorable environmental factors, a concentrated calving season and more homogeneous calf crop, increased opportunities to perform prebreeding management procedures and monitor nutrition, improved female replacement and culling procedures, and the ability to detect problems early (using herd pregnancy diagnosis and breeding season evaluation).

Pregnancy Testing: For most effective use, pregnancy testing should involve more than a simple sorting exercise of female cattle into pregnant and nonpregnant groups. The addition of information such as projected calving dates and patterns makes the service more attractive. The herd pregnancy diagnosis (HPD) represents an important starting point for beef herd diagnostics and advice and is a pivotal component for informed decision making. It allows analysis of group patterns for problem solving (breeding season evaluation, *see* below), as well as sorting of animals into groups for specific purposes such as strategic feeding, calving supervision, culling, or rebreeding. HPD facilitates the selection of replacement females and culling for infertility.

Breeding Soundness Evaluation: Reproductive performance is influenced by many factors including sire fertility, herd health aspects, and opportunities to mate. Breeding soundness evaluation is a technique for assessing the reproductive performance of the cow herd. It includes obtaining relevant information, its analysis and interpretation, and recommendations for improvement. One measure of reproductive performance is the number of exposed females that actually raise a live calf. Other valuable information may be obtained from an analysis of the distribution of pregnancies (and calvings) that resulted from a particular breeding season. This distribution may be studied on the basis of timing (eg, 21-day estrus periods), breeding groups, female age or parity, nutritional opportunity (eg, body condition score), etc. Such analyses provide the basis for evaluation of either the breeding or calving season. For evaluation of the breeding season, good records must be obtained at the time of pregnancy testing for the subsequent analysis to be valid.

Because reproductive performance is the single most important economic trait in the cow herd, the reproductive capabilities of breeding bulls assume great importance. The best assurance that a bull is likely to be fertile is a successful breeding soundness evaluation. (*See* BREEDING SOUNDNESS EXAMINATION OF THE MALE, p 1797.) Bulls that pass a breeding soundness examination can handle considerably more females in a breeding season than would be suggested by traditional recommendations.

Cull Cow Selection and Management

Culling of cattle in a beef operation usually implies removing those that cannot meet or maintain performance criteria for the herd. Other reasons may include physical or temperament problems in animals, as well as judicious culling during periods of environmental hardship or economic necessity. The judicious removal of nonperforming females is also important in maintaining or improving herd fertility. However, the assumption that cull cows are necessarily unproductive may not always be correct; recent surveys indicate that ~43% of cull cows in the USA are pregnant at the time of survey. In addition, "open" females are not necessarily infertile. Identification of appropriate candidates for culling is critical and should be an important component of pregnancy testing.

Nutritional Management

In general, nutrition is the most important limiting factor of beef breeding performance. An understanding of the principles underlying the nutritional management of breeding females is necessary, including a working knowledge of the different energy measuring systems that are commonly used and their applications for different classes of animals, activities, and feedstuffs. (*See* NUTRITION: CATTLE, p 1811.) Increasing stocking rate tends to cause increased gain per unit land area, but decreased gain per animal. This relationship generally holds true until lack of available forage leads to decreased intake. Optimal stocking rates are attained before this point is reached. Increasing stocking rate beyond this point leads to a decrease in both gains per animal and per land unit urea.

Nutritional requirements vary throughout the year. The most critical periods for reproduction are early postcalving, when maximal lactation is combined with the need for rebreeding, and immediately precalving, when fetal growth is maximal along with lactation preparation. (*See also* MANAGEMENT OF REPRODUCTION: CATTLE, p 1747.)

Environmental conditions can strongly influence the nutritional requirements and intake of cattle. For example, cold weather increases energy needs, whereas hot or inclement weather can reduce foraging opportunity. The quality and quantity of range forage varies greatly throughout the year and between years, influenced by moisture, plant species, and grazing pressure. Seasonal changes in the nutrient density of rangeland forages are mainly associated with the degree of plant maturity. In general, the greatest nutritional value of plants develops before maturity. Good nutritional management involves matching, as far as possible, the nutrient requirements of cows and nutrient density of the pasture by careful consideration of factors such as the types of animals involved, stocking rates, plant species available, season of grazing, fertilization, and grazing methods used.

Body Condition Score: Accurate and timely determination of nutritional status of grazing animals represents a challenge for beef producers, because many variables can influence a cow's response to a given level of nutrition. The use of a body condition score (BCS) is an effective indirect method for determining nutritional status in breeding females. The BCS represents a subjective assessment of body fat (or energy reserves) that is strongly related to female reproductive performance. BCS, and changes in BCS, appear to be more reliable indicators of nutritional status than is body weight, or changes in body weight, which can vary with gut fill and pregnancy status. In addition, BCS can often be assessed more conveniently than body weight can be measured. BCS is both repeatable and accurate in experienced hands. It is best done through visual appraisal, reinforced by palpation of body regions most likely to demonstrate fat deposits. Group observations of BCS made from a distance when animals are in the pasture or paddock are less accurate than those made when animals are nearby in the pen or chute.

BCS varies throughout the year and should be monitored regularly. In the 1-9 BCS system widely used in North America, the reference standard for beef females is a BCS of 5, which represents an average, moderately fleshed cow that is neither fat nor thin. However, the BCS for optimal female efficiency varies with breed and operation and may be higher or lower. In general, females should calve when they are between condition scores 4-6 and then gain slightly until breeding. It generally takes ~2 mo to gain 1 score under pasture conditions. Care should be taken not to rely on averages, as these can mask variations that might adversely affect herd fertility.

The BCS of females at calving can provide much information about their rebreeding prospects. However, assessment of BCS at this time provides a relatively short length of time in which to meet targets and necessitates either gathering cows with very young calves, which is often inadvisable, or using visual assessment from a distance, which is less reliable. Assessment of BCS in females at breeding should provide the most accurate prediction of herd fertility because it is done just before the predictive event. The disadvantage is that there is little opportunity to correct significant shortfalls in time to affect the current breeding season. Assessment of BCS at the time of pregnancy checking has the advantage of not requiring a separate animal handling. It also allows considerable time to remedy obvious deficiencies before calving and subsequent rebreeding. The disadvantage is that, although it can provide clues to explain current pregnancy patterns, it is too late to remedy them.

Health and Production Management Program

A cost-effective herd health and production management program is essential for the economic viability of most cow-calf operations. Such programs vary by region, relative economics, perceptions, and opportunity. A good herd health program manages risk of disease and lowered productivity at a number of levels, including considerations of biosecurity, nutrition, and the judicious use of biologics such as vaccines.

One starting point for such a program is to identify current production losses by comparing the performance of the particular herd with relevant standards, eg, from regional national surveys, which can also provide an economic estimate of losses.

The major disease risks for a given herd, and appropriate preventive measures, should be established in consultation with herd owners. The best times for herd intervention must be identified. These often coincide with other managerial tasks and can be synchronized to minimize herd disruption and labor costs. One approach is to devise a herd-health "calendar" in which the health events are coordinated with major operational events. Interventions for a particular herd vary based on factors such as breed types, normal herd working dates, calf weaning dates, calf management practices, source of bulls, and previous disease problems.

Vaccinations

Prebreeding vaccinations should be completed within 2-4 wk of the start of breeding and should be based on local patterns of disease and any state or national requirements. Replacement females should be vaccinated with the same vaccines given to females before breeding.

Precalving vaccinations are intended to protect the newborn calf through colostral transfer. Important antigens include those of the major clostridial diseases (particularly *Clostridium perfringens*) and leptospirosis, as well as those for calf scour pathogens, respiratory disease, and redwater, where these represent significant problems.

Preweaning is an important intervention that can help prepare calves for the stress of weaning and reduce the possibility that such stress will compromise the efficacy of biologicals. Common vaccinations include the clostridials, bovine respiratory disease complex (BRD), and leptospirosis. For BRD vaccinations, only products licensed for suckling calves should be given. A broad-spectrum anthelmintic may also be given at this time to ensure that calves cause minimal pasture infestation. At weaning, a second vaccination should be given for those products recommending 2 injections. Modified live viral products can be given at this stage. Another clostridial vaccination is not indicated if calves were previously vaccinated at working and preweaning. For areas where brucellosis is under regulatory control, appropriate heifer vaccination should be done within the age ranges stipulated.

Bulls should receive the same vaccines as the cow-calf herd, with some exceptions. Bulls should not be vaccinated for brucellosis. Also, the trichomoniasis vaccine currently approved for use in the USA is not approved for bull use. Caution is advised with modified live virus infectious bovine rhinotracheitis vaccines, because bulls may recrudesce this virus and shed it in semen. Also, semen shipment to other countries may be jeopardized. Otherwise, recommended bull vaccinations include leptospirosis and campylobacteriosis, in accord with recommendations for the cow herd.

Calf Management

Management of the calving season is critical to optimizing the weaned calf crop. Research indicates that 57% of mortality is seen in the first 24 hr and 75% within 7 days of birth. In addition, there are significant risk factors for increased calf morbidity at the time of calving that can lead to increased mortality and decreased calf performance. Factors to consider in calving management include dystocia management (of primary concern in replacement heifers), passive transfer, calving environment, and cow-calf pair management. (*See* MANAGEMENT OF REPRODUCTION: CATTLE, p 1747.) A visit to the farm ~4 wk before the onset of the calving season provides the opportunity to evaluate the preparations made by the producer and to recommend any changes.

Keeping records on calving ease and morbidity and mortality incidence allows for analysis of risks and risk groups and detection of any increased incidence of disease. At least one additional visit should be made to the farm 2-3 wk after calving has begun to assess the management and environment. Morbidity and mortality incidence levels may be established; if these are exceeded, the veterinarian should be called and an investigation begun.

The most common cause of calf morbidity in the neonatal period is diarrhea. (*See* DIARRHEA IN NEONATAL RUMINANTS, p 228.) It is generally not possible to differentiate diarrheas associated with different etiologic agents based on clinical signs. Control for pathogenic agents of neonatal diarrhea involves segregation of sick animals from the healthy nursery to decrease environmental contamination and transmission. In addition, *E coli* and *Salmonella* control involves biosecurity rules to prevent the purchase and introduction of new calves or cows during the calving season. Sick calves should be isolated quickly to prevent further environmental contamination. Once the environment is contaminated, moist cool conditions allow survival of infectious agents for an extended period. Cryptosporidia are especially suited to survival in the environment, and prevention of contamination in the healthy nursery is critical. Commercial vaccines for rotavirus, coronavirus, *Escherichia coli* K99, and *Clostridium perfringens* types B and C should be given to cows and heifers before calving to elevate specific immunoglobulin levels in colostrum. An initial vaccination and booster followed by a yearly booster is required. The booster vaccination should be given at least 2 wk and not more than 6 wk before calving. Clinical trial data are not consistent; some trials report no effect, whereas others report significant decreases in morbidity. Vaccination is likely a useful adjunct to proper management in controlling neonatal diarrhea.

Castration and Dehorning: Castration of male calves in early life is likely to be less stressful to calves than castration performed later when testicular size is dramatically increased. In addition, early castration raises less concern about humane treatment. A number of methods may be used, including the open surgical technique, the use of rubber rings, and the Burdizzo method. Calves castrated surgically initially exhibit more agitation compared with calves castrated with rubber rings, but both groups resume normal behavior soon after the operation is completed. Dehorning early in life is also less stressful than when performed later when horns have increased in size. Horns are mostly a problem for the feeding period (ie, horned calves require more bunk space), and they may cause bruising in penmates. Such problems are best managed by polled breeding or early dehorning.

Identification: Individual identification of cows and calves allows for selection based on performance as well as for tracing the animal to its herd of origin to track or contain disease. Plastic ear tags are the most commonly used method of individual identification. Branding as a method of herd identification is coming under increasing scrutiny for product quality and animal welfare reasons. Commercial products are currently on the market that allow individual electronic identification. Such initiatives may eventually replace current identification systems.

Vaccinations: Vaccines are available for viral and bacterial respiratory pathogens. Residual passive immunity in young calves may limit the detectable antibody response to vaccination at an early age. Calves vaccinated at branding time may be sensitized to the antigens and respond with an anamnestic response when given a booster vaccine at arrival in the feedlot. Recommended vaccination programs include clostridial and viral respiratory vaccination at the time of branding. A number of "value-added" calf programs have been initiated, some of which require a vaccination program at branding time. Pneumonia incidence is typically low during the summer grazing periods, making clinical effectiveness of a vaccination program against respiratory disease difficult to demonstrate. Primary sensitization to increase subsequent vaccination response preweaning may be the major benefit of such a vaccination program. A booster vaccination is often administered to calves before weaning for viral respiratory agents. Vaccination for *Mannheimia* (*Pasteurella*) has been recommended for inclusion in a preweaning or weaning vaccination program as well. Field trail data on the effectiveness of respiratory vaccines in decreasing morbidity and mortality in weaned calves are lacking.

Infectious keratoconjunctivitis (p 412) is a significant problem in suckling calves, although control has proved to be difficult. Vaccination has shown variable results. Challenge with a homologous strain after vaccination may provide some level of control, but challenge with a heterologous strain creates little protection.

Implant Strategies: Use of hormonal implants as a management practice for calves may increase weaning weights by 3-5%, but response is often variable. (*See* GROWTH PROMOTANTS AND PRODUCTION ENHANCERS, p 2168.)

Parasite Control: Egg burdens of calves are typically low at spring branding but may rise significantly by midsummer. Deworming of cows in late spring may lead to increased weaning weights in calves. Studies examining the effects of deworming calves only at branding have been few and results were inconsistent—some showed positive effects, while others found no effect. Deworming of calves in addition to cows in late spring appears to confer minimal additional benefit. External parasites of cattle are estimated to be an important cause of economic loss as well. Studies have generally shown a weight gain of 10-20 lb in suckling calves when fly control is provided. The most common method of fly control is the use of insecticide-impregnated ear tags. Cows are commonly the only animals tagged. With the widespread use of pyrethroid insecticides in ear tags, emerging resistance has become a problem. Insecticide sprays and back rubbers can also be effective (and less expensive), but cattle must be forced to use them.

Nutrition: Suckling beef calves are generally not supplemented during the summer grazing period, when milk and an increasing intake of forage provide their diet. Deficiency of trace minerals may be a concern in some areas. Proper nutrition of the herd before calving should provide the calf with adequate reserves at birth. Subsequent supplementation is difficult, however, as trace mineral mix intake is sporadic at best in calves. Creep feeding may increase the reliability of intake, but it is an expensive substitute for available forage and the response is highly variable. Creep feeding for 3-4 wk before weaning may be an effective way to reduce stress and disease at weaning. (*See also* NUTRITION: CATTLE, p 1811.)

Weaning: Weaning is stressful because the calf is removed from its dam and forced to adjust to a different diet; population density is increased, leading to potential for increased disease exposure and transmission. Management procedures should aim to minimize stress on calves while ensuring they are in sound condition nutritionally and immunologically. Castration and dehorning should be performed well before weaning. Completion of vaccination, deworming, and implant procedures before weaning allows calves to be weaned without handling.

Early weaning of beef calves at 30-170 days of age may create more efficient use of feed resources by directly supplementing calves to maintain weight gain rather than supplementing cows to produce milk. Weaning times as early as 30-60 days can increase reproductive performance of cows and heifers. Cows and heifers cycle and rebreed earlier in the calving season, and pregnancy rates are higher in a limited breeding season after early weaning. Nutritional needs of the weaned calves must be met carefully to ensure acceptable health and performance. Weaning at 150-170 days of age decreases lactational stress on cows when forage resources are limited and improves cow condition. Reproductive performance in the breeding season is not affected by weaning at this time. When forage resources are limited, weaning calves to decrease the nutritional requirements of the cows allows them to regain condition before winter with less or no supplementation. Calves can be supplemented more efficiently than cows.

Replacement Heifers

Replacement heifer development programs generally commence at weaning as the heifers begin preparation for the breeding season. However, decisions relating to use of hormonal growth-promoting implant programs (see p 2168) for replacements must be made beginning at the spring working of calves at 2-3 mo of age. In general, reimplanting heifers at weaning, or after 6 mo of age, is not recommended. Heifers that calve at 24 mo of age have increased lifetime production compared with heifers that calve first at 30 or 36 mo of age.

Heifer Selection: Selection of replacement heifer prospects begins at weaning, when heifers are typically 6-8 mo old, and is based on birth date, conformation, frame score, and dam production records. Selection of heifers born early in the calving season leads to replacement heifers that are older and heavier at the start of the breeding season. Heifers should be evaluated for conformation of the feet, legs, and udder. Unacceptable conformation should disqualify a heifer as a replacement prospect. Age-adjusted frame scores can be used to estimate the mature size of prospects. These scores provide an objective method of selecting replacements to maintain a constant cow size suitable for the environment and feed resources.

Once potential replacement heifers are selected, a nutrition and vaccination program should be instituted in preparation for breeding. If heifers are to calve by 24 mo of age, they must be bred by 15 mo of age. For optimal fertility, heifers should weigh ~65% of their mature body weight by 12-13 mo of age. The ration must be balanced to provide the required rate of gain to meet the target goal of 65% of mature body weight in the time available. Specific requirements vary with the weight and breed of the heifers and the amount of time available before breeding. (See also NUTRITION: CATTLE, p 1811.)

Vaccination: The vaccination program for replacement heifers should provide optimal protection from reproductive diseases and should include vaccination for *Brucella abortus*, infectious bovine rhinotracheitis (IBR), bovine viral diarrhea (BVD), *Campylobacter*, and *Leptospira*. *Brucella* vaccination is performed according to state or regional regulations. Modified live vaccines for IBR and BVD may give the broadest immunity to strain differences and should be given twice to ensure a high level of immunity. Some evidence suggests that modified live BVD and IBR vaccines may transiently infect the ovary and cause decreased fertility. For this reason, the second vaccination should be given ≥1 mo before breeding. A vaccine containing *Campylobacter fetus* and 5 strains of *Leptospira* is given twice before breeding. Vaccination of heifers with *Trichomonas* vaccine increases calving rate and decreases duration of infection in herds, but does not prevent infection. A vaccine for trichomoniasis may be useful in infected herds or in herds that are at high risk of infection, but it may not be economic in low-risk herds.

Management: Heifers should be well developed at the time of first breeding, and their management during gestation must ensure their continued growth. Pregnant heifers should be separated from the main cow herd at the time of pregnancy testing and maintained separately until reentry into the breeding herd after their first calving. Undernutrition during pregnancy in first-calf heifers commonly leads to an increased incidence of dystocia because of lack of weight and size, weakness at the time of parturition, insufficient colostrum, weak calves at birth, and a high incidence of prolonged postpartum anestrus, which leads to a high percentage of nonpregnant animals that may have to be culled. Thus, pregnant heifers should be fed and managed separately from cows and should be on a higher plane of nutrition than cows. Such management may increase calf birth weight, but most of the increase is in soft tissue and skeletal structure and should be more than offset by the increased size and vigor of the heifers. Heifers should be bred early to ensure that any increase in the postpartum anestrus period after their first, perhaps difficult, calving does not compromise their chances for cycling and rebreeding with the main cow herd.

General Health Management Considerations

The greatest risk for initial introduction of many infectious diseases into a herd is the addition of subclinically infected animals, although some risk is also attributable to wildlife carriers. Potential sources of infection may be seen with herd additions, or through intentional or inadvertent movements and contacts. Herds may be classified as "closed," "modified open," and "open," based on their potential for pathogen exposure. (*See also* BIOSECURITY, p 1679.) Closed herds restrict the introduction of animals (eg, only breeding bulls) as well as contact with other herds and animals, whereas modified open herds may replace animals from outside sources on a limited basis and allow other controlled contacts, such as at livestock exhibitions. Open herds have high risk of introducing pathogens through such practices as regular introduction of purchased replacements (especially from commingled sale groups), direct introduction of stressed stocker calves (especially into high population densities), and mingling of animals of different backgrounds, through either cooperative breeding programs or poor herd biosecurity.

In general, all purchased or introduced animals should be separated from the home herd for a reasonable observation period (eg, 4 wk); these animals should undergo the same health procedures as the home herd. It is preferable to obtain animals from herds in which the herd health history is known and to have a record of vaccinations and treatments. If the origin of the newcomers is unknown, they should be tested for bovine leukosis, paratuberculosis, and bovine viral diarrhea. Pubertal bulls should be tested for trichomoniasis and vibriosis. For artificial insemination (AI) programs, semen should only be used only if it was processed by an approved AI center with a comprehensive health program for minimizing the risk of transmission of venereal (and other) diseases through frozen semen.

BEEF FEEDLOTS

In beef feedlots, young growing cattle are fed a high-energy diet to produce marketable beef at the lowest cost and in the shortest time possible. Depending on the starting body weight and age of the cattle, the period of confinement and feeding varies from 60 days to 12 mo. The success of a modern feedlot depends on good management, a favorable economic climate, and relative freedom from unfortunate events such as disease epidemics or unexpected increases in costs (eg, feed) or decreases in the price received for the final product. The concept of disease should include all of the identifiable factors that cause suboptimal performance: inadequacies in feeds and feeding systems, the purchase of undesirable types of cattle, and clinical and subclinical disease.

The feedlot veterinarian is responsible for maintaining optimal animal health through the following activities: 1) Making regularly scheduled visits to the feedlot. The frequency of visits depends on the size of the feedlot, the time of year, the expertise of the feedlot personnel, whether animals have recently arrived, and the degree to which the veterinarian is contractually responsible for the total animal health program. 2) Being available for emergency visits to the feedlot when disease epidemics are seen. 3) Performing necropsies during visits and training feedlot personnel to do necropsies at other times. 4) Examining sick animals to ensure that reasonably accurate diagnoses are being made and rational therapy is being given according to the established treatment protocol. 5) Regularly examining, analyzing, and interpreting animal health and production data and making recommendations in a written report. The effectiveness of detection of sick animals, based on response and relapse rates and case fatality rates, should be determined, and the effectiveness of the processing program for new arrivals, which includes the vaccines used and the medications given, should be examined and analyzed regularly. 6) Selecting and prescribing all drugs used in the feedlot, giving specific advice about the use of drugs, and establishing a drug residue-avoidance program. 7) Discussing overall animal health and production performance with the feedlot manager and other consultants, setting animal health and production goals, and monitoring achievement. 8) Comparing the feedlot with other operations. The veterinarian should produce a monthly report that compares processing costs, treatment costs, and death loss by arrival weight and days on feed.

When the consulting veterinarian is not readily available, a local practitioner can serve as a valuable resource for the feedlot. Serving as part of the feedlot's health care team, the local veterinarian can make significant contributions to the animal health program.

Economic Impact of Disease

Disease may cause economic loss in feedlots through mortality, treatment cost, or effects on productivity. The impact of clinical and subclinical disease on production efficiency and economic returns may be greater than the losses associated with mortality. A thorough understanding of the impact of disease on animal performance and economic loss is essential to make cost-effective recommendations to feedlot managers. The costs associated with death loss, chronically ill cattle marketed prematurely at a discount, and treatment are obvious and easy to calculate. Hidden costs, such as reduced performance and lower carcass quality, are often overlooked.

Treatment costs are another source of economic loss. Factors influencing the average cost include the morbidity rate, retreatment rate, cost of the drug(s), combination versus single antimicrobial therapy, whether or not adjunct therapy is used, labor, and feedlot markup on the products used. The morbidity rate has the strongest influence on the average treatment cost for all cattle in the pen. When metaphylaxis is used to manage bovine respiratory tract disease, it must be added to the total medical cost for the pen.

Implementing a Feedlot Medicine Program

Regular Inspection: Regular inspection of all areas of the feedlot for possible health problems should be included in a feedlot health service. Errors in animal husbandry should be noted and recorded for discussion with personnel. Attention should be given particularly to the delivery of feed and water, the general well-being of cattle, and any unusual characteristics of each feeding pen. Many feedlot health problems can be attributed to errors in management.

Disease Surveillance: Continued disease surveillance through regular necropsy examination of all dead cattle and regular observations of sick cattle are necessary. In colder climates, carcasses may freeze solid before the veterinarian is available. Conversely, in warmer climates, carcasses may decompose beyond usefulness. When distance prevents the consulting veterinarian from performing a necropsy on every animal that dies, a more accessible veterinarian may be employed. In many cases, feedlot personnel can be trained to recognize common postmortem lesions.

A key to the management of disease in feedlots is fast, accurate diagnosis. This requires a good surveillance system, a careful full-time search for sick animals, appropriate facilities for examination and treatment, accurate identification of animals, and appropriate laboratory facilities, especially a necropsy service. Emphasis is placed on training and supervising feedlot employees in the detection and early treatment of sick cattle. Employees, particularly any personnel responsible for checking the cattle pens for sick cattle, should be given regular instruction in the clinical signs of common diseases. These include anorexia, depression, lameness or abnormal gait, stiff movement, coughing, nasal and ocular discharge, increased breathing rate, crusted muzzle, sunken eyes, rough hair coat, loose or extra-firm feces, abnormal abdominal fill, and straining. Cattle with these or other obvious signs of illness are examined more closely in the hospital area and, if necessary, treated. In some feedlots, treated cattle are immediately returned to their original pens, whereas in others cattle are kept in hospital pens until they recover. Most animals that do not recover or that relapse after the first treatment are retreated, although this decision depends on the nature of the disease and the economics involved. If the animal can still be sold and chances of recovery are slim, it is usual to cull it after 2 or 3 courses of treatment.

Pens from which sick animals are taken should be closely observed. A potential epidemic must be identified early so that pen-level intervention can be considered.

Despite its importance, pen surveillance is not highly reliable for the detection of sick feedlot animals, particularly calves in the first week after arrival. It is difficult to distinguish tired, gaunt calves that may have been weaned a few days earlier from calves in the early stage of acute undifferentiated respiratory disease. Up to 50% of animals pulled from a pen of recently arrived calves will not show clinical signs based on measurement of body temperature and a cursory clinical examination.

Treatment Protocols: The veterinarian must specify procedures for the clinical management of sick cattle and provide a standard protocol that outlines specific treatments for disease syndromes, including drug dosages, treatment intervals, routes of administration, and withdrawal times. The protocol should be followed strictly by all personnel so that the success or failure of therapy can be evaluated accurately and that chances of creating food safety hazards are minimized. The effectiveness of the treatment protocol should be evaluated regularly by determination of the response rates for the various treatment regimens. The failure to develop and implement appropriate treatment protocols often leads to the use of many different drugs indiscriminately, which then leads to excessive treatment costs and often an increase in the case fatality rate.

Feedlot Records

Records are essential to monitor the incidence of disease, response to treatment, and production performance, and they should be analyzed regularly by the veterinarian and feedlot manager. They can be maintained by hand or by using commercially available computer software. The necessary input records include the lot description, processing record, lot update, sale information, animal identification, and feed and animal health product purchases. The necessary output records include the numbers of animals pulled from each pen daily, from which an epidemic curve can be drawn; the treatment response report according to pen or drug used; the percentage of pulled animals that had a fever, which is an indication of how many are probably affected with an acute respiratory disease rather than a noninfectious disease such as grain overload; the daily mortality report, which should include the list of animals that died, along with their arrival dates, the dates of treatment, and the causes of death; a case abstract of the treatment history of each individual animal; and a close-out summary, which includes all of the costs of production, the health and production performance of the lot or pen of cattle (including morbidity, mortality, ratio of feed conversion to body weight gain, average daily gain), the costs of gain per unit of gain, the number of days on feed, and the profit or loss.

Individual Treatment Record: Each animal treated should be individually identified, if this was not done on entry, and the information recorded on the treatment card. Treatment personnel should record the feeding pen, lot number, body temperature, body weight, disease suspected, treatment given, and location of the animal after treatment (eg, which hospital pen). The severity of the illness should be assessed to properly evaluate response to treatment. Late treatment in advanced stages of disease, particularly respiratory disease, is a major cause of failure to respond, even when the treatment of choice is instituted. A card is filled out for each animal treated, and all subsequent treatments are recorded on the same card. The cards are filed and retrieved for animals that relapse or die. The cumulative information on the card can be used to decide whether an animal should be culled for chronic or recurring illnesses that are refractory to treatment, to decide on alternative treatments, to explain reasons for death, and to evaluate the effectiveness of the treatments recommended. Some feedlots record animals that are removed from the pen but sent back untreated because they failed to meet the temperature criterion in the case definition for a given disease. This information can be of value if the animal is removed again or dies.

Daily Morbidity and Mortality Record: This record contains the number of treated cattle by pen and lot number, the disease diagnosed, and the date. It provides both the manager and the veterinarian with a rapid assessment of the location of disease problems in the feedlot. It contains information on the number of animals removed and the number not treated and then classifies those treated according to diagnosis and whether they are a relapse or new case. By using this report in conjunction with an inventory report showing filling dates and numbers added to the pen on those dates, it is possible to generate epidemic curves.

Morbidity and Treatment Analysis Record: This aggregation of data summarizes the morbidity rate, the relapse rate, and the death rate for a lot or pen of cattle. It is especially important as a tool to evaluate the overall effectiveness of the treatment program for various diseases; the relapse rates and death rates are compared with goals set for the feed and with standards published in the literature. The disposition summary alerts the feedlot manager and consulting veterinarian when the chronic or culling rates are abnormally high, which can lead to significant economic losses.

Mortality Analysis: The causes of death as determined by necropsy should be summarized on a regular basis. A mortality analysis includes the number of days the animal was in the feedlot, any observed premonitory signs, and treatment (diagnosis, drug used, and when treated). The location of the animal in the feedlot at the time of death should also be considered.

Feedlot Performance Summary: Most feedlots complete a close-out summary for each group of cattle that have been finished and shipped to market. The performance record and feeding summary sections include average daily gain in body weight, total feed consumption, feed conversion ratios and cost per unit of body weight gain, mortality rates, culling rate, and medical costs. The financial summary provides the profit or loss on an individual and lot basis.

Vaccination Protocols

An important component of feedlot health programs is the planning of vaccination programs. Vaccination schedules vary depending on the prevalence of disease both in the feedlot area and in the area from which the cattle originated. The vaccines used and the vaccination schedule should be based on the expected incidence of the disease, the cost of the disease when it is seen, the cost of the preventive procedure (vaccine plus labor), the field efficacy of the vaccine, and other available control procedures.

Nutritional Advice

Feedlots frequently consult a qualified nutritionist to assist in the formulation of cost-effective diets. The veterinarian should communicate with the nutritionist regarding the composition of the diets and any changes that are being planned. Most of the emphasis in feedlot nutrition has been on the development of cost-effective diets that support a maximal growth rate without any deleterious effects. Considerable information is available on the nutrient requirements for feedlot cattle and on the feeds and feeding systems used. (*See also* NUTRITION: BEEF CATTLE, p 1811.)

Nutritional deficiency diseases are uncommon in feedlot cattle, because cattle usually receive a diet that contains the nutrients required for maintenance and promotion of rapid growth. Diets prepared according to published standards should meet all the requirements under most conditions. Specific nutrient deficiencies are extremely rare; however, such a situation may be seen in a small farm feedlot that prepares its own diet with little or no attention to the necessity for supplementation of homegrown feeds.

Although only a few nutritional diseases may affect a well-managed feedlot, these diseases may cause large economic losses when they develop. They include carbohydrate engorgement (grain overload or D-lactic acidosis), feedlot bloat or ruminal tympany, and feeding errors (ie, accidental incorporation of an excessive amount of a feed additive, such as monensin or urea, or sudden unintended changes in the ingredient composition of the diet).

Disease Epidemics

In spite of good management, unexpected disease epidemics are seen in feedlot cattle. When feeding accidents occur, many animals can be affected suddenly, ie, within 1 or 2 days. In outbreaks of acute infectious diseases, such as infectious bovine rhinotracheitis, pneumonic pasteurellosis, or *Haemophilus* meningoencephalitis, the first few cases are followed by a steady increase in the morbidity rate for several days and then a decline as the outbreak subsides 10-14 days after the index case.

In some cases, the diagnosis may be obvious (eg, carbohydrate engorgement caused by a feeding error). In other cases (eg, infectious diseases of the respiratory tract), the diagnosis may not be readily obvious, and a detailed epidemiologic, clinical, and laboratory investigation may be required. A complete investigation may require specialists from several disciplines. Every effort should be made to determine the specific source of the disease. The investigation should include a general description of the problem, a complete history of the disease outbreak (including details and date of index case, total number of sick animals, treatments, case fatality rate, population mortality rate, and vaccination history), and clinical examination of several affected animals (with appropriate samples) as well as necropsies. After the diagnosis is determined, the rationale for treatment is outlined. When outbreaks of infectious disease are encountered, the intensity of surveillance must be increased to detect new cases in the early stages of disease when response to treatment is usually good.

All of the details of the outbreak should be listed in chronologic order and then analyzed. Correlations can be made between exposure factors and the development of new cases during the course of the outbreak. Often epidemiologic determinants that explain disease occurrence can be identified and the information used to control future episodes. A detailed report of the outbreak, outlining the conclusion and recommendations, should be prepared by the veterinarian and submitted to the owner.

CONTROL AND PREVENTION OF DISEASE

Control and prevention of disease in feedlot cattle depends on purchasing healthy animals; providing a transportation system that minimizes stress, a comfortable feedlot pen environment, and an adequate feeding system; establishing a good surveillance system; and judiciously using vaccines and, when necessary, antimicrobial agents.

Feedlot Facilities

One of the most important considerations in the construction of a feedlot is good drainage. The pens and alleyways should be well drained and easily accessible for scraping the ground surface as necessary. Good drainage requires a 6% slope. To avoid overstocking, each animal should be provided with 18 m^2 of space in well-drained land and with 9 m^2 in a paved lot.

Cattle need protection from wind, rain, snow, excessive heat, and sunshine. Trees are planted as windbreaks, and buildings and fences are placed so that the wind is not deflected into feeding areas or sheds. An open-front shed provides protection from winter storms and hot summer sun. Each animal needs ~1-1.5 m^2 of cover. The shed should be open to the south or southeast, and the front should be high enough so that the sun strikes the ground at the back on the shortest day of the winter. The back of the shed should be ≥2.5 m high. A covered feed bunk protects feed from weather damage and affords cattle added comfort when eating. Feed remains dry and palatable, and waste is reduced. Shades to provide relief from extreme summer heat are useful in feedlots in the extreme southwestern USA.

Environmental concerns about feedlot operations have greatly increased in recent years. Stricter environmental laws require that all feedlot waste and run-off be contained in approved lagoon systems. Pollution prevention plans must be on file with the appropriate government agency. Monitoring, testing, and record-keeping requirements vary from country to country as well as regionally. In addition, foodborne illnesses, particularly those caused by *Escherichia coli* O157H:7 and *Salmonella*, have forced the meat-packing industry to change the way beef carcasses are processed. The packing industry has placed pressure on feedlots to provide animals that are as clean as possible.

Transportation of Cattle

Transportation or shipping of cattle has long been associated with increased bovine respiratory disease (BRD) in the feedlot, hence the term "shipping fever." With current improvements in transportation, however, there is no correlation between the distance cattle are shipped and the risk of fatal fibrinous pneumonia in the feedlot. Apparently factors such as level of immunity, commingling, and other stressors are more important in the risk of BRD than distance shipped.

Cattle lose considerable weight within the first 24-48 hr after weaning, during shipment, and after deprivation of feed and water. This loss in body weight (known as shrink) varies from a minimum of 4% in cattle deprived of feed and water for 24 hr up to 9% in animals that are transported long distances over a period of 2-4 days. Most of the fluid and electrolyte loss can be restored within a few days if the animals begin to eat and drink normally. Shrink >7% has been associated with increased health problems. The total loss in body weight may not be restored for up to 3 wk.

Transportation equipment and facilities should meet local standards and be able to transport cattle comfortably regardless of the season of the year. Some countries prohibit the transport of cattle over a certain length of time without unloading for rest, feed, and water. On arrival at their destination, cattle should be examined carefully for evidence of clinical disease or injury. Provision of fresh hay and water can help detect those that are anorectic and that should be examined more closely. This is particularly important if unexpected delays in transportation have occurred that increase the level of stress in the animals.

Cattle Purchase and Introduction to a Feedlot

Infectious diseases of the respiratory tract, particularly "shipping fever" pneumonia caused by *Pasteurella* spp, are major causes of morbidity and mortality during the first 30-45 days after arrival in the feedlot. Digestive diseases, especially carbohydrate engorgement, in cattle placed on a high-energy diet within 30 days after arrival in the feedlot are a major potential threat but can be controlled. The acute respiratory disease complex (p 1190) is much more difficult to control in feedlot cattle, even under good management conditions.

The major objective on arrival at the feedlot is to get the cattle onto a high-energy diet—which will result in rapid growth—as soon as possible, usually within 21 days, while minimizing the morbidity and mortality associated with acute respiratory disease, other common infections (eg, *Haemophilus* septicemia), and digestive diseases associated with adjustments to high-energy diets.

Preimmunization and Preconditioning

Preconditioning is the preparation of feeder calves for marketing and shipment; it may include vaccinations, castration, and training calves to eat and drink in pens. The concept of preconditioning is based in part on immunologic and nutritional principles. Preimmunization, or vaccination of calves 2-3 wk before shipment from the ranch to the feedlot, was the basis of preconditioning. In addition to vaccination, more recent efforts have been directed toward increasing the number of days weaned before movement and improving management procedures on the ranch, such as genetic selection and nutrition, that assist calves in making an easier transition to the feedlot.

In the USA, preconditioning has been defined by the following elements: 1) weaning at least 3 wk before sale, 2) training to eat from a feed bunk and to drink from a trough, 3) parasite treatment, 4) vaccination for blackleg, malignant edema, parainfluenza 3, infectious bovine rhinotracheitis, *Pasteurella*, and sometimes bovine viral diarrhea and *Haemophilus*, 5) castration and dehorning, 6) identification with an ear tag, and 7) sale through special auctions. When preconditioned calves are placed in a feedlot, they usually begin to eat and drink on arrival; if they have not been subjected to unusual stressors, the incidence of disease is minimal. However, daily surveillance is still necessary to identify cases of illness. Although preconditioning is profitable to some producers, on average, preconditioning is difficult to justify economically.

Backgrounding is a variation of preconditioning in which recently weaned calves are grown to yearling feeder cattle weight, usually in a smaller feedlot. The principal objective is to prepare yearling cattle to adjust to a high-energy finishing ration in a feedlot with minimal problems. This is achieved by feeding the calves a growing diet that yields rapid, efficient body weight gains without fattening. The spectrum of diseases that are seen in backgrounding operations during the first 45 days after arrival of the calves depends on whether the calves were preimmunized, preconditioned, or obtained from several different sources with no preconditioning. Infectious diseases of the respiratory tract (pneumonic pasteurellosis) and of the digestive tract (coccidiosis) account for most of the losses.

Recently arrived cattle of unknown backgrounds (eg, those from sales yards) require extra surveillance and care. Most of these cattle must be vaccinated as necessary, and some need to be castrated, dehorned, and given growth promotant implants. Nonpreconditioned stressed cattle of unknown backgrounds should be allowed to adjust to their new surroundings for up to 3 wk after arrival. During this adjustment period, the cattle are fed good-quality roughage along with a quantity of a highly palatable, nutrient-dense ration. They are checked carefully at least twice daily for evidence of illness, and sick cattle are identified and treated. Once the animals are healthy and the common infectious diseases are not a problem, the animals can be fed growing and finishing diets.

Vaccination against certain respiratory diseases within 24 hr of arrival is standard practice for the majority of feedlot and backgrounding operations. Vaccination should be limited to those products that actually reduce losses resulting from respiratory disease. Other procedures and product use should be delayed for ≥2-3 wk. The use of prophylactic antimicrobials against respiratory disease may be necessary in high-risk nonpreconditioned calves.

Regardless of the system used, immediately on arrival the cattle should be weighed as a group, examined for evidence of illness, and treated if necessary. Some feedlots administer antimicrobials to all calves considered to be at high risk of acute respiratory disease. If the illness appears different from the usual case of respiratory disease, diagnosis by a veterinarian should be sought at the earliest possible time. Close examination and surveillance are desirable for groups of cattle with a history of unusual stress. The youngest and smallest cattle often need special attention, and it may be necessary to separate them from older cattle. A reliable history of vaccination, vitamin injections, implants, and anthelmintic administration would be useful but is usually not available. The major objective during the first few days is to avoid unnecessary deaths from diseases that normally respond well to treatment. Depending on the condition of the cattle, it may be difficult during the first few days after arrival to easily distinguish sick cattle from healthy cattle, and careful clinical surveillance every few hours may be necessary. Observations at the time of feeding often reveal anorectic animals that should be pulled from the pen and examined.

Processing Procedures

Identification: Each animal must be identified immediately, preferably with a color-coded and numbered plastic ear tag that is easily visible from a distance. In many feedlots, each animal is not identified individually but instead receives a tag with a lot number (group) or pen number. Systems are now in place that individually identify animals with tags that can be read electronically from a distance of 8-10 in. Information that can be maintained on individual animals through this technology includes performance, vaccine, and treatment history. These tags remain on the animal until slaughter, at which time the identification from the ear tag can be transferred to the overhead trolley system.

Measurement of Body Temperature: On arrival, some animals may be affected with acute disease but show no obvious clinical signs. Others may appear fatigued and gaunt but are not affected with clinical disease. Identifing animals with acute infectious disease that should be treated early to minimize mortality can be difficult. The body temperature of high-risk cattle (eg, calves from auctions or calves that have been transported long distances over several days) is often measured at processing. Animals with a body temperature >104°F (40°C) are treated with an antimicrobial. Treated animals may be tagged and noted in the individual animal database, or the total number of animals treated (total amount of drug administered) in a group or pen may be recorded.

Vaccination: The value of vaccinating feedlot cattle for common infectious diseases, particularly those of the respiratory tract, has been controversial since the vaccines were introduced. Nevertheless, a wide variety of vaccines are used in feedlot health programs.

Vaccines are available for the following diseases or infections of feedlot cattle: infectious bovine rhinotracheitis, pneumonic pasteurellosis, parainfluenza 3 virus infection, bovine respiratory syncytial virus infection, *Histophilus somni* disease complex, bovine viral diarrhea, and clostridial disease. The vaccines available for clostridial diseases are highly effective. The number of antigens to be used (2- or 8-way) depends on local prevalence of clostridial diseases, including blackleg (*Clostridium chauvoei*), malignant edema (*C septicum*), bacillary hemoglobinuria (*C novyi*, type D [*haemolyticum*]), infectious hepatitis (*C novyi*, type B), tetanus (*C tetani*), enterotoxemia (*C perfringens*, types B, C, and D), and leptospirosis (*Leptospira* serovars *hardjo*, *pomona*, *grippotyphosa*, *canicola*, and *icterohaemorrhagiae*).

A basic vaccination schedule for receiving calves should include a 4-way respiratory viral vaccine plus a clostridial vaccine. Additional vaccines should be included only if 2 criteria can be met: the disease is enough of a risk that prevention is necessary (eg, leptospirosis in some areas), and data can be found to support the use of vaccines to prevent disease.

Castration and Dehorning: These surgical procedures are frequently performed at processing but are very stressful to cattle and may reduce performance for up to 90 days and increase the mortality rate. It is generally recommended that these procedures be delayed until the animals are adjusted to the feedlot.

Anthelmintics and Insecticides: Anthelmintics and insecticides are administered according to local conditions. The feedlot operator and veterinarian should be informed about feeder calves or yearling cattle that have originated from farms or areas in which intestinal parasitism is likely. When compared with treatment with a topical organophosphate, treatment with ivermectin can cause improved average daily weight gain and feed conversion in feedlot calves under commercial conditions. Young cattle raised on small farms in which the stocking rate on pasture is high may harbor helminths. Young cattle may also be affected by chronic verminous pneumonia caused by *Dictyocaulus viviparus*.

Growth-promoting Agents: Growth-promoting agents (p 2168) increase growth rate of animals without being used themselves to provide nutrients for growth. They are generally administered in small amounts—often via implants or in feed—to alter metabolism so that the animal increases body tissues and grows more rapidly. They include antibacterials, antimicrobials, steroids (eg, estrogens, androgens), and ionophores. They promote changes in composition, conformation, mature weight, or efficiency of growth, although these effects are frequently accompanied by changes in the rate of live weight gain. Vitamin injections are given in some processing schedules as a mixture of vitamins A, D, and E. This procedure prevents any possible development of hypovitaminosis A, which may be present in cattle that have originated from a dry, carotene-deficient pasture or diet. However, the vitamins may also be supplied in the feed at high concentrations during the conditioning period to increase levels in the liver.

BEEF QUALITY ASSURANCE AND BEEF SAFETY PROGRAMS

The purpose of a beef quality assurance (BQA) program is to identify and avoid areas in the feedlot where quality or safety defects can be seen. The goal of the BQA program is to assure the consumer that all cattle shipped from a feedlot are healthy, wholesome, and safe and that their management has met all government and industry standards.

The feedlot must be able to document all the steps of production. Critical points in production must be monitored to ensure no residue violations or carcass defects are seen. These critical points include, but are not limited to, incoming cattle, product and commodities, cattle handling, and evaluation of outgoing cattle. There is a built-in margin of safety for withdrawal times in the feedlot industry, because most withdrawal times for animal health products are shorter than the feeding periods. Feedlot personnel must be aware of high residue-risk situations. Nonperforming cattle could have organ damage, which could prevent normal clearance of a drug product, causing violative residues even after the preslaughter withdrawal time has elapsed.

The BQA program is based on the principles of the Hazard Analysis of Critical Control Points (HACCP) system. Each production step should be evaluated for potential quality or safety defects, including bacterial contamination, which can cause infectious disease in cattle or employees; chemical usage-contamination, which can lead to violative residues; and physical damage, such as injection site damage, bruising, or broken needles in animal tissues. The analysis should include sanitation standard operating procedures (eg, finding ways to prevent or minimize fecal-oral contamination).

All relevant government regulations on feedstuffs, feed additives, and medications (including route of administration and withdrawal times) must be closely followed. Extra-label drug use must be prescribed only by the feedlot veterinarian. All owners of cattle treated with medications administered extra-label must comply with prescribed, extended withdrawal times that have been set by the feedlot veterinarian under the guidelines of a valid veterinarian-client-patient relationship. The Food Animal Residue Avoidance Databank is the primary resource for determining the preslaughter withdrawal time when an animal has been treated in an extra-label manner.

Record Keeping: All records should be kept for ≥ 2 yr after cattle have been shipped from the feedlot. If a violative residue is found in any cattle shipped for slaughter, the feedlot must make applicable records available to the appropriate government agencies. The source and cause of violative residue should be determined and corrective action taken to prevent reoccurrence.

Individual Records: Treatment records should be maintained for all cattle treated individually. This can be done using hand-written records or a computerized record system. Essential information includes the individual animal identification, treatment date(s), diagnosis, drug administered, serial/lot number, dosage used, approximate weight of animal, route and location of administration, and earliest date the animal could clear the preslaughter withdrawal period. The treatment history of cattle with chronic medical problems, or of those that have a poor, unexplained growth rate, should be scrutinized carefully. In many cases residue screening, such as the live animal swab test, is advisable. Residue screening should be performed under the supervision of the feedlot veterinarian. The results of such testing determine whether an animal can be released for shipment.

Group Records: All animals treated as part of a group (processing or mass medication) should be identified by group or lot, and the treatment information should be recorded. Records should include the animal lot or group identification, product used, serial/lot number of the product, date treated, dosage used, route and location of administration, and withdrawal information. A preslaughter withdrawal time is assigned to the entire pen. Recording treatments under this system assumes that every animal in the lot or group received the treatment. The health records of cattle shipped to slaughter should be checked by feedlot personnel to ensure that treated animals have cleared the appropriate withdrawal times. All pesticides should be used in accordance with label directions, and their use and withdrawal time should be recorded.

Treatment Protocol Book: The feedlot veterinarian should provide a treatment protocol book specific to the feedlot operation. It should be reviewed regularly and updated at least every 90 days. One copy should be kept at the treatment facility and another copy should be maintained in the feedlot office. A written treatment protocol and current prescriptions are important documents that the feedlot must have if there is a government inspection of the feedlot facilities, drug usage procedures, and residue avoidance plans. It also provides written guidelines for animal health programs, thus minimizing chances of mistakes or misunderstandings.

Culling of Feedlot Cattle

Culling may be done at any point between examination of the cattle on arrival and a few weeks later, before the cattle are placed on a high-energy diet. Diseases that justify culling include chronic unthriftiness and inappetence of undetermined etiology, chronic laminitis, chronic lameness caused by footrot, chronic bloat, chronic pneumonia, acute and chronic pulmonary abscess, and bovine viral diarrhea. Each of these diseases leads to unthriftiness, and a clinical examination is necessary for diagnosis.

Animal Welfare in Feedlots

Good feedlot design is important to ensure animal comfort. Handling facilities must be modern and efficient and must not induce animal attendants to be cruel to animals when they are being moved from one location to another; excessive force should not be used to get the animals to move. The feedlot personnel must be educated about the signs of pain and discomfort associated with certain illnesses and how cattle can be handled humanely.

The veterinarian should emphasize good feedlot design and equipment that will ensure comfort for the animals and minimize pain and stress associated with handling procedures. The veterinarian must also be a vigilant guardian, denouncing inhumane practices and encouraging sound animal welfare management. (*See also* ANIMAL WELFARE, p 1330.)

DEVELOPMENT OF ANTIMICROBIAL-RESISTANT BACTERIA

The use of antimicrobials, particularly the subtherapeutic use of antimicrobials in the feed of feedlot cattle, is controversial because it may promote the development of antimicrobial-resistant strains of bacteria. The major concern is that these strains can then be transferred in the meat to humans, causing disease that may be difficult to treat because of drug resistance. It is also possible that resistance plasmids from animal enteropathogens can be transferred by the process of conjugation to human enteropathogens.

The bacteria of major concern in this context are *Campylobacter* and the *Salmonella* spp, which are enteric in cattle. The use of subtherapeutic levels of antimicrobials in the feed of cattle can result in the emergence of drug-resistant (and multidrug resistant) strains of bacteria in the intestinal flora of the animals. If these bacteria contaminate beef carcasses, they can become a foodborne pathogen for humans who handle the meat or eat meat that is not cooked adequately. In 1999, the American Association of Bovine Practitioners published *Prudent Drug Usage Guidelines*, which provide guidelines for antimicrobial usage in cattle feedlot operations.

DAIRY HERDS

In recent years, the structure of the dairy industry of developed countries has undergone remarkable changes. These changes include continued restructuring of the industry through reduced herd numbers, increased herd sizes, and adoption of specialized management practices that encourage higher productivity.

In the past, most dairy cows were housed in stall-barn facilities that were designed to maximize operator comfort. Today, most new free-stall facilities are built to maximize natural ventilation. Historically, barns were often placed in sheltered locations, while today they are usually located in open fields or on hilltops to ensure adequate airflow and to optimize cow comfort. The type of milking facility is also evolving; whereas many operations report using tie-stall or stanchion milking facilities, the majority of cows are now milked in parlors. Most parlors are highly mechanized and designed to minimize the amount of labor required.

Milk quality is traditionally defined by the somatic cell count (SCC) and bacterial count in prepasteurized bulk tank milk. In all developed nations, regulatory officials set allowable maximums for SCC. Since 1986, allowable limits for SCC and bacteria have been gradually lowered. The current upper limit for bulk tank SCC is 750,000 and 500,000 cells/mL in the USA and Canada, respectively. The SCC maximum in the EU is 400,000 cells/mL using geometric means as the basis for calculation.

Artificial insemination (AI) through the commercial distribution of frozen semen is the preferred method of reproductive management on most dairy operations. In fact, 45% of USA dairy operators in 1996 reported that no breeding bulls were present on their farms. The use of genetically elite sires has contributed to increases of >150 kg/yr in genetic merit for milk production. Declining fertility has accompanied advancements in genetic merit. Dairy farms commonly record herd conception rates of <50%. Technologies such as embryo transfer, rapid hormonal assays, controlled breeding programs that use reproductive hormones, and ultrasonography are used increasingly on modern dairy farms.

Nutritional research also has advanced rapidly, especially in areas such as rumen physiology and lipid metabolism. (*See* NUTRITION: CATTLE, p 1828.) Lactating dairy cows are generally fed either a component-based ration (forages and grain are fed separately) or a total mixed ration (TMR, forages and grain are mixed and fed together). The basis of a successful nutritional program is the determination of nutrient content of the ration ingredients through laboratory testing, formulation of nutritionally sound diets, and assurance of adequate intake of required nutrients through feed bunk management. Maintaining a stable, healthy rumen environment is difficult with component-based feeding systems. TMR diets are generally based on mixing stored forages (usually haylage or corn silage) with grains (such as high-moisture corn or soybeans) and byproducts such as cottonseed or locally available commodities such as citrus pulp, brewers grains, or bakery waste. On larger farms, cows are often grouped and fed diets specifically formulated to meet their production and metabolic needs. Many farms use the expertise of professional nutritionists to formulate rations.

Most producers raise their own replacement animals, but an increasing number of large dairy farms contract with specialized heifer growing operations. Virtually all newborn heifer calves are hand-fed colostrum within the first 24 hr of life to ensure adequate intake of immunoglobulins. The use of mastitic or antibiotic-containing waste milk has been related to high mortality rates. Many producers feed milk replacer to decrease the potential transmission of infectious disease. Holstein heifers are now heavier and taller at the withers than shown in published standards from years past. Efficient replacement programs endeavor to calve Holstein heifers that weigh 550 kg at 22.5-25 mo of age. Various health management programs are used to reach this goal, including deworming and the use of oral coccidiostats, supplemental selenium, and ionophores.

ANIMAL AND HERD PRODUCTIVITY

The productivity of an individual cow is the sum of the value of the milk she produces, the value of her offspring, and her individual market value when she leaves the herd. Many factors influence individual cow productivity, which is also based on longevity and the proportion of the cow's lifetime spent producing milk. Nonproductive periods include the period from birth until first parturition and dry periods before subsequent calvings. Heifers must be managed to reach appropriate breeding size by 13-15 mo of age to maximize lifetime production.

Milk yield is related to stage of lactation. Milk yield increases rapidly after calving, reaches a plateau ~40-60 days after calving, and then declines at a rate of ~5-10%/mo. The rate of decline is lower in younger animals compared with older cows. Good reproductive management ensures that the largest proportion of a cow's total lifetime production is spent during early high-producing stages of lactation rather than late lower-producing periods. Milk yield increases with age and parity until about the sixth lactation; these cows may produce up to 25% more milk volume compared with first lactation cows. Health disorders or other management problems that reduce longevity have a negative impact on productivity.

On small farms, veterinary care is often directed at individual animals and the veterinarian is the actual provider of technical services. As farms expand, the dairy practitioner must become involved in defining systems and standard operating procedures that allow the easy application of preventive health care programs to groups of animals. In many instances, technical services (such as vaccination, hoof care, and individual animal treatments) are performed by farm staff that have been trained to deliver treatments defined by the herd veterinarian. Another key role of veterinarians serving the dairy industry is to help producers evaluate the costs versus the relative benefits of production technologies, preventive health care programs, and management choices.

Nutritional Management

In most dairy herds, nutritional management is the most important determinant of herd productivity. The relationship between nutrition and productivity begins at birth. The feeding system must deliver the necessary nutrients to each cow at the correct stage of lactation to maintain optimal productivity. The choice of a feeding system is associated with both herd size and production level. Three general types of feeding systems are used currently by dairy farmers: total mixed rations (TMR), component feeding, and management-intensive grazing. Each of these systems, when implemented correctly, can deliver adequate nutrients for a highly productive dairy herd. Each system has its own inherent challenges in the achievement of optimal productivity.

The use of TMR feeding systems has increased as more herds have adopted free-stall or dry-lot housing. TMR diets have several advantages: cows consume the desired proportion of forages, risk of digestive upset is reduced, feed efficiency is increased, byproduct feeds may be used, accuracy of diet formulation is higher, and labor needs are reduced. The performance of herds using TMR diets can be lowered by errors in ration formulation and feed delivery. Some common errors include inadequate or nonexistent forage testing, variation in forage dry matter, variation in dry-matter intakes, overmixing of diets that causes inadequate fiber levels, and overfeeding or underfeeding energy to late lactation cattle. When TMR are fed, nutritional mistakes are often spread across the entire group or herd. Health management programs of herds that receive TMR diets should include systems to monitor the adequacy of the ration formulation and delivery.

Component-fed herds receive grain and forage separately. The successful operation of a component feeding system depends on maintaining a stable rumen environment while meeting the nutritional needs of modern, high-producing dairy cows. Advocates of component feeding emphasize the ability to meet the production and metabolic needs of individual cows throughout their production cycle.

Management-intensive grazing systems can be used to meet the needs of modern dairy cows. In some regions of the world (eg, New Zealand and Australia) pasture-based systems are the predominant method of feeding dairy cattle. In these truly pastoral systems, nutrition is often the most limiting factor in achieving optimal productivity. These regions may experience significant annual variation in productivity because of year-to-year differences in growing conditions. Some herds use seasonal dairying to match pasture conditions with the energy needs of early lactation cows. Attention to reproductive management is critical for herds that attempt to breed all cows within a defined period. Production management programs for herds using management-intensive grazing systems must include programs to control bloat, hypomagnesemia, and copper and selenium deficiency. Pastured cattle may walk considerable distances to harvest forages. Therefore a system to monitor and minimize lameness must be included in the health delivery system.

Reproductive Management

The reproductive program is the most common reason for scheduled herd visits by veterinarians. Veterinarians can improve herd productivity significantly by designing and implementing sound reproductive management programs that include cost-effective strategies to meet farm goals and reduce involuntary culling related to reproductive failure. Reproductive disorders are the most common and costly reason for premature culling of dairy cows. (*See* MANAGEMENT OF REPRODUCTION: CATTLE, p 1747.) In conventional dairy herds in which calving occurs throughout the year, reproductive management can influence productivity by minimizing production losses due to cows milked in later, lower-producing stages of lactation; long dry periods; culling losses; reproductive inefficiencies related to delayed age at first calving; and excessive labor and therapeutics costs associated with the reproductive program. Some herds have returned to extensive use of natural service sires to ensure that cows conceive promptly. In these herds, breeding soundness examinations and bull management programs should be included to ensure continued herd productivity. (*See also* BREEDING SOUNDNESS EXAMINATION OF THE MALE, p 1797.)

Replacement Management

Herd productivity can be affected negatively by high mortality of replacement animals. The highest morbidity and mortality rates on dairy farms generally are seen before weaning. On many farms, the most significant causes of preweaning death are infectious diseases of the digestive and respiratory systems. These disorders can be controlled by well-designed health management procedures that define the care and housing of the dam during the periparturient period, the calving process, and the application of proper preventive measures (including sound nutritional programs) for newborn calves.

Disease Incidence

Increased culling, reduced milk or protein yield, increased adult cow mortality, and reduced reproductive efficiency are all potential results of disease. Milk production is often profoundly reduced in cows with clinical disease. The duration of acute clinical syndromes is often short, but the effects of the disease may persist throughout the entire lactation. Early lactation is the highest risk period for many diseases. Disease during early lactation may reduce peak milk yields and therefore contribute to lower total lactational yields. Through advances in animal husbandry and health management programs, many farms have minimized clinical syndromes associated with infectious and metabolic disease.

While epidemics of clinical syndromes still are seen, the nature of disease has changed on many dairy farms. The trend toward larger units and shrinking profit margins has encouraged a shift toward optimizing herd or group productivity through reduction of subclinical disease, such as mastitis, acidosis, and laminitis, which can have a major impact on productivity.

Herd Size, Composition, and Culling

There is a well-demonstrated relationship between productivity and herd size. One reason for this relationship is the greater willingness for larger operations to adopt production-enhancing technologies. Government policies can also substantially influence herd size (eg, countries with supply management systems effectively limit the annual income that a farm can achieve from the sale of milk). The amount and productivity of pasture can influence the size of herds that use grazing. In these herds, productivity is determined by balancing the ability of the pasture to produce nutrients against the ability of the cows to produce milk. The size of both grazing and confinement herds are increasingly affected by competing demands for land.

The proportion of the herd producing milk compared with nonproductive stock (dry cows, calves, heifers, and bulls) has an effect on total herd productivity. Herd composition is the result of a number of interrelated management decisions, such as culling policy, rate of reproductive success, rate of disease, replacement management, and longterm goals regarding herd size. The ability of a herd manager to cull animals can have a significant impact on herd composition. When numerous replacement heifers are available, culling may intensify, leading to a younger herd. In countries where herd production is not limited, such as in the USA, longterm plans regarding expansion often influence herd composition. Some growing or start-up herds prefer to purchase only nonlactating cattle to reduce the risk of purchasing animals with infectious diseases such as contagious mastitis or BVD. These herds are often composed of almost all first lactation animals.

Decisions regarding cow removal can significantly impact productivity of the dairy herd. Culling rates vary between herds and may be related to disease rates or disease control programs. Fertility, mastitis, and lameness are commonly reported reasons for cow removal. Culling is an important aspect of controlling other diseases such as bovine tuberculosis, brucellosis, Johne's disease, and chronic mastitis caused by some contagious mastitis pathogens.

Environmental Conditions

Even with optimal housing situations, herd productivity can be affected by environmental conditions. High-producing cows have larger dry matter intakes, generate more internal heat, and are less tolerant of high ambient temperatures. Weather conditions that combine high ambient temperatures and high humidity without periods of cooling generally cause depressed dry-matter intakes and reductions in milk yield. The increased concentration of dairy farming in regions that experience considerable periods of high temperatures has resulted in more seasonal variation in milk output. Farmers have adopted a variety of systems to combat heat stress. Many new facilities are constructed with large open sides (often >4.3 m high) and ends and use fans and cooling systems to keep cows comfortable. Older enclosed facilities can be retrofitted with tunnel ventilation systems to provide adequate air movement. (See also VENTILATION, p 1699.)

Drying Off and Dry Cow Management

Risk factors for most postpartum diseases of dairy cows are seen during the dry period, with clinical signs of disease becoming evident after calving. Diseases such as hypocalcemia (milk fever), hypomagnesemia, udder edema, ketosis, displaced abomasum, and mastitis often begin during the dry period. Dairy health management programs focus on many preventive practices such as vaccination, hoof care, and nutritional monitoring during this period.

The length of the dry period influences milk yield in the subsequent lactation. The recommended dry period is 6-8 wk. Dry periods of <40 days have been demonstrated to reduce milk yield in the following lactation. Dry periods that are too long often lead to excessive weight gain and reduced production efficiency. Both short and long dry periods are most common when breeding dates are uncertain because of either bull breeding or inaccurate (or missing) reproductive records.

INTERACTIONS BETWEEN HEALTH AND PRODUCTION

An important factor that influences dairy herd productivity is the amount and type of disease in the herd. The basis of disease control programs includes knowledge of the frequency of disease, information about the biologic effect of disease, and information on the effectiveness of control procedures.

Most studies report incidence rates of only common, easily diagnosed, clinical diseases such as mastitis, lameness, milk fever, retained placenta, or displaced abomasum. The frequency of subclinical disease is much more difficult to discern. The cost of obtaining subclinical disease information is inflated by the need to use screening tests (eg, culture or somatic cell counts [SCC] for mastitis, fecal culture or ELISA for paratuberculosis) for diagnosis. The lack of repeated testing leads to the reporting of prevalence rather than incidence for many subclinical diseases. Estimates of the frequency of sporadic or endemic infectious diseases (such as listeriosis, infectious bovine rhinotracheitis, or leptospirosis) are also sparse. There is zero tolerance for some diseases that have serious consequences for public health. The diagnosis of even one case of bovine spongiform encephalopathy, brucellosis, rabies, or tuberculosis in areas thought to be free of those conditions is cause for immediate action.

Influence of Disease on Productivity

The effects of disease on productivity can be direct (such as mastitis causing a profound reduction in milk yield) or indirect (reduced locomotor ability leading to reduced feed intake, thus causing reduced milk yield). Diseases occurring in early lactation can also cause cascading effects that ultimately lower productivity. For example, periparturient disorders often are seen as a complex, and cows diagnosed with parturient paresis are at increased risk of retained placenta, complicated ketosis, and mastitis. Cows with dystocia and retained placenta are at increased risk of metritis. The best documented direct effect is the effect of mastitis on milk yield. A single case of clinical mastitis can result in a milk yield loss of 300-400 kg/lactation with variations from negligible to 1,050 kg. Mastitis during early lactation is associated with higher losses (450-550 kg) compared with cases that are seen later. (*See also* MASTITIS IN CATTLE, p 1121.)

Several common diseases of dairy cattle may affect lactational milk yields. Milk fever, retained placenta, abortion, and other diseases can be detrimental to milk production. Metritis and ovarian cysts had a positive effect on concurrent milk production because of increased number of days of lactation. Increased and decreased milk yields have been associated with lesions in specific regions of the hoof. A tendency for increased lameness in high-yielding cows has been noted in some studies.

Losses resulting from subclinical disease are often considerable. The best described relationship between subclinical disease and productivity is the effect of subclinical mastitis on milk yield. Each 2-fold increase in SCC >50,000 cells/mL caused a loss of 0.4 and 0.6 kg milk/day in primiparous and multiparous cows, respectively. Total lactational milk yields were estimated to be reduced by 80 kg for primiparous cows and 120 kg for multiparous cows for each 2-fold increase in the geometric mean SCC >50,000 cells/mL. Other subclinical diseases (eg, paratuberculosis) have also been related to reduced productivity.

Diseases that delay or prohibit conception have a negative effect on herd productivity by prolonging the time that cows spend in lower-producing stages of lactation, by reducing the number of offspring for replacements or for sale, and by increasing the likelihood that the animal will be culled prematurely. Several diseases have been associated with decreased conception rates. The likelihood of conception was reduced by 14%, 15%, and 21% for cows that experienced retained placenta, metritis, or ovarian cysts, respectively. Mastitis, metritis, and ovarian cysts reduced the likelihood of cattle being bred for the first time. Postpartum diseases that prolong negative energy balance in early lactation probably also have a negative effect on reproductive performance through alterations in hormonal activities.

The effect of disease on longevity has been investigated. A large proportion of cow culling is considered involuntary (driven by disease, injury, or death) rather than for reasons of low production. The premature removal of a cow from the herd reduces lifetime milk yield. Reproductive failure and mastitis are consistently recorded as the top 2 reasons for culling.

THE HEALTH MANAGEMENT PROGRAM

The goal of health management programs is to ensure the optimal care and well-being of the dairy animals and to reduce losses in productivity caused by disease and management errors. The health management program is generally developed based on comparisons of herd performance with predetermined performance goals. The selection of herd performance goals should be considered carefully based on the farm environment, producer motivation, and presence of adequate resources (labor, capital, and information sources) to succeed. The structure of health management programs is generally unique to each farm but is minimally composed of scheduled herd visits that combine routine reproductive examinations, review of selected herd performance records, and decisions and actions related to specific herd management issues.

Performance Targets

Performance targets reflect herd standards of performance that are perceived as indicators of successful herd management. They are useful as comparison values for herd performance and as a starting point to initiate discussions about potential areas for improvement. To use a performance target, it is necessary for a herd to have a record system that allows for the generation of comparable herd indices. In many instances, performance targets have been calculated as arithmetic averages, which are useful indicators of herd performance when the contributing data (such as milk, fat, and protein yields) are normally distributed and have a reasonable degree of variation. However, many reproductive indices and values such as SCC are not distributed normally, and erroneous conclusions about herd performance may be made if averages alone are used to make management decisions. Appropriate frequency distributions are more useful for these types of data.

Key indicators for the performance targets should be defined. The monitoring system should specify the indices used, the animals included, and the time interval for reassessing progress made toward reaching each target. When data are available, it is probably useful to review some data (such as daily milk weights or dry matter intakes) more frequently than once a month, depending on the schedule of routine herd visits. Typical performance indicators include milk production, reproductive performance, milk quality, replacement management, cow removal, animal health, and special reports. Performance targets should be reviewed at appropriate intervals with realistic expectations regarding the amount of time it takes to effect change in an index. For example, management actions taken to reduce days to first calving would require ≥9-10 mo to become apparent. A more timely value such as age at conception would more rapidly reflect current management changes.

Record Keeping

A system of unique individual cow identification is a prerequisite for a successful health management program. The most common methods of animal identification are ear tags, collars, and branding. Increasingly, farms are using electronic identification through the use of transponders on ankle bands or neck straps. At a minimum, data must be recorded on birth, breeding, and calving dates and periodic milk yield. Under ideal circumstances, summarized data should be available for the nutritional program, disease occurrence, and financial performance.

Record analysis is a necessary component of the health management cycle. Most or all dairy herd improvement (DHI) systems allow for electronic access to performance data, and various computerized systems for herd management are used throughout the industry. Most monitoring systems can be characterized broadly as one the following: 1) manual (handwritten) card systems, 2) on-farm computer programs, 3) DHI, or 4) DHI and on-farm computer. Regardless of the type of system used, it should be easy to use and relevant to the day-to-day operations of the dairy. One important function of record systems is the generation of "action" lists (due to calve, due to dry, etc). This function is critical in large herds in which cattle are not individually known by the animal handlers and can be overlooked easily. Most systems also provide for a minimal level of herd analysis, such as the generation of timely performance reports for production, reproduction, and disease. Some programs can also generate statistics. The record-keeping system should allow the producer and veterinarian to understand and modify the formulas that are used to generate herd performance indices.

The veterinarian should ensure that collected data are used in a timely manner. Accurate data collection is most likely when the producer is using the data frequently and understands its value. The validity of data generated from both manual and automated data collection systems should be reviewed and critically assessed. Unusual results and deviations from normal performance targets should be challenged. The producer and the veterinarian should agree on defined actions that are based on the herd status and goals. Actions are generally diagnostic, preventive, or treatment oriented. Records are often used to generate action lists. Typical activities might include listing animals for routine herd fertility or illness examinations, selection of cows to obtain milk samples for culture, animals to vaccinate, animals to consider culling, animals to breed, animals to receive body condition scoring, or animals requiring treatments.

Scheduled Farm Visits

The frequency of scheduled veterinarian visits is variable and somewhat dependent on herd size. In herds of <100 cows, 1 or 2 cows calve every week and a single scheduled monthly visit is probably appropriate. These herds may have more unscheduled visits for examination of sick cows compared with herds that are visited more regularly. Larger herds in which cows are calving daily warrant more frequent visits, and weekly scheduled visits are not uncommon for herds of >200 cows. A developing trend on extremely large dairy farms (>2,000 cows) is employment of a staff veterinarian to oversee and direct day-to-day issues regarding health and performance. The frequency of scheduled herd visits for grass-based seasonal dairy operations varies depending on the herd's stage of lactation. More frequent visits are necessary in early lactation and during the breeding period.

Activities at herd visits fall into 4 general categories: provision of individual animal health care and emergency services, scheduled technical activities, scheduled analytic and training activities, and the provision of quality control programs. The frequency of individual activities varies.

Individual Health Care and Emergency Services: The examination and treatment of individual animals is an important activity during scheduled dairy visits. Frequent herd visits allow practitioners to examine cows early in the course of disease when the likelihood of successful treatment is higher. Routine visits also allow veterinarians to monitor the outcome of treatments and modify treatment protocols as needed. Ideally, monitoring programs include a system to detect cows that are not performing as expected. Special attention should be paid to the highest-risk cows, including frequent observation of animals during the periparturient period. Some farms have adopted a system that includes routine daily monitoring of body temperature and rumen activity of cows during the first 7 days after calving. Animals that fall outside of normal limits are treated according to predefined criteria or detained for examination by the herd veterinarian. All treatments administered to dairy cows should be recorded in treatment logs (either computerized or handwritten) to ensure adherence to proper meat and milk withholding periods. The frequency of unscheduled visits for emergency medical services usually diminishes in herds that have adopted a health and production management program.

Scheduled, Traditional, Technical Activities: Routine reproductive examinations account for much of the veterinarian's time during scheduled herd visits. Attaining reproductive success is an essential determinant of herd productivity. Reproductive programs are described in MANAGEMENT OF REPRODUCTION: CATTLE (p 1747). The end point of fertility examinations should be to generate data that can be used to determine the success or failure of breeding programs. The implementation, success, and cost-effectiveness of scheduled breeding programs should be reviewed frequently.

It is also common to monitor the effect of the nutritional program by recording body condition scores (BCS) for selected animals. BCS are a good indicator of how the delivered diet meets the energy needs of the cows. While the process of body condition scoring focuses attention on the nutritional adequacy of the diet, a mechanism of summarizing BCS for groups of animals is necessary for full use of the data.

On smaller farms, it is often customary for the veterinarian to perform routine individual animal treatments (such as IV injections), prophylactic activities (such as vaccinations), and some technical tasks (such as dehorning calves) during scheduled herd visits. It is appropriate for the veterinarian to perform these tasks because the farm staff may not perform them often enough to become technically proficient. On larger farms, these tasks may be performed on a daily basis, and animal handlers may become quite competent.

Scheduled Analytic and Training Activities: Conducting scheduled or unscheduled technical activities will not be effective unless there is a system that captures the results of the activities and allows for analysis and ongoing revision. The structure of the health and production management program must include time for the farmer and the herd veterinarian to analyze and discuss herd management issues. In herds that are dependent on hired personnel to implement designated tasks, time must be scheduled to effectively train personnel that are ultimately responsible for performing the programs. Development of standard operating procedures is one method to ensure that agreed-on practices are implemented.

Treatment protocols are used to define standard treatments for common diseases on dairy farms and should be used when multiple people have responsibility for administering antibiotic treatments to dairy cattle or when extra-label drug use is prescribed. They provide a mechanism for increased communication about treatment plans between the veterinarian and client and allow the farm to partially fulfill requirements for legal extra-label drug use.

The avoidance of residues in food products is a major responsibility of dairy practitioners. Increased scrutiny regarding antimicrobial use in food-producing animals has arisen because of concern about the development of antimicrobial resistance in foodborne pathogens. Although the level of detected antibiotic residues in meat and milk products is extremely low, antibiotic residues in bulk milk and carcasses are seen occasionally. In the USA, contamination of bulk milk is rare because of an effective surveillance system based on rapid testing for selected antimicrobial agents of every load of raw milk. Milk that is contaminated with antibiotics is discarded, and the producer is fined.

The requirements for extra-label drug use in the USA have been defined by regulatory officials under the Animal Medicinal Drug Use Clarification Act and should be closely followed. The American Association of Bovine Practitioners also has responded to societal and regulatory concerns about the use of antimicrobial agents by adopting recommendations for the prudent and judicious use of antimicrobial agents in dairy cattle.

Quality Control Programs: Quality control refers to activities that ensure consistency in performing key management processes. Vital management areas for most herds include nutritional management, milking management, and young-stock programs. Some farms may also develop quality control processes for environment and housing and farm-specific management of breeding bulls.

Some dairy practitioners function as the nutritional specialists for the dairy farms they serve. They may collect feed samples for nutrient analysis, formulate rations, and advise the farmer regarding crop and harvesting conditions. These veterinarians often devote a considerable amount of their professional time to nutritional management (p 1828). Other farms employ a professional nutritionist or use a nutritionist employed by a feed company or local cooperative to formulate the rations and submit feed samples for nutrient analysis. However, the veterinarian can ensure that the diet described on paper is adequately formulated and delivered to the cows. Assessing pasture conditions by periodic inspection of pasture is an important component of managing the nutritional program of herds that use management-intensive grazing. These quality control activities should be conducted routinely as part of the health and production management program.

Milking management should be a standard element of quality control programs. Tasks such as observation of the milking routine and scoring the condition of teats should be performed at least quarterly. A scheduled system of routine screening for mastitis pathogens can be implemented as part of the milking management program. The veterinarian can teach farm personnel how to perform the California Mastitis Test as part of a surveillance program. Animals routinely screened may include cows at dry off, fresh cows and heifers, and newly purchased cows. Milk samples can be collected and submitted for culture from quarters that show positive reactions.

Newborn calves and replacement heifers are often housed separately from lactating cows and may not be observed routinely by the herd veterinarian. However, routine surveillance of critical management issues such as adequate delivery of colostrum to calves and growth rates of replacement heifers can be done as part of scheduled herd visits.

The environment of dairy cattle can have considerable influence on health and productivity. Some veterinarians routinely schedule "walkabouts" through the housing areas to assess factors related to animal comfort and hygiene. Udder cleanliness, hoof and hock lesions, and respiratory disease are often determined by housing conditions. Herd walkabouts should include areas that are often ignored, such as dry-cow and heifer housing.

Investigations of Health and Production Problems

Even on the best managed farms, unexpected health and production problems arise. Surveillance programs incorporated in health and production management programs should detect problems early before considerable financial damage has occurred. Systems of investigating herd outbreaks have been described. Epidemiologic concepts of disease investigation are useful to identify risk factors and to stimulate corrective action.

HEALTH-MANAGEMENT INTERACTION: GOATS

Management of goats depends on the type (eg, dairy, pygmy, meat, mohair, or cashmere) and the reasons for which they are kept (eg, companionship or commercial enterprise). However, all are ruminants, and the basic principles of livestock husbandry are applicable. Dairy goats and pygmies usually are raised intensively, with most of the feed being brought to the animals. Meat goats and fiber goats mainly are raised extensively with most of the diet coming from browse and occasionally from high-quality pasture at times of highest nutritional need, such as the first 18 mo of life and the last 6 wk of gestation. A pregnant Angora doe without adequate energy and protein continues to grow mohair, even if stressed until she aborts.

Of all farm animals, goats have the strongest social hierarchy; thus, adequate feeder space should be provided so that the dominant animals cannot guard the feeders and prevent others from eating. The amount of floor space available per doe affects the amount of aggressive behavior. A goat can become so subordinated to its penmates that it does not eat and loses condition. This behavioral component must be considered in cases of wasting goats. To maximize longevity and to avoid fighting injuries, adult males should be fed and housed individually, especially during the breeding season when fighting increases.

Goats are adventurous and are natural climbers, and efforts to control them are necessary. The ultimate control would be high-tensile, electric fences; goats stand and push on other fences and can be very destructive. Hazards that might contribute to broken legs and strangulations should be removed. Tethering goats is potentially dangerous because they are vulnerable to dog attacks; also if 2 goats are chained too close to each other, frequently one will strangle. Goats chew on painted surfaces, and lead poisoning is a potential hazard in old barns. An efficient layout of pens, easy access to well-designed feeders, and effective control minimize management-related problems.

It is extremely difficult to keep goats' feet, urine, and feces out of many types of grain feeders, hay racks, and waterers. Goats often refuse to eat soiled feed or water, hay that has fallen on the floor, and grain contaminated with urine and feces of farm pets or vermin. Design of hay feeders is critical to reduce feed wastage. Most dairy and pygmy goats are bedded on wasted hay. Wet bedding contributes to development of coccidiosis in kids and staphylococcal impetigo on the udder, commonly but erroneously known as "goatpox." Under similar conditions, joint-ill and navel infections of the newborn are likely. In certain areas, kids are susceptible to white muscle disease (p 897), which can be controlled by injection of vitamin E/selenium to the pregnant doe and/or newborn and by selenium supplements in the diet.

Housing of goats affects disease patterns. Angoras in the south and west of the USA are usually given access to shelter only during severe storms or for a few weeks after the twice yearly shearing, without which they may die of cold weather stress. Goats in the northern USA are housed in the winter, perhaps more for the owners' comfort than for optimal health of the goats. Combinations of manure packs, overhead hay-mows, or un-insulated ceilings lead to dampness and ammonia buildup, especially if the barn is closed tightly. Warm, wet, poorly ventilated barns are conducive to development of neonatal navel infections, mastitis, enteritis, pneumonia, and coccidiosis. Caseous lymphadenitis (the disease known as "abscesses"), caused by *Corynebacterium pseudotuberculosis (ovis)*, spreads rapidly in closely confined goats (*see also* p 52). The slow-growing, non-painful lymph node abscesses eventually rupture and contaminate the feeders, walls, and other animals. The infection is spread by contact with the pus, and the organism can penetrate intact skin. Isolating affected goats, preferably culling them, and preventing environmental contamination is important. In Australia, a vaccine is available. Intensive management of adult dairy goats may promote horizontal transmission of the virus that causes caprine arthritis and encephalitis (CAE, p 598).

Mature bucks develop a powerful characteristic odor that is most intense in the breeding season, and personnel are reluctant to handle them. This often leads to neglect of feet and failure to recognize heavy parasite loads. The sebaceous glands on top of the head can be removed surgically at any age or can be cauterized at the time of disbudding; however, this does not render the buck totally odorless. Does are attracted by this smell and may refuse to be bred by a descented buck if there is an odoriferous one nearby; therefore, the glands should not be removed inadvertently at the time of disbudding if male kids are to be kept for breeding. The habit of urinating on the face, beard, and forelegs also contributes to buck odor and often leads to ulcerating sores in cold weather. During the breeding season, most bucks lose weight, although this is not necessarily due to breeding too many does. Many bucks lose weight when housed close to does in heat, even when breeding is not allowed. One management strategy is to ensure that bucks are in prime physical condition before the breeding season. The dominant male in a group of bucks is usually in much better condition than some of the others.

The genetically homozygous polled doe usually is anatomically an intersex and, therefore, infertile. Aberrations vary from a slightly enlarged clitoris visible only after puberty, to a buck-like conformation with a scrotum, penis (often shortened), and ovo-testes. Some phenotypically male pseudohermaphrodites show male libido with breeding activity. Because these animals are infertile, early recognition and culling is advisable. Some homozygous polled males may be capable of siring kids but are likely to develop sperm granulomas as they mature. Most owners reduce the incidence of homozygous polled animals by never mating 2 polled animals. While most intersex goats are polled, similar anatomic aberrations are seen occasionally in horned goats. These would most probably be chimeras (freemartins), the result of anastomoses developing in utero between males and females. Such chimeras in goats are rare (considering the high frequency of twins) when compared with cattle.

For foot care, *see* LAMENESS IN GOATS, p 893.

Perinatal Management

Common problems in does are extra teats, double teats, and fish-tail teats with double orifices. In cattle, extra teats can be removed with impunity, but in dairy goats there is often a functional milk gland behind the spare teat.

Newborn goats must be fed colostrum, and if CAE is a problem, heat treatment is essential for control. Later, kids can be fed (in decreasing order of desirability) goat's milk, goat-milk replacer, lamb-milk replacer, or cow's milk. Any fresh milk fed should be pasteurized or from stock known to be free of CAE virus, mycoplasmas, and paratuberculosis. Newborn goats should be fed at 10-12% of their body wt per day. On average, they are fed 1 pt (500 mL) of milk twice daily, but often they are overfed.

Kids should have access to hay and a grain-based creep feed as early as 1 wk of age. They can be weaned when they are readily eating a large handful of grain per day; this should be no later than 8 wk of age in dairy breeds and at 6 wk in others. Weaning is delayed in many goat operations because there is no commercial outlet for doe's milk other than to feed it to kids.

Dairy goats should be disbudded as soon as the kid has good muscle tone. For bucks of the Swiss breeds, it is important to disbud at 1-2 days of age to have the best chance of inhibiting horn growth or subsequent development of abnormal regrowth (scurs). Nubian doe kids have the least vigorous horn growth, and disbudding can be delayed until 2-3 wk of age. Hot-iron disbudding is the method of choice, using either a restraint box and nerve block, or general anesthesia such as xylazine (1-2 mg/kid). Excessive applications of the hot iron can lead to brain damage or subsequent death of the kids. Disbudding kids with caustic paste is not recommended.

Angora goats in range operations are not disbudded because the horns are thought to be helpful against predators, and because owners handle the goats by their horns. When goats are housed in winter, disbudding is advantageous; it reduces trauma and prevents accidents in which goats are trapped by their horns in feeders and fence lines. Pygmies can be disbudded according to the owner's preference; it is not a cause for disqualification or discrimination in the show ring in the USA. Dairy goats generally are disbudded, and horned animals usually are barred from the show ring in the USA. Tetanus can be seen after disbudding or castration and, as a precaution, antitoxin (150 U/kid) can be given.

Dairy goats and pygmy bucks are castrated in the first few weeks; Angoras are castrated later, after they have attained good horn growth. In males to be kept as pets, castration should be delayed to allow maximal urethral development, which reduces the likelihood of urolithiasis (p 1259). To improve their desirability as pets, these goats also should have the scent glands, located caudomedially to the horn base, removed along with the horns.

Nutrition

Dairy goats should be fed similarly to dairy cattle (*see also* p 1866 and p 1811). A good-quality hay, preferably alfalfa, should be the basis of the ration, and a 14-16% protein concentrate should be fed as a supplement during lactation. Silage is not a common dietary constituent because most goats are kept in small groups, which does not justify the equipment. A common problem is overfeeding grain to does in late lactation. Goats store fat preferentially in the abdominal cavity, and by the time fat is grossly obvious, the internal deposits are substantial; this can lead to problems at parturition and to pregnancy toxemia.

Loose trace mineral salt (TMS) should be fed rather than block salt; its composition varies with the area of the country (eg, iodine and selenium supplements are necessary in some regions of the USA). Goats are highly susceptible to copper deficiency and, unlike sheep, fairly resistant to copper toxicity. Therefore, cattle TMS, rather than sheep salt with no copper, should be offered. Goats raised for fiber may require supplementation of sulfur for proper fiber production.

Pet wethers fed on substantial amounts of grain are prone to develop urinary calculi. Reducing grain consumption, adding ammonium chloride to the diet, keeping the calcium:phosphorus ratio ~2:1, and keeping the magnesium level low helps. A urethrostomy helps such animals, but recurrences and urethral scarring necessitate euthanasia for many. To encourage water consumption, clean, loose TMS should be fed and fresh water offered twice daily. To increase water consumption, especially for high-yielding does, their water should be fresh and warm in winter, and fresh and cool in summer.

Common Diseases

Goat kids harbor several species of **coccidia**, but not all have clinical coccidiosis (p 163). Signs are diarrhea or pasty feces, loss of condition, general frailness, and failure to grow. In peracute cases, the goat may die with no signs. Rotating all the kids through 1 or 2 pens is dangerous; adult goats shed coccidia and infect the newborn. As infection pressure builds up in the pens, morbidity in kids born later is increased. To help prevent coccidiosis in artificially reared dairy goats, the kids should be put in small, age-matched groups in outside portable pens that are moved to clean ground periodically. Eradication is not feasible, but infection can be controlled through good management practices. Coccidiostats added to the water or feed are adjuncts to a management control program and not substitutes. Chronic coccidiosis is one of the main causes of poor growth in kids and is responsible for the uneconomical practice of delaying breeding for a year until the goat has reached adequate size (70 lb [32 kg] for dairy breeds). In Angora goats kept extensively, the problem is seen at weaning, when the kids are kept in smaller lots and fed supplement on the ground.

In pastured and free-ranging goats, **helminthiasis** can assume great clinical significance. GI nematodiasis, liver fluke infestation, and lungworm infections all may be seen. Age-related resistance to parasitism in goats is weak relative to other ruminants. Although most common in yearlings during their first season at pasture, clinical disease may be seen in adults as well. Poor growth, weight loss, diarrhea, a scruffy hair coat, signs of anemia, and intermandibular edema (bottle jaw) may be seen with GI parasitism or liver fluke disease. Persistent coughing in late summer and autumn is the usual presentation of lungworms; secondary bacterial pneumonia with fever is a common sequela. Parasitism is insidious on hobby farms where the problem may not exist for several years and then suddenly explodes as goat numbers continue to increase and pastures become overstocked. Tapeworm proglottids are often noted in goat feces by owners. Although tapeworms are not generally considered to be of clinical importance, their discovery can be used to review the subject of helminthiasis with owners and develop an overall parasite control program.

Clostridium perfringens type D can be fatal, and it is not always associated with the classic "change in quality and quantity of feed." In problem herds, vaccination every 4-6 mo may be necessary. Vaccination prevents the acute death syndrome, but occasionally even vaccinated goats may develop acute enteritis. Affected goats develop severe diarrhea and profound depression; milk yield drops abruptly. Death may result in 24 hr. Treatment involves fluid therapy, correction of acidosis, and antibiotics.

Vaccination for **contagious ecthyma** (soremouth, p 697) is not indicated unless the disease exists in the herd. The main problems with infected kids are difficulty in nursing, spreading lesions to the does' udders or the assistants' hands, and attendance at goat shows being disallowed. Live virus vaccine is used by scarifying the skin (eg, inside the thighs or under the tail) and painting on the vaccine. Both natural lesions and those resulting from vaccination may last as long as 4 wk, but after the scabs have dropped off, the goats can go to shows.

Culling is vital to the overall productivity of the herd. **Wasting disease** is seen quite frequently; it is not a single disease, but a syndrome. Generally, if a goat is well fed, kept in a stress-free environment, and has good teeth and a low parasite load, it should thrive and produce. If it does not, and begins "wasting," it should be culled immediately. The major causes of wasting disease, in addition to poor nutrition, parasitism, and dental problems, are paratuberculosis, internal visceral abscesses due to *Corynebacterium pseudotuberculosis (ovis)* or *Arcanobacterium (Corynebacterium) pyogenes*, locomotor problems (particularly arthritis due to retrovirus infection [CAE virus]), and any chronic hidden infections (eg, metritis, peritonitis, or pneumonia). Tumors are rarely seen. None of these diseases is treatable, and many are contagious; this is the basis for the strict culling policy. **Paratuberculosis** in goats differs from that in cattle (p 612) in that there is no profuse diarrhea, and gross postmortem lesions are less pronounced. Consequently, many cases may go undiagnosed at necropsy. The ileocecal node is the most rewarding tissue for bacteriologic culture and histopathology. Agar gel immunodiffusion is a useful serologic test, but it can be used only on a herd basis for test and cull. Availability is limited, and it will not function as a prepurchase screening test. Use of ELISA for diagnosis of caprine paratuberculosis is increasing. The control program for paratuberculosis in goats is similar to that in cattle.

Caprine arthritis and encephalitis (CAE, p 598) virus has emerged as an important infectious agent of intensively raised dairy goats. The prevalence of the infection in nondairy goats is comparatively low and less clinically important. CAE infection in goats can manifest in numerous ways: subclinical, persistent infection; a progressive paresis of young goats 2-12 mo old; agalactia with a firm, noninflamed udder at parturition in bred females; and an arthritic condition with pain and swollen joints in adults. A chronic, progressive interstitial pneumonia or a wasting syndrome may also be seen in adults. CAE infection has been considered primarily to be spread from dam to offspring through virus-laden colostrum and milk, and control programs have been aimed at feeding of heat-treated colostrum and pasteurized milk. However, even in herds in which this is practiced, infection may persist. There is increasing epidemiologic evidence that horizontal transmission between adults is important in the spread of the disease. Regular testing and rigorous culling of all seropositive goats must be practiced if disease eradication is the goal.

For mastitis in goats, *see* p 1129.

HEALTH-MANAGEMENT INTERACTION: HORSES

Proper management can reduce the incidence of many disease conditions in horses. Informed management of the environment and diet, routine foot and dental care, and adherence to an appropriate deworming and vaccination program form the basis of a preventive health program. Client education is important for compliance. Owners are more likely to follow recommended changes in husbandry programs once they appreciate the advantages: diet manipulation reduces the incidence of certain types of colic and exercise-induced myopathies, good dental care improves feed utilization, minimizing exposure to barn dusts and molds reduces the risk of chronic obstructive pulmonary disease, and individually designed deworming and vaccination programs reduce morbidity and mortality rates due to parasitism and infectious disease.

Housing: Stabled horses are exposed to numerous respiratory and GI pathogens, including viruses, bacteria, mold spores, dust mites, and parasites. Stable environments affect disease transmission in terms of air quality and ventilation, population density, and general cleanliness. Barns should be constructed to optimize ventilation and light, minimize exposure to dust and molds, provide temperature regulation, facilitate cleaning and disinfection, and provide ample space for each horse. Windows and skylights provide sunlight and natural ventilation. Sunlight is a potent killer of many bacteria and viruses; it also promotes coat shedding and regular estrous cycles. Eight air changes per hour is considered adequate ventilation for temperate climates and average humidity. (*See also* VENTILATION, p 1699.) Ceiling or wall-mounted fans can be used to increase air circulation on hot humid days. Stall doors that are open at the top or made of heavy mesh screening provide better ventilation. Stalls should have nonslip flooring and walls or partitions that prevent direct contact between horses in adjacent stalls. Suggested stall dimensions for adult horses and mares with foals are 3.6 × 3.6 m and 5.0 × 5.0 m, respectively. Doorways should be at least 2.4 m high × 1.2 m wide.

Recurrent airway obstruction (chronic obstructive pulmonary disease, p 1213) is associated with airway hypersensitivity to environmental allergens and irritants. The most commonly incriminated allergens are fungal spores and pollens. The population of spores increases with the dustiness of the barn, bedding, and forage. Management changes that help prevent this condition include substituting wood chips, peat moss, or shredded paper for dusty straw bedding; avoiding dusty concentrates; using shallow rather than deep feed containers; and soaking hay before feeding at ground level. Air quality can be improved further if bedding and feed are not stored above the stalls. Riding areas and the dust they generate should be situated away from stalls to reduce exposure to dust.

Regular disinfection of stables and feed and water buckets helps reduce persistence of infectious agents in the environment. Organic debris inactivates most chemical disinfectants; therefore, disinfection should begin with physical cleaning (ie, hosing, scrubbing) of all surfaces followed by chemical disinfection. Phenols, quaternary ammonium compounds, and chlorine are the most commonly used disinfectants. To further reduce spread of infectious disease, stalls should have walls or partitions to prevent direct contact between horses in adjacent stalls. Pregnant mares, mares with foals, and weanlings should be kept separate from yearlings and adult horses. Ideally, new arrivals should be isolated from the resident horse population for 30 days to reduce introduction of contagious diseases, including respiratory viruses and bacterial infections (eg, influenza, rhinopneumonitis, and *Streptococcus equi*).

Feeds should be stored in dry containers to reduce contamination with molds and animal excreta. Moldy hay and silage feeding have been associated with cases of equine botulism. Opossum feces can transmit infective sporocysts of *Sarcocystis neurona*, the causative agent of equine protozoal myeloencephalitis (p 1031). Contamination of feeds by deer urine has been incriminated in the spread of certain strains of *Leptospira* (p 525).

Pasture: Ensuring that horses have ample time on good quality pasture provides optimal ventilation, a source of good forage, and the opportunity to graze and exercise. Exercise improves condition, prevents boredom-related abnormal behaviors (eg, cribbing and weaving), and reduces the risk of large-intestinal impactions. Grazing also helps reduce the incidence of gastric ulcers. Reducing the time spent in poorly ventilated barns reduces exposure to many inhalant allergens incriminated in the development of recurrent airway obstruction. Access to good forage provides a natural source of vitamins and fiber. If horses are fed in groups, sufficient space should be allowed to minimize competition and to ensure even the most submissive horse has access to an adequate diet. Feeding hay and grain in elevated feeders off the ground reduces ingestion of sand, infective parasite eggs, and animal excreta.

Safe, durable fencing should be used for pastures and paddocks to reduce the risk of self-trauma. Double fencing between paddocks minimizes transmission of contagious disease between horses. Overcrowding should be avoided. Overgrazed pastures, which result from overstocking, lead to extremes in ground conditions (eg, dust or mud), contribute to increased parasite burdens, and favor overgrowth of potentially toxic plants. Excessive dust increases the risk of respiratory infections among young horses by inhalation of soil saprophytes, such as *Rhodococcus equi* (p 1209). The risk of this potentially fatal bacterial pneumonia on farms where the disease is enzootic can be reduced by minimizing exposure of young (<4 mo old), susceptible foals to aerosolized *R equi* using environmental control strategies such as decreasing dust formation on pastures and paddocks, housing foals in well-ventilated areas, rotating pastures, reducing the size of mare-foal bands, irrigating and planting dirt areas with grass, and removing feces frequently from stalls, paddocks, indoor arenas, and pastures. Breeding mares earlier in the season to ensure foaling during colder weather may reduce the number of susceptible foals exposed to dry, dusty summer conditions. On farms where *R equi* is endemic and foal morbidity and mortality rates are high despite attempts at pasture management, the incidence of disease can be reduced with preventive administration of one dose of hyperimmune plasma containing high concentrations of antibodies against *R equi* to newborn foals within the first week of life followed by a second dose 25 days later.

Overstocking in barns and pastures favors outbreaks of other contagious respiratory infections caused by viral and bacterial pathogens spread between horses via aerosolization of respiratory tract secretions. Enteric infections with *Clostridium difficile* and *C perfringens* can become endemic on some farms. An increased incidence of *Clostridium* diarrhea in newborn foals has been associated with foaling on dirt, gravel, or sand surfaces, and stall confinement or limited turnout on dry lots during the first 3 days of life.

Whenever possible, horses should not be pastured on sandy soils because sand ingestion during grazing predisposes to colonic and rectal impaction, chronic diarrhea, and weight loss. If sandy pastures are unavoidable, the risk of sand colic can be reduced by feeding psyllium and by providing trace mineralized salt with equal parts of bone meal.

Horses grazing on pastures near water may be at increased risk of contracting certain diseases such as Potomac horse fever, caused by *Ehrlichia risticii* and disseminated by aquatic insects and snails (p 236). Pastures should be kept free of standing or stagnant water to reduce the breeding grounds for mosquitos carrying West Nile virus, another equine pathogen (p 1077).

Nutrition: Diet plays a role in the health of the horse from birth through old age and is an often overlooked method of disease control. (*See also* NUTRITION: HORSES, p 1872.) In young horses, developmental orthopedic disease (p 929) is the result of rapid growth, trauma to articular cartilage or growth plates, genetic predisposition, and nutritional imbalances. Dietary management involves regulating energy intake to avoid excessive rates of growth and weight gain. The proper balance of protein, calcium, phosphorus, zinc, and copper is important in supporting healthy endochondral ossification and in stabilizing bone collagen and elastin synthesis. The amount of nutrients required in the diet for normal bone development are dictated by rate of growth. Excessive energy intake contributes to osteochondrosis by decreasing bone density and cortical thickness.

Deficiency of protein must be severe to interfere with endochondral ossification. Rapidly increasing protein intake may produce faster bone growth; however, if the diet lacks adequate minerals to support this increased growth, altered endochondral ossification can be seen. Calcium and phosphorus balance affect bone density, rate of growth, and cartilage thickness. Inadequate amounts of copper and zinc have been associated with an increased incidence of osteochondrosis and osteodysgenesis.

Some of the most common mistakes made when feeding young horses include feeding excessive grain and leafy legumes (eg, alfalfa, which results in too high an energy intake), feeding a diet with too little zinc or copper to support rate of growth, and feeding a diet with an improper calcium:phosphorus ratio. Cereal grains and grass forages are low in calcium, phosphorus, protein, and lysine. Excess energy from cereal grains may be more detrimental than excess energy from grass forages; one reason may be that energy from grain is derived from starch, whereas energy from grass forage comes from microbial production of volatile fatty acids. Starch, but not volatile fatty acids, stimulates insulin secretion, which has been implicated in stimulating hormone changes that contribute to ostechondrosis. Older horses often have dental problems that compromise feed intake and mastication. Extruded or soft pelleted feeds are ideal. Hay should be good quality, leafy, and easy to chew.

Diet manipulation can help treat, control, and prevent other disease conditions. Horses with recurrent airway obstruction should be fed as dust-free a feed as possible. Adding water or oil to grains decreases dust. Hay should be thoroughly soaked and fed close to the ground. If complete pelleted feeds are fed, hay can be removed completely from the diet. On sandy soils, hay should be fed off the ground to reduce sand ingestion. Dietary management can be used to reduce the risk of gastric ulcers. Alfalfa hay, with its high calcium and protein concentration, acts as a buffering antacid and has a protective effect on the nonglandular squamous mucosa. Small hay meals fed frequently or access to pasture also reduces the risk of gastric ulceration.

Nutritional management for Quarter Horses with hyperkalemic periodic paralysis is focused on decreasing dietary intake of potassium and increasing renal potassium losses. Dietary manipulation includes avoiding high potassium feeds such as alfalfa hay, brome grass, canola oil, soybean meal or oil, and sugar or beet molasses and replacing them with timothy or bermuda grass, beet pulp, and grains such as oats, corn, wheat, or barley. Affected horses should be exercised regularly and have access to pasture.

Heavily muscled breeds of horses including Quarter Horses, draft horses, and warmbloods are prone to myopathies associated with elevated muscle glycogen stores and polysaccharide storage inclusions in type II muscle fibers. Successful management of this condition, known as polysaccharide storage myopathy, focuses on increasing the fat content of the diet and on eliminating or reducing grain intake.

Stall confinement, poor-quality or high-fiber feed, inadequate water intake, and ingestion of foreign material (eg, rubber fencing) predispose to intestinal impaction. Management practices to reduce the risk of impaction include ad lib access to fresh water (warm water may be preferred during cold weather), adequate exercise, good quality feed, and good dental care. If impaction has been a problem, poorly digestible feeds (eg, mature forages) should be placed with low-fiber, highly digestible forages (eg, growing grass or legume hays). A complete pelleted or extruded feed helps maintain soft feces.

Foot Care: Proper foot care is essential. Corrective trimming and shoeing maintains proper foot balance and helps reduce the risk of laminitis, thrush, white line disease, and hoof cracks. In young foals and weanlings, feet should be examined and trimmed regularly to ensure a proper weight-bearing axis. A balanced foot in a young horse minimizes the risk of angular limb deformities. (*See also* LAMENESS IN HORSES, p 897.)

Dental Care: Routine dental care reduces the incidence of dental disease. Sharp teeth and uneven dental wear predispose to tongue and cheek lacerations, poorly masticated feed, decreased feed intake, choke, and weight loss, and may contribute to mouth pain when the horse is bridled. Frequent dental examination allows early detection of tooth root abcessation before more serious complications (eg, sinusitis) develop. (*See also* DENTISTRY IN LARGE ANIMALS, p 140.)

Parasite Control: Parasites and the damage they cause to the intestinal vasculature and mucosa contribute to GI disturbances, including impactions, motility disorders, diarrhea, and peritonitis. Migrating ascarids contribute to pulmonary inflammation in foals. The principal internal parasites of horses are nematodes. With the advent of more effective anthelmintics, the nematode species of importance have shifted from large strongyles to cyathostomes. There is no single parasite control program that is ideal for all horses. Age of the horse, population density, and pasture size and quality can affect choice of programs. As horses age, they develop resistance to reinfection with certain parasites, such as *Strongyloides westeri* and *Parascaris equorum*. Resistance to other strongyles is incomplete.

The 3 major classes of anthelmintics commonly used are avermectins and milbemycins, benzimidazoles, and pyrimidines. Avermectins have a broad range of activity, are effective at low dosages, suppress fecal egg counts for long periods of time, and are active against adult and migrating larval nematodes and various ectoparasites including lice, mites, ticks, and bots (eg, *Gasterophilus* spp). Treatment of mares with ivermectin within 24 hr of foaling greatly reduces transmission of *S westeri* to foals via the dam's milk. Prompt deworming of the mare soon after delivery minimizes the newborn foal's potential exposure to parasite ova in the mare's manure as a result of coprophagy. Due to their efficacy against adult and migrating roundworms, avermectins should be included in the foal's anthelmintic schedule. Avermectins are not effective against tapeworms (*Anaplocephala*), *Onchocerca* adults, flukes, or encysted cyathostome larvae. Milbemycins are effective against encysted cyathostome larvae. Benzimidazoles are effective against most nematodes; however, cyathostomes have developed resistance to this class of anthelmintic. Increased dosages of this drug class are required to kill migrating immature large strongyles and encysted cyathostomes. The pyrimidines have reasonable efficacy against nematodes and good activity against tapeworms when used at increased dosages. A new combination anthelmintic, praziquantel/ivermectin, has demonstrated excellent efficacy against field strains of equine cestodes (ie, tapeworms) in addition to most nematodes. An effective deworming protocol for horses should incorporate ivermectin/praziquantel or a double dose of pyrantel pamoate during the fall to remove tapeworms and a larvicidal dose of anthelmintic (eg, 10 mg/kg fenbendazole, PO, SID for 5 days, or a single dose of moxidectin) during the winter months to remove encysted cyathostome larvae. (*See also* GASTROINTESTINAL PARASITES OF HORSES, p 265.)

Vaccination Program: The goal of vaccination is to develop and maintain both individual and herd immunity against infectious diseases. Commercial vaccines are available for rabies, encephalomyelitis (Eastern, Western, and Venezuelan), tetanus, influenza, equine herpesviruses 1 and 4, botulism, equine ehrlichiosis (Potomac horse fever), equine viral arteritis, rotavirus, West Nile virus, equine protozoal myelitis, and *Streptococcus equi* (strangles). Vaccination programs are formulated based on the animal's age, use, and level of exposure. Broodmare vaccination is important to provide active immunity for the mare and passive immunity for the foal via transfer of colostral antibodies. Vaccination guidelines for foals have been modified due to the interference of maternal antibodies with the initial vaccination response. In most instances, the primary vaccination series includes 3 doses.

The following vaccination recommendations assume that foals are born to vaccinated mares and have absorbed adequate colostral antibodies with IgG levels >800 mg/dL.

Tetanus: Recommended for all foals and horses. Initial vaccination at 6 mo of age, with a 3-dose series at 4- to 6-wk intervals, followed by annual boosters. Broodmares should receive a booster 4-6 wk before foaling. A horse with an unknown vaccination status that sustains an injury should receive a dose of tetanus antitoxin along with a dose of tetanus toxoid. A second dose of toxoid should be given 4 wk later.

Rhinopneumonitis (Equine Herpesvirus 1 and 4): Recommended for all foals and horses. Initial vaccination begins at 5 mo of age followed by 2 more doses at 4- to 6-wk intervals. Young horses are most susceptible and should be vaccinated at 3- to 4-mo intervals. Pregnant mares are vaccinated against EHV-1 during months 3, 5, 7, and 9 of gestation and 4-6 wk before foaling.

Encephalomyelitis (Eastern and Western): Recommended for all foals and horses. Initial vaccination between 4 and 5 mo of age (3-4 mo of age in highly endemic areas), with a 3-dose series at 4- to 6-wk intervals, followed by semiannual boosters. Broodmares should receive a booster 4-6 wk before foaling.

Influenza: Recommended for all foals and horses. Due to the persistence of maternally derived antibodies, initial vaccination using the IM vaccine should begin at 9-10 mo of age followed by 2 additional doses given at 4-wk intervals. If the intranasal vaccine is used, a single dose can be administered at 9 mo of age. Pregnant mares should receive an annual IM booster 4-6 wk before foaling. If the mare was not vaccinated during the last trimester of her pregnancy, then the 3-dose vaccination series for her foal can begin as early as 5 mo of age, with subsequent doses given at 4- to 6-wk intervals. Young performance horses should be vaccinated every 3-4 mo. Adult horses are usually vaccinated annually.

Rabies: Recommended for foals and horses in areas where rabies is prevalent. Vaccination of all horses should be encouraged. Initial vaccination should begin at 6 mo of age, followed by a second dose at 7 mo and a booster at 1 yr of age, followed by annual boosters. Broodmares can receive a booster before breeding or 4-6 wk before foaling.

Potomac Horse Fever: Vaccination is suggested in areas where the disease is endemic. Initial vaccination can begin at 5-6 mo of age, followed by a second dose in 3-4 wk and a booster at 1 yr of age. Annual boosters in the spring are recommended. Pregnant mares should receive a booster before foaling.

West Nile Virus: Vaccination of all foals and horses in the continental USA is recommended. Initial vaccination can begin at 5 mo of age followed by a second dose in 4 wk. A booster should be administered in late summer for fcals born early in the year. Pregnant mares should receive a booster 4-6 wk before foaling.

Botulism: Vaccination is recommended for horses in the mid-Atlantic states and other regions of the USA where the disease is common. Initial vaccination involves a series of 3 doses administered at 4-wk intervals followed by annual boosters. Foals from vaccinated mares can begin their primary vaccination series at 5 mo of age. Broodmares that have never been vaccinated should receive an initial series of 3 doses administered at 4-wk intervals during the last trimester, followed by annual boosters administered 4-6 wk before foaling.

Strangles: Use of this vaccine is restricted to farms where strangles is endemic. Initial immunization with the IM vaccine involves a 3-dose series administered 4 wk apart beginning at 5 mo of age. If the intranasal vaccine is used, vaccination can begin at 11 mo of age with a second dose given at 12 mo and annual boosters thereafter. Broodmares on endemic farms should receive an annual booster 4-6 wk before foaling.

Rotavirus: On farms where foal rotaviral diarrhea is a problem, pregnant mares should be given a 3-dose series at 3- to 4-wk intervals, during the last trimester of pregnancy. Foals obtain passive immunity through absorption of colostral antibodies.

Foals with failure of passive antibody transfer (ie, IgG levels <200 mg/dL) and/or foals born to unvaccinated mares can receive their initial vaccination for equine herpesvirus 1 and 4, tetanus, and Eastern and Western equine encephalomyelitis in a 3-dose series beginning at 3-4 mo of age. These foals can receive their first dose of rabies vaccine at 3 mo of age, followed by a booster at 12 mo. Influenza vaccination can be started at 9 mo of age. Foals born to mares that have never been exposed to or vaccinated against West Nile virus can receive their first vaccination at 3 mo of age.

Perinatal Mare and Foal Care: During the last trimester, pregnant mares should be on a slowly rising plane of nutrition that includes a concentrate containing at least 12-14% protein. The diet should be balanced in calcium, phosphorus, copper, and zinc. During the immediate prepartum period, bran or psyllium can be added to the diet as a laxative to keep feces soft and to reduce the risk of postpartum impactions.

In addition to routine deworming throughout pregnancy, mares should be dewormed within 24-48 hr of parturition to reduce the foal's exposure to parasite ova. Mares should receive annual booster vaccinations 4-6 wk prepartum to improve colostral quality. In addition to producing antibodies in response to vaccination, mares produce antibodies to pathogens indigenous to their environment. Because colostrum is produced during the last 3-5 wk of pregnancy, mares should not be moved to new premises during the immediate prepartum period, and mares and foals should remain in the foaling environment during the early postnatal period.

Prior to parturition, the mare's udder and perineum should be cleaned and fresh bedding added to the stall to optimize the hygiene of the foaling environment and reduce the neonate's exposure to bacterial pathogens. Ideally, the flooring in the foaling stall should be easy to disinfect. Immediately after birth, the foal's umbilicus should be dipped with either 2% iodine or chlorhexidine disinfectant to decrease the risk of ascending umbilical remnant infection and septicemia. A gravity enema is often administered prophylactically to stimulate meconium passage and reduce the likelihood of meconium impaction. Early colostrum ingestion is essential to ensure adequate absorption of colostral antibodies and to stimulate early gut closure and reduce uptake of potentially pathogenic bacteria via translocation across the intestinal mucosa. (*See also* MANAGEMENT OF THE NEONATE, p 1683.)

Foals are born virtually without gamma globulins and rely on passive immunity through absorption of colostral antibodies for protection against common equine infectious diseases during the first 4-8 wk of life. Intestinal absorption of colostral antibodies is optimal during the first 10 hr of life and ceases after 24 hr. A newborn foal's serum IgG concentration should be >800 mg/dL after colostrum ingestion. Foals with <400 mg/dL of serum IgG should be supplemented with additional colostrum if <18-20 hr old, or given a plasma transfusion if >20 hr old or if compromised GI function is suspected.

In general, foaling mares should be kept in an environment where they can be monitored frequently both before and after foaling. Attended foalings are mandatory to help avoid foal loss due to correctable periparturient problems (eg, dystocia, failure to rupture fetal membranes normally, and maternal rejection or aggression).

See also FEEDING THE ORPHAN FOAL, p 1888.

HEALTH-MANAGEMENT INTERACTION: PIGS

Proper management can increase reproductive performance and feed utilization and decrease mortality. Disease in farm animals is often the result of inadequate management, allowing for proliferation of commensal microflora or the introduction of a pathogen (eg, porcine reproductive and respiratory syndrome virus, PRRSV) to the population. Properly managing the interaction between pigs, people, and the environment has a positive effect on controlling the level of commensal organisms within the population, disease expression, and productivity of the herd. In many cases, clinical disease is merely the indicator of failure in one or more of these interactions. Treatment of disease through chemotherapy is a first step in disease control, but elimination of the underlying environmental or management problem is the most important one.

When large numbers of pigs are housed together, pig-to-pig and pig-to-environment interactions are enhanced, and manager-to-pig interaction is diminished. These are the bases of disease problems on intensive swine farms, and an understanding of their consequences is necessary to reduce health-related losses in modern pig enterprises.

On poorly managed farms, ~30% of pigs born alive do not survive to market weight. For example, ~15% die before weaning, 10% in the nursery, and 5% during the grower-finisher stages of production.

Survival of neonatal piglets during the first 7 days depends on 3 major factors: 1) adequate intake of energy, 2) suitable environmental temperature, and 3) passive transfer of immunity from the sow. Because piglets are born with limited glycogen reserves, they need to replace and add to their energy reserves within hours of birth. If energy (colostrum) is not acquired, mortality due to hypoglycemia follows. Hypoglycemia (p 1686) probably is the most common cause of piglet death. Several management procedures may reduce these starvation losses. For example, equalizing piglet weights within litters by cross-fostering in the first few hours of life eliminates or markedly reduces losses and can have a dramatic effect on overall mortality rates. Another important management factor is proper thermoregulation of the lactation area. During lactation, piglets are sensitive to low environmental temperatures, and should be born and maintained for 1 wk in environmental temperatures of 86-93°F (30-34°C).

In addition to its vital role in supplying energy, colostrum supplies piglets with antibodies to protect them against common infections. The most common fatal infection is intestinal colibacillosis; losses can be reduced by vaccinating the sow, which provides antibodies to the piglets via the colostrum and, especially against gut diseases, via the milk.

Any sow disease that results in decreased milk production increases susceptibility to *Escherichia coli* diarrhea, as does low environmental temperature, which slows gut motility. (*See also* POSTPARTUM DYSGALACTIA SYNDROME, p 1134, and MASTITIS, p 1120.) Slower passing of milk and its antibodies through the intestines enables *E coli* to adhere more readily to the intestinal wall and then produce enterotoxins that cause excess secretion of the intestinal cells and diarrhea.

Significant numbers of piglets die from crushing in the first few days after birth. The sow is likely to lie on piglets if she is clumsy, if the warmest spot in the farrowing pen is next to her, or if the piglets are hypoglycemic and sleepy. Suitably designed farrowing crates and correctly placed heat lamps can minimize losses from crushing, although they are unlikely to completely eliminate them.

Careful attention to these management factors usually reduces neonatal mortality to 5-10%. Even in extensive systems, at least some of the neonatal pig mortality is due to management and, to this extent, avoidable.

In today's swine industry, no agent has affected performance of nursery pigs more than PRRSV (p 581). Following introduction of the virus to the nursery through the entry of infected pigs at weaning, PRRSV circulates from room to room; older infected pigs become the source of virus for newly weaned piglets following loss of maternal immunity at 4-6 wk of age. Endemic PRRSV in the nursery has significantly reduced growth rate and increased mortality, feed conversion ratio, and vaccination and medication costs. However, management strategies such as partial depopulation and vaccination have been very effective at reducing the severity of the disease.

In farms that are free of PRRSV, fewer pigs die (2-3% nursery mortality is considered acceptable on a commercial basis). In the absence of PRRSV, the major infectious disease is diarrhea, but starvation and inadequate growth are also problems. Weaning is a particularly stressful period due to changes in diet and surroundings and often in social order. Generally, the earlier the weaning, the more important management becomes. At weaning, piglets should have enough trough space to allow them all to eat at the same time. The inclusion of feeding boards for the first 5-7 days after weaning enhances feeder space and promotes group feeding. Piglets should have ready and continuous access to acidified water but should be fed small amounts of feed frequently (3-5 times a day) for the first week after weaning. The quality of the feed enhances intake, and diets that are fortified with plasma protein and milk products are required. Environmental temperature is also critical—pigs maintained in suboptimal temperatures frequently succumb to diarrheal disease. Depending on the age of pigs to be weaned, environmental temperatures should be maintained at 77-80°F (25-27°C). Size at weaning is as important as age; small pigs are more likely to starve or have diarrhea. Oral fluid therapy is a good adjunct to antibiotics in the prevention and treatment of postweaning diarrhea.

Finally, due to the warm nursery environment, skin diseases such as exudative dermatitis (greasy pig disease) may be more prevalent, secondary to high humidity. *Streptococcus suis* and *Haemophilus parasuis* infections also develop in intensively maintained, recently weaned pigs.

Regarding the growing-finishing area, allowing for sufficient pen space is important to reduce crowding, stress, and pathogen transmission. Space recommendations for growing pigs are based on a report by the Nutrition Council of the American Feed Industry Association (TABLE 1). When maintained on slatted floors, each growing-finishing pig should be provided 4-6 sq ft of floor space from 50-125 lb, and 8 sq ft from 125-240 lb body wt. Pigs carried to heavier weights (eg, 270 lb) may be more efficient if allowed 10 sq ft, but that recommendation is difficult to justify economically.

The greatest economic losses due to inadequate management are seen in the grower-finisher stage of production. Respiratory diseases (such as *Actinobacillus* pleuropneumonia, enzootic pneumonia, and porcine respiratory and reproductive syndrome) and intestinal diseases (such as ileitis) significantly reduce growth rate and efficiency of feed utilization.

The most significant management technologies recently adapted in the nursery and grow-finish areas are "all-in/all-out" animal flow and segregated early weaning. All-in/all-out production systems greatly enhance grower-finisher productivity and disease control and can be adapted to room, building, or site. Segregated early weaning consists of segregation of the weaned pig from the sow at an early age (14-16 days). The principle behind this production system is simple. Most infections early in life are derived from sows during lactation. If each week's production of weaners is isolated from the sow, the chance of infection spreading to each batch of new pigs is reduced. Nursing pigs are protected, to some extent, from infections carried by their dams through colostral antibodies. Weaning at an early age, before the colostral antibodies have been lost, reduces the chance of the piglets being infected from their dams. Advanced systems combine segregated early weaning with all-in/all-out animal flow to prevent the transmission of pathogens from older, previously infected pigs to younger, more susceptible pigs. Finally, combining segregated early weaning with all-in/all-out animal flow and housing the sow herd, nurseries, and growing-finishing population on separate sites forms the basis for multisite production.

Together, these technologies represent a major development in production and disease control. They are not, however, completely foolproof. In some cases, they may merely delay the development of clinical disease to a later age group, particularly *S suis* and *H parasuis* infections. But in most herds, practicing this form of continuous depopulation and repopulation has notably improved productivity and disease control.

Finally, proper biosecurity is essential to protect the health and productivity of the farm. Selecting a breeding stock source that is free of PRRSV, *Actinobacillus* pleuropneumonia, *Brachyspira hyodysenteriae*, transmissible gastroenteritis virus, and sarcoptic

TABLE 1. Space Needs of Growing-Finishing Pigs

	Weaning to 75 lb (<34 kg)	75-125 lb (34-57 kg)	125 lb to Market Size (>57 kg)
Sleeping space or shelter per pig (square feet)	4	5-6	8
Pigs per linear foot of self-feeder space (or per hole)			
On dry lot	4	3	3
On pasture	4-5	3-4	3-4
Percent of feeder space for protein supplement			
On dry lot	25	20	15
On pasture	20-25	15-20	10-15
For hand-feeding or hand-watering, running feet of trough per pig (access from one side)	3/4	1	1/4

mange is critical. Following purchase, animals should be quarantined and tested prior to entry. Protocols should be in place to limit visitors, control rodents, and ensure the safe introduction of personnel (shower in/shower out) and shipments (fumigation rooms). Finally, a site and protocol for cleaning and disinfecting transport vehicles is necessary, particularly in multi-site systems that rely on frequent movement of pigs across the country. (*See also* BIOSECURITY, p 1679.)

HEALTH-MANAGEMENT INTERACTION: SHEEP

The major products from sheep are meat, wool, and hides; sheep milk is important in some areas of the world. Sheep are raised in many different environments, with great variation in efficiency. The type of production system in any area depends on many factors, primarily the availability and cost of pasture, the climate, and the interaction with other livestock and cropping systems.

Different areas of the world use different production systems. Extensive year-round grazing, with large flocks (>2,000 sheep) and minimal sheep handling, is the typical system of sheep management in the major wool-producing nations of Australia, New Zealand, South Africa, and parts of South America and the USA. Confinement and intensive feeding during the winter months, with access to pasture for the rest of the year, is the common system of sheep management in Europe and most of the USA. Close confinement in feedlots in the final growth stage of lambs for meat is virtually restricted to North America. Shepherding small flocks of sheep and goats along roadsides and common grazing areas is a typical management system in the Middle East and in Asia.

Extensive Grazing Systems: Economics are an essential consideration. In addition to animal welfare and public health considerations, veterinary services should aim to increase net farm income rather than just control disease. Although the diagnosis, treatment, and control of disease, including the investigation of outbreaks to solve a disease problem, are important on most farms, outbreaks of clinical disease are of minor importance to longterm profitability. Advice that is technically sound from a disease control perspective may be detrimental to the overall economic well-being of the farm. For example, a reduced stocking rate may mean better nutrition for the flock, fewer lamb mortalities, and lower burdens of GI parasites, but a significantly lower net farm income. Net income per hectare is generally very sensitive to changes in stocking rate.

A better approach involves a "flock health" program. These are designed to anticipate health and production problems and, when it is economic to do so, to implement appropriate prevention measures. A flock health program must be tailored to the needs of the specific farm. For most farms, key areas of flock health programs include: 1) controlling internal and external parasites; 2) preventing diseases for which there is a cost-effective vaccination program; 3) preventing the introduction of contagious diseases, such as footrot, brucellosis, and external parasites; and 4) improving the number of lambs weaned per ewe bred, with enhanced ewe and ram fertility and reduced lamb mortalities.

When wool is the major source of income, the economic outcome from an outbreak of disease or nutritional problem is not always obvious. For example, a moderate parasite burden may cause ill-thrift and a reduction in kilograms of wool cut per head, but a reduction in fiber diameter as well, which results in a more valuable fleece. A ewe that does not conceive or aborts in the first 3 mo of pregnancy may produce more wool than a ewe that rears a lamb, because a ewe rearing a lamb has a higher nutritional requirement and produces less wool than a dry ewe. Fiber and meat prices should be considered when providing advice.

Beyond a flock health program, veterinarians can also develop a comprehensive flock management advisory service. These programs adopt a whole farm approach that considers the physical and financial resources of the farm and the interaction of livestock production with other activities such as cropping and pasture production. The stocking rate, type of stock run, timing of husbandry procedures, marketing strategies, and risk management should be reviewed as part of the program. A financial analysis of the farm as a business and preparation of farm budgets and gross margin analyses is a key part of most programs.

Summer Grazing with Winter Confinement and Feeding: Veterinary services in these systems include clinical and preventive medicine and management recommendations. Clinical medicine becomes more cost-effective as the value of the individual sheep increases. Wool production is usually a minor concern, and lambs marketed per ewe joined is the major determinant of economic return. The greatest potential loss is caused by neonatal lamb mortality resulting from mismothering, starvation, cold stress, and hypothermia. Intensive management at lambing reduces this loss but is accompanied by increased risk of mortality from infectious neonatal disease. Labor-intensive lambing systems; intensive care of young lambs; and diagnosis, treatment, and surgery of individual sheep may be justified by the value of the animals. Preventive medicine programs should be developed to prevent the numerous husbandry-related diseases associated with pastoral practices in summer and close stocking during confinement in winter. Feed and labor are the largest production costs for housed or intensively fed sheep. Therefore, nutritional management can have a major impact on farm profitability. Management issues involve minimizing flock energy requirements during the winter months, using body fat reserves without incurring undue decreases in production, and using least-cost rations (including fodder produced on farm). Feed imbalances and close confinement with sheep in feedlots are major determinants of diseases such as pneumonia (p 1230), urolithiasis (p 1259), pulpy kidney disease (p 494), and polioencephalomalacia (p 1061).

Shepherding: Veterinary services to the small, shepherded sheep and goat flocks in the Middle East and Asia are primarily concerned with controlling clinical diseases and improving the survival rate of young lambs and kids. The restricted availability and low nutritional value of feed limit productivity. Sheep and goats are kept primarily as a source of meat and milk for the owner's family and for sale as a source of cash income. The value of animals in the flock is often high relative to the income of the owner, and funds available to invest in veterinary services are limited. The death or severe ill-health of a few animals can have a major impact on both the productivity of the flock and the well-being of the owner.

In Asia, the system of land use is often complex, with sheep and goats integrated with, but grazing around the fringes of, a more productive cropping or plantation enterprise. This may also be true in the Middle East, or sheep and goats may graze poorly productive arid areas that will support little else. In either case, opportunities for major changes to the management system are limited.

Management Practices and Predisposition to Disease: Management practices can be the primary determinant of cases or outbreaks of infectious or metabolic disease in all flocks of sheep.

Pregnancy toxemia (p 828) may be seen in late-pregnant ewes subjected to a falling plane of nutrition, especially ewes with twins or triplets. It is also associated with starvation, ewes that are too fat in early pregnancy, ewes that are fat in late pregnancy and voluntarily reduce feed intake, and ewes subjected to stress in late pregnancy, such as transport or other environmental changes. **Hypocalcemia** (p 808) is seen in pregnant ewes or ewes in early lactation subjected to a period of temporary starvation, especially ewes with twins or triplets; as a result of decreased food intake in late pregnancy; and in weaner sheep on a grain-based ration during drought conditions. **Hypomagnesemia** (p 812) may be seen during a period of temporary starvation in late pregnancy or early lactation, after movement of lactating ewes to lush growing pasture (especially green cereal crops), or among lactating ewes on rapidly growing pastures (eg, spring growth). **Dermatophilosis** (p 690) is associated with poor shearing practices leading to shearing cuts, dipping immediately after shearing with contaminated dip, and sheep in long wool at times of high rainfall. Some sheep are also genetically predisposed. **Caseous lymphadenitis** (p 52) may be associated with not shearing according to ascending age groups, not separating infected or discharging sheep before shearing, close confinement (nose to fleece) of sheep after shearing and dipping, and contaminated dip. **Pulpy kidney disease** (*Clostridium perfringens* type D infection, p 494) is seen in sheep on a rising plane of nutrition, such as those moved to better pasture, following a "flush" in pasture growth, or in sheep fed grain. *C perfringens* **type C infection** is seen in artificially reared "bummer" lambs. **Malignant edema** (p 489) and **blackleg** (p 488) may follow wounds (eg, improper shearing, vaccination). **Tetanus** (p 495) may also be seen after a wound associated with procedures, such as castration, docking, improper shearing, or vaccination, performed in contaminated permanent yards. **Black disease** (p 489) is seen among grazing sheep on pastures that support the intermediate host of *Fasciola hepatica*. **Erysipelas arthritis** (p 504) is associated with contaminated dip, and poor hygiene at docking, castration, and lambing. **Ovine posthitis** is seen in merino wethers on high protein pasture. **Squamous cell carcinoma** is seen on the vulva of short tail docked or mulesed sheep. **Actinobacillosis** (p 476) is seen in sheep grazing on abrasive, thorny pasture.

For disease risks associated with pasture or with specific plants (eg, the risk of bloat, polioencephalomalacia, hemolytic anemia, esophageal obstruction, and enterotoxemia in sheep, and goiter in the lambs of pregnant ewes grazing *Brassica* spp), *see* PLANTS POISONOUS TO ANIMALS, p 2432. For the risk for nutritional deficiency or toxic disease associated with formulated feeds, *see* NUTRITION:SHEEP, p 1902.

HEALTH-MANAGEMENT INTERACTION: SMALL ANIMALS

Proper management to prevent and control disease has historically been a higher priority in large animal medicine than in small animal medicine. However, appropriate management is just as important for small animals, whether their environment is that of a single or multiple-pet home or a more intensive housing situation such as a kennel or cattery.

Responsible pet ownership must be emphasized to all those owning and considering owning pets. Areas of client education that should be emphasized include the following: 1) routine care and grooming, 2) preventive health care, 3) parasite control, 4) nutrition, 5) household hazards, and 6) housing requirements and environmental factors.

Routine care and grooming not only help maintain pet health but also allow identification of health problems early in the course of disease. Close observation of pets allows for evaluation of changes in appetite, thirst, urination, defecation, ambulation, and general behavior. Any changes may suggest the need for a more thorough examination. Special attention should be given to hair coat, skin, ears, eyes, and teeth. Anal gland impaction and overgrowth of nails are common problems.

Preventive health care in small animals is dominated by vaccination. Vaccines are available for a variety of infectious diseases in dogs, including distemper, parvovirus, hepatitis, leptospirosis, tracheobronchitis, rabies, Lyme disease, and coronavirus. Vaccines are available against a number of infectious diseases in cats, including panleukopenia, rhinotracheitis, calicivirus, rabies, feline infectious peritonitis (FIP), and feline leukemia virus (FeLV).

Vaccination schedules vary but generally require an initial vaccination at 6-8 wk of age, followed by additional vaccinations at 3-wk intervals until the animal is 4-5 mo old. After this, most vaccines are given annually. Rabies vaccination is dictated by state law or local jurisdiction. First-time vaccination for diseases other than rabies in adult animals should include an initial vaccination followed by at least one booster.

Recently, there has been some question concerning the overvaccination or hyperimmunization of both dogs and cats. Vaccine-associated sarcomas, specifically fibrosarcoma, have been an increasing problem in cats (*see also* p 777). The etiology of this tumor is not completely understood, but it appears at vaccination sites of rabies and FeLV vaccines. In dogs, there has been some correlation between vaccination and immune-mediated disorders such as immune-mediated hemolytic anemia.

Current recommendations for vaccination sites follow the guidelines of the American Association for Feline Practitioners. This protocol can also be used for dogs. The guidelines suggest that cats be vaccinated in an area amenable to surgical resection, ie, distal limbs rather than torso. Vaccinating dogs and cats less frequently has also been suggested. A triannual vaccination protocol for vaccines other than rabies has been adopted at some institutions. It is also recommended to reserve vaccines for certain diseases such as FeLV, Lyme disease, leptospirosis, feline immunodeficiency virus, and FIP for at-risk animals.

Other preventive health care measures may include castration or ovariohysterectomy, and annual veterinary examinations. The current trend in preventive health care is to emphasize the annual examination and to uncouple this from visits for vaccination. The preventive health visits allow the veterinarian to see the animal frequently and detect disease at an earlier stage.

Parasite control continues to be important. The primary endoparasites include GI parasites such as roundworms, whipworms, and tapeworms (*see also* p 352 et seq). Heartworm disease (p 100), an important clinical entity in both dogs and cats, is preventable with prophylactic therapy. Although a treatment is currently available for heartworm disease in dogs, no safe or acceptable treatment is available for cats. The primary ectoparasites include fleas, ticks, and mites. Both oral and topical products are available for flea control in dogs and cats. Another important aspect of parasite control includes prevention of zoonotic diseases such as visceral larva migrans.

Nutrition is an important and often overlooked aspect of pet ownership. Most pet foods on the market have been formulated based on significant research and development. Specialty diets are available (both over-the-counter and from veterinarians) for young, growing, and geriatric pets, as well as for specific disease processes. Overfeeding and oversupplementation may lead to numerous problems, and feeding of table scraps should be kept to a minimum. (*See also* NUTRITION IN SMALL ANIMALS, p 1914.)

Water quality should not be overlooked, especially in rural areas and in kennels and catteries. Fresh water should be available to pets ad lib.

Household hazards provide a variety of dangers to dogs and cats. Potential hazards include electrical cords, lead-based paint, cleaning supplies, antifreeze (p 2357), houseplants, insecticides (p 2393), prescription drugs (p 2532), illicit and abused drugs (p 2537), alcoholic beverages, chocolate (p 2362), sewing needles, and many others. (*See also* HOUSEHOLD HAZARDS, p 2388.) Elements of house design, such as steep stairs, slippery floors, open windows, etc, may also be hazardous.

Housing requirements and environmental factors are an important consideration for pets. For companion animals sharing an owner's home, concerns are generally limited. However, outdoor housing must provide cover from direct sunlight, shelter from excessive wind and extreme temperatures, adequate ventilation, and an adequate supply of fresh water. These factors are critical in catteries and kennels. Drainage must be appropriate for proper sanitation, and surfaces must be suitable for cleaning and disinfection. Hazardous environmental conditions can result in hyperthermia, sunburn, dehydration, hypothermia, or frostbite. Housing must also be safe and keep pets away from dangers such as other animals, motor vehicles, and malicious mischief. If animals are restrained by a leash or a chain, care should be taken that self-trauma cannot be inflicted.

Miscellaneous considerations include obedience training, which may help reduce aggressive interactions with other animals and people. **Traveling** with pets is another important consideration. If crossing state lines, a health certificate should be issued. When international travel is planned, owners should be advised to become familiar with the appropriate health, quarantine, agriculture, and customs requirements. Animals should not be allowed to ride in the back of open vehicles such as pick-up trucks. Motion sickness (p 1047) and anxiety are common problems in dogs and cats when traveling. The phenothiazine tranquilizer acepromazine may be beneficial in this situation, and antihistamine therapy such as diphenhydramine may be useful. The potential disease-management interaction between pets and owners is important in prevention of **zoonotic diseases**, especially when pets are owned by immunocompromised people. Pet owners with human immunodeficiency virus or those being treated with chemotherapy can safely own animals but should consult both their veterinarian and physician. Most animal-associated infections, including those due to *Toxoplasma gondii, Cryptosporidium, Salmonella,* and *Campylobacter,* appear to be acquired by immunosuppressed individuals from sources other than exposure to animals. The possible exception may be *Bartonella* or cat scratch disease. Because the risk of zoonotic transmission is low, animals pose a minimal risk to immunocompromised people if basic precautions are followed. Precautions include avoiding the cleaning of litter boxes or using gloves when doing so, avoiding dog feces, avoiding young or unhealthy pets in favor of healthy or adult pets, having sick animals evaluated by a veterinarian, not allowing cats to hunt, not feeding pets undercooked meat, and preventing coprophagy or access to garbage.

MANAGEMENT OF REPRODUCTION: CATTLE*

A major and realistic goal of every cow/calf operator and dairy producer should be to raise or market 75-85 calves per 100 cows every year. Reproductive performance can be improved by the following: 1) properly identifying animals; 2) keeping records that enable determination of important herd indices, such as percent calf crop, pregnancy rate, length of calving season, culling rates, calf morbidity and mortality, breeding efficiency of bulls, and performance and production information; 3) meeting the nutritional requirements of various classes of livestock in the herd, emphasizing nutritional needs and cost efficiencies; 4) establishing a breeding program for heifer replacements and cows; 5) practicing sire selection and reproductive management; 6) adopting an immunization program for the cow/calf herd, bulls, and calves; 7) evaluating reproductive failure and abortions; 8) providing adequate facilities; and 9) ensuring that the calf is well cared for at birth and receives adequate colostrum.

NUTRITION

Nutrition is one of the most important management factors in reaching calf crop goals and in attaining a short calving season every year in beef breeding herds. The limiting nutrient related to reproduction in beef cattle is usually energy; this is not as significant in dairy cattle because most are fed rations that supply adequate energy during lactation. The level of energy before calving primarily influences when a cow returns to estrus, while level of energy after calving primarily influences subsequent conception. Feed requirements vary during the reproductive cycle (*see* NUTRITION: CATTLE, p 1811).

There are 4 periods of beef cow nutrient requirements, and generally 3 for dairy cows. **Period 1** is the interval from calving to breeding; it is ~82 days and is the period of greatest nutritional demand. The cow is at maximal milk production and recovering from the stress of parturition. During this period, she is expected to be ready to breed.

Period 2 is the interval from rebreeding to weaning the calf; it is ~123 days in beef cows. Periods 2 and 3 overlap in dairy cows and are not as easily separated as in beef cattle. The beef cow should gain weight while still milking. Although some dairy cows maintain body weight, most high producers continue to lose weight during this period.

Period 3 is from weaning to 50 days before calving; it is ~110 days and is the period of least nutritional demand. The beef cow has only to maintain her condition and continue fetal development. The dairy cow should gain body weight during the last months of lactation.

Period 4 is a critical stage and is the 50 days preceding calving. During the last 50 days of pregnancy, 75% of fetal growth occurs. Cow condition at calving is critical to rebreeding; the onset of estrus after calving is delayed in cows that lose weight or are thin and not gaining during late pregnancy.

*Adapted, in part, from a joint effort by the National Cattleman's Association and the American Association of Bovine Practitioners.

Dairy cows (see NUTRITIONAL REQUIREMENTS OF DAIRY CATTLE, p 1828) are usually fed for optimal milk production throughout their 305-day lactation. It is assumed that they will lose weight during heavy lactation (the early months) and regain the loss during the remainder of lactation. Dairy cows should not be overfed during the dry period because of the increased probability of metabolic diseases, eg, fatty liver disease (p 824) and ketosis (p 830), during early lactation.

The amount of cow feed required per pound of calf weaned is fairly constant, although larger cows require more feed than smaller cows. Cows that give more milk require more feed with a higher level of protein. Increased milk is produced at the expense of reproduction when feed is not adequate to meet all needs.

The protein requirement of young growing stock and heavy-milking cows is often a limiting factor, while mature dry cows are often overfed protein. Heifers must be fed adequately from weaning to breeding if they are to calve at 2 yr of age.

To provide the essential nutrient requirements during various stages of the reproductive cycle, major roughages and homegrown grains should be analyzed to monitor nutrient content and actual dollar value. Variation in amounts of trace minerals is common between and within different geographic areas. Two systems used to determine energy levels of the ration are the Total Digestible Nutrient System and the California Net Energy System. Both are commonly used, and application should be tailored to fit the individual operation.

Even within nutritional need categories, cattle benefit from feeding and handling in subgroups: lightweight heifers at weaning need to gain more than heavier heifers to reach puberty by breeding season; first-calf heifers require special attention from both an energy and competition standpoint if they are expected to breed and conceive at the proper time. These heifers are still growing, as well as lactating, and they may not have the rumen capacity to meet postcalving energy needs on roughage alone. Supplemental feeding of both high-energy and high-protein feeds to first-calf heifers may be required for optimal reproductive potential. Calves from first-calf beef heifers may be weaned 30-40 days earlier than calves from cows in the main herd to allow the heifer more time to grow and recover from demands associated with lactation.

Thin, old, and small cows may not compete favorably with heavier cows within the same herd and often benefit from being fed as a separate subgroup.

Lactating dairy cattle are usually fed according to milk production. They may be fed concentrate on an individual basis or divided into groups according to milk production and fed an appropriate complete blended ration.

BREEDING PROGRAM FOR HEIFER REPLACEMENTS AND COWS

If a cow is to calve consistently, she must deliver her first calf early. Puberty is a function of breed, age, and weight. Beef heifers that are bred at 13-15 mo and calve at 22-24 mo have 2 advantages—they get closer attention from caregivers by calving before the main herd starts to calve, and subsequently they have the extra time needed to rebreed with the mature cow herd. For heifers to breed at 14 mo, they should have attained at least 65-75% of their projected mature weight; therefore, adequate nutrition is of major importance. The breeding season for virgin beef heifers should start 3 wk before that of the main cow herd. The above considerations do not apply to dairy cattle, which calve throughout the year.

To compensate for the greater attrition rate usually seen with virgin heifers, a greater number should be bred than is needed to maintain or increase herd numbers, eg, 150%.

Irregularities of Estrus and Anestrus

Breeding will not occur if the cow is anestrous, or if estrus is undetected. Anestrus or irregular estrous cycles in the cow may result from a number of factors, including poor management or nutrition, disease, injury, or disturbances in endocrine functions. One of the most important management factors in artificially bred herds is failure to detect or observe estrus. The average duration of estrus is 18 hr, but in many cows it is appreciably shorter. A systematic program for detection of estrus is important if cows are to be bred at the right time. A producer must be familiar with signs of estrus. Cows or steers given an androgen, or bulls altered so they cannot inseminate cows, make excellent estrus detectors and are used in many herds bred by artificial insemination. Aids in estrus detection that are valuable adjuncts to the heat-detection program include chalk marks on the tailhead, chemically or electronically activated devices attached to the tailhead of the cow that reveal when other cows have mounted, and a vaginal probe that measures the electrical conductivity of the vaginal mucus. Accidental access of bulls to cows and failure to keep proper breeding records often result in anestrus due to pregnancy without a service history.

Silent heat refers to normal follicular development and ovulation without evident signs of estrus. Its frequency decreases as lactation progresses, so that incidence is low by 4 mo postpartum. Cows with true silent heats may be detected only through rectal palpation of the ovaries or the use of progesterone assay in milk or plasma.

The 21-day cyclic changes in the ovary—particularly in the 3-4 days before ovulation, at the time of ovulation, or 3-4 days after ovulation—generally can be recognized and the time of the cycle estimated. The corpus luteum (CL) regresses 3-4 days before the onset of estrus; it becomes smaller in size and changes from a diestrous, liver-like consistency to one that is more fibrous. Estrus is evidenced by the presence of a palpable follicle, an absent or regressed CL, and firm uterine tone. The vaginal mucosa is edematous, the cervix is relaxed and hyperemic, and a variable amount of clear serous mucus is frequently seen at the vulva, which is puffy and swollen. The immediate postovulatory period is characterized by blood in the mucous discharge and an ovary with a corpus hemorrhagicum, which on palpation is recognized as a soft area (5-15 mm in diameter) in the ovary. The CL is detectable by day 4-5 as a small and somewhat softer structure than the mature CL, which reaches maximal size by day 7.

During almost half the cycle, the examiner can predict the next estrus with reasonable accuracy. Thus, the cow can be watched closely for the next anticipated estrus. In cows that are approaching ovulation, the appropriate time can be estimated and the cow bred, regardless of whether she shows behavioral signs. Should the estimate be in error and the cow exhibit signs a few days later, she can be rebred. Because these cows lack only behavioral signs of estrus, endocrine treatments are not indicated.

Regimens have been developed for the administration of prostaglandins and their analogs to synchronize estrus and to reduce the dependence on estrus detection. Prostaglandins are effective only if a cow has a functional CL. For estrus synchronization, the prostaglandin or its analog is administered to all cows. In those in days 6-18 of the cycle, the CL will regress and estrus will occur in 2-7 days. The others may either have been in estrus recently or will be in a few days. Eleven days later, all cows will be between days 6 and 18 of their cycle, and prostaglandin is administered a second time. Most cows will be in estrus in 3-4 days and will ovulate in 4-5 days. Breeding is done either on signs of estrus, or heifers are bred once at 60 hr and lactating cows are bred once at 72 hr after prostaglandin injection. (See also HORMONAL CONTROL OF ESTRUS, p 1808.) Results with appointment breeding have been poor in some cases. Cystic ovary disease (p 1116) may be responsible for irregularities of the estrous cycle, eg, follicular cysts (anestrus, nymphomania, and shortened cycles) and luteal cysts (anestrus).

Under certain circumstances, ovaries are nonfunctioning. They can be recognized as smooth, small, bean-shaped structures on a single examination, or reveal no activity or change after several examinations over a period of 3 wk. The most common cause is low total energy intake during late winter or droughty summer pastures.

The stress of chronic or severe disease, injury, or ovarian tumors may interrupt ovarian activity and result in anestrus. Congenital defects, such as freemartinism and ovarian hypoplasia, result in estrual failure. Inactive ovaries are treated by correcting the basic cause; they usually do not respond to gonadotropin or steroid hormone treatment.

BULL REPRODUCTIVE MANAGEMENT

A desirable goal for beef producers is a 95% calf crop delivered within 45-65 days, with an optimal weaning weight obtained at the most efficient cost. Bull selection, management, and evaluation of performance are integral aspects of beef improvement. The bull can affect calving percentage as well as quality of calves. The use of performance-tested bulls (beef and dairy) is recommended for both natural breeding and artificial insemination.

A disease control program for bulls should include the following procedures: 1) Before using a bull, he should be checked for brucellosis, tuberculosis, trichomoniasis, and paratuberculosis (ie, from a herd free of paratuberculosis). Bulls previously used in other herds, particularly herds in which disease status is not known, may spread diseases, particularly campylobacteriosis and trichomoniasis. 2) Bulls should be vaccinated against infectious bovine rhinotracheitis, bovine viral diarrhea, clostridia, *Haemophilus*, campylobacteriosis, and leptospirosis. Vaccines should be administered at 6 mo and 1 yr of age and then annually, 1 mo before the breeding season. 3) Breeding soundness examinations should be performed annually at the most economically advantageous time for the producer (usually 1 mo before the breeding season).

All bulls should be on the premises 2 mo before the breeding season to allow them to adapt to the environment. Isolation of all new additions to the herd (bulls or cows) is recommended for proper adaptation and preparation. A breeding soundness examination consisting of a thorough physical examination including internal and external genitalia, measurement of scrotal circumference, and microscopic examination of semen for sperm motility and morphology should be conducted ~1 mo before the breeding season. (*See also* BREEDING SOUNDNESS EXAMINATION OF THE MALE, p 1797.)

During the breeding season, the bull should be watched closely for mating behavior. The standard recommendation is 25 cows/bull. There are some variations in this ratio, depending on the breeding soundness and libido of individual bulls, differences in terrain, and length of breeding season.

The weight loss that develops in bulls during the breeding season should be restored during the off-period, but overconditioning should be avoided.

BREEDING

The breeding program may be either artificial insemination (AI) or natural service. AI has been commercially available for ~60 yr; it is widely used in dairy cattle but is used much less in beef cattle because of confinement and labor costs. AI offers a selection of bulls known to sire calves that have low birth weights. When nutrition and heat detection are properly managed, satisfactory results are obtained. Failure to detect estrus is the major reason for unsuccessful AI. When cows are properly inseminated with good-quality semen at the proper time, 50-60% conceive on first service, the same percentage on second service.

Embryo transfer (p 1804) is frequently used to increase the number of progeny from the most valuable beef and dairy cows. Sexing of embryos has been adapted to field usage and is currently used. Cloning of embryos and sexing of spermatozoa are becoming more readily available and practical for field usage.

Heifers should be bred according to size and age at puberty; at first breeding they should be 65-70% of their projected mature body weight. Selection of bulls to be used for natural service should be based on likely size of the calf at birth; the bull's own birth weight (not his adult weight) is a useful guide.

Heat synchronization of heifers and cows is possible, but such programs depend on adequate management and cooperation. Also, sufficient skilled labor to breed and assist during calving is essential.

Artificial Insemination (AI)

In cattle, AI is used primarily for genetic improvement of livestock, although other conditions also warrant its use. The worldwide adoption of AI for genetic improvement in dairy cattle was made possible by development of a progeny test system and subsequent use of milk production records as an objective measure of performance on which to select superior bulls, techniques for freezing semen, and liquid nitrogen storage refrigerators.

The development of objective systems to measure economic traits in beef cattle (eg, growth rate, carcass conformation and composition, efficiency of feed conversion) and thus the more accurate selection of sires, as well as control of the estrous cycle, have led to an increase in use of AI in beef cattle.

Processing of frozen semen is a highly specialized technique. Attention to detail at each step is important to maintain semen quality. The freezability of semen varies among bulls. However, semen that is of high quality generally freezes well. Best results are obtained when semen is processed in a properly equipped laboratory by experienced staff at an AI center.

Collection and Handling of the Semen Sample: (*See also* p 1797.) Semen is collected using an artificial vagina or electroejaculation (electrical stimulation of the seminal vesicles and ampullae). As long as the sample is of high quality, freezability and fertility should be normal. These techniques should not be used if the bull is unable to naturally service a cow for reasons that could be genetic.

Most AI in cattle today is performed with frozen semen. Frozen semen may be maintained for years; extenders permit more insemination doses to be processed from one collection of semen, maintain the fertility of the semen longer, protect the spermatozoa from sudden temperature or pH change, and prolong viability. Semen is usually extended with citrate-buffered egg yolk or heat-treated skim milk plus glycerol, sugars, enzymes, and antibiotics. Final extension is designed to package 0.5 mL of semen containing 20-30 million spermatozoa at time of freezing.

Extenders are often divided into fraction A and fraction B. The initial extension of semen is done with fraction A at the same temperature, eg, 86°F (30°C). The extended semen is then cooled to 41°F (5°C) over 40-50 min, or more slowly. Holding the extended semen at this temperature for 3-4 hr enables the antibiotics in fraction A to complete their action before being inhibited by the cryoprotectant glycerol. Fraction B contains glycerol (eg, 14%) and is added at 5°C in equal quantity to the extended semen. Each AI center has its own standard extenders and processing procedures. Glycerol (11-13%) may be used with milk-based diluents. Before freezing, semen should be stored for 4-18 hr at 5°C.

For freezing, bull semen is usually packaged in appropriately identified plastic straws (0.25 or 0.5 mL). Optimal freezing rates are known for many cell types, and spermatozoa can withstand a wide range of rates. In practice, extended semen is frozen in liquid nitrogen vapor before being plunged into liquid nitrogen at -320°F (-196°C). Storage in liquid nitrogen tanks is safe for ≥20 yr, and semen is transported in such tanks. The level of liquid nitrogen in tanks must be monitored to avoid semen losses, which is seen when the tanks become defective or when liquid nitrogen gradually evaporates.

Because spermatozoa do not survive for long after thawing, the semen should be used immediately. Thawing is best done as quickly as possible without damaging the semen by overheating. In practice, straws may be thawed in warm water (95-98°F [35-36.5°C]) for ≥30 sec and immediately placed in the cow's reproductive tract. Recommendations by the AI center that processed the semen should be followed.

Insemination Technique: The rectovaginal method is used almost exclusively. After thoroughly cleaning the external genitalia with disposable toweling, one gloved hand is introduced into the rectum and grasps the cervix. The insemination pipette is introduced through the vulva and vagina to the external cervical os. By manipulating the cervix, along with light cranial pressure on the pipette, the pipette is advanced through the annular rings of the cervix to the junction of the internal cervical os and the body of the uterus. The semen should be expelled slowly (5 sec) to avoid sperm loss. If insemination records and consistency of the cervical mucus suggest possible pregnancy, the pipette should be advanced less than one-half of the way through the cervix, and the semen expelled. The optimal time to inseminate is between the last half of standing estrus and 6 hr thereafter.

If fertility problems arise when AI is being used, the semen should be investigated, although many factors other than semen are involved in attaining high fertility. Motility after thawing is an important criterion. An adequate number of motile spermatozoa at the time of insemination is critical. Morphologic examination also helps assess the role of semen in infertility cases. Comparisons within herds of diagnosable pregnancies resulting from the suspect semen and from semen from other bulls may be useful. Estrus detection continues to be the most important factor that influences AI efficiency. This factor should be investigated first, and inseminator proficiency second. The latter includes an evaluation of thawing temperature, time of thawing in relation to actual insemination, temperature changes from thawing to insemination, site and speed of semen deposition, and sanitary procedures. If semen is purchased from a reputable supplier, it is unusual for the cause of the infertility to be poor-quality semen.

PREGNANCY DETERMINATION

Pregnancy determination is recommended to maximize breeding efficiency. In beef herds, the breeding season (natural service or AI) is ideally fixed at a length of 60-70 days. This gives the average cow 2 or 3 services to conceive. Cows that are not pregnant or were bred late should be identified; if kept in the herd, they will calve later in the season. Maintenance costs are significant, although they vary widely by farm and by year.

Pregnancy determination of beef cows should be done shortly after the breeding season is over (eg, 45-60 days); if the breeding season starts June 1 and ends early in August, it can be done during late September while the cows still have plenty of flesh from summer pasture. It is then possible to profitably market nonpregnant cows before expensive winter feeding starts. Dairy cows should be examined within 1 mo after calving and again 6-9 wk after breeding.

Other herd health examinations should be considered while the cows are being checked for pregnancy. These include an accurate evaluation of body condition, the reproductive tract, teats and udder, feet and legs, teeth, and early cancer-eye lesions. Vaccinations, internal and external parasite control, and processing of beef calves also can be done at this time.

EMBRYONIC DEATH, ABORTION, AND ABNORMAL FETAL DEVELOPMENT

Pregnancy may be terminated prematurely, resulting in abortion due to death of the conceptus or failure of the uterine environment to support the fetus. Abnormal fetal development may result in abortion or in a calf that dies soon after birth. Many cases of bovine abortion are not diagnosed. (*See also* ABORTION IN LARGE ANIMALS, p 1097.)

Etiology: Viruses, bacteria (including rickettsia and chlamydiae), molds, protozoa, or other infectious agents may attack the placenta or the fetus, or both. Some of these microorganisms reach the uterus hematogenously; others (such as venereal infections) are contracted during mating.

Infectious abortion may be sporadic or a herd problem. Herd problems usually are associated with significant losses and may be caused by infectious bovine rhinotracheitis, bovine viral diarrhea, brucellosis, leptospirosis (various serotypes), campylobacteriosis, trichomoniasis, anaplasmosis, ureaplasmas, mycoplasmas, *Neospora*, and others not yet identified.

Mycotic abortion usually is caused by *Aspergillus* or *Mucor* spp, which reach the uterus hematogenously and cause abortion in late gestation. In many of these fetuses, the skin is not affected; in others, ringworm-like lesions are seen. The placenta frequently is severely affected with necrosis of the cotyledons and thickening of the intercotyledonary areas. Diagnosis is based on identification of the fungus through culture of the fetal or placental tissues, histologic examination of these tissues, or direct examination of cotyledons after clearing with potassium hydroxide solution. These abortions are almost always sporadic, and the only means of control is to reduce exposure to the fungi.

Sporadic losses may result from *Listeria* sp (a bacterium occasionally present in silage when pH is >7); miscellaneous bacteria such as *Haemophilus* sp, *Arcanobacterium* (*Actinomyces*) *pyogenes*, *Staphylococcus aureus*, *Bacillus cereus*, *Pasteurella multocida*,

Pseudomonas aeruginosa, Streptococcus bovis, Chlamydia sp, and others; or viruses (eg, bluetongue).

Noninfectious causes of abortion are numerous; the most common include: 1) recessive or lethal genes (or both), hydrocephalus, osteopetrosis ("marble bone" disease), arthrogryposis ("crooked calf" syndrome), and several others, some not fully identified; 2) toxins (eg, excessive nitrates from feed or water), certain pine needles, poisonous plants (eg, lupine, locoweed), or mycotoxins (moldy feeds); 3) hormonal imbalances in the pregnant dam; 4) injuries affecting the pregnant cow; and 5) nutritional deficiencies, particularly of vitamin A, vitamin E or selenium (or both), iodine, and manganese.

Diagnosis: Accurate diagnoses of reproductive loss contribute to the cumulative herd history and provide criteria for evaluating the impact on herd performance, and the need for implementation of preventive measures. Laboratory assistance is needed in most cases. Carefully selected, properly preserved, quality specimens should be submitted to a diagnostic laboratory for analysis. Even with these, the exact cause of an abortion may not be detected, especially if it is noninfectious. Many infectious causes can be excluded, however, which assists in formulating a preventive strategy. Laboratory diagnosis of abortion requires both serology and examination of the fetus and placenta. For serology, paired blood samples should be collected from the aborting dam, with the first sample taken at the time of abortion and the second 10-14 days later. An absolute diagnosis may be impossible because, in many cases, the causative agent may not be present when abortion occurs.

Defective newborn calves can be recognized only by a thorough examination and sometimes only after some time has passed.

Prevention and Control: Several factors are critical to prevent and control abortion and development of defective calves. A balanced nutritional program helps control losses associated with mineral or vitamin deficiencies and poor-quality feeds, including moldy grains and forages. Genetic selection and accurate record-keeping help to detect and eliminate bloodlines that prove to be carriers of recessive or lethal genes. Appropriate housing and handling facilities decrease the incidence of accidents and provide an environment conducive to health. The cattle producer and veterinarian should work together to assess the herd's reproductive performance, tailor a vaccination program to the herd's specific needs, and diagnose and control potential herd problems.

Regular Immunizations: Infectious diseases in a herd can disrupt and reduce reproductive efficiency by causing embryonic or fetal death, abortion, or illness and death of neonates. A complete vaccination program will not eliminate reproductive problems but may prevent or reduce losses associated with specific infections (*see* TABLE 2 and TABLE 3).

CALVING MANAGEMENT

Dystocia is expected to occur in ~10-15% of first-calf heifers and in 3-5% of mature cattle. Although dystocia cannot be eliminated from a herd, the incidence can be greatly reduced by management decisions made before the breeding season and during gestation.

Nutrition: Heifers and cows should be gaining weight before calving, but overconditioning causes excess fat deposition in the udder and results in lower milk production. Excessive fat deposition in the pelvis also may result in dystocia. Good body condition aids in calving and also milk production. If cows are placed on a ration to maintain or increase body weight after calving, breeding will be more uniform and the breeding season shorter.

Calving Facilities: Calving facilities may be needed in certain areas. They should be in good repair and functional before the calving season starts. Weather conditions, geographic differences, and local experience usually dictate how much attention and individual care calves will need immediately after birth. The calving environment (eg, calving

TABLE 2. Immunization Program to Protect Against Prepartum Diseases of the Breeding Herd

	Disease	When to Immunize
Heifers	Brucellosis	Calfhood
	IBR[*]	Before weaning and
	BVD[†]	before breeding
	Campylobacteriosis	Before breeding
	Leptospirosis	
	Trichomoniasis	
Cows	IBR	May booster early before breeding
	BVD	
	Campylobacteriosis	Each year, before
	Leptospirosis	breeding
	Trichomoniasis	
Bulls	IBR	Calfhood and booster
	BVD	before first breeding
	Campylobacteriosis	Each year, before
	Leptospirosis	breeding

[*]Infectious bovine rhinotracheitis
[†]Bovine viral diarrhea

sheds, small pastures) must be clean, dry, and protected from the weather. A clean area to handle dystocia problems is also needed. Calving in a clean area, separated from the rest of the herd, helps to reduce calfhood diseases, particularly scours. In large herds, several small calving pastures allow regular rotation to avoid buildup of disease-causing organisms. When calving stalls are used during inclement weather, they should be cleaned and disinfected between calvings.

Calving: Close observation of labor is necessary to determine when a delivery should be assisted. Labor is divided into 3 stages. Stage 1 begins with uterine contractions and dilation of the cervix and ends with passage of the amnion and part of the fetus into the vagina. Stage 1 may last 1-24 hr, with 1-4 hr being normal. Stage 2 is characterized by abdominal contractions due to the fetus in the vaginal canal and ends with the expulsion of the fetus through the vulva. Birth should be expected within 1-4 hr for heifers. A mature cow should calve in <3 hr if the presentation of the calf is normal; if no progress is seen within 1 hr, assistance may be required. Stage 3 is expulsion of the fetal membranes and the initiation of uterine involution. Expulsion of the fetal membranes normally occurs within 12 hr after parturition.

Feeding preparturient cows in the late morning (11:00 am-12:00 noon) and again at night (9:30-10:00 pm) encourages cows to calve during the day (7:00 am-7:00 pm), a period when a problem is more likely to be identified and assistance more likely to be available.

TABLE 3. Immunization Program to Protect Against Diseases of the Neonatal Calf

	Disease	When to Immunize
Heifers and cows	Rotaviruses and coronaviruses	As on label
	E coli bacterins	As on label
	Clostridial bacterins	As on label
Calves	Rotaviruses and coronaviruses (if indicated)	As on label

Parturition is often difficult for both fetus and dam. Many factors influence the degree of difficulty, including breed, age, nutrition, and pelvic area of the dam; breed and genotype of the sire; gestation length; and sex, size, position, and presentation of the fetus. Some, though not all, of these factors are directly influenced by management.

When dystocia (*see* below) develops, survival of both dam and calf depends on proper assistance. This requires identification of the problem, proper facilities, and adequate help. A delay in assisting may mean the loss of the calf or injury and even death of the cow. However, it is important to allow sufficient time for the dam to dilate before applying traction. Before assisting the delivery, the position of the fetus must be determined accurately, and any abnormal presentation corrected. If the calf is simply too large to pass through the birth canal without danger to the cow or calf, a cesarean section or other surgical assistance may be necessary.

Management After Calving: Muddy lots, crowding, filth, chilling, and inclement weather make the calf more vulnerable to disease organisms and may result in sickness and possibly death for both dam and calf. (*See also* HEALTH-MANAGEMENT INTERACTION: CATTLE, p 1707, and MANAGEMENT OF THE NEONATE, p 1683.)

Passive Transfer: Calves receive immunity passively from the dam through the ingestion of colostrum. The calf's immune system is immature at birth and depends on acquisition of passive immunity for disease protection in early life. Immunoglobulins (IgG and IgM) and lymphocytes are absorbed directly across the gut into the calf's circulation to provide immunity. The ability of the gut to absorb these large molecules and cells is a transient phenomenon; gut closure is complete by 24 hr, and absorption has decreased significantly by 6-8 hr of age. Ingestion of adequate amounts of quality colostrum as early as possible after birth is important for calf survival and growth. Calves with failure of passive transfer (FPT) are 3-9 times more likely to become sick before weaning, and 5 times more likely to die before weaning compared with calves with adequate passive transfer.

Minimizing the incidence of FPT should emphasize dystocia management, proper nutrition, and intervention for calves at high risk for FPT. Cows that have dystocia should be milked out immediately and the calf force-fed colostrum to ensure ingestion. Cows with poor udder conformation or mastitis should be milked and the colostrum fed to the calf to ensure timely intake. Colostrum supplements have not proved useful in controlled clinical trials in elevating serum IgG levels. Vaccination of the cow before calving with pathogens causing enteric disease in calves may be a useful adjunct to good overall management in reducing morbidity.

DYSTOCIA MANAGEMENT

Dystocia management must begin with proper heifer development. Fetopelvic disproportion is a major contributing cause of dystocia. Calf birth weight, the size of the pelvic area of the dam, and the interrelationships of these 2 factors are major determinants of dystocia. The weight of the calf is a function of genetic and environmental factors. Genetic factors include sex, length of gestation, breed, heterosis, inbreeding, and genotype. Nongenetic factors include age and parity of the dam, nutrition of the dam during various phases of gestation, and environmental temperature. Efforts to manage the dystocia rate and moderate its effects should focus on replacement heifer development, sire selection, and early dystocia intervention.

Replacement Heifer Development: Dystocia rates in beef heifers cannot be reduced by nutritional restriction during late pregnancy. On the contrary, the loss of 0.5 kg/ day during the last trimester of pregnancy in beef heifers is associated with weak labor, increased dystocia rate, reduced calf growth rate, prolonged postpartum anestrus, reduced pregnancy rate, and increased morbidity and mortality. It is recommended that heifers be fed to allow modest rates of gain (0.5 kg/day) during late pregnancy. Protein malnutrition in late pregnancy has been associated with weak calf syndrome and may be a factor contributing to neonatal mortality.

Measurement of the pelvic area of the dam to predict dystocia is used as a criterion for the selection of replacement heifers, even though pelvic area alone explains only a small proportion of the variability in dystocia. Pelvic area measurements before the breeding season or at the time of pregnancy examination have been used to estimate the pelvic area before calving. Those heifers with a small pelvic area before the breeding season may then be culled or selectively mated to easy calving bulls, and those with a small pelvic area at the time of pregnancy examination may be aborted, culled, or identified for careful observation at calving. Some evidence suggests that culling heifers with the narrowest pelvic width may be more effective than culling based on pelvic area.

Sire Selection: A combination of culling heifers with small pelvic areas and using bulls that sire calves with small birth weights may reduce dystocia significantly. Using only the sires' birth weight to control calf birth weight and dystocia is not effective. A large number of nongenetic influences affect birth weight, such as age of the dam, environment, and birth type. The ability to identify sires appropriate for use on replacement heifers has advanced significantly in recent years. The use of expected progeny differences (EPD) for birth weight is more effective than using only sire birth weight in selecting for acceptable birth weights. EPD are reported in the units of the trait that they reflect (eg, pounds for birth weight). Along with each EPD is reported an accuracy ranging from 0 to 1. Higher accuracies indicate a higher level of confidence that the stated EPD truly reflects the bull's effect. EPD are most effective for comparing bulls rather than identifying the specific effect a bull will have on a herd. For example, a bull with a birth weight EPD of 4.0 would be expected to sire calves 6 lb heavier on average than a bull with a birth weight EPD of -2.0 when bred to the same group of heifers. An attempt should be made to identify bulls with low birth-weight EPD for use on heifers while maintaining at least moderate weaning and yearling weight EPD. This is best achieved by the use of AI sires with high accuracy EPD. EPD can be calculated on yearling bulls with no progeny, but the accuracy is low. Until recently, EPD were useful only in comparisons within breeds; however, methods for across-breed EPD have now been developed. This is of particular use in selecting bulls to control dystocia in crossbreeding programs. Two recent innovations in the use of EPD for management of dystocia are the calving ease EPD and the maternal calving ease EPD. Calving ease EPD is related to birth weight EPD but may predict calving ease more effectively. Maternal calving ease is a measure of the effect of the maternal grandsire and the ease with which a bull's daughters will calve.

As the birth weight of the calf increases, the incidence of dystocia also increases. Calving difficulty is higher for male than female calves. Abnormal presentations of the calf accounted for 22% of dystocias and 4% of all births in one study. Most dystocias are seen in primiparous 2-yr-old heifers, and the frequency decreases with increasing age and weight of the cow. Some studies have suggested that cows that previously experienced dystocia are more likely to do so again. Environmental effects may also have an effect on calf birth weight and dystocia. Cold weather may increase birth weights and subsequently increase the incidence of dystocia.

Early Intervention: Despite the best efforts to avoid dystocia, some cases will be seen. Early intervention minimizes the effects of dystocia on calves. Heifers should be monitored regularly and provided with assistance promptly if stage II labor is prolonged (eg, 1 hr). Producers need to identify the level of dystocia and growth that is economically acceptable and select a bull to match. They must be well trained to intervene appropriately in dystocia and recognize when to call the veterinarian. A general rule of thumb is that if a heifer has not made significant progress in delivering her calf within 30 min, it is time to get help.

COW-CALF PAIR MANAGEMENT

Cows and heifers should be moved from winter grounds to calving grounds 2-3 wk before the calving season begins. They should be sorted into groups based on estimated calving date. This date can be determined at the time of pregnancy examination, when cows and heifers are grouped based on estimated duration of gestation. Separation of the herd into groups allows more concentrated observation of a smaller number of cows or heifers that are more likely to calve and potentially need help. Cows and heifers should be observed to ensure that they accept and mother their calves. Heifers especially are at risk for calf rejection, which increases the risk of calf disease. If heifers do not accept their calves and allow nursing within a short time, they should be brought into the calving barn and restrained to allow the calf to suck. Heifers that experience dystocia and human assistance are at increased risk for rejecting their calves. Cows or heifers that experience difficulty in calving or mothering should be moved to the calving barn for assistance and monitoring. Pairs entering the calving barn are at increased risk for disease because of dystocia, mismothering, hypothermia, and exposure to a higher population density. Once a pair enters the calving barn, they should not go to the general nursery pasture but to a separate high-risk nursery. Calves in the high-risk nursery can be monitored more closely for morbidity and treated promptly. Segregation of these high-risk calves also avoids exposure of the rest of the herd.

Once cows or heifers have calved, the pair should be moved out of the calving area to a nursery pasture within 24 hr. When the pair has bonded and passive transfer has occurred, movement to a nursery with decreased population density minimizes infection rates. Sick calves in the healthy nursery pasture should be removed and brought to the barn for treatment if necessary and placed in a morbidity nursery. Infectious agents can multiply in clinically ill calves and cause high levels of environmental contamination. The morbidity nursery may be combined with the high-risk nursery, but this increases exposure of the high-risk calves to pathogens. Ill calves should not be returned to the general nursery area. Treatment equipment should be disinfected thoroughly between calves to avoid transfer of infectious agents from calf to calf.

MANAGEMENT OF REPRODUCTION: GOATS

PUBERTY AND ESTRUS

In theory, goats cycle at 21-day intervals, but most dairy goats and Angoras in temperate regions are seasonal breeders and come in heat in the fall in response to decreasing day length. Pygmies and some individuals of other breeds (particularly Nubians) can cycle at other times of the year. Heat detection is based on behavioral signs, bleating, flagging of the tail, reddened vulva, vaginal discharge (which causes the tail hairs to stick together), and occasional "riding" by other does, although this last sign is far less common than in cattle. Shorter cycles can be seen at the onset of the breeding season and sometimes can be provoked by prostaglandin induction of estrus. Longer cycles are seen later in the season. Goats can show overt signs of estrus while pregnant; natural service will not interfere with pregnancy, but these does should not be artificially inseminated. Most dairy goat females can be bred at 70 lb (32 kg) or 7 mo, if they are born early in the year. Late-born kids may not cycle in the first season. Angora kids frequently are not bred until they are $1^1/_2$-$2^1/_2$ yr old. Puberty in well-grown bucks can be seen as early as 4 mo.

BREEDING SOUNDNESS EXAMINATION

The external genitalia of does should be examined for abnormalities that suggest intersex, a condition common in homozygous polled females. These include an enlarged clitoris and a hypotrophic vulva. Occasionally, a doe has a shortened vagina and no cervix, and segmental aplasia of various parts of the tract can be seen. Intersex goats are sterile and should be culled.

Physical examination of the buck before the breeding season should include evaluation of the penis and prepuce. The buck is set on his rump and the shoulders pushed down to curve the spine convexly; this makes it easier to protrude the penis. Shearing wounds (especially in Angoras), prior balanoposthitis, and old fly-strike wounds and scarring around the prepuce may make protrusion of the penis impossible. Based on data from other species, it would seem wise to eliminate those animals with testicles smaller and softer than their seasonal age-matched counterparts. Prior amputation of the urethral process to prevent obstruction by a calculus has no apparent deleterious effect on breeding ability. Occasionally, bucks develop functional udders but this does not preclude their siring kids.

Caseous lymphadenitis (p 52), spermatic granulomata, and calcification of the testicles (which also may be due to *Corynebacterium pseudotuberculosis* [*ovis*] infection) all reduce or eliminate the buck's fertility.

Anemia due to heavy parasite infections, chronic debilitating diseases (commonly pneumonia), and foot problems lead to loss of libido. Bucks with caprine arthritis and encephalitis virus infection (p 598) may have painful, enlarged stifles; they may mount does but are reluctant to ejaculate due to pain.

ARTIFICIAL INSEMINATION

In the dairy goat industry, most artificial insemination (AI) is done by the owners rather than by inseminators. Deep intracervical or intrauterine insemination is considered to give better conception rates than insemination just into the first cervical ring or onto the cervical os. The goat cervix has multiple rings, and the pipette must be maneuvered past each one. Frozen semen in 0.5 mL straws may be purchased directly from buck owners or custom collectors. There is no legislation or industry-wide standard in North America that governs the collection, processing, and sale of frozen semen. Natural service is the easiest, and most systems have bucks running with the does. Most hobby operations have a low doe:buck ratio (5:1) because of multiple breeds and different bloodlines. Bucks have a strong libido and can breed far more does than this, although as they get older, and especially during the off-season, they are less efficient.

Semen can be collected in an artificial vagina. Most bucks will mount a doe in estrus and ejaculate; with training they will ejaculate year round and even mount wethers. Old bucks are often reluctant to breed does that have had estrus induced outside the normal breeding season; therefore, collections are more successful when young bucks are used.

INDUCTION OF ESTRUS

Estrus can be induced in several ways, depending on the time of year and the relationship to the doe's natural breeding season. Out-of-season breeding is of interest to dairy goat owners because it reduces seasonal fluctuation in the herd's milk production.

The sudden introduction of an odoriferous buck often advances the onset of cycling by a few weeks, and the does also may show some synchronization. The buck should be housed well away from the does (out of their sight and smell) for ≥3 wk before he is introduced. Even if the whole group does not cycle, this method can get a few to conceive in the theoretically out-of-season period.

If the corpus luteum is functional, 2.5 mg prostaglandin (PG) $F_{2\alpha}$ will induce estrus (but this is not effective during anestrus); it also may provoke short cycles, which tend to be seen normally at the beginning of the season.

Providing 20 hr of light per day in January and February (northern USA), with a sudden return to available daylight on March 1, will bring goats into estrus several weeks later. In this system, it is more difficult for the owner to pick out the does that are in estrus; consequently, running a young, vigorous buck with the does gives the highest conception rate. If a portion of the herd is artificially synchronized, some of the remaining does also may come into estrus.

Progestagen treatment, combined with follicle-stimulating hormone or pregnant mare serum gonadotropin (PMSG), will cause out-of-season estrual activity. Good conception rates can be achieved with this system, and fixed-time insemination is feasible, but these products are not approved for use in goats. Progestagen treatment can be in the form of injections with an oily base every 3 days, impregnated vaginal sponges, or a CIDR—a form of impregnated plastic for vaginal use. A more readily available, but also unapproved, product now being widely used in conjunction with PMSG is a norgestomet ear implant (designed for cattle).

PREGNANCY TESTING

With the rectal Doppler ultrasonography machine, pregnancies can be diagnosed early with no false positives. The external Doppler can be used from mid- to late gestation. The sonic pregnancy machine also can be used, however, it may give false positives in midgestation and is not effective in late gestation.

Ultrasound scanners as used for sheep and racehorses are accurate with a skilled operator; they are also expensive. Scanners are best used between 40 and 90 days of pregnancy, and multiple pregnancies are diagnosed with 95% accuracy. Routine radiography can be used with 100% accuracy after day 70 and can detect the number of kids after day 75.

The progesterone test can be done on milk or serum, but samples must be collected precisely 1 cycle after the animal was bred. The progesterone test is good at detecting nonpregnancy but is not a positive pregnancy test because it cannot differentiate between midcycle, true pregnancy, or false pregnancy. The estrone sulfate test, performed on milk or urine, can determine pregnancy. Between 40 and 50 days after conception, the level of estrone sulfate increases substantially and stays increased throughout pregnancy. Abortion, fetal death, or resorption causes the estrone sulfate level to drop; therefore, the test also is a useful measure of fetal viability.

Precocious milking is common in heavy-milking strains of goats. It can be seen in a virgin doe or during the first pregnancy. Therefore, udder development is no guarantee of pregnancy.

False pregnancy is a problem in dairy goats. It can be shorter or longer than a true pregnancy. Usually, the udder enlarges, but true filling does not occur. The doe may show behavioral signs of impending parturition; she may even call or search for the nonexistent kid. Many of these does conceive the next year, but many are dried off and are economic losses for 1 yr.

PARTURITION

Parturition or kidding occurs 145-155 days (average 150) after breeding. Generally, first-kidding does have 1-2 kids, and in subsequent kiddings, >2. Quadruplets are not uncommon, especially in large, well-fed, heavy milkers. Quintuplets and sextuplets are rare. The flock average for range Angora goats in the USA and South Africa is ~100% but is higher in Australasia; the weaning average varies with the harshness of the environment, including the existence of predators. Induction of parturition is a useful technique to increase survival in dairy goat kids and to catch and separate kids from dams before they suckle in herds with control programs for caprine arthritis encephalitis virus and mycoplasma. Cloprostenol (125 mg) or $PGF_{2\alpha}$ (10 mg) injection usually results in delivery of kids ~30-35 hr after injection. Viability of multiple fetuses may be compromised if parturition is induced before day 144.

Retained placentas are uncommon in goats and usually are associated with the birth of a mummy or rotten fetus or a difficult delivery.

Pregnancy toxemia in goats is similar to that in sheep (p 828). Hypocalcemia or milk fever (p 806) is seen but not nearly so frequently, nor as severely, as in cattle. Often, there is only a tendency to fall off the milk stand. Lactational ketosis is seen.

In extremely cold weather, newborn kids should be dried (especially the ears) to prevent frostbite. Heat lamps are not necessary if the kids are dry, well fed, and out of a draft. Kids born in intensive systems should have their navels dipped in tincture of iodine to prevent infection. Angora, pygmy, and meat kids are raised on the dams. Dairy goat kids often are removed at birth and, after receiving colostrum, fed from a bottle or nipple-pail.

MANAGEMENT OF REPRODUCTION: HORSES

REPRODUCTIVE CYCLE

Nearly all mares are seasonally polyestrous and cycle when day length is long. Anestrus is seen during the winter when day length is short. During anestrus, the uterus is flaccid, and the ovaries are inactive with no significant follicles or corpora lutea. The cervix may be closed but not firm and tight, or it may be thin, short, and dilated. As day length increases, mares undergo a vernal transition and the ovaries become active, with numerous large (>25 mm) follicles. The cervix and uterus have minimal tone. Mares have 3-4 prolonged intervals of estrus (sexual receptivity) during the vernal transition, but ovulation does not occur. The end of vernal transition is marked by a surge of luteinizing hormone (LH) and subsequent ovulation. After this first ovulation, the first 21-day interovulatory period is seen and a regular estrous cycle is established. Although the mare then continues to ovulate regularly every 21 days throughout the breeding season, the length of estrus (receptivity to the stallion) varies, ranging from 2-8 days, and the length of diestrus varies accordingly. Early in the breeding season, estrus tends to be longer, whereas around the summer solstice the mare may be sexually receptive for only 2-3 days. Follicles enlarge on the ovary during estrus. Usually, one follicle becomes dominant and ovulates when it is ≥30 mm in diameter. The dominant follicle becomes tense and then softens before ovulation. The oocyte is released through the ovulation fossa. A corpus hemorrhagicum and subsequent corpus luteum form and produce progesterone, which simulates closure of the cervix and increases uterine tone. This corpus luteum will be mature and become responsive to prostaglandin at ~5 days. If pregnancy is not established, luteolysis develops at 14 days, and the mare returns to estrus and continues to cycle.

Artificial Manipulation of Photoperiod: After the winter anestrus and the vernal transition, cyclicity naturally commences some time in April, when breeding can begin. Because changes in the mare's genital tract are seen in response to day length, the onset of regular estrous cycles—and thus, the onset of the breeding season—can be hastened by exposing the mare to 16 h of artificial light per day; 8-10 wk are required for mares to respond. If the breeding season is scheduled to begin February 15, artificial lighting should be started December 1. It is recommended that mares experience a natural photoperiod of decreasing day length in the fall. Mares can be exposed to light abruptly for a 16-hr day, or the light can be gradually increased to 16 hr over 60 days. In a constant program, light is added from 4:30 pm until 11:00 pm daily. In a less expensive stepwise program, 3 hr of light are added in the evening during the first week, increasing by 30 min each additional week. An automatic timer aids compliance and saves on labor.

The supplemental light must be added at dusk; light added in the morning before dawn is not effective. A minimum of 10 foot-candles (107 lux) of incandescent or fluorescent light is necessary. The amount of light should allow one to comfortably read newsprint. A 3.7 × 3.7 m stall may require one 200-watt bulb or two 40-watt bulbs. Mares can be stimulated as a group in a lighted paddock.

Manipulation of Ovarian Activity: Ovarian activity is frequently manipulated to facilitate scheduling of breeding appointments and to allow many mares and stallions to remain in competition during the breeding season. Breedings should be spaced for stallions with large books of mares so that semen use is optimized. Geographic locations and transportation constraints also may necessitate scheduled breedings. Many situations can benefit from an ovulation control program. (*See also* HORMONAL CONTROL OF ESTRUS, p 1808.)

Administration of prostaglandin (PG) $F_{2\alpha}$, IM, to a mare in diestrus causes luteolysis and allows a follicle to develop and ovulate. The corpus luteum must be 5-14 days old to respond. The mare will come into estrus 2-5 days after administration of $PGF_{2\alpha}$. Time to ovulation is variable (3-10 days) and depends on the size and development of follicles at the time of PG administration.

Dinoprost, a naturally occurring $PGF_{2\alpha}$ (1 mg/45.5 kg, IM), may cause transient side effects such as lowered body temperature, increased heart and respiratory rates, sweating, muscle cramping, colic, ataxia, and weakness. Signs are seen within 15 min and usually subside within 1 hr. Synthetic preparations, eg, cloprostenol sodium (0.55 µg/kg, IM) have fewer side effects.

Human chorionic gonadotropin (hCG) 2,500-5,000 IU, IV or IM, can be used to hasten ovulation of a dominant follicle during estrus. If the mare has a preovulatory follicle ≥35 mm diameter, ovulation occurs within 36-48 hr after injection.

Deslorelin (SC implant), a gonadotropin-releasing hormone analog, causes ovulation of a 30-mm follicle in ~40-48 hr. As nonpregnant implanted mares may have a delay of 2-5 days before returning to estrus and ovulation, it is recommended that implants be removed 48 hr after insertion. It may be convenient to insert the implant in vulvar mucosa.

Ovulation can be timed accurately by using the following protocol: On days 1-10, 10 mg of estradiol 17-β and 150 mg of progesterone are administered IM. On day 10, dinoprost (1 mg/45.5 kg, IM) is administered. On day 16, mares come into estrus, and on days 19 or 20, insemination should be performed. On days 20, 21, or 22, most mares ovulate. This regimen is effective at any time in cycling mares except when a large, dominant follicle <48 hr from ovulation is present. If a mature follicle is present, the protocol should not begin until after ovulation.

Altrenogest is a synthetic progestin that suppresses the receptive behavior that develops during estrus. It is administered at 0.44 mg/kg, PO by dose syringe or top-dressed on feed for 12-15 days. Estrus occurs 4-5 days after treatment ends with variable timing of ovulation (8-15 days). Although altrenogest effectively suppresses estrus, it does not consistently control the time interval to ovulation.

Estrus Detection: A successful breeding management program revolves around a good estrus detection program. The mare should be presented to a stallion (teaser) daily or every other day during the breeding season, and an accurate interpretation and record should be made of her response. Mares in estrus raise their tail, squat, urinate, and evert the vulvar lips to expose the clitoris, and ultimately tolerate copulation. Mares in diestrus usually squeal, kick, bite, and reject the stallion's advances. Mares in seasonal anestrus may remain passive. Although anestrus mares are not receptive when confronted by a stallion, some will tolerate a stallion's sexual advances. This tolerance seems to be due to a lack of progesterone, similar to the tolerance seen in an ovariectomized mare used as a stimulus for mounting. Adequate exposure to and contact with the teaser should be allowed to thoroughly evaluate the mare's response; a mare in estrus may initially not appear receptive due to nervousness or inexperience. Some mares with foals by their side may not exhibit estrus to the teaser due to their protective nature. The mare's behavior when teased should be consistent with the findings on examination of her genital tract. Response to teasing can determine if estrus has begun and indicate when a mare should be palpated and bred. Failure to return to estrus 2-3 wk after breeding may suggest that the mare is pregnant. Prolonged, erratic periods of estrus are common and normal during the vernal and autumnal transitional breeding season.

BREEDING SOUNDNESS EXAMINATION OF THE MARE

A comprehensive reproductive evaluation is recommended for the mare that has questionable fertility. Abnormalities can be diagnosed and appropriate therapy instituted to correct any problem before breeding is scheduled. A coordinated plan of management should be developed based on the mare's history of reproductive performance, previous treatments, examination findings, laboratory test results, and the intended use of the mare.

Theriogenologists typically examine mares for breeding soundness before purchase or breeding or when a mare is barren. A complete breeding soundness examination includes examination of the external genitalia and mammary gland, palpation and ultrasonography per rectum of the internal genitalia, manual and visual vaginal examination (vaginoscopy), endometrial swab for aerobic culture, and biopsy of the endometrium for histologic evaluation.

In the case of a young maiden mare, palpation and ultrasonography per rectum to determine the presence of a uterus of normal size and consistency, normal active ovaries, and functional cervix may suffice. Perineal conformation should be evaluated. If there is evidence of pneumovagina or vaginitis, commonly present in slim, fit, racing fillies, an endometrial swab and biopsy are indicated.

In foaling mares, palpation and ultrasonography per rectum are required to evaluate uterine involution. A manual vaginal examination should be performed to ascertain whether the reproductive tract was traumatized during foaling. Thorough evaluation of the cervix requires direct manual palpation per vagina of the cervix after foal heat ovulation when the mare is in diestrus and under progesterone stimulation. Mares that had foaling problems (eg, dystocia, retained placenta) require a more extensive evaluation. All postpartum mares have a transient endometritis during uterine involution; therefore, uterine swab and biopsy typically provide more useful information if delayed for ≥3 wk after parturition.

Barren mares require a complete breeding soundness examination. Occasionally, hysteroscopy or endocrine assay may provide additional information.

Signalment and History: A standard breeding soundness examination form to record examination findings can be helpful in ensuring all areas are covered during the examination. The animal should be accurately identified.

Determination of stage of reproductive cycle and estrous cycle is essential for proper evaluation and interpretation of laboratory test results. The history should include previous length and character of estrus, breedings and their results, therapy, and specific reproductive problems. In particular, histologic findings of an endometrial biopsy sample reflect the stage of the mare's reproductive cycle and any recent intrauterine activities (breeding, treatment, foaling). Regardless of the history, the mare's nonpregnant status should be confirmed before performing any procedures (eg, endometrial swab, endometrial biopsy, direct manual cervical palpation) that would compromise an existing pregnancy (see PREGNANCY DETERMINATION, p 1752).

Restraint: The mare can be restrained in hand, in stocks, or positioned in a doorway. For fractious mares, a twitch may provide short-term restraint to allow completion of the examination. For the occasional situation in which the temperament of the mare poses risk of injury to the mare or examiner, chemical restraint may be used. A combination of acepromazine (0.02 mg/kg) and xylazine (0.3-0.5 mg/kg) administered IV works well for short procedures. If possible, the external genitalia should be evaluated before tranquilizers are administered because their use may alter the tone and competency of the perineum.

Physical Examination: The mare's tail should be wrapped and tied to one side. The tail and inner thighs should be examined for the presence of dried exudate indicative of genital infection or urine staining that may be associated with urine pooling or incontinence. The size and shape of the clitoris should be assessed. A mare with an excessively large clitoris may have been androgenized either by exogenous hormones or by endogenous hormones in an intersex condition (male pseudohermaphrodite or hermaphrodite). Normal vulvar lips have good tone and apposition and form the first barrier of the uterus against environmental contaminants. The vulvar lips should be parted to determine the competency of the fold. If air readily aspirates into the vagina, the mare may be prone to pneumovagina and may require a vulvoplasty (Caslick's operation).

For per rectum procedures, the examiner, wearing a clean examination sleeve with water-soluble lubricant, must first empty the rectum of feces. Palpation and ultrasonography per rectum permit assessment of the internal genital tract. Each part of the genital tract should be systematically palpated. Typically, a real-time 5-7.5 mHz linear probe, which produces a rectangular, cross-sectional image of the structure scanned, is used for ultrasonographic examinations of the reproductive tract. Ovarian size and character as well as the presence of an ovulation fossa should be noted. Anechoic follicles should be measured and counted, and the presence of a hyperechoic corpus luteum recorded. Normal oviducts are not routinely examined because their small size prevents palpation and imaging.

The size, shape, and contents of the uterus should be recorded. The mare's uterus is T-shaped with the horns perpendicular to the body of the uterus. It is suspended in the pelvic canal by the broad ligament, which is attached dorsally to the sublumbar region. Ultrasonography permits accurate assessment and measurement of the uterine horns. The uterus has several endometrial folds that increase the surface area of the uterine lumen. The endometrial folds should be carefully assessed during palpation per rectum by slipping the folds through the examiner's fingers along the entire length of each horn. The character of the uterus changes during the estrous cycle. During estrus, the endometrial folds become edematous, causing the uterine horns to have an echo texture characterized by alternating areas of hypo- and hyper-echogenicity when a cross section is viewed with ultrasonography. After ovulation and development of the corpus luteum, the uterus is stimulated by progesterone, uterine tone increases, and the endometrial folds are no longer edematous. After 14-18 days of gestation, the endometrial folds are not readily palpable because of the gradual but marked increase in uterine wall thickness. The size and character of any anechoic endometrial cysts should be recorded for reference during subsequent early pregnancy examinations.

The length, width, and shape of the cervix are palpable per rectum; however, thorough evaluation of the cervix requires direct palpation per vagina (see VAGINAL EXAMINATION, below). The cervix changes in response to the steroid hormone status of the mare. During anestrus, ovarian steroid concentrations are low, and the cervix is either short, thin, and open or closed but readily opened. After the first ovulation of the season and during subsequent periods of diestrus, progesterone concentrations are high and the cervix is closed, with a long cylindrical shape. During estrus, progesterone concentrations are low, and estrogen concentrations are high; the cervix is relaxed and edematous. It may be difficult to palpate its dimensions accurately per rectum at this time.

Urine in the vagina (urovagina) may be seen sporadically or be a chronic problem. Mares may have an abnormal voiding pattern, and the endometrium may show histologic evidence of chronic irritation. Using the neck of the bladder to indicate the caudal boundary of the vagina during ultrasonography, the vagina can be examined for any accumulation of echogenic fluid caudal to the cervix. A definitive diagnosis of urovagina requires direct observation of urine in the vagina on speculum examination.

Endometrial Swab: Before an endometrial swab, the nonpregnant status of the mare must be confirmed because the swabbing could lead to termination of a pregnancy (see PREGNANCY DETERMINATION, p 1752). The perineum is cleansed with povidone-iodine scrub, rinsed, and dried. The operator dons a sterile sleeve or clean examination sleeve with the hand encased in a sterile glove. A water-soluble lubricant that is free of bacteriostatic chemicals is placed on the back of the hand and lower arm. When obtaining an endometrial swab sample, the vestibule, vagina, and cervix must be passed. Care must be taken to avoid contamination of the swab by microorganisms in the structures caudal to the uterus that would hinder accurate interpretation of the culture results. A double-guarded occluded uterine swab is gently guided through the cranial end of the cervix, and the inner guard is inserted into the uterine lumen for 30-60 sec. The swab tip is carefully placed into a transport system, which is vital to maintain viability of the organisms from the time of sample collection until culture in the laboratory.

Most laboratories streak the swabs on 5% sheep blood agar for general growth and on MacConkey's agar for growth of gram-negative organisms, after which they are aerobically incubated at 37°C.

Organisms commonly isolated that are associated with endometritis include β-hemolytic streptococci (90% *Streptococcus zooepidemicus*, 10% *S equisimilis*), *Escherichia coli*, *Pseudomonas* (65% *P aeruginosa*), and *Klebsiella pneumoniae*. Organisms isolated that are commonly suspected to be contaminants include α-hemolytic streptococci, *Actinobacillus equuli*, *Salmonella enteritidis*, *Pasteurella*-like species, and *Staphylococcus*, *Enterobacter*, *Acinetobacter*, *Proteus*, *Citrobacter*, *Alcaligenes*, and *Aeromonas* spp.

In most cases, the growth of a few miscellaneous microorganisms is not significant. A heavy growth of any microorganism should be considered significant unless obvious contamination has occurred. Isolation of an organism transmitted venereally, such as *Taylorella equigenitalis* (requires a special culture system) and certain strains of *Pseudomonas* and *Klebsiella*, is considered a significant finding. Occasionally, microorganisms causing a pyometra may not be detected on aerobic culture due to products of the inflammatory reaction prohibiting their growth.

Culture results of the endometrial swab should be used as a diagnostic adjunct and not as the sole determinant in diagnosing a uterine infection. A positive culture result must be accompanied by evidence of inflammation for the diagnosis of endometritis to be made. Mares exhibiting clinical signs of infection (uterine fluid as seen on ultrasonographic examination per rectum, tail matting or uterine discharge, and the presence of inflammatory cells seen on a stained smear from a uterine swab) with a positive endometrial swab are likely to have endometritis. Inflammation seen on histologic evaluation of the endometrium confirms the diagnosis of endometritis. In these cases, the culture results are most useful in determining the sensitivity of the causative microorganism and developing an antimicrobial treatment plan.

The following antibiotics are commonly used for daily uterine infusion by diluting with sterile saline to an infusion volume of 60-100 mL: penicillin (sodium or potassium salt), 5 million U; ampicillin, 3 g; ticarcillin, 1-3 g; carbenicillin, 2-5 g; gentamicin sulfate (diluted with 20 mL sodium bicarbonate and 20 mL saline), 1 g; amikacin sulfate, 2 g; ceftiofur, 1 g; or clotrimazole, 500 mg.

Endometrial Biopsy: An endometrial biopsy is usually obtained after an endometrial swab has been procured. Preparation for biopsy is the same as for taking a swab (*see* above). The basket of the biopsy instrument should be kept closed during positioning to prevent accidental procurement of vagina, cervix, or examination glove. The instrument is manually guided with the gloved hand through the caudal genital tract into the uterine lumen. While keeping the instrument in place within the uterus with the non-gloved (external) hand, the gloved hand is carefully withdrawn from the genital tract and inserted into the rectum to allow positioning of the basket of the biopsy instrument at the ventral surface of the base of a uterine horn. The instrument jaws are then opened, the uterine wall is pressed into the side of the basket, and the jaws are closed. The jaws should be kept closed while the instrument is withdrawn from the genital tract. The tissue should be gently teased from the basket and placed into Bouin's fixative. If the sample will not be processed within a few days, it should be transferred into 70% ethanol or 10% formalin.

It is not unusual for a small amount of uterine bleeding to be seen after biopsy. The biopsy procedure does not seem detrimental to fertility, and mares can conceive from breedings during an estrus when biopsy was performed.

Histologic evaluation of the endometrium provides prognostic information about the mare's ability to carry a foal to term. The luminal contents may indicate the presence of uterine fluid or exudate. Epithelial cell type is related to hormone status; cells are cuboidal during anestrus and low to tall columnar during the breeding season. Transepithelial cells may indicate active inflammation. The pattern, character, and location of inflammation indicate the chronicity of response—neutrophils indicate an acute reaction, and lymphocytes and plasma cells indicate a chronic reaction. Focal or diffuse cellular distribution pattern, frequency of cells, and degree of infiltration (slight to severe) relate to severity of inflammation. Histologic evidence of significant inflammation, combined with a report of growth of microorganisms from culture of endometrial swab and the presence of clinical signs of infection (uterine fluid, uterine discharge), support the decision that an endometrium would benefit from therapy to decrease inflammation. The pattern of distribution and severity of periglandular fibrosis is prognostically useful. Fibrosis surrounding groups of glands ("fibrotic nest") is thought to be more clinically significant than fibrosis of individual glands. Periglandular fibrosis may interfere with endometrial gland function and may be a factor in early embryonic death. Glandular distention normally develops during pregnancy, but widespread cystic glandular distention in the nonpregnant mare is undesirable. Cystic glandular distention is often associated with periglandular fibrosis and may result from an occlusion of the endometrial glands by the fibrosis.

Endometria are classified in 4 categories. **Category I** indicates no significant changes are present in the endometrium and no treatment is required. The estimated foaling rate is 80-90%. An endometrium with any notable periglandular fibrosis cannot be classified as Category I. **Category II** is a broad category that includes most mares. It has been divided into **Category IIA**, for mares with less severe changes, and **Category IIB**, for mares with more severe changes. The estimated foaling rate is 50-80% in Category IIA and 10-50% in Category IIB. Often, therapy may improve the state of the endometrium by reducing inflammation, cystic glandular distention, and lymphatic lacunae. Improvement in the endometrium may allow for better classification at a later date. There is no effective treatment to decrease the severity of periglandular fibrosis. **Category III** is the poorest classification, and these endometria have widespread, severe changes that include periglandular fibrosis or inflammation. A widespread pattern of distribution of slight to moderate changes may be more deleterious than more severe changes that are infrequent and only involve individual glands. The estimated foaling rate of a Category III endometrium is <10%.

During interpretation of the findings on histologic evaluation of an endometrial biopsy sample, the extent of normal, unaffected endometrium is more significant than the presence of any particular lesion. In barren mares with a Category I or IIA endometrium, other reproductive abnormalities or poor breeding management should be investigated as the cause of infertility.

Vaginal Examination: The perineum is cleansed, rinsed, and dried before the visual vaginal speculum examination. The vulvar lips are separated, and the speculum is advanced cranially at a dorsal angle so as to pass over and through the transverse (vulvovaginal) fold of the vagina. Resistance against the speculum by this fold of tissue indicates good tone and function. A bright light is necessary to adequately view the cervix and vaginal wall. After the examination, it should be noted whether the vulvovaginal fold occludes the vagina as the speculum is withdrawn. The competency of the vulvovaginal fold is important to note because it forms the second barrier for the uterus against external contaminants. Thorough evaluation of the completeness and competency of the cervix can be accomplished only by direct palpation per vagina while the mare is under progesterone stimulation (ie, cervix closed). The cervix forms the third barrier for the uterus against external contaminants.

PREGNANCY DETERMINATION

The schedule for determination of pregnancy varies among breeding farms. One schedule is as follows: 1) days 14-18—check for twins; if open, mare can be rebred on days 19-20; 2) days 25-30—evaluate normal embryo development (heartbeat present at 24-25 days), recheck for twins; 3) days 40-60—evaluate normal fetal development; 4) fall check—confirm mare is still pregnant.

Palpation Per Rectum: The pregnant cervix should be tightly closed and elongated with a prominent portio vaginalis 14-21 days after ovulation. Uterine tone increases and the uterine wall thickens so that by 14-18 days, the endometrial folds can no longer be readily palpated.

The conceptus develops in a recognizable pattern of size and shape, allowing estimation of age based on palpable characteristics. In maiden and barren mares, at 25-28 days of gestation, a careful, experienced palpator may be able to feel the embryonic vesicle ventrally at the base of one uterine horn, producing a bulge 3.5 cm in diameter. At 30 days, the uterine horns are small with pronounced tone, and the conceptus can be felt as a ventral bulge 4 cm in diameter and positioned at the base of the gravid uterine horn. The uterine wall is thin over the expanding conceptus. At 42-45 days, the conceptus occupies about half of the gravid uterine horn and is 5-7 cm in diameter. By 48-50 days, the enlargement of the conceptus begins to involve the uterine body and is 6-8 cm in diameter and 8-10 cm long. At 60 days, nearly the entire gravid horn and half of the uterine body are filled with conceptus, but the nongravid horn remains small with considerable tone. The 60-day conceptus is 8-10 cm in diameter and 12-15 cm long. After 85 days, the turgidity of the conceptus decreases such that the fetus becomes palpable. At 90 days, the conceptus fills the entire uterus, and the cranial portion of the uterus may extend over the brim of the pelvis into the abdominal cavity. After 100-120 days of gestation, the gravid uterus is positioned cranial to the pelvic brim in the abdominal cavity. The ovaries are positioned cranially and ventrally and closer together because of the downward traction exerted by the enlarging uterus on the broad ligament.

Ultrasonography: The spherical shape of the equine embryo and the characteristic pattern of the development of the fetal membranes permit accurate estimation of stage of gestation by ultrasonography until 45 days after ovulation. The embryo may first be imaged in the uterus with a 5.0-MHz linear transducer at 9-10 days as a round nonechogenic conceptus 4 mm in diameter. The spherical conceptus moves throughout the lumen of the uterine horns as well as into the uterine body from day 6-16. Due to specular reflections, the early conceptus is seen to have a bright white (echogenic) line on the dorsal and sometimes the ventral aspect of its image. This specular reflection, embryonic motility, and linear growth rate may be helpful in differentiating an early <16 day, motile embryo from some uterine cysts. At day 17-18, the conceptus has a characteristic "guitar-pick" shape. At day 21, the embryo proper can be seen in the ventral aspect of the yolk sac. At day 25, a heartbeat should be present in the embryo proper, and the allantoic fluid is imaged as an anechoic space ventral to the embryo proper. As the allantoic cavity enlarges, the yolk sac comprises a decreasing portion of the conceptus. The position of the allantois and relative size of the allantoic cavity can indicate the stage of gestation between days 25 and 45. At 30 days, the allantoic cavity occupies one half of the conceptus so that the size of the yolk sac is the same as the size of the allantoic cavity. At 45 days, the only visible fluid cavity is the allantoic cavity, and the fetus hangs from the dorsal wall of the uterus by its umbilical cord and is positioned in dorsal recumbency.

Endocrine Tests: Cells from the conceptus invade the endometrium to form endometrial cups that produce equine chorionic gonadotropin (eCG, formerly called pregnant mare serum gonadotropin) between 40-120 days of gestation. Increased plasma concentrations of eCG (40-120 days) after ovulation are indicative of the presence of endometrial cups. Concentrations of eCG may remain elevated until 120 days, even if fetal death occurs (false positive). A false negative eCG pregnancy test can result if blood sampling is done in a pregnant mare before 40 or after 120 days.

Estrone sulfate is produced by the fetus and is a good indicator of fetal viability. Plasma and urine concentrations of estrone sulfate are elevated after 60 days and 150 days, respectively, of pregnancy.

PARASITE CONTROL DURING PREGNANCY

Most horse dewormers are safe for use throughout pregnancy, but precautions and contraindications on package inserts should be heeded. Ivermectin and oxibendazole have been used safely in pregnant mares. Cambendazole and organophosphates are contraindicated during the first trimester of pregnancy. In general, anthelmintics should not be administered to mares during the first 60 days of gestation (ie, organogenesis) or during the last few weeks before foaling. Otherwise, mares should be dewormed every 6-8 wk, and anthelmintics should be rotated. A low dose of pyrantel tartrate (1.2 mg/lb) can be administered daily throughout gestation. Anthelmintics effective against bots should be used in the fall. Mares can be dewormed 1-2 days after parturition to reduce "foal heat" diarrhea in foals, which is actually caused by small strongyles. Foals should be treated at 6-8 wk of age on the same day as the dam and again at weaning.

VACCINATIONS

Vaccination programs should follow a continuous year-round schedule based on local health problems. Vaccination against rhinopneumonitis should be performed at 3, 5, 7, and 9 mo of gestation. Vaccinations that require annual boosters should be administered 30 days before the due date to stimulate the dam to produce antibodies that will be transferred to the foal via the colostrum (TABLE 4).

ABORTION

See also ABORTION IN HORSES, p 1106. Twin pregnancy may be the most common cause of abortion in mares. It is thought that uterine capacity and subsequent placentation is inadequate to support 2 fetuses to term. Although twins may spontaneously reduce to a viable singleton early in gestation (<60 days), visible abortions tend to be seen after 7-9 mo. Premonitory clinical signs of impending abortion may be only premature mammary gland development. Fetal membranes should always be examined for large avillous areas typically located between twin conceptuses.

Because of the risk of abortion and dystocia in a mare carrying twins, if twins are detected by ultrasonography per rectum at <30 days, reduction to 1 twin by manual

TABLE 4. Example of Vaccination Schedule for Broodmares

Vaccine	Timing
Equine rhinopneumonitis (killed virus)	3, 5, 7, and 9 mo of gestation and after foaling
Tetanus (toxoid)	4-6 wk before foaling
Equine influenza	4-6 wk before foaling; every 2-3 mo during gestation for mares exposed to transient population
Eastern and Western equine encephalomyelitis	Usually administered to mares in late spring or early summer before onset of insect season; depends on location; if foaling late in season, should be administered again 4-6 wk before foaling
Rabies	4-6 wk before foaling; annual if endemic
Botulism (toxoid)	Initially 3 injections at 1 mo intervals, then annual booster 4-6 wk before foaling
Equine viral arteritis (modified live virus)	EVA titer should be documented prior to vaccination; pregnant mares should not be vaccinated; mares should be vaccinated before breeding to a positive stallion that is shedding the virus; mares must be isolated from other horses for 3 wk after vaccination; annual boosters recommended; positive titers may cause problems if mare is to be shipped overseas or to certain farms. (Stallions should also be vaccinated 3 mo before breeding.)
Strangles (bacterin)	Not routinely administered, used only if warranted for a specific mare and situation; occasional problems with abscesses and sore muscles; questionable efficacy
West Nile virus	Recommendations not yet available for pregnant mares; clinically, vaccination during pregnancy seems safe but efficacy is not known

crushing per rectum is recommended (85% success). Between 30-60 days of gestation, transvaginal aspiration of 1 conceptus may result in a viable singleton (20-25% success). After 110 days of gestation, 1 twin may be reduced by intracardiac injection of potassium chloride guided by transabdominal ultrasonography (50% success). Pregnancy should be monitored repeatedly by ultrasonography after twin reduction.

The most common infectious cause of abortion in mares is equine herpesvirus 1 (equine rhinopneumonitis). These abortions occur predominantly in the last trimester and usually are not associated with a respiratory infection. Mares should be vaccinated at 3, 5, 7, and 9 mo of gestation. Equine arteritis virus can also cause abortion. Seronegative mares scheduled to be bred to positive stallions that are shedding the virus should be vaccinated. Vaccinated horses must be isolated for 3 wk after vaccination.

Sporadic abortions due to placentitis can be caused by bacterial and mycotic infections of the placenta. These are predominantly ascending infections acquired through the caudal genital tract, but may also be focal or diffuse. Bacteria involved include *Streptococcus zooepidemicus*, *Escherichia coli*, *Klebsiella pneumoniae*, *Pseudomonas aeruginosa*, *Staphylococcus aureus*, *Rhodococcus equi*, and *Actinobacillus equuli*. Mycotic organisms include *Mucor* and *Aspergillus* spp. These abortions may be prevented by good breeding hygiene, treatment of genital disease before breeding, maintaining good body condition throughout pregnancy, and episioplasty (Caslick's operation) to prevent pneumovagina.

The fetus and fetal membranes should be submitted fresh or cooled to a diagnostic laboratory to attempt to determine the etiology of any abortion.

PARTURITION

Preparation of the Environment: The mare should be taken to the foaling location 3-4 wk before the expected foaling date so she can produce antibodies to the pathogens present in the environment. These antibodies will be sequestered in colostrum for passive immunity in the newborn.

Foaling box stalls should be large (at least 3.5 × 3 × 3.5 m). The foaling area should have good ventilation and be well bedded with clean, dry straw. The walls should be solidly constructed and free of sharp edges. Observation of the mare should be possible without disturbance.

Mammary Gland: Evaluation of the signs that precede parturition is useful but does not permit precise prediction of the time it will be seen. The mammary gland starts developing 3-6 wk before foaling and distends with colostrum in most mares 2-3 days before parturition. Colostrum drips from the teats and dries to form a waxy material at each teat orifice. This "waxing" develops in ~95% of mares 6-48 hr before foaling, but in some cases, it is not seen at all or it precedes parturition by many days. Before foaling, the calcium and potassium content of udder secretions increase, and the sodium content decreases. Water hardness chemical tests have been used on mammary gland secretions to predict imminent parturition.

Stages of Parturition: It is critical to understand the normal progression of events during parturition. This permits identification of abnormal events and whether and when intervention is needed. Parturition is divided into 3 stages.

Stage I is characterized by signs of abdominal pain and restlessness due to uterine contractions. Patches of sweat in the flank area and behind the elbows usually appear a few hours before foaling. The uterine contractions increase in frequency and intensity, causing the fetus to move into the pelvic canal, which causes the cervix to dilate. The fetus changes from a dorsopubic to dorsosacral position before parturition. Mares may roll during the first stage, which is thought to facilitate the rotation of the fetus. Increasing pressure in the uterus causes the allantochorion to protrude through the internal os of the cervix. The allantochorion over the cervix (cervical star) does not have microvilli and is thinner than the rest of the membranes. The allantochorion usually ruptures at the cervical star, and this marks the end of the first stage of parturition.

Stage II starts with the rupture of the allantochorion and ends when the fetus is delivered. Labor usually takes 10-30 min. Stimulation of the cervix by the fetus (Ferguson reflex) causes the mare to have abdominal contractions. The allantoic fluid lubricates the canal, facilitating expulsion of the amnion and fetus. Vaginal distention causes release of oxytocin and further myometrial and abdominal contractions. The amniotic membrane appears between the vulvar lips as a white, fluid-filled structure. The straining efforts of the mare consist of 3-4 strong contractions, followed by a short period of rest. The mare usually assumes lateral recumbency during delivery with her limbs extended. The foal is normally delivered in an anterior presentation and dorsosacral position with the head, neck, and forelimbs extended. One front hoof of the foal usually precedes the other by ~15 cm, facilitating passage of the elbows and shoulders through the pelvic canal. The foal is usually born with the umbilical cord intact and covered by the amnion, which is ruptured by movements of the mare or the foal. If amnion remains over the foal's nose, an attendant should remove it to prevent suffocation. If left undisturbed, the mare may lie for some time with the foal's hindlimbs in her vagina. If the foal has not been delivered within 30 min of the rupture of the chorioallantois and release of the tea-colored allantoic fluid, obstetric intervention is warranted.

Stage III involves expulsion of the fetal membranes. Normally, fetal membrane passage occurs rapidly (within 3 hr) after delivery of the foal. The weight of the amnion and cord helps the allantochorion separate from the endometrium. Progressive traction by the amnion and powerful uterine contractions originating at the tip of the horn cause complete separation of the allantochorion, which may become inverted during the process. The mare will stand with the amnion hanging from the vulva at the level of the hocks or below. If the mare kicks, which endangers the foal, the membranes should be tied above the hocks. If the fetal membranes have not been passed by 3 hr after parturition, oxytocin (20 IU, IV or IM) should be administered at 15- to 30-min intervals.

Premature Separation of the Placenta: Normally, the translucent white amnion appears first at the vulvar lips during the expulsion stage of labor. Premature separation of the placenta is characterized by the appearance of the bright red, velvety, intact chorioallantois between the vulvar lips before the foal is delivered. The presence of the chorion at the vulvar lips indicates that it has separated from the endometrium before the foal is able to breathe spontaneously. The chorioallantois must immediately be ruptured and the foal manually delivered, or the foal may asphyxiate. The severity and duration of asphyxia that results determines the severity of neurologic abnormalities displayed by the foal (peripartum asphyxia or neonatal maladjustment syndrome [p 1039]).

EXAMINATION OF THE PLACENTA

Normally, the membranes are ruptured by the foal over the avillous cervical star region of the chorioallantois. The chorion and allantois (containing many blood vessels) should be examined. Normally, the chorionic surface color ranges from red to brownish red. Patches of discolored, thick, chorioallantois at the cervical star or between the 2 horns may indicate an ascending or focal placentitis. The fetal membranes should be examined for completeness, paying particular attention to the presence of the edematous gravid horn tip and puckered nongravid horn tip.

The amnion has a white translucent appearance and contains many tortuous blood vessels. Small, pale amniotic plaques can normally be seen along the umbilical cord.

Fetal and neonatal foal deaths may be associated with pathologic changes present in the fetal membranes. Typically, the fetal membranes weigh ~10-11% of the foal's body weight. Placentitis or placental edema may increase the weight of the membranes. Integrity of the junction between the fetal and maternal components of the placenta is essential for normal fetal development. The mare has a diffuse eptheliochorial type of placentation, which directly reflects the presence of abnormalities in the endometrium.

Retained Fetal Membranes: Fetal membranes that are not expelled within 3 hr of parturition are considered to be retained. Fetal membrane retention may be complete, but commonly only the nongravid horn is retained. If the typically puckered nongravid tip is not observed, it is assumed to be retained. If any membranes are exposed, the amnion and cord should not be removed because they provide tension necessary for placental separation and expulsion to occur. Membranes not passed within 3-10 hr are considered to be pathologic and can lead to metritis, endotoxemia, and subsequently laminitis with fatal results. Accordingly, it is prudent to treat the condition as potentially serious. If dystocia or traumatic uterine manipulation has occurred, aggressive treatment for retained membranes should be instituted immediately after parturition. For early treatment (3-8 hr), oxytocin at 10-20 IU can be repeatedly administered IV or IM every 15 min until the placenta has passed. The dose of oxytocin should be decreased if the mare shows severe signs of colic or discomfort. Milking or sucking also stimulates endogenous release of oxytocin. Treatment for fetal membrane retention >8 hr should also include broad-spectrum antibiotics, such as potassium penicillin (22,000-44,000 IU/kg, IV, QID), gentamicin (2.2 mg/kg, IV, QID), and NSAID, such as flunixin meglumine (0.25-0.5 mg/kg, IV, TID). (*See also* p 2028.)

THE EARLY POSTPARTUM PERIOD

Uterine involution is characterized by expulsion of the fetal membranes and contraction of the uterus, cervix, and broad ligaments to normal nongravid dimensions. The maximal reproductive efficiency of a broodmare is when a foal is produced every year. Horses have an average gestation length of ~340 days. Therefore, to maintain a 12-mo foaling interval, the mare must be bred again within 25 days of foaling. Mares can be bred on "foal heat," which develops 5-11 days after foaling in most mares. However, mares that experienced dystocia or retained membranes and metritis should not be bred on foal heat. Foal heat pregnancy rates are higher for mares bred at least 10 days postpartum.

The fertility of the first breeding may be increased if breeding is delayed and dinoprost (1 mg/45.5 kg, IM) is administered at ~5 days after the foal heat (first) ovulation. The mare is then bred just prior to the next (second) ovulation.

BREEDING SOUNDNESS EXAMINATION OF THE STALLION

See also BREEDING SOUNDNESS EXAMINATION OF THE MALE, p 1797. The breeding soundness examination should begin with a thorough history, including information regarding libido, mating ability, fertility, prior illness or injury, and any medications administered. A general physical examination should be performed, noting lameness (particularly of the back and hindlimbs) and heritable conditions that may affect breeding ability or desirability as a sire. The penis and prepuce should be free of lesions. The testes and epididymides should be evaluated for size, shape, and consistency. The testes should be freely movable within the scrotum and have a total scrotal width >8 cm. The internal genitalia, inguinal rings, and aorta and iliac vessels are evaluated by palpation and ultrasonography per rectum. For semen collection and evaluation techniques, *see* p 1797.

If consistent heavy growth of potential pathogens such as *Pseudomonas aeruginosa*, *Klebsiella pneumoniae*, or *Streptococcus zooepidemicus* results from aerobic culture of swabs of the genital tract and there is a history of repeated infection in mares bred, it may be necessary to breed by artificial insemination using semen extender continuing an appropriate antibiotic. If natural service is required, semen extender containing an antibiotic may be infused into the mare's uterus before servicing. If *Taylorella equigenitalis* is present, the stallion should not be used for breeding (*see* CONTAGIOUS EQUINE METRITIS, p 1133). The isolation of *T equigenitalis* requires special culture conditions; the organism will not grow in routine aerobic cultures. Stallions with lesions of coital exanthema (p 1119) should not be used for breeding until skin ulcers are completely healed.

BREEDING

Natural Service: Mares are commonly bred by natural service. The proper time to breed is determined by teasing and palpation per rectum, which permits detection of estrus and the presence of a dominant follicle. Estrous mares should be bred when a follicle >30 mm is present or beginning on day 2-3 of estrus and every other day until ovulation occurs or the mare goes out of heat. Mares ovulate 0-48 hr before the end of estrus. Breeding should take place before ovulation.

A tail wrap should be applied, and the perineal area cleansed. The stallion's penis should be rinsed with water before breeding to remove smegma and to minimize contamination of the mare's reproductive tract. The mare should be slowly introduced to the stallion and teased until she displays obvious signs of receptivity (tail raise, abduction of hindlegs, eversion of vulvar lips, urination). A nose twitch may be used for additional restraint. During breeding, the stallion should be controlled adequately to prevent injury to the mare. After breeding, the penis can be rinsed with warm water to reduce potential contamination.

Artificial Insemination: Semen is obtained using an artificial vagina; motility, morphology, and concentration are determined; and the number of morphologically normal, progressively motile sperm is calculated. Semen extender containing an antibiotic is then added to semen to improve sperm survival. A commonly used semen extender is nonfat dry skim milk glucose extender (instant nonfat dry milk [2.4 g], glucose [4.9 g], sterile distilled water [100 mL]). One of the following antibiotics can be added: ticarcillin, 100 mg (1 mg/mL); gentamicin, reagent grade, must be buffered with 2 mL 8.4% $NaHCO_3$, 100 mg (1 mg/mL); or amikacin sulfate 100 mg (1 mg/mL).

The mare is prepared for insemination by application of a tail wrap and cleansing of the perineal area. If soap is used, it should be rinsed thoroughly to remove any residue. Mares should be inseminated with at least $250\text{-}500 \times 10^6$ progressively motile, morphologically normal spermatozoa prior to ovulation. Insemination is accomplished by depositing the semen into the body of the uterus using a sterile, plastic insemination pipette. Disposable equipment is recommended to prevent contamination. Normal sperm cells can be expected to remain viable in the mare's reproductive tract for at least 48 hr. Mares should be examined by palpation and ultrasonography per rectum to determine that ovulation occurs.

MANAGEMENT OF REPRODUCTION: PIGS

Management of commercial swine breeding herds involves a thorough understanding of reproductive physiology, genetics, nutrition, immunology, disease control, environment, and other factors. (*See also* ABORTION IN PIGS, p 1104.) The closed-herd concept, which emphasizes preventive medicine strategies along with herd protection, minimizes the risk of disease loss when combined with sound nutrition and genetic selection. The breeding program should be evaluated at specified intervals to ensure that progress in efficiency is being made. Efficiency parameters to review when analyzing herd reproductive performance include wean-to-estrus interval (WEI), wean-to-service interval (WSI), percent multiple matings, percent repeat services, abnormal returns to service, abortions, farrowing rate, piglets born alive/litter, piglets born dead (ie, stillborns, mummies), preweaning mortality, litters/mated sow/year, pigs weaned/mated sow/year, and nonproductive sow days (TABLE 5). The postweaning performance of a herd can be measured by feed conversion, feed efficiency, total days to market, and postweaning death loss.

Problems on a swine farm are usually caused by a combination of genetic, nutritional, environmental, health, and management factors. When investigating a swine herd problem, the practitioners should concentrate on the herd and not individual animals. Accurate, up-to-date records are essential when investigating a herd problem. When analyzing a herd and its records, one can and should expect a certain percentage of "abnormal" animals and/or reproductive problems.

TABLE 5.   Reproductive Indices Used in Swine Herds

Reproductive Index	Target	Interference Level
Wean-to-estrus interval (95% in estrus by 10 days postweaning)	<7 days	>10 days
Repeat services at 21 days	<10%	>15%
Abnormal returns to service (25-37 days)	<3%	>5%
Multiple matings	>85%	<75%
Abortions	<2%	>2%
Not-in-pig	1%	2.5%
Farrowing rate	>85%	<80%
Live births/litter	10-12	<10
Stillbirths	<5%	>10%
Mummies	<1%	>2%
Litter scatter (≤7 pigs/litter)	<10%	>15%
Weaned/litter	9.5	9
Preweaning mortality	<10%	>15%
Litters/mated sow/year	2.5	<2
Pigs weaned/mated sow/year	≥23	<20
Nonproductive sow days	40	>60
Culling rate	30-50%	>50%

SOW AND GILT MANAGEMENT

Selection: Gilt selection should be based on growth rate, disease status, sexual development, reproductive history (including dam's performance as to wean-to-service and wean-to-estrus intervals, litter size, milking ability, and pigs weaned), conformation, and underline (including teat number and placement). Of potential replacements, up to 30-40% may be culled because of problems such as delayed puberty, failure to conceive, defective teats, locomotor problems, or vulval abnormalities (indicative of intersexuality or genital hypoplasia). Prepubertal gilts are usually fed a grower-finisher ration ad lib until they reach 150-200 lb (68-90 kg) or are 3-5 mo old. At that time, they are usually separated and placed in gilt development, where they are fed a diet formulated specifically for replacement gilts.

Gilts selected for breeding should have exhibited estrus cyclicity by 8 mo. They should not have excessively straight legs or muscling. Their external genitalia should be well developed by 5 mo of age, and their udders and milk pads should be well developed with at least 6 pair of evenly spaced teats.

Disease Precautions: Porcine reproductive and respiratory syndrome (PRRS), parvovirus, pseudorabies, influenza, brucellosis, leptospirosis, and other infectious diseases can affect reproductive performance. The reproductive herd (gilts, sows, and boars) should be vaccinated, at a minimum, against leptospirosis, parvovirus, and erysipelas. Brought-in gilts should be isolated for a minimum of 45-60 days, during which visual observation and serial serologic testing for exposure to undesirable infectious diseases should be done. To minimize the number of days for introduction of these gilts into the breeding herd, the latter portion of the isolation period can be used for acclimatization to the herd's resident pathogens through the introduction of cull sows, market hogs, and manure exchange and/or feedback. This natural exposure to endemic herd pathogens can provide essential protection against diseases such as PRRS, parvovirus, and influenza.

Puberty: Early puberty is desirable to decrease production costs and is considered a good indicator of reproductive capability. First estrus usually is seen between 5-8 mo of age depending on genotype, liveweight, nutritional status, season, and management (including exposure to the boar). Exposure to a sexually mature boar, also known as the "boar effect," is the most influential of all management factors. The boar effect is strongest when females are exposed to the sight, sound, touch, and smell of a mature boar and decreases as the number of senses stimulated by the boar decrease. Consequently, the boar effect is greatest with direct contact using a mature sterile boar. Exposure of peripubertal gilts (5-8 mo old) to a mature boar for 10-15 min/day appears to provide an adequate stimulus. Along with the boar effect, other management tools for manipulating the onset of puberty include crossbreeding, changes in housing (eg, confinement to outside pens and vice versa), and forming new groups by mixing gilts from different pens. Gilts are usually not served until their second or third estrus to allow for uterine development and aid in an optimal ovulation rate and litter size.

Strict culling criteria should be established for the gilt pool. Gilts in which first visible estrus does not occur by 8 mo of age should be culled. Some producers may elect to use injectable gonadotropins to bring these reproductively inefficient gilts into estrus; if this is the case, the progeny should not be kept for breeding herd replacements. Gilts that have been serviced for 3 consecutive estrous cycles and do not conceive should also be culled.

Timing of estrus can be controlled by adding a progestagen to the feed (eg, altrenogest at 15-20 mg/day for 14 days); this is an unapproved use. Estrus will be seen in gilts 4-9 days after the last feeding. This allows estrus in gilts to be synchronized with that of a batch of weaned sows or formation of a group of gilts that will farrow together. Prostaglandins can also be used as an abortifacient to synchronize estrus when administered after day 12 and before day 55 of gestation; females generally come into heat 4-7 days later. The cost-benefit of these programs should be assessed before long-term implementation.

BOAR MANAGEMENT

Male fertility in the breeding program more often than not receives too little attention in herd health programs. As with other food animal species, boars should be examined for breeding soundness before introduction into a herd, whenever they show lack of libido or inability to copulate, or if an increased number of served females return to estrus ~3 wk later. At a minimum, a breeding soundness evaluation should include a history, general physical examination (including genital examination), a semen evaluation, and a behavior evaluation. (*See also* p 1797.)

Selection: When selecting a boar for a breeding program, factors such as origination from a specific disease-free herd, performance, soundness and conformation, age of puberty, and other pertinent parameters related to reproduction should be considered. All boars that are to be used in a breeding program should, at a minimum, be disease seronegative for brucellosis and pseudorabies (Aujeszky's disease). Additionally, all boars should be isolated and acclimatized for at least 45-60 days and be serologically retested for diseases naive to the herd before introduction into the herd. With respect to puberty, boars from large litters (>10 piglets) that reach puberty early ($5^1/2$-6 mo) tend to produce highly productive daughters who also reach puberty at an early age. Performance parameters such as feed efficiency, backfat, and average daily gain are also highly heritable. Skeletal conformation and examination for current or potential locomotor dysfunction should be assessed. Any unsoundness that may interfere with the boar's ability to approach, mount, and successfully breed should be determined. Acute or chronic musculoskeletal conditions may elicit pain that causes the boar to appear uninterested in the female. Boars are usually selected as breeding prospects at 3-8 mo. The genetic background of the boar should be consistent with the intended use. Selection of boars with heritable defects such as umbilical or inguinal hernias, cryptorchidism, rectal prolapse, and poor underlines can be avoided by careful analysis of the source herd production records.

History: A complete history should include the age and origin of the boar, source herd health, immunizations, previous disease problems and treatments, exposure to other animals and premises, as well as the time spent in isolation and exposure to the present premises and its breeding animals. It should also include a description of the boar's previous libido, mating behavior, conception rates, litter size, and performance of relatives and other boars in the herd. For young boars, observations of sexual behavior may be useful.

Physical and Genital Examinations: A general physical examination should be part of every fertility evaluation. Attention should be given to body condition and conformation, including the back and legs, and locomotor function. Osteomalacia, osteoarthrosis, and arthritis, which may result in lameness and reluctance to mount or bear weight on the rear legs, are serious problems.

The testicles, epididymides, and scrotum should be examined and palpated for size, symmetry (<1 cm difference in diameter), consistency, and pathologic changes. An appreciation of normal testicular consistency is necessary to detect subtle changes. The penis and prepuce should be examined for abnormalities during semen collection. Testicular size is directly correlated with genotype, age, and weight of boars between 142-282 days of age and 185-375 lb (84-171 kg) body wt. Testicular size increases until ~18 mo of age; testicular growth and sperm numbers increase at the greatest rate between 5 and 12 mo of age. Because age and testicular weight are important identifiers of early sexual development, boars should be ≥8 mo old before use in a breeding program.

The testicles can be affected by diseases (eg, brucellosis, actinobacillosis) and are vulnerable to trauma by handlers or other animals or as a result of improperly maintained facilities. They should contain no nodules or soft masses. The initial reaction of testicles to trauma or infection is swelling; if untreated, the longterm result is testicular atrophy, identified by increased firmness and loss of resiliency. Asymmetry, as a result of unilateral atrophy, is potentially deleterious to fertility, and semen evaluation may reveal azoospermia, oligospermia, asthenospermia, or morphologic changes indicative of testicular damage.

Behavioral Evaluation and Semen Collection: Collection allows evaluation of libido and ability to mate and ejaculate; in addition, it provides a sample ejaculate. Precopulatory behavior involves visual and olfactory stimulation. The boar grunts or barks rhythmically, chomps jaws, salivates, and typically engages in head-to-head contact with the sow or dummy, followed by nuzzling her flanks to test for voluntary immobilization. These activities should be observed because aberrant sexual behavior may result in infertility. Constant head mounting is a common problem with inexperienced boars.

Poor libido is likely caused by behavioral rather than endocrinologic problems. Fighting and domination by older boars and sows can inhibit libido in young boars. Breed and strain differences are also seen; the tendency to be timid, nervous, and nonaggressive can be influenced by selection in a breed over several generations and can result in boars with poor libido. Pain from genital lesions or musculoskeletal problems can have a strong negative effect. Libido can also be impaired by an unfamiliar environment, the presence of a feared person, or distractions such as available feed.

Once the boar has mounted, erection and protrusion of the penis occur as the boar searches for the vulva. Close observation is necessary to notice injuries and lesions of the penis as well as improper erection. Congenital and genetic problems include incomplete erection, penile hypoplasia, masturbation into the diverticulum (ie, "balling up"), and persistent frenulum.

There are basically 2 methods of semen collection in the boar—the gloved-hand method and electroejaculation. A third method using a water-jacketed artificial vagina is no longer in common use. Although satisfactory ejaculates can be obtained using either the gloved-hand or electroejaculation methods, the gloved-hand method is preferable because it is simpler and reproductive behavior can be simultaneously assessed. The boar is allowed to mount an estrous female and attempt to copulate. Boars used for artificial insemination are usually trained to mount a dummy sow. The boar should then be approached quietly from the rear without being touched or frightened. Preputial fluids are first evacuated by massaging the prepuce to prevent contamination of the ejaculate. The back of the gloved hand is then placed against the ventral abdomen of the boar just cranial to the preputial orifice, and the penis is allowed to thrust into the gloved hand. Digital pressure is applied to the distal 3-6 cm of the penis. If properly stimulated, the boar will fully extend the penis and become very quiet. This is followed immediately by ejaculation. Once the tip of the penis is firmly in the hand and ejaculation has begun, it continues for ≥3-7 min. If the boar dismounts when the attempt is made to grasp the penis, he should be allowed to make several false mounts until he is aggressively attempting intromission again.

A nervous boar may not allow the penis to be locked into the hand, even after several attempts. Semen can be collected from many such boars by allowing them to achieve natural intromission and lock the penis into the sow's cervix to begin the ejaculation, then quickly retrieving the penis and locking it into the hand. The boar will continue to ejaculate, and the major portion of the ejaculate can be collected.

A prewarmed (37°C) vacuum bottle or styrofoam cup is a convenient and economical collection vessel. The pre-sperm fraction, consisting of 5-15 mL of fluid, is usually ejaculated first and allowed to fall on the ground (ie, it is not collected). The boar then usually ejaculates a small amount of gel, which is filtered out of the ejaculate by a double layer of coarse gauze (placed over the mouth of the collection receptacle) because it coagulates into a semisolid mass that can interfere with subsequent evaluation of semen quality. The boar then ejaculates the milky to cream-colored, sperm-rich fraction. The final, sperm-poor, fraction contains the largest volume of fluid and gel. Care should be taken to let the boar complete the ejaculation, voluntarily withdraw the penis from the hand, and dismount. Some boars will go through ≥2 complete ejaculations before voluntarily dismounting.

Semen collection by electroejaculation is done only on an anesthetized boar. An injectable anesthetic that will allow for 15-30 min of general anesthesia is recommended. The rectum is cleaned out using a lubricated hand, and a lubricated rectal probe is inserted. The penis is then exteriorized with the aid of Bozeman sponge forceps and grasped with a surgical sponge wrapped around the penis 5-10 cm distal to the glans penis. Electrostimulation of the boar is performed as in the bull or ram, with the ejaculate collected in a clear, plastic bag that envelops the glans penis.

Semen Evaluation: Standard tests used to evaluate boar semen include sperm motility, morphology, concentration, and total numbers. The ejaculate should be protected from changes in temperature, osmotic pressure, and pH during handling and analysis. All equipment and materials that come into contact with semen should be warmed to 35-39°C.

Sperm motility should be evaluated as soon as possible after collection. Estimating sperm motility in an ejaculate by examining the mass activity or swirl motion of a drop of semen on a slide is of limited value and is not recommended. Gross sperm motility is best estimated on prepared samples in which a monolayer of individual sperm can be visualized using light microscopy. To do this, a 5-10 µL drop of semen is placed on a prewarmed slide and overlaid with a coverglass. Sample motility is then subjectively estimated to the nearest 5% by viewing several random fields under 20× magnification.

Sperm morphology can be a valuable indicator of fertility potential, especially in those ejaculates with a high percentage of abnormal sperm. When using bright-light microscopy, stained slides are necessary to provide adequate contrast for evaluating sperm morphology. When using higher resolution microscopy (ie, phase-contrast, differential interference contrast), glutaraldehyde or buffered formalin preserved samples can be used. A minimum of 100 (preferably 200) sperm should be assessed for morphology of the head, midpiece, and principal piece (ie, the tail distal to the midpiece). Sperm can be categorized into 3 groups: normal, sperm with abnormal heads, and sperm with abnormal tails (midpiece, principal piece, including cytoplasmic droplets). Samples with a high number of sperm defects can be examined further, and abnormalities classified as major and minor defects. Acrosome morphology should also be assessed if possible.

Several techniques are available for determining sperm concentration in a filtered boar ejaculate. A crude, subjective, qualitative estimation of sperm concentration can be done by assessing visual opacity of a raw ejaculate either by direct examination or with the aid of a Karras spermiodensimeter. Analytical determination of sperm concentration can be performed by measuring opacity via a calibrated spectrophotometer on a diluted semen sample. It is essential that the photometer be calibrated for boar semen. Even with a calibrated photometer, estimates of sperm numbers may be ±30% from that of the actual concentration; this can be attributed, in part, to improper technique, human error, and/or the inherent opacity of the secretions of the accessory sex glands present in the boar ejaculate. Photometric readings can also be inaccurate if the reading is outside the calibration curve or optimal operating range. A second, more direct method for measuring sperm concentration is with a hemocytometer or counting chamber. In this method, concentration can be determined by diluting a portion of the filtered ejaculate to a 1:200 ratio—most easily done using a Unopette® system. The hemocytometer should be charged, and the charged unit allowed to set for 5 min so that the sperm settle into one visual field. Using microscopy, a sperm count is performed and calculated as normally done for RBC determination. Determining sperm concentration using a counting chamber is tedious and time consuming, making its use on a routine basis impractical in most commercial operations.

After calculating sperm concentration/mL, total sperm numbers in an ejaculate can be calculated by multiplying sperm concentration with the total volume (in mL) of the gel-free ejaculate. Ejaculate volume can be measured by using a warmed measuring apparatus (eg, graduated cylinder, disposable plastic measuring cups) or by measuring the weight of the ejaculate (with 1 g equivalent to 1 mL).

Interpretation of Findings: Semen values can be affected by frequency of use, age, environment, disease, level of nutrition, genotype, and method of sperm cell fixation. Therefore, boars that do not have acceptable semen values are not necessarily subfertile or infertile. Spermiograms can change dramatically over a short period of time, and boars should not be culled on the evaluation of a single ejaculate. Breed differences in onset of puberty, libido, mating ability, and conception rate have been seen.

Environment can affect fertility over a short period of time, due primarily to disturbances in the thermoregulation of the testes. Boars exposed to cold or hot environmental temperatures may have abnormal spermiograms for ≥7 wk after the insult. Severe exposure may result in abnormal spermiograms for a longer time or may even lead to permanent spermatogenic disruption. Any disease that increases body temperature, and thus disrupts thermoregulation of the testes, also has the potential to cause temporary sub- or infertility.

Guidelines for Boar Evaluation: Ideally, libido, mating ability, semen quality (TABLE 6), and breeding results (conception rate and litter size) should be considered. The duration of spermatogenesis and spermatozoal maturation is ~51 days in the boar. If a boar produces an ejaculate of low or marginal quality when examined in vitro, additional ejaculates should be assessed at 3- to 4-wk intervals to ascertain whether quality has improved over time. Boars with spermiograms that do not improve over 2-3 mo are unlikely to ever improve. Boars with azoospermia on 2 complete ejaculates or that are unable to achieve complete erection should be culled immediately. Those that have penile lesions or blood in the semen should be sexually rested for ≥2-3 wk and reevaluated. For boars with persistent frenulum or that habitually masturbate in the diverticulum, surgical correction is recommended; however, the progeny should not be kept for breeding because these conditions are most likely heritable. All results of the fertility examination must be considered in relation to age, disease history, environmental stress, prior breeding usage, mating system, and the techniques of semen collection and handling.

BREEDING MANAGEMENT

Estrus: Sows and gilts are nonseasonal and polyestrous, with the estrous cycle lasting 18-24 (average 21) days. Sows are behaviorally anestrous during pregnancy. Ovulatory estrus usually is not seen during lactation except under conditions of group rearing, high feed levels, or boar contact. Partial weaning or gonadotropin treatment can induce estrus during lactation, but the results are inconsistent and not economical. Normal uterine physiology is reestablished by 20-25 days postpartum. Most sows exhibit estrus 3-7 days after weaning. Estrus in gilts and postweaning anestrous sows can be initiated with exogenous hormones. However, these hormones circumvent natural selection for reproductive efficiency, and this should be kept in mind when they are used in breeding management programs. Exogenous hormones should not be used as a longterm solution to address reproductive inefficiency in a herd.

Estrus lasts ~36-48 hr in gilts and ≥48-72 hr in sows. Time to estrus after weaning and duration of estrus in sows can be influenced by length of lactation, nutrition, body condition, genetics, and other management practices (TABLE 7). Estrus is characterized by behavioral (eg, mounting, fence walking, vocalizing, tilted ears, kyphosis) and sometimes physical (eg, vulvar swelling, vaginal discharge) changes. Ovulation generally occurs in mid to late estrus. During ovulation, ~15-24 ova are released over a 1- to 4-hr period. Ovulation rate increases over the first 4 parities, so that the fourth to sixth litters tend to be the

TABLE 6. Suggested Minimum Spermiogram Values for Breeding Boars

Parameter	Natural Service	Artificial Insemination
Color	Opaque to white	Opaque to white
Total sperm numbers	>35 × 10^9 sperm/ejaculate	>35 × 10^9 sperm/ejaculate
Gross motility (raw)	>60%	>70%
Abnormal morphology (including cytoplasmic droplets)	<25%	<20-25%
Cytoplasmic droplets (both proximal and distal)	<15%	<15-20%

TABLE 7. Factors Affecting Ovarian Activity of Pigs*

Proven or Suspected Factors	Stage of Breeding Affected		
	Puberty	After weaning	After service
Insufficient male stimulation	+[†]	+	−[‡]
Housing and social environment	+	+	−
High ambient temperature	+	+	+
Season of year (summer/fall)	+	+	+
Photoperiod	+	?[§]	
Genotype	+	+	+
Nutrition	+	+	+
Short lactation	−	+	−
Large litter reared	−	+	−

*Adapted, with permission, from Meredith MJ, *Pig News and Information* 5, 1984, published by CAB International, Wallingford, Oxon, UK.

[†]Effect has been demonstrated

[‡]No evidence for effect

[§]Effect uncertain

largest in number. Ovulation rate can decrease when gilts or sows are undernourished. Most gilts are on full feed, thereby averting the adverse affects of undernourishment on early reproductive performance. In countries in which gilts are not routinely provided full feed, increasing energy intake for 10 days before estrus (ie, "flushing") is performed. This has optimized ovulation rate under these circumstances. To prevent undernourishment in recently weaned sows, an energy-dense diet should be fed until after estrus and breeding.

Behavioral changes are most pronounced when the sow or gilt is exposed directly to the sight, sound, odor, and attention (nuzzling and grunting) of a mature boar. A sow or gilt in standing heat normally assumes a rigid, immobile, receptive stance when exposed to a boar. Physical changes such as vulvar swelling and discharge are often unreliable; they do, however, appear to be more marked in gilts than sows and commonly develop 2-3 days before estrus. The ultimate criterion of estrus is either standing to the boar or a positive response to the "riding test" (an attendant applies pressure with the hands in the loin area, then gently sits on the pig's back to elicit the standing reaction; this test is best conducted in the presence of a boar (eg, in an adjacent pen) or, as an alternative, after exposing the sow to a synthetic boar-odor aerosol or taint rag.

Anestrus is a common problem. Failure to detect estrus must be distinguished from true cases of ovarian inactivity. First-litter and early-weaned sows are particularly vulnerable to postweaning anestrus. The primiparous sow must support her own growth as well as maintenance and lactation demands while her feed intake capacity is not yet fully developed. This problem can be avoided by breeding only gilts in good condition; not overfeeding during the first gestation; and encouraging energy intake during the first lactation by frequent feeding of high-density diets, wet feeding, and avoiding high temperatures in the farrowing rooms. Management practices such as segregated early weaning, modified medicated early weaning, and medicated early weaning recommend weaning as early as 10 days postpartum; postweaning anestrus is not an uncommon sequela of these management techniques. General guidelines to minimize the negative effect of early weaning on sow reproduction recommend weaning at no less than 14-16 days into lactation for primiparous sows, at no less than 12-14 days into lactation for sows on their second litter, and at no less than 9-11 days into lactation for sows on their third or subsequent litters.

Breeding: The 3 methods of breeding are pen mating (boar run with females), hand mating (supervised natural mating), and artificial insemination (AI). Pen mating is generally found on smaller operations and works best in a pen of pigs in various stages of the estrous cycle. Pen mating with a group of recently weaned sows is less desirable because their estrous cycles may occur close together and lead to overuse of the boar. In hand mating, the female is usually mated 2-3 times during estrus, with the first service on the first day of standing estrus, and subsequent matings at 24-hr intervals; confirmed matings should be recorded. Many commercial producers breed the sow or gilt once daily as long as she will accept the boar. The use of 2 different boars may increase the number of pigs per litter but may mask infertility in one of the boars.

In AI programs, heat detection is performed either twice or once per day. If heat detection is performed twice per day, gilts should be inseminated twice, 8-12 hr after the onset of standing heat and again 12-16 hr later. Sows should be inseminated 24 hr after onset of standing heat and again 18-24 hr later. If heat detection is performed once per day, gilts should be inseminated within 4 hr and sows within 12-16 hr from when they were first seen in standing heat. A second insemination should be performed as described above for those animals that remain in standing heat. As a general guideline, timing of AI may need to be modified based on a particular farm's availability of labor, building design, or herd genetics. Some experienced users of AI obtain satisfactory results with a timed, single insemination; however, performing 2 inseminations is more common. Inseminations can be performed using either single-sire (sourced from 1 boar) or pooled (sourced from multiple [3-6] boar ejaculates) extended semen. In general, single-sire matings are performed when particular genetic (ie, breeding or show animals) offspring are desired, whereas matings with pooled semen are used as a means to produce market hog offspring. For extended semen used within 72 hr after collection, the recommended dose is 2-3 billion sperm ($2-3 \times 10^9$) in 60-80 mL; total sperm numbers in a dose of semen depend on quality and storage time of the semen.

Boars should not be overused (TABLE 8). If sows are weaned in groups, a boar-to-sow ratio of 1:4 for mature boars and 1:2 for young boars is recommended. In hand mating, a mature boar should be used for ≤2 breedings/day. When using natural service, a boar-to-sow ratio of 1:15-1:25 (average 1:17 or 18) is usually needed. When using AI, the boar-to-sow ratio can be increased to 1:150-1:250.

Pregnancy: Sperm cells reach the oviducts within 30 min of mating, and fertilization can occur within 2-6 hr. Fertilization rates approach 100% in sows, but embryo mortality up to 30-40% accounts for the usual litter size of 10-12 pigs. Embryos enter the uterus ~48-60 hr after ovulation. Embryos hatch from the zona pellucida and form blastocysts 144 hr after ovulation. Maternal recognition of pregnancy (embryos secreting estradiol) occurs by day 10-14 of gestation, with intrauterine migration and distribution of embryos. Embryo attachment begins by day 13-14, with implantation complete by day 40; a minimum of 4 embryos must be present at this time for pregnancy to continue. Skeletal mineralization develops by day 35, with fetuses immunocompetent by day 70-75. Fetal deaths that occur after day 35 can result in expulsion or retention of recognizable piglets.

TABLE 8.   Suggested Guidelines for Boar Usage Based on Breeding Program*

Artificial Insemination		Natural Mating		
Boar Age (mo)	Semen collection frequency[†]	Matings/day	Total matings/ week	Pen-breeding (females/mo)
6-8	1 time/wk	1	4	<8
8-12	1-2 times/wk	1	5-7	8-10
>13	≥4 times/2 wk	2 (spaced)	8-10	10-12

*Depends on boar libido

[†]Adapted from Althouse GC. *Animal Health and Production Compendium*, 2002, by CAB International, Wallingford, Oxon, UK.

Retained dead fetuses in this sterile environment become mummified and are usually expelled at the time of farrowing. The average gestation length is 114 ± 2 days and is somewhat shortened in sows with large litters.

Embryos are at greatest risk of dying during the first 30 days, and efforts should be directed toward avoiding stresses (eg, overfeeding, heat, handling or moving, immunization) during this critical period. Pregnancies of <16 days are especially sensitive to heat stress. Avoiding exposure to outside animals reduces disease risk. If the gilts have been flushed for breeding, the feed intake should be reduced to the limit feeding level of 4-5 lb (~2 kg) immediately after breeding to avoid embryo loss due to high energy intake. Farrowing <5 piglets is indicative of embryo death after the time of attachment.

To increase colostral antibodies, the gilt or sow should be immunized during the last 6 wk of gestation. An immunization program may include vaccination against *Escherichia coli*, atrophic rhinitis, erysipelas, and any other vaccines appropriate for the disease situation on the individual farm.

Pregnancy Determination: Several techniques are available for pregnancy determination (TABLE 9). Pregnancy is most commonly diagnosed by noting that the female does not return to estrus in 18-25 days; this is 75-85% accurate. Ultrasonography is another popular technique, and 3 types can be used: pulse echo (A-mode), Doppler, and real-time. Pulse echo or amplitude depth involves emitting ultrasonic waves from a hand-held transducer placed on the skin in the flank area. Reflected waves from a fluid-filled area (ie, developing conceptus or fetus) are picked up by the transducer and converted into either an audible or visual signal. Doppler ultrasonography detects changes in sound frequency (fluid movement) using an audible signal; movements indicative of pregnancy include blood flow in middle uterine or umbilical arteries, fetal heartbeat, and fetal movements. Real-time ultrasonography involves visualization of a 2-dimensional image of scanned tissues directly under the transducer. Ultrasonographic techniques are generally used at 22-75 days for determining pregnancy, with real-time ultrasonography being used as early as 18 days after breeding. Rectal palpation can be used to confirm pregnancy at >30 days gestation. The examiner palpates for fremitus, size, and position of the middle (medial) uterine artery in relation to the external iliac artery. The tone and tension of the cervix and weight and contents of the uterus can also be used to aid in confirming pregnancy. Other techniques such as hormonal assays (eg, estrone glucuronide, progesterone, prostaglandin) and vaginal biopsy can be used but are not economically feasible.

Parturition: The preparturient period involves restlessness and nest building the last 24 hr. Mammary glands become turgid, and the secretion changes from serous to milk as parturition approaches. Parturition is initiated by increased cortisol levels, which also stimulate release of prostaglandin (PG) $F_{2\alpha}$ from the uterus. $PGF_{2\alpha}$ causes luteolysis of the corpora lutea and release of relaxin, which causes relaxation of the birth canal and cervix. Oxytocin is released from the pituitary gland, which causes uterine contractions

TABLE 9.	Common Tests to Detect Pregnancy In Pigs	
Technique	Test Type	**Application of Test After Breeding (Accuracy)**
Estrus detection	Indirect	Daily testing 18-25 days (75-85%) and through gestation (98%)
External physical signs	Indirect	>55 days (gilts); >84 days (sows)
Rectal palpation (sows)	Indirect	30 days (94%), >60 days (100%)
Ultrasonography		
A-mode	Indirect	30-75 days (95%)
Doppler	Direct/Indirect	≥35 days (>85%)
Real-time (B-mode)	Direct	≥22 days (>95%)

and onset of labor. Piglets are usually delivered at frequent intervals (10-15 min; 5-45 min range). Uterine horn evacuation is random. The stillbirth rate usually is 5-10%; intrauterine deaths are due to infection, incorrect position in the uterine horn during delivery, or anoxia. Anoxia is seen when the umbilical cord ruptures or becomes constricted because of the extreme length of the uterine horn, or when there is a delay in transit along the birth canal. Stillborn and weak piglets also may be due to low temperatures in the farrowing house or low Hgb levels (<9 g/dL) in the sow. Any increase in the time interval between pigs born (eg, due to exhaustion, atony of the uterus, or dystocia) increases the chance of injury or death to the piglets still in the uterus. Piglets are born in both cranial (60%) and caudal (40%) presentation. Assistance can be provided in the form of oxytocin injections (10-30 IU) and manual removal of piglets. Walking the sow for a few moments also can be helpful. The number of pigs born alive can be increased by ~1/sow if an attendant is present to assist delivery (see PREWEANING MORTALITY, below).

Farrowing can be induced by IM injection of 10-15 mg of natural $PGF_{2\alpha}$ or equivalent dose of synthetic analogs. Farrowing generally occurs 18-36 hr later (most within 22-32 hr) in 80-90% of sows when $PGF_{2\alpha}$ is given at 112-113 days gestation. Induction can be used so that most farrowings take place during normal working hours, avoiding weekends and holidays. Good records are essential, and average days of gestation for the sow herd and individual breeding dates for each sow must be known. $PGF_{2\alpha}$ must be used within 72 hr of the expected farrowing date to prevent an increase in stillbirths. The slightly premature piglets require good environmental conditions, particularly in winter. Farrowings may be concentrated into an even shorter period by injecting 20 IU of oxytocin 15-24 hr after the $PGF_{2\alpha}$ injection. This shortens the interval to parturition but can be accompanied by an increase in dystocia.

Incidence of dystocia is low (1-2%) in sows. As with all polytocous species, uterine inertia accounts for most dystocia in swine. Other causes include fetal malposition, obstruction of the birth canal, deviation of the uterus, fetopelvic disproportion, and maternal excitement. A thorough digital examination of the birth canal is prerequisite to therapeutic intervention. Medical therapy for unobstructive dystocia may include use of an ecbolic agent (oxytocin at 20-30 IU every 30 min, up to 3 times). Administration of injectable calcium may be warranted if uterine inertia is suspected.

Lactation peaks at 3-4 wk postpartum. Sows that have been on an 8-wk lactation produce 400-700 lb of milk. Poor lactation is a significant cause of impaired productivity in pigs (see POSTPARTUM DYSGALACTIA SYNDROME, p 1134).

Preweaning Mortality: Supervised farrowing alone can help to reduce piglet mortality because it minimizes stillbirths, provides piglets with needed warmth, allows for observation of nursing activity, and prevents crushing and cannibalism. Other management techniques available for reducing piglet mortality include cross-fostering, split-suckling, well-designed farrowing crates and pens, prepartum vaccination of sows, appropriate feeding programs for lactating sows, and cleanliness.

MANAGEMENT OF REPRODUCTION: SHEEP

Both genetic and nongenetic factors can markedly affect the reproductive performance of sheep flocks. Breed differences have been recorded in the duration of anestrous periods, occurrence of photoperiod effect, conception rates, semen quality, embryo mortality, birth and weaning weights, percentage of multiple births, ovarian and behavioral response to hormones, and adaptation to environmental stress. Rapid changes, with improvements in some characteristics (including reproduction), can be achieved by crossbreeding, provided that the crosses are appropriate for the local conditions. In the USA and Australia, the introduction of Finnsheep and the Booroola (Australia) and Inverdale (New Zealand) genes has resulted in significant increases in the number of live lambs produced per ewe. This can be advantageous under intensive or semi-intensive conditions in which multiple births are of maximal advantage. Nongenetic factors that influence reproductive efficiency include season of mating and lambing, nutrition, the presence of phytoestrogens, disease, management techniques, male or female infertility, isolation or presence of the male, and environmental factors. These factors can interact within a flock to cause losses at many, but specific, stages of the reproductive cycle.

Reproductive efficiency in sheep is usually measured by weaning percentage (number of lambs surviving to weaning, divided by the number of ewes mated). Acceptable figures depend on the type of operation; weaning percentages range from 70-85% under range conditions with minimal shelter to 170-200% under intensive confinement systems. Lamb marking percentages are also used to measure reproductive efficiency. Lamb marking percentages in Merino flocks in western Australia over a 30-yr period varied between 57% and 75%, and average 72% in southern Australia. The major factors contributing to low marking percentage include those associated with low fertility combined with embryonic and fetal death or neonatal mortality seen mainly in the early postnatal period. Fertility can be increased by improved nutrition, mating during the fall, the use of teaser rams to hasten the onset of ovarian cyclicity (ram effect), improved preparation of rams before joining, reduction in the dietary intake of phytoestrogens and plant-associated toxins, pasture management, and control of diseases of the reproductive system of the ewe and ram.

REPRODUCTIVE PHYSIOLOGY

Ewes are seasonally polyestrous, cycling every 16-17 days during the breeding season. The major environmental factor controlling the estrous cycle is the photoperiod. Geographic location and environmental temperatures also modify the length of anestrus, as does the breed of sheep. Fine-wool breeds (eg, Rambouillet, Merino) and Dorsets have a shorter anestrous period than other breeds such as the Suffolk, Hampshire, Border Leicester, and Columbia. Regardless of this breed-related variation in the length of the breeding season, all breeds are most fertile in the fall, and anestrus is an unlikely problem associated with regular annual mating.

The duration of estrus (~30 hr) is also influenced by the breed and age of the ewe, the onset of puberty, the presence of the male, and the season. Estrous periods that occur in the fall are longer and more intense, and maiden ewes have a shorter and less intense estrus than mature ewes. In general, a ewe's reproductive performance is maximal at 4-5 yr. The optimal time to mate ewes (naturally or artificially) is in the first half of the estrous period or 12-18 hr after the onset of estrus. Ewes show no overt signs of estrus, and heat detection requires the presence of a ram or testosterone- or estrogen-treated wether.

The age of puberty of ewe lambs varies greatly and is influenced by breed, nutrition, presence of the ram, and season of birth. Well-grown ewe lambs, particularly of the meat breeds, can be mated at 7-8 mo of age and 75-100 lb (35-45 kg) body wt; maximal conception rates are seen in ewes with body condition score 3.5. Ewes that cycle as lambs may have higher twinning rates as adults; therefore, selecting such ewes for replacements increases the prolificacy of the flock. However, this will increase the nutritional demand of the flock, reducing the number of ewes that can be maintained at pasture. Ewes that breed as lambs are able to produce more lamb crops than those bred as 2-yr-olds, although the increase in lifetime lamb production may be small.

Follicle development and ovulation rates, which are major determinants of fertility, are influenced by breed and genetic factors, age, nutrition, body condition, and season. Breeds such as the Finnsheep consistently have multiple ovulations, while Merino ewes average 1.3 conceptus. Ovulation rate is a polygenic trait showing some breed difference; heritability estimates are low (0.3-0.5%). Single genes with a large effect have been determined in a number of breeds, most notably the Booroola Merino. In this strain, the gene, at an autosomal locus, has an additive effect on ovulation rate. This Fec-B gene (fecundity Booroola) has been introduced into other breeds, eg, Border Leicester. Ewes homozygous for the gene have a high ovulation rate (eg, 7) but low numbers of lambs born due to embryo death. Ewes heterozygous for the gene are the most fecund. Crossing British breed rams homozygous for the gene with Merino ewes produces heterozygous crossbred ewes that have high ovulation rates; in Australia and the USA, they are crossed with meat breeds to produce lambs for meat.

Ewe lambs have lower ovulation rates than mature ewes, and ovulation rates tend to be higher for all breeds in the fall. Nutrition affects ovulation rate; ewes that are relatively heavier or that have higher body condition scores generally have more ovulations than lighter ewes. Nutritional supplementation over a few weeks before mating ("flushing") may result in higher ovulation rates. However, flushing by itself may offer no benefit beyond that consistent with any increase in body weight or condition of the ewe, although in some cases ovulation rate increases before any change in body weight. Flushing with limited amounts of protein-rich supplements before and during mating increases ovulation rate and is generally required for ewes on protein-deficient pasture. Overfeeding of both energy and crude protein leads to decreased oocyte quality. Toxins associated with high-protein grains can increase liver metabolism, possibly increasing progesterone breakdown and reducing embryo implantation. Plant mycotoxins and the phytoestrogens present in some strains of subterranean clover can cause high- or low-grade infertility that may be temporary or permanent. Temporary phytoestrogen infertility is seen when ewes graze highly estrogenic pastures around the time of mating; it is due to reduced incidence of estrus and twin ovulations, transport of ova through the oviduct, and transport of sperm through the cervix (resulting in reduced conception rates). Permanent phytoestrogen infertility results from prolonged exposure to phytoestrogens. The basis is failure of fertilization resulting from failure of sperm transport through the cervix, reflecting estrogen-induced transdifferentiation of the cervix. The cervix histologically resembles the uterus, and the structure of the cervical mucus is altered, resulting in reduced ability to form mucus strands or threads and impairing passage of sperm. The wall of the uterus is also altered, preventing implantation and survival of the embryo.

Estrus Induction: Estrus, though not necessarily with a fertile ovulation, can be induced in acyclic and anestrous ewes by the introduction of rams (ram effect) or by treatment with progestagens, equine chorionic gonadotropin (eCG), and exogenous melatonin. (*See also* HORMONAL CONTROL OF ESTRUS, p 1808.)

The sudden introduction of rams or teasers (vasectomized or epididymectomized rams or testosterone-treated wethers) to ewes that have been isolated from rams, bucks, and their odor can induce the onset of ovarian cyclicity. The response to this "ram effect" depends on the depth of anestrus of the ewes (which is generally higher in British breeds), in the middle of the photoperiod anovulatory season, in nutritionally challenged ewes, in young ewes, and in the early postpartum period. Merino ewes respond readily throughout the photoperiod anovulatory season, while British breeds commonly respond only when the onset of the ovulatory season is close. Responding ewes commonly ovulate within 48 hr of ram introduction and may or may not display estrus. Ewes that do show estrus and that mate and ovulate in the first 4-5 days after ram introduction lack preovulatory progesterone and generally have poor conception rates. Some of these ewes may not continue to cycle. In ewes with a silent estrus, ovulation is followed by the formation of either a normal or a short-lived (5-6 days) corpus luteum (CL). After regression of a normal CL, most ewes display estrus (~19 days after ram introduction). After regression of a short-lived CL, ewes ovulate without displaying estrus and commonly form a normal CL. Regression of this CL results in estrus (~25 days after ram introduction). Pretreatment of acyclic ewes with progestagen pessaries—but not with a progesterone injection—for 7-10 days before ram introduction results in estrus accompanying the early ovulation. The ovulation rate is higher at this progesterone-supported estrus than at subsequent heats and may be fertile.

Estrus can also be induced by treatment with progestagen pessaries for 7-14 days, followed by eCG at 600-750 IU. Factors affecting fertility following the induction of estrus include breed, season, lactation, and postpartum period, as well as the ewe's dry/suckling status, mating by natural or artificial insemination, and number of inseminations (1 or 2).

Acyclic, seasonally anestrous ewes can be induced into estrus and to ovulate with exogenous melatonin. Ewes are given melatonin 6 wk prior to joining and are isolated from rams during that period. The joining period should cover 2 complete estrous cycles

(35 days). Exogenous melatonin is more successful toward the end of the seasonal anestrous period.

Estrus Synchronization: Estrus can be synchronized in estrous cyclic and acyclic ewes by inserting progestagen-containing pessaries or controlled intravaginal drug releasing devices (CIDR) into the vagina for 12-15 days. The longer period may yield tighter synchrony but lower conception rates. Synchronization and conception are improved by use of eCG or pregnant mare serum gonadotropin (PMSG) (200-400 IU) at the time of pessary or CIDR removal. They can be further improved with the use of prostaglandin (PG) $F_{2\alpha}$ or its analogs (either at, or 12-24 hr before, pessary or CIDR removal), which regresses remnant corpus luteal tissue. SC elastomer "plugs" containing norgestomet (2 mg) can be inserted under the skin of the ear for 14 days for the same effect. Estrous cyclic ewes can also be synchronized by 2 injections of $PGF_{2\alpha}$ or its analogs 8-14 days apart. Estrus commonly is seen 2-3 days after progestagen removal, with a shorter interval during the fall, or within 3 days of the second PG injection. Fertility is better using progestagen pessaries or CIDR than using PG alone, which are less reliable for fixed-time breeding programs.

Superovulation: Ovulation rates can be increased with the use of follicle stimulating hormones such as FSH, PMSG, or human chorionic gonadotropin (hCG) or with the use of vaccines against androgenic hormones. PMSG is the most common product used in natural and artificial insemination programs, while hCG is used in embryo transfer programs. Antiandrogenic vaccines result in a decreased level of plasma-free androgen and increased gonadotropin release. Vaccination given at 5 and 2 wk before a 5-wk joining results in an increase of 15-35% in lambs marked, with better results in higher conditioned ewes. Vaccination does not reduce the number of nonpregnant ewes in the flock. One vaccine, given to Romney ewes 8 wk and 4 wk prior to joining (with an annual booster 4 wk before joining), increased ovulation rate by 60%, with a 20% increase in lambs marked. Management of late pregnant and lambing ewes is critical in these expanded lambing systems.

PRENATAL LOSSES

Embryo mortality is seen up to the end of implantation—about day 40 in sheep. It is the main source of loss during pregnancy; deaths during the fetal period, after 40 days, are usually few. Because most embryonic deaths are seen sufficiently early in pregnancy to allow at least one more service before the rams are removed, early embryo mortality does not usually result in a dramatic fall in lambing percentages; however, it delays lambing, increases its time distribution, reduces twinning rates, leaves a few ewes barren, and is a problem with short joining periods of 5-6 wk (2 estrous cycles). Embryo death before day 12 does not disturb the normal cycle length, whereas embryo death after this time increases cycle length.

The basal level of embryonic mortality (ie, that occurring in the absence of recognized stress) has been estimated to be 20-30%. The causes of this loss are unknown, although environmental factors such as severe undernutrition or marked increase in nutrition, plant toxins, selenium deficiency, and high temperatures may increase embryonic loss above this basal level. Ureaplasmosis may also contribute to embryonic mortality.

Fetal death results most commonly from infectious processes, and the organisms responsible almost invariably have their effect in middle and late pregnancy.

PREGNANCY DETERMINATION

Accurate determination of pregnancy allows differential ewe management by allowing the separation of multiple pregnant ewes for supplementary feed and lambing supervision and for culling of nonpregnant ewes. Procedures for the diagnosis of pregnancy can involve detection of ewes that do not return to estrus (nonmarking by ram or teaser fitted with harness and crayon); transabdominal, real-time ultrasonographic scanning; rectoabdominal palpation (from 70 days); abdominal palpation (from 100 days); measurement of plasma progesterone concentrations 18 days after mating (detectable progesterone levels indicate an active CL); and laparoscopy (from 30 days). Real-time ultrasonography (from 20 days) is a rapid, highly sensitive and very specific test for pregnancy diagnosis of ewes and does. It involves placing the ultrasonographic transducer in the woolless area of both flanks and directing the beam forward and upward toward the last rib on the opposite side. It is possible to examine, at low cost, 100-150 ewes/hr and to accurately diagnose single and multiple fetuses.

RAM MANAGEMENT

To achieve maximum fertility, rams should be physically examined for reproductive fitness to detect any abnormalities that may limit mating. (*See also* BREEDING SOUNDNESS EXAMINATION OF THE MALE, p 1797.) The scrotum and its contents and the penis and prepuce must be carefully examined. The size and symmetry of both testes and epididymides should be assessed, and both testes should be firmly palpated for consistency and resilience. Any palpable lesions, particularly of the epididymides, should be considered potentially contagious (eg, *Brucella ovis* and *Actinobacillus seminis*). Appropriate tests should be performed to establish a flock diagnosis to initiate a test and eradicate program for infected rams. Semen can be collected and evaluated to screen potential sires, particularly in single-sire mating systems. All screening procedures should be done 6-8 wk before mating to allow management changes of the ram team or purchase of replacements for defective rams. Supplementary feeding of the rams can be started 6 wk prior to joining. High-protein grains, particularly lupines, increase both testicular size and the number of cells in the germinal layers of the testicle, resulting in increased sperm production.

Mating activity can be monitored by using a breeding harness on the rams and changing the crayon color every 14-17 days. When fewer than expected ewes are marked, poor ram libido, a low ram-to-ewe ratio, or anestrus is suggested. When ewes are serially marked with different colors, conception failure or early embryonic death is suspected.

Under flock conditions with multi-sire matings, mature rams usually make up 1-2% of the flock; single sires are used for stud flocks. Flock dispersion should be avoided at mating, but normal handling should not affect mating. Because younger ewes have a shorter, less intense estrous period, they are better mated separately from older ewes with experienced, though not necessarily older, rams.

Collection of Semen: The artificial vagina is used most commonly for collection of ram semen. It is prepared for collection by the introduction of warm water (100-130°F [40-55°C]) and air between the outer casing and soft inner sleeve, lubrication with petrolatum in the end where intromission of the penis occurs, and attachment of a graduated collecting glass at the opposite end. Rams quickly learn to mount a restrained ewe, and intromission and ejaculation are extremely rapid.

The second method of semen collection is by electroejaculation, for which the ram may be restrained on its side. The lubricated bipolar electrode is inserted into the rectum. The withdrawn penis is held with a piece of gauze to facilitate insertion of the glans into a 10- to 15-mm diameter graduated collecting tube. Ejaculation usually occurs after a few short electrical stimulations; "stripping" of the urethra may be helpful when expulsion of semen seems incomplete. Electroejaculation is less reliable than the artificial vagina; specimens vary in quality and can be contaminated with urine.

The volume of semen collected with the artificial vagina is 0.5-1.8 mL, and the concentration of the spermatozoa is $2.5\text{-}6.0 \times 10^9$/mL. Semen obtained by electroejaculation generally is of larger volume but lower concentration.

Evaluation of Semen: Immediately after collection, the semen is assessed for contamination, volume, concentration of spermatozoa, and sperm motility (wave motion and sperm progression).

Extension of Semen: Semen can be processed by extending or diluting, packaging, and storing. Semen may be extended 5-fold, depending on the initial concentration, the processing and storage method, and whether the semen will be used fresh, chilled, or frozen-thawed. Most semen extenders or diluents are based on Tris, egg yolk, and additional cryoprotectants such as glycerol. Commercial extender concentrates contain cryoprotectants and require the addition of egg yolk and double-distilled water. These extenders can be used for either fresh or frozen semen.

Extenders for fresh and chilled semen include whole, skimmed, or reconstituted cow's milk that has been heated to 92-95°C for 8-10 min in a water bath to inactivate toxic factors, egg yolk/glucose/citrate (15% egg yolk, 0.8% glucose [anhydrous], 2.8% sodium citrate dihydrate in glass-distilled water). The addition of Tris or glycerol improves the sperm survival of frozen-thawed semen. The reconstitution of frozen-thawed semen with fresh seminal plasma improves its fertilizing ability when used for intracervical insemination but not for intrauterine insemination. The number of motile spermatozoa and the volume of an insemination dose for the ewe depends on the site of insemination and the method of processing. For vaginal insemination, 0.3-0.5 mL with 300 million motile spermatozoa is used; for cervical insemination, 0.05-0.2 mL is used with 100, 150, and 180 million spermatozoa of fresh, liquid-stored, and frozen-thawed semen, respectively. Intrauterine insemination by laparoscopy requires 0.08-0.25 mL (with a total of 20 million motile spermatozoa) into each uterine horn.

Storage of Semen: Ram semen may be stored for up to 24 hr by cooling the extended semen to 35-41°F (2-5°C) over 90-120 min and by holding at this temperature. Fertility decreases rapidly and is low by 48 hr.

Freezing and storage of ram semen in 0.25-0.3 mL, 3-dose pellets or in 0.25 mL, single-dose synthetic straws at liquid nitrogen temperature (-320°F [-196°C]) is successful in maintaining sperm viability, but there may be a range in post-thaw motility and fertility between rams or processing batches. Use of frozen-thawed semen may result in lambing rates of 50% with cervical insemination and of 50-80% with intrauterine insemination.

Freeze-thawing reduces the numbers of motile sperm. Chilling results in membrane changes that reduce the longevity of sperm. The membrane changes are similar to capacitation and acrosome reactions, and affected sperm are thus ready to fertilize oocytes. Fresh seminal plasma mitigates the effects of some of the capacitation changes.

ARTIFICIAL INSEMINATION

The optimal time for insemination with nonfrozen semen is 12-18 hr after the onset of estrus. When estrus has been synchronized or induced using progestagens and gonadotropins and/or ram effect, most ewes are in estrus within 36-48 hr and ovulate at ~60 hr. Insemination should be done 48-58 hr after pessary removal for cervical insemination, or 48-60 hr for intrauterine insemination with frozen-thawed semen, with highest conception around 53-54 hr.

Extended fresh or chilled semen can be placed into the vagina or cervix, and extended fresh, chilled, or frozen-thawed semen can be placed into the uterus. Frozen-thawed semen reconstituted with fresh seminal plasma can be placed into the cervix with conception rates >50%.

Vaginal Insemination: An artificial insemination pipette with a 1-2 mL syringe attached is placed deep into the vagina. This method is quick and involves minimal restraint of the ewe. For cervical insemination, the ewe is restrained to limit movement and to present the hindquarters at a convenient height for easy access to the vagina. After cleaning the vulvar region, the cervix is located with the aid of a speculum and suitable illumination, and the insemination made as deeply as possible into the cervical canal. A long, thin inseminating tube with attached syringe or a semiautomatic inseminating device can be used. The relatively long, tortuous, and firm-walled cervical canal of the ewe usually precludes penetration by the tube for >1 cm. In old, multiparous ewes with cervical tissue distortion, the difficulty increases, and the semen is deposited into the posterior folds of the cervix. In periparturient ewes, the cervix may be fully penetrated. In maiden ewes, in which insertion of the speculum and dilation of the vagina can cause injury, the semen should be deposited in the anterior vagina.

Intrauterine Laparoscopic Insemination: Food and water should be withheld from the ewe for ~12 hr. Ewes should be sedated with 1.5-2 mg xylazine, IM, and placed in cradles that restrain and invert them—first in dorsal recumbency for preparation of the abdomen. Local anesthetic may be injected SC at 2 sites (~4 cm on each side of the ventral midline and ~6 cm anterior to the udder). The cradle is then raised at the posterior end of the ewe so she is tilted at ~45° with the lateral abdomen presented to the operator. The anesthetized sites allow for entrance of 2 trocars and cannulae; carbon dioxide is insufflated through the first cannula to distend the abdomen. The laparoscope is inserted through the near cannula, the uterine horns are visualized, and a glass or plastic inseminating pipette or sheathed inseminating gun is inserted through the second cannula. Semen is deposited into the lumen of the uterus. Conception rates are similar if semen is deposited into one or both horns of the uterus.

EMBRYO TRANSFER

Embryo transfer programs involve synchronization, superovulation, embryo recovery, and assessment and transfer of embryos. Programs may include short-term in vitro culture, cryopreservation, and nuclear manipulation, including sex determination.

Estrus synchronization of both donors and recipients is done as for artificial insemination with progestagen pessaries or CIDR. Superovulation can be induced in ewes during progestagen synchronization by the administration of preparations with gonadotropin activity (PMSG, horse anterior pituitary extract, human menopausal gonadotropin, and purified forms of FSH) to mimic the hormones and hormone pulses of the ovine estrous cycle. Factors affecting the ovulatory response to treatment include the nature and timing of treatment within the estrous cycle; age, breed, strain and fecundity of the ewe; nutritional and lactational status; and season. The time of ovulation after pessary removal is also affected by the treatment. (*See also* p 1804.)

Higher conception rates and more transferable embryos are obtained from a single intrauterine laparoscopic insemination than with mating by the ram or with 2 artificial inseminations. Embryos may be collected on days 5-7 after the uterus is exposed via either a midventral surgical laparotomy or through a modified laparoscopic approach. Embryos are flushed either by repeat, high-volume reverse flushing of the uterine horns or by through-flushing of the uterine horn and fallopian tube. Embryos are classified as "A," which can be immediately transferred or may be frozen, "B," which are immediately transferred, and "C," which are discarded.

Usually, 2 embryos are transferred into the ipsilateral horn of an active corpus luteum after laparoscopic-guided externalization of the uterus through a 2- to 3-cm midventral stab incision anterior to the udder.

MANAGEMENT OF REPRODUCTION: SMALL ANIMALS

BREEDING SOUNDNESS EXAMINATION

Female: The breeding soundness examination should begin with a thorough reproductive and medical history, including information on previous cycles (onset and regularity), breeding management (past and intended), outcome of any breeding, and relevant family history, as well as routine medical information (diet, medications, environment, health status). A thorough physical examination, with particular attention given to the genitalia and mammary glands, should be performed. Screening for hereditary defects common to the breed should be advised, which may require techniques such as radiography, ophthalmoscopy, or specific DNA testing. Digital vaginal examination and vaginoscopy of the bitch may detect strictures or other defects of the vulva or vagina that may hinder copulation or whelping. Vaginal strictures are more commonly congenital than acquired and may be in the form of either a septate or a circumferential band. They most commonly form at the vestibulovaginal junction, caudal to the urethral papilla. The heritability of such defects is unknown. Strictures of the vagina or vestibule are not uncommon in the bitch and usually prevent normal copulation, but if pregnancy ensues from mating without a tie or from artificial insemination, dystocia can result. Septate bands can be easily resected surgically, but circumferential strictures are difficult to resolve without episiotomy and major revision and tend to reform. Elective artificial insemination and cesarean section may be preferable if the bitch has outstanding breeding potential. Evaluation of the mammary glands should include inspection of the nipples for normal anatomy. Routine vaginal cultures are not advised because the vagina normally harbors a wide variety of bacteria, including β-hemolytic streptococci and *Mycoplasma* spp. Bitches should be screened for brucellosis before each estrus when breeding is planned. A negative *Brucella canis* screening test is reliable; positive results warrant serologic evaluation, as false positives are common. Queens should be tested annually for feline leukemia virus and feline immunodeficiency virus as medically indicated. Bitches and queens >5 yr of age should also have their general health assessed by performing a CBC, serum chemistries, and a urinalysis.

Before an anticipated breeding, females should be in optimal body condition to improve conception rate and whelping outcome. Breeders commonly skip cycles between breedings; this may not be optimal husbandry as the inevitable exposure to estrogen (queen) and progesterone (bitch, sometimes queen) during the estrous cycle promotes cystic endometrial hyperplasia and may result in pyometra. Bitches and queens kept in optimal health can be bred sequentially and should be ovariohysterectomized when production is finished. Proper nutrition and exercise strategies for pregnancy and lactation should be outlined.

Bitches should be currently vaccinated for core infectious diseases (canine distemper virus, parvovirus, adenovirus 2, and rabies virus). Other noncore vaccinations should be administered only according to good medical practice (appropriate for the dog's age, health status, home and travel environment, and lifestyle). Queens should similarly be vaccinated appropriately (based on duration of immunity recommendations) for feline distemper, rhinotracheitis, and calicivirus. Vaccination against rabies virus, feline leukemia virus, and other noncore diseases should be done when indicated by good medical practice, based on risk factors associated with the cat's age and husbandry. Unnecessary revaccination of bitches and queens prior to breeding is not advised, as little improvement in immunity can be expected and adverse effects may be seen. Vaccination during pregnancy is not advised.

The use of preventive medication for heartworm disease, and internal and external parasite control (according to manufacturers' recommendations) during pregnancy and lactation is advised. Appropriate isolation of the pregnant animal during the last half of pregnancy for infectious disease prevention is important (eg, avoiding exposure to canine herpesvirus in the bitch and upper respiratory infections in the queen). Client education concerning normal whelping and queening events and about the timely identification of dystocias is essential. Fetal and uterine monitoring systems developed for routine use in the bitch and queen result in improved neonatal survival with reduced morbidity and mortality for the dam.

Male: The breeding soundness examination for males should also begin with a thorough reproductive and general health history, including past and intended breeding management, outcome of any breedings already performed, relevant family history, as well as routine general history (diet, medication, environment, and health status). Screening for relevant heritable defects of concern for the breed should be advised. A thorough physical examination should be performed, with particular attention given to the genitalia. The penis should be fully extruded from the prepuce and examined. This may require sedation in toms. If hair accumulates around the base of the feline penis, it can prevent copulation and should be removed. Prostate size and symmetry should be assessed by simultaneous abdominal and rectal palpation in the dog; this is not generally necessary in cats because prostate disease is rare. Palpable abnormalities (pain or asymmetry) or semen abnormalities warrant ultrasonographic evaluation of the prostate. The testes and epididymi should be palpated carefully for symmetry and normalcy—abnormalities again warrant ultrasonographic evaluation. The scrotum should be evaluated for evidence of dermatitis or trauma, which can impact fertility. A small amount of mucoid discharge noted at the preputial opening is normal in the dog. (See also REPRODUCTIVE DISEASES OF THE MALE SMALL ANIMAL, p 1157.)

Cryptorchidism, a common genital defect in males, is diagnosed if either or both testes are not present in the scrotum at puberty; testicles normally descend into the scrotum by 6-16 wk of age. Unilateral cryptorchidism does not result in infertility. In dogs, cryptorchidism is hereditary, and affected animals should not be bred. Both parents of affected individuals should be implicated as carriers. Because retained testes have a higher incidence of neoplasia, bilateral orchiectomy is recommended. Attempts at medical therapy with gonadotropins or testosterone have been unsuccessful and are not ethical. Orchiopexy is also considered unethical. Failure of one testis to develop (true monorchidism) may be seen in dogs but is rare. A persistent penile frenulum prevents protrusion of the penis from the prepuce and thus copulation. Treatment is surgical. Deviation of the penis is uncommon; these animals require assistance in breeding or may be bred via artificial insemination. Hypospadias prevents normal sperm transport from the testes to the glans penis and is easily detected by physical examination. Small defects may close spontaneously, but some type of reconstructive surgery involving urethrostomy and penile amputation is usually necessary. Phimosis can be caused by stenosis of the preputial opening, which may be congenital or result from chronic inflammation (trauma or bacterial dermatitis). Any underlying cause should be treated and then, if necessary, the opening enlarged surgically.

Ideally, a complete semen evaluation should be performed in male dogs intended for breeding and repeated at least annually in an active stud dog. Semen is readily collected from most dogs by manual stimulation; the presence of a teaser bitch is advised to optimize results by improving libido. All equipment (artificial vagina, collecting tubes, pipettes, slides, and coverslips) should be room to body temperature, dry, and free of contaminants such as chemical disinfectants. The canine ejaculate consists of 3 fractions—the first and third are of prostatic origin, while the second is sperm-rich. Sperm production is related to testicular size, so large dogs should produce higher sperm counts than small dogs. Semen evaluation should include an assessment of libido, total sperm count per ejaculate (normal is 200-400 million), sperm motility (>90% progressively motile, with moderate to fast speed), and morphology (>90% normal). The sperm count (sperm/mL) is usually determined with a hemocytometer or by spectrophotometry. Sperm/ejaculate is calculated by multiplying the sperm count by the volume of semen collected. Motility is evaluated in an unstained sample as soon as the sample is collected, ideally using clean slides prewarmed on a slide warmer. Several commercially available stains are suitable for morphology examination; eosin-nigrosin and Giemsa stains are used most commonly. An adequate amount of the third fraction should be collected to ensure that the entire sperm-rich fraction has been acquired and to permit evaluation of the prostatic component, which should be clear (free of urine and cellular contamination). Subfertility or infertility should never be diagnosed based on one collection. If the sample is azoospermic, semen alkaline phosphatase can be measured in the ejaculate to assess whether the ejaculate was complete, as it is an epididymal marker. Levels >5,000 μg/dL indicate the ejaculate included the second, normally sperm-rich fraction. Levels <5,000 μg/dL indicate either bilateral obstructive disease or libido problems preventing the release of the second fraction. Sperm function is not assessed with routine semen evaluation. Acrosomal evaluation requires special techniques.

Collection of semen for evaluation is difficult in toms unless the cat has been trained to ejaculate into an artificial vagina or electroejaculation equipment is available. Sperm can be evaluated in the tom's urine obtained by cystocentesis after a breeding. Collecting a vaginal wash from the queen immediately after copulation can determine if the tom is producing sperm. (Sperm disappear from the vagina within 1-2 hr of copulation.) Warm saline is flushed into the vagina of the queen and aspirated, the sample is centrifuged, and the sediment examined (new methylene blue or routine hematologic stains are adequate). Fine-needle aspiration of the testes can also be used to demonstrate spermatogenesis, but both methods provide only crude information. Breeding a questionable tom to a proven queen may be the most practical method of assessing fertility.

BREEDING MANAGEMENT

Dogs

Bitches may be bred naturally, or artificially inseminated using fresh, chilled, or frozen-thawed semen. The practice of ovulation timing has become increasingly desirable to breeders. Popular stud dogs' owners commonly permit a limited number of breedings (usually 2), and may need to prioritize bitches based on their timing. Owners of bitches wish to minimize travel time to the stud dog facility. Boarding of bitches in season can be reduced with recognition of their fertile period. The use of extended and chilled semen and frozen semen, or subfertile stud dogs, necessitates ovulation timing for optimal conception. Proper ovulation timing permits accurate evaluation of gestational length and is essential in the evaluation of apparent infertility in the bitch. In addition, litter size is optimal with properly timed breedings.

Sound knowledge of the bitch reproductive cycle is essential. Individual bitches may vary from normal, be presented at variable times during their estrous cycle for evaluation, and sometimes exhibit pathologic variations in cycles. Each of these scenarios requires veterinary interpretation. The normal canine reproductive cycle can be divided into 4 phases, each having characteristic behavioral, physical, and endocrinologic patterns, although considerable variation exists. Bitches with normal estrous cycles but unexpected patterns must be differentiated from those with true abnormalities. Detection of individual variation within the normal range of events in a fertile bitch can be crucial to breeding management. Evaluation of the estrous cycle for true abnormalities is an important part of the evaluation of an apparently infertile bitch.

The interestrous interval is normally 4-13 mo, with 7 mo the average. The **anestrus** phase of the estrous cycle is marked by ovarian inactivity, uterine involution, and endometrial repair. An anestrous bitch is not attractive or receptive to male dogs. No overt vulvar discharge is present, and the vulva is small. Vaginal cytology is predominated by small parabasal cells, with occasional neutrophils and small numbers of mixed bacteria. The endoscopic appearance of vaginal mucosal folds is flat, thin, and red. The physiologic controls terminating anestrus are not well understood, but the deterioration of luteal function and the decline of prolactin secretion seem to be prerequisites. The termination of anestrus is marked by an increase in the pulsatile secretion of pituitary gonadotropins, follicle stimulating hormone (FSH), and luteinizing hormone (LH), induced by gonadotropin-releasing hormone (GnRH). Hypothalamic GnRH secretion is itself pulsatile, its intermittent secretion is a physiologic requirement of gonadotropin release. Mean levels of FSH are moderately elevated, and those of LH slightly elevated, during anestrus. At late anestrus, the pulsatile release of LH increases, causing the proestrous folliculogenesis. Estrogen levels are basal (2-10 pg/mL) and progesterone levels at nadir (<1 ng/mL) at late anestrus. Anestrus normally lasts 1-6 mo.

During **proestrus**, the bitch becomes attractive to male dogs but is still not receptive to breeding, although she may become more playful. A serosanguineous to hemorrhagic vulvar discharge of uterine origin is present, and the vulva is mildly enlarged. Vaginal cytology shows a progressive shift from small parabasal cells to small and large intermediate cells, superficial-intermediate cells, and finally superficial (cornified) epithelial cells, reflecting the degree of estrogen influence. RBC are usually, but not invariably, present. The vaginal mucosal folds appear edematous, pink, and round. FSH and LH levels are low during most of proestrus, rising during the preovulatory surge. Estrogen rises from basal anestrous levels (2-10 pg/mL) to peak levels (50-100 pg/mL) at late proestrus, while progesterone remains at basal levels (<1 ng/mL) until rising at the LH surge (2-4 ng/mL). Proestrus lasts from 3 days to 3 wk, with 9 days average. The follicular phase of the ovarian cycle coincides with proestrus and very early estrus.

During **estrus**, the normal bitch displays receptive or passive behavior, enabling breeding. This behavior correlates with decreasing estrogen levels and increasing progesterone levels. Serosanguineous to hemorrhagic vulvar discharge may diminish to variable degrees. Vulvar edema tends to be maximal. Vaginal cytology remains predominated by superficial cells; RBC tend to decrease but may persist throughout. Vaginal mucosal folds become progressively wrinkled (crenulated) in conjunction with ovulation and oocyte maturation.

Estrogen levels decrease markedly after the LH peak to variable levels, while progesterone levels steadily increase (usually 4-10 ng/mL at ovulation), marking the luteal phase of the ovarian cycle. Estrus lasts 3 days to 3 wk, with an average of 9 days. Estrous behavior may precede or follow the LH peak—its duration is variable and may not coincide precisely with the fertile period. Primary oocytes ovulate 2 days after the LH peak, and oocyte maturation is seen 2-3 days later; the lifespan of secondary oocytes is 2-3 days.

During **diestrus**, the normal bitch becomes refractory to breeding, with diminishing attraction of male dogs. Vulvar discharge diminishes and edema slowly resolves. Vaginal cytology is abruptly altered by the reappearance of parabasal epithelial cells and frequently neutrophils. The appearance of vaginal mucosal folds becomes flattened and flaccid. Estrogen levels are variably low, and progesterone levels steadily rise to a peak of 15-80 ng/mL before progressively declining in late diestrus. Progesterone secretion depends on both pituitary LH and prolactin secretion. Proliferation of the endometrium and quiescence of the myometrium develop under the influence of elevated progesterone levels. Diestrus usually lasts 2-3 mo in the absence of pregnancy. Parturition terminates pregnancy 64-66 days after the LH peak. Prolactin levels increase in a reciprocal fashion to falling progesterone levels at the termination of diestrus or gestation, reaching much higher levels in the pregnant state. Mammary ductal and glandular tissues increase in response to prolactin levels.

Estrogen, LH, and progesterone are important in ovulation timing. All may be assessed as part of a reproductive evaluation.

Estrogen: Increased estrogen causes an increased turnover rate of vaginal epithelial cells, resulting in the progressive cornification seen on vaginal cytology. Progressive edema of the vaginal mucosa also develops and can be visualized with endoscopic examination. Estrogen assays are performed by many commercial laboratories; however, the information is of little value for ovulation timing because peak estrogen levels vary from bitch to bitch, and even relative changes do not correlate to ovulation or the fertile period. Estrogen is best assessed by serial vaginal cytologies and vaginoscopy. Estrogen levels do not indicate the fertile period because ovulation is triggered by the LH surge, not an estrogen peak. Examination of the cells on the surface of the vaginal epithelium can provide information about the stage of the estrous cycle. Proper technique is important so that the cells obtained are representative of the hormonal changes occurring. The sample should be collected from the cranial vagina; cells from the clitoral fossa, vestibule, or caudal vagina are not as indicative of the stage of the cycle. Under the influence of rising estrogen levels, the number of layers composing the vaginal epithelium increases dramatically, presumably to provide protection to the mucosa during copulation. As estrogen rises during proestrus, the maturation rate of the epithelial cells increases, as does the number of keratinized, cornified epithelial cells seen on a vaginal smear. Full cornification continues throughout estrus until the "diestral shift" occurs 7-10 days after the LH surge, signifying the first day of diestrus. The vaginal smear then changes abruptly, with appearance of neutrophils and epithelial cells changing from full cornification to 40-60% immature (parabasal and intermediate) cells over the next 24-36 hr. If vaginal cytology is performed until the diestral shift is observed, the LH surge, ovulation, and the fertile period can be analyzed retrospectively.

Luteinizing Hormone: At the end of the follicular phase of the estrous cycle, a marked increase in LH over usual baseline values devlops over 24-48 hr, followed by a return to baseline values. This surge is thought to occur in response to the decline in estrogen levels and increase in progesterone levels. The LH surge triggers ovulation, making it the central endocrinologic event in the reproductive cycle of the bitch. Daily serial measurement of LH to identify the exact date of the LH surge is an accurate diagnostic tool for timing breedings. Affordable semiquantitative in-house kits are available for measuring serum LH levels in the dog and for identifying the preovulatory LH surge and thus the time of ovulation and the true fertile period. Blood samples must be drawn daily (at about the same time) for LH testing, as the LH surge may last only 24 hr in many bitches. The kits can be subject to variable interpretation, so the same person should run the tests if possible.

Progesterone: Progesterone levels begin to rise at approximately the time of the LH surge (prior to ovulation). Rising progesterone acts synergistically with declining estrogen to reduce edema of the vulva and vagina, which can be seen on vaginoscopic exam. Other observable clinical signs are minimal. Serial blood samples performed every 2 days may identify the initial rise in progesterone (usually >2 ng/mL), which indicates that the LH surge has occurred. Progesterone can be assayed by radioimmunoassay at most veterinary commercial laboratories. Several in-house semiquantitative kits are also available. No single absolute value of progesterone correlates to any particular stage of the cycle. Progesterone varies from 0.8-3.0 ng/mL at the point of the LH surge, from 1.0-8.0 ng/mL at ovulation, and from 4.0-20.0 ng/mL during the fertile period. However, if accurate serial quantitative progesterone assays are obtained, the LH surge may be estimated as the day a distinct increase in progesterone level is seen. While this is not as accurate as actual identification of the LH surge by assay, estimation by progesterone levels is still very useful and is often more widely available and convenient. When timing breeding using semiquantitative in-clinic progesterone assays, only a range of progesterone is obtained, which makes it difficult to accurately identify the day of the initial rise in progesterone or the true fertile period. Technical problems with these kits have also been seen. Therefore, these assays should be used only for routine breedings in which a wider margin of error is acceptable. A safe rule of thumb is that when progesterone is >2 ng/mL, breeding should begin. Optimal ovulation timing should use quantitative progesterone assays from commercial laboratories—the cost difference is minimal. Regardless of which assay is used, an additional test should always be performed 2-4 days after the first rise is detected to indicate that the cycle has progressed as expected, a functional corpus luteum has been formed, and ovulation has occurred.

Use of Hormonal Evaluation to Time Breeding: Owners of breeding animals should be advised to notify the clinic when they first notice that a bitch for which timing is planned is in season, based on vaginal discharge or vulvar swelling/attraction to males. Even the most astute owner may not notice the true onset of proestrus for a few days. Early proestrus should be documented with vaginal cytology (<50% cornification/superficial cells). A baseline progesterone level (usually 0-1 ng/mL) might be informative if the true onset of the cycle is unknown. Vaginal cytology should be performed every 2 days until cornification progresses significantly, usually >70% superficial cells. At that point, serial hormonal assays should begin. For routine breedings, progesterone testing may be done every other day, until a rise in progesterone >2 ng/mL is identified. The day of the initial rise in progesterone >2 ng/mL is identified as "day 0." Breedings are advised on days 2, 4, and 6.

When increased accuracy of ovulation timing is necessary (eg, frozen or chilled semen breedings, infertility cases, breedings with subfertile stud dogs), daily LH testing is recommended. Once the LH surge is identified, breeding days may be planned. The day of the LH surge is also "day 0." It is useful to perform vaginal cytology every 2-3 days until cornification is complete (>90% superficial cells). This maximal cornification usually develops before the fertile period and continues until the onset of dietrus, which is usually a few days after the end of the fertile period. Vaginal cytology may be continued until the diestral shift is identified, which gives a retrospective evaluation of the breeding just completed. In addition, at least 1 progesterone assay should be performed after day 0 is identified to document that levels continue to rise. This illustrates sustained corpus luteum function and strongly suggests that an ovulatory cycle has occurred. Insemination with extended, chilled semen should be done on days 4 and 6, or 3 and 5, after day 0. The days chosen can depend on overnight shipping possibilities and the schedules of all involved parties. Frozen semen breedings should be done on day 5 or 6.

Vaginoscopy may be performed throughout the cycle as an adjunct to vaginal cytology and hormonal assays, especially when evaluating an unusual cycle. Behavior and other observations should also be made. Ovulation timing is most accurate when information from several tests is pooled (vaginal cytologies, vaginoscopy, and progesterone or LH tests).

Artificial Insemination: Artificial insemination (AI) is becoming more common in canine reproduction, permitting the use of shipped semen, assistance for geriatric or subfertile males, coverage of dominant females, and advanced reproductive technology such as intrauterine deposition of semen. AI may be performed with fresh, chilled, or frozen semen. All instruments should be clean and free of any chemical contamination. After semen has been collected and evaluated (*see* p 1789), it can be deposited in the cranial vagina of the bitch using a rigid insemination pipette of appropriate length, or into the uterus via transcervical catheterization. Access to the uterus via laparoscopy or laparotomy is less desirable due to invasiveness. Semen (the second fraction) may be diluted with extenders and chilled for later or distant use (within 48 hr), or extended and frozen in liquid nitrogen (in straws or pellets) for longterm storage. Phosphate-buffered egg yolk diluent or Tris-buffered diluent is used most often; several commercial extenders are available. Chilled semen should be warmed for evaluation before use. Frozen semen should be thawed as directed by the cryopreservation center, evaluated, and immediately inseminated.

Cats

The queen should be taken to the tom when showing signs of estrus. The breeding area should be familiar to the tom, quiet, and have good footing and a minimum of interference, while permitting observation. The courtship should not be interrupted unless there is concern for the safety of either cat. Toms have been known to mate to the point of physical exhaustion, but queens normally go through a period of rolling and grooming after a breeding and may not let the tom remount for some time. Because ovulation is induced by vaginal-cervical stimulation, multiple breedings over 3 days are advised. Periods of separation between matings prevent exhaustion and diminish the chances of fighting. The stress of transportation may affect reproductive functions in nervous queens. Evaluation for pregnancy can be performed at 21-30 days gestation by abdominal palpation and ultrasonography.

MANIPULATION OF THE ESTROUS CYCLE

The estrous cycles of dogs and cats are not as easily manipulated as in other species. Controlled studies are lacking with most protocols, and their use in valuable breeding individuals is not advised. Although onset of a particular cycle may be delayed, return to normal cycling is highly variable. Induction of estrus is possible in late anestrus bitches using prolactin inhibitors (eg, bromocriptine, cabergoline).

Ovariohysterectomy is the best method to prevent estrus in the bitch and queen. Longterm suppression of estrus in the bitch may be accomplished with a synthetic compounded androgen. The dose is 3 µg/kg/day except for German Shepherds and their crosses, which require 6 µg/kg/day. Therapy must begin ≥1 mo before proestrus. Common side effects are clitoral hypertrophy, vaginitis (especially in prepubertal bitches), increased activity of skin sebaceous glands, mild epiphora, and alterations in hepatic function studies. Return to estrus after treatment is discontinued is variable but is ~70-90 days. Conception rates are reportedly normal by the second cycle after treatment. If given to pregnant bitches, synthetic androgens induce severe developmental anomalies in the urogenital system of female puppies. This synthetic androgen should not be given to cats.

The use of megestrol acetate, a synthetic progestagen, is not advised in breeding females due to the increased risk of cystic endometrial hyperplasia and pyometra, as well as other adverse effects (eg, mammary hyperplasia and neoplasia, hyperglycemia secondary to insulin resistance, and rebound hyperprolactinemia and lactation).

Ovulation can be induced in estrual queens physically or, more reliably, hormonally to produce a luteal phase (diestrus or metestrus) of ~45 days. Physical methods include mating with a vasectomized tom (very effective) or inserting a sterile swab or glass rod into the vagina. The latter should be performed repeatedly for best results. Hormonal methods include administration of human chorionic gonadotropin at 500 IU/cat or GnRH at 25 µg/cat. Both are given IM, SID for 2 days.

The safety and efficacy of injectable testosterone, as is practiced commonly in racing Greyhounds, has not been supported by controlled studies and is not advised.

PREGNANCY DETERMINATION

Fertilization occurs in the oviducts in both the bitch and queen. Implantation of zygotes in the uterus occurs at ~18 days in the bitch and 14 days in the queen. This is accompanied by the formation of small swellings along the uterine horns (deciduomata) by ~21 days. These are palpable, assuming the animal is cooperative, at this time. Fetal growth is rapid during early pregnancy, and these swellings double in diameter every 7 days. After day 35-38, they become indistinct, and palpation becomes difficult until late pregnancy when fetal heads and rumps are palpable as firm, nodular structures in the ventral posterior abdomen. A commercial relaxin assay, specific and sensitive for pregnancy diagnosis in the bitch after 30 days gestation, is available.

Although the fetal skeleton begins to calcify as early as day 28, it is not detectable by routine radiography until about day 42-45 and is quite prominent by day 47-48. Radiography at this time is not teratogenic. Late gestational radiography is the best method to determine litter size. Ultrasonography is also useful in pregnancy determination and permits evaluation of fetal viability. Ultrasonography is best performed at 25-35 days gestation. Before 21 days, "false negative" results are seen. Doppler-type instruments allow one to "hear" the fetal heart, which beats 2-3 times faster than that of the dam. Placental sounds may also be heard. Ultrasonography is especially helpful in differentiating pregnancy from other causes of uterine distention (eg, hydrometra, pyometra, mucometra).

PREVENTION OR TERMINATION OF PREGNANCY

Unplanned and unwanted mating of cats and dogs is a common concern. Pregnancy can be completely prevented or terminated by ovariohysterectomy. Sixty percent of misbred bitches do not conceive, so confirmation of an undesired pregnancy is advised before proceeding. Postcoital douches are of no value in preventing unwanted pregnancy. Although injectable estrogens, when administered appropriately, can prevent pregnancy, their use involves great risk for serious side effects, including pyometra and potentially fatal bone marrow suppression, and they are not advised. They must be administered soon after copulation, before potentially fertilized ova reach the uterus. Oral estrogens given during diestrus greatly increase the risk of pyometra, are unreliable in terminating pregnancy, and are not advised. Safe and effective termination of pregnancy is possible in both the bitch and queen by the administration of prostaglandin $F_{2\alpha}$ (natural hormone) dosed at 0.1 mg/kg, SC, TID for 48 hours followed by 0.2 mg/kg, SC, TID to effect (until all fetuses are evacuated as confirmed by ultrasonography). Treatment times can reach 14 days. In the bitch, treatment time can be reduced (usually by 48 hr) by the concurrent administration of prostaglandin E (misoprostol) intravaginally at 1-3 µg/kg, SID. The side effects of prostaglandins at this dosage (panting, trembling, nausea, and diarrhea) are mild and transient. The therapeutic window for prostaglandins is narrow and doses should be calculated carefully. Synthetic prostaglandins more specifically target the myometrium but are not approved in the USA for use in small animals. Pregnancy can also be reliably terminated in the bitch by the administration of dexamethasone at 0.2 mg/kg, PO, BID to effect. The owner should be informed of the side effects of corticosteroid administration (eg, panting, polyuria, polydipsia).

WHELPING AND QUEENING

Normal gestation in the bitch is 56-58 days from the first day of diestrus or 64-66 days from the initial rise in progesterone from baseline (generally >2 ng/mL), or 58-72 days from the first instance that the bitch permitted breeding. Predicting length of gestation without prior ovulation timing is difficult because of the disparity between estrual behavior and the actual time of conception in the bitch, and the length of time semen can remain viable in the reproductive tract (often ≥7 days). Breeding dates and conception dates do not correlate closely enough to permit accurate prediction of whelping dates. Additionally, clinical signs of term pregnancy are not specific—radiographic appearance of fetal skeletal mineralization varies at term, fetal size varies with breed and litter size. A drop in rectal temperature to a mean of 98.8°F (range 98.1-100.0°F) is seen in most bitches 8-24 hr before whelping. Breed, parity, and litter size can also influence gestational length. Prolonged gestation is a form of dystocia. Subtle signs of impending delivery include relaxation of the perineum, mammary engorgement, and a change in the appearance of the gravid abdomen, but these changes are not sensitive or specific. Because there is no means to effectively manage prematurely born puppies, premature intervention in the whelping process is undesirable. Unfortunately, an excessively conservative approach resulting in intrauterine fetal death is undesirable as well. Parturition in the queen occurs 64-66 days from the LH surge triggered by copulation.

Bitches typically enter stage I labor within 24 hr of a decline in serum progesterone to <2-5 ng/mL, which develops in conjunction with elevated circulating prostaglandins and is commonly associated with a transient drop in body temperature. Monitoring serial progesterone levels for impending labor is problematic due to the fact that in-house kits enabling rapid results are inherently inaccurate between 2-5 ng/mL. Commercial laboratories offering quantitative progesterone by radioimmunoassay typically have a 12-24 hr turnaround time, which is not rapid enough to make decisions about obstetric intervention. Clearly, it is beneficial to obtain information about ovulation timing, minimally by determining the onset of cytologic diestrus, for evaluating length of gestation at term.

A predictable and safe method of inducing parturition in the bitch and queen has not been determined.

LABOR AND DELIVERY

Normal Labor: Stage I labor in the bitch and queen normally lasts 12-24 hr, during which time the myometrial contractions of the uterus increase in frequency and strength and the cervix dilates. No abdominal efforts (visible contractions) are evident during stage I labor. Bitches and queens may exhibit changes in disposition and behavior during stage I labor, becoming reclusive, restless, and nesting intermittently, often refusing to eat and sometimes vomiting. Panting and trembling may be seen. Vaginal discharge is clear and watery.

Normal stage II labor is marked by visible abdominal efforts, which are accompanied by myometrial contractions that culminate in the delivery of a neonate. Typically, these efforts should not last >1-2 hr between puppies or kittens, although great variation exists. The entire delivery can take 1 to >24 hr; however, normal labor is associated with shorter total delivery time and intervals between neonates. Vaginal discharge can be clear, serous to hemorrhagic, or green (uteroverdin). Typically, bitches and queens continue to nest between deliveries and may nurse and groom neonates intermittently. Anorexia, panting, and trembling are common.

Stage III labor is defined as the delivery of the placenta. Bitches and queens typically vacillate between stages II and III of labor until the delivery is complete. During normal labor, all fetuses and placentae are delivered vaginally, although they may not be delivered together in every instance.

Dystocia: Dystocia can be objectively diagnosed if uterine contractility is inappropriate (generally infrequent, weak myometrial contractions) for the stage of labor, or if excessive fetal stress results from labor. Subjectively, dystocia is diagnosed if stage I labor is not initiated at term, if stage I labor is >24 hr without progression to stage II, if stage II labor does not produce a vaginal delivery within 1-4 hr, if fetal or maternal stress is excessive, if moribund or stillborn neonates are seen, or if stage II labor does not result in the completion of deliveries in a timely manner (within 12-24 hr). Dystocia results from maternal factors (uterine inertia, pelvic canal anomalies), fetal factors (oversize, malposition, malposture, anomalies) or a combination of both. Clinically, uterine inertia developing after the delivery of one or more neonates (secondary inertia) is the most common cause of dystocia.

Uterine and fetal monitors can be used to detect and monitor labor, as well as manage dystocia. Unresponsive uterine inertia, obstructive dystocia, aberrant uterine contractions, or progressive fetal distress without response to medical management are indications for cesarean section.

Medical management includes administration of calcium gluconate and oxytocin based on the results of monitoring. Drugs are given only after 8-12 hr of an established contraction pattern (stage I labor) as detected by the uterine monitor and only if inertia is detected when stage II labor is anticipated. Premature administration of drugs results in suboptimal response.

Generally, the administration of calcium increases the strength of myometrial contractions, while oxytocin increases the frequency. Calcium gluconate (10% solution, 1 mL/22 kg body wt, BID-QID) is given when uterine contractions are ineffective or weak. It can be given SC, avoiding the potential for cardiac irritability associated with IV administration. Oxytocin (0.5-2.0 U in bitches; 0.25-1.0 U in queens) is given when uterine contractions are less frequent than expected for the stage of labor. The most effective time for treatment is when uterine inertia begins to develop, before the contractions stop completely. High doses of oxytocin saturate the receptor sites and make it ineffective as a uterotonic. If fetal stress is evident (persistent bradycardia) and response to medications is poor, cesarean section is indicated.

POSTPARTUM CARE

Palpation and, if necessary, radiography should be used to determine that all puppies or kittens have been delivered. The routine postpartum administration of oxytoxin or antibiotics is unnecessary in healthy dams with nursing neonates, unless the placenta has been retained. The dam's body temperature and the character of the postpartum discharge or lochia and milk should be monitored. Normally, the lochia is dark red to black and is heavy for the first few days after parturition. It is not necessary that the dam consume the placentas. Disinfection of the neonatal umbilicus with tincture of iodine helps prevent bacterial contamination. The neonate should be weighed accurately as soon as it is dry and then twice daily for the first week. Any weight loss after the first 24 hr indicates a potential problem and should be given immediate attention (eg, supplemental feeding, assisted nursing, evaluation for sepsis).

PERIPARTURIENT PROBLEMS

Bitches and queens should deliver in a familiar area where they will not be disturbed. Unfamiliar surroundings or strangers may impede delivery, interfere with milk letdown, or adversely affect maternal instincts. This is especially true in young or primiparous animals. The dam's apprehension or nervousness may subside in a few hours, but in the meantime the neonates must receive colostrum and be kept warm.

A nervous dam may ignore the neonates or give them excess attention. The latter may result in nearly continuous licking and biting at the umbilical stump, which may cause hemorrhage or damage the abdominal wall, which may lead to evisceration. Excess grooming of the neonate may prevent it from nursing. If the dam's maternal instincts fail, she may assume sternal recumbency and not allow nursing, or leave the neonates unattended. It is not unusual for the dam to pick up the pups and to rearrange them in the box, especially after delivery of each pup; however, she should then assume the normal nursing position.

The principal metabolic disease associated with pregnancy is puerperal hypocalcemia (p 809). It is rare in cats and most common in dogs weighing <20 kg, exacerbated by improper perinatal nutrition (excessive calcium/phosphorus supplementation or an imbalanced prenatal diet).

Common inflammatory diseases in the postpartum period include metritis and mastitis. Retention of a placenta or its remnants usually leads to metritis. Signs include continued straining as if in labor, the presence of a fusiform mass associated with the uterus best identified by ultrasonographic evaluation, abnormal vulvar discharge, fever, and lethargy as the infection develops. If given within 24 hr of labor, oxytocin may cause passage of the placenta; if oxytocin is ineffective, prostaglandin $F_{2\alpha}$ (0.1 mg/kg, SC, SID-BID to effect) can usually induce passage of the placenta. Mastitis (p 1153) is more common in bitches than in queens. The bacteria associated with mastitis tend to be coliforms or *Staphylococcus* spp. Galactostasis can predispose bitches to mastitis, as can excessive human manipulation of the mammary glands.

Significant postpartum uterine hemorrhage is rare. Treatment with ergonovine (15 mg/kg, IV) may be tried; if it fails to stop the hemorrhage, ovariohysterectomy must be performed. An underlying coagulopathy should be suspected.

Uterine subinvolution results in hemorrhagic spotting for >12-16 wk (the normal period of involution in the bitch). Treatment is unnecessary unless blood loss is significant because the condition resolves spontaneously. Future fertility is unaffected.

Agalactia (other than that caused by severe illness) is uncommon in dogs and cats. Determination that lactation is adequate should be performed prior to elective cesarean section. If an emergency cesarean section is required, regardless of the status of lactation, intervention is indicated (*see* below). Bitches and queens with inadequate lactation at term should be thoroughly evaluated for metabolic or inflammatory disorders (metritis, eclampsia, mastitis), as well as for nutritional and hydration status, and treated appropriately. Evaluation of a hemogram, serum chemistries, vaginal discharge, and ultrasonographic evaluation of the uterus may be required. The normal presence of colostrum (typically not copious) should not be confused with agalactia. The level of neonatal contentment and daily weight gain (after the first 24 hr) indicates adequate lactation. Milk letdown is promoted by oxytocin release, a reflex triggered by nursing, therefore neonates must spend adequate time suckling. Disruption of the pituitary-ovarian-mammary gland axis can result in idiopathic agalactia. Agalactia can be associated with premature delivery of neonates. Because estrogen promotes lactogenesis, the adequacy of mammary development should be assessed prior to removal of the ovaries at cesarean section. Ovariohysterectomy should not have a negative effect on bitches and queens with adequate lactogenesis at term. If this is seen, a genetic component may be involved.

Lactation can be stimulated if treatment is prompt. Mini-dose oxytocin (0.5-2.0 U/dose, SC, every 2 hr) should be administered. The neonates should be removed from the dam prior to each injection and returned 30 min later. The neonates should be supplemented adequately to ensure survival, but not excessively, so that they will suckle vigorously. Gentle hand stripping of the mammary glands should take place if suckling is not vigorous. Concurrent administration of metoclopramide (0.1-0.2 mg/kg, SC, TID-QID) promotes prolactin release. Acepromazine at mild tranquilization dosages may also facilitate milk letdown. Therapy should continue until lactation is adequate, usually 12-24 hr later.

INFERTILITY

The most common cause of infertility in dogs and cats is related to husbandry problems. Breeding with a proven fertile male must occur at the optimal time for the female. Infectious, anatomic, metabolic, and functional problems associated with infertility are seen less frequently. (*See also* INFERTILITY, p 1092.)

The only confirmed infectious cause of infertility in the bitch is brucellosis (p 1159). This highly contagious disease caused by *Brucella canis* causes abortion and infertility in bitches and infertility in males. A rapid slide agglutination test (RSAT) kit to detect serum antibodies is commercially available. If the RSAT is negative, the bitch is presumed to be *Brucella*-free; if positive, the serum is treated with 2-mercaptoethanol (2ME) to eliminate nonspecific antibodies, and the RSAT repeated. If the 2ME-RSAT is positive, the bitch is presumed to be infected and further tests are indicated (serology and confirmatory blood and vaginal cultures). In cats, infectious causes of infertility include toxoplasmosis, feline leukemia virus infection, feline infectious peritonitis, and feline viral rhinotracheitis. These may cause abortion, neonatal death, fetal resorption, and apparent infertility.

Anatomic causes of infertility include acquired and congenital problems. Fibrosis of the oviducts or uterine horns, probably a result of inflammation after infection or trauma, leads to infertility. Diagnosis is via laparotomy with dye studies. There is no reliable treatment, although microsurgery may be attempted. Similarly, bilateral obstruction of the sperm ducts can cause azoospermia and infertility. High environmental temperature can induce either temporary or permanent azoospermia. Kennel or cattery management should allow for breeding males to remain cool during the summer. Scrotal dermatitis can have the same result. Disorders of sexual differentiation result in infertility (eg, hermaphrodite, pseudohermaphrodite).

Metabolic causes of infertility, other than in severely ill individuals, are rare. Hypothyroidism has no effect on male libido or semen quality. Hypothyroid bitches may not cycle or may have increased abortion rates.

Estrous cycle abnormalities can cause infertility. Prolonged anestrus may be congenital or acquired. Some large breeds of dogs may not have their first estrus until they are ≥2 yr old, and some individuals and some breeds typically have only one estrous cycle each year. Congenital forms of anestrus may be due to lack of function of the hypothalamic-pituitary axis or ovarian dysgenesis. The diagnosis of congenital anestrus is based on the age of the animal and exclusion of all other possible causes (including chromosomal defects, endocrine disorders, and previous oophorectomy). Because cyclicity in queens is determined by photoperiod, lighting conditions should be appropriate for several months before congenital anestrus is diagnosed and exogenous hormones are administered. One reported method for estrus induction in cats is FSH at 2 mg/cat, IM, SID until signs of estrus appear (not administered for >5 days).

Acquired anestrus may result from previous oophorectomy, exogenous hormonal treatment (including glucocorticoids), profound hypothyroidism, or ovarian disease (cysts or neoplasia). Diagnosis is based on history, physical examination, biochemical evaluation, ultrasonography, and laparotomy.

Prolonged estrus may be caused by ovarian cysts that produce estrogen, functional ovarian tumors, or exogenous estrogens. Exogenous hormones should be discontinued. Laparotomy with histopathology is usually indicated, as medical attempts at inducing ovulation (human chorionic gonadotropin, FSH, GnRH) are usually unrewarding. Prolonged diestrus can result from luteal cysts in the ovary. Medical manipulation with prostaglandins is usually unrewarding, and ovariectomy with histopathology indicated. Testicular neoplasia, commonly producing estrogen, usually causes infertility. Castration of the affected testis may allow the other testis to regain its ability to produce sperm, but the prognosis is guarded.

BREEDING SOUNDNESS EXAMINATION OF THE MALE

The major components of fertility in the male are desire to breed (libido), ability to breed, and semen quality. Semen quality is determined by assessing the motility of the sperm, the presence of epithelial or blood cells in the ejaculate, percentage of morphologically normal sperm present, and the total number of sperm in the ejaculate, which in some cases (eg, ruminants) is estimated by measuring scrotal circumference. Scrotal circumference is correlated with daily sperm output and therefore the serving capacity of a bull (ie, number of females he can settle in a limited time). High conception rates are the best evidence of normal fertility; eg, a bull that impregnates 95% of 50 cows over 9 wk, most of them in the first 3 wk, can be called highly fertile. Low conception rates, however, may be related to low male or female fertility or to poor management. The following are general guidelines for breeding soundness examinations.

Cattle

In bulls, assessment of libido is often not possible during a routine breeding soundness examination. However, if possible, the bull should be observed serving cows to allow assessment of his desire to breed, ease of mounting, ability to achieve erection and extend the penis, and presence of penile deviation or other abnormalities that may prevent successful service. Libido and serving capacity tests (scoring the number of services achieved during a set time that a bull is in a pen with a restrained cow) have been devised but are time consuming and difficult to standardize under field conditions. In addition, the results are difficult to interpret in light of the variety of stocking conditions used, eg, single versus multiple bulls or small paddocks versus large ranges.

Breeding soundness examination forms have been developed and should be used to ensure the systematic completion of the breeding soundness examination and accurate reporting of results. The bull should be restrained in a chute for the examination. Body condition should be scored, and a general physical examination conducted with special attention paid to the feet, legs, eyes, and sheath. The inguinal rings and internal genitalia should be palpated per rectum for the detection of any abnormalities, eg, seminal vesiculitis. The scrotum should be palpated to evaluate the testicles, epididymides, spermatic cord, and scrotal skin. Cryptorchidism is considered an undesirable heritable trait and renders a bull unsatisfactory for breeding even though his semen quality might be acceptable. Normal testicles have a smooth surface and are firm and resilient, without palpable lumps. The tail of the epididymis is located ventrally and the head dorsally. The body of the epididymis runs dorsally to ventrally on the caudal-medial surface, near the midline. The epididymis should have no palpable masses. The scrotal circumference should be measured at its maximal diameter; this should be ≥30 cm for bulls <15 mo old, 31 cm for bulls 16-18 mo, 32 cm for bulls 19-21 mo, 33 cm for bulls 22-23 mo, and 34 cm for bulls ≥2 yr old. Placing the thumb or fingers between the testicles during measurement can lead to a false increase in apparent circumference. Scrotal circumference is directly related to the number of sperm the bull is capable of producing, as well as to the percentage of morphologically normal sperm produced.

Semen is collected from most bulls by electroejaculation, although semen can be collected with an artificial vagina (AV) in bulls trained to use one (eg, those in bull studs). The penis usually extends during electroejaculation and should be examined at that time for any abnormalities. If it is not extended during electroejaculation, it should be gently exteriorized for examination by grasping the glans with a cotton gauze and, if necessary, by putting pressure on the sigmoid flexure immediately caudal to the scrotum. Preputial wash samples may be taken for culture of *Campylobacter* (using Clark's medium) or *Trichomonas* (using Diamond's medium or a commercially available diagnostic medium kit).

The electroejaculator consists of a rectal probe that has a series of linear banded electrodes connected to a variable current and voltage source. The bull is restrained in a chute, the rectum is emptied, and the entire probe is inserted rectally with the electrodes placed ventrally. A hand-operated rheostat permits intermittent pulses of current to be given as the voltage is gradually increased. The response varies considerably, but it is common to use 2- to 4-sec pulses repeated at 5- to 7-sec intervals. After a variable number of such stimulations, erection and protrusion of the penis may be seen, followed by a flow of seminal fluid, or the bull may ejaculate into the sheath without protruding the penis. The semen may be collected by any convenient method; typically a rubber AV cone inserted within a plastic cylinder attached to an 18-in. handle, with a test tube attached to the cone, is used. In some bulls, ejaculation is seen only after a final series of momentary pulses at 1- to 2-sec intervals. Older bulls usually require a higher voltage for ejaculation. In some large bulls, the probe may not reach the correct areas for stimulation; having 2 or more probe sizes is recommended if breeding soundness examinations are to be done on a variety of sizes of bulls. Although ejaculate volume and sperm concentration are variable, semen collected by electrical stimulation appears to be as fertile as that collected with an AV.

If an AV is to be used, bulls are induced to mount a teaser animal (eg, restrained steer, cow, or phantom), and the erect penis is directed into the AV by the collector as the bull mounts. In preparing the AV, the temperature, which is a critical factor in stimulating ejaculation, is maintained at 105-107°F (40.5-42°C). Temperatures up to 118°F (48°C) may assist collections in untrained bulls. The AV should be lubricated with nonspermicidal jelly. The typical volume of an ejaculate is 4-8 mL, and the concentration 1-1.5 billion sperm/mL. A semen sample can be collected from some bulls by transrectal massage of the accessory sex glands. With this technique, erection seldom occurs. After the rectum is completely emptied, the vesicular glands are massaged with a backward motion until a few mL of fluid drop from the sheath. The ampullae are then massaged, and an assistant collects the semen as for electroejaculation. This method is not always successful, and the quality of the semen emission is usually lower than the ejaculate collected by the other 2 methods.

Sperm concentration, ejaculate volume, and the total number of sperm in the ejaculate collected by electroejaculation are highly variable and should not be evaluated as they do not reflect a bull's potential breeding ability. The semen sample should be evaluated immediately for motility. The materials that contact the sperm should be at the same temperature as the sperm (to avoid temperature shock), clean, dry, and nontoxic. Motility evaluation is best when the temperature of the semen is either maintained at ~37°C during the short time before it is evaluated, or when the semen is gently warmed to 37°C before evaluation. Both gross motility ("swirl pattern") in the semen and motility of individual spermatozoa should be evaluated; the individual motility is the more accurate measure and should be used for classification of the bull. Gross motility is a function of sperm concentration and individual sperm motility and is evaluated in an undiluted drop of semen placed on a slide without a coverslip and examined at low power (~40×). The intensity of wave motion may be classified into 4 categories: very good—intense swirling, rapid dark and light waves; good—slower swirling, waves not as intense; fair—slow movement with fewer waves; or poor—very little or no swirl activity. Individual motility is assessed in a sample diluted with warmed saline or prepared semen extender. A drop of diluted sperm is placed on a slide, covered with a coverslip, and examined at 200-400×. The proportion of sperm that are moving progressively across the field of view is estimated by finding multiple groups of ~10 sperm and estimating how many sperm are progressive versus how many are not. The environments in which breeding soundness examinations are done are variable, and there is a high chance of temperature shock to sperm before they may be evaluated. Therefore, >30% individual progressive motility, or fair gross motility, is considered acceptable. If the examination is performed under optimal conditions, some associations (eg, the Canadian Bovine Practitioners Association) recommend a minimum of 60% motility for a bull to be classified as a satisfactory potential breeder.

The presence of cells other than spermatozoa in the sample should be investigated while estimating motility. RBC, WBC, and excess numbers of round epithelial cells and developing forms of spermatozoa may indicate a genital tract abnormality. Careful evaluation of the tract, especially the internal genitalia, may indicate the source of WBC. The most common cause is seminal vesiculitis. Round epithelial cells and immature spermatozoa with proximal cytoplasmic droplets may indicate immaturity or, alternatively, testicular degeneration.

A sample of the semen should be fixed in a buffered formaldehyde saline solution for evaluation of sperm morphology. This is best done with the fixed, unstained sperm examined under high power (1,000×) using a phase-contrast microscope. Morphology may also be assessed by using a vital sperm stain (eg, eosin-nigrosin), but this method may not be as accurate as phase-contrast microscopy. At least 100 sperm should be counted, and the proportion of sperm showing different types of abnormalities noted. However, the only number used in the evaluation of the bull is the proportion of normal sperm, which should be >70%. Use of a live-dead stain is no longer recommended because the percentage of morphologically normal sperm, scrotal circumference, and physical soundness are more highly correlated with fertility than the live:dead ratio of sperm in an ejaculate.

Bulls are classified as "satisfactory potential breeders" if they have no physical abnormalities that would prevent breeding and if they meet the minimal qualifications for scrotal circumference, sperm motility, and sperm morphology. Bulls that do not meet these criteria are classified as "unsatisfactory potential breeders" or, if the results are marginal or questionable, they are considered "classification deferred" and a retest should be recommended.

Sheep

In rams, the breeding soundness evaluation is performed much as for bulls, using the electroejaculator with a smaller (ram) probe. Body score is classified as 1-2, questionable (underconditioned); 3-4, satisfactory; and 5, questionable (overconditioned). Any major abnormalities of the external genitalia or lumps or irregularities of the testicles or epididymides render the ram unsatisfactory. Epididymal masses are commonly found to be sperm granulomas caused by infection with *Brucella ovis*, which is a major cause of reproductive loss in sheep. *B ovis* may also be associated with testicular atrophy. Scrotal circumference should be ≥28 cm for rams 8-14 mo old (>36 cm is exceptional) and ≥32 cm for rams >14 mo old (>40 cm is exceptional). Scrotal circumference lower than satisfactory is questionable. Motility of individual spermatozoa is evaluated as for bulls, with >70% progressive motility being exceptional, >30% satisfactory, 10-30% questionable, and 0% unsatisfactory. The percentage of morphologically normal sperm should be >50%; between 30 and 50% is questionable, and <30% unsatisfactory; >80% normal sperm is exceptional. Presence of >5 WBC per high power field is questionable (WBC are correlated with *B ovis* infection). An ELISA test for *B ovis* should be done on range rams and rams >9 mo old. A positive test renders the ram unsatisfactory. Suspect tests should be repeated.

Any ram with one unsatisfactory rating in any parameter is classified "unsatisfactory;" a ram with questionable rating in any parameter is "questionable." For a ram to be classified exceptional, he must have exceptional ratings in scrotal circumference, sperm motility, and sperm morphology. All other rams are considered "satisfactory."

Goats

Breeding soundness evaluation in bucks has not been detailed to the extent that it has in rams. Careful testicular palpation should be performed; *Brucella ovis* infection is rare, but sperm granulomas are frequently related to the polled condition. These are most often found in the head of the epididymis. Cryptorchidism is also common and heritable; as in other species, cryptorchid bucks should not be used for breeding. Testicular degeneration is a common cause of fertility loss in older bucks. Semen is collected using an artificial vagina (AV); bucks are easily trained for this method and do not tolerate an electroejaculator. Parameters for semen evaluation are similar to those for rams. Because the ejaculate is collected with an AV, sperm production may be measured rather than estimated from scrotal circumference. Semen volume should be 0.5-2.0 mL, and concentration 1.5-4.0 billion sperm/mL.

Horses

A complete breeding soundness examination of the stallion consists of the history, physical examination, culture of urethral and possibly penile swabs, and collection and evaluation of one or more ejaculates for total sperm number, sperm motility, and sperm morphology.

The history should include the stallion's prior fertility and the type of management used for breeding. If <10 mares were bred, individual mare fertility should be considered if pregnancy rates were low. If the stallion has been racing or training recently, he may have been receiving anabolic steroids or other drugs. Stallions recently retired from a performance career may be evaluated again in 3-6 mo if they fail the initial breeding soundness examination.

During the physical examination, the stallion should be evaluated for general body condition and the presence of any conditions that might interfere with breeding. Genetically inherited defects, including parrot mouth and cataracts, render the stallion unfit for breeding. Blindness, lameness or ataxia, penile paralysis, or other defects that prevent the stallion from breeding also render him unsatisfactory as a breeding prospect. Cryptorchidism has not been verified to be hereditary but is considered to render the stallion an unsatisfactory prospective breeder. The scrotum should be palpated for its contents (this may be done after the first ejaculation when the stallion may be more relaxed). Total scrotal width should measure >8 cm (preferably >9 cm), as measured with a blunt caliper across both testicles together. The testicles should be firm, resilient, and homogeneous on palpation. The tail of the epididymis is easily palpated on the caudal aspect of the testis, whereas the body and head of the epididymis tend to blend with the dorsal surface of the testis. Rotation of the testicle 180° (the tail of the epididymis being palpated on the cranial aspect of the testicle; also called torsion of the spermatic cord) is common and has no clinical significance in healthy stallions. The penis is usually examined while it is washed before the first semen collection. The penis can vary in size with no effect on fertility. It should be freely distensible from the sheath without large bumps and bends. Of the internal genitalia of the stallion, the ampullae, vesicular glands, and lobes of the prostate gland are palpable per rectum. The vesicular glands are difficult to palpate unless the stallion is first teased to a mare in estrus to stimulate filling of the glandular lumina with fluid. The bulbourethral glands are covered by muscle, making it impossible to palpate their structure. Because of the danger inherent in adequately restraining a stallion, some veterinarians perform palpation only if deemed necessary because of an abnormal finding on the remainder of the examination, such as blood or pus in the ejaculate. When performing palpation per rectum on a stallion, the internal inguinal rings should also be palpated to determine their size and presence of any abnormalities. They are felt as flaps of peritoneum that form pockets in the abdominal lining at the 3 o'clock and 9 o'clock locations at the entrance of the pelvis.

Semen is collected from the stallion using an artificial vagina (AV) filled with water at ~50°C, which typically cools to 40-45°C at the time of collection. The stallion is teased to an estrous (or ovariectomized) mare; when the penis is erect, it is washed with water with or without a nonbactericidal soap. If the penile skin is suspected to harbor potentially transmissible bacteria (eg, *Klebsiella pneumoniae* or *Pseudomonas aeruginosa*), a culture swab of the sheath and fossa glandis should be obtained before the penile area is washed and rinsed for semen collection. Smegma can fill the urethral fossa, dorsal to the urethral process, and harden to form a "bean." This can cause irritation and swelling and should be removed. After the penis is rinsed and dried, the glans is massaged to cause the stallion to expel some preseminal fluid, and a swab sample of the distal urethra is obtained. The stallion is then allowed to mount the mare or phantom (breeding dummy), and the semen is collected by diverting the penis into the AV. A second swab sample is taken from the distal urethra immediately after ejaculation. The stallion should be given 1 hr of rest if a second ejaculate is to be collected (based on semen quality and sperm numbers in the first ejaculate).

The culture results of the urethral swab samples can be difficult to interpret. Prewash penile cultures usually show moderate to heavy growth of mixed bacteria. Pre-ejaculate urethral swabs also may reveal growth of a mixed bacterial population. Growth of *Pseudomonas* or *Klebsiella* may indicate that the penis has been colonized by these organisms; in the USA these are the only bacteria (besides that of contagious equine metritis, p 1133) that, in some cases, may be passed to mares and cause endometritis. The postejaculate urethral swab should yield less bacterial growth because the urethra has been "washed" by the ejaculate. High numbers of bacteria, especially of a single species, on the postejaculate swab may indicate infection of the internal sexual organs.

The ejaculate should be evaluated for appearance, volume, sperm concentration, sperm motility, percentage of morphologically normal sperm, and percentages of specific spermatozoal morphologic abnormalities. The ejaculate should be free of pus, urine, or blood. The normal ejaculate may contain gel, a viscous, clear to cloudy material, that can be removed by having an in-line filter at the mouth of the collection bottle in the AV (preferred), or by aspiration with a syringe out of the collected ejaculate. The analysis of the semen is done on the gel-free fraction. Concentration may be determined using a hemocytometer or a properly calibrated photometric instrument. Several instruments specially designed for this purpose are commercially available. Sperm motility and morphology evaluations are performed as described for the bull (p 1797); however, the sperm concentration is much lower in stallions (typically 100-400 million/mL), so only individual sperm motility is evaluated. Assessment of motility should be performed with both raw semen and semen diluted with a good quality extender. Semen should be warmed to 35-38°C prior to assessing spermatozoal motility. Total number of spermatozoa are calculated as volume × concentration.

If the first ejaculate collected has high numbers of sperm with good motility and a high percentage of sperm that are morphologically normal or have defects that do not affect fertility, it may not be necessary to obtain a second ejaculate. If values obtained from the first ejaculate are marginal, a second or further ejaculates may be collected to obtain more information. The ejaculates are considered to be representative if the second ejaculate contains about half the number of sperm as the first. The second ejaculate should have about the same, or a slightly higher, percentage of morphologically normal sperm and each of the morphologic abnormalities noted, as well as the same motility as the first. If sperm numbers or quality differ from this guideline, then either prolonged sperm storage in the excurrent ducts has occurred (see below), or one of the ejaculates was not complete, and a third ejaculate should be obtained. The third ejaculate should have about half as many sperm as the second ejaculate, and the same morphology and motility. A third ejaculate may also be collected if the sperm evaluation does not appear to agree with the total scrotal width (eg, high sperm numbers from a stallion with small testes).

Prolonged storage of sperm in the excurrent ducts results in high numbers in the initial ejaculate, but these sperm may have poor motility and morphology. Some stallions with extreme sperm storage require daily collection for 7-10 days before representative ejaculates are obtained (sperm evaluation is consistent on successive collections).

Sperm may accumulate in the ampullae and inspissate, causing blockage of the ductuli deferentiae. This may result in no sperm or few sperm, typically with detached heads, present in the ejaculate. Multiple attempts at collection may be necessary before the blockage is cleared.

In a satisfactory potential breeding stallion, sperm numbers after >5 days of sexual rest should be ≥8-10 billion in the first ejaculate and ≥4 billion in the second ejaculate. Total spermatozoal motility should be ≥65% and progressive motility ≥45%. At least 50% of the sperm should be morphologically normal.

Stallions are classified as "satisfactory," "questionable," or "unsatisfactory" potential breeders based on the results of the examination. However, classification can be somewhat subjective, and an excellent finding in one category can balance a marginal finding in another. Satisfactory potential breeders should achieve a seasonal pregnancy rate of >80% when bred to 50 mares by natural breeding or to 120 mares by artificial insemination under normal management conditions. Questionable potential breeders may experience difficulty in doing the above; unsatisfactory breeders have problems that may profoundly reduce their fertility or have undesirable heritable traits that may be transmissible to their offspring. Some stallions may be used to inseminate a percentage of mares with transported semen. Under these circumstances, longevity of spermatozoal motility should be tested using commercial semen containers before a decision is rendered regarding a stallion's fertility.

Pigs

In postpubertal boars, testes should be symmetric (<1.0 cm difference), with each testicle having a minimum length and width of 8.0 and 5.0 cm, respectively. Semen is collected with the boar mounted on a phantom or an estrous sow. As the penis is extruded, the tip (incorporating the coiled part) is grasped with a gloved hand and compressed; this stimulates full erection and ejaculation. The opening of the urethra is slightly proximal to the tip of the glans. The volume of semen is high, and ejaculation occurs over a long period, so semen is usually collected into an insulated container to maintain a relatively constant temperature. A filter or opened gauze sponge is fastened across the opening of the container to filter out gel and debris. Normal semen values for the boar are volume, 50-500 mL; sperm concentration, >50×10^6/mL; progressive motility, >70%; total sperm per ejaculate, >60×10^9; and percentage of morphologically normal sperm, >80%.

Dogs

A complete breeding soundness examination in dogs consists of a history, physical examination, semen evaluation, and testing for *Brucella canis*. If infertility is suggested from the history, it should be established that adequate breeding management was practiced and that bitches had normal fertility when bred to other dogs. The time sequence of litters sired and bitches that did not conceive should be recorded, as should any recent illness during or before the time that the bitches were bred. These should be assessed to determine if the infertility may be transient (eg, fever can adversely affect semen production for >60 days after the initial insult).

A general physical examination should be performed. Dogs with abnormalities such as severe joint disease or spinal problems may not be able to mount. Endocrinopathies such as hyperadrenocorticism or hypothyroidism may reduce fertility; these may be associated with abnormalities in weight or hair coat. The penis and prepuce should be examined; problems such as persistent frenulum, growths, or swelling due to balanoposthitis may prevent normal intromission. Abrasions or lacerations on the penis may bleed during coitus, and blood may be seen in the semen. The prostate should be digitally palpated per rectum; prostatitis may be painful, causing the dog to be unable to finish a mating or appear to have lowered libido. In addition, WBC, RBC, and bacteria from an inflamed prostate may decrease sperm viability, and infection of the prostate can potentially ascend to cause orchitis. The scrotum, testicles, and epididymides should be palpated. Small, soft testicles are usually associated with poor semen quality; greatly enlarged testicles suggest orchitis or epididymitis. Lumps suggesting neoplasia may be palpable. Scrotal abnormalities such as dermatitis may adversely affect semen quality by decreasing scrotal thermoregulation. Length, width, and diameter of testicles should be measured with blunt calipers; these measurements are often of value for future comparison in cases of suspected testicular degeneration. Ultrasonographic examination of the scrotal contents is valuable to evaluate presence of testicular or epididymal masses.

Semen collection is performed with the dog on good footing (eg, a rug) rather than on a slippery surface or table. Care should be taken to intimidate the dog as little as possible; lifting the dog to an examination table, giving injections, etc, should be performed after the semen is collected. Semen may be collected in the absence of a bitch (although sperm numbers may be lower), but the presence of a bitch is preferable . The pheromone methyl paraben may be helpful for collection in the absence of a bitch; some veterinarians freeze swabs of estrous bitch urine for this purpose but the reaction of male dogs is variable. A collecting cone such as the liner of a bull artificial vagina (AV), lubricated with sterile nonspermicidal lubricant or petroleum jelly and attached to a test tube, is used. The penile sheath is gently pulled back and the cone is slipped over the penis. As soon as the bulbus glandis is exteriorized from the sheath and is within the cone, the penis is grasped through the cone, immediately caudal to the bulbus. Constant pressure is maintained caudal to the bulbus, and erection and eventually ejaculation should be achieved. Scratching the dog's chest and speaking encouragingly may be helpful. If a bitch in estrus is available, the penis should be diverted into the cone as the dog mounts. Contact of the penis with the lubricated cone typically stimulates the dog to thrust into the cone, and the penis is compressed through the cone caudal to the bulbus as described above.

If no cones are available, or it is suspected that the dog's semen is sensitive to the rubber in the cone, a gloved hand (using a non-latex glove) can be used to compress the unsheathed penis caudal to the bulbus glandis, and the semen collected into a urine specimen cup or waxed drinking cup. The rim of the specimen cup should be taped to prevent cutting the penis if it should contact the cup. Some breeders simply use a plastic bag held over the penis to collect semen.

The first (clear) fraction and the second (sperm-rich, cloudy) fraction should be collected. After these fractions are ejaculated, close inspection of the collection tube should demonstrate that clear fluid is starting to layer on the cloudy second fraction; at this point, the collection may be stopped. The dog may continue to ejaculate prostatic fluid for up to 10 min before the erection subsides. The sheath should be examined after the penis is retracted to ensure that the penis is situated normally within the sheath and that no hair is caught within the sheath. Residual protrusion may occur if the sheath rolls inward as the penis retracts.

Semen evaluation consists of determination of appearance, volume, concentration, motility, and percent morphologically normal sperm. Yellow, brown, or red samples may indicate the presence of blood or urine in the ejaculate. The volume is variable, depending on how much prostatic fluid was collected and the size of the dog; it ranges from <2 to >20 mL but is typically ~5 mL. Sperm motility should be evaluated immediately using warmed equipment; sperm should be >70% progressively motile spermatozoa. Sperm morphology is determined as for the bull (p 1797). At least 80% of the sperm should be morphologically normal. The concentration is determined using a hemocytometer. To do this, the sperm is diluted at 1:100, and the number of sperm in the large central square (made up of 25 smaller squares) on the hemocytometer is counted. The number of sperm counted $\times 10^6$ is the concentration of spermatozoa/mL. The total number of sperm in the ejaculate is calculated as volume × concentration. This should be $\geq 200 \times 10^6$, and closer to 400×10^6 in larger dogs.

Every dog investigated for infertility should be screened for *Brucella canis*. (*See also* BRUCELLOSIS, p 1159.)

Sperm quality may be normal or abnormal, or no sperm may be seen in the ejaculate. Infertility is rare in dogs with a normal sperm evaluation and, if seen, the history should be reviewed for mismanagement or bitch infertility. The presence of WBC or RBC in the ejaculate suggests inflammation of the tract, most commonly prostatitis; culture of prostatic fluid and appropriate treatment may help fertility. If sperm quality is abnormal, the history should again be reviewed to determine if the dog has been sick recently or has received any drugs, especially anabolic steroids. Other recognized causes of abnormal sperm quality include inflammation of the scrotum or other factors that may be causing a high scrotal temperature, testicular neoplasia (ultrasonography of the testicles is recommended because many neoplasms of the testes are not palpable), trauma to the area of the scrotum, or brucellosis. However, most cases of low sperm quality in dogs are idiopathic.

The dog's pituitary status can be investigated but is usually unrevealing. Luteinizing hormone and follicle-stimulating hormone are typically normal to high in dogs with abnormal semen quality because the degenerating testes are not able to provide the feedback mechanism to the pituitary. Because abnormal sperm quality may be induced by a recent transient disease or exposure to toxins, and spermatogenesis might resume, collections should be repeated about every 3 mo for ~1 yr before a definitive prognosis for breeding can be given.

Azoospermia is relatively common in dogs. It may be due to failure of the dog's testicles to produce sperm, or to failure of the sperm to exit the testicles because of epididymal blockage or incomplete ejaculation. The ejaculate may be tested for the presence of alkaline phosphatase, which is secreted by the epididymis. A high value (>5,000 IU/L [very high in comparison with blood]) indicates fluid from the epididymis was collected. High alkaline phosphatase values in sperm-free fluid suggest that the testes are not producing sperm or that sperm transit is blocked between the testes and epididymides. Low values suggest epididymal blockage or failure of ejaculation; semen collections should be repeated, using a strong stimulus such as a bitch in estrus. The urinary bladder should be catheterized to determine if retrograde ejaculation is occurring; swab samples of the vagina of a bitch after natural mating may also be performed to determine if the dog is not ejaculating due to aversion to manual collection. Careful palpation and ultrasonographic examination should be performed to detect any abnormality of the epididymides or spermatic cords, such as absence or blockage of the epididymis.

EMBRYO TRANSFER IN FARM ANIMALS

In farm mammals, early embryos can be removed from the uterus of their dam (the donor) and transferred to the uterus of other females (recipients) for development to term. The main use of embryo transfer is increased productivity of selected females; others are identification of potential artificial insemination (AI) bulls through contract matings, disease control, importation and exportation of livestock, rapid screening of AI sires for genetically recessive characteristics (eg, syndactyly), and treatment or circumvention of certain types of infertility. Embryo transfer also is a useful research tool for evaluating fetal and maternal interactions.

Cattle: In cattle, the day of the estrous cycle in donors and recipients is estimated by estrus detection (first day of estrus = day 0). Donors are induced to superovulate by treatment with equine chorionic gonadotropin (eCG; currently not available) or with follicle-stimulating hormone (FSH; activity varies, use according to label directions), typically given BID starting on day 9-14 of the cycle. Prostaglandin (PG) $F_{2\alpha}$, 25-35 mg, IM, is administered on the third or fourth day of gonadotropin treatment, and estrus should be seen 36-48 hr later. Although there appears to be no difference in pregnancy rates among recipients ovulating from 1 day before to 1 day after the donor, synchrony is considered to be optimal when the recipient ovulates on the same day as the donor. Recipients with a single growing follicle take longer to come into estrus after prostaglandin administration than do donors that have multiple follicles. For this reason, $PGF_{2\alpha}$ is often given to recipient cows in mid-diestrus the evening before the donor cow is treated with prostaglandin. Donors are typically inseminated with high-quality semen at 12 and 24 hr after the onset of estrus, or at 72, 84, and 96 hr after treatment with prostaglandin. Estrus may also be synchronized by use of progestagen and estrogen regimens or gonadotropin and prostaglandin regimens (*see* HORMONAL CONTROL OF ESTRUS, p 1808). While up to 90% of cows have been reported to respond to superovulatory treatments, 20-30% of cows flushed produce no transferable embryos. An average of 5 or 6 transferable embryos can be expected from each donor cow, but variability in response to superovulatory treatments is high. Induction of superovulation is particularly difficult in old or high-yielding, lactating dairy cows and may lead to loss of milk. Some practitioners use repeated single embryo collections during successive untreated cycles, while others superovulate and collect embryos from donor cows on the cycle before the cow is bred for pregnancy establishment (to initiate the next lactation) to maintain close to a 365-day calving interval. Cows can be successfully superovulated every 35-40 days.

To perform embryo collection, the rectum is evacuated (at this time the number of corpora lutea on the ovary may be estimated), and the cow is given an epidural anesthetic. The perineum is washed, and a 12- to 24-French Foley-type or 3-way catheter, stiffened by a stylet, is passed into the vagina. While palpating per rectum, the operator guides the catheter through the cervix into the uterus, about halfway up one uterine horn; the stylet is then withdrawn, and the cuff near the end of the catheter is inflated. In this way, the tip of each uterine horn is flushed separately. This may be done because cattle embryos do not migrate after descending into the horn.

About 20-35 mL of fluid (typically Dulbecco's phosphate buffered saline) with added antibiotics (eg, 60 IU penicillin and 60 μg streptomycin/mL) and either 1% fetal calf serum or bovine serum albumin (4 mg/mL) is placed into the horn during each flush. Complete flush medium is also available. Medium containing polyvinyl alcohol in place of protein may foam less when used for flushing and can be stored at room temperature. When the horn becomes mildly distended, as detected by transrectal palpation, the fluid is drained from the horn. The flushes are repeated ~10-15 times if using a fluid-in/fluid-out technique, or for a total of 800 mL if using a continuous flow technique. Alternatively, the entire uterus may be flushed at one time; the uterus may take up to 1 L of medium per flush. An embryo filter is placed in the outflow, and embryos are washed from the filter for examination. Ova or embryos are located using a dissecting microscope at ~10× magnification.

Once embryos are located, they are transferred to a smaller volume of transfer medium (Dulbecco's phosphate buffered saline with up to 20% serum or 0.4% bovine serum albumin; complete transfer medium is also available commercially) and examined morphologically at 50-100× magnification to evaluate their quality. Those selected as being viable and of transferable quality are held in the medium at room temperature until they are transferred to recipients or prepared for freezing, bisection ("splitting"), or more specialized treatment, such as sex determination. Alternatively, embryos can be refrigerated in transfer medium for up to 24 hr with no loss of viability. Splitting embryos into identical halves by microsurgery is practiced by a few commercial embryo transfer teams. The number of embryos to be transferred can be doubled with only a minor reduction in pregnancy rates. However, techniques of freezing manipulated embryos still need to be improved.

Almost exclusively, embryos are transferred nonsurgically. The embryo is loaded into a small pipette (embryo straw) in a specialized (Cassou-type) insemination "gun." This is placed into the vagina and, with the aid of manual palpation per rectum, is threaded through the cervix into the horn ipsilateral to the corpus luteum. Although it is desirable to place the embryo into the cranial uterine horn, it is better to place it quickly and atraumatically into the caudal horn than to manipulate the tract for a prolonged period of time. Surgical transfer is performed rarely; paravertebral or local anesthesia is used, and the flank ipsilateral to the recipient's corpus luteum is opened by a straight or grid incision. The uterus is grasped and a small puncture made, then a pipette holding the embryo is placed through the puncture, and the embryo is deposited into the horn with a minimal volume of medium. The flank incision is closed routinely.

After direct transfer of single fresh embryos, 60-70% of recipients become pregnant; frozen embryos result in pregnancy rates of 50-60%. When 2 embryos are transferred to each recipient, the pregnancy rate is 60-90%, with 40-60% embryo survival, but twin transfers are rarely performed commercially because of the risks of causing calving difficulties and of producing freemartins when the twins are not of the same sex. Splitting of embryos would overcome the latter problem.

Sheep and Goats: Techniques and results in sheep and goats are basically similar to those in cattle, except that surgical or laparoscopic methods are almost always used for collection and transfer. Ewe and doe recipients are synchronized so that ovulation occurs ~12 hr before donor ovulation. Transcervical collection of embryos in the doe has been attempted with variable success. Per rectum manipulation of the tract is not possible, so flushes generally involve the whole uterus rather than individual horns as in the cow. Although this method is possible in goats, it is much less repeatable in sheep because the more convoluted cervix is difficult to cannulate.

Pigs: Embryo collection and transfer in pigs is usually done surgically. Nonsurgical and endoscopic techniques for transfer have been reported but tend to result in lower pregnancy rates. Although sows can be superovulated, donors that are to be used repeatedly are typically allowed to cycle normally because the ovulation rate in sows is high and superovulation response can be variable. There is evidence of reduced embryo viability if superovulation response is too high. Survival of embryos from first-estrus gilts is ~20% lower than from older gilts. Embryos are collected via midventral laparotomy, under general anesthesia 4-6 days after the onset of estrus, by normograde flushing of the oviduct and collection of the flush fluid from the tip of the uterine horn. On day 4, embryos are in the 4- to 8-cell stage and are easily differentiated from unfertilized ova, whereas later stages are not. For surgical transfer, recipients should come into estrus 1 day before to 2 days after the donor; preference is given to those that come into estrus the same day or 1 day later than the donor. Methods of synchronization are more complicated than in cattle because the corpus luteum of swine is not responsive to prostaglandins until late in diestrus (*see* HORMONAL CONTROL OF ESTRUS, p 1808). Embryos >2 cells are placed in the tip of the uterine horn of the recipient under general anesthesia. Bleeding and adhesion formation may be minimized by puncturing the oviduct near the uterotubal junction and threading a narrow-gauge catheter (eg, tomcat catheter) through this opening into the uterus; embryos are expelled into the uterus through the catheter. Embryos will migrate throughout the uterus after transfer. Nonsurgical transfer involves threading a spiral pipette into the cervix of the recipient, expelling the embryos into the uterus, and flushing the catheter with 10-12 mL of medium. There is some evidence that using nonsedated recipients results in higher pregnancy rates with this method. With either method, ≥14 embryos should be transferred to help ensure that luteolysis is prevented.

Farrowing rate after surgical embryo transfer is ~70%. When transfers are done within 6 days of the onset of estrus, embryo survival rates in farrowing recipients are reported to be similar to those occurring naturally; about 30% of embryos fail to survive. Nonsurgical transfer resulted in a lower farrowing rate (~20%) and smaller litter size. Significant developments have been made with respect to the freezing of porcine embryos. These techniques, although still uncommonly used, include delipidating embryos prior to freezing and vitrification techniques.

Horses: In mares, embryo transfer is used to increase productivity of a given mare or to obtain a foal from a mare that is not able to carry a foal to term. Superovulation is of variable efficacy in mares. Recent work with BID administration of equine FSH resulted in an increased ovulation rate (3-4 ovulations/mare) and increased embryo recovery (>1.5 embryos/treated mare, compared with 0.5 embryos/control mare). Equine FSH is now commercially available in the USA. For fertile, naturally ovulating donors, an embryo recovery rate of 60-70% and a pregnancy rate after transfer of 70% can be expected; these rates are 30% and 50% for subfertile donors. Breeding of the donor mare is done as for a conventional pregnancy; however, ultrasonography is essential to determine the exact day of ovulation, on which the day of embryo recovery is based.

The recipient mare should ovulate from 1 day before to 3 days after the donor mare ovulates. If a large recipient mare herd is available, mares that have ovulated at the appropriate time may be selected from the herd. If small numbers of recipients are used, the time of ovulation of the donor and recipient mares must be synchronized. This may be done using a progesterone and estrogen regimen (*see* HORMONAL CONTROL OF ESTRUS, p 1808). The recipient mares should be started on the regimen 2 days after the donor to help ensure that they do not ovulate before the donor. Mares should be examined by ultrasonography daily to detect ovulation. To aid synchronization, ovulation may be speeded in the donor or recipient by administration of human chorionic gonadotropin (hCG) or deslorelin when a mature follicle is present. Two recipients should be synchronized for each donor to enable the recipient with the best synchronization to be chosen at the time of transfer; in addition, both recipients may be needed if the mare ovulates 2 follicles. Alternatively, ovariectomized or follicle-suppressed progesterone-treated mares may be used as recipients, eliminating the need for donor synchronization and for examination of recipient mares to detect ovulation. Recipients should be ovariectomized no more than 6 mo before transfer or should be treated with estrogen and then progesterone for a period (followed by at least 1 wk of no treatment) before being used as a recipient. Follicular suppression may be induced by administration of 2 deslorelin implants (2.2 mg, IM) to induce ovulation of a mature follicle, followed by prostaglandin administration when the resulting corpus luteum is 5-7 days old. This may result in up to 30 days of follicular suppression. The ovariectomized or suppressed recipient is untreated until donor ovulation is detected (day 0), or may be given estradiol (eg, 3.3 mg estradiol 17β, IM, SID) during this time. Starting on day 2, the recipient is given progesterone in oil, 300 mg, IM, SID. After embryo transfer, the recipient is continued on a progestagen daily until day 100 of gestation, after which placental progesterone is sufficient to maintain pregnancy. Recipients with intact ovaries may be able to discontinue progesterone sooner if secondary ovulations are seen after day 40 of pregnancy. Ovariectomized recipient mares have normal pregnancy rates after transfer, as well as normal parturition, lactation, and maternal behavior; they may also be used successfully again as embryo recipients after foaling. Fewer data are currently available on follicle-suppressed, hormone-treated mares, but no abnormalities in pregnancy or maternal function have been noted.

Embryos are usually recovered on day 7 or 8 after donor mare ovulation. Modified Dulbecco's phosphate buffered saline with 1% fetal calf serum, or a commercially available equine embryo flush solution, is used for embryo recovery. Three 1-L flushes are performed. The mare is restrained in stocks with the tail wrapped and tied to the side, and the perineum is scrubbed and dried. A Foley-type catheter is passed manually through the vagina and cervix and into the uterine body. The cuff is then inflated with 30-40 mL of air and is pulled caudally to rest against the internal cervical os. The flush medium (1 L) is infused by gravity flow into the uterus. The fluid is then drained from the uterus by gravity flow. A wait of 3 min before draining may increase embryo recovery rates; alternatively, the fluid may be massaged throughout the uterus by palpation per rectum before it is drained. The fluid may be collected into a 1-L container and then poured through an embryo filter, or the filter may be placed directly in the outflow line. The latter may limit the speed of the outflow, potentially reducing embryo recovery. After the 3 uterine flushes have been performed, the donor mare is given $PGF_{2\alpha}$, 10 mg, IM, to shorten the cycle and to reduce the chance of endometritis due to organisms introduced into the uterus during flushing.

The embryo is then located within the filter contents. Early embryos are similar to those of cattle, being still enclosed by the zona pellucida, appearing somewhat like a parasite egg ~200 μm in diameter. Later embryos have a hollow center and cellular rim or, if completely expanded, appear as a gray, semitranslucent sphere of up to 0.5 mm diameter on day 7 and 1 mm diameter on day 8. The embryo is transferred into a small (35 mm) Petri dish containing fresh medium with 10-20% neonatal calf serum or commercial handling medium, and is washed by transferring it at least 2 more times to droplets of fresh medium. As soon as the embryo is washed, it may be transferred, which should be done within 3 hr of collection.

For transcervical transfer, the recipient should be restrained and the perineum scrubbed as described above for the donor. Tranquilization of the recipient with xylazine or acepromazine, if necessary, does not appear to lower pregnancy rates. Tranquilization may relax the cervix and aid in a smooth transfer. The embryo is loaded into an insemination pipette or an embryo straw in the following sequence: medium, air, medium, air, medium containing the embryo, air, medium, air. If a straw is used, it is then loaded into an insemination gun. The pipette or insemination gun is passed manually into the vagina. The external os of the cervix is located but not cannulated with the finger. By stabilizing the cervix with the fingers, the pipette is passed into the external os, and the hand is withdrawn from the vagina. The pipette is manipulated through the cervix by palpation per rectum, and the embryo is expelled into the uterus. Surgical transfer may be done via flank incision as described for cattle (see above) but has no benefit over transcervical transfer.

Embryo freezing is still not widely used in horses because larger embryos (>6.5 days old) have poor viability after thawing. However, embryos in commercial handling media may be successfully cooled and stored for up to 24 hr in semen transport containers, allowing time for shipment to an embryo transfer facility, with no decrease in pregnancy rates after transfer.

HORMONAL CONTROL OF ESTRUS

The major areas in which administration of hormones may be used to manipulate the estrous cycle are to induce luteolysis, suppress estrus, induce cyclicity in anestrous animals, superovulate cyclic animals, and induce ovulation of a mature follicle. The most effective treatments for these manipulations vary among species. Some of the following treatments currently lack regulatory approval; label instructions should be followed.

Horses: Estrous behavior may be undesirable in performance horses and can be suppressed in mares by administration of progestagens, either progesterone in oil (150-300 mg, IM, SID) or altrenogest (0.44 mg/kg, PO, SID). The oral progestagen is preferable because of muscle irritation from the injectable preparation. Progesterone in a biorelease vehicle may be available by prescription from a compounding pharmacy. This preparation (1.5 g, IM) is administered once every 7-10 days. Treatment with progestagens for 15 days during the late transition season can advance the first ovulation of the year by ~10 days. Although these preparations suppress estrous behavior, they may not effectively suppress follicle growth and ovulation in cyclic mares.

Ovulation may be synchronized in mares by administration of progesterone in oil (150 mg) and estradiol 17β in oil (10 mg, IM, SID for 10 days) with prostaglandin (PG) $F_{2\alpha}$ (10 mg, IM) administered on the tenth day. Mares should come into estrus ~3 days after the end of treatment, and 85% of mares ovulate 9-13 days after the end of treatment.

Estrus may be induced in diestrous mares (having a corpus luteum that is 5 or more days postovulation) by treatment with $PGF_{2\alpha}$ (10 mg, IM) or cloprostenol (250 μg, IM) to lyse the corpus luteum. Mares should return to estrus in ~3 days and ovulate an average of 9-10 days after PG treatment. The time to ovulation is variable, however, depending on the size of the largest follicle on the ovary at the time of PG administration. $PGF_{2\alpha}$ causes numerous transient side effects in horses, including sweating, colic, and trembling. PG causes luteolysis of a mature corpus luteum and so is not effective in inducing estrus in anestrous mares.

Behavioral estrus may be induced in anestrous or ovariectomized mares by administration of estradiol 17β in oil (1-10 mg, IM) or estradiol cypionate (0.5 mg, IM). Mares should show estrus in 12-24 hr. This estrus is not associated with follicular growth and is not fertile. Treatment with estradiol cypionate is longlasting, but repeated or high doses may cause aggressive or defensive behavior when the mare is approached by a stallion. Treatment with estrogen in the presence of progesterone (eg, in a cyclic mare in diestrus) will not induce estrous behavior.

Ovulation may be induced in mares with mature preovulatory follicles (>33 mm diameter) by administration of human chorionic gonadotropin (hCG), 2,500 IU, IV; by administration of a deslorelin implant, 2.2 mg, SC; or by administration of deslorelin, 1-2 mg, IM, in a biorelease vehicle. Ovulation is seen in 85% of mares within 48 hr, typically 36-42 hr after hCG or injectable deslorelin treatment or 40-44 hr after treatment with a deslorelin implant. Repeated use of hCG over a long period may be associated with antibody formation and decrease in response to treatment; this should not be seen with deslorelin. Use of deslorelin in implant form has been associated with periods of anestrus in treated mares, especially if the corpus luteum of ovulation is lysed with PG. For this reason, many veterinarians remove the implant after ovulation is seen; this is easily performed if the implant is placed in the vulvar mucosa.

Techniques for superovulation have recently shown promise. Mares do not superovulate in response to equine chorionic gonadotropin (eCG), and they do not respond well to follicle-stimulating hormone (FSH) derived from other species, but they may be superovulated (average of 3-4 follicles ovulated) by treatment with equine FSH, which is now commercially available. Administration of 2-20 μg GnRH/hr (by infusion pump) over ~10 days is effective in inducing normal follicular growth and ovulation in anestrous mares; the larger dose induces superovulation (average of 3 follicles). Cyclicity has also been induced in anestrous mares by treatment with 200 μg GnRH every 6 hr, or by administration of a GnRH agonist every 12 hr.

Cattle: In cows, ovulation may be synchronized with a progestagen and estrogen combination treatment, a 2-dose PG regimen, or a GnRH and PG combination. An effective progestagen treatment is a commercially available combination of an IM injection of 5 mg estradiol valerate and 3 mg norgestomet, with an ear implant of 6 mg norgestomet that is left in for 9 days. Cows come into estrus 1-2 days after cessation of treatment and may be inseminated one time at 48-54 hr after the implant is removed for acceptable conception rates. Alternatively, a controlled intravaginal drug-release device may be used. This device contains progesterone and is labeled for estrus synchronization in beef and dairy cattle. It is inserted for 7 days, with an injection of $PGF_{2\alpha}$ on day 6 (or off-label, day 7); most heats are synchronized at ~48 hr after removal. Administration of $PGF_{2\alpha}$ (25 mg, IM) or PG analog (cloprostenol at 500 μg, IM) to cows with a corpus luteum 7 days after ovulation results in estrus in ~2-5 days. Two PG injections given 14 days apart synchronize estrus and ovulation in most cows. Time to estrus is more variable than with progesterone suppression, so insemination should be based on detection of estrus. Ovulation may also be synchronized by administration of GnRH, 100 μg, IM (day 1), followed by PG treatment on day 8 and a second GnRH treatment on day 10. Cows should be inseminated 0-20 hr after the second GnRH treatment. This GnRH and $PGF_{2\alpha}$ protocol is termed "ovsynch." There are many variations on this protocol, using additional steroids, PG, or GnRH treatments, that may increase the degree of synchrony or pregnancy rates after artificial insemination.

Ovulation may be induced in cows with mature follicles (10-15 mm diameter) by treatment with GnRH at 100-250 μg, IM; luteinizing hormone (LH) at 25 mg, IM; or hCG at 5,000-10,000 IU, IM. Because the endogenous LH peak develops at the onset of estrus, this administration will not speed the time of ovulation in estrous cows but may be used to ensure luteinization in cows with histories of cystic ovarian disease or to induce ovulation in anestrous postpartum cows.

Superovulation may be achieved in the cow by treatment with eCG (not currently commercially available) in mid-diestrus followed by PG-induced luteolysis 2-3 days later, or by treatment with FSH (potencies differ, refer to label instructions), typically IM, BID for 4-5 days, with administration of PG (25-35 mg, IM) usually on day 3 or 4 of treatment. FSH treatment is discontinued at the onset of estrus.

Goats and Sheep: In cycling goats, luteolysis may be induced by administration of $PGF_{2\alpha}$ (2.5-5 mg, IM) as early as day 4. In sheep, $PGF_{2\alpha}$ (5 mg) or cloprostenol (125 μg) is effective after day 5 of the cycle. Estrus may be synchronized by 2 doses of PG, 11 days apart in does or 9 days apart in ewes. Estrus may also be synchronized in cycling or anestrous does and ewes by administration of progestagens; impregnated vaginal pessaries have been the most widely used agents for control of ovulation but are not currently available for clinical use in the USA. A portion of a bovine norgestomet implant (3 mg/goat) or injection of progesterone in oil (10 mg/day, IM) has also been effective. Progestagen treatment is administered for 10-14 days in sheep and for 14-21 days in goats. Ewes should be joined with rams the day after cessation of treatment; does return to heat on the second or third day after treatment ends. Injection of eCG (500 IU; not currently commercially available) at the end of treatment increases synchronization of ovulation or ovulation rate, or both, but may result in superovulation and problems with multiple lambs or kids. Alternatively, in does, progestagens may be given for 11 days with eCG and PG administered on day 9, and insemination performed on days 12 and 13. In regimens involving treatments other than PG alone, fertility may be reduced on the first estrus after treatment.

Pigs: In pigs, estrus synchronization may be easily achieved by synchronized weaning of lactating sows; estrus is seen 4-10 days later. Administration IM of a commercially available combination of eCG (400 IU) and hCG (200 IU), given as a single injection within 12 hr after weaning, tightens the synchronization, and estrus is seen 4-5 days after weaning. This eCG and hCG combination also induces estrus in gilts with delayed puberty and in sows with postweaning anestrus. Exogenous PG induces luteolysis of the porcine corpus luteum only after day 12 of the estrous cycle and, therefore, is not a practical agent for estrous cycle control; however, estrus may be synchronized by induction of abortion in sows pregnant >15 days by administration of $PGF_{2\alpha}$ (15 mg, IM, then 10 mg, IM, 12 hr later) or cloprostenol (1 mg, followed 24 hr later by 0.5 mg); sows return to estrus 4-10 days after treatment. Estrus may also be synchronized by feeding altrenogest (15-20 mg, PO, SID for 14-18 days) or by using bovine norgestomet implants (one implant followed by addition of a second implant 9 days later) removed 19 days after initiation of treatment; neither treatment is currently approved in the USA for swine. Combination eCG and hCG may be given on the day of progestagen withdrawal to better synchronize estrus.

Dogs: In bitches, estrus may be suppressed by administration of mibolerone (an androgen, 30-180 μg, PO, SID, depending on the dog's weight) for no more than 24 mo. Treatment must be started at least 30 days before estrus. Estrus is variable but typically develops soon after cessation of treatment; fertility should be normal by the second estrus after treatment. The progestagen megestrol acetate (2.2 mg/kg, PO, SID for 8 days) may be used to stop a cycle when the bitch has already entered proestrus. Administration must start in the first 3 days of proestrus (vulvar bleeding). The next estrus usually develops 4-6 wk earlier than expected. To delay estrus, megestrol acetate treatment is begun in late anestrus (up to a few weeks before estrus is expected); the bitch is treated with 0.55 mg/kg, PO, SID for 32 days. Estrus is seen in 2-9 mo (typically 5-6 mo); fertility is not affected. Neither drug is recommended for use in bitches on their first estrus or in bitches primarily used for breeding. Side effects of megestrol acetate treatment are uncommon but include cystic endometrial hyperplasia and pyometra; longterm treatment may result in obesity, diabetes mellitus, and neoplasia of the uterus and mammary glands. Mibolerone may cause skin, vaginal, and clitoral changes. Extended-release implants of deslorelin have suppressed estrus for >1 yr in bitches without apparent side effects and with full return to fertility; clinical use of deslorelin for estrus suppression is currently under investigation.

Estrus induction in bitches is problematic; many methods have been proposed but repeatability is low. Recently, use of the dopamine agonists cabergoline (5 µg/kg, PO, SID until 2 days after onset of proestrus) and bromocriptine (0.3 mg/bitch for 3 days followed by 0.6-2.5 mg per bitch for 3-6 days after onset of proestrus) has been reported to induce fertile estrus. Average length of treatment was 16-19 days. Use of deslorelin implants may also be effective for induction of estrus but has been associated with low progesterone values during diestrus. Removal of the implant 10 days after insertion may overcome this problem. Induction of estrus with GnRH analogs is currently under investigation.

Cats: Megestrol acetate may be used to suppress estrus in queens by treating with 5 mg/cat daily for 3 days, then 2.5-5 mg once weekly for a maximum of 10 wk. The queen should be allowed an estrus before resuming therapy. Mibolerone is not approved for use in queens due to hepatotoxicity but is effective at 50 µg/cat, PO, SID. Longterm deslorelin implants have also suppressed estrus in cats, but the length of suppression is variable. Estrus may be induced in queens with FSH, 2 mg, IM, the first day, then 0.5-1 mg, IM, daily for 4 additional days. For queens with anovulation or for queens undergoing artificial insemination, ovulation of mature follicles (present on day 2 of estrus) may be induced by treatment with hCG at 250 mg, IM, or GnRH at 25 µg, IM.

NUTRITION: CATTLE

BEEF CATTLE

NUTRITIONAL REQUIREMENTS

Beef cattle production, whether on range, improved pasture, or in the feedlot, is most economic when roughages are used effectively. Young growing grass or other pasture crops usually supply ample nutrients, such that mature and young growing cattle can consume sufficient good-quality mixed pasture (grasses and legumes) for normal growth and maintenance. However, mature and weathered pasture, crop residues, or forage crops harvested in a manner that results in shattering, leaching, or spoilage may be so reduced in nutritive value (particularly protein, phosphorus, and provitamin A or β-carotene) that they are suitable only in a maintenance ration for adult cattle. Such feedstuffs should be supplemented if used for any other purposes.

The mineral content of forages may be influenced by the corresponding mineral levels in the soil or by excess levels of some minerals that reduce the availability of others. Mature forages may also be lower in mineral content, especially phosphorus. Normally, supplemental minerals are supplied in a free-choice mineral mix or force-fed in the total mixed ration.

Certain nutrients are required by beef cattle in the daily ration, whereas others can be stored in the body. When body stores of a nutrient are high, eg, vitamin A, dietary supplementation is unnecessary until such stores are depleted. However, it may be difficult to determine when body stores have been depleted until advanced signs of deficiency start to appear.

The following are dietary requirements for maintenance, growth, finishing, reproduction, and lactation in beef cattle.

Water: Water, although not considered a nutrient per se, is required for the regulation of body temperature, as well as for growth, reproduction, lactation, digestion, metabolism, excretion, hydrolysis of nutrients, transportation of nutrients and waste in the body, joint lubrication, plus many more functions. Restricting water intake results in impaired performance. An animal will expire more quickly from a water deficiency than from a deficiency of any other nutrient.

Because feeds themselves contain water, and the metabolism of ingested feeds releases water (called metabolic water), not all of the animal's water needs have to be met by drinking water. Thirst is the result of need, and animals drink to meet this need. The need for water results from an increase in the electrolyte concentration in the body fluids, which activates the thirst mechanism.

Many factors, including temperature and body weight, affect water consumption in cattle. An 800-lb (364-kg) heifer at an environmental temperature of 4.4°C (40°F) can be expected to consume 6.3 gal. (23 L) per day; at 21°C (70°F), this will increase to 9.2 gal. (34.8 L). At the same 40°F temperature, a 400-lb (182-kg) heifer will consume ~4 gal. (15.1 L). Note that water consumption and body weight are not correlated by a straight-line relationship. A 900-lb (409-kg) lactating cow at the 40°F temperature will consume 11.4 gal. (43.1 L) per day.

Energy: Productive animals need essentially 2 types of energy. Energy of maintenance is that needed for maintaining respiration, circulation, digestion, etc. Therefore, in calculating total energy needs, the net energy for maintenance, or NE_m, must be considered. The energy required for work, growth, lactation, and reproduction is called the net energy for production, or NE_g. (*See* TABLE 10, TABLE 11, TABLE 12, TABLE 13, and TABLE 14.)

Except for young calves, beef cattle can meet their maintenance energy requirements from roughages of reasonably good quality (green, leafy, fine-stemmed, free of mold and weeds). A shortage of energy may exist on overstocked pastures, with inadequate feed allowance or poor-quality forages, or during a drought. For production, additional energy from concentrates may be necessary, especially when forages of fair to poor quality are consumed.

Especially in cold weather, roughages of varying quality may have similar maintenance energy values. Heat released during digestion and assimilation—called "heat increment"—contributes to the maintenance of body temperature for wintering stock.

Protein: Protein requirements are currently evaluated as metabolizable protein, which is interchangeable with absorbed protein. Metabolizable protein defines the protein more nearly as that which is available to the animal for maintenance and production. It is defined as the combination of the true protein absorbed by the intestine, supplied by bacterial (microbial) synthesized protein plus undegraded intake protein (UIP). The latter often has been called "bypass" protein.

Except for energy deficiency due to low feed intake, protein deficiency is the most common deficiency that limits growth, development in heifers and bulls, milk production, and reproduction. Protein deficiency of long duration eventually depresses appetite with eventual weight loss and unthriftiness, even when ample energy is available.

Feedstuffs vary greatly in protein digestibility. For example, the protein of common grains and most protein supplements is ~75-85% digestible, that of alfalfa hay ~70%, and that of grass hays usually 35-50%. The protein of low-quality feeds, such as weathered grass hay or range grass and cottonseed hulls, is digested poorly. Thus, even though total protein intake may appear to be adequate, metabolizable protein might be deficient.

A lack of protein in the diet adversely affects the microbial protein production in the rumen, which in turn reduces the utilization of low-protein feeds. Thus, much of the potential nutritive value of roughages (especially energy) may be lost if protein levels are inadequate. There is little storage of metabolizable protein in the body; it must be present in the daily ration for optimal results.

Urea and other sources of nonprotein nitrogen (NPN) are commonly used in commercial protein supplements to supply one-third or more of the total nitrogen requirement. Such products are broken down readily by the ruminal microbial protein to ammonia and then synthesized to high-quality microbial protein. The use of NPN needs available sources of ample phosphorus, trace minerals, sulfur, and soluble carbohydrates for the microbial synthesis of utilizable protein. The amount of crude protein (%N × 6.25) supplied by NPN must be stated on the feed tag accompanying commercial supplements. Toxicity is not a serious problem when urea is fed at recommended levels and mixed thoroughly with the other ingredients of the ration. However, rapid ingestion of urea at levels >20 g/100 lb (45 kg) body wt may lead to toxicity (p 2426). Several urea-molasses liquid supplements, containing as much as 10% urea, currently are self-fed to beef cattle. Caution should be exercised when cattle are started on such supplements. It is safest to offer these supplements in a lick-wheel device.

Minerals: Qualitatively, beef cattle require the same mineral elements as do dairy cattle; however, the relative quantities of the several minerals are different (*see* TABLE 15). The minerals most likely to be deficient in beef cattle diets are sodium (as salt), calcium, phosphorus, and magnesium. In some areas, including the interior of the USA, iodine may be deficient in diets for pregnant cows; likewise, there may be regional deficiencies (probably reflecting soil deficiencies) of several trace minerals, including copper, cobalt, and selenium. However, there are areas where some mineral elements (eg, selenium, molybdenum) are present at toxic levels. Attempts have been made to correct natural soil deficiencies for trace minerals by soil fertilization practices. Thus, it is implied that a beef producer needs to know the mineral and trace mineral content of the feedstuffs used in cattle rations. A general approach to prevent such deficiencies is to feed trace mineralized salt, along with a mixture of calcium and phosphorus supplements.

The **salt** (NaCl) requirements for beef cattle are quite low (0.2% of the dry matter); however, there appears to be a satiety factor involved—almost all animals appear to seek out salt if it is not readily available. Range cattle may consume 2-2.5 lb (1 kg) salt/ head/mo when forage is succulent but about half that amount when forage is mature and drier. When salt is added to a free-choice protein feed to limit intake, beef cows might consume >1 lb salt/day over long periods of time without adverse effects if they have plenty of drinking water. Signs of a salt deficiency are rather nonspecific and include pica and reduced feed intake, growth, and milk production.

Calcium is the most abundant mineral element in the body; ~98% functions as a structural component of bones and teeth. The remaining 2% is distributed in extracellular fluids and soft tissues and is involved in such vital functions as blood clotting, membrane permeability, muscle contraction, transmission of nerve impulses, cardiac regulation, secretion of certain hormones, and activation and stabilization of certain enzymes. Most roughages are relatively good sources of calcium. Cereal hays and silages and such crop residues are relatively low in calcium. Although leguminous roughages are excellent sources of calcium, even nonlegume roughages may supply adequate calcium for maintenance of beef cattle. When cattle are fed such roughages produced on calcium-low soils, or when finishing cattle are fed high-grain diets with limited nonlegume roughage, a calcium deficiency may develop. Because lactating beef cows do not produce nearly the amount of milk that dairy cattle do, their calcium requirement is much less. Nevertheless, it is sound management to provide a free-choice mineral mixture of two-thirds dicalcium phosphate and one-third iodized or trace mineralized salt. In addition, free-choice iodized or trace mineralized salt may be provided in another compartment of the mineral feeder. The total ration should provide a calcium:phosphorus ratio of ~2:1, although it appears wider ratios are tolerated if the minimum requirements for each mineral element are met and if adequate vitamin D (exposure to sunlight) is available. Range cattle should be provided a mineral supplement that has as much or more phosphorus than calcium.

About 80% of the **phosphorus** in the body is found in the bones and teeth, with the remainder distributed among the soft tissues. Phosphorus may be deficient in ordinary beef cattle rations because roughages are often low in phosphorus, perhaps reflecting a soil deficiency. Furthermore, as forage plants mature, their phosphorus content declines, making mature and weathered forages a poor source. Phosphorus has been described as the most prevalent mineral deficiency for grazing cattle worldwide. Most natural protein

TABLE 10. Mean Nutrient Content of Feeds Commonly Used in Beef Cattle Diets*

Feedstuff	DE (Mcal/kg)	ME (Mcal/kg)	NE$_m$ (Mcal/kg)	NE$_g$ (Mcal/kg)
Alfalfa (*Medicago sativa*)				
Fresh	2.73	2.24	1.38	0.80
Fresh, late vegetative	2.91	2.39	1.51	0.92
Fresh, full bloom	2.22	1.81	0.97	0.42
Hay	2.65	2.17	1.31	0.74
Hay, sun-cured, early bloom	2.65	2.17	1.31	0.74
Hay, sun-cured, mid bloom	2.56	2.10	1.24	0.68
Hay, sun-cured, full bloom	2.43	1.99	1.14	0.58
Silage	2.78	2.28	1.41	0.83
Barley (*Hordeum vulgare*)				
Grain	3.84	3.03	2.06	1.40
Silage	2.65	2.17	1.31	0.74
Beet pulp, dried	3.26	2.68	1.76	1.14
Bermuda grass (*Cynodon dactylon*)				
Fresh	2.82	2.31	1.44	0.86
Hay, sun-cured	2.16	1.77	0.93	0.39
Brewer's grains, dried	2.39	2.39	1.51	0.91
Citrus pulp, dried	3.62	2.96	2.00	1.35
Corn (*Zea mays indentata*)				
Distiller's grains, dried	3.88	3.18	2.18	1.50
Gluten feed	3.53	2.89	1.94	1.30
Grain, cracked	3.92	3.25	2.24	1.55
Silage, well-eared	3.17	2.60	1.69	1.08
Cotton (*Gossypium spp*)				
Seed	3.97	3.25	2.24	1.55
Meal	3.31	2.71	1.79	1.16
Molasses, cane	3.17	2.60	1.70	1.08
Oats	3.40	2.78	1.85	1.22
Sorghum (*Sorghum bicolor*), grain	3.62	2.96	2.00	1.35
Soybeans (*Glycine max*), meal	3.70	3.04	2.06	1.40
Wheat (*Triticum aestivum*)				
Wheat bran	3.09	2.53	1.63	1.03
Fresh, early vegetative	3.22	2.64	1.73	1.11

*Dry-matter basis; DE, digestible energy; ME, metabolizable energy; NE$_m$, net energy for maintenance; NE$_g$, net energy for gain; NE$_l$, net energy for lactation; TDN, total digestible nutrients; NDF, neutral detergent fiber; ADF, acid detergent fiber.

Adapted, with permission, from *Nutrient Requirements of Beef Cattle*, 2000, National Academy of Sciences, National Academy Press, Washington, DC.

◀ **TABLE 10.** (continued)

TDN (%)	Crude Protein (%)	Crude Fiber (%)	Ash (%)	NDF (%)	ADF (%)	Ca (%)	P (%)	Dry Matter (%)
62	18.9	26.5	10.5	47.1	36.8	1.29	0.26	23.4
66	22.2	24.2	10.2	30.9	24.0	1.71	0.30	23.2
50	19.3	30.4	10.9	4.79	3.7	1.19	0.26	23.8
60	18.6	26.1	8.6	43.9	33.8	1.40	0.28	90.6
60	19.9	28.5	9.2	39.3	31.9	1.63	0.21	90.5
58	18.7	28.0	8.5	47.1	36.7	1.37	0.22	91.0
55	17.0	30.1	7.8	48.8	38.7	1.19	0.24	90.9
63	19.5	25.4	9.5	47.5	37.5	1.32	0.31	44.2
88	13.2	3.37	2.4	18.1	5.8	0.05	0.35	88.1
60	11.9	2.92	8.3	56.8	33.9	0.52	0.29	37.1
74	9.8	20.0	5.3	44.6	27.5	0.68	0.10	91.0
64	12.6	28.4	8.1	73.3	36.8	0.49	0.27	30.3
49	7.8	2.7	76.6	—	—	38.3	8.0	93.0
66	29.2	7.8	4.18	48.7	31.2	0.29	0.70	90.2
82	6.7	12.8	6.6	23.0	23.0	1.88	0.18	91.1
90	30.4	6.9	4.6	46.0	21.3	0.26	0.83	90.3
80	23.8	7.5	6.9	36.2	12.7	0.07	0.95	90.0
90	9.8	2.3	1.5	10.8	3.3	0.03	0.32	90.0
72	8.7	19.5	3.6	46.0	26.6	0.25	0.22	34.6
90	24.4	25.6	4.2	51.6	41.8	0.17	0.52	89.4
75	46.1	13.2	7.0	28.9	17.9	0.20	1.16	90.2
72	5.8	0.5	13.3	—	0.4	1.00	0.10	74.3
77	13.6	12.0	3.3	29.3	14.0	0.01	0.41	89.2
82	12.6	2.76	1.9	16.1	6.4	0.04	0.34	90.0
84	51.8	5.4	6.9	10.3	7.0	0.46	0.73	90.9
70	17.4	11.3	6.6	42.8	14.0	0.14	1.27	89
73	27.4	17.4	13.3	46.2	28.4	0.42	0.40	22.2

supplements are fairly good sources of phosphorus. Because adequate phosphorus is critical for optimal performance of beef cattle, including growth, reproduction, and lactation, a phosphorus supplementation program is recommended using either a free-choice mineral mixture or direct supplementation in the diet. In a phosphorus deficiency,

TABLE 11. Nutrient Requirements of Pregnant Replacement Beef Cows[*] ▶

	Months Since Conception			
	1	2	3	4
NE$_m$ required (Mcal/day)				
Maintenance	5.98	6.14	6.30	6.46
Growth	2.29	2.36	2.42	2.48
Pregnancy	0.03	0.07	0.16	0.32
Total	8.31	8.57	8.87	9.26
MP required (g/day)				
Maintenance	295	303	311	319
Growth	118	119	119	119
Pregnancy	2	4	7	18
Total	415	425	437	457
Calcium required (g/day)				
Maintenance	10	11	11	11
Growth	9	9	9	8
Pregnancy	0	0	0	0
Total	19	19	20	20
Phosphorus required (g/day)				
Maintenance	8	8	8	9
Growth	4	4	3	3
Pregnancy	0	0	0	0
Total	12	12	12	12
Average daily gain (kg/day)				
Growth	0.39	0.39	0.39	0.39
Pregnancy	0.03	0.05	0.08	0.12
Total	0.42	0.44	0.47	0.51
Body wt (kg)				
Shrunk body	332	343	355	367
Gravid uterus mass	1	3	4	7
Total (kg)	333	346	359	374
Total (lb)	733	761	790	823

[*]Mature weight, 533 kg (1,173 lb); calf birth weight, 40 kg (88 lb); age at breeding, 15 mo; breed code Angus; see TABLE 10 for abbreviations. The concentration of vitamin A in all diets should be 2,200 IU/kg (1,000 IU/lb) of dry matter.

Adapted, with permission, from *Nutrient Requirements of Beef Cattle*, 2000, National Academy of Sciences, National Academy Press, Washington, DC.

reduced growth and efficiency of feed conversion, decreased appetite, impaired reproduction, reduced milk production, and weak, fragile bones can be expected. There does not appear to be any advantage to feeding more phosphorus than is recommended. Furthermore, feeding excess phosphorus contributes to increased environmental pollution. Good sources of supplemental phosphorus include steamed bone meal, mono- and dicalcium phosphate, defluorinated rock phosphate, and phosphoric acid. Because most

TABLE 11. *(continued)*

Months Since Conception				
5	6	7	8	9
6.61	6.77	6.92	7.07	7.23
2.54	2.59	2.65	2.71	2.77
0.64	1.18	2.08	3.44	5.37
9.79	10.55	11.65	13.23	15.37
326	334	342	349	357
119	117	115	113	110
27	50	88	151	251
472	501	545	613	718
12	12	12	13	13
8	8	8	8	8
0	0	12	12	12
20	20	33	33	33
9	9	10	10	10
3	3	3	3	3
0	0	7	7	7
12	13	20	20	20
0.39	0.39	0.39	0.39	0.39
0.19	0.28	0.40	0.57	0.77
0.58	0.67	0.79	0.96	1.16
379	391	403	415	426
12	19	29	44	64
391	410	432	459	490
860	902	950	1,010	1,078

grains are relatively good sources of phosphorus, feedlot cattle rarely suffer a phosphorus deficiency, although phytic acid chelation of phosphorus in grains may render up to one-half of it unavailable—especially for monogastric animals such as swine and poultry.

Magnesium maintains electrical potentials across nerve endings. In a deficiency, the lack of control of muscles is obvious. However, deficiencies are not normally anticipated. A magnesium deficiency in calves results in excitability, anorexia, hyperemia, convulsions, frothing at the mouth, and salivation, but such a condition is uncommon. Usually, a magnesium deficiency is seen in the spring in more mature grazing cattle under field conditions (ie, grass tetany, p 812). The initial signs are nervousness, reduced feed intake, and muscular twitching about the face and ears. Animals are uncoordinated and walk with a stiff gait. In advanced stages, affected cows fall to the ground, convulse, and die shortly after. A blood sample from affected cows probably would show a serum

TABLE 12. Nutrient Requirements of Beef Cows[*]

	Months Since Calving			
	1	2	3	4
NE$_m$ required (Mcal/day)				
Maintenance	10.25	10.25	10.25	10.25
Lactation	4.78	5.74	5.17	4.13
Pregnancy	0	0	0.01	0.03
Total	15.03	15.99	15.43	14.41
MP required (g/day)[†]				
Maintenance	422	422	422	422
Lactation	349	418	376	301
Pregnancy	0	0	1	2
Total (g)	771	840	799	725
Total (lb)	1.7	1.9	1.8	1.6
Calcium required (g/day)[†]				
Maintenance	16	16	16	16
Lactation	16	20	18	14
Pregnancy	0	0	0	0
Total	32	36	34	30
Phosphorus required (g/day)[†]				
Maintenance	13	13	13	13
Lactation	9	11	10	8
Pregnancy	0	0	0	0
Total	22	24	23	21
Gain in weight from pregnancy/day[†]				
Grams	0	0	20	30
Pounds	0	0	0.04	0.07
Milk production/day				
Kilograms	6.7	8.0	7.2	5.8
Pounds	14.7	17.6	15.8	12.8
Weight of conceptus				
Kilograms	0	0	1	1
Pounds	0	0	2	2

[*]Mature weight, 533 kg (1,172 lb); calf birth weight, 40 kg (88 lb); age at calving, 60 mo; peak milk, 8 kg (17.6 lb); age of calf at weaning, 30 wk; breed code Angus; milk protein, 3.4%; calving interval, 12 mo; *see* TABLE 10 for abbreviations. Crystalline vitamin A should be added at a level of 2,200 IU/kg (1,000 IU/lb) dry matter feed.

[†]No allowance made for gain because these are mature cows.

Adapted, with permission, from *Nutrient Requirements of Beef Cattle*, 2000, National Academy of Sciences, National Academy Press, Washington, DC.

magnesium level of <2.0 mg/dL. This condition is sufficiently prevalent that many beef cow herd managers supplement in the spring with magnesium oxide at 28-56 g/head/day. Beef cows generally do not like magnesium oxide; dilution by mixing it with ground corn or incorporating it into a free-choice liquid supplement improves acceptability.

TABLE 12. (continued)							
Months Since Calving							
5	6	7	8	9	10	11	12
10.25	10.25	8.54	8.54	8.54	8.54	8.54	8.54
3.10	2.23	0	0	0	0	0	0
0.07	0.16	0.32	0.64	1.18	2.08	3.44	5.37
13.42	12.64	8.87	9.18	9.72	10.62	11.98	13.91
422	422	422	422	422	422	422	422
226	163	0	0	0	0	0	0
4	7	14	27	50	88	151	251
652	592	436	449	472	510	573	673
1.4	1.3	1.0	1.0	1.0	1.1	1.3	1.5
16	16	16	16	16	16	16	16
11	8	0	0	0	0	0	0
0	0	0	0	0	12	12	12
27	24	16	16	16	28	28	28
13	13	13	13	13	13	13	13
6	4	0	0	0	0	0	0
0	0	0	0	0	5	5	5
19	17	13	13	13	18	18	18
50	80	120	190	280	400	570	770
0.11	0.18	0.26	0.42	0.62	0.88	1.25	1.70
4.3	3.1	0	0	0	0	0	0
9.5	6.8	0	0	0	0	0	0
3	4	7	12	19	29	44	64
7	9	15	26	42	64	97	141

Potassium is the major cation in intracellular fluid and is important in acid-base balance; it is involved in regulation of osmotic pressure, water balance, muscle contractions, nerve impulse transmission, and several enzymatic reactions. Potassium deficiencies are normally not anticipated in cattle diets because most forages are good sources, containing 1-4%. In fact, the high potassium content of spring pasture grass has been a suspect cause for grass tetany (p 812). A potassium deficiency might be anticipated when diets extremely high in grain are fed (eg, in finishing cattle) because grains may contain <0.5% potassium. A marginal to deficient level of potassium in growing and finishing cattle results in decreased feed intake and rate of gain. However, this effect is subtle and would probably not be noticed other than by the very experienced cattle feeder. Body stores of potassium are small, and a deficiency may develop rapidly. It is good practice to supplement rations for growing and finishing cattle such that they will contain >0.6% potassium on a dry-matter basis.

TABLE 13. Nutrient Requirements of Growing and Finishing Beef Cattle[*] ▶

Body Weight in kg (lb)	200 (440)	250 (550)
Maintenance requirement		
NE_m (Mcal/day)	4.1	4.84
MP (g/day)	202	239
Calcium (g/day)	6	8
Phosphorus (g/day)	5	6
Growth requirement		
Average daily gain in kg (lb)		
NE_g required for gain (Mcal/day)		
0.5 (1.1)	1.27	1.50
1.0 (2.2)	2.72	3.21
1.5 (3.3)	4.24	5.01
2.0 (4.4)	5.81	6.87
2.5 (5.5)	7.42	8.78
MP required for gain (g/day)		
0.5 (1.1)	154	155
1.0 (2.2)	299	300
1.5 (3.3)	441	440
2.0 (4.4)	580	577
2.5 (5.5)	718	721
Calcium required for gain (g/day)		
0.5 (1.1)	14	13
1.0 (2.2)	27	25
1.5 (3.3)	39	36
2.0 (4.4)	52	47
2.5 (5.5)	64	59
Phosphorus required for gain (g/day)		
0.5 (1.1)	6	5
1.0 (2.2)	11	10
1.5 (3.3)	16	15
2.0 (4.4)	21	19
2.5 (5.5)	26	24

[*]Weight at small marbling, 533 kg (1,173); weight range, breed code Angus; *see* TABLE 10 for abbreviations. The concentration of vitamin A in all diets for finishing steers and heifers is 2,200 IU/kg (1,000 IU/lb) dry diet.

Copper and **cobalt** deficiencies usually are regional and associated with low soil levels. In the USA, problem areas include parts of Florida and possibly isolated areas in Michigan. Cobalt functions as a component of vitamin B_{12}. Cattle do not depend on dietary vitamin B_{12} because ruminal microorganisms can synthesize it from dietary cobalt. In cattle, therefore, a cobalt deficiency is a relative vitamin B_{12} deficiency, and such cattle show weight loss, unthriftiness, fatty degeneration of the liver, and pale skin and mucosa. Copper functions as an essential component of many enzyme systems, including

◄ **TABLE 13.** (continued)

300 (660)	350 (770)	400 (880)	450 (990)
5.55	6.23	6.89	7.52
274	307	340	371
9	11	12	14
7	8	10	11
NE_g required for gain (Mcal/day)			
1.72	1.93	2.14	2.33
3.68	4.13	4.57	4.99
5.74	6.45	7.13	7.79
7.88	8.84	9.77	10.68
10.06	11.29	12.48	13.64
MP required for gain (g/day)			
158	157	145	133
303	298	272	246
442	432	391	352
577	561	505	451
710	687	616	547
Calcium required for gain (g/day)			
12	11	10	9
23	21	19	17
33	30	27	25
43	39	35	32
53	48	43	38
Phosphorus required for gain (g/day)			
5	4	4	4
9	8	8	7
13	12	11	10
18	16	14	13
22	19	17	15

Adapted, with permission, from *Nutrient Requirements of Beef Cattle*, 2000, National Academy of Sciences, National Academy Press, Washington, DC.

those that involve the production of blood components. Recommended levels of cobalt and copper should be provided in the diet, either by supplementation of the total mixed ration or as part of the free-choice mineral mix or supplemental mix.

Iodine is an integral part of thyroxine and, as such, is largely responsible for control of many metabolic functions. Typically, coastal regions that are subjected to iodine-carrying winds off the ocean have abundant supplies of iodine; however, inland soils (in the USA, especially between the Allegheny and Rocky mountains), the soil generally does

TABLE 14. Nutrient Requirements Of Growing Beef Bulls[*] ▶		
Body Weight in kg (lb)	300 (660)	400 (880)
Maintenance requirement		
NE_m(Mcal/day)	6.38	7.92
MP (g/day)	274	340
Calcium (g/day)	9	12
Phosphorus (g/day)	7	10
Growth requirement		
Average daily gain in kg (lb)		
NE_g required for gain (Mcal/day)		
0.5 (1.1)	1.72	2.13
1.0 (2.2)	3.68	4.56
1.5 (3.3)	5.74	7.12
2.0 (4.4)	7.87	9.76
2.5 (5.5)	10.05	12.47
MP required for gain (g/day)		
0.5 (1.1)	158	145
1.0 (2.2)	303	272
1.5 (3.3)	442	392
2.0 (4.4)	577	506
2.5 (5.5)	710	617
Calcium required for gain (g/day)		
0.5 (1.1)	12	10
1.0 (2.2)	23	19
1.5 (3.3)	33	27
2.0 (4.4)	43	35
2.5 (5.5)	53	43
Phosphorus required for gain (g/day)		
0.5 (1.1)	5	4
1.0 (2.2)	9	8
1.5 (3.3)	13	11
2.0 (4.4)	18	14
2.5 (5.5)	22	17

[*]Weight at maturity, 890 kg (1,958 lb); breed code Angus; see TABLE 10 for abbreviations. Vitamin A should be added at a level of 2,200 IU/kg (1,000 IU/lb) feed dry matter.

not have sufficient iodine to meet most livestock needs. Iodine requirements in cattle can be adequately met by feeding stabilized iodized salt.

Selenium is part of the enzyme glutathione peroxidase, which catalyzes the reduction of hydrogen peroxide and lipid hydroperoxides, thus preventing oxidative damage to the body tissues. White muscle disease in calves (p 897), characterized by degeneration and necrosis of skeletal and heart muscles, is the result of a selenium deficiency. Vitamin E plays a role in preventing such conditions. Other signs of a selenium deficiency include unthriftiness, weight loss, reduced immune response, and decreased reproductive

◀ TABLE 14. (continued)			
500 (1,100)	**600 (1,320)**	**700 (1,540)**	**800 (1,760)**
9.36	10.73	12.05	13.32
402	461	517	572
15	19	22	25
12	14	17	19
NE_g required for gain (Mcal/day)			
2.52	2.89	3.25	3.59
5.39	6.18	6.94	7.67
8.42	9.65	10.83	11.97
11.54	13.23	14.85	16.41
14.74	16.90	18.97	20.97
MP required for gain (g/day)			
122	100	78	58
222	175	130	86
314	241	170	102
400	299	202	109
481	352	228	109
Calcium required for gain (g/day)			
9	7	6	4
16	12	9	6
22	17	12	7
28	21	14	8
34	25	16	8
Phosphorus required for gain (g/day)			
3	3	2	2
6	5	4	2
9	7	5	3
11	8	6	3
14	10	6	3

Adapted, with permission, from *Nutrient Requirements of Beef Cattle*, 2000, National Academy of Sciences, National Academy Press, Washington, DC.

performance. It is generally accepted that the selenium requirements for cattle can be met by 0.1 mg/kg of diet (0.1 ppm).

Vitamins: While cattle probably have a metabolic requirement for all the known vitamins, dietary sources of vitamins C and K and the B-vitamin complex are not necessary in all but the very young. Vitamin K and the B vitamins are synthesized in sufficient amounts by the ruminal microflora, and vitamin C is synthesized in the tissues of all cattle. However, if rumen function is impaired, as by starvation, nutrient deficiencies, or excessive levels of antimicrobials, synthesis of these vitamins may be impaired.

TABLE 15. Requirements and Maximum Tolerable Levels of Minerals for Beef Cattle[*]

Mineral	Requirement			Maximum Tolerable Level
	Growing and Finishing	Gestation	Early Lactation	
Chlorine (%)	—	—	—	—
Chromium (mg/kg)	—	—	—	1,000
Cobalt (mg/kg)	0.10	0.10	0.10	10
Copper (mg/kg)	10	10	10	100
Iodine (mg/kg)	0.50	0.50	0.50	50
Iron (mg/kg)	50	50	50	1,000
Magnesium (%)	0.10	0.12	0.20	0.40
Manganese (mg/kg)	20	40	40	1,000
Molybdenum (mg/kg)	—	—	—	5
Nickel (mg/kg)	—	—	—	50
Potassium (%)	0.60	0.60	0.70	3
Selenium (mg/kg)	0.10	0.10	0.10	2
Sodium (%)	0.06-0.08	0.06-0.08	0.10	—
Sulfur (%)	0.15	0.15	0.15	0.40
Zinc (mg/kg)	30	30	30	500

[*]Requirements for calcium and phosphorus are listed in the preceding nutrient requirement tables.

Adapted, with permission, from *Nutrient Requirements of Beef Cattle*, 2000, National Academy of Sciences, National Academy Press, Washington, DC.

Vitamin A can be synthesized from β-carotene contained in feedstuffs such as green forages and yellow corn. However, this ability varies among breeds; Holstein cattle are perhaps the most efficient converters of carotenes, whereas some of the beef breeds are much less efficient. Therefore, providing supplemental vitamin A to beef cattle should be considered. Vitamin A is one of the few vitamins that cattle store in their livers—as much as a 6-mo supply. Cattle on a diet deficient in vitamin A may not begin to show signs for several weeks. Newborn calves, which have small stores of vitamin A, depend on colostrum and milk to meet their needs. If the dam is fed a ration low in carotene or vitamin A during gestation (eg, in winter), severe deficiency signs may become apparent in the young suckling calf within 2-4 wk of birth, while the dam may appear normal.

It is sound practice to provide 2-5 lb (1-2 kg) of early-cut, good quality legume or grass hay, or 0.5 lb (0.25 kg) of dehydrated alfalfa pellets in the daily ration of stocker cattle and pregnant cows to prevent vitamin A deficiency. Most commercial protein and mineral supplements are fortified with dry, stabilized vitamin A. The daily requirements for beef cattle appear to be ~5 mg of carotene or 2,000 IU of vitamin A/100 lb (45 kg) body wt; lactating cows may require twice this amount to maintain high vitamin levels in the milk.

Vitamin A deficiency under feedlot conditions can cause considerable loss to cattle feeders, especially if high-concentrate and corn silage rations low in carotene have been fed. Destruction of carotene during hay storage or in the GI tract, or the failure of beef cattle to convert carotene to vitamin A efficiently, may increase the need for supplemental vitamin A. Growing and finishing steers and heifers fed low-carotene diets for several months require 2,200 IU of vitamin A/kg of air-dry ration. Commercial vitamin A supplements are not expensive and should be used when such rations are fed and any danger of a deficiency exists. An alternative method of supplying supplemental vitamin A is by IM injection; in nonpasture settings, an IM injection of 5 million IU of vitamin A once yearly will suffice.

Vitamin D deficiency is comparatively rare in beef cattle because they are usually outside in direct sunlight or fed sun-cured roughage. In northern latitudes during long winters, or in show calves that are kept in the barn or turned out only at night, a deficiency is possible. The ultraviolet rays of sunlight convert provitamin D found in the skin of animals (7-dehydrocholesterol) or in harvested plants (ergosterol) to active vitamin D. Direct exposure to sunlight, consumption of sun-cured feed, or supplementary vitamin D (300 IU/45 kg body wt) prevent a deficiency.

See MYOPATHIES, p 947, for the interrelationships of vitamin E and selenium in reproduction and in the etiology of various myopathies and the predisposition of a relative thiamine (vitamin B_1) deficiency. (*See also* POLIOENCEPHALOMALACIA, p 1061.)

FEEDING AND NUTRITIONAL MANAGEMENT

Feeds for beef cattle vary widely in quality, palatability, and essential nutrient content (TABLE 10). To be most effective, any supplement must be patterned to fit the kind and quality of roughage available. Chemical analyses of roughages are very useful to determine their nutrient deficiencies and adequacies. Under certain systems of management, beef cattle are wintered as economically as possible on low-quality roughages and thus may not receive the recommended nutrients for optimal performance. Low-quality roughages, such as cereal straw, especially if cut and fed to pregnant heifers during the prolonged period of very cold weather in northern climates during winter, may result in outbreaks of highly fatal abomasal impaction. This can be prevented by ensuring that adequate amounts of grain are fed to meet the energy and protein requirements of pregnant heifers during colder weather. This may be acceptable if no serious deficiency signs develop and if the cattle can make up for poor winter gains on abundant, high-quality summer pasture. However, when maximal performance is desired (cows nursing calves, rapid growth of calves, steers and heifers on full feed), nutrient requirements should be met (TABLE 11, TABLE 12, TABLE 13, TABLE 14).

Feeding and nutritional management for 3 systems of beef production are discussed separately. (*See* HEALTH-MANAGEMENT INTERACTION: BEEF CATTLE, p 1707.)

The Breeding Herd

In many areas, producers follow a spring calving program (February to May in the USA), depending on the available feed, growth of early pasture, and prevailing climate. Fall calving has become more prevalent, particularly in the south. Wintering the lactating cow presents a much greater nutritional problem than does wintering the pregnant, non-lactating cow. Spring-born calves commonly are weaned at 6-8 mo, and their dams bred again while on pasture. Heifers may be bred to calve first as 2-yr-olds (24-27 mo) if good winter feeding is practiced to ensure maximal development and prevent high death loss of dam or calf at parturition. Heifers of British breeds should weigh at least 600-650 lb (275-300 kg) at breeding time (exotic crossbreds should be heavier) and should be fed well thereafter to allow for continued growth, good milk production, and prompt rebreeding.

Mature cows have greater body reserves and lower nutrient requirements than heifers; therefore, they can be wintered on rations of poorer quality. Usually, they are fed hay, fodder, silage, or dry grass free choice. Their ration should provide a minimum of 8% total or crude protein in the dry matter; if it does not, then 1-2 lb (0.5-1 kg) of a 20-30% protein supplement or its equivalent should be fed daily. A mineral mix and salt should be provided.

Mature beef cows may lose >150 lb (67 kg) of body wt from fall until after calving in the spring. Although this weight loss is not desirable, it may not impair reproductive performance in mature cows if spring and summer pastures are adequate. Under most profitable systems of management, a mature beef cow should maintain her weight from fall to fall. Lactation requires more nutrients than gestation. However, feeding beef cows more than is necessary for satisfactory production, such as is frequently done in purebred herds and show herds, is also undesirable. Large accumulations of body fat may lead to lowered conception rates, difficult calving, a lower calf crop, and a shorter life span for the cow.

Often a system of "creep feeding" is practiced in which suckling calves are allowed access to a grain mixture in a self-feeder in an enclosure. A creep-feed mixture might consist of 6 parts shelled corn, 3 parts wheat bran, and 1 part protein supplement (preferably pelleted). The mixture should be rather large particles to prevent dustiness. A commercial 12-14% protein creep feed may be used as an alternative.

Growing bull calves and yearlings should receive ~2 lb (1 kg) of protein supplement, 3-5 lb (1.5-2 kg) of grain, and good-quality roughage. Mature bulls commonly are wintered in the same manner as the cow herd, with a greater feed allowance during the late winter. In highly fitted show bulls, a gradual reduction in the ration and much exercise are needed before they will be in suitable shape and condition for pasture breeding. Breeding stock should have adequate nutrients in their ration and be gaining weight before and during the breeding season. Deficiency of several nutrients, especially carotene, phosphorus, energy, and protein, reduces fertility. These nutrients should be present in adequate amounts in the ration at least 6-8 wk before breeding.

Stocker Cattle

It is common practice to feed calves and yearlings to make moderate gains in winter, with faster and less expensive gains on summer pasture. Such cattle may be sold as feeders in the spring or finished out in dry lot the following fall. The cost of winter gain on harvested feeds invariably is higher than summer gain on pasture; hence, it is advisable to winter cattle so as to make the greatest possible gains on pasture. To maintain good health, weanling calves should gain >1 lb (0.5 kg)/day. Two pounds (1 kg) of grain plus 1-2 lb (0.5-1 kg) of protein supplement are recommended in addition to nonlegume roughage. If legume roughage is fed, no protein supplement is needed. Older cattle, particularly if they enter the winter in fleshy condition, may do well just to maintain their weight. A free-choice mineral mixture and trace mineralized salt should be supplied. Limited amounts of grain fed to yearling cattle on pasture during the late summer may increase their market value.

Finishing Cattle

This phase of beef production consists of full feeding of grain with limited amounts of roughage until market weight and finish are reached. Older cattle may reach finish on pasture alone (or with only a few pounds of grain/day) or after 60-90 days in the feedlot on high-grain rations to improve market grade and to remove any yellow tinges from their body fat (due to stored carotene from pasture forage). Weanling calves commonly are shipped direct to the feedlot and after 120-150 days are fed finishing rations for 100-150 days; yearlings require ~150 days, and older steers 100-125 days. Grain consumption of cattle on full-feed is ~2-2.5 lb/100 lb (1 kg/45 kg) body wt. Roughage consumption usually is limited to about one-fourth to one-third of the total concentrate consumption after cattle are on full-feed. Cattle consume ~3% of their body wt/day when self-fed mixed rations. For calves, ~1.5-2 lb (<1 kg) of a 33% protein supplement is required daily for best gains and market grades when nonlegume roughage is fed.

The grain (concentrate) allowance for finishing cattle should be increased gradually over 2-3 wk from the time they are started on a finishing program to get them on full feed. Feeding too much grain to finishing cattle too rapidly can lead to lactic acidosis or founder. Self-fed, total mixed rations should contain >50% roughage as cattle are started on feed.

Corn or sorghum silages are very palatable, and cattle of lower grade may be finished principally on silage supplemented with protein and minerals. Alfalfa or grass silage is relatively high in protein, carotene, and minerals but is lacking in available energy. Alfalfa hay is an excellent roughage but may cause bloat in calves if fed as the only feed. Grains for finishing cattle have about the same relative value as indicated by their total digestible nutrient content. Plant-source proteins are equal in value and can be replaced in part by feeding supplements containing urea. For optimal performance, undegraded intake protein, also known as "bypass protein," should be provided (*see* PROTEIN, p 1918). Supplements should be fortified with minerals, vitamins, and desired feed additives. A small amount of molasses (1 lb [0.5 kg]/head/day) may improve rations that contain low-quality roughages, such as corn cobs, weathered hays, or cottonseed hulls.

PERFORMANCE MODIFIERS

See also GROWTH PROMOTANTS AND PRODUCTION ENHANCERS, p 2168.

There are 2 groups of performance modifiers used in beef cattle production—hormone-like growth enhancers (mostly subcutaneous implants) and ruminal chemistry modifiers, which alter ruminal fatty acid production in the rumen.

Hormone-like growth enhancers for finishing beef cattle were discovered in 1948, when it was shown that subcutaneous implantation of diethylstilbestrol (DES) caused an increase in growth rate of ~10%. The use of DES in finishing beef cattle was practiced for ~25 yr, until the FDA declared it illegal. However, other similar compounds were approved by the FDA by that time. The average increase in daily gain due to the use of effective implants is ~0.23 kg (0.5 lb), and the improvement in the feed to gain ratio is 0.56 kg feed/ kg gain.

Ionophores are antibiotics that alter the chemistry of the rumen by altering the rumen microflora to produce increased proportions of propionic acid and decreased proportions of acetic and butyric acids. These 3 acids, called volatile fatty acids (VFA), are the products of ruminal fermentation and can be absorbed from the digestive tract of the cow and used as energy sources. Because propionic acid releases more energy per unit weight to the host cow upon oxidation than do the other 2 VFA, it is important in beef cattle production. However, because butyric acid, especially, is involved in butterfat production, anything that decreases its proportions in ruminal fermentation is undesirable. Therefore, ionophores are not used in lactating dairy cattle management.

In a recent summary of 67 finishing trials and 55 pasturing beef cattle trials, ionophores improved feed:gain ratio and mean daily weight gain (*see* TABLE 16).

The consistent improvement in gain of cattle fed ionophores on high-roughage diets as compared with less consistent improvement for cattle fed high-energy diets is explained by energy availability between the 2 systems. On high-energy diets, cattle eat until they meet energy requirements; thus, ionophores help them derive more energy per unit of ingested feed, and they eat less. On high-roughage diets (less energy per unit weight) cattle consume feed until the rumen will hold no more. However, on the latter program, if ionophores are fed, such cattle derive more energy per unit of feed consumed, and thus gain more.

TABLE 16. Effects of Ionophores on the Performance of Beef Cattle

			Inophore			
	Control	Laidlomycin	Lasalocid	Monensin	Tylosin[*] + Monensin	Bamber-mycin
Feedlot						
Dose, mg/head/day	0	85.8	285.9	272.2	263.2	
Daily gain (kg)	1.39[†]	1.46[‡]	1.38[†]	1.38[†]	1.39[†]	
Feed:gain ratio	6.81[†]	6.48[‡]	6.52[‡]	6.44[‡]	6.35[‡]	
Grazing Cattle						
Dose, mg/head/day	0		188	167		25
Daily gain (kg)	0.64[†]		0.78[‡]	0.75[‡]		0.78[‡]

[*]Tylosin dose, 98 mg/head/day
[†,‡] = Means differ (P<0.05)

TABLE 17. Feeding Guidelines for Large-Breed Dairy Cattle[*] ▶

	Dry (Far Off)	Close (Close up)
Body wt, lb (kg)	1,500 (675)	1,500 (675)
DMI, lb (kg)	32 (14)	22 (10)
Milk, lb[†] (kg)		
CP (%)	9.9	12.4
RDP (%)	7.7	9.6
RUP (%)	2.2	2.8
MP (%)	6.0	8.0
NE$_l$, Mcal/lb (Mcal/kg)	0.60 (1.32)	0.65 (1.43)
ME, Mcal/lb (Mcal/kg)		
NDF (%)	40	35
ADF (%)	30	25
NFC (%)	30	34
Calcium (%)	0.44	0.48
Phosphorus (%)	0.22	0.26
Magnesium (%)	0.11	0.40
Chlorine (%)	0.13	0.20
Sodium (%)	0.10	0.14
Potassium (%)	0.51	0.62
Sulfur (%)	0.20	0.20
Vitamin A (IU)	80,300	83,270
Vitamin D (IU)	21,900	22,700
Vitamin E (IU)	1,168	1,200

[*]Adapted, with permission, from *Nutrient Requirements of Dairy Cattle*, 2001, National Academy of Sciences, National Academy Press, Washington, DC. DMI, dry matter intake; CP, crude protein; RDP, rumen degradable protein; RUP, rumen undegraded protein; MP, metabolizable protein; NE$_l$, net energy lactation; ME, metabolizable energy; NDF, neutral detergent fiber; ADF, acid detergent fiber; NFC, non-fiber carbohydrate. Trace mineral added to ration (expressed as ppm): cobalt: 0.11; copper 10-18; iodine: 0.3-0.4; iron: 13-130; manganese: 14-24; selenium: 0.30; zinc: 22-70.
[†]Milk components: 3.5% fat, 3.0% true protein, and 4.8% lactose.

DAIRY CATTLE

NUTRITIONAL REQUIREMENTS

The specific dietary needs of dairy cattle are greatly modified by rumen activity. For their first 3-5 wk, calves are essentially monogastric animals, have dietary requirements similar to those of pigs and dogs, and must obtain nutrients from milk or a milk replacer. They require high-quality, easily digested feeds to supply available energy, essential amino acids, essential minerals, and nearly all vitamins. Soon after 1 mo of age, as forage and grain consumption increases, microorganisms in the rumen become increasingly

TABLE 17. (continued)

	Cows			Heifers (age in mo)			24 (Close up)
Fresh	Early	Mid	Late	6	12	18	
1,500 (675)	1,500 (675)	1,500 (675)	1,500 (675)	440 (200)	660 (300)	1,000 (450)	1,375 (625)
34 (15)	66 (30)	52 (24)	45 (20)	11 (5)	16 (7)	25 (11)	23 (10)
77 (35)	120 (55)	77 (35)	55 (25)				
19.5	16.7	15.2	14.1	12.3	11.4	8.8	15.0
10.5	9.8	9.7	9.5	9.4	9.5	8.8	10.1
9.0	6.9	5.5	4.6	2.9	1.9	0.004	4.9
13.8	11.6	10.2	9.2	7.2	7.0	5.3	9.7
1.01‡ (2.22)	0.73 (1.61)	0.67 (1.47)	0.62 (1.36)	—	—	—	0.72 (1.58)
				0.93 (2.05)	1.03 (2.27)	0.82 (1.80)	
30	28	30	32	30	32	33	35
21	19	21	24	20	22	24	25
35	38	35	32	35	30	25	34
0.79	0.60	0.61	0.62	0.41	0.41	0.37	0.40
0.42	0.38	0.35	0.32	0.28	0.23	0.18	0.23
0.29	0.21	0.19	0.18	0.11	0.11	0.08	0.40
0.20	0.29	0.26	0.24	0.11	0.12	0.10	0.20
0.34	0.22	0.23	0.22	0.08	0.08	0.07	0.14
1.24	1.07	1.04	1.00	0.47	0.48	0.46	0.55
0.20	0.20	0.20	0.20	0.20	0.20	0.20	0.20
75,000	75,000	75,000	75,000	24,000	24,000	36,000	75,000
21,000	21,000	21,000	21,000	6,000	9,000	13,500	20,000
545	545	545	545	240	240	360	1,200

‡These cows will lose body weight (values >0.82 not feasible).

active in synthesizing the essential amino acids and B vitamins and in digesting cellulose. Functionally, ruminant dairy cattle can survive largely independently of a dietary supply of essential amino acids and B vitamins. However, for high-producing dairy cows early in lactation, degradability of dietary protein in the rumen should be considered. Supplemental niacin and biotin may be beneficial under some conditions. In common with other ruminants, mature cattle can use coarse feeds, high in cellulose and hemicellulose, that are less useful for nonherbivores. Veal calves, which are fed solely a milk or milk-replacer diet and no dry feed, are considered nonruminants in terms of their nutritional requirements.

For daily nutrient requirements of dairy cattle, *see* TABLE 17 for large breed growing heifers, dry cows, close up cows, fresh cows, and lactating cows. For nutrient requirements for maintenance, pregnant cows, and lactating cows, *see* TABLE 18.

Water: Because dairy cattle suffer more quickly from an inadequate water intake than from a deficiency of any other nutrient, clean, fresh drinking water should be available at

TABLE 18. Daily Nutrient Requirements for Dairy Cattle[*]

		NE$_l$ (Mcal)	MP		Calcium		Phosphorus	
			(lb)	(g)	(lb)	(g)	(lb)	(g)
Body Weight								
(lb)	**(kg)**							
900	409	6.3	0.868	394	0.029	13	0.022	9
1,000	454	7.9	0.898	408	0.032	15	0.023	10
1,100	500	8.4	0.908	412	0.035	16	0.023	10
1,200	545	9.0	0.919	417	0.038	17	0.023	10
1,300	591	9.6	0.929	421	0.041	19	0.023	10
1,400	636	10.1	0.939	426	0.045	20	0.023	10
1,500	682	10.7	0.947	430	0.048	22	0.024	11
Days Pregnant								
(1,400 lb cow)								
220		2.9	0.527	239	0.010	5	0.007	3
240		3.2	0.615	279	0.014	6	0.009	4
260		3.5	0.703	319	0.018	8	0.011	5
270		3.6	0.748	340	0.021	9	0.011	5
279		3.7	0.787	359	0.022	10	0.012	5
Milk Production (per lb of milk)								
(% fat/% true protein)								
3.0 / 2.8		0.288	0.042	19	0.00104	0.47	0.0009	0.41
3.5 / 3.0		0.314	0.045	20	0.00113	0.51	0.0009	0.41
3.5 / 3.2		0.319	0.048	22	0.00113	0.51	0.0009	0.41
3.7 / 3.0		0.322	0.045	20	0.00117	0.53	0.0009	0.41
4.0 / 3.2		0.340	0.048	22	0.00122	0.55	0.0009	0.41
4.0 / 3.4		0.345	0.051	23	0.00122	0.55	0.0009	0.41
4.5 / 3.4		0.366	0.051	23	0.00131	0.59	0.0009	0.41
5.0 / 3.6		0.393	0.054	25	0.00140	0.64	0.0009	0.41

[*]Adapted, with permission, from *Nutrient Requirements of Dairy Cattle*, 2001, National Academy of Sciences, National Academy Press, Washington, DC. *See* TABLE 10 for abbreviations.

all times. Milk production and feed intake will be depressed if free access to water is not allowed. Cows consume 3-5 kg of water for each kg of dry matter consumed, plus additional water for milk production. The following equation can be used to estimate the gallons of water a cow needs each day:

$$\text{water intake (gal./day)} = 4.2 + (0.19 \times \text{dry matter consumed [lb]})$$
$$+ (0.108 \times \text{milk produced [lb]})$$
$$+ (0.374 \times \text{sodium consumed [oz]})$$
$$+ (0.06 \times \text{minimum daily temperature} [°F])$$

On succulent feeds, water consumption is less. In winter, cows will drink more water if it is warmed slightly; in warm weather, intake may be tripled. Calves >1 wk of age and

TABLE 19. Water Intake of Dairy Cattle (gal./day)

Weight	Milk Yield	Temperature (°F)		
(lb)	(lb)	<40	60	80
Heifers				
200	NA*	2.0	2.5	3.3
400	NA	3.7	4.6	6.1
800	NA	6.3	7.9	10.6
1,200	NA	8.7	10.8	14.5
Dry Cows				
1,400	NA	9.7	12.0	16.2
1,600	NA	10.4	12.8	17.3
Lactating Cows				
1,400	60	12.0	14.5	17.9
1,400	80	27.0	31.9	38.7
1,400	100	32.0	37.7	45.7

*NA = not applicable

heifers should be offered water ad lib. TABLE 19 lists the water requirement for dairy cattle at various ages, milk yield, and environmental temperatures.

Energy: The principal use of feed by the body is as a source of energy. All organic nutrients (protein, carbohydrates, and fats) supply energy. The energy values of the organic components of a feedstuff are combined and expressed as total digestible nutrients (TDN), digestible energy (DE), metabolizable energy (ME), or net energy (net energy for maintenance, NE_m; net energy for gain, NE_g; net energy for lactation, NE_l). TDN and DE account for energy losses in the feces. ME accounts for energy losses from the feces, urine, and combustible gases from the gut. NE equals ME minus the heat increment or energy losses from the metabolism of feed nutrients for specific purposes. Net energy reflects a truer value of the feedstuffs for productive purposes and more accurately compares concentrates with forages. Consequently, it is the most commonly used method for calculating the energy value of feeds. In many laboratories, NE values are calculated from acid detergent fiber. Recently, an equation including digestible neutral detergent fiber (NDF) and other nutrients has been developed and reflects fiber digestibility, the higher energy of fats and oils, and the lower energy values of ash content.

Insufficient intake of energy is probably a more frequent cause of retarded growth, delayed puberty, or depressed milk production than any other nutritional deficiency. The energy requirements (*see* TABLE 17 and TABLE 18) serve as guides. Lower intakes than suggested reduce growth rates and decrease milk production.

Under rigid experimental conditions, calves have been shown to require essential fatty acids. However, under usual feeding conditions, even when low-fat milk replacers are used, essential fatty acid deficiency does not develop. A specific dietary fat requirement for ruminating cattle does not appear to exist, or at least is met by normal feedstuffs. High-producing cows may require an additional 2-3% added fat to meet energy needs and to minimize weight loss. Feeding polyunsaturated fatty acids (eg, linoleneic, linoleic, and 20-carbon polyunsaturated fatty acids) may enhance reproductive performance through effects on reproductive hormones such as progesterone. Oils in the form of whole cottonseed or soybeans are frequently added to rations of high-producing cows to improve energy balance. The amount of oil added should be limited to 1.0 lb or 0.45 kg/

cow/day. If higher levels of fat are needed, rumen inert sources should be considered (such as calcium salts of fatty acids).

Fiber: Although fiber is the most undigestible portion of the ration of a dairy cow, it is a necessary part of the overall feeding program. The actual amount to be included depends on several factors, including body condition, level of production, type of fiber fed, and physical characteristics of the fiber. Cows producing large amounts of milk are fed rations with less fiber, while those producing less milk, or during the growing or dry periods, are fed diets with more fiber from forage sources. The amount and type of fiber that is fed can significantly affect rumen function, which affects the amount of rumination, saliva production, rumen pH, and milk fat level.

The amount of fiber is expressed in terms of acid detergent fiber (ADF) or neutral detergent fiber (NDF). ADF consists of cellulose, lignin, acid-detergent-insoluble nitrogen, and acid-insoluble ash; NDF consists of the same plus hemicellulose. Generally, the ADF content of a ration is thought to be a good indicator of the overall digestibility of the diet, while the NDF content is considered to correlate well with total dry-matter intake. However, because both chemical and physical properties of feeds affect the fiber determination, it is difficult to completely predict the fiber quality and energy value of feeds.

Published recommendations for the levels of ADF and NDF vary widely. In general, it appears that levels of ADF in lactating cow rations should be 19-21% on a dry-matter basis, while the level of NDF should be 28-32%. Further, it is recommended that 75% of the NDF should be present in the forage fraction of the total ration. The Penn State Forage Box consists of a series of boxes that can be used to sieve or separate 400-500 g of forage or total mixed ration (TMR) to measure feed particle size. A TMR should have <50% by weight in the bottom 2 boxes of the 4-box unit. Feeds in the top 2 boxes are considered effective or long-feed particles that will form a forage mat in the rumen and lead to >9 hr of cud chewing daily.

Cows will consume 1.2% of their body wt/day as NDF or 0.9% of their body weight as forage NDF. Thus, given a level of 28% NDF in a given ration, a 1,300-lb (600-kg) cow might be expected to consume 55 lb (25 kg) of feed dry matter per day. If her production level suggests a higher or lower level of dry-matter intake is appropriate, reformulation of the feed, including the concentration of NDF, may be in order.

Protein: Crude protein and metabolizable protein (MP) values in TABLE 17 and TABLE 18 represent the approximate requirements. Additional protein may result in a marginal increase in milk production. However, gross excess of protein (>19%) in the ration of dry pregnant cows or lactating cows may prolong days open and services per conception after parturition.

Dairy cattle, like other animals, require essential amino acids that must be absorbed from the small intestine. These amino acids are derived from microbial protein produced in the ruminoreticulum and digested in the small intestine, as well as from dietary protein that escapes degradation in the rumen but is digested to amino acids postruminally. In recommendations published by the National Research Council (NRC) in 2001, a new term, metabolizable protein (MP), represents the amino acids from microbial sources and amino acids from undegraded feed sources. Under normal feeding conditions in which total MP requirements are met, growing heifers, dry cows, and cows in mid to late lactation can meet amino acid needs from microbial protein produced in the rumen. The amount of microbial protein synthesis depends on factors such as the level of nonstructural carbohydrate in the diet, physical density and form of the diet, level and frequency of feeding, availability in the rumen of sulfur and branched-chain fatty acids, and especially on the amount of rumen degradable protein (RDP). High-yielding cows, however, have amino acid requirements in excess of what can be supplied by rumen microbes even at high rates of synthesis. The diet of such cows should include proteins of relatively low degradability in the rumen that will escape breakdown until they reach the small intestine. This escape protein is known as rumen undegraded protein (RUP). Lysine and methionine are considered first-limiting amino acids and should be evaluated using a

TABLE 20. Estimates of Rumen Undegraded Protein in Common Feedstuffs at 4 x Maintenance*

Barley	0.24	Legume hay	0.20
Blood meal	0.78	Legume silage	0.21
Brewer's dried grains	0.57	Linseed meal	0.53
Canola meal	0.36	Meat and bone meal (pork)	0.60
Corn distiller's dried grains	0.51	Soybean meal	0.35
Corn gluten feed, dry	0.30	Soybeans, raw	0.30
Corn gluten meal	0.75	Wheat	0.26
Corn grain	0.47	Wheat midds	0.24
Corn silage	0.41		
Fishmeal	0.66		

*Adapted, with permission, from *Nutrient Requirements of Dairy Cattle*, 2001, National Academy of Sciences, National Academy Press, Washington, DC. Data are % rumen undegraded protein of total crude protein.

computer-based software program such as the 2001 Dairy NRC model. *See* TABLE 17 for estimates of RUP and RDP requirements. Because feedstuffs vary considerably in proportions of degradable and undegradable proteins, *see* TABLE 20 for selected values for use in balancing diets. To fine tune rations, an amino acid computer model can be used to calculate the rate of protein degradation related to feed intake, intestinal availability, and disassociation constants in rumen. Generally, a 3:1 ratio of lysine:methionine is an optimal amino acid balance for these 2 first-limiting amino acids.

Urea may be used in the ration to meet part of the RDP requirement of older heifers, dry cows, and low-producing cows, as long as adequate energy in the form of nonstructural carbohydrate is present in the rumen. Some urea may occasionally be justified in diets of high-yielding cows to meet soluble protein needs for the rumen microbes along with RUP sources. Urea should be introduced to the diet gradually over a 3-wk period and mixed thoroughly with palatable feeds, preferably in ways that will avoid excessive intakes over short periods of time. (*See also* NONPROTEIN NITROGEN POISONING, p 2426.) Common recommendations are to add urea at rates up to 7.5 kg/ton of corn silage, or up to 1% of the concentrates for a maximum intake of 0.2 kg (0.45 lb) of urea daily for a mature cow. If urea is added to a ration that is already more than adequate in degradable and soluble protein, it is not only wasted but can adversely affect feed intake, health, and production. Conversely, if rations are relatively high in RUP and starches, urea or other nonprotein nitrogen such as ammonia may be used to meet the nitrogen needs of rumen microorganisms.

Minerals: Dairy cattle need a dietary source of calcium, phosphorus, magnesium, sulfur, potassium, sodium, chlorine, iron, iodine, manganese, copper, cobalt, zinc, and selenium. Minerals needing special attention in practical feeding are discussed below.

Salt (sodium chloride) is not found in ordinary feeds in amounts sufficient to meet the needs of dairy cattle. The preferred method of feeding salt is to include it in concentrate mixtures or complete feeds at 0.46% of the total ration dry matter for lactating cows and at 0.25% of the total ration dry matter for dry cows and other nonlactating cattle. Allowing free access to salt is a practical way of meeting the requirement of cattle not receiving concentrates. Loose salt (which leads to higher intake) or block salt should be protected from the weather.

Calcium and **phosphorus** must be added to most dairy cattle diets. *See* TABLE 21 for the calcium and phosphorus contents of certain supplements. Legumes (such as alfalfa) are rich in calcium, but lower in phosphorus. Nonlegume forages are lower in calcium. Concentrate feeds used for dairy cattle are deficient in calcium. Wheat midds, corn distiller's grain with solubles, and soybean meal are common feeds rich in phosphorus but low in calcium.

TABLE 21. Sources of Supplemental Calcium and Phosphorus for Dairy Cattle[*]

Feed Ingredient	Calcium		Phosphorus	
	(%)[†]	% AC[‡]	(%)[†]	% AC
Ammonium phosphate (monobasic)	0	0	24.7	80
Bone meal	30.7	95	12.9	80
Defluorinated rock phosphate	30.0	70	14.0	30
Dicalcium phosphate	22.0	94	19.0	75
Limestone	39.4	75	0	0
Limestone, dolomitic	22.3	60	0	0
Monocalcium phosphate	16.4	95	21.6	80

[*]Adapted, with permission, from *Nutrient Requirements of Dairy Cattle*, 2001, National Academy of Sciences, National Academy Press, Washington, DC.
[†]100% dry-matter basis
[‡]Absorption coefficient (bioavailability)

Monocalcium phosphate and dicalcium phosphate are common supplements of calcium and phosphorus. Limestone (feed grade) is the least expensive single source of calcium. Levels of calcium, phosphorus, and vitamin D affect calcium and phosphorus use. A calcium:phosphorus ratio of 1.6-2.5:1 is recommended for growth, maintenance, and milk production. Milk fever (p 806) has been reduced by decreasing potassium intake to <1% for 3 wk before calving or using anionic salts (chloride and sulfur minerals) to lower the dietary cation-anion difference to -50 to -150 mEq/kg of ration dry matter. To guarantee satisfactory intakes, mineral supplements should be incorporated in the concentrate or total mixed ration at levels calculated to meet requirements. Free-choice feeding of minerals to heifers and dry cows is not recommended, as cattle will not balance their diets in this way.

Iodine is required for the synthesis of thyroxine, by which the thyroid gland exercises a degree of control over the basal metabolic rate and growth, reproduction, and lactation. In the newborn calf, simple goiter (p 465) is evident when maternal iodine intake was deficient. The iodine requirement is increased by goitrogenic substances in feeds, such as raw soybeans. Pasture plants vary greatly in their ability to take up iodine from the soil. Deficiencies can be prevented by providing stabilized iodized salt at 0.6 ppm of the total ration dry matter. Excessive quantities of iodine can lead to hyperthyroidism and high levels in milk. Iodine deficiency develops on deficient soils around the Great Lakes and westward to the Pacific coast of North America.

Cobalt is required for normal rumen metabolism. When the intake of cobalt is inadequate, the bacterial population in the rumen is altered, and the synthesis of vitamin B_{12} is greatly lowered. In some areas, particularly the southeastern seacoast of the USA, the soil is deficient in cobalt. Adding 0.10 ppm of cobalt to the ration dry matter for dairy cattle is recommended.

Copper plays a critical role in cellular functions, including enzyme activation, free radical removal, and blood cell maturation. Organic copper has been reported to reduce mastitis severity and duration. Fetal demands for copper are also high in the last trimester of pregnancy. The zinc to copper ratio should be 4:1 with a level of 13-16 ppm. Jersey cattle are more at risk of copper toxicity than other breeds. Copper antagonists such as sulfur, molybdenum, zinc, and iron increase the need for copper.

Zinc is an essential mineral for normal growth and health as it is needed for energy and protein metabolism, skin integrity and cell repair, and immune function. Low zinc status leads to lower quality milk with higher somatic cell counts and an increase in mastitis. Organic zinc can increase reproductive performance by increasing conception rate. Field studies also reveal an improvement in hoof hardness and less white line disease with supplemental organic zinc. Recommended levels of zinc vary from 20-75 ppm with one third from organic sources.

Selenium is required for managing reproduction and health as it plays a key role in immune function. Selenium deficiencies can lead to poor uterine involution, retained placenta, metritis, reduced fertility, and weak heats. Severely deficient animals develop white muscle disease. Vitamin E and selenium both impact immunity, but supplementation with one will not remedy a deficiency of the other. Signs of selenium toxicity seen in the plains states of the USA include lameness, sore feet, and loss of hair from the tail. The legal maximum limit for supplemental selenium is 0.3 ppm in the USA. Organic selenium was approved by the FDA in 2003 and should be included.

Vitamins: Calves up to 4-5 wk old should receive all known vitamins in their feed. Milk replacers should contain all the added fat and water-soluble vitamins.

As bacterial function develops in the rumen, the B vitamins are synthesized in large amounts, and a dietary supply is no longer needed. However, evidence suggests that under some conditions, high-yielding cows in early lactation may be less prone to ketosis when fed supplemental **niacin**. Supplementation of 6 g (prepartum) to 12 g (postpartum) of niacin/day from 2 wk before calving and continued 8-12 wk after calving may be beneficial in dairy herds with an above average incidence of ketosis and over-conditioned cows. Supplemental **biotin** (15-20 mg/cow/day) can improve hoof condition and health over several months while increasing milk yield by 2 kg (4-5 lb) within weeks.

A deficiency of **vitamin A, D, or E** is relatively rare in cattle fed natural mixtures of high-quality feeds. White muscle disease (p 897) due to a deficiency of vitamin E or selenium is not uncommon in dairy calves in areas where the soil is low in selenium. Injections of vitamins A, D, and E at the time of drying off and prior to calving are given on dairy farms, but researchers report limited value to cows fed normal diets. Milk replacers should be fortified with these vitamins.

When fed poor-quality, damaged forage for long periods, dairy cattle may show reproductive failure from vitamin A deficiency. Under such conditions, supplementation with synthetic vitamin A is desirable. Fresh pasture in summer is an excellent source of carotene, the precursor of vitamin A. Because properly cured hay or silage loses vitamin A with storage, most commercial concentrates now contain several thousand IU of vitamin A/kg to prevent deficiency.

All natural feeds except sun-cured hay have a low vitamin D content. Animals that are exposed to sunlight synthesize ample vitamin D in the skin and do not require high levels in their feed. Vitamin D deficiency may be seen in young calves that are confined with inadequate sunlight and that do not consume sun-cured roughage. Whole milk and skim milk are always low in vitamin D. Concentrate mixtures are also naturally low in vitamin D. Because vitamin D is relatively inexpensive and cattle may be exposed to little sunlight, it is commonly included in calf and cow rations.

Vitamin E is added to dairy rations at 500-1,200 IU/cow/day to minimize mastitis risk and severity, improve immune function, and improve reproductive performance.

β-**Carotene** has been suggested to be of value in minimizing reproductive problems, especially when blood levels are low in cows and heifers. However, research data are limited and conflicting, and routine supplementation is not recommended.

Vitamin K is ordinarily synthesized in the rumen in ample quantities. (*See also* SWEET CLOVER POISONING, p 2523.)

Nutrient Requirements of Dairy Cattle

The most recent NRC guidelines and recommendations for dairy cattle were published in 2001. The key changes or new additions are: 1) Metabolizable protein (MP) includes the grams of microbial protein and rumen undegraded proteins required by the animal. The NRC 2001 model estimates the grams of degraded protein converted to microbial protein and individual amino acids and grams of rumen undegraded protein and amino acids. Lysine and methionine should be provided in a ration of 3 parts lysine to 1 part methionine. MP is converted to a crude protein basis for users, but the level of crude protein represents the calculated MP and should not be interchanged with NRC 1989 crude protein values. 2001 NRC crude protein values are typically 0.5% crude protein units lower; for example, 17.2% using 2001 NRC compared with 17.7% using 1989 NRC crude protein values. 2) Dry-matter intake was calculated using experimental data increasing dry-matter intake by 4-5 lb (2 kg) compared with NRC 1989 values. Excellent feed bunk management is needed to achieve the higher values calculated by the 2001 NRC model. Accurate dry matter intake is critical as it impacts protein degradation and calculated energy prediction values. 3) Energy value for each feed ingredient and ration was calculated by the 2001 model based on dry-matter intake and feed ingredients selected. Feed energy values are unique to the 2001 model and should not be compared with NRC 1989 table values. 4) Mineral requirements are based on absorption coefficients (bioavailability) of each mineral in each feed ingredient. True mineral requirement is calculated and expressed as a percent of ration dry matter based on feed ingredient. No adjustment of organic trace minerals was included. 5) Nutrient requirements were refined for heifers using winter hair coat, mud, and wind chill effects for cold weather. Lactating cow nutrient requirement adjustments included new pasture recommendations (distance to the pasture and topography), body condition score changes, and milk components (level of milk fat, milk protein, and lactose). 6) The NRC model is a computer software program that adjusts for key factors resulting in a unique ration based on animal, environment, feed ingredients, and dry-matter intake. Model output includes nutrient concentration and values, feed ingredient values, amino acid flow, and mineral status. No balancing function is available when using the NRC 2001 model; the user must balance the ration manually.

FEEDING AND NUTRITIONAL MANAGEMENT

Dairy cattle require some concentrates until the age of 12 mo, although forage can supply an increasing percentage of the ration after 6 mo. In addition, concentrates are needed for lactating cows to complement forage nutrients. However, concentrates do not completely compensate for lack of quality in forages fed to high-yielding cows.

In determining the amount and kind of concentrate mixture needed, it is essential to know what types and amounts of forage are available; a concentrate can then be selected that will supply the amounts of additional nutrients needed at lowest cost.

See TABLE 10 for the amounts of nutrients furnished by some common cattle feeds. Hays and silages of the same species vary greatly in composition, depending on the stage of maturity at the time of cutting and curing and on preservation methods. Although the precise nutrient value of a hay or silage cannot be known without chemical analysis (or even a feeding experiment), its approximate value can be estimated, and a concentrate mixture of appropriate composition can be made or purchased to balance the forage available. Forage-testing services available either through commercial feed-testing laboratories or local feed companies can provide more precise information as to composition and should be used whenever possible.

High-protein feeds such as soybean meal, cottonseed meal, and canola meal usually are higher in price than cereal grains. Therefore, it is generally more economical to use concentrate mixtures as low in protein as possible while supplying an adequate amount of amino acids. Simple mixtures can be as effective as complex mixes, provided RUP, RDP, and amino acid balance are considered. Byproduct feeds (such as distiller's grain and brewer's grain) provide economic advantages.

Palatability and nutrient content, rather than the number of ingredients in a mixture, largely determine the value of feeds for dairy cattle. Minimizing dustiness and fine feed particles, mixing with silages, adding water or liquid molasses, and supplementing with oil can enhance feed palatability and dry-matter intake.

Calves should receive colostrum for at least the first 3 days, and then milk or milk replacer at the rate of 10-12% of body wt/day during the first few weeks after birth. A new liquid diet program for heifer calves (accelerated system) is an aggressive, growing approach. Calves receive milk replacer containing 28% protein and 15% fat, and consume >2 lb of milk replacer fed at 14-16% of body wt, resulting in growth rates > 2 lb (1 kg)/day. Traditional milk replacers contain 22% protein and 20% fat, and are fed at the rate of 1 lb of powder/calf/day. Heifers fed the new diet grow faster. However, the cost of the high quality and quantity milk replacer increases feed costs. Fermented colostrum (mixed 1:1 with water) is also an excellent liquid feed. Waste or discard milk from cows with mastitis or another illness is satisfactory if the milk is wholesome (avoid the first milking after udder treatment for mastitis).

Calves usually can be weaned at 4-8 wk of age or when they are regularly consuming 2 lb (1 kg) of starter daily. During the first week, a complete calf starter containing 20% protein (dry-matter basis) with no forage should be offered to young calves. They should be allowed free-choice starter up to a maximum of 5 lb (2.3 kg)/day. Calves do not like finely ground or dusty feeds; pelleted or textured grain with wet molasses is recommended. They will consume coarsely cracked or rolled grains and protein sources with minerals that are pelleted. Forage is not required during the first 2 mo of age if the starter contains a fiber source such as oats, barley, or soy hull (complete calf starter). With a coarse starter, calves begin to ruminate within 2 wk. When forage is provided, green, leafy, soft-stemmed legume grass mixed with hay is optimal for calves. They can be offered hay, but they must consume 5 lb of calf starter daily as an energy source ("hay belly" calves may develop if they eat only hay). After 3 mo of age, the calf starter can be replaced with a less expensive heifer grower ration containing 16% total protein. Pasture or corn silage can be fed to calves after 4-6 mo of age.

Well-grown heifers and young stock normally do not need concentrates after 12 mo of age if fed high-quality forage. More rapid growth or improved condition results from the addition of 2-3 lb (1-1.5 kg) of concentrates. Feeding 5-6 lb (2-3 kg) daily is advisable if the forage is of poor quality or limited in quantity.

Pregnant cows and heifers should receive as much attention just before calving as after. If too fat, they are predisposed to ketosis (p 830). If they are in good condition, and fed at a high level after calving, ketosis tends to be reduced. During most of the dry period, cows in good condition fed good-quality legume-grass forage or pasture require few or no concentrates. Feeding all-corn silage (plus protein supplements and minerals) can result in heifers that are too fat at parturition and an increased incidence of left displaced abomasum (p 193).

Two weeks before parturition, cows and heifers should be offered supplemental concentrate up to 6-10 lb (3-4 kg)/day to allow the rumen to adjust by calving time and to provide added nutrients for colostrum synthesis and fetal development. After calving, cows should be encouraged to increase feed intake to minimize negative energy balance and to produce to their genetic potential. Abrupt changes in types and amounts of feed offered should be avoided to minimize risk of displaced abomasums. Off-feed problems are less likely with complete feeds (total mixed rations). A fresh-cow ration (TABLE 17) can shift nutrient density gradually to minimize acidosis and twisted abomasal disorders. If grain is fed separately, an increase at the rate of 1 lb (0.45 kg)/day is optimal for production while minimizing digestive upsets. Greater feed intakes are possible if cows are fed concentrates more often (3-4 times a day with a maximum of 6 lb of dry matter per meal) and forages several times per day.

After the peak of lactation, the ration or amount of concentrate should be adjusted gradually, based on the amount and fat content of the milk produced and the quality of the forage consumed. Size and age of the cow and her feed intake capacity must be considered in deciding on concentrate allowance. Computer programs consider these factors to determine optimal levels of nutrition. Cows fed complete feeds or total mixed rations should be grouped by age and production and offered rations ranging from a maximum of 60% concentrate and 40% forage (dry-matter basis) for early lactation cows, to 20% concentrate and 80% forage for low-producing cows. When corn silage is a major forage ingredient, <50% concentrate and >50% forage is optimal for high-producing cows. For maximal fat test, the total ration should contain at least 19% acid detergent fiber (ADF) or 28% neutral detergent fiber (NDF). However, the optimal levels of ADF or NDF depend on level of milk production, type of forage, and processing of forages being fed. Feed consultants, company representatives, and extension personnel can assist in determining best-cost rations. All dairy producers should participate in some type of milk-testing association as a means of evaluating their herd and its feeding and management program.

Feed Additives: Feed additives are ingredients that cause a desired response in a non-nutrient role such as a shift in pH, rumen environment, or metabolic change. Several feed additives contain nutrients (eg, sodium in sodium bicarbonate, protein in yeast culture). Feed additives are not a requirement for or guarantee of high productivity. *See* TABLE 22 for properties that may help determine the use of various feed additives.

TABLE 22. Feed Additives

Additive	Function[*]	Level[†]	Benefit: cost Ratio[‡]	Feeding Strategy[§]	Status[¶]
Anionic salts and products	Acidify diet, raise blood calcium	Reduce DCAD to -50 mEq/kg using Cl⁻	10:1	Feed to dry cows 2-3 wk before calving; adjust dietary Ca levels to 120 g/day (40 g inorganic); raise dietary Mg levels to 0.4%	Recommended
Aspergillus oryzae	Stimulate fiber-digesting bacteria, stabilize rumen pH, reduce heat stress	3 g/day	6:1	High grain diets, low rumen pH conditions, heat stress (cows), calves receiving a liquid diet	Evaluative
Biotin	Reduce heel warts, claw lesions, white line separations, sand cracks, sole ulcers, and increase milk yield	10-20 mg/day for 6-12 mo	3:1	Herds with chronic foot problems; may require supplementation for 6 mo; begin supplementation at 15 mo of age	Experimental
β-carotene	Improve reproductive performance, immune response, and mastitis control	200-300 mg/day	NA[*]	In early lactation and during mastitis-prone periods	Not recommended
Calcium propionate	Increase blood glucose and Ca	120-225 g	NA	Feed 7 days prepartum to 7 days postpartum or until appetite responds; unpalatable	Recommended

TABLE 22. (continued)

Additive	Function[*]	Level[†]	Benefit: cost Ratio[‡]	Feeding Strategy[§]	Status[¶]
Pro-tected choline	Minimize fatty liver for-mation, improve fat mobilization	15-30 g/day	2:1 (when pro-tected)	Feed 2 wk prepartum to 8 wk postpartum to cows with ketosis, weight loss, and high milk yield	Experi-mental (rumen pro-tected)
Enzymes (fibrin-olytic)	Increase fiber digestibility	Not clearly defined	2:1	Treat 12 hr before feeding; spray-on product more effec-tive when applied to dry diets	Experi-mental
Magne-sium oxide	Increase rumen pH, increase uptake of blood metab-olites	45-90 g/day	NA	Feed with sodium-based buffers (ratio of 2-3 parts NaH_2CO_3 to 1 part MgO)	Recom-mended
Methio-nine hydroxy analog	Minimize fatty liver for-mation, con-trol ketosis, improve milk fat	30 g	2:1	Feed to cows in early lactation receiving high levels of concen-trate and limited dietary protein	Evalua-tive
Niacin	Improve energy bal-ance, control ketosis, stim-ulate rumen protozoa	6 g (preven-tive, prepartum), 12 g (treat-ment, post-partum	6:1 (6 g level)	Feed to high-produc-ing cows in negative energy balance, heavy dry cows, and cows prone to ketosis fed 2 wk prepartum to peak dry matter intake (10-12 wk postpartum)	Evalua-tive
Probiotics (direct-fed microbes)	Destroy undesirable organisms, improve nutrient availability, detoxify harmful metabolites	Not clearly defined	NA	Feed to calves on liquid diet, transition cows, and during stressful conditions	Evalua-tive for cows, recom-mended for milk-fed calves
Propyl-ene glycol	Stimulate insulin response, reduce fat mobilization	8-16 oz/day	NA	Drench cow starting 1 wk prepartum (pre-ventive) or after calv-ing when signs of ketosis appear (treat-ment); feeding not as effective as drenching	Recom-mended

(continued)

TABLE 22. Feed Additives (continued)

Additive	Function[*]	Level[†]	Benefit: cost Ratio[‡]	Feeding Strategy[§]	Status[¶]
Silage bacterial inoculants	Stimulate silage fermentation, reduce dry matter loss, decrease ensiling temperature, increase feed digestibility, improve forage surface stability, increase lactate production	100,000 CFU/g wet silage[**]	3:1 (feed recovery), 7:1 (milk improvement)	Apply to wet silage (>60% moisture), corn silage, haylage, and high-moisture corn; low natural bacteria counts (first and last legume/grass silage); and under poor fermentation conditions	Recommended
Sodium bentonite	Shifts volatile fatty acid patterns, slows rate of passage, exchanges mineral ions	450-700 g/day (rumen effect), 110 g/day (mycotoxin effect)	NA	Feed with high-grain diets, loose stool conditions, mold, low-fat test, and dirt eating	Evaluative
Sodium bicarbonate/ sodium sesquicarbonate	Increase dry-matter intake, stabilize rumen pH	0.75% of total ration dry matter intake	4:1 to 12:1	Feed 120 days postpartum with diets >50% corn silage, wet rations (>50% moisture), low-fiber rations (<19% ADF), little hay (<5 lb), finely chopped forage, pelleted grain, slug feeding, and heat stress conditions	Recommended
Yeast culture and yeast	Stimulate fiber-digesting bacteria, stabilize rumen environment, utilize lactic acid	10-120 g, depending on yeast culture concentration	4:1	Feed 2 wk prepartum to 10 wk postpartum and during off-feed and stressful conditions	Recommended
Yucca extract	Decrease urea nitrogen in plasma and milk	0.8-9 g/day, depending on source	NA	Feed to cows with high BUN and MUN levels	Evaluative

TABLE 22. *(continued)*

Additive	Function*	Level†	Benefit: cost Ratio‡	Feeding Strategy§	Status¶
Zinc methionine	Improve immune response, harden hooves, lower somatic cell count	9 g/day	14:1	Feed to cows with foot disorders, high somatic cell counts, and in wet environments	Recommended

*Intended effect of the additive
†Amount required to produce the effect, based on research results
‡Ratio of increased milk yield to cost of the additive
§Conditions under which additive should be used
¶Recommended, include as needed; evaluative, monitor effectiveness/research results variable; experimental, additional study needed; not recommended, lacks economic data to currently recommend.
*NA = not applicable
**Recommended, bacteria include *Lactobacillus plantaerium, L buchneri, L acidilacti, Pediococcus cereviseai, P pentacoccus,* and *Streptococcus faecium.*

NUTRITIONAL DISEASES OF CATTLE

Ataxia is found predominantly in calves and is most often attributed to a chronic manganese deficiency. Deformities of affected animals include weak legs and pasterns, enlarged joints, stiffness, twisted legs, general weakness, and reduced bone strength.

Blind staggers is a sign of acute selenium toxicity. Affected cattle show dullness, ataxia, rapid weak pulse, labored respiration, diarrhea, and lethargy; the head is lowered and the ears droop. Death is due to respiratory failure. In less severely affected cattle, there is lameness; loss of vitality; loss of appetite; emaciation; deformed, cracked, and elongated hooves; loss of hair from the tail; and liver cirrhosis. *(See also* p 2516.)

Bloat is seen when gases are produced in the rumen in too great quantity or the animal is not able to get rid of such gases as rapidly as they are produced. In either situation, the accumulation of gases causes inflation and swelling of the rumen, which is visible on the animal's left flank. Bloat can be seen in cattle grazing lush, young legumes or in those fed large amounts of concentrates. Whereas legume bloat may kill cattle within hours, feedlot bloat develops slowly over weeks and often becomes chronic. *(See also* p 183.)

Bone calcification retardation is generally attributed to a vitamin D deficiency but is rare because sunlight is so effective in converting the provitamin D (7-dehydrocholesterol) of the skin to active vitamin D.

Cardiac arrhythmia is usually associated with a long and severe deficiency of sodium in the diet.

Corneal lesions are usually associated with advanced vitamin A deficiency.

Delayed puberty is largely attributable to diets greatly decreased in energy fed to young, growing animals.

Depraved appetite is seen when cattle consume nonfeed materials such as dirt, sand, fine stone, and many other substances for no apparent reason. Many suggest that these habits can be explained on the basis of nutrient deficiency, but this has not been confirmed by research. One possible explanation for this habit is that such cattle are "bored."

Dermatitis can be seen in both calves and mature cows due to a zinc deficiency, usually in the range of <10 ppm of dietary zinc. Generally, it is most severe on the legs, neck, and head and around the nostrils. Wounds are slow to heal. Additional signs associated with zinc deficiency include decreased testicular growth, listlessness, development of swollen feet with open scaly lesions, and alopecia.

Displaced abomasum, in which the abomasum moves to the right of its normal position, can be seen in as many as 20% of older cows. The incidence is much higher in cows fed high-concentrate, low-forage diets and in those fed only finely chopped forage diets. Reduced appetite and feed intake, lower milk production, loss of weight, and mild secondary ketosis are typical. *See also* p 193.

Dystrophic tongue is most common in the overall selenium deficiency syndromes.

Fat cow syndrome can be recognized by the presence of very fat cows among the dry cow group. It is characterized by inappetence, reduced milk production, and extensive loss of condition. Measures to reduce the incidence include avoiding overconditioning of cows during late lactation and the dry period and formulating rations that maximize feed intake after calving. (*See also* p 824.)

Growth retardation can develop as a result of many nutritional factors, most commonly deprivation of energy. Additional factors may include salt (sodium chloride), cobalt, copper, iron, zinc, vitamin A, and some B vitamins in calves.

Hair coat roughness is a rather subjective evaluation but is related to deficiency of energy, phosphorus, salt, vitamin A, cobalt, or copper.

Heart failure is often associated with a selenium deficiency.

Hemoglobinemia most often is a manifestation of a copper deficiency.

Hemorrhaging (generalized) is usually due to a relative vitamin K deficiency.

Hypomagnesemic tetany (grass tetany) is due to a relative deficiency of magnesium— relative because the dietary magnesium may be tied up in such a manner that it is not available. Among the signs of experimentally produced magnesium deficiency in both young and mature cattle are anorexia, hyperemia, greatly increased excitability, and calcification of soft tissues in a chronic deficiency condition. An affected animal exhibits convulsions, falling on its side with its legs alternately extended and relaxed. Death may occur during the convulsions. Frothing at the mouth and profuse salivation are evident. The signs appear to progress much more rapidly in adult cows. (*See also* p 812.)

Ketosis is usually characterized by a dullness, typically during the first 6 wk after calving, and is seen primarily in dairy cows. Occasionally, such cows are highly excitable and blood glucose is decreased, whereas ketones and free fatty acids are increased. It is proposed that the major causative factor is an inadequate supply of glucose precursors to maintain adequate blood glucose levels. (*See also* p 830.)

Lactic acid acidosis, founder, and laminitis can develop when unadapted cattle consume a large quantity of concentrate over a short period of time. Acute indigestion often develops, introducing greatly increased levels of lactic acid into the rumen and lowering the rumen pH to a dangerous level. Frequently, lamina of the feet are severely damaged (laminitis), which is often permanent. Cattle in which the onset is severe may die. Some concentrates are broken down much more rapidly than others (eg, wheat is broken down much more rapidly than corn) and therefore are more likely to cause the condition. (*See also* p 873.)

Mastitis may possibly be alleviated by supplementation with β-carotene. (*See also* p 1120.)

Milk fever is characterized by low blood calcium and paralysis and is usually seen within 48 hr after calving in cows beyond their first lactation. High-calcium intake during the dry period increases the incidence; limiting calcium intake before calving but increasing it at calving time decreases the incidence. (*See also* p 806.)

Osteomalacia, which is characterized by weak, brittle bones that may fracture when stressed, can develop after demineralization of the bones of aged animals. Feeding a diet low in calcium to lactating cows over a long period of time may cause a depletion of calcium and phosphorus, resulting in fragile, easily fractured bones plus decreased milk production, without affecting calcium level in the milk produced.

Polioencephalomalacia is characterized by listlessness, muscular incoordination, progressive blindness, convulsions, and death. It is linked to some aspect of the diet that produces high levels of thiaminase, which deactivates thiamine. Affected cattle are very responsive to therapeutic levels of thiamine, preferably via IM injection. Thiamine is believed to be involved in the normal functioning of the CNS. (*See also* p 1061.)

The nutritional causes of **retained placenta** appear to be rather complex and include deficiencies of selenium, vitamin A, copper, and iodine. The incidence increases with parturient hypocalcemia and appears to be related to fat cow syndrome. Prepartum injection of selenium has reduced the incidence of retained placenta. There is a genetic implication, and such cows should be considered strong candidates for culling. (*See also* p 1141.)

Rickets is characterized by improper calcification of the organic matrix of bone, which results in weak, soft bones that lack density. Signs include swollen, tender joints; enlarged bone ends; an arched back; stiffness of the legs; and development of beads on the ribs. Rickets is a disease of young animals and may be caused by deficiencies of calcium, phosphorus, or vitamin D. (*See also* p 853.)

Thyroid gland enlargement (goiter) is the first sign of an iodine deficiency. Signs of a deficiency may not be seen for >1 yr on low-iodine diets. Iodine deficiency may be seen in cattle that are consuming an "adequate" level of iodine if they are also consuming fairly large quantities of crops of the cruciferae family, such as turnips or cabbage. Affected cows may give birth to hairless calves.

Udder edema, characterized by excessive accumulation of fluid in the intercellular spaces of the udder and in areas forward of the udder, usually develops at calving time. The causes are not well understood, but a reduction of blood proteins at calving time seems to reduce the incidence. Some studies have indicated that a high intake of sodium chloride may increase the severity of the condition. (*See also* p 1144.)

White muscle disease normally is seen in young calves (or lambs) and is associated with deficiencies of selenium or vitamin E, or both. Affected animals have chalky white striations, degeneration, and necrosis of cardiac and skeletal muscle. In addition, paralysis of the hindlimbs, a dystrophic tongue, and increased AST levels may be evident. (*See also* p 897.)

Xerophthalmia is a degenerative condition of the eye associated with a vitamin A deficiency.

NUTRITION: EXOTIC AND ZOO ANIMALS

The field of zoo and exotic animal nutrition has made significant advances in recent decades. Exotic animal nutritionists in zoos and in the feed industry are studying problems and generating information on proper nutritional management for many species.

All animals require nutrients and energy in a metabolizable form. The nutrients and energy must be properly balanced and in the correct form to accommodate particular tastes, digestive systems, and feeding methods. For example, large psittacines typically use their feet for holding food, while other species obtain or position food using other appendages (or they do not manipulate food). If a commercial extruded food is fed, the pieces must be large enough for the bird to grasp easily. Diets for exotic and zoo animals have been developed by considering food habits in the wild, oral and GI tract morphology, nutrient requirements established for domestic and laboratory animals and humans, nutritional research on exotic species, and practical experience. The ultimate criteria for evaluating the suitability of a diet for a given species are growth, reproductive success, and longevity.

The minimum nutrient requirements established by the National Research Council (NRC) for domestic and laboratory animals can be useful starting points in setting target nutrient levels for an exotic species. For many exotic species that have closely related domestic counterparts, diets can be formulated to contain nutrients that would meet the requirements established for ungulates, mustelids, canids, felids, rodents, primates, lagomorphs, gallinaceous and anseriform birds, and fish. However, nutrient requirements established by the NRC should be used only as guidelines because the goals of livestock producers in feeding their animals include rapid and efficient gain and high milk yield or egg production—goals that differ from the goals of zoo personnel. Although the NRC requirements are less directly applicable to other species, they can still serve as a useful general reference for evaluating the nutritional adequacy for most birds and mammals. The formulation and evaluation of diets for reptiles and amphibians is even more difficult because there are no domestic animal models and because metabolic rates of poikilothermic animals fluctuate with changes in ambient temperature. Once the nutrient concentrations for the diet have been established, the types and amounts of foodstuffs, methods of presentation, and feeding frequencies should be selected based on the physical and behavioral attributes of the species.

All food should be of good quality. Spoiled or moldy foods, or foods stored for long periods (eg, >1 yr for most bagged feeds and 6-12 mo for most frozen foods) should not be fed. The practice of "topping off" the feed bowl daily or every other day should be discouraged because uneaten food on the bottom can spoil. Food and water dishes should be thoroughly cleaned before adding food or water. Clean, fresh water should always be available to nonmarine species, although it is common practice to offer water to desert-adapted tortoises 2-3 times/wk. Trace mineral salt blocks, bricks, or "spools" are commonly offered to ungulates, psittacine birds, and some rodents.

Cafeteria-style feeding is strongly discouraged because captive animals rarely select a balanced diet if given a wide selection of foods. Usually, a nutritionally complete commercial product or in-house mixture that cannot be sorted should comprise the bulk of the diet, with components such as meat, fruit, and seeds comprising only a small percentage. Pelleted diets are especially important with psittacines, to avoid self-selection of calcium-deficient seeds. Muscle and organ meat, fruit, most grains and seeds, and most insects are poor sources of calcium, and excess consumption can result in calcium deficiency. Calcium gut-loading diets can be fed to insects intended for food, or items can be dusted with a balanced calcium-phosphorus powder. Other sources of calcium include oyster shell, cuttle bone, and ground calcium carbonate tablets (see also p 1865).

Obesity is more common than inadequate nutrient intake. Ungulates, primates, and carnivores can rapidly become overweight when excess amounts of a high-quality diet are offered, particularly when activity is limited. In some birds (eg, ratites, waterfowl), rapid growth rates increase the incidence of leg and wing problems. Both adult and growing animals should be routinely weighed to monitor changes. If a dietary change is contemplated due to suspected nutrient imbalances, deficiencies, or toxicities, the diet currently fed should first be computer-analyzed to assess nutrient concentrations. Ingredient or nutrient changes can then be made based on correcting a suspected or confirmed health problem. For captive, exotic animals, establishing and maintaining dietary histories can be particularly helpful in health assessment. Activity patterns of individuals are also important (eg, atherosclerosis is relatively common in obese birds).

Nutritional Supplements: The use of nutritional supplements is becoming increasingly popular among animal caretakers. While many keepers and pet owners use nutritionally complete feeds that require no supplementation, supplements are still often provided. Unfortunately, diets are rarely evaluated first to determine which nutrients (if any) are unbalanced. Excessive supplementation of some nutrients (eg, some fat-soluble vitamins, selenium, copper) can be just as harmful as not enough. Diets consisting primarily of cultivated fruits and vegetables may need micronutrient supplementation; however, supplements vary widely in their composition. Analysis of 5 commonly sold supplements revealed markedly different concentrations of nutrients: calcium was 6.3-32%; phosphorus 0-20%; vitamin A 222,000-6,600,000 IU/kg; and vitamin D 636-22,000 IU/kg. The nutrient content of the current diet should be established or estimated first to determine whether any supplement is needed or if a supplement should be discontinued. If a nutrient is deficient in a diet, a specific supplement in a specific amount should be recommended. The indiscriminate use of supplements should be discouraged because toxicities and nutrient imbalances may result.

Water: Water intake should be assessed routinely but especially in animals with compromised renal function, in lizards or birds prone to gout, and in animals under conditions of high temperature or low humidity in which evaporative losses can be expected. The salt content of water should be known because some species are less tolerant than others. Animals fed dry feeds (pellets, extrusions, hay, etc) require more water than those fed succulent feeds. Potable water should be available ad lib. Many animals in the wild consume much of their water in the foods they eat. When low-moisture foods are consumed (pellets, extrusions, etc), some animals, depending on how water is presented, may not maintain adequate hydration. Many free-ranging small and tropical lizards receive water from foods and from licking drops that accumulate after rainfall. When in captivity, they frequently do not drink readily from containers. Humidity may be especially important in maintaining hydration of many reptiles, especially tropical species. Daily misting with warm water is an important source of hydration for some lizards that may not be observed drinking standing water. Eye lesions in semiaquatic turtles (eg, box turtles) and some tortoises may be the result of low environmental humidity (or possibly upper respiratory tract disease) and not vitamin A deficiency. Conjunctivitis may respond better to supportive antibiotic therapy and higher humidity than to supplemental vitamin A. Dietary histories may be especially important in such cases because many captive turtles are fed commercial cat food that is high in vitamin A.

For a discussion of nutrition for orphaned animals, see p 1691.

BIRDS

Nutrient deficiencies in birds often do not become obvious until molt or unless breeding is attempted. Feather problems frequently are related to inadequate nutrition. Deficiencies of vitamin A, protein (sulfur amino acids in particular), calcium, zinc, folic acid, and pantothenic acid, as well as other nutrients, can cause abnormal and ragged feathering. Some birds (eg, flamingos, ibises, trogons, tanagers, woodpeckers) depend on dietary carotenoid pigments for natural feather coloration. Suitable pigment sources include carrots, carrot extract, alfalfa meal, shrimp meal, brine shrimp, and synthetic pigments such as canthaxanthin. Although most captive birds are fed the same diet year-round, many birds in the wild have evolved with diets that vary greatly with seasons. Little is known about the influence of seasonal dietary changes in the reproduction of exotic birds. Fruits and vegetables should always be washed thoroughly to remove residual pesticides. Uneaten soft foods should be discarded daily to prevent bacterial contamination. Birds do not use vitamin D_2 efficiently; vitamin D_3 should be used when vitamin D is added to avian diets. Seed-eating species should always have grit available for proper gizzard function, as well as calcium supplements, especially during breeding and egg-laying season. (See p 1850.)

Aquatic Birds

Penguins, pelicans, and other fish-eating species in the wild feed primarily on fish, crustaceans, and squid. In captivity, capelin, squid, smelt, herring, mackerel, and whiting are commonly fed. One of the most important aspects of feeding penguins and other fish-eating birds is fish quality (see MARINE MAMMALS, p 1529). All fish-eating birds should receive a mixed diet consisting of ≥2 fish species to ensure proper nutrition. Supplements commonly given to penguins include salt, polyunsaturated fatty acids, and vitamins. Dietary salt (NaCl) is provided to birds in freshwater exhibits to help maintain proper functioning of the salt glands; 0.5-1 g salt/bird/day should be adequate for most species. Providing a supplemental source of essential fatty acids has been recommended during reproduction and molting when monotypic diets of smelt are fed: 2-3 mL of corn oil/bird/day has been satisfactory. Thiamine and vitamin E supplementation (25 mg thiamine and 100 IU vitamin E/kg of fish, as fed) is recommended whenever fish that have been frozen are fed. Vitamin D_3 supplementation (250-500 IU/kg of fish, as fed) may be beneficial for birds not exposed to direct sunlight. Providing calcium carbonate or dicalcium phosphate to females during reproductive periods is a common practice to ensure proper eggshell formation. Penguins and pelicans should be fed individually by hand to ensure that each bird receives the proper amount of supplements and to better monitor intake. Generally, intake is 0.5-2 kg fish/day depending on the species of penguin, fat content of the fish, and molt status.

Recommendations for feeding other fish-eating birds (eg, cormorant, heron, gull, tern, loon, grebe, petrel) are similar to those for penguins. Some species will accept commercial bird-of-prey diets, trout pellets, and/or mice in the diet, as well as fish.

Flamingos can be fed commercial flamingo diets or a mixture of trout pellets (number 4 size), duck-grower or game-bird pellets, dry dog food, and a carotenoid pigment source (eg, canthaxanthin, carrot oil extract). Lack of a suitable pigment source in the diet results in faded feather coloration. Dry ingredients should be mixed with water, forming a slurry to permit natural filter feeding.

Most waterfowl can be fed commercial duck or game-bird pellets along with chopped greens. Dry dog food (<10% fat, dry-matter basis) or trout pellets are readily consumed by many species, particularly diving ducks, and can be included in the diet. Scratch grains can be fed in moderation (<25% of the diet dry matter) but should not be substituted for a nutritionally complete pelleted product.

Gallinaceous Birds

Most gallinaceous birds (eg, pheasant, quail, turkey, grouse, partridge) do well on commercial game-bird diets. Starter, grower, maintenance, and layer diets are available. Grit should always be available free-choice, with calcium supplements available during breeding season. Chopped lettuce or other green vegetation also can be provided. Some herbivorous grouse species are difficult to maintain in captivity and may require specific natural foods such as willow, heather, or blueberry leaves and buds. Artificial diets that have been used successfully for grouse often contain higher levels of fiber (eg, 10% crude fiber, dry basis) than rations for poultry and game birds. Growing chicks of some grouse species appear to require a dietary source of vitamin C. Diets of most young gallinaceous birds may be supplemented with crickets and mealworms (fed appropriate calcium gut-loading diets) to provide variety and to serve as a feeding stimulus.

Hummingbirds

Captive hummingbirds readily adapt to artificial nectar mixtures (TABLE 23). Nectar should always be available to satisfy their extremely high energy requirements. Satisfactory commercial nectar dry mixes that are fortified with protein, vitamins, and minerals also are available. Commercial nectar mixes that are simply sugar and food coloring are not adequate. A nutritionally complete nectar should be offered early each morning. At the end of each day, the morning nectar should be discarded to prevent bacterial contamination and fermentation; in hot weather, replacement during the day may be required. In the afternoon, morning nectar can be replaced with a sugar-water mixture that is less likely to sour overnight. Nectar can be dispensed in commercially available tube-type hummingbird feeders. Common backyard hummingbird feeders are not recommended for captive hummingbirds because they tend to clog with morning nectar and are difficult to clean. Feeding tubes should be colored (usually red) and must be an appropriate size and shape to accommodate the hummingbird's bill. Feeders should be cleaned thoroughly each day. Coloration of hummingbirds is not influenced by dietary pigments; therefore, pigmented nectars are not necessary. Fruit flies also should be included in the diet. Screen-covered containers (with screens of suitable size to permit fruit flies to exit but exclude insect pests) with fruit-fly cultures can be placed in the birds' enclosures and replaced as the flies are depleted.

Passerines

Passerines can be grouped into 5 categories based on their primary natural food habits: insect feeder, fruit eater, nectar feeder, seed eater, and omnivore. Insectivorous birds (eg, warbler, flycatcher, shrike) can be fed artificial insectivore mixtures supplemented with crickets, mealworms, maggots, house flies, and/or fruit flies. Many insectivore mixes have been devised (TABLE 23). Insects can be placed on top of the insectivore mixture to stimulate feeding.

Frugivorous birds (eg, waxwing, bellbird) can be fed fruit mixtures fortified with protein, minerals, and vitamins (TABLE 23).

TABLE 23. Avian Diets

Morning Nectar

Protein powder (soy-based)	25 g
Protein supplement (casein-based)	10 g
Multivitamin drops[*]	2.4 mL
Calcium, phosphorus, vitamin D_3 supplement	6.5 g
Canthaxanthin	0.5 g
Sugar	400 g
Water	1,920 mL

Nectar remaining at the end of each day should be discarded. Canthaxanthin is optional and is not required for birds that do not depend on carotenoids for feather pigmentation (eg, hummingbirds).

Evening Nectar

Sugar	400 g
Multivitamin drops[*]	2.4 mL
Water	1,440 mL

Insectivore

Ground dog food	23%
Steamed bone meal	5%
Ground trout pellets	4%
Protein supplement (casein-based)	2%
Ground mynah bird pellets	8%
"Super Caradee"	6%
Frozen bird-of-prey diet	52%

Bird-of-prey diet should be thawed, and all ingredients mixed thoroughly. The final product should have a crumbly texture and be refrigerated or frozen for storage.

Small Frugivore | **g/kg of diet**

Apple	470
Grape	110
Banana without skin	100
Currant	70
Tomato	50
Papaya	50
Blueberry	50
Frugivore base mix (see below)	100

Apples and grapes should be mixed in a food processor (until in small pieces but not soupy) and drained in a colander. Tomato, papaya, and banana should be blended in a food processor. Pieces should be small, but the mixture should not be soupy. All ingredients should be mixed thoroughly. The mixture can be refrigerated for up to 3 days. Calculated analysis (dry-matter basis): 24% dry matter, 26% crude protein, 4% fat, 3.6% crude fiber, 7.7% ash, 1.49% calcium, 0.76% phosphorus.

Large Frugivore | **g/kg of diet**

Apple	480
Banana without skin	200
Grape	100
Raisin (seedless)	50
Blueberry	50
Frugivore base mix (see below)	120

Apple and banana should be chopped into pieces ~15 mm wide and combined with all ingredients and mixed thoroughly until blended to a thin applesauce-like consistency. Calculated analysis (dry-matter basis): 31% dry matter, 24% crude protein, 3.7% fat, 2.6% crude fiber, 7.2% ash, 1.4% calcium, 0.71% phosphorus.

(continued)

TABLE 23. Avian Diets (continued)

Frugivore Base mix	g/kg of base mix
Corn gluten meal (60% crude protein)	359
Calcium caseinate	280
Soybean protein concentrate (70% crude protein)	100
Dicalcium phosphate	75
Corn oil	50
Brewer's yeast, dehydrated	45
Calcium carbonate	38
Iodized salt (NaCl)	13
L-lysine monohydrochloride	5.5
DL-methionine	4.5
Frugivore vitamin premix[†]	16
Frugivore mineral premix[‡]	14

Large Psittacine	
Seeds and nuts	20%
Fruit	25%
Greens	15%
Yellow vegetables	25%
Monkey biscuit or dry dog food	15%
Cuttlebone or mineral block	free-choice

Kiwi (per adult)	
Rolled oats	20 g
Water	160 mL
Vegetable oil	2.5 mL
Wheat germ	2 g
Vitamin-mineral premix[§]	2 g

Beef heart should have fat trimmed before slicing into thin, worm-like strips. Oats should be cooked in water. All ingredients should be combined to make a gruel and fed from a shallow dish. Earthworms also can be offered.

[*]Multivitamin drops (per mL): 1500 IU vitamin A, 400 IU vitamin D, 5 IU vitamin E, 0.5 mg vitamin B_1, 0.6 mg vitamin B_2, 8 mg niacin, 0.4 mg vitamin B_6, 1.5 μg vitamin B_{12}, 35 mg vitamin C

[†]Frugivore vitamin premix (g/kg of premix): 33.3 g retinyl acetate mix (30,000 IU/g), 0.4 g cholecalciferol mix (500,000 IU/g), 18.1 g DL-α-tocopherol acetate mix (276 IU/g), 576 g choline chloride mix (60% choline chloride), 1.38 g thiamine HCl (87.5% B_1), 1.3 g riboflavin (96% B_2), 10.1 g niacin (99.5% niacin), 1.55 g pyridoxine HCl (80.65% B_6), 5.43 g D-calcium pantothenate (92% pantothenate), 2.5 g biotin mix (2% biotin), 1.25 g folic acid mix (20% folic acid), 1.89 g vitamin B_{12} mix (600 mg/lb), 0.76 g menadione sodium bisulfite complex (33% menadione), and 346 g soybean protein concentrate

[‡]Frugivore mineral premix (g/kg of premix): 7 g $CuSO_4 \times 5H_2O$ (25.2% Cu), 42 g $ZnSO_4 \times H_2O$ (35.5% Zn), 60 g $MnSO_4 \times 5H_2O$ (28% Mn), 17 g $FeSO_4 \times H_2O$ (30% Fe), 150 g sodium selenite mix (0.02% Se), and 724 g calcium caseinate

[§]Vitamin-mineral premix for kiwis (per kg): 320 g calcium, 2.7 g iron, 2.7 g zinc, 2.7 g manganese, 0.27 g copper, 27 mg iodine, 27 mg cobalt, 16 mg selenium, 800,000 IU vitamin A, 60,000 IU vitamin D, 6,000 IU vitamin E, 0.43 g vitamin B_1, 0.32 g vitamin B_2, 0.27 g vitamin B_6, 40 g choline, 10.6 g inositol, 5.3 g ascorbic acid, 2.13 g nicotinic acid, 1.6 g pantothenic acid, 0.43 g vitamin K, 0.11 g folic acid, 21 mg biotin, 2.7 mg vitamin B_{12}, 1.06 g butylated hydroxytoluene

Nectar feeders (eg, sunbird, honeycreeper) can be maintained in captivity using artificial nectars (see HUMMINGBIRDS, above and TABLE 23). Most nectar-feeding species will also eat insects, insectivore mix, and/or frugivore mix.

Seed eaters (eg, finches, sparrows, cardinals) can be offered seed mixtures (primary seeds include canary seed and yellow, white, and red millet; secondary seeds include oat groats, flax, and niger or thistle). Chopped green vegetables, insects, insectivore and frugivore mixes, peanut butter, and cooked egg yolk also are readily accepted by most species and should be included in addition to seeds to provide a balanced diet. Cuttlebone (or other calcium sources) and grit should be available free-choice to seed-eating birds.

Omnivorous species (eg, corvid, tanager, starling, mynah, oriole, manakin, bird of paradise) can be fed frugivore mixes with insects, chopped green vegetables, and cooked egg yolk. Some of these species appear to accumulate hepatic iron that may be fatal. The etiology is unknown, but copper deficiency and the presence of dietary ascorbic acid are known to affect, in some animals, release of hepatic iron and gut absorption of iron, respectively. Diets containing high (available) iron concentrations or diets with heme iron, a highly available source of iron found in red meat, should be avoided. Commercial diets formulated with low iron concentrations (eg, <100 mg iron/kg diet dry matter) are available and should be used with susceptible species. Commercial soft-pelleted diets are available for mynahs. Some omnivorous passerines (eg, blackbird, meadowlark, horned lark) will also eat seed and grain mixtures.

Pigeons and Doves

Seed-eating pigeons and doves can be fed commercial pigeon pellets and pigeon grains (wheat, milo, corn, Canada peas [field peas], and millet). Fruit-eating pigeons and doves can be fed a large-frugivore mixture (TABLE 23).

Psittacines

Large seed-eating species (eg, macaw, parrot, cockatoo) commonly are maintained on diets of seeds (sunflower, hemp, millet, canary, safflower, oats), peanuts, monkey biscuits, dry dog food, fruits (apple, banana, grape, orange), vegetables (green vegetables, carrot, ear corn, sweet potato), and various supplements (cooked egg yolk, vitamins, minerals, wheat germ). (See TABLE 23.) The percentage of each ingredient fed varies widely. Some breeders have reported good success on diets consisting almost entirely of monkey biscuits, while others have recommended that no more than 10% of the diet consist of monkey biscuits.

Intake of each ingredient should be monitored closely whenever mixed diets are fed. Many birds preferentially select seeds and nuts. While differences in the nutrient concentrations of seeds and nuts do vary, they are almost all marginal to deficient in calcium, phosphorus, sodium, zinc, iron, iodine, selenium, the fat-soluble vitamins, and some B vitamins. Only a few types of seeds may provide enough protein for growth. In addition, seeds and nuts contain high concentrations of fat that promote obesity in many species. Seeds and nuts, if fed, should be offered in limited quantities and are inappropriate in diets of reproductively active females and growing chicks. When certain items are selected in unduly high amounts, they should be decreased in the diet to force consumption of other foods. Vitamin and mineral premixes can be added to the drinking water, and dusted over fruits and vegetables that have been cut into pieces that are easy for the birds to handle.

Several commercial diets are available for large psittacines. Some are simply mixes of seeds and other ingredients that still permit sorting by the birds. Others are fortified, pelleted, or extruded products that ensure the birds consume a specific concentration of nutrients. Although the pelleted or extruded diets are easier to feed than mixed diets, acceptability is often poor in older birds accustomed to a seed and fruit-based diet. With persistence, older birds can gradually be switched to commercial products. Young birds should accept an extruded or pelleted product readily; these are ideal for maintaining proper nutrition throughout life.

Some commercial diets marketed for psittacines may not be appropriately formulated. For recommended nutrient concentrations that promote reproduction and maintenance in many psittacine species, *see* TABLE 24. Products that meet, or are very similar to, these nutrient concentrations should be fed. The typical calculated analyses of nutrients of a product should be reviewed and compared with recommended nutrient concentrations before the product is fed. Although many products are marketed as nutritionally complete feeds, analyses of nutrient concentrations in various manufactured

TABLE 24. Recommended Nutrient Concentrations for Most Psittacines

Nutrient	Concentration
Protein	20-24%
Arginine	1.3%
Isoleucine	1.1%
Lysine	1.2%
Methionine	0.5%
Methionine + cysteine	0.9%
Threonine	0.95%
Tryptophan	0.24%
Linoleic acid	2.0%
Calcium	1.1%
Phosphorus	0.8%
Potassium	0.7%
Sodium	0.2%
Chlorine	0.2%
Magnesium	0.15%
Manganese	65 ppm
Zinc	120 ppm
Iron	150 ppm
Copper	20 ppm
Iodine	1 ppm
Selenium	0.3 ppm
Vitamin K	4 ppm
Riboflavin	6 ppm
Pantothenic acid	20 ppm
Niacin	55 ppm
Vitamin B_{12}	0.025 ppm
Choline	1,700 ppm
Biotin	0.3 ppm
Folacin	0.9 ppm
Thiamine	6 ppm
Pyridoxine	6 ppm
Vitamin A	8,000-10,000 IU/kg
Cholecalciferol (vitamin D_3)	2,000 IU/kg
Vitamin E	250 IU/kg

diets suggests that this may not be the case. Dietary ranges, on a dry-matter basis, were crude protein 15-30%; calcium 0.18-1.5%; phosphorus 0.29-1.06; calcium:phosphorus ratio 0.62-1.97; sodium 0.03-0.4%; iron 80-4,200 mg/kg; copper 8-132 mg/kg; zinc 31-939 mg/kg; manganese 15-1,055 mg/kg. Diets low in calcium, phosphorus, sodium, zinc, or manganese result in clinical signs of ill health, and diets high in iron, copper, zinc, or manganese may produce frank toxicity.

Smaller seed-eating psittacines (eg, cockatiel, budgerigar, lovebird) can be fed commercial seed mixtures (canary seed; red, yellow, and white millet; oat groats) along with chopped greens, bread, and fruit. There are also commercial diets (complete feeds) available in small sizes; these are more likely to provide well-balanced diets. Vitamin and mineral supplements can be added in the same manner as with the larger species. Unlike most psittacines, lories and lorikeets are primarily frugivorous. Various fortified fruit mixtures have been used successfully for these species.

Cuttlebone, oyster shell, or a mineral block should be available free-choice to all psittacines. Daily food intake is usually ~10-15% of body wt for most species, with higher relative intakes seen in smaller birds.

Raptors

Vultures, hawks, falcons, eagles, and owls can be fed whole-animal diets. Commonly fed items include chicks up to 5 wk old, *Coturnix* quail, mice, rats, and pigeons. Feeding a variety of prey items is preferred, although some species more readily accept certain kinds of prey, depending on natural food habits. Fish can be included in the diet of piscivorous species (eg, osprey, sea eagle, bald eagle), and calcium-fortified insects can be given to kestrels and falconettes. If fish or day-old chicks are fed, thiamine supplementation (30 mg/kg feed, as-fed basis) on alternate days is recommended. To ensure a nutritionally complete diet, prey items should not be eviscerated before feeding. Commercial bird-of-prey diets also can be used successfully by many species and often provide a simpler, more economical alternative to live-prey diets. A commercial diet suitable for a variety of species is 55-60% moisture and contains (dry-matter basis) 45-50% crude protein, 18-20% ether extract, 2.2-2.5% crude fiber, 1-1.5% calcium, and 0.7-1% phosphorus. Due to the soft consistency of these diets, whole-prey items should generally be provided twice a week to help prevent impaction and beak overgrowth and to ensure a complete diet. Small raptors can eat as much as 25% of their body wt/day; large species may eat as little as 4%. Captive raptors should be weighed regularly to monitor weight gain and loss, and food intake should be adjusted accordingly.

Ratites

All large ratite birds (emu, cassowary, ostrich, rhea) can be fed commercial pelleted ratite diets. Diets suitable for growth and maintenance contain 20-24% crude protein, 12-19% crude fiber, 1.2-2% calcium, 0.6-1.1% phosphorus, 10,000-15,000 of vitamin A/kg, and 1,500-2,500 IU/kg of vitamin D_3 (dry-matter basis). (*See* TABLE 25.) Breeding diets are similar except for a higher level of calcium (eg, 2.8% calcium in the pellet, or oyster shell free-choice). Mixtures of pelleted poultry or duck feed, dry dog food, rabbit pellets, and oyster shell also have been used. Green, leafy vegetables and, for cassowaries, chopped apple can be added to the diet. Young ratites are particularly susceptible to leg abnormalities that appear to be nutritionally related. Reducing the growth rate by feeding diets lower in metabolizable energy and higher in fiber appears to reduce the incidence of spraddled leg syndrome in young birds. A diet using beef heart cut into worm-like strips as a base item has been used successfully for kiwis (TABLE 23). (*See also* p 1555.)

Miscellaneous Birds

Most large, fruit-eating softbills, eg, hornbill, toucan, toucanet, and touraco, will eat a large-frugivore mixture (TABLE 23) along with insects, greens, and dry dog food or bird-of-prey diet. Because toucans also appear to store excessive hepatic iron, low-iron diets should be fed, and diets with heme iron should be avoided. Gelatin-based diets also have been used successfully for hornbills and toucans. Placing diet ingredients in gelatin

TABLE 25. Recommended Nutrient Concentrations for Ostriches, Rheas, and Emus

Nutrient	Concentration
Protein	20-24%
Arginine	1.3%
Lysine	1.2%
Methionine	0.35%
Methionine + cysteine	0.7%
Tryptophan	0.3%
Linoleic acid	1.0%
Calcium	1.6%
Phosphorus, total	1.0%
Phosphorus, available	0.8%
Potassium	1.1%
Sodium	0.2%
Magnesium	0.2%
Manganese	70 ppm
Zinc	120 ppm
Iron	150 ppm
Copper	20 ppm
Iodine	1 ppm
Selenium	0.3 ppm
Vitamin K	4 ppm
Riboflavin	9 ppm
Pantothenic acid	30 ppm
Niacin	70 ppm
Vitamin B_{12}	0.03 ppm
Choline	1,600 ppm
Biotin	0.3 ppm
Folacin	1 ppm
Thiamine	7 ppm
Pyridoxine	5 ppm
Vitamin A	8,000 IU/kg
Cholecalciferol (vitamin D_3)	1,600 IU/kg
Vitamin E	250 IU/kg
Vitamin K (menadione equivalent)	4 ppm

prevents sorting but requires careful formulation to compensate for the low tryptophan content of the gelatin. Frogmouths and kookaburras will eat mice and commercial bird-of-prey diets.

MAMMALS

Handrearing Mammals: Successful nutrition of handreared mammals requires: 1) selecting a formula that will support adequate growth and not cause GI upset; 2) offering it at proper intervals, in proper amounts, and in the proper way to ensure acceptance, and prevent overfeeding, underfeeding, or aspiration into the lungs; and 3) keeping all feeding utensils clean and disinfected. If success is judged in terms of survival and not in comparison with maternal-raised growth and health, most precocial species maintained in captive collections have been handreared successfully. Handrearing more altricial species (eg, marsupials, rodents, rabbits) is generally less successful unless the young have been dam-raised to a more advanced stage.

Whenever possible, data on milk composition and handrearing case histories should be consulted before attempting to bottle-raise a species for the first time. Unfortunately, milk composition data are not available for most species, and some of the published data are of dubious value. Lactose content of milk varies widely between different species. Animals (eg, pinnipeds, rabbits) that normally consume milk low in lactose generally produce little lactase and often develop severe GI problems and diarrhea when fed a high-lactose milk, eg, bovine. Similarly, adding sucrose to milk formulas is often contraindicated because many neonates produce little sucrase. Many species have been raised using diluted evaporated milk or commercial calf, lamb, foal, or doe milk replacers (eg, most ungulates), commercial dog milk replacer (eg, canids, procyonids, bears, bats, edentates, mustelids, rabbits, rodents), commercial cat milk replacer (eg, felids), human infant formulas in general (eg, most primates), and soy-based human infant formulas in particular (eg, rabbits, some marsupials). In some cases, these basic formulas can be modified to better suit the needs of a particular species by the addition of ingredients such as egg yolk, butterfat, and casein. Supplementation with vitamin and mineral products may be warranted.

Some species (eg, ungulates, marsupials, mink) must receive colostrum within 12-48 hr of birth to acquire immunoglobulins necessary for survival. Including some colostrum in the diet of ungulates for up to 2-3 wk after birth may provide additional local gut protection. Colostrum from domestic cows has proved satisfactory for many exotic ruminants and can be stored frozen. Recent studies suggest that conspecific serum, collected aseptically, can be given PO or SC as a substitute for colostrum. Many neonates (eg, artiodactyls, rodents, carnivores) must be stimulated to defecate and urinate by gently rubbing anal and genital areas.

Frequency of feeding and the amount fed depends on natural nursing behavior, formula composition, and the desired rate of gain as well as practical labor restrictions. The stomach capacity of most species can be estimated at 50 mL/kg. Overfilling the stomach leads to GI upset, decreased transit time, and diarrhea. Daily intake, as a rule, should not exceed 20% body wt per day, and should be divided into frequent feedings that do not exceed 35-40 mL/kg. As a general guide, most newborns should be fed every 2-4 hr, and daily metabolizable energy intake (kcal) should be ~210 × body wt (kg)$^{0.75}$. Appetite, condition of feces, and general health should be monitored closely. Body weights should be recorded at frequent intervals. Smaller, more altricial species often must be fed by stomach tube.

See also CARE OF ORPHANED NATIVE BIRDS AND MAMMALS, p 1691.

Bats

Captive insectivorous bats frequently are fed diets consisting primarily of mealworms. Crickets, fruit flies, blowfly larvae, and other insects also are commonly offered. Because insects typically are low in calcium, they should be maintained on a calcium-enriched diet so that the bat will consume the insect's high-calcium gut contents. A suitable mealworm diet can be formulated using 40% wheat middlings, 40% ground dry dog or cat food, and 20% ground calcium carbonate. Alternatively, calcium and vitamin supplements can be dusted on the insects just before feeding, and vitamin drops can be added to drinking water. Often, captive insectivorous bats must be fed by hand when flying insects are not available. Some bats can be trained to accept insects from a food dish by being placed directly on the live food. Various artificial diets have been used with insectivorous bats with mixed success.

Many frugivorous and insectivorous bats can be maintained successfully in captivity using artificial liquid or solid diets (TABLE 26). Liquid diet can be placed in shallow plastic trays positioned near wire or branches for the bats to land on and hang from while

TABLE 26. Diets of Selected Mammals

Freshwater Otter Diet	Percent (%)
Ground horsemeat	38
Ground beef heart	20
Ground dry cat food	13
Beet pulp	2.9
"Mirra Coat"	1.9
Calcium carbonate	0.8
Poultry fat	4.9
Water	16.9
Lactose	0.04
Yogurt	0.72
Mineral-vitamin mix	0.84

All ingredients should be combined in a large mixer, divided into daily portions, and frozen. Lactose for lactobacilli can be added in yogurt to help maintain freshness. Lactose and yogurt are optional.

Liquid Diet for Bats	Percent (%)
Dry mix:	
Mixed baby cereal	20.7
Wheat germ	4
Nonfat dried milk powder	9
Calcium caseinate	15.8
Sugar	45.5
Protein supplement (casein-based)	3
Mineral-vitamin mix	2

The dry mix (100 g) should be mixed with canned peach nectar (540 mL), water (260 mL), and corn oil (6 mL) and fed with peeled bananas.

Large Herbivore Pellet	Percent (%)
Wheat middlings	30
Alfalfa hay, sun-cured, ground (16% crude protein)	22
Corn grain, ground	19.1
Soybean meal without hulls (48% crude protein)	11.4
Alfalfa meal, dehydrated (17% crude protein)	10
Sugarcane molasses	5
Soybean oil	1
Phosphorus supplement	0.8
Sodium chloride	0.5
Mineral premix[*]	0.1
Vitamin premix[†]	0.1

Calculated composition (dry-matter basis): 89% dry matter, 19% crude protein, 4.3% fat, 16% acid detergent fiber, 12% crude fiber, 0.75% calcium, 0.7% phosphorus

[*]Mineral premix (mg/kg of premix): 75,000 Zn, 50,000 Fe, 30,000 Mn, 10,000 Cu, 800 I, 200 Se, and 100 Co
[†]Vitamin premix (per kg of premix): 5,000,000 IU vitamin A, 400,000 IU vitamin D_3, 200,000 mg vitamin E, 500,000 mg choline, 40,000 mg niacin, 20,000 mg pantothenic acid, 4,000 mg riboflavin, 20 mg vitamin B_{12}

feeding. Leftover liquid diet should be replaced daily. Solid diets usually include bananas as the major ingredient. Additional ingredients frequently offered include papaya, apple, pear, melon, grape, and cooked carrot and sweet potato. Fruit can be rolled in a supplement mixture that contains powdered milk, protein powder, corn oil, and a vitamin-mineral mix. Canned cat or dog food, chopped eggs, and mealworms also have been fed with the fruit.

Carnivores

Most zoos in the USA use nutritionally complete commercial diets for feeding exotic felids, canids, mustelids, and viverrids rather than attempting to prepare diets in-house. The incidence of nutritional problems in captive exotic carnivores has greatly declined, and problems previously commonplace when meat diets were fed (eg, calcium, vitamin A, and iodine deficiencies) have virtually been eliminated. Most commercial diets are based on horsemeat and its byproducts, but diets based on beef and poultry are also available. Typical lesser ingredients include fish meal, soybean meal, beet pulp, and ground corn, as well as mineral and vitamin supplements.

Exotic feline diets are usually higher in fat, protein, and vitamin A than canine diets. A diet suitable for most cat species contains 45-50% protein, 30-35% fat, 3-4% crude fiber, 1.2-1.5% calcium, 1-1.2% phosphorus, and 20,000-40,000 IU of vitamin A/kg diet (dry-matter basis). Apparently exotic cats, like domestic cats, are unable to convert carotene to vitamin A, tryptophan to niacin, and linoleic acid to arachidonic acid. They also probably cannot synthesize adequate taurine (a taurine deficiency has been reported in leopards) and would be susceptible to ammonia toxicity if fed an arginine-deficient diet. Therefore, these nutrients should be considered dietary essentials for all felids. Frozen and canned cat foods usually are more palatable than dry ones to exotic cats. Many zoos prefer to use frozen diets over canned products because generally they are less expensive, and large quantities are easier to feed. The soft, hamburger-like consistency of commercial diets can result in excess calculus deposits and periodontal disease if hard or unprocessed items are not also provided. All cats fed a soft diet should receive bones with some meat intact twice weekly. Horse or beef shank bones are suitable for large cat species; oxtails, rib bones, or whole rodents can be used for smaller cats. Mice, rats, and chicks are frequently included in the diets of smaller cats. Rodents, poultry, fish, and organ and chunk muscle meats can be offered as occasional treat items to administer medication or to stimulate appetite, but generally they are not required as dietary staples for large cats fed commercial diets.

Canids can be fed frozen, canned, or dry canine diets. Although most canids are less particular than cats, frozen and canned foods are generally preferred over dry ones. Bones should also be included in the diet when soft foods are fed. Small amounts of fruits and vegetables can be included in the diets of foxes and coyotes.

Most mustelids and viverrids do well on frozen feline diet or canned cat foods. Many species readily accept small amounts of fruits, vegetables, and cooked egg. Mice, fish, and chicks can be offered as occasional treat items and to stimulate appetite and activity. Rib bones can be given twice weekly to promote dental health. Commercial dry ferret diets and some premium feline diets formulated for kittens promote growth and reproduction in ferrets. Canned foods may be more palatable but are not recommended as a base diet, because ferrets may not be able to eat enough to meet their needs for calories and protein. *See* TABLE 26 for a diet used successfully for freshwater otter species.

Procyonids can be fed diets similar to those offered to small canids. Feeding a good-quality dry dog food along with apple, banana, and carrot is satisfactory for raccoons and helps minimize obesity problems that commonly result when frozen or canned diets are fed. The red or lesser panda has been maintained successfully on commercial high-fiber primate biscuits and bamboo.

Bears can be fed frozen canine diet, dry dog food, fish, and commercial omnivore biscuits. Polar and Kodiak bears do well on a diet of 25% frozen canine diet, 25% fish (eg, smelt), 15% dry dog food, 15% omnivore biscuits, 10% bread, and 10% apples. Commercial diets formulated especially for polar bears are available. Other bear species can be fed less fish and more omnivore biscuits, bread, and produce. Bananas and green vegetables can be included in the diet of sun, sloth, spectacled, and black bears. Food intake of captive bears varies widely with season. Intakes generally are maximal during summer and early fall and minimal during winter. The herbivorous food habits of the giant panda require large amounts of bamboo supplemented with high-fiber primate biscuits.

Insectivores, Edentates, and Aardvarks

Most shrews, hedgehogs, tenrecs, and moles can be fed frozen cat food supplemented with mealworms, earthworms, crickets, and mouse pups. Ground meat fortified with minerals and vitamins, canned dog food, cooked egg, and small amounts of fruits and vegetables also are readily accepted by many species. Bacterial hazards have been associated with the feeding of raw, horsemeat-based diets to some species. Carnivorous and insectivorous small mammals appear particularly susceptible, and septicemia and deaths have been reported from *Streptococcus zooepidemicus* cultured from horsemeat. Canned, meat-based products are a safer alternative.

Armadillos will eat frozen feline diet, moistened dry cat food, canned dog food, or ground meat fortified with minerals and vitamins. Milk, chopped egg, cooked sweet potato, diced banana, and other fruits also are consumed. Vitamin K supplementation of armadillos has been recommended to help prevent hemorrhages: 5 mg of menadione sodium bisulfite/kg dry diet should be adequate. Two-toed sloths will eat a variety of diced vegetables and fruits (eg, lettuce, kale, spinach, celery, green beans, carrot, cooked sweet potato, banana, apple) in combination with frozen feline diet, moistened dry dog food, canned primate diet, and/or monkey biscuits. Food pans should be placed such that the animal can hang from a perch while feeding.

In captivity, aardvarks, lesser anteaters, and giant anteaters readily accept semiliquid diets in place of termites, ants, and other natural foods. Artificial diets typically consist of milk, water, ground meat, and/or a meat-based product such as frozen feline diet, mink chow or dry dog food, hard-boiled egg, protein powder, baby cereal, and a mineral-vitamin supplement. All ingredients are mixed in a blender to the consistency of a thick gruel. Adult giant anteaters may develop loose feces when fed a semiliquid diet. In this case, milk and water can be withdrawn gradually from the formula. As a precaution, vitamin K often is added to all edentate diets.

Marine Mammals

See also MARINE MAMMALS, p 1529.

Fish are the primary food of captive marine mammals except for the herbivorous sirenians. The purchase and subsequent proper storage and handling of high-quality fish are the most important aspects of feeding cetaceans and pinnipeds. On receipt, fish should always be inspected for quality; the following are useful for evaluation: 1) the boxes should be checked to see if catch dates are indicated; 2) overall appearance of the fish should be good; 3) gills should be red (light pink gills indicate considerable time may have elapsed before the fish were frozen after being caught); 4) eyes should not be sunken, indicating dehydration; 5) flesh of thawed fish should be firm, skin should be intact and not discolored, and there should not be a bad odor; 6) there should not be excess water and blood pooled in the bottom of frozen cases, which indicates the fish have thawed and been refrozen; and 7) ideally, the lenses of frozen fish should be cloudy, which indicates the fish have been properly stored at or below -30°C before purchase (higher temperatures often result in clear lenses). To minimize peroxidative damage and nutrient destruction, fish should be stored at or below -30°C. Most fish species should not be stored >6 mo if at all possible. A maximum of 3-4 mo is recommended for fatty fish such as mackerel; lean fish such as smelt may remain in good condition for up to 9 mo. Ideally, fish should be thawed overnight under refrigeration. If this is not possible, thawing at room temperature is preferable to thawing in water, which can cause significant nutrient leaching. Individually quick frozen fish are preferred by many zoos because proper quantities can be thawed without waste.

As a general rule, marine mammals should be given marine fish. Composition of marine fishes can vary greatly between species and even within species depending on age, season, and catch location. Fish that have been used successfully include Atlantic and Pacific herring; Atlantic, Pacific, and Spanish mackerel; bluerunner; capelin; and anadromous smelt. Squid are readily consumed by many pinnipeds, and clams can be included in walrus diets. No commercial substitute for fish has been developed that will be accepted by cetaceans, but such products have been used with some success for pinnipeds. The regular diet of any marine mammal should consist of ≥2 fish species to help ensure a balanced diet.

Thiamine should be added (at 25 mg/kg fish, as fed daily) to any marine mammal feeding program because of the possibility of thiamine destruction by thiaminases that are found in several fish species. Supplemental vitamin E helps compensate for oxidative destruction of natural vitamin E in fish during storage and helps protect against the deleterious effects of peroxides formed in stored fish. Oily fish such as mackerel, which are high in unsaturated fatty acids, are particularly susceptible to vitamin E destruction and peroxidative damage. Vitamin E at 100 IU/kg fish, as fed per day, is generally recommended whenever fish are fed.

Salt (NaCl) supplementation of pinnipeds maintained in freshwater is recommended to prevent hyponatremia; 3 g salt/kg fish is adequate. Although supplemental vitamin C is frequently given to captive cetaceans, there is no conclusive evidence it is beneficial. Evidence indicates hepatic vitamin A levels in captive dolphins are often much lower than in their wild counterparts. Although specific recommendations cannot be made, vitamin A supplementation of some captive cetacean diets may be desirable.

Food intake in marine mammals varies considerably, depending on fat content of fish, water temperature, and activity. Performing Atlantic bottlenose dolphins generally eat 7-10 kg fish/day. Adult seals and sea lions consume ~5-8% of their body wt in fish/day. Captive sirenians can be maintained on a diet of lettuce, cabbage, alfalfa, and aquatic plants (eg, water hyacinth).

Marsupials

Most didelphid marsupials can be fed dry or canned dog or cat food. Smaller species can be fed canned primate diet. Hard-boiled egg, green vegetables, carrot, sweet potato, apple, and banana also can be offered. Dasyurids (eg, marsupial "mice," native cats, Tasmanian devil) and bandicoots can be fed canned or frozen feline diet. In addition, crickets, mealworms, and mouse pups can be given to smaller species; larger species can be given mice and shank or rib bones. Wombats and the larger macropod marsupials can be fed a combination of large herbivore pellets and rabbit pellets. Rat kangaroos will eat a combination of mouse pellets and rabbit pellets. In addition, green vegetables, carrot, sweet potato, apple, and banana can be offered to all herbivorous and omnivorous marsupials. Because of potential problems with lumpy jaw, feeding hay to macropods is generally discouraged unless high-quality, leafy hay that is free of weeds, awns, and coarse stems is available. Currently, captive koalas can be fed successfully only on leaves of certain species of eucalyptus.

Primates

Most primates can be fed a diet based on commercial monkey biscuits or canned primate or marmoset diet (TABLE 27). Moderate amounts of assorted green vegetables,

TABLE 27. Nutrient Requirements of Nonhuman Primates[*]

Nutrient	Concentration
Crude protein[†]	15-22%
Essential Ω-3 fatty acids	0.5%
Essential Ω-6 fatty acids	2%
Neutral detergent fiber[‡]	10-30%
Acid detergent fiber[‡]	5-15%
Calcium	0.8%
Total phosphorus[§]	0.6%
Nonphytate phosphorus	0.4%
Magnesium	0.08%
Potassium	0.4%
Sodium	0.2%
Chloride	0.2%
Iron[¶]	100 mg/kg

(continued)

TABLE 27. Nutrient Requirements of Nonhuman Primates* (continued)

Nutrient	Concentration
Copper	20 mg/kg
Manganese	20 mg/kg
Zinc	100 mg/kg
Iodine	0.35 mg/kg
Selenium	0.3 mg/kg
Trivalent chromium	0.2 mg/kg
Vitamin A	8,000 IU/kg
Vitamin D₃#	2,500 IU/kg
Vitamin E**	100 mg/kg
Vitamin K††	0.5 mg/kg
Thiamine	3.0 mg/kg
Riboflavin	4.0 mg/kg
Pantothenic acid	12.0 mg/kg
Available niacin‡‡	25.0 mg/kg
Vitamin B₆	4.0 mg/kg
Biotin	0.2 mg/kg
Folacin	4.0 mg/kg
Vitamin B₁₂	0.03 mg/kg
Vitamin C§§	200 mg/kg
Choline	750 mg/kg

*Based on primate research; nutrient requirements of other herbivorous, omnivorous, and carnivorous mammals published in the USA National Research Council nutrient requirement series; and composition of successful research and commercial primate diets. These nutrient concentrations have not been directly tested as a group with any primate and may not be appropriate for all species or all postweaning physiologic stages.

†Lactation and growth of young, particularly of smaller primates, can be more satisfactory when the higher protein concentrations are used. Required concentrations are greatly affected by protein quality (amounts and proportions of essential amino acids). Taurine appears to be a dietary essential for some primate species through the first postnatal year.

‡Although not nutrients, neutral detergent fiber and acid detergent fiber have been positively related to GI health.

§Much of the phytate phosphorus found in soybean meal and some cereals appears to be of limited bioavailability.

¶Because some primates appear to be susceptible to iron-storage disease, particularly in the absence of iron-binding polyphenols found in some plants and when large quantities of fruits are offered, it might be desirable to limit dietary iron concentrations to near or slightly below this concentration.

#There are anecdotal reports of higher vitamin D₃ requirements in callitrichids under certain circumstances.

**As all-rac-α-tocopherol acetate.

††As phylloquinone.

‡‡Niacin in corn, grain sorghum, wheat, and barley is poorly available, as is niacin in byproducts of these grains unless they have undergone fermentation or wet-milling.

§§Ascorbyl-2-polyphosphate is a source of vitamin C that is biologically active and relatively stable during diet extrusion and storage.

Adapted, with permission, from *Nutrient Requirements of Nonhuman Primates*, 2003, National Academy of Sciences, National Academy Press, Washington, DC.

carrot, sweet potato, apple, banana, and orange also can be offered. Monkey biscuits and the canned products should comprise ≥50% of the dry-matter intake of most species; fruits and treat items should comprise ≤25%. High-protein monkey biscuits (25% crude protein) should be fed to New World primates to ensure that their higher protein requirements are met. Regular or high-protein monkey biscuits can be fed to Old World species depending on other components in the diet, although many larger Old World species such as gibbons, orangutans, chimpanzees, and gorillas readily accept higher fiber products. The laboratory primate biscuits are typically formulated with very low fiber levels (eg, 5%). Because many of the natural foods consumed by these species appear to contain very high fiber levels (eg, >20%), increasing the dietary fiber intakes of larger primate species is widely practiced. High-fiber biscuits should comprise at least 50% of the dietary dry matter, with leafy and green vegetables making up at least 40% of the dietary dry matter.

Cultivated fruits should be used sparingly for great apes and leaf-eating species because, compared with cultivated green vegetables, they are typically high in sugars and simple carbohydrates and low in protein and calcium. Monkey biscuits can be made more palatable for some species by soaking them in water or fruit juice. To prevent leaching of nutrients, the biscuits should be placed in a thin film of liquid so that the liquid is drawn up into the biscuit.

Other items commonly included in primate diets include hard-boiled egg, yogurt, and bread. Grapes, raisins, peanuts, crickets, and mealworms are treat items well liked by most species. Mouse pups are favored items for many smaller primates. However, callitrichid hepatitis in tamarins and marmosets has been associated with the feeding of newborn mice infected with lymphocytic choriomeningitis virus. Most zoos have discontinued the feeding of mouse pups to these New World primates. Sunflower seeds, instant rice, cracked corn, and shredded coconut can be scattered around exhibit or holding areas to promote foraging activity. Hay should be provided for nesting materials and diversion and to act as a foraging substrate. Many zoos offer meat to their great apes; although meat is often relished by the animals, there is no evidence it is necessary if the diet is properly balanced. Because hypercholesterolemia is seen in many captive gorillas, the feeding of meat may be contraindicated. For most primates, meals should be offered at least twice daily. Smaller species may benefit from even more frequent feedings.

New World primates use vitamin D_2 poorly. It is particularly important that these species receive an adequate source of stabilized vitamin D_3 (cholecalciferol) in their diet if they are not exposed daily to direct sunlight. Marmosets require up to 4 times the amount of vitamin D_3 required by other New World primates. Because of potential vitamin D toxicity, commercial marmoset diets should be fed only to marmosets. Several cases of rickets in some Old World species at weaning have been reported. This may be due to replacement of barred, outdoor primate exhibits with more naturalistic, but indoor, exhibits. While most free-ranging primate species probably satisfy their requirement for vitamin D by exposure to ultraviolet B (UVB) from sunlight, captive animals may rely entirely on a dietary source. Infants at weaning appear particularly at risk because milk levels of vitamin D are probably quite low, and many foods the young begin to eat are not fortified with this vitamin. Exposing the infant or juvenile to natural sunlight may be the best solution, because assuring that a dietary supplement is consumed by a young primate may not be possible. Skylight materials that permit the transmission of UVB are available for installation in zoo habitats, but aging skylights may block adequate UVB transmission. Lights that emit energy in the UVB range are not practical for use with primates.

All primates require a source of vitamin C. Because vitamin C (except for a recently available, more stable form) added to commercial monkey biscuits can begin undergoing significant destruction within 6 mo of milling, a supplementary source should be included in the diet (eg, green vegetables, oranges, multiple vitamins, fruit juice, or fruit-juice powders with added vitamin C).

Members of the subfamily Colobinae are perhaps the greatest challenge in the proper feeding of captive primates. Pregastric fermentation, similar to that in ruminants, occurs in the complex stomach of these species. In the wild, leaves make up a major part of the diet of most colobines (the more frugivorous red colobus is an exception). Therefore, natural diets are usually moderately high in fiber, and animals spend much time foraging.

Offering a rich, rapidly consumable diet of monkey biscuits and fruit in captivity presents a situation quite different from that typically found in the wild and may be partly to blame for the frequent GI problems reported in these species. Also, some evidence suggests that a high percentage of colobus monkeys may be sensitive to gluten. A commercial, gluten-free, high-fiber monkey biscuit (25% neutral detergent fiber) has been developed for feeding captive colobines. A diet consisting of 50% high-fiber biscuit, 40% green vegetables and fresh browse, and 10% fruit is recommended for most colobines. Alfalfa pellets or good-quality alfalfa hay can be provided free-choice. If a suitable high-fiber biscuit is not available, fresh browse and/or high-fiber green vegetables such as kale, mustard greens, broccoli, celery, spinach, green beans, lettuce, and escarole should comprise ≥50% of the diet, with regular monkey biscuits and canned primate diet comprising ~25% of the dietary dry matter. If a gluten-sensitive enteropathy is suspected, any product that contains wheat, barley, rye, or oats should be removed from the diet. Dietary changes always should be made gradually in colobines to allow their stomach microflora time to adapt.

Rodents and Lagomorphs

Most rodent and lagomorph species do well on diets based on commercial laboratory rodent pellets or rabbit pellets. Rabbits, hares, pikas, marmots, and prairie dogs can be maintained on rabbit pellets, alfalfa or grass hay, and assorted vegetables. Most other sciurids can be fed rat pellets and a mixture of sunflower seeds, millet, corn, and rolled oats. Ground squirrels can also be offered green leafy vegetables, carrot, and apple. Most murids, cricetids, gophers, dormice, and jerboas do well on rat pellets; for smaller species, mouse pellets, a seed and grain mix, green leafy vegetables, carrot, and apple can be fed. Hay should be made available to voles and lemmings. Captive voles may be difficult to manage unless a high-fiber rabbit pellet is used. Muskrats, agoutis, and capybaras will eat a combination of rat and rabbit pellets along with alfalfa hay, carrot, and apple. Porcupines can be fed rat pellets, rabbit pellets, and dry dog food in equal portions along with some apple, carrot, and bread; evergreen and willow branches should be made available whenever possible. Beavers will eat a combination of rabbit pellets, large herbivore pellets, and dry dog food, regularly augmented with willow, poplar, aspen, or alder branches. Guinea pigs can be offered commercial guinea-pig pellets along with greens and carrot. Although guinea pigs and cavies are the only rodents known to require a dietary source of vitamin C, lagomorphs and rodents may benefit from it.

Subungulates and Ungulates

Hay comprises the bulk of the diet for most ungulates in captivity and should be available for most of the day rather than fed at intervals as meals. As a general rule, a leafy legume hay, eg, alfalfa, should be used for those species that are primarily browsers (eg, Giraffidae, Cervidae, sitatunga, bongo, duiker, tapir), whereas a good-quality grass hay is satisfactory for most grazers or bulk feeders (eg, zebra, elephant, bison, buffalo, wildebeest, camel). Legume hays are higher in nitrogen and calcium and, if of good quality, are more digestible than grass hays. Hay should be leafy and green, free of mold, dirt, excess weeds, and other foreign matter, and should not be overmature. Hay analysis can be very useful for evaluating quality and designing proper feeding programs.

In addition to hay, a pelleted diet that contains protein, minerals, and vitamins in concentrations adequate to meet the needs of domestic species and those wild species for which data are available (eg, white-tailed deer) should be offered. In the frequent situation in which animals are fed as a group rather than as individuals, it is preferable to use a pelleted diet that is not excessively high in digestible energy (~3 kcal DE/g dry matter is suggested) and that contains sufficient fiber to support proper rumen or colon function. This precaution reduces the possibility of untoward effects (eg, rumen acidosis, colic, obesity) caused by the overconsumption of concentrates. Some zoos prefer to use 2 pelleted diets: one high in fiber for grazers or bulk feeders, and one lower in fiber for browsers. Other zoos prefer to use one pelleted diet for all grazing and browsing species. In the latter case, the type of hay fed along with the pellet, and the percentage of pelleted diet offered, are used to adjust for differences between grazing and browsing species. See TABLE 26 for a pelleted diet. A $^3/_{16}$ in. pellet size is satisfactory for most artiodactyls, whereas a $^1/_2$ in. (~13 mm) pellet or cube size helps minimize waste when fed to larger perissodactyls and subungulates. Commercial equine products are not recommended for zoo herbivores because they often contain high levels of copper and lower than needed levels of vitamin E. Likewise, commercial cattle products should not be fed to zoo herbivores because vitamin E levels are very low and some products may contain nonprotein nitrogen sources (eg, urea) that are not tolerated by hindgut-fermenting species (eg, equids). Commercial omnivore biscuits are readily consumed by tapirs and can be used in combination with commercial hog pellets for peccaries.

As a general rule, most large ungulates (>250 kg) consume 1.5-2% of their weight in dry matter daily. Smaller species (<250 kg) generally consume 2-4%. Offering a pelleted diet at 25-50% of the dry-matter intake is adequate for most species if good-quality hay is fed. As hay quality declines, or for more delicate species, the percentage of pellets should be increased. Hay should be fed from a rack rather than off the ground for most species (elephants are an exception). Hay racks should be located at eye level for tall browsers such as giraffes and gerenuks. Pellets can be offered from a covered trough or rubber feed pans. Regularly feeding the pelleted diet in an animal's holding area can facilitate close observation and easy capture. At least 2 widely separated feeding stations may be necessary to reduce conflict and ensure that subordinate animals obtain their share of food.

Water should always be freely available. Also, in addition to hay and pelleted diet, assorted fruits and vegetables often are fed to exotic ungulates. For most species, these items usually are not necessary except as an occasional treat. The exception might be those species that regularly feed on fruits and succulents in the wild. It may be advisable to include some fruits and vegetables (~0.5 kg/100 kg body wt) in the diet of species such as okapi, duikers, dik diks, bongo, and tapirs. Fresh or frozen browse is consumed avidly by most captive ungulates and subungulates and can be offered to relieve boredom. Recent evidence also indicates that browse may improve rumen function.

REPTILES

See also REPTILES, p 1597.

Appropriate husbandry of reptiles is as important as is providing adequate nutrients. Photoperiod, temperature, humidity, substrate, and cage "furniture" can affect feeding behavior and, thus, nutrient intakes. Temperature and humidity gradients within a reptile enclosure allow the animal to select warm, dry spots or cooler, moist areas. Competition for preferred sites and for food pans in an enclosure with multiple animals should also be assessed. Sufficient numbers of warm spots, ultraviolet exposure spots, and food pans should be available for all animals within an enclosure. Visual barriers may be useful in reducing competition for preferred sites or food dishes.

Prey such as rabbits, rats, or mice should be offered dead to prevent injury to the reptile. Although it is rare, prey have been known to attack predators and can inflict bites. Offering dead prey can also reduce the chance of injury to the predator caused by striking the walls of the enclosure. However, some reptiles may initially need the stimulation of live prey, particularly if they are not adapted to captivity. The possibility of disease or parasite transmission from prey to predator should be considered. Vertebrate prey should also be fed nutritionally complete diets appropriate for the species (eg, mouse diet, rabbit diet, rat diet, etc). The nutrient content of the prey depends on what it is fed (eg, mice that are raised on a diet deficient in vitamin A have decreased liver storage of this essential nutrient). Additionally, if frozen mice or rats are routinely used for feeding carnivorous reptiles, freezer storage conditions should be optimal (eg, ≤6 mo and in thick, plastic bags to retard deterioration). Methods of thawing that minimize water loss are also important. Because many carnivorous reptiles rely on their prey not only as sources of nutrients, but also as sources of water, the state of hydration of the prey can be very important.

Familiarity with a species' food habits in the wild is essential if appropriate foods and nutrient levels are to be offered. Common practice has been to offer ≥2 different prey species because differences in nutrient content exist among vertebrate and invertebrate prey. Reduced dependence on a single food or prey species is desirable because some prey items may be periodically difficult to obtain. Dependence on a single prey item frequently is seen in snakes and may be unavoidable.

Increasing numbers of commercial diets for reptiles have appeared on the market in recent years. Many products for carnivorous, herbivorous, and omnivorous reptiles are now available in the USA in frozen, freeze-dried, canned, extruded, and pelleted forms. Acceptability may be better when the commercial diets are offered to young reptiles. Appropriately formulated, manufactured diets for reptiles are a potentially simpler and more economical alternative to feeding fresh produce or live prey. However, some of these diets may not be formulated rationally, and frequently little information concerning micronutrient concentrations is provided from the manufacturers. When selecting a commercial product, the purchaser should contact the manufacturer to obtain information about product formulation and specific nutrient concentrations. Unfortunately, little controlled research has been conducted on nutrient requirements of reptiles, and claims of product superiority may not have a scientific justification. *See* TABLE 28 for recommended nutrient concentrations for reptiles.

Ulcerative Stomatitis: Vitamin C synthesis has been reported in many reptile species. It has been suggested that ulcerative stomatitis seen in snakes and lizards may be associated with a vitamin C deficiency, although there is no supportive evidence. In controlled studies with garter snakes (*Thamnophis* sp) fed supplemental vitamin C,

TABLE 28. Recommended Nutrient Concentrations for Reptiles*

Nutrient	Concentration[†]	
	Carnivorous Reptiles	Omnivorous Reptiles
Crude protein[‡]	30-50%	20-25%
Arginine	1.0%	1.8%
Isoleucine	0.5%	1.3%
Lysine	0.8%	1.5%
Methionine	0.4%	0.4%
Methionine + cysteine	0.75%	0.75%
Threonine	0.7%	1.0%
Tryptophan	0.15%	0.3%
Linoleic acid[§]	1.0%	1.0%
Calcium	0.8-1.1%	1.0-1.5%
Phosphorus	0.5-0.9%	0.6-0.9%
Potassium	0.4-0.6%	0.4-0.6%
Sodium	0.2%	0.2%
Magnesium	0.04%	0.2%
Manganese	5 ppm	150 ppm
Zinc	50 ppm	130 ppm
Iron	60-80 ppm	200 ppm
Copper	5-8 ppm	15 ppm
Iodine	0.3-0.6 ppm	0.4 ppm
Selenium	0.3 ppm	0.3 ppm
Riboflavin	2-4 ppm	8 ppm
Pantothenic acid	10 ppm	60 ppm
Niacin	10-40 ppm	100 ppm
Vitamin B_{12}	0.020 ppm	0.025 ppm

TABLE 28. *(continued)*

Nutrient	Concentration[†]	
	Carnivorous Reptiles	**Omnivorous Reptiles**
Choline	1,250-2,400 ppm	3,500 ppm
Biotin	70-100 ppb	400 ppb
Folacin	200-800 ppb	6,000 ppb
Thiamine[¶]	1-5 ppm	5 ppm
Pyridoxine	1-4 ppm	10 ppm
Vitamin A[#]	5,000-10,000 IU/kg	15,000 IU/kg
Cholecalciferol (vitamin D_3)[**]	500-1,000 IU/kg	500-1,000 IU/kg
Vitamin E[††]	150 IU/kg	150 IU/kg

[*]Nutrient levels expressed on a dry-matter basis.

[†]Nutrient concentrations are recommended minimums for carnivorous reptiles and averages for herbivorous reptiles.

[‡]Taurine requirements have not been determined for reptiles (the requirement for cats is 400-500 mg taurine/kg dry diet).

[§]A dietary source of arachidonic acid at 200 mg/kg dry diet may be necessary.

[¶] Thiamine concentrations should be increased to 10-20 mg/kg if frozen, thawed fish constitute >25% of the diet offered.

[#]A source of preformed vitamin A may be required because it is not known if reptiles can convert carotenes to retinol (vitamin A), although it is likely that herbivorous reptiles can.

[**]Requirements for vitamin D may be partially or totally satisfied by exposure to sunlight or appropriate sources of artificial ultraviolet light. These suggested concentrations are not sufficient to prevent signs of vitamin D deficiency in green iguanas.

[††]300 IU/kg dry matter is advisable if the diet is high in fat, especially unsaturated fat.

tissue levels and body stores remained stable, while synthesis by the snakes was reduced.

Gout: Although most reptiles excrete nitrogen primarily as uric acid, aquatic reptiles typically excrete excess nitrogen as urea or ammonia. The relative proportions of various nitrogenous wastes may depend on the amount and composition of feed, frequency of feeding, and state of hydration. The excessive precipitation of urate crystals in joints, kidneys, or other organs (gout) can be a common condition in some species of captive reptiles. The etiology of gout is not clear, but it is commonly thought that diets high in protein may predispose reptiles to gout. Impaired renal function and dehydration have also been suggested as possible causes. If poor-quality protein is fed (unbalanced amino acids) or when tissue is catabolized for energy, uric acid excretion increases. While gout in some reptiles is associated with increased circulating levels, postprandial, transient increases in circulating uric acid may be seen in some species and confound the diagnosis. Assuring an adequate state of hydration in a susceptible animal may help prevent uric acid precipitation in joints and organs. Feeding diets low in protein to carnivorous reptiles is unwise because they are adapted to feeding on high-protein prey.

Vitamin D and Ultraviolet Light: Most vertebrates can either absorb vitamin D from the diet or synthesize it in the skin from 7-dehydrocholesterol using energy from ultraviolet (UV) light of certain wavelengths (290-315 nm) in a temperature-dependent reaction. Thus, vitamin D is required in the diet only when endogenous synthesis is inadequate, as develops when animals are not exposed to UV light of appropriate wavelengths. Many captive basking species appear susceptible to rickets or osteomalacia. Bone fractures, soft-tissue mineralization, renal complications, and tetany can develop. Reptiles frequently show few premonitory signs, although lethargy, inappetence, and reluctance to move are commonly reported. Serum calcium concentrations may not be diagnostically useful. Supplementation with injectable calcium and vitamin D may provide some short-term relief. However, exposure to UV light, or lack of it, may be an important, yet often overlooked, factor in the differential diagnosis. Complicating the diagnosis may be soft-tissue mineralization, seen radiographically or at necropsy.

In green iguanas, metastatic calcification may not result from vitamin D toxicity. Iguanas with both fractured bones and extremely low or undetectable levels of circulating 25-hydroxycholecalciferol also had calcified soft tissues. The etiology of the metastatic calcification is not understood and is contrary to conventional understanding of the signs of vitamin D deficiency and toxicity in domestic species. Dietary sources of vitamin D may not be sufficient to prevent rickets and osteomalacia. Diets with as much as 3,000 IU vitamin D_3/kg did not prevent bone fractures and cortical thinning in green iguanas. Weak UV bulbs placed over the lizards at ~12-18 in. for 12 hr/day appeared to reverse the signs in the least severely affected lizards. Because some lizards seek a warm spot to increase body temperature, placement of the warming bulb, usually incandescent, adjacent to a UV bulb helps ensure adequate exposure to UV light. Exposure to unfiltered natural sunlight during warmer months and use of UV bulbs during the rest of the year usually eliminates the risk of bone disease caused by insufficient absorption of calcium (due to a vitamin D deficiency).

Some lizard species may be unable to absorb sufficient dietary vitamin D_3, although the reason is poorly understood. New World primates are believed to have exceptionally high dietary requirements for vitamin D, which may be related to lower numbers of vitamin D cellular receptors than are present in Old World primates. Similar metabolic differences may exist in some basking lizard species, although this has not been established. UV bulbs are sold in pet stores, but label claims may not be reliable. Enlisting the assistance of a specialist is advised because there is no ideal UV bulb (*see also* p 1590).

Crocodilians

Captive alligators and crocodiles are usually fed a combination of rodents, poultry, fish, and meat-based diets. A varied diet is recommended. Diets consisting primarily of fish should include ≥3 different species of fish and should be supplemented with 25-30 mg of thiamine and 100 IU vitamin E/kg of fish, as fed. Signs of vitamin E deficiency (eg, steatitis) have been reported in crocodilians fed fish inadequately supplemented with vitamin E. Although previously reported otherwise, alligators can digest some carbohydrate; however, the total carbohydrate in the diet should not exceed 20%. Commercial, dry alligator diets are being marketed, largely to reduce the cost and to improve nutrient intakes of farmed alligators; their use is still uncommon in zoos.

Snakes

Snakes feed almost exclusively on vertebrate or invertebrate prey. A few species are specialized egg feeders. Most boids, pythons, vipers, colubrids, crotalids, and elapids are fed mouse pups, mice, chicks, hamsters, rats, guinea pigs, chickens, ducks, and rabbits. Frozen, thawed prey are usually used in zoos. Prey should not be fed cold, although thawing under refrigeration is recommended. After thawing, prey should be fed at room temperature, or preferably warmer. Some species (eg, king cobra, hognose snake, garter snake) feed primarily on other poikilotherms in the wild. Some of these species can be switched, at least in part, to homeothermic prey, which is often more available and less expensive.

The scent of preferred foods can be rubbed on the new item. Alternatively, the preferred foods can be inserted into, or attached to, the new food. Anoles, yellow rat snakes, frogs, and smelt, depending on natural feeding habits, can be fed when homeotherms are not accepted. Prey size is usually proportional to snake size and should not be much larger in diameter than the snake's head. Snakes that are routinely handled can be fed in a separate tank to reduce biting. To reduce the chance of regurgitation, snakes should not be handled for 3 days after feeding. Most species should be fed every 1-2 wk. Some large, less active snakes may typically go 6 wk between feedings. Force-feeding should be used only if necessary. Animals can be force-fed whole prey lubricated with egg white by gently inserting the food a few inches down the throat using forceps. Tube feeding is also possible using ground (homogenized) prey.

Turtles

Many freshwater turtles in the wild eat primarily animal matter but also consume some plant material. Some species may be carnivorous when young and shift to omnivorous or herbivorous feeding patterns as adults. Most aquatic turtles cannot be considered strict carnivores because they occasionally consume at least some plant material. Commercially available turtle feeds are available from many manufacturers, although nutrient content can vary widely. These products are usually manufactured as extruded or pelleted diets and are typically 30-50% protein. Such diets may be appropriate for carnivorous and omnivorous turtles, although the more omnivorous species would benefit from the addition of some fruits or vegetables.

A sample diet for carnivorous and omnivorous turtles consists of the following feed items: water (272 g), gelatin (unsweetened or dry, 34 g), corn oil (11 g), spinach (23 g), cooked sweet potato (23 g), Vionate® (a vitamin/mineral supplement, 5 g), trout pellets (50 g), vitamin E at 50 IU/g (1 g). This diet contains on a dry-matter basis: 47% protein, 14% fat, 1.5% calcium, 0.55% phosphorus, vitamin A at 10,000 IU/kg, vitamin D_3 at 1,000 IU/kg, vitamin E at 279 IU/kg, and vitamin C at 280 mg/kg.

Tortoises

Tortoises are herbivorous and, like herbivorous lizards (see below), must consume plant material to maintain healthy gut physiology. Microbial fermentation of plant fiber can be a significant source of nutrients for tortoises. While small tortoises consuming pelleted diets can use plant fiber effectively, they should be fed more frequently than larger animals. Small and large tortoises can be maintained on appropriately formulated, extruded, pelleted, or coarsely ground tortoise diets. Larger tortoises, such as Aldabra or Galapagos tortoises, can consume alfalfa hay along with a complete pelleted food formulated for tortoises or for exotic herbivores. A vegetable mix consisting of broccoli, green beans, leafy greens (such as romaine or green leaf lettuce) kale, and shredded carrots may be also fed as a supplement to a formulated tortoise diet. Tortoises consuming vegetable mixtures do not need additional vitamin or mineral supplementation if the vegetable mix contains the items listed above, which supply adequate protein, calcium, and micronutrients. Cultivated fruits are typically poorer sources of protein, calcium, and micronutrients. Some herpetologists offer oyster shell and pea gravel to tortoises because "mining" activity has been seen in free-ranging animals. Shell deformities in tortoises have been thought to result from rapid growth associated with the consumption of high-protein diets. However, scientific evidence to support this claim is lacking. Diets of tortoises in the wild often contain >15% protein (dry-matter basis) in plant materials consumed because natural vegetative materials are usually high in protein in the pre-seed stage.

Lizards

The feeding patterns of lizards are extremely diverse. Lizards may be insectivorous (eg, day and leopard gecko, whiptail lizard, anole, chameleon), carnivorous (eg, varanids such as monitor lizard, Gila monster, Mexican beaded lizard), omnivorous (eg, many iguanid and agamid species), or herbivorous (eg, iguanid species, prehensile-tailed skink). Insectivorous lizards in captivity are usually fed diets of mealworm larvae or crickets. Because calcium concentrations in these, and most insects, are extremely low (0.03-0.3% calcium with 0.8-0.9% phosphorus), the inverse calcium:phosphorus ratio must be corrected before the insects are fed to lizards. A diet containing 8% calcium as calcium carbonate can be fed to crickets or mealworm larvae 2-3 days before the insect is fed to the lizard. However, this diet should not be used to maintain a cricket colony. Within 2 days of feeding the high-calcium diet, the gut of the insect is filled with calcium, raising the calcium concentration of the insect to ~0.8-0.9% and resulting in a calcium:phosphorus ratio of

~1.2:1. A satisfactory high-calcium diet for crickets can be inexpensively made by using 29% wheat middlings, 10% corn meal, 40% ground dry cat or dog food, and 21% ground oyster shell or calcium carbonate (*see also* BATS, p 1853, for mealworm diet). Larger insectivorous lizards may also consume mouse pups and earthworms. Carnivorous lizards may be offered mouse or rat pups, adult mice and rats, chickens, and eggs. The size of prey should be appropriate for the lizard species. Omnivorous lizards are usually fed a combination of foods including insects, vertebrate prey, and a chopped vegetable mixture (*see* TORTOISES, above, for vegetable mix). Most lizards should be fed daily (juveniles and small species) or at least every other day. Large carnivorous species should be fed 1-2 times/wk.

Herbivorous lizards are adapted to ferment plant fiber in enlarged hindguts. The microbes in the cecum and colon digest plant fiber that the lizard could not otherwise use. As with tortoises, herbivorous lizards should be fed plant-based diets to assure healthy gut function. The use of insects, vertebrate prey, or diets high in fruits is not advised because these feeds are low in fiber and are inappropriate for herbivores. Diets for lizards may be commercial preparations formulated for herbivorous reptiles, or vegetable mixes (*see* TORTOISES, above).

NUTRITION: GOATS

Although goats and sheep have several similarities, their nutrient requirements differ in several ways. Goats exhibit significant differences from sheep in grazing habits, physical activities, feed selection, milk composition, carcass composition, and metabolic disorders. Goats browse more than sheep, while sheep tend to be true grazers. Still, many of the principles useful for sheep feeding and nutrition are applicable for goats. The basic assessment for nutritional well-being should be body condition or body fat covering. Goats in good flesh, or with normal fat stores, are usually being fed a diet with adequate energy and to a lesser extent, protein. (*See also* NUTRITION: SHEEP, p 1902.)

NUTRITIONAL REQUIREMENTS

Water: Goats should be provided unlimited access to fresh, clean water. Goats are among the most efficient of domestic animals in their use of water, approaching the camel in their low rate of water turnover per unit of body weight. Goats appear to be less subject to high temperature stress than other species of domestic livestock. In addition to a lesser need for body water evaporation for maintaining comfort in hot climates, they can conserve body losses of water by decreasing losses in urine and feces. Factors affecting water intake in goats include lactation, environmental temperature, water content of forage consumed, amount of exercise, and salt and mineral content of the diet.

Energy: Energy limitations may result from inadequate feed intake or from low quality of the diet; too high water content of the feed also may become a limiting factor. Energy requirements are affected by age, body size, growth, pregnancy, and lactation. Energy requirements also may be affected by the environment, hair growth, activity, and relationship with other nutrients in the diet. Increased temperature, humidity, sunshine, and wind velocity may decrease energy requirements. Shearing mohair from Angora goats and pashima from Cashmere goats decreases insulation and results in increased energy needs (at least in colder environments).

Good quality roughage furnishes ~2 Mcal metabolizable energy (ME) per kg dry matter. Roughage-concentrate mixtures that provide 2.5-3.0 Mcal ME/kg dry matter sometimes are necessary when feeding early weaned kids or high-producing dairy goats. Energy requirements for **maintenance** of goats have been derived from pooled means of experimental data reported in terms of kcal ME/kg body wt$^{0.75}$ (the mean value of which is 101.38 kcal). In addition to the maintenance requirement, requirements for activity, pregnancy, growth, lactation, and fiber production must be considered (TABLE 29).

Goats exhibit a wide range of grazing activity, ranging from light activity for goats under intensive management, through moderate activity on semiarid land, to great activity for goats grazing on sparsely vegetated grassland and on mountainous pastures that necessitate long-distance travel daily.

The best assessment of energy intake adequacy in the goat is proper body condition or fat covering the loin, brisket, inner thigh, and ribs. If animals are parasite- and disease-free, yet underconditioned, then they are usually being fed an energy-deficient diet; the reverse is true for obese animals. The energy values required for growth and lactation are very comparable to the numbers used for sheep and cattle, respectively. Therefore, sheep nutrition principles from an energy standpoint will probably suffice when dealing with all classes of goats, except for lactating dairy goats.

Protein: Protein is required for most normal functions of the body, including maintenance, growth, reproduction, lactation, and hair production. Protein deficiencies in the diet deplete stores in the blood, liver, and muscles and predispose animals to a variety of serious and even fatal ailments. Food intake and dietary digestibility are reduced if dietary crude protein is <6%, further compounding an energy-protein deficiency.

The protein requirement for maintenance, based on an average of published data, is ~4.15 g protein (TP)/kg body $wt^{0.75}$, with an average digestibility of ~68%. Information regarding requirements for growth are quite sparse; however, a mean of 0.284 g TP/g gain has been suggested. A value of 6.97 g TP/kg body $wt^{0.75}$ has been recommended for pregnancy. Protein requirements for lactation are presented on the basis of 96.90 g TP/kg of 4.5% butterfat milk. Data on protein requirements for different activities and also fiber production are too sparse to make definite recommendations.

Minerals: Requirements for minerals have not been established definitively for goats at either maintenance or production levels. Research has been conducted with goats in mineral metabolism studies, especially with calcium and phosphorus. In general, these data support assumptions that several mineral requirements for goats are similar to those for sheep. (*See* TABLE 29 and TABLE 40.) The addition of specific minerals (phosphorus for dry winter forages, selenium in deficient areas, etc) to salt (NaCl), preferably in granular form and offered free choice, helps prevent most mineral deficiencies and improves performance.

Meeting **calcium** requirements is seldom a problem under grazing conditions with either Angora or meat-type goats, but it should be checked in high-producing dairy goats because a deficiency can lead to reduced milk production. Adequate levels of calcium for lactating goats are necessary to prevent parturient paresis (milk fever). In browsing or grain-fed goats, the addition of a calcium supplement (dicalcium phosphate, limestone, etc) to the feed or to a salt or trace mineral-salt mixture usually meets calcium requirements. Legumes (eg, clover, alfalfa, kudzu) are also good sources of calcium.

Phosphorus deficiency results in slowed growth, unthrifty appearance, and occasionally a depraved appetite. Goats can maintain milk production on phosphorus-deficient diets for several weeks by using phosphorus from body reserves, but during long periods of phosphorus deficiency, milk production was shown to decline by 60%. The calcium:phosphorus ratio should be maintained between 1:1 and 2:1, preferably 1.2-1.5:1 in goats due to their predisposition for urinary calculi. Phosphorus deficiency in grazing goats is more likely than a calcium deficiency. In cases of struvite calculi, the ratio should be maintained at 2:1.

Magnesium deficiency is associated with hypomagnesemic tetany (grass tetany), but ordinarily this condition is less common in grazing goats than it is in cattle. Goats do have marginal ability to compensate for low magnesium by decreasing the amount of magnesium they excrete. Both urinary excretion and milk production are reduced in a magnesium deficiency.

TABLE 29. Daily Nutrient Requirements of Goats ▶

Body Weight		Feed Energy TDN		ME	Crude Protein
(kg)	(lb)	(g)	(lb)	(Mcal)	(g)
Maintenance at low activity, including early pregnancy					
10	22	199	0.44	0.71	27
30	66	452	1.00	1.62	62
50	110	662	1.46	2.38	91
70	154	852	1.88	3.07	118
90	198	1030	2.27	3.70	153
Maintenance at medium activity, slightly hilly pasture, and including early pregnancy					
10	22	239	0.53	0.86	33
30	66	543	1.20	1.95	74
50	110	795	1.75	2.86	110
70	154	1023	2.25	3.68	141
90	198	1236	2.72	4.44	170
Maintenance at high activity, mountainous pasture, and including early pregnancy					
10	22	278	0.61	1.00	38
30	66	634	1.40	2.28	87
50	110	928	2.04	3.34	102
70	154	1194	2.63	4.29	165
90	198	1442	3.18	5.18	198
Additional requirements for late pregnancy, all goat sizes					
		397	0.87	1.42	82
Additional requirements for growth at 50 g/day, all goat sizes					
		100	0.22	0.36	14
Additional requirements for growth at 150 g/day, all goat sizes					
		300	0.66	1.08	42
Additional requirements for milk production, per kg, at different fat percentages					
(% fat)					
3.0		337	0.74	1.21	64
4.5		351	0.77	1.26	77
6.0		365	0.80	1.31	90
Additional requirements for mohair production by Angora goats at different production levels					
Annual fleece yield (kg)					
4		34		0.12	17
8		66		0.24	34

◀ **TABLE 29.** *(continued)*

Ca (g)	P (g)	Vitamin A (1,000 IU)	Dry Matter/Animal			
			1 kg = 2.0 Mcal ME		1 kg = 2.4 Mcal ME	
			(kg)	(lb)	(kg)	(lb)
Maintenance at low activity, including early pregnancy						
1	0.7	0.5	0.36	0.79	0.30	0.66
2	1.4	1.2	0.81	1.78	0.67	1.47
4	2.8	1.8	1.19	2.62	0.99	2.18
5	3.5	2.3	1.54	3.39	1.28	2.82
6	4.2	2.8	1.85	4.07	1.54	3.39
Maintenance at medium activity, slightly hilly pasture, and including early pregnancy						
1	0.7	0.6	0.43	0.95	0.36	0.79
3	2.1	1.5	0.98	2.16	0.81	1.78
4	2.8	2.1	1.43	3.15	1.19	2.52
6	4.2	2.8	1.84	4.04	1.53	3.37
7	4.9	3.3	2.22	4.88	1.85	4.07
Maintenance at high activity, mountainous pasture, and including early pregnancy						
2	1.4	0.8	0.50	1.10	0.42	0.92
3	2.1	1.7	1.14	2.50	0.95	2.09
5	3.5	2.5	1.67	3.67	1.39	3.06
6	4.2	3.2	2.14	4.71	1.79	3.94
8	5.6	3.9	2.59	5.70	2.16	4.75
Additional requirements for late pregnancy, all goat sizes						
2	1.4	1.1	0.71	1.56	0.59	1.30
Additional requirements for growth at 50 g/day, all goat sizes						
1	0.7	0.3	0.18	0.40	0.15	0.33
Additional requirements for growth at 150 g/day, all goat sizes						
2	1.4	0.8	0.54	1.19	0.45	0.99
Additional requirements for milk production, per kg, at different fat percentages						
2	1.4	3.8				
3	2.1	3.8				
3	2.1	3.8				
Additional requirements for mohair production by Angora goats at different production levels						

Salt (NaCl) is usually recognized as a necessary dietary component but is often forgotten. Goats may consume more salt than is required when it is offered ad lib; this does not present a nutritional problem but may depress feed and water intakes in some arid areas where salt content of the drinking water is quite high. Salt formulations are used as carriers for trace minerals, as goats have a clear drive for sodium intake.

Potassium has an important role in metabolism. However, forages generally are quite rich in potassium, so a deficiency in grazing goats would be extremely rare. Marginal potassium intake is seen only in heavily lactating does fed diets composed predominately of cereal grains.

Iron deficiency is seldom seen in mature grazing goats. Such deficiency might be seen in young kids because of their minimal stores at birth, plus the low iron content of the dam's milk. This is more commonly seen in kids fed in complete confinement. Iron deficiency can be prevented by access to pasture or a good quality trace mineral salt containing iron. In severe cases, and for kids reared in confinement, iron dextran injections at 2- to 3-wk intervals (150 mg, IM) for the first few months may be curative.

Iodine deficiency in the soil, and in the crops produced thereon, is seen in some areas of the USA. Therefore, iodine should be provided in stabilized salt. Conditional iodine deficiency may develop with normal to marginal iodine intake in goats consuming goitrogenous plants. Marked deficiency of iodine results in an enlarged thyroid; poor growth; small, weak kids at birth; and poor reproductive ability.

Zinc deficiency results in parakeratosis, stiffness of joints, smaller testicles, and lowered libido. A minimal level of 10 ppm of zinc in the diet, or a trace mineral salt mixture of 0.5-2% zinc prevents deficiencies. Excessive dietary calcium (alfalfa) may increase the likelihood of zinc deficiency in goats.

Vitamins: Suggestions as to the vitamin requirements of goats are even more sparse than for mineral requirements. At best, almost all vitamin recommendations for goats must be based on those for sheep (p 1902).

HERBAGE AND BROWSE UTILIZATION

(For sample rations for kids and goats, *see* TABLE 30).

In contrast to other farm animals, except the llama, goats prefer shrubs and tree leaves, whether deciduous or evergreen. Because of this preference, goats have been used to control encroaching shrub-type growth in pastures. Goats consume approximately the same weight of forage as do sheep of similar size. Browse (leaves and twigs of trees and shrubs) generally contain higher levels of crude protein and phosphorus during their growing season than do grasses. However, some palatable browse species are limited in value because of one or more inhibitors that may bind or otherwise prevent use of nutrients contained in the plants. One such inhibitor is lignification of woody twigs and tree leaves, which physically binds (or encapsulates) the desirable nutrients. Certain oils (terpene-based compounds) are present in relatively high concentrations in some range shrubs and apparently inhibit growth of rumen bacteria. High concentrations of tannins are present in certain browse plants and depress digestion of feedstuffs by binding enzymes or by inhibiting enzymatic activity. Excessive tannins may also increase sulfur requirements, which may be more critical for hair-producing goats. However, in spite of these potential problems, when given the opportunity to choose, goats appear to be able to select more digestible and beneficial browse.

NUTRITIONAL DISEASES

Enterotoxemia is a feed-related malady that causes almost sudden death due to a toxin produced by *Clostridium perfringens* type D and sometimes type C. The organism appears to be widespread in nature. Under conditions of high carbohydrate consumption or high intake of immature succulent forage, the causative bacteria multiply rapidly and produce an ε toxin that increases intestinal permeability. (*See also* p 493.) Some cases of enterotoxemia are seen in goats, usually those fed diets with high concentrations of carbohydrates. Diarrhea, depression, lack of coordination, digestive upsets, coma, and death

TABLE 30. Example Rations for Goats*

For a 30-kg (66-lb) goat in a nonproductive state, minimal activity, maintenance only:
Chickpea straw 630 g (1.4 lb)
Alfalfa, fresh, 95 g (0.20 lb)

For a 50-kg (110-lb) goat in a nonproductive state, minimal activity, maintenance only:
Wheat straw 716 g (1.6 lb)
Alexandrian clover, fresh, 333 g (0.73 lb)

For a 20-kg (44-lb) kid gaining 50 g/day, minimal activity:
Alfalfa hay, full bloom, 80 g (0.18 lb)
Corn grain 360 g (0.79 lb)

For a 30-kg (66-lb) kid gaining 150 g/day (0.33 lb):
Chickpea straw 500 g (1.10 lb)
Corn grain 400 g (0.88 lb)
Linseed meal 65 g

For a 40-kg (88-lb) doe in late gestation with minimal activity:
Johnsongrass hay 960 g (2.11 lb)
Sorghum grain 350 g (0.77 lb)

For a 70-kg (154-lb) doe producing 5 kg (11 lb) of milk testing 3.5% butterfat:
Corn silage (dough stage) 1,000 g (2.2 lb)
Alfalfa hay, full bloom, 500 g (1.10 lb)
Corn grain 1,365 g (3.00 lb)
Soybean meal 280 g (0.62 lb)

*Dry-matter basis

may be seen after excessive carbohydrate feeding of both baby kids and mature goats. The best method to prevent enterotoxemia in stable-fed goats is frequent, small volume feeding of milk, grain, and forage. Large meals fed once a day should be avoided. Acute indigestion and a rumen pH of <4.8 indicates lactic acidosis, which can lead to the secondary complication of enterotoxemia.

In **polioencephalomalacia**, clinical signs include disorientation, dullness, aimless wandering, loss of appetite, circling, progressive cortical blindness, extensor spasms, and occasionally head pressing. Some animals become recumbent and may eventually die without treatment. Diets that produce a low rumen pH or that are high in grain and low in forages predispose ruminants to polioencephalomalacia. Such dietary conditions can result in depressed production of thiamine, the production of thiamine antimetabolites, or the production of thiaminases in the rumen. Affected animals can usually be treated successfully with thiamine (200-500 mg, IV, IM, or SC). Although response is dramatic and almost immediate, if significant brain damage has occurred, animals rarely return to a satisfactory level of production. Therefore, prompt treatment is critical. The diet should be modified to reduce grain and increase forage intake. During times of stress, or when predisposing diets are unavoidable, the inclusion of thiamine mononitrate in the diet may aid in prevention. (*See also* p 1061.)

Pregnancy disease is seen in late pregnancy, much more commonly in dams carrying multiple fetuses. Clinical features include abnormally increased blood levels of ketone bodies with concurrent hypoglycemia. Affected animals exhibit many of the signs described for enterotoxemia (*see* above). During late gestation, the developing fetuses have high demands for glucose; in an attempt to meet the glucose needs, the dam begins to metabolize adipose tissue (fat). The ability of the liver to metabolize this extra fat load is compromised, with a subsequent increase in the release of ketone bodies into the bloodstream. Signs include depression, dullness, opisthotonos, and eventually death. In early stages of the disease, when signs first appear, a drench of 200-300 mL of propylene glycol or glycerol can be used as an energy source for the dam to prevent so much body fat from being metabolized. However, the administration of glucose (5% dextrose or 50-120 mL of 23% calcium borogluconate solution into a liter of 5% dextrose IV) is the treatment of choice. Prevention should be aimed at maintaining a proper body condition score, identifying females with twins and triplets and feeding accordingly, reducing the incidence of chronic disease, shearing ewes in late gestation, and including niacin (1 g/day in the diet during late gestation) in the diet. (*See also* p 828.)

Urinary calculi result from mineral deposits in the urinary tract. Difficult and painful urination is evidenced by straining, slow urination, stomping of the feet, and kicking at the area of the penis. Blockage of the flow of urine generally is seen only in intact or castrated males. The blockage may rupture the urinary bladder, resulting in a condition known as waterbelly, and cause death. It is common when diets with high concentrations of cereal grains are fed (feedlot lambs, pet goats, etc). Affected animals excrete an alkaline urine that has a high phosphorus content. The incidence of urinary struvite calculi can be reduced by lowering phosphorus consumption to minimal levels and maintaining a calcium:phosphorus ratio >2:1. The use of anionic salts such as ammonium chloride (0.5% of the complete diet), dietary tetracycline, adequate vitamin A (or β-carotene) intake, and increased dietary intake of NaCl have proved beneficial. Affected animals drenched with ammonium chloride (7-14 g/day for 3-5 days) may show a good response. In range sheep and goats, the disease is associated with the consumption of forages having a high silica content. (*See also* p 1259.)

White muscle disease seems to develop less frequently in goats than in sheep. This condition is caused by low levels of selenium and possibly vitamin E. Signs include stiffness (especially in the hindquarters), tucked-up rear flanks, arched backs, pneumonia, and acute death. On necropsy, white striations are found in cardiac, diaphragmatic, and skeletal muscles. Levels of AST and lactic dehydrogenase are increased, indicating muscle damage. Blood levels of the selenium-containing glutathione peroxidase are reduced. (*See also* p 897.)

NUTRITION: HORSES

Horses are kept for a much longer time than most farm animals and have more varied uses as athletes, breeding animals, and pets. Feeding programs, therefore, must sustain a long, productive, and athletic life. The feeding recommendations given below are based on both practical experience and scientific research.

NUTRITIONAL REQUIREMENTS

Although horses can use hay and other roughage much more efficiently than do other nonruminants such as poultry or pigs, this ability is limited by the anatomy of the equine GI tract and is less efficient than that of ruminants. The site of fermentation in horses is the cecum and large intestine, where large numbers of microorganisms digest hemicellulose and cellulose, utilize protein and nonprotein nitrogen, and synthesize certain vitamins. Some of the products of fermentation, such as volatile fatty acids and vitamins, are absorbed and used. Microbial protein synthesized from nitrogen entering the cecum and colon undergoes only limited proteolysis, and the supply of essential amino acids from an unbalanced dietary nitrogen source is not satisfactorily balanced by microbial amino acids for optimal growth. Horses, therefore, depend more on the quality of the protein in the ration than do ruminants.

Water: Water requirements depend largely on environment, amount of work or physical activity being performed, nature of the feed, and physiologic status of the horse. The minimal daily water requirement of an adult horse is 33 mL/kg body wt/day (0.4 gal./100 lb/day) with average intakes of ~50 mL/kg body wt/day (0.65 gal./100 lb/day). Lactation or sweat losses, however, may increase the needs by 50-200%. Unlimited free access to clean water is usually recommended, although horses can easily adapt to only periodic access throughout the day if the amounts offered during the watering sessions are not limited.

Energy: Energy requirements may be classified into those needed for maintenance, growth, pregnancy, lactation, and work. Equations to estimate energy requirements at any state of performance or production have been derived primarily from studies of light horses (TABLE 31 and TABLE 32). However, the need for energy differs considerably among individuals; some horses require much greater amounts of feed than others under similar conditions, and digestibility of feeds often differs greatly from published values. Therefore the caloric recommendations these formulas provide should be considered only a starting point to determine the actual energy needs of a given horse.

Amounts fed should be adjusted to maintain a body condition score between 4 and 6 (*see* TABLE 33). Emaciated and very thin horses have decreased stress tolerance and increased susceptibility to infections. Obese horses have decreased tolerance of exercise and heat, increased risk of laminitis and lipoma strangulation colic, and, if fasted, hyperlipidemia and hypertriglyceridemia. Obesity is also associated with insulin resistance and glucose intolerance.

For **maintenance** of body weight and to support normal activity, the daily digestible energy (DE) requirement (in Mcal) of the nonworking adult horse in good body condition weighing <600 kg (1,320 lb) is estimated to be $1.4 + (0.03 \times BW)$, in which BW is the body weight in kg. The daily DE Mcal requirement for horses weighing >600 kg (1,320 lb) or draft and warmblood types of horses is estimated to be $1.82 + (0.0383 \times BW) - (0.000015 \times BW^2)$. For obese or emaciated horses, the estimated ideal body weight in kg should be used in the equation rather than current body weight.

Cold weather increases the energy requirement by 0.00082 Mcal DE/kg BW for each degree Celsius drop below the lower critical temperature (LCT) of the animal. However, the LCT of cold-adapted adult horses in Canada was estimated to be -15°C, whereas donkeys acclimatized to summer temperatures in Nevada had an LCT of 26°C. Wind, precipitation, and body condition also affect LCT. Therefore, LCT must be estimated based on regional average temperatures and conditions and perhaps type of horse. For example, draft breeds with thick hair coats would tolerate lower temperatures than a thin-haired, thin-skinned Thoroughbred.

For **growth**, the daily DE requirement of light horse breeds is estimated to be (maintenance DE Mcal/day) $+ (4.81 + 1.17X - 0.023X^2) \times ADG$, using the above equation(s) for the maintenance DE, and X as the age in months and ADG as the desired average daily gain in kg. For foals <6 mo old in ambient temperatures <10°C, the equation $1.1 \times (1.4 + 0.047 \times BW)$, in which BW is the body weight in kg, should be used instead of the one(s) listed above to calculate the maintenance DE requirement. Draft or draft-cross breeds may require less.

During **pregnancy**, if the mare is not exercised or exposed to extreme weather conditions, maintenance DE intakes are usually adequate until the last 90 days of gestation. Energy requirements during months 9, 10, and 11 of gestation are estimated by multiplying estimated maintenance requirements by 1.11, 1.13, and 1.20, respectively. Voluntary intake of roughage decreases as the fetus gets larger, and it may be necessary to increase the energy density of the ration by using supplemental concentrates in late pregnancy.

To support **lactation**, the National Research Council (NRC) has estimated that 792 kcal of DE/kg of milk produced per day (TABLE 34) should be added to maintenance needs. However, this recommended level of energy intake has increased body weight gain in lactating ponies, indicating that it may exceed the needs of some breeds.

The energy requirements of **work** are influenced by many factors, including type of work, condition and training of the horse, fatigue, environmental temperature, and skill of the rider or driver. As the duration of exercise increases and level of activity is maintained, the DE requirement per unit of time worked actually decreases. For these reasons, DE recommendations for various activities of light horses (TABLE 35) should be adjusted to meet individual needs and to maintain desirable body condition.

Protein and Amino Acids: Although some amino acid synthesis occurs in the cecum and large intestine, it is not sufficient to meet the amino acid needs of growing, working, or lactating horses; therefore, the protein quality of the feed is important. Weanlings require 2.1 g, and yearlings 1.9 g, of lysine/Mcal DE/day. Requirements for other dietary amino acids have not been established; however, the crude protein recommendations given

TABLE 31. Daily Nutrient Requirements of Growing Horses and Ponies ▶

Age (mo)	Body Weight kg (lb)	Fraction of Adult Weight	Daily Gain kg (lb)	Daily Feed* kg (lb)
Daily Nutrients Per Animal				
Adult weight 200 kg (440 lb) (Ponies)				
3	60 (132)	0.30	0.40 (0.88)	2.10 (4.6)
6	95 (209)	0.48	0.30 (0.66)	2.60 (5.7)
12	140 (309)	0.70	0.20 (0.44)	3.50 (7.7)
18	170 (375)	0.85	0.10 (0.22)	3.80 (8.4)
24	185 (408)	0.92	0.05 (0.11)	3.90 (8.6)
Adult weight 400 kg (880 lb) (Small horses)				
3	125 (276)	0.31	0.85 (1.87)	4.40 (9.7)
6	180 (397)	0.45	0.65 (1.43)	4.90 (10.9)
12	265 (584)	0.66	0.40 (0.88)	6.60 (14.6)
18	330 (728)	0.82	0.25 (0.55)	7.40 (16.4)
24	365 (805)	0.91	0.15 (0.33)	7.80 (17.1)
Adult weight 500 kg (1,100 lb) (Average horses)				
3	155 (342)	0.31	0.90 (1.98)	5.43 (12.0)
6	215 (474)	0.43	0.80 (1.76)	5.91 (13.0)
12	325 (716)	0.65	0.55 (1.21)	8.13 (17.9)
18	400 (882)	0.80	0.35 (0.77)	9.00 (19.8)
24	450 (992)	0.90	0.20 (0.44)	9.56 (21.1)
Adult weight 600 kg (1,320 lb) (Large horses)				
3	170 (375)	0.28	1.00 (2.2)	5.95 (13.1)
6	245 (540)	0.41	0.85 (1.87)	6.74 (14.9)
12	375 (827)	0.63	0.70 (1.54)	9.38 (20.2)
18	475 (1,042)	0.79	0.45 (0.99)	10.69 (23.6)
24	540 (1,190)	0.90	0.30 (0.66)	11.48 (25.3)

*90% dry matter. Assumes good-quality forage with or without additional concentrates. Maximal daily intake is estimated to be 2.5-3.0% body wt in dry matter.

in TABLE 31, and TABLE 32, should be adequate if good quality forages and concentrates are used in the ration.

Growing horses have a higher need for protein (14-16% of total ration) than mature horses (8-10% of total ration). Aged horses (>20 yr old) may require levels of protein equivalent to young, growing horses to maintain body condition; however, hepatic and renal function should be assessed before increasing the protein intake of old horses. Fetal growth during the last third of pregnancy increases protein requirements somewhat (10-11% of total ration), and lactation increases requirements still further (12-14% of total ration). Work apparently does not significantly increase the protein requirement, provided that the ratio of crude protein to DE in the diet remains constant and the increased energy requirements are met.

Minerals: Because the skeleton is of such fundamental importance to performance of the horse, macromineral requirements deserve careful attention (TABLE 31 and TABLE 32). Excessive intakes of certain minerals may be as harmful as deficiencies; therefore, mineral

TABLE 31. *(continued)*

Daily Nutrients Per Animal				
Digestible Energy (Mcal)	Crude Protein (g)	Ca (g)	P (g)	Vitamin A[†] (IU)
Adult weight 200 kg (440 lb)				
6.44	404	22	12	2,700
7.55	488	22	11	4,300
8.71	392	12	7	6,300
8.34	375	10	6	7,700
7.93	337	9	5	8,300
Adult weight 400 kg (880 lb)				
12.05	562	29	16	5,600
13.95	698	28	16	8,300
15.56	700	23	13	11,900
15.90	716	21	12	14,900
15.30	608	18	10	16,400
Adult weight 500 kg (1,100 lb)				
13.35	668	35	19	7,000
16.65	883	34	21	10,400
19.70	887	31	19	14,600
19.85	893	27	17	18,000
18.83	759	23	15	20,300
Adult weight 600 kg (1,320 lb)				
14.61	711	37	21	7,700
18.10	905	37	21	11,900
23.53	989	34	19	17,300
23.94	995	30	17	21,400
23.49	915	28	15	24,300

[†]One mg of β-carotene equals 400 IU of vitamin A for the horse.

Adapted, with permission, from *Nutrient Requirements of Horses*, 1989, National Academy of Sciences, National Academy Press, Washington, DC.

supplements should complement the composition of the basic ration. For example, if the horse is consuming mostly roughage with little grain, phosphorus is more likely to be in short supply than calcium. However, if little roughage and large amounts of grain are being consumed, a deficit of calcium is more common. The total mineral contribution and availability from all parts of the ration (forages and roughages, concentrates and all supplements) should be considered when evaluating the mineral intake. However, aside from actual feeding trials, no suitable test for availability of minerals exists.

Requirements for **calcium** and **phosphorus** are much greater during growth than for maintenance of mature animals. The last third of pregnancy and lactation also appreciably increase the requirement. Aged horses (>20 yr old) may require more phosphorus than is required for adult maintenance (0.3-0.4% of total ration). Excess calcium intake (>1.0% of total ration) should be avoided in aged horses, especially if renal function is reduced.

TABLE 32. Daily Nutrient Requirements of Mature Horses and Ponies

Body Weight kg (lb)	Daily Feed* kg (lb)	Digestible Energy (Mcal)	Crude Protein (g)	Ca (g)	P (g)	Vitamin A† (IU)	Daily Milk Production (kg)
Maintenance							
200 (441)	3.5 (7.7)	7.40	296	8	6	6,000	—
400 (882)	7.0 (15.4)	13.40	536	16	11	12,000	—
500 (1,102)	8.7 (19.3)	16.40	656	20	14	15,000	—
600 (1,323)	10.5 (23.1)	19.40	776	24	17	18,000	—
Last 90 Days of Gestation							
200 (441)	3.5 (7.7)	8.58	378	16	12	12,000	—
400 (882)	7.0 (15.4)	15.54	684	30	22	24,000	—
500 (1,102)	8.7 (19.3)	19.02	837	36	27	30,000	—
600 (1,323)	10.5 (23.1)	22.50	990	43	32	36,000	—
Lactating Mares, First 3 Mo							
200 (441)	5.0 (11.0)	13.74	688	27	18	12,000	8
400 (882)	10.0 (22.0)	22.90	1,141	45	29	24,000	12
500 (1,102)	12.5 (27.6)	28.28	1,427	56	36	30,000	15
600 (1,323)	15.0 (33.1)	33.66	1,711	67	43	36,000	18
Lactating Mares, 3 Mo to Weaning							
200 (441)	4.5 (9.9)	12.15	528	18	11	12,000	6
400 (881)	9.0 (19.8)	19.74	839	29	18	24,000	8
500 (1,102)	11.25 (24.8)	24.32	1,048	36	22	30,000	10
600 (1,323)	13.50 (29.8)	28.90	1,258	43	27	36,000	12

*90% dry matter. Assumes good-quality forage with or without additional concentrates. Maximal daily intake is estimated to be 2.5-3.0% body wt in dry matter.

†One mg of β-carotene equals 400 IU of vitamin A for the horse.

Adapted, with permission, from *Nutrient Requirements of Horses*, 1989, National Academy of Sciences, National Academy Press, Washington, DC.

For all horses, the calcium:phosphorus ratio, should be maintained at >1:1. A desirable ratio is ~1.5:1, although if adequate phosphorus is fed, foals tolerate a ratio of 3:1 and young adult horses a ratio of 6:1. Work does not appreciably increase calcium or phosphorus requirements as a portion of diet.

Salt (NaCl) requirements are markedly influenced by sweat losses. It is recommended that horse rations contain 0.5-1.0% salt, although there are limited data on the precise requirements. Sweat losses may cause NaCl losses >30 g (1 oz) in only 1-2 hr of hard work. However, NaCl is the only mineral for which horses are known to have true "nutritional wisdom." Horses voluntarily seek out and consume salt in amounts to meet their daily needs if given the opportunity. Salt blocks should be available free choice at all times. Supplemental salt may be provided by oral dosing or added to feed or water in addition to free-choice salt to replace acute losses during hard work. Some horses, usually those confined to stalls, ingest excessive amounts of salt, possibly due to restricted feed intake and/or boredom. However, salt poisoning is unlikely unless a deprived animal is suddenly allowed free access to salt, or if water is not available to horses force-fed salt (electrolyte mixtures dosed PO). Excessive salt content of feed or water will limit

TABLE 33. Body Condition Scores for Horses

Score		Description
1	Emaciated	Spinous processes, ribs, tailhead, tuber coxae, and ischii prominent. Bone structure of neck, withers, and shoulders easily visible. No fat palpable over lumbar vertebral transverse processes.
2	Very thin	Slight fat covering spinous processes and tailhead. Transverse processes slightly rounded. Ribs, tailhead, and tuber coxae and ischii prominent. Bone structure of neck, withers, and shoulders faintly discernible.
3	Thin	Fat buildup halfway on spinous process and tailhead; both prominent, but individual vertebrae in tailhead not visible. Transverse processes cannot be felt. Slight fat buildup over ribs and tuber coxae but easily visible. Tuber ischii not discernible. Withers, neck, and shoulder accentuated, but bone structure not visible.
4	Lean	Slight ridge visible over loin, faint outline of ribs visible. Tailhead prominence depends on conformation, but fat palpable around it. Tuber coxae not visible. Withers, shoulder, and neck not obviously thin.
5	Moderate	Loin is flat (no crease or ridge) Ribs not visible but easily felt. Fat around tailhead is spongy, withers rounded over spinous process, and shoulders and neck blend smoothly into body.
6	Moderately fleshy	May have slight crease down loin, ribs barely palpable with light pressure, and fat around tailhead soft. Some fat palpable on side of withers, neck, and behind shoulder.
7	Fleshy	May have crease down loin, and ribs difficult to feel. Fat deposited along withers, behind shoulder, and along neck.
8	Fat	Crease down loin. Ribs very difficult to feel; fat around tailhead very soft. Fat filling area over withers and behind shoulder with noticeable thickening of neck.
9	Obese	Obvious crease down loin. Patchy fat deposits over ribs. Fat bulging around tailhead, along withers, behind shoulders, and along neck. Flank filled with fat (no abdominal tuck).

TABLE 34. Average Milk Production of Mares

	Average Daily Milk Production (kg)		
Months After Foaling	Draft Horse	Light Horse	Shetland Pony
0-1	15.4	13.9	10.3
1-2	16.8	14.7	11.8
2-3	18.2	16.9	12.5
3-4	17.0	15.1	9.5
4-5	14.7	10.9	9.1

voluntary intakes, precluding toxicity but putting the horse at risk of dehydration or energy deficits.

The most satisfactory method of providing supplemental calcium, phosphorus, and salt is to furnish a mixture of one-third trace mineral or plain salt and two-thirds dicalcium

TABLE 35. Energy Requirements of Work for Light Horses[*] **and Desirable Body Condition Scores**

Activity	DE (Mcal/day)	Body Condition Score
Idle (maintenance)	$1.1 + (0.3 \times$ body wt [in kg])	4-6
Halter competition, pleasure trail riding	$1.25 \times$ DE for maintenance	5-6
Performance show (park, English, and Western pleasure, youth activity), equestrian instruction	$1.50 \times$ DE for maintenance	5-6
Ranch work, show cutting and roping, barrel racing, endurance trail ride, 3-day event (hunt course, stadium jumping, dressage)	$1.75 \times$ DE for maintenance	4-5
Polo, race training, and competitive racing	$2.00 \times$ DE for maintenance	4-5

[*]200-600 kg body wt

phosphate free choice. Trace mineral salt blocks do not contain additional calcium or phosphorus.

The daily **magnesium** requirement for maintenance has been estimated at 6.8 mg/lb (15 mg/kg) body wt based on limited equine studies. Working horses require 10-25% more magnesium for light to moderate exercise, respectively, due to sweat losses. The requirements for growth have not been well established but are estimated to be 0.07% of the total ration. Most feeds used for horses contain 0.1-0.3% magnesium. Though deficiencies are unlikely, hypomagnesemic tetany has been reported in lactating mares and stressed horses. Adding 5% magnesium oxide to the free-choice salt mixture has been reported to be protective in such cases. The upper limit of recommended intake is estimated to be 0.3% based on data from other species, but adult horses have been fed rations with higher magnesium content without apparent adverse affects.

Potassium requirements of foals fed a purified ration were determined to be 1% of the total ration. The requirement for sedentary adult horses is estimated to be 0.4% of the ration. Because most roughages contain >1.0% potassium, a ration containing ≥50% roughage provides sufficient potassium for maintenance animals. Working horses and horses receiving diuretics need more potassium due to sweat and urinary losses. Potassium may be supplemented by adding potassium salts such as KCl to the ration. Although upper safe limits have not been established, and excesses are usually efficiently excreted by the kidneys, acute hyperkalemia can induce potentially fatal cardiac arrhythmias. Therefore, excessive supplementation with potassium salts should be avoided.

The requirement for **sulfur** in horses is not established. However, sulfur-containing amino acids (methionine) and vitamins (biotin) are essential for healthy hoof growth. If the protein requirement is met, the sulfur intake of horses is usually ~0.15% dry-matter intake—a level that is apparently adequate for most individuals.

Most iodized salts fulfill the dietary **iodine** requirement (estimated to be 0.6 ppm). Iodine toxicity has been noted in pregnant mares consuming as little as 40 mg of iodine/day. Goiter due to excess iodine was noted in both mares and their foals, and several cases were associated with large amounts of dried seaweed (kelp) in the diet.

The dietary requirement for **cobalt** is apparently <0.05 ppm. It is incorporated into vitamin B_{12} by the microorganisms in the cecum and colon and, therefore, is an essential nutrient per se only if exogenous sources of B_{12} are not incorporated into the ration.

The dietary **copper** requirement for horses is probably 8-10 ppm, though many commercial concentrates formulated for horses contain >20 ppm. The presence of 1-3 ppm of molybdenum in forages, which would interfere with copper utilization in ruminants, does not cause problems in horses. Copper deficiency may cause osteochondritis dissecans in young, growing horses and is associated with a higher risk of aortic or uterine artery rupture in adults. Copper deficits may also cause hypochromic microcytic anemia and pigmentation loss. Horses are extremely tolerant of copper intakes that would be fatal to sheep. However, high copper intakes potentially reduce the absorption and utilization of selenium.

The dietary maintenance requirement for **iron** is estimated to be 40 ppm. For rapidly growing foals and pregnant and lactating mares, the requirement is estimated to be 50 ppm. Virtually all commercial concentrates formulated for horses and most forages contain iron well in excess of the recommended concentrations. Only horses suffering chronic blood loss (eg, parasitism) should be considered to be at risk of iron deficiency. Excess iron intake potentially interferes with copper utilization.

Manganese requirements for horses have not been well established; amounts found in the usual forages (40-140 ppm) are considered sufficient.

The **zinc** requirement is estimated to be 40 ppm of the ration. This mineral is relatively innocuous, and intakes several times the requirement are considered safe, although intakes >1,000 ppm have induced copper deficiency and developmental orthopedic disease in young horses.

Rock phosphates, when used as mineral supplements for horses, should contain <0.1% **fluorine**. Fluorine intake should not exceed 50 ppm in the diet or 0.45 mg/lb (1 mg/kg) body wt. Excessive ingestion can result in fluorosis (p 2359).

Although **molybdenum** is an essential cofactor for xanthine oxidase activity, no quantitative requirement for horses has been demonstrated. Excessive levels (>15 ppm) may interfere with copper utilization.

The dietary requirement for **selenium** is probably not >0.2 ppm, but there are regions of the world (including the lower Great Lakes states, the Pacific northwest, the Atlantic Coast, Florida, and part of New Zealand) where soils are deficient. In other areas (including parts of Colorado, Wyoming, and North and South Dakota), forages may contain 5-40 ppm of selenium and produce toxicity (p 2516). Exercise increases glutathione peroxidase (selenium-containing enzyme) activity and may indicate an increased need for supplementation in heavily exercised horses. No more than 0.002 mg/kg body wt should be supplemented on a daily basis; toxicity has been seen with as little as 5 ppm selenium intake.

Vitamins: The **vitamin A** requirement of horses can be met by β-**carotene**, a naturally occurring precursor, or by active forms of the vitamin (eg, retinol). Fresh green forages and good-quality hays are excellent sources of carotene, as are corn and carrots. It is estimated that 1 mg of β-carotene is equivalent to ~400 IU of active vitamin A. However, because of oxidation, the carotene content of forages decreases with storage, and hays that are stored >1 yr may not furnish sufficient vitamin A activity. Horses that have been consuming fresh green forage usually have sufficient stores of active forms of vitamin A in the liver to maintain inadequate plasma levels for 3-6 mo. The NRC has suggested that diets for all horses should provide 30-60 IU vitamin A/kg body wt (13.6-27.2 IU/lb). *See* TABLE 32. Prolonged feeding of excess active vitamin A (>10 times recommended amounts) may cause bone fragility, hyperostosis, epithelial exfoliation, and teratogenesis. The proposed upper safe concentration for chronic administration is 16,000 IU vitamin A/kg of dry ration. There is no known toxicity associated with β-carotene.

Horses that are exposed to ≥4 hr of sunlight per day or that consume sun-cured hay do not have dietary requirements for **vitamin D**. For horses deprived of sunlight, suggested dietary vitamin D concentrations are 365-455 IU/lb (800-1,000 IU/kg) for early growth and 227 IU/lb (500 IU/kg) for later growth and other life stages. Vitamin D toxicity is characterized by general weakness; loss of body weight; calcification of the blood vessels, heart, and other soft tissues; and bone abnormalities. Dietary excesses as small as 10 times the requirement may be toxic and are aggravated by excessive calcium intake.

No minimal requirement for **vitamin E** has been established. Selenium and vitamin E work together to prevent nutritional muscular dystrophy (white muscle disease, p 897).

Evidence of vitamin E deficiency is most likely to appear in foals that are nursing mares on dry winter pasture or given only low-quality hay unsupplemented with commercial concentrates. Horses forced to exert great physical effort and/or fed high-fat (>5%) rations may have increased needs for vitamin E. However, if selenium intakes are adequate, it is likely that 40-60 IU of vitamin E/kg (80-120 IU/lb) of ration is adequate for most stages of the life cycle and moderate activity. Supplementation with 500-1,000 IU vitamin E may, however, be necessary for horses that are working hard and/or are fed high-fat (>7%) rations.

Vitamin K is synthesized by the microorganisms of the cecum and colon in sufficient quantities to meet the normal requirements of horses. However, consumption of moldy sweet clover hay may induce vitamin K-dependent coagulation deficits (*see* p 2523). The synthetic form of vitamin K (menadione) is nephrotoxic if administered parenterally to dehydrated horses.

Mature horses synthesize adequate amounts of **ascorbic acid** for maintenance. Some horses may need supplemental ascorbic acid (5-20 g/day) during periods of stress. Oral availability is variable. Ascorbyl palmitate is reportedly more readily absorbed than ascorbic acid or ascorbyl stearate. Prolonged supplementation to nonstressed horses may reduce endogenous synthesis, resulting in deficiencies if supplementation is abruptly discontinued.

Although **thiamine** is synthesized in the cecum and colon by bacterial action and ~25% of this may be absorbed, thiamine deficiency has been seen in horses fed poor-quality hay and grain. While not necessarily a minimum value, 3 mg thiamine/kg ration dry matter has maintained peak food consumption, normal gains, and normal thiamine levels in skeletal muscle in young horses. As much as 5 mg/kg ration dry matter may be necessary for horses that are exercising strenuously. Occasionally, horses are poisoned by consuming certain plants that contain thiamine or antithiamines (*see* BRACKEN FERN POISONING, p 2349).

Under certain conditions, **riboflavin** may be required in the diet. Although some reports implicated riboflavin deficiency in equine recurrent uveitis (p 407), this has not been substantiated. Apparently, the dietary riboflavin requirement is not likely to be >2 mg/kg ration dry matter.

Intestinal synthesis of **vitamin B_{12}** is probably adequate to meet ordinary needs, provided there is sufficient cobalt in the diet; deficiencies of cobalt in horses have not been reported. Vitamin B_{12} is absorbed from the cecum, and feeding a ration essentially devoid of vitamin B_{12} for 11 mo had no effect on the normal hematology or apparent health of adult horses. Vitamin B_{12} injected parenterally into racehorses and foals is rapidly and nearly completely excreted via bile into the feces.

Niacin is synthesized by the bacterial flora of the cecum and colon and is synthesized in the liver from tryptophan. There is no known dietary requirement for niacin in horses.

Folacin, biotin, pantothenic acid, and vitamin B_6 probably are synthesized in adequate quantities in the normal equine intestine. Biotin supplementation (15-25 mg/day), however, has been documented to improve hoof quality in adult horses with soft, shelly hoofwalls.

FEEDING PRACTICES

Ideally, horses should be given access to hay and/or pasture forages with salt and water ad lib. Horses should not be offered >0.4% of their body weight in concentrates (textured grain, pellets, or extruded feed) in a single feeding. More than this in a single meal reduces digestive efficiency and predisposes to problems such as gastric ulcers and colic. If large amounts of concentrates are being fed, the total amount offered daily should be divided into 2 or more feedings. It has been documented that feeding >50% of the total ration in the form of concentrates increases the risk of colic and laminitis in adult horses. Large meals of concentrates should not be offered <1 hr before strenuous exercise, transport, or other stress, or to exhausted horses with poor gut motility.

Because horses are particularly sensitive to toxins found in spoiled feeds, all grains and roughages offered should be of good quality and free of mold. Grains should be stored at a moisture content of <13%. In humid areas, feeds should contain a mold inhibitor to preclude spoilage. On the other hand, excessively dry, dusty feeds tend to initiate or aggravate respiratory problems.

Feeds

Pasture: Good pasture provides both nutrients and the opportunity to exercise. The pasture should be kept free of weeds if possible by regular mowing or clipping. A legume-grass mixture offers the advantages of good nutrient supply, persistence, and durability. Ideal mixes vary with region, and local recommendations from specialists should be followed. Alsike clover (*Trifolium hybridum*) and kleingrass (*Panicum coloratum*) are hepatotoxic to horses, and Johnson grass (*Sorghum halepense*) and Sudan grass (*S sudanense*) contain cyanogenic glycosides. Buffel (*Cenchrus* spp), panic (*Panicum* spp), pangola (*Digitaria decumbens*), kikuyu (*Pennisetum* spp), and *Setaria* spp grasses all contain potentially harmful concentrations of oxalates. None of these potential forage species should be used for horse pastures.

In sandy areas, horses should be provided with supplemental hay when pasture is short (ie, overgrazed) to prevent sand ingestion and subsequent colic. The hay should be offered in feeders or on a platform to reduce sand ingestion. The use of psyllium products to enhance the elimination of sand from the equine GI tract is expensive and efficacy has not been proved.

Hay: Common types of hay used to feed horses include both grass hays, such as timothy, brome, coastal Bermuda, or orchard, and legumes such as alfalfa or clover. Legume-grass mixtures are generally high-yielding and contain considerably more protein, minerals, and vitamins than do grasses alone. However, they may be more difficult to cure in a humid climate. Moldy hay should not be fed to horses. Coastal Bermuda grass has been associated with an increased risk of impaction colic. Alfalfa may be contaminated with blister beetles and also tends to be more allergenic than grass hays or clover.

Concentrates and Other Supplements: Concentrates include all grains and byproduct feeds high in energy and/or protein. Processing them before feeding is often desirable to improve nutrient availability. However, grains that are cracked or rolled are more susceptible to mold. Horses should be slowly acclimated to ingestion of large amounts of concentrate over 1-2 wk. Due to differences in density, grains should be measured by weight, not volume.

Oats, one of the most traditional grains for horses, may be fed whole, rolled, or crimped, which increases the bulk 20-30% and improves digestibility by ~10%. Newly harvested oats may be dangerous due to development of molds if moisture content is >13%. "Hulled" or "naked" oats are more energy dense than regular oats and should be introduced slowly to reduce the risk of founder or colic.

Barley is a good grain for horses. It is higher in energy than regular oats but lower than corn. It may be fed as the only grain to horses that have a high energy need. It should be rolled or crimped. Palatability, however, is not as high as that of oats or corn.

Corn (maize) is a high-energy feed, useful for horses that are working hard or being fattened. However, the starch in corn is less digestible than that of oats and can more easily bypass small-intestinal digestion, resulting in colic and/or laminitis if fed in large amounts. To maximize digestibility, shelled corn may be cracked or rolled, but the moisture level should be low enough to avoid spoilage during storage. Moldy corn can cause fatal leukoencephalomalacia.

Sorghum grain (milo) and **wheat** should be fed with care. These grains must be cracked or rolled if fed to horses.

Other Supplements: **Wheat bran** and **rice bran** are byproduct supplements that are commonly fed to horses. However, both are very high in phosphorus (>1.2%), and the proper calcium:phosphorus ratio should be maintained when any form of bran is added to the diet. Wheat bran is not laxative, contrary to popular belief, but is extremely palatable to horses and often used as a "mash." Rice bran is a high-fat product that is added to rations of horses that need extra calories. Many rice bran products have added calcium to offset the high phosphorus content.

Beet pulp, a byproduct of the sugar beet industry, is added to horse rations as both a source of calories and fiber. It contains moderate amounts of calcium and protein and can be safely fed on a daily basis in larger amounts than the bran products. Shredded beet pulp should be soaked in water before feeding to horses. Beet pulp pellets do not require presoaking.

Fats may be added to the diet to increase the energy density. Corn and vegetable oils are commonly used. Diets containing 5-10% added fat have been associated with improved performance in some types of exercise. Oils should be introduced slowly to the ration to avoid diarrhea. Though highly digestible, animal fat is not commonly used in horse rations.

Soybean meal is a palatable protein supplement with good amino acid balance for use with grains. It may be fed when pastures or hay are low in protein and are of poor quality or when protein requirements are greatest, such as during early growth or lactation. **Linseed meal** or **cottonseed meal** should not be used as a protein supplement for young foals due to their low lysine content, but they are adequate for adult horses.

Cane molasses is frequently added to grain mixtures (sweet feeds). It is highly palatable, minimizes separation of "fines" and reduces dustiness of concentrate mixtures. It is also high in potassium. The readily fermentable carbohydrates and moisture that cane molasses contains may increase mold growth in hot weather and freeze solid in cold winter weather.

Limestone of a high grade (38% calcium) may be used as a supplemental source of calcium. When both supplemental calcium and phosphorus are needed, dicalcium phosphate, steamed bone meal, or defluorinated rock phosphate is recommended. Dicalcium phosphate is particularly good because the cost per unit of phosphorus is low, the elements are quite available, and there is no danger of anthrax (p 479), as there might be in improperly processed bone meal. Monocalcium-dicalcium phosphate mixtures supply relatively more phosphorus than calcium and are recommended when the need for supplemental phosphorus is greater than that for calcium.

Salt (NaCl) should be provided in a block or in granular form ad lib. It may be desirable to use a trace mineralized salt that contains added iodine, iron, copper, cobalt, manganese, zinc, and selenium. The need for these additional minerals varies with the locality.

Succulent Feeds: These feeds are high in water and tend to be highly palatable. Horses fed good-quality hay and water ad lib have no need for succulent forages. If used, succulent feeds should be introduced gradually when offered for the first time. Carrots and apples are commonly used as treats. A daily allowance of 0.5-1.5 kg (1-3 lb) is common.

Well-preserved, mold-free silage or haylage of good quality affords a highly nutritious succulent forage. However, horses are extremely sensitive to mold in silage, and its use is not recommended, especially in hot, humid climates. Mechanical silo unloaders may blend good and spoiled silage together, and the spoilage may go undetected until signs of toxicity (eg, sudden death) appear. Various types of silages may be used, but corn silage and grass-legume silage are the most common. Silage should not replace more than one-third to one-half of the roughage ration and should be used with extreme caution.

Feeding Rates

Individual differences in the need for energy and nutrients and gross variations in nutrient contents of feedstuffs make it difficult to generalize about the amount of feed to provide. The amounts given in TABLE 36 and TABLE 37 can be used as guidelines, but body condition should be monitored and amounts adjusted accordingly. The maximal dry matter intake in 24 hr is only 3-3.5% of a horse's body wt, and many horses voluntarily consume only 2.5% of their body wt in dry matter in 24 hr.

The need for concentrate supplementation while on pasture depends on pasture quality, but is more important for young horses and lactating mares. If the pasture is of good to excellent quality, no supplementation other than water and salt are needed by most adult horses at maintenance or in light work. It is desirable to creep-feed nursing foals at the rate of 0.5-1.0% body wt with concentrates formulated specifically for growth. Good-quality hay may be needed even when on pasture, especially in winter.

Complete feeds, incorporating both concentrate and roughage, have been developed for horses. These can be textured, pelleted, cubed, or extruded products. They have the advantage of uniform quality, complete control over nutrient intake, suitability for horses with bad teeth, less dustiness (which reduces repiratory problems), and reduced bulk for storage and transport. Disadvantages include an increased risk of choke and increased wood chewing. Wood chewing and boredom can be minimized by feeding long-stem hay with these products. Damage to stables and fences can be reduced by treating wood with foul-tasting substances or by covering or replacing wood with metal in vulnerable areas.

NUTRITIONAL DISEASES

Descriptions of uncomplicated nutrient deficiencies in horses are rare. The nutrients most likely to be deficient are caloric sources, protein, calcium, phosphorus, copper, sodium chloride, and selenium, depending on age and type of horse and geographic area. Signs of deficiency are frequently nonspecific, and diagnosis may be complicated by deficiencies of several nutrients simultaneously. The consequences of increased susceptibility to parasitism and bacterial infections may be superimposed over still other clinical signs. Simple excesses are more common. Nutrients most commonly given in excess of needs, leading to toxicity or induced deficits of other nutrients, are: energy, phosphorus, iron, copper, selenium, and vitamin A.

Energy Deficiency: Many nonspecific changes found in horses with nutritional deficiencies are related to caloric deficiency and can result from inadequate intake, maldigestion, or malabsorption. In partial or complete starvation, most internal organs exhibit some atrophy. The brain is least affected, but the size of the gonads may be strikingly decreased, and estrus may be delayed. The immune system is adversely affected, resulting in increased risk of viral diseases. The young skeleton is extremely sensitive, and growth slows or may completely stop. A decrease in adipose tissue is an early and conspicuous sign and is seen not only in the subcutis but also in the mesentery; around the kidneys, uterus, and testes; and in the retroperitoneum. Low-fat content of the marrow in the long bones is a good indicator of prolonged inanition. The ability to perform work is impaired, and endogenous nitrogen losses increase as muscle proteins are metabolized for energy.

Energy Excess: Overfeeding of high-calorie feeds results in obesity in horses and may contribute to developmental orthopedic disease in growing horses. Obesity increases the risk of laminitis and colic due to strangulation of the small intestine by pedunculated mesenteric lipomas. Obese horses and ponies have decreased insulin sensitivity and reduced heat and exercise tolerance.

Protein Deficiency: A deficiency of dietary protein may represent either an inadequate intake of high-quality protein or the lack of a specific essential amino acid. The effects of deficiency are generally nonspecific, and many of the signs do not differ from the effects of partial or total caloric restriction. In general, the horse will have poor quality hair and hoof growth, weight loss, and inappetence. In addition, there may be decreased formation of Hgb, RBC, and plasma proteins. Milk production is decreased in lactating mares. The following liver enzymes have shown decreased activity: pyruvic oxidase, succinoxidase, succinic acid dehydrogenase, D-amino acid oxidase, DPN-cytochrome C reductase, and uricase. Corneal vascularization and lens degeneration have been noted. Antibody formation is also impaired.

Mineral Deficiencies and Excesses: Nutritional Secondary Hyperparathyroidism (Bighead, Bran disease): Horses of all ages fed grass hay or pasture and supplemented with large amounts of grain-based concentrates or wheat bran are most likely to develop relative or absolute calcium deficiencies leading to nutritional secondary

TABLE 36. Recommended Nutrient Concentrations in Rations for Horses and Ponies* ▶

	Digestible Energy (Mcal/kg)	Crude Protein (%)	Ca (%)	P (%)	Vitamin A[†] (IU/kg)
Mature horses and ponies, maintenance	1.80	7.2	0.21	0.15	1,650
Mares, last 90 days of gestation	2.15	9.5	0.41	0.31	3,280
Lactating mares, first 3 mo	2.35	12.0	0.47	0.30	2,480
Lactating mares, 3 mo to weaning	2.20	10.0	0.33	0.20	2,720
Stallions, breeding season	2.15	8.6	0.26	0.19	2,370
Creep fed	2.80	16.0	0.65	0.35	1,800
Foal (3 mo old)	2.70	14.0	0.65	0.35	1,500
Weanling (6 mo old)	2.60	13.1	0.55	0.30	1,680
Yearling (12 mo old)	2.50	11.3	0.40	0.22	1,950
Long yearling (18 mo old)	2.35	10.4	0.32	0.18	2,050
2-yr-old (light training)	2.40	10.1	0.31	0.17	2,380
Mature working horses					
light work[#]	2.20	8.8	0.27	0.19	2,420
moderate work[**]	2.40	9.4	0.28	0.22	2,140
intense work[††]	2.55	10.3	0.31	0.23	1,760

*90% dry matter
[†]One mg of β-carotene equals 400 IU of vitamin A for the horse.
[‡]Good quality legume-grass hay; DE = digestible energy
[§]Grass hay
[¶]Concentrate containing 3.2 Mcal DE/kg; A or B refers to suitable concentrates (see TABLE 37).

hyperparathyroidism. Excess phosphorus intake (Ca:P ratio <1.0) causes the same clinical signs,. Blood concentrations of calcium do not reflect intake due to homeostatic mechanisms, though blood inorganic phosphorus may be elevated due to mobilization of bone mineral content. Serum alkaline phosphatase activity is usually increased, and clotting time may be prolonged slightly. Young, growing bone is frequently rachitic and brittle. Fractures may be common and heal poorly. Swelling and softening of the facial bones and alternating limb lameness are frequently reported. (*See also* OSTEOMALACIA, p 854.)

Phosphorus Deficiency: This is most likely in horses being fed poor-quality grass hay or pasture without grain. Serum inorganic phosphorus concentrations may be decreased and serum alkaline phosphatase activity increased. Occasionally, serum calcium levels may be increased. An insidious shifting lameness may be seen. Bone changes resemble those described for calcium deficiency. Affected horses may start to consume large quantities of soil or exhibit other manifestations of pica before other clinical signs are apparent.

Salt Deficiency: Horses are most likely to develop signs of salt (NaCl) deficiency when worked hard in hot weather. Sweat and urinary losses are appreciable. Horses deprived of salt tire easily, stop sweating, and exhibit muscle spasms if exercised strenuously. Hemoconcentration and acidosis may be expected. Anorexia and pica may be evident in chronic deprivation, although these are not specific signs of salt deficiency. In

◀ **TABLE 36.** (*continued*)

Example Diet Proportions			
Hay Containing 2.0 Mcal DE/kg[‡]		Hay Containing 1.8 Mcal DE/kg[§]	
Concentrate%[¶]	Roughage%	Concentrate%[¶]	Roughage%
0	100	0	100
20B	80	25A	75
40A	60	50A	50
30B	70	40A	60
25A	75	30A	70
70A	30		
50A	50	70A	30
50A	50	60A	40
40B	60	50A	50
30B	70	40B	60
40B	60	50B	50
0-25B	75	25B	75
40B	60	50B	50
50B	50	60B	40

[#]Western pleasure, bridle path hack, equitation
[**]Ranch work, roping, cutting, barrel racing, jumping
[††]Race training, polo

Adapted, with permission, from *Nutrient Requirements of Horses*, 1989, National Academy of Sciences, National Academy Press, Washington, DC.

lactating mares, milk production seriously declines. Polyuria and polydipsia secondary to renal medullary washout may be seen in prolonged deficits.

Potassium: Chronic dietary deficiency of potassium results in a decreased rate of growth, anorexia, and perhaps hypokalemia. However, most forages contain more than sufficient potassium for the average horse. Acute deficits due to sweat losses are more likely and may cause muscle tremors, cardiac arrhythmias, and weakness. Excess potassium intake, especially if given as a bolus PO or IV, also will induce cardiac arrhythmias such as atrial fibrillation.

Magnesium: Foals fed a purified diet containing magnesium at 8 mg/kg (3.6 mg/lb) exhibited hypomagnesemia, nervousness, muscular tremors, and ataxia followed by collapse, with increased respiratory rates, sweating, convulsive paddling, and death after a few weeks. However, most commonly used feeds contain Mg well in excess of the 70-100 mg/kg dry ration currently recommended. Oversupplementation of this mineral is more likely. Though the effects of excessive Mg intake in horses have not been determined, based on data from other species it may cause clinical signs of calcium deficiency.

Iron: Iron deficiency may be secondary to parasitism or chronic blood loss and results in microcytic, hypochromic anemia. However, it is highly unlikely that even anemic horses are iron deficient. Iron excess interferes with copper metabolism and also causes microcytic, hypochromic anemia. Blood transferrin concentrations are the most reliable method to determine the iron status of a horse.

TABLE 37. Concentrates Satisfactory for Use with Hays as Indicated in TABLE 36

Ingredient[*]	Formula A	Formula B
Corn[†] or sorghum grain, rolled or cracked	45	55
Oats[†], rolled or crimped	24	24
Soybean meal (44% crude protein)	20	10
Cane molasses[‡]	8	8
Limestone (34% Ca)	0.5	0.5
Calcium phosphate, monobasic (16% Ca, 22% P)	1.5	1.5
Trace mineral salt[§]	1	1
	100	100
Analysis		
Digestible energy (Mcal/kg)	3.2	3.2
Crude protein (%)	16	12
Digestible protein (%)	12	8.5
Calcium (%)	0.60	0.58
Phosphorus (%)	0.67	0.62

[*]Except for the cane molasses, all figures are on a 90% dry-matter basis.
[†]Barley may be used to replace the corn or sorghum and the oats, by using weights of barley equal to the combined weights of the grains replaced.
[‡]Cane molasses is not an essential part of a concentrate mixture, but it may help to minimize separation of "fines" and reduce dustiness.
[§]Providing NaCl, Fe, Cu, Mn, Co, I, Zn, and Se (from sodium selenite) to provide 0.2 mg selenium/kg concentrate.

Zinc: Zinc deficiency in foals causes reduced growth rate, anorexia, cutaneous lesions on the lower extremities, alopecia, decreased blood levels of zinc, and decreased serum alkaline phosphatase activity. Excesses (>1,000 ppm) were associated with developmental orthopedic disease in young horses. The effects of excesses or deficits of zinc have not been documented in adult horses.

Copper: An apparent relationship between low blood copper concentrations and uterine artery rupture in aged parturient mares suggests reduced copper absorption with age or reduced ability to mobilize copper stores. Dietary deficiency may cause aortic aneurysm, contracted tendons, and improper cartilage formation in growing foals. Excessive copper intake may interfere with selenium and/or iron metabolism.

Selenium: Selenium deficiency results in reduced serum selenium, increased AST activity, white muscle disease, and perhaps rhabdomyolysis in working horses. (*See also* NUTRITIONAL MYOPATHIES, p 948.) Selenium excesses of as little as 5 ppm in the ration cause loss of mane and tail hairs and sloughing of the distal portion of the hoof.

Vitamins: A **Vitamin A** deficiency may develop if dried, poor-quality roughage is fed for a prolonged period. If body stores of vitamin A are high, signs may not appear for several months. The deficiency is characterized by nyctalopia, lacrimation, keratinization of the cornea, susceptibility to pneumonia, abscesses of the sublingual gland, incoordination, impaired reproduction, capricious appetite, and progressive weakness. Hooves are frequently deformed, with the horny layer unevenly laid down and unusually brittle. Metaplasia of the intestinal mucosa and achlorhydria have been reported. Genitourinary mucosal metaplasia may be expected. Bone remodeling is defective. The foramina do not enlarge properly during early growth, and skeletal deformities are evident. The latter may be seen in foals of vitamin A-deficient mares.

If sun-cured hay is consumed or the horse is exposed to sunlight, it is doubtful that a **vitamin D** deficiency will develop. Prolonged confinement of young horses offered only limited amounts of sun-cured hay may result in reduced bone calcification, stiff and swollen joints, stiffness of gait, irritability, and reduced serum calcium and phosphorus.

Signs of experimental **thiamine** deficiency include anorexia, weight loss, incoordination, decreased blood thiamine, and increased blood pyruvate. At necropsy, the heart is dilated. Similar signs have been seen in bracken fern poisoning (p 2349). Under normal circumstances, the natural diet plus synthesis by microorganisms in the gut probably meet the need for thiamine. However, needs may be increased by stress.

Although natural feeds plus synthesis within the gut normally provide adequate **riboflavin**, limited evidence indicates an occasional deficiency when the diet is of poor quality. The first sign of acute deficiency is catarrhal conjunctivitis in one or both eyes, accompanied by photophobia and lacrimation. The retina, lens, and ocular fluids may deteriorate gradually and result in impaired vision or blindness. Equine recurrent uveitis (p 407) has been linked to riboflavin deficiency but may be a sequela of leptospirosis (p 525) or onchocerciasis (p 736).

The normal feedstuffs of horses generally contain very little **vitamin B_{12}**. However, the horse can synthesize this vitamin in the gut, from which it is absorbed.

FEEDING THE SICK HORSE

Nutrition is an important part of the management and treatment of sick horses. Stresses (eg, surgery, severe orthopedic problems, or infection) can significantly increase caloric needs due to an increase in catabolism. In addition, anorexia or dysphagia can lead to inadequate intake of the proper nutrients. The consequences of not providing proper nutrition include impairment of the immune system, delayed wound and fracture healing, hypoproteinemia, muscle wasting, and weakness. Generally, supportive nutritional therapy should be considered if an adult horse has been hypophagic for ≥3 days. Neonatal foals require some energy source within 24 hr of decreased intake.

The order of nutrient priorities is water, energy, electrolytes, and protein. Some water-soluble vitamins are poorly stored in the body and should be supplemented. The basal energy requirement (BER) in kcal/day can be calculated by the following formula: BER = 70 (body wt in kg)$^{0.75}$. For example, BER is ~6,800 kcal/day for a 450-kg horse and 1,300 kcal/day for a 50-kg foal. Severe illness or trauma (eg, barn fire burns) significantly increase these needs.

There are several methods of providing nutritional support to a sick horse. The simplest method is to encourage the horse to eat on its own. Unusual feed preferences may be seen. Offering a variety of feeds and letting the horse choose can best determine what is most palatable to the animal. Many horses will eat fresh, green grass even though they refuse other feeds. Alfalfa hay is more palatable than grass hays. Whole oats and sweet-feed mixtures of rolled grains and molasses are the most appetizing of grains. Bran mashes are usually palatable, but the addition of molasses, applesauce, and salt may increase their acceptance in anorectic horses.

When horses experience pain or fever, analgesics can improve food intake; NSAID, such as dipyrone, flunixin meglumine, meclofenamic acid, and phenylbutazone, can be used. Prolonged use of phenylbutazone should be avoided because of the side effects of gastric and small-intestinal ulceration and renal papillary necrosis.

Tube feeding is a second method of providing nutrition to horses that will not (or cannot) eat voluntarily. A normal stomach tube may be passed several times a day or may be sutured to the nostril and left as an indwelling feeding tube. This is an effective method of providing nutrients to sick neonates. It is also an inexpensive method of replacing fluid and electrolyte losses. Enteral nutritional supplements used in human medicine are particularly useful in providing sufficient caloric intake to adult horses. These products have a known caloric content, which facilitates calculation of the animal's needs. Soaking a complete pelleted feed in water can make a slurry for tube feeding; however, when feeding a slurry in this manner, the stomach tube may clog with feedstuff.

The third method of providing energy and protein to sick horses is through use of total or partial parenteral nutrition (TPN or PPN). Fluid administration (IV) can maintain hydration in horses that are unable either to drink or absorb fluids. Common replacement solutions include sodium chloride, lactated Ringer's, and 5% dextrose. The nutritional value of these fluids is insignificant. Fat and amino acid solutions are also available. The components of parenteral nutrition are glucose, amino acids, lipid, trace minerals, and multivitamins. The resultant solution is hypertonic and is delivered by constant infusion through a jugular catheter. Delivery is optimized through use of a fluid pump. Blood and urine glucose should be monitored twice daily to regulate the rate of infusion. TPN is costly and requires intensive care and monitoring, which limits its usefulness in adult horses.

Nutrition for Specific Diseases

Horses with **recurrent airway obstruction** (p 1213) are frequently sensitive to the dust and molds found in normal hay. They often improve when hay is removed from their diet and they are placed on a complete ration that is pelleted or contains a roughage source such as beet pulp. They do best on pasture. Another source of dust-free roughage is haylage.

Diarrhea in horses is primarily a colonic disease. Traditionally, affected horses are fed less grain and more hay. This increase in dietary fiber can bind water and may result in better formed feces. If weight loss is a concurrent problem, it may be better to maintain grain intake. Grain is digested mainly in the small intestine, and hay in the large intestine. Unless the small intestine is also affected, feeding grain helps maintain body mass. (*See also* COLIC IN HORSES, p 202, and INTESTINAL DISEASES IN HORSES AND FOALS, p 233.)

The role of nutrition in horses with **liver disease** (p 277) is to provide adequate energy, thus easing the liver's role in energy production and decreasing the amount of metabolic waste to which the liver is exposed. Parenteral or enteral glucose administration may be important as an energy source in anorectic horses. In horses that are eating, cereal grains should provide adequate carbohydrates. Corn is the grain of choice due to its low-protein, high-carbohydrate content. High-protein feeds, such as alfalfa hay, should be avoided.

Horses excrete significant amounts of calcium in their urine. In cases of **renal disease**, low-protein, low-calcium diets should be fed. Corn and grass hay are the feeds of choice.

FEEDING THE AGED HORSE AND THE ORPHAN FOAL

Aged horses often lose weight due to dental wear. Their teeth lose the grinding surface, which results in poor mastication of food. Aged horses also may have reduced protein, fiber, and phosphorus digestion. Feeding a moistened, complete pelleted ration designed for aged horses may improve the horse's well-being.

If an **orphan foal** has not received colostrum from its dam, it must receive either colostrum from another mare or frozen-stored colostrum within 24 hr of birth—preferably within the first 3-12 hr. Antibody-rich plasma replacement products for IV administration are available but are expensive and provide protection of questionable duration.

A nurse mare, preferably with a good disposition, is best for the overall care of an orphan foal. The amnion and/or placenta of a mare who has lost a newborn foal can be placed over the orphan foal to increase the mare's acceptance of the foal. The mare and foal should not be left unattended until the mare has accepted the orphan; physical or chemical restraint of the mare may be required initially and repeated on several occasions before she will accept the new foal.

If a nurse mare is not available, a lactating dairy goat (positioned on a stand or bale of hay or straw) may serve as an alternative. Constant monitoring is necessary because the foal should be fed every 4 hr.

Artificial mare's milk diets and goat's milk have also been used successfully to feed orphan foals. Foals should be fed every 1-2 hr for the first 1-2 days of life, then every 2-4 hr for the next 2 wk at the rate of 250-500 mL per feeding, using a warmed milk container and an artificial nipple. Of the various artificial nipples available, those designed for use by lambs are best suited for foals. The feeding intervals may be lengthened gradually after 2 wk; however, the amount per feeding also should be increased so that the foal consumes 10-15% of its body wt/day. A foal should be encouraged to drink freshly prepared milk out of a bucket, ad lib, early in life. After 1 mo, the foal can be encouraged to eat grain mixes (with ≥18% crude protein designed for growing foals) and good-quality hay in addition to the milk or milk replacer. The foal can be weaned off the milk replacer at 3 mo of age. Fresh water should be available to the foal at all times from birth. *See also* PERINATAL MARE AND FOAL CARE, p 1739.

A heat lamp in an enclosed stall should be available, particularly for the first few weeks of life so that the foal may rest in a warm environment 68°F (20°C). Another alternative during cold weather is a comfortably fitted down vest.

NUTRITION: PIGS

NUTRITIONAL REQUIREMENTS

Nutrition and feeding management are very important aspects of modern swine production. Feeding practices and diet formulation continue to become more precise as new knowledge is gained. Pigs require a minimal amount of a number of essential nutrients to meet their needs for maintenance, growth, reproduction, lactation, and other functions. The National Research Council (NRC) provides estimates of the amounts of these nutrients for various classes of swine under standard conditions. However, factors such as genetic variation, environment, availability of nutrients in feedstuffs, disease levels, and other stressors may increase the needed level of some nutrients for optimal performance and reproduction. Although the NRC attempts to address factors such as lean growth rate, gender, energy density of the diet, environmental temperature, crowding, and sow productivity in estimating nutrient requirements of growing-finishing pigs and of gestating and lactating sows, nutritionists, feed manufacturers, veterinarians, or swine producers may wish to include higher levels of nutrients than those listed by NRC to ensure adequate intake. Any negative effects from oversupplementing diets are generally minimal except in cases of extreme imbalance.

Swine require 6 general classes of nutrients: water, carbohydrates, fats, protein (amino acids), minerals, and vitamins. Energy, though not a specific nutrient, is an important nutritional component and is primarily derived from the oxidation of carbohydrates and fats. In addition, amino acids (from protein) that exceed the animal's requirements for maintenance and tissue protein synthesis provide energy when their carbon skeletons are oxidized. Antibiotics, chemotherapeutic agents, and other feed additives are commonly added to swine diets to increase the rate and efficiency of gain and for other purposes, but they are not considered nutrients. NRC estimates of nutrient requirements for pigs of 3-120 kg body wt, expressed as dietary concentrations, are shown in TABLE 38. Requirements for gestating and lactating sows, expressed as dietary concentrations, are shown in TABLE 39.

Water: Pigs should have free and convenient access to water, beginning before weaning. The amount required varies with age, type of feed, environmental temperature, status of lactation, fever, high urinary output (as from high salt or protein intake), or diarrhea. Normally, growing pigs consume 2-3 kg of water for every kg of dry feed. Lactating sows consume more water because of the high water content of the milk that they produce. Water restriction reduces performance and milk production and may result in death if the restriction is severe.

Energy: Energy requirements are expressed as kilocalories (kcal) of digestible energy (DE), metabolizable energy (ME), or net energy (NE). DE and ME values are used most

TABLE 38. Dietary Nutrient Requirements of Growing Pigs Allowed Ad Lib Feed (90% dry matter)

	Body Weight (kg)					
	3-5	5-10	10-20	20-50	50-80	80-120
DE content of diet (kcal/kg)	3,400	3,400	3,400	3,400	3,400	3,400
ME content of diet (kcal/kg)[†]	3,265	3,265	3,265	3,265	3,265	3,265
Estimated DE intake (kcal/day)	855	1,690	3,400	6,305	8,760	10,450
Estimated ME intake (kcal/day)[†]	820	1,620	3,265	6,050	8,410	10,030
Estimated feed intake (g/day)	250	500	1,000	1,855	2,575	3,075
Crude protein (%)[‡]	26.0	23.7	20.9	18.0	15.5	13.2
Amino acids, total (%)[§]						
Arginine	0.59	0.54	0.46	0.37	0.27	0.19
Histidine	0.48	0.43	0.36	0.30	0.24	0.19
Isoleucine	0.83	0.73	0.63	0.51	0.42	0.33
Leucine	1.50	1.32	1.12	0.90	0.71	0.54
Lysine	1.50	1.35	1.15	0.95	0.75	0.60
Methionine	0.40	0.35	0.30	0.25	0.20	0.16
Methionine + cystine	0.86	0.76	0.65	0.54	0.44	0.35
Phenylalanine	0.90	0.80	0.68	0.55	0.44	0.34
Phenylalanine + tyrosine	1.41	1.25	1.06	0.87	0.70	0.55
Threonine	0.98	0.86	0.74	0.61	0.51	0.41
Tryptophan	0.27	0.24	0.21	0.17	0.14	0.11
Valine	1.04	0.92	0.79	0.64	0.52	0.40
Minerals						
Calcium (%)[¶]	0.90	0.80	0.70	0.60	0.50	0.45
Phosphorus, total (%)[¶]	0.70	0.65	0.60	0.50	0.45	0.40
Phosphorus, available (%)[¶]	0.55	0.40	0.32	0.23	0.19	0.15
Sodium (%)	0.25	0.20	0.15	0.10	0.10	0.10
Chlorine (%)	0.25	0.20	0.15	0.08	0.08	0.08
Magnesium (%)	0.04	0.04	0.04	0.04	0.04	0.04
Potassium (%)	0.30	0.28	0.26	0.23	0.19	0.17
Copper (mg)	6.00	6.00	5.00	4.00	3.50	3.00
Iodine (mg)	0.14	0.14	0.14	0.14	0.14	0.14
Iron (mg)	100	100	80	60	50	40
Manganese (mg)	4.00	4.00	3.00	2.00	2.00	2.00
Selenium (mg)	0.30	0.30	0.25	0.15	0.15	0.15
Zinc (mg)	100	100	80	60	50	50

TABLE 38. (*continued*)

	Body Weight (kg)					
	3-5	5-10	10-20	20-50	50-80	80-120
Vitamins and fatty acids						
Vitamin A (IU)[#]	2,200	2,200	1,750	1,300	1,300	1,300
Vitamin D_3 (IU)[#]	220	220	200	150	150	150
Vitamin E (IU)[#]	16	16	11	11	11	11
Vitamin K (menadione, mg)	0.50	0.50	0.50	0.50	0.50	0.50
Biotin (mg)	0.08	0.05	0.05	0.05	0.05	0.05
Choline (g)	0.60	0.50	0.40	0.30	0.30	0.30
Folacin (mg)	0.30	0.30	0.30	0.30	0.30	0.30
Niacin, available (mg)[**]	20.00	15.00	12.50	10.00	7.00	7.00
Pantothenic acid (mg)	12.00	10.00	9.00	8.00	7.00	7.00
Riboflavin (mg)	4.00	3.50	3.00	2.50	2.00	2.00
Thiamine (mg)	1.50	1.00	1.00	1.00	1.00	1.00
Vitamin B_6 (mg)	2.00	1.50	1.50	1.00	1.00	1.00
Vitamin B_{12} (µg)	20.00	17.50	15.00	10.00	5.00	5.00
Linoleic acid (%)	0.10	0.10	0.10	0.10	0.10	0.10

[*]Adapted, with permission, from *Nutrient Requirements of Swine*, 1998, National Academy of Sciences, National Academy Press, Washington, DC. Estimates are for the midpoint of the weight range as determined by the NRC growth model for pigs of mixed gender (1:1 ratio of barrows and gilts) with high-medium lean growth rate (325 g/day of fat-free carcass lean) from 20-120 kg body wt. DE = digestible energy, ME = metabolizable energy.

[†]ME is assumed to be 96% of DE.

[‡]Crude protein levels apply to corn-soybean meal diets. In 3- to 10-kg pigs fed diets with dried plasma and/or dried milk products, protein levels will be 2-3% less than shown.

[§]Total amino acid requirements are based on the following types of diets: 3- to 5-kg pigs, corn-soybean meal diet that includes 5% dried plasma and 25-50% dried milk products; 5- to 10-kg pigs, corn-soybean meal diet that includes 5-25% dried milk products; 10- to 120-kg pigs, corn-soybean meal diet.

[¶]The percentages of calcium, phosphorus, and available phosphorus should be increased by 0.05-0.10 percentage points for developing boars and replacement gilts from 50-120 kg body wt.

[#]Conversions: 1 IU vitamin A = 0.344 µg retinyl acetate; 1 IU vitamin D_3 = 0.025 µg cholecalciferol; 1 IU vitamin E = 0.67 mg of D-α-tocopherol or 1 mg of DL-α-tocopherol acetate.

[**]The niacin in corn, grain sorghum, wheat, and barley is unavailable. Similarly, the niacin in byproducts made from these cereal grains is poorly available unless the byproducts have undergone a fermentation or wet-milling process.

commonly, but there is increasing interest in the use of NE. On average, ME is ~96% of DE. Energy requirements of pigs are influenced by their weight (which influences the maintenance requirement), their genetic capacity for lean tissue growth or milk production, and the environmental temperature at which they are housed. The amount of feed consumed by growing pigs fed ad lib is controlled principally by the energy content of the diet. If the energy density of the diet is increased by including supplemental fat, voluntary feed consumption decreases. Pigs fed such a diet generally will gain faster and efficiency of gain will improve, but carcass fat may increase. If the diet contains excessive amounts of fiber (>5-7%) without commensurate increases in fat, the rate—and especially the efficiency—of gain are decreased.

TABLE 39. Dietary Nutrient Requirements of Gestating and Lactating Sows (90% dry matter)[*]

	Gestation[†]	Lactation[‡]
DE content of diet (kcal/kg)	3,400	3,400
ME content of diet (kcal/kg)[§]	3,265	3,265
Estimated DE intake (kcal/day)	6,405	18,205
Estimated ME intake (kcal/day)[§]	6,150	17,475
Estimated feed intake (kg/day)	1.88	5.35
Crude protein (%)[¶]	12.4	17.5
Amino acids, total (%)[#]		
Arginine	0.00	0.48
Histidine	0.17	0.36
Isoleucine	0.31	0.50
Leucine	0.46	0.97
Lysine	0.54	0.91
Methionine	0.14	0.23
Methionine + cystine	0.37	0.44
Phenylalanine	0.30	0.48
Phenylalanine + tyrosine	0.51	1.00
Threonine	0.44	0.58
Tryptophan	0.11	0.16
Valine	0.36	0.76
Minerals		
Calcium (%)	0.75	0.75
Phosphorus, total (%)	0.60	0.60
Phosphorus, available (%)	0.35	0.35
Sodium (%)	0.15	0.20
Chlorine (%)	0.12	0.16
Magnesium (%)	0.04	0.04
Potassium (%)	0.20	0.20
Copper (mg)	5.00	5.00
Iodine (mg)	0.14	0.14
Iron (mg)	80	80
Manganese (mg)	20	20
Selenium (mg)	0.15	0.15
Zinc (mg)	50	50
Vitamins and fatty acids		
Vitamin A (IU)[**]	4,000	2,000
Vitamin D_3(IU)[**]	200	200
Vitamin E (IU)[**]	44	44
Vitamin K (menadione, mg)	0.50	0.50
Biotin (mg)	0.20	0.20
Choline (g)	1.25	1.00

TABLE 39. *(continued)*

	Gestation[†]	Lactation[‡]
Folacin (mg)	1.30	1.30
Niacin, available (mg)[††]	10	10
Pantothenic acid (mg)	12	12
Riboflavin (mg)	3.75	3.75
Thiamine (mg)	1.00	1.00
Vitamin B_6 (mg)	1.00	1.00
Vitamin B_{12} (µg)	15	15
Linoleic acid (%)	0.10	0.10

[*]Adapted, with permission, from *Nutrient Requirements of Swine*, 1998, National Academy of Sciences, National Academy Press, Washington, DC. DE = digestible energy; ME = metabolizable energy.

[†]Estimates for gestation are for a sow weighing 175 kg breeding and gaining 40 kg body wt during gestation (includes maternal tissue and products of conception) with an anticipated litter size of 12 piglets.

[‡]Estimates for lactation are for a sow weighing 175 kg post- farrowing and losing no weight during a 21-day lactation while nursing 10 piglets that each gain 200 g/day.

[§]ME is assumed to be 96% of DE.

[¶]Crude protein levels are based on corn-soybean meal diets.

[#]Total amino acid requirements are based on corn-soybean meal diets.

[**]Conversions: 1 IU vitamin A = 0.344 µg retinyl acetate; 1 IU vitamin D_3 = 0.025 µg cholecalciferol; 1 IU vitamin E = 0.67 mg of D-α-tocopherol or 1 mg of DL-α-tocopherol acetate.

[††]The niacin in corn, grain sorghum, wheat, and barley is unavailable. Similarly, the niacin in byproducts made from these cereal grains is poorly available unless the byproducts have undergone a fermentation or wet-milling process.

Protein and Amino Acids: Amino acids, normally supplied by dietary protein, are required for maintenance, muscle growth, development of fetuses and supporting tissues in gestating sows, and milk production in lactating sows. Of the 22 amino acids, 12 are synthesized by the animal; the other 10 must be provided in the diet for normal growth. The 10 dietary essential amino acids for growing pigs are arginine, histidine, isoleucie, leucine, lysine, methionine, phenylalanine, threonine, tryptophan, and valine. Cystine and tyrosine can meet a portion of the requirement for methionine and phenylalanine, respectively. The levels of crude protein listed in TABLE 38 provide the required levels of amino acids when diets are based on corn and soybean meal.

The amino acids of greatest practical importance are lysine, tryptophan, threonine, and methionine. Corn, the basic grain in most swine diets, is markedly deficient in lysine and tryptophan. The other principal grains for pigs (grain sorghum, barley, and wheat) are low in lysine and threonine. The first limiting amino acid in soybean meal is methionine, but sufficient amounts are provided when soybean meal is combined with cereal grains into a complete diet that meets the lysine requirement. An exception might be in young pigs that have high levels of soybean meal or in diets containing dried blood products that are low in the sulfur-amino acids. Milk protein is well balanced in essential amino acids but usually is too expensive to be used in swine diets, except for very young pigs. Dried whey, commonly used in starter diets, contains protein with an excellent profile of amino acids, but the total protein content of whey is low. Diets based on corn and animal-protein byproducts (eg, meat meal, meat and bone meal) are inferior to corn-soybean meal diets, but they can be improved significantly by adding tryptophan or supplements that are good sources of tryptophan.

Recent research indicates that diets formulated for medicated or segregated early weaned pigs, which contain high levels of dried animal plasma or dried blood cells, may be deficient in methionine. However, high levels of methionine can depress growth, so methionine should not be added indiscriminately to diets. Supplemental valine may be of value in corn-soybean meal diets fed to lactating sows, but it is still too expensive to be considered as a dietary supplement.

Lysine is generally the first limiting amino acid in almost all practical diets, so if diets are formulated on a lysine basis, the other amino acid requirements should be met. However, caution must be exercised when a crystalline lysine supplement is included in the diet to meet a portion of the pig's lysine requirement. A general rule of thumb is that crude protein content can be reduced by 2 percentage points and supplemented with 0.15% lysine (0.19% lysine•HCl). However, greater reductions in dietary protein coupled with additional lysine may result in deficiencies of tryptophan, threonine, and/or methionine unless they are also supplemented.

Several feed manufacturers now formulate swine diets based on the concept of "ideal" protein. In this method, all essential amino acid requirements are expressed as a specific ratio to, or a percent of, the lysine requirement. Additionally, some swine diets are formulated on the basis of true or apparent digestible amino acids. This method is particularly advantageous when substantial amounts of byproduct feeds are included in the diet.

Minerals: These nutritional elements have many important functions in the body. The dietary requirements for the essential macro- and trace minerals are listed in TABLE 38 and TABLE 39.

Calcium and Phosphorus: Although used primarily in skeletal growth, calcium and phosphorus play important metabolic roles in the body and are essential for all stages of growth, gestation, and lactation. The NRC estimates requirements of 0.6% calcium and 0.5% phosphorus for growing pigs of 20-50 kg body wt. The requirements are higher for younger pigs and lower for finishing pigs, but the ratio is approximately the same for all weight groups. These levels are adequate for maximal growth (rate and efficiency of gain), but they do not allow for maximal bone mineralization. Generally, maximal bone ash and strength can be achieved by including 0.10-0.15% additional calcium and phosphorus in the diet.

For gestating and lactating sows, calcium and phosphorus requirements are estimated at 0.75% and 0.60%, respectively. Swine producers often feed slightly higher levels to sows to ensure adequacy of these minerals and to prevent posterior paralysis in heavy milking sows. These requirements are based on daily feed intakes of at least 4 lb (1.8 kg) of feed during gestation and 12 lb (5.5 kg) of feed during lactation. If less feed is consumed per day, the percentages of calcium and phosphorus may need to be adjusted upwards.

The ratio of total calcium:total phosphorus should be kept between 1.25:1 and 1:1 for maximal utilization of both minerals. A wide calcium:phosphorus ratio reduces phosphorus absorption, especially if the diet is marginal in phosphorus. The ratio is less critical if the diet contains excess phosphorus. When based on available phosphorus, the ideal ratio of calcium to available phosphorus is 2-3:1.

Most of the phosphorus in cereal grains and oilseed meals is in the form of phytic acid (organically bound phosphorus) and is poorly available to pigs, whereas the phosphorus in protein sources of animal origin, such as meat meal, meat and bone meal, and fish meal, is in inorganic form and is highly available to pigs. Even in cereal grains, availability of phosphorus varies. For example, the phosphorus in corn is only 10-20% available, whereas the phosphorus in wheat is 50% available. Therefore, swine diets should be formulated on an "available phosphorus" basis to ensure that the phosphorus requirement is met.

Phosphorus supplements such as monocalcium or dicalcium phosphate, defluorinated phosphate, and steamed bone meal are excellent sources of highly available phosphorus. These supplements also are good sources of calcium. Ground limestone also is an excellent source of calcium.

Phosphorus is considered a potential environmental pollutant, so many swine producers are now feeding diets with less excess phosphorus than in the past to reduce phosphorus excretion. Supplemental phytase, an enzyme that degrades some of the phytic acid in feedstuffs, can be added to diets to further reduce phosphorus excretion. The general recommendation is that dietary calcium and phosphorus can both be reduced by 0.05-0.10% when ≥500 units of phytase per kg of diet are included.

Sodium and Chloride: These minerals are provided by common salt, which contains 40% sodium and 60% chloride. The recommended level of salt is 0.25% in growing and finishing diets, 0.40-0.50% in starter diets, and 0.50% in sow diets. These levels should provide ample sodium and chloride to meet the animal's requirements. Animal, fish, and milk byproducts can contribute some of the requirement.

Potassium, Magnesium, and Sulfur: Practical diets contain ample amounts of these minerals from the grain and protein sources, and supplemental sources are not needed. Magnesium oxide supplementation has been used to prevent cannibalism, but controlled studies do not support this practice.

Iron and Copper: These minerals are involved in many enzyme systems. Both are necessary for formation of hemoglobin and, therefore, for prevention of nutritional anemia. Because the amount of iron in milk is very low, suckling pigs should receive supplemental iron preferably by IM injection of 100-200 mg of iron in the form of iron dextran, iron dextrin, or gleptoferron during the first 3 days of life (*see also* IRON TOXICITY IN NEWBORN PIGS, p 2403). Giving oral or injectable iron and copper to sows will not increase piglet stores at birth nor will it increase colostrum and milk iron sufficiently to prevent anemia in neonatal pigs. High levels of iron in lactation feed results in iron-rich sow feces that pigs can obtain from the pen. Iron can also be supplied by mixing ferric ammonium citrate with water in a piglet waterer or by frequently placing a mixture or iron sulfate and a carrier, such as ground corn, on the floor of the farrowing stall.

Copper at pharmaceutical levels in the diet (100-250 mg/kg) is an effective growth stimulant for weanling and growing pigs. The action of copper at high levels appears to be independent of, and additive to, the growth-stimulating effect of antibiotics.

Iodine: The thyroid gland uses iodine to produce thyroxine, which affects cell activity and metabolic rate. The iodine requirement of all classes of pigs is 0.14 mg/kg of diet. Stabilized iodized salt that contains 0.007% iodine; when it is fed at sufficient levels to meet the salt requirement, it will also meet the iodine needs of pigs.

Manganese: Although essential for normal reproduction and growth, the quantitative requirement for manganese is not well defined. Manganese at 2-4 mg/kg in the diet is adequate for growth, but a higher level (20 mg/kg) is needed by sows during gestation and lactation.

Zinc: Zinc is an important trace mineral with many biologic functions. Grain-soybean meal diets must contain supplemental zinc to prevent parakeratosis (p 793). Higher levels of zinc may be needed when dietary calcium is excessive, especially in typical high-phytic acid diets such as corn-soybean meal diets. Pharmacologic levels of zinc (1,500-3,000 mg/kg) as zinc oxide have been consistently found to increase pig performance during the postweaning period. In some instances, high levels of zinc oxide have been reported to reduce the incidence and severity of postweaning diarrhea.

Selenium: The selenium content of soils and, ultimately, crops is quite variable. In the USA, areas west of the Mississippi River generally contain higher amounts of selenium, while areas east of the river tend to yield crops deficient in selenium. Under most practical conditions, 0.2-0.3 mg of added selenium/kg of diet should meet the requirements. This trace mineral is regulated by the FDA, and the maximal amount of selenium that can be added to swine diets is 0.3 mg/kg.

Chromium: This trace mineral, which is a cofactor with insulin, is required by pigs, but the quantitative requirement has not been established. In some studies, chromium at a supplemental level of 200 µg/kg (ppb) improved carcass leanness in finishing pigs and improved reproductive performance in gestating sows, but these effects have been somewhat inconsistent.

Cobalt: Cobalt is present in the vitamin B_{12} molecule and has no benefit when added to swine diets in the elemental form.

Vitamins: These micronutrients serve many important roles in the body. The estimated requirements for the essential vitamins are given in TABLE 38 and TABLE 39.

Vitamin A: This fat-soluble vitamin is essential for vision, reproduction, growth and maintenance of epithelial tissue, and mucous secretions. Vitamin A is found as carotenoid precursors in green plant material and yellow corn. β-carotene is the most active form of the various carotenes. Unfortunately, only about one-fourth of the total carotene in yellow corn is in the form of β-carotene. The NRC suggests that for pigs, 1 mg of chemically determined carotene in corn or a corn-soybean mixture is equal to 267 IU of vitamin A. The use of stabilized vitamin A is common in manufactured feeds and in vitamin supplements or premixes. Concentrates containing natural vitamin A (fish oils most often) may be used to fortify diets. Green forage, dehydrated alfalfa meal, and high-quality legume hays are good sources of β-carotene. Both natural vitamin A and β-carotene are easily destroyed by air, light, high temperatures, rancid fats, organic acids, and certain mineral elements. For these reasons, natural feedstuffs probably should not be entirely relied on as sources of vitamin A, especially as synthetic vitamin A is very inexpensive. An international unit of vitamin A is equivalent to 0.344 μg of retinyl acetate.

Vitamin D: This antirachitic, fat-soluble vitamin is necessary for proper bone growth and ossification. Vitamin D is seen as ergocalciferol (vitamin D_2) or cholecalciferol (vitamin D_3). Although pigs can use vitamin D_2 (irradiated plant sterol) or vitamin D_3 (irradiated animal sterol), they seem to preferentially use D_3. Some of the vitamin D requirement can be met by exposing pigs to direct sunlight for a short period each day. Sources of vitamin D include irradiated yeast, sun-cured hays, activated plant or animal sterols, fish oils, and vitamin premixes. For this vitamin, 1 IU is equivalent to 0.025 μg of cholecalciferol.

Vitamin E: This fat-soluble vitamin serves as a natural antioxidant in feedstuffs. There are 8 naturally occurring forms of vitamin E, but D-α-tocopherol has the greatest biologic activity. Vitamin E is required by pigs of all ages and is closely interrelated with selenium. The vitamin E requirement is 11-16 IU/kg of diet for growing pigs and 44 IU/kg for sows. Some nutritionists recommend higher dietary levels for sows in the eastern corn belt of the USA where selenium levels in feeds are likely to be low. Vitamin E supplementation can only partially obviate a selenium deficiency. Green forage, legume hays and meals, cereal grains, and especially the germ of cereal grains contain appreciable amounts of vitamin E. Activity of vitamin E is reduced in feedstuffs when exposed to heat, high-moisture conditions, rancid fat, organic acids, and high levels of certain trace elements. One IU of vitamin E activity is equivalent to 0.67 mg of D-α-tocopherol or 1 mg of DL-α-tocopherol acetate.

Vitamin K: This fat-soluble vitamin is necessary to maintain normal blood clotting. The requirement for vitamin K is low, 0.5 mg/kg of diet. Bacterial synthesis of the vitamin and subsequent absorption, directly or by coprophagy, generally will meet the requirement for pigs. However, hemorrhages have been reported in newborn as well as growing pigs. In such cases, supplemental vitamin K has been recommended at 2 mg/kg of diet as a preventive measure.

Riboflavin: This water-soluble vitamin is a constituent of 2 important enzyme systems that are involved with carbohydrate, protein, and fat metabolism. Swine diets are normally deficient in this vitamin, and the crystalline form is included in premixes. Natural sources include green forage, milk byproducts, brewer's yeast, legume meals, and some fermentation and distillery byproducts.

Niacin (Nicotinic Acid): Niacin is a component of coenzymes involved with metabolism of carbohydrates, fats, and protein. Pigs can convert excess tryptophan to niacin, but the conversion is inefficient. The niacin in most cereal grains is completely unavailable to pigs. Swine diets are normally deficient in this vitamin, and the crystalline form is included in premixes. Natural sources of niacin include fish and animal byproducts, brewer's yeast, and distiller's solubles.

Pantothenic Acid: This vitamin is a component of coenzyme A, an important enzyme in energy metabolism. Swine diets are deficient in this vitamin, and the crystalline salt, D-calcium pantothenate, is included in vitamin premixes. Natural sources of pantothenic acid include green forage, legume meals, milk products, brewer's yeast, fish solubles, and certain other byproducts.

Vitamin B$_{12}$: This vitamin, also called cyanocobalamin, contains cobalt and has numerous important metabolic functions. Feedstuffs of plant origin are devoid of this vitamin, but animal products are good sources. Although some intestinal synthesis of this vitamin occurs, vitamin B$_{12}$ is generally included in vitamin premixes for swine.

Thiamine: This vitamin has important roles in the body, but it is of little practical significance for swine because grains and other feed ingredients supply ample amounts to meet the requirement in pigs.

Vitamin B$_6$: A group of compounds called the pyridoxines have vitamin B$_6$ activity and are important in amino acid metabolism. They are present in plentiful quantities in the natural feed ingredients usually fed to pigs.

Choline: Choline is essential for the normal functioning of all tissues. Pigs can synthesize some choline from methionine in the diet. Sufficient choline is found in the natural dietary ingredients to meet the requirements of growing pigs. However, in some studies, choline supplemented at 440-800 mg/kg of diet increased litter size in gilts and sows. Natural sources of choline include fish solubles, fish meal, soybean meal, liver meal, brewer's yeast, and meat meal. Choline chloride, which is 75% choline, is the common form of supplemental choline used in feeds. If choline is added as a supplement to sow diets, it should not be combined with other vitamins in a premix, especially if trace minerals are present, because choline chloride is hygroscopic and destroys some of the activity of vitamin A and other less stable vitamins.

Biotin: This vitamin is present in a highly available form in corn and soybean meal, but the biotin in grain sorghum, oats, barley, and wheat is less available to pigs. There is evidence that when these latter cereal grains are fed to swine, especially breeding animals, biotin may be marginal or deficient. Reproductive performance in sows appears to improve with biotin additions. Though not as clear, there is evidence that reproductive performance also is improved with addition of biotin to corn-soybean meal diets. In some instances, biotin supplementation decreased footpad lesions in adult pigs. For insurance, biotin supplementation is recommended, especially for sow diets. Raw eggs should not be fed to pigs because the egg white contains a protein, avidin, that complexes with biotin and renders it unavailable.

Folacin: This group of compounds has folic acid activity. Sufficient folacin is present in natural feedstuffs to meet the requirement for growth, but recent studies have shown a benefit in litter size when folic acid was added to sow diets.

Ascorbic Acid (Vitamin C): Pigs are thought to synthesize this vitamin at a rapid enough rate to meet their needs under normal conditions. However, a few studies have shown benefits in performance of early-weaned pigs under stressful conditions when this vitamin was added to the diet.

Fatty Acids: Linoleic acid, arachidonic acid, and probably other long-chain, polyunsaturated fatty acids are required by pigs. However, the longer chain fatty acids can be synthesized in vivo from linoleic acid, so linoleic acid is considered the dietary essential fatty acid. The NRC estimates the linoleic acid requirement at 0.10% for growing and breeding swine. The requirement is generally met by the fat present in natural dietary ingredients.

FEEDING LEVELS AND PRACTICES

Performance of weanling, growing, and finishing pigs; gestating sows; and lactating sows and their nursing pigs is related to both the quality of the diet and the amount that is consumed on a daily basis. Knowing the amount of feed that animals consume is important in the overall feeding management process. Weanling, growing, and finishing pigs are ordinarily allowed to consume feed on an ad lib basis, and the amount consumed is affected by the energy density of the diet, environmental temperature, gender, and feed quality (eg, absence of molds), as well as a host of other management factors such as feeder design, crowding, etc.

Daily feed intakes of 6 weight classes of **growing-finishing pigs** fed a diet containing 3,400 kcal of DE/kg (typical of a corn-soybean meal diet) as estimated by the NRC growth model are shown in TABLE 38. These intake levels represent an average for barrows and gilts. Feed intakes will be slightly higher for barrows and slightly less for gilts weighing 50-120 kg. Preventing overcrowding and cooling pigs with automatic water sprayers during hot weather help to alleviate reduced feed intake. These intake levels can be used as a guide to project total feed requirements or prescribe in-feed medication.

For **gestating gilts and sows**, the NRC estimates that a feeding level of 4-4.5 lb/day (1.8-2.0 kg/day) of a corn-soybean meal diet (3,400 kcal DE/kg) provides sufficient energy for maintenance, some lean and fat tissue accretion (particularly in gilts), and the energy needs of the developing fetuses, placenta, and other supporting tissues. Mature sows do not need more energy than that required for maintenance and some increase in body weight. If gestation diets contain oats, alfalfa meal, or other energy diluents, higher feeding levels will be needed to meet the sow's energy requirement. Voluntary intake cannot be limited during gestation even with extremely high-fiber diets; invariably, excess weight gain develops.

Swine managers should adjust the feeding level of pregnant gilts and sows to keep them in good condition. Excess body condition at the end of gestation is often associated with reduced feed intake during lactation and sometimes results in reduced litter size, greater incidence of dystocia, more pig overlay, and a greater incidence of postpartum dysgalactia syndrome (p 1134). Poor body condition results in a greater incidence of shoulder sores in sows, lower birth weights, and thin sows at weaning with delayed return to postweaning estrus (or even anestrus). Litter size at the subsequent farrowing can also be negatively affected if sows are in poor condition at breeding.

The NRC estimates that **lactating sows** require 10-13 lb (4.3-5.7 kg) of feed (3,400 kcal/kg) daily to meet their energy requirements. The amount of energy and feed depends on number of pigs nursed, weight gain of the pigs (both of these factors influence milk production), and weight loss of the sow. High-energy diets should be self-fed to sows during lactation or sows should be hand-fed all they will consume 3 times daily. Proper temperature regulation in the farrowing room and the use of drip-coolers during hot weather help to alleviate low feed intake. If feed intake is too low, sows will lose excessive weight during lactation (*see* above). If this is a problem, including 3-6% fat in the lactation diet or top-dressing the lactation feed with additional fat should be considered. If problems persist, more energy during the trimester of pregnancy may be helpful.

Diets high in protein and amino acids should be fed to prolific sows nursing large litters to maximize milk production and to prevent excessive weight loss of the sow. Such sows may require diets containing 18% or more crude protein (0.90.% lysine). If energy intake is sufficient, these high-protein diets will minimize or even eliminate weight loss in sows during lactation.

Major Feed Ingredients: A fundamental principle of the economics of pork production is to feed the most economical cereal grains and to correct the deficiencies by supplementation with good-quality protein sources, minerals, and vitamins. Dependable mineral and vitamin premixes or complete manufactured supplements are commercially available. Fortified corn-soybean meal diets are very popular in pig operations, but other cereals and protein sources can be used.

Corn (maize) is by far the most widely used grain for feeding pigs in the USA. It is very palatable and high in energy, but is relatively low in crude protein. In addition, corn is deficient in lysine, tryptophan, threonine, and several other essential amino acids, as well as vitamins and minerals.

Grain sorghum is a major energy source for pigs in western and southwestern USA. The protein content is variable depending on factors such as variety, whether the crop was grown on irrigated or dry land, amount of fertilizer used, and other environmental factors. In general, grain sorghum can be substituted for corn on an equal-weight basis, but because the ME value is slightly lower than that of corn, a poorer feed conversion should be expected.

Wheat has about the same energy content as corn and contains 2-3% more protein and 0.05-0.10% more lysine than corn. Wheat can be substituted for corn on either an equal-weight basis or on a lysine basis, but not on a crude protein basis or it will result in a lysine deficiency. Wheat can constitute all of the grain in a swine diet.

Barley has ~85-90% of the feeding value of corn, even though it usually contains 2-3% more protein. Scabby barley should not be fed to pigs.

Oats have a relatively low energy content and, therefore, should not account for more than 20-25% of the cereal grain in the diet. Generally, when oats are included in the diet, the rate and efficiency of gain should be expected to decline. Rolled oats groats are sometimes used in starter diets because of their excellent palatability.

Cereal grains should be ground or rolled to maximize their feeding value. Corn and grain sorghum should be reduced to a medium-fine particle size (550-600 microns). Wheat should be ground more coarsely (650-700 microns) to prevent pasting. Fine grinding improves feed conversion, but excessive reduction in particle size may lead to an increased incidence of gastric ulcers. Pelleting of diets may result in a small improvement in gain and especially feed efficiency. In general, the benefit is greatest with pelleted diets that contain high levels of fiber. Response to pelleted barley-based diets is excellent. Cereal grains should be as free as possible from mycotoxins. Aflatoxins, vomitoxin, zearalenone, fumonisin, and other mycotoxins can reduce animal performance, depending on level in the feed, and can especially cause reproductive problems in breeding animals.

Soybean meal accounts for >90% of the supplemental protein fed to pigs in the USA. It is very palatable and has an excellent amino acid profile that complements the amino acid pattern in cereal grains. Ground, full-fat soybeans can also be fed to swine, but only after they are heated (by extrusion or roasting) to inactivate the trypsin inhibitors and other heat-labile antinutritional factors. Canola meal also is a good protein source. Cottonseed meal, peanut meal, sunflower meal, and other oilseed-based meals can be used in swine feed, but generally not as the sole source of supplemental protein. Animal protein sources such as meat meal, meat and bone meal, or fish meal can supply a portion of the supplemental protein in swine diets.

Feeding Management of Sows and Litters: Gestation diets adequate in all nutrients should be fed to sows to produce healthy, vigorous pigs. Sows should be fed so that they are in good body condition at farrowing—not too fat or too thin. After farrowing, the sow should be returned to full feed as soon as possible. Constipation in sows is generally not a problem if the sow is eating well. Wheat bran or dried beet pulp can be included in the farrowing diet at 5-10% if constipation is a problem, or chemical laxatives such as potassium chloride or magnesium sulfate can be included in the diet at 0.75-1.0%. Newly farrowed pigs should be checked to ensure that each has nursed. If necessary, milk flow may be stimulated by giving oxytocin. If the sow is slow in coming into milk, weak pigs may benefit from receiving artificial milk, but success depends on good management and sanitation. Nutritional anemia should be prevented. A palatable pig starter diet should be provided beginning at 2-3 wk if pigs are weaned later than 3 wk of age. (*See also* HEALTH-MANAGEMENT INTERACTION: PIGS, p 1740, and MANAGEMENT OF REPRODUCTION: PIGS, p 1771.)

Feeding Management of Weanling Pigs: Pigs weaned at an early age (3-4 wk) perform best if fed a complex starter diet for 1-2 wk after weaning. Typically, the starter diet contains dried whey and/or lactose, dried blood products, and a high level of lysine. The current trend in the swine industry is toward medicated early weaning or segregated early weaning to produce healthier pigs. This entails weaning at 10-16 days of age and requires excellent nutritional management. Such diets should contain even higher levels of lysine as well as high levels of lactose (as the sugar or from dried whey) and 3-7% dried animal plasma. A gradual transition should eventually be made to less expensive starter diets and then to corn-soybean meal diets.

The nutritional needs of growing-finishing pigs are best met by a full-feeding program. Limit-feeding reduces the rate and efficiency of gain but may improve carcass quality of finishing pigs. Proper design and adjustment of self feeders is necessary to prevent feed wastage or restricted growth.

Growth Stimulants: Antibiotics and other chemotherapeutic agents are commonly added to swine diets to promote growth. The greatest response to these growth enhancing agents is in young pigs, with lesser responses as pigs progress in age and weight. The levels of antibiotics fed and drug withdrawal requirements should be in accordance with manufacturers' recommendations and legal restrictions. (*See also* GROWTH PROMOTANTS AND PRODUCTION ENHANCERS, p 2168.)

The inclusion of effective antibiotics in diets for starter pigs increases rate of gain by ~15% and feed efficiency by ~7%; for grower-finisher pigs, improvements of ~4% in rate of gain and ~2% in feed efficiency can be expected. The antibiotics approved for swine include apramycin, bacitracin, bambermycins, chlortetracycline, lincomycin, neomycin, oxytetracycline, penicillin, tiamulin, tylosin, and virginiamycin. Chemotherapeutic agents include arsanilic acid, carbadox, roxarsone, sulfamethazine, and sulfathiazole. Several of these are approved only in combination with certain other additives. In addition, pharmaceutical levels of zinc (1,500-3,000 ppm) as zinc oxide, or copper (100-250 ppm) as copper sulfate or copper chloride are effective growth stimulants in young pigs.

For best results, antibiotics should be included in the diet throughout the growing-finishing period. It may help to reduce the number of runts and unthrifty pigs and allow such pigs to make more rapid and efficient gains. Antibiotics also help to prevent and control scours and certain forms of enteritis. Feeding a high level of certain antimicrobial agents at breeding time and at farrowing results in improved reproductive performance. The feeding of antimicrobials to pigs should not be considered a substitute for good management.

Microbials that are directly fed (once referred to as probiotics) such as live cultures of *Lactobacillus acidophilus*, *Streptococcus faecium*, and *Saccharomyces cerevisiae* have been evaluated as possible substitutes for antibiotics, but controlled studies have not shown consistent, beneficial responses from their inclusion. In some instances, inclusion of specific sugars (mannanoligosaccharides, fructooligosaccharides) have shown promise as possible alternatives to antibiotics for young pigs, but growth responses are less consistent and of lower magnitude than from the inclusion of antibiotics.

Certain "repartitioning agents" have been tested with finishing swine and found to be very effective in improving growth rate, feed conversion, and carcass leanness. Examples are β-agonists, such as ractopamine and porcine somatotropin. Presently, ractopamine is the only such agent approved for use in pigs in the USA. These agents affect nutrient requirements; in particular, they increase the dietary requirements for amino acids.

NUTRITIONAL DISEASES

Diagnosis of nutritional deficiencies by observation is difficult. Quite often, the clinical signs are the result of a complex of mismanagement and infectious diseases, including parasitism, as well as malnutrition. For most nutritional deficiencies, the signs are not specific, eg, poor appetite, reduced growth, and unthriftiness. Deficiency of a single nutrient may bring about inanition; the subsequent starvation may cause multiple deficiencies. Then, too, a nutritional deficiency may exist without the appearance of definite signs. In the field, the deficiency may be only slight or borderline, which makes diagnosis difficult.

Diagnosis of a deficiency by observing the response to nutritional therapy is not always clear, particularly for longterm deficiencies, the lesions of which may be irreversible. A nutritional deficiency should be diagnosed positively only after observance of several of the expected clinical signs and a careful review of the dietary, disease, and management history of the animals.

Protein Deficiency: Protein deficiency, which may result from suboptimal feed intake or a deficiency of one or more of the essential amino acids, causes reduced gains, poor feed conversion, and fatter carcasses in growing and finishing pigs. In lactating sows, milk production is reduced, excess weight loss is seen and sows may fail to show estrus or have delayed return to estrus. For optimal use of protein, all essential amino acids must be liberated during digestion at rates commensurate with needs. Therefore, protein supplements should not be handfed at infrequent intervals but should be mixed with the grain or be available at all times with grain on a free-choice basis.

No evidence has been presented to support the theory of "protein poisoning." Diets containing as much as 35-50% protein were found to be laxative and less efficiently used, but no toxic effects were noted.

Fat Deficiency: Certain long-chain polyunsaturated fatty acids are essential for swine. Linoleic acid is essential in the diet and is used to produce longer-chain fatty acids that are probably also essential. A linoleic acid deficiency induces hair loss, scaly dermatitis, skin necrosis on the neck and shoulders, and an unthrifty appearance in growing pigs. Conventional swine diets generally contain adequate fat from the natural ingredients to furnish ample amounts of essential fatty acids.

Mineral Deficiency: Deficiencies of **calcium** or **phosphorus** result in rickets (p 853) in growing pigs and osteomalacia in mature pigs. Signs include deformity and bending of long bones and lameness in young pigs, and fractures and posterior paralysis (a result of fractures in the lumbar region) in older pigs. Sows that produce high levels of milk and nurse large litters are particularly susceptible to posterior paralysis toward the end of lactation or after weaning if dietary calcium or phosphorus is deficient. These signs can also result from a deficiency of vitamin D, but phosphorus deficiency is the most common cause.

Pigs fed diets low in **salt** (NaCl) grow poorly and inefficiently, due largely to a marked reduction in feed intake. Though not specific for salt deficiency, poor hair and skin condition may also develop. There have been reports of salt-deficient pigs attempting to consume urine of other pigs.

Sows fed diets deficient in **iodine** produce hairless pigs that are weak or stillborn. With a borderline deficiency, the newborn pigs may only be weak at birth, but their thyroids are enlarged and have histologic abnormalities. (*See also* GOITER, p 465.) Some feedstuffs (including soybeans and soybean meal) contain goitrogens that may cause marginal goiter if iodine is not included in the diet. Iodized salt at recommended levels prevents this deficiency.

Deficiencies of **iron** and **copper** reduce the rate of Hgb formation and produce typical nutritional anemia. Signs of nutritional anemia in suckling pigs include low Hgb and RBC count, pale mucous membranes, enlarged heart, skin edema about the neck and shoulders, listlessness, and spastic breathing (thumps). Iron deficiency is more common than copper deficiency and is most common in nursing pigs that do not receive an iron injection or oral iron early in life.

A deficiency of **zinc** results in parakeratosis (p 192) in growing pigs, particularly when fed diets high in phytic acid (or phytate, the primary form of phosphorus in cereal grains and oilseed meals) and more than the recommended amount of calcium. The exact mode of action of zinc in the prevention of parakeratosis is not known.

Deficiencies of **selenium** and/or **vitamin E** can cause sudden death of young, rapidly growing pigs (*see* HEPATOSIS DIETETICA and MULBERRY HEART DISEASE, p 950). In addition, selenium/vitamin E deficiency in nursing pigs makes them more susceptible to iron toxicosis from iron injections. (*See* IRON TOXICITY IN NEWBORN PIGS, p 2403.)

Vitamin Deficiency: Most commercial diets are fortified with vitamins, so deficiencies are less common than they were years ago. Deficiency of **vitamin A** results in disturbances of the eyes and the epithelial tissues of the respiratory, reproductive, nervous, urinary, and digestive systems. Reproduction is impaired in sows, and they may farrow blind, eyeless, weak, or malformed pigs. Herniation of the spinal cord in fetal pigs is reported as a unique sign of vitamin A deficiency in pregnant sows. Growing pigs deficient in vitamin A show incoordination and develop night blindness and respiratory disorders. Vitamin A deficiency is rare due to the ability of the liver to store this vitamin.

Signs of **vitamin D** deficiency include rickets, stiffness, weak and bent bones, and posterior paralysis. These signs are indistinguishable from those of a calcium or phosphorus deficiency (*see* above).

Vitamin E deficiency can result in poor reproduction and impaired immune system. Many of the signs of vitamin E deficiency are similar to those of selenium deficiency (*see* above).

Pigs deficient in **vitamin K** have prolonged blood clotting time and may die from hemorrhages. Certain components in moldy feed can interfere with vitamin K synthesis. Also excessive levels of dietary calcium interfere with vitamin K activity, causing these signs.

In pigs deficient in **riboflavin**, reproduction is impaired; postpubertal gilts fail to cycle but show no other clinical signs. Deficient sows are anorectic and farrow dead pigs 4-16 days prematurely. The stillborn pigs have very little hair, often are partially resorbed, and may have enlarged forelegs. Growing pigs fed diets low in riboflavin gain weight slowly and have a poor appetite, a rough coat, an exudate on the skin, and possibly cataracts.

Pigs deficient in **niacin** have inflammatory lesions of the digestive tract and exhibit diarrhea, weight loss, rough skin and coat, and dermatitis on the ears. Intestinal conditions can be due to niacin deficiency or bacterial infection. Deficient pigs respond readily to niacin therapy and, although not a cure for infectious enteritis, adequate dietary niacin probably allows the pig to maintain its resistance to bacterial invasion.

Growing pigs and pregnant sows develop a typical "goose-stepping" gait, ataxia, and a noninfectious bloody diarrhea when maintained on diets deficient in **pantothenic acid**. When the deficiency becomes severe, anorexia develops.

Pigs with a **choline** deficiency exhibit incoordination and an abnormal shoulder conformation. At necropsy, they may have fatty livers and usually show kidney damage. Sows deficient in choline have reduced litter size and may give birth to spraddle-legged pigs.

Biotin deficiency includes excessive hair loss, skin ulcerations and dermatitis, exudates around the eyes, inflammation of the mucous membranes of the mouth, transverse cracking of the hooves, and cracking or bleeding of the footpads.

Neonatal pigs fed synthetic diets low in **vitamin B_{12}** show hyperirritability, voice failure, and pain and incoordination in the hindquarters. Histologic examination of the bone marrow reveals an impaired hematopoietic system. Fatty livers are also noted at necropsy.

NUTRITION: SHEEP

The economical and efficient production of lamb and wool is contingent on maximal production per ewe. Economical maintenance of breeding animals, a high percentage of the lamb crop weaned, continuous and rapid growth of lambs, heavy weaning weights, and a heavy fleece weight are important to efficiency. All of these are influenced by nutrition. Quantifying the nutritional requirements for maintenance, reproduction, growth, finishing, and wool production is complex because sheep are maintained under a wide variety of environmental conditions.

NUTRITIONAL REQUIREMENTS

An adequate diet for optimal growth and production must include water, energy (carbohydrates and fats), proteins, minerals, and vitamins (TABLE 40). Under field conditions of particular stress, additional nutrients may be needed.

Water: The usual recommendations are ~1 gal. (3.8 L) of water/day for ewes on dry feed in winter, $1^1/2$ gal./day for ewes nursing lambs, and $^1/2$ gal./day for finishing lambs. In many range areas, water is the limiting nutrient; even when present, it may be unpotable because of filth or high mineral content. For best production, range sheep should be watered daily during warm weather. However, the cost of supplying water often makes it economical to water range sheep every other day. When soft snow is available, range sheep do not need additional water except when dry feeds such as alfalfa hay and pellets are fed. If the snow is crusted with ice, the crust should be broken to allow access. Still, when possible, sheep should be allowed unlimited access to fresh, clean water.

Energy: Because so much of the diet can depend on grass and forage that is either sparse or of poor quality, the provision of adequate energy is important. Poor-quality forage, even in abundance, may not provide sufficient available energy for maintenance and production. The energy requirement of ewes is greatest during the first 8-10 wk of lactation. Because milk production declines after this period and the lambs have begun foraging, the requirement of the ewe is then reduced to prelambing levels.

Protein: Good-quality forage and pasture generally provide adequate protein for mature sheep. However, sheep do not digest poor-quality protein as efficiently as do cattle, and there are instances when a protein supplement should be fed with mature grass and hay, or when on winter range.

Sheep can convert nonprotein nitrogen (such as urea, ammonium phosphate, and biuret) into protein in the rumen, but possibly less efficiently than beef cattle. This source of nitrogen can provide at least a part of the necessary supplemental nitrogen in high-energy diets with a nitrogen:sulfur ratio of 10:1. In lamb-finishing diets, the inclusion of alfalfa, approved growth stimulants, and a source of fermentable carbohydrates (eg, ground corn, ground milo) enhance nitrogen utilization.

Minerals: Sheep require the major minerals sodium, chlorine, calcium, phosphorus, magnesium, sulfur, potassium, and trace minerals including cobalt, copper, iodine, iron, manganese, molybdenum, zinc, and selenium. Trace mineralized salt provides an economical method of preventing deficiencies of sodium, chlorine, iodine, manganese, cobalt, copper, iron, and zinc. Selenium is approved by the FDA for inclusion in salt mixtures, and such formulations should be used in deficient areas. Sheep diets usually contain sufficient potassium, iron, magnesium, sulfur, and manganese. Of the trace minerals, iodine, cobalt, and copper status in ewes are best assessed via analysis of liver biopsy tissue. Zinc adequacy can be assessed from the careful collection of non-hemolyzed blood placed in trace element-free collection tubes. Selenium status is easily assessed by collection of whole, preferably heparinized, blood.

Salt: In the USA, except on certain alkaline areas of the western range and along the seacoast, sheep should be provided with ad lib salt (sodium chloride). Sheep need salt to remain thrifty, make economical gains, lactate, and reproduce. Mature sheep will consume ~0.02 lb (9 g) of salt daily, and lambs one-half this amount. Range operators commonly provide 0.5-0.75 lb (225-350 g) of salt/ewe/mo. Salt as 0.2-0.5% of the dietary dry matter is usually adequate.

Calcium and Phosphorus: In plants, generally the leafy parts are relatively high in calcium and low in phosphorus, whereas the reverse is true of the seeds. Legumes, in general, have a higher calcium content than grasses. As grasses mature, phosphorus is transferred to the seed (grain). Furthermore, the phosphorus content of the plant is influenced markedly by the availability of phosphorus in the soil. Therefore, low-quality pasture devoid of legumes and range plants tends to be naturally low in phosphorus, particularly as the forage matures and the seeds fall. Consequently, sheep subsisting on mature, brown, summer forage and winter range sometimes develop a phosphorus deficiency. Sheep kept on such forages or fed low-quality hay with no grain should be provided a phosphorus supplement (ie, defluorinated rock phosphate) added to a salt-trace mineral mixture. Because most forages have a relatively high calcium content, particularly if there is a mixture of legumes, diets usually meet maintenance requirements for this element. However, when corn silage or other feeds from the cereal grains are fed exclusively, ground limestone should be fed daily at the rate of 0.02-0.03 lb (9-14 g). Sheep seem to be able to tolerate wide calcium:phosphorus ratios as long as their diets contain more calcium than phosphorus. However, an excess of phosphorus may be conducive to development of urinary calculi or osteodystrophy. A calcium:phosphorus ratio of 1.5:1 is appropriate for feedlot lambs. For pregnant ewes, the diet should contain ≥0.18% and, for lactating ewes, ≥0.27%. A content of 0.2-0.4% calcium is considered adequate, as long as the ratio is maintained between 1:1 and 2:1.

Iodine: Sometimes, either as a consequence of low availability of iodine from the soil or goitrogenic substances in the feed, the iodine requirements of sheep are not met in the natural diet and iodine supplements must be fed. Goitrogenic substances are found in many types of plants (eg, *Brassica* spp) and interfere with the use of iodine by the thyroid. Regions naturally deficient are found throughout the western USA, in the Great Lakes area, and in other parts of the world. A deficiency of iodine (manifested as goiter in the adult and as lack of wool and/or goiter in lambs) can be prevented by feeding stabilized iodized salt to pregnant ewes. The young of iodine-deficient ewes may be aborted, stillborn, or born with goiters. Diets of 0.2-0.8%

TABLE 40. Daily Nutrient Requirements of Sheep ▶

Body Weight		Weight Change/Day		Dry Matter per Animal*		
(kg)	(lb)	(g)	(lb)	(kg)	(lb)	(% body wt)
Ewes Maintenance‡						
50	110	10	0.02	1.0	2.2	2.0
60	132	10	0.02	1.1	2.4	1.8
70	154	10	0.02	1.2	2.6	1.7
80	176	10	0.02	1.3	2.9	1.6
90	198	10	0.02	1.4	3.1	1.5
Nonlactating—first 15 wk gestation						
50	110	30	0.07	1.2	2.6	2.4
60	132	30	0.07	1.3	2.9	2.2
70	154	30	0.07	1.4	3.1	2.0
80	176	30	0.07	1.5	3.3	1.9
90	198	30	0.07	1.6	3.5	1.8
Last 4 wk gestation (130-150% lambing rate expected) or last 4-6 wk lactation suckling singles§						
50	110	180 (45)	0.40 (0.10)	1.6	3.5	3.2
60	132	180 (45)	0.40 (0.10)	1.7	3.7	2.8
70	154	180 (45)	0.40 (0.10)	1.8	4.0	2.6
80	176	180 (45)	0.40 (0.10)	1.9	4.2	2.4
90	198	180 (45)	0.40 (0.10)	2.0	4.4	2.2
Last 4 wk gestation (180-225% lambing rate expected)						
50	110	225	0.50	1.7	3.7	3.4
60	132	225	0.50	1.8	4.0	3.0
70	154	225	0.50	1.9	4.2	2.7
80	176	225	0.50	2.0	4.4	2.5
90	198	225	0.50	2.1	4.6	2.3
First 6-8 wk lactation suckling singles or last 4-6 wk lactation suckling twins§						
50	110	-25 (90)	-0.06 (0.20)	2.1	4.6	4.2
60	132	-25 (90)	-0.06 (0.20)	2.3	5.1	3.8
70	154	-25 (90)	-0.06 (0.20)	2.5	5.5	3.6
80	176	-25 (90)	-0.06 (0.20)	2.6	5.7	3.2
90	198	-25 (90)	-0.06 (0.20)	2.7	5.9	3.0
First 6-8 wk lactation suckling twins						
50	110	-60	-0.13	2.4	5.3	4.8
60	132	-60	-0.13	2.6	5.7	4.3
70	154	-60	-0.13	2.8	6.2	4.0
80	176	-60	-0.13	3.0	6.6	3.8
90	198	-60	-0.13	3.2	7.0	3.6

◀ **TABLE 40.** (*continued*)

TDN		Energy[†]		Crude Protein		Ca	P	Vitamin A Activity	Vitamin E Activity
(kg)	(lb)	DE (Mcal)	ME (Mcal)	(g)	(lb)	(g)	(g)	(IU)	(IU)
Ewes Maintenance[‡]									
0.55	1.2	2.4	2.0	95	0.21	2.0	1.8	2,350	15
0.61	1.3	2.7	2.2	104	0.23	2.3	2.1	2,820	16
0.66	1.5	2.9	2.4	113	0.25	2.5	2.4	3,290	18
0.72	1.6	3.2	2.6	122	0.27	2.7	2.8	3,760	20
0.78	1.7	3.4	2.8	131	0.29	2.9	3.1	4,230	21
Nonlactating—first 15 wk gestation									
0.67	1.5	3.0	2.4	112	0.25	2.9	2.1	2,350	18
0.72	1.6	3.2	2.6	121	0.27	3.2	2.5	2,820	20
0.77	1.7	3.4	2.8	130	0.29	3.5	2.9	3,290	21
0.82	1.8	3.6	3.0	139	0.31	3.8	3.3	3,760	22
0.87	1.9	3.8	3.2	148	0.33	4.1	3.6	4,230	24
Last 4 wk gestation (130-150% lambing rate expected) or last 4-6 wk lactation suckling singles[§]									
0.94	2.1	4.1	3.4	175	0.38	5.9	4.8	4,250	24
1.00	2.2	4.4	3.6	184	0.40	6.0	5.2	5,100	26
1.06	2.3	4.7	3.8	193	0.42	6.2	5.6	5950	27
1.12	2.4	4.9	4.0	202	0.44	6.3	6.1	6,800	28
1.18	2.5	5.1	4.2	212	0.47	6.4	6.5	7,650	30
Last 4 wk gestation (180-225% lambing rate expected)									
1.10	2.4	4.8	4.0	196	0.43	6.2	3.4	4,250	26
1.17	2.6	5.1	4.2	205	0.45	6.9	4.0	5,100	27
1.24	2.8	5.4	4.4	214	0.47	7.6	4.5	5,950	28
1.30	2.9	5.7	4.7	223	0.49	8.3	5.1	6,800	30
1.37	3.0	6.0	5.0	232	0.51	8.9	5.7	7,650	32
First 6-8 wk lactation suckling singles or last 4-6 wk lactation suckling twins[§]									
1.36	3.0	6.0	4.9	304	0.67	8.9	6.1	4,250	32
1.50	3.3	6.6	5.4	319	0.70	9.1	6.6	5,100	34
1.63	3.6	7.2	5.9	334	0.73	9.3	7.0	5,950	38
1.69	3.7	7.4	6.1	344	0.76	9.5	7.4	6,800	39
1.75	3.8	7.6	6.3	353	0.78	9.6	7.8	7,650	40
First 6-8 wk lactation suckling twins									
1.56	3.4	6.9	5.6	389	0.86	10.5	7.3	5,000	36
1.69	3.7	7.4	6.1	405	0.89	10.7	7.7	6,000	39
1.82	4.0	8.0	6.6	420	0.92	11.0	8.1	7,000	42
1.95	4.3	8.6	7.0	435	0.96	11.2	8.6	8,000	45
2.08	4.6	9.2	7.5	450	0.99	11.4	9.0	9,000	48

(*continued*)

TABLE 40. Daily Nutrient Requirements of Sheep (*continued*) ▶

Body Weight		Weight Change/Day		Dry Matter per Animal*		
(kg)	(lb)	(g)	(lb)	(kg)	(lb)	(% body wt)
Replacement ewe lambs¶						
30	66	227	0.50	1.2	2.6	4.0
40	88	182	0.40	1.4	3.1	3.5
50	110	120	0.26	1.5	3.3	3.0
60	132	100	0.22	1.5	3.3	2.5
70	154	100	0.22	1.5	3.3	2.1
Replacement ram lambs¶						
40	88	330	0.73	1.8	4.0	4.5
60	132	320	0.70	2.4	5.3	4.0
80	176	290	0.64	2.8	6.2	3.5
100	220	250	0.55	3.0	6.6	3.0
Lambs finishing—4-7 mo old#						
30	66	295	0.65	1.3	2.9	4.3
40	88	275	0.60	1.6	3.5	4.0
50	110	205	0.45	1.6	3.5	3.2
Early weaned lambs—moderate growth potential#						
10	22	200	0.44	0.5	1.1	5.0
20	44	250	0.55	1.0	2.2	5.0
30	66	300	0.66	1.3	2.9	4.3
40	88	345	0.76	1.5	3.3	3.8
50	110	300	0.66	1.5	3.3	3.0

*To convert dry matter to an as-fed basis, divide dry-matter values by the percentage of dry matter in the particular feed.

†One kg TDN (total digestible nutrients) = 4.4 Mcal DE (digestible energy), and ME (metabolizable energy) = 82% of DE

‡Values are applicable for ewes in moderate condition. Fat ewes should be fed according to the next lower weight category and thin ewes at the next higher weight category. Once desired or moderate weight condition is attained, that weight category should be used through all production stages.

ppm are usually sufficient, depending on the animals' level of production (maintenance/growth, lactation, etc).

Cobalt: Sheep require ~0.1 ppm of cobalt in their diet. Cobalt-deficient soils are found in North America, but are relatively rare compared with other parts of the world. Normally, legumes have a higher content than grasses. Because cobalt levels of the feedstuffs are seldom known, a good practice is to feed trace mineralized salt that contains cobalt.

Copper: Pregnant ewes require ~5 mg of copper (Cu) daily, which is the amount provided when the forage contains ≥5 ppm. However, the amount of copper in the diet necessary to prevent copper deficiency is influenced by the intake of other dietary constituents, notably molybdenum (Mo), inorganic sulfate, and iron. High intake of molybdenum in the presence of adequate sulfate increases copper requirements. Because sheep are more susceptible than cattle to Cu toxicity, care must be taken to avoid excessive copper intake (p 2353). Toxicity may be produced in lambs being fed diets with 10-20 ppm of copper, particularly if the Cu:Mo ratio is >10:1. The Cu:Mo ration should be maintained between 5:1 and 10:1.

◀ **TABLE 40.** (*continued*)

TDN		Energy[†]		Crude Protein		Ca	P	Vitamin A Activity	Vitamin E Activity
(kg)	(lb)	DE (Mcal)	ME (Mcal)	(g)	(lb)	(g)	(g)	(IU)	(IU)
Replacement ewe lambs[¶]									
0.78	1.7	3.4	2.8	185	0.41	6.4	2.6	1,410	18
0.91	2.0	4.0	3.3	176	0.39	5.9	2.6	1,880	21
0.88	1.9	3.9	3.2	136	0.30	4.8	2.4	2,350	22
0.88	1.9	3.9	3.2	134	0.30	4.5	2.5	2,820	22
0.88	1.9	3.9	3.2	132	0.29	4.6	2.8	3,290	22
Replacement ram lambs[¶]									
1.1	2.5	5.0	4.1	243	0.54	7.8	3.7	1,880	24
1.5	3.4	6.7	5.5	263	0.58	8.4	4.2	2,820	26
1.8	3.9	7.8	6.4	268	0.59	8.5	4.6	3,760	28
1.9	4.2	8.4	6.9	264	0.58	8.2	4.8	4,700	30
Lambs finishing—4-7 mo old[#]									
0.94	2.1	4.1	3.4	191	0.42	6.6	3.2	1,410	20
1.22	2.7	5.4	4.4	185	0.41	6.6	3.3	1,880	24
1.23	2.7	5.4	4.4	160	0.35	5.6	3.0	2,350	24
Early weaned lambs—moderate growth potential[#]									
0.40	0.9	1.8	1.4	127	0.38	4.0	1.9	470	10
0.80	1.8	3.5	2.9	167	0.37	5.4	2.5	940	20
1.00	2.2	4.4	3.6	191	0.42	6.7	3.2	1,410	20
1.16	2.6	5.1	4.2	202	0.44	7.7	3.9	1,880	22
1.16	2.6	5.1	4.2	181	0.40	7.0	3.8	2,350	22

[§]Values in parentheses are for ewes suckling lambs the last 4-6 wk of lactation.
[¶]Lambs intended for breeding; thus, maximal weight gains and finish are of secondary importance.
[#]Maximal weight gains expected

Adapted, with permission, from *Nutrient Requirements of Sheep*, 1985, National Academy of Sciences, National Academy Press, Washington, DC.

Selenium: Selenium is effective in at least partially controlling nutritional muscular dystrophy. Areas east of the Mississippi River and in the northwestern USA appear to be low in selenium. The dietary requirement is ~0.3 ppm. Providing selenium-containing mineral mixture may prevent selenium deficiency if animals are allowed free access. Levels of 7-10 ppm or higher may be toxic.

Zinc: Growing lambs require ~30 ppm of zinc in the diet on a dry-matter basis. The requirement for normal testicular development is somewhat higher. Classic zinc deficiency (parakeratosis) is more common in other small ruminants (goats), but is occasionally encountered in sheep, particularly if fed excessive quantities of dietary calcium (legumes).

Vitamins: Sheep diets usually contain an ample supply of vitamins A (provitamin A), D, and E. Under certain circumstances, however, supplements may be needed. The B vitamins and vitamin K are synthesized by the rumen microorganisms and, under practical conditions, supplements are unnecessary. However, polioencephalomalacia can be seen and is due to aberrations in ruminal thiamine metabolism, secondary to altered ruminal pH and/or microflora content. Vitamin C is synthesized in the tissues of sheep. On diets rich in carotene, such as high-quality pasture or green hays, sheep can store large quantities of vitamin A in the liver, often sufficient to meet their requirements for up to 6 mo.

Vitamin D_2 is derived from sun-cured forage, and vitamin D_3 from exposure of the skin to ultraviolet light. When exposure of the skin to sunshine is reduced by prolonged cloudy weather or confinement rearing, and when the vitamin D_2 content of the diet is low, the amount supplied may be inadequate. The requirement for vitamin D is increased when the amounts of either calcium or phosphorus in the diet are low or when the ratio between them is wide. But such dietary modification should be done cautiously, as vitamin D toxicity is a severe syndrome. Fast-growing lambs kept in sheds away from direct sunlight or maintained on green feeds (high carotene) during the winter months (low irradiation) may have impaired bone formation and show other signs of vitamin D deficiency. Normally, sheep on pasture seldom need vitamin D supplements.

The major sources of vitamin E in the natural diet of sheep are green feeds and the germ of seeds. As vitamin E is poorly stored in the body, a daily intake is needed. When ewes are being fed poor-quality hay or forage, supplemental vitamin E may result in improved production, lamb weaning weights, and colostrum quality. Vitamin E deficiency in young lambs may contribute to nutritional muscular dystrophy if selenium intake is low.

FEEDING PRACTICES

Feeding Farm Sheep

See TABLE 40 for nutrient requirements of sheep. Using these data and the results of practical experience, suggestions for feeding sheep are outlined below.

Use of Forage: Sheep make excellent use of high-quality roughage stored either as hay or low-moisture, grass-legume silage or occasionally chopped green feed. Good-quality hay or stored forage is a highly productive feed; poor-quality forage, no matter how much is available, is suitable only for maintenance. Hay quality is determined primarily by the following: 1) its botanic composition, eg, a mixture of palatable grasses and legumes such as brome/alfalfa or bluegrass/clover; 2) the stage of maturity when cut, eg, the grass before heading and alfalfa before one-tenth bloom; 3) method and speed of harvesting because they affect loss of leaf, bleaching by sun, and leaching by rain; and 4) spoilage and loss during storage and feeding. In general, the same factors influence the quality of silage. Complete analysis of cut-stored forages enhances the utilization of these feedstuffs and allows for the most efficient use of supplemental grains and minerals.

Feeding Ewes

The period from weaning to breeding of ewes is critical if a high twinning rate is desired. Ewes should not be allowed to become excessively fat but should make daily gains from weaning to breeding. The rate of gain depends on the desired weight, but should be ~60-70% of projected mature weight at breeding and 80-90% of projected mature weight at lambing. If pasture production is inadequate, ewes may be confined and fed high-quality hay and a small amount of grain if necessary. Breeding while grazing legume pastures (eg, sage, white clovers) may tend to depress the size of the lamb crop, lowering the intake of certain feedstuffs. After mating, ewes can be maintained on pasture, thus allowing feed to be conserved for other times of the year. Good pasture for this period allows the ewes to enter the winter feeding period in good condition. When pasture is unavailable, an appropriate ration should be formulated (TABLE 41).

During the last 6-8 wk of pregnancy, growth of the fetus is rapid. This is a critical period nutritionally, particularly for ewes carrying more than one fetus. Beginning 6-8 wk before lambing, the plane of nutrition should be increased gradually and continued without interruption until after lambing. The amount offered depends on the condition or fat covering of the ewes and quality of the forage. If ewes are in fair to good condition, 0.5-0.75 lb (225-350 g) daily is usually sufficient. The roughage content of the ration should provide all the protein required for all nonlactating ewes. If necessary, the ewes may be classified according to age, condition, and number of fetuses and divided into groups for different treatment.

Lactating Ewes: Succulent pasture furnishes adequate energy, protein, vitamins, and minerals for ewes and lambs; no added grain is necessary. When pasture is not being

TABLE 41. Rations for Pregnant Ewes up to 6 Wk Before Lambing

Feed	Ration No.			
	1	2	3	4
	lb (kg)	lb (kg)	lb (kg)	lb (kg)
Legume hay, such as alfalfa, clover, or lespedeza	3.0-4.5 (1.36-2.04)	1.5-2.0 (0.68-0.91)	—	—
Corn or sorghum silage	—	4-5 (1.81-2.27)	—	—
Legume grass, low-moisture silage (50%)	—	—	6-8 (2.72-3.63)	—
Cottonseed, soybean, linseed, or peanut meal (90%); limestone (10%)	—	—	—	0.25 (0.112)
Minerals[*]	ad lib	ad lib	ad lib	ad lib

[*]Mineral mix: 2 parts dicalcium phosphate to 1 part trace mineralized salt

TABLE 42. Grain Mixture for Pregnant Ewes

Feed	Mixture No.			
	1	2	3	4
	%	%	%	%
Whole barley, corn, or wheat	60	75	75	50
Whole oats	30	—	25	50
Beet pulp, dried	—	25	—	—
Wheat bran	10	—	—	—

used (confinement rearing), ewes should be fed one of the rations outlined for pregnant ewes in TABLE 41, and 1-1.5 lb (450-675 g) of one of the grain mixtures in TABLE 42. Ewes should have access to a mixture of trace mineralized salt and dicalcium phosphate. Ewes with twin or triplet lambs should be separated from those with single lambs and fed more concentrates (grain) and/or better-quality forages. Ewes nursing twin lambs produce 20-40% more milk than those with singles. Under confinement rearing or accelerated lambing, lambs are commonly weaned at 2 mo of age. The ewe's milk production declines rapidly after this period, and creep feed is more efficiently converted into weight gains when fed to lambs than to the ewe.

Feeding Lambs

From ~2 wk of age, lambs should have free access to creep feed unless they are born and raised on succulent pasture. Where pasture is limited, they should be creep-fed for 1-2 mo until adequate forages are available. If pasture will not be available until the lambs are 3-4 mo old, they can be finished in a dry lot. The grain used should be ground coarse or rolled, but as the feeding period progresses, whole grains may be used. Small amounts of fresh, clean grain should be slowly introduced to the lambs' diet. The amount of grain is increased gradually until the lambs are on full feed.

Feeding lambs from birth to market in a dry lot, together with early weaning at 2-3 mo of age, has become more popular throughout the USA. A complete diet of hay, grain, and vitamin-mineral supplement is ground, mixed, and either fed as is or pressed into pellets

TABLE 43. Creep Rations for Suckling and Early-weaned Lambs

Feed	Mixture No.			
	1	2	3	4
	%	%	%	%
Alfalfa hay, leafy ground	25	30	40	—
Dehydrated alfalfa leaf meal	53.5	—	20	48
Corn, shelled	—	—	—	35
Corn or wheat	—	55	—	—
Oats or barley	—	—	20	—
Soybean, linseed, or cottonseed meal	19	10	10	10
Molasses	—	3.5	8.5	5.5
Bone meal or dicalcium phosphate	1	1	1	1
Limestone	1	—	—	—
Trace mineralized salt	0.5	0.5	0.5	0.5
Antibiotic	—	—	0.002	0.002

$^3/_{16}$- or $^3/_8$-in. (5-10 mm) long. Such lambs usually reach market weight in $3^1/_2$-4 mo. *See* TABLE 43 for some examples of creep rations used in dry lot feeding.

Rearing Lambs on Milk Replacer: Orphaned lambs, extras, triplets, or those from poor-milking ewes can be raised on milk replacers to improve productivity. Such lambs should receive 10-20% of their body wt in colostrum divided into multiple feedings within 18-24 hr of birth. If ewe colostrum is unavailable, a frozen, pooled supply from several cows can be used. Milk replacers designed specifically for lambs are available and contain ~30% fat, 25% protein, and a high level of antibiotic. Under certain conditions it may be advisable to inject orphaned lambs with vitamins A, D, and E and selenium. In hand-drearing systems, milk replacer should be fed at 10-20% of the lamb's body wt, divided into 4-6 feedings/day during the first week of life. The number of feedings can be reduced over time to only 2/day by 3-4 wk of age.

Multiple-nipple pails or containers can be used. Cold milk replacer can be used by older lambs who nurse more often. By 9-10 days of age, lambs should be given water in addition to the milk if a creep ration is offered. They can be weaned abruptly at 4-5 wk of age if consumption of creep feed and water intake is at a reasonable level.

Finishing Feeder Lambs: Lambs should be preconditioned before they leave the producer's property. This includes starting on feed, vaccinating, worming, and under some conditions, shearing. If this is not done, the lambs should be rested for several days and fed dry, average-quality hay after arrival at the feedlot. See TABLE 44 for some recommended formulas for finishing lambs.

Feeding Method: There is no best method or diet for finishing lambs. They may be finished on good to excellent quality forage (alfalfa, wheat) with no supplemental grain. They may be started on pasture or crop residue and moved to grain feeding systems as the forage is used up. When fed in a dry lot, they are usually allowed free access to feedstuffs. These diets may be completely pelleted, ground and mixed, a mixture of ground forage (alfalfa) pellets and grain, and/or high-concentrate type. Self-feeding usually results in maximal feed intake and gain, and labor costs may be reduced. Hand-feeding can be mechanized with an auger system or self-unloading wagon. It involves feeding at regular intervals so that the lambs consume all the feed before more feed is offered. Feed consumption and gain can be controlled. When used, corn silage should be hand-fed to minimize spoilage.

TABLE 44. Recommended Formulas for Finishing Lambs*

Feed	Starter 10-day Period		High Roughage		High Concentrate	Corn Silage
	Loose	Pelleted	Loose	Pelleted		
Grain (corn, barley, or milo)[†]	500	200	780	400	1,500	540
Alfalfa hay	1,280	1,700	1,000	1,400	200	
Molasses	100	100	100			
Oilseed meal	100		100			100
Urea					45	
Beet pulp			200	200		
Silage						1,350
Limestone	10				35	10
Trace mineralized salt	10		20	20	35	
Antibiotic (g)	50	20	20	10	20	10
Vitamin A (IU/ton)						1,000,000

*Lb/ton or kg/metric ton; feeder lambs should have ~14% crude protein in rations (dry basis).
[†]Wheat can be substituted for other grains, but a period of time should be allowed for adaptation.

Starting on Feed: Feeders who feed lambs year-round, or feed heavy lambs, usually prefer to place the lambs on full feed as soon as possible (10-14 days). Lambs can be started safely on self-fed, ground, or pelleted diets containing 60-70% hay. Within 2 wk the hay can be reduced to 30-40% when the ration is not pelleted. Other roughages such as cottonseed hulls or silage can be used in a similar manner.

Vaccinating against enterotoxemia (*Clostridium perfringens* types C and D) and feeding tetracyclines (22 mg/kg/day) in diets are useful in starting lambs on feed more rapidly and controlling *Pasteurella multocida* and *Escherichia coli* enteritis infections.

Feeds: Corn, sorghum, or alfalfa silage can replace about half the hay with hand-feeding, but finish and yield will be decreased to some extent. *See* TABLE 45 for rations that can be used in self-feeding. Corn, barley, milo, wheat, or a mixture of these are used; 0.5% salt and 0.5% bone meal or equivalent should be added to the grain. Pelleting of rations for finishing lambs is beneficial when low-grade roughages or high-roughage rations are used. Caution should be used when feeding large amounts of wheat; lambs not adapted to it are more apt to develop acute indigestion than if fed grains such as corn, sorghum, or barley.

Mineral supplements, including salt, should be offered separately whether or not they are included in the grain mixture. Approved growth stimulants usually increase growth rate 10-15% and feed efficiency 8-10% but may decrease carcass quality.

Feeding Mature Breeding Rams

Mature breeding rams should be grazed on pasture when available, or fed rations 1, 2, or 3 according to TABLE 41. If rams are in a thrifty condition at breeding time and the ewes are on a good flushing pasture, it should not be necessary to grain-feed the rams while with the ewes. Rams should be maintained at a good body condition (3-3.5 on a 1-5 scale) prior to the breeding season. When daytime temperatures are >90°F (32°C), rams should be shorn before mating and turned out with the ewes at night only.

Feeding Range Sheep

The condition of the sheep, the amount and kind of forage on the range, and the climatic conditions determine the kind and amount of supplement to feed. Supplements

TABLE 45. Pattern for Range Supplements for Sheep

Supplement Group	Supplement Subgroup	Feedstuff	Suggested Maximum %	Recommended Amount of Protein		
				high %	medium %	low %
Energy feeds	Grains	Barley	75		33.0	57.5
		Corn	60	5.0	10.0	15.0
		Wheat	60			
		Milo	60			
		Oats	15			
		Screenings No. 1	10			
	Mill feeds	Wheat mixed feed	10			
		Shorts	10			
		Molasses	15	5.0	5.0	10.0
		Beet pulp	10			10.0
Protein supplements	30-40% Protein feeds	Cottonseed meal	75	62.5	32.5	5.0
		Linseed meal	25			
		Soybean meal	75	10.0	10.0	
		Peanut meal	25			
	20-30% Protein feeds	Corn gluten feed	15			
		Corn distiller's dried grains	10			
		Wheat distiller's grains	10			
		Brewer's dried grains	5			
		Safflower meal	25			
		Cull beans	15			
Mineral supplements		Bone meal or defluorinated phosphate		4.0	3.0	2.0
		Dicalcium phosphate		1.0	0.5	0.5
		Disodium phosphate				
		Monocalcium phosphate				
		Monosodium phosphate				
		Salt or trace mineralized salt				
Vitamin supplements		Dehydrated alfalfa meal	20	12.5	6.0	
		Sun-cured alfalfa meal	20			
		Vitamin A and carotene concentrates				
Total				100.0	100.0	100.0
Suggested composition						
		Total crude protein (%)		36.0	24.0	12.0
		Phosphorus (%)		1.5	1.0	0.5
		Carotene (mg/kg)		35.0	17.0	—
		Rate of feeding (g/day)—ewes		115	150-225	90-450

usually consist of high-protein pellets or cottonseed meal and salt, medium-protein pellets, low-protein pellets or corn, alfalfa hay, and minerals. When the diets of sheep on the western winter range are supplemented properly, the lamb crop can be increased 10-15% and wool production increased by ~1 lb (400-500 g) per ewe. One recommended practice is to feed ~0.25 lb (115 g) of high-protein (36%) supplement or 0.33-0.5 lb (150-225 g) of medium-protein (24%) pellets ~3 wk before and during the breeding season, during extremely cold weather, and for ~1 mo before green feed starts in the spring. In addition, small lambs, small yearling ewes, old ewes with poor teeth, and thin ewes should be separated from the main flock and fed one of the above supplements from about December 1 until shearing time. In many instances, the old ewes, lambs, and yearlings from more than one band can be maintained in a flock for special dietary supplementation. When sheep are unable to obtain a full ration of forage because of deep snow or other weather conditions, 1-3 lb (450-1,350 g) of alfalfa hay and 0.2-0.3 lb (90-150 g) of a low-protein pellet mixture or corn should be fed (TABLE 45). If alfalfa hay is not available, 0.5-1 lb (225-450 g) per head of a low-protein pellet mixture should be fed daily for emergency feeding periods.

Deficiencies of Range Forages: Deficiencies most apt to be seen among range forages are protein, energy, and phosphorus. These are most prevalent as the forages approach maturity or are dormant, and they may appear singly or in combination. Range sheep often travel long distances and are exposed to cold weather, resulting in higher energy requirements. Protein supplements (soybean or cottonseed meal, alfalfa pellets, etc) increase digestibility and use of poor-quality forages. When possible, the inclusion of a phosphorus supplement (eg, dicalcium phosphate, monocalcium phosphate, defluorinated rock phosphate) to a salt or trace mineral salt mixture may greatly improve productivity. Most ranges used for winter grazing are considered adequate in carotene, as many species of browse furnish as much carotene as sun-cured alfalfa hay. However, when sheep are required to graze dry grass ranges for >6 mo without intermittent periods of green feed, vitamin A supplements are recommended. The addition of 45-50 IU of vitamin A/kg/day improves productivity in cases of extended consumption (>2 mo) of dry or weathered forages.

Mineral Mixtures: On the range, portable mineral boxes are convenient for sheep. One of these mineral mixtures should be fed free choice. A salt and bone meal or phosphorus supplement is used if there are no iodine or trace-mineral deficiencies. Iodized salt is substituted for regular salt when an iodine deficiency exists, and trace mineralized salt is substituted if deficiencies of trace minerals are present.

Under winter range conditions, the amount of phosphorus supplement that should be added to range pellets varies with the type of range forage available, the rate of feeding, and the ingredients used in the pellets. It is suggested that 36, 24, and 12% protein pellets contain 1.5, 1.0, and 0.5% phosphorus, respectively. When feeding supplemental protein, 36% protein pellets should be fed at the rate of 0.25 lb (115 g) per head daily, the 24% protein pellets at 0.33-0.5 lb (150-225 g), and the 12% protein pellets at 0.2-0.5 lb (90-225 g), together with alfalfa or clover hay.

NUTRITIONAL DISEASES

Nutritional diseases in sheep are for the most part the same as those seen in goats (*see* p 1870).

Enterotoxemia is a feed-related malady that causes almost sudden death in sheep due to a toxin produced by *Clostridium perfringens* type D and sometimes type C. The organism appears to be widespread in nature. Under conditions of high carbohydrate consumption or high intake of immature succulent forage, the causative bacteria multiply rapidly and produce an ε toxin that increases intestinal permeability. Protection of lambs is possible by vaccinating twice at least 10 days apart with *C perfringens* type D toxoid, or by administering antitoxin at birth. (*See also* p 493.)

White muscle disease is caused by low levels of selenium and possibly vitamin E. Signs include stiffness (especially in the hindquarters), tucked-up rear flanks, arched backs, pneumonia, and acute death. On necropsy, white striations are found in cardiac, diaphragmatic, and skeletal muscles. Levels of AST and lactic dehydrogenase are increased, indicating muscle damage. Blood levels of the selenium-containing glutathione peroxidase are reduced. Although several feedstuffs are fairly rich in selenium and vitamin E, it may be a good management practice in deficient areas to inject lambs shortly after birth with a preparation of vitamin E and selenium designed for parenteral use. The use of a selenium and/or vitamin E supplemented trace mineral mixture (90 ppm) as the only source of salt fed may be useful as a preventive measure. (*See also* p 948.)

NUTRITION: SMALL ANIMALS

Domestic dogs and cats are both members of the order Carnivora. Observations of feral canids indicate that their feeding habits are broad and include various parts of plants as well as both small and large prey. By comparison, cats show no omnivorous feeding behaviors and require nutrients that are produced exclusively by other animals and not plants (eg, vitamin A, arachidonic acid, and taurine). Thus, dogs are described as omnivores, while cats are regarded as true carnivores.

Using appropriate feeding practices is one of the most important components of maintaining companion animal health. Nutritional management is also important as an integral part of both preventive health care and treatment protocols for medical and surgical patients. Feeding an appropriately formulated and tested complete and balanced commercial diet is the simplest method of meeting the nutritional requirements of dogs or cats. Numerous products are available, and many are formulated for specific life stages. However, dogs and cats can thrive well eating a variety of commercial or home-prepared foods, which may include vegetables and synthetic supplements.

In recent years, companion animal obesity (ie, overnutrition) has become as much of a problem as undernutrition; thus, a systematic method of assessment of an animal's overall condition is necessary. Body condition scoring is used in many species to provide an estimate of nutritional adequacy of a diet and amount of food intake. To perform this assessment, dogs and cats should be weighed and a body condition score of 1-5 assigned as follows: 1) Emaciated: ribs, lumbar vertebrae, pelvic bones, and all body prominences evident from a distance. No discernible body fat. Obvious absence of muscle mass. 2) Thin: ribs easily palpated and may be visible with no palpable fat. Tops of lumbar vertebrae visible. Pelvic bones less prominent. Obvious waist and abdominal tuck. 3) Moderate: ribs palpable without excess fat covering. Abdomen tucked up when viewed from side. 4) Stout: general fleshy appearance. Ribs palpable with difficulty. Noticeable fat deposits over lumbar spine and tail base. Abdominal tuck may be absent. 5) Obese: large fat deposits over chest, spine, and tail base. Waist and abdominal tuck absent. Fat deposits on neck and limbs. Abdomen distended.

NUTRITIONAL REQUIREMENTS AND RELATED DISEASES

Dogs are a biologically diverse species, with normal body weight of 4-80 kg (2-175 lb). Normal birth weight of pups depends on breed type (120 to 550 g). The first 2 wk of a puppy's life is spent eating, seeking warmth, and sleeping. External food sources beyond bitch's milk is rarely needed unless the bitch cannot produce enough milk or the puppy is orphaned. In these cases, the puppy must be hand-reared. Growth rates of puppies are rapid for the first 5 mo; in this period, pups gain an average of 2-4 g/day/kg of their anticipated adult weight. The growth rate begins to plateau after 6 mo, and growth may be completed by 9-12 mo of age in small breeds and by 12-18 mo in large breeds. By comparison, the average mature body weight of domestic cats is 3.2 kg (7 lb) for toms, and 2.8 kg (6 lb) for queens. Normal birth weight of kittens is 90-100 g. The growth rate is exceptionally rapid for the first 3-4 mo, and kittens gain 50-100 g/wk. The growth rate begins to plateau at 150-160 days of age, and growth is completed within 200-220 days.

Dogs and cats require specific dietary nutrient concentrations based on their life stage. The Association of American Feed Control Officials (AAFCO) publishes dog and cat nutrient profiles for growth, maintenance, and reproduction. These are based in part on the 1974 and 1985 National Research Council (NRC) nutrient requirements for these species (TABLE 46 and TABLE 47). Updated NRC requirements have recently been established and will be published soon. These provide a comprehensive review of the nutrient requirements for various life stages and may be used by AAFCO to modify their profiles.

In developed countries, nutritional diseases are rarely seen in dogs and cats especially when they are fed good quality commercial rations or nutritionally balanced home-made diets. Dog or cat foods or homemade diets derived from a single food item are inadequate. For example, feeding predominately meat or even an exclusive hamburger and rice diet to dogs can induce calcium deficiency and secondary hypoparathyroidism.

TABLE 46. AAFCO Nutrient Requirements for Dogs*

Nutrient	Growth and Reproduction Minimum	Adult Maintenance Minimum	Adult Maintenance Maximum
Protein (%)	22.0	18.0	
Arginine (%)	0.62	0.51	
Histidine (%)	0.22	0.18	
Isoleucine (%)	0.45	0.37	
Leucine (%)	0.72	0.59	
Lysine (%)	0.77	0.63	
Methionine + cystine (%)	0.53	0.43	
Phenylalanine + tyrosine (%)	0.89	0.73	
Threonine (%)	0.58	0.48	
Tryptophan (%)	0.20	0.16	
Valine (%)	0.48	0.39	
Fat (%)	8.0	5.0	
Linoleic acid (%)	1.0	1.0	
Minerals			
Calcium (%)	1.0	0.6	2.5
Phosphorus (%)	0.8	0.5	1.6
Ca:P ratio	1:1	1:1	2:1
Potassium (%)	0.6	0.6	
Sodium (%)	0.3	0.06	
Chloride (%)	0.45	0.09	
Magnesium (%)	0.04	0.04	0.3
Iron (mg/kg)	80	80	3,000
Copper (mg/kg)	7.3	7.3	250
Manganese (mg/kg)	5.0	5.0	
Zinc (mg/kg)	120	120	1,000
Iodine (mg/kg)	1.5	1.5	50
Selenium (mg/kg)	0.11	0.11	2
Vitamins			
Vitamin A (IU/kg)	5,000	5,000	250,000
Vitamin D (IU/kg)	500	500	5,000
Vitamin E (IU/kg)	50	50	1,000
Thiamine (mg/kg)	1.0	1.0	
Riboflavin (mg/kg)	2.2	2.2	
Panthothenic acid (mg/kg)	10	10	
Niacin (mg/kg)	11.4	11.4	
Pyridoxine (mg/kg)	1.0	1.0	
Folic acid (mg/kg)	0.18	0.18	
Vitamin B_{12} (mg/kg)	0.022	0.022	
Choline (mg/kg)	1,200	1,200	

*Nutrient requirements are indicated on a dry-matter basis. These AAFCO nutrient profiles for dog foods presume an energy density of 3.5 kcal ME/g dry matter. Rations >4.0 kcal/g should be corrected for energy density.

Feeding raw, freshwater fish to cats can induce a thiamine deficiency. Feeding liver can induce a vitamin A toxicity in both dogs and cats. Malnutrition has been seen in dogs and cats fed "natural," "organic," or "vegetarian" diets produced by owners with good intentions, and most published recipes have been only crudely balanced (by computer) using nutrient averages. Because the palatability, digestibility, and safety of these recipes have

TABLE 47. AAFCO Nutrient Requirements for Cats[*]

Nutrient	Growth and Reproduction Minimum	Adult Maintenance Minimum	Adult Maintenance Maximum
Protein (%)	30.0	26.0	
Arginine (%)	1.25	1.04	
Histidine (%)	0.31	0.31	
Isoleucine (%)	0.52	0.52	
Leucine (%)	1.25	1.25	
Lysine (%)	1.20	0.83	
Methionine + cystine (%)	1.10	1.10	
Methionine (%)	0.62	0.62	1.5
Phenylalanine + tyrosine (%)	0.88	0.88	
Phenylalanine (%)	0.42	0.42	
Taurine (extruded, %)	0.10	0.10	
Taurine (canned, %)	0.20	0.20	
Threonine (%)	0.73	0.73	
Tryptophan (%)	0.25	0.16	
Valine (%)	0.62	0.62	
Fat (%)	9.0	9.0	
Linoleic acid (%)	0.5	0.5	
Arachidonic acid (%)	0.02	0.02	
Minerals			
Calcium (%)	1.0	0.6	
Phosphorus (%)	0.8	0.5	
Potassium (%)	0.6	0.6	
Sodium (%)	0.2	0.2	
Chloride (%)	0.3	0.3	
Magnesium (%)	0.08	0.04	
Iron (mg/kg)	80	80	
Copper (mg/kg)	5	5	
Iodine (mg/kg)	0.35	0.35	
Zinc (mg/kg)	75	75	2,000
Manganese (mg/kg)	7.5	7.5	
Selenium (mg/kg)	0.1	0.1	
Vitamins			
Vitamin A (IU/kg)	9,000	5,000	750,000
Vitamin D (IU/kg)	750	500	10,000
Vitamin E (IU/kg)	30	30	
Vitamin K (mg/kg)	0.1	0.1	
Thiamine (mg/kg)	5.0	5.0	
Riboflavin (mg/kg)	4.0	4.0	
Pyridoxine (mg/kg)	4.0	4.0	
Niacin (mg/kg)	60	60	
Panthothenic acid (mg/kg)	5.0	5.0	
Folic acid (mg/kg)	0.8	0.8	
Biotin (mg/kg)	0.07	0.07	
Vitamin B_{12} (mg/kg)	0.02	0.02	
Choline (mg/kg)	2,400	2,400	

[*]Nutrient requirements are indicated on a dry-matter basis. These AAFCO nutrient profiles for cat foods presume an energy density of 4.0 kcal ME/g dry matter. Rations >4.5 kcal/g should be corrected for energy density.

not been adequately or scientifically tested, it is difficult to characterize all of these homemade diets. Generally, most formulations contain excessive protein and phosphorus and are deficient in calcium, vitamin E, and microminerals such as copper, zinc, and potassium. Also, the energy density of these diets may be unbalanced relative to the other nutrients. Commonly used meat and carbohydrate ingredients contain more phosphorus than calcium. Homemade feline diets that are not actually deficient in fat or energy usually contain a vegetable oil that cats do not find palatable; therefore, less food is eaten causing a calorie deficiency. Rarely are homemade diets balanced for microminerals or vitamins.

Some nutritional diseases are seen secondary to other pathologic conditions or anorexia, or both. Owner neglect is also a frequent contributing factor in malnutrition.

Water: Clean fresh water should be available at all times. Multiple water sources encourage consumption. Several approaches have been used to estimate daily water needs. In a thermoneutral environment, most mammalian species need ~44-66 mL/kg body wt. Another approach takes into account the fact that water needs appear to be highly associated with the amount of food consumed. In this case, daily maintenance fluid requirements in mL should equal the animal's maintenance energy requirement in kcal of metabolizable energy (ME). A third technique sets daily water intake as 2-3 times the dietary dry matter intake. When provided ample amounts of water, healthy animals can effectively self-regulate their intake. Water deficiency can be seen as a result of poor husbandry or disease. Dehydration is a serious problem in disorders of the GI, respiratory, and urinary systems. During anorexia or increased fluid losses, a 2-5% (dogs) or 1-2% (cats) glucose and electrolyte solution should be administered PO, SC, or IV to adult dogs or cats at 60-80 mL/kg body wt/day (80-100 mL/kg in puppies and kittens) to maintain normal fluid balance.

Energy: The most useful measure of energy for nutritional purposes is ME, which is defined as that portion of the total energy of a diet that is retained within the body. It is typically measured in calories or joules. Dogs and cats require sufficient energy to allow for optimal use of proteins and to maintain optimal body weight and condition through growth, maintenance, activity, pregnancy, and lactation. Of the 6 nutrient groups, only protein, fat, and carbohydrate provide energy, whereas vitamins, minerals, and water do not. Dogs and cats not consuming sufficient calories lose body weight and condition. Energy requirements for dogs and cats are not a linear function of body weight. Recent evidence indicates that pets maintained in households require fewer calories per day compared with dogs held in kennels, but considerable variability exists. Breed differences also affect caloric needs independent of body size. For example, Newfoundlands appear to require fewer calories/day than Great Danes. Other factors that determine daily energy needs include activity level, life stage, percent lean body mass, age, and environment. Even when specific formulae are used, any given animal may require up to 30% more or less of the calculated amount. Consequently, general recommendations may need to be modified within this 30% range, and body condition scoring should be regularly performed. In view of this variability, energy requirements for dogs are ~65 kcal/kg body wt for kennel or active adult dogs, ~50 kcal/kg body wt for inactive adults, ~120 kcal/kg for growing puppies, ~200 kcal/kg for lactating bitches (depending on litter size), and ~450 kcal/kg for heavily worked dogs. For cats, energy requirements are ~70 kcal/kg for lean adults, ~200 kcal/kg for growing kittens, and ~150 kcal/kg for lactating queens.

The precise ME values for many dog food ingredients have not been experimentally determined and are often estimated using those for other monogastric species (such as pigs) or calculated using Atwater physiologic fuel values modified for use with typical dog food ingredients. The precise ME values for many cat foods are not known, although it is believed that the factors used for dogs may apply. The modified Atwater ME values for dogs are 3.5 kcal/g for carbohydrate or protein and 8.5 kcal/g of fat. The impact of various environmental temperatures is described in the recent NRC publication on nutrient requirements of dogs and cats and has been documented under certain conditions. For example, energy requirements increased from 120 to 205 $kcal/kg^{0.75}$ in Huskies as ambient temperatures decreased from 14°C in summer to -20°C in winter. Effects of environmental temperature are not well characterized in cats because most of the research has been done under thermoneutral (68-72°F [20-22°C]) conditions. However, unacclimatized adult cats increased their daily caloric intakes by nearly 2-fold when environmental temperatures of 23°C and 0°C were studied.

Protein: Protein is required to increase and renew the nitrogenous components of the body. A primary function of dietary protein is as a source of essential amino acids and nitrogen for the synthesis of nonessential amino acids. Amino acids supply both nitrogen for the synthesis of all other nitrogenous compounds and a variable amount of energy when catabolized. The amount of protein required depends on the age of the animal and protein quality and is different for dogs and cats.

Healthy adult dogs need ~2 g of protein of high biologic value per kg body wt/day. The cat has a higher protein requirement than most species, and healthy adult cats need ~4 g of protein of high biologic value per kg body wt/day. The biologic value of a protein is related to the number and types of essential amino acids it contains and to its digestibility and metabolizability. The higher the biologic value of a protein, the less protein needed in the diet to supply the essential amino acid requirements. Egg has been given the highest biologic value, and organ and skeletal meats have a higher biologic value than do vegetable proteins.

The dietary requirement for protein is satisfied when the dog's metabolic need for amino acids and nitrogen is satisfied. Optimal diets should contain 22-25% protein as dry matter for growing puppies, and 10-14% for adult dogs. Optimal diets should contain at least 24-28% ME as protein for growing kittens, and ~20% for adult cats. Growing kittens are more sensitive to the quality of dietary protein and amino acid balance than are adults. Protein suitable for cats must supply >500 mg of taurine/kg diet dry matter. Unless synthetic essential amino acids are added, some animal protein is necessary in the diet to prevent taurine depletion and development of feline central retinal degeneration or dilated cardiomyopathy.

Without sufficient energy from dietary fat or carbohydrate, dietary protein ordinarily used for growth or maintenance of body functions is less efficiently converted to energy. Too little high biologic protein in the diet, relative to the energy density, can cause an apparent protein deficiency.

Protein requirements of animals vary with age, activity level, temperament, life stage, and health status. Most commercial dog foods contain a combination of cereal and meat proteins, with protein digestibilities of 75-90%. Digestibility is less for protein ingredients of poor biologic value and for poor-quality diets. If excessive heat is used in processing, proteins can become chemically unavailable for digestion and absorption. The signs produced by protein deficiency or an improper protein to calorie ratio may include any or all of the following: weight loss, skeletal muscle atrophy (dogs), dull unkempt coat, anorexia, reproductive problems, persistent unresponsive parasitism or low-grade microbial infection, impaired protection via vaccination, rapid weight loss after injury or during disease, and failure to respond properly to treatment of injury or disease. High protein intakes per se do not cause skeletal abnormalities in dogs (including osteochondrosis in large breeds) or renal insufficiency later in life in cats.

Fats: Dietary fat consists mainly of triglyceride with varying amounts of sterols and phospholipids. Fat is a concentrated source of energy, yielding ~2.25 times the ME (as an equal dry-weight portion) of soluble carbohydrate or protein. As much as 60% of the calories in a cat's diet may come from fat, and diets that contain 8-40% fat (dry-matter basis) have also been fed successfully. Triglycerides are divided into short, medium, and long chain based on the number of carbon atoms in the fatty acid chain. Fatty acids are either saturated, indicating there are no double bonds, or unsaturated, indicating there are one or more double bonds. Dietary fatty acid profiles are reflected in the fatty acid composition of tissues and cell membranes. In general, as the fat content of a diet increases, so does the caloric density and palatability, which promotes excess consumption that results in obesity. Dietary fat also facilitates the absorption, storage, and transport of fat-soluble vitamins such as vitamins A, D, E, and K. They are also a source of essential fatty acids (EFA), which maintain functional integrity of cell membranes and are precursors of prostaglandins and leukotrienes. Animal fats are the most digestible component of the diet, and dogs can tolerate quite high dietary concentrations. However, the addition of too much dietary fat may result in excessive energy intake and subsequent suboptimal intakes of protein, minerals, and vitamins.

Dietary fats, especially the unsaturated variety, require a protective (natural or synthetic preservatives) antioxidation system. If antioxidant protection from a natural preservative system (eg, vitamin C or mixed tocopherols) or from synthetic preservatives (eg, BHA, BHT, ethoxyquin) in the diet is insufficient, dietary and body polyunsaturated fats become oxidized and lead to steatitis. Canine diets typically contain 5-15% fat (dry-matter basis) for adults. Puppy diets usually contain 8-20% fat (dry-matter basis). One reason for the wide range of fat content seen in commercial dog foods is the purpose of the diet—work, stress, growth, and lactation require higher levels than maintenance. However, because fat can add considerably more calories to a finished diet, it is important to remember that the amount of protein relative to energy must be balanced appropriately to the life stage and typical intakes expected for an animal's size and needs.

Cats cannot readily convert linoleic acid to arachidonic acid, which must be obtained from animal sources. Recommendations include both linoleic acid and arachidonic acid at ~5 g and 0.2 g/kg diet, respectively.

Dogs have a dietary requirement for linoleic acid, an unsaturated EFA that is found in appreciable amounts in corn and soy oil. Recent studies suggest that α-linolenic acid (ALA, an omega-3 fatty acid) is also essential in dogs and possibly cats. In addition, the longer chain omega-3 fatty acid, docosahexaenoic acid, may be conditionally essential for normal neurologic growth and development of puppies and kittens. The amount of dietary ALA needed likely depends on the linoleic acid content. Although required amounts of these omega-3 fatty acids are presently unknown, current minimal recommendations include 0.8 g/kg diet of ALA when linoleic acid is 13 g/kg diet (dry-matter basis) for puppies and 0.44 g/kg diet ALA when linoleic acid is 11 g/kg diet (dry-matter basis) for adults. Amounts for cats are currently unspecified. EFA deficiencies are extremely rare in dogs and cats fed complete and balanced diets formulated according to AAFCO profiles. Deficiencies of EFA induce one or several signs, such as a dry, scaly, lusterless coat; inactivity; or reproductive disorders such as anestrus, testicular underdevelopment, or lack of libido. Fatty acid supplements are often recommended for dogs with dry, flaky skin and dull coats, but underlying metabolic conditions should always be evaluated first.

Carbohydrates and Crude Fiber: Carbohydrates in pet foods include low- and high-molecular-weight sugars, starches, and various cell wall and storage nonstarch polysaccharides or dietary fibers. The 4 carbohydrate groups functionally are absorbable (eg, monosaccharides such as glucose and fructose), digestible (eg, disaccharides, some oligosaccharides), fermentable (eg, lactose, some oligosaccharides), and nonfermentable (eg, fibers such as cellulose, which is an insoluble fiber). Different carbohydrate sources have varying physiologic effects. In cats, carbohydrates apparently are not essential in the diet when ample protein and fats supply glucogenic amino acids and glycerol. Properly cooked nonfibrous carbohydrates are utilized well by dogs. In both dogs and cats, if starches are not cooked, they are poorly digested and may result in flatulence or diarrhea. Except for the occasional case of lactose or sucrose intolerance, most cooked carbohydrates are well tolerated. There is evidence that fermentable sources of carbohydrates (ie, digestible or soluble fibers) are useful in dogs; digestible versus nondigestible carbohydrate sources must be evaluated for their unique characteristics and intended purposes. Beet pulp, for example, contains both soluble and insoluble fiber and provides good stool quality in dogs without affecting other nutrient digestibility when included at ≤7.5% (dry-matter basis).

There are several chemical methods to determine the fiber level of a food; all extract the components of fiber to different degrees, which results in different estimates of fiber level for the same feedstuff. Crude fiber consists mainly of cellulose and lignin. It is resistant to hydrolysis by mammalian digestive secretions but is not an inert traveler through the GI tract. Increased levels of crude fiber in feline rations increase fecal output, normalize transit time, alter colonic microflora and fermentation patterns, alter glucose absorption and insulin kinetics, and at high levels, can depress diet digestibility.

Vitamins: Most commercial dog and cat foods are fortified with vitamins to levels that exceed minimal requirements. There is no AAFCO dietary requirement for vitamins C or K for dogs. Cats have no documented dietary requirement for vitamin C. Deficiencies of fat-soluble vitamins (A, D, and E in dogs; A, D, E, and K in cats) and some of the 11 water-soluble B-complex vitamins have been produced experimentally. Water-soluble vitamins are usually readily excreted if excess amounts are consumed and are thought to be far less likely to cause toxicity or side effects when ingested in megadoses. Vitamin B_{12} is the only water-soluble vitamin stored in the liver, and dogs may have a 2- to 5-yr depot. Fat-soluble vitamins (except for vitamin K in cats) are stored to an appreciable extent in the body, and when vitamins A and D are ingested in large amounts (10-100 times daily requirement) over a period of months, toxic reactions may be seen. Only clinically relevant vitamin-related imbalances are described below.

Vitamin A: Excessive consumption of liver can lead to hypervitaminosis A and may produce skeletal lesions, including deforming cervical spondylosis, osseocartilaginous hyperplasia, osteoporosis, inhibited collagen synthesis, and decreased chrondrogenesis in growth plates of growing dogs.

Unlike most other mammals, cats cannot convert β-carotene to vitamin A because they lack intestinal carotenase. Therefore, cats require a preformed source in their diet, such as that supplied by liver, fish liver oils, or synthetic vitamin A. Signs of a vitamin A deficiency in cats are similar to those in other species, except that classic xerophthalmia, follicular hyperkeratosis, and retinal degeneration are rarely seen and usually are associated with concomitant protein deficiency. Nonetheless, cats fed diets deficient in vitamin A exhibited conjunctivitis, xerosis with keratitis and corneal vascularization, retinal degeneration, photophobia, and slowed pupillary response to light. Certain of these alterations also result from the retinal degeneration that is seen in taurine deprivation. Hypovitaminosis A in cats may exhaust vitamin A reserves of the kidneys and liver; affect reproduction causing stillbirths, congenital anomalies (hydrocephaly, blindness, hairlessness, deafness, ataxia, cerebellar dysplasia, intestinal hernia), and resorption of fetuses; and cause the same changes in epithelial cells noted in other animals. Squamous metaplasia of the respiratory tract, conjunctiva, endometrium, and salivary glands has been noted. Changes such as subpleural cysts lined by keratinizing squamous epithelium and extensive infectious sequelae are frequent in the lungs and are occasionally noted in the conjunctiva and salivary glands. Focal dysplasia of pancreatic acinar tissue and marked hypoplasia of seminiferous tubules, depletion of adrenal lipid, and focal atrophy of the skin have been reported. Borderline deficiency is more common, especially in chronic ill health. Retinol at 9,000 IU/kg of diet should meet dietary needs for vitamin A during gestation and lactation and exceed the needs of the growing kitten. Excessive consumption of liver can lead to hypervitaminosis A, which is characterized by new bone formation without osteolysis. Vitamin A toxicosis produces skeletal lesions of deforming cervical spondylosis, ankylosis of vertebrae and large joints, osseocartilagenous hyperplasia, osteoporosis, epiphyseal plate damage, and a narrowing of the intervertebral foramina.

Vitamin D: Vitamin D deficiency results in rickets in young animals and osteomalacia in adult animals. Classic signs of rickets are rare in puppies and kittens and most often are seen when homemade diets are fed without supplementation. Rickets has been reported in kittens fed diets deficient in vitamin D, even though dietary amounts of calcium and phosphorus were normal. In rickets, serum calcium and phosphorus are decreased or low normal with a corresponding high parathyroid hormone level; bone mineralization is decreased, and the metaphyseal areas are enlarged. Osteomalacia rarely causes clinical signs in dogs or cats. Hypervitaminosis D causes hypercalcemia and hyperphosphatemia with irreversible soft-tissue calcification of the kidney tubules, heart valves, and large-vessel walls. Death in dogs is either related to chronic renal failure or acutely due to a massive aortic rupture. Death in cats is related to chronic renal failure.

Vitamin E: In cats, steatitis results from a diet high in polyunsaturated fatty acids, particularly from marine fish oils when these are not protected with added antioxidants. Kittens or adult cats develop anorexia and muscular degeneration; depot fat becomes discolored by brown or orange ceroid pigments. Lesions are seen in cardiac and skeletal muscles and are similar to those described for other species.

Thiamine: Deficiency generally does not develop in cats fed properly prepared commercial diets. Thiaminase, which tends to be high in uncooked freshwater fish, can produce a deficiency by rapid destruction of dietary thiamine. Although canned commercial cat foods may contain fish, the heat associated with canning is sufficient to destroy thiaminase. Destruction of thiamine has also resulted from treatment of food with sulfur dioxide or overheating during drying or canning, but deficiencies are now rare. Thiamine-deficient cats develop anorexia, an unkempt coat, a hunched position, and with time, convulsions that become more severe, leading later to prostration and death. At necropsy, small petechiae may be found in the cerebrum and midbrain. Diagnosis can be confirmed in the early stages by giving 100-250 mg thiamine, PO or IM, BID for several days. Recovery occurs in minutes to hours but, if the diet is not supplemented after this treatment, relapse can be expected. Thiamine deficiency may cause a number of other neurologic disorders, including impairment of labyrinthine righting reactions, seen as head ventroflexion and loss of the ability to maintain equilibrium when moving or jumping; impairment of the pupillary light reflex; and dysfunction of the cerebellum, suggested by asynergia, ataxia, and dysmetria.

Minerals: Minerals can be classified into 3 major categories: macrominerals (sodium, potassium, calcium, phosphorus, magnesium) required in gram amounts/day, trace minerals of known importance (iron, zinc, copper, iodine, fluorine, selenium, chromium) required in mg or µg amounts/day, and other trace minerals important in laboratory animals but that have an unclear role in companion animal nutrition (cobalt, molybdenum, cadmium, arsenic, silicon, vanadium, nickel, lead, tin). A balanced amount of the necessary dietary minerals in relation to the energy density of the diet is important. As intake of a mineral exceeds the requirement, an excessive amount may be absorbed, or a large amount of the unabsorbed mineral may prevent intestinal absorption of other minerals in adequate amounts. Indiscriminate mineral supplementation should be avoided due to the likelihood of causing a mineral imbalance. Mineral deficiency is rare in well-balanced diets. Manipulation of dietary intake of calcium, phosphorus, sodium, magnesium (dogs and cats), and copper (dogs) for therapeutic effect is common. Limited evidence exists for the recommendations of dietary mineral requirements for cats made in TABLE 47; many are based on the mineral content of successfully fed diets.

Macrominerals: Calcium and phosphorus deficiency is uncommon in well-balanced growth diets. Exceptions may include high-meat diets that are high in phosphorus and low in calcium and diets high in phytates, which inhibit absorption of trace minerals. In both dogs and cats, the requirements for dietary calcium and phosphorus are increased over maintenance during growth, pregnancy, and lactation. In dogs, the calcium:phosphorus ratio should be ~1.2-1.5:1; a range of 1:1 to 2.5:1 is sufficient. Less phosphorus is absorbed at the higher ratios, so an appropriate balance of these 2 minerals is necessary. Also, insufficient supplies of calcium or excess phosphorus decrease calcium absorption and result in irritability, hyperesthesia, and loss of muscle tone with temporary or permanent paralysis associated with nutritional secondary hyperparathyroidism. Skeletal demineralization, particularly of the pelvis and vertebral bodies, develops with calcium deficiency. By the time there is a pathologic fracture and the condition can be confirmed radiographically, bone demineralization is severe. Often, there is a history of feeding a diet composed almost entirely of meat, liver, fish, or poultry. Excess intakes of calcium are more problematic for growing (weaning to 1 yr) large- and giant-breed dogs. Excessive supplementation (>3% calcium [dry-matter basis]) causes more severe signs of osteochondrosis and decreased skeletal remodeling in young, rapidly growing large-breed dogs than in dogs fed diets with lower dietary calcium (1-3% [dry-matter basis]). The clinical signs of lameness, pain, and decreased mobility have not been reported in small-breed dogs or more slowly growing breeds fed the higher calcium amounts.

Magnesium is an essential cofactor of many intercellular metabolic enzyme pathways and is rarely deficient in complete and balanced diets. However, when calcium or phosphorus supplementation is excessive, insoluble and indigestible mineral complexes form within the intestine and may decrease magnesium absorption. Clinical signs of magnesium deficiency in puppies are depression, lethargy, and muscle weakness. Excessive magnesium is excreted in the urine. In cats, there is evidence that magnesium concentrations >0.3% (dry-matter basis) may be detrimental if the diet is too alkaline.

Trace Minerals: Iodine deficiency is rare when complete and balanced diets are fed but may be seen when high-meat diets are used (dogs and cats) or when diets contain saltwater fish (cats). Deficient kittens show signs of hyperthyroidism in the early stages, with increased excitability, followed later by hypothyroidism and lethargy. Abnormal calcium metabolism, alopecia, and fetal resorption have been reported. The condition can be confirmed by thyroid size (>12 mg/100 g body wt) and histopathology at necropsy. The etiology of hyperthyroidism that develops in older cats with increased blood thyroxine and triiodothyronine is unknown.

Iron and copper found in most meats are utilized efficiently, and nutritional deficiencies are rare except in animals fed a diet composed almost entirely of milk or vegetables. Deficiency of iron or copper is marked by a microcytic, hypochromic anemia and, often, by a reddish tinge to the hair in a white-haired animal. Deficiency of zinc results in emesis, keratitis, achromotrichia, retarded growth, and emaciation. Decreased zinc availability has been noted in canine diets containing excessive levels of phytate, which emphasizes the value of feeding trial tests over laboratory nutrient analyses of pet foods. Manganese toxicity has been reported to produce albinism in some Siamese cats; a deficiency of manganese in other species results in bone dyscrasia.

DOG AND CAT FOODS

Pet Food Labels

Manufacturers of all commercial dog and cat foods are legally required to provide certain information on the label, including name of product, guaranteed analysis, ingredient guarantee, net weight, and name and address of the manufacturer or distributor. The most important nutritional information on the label is the guaranteed analysis, ingredient list, and the statement of nutritional adequacy. In the USA, all pet foods sold must be registered with state feed control officials and must contain approved ingredients generally regarded as safe, unless they are for specialized purposes such as the amelioration or prevention of disease. Such foods are considered to be drugs and must be approved by the FDA.

Guaranteed Analysis: This part of the label lists the minimal amounts of crude protein and crude fat and the maximal amounts of water and crude fiber on an as-fed (not dry-matter) basis. This analysis does not specify the actual amount of protein, fat, water, and fiber in the product. Instead, it indicates the legal minimums of protein and fat and the legal maximums of water and crude fiber content contained in the product. A laboratory proximate analysis lists the actual nutrient concentrations in the food, and 2 foods that have identical guaranteed analyses may have very different proximate analyses. A guaranteed analysis for protein may list a minimal level of 25%, while the product may (and usually does) contain >25%. A certain variance above or below a minimum or maximum should be expected. Consequently, whenever possible, the manufacturer's average nutrient profile should be used to evaluate a food. Direct product comparisons made between like (similar water content) products (ie, dry vs dry, or canned vs canned) are generally valid. However, comparisons across different food types should be made on a dry-matter or caloric basis. As a rule of thumb, dry-food analyses can be converted to a dry-matter basis by simply adding 10% to the as-is value because most dry foods contain ~10% water (eg, a dry-food protein content of 25% on an as-fed basis is equal to 27.5% dry-matter basis). Canned food analyses can be converted to a dry-matter basis by simply multiplying by 4 because most canned foods contain ~75% water (ie, a canned food protein content of 6% on an as-fed basis is equal to 24% dry-matter basis).

Ingredient List: Ingredients are listed in descending order of weight, on an as-fed basis, in the food. Although a food ingredient (eg, chicken) may be listed first, if that ingredient is 75% moisture, it will contribute a much smaller percentage of total nutrients to the food dry matter. In addition, an ingredient such as corn may be listed by individual types, eg, flaked corn, ground corn, screened corn, kibbled corn, etc. In this case, the total corn amount may be a significant amount of the total food dry matter, but when presented as individual types, each type appears lower on the ingredient list. No reference to quality or grade of an ingredient is allowed to be listed; therefore, it is difficult to evaluate a product solely on the basis of the ingredient list. The value of this list is limited to determining the sources of the proteins and carbohydrates for dogs or cats. This kind of information is useful when evaluating animals that are having an adverse reaction to a food, possibly due to an allergy or intolerance to one or more ingredient sources such as beef, poultry, rice, corn, etc.

Product formulations can be either fixed or open. In a fixed formula, combinations of ingredients and nutrient profiles do not change regardless of fluctuating market prices of the ingredients. In an open formula, ingredients, and possibly actual nutrient profiles, change depending on availability and market prices.

Statement of Nutritional Adequacy: This statement indicates how the food was tested (feeding versus laboratory analysis or formulation) and for which life stage the food is intended. AAFCO recognizes only 4 life stages: growth, maintenance, gestation, and lactation. The term "all life stages" is frequently used on a label and indicates that the product has been either formulated or tested for growth. By default, it is anticipated that such a food would also pass a maintenance protocol because testing a food for growth generally includes gestation and lactation. There are no AAFCO-approved nutrient profiles for geriatric, senior, or weight loss stages.

The statement "complete and balanced" indicates the product contains all nutrients presently known to be required by dogs or cats and that these nutrients are properly balanced to the energy density of the diet. The "complete and balanced" claim must be substantiated by successfully completing AAFCO feeding trials, or the food must contain at least the minimal amount of each nutrient recommended by AAFCO. There are cautions "against the use of these requirements (levels) without demonstration of nutrient availability" because some of the requirements are based on studies in which the nutrients were supplied as purified ingredients and, therefore, are not representative of ingredients used in commercial pet foods. Laboratory analysis does not address the issue of bioavailability. Supplements, snacks, treat products (ie, those intended for intermittent or supplemental feeding), and therapeutic or dietary products (ie, those intended for use under the direction of a veterinarian) are exempted from AAFCO testing.

Pet Food Product Types

Commercial dog and cat foods are available in 3 principal forms: canned, dry, and semimoist. The classifications used depend on the processing method and water content more than on the ingredient content or nutrient profile. Complete and balanced commercial dog and cat diets are formulated to provide adequate quantities of each required nutrient without an intolerable excess of any nutrient. Supplementation of particular nutrients to commercially produced complete and balanced dog and cat foods should be done carefully and only with appropriate justification. Dog foods are not satisfactory for cats because most dog foods are lower in protein, often do not contain assured concentrations of taurine, and are not designed to produce a urinary pH of <6.5 (which helps prevent the crystallization of struvite or magnesium-ammonium-phosphate in the feline urinary tract (*see also* FELINE UROLITHIASIS AND FELINE LOWER URINARY TRACT DISEASE, p 1930).

Dry Food: This is the most popular category of pet food in the USA and some other countries. Dry foods generally contain ~90% dry matter and 10% water. About 95% of dry dog and cat foods are extruded, ie, they are made by combining and cooking ingredients (grains, meat and meat byproducts, fats, minerals, and vitamins), then forcing the mixture through a die. During cooking and extrusion, a temperature of ~150°C converts the starches into a form more easily digested, destroys toxins and inhibitory substances, and flash sterilizes the product. The food is then enrobed with fat and/or digest (material derived from controlled degradation of animal tissues, eg, chicken digest) during drying to increase palatability. Advantages of dry food include a lower cost than canned or soft-moist food, and refrigeration of unused portions is not needed. Dry food may also provide beneficial massage of the teeth and gums to help decrease periodontal disease.

Canned Food: Canned dog and cat foods contain 68-78% water and 22-32% dry matter. Many of the same ingredients are used in canned pet foods as in dry-extruded types but usually not at the same levels of inclusion. Given their high moisture content, canned foods typically contain higher amounts of fresh or frozen meat, poultry, or fish products and animal byproducts. Many canned pet foods contain textured proteins derived from grains, such as wheat or soy. These materials function as meat analogs having a physical structure similar to meat and high nutritional quality. The use of meat in combination with some of the textured proteins not only holds costs down but can improve the overall nutritional profile of the final product.

Canned pet food processing begins with blending meat or meat analogs and fat ingredients with water and dry ingredients, such as vitamins and minerals, for proper nutrient content. The mixture is blended and sometimes ground to produce a fine slurry depending on product profile. After cans are filled, they are sealed and retorted (a heat and pressure-cooking process that also sterilizes the contents) assuring destruction of foodborne pathogens. Advantages of canned food include a long shelf life in a durable container and high palatability. However, canned food is more expensive than dry food.

Soft-moist Food: Soft-moist dog and cat foods contain 25-40% water and 60-75% dry matter. They do not require refrigeration and are preserved using humectants—substances that bind water so that it is unavailable for bacteria and mold growth and assure shelf life. They include simple sugars (usually sucrose), sorbitol, propylene glycol, and salts. Reports of an increased risk of Heinz body anemia in cats that consume soft-moist foods preserved with propylene glycol have raised concerns over the use of propylene glycol in cat foods, and it has been removed from the generally recognized as safe list for cat foods. Many soft-moist foods are acidified using phosphoric, malic, or hydrochloric acid to further retard spoilage. Advantages of soft-moist foods include convenience, high energy digestibility, and palatability. However, soft-moist food is more expensive than dry food.

Home-cooked Diets: Dogs can be successfully maintained on properly formulated home-cooked diets; this is much more difficult in cats. Advantages of home-cooked diets include the use of fresh, high-quality ingredients chosen by the owner. Disadvantages include preparation time, variable quality control and diet consistency, higher cost, and the difficulty in formulating and preparing a nutritionally complete and balanced diet. It is most difficult to formulate a nutritionally complete and balanced diet with sufficient nutrient density in a small volume of food that is palatable for cats. Many home-cooked diets result in foods that are high in protein and caloric density and have inappropriate calcium:phosphorus ratios and inadequate levels of calcium, copper, iodine, fat-soluble vitamins, and several of the B vitamins. Many published recipes for feline diets have very high ash or mineral levels due to the extent of synthetic nutrient supplementation required.

FEEDING PRACTICES

Domestication and use of dogs and cats as companions may have modified eating patterns of these animals to varying extents. Easier access to food and consistency of food quality has led to increased food consumption and the possibility of decreased energy expenditure overall. Hence, there is greater risk of obesity. At the same time, longevity of companion animals has also increased and, along with it, the emergence of other chronic progressive diseases such as osteoarthritis, cancer, and immune and cognitive disorders. Healthy dogs and cats eat a variety of foods. During a 24-hr period, most dogs will eat 1-3 meals, while most cats will eat frequent small meals.

While odor, consistency, taste, and learned dietary habits determine which foods a dog will eat, most are indiscriminate eaters. Finicky, begging dogs have learned such behaviors. Likewise, odor, consistency, taste, and learned dietary habits determine which foods a cat prefers, but how much a cat will eat is affected by such things as noises, lights, food containers, the presence or absence of humans or other animals (including other cats), physiologic state, and disease. Cats can and will refuse to eat to the point of starving themselves under stressful conditions. These cats are at risk of developing hepatic lipidosis, which can be fatal if not treated early and aggressively. Some dogs and cats have adequate appetite controls and maintain an optimal body condition, even with dietary changes. By contrast, other dogs and cats overeat, consume excessive calories, and become obese. The thickness of the fat layer over the rib cage and pelvic bones is a good indicator of obesity, as is regular body condition scoring over time. Normally, the ribs and hip bones should be easily felt but not seen; these cannot be easily palpated in an obese animal. A pendulous abdomen, a waddling gait, and sluggish behavior are also seen in some obese animals.

Dietary modifications are required by changes in life stage, environment, body weight and condition, and disease. Energy density varies from 2,500 to >5,000 kcal/kg dry matter for dog foods and from 3,000 to >5,000 kcal/kg dry matter for cat foods. Therefore, general feeding recommendations cannot be given for all dogs and cats on any particular food. Instead, feeding recommendations should be individualized. The best feeding method is one that maintains optimal body weight and condition, bearing in mind that disease conditions may require dietary changes.

When a dietary change is necessary, it should not be done abruptly. New food should be introduced gradually over 3-5 days. Also, it is better to offer slightly less than the calculated new food amount. Overindulgence and abrupt changes are frequently the inciting cause of GI disorders that may ultimately lead to diet refusal. In dogs, the new food should be introduced slowly by replacing 25% more of the old food every day or two until the new diet makes up the entire amount fed. Cats can easily become habituated to a particular food and may resist any dietary change. In cats, new food should also be introduced slowly. Some cats have definitive preferences for dry food, while others prefer the same food moistened or canned. If the dog or cat is to be switched from a canned to a dry diet, it may be useful to moisten the product by adding sufficient warm water, and the food can be warmed to release odors and flavors that encourage consumption. Dry-matter digestibilities are 60-90% for dog food and from 75-90% for cat food due to ingredient quality, crude-fiber content, processing, and level of intake. Small, firm, dark feces suggest high nutrient digestion and absorption, while large volumes of pale feces indicate less dietary utilization. High digestibility is not always the dietary goal, as in weight loss programs and diabetes mellitus.

Maintenance: After a dog has reached ~90% of its expected adult weight, a diet that is less nutrient dense than the growth diet is recommended. The dietary goal is to maintain optimal body weight and condition for that particular dog. Most adult dogs can be fed a maintenance diet either ad lib or as several meals/day. Ad lib feeding may not be possible for dogs that overeat or for multiple-dog households. Overfeeding dogs by providing excessive calories and food amounts relative to energy expenditure is the most common error in feeding adult dogs and promotes obesity. More than 40% of owners feed treats and snacks, which are often an important aspect of the human-animal bond. Complete and balanced treat products that use low-fat, high-fiber ingredients are available. Nutritional supplements are not required and, in fact, may be harmful. In an animal prone to obesity, the caloric content of all treats fed should be considered in an effort to match energy intake to expenditure. Regular assessment of the animal's body condition helps ensure minimal weight gain beyond optimal adult values throughout life.

Most inactive, neutered adult cats can be fed a reduced fat diet (6-9% dry-matter basis) ad lib, but in some animals increasing the insoluble fiber content may be necessary to satisfy hunger. Cats exposed to variations in temperature (eg, cats that remain outdoors year-round or at night) may eat more during the winter. The need for a different nutritional profile in older cats versus middle-aged cats has not been documented. However, depending on activity level, feeding a food with a different fat and fiber content (increased or decreased as needed) may be needed to maintain optimal body weight and condition.

Growth and Reproduction in Dogs: Growth, pregnancy, and lactation greatly increase nutrient demands over those of maintenance. Growth diets have increased nutrient density, digestibility, and bioavailability to provide nutrients necessary in a smaller volume of food. Supplementation of calcium, phosphorus, and vitamin D beyond amounts present in complete and balanced diets designed for growth and reproduction is rarely necessary and may be contraindicated if calcium is >3.0% (dry-matter basis) or the calcium:phosphorus ratio is outside the ratio of 1:1 to 3:1.

Growth: Overfeeding during growth increases growth rate. This is not desirable because it is incompatible with proper skeletal development and also contributes to obesity later in life. Feeding methods for growing puppies should be individualized for the puppy and owner. General recommendations are that puppies between weaning and 6 mo of age should be fed 3 times a day; puppies 6-12 mo old should be fed twice daily. Large- and giant-breed puppies should be fed complete and balanced growth diets that have been tested in feeding trials and that contain calcium, fat, and protein at levels closer to the minimums stated by AAFCO. Small-breed puppies may have to be fed more than 3 times a day using a tested diet that contains calcium, fat, and protein at levels greater than the minimums stated by AAFCO.

Only limited data have been published with respect to breed growth curves. Nonetheless, a slow growth rate is preferable to a fast growth rate. Weight gains should be closely monitored (weekly), and feeding recommendations adjusted such that the puppy gains a small amount of weight each week. When growing large-breed puppies were fed 50-70% of their littermate's ad lib intake, adult height, length, and bone or muscle mass were not stunted; only total body fat was affected. It is difficult to stunt the growth of a puppy being fed a complete and balanced growth diet that has passed an approved AAFCO feeding trial using meal feeding of an appropriate amount for 2-3 times/day.

Gestation: Feeding recommendations for pregnant bitches through the first two-thirds of gestation are the same as those for maintenance. A common mistake is to overfeed during early gestation and to underfeed during lactation. In the last third of gestation, the total amount of food offered should be increased at least 20-30% over the amount for maintenance. Growth diets are often used during gestation because of their higher energy density and smooth transition after parturition to support lactation.

Lactation: Lactating bitches often require energy levels 2-4 times those of maintenance to avoid excessive loss of body condition. Ad lib feeding using a complete and balanced growth diet containing 10-20% fat (dry-matter basis) that has passed an approved AAFCO feeding trial is recommended to maintain lactation and to permit optimal body weight and condition to be required by weaning. If a bitch loses significant body condition during lactation, the fat content of the diet should be increased to 20-30% fat (dry-matter basis), and she should be fed ad lib.

Growth and Reproduction in Cats: The pattern of weight changes during gestation and lactation differs between bitches and queens. Because queens tend to lose weight during lactation regardless of diet fed, it has been assumed that net tissue reserves should increase somewhat in preparation for lactation. A kitten/growth diet that contains 10-35% fat, 30-40% protein, and low (<5%) fiber (dry-matter basis) should be fed. Growing kittens and pregnant and lactating queens can be fed ad lib or several times a day to meet their daily needs. During the latter third of gestation, the amount of food and level of nutrient intake normally increases an average of 25%, although energy intakes for cats during pregnancy have been estimated to be as much as 40% greater than for maintenance. Some queens may eat less early in gestation and immediately before parturition; such changes are of concern only if prolonged. Queens require 2-3 times the normal food intake during lactation, depending on litter size. Supplementing an already balanced diet is not necessary and should be discouraged.

Geriatric: Older dogs have not been documented to have different nutritional requirements than middle-aged dogs. Some dogs begin old age considerably overweight, while others may show some loss of condition. Feeding an appropriate food with a different nutrient profile with respect to energy, fat, or fiber content (increased or decreased) may be needed to maintain optimal body weight and condition. Geriatric dogs and cats should be monitored in a preventive health program that includes periodic assessments of body weight and condition. The incidence of chronic degenerative organ disease increases with age, and early diagnosis fosters earlier treatment and more effective nutritional management.

Work or Stress: The caloric needs of working or stressed dogs may exceed the levels of a maintenance diet, depending on the animal and extent of work performed. Most diets designed for work or stress have increased levels of animal fats, with the other nutrients appropriately balanced to the increased energy density. At extreme levels of stress (eg, an Alaskan sled dog requiring 10,000 kcal/day), many recommend not only increasing the percent ME from fat, but also from protein, while minimizing the contribution of carbohydrate. Any daily feeding recommendation should be considered an estimate or starting point and should be modified based on continual evaluation of the dog's weight and condition, skin and coat, performance, and general attitude. Feeding a smaller amount of the daily ration (eg, $^1/_3$ of the daily amount) prior to beginning a work shift is recommended with the remainder being fed thereafter. Plenty of fresh water should be available, and opportunities to stop work for a water break should be scheduled in any daily work routine for these dogs.

NUTRITION IN DISEASE MANAGEMENT

Nutrition is an important part of disease management, even though few disorders can be cured solely with diet. The interaction between illness, health, and nutritional status is multifactorial and complex. The nutritional requirements of sick dogs and cats are qualitatively the same as those of healthy ones; however, they differ in the amounts required—certain nutrients may be needed in greater amounts or may need to be restricted.

Adverse Reaction to Foods: Food reactions are classified using specific terminology. An adverse reaction to a food is a clinically abnormal response to any type of food ingested. Food intolerance is a type of adverse reaction that does not involve the immune system, eg, food poisoning. A food allergy is a type of adverse reaction that does involve the immune system, eg, colitis or atopy. *See also* p 688 and p 649.

Dogs and cats with food allergy usually have GI signs (eg, vomiting or diarrhea, or both) or a pruritic skin condition. The prevalence of true food allergies is very small. Most dogs and cats with nonseasonal pruritus are having an adverse reaction to food. Unfortunately, food allergy cannot be differentiated from intolerance. Hence, given all the possible etiologies and limited diagnostics available, any animal suspected of having an adverse reaction to food should be fed a single novel protein, single novel carbohydrate diet with little or no known additives for a 2-mo trial period. If the owner elects to feed a commercially prepared food, several products are available that use single novel protein sources (eg, venison, rabbit, duck, or fish) and a single carbohydrate source (eg, potato). Fish is not a novel option for most cats. A careful dietary history must be obtained from the pet owner prior to selecting the type of diet. There is a possible, but yet unclear, relationship between adverse food reactions in cats fed foods containing scombroid fish and histamine content. Most importantly, the formulation of whatever product or diet is fed must be fixed to ensure that the ingredient composition is consistent from batch to batch. These products are more expensive not only because of their unique and limited sources of protein but also because of the quality control procedures required to ensure fixed formulations and to eliminate cross-contamination with previous production batches of different foods.

Simplified homemade diets are also possible using the same protein and carbohydrate sources suggested above (or other ingredient sources the owner wants to test). Homemade diets actually allow for a wider selection of source ingredients. Beef, lamb, pork, mutton, tofu (soybean), egg, and dairy products should be discouraged as protein sources because animals have likely been exposed to these sources if previously fed foods with an open formulation. Likewise, corn, wheat, barley, and rice should be discouraged as carbohydrate sources. The basic recipe should closely resemble "complete and balanced," but single sources of protein and carbohydrate can be sequentially tested and replaced. The owner is responsible for quality control and consistency and must be willing to make such a diet for ~2 mo. On average, there is no price advantage in making a homemade diet over using commercially prepared foods.

The trial diet should be exclusively fed for the 2-mo period, eliminating all treats, snacks, and table foods unless made of the exact same ingredients as the trial diet. All chewable medications and supplements must be eliminated from the trial diet because most contain the same protein and additive ingredients as pet foods and treats. A positive diagnosis of adverse reaction to food is made when there is ~50% improvement within 3 mo of eating the trial diet. Other therapies such as hyposensitization and flea control are necessary in animals with concurrent disease. Testing various suspect ingredients by reintroducing them to the diet one at a time followed by recurrence of clinical signs is affirmation of an adverse reaction to that ingredient. Dietary ingredients reintroduced could reproduce clinical signs as early as 12 hr after ingestion but could take as long as 10 days. Lifelong treatment is dietary avoidance, which may be difficult if the offending ingredients are not positively identified.

Anemia: Iron or copper deficiency (or both) is the major cause of hypochromic, microcytic anemia. A folic acid and B_{12} deficiency also produces anemia. Most commercial diets have more than required amounts of iron, copper, and vitamins; therefore, secondary causes such as hemorrhage or heavy parasite infection should be investigated. Feeding large proportions of a single item food or an unbalanced homemade diet may result in anemia. The objective of dietary management of anemia is to feed a diet that is known to support RBC production; this avoids the possibility of a particular nutrient acting as the limiting factor. Ample amino acids must be available for the synthesis of Hgb, iron for heme synthesis, and copper for the proper mobilization of iron. Folic acid and vitamin B_{12} are necessary to support normal cell division, although there is probably a 2-5 yr hepatic supply of B_{12} in previously normal animals. Anemic dogs or cats should be fed a growth diet to provide adequate nutrition rather than individual synthetic nutritional supplements. Adding cooked liver to the existing diet is another major source of these nutrients but should not be included at >10-15% of the total food fed.

Anorexia: Anorexia (partial or complete) accompanies many disorders, including drug reactions or reactions to environmental changes. Learned food aversions may also contribute to anorexia. Pain may also be a significant contributor to anorexia, and in most cases when the pain is adequately controlled, the anorexia resolves. The nutritional goal is to stimulate normal appetite and maintain adequate food intake. Partial anorexia is seen when the animal is eating some food but not enough to provide at least 30 kcal/kg body wt in dogs and 40 kcal/kg body wt in cats. Complete anorexia is when the animal eats nothing for ~3 days. Anorectic dogs and cats can sometimes be persuaded to eat by adding highly flavored substances to the diet (eg, animal fat, meat drippings, fish [fish juices or oils for cats]). Nutrition can be provided by several methods for anorectic dogs and cats that are hospitalized. Tube feeding using either a nasogastric or gastric tube is most common. Nasogastric tubes are used more commonly for short durations (1-7 days), while gastric tubes are more convenient for longer durations (weeks or months). Dogs and cats can be maintained at home with tube feedings after the procedure has been accepted by the animal and fully explained to the owner. The liquid tube feeding diet should be nutritionally dense to provide at least 30 kcal/kg body wt/day (dogs) or 40 kcal/kg body wt (cats) in a total daily volume tolerated by the animal. It is possible to feed a 20-kg dog three 200-mL meals/day or a cat three 60-mL meals/day and adequately meet nutritional requirements. If anorexia has been persistent for >1 wk, it is advisable to begin feeding smaller volumes more frequently. For example, most dogs can be started with 30-60 mL meals, and most cats with six 20-30 mL meals/day. Several commercially available canned products are calorically dense and (when blended with water) will pass through an 8 French or larger nasogastric or gastric tube. Nasogastric tubes smaller than 8 French require a commercially prepared homogenized liquid. If for some reason a tube cannot be placed, dogs and cats can be maintained by IV solutions that provide adequate calories, protein, electrolytes, B vitamins, and selected trace minerals until access to the small intestine is possible.

Cachexia: Cachexia, usually present in cases of neoplasia or chronic renal or cardiac disease, appears to be a response to increased catabolism with either normal or decreased appetite. The deterioration of the animal's condition clearly indicates that nutritional requirements are not being met, and the dietary goal is to increase the caloric density and palatability of the food while meeting the animal's requirements for protein and other nutrients. The usual management of cachexia is to feed smaller amounts of a more calorically dense (ie, higher fat content) but complete and balanced food more frequently (3-6 meals/day). The form of food (dry or canned) that the dog or cat prefers should be fed. Tube feeding and IV nutritional support (*see* above) should also be considered if the dog or cat continues to lose weight and condition.

Diarrhea: This results from increased fluid secretion into, or decreased resorption from, the colon. The etiology should be established, and any intestinal infection or parasites treated. Diarrhea often resolves with the addition of fiber (>10% dry-matter basis in dogs, 5-10% in cats), which modulates intestinal motility, rate of passage, fecal water content, and intracolonic pressure. If dehydrated, the animal should be rehydrated with oral or parenteral fluids, and lost electrolytes replaced. Fat content of the diet is not an issue if there is no steatorrhea, which is rare. Dietary fat content should be adjusted for body condition; however, diets with >12-16% fat (dry-matter basis) should not be necessary. Animals with diarrhea should be offered small, frequent meals (3-6/day). If the animal does not respond within 3-6 wk, a highly digestible, novel protein and carbohydrate diet should be tried.

Congestive Heart Failure (CHF): One objective in managing CHF is to reduce water retention; restricting sodium intake and lowering sodium levels encourage diuresis. Typical commercial dog and cat foods have a sodium content of 0.45-0.90% (450-900 mg sodium/100 g diet dry matter). Dietary sodium restriction is classified as mild (400 mg sodium/100 g diet dry matter) to severe (240 mg sodium/100 g diet dry matter). In view of these values, commercial dog and cat diets cannot even be classified as mild sodium restriction. Therefore, commercially prepared low-sodium diets or recipes that use low-sodium foods must be substituted. Sodium restriction often requires a special diet, although some manufacturers provide veterinary therapeutic diets for heart disorders. When using a home-prepared diet, all processed meats, cheeses, bread, heart, kidney, liver, salted fats, whole eggs, and snack foods should be avoided. Foods that are reasonably low in sodium include beef, rabbit, chicken, horsemeat, lamb, freshwater fish, oatmeal, corn, and rice.

Failed cardiac contractility may contribute to CHF, and taurine supplementation should be used to exclude a possible depletion of this amino acid in cardiac muscle. Obesity can also be a contributing factor in CHF. Such animals should be placed on a weight management program in addition to sodium restriction. In some instances, edema may give the appearance of obesity and mask emaciation. The edema should first be resolved so that body weight and condition can be evaluated. If the animal is underweight, the food intake should be increased or the caloric content of the diet increased. If renal failure is also present, protein and phosphorus intake must be restricted. Supplementation of carnitine remains somewhat controversial and expensive for longterm use.

Constipation: This results from impaired peristalsis or increased water absorption from the large intestine. The objective of dietary management is to provide a balanced diet with increased amounts of insoluble fiber (10-25% dry-matter basis to effect) in dogs or a balanced diet that is reasonably high in fiber in cats. Such diets increase intestinal volume, stimulate peristalsis, and hold water within the colon. Animals should be fed 2-4 times/day. In dogs, sometimes adding a high-fiber breakfast cereal to the existing diet, 1-10 tbsp to effect depending on the size of the dog, is also effective. In cats, administration of petroleum jelly, 1 tsp (5 mL), PO, once weekly or more often, is helpful in preventing constipation, particularly in cats prone to hairball production. Commercial diets are also available to help manage hairballs and generally contain increased amounts of insoluble fiber.

Diabetes Mellitus: Most cases of diabetes in dogs and cats are mature onset (type II) and believed due to insulin insensitivity, although insulin-dependent diabetes mellitus is seen. The objective of dietary management is to reduce food consumption and to balance carbohydrate intake with insulin dosage, while slowing the rate of carbohydrate absorption. Reducing diets that are available for dogs and cats are usually high in protein and low in fat and carbohydrates and may help in diabetes mellitus management. To ensure a reasonably constant intake of carbohydrates or nutrients that contribute to blood glucose, a fixed formulation food should be fed. Some believe that minimal carbohydrate should be present in the diet overall, but this approach remains controversial. Because removal of both fat (triglycerides) and carbohydrate (glucose) from the circulation depends on insulin, blood concentrations of these macronutrients are known to affect the amount of insulin required. Consequently, meals should be timed to coincide with peak insulin action, and more than 1-2 meals/day may be required. Many diabetic dogs and cats are overweight and benefit from a weight management program, which is especially useful in cases of type II diabetes.

Feline Lower Urinary Tract Disease (FLUTD): In this condition, magnesium-ammonium-phosphate crystals accumulate in the urinary tract, together with mucous-like material. There are other etiologic factors, but providing the cat with a diet that has a low magnesium content and that maintains a urine pH of <6.4 helps limit the development of crystals and uroliths. Because prevention of FLUTD depends largely on control of urine dilution and whole body acid-base balance, dietary management is an important component of urinary tract health in cats. Watering dishes and litter boxes should be cleaned daily (without using any phenolic disinfectants or phenolic-based soaps) to encourage maximal water intake and urination. If more than one cat uses the litter box, pheromones or other odors may tend to repel one of them. Thus, when multiple cats are confined together, having several litter boxes may be helpful in controlling FLUTD. Some cats with signs of FLUTD produce calcium oxalate crystals and uroliths; in this case, dietary management should minimize calcium intake and produce a more alkaline urine pH.

Fever: Fever increases energy requirements due to increased metabolic activity—a 1°F (0.5°C) rise causes an increase in caloric need of ~7 kcal/kg body wt/day. A highly palatable diet should be fed in quantities that can be consumed easily, and the caloric content should be increased by feeding a higher fat diet. Because animals with fever generally have a decreased appetite, offering smaller meals more frequently with personal attention and encouragement may help stimulate intake. Feeding a feline growth diet or a calorically dense recovery-type diet also increases protein and energy intake in smaller feedings.

Gastric Dilatation (Bloat): Currently, there is little evidence to suggest that certain nutritional practices (eg, feeding soy protein diets or canned versus dry food) lead to the development of gastric dilatation in susceptible dogs. (*See also* p 325.)

Head Trauma, Burns, and Respiratory Diseases: It is unknown whether the metabolic effects and energy expenditure in dogs and cats with severe head trauma, burns with ≥50% loss of skin, or prolonged dyspnea are the same as those in humans with similar conditions. However, it is anticipated that they are. Thus, providing aggressive nutritional support early is essential. Head trauma significantly alters neurologic control of metabolic rate, which is usually increased. Burns and other causes of significant areas of skin loss increase heat loss to the environment, thereby increasing energy needs.

Increased respiratory rate and dyspnea are deceptively intense work that also result in increased energy needs. If a dog or cat is in an oxygen cage for >1 day, nutritional support (feeding IV or via gastric tube) must be instituted. In all cases, energy is provided minimally at 30 kcal/kg body wt (dogs) or 40 kcal/kg body wt (cats) and increased in increments of 5 kcal/kg as the condition progresses and if weight loss is apparent. The energy source should be predominately fat (60-90% calories from fat, 10-40% from glucose) because the body metabolism is predominately lipolytic under these conditions, with the liver utilizing fat better than glucose during response to burns or trauma. Protein intake must also be matched with the energy intake to avoid net protein and muscle catabolism. Food that is 30-45% protein and 25-30% fat (dry-matter basis) that is complete and balanced for all other nutrients should be fed using tube feeding. Human baby foods are not suitable for this purpose. These nutritional goals can also be met by parenteral (IV) nutrition.

Hepatic Disease: Liver disorders are managed by reducing the need for liver function and providing the nutrients necessary for healing and regeneration. In general, diets should provide a protein source of high biologic value and be limited to an amount consistent with the animal's maintenance needs. Sufficient energy from fat and carbohydrate are needed to minimize dietary protein transamination and deamination for energy and to reduce toxic nitrogenous waste products of protein metabolism. Foods that contain purines and uric acid, such as shellfish, fish meal, spleen, thymus, liver, brain, etc, should be restricted in a further effort to decrease the load of uric acid precursors, which require hepatic metabolism. Frequent feeding of small meals (4-6/day) lowers the amount of nutrients or metabolites requiring hepatic processing at a single time, thereby imposing less metabolic demand on the liver. In general, protein sources equivalent to egg or milk protein in quality are provided at 2-3 g/kg body wt in dogs and 5 g/kg body wt in cats. If ascites or edema is present, the animal should be placed on a restricted sodium diet that contains ~240 mg sodium/100 g diet (dry-matter basis). If blood ammonia levels are increased (hepatic encephalopathy), the protein intake should be restricted to 1-1.5 g protein/kg body wt in dogs and 3-4 g protein/kg body wt in cats. In practice, protein intake is reduced, and the serum ammonia levels are monitored until they return to normal. Arginine is important in the conversion of ammonia to urea. It is present in adequate amounts in most commercial diets. Animals with liver disorders are frequently anorectic. Thus, food consumption and body weight and condition should be monitored. For dogs, a diet high in fat and low in residue should be selected initially, although fat restriction may be necessary to maintain normal feces. Dietary fats are not a source of short-chain fatty acids, which may exacerbate hepatic encephalopathy. Soluble fiber-containing diets may be a problem, depending on the extent of encephalopathy present. Copper should be restricted in dogs at risk of developing copper-induced hepatopathy, and water-soluble vitamins should be increased above maintenance levels. The effectiveness of manipulation of branched chain and aromatic amino acids in dogs with chronic liver disease has not been demonstrated.

Hyperlipidemia in Dogs: This can be primary or secondary to hypothyroidism, pancreatitis, hepatic disease, diabetes mellitus, nephrotic syndrome, hyperadrenalism, or high-fat diets. Hyperlipidemia is present when blood lipids are increased with or without gross lipemia and probably results from abnormalities in the synthesis or use of plasma lipoproteins. In primary hyperlipidemia, the abnormalities can be familial and might be genetic, as has been suggested in Miniature Schnauzers. Some dogs with hyperlipidemia are asymptomatic. Clinically affected dogs may have recurrent seizures, depression, recurrent pancreatitis, vomiting, acute blindness, corneal opacity, and xanthogranulomas. The goal of dietary management is to decrease the digestion and absorption of fat by feeding a diet restricted in fat (<10% dry-matter basis). The use of fish oil capsule supplements at a dosage of 1 g/4.5 kg body wt either once a day or in divided doses, depending on the number of capsules needed, help reduce serum triglyceride concentrations. Although fish oil supplements generally do not return serum triglycerides to normal values, partial reduction is believed to mitigate the risk of pancreatitis or other problems related to marked elevations of this lipid.

Malabsorption and Maldigestion in Dogs: Diseases of the small intestine and pancreas often lead to a vague clinical syndrome characterized by weight loss, vomiting, diarrhea (with or without steatorrhea), and changes in appetite. In such cases, a highly digestible diet that is low in fiber (0-5%), moderate in fat (10-15%) and protein (20-25%), and contains carbohydrate from noncereal byproduct sources is recommended. Supplemental water-soluble vitamins should also be used. In exocrine pancreatic insufficiency, supplementation with a powdered enzyme supplement, mixed with the food a few minutes before feeding, should be considered. (*See also* MALABSORPTION SYNDROMES, p 339.)

Obesity: It is estimated that 40-50% of dogs and 20% of cats seen by veterinarians are overweight and that 25% of dogs and 5% of cats are obese. Obesity, or the storage of excess fat, results from an imbalance between calorie intake and expenditure. The principal cause is excessive food intake combined with inadequate exercise. Obesity is regarded as the most common nutritional disorder in dogs. Its incidence increases with age and neutering because there is a reduction of both metabolic rate and physical activity. Similarly, obesity is a common nutritional disorder of neutered, male indoor cats ~6-11 yr old. Some breeds of dogs, including Labrador Retrievers, Dachshunds, and Beagles, are more prone to obesity. Dogs fed homemade meals, table scraps, and snacks have a greater tendency to be overweight than those on an exclusive diet of commercial pet food. Obesity appears to be increasing in frequency, probably due to increased dietary fat levels and caloric density of some foods in conjunction with improved palatability of commercial pet foods. An increasing number of neutered dogs and cats confined to living indoors may exacerbate the problem. Pathologic conditions in dogs that may be associated with obesity include hypothyroidism, hyperadrenocorticism, diabetes mellitus, and insulinoma. Obesity predisposes dogs to other problems, including ruptured cruciate ligaments, dyspnea and fatigue, impaired reproductive efficiency, and dystocia. Pathologic conditions in cats that may be associated with obesity include diabetes mellitus, nonallergic skin conditions, and lameness (ruptured cruciate ligaments). Obesity may also predispose cats to other problems including impaired reproductive efficiency and dystocia.

Dietary management of obesity requires a significant reduction of caloric intake until a normal body weight is achieved. In addition, activity level or exercise should be increased (eg, a regular exercise program for dogs or outdoors regularly for cats) to expend energy and possibly reduce appetite. To begin a weight loss program for canine obesity, the normal or ideal weight for the animal should be estimated and enough food provided to meet 60% of the requirement for the animal's ideal or normal weight (75% of the necessary caloric requirement for cats). An accurate dietary history should also be obtained to determine the animal's present daily caloric intake. The most effective diets are those that are nutritionally complete, balanced, and formulated as a reducing diet. These diets should be low in calories and fat (5-8% dry-matter basis). High-fiber diets are also often used to dilute caloric density (10-25% dry-matter basis for dogs, 20-30% for cats). Commercial or homemade reducing diets are preferable to feeding smaller quantities of the normal diet so that dilution of other important nutrients such as protein, vitamins, and minerals does not develop. Small meals may be fed frequently during the day. Table food should be eliminated because it tends to be high in calories; other snacks should be accounted for as part of the total daily ration. When the diet is changed, the new diet should be introduced slowly (over several weeks) replacing 25-30% of the old food weekly and then restricting the volume fed into multiple meals per day. Cats should also be introduced to a new diet slowly, replacing 25-30% of the old food weekly until 100% of the new food is accepted. Afterward, ad lib access to the new food for 2-3 mo is followed by the appropriate restricted amount of food fed as multiple meals per day. In dogs, the rate of weight loss should be ≤2% of body wt/wk for the first few weeks. In cats, the rate of weight loss should be 1-3% of body wt/wk, or more commonly 5% body wt/mo for the first few weeks. As the cat approaches optimal weight, the rate of weight loss per week will decrease. It may be more difficult to reduce the weight of cats that weigh ≥20 lb initially, and owners should be aware that a weight-loss program may take ≥1 yr. Progress should be monitored by weighing monthly, and dietary modifications made if necessary. Frequent monitoring and communication help the owner maintain enthusiasm for a weight-loss program, as does a commitment on the part of the owner to increase the frequency of exercise for their pet (eg, walking, running off leash). The burden of resisting the constantly begging dog or cat under these circumstances can be lessened by feeding small amounts (1 tbsp) several times a day and carefully monitoring future food allotments once the desired body weight is attained. Another tip is to have owners make sure that all the food (including any snacks) offered is placed in the animal's regular food bowl rather than given by hand. This forces the owner to go to the food dish each time a treat is offered and may reduce the number of between-meal snacks.

Pancreatitis and Parvovirus Enteritis in Dogs: The goal in treating pancreatitis is to minimize stimulation of the exocrine function of the pancreas until inflammation has decreased. Cases of parvovirus enteritis, which is more common in puppies 3-8 mo old, are often treated similarly. In either case, the dog has multiple episodes of vomiting. A standard treatment is nothing per os (NPO) until vomiting ceases, which can last from 3-15 days. Antibiotic, fluid, and electrolyte therapy during NPO treatment is essential, and IV nutritional support should be instituted if NPO therapy continues for ≥3 days. Adult and young dogs can be nutritionally maintained by IV parenteral solutions that provide adequate calories, protein, electrolytes, B vitamins, and selected trace minerals until oral feeding is possible. When oral feeding can be resumed, a commercially prepared, homogenized liquid diet fed as small, frequent meals (1-2 mL/kg, 3-6 times/day) is the next least stimulatory to the pancreas and best used by a small intestine with an abnormal or absent mucosal surface. The liquid can be fed by syringe by placing the syringe tip in the cheek pouch, lateral to the teeth and gums, with the head in a normal or slightly down position. This method encourages voluntary swallowing with less risk of aspiration. When oral feedings of the liquid diet have been well tolerated for 1-2 days, a moderate-fiber diet (10-15% dry-matter basis), low in fat (5-10%) for pancreatitis or moderate in fat (10-15%) for parvovirus, can be fed in increasing amounts until maintenance intakes have been achieved. Pups with parvovirus should not be fed food sufficient to support growth until feces are normal. Also, because recurrent episodes of pancreatitis are common, feeding a complete and balanced low-fat diet on a continual basis is recommended for longterm management. Obesity and hyperlipidemia are common concurrent problems in pancreatitis cases and should be investigated and resolved.

Renal Insufficiency: Numerous metabolic abnormalities that may alter an animal's nutritional status develop in progressive renal failure. These include impaired clearance of nitrogenous products of protein metabolism; impaired regulation of sodium, potassium, and phosphorus; impaired vitamin D metabolism; and often anorexia. The objective of dietary management in renal failure is to lessen the metabolic demands on the kidneys and to diminish metabolic end-products that cannot be readily excreted. The first consideration is to ensure normal water homeostasis. Regardless of whether the animal is polyuric, oliguric, or anuric, water should always be readily available. Increased BUN is lowered by reducing dietary components that produce nitrogen (and urea) as a consequence of hepatic deamination. Supplying energy primarily via feeding relatively more digestible fats and carbohydrates and less protein is recommended. The amount of protein in the diet should be the minimum that meets the requirements imposed by turnover of enzymes and tissue repair and maintains a slightly positive nitrogen balance. In addition, phosphorus intake should be restricted. Diets should have high energy density, with a moderate amount of protein of high biologic value (15-20% in dogs and ~28% in cats). No more than 0.4-0.6% phosphorus and 0.2-0.4% sodium (dry-matter basis), with a balanced calcium level and increased levels of water-soluble vitamins, should be included. These amounts are less than those ordinarily found in many commercial diets, which often necessitates a dietary change. If renal failure becomes more advanced, and the BUN and serum phosphorus concentration can no longer be maintained near normal limits, more energy from fat should be included. Adding $^1/_2$ cup of fat as cooked beef fat, chicken skin, fat drippings, or fish oil to the diet increases caloric density and improves palatability. This helps to meet the animal's energy needs with less total food consumed and, therefore, less protein. The criteria used (eg, serum creatinine concentration, BUN) to define when dietary modifications should be made are currently being debated. However, it is easier to change the diet when the animal is feeling reasonably well as opposed to when the animal is anorectic. There is likely to be little harm in changing the diet early in the course of renal disease. Some therapeutic renal diets tend to alkalinize blood pH as acidosis begins, which may minimize the effects of acidosis and help the animal feel more energetic and eat better.

Urolithiasis in Dogs: Uroliths in dogs most commonly are struvite (magnesium-ammonium-phosphate), calcium oxalate, urate, or cysteine. A definitive diagnosis can be obtained only by stone analysis. A medical protocol using antimicrobials and a calculolytic diet for prevention or dissolution of recurrent stones is an effective alternative to surgery once the stone type is known. The dietary goal is to decrease intake of the mineral constituents and to modify urine pH to discourage stone formation. The dietary profile includes a reduced amount of protein of high biologic value (low in nucleic acids), calcium, phosphorus, and magnesium, with increased salt to encourage frequent urination. An acidic (<7) urine pH is recommended for struvite uroliths, whereas an alkaline (>7) urine pH is recommended for calcium oxalate, urate, or cysteine uroliths. These nutritional formulations should be used with caution during growth, lactation, and gestation, and in cases of azotemic primary renal failure, congestive heart failure, or liver disease. (*See also* p 1259.)

Steatitis in Cats: Steatitis (pansteatitis, yellow fat disease) is seen most often in kittens fed exclusively large amounts of unsaturated fatty acids, oily fish such as tuna or mackerel (packed in oil not water), or diets that do not have an appropriate balance of antioxidants relative to polyunsaturated fats. Clinical signs are anorexia, pyrexia, pain over the thorax and abdomen, neutrophilia, and subcutaneous nodules of necrotic fat. Cats with steatitis should be fed diets restricted in polyunsaturated fatty acids (monounsaturated and saturated fats are permitted) and given vitamin E supplementation at 10-20 mg, BID for 5-7 days. The diet of choice is a commercial food to which vitamin E (α-tocopherol) or other antioxidants have been added.

PHARMACOLOGY

CHEMOTHERAPEUTICS

INTRODUCTION   2049

ANTIBACTERIAL AGENTS   2056

ANTIFUNGAL AGENTS   2098

ANTIVIRAL AGENTS AND BIOLOGIC RESPONSE MODIFIERS   2107

ECTOPARASITICIDES 2158

GROWTH PROMOTANTS AND PRODUCTION ENHANCERS 2168

VACCINES AND IMMUNOTHERAPY 2176

PHARMACOLOGY
INTRODUCTION

Once a diagnosis has been made and medical treatment is deemed necessary, safe and effective pharmacologic agents that exert the appropriate actions should be selected. Factors to be considered include dose and frequency of administration of the chosen drugs, the optimal routes for delivery, the particular pharmaceutical forms to be used, any public health or environmental implications, and regulatory constraints. For selected therapies, such as antimicrobials, distribution to the site of action also should be considered.

Although the Animal Drug Medicinal Use Act of 1994 legalizes extra-label drug use in the USA, selected states or other countries may have additional or complementary regulatory or legal restrictions. In all instances, it is important to read carefully the label instructions for use of specific drugs.

DISPOSITION AND FATE OF DRUGS

Once a drug has been administered by any route other than IV, it must be absorbed into the bloodstream from the site of administration. The drug then is distributed into various body fluids and tissues to attain an effective, yet safe, concentration for a sufficient period of time at the site of action. Subsequently, the drug is inactivated or eliminated from the body, generally by metabolism (usually lipid-soluble drugs) and excretion (mainly renal and biliary routes). The effectiveness of these processes with respect to time (pharmacokinetics) varies with the particular drug and species of animal. It is equally influenced by disease and the effects of concurrently administered agents (drug interactions).

Drug Absorption

Passage of Drugs Across Cellular Membranes: Regardless of the route of administration, a drug usually must cross a number of membranes before it reaches its site of action. Membrane barriers may be composed of several layers of cells (eg, skin, vagina, cornea, placenta) or a single layer of cells (eg, enterocytes, renal tubular epithelial cells), or they may consist only of a boundary <1 cell in thickness (eg, hepatic sinusoids, single cell membrane, mitochondrion, nucleus).

Drugs and other molecules can cross cellular membranes by several processes. Passive transfer or simple diffusion is the most important for xenobiotics, although specialized transport systems are used for a limited number of therapeutic agents.

In simple diffusion, movement of the drug is due to and directly related to its concentration gradient across the membrane. In the case of lipid diffusion, lipid-soluble substances dissolve in the lipid phase of the membrane and diffuse down their concentration gradients into the aqueous phase on the other side of the barrier. Thus, the ability of a compound to cross a membrane by simple lipid diffusion is a function of its degree of lipid solubility (lipid-to-water partition coefficient). The molecular mass of the drug, the thickness of the membrane(s), and the surface area available also influence the rate of diffusion.

Many agents of pharmacologic interest are weak organic electrolytes. At physiologic pH, these weak acids or bases may be present partly in the ionized (dissociated) and partly in the nonionized (undissociated) form. The ratio between the respective forms depends on the drug's dissociation constant (pK_a) and the pH of the solution in which it is dissolved. The nonionized fraction may penetrate biologic membranes by lipid diffusion and become distributed across the membrane according to the degree of ionization on each side of the membrane and the extent to which the drug is bound to proteins or other macromolecules in the solutions bathing either side of the membrane. Membranes are more permeable to the undissociated molecule than to the ionized form, simply because the nonionized form is much more lipid soluble. Although a compound may be nonionized, it also may be so poorly soluble in lipids that it penetrates biologic membranes only to a limited extent. A degree of aqueous solubility is also necessary for a drug to be in solution in the body fluids on either side of a cellular membrane.

It is supposed that aqueous pores exist in lipoproteinaceous biologic membranes. Lipid-insoluble compounds can easily diffuse through these pores, as well as directly through the membrane, at rates that depend on their molecular masses and concentration gradients. However, with ions or other polar compounds, the speed of transfer is determined by both the charge and molecular dimensions of the drug. When a hydrostatic or osmotic pressure difference exists across a membrane, water flows through the aqueous pores; this bulk fluid movement carries or "drags" solute molecules through the pores in the moving stream, provided that the solute molecules are smaller than the aqueous channels.

Several specialized transfer processes account for the passage of certain organic ions and other large lipid-insoluble substances across biologic membranes. Active transport, facilitated diffusion, and exchange diffusion are 3 distinct types of carrier-mediated systems used for moving specific substances across cellular membranes. The highly selective carrier-mediated systems are principally used for transporting nutrients and natural substrates across biologic membranes.

Pinocytosis is an important transport process in mammalian cells, particularly intestinal epithelial cells and renal tubular cells. Drugs that exist in solution as molecular aggregates, have large molecular masses themselves, or are bound to macromolecules may be transferred across membranes by pinocytosis.

Drug Absorption from the GI Tract: Although the basic principles governing the absorption of drugs from the GI tract are understood, many confounding factors may play a role in modifying the process, and erratic responses may result. Some of the more important factors to be considered include the following: 1) molecular size and shape of the drug and its concentration, 2) degree of ionization at specific pH values (depends on pK_a of the drug), 3) lipid solubility of the neutral or nonionized form of the drug, 4) chemical or physical interactions with coadministered drug preparations or even food constituents, 5) the pharmaceutical preparation and characteristics of the dosage form (especially the disintegration and dissolution rates of solid dosage forms), 6) morphologic and functional differences of the GI tract among the various animal species, 7) gastric motility, secretion, and the rate of gastric emptying, 8) intestinal motility and secretions as well as the intestinal transit time, 9) fluid volume within the GI tract, 10) osmolality of intestinal content, 11) intestinal blood and lymph flow, 12) disruption of the structural and functional integrity of the gastric and intestinal epithelium, and 13) drug biotransformation within the intestinal lumen by microflora, or within the mucosa by host enzyme systems.

Bioavailability: This term is used to define the rate and extent to which a drug administered in a particular dosage form enters the systemic circulation intact. All of the considerations outlined above, as well as the particular product used, can influence bioavailability. Biotransformation by intestinal epithelial cells, and particularly by liver cells, can substantially reduce the amount of unchanged drug that enters the systemic circulation after administration PO. This is known as the "first-pass" effect and is significant for a number of drugs.

Drug Absorption from Topical Administration: Drugs may be absorbed through the skin after topical application; however, the stratum corneum presents an effective barrier to movement of most drugs. The intact skin allows the passage of small lipophilic substances but efficiently retards the diffusion of water-soluble molecules in most cases. Lipid-insoluble drugs generally penetrate the skin slowly in comparison with their rates of absorption through other body membranes. Absorption of drugs through the skin may be enhanced by inunction or more rarely by iontophoresis if the compound is ionized. Certain solvents (eg, dimethyl sulfoxide [DMSO]) may facilitate the penetration of drugs through the skin. Damaged, inflamed, or hyperemic skin allows many drugs to penetrate the dermal barrier much more readily. The same principles that govern the absorption of drugs through the skin also apply to the application of topical preparations on epithelial surfaces.

Drug Absorption from Tracheobronchial Surfaces and Alveoli: Because volatile and gaseous anesthetics have relatively high lipid-to-water partition coefficients and generally are rather small molecules, they diffuse practically instantaneously into the blood in the alveolar capillaries. Particles contained in aerosols can be deposited, depending on the size of the droplets, on the mucosal surface of the bronchi or bronchioles, or even in the alveoli. Most drugs are usually absorbed quite rapidly from these sites according to the principles discussed above.

Drug Absorption from Parenteral Delivery Sites: After a drug has penetrated the skin, GI epithelium, or other absorbing surface, or has been deposited by injection into a body tissue, it comes into the immediate vicinity of capillaries. Solutes traverse the capillary wall by a combination of 2 processes: diffusion and filtration. Diffusion is the predominant mode of transfer for lipid-soluble molecules, small lipid-insoluble molecules, and ions. All drugs, whether lipid-soluble or not, cross the capillary wall at rates that are extremely rapid compared with their rates across other body membranes. In fact, the movement of most drug molecules in various tissues is limited only by the rate of blood flow rather than by the capillary wall. However, some endothelial cells, such as the blood-brain barrier, have much tighter intercellular junctions than others and, therefore, restrict drug movement more significantly.

Aqueous solutions of drugs are usually absorbed from an IM injection site within 10-30 min, provided blood flow is unimpaired. Faster or slower absorption is possible, depending on the concentration and lipid solubility of the drug, vascularity of the site (there are differences between various muscle groups), the volume of injection, the osmolality of the solution, and other pharmaceutical factors. Substances with molecular weights >20,000 daltons are principally taken up into the lymphatics.

Absorption of drugs from subcutaneous tissues is influenced by the same factors that determine the rate of absorption from IM sites. Some drugs are absorbed as rapidly from subcutaneous tissues as from muscle, although absorption from injection sites in subcutaneous fat is always significantly delayed.

Increasing blood supply to the injection site by heating, massage, or exercise hastens the rate of dissemination and absorption. Spreading and absorption of a large fluid volume that has been injected SC may be facilitated by including hyaluronidase in the solution.

The rate of absorption of an injected drug may be prolonged in a number of ways, including immobilization of the site, local cooling, a tourniquet, incorporation of a vasoconstrictor, an oil base, and implant pellets and other insoluble "depot" preparations. Among these depot preparations are drugs that are converted to less soluble salts (eg, procaine and benzathine penicillin) or less soluble complexes (eg, protamine zinc insulin), or that are administered as insoluble microcrystalline suspensions (eg, methylprednisolone acetate).

Drug Distribution

After absorption into the bloodstream, drugs become disseminated to all parts of the body. Compounds that permeate freely through cell membranes become distributed, in time, throughout the body water, both extracellular and intracellular. Substances that pass readily through and between capillary endothelial cells, but do not penetrate other cell membranes, are distributed into the extracellular fluid space. Occasionally, the drug molecule may be so large (>65,000 daltons) or so highly bound to plasma proteins that it remains in the intravascular space after IV administration. Drugs may also undergo redistribution in the body after initial high levels are achieved in tissues that have a rich vascular supply, eg, the brain. As the plasma concentration falls, the drug readily diffuses back into the circulation to be quickly redistributed to other tissues with high blood-flow rates, such as the muscles; then, over time, the drug also becomes deposited in lipid-rich tissues with poor blood supplies, such as the fat depots. Most drugs are not distributed equally throughout the body but tend to accumulate in certain specific tissues or fluids. The general principles that govern the passage and distribution of drugs across cellular membranes (*see* above) are applicable. Basic drugs tend to accumulate in tissues and fluids with pH values lower than the pK_a of the drug; conversely, acidic drugs concentrate in regions of higher pH, provided that the free drug is sufficiently lipid soluble to be able to penetrate the membranes that separate the compartments. Even small differences in pH across boundary membranes, such as those that exist between CSF (pH 7.3) and plasma (pH 7.4), milk (pH 6.5-6.8) and plasma, renal tubular fluid (pH 5.0-8.0) and plasma, and inflamed tissue (pH 6.0-7.0) and healthy tissue (pH 7.0-7.4), can lead to unequal distribution of drugs with pK_a values close to those of the pH of the fluid. Only freely diffusible and unbound drug molecules are able to pass from one compartment to another. Binding to macromolecules such as protein components of cells or fluids, dissolution in adipose tissue, formation of nondiffusible complexes in tissues such as bone, incorporation into specific storage granules, or binding to selective sites in tissues all impede movement of drugs in the body and account for differences in the cellular and organ distribution of particular drugs. Therapeutic agents may also be transported by carrier-mediated systems across certain cellular membranes, which leads to higher concentrations on one side than the other. Examples of such nonspecific transport mechanisms are found in renal tubular epithelial cells, hepatocytes, and the choroid plexus.

Only the unbound or free fraction of a drug can diffuse out of capillaries into tissues. The most important binding of drugs in circulation is to plasma albumin, although the globulins and, especially, α-1 acid glycoprotein (for bases) may also play a significant role. A drug may become bound to plasma proteins to a greater or lesser degree, depending on a number of factors, eg, plasma pH, concentration of plasma proteins, concentration of the drug, the presence of another agent with a greater affinity for the limited number of binding sites, and the presence of acute-phase proteins during active inflammatory conditions. The degree of plasma-protein binding and the affinity of a drug for the nonspecific protein-binding sites is of great clinical significance in some instances and much less so in others. For example, a potentially toxic compound (such as dicumarol) may be 98% bound, but if for any reason it becomes only 96% bound, then the concentration of the free active drug that becomes available in the plasma is doubled, with potentially harmful consequences. The concentration of a drug administered in overdose may exceed the binding capacity of the plasma protein and lead to an excess of free drug, which can diffuse into various target tissues and produce exaggerated effects. Of equal importance is the readiness with which drugs dissociate from plasma proteins. Those that are more tightly bound tend to have much longer elimination half-lives because they are released gradually from the plasma protein reservoir. The long-acting sulfonamides are good examples of this phenomenon. Most unbound drugs distribute easily to extracellular fluid. All membranes are transversed only by the more lipid-soluble drugs. During distribution and elimination from the body, a drug may or may not penetrate certain "physiologic" (eg, blood-brain, placental, and mammary) barriers. A drug may gain access to the CNS by 2 distinct routes—the capillary circulation and the CSF. Drugs penetrate into the cortex more rapidly than into white matter, probably because of the greater delivery rate of drug via the bloodstream to the tissue. The pharmacologic factors and consequences of the diverse rates of entry of different drugs into the CNS include the following: 1) water-soluble ionized drugs will not enter the CNS; 2) low ionization, low plasma-protein binding, and a fairly high lipid-water partition coefficient confer ready penetration; 3) direct injections into the CSF often produce unexpected effects; and 4) meningoencephalitis can substantially alter the permeability of the blood-brain barrier.

The placental barrier should be considered when selecting an agent to treat a pregnant animal. The potential teratogenicity of any drug needs to be known before its administration; if it is to be used during late gestation, its effects on the fetus and on the process of parturition should be considered. Nutrients, such as glucose, amino acids, minerals, and even some vitamins, are actively transported across the placenta. The passage of drugs across the placenta is largely by lipid diffusion, and the factors discussed above play a role. The distribution of drugs within the fetus follows essentially the same pattern as in the adult, with some differences with respect to the volumes of drug distribution, plasma-protein binding, blood circulation, and greater permeability of interceding membranous barriers.

The mammary gland epithelium, like other biologic membranes, acts as a lipid barrier, and many drugs readily diffuse from the plasma into milk. The pH of milk varies somewhat, but in goats and cows it is generally 6.5-6.8 if mastitis is not present. Weak bases tend to accumulate in milk because the fraction of ionized, nondiffusible drug is higher. The opposite is true for acidic drugs. Agents delivered by intramammary infusion can diffuse into plasma to a greater or lesser degree by the same processes noted earlier.

Drug Biotransformation

Drugs and foreign chemicals that are lipid soluble are converted by enzymatic processes to compounds of ever-increasing water-solubility until they can be excreted via one or several of the routes available. Metabolism or biotransformation and the subsequent excretion of drugs is known as "elimination." Metabolism generally occurs in 2 phases: Phase I induces a chemical change (most frequently oxidation, but also reduction) that renders the drug more conducive to phase II. Phase II is a conjugative or synthetic addition of a large, polar molecule that renders the drug water soluble and amenable to renal excretion.

There are several possible consequences of the biochemical transformation of drugs: 1) inactivation, during which an active drug is converted to inactive metabolite(s); 2) activation, during which an inactive drug (or pro-drug) is converted to a pharmacologically active primary metabolite; 3) modification of activity after the conversion of an active drug to a metabolite that also has pharmacologic activity; 4) lethal synthesis (or intoxication), in which a drug is incorporated into a normal cellular metabolic pathway that ultimately leads to failure of the reaction sequence because of the presence of spurious substrate (cell death then occurs).

Several aspects of the biotransformation of drugs have direct clinical significance. These include microsomal enzyme induction and inhibition, nutritional state, age, disease conditions, and species differences.

Because drug biotransformation is negligible in early life, neonates are much more sensitive to lipid-soluble drugs than are adults of any species. The postnatal development of drug-metabolizing enzymes in the liver appears to be biphasic, consisting of a rapid and nearly linear increase in activity during the first 3-4 wk, followed by slower development up to the tenth week postpartum; dose or interval for the very young must be reduced accordingly. Hepatic mass, hepatic blood flow, and microsomal enzyme activity may decrease in older animals.

Many disease states impair the normal activity of the hepatic microsomal enzyme system, which in turn prolongs the half-lives of many drugs. Frank hepatotoxicity, acute hepatitis, or other extensive liver lesions invariably depress enzyme activity. Changes in hepatic blood flow, with similar consequences, may be encountered in congestive heart failure, circulatory shock, and cirrhosis. Hypothyroidism tends to reduce microsomal enzyme function, and hyperthyroidism tends to increase activity.

Species variations in the biotransformation patterns of lipid-soluble drugs are common. Differences in the duration of action of these drugs in various species frequently can be attributed to differences in their rates of biotransformation. This must be remembered when either dosages or withdrawal times are extrapolated from one species to another.

Drug and Metabolite Excretion

The concentration of a drug in the plasma or at its receptor sites may be reduced in 3 ways: 1) distribution or redistribution into various tissue compartments, 2) metabolic inactivation, and 3) excretion from the body. The kidneys are the principal organ of excretion, but the liver, GI tract, and lungs also may play important roles. Milk, saliva, and sweat are usually of less importance, although the presence of an active drug in milk may affect nursing young.

Renal excretion of foreign compounds involves glomerular filtration, passive diffusion into and out of the tubular lumen, and carrier-mediated secretion, mainly in the proximal convoluted tubule. Only unbound molecules <66,000 daltons are readily filtered through the glomerular membranes into the tubular lumen. Acidification or alkalinization of the urine may alter the rate of excretion of some drugs because of ion-trapping in the tubular fluid.

Binding to plasma proteins usually does not hinder tubular excretion of drugs because of the dynamic equilibrium that exists between free and bound drug. As free drug is removed and transported across the tubular epithelium, immediate dissociation of the drug-albumin complex usually occurs. Concurrent administration of either acidic or basic drugs that are substrates for carrier-mediated secretion processes prolongs the elimination of the drug that has the lesser affinity for the carrier sites, thus increasing its duration of action.

Drugs and their metabolites may also be excreted either passively or actively by hepatocytes into the bile canaliculi and, ultimately, into the duodenum in the bile. Drugs may become unconjugated by intestinal microflora. Released drug can be reabsorbed into the systemic circulation. Enterohepatic cycles often account for prolonged half-lives of drugs that are primarily excreted in bile. Impairment of the excretory functions of the hepatocytes or obstruction of bile flow due to any cause interferes with the biliary excretion of drugs. Dose or interval should then be adjusted accordingly. The normal kinetics of a drug's enterohepatic cycle may change in such cases, or may be modified by disruption or elimination of the intestinal flora.

The other routes of excretion are of lesser clinical importance. However, several drugs may diffuse directly into the GI tract and then be eliminated in the feces. The ruminoreticulum can act as a drug reservoir or "sink." The tracheobronchial tree also may be a potential avenue of excretion. Many drugs that are administered parenterally are found in bronchial secretions. Alveolar elimination is of major significance when inhalant anesthetics are used. The main factors governing elimination by this route are the same as those determining the uptake of inhalant anesthetics—the concentrations in plasma and alveolar air and the blood/gas partition coefficient. The mammary and salivary glands excrete drugs by nonionic passive diffusion. The salivary route of excretion is important in ruminants because they secrete such voluminous amounts of alkaline saliva.

If the excretory functions of those organs concerned with drug elimination are impaired or altered in any way (eg, disease, very young or very old animal), prolonged elimination patterns result. Moreover, several nutritional and pharmacokinetic interactions have the potential to change the rates of drug excretion.

When urinary excretion is an important route of elimination, renal failure results in decreased drug clearance and, thus, slower removal of the drug from the body. A usual dosage regimen in such cases tends to lead to accumulation and, ultimately, toxicity. A number of disturbances may occur within failing kidneys, all of which may influence the excretion of drugs: renal ischemia, glomerular involvement, tubular damage, impaired intrarenal perfusion, functional disabilities of the tubular cells, failed homeostatic mechanisms, and obstructive lesions in the tubules or collecting ducts (or even the ureters or urethra). Changes in the pH of the filtrate also alter the excretion rates of drugs with appropriate pK_a values. In addition to the direct effect on renal excretory mechanisms, pathologic changes in the kidneys can influence the disposition and elimination of drugs. In most instances, drug toxicity is increased. The binding of many drugs to plasma proteins is decreased in uremic animals. The rate of metabolic reactions may be depressed in renal failure, impairing effective elimination of agents that require biotransformation. Associated clinical signs and pathophysiologic changes, often encountered in renal failure, can also alter pharmacodynamic responses to particular drugs. Derangements of acid-base balance, hyper- and hypokalemia, hyper- and hyponatremia, dehydration, and hyper- and hypotension are examples of systemic conditions that may radically modify a drug's fate or action.

PHARMACOKINETICS

The pharmacokinetic characteristics of a particular drug (rates of absorption, distribution, biotransformation, and excretion) determine its concentration in the plasma. Because the intensity of the tissue response is usually determined by the concentration of the drug in the direct environment of the receptors, a drug's concentration in plasma is generally assumed to be correlated with the time course of its action. Dosage regimens are derived from pharmacokinetic studies in normal animals but often require modification in diseased, young, old, obese, thin, or pregnant animals. A large number of pharmacokinetic measures can be determined from time-course studies of drug concentrations in plasma, but only the more clinically useful features and values are emphasized below.

Drug Concentration in Blood

Drug concentrations in the blood can be determined and graphed against time. In most instances, the time course of a drug's concentration in the plasma correlates well with the onset, intensity, and duration of the pharmacologic effect. Thus, the measurement of sequential plasma concentration of drugs after their administration is used to establish dosage regimens that are likely to produce the desired therapeutic levels for appropriate periods of time, without the risk of drug failure or toxicity.

Single-dose Concentration Curves After Extravascular Administration: When a drug is administered by an extravascular route, it usually appears in the plasma within a short time, and its concentration rises steadily until it peaks. Once absorbed into the circulation, it is subjected simultaneously to distribution, biotransformation, and excretion. During the initial period, the rate of absorption and distribution exceeds the rate of elimination. The peak plasma concentration is reached when absorption and elimination rates are equal. Thereafter, the elimination rate exceeds the rate of absorption because less drug remains available at the site of administration, and plasma drug levels begin to fall.

The term "bioavailability" is used to express the rate and extent of absorption of a drug, usually from the GI tract after administration PO. Bioavailability is determined by administering equal doses of a drug by the IV (absorption effectively 100%) and PO routes and then comparing the areas under the 2 curves. Bioavailability is expressed as a percentage. The same principles can be applied to calculation of the bioavailability of drugs administered by other routes.

Single-dose Concentration Curves After Intravascular Administration: When a drug is administered by rapid IV injection, the maximum concentration in the blood is reached almost at once and immediately begins to fall. The profile of this decline can be determined by monitoring blood levels at periodic intervals and then plotting these concentrations against time.

From the single-dose concentration curves (extravascular and intravascular), a number of pharmacokinetic parameters can be calculated. These include the transfer rate constants between central and peripheral compartments; the elimination rate constant (K_{el}) for disappearance of drug from the central compartment; and the elimination half-life ($t_{1/2}$), which has important clinical significance when determining dosing interval.

Apparent Volume of Distribution

The pharmacokinetic measure used to indicate the pattern of distribution of a drug in plasma and in the different tissues, as well as the size of the compartment into which a drug would seem to have distributed in relation to its concentration in plasma, is known as the apparent volume of distribution (Vd). It is usually reported as liters (L) or as liters per kilogram (L/kg) if corrected for the body weight of the animal. The apparent Vd for a drug is determined by its degree of water or lipid solubility, the extent of plasma- and tissue-protein binding, and the perfusion of tissues. Drugs that tend to maintain high concentrations in the plasma because of low lipid solubility, extensive binding to plasma proteins, and diminished tissue binding have low Vd. The reverse is true for drugs with high apparent Vd. The value of Vd is characteristic for a drug and is usually constant over a wide dose range for a given species of animal. However, a number of clinically significant factors can influence the Vd. Included among these are age; functional status of the kidneys, liver, and heart; fluid accumulations; concentration of plasma proteins; acid-base status; inflammatory processes or necrosis; and any other causes for alteration in the degree of plasma-protein binding. Vd is used to determine dose. A dose necessary to achieve desired plasma concentration can be calculated from the formula $D = C \times Vd \times$ body wt (in kg), in which D is the dose and C is the required plasma concentration for a given drug.

Drug Clearance (Elimination)

Once a drug is absorbed and distributed among the tissues and body fluids, it is then eliminated, or cleared, mainly by the liver and kidneys. Consequently, the plasma concentration of a drug decreases steadily, although at different rates for various drugs in different species. After a single dose, only ~3% of a given dose remains in the body after

5 half-lives because 96.87% has been cleared by this time. Drug clearance (Cl) is defined as the volume of plasma that would contain the amount of drug excreted per minute or, alternatively, the volume of plasma that would have to lose all of the drug that it contains within a unit of time (usually 1 min) to account for an observed rate of drug elimination. Thus, clearance expresses the rate or efficiency of drug removal from the plasma but not the amount of drug eliminated. The concept of drug clearance is of great clinical significance.

Renal clearance is defined as the volume of plasma that is totally cleared of a drug in 1 min during passage through the kidneys. The renal clearance of drugs depends on urine pH, extent of plasma-protein binding, and renal plasma flow. These factors may vary from animal to animal as well as among species, because of differences in diet, environmental temperature, physical activity, disease, and concomitant use of certain drugs. For drugs that are excreted primarily by glomerular filtration, the animal's creatinine clearance may serve as an indicator of drug clearance because creatinine undergoes complete glomerular filtration while being subjected to minimal tubular reabsorption. Consequently, creatinine clearance rate can be used for adjusting dosage schedules of some drugs in animals with impaired renal function.

Hepatic clearance is defined as the volume of plasma that is totally cleared of drug in 1 min during passage through the liver. Most drugs, except highly hydrophilic compounds, are cleared from the plasma mainly by biotransformation in the liver, although biliary excretion can also contribute to the hepatic clearance of a drug. The main factors that determine hepatic clearance include hepatic blood flow (delivery of drug to the liver), uptake of the unbound drug by the hepatocytes from the blood, metabolic transformation of the drug by microsomal or other enzyme systems, and rate of biliary secretion.

Some drugs undergo substantial removal from the portal circulation by the liver after administration PO. This "first-pass" effect can significantly reduce the amount of parent drug that reaches the systemic circulation. A number of factors can modify the magnitude of the first-pass effect for a particular drug. Hepatic clearance can be impaired by liver disease, biliary stasis, decreased hepatic blood flow, and drugs that inhibit microsomal enzyme systems. Microsomal enzyme inducers often increase hepatic clearance of a concurrently administered drug. There is no reliable liver function test to assess the impediment of hepatic clearance of drugs (as creatinine clearance does for the kidneys). The dose rates for drugs used in animals with liver disease must be adjusted on clinical judgment alone.

Steady State Plasma Concentration (Repeated Administration or Constant IV Infusion): In some cases, the desired therapeutic effect of a drug is produced with a single dose. However, to achieve a satisfactory response, it is frequently necessary to maintain drug concentrations in the therapeutic range for a longer time. Rather than administering large doses, which could be potentially toxic, repeated safe doses at regular intervals or continuous IV delivery are generally necessary.

When a drug is infused IV, the plasma concentration continues to rise until elimination equals the rate of delivery into the body. Regardless of the drug, 50% of the plateau concentration is attained in 1 half-life of the drug; for 2, 3, and 4 half-lives, 75%, 87.6%, and 93.6% of the plateau concentration are reached, respectively. For practical purposes, steady state is achieved by 3-5 half-lives. The time required to reach steady state depends only on the drug's half-life. The shorter the half-life, the more rapidly steady state is reached. The size of the dose and the route of administration have little effect. Consequently, whether a drug is delivered by constant or intermittent IV injection, by other parenteral routes (provided there is no pharmaceutical manipulation to delay absorption), or PO, a steady state concentration is reached after at least 5 half-lives. The magnitude of drug concentrations at steady state compared with the first dose is determined by the relationship between dosing interval and the half-life. For drugs with a long half-life compared with the dosing interval, the drug will markedly accumulate. For drugs with a short half-life compared with the dosing interval, most of the drug is eliminated between doses, with little accumulation.

A drug normally requires some time to reach steady state. When some haste is necessary, plasma levels may be achieved more rapidly by the administration of a loading dose or doses. This entails the administration of a single large dose or smaller doses at frequent intervals to bring the concentration in plasma quickly to the level desired during the steady state. The loading dose required to achieve the plasma levels present at steady state can be determined from the fraction of drug eliminated during the dosing interval and the maintenance dose.

An appropriate dosing interval for most drugs depends on the distance between the maximum and the minimum target drug concentration (ie, therapeutic range). Shorter dosing intervals compared with half-life increase the risk of drug-induced toxicity because of increased blood levels. Prolonged dosing intervals diminish the drug's efficacy because of decreased blood levels. Often, however, dosing intervals equal to the half-lives are impractical for drugs with short half-lives. In most cases, either high doses of a relatively nontoxic drug are given to attain therapeutic concentrations for a sufficient time period, or potentially harmful drugs are administered by careful IV infusion. Another approach is to use dosage formulations or devices that allow for a more gradual release of the active principle into the systemic circulation.

DRUG ACTION AND PHARMACODYNAMICS

Pharmacodynamics is the study of the biochemical and physiologic effects of drugs and their mechanisms of action. It considers both drug action, which refers to the initial consequence of a drug-receptor interaction, and drug effect, which refers to the subsequent effects. The drug action of digoxin, for example, is inhibition of membrane Na^+/K^+-ATPase; the drug effect is augmentation of cardiac contractility.

Not all drugs exert their pharmacologic actions via receptor-mediated mechanisms. The action of some drugs—including inhalation anesthetic agents, osmotic diuretics, purgatives, antiseptics, antacids, chelating agents, and urinary acidifying and alkalinizing agents—is attributed to their physicochemical properties. Certain cancer and antiviral chemotherapeutic agents, which are analogs of pyrimidine and purine bases, elicit their effects when they are incorporated into nucleic acids and serve as suicide substrates for DNA or RNA synthesis. The effect of most drugs, however, results from their interactions with receptors. These interactions and the resulting conformational changes in the receptor initiate biochemical and physiologic changes that characterize the drug's response.

Drug Concentration and Effect

Drug therapy is intended to result in a particular pharmacologic response of desired intensity and duration while avoiding adverse drug reactions. The relationship between the administered dose and the clinical response has been investigated for some drugs using a pharmacokinetic/pharmacodynamic (PK/PD) modeling approach. However, a simpler relationship between the concentration of a drug and its effect in an idealized in vitro system is modeled mathematically to conceptualize receptor occupancy and drug response. The model assumes that the drug interacts reversibly with its receptor and produces an effect proportional to the number of receptors occupied, up to a maximal effect when all receptors are occupied. The reaction scheme for the model is:

$$\text{Drug (D)} + \text{Receptor (R)} \underset{k_1}{\overset{k_2}{\longleftrightarrow}} \text{DR} \rightarrow \text{Effect}$$

The relationship between effect and the concentration of free drug for the model can be written:

$$E = \frac{E_{max} \times C}{EC_{50} + C}$$

where E is the effect observed at concentration C, E_{max} is the maximal response that can be produced by the drug, and EC_{50} is the concentration of drug that produces 50% of maximal effect.

The above equation describes a rectangular hyperbola. It is generally more convenient to plot dose-response data as the drug effect (ordinate) against log dose or concentration (abscissa). The transformation yields a sigmoidal curve that allows the potency of different drugs to be readily compared. In addition, the effect of drugs used at therapeutic concentrations commonly falls on the portion of the sigmoidal curve that is approximately linear, ie, between 20% and 80% of maximal effect. This makes for easier interpretation of the plotted data.

Agonists and Antagonists

An **agonist** is a drug that binds to receptors and thereby alters (stabilizes) the proportion of receptors that are in the active conformation, resulting in a biologic response. A full agonist results in a maximal response by occupying all or a fraction of receptors. A partial agonist results in less than a maximal response even when the drug occupies all of the receptors. A partial agonist produces an effect if no full agonist is present, but acts as an antagonist in the presence of a full agonist. Concentration-effect curves of partial agonists resemble curves of full agonists in the presence of a noncompetitive antagonist.

An **antagonist** is a drug that blocks the response produced by an agonist. It interacts with the receptor or other component of the effector mechanism, but is devoid of intrinsic activity (ie, the ability to elicit a response upon binding to a receptor). A competitive antagonist results in reversible inhibition that can be overcome by increasing the concentration of agonist. The presence of a competitive antagonist causes a parallel shift of the log dose-effect curve to the right, without altering the E_{max} or EC_{50} of the agonist. A noncompetitive antagonist results in irreversible inhibition that generally prevents the agonist from producing a maximal effect (ie, E_{max} and EC_{50} are lowered). However, at low concentrations, a noncompetitive antagonist may cause a parallel shift of the log dose-effect curve to the right without reducing the maximal response of the agonist.

Agonists, but not antagonists, elicit an effect even when they bind to the same site on the same receptor. An explanation is provided by both structural and functional studies, which indicate that receptors exist in at least 2 conformations, active and inactive, and these are in equilibrium. Because agonists have a higher affinity for the receptor's active conformation, agonists drive the equilibrium to the active state, thereby activating the receptor. Conversely, antagonists have a higher affinity for the receptor's inactive conformation and push the equilibrium to the inactive state, producing no effect.

The concept of **spare receptors** is implicit in the definition of a noncompetitive antagonist; the latter effectively removes receptors irreversibly from the system. Yet low concentrations of a noncompetitive antagonist may result in a parallel shift of the log dose-effect curve to the right without reducing the maximal response of the agonist. This observation is attributed to a maximum response being elicited without all receptors being occupied, in which case the tissue is said to possess spare receptors. From a functional perspective, spare receptors are significant because they increase both the sensitivity and speed of a tissue's responsiveness to a ligand.

Structure-activity Relationships

The chemical structure of a drug determines its affinity for the receptor and ability to elicit a response (ie, intrinsic activity). Structure-activity relationships are exploited in drug design; relatively minor modifications to drug structure can potentially result in more favorable therapeutic profiles and/or pharmacokinetic properties.

Signal Transduction and Drug Action

Most receptors are proteins. The best characterized of these are regulatory proteins, enzymes, transport proteins, and structural proteins. Nucleic acids are also important drug receptors, particularly for cancer chemotherapeutic agents.

The receptors for several neurotransmitters modulate ion channel opening and closing through ligand gating or voltage gating. The nicotinic acetylcholine receptor is an example of a ligand-gated receptor, which allows Na^+ to flow down its concentration gradient into cells, resulting in depolarization. Most of the clinically useful neuromuscular blocking drugs used by anesthetists compete with acetylcholine for the receptor but do not initiate ion-channel opening. Other ligand-gated ion channels include the receptors for the excitatory amino acids (glutamate and aspartate), the inhibitory amino acids (γ-amino butyric acid [GABA] and glycine), and certain serotonin ($5\text{-}HT_3$) receptors. The sodium channel receptor is an example of a voltage-gated receptor; these are present in the membranes of excitable nerve, cardiac, and skeletal muscle cells. In the resting state, the Na^+/K^+-ATPase pump in these cells maintains an intracellular Na^+ concentration much lower than that in the extracellular environment. Membrane depolarization causes channel opening and a transient influx of Na^+ ions, followed by inactivation and return to the resting state. The action of local anesthetics is due to their direct interaction with voltage-gated Na^+ channels.

Many transmembrane receptors are linked to guanosine triphosphate binding proteins, which activate second messenger systems. Two important second messenger systems are cyclic adenosine monophosphate (cAMP) and the phosphoinositides. In cAMP second messenger systems, binding of the ligand to the receptor increases or decreases adenylyl cyclase activity, which in turn regulates the formation of cAMP from adenosine triphosphate. The activation of protein kinase A by cAMP results in the phosphorylation of proteins and a physiologic effect. From a therapeutic standpoint, drug binding to β-adrenergic, histamine H_2, or dopamine D_1 receptors activates adenylyl cyclase, whereas binding to muscarinic M_2, α_2-adrenergic, dopamine D_2, opiate μ and δ, adenosine A_1, or GABA type B receptors inhibits adenylyl cyclase. In phosphoinositide second messenger systems, membrane phosphatidylinositol 4,5-biphosphate is hydrolyzed to 1,4,5-trisphosphate (IP3) and 1,2-diacylglycerol (DAG) by activation of a phospholipase C. Both IP3 and DAG activate kinases, and in the case of IP3, this involves the mobilization of calcium from intracellular stores. The action of numerous drugs is due to their interaction with receptors that rely on these second messengers, which include α_1-adrenergic, muscarinic M_1 or M_2, serotonin $5\text{-}HT_2$, and thyrotropin-releasing hormone receptors.

Protein tyrosine kinase receptors are generally transmembrane enzymes that phosphorylate proteins exclusively on tyrosine residues, rather than on serine or threonine residues. They include endocrine hormone receptors for insulin and receptors for several growth hormones.

Intracellular receptors mediate the action of hormones such as glucocorticoids, estrogen, and thyroid hormone. These hormones, which regulate gene expression in the nucleus, are lipophilic and freely diffuse through the cell membrane to reach the receptor. Glucocorticoid receptors reside predominantly in the cytoplasm in an inactive form until they bind to the glucocorticoid steroid ligand. This results in receptor activation and translocation to the nucleus, where the receptor interacts with specific DNA sequences. Unlike glucocorticoid receptors, the receptors for estrogen and thyroid hormone reside in the nucleus.

Drug Dose and Clinical Response

To make rational therapeutic decisions, veterinarians must understand the fundamental concepts linking drug doses to clinical responses. The dose-response relationships for drugs may be graded or quantal. A **graded dose-response curve** can be constructed for responses that are measured on a continuous scale, eg, heart rate. Graded dose-response curves relate the intensity of response to the size of the dose, and hence are useful for characterizing the actions of drugs. A **quantal dose-response curve** can be constructed for drugs that elicit an all-or-none response, eg, presence or absence of epileptic seizures. For most drugs, the doses that are required to produce a specified quantal effect in a population are log normally distributed, so that the frequency distribution of responses plotted against log dose is a gaussian normal distribution curve. The percentage of the population requiring a particular dose to exhibit the effect can be determined from this curve. When these data are plotted as a cumulative frequency distribution, a sigmoidal dose-response curve is generated.

The **equilibrium dissociation constant of the receptor-drug complex, K_D,** is the ratio of rate constants for the reverse (k_2) and forward (k_1) reaction between the drug and receptor and the drug-receptor complex (*see* above). K_D is also the drug concentration at which receptor occupancy is half of maximum. Drugs with a high K_D (low affinity) dissociate rapidly from receptors; conversely, drugs with a low K_D (high affinity) dissociate slowly from receptors. These effects impact the rate at which biologic responses end.

The **affinity** of a drug for a receptor describes how avidly the drug binds to the receptor (ie, the K_D).

Potency refers to the concentration (EC_{50}) or dose (ED_{50}) of a drug required to produce 50% of the drug's maximal effect. EC_{50} equals K_D when there is a linear relationship between occupancy and response. Often, signal amplification occurs between receptor occupancy and response, which results in the EC_{50} for response being much less (ie, positioned to the left on the abscissa of the log dose-response curve) than K_D for receptor occupancy. Potency depends on both the affinity of a drug for its receptor, and the efficiency with which drug-receptor interaction is coupled to response. The dose of drug required to produce an effect is inversely related to potency. In general, low potency is important only if it results in a need to administer the drug in large doses that are impractical. The ED_{50} for a quantal dose-response relationship is the dose at which 50% of individuals exhibit the specified quantal effect.

Efficacy (also referred to as intrinsic activity) of a drug is the ability of the drug to elicit a response when it binds to the receptor. In some tissues, agonists demonstrating high efficacy can result in a maximal effect, even when only a small fraction of the receptors are occupied. Efficacy is not linked to potency of a drug.

The **median inhibitory concentration** or IC_{50} is the concentration of an antagonist that reduces a specified response to 50% of the maximal possible effect.

Selectivity refers to a drug's ability to preferentially produce a particular effect and is related to the structural specificity of drug binding to receptors. For example, propranolol (a β-blocker) binds equally well to β_1- and β_2-adrenoceptors; metoprolol (a cardioselective β-blocker) binds selectively to β_1-adrenoceptors; and salbutamol (a β-agonist used for treating asthma) binds selectively to β_2-adrenoceptors. The selectivity of salbutamol may be further enhanced by administering it directly to the lungs.

Specificity of drug action relates to the number of different mechanisms involved. Examples of specific drugs include atropine (a muscarinic antagonist), salbutamol (a β_2-adrenoceptor agonist), phenoxybenzamine (an α-adrenergic blocking agent), and cimetidine (an H_2-receptor antagonist). By contrast, nonspecific drugs result in drug effects through several mechanisms of action. A case in point is phenothiazine, which causes blockade of D_2-dopamine receptors, α-adrenergic receptors, and muscarinic receptors.

The **therapeutic index** of a drug is the ratio of the dose that results in an undesired effect to that which results in a desired effect. The therapeutic index of a drug is usually defined as the ratio of LD_{50} to ED_{50}, which indicates how selective the drug is in resulting in its desired effect. Values of LD_{50} and ED_{50} for this purpose are derived from quantal dose-response curves generated in animal studies.

The information obtained from dose-response curves is critically important when choosing between drugs and when determining the dose to administer. A drug is chosen largely on the basis of its clinical effectiveness for a particular therapeutic indication. In this context, the drug concentration at the receptor (determined by the pharmacokinetic properties of the drug) and the efficacy of the drug-receptor complex are the primary determinants of a drug's clinical effectiveness. The administered dose of a drug, by comparison, depends to a greater extent on potency than on maximal efficacy.

The maximal efficacy of the drug-receptor complex to result in a graded effect is E_{max} on a graded dose-response curve. E_{max} is derived from a quantitative dose-response relationship for a single animal and varies among individuals. The extrapolation of this value of E_{max} to a clinical case is only an estimate, but it facilitates a comparison of the maximal efficacy of drugs that result in a specified effect by identical receptors. A drug's potency (ie, EC_{50} or ED_{50}) obtained from either graded or quantal dose-response curves is used to determine the dose that should be administered. The slope of the graded dose-response curve provides information concerning the dose range over which a drug elicits its effect. Other information concerning the selectivity of drug action and the therapeutic index is also obtained from the graded dose-response curve. When quantal effects are being considered, information concerning pharmacologic potency, selectivity of drug action, the margin of safety, and the potential variability of responsiveness among individuals is obtained from quantal dose-response curves.

An indication of the ability of drugs to reach the receptor is obtained from pharmacokinetic parameters that characterize the absorption, distribution, and clearance of a drug. There may not be a simple temporal correlation between plasma concentration of a drug and its therapeutic effect, in which case plotting plasma concentrations of a drug (abscissa) versus therapeutic effect (ordinate) in chronologic order displays the data as a loop. This phenomenon is referred to as hysteresis in the concentration-effect relationship. A counterclockwise hysteresis loop is observed for a drug such as digoxin, which distributes slowly to its site of action. The extent and duration of action of a competitive antagonist depends on its concentration in plasma, which depends (in part) on its rate of elimination. This requires that the dose be adjusted accordingly to maintain plasma concentrations in the therapeutic range. By contrast, the duration of action of an irreversible antagonist is relatively independent of its rate of elimination, and therefore plasma concentration, and more dependent on the rate of turnover of receptor molecules.

The density of most receptors is not constant with time, which has important therapeutic implications. Down-regulation of receptors may occur as a result of continual stimulation by an agonist, and manifests as the development of tachyphylaxis, which demonstrates a clockwise hysteresis loop in the concentration-effect relationship. Conversely, additional receptors can be synthesized in response to chronic receptor antagonism—a phenomenon known as up-regulation. Because more receptors are now available, a hyperreactive response occurs when the cell is exposed to an agonist.

DOSAGE FORMS AND DELIVERY SYSTEMS

A diverse range of dosage forms and delivery systems has been developed to provide for the care and welfare of animals. The development of dosage forms draws on the discipline of biopharmaceutics, which integrates an understanding of formulations, dissolution, stability and controlled release (pharmaceutics); absorption, distribution, metabolism, and excretion (pharmacokinetics, PK); concentration-effect relationships and drug-receptor interactions (pharmacodynamics, PD), and treatment of the disease state (therapeutics). Formulation of a dosage form typically involves combining an active ingredient and one or more excipients; the resultant dosage form determines the route of administration and the clinical efficacy and safety of the drug. Optimization of drug doses is also critical to achieving clinical efficacy and safety. Increasingly, a PK/PD model that describes the drug response is the basis of dose optimization. The PK and PD phases are linked by the premise that free drug in the systemic circulation is in equilibrium with the receptors. The PD phase involves interaction of the drug with receptor, which triggers post-receptor events, and eventually leads to a drug effect (*see* p 1949).

Drug delivery strategies for veterinary formulations are complicated by the diversity of species and breeds treated, the wide range in body sizes, different husbandry practices, seasonal variations, cost constraints associated with the value of the animal being treated, the persistence of residues in food and fiber (wool, mohair), and the level of convenience, among other factors. Innovative solutions have been developed to meet many of these challenges (eg, the convenient dosing option offered by topical spot-on formulations for treating external and internal parasites on dogs and cats, the microencapsulation of NSAID as a means of masking taste when these agents are added to the rations of horses). Unique opportunities also exist for controlled-release drug delivery systems in veterinary medicine, and many such systems are on the market. For example, a range of controlled-release boluses have been developed for delivering antimicrobials, anthelmintics, production enhancers, nutritional supplements, and other drugs to ruminants.

Oral Dosage Forms and Delivery Systems

Oral dosage forms comprise liquids (solutions, suspensions, and emulsions), semi-solids (pastes), and solids (tablets, capsules, powders, granules, premixes, and medicated blocks).

A **solution** is a mixture of 2 or more components that form a single phase that is homogeneous down to the molecular level. Solutions offer several advantages over other dosage forms. Compared with solid dosage forms, solutions are absorbed faster and generally cause less irritation of the GI mucosa. Moreover, phase separation on storage is not a concern with solutions, as it may be for suspensions and emulsions. The disadvantages of solutions include susceptibility to microbial contamination and the hydrolysis in aqueous solution of susceptible active ingredients. In addition, the taste of some drugs is more unpleasant when in solution. A range of additives is used in the formulation of oral solutions, including buffers, flavors, antioxidants, and preservatives. Oral solutions provide a convenient means of drug administration to neonates and young animals.

A **suspension** is a coarse dispersion of insoluble drug particles, generally with a diameter exceeding 1 μm, in a liquid (usually aqueous) medium. Suspensions are useful for administering insoluble or poorly soluble drugs or in situations when the presence of a finely divided form of the material in the GI tract is required. An example of the latter is the treatment of "frothy bloat" with dimethyl polysiloxanes, which relies on a dispersion of finely divided silica in the forestomach of ruminants. The taste of most drugs is less noticeable in suspension than in solution, due to the drug being less soluble in suspension. Particle size is an important determinant of the dissolution rate and bioavailability of drugs in suspension. In addition to the excipients described above for solutions, suspensions include surfactants and thickening agents. Surfactants wet the solid particles, thereby ensuring the particles disperse readily throughout the liquid. Thickening agents reduce the rate at which particles settle to the bottom of the container. Some settling is acceptable, provided the sediment can be readily dispersed when the container is shaken. Because hard masses of sediment do not satisfy this criterion, caking of suspensions is not acceptable.

An **emulsion** is a system consisting of 2 immiscible liquid phases, one of which is dispersed throughout the other in the form of fine droplets; droplet diameter generally ranges from 0.1-100 μm. The 2 phases of an emulsion are known as the dispersed phase and the continuous phase. Emulsions are inherently unstable and are stabilized through the use of an emulsifying agent, which prevents coalescence of the dispersed droplets. Creaming, as occurs with milk, also occurs with pharmaceutical emulsions. However, it is not a serious problem because a uniform dispersion returns upon shaking. Creaming is, nonetheless, undesirable because it is associated with an increased likelihood of the droplets coalescing and the emulsion breaking. Other additives include buffers, antioxidants, and preservatives. Emulsions for oral administration are usually oil (the active ingredient) in water, and facilitate the administration of oily substances such as castor oil or liquid paraffin in a more palatable form.

A **paste** is a 2-component semi-solid in which drug is dispersed as a powder in an aqueous or fatty base. The particle size of the active ingredient in pastes can be as large as 100 μm. The vehicle containing the drug may be water; a polyhydroxy liquid such as glycerin, propylene glycol, or polyethylene glycol; a vegetable oil; or a mineral oil. Other formulation excipients include thickening agents, cosolvents, adsorbents, humectants, and preservatives. The thickening agent may be a naturally occurring material such as acacia or tragacanth, or a synthetic or chemically modified derivative such as xanthum gum or hydroxypropylmethyl cellulose. The degree of cohesiveness, plasticity, and syringeability of pastes is attributed to the thickening agent. It may be necessary to include a cosolvent to increase the solubility of the drug. Syneresis of pastes is a form of instability in which the solid and liquid components of the formulation separate over time; it is prevented by including an adsorbent such as microcrystalline cellulose. A humectant (eg, glycerin or propylene glycol) is used to prevent the paste that collects at the nozzle of the dispenser from forming a hard crust. Microbial growth in the formulation is inhibited using a preservative. It is critical that pastes have a pleasant taste or are tasteless. Pastes are a popular dosage form for treating cats and horses, and can be easily and safely administered by owners.

A **tablet** consists of one or more active ingredients and numerous excipients and may be a conventional tablet that is swallowed whole, a chewable tablet, or a modified-release tablet (more commonly referred to as a modified-release bolus due to its large unit size). Conventional and chewable tablets are used to administer drugs to dogs and cats, whereas modified-release boluses are administered to cattle, sheep, and goats. The physical and chemical stability of tablets is generally better than that of liquid dosage forms. The main disadvantages of tablets are the bioavailability of poorly water-soluble drugs or poorly absorbed drugs, and the local irritation of the GI mucosa that some drugs may cause.

A **capsule** is an oral dosage form usually made from gelatin and filled with an active ingredient and excipients. Two common capsule types are available: hard gelatin capsules for solid-fill formulations, and soft gelatin capsules for liquid-fill or semi-solid-fill formulations. Soft gelatin capsules are suitable for formulating poorly water-soluble drugs because they afford good drug release and absorption by the GI tract. Gelatin capsules are frequently more expensive than tablets but have some advantages. For example, particle size is rarely altered during capsule manufacture, and capsules mask the taste and odor of the active ingredient and protect photolabile ingredients.

A **powder** is a formulation in which a drug powder is mixed with other powdered excipients to produce a final product for oral administration. Powders have better chemical stability than liquids and dissolve faster than tablets or capsules because disintegration is not an issue. This translates into faster absorption for those drugs characterized by dissolution rate-limited absorption. Unpleasant tastes can be more pronounced with powders than with other dosage forms and can be a particular concern with in-feed powders, in which it contributes to variable ingestion of the dose. Moreover, sick animals often eat less and are therefore not amenable to treatment with in-feed powder formulations. Drug powders are principally used prophylactically in feed, or formulated as a soluble powder for addition to drinking water or milk replacer. Powders have also been formulated with emulsifying agents to facilitate their administration as liquid drenches.

A **granule** is a dosage form consisting of powder particles that have been aggregated to form a larger mass, usually 2-4 mm in diameter. Granulation overcomes segregation of the different particle sizes during storage and/or dose administration, the latter being a potential source of inaccurate dosing. Granules and powders generally behave similarly; however, granules must deaggregate prior to dissolution and absorption.

A **premix** is a solid dosage form in which an active ingredient, such as a coccidiostat, production enhancer, or nutritional supplement, is formulated with excipients. Premix products are mixed homogeneously with feed at rates (when expressed on an active ingredient basis) that range from a few milligrams to ~200 g/ton of feed. They are administered to poultry, pigs, and ruminants. The density, particle size, and geometry of the premix particles should match as closely as possible those of the feed in which the premix will be incorporated to facilitate uniform mixing. Issues such as instability, electrostatic charge, and hygroscopicity must also be addressed. The excipients present in premix formulations include carriers, liquid binders, diluents, anti-caking agents, and anti-dust agents. Carriers, such as wheat middlings, soybean mill run, and rice hulls, bind active ingredients to their surfaces and are important in attaining uniform mixing of the active ingredient. A liquid binding agent, such as a vegetable oil, should be included in the formulation whenever a carrier is used. Diluents increase the bulk of premix formulations, but unlike carriers, do not bind the active ingredients. Examples of diluents include ground limestone, dicalcium phosphate, dextrose, and kaolin. Caking in a premix formulation may be caused by hygroscopic ingredients and is addressed by adding small amounts of anti-caking agents such as calcium silicate, silicon dioxide, and hydrophobic starch. The dust associated with powdered premix formulations can have serious implications for both operator safety and economic losses, and is reduced by including a vegetable oil or light mineral oil in the formulation. An alternate approach to overcoming dust is to granulate the premix formulation.

A **medicated block** is a compressed feed material that contains an active ingredient, such as a drug, anthelmintic, surfactant (for bloat prevention), or a nutritional supplement, and is commonly packaged in a cardboard box. Ruminants typically have free access to the medicated block over several days, and variable consumption may be problematic. This concern is addressed by ensuring the active ingredient is nontoxic, stable, palatable, and preferably of low solubility. In addition, excipients in the formulation modulate consumption by altering the palatability and/or the hardness of the medicated block. For example, molasses increases palatability and sodium chloride decreases it. Additionally, the incorporation of a binder such as lignin sulfonate in blocks manufactured by compression or magnesium oxide in blocks manufactured by chemical reaction, increases hardness. The hygroscopic nature of molasses in a formulation may also impact the hardness of medicated blocks and is addressed by using appropriate packaging.

Oral Modified-release Delivery Systems

Several modified-release delivery systems have been developed that take advantage of the unique anatomy of the ruminant forestomach. These systems generally comprise intraruminal boluses with a controlled rate of release and are administered using a balling gun. Release of the active ingredient generally relies on erosion, diffusion from a reservoir, dissolution of a dispersed matrix, or an osmotic "driver." Regurgitation during rumination is prevented by the bolus having a density of ~3 g/cm^3 or a variable geometry.

Several sustained-release boluses containing sulfonamides are available for treating cattle. These provide for the delivery of the active ingredient over a period of ~72 hr. Sustained-release boluses, which contain methoprene or diflubenzuron, are approved for the control of manure-breeding flies in cattle.

The intraruminal devices for supplementing cattle and sheep with copper, cobalt, or selenium are erodible systems that include intraruminal pellets (also known as bullets) and soluble glass boluses. Limitations of these systems include loss via regurgitation during rumination and the formation of calcium phosphate coatings on the surface of the pellets. Copper oxide needles encapsulated in gelatin are also available for supplementing sheep and cattle with copper. The gelatin capsule dissolves in the rumen; however, they are not strictly intraruminal devices because the particles progress into the abomasum where some are trapped in the mucosal folds and release copper. Boluses of soluble glass containing copper, cobalt, and selenium are designed to dissolve in ruminal fluids, thereby releasing the incorporated elements. The composition of the glass determines the solubility of the bolus, with an increase in the ratio of monovalent to divalent cations resulting in an increase in solubility. The glass boluses are retained in the rumen for up to 9 mo.

Most commercially available intraruminal boluses are continuous-release devices. A number of these depend on erosion for release of the active ingredient.

Parenteral Dosage Forms and Delivery Systems

Parenteral dosage forms and delivery systems include injectables (ie, solutions, suspensions, emulsions, and dry powders for reconstitution), intramammary infusions, intravaginal delivery systems, and implants.

A **solution** for injection is a mixture of 2 or more components that form a single phase that is homogeneous down to the molecular level. "Water for injection" is the most widely used solvent for parenteral formulations. However, a nonaqueous solvent or a mixed aqueous/nonaqueous solvent system may be necessary to stabilize drugs that are readily hydrolyzed by water or to improve solubility. A range of excipients may be included in parenteral solutions, including antioxidants, antimicrobial agents, buffers, chelating agents, inert gases, and substances for adjusting tonicity. Antioxidants maintain product stability by being preferentially oxidized over the shelf life of the product.

Antimicrobial preservatives inhibit the growth of any microbes that are accidentally introduced while doses are being withdrawn from multiple-dose bottles and act as adjuncts in aseptic processing of products. Buffers are necessary to maintain both solubility of the active ingredient and stability of the product. Chelating agents are added to complex and thereby inactivate metals, including copper, iron, and zinc, which generally catalyze oxidative degradation of drugs. Inert gases are used to displace the air in solutions and enhance product integrity of oxygen-sensitive drugs. Isotonicity of the formulation is achieved by including a tonicity-adjusting agent. Failing to adjust the tonicity of the solution can result in the hemolysis or crenation of erythrocytes when hypotonic or hypertonic solutions, respectively, are given IV in quantities >100 mL. Injectable formulations must be sterile and free of pyrogens. Pyrogenic substances are primarily lipid polysaccharides derived from microorganisms, with those produced by gram-negative bacilli generally being most potent. Injectable solutions are very commonly used, and aqueous solutions given IM result in immediate drug absorption, provided precipitation at the injection site does not occur.

A **suspension** for injection consists of insoluble solid particles dispersed in a liquid medium, with the solid particles accounting for 0.5-30% of the suspension. The vehicle may be aqueous, oil, or both. Caking of injectable suspensions is minimized through the production of flocculated systems, comprising clusters of particles (flocs) held together in a loose open structure. Excipients in injectable suspensions include antimicrobial preservatives, surfactants, dispersing or suspending agents, and buffers. Surfactants wet the suspended powders and provide acceptable syringeability while suspending agents modify the viscosity of the formulation. The ease of injection and the availability of the drug in depot therapy are affected by the viscosity of the suspension and the particle size of the suspended drug. These systems afford enhanced stability to active ingredients that are prone to hydrolysis in aqueous solutions. Injectable suspensions are commonly used. Compared with that of injectable solutions, the rate of drug absorption of injectable suspensions is prolonged because additional time is required for disintegration and dissolution of the suspended drug particles. The slower release of drug from an oily suspension compared with that of an aqueous suspension is attributed to the additional time taken by drug particles suspended in an oil depot to reach the oil/water boundary and become wetted before dissolving in tissue fluids.

An **emulsion** for injection is a heterogeneous dispersion of one immiscible liquid in another; it relies on an emulsifying agent for stability. Parenteral emulsions are rare because it is seldom necessary to achieve an emulsion for drug administration. Untoward physiologic effects following IV administration may occur, including emboli in blood vessels if the droplets are >1 μm in diameter. Formulation options for injectable emulsions are also severely restricted because suitable stabilizers and emulsifiers are very limited. Examples of parenteral emulsions include oil-in-water sustained-release depot preparations, which are given IM, and water-in-oil emulsions of allergenic extracts, which are given SC.

A **dry powder** for parenteral administration is reconstituted as a solution or as a suspension immediately prior to injection. The principal advantage of this dosage form is that it overcomes the problem of instability in solution.

Mastitis **intramammary infusion products** are available for lactating and nonlactating (dry) cows. Lactating cow intramammary infusions should demonstrate fast and even distribution of the drug and a low degree of binding to udder tissue. These properties result in lower concentrations of drug residues in the milk. By comparison, it is desirable for nonlactating cow formulations to demonstrate prolonged drug release and a high degree of binding to mammary secretions and udder tissues. Particle size is particularly important because it affects both the rate of release of the active ingredient and irritancy to the udder tissue. Drug particle size in nonlactating intramammary formulations is usually smaller than in those for lactating cows, which is critical in reducing irritancy during prolonged retention in the udder. Thickening agents are added to modify the rate of release of the suspended particles from oil formulations, and antioxidants are commonly incorporated in the formulations to prevent rancidity. Mastitis infusion products are often terminally sterilized by irradiation.

Intravaginal delivery systems include controlled internal drug release (CIDR) devices, progesterone-releasing intravaginal devices (PRID), and vaginal sponges. These systems are used for estrus synchronization in sheep, goats, and cattle. Silicone is used in the manufacture of the T-shaped CIDR device and the coil-shaped PRID, whereas intravaginal sponges are made from polyurethane. The active ingredients in these systems are synthetic or natural hormones such as progesterone, methylacetoxy progesterone, fluorogestone acetate, or estradiol benzoate. An applicator consisting of a speculum and a separate plunger is used to insert sponges into the vaginal cavities of sheep and goats, and PRID into the vaginal cavities of cattle. A different type of applicator is used for inserting CIDR devices into the vaginal cavities of sheep, goats, and cattle. Retention in the vagina depends on either the entire device (sponges and PRID), or the wings (CIDR device), expanding. With all 3 devices, gentle pressure exerted on the vaginal wall is responsible for retention of the device, which is >95%.

The majority of **implants** used in veterinary medicine are compressed tablets or dispersed matrix systems in which the drug is uniformly dispersed within a nondegradable polymer. Drug release from dispersed matrix systems involves dissolution of the drug into the polymer, followed by diffusion of the drug through the polymer, and partitioning from the surface of the polymer into the surrounding aqueous environment. Implants are available to increase weight gain and feed conversion efficiency in food-producing animals. These implants are typically prepared in a manner similar to tablets. One controlled-release implant consists of a cylindrical core of silicone, surrounded by an outer layer of estradiol-loaded silicone. A range of implants is available to enhance reproductive performance in breeding animals. These include ear implants containing norgestomet dispersed in polyethylene methacrylate or silicone, a biocompatible tablet implant containing deslorelin (a GnRH agonist) for use in mares that does not require removal, and a sustained-release pellet of melatonin, which is implanted in the ear of ewes to enhance breeding performance. Testosterone pellets are available for implanting in the ears of wethers at doses of 70-100 mg every 3 mo for the prevention of ulcerative posthitis.

Topical Dosage Forms and Delivery Systems

The topical dosage forms available for treating animals include solids (dusting powders), semisolids (creams, ointments, and pastes), and liquids (solutions, suspension concentrates, suspoemulsions, and emulsifiable concentrates). Of special interest are transdermal delivery systems that elicit clinical responses by carrying medications across the skin barrier to the bloodstream. Examples of these are transdermal gels and patches that are used in companion animals. Also of interest are dosage forms that are unique to veterinary medicine, such as spot-on, pour-on, and backliner formulations developed for the control of parasites.

A **dusting powder** is a finely divided insoluble powder containing ingredients such as talc, zinc oxide, or starch. Coarse powders often have a gritty feel, whereas powders containing particles that are <20 μm in all dimensions have a smooth feel. Some dusting powders absorb moisture, which discourages bacterial growth. Others are used for their lubricant properties. The use of dusting powders is indicated on skin folds and contraindicated on wet surfaces, as caking is likely to result.

A **cream** is a semisolid emulsion formulated for application to the skin or mucous membranes. Droplet diameter in topical emulsions generally ranges from 0.1-100 μm. Cream emulsions are most commonly oil-in-water but may be water-in-oil. The former readily rub into the skin (hence the term "vanishing" cream), and are readily removed by licking and washing. By comparison, water-in-oil emulsions are emollient and cleansing. Water-in-oil emulsions are also less greasy and spread more readily than ointments, and soothe inflamed skin as a consequence of the water in the formulation evaporating.

An **ointment** is a greasy, semisolid preparation that contains dissolved or dispersed drug. A range of ointment bases is used, including hydrocarbons, vegetable oils, silicones, absorption bases consisting of a mixture of hydrocarbons and lanolin, emulsifying bases consisting of a mixture of hydrocarbons and an emulsifying agent, and water-soluble bases. Ointment bases influence topical drug bioavailability via 2 mechanisms.

First, their occlusive properties are responsible for hydrating the stratum corneum, which enhances the flux of drug across the skin. Second, they affect drug dissolution within the ointment and drug partitioning from the ointment into the skin. Ointments are effective emollients due to their occlusive nature. Ointments are indicated for chronic, dry lesions and contraindicated in exudative lesions.

A **paste** for topical use is a stiff preparation containing a high proportion of finely powdered solids such as starch, zinc oxide, calcium carbonate, and talc. Pastes are less greasy than ointments because much of the fluid hydrocarbon fraction is absorbed onto the solid particles. Pastes are also less occlusive than ointments. Pastes are indicated for ulcerated lesions.

A **solution** for topical use is a mixture of 2 or more components that form a single phase down to the molecular level. Topical solutions include eye drops, ear drops, and lotions. **Eye drops** are sterile liquids that contain a range of drugs, including local anesthetics, antibiotics, anti-inflammatory agents, and drugs acting on the autonomic nervous system of the eye. They are instilled onto the eyeball or within the conjunctival sac. **Ear drops** are solutions of drugs such as antibiotics, insecticides, or anti-inflammatory agents. The vehicle may be water, glycerol, propylene glycol, or alcohol/water mixtures. They are applied to the external auditory canal. A **lotion** is usually an aqueous solution (or suspension) for application to inflamed, ulcerated skin. Lotions cool the skin by evaporation of solvents, leaving a film of dry powder. Lotions are suitable for use on hairy areas and for lesions with minor exudation and ulceration.

A **suspension concentrate** for topical use is a mixture of insoluble, solid active ingredients, which are normally at high concentrations, in water or oil. Suspension concentrate formulations are generally water-based; the water-insoluble active ingredients and inert ingredients are of very small particle size (0.1-5 μm). Other formulation additives include suspending agents, surfactants, and other excipients to ensure the production of a shelf-stable, pourable product. Surfactants serve to wet, disperse, and stabilize the solid particles in the continuous phase, prevent flocculation, and prevent changes in particle size. Thickening agents are included to increase the viscosity of the formulation, thereby overcoming sedimentation of the suspended particles and affording good long-term stability. Suspension concentrates are used topically as pour-ons, plunge and shower dip concentrates, and jetting fluids.

A **suspoemulsion** combines the elements of an emulsion and a suspension, allowing active ingredients with widely varying physical properties to be formulated in a single product. Typically, a suspoemulsion contains one or more solvent-soluble active ingredients in an emulsion phase, combined with one or more low solubility active ingredients in a continuous aqueous suspension phase.

Following dilution, an **emulsifiable concentrate** for topical use produces a 2-phase system involving 2 immiscible liquids, a dispersed phase consisting of fine oil droplets ranging in size from 0.5 μm to several hundred microns, and a continuous phase. Addition of an emulsifiable concentrate formulation to water results in the formation of an emulsion, which relies on surface-active agents concentrating at the oil/water interface. Active ingredients that are soluble in water-immiscible organic solvents are frequently formulated as emulsifiable concentrates. The flocculation of oil droplets in emulsifiable concentrate formulations leads to a layer of cream that can be readily dispersed by mild agitation, whereas the coalescence of droplets leads to the inversion or "breaking" of the emulsion. Water with a high content of Ca^{2+} and/or Mg^{2+} reacts with anionic surfactants in the emulsifiable concentrate formulation; this affects both spontaneity of emulsification and stability. Zinc sulfate, which is used as a dip additive to minimize the spread of dermatophilosis in sheep, also adversely affects emulsions.

A **transdermal delivery gel** consists of a vehicle, most commonly pluronic lecithin organogel (PLO gel), which delivers drug via the transdermal route to the bloodstream. The micellar composition of PLO gel enhances skin penetration of the pharmaceutical agent present in the formulation. PLO gel is generally well tolerated and is nontoxic if ingested. However, not all drugs are suitable for transdermal application and there are relatively few studies of the bioavailability of drugs from compounded transdermal gels. Transdermal gels are used to deliver drugs to treat several diseases in dogs and cats, including undesirable behavior, cardiac disease, and hyperthyroidism. The dose is applied to the inner surface of the pinnae, thereby offering ease of administration, especially in cats.

A **transdermal delivery patch** typically consists of a drug incorporated into a reservoir, a protective backing layer, a rate-limiting release membrane, and an adhesive layer for securing the patch to the skin. The physicochemical properties of a drug suitable for transdermal delivery ideally include low molecular weight (<500 daltons), high potency, water solubility (to facilitate movement of the drug out of the reservoir and to allow passage through the epidermal and dermal layers of the skin), and lipid solubility (to permit penetration of the stratum corneum of the skin). Fentanyl, a synthetic opioid agonist, is delivered by transdermal patch in dogs, cats, and horses.

Specialized Topical Dosage Forms, Delivery Systems, and Application Methods for Parasite Control: The control of internal and external parasites of companion and food-producing animals has led to the development of specialized dosage forms, delivery systems, and application methods that are unique to veterinary medicine.

A **spot-on** formulation is a solution of active ingredient(s), which typically contains a cosolvent and a spreading agent. The active ingredients in spot-on products for flea, GI parasite, and heartworm control in dogs and cats include fipronil, imidacloprid, selamectin, pyriproxyfen, ivermectin, and moxidectin. Spot-on formulations are also available to control lice in cattle. The physicochemical properties of the active ingredient(s) are important determinants of topical or transdermal behavior. Topical activity against ectoparasites depends to some extent on the active ingredient spreading, mixing with the sebum coating the skin and hair, and forming depots in the pilosebaceous units. The mechanism of percutaneous drug absorption varies between species and is not completely understood. However, low molecular weight and a high lipid/water partition coefficient tend to favor passage of the drug through the skin.

Backliner products for sheep consist of pour-on and spray-on formulations for the control of lice and sheep blowflies. Sheep lousicides include synthetic pyrethroids, organophosphates, and insect growth regulators. These products are formulated for pour-on application within 24 hr after shearing or spray-on application (sheep with wool growth >6 wk). Their efficacy against lice depends on topical activity and not on percutaneous absorption of the active ingredient into the bloodstream. Translocation of the pesticide from the application site to remote sites at concentrations lethal to lice is critical to the efficacy of these products and is facilitated by the increased secretion of wool grease that occurs after shearing.

The active ingredients in sheep blowfly products include insect growth regulators, synthetic pyrethroids, and organophosphates. Following their topical application, sheep blowfly larvicides form follicular depots at the time of application and subsequently translocate as a coating on new wool growing out of the follicles.

Hand-jetting of long-wool sheep (wool growth >6 wk) is done to control lice, keds, mites, and sheep blowflies. The pesticides used include rotenone, synthetic pyrethroids, organophosphates, insect growth regulators, and macrocyclic lactones. Hand-jetting involves the use of a handpiece (or wand) to "rake" a pesticide solution into the wool along the dorsal midline and sometimes into the breech or crutch, as well as the poll. The solution penetrates to the skin.

Some of the **pour-on** products on the market are formulated to deliver an active ingredient percutaneously. The macrocyclic lactones ivermectin, moxidectin, doramectin, and eprinomectin are formulated as pour-on preparations for application to cattle. These formulations are usually solutions or emulsifiable concentrates for dilution with water prior to use. The principal route of percutaneous absorption for most drugs in humans is the intercellular pathway, making the intercellular lipid matrix the primary barrier to absorption. However, this may not be the case in species (eg, cattle and sheep) in which the emulsifying properties of skin secretions and the large numbers of follicles and glands per unit surface area must be taken into account. Ionized solutes, for example, are reported to cross the skin of animals via shunt pathways (sweat ducts, follicles). Pour-on products are formulated to spread without run-off when applied to the skin and to be resistant to rain. The formulation also facilitates the partitioning of the drug out of the vehicle and into the skin and transport of the drug across the skin. The control of these processes is critical because some drug is required to remain at the skin if the drug is to be active against external parasites. In addition, too rapid passage of drug through the skin may result in unacceptable chemical residues in tissues or milk.

The **plunge dipping** of sheep and cattle for external parasites requires a dipping vat, which may be a portable unit or a permanent in-ground structure shielded from direct sunlight by roofing. A draining pen located at the exit of the vat allows dip wash draining off treated animals to return to the vat. Dip chemicals are usually formulated as aqueous solutions, emulsifiable concentrates, or suspension concentrates, all of which are diluted with water prior to use. The high costs associated with plunge dipping relate principally to the costs of chemicals for charging large vats, labor, and the disposal of the hazardous wastes. Plunge dips must be managed properly, and the pesticide maintained at the concentration recommended by the manufacturer. Dipping of sheep and cattle is associated with "stripping" of the active ingredient from the dip wash, eg, pesticide loss from the dip wash occurring at a greater rate than water loss, and is categorized as mechanical or chemical. In the case of sheep, mechanical stripping results from the fleece acting as a sieve toward the active ingredient, with the degree of filtration being primarily determined by particle size. Chemical stripping is due to the preferential absorption of pesticide by the fleece. To counteract stripping, a complex dip management regimen that involves reinforcement and "topping-up" is used. Reinforcement refers to the addition of undiluted chemical product to the dip without the addition of water, whereas topping-up refers to the addition of water and undiluted chemical product to the dip vat to return the volume to the starting level. Proper dip management also minimizes the contamination of the dip with organic matter. This requires that the race leading to the vat is constructed of concrete or slats to remove dirt from the animals' feet and for animals to be held in a yard overnight prior to dipping, during which time they are offered water but no food.

Hand spraying generally results in uneven coverage of animals and is considered an inefficient method of application. By comparison, recirculating and nonrecirculating **spray races** facilitate whole body spraying and wet cattle to the skin. The situation with sheep is different— the very short contact time in a spray race limits the uptake of insecticide, which means that the fleece seldom becomes saturated. Because of this, spray races should be used as an adjunct to shower or plunge dipping of sheep.

Shower dips are less labor intensive than plunge dips and are cheaper to operate. A typical shower dip consists of a sump containing the dip wash, a pump, and a showering pen constructed with a concrete floor and fitted with an overhead rotating boom with nozzles and fixed nozzles near ground level. There are 2 types of shower dips: a conventional shower dip in which the sump volume is periodically maintained by adding fresh dip wash, and a constant replenishment shower dip in which a small-volume sump is continuously filled from a large-volume supply tank to maintain dip levels. Proper dip management requires attention to the factors described above for plunge dipping. In addition, all equipment must be functioning properly for the fleece to become saturated. Sheep should not be dipped (by either the plunge or shower method) until shearing wounds have healed to avoid clostridial infections or caseous lymphadenitis caused by *Corynebacterium pseudotuberculosis*. Moreover, the correct use of bacteriostats is recommended to prevent post-dipping lameness caused by *Erysipelothrix insidiosa*.

Insecticidal collars are plasticized polymer resins impregnated with an active ingredient. Collars for the control of ticks and fleas on dogs and cats release the active ingredient as a vapor, a dust, or a liquid, depending on the physicochemical properties of the chemical. Volatile liquid insecticides such as dichlorvos or naled are used in vapor-release collars. The insecticide distributes through the collar matrix as a vapor before being released. Powdered insecticides such as phosmet, stirofos, carbaryl, and propoxur are used in dust-release collars. Translocation of the active ingredient within the collar matrix leads to deposits forming at the surface; distribution of the insecticide to the animal depends on the physical activity of the animal. Nonvolatile liquid insecticides such as chlorfenvinphos or diazinon are used in liquid-release collars. The active ingredient distributes as a liquid in the collar matrix and to the surface, where it is released. The animal's activity plus the dissolution of lipophilic insecticides in skin secretions are important factors in the translocation of the insecticide from the collar to the animal.

Two types of insecticide-releasing **ear tags** for controlling flies on cattle are available. One is constructed from a polymer that provides structural support and acts as a release rate-controlling matrix. The other is a membrane-based ear tag that consists of an insecticidal reservoir with a relatively impermeable backing on one side and a rate-controlling membrane on the other. Both types rely on the animal's ear and head movements and grooming to transfer insecticide from the surface of the ear tag to the animal's skin or to other animals.

Back rubbers typically consist of burlap supported across lanes, gateways, or areas where cattle congregate. Back rubbers are charged by soaking thoroughly in oil-containing pesticide, typically a synthetic pyrethroid, an organophosphate, or a combination of the two. The oil retards evaporation of the insecticide and enhances adherence to the animal's coat.

Dust bags facilitate the self-treatment of cattle in the control of flies and lice. They are constructed of an inner porous bag containing the active ingredient, which is commonly a synthetic pyrethroid or an organophosphate, and an outer weatherproof skirt. Dust bags are hung in lanes or gateways so that passing cattle brush against them and receive a topical application of pesticide.

CHEMICAL RESIDUES IN FOOD AND FIBER

Veterinary drugs and pesticides are used routinely in animal production to manage diseases and control parasites, and crop protection chemicals are used in the production of animal feeds. It is possible, therefore, for foodstuffs of animal origin to be adulterated with residues of veterinary drugs and pesticides, and for animal fibers to be contaminated with pesticide residues. The veterinarian must consider the implications of both possibilities when providing for the health and welfare of animals. First, animals and animal products destined for human consumption must not contain residues of drugs or pesticides that exceed legally permitted concentrations. Second, pesticide residues in fiber have potential implications for public health, occupational health and safety, and environmental safety.

Chemical Residues in Foodstuffs of Animal Origin

Chemical residues may be found in animal tissues, milk, or eggs following the administration of veterinary drugs and medicated premixes, the application of pesticides to animals, or the consumption of stockfeeds previously treated with agricultural chemicals.

Residues Resulting from Veterinary Drugs, Medicated Feeds, or Application of Pesticides: Extensive regulatory and monitoring systems have been established to ensure that chemical residues in food do not constitute an unacceptable health risk. The premarket approval process undertaken by regulatory authorities for new veterinary drugs and medicated feeds evaluates the quality, safety, and efficacy of these products. For those veterinary medicines intended for administration to food-producing animals, an additional consideration is the safety of products derived from treated animals for human consumption. Maximum residue limits (MRL) or tolerances are established, and withdrawal times are set in a manner that ensures residues of the active constituent will not exceed the MRL when the label instructions for the product are followed.

Residue programs consist of 2 principal activities: monitoring and surveillance. Residue-monitoring programs randomly sample tissues from animals at slaughter. Tissue samples are assayed for residues of specific veterinary drugs, pesticides, and environmental contaminants, and the residues are assessed for compliance with the applicable MRL or environmental standard. The sample size chosen for monitoring purposes typically provides a 95% probability of detecting at least 1 violation when 1% of the animal population contains residues above the MRL. Surveillance programs, by comparison, sample tissues from animals suspected of violative residues on the basis of clinical signs or herd history. Animals identified with violative residues of veterinary drugs or pesticides do not enter the food chain.

Residue monitoring is also a trade requirement, either mandatory or as an expectation, of importing countries allowing market access to food products derived from animals. Governments adopt health standards, regulatory policies, and MRL-setting approaches that may differ between countries. The situation is often exacerbated when patterns of use differ across countries or where the minor status of a disease or pest in a country does not warrant product registration, in which case MRL are unlikely to be established. In addition to confounding international trade by requiring exporting countries to comply with a diverse range of standards imposed by importing countries, differing national standards may have implications for the protection of public health.

Regulatory authorities undertake premarket approval assessments of applications in support of new veterinary drugs and medicated feeds. These assessments consider scientific data submitted by the sponsor. In the case of veterinary medicines proposed for use in food-producing animals, the data must demonstrate the safety of any residues remaining in the edible products of treated animals. These data describe the compound's toxicology, metabolism, pharmacokinetics, residue depletion, and dietary exposure. The key parameters derived in the safety and residue evaluations are defined below.

The **acceptable daily intake (ADI)** is the amount of a veterinary drug, expressed on a body weight basis, that can be ingested daily over a lifetime without an appreciable risk to human health. The ADI is established based on a review of animal studies on toxicologic, pharmacologic, or microbiologic effects as appropriate. Conservative safety factors are built into the ADI.

The **safe concentration** is the maximal allowable concentration of total residues of toxicologic concern in edible tissue. The safe concentration is calculated from the ADI and considers the weight of an average person and the amount of meat, milk, or eggs consumed daily by a high-consuming individual.

An **MRL** or **tolerance** is the maximal concentration of residue resulting from the use of a veterinary drug (expressed in mg/kg or µg/kg on a fresh-weight basis) that is legally permitted as acceptable in or on a food. It is based on the type and amount of residue considered to be without any toxicologic hazard for human health as expressed by the ADI. Other relevant public risks and aspects relating to food technology, good practice in the use of veterinary drugs, and analytical methodologies are also considered when establishing MRL.

The concentration of the **marker residue** decreases in a known relationship to the level of total residues in tissues, eggs, milk, or other animal tissues.

The **target tissue** is the edible tissue with residues that deplete to a concentration below the MRL at a slower rate compared with other edible tissues. It is considered suitable for monitoring compliance with the MRL of the whole carcass of the animal. The target tissue is frequently liver or kidney for the purpose of domestic monitoring and muscle or fat for monitoring meat or carcasses in international trade.

The **withdrawal time** is the period of time between the last administration of a drug and the collection of edible tissue or products from a treated animal that ensures the total residues deplete to below the safe concentration, and the marker residue depletes to below the MRL. Failure to observe the correct withdrawal time for the drug is the most common cause of violative residues of veterinary drugs in food. To ensure that withdrawal times are observed, the veterinarian must understand the clinical utility of withdrawal times in product labeling and the pharmacokinetic basis of assigning a significantly extended withdrawal time when treating certain unhealthy animals or when using veterinary drugs extra-label.

Regulatory authorities determine withdrawal times on the basis of residue depletion data generated using healthy animals representative of those normally treated with the product. The drug formulation used in these trials is identical to the market formulation, which is administered at the maximal label rate. The withdrawal time is determined using a statistical approach, taking into account variability among animals in drug disposition.

Unlike an MRL, which applies to a veterinary drug regardless of the dosage form, route of administration, or dosage regimen, the withdrawal time stated in the product labeling applies only to that particular formulation when administered by the recommended route and in accordance with the dosage regimen. Alteration to any of these factors modifies the pharmacokinetic behavior of the drug in the animal and invalidates the withdrawal time. In addition, a range of physiologic and pathologic factors may modify the drug's disposition in the animal and prolong its elimination. The withdrawal time in the product labeling, which is based on studies in healthy animals, is likely to underestimate the time required for residues to decline below the MRL in these situations.

In the USA, some veterinary or human drugs can be used extra-label (off-label) in food-producing animals under the Animal Medicinal Drug Use Clarification Act, provided certain conditions are met. The veterinarian must be mindful, however, that the extra-label use of a small number of veterinary drugs is prohibited by the FDA. Extra-label use refers to use in a species not included in the product labeling or at a dosage rate higher than those stated in the product labeling. For drugs used in this manner, data are inadequate to demonstrate the safety of food products derived from the treated animal. An understanding of pharmacokinetic principles allows extended withdrawal times to be estimated both when veterinary drugs are used in an extra-label manner and in situations that may lead to changes in the kinetic behavior of a drug in an individual animal.

The elimination half-life is the time required for the concentration of a drug to be reduced by 50%. It follows that 99.9% of an administered dose is eliminated over 10 half-lives. In food-producing animals, the residues of drugs with longer terminal elimination half-lives take longer to deplete to below the MRL. The pharmacokinetic behavior of the drug determines if the elimination half-life in tissues will exceed the elimination half-life in plasma. In food-producing animals, the terminal elimination half-life for the slow elimination phase, or γ phase, of the residue concentration versus time profile determines the withdrawal time. Half-life is determined by both clearance (Cl) and volume of distribution (Vd) as shown by the relationship:

$$t_{1/2} = 0.693 \times \frac{Vd}{Cl}$$

Clearance is the blood volume cleared of drug per unit time and refers to the irreversible elimination of a drug from the body. The principal organs of elimination are the liver and kidneys; organ clearance is related to blood flow and the efficiency of drug removal.

Hepatic clearance (Cl_H) = Hepatic blood flow (Q_H) $\times$ Hepatic extraction ratio(E_H)

Factors that affect hepatic clearance include hepatic function, hepatic microsomal enzyme activity, and hepatic blood flow.

Volume of distribution relates the amount of drug in the body to the concentration of drug in plasma according to the relationship:

$$Vd = \frac{\text{Amount of drug in body (dose)}}{\text{Concentration } (C_{max})}$$

Vd is a characteristic property of the drug rather than the biologic system. A drug confined to the vascular compartment has a minimal value of Vd equal to plasma volume. Factors influencing Vd include the size of the drug molecule, lipid solubility, drug pK_a, and tissue blood flow. Certain disease states effect changes in volume of distribution for a drug, and changes in drug binding, in particular, usually alter Vd.

The following examples demonstrate the use of these pharmacokinetic principles to estimate an extended withdrawal time: 1) Administration of a veterinary drug to a healthy animal at twice the recommended rate—in this situation, the elimination half-life of the drug is unchanged. Assuming the pharmacokinetic behavior of the drug demonstrates first-order kinetics, which is generally the case, doubling the administered dose will increase the depletion time by one half-life. Thus, the withdrawal time should be extended by one half-life to arrive at the same concentration as observed for the recommended rate. 2) Administration of a veterinary drug to an unhealthy animal with impaired drug excretion in which clearance is reduced by 50%—from the relationship for half-life shown above, it can be seen that reducing clearance by 50% will double the half-life. Accordingly, the withdrawal time should be doubled to arrive at the same concentration as observed for an animal with a fully functional drug excretory system.

The predicted result should always be verified using a rapid-screening test. The detection of residues is likely to signal that the withdrawal time should be extended and the rapid-screening test repeated.

Residues Resulting from Consumption of Stockfeeds Treated with Agricultural Chemicals: The use of agricultural chemicals can result in residues in crops and pastures, which are subsequently consumed by animals. During drought conditions, the feeding of potentially contaminated crop byproducts, such as stubbles and fodder, and processed fractions, including grape marc, citrus pulp, fruit pomace, and cannery wastes, is likely to become more prevalent. Chemical residues may be found in animal tissues, milk, or eggs in all cases. For approved uses of crop protection chemicals that are likely to result in dietary exposure of food-producing animals, regulatory authorities establish animal commodity MRL. The approach adopted for establishing these MRL is fundamentally different from the one that applies to veterinary drugs. Animal transfer studies, which allow determination of the relationship between the level of chemical in the animal diet and the concentration of residue found in edible tissues, milk, and eggs, are pivotal in determining MRL. MRL for animal tissues, milk, and eggs are established at concentrations that cover the highest residues expected to be found from the estimated livestock dietary exposure. Human dietary exposure assessments are also performed to verify that food complying with MRL is safe for consumption. In animal production systems, compliance with animal commodity MRL relies on adherence to a stipulated period to allow residues in the crop to deplete prior to the commencement of animal feeding, a stipulated period to allow residues in the animal to deplete prior to slaughter, or a combination of both.

Chemical Residues in Animal Fibers

From an economic standpoint, the major animal fibers are wool and mohair. Although the primary focus of this section is pesticide residues in wool, many of the concepts discussed apply equally to mohair.

Flies, lice, keds, and mites adversely affect wool production and have animal welfare implications for the sheep industry. Ectoparasiticides have been the mainstay for managing infestations of these parasites in sheep flocks for many years. Two important manifestations of chemical application to sheep are the emergence of strains of parasites resistant to chemicals and the contamination of wool with pesticide residues. A particular concern is the application of pesticides to resistant strains of flies or lice, which increases the likelihood of treatment failure and the need to re-treat later in the wool-growing season. Higher residues in both the wool on treated sheep and in harvested fleeces are possible consequences. Nonetheless, there are some situations in which late-season applications are justified on animal health or economic grounds. In view of community health and safety expectations and changing environmental standards, wool producers are seeking methods of managing external parasites on sheep that rely less on chemicals. Integrated pest management (IPM) approaches have been adopted to achieve this objective. IPM may involve various husbandry options such as shearing, mulesing, and crutching to combat flystrike; genetic improvements such as selecting against animals susceptible to fleece rot; biologic and environmental controls such as the use of fly traps; and the selective use of chemicals.

Pesticide residues in wool are influenced by many factors, including the chemical and formulation used, the method of application, the rate and timing of the chemical application, and the length of wool at the time of application. (See also DOSAGE FORMS AND DELIVERY SYSTEMS, p 1953.) The product types and chemical groups commonly used in the management of flies and lice on sheep include off-shears backline or spray-on products containing insect growth regulators (IGR), organophosphate pesticides (OP), and synthetic pyrethroid pesticides; short-wool plunge or shower dips that use IGR, magnesium fluorosilicate, OP, and spinosad; long-wool backline or spray-on products containing

IGR; and long-wool jetting products containing IGR, macrocyclic lactones, OP, or spinosad. Wool producers must ensure that pesticides are applied in accordance with the label directions. Unacceptably high residues remain in wool to the next shearing when some chemicals are applied to sheep with >6 wk wool growth. Repeat applications of pesticides may also result in higher wool residues at the next shearing, and backline products commonly leave higher residues at the site of application. Wool producers must be in compliance with stated rehandling periods and wool withholding periods. The rehandling period is the time that must elapse before treated sheep are shorn. It takes precedence over all other applicable standards and ensures the wool meets occupational health and safety standards to protect shearers and other wool handlers. The wool-harvesting interval (or wool withholding period) is the time that must elapse before treated sheep are shorn. It ensures that harvested wool meets the prescribed environmental residue limits. When determining the wool-harvesting interval, the percentage of the national flock likely to be treated with the product is considered.

Pesticide residues in wool have possible implications for public health, occupational health and safety, and environmental safety. Processed wool used in the manufacture of garments is unlikely to pose a human health hazard because any residual pesticide is removed during the scouring process. Of greater concern is residual pesticide that remains associated with the wax component of lanolin, which requires expensive refining techniques to remove. Additional assurance as to the quality of low pesticide grades of lanolin stems from regulatory standards that apply to the lanolin used in pharmaceuticals and cosmetics for use on human skin and to lanolin used as a nipple emollient by nursing mothers.

Another concern relates to possible occupational health and safety implications. Residual pesticide in wool wax poses an occupational hazard to shearers and other wool handlers through dermal absorption. Nervous disorders and dermal irritation have allegedly occurred in shearers after shearing sheep treated with certain OP and synthetic pyrethroid (SP) pesticides, respectively. Long-wool backline applications of SP pesticides can result in residue concentrations at the tips of backline staples high enough to cause dermal erythema in shearers and wool handlers. To protect workers from unacceptable exposure to chemical residues in wool, it is important that rehandling periods for products are observed.

A third major issue is the environmental impact of pesticides that remain in scour effluent. Environmental legislation relating to the discharge of pesticides into aquatic ecosystems has been enacted to protect the environment. For some pesticides, environmental quality standards have been established and represent concentrations that will not harm the most sensitive organisms in aquatic ecosystems. The EU has also included textile products as part of its eco-label requirements, which labels garments that have been manufactured from low-residue wools and have been processed in accordance with stringent environmental regulations.

The depletion of pesticide residues in wool has been mathematically modeled to predict the likely consequences of treatments at different times during the wool-growing season and to determine how late a pesticide may be applied to sheep without creating excessive residues at shearing. Modeling is a useful tool for determining wool-harvesting intervals and for assisting wool growers when choosing a pesticide and method of application. Finally, test kits are available for establishing the status of pesticide residues in wool.

SYSTEMIC PHARMACOTHERAPEUTICS OF THE CARDIOVASCULAR SYSTEM

See also PRINCIPLES OF THERAPY, THE CARDIOVASCULAR SYSTEM, p 64; HEART FAILURE MANAGEMENT, p 85; FLUID THERAPY, p 1404; and MACROCYCLIC LACTONES, p 2115.
See TABLE 1 for a listing of commonly used cardiovascular drugs and dosages.

POSITIVE INOTROPES

Positive inotropes increase the strength of cardiac muscle contraction by increasing the quantity of intracellular calcium available for binding by muscle proteins. This, in turn, augments contractile protein interaction in the myocardial cell. Intracellular calcium can be increased by altering the Na^+/Ca^{2+} exchange pump, by increasing production of cyclic adenosine monophosphate (cAMP) via stimulation of adenylate cyclase, or by decreasing degradation of cAMP via inhibition of phosphodiesterases. A new class of inotropic agents increases the sensitivity of contractile protein to calcium.

TABLE 1. Commonly Used Cardiovascular Drugs and Dosages

Drug	Dose
Amrinone	Dog and cat: 1-3 mg/kg, IV, loading dose, then 30-100 µg/kg/min, IV, CRI[*]
Amlodipine	Dog: 0.1 mg/kg, PO, SID Cat: 0.18 mg/kg, PO, SID (0.625-1.25 mg/cat, PO, SID)
Aspirin, antiplatelet	Dog: 5-10 mg/kg, PO every 24-48 hr Cat: 80 mg, PO every 48-72 hr
Atenolol	Dog: 0.25-1 mg/kg, PO, SID-BID Cat: 2-3 mg/kg, PO, BID
Benazepril	Dog and cat: 0.25-0.5 mg/kg, PO, SID
Boldenone undecylenate[†]	Horse: 1.1 mg/kg, IM, every 3 wk
Desmopressin	Dog: 0.4 µg/kg, SC; 1 µg/kg in 20 mL saline, IV over 10 min
Diltiazem	Dog: 0.5-1.5 mg/kg, PO TID Cat: 0.5-2.5 mg/kg, PO, TID
CARDIZEM® CD (diltiazem)	Cat: 10 mg/kg, PO, BID
DILACOR XR® (diltiazem)	Cat: 15-30 mg/kg, PO, SID
Digoxin[‡]	Dog: 0.0055-0.011 mg/kg, PO, BID; 0.22 mg/m², PO, BID Cat: 0.005-0.01 mg/kg, PO, every 24-48 hr
Dobutamine	Dog: 2-20 µg/kg/min, IV, CRI Cat: 0.5-10 µg/kg/min, IV, CRI
Dopamine	Dog: 2-15 µg/kg/min, IV, CRI
Enalapril[§]	Dog and cat: 0.5 mg/kg, PO, SID-BID[¶]
Epoetin alfa	Dog and cat, initial: 100 U/kg, SC, 3×/wk Dog and cat, maintenance: 75-100 U/kg, SC, 2-3×/wk
Folic acid	Dog: 5 mg, PO, SID Cat: 2.5 mg, PO, SID
Heparin, high dose	Dog: 150-250 U/kg, SC, TID Cat: 250-375 U/kg, SC, BID
Heparin, low dose	Dog and cat: 75 U/kg, SC, TID Horse: 25-100 U/kg, SC, TID
Hydralazine	Dog: 0.5-3 mg/kg, PO, BID Cat: 0.5-0.8 mg/kg, PO, BID
Iron (dextrans)[#]	Pig, neonate: 100 mg, IM[¶]
Iron (ferrous sulfate)	Dog: 100-300 mg, PO, SID Cat: 50-100 mg, PO, SID
Lidocaine[**]	Dog: 1-2 mg/kg, IV; 40-80 µg/kg/min, IV, CRI
Mexiletine	Dog: 4-10 mg/kg, PO, TID

(*continued*)

TABLE 1. Commonly Used Cardiovascular Drugs and Dosages (*continued*)

Drug	Dose
Nandrolone decanoate	Dog: 1-1.5 mg/kg, IM, weekly Cat: 1 mg/kg, IM, weekly Horse: 1 mg/kg, IM, every 4 wk
Nitroglycerin ointment (1 in. = 15 mg)	Dog: 4-15 mg, topically, TID Cat: 2-4 mg, topically, TID
Nitroprusside	Dog: 1-10 µg/kg/min, IV, CRI
Oxymetholone	Dog and cat: 1-5 mg/kg, PO, every 18-24 hr
Phenytoin	Dog: 30-50 mg/kg, PO, TID
Pimobendan	Dog: 0.1-0.3 mg/kg, PO, BID
Procainamide	Dog: 10-30 mg/kg, PO, QID; 10-40 µg/kg/min, IV, CRI Cat: 3-8 mg/kg, PO, TID-QID; 10-20 µg/kg/min, IV, CRI Horse: 25-35 mg/kg, PO, TID; 1 mg/kg/min, IV to a maximum of 20 mg/kg
Propranolol	Dog: 0.1-2 mg/kg, PO, TID Cat: 2.5-5 mg/cat, PO, TID
Quinidine sulfate	Dog and cat: 4-20 mg/kg, PO, TID-QID Horse: 22 mg/kg, PO every 2 hr
Quinidine gluconate	Horse: 1-1.5 mg/kg, IV every 5-10 min
Stanozolol[††]	Dog: 1-4 mg, PO, BID; 25-50 mg, IM, weekly[¶] Cat: 1 mg, PO, BID; 25 mg, IM, weekly[¶] Horse: 0.55 mg/kg, IM, weekly for up to 4 wk[¶]
Tocainide	Dog: 15-20 mg/kg, PO, TID
tPA	Cat: 0.25-1 mg/kg/hr, IV (total dose 1-10 mg/kg)
Vitamin B_{12}[#]	Dog: 100-200 µg, PO or SC, SID Cat: 50-100 µg, PO or SC, SID
Warfarin sodium	Dog and cat: 0.1-0.2 mg/kg, PO, SID Horse: 0.067-0.167 mg/kg, PO, SID

[*]CRI = continuous rate infusion
[†]Approved by FDA for adjunctive therapy in treating debilitated horses.
[‡]Approved by FDA for initial and chronic treatment of heart failure and supraventricular tachycardia, atrial flutter, and atrial fibrillation in dogs.
[§]Approved by FDA for treatment of mild, moderate, or severe heart failure in dogs due to mitral regurgitation and/or reduced ventricular contractility.
[¶]FDA/CVM approved dosage regimen
[#]Several FDA-approved products are available.
[**]Several FDA-approved products are available; however, none are specifically approved for control of cardiac arrhythmias.
[††]Approved by FDA as a sterile suspension and oral tablets for use in dogs, cats, and horses.

Cardiac Glycosides

The most probable mechanism of action for the inotropic effect of digitalis is inhibition of the membrane-bound Na^+/K^+-ATPase pump; when this occurs, Na^+ increases in the cell, the exchange of Na^+ for Ca^{2+} is augmented, and calcium influx is increased. The increased intracellular calcium in turn leads to increased release of Ca^{2+} from the sarcoplasmic reticulum and increased contractility of the cardiac muscle. Changes in the ratio of intracellular and extracellular electrolytes can result in increased automaticity and cardiac arrhythmias.

Digitalis also has a negative chronotropic effect due to decreased conduction velocity in the atrioventricular (AV) node. In addition, digitalis potentiates vagal (cholinergic) activity in the heart. Changes in conduction can ultimately result in AV nodal blockade. At toxic levels, digitalis also can directly slow sinus nodal activity due to increased sensitivity to acetylcholine. Because the atria are sensitive to acetylcholine, atrial conduction is also enhanced in the diseased heart, which can then lead to atrial arrhythmias. Digitalis may also improve vascular baroreceptor responsiveness, thereby minimizing sympathetic activation in heart failure states.

Preparations: Digoxin and digitoxin are the 2 most widely used preparations. Digoxin is available for administration IV or PO. Administration IV results in pharmacologic effects in 5-30 min with a maximal effect in 2 hr. However, toxic drug concentrations are more difficult to avoid with this route. Digoxin should not be given IM because it causes pain and muscle necrosis. Administration PO results in pharmacologic effects in 1-2 hr.

Disposition: Absorption of digoxin varies with the preparation. Absorption of the alcohol (elixir) form is best. Variation in bioavailability of tablets results from differences in dissolution between products. Absorption is slowed by food, but the absorption of digitoxin is more complete because it is more lipid soluble. Both drugs are distributed slowly and are concentrated in cardiac tissues. Only 25% of digoxin is bound to plasma proteins, while ~90% of digitoxin is protein bound. Digoxin is primarily eliminated unchanged by the kidneys; its half-life (~1.7 days in dogs) is strongly influenced by renal function. Digitoxin is metabolized by the liver (one of the metabolites is digoxin); its half-life in dogs is 8-12 hr.

Drug Interactions: The concurrent administration of quinidine increases plasma concentrations of digoxin, probably due to displacement from tissue-binding sites. Verapamil, spironolactone, and captopril also may increase plasma digoxin concentrations. Interactions between digitalis and diuretics (eg, furosemide) stem primarily from the effects on potassium (hypokalemia). Administration of β-adrenergic agonists increases the likelihood of arrhythmias. Amphotericin B and glucocorticoids deplete body K^+ and thus potentiate digitalis intoxication.

Toxicity: Toxic effects with digitalis glycosides are frequent and can be lethal. Cats are more sensitive to digoxin than dogs. Probably the most frequent cause of toxicity is overdosing. The potential for toxicity is increased with hypokalemia. The likelihood and severity of toxicity are related to the severity of cardiac disease. Any type of cardiac arrhythmia can be induced by digitalis. Other signs of toxicity include diarrhea, anorexia, and nausea and vomiting due to direct stimulation of the chemoreceptor trigger zone. Frequently, these are the earliest indications of toxicity. Neurologic effects include malaise and drowsiness. Digitalis toxicity can be diagnosed (and avoided) by monitoring plasma drug concentrations. Treatment of intoxication includes discontinuing therapy with digitalis and potassium-depleting diuretics and administering phenytoin (blocks AV nodal effects of digitalis), lidocaine (for ventricular arrhythmias), and if indicated, potassium (preferably PO). Atropine may be useful to treat both sinus bradycardia and second- or third-degree heart block induced by cholinergic augmentation.

Clinical Use: Digitalis is used for restoring adequate circulation in animals with congestive heart failure (CHF) due to poor systolic (ie, contractile) function or for slowing the ventricular rate during supraventricular tachyarrhythmias, such as atrial fibrillation or flutter. Both syndromes require longterm treatment. Digoxin is the cardiac glycoside more commonly used except in animals with renal disease, in which digitoxin is preferred. The maintenance dosage schedules are 0.0055-0.011 mg/kg, PO, BID, for dogs, and 0.005-0.01 mg/kg, PO, every 24-48 hr for cats. Calculation of digoxin doses should be based on lean body weight, and dosages should be reduced in obese or cachectic animals and in the presence of ascites. The calculated dose should be multiplied by 0.75 for elixir and by 0.85 for tablet formulations of digoxin. Alternatively, dosing of digoxin on the basis of body surface area (0.22 mg/m^2, BID) is best for large and giant breeds of dogs. *See* TABLE 9, p 2589, for weight to body surface area (in m^2) conversion. Electrolyte disorders should be corrected before digitalis glycosides are administered.

β-Adrenergic Agonists

These drugs cause their positive inotropic effect by activating β-receptors with subsequent stimulation of adenylate cyclase and increased cAMP.

Dopamine is an endogenous catecholamine precursor with selective β_1 activity. However, it also stimulates the release of norepinephrine. At low doses, it stimulates renal dopaminergic receptors, which causes increased renal blood flow and diuresis. Dopamine is not effectively absorbed if given PO. It is rapidly metabolized by the body and has a half-life of <2 min. Dopamine is available as a solution, which is further diluted with saline or dextrose. It is administered IV, usually by constant infusion (2-15 μg/kg/min). Cardiac arrhythmias may develop due to β-adrenergic activity. Indications include cardiogenic or endotoxic shock and oliguria.

Dobutamine is a synthetic drug similar to dopamine, but it does not cause release of norepinephrine and therefore has minimal effects other than β_1-activity. Dobutamine is a more effective positive inotrope than dopamine with less chronotropic effects, although it does not dilate the renal vascular bed. Like dopamine, dobutamine is not effective if given PO and has a plasma half-life of ~2 min. Dobutamine is also prepared as a solution to be diluted with 5% dextrose or normal saline. It is the preferred drug for short-term therapy of refractory CHF. Dobutamine causes an immediate increase in blood pressure due to increased cardiac output. It is given as a constant rate IV infusion at 2-20 μg/kg/min; heart rate, blood pressure, and cardiac output should be monitored. In cats, dobutamine has a longer half-life and causes CNS stimulation, so lower infusion rates (≤10 μg/kg/min) should be used.

Compared with other inotropic drugs, **epinephrine** causes the greatest increase in the rate of energy usage and myocardial oxygen demand. This increase in oxygen need may be detrimental to the failing heart. Epinephrine also causes vasoconstriction and bronchodilation. Epinephrine is rapidly metabolized in the GI tract and is not effective after administration PO. Absorption is more rapid after IM versus SC administration. Epinephrine is available in several preparations and is effective after IV, pulmonary, and nasal administration. However, because of the decreased efficiency of cardiac work, epinephrine is not used as a positive inotropic agent but rather for emergency therapy of cardiac arrest and anaphylactic shock. Ventricular arrhythmias can be expected.

Isoproterenol is a nonspecific β-agonist that, like epinephrine, increases myocardial oxygen demand. Tachycardia and the potential for other arrhythmias excludes its use in the cardiac patient except for short-term therapy of bradyarrhythmias or AV block.

Calcium is also a positive inotrope but must be given as a slow IV injection or infusion. Calcium must be administered carefully because it can cause cardiac rigor and standstill at high doses. The gluconate form is preferred to calcium chloride.

Phosphodiesterase Inhibitors

Phosphodiesterase (PDE) inhibitors block the breakdown of cAMP and therefore increase intracellular cAMP concentrations. The result is an increase in myocardial contractility. Methylxanthine derivatives have been classified as PDE inhibitors, but this is controversial. Of the methylxanthines, theophylline is the most cardiopotent. In addition to their cardiac effects, these drugs have significant CNS, renal, and smooth muscle effects. Their use for cardiac disease is limited to conditions that accompany respiratory disease that would benefit from bronchodilation.

The mechanism of action of the bipyridine derivatives **amrinone** and **milrinone** is probably inhibition of PDE and increased levels of intracellular cAMP. These effects appear to occur without a dramatic rise in myocardial oxygen consumption. Peripheral vasodilation is another major therapeutic benefit of these drugs. Arrhythmias may be exacerbated in some animals, and milrinone has been associated with decreased long-term survival in chronic heart failure in humans. Both amrinone and milrinone are available for IV administration and are suitable only for short-term management of CHF. Experience is limited with both drugs in dogs and cats, particularly with the IV administration of milrinone. Amrinone can be diluted for administration in normal or half-strength saline, but not dextrose; a loading dose of 1-3 mg/kg is followed by constant rate infusion of 10-100 μg/kg/min, starting at the low end of the range and titrating upward as needed.

Pimobendan is a benzimidazole pyridazinone derivative approved in Europe for treatment of CHF due to dilated cardiomyopathy and mitral valve insufficiency in dogs. At present it is not approved for use in the USA. Like amrinone and milrinone, pimobendan is a PDE inhibitor and has both positive inotropic and vasodilating properties. In addition, pimobendan increases myocardial contractility by increasing the sensitivity of contractile proteins to calcium. Calcium-sensitizing agents may increase contractility without increasing myocardial oxygen consumption. In humans with heart failure, pimobendan has been associated with an increase in death due to arrhythmias. The dose of pimobendan for treating CHF in dogs is 0.1-0.3 mg/kg, PO, BID.

ANGIOTENSIN-CONVERTING ENZYME INHIBITORS

Angiotensin-converting enzyme (ACE) inhibitors are widely used in treating chronic CHF in dogs. In the pathogenesis of CHF, the proteolytic enzyme renin is released by the kidneys and acts on angiotensinogen, which is produced by the liver and distributed in the blood, to produce angiotensin I. The formation of angiotensin II from angiotensin I occurs through the action of ACE. Angiotensin II causes retention of Na^+ and water, in part through stimulation of the synthesis and release of aldosterone by the adrenal cortex. Angiotensin II also causes vasoconstriction, thus increasing vascular resistance. By inhibiting the formation of angiotensin II, ACE inhibitors prevent vasoconstriction and reduce the retention of Na^+ and water in animals with CHF. ACE inhibitors are balanced vasodilators, reducing both preload and afterload. The effects during CHF include decreased vascular resistance and cardiac filling pressures and increased cardiac output and exercise tolerance.

Preparations: Enalapril maleate is a widely used ACE inhibitor and is available in various sized tablets for oral administration. It can delay mortality while improving quality of life in dogs with CHF. Captopril was the first ACE inhibitor developed for people and had been used extra-label in dogs and cats. Compared with enalapril, captopril has a greater propensity for GI side effects and a shorter half-life in dogs, necessitating more frequent dosing. Benazepril is approved in several countries outside the USA for treating CHF in dogs.

Disposition: After absorption from the GI tract, enalapril is converted in the liver to the active metabolite enalaprilat. Therefore, enalapril has a delayed onset of action (4-6 hr) but a duration of action of 12-14 hr. The half-life of enalapril (enalaprilat) is increased in animals with severe CHF or renal failure.

Drug Interactions: Hypotension may develop with concurrent use of ACE inhibitors and other vasodilators or diuretics. Concurrent use of potassium-sparing diuretics (ie, spironolactone) may cause hyperkalemia.

Toxicity: Relative to other drugs used to treat CHF, ACE inhibitors have a better safety profile. However, azotemia may develop, and monitoring of BUN and creatinine (with possible dosage adjustments) is warranted. Other possible adverse effects include GI disturbances (anorexia, vomiting, diarrhea), hypotension, and renal dysfunction.

Clinical Use: ACE inhibitors are indicated in the treatment of CHF in dogs and cats stemming from valvular heart disease and dilated cardiomyopathy. While ACE inhibitors may delay the onset of CHF in asymptomatic animals with cardiac disease, this has yet to be proved. ACE inhibitors may also be considered for management of hypertension in cats. The approved use of enalapril in dogs is as adjunctive therapy with furosemide and digoxin for dilated cardiomyopathy, or with furosemide with or without digoxin for chronic valvular insufficiency. The dose of enalapril for treating CHF in dogs is 0.5 mg/kg, SID. If, after 14 days, the clinical response is inadequate, enalapril may be administered at 0.5 mg/kg, BID. Alternatively, therapy with enalapril alone at 0.5 mg/kg, SID, may be initiated in asymptomatic animals or in animals with mild signs related to heart failure. In animals with moderate to advanced signs, enalapril can be administered at 0.5 mg/kg, BID, with or without furosemide or digoxin (or both).

Like enalapril, benazepril is a prodrug that undergoes metabolism by the liver to the active benazeprilat. Benazepril is indicated for treatment of CHF in dogs. Benazeprilat inhibits plasma ACE for >24 hr after a single dose. About half of benazeprilat undergoes hepatic excretion, a possible advantage in animals with renal failure. The dose of benazepril for dogs and cats is 0.25-0.5 mg/kg, PO, SID.

Lisinopril is another ACE-inhibitor occasionally used to treat CHF in dogs; however, efficacy and safety in dogs and cats have yet to be established. Unlike enalapril, lisinopril does not require hepatic activation. A suggested dose for dogs is 0.5 mg/kg, PO, SID.

VASOACTIVE DRUGS

Vasodilator drugs can be categorized as afterload reducers or preload reducers according to the type of vessels that they dilate. Afterload is reduced by dilation of arterioles (ie, resistance vessels), while preload is reduced by dilation of veins (ie, capacitance vessels).

Arterial Dilators

Hydralazine is an arteriolar vasodilator. It relaxes arteriolar smooth muscle by inhibiting calcium fluxes into the cell or by increasing local prostacyclin concentrations. The result is a decrease in peripheral vascular resistance without a decrease in myocardial contractility. Hydralazine is bound to smooth muscle, which results in a biologic half-life that is longer than plasma half-life. The drug is well absorbed after administration PO but (in humans) is subject to first-pass metabolism. The incidence of toxicity caused by hydralazine may be significant. Hypotension may develop, leading to reflex tachycardia; this effect may be detrimental to animals with CHF because of increased myocardial oxygen demand. Hydralazine (dogs: 0.5-3 mg/kg, PO, BID; cats: 0.5-0.8 mg/kg, PO, BID) is used to reduce afterload in animals with CHF due to chronic mitral regurgitation. It can decrease regurgitant volume and left atrial compression of the left main stem bronchus. The drug should be titrated to the response of the individual animal.

Calcium-channel blockers primarily have arterial effects with little to no venodilator effects. Coronary vasodilation can be significant. Calcium-channel blockers are of value in treating hypertrophic cardiomyopathy and certain arrhythmias. The dihydropyridine calcium-channel blocker amlodipine besylate has been recommended for treating hypertension in cats and dogs. The suggested dose for dogs is 0.1 mg/kg, PO, SID; for cats, the suggested dose is 0.18 mg/kg, PO, SID (0.625-1.25 mg/cat, PO, SID).

Arterial and Venous Dilators

Organic nitrates and nitrites relax both arterial and venous smooth muscle. These drugs directly dilate coronary vessels. At low concentrations, which are generally used clinically, venular dilation predominates, and net systemic vascular resistance is usually not affected. Pharmacologic effects occur rapidly. First-pass metabolism limits the use of these drugs to IV, sublingual, and topical (ointment) administration.

Nitroglycerin, an organic nitrate, relaxes vascular smooth muscle. However, the dose of nitroglycerin used results in predominantly venous dilation and preload reduction. Preferential mesenteric venous dilation results in a shift in blood from the pulmonary to the systemic vasculature. Myocardial workload is reduced. Nitroglycerin is indicated for acute (emergency) treatment of CHF, particularly that associated with fulminant pulmonary edema. It is available for IV and sublingual use and as an ointment. The 2% ointment preparation is the most commonly used; it is applied (dog: 4-15 mg, TID; cat: 2-4 mg, TID; 1 in. = 15 mg) to the hairless portion of the animal's skin (abdomen or ear).

Nitroprusside is one of the most potent vasodilators available. It is an organic nitrate and reduces preload and afterload. The advantages of this drug include potency, both preload and afterload reduction, immediate hemodynamic effects, short half-life, and low cost. The major disadvantage is that it must be administered by constant IV infusion (1-10 μg/kg/min). Nitroprusside is useful in dogs for emergency reduction of blood pressure and for immediate afterload reduction (severe CHF). Hypotension is the major complication and necessitates close monitoring of blood pressure.

Prazosin is an α_1-adrenergic receptor blocker and thus considered to be both a preload and afterload reducer. Prazosin is effective when given PO, but tolerance develops rapidly. In addition, prazosin undergoes significant first-pass metabolism. Prazosin is rarely used clinically in small animals.

ANTIARRHYTHMICS

Antiarrhythmics have been grouped into 4 main classes according to their dominant electrophysiologic effect on myocardial cells.

Class I Drugs

Class I agents comprise the standard membrane-stabilizing drugs such as quinidine, procainamide, and lidocaine. These agents work by selectively blocking the fast sodium channels and depressing phase 0 of the action potential. This is caused by a direct membrane-stabilizing or "local anesthetic" effect. The decrease in phase 0 depolarization results in decreased conduction velocity. In addition, the class I drugs increase the threshold of excitability and decrease the rate of spontaneous phase 4 depolarization, thus reducing the emergence of ectopic foci. Some of these drugs also are useful in treating re-entrant arrhythmias.

Class I agents can be further subdivided based on their effects on the refractory period and the rate of repolarization. Class IA drugs include quinidine, procainamide, and disopyramide.

Quinidine is related to the antimalarial drug quinine. It has efficacy against supraventricular and ventricular arrhythmias. It is useful in the treatment of re-entrant arrhythmias, eg, atrial fibrillation. In the atria, quinidine also has indirect, antivagal ("atropine-like") effects. The sulfate preparation of quinidine is absorbed rapidly after administration PO. The gluconate form is absorbed more slowly. It can be given IM but is painful. Although 90% of quinidine is protein-bound, distribution is rapid to most tissues. The half-life varies among species and is ~6 hr in dogs and ~8 hr in horses.

Quinidine (dogs and cats: 4-20 mg/kg, PO, TID-QID; horses: 22 mg/kg, PO, every 2 hr, or quinidine gluconate at 1.0-1.5 mg/kg, IV, every 5-10 min) can be used to treat supraventricular and ventricular arrhythmias. Individualized therapy is necessary because of significant pharmacodynamic variation among animals. Cardiotoxicity may result in AV blockade or ventricular arrhythmias. The atropine-like effects of quinidine may result in increased impulse conduction through the AV node to the ventricles and paradoxical acceleration. Quinidine, particularly in the sulfate form, can cause vasodilation and GI side effects. In horses, swelling of the nasal mucosa, urticarial wheals, and laminitis are other potential side effects. Monitoring the ECG and serum quinidine concentration can reduce the likelihood of adverse drug effects.

Procainamide affects cardiac automaticity, excitability, responsiveness, and conduction similarly to quinidine. However, its effects on the autonomic nervous system are significantly weaker. It does not cause α-adrenergic blockade or paradoxical acceleration. Procainamide is rapidly and almost completely absorbed after administration PO. Only ~20% is protein bound. Procainamide is extensively biotransformed by the liver to metabolites that are generally inactive in dogs. It is available as oral capsules and tablets for longterm use. IV preparations are available for acute therapy and can also be administered IM.

Procainamide (dogs: 10-30 mg/kg, PO, QID; 2-8 mg/kg, IV over 5 min, then 10-40 µg/kg/min constant rate infusion; cats: 3-8 mg/kg, PO, TID-QID; 1-2 mg/kg, IV over 5 min, then 10-20 µg/kg/min, IV; horses: 25-35 mg/kg, PO, TID; 1 mg/kg/min, IV, to a maximum of 20 mg/kg) is generally more effective in controlling ventricular arrhythmias than atrial arrhythmias. Its actions parallel those of quinidine, and it is useful in animals that have not responded to quinidine therapy. Toxicities include cardiotoxicity similar to that induced by quinidine, hypotension with rapid IV administration (bolus), GI disturbances (anorexia, nausea, vomiting, and diarrhea), and possibly a systemic lupus erythematosus-like syndrome.

Disopyramide has limited use in small animals.

Class IB drugs include lidocaine, tocainide, mexiletine, and phenytoin.

Lidocaine is used predominantly for emergency treatment of ventricular arrhythmias. Lidocaine has minimal effects on the autonomic nervous system. It counteracts arrhythmias in abnormal Purkinje and ventricular fibers without affecting normal cardiac tissues. Although well absorbed if given PO, lidocaine is subject to first-pass metabolism and only one-third of the drug reaches the systemic circulation. Absorption is complete after IM administration. Distribution of lidocaine to extravascular tissues is rapid. Lidocaine is extensively metabolized by the liver; hepatic disease and reduced hepatic blood flow prolong the half-life, which is normally <1 hr in dogs.

Lidocaine is prepared for IV administration; no other drug should be included in the solution prepared for treatment of cardiac arrhythmias. It can be administered IV as a rapid bolus or as a continuous infusion (dogs: 1-2 mg/kg, IV bolus, followed by 40-80 μg/kg/min). Lidocaine has few undesirable effects. Toxicity is manifest in dogs primarily as CNS signs. Drowsiness or agitation may progress to muscle twitching and convulsions at higher plasma concentrations. Hypotension may develop if the IV bolus is given too rapidly. In cats, which are more susceptible to toxicity, cardiac suppression and CNS excitation may be seen.

Mexiletine is an analog of lidocaine that is used to treat ventricular arrhythmias in dogs (4-10 mg/kg, PO, TID). After oral administration, it undergoes minimal first-pass hepatic metabolism. Potential adverse effects include GI disturbances and tremor. Mexiletine may be combined with other class I antiarrhythmic agents in treating refractory ventricular arrhythmias.

Tocainide is an analog of lidocaine that does not undergo extensive first-pass metabolism and thus is effective after administration PO. Tocainide has been used in dogs (15-20 mg/kg, PO, TID) for the longterm control of ventricular arrhythmias that respond to lidocaine. Potential adverse effects include CNS and GI disturbances, hypotension, bradycardia, tachycardia, other arrhythmias, and progressive corneal edema. Because of these adverse effects, tocainide has limited use.

Phenytoin has a limited spectrum of antiarrhythmic activity. Its primary usefulness is for the management of digitalis-induced arrhythmias because it abolishes digitalis-induced abnormal automaticity. The recommended dosage in dogs is 30-50 mg/kg, PO, TID.

Class II Drugs

Class II antiarrhythmic drugs are the β-adrenergic receptor blocking agents.

Propranolol, the prototype, is competitive and nonselective, blocking both β_1 and β_2 receptors. As a β_1 blocker, propranolol has a negative chronotropic effect in conditions of supraventricular tachycardia. Propranolol is also a negative inotrope. This pharmacologic effect can be detrimental in animals with limited cardiac reserve (eg, animals with severe CHF) but is beneficial in cats with hypertrophic cardiomyopathy.

Clinical indications for propranolol include reduction of ventricular rate in cases of supraventricular tachycardia, atrial fibrillation, or atrial flutter, and treatment of hypertrophic cardiomyopathy, hypertension, and thyrotoxicosis. Propranolol (dogs: 0.1-2 mg/kg, PO, TID; cats: 2.5-5 mg/cat, PO, TID) is used clinically as a negative chronotrope in dogs and cats with supraventricular arrhythmias and as a negative chronotrope and negative inotrope in cats with hypertrophic cardiomyopathy. Digitalization may be necessary before propranolol is used in dogs with CHF. β-Blockers may be preferred over calcium-channel blockers in treating the obstructive form of hypertrophic cardiomyopathy in cats. Use of propranolol should be avoided in cats with evidence of respiratory disease (eg, asthma).

The toxic effects of propranolol are the result of β-receptor blockade and include bradyarrhythmias, hypotension, heart failure, bronchospasm, and hypoglycemia, particularly in diabetic animals. Administration of a β-blocker to an animal with little myocardial reserve must be done cautiously by initiating therapy at the low end of the dose range.

Atenolol is a β_1-selective blocking agent that may be effective in treating supraventricular tachyarrhythmias, systemic hypertension, and hypertrophic cardiomyopathy. In addition to relative safety in animals with bronchospastic disease, atenolol requires less frequent dosing than propranolol (dogs: 0.25-1 mg/kg, PO, SID-BID; cats: 2-3 mg/kg, PO, BID).

Class III Drugs

Class III drugs prolong the cardiac action potential and refractory period. They have no effect on the fast sodium conductance. There are 3 drugs in this class—bretylium, amiodarone, and sotalol. At present, none have practical clinical application in veterinary medicine. In addition to the Class III effect on action potential, sotalol is a nonselective β-adrenergic blocker.

Class IV Drugs

Class IV antiarrhythmic drugs are referred to as calcium antagonists or calcium-channel blocking drugs. Those used in veterinary medicine include diltiazem, amlodipine, and verapamil.

Calcium-channel blockers inhibit the entry of calcium into the cell or inhibit its mobilization from intracellular stores in both cardiac and smooth muscle cells. Cardiac and vascular smooth muscle depend on calcium for contraction. In addition, specialized cardiac tissues capable of automaticity and AV conduction depend, in part, on calcium entry or mobilization for depolarization. Calcium-channel blockers slow the sinus rate and AV conduction; the ventricular rate is reduced in animals with atrial fibrillation or flutter. Ventricular arrhythmias are generally unresponsive. Cardiovascular side effects of calcium-channel blockers include hypotension, bradycardia, various degrees of heart block, and exacerbation of CHF due to negative inotropic effects.

Diltiazem is indicated for the treatment of atrial fibrillation, supraventricular tachycardias, hypertrophic cardiomyopathy, and hypertension. The dosage for dogs is 0.5-1.5 mg/kg, PO, TID, and for cats 0.5-2.5 mg/kg, PO, TID, with middle range to high-end dosages for hypertrophic cardiomyopathy. Alternatively, sustained-release formulations of diltiazem are available for administration to cats. The benefits of diltiazem for hypertrophic cardiomyopathy include decreased heart rate, edema formation, and possibly ventricular wall thickness, and improved diastolic relaxation and ventricular compliance. To slow the ventricular response to supraventricular tachyarrhythmias, generally a lower dosage is initially administered and increased in 2-3 days as needed to achieve the desired ventricular rate. Diltiazem is well tolerated by dogs and cats. Noncardiovascular adverse effects might include GI or CNS disturbances and increases in liver enzymes. Diltiazem increases the bioavailability of propranolol; concurrent therapy with β-blockers increases the propensity for cardiovascular side effects.

Amlodipine is selective for calcium-channel blockade in vascular smooth muscle with minimal effects on cardiac calcium transport. Amlodipine is recommended for hypertension in cats and dogs.

DRUGS ACTING ON THE BLOOD OR BLOOD-FORMING ORGANS

Hematinics

Anemia can be treated pharmacologically by providing components needed for RBC production, including Hgb synthesis, and by stimulating bone marrow formation of RBC.

Vitamin B_{12} is essential for DNA synthesis. Deficiency causes inhibited nuclear maturation and division. RBC maturation arrest in the bone marrow leads to megaloblastic or pernicious anemia. Vitamin B_{12}, a porphyrin-like compound consisting of a ring structure that contains a centrally located cobalt, is derived from the diet and microbial synthesis in the GI tract. However, except for ruminants, microbial production occurs in the large intestine, from which vitamin B_{12} is not readily absorbed. Dietary deficiency of B_{12} is rare; deficiency usually results from poor absorption from the GI tract.

Vitamin B_{12} absorption is complex and depends on gastric acid, pepsin, and intrinsic factor secreted from gastric parietal cells or pancreatic duct cells. Intrinsic factor binds to and protects vitamin B_{12} from digestion. In this form, B_{12} binds to highly specific receptor sites in the brush border of the ileum, where it enters enterocytes by pinocytosis. Interference with its absorption in the ileum results in continuous depletion, although many months of defective absorption are necessary before deficiency develops. Vitamin B_{12} is bound in the plasma to transcobalamin. It is stored in large quantities in the liver and slowly released as needed. It is excreted into the bile but undergoes enterohepatic cycling.

Vitamin B_{12} (dogs: 100-200 μg, PO, SC, SID; cats: 50-100 μg, PO, SC, SID) is available in oral and parenteral preparations of cyanocobalamin. There are no significant toxicities associated with therapy. Indications for therapy are limited to cases of vitamin B_{12} malabsorption, such as ileectomy, gastrectomy, or deficiency malabsorption syndromes (eg, exocrine pancreatic insufficiency). Chronic administration of H_2-receptor blockers (cimetidine, ranitidine, famotidine) can also lead to vitamin B_{12} deficiency because an acid environment is necessary for its absorption.

Folic acid is needed for DNA and RNA synthesis. Anemia associated with folic acid deficiency is characterized as megaloblastic. Sources of folic acid in the diet include yeast, liver, kidney, and green vegetables, although it can also be formed by microbes. Folic acid is stored in the liver but not as avidly as vitamin B_{12}. Because folic acid is destroyed by catabolic processes every day, serum levels decrease rapidly in the presence of deficient diets. Absorption of folic acid is not as sensitive as that of vitamin B_{12}, although jejunal pathology can result in folate deficiency.

Folic acid (dogs: 5 mg, PO, SID; cats: 2.5 mg, PO, SID) is available in both oral and parenteral formulations. Significant toxicity is not associated with therapy. Indications for therapy include inadequate intake due to administration of selected drugs (eg, methotrexate, potentiated sulfa drugs, some anticonvulsants [eg, primidone and phenytoin]), liver disease, malabsorption, or other chronic debilitating diseases.

Iron is necessary for Hgb formation. It is available in the diet either as a heme form, which is a small percent of the total but readily absorbed, or a nonheme form. Absorption of the nonheme form is profoundly affected by diet. Iron is absorbed from the proximal jejunum, where it immediately combines in the enterocyte to the globulin transferrin. It is transported in the plasma in this form, but the binding is loose and iron can be easily transferred to tissues. Iron enters cells via specific receptors that interact with transferrin. In the cell, iron combines with the protein apoferritin to become ferritin, the soluble form of iron storage. Smaller quantities are also stored as the insoluble hemosiderin; the amount of this storage form increases when the total amount of iron in the body is much more than apoferritin can accommodate. There is no mechanism for the excretion of iron other than via the GI tract. GI elimination occurs by exfoliation of enterocytes containing iron, biliary elimination, and elimination of dietary iron that has not been absorbed. Indications for iron therapy are limited to treatment or prevention of iron deficiency (eg, blood loss, pregnancy). Iron is available in both oral and parenteral preparations. Oral preparations should be ferrous salts, such as sulfate (dogs: 100-300 mg, SID; cats: 50-100 mg, SID), gluconate, and fumarate. Therapy can be continued for several months to replenish body iron stores. Response to iron therapy can be assessed by monitoring circulating Hgb concentrations. Side effects are dose-related. Parenteral preparations are indicated for initial treatment of iron deficiency or if oral preparations cannot be tolerated or are not feasible (ie, neonatal pigs). Iron dextrans can be given as a single IM injection (100 mg) at 2-3 days of age in newborn piglets. Toxicity may be seen and is manifest as pale skin, bloody diarrhea, and shock (*see* p 2403). When efficacy of parenteral preparations is compared, dextran complexes and hydrogenated dextrans are more efficient than dextrins. Hgb formation requires pyridoxine and the trace elements copper and cobalt (necessary for B_{12} synthesis by ruminal microflora). "Shotgun" preparations contain a combination of hematinic agents; the efficacy of such products is questionable. As with any hematinic preparation, provision of these compounds will be ineffective if the nutritional status of the animal is poor.

Epoetin alfa is the synthetic form of the human glycoprotein erythropoietin (ERP). Epoetin alfa is indicated in the treatment of anemia associated with chronic renal failure in dogs and cats. The initial dosage is 100 U/kg, SC, 3 times/wk for 4 mo, while monitoring PCV, followed by a maintenance dosage of 75-100 U/kg, SC, 2-3 times/wk. The most significant adverse effects in dogs and cats are the development of antibodies to ERP, resistance to treatment, and worsening of anemia. Other potential adverse effects include iron deficiency, hypertension, fever, local cellulitis, arthralgia, mucocutaneous ulcers, polycythemia, and CNS disturbances (seizures).

Anabolic steroids are compounds structurally related to testosterone that have similar protein-anabolic activity but minimal androgenic effects, such as masculinization.

As part of their anabolic activity, these compounds increase the circulating RBC mass and possibly granulocytic mass. Clinical indications for use of anabolic steroids include chronic, nonregenerative anemias. Response to therapy is variable, and the time to clinical improvement is long, frequently ≥3 mo. The proposed mechanisms of action include increased ERP production via ERP-stimulating factor, differentiation of stem cells into ERP-stimulating factor-sensitive cells (eg, hemocytoblasts), and direct stimulation of erythroid-progenitor cells. The effect of anabolic steroids requires adequate ERP levels and sufficient cells in the bone marrow. Thus, the effectiveness of anabolic steroids in treating anemia may be limited, depending on the cause.

Anabolic steroids can be divided into 2 categories depending on the presence or absence of an alkyl group at the 17-carbon position. They are available as oral and parenteral preparations, including oil-based products intended for slow release. The absorption and disposition of anabolic steroids depend on the type of preparation and the animal species. Most are eliminated after hepatic metabolism. The alkylated products are more effectively absorbed when given PO and are more effective stimulants of bone marrow. Alkylated anabolic steroids include oxymetholone (dogs and cats: 1-5 mg/kg, PO, every 18-24 hr) and stanozolol (dogs: 1-4 mg, PO, BID; 25-50 mg, IM/wk; cats: 1 mg, PO, BID; 25 mg, IM/wk; horses: 0.55 mg/kg, IM, weekly for up to 4 wk). Nonalkylated anabolic steroids include nandrolone decanoate (dogs: 1-1.5 mg/kg, IM/wk; cats: 1 mg/kg, IM/wk; horse: 1 mg/kg, IM, once every 4 wk). Boldenone undecylenate is approved for horses at 1.1 mg/kg, IM, every 3 wk. Side effects of anabolic steroids include sodium and water retention, virilization, and hepatotoxicity. The alkylated products are more hepatotoxic than the nonalkylated products, particularly in cats. Cholestatic liver damage develops early and can be significant but frequently is reversible.

Hemostatics

Lyophilized concentrates of one or more clotting factors are available as topical or local hemostatics. Most act to provide an artificial factor or structural matrix that facilitates control of capillary bleeding. An intact hemostatic mechanism is necessary. These absorbable products are indicated for capillary oozing from small, superficial vessels. Concentrated factors include thromboplastin, thrombin (available as a powder, solution, or sponge), collagen, and fibrinogen. Artificial matrices include fibrin foam, absorbable gelatin sponge, and oxidized cellulose.

Astringents act locally by precipitating proteins. These agents do not penetrate tissues and, thus, are restricted to surface cells. They can be damaging to surrounding tissues. Examples include ferric sulfate, silver nitrate, and tannic acid.

Epinephrine and **norepinephrine** are hemostatics by virtue of their vasoconstrictive effects. They may be included in topical medications to decrease blood flow to the tissues, or applied intranasally in tampons to decrease epistaxis.

Systemic hemostatics include fresh blood or blood components administered to animals that have a coagulation factor deficiency. Examples include fresh plasma, fresh frozen plasma, cryoprecipitate, and platelet-rich plasma.

Vitamin K is a hemostatic only in instances of vitamin K deficiency. It is necessary for hepatic synthesis of coagulation factors II, VII, IX, and X. The principal indication is treatment of rodenticide toxicity, moldy sweet clover poisoning (dicumarol), and sulfaquinoxaline toxicity.

Vitamin K_1 (phytonadione) is a plant form of vitamin K that is safer and more effective with more rapid restoration of coagulation factors than other analogs such as vitamin K_3 (menadione). The preferred routes for administering phytonadione are SC and PO, although it can be given by slow IV (anaphylactic reactions have been reported) or IM injections. After IM administration, bleeding could be seen at the injection site. The dosage regimen selected depends on the nature of the anticoagulant toxicity. Vitamin K_1 must be given as long as the anticoagulant is present in the body at toxic levels; this duration varies depending on the rodenticide. Second-generation coumarin derivatives or indanediones are potent and have long half-lives. Several weeks of vitamin K_1 therapy may be necessary after ingestion of these long-acting rodenticides. Coagulation status should be monitored during therapy. The lag period after administration of phytonadione and synthesis of new clotting factors is 6-12 hr.

Desmopressin is a synthetic analog of vasopressin and is used to treat diabetes insipidus. In animals with von Willebrand's disease, desmopressin transiently elevates von Willebrand's factor and shortens bleeding time. It may be useful in dogs with von Willebrand's disease (0.4 µg/kg, SC; 1 µg/kg, IV, diluted in 20 mL of saline and given over 10 min), permitting surgical procedures or controlling capillary bleeding.

Anticoagulants

Anticoagulants interfere either directly or indirectly with the clotting cascade.

Heparin is a heterogeneous mixture of sulfated (anionic) mucopolysaccharides named because of its initial discovery in high concentrations in the liver. It is prepared from porcine intestinal mucosa and bovine lung. It acts indirectly to facilitate endogenous anticoagulants, specifically antithrombin III and heparin cofactor II. These molecules form stable complexes with (and thus inactivate) clotting factors, especially thrombin. Heparin is released in its active form after inactivation of the clotting factor and thus can interact with other molecules. The effect is greater with low concentrations of heparin. Heparin is also antithrombotic due to binding to endothelial cell walls, thus impairing platelet aggregation and adhesion.

Clinical indications for heparin therapy include the prevention or treatment of venous or pulmonary embolism and embolization associated with atrial fibrillation. It is also used as an anticoagulant for diagnostic use and blood transfusions. Heparin is used in conjunction with blood and/or plasma for the treatment of disseminated intravascular coagulopathy (DIC) and other hypercoagulable conditions. Heparin has also been used to clear hyperlipidemia.

Heparin is available as a sodium or calcium salt. Absorption and distribution of heparin are limited by the large size and polarity of the molecule. Oral absorption is poor; hence, it is a parenteral anticoagulant. Although anticoagulant activity is first order, half-life of the drug is dose-dependent, steady-state concentrations are difficult to achieve, and pharmacokinetics vary among individuals. Heparin is metabolized by heparinase in the liver and by reticuloendothelial cells. Metabolites of heparinase activity are excreted in the urine. The half-life is prolonged in renal or hepatic failure.

Heparin can be given IV (either intermittently or as a constant infusion) or SC. Deep SC or intrafat injection prolongs persistence of therapeutic concentrations. Large hematomas can develop after deep IM injection. High-dose heparin therapy (dogs: 150-250 U/kg, TID; cats: 250-375 U/kg, BID) has been recommended for established thromboembolism. Lower dosages (dogs and cats: 75 U/kg, TID; horses: 25-100 U/kg, TID) are indicated in the management of DIC. Blood coagulation times (eg, activated partial thromboplastin time) should be monitored during therapy. Side effects and toxicities of heparin are limited to potential hemorrhage, and because heparin is a foreign protein, possible allergic reactions. Heparin is contraindicated in bleeding animals and in DIC unless replacement blood or plasma therapy is also given.

Vitamin K antagonists (oral anticoagulants) differ from heparin primarily in their duration of activity and magnitude of effect. Their primary importance has been because of their toxic rather than therapeutic effects. Therapeutic indications include oral long-term treatment and prevention of recurrence of thrombotic conditions (eg, aortic or pulmonary thromboembolism and venous thrombosis) in cats, dogs, and horses.

There are several groups of vitamin K antagonists. They interfere with the hepatic synthesis of vitamin-K-dependent clotting factors by blocking the reduction of vitamin K epoxide after clotting factor synthesis, thus effectively reducing the concentration of vitamin K. Their anticoagulant activity (and therefore therapeutic or toxic effect) is delayed for 8-12 hr after administration or accidental ingestion because of the persistence of factors synthesized before administration. Factor VII has the shortest half-life and is the first factor to become deficient.

The vitamin K antagonists are rapidly and completely absorbed after administration PO. Levels peak in 1 hr. They are almost totally protein bound in the plasma, and their volume of distribution is limited to the plasma volume. They are metabolized by the liver to primary metabolites and then conjugated to glucuronides. They undergo an enterohepatic cycle. A variety of factors can increase the activity of these drugs, including hypoproteinemia, antimicrobial therapy, hepatic disease, hypermetabolic states, pregnancy, and the nephrotic syndrome. The potential for drug interactions is significant. Because they are highly protein bound, they can be displaced by other drugs that are protein bound (eg, acetylsalicylic acid and phenylbutazone), and their anticoagulant effects can be increased to the point of toxicity. Drug interactions also are seen with other antihemostatics.

Warfarin sodium is the most commonly used therapeutic preparation. The dosage is 0.1-0.2 mg/kg, PO, SID, for dogs and cats, and 0.067-0.167 mg/kg, PO, SID, for horses. Toxicity, manifest as hemorrhage, is a major concern with vitamin K antagonists. Coagulation times (particularly prothrombin time), CBC, and clinical evidence of bleeding (eg, occult blood in feces and urine) must be monitored carefully during warfarin therapy.

Fibrinolytic agents increase the activity of plasmin (fibrinolysin), the endogenous compound that is responsible for dissolving clots. The inactive precursor of plasmin is plasminogen, which exists in 2 forms: plasma soluble form and fibrin (clot) bound form. Streptokinase and streptodornase are synthesized by streptococci and activate both forms of plasminogen. They are used locally as a powder, infusion, or irrigation in the treatment of selected chronic wounds (eg, burns, ulcers, chronic eczemas, ear hematomas, otitis externa, osteomyelitis, chronic sinusitis, or other chronic lesions) that have not responded to other therapy. Tissue-type plasminogen activator (tPA) preferentially activates the fibrin-bound form of plasminogen. Unlike parenterally administered streptokinase, tPA does not induce a systemic proteolytic state. Selective clot lysis occurs without increasing circulating plasmin; thus, tPA has a lower risk of bleeding than does parenteral streptokinase. While tPA has been used to treat aortic thromboembolism in cats (0.25-1.0 mg/kg/hr, IV, for a total dosage of 1-10 mg/kg), both the risk of death due to reperfusion (and release of toxic metabolites) and the expense of this genetically engineered product may limit its use.

Antithrombotic drugs affect platelet activity, which is normally controlled by substances (such as prostaglandins) generated both outside and within the platelet. Platelet activity can be modulated by interacting with these substances. NSAID inhibit the formation of cyclooxygenase, the enzyme responsible for the synthesis of prostaglandin products from arachidonic acid that has been released into cells and platelets. The formation of all prostaglandins is inhibited, including that of thromboxane, a potent platelet aggregator and vasoconstrictor. In addition to its inhibitory effects on cyclooxygenase, aspirin irreversibly acetylates thromboxane synthetase, the specific enzyme responsible for the synthesis of thromboxane. Aspirin is a potent inhibitor of platelet activity; new platelets must be generated before the effects of aspirin on platelet activity disappear. At higher dosages, aspirin inhibits prostacylin, a prostaglandin product that counteracts the thrombogenic effects of thromboxane. Thus, the drug must be used cautiously for antiplatelet effects. The antiplatelet dosage for dogs is 5-10 mg/kg, every 24-48 hr, and for cats 80 mg, every 48-72 hr.

SYSTEMIC PHARMACOTHERAPEUTICS OF THE DIGESTIVE SYSTEM

See also PRINCIPLES OF THERAPY, THE DIGESTIVE SYSTEM, p 130.

THE MONOGASTRIC DIGESTIVE SYSTEM
DRUGS AFFECTING APPETITE

Disorders of appetite are very common in animals. Obesity as a result of overeating is common in companion animals and is best managed by educating the owner and regulating the animal's diet. Anorexia is a common clinical problem seen with many systemic diseases and exacerbates disease-induced catabolism. In the anorectic animal that does not respond to coaxing with small amounts of highly palatable foods, drug therapy may

TABLE 2. Drugs Used to Stimulate Appetite

Drug	Dosage
Prednisone	1 mg/kg, PO, every other day
Stanozolol	0.25-3 mg/kg, PO, SID; 2-10 mg/kg, IM, once weekly
Boldenone undecylenate	2.5 mg/kg, IM, every 2-4 wk
Diazepam	Cats: 0.005-0.4 mg/kg, IM or IV, SID; 1 mg/kg, PO, SID
Oxazepam	Cats: 2 mg, PO, BID
Cyproheptadine	Cats: 1-4 mg, PO, BID
Megestrol acetate	Dogs: 5 mg/kg, PO, SID

be used to stimulate appetite. If such therapy is unsuccessful, more invasive procedures, such as nasogastric or gastrotomy tube feeding, or total parenteral nutrition may be necessary to provide sufficient nutrition.

Drugs used as appetite stimulants in monogastrics include B vitamins, glucocorticoids, anabolic steroids, benzodiazepines, and cyproheptadine (see TABLE 2). B vitamin preparations have been administered PO and parenterally to debilitated animals, especially horses, to promote appetite.

Glucocorticoids increase gluconeogenesis and antagonize insulin for an overall hyperglycemic effect. Appetite is stimulated by the steroid-induced euphoria. Continued use of glucocorticoids has catabolic effects because skeletal muscle and collage proteins are broken down to provide the precursors for gluconeogenesis.

The anabolic steroids are synthetic derivatives of testosterone that have enhanced anabolic effects with reduced androgenic effects. Anabolic steroids antagonize the catabolic effect of glucocorticoids and the negative nitrogen balance associated with surgery, illness, trauma, and aging. In all cases, improved nitrogen balance depends on adequate intake of protein and calories and on treatment of the underlying disease. Anabolic steroids stimulate hematopoiesis, appetite, and weight gain. The adverse effects of anabolic steroid therapy include hepatotoxicity, masculinization, and early closure of bony epiphyses in young animals. Anabolic steroids are contraindicated in animals with congestive heart failure because of sodium and water retention. Because of the potential for abuse by people, anabolic steroids are controlled substances. Stanozolol is approved for use in small animals and horses, and boldenone undecylenate is approved for use in horses.

The benzodiazepines are effective appetite stimulants in cats (but not dogs) by effects induced by γ-aminobutyric acid (GABA) and by central inhibition of the satiety center in the hypothalamus. Diazepam can be administered IV, IM, or PO, SID. Cats that respond begin eating within a few seconds of IV administration, so palatable food should be promptly available. Oxazepam, a metabolite of diazepam, can be given PO. Diazepam is the more effective appetite stimulant but also has a greater sedative effect than oxazepam.

Cyproheptadine is an antihistamine with antiserotonin action. It promotes appetite by inhibition at the serotoninergic receptors, which control satiety. It is used clinically in cats as an appetite stimulant. CNS excitement and aggressive behavior may be seen in some cats.

Megestrol acetate is a synthetic progestin. It has significant antiestrogen and glucocorticoid activity, with resulting adrenal suppression. It is used to stimulate appetite and promote weight gain in people with cancer and cachexia (related to acquired immunodeficiency syndrome) and may have a similar effect in anorectic cats and dogs. Megestrol acetate is contraindicated in pregnant animals and in animals with uterine disease, diabetes mellitus, or mammary neoplasia. In cats, megestrol acetate can induce a profound adrenocortical suppression, adrenal atrophy, and diabetes mellitus, which may or may not be reversible.

DRUGS TO CONTROL OR STIMULATE VOMITING

The vomiting reflex is initiated by conditions that stimulate the emetic center of the medulla. (*See also* p 389.) Emetics stimulate either peripheral receptors or directly stimulate central vomiting centers. The peripheral-acting emetics directly stimulate the pharynx, which triggers the emetic center via the ninth cranial nerve, or the visceral afferent nerves of the stomach and intestines by causing irritation, inflammation, or distention. Vomiting can be initiated centrally by intracranial stimuli (head trauma, increased intracranial pressure, or psychic stimuli) or by stimulation of the vestibular apparatus (motion sickness, vestibulitis). Toxins or drugs, such as digoxin and anticancer drugs, directly stimulate the chemoreceptor trigger zone (CTZ) because it is not protected by a complete blood-brain barrier. Acetylcholine is the primary neurotransmitter acting on the emetic center. The CTZ is stimulated by dopamine, α_2-adrenergic drugs, serotonin, and histamine.

Emetic Drugs: These are usually administered in emergency situations after ingestion of a toxin (TABLE 3). They generally remove <80% of the stomach contents.

Apomorphine is an opiate drug that acts as a potent central dopamine agonist to directly stimulate the CTZ. It can be administered PO, IV, or SC; the IM route is not as effective. It can also be applied directly to conjunctival and gingival membranes, using the tablet formulation, which can easily be removed once emesis is initiated. Vomiting usually occurs in 5-10 min. Although apomorphine directly stimulates the CTZ, it has a depressant effect on the emetic center. Therefore, if the first dose does not induce emesis, additional doses are not helpful. Because the vestibular apparatus may also be involved in apomorphine-induced vomiting, animals that are sedate and motionless will not vomit as readily as animals that are active. Because it can cause CNS stimulation, apomorphine is used cautiously in cats. Opiate-induced excitement in cats can be treated with naloxone (an opiate antagonist).

Xylazine is an α_2-adrenergic agonist used primarily for its sedative and analgesic action. It is a reliable emetic, particularly in cats, in which it stimulates the CTZ. Because xylazine can produce profound sedation and hypotension, animals should be closely monitored after administration. The IV route is preferred over IM administration.

Syrup of ipecac is an over-the-counter preparation that contains emetine, a toxic alkaloid that produces vomiting by acting as a stomach irritant. It usually, but not consistently, produces vomiting in 15-30 min. If repeated use fails to induce emesis, then gastric lavage is necessary to remove the emetine to prevent additional toxicosis.

Hydrogen peroxide (3%) or salt applied to the back of the pharynx stimulates vomiting via the ninth cranial nerve. Small doses (5-10 mL) of hydrogen peroxide can be administered via oral syringe until emesis occurs. It should be administered cautiously, especially in cats, because aspiration of hydrogen peroxide foam causes severe aspiration pneumonia.

Antiemetic Drugs: Protracted vomiting is physically exhausting and can cause dehydration, acid-base and electrolyte disturbances, and aspiration pneumonia. Antiemetic drugs are used to control excessive vomiting once an etiologic diagnosis has been made, to prevent motion sickness and psychogenic vomiting, and to control emesis from radiation

TABLE 3.   Emetic Drugs

Drug	Dosage
Apomorphine	Dogs: 4 mg/kg, PO; 0.02 mg/kg, IV; 0.3 mg/kg, SC; 0.25 mg in the conjunctival sac
Xylazine	Cats: 0.4-0.5 mg/kg, IV or IM
Syrup of ipecac	3-6 mL/kg, PO
Hydrogen peroxide	Dogs: 5-10 mL, PO
Salt	Dogs: 1 tsp of table salt into pharynx

TABLE 4. Antiemetic Drugs

Drug	Dosage
Acepromazine	0.025-0.2 mg/kg, IV, IM, SC, maximum 3 mg; 1-3 mg/kg, PO
Chlorpromazine	0.5 mg/kg, IV, IM, SC, TID-QID
Prochlorperazine	0.1 mg/kg, IM, TID-QID; 1 mg/kg, PO, BID
Isopropamide	0.2-1.0 mg/kg, PO, BID
Propantheline	0.25 mg/kg, PO, TID
Dimenhydrinate	4-8 mg/kg, PO, TID
Diphenhydramine	2-4 mg/kg, PO, TID
Cyclizine	4 mg/kg, PO, TID
Meclizine	4 mg/kg, PO, SID
Butorphanol	0.2-0.4 mg/kg, IM, SID-BID
Metoclopramide	0.1-0.5 mg/kg, IM, SC, or PO, TID; 0.01-0.02 mg/kg/hr, IV infusion
Ondansetron	0.1-0.2 mg/kg, PO, SID-BID; 0.22 mg/kg, IV, BID-TID
Dolasetron	0.6 mg/kg, IV, SID

and chemotherapy (TABLE 4). Antiemetics may act peripherally to reduce afferent input from receptors or to inhibit efferent components of the vomiting reflex response. They may also act centrally to block stimulation of the CTZ and emetic center.

The phenothiazine tranquilizers antagonize the CNS stimulatory effects of dopamine, thereby decreasing vomiting from many causes. These drugs also have antihistaminic and weak anticholinergic action. Phenothiazine tranquilizers used as antiemetics include aceromazine, chlorpromazine, and prochlorperazine. Potential side effects include hypotension due to α-adrenergic blockade, excessive sedation, extrapyramidal signs, and a lowering of the seizure threshold in epileptics. Extrapyramidal signs can be counteracted with an antihistamine (such as diphenhydramine).

The anticholinergic drugs block cholinergic afferent pathways from the GI tract and the vestibular system to the vomiting center. Alone, they are less effective than the other emetics. Atropine, scopolamine, and isopropamide cross the blood-brain barrier. They tend to have a brief duration of effect and cause excitement in cats. Peripherally acting anticholinergic drugs include glycopyrrolate, propantheline, and methscopolamine. Only isopropamide and propantheline are commonly used in small animals for vomiting related to vestibular stimulation (*see also* MOTION SICKNESS, p 1047).

The antihistamines can block both cholinergic and histaminic nerve transmission responsible for transmission of the vestibular stimulus to the vomiting center. The histamine (H_1)-blocking drugs include diphenhydramine, dimenhydrinate, promethazine (a phenothiazine with H_1-blocking effects), cyclizine, and meclizine. They may cause mild sedation, especially diphenhydramine, dimenhydrinate, and promethazine. Cyclizine and meclizine are potentially teratogenic at high doses.

Metoclopramide exerts its antiemetic effects via 3 mechanisms. At low doses, it inhibits dopaminergic transmission in the CNS, while at high doses, it inhibits serotonin receptors in the CTZ. Peripherally, metoclopramide increases gastric and upper duodenal emptying. Metoclopramide is a popular antiemetic for small animals. It is used to control emesis induced by chemotherapy, nausea and vomiting associated with delayed gastric emptying, reflux gastritis, and viral enteritis. There is tremendous individual variability in metoclopramide pharmacokinetics, and oral bioavailability is only ~50% due to a significant first-pass effect. At high doses or with rapid IV administration, metoclopramide causes CNS excitement by dopamine antagonism (similar to the phenothiazine tranquilizers). Extrapyramidal signs can be counteracted with an antihistamine such as diphenhydramine. Metoclopramide should not be administered if a GI obstruction or perforation is suspected.

The serotonin antagonists ondansetron and dolasetron are specific inhibitors of serotonin subtype 3 receptors in the CTZ. These receptors are located peripherally on vagal nerve terminals and centrally in the area postrema of the brain. Cytotoxic drugs and radiation damage the GI mucosa, causing release of serotonin. These are the most effective antiemetics used in people undergoing radiation and chemotherapy, and they have been used in dogs receiving chemotherapy. Ondansetron is not effective for emesis caused by motion sickness. Side effects of dolasetron include ECG changes (PR and QT prolongation, QRS widening) caused by dolasetron metabolites that block sodium channels.

Butorphanol is an effective antiemetic for dogs receiving cisplatin chemotherapy. It causes only mild sedation. It is believed to exert its antiemetic effect directly on the vomiting center.

THERAPY OF GASTROINTESTINAL ULCERS

GI ulceration is a common problem in small and large animals, in association with physiologic stress (endogenous cortisol), dietary management, or as a sequela of administration of ulcerogenic drugs (see also p 333 and p 175). Helicobacter organisms, incriminated as the most frequent cause of ulcers in humans, appear to be involved in some cases of gastritis in animals (see p 335). Antiulcerative drugs are listed in TABLE 5.

Antacids: The common antacids are bases of aluminum, magnesium, or calcium (aluminum hydroxide, magnesium oxide or hydroxide, and calcium carbonate). These drugs neutralize stomach acid to form water and a neutral salt. They are usually not absorbed systemically. In addition to their acid-neutralizing ability, antacids decrease pepsin activity, binding to bile acids in the stomach and stimulating local prostaglandin (PGE_1) production. Over-the-counter antacid preparations are combinations of magnesium hydroxide and aluminium hydroxide; such combinations optimize the buffering capabilities of each compound and balance the constipating effect (from aluminum hydroxide) and the laxative effect (from magnesium hydroxide). Up to 20% of the magnesium can be absorbed after administration PO and can cause hypermagnesemia in animals with renal insufficiency. Antacids frequently interfere with the GI absorption of concurrently administered drugs (eg, digoxin, tetracyclines, fluoroquinolones). Aluminum-containing antacids impair absorption of phosphate. Because they are difficult to administer and require frequent dosing in small animals, they are not as popular as newer therapies.

TABLE 5.   Antiulcerative Drugs

Drug	Dosage
Antacids	2-10 mL, PO, every 2-4 hr
Cimetidine	Dogs: 5-10 mg/kg, PO, QID Horses: 4 mg/kg, IV, BID; 18 mg/kg, PO, BID
Ranitidine	Dogs: 0.5 mg/kg, PO, SC, or IV, BID Horses: 1.3 mg/kg, IV, BID; 11 mg/kg, PO, BID
Famotidine	Dogs: 0.5-1 mg/kg, PO or IV, SID Horses: 0.4 mg/kg, IV, BID; 3 mg/kg, PO, BID
Sucralfate	Cats: 250 mg, BID-TID Dogs: 500 mg to 1 g, TID-QID Foals: 1-2 g, QID
Omeprazole	Dogs: 0.5-1 mg/kg, PO, SID Horses: 4 mg/kg, PO, SID for treatment; 2 mg/kg, PO, SID to prevent recurrence
Misoprostol	Dogs: 2-5 µg/kg, PO, TID-QID

Histamine (H_2)-receptor Antagonists: Acid secretion by the parietal cells of the stomach is controlled by stimulation of 3 receptors: gastrin, muscarinic (cholinergic), and histamine (H_2). Normal acid secretion is from an interrelationship of all 3 receptors, but inhibition of a single receptor can effectively inhibit all acid secretion. H_2-receptor antagonists effectively block gastric acid secretion from parietal cells by blocking the H_2 receptor.

Cimetidine, ranitidine, and famotidine are the commonly used H_2-receptor antagonists. Ranitidine is 3-13 times as potent on a molar basis as cimetidine in inhibiting gastric acid secretion. Famotidine is 20-150 times as potent as cimetidine. In people, food tends to delay the absorption of cimetidine, has minimal effect on ranitidine, and slightly enhances absorption of famotidine. Some evidence suggests that cimetidine strengthens the gastric mucosal defenses against ulceration and enhances cytoprotection. Cimetidine reduces the metabolism of other drugs (warfarin, phenytoin, lidocaine, metronidazole, theophylline) by inhibiting hepatic microsomal enzyme systems. Ranitidine interacts differently than cimetidine and only minimally (10%) inhibits hepatic metabolism of some drugs. Famotidine seems to have no effect on metabolism of other drugs. Antacids should be given 1 hr before or after cimetidine to avoid interactions. Famotidine may be given with antacids; ranitidine may be given with low doses of antacids. Sucralfate may alter absorption of cimetidine and ranitidine.

Cimetidine suppresses gastric acid secretion in dogs for 3-5 hr. Because ranitidine has a longer elimination half-life, it suppresses acid for up to 8 hr, so it may be administered less frequently. Famotidine can be administered once daily. Oral bioavailability in horses for these drugs is only 10-30%, so large oral doses must be administered.

Sucralfate is an antiulcerative drug that has a cytoprotective effect on GI mucosa. It disassociates in the acid environment of the stomach to sucrose octasulfate and aluminum hydroxide. Sucrose octasulfate polymerizes to a viscous, sticky substance that creates a protective effect by binding to ulcerated mucosa. This prevents "back diffusion" of hydrogen ions, inactivates pepsin, and adsorbs bile acid. In addition, sucralfate increases the mucosal synthesis of prostaglandins, which have a cytoprotective role. Because sucralfate is not absorbed, it causes virtually no side effects. Dosage regimens are extrapolated from human dosages.

Omeprazole is a proton-pump inhibitor. It inhibits the sodium/potassium proton pump at the luminal surface of the parietal cell that secretes hydrogen ions into the gastric lumen. In dogs, a single dose inhibits acid secretion for 3-4 days, despite a relatively short plasma half-life. Omeprazole also reduces gastric acid production and allows healing of gastric ulcers in horses. A specific horse product has been developed, as oral bioavailability of the human omeprazole formulation is poor in horses. Its use in cats has not been reported. In humans, adverse effects from suppression of gastric acid secretion include hypergastrinemia, which causes mucosal cell hyperplasia, hypertrophy of the gastric rugae, and eventually development of carcinoids. Therefore, omeprazole is contraindicated for chronic therapy. Omeprazole is also a microsomal enzyme inhibitor (to a similar extent as cimetidine).

Misoprostol is a synthetic prostaglandin E_1 analog used in dogs to reduce the risk of GI ulcers induced by chronic NSAID therapy. Misoprostol suppresses gastric acid secretion by inhibiting the activation of histamine-sensitive adenylate cyclase. It has a cytoprotective effect from stimulation of bicarbonate and mucus secretion, increased mucosal blood flow, decreased vascular permeability, and increased cellular proliferation and migration. Misoprostol is clinically effective in preventing GI bleeding and ulceration from NSAID therapy but is less efficacious than H_2-blockers for treatment of ulcers. Side effects of misoprostol are mainly limited to diarrhea and flatulence. Magnesium-containing antacids may aggravate the diarrhea. Misoprostol is contraindicated in pregnant dogs because it can induce abortion.

DRUGS USED IN TREATMENT OF DIARRHEA

Therapy for diarrhea includes fluids, electrolyte replacement, maintenance of acid/base balance, and control of discomfort. Antiparasitic drugs or dietary therapy can also play an important role in the treatment of some types of diarrhea. Additional therapy may

TABLE 6. Antidiarrheal Drugs

Drug	Dosage
Kaolin-pectin	1-2 mL/kg, PO, QID
Activated charcoal	2-8 g/kg, PO
Bismuth subsalicylate	1-3 mL/kg/day in divided doses, PO
Aminopentamide	0.1-0.4 mg, IM, SC, or PO, BID
Isopropamide	0.2-1.0 mg/kg, PO, BID
Propantheline	0.25-0.5 mg/kg, PO, BID-TID
Paregoric	0.06 mg/kg, PO, TID
Diphenoxylate	0.05-0.1 mg/kg, PO, QID
Loperamide	0.08 mg/kg, PO, TID-QID

include intestinal protectants, motility modifiers, antimicrobials, anti-inflammatory drugs, and antitoxins (TABLE 6).

Mucosal Protectants and Adsorbents: Kaolin-pectin formulations are popular for symptomatic therapy of diarrhea. Kaolin is a form of aluminum silicate and pectin (a carbohydrate extracted from the rind of citrus fruits). Although kaolin-pectin is claimed to act as a demulcent and adsorbent in the treatment of diarrhea (related to the binding of bacterial toxins [endotoxins and enterotoxins] in the GI tract), clinical studies have not demonstrated any benefit from its administration. It may change the consistency of the feces but neither decreases the fluid or electrolyte loss, nor shortens the duration of the illness. Nevertheless, it is often administered to small animals, foals, calves, lambs, and kids. Kaolin-pectin products may adsorb or bind other drugs administered PO and reduce bioavailability.

Activated charcoal is derived from wood, peat, coconut, or pecan shells. The material is heated and treated in such a way that many large pores are formed, which dramatically increases the internal surface area. Activated charcoal is available in a variety of pore sizes. The formulations that are sold for drug and toxicant adsorption typically have pore sizes of 10-20 Å. Activated charcoal is very effective for adsorbing bacterial enterotoxins and endotoxins that cause some types of diarrhea. It also adsorbs many drugs and toxins and prevents GI absorption, so it is a common nonspecific treatment for intoxications. Activated charcoal is not absorbed, so overdose is not a problem.

Although other "mucosal protectants" have questionable efficacy, bismuth subsalicylate is considered by many human gastroenterologists to be the symptomatic treatment of choice for acute diarrhea. Its efficacy has been proved in controlled clinical trials in people with acute diarrhea (enterotoxigenic *Escherichia coli* or "traveller's diarrhea"). Bismuth adsorbs bacterial enterotoxins and endotoxins and has a GI protective effect. The salicylate component has antiprostaglandin activity. Practically all of the salicylate is absorbed systemically when administered to dogs and cats. Some animals may resent the taste of bismuth subsalicylate, and owners should be warned that it will turn the feces black. This may interfere with evaluating the feces for hemorrhage. Salicylate toxicosis is possible, especially in cats.

Motility-modifying Drugs: Anticholinergic drugs are common ingredients in antidiarrheal preparations because they significantly decrease intestinal motility and secretions. Their parasympatholytic effects decrease segmental and propulsive intestinal smooth muscle contractions and relax spasms of smooth muscle. Although they do not alter the course of the disease, anticholinergic drugs decrease the urgency associated with some forms of diarrhea in small animals, the amount of fluid secreted into the intestine, and abdominal cramping associated with hypermotility. Because few of the types of diarrhea seen in animals can be classified as "hypermotile," use of anticholinergic drugs is limited in veterinary medicine. Intestinal motility is already impaired in many animals with diarrhea, and these drugs may actually worsen the diarrhea. The anticholinergic drugs also have profound systemic pharmacologic effects. If they are administered in sufficient doses to affect intestinal motility, possible side effects include severe ileus, xerostomia, urine retention, cycloplegia, tachycardia, and CNS excitement. Chronic administration may lead to serious intestinal atony.

Atropine is the best known anticholinergic drug, but because it has many other systemic effects, it is not ordinarily used for an antidiarrheal effect. To avoid CNS excitement, quaternary amines such as aminopentamide, isopropamide, and propantheline are preferred because they do not cross the blood-brain barrier readily.

Opiates have both antisecretory and antimotility effects. They decrease propulsive intestinal contractions and increase segmentation for an overall constipating effect. They also increase GI sphincter tone. There is some evidence that opiates inhibit colonic motor activity in horses. In addition to affecting motility, opiates stimulate absorption of fluid, electrolytes, and glucose. Their effects on secretory diarrhea are probably related to inhibition of calcium influx and decreased calmodulin activity. They are frequently used for diarrhea in dogs, but their use in cats is controversial because they may cause excitement. The constipating effects of morphine and codeine have been known for many years, but they are not used clinically as antidiarrheal drugs. Paregoric is a tincture of opium product and a controlled substance (5 mL of paregoric corresponds to ~2 mg of morphine). Diphenoxylate and loperamide are 2 synthetic opiates that have specific action on the GI tract, without causing other systemic effects. They have been used in small animals and large animal neonates. Diphenoxylate is a controlled substance in a formulation that contains atropine to discourage abuse; at therapeutic doses, there is no effect from the atropine. Opiates can have potent effects on the GI tract and should be used cautiously. Loperamide is available over-the-counter. These drugs are contraindicated in infectious diarrhea because slowing GI transit time may increase the absorption of bacterial toxins. In dogs, constipation and bloat are the most common adverse effects. Potentially, paralytic ileus, toxic megacolon, pancreatitis, and CNS effects can develop, especially in cats.

Antimicrobial Therapy: The efficacy of antimicrobials in the therapy of diarrhea is unknown or unproved in most clinical situations. In most cases of diarrhea in small animals, a bacterial etiology is not identified. In large animals, antimicrobial therapy has not been shown to alter the course of bacterial enteritis, and in some cases, is thought to perpetuate the disease by producing "carrier" animals (eg, salmonellosis). Nonabsorbed antimicrobials are frequently combined with motility modifiers, adsorbents, and intestinal protectants in some preparations. Many of these combinations are irrational. Antimicrobials frequently are a treatment for diarrhea in animals, but there are few conditions that have a known etiology for which antimicrobial therapy is indicated. *Campylobacter* enteritis, from infection with *Campylobacter jejuni*, is seen in cats and dogs and can be zoonotic. Treatment alleviates clinical signs, but animals usually remain carriers. Suggested antimicrobial therapy includes erythromycin, enrofloxacin, clindamycin, tylosin, tetracycline, or chloramphenicol. Intestinal bacterial overgrowth is usually due to *Escherichia coli* or *Clostridium* spp, so therapy is initiated with an oral drug effective in the GI lumen with anaerobic activity, eg, metronidazole, amoxicillin, ampicillin, tylosin, or clindamycin. Equine monocytic ehrlichiosis (POTOMAC HORSE FEVER, p 236) is caused by the rickettsial organism *Ehrlichia risticii* but clinically resembles salmonellosis. Treatment of choice is IV oxytetracycline.

Enteritis from a variety of pathogens is common in young animals. When integrity of the intestinal mucosa is lost, septicemia or endotoxemia is likely. Signs of sepsis include severe bloody diarrhea, fever, scleral injection, dehydration, and alteration in the leukogram (early leukopenia in endotoxic shock, followed by leukocytosis). If septicemia or endotoxemia is suspected, systemic antimicrobials are warranted along with NSAID. Neonates with diarrhea deteriorate rapidly before culture and sensitivity results are available. Therefore, broad-spectrum antimicrobial therapy should be initiated. Suggested antimicrobials (depending on species) include fluoroquinolones, a penicillin or cephalosporin plus an aminoglycoside (gentamicin, amikacin), ampicillin or amoxicillin, tetracyclines, potentiated sulfonamides, chloramphenicol, or florfenicol. In septic animals, GI absorption is likely to be altered, so parenteral administration is preferred.

Nonsteroidal Anti-inflammatory Drugs (NSAID): The antiprostaglandin activity of NSAID may be beneficial with some types of diarrhea and may be important in the treatment of septicemia or endotoxemia. Prostaglandins are important intracellular messengers for stimulating hypersecretion by the intestinal mucosa, possibly by stimulating an increase in cAMP. Antiprostaglandin drugs may directly inhibit fluid and electrolyte hypersecretion by the intestinal cells. NSAID should be administered cautiously because they have adverse GI, hepatic, and renal effects.

Antitoxins: Antiendotoxin antiserum is available for treatment of equine and canine endotoxemia. This hyperimmune serum appears to improve the clinical condition of horses exhibiting signs of endotoxemia and reduces mortality from parvovirus enteritis in dogs.

DRUGS USED IN TREATMENT OF CHRONIC COLITIS

The specific cause of chronic colitis in animals is frequently unknown; therefore, it is difficult to prescribe a specific treatment for the underlying disorder (TABLE 7). The goal of colitis therapy is to restore normal intestinal motility and to relieve inflammation, spasm, or ulceration. In small animals, dietary therapy is a major component of therapy for chronic colitis (p 320).

Sulfasalazine is composed of sulfapyridine and 5-aminosalicylic acid (mesalamine) joined by an azo bond. The bond is broken by bacteria in the colon to release the 2 drugs. The sulfonamide component is absorbed into the circulation, while the salicylic acid component is active locally in the GI tract. Less than half of the salicylate component is absorbed systemically. Clinical efficacy appears to be primarily due to the anti-inflammatory effect of the salicylate component. There is evidence for antilipoxygenase activity, decreased interleukin-1, decreased prostaglandin synthesis, and oxygen radical scavenging activity. Sulfasalazine is commonly used in small animals in the therapy of ulcerative or idiopathic colitis or of plasmacytic-lymphocytic colitis once dietary causes have been excluded. As the salicylate component is only minimally absorbed, its systemic effects are minimal. The sulfonamide component may cause keratoconjunctivitis sicca in dogs, and the salicylate component may cause toxicity in cats. Dose recommendations for sulfasalazine vary widely, and the dosage is gradually reduced after an initial response. New products have been developed to overcome the difficulty of the 5-aminosalicylic acid reaching the colon and the systemic side effects. Mesalamine is a pH-sensitive, coated 5-aminosalicylic acid. The polymer coating prevents release of the active drug until it reaches the colon. Olsalazine consists of 2 molecules of 5-aminosalicylic acid joined together with an azo bond. Mesalamine is also available as an enema. Rectal administration allows delivery of active drug to the colon. It appears useful in dogs with chemotherapy-induced hemorrhagic colitis or with idiopathic distal proctitis. It may also be useful in dogs with perianal fistulas.

TABLE 7. Drugs Used for Chronic Colitis	
Drug	**Dosage**
Sulfasalazine	10-30 mg/kg, PO, BID-TID
Tylosin	40-80 mg/kg, SID
Metronidazole	10-30 mg/kg, PO, SID-TID
Prednisone	2-4 mg/kg, PO, every other day
Raw linseed oil	1 oz/day in the feed
Azathioprine	50 mg/m^2, PO, SID for 2 wk, then every other day

Tylosin is a macrolide antimicrobial that is used successfully in some animals with colitis. It is commonly administered on a chronic basis as an alternative to sulfasalazine therapy. The mechanism of action is unknown, but it is suspected that its activity against *Mycoplasma*, spirochetes, and *Chlamydia* is important. Best results are attained when the powdered form, labeled for use in swine, is mixed with food or added to water. Some animals may find the bitter taste unpalatable.

Metronidazole has fair efficacy against *Giardia*, and it is also efficacious in some cases of diarrhea in which giardiasis was not definitively diagnosed. It is suspected that this efficacy is related to the activity of metronidazole against anaerobic bacteria. Metronidazole also has an immunosuppressive effect on the GI mucosa by decreasing the cell-mediated response. Adverse neurologic effects have been reported in dogs.

The efficacy of glucocorticoids for treating colitis is probably related to their anti-inflammatory and immunosuppressive capabilities. Some cases of colitis may be due to autoantibodies and T lymphocytes directed against colonic epithelial cells. Glucocorticoids suppress the immune reaction and are used when biopsy results suggest eosinophilic or plasmacytic-lymphocytic colitis. They are used in dogs, cats, and horses, often when all other forms of therapy have failed. Immunosuppressive doses of oral prednisone are usually administered and slowly tapered to every-other-day therapy with the lowest effective dose.

N-3 fatty acids have been suggested for therapy in people with ulcerative colitis or Crohn's disease. The addition of n-3 fatty acids to the diet makes fewer n-6 fatty acids available for the arachidonic acid cascade. Several formulations are available for small animals, and raw linseed oil may be added to horses' grain for this effect.

Potent immunosuppressive drugs such as azathioprine are used to manage some forms of colitis. Azathioprine is metabolized to 6-mercaptopurine, which is immunosuppressive by interfering with nucleic acid synthesis and by impairing lymphocyte proliferation.

GASTROINTESTINAL PROKINETIC DRUGS

Prokinetic drugs increase the movement of ingested material through the GI tract (TABLE 8). They are useful in the treatment of motility disorders in humans and other animals because they induce coordinated motility patterns. Unfortunately, some prokinetic drugs may produce a number of serious side effects that complicate their use.

TABLE 8.   Prokinetic Drugs

Drug	Dosage
Metoclopramide	Dogs and cats: 0.2-0.5 mg/kg, PO or SC, TID; 0.01-0.02 mg/kg/hr, IV infusion Horses: 0.125-0.25 mg/kg, diluted in 500 mL of polyionic solution and administered IV over 60 min
Domperidone	0.1-0.5 mg/kg, IM; 0.5-1.0 mg/kg, PO
Cisapride	Dogs: 0.1 mg/kg, PO, TID Cats: 2.5 mg/cat, TID for cats <5 kg, and 5.0 mg/cat for cats >5 kg Horses: 0.1 mg/kg, PO, TID
Erythromycin	0.5-1.0 mg/kg, PO, BID-TID
Ranitidine	1-2 mg/kg, PO, BID
Nitazidine	2.5-5 mg/kg, PO, BID
Neostigmine	0.02 mg/kg, SC, as needed
Lidocaine	Horses: 1.3 mg/kg as a bolus followed by a continuous infusion of 0.05 mg/kg/min

Metoclopramide is a dopaminergic antagonist and peripheral serotonin receptor antagonist with GI and CNS effects. In the upper GI tract, metoclopramide increases both acetylcholine release from neurons and cholinergic receptor sensitivity to acetylcholine. Metoclopramide stimulates and coordinates esophageal, gastric, pyloric, and duodenal motor activity. It increases lower esophageal sphincter tone and stimulates gastric contractions; while relaxing the pylorus and duodenum. Inadequate cholinergic activity is incriminated in many GI motility disorders; therefore, metoclopramide should be most effective in diseases where normal motility is diminished or impaired. Metoclopramide speeds gastric emptying of liquids, but may slow the emptying of solids. It is effective in treating postoperative ileus in dogs, which is characterized by decreased GI myoelectric activity and motility. Metoclopramide has little or no effect on colonic motility.

Metoclopramide is primarily indicated for the relief of nausea and vomiting associated with chemotherapy and as an antiemetic for dogs with parvoviral enteritis and for the treatment of gastroesophageal reflux and postoperative ileus. GI obstruction, such as intussusception in puppies with parvoviral enteritis, must be excluded prior to initiating metoclopramide therapy. Its prokinetic action is negated by narcotic analgesics and anticholinergic drugs, such as atropine. Drugs that dissolve or are absorbed in the stomach, such as digoxin, may have reduced absorption. Bioavailability may be increased for drugs that are absorbed in the small intestine. Due to accelerated food absorption, metoclopramide therapy may increase the insulin dose required in diabetics. Concurrent use of phenothiazine and butyrophenone tranquilizers should be avoided because they also have central antidopaminergic activity, so they increase the potential for extrapyramidal reactions.

Metoclopramide readily crosses the blood-brain barrier, where dopamine antagonism at the CTZ produces an antiemetic effect. However, dopamine antagonism in the striatum causes adverse effects known collectively as extrapyramidal signs, which include involuntary muscle spasms, motor restlessness, and inappropriate aggression. If recognized in time, the extrapyramidal signs can be reversed by restoring an appropriate dopamine:acetylcholine balance with the anticholinergic action of an antihistamine, such as diphenhydramine hydrochloride given IV at a dosage of 1.0 mg/kg.

Cisapride is chemically related to metoclopramide, but unlike metoclopramide, it does not cross the blood-brain barrier or have antidopaminergic effects. Therefore, it does not have antiemetic action or cause extrapyramidal effects (extreme CNS stimulation). Cisapride enhances the release of acetylcholine from postganglionic nerve endings of the myenteric plexus and antagonizes the inhibitory action of serotonin on the myenteric plexus, resulting in increased GI motility and heart rate. Cisapride is more potent and has broader prokinetic activity than metoclopramide, increasing the motility of the colon, as well as that of the esophagus, stomach, and small intestine.

Although availability is now restricted (see below), cisapride was especially useful in animals that experienced neurologic side effects from metoclopramide. It was also useful in managing gastric stasis, idiopathic constipation, gastroesophageal reflux, and postoperative ileus in dogs and cats. Cisapride was especially useful in managing chronic constipation in cats with megacolon; in many cases, it alleviated or delayed the need for subtotal colectomy. Cisapride was also useful in managing cats with hairball problems and dogs with idiopathic megaesophagus that continued to regurgitate frequently despite a carefully managed, elevated feeding program. In horses, cisapride increases motility of the left dorsal colon and improves coordination of the ileocecal-colonic junction. There is some evidence that cisapride is useful in preventing postoperative ileus, but clinical use has so far been limited. In comparative studies of GI motility in humans and animals, cisapride was clearly superior to other treatments.

Initially, the only adverse effects reported in humans were increased defecation, headache, abdominal pain, and cramping and flatulence; cisapride appeared to be well tolerated in animals. As cisapride became widely used in the management of gastroesophageal reflux in humans, cases of heart rhythm disorders and deaths were reported to the FDA. These cardiac problems in humans were highly associated with concurrent drug therapy or specific underlying conditions. In veterinary medicine, adverse reactions to clinical use of cisapride have not been reported. But because of the cardiovascular side effects in humans, the manufacturer of cisapride voluntarily placed it under a limited-access program. Cisapride for animals can still be obtained through compounding veterinary pharmacies.

Domperidone is a peripheral dopamine receptor antagonist that has been marketed outside the USA since 1978. It is available in Canada as a 10-mg tablet. Currently, it is available in the USA only as an investigational new drug (as a 1% oral domperidone gel) for the treatment of agalactia in mares due to fescue toxicosis. Domperidone regulates the motility of gastric and small-intestinal smooth muscle and has some effect on esophageal motility. Domperidone appears to have very little physiologic effect in the colon. It has antiemetic activity from dopaminergic blockade in the CTZ. But because very little domperidone crosses the blood-brain barrier, reports of extrapyramidal reactions are rare, and treatment is the same as for metoclopramide. Domperidone failed to enhance gastric emptying in healthy dogs in one study. In other studies, however, domperidone was superior to metoclopramide in stimulating antral contractions in dogs but not cats and improved antroduodenal coordination in dogs. Because of its favorable safety profile, domperidone appears to be an attractive alternative to metoclopramide.

Macrolide antibiotics, including erythromycin and clarithromycin, are motilin receptor agonists. They also appear to stimulate cholinergic and noncholinergic neuronal pathways to stimulate motility. At microbially ineffective doses, some macrolide antibiotics stimulate migrating motility complexes and antegrade peristalsis in the proximal GI tract. Erythromycin therapy has been effective in the treatment of gastroparesis in human patients in whom metoclopramide or domperidone was ineffective. Erythromycin increases gastric emptying rate in healthy dogs, but large food chunks may enter the small intestine and be inadequately digested. Erythromycin induces contractions from the stomach to the terminal ileum and proximal colon, but the colon contractions do not appear to result in propulsive motility. Therefore, erythromycin is unlikely to benefit patients with colonic motility disorders.

Human pharmacokinetic studies indicate that erythromycin suspension is the ideal dosage form for administration of erythromycin as a prokinetic agent. Other macrolide antibiotics have prokinetic activity with fewer side effects than erythromycin and may be suitable for use in small animals. While causing less GI distress than erythromycin, clarithromycin (250 mg, IV) increased gastroduodenal motility in patients being treated for functional dyspepsia and *Helicobacter pylori* gastritis. Both erythromycin and clarithromycin are metabolized by the hepatic cytochrome P450 enzyme system and inhibit the hepatic metabolism of other drugs including theophylline, cyclosporine, and cisapride. Nonantibiotic derivatives of erythromycin are being developed as prokinetic agents.

Ranitidine and nizatidine are 2 histamine H_2-receptor antagonists that are prokinetics in addition to inhibiting gastric acid secretion in dogs and rats. Their prokinetic activity is due to acetylcholinesterase inhibition, with the greatest activity in the proximal GI tract. Cimetidine and famotidine are not acetylcholinesterase inhibitors and do not have prokinetic effects. Ranitidine and nizatidine stimulate GI motility by increasing the amount of acetylcholinesterase available to bind smooth muscle muscarinic cholinergic receptors. They also stimulate colonic smooth muscle contraction in cats through a cholinergic mechanism. Ranitidine is available as tablets (75, 150, and 300 mg), a syrup (15 mg/mL), and an injectable solution (25 mg/mL). An oral dose of 1-2 mg/kg, BID, inhibits gastric acid secretion and stimulates gastric emptying. Nizatidine is available as capsules (75, 150, and 300 mg). Like ranitidine, at gastric antisecretory dosages of 2.5-5 mg/kg, nizatidine also has prokinetic effects. Ranitidine causes less interference with cytochrome P450 metabolism of other drugs than does cimetidine, and nizatidine does not affect hepatic microsomal enzyme activity, so both drugs have a wide margin of safety.

Neostigmine inactivates acetylcholinesterase and, therefore, prolongs the action of acetylcholine. It may also directly stimulate cholinergic receptors. It is recommended for use in large animals for treatment of paralytic ileus; however, it is short acting (15-30 min). It may cause increased secretion into the GI tract, so it is contraindicated in small-intestinal disease. In horses, it may actually decrease small-intestinal propulsive contractions and delay gastric emptying.

IV lidocaine is used in the treatment of postoperative ileus in humans, and has recently been shown to be useful in treating ileus and proximal duodenitis-jejunitis in horses. It is thought to suppress the firing of primary afferent neurons, as well as to have anti-inflammatory properties and direct stimulatory effects on smooth muscle. The dosage is 1.3 mg/kg as a bolus, followed by a continuous infusion of 0.05 mg/kg/min. Most horses respond within 12 hr of starting the infusion.

CATHARTIC AND LAXATIVE DRUGS

Cathartics and laxatives increase the motility of the intestine or increase the bulk of feces. The dosages for all of these drugs are highly empirical and usually extracted from human dosages (TABLE 9). Clinically, these drugs are administered to increase passage of gut contents associated with intestinal impaction, to cleanse the bowel before radiography or endoscopy, to eliminate toxins from the GI tract, and to soften feces after intestinal or anal surgery.

Stimulant Cathartics: Stimulant (irritant) cathartics appear to stimulate intestinal motility via an irritant effect on the mucosa or stimulation of intramural nerve plexi. They also activate secretory mechanisms, provoking fluid accumulation in the GI lumen. These drugs can have potent effects, and excessive fluid and electrolyte loss can result. They act directly or indirectly (if a metabolic conversion is necessary before the compound is active).

Emodin is an irritant glycoside that is an active ingredient in several products. Its action is limited to the large intestine, and it may take 4-6 hr for an effect to be seen. Repeat dosages should be avoided in horses because of the long latent period and risk of severe superpurgation. The naturally occurring emodins (eg, senna) are found in human formulations.

The vegetable oils are indirect-acting cathartics. They are hydrolyzed by pancreatic lipase in the small intestine to irritating fatty acids. Castor oil is a potent cathartic. It is hydrolyzed to release ricinoleic acid, which causes increased water secretion in the small intestine. It is used mainly in nonruminants and preruminant calves. Raw linseed oil (cooked linseed oil is toxic) is hydrolyzed to release linoleates, which are less irritating than ricinoleic acid. In smaller daily doses, linseed oil is a mild lubricant laxative and a source of fatty acids for horses.

Phenolphthalein and bisacodyl are diphenylmethane compounds that affect the large intestine and are found in many over-the-counter human laxative formulations. Phenolphthalein is effective only in primates and pigs. Bisacodyl appears to inhibit glucose

TABLE 9.   Cathartic and Laxative Drugs

Drug	Dosage
Castor oil	Dogs: 5-25 mL, PO Foals: 25-50 mL, PO
Bisacodyl	Dogs: 5-20 mg, PO, SID-BID Cats: 2.5-5.0 mg, PO, SID-BID
Magnesium sulfate (Epsom salts)	Dogs: 5-25 g, PO Cats: 2-5 g, PO Horses: 30-100 g, PO
Magnesium hydroxide (milk of magnesia)	Dogs: 5-10 mL, PO Cats: 2-6 mL, PO Horses: 1-4 L, PO
Lactulose	Dogs: 5-15 mL, PO, TID Cats: 2-3 mL, PO, TID
Docusate sodium, docusate calcium, docusate potassium	Dogs and cats: 2 mg/kg, PO, SID Horses: 10-20 mg/kg in 2 L water, PO, every other day

absorption and Na^+/K^+-ATPase activity and to alter the motor activity of visceral smooth muscle. It is administered by mouth or by enema, and only 5% of any dose is absorbed.

Hyperosmotic Cathartics: These drugs are poorly absorbed from the GI tract and draw fluid into the intestine by osmosis. The fluid content of the feces increases, which causes intestinal distention and promotes peristalsis. Although hyperosmotic cathartics are relatively safe, overdoses can cause excessive fluid loss and dehydration, so adequate water intake must be assured. Examples of hyperosmotic cathartics include magnesium salts, sodium salts, and sugar alcohols.

Magnesium salts are frequently used PO as saline purgatives. Normally, only 20% of the magnesium is systemically absorbed and eliminated by the kidneys. If absorption is excessive or renal elimination is impaired, then severe hypermagnesemia and metabolic alkalosis may develop.

Sodium salts can be given PO as saline cathartics but are more commonly administered as sodium biphosphate or sodium phosphate enemas. These should not be used in cats because fatal hyperphosphatemia, hypocalcemia, and hypernatremia may result.

Sugar alcohols, such as mannitol and sorbitol, are poorly absorbed and fermented in the terminal ileum and large intestine. Lactulose is a synthetic disaccharide that is fermented in the large intestine to produce acetic, lactic, and other organic acids that have an osmotic effect. Lactulose is used to treat chronic constipation in cats with megacolon. It is also used in the management of hepatic encephalopathy, in which acidification of the large intestine promotes formation of nonabsorbable ammonium ions and quaternary amines, thereby reducing the need for detoxification by the liver.

Hydrophilic Colloids ("Bulk Laxatives"): These are composed of nonabsorbed synthetic or natural polysaccharide cellulose derivatives. These compounds imbibe water and increase the mass of nondigestible material in the intestine. Examples include methylcellulose, psyllium, prunes, wheat bran, and canned pumpkin.

Lubricant Laxatives: These act by coating the surface of the feces with a water-immiscible film and by increasing the water content of the feces to provide a lubricant action. Lubricant laxatives usually contain mineral oil or white petroleum. Chronic use may reduce intestinal absorption of fat-soluble vitamins and cause a granulomatous enteritis. Mineral oil is very commonly used in horses and cattle, and commercial products are available to promote passage of hairballs in cats.

Fecal Softeners (Surfactants): Docusate sodium, docusate calcium, and docusate potassium are salts that decrease surface tension and allow water to accumulate in the feces. Docusate also increases cAMP in colonic mucosal cells, which increases ion secretion and fluid permeability. When docusate is used concurrently with mineral oil, soaps are formed and mineral oil absorption is increased.

DRUGS AFFECTING DIGESTIVE FUNCTIONS

Pancrealipase contains the pancreatic enzymes lipase, amylase, and protease. It is derived from the pancreatic tissues of swine. These enzymes help to digest and absorb fats, proteins, and carbohydrates. Pancrealipase is used to treat dogs and cats with exocrine pancreatic insufficiency. There are several formulations available, including oral capsules, tablets, and delayed-release capsules and tablets. The powdered forms can be added to food, and the dosage adjusted to maintain normal feces. Antacids may diminish the efficacy of pancrealipase, while H_2-receptor antagonists may increase the amount of pancrealipase that reaches the duodenum.

Ursodiol, also known as ursodeoxycholic acid, is a naturally occurring bile acid. It suppresses hepatic synthesis and secretion of cholesterol and decreases intestinal absorption of cholesterol. Reducing cholesterol saturation allows solubilization of cholesterol-containing gallstones. Ursodiol also increases bile flow and reduces the hepatotoxic effect of bile salts by decreasing their detergent action. In small animals, ursodiol may be useful in the treatment of cholesterol-containing gallstones, idiopathic hepatic lipidosis, and chronic active hepatitis. The dosage in dogs and cats is 15 mg/kg, PO, SID.

S-Adenosylmethionine (SAMe) is an endogenous molecule synthesized by cells throughout the body. Formed from the amino acid methionine and ATP, SAMe is an essential part of 3 major biochemical pathways: transmethylation, transsulfuration, and aminopropylation. Deficiency of SAMe is associated with cellular derangements in hepatocytes, and there is evidence that a SAMe deficiency may contribute to abnormalities of cellular structure and function in many body tissues, including the liver. Exogenous administration of SAMe appears to improve hepatocellular function in in vivo and in vitro studies, without cytotoxicity or significant side effects. SAMe increases hepatic glutathione levels in cats and dogs. Glutathione is a potent antioxidant that protects hepatic cells from toxins and death. The daily dosage is 18 mg/kg, rounded to the nearest size of enteric-coated tablet, and given on an empty stomach.

THE RUMINANT DIGESTIVE SYSTEM

Other than the forestomachs (rumen, reticulum, omasum), the components of the ruminant GI tract are similar to those of monogastric mammals, and the use of pharmacologic agents to treat diseases of the glandular stomach (abomasum) and intestine follows principles common to both monogastric and ruminant species. Ruminants differ significantly from other mammals in that much of their feed undergoes microbial predigestion in the forestomachs, chiefly in the rumen and reticulum. There is also postgastric fermentation in the cecum and colon, but this is much less important than in some other herbivores, eg, horses.

Ruminoreticular motility or fermentation is depressed in many conditions, including improper feeding (overload or deficiency of specific nutrients), lack of water, infectious diseases, intoxications, lesions of any part of the upper GI tract, metabolic states (eg, hypocalcemia), or reduced flow of alkaline saliva that allows pH to fall and the microbial population to be altered to an extent that is harmful to the animal. (*See also* DISEASES OF THE RUMINANT FORESTOMACH AND ABOMASUM, p 177.)

The primary objectives of pharmacotherapy are to remove the cause and to promote the return of normal digestive function by meeting or reestablishing the requirements for optimal ruminoreticular function as quickly as possible. This may include any of the following: 1) ensuring an appropriate substrate for microbial fermentation; 2) providing any cofactors (eg, phosphorus, sulfur) that are necessary for microbial fermentative processes; 3) removing any soluble end-products, undigested solid residues, and gas; 4) maintaining continual flow culture of ruminal microorganisms; 5) ensuring that the contents of the ruminoreticulum are fluid; 6) maintaining optimal intraruminal pH (generally between 6 and 7); and 7) promoting active ruminoreticular activity.

DRUGS FOR SPECIFIC PURPOSES

Esophageal Obstruction: Esophageal obstruction due to a foreign body (p 174) leads to severe discomfort and acute free-gas bloat. Physical removal of the object may be hampered by marked spasm of the surrounding muscle. Specific spasmolytic drugs such as acepromazine may be used. Alternatively, the moderate sedative and muscle relaxant effects of a low dose of xylazine (0.05 mg/kg, IM in cattle) aid the removal of obstructions.

Ruminotorics: Agents and mixtures that promote forestomach function (fermentation and motility) are known as ruminotorics. Formulations that contain glucogenic substrates, minerals, cofactors, and bitters (eg, nux vomica) have limited application in current therapy of ruminoreticular indigestion. Generally, restoration of the normal ruminoreticular environment using a physiologic approach is much more satisfactory. The mild laxative and antacid effects of magnesium hydroxide may be beneficial in those animals that do not already have alkaline ruminoreticular fluid.

Mineral oil (1-2 L) or dioctyl sodium sulfosuccinate (DSS, 90-120 mL in 1-2 L of water) administered PO or via nasogastric tube followed by gentle ruminal massage can be helpful in promoting the dissolution and passage of impacted fibrous ruminal contents.

DSS can markedly depress rumen protozoa; thus, ruminal transfaunation should follow the use of this agent if ruminal hypomotility continues.

Ruminal Fluid Transfer: Fresh ruminal fluid is considered to be the best available "ruminotoric" because it contains viable ruminal bacteria (1×10^8-10^{11}/mL) and protozoa (1×10^5-10^6/mL) as well as many useful fermentation factors (volatile fatty acids, microbial protein, minerals, vitamins, buffers). Strained fresh ruminal juice (at least 3 L; 8-16 L is ideal in cattle; sheep require ~1 L) given PO or by tube is indicated in cases of ruminoreticular stasis. Ruminal fluid can be aspirated through a stomach tube from the ruminoreticulum of healthy animals using an extractor pump or by siphoning, or it can be collected at slaughterhouses. A rumen-cannulated donor animal is particularly convenient. It is best for the donor to be on a ration similar to that of the recipient because the ruminal microflora will then be more appropriately adapted. Provided the initiating condition or lesion is responding favorably, improvement almost invariably follows the reestablishment of normal ruminal microflora, with consequent normalization of the fermentation process and ruminoreticular motility. When the ruminoreticular contents are putrified, ingesta must first be removed prior to transfer of fresh ruminal fluid. This can be accomplished using a large-bore stomach tube or by performing a ruminotomy. (*See also* p 123.)

Antifoaming Agents: The therapeutic approaches to the control of acute frothy bloat involve the administration of antifoaming agents to reduce foam stability and to promote release of free gas, which is then promptly eructated. (*See also* BLOAT, p 183.)

Acute frothy bloat in cattle should be treated with poloxalene, which may be administered as a drench or by stomach tube (25-50 g). Frothy bloat can be prevented by administering poloxalene as a top dressing to feed (1 g/45 kg body wt/day) or in a molasses block (1.5 g/45 kg body wt/day). The direct intraruminal injection of poloxalene often does not give satisfactory results. Polymerized methyl silicone (3.3% emulsion [cattle: 30-60 mL; sheep: 7-15 mL]) may be used in a similar manner as poloxalene, although direct intraruminal injection via a needle or cannula may be more satisfactory in this case. Administration of docusate sodium in emulsified soybean oil (6-12 fl oz containing 240 mg/mL) or administration of vegetable oils alone, such as peanut oil, sunflower oil, or soybean oil (cattle: 60 mL; sheep: 10-15 mL), also relieve acute frothy bloat when given PO. The incidence of frothy bloat in feedlot cattle may be reduced by including ionophores (such as monensin) in the ration or administering these as controlled-release capsules.

Ruminoreticular Antacids: Ruminal alkalinizing agents are principally used to treat ruminal lactic acidosis (pH <6) due to grain engorgement or soluble carbohydrate overload. (*See also* SUBACUTE RUMINAL ACIDOSIS, p 181.) The resultant systemic dehydration and acidosis necessitate immediate correction of fluid and electrolyte balance and restoration of a viable microbial population. Often, the latter involves removal of ruminoreticular contents and replacement with fresh ruminoreticular fluid. Antacids that may be given PO, BID-TID, include magnesium hydroxide (cattle: 100-300 g; sheep: 10-30 g) and magnesium carbonate (cattle: 10-80 g; sheep: 1-8 g). Antacids should be mixed in ~10 L of warm water to ensure adequate dispersion through the ruminoreticular contents. Administration PO of activated charcoal (2 g/kg) is believed to protect the ruminoreticular mucosa from further injury by inactivating toxins.

Ruminoreticular Acidifying Agents: Ruminal acidifying agents are used to treat ruminal stasis or simple indigestion as well as acute ammonia poisoning. In ruminal stasis, the intraruminal pH often increases to >7.5 because of the constant inflow of bicarbonate-rich saliva in the absence of active ruminal fermentation and formation of volatile fatty acids. In acute ammonia intoxication, the elevated intraruminal pH increases the activity of urease and facilitates the absorption of free ammonia (pK_a of ammonium is 9.1). Administration of weak acids in cold water returns the pH of ruminoreticular content toward physiologic levels, promotes the uptake of volatile fatty acids, depresses the absorption of ammonia, and inhibits excessive urease activity. Acetic acid (4-5%) or vinegar (cattle: 4-8 L; sheep: 250-500 mL) is the most common acidifying agent used.

Modulators of Ruminoreticular Motility: A number of factors may exert a detrimental influence on forestomach motility and result in ruminoreticular hypomotility or atony. The most effective strategy for reestablishing motility is to restore the normal ruminoreticular environment, which often requires transfaunation. The use of parasympathomimetic agents (eg, neostigmine, physostigmine, carbachol, or bethanechol) is seldom appropriate. All these drugs have cholinergic effects, which are potentially hazardous. Neostigmine (cattle: 0.02 mg/kg, SC; sheep: 0.01-0.02 mg/kg, SC) generally produces the fewest side effects but tends to increase frequency, rather than strength, of ruminoreticular contractions. This is particularly true in ruminal atony. The stimulatory effect of neostigmine is not always reliable, and some inhibition of motility can be seen. This may be due to the adrenergic component associated with ganglion stimulation by cholinergic agents. Metoclopramide has been reported to be useful in correcting disorders of ruminoreticular motility, but few definitive studies are available; it does produce powerful abomasal contractions.

Conditioned responses to the presence of feed and feeding itself are 2 physiologic means by which ruminoreticular motility can be notably enhanced.

Several pharmacologic agents such as anticholinergics, adrenergics, opiate analgesics, CNS depressants, and several toxic compounds (eg, cyanide) can result in ruminoreticular paresis.

DRUG DISPOSITION IN THE RUMINORETICULUM

Morphologic and functional characteristics of the ruminoreticulum that make it suitable for fermentative digestion of plant material also affect the activity, distribution, and absorption of many drugs, particularly when given PO. The anaerobic and reductive environment of the ruminoreticulum and the presence of many microbial enzymes result in inactivation of drugs such as chloramphenicol, trimethoprim, and cardiac glycosides. Slow and inefficient mixing of drugs in the large volume of the ruminoreticular fluid delays attainment of uniform concentrations throughout the multiphasic ingesta and retards absorption from the ruminoreticulum. Absorption is also affected by the polarity and ionization status of the drug, which is determined by the pK_a of the drug and the pH of the ruminoreticular fluid. The latter depends on the diet and the relative contributions of alkaline saliva and acidic ruminoreticular fluid. Aside from the many effects that the ruminoreticular environment can have on the activity and disposition of drugs, the drugs themselves may have unintended effects on ruminoreticular function. In particular, broad-spectrum antibacterial agents and antiprotozoal agents can disrupt the normal balance of microflora in the ruminoreticulum.

These factors affecting the activity and disposition of drugs in the ruminoreticulum, together with the possible effects of drugs on ruminoreticular function, complicate oral administration of drugs to ruminants. In young animals, these undesirable effects can be avoided by making use of the esophageal groove reflex. This reflex, which is elicited by receptors in the mouth and pharynx, is well developed in suckling neonates but becomes less reliable in older animals. After ~2 yr in cattle and ~18 mo in sheep, provoked reticular groove closure is often irregular, incomplete, or absent. Administration PO of medicaments intended for local intestinal effect (eg, purgatives, antidiarrheals, contrast media, and some anthelmintics) can be preceded by administration of an appropriate salt solution to close the reticular groove and, therefore, avoid ruminoreticular dispersion. In cattle, closure of the groove can be elicited with 60 mL of 5% copper sulfate, 5% zinc sulfate, 10% sodium bicarbonate, or 10% sodium sulfate; in sheep, 1-2% copper sulfate is effective. Onset of the reflex response takes 5-10 sec, and the groove may remain closed for up to 60 sec.

Ruminoreticular morphology and function has less influence on drug disposition in neonatal ruminants than in adults. At birth, the forestomachs are underdeveloped, and the newborn ruminant is essentially monogastric. Drugs that are usually destroyed in the ruminoreticulum of adults (eg, trimethoprim) may be well absorbed during the first 2-3 wk of life. This developmental pattern depends on the period between birth and initiation of a roughage diet and exposure to microbes in the environment.

SYSTEMIC PHARMACOTHERAPEUTICS OF THE EYE

See also OPHTHALMOLOGY, p 394.

The eye is unique in the opportunities for topical and systemic medical treatment of neural tissue. Like the brain, the eye has protective barriers from the vascular system. These are known as the blood-ocular barriers (ie, the blood-aqueous and blood-retinal barriers). They allow the eye to control entry of inflammatory cells, protein, and low-molecular-weight compounds from the systemic circulation.

The **blood-aqueous barrier** is a function of the iris and ciliary body epithelium. In the iris, the capillary endothelium is not fenestrated, but there are tight junctions. In the ciliary body, there are tight connections between the apical ends of the nonpigmented epithelial cells. Breakdown of this barrier results in entry of protein and cells into the anterior chamber and is seen as aqueous flare or plasmoid aqueous. The **blood-retinal barrier** is composed of 2 layers—an endothelial and epithelial portion. The endothelial part is composed of the endothelium of the retinal capillaries, which are also nonfenestrated. The epithelial portion is the retinal pigment epithelium. When treating the eye via the systemic circulation, these barriers can limit the entry and amount of medications into the eye, especially highly water-soluble compounds. They are less effective in the face of inflammation, and many drugs gain increased access to the intraocular structures when the eye is inflamed. The time for drugs to reach their peak concentrations in the eye depends highly on the physicochemical properties of the particular drug.

The presence of barriers such as the iris, ciliary body, and lens, as well as normal movement of aqueous humor through the pupil and out the trabecular and uveoscleral meshwork can further limit the distribution of drugs. A number of enzymes present in the cornea and ciliary body can metabolize drugs to inactive metabolites before and after the compound reaches the anterior chamber. Drugs predominantly leave the anterior chamber with the aqueous humor via the corneal trabecular and uveoscleral meshwork, although small amounts may move posteriorly into the vitreous.

ROUTES OF ADMINISTRATION

The 3 primary methods of delivery of ocular medications to the eye are topical, local ocular (ie, subconjunctival, intravitreal, retrobulbar, intracameral), and systemic. The most appropriate method of administration depends on the area of the eye to be medicated—extraocular structures, cornea, anterior segment (anterior chamber and iris), posterior segment (ciliary body, retina, vitreous), and retrobulbar or orbital tissues. The conjunctiva, cornea, anterior chamber, and iris are usually best treated with topical therapy. In contrast, the eyelids can be treated with topical therapy but more frequently require systemic therapy. The posterior segment always requires systemic therapy, as most topical medications do not penetrate to the posterior segment. Retrobulbar and orbital tissues are most frequently treated systemically.

Subconjunctival or sub-Tenon's therapy, while not a true form of systemic medication, has potentially increased drug absorption and contact time. Medications both leak onto the cornea from the entry hole of injection and diffuse through the sclera into the globe. Drugs with low solubility such as corticosteroids may provide a repository of drug lasting days to weeks. Appropriate amounts of medication must be used, as large amounts, especially of long-acting salts, can cause a significant inflammatory reaction. For sub-Tenon's injections, 0.5 mL/site is usually safe and effective in small animals and ≤1 mL in large animals such as the horse and cow.

Retrobulbar medications are used infrequently for therapeutics. In cattle, the retrobulbar tissues can be anesthetized with local anesthetic (lidocaine) for enucleations using either a Peterson block (15-20 mL) or a 4-point block of the orbit (5-10 mL/site). Whenever any medication is placed into the orbit, extreme care must be taken to ensure that the medication is not inadvertently injected into a blood vessel, the optic nerve, or one of the orbital foramen. Retrobulbar injection has a high risk of adverse effects and should not be used unless the clinician is experienced and the animal is appropriately restrained.

Systemic medication is required for posterior segment therapy and to complement topical therapy for the anterior segment. The blood-ocular barriers can limit absorption of less lipophilic drugs, but inflammation initially allows greater drug concentrations to reach the site. As the eye starts to heal, these barriers become more effective and can limit further drug penetration. This should be considered when treating posterior segment disease, eg, blastomycosis in small animals with hydrophilic drugs such as itraconazole.

Following topical administration, up to 80% of the applied drug(s) is absorbed systemically across the highly vascularized nasopharyngeal mucosa. Because absorption via this route bypasses the liver, there is not the large first-pass metabolism seen after administration PO. Depending on the drugs used, this may result in systemic side effects. Topically applied β-blockers used in the treatment of glaucoma can cause heart block, atrial tachycardia, congestive heart failure, bronchospasm, dyspnea, and decreased exercise tolerance. These drugs should be used very carefully in older animals or in those with cardiac or respiratory disease. Cushing's syndrome can be easily induced in small or medium-sized dogs with chronic use of potent topical steroids.

LOCAL ANESTHETICS

Parenterally, local nerve blocks are an excellent aid for routine equine ocular evaluation and diagnostic procedures. The auriculopalpebral block helps limit blepharospasm during ocular examinations. This procedure blocks some of the motor nerves of the upper eyelid and enables the examiner to control the horse's upper eyelid. The auriculopalpebral nerve is a branch of the facial nerve and can be palpated as it runs across the superior margin of the zygomatic arch. To block sensory input, a supraorbital nerve block or a ring block is used. The supraorbital nerve is a branch of the frontal nerve that traverses the supraorbital foramen of the upper orbit. If placed correctly, a dose of 1-2 mL of lidocaine is usually sufficient to block either the auriculopalpebral or supraorbital nerve. The block is usually effective within 3-5 min and can last up to 2-3 hr.

The same principles are used in food animals, such as cattle, in which both a retrobulbar and ring block may be used. A correctly placed retrobulbar block blocks cranial nerves II, III, IV, VI, and the ophthalmic branch of V. The ring block is needed to inhibit sensory input from the skin around the eye.

DRUGS USED IN TREATMENT OF GLAUCOMA

Topical medications, such as prostaglandins, miotics, β-blocking adrenergics, and topical carbonic anhydrase inhibitors, are the primary drugs for treatment of glaucoma (see p 399), but these are often supplemented with systemic drugs.

Osmotic Diuretics: In the emergency treatment of acute glaucoma, intraocular pressure must be reduced urgently. This is done pharmacologically using osmotic diuretics such as mannitol or glycerol in combination with other topical and systemic drugs. Osmotic diuretics are high molecular weight molecules that increase the osmotic pressure of plasma relative to the aqueous and vitreous. Most of the water in the eye is in the vitreous. Dehydration of the vitreous allows the lens and iris to move posteriorly, opening the iridocorneal angle. The other effect is to decrease formation of aqueous humor. Mannitol is given IV (1-1.5 g/kg slowly over 10-15 min) with the effect peaking in 2-3 hr and lasting up to 5 hr. Mannitol is not metabolized and thus can be used in diabetics. Oral glycerol (1-2 g/kg) can be used but is unpalatable and most dogs vomit. With both drugs, water should be withdrawn for 3-5 hr, and the animal should have an opportunity to urinate. Kidney function should be checked prior to initiating therapy, and cardiac function monitored during treatment. Mannitol can be used again if initial control of intraocular pressure is not maintained; longterm control is unlikely if intraocular pressures do not stay within the normal range after 2 treatments.

Carbonic Anhydrase Inhibitors: Other compounds used in the treatment and management of acute glaucoma include oral carbonic anhydrase inhibitors. These inhibit the enzyme carbonic anhydrase in the nonpigmented ciliary epithelium responsible for catalyzing the following reaction: $CO_2 + H_2O \leftarrow$ carbonic anhydrase $\rightarrow H_2CO_3 \leftrightarrow H^+ + HCO_3^-$ The bicarbonate and sodium ions are actively transported into the anterior chamber, and there is passive movement of water. This mechanism produces 40-60% of aqueous humor. Compounds used include acetazolamide (5-8 mg/kg, PO, BID-TID), methazolamide (5 mg/kg, PO, BID-TID), and dichlorphenamide (2-4 mg/kg, PO, BID-TID). The effect peaks 3-6 hr after administration PO. The most common side effect is a metabolic acidosis, seen as panting. Other effects can include vomiting, diarrhea, and hypokalemia. Acetazolamide commonly causes anorexia; methazolamide is the drug of choice. Potassium supplementation can be given with potassium bicarbonate or citrate (1-2 g/day) added to the food.

DRUGS USED IN TREATMENT OF INFECTIOUS DISEASE

Feline Herpesvirus Keratitis and Conjunctivitis: Systemic antiviral drugs for the treatment of feline ocular herpesvirus are needed only in extreme circumstances when topical antiviral therapy is not effective. Acyclovir has been used at 200 mg, PO, BID-TID, although toxicity should be monitored. Oral L-lysine (250-500 mg/day) can prevent or reduce the severity of recurrent feline herpesvirus infections in cats by suppressing viral replication, but when used in vitro requires low arginine levels. L-Lysine can cause gastric upset. Recombinant human α-interferon 5-25 U/day, PO and topically, has also been recommended and may work by inhibiting replication of herpesvirus and stimulating lymphocytes for antiviral responses via enhanced macrophage activation and lymphocyte-mediated cytotoxicity.

Feline Chlamydial Conjunctivitis: Refractory feline conjunctivitis caused by *Chlamydophila* (*Chlamydia*) *psittaci* (p 406) that is nonresponsive to topical therapy can be treated with oral doxycycline (5-10 mg/kg, SID). All cats in the household should be treated for at least 4 wk, or for 2 wk after clinical signs have resolved. Systemic macrolides such as erythromycin (15-25 mg/kg, PO, BID, or 10-15 mg/kg, PO, TID) or azithromycin (5-10 mg/kg, PO, SID for 3-5 days) are also effective.

Feline Toxoplasmosis: Feline anterior uveitis with increasing *Toxoplasma gondii* titers as shown by serology and anterior chamber centesis may be treated with oral clindamycin at 8-17 mg/kg, PO, TID or 10-12.5 mg/kg, PO, BID for 2-4 wk, in association with topical corticosteroids (0.5-1% prednisolone acetate or 0.01% dexamethasone alcohol TID-QID). Systemic corticosteroids have been used (0.25 mg/kg divided doses daily) in conjunction with oral clindamycin and can improve therapeutic response. Side effects of clindamycin include anorexia, vomiting, and diarrhea, mainly at the higher doses. Other systemic antibiotics used include the synergistic combination of sulfonamides (sulfadiazine, sulfamethazine, sulfamerazine, 100 mg/kg, PO, SID) and pyrimethamine (2 mg/kg, PO, SID) for 1-2 wk. Side effects include bone marrow suppression. Frequent hematologic monitoring is recommended if therapy is to be >2 wk.

Feline and Canine Rickettsial Infection: Anterior and posterior uveitis and chorioretinitis secondary to infection with *Ehrlichia* or *Rickettsia* spp (*see* RICKETTSIAL DISEASES, p 638) is common. Tetracyclines are the drugs of choice and have excellent intraocular penetration. Doxycycline is given at 5-10 mg/kg, SID-BID for dogs and 10 mg/kg, BID for cats for 10-21 days. In cases of uveitis of unknown cause in dogs from a geographic area associated with rickettsial disease, animals may be empirically treated with doxycycline pending serology. The use of chloramphenicol is not recommended because this drug directly interferes with heme and bone marrow synthesis. Appropriate topical and systemic NSAID therapy is also recommended to control ocular inflammation. When the intraocular inflammation is severe or there is a serous retinal detachment, short-term (2-7 days) oral corticosteroids may be used concurrently 24-48 hr after the start of oral antibiotic therapy. Animals can regain vision following reattachment of the retina.

Canine and Feline Ocular Mycoses: Dogs and cats diagnosed with ocular mycoses require systemic treatment. Along with systemic antifungals, topical and systemic anti-inflammatories, and topical mydriatics and cycloplegics are needed to control the secondary and potentially blinding intraocular inflammation.

Blastomycosis (p 518) is more common in dogs than in cats. Up to 40% have ocular signs, usually anterior uveitis. Treatment options include parenteral amphotericin B deoxycholate or PO or IV triazoles. In dogs, itraconazole is used at 5 mg/kg, PO, BID for 5 days, after which the dose is reduced to 5 mg/kg, PO, SID. Treatment should continue for a minimum of 60 days or 1 mo after all clinical signs of the disease have resolved. Side effects include anorexia, which is associated with liver toxicity. Cats can be treated with 10 mg/kg, SID or 5 mg/kg, BID. Ketoconazole may also be used to treat blastomycosis, but because the onset of effect is so slow, other triazoles should be used initially. Amphotericin B deoxycholate is also effective but is nephrotoxic. The dosage is 0.5 mg/kg, IV, in dogs and 0.25 mg/kg, IV, in cats 3 times weekly until the animal becomes azotemic or until reaching a cumulative dose of 4-6 mg/kg in dogs or 4 mg/kg in cats. Amphotericin B lipid complex used at the same or a slightly higher dose is less nephrotoxic.

The predominant lesion of histoplasmosis (p 516) is granulomatous choroiditis. Treatment can be with itraconazole (10 mg/kg, PO, SID-BID) or fluconazole (2.5-5 mg/kg, PO, SID-BID) for 4-6 mo, or amphotericin B deoxycholate (0.25-0.5 mg/kg, IV, every 48 hr) until a cumulative dose of 5-10 mg/kg (dogs) or 4-8 mg/kg (cats) is reached. Because of its lipophilic nature and ability to cross the blood-ocular barriers, fluconazole is recommended for use in ocular disease, although animals have also had complete resolution when treated with the more hydrophilic itraconazole.

Ocular signs are present in 15% of cryptococcosis (p 514) cases and are more common in cats than in dogs. Treatment can be with amphotericin B deoxycholate (0.1-0.5 mg/kg, IV, 3 times/wk) alone or in combination with flucytosine (30-75 mg/kg, BID-QID for up to 9 mo). Ketoconazole, itraconazole, and fluconazole are also effective. Ketoconazole is administered PO at either 5-10 mg/kg, BID or 10-20 mg/kg, SID for 6-10 mo. If toxicity occurs, the dosage can be changed to 50 mg/kg/cat, PO, every other day. In dogs, dosages are either 5-15 mg/kg, PO, BID or 30 mg/kg, PO, SID, also for 6-10 mo. Systemic absorption from the GI tract is significantly enhanced by food. Side effects of ketoconazole include anorexia, diarrhea, vomiting, and elevated liver enzymes. Because of poor CNS penetration, ketoconazole is not recommended for use as the sole agent in ocular cryptococcosis. Itraconazole (cat, 5-10 mg/kg, PO, BID or 20 mg/kg, PO, SID) has fewer adverse effects than ketoconazole, and its GI tract bioavailability is also enhanced by food. Like ketoconazole, its hydrophilic nature leads to poor distribution into the CNS, but it has been successful in treating CNS and ocular cryptococcosis. Side effects are mainly associated with the GI tract (anorexia and vomiting), but liver disease can also develop. Liver enzymes (alanine aminotransferase) should be monitored regularly (every 2 wk) for the first month of treatment and monthly after that. Fluconazole is more lipophilic and has better bioavailability than itraconazole. It also penetrates the CNS better (60-80% of serum levels) and has fewer side effects than itraconazole. The dosage for cats and dogs is 5-15 mg/kg, PO, SID-BID for 6-10 mo.

Ocular coccidioidomycosis (p 513) is more common in dogs than in cats. Treatment is ketoconazole (dog, 15-20 mg/kg, PO, BID; cat, 15-20 mg/kg, PO, SID-BID) for 8-12 mo, although CNS and ocular penetration is poor. Amphotericin B deoxycholate can also be used (0.4-0.5 mg/kg, IV, every 48-72 hr) until the cumulative dose is 8-11 mg/kg.

Infectious Keratoconjunctivitis: Treatment of infectious keratoconjunctivitis (p 412) associated with *Moraxella bovis* in cattle is often systemic, involving oxytetracycline or florfenicol. Two doses of parenteral long-acting oxytetracycline (20 mg/kg, IM or SC) 48-72 hr apart is effective, although care should be taken using tetracyclines in endemic anaplasmosis areas. Florfenicol, at a single dose of 40 mg/kg, SC or 2 doses of 20 mg/kg, IM, 48 hr apart, is also effective. The organism is usually sensitive to trimethoprim-sulfonamide (15-30 mg/kg, IM or IV, SID-BID) but resistant to macrolides, lincosamides, and often penicillins.

Chlamydial keratoconjunctivitis in sheep and goats and nonchlamydial keratoconjunctivitis caused by *Mycoplasma* spp in goats can be treated with systemic antibiotics in addition to topical therapy. These include oxytetracycline (6-11 mg/kg, IV or IM), florfenicol (20 mg/kg, IM or SC), tylosin (10mg/kg, IM), erythromycin base (2.2-15 mg/kg, IM, SID-BID), or tilmicosin (10 mg/kg, IM). Most animals are treated with a single dose because of management issues involved in treating flock outbreaks.

Penetrating Trauma: All penetrating wounds of the eye should be considered infected, and animals should be treated aggressively with systemic broad-spectrum bactericidal antibiotics. For dogs and cats, oral amoxicillin-clavulanic acid (10-20 mg/kg, BID) is appropriate. When feasible, culture and sensitivity and cytology performed on anterior chamber centesis samples best guide appropriate antibiotic selection. Treatment should continue for a minimum of 14-21 days. In horses, the combination of systemic penicillin G procaine (22,000-44,000 U/kg, IM, BID) and gentamicin (6.6 mg/kg, IM or IV, SID) is an appropriate choice.

In all cases, intensive systemic NSAID (flunixin 0.5-1 mg/kg, IV or PO, SID-BID; ketoprofen 1.1-2.2 mg/kg, PO or IV, SID) are warranted to control the severe inflammation usually associated with these injuries. Because treatment duration in these cases extends beyond label recommendations of 5 days, an appropriate H$_2$-blocker (ranitidine, famotidine) or proton pump inhibitor (omeprazole) should be used prophylactically to prevent gastric ulceration. When the inflammation is also associated with leakage of lens material into the anterior chamber, the only treatment to control the inflammation is removal of the lens.

DRUGS USED IN TREATMENT OF INTRAOCULAR INFLAMMATION

Many infectious and noninfectious diseases cause intraocular inflammation. Unless it is controlled early, irreversible damage and blindness may result. Both topical and systemic corticosteroids and NSAID are used to control inflammation, depending on the cause. Care should be taken when using longterm treatment. Adrenocortical suppression develops and, following resolution of inflammation, animals need to be weaned off treatment slowly. In all species, control of noninfectious intraocular inflammation involves high initial doses of systemic corticosteroids (prednisone, 1-2 mg/kg) in combination with topical corticosteroids (0.5% or 1.0% prednisolone acetate or 0.1% dexamethasone alcohol), TID-QID. Some cases of infectious disease (eg, rickettsial infections) can be treated with low doses of systemic corticosteroids, but only after antibiotic therapy has been started for 24-48 hr. Topical steroids can be initiated at the same time as systemic antibiotic therapy. When the cause of intraocular inflammation is unknown, a combination of topical corticosteroids and systemic NSAID is also appropriate. Use of H$_2$-blockers or proton pump inhibitors should be considered when starting therapy; GI and renal parameters should be routinely monitored.

Canine Immune-mediated Disease: Nodular granulomatous episclerokeratitis (NGE) is often seen in Collies as a raised granulomatous lesion involving the episclera and third eyelid and infiltrating into the cornea. In addition to infectious anterior and posterior uveitis, immune-mediated uveitis (uveodermatologic syndrome) associated with an immune reaction to melanin is seen in a number of breeds, most commonly those of Arctic origin. Both are treated with either combined topical and oral corticosteroids (prednisone, 0.5-1 mg/kg, BID) or a lower corticosteroid dose in combination with oral azathioprine (1.5-2 mg/kg, SID, reducing the dose after 3-5 days). Some cases of NGE can be kept in remission with azathioprine, 1-2 mg/kg, PO, every 3-7 days for 1-8 mo. An alternative treatment for dogs >10 kg is administration PO of 500 mg niacinamide and 500 mg tetracycline, TID, decreasing to SID or BID once improvement is seen. Side effects of azathioprine include pancreatitis, liver disease, and bone marrow suppression. Frequent hematology and serum biochemistry monitoring is recommended.

Canine Optic Neuritis: Inflammation of the optic nerve is more common in dogs than in other species. Systemic corticosteroids (prednisone, 1-2 mg/kg, PO) for extended periods (often weeks) are used in an attempt to retain vision. Granulomatous encephalomyelitis is responsive to early treatment with systemic corticosteroids.

Damage to the optic nerve as a result of trauma is treated with systemic corticosteroids at similar dose rates as above.

Equine Uveitis: The principles of anti-inflammatory treatment for equine uveitis (p 407) are very similar regardless of the cause. In acute uveitis, systemic NSAID (flunixin meglumine, 0.25-1.0 mg/kg, IV or PO, BID) are used in conjunction with topical corticosteroids to control the intraocular inflammation. Phenylbutazone does not seem to be as effective in the initial treatment of equine uveitis. Horses are often treated with high doses of NSAID for longer than label recommendations (often 7-10 days); once the uveitis is controlled, the dose is slowly tapered down over 1-2 wk. Concurrent gastric protection with either an H$_2$-blocker (ranitidine, 6.6 mg/kg, PO, TID, or 1 mg/kg, IV, TID, or famotidine, 0.23-0.35 mg/kg, IV, BID-TID or 1.88-2.8 mg/kg, PO, BID-TID) or a proton pump inhibitor (omeprazole, 4 mg/kg, PO, SID) is recommended. Renal function should be monitored, and extreme care taken if the horse is also being treated with gentamicin. Oral aspirin (25 mg/kg/day) has been used longterm to prevent recurrence in horses diagnosed with equine recurrent uveitis.

Equine Optic Neuritis: Trauma to the equine poll is associated with overextension or shearing of the optic nerve within the optic canal secondary to movement of the brain in the skull. Treatment is systemic anti-inflammatory agents, usually NSAID at higher dose rates (flunixin meglumine, 0.5-1.1 mg/kg, IV or PO) and for longer than label recommendations. Prophylactic use of H$_2$-blockers or a proton pump inhibitor is recommended. In addition, dimethyl sufoxide (DMSO), 1 g/kg, IV as a 20% solution in saline or 5% dextrose in water given SID for 3 days, then every other day for 6 days, can be used. When given IV, DMSO can cause hemolysis and hemoglobinuria. No return of vision after 72 hr indicates a poor prognosis for vision restoration.

DRUGS USED IN TREATMENT OF MISCELLANEOUS FELINE CONDITIONS

Feline Eosinophilic Keratitis: Treatment with topical steroids usually is sufficient, but some cases do not respond. Oral megestrol acetate (0.5 mg/kg, SID until a response is noted, then 1.25 mg, PO, 2-3 times weekly as required) helps to improve or resolve the corneal inflammation via an unknown mechanism. However, its use is associated with side effects such as diabetes mellitus, adrenocortical suppression, and uterine hyperplasia, and it should be used with extreme caution. Megestrol acetate can also be dangerous to women handling the pills.

Feline Hypertensive Retinopathy: Older cats can present with sudden blindness due to serous retinal detachments secondary to systemic hypertension. Treatment is with the calcium channel blocker amlodipine (0.625 mg/cat) and systemic corticosteroids (prednisone, 0.5-1 mg/kg, PO) to help control the posterior inflammation. Retinas can reattach once blood pressure returns to the normal range. At least 50% of cats regain some clinical vision if treated early.

SYSTEMIC PHARMACOTHERAPEUTICS OF THE INTEGUMENTARY SYSTEM

See also PRINCIPLES OF TOPICAL THERAPY, THE INTEGUMENTARY SYSTEM, p 677.

Drugs that may be used in the integumentary system fall into several therapeutic categories—antimicrobials (antibacterials, antifungals), antiparasitics, NSAID, immunomodulators, hormones, psychotropic agents, and vitamin and mineral supplements.

Several factors may contribute to the development of the particular clinical presentation. Each factor should be identified and treated for therapy to succeed. For example, recurrent otitis may have a primary underlying skin disease but be complicated by both predisposing and perpetuating factors. Further, successful treatment of skin disease may require longterm or lifelong therapy and is frequently a matter of successful control rather than "cure."

ANTIBACTERIALS

Most canine skin infections are caused by coagulase-positive *Staphylococcus intermedius*, which commonly produce β-lactamase. Occasionally, *Proteus* spp, *Pseudomonas* spp, and *Escherichia coli* are secondary invaders of the dermis. *Pasteurella multocida* and β-hemolytic streptococci are the most common bacteria isolated from the epidermis of cats. Actinomycetes and mycobacteria are rare opportunistic invaders in dogs and cats. Bactericidal drugs expected to be effective against these bacteria should be used when treating the first occurrence of pyoderma in an animal (TABLE 10).

Bacterial skin disease in large animals may be caused by *Dermatophilus congolensis*, staphylococci, *Corynebacterium* spp, *Actinomyces*, and rarely *Bacillus* spp or *Pseudomonas* spp. Draining tracts or abscesses in the skin of sheep or goats may be caused by *Corynebacterium pseudotuberculosis*. *Fusobacterium* spp and *Bacteroides* spp are the primary invaders in interdigital necrobacillosis (footrot). The spirochete *Borrelia suilla* is a secondary invader of skin lesions caused by sarcoptic mange or ear biting in swine. Clostridial diseases in cattle and erysipelas in swine are disorders that involve the integumentary system and cause serious economic losses.

Numerous studies have investigated the sensitivity of *Staphylococcus intermedius* in dogs and failed to show any pattern of increasing resistance over time. Thus, if the exudative cytology shows the presence of an active infection with coccoid organisms, empirical antibiotic treatment should begin. In most clinics worldwide, canine isolates of *S intermedius* have excellent (>95%) sensitivity to oral cephalosporins, fluoroquinolones, antistaphylococcal penicillin (cloxacillin, oxacillin), and amoxicillin-clavulanate.

TABLE 10. Dosages of Antistaphylococcal Antibiotics

Drug	Dosage
Cephalosporins	
Cephalexin	20-30 mg/kg, BID
Cephadroxil	Dogs: 20 mg/kg, BID
	Cats: 20 mg/kg, SID
Cefaclor	10-25 mg/kg, BID
Penicillins	
Amoxicillin-clavulanate	13.75 mg/kg, BID
Oxacillin	22 mg/kg, TID
Fluoroquinolones	
Enrofloxacin	5 mg/kg, SID
Marbofloxacin	2 mg/kg, SID
Orbifloxacin	2.5 mg/kg, SID
Sulfonamides	
Trimethoprim-sulfadiazine	15-30 mg/kg, BID
Trimethoprim-sulfamethoxazole	15-30 mg/kg, BID
Macrolides and lincosamide	
Erythromycin	15-30 mg/kg, TID
Clindamycin	Dogs: 10-20 mg/kg, BID
	Cats: 12.5-25 mg/kg, BID
Lincomycin	10-20 mg/kg, BID

Erythromycin, lincomycin, clindamycin, and chloramphenicol have good (>75%) efficacy, while potentiated sulfonamides have shown variable efficacy.

Duration of therapy varies with the type of infection present. In general, superficial infections should be treated for 7 days beyond surface healing; deep infections should be treated 7-21 days beyond resolution, which may require treatment durations of 8-12 wk if continued improvement is seen. Culture and sensitivity testing should be done in all cases of refractory or recurrent pyodermas or if exudative cytology shows a mixed infection.

ANTIFUNGALS

The antifungal drugs used most commonly to treat integumentary diseases are listed in TABLE 11.

Griseofulvin: Griseofulvin has a very low solubility in water; GI absorption is variable and incomplete with the micronized form. Absorption may be enhanced by administration with a fat-containing meal or by formulations using polyethylene glycol or very small particles (micronization). The ultramicronized form is nearly 100% absorbed.

Griseofulvin is concentrated in skin (the highest concentration is in the stratum corneum), hair, nails, fat, skeletal muscle, and liver and can be found in the stratum corneum within 4 hr of dosing. It is also secreted in sweat and is deposited in keratinocytes and remains tightly bound during differentiation, so new skin growth is the first to be clear of infection. It is effective only against dermatophytes, eg, *Microsporum*, *Trichophyton*, and *Epidermophyton*.

In dogs, side effects (eg, vomiting, diarrhea) and elevated liver enzymes predominate. In cats, anemia, leukopenia, vomiting, diarrhea, depression, pruritus, fever, and ataxia have been described. Bone marrow suppression (usually manifest as neutropenia) may occur idiosyncratically, especially in FIV-positive cats and in kittens. FIV status should be determined before use and griseofulvin avoided in kittens <8 wk old. The reactions may also be more common and severe in Persian, Himalayan, Siamese, and Abyssinian cats. Teratogenicity is a major problem in all species.

Hemograms should be collected every 2 wk and close observation maintained. Leukopenia is more common in FIV-positive cats, so screening should be done before initiating treatment.

Ketoconazole: Ketoconazole is a synthetic, broad-spectrum antifungal drug belonging to the imidazole family. It is a potent inhibitor of ergosterol synthesis (a main membrane lipid of fungi). Fungal cells are thus unable to maintain the integrity of plasma membranes, which leads to cell wall rupture.

TABLE 11. Dosages of Antifungal Medications

Drug	Dosage
Griseofulvin	
Microsize	25-60 mg/kg, PO, BID
Ultramicrosize	2.5-15 mg/kg, PO, BID
Ketoconazole	10 mg/kg, PO, SID; 20 mg/kg, PO, every 48 hr
Itraconazole	5-10 mg/kg, PO, SID
Fluconazole	10-20 mg/kg, PO, BID
Amphotericin B	Dogs: 0.25-0.75 mg/kg, IV, 3 times/wk to total cumulative dose of 4-8 mg/kg or until azotemia develops Cats: 0.1-0.25 mg/kg, IV, 3 times/wk to cumulative dose of 4-6 mg/kg
Flucytosine	25-50 mg/kg, PO, TID-QID
Potassium iodine	Dogs: 40 mg/kg, PO, SID-BID with food Cats: 20 mg/kg, PO, SID-BID with food

Because the therapeutic effect of ketoconazole is delayed, amphotericin B is often used in combination for cases of serious systemic disease.

For dermatophytosis, ketoconazole is active against *Trichophyton verrucosum*, *T equinum*, *T mentagrophytes*, *Microsporum canis*, and *M nanum*. It is also active against the yeast *Malassezia pachydermatis* and *Cryptococcus neoformans* and is normally used at 10 mg/kg, PO, SID. For candidiasis, the dosage is 10 mg/kg for 6-8 wk. In some chronic cases, a maintenance dosage of 2.5-5 mg/kg can be used. Coccidioidomycosis responds better to ketoconazole than to amphotericin B in many instances, with a minimal treatment period of 12 mo in animals with disseminated disease. Blastomycosis, histoplasmosis, and cryptococcosis may be treated with a combination of ketoconazole and amphotericin B (the combination is not more effective than the latter alone, but there are fewer nephrotoxic signs). For blastomycosis, a 4-6 mg/kg total dose of amphotericin B is combined with ketoconazole (20 mg/kg, SID in dogs, and 10 mg/kg, SID in cats). For histoplasmosis, a 2-4 mg/kg total dose of amphotericin B is combined with ketoconazole (20 mg/kg, SID in dogs, and 10 mg/kg, SID in cats).

Ketoconazole inhibits cortisol synthesis and has been used to treat canine hyperadrenocorticism at 10 mg/kg, SID. If the cortisol level is still above resting levels after 10 days, the dosage may be increased to 15 mg/kg, SID.

Ketoconazole requires an acidic environment for optimal absorption, so H_2-blockers or antacids should not be concurrently administered.

In dogs, the most common side effects are inappetence, vomiting, pruritus, alopecia, and reversible lightening of the hair coat. Anorexia may be reduced by administering the dose with food. Cats appear to be more sensitive to ketoconazole. Clinical signs of toxicity include anorexia, fever, depression, diarrhea, and elevated liver enzymes. Dosages >10 mg/kg/day are rarely given. Hepatotoxicity (cholangiohepatitis and elevated liver enzymes) has also been reported.

Itraconazole: The primary antifungal mechanism of action of itraconazole seems to be the same as that of ketoconazole; however, it has a greater potency, decreased toxicity, and a wider spectrum of activity. Even at high dosages, it does not alter hormone levels in rats, dogs, or humans. Itraconazole should be administered with food; the concurrent administration of antacids, H_2-blockers, and cholinergics is contraindicated.

Itraconazole is effective against dermatophytes, *Candida*, *Cryptococcus*, *Histoplasma*, *Blastomyces*, and *Sporotrichum* spp, and the protozoans *Leishmania* and *Trypanosoma*. For dermatophytosis in dogs, the dosage is 5 mg/kg, SID. For systemic mycoses, the dosage is 5-10 mg/kg, SID, but the addition of amphotericin should be considered in rapidly progressing infections. For treatment of dermatophytosis and systemic mycoses in cats, the dosage is 10 mg/kg, SID.

A severe, dose-related ulcerative dermatitis (due to vasculitis) has been seen in 5-10% of dogs given 10 mg/kg doses of itraconazole. If the condition is identified early, drug withdrawal leads to resolution; if not recognized early, severe, extensive necrosis and sloughing can develop.

Fluconazole: Fluconazole is a fungistatic triazole compound with a mode of action similar to that of ketoconazole. However, it does not affect mammalian hormone synthesis. Because of its small molecular size and low lipophilicity, it may be more useful in treating CNS mycoses.

Fluconazole is effective against superficial dermatophytes and *Candida*, *Cryptococcus*, *Histoplasma*, and *Blastomyces* spp. The dosage is 2.5-10 mg/kg, SID in dogs. Cats with cryptococcosis can be given 2.5-10 mg/kg, BID.

Fluconazole has had limited use in small animals. In humans, it can cause occasional GI effects (eg, vomiting, diarrhea, anorexia, nausea).

Amphotericin B: Amphotericin is a lipophilic polyene from *Streptomyces nodosus* that binds to sterols (especially ergosterol), causing increased permeability and leakage of nutrients and electrolytes. It is poorly absorbed from the GI tract and must be given parenterally. IV administration gives good penetration, except into muscle, bone, eye, or synovial fluid.

Amphotericin B is used in progressive or disseminated deep mycosis. It may be combined with flucytosine or minocycline for treatment of *Candida* and *Cryptococcus*. Rifampin potentiates the effect of amphotericin on *Aspergillus* (which is usually resistant against amphotericin alone), *Candida*, and *Histoplasma*.

Amphotericin B is insoluble in water and is prepared as an IV solution by forming a colloidal dispersion with sodium deoxycholate. Because it is inactivated by sunlight, it should be stored in the dark. Dilution with large volumes of 5% glucose (10 mg amphotericin B/100 mL fluid) is recommended to reduce nephrotoxicity. The dilution should be given over 2-6 hr. If a bolus is given in 10-60 mL of dextrose (via a butterfly catheter), supplemental fluid diuresis is helpful. Amphotericin B is given at 0.15-0.5 mg/kg every 48 hr until a total cumulative dose of 4-12 mg/kg is reached. Renal toxic effects are monitored by electrolytes or urinalysis at least weekly (urinalysis detects toxicity earlier than biochemistry); BUN, creatinine, PCV, and total plasma proteins should be checked before the administration of each dose. Monthly maintenance therapy is recommended to avoid relapses.

The major adverse effect seen with amphotericin B is nephrotoxicity—most dogs incur some kidney damage. The damage is not correlated with either total dose or duration of therapy. The causes of toxicity include vasoconstriction, impaired acid excretion, and direct tubular injury. Cats are more sensitive, so lower doses are recommended. Side effects such as fever, nausea, and vomiting are less severe if diphenhydramine (0.5 mg/kg, IV), aspirin (10 mg/kg, PO), or hydrocortisone sodium succinate (0.5 mg/kg, IV) is given prior to administration of amphotericin B.

Flucytosine: This fluorinated pyrimidine was developed as an antineoplastic agent. It interferes with RNA metabolism and protein sythesis in fungal cells. It is well absorbed and enters the CNS in high concentrations. Most of the drug is excreted unchanged in the urine.

Flucytosine is effective against *Cryptococcus neoformans*, *Candida*, and other yeasts but has little or no effect on other fungi. Resistance develops frequently, thus it is given in combination with amphotericin B. It is used almost exclusively for treatment of cryptococcosis. The dosage in dogs and cats is 25-50 mg/kg, TID-QID.

GI tract disturbances (vomiting, diarrhea, anorexia), bone marrow suppression (anemia, leukopenia, thrombocytopenia), and cutaneous eruption (depigmentation, ulceration, exudation, and crust formation) are the most common adverse effects.

Terbinafine: Terbinafine is an allylamine compound that interferes with fungal sterol biosynthesis at an early stage, causing deficiency of ergosterol, intracellular accumulation of squalene, and fungal cell death. It achieves high concentrations in hair follicles, hair, sebum-rich skin, nail plates and nails. In humans, levels exceeding the minimum inhibitory concentration may be found for up to 3 wk after treatment has ended. There are anecdotal reports of its use against *Trichophyton*, *Microsporum*, and *Epidermophyton*. The dosage in cats is 10-30 mg/kg, SID. In humans, rare cases of hepatic toxicity are seen, along with GI tract signs (eg, nausea, vomiting, diarrhea) and skin signs (eg, urticaria, itch, erythema).

Systemic Iodine: The mechanism of action of systemic iodine is unknown; no fungicidal effects are seen in vitro. It is used in small animals for sporotrichosis; in cattle for actinomycosis and actinobacillosis; and in horses for mycetomas, zygomycosis, and *Sporotrichum schenckii*. Dogs are treated with potassium iodide 40 mg/kg, PO, BID; cats with potassium iodide 20 mg/kg, PO, SID-BID; cattle with sodium iodide 60 mg/kg, IV, weekly; and horses (sporotrichosis) with sodium iodide, 40 mg/kg, IV, SID for 2-5 days, followed by potassium iodide, 2 mg/kg, PO, SID for 60 days.

In small animals, vomiting, diarrhea, depression, and inappetence (cats especially) may develop. Ocular and nasal discharge, scaling, and a dry hair coat also may be seen in dogs. In large animals, seromucoid discharge, lacrimation, cough, variable appetite, joint pain, and seborrhea sicca with partial alopecia may develop. Systemic iodine may also cause abortion and should not be used in pregnant or lactating animals.

ANTIPARASITICS

Ivermectin: Ivermectin is an avermectin and a fermentation product of *Streptomyces avermitilis* (*see also* MACROCYCLIC LACTONES, p 2115). It acts as a GABA agonist, causing paralysis in susceptible arthropods and nematodes. It is used in small animals for treatment of *Sarcoptes scabeii, Otodectes cynotis, Cheyletiella blakei, C yasguri*, and *Demodex canis*; in cattle for psoroptic mange, lice, and *Hypoderma* larvae; in horses for equine filarial dermatitis from *Onchocerca cervicalis*; and in swine for *Sarcoptes scabeii*.

In small animals, all use for skin conditions is extra-label in the USA. For *Demodex*, the dosage is 0.3-0.6 mg/kg, PO, SID until 2 negative skin scrapings 1 mo apart. For *Sarcoptes, Otodectes*, and *Cheyletiella*, the dosage is 0.3 mg/kg, PO, repeated in 2 wk. In cattle, 0.2 mg/kg is given as a single SC injection for *Psoroptes* and lice. In horses, 0.2 mg/kg, PO, kills microfilariae but not adult *Onchocerca cervicalis*, so relapse may be noted within 2 mo of treatment. In swine, the dosage is 0.3 mg/kg, SC, repeated in 2 wk, or 0.1-0.2 mg/kg in feed for 7 days.

In mammals, GABA is found only in the CNS and does not readily cross the blood-brain barrier. At least 10 times the normal dose of ivermectin is needed for toxic reactions. Ataxia, depression, and visual impairment develop in horses given 2 mg/kg, PO. In cattle, 4 mg/kg by drench or 8 mg/kg, SC, leads to listlessness and ataxia; 30 mg/kg induces ataxia in swine.

Some dog breeds (Collies, Shetland Sheepdogs, Old English Sheepdogs, Australian Collies, and their crosses) seem to have greater penetration of ivermectin through the blood-brain barrier. The critical point seems to be 120-150 µg/kg, at which transient, nonfatal clinical signs (mydriasis, ataxia, tremors) are seen. At higher doses, collapse, coma, and respiratory collapse may develop. Similar idiosyncratic reactions may develop in any breed, so a gradually increasing dose (daily progression of 50, 100, 150, 200, then 300 µg/kg) should be given to identify susceptible individuals. Administration should be stopped if any side effects are seen. One cat treated with 4 mg of the oral paste (~70 µg/kg) showed ataxia, blindness, tremors, and mydriasis, with retinal atrophy in one eye 10 hr later.

Milbemycin: Milbemycin is derived from fermentation products or *Streptomyces hygroscopicus* and, like ivermectin, acts as a GABA agonist but with a wider spectrum of activity against intestinal parasites. It has been used extra-label in dogs to treat nasal mites, scabies, and generalized demodicosis. No adverse effects have been seen in ivermectin-sensitive breeds. The dosage in dogs is 1-2 mg/kg every 7 days for 3-5 treatments for nasal mites and scabies and 1-2 mg/kg, SID for *Demodex*.

Moxidectin: Moxidectin belongs to the milbemycin class of compounds. It is registered for heartworm control (*Dirofilaria immitis*) but has also been used extra-label for treatment of *Otodectes* and demodicosis in dogs. In cattle, it is used to treat lice (*Linognathus vituli, Solenopotes capillatus, Bovicola bovis*), mites (*Psoroptes, Chorioptes bovis*), ticks (*Boophilus microplus*), and fly warbles and grubs (*Hypoderma bovis, H lineatum*). In sheep, it is used for *Psorergates ovis* infestation. The dosage is 0.2-0.4 mg/kg, PO, SID in dogs and 0.2 mg/kg in cattle and sheep.

Selamectin: This novel semisynthetic macrocyclic lactone is applied topically, but acts systemically. It is effective against *Ctenocephalides* spp (both adults and larvae), *Sarcoptes scabeii, Otodectes cynotis*, and *Dermacentor variabilis*. The dosage in dogs and cats is 6 mg/kg, applied topically.

Lufenuron: Lufenuron is an insect growth regulator that inhibits the synthesis of chitin—a critical component of insect exoskeletons. It is taken up by adult fleas while feeding. While it has no effect on adult fleas, it prevents development of the intermediate stages of the flea life cycle (ie, eggs, larvae, pupae). It is effective against *Ctenocephalides* spp in dogs and cats at a dosage of 10 mg/kg, PO, once a month. Chitin is also a component in the fungal cell wall of dermatophytes, and an initial study showed efficacy of lufenuron in treating small animal dermatophytosis. Additional studies have not confirmed this result.

Nitenpyram: Nitenpyram inhibits the nicotinic acetylcholine receptor. It is used to treat *Ctenocephalides* spp in dogs and cats at a dosage of 1 mg/kg, PO. Nitenpyram has a short half-life and kills fleas on the animal within 30 min of administration. It is toxic to fleas for only 24-48 hr and is normally used in combination with an insect growth regulator to provide continuous flea control.

Cythioate: Cythioate is an organophosphate that kills via anticholinesterase activity. It is indicated for *Ctenocephalides* spp infestations at a dosage of 3 mg/kg, PO, twice weekly (dogs) or 1.5 mg/kg, PO, twice weekly (cats). Although effective blood levels are maintained for <12 hr, serum cholinesterase activity may be decreased for >1 mo after dosing.

ANTIHISTAMINES

Antihistamines block either H_1 or H_2 receptors. H_1 receptors are responsible for pruritus, increased vascular permeability, release of inflammatory mediators, and attraction of inflammatory cells. H_1 blockers act by competing with histamine for H_1-receptor sites on effector cells (they do not block release of histamine but can antagonize its effects). They also have anticholinergic, sedative, and local anesthetic effects and vary greatly in their potency, dosage, incidence of side effects, and cost.

Second-generation H_1 blockers (eg, terfenadine, cetirazine, loratadine, astemazole) are less likely to cross the blood-brain barrier, or they have a low affinity for brain compared with peripheral H_1 receptors. They have not proved useful to date in controlling pruritus in small animals. Responses to antihistamines vary considerably, and several may need to be tried to find one that is effective for an animal (TABLE 12). Antihistamines may act synergistically with NSAID, glucocorticoids, or fatty acid supplements and may allow dosages of these agents to be reduced in some cases.

First-generation antihistamines may cause drowsiness or GI signs (eg, vomiting, diarrhea). Overdoses may cause CNS hyperexcitability and may be fatal. Anticholinergic properties lead to hypertension (thus they are contraindicated in cardiac patients), dry mouth, blurred vision (they are contraindicated in glaucoma), and urinary retention. Hydroxyzine is teratogenic. They may also stimulate appetite (particularly cyproheptadine).

Second-generation antihistamines are cardiotoxic at high doses. High doses of terfenadine and astemizole lead to prolonged QT intervals and arrhythmias (eg, ventricular tachycardia, cardiac arrest). Cardiotoxicity has been reported only as a result of overdose in animals with impaired hepatic metabolism.

ESSENTIAL FATTY ACIDS

Fatty acids are essential components of cell membranes and are an integral component of the intercellular barrier in the stratum corneum. Essential fatty acids cannot be synthesized and therefore must be supplied in the diet. The essential fatty acids most

Drug	**Dosage**
Diphenhydramine	2-4 mg/kg, BID-TID
Hydroxyzine	0.5-2 mg/kg, TID-QID
Clorpheniramine	Cats: 2-4 mg, BID Dogs (<20 kg): 4 mg, TID Dogs (>20 kg): 8 mg, TID; 0.25-0.5 mg/kg, TID
Cyproheptadine	0.25-0.5 mg/kg, TID; 1.1 mg/kg, BID
Terfenadine	5 mg/kg, BID
Clemastine	Cats: 0.05 mg/kg, BID Dogs: 0.1 mg/kg, BID
Trimeprazine	1 mg/kg, BID

TABLE 12. Antihistamine Dosages

important for homeostasis of the skin in dogs and cats are linoleic acid and linolenic acid. The anti-inflammatory properties of fatty acids are thought to be due both to competitive inhibition of arachidonic acid metabolism, leading to a reduction in inflammatory leukotriene and prostaglandin sythesis and activity, and to the formation of metabolic byproducts of normal fatty acid metabolism that have direct anti-inflammatory properties.

Essential fatty acids are indicated for pruritic inflammatory diseases (eg, allergies, feline eosinophilic granuloma), crusting diseases (eg, discoid lupus erythematosus), and onychodystrophy. Many commercial products are available and may be used at the manufacturer's recommended dose. Failure to respond to one product does not preclude response to another, and increasing the dose to several times the label recommendation can help in some cases. Approximately 20% of dogs and 50% of cats with allergic pruritus will show some improvement. There are few side effects; however, pancreatitis has been rarely reported. Large doses may also cause weight gain or diarrhea.

HORMONAL THERAPY

Glucocorticoids: Glucocorticoids have profound effects on nearly all cell types and organ systems, particularly immunologic and inflammatory activity. They may be used in either an anti-inflammatory or immunosuppressive capacity, depending on the dosage selected. Glucocorticoids are used for hypersensitivity dermatoses, contact dermatitis, immune-mediated diseases (eg, pemphigus, pemphigoid, lupus erythematosus), and neoplasia (eg, mast cell tumor, lymphoma). Glucocorticoids may be classified according to their duration of effect and relative potency (TABLE 13). They may be administered PO, IV, IM, or SC. The anti-inflammatory dosage of prednisolone is 0.5-1.0 mg/kg, SID in dogs (severe cases may require 2 mg/kg, SID) and 1-2 mg/kg, SID in cats.

This dosage is given for an induction period of 5-7 days and then reduced to the lowest possible maintenance dose (ideally 0.25 mg/kg, every 48-72 hr or lower in dogs). Maintenance doses must be given ≥48 hr apart to minimize adrenal suppression and chronic side effects. The immunosuppressive dosage of prednisolone is 2.2 mg/kg, SID in dogs (up to 6.6 mg/kg, SID, may be required in severe disease) and 4.4 mg/kg, SID in cats.

The induction period is generally longer (10-20 days) than with anti-inflammatory dosing, but is then gradually tapered in a stepwise fashion to an alternate-day dosing regimen once there is evidence of disease remission. Treatment should never be stopped abruptly, as there is a risk of inducing signs of hypoadrenocorticism. If relapse occurs during the tapering process, the dose is increased to at least 1 step above the point at which the relapse occurred and tapered again if possible. In many cases, therapy may be withdrawn entirely without relapse, while others require lifelong treatment.

Administration PO is preferred because dosing can be more closely regulated and physiologic processes are disrupted less than with reposital forms. In some cases, difficulties with animal handling or owner adherence may require injectable therapy. This is normally satisfactory for acute, short-term disease that does not require repeated

TABLE 13. Glucocorticoids

Drug	Relative Potency	Duration of Effect
Hydrocortisone (cortisol)	1	<12 hr
Prednisolone	4	12-36 hr
Prednisone	4	12-36 hr
Methylprednisolone	5	12-36 hr
Triamcinolone	5	12-36 hr
Flumethasone	15-30	36-48 hr
Betamethasone	25	>48 hr
Dexamethasone	30	>48 hr

administration (eg, a single injection of methylprednisolone acetate alters adrenocortical function in dogs for up to 10 wk).

Side effects include polyuria, polydipsia, polyphagia, weight gain, increased susceptibility to infection, GI ulceration, pancreatitis, osteoporosis, hyperglycemia, steroid myopathy, and calcinosis cutis. The extent and severity of side effects are related to the dose, duration, and type of glucocorticoid used, along with individual animal sensitivity. The most commonly encountered infections are urinary tract infections, pyoderma, and pulmonary infections. Urinary tract infections may develop in many animals on longterm glucocorticoid therapy (68% in one study), and these animals may show no clinical signs of the infection. Urine should be cultured for bacterial growth every 3-6 mo in all animals on longterm therapy.

Progressive hepatocellular swelling due to glycogen accumulation may develop during glucocorticoid therapy. Alkaline phosphatase (ALP), ALT, and γ-glutamyl transferase all show progressive increases. In dogs, the initial ALP increase is due to hepatic ALP but later is due to a cortisone isoenzyme.

Most injectable forms are labeled for IM use; however, they are commonly given SC. Local areas of alopecia, pigmentation, and epidermal and dermal atrophy may be seen with SC injection.

Thyroid Hormone: Thyroid hormones are indicated as replacement therapy for primary, secondary, and tertiary hypothyroidism. Most cases of canine hypothyroidism are primary in nature and are due to autoimmune destruction of the thyroid gland. Drug-induced low hormone levels or "euthyroid sick syndrome" are not indications for supplementation with thyroid hormones.

Synthetic levothyroxine (T_4) is the drug of choice for canine hypothyroidism. Most dogs respond clinically to a dosage of 0.02 mg/kg, BID. Insufficient serum levels after 4-6 wk of treatment or lack of a clinical response after 12 wk are indications for increasing the dose. Synthetic liothyronine (T_3) may be used for those rare animals that cannot convert T_4 to T_3. It should not be used for routine treatment of hypothyroidism because it bypasses the normal cellular regulatory pathways and has a short half-life. Dosage is 4-6 µg/kg, PO, BID-TID. Crude preparations from thyroid tissue and synthetic thyroid hormone combinations that mimic the T_4:T_3 ratio in humans should not be used in animals.

Signs of thyrotoxicosis in cats and dogs are rare. They include polyuria, polydipsia, nervousness, aggressiveness, panting, diarrhea, tachycardia, pyrexia, and pruritus. Complications in dogs are usually related to concurrent cardiac or adrenal insufficiencies. In animals with a marginal cardiac reserve, T_4 medication should be initiated at one-fourth the recommended dosage and gradually increased to full dosage over a 1-mo period.

Progesterones: The 2 most commonly used forms of progesterone are megestrol acetate and medroxyprogesterone acetate. Megestrol acetate has a quick onset of action, potent glucocorticoid and slight mineralocorticoid activity, and may be given PO. Medroxyprogesterone acetate is antiestrogenic and has significant glucocorticoid activity. Neutered male and female cats with bilateral alopecia suspected to be caused by sex hormone imbalances may respond to treatment. The dosage of megestrol acetate is 2.5-5.0 mg/cat, PO, every 48 hr, decreasing to every 1-2 wk for maintenance. Medroxyprogesterone acetate is given at a dosage of 50-100 mg/cat, IM, and may be repeated in 3-6 mo.

Progestagens should be avoided whenever possible because of side effects; severe, prolonged adrenocortical suppression is seen even with low doses. Diabetes mellitus has been reported in cats treated with megestrol acetate. Decreased spermatogenesis, pyometra, increased levels of growth hormone with acromegaly, mammary gland hyperplasia and tumors, and behavioral changes may be seen.

Growth Hormone: Growth hormone (somatotropin) is a polypeptide produced by the anterior pituitary that acts either directly on target tissues or indirectly through insulin-like growth factors (somatomedins) produced by the liver (*see also* THE PITUITARY GLAND, p 451). It is necessary for hair growth and for development of elastin fibers in the skin. It is used to treat growth hormone-responsive alopecia in dogs. Either bovine, porcine, or human growth hormone (0.1 IU/kg, 3 times/wk for 4-6 wk) is effective. Hair usually regrows in 2-3 mo, and remission may last from 6 mo to 3 yr. Growth hormone is diabetogenic, and dogs can develop transient or permanent diabetes mellitus during therapy. Weekly monitoring of blood glucose before and during therapy is recommended.

Sex Hormones: Several clinical syndromes in dogs and cats have been attributed to imbalances of sex hormones; however, the etiopathogenesis of these disorders is generally poorly documented. Hypoestrogenism in spayed female dogs, hypoandrogenism in male dogs, and feline acquired symmetric alopecia may respond to sex-hormone therapy. Dosages for sex-hormone replacement therapy are empirical. Hypoestrogenism in spayed female dogs may be treated with diethylstilbestrol (0.02 mg/kg, SID for 3 wk of every month until hair regrows or for a maximum total dose of 1.0 mg/dog). After hair regrows, the maintenance dosage should be given 1-2 times /wk. An alternative protocol is to treat every other day or twice weekly until a clinical response is seen. Hair regrowth should be evident in 3-4 wk, with a complete response within 4 mo. Exogenous estrogen can cause bone marrow hypoplasia, so a CBC and platelet count should be performed weekly during therapy. Other potential side effects include induction of estrus, hepatotoxicity, nymphomania, abortion, pyometra, or prostatic hyperplasia. Cats are highly sensitive to estrogens, and a total dose of 10 mg of diethylstilbestrol can be lethal.

Hypoandrogenism of male dogs may be treated with methyltestosterone, 0.5-1.0 mg/kg, PO, up to a total maximal dose of 30 mg every 48 hr. Alternatively, testosterone proprionate can be given IM once weekly at dosages of 0.5-1.0 mg/kg, or every 4-16 wk at 2 mg/kg. Complications include aggressive behavior, greasy hair coat, prostatic hypertrophy, and hepatotoxicity. Liver function should be evaluated before treatment and monthly during therapy.

Repositol testosterone, 12 mg/cat, IM, may be given once for treatment of feline acquired symmetric alopecia or may be combined with a low dose of diethylstilbestrol, 0.625 mg/cat, IM, or with a low dose of estradiol, 0.5 mg/cat, IM. Hepatobiliary disease has also been reported in cats given testosterone.

Melatonin: Melatonin is produced in the pineal gland and is involved in the control of photoperiod-dependent molting of some mammals. Secretion is inversely related to daylight length and is highest during the winter. Various canine hair-growth disorders including recurrent flank alopecia, pattern baldness, and excessive tricholemmal keratinization have improved with melatonin supplementation. Recurrent flank alopecia may be treated with 36 mg SC implants. Oral melatonin is also available; an empirical dosage of 3-6 mg/dog, TID-QID, has been used successfully.

IMMUNOMODULATORS

Immunostimulants

Immunostimulation is used to enhance a deficient immunologic response; however, animals that appear to benefit from these agents are not severely immunosuppressed. The most common use of immunostimulants in dogs is for chronic, recurrent staphylococcal pyoderma. For primary therapy, immunomodulatory bacterins should not be substituted for antibiotics; they should be used concurrently with an appropriate antibiotic until the infection has been resolved. The immunomodulator is then continued and success judged on the time to and severity of any infection relapse. They are clearly helpful as adjunct agents or for maintenance therapy for some dogs with recurrent pyoderma but have no benefit in other cases.

Staphage lysate is a preparation of *Staphylococcus aureus* and polyvalent staphylococcus bacteriophage. When given concurrently with antibiotics, staphage lysate (0.5 mL, SC, twice weekly, or 1.0 mL, SC, weekly) has improved the response of dogs with superficial staphylococcal pyoderma compared with antibiotics alone. The mechanism of action is believed to be stimulation of T lymphocytes and activation of phagocytic cells. Deficient IgM levels—but not IgA or IgG levels—may be normalized with treatment.

S aureus bacterin-toxoid, used for prevention of staphylococcal mastitis in cattle, has been used with some success in cases of canine bacterial hypersensitivity. Various treatment protocols have been advocated. One schedule consists of 0.1 mL, intradermally,

SID for 5 days, then weekly for 1 mo, then at monthly intervals. At corresponding times, doses given SC increase from 0.15 mL to 1.9 mL. Local swelling at the injection site, fever, and malaise are common side effects in dogs.

Propionibacterium acnes bacterin is labeled for use in dogs (0.25-2.0 mL, IV, 1-2 times/wk) and appears to have some benefit as adjunct treatment for recurrent pyoderma.

Many other immunostimulants have been described for use; however, responses in dermatologic disorders have been equivocal.

Immunosuppressants

Glucocorticoids: Glucocorticoids are the immunosuppressive agents most commonly used to treat immune-mediated skin disease (p 653). A range of other immunosuppressants may be used either concurrently with glucocorticoids or alone for the treatment of various immune-mediated dermatoses, including systemic lupus erythematosus (SLE), pemphigus complex, bullous pemphigoid, and vasculitis.

Azathioprine: Azathioprine is converted to 6-mercaptopurine in the liver. It competes with purines in the synthesis of nucleic acids and prevents proliferation of rapidly dividing cells. It is used for treatment of pemphigus disorders, bullous pemphigoid and SLE in dogs, ocular inflammation in the uveodermatologic syndrome, and histiocytomas. There is a 3- to 5-wk lag period before its effects are evident, so it is often initially combined with glucocorticoids. The dosage is 2.2 mg/kg (50 mg/m^2), SID until there is a clinical response, then it is reduced to every 48 hr. In dogs, it may be used in combination with metronidazole (10 mg/kg, SID) for perianal furunculosis, although surgery may be necessary to remove residual scarring.

GI side effects (vomiting, diarrhea) may be avoided by administering with food or lowering the dose. Bone marrow suppression may also develop. All 3 cell lines can be affected, but leukopenia is the most common. CBC should be monitored every 2 wk during induction and at least every 4 mo during maintenance therapy. Acute pancreatitis and hepatotoxicity has been reported in dogs. Azathioprine is contraindicated in cats, due to rapid, lethal bone marrow suppression.

Cyclophosphamide: Cyclophosphamide is an alkylating agent used to treat a wide variety of cancers, especially lymphoreticular neoplasms, and is usually given in combination with other drugs. It may also be used short-term in severe cases of SLE, rheumatoid arthritis, pemphigus complex, and vasculitis. The dosage for immunosuppression is 1.5-2.5 mg/kg, every 48 hr. The dose should be given in the morning so that it does not remain in the bladder overnight. Because most animals treated with cyclophosphamide are also receiving corticosteroids, polyuria induced by the steroids may be somewhat protective. The potential for hemorrhagic cystitis and bladder fibrosis limits the use of cyclophosphamide to no more than 3-4 mo. GI tract toxicity, bone marrow suppression, alopecia, infertility, and teratogenic effects may also be seen.

Chlorambucil: Chlorambucil is an alkylating agent similar to cyclophosphamide. However, it is slower acting and the least toxic of the group. It may be used for treatment of immune complex diseases in which azathioprine or cyclophosphamide are not tolerated and may be given to cats. The dosage is 0.1-0.2 mg/kg, SID, reduced to every 48 hr once a clinical response is seen. It is mostly used in combination with glucocorticoids but can be used with azathioprine (dogs only) in particularly refractive cases. It may also be used to replace cyclophosphamide if hemorrhagic cystitis develops. Adverse effects are rare and include bone marrow suppression, which generally develops within 7-14 days of starting treatment and resolves in 7-14 days, GI irritation, and seizures. Delayed hair regrowth has been reported in shaved dogs.

Crysotherapy: Gold salts have anti-inflammatory, antirheumatic, immunomodulating, and antimicrobial (in vitro) effects. Two forms are available—parenteral and oral. Aurothioglucose is given parenterally. It is absorbed rapidly and reaches peak levels in 4-6 hr. Rising serum values are noted for 5-10 wk. Beneficial effects are seen 6-12 wk after the start of treatment. The oral form is auranofin. Only 25% is absorbed, and lower and more predictable plasma concentrations are found. The half-life is ~21 days, but the retention and tissue accumulation are only 1% (parenteral gold 30%). Results with this compound are equivocal in dogs. Gold salts are indicated for canine and feline pemphigus unresponsive to glucocorticoids and feline plasma cell pododermatitis.

Routine protocols start with a test dose IM (1 mg if <10 kg, 5 mg if >10 kg body wt). The next week a second test dose is given IM (2 or 10 mg), and if no adverse reactions are seen treatment continues at 1 mg/kg, IM, weekly until remission. Once in remission, the dose is given every 2 wk and may later be reduced to monthly injections. Occasionally, a higher dosage (1.5-2.0 mg/kg) may be required to induce remission. Treatment effects are not seen for 6-12 wk, so other medications (commonly glucocorticoids) must be given at therapeutic doses during this time. Gold salts should not be administered with other cytotoxic drugs as there is an increased risk of toxic reactions. Adverse effects include allergic reactions (skin eruption, oral reactions), nephrotoxicity, and bone marrow suppression. Toxic epidermal necrolysis has been reported in dogs starting gold therapy immediately after azathioprine, so a 4-wk washout period is recommended in these cases.

Cyclosporine: Cyclosporine impairs the proliferation of activated T cells by inhibiting transcription of interleukin-2, gene activation, and RNA transcription. This early inhibition of T cells also leads to reduced production of other cytokines, mast cells, and eosinophils, and inhibition of mononuclear cells, antigen presentation, histamine release from mast cells, neutrophil adherence, natural killer cell activity, and B cell growth and differentiation. Cyclosporine is used for treatment of atopic dermatitis and anal furunculosis. Extra-label use for the treatment of immune-mediated disorders (pemphigus, SLE) and epitheliotropic lymphoma has been less successful. Response has been good when used for sebaceous adenitis. The dosage for atopic dermatitis is 5 mg/kg, SID. This may be reduced to alternate-day or even third-day dosing in some individuals. The dosage for anal furunculosis is 7.5 mg/kg, SID.

Adverse effects include GI signs (nausea, vomiting, soft stools, diarrhea), gingival hypertrophy, hirsutism, and papillomatosis (which generally decreases when the dose is decreased). Drugs that inhibit cytochrome P450 (eg, ketoconazole) potentiate cyclosporine toxicity significantly. If ketoconazole (10 mg/kg, BID) is administered in addition to animals with anal furunculosis, the dosage of cyclosporine can be reduced to 1 mg/kg, BID. This induction dose is maintained for 4 wk and then reduced if clinical response is adequate or side effects (vomiting, lethargy) develop.

Sulfones: Dapsone is an anti-inflammatory, antibacterial sulfone that inhibits neutrophil chemotaxis and adhesion to basement membrane zone antibodies, degranulation of mast cells, action of lysosomal enzymes, and activation of the alternative complement pathway. Dapsone also inhibits synthesis of IgG, IgA, and prostaglandins, as well as T-cell responses. Although it is used for a variety of diseases characterized by accumulation of neutrophils in humans, the results are more equivocal in dogs. However, it has been used for pemphigus foliaceus and erythematosus, subcorneal pustular dermatosis, leukocytoclastic vasculitis, and IgA dermatosis. The dosage is 1 mg/kg, TID (dogs only) for 2-4 wk or until a clinical response is seen, then every 24-48 hr. Longterm therapy is not recommended. Mild anemia or severe leukopenia, blood dyscrasias, hepatotoxicity, or skin reactions may develop. Animals should be monitored by CBC, urinalysis, BUN, and ALT every 2 wk during induction. Cats are particularly sensitive to toxicity, and a dosage of 1 mg/kg, SID is recommended. Concurrent use may allow the dosage of glucocorticoids to be reduced.

Tetracycline and Niacinamide: Although the precise mechanism of action is unknown, tetracyclines may inhibit in vitro lymphocyte blastogenic transformation and antibody production, activation of complement (component C3), prostaglandin synthesis, lipases and collagenases, and suppress leukocyte chemotaxis in vitro and in vivo. Niacinamide blocks IgE-induced histamine release, inhibits phosphodiesterases, and decreases protease release by leukocytes. The combination is indicated for discoid lupus erythematosus and pemphigus erythematosus. These diseases are characterized by leukocyte chemotaxis secondary to complement activation by antigen-antibody complexes and by release of proteases. Dogs weighing >10 kg are given 500 mg of each drug TID. If a clinical response is seen, the frequency may be decreased to SID-BID. Vomiting, diarrhea, and anorexia are the most common side effects.

Pentoxifylline: Pentoxifylline results in a range of immunologic and rheologic effects, including increases in RBC and WBC deformability; decreases in RBC and platelet aggregation, leukocyte endothelial adherence, natural killer cell activity, neutophil degranulation, and production of monocyte TNF-α, IL-1, IL-4, and IL-12; and inhibition of T- and B-cell activation. It has been used in limited numbers of animals for a variety of conditions including vasculitis, canine familial dermatomyositis, ulcerative dermatitis of Shetland Sheepdogs and Collies, rabies vaccine-induced ischemic alopecia, ear margin dermatosis, contact allergy, and atopic dermatitis. The dosage is 10 mg/kg, SID-TID. Once a response is seen, the dose may be tapered to SID-BID. GI-related adverse effects have been reported (eg, nausea, vomiting).

PSYCHOTROPIC AGENTS

Psychotropic drugs have been used extra-label for treatment of feline psychogenic alopecia and canine acral lick dermatitis, syndromes characterized by excessive self-licking (*see also* OTHER CANINE BEHAVIORAL PROBLEMS, p 1314, and OTHER FELINE BEHAVIORAL PROBLEMS, p 1325). Classes of drugs used include antidepressants, antipsychotics, opiate antagonists, anxiolytics, and mood stabilizers (TABLE 14).

Sedation is the most common side effect of diazepam. It is also an appetite stimulant in cats. Idiosyncratic fatal hepatic necrosis has been reported in several cats treated for as little as 8-14 days. Tricyclic antidepressants are potent H_1 blockers in addition to inhibiting uptake of serotonin and norepinephrine. These drugs can induce cardiac arrhythmias and lower the seizure threshold. Other side effects include dry mouth, hypersalivation, vomiting, constipation, urinary retention, ataxia, disorientation, depression, and anorexia. Tricyclic antidepressants should not be used concurrently with monoamine oxidase inhibitors, including amitraz dips for demodicosis. Dosages should be tapered slowly when discontinued.

VITAMINS AND MINERALS

Retinoids: Those naturally occurring and synthetic compounds with vitamin A activity include retinol, retinoic acid, and retinol derivatives or analogs. At the molecular level, retinoids are important in regulation of proliferation, growth, differentiation, and

---

TABLE 14. Psychotropic Drugs Used for Skin Disorders

Drug	Dosage
Antidepressants	
Clomipramine	Dogs: 1-3 mg/kg, BID
	Cats: 0.5-1.5 mg/kg, SID
Amitriptyline	1-3 mg/kg, BID
Doxepin	0.5-2 mg/kg, BID
Fluoxetine	1 mg/kg, SID
Anxiolytics	
Diazepam	1-2 mg/kg, BID
Phenobarbital	0.5-2.2 mg/kg, BID
	15 mg/cat, twice weekly
Hydroxyzine	2.2 mg/kg, TID
Opiate Antagonist	
Naltrexone	2.2 mg/kg, SID

maintenance of epithelial tissues. Retinoids also affect proteases, biosynthesis of mucopolysaccharides, prostaglandins, cellular adhesion, cellular communication, and immunity. They prevent tumor promotion by inhibition of ornithine decarboxylase, a key enzyme for cell proliferation and differentiation. Vitamin A (1,000 IU/kg) has been used for follicular keratosis in cats. However, the retinoids used most commonly are isotretinoin (13-cis-retinoic acid) and etretinate (no longer available but replaced with acitretin, a metabolically active metabolite of etretinate).

Isotretinoin is indicated for Schnauzer comedo syndrome, ichthyosis, feline acne, sebaceous adenitis, epitheliotropic lymphoma, keratoacanthoma, and sebaceous gland hyperplasias and adenomas. The dosage is 1-3 mg/kg, SID. Adverse effects include conjunctivitis, mucocutaneous drying, alopecia, pruritus, hyperactivity, vomiting, and diarrhea. In dogs, blood chemistry increases not normally associated with clinical disease include plasma cholesterol, triglycerides, ALT, AST, and alkaline phosphatase. Rarely, keratoconjunctivitis sicca may develop in dogs. Conjunctivitis, anorexia, diarrhea, and vomiting are the major side effects in cats. All retinoids are potent teratogens, and teratogenicity may persist for up to 2 yr after treatment with etretinate because the half-life is ~100 days. Skeletal abnormalities, including premature closure of the epiphyses in growing animals, cortical hyperostosis, periosteal calcification, and long-bone demineralization, that may be seen with longterm therapy are less common with etretinate than with isotretinoin. Monitoring during longterm therapy should include complete physical examinations and serum chemistry profiles at monthly intervals for the first 3-4 mo and then every 4-6 mo.

Zinc: Zinc is an important factor of many enzyme systems and is necessary for maintenance of growth, metabolism, normal reproduction, and hormonal regulation. It is essential for keratinization and immune function. Zinc supplementation is given in cases of insufficient intestinal absorption, including deficiency syndrome I (Siberian Huskies, Alaskan Malamutes) and syndrome II (rapidly growing dogs on zinc-deficient diets). Dietary deficiency may be either absolute or relative—diets high in phytates or minerals may inhibit zinc absorption. For syndrome I, zinc supplementation is given at 1 mg elemental zinc/kg, PO, SID (10 mg zinc sulfate/kg, 5 mg zinc gluconate/kg, or 1.7 mg zinc methionine/kg). Supplementation is typically lifelong. If response is insufficient after 4 wk, the dose should be increased by 50%. Low-dose corticosteroids may also enhance zinc absorption through induction of metallothionein in some nonresponsive cases. Animals with syndrome II normally respond to correction of the diet with resolution within 2-6 wk, although supplementation speeds this process.

Hereditary zinc deficiency associated with deficient intestinal absorption has also been reported in Friesian, Danish Black Pied, and Shorthorn cattle. There is a rapid response to zinc oxide given at 0.5 g, PO, SID, or zinc sulfate at 2 g, PO, given weekly. Response to zinc supplementation is usually rapid (a few days) except for cases of achromotrichia, which requires several weeks for resolution.

SYSTEMIC PHARMACOTHERAPEUTICS OF THE MUSCULAR SYSTEM

Drugs that affect skeletal muscle function fall into several therapeutic categories. Some are used during surgical procedures to produce paralysis (neuromuscular blocking agents); others reduce spasticity (skeletal muscle relaxants) associated with various neurologic and musculoskeletal conditions. In addition, there are several therapeutic agents that influence metabolic and other processes in skeletal muscle. Included among these are the nutrients that are required for normal muscle function and that are used to prevent or mitigate degenerative muscular conditions. For example, selenium and vitamin E are used to prevent or treat muscular dystrophies such as white muscle disease (p 948). The steroidal, nonsteroidal, and various other anti-inflammatory agents (eg, dimethyl sulfoxide) are also commonly used to treat acute and chronic inflammatory conditions involving skeletal muscle. Anabolic steroids promote muscle growth and development and are administered in selected cases in which serious muscle deterioration has developed as a complication of a primary disease syndrome.

The clinical pharmacology of the neuromuscular blocking agents, skeletal muscle relaxants, and anabolic steroids are discussed below. For anti-inflammatory agents, *see* p 2125.

NEUROMUSCULAR BLOCKING AGENTS

The peripherally acting skeletal muscle relaxants characteristically interfere with the transmission of impulses from motor nerves to skeletal muscle fibers at the neuromuscular junction, thus reducing or abolishing motor activity. The skeletal muscle paralysis that ensues is not associated with depression of the CNS. Animals are fully conscious throughout the period of immobilization unless an anesthetic or hypnotic agent is administered concurrently.

Neuromuscular transmission can be modified either at the axonal membrane (prejunctional blockade) or at the cholinergic receptors in the sarcolemma (postjunctional blockade).

There are no clinically useful drugs that act prejunctionally, but a number of important substances can impair the synthesis, storage, and release of acetylcholine, thus resulting in prejunctional blockade at the motor endplate and consequently paralysis. Examples of prejunctional blocking agents include biotoxins, electrolytes, local anesthetics or other drugs, and antibiotics. **Biotoxins** include black widow spider venom, which depletes acetylcholine stores; botulinum toxin, which decreases acetylcholine release; tetradotoxin from the puffer fish and saxitoxin from shellfish, which block Na^+-conducting channels; and grayanotoxin found in rhododendrons, which facilitates excessive Na^+ entry through the sarcolemma leading to constant depolarization of the membrane. **Electrolytes** include excess Mg^{2+}, which inhibits release of acetylcholine from the axon and uncouples the excitation-contraction process by competing with Ca^{2+}; and depleted Ca^{2+} levels, which decrease release of acetylcholine and impairment of excitation-contraction coupling. **Local anesthetics** in high concentration can stabilize membranes by blocking both Na^+ and K^+ channels; **hemicholinium** can inhibit synthesis of acetylcholine by blocking choline uptake into the nerve. **Antibiotics**, such as the aminoglycosides, polymyxins, tetracyclines, and lincosamides, appear to act by decreasing the availability of Ca^{2+} at membrane-binding sites on the axonal terminal and perhaps by reducing the sensitivity of the nicotinic receptors to acetylcholine.

Postjunctional blocking agents are used clinically and act either by blocking the nicotinic receptors in a competitive fashion (nondepolarizing agents) or by interacting with these receptors in a manner that does not allow the membrane to repolarize so that paralysis results (depolarizing agents). The mechanisms involved in the latter case are not fully understood. All of the neuromuscular blocking agents are structurally similar to acetylcholine (actually 2 molecules linked end-to-end). The depolarizing agents are usually simple linear structures, and the nondepolarizing agents are more complex bulky molecules. With a single exception (vecuronium), all have a quaternary nitrogen in their structure, which makes these drugs poorly lipid soluble.

Competitive Nondepolarizing Agents: The members of this group of peripherally acting skeletal muscle relaxants are often referred to as curarizing agents because of their relationships with the curare alkaloids that were first used clinically. The currently available drugs, which interact with nicotinic cholinergic receptors on skeletal muscle cells and render them inaccessible to the transmitter function of acetylcholine (and thus produce a flaccid paralysis), include tubocurarine, metocurine (dimethyltubocurarine), gallamine, pancuronium, alcuronium, atracurium, vecuronium, and fazadinium.

In general, nondepolarizing muscle relaxants are not absorbed from the GI tract and must be administered parenterally, usually IV. Plasma-protein binding is insignificant, and there is rapid equilibration but only within the extracellular fluid. The blood-brain and blood-placental barriers are rarely crossed. Tubocurarine, metocurine, and gallamine are not biotransformed to any extent and are excreted unchanged, principally in the urine but sometimes in bile. The other members of the group undergo metabolic transformation to some degree, and the metabolites are excreted by both renal and biliary routes in most instances. The elimination half-lives at standard dosages are 60-100 min, and the duration of paralysis is 30-60 min, except in the case of atracurium and vecuronium, which have shorter actions of ~20-30 min.

After IV administration of these agents, the skeletal muscles become totally flaccid and nonresponsive to neuronal stimulation. Muscles capable of rapid movement, such as those of the eye, are paralyzed before the larger muscles of the head and neck, which are followed by those of the limbs and body. Lastly, the diaphragm becomes paralyzed, and respiration ceases. If ventilation is controlled (tracheal intubation and positive pressure ventilation), there are no adverse effects and full recovery ensues in reverse order, with the diaphragm regaining function first. All of the currently used nondepolarizing muscle relaxants have cardiovascular effects, many of which are mediated by autonomic and histamine receptors. Tubocurarine and, to a much lesser extent, metocurine result in hypotension, which probably results from the liberation of histamine and, in larger doses, from ganglionic blockade. Premedication with an antihistamine reduces tubocurarine-induced hypotension. Pancuronium causes a moderate increase in heart rate and, to a lesser degree, cardiac output. Gallamine increases heart rate by both a vagolytic action and sympathetic stimulation.

A number of agents can potentiate the activity of neuromuscular blockers. These include other peripherally acting skeletal muscle relaxants, inhalant anesthetics (halothane, methoxyflurane), antibiotics (aminoglycosides, polymyxins, tetracyclines, and lincosamides), and various other drugs (quinidine, procaine, lidocaine, diazepam, and barbiturates). Several states such as hyper- and hypomagnesemia, hypokalemia, acidosis, and hypothermia also prolong the action of this group of drugs. Animals with myasthenia gravis are much more susceptible to the action of muscle relaxants.

Indications for the use of nondepolarizing neuromuscular blocking agents include muscle relaxation of the operative field, hypoxemic animals resisting mechanical ventilation, tracheal intubation, animals with unstable cardiovascular function that require anesthesia but cannot tolerate cardiac depression, cesarean section in toxic or high-risk animals, epileptiform convulsions not controllable with usual anticonvulsant agents, tetanus, strychnine poisoning, shivering animals in which the metabolic demand for oxygen should be reduced, and capture of certain exotic species (eg, gallamine used for immobilization of crocodiles). Animals should *always* be carefully monitored when under the influence of neuromuscular blocking drugs, and support of ventilation is essential.

The action of the competitive relaxants can be reversed by anticholinesterase drugs, especially neostigmine, after the administration of atropine, which eliminates excessive muscarinic responses. This attribute is a great advantage for this group of peripherally acting muscle relaxants.

The selection of dose rates (*see* TABLE 15) serves only as general guidelines for the use of competitive blocking agents.

TABLE 15. Competitive Nondepolarizing Agents and Antagonists

Drug	Dosage
Tubocurarine chloride	Horses: ≤0.22-0.25 mg/kg, IV
	Dogs, cats: ≤0.4 mg/kg, IV
Gallamine triethiodide	All species (except pigs): 0.8-1 mg/kg, IV
Pancuronium bromide	Dogs, cats: 0.6 mg/kg, IV
Alcuronium chloride	Dogs, cats: 0.1 mg/kg, IV
Atracurium besylate	Dogs, cats: 0.5 mg/kg, IV
Antagonists	
Neostigmine	0.04 mg/kg, with atropine at 0.04 mg/kg, IV
Pyridostigmine	0.2-0.25 mg/kg, with atropine at 0.04 mg/kg, IV
Edrophonium	0.125 mg/kg, IV

Depolarizing Agents: Succinylcholine (suxamethonium) is the only commonly used peripherally acting muscle relaxant that is a depolarizing agent. Decamethonium, the other member of the group, is rarely used clinically.

Depolarizing blocking drugs occupy the postjunctional cholinergic receptors and, by mechanisms that remain obscure, elicit prolonged depolarization of the endplate region. This prevents the synaptic membrane from completely repolarizing, thus rendering the motor endplate unresponsive to the normal action of acetylcholine. Characteristically, succinylcholine elicits transient muscle fasciculations before causing neuromuscular paralysis. The onset of action of succinylcholine is rapid after IV injection (20-50 sec), and the duration of the effect is usually 5-10 min in most species. Succinylcholine is rapidly hydrolyzed by pseudocholinesterases in the plasma and liver in most species, but substantial genetic differences exist.

Other pharmacologic effects are associated with the depolarizing muscle relaxants. After IV administration of succinylcholine, transient muscle fasciculations are usually evident, although general anesthesia tends to attenuate them. Succinylcholine-induced cardiac arrhythmias are many and varied. Succinylcholine stimulates all autonomic cholinergic receptors—both nicotinic and muscarinic. Sudden hyperkalemia may be precipitated by succinylcholine, and muscle pain is seen with the use of succinylcholine in the absence of anesthesia. After recovery from succinylcholine-induced muscle paralysis, muscle damage and even myoglobinuria can develop. Malignant hyperthermia (p 832) or clinical signs related to this syndrome may also follow the use of succinylcholine in susceptible animals.

Factors that can alter the activity of competitive blocking agents (*see* above) can also affect the action of succinylcholine. In addition, previous (within 1 mo) or concurrent use of organophosphate anthelmintics or external parasiticides can have a significant impact on the recovery time from succinylcholine immobilization, because of prolonged inhibition of the pseudocholinesterase enzyme systems. A genetically mediated deficiency of pseudocholinesterases also has been identified in certain strains of sheep. Cattle are much more susceptible to the effects of succinylcholine than other species.

The indications for the clinical use of succinylcholine are similar to those for the nondepolarizing agents. However, it must be emphasized that succinylcholine should never be used as an agent for euthanasia or for immobilization for castration without local or general analgesia. The use of succinylcholine for game-cropping procedures is also highly undesirable.

No antagonists are available to reverse the action of the depolarizing muscle relaxants. Continued positive-pressure ventilation until recovery occurs is the only therapy in cases of overdosage.

The IV dose rates for succinylcholine by species are as follows: horses: 0.125-0.20 mg/kg (~8 min recumbency); cattle: 0.012-0.02 mg/kg (~15 min recumbency); dogs: 0.22-1.1 mg/kg (~15-20 min paralysis); and cats: 0.22-1.1 mg/kg (~3-5 min paralysis).

SKELETAL MUSCLE SPASMOLYTICS

Muscle spasticity is a characteristic of many clinical conditions, including trauma, myositis, muscular and ligamentous sprains and strains, intervertebral disk disease, tetanus, strychnine poisoning, neurologic disorders, and exertional rhabdomyolysis. An increase in tonic stretch reflexes originates from the CNS with involvement of descending pathways and results in hyperexcitability of motor neurons in the spinal cord. Drug therapy alleviates muscle spasms by modifying the stretch reflex arc or by interfering with the excitation-coupling process in the muscle itself (TABLE 16). Centrally acting muscle relaxants block interneuronal pathways in the spinal cord and in the midbrain reticular activating system. Some drugs also have sedative effects, which are beneficial to anxious, painful animals. The hydantoin derivatives have a direct action on muscle.

Methocarbamol is a centrally acting muscle relaxant chemically related to guaifenesin. Its exact mechanism of action is unknown, and it has no direct relaxant effect on striated muscle, nerve fibers, or the motor endplate. It also has a sedative effect. In dogs, cats, and horses, methocarbamol is indicated as adjunct therapy of acute inflammatory and traumatic conditions of skeletal muscle and to reduce muscle spasms. Because

TABLE 16. Skeletal Muscle Relaxants

Drug	Dosage
Methocarbamol	Dogs, cats: 44 mg/kg, IV, up to 330 mg/kg/day for tetanus or strychnine poisoning; 132 mg/kg/day, PO, divided BID-TID Horses: 4.4-55 mg/kg, IV
Guaifenesin	Dogs: 44-88 mg/kg, IV Horses, ruminants: 66-132 mg/kg, IV
Diazepam	Cats: 2-5 mg, PO, TID, for urethral obstruction
Dantrolene	Horses: 15-25 mg/kg, slow IV, QID; 2 mg/kg, PO, SID, for prevention of exertional rhabdomyolysis Swine: 3.5 mg/kg, IV
Phenytoin	Horses: 6-8 mg/kg, PO, SID, increase by 1 mg/kg every 3 days until rhabdomyolysis is prevented or the horse appears sedated

methocarbamol is a CNS depressant, it should not be given with other drugs that depress the CNS. Overdosage is generally characterized by CNS depression, but emesis (small animals), salivation, weakness, and ataxia may be seen.

Guaifenesin (glyceryl guaiacolate) is a centrally acting muscle relaxant that is believed to depress or block nerve impulse transmission at the internuncial neuron level of the subcortical areas of the brain, brain stem, and spinal cord. It also has mild analgesic and sedative actions. Guaifenesin is given IV to induce muscle relaxation as an adjunct to anesthesia for short procedures. It relaxes both laryngeal and pharyngeal muscles, allowing easier intubation, but has little effect on diaphragm and respiratory function. It may cause transient increases in cardiac rate and decreases in blood pressure. It is also used in treatment of horses with exertional rhabdomyolysis and in dogs with strychnine intoxication. Overdose results in apneustic breathing, nystagmus, hypotension, and contradictory muscle rigidity. Treatment of overdose is supportive until the drug is cleared to nontoxic levels.

Benzodiazepines, such as diazepam, affect polysynaptic reflexes at the supraspinal level, act as a spinal cord depressant at the interneuronal level, and inhibit presynaptic acetylcholine release. Clinically, diazepam is used as an adjunct to anesthesia, in the management of clinical signs of tetanus, and in the treatment of functional urethral obstruction and urethral sphincter hypertonus in cats.

Dantrolene is a hydantoin derivative that is structurally and pharmacologically different from other skeletal muscle relaxants. Dantrolene has a direct action on muscle, probably by interfering with the release of calcium from the sarcoplasmic reticulum. It has no discernible effects on respiratory and cardiac function but can cause dizziness and sedation. In veterinary medicine, dantrolene is used in the treatment of malignant hyperthermia in various species, porcine stress syndrome, equine postanesthetic myositis, and equine exertional rhabdomyolysis (see also p 832 and p 947).

Phenytoin is a hydantoin derivative, primarily used as an anticonvulsant in humans. Phenytoin has shown efficacy in some horses susceptible to exertional rhabdomyolysis. Phenytoin may alter the function of neurotransmitters at the neuromuscular junction, the release of calcium from the sarcoplasmic reticulum, and sodium flux at the sarcolemma. Dosages are adjusted in horses to maintain serum concentrations of 5-10 µg/mL.

ANABOLIC STEROIDS

Anabolic steroids are synthetic derivatives of testosterone with enhanced anabolic activity and reduced androgenic activity (TABLE 17). Testosterone or its derivatives diffuse through cell membranes of target organs and combine with specific receptor proteins in the cytoplasm. The receptor-hormone migrates into the cell nucleus and binds to nuclear chromatin, stimulating the production of specific messenger RNA. The messenger

TABLE 17. Anabolic Steroids

Drug	Dosage
Boldenone undecylenate	Horses: 1.1 mg/kg, IM, every 3 wk
Nandrolone decanoate	Dogs: 1-5 mg/kg, IM, once/wk Cats: 10-20 mg, IM, once/wk
Stanozolol	Dogs: 1-4 mg, PO, BID; 25-50 mg, deep IM, once/wk Cats: 1-2 mg, PO, BID; 25 mg, deep IM, once/wk Horses: 0.55 mg/kg, deep IM, once/wk

RNA then regulates the enzyme synthesis responsible for the physiologic activity of the anabolic steroid.

Anabolic steroids stimulate and maintain a positive nitrogen balance by reducing renal elimination of nitrogen, sodium, potassium, chloride, and calcium. Production of myosin, sarcoplasm, and myofibrillar protein is enhanced. Anabolic steroids promote appetite, weight gain, and improved mental attitude, so they are used to reverse debilitation associated with surgery, trauma, illness, glucocorticoid-induced catabolism, and aging. In all cases, improved well-being depends on adequate intake of protein and calories and on treatment of the underlying disease.

Anabolic steroids have a variety of undesirable effects. They induce androgenic effects, such as increased libido in males and abnormal sexual behavior in females, along with adverse reproductive effects, including azoospermia, anestrus, testicular atrophy, and clitoral hypertrophy. They promote edema formation due to sodium and water retention. Icterus can develop due to intrahepatic cholestasis. Anabolic steroids can induce epiphyseal plate closure, thereby retarding growth. Anabolic steroids are used in the treatment of debilitated animals; however, they are often misused to gain a competitive advantage in performance animals.

SYSTEMIC PHARMACOTHERAPEUTICS OF THE NERVOUS SYSTEM

See also PRINCIPLES OF THERAPY, NERVOUS SYSTEM, p 990.

ANTICONVULSANTS

During a seizure episode or status epilepticus, the route of administration for anticonvulsants is IV. The oral route is preferred for longterm maintenance therapy, although absorption may be limited or variable depending on the drug used (TABLE 18). SC or IM injections are seldom used because of the variability in drug absorption.

Maintenance anticonvulsant therapy should be initiated in animals that have more than one seizure monthly or more than one seizure on any particular day, if the first episode is protracted or severe, or during an episode of status epilepticus (as a followup to emergency treatment, *see* below). Treatment should begin with a single drug at the minimal required level for effect and with an interim period equal to the interval between past episodes. (Owners should keep a calendar to document the frequency and pattern of seizures as a guide for treatment strategy.) This regimen is maintained if seizures are controlled without toxic effects. If control is unsatisfactory, the dose should be increased over multiple steps before adding or switching to a new drug. Doses may be doubled in early stages and increased by 50% in later stages. To discontinue a drug, even when changing drugs, the dose should be tapered gradually to avoid precipitating a seizure.

In status epilepticus, treatment is essential to prevent death from hyperthermia, acidosis, hypoperfusion, and hypoxia (TABLE 19). A benzodiazepine should be used first,

TABLE 18. Anticonvulsant Drugs

Anticonvulsant Drug	Dosage and Frequency	Half-life
First-line Anticonvulsant Drugs		
Phenobarbital	Dogs: 2-4 mg/kg, PO, BID (starting dose); up to 10 mg/kg, BID	40-90 hr (Beagles 25-38 hr)
	Cats: 1-2 mg/kg, PO, BID (starting dose) Horses: 3-5 mg/kg, PO, SID; up to 11 mg/kg, PO, SID Foals: 20 mg/kg diluted to 30 mL with normal saline IV over 30 min, then 9 mg/kg diluted and infused as above TID; 8 mg/kg, PO, TID	34-43 hr 18 hr 13 hr
Bromide (potassium salt)	Dogs, horses: 20-40 mg/kg, PO, SID or divided BID if GI upset. Dogs: loading dose 400-600 mg/kg, PO or per rectum, divided into 4 doses, given over 24 hr	Dogs: 20-46 days Cats: 10 days Horses: 5 days
Bromide (sodium salt)	17-30 mg/kg, PO, SID or divided BID if GI upset	
Diazepam	Dogs: 0.5-2 mg/kg per rectum at onset of seizure; repeat up to 3 times in 24 hr Cats: 0.25-2.0 mg/kg, PO, divided BID-TID Horses: 25-50 mg/kg, IV; repeat in 30 min if necessary Foals: 0.02-0.4 mg/kg, IV; repeat in 30 min if necessary	Dogs: 2.5-3.2 hr Cats: 5.5 hr Horses: 7-22 hr
Second-line (Add-on) Anticonvulsant Drugs		
Clonazepam	Dogs: 0.1-0.5 mg/kg, PO, BID-TID	1.5-3 hr
Clorazepate	Dogs: 2-6 mg/kg, PO, BID	5-6 hr
Felbamate	Dogs: 15 mg/kg, PO, TID; increase by 15 mg/kg biweekly until seizures controlled; maximal (toxic) dosage 300 mg/kg	5-6 hr
Gabapentin	Dogs: 25-60 mg/kg, PO, divided TID-QID; 100-300 mg/dog, TID	3-4 hr
Levetiracetam	Dogs: 20 mg/kg, PO, TID; 500-4,000 mg/day	4-10 hr
Topiramate	Dogs: 5-10 mg/kg/day, PO, divided BID	12-30 hr

TABLE 18. (continued)		
Time to Steady State	**Therapeutic Level**	**Adverse Effects/Comments**
First-line Anticonvulsant Drugs		
10-24 days	15-45 µg/mL (66-200 µmol/L), preferably keep values within 20-35 µg/mL (85-150 µmol/L)	Sedation, polydipsia, induces P450 system, increase in liver enzymes; liver disease is uncommon. Adjust dosage by monitoring serum levels.
	10-30 µg/mL	Liver enzymes do not increase in cats. Adjust dose in all species by
	10-40 µg/ml (43-175 µmol/L)	monitoring serum levels.
Dogs: 100-200 days Cats: 6 wk	Bromide alone: 1-3 mg/mL (15-20 µmol/L) Bromide/phenobarbital combined: 1-2 mg/mL	Sedation, weakness, polydipsia vomiting, polyphagia, skin rash. Respiratory problems occur in cats (may be fatal). Use with extreme caution in cats and monitor with thoracic radiographs.
		Reduce dose with renal insufficiency. High chloride intake increases bromide elimination. Chloride content of diet should be stable. Decrease the dose by 15% for the sodium salt to account for the higher bromide content.
		Client treatment at home for cluster seizures or status epilepticus. Sedation, liver failure in cats.
Second-line (Add-on) Anticonvulsant Drugs		
	22-77 ng/mL	Extremely potent benzodiazepine; sedation, withdrawal signs if drug stopped abruptly.
1-2 days	20-75 µg/L	15 times less potent than clonazepam; sedation, withdrawal seizures.
1 day	125-250 µmol/L[*]	Blood dyscrasia; induces P450 system, liver disease. Use with care with other potentially hepatotoxic drugs.
<24 hr	4-16 mg/L[*] (70-120 µmol/L)	Sedation, dizziness, ataxia, fatigue, diarrhea; reduce dose with renal dysfunction.
2-3 days	35-120 µmol/L[*]	Restlessness, vomiting, ataxia at dosages >400 mg/kg/day.
3-5 days	2-25 mg/L (15-60 µmol/L)[*]	GI upset, irritability

(*continued*)

TABLE 18. Anticonvulsant Drugs (continued) ▶

Anticonvulsant Drug	Dosage and Frequency	Half-life
Second-line (Add-on) Anticonvulsant Drugs		
Valproic acid	Dogs: 10-60 mg/kg, PO, TID	90-120 min
Zonisamide	Dogs: 4-8 mg/kg/day, PO, divided; up to 10 mg/kg, BID	15-20 hr

because its transient effect permits a rapid shift in the therapeutic approach. For dogs, an initial IV bolus of diazepam (0.5-2 mg/kg) or, alternatively, clonazepam (0.05-0.2 mg/kg) may be necessary to reduce motor activity and permit placement of an IV catheter. Fluids are then infused to correct any detectable metabolic disturbances, and diazepam is added at 5-20 mg/hr. Alternatively, IV boluses of diazepam may be repeated up to a total of 3 times at intervals of 5-10 min before switching to phenobarbital (to begin the maintenance phase of therapy in dogs). Phenobarbital may be given at 2-4 mg/kg, as a slow IV bolus every 20-30 min, up to a total of 20 mg/kg. As a safer alternative in dogs, phenobarbital may be infused IV to effect at 3-10 mg/hr. If phenobarbital is effective in controlling seizures, a maintenance regimen may be initiated with phenobarbital, and the anticonvulsant infusion discontinued 2-4 hr later. In small breeds, infusion with diazepam alone is continued after the oral administration of phenobarbital. Cats in status epilepticus are best treated with diazepam only (0.5-2 mg/kg, IV) and seldom need any other anticonvulsant.

To initiate maintenance anticonvulsant therapy in dogs, the drug of choice is phenobarbital (starting dosage 2-4 mg/kg, BID). Most dogs develop tolerance to side effects within 2 wk (sedation, polydipsia, polyuria, and polyphagia). The dosage should be adjusted on the basis of serum concentration monitoring (15-45 µg/mL) after 2 wk of treatment. Tolerance to anticonvulsant therapy may develop in dogs treated continually for months to years. Minimal dosage and periodic medication withdrawal (gradual) are recommended to minimize development of tolerance.

Diazepam is generally continued as maintenance treatment in cats, with dosages ranging from 0.25-0.5 mg/kg, PO, BID-TID. Phenobarbital is a second drug of choice for maintenance, given at 3-6 mg/kg, divided into 2-3 daily doses.

Preliminary studies suggest that acupuncture and resective surgery (callosotomy) may offer alternative therapies in dogs with idiopathic epilepsy that is poorly controlled by medication.

For treatment of acute convulsions in foals (eg, with neonatal maladjustment syndrome or idiopathic epilepsy), seizures are best treated with diazepam, 0.02-0.40 mg/kg, given slowly IV. This dose may be repeated, and with a few doses, convulsions do not recur in some foals. However, if seizures recur, treatment with diazepam or another anticonvulsant should be continued for 1-4 wk before being gradually withdrawn. After diazepam treatment, phenobarbital may be administered at 20 mg/kg by slow IV injection, followed by a maintenance dosage of 9 mg/kg, BID or TID. Alternatively, treatment of foals can be initiated and later maintained with phenytoin (for dosages, *see* below). If seizures are otherwise uncontrollable, sodium pentobarbital (2-4 mg/kg, IV) can be given to effect (in all species). In foals, chloral hydrate/magnesium sulfate (3-10 g/50 kg) may be used instead. Also, if cerebral edema is suspected, *see* PRINCIPLES OF THERAPY, NERVOUS SYSTEM, p 990.

Horses with seizures induced by toxins or adverse drug effects (eg, xylazine) can be treated with diazepam (0.1-0.15 mg/kg, IV). Alternatively, a mixture of guaifenesin (5%) and thiamylal (2 mg/mL) may be given at 1 mL/kg to effect.

◀ TABLE 18.	(continued)	
Time to Steady State	**Therapeutic Level**	**Adverse Effects/Comments**
Second-line (Add-on) Anticonvulsant Drugs		
<24 hr		Probably ineffective due to very short half-life; liver toxicity and pancreatitis.
3-4 days	10-40 mg/L (45-180 μmol/L)[*]	Sedation, ataxia, loss of appetite

[*]Therapeutic range established for humans

TABLE 19.	Drugs Used for Treatment of Status Epilepticus
Drug	**Dosage and Frequency**
Diazepam	0.5-1.0 mg/kg, IV bolus; can repeat 2-3 times at intervals of 5-10 min
Phenobarbital	2-4 mg/kg/ IV bolus; can repeat at 20- to 30-min intervals to a total dosage of 20 mg/kg
Pentobarbital	2-15 mg/kg, IV, to effect to stop motor activity
Propofol	1-2 mg/kg, IV, to effect to stop motor activity; constant rate infusion: 0.1-0.6 mg/kg/min to effect

Phenothiazine tranquilizers should be avoided in epileptic treatment in all species because they lower the seizure threshold. Also, xylazine should not be used during seizures because it severely depresses cardiovascular and respiratory function; even at low doses, it can cause prolonged sedation and death.

Diazepam is the most commonly used benzodiazepine. Injectable solutions should not be left in plastic containers, including syringes, because of rapid inactivation (over minutes). Diazepam is not suitable for oral maintenance therapy in dogs because it is absorbed poorly and eliminated rapidly, and a tolerance to anticonvulsant effects develops rapidly. However, it is a drug of choice for controlling status epilepticus in dogs. Diazepam given per rectum (0.5-2 mg/kg, up to 3 times in 24 hr) may be used as an adjunct to phenobarbital and bromide in dogs exhibiting antiepileptic drug tolerance, which is recommended for emergency administration by the owner at the start of a seizure. Diazepam is the anticonvulsant of choice for cats, either for maintenance therapy (0.25-0.5 mg/kg, PO, BID-TID) or for status epilepticus (0.5-2 mg/kg, IV). Cats not only have a slower elimination rate than dogs but also do not develop a tolerance to the anticonvulsant effects. Diazepam has a long elimination half-life in horses and, therefore, is the anticonvulsant of choice (5-20 mg/dose, IV) in foals with neonatal maladjustment syndrome (p 1039). Higher doses can be fatal to neonates. For seizures in adult horses, diazepam can be given at 25-50 mg/kg, IV.

Clonazepam, unlike diazepam, can be used in dogs for oral maintenance therapy because anticonvulsant tolerance develops less rapidly, the saturatability of its metabolism reduces the elimination rate at therapeutic concentrations, and it is more highly absorbed orally (particularly in micronized formulations). In maintenance therapy in dogs, it is best used as an adjunct to phenobarbital at dosages of 0.1-0.5 mg/kg/day, or it may be used alone at 0.5 mg/kg, TID. Diarrhea sometimes develops with clonazepam, but this may be avoided by increasing the dose frequency from 1 to 3 times/day over a period of several days.

Chlorazepate dipotassium (2-6 mg/kg, BID) has been proposed as an adjunct to phenobarbital treatment in dogs.

Phenobarbital is the preferred maintenance drug for dogs due to safety, efficacy, low cost, and convenience for monitoring serum concentrations. Because of a long half-life in all species, 2 wk are required to approach steady state in plasma concentration, and dosage adjustment should be attempted only at 2-wk intervals. In dogs, it is used as a followup to diazepam in status epilepticus by an IV infusion (3-10 mg/hr to effect) or a slow IV bolus (2-4 mg/kg every 20-30 min up to a total of 20 mg/kg). As in all species, caution is necessary in switching from diazepam to phenobarbital because a potentiation of their effects increases the risk of respiratory and cardiovascular collapse. For longterm maintenance in cats and dogs, phenobarbital may be given at 2-4 mg/kg/day, PO, divided in 2, sometimes 3, daily doses. Phenobarbital has also been used to treat episodic dyscontrol syndrome (rage) in dogs when seizure activity is demonstrable (1.5-3.0 mg/kg, PO, BID). In foals, phenobarbital may be started as a followup to diazepam, with 20 mg/kg administered IV over 20 min, and then maintained at a dosage of 9 mg/kg, BID or TID. In all species, oral absorption is extremely variable and drug levels should be monitored 3 wk from initiation of therapy, 2 wk after dosage changes, and then every 6-12 mo. Therapeutic concentrations are 15-45 µg/mL. In dogs, incidence of sedation is low; when sedation does occur, it disappears within the first week of treatment. Other adverse effects include transient polyuria, polydipsia, and polyphagia; physical dependence and withdrawal-induced seizures; hepatotoxicity associated with high serum concentrations (>35 µg/mL); idiosyncratic hyperexcitability; and rarely dermatitis, anemia, gingival hyperplasia, and osteomalacia. If foals become highly sedated, the dose of phenobarbital should be reduced.

Primidone is less preferred than phenobarbital because most of its anticonvulsant activity is due to its metabolism to phenobarbital. It requires a TID vs BID administration, and it can be hepatotoxic. Nevertheless, one report indicates that dogs that are not well controlled by phenobarbital may respond better to primidone (eg, psychomotor seizures). ALT, serum alkaline phosphatase, or bile acids should be monitored. The initial dosage (dogs only) is 5-15 mg/kg/day in 3 divided doses, increased over time to a maximum of 35 mg/kg/day. If treatment is switched to phenobarbital, the initial dose should be one-fifth the previous primidone dose to achieve a comparable concentration of phenobarbital. Primidone is not recommended for use in cats because of toxicity concerns. However, preliminary studies suggest primidone (40 mg/kg/day for 90 days) may be acceptable in cats.

Bromide (potassium or sodium salt) is recommended as a treatment in dogs for refractory seizure disorders or unacceptable side effects related to phenobarbital or primidone. Where it is not available as a pharmaceutical formulation (USA), an analytical grade may be obtained from a chemical supply company, although caution is recommended in handling and packaging. As adjunct therapy with phenobarbital, bromide can be administered at 20-40 mg/kg, PO, SID, or BID in divided doses (potassium salt) or 17-30 mg/kg, PO, SID or BID in divided doses (sodium salt). It has been used as the first and sole drug treatment for epilepsy in dogs at dosages of 50-80 mg/kg/day, divided for BID treatment. It should be administered with food in gelatin capsules or in a 100 mg/mL solution. Bromide is reported to be effective in cats but must be used with caution as it has been associated with pneumonitis (bronchial asthma) that is usually reversible on drug withdrawal. However, deaths have been reported. Bromide is generally well tolerated by dogs, but side effects include bitter taste, gastric irritation, nausea (particularly potassium form), polyuria, polydipsia, polyphagia, sedation, ataxia, and rarely pancreatitis (when administered concurrently with phenobarbital). Bromide toxicosis (bromism) is characterized by neurologic signs of lethargy, disorientation, delirium, and ataxia. Bromide should not be used in dogs with renal dysfunction; if azotemia is present, the initial dose should be reduced by half, and serum concentrations monitored. Bromide intoxication should be treated with an IV infusion of normal saline to promote renal excretion.

Valproic acid (10-60 mg/kg, TID) has been used as an adjunct to phenobarbital and primidone in dogs with refractory seizures. It has also been used to treat aggressive behavior problems (*see* PSYCHOTROPIC AGENTS, p 2013). Common side effects are a transient GI distress, sedation, and tremor. Hepatic failure is rare.

Carbamazepine is not recommended for use in dogs due to a rapid induction of hepatic enzymes eliminating the drug. Accordingly, plasma concentrations declined rapidly in dogs on a 1-wk regimen of 30 mg/kg, TID. However, one case report described adequate seizure control despite undetectable drug concentrations in plasma, possibly due to either an active metabolite or to a highly sensitive drug reaction. Carbamazepine has been used to treat aggressive behavior problems in cats (*see* PSYCHOTROPIC AGENTS, p 2013).

Phenytoin (diphenylhydantoin) is no longer recommended for use in dogs, cats, or foals due to undesirable pharmacokinetic properties (too rapid metabolism in dogs, reducing its effectiveness; too slow metabolism in cats, increasing the risk for toxicity [salivation, vomiting, weight loss]; and erratic plasma concentrations in foals). Its careful use (at 15-40 mg/kg, PO, TID) may be considered as an alternative in dogs that have not responded to phenobarbital or primidone, and it may still be used in status epilepticus (dogs) as a slow IV injection of 2-5 mg/kg. If used in foals with acute seizures, phenytoin has been used at 5-10 mg/kg, IV, with subsequent treatments of 1-5 mg/kg, IV, IM, or PO, every 2-4 hr for 12 hr. Afterward, doses should be given BID-QID. The dose may need to be reduced if sedation is seen.

Mephenytoin, although related to phenytoin, has been effective in dogs (10 mg/kg, TID) due to a slower rate of elimination. It may be combined with phenobarbital or bromide. Side effects consist of sedation only, but periodic hematologic monitoring is advised because blood dyscrasias and hepatoxicity are reported in humans.

Sodium pentobarbital is generally reserved for the treatment of uncontrollable status epilepticus in dogs and cats, when diazepam and phenobarbital have failed (TABLE 19). In these species, it is administered at 2-15 mg/kg to effect for anesthesia. In foals, as an alternative to diazepam and phenobarbital, it may be given at 2-4 mg/kg, IV to effect for controlling convulsions; sedation is likely at these dosages.

Several newer human antiepileptic drugs have been tried in dogs and may be useful as "add-on" drugs (polytherapy) when phenobarbital and bromide do not adequately control seizures. **Felbamate** may improve seizure control in dogs refractory to phenobarbital and bromide. It is metabolized 30% in the liver; the remainder is excreted in the urine. Felbamate is well tolerated in dogs, but there is no clinical information on its use in cats. It is nonsedating and side effects are uncommon. In humans, felbamate has been associated with aplastic anemia and liver toxicity. The risk of liver dysfunction is increased when used with other potentially hepatotoxic drugs, such as phenobarbital. Regular monitoring for anemia and liver dysfunction in dogs is recommended. **Gabapentin** is sometimes used in dogs with seizures refractory to other drugs. In dogs, it is metabolized 30% in the liver; the remainder is excreted by the kidneys. Food has no effect on its rate and extent of absorption. In dogs, side effects are uncommon and it is not sedating. In people, side effects include sedation, dizziness, ataxia, fatigue, and diarrhea. No drug interactions have been reported. There is no information on the use of gabapentin in cats. **Levetiracetam** is a new pyrrolidine-based anticonvulsant that has been tried as an adjunct antiepileptic drug for dogs. Its clinical usefulness has not yet been reported. There is no hepatic metabolism; 70% of the drug is eliminated unchanged by the kidneys. Levetiracetam is safe in dogs with the reported side effects of salivation, restlessness, vomiting, and ataxia at dosages >400 mg/kg/day. These resolved within 24 hr of discontinuing the drug. There are no reports of its use in cats. **Topiramate** is a new antiepileptic drug, well tolerated by humans and increasingly being used for neuropathic pain. In one report it was listed as an adjunct antiepileptic drug for dogs, but its effectiveness is not yet known. **Zonisamide** is a new sulfonamide-based anticonvulsant used for both focal and generalized seizures. It restricts the propagation and spread of seizures and suppresses epileptogenic focus activity. Zonisamide is metabolized by the liver. It has been used as an adjunct antiepileptic drug in dogs not adequately controlled by phenobarbital and bromide. Side effects are drowsiness, ataxia, loss of appetite and GI upset; no serious adverse effects have been reported. It has been used as effective monotherapy in humans. **Propofol** is a short-acting IV hypnotic anesthetic agent useful for control of refractory status epilepticus. Propofol may have anticonvulsant activity, as it is GABA-mimetic, stabilizing GABA-inhibitory neurotransmitter sites. During induction, transient seizure-like signs of excitement, paddling, nystagmus, muscle twitching, and opisthotonos may be seen in unsedated animals. Therefore, this agent should be used cautiously in animals with a history of seizure disorders.

TRANQUILIZERS, SEDATIVES, AND ANALGESICS

Tranquilization reduces anxiety and induces a sense of tranquility without drowsiness. Drug-induced sedation has a more profound effect and produces drowsiness and hypnosis. Analgesia is the reduction of pain, which according to a drug's effect, may be more pronounced in either the viscera or the musculoskeletal system. Many drugs cannot be categorized by only one pharmacologic effect, ie, as tranquilizers, sedatives, or analgesics. For example, many psychotropic drugs can either tranquilize or sedate according to the dose administered, and many sedatives are also analgesics. Also, drugs classified as tranquilizers, sedatives, and/or analgesics may have additional effects in behavioral modification, antiemesis, etc.

For drugs commonly used in various species for tranquilization, sedation, or analgesia, see TABLE 20 and TABLE 21. Drugs that have some of these effects but are used mainly for other properties (eg, as antispasmodics, antiemetics, or preanesthetics) are not listed. Single-use doses are emphasized because many situations require only a brief duration of effect, but frequency of administration is also provided for drugs likely to be used for multiple-dose therapy. The dosages listed serve only as a general guideline and apply to the use of each drug alone, not to a combination for anesthesia or neuroleptanalgesia. No reference is made to schedule restrictions, extra-label use, or precautions in the use of these drugs, and the product label and referenced texts should be consulted for information on the pharmacology and alternative applications of each drug.

TABLE 20. Tranquilizers and Sedatives without Analgesic Effects ▶

Drug	Dogs	Cats	Ferrets
Benzodiazepines			
Diazepam	1 mg/kg, IV or PO	1 mg/kg, IV	2 mg/kg, IM
Midazolam			
Butyrophenone			
Azaperone			
Phenothiazines			
Acepromazine maleate	0.05-0.1 mg/kg, IV, IM, or SC; 0.55-2.2 mg/kg, PO, TID-QID	0.11-0.22 mg/kg, IV, IM, or SC; 1.1- 2.2 mg/kg, PO, BID-TID	0.1-0.25 mg/kg, IM or SC
Chlorpromazine hydrochloride	0.55-4.4 mg/kg, IV; 1.1- 6.6 mg/kg, IM; 3.2 mg/kg, PO, TID-QID as needed	1-2 mg/kg, IV or IM, BID	
Promazine hydrochloride	2-6 mg/kg, IV, IM, or PO, TID-QID	2-4.4 mg/kg, IV, IM, or PO, TID-QID	
Triflupromazine hydrochloride	1.1-2.2 mg/kg, IV; 2.2-4.4 mg/kg, IM	4.4-8.8 mg/kg, IM	

PSYCHOTROPIC AGENTS

Anxiolytics, antipsychotics, antidepressants, and mood stabilizers used to treat human behavioral disorders are being used more commonly in veterinary medicine as adjuncts to behavioral modification therapy (*see also* PRINCIPLES OF PHARMACOLOGIC TREATMENT, p 1297). Few veterinary clinical studies have been reported, and guidelines for veterinary use are grounded on therapeutic applications in human medicine.

Anxiolytics, including the benzodiazepines and an azapirone (buspirone), have been used to treat generalized anxiety and panic disorder in humans. Diazepam has been recommended to alleviate fear-related behaviors in animals, eg, thunderstorm anxiety in dogs and social anxiety in cats. However, benzodiazepines may not alleviate fear-related aggression in certain animals, but instead may cause a paradoxical increase in such behaviors. Diazepam has been reported to diminish urine-spraying behavior in cats, although most cats resumed urine spraying when the drug was withdrawn. Additional reported usages for diazepam include taming effects on wild animals, correcting sleep disorders in dogs, and stimulating appetite in cats. Diazepam, clonazepam, and chlorazepate dipotassium also have antiepileptic properties (*see* above) and may be useful in treating behaviors based on nonconvulsive seizures. Buspirone differs from the benzodiazepines in pharmacologic properties, ie, basis of receptor interactions, delayed onset of antianxiety effect (≥1 wk), and lack of sedative effect. Buspirone appears to offer no greater control for anxiety-related behaviors than the benzodiazepines.

Antipsychotics are classified as low-potency agents (acepromazine, chlorpromazine, and thioridazine hydrochloride) and high-potency agents (haloperidol, fluphenazine, trifluoperazine hydrochloride, prochlorperazine, thiothixene, risperidone). Low-potency agents are administered at dosages of 1-3 mg/kg and have side effects of sedation, anticholinergic effects, and α-adrenergic blockade. The high-potency agents are administered at dosages of 0.5-1.0 mg/kg and result in less sedation and fewer autonomic side effects but commonly result in extrapyramidal effects of parkinsonism, dystonia, dyskinesia, and akathisia. All the antipsychotics are used for nonselective tranquilization

◀ **TABLE 20.** *(continued)*

	Dosage		
Rabbits	**Horses**	**Cattle**	**Pigs**
2 mg/kg, IV; 5-10 mg/kg, IM or IP	0.05-0.4 mg/kg, IV	0.5-1.5 mg/kg, IV	0.5-10 mg/kg, IM; 0.5-1.5 mg/kg, IV
2 mg/kg, IM or IV			
	0.4-0.8 mg/kg, IM		2.2 mg/kg, IM
1-5 mg/kg, IM	0.04-0.1 mg/kg, IV, IM, SC, or PO, SID	0.05-0.1 mg/kg, IV, IM, or SC	0.1-0.2 mg/kg, IV, IM, or SC
3 mg/kg, IV or IM (may produce myositis)			0.5-4.0 mg/kg, IM
	0.4-1 mg/kg, IV or IM; 1-2 mg/kg, PO	0.4-1 mg/kg, IV or IM; 1.6-2.8 mg/kg, PO	0.4-1 mg/kg, IV or IM
	0.22-0.33 mg/kg, IV or IM (maximum 100 mg/horse/day)		

TABLE 21. Analgesics ▶

Drug	Dosage		
	Dogs	Cats	Ferrets
Opioid Analgesics*			
Buprenorphine	0.01-0.02 mg/kg, SC, BID	0.005-0.01 mg/kg, SC or IM, BID	0.01-0.03 mg/kg, IV, IM, or SC, BID-TID
Butorphanol tartrate	0.2-0.4 mg/kg, IM or SC; 0.55 mg/kg, PO, every 4 hr	0.1-0.2 mg/kg, IV; 0.2-0.4 mg/kg, IM or SC, every 4 hr	0.4 mg/kg, IM, every 4-6 hr
Meperidine hydrochloride	2-10 mg/kg, IM or SC, every 2 hr	2-10 mg/kg, IM or SC, every 2 hr	5-10 mg/kg, IM or SC, every 2-4 hr
Morphine sulfate	0.22-0.88 mg/kg, IM or SC, every 4-6 hr as needed	0.1 mg/kg, IM or SC, as needed	0.5-5 mg/kg, IM or SC, QID
Nalbuphine	0.5-2.0 mg/kg, SC, every 4-8 hr	1.5-3.0 mg/kg, IV, every 3 hr	
Oxymorphone hydrochloride	0.22 mg/kg, IV, IM, or SC, SID	0.1-0.2 mg/kg, IV, IM, or SC, SID	
Pentazocine lactate	2-3 mg/kg, IM, every 4 hr; 15 mg/kg, PO, TID	2.2-3.3 mg/kg, IV, IM, or SC	
Nonopioid Sedative Analgesics			
Xylazine hydrochloride	0.5-1 mg/kg, IV; 1-2 mg/kg, IM or SC	0.5-1 mg/kg, IV; 1-2 mg/kg, IM or SC	1 mg/kg, IM or SC
Detomidine			
Nonpsychotropic Analgesics			
Acetaminophen	15 mg/kg, PO, QID as needed	Contraindicated	
Aspirin	10-25 mg/kg, PO, BID	10 mg/kg, PO, every 48 hr	0.5-20 mg/kg, PO, SID-TID
Carprofen	4 mg/kg, IV or SC, SID	4 mg/kg, IV or SC, SID	
Dipyrone	28 mg/kg, IV, IM, SC, or PO, TID	28 mg/kg IV, IM, SC, or PO, TID	
Flunixin meglumine	1-2 mg/kg, PO, IV, or IM, SID up to 3 days	1 mg/kg, PO; 0.3-1 mg/kg, IM or SC, SID up to 5 days	0.5-2 mg/kg, SC, SID-BID
Ibuprofen	5-10 mg/kg, PO, SID-BID	5 mg/kg, PO, SID	
Indomethacin	10 mg/kg, PO, SID		
Ketoprofen	2 mg/kg, SC, IM, or IV, SID up to 3 days; 1 mg/kg, PO, SID up to 5 days	1 mg/kg, SID, SC up to 3 days, or PO up to 5 days	
Meclofenamic acid	2.2 mg/kg, PO, SID	2.2 mg/kg, PO, SID	

◀ **TABLE 21.** (continued)

	Dosage		
Rabbits	**Horses**	**Cattle**	**Pigs**
*Opioid Analgesics**			
0.02-0.05 mg/kg, SC, IM, or IV, BID			0.005-0.02 mg/kg, IM or IV, BID-QID
0.1-0.5 mg/kg, IV, every 4 hr	0.05-0.1 mg/kg, IV, IM, or SC		0.1-0.3 mg/kg, IM
10-20 mg/kg, IM or SC, every 2-3 hr	0.2-0.4 mg/kg, IV; 1-3 mg/kg, IM or SC	500 mg/cow, IV	4-10 mg/kg, IM or IV
2-5 mg/kg, SC or IM, every 2-4 hr	0.2 mg/kg, IV; 0.2-0.4 mg/kg, IM		0.2-1 mg/kg, IM, every 4 hr
1-2 mg/kg, IV, every 4 hr			
5-10 mg/kg, SC, IM, or IV, every 4 hr	0.02-0.03 mg/kg, IV or IM		0.15 mg/kg, IM
10-20 mg/kg, SC or IM, every 4 hr; 5 mg/kg, IV, every 2-4 hr	0.33 mg/kg, IV; 1-3 mg/kg, SC or IM		2-5 mg/kg, IM, every 4 hr
Nonopioid Sedative Analgesics			
	0.1-1 mg/kg, IV; 0.5-1.0 mg/kg, IM or SC	0.05-0.1 mg/kg, IV; 0.1-0.2 mg/kg, IM	2 mg/kg, IM
	0.02-0.04 mg/kg, IV		
Nonpsychotropic Analgesics			
5-20 mg/kg, PO, SID	30-47.5 mg/kg, PO, BID-QID	26 mg/kg, IV; 100-124 mg/kg, PO, BID	10-20 mg/kg, PO, every 4 hr as needed
1.5 mg/kg, PO, BID	0.7 mg/kg, IV, IM, or SC, SID	0.7 mg/kg, IV, IM, or SC, SID	
	5-10 g/horse, IV or IM, TID as needed	50 mg/kg, IV, IM, or SC	50 mg/kg, IV, IM, or SC
1.1 mg/kg, SC or IM, BID	1-2.2 mg/kg, IV; 2.2 mg/kg, IM or PO, SID	1.1-2.2 mg/kg, IM or PO, SID-TID	1-2 mg/kg, IV or IM, SID
10-20 mg/kg, IV, every 4 hr			
10 mg/kg, IV or PO, every 4 hr		1.5 mg/kg, SID	
3 mg/kg, IM	2.2 mg/kg, IV, SID	2.2 mg/kg, IV; 3 mg/kg, IM, SID	
	2.2 mg/kg, PO, SID		

(continued)

TABLE 21. Analgesics (*continued*) ▶

	Dosage		
Drug	**Dogs**	**Cats**	**Ferrets**
Naproxen	5 mg/kg, PO, initial dose; 1.2-2.8 mg/kg, PO, SID for maintenance		
Phenylbutazone	22 mg/kg, PO; 15 mg/kg, IV, TID (maximum 0.8 g/dog/day)	15 mg/kg, IV, TID; 10-14 mg/kg, PO, BID	

and diminishing behavioral arousal. Acepromazine is commonly used for infrequent anxietal episodes, but it may induce a paradoxical hyperactivity in some dogs and cats. In one report, a dog with aberrant behavior (tail chewing, growling, snapping, barking) was controlled with thioridazine at 1.1 mg/kg.

Mood-stabilizing drugs (lithium, carbamazepine, and valproic acid) are unrelated chemical compounds that are used in human medicine to treat bipolar disorder, impulsivity, emotional reactivity, and aggression. Carbamazepine and valproic acid are also antiepileptic. Carbamazepine has been used in cats (25 mg/cat, PO, BID) to decrease fear-related aggression against people, but it may paradoxically increase aggression against conspecifics. Lithium is excreted unmetabolized via the urine. Serum concentration monitoring is necessary due to its narrow therapeutic index (recommended range: 0.8-1.2 mEq/L). Side effects include polyuria, polydipsia, memory problems, weight gain, and diarrhea. In one report, lithium (75 mg total dose, BID) was used to treat dominance-related aggression and psychotic behavior (random air-snapping, pawing) in a Cocker Spaniel.

Antidepressants can be used to treat behavioral disorders, including obsessive-compulsive behaviors, stereotypies, aggression, and inappropriate elimination. These drugs are classified as tricyclic compounds (tertiary amines, secondary amines), selective serotonin-reuptake inhibitors, and atypical antidepressants.

The **tricyclic antidepressants** have been commonly used in veterinary medicine. Case reports indicate that treatment success for behavioral disorders is highly variable among drugs within the same chemical class. The antihistaminic effect of these agents may be a useful adjunct in controlling pruritus due to atopy and food allergies. Side effects include vomiting, diarrhea, hyperexcitability, sedation, arrhythmias including tachycardia, orthostatic hypotension, mydriasis, reduced lacrimation and salivation, urine retention, constipation, and weight gain. Widening of the QRS complex on an ECG has been used as an early indication of toxicity. Amitriptyline hydrochloride has been used in dogs at 1-2 mg/kg for separation anxiety, anxiety-related aggression, urination due to submission or excitement, and allergy-related pruritus, and in cats at 0.5-1 mg/kg for urine marking and hypervocalization. Imipramine hydrochloride has been used in dogs at 2.2-4.4 mg/kg, BID-TID, for urination due to submission or excitement. Clomipramine hydrochloride has been used in dogs at 1-3 mg/kg for reducing lick behavior for canine lick granuloma and for stereotypies such as circling and tail chasing, and in cats at 0.5 mg/kg. In some countries it is approved for treatment of separation anxiety in dogs. Doxepine has been used in dogs at 3-5 mg/kg.

Selective serotonin-reuptake inhibitors, including fluoxetine, sertraline, and paroxetine, have been used for treating psychogenic alopecia, allergy-related pruritus, dominance-related aggression, fearful behaviors, obsessive-compulsive behaviors, and urine marking. Dosages for fluoxetine are 1 mg/kg, PO, SID for dogs, and 0.5-1.0 mg/kg, PO, SID for cats.

TABLE 21. (continued)			
Dosage			
Rabbits	**Horses**	**Cattle**	**Pigs**
	5 mg/kg, IV; 10 mg/kg, PO, BID		
	4.4 mg/kg, PO, BID on day 1; 2.2 mg/kg, PO, BID for 4 days; 2.2 mg/kg, PO, SID or every other day	2-5 mg/kg, IV; 4-8 mg/kg, PO	2-5 mg/kg, IV; 4-8 mg/kg, PO

*Recommended dosages of opiates may produce excitement in cats and horses.

SYSTEMIC PHARMACOTHERAPEUTICS OF THE REPRODUCTIVE SYSTEM

See also PRINCIPLES OF THERAPY, REPRODUCTIVE SYSTEM, p 1092.

Drugs used for regulating or controlling the reproductive system are often naturally occurring hormones or chemical modifications of hormones. **Gonadotropin-releasing hormone** and its analogs are used for treatment of ovarian cysts in cattle, for estrus induction (by pulsatile administration) in mares and bitches, and for stimulation of testicular function (eg, in testing for cryptorchidism). Implants of slow-release analogs (eg, deslorelin) are effective for induction of estrus and ovulation in mares and bitches. **Follicle-stimulating hormone** (FSH), usually extracted from animal pituitary glands, stimulates follicular growth and estrogen production in the female and spermatogenesis in the male. It is used for superovulation of several domestic species. It has also found application in induction of fertile estrus in bitches and queens. Prolonged FSH use or higher doses can cause adverse effects such as cystic endometrial hyperplasia and follicular cysts. **Human chorionic gonadotropin** (hCG), which exerts mainly luteinizing-hormone-like effects in domestic animals, is used for stimulation of gonads (as a test for cryptorchidism and also for the treatment of ovarian cysts in cattle or dogs). hCG is given parenterally; plasma levels peak in ~6 hr. It is primarily distributed to the ovaries in females and the testes in males, although some is also distributed to the renal proximal tubules. **Equine chorionic gonadotropin** has FSH activity in most species and is used to induce ovarian follicular growth, both for superovulation and for estrus induction. *See also* HORMONAL CONTROL OF ESTRUS, p 1808, and MANAGEMENT OF REPRODUCTION, p 1747 et seq.

Estradiol esters (eg, valerate, cypionate, or propionate) have a longer duration of action than the parent compound. These compounds are used in bitches, mares, and cows for induction of fertile estrus; treatment of urinary incontinence in bitches; and for antitumor activity in prostatic and perianal tumors. Estrogenic therapy may cause bone marrow suppression and potentially fatal aplastic anemia in dogs and cats; its use is also associated with development of cystic endometrial hyperplasia in these species, and it may have teratogenic effects in pregnant animals. Because of these potential complications, estrogens are no longer recommended for termination of pregnancy in cases of mismating. The nonsteroidal synthetic compound **diethylstilbestrol** also has estrogenic activity; its use is prohibited in food animals in the USA. Estrogen antagonists, such as tamoxifen, have been proposed for treatment of metastatic mammary carcinoma in dogs.

Progesterone and **synthetic progestins** are used for suppression or postponement of estrus in bitches and queens. They have also been used in behavior modification and for treatment of dermatologic disorders. Progesterone supplementation is used to support pregnancies regarded as at risk (eg, in pregnant mares with potentially endotoxemic conditions). Side effects of progestin administration in small animals include induction of cystic endometrial hyperplasia, adrenocortical suppression, induction or exacerbation of diabetes mellitus, and mammary gland development. Mifepristone (a progesterone-receptor antagonist) has been used experimentally as a canine abortifacient; epostane, a progesterone-synthesis inhibitor, also terminates canine pregnancy.

Testosterone is used for estrus suppression (particularly in racing Greyhounds). Mibolerone, a weak androgenic steroid, is used to prevent estrus in bitches. It should not be used in Bedlington Terriers or cats, and it may exacerbate perianal tumors. Following PO administration, mibolerone is absorbed from the intestine, metabolized in the liver, and excreted in the urine and feces. Chronic administration of testosterone may cause testicular degeneration in male animals. Finasteride, a 5α-reductase inhibitor, prevents the conversion of testosterone to 5α-dihydrotestosterone, the active androgen in male accessory sex glands. It is useful in the treatment of benign prostatic hyperplasia of dogs (0.1-0.5 mg/kg, PO, SID). Flutamide blocks dihydrotestosterone receptors and is used for the same purpose. Chemical modifications of testosterone potentiate its anabolic actions while minimizing virilizing effects. These compounds (eg, boldenone undecylenate, stanozolol, nandrolone decanoate) are used for their anabolic effects in convalescing or athletic animals. Protracted use may cause at least temporary infertility in both sexes.

Prostaglandin (PG) $F_{2\alpha}$ and its analogs are used mainly for their luteolytic effects to induce predictable onset of estrus (or synchronization of estrus) in a variety of species. They may also be used for termination of pregnancy either alone, or in combination with corticosteroids (cattle, sheep) or dopaminergic agents (dogs). These compounds also cause marked uterine contractions, which may be useful for expulsion of uterine contents in pathologic conditions (eg, pyometra).

Oxytocin is used to promote milk letdown, to treat agalactia, as an adjunctive treatment of mastitis, and to cause contraction of the uterus either to induce (or supplement) labor or to enhance postpartum uterine contraction and expulsion of uterine fluid or fetal membranes. It is administered parenterally (IV, IM, or SC). Oxytocin may be given intranasally but absorption can be erratic. Uterine relaxation is caused by β_2-mimetic agents, such as clenbuterol. Such agents have been used for postponing parturition (to reduce obstetrical complications in heifers) and for facilitating obstetrical manipulations in large domestic animals. Clenbuterol use in animals is illegal in the USA.

Dopaminergic agents, such as bromocriptine or cabergoline, cause decreased serum prolactin concentrations. They are useful in treatment of pseudopregnancy in dogs (bromocriptine: 10 µg/kg, PO, for 10 days, or 30 µg/kg for 16 days) and as an adjunct to $PGF_{2\alpha}$ in terminating pregnancy, although not approved in the USA for this use. Prolactin is luteotrophic in some species, including dogs. **Dopamine antagonists**, such as sulpiride, have shown promise in the manipulation of seasonal breeding species—their use hastens the onset of estrous cycles in mares in the spring. In the UK and New Zealand, **melatonin** is labeled for use in sheep (and goats in New Zealand) to improve early breeding and ovulation rates. It is available as an 18-mg SC implant; combined with exposure to rams, its use is associated with hastened onset of the breeding season and increased prolificacy.

Glucocorticoids, especially the C-16 substituted steroids dexamethasone, betamethasone, and flumethasone, are used for induction of parturition in ruminants (eg, dexamethasone 20-30 mg, IM, given within 2 wk of normal term). Their therapeutic administration may inadvertently lead to abortion. Xylazine and other α_2-adrenergic agents cause myometrial contraction that may harm the fetus or impede obstetrical manipulations.

Effect of Reproductive Therapy on the Fetus or Neonate

An important component of reproductive pharmacology encompasses the effect of treatment on the fetus or neonate of medication administered to pregnant or lactating animals that are nursing. Many factors influence the ability of a drug to cross the placenta, including placental architecture of the particular species, but in general, drugs that are lipid-soluble, nonionized, and of low molecular weight can be expected to cross the placenta readily. Among antimicrobials, aminoglycosides are associated with nephrotoxicity and ototoxicity in the fetus, fluoroquinolones may affect developing cartilage, and tetracyclines affect bone and tooth development. Teratogenicity has been associated with the use of the antifungal agents griseofulvin and ketoconazole in pregnant animals. All cancer chemotherapeutic agents are potentially harmful to developing fetuses. Glucocorticoids may induce palatoschisis or other defects in puppies.

Any administration of medication to lactating animals requires consideration of the excretion of the drug or its metabolites in milk and of the effects on suckling neonates. Milk produced for human consumption must be free of potentially harmful residues, and all relevant laws and regulations regarding usage and appropriate withdrawal times should be followed.

SYSTEMIC PHARMACOTHERAPEUTICS OF THE RESPIRATORY SYSTEM

See also PRINCIPLES OF THERAPY, RESPIRATORY SYSTEM, p 1175.

Drugs used to treat respiratory conditions fall into several categories: antitussives, bronchodilators, expectorants, decongestants, and respiratory stimulants. In addition, antimicrobials and anti-inflammatory drugs are important in the therapy of many respiratory diseases.

ANTITUSSIVE DRUGS

The afferent arc of the cough reflex receives input from sensory nerves in the bronchial and tracheal airways. Airway irritation and inflammation stimulate the afferent nerves, which in turn activate the cough center located in the medulla oblongata. Most of the antitussive drugs are opiates or opioids that directly suppress the cough center in the medulla oblongata (TABLE 22). The antitussive effect does not appear to be related to the binding of traditional opiate receptors. For example, dextromethorphan is an opiate derivative with good antitussive activity, but it does not have activity at opiate receptors and is not analgesic or addictive.

Morphine is an effective antitussive at doses lower than the doses that produce analgesia and sedation. It is not commonly used for antitussive activity due to side effects and the potential for abuse and addiction. Morphine has poor oral bioavailability due to a significant first-pass effect by the liver.

Codeine is methylmorphine; methylation of morphine significantly improves the oral bioavailability by reducing the first-pass effect. Codeine phosphate and codeine sulfate are found in many preparations, including tablets, liquids, and syrups. Codeine has

TABLE 22. Antitussive Drugs	
Drug	**Dosage**
Morphine	Dogs: 0.1 mg/kg, IM,TID-QID
Codeine	Dogs: 1-2 mg/kg, PO, BID-QID
Hydrocodone	Dogs: 0.25 mg/kg, PO, BID-QID
Dextromethorphan	Dogs, cats: 0.5-1 mg/kg, PO, TID-QID
Butorphanol	Dogs: 0.055-0.11 mg/kg, SC, BID-QID; or 0.055-1.1 mg/kg, PO, BID-QID

analgesic effects that are about one-tenth that of morphine, but its antitussive potency is about equal to that of morphine. The side effects of codeine are significantly less than those seen with morphine at antitussive doses. Toxicity (especially in cats) is exhibited as excitement, muscular spasms, convulsions, respiratory depression, sedation, and constipation. Codeine should not be used after GI tract surgery. The potential for addiction and abuse of codeine is considerably lower than that for morphine.

Hydrocodone is chemically and pharmacologically similar to codeine but more potent. It is combined with an anticholinergic drug (homatropine) to discourage abuse by people. It can be prescribed for small animals but should be used with caution in cats.

Dextromethorphan is technically not considered an opiate because it does not bind to traditional opiate receptors and is not addictive or analgesic. It is the D-isomer of levorphanol. The L-isomer of levorphanol has addictive and analgesic properties. Dextromethorphan is the safest antitussive to use in cats and is reported to be more efficacious in cats than codeine.

Butorphanol, an opioid agonist-antagonist, is used as an analgesic and antitussive in dogs. It is more potent than morphine as an analgesic and more potent than codeine or dextromethorphan as an antitussive. It may produce considerable sedation. Because butorphanol has poor bioavailability, the oral dose in dogs is 10 times the SC dose. Its use in cats is controversial.

SYSTEMIC THERAPY OF AIRWAY DISEASE

β-Adrenergic Agonists

The β-adrenergic agonists have beneficial effects in the treatment of bronchoconstrictive respiratory tract diseases (TABLE 23). Bronchial smooth muscle is innervated by β_2-adrenergic receptors. Stimulation of these receptors leads to increased activity of the enzyme adenylate cyclase, increased cAMP, and relaxation of bronchial smooth muscle. Stimulation of β receptors on mast cells decreases the release of inflammatory mediators from mast cells, but other inflammatory cells are not suppressed. There is some evidence that β-adrenergic receptor agonists increase mucociliary clearance in the respiratory tract.

Epinephrine (adrenaline) stimulates α and β receptors, resulting in pronounced vasopressive and cardiac effects in addition to bronchodilation. Epinephrine is reserved for emergency treatment of life-threatening bronchoconstriction (eg, anaphylaxis). The nonspecific stimulation of other receptors and its short duration of action make it unsuitable for longterm use. Epinephrine is available as a 1 mg/mL solution. Its onset of action is immediate, and the duration of effect is 1-3 hr.

Isoproterenol is a potent β-receptor agonist. It is selective for β receptors, but cardiac (β_1) effects make it unsuitable for longterm use. It is administered by inhalation or

TABLE 23. β-Adrenergic Receptor Agonist Drugs

Drug	Dosage
Epinephrine	Dogs: 0.05-0.5 mg, intratracheally or IV Cats: 0.1 mg, IV or IM Large animals: 0.1 mg/kg, IV, SC, or IM
Isoproterenol	Dogs: 0.1-0.2 mg, IM or SC, QID Cats: 4-6 µg, IM, every 30 min as needed Horses: 0.4 µg/kg, IV (diluted)
Terbutaline	Dogs, cats: 0.1 mg/kg, SC, every 4 hr, or 0.03 mg/kg, PO, TID Horses: 0.0033 mg/kg, IV, or 0.2-0.6 mg/kg, PO, BID
Albuterol	Dogs: 0.05 mg/kg, PO, TID Horses: 8 µg/kg, PO, BID
Clenbuterol	Horses: 0.8-3.2 µg/kg, PO, BID

injection and has a short duration of action (<1 hr). For emergency relief of bronchoconstriction in horses, it is given by slow IV solution at a dilution of 0.2 mg/50 mL of saline. Administration is discontinued when the heart rate doubles.

Terbutaline is a β_2-receptor agonist, similar to isoproterenol but longer acting (6-8 hr). For cats that experience frequent, severe bronchoconstrictive episodes while on chronic glucocorticoid therapy, injectable terbutaline can be dispensed to clients with instructions to administer 0.01 mg/kg, SC, to abort episodes at home within ~15 min. An increase in the cat's heart rate to 240 bpm and a 50% decrease in respiratory rate indicates a positive effect. Terbutaline can also be given as chronic oral therapy at 0.625 mg/cat, BID ($\frac{1}{4}$ of a 2.5 mg tablet). It should not be used in cats with hypertrophic cardiomyopathy or glaucoma, in which β_2-receptor stimulation would be detrimental. It may be used concurrently with methylxanthine bronchodilators. **Albuterol** (salbutamol) is similar to terbutaline and is used systemically in dogs and horses.

Clenbuterol is used in the treatment of recurrent airway inflammation (RAI) in horses. Results of efficacy studies for bronchoconstriction have been conflicting, but clenbuterol appears to significantly increase mucociliary transport in horses with RAI. The dosage is increased gradually until a satisfactory clinical response is seen. If there is no response at the highest recommended dose, the horse is considered to have irreversible bronchospasm. The most common adverse effects are tachycardia and muscle tremors. Clenbuterol inhibits uterine contractions, so it should be used during late pregnancy only if this effect is desired for obstetric manipulations. Clenbuterol is also a repartitioning agent; it directs nutrients away from adipose tissue and toward muscle. The result is increased carcass weight, increased ratio of muscle to fat, and increased feed efficiency. Because there is a significant human health risk from clenbuterol residues, it is banned in food animals and should not be used in horses that may be sent to slaughter.

Methylxanthines

The methylxanthines, particularly theophylline, are used as bronchodilators (TABLE 24). Once the mainstay of human asthma therapy, theophylline has a high incidence of side effects, and its use has diminished with the development of local drug delivery by metered dose or disk inhalers. The methylxanthines have a variety of pharmacologic effects on various organ systems, including bronchial smooth muscle relaxation, CNS stimulation, mild diuresis, and mild cardiac stimulation.

The respiratory effects of methylxanthines are due to several cellular mechanisms. Antagonism of adenosine is currently thought to be the most important action. Adenosine induces bronchoconstriction in asthmatic animals and antagonizes adenylate cyclase. Adenylate cyclase is responsible for the synthesis of cAMP, which controls bronchial smooth muscle relaxation and inhibits the release of inflammatory mediators from mast cells. Methylxanthines also inhibit phosphodiesterase, which further increases intracellular cAMP. They also inhibit calcium mobilization in smooth muscle, inhibit prostaglandin production, augment the release of catecholamines from storage granules, and increase the availability of calcium to contractile proteins of the heart and diaphragm. In addition to promoting bronchial smooth muscle relaxation, methylxanthines decrease the release of inflammatory mediators from mast cells and increase mucociliary transport.

Theophylline is available in several formulations including injectable, aqueous solutions, elixirs, tablets, and capsules. Theophylline base is poorly soluble in water and often results in GI irritation when administered PO. Aminophylline is a theophylline salt that is 78-86% theophylline. It is more water soluble and results in less GI irritation. Other theophylline salts, such as oxytriphylline (a choline salt), are available, and their theophylline content must be considered when developing a drug dosage regimen. Several sustained-release formulations of theophylline are suitable for use in dogs and cats and may be administered less frequently than the regular formulations. After oral administration, theophylline is rapidly and completely absorbed. Therapeutic plasma concentrations, extrapolated from people, are 5-20 μg/mL. Animals are sensitive to high concentrations of theophylline, especially after rapid IV administration, and toxicity may be seen with concentrations <20 μg/mL. Theophylline tablets may become trapped in bezoars (such as hair balls in cats), and

TABLE 24. Methylxanthine Bronchodilators

Drug	Dosage
Theophylline (parenteral)	Dogs: 10 mg/kg, IV (slow) or IM Horses: 15 mg/kg, IV (slow)
Theophylline (oral)	Dogs: 5-7 mg/kg, PO, TID Cats: 3 mg/kg, PO, BID Horses: 10-15 mg/kg, PO, BID
Theophylline (extended-release tablets)	Dogs: 20 mg/kg, PO, SID Cats: 25 mg/kg, PO, SID Horses: 15 mg/kg, PO, SID
Aminophylline (parenteral)	Dogs: 10 mg/kg, IV (slow) Cats, horses: 5 mg/kg, IV (slow)
Aminophylline (oral)	Dogs: 10 mg/kg, PO, TID Cats: 5 mg/kg, PO, BID Horses: 15 mg/kg, PO, BID

continued absorption can result in toxicity. Cardiac arrhythmias, CNS excitement, tremors, convulsions, and GI irritation may be seen. Theophylline undergoes enterohepatic recirculation, so activated charcoal is recommended if clinical signs are present, no matter how long after the drug was administered. Theophylline metabolism is inhibited by erythromycin, cimetidine, propranolol, and fluoroquinolones; concomitant therapy can result in theophylline toxicity. Theophylline metabolism is induced by rifampin and phenobarbital, which may necessitate increasing the dose of theophylline.

Theophylline is used for the treatment of both cardiac and respiratory diseases in dogs and cats. Theophylline is also used in the management of intrathoracic collapsing trachea and various forms of bronchitis in dogs. Theophylline and aminophylline were used in horses in the management of RAI, but efficacy was often poor and their use has been replaced by β-agonist bronchodilators. There is little clinical experience with the use of theophylline in cattle; experimental evidence suggests that it is a poor bronchodilator in this species.

Anticholinergic Drugs

The anticholinergic (parasympatholytic) drugs are effective bronchodilators that act by reducing the sensitivity of irritant receptors and by inhibiting vagally mediated cholinergic smooth muscle tone in the respiratory tract. Cholinergic stimulation causes bronchoconstriction; asthmatic individuals appear to have excessive stimulation of cholinergic receptors.

Atropine is primarily used as a preanesthetic, to prevent bradycardia and reduce airway secretions, and as emergency therapy of dyspneic animals with organophosphate intoxication. Atropine is also used for acute bronchodilation in horses, in which a low IV dosage (0.014 mg/kg) is more effective and less toxic than IV theophylline. A test dose of 0.022 mg/kg may also be used to determine prognosis in horses with RAI; if pulmonary function does not improve with a test dose of atropine, successful management with bronchodilators is unlikely. Atropine should be used with caution, as even low doses may cause tachycardia, ileus, neurologic derangement, and blurred vision in horses.

Glycopyrrolate is twice as potent as atropine in people and does not cross the blood-brain barrier. Its onset of action is slower than atropine, but its duration of effect is longer. Information about use in horses is sparse, but doses of 2-3 mg can be given IM, BID-TID.

Glucocorticoids

The glucocorticoids inhibit the release of inflammatory mediators from macrophages and eosinophils but do not inhibit the release of granules from mast cells. Glucocorticoids decrease synthesis of prostaglandins, leukotrienes, and platelet-activating factor, which play important roles in the pathophysiology of respiratory tract diseases. Studies suggest glucocorticoids enhance the action of adrenergic agonists on β_2 receptors in the bronchial smooth muscle. Because of immunosuppressive effects, glucocorticoids are generally avoided in infectious respiratory diseases.

For severe attacks of allergic bronchitis, asthma, or RAI, parenteral injection of glucocorticoids usually provides rapid relief. For chronic therapy in small animals, oral prednisone is usually the drug of choice. Prednisone is a prodrug, as it is hepatically metabolized to the active drug prednisolone. Only animals with severe hepatic impairment and horses are unable to metabolize prednisone to prednisolone. A typical anti-inflammatory dosage is 0.5-1.0 mg/kg, with chronic therapy on an every-other-day basis. Cats are somewhat resistant to the effects of glucocorticoids, and dosages of prednisone of 1.0 mg/kg/day may be necessary for chronic therapy of feline asthma. Alternatively, 20 mg of methylprednisolone acetate can be administered IM to asthmatic cats every 3 wk. For emergency treatment of dyspneic cats, a shock dose of an IV glucocorticoid (prednisone sodium succinate, 5-10 mg/kg; or dexamethasone sodium phosphate, 1-2 mg/kg) should be used. Prednisone has a low oral bioavailability in horses. After administration of prednisone, only negligible plasma concentrations of prednisone or prednisolone are measured. While prednisolone can be administered to horses, the small tablet sizes available make it inconvenient, so equine formulations of oral dexamethasone are recommended. The injectable formulation of dexamethasone can be given IV to horses with acute bronchoconstriction and dyspnea.

Cyproheptadine

Because of serotonin's role in allergen-induced bronchoconstriction in cats, the serotonin antagonist cyproheptadine (2 mg, PO, SID-BID) may be used as an adjunct to glucocorticoids and bronchodilators to block bronchoconstriction in chronically asthmatic cats. Because of its long elimination half-life (12 hr), it requires several days to reach steady-state concentrations and may take 4-7 days to be clinically effective. Cyproheptadine's serotonin antagonism in the appetite center stimulates appetite, so weight gain may be a problem. Lethargy, depression, and increased appetite may be seen within 24 hr of initiating therapy.

Cyclosporine

Cyclosporine can be administered to asthmatic cats as an adjunct to glucocorticoid therapy because of its inhibitory effect on activated T lymphocytes. Although its adverse effects are less severe in cats than in humans, cyclosporine is typically reserved for use in cats with severe signs despite high-dose glucocorticoid therapy. It is initially given at 10 mg/kg, PO, BID, but oral absorption is unpredictable, so weekly therapeutic drug monitoring needs to be performed until trough blood concentrations of 500-1,000 ng/mL are reached. Therapeutic drug monitoring for cyclosporine can be done at most human hospitals.

Antileukotriene Drugs

Leukotriene receptor antagonist and 5-lipoxygenase inhibitor drugs are available for chronic asthma therapy in humans. These drugs are not bronchodilators and are not used for acute bronchoconstriction. They antagonize or inhibit 5-lipoxygenase, the enzyme that catalyzes the formation of leukotrienes from arachidonic acid. Leukotrienes produce numerous biologic effects that contribute to inflammation, edema, mucus secretion, and bronchoconstriction in the airways of human asthmatics. In normal cats, however, leukotrienes do not cause bronchoconstriction. In an experimental asthmatic cat model, a 5-lipoxygenase inhibitor had no effect on bronchoconstriction, suggesting that the antileukotriene drugs are of questionable benefit to asthmatic cats. These drugs may be beneficial in horses or dogs, but clinical trials have not been reported in the veterinary literature.

Antimicrobial Therapy

Antimicrobial therapy may or may not be necessary in the treatment of airway inflammatory diseases. Antimicrobial therapy should only be started for cats with tracheobronchial cultures suggestive of a true bacterial infection or those positive for *Mycoplasma*. *Mycoplasma* spp can be isolated from normal dogs but are not found in normal cats. Doxycycline, azithromycin, and fluoroquinolones are effective for treating *Mycoplasma* infections. Secondary bacterial infection from *Streptococcus zooepidemicus* may exacerbate inflammatory airway disease in horses and can easily be treated with penicillin, ceftiofur, or a trimethoprim/sulfonamide.

INHALATION THERAPY OF AIRWAY DISEASE

With inhalation therapy, high drug concentrations are delivered directly to the lungs via nebulizers or metered-dose inhalers (MDI), and systemic side effects are avoided or minimized. The onset of action for inhaled bronchodilators and anti-inflammatory drugs is substantially shorter than that of oral or parenteral formulations. Nebulizers have long been used in animals, but the overall efficiency of dug delivery is low and the equipment is cumbersome and inconvenient for owners. Administration of medications via MDI is now commonplace in the treatment of human asthma and appears to be beneficial in the management of animals as well. Human MDI are designed to provide optimal lung delivery following actuation during a slow, deep inhalation. The addition of spacers enables MDI to be used in young children and small animals. Spacers decrease the amount of drug deposited in the oropharynx (up to 80% of the actuated dose with the MDI alone), reducing systemic drug absorption. Equine delivery devices allow MDI to be used in horses. Clinical use in asthmatic cats, dogs with chronic bronchitis, and horses with RAI is promising but anecdotal; clinical trials are needed to determine the most effective therapies. Drugs available in MDI formulations include β_2 agonists, glucocorticoids, ipratropium bromide, cromolyn sodium, and nedocromil.

β_2 Agonists

Short-acting β_2 agonists such as **albuterol** (salbutamol) in MDI are the medications of choice for treating acute exacerbations of bronchoconstriction, as they relax smooth muscle and promptly increase airflow. While effective for symptomatic relief, β_2 agonists do not control inflammation. Monotherapy may exacerbate airway disease and has been proved to increase morbidity and mortality in human asthmatics. Tolerance may develop with chronic therapy.

Salmeterol is a long-acting β_2 agonist; its onset of action is slow (15-30 min) but its duration of action is >12 hr. It is not recommended for use in acute bronchoconstriction, but daily use with glucocorticoids provides better control than just increasing the glucocorticoid dose.

Glucocorticoids

Inhaled glucocorticoids are the most potent inhaled anti-inflammatory drugs available. In humans, early intervention with inhaled glucocorticoids improves asthma control, normalizes ling function, and may prevent irreversible airway damage. The potential risk of adverse effects is well balanced by their efficacy in management of chronic inflammation. Oral candidiasis (thrush), dysphonia, and reflex cough and bronchospasm are the most common adverse effects in humans; all of these effects are reduced by the use of a spacer. The risk of systemic side effects, such as suppression of the hypothalamic-pituitary axis, is less than with oral prednisone therapy. Inhaled glucocorticoid formulations include fluticasone, beclomethasone, flunisolide, and triamcinolone. Currently, fluticasone is considered the most potent formulation with the longest duration of action.

Ipratropium Bromide

Ipratropium bromide is a quaternary derivative of atropine that lacks its adverse effects and is available in an MDI (500 µg/actuation). In asthmatic humans, ipratropium bromide is used as an additional reliever medication to reverse bronchoconstriction when inhaled short-acting β_2 agonists do not provide enough relief. Its anticholinergic action also decreases mucous secretions. In an experimental model of feline asthma, longterm antigen senstization caused an augmented muscarinic receptor response to acetylcholine. Modulation of muscarinic receptors with anticholinergic drugs may be useful for treatment of asthmatic cats. Currently, there are no published reports of the use of ipratropium in cats, however it has shown efficacy for RAI in horses. It is not well absorbed after inhalation and, therefore, does not cause systemic cholinergic effects.

Cromolyn Sodium and Nedocromil

Cromolyn sodium and nedocromil sodium are chloride-channel blockers that modulate mast cell mediator release and eosinophil recruitment. They are both available in MDI. Cromolyn sodium and nedocromil sodium have strong human safety profiles, but nedocromil sodium has been reported to have a broader spectrum of efficacy. In humans, the clinical response to both drugs is less predictable than the response to glucocorticoids. There are no published reports of the use of cromolyn or nedocromil in asthmatic cats or dogs with bronchitis; however, pretreatment with nedocromil sodium aerosols attenuated viral-induced airway inflammation in Beagle puppies. Further investigation of these drugs in asthmatic cats seems warranted given the sensitivity of cats to serotonin released from degranulating mast cells.

EXPECTORANTS AND MUCOLYTIC DRUGS

Expectorants and mucolytic drugs are used to increase the output of bronchial secretions, enhance the clearance of bronchial exudate, and promote a productive cough. Saline expectorants are promoted to stimulate bronchial mucous secretions via a vagally mediated reflex action on the gastric mucosa. However, there are no well-designed studies that support these claims. Examples of these drugs include ammonium chloride, ammonium carbonate, potassium iodide, calcium iodide, and ethylenediamine dihydroiodide. Iodine-containing products should not be administered to pregnant, hyperthyroid, or milk-producing animals.

Direct stimulants of respiratory secretions include the volatile oils, such as eucalyptus oil and oil of lemon. They are believed to directly increase respiratory tract secretions. Their efficacy in animals is unknown.

Guaifenesin (glyceryl guaiacolate) is a centrally acting muscle relaxant that may also have an expectorant effect. It may stimulate bronchial secretions via vagal pathways. The volume and viscosity of bronchial secretions does not change, but particle clearance from the airways may accelerate. It is a common component of human cold remedies in combination with dextromethorphan.

N-acetylcysteine is available as a 10% solution that can be nebulized. Its mucolytic effect is due to the exposed sulfhydryl groups on the compound, which interact with disulfide bonds on mucoprotein. Acetylcysteine helps to break down respiratory mucus and enhance clearance. Acetylcysteine may also increase the levels of glutathione, which is a scavenger of oxygen-free radicals. Aerosolization of acetylcysteine can cause reflex bronchoconstriction due to irritant receptor stimulation, so its use should be preceded by bronchodilator therapy.

Dembrexine is a phenolic benzylamine available in some countries for respiratory disease in horses. The proposed effect is through an alteration of the constituents and viscosity of abnormal respiratory mucus and an improved efficiency of respiratory clearance mechanisms. It also has an antitussive action and enhances concentrations of antibiotics in lung secretions. It is supplied as a powder that is sprinkled on the feed at a dosage of 0.33 mg/kg, BID.

DECONGESTANTS

Decongestants are commonly used in people for allergic rhinitis, but they are rarely used for this purpose in animals. The α-adrenergic agonist drugs cause local vasoconstriction in mucous membranes, which reduces swelling and edema. They are used topically as nasal decongestants in allergic and viral rhinitis, or systemically in combination with antihistamines as respiratory tract decongestants. Antihistamines are effective for treatment of allergic rhinitis in people when combined with the α-adrenergic agonist drugs, but their effectiveness in animals has not been demonstrated. The topical α-adrenergic agonist drugs act within minutes with few side effects, but extended use may cause rebound hyperemia and mucosal damage. Systemic administration can result in hypertension, cardiac stimulation, urinary retention, CNS stimulation, and mydriasis. Systemic administration of antihistamines often causes sedation.

RESPIRATORY STIMULANTS

Doxapram stimulates the medullary respiratory center and the chemoreceptors of the carotid artery and aorta to increase tidal volume. Other portions of the CNS are stimulated only when high doses are administered. Doxapram is primarily used in emergency situations during anesthesia or to decrease the respiratory depressant effects of opiates and barbiturates. Recommended dosages are 1-5 mg/kg, IV, in dogs and cats, or 1-2 drops under the tongue of apneic neonates. In adult horses, the dosage is 0.5-1.0 mg/kg, IV, while foals are dosed carefully at 0.02-0.05 mg/kg/min, IV.

SYSTEMIC PHARMACOTHERAPEUTICS OF THE URINARY SYSTEM

See also PRINCIPLES OF THERAPY, URINARY SYSTEM, p 1252.

BACTERIAL URINARY TRACT INFECTIONS

Bacterial urinary tract infections (UTI) typically result from normal skin and GI tract flora ascending the urinary tract and overcoming the normal urinary tract defenses that prevent colonization. Bacterial UTI is the most common infectious disease of dogs, affecting 14% of all dogs during their lifetime. It is less common in cats, and is seen only infrequently in large animals. Young cats with feline lower urinary tract disease usually have bacteriologically sterile urine. However, 50% of geriatric cats with urinary tract disease have a bacterial UTI. Approximately two-thirds of those cats also have renal failure. Unlike humans, animals are often asymptomatic, and the UTI may be an incidental finding. The consequences of untreated UTI include lower urinary tract dysfunction, urolithiasis, prostatitis, infertility, septicemia, and pyelonephritis with scarring and eventual kidney failure. Coagulase-positive staphylococci are involved in the formation of struvite ($MgNH_4PO_4$) calculi in dogs. In intact male dogs, UTI frequently extends to the prostate gland. Due to the blood-prostate barrier, it is difficult to eradicate bacteria from the prostate, and the urinary tract may be reinfected following appropriate treatment, causing a systemic bacteremia, infecting the rest of the reproductive tract, or causing an abscess within the prostate.

Antimicrobials are the cornerstone of UTI therapy, and many animals with recurring UTI are managed empirically with repeated courses (TABLE 25). This approach fails if the underlying pathophysiology predisposing the animal to the UTI is not addressed; as well, it encourages the development of resistant bacteria. With chronic UTI from highly resistant bacteria, therapeutic options are extremely limited.

Antimicrobial Therapy

Urine concentrations of antimicrobials are more important than plasma concentrations. Clinical efficacy correlates with maintaining urine antimicrobial concentrations that are 4 times the minimum inhibitory concentration (MIC) of the pathogen(s) throughout the dosage interval. Most antimicrobials undergo renal elimination to a great extent, so urine concentrations may be up to 100 times peak plasma concentrations. Drugs

TABLE 25. Drugs Commonly Used to Treat Urinary Tract Infections in Small Animals

Drug	Dosage	Typical Antimicrobial Activity	Mean Urine Concentration (µg/mL)
Amoxicillin	11 mg/kg, PO, TID	Staphylococci, streptococci, enterococci, *Proteus*	201
Ampicillin	25 mg/kg, PO, TID	Staphylococci, streptococci, enterococci, *Proteus*	309
Amoxicillin/ clavulanic acid	25 mg/kg, PO, TID	Staphylococci, streptococci, enterococci, *Proteus*	201
Cephalexin/ cefadroxil	30 mg/kg, PO, TID	Staphylococci, streptococci, *Proteus*, *Escherichia coli*, *Klebsiella*	500
Ceftiofur	2.0 mg/kg, SC, SID	*E coli*, *Proteus*	8
Enrofloxacin	5 mg/kg, PO, SID	Staphylococci, some strepto-cocci, some enterococci, *E coli*, *Proteus*, *Klebsiella*, *Pseudomonas*, *Enterobacter*	200
Gentamicin	4-6 mg/kg, SC, SID	Staphylococci, some strepto-cocci, some enterococci, *E coli*, *Proteus*, *Klebsiella*, *Pseudomonas*, *Enterobacter*	107
Nitrofurantoin	5 mg/kg, PO, TID	Staphylococci, some strepto-cocci, some enterococci, *E coli*, *Klebsiella*, *Enterobacter*	100
Tetracycline	18 mg/kg, PO, TID	Streptococci, some activity against staphylococci and enterococci at high urine con-centrations	300
Trimethoprim/ sulfa	15 mg/kg, PO, BID	Streptococci, staphylococci, *E coli*, *Proteus*, some activity against enterococci and *Kleb-siella*	55/246

such as the penicillins and tetracycline may be effective against gram-negative pathogens in the urinary tract, even when they would be ineffective elsewhere in the body.

In addition to having the appropriate antimicrobial activity and achieving effective concentrations in urine, the selected antimicrobial should be easy for clients to administer, have few adverse effects, and be relatively inexpensive. Once urine culture and sensitiv-ity results are known, the bacterial MIC can be compared with the mean urinary concen-tration of the drug and an appropriate antimicrobial chosen.

Amoxicillin and **ampicillin** are bactericidal and relatively nontoxic, with a spec-trum of antibacterial activity greater than that of penicillin G. They have excellent activ-ity against staphylococci, streptococci, enterococci, and *Proteus*, and may achieve urinary concentrations high enough to be effective against *E coli* and *Klebsiella*. *Pseudomonas* and *Enterobacter* are resistant. Amoxicillin is more bioavailable in dogs and cats (better absorbed from the GI tract) than ampicillin, hence the lower dosage. Absorption of ampi-cillin is also affected by feeding, so therapeutic success may be easier to achieve with amoxicillin. As penicillins, they are weak acids with a low volume of distribution, so they do not achieve therapeutic concentrations in prostatic fluid of dogs or accessory sex glands of large animals.

Amoxicillin/clavulanic acid has an increased spectrum of activity against gram-negative bacteria due to the presence of clavulanic acid. Clavulanic acid irreversibly binds to β-lactamases, allowing the amoxicillin fraction to interact with the bacterial pathogen. This combination usually has excellent batericidal activity against β-lactamase producing staphylococci, *E coli*, and *Klebsiella*. *Pseudomonas* and *Enterobacter* remain resistant. However, clavulanic acid undergoes some hepatic metabolism and excretion, so much of the antimicrobial activity in the bladder may be due to the high concentrations of amoxicillin achieved in urine. Thus, despite an unfavorable susceptibility report for amoxicillin, clinically it may be as effective as amoxicillin/clavulanic acid in treating UTI.

Cefadroxil and **cephalexin** are first-generation cephalosporins. Both are available in tablet and liquid formulations that are used in small animals. Cefadroxil is the veterinary-labeled product, while cephalexin is a human formulation. Like the penicillins, they are bactericidal, acidic drugs with a low volume of distribution and are relatively nontoxic. Vomiting and other GI signs may develop in dogs and cats treated with cephalosporins. Cephalosporins have greater stability to β-lactamases than penicillins, so they have greater activity against staphylococci and gram-negative bacteria. They have excellent activity against *Staphylococcus*, *Streptococcus*, *E coli*, *Proteus*, and *Klebsiella*. *Pseudomonas*, enterococci, and *Enterobacter* are resistant.

Ceftiofur is an injectable cephalosporin approved for respiratory disease in horses and cattle and for treatment of canine UTI caused by *E coli* and *Proteus*. Ceftiofur has pharmacokinetic properties that are very different from other cephalosporins. After injection, ceftiofur is immediately metabolized to desfuroylceftiofur, which has different antimicrobial activity than the parent compound. Desfuroylceftiofur has equivalent activity to ceftiofur against *E coli* (MIC 4 µg/mL), but is much less active against *Staphylococcus* and has variable activity against *Proteus* (MIC 0.5-16 µg/mL). Due to instability of desfuroylceftiofur, microbiology services use a ceftiofur disk when performing susceptibility testing, so a false expectation of therapeutic efficacy may result for some pathogens. *Pseudomonas*, enterococci, and *Enterobacter* are resistant to ceftiofur and desfuroylceftiofur. Ceftiofur is associated with a duration and dose-related thrombocytopenia and anemia in dogs, which would not be expected with the recommended dosage regimen.

Enrofloxacin, orbifloxacin, difloxacin, and **marbofloxacin** are all fluoroquinolones approved for UTI in dogs; although all are used in cats, only some are approved for this use. The fluoroquinolones are bactericidal, amphoteric drugs. They possess acidic and basic properties but are very lipid soluble at physiologic pH (pH 6.0-8.0) and thus have a high volume of distribution. All fluoroquinolone drugs usually have excellent activity against staphylococci and gram-negative bacteria, but may have variable activity against streptococci and enterococci. The therapeutic advantages of these drugs are their gram-negative antimicrobial activity and high degree of lipid solubility. They are the only orally administered antimicrobials with efficacy against *Pseudomonas*. Therefore, fluoroquinolones should be reserved for UTI that involve gram-negative bacteria, especially *Pseudomonas*, and for UTI in intact male dogs because of their excellent penetration into the prostate gland and activity in abscesses. They are concentration-dependent killers with a long post-antibiotic effect, so once daily, high-dose therapy for a relatively short duration of treatment is effective. Fluoroquinolones should be avoided for chronic, low-dose therapy, as this encourages the emergence of resistant bacteria that are cross-resistant to other antimicrobial drugs as well. Cases that involve *Pseudomonas* should be carefully investigated for underlying pathology, which must corrected if at all possible. Once *Pseudomonas* spp become resistant to the fluoroquinolones, there are no other therapeutic options that are convenient for the animal and owner.

Gentamicin and the other aminoglycosides are very large polar (water soluble) molecules, so they have a low volume of distribution and do not penetrate the blood-prostate barrier. They are not absorbed orally and must be given by SC, IM, or IV injection. The aminoglycosides have a similar spectrum of activity to that of the fluoroquinolones, but their use for UTI is limited because of the necessity of parenteral injections and the risk of toxicity with anything but short-term use. Like the fluoroquinolones, the aminoglycosides are concentration-dependent, bactericidal killers with a long post-antibiotic effect, so once-daily therapy of short duration is effective and minimizes the risk of nephrotoxicity. They can be considered for in-hospital or outpatient treatment of UTI due to fluoroquinolone-resistant pathogens; however, the importance of identifying and correcting underlying pathology must be emphasized.

Nitrofurantoin is a human product available as tablets, capsules, and a pediatric suspension. It is not commonly used in veterinary medicine. It has a very low volume of distribution, and therapeutic concentrations are attained only in urine. It is used for infections caused by *E coli*, enterococci, staphylococci, *Klebsiella*, and *Enterobacter*.

Tetracyclines are bacteriostatic, amphoteric drugs with a high volume of distribution. Tetracyclines are broad-spectrum antmicrobials, but because of plasmid-mediated resistance, susceptibility is variable in staphylococci, enterococci, *Enterobacter*, *E coli*, *Klebsiella*, and *Proteus*. In most tissues, *Pseudomonas* spp are resistant. However, the tetracyclines are excreted unchanged in urine, so high urinary concentrations may result in therapeutic efficacy. Doxycycline is a very lipid-soluble tetracycline that is better tolerated in cats and achieves therapeutic concentrations in the prostate, but it is eliminated in bile and directly excreted into the intestine, so is not useful for most UTI.

Trimethoprim/sulfonamides (TMP/sulfas) are combinations of 2 very different drugs that act synergistically on different steps in the bacterial folic acid pathway. Trimethoprim is a bacteriostatic, basic drug that has a high volume of distribution and a short elimination half-life, while the sulfonamides are bacteriostatic, acidic drugs with a medium volume of distribution and long half-lives (ranging from 6 to >24 hr). These drugs are formulated in a 1:5 ratio of TMP to sulfa, although the optimal bactericidal concentration is a ratio of 1:20 TMP:sulfa. Microbiology services use the 1:20 ratio in susceptibility testing, however the widely varying pharmacokinetic properties of this drug combination make it difficult to determine a therapeutic regimen that achieves the 1:20 ratio at the infection site. Although the combination does penetrate the blood-prostate barrier, sulfa drugs are ineffective in purulent material because of freely available para-aminobenzoic acid from dead neutrophils. The combination of TMP/sulfa is synergistic and bactericidal against staphylococci, streptococci, *E coli*, and *Proteus*. Activity against enterococci and *Klebsiella* is variable and *Pseudomonas* is resistant. TMP/sulfas are associated with a number of adverse effects, and chronic low-dose therapy may result in bone marrow suppression and keratoconjunctivitis sicca in dogs.

Dosage Regimens for UTI

Therapy for a UTI is usually recommended for 7-21 days, depending on the animal (eg, intact vs neutered male dog), activity of the antimicrobial and concentration attained in the urine, and the relationship of patient pathology and pathogen virulence. The fluoroquinolones and aminoglycosides are generally effective with a short course of therapy, while the antimicrobials with time-dependent killing activity usually require a more prolonged course. Dogs with prostatitis or animals with complicating pathology (eg, pyelonephritis, cystic calculi) require 4-6 wk of treatment for microbiologic cure. In dogs, antimicrobials should be administered just before bedtime or confinement, to maintain high urine concentrations for the longest possible time.

A followup urine culture should be performed after 4-7 days, while the animal is still on therapy, to determine antimicrobial efficacy. If the same or a different pathogen is observed, then an alternative therapy should be chosen and the culture repeated again after 4-7 days. Urine should also be cultured 7-10 days after completing antimicrobial therapy to determine if the UTI is cured or has recurred.

Managing Multiple Episodes of UTI

If episodes occur only once or twice yearly, each may be treated as an acute, uncomplicated UTI. If they occur more often, and predisposing causes of UTI cannot be identified or corrected, chronic low-dose therapy may be necessary to manage the animal. Low antimicrobial concentrations in the urine may interfere with fimbriae production by some pathogens and prevent their adhesion to the uroepithelium.

Recurrent UTI are due to a different strain or species of bacteria about 80% of the time; therefore, antimicrobial culture and susceptibility testing is still indicated. Therapy should be started when urine culture is negative, and antimicrobial therapy should be continued SID at $^1/_3$ of the total daily dose. The antimicrobial should be administered at night to maximize antimicrobial concentration in the bladder. Appropriate antimicrobials for chronic, low-dose therapy include amoxicillin, ampicillin, amoxicillin-clavulanic acid, cephalexin, and cefadroxil. A trimethoprim/sulfa can be used in dogs, but folate supplementation should be provided (15 mg/kg, BID) to prevent bone marrow suppression, and there is the risk of keratoconjunctivitis sicca developing with chronic use. During chronic therapy, urine culture should be repeated every 4-6 wk. As long as the culture is negative, therapy is continued for 6 mo. If bacteriuria occurs, the infection is treated as an acute episode with an appropriate antimicrobial. After 6 mo of bacteria-free urine, the chronic low-dose antimicrobial therapy may be discontinued and many animals will not have additional recurrences. In some cases, chronic therapy may be continued for years in animals with recurrent UTI.

Therapeutic Failures

Although most UTI respond readily to initial antimicrobial therapy, some animals do not respond or suffer recurrent episodes. It should be considered whether the UTI is due to a relapse or a reinfection. Relapses are recurrences due to the same species of bacteria shortly after discontinuing antimicrobial therapy. Reasons for relapses include inappropriate antimicrobial choice, development of bacterial resistance, a mixed UTI in which all organisms were not eliminated, an inadequate dosage regimen (dose, duration, or frequency), or poor client adherence to the treatment regimen. In cases with sequestered infections, such as prostatitis or pyelonephritis, an appropriate antimicrobial may fail to reach adequate tissue concentrations. Reinfections are recurrent infections caused by different species of bacteria than previously involved in the UTI. Reasons for reinfection include impaired bacteriostatic nature of urine (eg, glucosuria), disruption of the uroepithelial barrier, reduced immunocompetence, altered urethral function or structure, and urinary retention. If these problems cannot be corrected, chronic antimicrobial therapy is required to prevent further episodes of UTI. Following cessation of antimicrobial therapy, reinfections usually occur at a longer interval than relapses.

Fungal Urinary Tract Infections

Although uncommon, most fungal UTI in dogs and cats are caused by *Candida* spp. Finding *Candida* organisms in the urine may indicate sample contamination; however, finding *Candida* organisms in 2 serial urine samples collected by cystocentesis is consistent with infection and warrants culture and definitive identification. Treatment includes eliminating potential predisposing factors (eg, excessive endogenous or exogenous corticosteroids, urinary catheters) and administering antifungal drugs with or without urinary alkalinization. Fluconazole is the antifungal drug of choice for the treatment of candidal cystitis. The dose in cats is 50 mg/cat, PO, SID-BID, and in dogs is 2.5-5.0 mg/kg/day, PO, divided BID. The duration of treatment needed to eliminate infection is unknown but may be as short as 7 days.

DIURETICS

Diuretics are used to remove inappropriate water in animals with edema or volume overload, correct specific ion imbalances, and reduce blood pressure and pulmonary capillary wedge pressure (TABLE 26). They are classified by their mechanism of action as loop diuretics, carbonic anhydrase inhibitors, thiazides, osmotic diuretics, and potassium-sparing diuretics. The efficacy and use of each class of diuretic depends on the mechanism and site of action. Patterns of electrolyte excretion vary between classes, while maximal response is the same within a class. Therefore, if one drug within a class is ineffective, a different drug from the same class will likely be ineffective as well. Combining diuretics from different classes lead to additive and potentially synergistic effects.

TABLE 26. Dosages of Diuretics

Drug	Dosage
Furosemide	4-6 mg/kg IV, IM, or SC for acute therapy Dogs: 2-4 mg/kg, PO, SID-TID Cats:1-2 mg/kg, PO, SID-BID Large animals: 0.5-1.0 mg/kg, IV or IM, SID
Hydrochlorothiazide	Dogs and cats: 2-4 mg/kg, PO, SID-BID
Chlorothiazide	Dogs and cats: 20-40 mg/kg, PO, SID-BID
Spironolactone	Dogs: 2-4 mg/kg, PO, BID
Mannitol	0.25-0.50 g/kg, IV
Dimethyl sulfoxide	Large animals: 1 g/kg, IV or via nasogastric tube

Furosemide

Furosemide is a sulfonamide derivative that is the most commonly administered diuretic. It is a loop diuretic—it inhibits the reabsorption of sodium and chloride in the thick, ascending loop of Henle, resulting in loss of sodium, chloride, and water into the urine. Furosemide induces beneficial hemodynamic effects prior to the onset of diuresis. Vasodilation increases renal blood flow, thereby increasing renal perfusion and lessening fluid retention. It appears that renal vasodilation depends on synthesis of local prostaglandins.

The elimination half-life of furosemide is short in most animals (~15 min). The effect peaks 30 min after IV administration and 1-2 hr after PO administration. The duration of diuretic action is 2 and 6 hr following IV and PO administration, respectively. Furosemide is highly protein bound (91-97%), almost totally to albumin. It is cleared through the kidneys by renal tubular secretion. Bioavailability of oral furosemide is low (only 50% is absorbed).

Furosemide is usually dosed to effect. For acute, short-term therapy, single IV, IM, or SC doses of 4-6 mg/kg are given. The major adverse effect from acute administration of large doses is acute intravascular volume reduction, which worsens cardiac output and hypotension and may precipitate acute renal failure. Chronic therapy in cats and some dogs can be accomplished by therapy every second or third day. Higher than normal doses may be required in animals with renal disease due to functional abnormalities of the renal tubule and binding of furosemide to protein in the urine. If the animal requires escalating doses of furosemide to control fluid retention, adding other types of volume-modifying medications, such as a potassium-sparing diuretic or an angiotensin-converting enzyme (ACE) inhibitor, may help avoid adverse effects.

Furosemide therapy is associated with a number of adverse effects. By nature of its mechanism of action, it causes dehyration, volume depletion, hypokalemia, and hyponatremia, which may be excessive and detrimental. The high degree of protein binding can lead to interactions with other highly protein-bound drugs, and any condition that alters albumin concentrations affects the concentration of free drug available for diuretic action. Furosemide's most important drug interaction is with the digitalis glycosides digoxin and digitoxin. The hypokalemia induced by furosemide diuresis potentiates digitalis toxicity. As long as animals continue to eat, hypokalemia does not usually develop. Hypokalemia also predisposes animals to hyponatremia by enhancing antidiuretic hormone secretion and the exchange of sodium ions for lost intracellular potassium ions. Concurrent administration of NSAID may interfere with prostanglandin-controlled renal vasodilation. Furosemide-induced dehydration of airway secretions may exacerbate respiratory disease.

Thiazide Diuretics

The thiazide diuretics, **hydrochlorothiazide and chlorothiazide**, are not as potent as furosemide and thus are infrequently used. The thiazides act on the proximal portion of the distal convoluted tubule to inhibit sodium resorption and promote potassium excretion. They may be administered to animals that cannot tolerate a potent loop diuretic such as furosemide. They should not be administered to azotemic animals, as they decrease renal blood flow. Because the thiazides act on a different site of the renal tubule than other diuretics, they may be combined with a loop diuretic or potassium-sparing diuretic in treating refractory fluid retention. Adverse effects are electrolyte and fluid balance disturbances, similar to furosemide.

Potassium-sparing Diuretics

Potassium-sparing diuretics include **spironolactone, amiloride**, and **triamterene** (available only in Canada). Spironolacton is used most frequently and is a competitive antagonist of aldosterone. Aldosterone is elevated in animals with congestive heart failure in which the renin-angiotensin system is activated in response to hyponatremia, hyperkalemia, and reductions in blood pressure or cardiac output. Aldosterone is responsible for increasing sodium and chloride reabsorption and potassium and calcium excretion from renal tubules. Spironolactone competes with aldosterone at its receptor site, causing a mild diuresis and potassium retention. Spironolactone is well absorbed after PO administration, especially if given with food. It is highly protein bound (>90%) and extensively metabolized by the liver to the active metabolite, canrenone. It is primarily eliminated by the kidneys. The onset of action for spironolactone is slow, and effects do not peak for 2-3 days. Spironolactone is not recommended as monotherapy, but can be added to furosemide or thiazide therapy to treat refractory heart failure cases. Because of the potential for hyperkalemia, spironolactone should not be administered concurrently with potassium supplements or ACE inhibitors.

Carbonic Anhydrase Inhibitors

Carbonic anhydrase inhibitors act in the proximal tubule to noncompetitively and reversibly inhibit carbonic anhydrase, which decreases the formation of carbonic acid from carbon dioxide and water. Reduced formation of carbonic acid results in fewer hydrogen ions within proximal tubule cells. Because hydrogen ions are normally exchanged with sodium ions from the tubule lumen, more sodium is available to combine with urinary bicarbonate. Diuresis occurs when water is excreted with sodium bicarbonate. As bicarbonate is eliminated, systemic acidosis results. Because intracellular potassium can substitute for hydrogen ions in the sodium resorption step, carbonic anhydrase inhibitors also enhance potassium excretion.

Osmotic Diuretics

Osmotic diuretics include **mannitol, dimethyl sulfoxide (DMSO), urea, glycerol**, and **isosorbide**. Mannitol is commonly used in small animals, but is expensive for use in adult large animals, so DMSO is often used. Mannitol acts as a protectant against further renal tubular damage and initiates an osmotic diuresis. The initial dosage is 0.25-0.50 g/kg, given IV over 3-5 min. A response should be noted within 20-30 min. If a response is seen, the dose can be repeated every 6-8 hr, or a constant rate infusion of 2-5 mL/min of a 5-10% solution can be given. The total daily dose should not exceed 2 g/kg. If a diuresis is not seen, the initial dose can be repeated up to a total dosage of 1.5-2 g/kg. However, repeated doses usually are not more effective and increase the likelihood of complications (eg, edema).

DMSO is an oxygen-derived free radical scavenger and an osmotic diuretic. It is used in large animals to treat inflammatory and edematous conditions. It is a very potent solvent and can penetrate intact skin and carry other chemicals along with it. It penetrates all body tissues and produces an odor that many people cannot tolerate. The dosage is 1 g/kg, IV or via nasogastric tube, as a 10% solution diluted in 5% dextrose or lactated Ringer's solution (higher concentrations can cause intravascular hemolysis).

DOPAMINE

Dopamine, an adrenergic neurotransmitter with specific receptors in the renal vasculature, is frequently used to combat reductions in renal blood flow that may contribute to acute renal failure. It also increases glomerular filtration and sodium excretion. Dopamine has a very short half-life and is administered as a constant rate infusion of 2-5 μg/kg/min. Higher dose rates cause tachycardia, cardiac arrhythmias, and peripheral vasoconstriction. Animals that do not produce urine with dopamine alone may respond to a combination of dopamine and furosemide. Dopamine is given as above, and furosemide is given at 1 mg/kg/hr, by IV bolus. If no improvement occurs within 6 hr, conversion is unlikely, and infusion should be discontinued. Dialysis (hemodialysis or peritoneal dialysis) may be required to maintain these animals.

GLOMERULAR DISEASE

Enalapril, an ACE inhibitor, may lead to reduction in proteinuria in some animals. The dosage is 0.5 mg/kg, PO, SID-BID. Dimethyl sulfoxide has been used in dogs with amyloidosis with variable results. It is given at a dosage of 80 mg/kg/day, divided TID, and given as a 10% solution either PO or SC. Thromboembolism and systemic hypertension are frequent complications of glomerular diseases in dogs, and to a lesser extent in cats, and should be managed as the need arises. Thromboembolism may be prevented by giving aspirin at 0.5-5 mg/kg, BID, to high-risk animals, such as those with serum albumin <2.0 g/dL, plasma fibrinogen >400 mg/dL, or plasma antithrombin III activity <70%.

DIABETES INSIPIDUS

Nephrogenic diabetes insipidus is a physiologic condition in which the kidneys fail to concentrate urine despite adequate amounts of antidiuretic hormone (ADH). Central, or pituitary-dependent, diabetes insipidus develops when there is a lack of ADH production. Animals with central diabetes insipidus can be given **desmopressin acetate**. The nasal spray formulation can be used, with 1-4 drops administered into the conjunctival sac SID-BID. Alternatively, the parenteral form can be given at 0.5-2 μg, SC, SID-BID. **Thiazide diuretics** may reduce polyuria by 30-50% in animals with nephrogenic or central diabetes insipidus. Inhibition of sodium resorption in the ascending loop of Henle leads to decreased total body sodium and contraction of the extracellular fluid volume. The net effect is to increase sodium and water resorption in the proximal renal tubule. Chlorothiazide is given at 20-40 mg/kg, PO, BID.

CONTROLLING URINE pH

The ideal urine pH should be 7-7.5 in dogs or 6.3-6.6 in cats. If the urine pH remains below these values after diet modification, **potassium citrate** at 80-150 mg/kg/day, PO, divided BID-TID, can be given to increase the pH. **Ammonium chloride** (200 mg/kg/day, PO, divided TID) and **DL-methionine** (1,000-1,500 mg/cat/day, PO) are the urinary acidifiers of choice. Chronic urine acidification, and ensuing acidosis, can be harmful and should not be instituted without complete evaluation of the animal.

CYSTINE-BINDING AGENTS

Cystinuria, with subsequent cystine urolith formation, results from an inherited disorder of renal tubular transport. Cystine stones are dissolved by dietary modification, urinary alkalinization or neutralization, and the use of cystine-binding agents. Urinary alkalinization or neutralization is accomplished as described above. **Tiopronin** at 15 mg/kg, PO, BID, or **D-penicillamine** at 15 mg/kg, PO, BID, given with food, are both cystine-binding agents. Tiopronin has fewer side effects and is the recommended choice. Both agents can cause Coombs'-positive anemia, thrombocytopenia, increased liver enzyme activity, glomerulonephritis, lymphadenopathy, cutaneous hypersensitivity, and delayed wound healing. Penicillamine also causes vomiting. Once stones are dissolved, a prevention protocol can be instituted. Dietary modification with or without urinary alkalinization may be all that is needed to prevent stone formation; however, tiopronin may also be needed if uroliths recur.

URINARY INCONTINENCE

Urinary incontinence is most commonly caused by urethral sphincter incompetence. It is most common in large breed, spayed female dogs (11-20% incidence) but may be seen in intact females, male dogs, and cats. Estradiol-17β concentrations decrease after ovariohysterectomy in bitches, resulting in deterioration of urethral closure within 3-6 mo. Currently, there are no approved drugs for the treatment of incontinence in animals, and most of the human products traditionally used have been removed from the market due to toxicity concerns. Some estrogen compounds and α-adrenergic drugs may still be available to veterinarians through compounding pharmacies (TABLE 27).

Diethylstilbestrol (DES) is a nonsteroidal estrogen derivative that closely resembles the natural estrogen, estradiol. Because it is inexpensive and infrequently administered, it is the first choice for treating urinary incontinence in female dogs. It is orally bioavailable and in dogs reaches peak plasma concentrations in 1 hr; it has an elimination half-life of 24 hr due to enterohepatic recirculation. Estrogens sensitize the urethral sphincter to α-adrenergic stimulation; therefore DES therapy is synergistic with α-adrenergic drugs. DES is given as a daily loading dose for 7-10 days, and then reduced to once weekly dosing, if possible, to avoid toxicity. Treated dogs are extremely susceptible to bone marrow suppression from estrogen, typified by early thrombocytopenia and potentially fatal aplastic anemia. Hematopoietic toxicity is rarely seen in cats. Other adverse effects seen in dogs include alopecia, cystic ovaries, cystic endometrial hyperplasia, pyometra, prolonged estrus, and infertility. When used once weekly in spayed female dogs, adverse effects from DES are rare.

α-Adrenergic agonists such as phenylpropanolamine (PPA), ephedrine, pseudoephedrine, and phenylephrine act directly on smooth muscle receptors to increase urethral tone and maximal urethral closure pressure. Although often more clinically effective than DES, their action is short lived, usually requiring dosing 2-3 times/day. Of this class of drugs, PPA is the most effective and produces fewer cardiovascular side effects. Previously available in over-the-counter cold medications and appetite suppressants, it has been withdrawn from the human market because of toxicity associated with overuse as a diet aid. It may still be available from some compounding pharmacies. Ephedrine, pseudoephedrine, or phenylephrine may be tried if PPA is unavailable. Adverse effects of α-adrenergic drugs include excitability, restlessness, hypertension, and anorexia.

In male dogs, testosterone injections are used to treat urinary incontinence but are generally less effective than estrogen therapy in female dogs.

URINE RETENTION

Disorders of micturition characterized by urine retention and a distended bladder are usually caused by hypocontractility of the bladder or by urethral obstruction. Prolonged bladder distention leads to breakdown of the tight junctions between detrusor muscle cells of the bladder, which prevents normal depolarization and contraction of the detrusor muscles.

TABLE 27. Drugs Used to Treat Urinary Incontinence

Drug	Dosage
Diethylstilbestrol	Dogs: 0.1-0.3 mg/kg/day, PO, for 7-10 days, followed by 1 mg/dog/wk
Phenylpropanolamine	Dogs: 1.5-2 mg/kg, PO, SID-TID
Ephedrine	Dogs: 1.2 mg/kg, PO, BID-TID Cats: 2-4 mg/kg, PO, BID-TID
Pseudoephedrine	Dogs >25 kg: 30 mg/dog, PO, TID Dogs <25 kg: 15 mg/dog, PO, TID
Testosterone propionate	Dogs: 2.2 mg/kg, IM, every 2-3 days
Testosterone cypionate	Dogs: 2.2 mg/kg, IM, every 30-60 days

An adrenergic antagonist may be indicated when manual expression or voluntary voiding is nonproductive because urethral sphincter tone is excessive, as is often the case in cats after relief of obstruction. **Phenoxybenzamine**, an irreversible antagonist, has been used with some success. The dosage for dogs or cats is 0.25 mg/kg, PO, BID.

Diazepam is a benzodiazepine anxiolytic that is also a central muscle relaxant. Dosages sufficient to allow for urethral relaxation may also cause sedation. The dosage in dogs is 0.2 mg/kg, PO, TID, and in cats is 0.5 mg/kg, IV. Diazepam given PO may cause idiosyncratic acute hepatic necrosis in cats.

In animals with detrusor hyporeflexia or bladder atony, **bethanechol chloride** may be of some benefit. This cholinergic agonist stimulates the initiation of the detrusor muscle contraction. The dosage for dogs is 5-25 mg/dog, PO, TID, and for cats is 2.5-7.5 mg/cat, PO, TID.

CHEMOTHERAPEUTICS
INTRODUCTION

Treatment with any chemotherapeutic agent involves the interrelationships among the host animal, the pathogen, and the drug. These relationships comprise the chemotherapeutic triangle (*see* below). An understanding of this triangle and the interactions among the "points" is critical to therapeutic success. The advent of professional flexible labeling places further emphasis on consideration of these factors when selecting a dosing regimen.

The chemotherapeutic armamentarium includes antibacterial, antiviral, antifungal, antiparasitic, and antineoplastic compounds. The basic mechanisms through which many of these agents exert their effects against pathogens are known. More importantly, the methods by which harmful organisms may protect themselves against the action of specific drugs are also becoming better understood. The pharmacologic modulation of these processes has added new dimensions to modern chemotherapeutics.

Chemotherapeutic agents may be selectively toxic to invading micro- or macroorganisms, but in many cases, they can also result in adverse effects in the host. To avoid toxic manifestations, the dose rate often becomes critical; additionally, the clinical condition of the animal and concurrently administered drugs can be responsible. Chemotherapeutic agents that are absorbed or injected into the body are eliminated by the same processes as all xenobiotics. The effect that disease may have on the absorption, distribution, biotransformation, and excretion of a therapeutic agent may be of notable clinical significance.

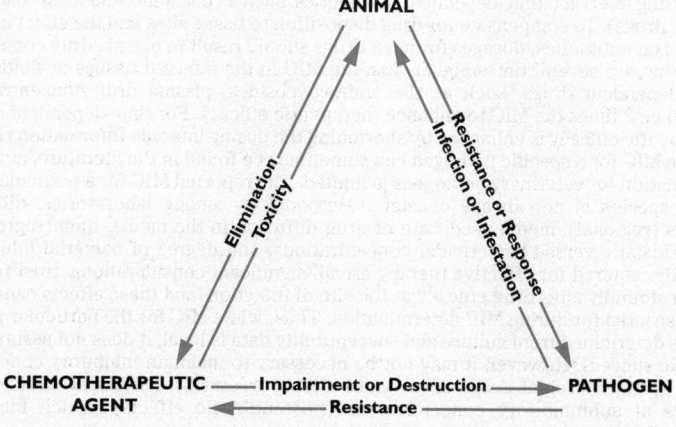

The effect of the pathogen on the host and its response to infection are also important components of the chemotherapeutic triangle. The pathogenesis of the disease, the pathophysiologic reactions, and the resultant lesions may have important bearings on clinical management; in addition to appropriate chemotherapy, supportive and adjunctive treatment may be crucial for success. Therapeutic measures such as fluids, blood transfusion, antisera, anti-inflammatory drugs, positive inotropic agents, and bronchodilators could well be life-saving, depending on the particular case.

Also, nonspecific and specific immune mechanisms play a vital role as part of the animal's response to an invading pathogen. Host defense mechanisms should be sustained by whatever means possible when treating an infectious or parasitic disease; otherwise, protracted recovery or relapses are likely inevitable. Minimizing stress, providing quality nutritional support, administering specific immunoglobulins, and using immunopotentiators are some of the approaches that may be used. These general principles apply to all classes of chemotherapeutic agents.

GUIDELINES FOR CLINICAL USE OF ANTIMICROBIAL AGENTS

The rational therapeutic management of infection is based on selection of an appropriate antimicrobial agent and course of treatment that will inhibit or destroy the specific pathogens without compromising the animal's response. The pathogen should be destroyed, or at least inhibited swiftly, to permit the host to begin recovery without relapse and to avoid emergence of microbial resistance and drug-induced toxicity. Factors related to the animal, the antimicrobial agent, and the pathogenic organism all play significant roles.

Successful antimicrobial therapy is based on 4 principles: 1) Identification and characterization of the pathogen(s), including its antimicrobial sensitivity, and selection of a drug based on the sites of infection and the lesions. 2) Effective concentrations of the indicated antimicrobial agent for a sufficient period at the site(s) of infection. 3) A dose rate, frequency, and route of administration of the antimicrobial agent, as well as a duration of therapy, that maximizes the likelihood of a cure, prevents relapse, and minimizes the risk of resistance without causing any harmful drug-induced effects in the animal. 4) Specific and appropriate supportive therapy to enhance the animal's ability to overcome the infection and associated disease conditions.

Ideally, a dosing regimen is based on the minimal inhibitory concentration (MIC) or even the minimal antibiotic concentration (MAC) of an antibacterial agent for a particular pathogen. Depending on the antimicrobial, plasma or tissue drug concentrations should either markedly exceed the MIC (for "dose-dependent" antimicrobials, such as the aminoglycosides and the fluorinated quinolones) or be above the MIC for most of the dosing interval ("time-dependent" antibiotics, such as β-lactams and most "bacteriostatic" drugs). To compensate for drug disposition to tissue sites and the effect of host factors on antibiotics, dosages for most drugs should result in plasma drug concentrations that are several times higher than the MIC in the infected tissues or fluids. For dose-dependent drugs, such as the aminoglycosides, plasma drug concentrations should be 8 times the MIC to enhance therapeutic efficacy. For time-dependent drugs, therapeutic efficacy is enhanced by shortening the dosing interval. Information regarding the MIC for a specific pathogen can sometimes be found in the literature, although information for veterinary pathogens is limited. The reported MIC for a particular bacterial species is not always constant. Methodology among laboratories, different strains (regional), media used, rate of drug diffusion in the media, time (regrowth), bacteriostatic versus bactericidal concentrations, and degree of bacterial inhibition actually required for effective therapy are all significant considerations. Host factors can profoundly alter drug efficacy at the site of infection, and these effects cannot be compensated for during MIC determination. Thus, while MIC for the particular pathogen as determined from culture and susceptibility data is ideal, it does not assure therapeutic success. However, it may not be necessary to maintain inhibitory concentrations of antimicrobial drugs at all times during treatment. Persistent antibacterial effects at subinhibitory concentrations (postantibiotic effects), which facilitate removal of affected bacteria by host defense mechanisms, have been demonstrated for penicillins, cephalosporins, macrolides, tetracyclines, aminoglycosides, and several other antibacterial agents. Organisms damaged by antibiotics are more susceptible to leukocidal activity.

The immunocompetence of the animal should always be assessed, recognizing that extraneous factors, stress, disease, malnutrition, and the effects of concurrently administered drugs may influence the animal's ability to resist infection. Host defense systems are seriously compromised in bone marrow depression, hypogammaglobulinemia, conditions in which alveolar macrophages are incapacitated, tracheobronchitis, necrotic enteritis, starvation, and other conditions. In addition, immunosuppressants (eg, corticosteroids and antineoplastics) compromise immune response. Any depression of immune capabilities can be expected to modify the effectiveness of many antimicrobial agents, especially those with only bacteriostatic activity.

The use of combinations of antibacterial drugs to treat or prevent infections is widespread and may be beneficial. However, many factors may confound the synergistic or additive effects of antimicrobial agents, and antagonism does occur between specific drugs, both in vitro and in vivo. As a rule, antibacterial agents should not be used in combination indiscriminately or without justification.

Requirements for Successful Antimicrobial Therapy

Clinical Diagnosis: Successful chemotherapy usually requires a specific diagnosis, even though a reasonable preliminary diagnosis is often all that is possible, at least initially.

Microbiologic Diagnosis: Treatment should be aimed at a specific pathogen whenever feasible. However, polymicrobial infections are common. The ideal is a conclusive microbiologic diagnosis, but frequently this must be presumptive (at least initially), and treatment must be based on experience. Rational deduction may be necessary under field conditions. The examination of a direct smear stained with Wright's or Gram's stain may help to establish what types of pathogens are involved (gram-positive or gram-negative rods or cocci).

Culture and Susceptibility Testing: Isolation and characterization of the causative pathogen, susceptibility testing, and determination of the MIC provide a sound foundation from which to select the antimicrobial drug, as well as the dosage regimen. However, under field conditions, it is often difficult to attain laboratory support for antimicrobial therapy.

Appropriate Selection of Antimicrobial Agents: Among the factors to be considered are the causative microorganism(s), results of sensitivity tests, pathogenicity of organisms, pathologic lesions, acuteness of infection, pharmacokinetics of the drug(s) indicated, expense, potential drug toxicity, organic dysfunctions (especially kidney and liver function), and possible interactions with drugs administered concurrently.

Correct Dosage and Route of Administration: The dosage selected should result in adequate therapeutic concentrations at the site(s) of infection for sufficient time without causing side effects or toxicity. For dose-dependent drugs, higher dosages are more likely to enhance therapeutic success than are shorter intervals. For β-lactam and other time-dependent drugs, therapeutic success appears to be greater if the concentration remains above the MIC for about one-half to two-thirds of the dosage interval, and efficacy is likely to be improved more by decreasing the interval than by increasing the dose. The advocated dosage schedules should be carefully followed for at least 7 days (although response should be apparent in 3-4 days for most infections), or longer if needed, to ensure elimination of the pathogen and to prevent relapse, reinfection, or development of antimicrobial resistance.

Ancillary Treatment, Nutritional Support, and Nursing Care: Supportive treatment, optimal nutrition, and general nursing care are often critical for successful management of infectious disease. Ancillary treatment might include the use of anti-inflammatory agents, antidiarrheal preparations, expectorants, bronchodilators, inotropic agents, urinary acidifiers and alkalinizers, immunopotentiators, and fluid and electrolyte replacement. Attention should be given to caloric and nutrient intake, especially of protein and vitamins. These nutrients play a cardinal role in immune responsiveness.

Combination Therapy

Treatment with antimicrobial combinations may be necessary in certain cases. The administration of 2 or more agents may be beneficial in the following situations: 1) to treat mixed bacterial infections in which the organisms are not susceptible to a common agent, 2) to achieve synergistic antimicrobial activity against particularly resistant strains (eg, *Pseudomonas aeruginosa*), 3) to overcome bacterial tolerance, 4) to prevent the emergence of drug resistance, 5) to minimize toxicity, or 6) to prevent inactivation of an antibiotic by enzymes produced by other bacteria that are present.

Additive or synergistic effects are seen when antibacterial agents are used in combination, but antagonism may also emerge, sometimes with serious consequences. Generally, bacteriostatic agents act in an additive fashion, whereas bactericidal agents are often synergistic. However, the effects of several bactericidal antibiotics are substantially impaired by simultaneous use of drugs that impair microbial growth or "bacteriostatic" drugs (eg, most ribosomal inhibitors). This is a general guideline only; many exceptions are known, and confounding factors also play a role. Classification of antimicrobials as bactericidal or bacteriostatic can also be misleading because "bactericidal" drugs can be rendered bacteriostatic if sufficient drug concentrations are not achieved at the site of infection. However, in general, the following common antimicrobials at usual concentrations are bactericidal: penicillins, cephalosporins, aminoglycosides, trimethoprim/sulfonamides, nitrofurans, metronidazole, and quinolones. The following antimicrobials at usual concentrations are generally bacteriostatic: tetracyclines, chloramphenicol, macrolides, lincosamides, spectinomycin, and the sulfonamides.

Ideally, antimicrobial selection should be based on mechanisms of action that are different and on spectra of activity that are complementary. β-Lactams are often selected because their action is unique and not only complements other drugs but also facilitates movement of other drugs through the damaged cell wall into the microbe. Examples of combination therapy for mixed infections include the use of clindamycin, metronidazole, or the semisynthetic penicillins for their anaerobic coverage in combination with aminoglycosides for their gram-negative efficacy. Synergism against certain bacterial pathogens frequently can be achieved with combinations of penicillins or cephalosporins and aminoglycosides. The combined use of trimethoprim with selected sulfonamides or clavulanic acid with other β-lactams are other examples of synergistic effects.

Preventing the development of resistance with combination antimicrobial therapy is best exemplified by the use of carbenicillin or amikacin together with gentamicin or tobramycin for the treatment of *Pseudomonas* infections.

Bacterial enzymatic inactivation of β-lactam antibiotics, such as the penicillins and cephalosporins, can be decreased by concurrent administration of a β-lactamase inhibitor, such as clavulanic acid or sulbactam.

Mechanisms of Action

Antimicrobial agents affect susceptible organisms in various ways, and bacteria sometimes protect themselves from these destructive effects by a variety of means. The major mechanisms of action of antimicrobial agents, with examples of each type, are as follows (*see also* the discussion of specific classes in ANTIBACTERIAL AGENTS, p 2056): 1) inhibition of cell wall synthesis: penicillins, cephalosporins and cephamycins, vancomycin, bacitracin, cycloserine; 2) impairment of cell membrane function: polymyxin B, colistin, tyrocidin, amphotericin, nystatin; 3) inhibition of protein synthesis: tetracyclines, aminoglycosides, spectinomycin, chloramphenicol, macrolides, lincosamides; 4) inhibition of DNA synthesis and replication: novobiocin, quinolones, griseofulvin; 5) inhibition of DNA-dependent RNA polymerase: rifamycins; 6) inhibition of folinic acid and consequently DNA synthesis: sulfonamides, trimethoprim.

Reasons for Failure of Antibacterial Therapy

Possible reasons for failure of antibacterial therapy include the following: 1) The diagnosis was incorrect, eg, viral and not bacterial infection. 2) The organisms were not susceptible to the action of the antibiotic that was selected, or they were in static phase and therefore refractory ("persisters"). 3) Although originally susceptible, the bacteria developed resistance. 4) The antibiotic(s) was insufficient for multiple pathogens. 5) A combination of incompatible antibiotics was administered. 6) Superinfection by a resistant opportunistic pathogen occurred. 7) Reinfection by the original or by other pathogenic bacteria occurred. 8) Drainage was inadequate in surgical infections, or a foreign body was present. 9) Perfusion and penetration to the site of infection was impaired because of inflammation, cellular debris, tissue destruction, abscessation, etc. 10) The organism is intracellular in location and able to avoid detrimental effects by phagocytic cells. 11) Defense mechanisms (specific and nonspecific) of the animal were compromised by disease, malnutrition, or concurrent therapy. 12) Detrimental changes, such as hypoxia, acidosis, or accumulation of tissue debris, developed in infected tissue, which reduced the effectiveness of the antibiotic or sulfonamide. 13) An inappropriate route of administration was selected or an incorrect dosage regimen was followed because the pharmacokinetic characteristics of the antimicrobial drug were not appreciated. 14) Expired or substandard products were used. 15) The selected agent had to be withdrawn because of adverse effects. 16) Interaction of the selected antimicrobial agent(s) with other concurrently administered drugs occurred, which diminished the antimicrobial effect or altered the pharmacokinetics of the agent(s). 17) The prescribed dosage regimen was not reliably followed (lack of owner compliance). 18) Supportive therapy was inadequate. 19) Nutritional deficits were not corrected. 20) Nursing care was substandard, and the stress associated with the disease process was not reduced. 21) Predisposing management factors were not corrected.

Resistance of Microorganisms to Antibacterial Agents

The emergence of bacteria resistant to antimicrobial agents within an animal population or during therapy is of great concern. Resistance requires that a previously successful therapeutic approach be discarded, especially if suitable alternative antimicrobial drugs are available; additionally, there frequently is concern from an epidemiologic and public health point of view.

There are differences in use of the term "antibiotic resistance." Natural resistance implies an intrinsic property in an organism that confers resistance, whereas acquired resistance suggests that an organism has obtained, by one mechanism or another, the means to survive exposure to an antimicrobial agent. Chromosomal, extrachromosomal, and transpositional resistance are terms used when the genetic determinants are on chromosomes, plasmids, or transposons, respectively. Phenotypic resistance, due to differences in physical and functional characteristics, is best exemplified by the bacterial-wall-defective variants (such as L-forms, spheroblasts, and protoplasts) and by the impermeability of the cell walls of some gram-negative bacteria due to very narrow conduits or porins. Microbiologic resistance implies an increase in the usual MIC range to levels that are too high to be reached at standard therapeutic dose rates. Clinical resistance, for which there may be many causes, is a general term used to describe unexpected lack of response to treatment in a clinical case.

Causes of conditional resistance include the physiologic state of the organism (eg, quiescent, as in "persisters"), antagonism or inactivation by a second agent, inactivation of the drug by enzymes produced by other bacteria at the site of infection, antagonism of the effect of the antimicrobial agent due to tissue debris or a foreign body, and inhibition of antibacterial action because of a low pH or hypoxia.

Resistance may also be classified in terms of the mechanisms of acquisition. Examples include selection of resistant clones, chromosomal mutation, phage transduction, and R-factor acquisition by conjugation.

The biochemical basis for microbial resistance to antibacterial agents permits a further approach to distinguishing various forms of resistance. Examples include the synthesis of destructive enzymes, altered receptor site or enzyme specificity, alternate metabolic pathways, modified carrier systems, and various barriers to penetration.

The means by which bacteria can protect themselves against antimicrobials include the following: 1) increased production of inactivating enzymes, which may be constitutive or inducible, eg, penicillins, cephalosporins, aminoglycosides, chloramphenicol; 2) defective production of autolytic enzymes ("tolerance"), eg, penicillins and cephalosporins; 3) alteration of the specific configuration of target sites, eg, oxacillin, cloxacillin, macrolides, lincomycin, streptomycin; 4) decreased enzyme affinity, eg, trimethoprim; 5) induction of membrane transport systems to remove the antibacterial, eg, tetracyclines; 6) inhibition or changes in membrane transport systems to prevent entry of the antibacterial, eg, aminoglycosides; 7) utilization of alternative metabolic pathways, eg, sulfonamides, trimethoprim; 8) increased synthesis of a key metabolic intermediate, eg, para-aminobenzoic acid in sulfonamide resistance; and 9) development of impermeable cell walls with extremely narrow porins, eg, *Pseudomonas aeruginosa* in response to many antibiotics.

In each of these cases, a modification of protein synthesis and enzyme activity is necessary to confer resistance; thus, this adaptation is genetically determined.

Bacteria have 2 types of genetic structures that may confer resistance—chromosomes and plasmids. Both consist of double-stranded DNA, and both are associated with the bacterial inner cell membrane at some time. Plasmids are not essential for survival but do carry genetic determinants that confer both antibiotic resistance and virulence on bacteria. There is always only 1 plasmid of its type in a cell (called "incompatibility").

Chromosomal resistance to antibacterial agents depends on a mutation in the bacterial genes that leads to resistance to particular antimicrobial agents. In this case, the antibacterial drugs act only as selective agents that allow the resistant mutants to emerge either by a single step or sequential mutations. Their genesis is independent of the presence of the agent. Mutated bacteria are often metabolically deranged and are at a selective growth disadvantage; they usually disappear with time in the absence of the antimicrobial agent.

Plasmid-mediated resistance (R-factor or acquired resistance) is far more complex. Plasmids may contain 20-500 genes that can carry resistance to a number of different antibacterial agents (3-6 is common; up to 9 have been recorded) and specific virulence factors. Many specific plasmids have been isolated, characterized, and identified. The 3 possible mechanisms by which plasmids may migrate from one bacterium to another are transformation, transduction, and conjugation. In **transformation**, naked DNA seems to pass from the donor to the recipient through the growth medium. This process appears to be confined to a limited range of bacteria. In **transduction**, the transfer is mediated by a bacteriophage that makes use of its specialized molecular equipment adapted for inserting DNA into recipient bacteria. Normally, it is phage DNA that is transferred; in certain cases, however, some DNA from the episome in the bacterial cell replaces the proper phage nucleic acid sequence. Phage-mediated transduction occurs in some gram-positive (especially *Staphylococcus aureus*) as well as gram-negative species. In **conjugation**, the DNA passes from the donor cell to the recipient via a bridge formed during direct cell-to-cell contact. This is the most sophisticated form of transmission because, for transfer to occur at all, the donor must have the necessary surface appendage (sex pilus) to form the bridge. This pilus is coded for by a resistance transfer factor on the plasmid and is called a conjugative sequence (vs a nonconjugative plasmid without a resistance transfer factor).

General facets of conjugation make it an important process for gene transfer under natural conditions. Many types of bacteria can act as recipients, and resistance can pass freely from organisms normally saprophytic in the gut of animals to pathogenic bacteria. Transfer among *Pasteurella* and *Pseudomonas* spp seems to be less efficient. In general, transfer occurs more frequently between gram-negative bacteria and only rarely between gram-positive organisms. Conjugation allows the passage of a number of distinct genes at one time. Thus, resistance to several antibiotics, all mediated by different biochemical means, may be acquired in a single step. The great efficiency of the conjugation process makes the probability of gene transfer to a super-infecting pathogen high.

Genetic sequences capable of coding for resistance can migrate from a plasmid to a chromosome and then back to the plasmid. These sequences are then transpositional and are known as transposons. A number of transposons responsible for the transfer of R-factor resistance also have been isolated, characterized, and identified.

The clinical relevance of plasmid-mediated resistance principally concerns the following: 1) intestinal infections, in which the reservoir of R-factors may be carried by saprophytic flora in the gut; 2) the use of low levels of antibiotics (as in animal feeds) or improper dosing regimens, which may lead to a high incidence of R-factors in a given population; and 3) the indiscriminate use of antibiotics, which may eliminate the effectiveness of many antimicrobial agents in the future.

The following guidelines will help to minimize the emergence of bacterial resistance: 1) A broad-spectrum antibacterial agent should not be used if a narrow-spectrum agent is also active against the causative organism(s). 2) Information regarding endemic infections and sensitivity patterns should be obtained and considered when choosing an antibiotic. 3) Appropriate dose rates should always be followed. 4) When a combination regimen is used to prevent the development of resistant strains, individual agents should be used at full dosage. 5) Antibacterials for topical application should be selected from those against which development of resistance is uncommon. 6) For prophylaxis, an antibacterial agent that prevents colonization of a specific organism or eradicates it shortly after it has become established should be used. 7) To the extent that it is consistent with reasonable practice, every effort should be made to use antibiotics only when the medical indications are clear and to avoid overuse of newer agents when already available agents are effective.

Role of Veterinarians in Antimicrobial Resistance

Two major aspects of antimicrobial use concern veterinarians—the likelihood of causing a pathogenic organism to become resistant to current antimicrobial therapy and the likelihood of commensal organisms (generally GI) becoming resistant to future antimicrobial therapy. The former largely can be prevented by assuring that adequate concentrations of the appropriate drug reach the targeted site. The latter concern is less problematic in small animals because the risk of transfer of resistant commensal organisms to humans is not as obvious as with the use of antibiotics in food production. However, even the latter risk is difficult to quantitate. The use of antibiotics in food animals, including use as growth promotants, may contribute to the transfer of resistance genes among bacteria and ultimately from food animals to humans, where the organisms become pathogenic. Additionally, contamination of food with resistant pathogenic bacteria during the processing of food is a concern. Carcasses may be contaminated at slaughter and processing, and subsequent improper handling or cooking of the product may lead to infection in people. The development of resistant pathogenic bacteria in poultry treated with fluoroquinolones has been documented. Infection of the human population is of particular concern because the bacterial resistance created in the animal following veterinary use of a drug or drug class may result in resistance to human drugs of the same class. Whereas the organism developing resistance might be nonpathogenic, transfer of the resistance gene to other bacteria in the human intestinal tract may result in a pathogenic organism becoming resistant and ultimately in therapeutic failure in the human patient.

When selecting drug therapies for food animals, veterinarians must be aware of the potential for resistance. Use of antibacterial drugs should be in the context of a valid veterinarian-client-patient relationship. Selection should be based on all information available (clinical signs, experience, laboratory data, physical examination findings, culture and sensitivity data). Pathogens should be identified, and drugs with the narrowest spectrum of activity with known effectiveness against the pathogen should be used. Client education is important in preventing unnecessary use of antibacterial agents (such as using "leftover" antibacterial drugs to treat a new occurrence of disease). In addition to judicious use, veterinarians should be proactive in the education of their clients, including proper withdrawal guidelines of any prescribed drugs, and should administer drugs in the proper classes, at proper doses, and through appropriate routes. (*See also* ANTIMICROBIAL FEED ADDITIVES, p 2175.)

ANTIBACTERIAL AGENTS

PENICILLINS

The penicillins are a large and commonly used class of β-lactam antibiotics that share many features, including chemistry, mechanism of action, pharmacologic properties, clinical effects, and immunologic characteristics.

Classes

Several subclassifications of the penicillins, based mainly on differences in antibacterial spectra, are recognized.

Narrow-spectrum β-Lactamase-sensitive Penicillins: This group includes naturally occurring penicillin G (benzylpenicillin) in its various pharmaceutical forms and a few biosynthetic acid-stable penicillins intended for oral use (penicillin V [phenoxymethylpenicillin] and phenethicillin). Penicillins in this class are active against many gram-positive and a limited number of gram-negative bacteria, but they are susceptible to β-lactamase (penicillinase) hydrolysis.

Narrow-spectrum β-Lactamase-resistant Penicillins: This group, through substitution on the penicillin nucleus (6-aminopenicillanic acid [6-APA]), is refractory to a greater or lesser degree to the effects of various β-lactamase enzymes produced by resistant gram-positive organisms, particularly *Staphylococcus aureus*. However, penicillins in this class are not as active against many gram-positive bacteria as penicillin G and are inactive against almost all gram-negative bacteria. Acid-stable members of this group (that are used PO) include isoxazolyl penicillins, such as oxacillin, cloxacillin, dicloxacillin, and flucloxacillin. Methicillin and nafcillin are available as parenteral preparations. Temocillin is a semisynthetic penicillin that is β-lactamase stable but also active against nearly all isolates of gram-negative bacteria except *Pseudomonas* spp.

Broad-spectrum β-Lactamase-sensitive Penicillins: Penicillins in this class are derived semisynthetically and are active against many gram-positive and gram-negative bacteria. However, they are readily destroyed by the β-lactamases (produced by many bacteria). Many members of the group are acid stable and are administered either PO or parenterally. Of those used in veterinary medicine, aminopenicillins, eg, ampicillin and amoxicillin, are the best known. Several ampicillin precursors that are more completely absorbed from the GI tract also belong to this class (eg, hetacillin, pivampicillin, talampicillin). Mecillinam is less active than ampicillin against gram-positive bacteria but is highly active against many intestinal organisms (except *Proteus* spp) that do not produce β-lactamases.

Broad-spectrum β-Lactamase-sensitive Penicillins with Extended Spectra: Several semisynthetic broad-spectrum penicillins are also active against *Pseudomonas aeruginosa*, certain *Proteus* spp, and even strains of *Klebsiella, Shigella,* and *Enterobacter* spp in certain cases. Examples of this class include carboxypenicillins (carbenicillin, its acid-stable indanyl ester, and ticarcillin), ureido-penicillins (azlocillin and mezlocillin), and piperazine penicillins (piperacillin).

β-Lactamase-protected Broad-spectrum Penicillins (Potentiated Penicillins): Several naturally occurring and semisynthetic compounds can inhibit many of the β-lactamase enzymes produced by penicillin-resistant bacteria. When used in combination with broad-spectrum penicillins, there is a notable synergistic effect because the active penicillin is protected from enzymatic hydrolysis—and thus is fully active against a wide variety of previously resistant bacteria. Examples of this chemotherapeutic approach include clavulanate-potentiated amoxicillin and ticarcillin as well as sulbactam-potentiated ampicillin.

Carbapenems: Imipenem is one of the most active drugs against a wide variety of bacteria. It is derived from a compound produced by *Streptomyces cattleya*. Aztreonam is a related (monobactam) compound.

General Properties

The penicillins are somewhat unstable, being sensitive to heat, light, extremes in pH, heavy metals, and oxidizing and reducing agents. Also, they often deteriorate in aqueous solution and thus require reconstitution with a diluent just before injection. Penicillins are poorly soluble, weak organic acids that are administered parenterally either as suspensions in water or oil, or as water-soluble salts. For example, sodium or potassium salts of penicillin G are highly water soluble and are absorbed rapidly from injection sites, whereas organic salts in microsuspension such as procaine penicillin G or benzathine penicillin G are gradually absorbed over 1-3 (or even more) days, respectively. The trihydrate forms of the semisynthetic penicillins have greater aqueous solubility than the parent compounds and are usually preferred for both parenteral and oral use.

Penicillins contain a β-lactam nucleus that when cleaved by a β-lactamase enzyme (penicillinase) produces penicilloic acid derivatives that are inactive but which may act as the antigenic determinants for penicillin hypersensitivity. Modification of the 6-aminopenicillanic acid nucleus, either by biosynthetic or semisynthetic means, has produced the array of penicillins used clinically. These differ in their antibacterial spectra, pharmacokinetic characteristics, and susceptibility to microbial enzymatic degradation.

Antimicrobial Activity

Mode of Action: Penicillins impair the development of bacterial cell walls by interfering with transpeptidase enzymes responsible for the formation of the cross-links between peptidoglycan strands. These enzymes are associated with a group of proteins in both gram-positive and gram-negative bacteria called the penicillin-binding proteins (PBP). During bacterial cell growth, while the peptidoglycan structure is being formed, autolysins continuously cleave the lattice to provide acceptor sites for new strands. Normal bacterial growth depends on a balance between cell wall deposition and autolysis. When a penicillin interacts with PBP and inhibits the synthetic enzymes, defective cell walls are formed, which lead to abnormal elongation of cells, formation of spheroplasts, or osmotic lysis. The effect of the penicillins is generally bactericidal. At concentrations lower than minimal inhibitory concentrations (MIC [at so-called minimal antibiotic concentrations]), β-lactam antibiotics do exert residual effects on bacterial structure and function that, in turn, promote phagocytosis.

β-Lactam antibiotics have little influence on formed bacterial cell walls, and even susceptible organisms must be actively multiplying or growing. Penicillins are most active during the logarithmic phase of bacterial growth. They also tend to be somewhat more active in a slightly acidic environment (pH 5.5-6.5), perhaps because of enhanced membrane penetration.

Efficacy of the β-lactams is related to the time that plasma or tissue drug concentrations exceed the MIC of the infecting organism. Generally, concentrations should remain above the MIC for about two-thirds of the dosing interval.

Bacterial Resistance: Only microorganisms that have cell walls are susceptible to the action of penicillins and other β-lactam antibiotics. Within this range of bacteria, resistance to penicillins is well recognized and takes a number of forms.

Permeability Barrier: In gram-positive organisms, capsular materials may hinder access to the cytoplasmic membrane, but this rarely limits the diffusion of the cell-wall inhibitors. Gram-negative bacteria have a restricting sieving mechanism in their outer membranes, which reduces the penetration of several types of antibiotics. Different species of gram-negative bacteria exhibit varying permeability barriers to β-lactam antibiotics, and these impair access of the antibiotics to the membrane-associated binding proteins. For example, the permeability barrier of *Haemophilus influenzae* is readily crossed by β-lactam antibiotics, *Escherichia coli* presents a greater obstacle to these agents, and the outer membranes of *Pseudomonas aeruginosa* are penetrated with great difficulty by most β-lactam compounds. The chemical nature of β-lactams (penicillins, cephalosporins, and the β-lactamase inhibitors), as well as their concentration gradients, also greatly influence their penetration of bacteria to their targets at the surface of the cytoplasmic membrane, giving rise to the differences between antibacterial spectra of the various classes of penicillin. Penicillins are also often used in combination with other antibiotics that disrupt the integrity of the membranes and thereby facilitate access by penicillins. The genetic loci controlling permeability generally have been considered to be chromosomally located, but they also may be plasmid-specified genes.

Specific Bacterial Binding Proteins: Resistance to β-lactam antimicrobial agents can be acquired by alterations in the PBP targets of these drugs. A loss or decrease in affinity of crucial PBP can lead to a significant increase in penicillin resistance.

L-forms of Bacteria: A phenotypic form of resistance can occur when spheroplasts (incomplete cell wall) or protoplasts (absence of cell wall) are present. These so-called "L-forms" must be present in a hyperosmotic environment (eg, the renal medulla) to survive; otherwise, they will lyse. The clinical significance of this form of resistance is unclear.

Quiescent Organisms: In any bacterial population, a few organisms will always be quiescent. Because the penicillins are active only against growing bacteria, the static organisms are unaffected and may persist. These "persisters" may then develop normally after the antibiotic is removed.

Tolerance: Some bacterial isolates, when treated with inhibitors of cell-wall synthesis, undergo inhibition of growth but not lysis at usual concentrations. These "tolerant" organisms are defective in their production or use of autolytic enzymes and can survive exposure to β-lactam antibiotics. Clinically, relapses and failures in serious infections due to tolerant organisms may be prevented by the frequently synergistic effect of the aminoglycosides with β-lactam antibiotics.

β-Lactamase (Penicillinase) Resistance: The most important mechanism of bacterial resistance to penicillins and the other β-lactam antibiotics is enzymatic inactivation. There are at least 6 major types of β-lactamase enzymes that can cleave the β-lactam ring, which renders the drug inactive. β-Lactamases are produced by gram-positive organisms (*Staphylococcus aureus*, *S epidermidis*), and 5 of the 6 types of β-lactamases are produced by gram-negative organisms. Some of these enzymes are active exclusively against penicillins, others are principally active against cephalosporins, and several types hydrolyze both equally. The type and concentration of β-lactamases are also bacterial species-specific. Gram-positive β-lactamases are generally excreted into the external environment as exoenzymes, produced in large quantity, plasmid-mediated (single determinant), usually inducible (rarely constitutive), unable to initiate self-transmission (rely principally on transduction), and active primarily against penicillins. Staphylococcal strains are the main gram-positive bacteria in which β-lactamase resistance develops, often very quickly. Gram-negative β-lactamases are generally heterogenous (wide range), retained within the periplasmic space, produced in small quantity, often constitutive (less often inducible), able to initiate self-transmission (conjugation mechanisms), and active against both penicillins and cephalosporins. Gram-negative bacteria capable of resistance as a result of β-lactamase production include *Escherichia*, *Haemophilus*, *Klebsiella*, *Pasteurella*, *Proteus*, *Pseudomonas*, and *Salmonella* spp; resistance may take longer to develop in some of these strains.

β-Lactamase-induced resistance is widespread. Of veterinary isolates, ~50-60% of *Staphylococcus* spp strains and 40-70% of *E coli* strains are resistant to penicillin G; 15-40% of *E coli* strains from farm animals may also be resistant to ampicillin.

Antibacterial Spectra: Penicillin G and its oral congeners (eg, penicillin V) are active against both aerobic and anaerobic gram-positive bacteria and, with a few exceptions (*Haemophilus* and *Neisseria* spp and strains of *Bacteroides* other than *B fragilis*), are inactive against gram-negative organisms at usual concentrations. Organisms usually sensitive in vitro to penicillin G include streptococci, penicillin-sensitive staphylococci, *Corynebacterium pyogenes*, *Clostridium* spp, *Erysipelothrix rhusiopathiae*, *Actinomyces ovis*, *Leptospira canicola*, *Bacillus anthracis*, *Fusiformis nodosus*, and *Nocardia* spp.

The semisynthetic β-lactamase-resistant penicillins, such as oxacillin, cloxacillin, floxacillin, and nafcillin, have spectra similar to those noted above (although often at higher MIC) but also include many of the β-lactamase-producing strains of staphylococci (especially *S aureus* and *S epidermidis*).

A large number of gram-positive and gram-negative bacteria (but not β-lactamase-producing strains) are sensitive to the semisynthetic broad-spectrum penicillins (ampicillin and amoxicillin). Susceptible genera include *Staphylococcus*, *Streptococcus*, *Corynebacterium*, *Clostridium*, *Escherichia*, *Klebsiella*, *Shigella*, *Salmonella*, *Proteus*, and *Pasteurella*. While bacterial resistance is widespread, the combination of β-lactamase inhibitors and broad-spectrum penicillins markedly enhances the spectrum and efficacy against both gram-positive and gram-negative pathogens. Clavulanate-potentiated amoxicillin is an excellent example of such a synergistic association.

The anti-*Pseudomonas* and other extended-spectrum penicillins are active against most of the usual penicillin-sensitive bacteria. They often have a degree of β-lactamase resistance and are usually active against one or more characteristic penicillin-resistant organisms. Yet, as a class, they remain susceptible to destruction by β-lactamases. Examples include the use of carbenicillin, ticarcillin, and piperacillin against *Pseudomonas aeruginosa* and several *Proteus* strains, and the use of piperacillin against *Pseudomonas aeruginosa*, several *Shigella* and *Proteus* strains, and some *Citrobacter* and *Enterobacter* spp. *Streptococcus faecalis* is often resistant to these new extended-spectrum penicillins. Imipenem is relatively resistant to β-lactamase destruction. Its spectrum includes a wide variety of aerobic and anaerobic microorganisms, including most strains of *Pseudomonas*, streptococci, enterococci, staphylococci, and *Listeria*. Anaerobes, including *Bacteroides fragilis*, are highly susceptible.

Pharmacokinetic Features

The pharmacokinetics of the many penicillins differ substantially. The general guidelines below emphasize singularly significant aspects.

Absorption: Most penicillins in aqueous solution are rapidly absorbed from parenteral sites. Absorption is delayed when the inorganic penicillin salts are suspended in vegetable oil vehicles or when the sparingly soluble repository organic salts (eg, procaine penicillin G and benzathine penicillin G) are administered parenterally. Although prolonged absorption results in longer persistence of plasma and tissue drug concentrations, peak concentrations may not be sufficiently high to be effective against organisms unless MIC are low. The penicillin G repositol salts should never be injected IV. Only some penicillins are acid stable and can be administered PO at standard doses. Absorption occurs from the upper GI tract, but the degree and rate of absorption differs greatly among the various penicillins. Penicillin V must be given at high oral doses. The aminopenicillins are orally bioavailable, although food impairs the absorption of ampicillin. The indanyl form of carbenicillin is orally bioavailable, but effective concentrations are likely to be achieved only in the urine. Serum concentrations of penicillins generally peak within 2 hr of PO administration. Penicillins may also be absorbed after intrauterine infusion.

Distribution: After absorption, penicillins are widely distributed in body fluids and tissues. The volume of distribution tends to reflect extracellular compartmentalization, although some penicillins do penetrate into tissues quite well. Significant levels of the various penicillins are generally found in the liver, bile, kidneys, intestines, muscle, and lungs, but only very low concentrations are found in poorly perfused areas such as the cornea, bronchial secretions, cartilage, and bone. The diethylamino salt of penicillin G produces particularly high levels in pulmonary tissue. The penicillins usually do not readily cross the normal blood-brain, placental, mammary, or prostatic barriers; however, massive doses or inflammation often allow diffusion into the respective fluids. Inflammation also permits effective levels of some penicillins to be reached in abscesses (except when very chronic) as well as pleural, peritoneal, and synovial fluids. Penicillins are reversibly and loosely bound to plasma proteins. The extent of this binding varies with particular penicillins and their concentration, eg, ampicillin is usually ~20% bound, and cloxacillin may be ~80% bound. Pregnancy increases the volume of distribution, which has the effect of lowering the concentration of drug produced by a given dose.

TABLE 28. Elimination, Distribution, and Clearance of Penicillins

Penicillin	Species	Elimination Half-life (min)	Volume of Distribution (mL/kg)	Clearance (mL/kg/min)
Penicillin G	Dogs	30	156	3.6
	Horses	38	301	5.5
Ampicillin	Dogs	48	270	3.9
Amoxicillin	Cattle	84	493	4.0
Ticarcillin	Dogs	48	347	4.9
Carbenicillin	Cattle	122	330	5.5

Biotransformation: Penicillins are generally excreted unchanged, but fractions of a given dose may undergo metabolic transformations by unknown mechanisms (usually <20% metabolized). Penicilloic acid derivatives that are formed tend to be allergenic.

Excretion: Most (60-90%) of a parenterally administered penicillin is eliminated in the urine within a short time (eg, up to 90% of penicillin G within 6 hr), which results in high levels in urine, often sufficient to suppress not only gram-positive but also many gram-negative bacteria. About 20% of renal excretion occurs by glomerular filtration and ~80% by tubular secretion—a process that may be deliberately inhibited (to prolong effective levels in the body) by probenecid and other weak organic acids. Anuria may increase the half-life of penicillin G (normally ~30 min) to 10 hr. The biliary route also may be a major excretory pathway for the broad-spectrum semisynthetic penicillins. Clearance values for penicillins are considerably lower in neonates than in adults. Penicillins are also eliminated in milk, although often only in trace amounts in the normal udder, and may persist for up to 90 hr. Penicillin residues in milk also have been found after intrauterine infusion.

Pharmacokinetic Values: Selected pharmacokinetic values for some penicillins in a few species are listed in TABLE 28. Dosage modifications may be necessary because of age or disease.

Therapeutic Indications and Dose Rates

The penicillins are commonly used to treat or prevent local and systemic infections caused by susceptible bacteria. There are several acute infectious disease syndromes that are specifically responsive. Penicillins are also used topically in the eye and ear as well as on the skin; intramammary administration to treat or prevent bovine mastitis is widespread.

A selection of general dosages for some penicillins is listed in TABLE 29. The dose rate and frequency should be adjusted as needed for the individual animal.

Special Clinical Concerns

Side Effects and Toxicity: Organ toxicity is rare. Hypersensitivity reactions do occur (particularly in cattle) and include skin reactions, angioedema, drug fever, serum sickness, vasculitis, eosinophilia, and anaphylaxis. Cross-sensitivity between penicillins is well recognized. Intrathecal administration may result in convulsions. Guinea pigs, chinchillas, birds, snakes, and turtles are sensitive to procaine penicillin. The use of broad-spectrum penicillins may lead to superinfection, and GI disturbances may occur after PO administration of ampicillin. Potassium penicillin G should be administered IV with some caution, especially if hyperkalemia is present. The sodium salt of penicillin G may also contribute to the sodium load in congestive heart failure.

TABLE 29. Dose Rates of Penicillins

Penicillin	Dosage, Route, and Frequency
Sodium penicillin G	10,000-20,000 IU/kg, IV or IM, QID
Potassium penicillin G	25,000 IU/kg, PO, QID
Procaine penicillin G	10,000-30,000 IU/kg, IM or SC, SID-BID
Benzathine penicillin G	10,000-40,000 IU/kg, IM (horses) or SC (cattle), every 48-72 hr
Penicillin V	15,000 IU/kg or 8-10 mg/kg, PO, TID
Cloxacillin	10 mg/kg, IM or PO, QID
Ampicillin	5-10 mg/kg, IV, IM, or SC, BID-TID 10-25 mg/kg, PO, BID-QID
Amoxicillin	4-7 mg/kg, IM, SID-BID 11 mg/kg, PO, BID (dogs) or SID-BID(cats)
Sodium carbenicillin	10-20 mg/kg, IV or IM, BID-TID
Potassium clavulanate:amoxicillin (1:4)	10-20 mg/kg (amoxicillin) and 2.5-5 mg/kg (clavulanate), PO, BID
Probenecid (prolongs blood levels of penicillins that have short plasma half-lives or that are costly)	1-2 mg/1,000 IU penicillin G (dogs), PO, QID
Amoxicillin-clavulanic acid	10-20 mg/kg, PO, BID-TID
Imepenem	1-7 mg/kg, IV or IM, TID-QID
Ticarcillin	15-110 mg/kg, IM or IV, every 4-8 hr

Interactions: Penicillins are displaced from plasma-protein binding sites and tubular secretion is delayed when drugs such as salicylates, phenylbutazone, sulfonamides, and other weak acids are administered concurrently. Gut-active penicillins potentiate the action of anticoagulants by depressing vitamin K production by gut flora. Absorption of ampicillin is impaired by the presence of food. Carbenicillin and ticarcillin interact chemically with the aminoglycosides and should not be mixed in vitro. Ampicillin and penicillin G are incompatible with many other drugs and solutions and should not be mixed.

Effects on Laboratory Tests: Laboratory determinations may be altered, depending on the penicillin used. Alkaline phosphatase, AST, ALT, and eosinophil count may be increased. A false positive Coombs' test may also result after penicillin therapy. A positive test for urine glucose and protein is also possible. Procaine is detectable in the urine of horses for several days after the administration of procaine penicillin; the pre-race withdrawal time may be up to 6 days.

Drug Withdrawal and Milk Discard Times: Regulatory requirements for withdrawal times for food animals and milk discard times vary among countries. These must be followed carefully to prevent food residues and consequent public health implications. The selection of times listed in TABLE 30 serve only as general guidelines.

CEPHALOSPORINS AND CEPHAMYCINS

The cephalosporins, and the closely related cephamycins, are a class of β-lactam antibiotics that has proliferated rapidly. They are similar to the penicillins in several respects and also share many pharmacologic features as a group. Ceftiofur is approved for use in cows and dogs, and cefadroxil is approved for use in dogs and cats.

TABLE 30. Drug Withdrawal and Milk Discard Times of Pencillins*

Penicillin	Species	Withdrawal Time (days)	Milk Discard Time (days)
Procaine penicillin G	Cattle	10 (at label dosage) 30 (at 20,000 IU/kg, BID)	3
	Sheep	9	
	Pigs	7	
Benzathine penicillin G	Cattle	30	
Ampicillin	Cattle	6	
	Preruminant calves	15	
Amoxicillin	Cattle	30	2

*All administered IM

Classes

The early cephalosporins differed mainly with respect to pharmacokinetic characteristics; the newer generations have much broader ranges of activity, and the modern classification of the group is based mainly on antibacterial spectra.

First-generation Cephalosporins: This group includes cephalothin, cephaloridine, cephapirin, cefazolin, cephalexin, cephradine, and cefadroxil. Cephalosporins in this group are usually quite active against many gram-positive bacteria but are only moderately active against gram-negative organisms. They are relatively susceptible to β-lactamases (cephalosporinases) and are not as effective against anaerobes as are the penicillins.

Second-generation Cephalosporins: This group includes cefamandole, cefoxitin (a cephamycin), cefotiam, cefachlor, cefuroxime, and ceforanide. These agents are generally active against both gram-positive and gram-negative bacteria. Moreover, they are relatively resistant to β-lactamase. They are ineffective against enterococci, *Pseudomonas aeruginosa*, *Actinobacter* spp, and many obligate anaerobes.

Third-generation Cephalosporins: This group includes ceftiofur, ceftriaxone, cefsulodin, cefotaxime, cefoperazone, moxalactam (not a true cephalosporin), and several others. Typically, these have only moderate activity against gram-positive bacteria but are active against a wide variety of gram-negative bacteria, including in certain instances *Pseudomonas* spp, *Proteus vulgaris*, *Enterobacter* spp, and *Citrobacter* spp. They are usually highly resistant to β-lactamase enzymes. Third-generation cephalosporins are often able to penetrate the blood-brain barrier and are frequently indicated in bacterial meningitis caused by susceptible pathogens. Ceftiofur has been specifically approved for use in cattle with bronchopneumonia, especially if caused by *Pasteurella haemolytica* or *P multocida*.

Fourth-generation Cephalosporins: A fourth generation of cephalosporins includes new drugs such as cefpodoxime and cefixime. The spectrum of third- and fourth-generation cepaholosporins varies and should be confirmed before using a drug for a targeted organism.

General Properties

The physical and chemical properties of the cephalosporins are similar to those of the penicillins, although the cephalosporins are somewhat more stable to pH and temperature changes. Cephalosporins are weak acids derived from 7-aminocephalosporanic acid. They are used either as the free base form for PO administration (if acid stable) or as sodium salts in aqueous solution for parenteral delivery (sodium salt of cephalothin contains 2.4 mEq sodium/g). Cephalosporins also contain a β-lactam nucleus that is susceptible to β-lactamase (cephalosporinase) hydrolysis. These β-lactamases may or may not also attack penicillins. Modifications of the 7-aminocephalosporanic acid nucleus and substitutions on the sidechains by semisynthetic means have produced differences among cephalosporins in antibacterial spectra, β-lactamase sensitivities, and pharmacokinetics.

Antimicrobial Activity

Mode of Action: This is similar to that of the penicillins. Cephalosporins also bind to penicillin-binding proteins located beneath the cell wall and thereby interfere with the action of transpeptidase and other cell-wall enzymes. A residual antibacterial effect is also evident with the cephalosporins. As a group, these antibiotics are most stable and effective at a pH of 6-7.

Bacterial Resistance: Resistance to the cephalosporins may be mediated in several ways that are comparable to those associated with penicillin resistance.

Permeability Barrier: There may be lack of bacterial permeability to the particular cephalosporin. First- and second-generation cephalosporins cannot penetrate the outer membrane of *Pseudomonas aeruginosa*.

Specific Bacterial Binding Proteins: Alteration in structure of target sites mediated by genetic mechanisms identical to those of penicillin resistance may lead to reduced sensitivity to the cephalosporins.

β-Lactamase (Cephalosporinase) Resistance: Cephalosporins generally are stable against the plasmid-mediated β-lactamases produced by gram-positive bacteria such as *Staphylococcus aureus*. Several types of inducible β-lactamases produced by gram-negative organisms may be mediated by either plasmids or chromosomally and may hydrolyze either or both penicillins and cephalosporins (cross-resistance). Second- and particularly third-generation cephalosporins have greater stability against gram-negative β-lactamases.

L-forms, Persisters, and Tolerance: These forms of resistance are also encountered against the cephalosporins (*see* PENICILLINS, p 2056).

Antibacterial Spectra: The first-generation cephalosporins are generally effective against most gram-positive aerobic cocci and several of the gram-negative bacteria, including *E coli* and *Proteus, Klebsiella, Salmonella, Shigella,* and *Enterobacter* spp. Cephalosporinase-producing organisms are not susceptible. The second-generation cephalosporins have greater activity against gram-negative organisms but are somewhat less active against gram-positive species. This trend continues with the third-generation cephalosporins, which may even be active against *P aeruginosa*. The newest members of this group are also highly resistant to β-lactamase. Ceftiofur is a third-generation cephalosporin, but unlike other members of this class, it has a gram-negative spectrum that is more similar to first-generation cephalosporins. However, unlike first-generation cephalosporins, efficacy against *Staphylococcus* spp is not predictable. The cephalosporins may be effective against anaerobic bacteria except *Bacteroides fragilis,* which is susceptible only to certain cephalosporins.

Pharmacokinetic Features

Not much information is available on the fate of the cephalosporins in animals; many of the recommendations are based on extrapolation from human data.

Absorption: Only a few cephalosporins are acid stable and thus effective when administered PO (cephalexin, cephradine, cefadroxil, and cefachlor). They are usually well absorbed, and bioavailability values are 75-90%. The others are administered either IV or IM, with plasma concentrations peaking ~30 min after injection.

Distribution: Cephalosporins are widely distributed through most body fluids and tissues, including kidneys, lungs, joints, bone, soft tissues, and the biliary tract, but in general, the volume of distribution is <0.3 L/kg. However, poor penetration into the CSF,

TABLE 31. Elimination, Distribution, and Clearance of Cephalosporins

Cephalosporin	Species	Elimination Half-life (min)	Volume of Distribution (mL/kg)	Clearance (mL/kg/min)
Cefazolin	Horses	45	188	5.5
Cefotaxime	Sheep	25	134	9.0
Cephalexin	Dogs	84	—	—
Cefadroxil	Dogs	120	—	—
	Cats	150-180	—	—
Ceftiofur	Cattle	~360	—	—

even in inflammation, is a notable feature of the standard cephalosporins. The third-generation cephalosporins (eg, moxalactam) may achieve good penetration into the CSF. The degree of plasma-protein binding is variable (eg, 20% for cefadroxil and 80% for cefazolin).

Biotransformation: Several cephalosporins (such as cephalothin, cephapirin, cephacetrile, and cefotaxime) are actively deacetylated, primarily in the liver but also in other tissues. The deacetylated derivatives are much less active with the exception of ceftiofur. Ceftiofur is metabolized to several active metabolites that can contribute significantly to efficacy. Few of the other cephalosporins are metabolized to any appreciable extent.

Excretion: Most cephalosporins are excreted by renal tubular secretion, although glomerular filtration is important in some cases (cephaloridine, cephalexin, and cefazolin). In renal failure, dose rates should be reduced. Biliary elimination of the newer cephalosporins (eg, cefoperazone) may be significant. Generally, these β-lactam antibiotics maintain effective blood levels for only 6-8 hr.

Pharmacokinetic Values: Plasma half-lives are often 30-120 min, but there are exceptions. Third-generation cephalosporins tend to have longer plasma half-lives in humans, but this is not always the case in other animals—substantial species differences exist. A selection of pharmacokinetic values for cephalosporins is listed in TABLE 31 to serve as a guide. Dosage modifications are often required in hepatic and renal disease.

Therapeutic Indications and Dose Rates

The cost of cephalosporins has limited their use in veterinary medicine. However, first-generation cephalosporins have proved useful, particularly for infections involving *Staphylococcus* spp (eg, oral cephalexin for dermatitis) and for surgical prophylaxis (eg, cefazolin). Ceftiofur is approved for use in bovine respiratory disease principally caused by *Pasteurella* spp and in urinary tract infections in dogs. Use of ceftiofur for treatment of soft-tissue infections in dogs is not recommended because proper dosages and safety have not been documented. Cephalosporins are particularly useful for treating infections of soft tissue and bone due to bacteria that are resistant to other commonly used antibiotics. Because of their favorable pharmacokinetic characteristics and effectiveness, they are often administered IV, 1 hr before surgery. Because of their ability to penetrate tissues and fluids so readily (the CSF being an exception for most), they are often effective in the management of osteomyelitis, prostatitis, and arthritis. Oral cephalosporins are also usually effective in the management of urinary tract infections, except those due to *Pseudomonas aeruginosa*. Cephapirin benzathine is used for dry-cow therapy, and cephapirin sodium is used in treatment of mastitis.

A selection of general dosages for some cephalosporins is listed in TABLE 32. The dose rate and frequency should be adjusted as needed for the individual animal.

TABLE 32. Dose Rates of Cephalosporins*

Cephalosporin	Dosage, Route, and Frequency
Cephalothin	20-35 mg/kg, IM or IV, TID-QID
Cephapirin	30 mg/kg, IM or IV, every 4-6 hr
Cefazolin	20-25 mg/kg, IM or IV, TID-QID
Cephalexin	10-30 mg/kg, PO, TID-QID
Cefadroxil	22 mg/kg, PO, BID
Ceftiofur	1.1 mg/kg, IM, SID

*All for use in small animals, except ceftiofur, which is for use in cattle.

Special Clinical Concerns

Side Effects and Toxicity: The cephalosporins are relatively nontoxic, although cephaloridine may be nephrotoxic in some species. IM injections can be painful, and repeated IV administration may lead to local phlebitis. Nausea, vomiting, and diarrhea may occasionally be seen. Hypersensitivity reactions of several forms have been seen, particularly in animals with a history of acute penicillin allergy. Superinfection may arise with the use of cephalosporins, and *Pseudomonas* or *Candida* spp are likely opportunistic pathogens.

Interactions: In vitro incompatibilities are quite common for cephalosporin and cephamycin preparations. Potential pharmacokinetic interactions are similar to those of the penicillin group. Aminoglycosides may enhance cephaloridine nephrotoxicity, but there is some doubt about this particular interaction. Furosemide and ethacrynic acid, however, do appear to potentiate the nephrotoxic action of cephaloridine.

Effects on Laboratory Tests: Several laboratory determinations may be altered by the cephalosporins. Alkaline phosphatase, AST, ALT, lactate dehydrogenase, and BUN may be increased. A false-positive Coombs' test and a false-positive urine glucose may also be present. Hypernatremia may be caused by the sodium salts of various cephalosporins.

Drug Withdrawal and Milk Discard Times: Although prolonged tissue residues for most cephalosporins are not anticipated, withdrawal times are not available for most of the cephalosporins because they are not approved for use in food animals in most countries (TABLE 33).

AMINOGLYCOSIDES
(Aminocyclitols)

These are mostly bactericidal drugs that share chemical, antimicrobial, pharmacologic, and toxic characteristics.

TABLE 33. Drug Withdrawal and Milk Discard Times of Cephalosporins

Cephalosporin	Withdrawal Time	Milk Discard Time
Ceftiofur	0 days	
Sodium cephapirin (intramammary)	4 days before slaughter	4 days
Benzathine cephapirin (dry-cow treatment)	42 days after latest infusion	3 days after calving—milk not used for food

Classes

Narrow-spectrum Aminoglycosides: Included in this group are streptomycin and dihydrostreptomycin, which are mainly active against aerobic, gram-negative bacteria.

Expanded-spectrum Aminoglycosides: Neomycin, framycetin (neomycin B), paromomycin (aminosidine), and kanamycin have broader spectra than streptomycin that often include several gram-positive as well as many gram-negative aerobic bacteria. Gentamicin, tobramycin, amikacin, sisomicin, and netilmicin are aminoglycosides with extended spectra that include *Pseudomonas aeruginosa*.

Miscellaneous Aminoglycoside Antibiotics: The chemical structure of apramycin differs somewhat from that of the typical aminoglycosides but is similar enough to be included in this class. The structure of spectinomycin is unusual, but it is fairly comparable to other aminocyclitols with regard to its mechanism of action and antibacterial spectrum.

General Properties

Chemically, the aminoglycoside antibiotics are characterized by an aminocyclitol group, with aminosugars attached to the aminocyclitol ring in glycosidic linkage. Because of minor differences in the position of substitutions on the molecules, there may be several forms of a single aminoglycoside. For example, gentamicin is a complex of gentamicins C_1 and C_2, and neomycin is a mixture of neomycins B, C, and fradiomycin. The amino groups contribute to the basic nature of this class of antibiotics, and the hydroxyl groups on the sugar moieties to high aqueous solubility and poor lipid solubility. If these hydroxyl groups are removed (eg, tobramycin), antibiotic activity is markedly increased. Differences in the substitutions on the basic ring structures within the various aminoglycosides account for the relatively minor differences in antimicrobial spectra, patterns of resistance, and toxicities. Aminoglycosides are typically quite stable. When the water solubility of an aminoglycoside is marginal, it is usually the sulfate salt that is used for PO or parenteral administration.

Antimicrobial Activity

Mode of Action: Aminoglycosides are more effective against rapidly multiplying organisms, and they affect and ultimately destroy bacteria by several mechanisms. They need only a short contact with bacteria to kill them. Their main site of action is the membrane-associated bacterial ribosome through which they interfere with protein synthesis. To reach the ribosome, they must first cross the bacterial cell wall and then the cell membrane. Because of the polarity of these compounds, a specialized transport process is required. The first concentration-dependent step requires binding of the aminoglycoside to anionic components in the cell membrane. The subsequent steps are energy-dependent and involve the transport of the polar, highly charged aminoglycoside across the cytoplasmic membrane, followed by interaction with the ribosomes. The driving force for this transfer is probably the membrane potential. These processes are much more efficient if the energy used is aerobically generated.

Several features of these mechanisms are of clinical significance: 1) The antibacterial activity of the aminoglycosides depends on an effective concentration of antibiotic outside the cell. 2) Anaerobic bacteria and induced mutants are generally resistant because they lack appropriate transport systems. 3) With low oxygen tension, as in hypoxic tissues, transfer into bacteria is diminished. 4) Divalent cations, eg, calcium and magnesium, can interfere with transport into bacteria because they can combine with the specific anionic sites and exclude the cationic aminoglycosides. 5) Transport of aminoglycosides across bacterial cell membranes is facilitated by an alkaline pH; a low pH may increase membrane resistance >100-fold. 6) Changes in osmolality also can alter the uptake of aminoglycosides. 7) Some aminoglycosides are transported more efficiently than others, and thus tend to have greater antibacterial activity. 8) Synergism is common when aminoglycosides and β-lactam antibiotics (penicillins and cephalosporins) are used in combination. The cell-wall injury induced by the β-lactam compounds allows increased uptake of the aminoglycoside by the bacteria because of easier accessibility to the bacterial cell membrane.

The intracellular site of action of the aminoglycosides is the ribosome, which has binding sites at both the 30 S and 50 S subunits, although they bind particularly to the former. There is some variation between aminoglycosides with respect to their affinity and degree of binding. A number of steps in protein synthesis appear to be affected, but this too varies among aminoglycosides. Spectinomycin lacks the ability to produce misreading of the mRNA and often is not bactericidal, in contrast to the other members. At low concentrations, all aminoglycosides may be only bacteriostatic.

A cell-membrane effect is also seen. The functional integrity of the bacterial cell membrane is lost during the late phase of the transport process, and high concentrations of aminoglycosides may cause nonspecific membrane toxicity, even to the point of bacterial cell lysis.

Efficacy of aminoglycosides is enhanced if peak plasma or tissue drug concentrations exceed MIC by 4-8 times. Once-daily dosing has been used to enhance both efficacy and safety.

Bacterial Resistance: Several mechanisms of resistance to the aminoglycoside antibiotics have been described. These may be plasmid-mediated or due to mutation.

Impaired transport across the cell membrane is one mechanism of nonplasmid-mediated resistance. Because the transport process is active and oxygen-dependent, anaerobic bacteria (eg, *Bacteroides fragilis* and *Clostridium perfringens*) and facultative anaerobes (eg, enterobacteria and *Staphylococcus aureus*) are more resistant to the aminoglycosides when in an anaerobic environment. Resistance due to impaired transport can be induced by exposure to sublethal concentrations of these antibiotics. Examples of this form include streptomycin resistance among strains of *Pseudomonas aeruginosa*, low-level aminoglycoside resistance among enterococci, and gentamicin resistance in *Streptococcus faecalis*.

Impaired ribosomal binding may not be a clinically important form of resistance. Examples include *Escherichia coli* strains in which a single-step mutation prevents the binding of streptomycin to the ribosome. The same mechanism has been described in *Pseudomonas aeruginosa*.

Enzymatic modification of aminoglycosides may be plasmid-encoded and chromosomally mediated. The enzymes are found in both gram-negative and gram-positive bacteria. There are 3 major types of enzymes involved, with several subclasses in each case. The main groups are acetylating enzymes (acetyltransferases), adenylating enzymes (nucleotidyltransferases), and phosphorylating enzymes (phosphotransferases). The susceptibility of the aminoglycosides to specific enzymatic attack is quite variable, and the substrate profiles differ for each subclass. This explains the common incidence of cross-resistance yet the frequent differences in susceptibility patterns. Chemical alteration of an aminoglycoside may render it relatively stable to enzymatic hydrolysis (eg, kanamycin modified to amikacin is relatively resistant to inactivating enzymes).

Several **other mechanisms of resistance** are recognized: 1) Increasing the concentration of divalent cations (especially Ca^{2+} and Mg^{2+}) in the media increases resistance in *Pseudomonas aeruginosa*. 2) Mutants of *P aeruginosa* produce an excess of outer cell membrane protein, called H1, that confers relative resistance to gentamicin. 3) A low pH, as found in acidic urine or in abscess cavities, leads to persistent viability of microorganisms even with relatively high concentrations of aminoglycosides.

Antibacterial Spectra: Streptomycin and dihydrostreptomycin have relatively narrow spectra, and bacterial resistance is becoming prevalent. However, some staphylococci and a number of gram-negative bacilli are still susceptible, among which are strains of *Actinomyces bovis*, *Pasteurella* spp, *E coli*, *Salmonella* spp, *Campylobacter fetus*, *Leptospira* spp, and *Brucella* spp. *Mycobacterium tuberculosis* is also sensitive to streptomycin.

Neomycin, framycetin, and kanamycin have broader spectra than streptomycin, and their clinical use is most often directed against gram-negative species such as *E coli* and

Salmonella, Klebsiella, Enterobacter, Proteus, and *Acinetobacter* spp. The aminoglycosides with broader spectra that include *P aeruginosa* (gentamicin, tobramycin, amikacin, sisomicin, and netilmicin) are often highly effective against a wide variety of aerobic bacteria. Anaerobic bacteria and fungi are not appreciably affected; streptococci are usually only moderately sensitive or quite resistant.

Pharmacokinetic Features

The pharmacokinetic features of the aminoglycosides are similar in most species.

Absorption: Aminoglycosides are poorly absorbed (usually <10%) from the healthy GI tract. However, enteritis and other pathologic changes may allow absorption to be significantly greater and, in renal failure, toxic levels can accumulate. Absorption from IM injection sites is rapid and nearly complete (>90% availability), except in severely hypotensive animals. Blood levels usually peak within 30-90 min after IM administration. Absorption after SC injection may be protracted. Absorption after IP administration can be rapid and substantial and has the potential to result in serious side effects. Aminoglycosides can be administered IV by bolus injection or by intermittent or continuous infusions. However, bolus injections and continuous infusions have a high risk of toxicity (*see* SPECIAL CLINICAL CONCERNS, below); intermittent (once daily) infusions are safer. Serum levels of aminoglycosides may reach bactericidal levels after repeated intrauterine infusion, particularly in endometritis.

Distribution: Because of their polarity at physiologic pH, the aminoglycosides distribute into the extracellular fluid space with minimal penetration into most tissues except the kidneys (where they accumulate in the renal cortex) and the endolymph of the inner ear. The extracellular fluid compartment approximates 25% of body weight, but this volume can change substantially and significantly influence the concentration of an aminoglycoside. The extracellular fluid space contracts with dehydration of any cause and during gram-negative sepsis. The distribution volume of aminoglycosides can increase in animals with congestive heart failure or ascites. Neonates also have a large extracellular fluid compartment relative to body weight. Although aminoglycosides are not appreciably bound to plasma proteins (usually <20%), they do attain therapeutic concentrations in the synovial, pleural, and even peritoneal fluids, especially if inflammation is present. However, effective levels are not reached in CSF, ocular fluids, milk, intestinal fluids, or prostatic secretions. Fetal tissue and amniotic fluid concentrations are very low in most species.

Biotransformation, Excretion, and Pharmacokinetic Values: The aminoglycosides are not metabolized in the body. They are eliminated unchanged in the urine by glomerular filtration, with 80-90% of administered drug recoverable from the urine within 24 hr of IM administration. A variable fraction of filtered aminoglycoside is absorbed onto the brush border of the proximal tubule and loop of Henle cells. After binding, they are transported into the cell and sequestered in lysosomes and subsequently redistributed into the cytosol. Excessive accumulation (mainly in the renal cortex) leads to a characteristic tubular cell necrosis. Glomerular filtration rates differ between species and are often less in neonates, which may explain the greater sensitivity to aminoglycosides in newborn foals and puppies.

Elimination depends on cardiovascular and renal function, age, volume of distribution, fever, and several other factors. The volume of distribution is usually represented by the volume of the extracellular fluid compartment. The aminoglycosides have relatively short plasma half-lives (~1 hr in carnivores and 2-3 hr in herbivores). The elimination kinetics often follow those of a 3-compartment model. About 90% of the injected drug is excreted unchanged through the kidneys during the β phase of elimination. The remainder is excreted over a protracted period, or γ phase, probably due to the gradual release of the antibiotic from renal intracellular binding sites (terminal elimination half-life often 20-200 hr). The limited selection of pharmacokinetic values for 2 typical aminoglycosides (TABLE 34) serves as a basis for any required dosage modifications that may

TABLE 34. Elimination, Distribution, and Clearance of Aminoglycosides

Aminoglycoside	Species	Elimination Half-life (min)	Volume of Distribution (mL/kg)	Clearance (mL/kg/min)
Gentamicin	Dogs	75	335	3.10
	Horses	110	190	1.23
	Foals	200	300	1.04
Kanamycin	Dogs	60	255	3.05
	Horses	85	174	1.43
	Sheep	110	217	1.52

be necessary due to age or renal insufficiency. The best way to alter a dosage regimen of aminoglycosides is to monitor plasma concentrations.

Therapeutic Indications and Dose Rates

Despite their potential to cause nephrotoxicity, the aminoglycosides are commonly used to control local and systemic infections caused by susceptible aerobic bacteria (generally gram-negative) because of their effectiveness. Examples include septicemia; tracheobronchitis; pneumonia; osteoarthritis; and infections of the urinary tract, GI tract, and skin and wounds. Several aminoglycosides are used topically in the ears and eyes. Intrauterine infusion to treat endometritis is also frequent. Occasionally, aminoglycosides are infused into the udder to treat mastitis.

A selection of general dosages for some aminoglycosides is listed in TABLE 35. The dose rate and frequency should be adjusted as needed for the individual animal (*see* below).

While a nomogram based on creatinine clearance values or the creatinine clearance values themselves could be used to calculate appropriate dosage modifications in renal insufficiency, such an approach is rarely practical, and generally is unnecessary with once-daily dosing. The ideal is to monitor both plasma aminoglycoside concentrations and renal function during therapy. As a precaution, the following general guidelines may be followed in cases of renal failure in which plasma creatinine values are increased (TABLE 36).

The treatment interval should be increased in neonates (especially puppies and foals), in renal failure, and in obese animals. Doses may be increased in animals with edema, hydrothorax, or ascites, provided their renal function is unimpaired.

Special Clinical Concerns

Side Effects and Toxicity: Ototoxicity, neuromuscular blockade, and nephrotoxicity are reported most frequently; these effects may vary with the aminoglycoside and dose or

TABLE 35. Dose Rates of Aminoglycosides

Aminoglycoside	Dosage, Route, and Frequency
Gentamicin	3-6 mg/kg, IM or SC, SID-BID
Kanamycin	12-15 mg/kg, IM or SC, SID-BID
Streptomycin/dihydrostreptomycin	7.5-12.5 mg/kg, IM or SC, BID
Amikacin	5-7.5 mg/kg, IM or SC, BID
Netilmicin	3-6 mg/kg, IM or SC, SID-BID
Neomycin	15 mg/kg, PO, SID-BID 0.5-1 g/quarter, intramammary, SID

TABLE 36. Dosage Modifications of Aminoglycosides in Renal Failure

Plasma creatinine (mg/dL)	Dose and Dosage Interval
<1	Full dose at usual dosage interval
2	Full dose doubling the usual dosage interval
3	Full dose tripling the usual dosage interval
4	Half dose doubling the usual dosage interval, or full dose quadrupling the usual dosage interval
>5	Aminoglycosides contraindicated

interval used, but all members of the group are potentially toxic. Nephrotoxicity is of major concern and may result in renal failure due to acute tubular necrosis with secondary interstitial damage. Aminoglycosides accumulate in proximal tubular epithelial cells, where they are sequestered in lysosomes and interact with ribosomes, mitochondria, and other intracellular constituents to cause cell injury. Persistence of aminoglycosides in plasma and thus urine is likely to predispose the tubular cells to toxicity, and the risk may by reduced by allowing plasma drug concentrations to drop below recommended levels (generally 1-2 μg/mL) before the next dose. Nonoliguric renal failure is the usual observation; it is generally reversible, although recovery may be prolonged. Any failure in glomerular filtration results in excessively high concentrations of aminoglycoside, which in turn result in further renal damage. Renal function should be monitored during therapy. Polyuria, decreased urine osmolality, enzymuria, proteinuria, cylindruria, and increased fractional sodium excretion are indicative of aminoglycoside nephrotoxicity. Later, BUN and creatinine concentrations may be increased. Early changes or evidence of nephrotoxicity can be detected in 3-5 days, with more overt signs in 7-10 days. Several factors predispose to aminoglycoside nephrotoxicosis, including age (with young [especially the newborn foal] and old animals being sensitive), compromised renal function, total dose, duration of treatment, dehydration and hypovolemia, aciduria, acidosis, severe sepsis or endotoxemia, concurrent administration of furosemide, and exposure to other potential nephrotoxins (eg, methoxyflurane, amphotericin B, cis-platinum, and perhaps some cephalosporins). In renal insufficiency, generally the interval between doses is prolonged (rather than reducing the dose) to minimize toxicity.

The risk of aminoglycoside-induced nephrotoxicity can be reduced by maintaining patient hydration and an alkaline urine pH, dosing once daily, and avoiding nephroactive drugs (eg, NSAID, diuretics).

Aminoglycosides can result in ototoxicity, which manifests as auditory or vestibular dysfunction. Vestibular injury leads to nystagmus, incoordination, and loss of the righting reflex. The lesion is often irreversible, although physiologic adaptation can occur. Cats are particularly sensitive to the toxic vestibular effects. Hearing impairment is produced by permanent damage and loss of the hair cells in the organ of Corti. High-frequency hearing is impaired first, and deafness may not be complete, depending on the dosage used. Such an impediment could be of enormous importance (eg, in guide dogs), and aminoglycosides should not be administered to such animals except under extenuating circumstances. Aminoglycosides should not be instilled into the ear unless the tympanic membrane is intact, because diffusion of the drug into the inner ear could cause damage. Several risk factors may predispose to vestibular and cochlear damage by aminoglycosides (in addition to those for nephrotoxicity), including preexisting acoustical or vestibular impairment and previous treatment with potentially ototoxic drugs or loop-acting diuretics (eg, furosemide, ethacrynic acid). The ototoxic potential is highest for gentamicin, sisomicin, and neomycin, and lowest for netilmicin.

All aminoglycosides, when administered in doses that result in high plasma levels, have been associated with muscle weakness and respiratory arrest attributable to neuromuscular blockade. The effect is more pronounced when aminoglycosides are used with other drugs that cause neuromuscular blockade and with gas anesthetics. Neomycin, kanamycin, amikacin, gentamicin, and tobramycin are listed in order of most to least potent for these neuromuscular effects. The effect is due to the chelation of calcium and competitive inhibition of the prejunctional release of acetylcholine in most instances (there are some differences among aminoglycosides). The blockade is antagonized by calcium gluconate and somewhat less consistently by neostigmine.

Other forms of toxicity and side effects include CNS disturbances and even convulsions, collapse after rapid IV administration, superinfection when used topically or PO, a malabsorption syndrome due to allocation of intestinal villous function when used PO in neonates, occasional hypersensitivity reactions, contact dermatitis, cardiovascular depression, and inhibition of some WBC functions (eg, neutrophil migration and chemotaxis and even bactericidal activity at high concentrations).

Interactions: Enhanced nephrotoxicity may become evident with concurrent administration of aminoglycosides and other potentially nephrotoxic agents. Neuromuscular blockade is more likely when aminoglycosides are administered at the same time as skeletal muscle relaxants and gas anesthetics. Aminoglycoside ototoxicity is enhanced by the loop-acting diuretics, especially furosemide. Cardiovascular depression may be aggravated by aminoglycosides when administered to animals under halothane anesthesia. High concentrations of carbenicillin, ticarcillin, and piperacillin inactivate aminoglycosides both in vitro and in vivo in the presence of renal failure.

Effects on Laboratory Tests: BUN, serum creatinine, serum transaminases, and alkaline phosphatase values may be increased. Proteinuria is a significant laboratory finding.

Drug Withdrawal and Milk Discard Times: Regulatory requirements for withdrawal times for food animals and milk discard times vary among countries. These must be followed carefully to prevent food residues and consequent public health implications. The selection of times listed serve only as general guidelines (TABLE 37).

Miscellaneous Aminocyclitol Antibiotics

Apramycin is used to control gram-negative infections, particularly *Escherichia coli* and salmonellae in calves and piglets. It also is active against *Proteus, Klebsiella, Treponema,* and *Mycoplasma* spp. There is little cross-resistance within the aminoglycosides, and plasmid-mediated resistance is yet to be confirmed. Apramycin is poorly absorbed after administration PO (<10%). It is rapidly absorbed from parenteral injection sites. Plasma levels peak within 1-2 hr of IM administration. Apramycin distributes only into the extracellular fluid and is excreted unchanged in the urine (95% within 4 days). The elimination half-life in calves is ~4-5 hr. Apramycin is toxic in cats but is considered safe in most other species (3-6 times the recommended oral dose rarely produces toxicity). The oral dose rate is 20-40 mg/kg, SID for 5 days. The parenteral dose rate is 20 mg/kg, BID. The withdrawal time in pigs and calves (Europe) is 28 days after oral use.

The structure of spectinomycin differs from that of the aminoglycosides, but it also binds to bacterial ribosomes and interferes with protein synthesis. However, the effect is bacteriostatic rather than bactericidal. Spectinomycin can be inactivated by an enzyme coded for by an R factor, but mutant resistance due to diminished ribosomal binding is perhaps more common. It is active against several strains of streptococci, a wide range

---

TABLE 37. Drug Withdrawal and Milk Discard Times of Aminoglycosides

Route	Approximate Withdrawal Time (days)
Oral	20-30 (3 for neonatal pigs)
Parenteral	100-200 (40 for neonatal pigs [often not approved for food animals])
Udder infusion	2-3[*] (often not approved for food animals)

[*]Milk discard time

of gram-negative bacteria, and *Mycoplasma* spp; most *Chlamydia* spp are resistant. It is poorly absorbed from the GI tract but is rapidly absorbed after IM administration, with blood levels peaking within 1 hr. Like aminoglycosides, spectinomycin penetrates tissues rather poorly and distributes principally into extracellular fluid. Metabolic transformation of spectinomycin is limited, and 80% can be recovered unchanged in the urine over 24-48 hr. About 75% is eliminated by glomerular filtration in ~4 hr. At usual doses, no major toxic reactions have been reported. It is administered both PO at 20 mg/kg, BID, and IM at 5-10 mg/kg, BID. Withdrawal time for pigs is usually ~3 wk.

QUINOLONES

Quinolone carboxylic acid derivatives are synthetic antimicrobial agents. Nalidixic acid and its congener oxolinic acid have been used for treatment of urinary tract infections for years, while flumequine has been used successfully in several countries to control intestinal infections in livestock. Many broad-spectrum antimicrobial agents have been produced by modification of the various 4-quinolone ring structures.

Classes

Known generically as quinolones or 4-quinolones, these drugs are derived from several closely related ring structures that have certain common features. The major classes are presented in TABLE 38 with several clinically useful examples of each.

General Properties

Within the diversity of their various ring structures, the quinolones have a number of common functional groups that are essential for their antimicrobial activity. In addition, various modifications have produced compounds with differing physical, chemical, pharmacokinetic, and antimicrobial properties. For example, substitution at position 6 with a fluorine moiety markedly enhances activity against both gram-negative and gram-positive bacteria, as well as mycoplasmas and chlamydiae. These so-called fluoroquinolones, which are generally the most efficacious within each class, include enrofloxacin, norfloxacin, ciprofloxacin, orbifloxacin, ofloxacin, danofloxacin, flumequine, difloxacin, marbofloxacin, and other newer drugs. In addition, substitution with a piperazine ring at position 7 significantly increases tissue and bacterial penetration with consequent enhancement of activity; substitution with an oxygen atom at position 8 improves activity against gram-positive and anaerobic organisms without affecting the bactericidal profile.

The quinolones are amphoteric and, with a few exceptions, generally exhibit poor water solubility between pH 6 and 8. In concentrated acidic urine, such as may be found in dogs and cats, some quinolones form needle-shaped crystals. Liquid formulations of various quinolones for PO or parenteral administration usually contain freely soluble salts in stable aqueous solutions. Solid formulations (eg, tablets, capsules, or boluses) contain the active ingredient either in its betaine form or, occasionally, as the hydrochloride salt.

TABLE 38. Classes of Quinolones

Quinolone carboxylic acids:	Enrofloxacin, norfloxacin, ciprofloxacin, orbifloxacin, pefloxacin, danofloxacin, difloxacin, marbofloxacin, rosoxacin, acrosoxacin, oxolinic acid
Naphthyridine carboxylic acids:	Enoxacin, nalidixic acid
Cinnoline carboxylic acids:	Cinoxacin
Pyridopyrimidine carboxylic acids:	Pipemidic acid, piromidic acid
Quinolizine carboxylic acids:	Ofloxacin, flumequine

Antimicrobial Activity

Mode of Action: The quinolones inhibit the bacterial enzyme DNA-gyrase (topo-isomerase), which is responsible for the supercoiling of DNA so that the DNA can twist in a number of chromosomal domains and seal around an RNA core. To do this, the chromosome also must be transiently nicked before sealing. When DNA-gyrase is inhibited by quinolones, a reduction in the supercoiling occurs with a consequent disruption of the spatial arrangement of DNA. The exposed nicks induce exonucleases that degrade chromosomal DNA into small fragments. Mammalian topoisomerases with nicking activity exist, but these enzymes are fundamentally different from bacterial gyrase and are not susceptible to quinolone inhibition. The quinolones are usually bactericidal; susceptible organisms lose viability within 20 min of exposure to optimal concentrations of the newer fluoroquinolones. Typically, clearing of cytoplasm at the periphery of the affected bacterium occurs and is followed by lysis. Affected bacteria are then recognizable only as ghosts.

Quinolones are known to produce a postantibiotic effect in a number of bacteria (eg, *Escherichia coli, Klebsiella pneumoniae, Pseudomonas aeruginosa*). The effect generally lasts 4-8 hr after exposure.

Ideal bactericidal concentrations of the quinolones are often 0.1-10 μg/mL; efficacy tends to diminish at higher concentrations. This unusual biphasic effect is thought to be due to suppression of RNA synthesis at higher quinolone concentrations. Efficacy of the fluorinated quinolones depends on concentrations in plasma that exceed the MIC of the infecting organism by 4- to 10- fold.

The fluoroquinolones often have significant antibacterial activity at extraordinarily low concentrations. The MIC (μg/mL) for enrofloxacin against some common veterinary pathogens are <0.01-0.5 for *E coli*, <0.03-0.5 for *Klebsiella* spp, 0.003-0.5 for *Salmonella* spp, 0.25-2 for *P aeruginosa*, <0.008-0.12 for *Mannheimia (Pasteurella) haemolytica*, 0.03-1 for *Staphylococcus aureus*, 0.06-4 for *Streptococcus* spp, and 0.01-1 for *Mycoplasma* spp.

Bacterial Resistance: Although resistance develops quite rapidly to nalidixic acid and some older quinolones, only low-frequency chromosomal mutational resistance to the newer quinolones has been recognized, and it is not regarded as a significant problem. Resistance is due to modification of the target gyrase enzyme. Plasmid-mediated resistance is rare. Fortunately, the virulence of refractory mutants diminishes substantially, and these bacterial populations tend to disappear because of growth deficiencies. Cross-resistance does occur between some closely related quinolones.

Antimicrobial Spectrum: The fluoroquinolones are active against a wide range of gram-negative and a number of gram-positive aerobes. They are highly effective against all intestinal bacterial pathogens, as well as several intracellular pathogens, eg, *Brucella* spp. These newer quinolones also have significant activity against *Mycoplasma* and *Chlamydia* spp. Obligate anaerobes tend to be resistant to most quinolones, as are most enterococcal group D *Streptococcus* spp (*S faecalis* and *S faecium*).

The older quinolones (eg, nalidixic acid and oxolinic acid) and the nonfluorinated quinolones (eg, cinoxacin) tend to have only a moderately extended gram-negative spectrum.

A synergistic effect of quinolones with the β-lactams, aminoglycosides, clindamycin, and metronidazole has been demonstrated in vitro.

Pharmacokinetic Features

Among the few quinolones that have been studied to any degree in domestic animals, pharmacokinetic differences are significant. Because of the physicochemical nature of the group, this is to be expected. A general overview follows, but some diversity should be anticipated.

Absorption: Quinolones are commonly administered PO, although forms of enrofloxacin and ciprofloxacin are available for IV, IM, and SC administration. Absorption into the blood after IM or SC delivery is rapid; after administration PO, peak blood concentrations are usually attained within 1-3 hr. Bioavailability is often >80% for most quinolones, except for ciprofloxacin and in ruminants with functional forestomachs, in which bioavailability may be as low as 20%. The presence of food may delay absorption in monogastric animals. The bioavailability of ciprofloxacin after administration PO in dogs is variable and can be as little as 40%.

Distribution: The quinolones, with few exceptions (eg, cinoxacin), penetrate all tissues well and quickly. Particularly high levels are found in the kidneys, liver, and bile, but levels found in prostatic fluid, bone, endometrium, and CSF are also quite notable. Most quinolones also cross the placental barrier. The apparent volume of distribution of most quinolones is large. The degree of plasma-protein binding is extremely variable, from ~10% for norfloxacin to >90% for nalidixic acid.

Biotransformation: Some quinolones are eliminated unchanged (eg, ofloxacin), some are partially metabolized (eg, cinoxacin, ciprofloxacin, enrofloxacin), and a few are completely degraded (eg, acrosoxacin, pefloxacin). Metabolites are sometimes active; enrofloxacin is de-ethylated to form ciprofloxacin. Characteristically, phase I reactions result in a number of primary metabolites (up to 6 have been described for some quinolones) that retain some antibacterial action. Conjugation with glucuronic acid then ensues, followed by excretion.

Excretion: Renal excretion is the major route of elimination for most quinolones. Both glomerular filtration and tubular secretion are involved. Urine concentrations are often high for 24 hr after administration, and crystals may form in concentrated acidic urine. The clinical significance of this finding is unclear. In renal failure, clearance is impaired, and reductions in dose rates are essential. Biliary excretion of parent drug, as well as conjugates, is an important route of elimination in some cases (eg, ciprofloxacin, pefloxacin, nalidixic acid). Quinolones appear in the milk of lactating animals, often at high concentrations that persist for some time.

Pharmacokinetic Considerations: The plasma half-lives are quite variable among species and the different quinolone classes: 3-6 hr are common, but prolonged plasma half-lives are seen (eg, 10 hr for pefloxacin in humans). Plasma concentrations attained are usually directly proportional to the dose administered. Although somewhat lower, the plasma drug concentration after administration PO is not greatly different from that after SC injection. The elimination patterns are also quite similar for PO and parenteral routes.

Therapeutic Indications and Dose Rates

Quinolones are indicated for the treatment of local and systemic infections caused by susceptible microorganisms, particularly against deep-seated infections and intracellular pathogens. Therapeutic success has been obtained in respiratory, intestinal, urinary, and skin infections, as well as in bacterial prostatitis, meningoencephalitis, osteomyelitis, and arthritis.

A selection of general dosages for some quinolones is listed in TABLE 39. The dose rate and frequency should be adjusted as needed for the individual animal.

Special Clinical Concerns

Side Effects and Toxicity: Although side effects with the older quinolones (nalidixic and oxolinic acids) were relatively common, the newer ones seem to be well tolerated. Quinolones tends to be neurotoxic, and convulsions can occur at high doses. Vomiting and diarrhea rarely develop with fluoroquinolones. Dermal reactions and photosensitization have been described in humans, but the occurrence seems low. Hemolytic anemia has also been seen. Administering large doses of quinolones for any length of time during pregnancy has resulted in embryonic loss and maternal toxicity. Because high prolonged dosages in growing dogs have produced cartilaginous erosions leading to permanent

TABLE 39. Dose Rates of Quinolones*

Quinolone	Species	Dosage, Route, and Frequency
Nalidixic acid	Cats, dogs	3 mg/kg, PO, QID
Norfloxacin	Dogs	10-20 mg/kg, PO, BID
Enrofloxacin	Cats	5 mg/kg, PO, SID or divided BID
	Dogs	5-20 mg/kg, PO, SID or divided BID
		2.5 mg/kg, SC, once then PO
	Beef cattle (not veal or dairy)	7.5-12.5 mg/kg, SC, once
		2.5-5 mg/kg, SC, SID
	Pigs	2.5-5 mg/kg, PO or IM, SID
	Preruminant calves	2.5-5 mg/kg, PO or SC, SID
Marbofloxacin	Cats, Dogs	2.75-5.5 mg/kg, PO, SID
Difloxacin	Dogs	5-10 mg/kg, PO, SID
Orbifloxacin	Cats, dogs	2.5-7.5 mg/kg, PO, SID

*Use of fluorinated quinolones in food-producing animals is extra-label in the USA.

lameness, excessive use of quinolones should be avoided in immature animals. Quinolone administration in horses has not yet been extensively studied, but there is some indication that damage to the cartilage in weightbearing joints may be seen. Otherwise, the safety of quinolones (especially enrofloxacin) has been established in laboratory animals, calves, pigs, dogs, cats, and poultry.

Interactions: The likelihood of interactions has not yet been clearly established. Antacids probably interfere with the GI absorption of the quinolones. It also seems that nitrofurantoin impairs the efficacy of quinolones if used concurrently for urinary tract infections. Quinolones do inhibit the biotransformation of theophylline, leading to prolonged and potentially toxic plasma levels.

Effects on Laboratory Tests: AST, ALT, alkaline phosphatase, and BUN may be increased. Urinalysis may reveal needle-shaped crystals.

SULFONAMIDES AND SULFONAMIDE COMBINATIONS

Sulfonamides remain among the most widely used antibacterial agents in veterinary medicine, chiefly because of low cost and their relative efficacy in some common bacterial diseases. The synergistic action of sulfonamides with specific diaminopyrimidines has added a significant dimension to sulfonamide therapy.

Classes

The many sulfonamides and sulfonamide derivatives available for clinical use can be categorized into several types, based mainly on their indications and duration of action in the body.

Standard Use Sulfonamides: In most species, members of this large group are administered 1-4 times/day, depending on the drug, to control systemic infections caused by susceptible bacteria. In some instances, administration of the sulfonamide every second or even third day may be sufficient to maintain blood levels if the drug is eliminated particularly slowly in the species being treated. Sulfonamides included in this class are sulfathiazole, sulfamethazine (sulfadimidine), sulfamerazine, sulfadiazine, sulfapyridine, sulfabromomethazine, sulfaethoxypyridazine, sulfamethoxypyridazine, sulfadimethoxine, and sulfachlorpyridazine.

Highly Soluble Sulfonamides Used for Urinary Tract Infections: A few very water-soluble sulfonamides, eg, sulfisoxazole (sulfafurazole) and sulfasomidine, are rapidly excreted via the urinary tract (>90% in 24 hr) mostly in an unchanged form; because of this, they are primarily used for the treatment of urinary tract infections.

Poorly Soluble Sulfonamides Used for Intestinal Infections: Some sulfonamide derivatives, such as sulfaguanidine, are so insoluble that they are not absorbed from the GI tract (<5%). Phthalylsulfathiazole and succinylsulfathiazole undergo bacterial hydrolysis in the lower GI tract with the consequent release of active sulfathiazole. Salicylazosulfapyridine (sulfasalazine) is also hydrolyzed in the large intestine to sulfapyridine and 5-aminosalicylic acid, an anti-inflammatory agent. This drug is used for the management of ulcerative colitis in dogs.

Potentiated Sulfonamides: Certain diaminopyrimidines when used in combination with sulfonamides cause a sequential blockade of microbial tetrahydrofolate synthesis, which ultimately kills the organism. Sulfonamides are used in combination with pyrimethamine to treat protozoal diseases such as leishmaniasis and toxoplasmosis. (*See also* POTENTIATED SULFONAMIDES, p 2080.)

Topical Sulfonamides: Several sulfonamides are used topically for specific purposes. Sulfacetamide is not highly efficacious but is occasionally used to treat ophthalmic infections. Mafenide and silver sulfadiazine are used on burn wounds to prevent invasion by many gram-negative and gram-positive organisms. Sulfathiazole is commonly included in wound powders for the same purpose.

General Properties

The sulfonamides are derivatives of sulfanilamide. All have the same nucleus to which various functional groups have been added to the amido group or in which various substitutions on the amino group are made. These changes produce compounds with varying physical, chemical, pharmacologic, and antibacterial properties. Although amphoteric, sulfonamides generally behave as weak organic acids and are much more soluble in an alkaline than in an acidic environment. Those of therapeutic interest have pK_a values between 4.8 and 8.6. Water-soluble sodium or disodium salts are used for parenteral administration. Such solutions are highly alkaline, somewhat unstable, and readily precipitate out with the addition of polyionic electrolytes. In a mixture of sulfonamides (eg, the sulfapyrimidine group), each component drug exhibits its own solubility; therefore, a combination of sulfonamides is more water-soluble than a single drug at the same total concentration. This is the basis of triple sulfonamide mixtures used clinically. The N-4 acetylated sulfonamides, except for the sulfapyrimidine group (sulfamethazine, sulfamerazine, sulfadiazine), are less water-soluble than their nonacetylated forms. This has bearing in the development of sulfonamide crystalluria. The highly insoluble sulfonamides (phthalylsulfathiazole and succinylsulfathiazole) are retained in the lumen of the GI tract for prolonged periods and are known as "gut-active" sulfonamides.

Antimicrobial Activity

Mode of Action: The sulfonamides are structural analogs of para-aminobenzoic acid (PABA) and competitively inhibit an enzymatic step (dihydropterate synthetase) during which PABA is incorporated into the synthesis of dihydrofolic acid (folic acid). Because dihydrofolate synthesis is reduced, the levels of tetrahydrofolate (folinic acid) formed from dihydrofolate diminish. Tetrahydrofolate is an essential component of the coenzymes responsible for single carbon metabolism in cells. Acting as antimetabolites to PABA, sulfonamides eventually block, in a complex fashion, several enzymes. These enzymes include those needed for the biogenesis of purine bases; for the transfer of desoxyuridine to thymidine; and for the biosynthesis of methionine, glycine, and formylmethionyl-transfer-RNA. This results in suppression of protein synthesis, impairment of metabolic processes, and inhibition of growth and multiplication of those organisms that cannot use preformed folate. The effect is bacteriostatic, although a bactericidal action is evident at the high concentrations that may be found in urine.

Sulfonamides are most effective in the early stages of acute infections when organisms are rapidly multiplying. They are not active against quiescent bacteria. Typically, there is a latent period before the effects of sulfonamide therapy become evident. This lag period occurs because the bacteria use existing stores of folic acid, folinic acid, purines, thymidine, and amino acids. Once these stores are depleted, bacteriostasis occurs. Bacterial growth can resume when the concentration of PABA increases or when the level of sulfonamide falls below an enzyme-inhibitory concentration. Adequate cellular and humoral defense mechanisms are critical for successful sulfonamide therapy.

Although all of the sulfonamides have the same mechanism of action, differences are evident with respect to activity, pharmacokinetic fate, and even antimicrobial spectrum at usual concentrations. The differences are due to the variety of physiochemical characteristics seen among the sulfonamides.

The bacteriostatic efficacy of sulfonamides can be reduced radically by excess PABA, folic acid, thymine, purine, methionine, plasma, blood, albumin, tissue autolysates, and endogenous protein-degradation products.

Bacterial Resistance: Both chromosomal and R-factor-mediated resistance to sulfonamides have been attributed to altered forms of dihydropterate synthetase (for which sulfonamides have a lowered affinity). Another mechanism of resistance is the overproduction of PABA, which overcomes the metabolic block imposed by the inhibition of dihydropterate synthetase. Cross-resistance between sulfonamides is the general rule. Resistance does emerge gradually and is widespread in many animal populations; continued use of sulfonamides increases the incidence. Plasmid-mediated sulfonamide resistance in intestinal gram-negative bacteria is often linked with ampicillin and tetracycline resistance.

Antimicrobial Spectrum: Different sulfonamides may show quantitative but not necessarily qualitative differences in antimicrobial activity. Sulfonamides inhibit both gram-positive and gram-negative bacteria, a few *Chlamydia*, *Nocardia*, and *Actinomyces* spp, and some protozoa such as coccidia and *Toxoplasma* spp. More active sulfonamides may include several species of *Streptococcus*, *Staphylococcus*, *Salmonella*, *Pasteurella*, and even *Escherichia coli* in their spectra. Strains of *Pseudomonas*, *Klebsiella*, *Proteus*, *Clostridium*, and *Leptospira* spp are most often highly resistant, as are rickettsiae.

Pharmacokinetic Features

There are notable differences among the many sulfonamides with respect to their pharmacokinetic fate in the various species. The standard classification of short-, medium-, and long-acting sulfonamides that is used in human therapeutics is usually inappropriate in veterinary medicine because of species differences in disposition and elimination.

Absorption: Sulfonamides may be administered PO, IV, IP, IM, intrauterine, or topically, depending on the specific preparation. Except for the poorly absorbed sulfonamides intended for intestinal use, most are rather rapidly and completely absorbed from the GI tract of monogastric animals. Absorption from the ruminoreticulum is delayed, especially if ruminal stasis is present. Therapeutic doses of sulfonamides are usually administered PO except in acute life-threatening infections when IV infusions are used to establish adequate blood levels as rapidly as possible. Sulfonamides are frequently added to drinking water or feed either for therapeutic purposes or to improve feed efficiency. A few highly water-soluble preparations may be injected IM (eg, sodium sulfadimethoxine) or IP (some irritation of the peritoneum can be seen). Absorption is rapid from these parenteral sites. Generally, sulfonamide solutions are too alkaline for routine parenteral use.

Distribution: Sulfonamides are distributed throughout all body tissues. The distribution pattern depends on the ionization state of the sulfonamide, the vascularity of specific tissues, the presence of specific barriers to sulfonamide diffusion, and the fraction of the administered dose bound to plasma proteins. The unbound drug fraction is freely diffusible. Sulfonamides are bound to plasma proteins to a greater or lesser extent, and levels in pleural, peritoneal, synovial, and ocular fluids may be 50-90% of that in blood. Sulfadiazine is 90% or more bound to plasma proteins. Concentrations in the kidneys exceed plasma levels, and those in the skin, liver, and lungs are only slightly less than the corresponding plasma levels. Concentrations in muscle and bone are ~50% those in the plasma, and those in the CSF may be 20-80% of blood levels, depending on the particular sulfonamide. Low levels are found in adipose tissue. After parenteral administration, sulfamethazine is found in jejunal and colonic contents at about the same concentration as in blood. Passive diffusion into milk also occurs; although the levels achieved are usually inadequate to control infections, sulfonamide residues may be detected in milk.

Biotransformation: Sulfonamides are usually extensively metabolized, mainly by several oxidative pathways, acetylation, and conjugation with sulfate or glucuronic acid. Species differences are marked in this regard. The acetylated, hydroxylated, and conjugated forms have little antibacterial activity. Acetylation (poorly developed in dogs) reduces the solubility of most sulfonamides except for the sulfapyrimidine group. The hydroxylated and conjugated forms are less likely to precipitate in urine.

Excretion: Most sulfonamides are excreted primarily in the urine. Bile, feces, milk, and sweat are excretory routes of lesser significance. Glomerular filtration, active tubular secretion, and tubular reabsorption are the main processes involved. The proportion reabsorbed is influenced by the inherent lipid solubility of individual sulfonamides and their metabolites and by urinary pH. Urinary pH, renal clearance, and the concentration and solubility of the respective sulfonamides and their metabolites determine whether solubilities are exceeded and crystals precipitate. This can be prevented by alkalinizing the urine, increasing the fluid intake, reducing dose rates in renal insufficiency, and using triple-sulfonamide or sulfonamide-diaminopyrimidine combinations.

Pharmacokinetic Considerations: There are great differences between the pharmacokinetic values of various sulfonamides in animals, and extrapolation of these values is rarely appropriate; for example, the plasma half-life of sulfadiazine is 10.1 hr in cattle and 2.9 hr in pigs. The recommended dose rates and frequencies reflect this disparity in elimination kinetics.

Therapeutic Indications and Dose Rates

The sulfonamides are commonly used to treat or prevent acute systemic or local infections. Disease syndromes treated with sulfonamides include actinobacillosis, coccidiosis, mastitis, metritis, colibacillosis, pododermatitis, polyarthritis, respiratory infections, and toxoplasmosis.

Sulfonamides are more effective when administered early in the course of a disease. Chronic infections, particularly with large amounts of exudate or tissue debris present, often are not responsive. In severe infections, the initial dose should be administered IV to reduce the lag time between dose and effect. In many instances, the initial dose should be double the maintenance dose. Adequate drinking water should be available at all times, and urine output monitored. A course of treatment should not exceed 7 days under usual circumstances. If a favorable response is seen within 72 hr, treatment should be continued for 48 hr after remission to prevent relapse and the emergence of resistance. The ability to mount an immune response must be intact for successful sulfonamide therapy.

A selection of general dosages for some sulfonamides is listed in TABLE 40. The dose rate and frequency should be adjusted as needed for the individual animal.

Special Clinical Concerns

Side Effects and Toxicity: Adverse reactions to sulfonamides may be due to hypersensitivity or direct toxic effects. Possible hypersensitivity reactions include urticaria, angioedema, anaphylaxis, skin rashes, drug fever, polyarthritis, hemolytic anemia, and agranulocytosis. Crystalluria with hematuria, and even tubular obstruction, can be seen

TABLE 40. Dose Rates of Sulfonamides

Sulfonamide	Species	Dosage, Route, and Frequency
Sulfathiazole	Horses	66 mg/kg, PO, TID
	Cattle, sheep, pigs	66 mg/kg, PO, every 4 hr
Sulfamethazine	Cattle	220 mg/kg, PO or IV, SID (initial dose; half for subsequent doses)
Sulfadiazine	All	50 mg/kg, PO, BID
Sulfadimethoxine	All	55 mg/kg, PO, SID (initial dose; half for subsequent doses)
Sulfaethoxypyridazine	Cattle	55 mg/kg, PO, SID
	Pigs	110 mg/kg, PO, SID (initial dose, half for subsequent doses)
Sulfapyridine	Cattle	132 mg/kg, PO, BID (initial dose, half for subsequent doses)
Succinylsulfathiazole	All	160 mg/kg, PO, BID (initial dose, half for subsequent doses)

but is not common in veterinary medicine. Sulfonamides with prolonged plasma half-lives and high solubilities tend not to cause crystalluria, particularly if water intake is high and the urine is alkaline. Acute toxic manifestations may be seen after too rapid IV administration or if an excessive dose is injected. Clinical signs include muscle weakness, ataxia, blindness, and collapse. GI disturbances, in addition to nausea and vomiting, may occur when sulfonamide levels are sufficiently high in the tract to disturb normal microfloral balance and vitamin B synthesis. Sulfonamides depress the cellulolytic function of ruminal microflora, but the effect is usually transient (unless excessively high levels are reached). Several adverse effects have been reported after prolonged treatment, including bone marrow depression (aplastic anemia, granulocytopenia, thrombocytopenia), hepatitis and icterus, peripheral neuritis and myelin degeneration in the spinal cord and peripheral nerves, photosensitization, stomatitis, conjunctivitis, and keratitis sicca. Mild follicular thyroid hyperplasia may be associated with prolonged administration of sulfonamides to sensitive species such as dogs, and reversible hypothyroidism can be induced after treatment with high doses in dogs. Several sulfonamides can lead to decreased egg production and growth. Topically, the sulfonamides retard healing of uncontaminated wounds.

Interactions: Sulfonamide solutions are incompatible with calcium- or other polyionic-containing fluids as well as many other preparations. Sulfonamides may be displaced from their plasma-protein-binding sites by other acidic drugs with higher binding affinities. Antacids tend to inhibit the GI absorption of sulfonamides. Alkalinization of the urine promotes sulfonamide excretion, and urinary acidification increases the risk of crystalluria. Some sulfonamides act as microsomal enzyme inhibitors, which may lead to toxic manifestations of concurrently administered drugs such as phenytoin.

Effects on Laboratory Tests: Bilirubin, BUN, sulfobromophthalein (BSP®), eosinophils, methemoglobin, AST, and ALT may be increased. Platelet, RBC, and WBC counts are often decreased. Urinalysis may show a change in color, glucose, porphyrins, and urobilinogen. Sulfonamide crystals may also be found.

Drug Withdrawal and Milk Discard Times: Regulatory requirements for withdrawal times for food animals and milk discard times vary among countries. These must be followed carefully to prevent food residues and consequent public health implications. The selection of times listed in TABLE 41 serve only as general guidelines.

TABLE 41. Drug Withdrawal and Milk Discard Times of Sulfonamides

Sulfonamide	Species	Withdrawal Time (days)	Milk Discard Time (hr)
Sulfamethazine	Cattle	10[*]	96
	Pigs	14	
Sulfabromethazine	Cattle	10	96
Triple sulfonamide solution[†]	Cattle	10	96
Sulfadimethoxidine	Cattle	7	60

[*]28 days for slow-release bolus
[†]8% sodium sulfamethazine, 8% sodium sulfapyridine, 8% sodium sulfathiazole

Potentiated Sulfonamides

A group of **diaminopyrimidines** (trimethoprim, methoprim, ormetoprim, aditoprim, pyrimethamine) inhibit dihydrofolate reductase in bacteria and protozoa far more efficiently than in mammalian cells. Used alone, these agents are not particularly effective against bacteria, and resistance develops rapidly. However, when combined with sulfonamides, a sequential blockade of microbial enzyme systems occurs with bactericidal consequences. Examples of such potentiated sulfonamide preparations include trimethoprim/sulfadiazine (co-trimazine), trimethoprim/sulfamethoxazole (co-trimoxazole), trimethoprim/sulfadoxine (co-trimoxine), and ormetoprim/sulfadimethoxine.

General Properties: Trimethoprim and ormetoprim are basic drugs that tend to accumulate in more acidic environments such as acidic urine, milk, and ruminal fluid.

Antimicrobial Features: In susceptible bacteria, the sulfonamide component blocks the synthesis of dihydrofolic acid, and the particular diaminopyrimidine used in combination inhibits the next enzyme in the sequence (dihydrofolate reductase) to prevent the formation of tetrahydrofolic acid (folinic acid). Folinic acid is required for the synthesis of DNA. This sequential blockade produces a bactericidal rather than bacteriostatic effect under usual conditions, but in the presence of thymidine, only bacteriostasis is evident because the block is circumvented.

The optimal ratio in vitro for the combination of trimethoprim or ormetoprim and a sulfonamide depends on the type of microorganism but is usually ~1:20. However, the commercially available preparations use a ratio of 1:5 because of pharmacokinetic considerations.

Bacterial resistance to trimethoprim readily develops, but resistance to the combination is not common—the presence of a sulfonamide appears to delay the emergence of bacterial resistance. Resistance may take 2 forms: mutant resistance, with bacteria becoming dependent on exogenous folinic acid or thymidine; and plasmid-mediated resistance, based on enzyme modification.

Antibacterial Spectrum: Sulfonamide-diaminopyrimidine combinations are active against gram-negative and gram-positive organisms, including *Actinomyces, Bordetella, Clostridium, Corynebacterium, Fusobacterium, Haemophilus, Klebsiella, Pasteurella, Proteus, Salmonella, Shigella,* and *Campylobacter* spp, as well as *Escherichia coli,* streptococci, and staphylococci. Some streptococcal strains are only moderately sensitive, as are *Brucella, Erysipelothrix, Nocardia,* and *Moraxella* spp. The antibacterial spectrum does not include *Pseudomonas* or *Mycobacterium* spp.

Pharmacokinetic Features: Trimethoprim is rapidly absorbed after administration PO (plasma levels peak in ~2-4 hr) except in ruminants, in which it tends to be trapped in the ruminoreticulum and appears to undergo a degree of microbial degradation. Absorption occurs readily from parenteral injection sites; effective antibacterial concentrations are reached in <1 hr, and peak levels in ~4 hr. Trimethoprim diffuses extensively into

TABLE 42. Dose Rates of Potentiated Sulfonamides

Combination	Dosage, Route, and Frequency
Trimethoprim/sulfadiazine	15-60 mg/kg, PO, IV, or IM, SID
Ormetoprim/sulfadimethoxine	55 mg/kg, PO, SID (initial dose; half for subsequent doses)

tissues and body fluids. Tissue concentrations are often higher than the corresponding plasma levels, especially in lungs, liver, and kidneys. About 30-60% of trimethoprim is bound to plasma proteins. The extent of metabolic transformation of trimethoprim has not yet been established, although there is a suggestion that hepatic biotransformation can be extensive, at least in ruminants. This may not be the case in all species; >50% of a dose is excreted unchanged in many instances. Trimethoprim is largely excreted in the urine by glomerular filtration and tubular secretion. A substantial amount may also be found in the feces. The concentrations in milk are often 1-3.5 times higher than those in plasma. The plasma half-life of trimethoprim is quite prolonged in most species; effective levels may be maintained for >12 hr, with the result that the frequency of administration is usually 12-24 hr. The elimination rates of trimethoprim in sheep seem to be much shorter than for monogastric species.

Elimination of ormetoprim appears to be prolonged.

Dose Rates: A selection of general dosages is listed in TABLE 42. The dose rate and frequency should be adjusted as needed for the individual animal.

Side Effects and Toxicity: Side effects due to the potentiated sulfonamides are quite rare, although adverse reactions to the sulfonamide components still occur. Up to 10 times the recommended dose of trimethoprim has been given with no adverse effects. Prolonged administration of trimethoprim at reasonably high levels leads to maturation defects in hematopoiesis due to impaired folinic acid synthesis. This effect is readily reversible by supplementation with folinic acid.

Drug Withdrawal and Milk Discard Times: Regulatory requirements for withdrawal times for food animals and milk discard times vary among countries. These must be followed carefully to prevent food residues and consequent public health implications. The selection of times in TABLE 43 serve only as general guidelines.

TETRACYCLINES

The tetracyclines are broad-spectrum antibiotics with similar antimicrobial features, but they differ somewhat from one another in terms of their spectra and pharmacokinetic disposition.

Classes

There are 3 naturally occurring tetracyclines (oxytetracycline, chlortetracycline, and demethylchlortetracycline) and several that are derived semisynthetically (tetracycline, rolitetracycline, methacycline, minocycline, doxycycline, lymecycline, etc). Elimination

TABLE 43. Drug Withdrawal and Milk Discard Times of Potentiated Sulfonamides

Combination	Withdrawal Time (days)	Milk Discard Time (days)
Trimethoprim/sulfadiazine	3	7
Trimethoprim/sulfadoxine	5 (PO) 28 (parenteral)	

times permit a further classification into short-acting (tetracycline, oxytetracycline, chlortetracycline), intermediate-acting (demethylchlortetracycline and methacycline), and long-acting (doxycycline and minocycline).

General Properties

All of the tetracycline derivatives are crystalline, yellowish, amphoteric substances that, in aqueous solution, form salts with both acids and bases. They characteristically fluoresce when exposed to ultraviolet light. The most common salt form is the hydrochloride, except for doxycycline, which is available as doxycycline hyclate. The tetracyclines are stable as dry powders but not in aqueous solution, particularly at higher pH ranges (7-8.5). Preparations for parenteral administration must be carefully formulated, often in propylene glycol or polyvinyl pyrrolidone with additional dispersing agents, to provide stable solutions. Tetracyclines form poorly soluble chelates with bivalent and trivalent cations, particularly calcium, magnesium, aluminum, and iron. Doxycycline and minocycline exhibit the greatest liposolubility and better penetration of bacteria such as *Staphylococcus aureus* than does the group as a whole.

Antimicrobial Activity

Mode of Action: The exact site involved in the antimicrobial activity of tetracyclines has not been clarified, but these antibiotics bind reversibly to bacterial 30 S ribosomes and inhibit protein synthesis, perhaps by several mechanisms. Mainly, the binding of aminoacyl-tRNA to the acceptor site on the mRNA-ribosome complex seems to be impaired. This effect also is evident in mammalian cells, although microbial cells are selectively more susceptible because of the greater concentrations that are seen. Tetracyclines enter microorganisms in part by diffusion and in part by an energy-dependent, carrier-mediated system that is responsible for the high levels achieved in susceptible bacteria. The tetracyclines are generally bacteriostatic, and a responsive host-defense system is essential for their successful use. At high concentrations, as may be attained in urine, they become bactericidal because the organisms seem to lose the functional integrity of the cytoplasmic membrane. Tetracyclines are more effective against multiplying microorganisms and tend to be more active at a pH of 6-6.5.

Bacterial Resistance: Microbial resistance to tetracyclines is based almost exclusively on decreased penetration of the drug into previously susceptible organisms. Two forms are recognized: 1) impaired uptake into bacteria, seen in mutant strains that do not have the necessary transport system, and 2) plasmid-mediated resistance, which confers the property of either diminished uptake or active efflux of tetracycline from the bacterial cell. The genomes for these capabilities may be transferred either by transduction (as in *Staphylococcus aureus*) or by conjugation (as in many enterobacteria). Resistance develops slowly in a multistep fashion but is widespread because of the extensive use of low levels of tetracyclines.

Antimicrobial Spectra: All tetracyclines are about equally active and typically have about the same broad spectrum, which comprises both aerobic and anaerobic grampositive and gram-negative bacteria, mycoplasmas, rickettsiae, chlamydiae, and even some protozoa (amebae). Strains of *Pseudomonas aeruginosa, Proteus, Serratia, Klebsiella,* and *Corynebacterium* spp frequently are resistant, as are many pathogenic *E coli* isolates. Even though there is general cross-resistance among tetracyclines, doxycycline and minocycline usually are more effective against staphylococci.

Pharmacokinetic Features

Absorption: After usual oral dosage, tetracyclines are absorbed primarily in the upper small intestine, and effective blood levels are reached in 2-4 hr. GI absorption can be impaired by sodium bicarbonate, aluminum hydroxide, magnesium hydroxide, iron, calcium salts, milk, and milk products. For doxycycline and minocycline, the latter applies only to a lesser extent. Tetracyclines at therapeutic levels should not be administered PO to ruminants: they are poorly absorbed and can substantially depress ruminal microfloral activity. Specially buffered tetracycline solutions can be administered IM and IV. Through chemical manipulation (especially choice of carrier and high magnesium content), the absorption of oxytetracycline from IM sites may be delayed, which produces a long-acting effect. Tetracyclines can cause tissue necrosis at injection sites, in which residues may remain for several weeks. Tetracyclines can also be absorbed from the uterus and udder, although plasma levels remain low.

Distribution: Tetracyclines distribute rapidly and extensively in the body, particularly after parenteral administration. They enter almost all tissues and body fluids; high concentrations are found in the kidneys, liver, bile, lungs, spleen, and bone. Lower levels are found in serosal fluids, synovia, CSF, ascitic fluid, prostatic fluid, and vitreous humor. The more lipid-soluble tetracyclines (doxycycline and minocycline) readily penetrate tissues such as the blood-brain barrier, and CSF levels reach ~30% of the plasma concentrations. They also are present in saliva and tears. Because tetracyclines tend to chelate calcium ions (less so for doxycycline), they are deposited irreversibly in the growing bones and in dentin and enamel of unerupted teeth of young animals, or even the fetus if transplacental passage occurs (*see* SPECIAL CLINICAL CONCERNS, below). Drug bound in this fashion is pharmacologically inactive. Because of this property, they may serve as markers in developing bone or in proliferating bone tissue. Tetracyclines are bound to plasma proteins to varying degrees (eg, oxytetracycline, 30%; tetracycline, 60%; doxycycline, 90%).

Biotransformation: Biotransformation of the tetracyclines seems to be limited in most domestic animals, and generally about one-third of a given dose is excreted unchanged. Rolitetracycline is metabolized to tetracycline. Doxycycline and minocycline may be more extensively biotransformed than other tetracyclines (up to 40% of a given dose).

Excretion: Tetracyclines are excreted via the kidneys (glomerular filtration) and the GI tract (biliary elimination and directly). Generally 50-80% of a given dose is recoverable from the urine, although several factors may influence renal elimination, including age, route of administration, urine pH, glomerular filtration rate, renal disease, and the particular tetracycline used. Intestinal (biliary) elimination is always significant, commonly ~10-20%, even with parenteral administration; for doxycycline and its metabolites, this is the major route of excretion. Tetracyclines are also eliminated in milk; concentrations peak 6 hr after a parenteral dose, and traces are still present up to 48 hr later. Levels in milk usually attain ~50-60% of the plasma concentration and are often higher in mastitic milk.

Pharmacokinetic Values: The plasma half-lives of tetracyclines are 6-12 hr and even longer depending on age (slower elimination in animals <1 mo old), disease, and the tetracycline itself (*see* TABLE 44). In large animals, daily injections of standard dosages usually are sufficient to maintain effective inhibitory concentrations. Long-acting formulations

TABLE 44. Elimination, Distribution, and Clearance of Tetracyclines

Tetracycline	Species	Elimination Half-life (hr)	Volume of Distribution (mL/kg)	Clearance (mL/kg/min)
Oxytetracycline	Dogs	6	3,000	4.23
	Calves (<3 mo old)	10-13	1,500-2,400	3.45
	Cattle	7-10	800-1,000	3.33
	Horses	8-10	1,100	2.89
Minocycline	Dogs	7	2,000	3.21

of oxytetracycline, when injected IM, generally produce plasma concentrations >0.5 μg/mL for ~72 hr. Tetracyclines usually are administered PO every 8-12 hr, or every 12-24 hr for doxycycline and minocycline.

Therapeutic Indications and Dose Rates

The tetracyclines are used to treat both systemic and local infections. General organ infections include bronchopneumonia, bacterial enteritis, urinary tract infections, cholangitis, metritis, mastitis, prostatitis, and pyodermatitis. Specific conditions include infectious keratoconjunctivitis in cattle, chlamydiosis, heartwater, anaplasmosis, actinomycosis, actinobacillosis, nocardiosis (especially minocycline), ehrlichiosis (especially doxycycline), eperythrozoonosis, and haemobartonellosis. Minocycline and doxycycline are often effective to a somewhat lesser degree against resistant strains of *Staphylococcus aureus*.

In addition to antimicrobial chemotherapy, the tetracyclines are used for other purposes. As additives in animal feeds, they serve as growth promoters. Because of the affinity of tetracyclines for bones, teeth, and necrotic tissue, they can be used to delineate tumors by fluorescence. Demethylchlortetracycline has been used to inhibit the action of antidiuretic hormone in cases of excessive water retention and to "stretch" flexor digital tendons in neonatal foals.

A selection of general dosages for some tetracyclines is listed in TABLE 45. The dose rate and frequency should be adjusted as needed for the individual animal.

Special Clinical Concerns

Side Effects and Toxicity: Because several diverse effects may result from the administration of the tetracyclines, caution should be exercised. Superinfection by nonsusceptible pathogens such as fungi, yeasts, and resistant bacteria is always a possibility when broad-spectrum antibiotics are used. This may lead to GI disturbances after either PO or parenteral administration or to "persistent infection" when they are applied topically (eg, in the ear). Severe and even fatal diarrhea can occur in horses receiving tetracyclines, especially if the animals are severely stressed or critically ill.

High doses administered PO to ruminants seriously disrupt microfloral activity in the ruminoreticulum, eventually producing stasis. Elimination of the gut flora in monogastric animals reduces the synthesis and availability of the B vitamins and vitamin K from the large intestine. With prolonged therapy, vitamin supplementation is a useful precaution.

Tetracyclines chelate calcium in teeth and bones; they become incorporated into these structures, inhibit calcification (eg, hypoplastic dental enamel), and cause yellowish then brownish discoloration. At extremely high concentrations, the healing processes in fractured bones is impaired.

Rapid IV injection of a tetracycline can result in hypotension and sudden collapse. This appears to be related to the ability of the tetracyclines to chelate ionized calcium,

TABLE 45. Dose Rates of Tetracyclines

Tetracycline	Species	Dosage, Route, and Frequency
Tetracycline	Cats, dogs	7 mg/kg, IM or IV, BID 20 mg/kg, PO, TID
Oxytetracycline	Cats, dogs	7 mg/kg, IM or IV, BID 20 mg/kg, PO, TID
	Cattle, sheep, pigs	5-10 mg/kg, IM or IV, SID
	Calves, foals, lambs, piglets	10-20 mg/kg, PO, BID-TID
	Horses	5 mg/kg, IV, SID-BID
Doxycycline	Dogs	5-10 mg/kg, PO, SID 5 mg/kg, IV, SID

although a depressant effect by the propylene glycol carrier itself may also be involved. This effect can be avoided by slow infusion of the drug (>5 min) or by pretreatment with IV calcium gluconate.

The IV administration of undiluted propylene-glycol-based preparations leads to intravascular hemolysis, which results in hemoglobinuria, and possibly other reactions such as hypotension, ataxia, and CNS depression.

Because tetracyclines interfere with protein synthesis even in host cells and therefore tend to be catabolic, an increase in BUN can be expected. The combined use of glucocorticoids and tetracyclines often leads to a significant weight loss, particularly in anorectic animals.

Hepatotoxic effects due to large doses of tetracyclines have been reported in pregnant women and in other animals. The mortality rate is high.

The tetracyclines are also potentially nephrotoxic and are contraindicated (except for doxycycline) in renal insufficiency. Fatal renal failure has been reported in septicemic and endotoxemic cattle given high doses of oxytetracycline. The administration of expired tetracycline products may lead to acute tubular nephrosis.

Swelling, necrosis, and yellow discoloration at the injection site almost inevitably are seen. Phototoxic dermatitis may be seen in human patients treated with demethylchlortetracycline and other analogs, but this reaction is rare in other animals. Hypersensitivity reactions do occur; for example, cats may show a "drug fever" reaction, often accompanied by vomiting, diarrhea, depression, inappetence, and eosinophilia.

The tetracyclines can inhibit WBC chemotaxis and phagocytosis when present in high concentrations at sites of infection. This clearly hinders normal host defense mechanisms. The addition of glucocorticoids to the therapeutic regimen would impair immunocompetence even further.

Interactions: The absorption of tetracyclines from the GI tract is decreased by milk and milk products (less so for doxycycline and minocycline), antacids, kaolin, and iron preparations. Tetracyclines gradually lose activity when diluted in infusion fluids and exposed to ultraviolet light. Vitamins of the B-complex group, especially riboflavin, hasten this loss of activity in infusion fluids. Tetracyclines also bind to the calcium ions in Ringer's solution.

Methoxyflurane anesthesia combined with tetracycline therapy may be nephrotoxic. Microsomal enzyme inducers such as phenobarbital and phenytoin shorten the plasma half-lives of minocycline and doxycycline. Except for minocycline and doxycycline, the presence of food can substantially delay the absorption of tetracyclines from the GI tract. The tetracyclines are less active in alkaline urine, and urine acidification can increase their antimicrobial efficacy.

Effects on Laboratory Tests: Tetracyclines may increase amylase, BUN, sulfobromophthalein (BSP®), eosinophil count, AST, and ALT. Tetracyclines used in combination with diuretics are often associated with a marked rise in the BUN. Cholesterol, glucose, potassium, and prothrombin time may be decreased. A false-positive urine glucose test is also possible.

Drug Withdrawal and Milk Discard Times: Regulatory requirements for withdrawal times for food animals and milk discard times vary among countries. These must be followed carefully to prevent food residues and consequent public health implications. The selection of times listed in TABLE 46 serve only as general guidelines.

CHLORAMPHENICOL AND CONGENERS

Chloramphenicol is a highly effective and well-tolerated broad-spectrum antibiotic. However, it does have several features that demand careful use in companion animals and that have led to prohibition of its use in food-producing animals in several countries, including the USA and Canada.

TABLE 46. Drug Withdrawal and Milk Discard Times of Tetracyclines

Tetracycline	Species	Withdrawal Time (days)
Oxytetracycline*	Cattle	15-22
	Pigs	22
	Poultry	5
Oxytetracycline (long-acting)*	Cattle	28
Chlortetracycline	Cattle	10
	Pigs	1-7

*Not for use in lactating dairy cows

Classes

Chloramphenicol is a unique antimicrobial agent; however, because of its tendency to cause blood dyscrasias in humans, 2 related drugs have been developed. Thiamphenicol is less effective but safer than chloramphenicol; florfenicol, a thiamphenicol derivative, is significantly more active in vitro than chloramphenicol against many pathogenic strains of bacteria. Florfenicol is approved for use in cattle.

General Properties

Chloramphenicol is a relatively simple neutral nitrobenzene derivative with a bitter taste. It is highly lipid soluble and is used either as the free base or in ester forms (eg, the neutral-tasting palmitate for administration PO and the water-soluble sodium succinate for parenteral injection). Chloramphenicol is a relatively stable compound and is unaffected by boiling, provided that a pH of 9 is not exceeded. The nitrophenol group of chloramphenicol is replaced by a methyl sulfonyl group for thiamphenicol and florfenicol; florfenicol also contains a fluorine molecule. These structural changes improve efficacy, reduce toxicity, and for florfenicol, the fluorine molecule reduces bacterial destruction.

Antimicrobial Activity

Mode of Action: Chloramphenicol and its congeners inhibit microbial protein synthesis by binding to the 50 S subunit of the 70 S ribosome and impairing peptidyl transferase activity. The binding of aminoacyl-tRNA to the active site of peptidyl transferase is also prevented. The effect is usually bacteriostatic but, at high concentrations, chloramphenicol may be bactericidal for some species. Chloramphenicol inhibits protein synthesis in both prokaryotic and eukaryotic (mitochondrial) ribosomes.

Bacterial Resistance: Resistance against chloramphenicol develops slowly and in a step-wise fashion. In clinical bacterial isolates, resistance is generally plasmid-mediated and is due to the production of chloramphenicol acetyltransferase, although other inactivating enzymes also may be involved. In resistant gram-negative bacteria, chloramphenicol acetyltransferase is a constitutive enzyme; in gram-positive organisms, the enzyme is inducible. In *Pseudomonas aeruginosa* and in strains of *Proteus* and *Klebsiella* spp, resistance is also nonenzymatic and is based on an inducible permeability block that is both chromosomal and plasmid-mediated. Resistance to chloramphenicol often develops together with resistance to tetracycline, erythromycin, streptomycin, ampicillin, and other antibiotics.

Antimicrobial Spectrum: Many genera of gram-positive and gram-negative bacteria and several anaerobes such as *Bacteroides fragilis*, as well as *Rickettsia* and *Chlamydia* spp are susceptible. Of special note is the efficacy against many *Salmonella* spp and the resistance of most strains of *P aeruginosa*. Florfenicol also has a broad antimicrobial spectrum.

Pharmacokinetic Features

Absorption: Absorption occurs promptly and rapidly from the upper GI tract when chloramphenicol base is administered PO to nonruminant animals. Blood levels usually are maximal in 1-3 hr. Because ruminal microflora readily reduce the nitro group, chloramphenicol is inactivated in the ruminoreticulum and is not available for absorption. The larger ester forms of chloramphenicol require hydrolysis by lipases to release the antibiotic for absorption from the GI tract; thus, the systemic availability of chloramphenicol is delayed when the palmitate and other ester preparations are used. Generic inequivalence has been seen with oral dosage forms. The presence of food and intestinal protectants does not interfere with the absorption of chloramphenicol, although drugs that depress GI motility do. Florfenicol is rapidly absorbed after administration PO, although milk interferes with absorption.

Chloramphenicol sodium succinate may be injected both IV and IM. However, hydrolysis is required in the body because only free chloramphenicol base is active. The kinetics of this hydrolysis reaction may be slow and incomplete, with considerable individual and species variability. The absorption of chloramphenicol base itself from IM injection sites is notably restricted. For example, in horses, the therapeutic blood concentration of 5 mg/mL is achieved at a dosage of 50 mg/kg body wt, IM, after only 6-8 hr. Chloramphenicol base is absorbed after IP injection. Florfenicol is available as an injectable solution intended for IM use.

Distribution: About 40-60% of chloramphenicol in plasma is reversibly bound to albumin, and the free fraction readily diffuses into almost all tissues (including the brain); highest concentrations are reached in the kidneys, liver, and bile. Substantial levels (~50% of plasma values) are also reached in many body fluids such as the CSF and aqueous humor. Milk concentrations are ~50% those of plasma but may be higher in mastitis. Transplacental diffusion is seen in all species, with levels of ~75% being reached in the fetus as compared with the dam. Chloramphenicol does not attain effective concentrations in normal synovial fluid but does so in septic arthritis. The blood-prostate barrier is an exception to the extensive intracorporeal distribution of chloramphenicol—levels in the inflamed prostate are low to nil. About 15-20% of peak serum concentrations are seen within abscesses. Florfenicol also penetrates most body tissues, although penetration of CSF and aqueous humor is less than that of chloramphenicol. Florfenicol does penetrate the milk of lactating cows.

Biotransformation: Unlike many other antibacterial agents, chloramphenicol undergoes extensive hepatic metabolism. Although some nitroreduction and other phase I reactions occur, free chloramphenicol is biotransformed primarily by glucuronide conjugation. Urinary products after administration of chloramphenicol sodium succinate include inactive forms, mainly the unhydrolyzed sodium succinate and the glucuronide; only 5-15% appears as biologically active chloramphenicol. There are several clinical concerns with respect to the biotransformation of chloramphenicol. In cats, a characteristic genetic deficiency in glucuronyl transferase activity leads to plasma half-lives that are often considerably longer than those in other species (eg, cats, 5.1 hr; ponies, 54 min), and dosages need to be adjusted accordingly. Very young animals frequently do not have full microsomal enzyme capabilities, and the plasma half-lives of chloramphenicol in the young (<4 wk) of many species are often much longer than those of adults. Foals appear to be a notable exception to this generalization. Liver disease also prevents chloramphenicol from undergoing normal metabolic degradation, and active antibiotic accumulates in the body.

Excretion: The principal route of excretion is renal. Free chloramphenicol and the chloramphenicol sodium succinate dosage form undergo glomerular filtration (5-10%), whereas the glucuronide metabolite is eliminated by tubular secretion (90-95%). Only 5-15% of chloramphenicol is present in the urine in the active, unchanged form. The biliary route also plays a part in excretion, but enterohepatic cycling is often pronounced, and usually only a small amount of chloramphenicol is recoverable in feces. Enterohepatic cycling prolongs blood levels to some degree in herbivores.

TABLE 47. Elimination and Distribution of Chloramphenicol and Florfenicol

Drug	Species	Elimination Half-life (hr)	Volume of Distribution (mL/kg)
Chloramphenicol	Cats	5.1	2,360
	Dogs	4.2	1,700
	Calves (<1 wk old)	5.0	1,080
	Cattle	3.0	1,580
	Horses	0.9	950
Florfenicol	Cattle	18.3	700

Pharmacokinetic Values: The plasma half-life of chloramphenicol varies among species and depends on age in some species. The specific volumes of distribution usually reflect the extensive diffusion into tissues (TABLE 47). Dose rates and frequencies are typically adjusted for the species and age of the animal. Florfenicol is eliminated by the kidneys.

Therapeutic Indications and Dose Rates

Chloramphenicol is used to treat both systemic and local infections. Chronic respiratory infections, bacterial meningoencephalitis, brain abscesses, ophthalmitis and intraocular infections, pododermatitis, dermal infections, and otitis externa are types of bacterial infections that are often responsive to chloramphenicol. Salmonellosis and *Bacteroides* sepsis are fairly specific indications. Urinary tract infections are often successfully treated with chloramphenicol, notwithstanding the fairly low concentration of active antibiotic present in the urine. Hematogenous delivery of chloramphenicol to the site of infection may play a role in these cases. Florfenicol is approved for use in treatment of bovine respiratory disease.

General dosages for chloramphenicol and florfenicol are listed in TABLE 48. The dose rate and frequency should be adjusted as needed for the individual animal.

Special Clinical Concerns

Side Effects and Toxicity: In humans, chloramphenicol (but not florfenicol) can produce 2 distinctive syndromes of bone marrow suppression. One form is characterized by nonregenerative anemia (with or without thrombocytopenia or leukopenia), increased serum iron, bone marrow hypocellularity, cytoplasmic vacuolization of blast cells and lymphocytes, and maturation arrest of erythroid and myeloid precursors. This suppression is dose-dependent and reversible. Daily doses of 50 mg/kg for 3 wk can produce similar effects in cats. Milder hematologic effects are evident in dogs at much higher daily dosages (225 mg/kg). Such blood dyscrasias may also be seen in susceptible neonatal animals given standard adult doses of chloramphenicol. This toxic effect is postulated to be due to interference with mRNA and protein synthesis in rapidly multiplying cells.

The second form of bone marrow suppression is much more serious. It is a usually irreversible aplastic anemia that is not related to dose and that often appears after the

TABLE 48. Dose Rates of Chloramphenicol and Florfenicol

Drug	Species	Dosage, Route, and Frequency
Chloramphenicol	Cats	45-60 mg/kg, PO, IV, or IM, BID
	Dogs	45-60 mg/kg, PO, IV, or IM, TID-QID
	Horses	50 mg/kg, PO, TID-QID, or IV, every 2-4 hr
Florfenicol	Cattle	20 mg/kg, IM, repeated in 48 hr

drug has been discontinued. The peripheral blood shows pancytopenia, and the bone marrow may be hypoplastic or aplastic. Usually, a hemorrhagic diathesis and secondary infection are also evident. The incidence is ~1:25,000-40,000. The aplastic anemia may result from toxic intermediates associated with the nitro group; thiamphenicol and florfenicol, without the nitro group, do not produce aplastic anemia, an observation that supports the theory. Due to the possibility that tissue residues in food animals might induce aplastic anemia in humans, use of chloramphenicol in food animals is prohibited in the USA and several other countries. A form of aplastic anemia, apparently a type of hypersensitivity reaction to chloramphenicol, has been recognized in dogs and cats.

GI disturbances can develop in all nonruminant animals treated with oral chloramphenicol. Use in neonatal calves leads to a malabsorption syndrome associated with ultrastructural and functional changes of the small-intestinal enterocytes. Anorexia and depression have been seen in cats treated for >1 wk.

Because chloramphenicol can suppress anamnestic immune responses, animals should not be vaccinated while being treated with this antibiotic. Because of its ability to inhibit protein synthesis, excessive topical application on wounds may delay healing.

In both male and female rats, chloramphenicol has adversely affected the structure and functions of the gonads. In large animals, adverse signs are most often associated with propylene-glycol-based preparations that, when infused rapidly IV, may result in collapse, hemolysis, and death.

Notwithstanding the severity of the chloramphenicol-associated side effects noted above, chloramphenicol is relatively safe, provided overdosage is avoided, courses of therapy are limited to 1 wk, the dose is reduced for newborn animals and for animals with impaired liver function, and there is no evidence of a preexisting bone marrow depression.

Interactions: Chloramphenicol is a potent noncompetitive microsomal enzyme inhibitor that can substantially prolong the duration of action of several drugs administered concurrently. Frank toxic effects are likely if administration is repeated. Examples of such drugs include pentobarbital, codeine, phenobarbital, phenytoin, NSAID, and coumarins.

In combination with sulfamethoxypyridazine, chloramphenicol can cause hepatic damage. Chloramphenicol also delays the response of anemia to iron, folic acid, and vitamin B_{12}. It interferes with the actions of many bactericidal drugs, such as the penicillins, cephalosporins, and aminoglycosides, and such combinations should not be used under most circumstances. Aqueous solutions of chloramphenicol sodium succinate should not be mixed with other preparations before administration because of a high incidence of incompatibility.

Chloramphenicol should not be administered concurrently with other antibacterial agents that bind to the 50 S ribosomal subunit (eg, the macrolides and lincosamides).

Effects on Laboratory Tests: Chloramphenicol may cause increased alkaline phosphatase levels and prothrombin times. WBC and thrombocyte counts may be decreased. Anemia becomes evident in extreme cases. A false glucosuria test is possible.

Drug Withdrawal and Milk Discard Times: The use of chloramphenicol in food animals is prohibited in several countries including the USA; in others, withdrawal times vary considerably and may be as long as 2 wk. Withdrawal time for florfenicol is 28 days. Florfenicol should not be used in dairy cattle ≤20 mo old, veal calves, calves <1 mo old, or calves on an all-milk diet.

MACROLIDES

The macrolide antibiotics typically have a large lactone ring in their structure and are much more effective against gram-positive than gram-negative bacteria. They are also active against mycoplasmas and some rickettsiae. (*See also* POLYENE MACROLIDE ANTIBIOTICS, p 2098.)

Classes

Macrolides fall into 3 classes, depending on the size of the lactone ring. None of the 12-membered ring group is used clinically. Erythromycin and the closely related oleandomycin and troleandomycin belong to the 14-membered ring group. Of the 16-membered ring group, spiramycin, josamycin, and tylosin are used clinically.

General Properties

A macrolide is actually a complex mixture of closely related antibiotics that differ from one another with respect to the chemical substitutions on the various carbon atoms in the structure, and in the aminosugars and neutral sugars. For example, erythromycin is mostly erythromycin A, but B, C, D, and E forms may also be included in the preparation. The macrolide antibiotics are colorless, crystalline substances. They contain a dimethylamino group, which makes them basic. Although they are poorly water soluble, they do dissolve in more polar organic solvents. Macrolides are often inactivated in basic (pH >10) as well as acidic environments (pH <4 for erythromycin). The multiple functional groups make it possible for them to undergo a large number of chemical reactions. More stable ester forms are commonly used in pharmaceutical preparations—eg, acetylates, estolates, lactobionate, succinates, propionates, and stearates.

Antimicrobial Activity

Mode of Action: The antimicrobial mechanism seems to be the same for all of the macrolides. They interfere with protein synthesis by reversibly binding to the 50 S subunit of the ribosome. They appear to bind at the donor site, thus preventing the translocation necessary to keep the peptide chain growing. The effect is essentially confined to rapidly dividing bacteria and mycoplasmas. Macrolides are regarded as being bacteriostatic, but at high concentrations, erythromycin is bactericidal. Macrolides are significantly more active at higher pH ranges (7.8-8).

Bacterial Resistance: Resistance to macrolides in gram-positive organisms results from alterations in ribosomal structure and loss of macrolide affinity. The resistance may be intrinsic or plasmid-mediated and constitutive or inducible; it may develop rapidly (erythromycin) or slowly (tylosin). Cross-resistance between macrolides has been reported. Gram-negative organisms are probably resistant because macrolides cannot penetrate their cell walls. There are a few exceptions, and gram-negative forms without cell walls are usually sensitive.

Antimicrobial Spectra: Macrolides are active against most aerobic and anaerobic gram-positive bacteria, although there is considerable variation as to potency and activity. In general, macrolides are not active against gram-negative bacteria, but some strains of *Pasteurella, Haemophilus,* and *Neisseria* spp may be sensitive. An exception is tilmicosin, the spectrum of which is characterized as broad and includes *Mannheimia (Pasteurella) haemolytica* and *P multocida. Bacteroides fragilis* strains are moderately susceptible to macrolides. Macrolides are active against atypical mycobacteria, *Mycobacterium, Mycoplasma, Chlamydia,* and *Rickettsia* spp but not against protozoa or fungi. In vitro synergism is seen with cefamandole (against *Bacteroides fragilis*), ampicillin (against *Nocardia asteroides*), and rifampin (against *Rhodococcus equi*).

Pharmacokinetic Features

Absorption: Macrolides are readily absorbed from the GI tract if not inactivated by gastric acid. Oral preparations are often enteric-coated, or stable salts or esters (such as stearate, lactobionate, glucoheptate, propionate, and ethylsuccinate) are used. Plasma levels peak within 1-2 hr in most cases, although absorption patterns may be erratic due to the presence of food and may depend on the salt or ester used. Absorption from the ruminoreticulum is usually delayed and is unreliable. Erythromycin and tylosin may also be administered IV or IM. Tilmicosin is administered SC. Absorption after injection is rapid, but pain and swelling can develop at the injection sites.

Distribution: Macrolides become widely distributed in tissues, and concentrations are about the same as in plasma, or even higher in some instances. They actually accumulate within many cells, including macrophages, in which they may be ≥20 times the plasma concentration. This accumulation accounts in part for the long dosing interval that characterizes some macrolides (eg, tilmicosin). With spiramycin, the tissue concentrations remain especially high even though plasma concentrations are rather low. Macrolides tend to concentrate in the spleen, liver, kidneys, and particularly the lungs. They enter pleural and ascitic fluids but not the CSF (only 2-13% of plasma concentration unless the meninges are inflamed). They concentrate in the bile and milk. Up to 75% of the dose is bound to plasma proteins, and they bind to α1-acid glycoproteins rather than to albumin.

Biotransformation: Metabolic inactivation of the macrolides is usually extensive, but the relative proportion depends on the route of administration and the particular antibiotic. After administration PO, 80% of an erythromycin dose undergoes metabolic inactivation, whereas tylosin appears to be eliminated in an active form.

Excretion: Macrolide antibiotics and their metabolites are excreted mainly in bile (>60%) and often undergo enterohepatic cycling. Urinary clearance may be slow and variable (often <10%) but may represent a more significant route of elimination after parenteral administration. The concentration of macrolides in milk often is several times greater than in plasma, especially in mastitis.

Pharmacokinetics: The plasma half-lives of macrolides usually are 1-3 hr, and apparent volumes of distribution of 1,000-2,000 mL/kg reflect the extensive tissue distribution. Effective inhibitory concentrations are maintained for ~8 hr after administration PO and for ~12-24 hr after IM injection. Dosage frequencies are commonly 2-3 times/day, PO, or 1-2 times/day, parenterally.

Therapeutic Indications and Dose Rates

The macrolides are used to treat both systemic and local infections. They are often regarded as alternatives to penicillins for the treatment of streptococcal and staphylococcal infections. General indications include upper respiratory tract infections, bronchopneumonia, bacterial enteritis, metritis, pyodermatitis, urinary tract infections, arthritis, and others. Formulations for treating mastitis are also available and often have the advantage of a short withholding time for milk. Tilmicosin is approved for use in the treatment of bovine respiratory diseases associated with *Mannheimia (Pasteurella) haemolytica*.

A selection of general dose rates for some macrolides is listed in TABLE 49. The dose rate and frequency should be adjusted as needed for the individual animal.

Special Clinical Concerns

Side Effects and Toxicity: Toxicity and side effects are uncommon for most macrolides (except tilmicosin), although pain and swelling may develop at injection sites.

TABLE 49. Dose Rates of Macrolides

Macrolide	Species	Dosage, Route, and Frequency
Erythromycin	Cattle	8-15 mg/kg, IM, SID-BID
	Cats	15 mg/kg, PO, TID
	Foals	25 mg/kg, IM, TID
Tylosin	Cattle	10-20 mg/kg, IM, SID-BID
	Pigs	10 mg/kg, IM, SID-BID
		7-10 mg/kg, PO, TID
	Cats	10 mg/kg, IM, BID
Tilmicosin	Cattle	10 mg/kg, SC, once

TABLE 50. Drug Withdrawal and Milk Discard Times of Macrolides

Macrolide	Species	Withdrawal Time (days)	Milk Discard Time (hr)
Erythromycin	Cattle	14	36-72
	Pigs	7	
Tylosin	Cattle	21	96
	Pigs	14	
Tilmicosin	Cattle	28	0

Hypersensitivity reactions have occasionally been seen. Erythromycin estolate may be hepatotoxic and cause cholestasis; it may also induce vomiting and diarrhea, particularly when high doses are administered. Horses are sensitive to macrolide-induced GI disturbances that can be serious and even fatal. In pigs, tylosin may cause edema of the rectal mucosa, mild anal protrusion with diarrhea, and anal erythema and pruritus. After 5 mg/kg/day, dogs had a greater tendency to develop ventricular tachycardia and fibrillation during acute myocardial ischemia. Tilmicosin is characterized by cardiac toxicity (tachycardia and decreased contractility). It is contraindicated in swine and should not be used in an extra-label manner. Cattle have died after IV injection of tilmicosin.

Interactions: Macrolide antibiotics probably should not be used with chloramphenicol or the lincosamides because they may compete for the same 50 S ribosomal binding site, although the in vivo significance of this potential interaction is unclear. Activity of macrolides is depressed in acidic environments. Macrolide preparations for parenteral administration are incompatible with many other pharmaceutical preparations. Erythromycin and troleandomycin are microsomal enzyme inhibitors that depress the metabolism of some drugs.

Effects on Laboratory Tests: Alkaline phosphatase, bilirubin, sulfobromophthalein (BSP®), total WBC count, eosinophil count, AST, and ALT may increase. Cholesterol levels may decrease.

Drug Withdrawal and Milk Discard Times: Regulatory requirements for withdrawal times and milk discard times vary among countries. These should be followed carefully to prevent food residues and consequent public health implications. The selection of times listed in TABLE 50 serve only as general guidelines. Tilmicosin is characterized by a 28-day withdrawal time and should not be used in any species other than adult cattle (but not in dairy cows >20 mo old).

LINCOSAMIDES

General Properties

Lincosamides are derivatives of an amino acid and a sulfur-containing octose. They are monobasic and more stable in salt forms (hydrochlorides and phosphates).

Antimicrobial Activity

Mode of Action: Lincomycin and clindamycin bind exclusively to the 50 S subunit of bacterial ribosomes and suppress protein synthesis. Lincosamides, macrolides, and chloramphenicol, although not structurally related, seem to act at this same site. The lincosamides are bacteriostatic or bactericidal depending on the concentration. Activity is enhanced at an alkaline pH.

Bacterial Resistance: Resistance to lincosamides appears slowly, perhaps as a result of chromosomal mutation. Plasmid-mediated resistance has been found in strains of *Bacteroides fragilis*. Resistance appears to be due to an alteration in the 50 S ribosomal subunit. Cross-resistance with other antibiotics has been shown in vitro but not in vivo with erythromycin.

Antimicrobial Spectra: Lincomycin has a limited spectrum against aerobic pathogens but a fairly broad spectrum against anaerobes. Clindamycin is a more active analog with somewhat different pharmacokinetic patterns. Many gram-positive cocci are inhibited by lincosamides, but most gram-negative organisms are resistant, as are most mycoplasmas. *Bacteroides* spp and other anaerobes are usually susceptible. *Clostridium difficile* strains appear to be regularly resistant.

Pharmacokinetic Features

Absorption: Lincomycin is incompletely absorbed from the GI tract, especially if administered soon after feeding; plasma levels peak within 2-4 hr. Absorption from IM injection sites is good; plasma levels peak in 1-2 hr. About 90% of an oral dose of clindamycin is absorbed, and effective plasma concentrations are achieved more rapidly than with lincomycin. Absorption is not significantly affected by the ingestion of food. Clindamycin palmitate is used PO, and clindamycin phosphate IM; the latter reaches peak plasma concentration in 1-3 hr.

Distribution: Lincosamides are widely distributed in many fluids and tissues, including bone, but significant concentrations are not attained in the CSF even when the meninges are inflamed. They diffuse across the placenta in many species. About 90% of clindamycin is bound to plasma proteins. It also accumulates in polymorphonuclear WBC and alveolar macrophages such that concentrations exceed those of plasma 50-fold, but the clinical relevance of this phenomenon is unclear.

Biotransformation: After administration PO, ~50% of a dose of lincomycin and 80-90% of a dose of clindamycin are metabolically altered in the liver. Metabolites often retain activity. Liver disease impairs the biotransformation of lincosamides.

Excretion: Unchanged antibiotic and several metabolites may be excreted in bile and urine. The proportions depend on the route of administration. Levels remain high in the feces for some days, and growth of sensitive microorganisms in the large intestine may be suppressed for up to 2 wk. Milk is also an important excretory route.

Pharmacokinetics: The elimination half-life of lincosamides is frequently >3 hr, and the apparent volume of distribution is >1 L/kg. They are usually administered BID. In dogs, clindamycin has an elimination half-life of 3.9 hr and a volume of distribution of 1.4 L/kg.

Therapeutic Indications and Dose Rates

The lincosamides are indicated for infections caused by susceptible gram-positive organisms, particularly streptococci and staphylococci, and for those caused by anaerobic pathogens.

A selection of general dosages for some lincosamides is listed in TABLE 51. The dose rate and frequency should be adjusted as needed for the individual animal.

TABLE 51. Dose Rates of Lincosamides

Lincosamide	Species	Dosage, Route, and Frequency
Lincomycin	Cattle	10 mg/kg, IM, BID
	Pigs	10 mg/kg, IM, BID
		7 mg/kg, in-feed
	Dogs	20 mg/kg, PO, SID
	Cats	10 mg/kg, IM, BID
		25 mg/kg, PO, BID
Clindamycin	Dogs, cats	5-10 mg/kg, PO, BID

Special Clinical Concerns

Side Effects and Toxicity: No serious organ toxicity has been reported, but GI disturbances do occur. Clindamycin-induced pseudomembranous enterocolitis (caused by toxigenic *Clostridium difficile*) is a serious adverse reaction seen in humans. Lincosamides are contraindicated in horses because severe and even fatal colitis may develop. Skeletal muscle paralysis may be seen at high concentrations. Hypersensitivity reactions occasionally are seen. Lincosamides should not be used in neonates because of their limited ability to metabolize drugs.

Interactions: Lincosamides have additive neuromuscular effects with anesthetic agents and skeletal muscle relaxants. Kaolin-pectin prevents their absorption from the GI tract. They should not be combined with bactericidal agents or with the macrolides.

Effects on Laboratory Tests: Alkaline phosphatase, AST, and ALT may be increased.

Drug Withdrawal Times: In several countries, there is a 2-day withdrawal time for pigs.

MISCELLANEOUS ANTIMICROBIAL AGENTS

A number of antimicrobial agents are used periodically for several diverse purposes. Several of these are discussed below.

Polymyxins

Of this group of polypeptide antibiotics, polymyxin B and polymyxin E, or colistin, are most commonly used topically and PO. Colistimethate is a form of colistin intended for parenteral administration. Polymyxins are bactericidal; they interact strongly with phospholipids in bacterial cell membranes and radically disrupt their permeability and function. The polymyxins are more effective against gram-negative than gram-positive bacteria. Their rather narrow spectrum includes *Enterobacter, Klebsiella, Salmonella, Pasteurella, Bordetella,* and *Shigella* spp, and *Escherichia coli.* Most *Proteus* spp are not susceptible. Although intrinsic bacterial resistance to polymyxins is recognized, resistance is uncommon and is chromosome-dependent only. Polymyxins act synergistically when combined with potentiated sulfonamides, tetracyclines, and some other antibacterials; they also reduce the activity of endotoxins in body fluids and may be beneficial in endotoxemia. Their action is inhibited by divalent cations, unsaturated fatty acids, and quaternary ammonium compounds.

Polymyxins are not absorbed after PO or topical administration; plasma levels peak ~2 hr after parenteral administration. Blood levels usually are low because polymyxins bind to cell membranes as well as tissue debris and purulent exudates. The polymixins undergo renal elimination mostly as degradation products, and their plasma half-lives are 3-6 hr. They are notably nephrotoxic and neurotoxic. Neuromuscular blockade can be seen at higher concentrations. Intense pain at sites of injection and hypersensitivity reactions also can be expected. Polymyxin B is a potent histamine releaser. The main indication for parenteral use of polymyxins is life-threatening infection due to gram-negative bacilli or *Pseudomonas* spp that are resistant to other drugs. Polymyxins are also used PO against susceptible intestinal infections. Topical application is common, eg, for otitis externa.

Recommended dose rates for polymyxins vary considerably. A general guideline is 20,000 U/kg, PO, BID; 5,000 U/kg, IM, BID; 50,000-100,000 U by intramammary infusion; 100,000 U intrauterine in cattle. IV administration of polymyxins is potentially dangerous.

Bacitracins

Bacitracins are branched, cyclic, decapeptide antibiotics. Bacitracin A is the most active of the group and the main component of the commercial bacitracin preparations that are used either topically or PO. These antibiotics are bactericidal. They interfere with cell membrane function, suppress cell wall formation by preventing the formation of peptidoglycan strands, and inhibit protein synthesis. Bactericidal activity requires the presence of divalent cations, such as zinc. The spectrum of bacitracins is similar to that of penicillin G and is mostly limited to gram-positive and a few gram-negative bacteria, as well as some spirochetes. Most gram-negative organisms are not susceptible, probably due to lack of penetration of the drug through the outer membrane. Resistance is rare. Bacitracins are often used in combination with neomycin and polymyxins to enhance the antibacterial spectrum. Bacitracins are not appreciably absorbed from the GI tract and are not used systemically because of their pronounced nephrotoxicity. However, they are used locally in wound powders and ointments, dermatologic preparations, eye and ear ointments, and as feed additives in swine and poultry rations for growth promotion. In antibiotic-associated pseudomembranous colitis caused by *Clostridium difficile* cytotoxin, bacitracin (given PO) is considered an alternative to vancomycin. Hypersensitivity reactions to bacitracins are seen occasionally.

Vancomycin

Vancomycin is a complex glycopeptide that binds to precursors of the peptidoglycan layer in bacterial cell walls. This effect prevents cell wall synthesis and produces a rapid bactericidal effect in dividing bacteria. Vancomycin is active against most gram-positive bacteria but is not effective against gram-negative cells because of their large size and poor penetrability. Resistance to vancomycin does not readily develop. The drug is widely distributed in the body. Excretion (in active form) is via the kidneys; in renal insufficiency, striking accumulations may develop. The plasma half-life in dogs is 2-3 hr. The only indication for the use of parenteral vancomycin is serious infection due to methicillin-resistant *Staphylococcus aureus*. Although poorly absorbed, oral vancomycin is used to treat antibiotic-associated enterocolitis, especially if caused by *Clostridium difficile*. Febrile reactions and thrombophlebitis (because of tissue irritation) at injection sites may be seen. Hypersensitivity reactions are seen infrequently. Ototoxicity and nephrotoxicity were fairly common in the past but are rare today because of fewer impurities in the final form.

Novobiocin Sodium

Novobiocin is a narrow-spectrum antibiotic that may be bacteriostatic or bactericidal at higher concentrations. It is active mostly against gram-positive bacteria but also against a few gram-negative bacteria. There is a synergistic effect with tetracyclines. Many species of bacteria can develop resistance to novobiocin. Adverse reactions are quite frequent after administration. Its main use is in combination with other agents for the treatment of bovine mastitis.

Tiamulin Fumarate

Tiamulin is active against gram-positive bacteria, mycoplasmas, and anaerobes, including *Treponema hyodysenteriae*. It is also clinically effective in the treatment of swine dysentery and mycoplasmal arthritis. Tiamulin is well absorbed when administered PO. The dosage is 8.8 mg/kg, daily for 3-5 days, in either food or water. The parenteral dosage for mycoplasmal pneumonia in pigs is 15 mg/kg. In poultry, tiamulin interferes with monensin and salinomycin metabolism, and if the drugs are fed together, they become toxic. Generally, however, tiamulin has few side effects.

Rifamycins

Several semisynthetic derivatives (rifamycin SV, rifampin [rifampicin], rifamide) of natural rifamycins have been used as extended-spectrum antibiotics. Rifamycins interfere with the synthesis of RNA in microorganisms by binding to subunits of sensitive DNA-dependent RNA polymerase. They are active against gram-positive organisms, some mycobacteria, a few strains of gram-negative bacteria (mostly cocci; bacilli are more resistant), some anaerobes, and chlamydiae. At high concentrations, they are also active against several viruses. Fungal and yeast infections resistant to rifampin alone often respond when a rifamycin is added to an antifungal agent (eg, amphotericin B).

Resistance to rifamycins may develop rapidly as a 1-step process. For this reason, they are often administered in combination with other antimicrobials, such as penicillins, erythromycin, miconazole, and amphotericin B. The primary use of the rifamycins in humans has been for the treatment of tuberculosis. Rifampin has been used in foals to control pneumonia induced by *Rhodococcus equi*. Because rifamycins penetrate tissues and cells to a substantial degree, they are particularly effective against intracellular organisms. Rifampin is readily but incompletely (~40%) absorbed from the GI tract, and plasma levels peak within 2-4 hr. Concurrent feeding may reduce or delay absorption. Rifampin may also be administered IM or IV. About 75-80% of rifampin is bound to plasma proteins. It is widely distributed in body tissues and fluids because of its high lipid solubility. Rifampin is biotransformed to several metabolites, some of which are active, and is primarily excreted in bile (used for cholangitis in humans) and to a lesser degree in urine. Enterohepatic cycling of the parent drug and its main metabolite (desacetylrifampin) commonly occurs. The elimination half-life of rifampin is dose-dependent: in horses, it is ~6 hr; in dogs, ~8 hr. The plasma half-life progressively shortens by ~40% during the first 2 wk of treatment due to the induction of hepatic microsomal enzymes; conversely, it is increased with hepatic dysfunction. Rifampin is usually well tolerated and produces few side effects. GI disturbances and abnormalities in liver function (icterus) have been reported in humans. Hypersensitivity reactions can also result from rifampin administration, and renal failure is a possible consequence when intermittent dosage schedules are followed. Partial, reversible immunosuppression of lymphocytes develops. Urine, feces, saliva, sputum, sweat, and tears are often colored red-orange by rifampin and its metabolites. CNS depression after IV administration and temporary inappetence are seen in horses. The dose range for rifampin in horses is 10-25 mg/kg, PO or parenterally, SID.

Nitrofurans

Nitrofurans are synthetic chemotherapeutic agents with a broad antimicrobial spectrum; they are active against both gram-positive and gram-negative bacteria, including *Salmonella* and *Giardia* spp, trichomonads, amebae, and some coccidial species. However, when compared with other antimicrobial chemotherapeutic agents, their potency is not particularly great. The nitrofurans appear to inhibit a number of microbial enzyme systems, including those involved in carbohydrate metabolism, and they also block the initiation of translation. However, their basic mechanism of action has not yet been clarified. Their primary action is bacteriostatic, but at high doses they are also bactericidal. They are much more active in acidic environments (pH 5.5 is optimal for nitrofurantoin activity). Resistant mutants are rare, and clinical resistance emerges slowly. Among themselves, nitrofurans show complete cross-resistance, but there is no cross-resistance with any other antibacterial agents. Because of very slight water solubility, the nitrofurans are used either PO or topically. No nitrofuran is effective systemically. They are either not absorbed at all from the GI tract or are so rapidly eliminated that they reach inhibitory concentrations only in the urine. Toxic signs seen with excessive doses of nitrofuran derivatives include CNS involvement (excitement, tremors, convulsions, peripheral neuritis), GI disturbances, poor weight gain, and depression of spermatogenesis. Various hypersensitivity reactions can also be seen. Some nitrofurans are carcinogenic, and their future use is in doubt.

Nitrofurantoin: Nitrofurantoin is used to treat urinary tract infections caused by susceptible bacteria, such as *Escherichia coli*, *Staphylococcus aureus*, *Streptococcus pyogenes*, and *Aerobacter aerogenes*. *Proteus* spp, *Pseudomonas aeruginosa*, and *Streptococcus faecalis* are usually resistant. After administration PO, nitrofurantoin is rapidly and completely absorbed (the macrocrystal form takes longer) and is swiftly eliminated by the kidneys, mainly by tubular secretion (~40% in the unchanged form). Serum concentrations are low, and little unbound drug is available for diffusion into the tissues. The plasma half-life is only ~20 min. Nitrofurantoin is concentrated in acid urine. When the pH reaches ~5, the drug becomes supersaturated without precipitation and its antibacterial action is maximal. Nitrofurantoin can be administered PO or parenterally. The dosage for dogs and cats is 4.4 mg/kg, PO, TID for 4-10 days. Side effects are not common at usual dosages, but nausea, vomiting, and diarrhea can develop. CNS disorders have been seen, and polyneuropathy is a serious effect that is seen in humans. Animals with decreased renal function have a predisposition for polyneuritis. Various manifestations of hypersensitivity reactions can be seen. Yellow discoloration of teeth occasionally has been reported in very young animals.

Nitrofurazone: Nitrofurazone is only slightly soluble in water but, in general, corresponds to nitrofurantoin in terms of its mechanism of action, antimicrobial spectrum, potency, and physicochemical characteristics. Its main indications include the treatment of bovine mastitis, bovine metritis, and wounds. However, pus, blood, and milk reduce the antibacterial activity. Nitrofurazone is also used as a feed additive (0.05%) to control intestinal bacterial and coccidial infections. The withdrawal time for nitrofurazone in pigs is 5 days.

Furazolidone: This is a nitrofuran with a wide range of antimicrobial activity that includes *Clostridium, Salmonella, Shigella, Staphylococcus* and *Streptococcus* spp, and *E coli*. It is also active against *Eimeria* and *Histomonas* spp. It is usually administered PO to treat intestinal infections but may also be applied topically. The usual oral dose of furazolidone in calves is 10-12 mg/kg, BID for 5-7 days. Caution should be exercised when treating small calves (eg, Jersey breed) to avoid excessive dose rates, lest neurotoxicity result; signs include head tremors, ataxia, visual impairment, and convulsions.

Miscellaneous Nitrofurans: Nifuraldezone, like furazolidone, is used to control bacterial enteritis in calves. Nifurprazine is used only topically as an antibacterial agent. Furaltadone is used both PO to prevent intestinal infections and directly into the teat to treat mastitis.

Nitroimidazoles

The 5-nitroimidazoles are a group of drugs that have both antiprotozoal and antibacterial activity. Nitroimidazoles with activity against trichomonads and amebae include metronidazole, tinidazole, nimorazole, flunidazole, and ronidazole. Metronidazole and nimorazole are effective in the treatment of giardiasis, while dimetridazole, ipronidazole, and ronidazole control histomoniasis in poultry. Several nitroimidazoles have activity against trypanosomes. Metronidazole, ronidazole, and other nitroimidazoles are active against anaerobic bacteria. Metronidazole is the compound that has been the most studied and is discussed as the prototype of the group.

Metronidazole: This has been used for many years in the therapeutic management of trichomoniasis, giardiasis, and amebiasis. It is active against obligate anaerobic bacteria. It is not active against facultative anaerobes, obligate aerobes, or microaerophilic bacteria other than *Campylobacter fetus* and *Corynebacterium vaginalis*. At concentrations readily attained in serum after PO or parenteral administration, metronidazole is active against *Bacteroides fragilis, B melaninogenicus, Fusobacterium* spp, and *Clostridium perfringens* and other *Clostridium* spp. It is generally less active against nonsporeforming, gram-positive bacilli such as *Actinomyces, Propionibacterium, Bifidobacterium*, and *Eubacterium* spp. Metronidazole is also somewhat less active against gram-positive cocci such as *Peptostreptococcus* and *Peptococcus* spp, but the less sensitive strains are usually not obligate anaerobes.

Metronidazole is bactericidal at concentrations equal to or slightly higher than the minimal inhibitory concentration. The precise mode of action is unclear, but it seems that after the drug enters a susceptible organism it is first reduced and then binds to DNA, causing loss of the helical structure, strand breakage, and impairment of DNA function. Only susceptible organisms (bacteria and protozoa) appear to be capable of metabolizing the drug.

The pharmacokinetic pattern of metronidazole generally follows that expected of a highly lipid-soluble basic drug. It is readily but variably absorbed from the GI tract (bioavailability 60-100%), with serum concentrations peaking within 1-2 hr, and becomes widely distributed in all tissues. Metronidazole penetrates the blood-brain barrier and also attains therapeutic concentrations in abscesses and in empyema fluid. It is only slightly bound to plasma proteins. Biotransformation is quite extensive, and parent drug and metabolites are excreted by both the renal and biliary routes. The elimination half-life in dogs is ~4.5 hr, and in horses, 1.5-3.3 hr.

The principal clinical indications for metronidazole include the treatment of specific protozoal infections (amebiasis, trichomoniasis, giardiasis, and balantidiasis) and anaerobic bacterial infections such as those that may be seen in abdominal abscesses, peritonitis, empyema, genital tract infections, periodontitis, otitis media, osteitis, arthritis, and meningitis, and in necrotic tissue. Metronidazole has been successfully used to prevent infection after colonic surgery. Nitroimidazoles also act as radiosensitizers, and metronidazole has been used as an adjunct to the radiotherapy of solid tumors.

Side effects are not commonly associated with metronidazole. High doses may induce signs of neurotoxicity in dogs, such as tremors, muscle spasms, ataxia, and even convulsions. Reversible bone marrow depression has been reported. The drug should not be used in pregnant animals, particularly during the first trimester, although the evidence for carcinogenicity and mutagenicity is still tenuous. Metronidazole may produce a reddish brown discoloration of the urine due to unidentified pigments.

Recommended dose rates for metronidazole in dogs are 44 mg/kg, PO, followed by 22 mg/kg, QID for anaerobic infections; 25 mg/kg, PO, BID for giardiasis; and 66 mg/kg, PO, SID for trichomoniasis. Courses of therapy are generally 5-7 days. Both PO and IV preparations are available.

Hydroxyquinolines

The 8-hydroxyquinolines are a group of synthetic compounds with antibacterial, antifungal, and antiprotozoal activity. The best known compounds of this class are iodochlorhydroxyquin (clioquinol), diiodohydroxyquin (iodoquinol), broxyquinoline, and hydroxyquinoline. Because they are not absorbed from the GI tract to any degree, their main use has been for the treatment of intestinal infections caused by bacteria or protozoa (such as *Giardia*). Hydroxyquinolines are also used topically for skin infections caused by bacteria and fungi. Hydroxyquinolines are potentially neurotoxic when used for prolonged periods. The dose for a 455-kg horse is 10 g, PO, SID, using a decreasing dosage regimen to end medication.

ANTIFUNGAL AGENTS

Topical infections caused by a large variety of fungi may become established on the skin and adnexa or mucous membranes (buccal, GI, ruminal, vaginal). The external auditory canal and cornea may also be invaded by yeasts and fungi that are opportunistic pathogens. Locally active antifungal drugs (p 2106) are used to treat such topical infections.

A number of serious systemic fungal diseases are well recognized in several parts of the world. (*See* FUNGAL INFECTIONS, p 510.) Antifungal agents have greatly reduced earlier mortality rates due to systemic mycoses in humans. A relatively narrow selection of drugs is used in these cases.

POLYENE MACROLIDE ANTIBIOTICS

A number of polyene antifungal antibiotics has been isolated from various strains of *Actinomyces*, but only amphotericin B, nystatin, and pimaricin (natamycin) are used in veterinary medicine. The polyenes are poorly soluble in water and the common organic solvents. They are reasonably soluble in highly polar solvents such as dimethylformamide and dimethyl sulfoxide. In combination with bile salts, such as sodium deoxycholate, amphotericin B is readily soluble (micellar suspension) in 5% glucose. This colloidal preparation is used for IV infusion. The polyenes are quite unstable in aqueous, acidic, or alkaline media but in the dry state, in the absence of heat and light, they remain stable for indefinite periods. They should be administered parenterally (diluted in 5% dextrose) as freshly prepared aqueous suspensions (stable for 1 wk if refrigerated).

Antifungal Activity

Mode of Action: The polyenes bind to sterol components in the phospholipid-sterol membranes of fungal cells to form complexes that induce physical changes in the membrane. The number of conjugated bonds and the molecular size of a particular polyene macrolide influence its avidity for different sterols in fungal cell membranes. Amphotericin B, because of its greater affinity, binds to ergosterol, the major sterol in fungal membranes, rather than to the cholesterol in host cells. The disruption of membrane function results in potassium ion efflux from the fungal cell and hydrogen ion influx, producing internal acidification and a halt in enzymatic functions. Sugars and amino acids also eventually leak from an arrested cell. Fungistatic effects are most often evident at usual polyene concentrations. High drug concentrations and pH values between 6.0 and 7.3 in the surrounding medium may lead to fungicidal rather than fungistatic action. In addition to these direct effects on susceptible yeasts and fungi, evidence suggests that amphotericin B may also act as an immunopotentiator (both humoral and cell-mediated), thus enhancing the host's ability to overcome mycotic infections.

Fungal Resistance: Resistance to the polyene antifungal macrolides is rare both clinically and in vitro. Resistance develops slowly and does not reach high levels, even after prolonged treatment.

Antifungal Spectra: The polyene antibiotics have broad antifungal activity against organisms ranging from yeasts to filamentous fungi and from saprophytic to pathogenic fungi, but there are great differences between the sensitivities of the various species and strains of fungi. In vitro sensitivities (both resistant and highly susceptible) do not always correlate well with the clinical response, which suggests that host factors may also play a role. Many algae and some protozoa (*Leishmania, Trypanosoma, Trichomonas,* and *Entamoeba* spp) are sensitive to the polyenes, but these compounds have no significant activity against bacteria, actinomycetes, viruses, or animal cells. Amphotericin B is effective against yeasts (eg, *Candida* spp, *Rhodotorula* spp, *Cryptococcus neoformans*), dimorphic fungi (eg, *Histoplasma capsulatum, Blastomyces dermatitidis, Coccidioides immitis*), dermatophytes (eg, *Trichophyton, Microsporum,* and *Epidermophyton* spp), and molds. The drug also has been used successfully to treat disseminated sporotrichosis, pythiosis, and zygomycosis, although it may not always be effective. The polyenes are not effective against dermatophytes. Nystatin is mainly used for the treatment of mucocutaneous candidiasis, but it is effective against other yeasts and fungi. The antimicrobial activity of pimaricin is similar to that of nystatin, though it is mainly used for the local treatment of candidiasis, trichomoniasis, and mycotic keratitis.

Pharmacokinetic Features

Absorption: The polyene macrolide antibiotics are poorly absorbed from the GI tract, although amphotericin B has reached reasonable blood levels in some experimental animals. Amphotericin B is usually administered IV (occasionally intrathecally or intraocularly) or topically. Nystatin and piramycin are mostly applied topically. Nystatin is given PO to treat intestinal candidiasis. Absorption is minimal from sites of local application.

Distribution: Amphotericin B becomes widely distributed in the body after IV infusion. It appears to become associated with cholesterol-containing membranes in many different tissues from which it is slowly released into the circulation. Penetration into the CSF, saliva, aqueous humor, vitreous humor, and hemodialysis solutions is generally poor. Amphotericin B becomes highly bound to plasma lipoproteins (~95%).

Biotransformation and Excretion: About 5% of a total daily dose is excreted unchanged in the urine. Over a 2-wk period, ~20% of the drug may be recovered in the urine.

TABLE 52. Dose Rates of Polyene Macrolide Antibiotics

Polyene Macrolide	Dosage, Route, and Frequency
Amphotericin B (0.1 mg/mL in 5% dextrose)	0.1-1 mg/kg, given IV slowly, 3 times/wk Total dose: 4-11 mg/kg
Nystatin	50,000-150,000 U, PO, TID (dogs)
Pimaricin (5% ophthalmic solution)	1 drop, instilled into the eye, every 1-2 hr

The hepatobiliary system accounts for 20-30% of the excretion process. The fate of the remainder of amphotericin B is unknown.

Pharmacokinetics: Amphotericin B has a biphasic elimination pattern. The initial phase lasts 24 hr, during which levels fall rapidly (70% for plasma and 50% for urine). The second elimination phase has a 15-day half-life, during which plasma concentrations decline very slowly. Amphotericin B is usually infused IV, every 48-72 hr, until the total cumulative dosage has been reached.

Therapeutic Indications and Dose Rates

Amphotericin B is used principally in the treatment of systemic mycotic infections. Despite its ability to cause nephrotoxicity (*see* below), amphotericin B remains a commonly used antifungal agent because of its effectiveness. Nystatin is primarily indicated for the treatment of mucocutaneous (skin, oropharynx, vagina) or intestinal candidiasis; pimaricin is mainly used in therapeutic management of mycotic keratitis.

A selection of general dosages for some polyene macrolide antibiotics is listed in TABLE 52. The dose rate and frequency should be adjusted as needed for the individual animal.

Special Clinical Concerns

Side Effects and Toxicity: Oral administration of nystatin can lead to anorexia and GI disturbances. The IV infusion of amphotericin B is potentially harmful, but the main concern is nephrotoxicity. Within 15 min of IV administration, renal arterial vasoconstriction occurs and lasts for 4-6 hr. This leads to diminished renal blood flow and glomerular filtration. Because amphotericin B binds to the cholesterol component in the membranes of the distal renal tubules, a change in permeability occurs in these cells, leading to polyuria, polydipsia, concentration defects, and acidification abnormalities. The net result is a distal renal tubular acidosis syndrome. The metabolic acidosis leads to bone buffering, the excessive release of calcium into the circulation, and ultimately, nephrocalcinosis due to calcium precipitation in the acidic environment of the distal tubules. Almost every animal treated with amphotericin B suffers some degree of renal impairment, which may become permanent depending on the total cumulative dose. The administration of amphotericin B can lead to a number of other adverse effects, including anorexia, nausea, vomiting, hypersensitivity reactions, drug fever, normocytic normochromic anemia, cardiac arrhythmias and even arrest, hepatic dysfunction, CNS signs, and thrombophlebitis at the injection site.

The incidence of serious adverse effects of amphotericin B therapy can be reduced. Pretreatment with antiemetic and antihistaminic agents prevents the nausea, vomiting, and hypersensitivity reactions. Giving corticosteroids IV also limits severe hypersensitivity reactions. Mannitol (1 g/kg, IV) with each dose of amphotericin B, and sodium bicarbonate (2 mEq/kg, IV or PO, daily) may help prevent acidification defects, metabolic acidosis, and azotemia; however, clinical evidence of efficacy has not been proved. Saralasin (6-12 µg/kg/min, IV) and dopamine (7 µg/kg/min, IV) infusions have prevented oliguria and azotemia induced by amphotericin B in dogs. Administering IV fluids or furosemide before amphotericin B prevents pronounced decreases in renal blood flow and glomerular filtration rate. Newer preparations in which amphotericin B is mixed with lipid or liposo-mal vehicles are safer (particularly liposomes) and have maintained efficacy.

Interactions: Amphotericin B may be combined with other antimicrobial agents with synergistic results. This often allows both the total dose of amphotericin B and the length of therapy to be decreased. Examples include combinations of 5-flucytosine and ampho-tericin B for the treatment of cryptococcal meningitis, minocycline and amphotericin B for coccidioidomycosis, and imidazole and amphotericin B for several systemic mycotic infections. Rifampin may also potentiate the antifungal activity of amphotericin B.

Drugs that should be avoided during amphotericin B therapy include aminoglyco-sides (nephrotoxicity), digitalis drugs (increased toxicity), curarizing agents (neuromus-cular blockade), mineralocorticoids (hypokalemia), thiazide diuretics (hypokalemia, hy-ponatremia), antineoplastic drugs (cytotoxicity), and cyclosporine (nephrotoxicity).

Effects on Laboratory Tests: Plasma bilirubin, CK, AST, ALT, BUN, and eosinophil count increase. Plasma potassium and platelet count decrease. Urine protein increases.

IMIDAZOLES

Imidazoles may have antibacterial, antifungal, antiprotozoal, and anthelmintic activ-ity. Several distinct phenylimidazoles are therapeutically useful antifungal agents with wide spectra against yeasts and filamentous fungi responsible for either superficial or systemic infections. The anthelmintic thiabendazole is also an imidazole with antifungal properties. Clotrimazole, miconazole, econazole, ketoconazole, itraconazole, and flu-conazole are the most clinically important members of this group.

Imidazoles generally are poorly soluble in water but can be dissolved in organic sol-vents, such as chloroform, propylene glycol, and polyethoxylated castor oil (preparation for IV use but dangerous in dogs). An exception is fluconazole. Imidazoles are weak di-basic agents. Alterations in side-chain structure determine antifungal activity as well as the degree of toxicity.

Antifungal Activity

Mode of Action: Imidazoles alter the cell membrane permeability of susceptible yeasts and fungi by blocking the synthesis of ergosterol (demethylation of lanosterol is inhib-ited), the primary cell sterol of fungi. Other enzyme systems are also impaired, such as those required for fatty acid synthesis. Because of the drug-induced changes of oxidative and peroxidative enzyme activities, toxic concentrations of hydrogen peroxide develop intracellularly. The overall effect is cell membrane and internal organelle disruption and cell death. The cholesterol in host cells is not affected by the imidazoles, although some drugs impair synthesis of selected steroids and drug-metabolizing enzymes in the host.

Fungal Resistance: Sensitivity to the imidazoles varies greatly between various strains of yeasts and fungi, but neither natural nor acquired resistance appears to be prevalent.

Antimicrobial Spectra: The antifungal imidazoles also have some antibacterial ac-tion but are rarely used for this purpose. Miconazole has a wide antifungal spectrum against most fungi and yeasts of veterinary interest. Sensitive organisms include *Blasto-myces dermatitidis*, *Paracoccidioides brasiliensis*, *Histoplasma capsulatum*, *Candida* spp, *Coccidioides immitis*, *Cryptococcus neoformans*, and *Aspergillus fumigatus*. Some *Aspergillus* and *Madurella* spp are only marginally sensitive. Ketoconazole has an antifungal spectrum similar to that of miconazole, but it is more effective against *C im-mitis* and some other yeasts and fungi. Itraconazole and fluconazole are the most active of the antifungal imidazoles. Their spectrum includes dimorphic fungal organisms and dermatophytes. They are also effective against some cases of aspergillosis (60-70%) and cutaneous sporotrichosis. Clotrimazole and econazole are used for superficial mycoses (dermatophytosis and candidiasis); econazole also has been used for oculomycosis. Thia-bendazole is effective against *Aspergillus* and *Penicillium* spp, but its use has largely been replaced by the more effective imidazoles.

Pharmacokinetic Features

Absorption and Distribution: The imidazoles are rapidly but sometimes erratically absorbed from the GI tract; plasma levels peak within 2 hr after administration PO. Fluconazole is an exception, being close to 100% bioavailable after administration PO. Except for fluconazole, an acidic environment is required for the dissolution of the imidazoles, and a decrease in gastric acidity can reduce the bioavailability after administration PO. The rate of absorption appears to be increased when the drug is given with meals, but reports are conflicting.

Imidazoles appear to be widely distributed in the body with detectable concentrations in saliva, milk, and cerumen. CSF penetration is poor except for fluconazole, which reaches 50-90% of plasma concentrations. Most imidazoles (except fluconazole) are highly protein bound in the circulation (>95%), most to albumin. The highest concentrations of imidazoles are found in the liver, adrenal glands, lungs, and kidneys.

Biotransformation and Excretion: Hepatic metabolism is the primary route of elimination. Metabolism of ketoconazole and most other imidazoles by oxidative pathways is extensive. Only ~2-4% of a dose administered PO appears unchanged in the urine. Itraconazole is metabolized to an active metabolite that may contribute significantly to antimicrobial activity. The biliary route is the major excretory pathway (>80%); ~20% of the metabolites are eliminated in the urine. Fluconazole (in people) is eliminated (≥90%) unchanged in the urine.

Pharmacokinetics: The rate of elimination of ketoconazole appears to be dose dependent—the greater the dose, the longer the elimination half-life. There is also a biphasic elimination pattern with rapid elimination in the first 1-2 hr, then a slower decline over the next 6-9 hr. Ketoconazole is usually administered BID. The half-life of itraconazole is longer (up to 48 hr in cats), thus allowing treatment SID-BID. Because of the long half-life and mechanism of action (impaired synthesis of the fungal cell membrane), time to efficacy may take longer than drugs that have more rapid actions (such as amphotericin B).

Therapeutic Indications and Dose Rates

The imidazoles are used to treat systemic fungal diseases, dermatomycoses that have not responded to griseofulvin or topical therapy, *Malassezia* in dogs, aspergillosis, and sporotrichosis in animals that cannot tolerate or do not respond to sodium iodide. For serious infections, combination with amphotericin B is strongly recommended. Among the imidazoles, fluconazole is most indicated for tissues that are tough to penetrate. Both itraconzaole and fluconazole are generally preferred to other imidazoles for treatment of systemic fungal infections, including aspergillosis and sporotrichosis. Topically applied imidazoles (clotrimazole, miconazole, econazole) are used for local dermatophytosis. Thiabendazole is included in some otic preparations for treatment of yeast infections.

Enilconazole is an imidazole that can be applied topically for the treatment of dermatophytosis and aspergillosis. It has been used safely in cats, dogs, cattle, horses, and chickens and is prepared as a 0.2% solution for the treatment of fungal skin infections. When infused into the nasal turbinates of dogs with aspergillosis, enilconazole treated and prevented the recurrence of fungal disease. When applied topically to dog and cat hairs enilconazole inhibits fungal growth in 2 rather than 4-8 treatments, as is necessary with other topically administered antifungal agents.

General dosages for the antifungal imidazoles are listed in TABLE 53. The dose rate and frequency should be adjusted as needed for the individual animal.

Special Clinical Concerns

Side Effects and Toxicity: The imidazoles given PO result in few side effects, but nausea, vomiting, and hepatic dysfunction can develop, particularly with ketoconazole. Altered testosterone and cortisol metabolism, as well as blunted adrenal responsiveness to ACTH, have been reported, particularly with ketoconazole. Reproductive disorders

TABLE 53. Dose Rates of Imidazoles

Imidazole	Dosage, Route, and Frequency
Enilconazole	10 mg/kg in 5-10 mL, BID for 7-14 days
Fluconazole	5-10 mg/kg, PO, SID-BID
Itraconazole	5-10 mg/kg, PO, SID-BID
Ketoconazole	5-20 mg/kg, PO, BID (dogs)
Thiabendazole	44 mg/kg, PO, SID, or 22 mg/kg, PO, BID

related to ketoconazole administration may be seen in dogs. The other antifungal imidazoles are now used topically only.

Interactions: The imidazoles may be used concurrently with amphotericin B or 5-flucytosine to potentiate its antifungal activity. The absorption of the imidazoles, except for that of fluconazole, is inhibited by concurrent administration of cimetidine, ranitidine, anticholinergic agents, or gastric antacids. Rifampin decreases the serum levels of active ketoconazole because of microsomal enzyme induction. The risk of hepatotoxicity is increased if ketoconazole and griseofulvin are administered together. Ketoconazole inhibits the metabolism of some drugs and, if administered concurrently, their concentrations may be higher than anticipated.

Effects on Laboratory Tests: AST, ALT, plasma bilirubin, and plasma cholesterol increase. Adrenal responsiveness is altered.

FLUCYTOSINE

Flucytosine (5-fluorocytosine) is a fluorinated pyrimidine related to fluorouracil that was initially developed as an antineoplastic agent. It should be stored in airtight containers protected from light. Solutions for infusion are unstable and should be stored at 15-20°C. Usually, it is given PO in capsules.

Antifungal Activity

Mode of Action: Flucytosine is converted by cytosine deaminase in fungal cells to fluorouracil, which then interferes with RNA and protein synthesis. Fluorouracil is metabolized to 5-fluorodeoxyuridylic acid, an inhibitor of thymidylate synthetase. DNA synthesis is then also halted. Mammalian cells do not convert large amounts of flucytosine to fluorouracil and, thus, are not affected at usual dosage levels.

Fungal Resistance: Resistance to flucytosine can develop rapidly even during the course of treatment; this has restricted its use as the sole treatment for mycotic infections. The mechanisms of resistance are not completely understood.

Antifungal Spectrum: The following are the main organisms usually sensitive to flucytosine: *Cryptococcus neoformans*, *Candida albicans*, other *Candida* spp, *Torulopsis glabrata*, *Sporothrix schenckii*, *Aspergillus* spp, and agents of chromoblastomycosis (*Phialophora*, *Cladosporium*). The other fungi responsible for systemic mycoses and dermatophytes are resistant to flucytosine.

Pharmacokinetic Features

Absorption and Distribution: Flucytosine is rapidly and well absorbed from the GI tract with plasma levels peaking in 1-2 hr in animals that have received the drug for several days. The drug is widely distributed in the body with a volume of distribution approximating the total body water. Flucytosine is minimally bound to plasma proteins. There is excellent penetration into body fluids such as the CSF, synovial fluids, and aqueous humor.

Biotransformation and Excretion: Nearly all of an oral dose (85-95%) is excreted unchanged. Flucytosine is principally excreted by glomerular filtration (>80%). The clearance of flucytosine is approximately equivalent to that of creatinine. In renal failure, elimination of flucytosine is markedly impaired.

Pharmacokinetics: With normal renal function, the plasma half-life of flucytosine is usually 2-4 hr but may be up to 200 hr with oliguria. Serum levels of 50-100 μg/mL are usually in the therapeutic range.

Therapeutic Indications and Dose Rates

The more common indications for flucytosine include cryptococcal meningitis, used together with amphotericin B (~30% of the isolates develop resistance during the course of treatment); candidiasis (~90% of isolates are usually sensitive); aspergillosis (some strains are sensitive at <5 μg/mL); chromomycosis (some strains are very sensitive); and sporotrichosis (some cases may respond).

General dosages for flucytosine are 25-50 mg/kg and 30-40 mg/kg, PO, TID-QID in dogs and cats, respectively. The dose rate and frequency should be adjusted as needed for the individual animal. Dosage modification is essential in renal failure. Flucytosine serum levels should be monitored if possible.

Special Clinical Concerns

Side Effects and Toxicity: Flucytosine is often well tolerated over long periods, but toxic effects may be seen when serum levels are high (>100 μg/mL). These include GI signs (nausea, vomiting, diarrhea) and reversible hepatic and hematologic effects (increased liver enzymes, anemia, neutropenia, thrombocytopenia). In dogs, erythemic and alopecic dermatitis may be seen but subsides when the drug is discontinued.

Interactions: There is synergistic antifungal activity between amphotericin B and ketoconazole, and the combination may retard the emergence of strains resistant to flucytosine. The renal effects of amphotericin B prolong elimination of flucytosine. If flucytosine is used together with immunosuppressive drugs, severe depression of bone marrow function is possible.

Effects on Laboratory Tests: Alkaline phosphatase, AST, ALT, and other liver leakage enzymes increase. RBC, WBC, and platelet counts decrease.

GRISEOFULVIN

Griseofulvin is a systemic antifungal agent that is effective against the common dermatophytes. It is practically insoluble in water and only slightly soluble in most organic solvents. Particle sizes of griseofulvin vary from 2.7 μm (ultramicrosized) to 10 μm (microsized).

Antifungal Activity

Mode of Action: Dermatophytes concentrate griseofulvin by an energy-dependent process. The drug then disrupts the mitotic spindle by interacting with the polymerized microtubules in susceptible dermatophytes. This leads to the production of multinucleate fungal cells. The inhibition of nucleic acid synthesis and the formation of hyphal cell wall material may also be involved. The result is distortion, irregular swelling, and spiral curling of the hyphae. Griseofulvin is fungistatic rather than fungicidal, except in young active cells.

Fungal Resistance: Dermatophytes can be made resistant to griseofulvin in vitro.

Antifungal Spectrum: Griseofulvin is active against *Microsporum*, *Epidermophyton*, and *Trichophyton* spp. It has no effect on bacteria, including *Actinomyces* and *Nocardia* spp, other fungi, or yeasts.

Pharmacokinetic Features

Absorption: Plasma levels peak in ~4 hr after administration PO, but absorption from the GI tract continues over a prolonged period. Absorption is highly variable, being influenced by a number of factors. The rates of disaggregation and dissolution in the GI tract limit the bioavailability of griseofulvin; thus, microsized and ultramicrosized particles are usually used. High-fat meals, margarine, or propylene glycol significantly enhance GI absorption of griseofulvin and are indicated if the microsized particles are used.

Distribution: Griseofulvin is deposited in keratin precursor cells within 4-8 hr of administration PO. Sweat and transdermal fluid loss appear to play an important role in griseofulvin transfer in the stratum corneum. When these cells differentiate, griseofulvin remains bound and persists in keratin, making it resistant to fungal invasion. For this reason, new growth of hair, nails, or horn is the first to become free of fungal infection. As the fungus-containing keratin is shed, it is replaced by normal skin and hair. Only a small fraction of a dose of griseofulvin remains in the body fluids or tissues.

Biotransformation and Pharmacokinetics: Depending on the species, 10-50% of a griseofulvin dose is excreted almost exclusively as metabolites in the urine, and the remainder in the feces for ~4-5 days after administration. The elimination half-life of griseofulvin is ~24 hr in several species. The drug can be detected in 48-72 hr at the base level of the skin, in 6-12 days in the lower quarter, and in 2-19 days in the middle section of the horny layer.

Therapeutic Indications and Dose Rates

Griseofulvin is used for dermatophyte infections in dogs, cats, calves, horses, and other domestic and exotic animal species. Most dermatophytes are sensitive, but certain species present greater therapeutic challenges than others. Several may require higher dose rates for satisfactory control.

General dosages for griseofulvin are listed in TABLE 54. The dose rate and frequency should be adjusted as needed for the individual animal.

Special Clinical Concerns

Side Effects and Toxicity: Side effects induced by griseofulvin are rare. Nausea, vomiting, and diarrhea have been seen. Hepatotoxicity has also been reported. Animals with impaired liver function should not be given griseofulvin because its biotransformation will be reduced and toxic levels may be reached. Idiosyncratic toxicity in cats has been reported. Griseofulvin is contraindicated in pregnant animals (especially mares and queens) because it is teratogenic.

Interactions: Lipids increase the GI absorption of griseofulvin. Barbiturates decrease its absorption and antifungal activity. Griseofulvin is a microsomal enzyme inducer and promotes the biotransformation of many concurrently administered drugs. The combined use of ketoconazole and griseofulvin may lead to hepatotoxicity.

Effects on Laboratory Tests: Alkaline phosphatase, AST, and ALT increase. Proteinuria may be detected.

TABLE 54. Dose Rates of Griseofulvin

Species	Dosage, Route, and Frequency
Dogs, cats	Microsized: 10-30 (up to 130) mg/kg, PO, SID or divided BID-TID; Ultramicrosized: 5-10 (up to 50) mg/kg, PO, SID
Horses, cattle	5-10 mg/kg, PO, SID for 3-6 wk, or longer if required

IODIDES

Sodium and potassium iodide have both been used to treat selected bacterial, actino-mycete, and fungal infections, although sodium iodide is preferred. The in vivo effects of iodides against fungal cells are not well understood. Iodide is readily absorbed from the GI tract and distributes freely into the extracellular fluid and glandular secretions. Iodide concentrates in the thyroid gland (50 times corresponding plasma level) and to a much lesser degree in salivary, lacrimal, and tracheobronchial glands. Longterm use at high levels leads to accumulation in the body and to iodinism. Clinical signs of iodinism include lacrimation, salivation, increased respiratory secretions, coughing, inappetence, dry scaly skin, and tachycardia. Cardiomyopathy has been reported in cats. Host defense systems, such as decreased immunoglobulin production and reduced phagocytic ability of leukocytes, are also impaired. Iodinism may also lead to abortion and infertility.

Sodium iodide has been used successfully to treat cutaneous and cutaneous/lymphadenitis forms of sporotrichosis; attempts to control various other mycotic infections with iodides often have had equivocal results.

The dosage for sodium iodide (20% solution) is 44 mg/kg, PO, SID for dogs, and 22 mg/kg, PO, SID for cats. The dose for horses is 125 mL of 20% sodium iodide solution, IV, SID for 3 days, then 30 g, PO, SID for 30 days after clinical remission. The dosage rate for treating actinomycosis and actinobacillosis in cattle is 66 mg/kg, by slow IV, repeated weekly. Potassium iodide should *never* be injected IV.

TOPICAL ANTIFUNGAL AGENTS

A large number of agents that have antifungal activity are applied topically, either on the skin, in the ear or eye, or on mucous membranes (buccal, nasal, vaginal) to control superficial mycotic infections. Concurrent systemic therapy with griseofulvin is often helpful for therapeutic management of dermatophyte infections. The hair should be clipped from affected areas and the nails trimmed to fully expose the lesions before antifungal preparations are applied. Bathing the animal may also be helpful. Isolation or restricted movement of infected animals is wise, especially when dealing with zoonotic fungi.

Preparations may be used in the form of solutions, lotions, sprays, powders, creams, or ointments for dermal application, or in the form of irrigant solutions, ointments, tablets, or suppositories for intravaginal use. The concentration of the active principle in these preparations varies and depends on the activity of the specific agent.

The clinical response to local antifungal agents is unpredictable. Resistance to many of the available drugs is common. Spread of infection and reinfection add to the difficulty of controlling superficial infections. Perseverance is often an essential element of therapy.

Some topical antifungal agents that have been used with success in various conditions and species include iodine preparations (tincture of iodine, potassium iodide, iodophors), copper preparations (copper sulfate, copper naphthenate, cuprimyxin), sulfur preparations (monosulfiram, benzoyl disulfide), phenols (phenol, thymol), fatty acids and salts (propionates, undecylenates), organic acids (benzoic acid, salicylic acids), dyes (crystal [gentian] violet, carbolfuchsin), hydroxyquinolines (iodochlorhydroxyquin), nitrofurans (nitrofuroxine, nitrofurfurylmethyl ether), imidazoles (miconazole, ticonazole, clotrimazole, econazole, thiabendazole), polyene antibiotics (amphotericin B, nystatin, pimaricin, candicidin, hachimycin), allylamines (naftifene, terbinafine), thiocarbamates (tolnaftate), and miscellaneous agents (tolnaftate, acrisorcin, haloprogin, ciclopirox, olamine, dichlorophen, hexetidine, chlorphenesin, tiacetin, polynoxylin, amorolfine).

Amorolfine is a topical antifungal agent used to treat onychomycosis and dermatophytosis. It is prepared as a cream or nail lacquer. Amorolfine is a morpholine derivative that appears to act by interfering with the synthesis of sterols essential for the functioning of fungal cell membranes. In vitro, activity has been shown against some yeasts and dimorphic, dematiaceous, and filamentous fungi (*Blastomyces dermatitidis, Candida* spp, *Histoplasma capsulatum, Sporothrix schenckii*, and *Aspergillus* spp). Despite its in vitro activity, amorolfine is inactive when given systemically and thus is limited to topical use in the treatment of superficial infections. Its role in the treatment of fungal infection in animals is not clear.

Terbinafine is an allylamine antifungal agent available as a topical cream or as tablets. It decreases synthesis of ergosterol by inhibiting squalene epoxidase and is used in the treatment of dermatophytes (eg, *Trichophyton, Microsporum,* and *Aspergillus* spp). Terbinafine is also active against yeasts (eg, *Blastomyces dermatitidis, Cryptococcus neoformans, Sporothrix schenckii, Histoplasma capsulatum, Candida,* and *Pityrosporum* spp). The use of this drug in animals is limited due to the lack of efficacy and safety studies, and it is used only occasionally in dogs and cats.

Because of its ability to inhibit chitin synthesis, **lufenuron** has been used to treat dermatophytosis and selected uterine fungal infections in mares.

ANTIVIRAL AGENTS AND BIOLOGIC RESPONSE MODIFIERS

The conventional approach to the control of viral diseases is to develop effective vaccines, but this is not always possible. The objective of antiviral activity is to eradicate the virus while minimally impacting the host and to prevent further viral invasion. However, because of their method of replication, viruses present a greater therapeutic challenge than do bacteria.

Viruses comprise a core genome of nucleic acid surrounded by a protein shell or capsid. Some viruses are further surrounded by a lipoprotein membrane or envelope. Viruses cannot replicate independently and, as such, are obligate intracellular parasites. The host's pathways of energy generation, protein synthesis, and DNA or RNA replication provide the means of viral replication. Viral replication occurs in 5 sequential steps: host cell penetration, disassembly, control of host protein and nucleic acid synthesis such that viral components are made, assembly of viral proteins, and release of the virus.

Drugs that target viral processes must penetrate host cells; in doing so, they are likely to negatively impact normal pathways of the host. Antiviral drugs are characterized by a narrow therapeutic margin. Therapy is further complicated by viral latency, ie, the ability of the virus to incorporate its genome in the host genome, with clinical infection becoming evident without reexposure to the organism. In vitro susceptibility testing must depend on cell cultures, which are expensive. More importantly, in vitro inhibitory tests do not necessarily correlate with therapeutic efficacy of antiviral drugs. Part of the discrepancy between in vitro and in vivo testing occurs because some drugs require activation (metabolism) to be effective.

Only a few agents have been found to be reasonably safe and effective against a limited number of viral diseases, and most of these have been developed in humans. Few have been studied in animals, and widespread clinical use of antiviral drugs is not common in veterinary medicine. Only a selection of the more promising agents and their purported attributes are briefly discussed.

Most antiviral drugs interfere with viral nucleic acid synthesis or regulation. Such drugs generally are nucleic acid analogs that interfere with RNA and DNA production. Other mechanisms of action include interference with viral cell binding or interruption of virus uncoating. Some viruses contain unique metabolic pathways that serve as a target of drug therapy. Drugs that simply inhibit single steps in the viral replication cycle are virustatic and only temporarily halt viral replication. Thus, optimal activity of some drugs depends on an adequate host immune response. Some antiviral drugs may enhance the immune system of the host. TABLE 55 lists the dosage rates for some commonly used antiviral drugs.

Pyrimidine Nucleosides

A variety of pyrimidine nucleosides (both halogenated and nonhalogenated) effectively inhibit the replication of herpes simplex viruses with limited host-cell toxicity. The exact mechanism of action of these compounds appears to reflect substitution of pyrimidine for thymidine, causing defective DNA molecules. Idoxuridine (IDU) is effective for

TABLE 55. Dosage Rates of Antiviral Drugs*

Drug	Preparation	Dose, Route, and Frequency	Indication
Idoxuridine	0.1% ophthalmic solution	1 drop, topical, every 5-6 hr	
	0.5% ophthalmic solution	1 drop, topical, every 1-2 hr	
Trifluridine	1% ophthalmic solution	1 drop, topical, every 2 hr initially (2 days) then 3-8 times daily	Ocular herpes-virus infection
Vidarabine	3% ophthalmic solution	0.4-1 cm ointment, topical, every 5-6 hr; 3-6 times daily	Ocular herpes-virus infection
	200-mg/mL suspension for injection	10-30 mg/kg, IV, SID as CRI for 12-24 hr	
Acyclovir	200-mg capsules or tablets	200 mg, PO, QID, every 4 hr, or 5 times/day	Feline herpesvirus
	5% cutaneous ointment	Cover lesion, topical, every 3 hr, 6 times/day	
	200 mg/5 mL suspension	80 mg/kg (mixed with peanut butter), PO, SID for 7-14 days	Pacheco's disease in birds
	500 mg/vial powder	250-500 mg/m², IV, TID, infused over at least 1 hr	
Ganciclovir	500 mg/vial powder	2-5 , IV, BID-TID	
Ribavirin		11 mg/kg, IV, SID for 7 days	Susceptible viral infections
	6 g/100 mL vial powder	Using SPAC-2 nebulizer only, inhalation, 8-18 hr period daily	
Amantadine	100- and 500-mg capsules	100 mg total (humans), PO, SID-BID	
	Syrup 10 mg/mL	100 mg total (juveniles), PO, SID	
Rimantadine		200-300 mg total (humans), PO, SID	
Interferon α-2	3 × 10⁶ IU/vial	3×10⁶ IU/human, SC, IM, SID	FeLV-associated disease
		0.5-5.0 U/kg, PO, SID	
		100,000 U/kg, SC, SID	FeLV-associated disease
		1 U, PO, SID	FeLV appetite stimulant
		15-30 U, PO, IM, SC, SID on alternate weeks	FIP, FIV

*CRI = controlled-rate infusion; FeLV = feline leukemia virus; FIP = feline infectious peritonitis; FIV = feline immunodeficiency virus

the treatment of herpesvirus infection of the superficial layers of the cornea (herpesvirus keratitis) and of the skin, but is toxic when administered systemically.

Trifluridine, also an analog of deoxythymidine, is currently the agent of choice for the treatment of herpesvirus keratitis in humans. The other antiviral pyrimidine nucleosides have not been used clinically to any notable extent.

Purine Nucleosides

Certain purine nucleosides have proved to be effective antivirals and are used as systemic agents. Two of these antiviral drugs deserve special mention. Vidarabine, or araA, is used topically for ocular herpes and systemically for herpetic encephalitis as well as for neonatal herpesvirus infections. This drug is an adenosine derivative that is phosphorylated by cellular enzymes to a triphosphate compound that inhibits many viral and human DNA polymerases and thus DNA synthesis. Herpesviral enzymes are ~20-fold more susceptible to the drug compared with host DNA. Vidarabine is administered IV in large volumes of fluid and is rapidly inactivated. It may produce bone marrow suppression and CNS side effects when high blood levels are reached.

Acyclovir (acycloguanosine) represents a new generation of antiviral agents, mainly because of its unique mechanism of action. This purine nucleoside is phosphorylated more efficiently by virus-induced thymidine kinase compared with host thymidine kinase. Once in the triphosphate form, it is a better substrate and inhibitor of viral, compared with host, DNA polymerase. Binding to DNA polymerase is irreversible. Once incorporated into viral DNA, the DNA chain is terminated. Acyclovir is relatively safe (probenecid renders the drug safer) and is useful against a variety of infections caused by DNA viruses, especially the herpesvirus family. However, resistance is increasing. Acyclovir is unable to eliminate latent infections. It is available as an ophthalmic ointment, a topical ointment and cream, an IV preparation, and various oral formulations. The prodrug deoxyacyclovir is more readily absorbed from the GI tract than acyclovir. Another similar antiviral purine nucleoside analog is ganciclovir, a synthetic guanine that is effective against human cytomegalovirus. Its mechanism of action is similar to that of acyclovir.

Ribavirin

Ribavirin is a synthetic triazole nucleoside (an analog of guanosine) with a broad spectrum of activity against many RNA and DNA viruses, both in vitro and in vivo. Susceptible viruses include adenoviruses, herpesviruses, orthomyxoviruses, paramyxoviruses, poxviruses, picornaviruses, rhabdoviruses, rotaviruses, and retroviruses. Viral resistance to ribavirin is rare. The action of ribavirin involves specific inhibition of viral-associated enzymes, inhibition of the capping of viral mRNA, and inhibition of viral polypeptide synthesis. It is well absorbed, widely distributed in the body, eliminated by renal and biliary routes as both parent drug and metabolites, and has a plasma half-life of 24 hr in humans. It does not have a wide margin of safety in domestic animals. Toxicity is manifest by anorexia, weight loss, bone marrow depression and anemia, and GI disturbances. It has been successfully administered by topical, parenteral, oral, and aerosol routes. Efficacy depends on the site of infection, method of treatment, age of the animal, and the infecting dose of virus. Results of human influenza studies with ribavirin have been equivocal.

Zidovudine

Zidovudine (azidothymidine, AZT) is a thymidine analog. Within the virus-infected cell, the 3′-azido group is used by retroviral reverse transcriptase and incorporated into DNA transcription, preventing viral replication. The shared mechanism of action is inhibition of RNA-dependent DNA polymerase (reverse transcriptase). This enzyme is responsible for conversion of the viral RNA genome into double-stranded DNA before it is integrated into the cell genome. Because these actions occur early in replication, the drugs tend to be effective for acute infections but are relatively ineffective for chronically infected cells. Cellular α-DNA polymerases are inhibited only at concentrations 100-fold greater than those necessary to inhibit reverse transcriptase, thus rendering this drug relatively safe to host cells. Cellular γ-DNA polymerase, however, is inhibited at lower concentrations.

AZT is effective against a variety of retroviruses at low concentrations. Resistance to AZT is associated with point mutations resulting in amino acid substitutions in the reverse transcriptase. Prolonged use of AZT can facilitate viral resistance. The risk of resistance also appears to correlate with CD4 cell count and the state of infection. Viral susceptibility to AZT may return after the drug has been discontinued for a period of time. Little information regarding the disposition of AZT is available in animals. Granulocytopenia and anemia are the major adverse effects of AZT in human patients. The risk of toxicity increases in human patients with low (CD4) lymphocyte counts, high doses, and prolonged therapy. Granulocyte colony-stimulating factor is indicated for management of granulocytopenia. CNS side effects are more likely as therapy is begun. The risk of myelosuppression is increased by drugs that inhibit glucuronidation or renal excretion and may be increased in cats. Studies in cats regarding the efficacy of AZT (10-20 mg/kg, BID for 42 days) for feline leukemia virus infection indicated that AZT prevents retroviral infection if administered immediately after viral exposure and may reduce replication if administered to previously infected animals. Serum-neutralizing antibodies developed in some of the infected cats, and the cats became resistant to subsequent viral challenge. There was no altered progression of disease in cats when treatment was withheld until 28 days after infection, although the level of viremia was much lower than in untreated cats. AZT appeared to be nontoxic in uninfected cats, although 3 of 12 infected kittens became anorectic and icteric and were vomiting after 40 days of treatment. AZT may cause Heinz body anemia. CBC should be performed on cats receiving AZT.

Amantadine

Amantadine, and its derivative rimantadine, are synthetic antiviral agents that appear to act on an early step of viral replication after attachment of virus to cell receptors. The effect seems to lead to inhibition or delay of the uncoating process that precedes primary transcription. Amantadine may also interfere with the early stages of viral mRNA transcription. Amantadine at usual concentrations inhibits replication of different strains of influenza A virus, influenza C virus, Sendai virus, and pseudorabies virus. It is almost completely absorbed from the GI tract, and ~90% of a dose administered PO is excreted unchanged in the urine over several days (human data). The main clinical use has been to prevent infection with various strains of influenza A viruses. However, in humans, it also has been found to produce some therapeutic benefit if taken within 48 hr after the onset of illness. Amantadine and its derivatives may be given by the PO, intranasal, SC, IP, or aerosol routes. It produces few side effects, most of which are related to the CNS; stimulation of the CNS is evident at very high doses.

Biologic Response Modifiers

Cytokines (polypeptides released mainly by immune cells) regulate cell growth and differentiation, apoptosis, inflammation, immunity, and repair and are important in the pathogenesis and treatment of disease. The complexities of cytokine nomenclature have been addressed by the World Health Organization, which provides a nomenclature system that includes cytokines of veterinary interest. Cytokines with application in companion animal medicine include interferons (IFN), interleukins (IL), and hematopoietic, growth factors.

Most cytokines are secreted by a variety of cells activated by viral, bacterial, and parasitic infections. Production is normally short lived, usually for hours to a few days, and is seldom accompanied by detectable circulating concentrations. Several cytokines may cause the same response, and often cytokines are modulated (synergistic, antagonistic, or additive effects) by other cytokines. Actions often reflect cascade effects. Cytokine interaction results from binding to specific high affinity cell surface receptors and intracellular signal transduction cascades. The cytokine effect ultimately results in the production of DNA-binding proteins that influence gene transcription. Recombinant DNA technology has led to the commercial availability of some (generally human) cytokines. By convention, recombinant products are designated by an "r" preceding the name of the cytokine and a designation of the species of origin (eg, rhIL indicating human origin, and rfe-IFN indicating feline origin). Because cytokines tend to be conserved, human recombinant products often stimulate similar effects in animals. However, because systemic concentrations of a given cytokine impact many cytokine cascades, side effects and toxicity are not uncommon. The magnitude of the dose may be critical, eg, low doses of IFN appear to immunostimulate, whereas higher doses appear to be immunosuppressive. Except for rfeIFN-α (in cats) and rhIL-1 (in dogs), the pharmacokinetics of cytokines in dogs and cats have not been determined. Current doses generally are empirically derived.

Interferons: Interferons are secreted by viral-infected cells. They bind to receptors on other cells and induce antiviral proteins that protect the cell from infection. However, IFN also have antiviral, antitumor, antiparasitic, and immunomodulatory effects.

Two classes of IFN exist. Class I includes α, ω, and β interferons, whereas Class II includes γ interferons. IFN-γ, IFN-α, and IFN-ω appear to be produced by all nucleated cells. Cloned feline IFN-α cDNA appears to have similar pharmacokinetic properties to human IFN. IFN-β was originally described as being produced by fibroblasts but is secreted by many other cells. IFN-γ is produced by activated T and natural killer (NK) cells. Canine IFN-γ has been characterized, and a recombinant form has been produced; feline IFN-γ cDNA has also been cloned. IFN is produced on a large scale either through recombinant methods or by culturing stimulated cells, leading to the production of "natural" or "native" IFN products (denoted by "N"). Natural IFN are less concentrated and may contain a mixture of IFN types, as well as other cytokines.

Interferons interfere with viral RNA and protein synthesis, resulting in resistance to viral infections that occurs within a few minutes and peaks within a few hours. Their role in veterinary medicine is currently being defined. IFN-γ inhibits viral replication by stimulating the release of other IFN. Anecdotal data suggest that rhIFN-α confers clinical benefit to cats symptomatic for FeLV infection; however, there are no controlled studies with naturally occurring infections. The dosage of IFN is 30 IU rhIFN-α/cat, PO, SID for 7 days, on a 1-wk on, 1-wk off schedule. The optimal dose of other recombinant and natural hIFN is unknown, but likely different. IFN also are induced by bacteria, fungi, and some protozoa; they facilitate activation of and intracellular and extracellular phagocytic killing of these organisms. IFN induce expression of class I and class II major histocompatibility molecules on antigen-presenting cells and thus enhance antigen presentation. IFN, and particularly IFN-γ, also influence T, B, and NK cell function. Oncogene expression is modulated in neoplastic cells. IFN inhibit cell proliferation of both normal and malignant cells and have numerous immunomodulating effects. Several human cancers respond to IFN therapy. At present, there are only preclinical data suggesting that IFN may be useful in the treatment of animal cancer.

Miscellaneous Antiviral Agents

Several drug classes continue to be investigated mainly because of their in vitro antiviral activities. Their potential clinical usefulness remains obscure in most instances. Included among these agents are thiosemicarbazones, guanidine, benzimidazoles, arildone, phosphonoacetic acid, rifamycins and other antibiotics, and several natural products.

ANTHELMINTICS

Many highly effective and selective anthelmintics are available, but such compounds must be used correctly and judiciously to obtain a favorable clinical response, accomplish good control, and minimize selection for anthelmintic resistance. It is impossible to list all claims and precautions regarding all drugs in all countries; the label should always be read before using any drug. Additional information is found under relevant disease headings. Any modification of the recommended dose rate must be discouraged, as this is likely to result in lowered efficacy and possibly increased pressure for development of resistance.

Modern anthelmintics generally have a wide margin of safety, considerable activity against immature (larval) and mature stages of helminths, and a broad spectrum of activity. Nonetheless, the usefulness of any anthelmintic is limited by the intrinsic efficacy of the drug itself, its mechanism of action, its pharmacokinetic properties, characteristics of the host animal (eg, operation of the esophageal groove reflex), and characteristics of the parasite (eg, its location in the body, its degree of hypobiosis, or whether it has developed anthelmintic resistance). The "ideal" anthelmintic should have a broad spectrum of activity against mature and immature parasites (including hypobiotic larvae), be easy to administer, inhibit reinfection for extended periods of time, have a wide margin of safety and be compatible with other compounds, not require long withholding periods because of residue(s), and be cost effective.

There are several classes of anthelmintics, eg, benzimidazoles and probenzimidazoles, salicylanilides and substituted phenols, imidazothiazoles, organophosphates, and macrocyclic lactones. Because of their broad spectrum, high efficacy against all parasitic stages, and their persistent activity, macrocyclic lactones now dominate the treatment and control of nematodes. Although it may be thought that chemotherapeutic control of helminth infections is currently satisfactory, parasite resistance against all important anthelmintics is a significant problem in some animal hosts.

Mechanisms of Action

Anthelmintics must be selectively toxic to the parasite. This is usually achieved either by inhibiting metabolic processes that are vital to the parasite but not vital to or absent in the host, or by inherent pharmacokinetic properties of the compound that cause the parasite to be exposed to higher concentrations of the anthelmintic than are the host cells. While the precise mode of action of many anthelmintics is not fully understood, the sites of action and biochemical mechanisms of many of them are generally known. Parasitic helminths must maintain an appropriate feeding site, and nematodes and trematodes must actively ingest and move food through their digestive tracts to maintain an appropriate energy state; this and reproductive processes require proper neuromuscular coordination. Parasites must also maintain homeostasis despite host immune reactions. The pharmacologic basis of the treatment for helminths generally involves interference with the integrity of parasite cells, neuromuscular coordination, or protective mechanisms against host immunity, which lead to starvation, paralysis, and expulsion of the parasite.

Cellular Integrity: There are several classes of anthelmintics that impair cell structure, integrity, or metabolism: 1) inhibitors of tubulin polymerization—benzimidazoles and probenzimidazoles (which are metabolized in vivo to active benzimidazoles and thus act in the same manner); 2) uncouplers of oxidative phosphorylation—salicylanilides and substituted phenols; and 3) inhibitors of enzymes in the glycolytic pathway—clorsulon.

The benzimidazoles inhibit tubulin polymerization; it is believed that the other observed effects, including inhibition of cellular transport and energy metabolism, are consequences of the depolymerization of microtubules. Inhibition of these secondary events appears to play an essential role in the lethal effect on worms. Benzimidazoles progressively deplete energy reserves and inhibit excretion of waste products and protective factors from parasite cells; therefore, an important factor in their efficacy is prolongation of contact time between drug and parasite. Cross-resistance can exist among all members of this group because they act on the same receptor protein, β-tubulin, which is altered in resistant organisms such that none of the benzimidazoles can bind to the receptor with high affinity.

Uncoupling of oxidative phosphorylation processes has been demonstrated for the salicylanilides and substituted phenols, which are mainly fasciolicides. These compounds act as protonophores, allowing hydrogen ions to leak through the inner mitochondrial membrane. Although isolated nematode mitochondria are susceptible, many fasciolicides are ineffective against nematodes in vivo, apparently due to a lack of drug uptake. Exceptions are the hematophagous nematodes, eg, *Haemonchus* and *Bunostomum*.

Clorsulon is rapidly absorbed into the bloodstream. When *Fasciola hepatica* ingest it (in plasma and bound to RBC), they are killed because glycolysis is inhibited and cellular energy production is disrupted.

Neuromuscular Coordination: Interference with this process may occur by inhibiting the breakdown or by mimicking or enhancing the action of neurotransmitters. The result is paralysis of the parasite. Either spastic or flaccid paralysis of an intestinal helminth allows it to be expelled by the normal peristaltic action of the host. Specific categories include: 1) cholinesterase inhibitors—organophosphates such as coumaphos, crufomate, dichlorvos, haloxon, naftalofos, trichlorfon; 2) cholinergic agonists—imidazothiazoles (levamisole, tetramisole) and pyrimidines (morantel, oxantel, pyrantel); 3) muscle hyperpolarization—piperazine; and 4) potentiation of inhibitory transmitters—macrocyclic lactones (ivermectin, abamectin, doramectin, moxidectin, milbemycin oxime, eprinomectin, selamectin).

Organophosphates inhibit many enzymes, especially acetylcholinesterase, by phosphorylating their esterification sites. This blocks cholinergic nerve transmission in the parasite, which results in spastic paralysis. The cholinesterases of host and parasite and those of different species of parasites vary in their susceptibility to organophosphates.

The imidazothiazoles are nicotinic anthelmintics that act as agonists at nicotinic acetylcholine receptors of nematodes. Their anthelmintic activity is mainly attributed to their ganglion-stimulant (cholinomimetic) activity, whereby they stimulate ganglion-like structures in somatic muscle cells of nematodes. This stimulation first results in sustained muscle contractions, followed by a neuromuscular depolarizing blockade resulting in paralysis. Hexamethonium, a ganglionic blocker, inhibits the action of levamisole.

Piperazine acts to block neuromuscular transmission in the parasite by hyperpolarizing the nerve membrane, which leads to flaccid paralysis. It also blocks succinate production by the worm. The parasites, paralyzed and depleted of energy, are expelled by peristalsis.

The macrocyclic lactones act by binding to glutamate-gated chloride channel receptors in nematode and arthropod nerve cells. This causes the channel to open, allowing an influx of chloride ions. Different chloride channel subunits may show variable sensitivity to macrocyclic lactones and different sites of expression, which could account for the paralytic effects of macrocyclic lactones on different neuromuscular systems at different concentrations. The macrocyclic lactones paralyze the pharynx, the body wall, and the uterine muscles of nematodes. Paralysis (flaccid) of body wall muscle may be critical for rapid expulsion, even though paralysis of pharyngeal muscle is more sensitive. As the macrocyclic lactone concentration decreases, motility may be regained, but paralysis of the pharynx and resultant inhibition of feeding may endure longer than body muscle paralysis and contribute to worm deaths. In filarial nematodes living in the tissues, females move very little and nutrients are absorbed through the cuticle. A major effect of macrocyclic lactones on adult worms of these species is probably paralysis of uterine muscles, resulting in disruption of reproduction. None of the macrocyclic lactones are active against cestodes or trematodes, presumably because these parasites do not have a receptor at a glutamate-gated chloride channel.

Pharmacokinetics

After administration, anthelmintics are usually absorbed into the bloodstream and transported to different parts of the body, including the liver, where they may be metabolized and eventually excreted in the feces and urine. It should be emphasized that the disposition of anthelmintics in the "whole body" situation is considerably more complex than can be described by a set of pharmacokinetic parameters in the peripheral circulation. Improved drug performance requires knowledge of drug behavior in the multicompartmental system, including the complex interaction between formulation and route of administration, physicochemical properties of the compound, and physiology of the compartment into which the drug is distributed.

While many helminth parasites reside in the lumen or close to the mucosa, others live at sites such as the liver and lungs; for action against these, absorption of drug from the GI tract, injection site, or skin is essential. Intestinal parasites come in contact not only with the unabsorbed drug passing through the GI tract but also with the absorbed fraction in the blood as they feed on the intestinal mucosa, and with any that is recycled into the gut. This is an important aspect of efficacy of many of the benzimidazoles.

The pharmacokinetics of an anthelmintic, its rate of metabolism and excretion, and its safety profile determines the length of the withdrawal time; this speed can vary among species and can also be affected by the route of administration and the dose. The usual site of metabolism of anthelmintics is the liver, where oxidation and cleavage reactions commonly occur.

Benzimidazoles and Probenzimidazoles: With a few exceptions, eg, albendazole, oxfendazole, and triclabendazole, only limited amounts of any of the benzimidazoles are absorbed from the GI tract of the host. The limited absorption is probably related to the poor water solubility of these drugs. The little absorption that occurs is generally rapid, 2-7 hr after dosing with flubendazole and 6-30 hr after dosing with albendazole, fenbendazole, and oxfendazole, depending on the species. Many of the benzimidazoles and their metabolites re-enter the GI tract by passive diffusion, but the biliary route is the most important pathway for secretion and recycling of benzimidazoles to the GI tract.

A number of benzimidazoles (eg, febantel, thiophanate, netobimin) exist in the form of prodrugs that must be metabolized in the body to the biologically active benzimidazole carbamate nucleus. Febantel is hydrolyzed to the active metabolite fenbendazole, and netobimin undergoes processes of reduction, cyclization, and oxidation to yield albendazole sulfoxide. Benzimidazole sulfoxides such as oxfendazole and albendazole sulfoxide bind poorly to parasite β-tubulin and probably act as prodrugs for fenbendazole and albendazole, respectively. The thiometabolites have high affinity for helminth tubulin.

Metabolism of the benzimidazoles is variable and may alter their activity, eg, albendazole is rapidly and reversibly oxidized to its sulfoxide. The sulfoxide may be irreversibly oxidized to its sulfone, which is significantly less active than the sulfoxide. Similarly, fenbendazole and oxfendazole (fenbendazole sulfoxide) are interchangeable, but the oxidation product fenbendazole sulfone is less active and is not reduced back to the sulfoxide or thio metabolites.

In ruminants, the benzimidazoles are most effective if deposited directly into the rumen. Administration directly into the abomasum, via the esophageal groove, may shorten the duration for drug absorption and increase the rate of excretion in the feces, which may reduce efficacy. For example, immediate arrival of oxfendazole in the abomasum after dosing reduces its efficacy from 91% to 45% against thiabendazole-resistant strains of *Haemonchus contortus*. The rumen acts as a drug reservoir from which plasma concentrations can be sustained for long periods; it also slows the passage of unabsorbed drug through the GI tract.

Imidazothiazoles: The absorption and excretion of levamisole is rapid and not affected by the route of administration or ruminal bypass because it is highly soluble. In cattle, blood levels of levamisole peak <1 hr after SC administration. These concentrations decline rapidly; 90% of the total dose is excreted in 24 hr, largely in the urine.

Tetrahydropyrimidines: Pyrantel tartrate (or citrate) is well absorbed by pigs and dogs, less well by ruminants. The pamoate salt of pyrantel is poorly soluble in water; this offers the advantage of reduced absorption from the gut and allows the drug to reach and be effective against parasites in the large intestine, which makes it useful in horses and dogs. Metabolism of pyrantel is rapid, and the metabolites are excreted rapidly in the urine (40% of the dose in dogs); some unchanged drug is excreted in the feces (principally in ruminants). Blood levels usually peak 4-6 hr after PO administration.

Morantel is the methyl ester analog of pyrantel and, in ruminants, it tends to be safer and more effective than pyrantel. It is absorbed rapidly from the upper small intestine of sheep and metabolized rapidly in the liver; ~17% of the initial dose is excreted in the urine as metabolites within 96 hr after dosing.

Macrocyclic Lactones: Macrocyclic lactones are lipophilic, an important characteristic of this class of anthelmintics. Regardless of their route of administration, macrocyclic lactones are distributed throughout the body and concentrate in adipose tissue. While the magnitude of lipophilicity differs among chemical types, the limited vascularization and slow turnover rate of body fat and the slow rate of release or exchange of drug from these lipid reserves prolongs the residence of drug in the peripheral plasma. Ivermectin is arguably the least lipophilic macrocyclic lactone, with the possible exception of eprinomectin. Moxidectin is ~100 times more lipophilic than ivermectin. Doramectin is less lipophilic than moxidectin, but more than ivermectin or eprinomectin, and as an injectable is available in an oil-based formulation, which can significantly affect drug availability.

Ivermectin was the first commercially available macrocyclic lactone and has been the most extensively studied. When given IV, ivermectin has a general elimination half-life of 32-65 hr. Despite the higher dose rate of the injectable formulation in pigs (300 μg/kg) than cattle (200 μg/kg), the maximum concentration (C_{max}) and area under curve (AUC) in peripheral plasma in pigs are about one third those in cattle. This may be due to a more extensive time for recycling of drug from the slower flowing digesta of a ruminant compared with a monogastric animal. While the elimination half-life after SC and IV administration of ivermectin is of similar duration, the extended release of drug from lipid broadens the concentration-time profile, with C_{max} in peripheral plasma of cattle occurring as late as 96 hr. The C_{max} and AUC in pigs and goats are considerably lower than those in cattle, horses, and sheep. Pigs, and possibly goats, may metabolize ivermectin faster than other species.

In ruminants, the macrocyclic lactones are, like benzimidazoles, most effective if deposited directly into the rumen. A 3- to 4-fold increase in C_{max} and AUC of ivermectin after intra-abomasal compared with intraruminal administration has been reported. Significantly, time to maximal concentration of ivermectin was reduced from 23 hr to 4 hr with the former route of delivery.

Concentrations of ivermectin are high in digesta sampled from the distal intestine, indicating that biliary secretion is an important pathway for clearance of macrocyclic lactones. This pathway also has been conclusively demonstrated for clearance of benzimidazole compounds. The extended high concentration in bile is influenced by prolonged exchange of drug from lipid reserves and the enterohepatic recycling of biliary compounds through the portal and biliary pools. The macrocyclic lactones are mostly excreted in the feces, the remainder (<10%) in the urine. Most macrocyclic lactones are also excreted in milk.

Salicylanilides and Substituted Phenols: Secretion via the liver and bile is especially important for drugs active against adult *Fasciola* spp. The fasciolicidal effects of salicylanilides (such as rafoxanide) in sheep depend on persistence of the drug in plasma, which influences their transport throughout the body and rate of elimination. Closantel, rafoxanide, and oxyclozanide have long terminal half-lives in sheep (14.5, 16.6, and 6.4 days, respectively), which are related to the high plasma-protein binding (>99%) of these 3 drugs. Residues in liver are detectable for weeks after administration. Associated with persistence, however, is the need for longer withholding periods. Oxyclozanide also is bound to plasma protein and then metabolized in the liver to the anthelmintically active glucuronide and excreted in high concentration in the bile duct, where it encounters the mature flukes.

Immature flukes in the liver parenchyma ingest mainly liver cells, which contain little anthelmintic; plasma-protein binding limits entry of the drug into the tissue cells. As the flukes grow and migrate through the liver, they cause extensive hemorrhaging and come into contact with anthelmintic bound to plasma protein. When they reach the bile ducts, they are in the main excretory channels for the active metabolites of the fasciolicides and are exposed to toxic concentrations. This may explain why mature flukes are more vulnerable to most fasciolicides than immature ones. The higher concentrations of fasciolicides and their metabolites in feces than in urine suggest that the bile ducts are their main excretory pathways. Diamfenetide is metabolized in the gut, and to a greater extent in the liver, to an active metabolite that can enter hepatic cells and exert its antiparasitic effect against very young stages of the fluke.

Because rumen bacteria metabolize and destroy the activity of nitroxynil, it must be injected.

Withholding Periods

Most anthelmintics have withholding periods if milk or meat from treated animals is intended for human consumption; the specific requirements for each must be observed. Thiabendazole is absorbed and excreted most quickly; fenbendazole, oxfendazole, and albendazole are absorbed and excreted over a longer period, which necessitates withholding periods of 8-14 days before slaughtering for meat, and 3-5 days before milking for human consumption. Other members of the group have withholding periods between these extremes, but are longer for bolus formulations.

A similar relationship between the rate of metabolism and activity against immature parasites also exists with certain fasciolicides. Closantel, rafoxanide, and nitroxynil bind more strongly to blood proteins than does oxyclozanide, and therefore remain in the blood for longer periods. While this greater persistence is associated with greater activity against immature liver flukes, the withholding period for slaughter is also longer: 21-30 days for closantel, rafoxanide, and nitroxynil, compared with 7-14 days for oxyclozanide. The low plasma-protein binding of diamfenetide, coupled with the rapid excretion of its active metabolite, necessitates only a short withdrawal time.

Levamisole and morantel are rapidly excreted; thus, withholding periods for meat are short, and frequently there is no, or only a short, withholding period for milk.

Ivermectin and doramectin are excreted in milk and are not recommended when milk is intended for human consumption; commensurate with their long period of activity, they have significant withholding periods before slaughter (eg, 35 days), which vary with the formulations (and local regulations). Moxidectin has a relatively low mammalian toxicity, and residual concentrations in milk after topical administration are below threshhold limits resulting in no withholding period in many countries. The chemical structure of the macrocyclic lactone molecule can be manipulated to change the milk partitioning coefficients in lactating dairy animals. This led to the development of eprinomectin, of which only 0.1% of the total dose is eliminated in the milk, resulting in no withholding period for milk worldwide.

Safety

Most modern anthelmintics have wide safety margins, ie, the dosage that can be given to an animal before adverse effects are induced is much higher than the dosage recommended for use. The wide safety margin of benzimidazoles is due to their greater selective affinity for parasitic β-tubulin than for mammalian tissues. Nonetheless, this selective toxicity is not absolute; some toxic effects based on antimitotic activity (teratogenicity or embryotoxicity) can occur in some target species, and some benzimidazoles, depending on the dose rate, are contraindicated in early pregnancy.

The safety index (SI) is not as wide for levamisole (SI = 4-6), nor for most of the chemicals active against liver flukes (SI = 3-6). Mammalian toxicity with levamisole is seen more often than with benzimidazoles, although toxic signs are unusual unless the normal therapeutic dosage is exceeded. Levamisole toxicity in the host animal is largely an extension of its antiparasitic effect, ie, cholinergic-type signs of salivation, muscle tremors, ataxia, urination, defecation, and collapse. In fatal levamisole poisoning, the immediate cause of death is asphyxia due to respiratory failure. Atropine sulfate can alleviate such signs. Levamisole may cause some inflammation at the site of SC injection, but usually this is transient.

The margin of safety for organophosphates is generally less than that of the benzimidazoles, and strict attention to dosage is necessary. Generally, their toxicity is additive;

thus, concurrent use of other cholinesterase-inhibiting drugs should be avoided. Atropine and 2-PAM are used as antidotes to organophosphate toxicity (*see also* ORGANO-PHOSPHATES, p 2398). Organophosphates also can be hazardous to humans. Being lipid soluble, they are readily absorbed through unbroken skin. Sprays, collars, and washes of organophosphates used for small animals can present significant hazards to young infants after ingestion, inhalation, or transcutaneous absorption.

Mammals are generally not adversely affected by macrocyclic lactones. The SI for the macrocyclic lactones is typically wide, but both abamectin and moxidectin are contraindicated in calves and foals <4 mo old, respectively, because of narrow safety margins in these classes of stock. Otherwise, single administration at ~10 times and multiple administration at 3 times the recommended therapeutic dose levels do not have any secondary effects on healthy host animals. Mammalian safety appears to depend on p-glycoprotein activity in the blood-brain barrier. P-glycoproteins pump out macrocyclic lactones from CNS cells, and animals with defective p-glycoprotein levels in the blood-brain barrier are susceptible to macrocyclic lactone toxicity. There have been cases of CNS depression in cattle breeds (Murray Grey) and purebred and crossbred Collies. Nervous signs (idiosyncratic reactions) including depression, muscle weakness, blindness, coma, and death were observed, especially in Collies. It is thought that p-glycoprotein deficiency in certain animals of this breed allows avermectins to penetrate and accumulate in the CNS more readily than would normally be expected, causing unusual signs at dose levels considerably below those required to produce toxicity in healthy animals.

Because salicylanilides, substituted phenols, and aromatic amides, with the possible exception of diamfenetide, are general uncouplers of oxidative phosphorylation, their SI are lower than those of many other anthelmintics. Nonetheless, they are safe if used as directed. Adverse effects are most commonly seen in animals that are severely stressed, in poor condition nutritionally or metabolically, or that have severe parasitic infections. Mild anorexia and unformed feces may be seen after treatment at recommended dosages. High dosages may cause blindness, hyperthermia, convulsions, and death—classic signs of uncoupled phosphorylation.

Resistance

The development of nematode and trematode resistance to various groups of anthelmintics is a major problem. Compared with development of antibiotic resistance in bacteria, resistance to anthelmintics in nematodes has been slow to develop under field conditions. However, resistance is becoming widespread because relatively few chemically dissimilar groups of anthelmintics have been introduced over the past several decades. Most of the commonly used anthelmintics belong to one of 3 chemical classes (benzimidazoles, imidazothiazoles, and macrocyclic lactones), within which all individual compounds act in a similar fashion. Thus, resistance to one particular compound may be accompanied by resistance to other members of the group (ie, cross-resistance). Resistance to an anthelmintic is expressed by passage of increased numbers of parasite eggs, higher survival rates of adults in the host, and greater numbers of larvae on the pasture after treatment than would be seen if the parasites were susceptible to the drug.

In nematodes of small ruminants, and especially in *Haemonchus contortus*, resistance to all classes of broad-spectrum anthelmintics has reached catastrophic proportions in many parts of the world, and reports of multiple resistance to all major classes of anthelmintics are increasing. Resistance also has been found in *Trichostrongylus* spp, *Cooperia* spp, and *Telodorsagia* spp in sheep and goats. Resistance to benzimidazoles is widespread in cyathostome nematodes of horses. There are limited reports of anthelmintic resistance in *Oesophogostomum dentatum* in pigs. Although resistance to benzimidazoles, levamisole, and macrocyclic lactones has been reported for nematodes of cattle, the problem is still not considered to be serious. However, there are reports of ivermectin resistance in *Cooperia oncophora, C punctata*, and *Haemonchus placei*. Anthelmintic resistance among nematode parasites of cattle is possibly more widespread than realized and needs more investigation.

The development of significant levels of resistance seems to require successive generations of helminths exposed to the same class of anthelmintic. However, evidence suggests that genes for resistance are invariably present, at a low frequency, before any given anthelmintic. Selection for resistance simply requires the preferential killing of the susceptible parasites and survival of the parasites with the resistance genes. Cross-resistance is frequently seen between members of the benzimidazole group because of their similar mechanisms of action; control of benzimidazole-resistant parasites by levamisole can be expected because of its different mode of action. Although there is no evidence for cross-resistance between levamisole and benzimidazoles, this does not mean that worms resistant to both kinds of drugs will not evolve if both types of anthelmintics are used frequently. Nematodes resistant to levamisole are cross-resistant to morantel due to the similarities of their mechanisms of action. When resistance to the recommended dose rate of ivermectin appears, moxidectin, at its recommended dose rate, is usually still effective. However, there is cross-resistance between the avermectins and the milbemycins, and the use of either subgroup will select for macrocyclic lactone resistance.

Every exposure of a target parasite to an anthelmintic exerts pressure for development of resistance. Management practices designed to reduce exposure to parasites and to minimize the frequency of anthelmintic use should be recommended. The development of an anthelmintic resistance problem may theoretically be delayed by rotating chemicals with different modes of action annually between dosing seasons. Drug combinations may be another appropriate, although expensive, choice, provided the anthelmintics used in the combination are both effective and select for different resistance mechanisms. Refugia should be considered above all when worm management in domestic animals is planned.

In parasite control, economic benefit is best obtained by careful management practices. Planned treatment of a whole flock or herd should be based on the biology, ecology, and epidemiology of the parasite(s), with particular reference to climatic conditions.

BENZIMIDAZOLES

The benzimidazoles are a large chemical family used to treat nematode and trematode infections in domestic animals. However, with the widespread development of resistance and the availability of more efficient and easier to administer compounds, their use is rapidly decreasing. They are characterized by a broad spectrum of activity against roundworms (nematodes), an ovicidal effect, and a wide safety margin. Those of interest are mebendazole, flubendazole, fenbendazole, oxfendazole, oxibendazole, albendazole, albendazole sulfoxide, thiabendazole, thiophanate, febantel, netobimin, and triclabendazole. Netobimin, albendazole, and triclabendazole are also active against liver flukes; however, unlike all the other benzimidazoles, triclabendazole has no activity against roundworms.

Because most benzimidazoles are sparingly soluble in water, they are given PO as a suspension, paste, or bolus. Differences in the rate and extent of absorption from the GI tract depend on such factors as species, dosage, formulation, solubility, and operation of the esophageal groove reflex.

The most effective of the group are those with the longest half-life, such as oxfendazole, fenbendazole, albendazole, and their prodrugs, because they are not rapidly metabolized to inactive products. Effective concentrations are maintained for an extended period in the plasma and gut, which increases efficacy against immature and arrested larvae and adult nematodes, including lungworms.

They are more effective in ruminants and horses, in which their rate of passage is slowed by the rumen or cecum. Because the nature of their antiparasitic action depends on prolongation of contact time, repeated (2-3 times) PO administration of a full dose at 12-hr intervals increases their efficacy, even against benzimidazole-resistant worms. In addition, a reduced feed intake, which reduces the flow rate of digesta, increases the availability of benzimidazoles.

In the case of oxfendazole, and probably other benzimidazoles, the major route of exposure is biliary metabolites, followed by enterohepatic recycling of the drug after absorption from the small and large intestine. Worms in the mucosa of the small intestine may be exposed to more recycled anthelmintic than to drug contained in the passing ingesta in the GI tract.

Ruminants: In ruminants, PO treatment with the benzimidazoles removes most of the major adult GI parasites and many of the larval stages. The relative rates of oxidation in the liver and reduction in the GI tract vary between cattle and sheep, with the metabolism and excretion of benzimidazole compounds being more extensive in cattle than in sheep. Consequently, the systemic anthelmintic activity of most benzimidazoles is greater in sheep than in cattle, and dose rates in cattle are often higher than those in sheep. Albendazole, fenbendazole, oxfendazole, and febantel are active against inhibited fourth-stage larvae of *Ostertagia* spp; however, inconsistent efficacy has been reported. Efficacy against *Dictyocaulus viviparus* has also been noted for these insoluble benzimidazoles. Oxfendazole, albendazole, and febantel are minimally teratogenic in sheep, whereas fenbendazole, mebendazole, and oxibendazole are not. An oxfendazole pulse-release bolus for intraruminal use has been developed for cattle—5 therapeutic doses of oxfendazole (750 or 1,250 mg/tablet) are released approximately each 3 wk in the rumen. A sustained-release fenbendazole bolus is also available in some countries; it contains 12 g fenbendazole and has a release profile of 140 days. An albendazole slow-release capsule has been marketed for small ruminants. This device contains 3.85 g of albendazole and delivers a daily dose of 36.7 mg for 105 days. It is an efficient device for controlling benzimidazole-susceptible nematodes. It may also prevent infection with benzimidazole-resistant larvae, but does not reduce existing infections.

In cattle and sheep, triclabendazole at 10 mg/kg, PO, is highly effective against immature *Fasciola hepatica* in the liver parenchyma and against the mature stage in the bile ducts. Albendazole and netobimin at 20 mg/kg are active against mature *F hepatica*; the other benzimidazoles and probenzimidazoles used for nematode control have only a marginal efficacy against liver flukes. Because of the lack of efficacy against the immature stages, most benzimidazoles are not indicated for treatment of acute fascioliosis.

Horses: In horses, the benzimidazoles are characterized by effective removal (90-100%) of almost all mature strongyles, but third- and fourth-stage larvae are more difficult to eliminate. High levels and repeated administration may be necessary for extraintestinal migrating stages of large strongyles and for small-strongyle larvae embedded or encysted in the wall of the intestine. However, widespread resistance to benzimidazoles in cyathostome nematodes of horses limits their usage. Repeated doses are thought to be advantageous because the lethal effect of benzimidazoles is a slow process—hence, their recent incorporation into feed supplements. Ascarid removal in horses varies with various members of the benzimidazole group. Activity against *Strongyloides westeri* varies also, but *Oxyuris equi* is usually removed by any of the benzimidazoles at the recommended dose.

Swine: Benzimidazoles (eg, fenbendazole, flubendazole) show high efficacy against both adult and immature stages of *Ascaris suum*. Benzimidazoles are also highly effective against most other swine nematodes. Resistance to benzimidazoles has been reported only on a limited scale (Denmark) in *Oesophagostomum* spp.

Dogs and Cats: In dogs and cats, mebendazole, fenbendazole, febantel, and flubendazole are used for treatment of roundworms, hookworms, and tapeworms. However, treatment must be given BID for 3 days. Fenbendazole has been used in a divided dose regimen in bitches against tissue-dwelling larvae of *Toxocara canis* and *Ancylostoma caninum*; daily administration of 50 mg/kg to bitches from day 40 of pregnancy through day 14 after parturition resulted in pups free of both parasites, although this has limited application in practice.

Birds: Mebendazole, flubendazole, and fenbendazole can be used effectively against nematodes of the GI and respiratory tracts of birds.

IMIDAZOTHIAZOLES

The anthelmintic activity of tetramisole, a racemic mixture, resides in the L-isomer, levamisole. It is commonly used in cattle, sheep, pigs, goats, and poultry to treat nematode infections; it has no activity against flukes and tapeworms. It is normally administered PO or SC, and efficacy is generally considered equivalent with either route. Topical preparations for cattle have been developed.

Levamisole acts on the roundworm nervous system and is not ovicidal. Its broad spectrum of activity, ease of use (being water soluble), reasonable safety margin, and lack of teratogenic effects have allowed it to be used successfully. Because of its mechanism of action, the peak blood concentration is more relevant to its antiparasitic activity than the duration of concentration. Levamisole resistance appears to be associated with a loss of cholinergic receptors. Levamisole has immunostimulant effects at dosage rates higher than those used for anthelmintic activity, and it has been used in humans and to a limited extent in other animals in several diseases.

Ruminants: In ruminants, levamisole is highly effective against the common adult GI nematodes and lungworms and many larval stages. It lacks efficacy against arrested larvae, such as those of *Ostertagia ostertagi*. Levamisole slow-release boluses are available in some countries and contain 22.05 mg levamisole. They release 2.5 mg during the first 24 hr and the remainder over a 90-day period.

Swine: Levamisole, similar to the benzimidazoles, is highly effective against both adult and immatures stages of *Ascaris suum*. Levamisole is also highly effective against other adult swine nematodes, except for *Trichuris suis*.

Birds: In poultry, levamisole is mainly used to remove ascarid infections.

TETRAHYDROPYRIMIDINES

Pyrantel was first introduced as a broad-spectrum anthelmintic against GI nematodes of sheep and has also been used in cattle, horses, dogs, and pigs. It is available as a citrate, tartrate, embonate, or pamoate salt.

Aqueous solutions are subject to isomerization on exposure to light, with a resultant loss in potency; therefore, suspensions should be kept out of direct sunlight. It is not recommended for use in severely debilitated animals because of its levamisole-type pharmacologic action.

Pyrantel is used PO as a suspension, paste, drench, or tablets. Both pyrantel and morantel are effective against adult gut worms and larval stages that dwell in the lumen or on the mucosal surface.

Ruminants: Pyrantel tartrate is effective as a broad-spectrum anthelmintic in ruminants; however, its activity is mainly limited to the adult GI nematodes.

Horses: Pyrantel is effective against adult ascarids, large and small strongyles, pinworms, and at double the recommended dose, the ileocecal tapeworm *Anoplocephala perfoliata*.

Swine: Pyrantel tartrate is used in swine for the treatment of *Ascaris* and *Oesophagostomum*.

Dogs and Cats: Pyrantel pamoate is effective against the common GI nematodes, except for whipworms. Oxantel, a phenol analog of pyrantel, is combined with pyrantel in some anthelmintic preparations for dogs (and humans) to increase activity against whipworms.

ORGANOPHOSPHATES

A number of organophosphates have been used as anthelmintics; however, due to their relative toxicity, limited efficacy against immature stages, narrow margin of safety, and contamination of the environment through fecal excretion, their use is declining. Dichlorvos is used as an anthelmintic in horses, pigs, dogs, and cats; trichlorfon in horses and dogs; and coumaphos, crufomate, haloxon, and naftalofos in ruminants.

Because of its high volatility, dichlorvos is a particularly versatile organophosphate that can be incorporated as a plasticizer in vinyl resin pellets; it is released slowly from the inert pellets as they pass through the GI tract, providing a therapeutic concentration along the tract. This controlled release governs the concentration available to the host as well as to the parasites and thereby increases the safety margin. When passed in the feces, the pellets still contain ~45-50% of the original drug. Dichlorvos is rapidly absorbed and metabolized in the body.

Ruminants: Haloxon and naftalofos have been the primary organophosphates used in cattle and sheep. However, their use is becoming limited because of their contraindications.

Horses: Trichlorfon (metrifonate) is still used in horses because of its high degree of activity against bots, ascarids, and oxyurids.

Swine: Dichlorvos is particularly useful in pigs against all major adult nematodes and was one of the first broad-spectrum anthelmintics to be used in this species. There is little or no activity against larval migrating nematodes.

MACROCYCLIC LACTONES

The macrocyclic lactones (avermectins and milbemycins) are products, or chemical derivatives thereof, of soil microorganisms belonging to the genus *Streptomyces*. The avermectins in commercial use are ivermectin, abamectin, doramectin, eprinomectin, and selamectin. Commercially available milbemycins are milbemycin oxime and moxidectin. The macrocyclic lactones have a potent, broad antiparasitic spectrum at low dose levels. They are active against many immature nematodes (including hypobiotic larvae) and arthropods. The published literature contains reports of use to treat infections of >300 species of endo- and ectoparasites in a wide range of hosts. Moreover, a single therapeutic dose can persist in concentrations sufficient to be effective against incumbent nematode infections for prolonged periods after treatment.

The macrocyclic lactones are well absorbed when administered PO, parenterally, or as pour-on formulations. Regardless of the route of administration, macrocyclic lactones are extensively distributed throughout the body and concentrate particularly in adipose tissue. However, the route of administration and formulation may affect disposition. The residence time of macrocyclic lactones administered SC may also be influenced by the body condition of the animal.

Effective levels are reached in the GI system, lungs, and skin regardless of the route of administration. There is, however, a very complex interaction between pharmacokinetic compartments and the quantitative and qualitative availability of drug/metabolite in one compartment. For example, the association of macrocyclic lactones with digesta affects absorption; systemic availability and elimination of ivermectin given PO may differ significantly with feed quantity or composition in sheep. Also, the practice of feed withdrawal before PO treatment broadens the pharmacokinetic profile, significantly increasing anthelmintic efficacy.

Environmental Effects

Although there has long been concern over the use of chemical additives in livestock feed (eg, potential consequences of insect-free manure), the effects on nontarget dung insects and dung dispersal primarily became a concern with the macrocyclic lactones. The commercially available macrocyclic lactones are primarily excreted in the feces, and a broad range of insecticidal activities have been observed against dung-inhabiting insect species.

Extensive fate and effects studies have been conducted with the macrocyclic lactones, with most data reported for ivermectin. Ivermectin in feces or soil degrades at a slow but significant rate. In a winter environment, decomposition is slow (half-life of 91-217 days); when exposed to an outdoor summer environment, ivermectin in soil has a half-life of 7-14 days.

Although highly toxic to aquatic organisms, tight soil-binding by macrocyclic lactones mitigates against aquatic exposure via run-off or leaching. Macrocyclic lactones have little adverse effect on freshwater algae and virtually none on germination or growth of plants; however, residues in animal feces have the potential to affect arthropod development in a variety of ways. The larvae of cyclorrhaphous Diptera are generally more sensitive to ivermectin and other macrocyclic lactones than are Coleopteran larvae. Mature adult Coleoptera are usually unaffected by macrocyclic lactone residues found in dung, probably because they are exposed to less macrocyclic lactone residue than their bulk-feeding larvae. Overall, the commercially available milbemycins appear to be less harmful to fly and beetle larvae tested than the avermectins. There is no evidence that ivermectin residues exert any direct effect on the development or survival of earthworms; however, effects on other dung-feeding organisms, in particular fly and beetle larvae, may disturb the processes of succession.

While macrocyclic lactones have the potential to disrupt the ecology of dung fauna if given in persistent formulations or sustained-release devices, there is no evidence for longterm adverse effects of macrocyclic lactone residues on the degradation of dung pats or on the accumulation of dung on pasture. In most husbandry systems, a large proportion of the feces will not contain residues of macrocyclic lactones, thus providing a large reservoir of safe habitat for dung insects. Therefore, it is unlikely that use of macrocyclic lactones will have a significant ecotoxicologic impact on a global or regional scale.

Persistent Efficacy

A single therapeutic dose of an avermectin can persist in concentrations sufficient to be effective against incumbent susceptible nematode infections for prolonged periods. The clinical significance of prolonged efficacy is important. Sustained availability protects animals from reinfection by some nematode (and arthropod) species for several weeks, which helps control pests that intermittently or constantly challenge livestock. Large variations in the persistent efficacy of a particular macrocyclic lactone against a particular worm species have been reported. Potential reasons for these variable results include study design and host- and parasite-related factors. Persistent efficacy has been investigated mainly against the 3 major cattle nematodes, *Ostertagia ostertagi*, *Cooperia oncophora*, and *Dictyocaulus viviparus*, and the sheep nematode, *Haemonchus contortus*. The duration of persistent efficacy varies according to the macrocyclic lactone and formulation used and may be 14-45 days for *Ostertagia*, 0-35 days for *Cooperia*, and 21-42 days for *Dictyocaulus*. The persistent efficacy of oral moxidectin (2-5 wk) gives it a special role in control of haemonchosis in sheep.

Cattle: Ivermectin, eprinomectin, abamectin, doramectin, and moxidectin are variously available as PO, SC, and pour-on formulations for use in cattle. The SC and PO formulations are given at 0.2 mg/kg, whereas the pour-on formulation is used at 0.5 mg/kg. Pour-on formulations are more convenient but exhibit greater variability between animals compared with SC or PO administration. Grooming behavior of cattle has a major influence on the plasma disposition of topical ivermectin. Allogrooming might result in cross-contamination of animals, giving rise to unexpected drug residues in edible tissues of untreated cattle. Undesirable subtherapeutic concentrations in both treated and untreated cattle may contribute to development of drug resistance. The macrocyclic lactones have a very high (>98%) efficacy against all stages (including inactive forms) of the common cattle nematodes. The least susceptible nematodes are *Cooperia* and *Nematodirus* spp. Due to their high potency and elimination through milk, the macrocyclic lactones are not recommended for use in animals that produce milk for human consumption. Eprinomectin and moxidectin are exceptions and have no milk withdrawal time in many countries. A wide range of effective chemoprophylactic systems has been developed to prevent outbreaks of parasitic gastroenteritis and control infections in first-season grazing calves. Suppressive anthelmintic medication during the first half of the grazing season, using carefully timed administration of macrocyclic lactones, has proved to be highly effective in western Europe for the control of GI nematodes of grazing calves during their first year. Due to differences in management, pasture infectivity, and climate, it is difficult to identify which program is most effective. Any chemoprophylactic program should be beneficial, as long as it is adapted to the epidemiologic situation.

Small Ruminants: Ivermectin, doramectin, and moxidectin are variously available as PO, SC, and IM formulations for use in small ruminants. As for cattle, the macrocyclic lactones have a very high (>98%) efficacy against all stages, including inactive forms, of the common sheep and goat nematodes. However, because of the widespread prevalence of resistance to macrocyclic lactones among nematodes of small ruminants, mainly in the southern hemisphere, their use is more problematic (*see* RESISTANCE, p 2117). Although moxidectin, at its recommended dose rate, is usually still effective when resistance to ivermectin is present, there is cross-resistance between the avermectins and the milbemycins. Continued use of either avermectins or milbemycins selects for resistance to macrocyclic lactones. Ivermectin controlled-release capsules have been used by sheep producers. The delivery rate, maintained for 100 days, is 0.8 mg ivermectin/day for sheep 20-40 kg in weight and 1.6 mg/day for sheep weighing 41-80 kg.

Swine: In pigs, ivermectin and doramectin are given at 0.3 mg/kg body wt, SC, or ivermectin is given in feed for 7 days at 0.1 kg body wt/day for the treatment of all adult and larval stages of the common swine parasites, including the kidney worm *Stephanurus*. The exception is *Trichuris suis*, in which efficacy is ~80%.

Horses: Ivermectin and moxidectin are the only macrocyclic lactones available for use in horses. Ivermectin is used in horses at a dosage of 200 µg/kg, whereas moxidectin is used at 400 µg/kg. Both ivermectin and moxidectin are effective against a broad range of adult and migrating larval stages of nematode and arthropod parasites. These include the spirurid stomach worms (*Trichostrongylus axei, Parascaris equorum, Oxyuris equi,* and *Strongyloides westeri*), bots (*Gasterophilus* spp), adult and immature large strongyles (*Strongylus vulgaris, S edentatus,* and *S equinus*), and adult Cyathostominae. The only reported difference in efficacy of the 2 products is that at therapeutic dosages, ivermectin has not shown significant efficacy against the intramucosal developing stages of the cyathostomes, and moxidectin appears less potent against stomach bots (*Gasterophilus* spp). Efficacy against the arrested stages is low for both anthelmintics. The persistence of moxidectin in circulation can provide horses with 2-3 wk of protection from infective cyathostome larvae.

Dogs and Cats: Ivermectin, selamectin, moxidectin, and milbemycin oxime may be used in dogs for the prevention of heartworm disease and control of GI roundworms. Many canine parasites are susceptible to ivermectin at the dosages used in other animals; however, because some dogs are adversely affected at these levels, ivermectin is used in dogs at only 6 µg/kg body wt, given at 1-mo intervals, to prevent development of *Dirofilaria immitis*, the cause of heartworm disease. At higher dosages (>100 µg/kg), some Collies are adversely affected by ivermectin. At a dosage of 0.5 mg/kg, PO, milbemycin oxime is used for prevention of heartworm infection and for treatment of hookworms, ascarids, and whipworms in dogs. Moxidectin is also effective for the prevention of heartworm infection at a dose rate of 3 µg/kg. The margin of safety of milbemycin and moxidectin in dogs, including those sensitive to ivermectin, appears to be similar to that of ivermectin.

Selamectin, an avermectin monosaccharide, is available in a topical formulation, thereby avoiding some of the problems associated with PO administration. Selamectin is also a true endectocide, as its activity encompasses most of the common intestinal parasites (eg, *Toxocara, Toxascaris, Uncinaria, Ancylostoma*), heartworms, and external parasites (fleas). Selamectin may also be given to pregnant and lactating bitches for treatment and prevention of *Toxocara canis* infection.

Other Species: Ivermectin and other avermectin/milbemycin compounds have been used extensively as antiparasitic agents in a wide variety of exotic pets including ferrets, rabbits, rodents, birds, and reptiles. Although the activity of these compounds was first established in laboratory animal parasite systems, their use in rodents and other exotic pets is extra-label, and treatment protocols are often established through empirical clinical experience rather than controlled studies.

SALICYLANILIDES, SUBSTITUTED PHENOLS, AROMATIC AMIDE

The members of this chemical grouping include salicylanilides (brotianide, clioxanide, closantel, niclosamide, oxyclozanide, rafoxanide), substituted phenols (bithionol, disophenol, hexachlorophene, niclofolan menichlopholan, nitroxynil), and the aromatic amide diamfenetide (diamphenethide). All members of these groups are active mainly against adult stages of liver flukes. They are used extensively against fasciolosis and haemonchosis in sheep and cattle. Diamfenetide is unique in that it has exceptionally high activity against the youngest immature stages of the liver fluke in sheep, with a diminution of activity as the flukes mature. The lowered efficacy of a number of the salicylanilides and substituted phenols against immature flukes may be due to the high protein binding of these drugs in the blood. A number of these compounds, however, appear to have activity against 6-wk-old flukes in cattle and sheep, by affecting them either at the time of administration or, more probably, by persisting in blood until the flukes start to ingest blood and become exposed to higher drug concentrations. They are all given PO, except nitroxynil, which is normally given SC.

MISCELLANEOUS ANTHELMINTICS

Piperazine is rapidly absorbed from the GI tract, and piperazine base can be detected in the urine as early as 30 min after administration. The excretion rate is maximal at 1-8 hr, and excretion is practically complete within 24 hr. The spectrum of activity of piperazine is largely against ascarid parasites in all animal species (including humans). The safety margin is wide.

Diethylcarbamazine (DEC), a derivative of piperazine, also acts to paralyze nematodes by interfering with nerve function. It is used for heartworm prevention in dogs; however, its use is declining. In existing infections, the dogs must first be cleared of adult heartworms and microfilariae to avoid reaction, then are given DEC daily PO throughout the mosquito season to prevent reinfection. DEC has also been used to treat prepatent *Dictyocaulus viviparus* infections (*see* LUNGWORM INFECTION, p 1181) in cattle, although it is relatively ineffective against the adult worms. It is routinely given IM at 22 mg/kg body wt for 3 consecutive days, although it is reported that 1 injection at 44 mg/kg provides better respiratory relief.

Praziquantel and epsiprantel are closely related analogs that have high efficacy against cestode parasites at relatively low dose rates but no effect on nematodes. Praziquantel exerts its antiparasitic effects by interfering with the regulation of intracellular Ca^{2+} concentrations, impairing both motility and function of the suckers of the cestode. In vivo studies have indicated that it induces spastic paralysis of the parasite; thus, praziquantel acts, as many anthelmintics, primarily on neuromuscular coordination. Praziquantel is rapidly and almost completely absorbed from the GI tract. After absorption, the drug is distributed to all organs; it is believed to reenter the intestinal lumen via the mucosa and bile of dogs. Praziquantel is rapidly hydroxylated into inactive forms in the liver and secreted in bile. It has a wide safety margin.

Praziquantel PO is highly effective against cestodes of ruminants (eg, *Moniezia* spp, *Stilesia*), horses (*Anoplocephala perfoliata*), and poultry. The PO (5 mg/kg) or SC (5.8 mg/kg) administration of praziquantel in dogs and cats is 100% effective against *Taenia* spp and *Echinococcus granulosus* (both adult and immature forms). Praziquantel at a dosage of 40 mg/kg is also effective against *Schistosoma* infections in cattle (and humans).

Epsiprantel at 5 mg/kg is used specifically for the treatment of the common tapeworms of dogs and cats, including adult *E granulosus*.

Clorsulon is a sulfonamide given PO as a suspension for infections with (mainly) adult liver flukes in sheep and cattle and as a SC injection for cattle, in combination with ivermectin. In plasma, clorsulon is bound to protein and, when ingested by liver flukes, inhibits enzymes of the glycolytic pathway. Although its safety margin is wide, clorsulon is not licensed for use in lactating dairy cows producing milk for human consumption.

Bunamidine is an anticestodal compound. It is used in small animals and is most effective if given after fasting. It is absorbed and metabolized in the liver and leads to digestion of tapeworms in the gut of the host. Vomiting and mild diarrhea may be seen, and exercise or excitement should be avoided in dogs soon after administration.

Nitroscanate, like the substituted phenols, probably acts by uncoupling oxidative phosphorylation. It is used in small animals against *Toxocara, Toxascaris, Taenia, Dipylidium, Ancylostoma, Uncinaria,* and *Echinococcus* spp. Vomiting occasionally occurs after treatment.

ANTI-INFLAMMATORY AGENTS

Inflammation is the complex pathophysiologic response of vascularized tissue to injury. The injury may result from various stimuli including thermal, chemical, or physical damage; ischemia; infectious agents; antigen-antibody interactions; and other biologic processes. The inflammatory response is typically characterized by the 5 classic clinical signs: heat, redness, swelling, pain, and loss of function. The desired outcome of the inflammatory response is isolation and elimination of the injurious agent, repair of tissue damage at the site of injury, and restoration of function.

PATHOPHYSIOLOGY OF INFLAMMATION

See also IMMUNOPATHOLOGIC MECHANISMS, p 645.

Inflammation occurs in 3 distinct phases—acute, subacute, and chronic (or proliferative). The acute response to tissue injury occurs in the microcirculation at the site of injury. Initially there is a transient constriction of arterioles; however, within several minutes, chemical mediators released at the site cause relaxation of arteriolar smooth muscle, vasodilation, and increased capillary permeability. Protein-rich fluid then exudes from capillaries into the interstitial space. This fluid contains many of the components of plasma, including fibrinogen, kinins, complement, and immunoglobulins that mediate the inflammatory response. The subacute phase is characterized by movement of phagocytic cells to the site of injury. In response to adhesion molecules released from activated endothelial cells, leukocytes, platelets, and RBC in injured vessels become sticky and adhere to the endothelial cell surfaces. Polymorphonuclear leukocytes such as neutrophils are the first cells to infiltrate the site of injury. Basophils and eosinophils are more prevalent in allergic reactions or parasitic infections. As the inflammatory process continues, macrophages predominate, actively removing damaged cells or tissue. If the cause of injury is eliminated, acute inflammation may be followed by a period of tissue repair. Blood clots are removed by fibrinolysis, and damaged tissues are regenerated or replaced with fibroblasts, collagen, or endothelial cells. However, inflammation may become chronic, leading to further tissue destruction and fibrosis.

CHEMICAL MEDIATORS OF INFLAMMATION

Biochemical mediators released during inflammation intensify and propagate the inflammatory response (TABLE 56). These mediators are soluble, diffusible molecules that can act locally and systemically. Mediators derived from plasma include complement and complement-derived peptides and kinins. Released via the classic or alternative pathways of the complement cascade, **complement-derived peptides** (C3a, C3b, and C5a) increase vascular permeability, cause smooth muscle contraction, activate leukocytes, and induce mast-cell degranulation. C5a is also a potent chemotactic factor for neutrophils and mononuclear phagocytes. The kinins are also important inflammatory

TABLE 56. Actions of Inflammatory Mediators

Action	Mediators[*]
Vasodilation, increased vascular permeability	Histamine, serotonin, bradykinin, C3a, C5a, LTC_4, LTD_4, PGI_2, PGE_2, PGD_2, PGF_2, activated Hageman factor, kinonogen fragments, fibrinopeptides
Vasoconstriction	TXA_2, LTB_4, LTC_4, LTD_4, C5a
Smooth muscle contraction	C3a, C5a, histamine, LTB_4, LTC_4, LTD_4, TXA_2, serotonin, PAF, bradykinin
Mast cell degranulation	C5a, C3a
Stem cell proliferation	IL-3, G-CSF, GM-CSF, M-CSF
Chemotaxis	C5a, LTB_4, IL-8, PAF, 5-HETE, histamine, others
Lysosomal granule release	C5a, IL-8, PAF
Phagocytosis	C3b, iC3b
Platelet aggregation	TXA_2, PAF
Endothelial cell stickiness	IL-1, TNF-α, LTB_4
Granuloma formation	IL-1, TNF-α
Pain	PGE_2, bradykinin, histamine, serotonin
Fever	IL-1, IL-6, TNF-α, PGE_2

[*]C = complement, LT = leukotriene, PG = prostaglandin, TX = thromboxane, PAF = platelet activating factor, IL = interleukin, CSF = colony stimulating factor, HETE = hydroxyeicosatetranoate, TNF = tumor necrosis factor

mediators. The most important kinin is **bradykinin**, which increases vascular permeability and vasodilation and, importantly, activates phospholipase A_2 (PLA_2) to liberate arachidonic acid (AA). Bradykinin is also a major mediator involved in the pain response.

Other mediators are derived from injured tissue cells or WBC recruited to the site of inflammation. Mast cells, platelets, and basophils produce the vasoactive amines serotonin and histamine. **Histamine** causes arteriolar dilation, increased capillary permeability, contraction of nonvascular smooth muscle, and eosinophil chemotaxis and can stimulate nociceptors responsible for the pain response. Its release is stimulated by the complement components C3a and C5a and by lysosomal proteins released from neutrophils. Histamine activity is mediated through the activation of 1 of 3 specific histamine receptors, designated H_1, H_2, or H_3, in target cells. Most histamine-induced vascular effects are mediated by H_1 receptors. H_2 receptors mediate some vascular effects, but are more important for their role in histamine-induced gastric secretion. Less is understood regarding the role of H_3 receptors, which may be localized to the CNS. **Serotonin** (5-hydroxytryptamine) is a vasoactive mediator similar to histamine found in mast cells and platelets in the GI tract and CNS. Serotonin also increases vascular permeability, dilates capillaries, and causes contraction of nonvascular smooth muscle. In some species, including rodents and domestic ruminants, serotonin may be the predominant vasoactive amine.

Cytokines, including interleukins 1-10, tumor necrosis factor α (TNF-α), and interferon γ (INF-γ) are produced predominantly by macrophages and lymphocytes, but can be synthesized by other cell types as well. Their role in inflammation is complex. These polypeptides modulate the activity and function of other cells to coordinate and control the inflammatory response. Two of the more important cytokines, interleukin-1 (IL-1) and TNF-α, mobilize and activate leukocytes, enhance proliferation of B and T cells and natural killer cell cytotoxicity, and are involved in the biologic response to endotoxins. IL-1, IL-6, and TNF-α mediate the acute phase response and pyrexia that may accompany infection and can induce systemic clinical signs including sleep and anorexia. In the acute phase response, interleukins stimulate the liver to synthesize acute phase proteins including complement components, coagulation factors, protease inhibitors, and metal-binding proteins. By increasing intracellular Ca^{2+} concentrations in leukocytes, cytokines are also important in the induction of PLA_2. Colony-stimulating factors (GM-CSF, G-CSF, and M-CSF) are cytokines that promote expansion of neutrophil, eosinophil, and macrophage colonies in bone marrow. In chronic inflammation, cytokines IL-1, IL-6, and TNF-α contribute to the activation of fibroblasts and osteoblasts and to the release of enzymes such as collagenase and stromelysin that can cause cartilage and bone resorption. Experimental evidence also suggests that cytokines stimulate synovial cells and chondrocytes to release pain-inducing mediators.

Lipid-derived autacoids play important roles in the inflammatory response and are a major focus of research into new anti-inflammatory drugs. These compounds include the eicosanoids such as prostaglandins (PG), prostacyclin, leukotrienes, and thromboxane A and the modified phospholipids such as platelet activating factor (PAF). Eicosanoids are synthesized from 20-carbon polyunsaturated fatty acids by many cells including activated leukocytes, mast cells, and platelets and are therefore widely distributed. Hormones and other inflammatory mediators (TNF-α, bradykinin) stimulate eicosanoid production either by direct activation of PLA_2, or indirectly by increasing intracellular Ca^{2+} concentrations, which in turn activate the enzyme. Cell membrane damage can also cause an increase in intracellular Ca^{2+}. Activated PLA_2 directly hydrolyzes AA, which is rapidly metabolized via 1 of 2 enzyme pathways—the cyclooxygenase pathway leading to the formation of PG and thromboxanes, or the lipoxygenase pathway that produces the leukotrienes.

Fatty acid cyclooxygenase (COX) catalyzes the oxygenation of AA to form the cyclic endoperoxide PGG_2, which is converted to the closely related PGH_2. Both PGG_2 and PGH_2 are inherently unstable and are rapidly converted to various prostaglandins, thromboxane A_2 (TXA_2), and prostacyclin (PGI_1). In vascular beds of most animals, PGE_1, PGE_2, and PGI_1 are potent arteriolar dilators and enhance the effects of other mediators by increasing small vein permeability. Other PG, including $PGF_{2\alpha}$ and thromboxane, cause smooth muscle contraction and vasoconstriction. PG sensitize nociceptors to pain-provoking mediators such as bradykinin and histamine, and in large concentrations can directly stimulate sensory nerve endings. TXA_2 is a potent platelet aggregating agent involved in thrombus formation.

Found predominately in platelets, leukocytes, and in the lung, 5-lipoxygenase catalyzes the formation of unstable hydroxyperoxides from AA. These hydroxyperoxides are subsequently converted to the peptide **leukotrienes**. Leukotriene B_4 (LTB_4) and 5-hydroxyeicosatetranoate (5-HETE) are strong chemoattractants stimulating polymorphonuclear leukocyte movement. LTB_4 also stimulates the production of cytokines in neutrophils, monocytes, and eosinophils and enhances expression of C3b receptors. Other leukotrienes facilitate the release of histamine and other autacoids from mast cells and stimulate bronchiolar constriction and mucous secretion. In some species, leukotrienes C_4 and D_4 are more potent than histamine in contracting bronchial smooth muscle.

Platelet activating factor (PAF) is also derived from cell membrane phospholipid by the action of PLA_2. PAF, synthesized by mast cells, platelets, neutrophils, and eosinophils, induces platelet aggregation and stimulates platelets to release vasoactive amines and synthesize thromboxanes. PAF also increases vascular permeability and causes neutrophils to aggregate and degranulate.

The role of the free radical gas **nitric oxide** (NO) in inflammation is also a focus of ongoing research. NO is an important cell-signaling messenger in a wide range of physiologic and pathophysiologic processes. Small amounts of NO play a role in maintaining resting vascular tone, vasodilation, and anti-aggregation of platelets. In response to certain cytokines (TNF-α, IL-1) and other inflammatory mediators, the production of relatively large quantities of NO is stimulated. In larger quantities, NO is a potent vasodilator, facilitates macrophage-induced cytotoxity, and may contribute to joint destruction in some types of arthritis.

ANTIHISTAMINES

Antagonists that selectively block specific histamine receptors have been developed. H_1 antagonists block the actions of histamine responsible for increased capillary permeability and wheal and edema formation. H_1 antihistamines may be useful in the treatment of the immediate hypersensitivity reactions such as anaphylaxis by blocking bronchoconstriction and vasodilation. H_1 antagonists may be less effective in the treatment of inflammatory diseases and allergic reactions such as atopy, primarily because mediators other than histamine play important roles in such conditions. H_2 antagonists are routinely used to block the gastric secretory effects of histamine and have limited anti-inflammatory effects.

CORTICOSTEROIDS

Two classes of steroid hormones, mineralocorticoids and glucocorticoids, are naturally synthesized in the adrenal cortex from cholesterol. (*See also* THE ADRENAL GLANDS, p 435.)

Mineralocorticoids are important in maintaining electrolyte homeostasis, whereas glucocorticoids play significant roles in carbohydrate, protein, and lipid metabolism; the immune response; and the response to stress. Glucocorticoids also have some mineralocorticoid activity, and therefore affect fluid and electrolyte balance.

Corticosteroids are the most commonly used anti-inflammatory drugs. However, their pharmacologic and physiologic effects are broad and the potential for misuse is great. While corticosteroids can be highly effective in suppressing or preventing inflammation, their anti-inflammatory effects are inherently linked with suppression of the immune response and associated consequences.

All therapeutic corticosteroids have a 21-carbon steroid skeleton, similar to cortisol. Modifications to this skeleton alter the degree of anti-inflammatory and metabolic effects and vary the duration of activity and protein-binding affinity of the resultant compound. This has led to the synthesis of a number of corticosteroids with increased anti-inflammatory potency but reduced mineralocorticoid effects. Therapeutic corticosteroids are typically classified based on their relative glucocorticoid and mineralocorticoid potency as well as duration of biologic effect (TABLE 57). In general, those compounds with the most potent glucocorticoid activity are also potent suppressors of the hypothalamic-pituitary-adrenal axis (HPAA).

Mode of Action: Glucocorticoids are capable of suppressing the inflammatory process through numerous pathways. They interact with specific intracellular receptor proteins in target tissues to alter the expression of corticosteroid-responsive genes. Glucocorticoid-specific receptors in the cell cytoplasm bind with steroid ligands to form hormone-

TABLE 57. Relative Potencies of Commonly Used Corticosteroids

Compound	Relative Glucocorticoid Activity	Relative Mineralocorticoid Activity	Biological Half-life (hr)
Cortisol	1	1	8-12
Cortisone	0.8	0.8	8-12
Prednisone	5	0.8	12-36
Prednisolone	5	0.8	12-36
Methylprednisolone	5	0.5	12-36
Triamcinolone	5+	0	24-48
Dexamethasone	25	0	36-72
Betamethasone	25	0	36-72

receptor complexes that eventually translocate to the cell nucleus. There these complexes bind to specific DNA sequences and alter their expression. The complexes may induce the transcription of mRNA leading to synthesis of new proteins. Such proteins include lipocortin, a protein known to inhibit PLA_{2a} and thereby block the synthesis of prostaglandins, leukotrienes, and PAF. Glucocorticoids also inhibit the production of other mediators including AA metabolites such as COX, cytokines, the interleukins, adhesion molecules, and enzymes such as collagenase.

Physiologic and Pharmacologic Effects: Peripherally and in the liver, glucocorticoids have important effects on carbohydrate, protein, and lipid metabolism. In the periphery, glucocorticoids stimulate lipolysis and protein breakdown, releasing glycerol and amino acids that act as substrates for gluconeogenesis. As a result, chronic exposure to excessive glucocorticoids may lead to muscle wasting and redistribution of body fat typical in animals with hyperadrenocorticism. In the liver, glucocorticoids stimulate hepatic gluconeogenesis and increase the hepatic synthesis and storage of glycogen. It is believed gluconeogenesis is stimulated through the transcription of enzymes such as glucose-6-phosphatase and phosphoenolpyruvate carboxykinase. Glucocorticoids also decrease glucose uptake in peripheral tissues, including adipose tissue, further contributing to increases in blood glucose. In response to elevated blood glucose, there is a compensatory increase in insulin. However, glucocorticoids inhibit the suppression of gluconeogenesis by insulin and cause insulin resistance in peripheral tissues, further contributing to hyperglycemia.

Although not as potent as the mineralocorticoid aldosterone, glucocorticoids do have effects on water and electrolyte balance, primarily due to their activity in the kidney. Polyuria/polydipsia associated with glucocorticoid use results from inhibition of antidiuretic hormone (ADH) secretion and decreased renal sensitivity to ADH. Glucocorticoids also enhance potassium excretion and sodium retention by the kidney. They can increase renal excretion and decrease intestinal absorption of calcium, causing depletion of calcium stores. Glucocorticoids also inhibit osteoblasts, stimulate osteoclasts, and increase parathyroid secretion, which could affect bone healing.

A number of mechanisms are responsible for the anti-inflammatory and immunosuppressive actions of glucocorticoids. In homeostasis, glucocorticoids help maintain normal vascular permeability and microcirculation and stabilize cellular and lysosomal membranes. However, in acute inflammation, glucocorticoids decrease vascular permeability and inhibit the migration and egress of polymorphonuclear lymphocytes into tissues. Glucocorticoids suppress cell-mediated immunity by inducing apoptosis in normal lymphoid cells, inhibiting the clonal expansion of T and B lymphocytes, and reducing the number of circulating eosinophils, basophils, and monocytes. In contrast, glucocorticoids inhibit margination of neutrophils and increase the release of mature neutrophils from the bone marrow. Inflamed tissue, phagocytosis and toxic oxygen-free radical production are inhibited in macrophages and monocytes. In later stages of inflammation, glucocorticoids inhibit the activity of fibroblasts, reducing fibrosis and the formation of scar tissue. However, they may also slow wound healing.

Glucocorticoids modulate the synthesis and release of a number of chemical mediators of inflammation, including prostaglandins, leukotrienes, histamine, cytokines, complement, and PAF and also suppress the production of inducible NO synthase and chondrodestructive enzymes such as collagenase.

Glucocorticoids have effects on other hormone systems. All anti-inflammatory glucocorticoid drugs in use today inhibit the HPAA, which can result in clinically significant adverse effects.

Administration and Pharmacokinetics: Steroid formulations are available for oral, parenteral, and topical use. Many, including prednisone, prednisolone, methylprednisolone, and dexamethasone are well absorbed when administered PO and are particularly useful when anti-inflammatory treatment is required for a period of one to several weeks. Other preparations are available for parenteral use. The sodium phosphate and succinate salts are highly water soluble, providing a rapid onset of action when given IV, and are often used in shock therapy. Other injectable formulations include esters such as methylprednisolone acetate and triamcinolone acetonide, which have limited water solubility. The release of corticosteroids from these preparations is very slow and may result in anti-inflammatory effects and associated HPAA suppression for several weeks. Corticosteroid preparations available for topical or intralesional administration can be effective in treating inflammation of the skin, eyes, or ears. Although controversial, intra-articular administration of glucocorticoids has been used in humans and animals, particularly horses, to manage inflammatory joint disease. Glucocorticoids are absorbed systemically from sites of local administration in amounts that may be sufficient to suppress the HPAA.

Following absorption, ~90% of cortisol (or its synthetic analogs) is reversibly bound to plasma proteins, primarily corticosteroid binding globulin and albumin. Only the unbound portion is available to exert physiologic and pharmacologic effects. At very high steroid concentrations, protein-binding capacity may be exceeded. Generally glucocorticoids are metabolized in the liver, where they are reduced and conjugated, forming inactive water-soluble derivatives that are excreted by the kidney.

Side Effects: Adverse or toxic effects of glucocorticoids commonly result from the longterm use of supraphysiologic doses to control inflammatory or immunologic disorders. Longterm administration may lead to iatrogenic Cushing's syndrome, characterized by polyuria, polydipsia, bilaterally symmetric alopecia, increased susceptibility to infection, peripheral myopathy and muscle atrophy, and redistribution of body fat. The gluconeogenic and insulin antagonistic effects of glucocorticoids may precipitate the onset of diabetes mellitus or exacerbate diabetes in animals with existing disease. Longterm suppression of the HPAA may cause adrenal gland atrophy and resultant iatrogenic secondary hypoadrenocorticism. In affected animals, abrupt discontinuation of glucocorticoid therapy may lead to an Addisonian-like crisis characterized by lethargy, weakness, vomiting, and diarrhea. In severe cases, circulatory shock and death may result.

Glucocorticoids induce glycogen accumulation in hepatocytes, resulting in hepatopathy and hepatomegaly, and stimulate the production of the steroid-specific isoenzyme of alkaline phosphatase. Slow turnover of enterocytes and inhibition of protective PG in the gut due to glucocorticoids may contribute to the development of GI ulceration. Further, glucocorticoids potentiate the ulcerogenic effects of NSAID. Glucocorticoids reduce collagen synthesis and may lead to thinning and increased fragility of the skin. Alterations in fluid and electrolyte balance may result in sodium and fluid retention and hypokalemic alkalosis. In horses, high doses of glucocorticoids may induce or exacerbate laminitis. Significant mood and behavioral changes have been described in humans receiving corticosteroid therapy and may be seen in animals as well.

Although immunosuppression may be a desired effect of glucocorticoid therapy, susceptibility to infection may increase or latent infections may be reactivated. Urinary tract infections are common in animals receiving glucocorticoids for longterm therapy of inflammatory or immunologic disease. In joints, glucocorticoids may reduce the formation of chondrocyte collagen and synovial fluid and contribute to the development of septic arthritis. Strict aseptic technique must be observed when administering intra-articular injections of steroids.

The side effects of longterm (>2 wk) glucocorticoid therapy can be diminished using an alternate-day treatment regimen. Once inflammation has been controlled using daily therapy with a drug with intermediate duration of activity (prednisolone or prednisone), a gradual change to alternate-day therapy can be made.

Therapeutic Uses: Short-acting soluble steroids such as the succinate esters are routinely used in the treatment of circulatory shock. When given IV in the early stages of shock, glucocorticoids and aggressive fluid therapy may improve hemodynamics and survival rates. Glucocorticoids are also routinely used in the treatment of cerebral edema, although controlled clinical trials supporting their effectiveness are lacking.

Glucocorticoids are used commonly to treat allergy and inflammation such as pruritic dermatoses and allergic lung and GI diseases. In acute cases of atopic or flea allergy dermatitis, anti-inflammatory dosages (prednisolone, 0.5-1 mg/kg, SID) alleviate pruritus and limit self-trauma from scratching until the underlying cause can be addressed. Similar dosages are used in the management of chronic allergic bronchitis and feline asthma.

Short-acting corticosteroids have also been used in the treatment of acute respiratory distress syndrome in cattle and chronic obstructive pulmonary disease in horses. Corticosteroids have been used to treat several musculoskeletal disorders including osteoarthritis, myositis, and immune-mediated arthritis. In most inflammatory conditions, glucocorticoids should be used in conjunction with therapies that target the underlying cause.

NONSTEROIDAL ANTI-INFLAMMATORY DRUGS

The importance of pain management and the use of NSAID in animals has recently increased significantly. NSAID have the potential to relieve pain and inflammation without the immunosuppressive and metabolic side effects associated with corticosteroids. However, all NSAID have the potential for other adverse effects that should be considered in the overall management of the inflammatory process.

Mode of Action: Generally, the classification NSAID is applied to drugs that inhibit one or more steps in the metabolism of arachidonic acid (AA). Unlike corticosteroids, which inhibit numerous pathways, NSAID act primarily to reduce the biosynthesis of prostaglandins (PG) by inhibiting cyclooxygenase (COX). In general, NSAID do not inhibit lipoxygenase (and hence leukotriene) formation, or the formation of other inflammatory mediators, although tepoxalin, a recently introduced NSAID does inhibit lipoxygenase.

The discovery of the 2 isoforms of COX (COX-1 and COX-2) has advanced understanding of the mechanism of action and potential adverse effects of NSAID. COX-1, expressed in virtually all tissues of the body, catalyzes the formation of constitutive PG, which mediate a variety of normal physiologic effects including hemostasis, GI mucosal protection, and protection of the kidney from hypotensive insult. In contrast, COX-2 is activated in damaged and inflamed tissues and catalyzes the formation of inducible PG, including PGE_2, associated with intensifying the inflammatory response. COX-2 is also involved in thermoregulation and the pain response to injury. Therefore, COX-2 inhibition by NSAID is thought to be responsible for the antipyretic, analgesic, and anti-inflammatory actions of NSAID. However, concurrent inhibition of COX-1 may result in many of the unwanted effects of NSAID including gastric ulceration and renal toxicity. Because NSAID vary in their ability to inhibit each COX isoform, a drug that inhibits COX-2 at a lower concentration than that necessary to inhibit COX-1 might be considered safer. This concept has propelled the development of the so-called "COX-2 selective" NSAID. Although ratios of COX-1:COX-2 activity for various NSAID in humans and animals have been reported, caution is advised when interpreting such ratios, as they vary greatly depending on the selectivity assay used. The COX selectivity of NSAID also varies by species; COX selectivity ratios reported for humans do not apply to other animals.

In general, drugs with ratios suggesting preferential activity against COX-2 may have fewer adverse effects due to COX-1 inhibition. In dogs, favorable ratios have been reported for carprofen, meloxicam, deracoxib, and firocoxib, while unfavorable ratios have been reported for aspirin, phenylbutazone, and piroxicam. COX-1-sparing drugs are associated with less GI ulceration and less platelet inhibition; however, it may be overly simplistic to assume that complete COX-2 inhibition is without potential risk. Recent research has suggested that COX-2 can be induced constitutively in various organs including the brain, spinal cord, ovary, and kidney. In dogs, COX-2 mRNA is present in the loop of Henle and the maculae densa and may play an important role in the protective response to hypotension. However, a recent study failed to demostrate COX-2 expression in canine kidneys, raising questions regarding its role. COX-2 also appears to be important in the healing of GI ulcers in humans, and certain COX-2-specific inhibitors delay ulcer healing experimentally. Although COX-1 plays a primary role in regulating homeostasis, it may play a more significant role in inflammation than originally proposed.

NSAID also vary in their mechanism of COX inhibition. Aspirin irreversibly acetylates a serine residue of COX, resulting in a complete loss of COX activity. The duration of the effect depends on the turnover rate of COX; activity is lost for the life of the platelet (7-10 days) following aspirin administration. Unlike aspirin, most other NSAID are reversible competitive COX inhibitors; their duration of inhibition is primarily determined by the elimination pharmacokinetics of the drug.

Pharmacologic Effects: All NSAID, except for acetaminophen, are antipyretic, analgesic, and anti-inflammatory. They are routinely used for the relief of pain and inflammation associated with osteoarthritis in dogs and horses and for colic, navicular disease, and laminitis in horses. The use of NSAID for the relief of perioperative pain in companion animals is increasing. In general, NSAID provide only symptomatic relief from pain and inflammation and do not significantly alter the course of pathologic damage. As analgesics, they are generally less potent than opioids and are therefore more effective against mild to moderate pain.

As antipyretics, NSAID reduce body temperature in febrile states. Although the beneficial effects of the febrile response usually outweigh the negative effects, NSAID inhibition of PGE_2 activity in the hypothalamus may provide symptomatic relief and improve appetite. In Europe, NSAID have been used in conjunction with antibiotics for treatment of acute respiratory diseases in cattle and may reduce morbidity through their antipyretic and anti-inflammatory effects.

The effects of some NSAID on chondrocyte metabolism have been investigated. Some, including aspirin, naproxen, and ibuprofen, are considered chondrotoxic because they inhibit the synthesis of cartilage proteoglycans. Others, including carprofen and meloxicam, may be considered chondroneutral, or depending on dose, actually stimulate the production of cartilage matrix. The potential beneficial or deleterious effects of NSAID on chondrocyte metabolism remain to be clarified.

A therapeutic area in which NSAID use may become important is in the treatment and prevention of cancer. Epidemiologic studies in humans show that aspirin use is associated with a significant reduction in the incidence of colon cancer. Newer evidence suggests that the therapeutic effect of NSAID on colon cancer is mediated by inhibition of COX-2, which may be up-regulated in many premalignant and malignant neoplasms. In veterinary medicine, piroxicam has been shown to reduce the size of tumors such as transitional cell carcinoma in dogs. Specific COX-2 inhibitors may prove useful as a primary or adjunctive therapy in the management of cancer.

Administration and Pharmacokinetics: Most NSAID are weak organic acids that are well absorbed following PO administration. However, food can impair the oral absorption of some NSAID (eg, phenylbutazone, meclofenamate, flunixin meglumine) in horses and ruminants. Several NSAID are available as parenteral formulations for IV, IM, or SC administration. Some parenteral formulations are highly alkaline and may cause tissue necrosis if injected perivascularly. Once absorbed, most NSAID are extensively (up to 99%) bound to plasma proteins, with only a small proportion of unbound drug available to be active in the tissues. NSAID administration to animals with low serum albumin can result in higher than anticipated available drug levels and associated toxic effects. NSAID may also compete for binding sites with other highly protein-bound compounds.

Most NSAID are biotransformed in the liver to inactive metabolites that are excreted by the kidney via glomerular filtration and tubular secretion. Biotransformation and elimination half-lives vary significantly by species (and in some cases by breed), so it is not possible to safely extrapolate dosages from one species or animal to another. Some NSAID, including naproxen, etodolac, and meclofenamic acid, undergo extensive enterohepatic recirculation in some species, resulting in prolonged elimination half-lives.

Side Effects: All NSAID have the potential to induce adverse reactions, some of which can be life threatening. Many reactions to NSAID are dose-related and are typically reversible with discontinuation of therapy and supportive care.

GI ulceration is the most common side effect. Loss of GI protective mechanisms results from inhibition of constitutive PG that regulate blood flow to the gastric mucosa and stimulate bicarbonate and mucus production. This disrupts the alkaline protective barrier of the gut, allowing diffusion of gastric acid back into the mucosa, injuring cells and blood vessels and causing gastritis and ulceration. As organic acids, NSAID, especially aspirin, may also cause direct chemical irritation of the GI mucosa. The enterohepatic recirculation of certain NSAID may result in high biliary concentrations that increase ulcerogenic potential in the gut. NSAID-induced GI bleeding may be occult, leading to iron-deficiency anemia, or more severe, resulting in vomiting, hematemesis, and hematochezia. Horses may develop oral, lingual, or gastric ulceration with accompanying signs of colic, weight loss, or loose manure. In addition, an idiosyncratic predisposition for ulceration of the right dorsal colon has been associated with NSAID therapy in horses.

GI blood loss may be further complicated by impaired platelet function. Platelet function is inhibited because NSAID prevent platelets from forming TXA_2, a potent aggregating agent. Because TXA_2 inhibition causes prolonged bleeding, evaluation of buccal mucosal bleeding time is advised in animals receiving NSAID for which surgery is anticipated. Blood dyscrasias after longterm NSAID therapy have been reported in cats, dogs, and horses. Acetaminophen administration in cats is associated with Heinz body anemia, methemoglobinemia, hepatic failure, and death. Bone marrow dyscrasias associated with phenylbutazone administration have also been reported.

Nephropathies associated with chronic NSAID use are common in humans. Animals with underlying renal compromise receiving NSAID could experience exacerbation or decompensation of their disease. It is important to maintain hydration and renal perfusion in animals receiving NSAID, especially those undergoing anesthesia or surgery.

Hepatopathies are relatively common in both humans and animals receiving NSAID. NSAID administration routinely induces mild hepatic changes characterized primarily by elevation in liver enzymes without clinical signs or hepatic dysfunction. Rare reports of idiosyncratic reactions resulting in hepatic dysfunction or failure have been reported in humans (acetaminophen and other), dogs (acetaminophen, carprofen, etodolac), and horses (phenylbutazone). Cytopathic (hepatocellular injury, necrosis), cholestatic, and mixed histopathologic patterns of injury have been documented. NSAID should be used with caution in animals with preexisting hepatic disease.

Specific Nonsteroidal Anti-inflammatory Drugs

Based on structure, most NSAID can be divided into 2 broad groups—carboxylic acid and enolic acid derivatives. The main subgroups of enolic acids are the pyrazolones (phenylbutazone, oxyphenbutazone, and ramifenazone) and the oxicams (meloxicam, piroxicam, and tenoxicam). Carboxylic acid subgroups include the salicylates (aspirin), proprionic acids (ibuprofen, naproxen, carprofen, ketoprofen, and vedaprofen), anthranilic acids (tolfenamic and meclofenamic acids), phenylacetic acids (acetaminophen), aminonicotinic acids (flunixin), and indolines (indomethacin). The newer coxib class of selective COX-2 inhibitors includes a diaryl-substituted furanone (rofecoxib), a diaryl-substituted pyrazole (celecoxib), and a diaryl-substituted isoxazole (valdecoxib), all available for human use. Two NSAID of the coxib class, deracoxib and firocoxib, have been introduced in veterinary medicine.

Aspirin: By far the most widely used anti-inflammatory drug in humans, aspirin is frequently used in veterinary medicine. The salicylic ester of acetic acid, aspirin (acetylsalicylic acid) is available in several different pharmaceutical preparations including plain, buffered, and enteric-coated formulations as well as topical and rectal preparations. Following PO administration, aspirin is rapidly absorbed from the stomach and upper small intestine, reaching peak plasma concentrations in most species (except ruminants) within 1-2 hr. Most aspirin is absorbed directly, but is rapidly hydrolyzed to salicylic acid. After absorption, both aspirin and salicylic acid are widely distributed through most tissues and fluids and readily cross the placental barrier. About 80-90% of the absorbed salicylate is bound to plasma proteins. Metabolism and elimination is via hepatic conjugation with glucoronic acid, followed by renal excretion. Cats, which lack glucuronyl transferase, have difficulty metabolizing aspirin. The elimination half-life of aspirin in cats approaches 40 hr, compared with 7.5 hr in dogs. In veterinary medicine, aspirin is used primarily for the relief of mild to moderate pain associated with musculoskeletal inflammation or osteoarthritis. Because aspirin is not approved for veterinary use, definitive efficacy studies have not been performed to establish effective dosages. Recommended dosages in dogs are 10-40 mg/kg, PO, BID-TID. Aspirin has been used in the treatment of laminitis in horses at a dosage of 10 mg/kg, PO, SID. In cats, aspirin may be used for its anti-platelet effects in thromboembolic disease at a dosage of 10 mg/kg, PO, every

48 hr, to allow for prolonged metabolism. Adverse effects are common following aspirin administration and appear to be dosage dependent. Even at therapeutic dosages of 25 mg/kg, plain aspirin may induce mucosal erosion and ulceration in dogs. Vomiting and melena may be seen at higher doses. The PGE_1 analog misoprostol may be effective in decreasing GI ulceration associated with aspirin and other NSAID. Aspirin overdose in any species can result in salicylate poisoning, characterized by severe acid-base abnormalities, hemorrhage, seizures, coma, and death.

Acetaminophen: Acetaminophen is a para-aminophenol derivative with antipyretic and analgesic activity, but minimal anti-inflammatory effects. Acetaminophen does not inhibit neutrophil activation, has little ulcerogenic potential, and has no effect on platelets or bleeding time. The pharmacologic effect of acetaminophen may vary from that of other NSAID because acetaminophen is more effective in inhibiting COX in the brain rather than in the periphery. It has recently been suggested that acetaminophen may act by inhibiting COX-3, a splice variant of COX-1. The recommended dosage of acetominophen in dogs is 10-15 mg/kg, PO, TID. Dose-dependent adverse effects include depression, vomiting, and methemoglobinemia. Use in cats is contraindicated due to a lack of glucuronosyl transferase and the potential for hemolytic anemia and centrilobular hepatic necrosis.

Phenylbutazone: One of the earliest NSAID approved for use in horses and dogs, phenylbutazone is a pyrazolone derivative available in tablet, paste, gel, and parenteral formulations. The plasma half-life of phenylbutazone is 5-6 hr in horses and dogs and >30 hr in cattle. When given PO, phenylbutazone absorbs to hay in the diet, which may reduce GI absorption and bioavailability. Once absorbed, binding to plasma proteins is high (99% in horses, 93% in cattle). Phenylbutazone is metabolized by the liver to several active and inactive metabolites, which are excreted in urine. One of the major therapeutic uses of the drug is the treatment of acute laminitis in horses. Laminitis is treated initially with injectable phenylbutazone at dosages up to 8.8 mg/kg, followed by therapy PO at 2.2-4.4 mg/kg, BID. Because the therapeutic index for phenylbutazone is relatively narrow, dosage should be adjusted to the minimum possible to maintain comfort and avoid toxicity. The ulcerogenic potential of phenylbutazone in horses is greater than that of flunixin meglumine and ketoprofen. Phenylbutazone dosages of 3-7 mg/kg, PO, TID, are recommended in dogs. In dogs, phenylbutazone has been associated with bleeding dyscrasias, hepatopathies, nephropathies, and rare cases of irreversible bone marrow suppression.

Meclofenamic Acid: This anthranilic NSAID is available for horses as a granular preparation and for dogs as an oral tablet. The recommended dosage is 2.2 mg/kg, SID for 5-7 days in horses and 1.1 mg/kg, SID, for 5-7 days in dogs. In cattle, administration of meclofenamic acid results in a biphasic pattern of absorption, with an initial peak plasma concentration reached at ~30 min and a secondary peak 4 hr after dosing. The second peak is presumed to be due to enterohepatic recirculation. In horses, meclofenamic acid is rapidly absorbed; however, the onset of action is slow, requiring 2-4 days of dosing for clinical effect. While it is effective in the treatment of chronic laminitis, meclofenamic acid has a therapeutic index that may be lower than that of other NSAID, possibly due to enterohepatic recirculation.

Flunixin Meglumine: In the USA, the nicotinic acid derivative flunixin meglumine is approved for use in horses as PO and parenteral formulations. The recommended dosage is 1.1 mg/kg, IV or PO, SID for 5 days. Flunixin meglumine is rapidly absorbed following PO or IM administration, and the elimination half-life is short (~2-3 hr). Elimination is primarily by renal excretion. Flunixin meglumine is highly effective for treatment of visceral pain associated with equine colic and may have anti-endotoxic effects. The dosage recommended in horses is 1.1 mg/kg, BID, or 0.25 mg/kg, TID. Toxicity in horses is relatively uncommon, but GI ulceration and erosion may develop. Flunixin has been used to treat mastitis and acute pulmonary emphysema in cattle although it is not approved for these indications. Chronic administration of flunixin meglumine to dogs results in severe GI ulceration and renal damage and use in this species is not recommended.

Carprofen: This NSAID of the arylpropionic acid class is available in the USA in caplet and chewable tablet formulations. An injectable formulation is also available in the USA and Europe. Carprofen is approved by the FDA to manage pain and inflammation associated with osteoarthritis and acute pain associated with soft-tissue and orthopedic surgery in dogs. The recommended dosage is 4.4 mg/kg, PO, SID or divided BID. In Europe and other countries, carprofen is also registered for use in cattle and for short-term therapy in cats. In dogs, oral bioavailability is high (90%) and plasma concentrations peak ~2-3 hr after dosing. The elimination half-life is ~8 hr. As with other NSAID, carprofen is highly (99%) protein bound. Elimination is via hepatic biotransformation with excretion of the resulting metabolites in feces and urine. Some enterohepatic recycling occurs. The exact mechanism of action of carprofen is unclear. Although it has greater selectivity for COX-2 over COX-1, carprofen is considered a weak COX inhibitor. In vitro canine cell line assays indicate that it is 129-fold selective for COX-2, whereas in vitro canine whole blood assays indicate it is 7- to 17-fold selective for COX-2, equine whole blood assays indicate it is 1.6-fold selective for COX-2, and feline whole blood assays indicate it is 5.5-fold selective for COX-2. Other mechanisms of action, including inhibition of PA_2 may be responsible for its anti-inflammatory effects. Carprofen has been used extensively in dogs since its introduction, and adverse events have been comparable to those of other NSAID (ie, ~2 events/1,000 dogs treated). Approximately one fourth of the adverse reactions reported were GI signs, including vomiting, diarrhea, and GI ulceration. Renal and hepatic side effects are rare, as with other NSAID. Potentially serious idiosyncratic hepatopathies, characterized by acute hepatic necrosis, have been reported in some dogs. Approximately one third of the dogs developing hepatopathies while receiving carprofen were Labrador Retrievers, although a true breed predisposition has not been established. As with any NSAID therapy, clinical laboratory monitoring for hepatic damage is advised, especially in geriatric animals that may be predisposed to more serious complications.

Ketoprofen: Ketoprofen is another propionic acid derivative available in the USA and other countries as a 10% injectable solution for horses, and in Europe and Canada as tablets and a 1% injectable solution for dogs and cats. Ketoprofen is recommended for acute pain (up to 5 days) in both dogs and cats. In horses, it is used for pain and inflammation associated with osteoarthritis and for visceral pain associated with colic. The recommended dosage is 1 mg/kg, IV or PO, SID for up to 5 days in dogs and cats, 2.2 mg/kg, IV, SID for up to 5 days in horses, and 3 mg/kg, IV or IM, SID for 1-3 days in cattle. Ketoprofen is a potent inhibitor of COX and bradykinin and may also inhibit some lipoxygenases. Its efficacy is comparable to that of opioids in the management of pain following orthopedic and soft-tissue surgery in dogs. Following administration PO, ketoprofen is rapidly absorbed and has a terminal half-life in cats and dogs of 2-3 hr. As with other NSAID, ketoprofen is metabolized in the liver to inactive metabolites that are eliminated by renal excretion. Adverse effects, including GI upset, are similar to those of other NSAID. Other side effects, including hepatopathies and renal disease, have been reported in animals. Due to potential antiplatelet effects, care should be exercised when using ketoprofen perioperatively.

Etodolac: The pyranocarboxylic acid etodolac is approved for use in dogs in the USA. The elimination half-life is ~8-12 hr, allowing dosing at 10-15 mg/kg, PO, SID. Extensive enterohepatic recirculation has been reported in dogs, followed by elimination of etodolac and its metabolites in the liver and feces. In in vitro studies, etodolac was more selective in inhibition of COX-2 than COX-1, although in vitro canine whole blood assays have also shown it to be nonselective. Etodolac has been shown to inhibit macrophage chemotaxis and has demonstrated efficacy for the treatment of lameness associated with hip dysplasia. Although the risk of GI ulceration is low at therapeutic doses, administration of 3 times the label dosage resulted in GI ulceration, vomiting, and weight loss in toxicity studies. GI, hepatic, and renal adverse reactions have been reported after administration of etodolac, similar to other NSAID.

Vedaprofen: The arylpropionic acid derivative vedaprofen is available in Europe in a gel formulation for horses and dogs and in an injectable formulation for horses. The drug is indicated for the treatment of pain and inflammation associated with musculoskeletal disorders in dogs (0.5 mg/kg, SID) and horses (1 mg/kg, BID) and for the treatment of pain associated with colic in horses (2 mg/kg, IV, as a single injection). Following administration PO, vedaprofen is rapidly absorbed. Biovailability is generally high, but may be reduced if the drug is administered with food. The terminal half-life is 10-13 hr in dogs and 6-8 hr in horses. Vedaprofen undergoes extensive biotransformation to hydroxylated metabolites, which are excreted in urine and feces.

Meloxicam: Approved for use in Canada and Europe in dogs, cats, and cattle, the oxicam NSAID meloxicam is available as an oral syrup and injectable solution. Meloxicam is also approved for human use in the USA and Canada and was recently approved for use in dogs in the USA. A potent inhibitor of prostaglandin synthesis, meloxicam is used for the treatment of acute and chronic inflammation associated with musculoskeletal disease, and for the management of postoperative pain. In dogs, a one-time loading dosage of 0.2 mg/kg, PO, is recommended, followed by 0.1 mg/kg, PO, SID. Once a therapeutic effect is seen, the dosage can be titrated to the lowest possible dose. COX-1:COX-2 ratios reported for meloxicam suggest the drug is COX-2 selective, with in vitro canine whole blood assays indicating it is 2.7- to 10-fold selective for COX-2. Once absorbed, meloxicam is highly protein bound (97%) and has a relatively long elimination half-life (12+ hr). GI safety appears to be greater for meloxicam than for nonspecific NSAID, and meloxicam has been shown to be chondroneutral in rodent studies.

Deracoxib: Deracoxib, the first NSAID of the coxib class approved for use in dogs, is available in a beef-flavored chewable tablet formulation in the USA. Deracoxib has been shown to inhibit COX-2-mediated PGE_2 production. COX-1:COX-2 ratios reported for deracoxib in in vitro cloned canine cell assays indicate it is 1,275-fold selective for COX-2, whereas in in vitro canine whole blood assays it is 12- to 37-fold selective for COX-2. The drug is indicated for the control of postoperative pain and inflammation associated with orthopedic surgery at a dosage of 3-4 mg/kg, PO, SID for up to 7 days and for the control of pain and inflammation associated with osteoarthritis at a dosage of 1-2 mg/kg, PO, SID. Once absorbed, protein binding is >90%, and the elimination half-life is 3 hr.

Firocoxib: Firocoxib is a coxib-class NSAID that was recently approved in the USA and Europe for the control of pain and inflammation associated with osteoarthritis in dogs. It is available in a chewable tablet formulation. Following administration PO, firocoxib is rapidly absorbed and then eliminated by hepatic metabolism and fecal excretion. The elimination half-life is ~8 hr, allowing dosing at 5 mg/kg, PO, SID. COX-1:COX-2 ratios from in vitro canine whole blood assays indicate it is 384-fold selective for COX-2. Like other NSAID, protein binding is high, at ~96%. GI safety appears to be greater than that of nonspecific NSAID.

Other NSAID: A large number of prescription and nonprescription NSAID are available for human use. However, due to species differences in metabolism, efficacy, and toxicity, many are not recommended for use in animals. For example, in dogs, indomethacin is highly toxic to the GI tract and may result in severe ulceration, hematemesis, and melena at therapeutic doses. Piroxicam undergoes extensive enterohepatic recycling in dogs, resulting in a prolonged plasma half-life. GI ulceration and bleeding and renal papillary necrosis have been observed in dogs receiving piroxicam dosages of 0.3-1 mg/kg, SID. Ibuprofen is an arylpropionic acid derivative that has been used in dogs as an anti-inflammatory agent. However, dogs are much more sensitive to the development of GI side effects from ibuprofen administration than are humans. At therapeutic doses, adverse effects observed in dogs include vomiting, diarrhea, GI bleeding, and renal infection. Ibuprofen is not recommended for use in dogs or cats. Naproxen has been used in horses at a dosage of 5-10 mg/kg, SID-BID. Bioavailability is lower (~50%) for naproxen than for other NSAID, and the elimination half-life is ~5 hr in horses. In dogs, the elimination half-life of naproxen is 35-74 hr, presumably due to extensive enterohepatic recirculation. The pharmacokinetics in dogs also appear to be breed dependent. Due to the prolonged half-life of naproxen, dogs are extremely sensitive to its toxic effects.

Coxib class drugs, including rofecoxib, celecoxib, and valdecoxib, recently introduced in human medicine, are COX-2 selective. The drugs are widely prescribed in humans because they do not inhibit COX-1 at therapeutic dosages. In clinical studies, the incidence of GI ulceration in patients receiving valdecoxib or celecoxib was significantly less than that of those receiving naproxen. The use of these drugs in animals has yet to be fully investigated. One pharmacokinetic study with celecoxib in Beagles demonstrated variability in drug elimination between dogs. In that study, one subgroup of Beagles metabolized celecoxib much more rapidly than the other, with elimination half-lives of ~2 and 18 hr, respectively. Until further data are available regarding the pharmacokinetics and safety of these drugs in animals, their use in veterinary medicine is not recommended.

CHONDROPROTECTIVE AGENTS

Polysulfated Glycosaminoglycan (PSGAG): PSGAG is a semisynthetic glycosaminoglycan prepared from bovine tracheal cartilage and composed of a polymeric chain of repeating disaccharide units. The primary glycosaminoglycan in PSGAG is chondroitin sulfate. PSGAG is approved for IM use in dogs and intra-articular and IM use in horses for the control of signs associated with noninfectious degenerative or traumatic arthritis. In horses, the recommended dosage is 500 mg, IM, every 4 days for 28 days, or 250 mg by intra-articular injection once weekly for 5 wk. In dogs, the recommended dosage is 2 mg/lb, IM, twice weekly for up to 4 wk. Following IM injection, PSGAG is absorbed into the systemic circulation and eventually incorporated into both normal and damaged cartilage. The exact mechanism of action is unknown, but in vitro studies show that PSGAG inhibits PGE_2 and catabolic enzymes such as stromelysin, elastase, the metalloproteases, and others. PSGAG also increases the synthesis of hyaluronic acid, proteoglycan, and collagen in vitro. Toxicity associated with the administration of PSGAG has been minimal. Because PSGAG is chemically similar to heparin, overdosage may inhibit coagulation, and concurrent use of aspirin may prolong bleeding times. The use of PSGAG is contraindicated in septic joints.

Pentosan Polysulfate Sodium (PPS): PPS is a polysulfate ester of xylan, a polymer prepared semisynthetically from beechwood plant material. PPS is chemically and structurally similar to heparin and glycosaminoglycan. The compound is approved by the FDA for use as an oral capsule for the treatment of interstitial cystitis in humans. An injectable product is available for use in humans, dogs, and horses in Australia and other countries. The mechanism of action is unknown. PPS stimulates hyaluronic acid and GAG synthesis in damaged joints, inhibits proteolytic enzymes including metalloproteinases, and scavenges free radicals. PPS may also decrease cytokine activity. In canine models of osteoarthritis, IM administration of PPS significantly decreased overall cartilage damage. Because PPS has a heparin-like structure, coagulopathies may be observed.

Hyaluronic Acid: Hyaluronic acid, a polydisaccharide of glucoronic acid and glucosamine, is a component of synovial fluid and articular cartilage. In the USA, a purified fraction of the sodium salt of hyaluronic acid extracted from rooster combs is available for the treatment of horses with osteoarthritis. Hyaluronic acid is responsible for the viscosity of the synovial fluid and contributes to its lubricating function in joint movement. As with other chondroprotective agents, the mode of action is unclear. However, because synovial fluid viscoelasticity is decreased in osteoarthritis, the intra-articular administration of hyaluronic acid may improve joint lubrication. Hyaluronic acid inhibits PGE_2 synthesis in vitro and in vivo and may inhibit inflammatory enzymes and reduce pain. Most clinical use has been in horses, in which hyaluronic acid appears to have minimal side effects.

Orgotein: Orgotein is a water-soluble metalloprotein containing copper and zinc. Found in low concentrations throughout the body, orgotein has superoxide dismutase activity scavenging free oxygen radicals. Orgotein, available as an injectable formulation, has been used for the treatment of soft-tissue inflammation in horses and of arthritis in dogs. Although it has been used as an IM or SC injection, orgotein is typically administered as an intra-articular injection, as its large molecular size may limit absorption via other routes. Intra-articular administration is effective in cases of acute lameness in horses, although the onset of therapeutic response may be slow (2-6 wk). Reports indicate that orgotein apparently has a wide safety margin.

ANTINEOPLASTIC AGENTS

Antineoplastic chemotherapy is an important component of small animal practice and is routinely used for selected tumors of horses and cattle. Effective use of antineoplastic chemotherapy depends on an understanding of basic principles of cancer biology, drug actions and toxicities, and drug handling safety.

Tumor Growth and Response to Chemotherapy: The fundamental biochemical and genetic differences between cancer cells and normal cells are not clearly understood. None of the empirically developed antineoplastic drugs appears to act on a process or component that is entirely unique to cancer cells. Clinically useful drugs achieve a degree of selectivity on the basis of certain characteristics of cancer cells that can be used as pharmacologic targets. These characteristics include rapid rate of division and growth, variations in the rate of drug uptake or in the sensitivity of different types of cells to particular drugs, and retention in the malignant cells of hormonal responses characteristic of the cells from which the cancer is derived, eg, estrogen responsiveness of certain breast carcinomas.

Aspects of normal cell growth and the cell cycle provide the rationale for and are of major importance in the successful application of antineoplastic chemotherapy. In the S phase, DNA synthesis occurs; the M phase begins with mitosis and ends with cytokinesis; and the G_0 phase is a dormant or nonproliferative phase of the cell cycle. Tumor doubling time is related to the length of the cell cycle and the growth fraction (the proportion of a population of cells undergoing cell division). Antineoplastic agents can be classified according to a number of schemes relative to effects at different stages of the cell cycle. In the simplest sense, cycle-nonspecific agents are considered to be lethal to cells in all phases of the cell cycle. Cells are killed exponentially with increasing drug levels, and the dose-response curves follow first-order kinetics. Phase-specific agents exert their lethal effects exclusively or primarily during one phase of the cell cycle, usually S or M; the greater the rate of cell division, the more effective the drug. The G_0 phase of the cell cycle is important, not as a target for chemotherapeutic agents, but as a time during which dormant tumor cells can escape the effects of drug therapy.

Principles of Antineoplastic Chemotherapy: The decision to use antineoplastic chemotherapy depends on the type of tumor to be treated, the stage of malignancy, the condition of the animal, and financial constraints. Chemotherapy can be used as an adjuvant to surgery and irradiation and can be administered immediately after or before the primary treatment. Neo-adjuvant therapy is administered before surgery or irradiation and is intended to improve the effectiveness of the primary therapy by possibly decreasing tumor size, stage of malignancy, or presence of micrometastatic lesions. Responses to cancer chemotherapy can range from palliation (remission of secondary signs, generally without increase in survival time) to complete remission (in which clinically detectable tumor cells and all signs of malignancy are absent). The percentage and duration of complete remissions are criteria for the success of a particular chemotherapeutic protocol.

Effective clinical use of antineoplastic drugs depends on the ability to balance the killing of tumor cells against the inherent toxicity of many of these drugs to host cells. Because of their narrow therapeutic indices, dosages for antineoplastics are frequently calculated based on body surface area (BSA) rather than body mass. However, evidence suggests that small dogs and cats may best be treated based on body weight to avoid overdosage. This is especially true if the primary toxicity is bone marrow suppression. Apparently, BSA does not correlate well with either stem cell number in the bone marrow or resulting hematopoietic toxicity. Correlation is better between body weight and these toxicities. Antineoplastic agents are administered by the PO, IV, SC, topical, intracavitary, intralesional, intravesicular, or arterial routes. The route chosen depends on the individual agent and is determined by drug toxicity; location, size, and type of tumor; and physical constraints.

Antineoplastic agents are commonly administered in various combinations of dosages and timing; the specific regimen is referred to as a protocol. A protocol may use 1 or as many as 5 or 6 different antineoplastic agents. Selection of an appropriate protocol should be based on type of tumor, grade or degree of malignancy, condition of the animal, and financial constraints. Preferences of individual clinicians for treatment of specific neoplastic conditions may also vary. Regardless of the protocol chosen, a thorough knowledge of the mechanism of action and toxicities of each individual therapeutic agent are essential.

Combination antineoplastic chemotherapy offers many advantages. Drugs with different target sites or mechanisms of action are used together to enhance destruction of tumor cells. If the side effects of the component agents are different, the combination may be no more toxic than the individual agents given separately. Combinations that include a cycle-nonspecific drug administered first, followed by a phase-specific drug, may offer the advantage that cells surviving treatment with the first drug are provoked into mitosis and, therefore, are more susceptible to the second drug. Another advantage of combination therapy is the decreased possibility of development of drug resistance.

Special considerations associated with administration of antineoplastic drugs include evaluation of the animal's quality of life, medical and nutritional support, control of pain, and psychological comfort for the owner. Many owners who choose to treat neoplasia in their pets have experienced cancer themselves or have been involved with individuals or family members who have had cancer. Discussion of neoplasia in pets should be handled tactfully and should provide the owners with appropriate information for decision-making.

Resistance to Antineoplastic Agents: Failure to respond, or resistance to antineoplastic agents, can be seen for several reasons. Pharmacokinetic resistance is seen when the concentration of a drug in the target cell is below that required to kill the cell. This may be due to altered rates of drug absorption, distribution, biotransformation, or excretion. In addition, marginal blood flow to a tumor may not provide sufficient drug, resulting in inadequate therapeutic drug concentrations and creation of a population of quiescent, less susceptible cells. Cytokinetic resistance is seen when the tumor cell population is not completely eradicated; this may be a result of dormant tumor cells, dose-limiting host toxicity associated with drug therapy, or the inability to achieve a 100% kill rate even at therapeutic drug dosages. Resistance can also develop via biochemical mechanisms within the tumor cell itself that block transport mechanisms for drug uptake, alter target receptors or enzymes critical to drug action, increase concentrations of normal metabolites antagonized by the antineoplastic drug, or cause genetic changes that result in protective gene amplification or altered patterns of DNA repair. Acquired multidrug resistance can result from amplification and overexpression of a multidrug resistance gene. This gene encodes a cell membrane protein that effectively pumps a variety of structurally unrelated antineoplastic agents out of the cell. As intracellular drug concentrations decline, tumor cell survival and resistance to therapy increase.

Patterns of Toxicity: Antineoplastic agents that act primarily on rapidly dividing and growing cells produce multiple side effects or toxicities, including bone marrow or myelosuppression, GI complications, and immune suppression. Patterns of toxicity may be either acute or delayed. Acute toxicities often include GI complications such as nausea, vomiting, anorexia, and diarrhea. Allergic reactions and anaphylaxis may also be of immediate concern with selected drugs. Delayed toxicities may develop days to weeks after antineoplastic therapy. Myelosuppression, a common delayed toxicity, can be life-threatening due to the increased incidence of infection associated with leukopenia, increased risk of hemorrhage associated with thrombocytopenia, and anemia. Other important delayed toxicities include tissue damage associated with extravasation of selected drugs, alopecia caused by hair follicle damage, and stomatitis or ulcerative enteritis. Adverse effects on spermatogenesis and teratogenesis may be of concern in breeding animals.

Prevention and management of toxicities is key to successful antineoplastic therapy. Collection of an adequate database before treatment can identify potential problems so that contraindicated drugs can be avoided. Several antineoplastic agents should not be used in the presence of specific organ impairment. For example, doxorubicin should not be used in animals with cardiac abnormalities, and cisplatin is contraindicated in animals with impaired renal function.

When a drug is chosen, supportive or preventive therapy aimed at ameliorating toxic side effects may be required. Concurrent administration of antiemetics may be indicated for acute GI toxicities. Active diuresis should accompany administration of nephrotoxic agents (eg, cisplatin). Administration or availability of appropriate antihistamines may be indicated with L-asparaginase and doxorubicin therapy.

The availability of recombinant products has added an additional resource for managing myelosuppression and immunosuppression induced by antineoplastic chemotherapy. Recombinant human erythropoietin (rhEPO) has been used in treatment of anemia related to chronic malignancy. Recombinant human (rhG-CSF) and canine (rcG-CSF) granulocyte colony-stimulating factor have been used effectively in management of cytopenias induced by chemotherapy and radiation. Administration of rcG-CSF results in a rapid, significant increase in neutrophil numbers that is sustainable as long as the factor is administered. Neutrophil counts drop quickly when therapy is discontinued. Neutrophil phagocytosis, superoxide generation, and antibody-dependent cellular cytotoxicity all increase with G-CSF treatment. A related cytokine, granulocyte-macrophage colony-stimulating factor (GM-CSF), has also shown promise for treatment of neutropenia induced by chemotherapy. Longterm (>2-3 wk) use of recombinant human products in dogs and cats results in anti-factor antibody formation and a decline in cell numbers.

Biologic Response Modifiers in Cancer Therapy: In recent years, a number of alternative modes of cancer therapy have been investigated. Foremost among these has been the development of biologic response modifiers aimed at enhancing innate antitumor defense mechanisms of the host. Nonspecific immunomodulators, including BCG, levamisole, and cimetidine, have been used to enhance immune responsiveness and improve outcomes after surgery or antineoplastic chemotherapy.

Development of lymphokines and cytokines (eg, interleukins, interferon, and tumor necrosis factor) for clinical use in cancer patients has long been an attractive goal. The clinical potential of these potent immunomodulators has not been fully realized, and they are not commonly used in veterinary medicine at this time. An exception to this is the use of selected cytokines (eg, G-CSF) to manage toxic side effects associated with antineoplastic chemotherapy (see above).

Anti-tumor antibody therapy has also been a cancer research focus for several years. Only one monoclonal antibody is approved and marketed for veterinary use—CL/MAb 231 recognizes canine lymphoma cells and is thought to mediate antibody-dependent cellular cytoxicity therapy has prolonged duration of remission when used in combination with chemotherapy.

Safe Handling of Antineoplastic Chemotherapeutic Agents: Most antineoplastic chemotherapeutic agents are potentially toxic as mutagens, teratogens, or carcinogens. Handling of these agents can result in unhealthy personal or environmental exposure in a number of different ways.

A common route of exposure is inhalation due to aerosolization during mixing or administration of cytotoxic drugs. This may occur when a needle is withdrawn from a pressurized drug container or upon expulsion of air from a drug-filled syringe. Transferring drugs between containers, opening drug-filled glass ampules, or crushing or splitting oral medications may also aerosolize drug residues.

The best way to prepare cytotoxic drugs to avoid aerosolization is in a biologic safety cabinet or hood; a Class II, type A vertical laminar air flow hood exhausted outside the building is recommended. If a hood is not available, drugs should be prepared in a specified low-traffic area with proper ventilation where no food, drink, or tobacco products are allowed. This area should be equipped with supplies needed for drug reconstitution, including a disposable, plastic-backed liner for the working surface; latex gloves; gown;

goggles; and mask with a filter. Disposal of contaminated vials, syringes, needles, and gloves in this area should be anticipated, and the proper containers provided. Aerosol exposures can be further decreased through the use of chemotherapy-dispensing pins ("chemo-pins") or hydrophobic filters that limit escape of air from drug vials into the environment.

Another potential route of exposure to antineoplastic agents is by absorption of drug through the skin. This could occur during preparation or administration of drug, cleaning of the drug preparation area, or handling of excreta from animals that have received selected cytotoxic drugs. Most exposure of this type may be avoided by conscientious wearing of latex gloves and careful handling of drug-contaminated needles or catheters. Re-capping of needles containing drug residues is discouraged to avoid accidental self-inoculation.

Finally, antineoplastic agents can be inadvertently ingested if food, drink, or tobacco products are allowed in the vicinity of drug preparation areas, treatment areas, or kennels housing treated animals. Any ingestible materials should be restricted to a separate area that is far enough away to avoid any possible contamination with these agents.

All personnel should handle antineoplastic agents with care. Women of child-bearing age should be particularly cautious, and pregnant women should not handle antineoplastic drugs.

Classification of Antineoplastic Chemotherapeutic Agents: Antineoplastic agents can be grouped by biochemical mechanism of action into the following general categories: alkylating agents, antimetabolites, mitotic inhibitors, antineoplastic antibiotics, hormonal agents, and miscellaneous. The clinically relevant drugs used in veterinary medicine are discussed below and the indications, mechanism of action, and toxicities of selected agents are summarized in TABLE 58.

ALKYLATING AGENTS

Alkylating agents form highly reactive intermediate compounds that are able to transfer alkyl groups to DNA. Alkylation can result in miscoding of DNA strands, incomplete repair of alkylated segments (which leads to strand breakage or depurination), excessive cross-linking of DNA, and inhibition of strand separation at mitosis. Monofunctional alkylating agents transfer a single alkyl group and usually result in miscoding of DNA, strand breakage, or depurination. These reactions can result in cell death, mutagenesis, or carcinogenesis. Polyfunctional alkylating agents typically cause strand cross-linking and inhibition of mitosis with consequent cell death. Resistance to one alkylating agent often implies resistance to other similar drugs and can be caused by increased production of nucleophilic substances that compete with the target DNA for alkylation. Decreased permeation of alkylating agents and increased activity of DNA repair systems are also common mechanisms of resistance.

Individual alkylating agents are generally cell-cycle nonspecific and can be subgrouped according to chemical structure into nitrogen mustards, ethyleneamines, alkyl sulfonates, nitrosoureas, and triazene derivatives.

Nitrogen Mustards: The most common subgroup of alkylating agents used is the nitrogen mustard group. Mechlorethamine hydrochloride is the prototype of the nitrogen mustards and has been used to treat Hodgkin's disease in humans, mycosis fungoides, lymphoreticular neoplasia, and pleural and peritoneal effusions. Because of its highly unstable nature and extremely short duration of action, mechlorethamine is not widely used in veterinary medicine. Derivatives of mechlorethamine that are commonly used include cyclophosphamide, chlorambucil, and less frequently, melphalan.

Cyclophosphamide is a cyclic phosphamide derivative of mechlorethamine that requires metabolic activation by the cytochrome P450 oxidation system in the liver. Cyclophosphamide is given PO or IV, and dose-limiting leukopenia associated with bone marrow suppression is the primary toxicity. Sterile hemorrhagic cystitis caused by acrolein, a metabolite of cyclophosphamide, can develop and should be treated by active diuresis and intravesicular administration of N-acetylcysteine. Mesna, a drug that acts to detoxify metabolites of cyclophosphamide, has been used in human medicine to preclude hemorrhagic cystitis. An analog of cyclophosphamide, ifosfamide, is available but is not currently used as a front-line drug in veterinary medicine.

TABLE 58. Mechanisms of Action, Indications, and Toxicities of Selected Antineoplastic Agents ▶

Drug	Mechanism of Action	Major Indications
Alkylating Agents		
Cyclophosphamide	Undergoes hepatic biotransformation to active metabolites that alkylate DNA; alkylation leads to miscoding of DNA and cross-linking of DNA strands	Lymphoma, sarcomas, mammary adenocarcinoma, lymphocytic leukemia
Melphalan	Alkylates DNA causing miscoding and cross-linking of DNA strands	Multiple myeloma
Chlorambucil	Alkylates DNA causing miscoding and cross-linking of DNA strands; slowest-acting alkylating agent	Chronic lymphocytic leukemia, lymphoma
Carmustine	Alkylates DNA causing miscoding and cross-linking of DNA strands; inhibits both DNA and RNA synthesis; not cross resistant with other alkylating agents	CNS neoplasias (astrocytomas and gliomas), GI carcinomas, multiple myeloma
Streptozocin	Inhibits DNA synthesis; high affinity for pancreatic β cells	Temporary remission of hypoglycemia resulting from functional pancreatic islet cell tumor
Dacarbazine	Undergoes hepatic biotransformation to active metabolites that alkylate DNA; inhibits RNA synthesis	Lymphoma (for use in protocols after relapse)
Busulfan	Alkylates DNA, causing miscoding and cross-linking of DNA strands	Chronic myelogenous leukemia, polycythemia vera
Antimetabolites		
Methotrexate	Inhibition of dihydrofolate reductase that is required for formation of tetrahydrofolate, a necessary cofactor in thymidylate synthesis; thymidylate essential for DNA synthesis and repair	Lymphoma, Sertoli cell tumor, osteosarcoma, metastatic transmissible venereal tumor
5-Fluorouracil	Pyrimidine analog; interferes with DNA synthesis and may be incorporated into RNA to cause toxic effects	GI, lung, liver, and mammary carcinomas (systemic); cutaneous carcinomas (topical)
Cytarabine	Pyrimidine analog; incorporates into DNA causing steric hindrance and inhibition of DNA synthesis	Lymphoma (including CNS), leukemias

◀ **TABLE 58.** (continued)

Acute Toxicities	Delayed Toxicities
Alkylating Agents	
Nausea, vomiting, anorexia	Severe myelosuppression, alopecia, sterile hemorrhagic cystitis
Nausea, vomiting, anorexia (infrequent)	Moderate myelosuppression, alopecia (infrequent)
Nausea, vomiting, anorexia	Moderate myelosuppression
Nausea, vomiting, anorexia	Moderate myelosuppression (may be delayed for 4-6 wk), nephrotoxicity, hepatotoxicity, pulmonary toxicity
Severe, potentially fatal nephrotoxicity and hepatotoxicity; nausea, vomiting, anorexia[*]	Mild myelosuppression, renal toxicity
Nausea, vomiting, anorexia; extravasation results in tissue damage; hepatotoxic	Moderate myelosuppression, alopecia, hepatotoxicity
Nausea, vomiting, anorexia (may be less severe than others in class)	Moderate myelosuppression (may persist for 1-2 yr), pulmonary toxicity
Antimetabolites	
Nausea, vomiting, anorexia; ulceration; stomatitis; hepatotoxicity; pulmonary toxicity	Moderate myelosuppression, alopecia
Systemic: nausea, vomiting, anorexia; GI ulceration; neurotoxicity; hepatotoxicity Topical: local irritation, pain, hyperpigmentation[†]	Moderate myelosuppression, oral and enteric ulcers, neurotoxicity
Nausea, vomiting, anorexia, nephrotoxicity, hepatotoxicity	Moderate myelosuppression, alopecia

(continued)

TABLE 58. Mechanisms of Action, Indications, and Toxicities of Selected Antineoplastic Agents (*continued*) ▶

Drug	Mechanism of Action	Major Indications
Antibiotic Antineoplastics		
Dactinomycin (Actinomycin D)	Intercalates and binds to DNA, disrupting helical structure and DNA template; inhibits RNA and DNA polymerases; causes DNA topoisomerase II-mediated chain scission; generates free radicals that cause DNA scission and cell membrane damage	Choriocarcinoma, testicular carcinoma, rhabdomyosarcoma, lymphoma
Doxorubicin	Intercalates and binds to DNA, disrupting helical structure and DNA template; inhibits RNA and DNA polymerases; causes DNA topoisomerase-II-mediated chain scission; generates free radicals that cause DNA scission and cell membrane damage	Lymphoma, acute lymphocytic and granulocytic leukemia, sarcomas (osteosarcoma, hemangiosarcoma, rhabdomyosarcoma) and carcinomas (mammary, ovarian, small cell lung, thyroid, testicular, prostatic, transitional cell, squamous cell of the head and neck, cervical), plasma cell myeloma, hepatoma, neuroblastoma
Mitoxantrone	Topoisomerase-II-mediated chain scission; DNA aggregation, oxidation, and strand breakage	Lymphoma, carcinomas (squamous cell, transitional cell, mammary, thyroid, renal), fibrosarcoma, hemangiopericytoma
Bleomycin	Mixture of glycopeptides; generates oxygen radicals that cause chain scission and fragmentation of DNA	Carcinomas (testicular, squamous cell of head and neck, cervical, penile) lymphoma, seminoma, malignant teratoma
Mitotic Inhibitors		
Vinblastine	Binds to tubulin, leading to disruption of mitotic spindle apparatus and arrest of cell cycle	Lymphoma and leukemias, mastocytoma
Vincristine	Binds to tubulin, leading to disruption of mitotic spindle apparatus and arrest of cell cycle	Transmissible venereal cell tumors, lymphoma and leukemias, CNS tumors, mast cell tumors, mammary adenocarcinoma, soft-tissue sarcomas, immune-mediated thrombocytopenia
Miscellaneous		
Cisplatin	Reacts with proteins and nucleic acids; forms cross-links between DNA strands and between DNA and protein; disrupts DNA synthesis	Osteosarcoma, carcinomas (transitional cell, testicular, squamous cell of head and neck, ovarian, cervical, bladder, and lung), mesothelioma

◀ **TABLE 58.** (continued)

Acute Toxicities	Delayed Toxicities
Antibiotic Antineoplastics	
Nausea, vomiting, anorexia, phlebitis, severe tissue reaction if extravasated	Severe myelosuppression, alopecia, stomatitis
Nausea, vomiting, anorexia, hemorrhagic colitis, red urine (not hematuria), transient ECG changes, arrhythmias, nephrotoxicity, urticaria, pruritus, anaphylactoid reactions, severe tissue reaction if extravasated	Cumulative, dose-related, digitalis-unresponsive congestive heart failure, severe myelosuppression, alopecia, stomatitis, anorexia and GI irritation, cutaneous reactions
Nausea, vomiting, anorexia, diarrhea, depression, less severe side effects than others in this group	Moderate myelosuppression
Nausea, vomiting, anorexia, fever, allergic reactions including anaphylaxis	Pneumonitis, pulmonary fibrosis, mild myelosuppression, alopecia, hyperpigmentation, skin ulceration, stomatitis
Mitotic Inhibitors	
Mild nausea, vomiting, anorexia, phlebitis, severe tissue reaction if extravasated	Severe myelosuppression, neurotoxicity with high doses, stomatitis, paralytic ileus, alopecia, inappropriate secretion of antidiuretic hormone
Mild nausea, vomiting, anorexia, phlebitis, severe tissue reaction if extravasated	Slowly reversible sensorimotor peripheral neuropathy and muscle weakness, constipation, paralytic ileus, alopecia, inappropriate secretion of antidiuretic hormone, mild myelosuppression
Miscellaneous	
Intense nausea, vomiting, anorexia, diarrhea, anaphylaxis, severe tissue reaction if extravasated	Extreme nephrotoxicity, renal potassium and calcium wasting, ototoxicity, moderate to severe myelosuppression, peripheral neuropathy, hyperuricemia, hypermagnesemia[‡]

(continued)

TABLE 58. Mechanisms of Action, Indications, and Toxicities of Selected Antineoplastic Agents (*continued*) ▶

Drug	Mechanism of Action	Major Indications
Miscellaneous (***continued***)		
L-Asparaginase	Inhibits protein synthesis by hydrolyzing tumor cell supply of asparagine	Acute lymphocytic and lymphoblastic leukemia and lymphoma
Mitotane (o,p'DDD)	Destroys adrenal zona fasciculata and zona reticularis	Pituitary hyperadrenocorticism, palliation of adrenal cortical tumors
Hydroxyurea	Inhibits conversion of ribonucleotides to deoxyribonucleotides by destroying ribonucleoside diphosphate reductase	Polycythemia vera, mastocytoma, granulocytic and basophilic leukemia, thrombocythemia
Etoposide	Causes topoisomerase-II-mediated DNA scission	Carcinomas (testicular, small cell lung)
Hormones		
Prednisolone	Lympholytic; inhibits mitosis in lymphocytes	Lymphoma, mast cell tumors, palliative treatment of brain tumors
Tamoxifen	Anti-estrogenic; blocks the effects of estrogen on target tissues	Estrogen-receptor-positive mammary carcinomas
Flutamide	Anti-androgenic; competes with testosterone for binding to androgen receptors	Testosterone-receptor-positive prostatic tumors; surgical castration preferred
Leuprolide	GnRH analog that initially stimulates, then decreases, the secretion of FSH and LH; reduced FSH and LH lead to decreased concentration of testosterone (males) and estrogen (females)[§]	Testosterone-receptor positive prostatic carcinomas or perianal tumors; surgical castration preferred

[*]Toxicities are so severe that use is very limited.
[†]Topical administration in cats has resulted in fatal neurotoxicity and hepatotoxicity.

Chlorambucil, the slowest-acting nitrogen mustard, achieves effects gradually and often can be used in animals with compromised bone marrow. It can cause bone marrow suppression, but this is usually late in onset and rapidly reversible. This drug is given PO and is most commonly used in treatment of chronic, well-differentiated cancers; it is considered ineffective in rapidly proliferating tumors.

Melphalan, an L-phenylalanine derivative of mechlorethamine, is given PO or IV and is primarily used in veterinary medicine to treat multiple myeloma.

Other Alkylating Agents: Of the other subgroups of alkylating agents, several have limited but specific uses. **Triethylenethiophosphoramide**, an ethylenimine, may be used intravesicularly in the treatment of transitional cell carcinoma of the bladder or as an intracavitary treatment for pleural and peritoneal effusions. **Busulfan**, an alkyl

◀ **TABLE 58.** *(continued)*

Acute Toxicities	Delayed Toxicities
Miscellaneous (continued)	
Nausea, vomiting, anorexia, abdominal pain, hypersensitivity reactions, anaphylaxis especially after repeated doses	Hepatotoxicity, nephrotoxicity, pancreatitis, CNS effects, inhibition of coagulation and immune responsiveness (B and T cells), mild myelosuppression
Nausea, vomiting, anorexia, diarrhea	Adrenal insufficiency, CNS depression, dermatitis
Nausea, vomiting, anorexia	Mild myelosuppression, alopecia, sloughing of claws, stomatitis, dysuria
Nausea, vomiting, anorexia, diarrhea, hypotension, anaphylaxis, cutaneous reactions, fever	Myelosuppression, peripheral neuropathy, allergic reactions, hepatotoxicity, alopecia
Hormones	
Sodium retention, GI ulceration, pancreatitis	Protein catabolism, muscle wasting, delayed wound healing, suppression of hypothalamic-pituitary-adrenal axis, immunosuppression
Vomiting, abnormalities in estrous cycle	—
—	—
—	—

[‡]Severe, potentially fatal pulmonary edema may develop in cats.
[§]GnRH = gonadotropin-release hormone, FSH = follicle-stimulate hormone, LH = luteinizing hormone

sulfonate, is used specifically in the treatment of chronic myelocytic leukemia and polycythemia vera. **Streptozotocin,** a naturally occurring nitrosourea, is used for palliation of malignant pancreatic islet-cell tumors or insulinomas. Other nitrosoureas, **carmustine** and **lomustine,** readily cross the blood-brain barrier and have been useful in management of CNS neoplasias. **Dacarbazine,** a triazene derivative, has been used in combination with doxorubicin for treatment of relapsed canine lymphoma.

ANTIMETABOLITES

Antimetabolites resemble normal cellular metabolites and so can subvert normal metabolic pathways in a toxic manner. Three subgroups of antimetabolites are used—folic acid, pyrimidine, and purine analogs.

Folic Acid Analogs: The prototype folic acid analog is methotrexate, an inhibitor of dihydrofolate reductase, the enzyme that catalyzes conversion of folic acid to tetrahydrofolate. Tetrahydrofolate deficiency blocks reactions requiring folate coenzymes, disrupting both DNA and RNA synthesis. Methotrexate is an S phase-specific drug that must be actively transported across cell membranes. It can be given PO, IV, or IM. Methotrexate is excreted in the urine and at high doses may precipitate in renal tubules. Folinic acid can be used to bypass the metabolic blockade produced by folic acid analogs and thus result in rescue of treated cells. Because tumor cells appear less efficient at transport of folinic acid, some degree of selectivity is achieved in the rescue. Resistance to methotrexate may develop due to impaired transport of the drug into cells, production of altered forms, or increased concentrations of dihydrofolate reductase.

Pyrimidine Analogs: Two pyrimidine analogs, 5-fluorouracil and cytarabine, are commonly used. **5-Fluorouracil** must be converted to an active 5-fluoro-2'-deoxyuridine-5'-phosphate form to bind the enzyme thymidylate synthetase and block or inhibit DNA and RNA synthesis. This drug is considered S phase-specific. It is used IV but is also available for topical use. Metabolism is via the liver, and the drug readily enters CSF. Occasional CNS reactions have been reported in dogs, and severe irreversible neurotoxicity and sudden death have been described in cats. Although 5-fluorouracil is thought to be effective in treatment of squamous cell carcinoma in cats, toxicity appears to preclude its use in this species. Resistance may develop by decreased activation of the drug or acquisition of altered thymidylate synthetase that is not inhibited.

Cytarabine (cytosine arabinoside) is an analog of 2'-deoxycytidine and must be activated by conversion to a 5'-monophosphate nucleotide. The nucleotide analog, AraCTP, inhibits DNA synthesis by substitution of arabinose for deoxyribose in the sugar moiety of DNA; cytarabine may also inhibit DNA repair enzymes. This drug is S phase-specific, and its effectiveness is directly proportional to exposure of cells to the drug; continuous infusion or repeated injections are usually required. Inhibition of conversion to AraCTP or increased degradation of AraCTP can account for development of resistance.

Purine Analogs: Two purine analogs, **6-mercaptopurine** (6-MP) and **6-thioguanine** (6-TG), are used occasionally. 6-MP is a sulfhydryl-substituted analog of hypoxanthine that must be converted to an active form by hypoxanthine-guanine phosphoribosyltransferase (HGPRT). The active drug inhibits synthesis and metabolism of purine nucleotides and thus disrupts synthesis and function of DNA and RNA. This S phase-specific drug can be administered PO or IV and undergoes rapid metabolic degradation and some renal excretion. Bone marrow suppression is gradual and infrequent with 6-MP; acute GI disturbances are also infrequent but do occur. Resistance may develop by diminished activation of the drug by HGPRT. 6-MP may be used to maintain remission in acute lymphocytic leukemia and has been used to treat granulocytic leukemia.

6-TG is a sulfhydryl-substituted analog of guanine and, like 6-MP, is converted by HGPRT to an active form capable of altering synthesis and metabolism of purine nucleotides and synthesis and function of DNA and RNA. 6-TG is also an S phase-specific drug. It is given PO and has side effects and mechanisms of resistance similar to those of 6-MP, except that leukopenia may be more severe and GI disturbances less common. 6-TG may be used to treat acute lymphocytic and granulocytic leukemia.

MITOTIC INHIBITORS

Vinca Alkaloids: The vinca alkaloids are large, complex molecules derived from the periwinkle plant. Binding to tubulin, the major component of cellular microtubules, accounts for the antineoplastic effects of these drugs. Vinca alkaloids inhibit microtubule polymerization and increase microtubule disassembly. The mitotic spindle apparatus is disrupted, and segregation of chromosomes in metaphase is arrested. These effects account for the primary M-phase action of vinca alkaloids, although other antitubulin effects related to cytoskeletal maintenance and protein trafficking may be seen. The 2 drugs of importance in this class are **vincristine** and **vinblastine**. Both are given IV, and both cause severe local vesication if injected perivascularly. Drug extravasation may cause deep, indolent ulceration and exposure of underlying tendons and bone. The vinca alkaloids are metabolized primarily in the liver but may be partially excreted in an unchanged form in the urine. Although vinca alkaloids are related structurally, resistance to one does not imply resistance to all drugs in this category. Vincristine use is limited by neurologic toxicity that may include a slowly reversible sensorimotor peripheral neuropathy and muscle weakness. In comparison, the dose-limiting toxicity associated with vinblastine is related to myelosuppression and leukopenia; neurologic toxicity develops only at high doses.

Taxanes: Paclitaxel and **docetaxel** are antimicrotubule agents extracted from the Pacific and European yew trees, respectively. Taxanes bind to tubulin subunits, enhance microtubule polymerization, and inhibit microtubule depolymerization. Formation of stable microtubule bundles disrupts tubulin equilibrium and blocks normal progression through the cell cycle. These agents are actively used in human medicine and are being investigated for use in treatment of lymphoma and mammary carcinoma in veterinary medicine. Myelosuppression, anaphylactoid reactions (probably related to the drug vehicle), and GI effects (diarrhea, mucosal ulceration, and emesis) have been reported in dogs treated with paclitaxel.

ANTINEOPLASTIC ANTIBIOTICS

The antineoplastic antibiotics are products of *Streptomyces*. The important drugs in this group include actinomycin D (dactinomycin), doxorubicin, mitoxantrone, and bleomycin. Drugs less commonly used include daunorubicin, mithramycin, and mitomycin.

Actinomycin A was the first *Streptomyces* antibiotic isolated and was followed by related antibiotics, including actinomycin D. Actinomycin D binds with double-stranded DNA and blocks the action of RNA polymerase, which prevents DNA transcription. Actinomycin D is considered cell-cycle nonspecific and is given IV but does not cross the blood-brain barrier. Resistance may develop due to decreased cellular uptake of the drug.

The anthracycline antibiotics, daunorubicin and doxorubicin, have become important antineoplastic antibiotics. These drugs intercalate and bind to DNA between base pairs on adjacent strands. This causes the DNA helix to uncoil, which destroys the DNA template and inhibits RNA and DNA polymerases. Scission of DNA is thought to be mediated by either the enzyme topoisomerase II or by generation of free radicals. Intracellular interactions of anthracycline antibiotics result in the formation of semiquinone radical intermediates capable of generating hydrogen peroxide and hydroxyl radicals. Considered cell-cycle nonspecific because of the damage associated with radical formation, these drugs probably have their maximal effect during the S phase of the cell cycle. The anthracycline antibiotics are given IV; they are severe vesicants if administered perivascularly and may cause a severe, delayed phlebitis. Urticaria may be seen in the area of the injection and, shortly after administration, erythematous areas may appear along the vein. Recurrence of this response may be prevented by premedication with corticosteroids and antihistamines. The anthracycline antibiotics are metabolized in the liver to a variety of less active and inactive products.

Doxorubicin toxicity can be manifested in a variety of acute and delayed reactions. Delayed toxicities can be severe, with the major problem being cumulative, dose-related, cardiac toxicity associated with binding of the drug to cardiac DNA and free radical damage to myocardial membranes. A nonspecific decrease in cardiac fibrils occurs, which leads to congestive heart failure that is unresponsive to digitalis. A dose-limiting toxicity of doxorubicin is severe myelosuppression. If doxorubicin is used in conjunction with radiation therapy, damage by radiation may be augmented. This radiation recall effect may necessitate reduction in radiation or drug dosages, or both. Because of the significant toxicity associated with the use of doxorubicin, newer-generation drugs specifically aimed at reduction of cardiac toxicity have been developed and are available in human medicine. Two of these, idarubicin and epirubicin, have been studied, but neither is in common use in veterinary medicine.

Mitoxantrone, an anthracenedione related to the anthracycline antibiotics, has shown promise in veterinary medicine for treatment of lymphoma and various carcinomas. The mechanism of action of mitoxanthrone is similar to that of the anthracyclines, but side effects are less severe than those of doxorubicin.

Bleomycin is actually a mixture of bleomycin glycopeptides that differ only in their terminal amine moiety. The cytotoxic action of these glycopeptides depends on their ability to cause chain scission and fragmentation of DNA molecules. Cells accumulate in the G_2 phase of the cell cycle, which accounts for the classification of bleomycin as a G_2 and M phase-specific agent. Bleomycin may also affect DNA repair enzymes. Given IV or SC, bleomycin does not cross the blood-brain barrier; a large portion is excreted via the kidneys. Bleomycin has minimal myelosuppressive and immunosuppressive activities but does have an unusual delayed pulmonary toxicity. Pulmonary toxicity may begin as a nonspecific pneumonitis that progresses to pulmonary fibrosis. Dangers from pulmonary complications are especially important in older animals with preexisting pulmonary disease.

HORMONAL AGENTS

Hormonal therapy for neoplasia commonly involves the use of glucocorticoids. Direct antitumor effects are related to their lympholytic properties; glucocorticoids can inhibit mitosis, RNA synthesis, and protein synthesis in sensitive lymphocytes. Glucocorticoids are considered cell-cycle nonspecific and are often used in chemotherapeutic protocols after induction by another agent. Unfortunately, resistance to a given glucocorticoid may develop rapidly and typically extends to other glucocorticoids. Toxic effects of glucocorticoid therapy can include peptic ulceration, glucose intolerance, polydipsia and polyuria, immunosuppression, necrotizing pancreatitis, osteoporosis, hypokalemia, cataracts, muscle atrophy, and Cushing's disease. Prednisone and prednisolone are commonly used to treat lymphoreticular neoplasms in combination with other drugs. Because they readily enter the CSF, dexamethasone, prednisone, and prednisolone are especially useful in treatment of leukemias and lymphomas of the CNS.

Indirect benefits of glucocorticoid therapy in cancer include symptomatic improvements in appetite and attitude, suppression of noninfectious fevers, management of hypercalcemia of malignancy, and relief of edema associated with spinal cord and brain tumors. However, evidence from several sources suggests that treatment of certain lymphomas with prednisone may increase resistance of neoplastic cells to subsequent cycles of antineoplastic chemotherapy.

Estrogen has also been used in antineoplastic therapy, but complications can be severe. Toxicities have effectively eliminated the use of estrogen in veterinary cancer therapy. Complications of estrogen therapy can include life-threatening myelosuppression, aplastic anemia, and thrombocytopenia. Anti-estrogen therapy with drugs such as tamoxifen may also be used in estrogen-receptor-positive mammary carcinomas to block growth-stimulatory hormonal activities in these cells. In addition, anti-estrogens have been used in the treatment of endometrial carcinomas.

Progestins have been used to oppose growth stimulatory effects of hormones in endometrial, prostatic, breast, renal cell, and ovarian carcinomas. Toxic side effects of the progestins include fluid retention, hypercalcemia, thromboembolism, and cholestatic jaundice.

Anti-androgens, such as **flutamide**, have been used experimentally in the treatment of prostatic and perianal neoplasia. Leuprolide, an analog of gonadotropin-releasing hormone (GnRH) initially stimulates, then decreases the secretion of follicle-stimulating hormone (FSH) and leuteinizing hormone (LH). Reduced FSH and LH lead to decreased concentration of testosterone in males and estrogen in females. Leuprolide has been used in the treatment of testosterone-receptor-positive prostatic carcinomas and perianal tumors. In veterinary medicine, surgical castration is the treatment of choice for testosterone-responsive neoplasias.

MISCELLANEOUS ANTINEOPLASTIC AGENTS

Several drugs used as antineoplastics do not fall into any of the categories mentioned thus far. These include L-asparaginase, cisplatin, mitotane (o,p′DDD), hydroxyurea, etoposide, and piroxicam.

L-Asparaginase is an enzyme derived from *Escherichia coli* that catalyzes hydrolysis of asparagine. Because some tumor cells are unable to produce asparagine, treatment with this drug deprives these cells of exogenously supplied asparagine and ultimately limits protein synthesis. Because protein synthesis is active in the G_1 phase of the cell cycle, L-asparaginase is considered to be a G_1 phase-specific drug. L-Asparaginase may be given IV, SC, IM, or by intraperitoneal injection. Anaphylaxis on repeated administration of L-asparaginase may occur as a result of host anti-asparaginase antibody production; pretreatment of animals with antihistamine helps prevent this acute toxic reaction. Anti-asparaginase antibody production may also account for the development of tumor resistance, as can a decreased tumor cell requirement for asparagine. A related drug, pegaspargase, is modified from L-asparaginase by covalent modification with monomethoxypolyethylene glycol. The conjugated drug produces fewer hypersensitivity reactions than does L-asparaginase.

Cisplatin (cis-diamine-dichloroplatinum) functions primarily as a bifunctional alkylator but is included in the miscellaneous category because of its unusual structure. It is a platinum ion complexed to 2 chloride ions and 2 ammonium molecules. Cisplatin causes inter- and intrastrand DNA cross-linking that disrupts DNA helices and prevents DNA synthesis. Cisplatin is cell-cycle nonspecific and is administered by IV drip in combination with fluids and mannitol to promote diuresis. Excretion is prolonged, with up to 50% of a dose still present in the body 5 days after administration. Extreme, dose-limiting, proximal tubular renal necrosis typifies the delayed side effects of cisplatin along with other responses that may include ototoxicity, moderate to severe bone marrow suppression, peripheral neuropathy, and renal potassium and magnesium wasting. Because of the extreme toxic adverse effects of cisplatin, newer generation derivatives such as carboplatin and iproplatin have been developed. Carboplatin is effective as an adjunct to surgery for treatment of osteosarcoma. Nausea and vomiting are less severe than with cisplatin, and carboplatin is not considered nephrotoxic. It is, however, myelosuppressive, with neutropenia being the dose-limiting toxicity. Carboplatin is considered safe for administration to cats.

Mitotane (o,p'DDD), a derivative of the insecticides DDT and DDD, causes selective destruction of normal and neoplastic adrenal cortical cells. Mitotane may act by inhibiting production of steroids induced by adrenocorticotropic hormone, which causes atrophy of the inner zones of the adrenal cortex. Mitotane is administered PO, and plasma concentrations can be detected for several weeks.

Hydroxyurea, a simple hydroxylated derivative of urea, is most commonly used in the treatment of polycythemia vera. Hydroxyurea inhibits ribonucleoside diphosphate reductase (RNDR), limits the conversion of ribonucleotides to deoxyribonucleotides, and blocks DNA synthesis. Cells are arrested in the G_1-S interface. Mechanisms of resistance include amplification of the RNDR gene or development of RNDR with reduced sensitivity to hydroxyurea. Painful loss of claws has been associated with hydroxyurea use in animals.

Epipodophyllotoxins are semisynthetic glycosides of podophyllotoxin derived from the mandrake plant. Although these toxins bind tubulin, their mechanism of action is unrelated to disruption of microtubules. Instead, they are thought to stimulate DNA cleavage mediated by topoisomerase II. Of the 2 drugs in this class, etoposide and teniposide, the former has been used primarily in the treatment of testicular carcinoma.

Piroxicam, an NSAID, has been used in treatment of transitional cell carcinoma. Like that of other NSAID, reported anti-tumor activity of piroxicam is not considered a result of direct cytotoxicity.

TREATMENT OF CANINE LYMPHOMA

Lymphoma (also referred to as lymphosarcoma) is the canine tumor most frequently treated with chemotherapy. It is the most common hematopoietic neoplasia of dogs and cats and is also among the most responsive to chemotherapy. Three antineoplastic agents, vincristine, cyclophosphamide, and prednisone, form the basis for many lymphoma treatment protocols. Treatments based on these 3 drugs, plus or minus additional drugs, are often abbreviated as COP or COP plus the additional drug (TABLE 59). Information in TABLE 59 is intended to provide a typical treatment approach, bearing in mind that

TABLE 59. Chemotherapy Protocols for Treatment of Canine Lymphoma[*]

Protocol	Drug	Dosage	Schedule
COP			
Induction	Vincristine	0.5-0.7 mg/m^2, IV	Day 1 of each week
		50 mg/m^2, PO, SID	Days 4-7 of each week
	Prednisone	20 mg/m^2, PO, BID	For 6 consecutive wk
Maintenance	Methotrexate	5 mg/m^2, PO, SID	Days 1 and 5 of each week
	Cyclophosphamide	100 mg/m^2, PO, SID	Day 3 of each week
	Prednisone	20 mg/m^2, PO, every other day	For 6 consecutive wk
COPLA			
Induction	L-Asparaginase	10,000 IU/m^2, SC	Day 1 of weeks 1 and 2
	Vincristine	0.5-0.7 mg/m^2, IV, every other day	Day 1 of each week for 8 wk
	Cyclophosphamide	50 mg/m^2, PO, every other day	For 8 wk
	Prednisone	20 mg/m^2, PO, SID	For 1st week, then every other day for 2-5 wk, then 10 mg/m^2, PO, every other day for weeks 6-12
	Doxorubicin	30 mg/m^2, IV, for dogs >10 kg; 1 mg/kg for dogs <10 kg	Given day 1 on weeks 6, 9, 12
Maintenance	Vincristine	0.5-0.7 mg/m^2, IV	Day 1 every other week for 2 times, then day 1 every 3rd week for 3 times, then day 1 every 4th week for 4 times, then day 1 every 6th week for 1 yr
	Chlorambucil	4 mg/m^2, PO, every other day	Start on week 9 and continue for up to 2 yr if complete remission maintained
Single Agent Doxorubicin			
	Doxorubicin	30 mg/m^2, IV, for dogs >10 kg; 1 mg/kg for dogs <10kg	Given as bolus with 5% dextrose and water drip on day 1 every 3 wk for 4-6 treatments

[*]Adapted, with permission, from Hahn, K.A. Lymphoma: good cop, bad cop. In: *Proceedings of the 20th Forum of the American College of Veterinary Internal Medicine*, 2002, p 45.

there are nearly 40 published protocols for the management of lymphoma in dogs. Likewise, COP provides the basis for most lymphoma chemotherapy protocols in cats. In general, fewer studies document the clinical effectiveness of various COP combinations in cats than in dogs.

ANTISEPTICS AND DISINFECTANTS

Antiseptics and disinfectants are nonselective, anti-infective agents that are applied topically. Their activity ranges from simply reducing the number of microorganisms to within safe limits of public health interpretations (sanitization), to destroying all microbes (sterilization) on the applied surface. In general, antiseptics are applied on tissues to suppress or prevent microbial infection. Disinfectants are germicidal compounds usually applied to inanimate surfaces. Sometimes the same compound may act as an antiseptic or as a disinfectant, depending on the drug concentration, conditions of exposure, number of organisms, etc. To achieve maximal efficiency, it is essential to use the proper concentration of the drug for the purpose intended. The logic that "if a little is good, twice as much is better" is not only uneconomical but often has toxicologic implications.

Topical anti-infective agents are extensively used in surgery for antisepsis of the surgical site and surgeon's hands and to disinfect surgical instruments, apparel, and hospital premises. Other common uses are as disinfectants for home and farm premises, food processing facilities, in water treatment, in public health sanitation, and as antiseptics in soaps, teat dips, dairy sanitizers, etc. Antiseptics also have been used for treating local infections. However, in most cases, systemic chemotherapeutic agents are preferred because they often penetrate better into the foci of infection and are less likely than the topical anti-infectives to lose their potency when in contact with body fluids and debris in the infected area.

Ideally, antiseptics and disinfectants should have a broad spectrum and potent germicidal activity, with rapid onset and long-lasting effect. They should withstand a range of environmental factors (eg, pH, temperature, humidity) and must retain activity even in the presence of pus, necrotic tissue, soil, and other organic material. High lipid solubility and good dispersibility increase their effectiveness. Antiseptic preparations should not be toxic to the host tissues and should not impair healing. Disinfectants should be nondestructive to applied surfaces. Offensive odor, color, and staining properties should be absent or minimal.

Most of these compounds exert their antimicrobial effect by denaturation of intracellular protein, alteration of cellular membranes (often through extraction of membrane lipids), or enzyme inhibition.

Acids and Alkalies

Acids: Hydrogen ion is bacteriostatic at pH ~3-6 and bactericidal at pH <3. Strong mineral acids (HCl, H_2SO_4, etc) in concentrations of 0.1-1 N have been used as disinfectants; however, their corrosive action limits their usefulness. Un-ionized weak organic acids can readily penetrate and disrupt bacterial cell membranes. Acids are used as food preservatives (eg, benzoic acid), antiseptics (eg, boric acid, acetic acid), fungicides (eg, salicyclic acid, benzoic acid), spermatocides (eg, acetic acid, lactic acid), and cauterizing agents (strong mineral acids).

Acetic acid, 1%, can be used in surgical dressings, and 0.25% acetic acid is a useful antibacterial agent for irrigation of the urinary tract. At 5%, it is bactericidal to many bacteria and has been used to treat otitis externa produced by *Pseudomonas*, *Candida*, *Malassezia*, or *Aspergillus* spp. Skin and hides that have been contaminated by anthrax spores can be disinfected with 2.5% HCl.

Alkalies: Hydroxyl ion also exerts antimicrobial activity. At a pH >9, it inhibits most bacteria and many viruses. Hydroxides of sodium and calcium are used as disinfectants. Their irritant or caustic property usually precludes their application on tissues.

A 2% solution of soda lye (contains 94% sodium hydroxide [NaOH]) in hot water is used as a disinfectant against many common pathogens, such as those causing fowl cholera and pullorum disease. It is a potent caustic and must be handled with care.

Calcium oxide (CaO), ie, lime (hydrated or air-slaked lime), soaked in water produces $Ca(OH)_2$. Aqueous suspensions of slaked lime are used to disinfect premises.

Alcohols

Primary aliphatic alcohols are germicidal. Their potency increases but water solubility decreases with chain length until amyl alcohol (6 carbons) is reached. Antimicrobial effect is related to their lipid solubility (damages bacterial membranes) and their ability to precipitate cytoplasmic proteins. However, they do not destroy bacterial spores. Ethyl alcohol (ethanol) and isopropyl alcohol (isopropanol) are the most widely used alcohols. They can be used in concentrations of 30-90% in aqueous solutions; best results are usually obtained with 70% ethanol or 50% isopropanol. Higher concentrations tend to be less effective. Isopropanol is slightly more potent than ethanol due to its greater depression of surface tension. "Rubbing alcohol" is a mixture of alcohols, with isopropanol as its principal ingredient. It is used as a skin disinfectant and rubefacient. Alcohol-based hand rinses have rapid-acting antiseptic effects. This makes them useful in minimizing the transmission of transient flora acquired from infected patients and reducing nosocomial diseases.

Biguanides

Chlorhexidine is the most popular antiseptic of this group. It has potent antimicrobial activity against most gram-positive and some gram-negative bacteria but not against spores. A 0.1% aqueous solution is bactericidal against *Staphylococcus aureus*, *Escherichia coli*, and *Pseudomonas aeruginosa* in 15 sec. However, it is relatively ineffective against other gram-negative organisms, spores, fungi, and most viruses. Nosocomial infections by *Pseudomonas* spp have developed from the use of contaminated chlorhexidine solutions in which the bacteria persisted. In susceptible organisms, chlorhexidine disrupts the cytoplasmic membrane. Its activity is unaffected or enhanced by alcohols, quaternary ammonium compounds, and alkaline pH, and is somewhat depressed by high concentrations of organic matter (pus, blood, etc), hard water, and contact with cork. It is incompatible with anionic compounds, including soap. It is one of the most commonly used surgical and dental antiseptics. A 4% emulsion of chlorhexidine gluconate is used as a skin cleanser, a 0.5% (w/v) solution in 70% isopropanol as a general antiseptic, and a 0.5% solution in 70% isopropanol with emollients as a hand rinse. Chlorhexidine soaps have good residual activity, which may be advantageous when applied as a presurgical scrub for prolonged surgical procedures. Chlorhexidine-alcohol mixtures are particularly effective in that they combine the antiseptic rapidity of alcohol with the persistence of chlorhexidine. Because of its antiseptic properties and low potential for systemic or dermal toxicity, chlorhexidine has been incorporated into shampoos, ointments, skin and wound cleansers, teat dips, surgical scrubs, etc. A 1% chlorhexidine acetate ointment is used as a topical antiseptic in treatment of external wounds in dogs, cats, and horses.

Oxidizing Agents

Peroxides: These compounds generally exert a short-acting germicidal effect on most organisms through release of nascent oxygen, which irreversibly alters microbial proteins. Most have little or no action on bacterial spores. Nascent oxygen is rendered inactive when it combines with organic matter.

Hydrogen peroxide solution (3%) liberates oxygen when in contact with catalase present on wound surfaces and mucous membranes. The effervescent action mechanically helps remove pus and cellular debris from wounds and is valuable for cleaning and deodorizing infected tissue. However, the antimicrobial action is of short duration and is limited to the superficial layer of the applied surface because there is no penetration of the tissue. Although its usefulness as an antiseptic is limited, hydrogen peroxide is finding increased application as a disinfectant in water treatment and food processing facilities and for sterilization of dental and surgical instruments.

Peracetic acid has been recognized only recently as a useful sterilant and antiseptic, combining the broad antimicrobial spectrum and lack of harmful decomposition products of hydrogen peroxide with greater lipid solubility and freedom from inactivation by tissue catalase and peroxidase. It has been accepted worldwide in the food industry, including meat and poultry processing plants and dairies. It is effective against bacteria, yeasts, fungi, and viruses at concentrations of 0.001-0.003% and is sporicidal at 0.25-0.5%. Solutions of 0.2% peracetic acid applied to compresses are effective at reducing microbial populations in severely contaminated wounds.

Sodium perborate, used in antiseptic solutions and in mouthwashes, acts by decomposing into sodium metaborate and hydrogen peroxide, which then gradually liberates oxygen.

Benzoyl peroxide slowly releases oxygen to act as an antiseptic. However, it can cause skin irritation. It also has keratolytic and antiseborrheic activity, which makes it useful in treating pyoderma in dogs.

Potassium permanganate has broad antimicrobial properties, but its intense purple color in solution, which stains tissues and clothing brown, is a disadvantage. It is an effective algicide (0.01%) and virucide (1%) for disinfection, but concentrations >1:10,000 tend to irritate tissues. Old solutions turn chocolate brown and lose their activity.

Halogens and Halogen-containing Compounds: Iodine and chlorine are used as topical antimicrobial agents. They owe their activity to high affinity for protoplasm, where they are believed to oxidize proteins and interfere with vital metabolic reactions.

Iodine: Elemental iodine is a potent germicide with a wide spectrum of activity and low toxicity to tissues. A solution containing 50 ppm iodine kills bacteria in 1 min and spores in 15 min. It is poorly soluble in water but readily dissolves in ethanol, which enhances its antibacterial activity.

Iodine tincture contains 2% iodine and 2.4% sodium iodide (NaI) dissolved in 50% ethanol; it is used as a skin disinfectant. Strong iodine tincture contains 7% iodine and 5% potassium iodide (KI) dissolved in 95% ethanol; it is more potent but also more irritating than tincture of iodine. Iodine solution contains 2% iodine and 2.4% NaI dissolved in aqueous solution; it is used as a nonirritant antiseptic on wounds and abrasions. Strong iodine solution (Lugol's solution) contains 5% iodine and 10% KI in aqueous solution.

Iodophores (eg, povidone-iodine) are water-soluble combinations of iodine with detergents, wetting agents that are solubilizers, and other carriers. They slowly release iodine as an antimicrobial agent and are widely used as skin disinfectants, particularly before surgery. They do not sting or stain. They are nontoxic to tissues but may be corrosive to metals. They are effective against bacteria, viruses, and fungi but less so against spores. Iodophor solutions retain good antibacterial activity at pH <4, even in the presence of organic matter, and often change color when the activity is lost. Phosphoric acid is often mixed with iodophores to maintain an acidic medium. They have been used in teat dips to control mastitis, as dairy sanitizers, and as a general antiseptic or disinfectant for various dermal and mucosal infections.

Chlorine: Chlorine exerts a potent germicidal effect against most bacteria, viruses, protozoa, and fungi through formation of undissociated hypochlorous acid (HOCl) in water at acid to neutral pH. It is effective against most organisms at a concentration of 0.1 ppm, but much higher concentrations are required in the presence of organic matter. Alkaline pH ionizes chlorine and decreases its activity by reducing its penetrability. Chlorine has a strong acid smell and is irritant to the skin and mucous membranes. It is widely used to disinfect water supplies and inanimate objects (eg, utensils, bottles, pipelines) in dairies, creameries, and milk houses.

Inorganic chlorides include sodium hypochlorite solutions (bleach). A 5% NaOCl solution decomposes on exposure to light. A 2-5% NaOCl solution can be used as a disinfectant, and a more diluted form (0.5%) can be used for irrigating suppurating wounds, but it dissolves blood clots and delays clotting. Calcium hypochlorite is used as a disinfectant.

Organic chlorides contain chlorine weakly bonded to nitrogen, which is slowly released for germicidal activity. They are generally less irritant, more stable, and more convenient to use than hypochlorite solutions.

Metals

Mercuric bichloride, one of the early antiseptics, was later replaced by the less irritant and less toxic organic mercurials, eg, merbromin, thimerosal, nitromersol, and phenylmercuric nitrate. At moderate concentrations, the organic mercurials are bacteriostatic and act by inhibiting bacterial enzymes through their affinity for sulfhydryl groups. This effect can be reversed by sulfur-containing compounds, eg, cysteine or glutathione. Mercurials are not effective against spores. Use of mercurial antiseptics or disinfectants has decreased, due, in part, to their environmental persistence and contaminant potential.

Silver compounds can have caustic, astringent, and antibacterial effects. Silver ions combine with sulfhydryl, amino, phosphate, and carboxyl groups, and thus precipitate proteins, in addition to interfering with essential metabolic activities of microbial cells.

A 0.1% aqueous silver solution is bactericidal and somewhat irritating, whereas a 0.01% solution is bacteriostatic. A 0.5% solution is sometimes applied as a dressing on burns to reduce infection and induce rapid eschar formation. Colloidal silver compounds, which release silver ions slowly, are bacteriostatic and have a more sustained effect. They do not irritate the tissues and have little astringent or caustic effect. They are generally used as mild antiseptics and in ophthalmic preparations.

Phenols and Related Compounds

Phenolic compounds used as antiseptics or disinfectants include pure phenol and substitution products with halogens and alkyl groups. They act to denature proteins and are general protoplasmic poisons.

Phenol (carbolic acid) is bacteriostatic at concentrations of 0.1-1% and is bactericidal/fungicidal at 1-2%. A 5% solution kills anthrax spores in 48 hr. The bactericidal activity is enhanced by ethylenediamine tetraacetic acid (EDTA) and warm temperatures and decreased by alkaline medium (through ionization), lipids, soaps, and cold temperatures. Concentrations >0.5% exert a local anesthetic effect, whereas a 5% solution is strongly irritating and corrosive to tissues. Oral ingestion or extensive application to skin can cause systemic toxicity, manifested primarily by CNS and cardiovascular effects; death may result.

Phenol has good penetrating power into organic matter and is mainly used for disinfection of equipment or organic materials that are to be destroyed (eg, infected food and excreta). Because of its irritant and corrosive properties and potential systemic toxicity, it is not used much as an antiseptic except to cauterize infected areas, eg, infected umbilicus of neonates. It is also incorporated into cutaneous applications for pruritus, stings, bites, burns, etc, because of its local anesthetic and antibacterial properties to relieve itching and control infections.

Cresol (cresylic acid) is a mixture of ortho-, meta-, and paracresols and their isomers. It is a colorless liquid; however, after exposure to light and air, it turns pink, then yellowish, and finally dark brown. A 2% solution of either pure or saponated cresol "lysol" in hot water is commonly used as a disinfectant for inanimate objects.

Hexachlorophene has a strong bacteriostatic action against many gram-positive organisms (including staphylococci) but only a few gram-negative ones. It is used widely in medicated soaps. Frequent washings every day with hexachlorophene soaps lead to sufficient retention of residue on the skin to provide prolonged bacteriostatic action. Washing with other soaps promptly removes these residues. Repeated exposure of skin to high concentrations of hexachlorophene may lead to sufficient absorption of the antiseptic to cause spongiform degeneration of the white matter in the brain and cause nervous disorders. To prevent such neurotoxicity, products containing >0.75% hexachlorophene are available only by prescription. Accidental oral ingestion of hexachlorophene results in acute poisoning.

Pine tar is a viscid blackish brown liquid, used primarily for antiseptic bandaging of wounds of the hoof and horn. Pine tar contains phenol derivatives that provide antimicrobial properties.

Chloroxylenols are broad-spectrum bactericides with more activity against gram-positive than gram-negative bacteria. They are active in alkaline pH; however, contact with organic matter diminishes their activity. Streptococci are more suscepti- ble than staphylococci. **Parachlorometaxylenol (PCMX)** and **dichlorometaxyle- nol (DCMX)** are the 2 most commonly used members of this group. DCMX is more active than PCMX. Strong solutions of these compounds can cause irritation and have a disagreeable odor. A 5% chloroxylenol (eg, PCMX) solution (in α-terpineol, soap, alcohol, and water) is diluted with water (1:4) for skin sterilization and (1:25 to 1:50) for wound cleansing and irrigation of the uterus and vagina. PCMX is also combined with hexachlorophene to enhance its antibacterial spectrum and to prevent contami- nation by gram-negative organisms.

Reducing Agents

Formaldehyde is a gas, whereas **glutaraldehyde** is an oil at room temperature. However, both are readily soluble in water. Their solutions are irritating or caustic to tissues but have potent germicidal properties against all organisms, including spores. Their solutions do not lose appreciable antimicrobial properties in the presence of or- ganic matter and are noncorrosive to metals, paints, and fabric. Both are used as disin- fectants. **Formalin** contains 37% formaldehyde gas in aqueous solution with variable amounts of methyl alcohol to prevent polymerization. A 1-10% solution of formaldehyde is commonly used as a disinfectant. Glutaral (glutaraldehyde), a 1-2% alkaline solution (pH 7.5-8.5) in 70% isopropanol, is a more potent germicide than 4% formaldehyde. It is often used to sterilize surgical and endoscopic instruments and plastic and rubber appa- ratus. It is a known sensitizer, causing occupational contact dermatitis, as well as bron- chial and laryngeal mucous membrane irritation.

Sulfur dioxide, as a gaseous fumigant, is produced by burning sulfur in closed spaces. For maximal effect, the surface should be moist as the gas dissolves in water to form sulfurous acid, which is bactericidal. However, this reducing effect of the acid can also corrode metals, rot fabrics, and bleach dyes.

Surface-active Compounds

Surfactants lower the surface tension of an aqueous solution and are used as wetting agents, detergents, emulsifiers, antiseptics, and disinfectants. As antimicrobials, they al- ter the energy relationship at interfaces. Based on the position of the hydrophobic moi- ety in the molecule, surfactants are classified as anionic or cationic.

Anionic Surfactants: Soaps are dipolar anionic detergents with the general for- mula RCOONa/K, which dissociate in water into hydrophilic K^+ or Na^+ ions and lipo- philic fatty acid ions. Because NaOH and KOH are strong bases (whereas most fatty ac- ids are weak acids), most soap solutions are alkaline (pH 8-10) and may irritate sensitive skin and mucous membranes. Soaps emulsify lipoidal secretions of the skin and remove, along with most of the accompanying dirt, desquamated epithelium and bacteria, which are then rinsed away with the lather. The antibacterial potency of soaps is often en- hanced by inclusion of certain antiseptics, eg, hexachlorophene, phenols, carbanilides, or potassium iodide. They are incompatible with cationic surfactants.

Cationic Surfactants: Cationic detergents are a group of alkyl- or aryl-substituted quaternary ammonium compounds (eg, benzalkonium chloride, benzethonium chloride, cetylpyridinium chloride) with an ionizable halogen, such as bromide, iodide, or chloride. The major site of action of these compounds appears to be the cell membrane, where they become adsorbed and cause changes in permeability. Their activity is reduced by porous or fibrous materials (eg, fabrics, cellulose sponges) that adsorb them. They are inacti- vated by anionic substances (eg, soaps, proteins, fatty acids, phosphates). Therefore, they are of limited value in the presence of blood and tissue debris. They are effective against most bacteria, some fungi (including yeasts), and protozoa but not against viruses and spores. Aqueous solutions of 1:1,000 to 1:5,000 have good antimicrobial activity, especially at slightly alkaline pH. When applied to skin, they may form a film under which microorganisms can survive, which limits their reliability as antiseptics. Concen- trations >1% are injurious to mucous membranes.

Other Antibacterial Agents

The antibacterial activity of **dyes** was first reported in 1913. Interestingly, the discovery of sulfonamides as chemotherapeutic agents ensued from the antibacterial activity observed in the dye prontosil.

Azo dyes (eg, scarlet red and phenazopyridine HCl) are most active in an acidic medium and are effective against gram-negative organisms. Scarlet red is often used as a 5% ointment on sores, ulcers, and wounds. Pyridium is often incorporated as an analgesic with sulfonamides for the treatment of urinary tract infections.

Acridine dyes (eg, acriflavine, proflavine, aminacrine) are more active against gram-positive bacteria. Their activity is enhanced in alkaline medium and antagonized by hypochlorites. Impregnated bandages and gauze and acriflavine jelly have been used extensively for treatment of burns.

Vapor-phase Disinfectants

Alkylating agents such as formaldehyde, ethylene oxide, and propylene oxide are broad-spectrum biocides active against bacteria, viruses, and fungi, including spores.

Ethylene and propylene oxides are highly reactive gaseous fumigants used for sterilizing animal feed, human food, surgical equipment that cannot be autoclaved (eg, endoscopes, gloves, syringes, catheters, tubing, implantable devices), laboratory equipment, etc. Both are noncorrosive. However, ethylene oxide has better penetrability than propylene oxide and, therefore, is more commonly used. For this application, ethylene oxide is mixed with chlorofluorocarbons or carbon dioxide and sold in gas cylinders.

Other gaseous disinfectants (eg, formaldehyde, sulfur dioxide, methylbromide) have been used infrequently because of their toxic or corrosive properties.

ECTOPARASITICIDES

ECTOPARASITICIDES USED IN LARGE ANIMALS

Arthropod parasites (ectoparasites) are a major cause of production losses in livestock throughout the world. In addition, many arthropod species act as vectors of disease for both animals and humans. Treatment with various drugs to reduce or eliminate ectoparasites is therefore often required to maintain health and to prevent economic loss in food animals. The choice and use of ectoparasiticides depends to a large extent on husbandry and management practices, as well as on the type of ectoparasite causing the infestation. Accurate identification of the parasite or correct diagnosis based on clinical signs is necessary for selection of the appropriate drug. The selected agent can be administered or applied directly to the animal, or introduced into the environment to reduce the arthropod population to a level that is no longer of economic or health consequence.

Parasites that live permanently on the skin, such as lice, keds, and mites, are controlled by directly treating the host. Some mange mites burrow into the skin and are therefore more difficult to control with sprays or dips than are lice and keds, which are found on the surface of the skin. However, once these obligate parasites are eradicated, reinfection occurs only from contact with other infected animals.

Nonpermanent parasites (ticks, flies, etc) are less easily controlled because only a small proportion of the population can be treated at any one time, and other hosts may maintain them. Some tick and mite species stay on the host only long enough to feed, which may be as short as 30 min, or as long as 21 days. Biting flies, such as the horn fly, can be found continuously on the backs and undersides of cattle, where they suck blood up to 20 times a day; other biting flies (such as stable flies and horse flies) and mosquitos feed to repletion, then leave the animal to lay eggs. Nonbiting flies, such as the face fly or the house fly, may visit infrequently but can be very annoying and may transmit disease agents. Larvae of certain blowflies live on the skin or in tissues of sheep and other animals and cause cutaneous myiasis. Larvae of other flies spend several months inside animals, eg, nasal bots in the nasal passages of sheep and goats, bots in the stomach of horses, and cattle grubs or warbles in the spinal canal, back, or esophageal tissues. (*See also* FLIES, p 715.)

Many ectoparasite infestations are seasonal and predictable and can be countered by prophylactic use of ectoparasiticides. For example, in temperate countries flies are seen predominantly from late spring to early autumn, tick populations increase in the spring and autumn, and lice and mites during the autumn and winter months. Treatments can therefore be targeted at anticipated times of peak activity as a means of limiting disease and parasite populations.

Chemotherapeutic Agents

Most ectoparasiticides are neurotoxins, exerting their effect on the nervous system of the target parasite. Those used in large animals can be grouped according to structure and modes of action into the organochlorines, organophosphates and carbamates, pyrethrins and pyrethroids, avermectins and milbemycins, formamidines, insect growth regulators, and a number of miscellaneous compounds, including synergists (eg, piperonyl butoxide). There are also a number of useful compounds that have repellent activity rather than insecticidal activity, including MGK-264, butoxypolypropylene-glycol, and DEET.

Organochlorines: Organochlorine compounds have been withdrawn in many parts of the world due to concerns regarding environmental persistence. However, some compounds, including lindane (γ benzene hexachloride) and methoxychlor, are still used for topical application and have excellent activity and apparent safety.

Organochlorines fall into 3 main groups: 1) chlorinated ethane derivatives such as DDT (dichlorodiphenyltrichloroethane), DDE (dichlorodiphenyldichloroethane), and DDD (dicofol, methoxychlor); 2) cyclodienes, including chlordane, aldrin, dieldrin, hepatochlor, endrin, and tozaphene; and 3) hexachlorocyclohexanes such as benzene hexachloride (BHC), which includes the γ-isomer, lindane.

Chlorinated ethanes cause inhibition of sodium conductance along sensory and motor nerve fibers by holding sodium channels open, resulting in delayed repolarization of the axonal membrane. This state renders the nerve vulnerable to repetitive discharge from small stimuli that would normally cause an action potential in a fully repolarized neuron.

The cyclodienes appear to have at least 2 component modes of action—inhibition of γ-amino butyric acid (GABA)-stimulated Cl⁻ flux and interference with Ca^{2+} flux. The resultant inhibitory postsynaptic potential leads to a state of partial depolarization of the postsynaptic membrane and vulnerability to repeated discharge. A similar mode of action has been reported for lindane, which binds to the picrotoxin side of GABA receptors, resulting in an inhibition of GABA-dependent Cl⁻ flux into the neuron.

DDT and BHC were used extensively for flystrike control but were subsequently replaced in many countries by more effective cyclodiene compounds, such as dieldrin and aldrin. The development of resistance, as well as environmental concerns, have largely led to their withdrawal. DDT and lindane were widely used in dip formulations for the control of sheep scab, but the organophosphates and subsequently the synthetic pyrethroids have mostly replaced them.

Organophosphates and Carbamates: The organophosphates comprise a large group, many of which are available for topical application and in ear tags as well as for premise control of parasites. There have been many products available worldwide for use in domestic animals, although only a few of the available compounds continue to be used for on-animal treatment.

Organophosphates are neutral esters of phosphoric acid or its thio analog that inhibit the action of acetylcholinesterase (AChE) at cholinergic synapses and at muscle endplates.

The compound mimics the structure of acetylcholine (ACh); when it binds to AChE it causes transphosphorylation of the enzyme. The transphorylated AChE is unable to break down accumulating ACh at the postsynaptic membrane, leading to neuromuscular paralysis. The degree of transphosphorylation of the enzyme helps to determine the activity of the organophosphate. This is not an irreversible process; eventually the AChE is metabolized by oxidative and hydrolytic enzyme systems.

Organophosphates can be extremely toxic in animals and humans, causing an inhibition of AChE and other cholinesterases (see p 2398). Chronic toxicity results from inhibition of the enzyme neurotoxic esterase and is associated with particular compounds. The physiologic function of this enzyme is unknown; however, its inhibition appears to cause structural changes in neuronal membranes and a reduction in conduction velocity, which may be manifest as posterior paralysis in some animal species. Cases of organophosphate toxicity are treated with oximes or atropine.

Organophosphates used topically include coumaphos, diazinon, dichlorvos, famphur, fenthion, malathion, trichlorfon, stirofos, phosmet, and propetamphos. Ear tags containing fenthion, chlorpyrifos, and diazinon are available in some countries. These compounds are generally active against fly larvae, flies, lice, ticks, and mites on domestic livestock, although activity varies between compounds and differing formulations. Chlorpyrifos is best used in the microencapsulated form for residual activity and improved safety. Diazinon and propetamphos have been available in dip formulations for the control of psoroptic mange in sheep. Both eliminate mites and protect in a single application when correctly applied. Diazinon provides longer residual protection than propetamphos. In cattle, a number of compounds have been used for the systemic control of warble fly grubs and lice as pour-on applications or in hand sprays, spray races, or dips for tick control.

Products containing haloxon and metriphonate have been used PO for the control of stomach bot fly larvae and helminths in horses.

Carbamate insecticides are closely related to organophosphates and are anticholinesterases. Unlike organophosphates, they appear to cause a spontaneously reversible block on AChE without changing it. The 2 main carbamate compounds used are carbaryl and propoxur. Carbaryl has low mammalian toxicity but may be carcinogenic and is often combined with other active ingredients.

Pyrethrins and Synthetic Pyrethroids: A number of pyrethroids are available in many countries as pour-on, spot-on, spray, and dip formulations with activity against biting and nuisance flies, lice, and ticks on a domestic livestock. Flumethrin and high cis-cypermethrin are also active against mites and are used for the treatment of psoroptic mange of sheep.

Natural pyrethrins are derived from pyrethrum, a mixture of alkaloids from the chrysanthemum plant. Pyrethrum extract, prepared from pyrethrum flower, contains ~25% pyrethrins. The pyrethrins and pyrethroids are lipophilic molecules that generally undergo rapid absorption, distribution, and excretion. They provide excellent knockdown (rapid kill) but have poor residual activity due to instability. Pyrethrin I is the most active ingredient for kill, and pyrethrin II for rapid insect knockdown.

Synthetic pyrethroids are synthesized chemicals modeled on the natural pyrethrin molecule. They are more stable and have a higher potency than natural pyrethrins.

The mode of action of pyrethrins and synthetic pyrethroids appears to be interference with sodium channels of the parasite nerve axons, resulting in delayed repolarization and eventual paralysis. Synthetic pyrethroids can be divided into 2 groups (types I and II, depending on the presence or absence of an α-cyano moiety). Type I compounds have a mode of action (similar to that of DDT) that involves interference with the axonal Na^+ gate leading to delayed repolarization and repetitive discharge of the nerve. Type II compounds also act on the Na^+ gate but do so without causing repetitive discharge. The lethal activity of pyrethroids seems to involve action on both peripheral and central neurons, while the knockdown effect is probably produced by peripheral neuronal effects only. Some preparations contain piperonyl butoxide, which acts as a synergist by helping to prevent the pyrethrin or pyrethroid breakdown by microsomal mixed-function oxidase systems in insects.

Pyrethroids are generally safe in mammals and birds but are highly toxic to fish and aquatic invertebrates. Concerns have been expressed over their environmental effects, particularly in relation to the aquatic environment.

Some of the more common pyrethroids used include bioallethrin, cypermethrin, deltamethrin, fenvalerate, flumethrin, lambdacyhalothrin, phenothrin, and permethrin. The content of some synthetic pyrethroids is also expressed in terms of the drug isomers, eg, cypermethrin preparations may contain varying proportions of their cis and trans isomers. Thus, cypermethrin (cis:trans 60:40) 2.5% is equivalent to cypermethrin (cis:trans 80:20) 1.25%. In general, cis isomers are more active than the corresponding trans isomers.

Macrocyclic Lactones (Avermectins and Milbemycins): Avermectins and the structurally related milbemycins, collectively referred to as macrocyclic lactones, are fermentation products of *Streptomyces avermilitis* and *Streptomyces cyanogriseus*, respectively. Avermectins differ from each other chemically in side chain substitutions on the lactone ring, while milbemycins differ from the avermectins through the absence of a sugar moiety from the lactone skeleton. A number of macrocyclic lactone compounds are available for use and include the avermectins abamectin, doramectin, eprinomectin, ivermectin, and selamectin, and the milbemycins moxidectin and milbemycin oxime. These compounds are active against a wide range of nematodes and arthropods and, as such, are often referred to as endectocides.

Endectocidal activity, particularly against ectoparasites, is variable and depends on the active molecule, the product formulation, and the method of application. Macrocyclic lactones can be given PO, parenterally, or topically (as pour-ons). The method of application depends on the host and, to some degree, on the target parasites. In cattle, eg, available endectocide products can be given PO, by injection, or topically using pour-on formulations. The latter are generally more effective against lice (*Lignonathus, Haematopinus,* and to some extent *Bovicola*) and headfly (*Haematobia/Lyperosia*) infestations, when compared with equivalent compounds administered parenterally. In sheep, PO administration of some endectocides has little effect against psoroptic mite infestations (*Psoroptes ovis*), but parenteral administration increases activity.

The route of administration and product formulation all influence rates of absorption, metabolism, excretion, and subsequent bioavailability and pharmacokinetics of individual compounds. Avermectins and milbemycins are highly lipophilic, a property that varies with only minor modifications in molecular structure or configuration. Following administration, macrocyclic lactones are stored in fat, from which they are slowly released, metabolized, and excreted. Ivermectin is absorbed systemically following PO, SC, or dermal administration; it is absorbed to a greater degree and has a longer half-life when given SC or dermally. Excretion of the unaltered molecule is mainly via the feces, with <2% excreted in the urine in ruminants. In cattle, the reduced absorption and bioavailability of ivermectin given PO may be due to its metabolism in the rumen. The affinity of these compounds for fat explains their persistence in the body and the extended periods of protection afforded against some species of internal and external parasites. The prolonged half-life of these compounds also determines residue levels in meat and milk, and subsequent compulsory withdrawal periods following treatment in food-producing animals.

The mode of action of avermectins and milbemycins is still not completely understood. Ivermectin is known to act on GABA neurotransmission at 2 or more sites in nematodes, blocking interneuronal stimulation of excitatory motor neurons, leading to flaccid paralysis. It appears to achieve this by stimulating the release of GABA from nerve endings and by enhancing the binding of GABA to its receptor on the postsynaptic membrane of an excitatory motor neuron. The enhanced GABA binding results in an increased flow of Cl⁻ ions into the cell, leading to hyperpolarization. In mammals, GABA neurotransmission is confined to the CNS; the lack of effect of ivermectin on mammalian nervous systems at therapeutic concentrations is probably because it does not readily cross the blood-brain barrier. More recent evidence suggests that ivermectin may exert its effect through action on glutamate-gated Cl⁻ ion conductance at the postsynaptic membrane or neuromuscular endplate.

Formamidines: Amitraz is the only formamidine used as an ectoparasiticide. It appears to act by inhibition of the enzyme monoamine oxidase and as an agonist at octopamine receptors. Monoamine oxidase metabolizes amine neurotransmitters in ticks and mites, and octopamine is thought to modify tonic contractions in parasite muscles. Amitraz has a relatively wide safety margin in mammals; the most frequently associated side effects include sedation, which may be associated with an agonist activity of amitraz on α_2-receptors in mammalian species.

Amitraz is available as a spray or dip for use against mites, lice, and ticks in domestic livestock. It is contraindicated in horses.

Chloronicotinyls and Spinosyns: Imidacloprid is a chloronicotinyl insecticide, a synthesized chlorinated derivative of nicotine. Spinosad is a fermentation product of the soil actinomycete *Saccharopolyspora spinosa*. Both compounds bind to nicotinic acetylcholine receptors (but at different sites) in the insect's CNS, leading to inhibition of cholinergic transmission, paralysis, and death. Spinosad has been developed in some countries for use on sheep in the control of blowfly strike and lice.

Insect Growth Regulators: Insect growth regulators are used throughout the world and represent a relatively new category of insect control agents. They constitute a group of chemical compounds that do not kill the target parasite directly, but interfere with growth and development. They act mainly on immature parasite stages and are not usually suitable for the rapid control of established adult parasite populations. Where parasites show a clear seasonal pattern, insect growth regulators can be applied prior to any anticipated challenge as a preventive measure. They are widely used for blowfly control in sheep but have limited use in other livestock.

Based on their mode of action, insect growth regulators can be divided into chitin synthesis inhibitors (benzoylphenyl ureas), chitin inhibitors (triazine/pyrimidine derivatives), and juvenile hormone analogs. Several benzoylphenyl ureas have been introduced for the control of ectoparasites. Chitin is a complex aminopolysaccharide and a major component of the insect's cuticle. During each molt, it has to be newly formed by polymerization of individual sugar molecules. The exact mode of action of the benzoylphenyl ureas is not fully understood. They inhibit chitin synthesis but have no effect on the enzyme chitin synthetase. It has been suggested that they interfere with the assembly of the chitin chains into microfibrils. When immature insect stages are exposed to these compounds, they are not able to complete ecdysis and die during molting. Benzoylphenyl ureas also appear to have a transovarial effect. Exposed adult female insects produce eggs in which the compound is incorporated into the egg nutrient. Egg development proceeds normally, but the newly developed larvae are incapable of hatching. Benzoylphenyl ureas show a broad spectrum of activity against insects but have relatively low efficacy against ticks and mites. The exception is fluazuron, which has greater activity against ticks and some mite species.

Benzoylphenyl ureas are highly lipophilic molecules. When administered to the host, they build up in body fat, from which they are slowly released into the bloodstream and excreted largely unchanged. Diflubenzuron and flufenoxuron are used for the prevention of blowfly strike in sheep. Diflubenzuron is available in some countries as an emulsifiable concentrate for use as a dip or shower. It is more efficient against first-stage larvae than second and third instars and is therefore recommended as a preventive, providing protection for 12-14 wk. It may also have potential for the control of a number of major insect pests such as tsetse flies. Fluazuron is available in some countries for use in cattle as a tick development inhibitor. When applied as a pour-on, it provides longterm protection against the 1-host tick *Boophilus microplus*.

Triazine and pyrimidine derivatives are closely related compounds that are also chitin inhibitors. They differ from the benzoylphenyl ureas both in chemical structure and mode of action, in that they appear to alter the deposition of chitin into the cuticle rather than its synthesis.

Cyromazine, a triazine derivative, is effective against blowfly larvae on sheep and lambs and also against other *Diptera* such as houseflies and mosquitos. At recommended dose rates, cyromazine shows only limited activity against established strikes and must therefore be used preventively. Blowflies usually lay eggs on damp fleece of treated sheep. Although larvae are able to hatch, the young larvae immediately come into contact with cyromazine, which prevents the molt to second instars. The efficacy of a pour-on preparation of cyromazine does not depend on factors such as weather, fleece length, and whether the fleece is wet or dry. Control can be maintained for up to 13 wk after a single pour-on application, or longer if cyromazine is applied by dip or shower.

Dicyclanil, a pyrimidine derivative, is highly active against dipteran larvae. A pour-on formulation, available in some countries for blowfly control in sheep, provides up to 20 wk of protection.

The juvenile hormone analogs mimic the activity of naturally occurring juvenile hormones and prevent metamorphosis to the adult stage. Once the larva is fully developed, enzymes within the insect's circulatory system destroy endogenous juvenile hormones, prompting development to the adult stage. The juvenile hormone analogs bind to juvenile hormone receptor sites, but because they are structurally different, are not destroyed by insect esterases. As a consequence, metamorphosis and further development to the adult stage does not proceed. Methoprene is a terpenoid compound with very low mammalian toxicity that mimics a juvenile insect hormone and is used as a feed-through larvicide for hornfly (*Haematobia*) control on cattle.

Miscellaneous Compounds: Piperonyl butoxide is a methylenedioxyphenyl compound that has been widely used as a synergistic additive in the control of arthropod pests. It is commonly used as a synergist with natural pyrethrins. The degree of potentiation of insecticidal activity is related to the ratio of components in the mixture; as the proportion of piperonyl butoxide increases, the amount of natural pyrethrins required to evoke the same level of kill decreases. The insecticidal activity of other pyrethroids, particularly of knockdown agents, can also be enhanced by the addition of piperonyl butoxide. The enhancement of activity of synthetic pyrethroids is normally less dramatic. Piperonyl butoxide inhibits the microsomal enzyme system of some arthropods and is effective against some mites. In addition to having low mammalian toxicity and a long record of safety, it rapidly degrades in the environment.

Various products from natural sources, as well as synthetic compounds, have been used as insect repellents. Such compounds include cinerins, pyrethrins and jasmolins (*see* PYRETHRINS AND SYNTHETIC PYRETHROIDS, p 2160), citronella, indalone, garlic oil, MGK-264, butoxypolypropylene-glycol, DEET, and DMP (dimethylphthalate). The use of repellents is advantageous as legislative and regulatory authorities become more restrictive toward the use of conventional pesticides. They are used mainly to protect horses against blood-sucking arthropods, particularly midges (*Culicoides*).

Insecticides may be used to provide environmental control of some insects by application to premises. The insect pheromone (Z)-9-tricosene is incorporated into some products to attract insects to the site of application.

Methods of Treatment

Products are available for both parenteral administration and for topical application by various methods including dips, sprays, pour-ons, spot-ons, dusting powders, and ear tags. The method used depends on the target parasite and host.

Ectoparasiticides that act systemically may be given parenterally or applied topically to the skin, where the active ingredient is absorbed percutaneously and taken up into the circulation. Many of the endectocides are now available as either SC or IM injections or as pour-on preparations acting systemically.

Dusting powders have been widely used for the topical treatment of ectoparasite infestation but have been largely superseded by other methods of application. Many of the earlier organochlorine, organophosphate, and pyrethroid insecticides were formulated with an inert base, or bulking agent, for direct topical application. Accurate dosing may be difficult as the recommended dose rates are often loosely based on the size of the animal. Powders also have limited residual activity, necessitating frequent reapplication. Hand application of insecticides as washes, ointments (especially to skin or wounds to control cutaneous myiasis), dusts, spray foams, aerosols, etc, can also be done. To avoid gathering range animals for treatment, self-treatment devices, such as "back rubbers" or dust bags, may be placed in areas where cattle can rub against them.

Another widely used method is spray application of aqueous emulsions or suspensions. Cattle sheds, barns, stables, and dairies are typically sprayed or misted with insecticidal sprays. The animals may be sprayed with insecticide, both to kill and repel flies. A range of formulations is available as liquid concentrates that require dilution with water to produce an emulsion for application by spray. The use of microencapsulation techniques, in which a thin coat of chemical is applied around the active ingredients, can enhance the residual activity of sprays.

Dips are used for the control of mites, ticks, lice, keds, and flies in sheep, cattle, goats, and horses. These may either be by full-body immersion or more shallow baths that cover only the legs and lower body. With immersion or plunge dipping, animals are either made to swim in straight swim-through or circular dip baths or are cage dipped for a prescribed period of time in strict accordance to manufacturer's instructions. Sheep dip formulations may deplete from the vat faster than the carrier fluid ("stripping dips"); to maintain therapeutic or prophylactic concentrations, the vat must be topped up with a higher than initial concentration of dip. Systems are now available for the automatic replenishment of the dip concentrate and carrier in the desired proportions. Dipping baths should be cleaned out and recharged after a certain number of animals have been dipped, (the number depends on factors such as the capacity of the dip, inclement weather conditions, and the amount of organic material deposited). Dip wash is considered hazardous waste and must be disposed of in accordance with applicable laws. Dip neutralizers can be added to break down the insecticide prior to disposal.

Impregnated devices include ear tags, tapes, bands, and collars in which a medium, usually plastic or some form of fabric, is impregnated with the chemical, which is then slowly released onto the animal's coat. A residual life of several months may be expected from such devices. Ear tags on cattle, eg, can provide almost season-long control of biting and nuisance flies. Horses may be treated with such tags attached to halters or with strips attached to halters or to tails. Unfortunately, in a number of areas, horn flies have become resistant to the pyrethroid insecticides that are commonly used in insecticide-impregnated ear tags.

Pour-ons and spot-ons contain the pesticide chemicals at relatively high concentration and are formulated to either penetrate the skin and act systemically or spread over the skin surface and act by contact. Pour-on treatments are usually applied along the backline of an animal or at a single spot on the shoulder blades using a specially designed applicator. They offer the obvious advantages of ease of use, speed, and accuracy of dose. Spot-on formulations offer a convenient and simple method of application of a small amount of the active ingredient to one or more sites.

Safety Restrictions

It is important to be aware of and follow safety restrictions to prevent poisoning or injury to treated animals. All organophosphates available for use on animals are cholinesterase inhibitors. They should not be used simultaneously or within a few days before or after treatment or exposure to other cholinesterase-inhibiting drugs, pesticides, or chemicals. They should not be applied to animals that are young, sick, convalescent, or stressed.

Pyrethroid insecticides available for use on large animals are considered safe but have general precautionary statements on their labels, particularly in relation to disposal and their potential ectoxicologic effects.

Some parasiticides may be used only by or under the supervision of a veterinarian; others are available via agricultural suppliers and pharmacists directly to the public. Approvals vary from country to country. Labels for pesticides contain explicit information on hazards to animals, humans, and the environment; storage of unused insecticide; and disposal of the container. For each insecticide, the label is the primary source of information on uses and safety instructions, which should be carefully followed.

Restrictions are applied to many of the ectoparasiticides indicated for use in food-producing animals to ensure that unacceptable residues are not present in products intended for human consumption. These restrictions may require that animals are not slaughtered for prescribed periods after administration of the product or that the product is not used in animals producing milk for human consumption. Labels and data sheets on all products contain specific instructions on restrictions, including withdrawal periods, and must be followed.

ECTOPARASITICIDES USED IN SMALL ANIMALS

Flea and tick infestation of dogs and cats is a major health problem to the animals and an economic burden to their owners. Traditionally, a wide array of ectoparasiticides has been available, and switching among brands was frequent, leading to problems in achieving acceptable external parasite control. Veterinarians are uniquely qualified to provide key advice on host/parasite interrelationships and selection of the most suitable program. However, many pets owners have historically purchased their flea and tick products in supermarkets or pet supply shops where professional advice is not available. Fortunately, recent advances in product technology and in our understanding of flea and tick epidemiology have dramatically altered the purchasing patterns of pet owners. Veterinarians should become aware of these technological improvements in both insecticidal chemistry and delivery systems and encourage client education by their staff.

Active Chemical Ingredients

Nomenclature can be confusing if the shorter approved name is not used and the full chemical name is written (eg, chlorpyrifos versus 0, 0-diethyl 0-[3,5,6 trichloro 2 pyridyl] phosphorothioate). The use of chemical trade names can cause added confusion (eg, Dursban® versus chlorpyrifos). Although most commercial products contain only 1 active ingredient, it is not uncommon for 2 or more to be combined. All labels should be read carefully for ingredients and directions for use.

Avermectins: Currently the only FDA-approved semisynthetic avermectin developed specifically to control internal and external parasites in dogs and cats is selamectin. While the exact mode of action of avermectins is controversial, it is believed that selamectin binds to glutamate-gated chloride channels in the parasites' nervous system, increasing their permeability and allowing for the rapid and continued influx of chloride ions into the nerve cell. This inhibits nerve activity and causes paralysis. Selamectin is applied topically, is rapidly absorbed through the skin, and is distributed via the blood. It has activity against both internal and external parasites.

Cholinesterase Inhibitors: Two groups of compounds, organophosphates and carbamates, share the same mechanism of action—inhibition of acetylcholinesterase. This enzyme normally is responsible for acetylcholine (neurotransmitter) destruction. Applications of organophosphates or carbamates to insects produce spontaneous muscular contractions followed by paralysis. The reaction between organophosphates and acetylcholinesterase is more persistent, if not permanent, than the reaction with carbamates, which is reversible. These compounds were once very popular for their prolonged action and potency. However, the use of organophosphates has declined because their systemic persistance creates a low margin of safety and slight variance from approved use or continued use may lead to toxicity. When these compounds are used for flea or tick control, it should be determined before treatment if any other cholinesterase inhibitor has been used on the animal or in its environment. Organophosphates for small animal therapy include chlorpyrifos, dichlorvos, malathion, diazinon, phosmet, fenthion, chlorfenvinphos, and cythioate. Carbamates include carbaryl and propoxur.

Chlorinated Hydrocarbons: These compounds are becoming less popular because of their persistence in the environment, although this factor brought the benefit of prolonged action. Lindane and methoxychlor are still occasionally used. (*See also* CHLORINATED HYDROCARBON COMPOUNDS, p 2395.)

Chloronicotinyls: The nicotinoids are a new class of insecticides that are referred to as nitro-quanidines, neonicotinyls, neonicotinoids, chloronicotines, and recently as chloronicotinyls. The nicotinoids are modeled after natural nicotine. Two compounds in this category are currently available for veterinary use—imidacloprid and nitenpyram. Imidacloprid works by binding to postsynaptic nicotinic acetylcholine receptors in insects. This inhibits cholinergic transmission, resulting in paralysis and death. Imidacloprid is applied as a 10% spot-on topical product and is used primarily to control fleas on both dogs and cats. It also has excellent activity against lice. While it has potent residual activity, swimming and repeated bathing may compromise its duration of activity. Nitenpyram is administered PO in pill form to kill fleas in both dogs and cats. It is absorbed rapidly, with maximal blood concentrations reached within 1.2 hr and 0.6 hr in dogs and cats, respectively. Fleas begin to die within 20-30 min of administration, with 100% flea mortality within 3-4 hr. The compound is rapidly eliminated, with >90% excreted in the urine within 24-48 hr, primarily as unchanged nitenpyram. Even though imidacloprid and nitenpyram are classified similarly, their mechanisms of action appear to be different. While imidacloprid is described as a paralytic, nitenpyram produces hyperexcitability in fleas prior to death.

Citrus Extracts: D-limonene and linolool are products extracted from fresh peels of citrus fruits. They have insecticidal activity that can be enhanced when synergized with piperonyl butoxide.

Formamidines: This small group of acaricidal compounds has the proposed mode of action of inhibiting monoamine oxidase. In veterinary medicine, the only approved formamidine is amitraz. It is used primarily as an acaricide to control ticks and mites. It is available as a dip for control of canine demodicosis and will also control scabies. An amitraz-impregnated collar is also marketed for the control of ticks on dogs. Amitraz is not approved for use on cats.

Insect Growth Regulators: These compounds inhibit the development of immature stages of insects. They are generally classified as either juvenile hormone analogs (or mimics) or as chitin synthesis inhibitors (insect development inhibitors). Methoprene, fenoxycarb, and pyriproxyfen mimic the activity of juvenile hormone and are classified as juvenile hormone analogs. When these compounds are applied to flea larvae or into their environment, they are absorbed by the larvae and act like natural insect juvenile hormone, maintaining the genetic transcription of larval morphologic characteristics. Juvenile hormone analogs bind to juvenile hormone receptor sites; larvae are prevented from completing metamorphosis and subsequently die. In addition, these compounds have ovicidal and embryocidal activity when applied topically to dogs and cats. Female fleas in the hair coat absorb the juvenile hormone analog, which kills developing eggs. While these compounds have been developed as control agents for fleas, they are active against a wide range of beneficial insect species. Therefore, their use outdoors should be limited to specific flea habitats to avoid adverse effects on beneficial insect species.

Lufenuron, a benzoylphenyl urea, inhibits the formation of chitin (a polymer of N-acetyl glucosamine), which is a major component of insect exoskeletons. During each larval molt, chitin is reformed by polymerization. Lufenuron interferes with polymerization and deposition of chitin, killing developing larvae either within the egg or after hatching. Lufenuron is administered PO to dogs or cats or by injection to cats. Female fleas feeding on treated animals are prevented from producing viable eggs or larvae. Other insect development inhibitors, such as diflubenzuron and cyromazine, also have considerable activity against developing fleas. Insect growth regulators affect many insect species that undergo complete metamorphosis, but have little or no activity against ticks or other Acari, which undergo incomplete metamorphosis.

Phenylpyrazoles: This group of compounds has broad-spectrum insecticidal and acaricidal activity. The only member of this group currently available for use in the USA is fipronil. Fipronil binds to γ-aminobutyric acid receptors of insects, inhibiting the flux of Cl⁻ ions into nerve cells, which results in hyperexcitability. Fipronil is a broad-spectrum pesticide with activity against fleas, ticks, mites, and lice. Three formulations are available in the USA—a 0.25% alcohol base spray, a 10% spot-on, and a combination spot-on with the insect growth regulator methoprene. Fipronil is absorbed and accumulates in the sebaceous glands, has very low solubility in water, and has prolonged residual activity on both dogs and cats.

Pyrethrins and Pyrethroids: These compounds disrupt sodium and potassium ion transport in nerve membranes, resulting in spontaneous depolarizations, augmented neurotransmitter secretion, and neuromuscular blockade. The action is extremely rapid, but paralyzed insects can also recover rapidly. The synergists piperonyl butoxide and N-octyl bicycloheptene dicarboxymide interfere with the insect detoxification mechanism. Natural pyrethrum is extracted from chrysanthemum flowers and is notable for its rapid but brief action and relative lack of toxicity in dogs and cats.

Synthetic pyrethroids are pyrethrum-like compounds that generally have greater potency and residual effects but are less well tolerated in cats. Some pyrethroids, such as permethrin, can be highly toxic to cats. Pyrethroids are generally classified by developmental generation. First-generation pyrethroids are unstable in heat and sunlight (eg, allethrin); second-generation are photostable, isomeric mixtures (eg, cypermethrin, permethrin); third-generation are photostable, more active isomers obtained by isomeric enrichment (eg, λ-cyhalothrin, β-cyfluthrin); and fourth-generation are nonester pyrethroids (eg, MTI 800, flufenprox, etofenprox).

Repellents: N,N-diethyl-3-methylbenzamide (DEET, previously called N,N-diethyl-meta-toluamide) remains the most effective among currently available insect repellents for humans. It is a broad-spectrum repellent that is effective against mosquitos, biting flies, chiggers, fleas, and ticks. However, the effectiveness of DEET formulations for dogs and cats has not been proved, and concentrated formulations containing DEET have caused weakness, paralysis, liver disease, and seizures in pets. The synthetic pyrethroid permethrin (*see* above), while not a true repellant, is a rapidly acting contact insecticide that affects arthropod nervous systems. This leads to death or "knockdown," thereby producing a repellent-like activity against fleas, ticks, and mosquitos.

Synergists: Synergists are generally not considered toxic or insecticidal, but are used with insecticides to enhance their activity. They are used primarily to increase the effectiveness of pyrethrum or pyrethroids. Synergists inhibit cytochrome P450-dependent monooxygenases or glutathione s-transferases, enzymes produced by microsomes in insect tissues. They bind the oxidative enzymes and prevent them from degrading the toxicant. Piperonyl butoxide and N-octyl bicycloheptene dicarboxamide are 2 common synergists.

Target Parasite Efficacy

Due to specific formulation and drug delivery technology, certain insecticides are used in a wide variety of ectoparasite control products. Efficacy of specific compounds can vary against target species, and tolerance to insecticides may develop in specific locations, especially with product use. It cannot be assumed that ticks and fleas are controlled by the same active compounds; product labels should be carefully read. Products that contain compounds specifically active against the target parasite should be chosen, whether the concern is fleas, ticks, mites, or a combination of these parasites.

Duration of activity (ie, "knockdown" or sustained effects) are often the primary concern in product choices. Some products allow for parasite recovery, while others are so slow that parasite loads on the host are not reduced because the rate of reinfestation exceeds the kill rate.

Safety

Although LD_{50} data concerning the safety or toxicity of an insecticidal product is often helpful, LD_{50} values frequently are misleading when safety of insecticides applied to pets or premises is considered. Consideration must also be given to the concentration of product as it is supplied (mg/mL), application rate (mg or g/m^2 for environmental products, and mL or g/kg for topicals), route of exposure (dermal or oral), and species exposed. The actual risk of exposure during treatment, after treatment, or following accidental ingestion can be assessed only after evaluation of these criteria.

Because animal toxicity can be modified by formulation technology, active ingredients are not the sole guide to safety assessment. Most commercial products have undergone adequate safety evaluation for regulatory approval, and the label remains the best source of information. Cats are sensitive to many insecticides, and use of insecticides on or near cats must be done with caution. Human and environmental safety also should be considered, especially when treating premises. The safety of older insecticidal compounds is sometimes questioned; the compound may break down into more toxic components, or regulatory approval may be withdrawn due to new testing data (eg, carcinogenicity or environmental concerns). Generalizations should not be made, as formulations that are generally safe may induce skin reactions, or even fatal reactions, in individuals and certain sensitive breeds of dogs and cats.

Delivery Systems

Consumer convenience is an important factor in product choice, especially for flea and tick control. A bewildering array of systems has historically been available—powders, aerosols, sprays, shampoos, rinses, dips, spot-ons, mousses, oral tablets or liquids, and impregnated collars. However, the safety, efficacy, and ease of use of the newer spot-on, injectable, and oral application systems have rendered many of the older application technologies essentially obsolete.

GROWTH PROMOTANTS AND PRODUCTION ENHANCERS

Achieving increased efficiency of feed conversion into edible human food products of high quality, without posing any significant risk to the consumer, is an important goal of livestock producers worldwide. The physiologic mechanisms involved in converting feed into muscle, fat, and bone by animals are increasingly being elucidated. Recently, consumer concerns about additives for food production have focused on animal safety, organoleptic quality, and the potential human health hazards of the food we eat.

A number of different approaches may be taken to improve conversion of animal feed into meat; two of the more practical approaches are hormonal treatments and antimicrobial feed additives. The hormonal approach includes administration of anabolic sex steroid hormones to either boost the animal's steroid production rate or to replace steroids lost through castration; use of growth hormone (GH) or insulin-like growth factor (IGF) 1 to augment endogenous GH levels; and use of β-adrenergic agonists (βAA) to preferentially increase nutrient partitioning to muscle (TABLE 60). The antimicrobial feed additives approach includes feeding of antibiotics to decrease populations of pathologic bacteria in host GI tracts, use of compounds to manipulate ruminal fermentation by changing the ruminal microflora population in healthy animals, and use of probiotics to promote beneficial microflora in the GI tract. The antimicrobial feed additives approach is currently under debate due to concerns surrounding the potential development of antibiotic-resistant strains in humans.

STEROID HORMONES

In general, the principle that dictates which type of **hormone** to be used is the need to supplement or replace the particular hormone type that is deficient in the animals to be treated. Females produce estrogens normally, so better results are obtained from the administration of male androgens, eg, trenbolone acetate (TBA). However, anabolic responses are obtained by giving supplemental estrogens, eg, cull cows. Estrogens should not be used in males (or androgens in females) retained for breeding purposes.

Manufacturers' instructions must be followed to ensure proper implant placement and dose administration. Anabolic hormones should not be administered by IM injection for growth-promoting purposes. Additionally, steroid hormones must not be used for anabolic or other purposes unless the indication is specifically approved by the appropriate regulatory body. The EU has banned the use of hormonal growth promoters in meat production. Appropriate surveillance programs have been established to ensure compliance by producers.

Endogenous Steroids: The steroidal compounds used for anabolic purposes in food animals are estradiol, progesterone, and testosterone. Gender and maturity of an animal influences its growth rate and body composition. Bulls grow 8-12% faster than steers, have better feed efficiencies, and produce leaner carcasses. Superior performance of bulls is due to the steroids produced in the testes (mainly testosterone but also estradiol, which in ruminants is also anabolic and is produced in relatively large quantities). Testosterone, or one of its physiologically active metabolites, binds to receptors in muscle and stimulates increased incorporation of amino acids into protein, thereby increasing muscle mass without a concomitant increase in adipose tissue. Estradiol, on the other hand, may act by stimulation of the somatotropic axis to increase growth hormone and thus IGF-1 production and availability by modulation of the IGF binding proteins. Naturally produced endogenous steroids are not orally active, require picogram concentrations of estradiol and nanogram concentrations of testosterone in blood for physiologic effects, and can transiently affect the behavior of treated animals (*see* TABLE 60).

Estradiol: A potent anabolic agent in ruminants at blood concentrations of 5-100 pg/mL, estradiol is administered as an ear implant, either as compressed tablets or silastic rubber implants. When estradiol is formulated as compressed tablets, a second steroid (usually testosterone or progesterone) is typically present, in a ratio of ~1 part estradiol to 10 parts of the other steroid. The purpose of the second steroid is to reduce the release rate of estradiol and thereby prolong the effective life span of the implant to 100-120 days. The release of hormones from compressed pellets is relatively rapid within 2-4 days after insertion (50-100 times higher than baseline), followed by a slower rate of release for the next 30-50 days (5-10 times higher than baseline). Hormone concentrations gradually decline up to day 80-100, when concentrations are no different from those in control animals.

Estradiol formulated in silastic rubber enhances the effective life span of the implant relative to pelleted formulations. The pattern of release includes a short-lived spike in plasma estrogen concentration for 2-5 days after insertion, followed by a stable but modest increase (5-10 times greater than baseline). Toward the end of the effective life span of the implant, there is a gradual decline to estradial concentrations found in control animals.

Estradiol, on its own, increases nitrogen retention, growth rate by 10-20% in steers, lean meat content by 1-3%, and feed efficiency by 5-8%. It can be used in steers to best advantage, but it has some anabolic effects in heifers and veal calves. It works best in lambs in conjunction with androgens. It is not effective as an anabolic agent in pigs.

Testosterone: A potent anabolic agent at the relatively high concentrations of 1-5 ng/mL in peripheral circulation, testosterone is not used on its own as an anabolic agent in farm animals, because it is very difficult to achieve the effective physiologic concentrations for long periods (up to 100 days) with current delivery systems. It is generally used as a propionate formulation in conjunction with 20 mg estradiol benzoate (EB) in a compressed tablet implant; its major role in the compressed pellet may be to slow down the release rate of estradiol. In high concentrations in blood, testosterone induces male sexual behavior (eg, aggression and mounting), but this is not observed with the concentrations delivered by compressed pellets in the ear (1 ng/mL). Behavior resulting from use of 20 mg EB and 200 mg progesterone is not different from that observed after the use of 20 mg EB and 200 mg testosterone propionate.

Progesterone: Unambiguous data suggesting progesterone is anabolic in farm animals does not exist. Its major use is to slow the release of estradiol from compressed pellet implants.

Synthetic Steroids: Synthetic steroids are commercially available in some countries because of their efficacy, their relatively mild androgenicity, and because they cause few behavioral anomalies (TABLE 61). Commercial synthetic steroids are androgenic, (TBA), or progestogenic (melengestrol acetate, MGA).

TABLE 60. Natural Steroid Hormones for Consideration as Growth Promoters ▶

Hormone		Form*	Content of Implant	Duration of Effect (days)
Estradiol	1	Pellet	20 mg EB[†] + 200 mg P4[‡]	100-120
	2	Pellet	20 mg EB + 200 mg testosterone propionate	100-120
	3	Pellet	10 mg EB + 100 mg P4	100-120
	4	Silastic rubber	45 mg estradiol	365
	5	Silastic rubber	24 mg estradiol	200
	6	Polylactic acid	28 mg estradiol	365
Progesterone		See 1 and 3 above		
Testosterone		See 2 above		

*Implants must be placed SC between the ear cartilage and skin to comply with label instructions so that consumption of residues may be avoided.
[†]Estradiol benzoate
[‡]Progesterone

Synthetic steroidal androgens are not commonly used as anabolic agents except for TBA. TBA is currently the only synthetic androgen approved for use for growth promotion in cattle; it is used to a lesser extent in sheep and not in pigs or horses. It has weak androgenic activity but has greater anabolic activity than testosterone. There are no obvious side effects in males. TBA has significant anabolic effects on its own in female cattle and sheep, but in castrated males, it gives maximal response when used in conjunction with estrogens. It is administered as a pellet-type implant containing 140-300 mg TBA for heifers and cull cows, and it can be used with estradiol in doses ranging from 140-200 mg TBA as either combined or separate implants.

Melengestrol acetate is an orally active synthetic progestagen. It is fed at doses of 0.25-0.5 mg per heifer per day in the feed. It suppresses recurrent estrus in feedlot heifers and increases growth rate and feed efficiency (TABLE 61). It is not effective in pregnant or spayed heifers or in steers. Its mode of action is to suppress ovulation presumably by suppressing luteinizing hormone (LH) pulse frequency; however, large follicles develop,

TABLE 61. Synthetic Steroid Hormones for Consideration as Growth Promoters ▶

Hormone	Method of Administration	Content of Implant
TBA*	Pellet implant	140, 200, or 300 mg
TBA + EB[†]	Pellet implant	140 mg TBA + 20 mg EB
Zeranol	Pellet implant	36 mg zeranol
Zeranol	Pellet implant	12 mg zeranol
MGA[‡]	In feed	0.25-0.5 mg/day, PO

*Trenbolone acetate
[†]Estradiol benzoate
[‡]Melengestrol acetate

◄ **TABLE 60.** (*continued*)

Animal	Growth Response	Potential Side Effects
Steers	10-15%	Transient increase in sexual behavior
Heifers, cull cows	5-15%	Udder development
Veal calves	0-8%	
Steers	10-15%	Transient increase in sexual behavior
Steers	10-15%	Transient increase in sexual behavior
Steers	10-15%	Transient increase in sexual behavior

which can increase concentrations of estradiol and growth hormone, and hence growth. There is generally a 48-hr withdrawl period prior to slaughter. Melengestrol is permitted for use in the USA but not in the EU.

Synthetic Nonsteroidal Estrogens: Two major classes of synthetic nonsteroidal estrogens have been used as production enhancers in food animals. **Stilbene estrogens** (either diethylstilbestrol [DES] or hexestrol) have been banned in most countries as anabolic agents because of residue and food safety concerns.

The discovery of a naturally occurring estrogen, zearalenone (produced by the fungi *Fusarium* spp) led to the development of the synthetic analog zeranol. Zeranol is estrogenic and has a weak affinity for the uterine estradiol receptor. It is used in animal production as a SC ear implant at a dose of 36 mg for cattle and 12 mg for sheep, with a duration of activity of 90-120 days. In steers, zeranol increases nitrogen retention, growth rate by 12-15% and feed conversion by 6-10%. However, lower responses are seen in heifers. Its effects are additive to those of androgens (generally TBA).

Use in Cattle: Calves have a high conversion of feed into animal tissue. Therefore, their responses to anabolic agents are variable. Responses of 0-10% have been obtained when zeranol was given to 3-mo-old castrated male calves. No significant response has

◄ **TABLE 61.** (*continued*)

Duration of Effect (days)	Animal	Growth Response	Potential Side Effects
60-90	Heifers, cull cows, steers	5-12%	
60-100	Steers, veal calves	10-20%	Transient increase in sexual behavior
90-120	Cattle	10-15%	
90-120	Lambs	10-15%	
As long as it is given	Heifers, cull cows	3-10%	Increased mammary development after longterm administration

been obtained from TBA. Bull calves in an intensive bull beef system can be given an estrogen implant at 1-2 mo of age to suppress testicular development, which may lead to subsequent reduction in mounting and aggression. A growth response of ~5-8% is also sometimes obtained from this implant. Reimplantation every 100 days is necessary if compressed pellet implants are used. The value of implanting heifer calves is doubtful because of the low and variable responses obtained.

A major limitation to the use of anabolic agents in weanlings is the low liveweight gain they may achieve because of poor feeding. Hence, anabolic agents should be considered only if the weanlings are expected to gain >0.5 kg/day. Zeranol can be used in male castrates. Dairy heifer replacements cannot be given steroid implants as weanlings.

Higher and more consistent responses are obtained in yearling and older cattle than in calves or weanlings. This is partly related to age and partly to the higher plane of nutrition. In the case of pellet-type implants with effectiveness of 90-100 days, consideration can be given to reimplanting cattle in midsummer, provided gains >0.5 kg/day are maintained. Silastic implants of estradiol are effective for 200-400 days, depending on dose used. Daily gains have increased 20-30% after implantation of male castrates with an estrogen and an androgen. Less research has been done in yearling beef heifers, so a definite recommendation cannot be given. However, TBA could be considered for use in these animals.

The choice of implant to use in finishing beef cattle is governed to some extent by which implants, if any, have been previously used. Responses are good when animals are on a high plane of nutrition. Feed conversion efficiency is improved, and lean meat content of the carcass is generally increased. Feed additives do not affect carcass composition. Although less clear, conformation of implanted cattle tends to improve, but repeated use of implants in older cattle can decrease the percentage of choice and prime carcasses produced.

In steers, an androgen plus an estrogen hormone combination can be used. Pellet-type implants are effective for 90-100 days; in a 4- to 5-mo finishing period, a silastic implant or reimplanting cattle after 70-80 days should be considered due to decreased response from the pellet-type implants. In a prolonged finishing phase, long-acting implants obviate the need to reimplant the estrogen component of the combination treatment. The other major alternative is to use a hormonal implant and a feed additive.

Heifers should be given TBA or a feed additive. They can be given estradiol, but 20-40% of the heifers so treated show mammary development and can be classified as "cow heifers" after slaughter. Cull cows can be given TBA, estradiol, or a feed additive, as mammary development is of no concern. TBA may play some role in drying off cull cows still in milk.

In some studies in which bulls were treated with estrogens, growth rate increased by 2-10%, and testicular growth was suppressed with a consequent reduction in mounting and aggression. This would make the bulls easier to manage on the farm and less subject to "dark cutting" after slaughter. The mechanism involved appears to be the reduction of gonadotropic hormones LH and follicle-stimulating hormone (FSH) from the pituitary gland by estrogen, which has a strong negative feedback effect on LH and FSH secretion. This reduction in LH and FSH results in decreased testicular size and lower testosterone levels, with a consequent reduction in aggressive behavior. However, there appears to be sufficient testosterone secreted to maintain an anabolic effect. Therefore, the repeated use of estrogens in bulls beginning at 1-3 mo of age may lead to a hormonal castration effect with increased growth rate.

Use in Horses: The use of anabolic agents in horses is not recommended because of adverse effects on the reproductive system. Administration of a steroid hormonal androgen analog decreases testicular size in stallions. Decreased hormonal concentrations, especially LH, testosterone, and inhibin, adversely affect testicular histology and spermatogenesis and transiently decrease sperm output and quality. One of the most commonly used compounds is 19-nortestosterone for therapy in debilitated and anemic horses. However, use of these compounds is contraindicated, and longterm treatment or large doses have serious side effects on reproductive tract function.

Use in Other Species: In **pigs**, the growth responses from the use of estradiol, progesterone, and zeranol are variable but generally low. TBA seems to increase lean meat content of pig carcasses.

In **sheep**, the responses to anabolic agents parallel those obtained in cattle. The most consistent responses have been obtained in lambs finished on high-concentrate diets; a 10-15% increase in daily gain can be expected. Anabolic steroids should not be used in lambs to be retained for breeding. Also, implantation with zeranol reduces testicular development in ram lambs and delays the onset of puberty and reduces the ovulation rate in female sheep. Moreover, the short finishing period and the extensive nature of some production systems militate against widespread practical use of growth promotants in sheep on economic grounds.

In **poultry**, responses to estrogens include increased fat deposition. Androgens, however, have given conflicting responses. Hence, their use is of no practical significance at this time.

In **fish**, methyl testosterone can induce sex reversal in rainbow trout, thereby promoting growth and improved feed conversion efficiency.

Possible Complications: Any hormonal implant has a negative feedback effect on pituitary gonadotropins, thereby reducing LH and FSH secretion. Therefore, they can affect the onset of puberty and the regularity of estrous cycles, as well as reduce conception rate in females and testicular development (and thus sperm output) in males. Hormonal growth promotants should never be used in animals that are or may be used for breeding purposes; nor should they be used before puberty to increase growth in yearling thoroughbreds or young pedigree bulls for show purposes. If given to pregnant heifers, TBA results in increased incidence of severe dystocia, masculinization of female genitalia of the fetus, increased calf mortality, and reduced milk yield in the subsequent lactation.

In general, no undue behavioral side effects have been reported after the use of either zeranol or TBA alone or in combination in cattle. However, cattle that have implants may succumb to stress more easily than cattle that do not. The major problem arises from the use of estradiol as a growth promotant. Its use in various implants has been associated with transient increased mounting behavior and aggression. These effects generally last for 1-10 days after implantation and then subside. In some cases, the size of rudimentary teats can be increased. However, there have been a few reports of undesirable behavior in steers that lasted for 4-10 wk. The cause of this unpredictable adverse behavior is not clear, but it is generally more severe in dairy cattle used for beef production. To minimize the adverse behavior after implantation, it is important to avoid crushing the pellet-type implants during insertion and to not mix new cattle with those that have implants. If the problem is severe, the buller steers should be identified and removed; if very severe, removal of the implants or administration of 50-100 mg progesterone in oil for a number of days to suppress behavior should be considered.

Factors Affecting Response: A number of factors affect the response, including genetic make-up, plane of nutrition, the sex and age of the animal, and prior implantation.

Animals should be gaining a minimum of 0.5 kg/day before an economic response is obtained. Implants are best used in animals on a high plane of nutrition and under good husbandry conditions. They are an aid to, but not a substitute for, good husbandry. Consequently, there is no point in implanting cattle destined for a 3- to 4-mo "store period." Responses are also lower in animals of high genetic merit (eg, growth rate >1.4 kg/day). The quality of the diet may influence the growth response, with higher crude protein (up to 18% of diet) yielding improved responses.

Steers show the maximal response. Responses are reduced in calves, and responses are good in yearlings and older animals. Maximal responses are probably obtained in older beef cattle at the beginning of an intensive winter finishing period. Females do respond, probably better to androgens such as TBA.

Prior implantation does not affect the response to the next implantation. Also, once the implant effect has ceased, the rate of gain reverts back to the rate that was obtained before implantation, assuming the level of feeding has not changed. Also, extra weight induced by implants in early life is transferred through to extra carcass weight at slaughter.

GROWTH HORMONE

The peptide most commonly used to enhance growth and production is growth hormone (GH). Its chemical structure is species-specific and it has a short half-life (20-30 min). It is not orally active and is rapidly digested and cleared by the gut, liver, and kidney; thus, it must be administered via a parenteral route. Sustained-release (14-28 days) formulations have been developed for use in cattle to obviate the need for daily injections. When administered to cattle, GH increases growth rate (5-10%), feed conversion efficiency, and the carcass lean to fat ratio. Gender has little effect on response in cattle. Response to GH is lower in older cattle with greater fat deposition. There is an interaction between magnitude of response and nutritional level; protein content and specific amino acid composition may be important to achieve maximal responses. The effects of GH are largely additive to those obtained from steroid implants. GH improves growth and feed efficiency in sheep but not in poultry. Recombinant GH in pigs has dramatic effects, resulting in an increase in daily gain (20%), decrease in feed intake (5%), and a decrease in the feed:gain ratio (20%). A 10% increase in lean content and a 35% decrease in adipose tissue may be realized in swine. Administration of 25 mg/day of bovine GH to lactating cattle increases milk yields of dairy cows by up to 20%. GH has been approved for commercial use in some countries to increase milk production.

β-ADRENOCEPTOR AGONISTS

Phenethanolamine β-adrenoceptor agonists (βAA) are chemically similar in structure to epinephrine and norepinephrine and have paracrine, neurotransmitter, and endocrine (hormonal) effects. There is a range of βAA compounds resulting from structural modifications and aromatic ring substitution. The βAA bind to β-adrenergic receptors, which have been classified into β1, β2, and β3 subtypes based on the physiologic response obtained. β1 receptors are located primarily in cardiac muscle, β2 receptors in tracheal and skeletal muscle, and β3 receptors in brown adipose tissue. In general, βAA have specificity for receptor subtypes, thereby providing specificity regarding their physiologic actions. However, there are multiple receptor subclasses in most tissues, and the relative concentrations of β1 and β2 receptors in a tissue determine the physiologic response. Muscle and adipose cells have predominantly β2 receptors. β-Adrenergic agonist use leads to an increase in muscle mass caused by increased protein synthesis with a concomitant decrease in protein degradation, and a decrease in carcass fat due to decreased rates of lipid accretion. The exact proportion of receptor subtypes varies between tissues and also across species, resulting in species-specific responses to selected βAA. The physiologic activity of βAA depends on the dose, receptor binding specificity, mode of administration, rate of absorption, and metabolic clearance rate in treated animals.

The major use of βAA in food animal production is to increase carcass leanness. In cattle and sheep, weight gain, gain:feed ratio, and meat content are increased by 10-20% and lipid content is decreased by 7-20%. In swine and chickens, responses are much lower, with pigs responding better than chickens. Weight gain is increased by 2-4%, and gain:feed ratio is slightly improved in chickens but not in pigs. Meat content is increased by 2-4% and lipid content decreased by 7-8% in chickens and pigs.

Side effects depend on compound administered, dose used, and species treated, but those selected for commercial use have minimal side effects. They are orally active. Dosage level of the compound used affects the response obtained; the optimal dose often varies for different production variables measured. The most consistent effects are increased proportion of lean meat, but the effects on meat quality vary with compound used, dosage given, duration of treatment, and species treated. Certain compounds have been reported to increase toughness of meat in cattle. Due to potential side effects and adverse effects on meat quality, many compounds are unlikely to be approved for use as growth promotants, although some countries do allow the use of specific compounds in pig production (ractopamine). The use of β-agonists as growth promoters is banned in the EU. Illegal use of clenbuterol in cattle and certain βAA in poultry is a threat in some countries, requiring vigilance by regulatory authorities. The longterm accumulation of these compounds in hair and ocular tissue has been used to screen for their presence in some countries.

ANTIMICROBIAL FEED ADDITIVES

Maintenance of healthy animals requires prevention of infection by pathogenic organisms. In addition, specific alteration of a host's microflora may have beneficial effects on animal production by alteration of ruminal flora, resulting in changes in the proportions of volatile fatty acids produced during ruminal digestion. Thus, antimicrobial compounds may improve production efficiency of healthy animals fed optimal nutritional regimens. Production-enhancing antimicrobial compounds can be classified as ionophore or nonionophore antibiotics. Antimicrobial compounds are administered in the feed at low dose rates relative to high doses required for therapeutic effects. Feed additives can be given once the rumen is functioning, although some antibiotic compounds can be fed to calves prior to this point.

Antimicrobial growth promotants commonly used in livestock are detailed in TABLE 62. Antimicrobials are used in male and female animals without adverse effects on ovarian and testicular development or function because they are poorly absorbed. Unlike anabolic steroids, they do not affect carcass composition. Antimicrobials are commonly used in conjunction with estradiol, zeranol, or TBA, and generally their combined effects are additive.

Ionophore Antibiotics: Ionophores (eg, monensin and lasalocid) modify the movement of monovalent (sodium and potassium) and divalent (calcium) ions across biologic membranes, modify the rumen microflora, decrease acetate and methane production, increase propionate, may improve nitrogen utilization, and can increase dry matter digestibility in ruminants. Their main effect is to increase feed efficiency, but they may also improve growth rates of ruminants on high-roughage diets. Administration of monensin to cattle results in 2-10% improvement in liveweight gain (in animals on a high-roughage diet), 3-7% increase in feed conversion efficiency, and up to a 6% decrease in food consumption. Initially, monensin was used only as a feed additive, but with the introduction of controlled-release formulations, its use has been extended to grazing animals. Other ionophores generally have similar effects. Doses range from 6-30 ppm in the diet. Ionophores are absorbed from the gut, rapidly metabolized by the liver, and reenter the gut from bile. Some ionophores also have a therapeutic use (eg, monensin for prevention of coccidiosis in poultry).

Nonionophore Antibiotics: These compounds are used to selectively modify microbial populations within animals to improve production efficiency and to maintain health

TABLE 62. Antibacterial Growth Promoters for Potential Use in Livestock Production

Compound	Class	Absorption	Effects
Bambermycins	Phosphogly-colipid	Not absorbed	Increase FCE[*], growth promotion in poultry, cattle
Lasalocid sodium	Ionophore		Increase FCE in cattle
Monensin sodium	Ionophore	Poorly absorbed	Increase FCE, increase DLWG[†] in cattle and lambs
Salinomycin	Ionophore		Increase DLWG and FCE
Virginiamycin	Peptide	Not absorbed	Growth promotion in poultry
Zinc bacitracin	Peptide	Not absorbed	Growth promotion in poultry

[*]Feed conversion efficiency
[†]Daily liveweight gain

by combating low-level infections, particularly in intensive systems. Phosphoglycolipid antibiotics (eg, flavophospholipol) alter ruminal flora by inhibiting the action of some gram-positive gut microorganisms and peptoglycan formation, yielding similar production responses to those produced by ionophores. The means by which specific compounds exert their antimicrobial effect differ. Antibiotics may have a nitrogen-sparing effect, thereby increasing the availability of amino acids to the animal.

Most feeds for broiler and pig production in some countries contain antimicrobial growth promoters. These compounds can also be administered to calves, yearlings, and finishing cattle either in milk replacer or in supplementary concentrates. Antibiotic compounds, in general, increase growth rate by 2-10% and feed conversion efficiency by 3-9%. Their effects are greater in young animals, and production responses are reduced when production conditions are optimized (good housing, optimal health, and hygiene). They have minimal effects on carcass composition other than that due to better growth rate.

The development of microbial resistance to antibiotics in treated animals, which can then be spread to humans, is an important concern regarding the widespread use of antimicrobial feed additives in food production. There is circumstantial evidence that use of subtherapeutic doses of antimicrobials creates selective pressure for the emergence of antimicrobial resistance, which may be transmitted to the consumer from food or through contact with treated animals or animal manure. A ban on the use of antibiotics as feed additives decreased drug-resistant bacteria in a Danish study. While overall mortality rates of chickens were not affected, more feed was consumed per kg of weight. Therapeutic use of antibiotics was increased, but the total volume of antibiotic use was significantly decreased. The EU has banned bacitracin, carbodox, olaquindox, tylosin, and virginiamycin; it is also phasing out the use of avilamycin, flavophospholipol, lasalocid sodium, monensin sodium, and salinomycin by 2006.

PROBIOTICS

Probiotics promote the establishment and development of a desirable intestinal microbial balance in the animal. There is a delicate balance between normal and pathogenic microorganisms. This balance can be upset by poor husbandry conditions, disease, or stressors (eg, transport). Bacteria that produce lactic acid can, in general, be beneficial to the animal; certain yeasts may also be beneficial. Their ability to increase growth and promote health are claimed to be due to one or more of the following factors: preventing colonization of the gut by pathogenic coliforms, altering GI absorption rate, and inhibiting bacterial growth and influencing the balance of bacteria in the gut. The probiotic feed additives consist of selected strains of lactobacilli and streptococci that alter the microbial species present in the GI system to the benefit of the treated animal. Unicellular yeasts are also used. The production benefits are variable, and positive responses are more likely when a stressful management change may result in a change in balance of gut microflora. Probiotics can help overcome the negative effects of certain conditions that detrimentally modify the gut flora. Thus, they are useful in some cases to minimize GI upsets or to help overcome stress due to weaning or transport. The unicellular yeast fungus may also have beneficial effects on rumen fermentation and thereby improve digestion and feed efficiency. The effect of probiotics in older animals may be reduced due to the well-established, balanced population of microflora that is less sensitive to minor detrimental husbandry challenges.

VACCINES AND IMMUNOTHERAPY

The acquired immunologic defenses of the body respond to antigen by producing antibodies or effector T cells, or both. Administration of a specific antigen (as in a vaccine) may result in the development of an immune response to the inducing antigen. As a result, vaccines can provoke effective, and often very specific, longterm immunity. In addition, some microbial molecules can stimulate the development of innate immune responses such as the production of acute-phase proteins or stimulation of cytokines and other soluble mediators of inflammation. On occasion, this nonspecific immuno-stimulation may enhance resistance to infection and may itself be therapeutically useful.

SPECIFIC IMMUNOTHERAPY

Active Immunization

Active immunization involves administration of antigen(s) derived from an infectious agent so that an animal mounts an acquired immune response and achieves resistance to that agent. When properly used, vaccines are highly effective in controlling infectious diseases. Several criteria determine whether a vaccine can or should be used. First, the actual cause of the disease must be determined. Although this appears self-evident, it has not always been followed in practice. For example, in the bovine respiratory disease complex, although *Mannheimia (Pasteurella) haemolytica* can be isolated consistently, these bacteria are not the sole cause of this syndrome. In some viral diseases (eg, equine infectious anemia, feline infectious peritonitis, Aleutian disease in mink) antibodies contribute to the disease process, and vaccination may make it more severe. Therefore, vaccination must be governed by the principle of informed consent. The risks of vaccination must not exceed those caused by the disease itself.

When vaccines are used to control disease in a population rather than in individuals, the concept of herd immunity must be considered. Herd immunity refers to increased resistance of a group because of the presence of some immune animals within the group, which reduces the probability of a susceptible animal encountering an infected one. As a result, spread of infectious disease is slowed or blocked.

An ideal vaccine for active immunization should confer prolonged, strong immunity in the vaccinated animal. It should not cause adverse side effects and should be inexpensive, stable, and adaptable to mass vaccination. It should also stimulate an immune response distinguishable from that due to natural infection so that vaccination and eradication may proceed simultaneously.

Vaccines Containing Nonreplicating Antigens

Killed Vaccines: Vaccines may contain either living or killed organisms. Killed organisms are commonly much less immunogenic than living ones. As a result, vaccines that contain killed organisms or their products usually require the use of adjuvants to increase their effective antigenicity. These adjuvants may, however, cause local inflammation, and multiple doses or high individual doses of antigen increase the risks of producing hypersensitivity.

Inactivated vaccines should resemble the living organisms as closely as possible. Chemical inactivation is usually used under conditions that cause minimal change to the antigens. Compounds used in this way include formaldehyde, ethylene oxide, ethyleneimine, acetylethyleneimine, and β-propiolactone.

While whole killed organisms are economical to produce, they contain many antigens that do not contribute to protective immunity. They may also contain toxic molecules that can provoke adverse effects. Thus, it is often advantageous to use subunits or subcomponents of microorganisms as vaccine antigens.

Subunit Vaccines: When the immunogenic portion of an organism can be identified, it can be used in a vaccine by itself. These fractions may be derived by purifying individual components of a whole cell culture. Thus, purified tetanus toxin, inactivated by treatment with formalin (tetanus toxoid), is used for active immunization against tetanus. The attachment pili of enteropathogenic *Escherichia coli* can be isolated, and the purified pilus proteins incorporated into vaccines. The antipilus antibodies thus protect animals by preventing bacterial attachment to the intestinal wall.

If quantities of purified antigen cannot be produced economically by fractionation, genetic material that codes for antigens can be isolated by recombinant DNA techniques. This DNA is then inserted into an expression vector such as a bacterium or yeast, which then expresses that protein. Subunit vaccines can then be derived from recombinant organisms into which a foreign gene from a specific pathogen has been inserted. The recombinant organism is propagated, and the protein encoded by the inserted gene is harvested, purified, and administered as a vaccine. An example of a subunit vaccine is one directed against the cloned subunit of *E coli* enterotoxin. Subunits are immunogenic and function as effective toxoids. The gene has been cloned, linked with a powerful promoter, and transfected into a nonpathogenic strain of *E coli*. A purified subunit protein vaccine, OspA, encoded by a single gene obtained from *Borrelia burgdorferi* has been highly effective in protecting dogs against Lyme disease. Recombinant DNA techniques are useful when protein antigens need to be synthesized in large, pure quantities.

Although antigens may be large molecules, they usually have only a small number of sites (epitopes) that are important in inducing protective immunity. If the structure of a protective antigen is known, its important epitopes may be identified, and their structure analyzed and then artificially synthesized. In theory, these synthetic epitopes may then be used in a vaccine if they are large enough to be immunogenic. In practice, they are usually uneconomical to produce commercially.

Vaccines Containing Replicating Antigens

Attenuated Vaccines: Vaccines that contain only killed organisms or subunits will not cause disease and are relatively easy to store. Some live vaccines, conversely, may have a limited ability to cause disease (residual virulence) in vaccinated animals. There is a risk of contamination with unwanted organisms in live vaccines. They also require considerable care in their preparation, storage, and handling to avoid temperature extremes that can affect the organisms.

As a compromise, the virulence of an organism can be reduced (attenuated) so that it is able to replicate but is no longer pathogenic. Attenuation has traditionally involved adapting organisms to unusual conditions. Bacteria can be attenuated by culture under abnormal conditions, and viruses can be attenuated by growth in species to which they are not naturally adapted. For example, rinderpest vaccine virus has been adapted to tissue culture to produce a safe vaccine. Other examples are adaptation of African horse sickness virus to mice and of canine distemper virus to ferrets, however, vaccines attenuated this way are not commonly used.

Vaccine viruses may also be attenuated by growth in alternative media, such as tissue culture or eggs. This has been done for canine distemper, bluetongue, and rabies vaccines. The most common method is prolonged tissue culture. Usually, cells from the species to be vaccinated are used to reduce the problems caused by the administration of foreign tissue. In these cases, the virus is attenuated by growing it in cells that it would not normally infect. For example, canine distemper virus normally infects lymphoid cells, but for attenuation purposes, the virus is repeatedly cultured in canine kidney cells.

Attenuation eventually results in the production of a genetically stable, avirulent agent. This may be difficult to achieve, and reversion to virulence is a concern. Rigorous reversion to virulence studies are performed to demonstrate stability of the attenuation. In addition, modern molecular techniques are increasingly used to ensure loss of virulence.

For some diseases, related organisms normally adapted to another species can impart limited immunity. Examples include measles virus, which can protect dogs against distemper, and bovine viral diarrhea virus, which can protect against classical swine fever.

Under some circumstances, fully virulent organisms can be used in vaccination procedures, eg, vaccination against contagious ecthyma (orf) of sheep. Lambs are vaccinated by rubbing dried, infected scab material into scratches made on the inner thigh, which produces local infection with only limited effects on the lambs; they become solidly immune. Because the vaccinated animals may spread the disease, however, they must be separated from unvaccinated stock for a few weeks.

Gene-deleted Vaccines: Because attenuated organisms may revert to virulence, deliberate deletion of genes associated with microbial or viral virulence is an increasingly attractive procedure. Gene-deleted vaccines were first used against the pseudorabies herpesvirus in swine, eg, development of a vaccine in which the thymidine kinase gene was removed from the virus. Herpesvirus requires thymidine kinase to return from latency. Viruses from which this gene has been removed can infect neurons but cannot replicate and cause disease. This vaccine not only confers effective protection but also blocks cell invasion by virulent pseudorabies virus and prevents development of a persistent carrier state. It is also possible to alter surface antigens so that a virus induces an antibody response distinguishable from that caused by wild strains. This concept is referred to as DIVA, or distinguishing infected from vaccinated animals.

Live Vectored Vaccines: An alternative method of inducing strong immunity is to place the genes for a protective immunogen in an avirulent "vector" organism. The most widely used viral vectors are poxviruses such as fowlpox, canarypox, and vaccinia. Vectored vaccines are commercially available for avian influenza in poultry, canine distemper, rabies in dogs and cats, West Nile virus infection in horses, and for use in vaccinating wildlife against rabies. These vaccines are free of adverse effects, stable, adaptable to mass vaccination, nonadjuvanted, and like the gene-deleted vaccines, allow for DIVA. They are created by recombinant technology, wherein one or more genes are deleted from the vector and replaced by one or more protective genes from the pathogen. The vector is then administered as the vaccine, and the inserted gene products are produced by the vaccinate's own body cells when infected by the vector. The vector may be severely attenuated so that it will not be shed from the vaccinate, or it may be host-restricted so that it will not replicate itself within the tissues of the vaccinate. Field data collected on these vaccines indicate strong immunity, limited side effects, and no shedding into the environment when used in a bait and distributed into the habitat of a wildlife species being immunized.

In the recombinant avian influenza vaccine, the hemagglutinin gene from the influenza virus has been incorporated into a gene-deleted vaccine strain of fowlpox. The immune system of the vaccinate reacts against the poxvirus, and the gene encodes proteins from the influenza virus, inducing protection against both diseases. The vaccine has been shown to be effective in the field against morbidity and shedding of the influenza virus, when used as a primary vaccination. In the recombinant-vectored rabies vaccine, the gene encoding the rabies glycoprotein has been incorporated into an attenuated vaccinia virus. Because this virus is taken up by mammalian cells nonselectively, many different wildlife species can be protected against rabies with this vaccine. Canarypox vector-containing genes obtained from canine distemper virus is now used to immunize dogs, and a similar vector containing the gene encoding rabies glycoprotein is effective in protecting dogs and cats against rabies.

DNA Vaccines: It is possible to immunize an animal simply by injecting it with bacterially derived DNA coding for an antigen. If the DNA is incorporated into an appropriate plasmid, it is able to express the protective antigen and trigger an immune response. Although no DNA vaccines are currently commercially available, they are likely to enter the veterinary market in the near future in preventative and therapeutic forms.

Administration of Vaccines

The simplest and most common method is SC or IM injection. This approach is excellent for relatively small numbers of animals and for diseases in which systemic immunity is important. However, local immunity is sometimes more important than systemic immunity, and in these cases, it is more appropriate to administer the vaccine at the site of microbial invasion. For example, intranasal vaccines are effective in protecting cattle against infectious bovine rhinotracheitis, cats against feline rhinotracheitis and calicivirus infections, and poultry against infectious bronchitis and Newcastle disease. Unfortunately, these techniques require handling each individual animal. Aerosolization of vaccines enables them to be inhaled by all the animals in a herd, group, or flock—an obvious advantage when the unit is large. This method is commonly used in the poultry industry. Alternatively, a vaccine may be administered in feed or drinking water, eg, vaccination of poultry for Newcastle disease and avian encephalomyelitis. Fish and shrimp may be vaccinated by immersion in a solution of antigen, which is absorbed through their gills. Advances in transdermal, needle-free injections make additional routes available.

Mixed Vaccines: Because of the complexity of many disease syndromes, and to avoid giving animals multiple injections, it is common to use mixtures of organisms in single vaccines. For example, for bovine respiratory disease complex, combined vaccines are available for bovine respiratory syncytial virus, infectious bovine rhinotracheitis virus, bovine viral diarrhea virus, parainfluenza 3 virus, and *Mannheimia (Pasteurella) haemolytica*. Mixed vaccines that save considerable time and effort are also commonly used in dogs and cats. Mixed vaccines are often used to protect animals against several different agents with economy of effort, but it may be wasteful to use vaccines against organisms that are not causing problems. In addition, when a mixture of different antigens is inoculated simultaneously, they may compete with one another. However, manufacturers have recognized this and modified vaccines accordingly. Vaccines should never be mixed indiscriminately because one component may dominate and interfere with responses to the other components.

Vaccination Schedules: Although it is not possible to devise precise schedules for each vaccine, certain principles are common to all methods of active immunization. Newborn animals are passively protected by maternal antibodies and, in general, cannot be vaccinated. If stimulation of immunity is deemed necessary at this stage, the mother may be vaccinated during late pregnancy, timing the doses so that peak antibody levels are reached at the time of colostrum formation. Successful active vaccination was previously thought to be possible only after passive immunity had waned. Neonatal animals with certain levels of pathogen-specific, detectable antibodies were thought to be protected against disease caused by that pathogen. However, studies in puppies born to bitches immunized against rabies during pregnancy have shown that passive antibody titers decrease significantly by 6 wk of age. In fact, when challenged with virulent rabies virus at 6 wk of age, >90% of these puppies succumbed. Similar puppies vaccinated at 7 and 11 wk of age with a recombinant vectored rabies virus were all solidly protected against rabies, even though many of them had high levels of maternal antibody when vaccinated. This has also been demonstrated with canine distemper virus and recombinant vaccines. It is now known that an antigen can impart memory to the immune system even when passive maternal antibody is present. With the availability of recombinant vaccines, the age of and interval between vaccinations may have to be reconsidered. Because the exact time of loss of maternal immunity cannot be predicted, young animals are often vaccinated at least twice to ensure successful immunization.

The interval between vaccine doses depends on an animal's immunologic memory. The duration of this memory depends on multiple used, such as the nature of the antigen, the use of live or dead organisms, adjuvants used, and the route of administration. Modern vaccines may induce immunity that persists for an animal's lifetime. Other vaccines may require boosting only once every 2-3 yr. Even killed viral vaccines may protect some animals against disease for many years. Unfortunately, the minimal duration of immunity has, until recently, rarely been reliably measured. Annual revaccination has been the rule because this approach is administratively simple and has the advantage of ensuring that an animal is regularly seen by a veterinarian. It is likely that this is more than sufficient for most vaccines.

Individual animal and vaccine variability make it difficult to estimate the duration of immunity. Within a group of animals, there may be a great difference between the shortest and longest duration of protection. Vaccines may differ significantly in their composition, and although all may induce immunity in the short term, it cannot be assumed that they confer equal longterm immunity. A significant difference likely exists between the minimal level of immunity required to protect most animals and the level of immunity required to ensure protection of all animals.

Unfortunately, there is insufficient information available for most vaccines to determine minimal vaccination intervals. A veterinarian should always assess the relative risks and benefits to an animal when determining the frequency of revaccination. Owners should be made aware that protection can be maintained reliably only when vaccines are used in accordance with the protocol approved by vaccine licensing authorities. The duration of immunity claimed by a vaccine manufacturer is the minimal duration that is supported by the data available at the time of approval.

Failures in Vaccination

There are many reasons why vaccination may fail. In some cases, the vaccine may not be effective because it contains strains of organisms or antigens that are different from the disease-producing agent. In other cases, the method of manufacture may have destroyed the protective epitopes, or there may simply be insufficient antigen. Such problems are relatively uncommon and generally can be avoided by using vaccines from reputable manufacturers. An effective vaccine may fail due to unsatisfactory administration. For example, a live vaccine may be inactivated as a result of improper storage, use of antibiotics in conjunction with a live bacterial vaccine, chemical sterilization of syringes, or excessive use of alcohol on the skin. Administration by nonconventional routes may also affect efficacy. When vaccine is administered to poultry or mink by aerosol or in drinking water, the aerosol may not be evenly distributed throughout a building, or some animals may not drink adequate amounts. Also, chlorinated water may inactivate vaccines. If an animal is incubating the disease before vaccination, the vaccine may not be protective; vaccination against an already contracted disease is usually impossible.

The immune response, being a biologic process, never confers absolute protection nor is equal in all individuals of a vaccinated population. Because the response is influenced by many factors, the range in a random population tends to follow a normal distribution: the response will be average in most animals, excellent in a few, and poor in a few. Those with a poor response may not be protected by an effective vaccine; it is difficult to protect 100% of a random population by vaccination. The size of this unresponsive population varies among vaccines, and its significance depends on the nature of the disease. For highly infectious diseases in which herd immunity is poor and infection is rapidly and efficiently transmitted (eg, foot-and-mouth disease), the presence of unprotected animals can permit the spread of disease and disrupt control programs. Problems also can arise if the unprotected animals are individually important, as in the case of companion animals or breeding stock. In contrast, for diseases that are inefficiently spread (eg, rabies), 60-70% protection in a population may be sufficient to effectively block disease transmission within that population and therefore may be satisfactory from a public health perspective.

The most important cause of vaccine failure in young animals is the inability of an antigen to impart immunologic memory whether or not passive maternal antibodies are present. Vaccines also can fail when the immune response is suppressed, eg, in heavily parasitized or malnourished animals (such animals should not be vaccinated). Stress, including pregnancy, extremes of cold and heat, and fatigue or malnourishment, may reduce a normal immune response, probably due to increased glucocorticoid production.

Adverse Consequences of Vaccination

Modern, commercially produced, government-approved vaccines are generally very safe. Nevertheless, they are not always innocuous. The more common risks associated with vaccines include residual virulence and toxicity, which may cause injection-site reactions, allergic responses, incomplete inactivation, disease in immunodeficient hosts (modified-live vaccines), neurologic complications, and, rarely, contamination with other live agents. For example, lesions of mucosal disease may be seen in calves vaccinated against bovine viral diarrhea. Vaccines that contain killed gram-negative organisms may also contain endotoxins, which stimulate release of interleukin-1 and can cause stress with fever and leukopenia. Although such a reaction is usually only a temporary inconvenience to males, it may be sufficient to induce abortion in females. In general, it is prudent to avoid vaccinating pregnant animals unless the risks of not vaccinating are greater. Certain modified-live virus Bluetongue vaccines have been reported to cause congenital anomalies when given to pregnant ewes. The stress from a vaccination reaction may be sufficient to activate latent infections. For example, activation of equine herpesvirus has been demonstrated after vaccination against African horse sickness. Another adverse reaction is the "sting" that occurs when some vaccines are administered. This can cause problems for the vaccinator if the vaccinated animal objects strenuously. Some vaccines cause mild immunosuppression.

In addition to potential virulence or toxicity, vaccines, like any antigen, may provoke hypersensitivity reactions. For example, type I hypersensitivity may be seen in response to any of the antigens found in vaccines, including those from eggs or tissue-culture cells. All forms of hypersensitivity are more commonly associated with multiple injections of antigen; therefore, they tend to be associated with use of inactivated products. Type III hypersensitivity reactions are also potential hazards of vaccination. These may cause an intense local inflammatory reaction or a generalized vascular disturbance such as purpura. An example of a type III reaction is clouding of the cornea in dogs vaccinated against infectious canine hepatitis. Type IV hypersensitivity reactions, expressed as granuloma formation, may be seen at the site of inoculation in response to the use of depot adjuvants. Some adjuvanted feline vaccines are associated with the subsequent development of a fibrosarcoma at the site of injection.

Production of Vaccines

In most countries, the production of biologics is regulated by government authorities. In general, regulatory authorities have the right to license establishments that produce vaccines and to inspect those premises to ensure that the facilities and the methods used are satisfactory. All vaccines are checked for safety and potency. Safety tests include confirmation of the identity of the organism used, freedom of the vaccine from contamination with extraneous organisms, and host safety toxicity tests. Because the living organisms found in vaccines normally die over time, it is necessary to ensure that they will be effective even after storage. Although properly stored vaccines may still be potent after the expiration of their designated shelf life, this should never be assumed; expired vaccines should not be used.

Passive Immunization

Passive immunization involves the production of antibodies in one animal by active immunization, followed by transfer of these antibodies to susceptible animals to confer immediate protection. The transfer of maternal antibody to offspring via the placenta or colostrum is the natural (and very important) form of passive immunization. Antisera may be produced in cattle against anthrax, in dogs against distemper, and in cats against panleukopenia. Their most important role is in protection against toxigenic organisms, eg, *Clostridium tetani* or *C perfringens*. Such antisera are known as immune globulins and are generally produced in young horses by a series of immunizing inoculations.

To check the potency of preparations of immune globulin, comparison is made with an international biological standard. An International Unit (IU) of tetanus immune globulin is the specific neutralizing activity contained in 0.03384 mg of the international standard. The USA Standard Unit (AU) is twice the IU.

Tetanus immune globulin (tetanus antitoxin) is given to animals to confer immediate protection against tetanus. At least 1,500-3,000 IU of immune globulin should be given to horses and cattle; at least 500 IU to calves, sheep, goats, and pigs; and at least 250 IU to dogs. The exact amount varies with the amount of tissue damage, degree of wound contamination, and time elapsed since injury. Tetanus immune globulin is of little use once clinical signs appear, although massive doses of up to 300,000 IU may help.

To reduce their antigenicity for other species, immune globulins of equine origin are usually treated with pepsin.

Monoclonal Antibodies: Antibodies produced by the normal immune response are derived from many different plasma cells. As a result, although they combine with a specific antigen, they are a heterogeneous mixture. Homogeneous antibodies can be generated through the use of cell lines called hybridomas; these, called monoclonal antibodies, represent an alternative source of passive protection. Currently, however, these are mainly made by mouse hybridomas (and thus consist of mouse antibodies) and may sensitize other animal species. Nevertheless, mouse monoclonal antibodies against the K99 pilus antigens of *E coli* can be given PO to calves to protect them against diarrhea caused by this organism, although this product is no longer commercially available.

Monoclonal antibodies also are used in diagnosis. Because they are homogeneous and specific, they have the ability to differentiate between closely related infectious agents in a manner that is impossible with conventional antibodies. For example, they can differentiate between the rabies viruses obtained from skunks, bats, or dogs.

NONSPECIFIC IMMUNOTHERAPY

In many situations, it is desirable to enhance the activity of an animal's immune system. This may include stimulation of the normal immune response to enhance protection and treatment of immunosuppressive conditions. The several different types of immunostimulators vary according to their origin, mode of action, and use.

Adjuvants

To maximize the effectiveness of vaccines, especially those containing killed organisms, adjuvants are commonly added. Adjuvants can greatly enhance the body's response to vaccines and are essential if longterm memory is to be established against soluble antigens. Adjuvants work in 1 of 3 ways: 1) depot adjuvants that protect antigens from rapid degradation and thus prolong immune responses, 2) particles that effectively deliver antigen to antigen-presenting cells, and 3) molecules that stimulate immune responses by mechanisms such as signaling through toll-like receptors.

Depot adjuvants delay the elimination of antigens and thus permit an immune response to last longer. Examples include aluminum salts such as aluminum hydroxide, aluminum phosphate, and aluminum potassium sulfate (alum). Some depot adjuvants incorporate the antigen in a water-in-oil emulsion. These depot adjuvants can cause significant tissue irritation and destruction. Mineral oils are especially irritating. Nonmineral oils, while less irritating, are also less effective and are now more widely used.

Particulate adjuvants include emulsions, microparticles, iscoms, and liposomes. All are designed to deliver antigen efficiently to antigen-presenting cells. They commonly are of similar size to bacteria and are readily endocytosed by antigen-presenting cells. They are not yet widely used in veterinary vaccines due to complexities in the manufacturing process.

Immunostimulatory adjuvants promote cytokine production by activating antigen-processing cells. They include lipopolysaccharides, killed anaerobic corynebacteria (especially *Propionibacterium acnes* and *Bordetella pertussis*), microbial cytidylate-phosphate-guanylate DNA, and saponins. Very powerful adjuvants can be constructed by combining a particulate or depot adjuvant with an immunostimulatory agent.

Immunostimulants

In contrast to adjuvants, immunostimulants do not need to be administered together with antigen to enhance immunity. They are generally given to induce a short-term, nonantigen-specific enhancement of the immune system. They appear to be most useful when treating chronic diseases in which there is good evidence of immunosuppression. They are used in the therapy of equine sarcoid, bovine papilloma, equine respiratory disease, equine endometritis, chronic skin diseases (eg, staphylococcal pyoderma or demodicosis), certain tumors of dogs and cats, and immunosuppressive viral diseases (eg, feline leukemia).

Many bacteria have been utilized as immunostimulants. The most potent of these is BCG, the live attenuated vaccine strain of *Mycobacterium bovis*. BCG produces a generalized enhancement of both B- and T-cell-mediated responses and of phagocytosis, graft rejection, and resistance to infection. Because BCG causes tuberculin sensitivity, these organisms must be fractionated to remove the reactive material. Thus, mycobacterial cell wall fractions, muramyl dipeptide (MDP), and trehalose dimycolate have all been used as immunostimulants. MDP, the most potent factor from mycobacteria, enhances antibody production and stimulates and activates macrophages.

Another organism, *Propionibacterium acnes* also promotes a generalized enhancement of nonspecific immunity. The cell wall of *P acnes* contains MDP and lipid compounds that are immunostimulatory. This material has a complex activity because it stimulates phagocytosis by macrophages and neutrophils; increased activity of natural killer cells; development of T and B lymphocytes; and increased production of interleukin-1, interferons, and tumor necrosis factor. *P acnes* also increases resistance to infection by many pathogenic bacteria and viruses. It is administered into the circulatory system and is used in therapy of dogs with pyoderma, cattle with bovine papilloma, and horses with respiratory disease and chronic endometritis. Clinical reports indicate some success in the treatment of symptomatic feline leukemia and as an adjunct to surgery in the treatment of oral melanoma in dogs.

Cell wall components of *Staphylococcus aureus* administered SC in dogs stimulate the production of interleukin-1, interleukin-6, tumor necrosis factor, and γ interferon. This product is used successfully in the treatment and management of *Staphylococcus*-associated pyoderma in dogs. Dogs occasionally become sensitized to this material.

Acemannan is a long-chained mannan extracted from *Aloe vera (barbadensis)*. It stimulates macrophages, induces cytokine production, and enhances cellular immunity. It is indicated for wound healing, as adjunct therapy for fibrosarcoma of dogs and cats, and in the management of feline retroviral diseases.

Endotoxins from gram-negative bacteria enhance antibody formation if given at about the same time as the antigen. They have a general immunostimulatory activity because they act through toll-like receptors to induce innate resistance to bacterial infections.

Certain complex carbohydrates, eg, zymosan, glucan, dextran sulfate, and lentinans, are immunostimulants and can activate macrophages.

■ ■ ■

CIRCULATORY SYSTEM

DIGESTIVE SYSTEM

INTEGUMENTARY SYSTEM

MUSCULOSKELETAL SYSTEM

VIRAL ARTHRITIS   2284

NERVOUS SYSTEM

AVIAN ENCEPHALOMYELITIS   2285

BOTULISM   2286

VIRAL ENCEPHALITIDES   2287

WEST NILE VIRUS INFECTION   2289

REPRODUCTIVE SYSTEM

ARTIFICIAL INSEMINATION   2290

DISORDERS OF THE REPRODUCTIVE SYSTEM   2291

EGG DROP SYNDROME   2294

RESPIRATORY SYSTEM

AIR SAC MITE   2296

ASPERGILLOSIS   2296

AVIAN INFLUENZA (Fowl Plague)   2297

AVIAN PNEUMOVIRUS   2299

BORDETELLOSIS   2300

BLOODBORNE ORGANISMS

Avian blood may contain various disease agents including viruses, bacteria, rickettsiae, protozoa, microfilariae, and rarely fungi. Except for viruses, these organisms often can be identified by microscopic examination of wet mounts, buffy coat, or blood smears; appropriate culturing techniques; or subinoculation of blood into susceptible birds. Microscopically, some are within blood cells (*Plasmodium, Haemoproteus, Leucocytozoon, Atoxoplasma, Hepatocystis, Babesia, Aegyptianella*), while others are free in the plasma (*Trypanosoma*, microfilariae, bacteria, spirochetes). None lives exclusively in the blood; most are found in tissues but are present in blood during part of their life cycle. Some, such as microfilariae and *Plasmodium*, may have a periodicity when numbers or stages of parasites are present at different times. In such cases, examining multiple smears at intervals will increase the likelihood of obtaining a diagnosis. Seasonal variations in infection rates relate to the activity of arthropod vectors. When possible, tissue cytology is also a useful adjunct to examination of blood. Several bloodborne organisms are either uncommon or not associated with clinical disease. However, weakened or injured raptors infected with hemoprotozoa had higher mortality and delayed recovery compared with uninfected birds. Routine examination for bloodborne organisms should be included in the clinical and diagnostic procedures for any ill bird.

Thin blood smears should be made with blood directly from the bird if possible. Anticoagulants, storage, and cooling of the blood can distort protozoan morphology and introduce artifacts. A small drop of blood can be collected using a syringe and needle, or by selecting a small vessel in the wing web and, after cleaning the site thoroughly with alcohol and letting it dry, puncturing the vessel with a lancet so that a small drop of blood wells up from the wound. The drop should be picked up without touching the skin and spread on a clean glass slide at a 30° angle to make a thin smear. A good quality Romanowsky-type stain that gives good polychromatic coloration (eg, Giemsa stain) should be used. At least 200 oil-immersion fields (~20,000 RBC) for single smears or 100 for multiple smears from the same bird should be examined. *Leucocytozoon* and microfilariae are found around the periphery of smears and can be easily seen on low-power magnification.

Bloodborne organisms in plasma or WBC are concentrated in the buffy coat. A diamond-tipped pencil can be used to cut the microhematocrit tube just below the buffy coat above the packed RBC. The buffy coat should be expressed from the cut end with a small amount of plasma to make a suspension, and a thin smear prepared. Stained buffy coat smears are recommended for detecting bacteremia, spirochetes, and chronic *Leucocytozoon, Trypanosoma,* or *Atoxoplasma* infections. An excellent technique for identifying low numbers of motile organisms such as spirochetes and microfilariae is direct examination of the buffy coat by darkfield or phase contrast microscopy. The buffy coat and all of the plasma should be expressed onto a glass slide, and covered with a coverglass, which is depressed slightly to spread the buffy coat. The buffy coat/plasma interface should be examined with darkfield or reduced light microscopy to detect motile organisms.

Plasmodium infections can be determined by subinoculation. Ideally, birds of the same or a known susceptible avian species should be used, but this is often not practical. In general, canaries are used for detecting passerine infections, and turkeys are susceptible to most plasmodia that infect other gallinaceous birds. Parasites remain viable in blood stored at 32°F (in ice) for at least 7 days. Inoculation IV is preferred and will result in earlier parasitemia, but any parenteral route can be used. Recipients should be examined twice weekly for a minimum of 4 wk if exposed IV; longer times are needed if other routes of inoculation are used. Spirochete, *Aegyptianella*, and bacterial infections can also be detected by subinoculation of infectious blood; bacteria can usually be identified by blood culture.

To make a diagnosis of infection with an intracellular blood protozoan on a thin blood film, it first should be determined that the "parasites" in question are neither normal nor artifact. The following should then be determined: the host cell and whether it is normal or deformed beyond identification, whether pigment granules are present or absent, and whether merogony is occurring (TABLE 1). Identification of an organism beyond genus (or subgenus in the case of *Plasmodium* spp) is difficult and usually unnecessary for clinical purposes.

TABLE 1. Characteristics of Protozoa Encountered in Avian Blood

Protozoan	Host Cell	Pigment Present	Merogony in Blood
Plasmodium	RBC	Yes	Yes
Haemoproteus	RBC	Yes	No
Leucocytozoon	RBC or WBC; distorted and enlarged often beyond recognition	No	No
Atoxoplasma	WBC; in nuclear indentation	No	No[*]
Hepatozoon[†]	WBC, large, elongated oval shape	No	No
Babesia[†]	RBC	No	No[‡]

[*]Multiple intracellular parasites may be seen in acute infections.
[†]Uncommon to rare.
[‡]*Babesia* are pyriform and may be in a V, X, or fan pattern.

AEGYPTIANELLOSIS

Aegyptianellosis is an acute, tickborne, febrile disease caused by *Aegyptianella* spp, a rickettsia in the family Anaplasmataceae. Infection of avian species, including chickens, turkeys, guineafowl, quail, pigeons, crows, waterfowl, ratites, passerines, and psittacines has been described. Ticks, especially *Argas* spp, transmit the organism; infection can also be reproduced by blood inoculation. Organisms appear as single or multiple, round, "signet-ring" (0.5-4 μm) or irregular oval bodies in RBC often lateral to the nucleus. Infections are most common in tropical and subtropical areas of Africa, Asia, and Europe; infection of wild turkeys in Texas has also been reported.

In endemic areas, infection is mild or asymptomatic. Ruffled feathers, anorexia, droopiness, diarrhea, fever, jaundice, and high mortality in younger birds occur in introduced or otherwise susceptible birds. Anemia, which can lead to right heart failure and ascites, enlargement of the liver and spleen, enlarged discolored kidneys, and pinpoint serosal hemorrhages are seen. Infestation with larval argasid ticks and *Borrelia* infection (SPIROCHETOSIS, p 2219) may accompany the disease.

Tetracyclines, especially doxycycline, are effective in controlling the disease and eliminating the organism from chronically infected birds. Tick control is an important adjunct to treatment.

ATOXOPLASMOSIS
(Isosporosis, Lankesterellosis)

Atoxoplasma are pale-staining, nonpigmented, oval, intracytoplasmic bodies within mononuclear cells currently thought to be lymphocytes. Usually, cells contain a single parasite, but multiple organisms can be seen in severe, acute infections. Presence of the protozoan causes the nucleus to curve around it giving the appearance that the organism is located within an indentation of the nucleus. At least 2 different genera of coccidian protozoa (*Isospora, Lankesterella*) have merozoites in the lymphocytes that are indistinguishable from each other and have been called *Atoxoplasma*. Passerine birds, especially canaries, finches, sparrows, and species of the Sturnidae family (starlings, mynahs) are affected by both protozoa. Poultry are not known to be affected.

Isospora has a direct life cycle that includes an extra-intestinal, systemic phase in some species. Merogony occurs in the intestine and oocysts are passed in the feces. The systemic part of the life cycle was initially not recognized, leading to the description of the intestinal stages and oocysts as *Isospora serini*. Transmission is fecal-oral via ingestion of oocysts in droppings from infected birds. Infected canaries can shed oocysts for at least 2 yr. Most species of avian *Isospora* do not have extra-intestinal stages. In canaries, *I serini* has a systemic phase while *I canaria* infects only the intestinal tract.

Lankesterella has stages in the blood indistinguishable from those caused by systemic *Isospora* spp, but merogony occurs in tissues other than the intestine, especially the lungs. The life cycle is indirect. Bloodsucking arthropods, particularly mites, become infected during feeding and transmit the protozoan when it refeeds on a susceptible bird.

Signs include listlessness, diarrhea, and anorexia. Mortality can be high (up to 80%) in young birds. In acutely affected birds, there is marked hepatomegaly and splenomegaly, often with multifocal necrosis. The enlarged liver and gallbladder can be seen through the abdominal wall, especially if it is moistened with alcohol, which provides the basis for the common name black spot disease. High numbers of parasites infecting lymphocytes are present in blood and organ impression smears. Nearly spherical oocysts averaging 19×21 μm are present in droppings of canaries infected with *Isospora*. Oocysts of *I serini* need to be distinguished from those of *I canaria*, which are slightly larger and more oval.

Diagnosis is difficult in chronically infected older birds. Very few parasites are present in blood and tissues, and oocysts are shed intermittently, although sometimes in high numbers. Buffy coat and organ smears are preferred. Negative findings should not be interpreted to mean that infection is not present. Hepatic and splenic enlargement persists because of infiltrations with high numbers of large lymphoid cells that serve as host cells for the parasite. Histopathologically, organisms are difficult to find and identify. Lesions may be mistaken for lymphosarcoma.

There is no known effective treatment. Anticoccidial drugs do not affect parasites in the tissues. Use of antimalarial drugs has been suggested. Good management procedures, including prevention of exposure to mites, isolation of age groups, and scrupulous cleanliness (particularly daily cleaning before oocysts sporulate) help control the disease. Disinfectants have little effect on oocysts.

FILARIASIS

Microfilariae are commonly found in the blood of wild birds but are rare to absent in poultry except in southeast Asia where infections in chickens and waterfowl occur. A high percentage of imported cockatiels have microfilariae. At least 16 genera of filarids are found in avian species. All have an indirect life cycle with bloodsucking insects (eg, lice, mosquitos, midges) serving as intermediate hosts. Adults are relatively short lived and mature in body cavities, including the eye and ventricles of the brain, respiratory system, cardiovascular system, or connective tissues; some produce characteristic subcutaneous nodules. In contrast, microfilariae are long lived and may be numerous in the skin as well as in the circulation. Increased numbers of microfilariae have been seen in stressed individuals, but they rarely cause clinical disease or mortality. A possible exception is infection of emus with *Chandlerella*, a common filarid of the brain of free-living grackles. Parasites apparently do not produce microfilariae in emus. Affected emus show signs of CNS disease. Treatment with ivermectin, levamisole, or injection of nodules with 0.5% potassium permanganate solution, and surgical removal of adults have been used.

HAEMOPROTEUS INFECTION

Infections with *Haemoproteus* spp are common in nondomestic birds. Pigeons and doves are frequently infected. Species are found in free-living ducks, quail, and turkeys but are rare to absent in commercial flocks probably because of very specific feeding habits of *Culicoides* spp and hippoboscid flies, the invertebrate vectors. In free-living bird populations, females are more frequently infected than males. Until recently, *Haemoproteus* was considered relatively innocuous and of little clinical significance. Fatal infections can occur because of extensive widespread necrosis accompanying development of large exoerythrocytic megalomeronts in muscle, heart, liver, and lung. Mortality as high as 78% has occurred in bobwhite quail infected with *Isospora lophortyx*. Similar meronts and lesions have been reported previously in cases of "aberrant leucocytozoonosis" and arthrocystosis. The diagnostic presence of large, pigmented gametocytes in mature RBC that often partially or completely encircle the nucleus without merogony can follow or occur simultaneously with systemic involvement. Sudden death without clinical signs or a prolonged course of weakness, lameness, dyspnea, lethargy, poor growth, and anemia may be seen. Little is known about effective treatment, although antimalarial drugs may be tried. Chloroquine (5 mg/kg) and buparvaquone (2.5 mg/kg) have been reported to be effective in treating pigeons; diminazene and quinapyramine were either ineffective or toxic. Measures to control invertebrate hosts should help prevent heavy infections.

LEUCOCYTOZOONOSIS

Infections with *Leucocytozoon* spp range from subclinical to fatal. Mortality may approach 100% but varies greatly with species and strain of parasite, host species, degree of exposure, and other factors. Acute outbreaks of leucocytozoonosis have been reported in chickens (Asia, Africa), turkeys (North America), waterfowl (North America, Europe), and a number of free-living and captive avian species throughout the world. Species in domestic birds include *L simondi* in waterfowl; *L smithi* in turkeys; and *L caulleryi*, *L sabrazesi*, *L andrewsi*, and *L schoutedeni* in chickens. *L caulleryi* can be highly pathogenic, causing a lethal hemorrhagic disease of chickens in southeast Asia. Numerous *Leucocytozoon* spp infect nondomestic birds (eg, blood smears from raptors often contain gametocytes). Clinical disease and mortality result from anemia caused by anti-erythrocytic factors produced by the parasite, high numbers of the large gametocytes blocking pulmonary capillaries, or parasites invading the endothelium of vessels in vital tissues (brain, heart, etc) where they form megalomeronts that occlude vessels and result in multifocal necrosis.

Wild birds are reservoirs in some areas and are responsible for initiating infection in young birds each year. Parasitemia often increases dramatically in late April and early May (called spring rise), just before arthropod vectors, black flies (*Simulium* spp), or biting midges (*Culicoides* spp) increase. Ducks that have recovered from infection with *L simondi* relapse when light cycles are manipulated to increase egg production. Increased levels of prolactin have been suggested as a possible cause.

Acute disease is seen more often in the young when they have high parasitemia and when black flies or biting midges are most abundant. Subacute or chronic disease is seen in the young outside fly season and in older birds at any season; parasitemia is usually low. Recovered birds remain carriers and serve as a reservoir for young, susceptible birds.

Clinical Findings, Lesions, and Diagnosis: Acutely affected birds are listless and have anemia, leukocytosis, tachypnea, anorexia, diarrhea with green droppings, and often CNS signs. Egg production is impaired in laying chickens infected with *L caulleryi*. Signs are evident ~1 wk after infection and coincide with the onset of parasitemia. Visibly affected birds die after 7-10 days or may recover with sequelae of poor growth and egg production. Hemorrhages, splenomegaly, and hepatomegaly are seen. Grossly visible white dots in affected organs are megalomeronts.

In thin blood smears, gametocytes may be seen along the edges and tail of the smear. *Leucocytozoon* is identified by large gametocytes that lack pigment and distort the host cell (RBC or WBC), making it no longer identifiable. Shape of gametocytes varies with the species—some are elongated with long tapering extremities, while others are round. Serology may detect prior infection.

Treatment and Control: Treatment usually is not effective. Preventive medication with combined pyrimethamine (1 ppm) and sulfadimethoxine (10 ppm) combined in the feed controls *L caulleryi*; clopidol (0.0125-0.025%) controls *L smithi*. Measures to control invertebrate vectors are helpful. Humoral immunity resulting from vaccination will protect against *L caulleryi* infection.

PLASMODIUM INFECTION

Plasmodium spp, which often are not host-specific, infect a wide variety of domestic and wild birds in most areas of the world and can cause high losses. *P gallinaceum* infects chickens in Asia and Africa and causes low mortality in indigenous chickens but rates may be as high as 80-90% in commercial birds. *P juxtanucleare* infects chickens in Asia, Africa, and South America; most infections are mild or asymptomatic. *P durae* infects turkeys and gallinaceous birds other than chickens in Africa; mortality in turkeys can approach 100%. Clinical malaria has not been reported from poultry in North America, but indigenous wild turkeys can become infected with at least 4 different *Plasmodium* species. Asymptomatic infections in endemic or introduced birds can be spread via mosquitos and cause fatal disease in introduced (eg, zoo penguins) or resident (eg, Hawaiian avifauna) birds, respectively. Invertebrate hosts are ornithophilic mosquitos, usually *Culex*, *Culiseta*, or *Aedes* spp.

Clinical Findings, Lesions, and Diagnosis: Infection with *Plasmodium* spp may be nonclinical or cause illness characterized by weakness, lassitude, dyspnea, anemia, abdominal distention, increased right heart weight, ocular hemorrhage, and death. Death results from severe anemia or blockage of capillaries in the brain or other vital organs by exoerythrocytic meronts in endothelial cells. Liver and spleen are markedly enlarged and often discolored (dark brown to black). Pigmented parasites including meronts are found in both immature and mture RBC. Infrequently, parasites are found in thrombocytes and WBC. In birds that die acutely, organisms may be sparse or absent in blood, but numerous meronts can be found in capillaries by examining squash or impression smears of brain, lung, liver, and spleen. Serologic and molecular diagnostic methods are under development but are not yet available for general use. Serology can detect infection when parasites are too few to be identified in blood smears.

Treatment and Control: Chemotherapy is variably effective in treating infected birds or flocks. Chloroquine (5-10 mg/kg) potentiated with primaquine (0.3 mg/kg), or chloroquine in drinking water (250 mg/120 mL) has been used. Grape or orange juice can disguise chloroquine's bitterness. Other antimalarial drugs have been used with success; quinacrine at 1.6 mg/kg/day for 5 days was successful for treating an infected peacock. Treatment with a combination of sulfamonomethoxine and sulfachloropyrazine is effective; halofuginone can be used for chemoprophylaxis in endemic areas. Persistent parasitemia or relapse may occur during and after treatment. Treatments should be evaluated on prevention of mortality and improvement of clinical disease. Birds that survive initial infection are generally refractory to subsequent infections. Prevention of exposure to mosquitos is a useful adjunct. Parasite development is reduced in mosquitos that survive previous infection with *Bacillus thuringiensis israelensis*.

OTHER BLOODBORNE ORGANISMS

Trypanosomes have been described in several avian species but rarely if ever cause clinical disease. They are more commonly identified in organ smears, especially bone marrow, than in peripheral blood, and can be cultured. Invertebrate hosts are thought to be any of several bloodsucking insects. Treatment is not warranted.

Borreliae are tickborne (*Argas* spp) spirochetes that can cause fatal systemic disease. Tetracyclines, penicillin, and tick control are used for prevention and treatment. (*See* AVIAN SPIROCHETOSIS, p 2219.)

Small, punctate, or rarely ring-shaped, rickettsia-like basophilic bodies resembling *Pirhemocyton*, an organism that infects reptiles, are frequently seen in avian erythrocytes. Their identity and significance are unknown. They tend to be smaller and morphologically distinct from *Aegyptianella*.

Babesia spp are uncommon, nonpigmented, pyriform-shaped, erythrocytic protozoan parasites of birds. Natural infections of penguins, falcons, cranes, and several Asian avian species occur. Ticks are considered to be the invertebrate hosts. V, X, or fan shapes characterize dividing forms. Nothing is known of their significance, treatment, or control.

Haemogregarina and *Hepatozoon* are protozoan parasites that are infrequently identified in birds. Both produce relatively large, nonpigmented, elongated gametocytes that can be found in RBC and WBC respectively. Gametocytes of *Haemogregarina* resemble gametocytes of *Haemoproteus* but lack pigment and are smaller, rarely if ever extending around or encircling the nucleus. Gametocytes of *Hepatozoon* are elongated with rounded ends and usually not located within an indentation of the nucleus, whereas *Atoxoplasma* is oval and partially encircled by the nucleus.

Zoites of other sporozoa (eg, *Toxoplasma*, *Sarcocystis*) and organisms normally in the digestive tract (eg, trichomonads, coccidia, histomonads) may be transiently found in blood. The latter often also produce liver lesions. (*See also* TRICHOMONIASIS, p 1142, and HISTOMONIASIS, p 2238.)

CHICKEN ANEMIA VIRUS INFECTION

(Chicken infectious anemia, Blue wing disease, Anemia dermatitis syndrome, Hemorrhagic aplastic anemia syndrome)

Etiology, Epidemiology, and Pathogenesis: Chicken anemia virus (CAV), a 25 nm, nonenveloped, icosahedral virus with a single-stranded, circular DNA genome, is the only member of the genus Gyrovirus of the Circoviridae family. The genome codes for 3 viral proteins (VP). VP1 is the capsid protein, but VP2 may be needed as a scaffold protein to allow proper folding of VP1. VP3, or apoptin, is a nonstructural protein that induces apoptosis in infected cells. CAV infects only chickens, although antibodies have been detected in Japanese quail. The virus is present worldwide based on serology and virus isolation. The disease, chicken infectious anemia, has been described in most countries where chickens are raised commercially.

Horizontal transmission of CAV is by the fecal-oral route and perhaps by the respiratory route. Vertical transmission occurs when seronegative hens become infected and continues until neutralizing antibodies develop. Chicks hatched from these eggs are viremic, and CAV can rapidly spread horizontally from these chicks to susceptible, maternal antibody-negative hatchmates. Roosters shedding CAV in the semen are another source of vertical transmission. Vaccination of seronegative flocks prior to the onset of egg production is recommended to prevent vertical transmission.

Maternal antibody-negative chicks are susceptible to infection and disease until 1-2 wk of age. In contrast, maternal antibody-positive chicks are protected from disease and probably from infection. Age resistance to clinical disease, but not infection, begins at approximately 1 wk of age. The age resistance can be overcome by coinfection of CAV with immunosuppressive agents such as infectious bursal disease virus (p 2239), Marek's disease herpesvirus (p 2248), and reticuloendotheliosis virus (p 2253).

Many SPF flocks developed antibodies to CAV during or after the onset of sexual development. Spread of infection by CAV-contaminated embryo- or cell-culture-derived vaccines is possible.

When day-old susceptible chicks are inoculated IM with CAV, viremia occurs within 24 hr. Virus can be recovered from most organs and rectal contents up to 35 days after inoculation. The principal sites of CAV replication are hemocytoblasts in the bone marrow, precursor T cells in the cortex of the thymus, and CD8 cells in the spleen. Replication in the first leads to anemia, while replication in the latter two causes immunosuppression. Neutralizing antibodies are detectable 21 days after infection and clinical, hematologic, and pathologic parameters return to normal ~35 days after infection. CAV infection has adverse effects on proliferative responses of spleen lymphocytes and on the production of interleukin-2 and interferons by splenocytes. Infection can cause a marked decrease in generation of antigen-specific cytotoxic T cells directed against other pathogens. In addition to T-cell defects, macrophage functions such as Fc-receptor expression, phagocytosis, and antimicrobial activity may be impaired. Subclinical, horizontally acquired infection with CAV in broiler progeny of seropositive parent flocks may be associated with impaired economic performance.

Clinical Findings: Signs of illness or adverse effects on egg production do not occur when seronegative adult chickens become infected. However, vertical transmission or infection of maternal antibody-negative chicks before 1 wk of age can cause clinical disease 12-17 days after hatching or infection. Chicks are anorectic, lethargic, depressed, and pale. PCV is low (in chicks, anemia is defined as a PCV of ≤27), and blood smears often reveal anemia, leukopenia, or pancytopenia depending on the state of the disease. Blood may be watery and clot slowly. Mortality rates are variable but may be high with secondary complicating infections.

Lesions: Organs are pale; the thymus is generally atrophied, and the bursa of Fabricius may be small. Bone marrow is pale or yellow. Hemorrhage may be present in or under the skin, muscle, and other organs. Histologically, lymphoid cell populations are depleted in primary and secondary lymphoid organs. Granulocytic and erythrocytic compartments in the bone marrow are atrophic or hypoplastic.

Diagnosis: A tentative diagnosis is based on history, signs, and gross and histopathologic lesions. Confirmation requires detection of virus or viral DNA in the thymus or bone marrow. PCR and quantitative PCR techniques are commonly used to demonstrate the presence of CAV. Viral isolation can be used but is slow and expensive. To isolate CAV, chloroform-treated extracts of tissues are inoculated in MDCC-MSB1 or MDCC-147 cultures (a lymphoblastoid cell line derived from Marek's disease tumor) or into susceptible, immunocompromised (antigen- and antibody-negative), day-old chicks. Commercial ELISA kits are available to detect serum antibodies to CAV and can be used to identify breeder flocks that are seronegative prior to egg production and to monitor the efficacy of vaccination.

Treatment and Prevention: There is no specific treatment. Secondary bacterial infections may be treated with antibiotics. Live vaccines are available for vaccination of antibody-negative breeder flocks prior to the start of egg production. Administration is by injection or by addition to the drinking water depending on the type of vaccine available in individual countries. In some areas, transfer of litter to noncontaminated premises and the addition of crude homogenates of tissues from affected chickens to the drinking water have been used to ensure infection and seroconversion of parent flocks before they begin to lay, thereby diminishing the risk of egg transmission. However, these procedures are risky and not recommended. Because of the synergism between CAV and other immunosuppressive viruses, control of the latter is also important.

At present, there is no vaccine available to prevent subclinical losses in broilers.

DISSECTING ANEURYSM

(Aortic rupture, Internal hemorrhage)

Dissecting aneurysm is a fatal disease of turkeys characterized by sudden death of rapidly growing birds with massive internal hemorrhage resulting from rupture of aneurysms formed in various parts of the vascular system. The frequency with which the posterior aorta is affected has given rise to the term "aortic rupture." The disease has been reported in North America, Europe, and Israel. Most breeds of turkeys are susceptible, and the largest and most rapidly growing males, 8-24 wk old, are affected most often; females are also affected but at a lower incidence.

Etiology: The cause is unknown. Probably several factors contribute to the development of fatal cases. For the disease to occur, birds must be fed and managed in such a way that they are growing rapidly, and they must have a genetic susceptibility. A prolonged lipemia generally develops during the period of rapid growth, and the period of greatest mortality typically corresponds to a sharp rise in blood pressure, with dissecting aneurysms developing at the site of arteriosclerotic plaques. The lipemia may result from a high dietary intake of fat or from the effects of hormonal factors, such as high dietary concentrations of estrogens. Although β-aminopropionitrile, the toxic agent in *Lathyrus odoratus*, is capable of producing the disease, there is no evidence that this or other nitriles are responsible for dissecting aneurysms in turkeys under natural conditions. The enzyme lysyloxidase, isolated from turkey aortas and active on tropelaston and collagen cross-linking, was found to be much lower in males than females; this may be a factor in the development of spontaneous aortic aneurysms in male turkeys.

Clinical Findings: Affected birds that had shown no premonitory signs are found dead with marked pallor of the head and neck. Occasionally, a caretaker observes an apparently healthy bird die within a few minutes. The incidence is usually <1% but may be as great as 10%. Formerly, when male turkeys were implanted with stilbestrol, the incidence was as high as 20%.

Lesions: The carcass is markedly anemic with large quantities of clotted blood in the peritoneal cavity and over the kidneys, or in the pericardial sac. The rupture in the ventral wall of the posterior aorta at about the position of the testes, or in the cardiac atrium, can be located readily by carefully washing away the blood clot. The aortic lumen may contain an organized, adherent thrombus at the site of rupture. Ruptures in smaller blood vessels are more difficult to locate. Almost always, an intimal thickening or a large, fibrous plaque is present in the region of the rupture. The tunicas intima and media are thrown into deep folds and separated from the tunica adventitia. Marked accumulation of lipids in the thickened intima and in the fibrous plaques can be identified by stains. Fibers of the tunica media may show degenerative changes and infiltration with heterophils and macrophages.

Diagnosis: The diagnosis is made by finding large clots of blood in the coelomic cavity (aortic rupture) or within the pericardial sac (auricular rupture) of rapidly growing male turkeys. The condition should be differentiated from hypertensive angiopathy (p 2199), which is also seen in rapidly growing turkeys. In hypertensive angiopathy, the major lesions include pulmonary edema and supcapsular perirenal hemorrhage.

Treatment, Control, and Prevention: There is no known treatment. Coagulants and vitamin K are useless because there is no defect in the clotting mechanism. Losses sometimes may be reduced during the critical period between 16 and 23 wk of age by limiting feed intake or slowing growth rate by reducing the energy level of the diet. High-fat diets should not be fed during this period. Some studies have indicated that the incidence of aortic rupture can be reduced by adding copper at 125-250 ppm to the diet from at least 4 wk of age until market.

INCLUSION BODY HEPATITIS/ HYDROPERICARDIUM SYNDROME

(Hepatitis hydropericardium)

Adenoviruses are widespread throughout all avian species. Studies have demonstrated the presence of antibodies in healthy poultry, and viruses have been isolated from normal birds. Despite their widespread distribution, the majority of adenoviruses cause no or only mild disease; however, some are associated with specific clinical conditions. Avian adenoviruses (AAV) in chickens are the etiologic agents of 2 important diseases known as inclusion body hepatitis (IBH) and hydropericardium syndrome (HP). Although in some cases each condition is observed separately, during the last decade the 2 conditions have been frequently observed as a single entity; therefore, the name hepatitis hydropericardium has been widely used to describe the pathologic condition. The syndrome is an acute disease of young chickens associated with anemia, hemorrhagic disorders, and hydropericardium. It is a common disease in several countries, where broilers are severely affected, resulting in high mortality rates.

Etiology, Transmission, and Pathogenesis: The AAV of group I are the etiologic agents of this condition. Although there are 12 different serotypes of AAV, the most common viruses isolated in cases of IBH/HP belong to serotypes 4 and 8. These AAV are capable of producing the disease without the immunosuppressive effects of associated viruses such as infectious bursal disease (IBDV, p 2239) or other immunosuppressive agents. However, the association with immunosuppressive viruses such as IBDV and chicken anemia virus (CAV, p 2196) will result in a more severe disease.

Horizontal and vertical transmission play an important role in IBH/HP. Vertical transmission has been described in progeny from breeder flocks infected with AAV serotypes 4 and 8. Horizontal transmission has also been demonstrated; young chicks in contact with infected chicks can die of peracute IBH/HP. Chicks and young chickens are commonly affected. Infection with some strains of AAV may result in minimal hepatic disease; however, if birds have been infected with immunosuppressive viruses (IBD, CAV, Marek's disease), the clinical disease becomes evident.

Clinical Findings, Lesions, and Diagnosis: Sudden mortality usually is seen in chickens <6 wk old and as young as 4 days of age. Mortality normally ranges from 2-40%, especially when birds are <3 wk of age. However, there have been outbreaks in which mortality has reached 80%. Mortality rates also vary depending on the pathogenicity of the virus and infection with other viral or bacterial agents. Signs associated with diseases caused by other pathogens (eg, bacteria, fungi, or viruses) commonly occur if birds are immunosuppressed.

Flocks of 3- to 5-wk-old broilers with HP may not show specific clinical signs, but abrupt onset of mortality, lethargy, huddling with ruffled feathers, and yellow, mucoid droppings may be seen. The duration of the infection usually ranges from 9-14 days with morbidity of 10-30% and a daily mortality of 3-5%. Gross lesions include up to 10 mL of a straw-colored transudate in the pericardial sac, generalized congestion, and an enlarged, pale, friable liver. Histopathologic lesions include myocardial edema in the heart with degeneration, necrosis, and mild mononuclear cell infiltration. Basophilic intranuclear inclusion bodies may be present in the liver. A tentative diagnosis is based on typical microscopic findings and confirmed by isolating adenoviruses from the liver. Serology, restriction enzyme analysis and PCR are used to classify adenoviruses isolated from clinical cases. This information is used for epidemiologic studies.

Treatment and Prevention: As with many other viral diseases, there is no treatment. Antibiotics may help prevent secondary bacterial infections. Sulfonamides are contraindicated if evidence of hematologic disease or immunosuppression is seen.

Vaccines against IBH/HP are not commercially available in the USA; however, in other countries both live and inactivated vaccines are used to control the syndrome. The AAV serotypes most frequently used to prepare commercial vaccines are serotypes 4 and 8. Primary breeders with stringent biosecurity practices sometimes use autogenous inactivated vaccines to ensure the transfer of maternal immunity from breeding flocks to their progeny. In Australia, a live vaccine given via drinking water was developed for breeders between 10-14 wk of age. In other countries, including Mexico, Pakistan, and Peru, inactivated vaccines are routinely used to vaccinate breeders and broilers. When breeders are properly vaccinated, antibodies generated by the vaccine are transmitted to the progeny, providing protection against field infections and clinical disease. Broilers are vaccinated at <10 days of age when their parents either do not have serotype-specific adenovirus antibodies or maternal antibody transmission is erratic due to improper vaccination procedures that result in a substantial number of unvaccinated birds.

PERIRENAL HEMORRHAGE SYNDROME OF TURKEYS

(Hypertensive angiopathy, Sudden death syndrome of turkeys)

Perirenal hemorrhage syndrome (PHS) is a noninfectious cardiovascular disease usually affecting rapidly growing male turkeys 8-15 wk old characterized by sudden death, perirenal hemorrhage, and hypertrophic cardiomyopathy. Mortality is usually 0.5-2% but can be higher; there is no morbidity. Healthy, rapidly growing flocks are more likely to be affected.

The pathogenesis is unknown, but PHS is apparently unrelated to pulmonary function or hypertension. Inadequate or inappropriate cardiac response to exercise, resulting in hypotension, vasodilation, arrhythmias, and sudden death, appears most likely. Acute congestive heart failure secondary to cardiac hypertrophy has also been suggested as a potential cause. Renal hemorrhage may occur due to severe passive congestion.

Gross lesions include good to excellent body condition, food in crop and stomach, enlarged dark red to purple spleen, variable retroperitoneal hemorrhage around one or both kidneys, generalized congestion, and pulmonary edema occasionally accompanied by hemorrhage. Cardiac hypertrophy involving the left ventricle and intraventricular septum may also be seen. Microscopic changes are consistent with gross findings; proliferative arterial and arteriolar lesions and ruptured renal veins also are often present. PHS has several characteristics in common with aortic rupture (p 2197) and flip-over in broilers (p 2227).

Diagnosis is based on history, typical gross lesions, and absence of infectious agents. Extensive PHS lesions may resemble aortic rupture.

There is no specific treatment. Factors that decrease growth rate and activity also tend to decrease PHS. Reserpine (0.5 ppm feed) decreases PHS, but aspirin (0.005%) or increased calcium has no effect. Reserpine is not listed in the Feed Additive Compendium as approved for use in feed for turkeys. Increased room temperature and various lighting programs have also reduced PHS. Activities that increase cardiovascular stress (eg, moving birds, tilling litter, noise) should be minimized, especially between 7 and 15 wk of age. Lower ambient temperatures (55°F [13°C]), intermittent lighting, and leaving toes unclipped increase mortality from PHS.

PHS may occur in healthy commercial male turkey flocks regardless of management practices used to prevent its occurrence.

ROUND HEART DISEASE OF TURKEYS

(Spontaneous cardiomyopathy)

Spontaneous cardiomyopathy of young turkeys is characterized by sudden death due to cardiac arrest. It has been suggested that the condition should be called spontaneous cardiomyopathy to distinguish it from round heart disease of chickens, a different syndrome that is rarely recognized today.

The exact etiology of spontaneous cardiomyopathy in turkeys is unknown. However, studies using furazolidone to produce dilated cardiomyopathy in turkeys have indicated altered membrane transport resulting in myocardial failure. Creatine kinase, glycolysis, glycogen, myofibril, Krebs cycle enzymes, fatty acid oxidation, and soluble proteins are all reduced. The calcium-transport ATPase activity of the sarcoplasmic reticulum is increased. This pattern of biochemical changes is consistent with ischemia playing a role in the pathogenesis of spontaneous cardiomyopathy in turkeys.

While most deaths occur during the brooding period, the ratio of heart weight to body weight of affected birds is increased throughout the growing period. Market body weights of affected birds are reduced an average of 3 lb (1.4 kg). Some outbreaks of the condition have been associated with hypoxia during incubation of the eggs or during transportation of poults from the hatchery to the brood farm.

Most deaths from spontaneous cardiomyopathy occur during the first 4 wk of life, with mortality peaking at 2 wk. Many poults die suddenly, but some may have ruffled feathers, drooping wings, and a general unthrifty appearance. They may show labored, gasping breathing before death. After 3 wk of age, mortality is sporadic. Characteristically, the affected poult in the first 4 wk of life has a greatly enlarged heart due to dilatation of both ventricles, congested lungs, and a swollen liver. Ascites, anasarca, pulmonary edema, and hydropericardium may or may not be present. In older poults, enlarged hearts are due to marked hypertrophy of the ventricles in addition to dilatation. Histologically, lesions of abnormal hearts are nonspecific and include congestion, damage of the myofibrils of the cardiocytes, and focal infiltration by lymphocytes.

Generally, diagnosis is based on history and gross findings at necropsy; although an ECG can be used, it is of little practical use. Sodium and polychlorinated biphenyls or related compounds may produce similar syndromes.

No treatment is available. Good brooding practices may reduce mortality. Any toxins should be eliminated. Incubation, transportation, and early brooding ventilation conditions should be reviewed.

CANDIDIASIS

(Thrush, Crop mycosis, Sour crop)

Candidiasis is a mycotic disease of the digestive tract of chickens and turkeys caused by *Candida albicans*. Lesions are most frequently found in the crop and consist of thickened mucosa and whitish, raised pseudomembranes. The same lesions may be seen in the mouth and esophagus. Occasionally, shallow ulcers and sloughing of necrotic epithelium may be present. Listlessness and inappetence may be the only clinical signs. A presumptive diagnosis may be made on observation of gross lesions. This diagnosis can be confirmed by demonstrating tissue invasion histologically and by culture of the organism. However, culture alone is not diagnostic of disease as the yeast-like fungus is commonly isolated from clinically normal birds. Young chicks and poults are most susceptible. Candidiasis is common after use of therapeutic levels of various antibiotics or unsanitary drinking facilities.

Improving sanitation and minimizing antibiotic use in poultry help reduce the incidence of candidiasis. Affected birds can be treated with copper sulfate at 0.5 mg/L of drinking water, or 0.5 mg copper sulfate per kg of feed. Vinegar is used as a treatment for candidiasis at 15 mL/L of drinking water. Chlorhexidine is used for prevention or treatment at 2.5 mL/L of drinking water. Chlorine bleach at 0.1 mL/L of drinking water may help control the infection. All of these treatments lack FDA approval.

COCCIDIOSIS

Coccidiosis is caused by protozoa of the phylum Apicomplexa, family Eimeriidae. In poultry, most species belong to the genus *Eimeria* and infect various sites in the intestine. The infectious process is rapid (4-7 days) and is characterized by parasite replication in host cells with extensive damage to the intestinal mucosa. Poultry coccidia are strictly host-specific, and the different species parasitize specific parts of the intestine. Coccidia are distributed worldwide in poultry and wild birds. (*See also* CRYPTOSPORIDIOSIS, p 168.)

Etiology: Coccidia are almost universally present in poultry-raising operations, but clinical disease occurs only after ingestion of relatively large numbers of sporulated oocysts by susceptible birds. Both clinically infected and recovered birds shed oocysts in their droppings, which contaminate feed, dust, water, litter, and soil. Oocysts may be transmitted by mechanical carriers (eg, equipment, clothing, insects, and other animals). Fresh oocysts are not infective until they sporulate; under optimal conditions (70-90°F [21-32°C] with adequate moisture and oxygen), this requires 1-2 days. The prepatent period is 4-7 days. Sporulated oocysts may survive for long periods, depending on environmental factors. Oocysts are resistant to some disinfectants commonly used around livestock but are killed by freezing or high environmental temperatures. (*See also* COCCIDIOSIS IN MAMMALS, p 163.)

Pathogenicity is influenced by host genetics, nutritional factors, concurrent diseases, and species of the coccidium. *Eimeria necatrix* and *E tenella* are the most pathogenic in chickens because schizogony occurs in the lamina propria and crypts of Lieberkühn of the small intestine and ceca, respectively, and causes extensive hemorrhage. Most species develop in epithelial cells lining the villi. Protective immunity usually develops in response to moderate and continuing infection. True age-immunity does not occur, but older birds are usually more resistant than young birds because of earlier exposure to infection.

Clinical Findings: Signs range from decreased growth rate to a high percentage of visibly sick birds, severe diarrhea, and high mortality. Feed and water consumption are depressed. Weight loss, development of culls, decreased egg production, and increased mortality may accompany outbreaks. Mild infections of intestinal species, which would otherwise be classed as subclinical, may cause depigmentation. Survivors of severe infections recover in 10-14 days but may never recover lost performance.

Chickens: *E tenella* infections are found only in the ceca and can be recognized by accumulation of blood in the ceca and by bloody droppings. Cecal cores, which are accumulations of clotted blood, tissue debris, and oocysts, may be found in birds surviving the acute stage.

E necatrix produces major lesions in the anterior and middle portions of the small intestine. Small white spots, usually intermingled with rounded, bright- or dull-red spots of various sizes, can be seen on the serosal surface. The white spots are diagnostic for *E necatrix* if clumps of large schizonts can be demonstrated microscopically. In severe cases, the intestinal wall is thickened, and the infected area dilated to 2-2.5 times the normal diameter. The lumen may be filled with blood, mucus, and fluid. Fluid loss may result in marked dehydration. Although the damage is in the small intestine, the sexual phase of the life cycle is completed in the ceca. Oocysts of *E necatrix* are found only in the ceca. Due to concurrent infections, oocysts of other species may be found in the area of major lesions, misleading the diagnostician.

E acervulina, the most common infection, is characterized by numerous, whitish, oval or transverse patches in the upper half of the small intestine and may be easily distinguished on gross examination. The clinical course in a flock is usually protracted and results in poor growth, an increase in culls, and slightly increased mortality.

E brunetti is found in the lower small intestine, rectum, ceca, and cloaca. In moderate infections, the mucosa is pale and disrupted but lacking in discrete foci, and may be thickened. In severe infections, extensive coagulative necrosis and sloughing of the mucosa occurs throughout most of the small intestine.

E maxima develops in the small intestine, where it causes dilatation and thickening of the wall; petechial hemorrhage; and a reddish, orange, or pink viscous mucous exudate and fluid. The oocysts and gametocytes (particularly macrogametocytes), which are present in the lesions, are distinctly large.

E mitis is recognized as pathogenic in the lower small intestine. Lesions resemble moderate infections of *E brunetti* but can be distinguished by finding small, round oocysts associated with the lesion.

E praecox, which infects the upper small intestine, does not cause distinct lesions but may decrease rate of growth. It is considered to be of less economic importance than the other species.

E hagani and *E mivati* are of dubious status but are thought to develop in the anterior part of the small intestine.

Turkeys: Only 4 of the 7 species of coccidia in turkeys are considered pathogenic— *Eimeria adenoeides*, *E dispersa*, *E gallopavonis*, and *E meleagrimitis*. *E innocua*, *E meleagridis*, and *E subrotunda* are considered nonpathogenic. Oocysts sporulate within 1-2 days after expulsion from the host; the prepatent period is 4-6 days.

E adenoeides and *E gallopavonis* infect the lower ileum, ceca, and rectum. The developmental stages are found in the epithelial cells of the villi and crypts. The affected portion of the intestine may be dilated and have a thickened wall. Thick, creamy material or caseous casts in the gut or excreta may contain enormous numbers of oocysts. *E meleagrimitis* chiefly infects the upper and mid small intestine. The lamina propria or deeper tissues may be parasitized, which may result in necrotic enteritis (p 2210). *E dispersa* infects the upper small intestine and causes a creamy, mucoid enteritis that involves the entire intestine, including the ceca. Large numbers of gametocytes and oocysts are associated with the lesions.

Common signs in infected flocks include reduced feed consumption, rapid weight loss, droopiness, ruffled feathers, and severe diarrhea. Wet droppings with mucus are common. Clinical infections are seldom seen in poults >8 wk old. Morbidity and mortality may be high.

Ducks: A large number of specific coccidia have been reported in both wild and domestic ducks, but validity of some of the descriptions is questionable. Presence of *Eimeria, Wenyonella,* and *Tyzzeria* spp has been confirmed. *T perniciosa* is a known pathogen that balloons the entire small intestine with mucohemorrhagic or caseous material. *Eimeria* spp also have been described as pathogenic. Some species of coccidia of domestic ducks are considered relatively nonpathogenic. In wild ducks, infrequent but dramatic outbreaks of coccidiosis occur in ducklings 2-4 wk old; morbidity and mortality may be high.

Geese: The most striking coccidial infection of geese is that produced by *Eimeria truncata,* in which the kidneys are enlarged and studded with poorly circumscribed, yellowish white streaks and spots. The tubules are dilated with masses of oocysts and urates. Mortality may be high. At least 5 other *Eimeria* spp have been reported to parasitize the intestine.

Diagnosis: The location in the host, appearance of lesions, and the size of oocysts are used in determining the species present. Coccidial infections are readily confirmed by demonstration of oocysts in feces or intestinal scrapings; however, the number of oocysts present has little relationship to the extent of clinical disease. Severity of lesions as well as knowledge of flock appearance, morbidity, mortality, feed intake, growth rate, and rate of lay are important for diagnosis. Necropsy of several fresh specimens is advisable. Classical lesions of *E tenella* and *E necatrix* are pathognomonic, but infections of other species are more difficult to diagnose. Comparison of lesions and other signs with diagnostic charts allows a reasonably accurate differentiation of the coccidial species. Mixed coccidial infections are common.

A diagnosis of clinical coccidiosis is warranted if oocysts, merozoites, or schizonts are demonstrated microscopically and if lesions are severe. Subclinical coccidial infections may be unimportant, and poor performance may be caused by flock disorders.

Control: Practical methods of management cannot prevent infection. Poultry that are maintained at all times on wire floors to separate birds from droppings have fewer infections; clinical coccidiosis is seen only rarely under such circumstances. Other methods of control are vaccination or prevention with anticoccidial drugs.

Vaccination: A species-specific immunity develops after natural infection, the degree of which largely depends on the extent of infection and the number of reinfections. Protective immunity is primarily a T-cell response.

Commercial vaccines consist of low doses of live, sporulated oocysts of the various coccidial species administered at low doses to day-old chicks. Because the vaccine serves only to introduce infection, chickens are reinfected by progeny of the vaccine strain on the farm. The vaccine strains of coccidia may or may not be attenuated. The self-limiting nature of coccidiosis is used as a form of attenuation for some vaccines, rather than biological attenuation.

Layers and breeders that are maintained on floor litter must have protective immunity. Often, they are given a suboptimal dosage of an anticoccidial drug during early growth, with the expectation that immunity will continue to develop from repeated exposure to wild types of coccidia. This method has never been particularly successful because of the difficulty in controlling all of these factors. Immunity is not necessary in broiler chickens or cage layers. Prevention of infection by anticoccidial drugs is preferred.

Anticoccidial Drugs: Many products are available for prevention or treatment of coccidiosis in chickens and turkeys (*see* TABLE 2 and TABLE 3). Detailed instructions for use are provided by all manufacturers to help users comply with regulatory approvals

TABLE 2. Drugs for Prevention of Coccidiosis in Poultry*

	Use Level (% in feed)		Withdrawal Time (days)
	Chickens	Turkeys	
Amprolium	0.0125-0.025	0.0125-0.250	0
Amprolium + ethopabate	0.0125-0.025 + 0.0004-0.004	—	0
Chlortetracycline	0.022	—	0
Clopidol or meticlorpindol	0.0125-0.025	—	0
Decoquinate	0.003	—	0
Diclazuril	0.0001	0.0001	0
Dinitolmide (zoalene)	0.004-0.0125	0.0125-0.01875	0
Halofuginone hydrobromide	0.0003	0.00015-0.0003	4-7
Lasalocid sodium	0.0075-0.0125	—	3
Maduramicin ammonium	0.0005-0.0006	—	5
Monensin sodium	0.01-0.0121	0.006-0.01[†]	0
Narasin	0.006-0.008	—	0
Narasin + nicarbazin	0.003-0.005 (of the combination)	—	5
Nicarbazin	0.0125	—	4
Oxytetracycline	0.022	—	3
Robenidine hydrochloride	0.0033	—	5
Salinomycin sodium	0.0044-0.0066	—	0
Semduramicin	0.0025	—	0
Sulfadimethoxine + ormetoprim	0.0125 + 0.0075	0.00625 + 0.00375	5

*Approved in the USA; anticoccidials not approved in the USA but available in various other countries include the purine derivative arprinocid, a combination of clopidol plus methylbenzoquate, and various combinations of ionophores with nicarbazin.

[†]Up to 10 wk of age.

Compiled from various sources, including, with permission, the *Feed Additive Compendium*, The Miller Publishing Co., 1994.

and management considerations. High dosages may sometimes be used over short periods for treatment or if a high level of exposure is anticipated.

Anticoccidials are given in the feed to prevent disease and the economic loss often associated with subacute infection. Prophylactic use is preferred because most of the damage occurs before signs become apparent, and because drugs cannot completely stop an outbreak. Water medication is generally preferred over feed medication for therapeutic treatment. Antibiotics and increased levels of vitamins A and K are sometimes used in the ration to improve rate of recovery and prevent secondary infections.

TABLE 3. Drugs for Treatment of Coccidiosis in Chickens*

	Feed or Water	Active Ingredient: Treatment, Duration	Withdrawal Time (days)
Amprolium	Water	0.012-0.024%, 3-5 days; 0.006%, 1-2 wk	0
Chlortetracycline	Feed	0.022% + 0.8% calcium; not more than 3 wk	0
Oxytetracycline	Feed	0.022% + 0.18-0.55% calcium; not more than 5 days	3
Sodium sulfachloropyrazine monohydrate	Water	0.03%, 3 days	4
Sulfadimethoxine	Water	0.05%, 6 days	5
Sulfamethazine (sulfadimidine)	Water	0.1%, 2 days; 0.05%, 4 days	10
Toltrazuril	Water	25 ppm, 2 days	NA[†]

*Approved in the USA, except for toltrazuril
[†]Not applicable

Continuous use of anticoccidial drugs promotes the emergence of drug-resistant strains of coccidia. Various programs are used in attempts to slow or stop selection of resistance. For instance, producers may use one anticoccidial continuously through succeeding flocks, rotate anticoccidials every 4-6 mo, or change anticoccidials during a single growout (ie, a shuttle program). While there is little cross-resistance to anticoccidials with different modes of action, there is widespread resistance to most drugs. Change of drug may be beneficial when resistance has been established. "Shuttle programs," in which 1 group of chickens is treated sequentially with different drugs (usually a change between the starter and grower rations), are common practice in many countries, and offer some benefit in reducing emergence of resistance. In the USA, the FDA considers shuttle programs as extra-label usage, but producers may use such programs on the recommendation of a veterinarian.

The effects of anticoccidial drugs may be coccidiostatic, in which growth of intracellular coccidia is arrested but development may continue after drug withdrawal, or coccidiocidal, in which coccidia are killed during their development. Some anticoccidial drugs may be coccidiostatic when given short-term but coccidiocidal when given long-term. Most anticoccidials currently used in poultry production are coccidiocidal.

The natural development of immunity to coccidiosis can be slowed by use of some highly effective anticoccidials. In the production of broilers during a short growout of 37-44 days, this may be of little consequence. However, natural immunity is important in replacement layers because they are likely to be exposed to coccidial infections for extended periods after terminating anticoccidial drugs. Anticoccidial programs for layer and breeder flocks are aimed at allowing immunizing infection while guarding against acute outbreaks.

Anticoccidials are commonly withdrawn from broilers 3-7 days before slaughter to meet regulatory requirements and to reduce production costs. Because broilers have varying susceptibility to infection at this point, the risk of coccidiosis outbreaks is increased with longer withdrawal.

Turkeys are given a preventive anticoccidial for confinement-reared birds up to 8-10 wk of age. Older birds are considered less susceptible to outbreaks.

The modes of action of anticoccidial drugs are poorly understood. Some that are better known are described below. Knowledge of mode of action is important in understanding toxicity and side effects.

Amprolium is structurally similar to and is a competitive antagonist of thiamine (vitamin B_1). Because rapidly dividing coccidia have a relatively high requirement for thiamine, amprolium has a safety margin of ~8:1 when used at the highest recommended level in feed. Maximal effect occurs about day 3 of the life cycle of coccidia. Because amprolium has poor activity against some *Eimeria* spp, its spectrum has been extended by using it in mixtures with the folic acid antagonists, ethopabate and sulfaquinoxaline.

Clopidol and **quinolines** (eg, decoquinate, methylbenzoquate) halt development of the sporozoites or trophozoites of *Eimeria* spp by inhibiting the electron transport system within parasite mitochondria. This action is coccidiostatic. Clopidol and quinolines have a broad species spectrum, but resistance may develop rapidly.

Folic acid antagonists include the sulfonamides, 2,4-diaminopyrimidines and ethopabate. These compounds are structural antagonists of folic acid or of para-aminobenzoic acid (PABA), which is a precursor of folic acid. (The host does not synthesize folic acid and has no requirement for PABA.) Coccidia rapidly synthesize nucleic acids, especially during schizogony, which accounts for activity against these stages. Although resistance to antifolate compounds is widespread, they are commonly used for water treatment when clinical signs are already evident. Diaveridine, ormetoprim, and pyrimethamine are active against the protozoan enzyme dihydrofolate reductase. They have synergistic activity with sulfonamides and often are used in mixtures with these compounds.

Halofuginone hydrobromide is related to the antimalarial drug febrifuginone and is effective against asexual stages of most species of *Eimeria*. It has both coccidiostatic and coccidiocidal effects.

The **ionophores** (**monensin, salinomycin, lasalocid, narasin, maduramicin,** and **semduramicin**) form complexes with various ions, principally sodium, potassium, and calcium, and transport these into and through biological membranes. The ionophores affect both extra- and intracellular stages of the parasite, especially during the early, asexual stages of parasite development. Drug tolerance was initially slow to emerge, probably because of the biochemically nonspecific way these fermentation products act on the parasite. Recent surveys suggest that drug tolerance is now widespread, but these products remain the most important class of anticoccidials.

Some ionophores depress weight gain when given at or slightly above the recommended levels. Primarily, this is the result of reduced feed consumption, but the reduced growth may be offset by improved feed conversion.

Nicarbazin was the first product to have truly broad-spectrum activity that is still in common use. While not completely understood, the mode of action is thought to be via inhibition of succinate-linked nicotinamide adenine dinucleotide reduction and the energy-dependent transhydrogenase, and the accumulation of calcium in the presence of ATP. Nicarbazin is toxic for layers, and a 4-day withdrawal period is required in broilers. Medicated birds are at increased risk of heat stress in hot weather.

Nitrobenzamides (eg, dinitolmide) exert their greatest coccidiostatic activity against the asexual stages. Efficacy is limited to *E tenella* and *E necatrix* unless combined with other products.

Robenidine, a guanidine compound, allows initial intracellular development of coccidia but prevents formation of mature schizonts. It is both coccidiostatic when given short term and coccidiocidal long term. Drug resistance may develop during use. A 5-day withdrawal period is needed to eliminate untoward flavor caused by residues in poultry meat.

CRYPTOSPORIDIOSIS

Cryptosporidiosis is caused by protozoa (phylum Apicomplexa) that are members of the family Cryptosporidiidae and are related to coccidia of the genera *Eimeria, Isospora, Sarcocystis,* and *Toxoplasma*. Until recently, it was thought that there were 19 species in the genus *Cryptosporidium*, but recent research has shown that most are merely species that lack host specificity. Cryptosporidia are parasitic in the intestine of mammals (*see* p 168), but in birds they are commonly found in the bursa and in the respiratory tract.

Cryptosporidiosis is more severe in turkeys than in chickens and is frequently fatal in quail.

The life cycle of *Cryptosporidium* is similar to that of other coccidia, involving asexual and sexual phases, and culminates in oocyst production. In the host, the oocyst forms four sporozoites without sporocysts. The life cycle is not self-limiting (as with other coccidia) because some oocysts are thin-walled and release sporozoites (after trypsin/bile stimulation) that reinfect adjacent tissues. The endogenous cycle is short (4-7 days), the endogenous stages are small (4-7 μm), and the parasites are just beneath the epithelial cell membranes.

In turkeys and chickens, *Cryptosporidium* have been found in the sinuses, trachea, bronchi, cloaca, and bursa. The respiratory disease causes coughing, gasping, and airsacculitis. Lungs become gray and wet. Signs last several weeks, and death may occur.

Examining tissue scrapings from the bursa, cloaca, and trachea, and finding the characteristic small (5 μm) oocysts can be diagnostic. Concentration of intestinal scrapings using saturated sugar solution and examination by phase-contrast or interference-contrast microscopy is preferred.

There are no satisfactory control measures except isolation and good sanitation. All known anticoccidial drugs are ineffective against *Cryptosporidium* spp. Unlike *Cryptosporidium* spp of other mammals, the avian species are not infectious to people.

CORONAVIRAL ENTERITIS OF TURKEYS

(Bluecomb, Transmissible enteritis)

Coronaviral enteritis is an acute, highly contagious disease of turkeys characterized by sudden onset, marked depression, anorexia, diarrhea, dehydration, and weight loss. Mortality may be high, particularly in poults, but failure to gain body weight in adult birds may be more important economically.

Etiology and Epidemiology: The causative agent is a coronavirus, but the clinical disease is often complicated by other intestinal viral, bacterial, and protozoal infections. Spread is by direct or indirect contact with infected birds or contaminated premises. Droppings of acutely infected birds are rich in virus, and recovered birds may continue to shed lower levels of virus for months. Environmental factors do not appear to influence the occurrence; however, cold temperatures may contribute to the severity of the disease. Cold weather, especially freezing, and high litter moisture increase survival of the virus.

Clinical Findings: A short incubation period, often 48-72 hr, is followed by general depression, anorexia, and diarrhea in the flock. Young poults appear cold, chirp constantly, and seek heat. Feed and water consumption drop markedly, and poults lose weight rapidly. Morbidity and mortality may approach 100% in uncontrolled outbreaks.

Morbidity and mortality are variable in growing and adult turkeys. Profuse diarrhea, with mucoid threads or casts in the droppings, is common. Dehydration and weight loss are often pronounced, and several weeks may be required for normal growth to resume. Cyanosis of the head is common. Breeder hens experience a severe drop in egg production and produce abnormal eggs with chalky shells. Vertical transmission does not occur.

Lesions: Young birds have few lesions other than flaccid, distended intestines that contain excess fluid and gas. Ceca are distended with foamy, pale brown, fetid fluid. Lesions in older birds are more extensive. Skin and musculature are dehydrated, and petechial hemorrhages may be seen on the viscera. Kidneys frequently are swollen and contain an excess of urates, and the pancreas may have multiple, chalky white areas. Severe catarrhal enteritis is common and mucoid casts may be present. The crop may be distended and contain sour-smelling fluid. The spleen is often small and pale gray.

Diagnosis: Although clinical findings and lesions are suggestive, definitive diagnosis requires laboratory techniques including demonstration of coronaviral antigen in intestines of affected birds by direct fluorescent antibody techniques, detection of coronavirus particles in intestinal contents by electron microscopy, reproduction of the disease in naive poults with bacteria-free intestinal filtrates, and negative findings for common bacterial and protozoal infections. Other conditions that may produce similar signs in poults include hexamitiasis (p 2209), salmonellosis (p 2262), inanition, and water deprivation. Other intestinal viruses (which are common in commercial flocks, including rotavirus, reovirus, astrovirus, enterovirus, and possibly others) can cause disease that resembles mild coronaviral enteritis. In older birds, severe larval ascarid infection may cause diagnostic confusion.

Prevention and Treatment: Introduction of virus should be minimized by good management and sanitation practices. Depopulation of problem premises followed by thorough cleaning and disinfection of buildings and equipment is effective in breaking the cycle of infection. Such farms are best cleaned during summer and should be left vacant for ≥1 mo.

A commercial vaccine is not available. "Controlled" exposure programs have been used with variable success on some problem farms, but such procedures are not recommended because carrier states may be induced.

The course of disease outbreaks may be altered by good nursing care and judicious use of antibiotics and other drugs to combat secondary bacterial infections and dehydration. Birds in brooder houses should be provided with supplemental heat, and birds on range should be protected from adverse environmental conditions. Antibiotic administration decreases mortality but not the growth suppressant effects. The selection of an antibiotic is empiric at best, but tetracyclines, neomycin, streptomycin, lincomycin, penicillin, and bacitracin are among those used with variable success. Antibiotics may be added to drinking water in combination with calf milk-replacer and electrolyte, eg, 25 lb (11.4 kg) of calf milk-replacer and 450 g of potassium chloride to 100 gal. (380 L) of water. Birds should be medicated for 7-10 days. During and after treatment, birds should be observed closely for secondary crop mycosis, a common sequela of longterm antibiotic therapy.

DUCK VIRAL ENTERITIS

(Duck plague)

Duck viral enteritis (DVE) is an acute, highly contagious disease of ducks, geese, and swans of all ages, characterized by sudden death, high mortality (particularly among older ducks), and hemorrhages and necrosis in internal organs. It has been reported in domestic and wild waterfowl in Europe, Asia, North America, and Africa, resulting in limited to serious economic losses on domestic duck farms and sporadic, limited to massive die-offs in wild waterfowl.

Etiology, Epidemiology, and Transmission: Field strains of the causative herpesvirus are antigenically similar but vary considerably in pathogenicity. The virus is relatively sensitive to heat and pH; lipid solvents, trypsin, and chymotrypsin inactivate it. It causes intranuclear inclusion bodies in infected tissues and in inoculated cell cultures. In nature, the virus is mainly transmitted from infected to susceptible ducks by direct contact or water and is acquired mainly by the oral route. Parenteral, intranasal, or oral administration of infected tissues can establish experimental infection. Recovered birds may remain carriers, serving as uncontrolled sources of the virus for susceptible ducks.

Clinical Findings: The incubation period is 3-7 days. Sudden high and persistent mortality is often the first sign of the disease. Mortality varies from 5-100% depending on the virulence of the infecting viral strain. Adult ducks usually die in higher proportions than young ones, increasing the economic significance of the disease. Dead males may have prolapse of the penis. Photophobia, inappetence, extreme thirst, droopiness, ataxia, nasal discharge, soiled vents, and watery or bloody diarrhea may be seen. Adult ducks may die in good flesh. In contrast, ducklings frequently show dehydration and weight loss, as well as blue beaks and blood-stained vents. In laying flocks, egg production may drop sharply.

Lesions: Hemorrhages in various tissues and free blood in body cavities indicate severe damage to blood vessels throughout the body. Petechial and ecchymotic hemorrhages on the heart ("paint brush" appearance), liver, pancreas, mesentery, and other organs are characteristic. Specific mucosal eruptions, found in the oral cavity, esophagus, ceca, rectum, and cloaca, undergo progressive alterations during the course of the disease. Macular hemorrhages initially develop into elevated, yellowish, crusted plaques and organize into green, superficial scabs, which may coalesce into large, patchy, diphtheritic membranes. The mucosal lesions align parallel with the longitudinal folds in the esophagus and with the annular bands in the intestines. All lymphoid organs are affected; necrosis and hemorrhages are apparent. A lesion that can be easily detected on necropsy is a clear, yellow fluid that infiltrates and discolors the subcutaneous tissues from the thoracic inlet to the upper third of the neck. Ruptured yolk and free blood may be found in the abdominal cavity of laying ducks.

Diagnosis: Presumptive diagnosis is based on disease history and lesions. Definitive diagnosis requires laboratory work. Isolation of the virus from liver, spleen, or kidney tissues may be attempted in various cell cultures (preferably primary Muscovy duck embryo fibroblasts or Muscovy duck embryo liver cultures), duck embryos, or ducklings. Inoculating the chorioallantoic membrane of 9- to 14-day-old embryonated Muscovy duck eggs may result in isolation of the virus, but this method is not as sensitive as intramuscular inoculation of day-old ducklings. Muscovy ducklings are more susceptible than White Pekin ducklings. Neutralization with specific antiserum in these systems confirms the identity of the virus. Fluorescent antibody test can demonstrate DVE viral proteins, and PCR, using DVE virus-specific primers, can amplify the viral DNA in duck tissues or inoculated cultured cells. Serologic tests have little value in the diagnosis of acute infections.

Differential diagnoses include duck viral hepatitis, pasteurellosis, necrotic and hemorrhagic enteritis, trauma, drake damage, and various toxicoses. Newcastle disease, avian influenza, and fowlpox may cause similar lesions but are rarely reported in ducks. Established cases should be reported to the appropriate regulatory agency.

Prevention, Treatment, and Control: There is no treatment. Contact with wild, free-flying waterfowl and direct or indirect contact with contaminated birds or material (free-flowing water) should be avoided. Control is effected by depopulation, removal of birds from the infected environment, sanitation, and disinfection. Prevention is based on maintaining susceptible birds in a disease-free environment or immunization. A chicken-embryo-adapted, modified live virus vaccine has been approved for use in domestic ducks, in zoological aviaries, and by private aviculturists. A 0.5 mL dose is administered subcutaneously or intramuscularly to domestic ducklings >2 wk of age with a booster inoculation a year later. The vaccine is not approved for use in wild ducks. An inactivated vaccine, which appears to be efficacious as the modified live vaccine, has not been tested on a large scale and is not currently licensed.

HEXAMITIASIS

Hexamitiasis is an acute, catarrhal enteritis of turkeys, pheasants, quail, chukar partridges, and peafowl. The highest mortality occurs in birds 1-9 wk old. Natural infection has not been observed in chickens. Pigeons are susceptible to another species of *Hexamita* (*H columbae*). Hexamitiasis is rare in North America.

Etiology: The causative protozoan parasite in turkeys, *Hexamita meleagridis*, is spindle-shaped, averages 8×3 µm, and has 6 anterior and 2 posterior flagella. It has not yet been cultured in experimental media, although it has been grown in the allantoic cavity of developing chicken and turkey embryos. It is transmitted directly by ingestion of contaminated feces. Encysted hexamitids may be more important in transmission than free flagellates. Many survivors become carriers and shed parasites in their droppings.

Clinical Findings and Lesions: The nonspecific signs include watery diarrhea, dry unkempt feathers, listlessness, and rapid weight loss despite the fact that the birds continue to eat. Birds may die in convulsions. Bulbous dilatations of the small intestine (especially duodenum and upper jejunum) filled with watery contents are characteristic. The crypts of Lieberkühn contain myriad *H meleagridis*, which attach to the epithelial cells by their posterior flagella.

Diagnosis: Diagnosis depends on finding the flagellates by microscopic examination of scrapings of the duodenal and jejunal mucosa. *Hexamita* spp move with a rapid, darting motion (in contrast to the jerky motion of trichomonads). To avoid contamination of instruments with other cecal protozoa, the duodenum should be opened first. *Hexamita* spp may be demonstrated in poults that have been dead for several hours if the scrapings are placed in a drop of warm (104°F [40°C]), isotonic saline solution on the slide. Presence of a few *Hexamita* in birds >10 wk old may be unimportant.

Prevention and Treatment: Because many birds remain carriers, breeder turkeys and poults should be raised on separate premises if possible, preferably with separate attendants. Wire platforms should be used under feeders and waterers. Pheasants and quail may also be carriers.

There is no effective treatment for hexamitiasis, although oxytetracycline (0.22% in the feed for 2 wk) or chlortetracycline (0.022-0.044% in the feed for 2 wk) may be of some benefit.

NECROTIC ENTERITIS

Necrotic enteritis is an acute enterotoxemia. The clinical illness is usually very short and often the only signs are a sudden increase in mortality. The disease primarily affects broiler chickens (2-5 wk old) and turkeys (7-12 wk old) raised on litter but can also affect commercial layer pullets raised in cages.

Etiology and Pathogenesis: The causative agent is the gram-positive, obligate, anaerobic bacteria *Clostridium perfringens*. It is usually isolated on blood agar, incubated anaerobically at 37°C, on which it produces a double zone of hemolysis. There are 2 primary *C perfringens* types, A and C, associated with necrotic enteritis in poultry. Toxins produced by the bacteria cause damage to the small intestine, liver lesions, and mortality.

C perfringens is a nearly ubiquitous bacteria readily found in soil, dust, feces, feed, and used poultry litter. It is also a normal inhabitant of the intestines of healthy chickens. The enterotoxemia that results in clinical disease most often occurs either following an alteration in the intestinal microflora or from a condition that results in damage to the intestinal mucosa (eg, coccidiosis, mycotoxicosis, salmonellosis, ascarid larvae). High dietary levels of animal byproducts (eg, fishmeal), wheat, barley, oats, or rye predispose birds to the disease. Anything that promotes excessive bacterial growth and toxin production or slows feed passage rate in the small intestine could promote the occurrence of necrotic enteritis.

Clinical Findings and Lesions: Most often the only sign of necrotic enteritis in a flock is a sudden increase in mortality. However, birds with depression, ruffled feathers, and diarrhea may also be seen. The gross lesions are primarily found in the small intestine (jejunum), which may be ballooned, friable, and contain a foul-smelling, brown fluid. The mucosa is usually covered with a tan to yellow pseudomembrane often referred to as a "Turkish towel" in appearance. This pseudomembrane may extend throughout the small intestine or be only in a localized area. The disease persists in a flock for 5-10 days, and mortality is 2-50%.

Diagnosis: A presumptive diagnosis is based on gross lesions and a gram-stained smear of a mucosal scraping that exhibits large, gram-positive rods. Histologic findings consist of coagulative necrosis of one-third to one-half the thickness of the intestinal mucosa and masses of short, thick bacterial rods in the fibrinonecrotic debris. Isolation of large numbers of *C perfringens*, from intestinal contents that produce the double zone of hemolysis as described above, can confirm the diagnosis. Double zone hemolysis should not be used as the sole criteria for identification of *C perfringens* because some strains do not produce both toxins responsible for the hemolysis characteristics. Differential media specifically designed for isolation of *C perfringens* is available and may be useful for diagnosis.

Necrotic enteritis must be differentiated from lesions produced by *Eimeria brunetti* and also from ulcerative enteritis. Uncomplicated coccidiosis rarely produces lesions as acute or severe as those seen with necrotic enteritis. Ulcerative enteritis caused by *C colinum* usually produces focal lesions from the distal portion of the small intestine (ileum) to the ceca and is almost always accompanied by hepatic necrosis.

Prevention, Control, and Treatment: Because *C perfringens* is nearly ubiquitous, it is important to prevent changes in the intestinal microflora that would promote its growth. This can be accomplished by adding antibiotics in the feed such as virginiamycin (20 g/ton feed), bacitracin (50 g/ton feed), and lincomycin (2 g/ton feed). The addition of anticoccidial compounds, especially of the ionophore class, has been extremely helpful in preventing the coccidial damage that leads to necrotic enteritis. Avoiding drastic changes in feed and minimizing the level of fishmeal, wheat, barley, or rye in the diet can also aid in the prevention of necrotic enteritis. Administration of probiotics or competitive exclusion cultures has been used to both prevent and treat clinical necrotic enteritis (presumably by preventing the proliferation of *C perfringens*). Treatment for necrotic enteritis is most commonly administered in the drinking water, with bacitracin (200-400 mg/gal. for 5-7 days), penicillin (1,500,000 u/gal. for 5 days), and lincomycin (64 mg/gal. for 7 days) most often used. In each case, the medicated drinking water should be the sole source of water. Moribund birds should be removed promptly, as they can serve as a source of toxicosis or infection due to cannibalism.

ROTAVIRAL INFECTIONS IN CHICKENS, TURKEYS, AND PHEASANTS

Rotaviral infections are characterized by enteritis and diarrhea in young birds, but chickens have been infected without showing clinical signs.

Avian rotaviruses consist of 4 distinct serotypes (A-D). Group A rotaviruses share a common group antigen with mammalian rotaviruses. Group D rotaviruses have been identified only in avian species. The relationships of the other 2 avian serotypes to mammalian serotypes have not been established. Transmission is horizontally by the oral route. Egg transmission has not been reported.

Early signs of diarrhea (wet litter), depression, and poor or abnormal appetite can be seen 2-5 days after infection. Dehydration occurs rapidly, and mortality can be as high as 30-50% in pheasants and turkeys. The survivors appear healthy but smaller than normal. Lesions consist of dilated intestines filled with yellowish, watery contents with gas bubbles. Often, the carcass is dehydrated. Mortality is variable and is usually due to dehydration and emaciation.

Early diarrhea and inappetence that sometimes end with death are indicative but not pathognomonic of rotaviral infection. Fecal samples or intestinal contents can be examined by electron microscopy with negative staining, either directly or after ultracentrifugation.

Numerous rotaviral particles ~70 nm in diameter, with double-shelled capsids, can be seen and are distinguishable from reovirus by their more sharply defined outer edges. For viral isolation in chicken-embryo liver cells or chick kidney cells, fecal material must be treated with trypsin. Isolated rotaviruses belong mostly to serotype A and, in general, do not cause cytopathic effects on primary isolation. The presence of virus can be demonstrated 2-3 days after inoculation by immunofluorescent staining.

No commercial vaccines are available. Thorough cleaning and disinfection of infected houses is advisable to limit infection. There is no specific treatment.

TRICHOMONIASIS

Trichomoniasis in domestic fowl, pigeons, doves, and hawks is characterized, in most cases, by caseous accumulations in the throat and usually by weight loss. It has been termed "canker," "roup," and, in hawks, "frounce."

Etiology: The causative organism is *Trichomonas gallinae*, a flagellated protozoan that lives in the sinuses, mouth, throat, esophagus, and other organs. It is more prevalent among domestic pigeons and wild doves than among domestic fowl, although severe outbreaks have been reported in chickens and turkeys. Some strains of *T gallinae* cause high mortality in pigeons and doves. Hawks may become diseased after eating infected birds and commonly show liver lesions, with or without throat involvement. Pigeons and doves transmit the infection to their offspring in contaminated pigeon milk. Contaminated water is probably the most important source of infection for chickens and turkeys.

Clinical Findings: The disease course is rapid. The first lesions appear as small, yellowish areas on the oral mucosa. They grow rapidly and coalesce to form masses that frequently completely block the esophagus and may prevent the bird from closing its mouth. Much fluid may accumulate in the mouth. There is a watery ocular discharge and, in more advanced stages, exudate about the eyes that may result in blindness. Birds lose weight rapidly, become weak and listless, and sometimes die within 8-10 days. In chronic infections, birds appear healthy, although trichomonads can usually be demonstrated in scrapings from the mucous membranes of the throat.

Lesions: The bird may be riddled with caseous, necrotic foci. The mouth and esophagus contain a mass of necrotic material that may extend into the skull and sometimes through the surrounding tissues of the neck to involve the skin. In the esophagus and crop, the lesions may be yellow, rounded, raised areas, with a central conical caseous spur, often referred to as "yellow buttons." The crop may be covered by a yellowish, diphtheritic membrane that may extend to the proventriculus. The gizzard and intestine are not involved. Lesions of internal organs are most frequent in the liver; they vary from a few small, yellow areas of necrosis to almost complete replacement of liver tissue by caseous necrotic debris. Adhesions and involvement of other internal organs appear to be contact extensions of the liver lesions.

Diagnosis: Lesions of *T gallinae* infection are characteristic but not pathognomonic; those of pox and other infections can be similar. Diagnosis should be confirmed by microscopic examination of a smear of mucus or fluid from the throat to demonstrate the presence of trichomonads. Trichomonads can be cultured easily in various artificial media such as 0.2% Loeffler's dried blood serum in Ringer's solution or a 2% solution of pigeon serum in isotonic salt solution. Good growth is obtained at 98.6°F (37°C). Antibiotics may be used to reduce bacterial contamination.

Control: Because *T gallinae* infection in pigeons is so readily transmitted from parent to offspring in the normal feeding process, chronically infected birds should be separated from breeding birds. In pigeons, recovery from infection with a less virulent strain of *T gallinae* appears to provide some protection against subsequent attack by a more virulent strain. Successful treatments include metronidazole (60 mg/kg body wt) and dimetridazole (50 mg/kg body wt, PO; or in the drinking water at 0.05% for 5-6 days). Neither of these drugs is approved for use in birds in the USA.

ULCERATIVE ENTERITIS

(Quail disease)

Ulcerative enteritis was first diagnosed in bobwhite quail (*Colinus virginianus*). It also affects chickens, turkeys, pheasants, grouse, and other gallinaceous birds. The disease has also been reported in pigeons. Japanese quail (*Coturnix coturnix japonica*) are resistant, as only experimentally induced cases were reported in highly inbred populations. Marked differences in mortality between males and females suggest that susceptibility is an inheritable trait in *Coturnix* quail. Ulcerative enteritis occurs worldwide and may be acute or chronic.

Etiology: *Clostridium colinum* is the etiologic agent. It is an anaerobic, fastidious to culture, gram-positive, spore-forming, slightly curved rod, ~1 × 3-4 μm wide, with subterminal, oval spores. In chickens, the disease is a complex that is linked to stress, coccidiosis, infectious bursal disease, and other predisposing factors. To induce experimental disease in quail, >10^6 viable bacterial cells must be administered PO; chickens inoculated at the same levels are not affected.

Epidemiology: Birds that develop chronic ulcerative enteritis or have recovered from the disease remain carriers. Infection can be introduced by flies feeding on contaminated fecal material or by recovered carrier birds. Infected birds shed the bacterium in their droppings. Bobwhite quail are the most susceptible to this highly contagious disease. Most cases are reported in captive populations of bobwhite quail, suggesting that management plays a role in the incidence of ulcerative enteritis. *C colinum* spores can survive in the premises for months.

Pathogenesis: After oral infection, the bacterium adheres to the intestinal villi, producing enteritis and ulcers in portions of the small intestine and upper large intestine. Bacilli migrate to the liver via portal circulation, producing necrotic foci that later coalesce into extensive hepatic necrosis. Infarcts of the spleen are common. Stained smears of the lesions reveal the rod-shaped *C colinum* microorganism. Although toxigenicity tests in mice have been negative, the role of an in situ-produced toxin in the pathogenesis has been suggested but not demonstrated.

Clinical Findings: In susceptible bobwhite quail, sudden death occurs without signs or weight loss and with up to 100% mortality in just 2-3 days. Acute lesions include hemorrhagic enteritis of the duodenum. In chickens, as well as other game birds, the course of the disease is less severe and is accompanied by anorexia. Signs are similar to those seen in coccidiosis—depressed, listless birds with humped backs, ruffled feathers, diarrhea, sometimes bloody or watery white droppings, especially in quail in the prolonged course. Chickens recover within 2-3 wk and mortality rarely exceeds 10%.

Lesions: In early disease stages, the most common lesions include small, round ulcers surrounded by hemorrhages in the small intestine, ceca, and upper large intestine. Small ulcers later coalesce to form larger, sometimes perforating ulcers, producing local or diffuse peritonitis. The presence of blood in the gut resembles coccidiosis. Characteristic yellow to gray necrotic foci are the predominant lesions in the hepatic parenchyma. Spleen enlargement with hemorrhages and nectrotic areas may be present.

Diagnosis: Gross postmortem lesions including intestinal ulcerations and yellow to gray necrotizing lesions in the liver assist in diagnosis. *C colinum* can be seen in gram-stained smears of the liver and intestinal lesions. In bacteremic birds, the microorganism can also be found in blood and spleen smears. In chickens, differentiating ulcerative enteritis from coccidiosis (p 2201) may be difficult as both diseases may be present simultaneously.

Necrotic enteritis (p 2210) and histomoniasis (p 2238) may also present a diagnostic problem, but the hepatic lesions of ulcerative enteritis help differentiate it from these diseases. *C colinum* can be isolated from liver samples cultured in strict anaerobic conditions in prereduced blood glucose-yeast horse plasma medium. A fluorescent antibody test also has been used to accurately diagnose ulcerative enteritis.

Prevention, Treatment, and Control: Bacitracin in the feed at 200 g/ton is used for prevention in quail. Streptomycin (0.006%) and furazolidone (0.02%s) in the feed are effective for treating the disease. Prevention must start with good management practices (eg, avoiding the introduction of new birds into existing flocks. High population density is a predisposing factor. The use of cages is recommended in quail breeding. Sick or dead birds should be removed promptly. Total cleanup between flocks and pest control in and around the premises are good preventive measures.

AVIAN *CAMPYLOBACTER* INFECTION

Campylobacteriosis is a significant enterocolitis of humans acquired through consumption of undercooked poultry meat contaminated with *Campylobacter jejuni*. This organism colonizes the intestine of chickens, turkeys, and waterfowl but is generally nonpathogenic in mature poultry. Some strains of *C jejuni* can cause enteritis and death in newly hatched chicks and poults; however, it has not been possible to satisfy Koch's postulates and reproduce the syndrome previously termed "avian vibrionic hepatitis" by administering isolates of *C jejuni* to chickens.

Commercial poultry and free-living birds are natural reservoirs of the thermophilic campylobacters (*C jejuni*, *C coli*, and *C lari*) and other poorly defined species. It is estimated that over half of all commercial broiler and turkey flocks harbor *C jejuni*. The organism has been isolated from numerous birds, including Columbae and domestic and free-living Galliformes and Anseriformes.

C jejuni has been demonstrated in all areas of commercial poultry production. Isolation of the organism is a function of surveillance and ability of laboratory personnel to culture and identify *Campylobacter* spp.

Etiology and Epidemiology: *Campylobacter jejuni* is the predominant species associated with foodborne infection derived from poultry. *Campylobacter coli* and *C lari* are occasionally recovered from the intestinal tract of poultry and have also been implicated in foodborne infection.

Environmental contamination is the source of infection for poults, chicks, and ducklings. Litter can remain infective for long periods, subject to at least a 10% moisture level and neutral pH. Infected chicks and poults become colonized and can continue to excrete *C jejuni* for their lifetimes. Contaminated water may introduce infection into poultry flocks, and nonchlorinated water derived from a dam, river, or shallow well should be regarded as a possible source. Rats, wild birds, and houseflies can infect flocks; equipment and footwear contaminated with feces from an infected source may also serve as a vehicle of transmission. Once *C jejuni* has been introduced into the environment, rapid transmission within the flock occurs, with subsequent colonization of a high proportion of exposed breeders, commercial-meat, or laying-strain poultry. It is unclear whether *C jejuni* can be transmitted vertically, either on the surface of eggs or by transovarial transmission. It can be isolated from the reproductive tracts of hens and roosters.

Clinical Findings: Many chicks are colonized with *Campylobacter* spp early in life with no associated clinical signs or pathology. Highly pathogenic isolates derived from people with enterocolitis may induce some mortality in chicks.

Lesions: Gross lesions in challenged chicks include distention of the jejunum, disseminated hemorrhagic enteritis, and in some cases, focal hepatic necrosis. Microscopic lesions include edema of the mucosa of the ileum and cecum with *C jejuni* in the brush border of enterocytes. Mononuclear infiltration of the submucosa and villous atrophy occur, with intraluminal accumulation of mucus, erythrocytes, and both mononuclear and polymorphonuclear cells. It is unclear whether these findings represent a true clinical syndrome in chicks.

Diagnosis: Fecal specimens should be collected using rayon-tipped swabs, then placed in semisolid Cary-Blair transport medium. Enrichment culture of specimens in semisolid motility medium facilitates isolation when small numbers of *C jejuni* are present in a sample. *Campylobacter* should be cultured on selective media containing brucella agar base and bovine blood with up to 7 antibiotics that inhibit overgrowth of other Enterobacteriaceae. Thermophilic *Campylobacter* spp should be cultured at 42°C under microaerophilic conditions for 48 hr. The microaerophilic conditions generally consist of 85% nitrogen, 10% carbon dioxide, and 5% oxygen; however, some strains require a hydrogen-enriched atmosphere (5%). *Campylobacter* spp of significance in poultry are oxidase- and catalase-positive, indole-negative, and reduce selenite. The thermophilic species may be characterized on the basis of hippurate hydrolysis; nalidixic acid sensitivity is no longer reliable due to the increasing prevalence of fluoroquinolone-resistant *C jejuni*. The Penner or Lior serotyping schemes can be used to classify *C jejuni* ribotyping, or pulsed-field gel analysis can distinguish among various *C jejuni* isolates.

Control and Prevention: Because *C jejuni* does not occur as a specific pathogen under commercial conditions, treatment of poultry flocks is not a consideration. If *C jejuni* is considered a problem in companion bird aviaries or in exotic species, antibiotics such as erythromycin can be administered in drinking water. Galliformes should receive a dosage of 10-30 mg/kg for 4 consecutive days, and Psittaciformes and exotics should be medicated at 30-40 mg/kg.

Preharvest prevention of *Campylobacter* infection in commercial species is based on strict biosecurity, decontamination of housing between successive flocks, exclusion of rodents and wild birds, and insect eradication. Chlorination of drinking water to 2 ppm and operation of farms on a strict "all-in/all-out" basis occasionally reduces the prevalence of infection. In the context of commercial production in the USA where earth-floored housing is used and litter is recycled, preharvest control of *C jejuni* is impractical. Innovative methods of prevention, such as competitive inhibition or the use of vaccines, are under intensive investigation, but are unlikely to be available for commercial application in the near future. Withholding feed from broilers and turkeys for at least 12 hr before slaughter and thorough decontamination of transport coops and modules reduce fecal contamination and lower the level of *C jejuni* introduced into processing plants.

Zoonotic Risk: *C jejuni* is a major source of foodborne enteritis in consumers; contaminated, undercooked poultry is responsible for >50% of cases investigated. The condition was recognized in the mid-1970s, and the significance of the organism has become apparent with improved methods of isolation and identification. Nonchlorinated ground water, unpasteurized milk, young diarrheic pets, and contaminated beef and pork products may also be responsible for infection of people.

Improved washing of carcasses, use of counter-flow scalding, elimination of immersion chillers, and reduction in manual handling by installation of advanced automated equipment can reduce *C jejuni* contamination. Chemical disinfectants, such as glutaraldehyde (0.125%) and succinic acid (3%), and organic compounds, such as lactic and acetic acids, may be used to destroy *C jejuni*.

Gamma irradiation at levels of 1-3 kGy effectively eliminates *C jejuni* from poultry carcasses and products. Irradiation using cobalt 60 and electron beam generation are cost-effective procedures, which are endorsed by a joint United Nations Committee of the Food and Agricultural Organization, the International Atomic Energy Agency, and the World Health Organization. However, irradiation is not well accepted by American consumers. Currently, the only measure to reduce the risk of *C jejuni* infection to consumers is thorough cooking of poultry to achieve a core temperature of 74°C for 1 min. This ensures destruction of *C jejuni*. Concurrent hygienic storage, handling, and preparation are necessary to prevent contamination of prepared foods, work surfaces, and utensils by raw poultry and other meats.

AVIAN CHLAMYDIOSIS

(Psittacosis, Ornithosis, Parrot fever)

Avian chlamydiosis can be an inapparent subclinical infection or acute, subacute, or chronic disease of wild and domestic birds characterized by respiratory, digestive, or systemic infection. Infections occur worldwide and have been identified in at least 150 avian species, particularly colonial nesting birds (eg, egrets, herons), ratites, caged birds (primarily psittacines), raptors, and poultry. Among poultry, turkeys, ducks, and pigeons are most often affected; infection of chickens is infrequent. The disease is a significant cause of economic loss and human exposure in European duck flocks. Longterm inapparent infections lasting for months to years are common and considered the normal chlamydia-host relationship; 10-30% of surveyed avian populations may be found positive. The same strain may cause mild disease or asymptomatic infection in one species, but severe or fatal disease in another species.

Avian chlamydiosis is a zoonotic disease that can affect people following exposure to air- or dustborne organisms when infected birds are in flocks or processed, or when organisms are shed from the digestive or respiratory tracts of infected birds confined in breeding aviaries, lofts, or wholesale or retail outlets. Human disease most often results from exposure to psittacines or pigeons and can occur even if there is only brief proximity to a single infected bird. When workers are exposed to infected turkeys or ducks at processing, increased absenteeism due to acute respiratory disease often occurs ~1 wk after a flock with a high condemnation rate due to airsacculitis has been processed. Some individuals, especially pregnant women and those with impaired immunity, are more susceptible than others. The illness in people is usually respiratory and characterized by abrupt onset of flu-like symptoms; pneumonia, organ failure, and death can result if the disease is severe or left untreated. Precautions should be taken when examining a dead infected bird (eg, detergent disinfectant to wet feathers, fan-exhausted examining hood, dust mask or plastic face shield, and gloves) to avoid exposure.

Etiology and Epidemiology: A recent taxonomic revision resulted in the causative organism being renamed *Chlamydophila psittaci* (formerly *Chlamydia psittaci*). The name of the disease resulting from infection with *C psittaci* remains avian chlamydiosis. *C psittaci* is an obligate intracellular bacterium. All strains of chlamydia share an identical genus-specific antigen in their lipopolysaccharide but often differ in the composition of other cell-wall antigens, providing a basis for serotypic identification. Currently, 8 serotypes are recognized; 6 (A-F) infect avian species and are distinct from mammalian chlamydia serotypes. Each avian serotype tends to be associated with certain types of birds (TABLE 4). Serotype D is highly virulent for turkeys and can cause mortality of 30% or higher. Serotypes B and E are most frequently recovered from wild birds. Avian serotypes are capable of infecting people and other mammals.

Respiratory discharges or feces from infected birds contain elementary bodies that are resistant to drying and can remain infective for several months. Airborne particles and dust spread the organism. After inhalation or ingestion, elementary bodies attach to microvilli on mucosal epithelial cells and are internalized by endocytosis. Elementary bodies within endosomes in the cell cytoplasm differentiate into metabolically active, noninfectious reticulate bodies that divide and multiply, eventually forming numerous infectious, metabolically inactive elementary bodies. Newly formed elementary bodies are released from the host cell by lysis.

TABLE 4. Associations Between Avian Serotypes of *C psittaci* and Types of Birds

	A	B	C	D	E	F*
Psittacines	+++					+
Pigeons, doves		+++			+++	
Waterfowl			+++			
Turkeys	+	+		+++	+	
Gulls, egrets			+++			
Ratites					+++	
Wild birds		+++			+++	

*Rarely isolated

Possible sources of *C psittaci* include infected birds, asymptomatic carriers, vertical transmission from infected hens, infected rodents, and contaminated feed. Stressors and concurrent infections, especially those causing immunosuppression, can initiate shedding in latently infected birds and may cause recurrence of clinical disease. Carriers often shed the organism intermittently for extended periods. Persistence of *C psittaci* in the nasal glands of chronically infected birds may be an important source of organisms. Transmission is fecal-oral or by inhalation. The incubation period typically is 3-10 days but may be up to 2 mo in older birds or following low exposure.

Host and microbial factors, route and intensity of exposure, and treatment determine clinical course.

Clinical Findings and Lesions: Severity of clinical signs and lesions depends on the virulence of the organism and susceptibilty of the bird; asymptomatic infections are common. Nasal and ocular discharges, conjunctivitis, sinusitis, green to yellow-green droppings, fever, inactivity, ruffled feathers, weakness, inappetence, and weight loss can be seen in clinically affected birds. Necropsy findings in acute infections include serofibrinous polyserositis (airsacculitis, pericarditis, perihepatitis, peritonitis), pneumonia, hepatomegaly, and splenomegaly. Multiple pale foci and/or petechial hemorrhages can be seen in the liver and spleen. Similar lesions are seen in other systemic bacterial infections and are not specific for avian chlamydiosis. Multifocal necrosis in the liver and spleen is associated with large, granular, basophilic intracytoplasmic inclusions, occasional heterophils, and increased mononuclear cells (macrophages, lymphocytes, plasma cells) in hepatic sinusoids and splenic sinuses. Necrosis results from direct cell lysis or vascular damage. The latter is also the source of the generalized serofibrinous exudation. Enlargement and discoloration of the spleen or liver characterize chronic infections. Necrosis and inclusions are not seen, but the mononuclear cell response is present in these birds. Lesions are usually absent in latently infected birds, even though *C psittaci* is often being shed.

Diagnosis: Because of the variety of clinical presentations and common occurrence of latently infected carriers, no single diagnostic test can reliably determine infection. Procedures to detect the organism or antibodies are used. In general, the more acute the disease, the greater the number of infective organisms and the easier it is to make a diagnosis. When birds are acutely ill, clinical findings, including hematology, clinical chemistries, and radiology or typical gross lesions, are adequate for a tentative diagnosis. The organism can often be identified in impression smears of affected tissues stained by Giemsa, Gimenez, or Macchiavello's methods.

Antigen detection methods include immunohistochemistry (immunofluorescence, immunoperoxidase), ELISA, and PCR. Immunohistochemistry is accurate when done by a skilled person and the number of organisms is sufficient for detection. ELISA kits are available commercially and are relatively inexpensive, easy to use, and have good specificity, but low sensitivity. They are most useful when birds are clinically ill. PCR tests have been developed but are not widely available and require further evaluation. Multiple samples collected for 3-5 days are recommended for detection of intermittent shedding by asymptomatic birds.

Confirmation requires isolation and identification of *C psittaci* in chick embryos or cell cultures (BGM, L929, Vero) at a qualified laboratory. Cloacal, choanal, oropharyngeal, conjunctival, or fecal swabs from live birds or tissues (eg, liver, spleen, serosal membranes) from dead birds should be submitted. Sampling from mutiple sites and over several days will increase detection of intermittent shedding. Freezing, drying, improper handling, and certain transport media can affect viability. Refrigeration; placing specimens in sealed plastic bags or other containers; using a special buffer prepared from sucrose, phosphate, and glutamase (SPG buffer); and prompt delivery of fresh specimens are preferred. The laboratory should be contacted for directions on submitting samples before they are sent. Concurrent infections with other more easily diagnosed diseases (eg, colibacillosis, pasteurellosis, herpesvirus infections, mycotic diseases, etc) may mask chlamydial infection. Laboratory and clinical findings should be correlated with each other. Chlamydiosis must be distinguished from other respiratory and systemic diseases of birds.

Antibodies may or may not be detectable depending on the test used, degree and stage of infection, and treatment of the bird. Interpretation of titers from single serum samples is difficult. A 4-fold increase in titers between paired acute and convalescent samples is diagnostic, and high titers in a majority of samples from several birds in a population are sufficient for a presumptive diagnosis. Serologic methods include direct and modified direct complement fixation, latex agglutination, elementary body agglutination, and direct and competitive ELISA. ELISA provides the greatest sensitivity and specificity compared with culture. The elementary body agglutination test detects IgM and is useful for determining recent infection.

Prevention and Treatment: Local governmental regulations should be followed wherever applicable. No effective vaccine for use in birds is available. Treatment will prevent mortality and shedding but cannot be relied on to eliminate latent infection; shedding may recur. Tetracyclines (chlortetracycline, oxytetracycline, doxycycline) are the antibiotics of choice. Drug resistance to tetracyclines is rare, but reduced sensitivity requiring higher dosages is becoming more common. Tetracyclines are bacteriostatic and only effective against actively multiplying organisms, making extended treatment times (from 2-6 wk, during which minimum-inhibitory concentrations in blood are consistently maintained) necessary.

Outbreaks in poultry flocks are not common. Treating infected flocks with chlortetracycline at 400-750 g/ton for a minimum of 2 wk before processing has effectively eliminated potential risk of infection for plant employees.

In companion birds, use of chlortetracycline-medicated feeds for 45 days is a standard recommendation for imported birds (*see* CHLAMYDIOSIS, p 1459). Difficulties in palatability of the feed itself or high level of antibiotic necessary for adequate blood levels have limited its use. Long-acting oxytetracycline at 50-100 mg/kg, IM, every 2-3 days for 30 days, provides adequate continuous blood levels and results in elimination of shedding within 24 hr. However, muscle necrosis at injection sites may be extensive, which limits the usefulness of this treatment. Doxycycline in a formulation for IM use has been given at 75-100 mg/kg as a series of 7 injections over a 6-wk period. Addition of doxycycline to feeds can also result in adequate blood levels and has less effect on normal intestinal flora than does chlortetracycline. Supportive care for acutely affected birds also aids recovery.

Appropriate biosecurity practices are necessary for controlling the introduction and spread of chlamydiae in an avian population. Minimal standards include quarantine and examination of all new birds, traffic control to minimize cross-contamination, isolation and treatment of affected and contact birds, thorough cleaning and disinfection of premises and equiment (preferably with small units managed on an all-in/all-out basis), provision of uncontaminated feed, maintenance of records on all bird movements, and continual monitoring for presence of chlamydial infection.

The organism is susceptible to heat and most disinfectants (eg, 1:1,000 quaternary ammonium chloride, 1:100 bleach solution, 70% alcohol, etc), but is resistant to acid and alkali. A voluntary cooperative improvement plan leading to certification of companion birds derived from chlamydia-free breeders has been developed.

AVIAN NEPHRITIS VIRAL INFECTIONS

Avian nephritis viral infections are contagious infections of chickens and turkeys characterized by renal damage and visceral urate deposits, growth retardation, runting-stunting syndrome, and limited mortality (2-6%). They are seen mainly in chickens <7 days old, but interstitial nephritis can be observed in chicks up to 4 wk old. These infections have been reported worldwide. Subclinical infections are common and have been detected by serologic surveys in some SPF flocks.

Etiology and Transmission: The causal viruses are avian nephritis virus (ANV, an astrovirus), ANV-like viruses, and related enterovirus-like viruses (ELV). Strains vary in virulence and in antigenicity. Transmission occurs by direct or indirect contact. Indirect evidence suggests that egg transmission may occur. Infection can be transmitted by oral administration of virus to day-old birds. Virus is consistently isolated from the kidneys or the feces during the first 10 days after infection.

Nephropathogenic strains of infectious bronchitis virus (p 2302) also cause interstitial nephritis. Therefore, when nephritis is diagnosed, it is necessary to isolate the causative agent.

Clinical Findings: Clinical signs vary from none to the so-called runting-stunting syndrome. Diarrhea and growth retardation are common in broilers. Outbreaks with mortality of 2-6% can occur in chicks newly hatched up to 7 days old; cardinal necropsy findings are renal damage and visceral urate deposits (baby chick nephropathy).

Lesions: Nephritis is a common necropsy finding. Gross and microscopic lesions are often seen in the kidneys. Swelling, paleness, or yellowish discoloration with excessive urate deposition is frequent. Histologic lesions consist of a degeneration of the epithelial cells with infiltration of granulocytes, interstitial lymphocyte infiltration, and moderate fibrosis. In the latter stages, lymphoid follicles develop.

Some ELV induce only intestinal lesions varying from decreased length of the microvillus border to total desquamation of the intestinal epithelium.

Diagnosis: ANV and related viruses may be isolated by inoculation of suspected material (kidney or rectal contents) in the yolk sac of SPF chick embryos and in chick kidney cells. However, many ANV, ANV-like, and ELV viruses are difficult to isolate. The best method of detection is by electron microscopic examination of fecal preparations. Direct immunofluorescence performed on kidney sections is also a useful diagnostic procedure and allows quick differentiation from infectious bronchitis virus.

Serologic diagnosis can be made using indirect immunofluorescence, seroneutralization, or ELISA tests.

Treatment and Prevention: There is no effective treatment. General hygienic precautions are the only applicable preventive measures.

AVIAN SPIROCHETOSIS

(Avian borreliosis)

Avian spirochetosis is an acute, febrile, septicemic, bacterial disease that affects a wide variety of birds.

Etiology, Epidemiology, and Transmission: The causal organism, *Borrelia anserina*, is an actively motile spirochete, ~0.2-0.3 μm × 8-20 μm, and consists of 5-8 loosely arranged coils. Cultivation in vitro is difficult. *Borrelia* will grow on Barbour-Stoenner-Kelly medium, but loses virulence after 12 passages. It can also be propagated in embryonating duck or chick embryos or in young ducks or chicks.

Spirochetosis is found in temperate or tropical regions, wherever the biologic vectors are found. The most common vector is *Argas (Persicargas) persicus*, the "cosmopolitan" fowl tick, but other *Argas* spp transmit the disease in different geographic areas. In the western USA, a highly efficient vector is *A sanchezi*.

Diverse immunologic and serologic types of *B anserina* have been demonstrated in many areas. Recovery from one type confers solid immunity against the homologous types for ≥1 yr, but not against heterologous strains. Relapses, such as occur with some human *Borrelia* infections, are unknown in *B anserina* infection of birds; any reinfection can be attributed to a heterologous type.

Generally, an infected *Argas* tick can transmit the disease at every feeding and maintains the infection throughout larval, nymphal, and adult stages. The ticks also transmit the infection transovarially, ie, the F_1 larvae are infective. Ticks remain infected despite feeding on chicks hyperimmune to *B anserina* or on chicks with high blood levels of chemotherapeutic agents effective against *Borrelia*. Other vectors (lice, mosquitos, some species of ticks, inanimate objects) can transmit the spirochete mechanically to a susceptible host whenever the piercing apparatus becomes contaminated with blood that contains *Borrelia*. Ingestion of bile-stained fecal droppings containing the spirochete, contamination of feed or water, and cannibalism during spirochetemia can result in infection. After the bite of an infected tick, the incubation period is ~3-12 days.

Clinical Findings: Marked enlargement and mottling of the spleen is the most characteristic lesion. Signs are highly variable, depending on the virulence of the spirochete, and may be absent. Signs include listlessness, depression, somnolence, moderate to marked shivering, and increased thirst. Young birds are affected more severely than older ones. During the initial stages of the disease, there is usually a green or yellow diarrhea with increased urates. The course of the disease is 1-2 wk. Mild strains are common. However, in many tick-infested geographic areas, morbidity can approach 100% and mortality may be 33-77%. Egg production in layers or breeders may be reduced by 5-10%, with a higher number of small eggs.

Lesions: An enlarged spleen with petechial or ecchymotic hemorrhages, not unlike spleens in marble spleen disease of pheasants (p 2236), is present. However, a contrasting situation may be seen in Mongolian pheasants, in which the spleen is reported to be small and pale. Occasionally, the liver may be swollen and contain focal areas of necrosis. Kidneys may be enlarged and pale. A green, catarrhal enteritis is common.

Diagnosis: Diagnosis depends on demonstration of *Borrelia* in the blood, either as actively motile during darkfield microscopy, or as stained spirochetes in Giemsa-stained blood smears. In young birds, the *Borrelia* may reach vast numbers per oil-immersion field and persist for several days. Older birds usually have low numbers of *Borrelia* that are detected only with difficulty, or not at all, and that persist for only 1-2 days. Anemia is common and results in increased numbers of immature RBC.

Agar-gel diffusion and various serologic tests have been described but are of questionable value due to diverse serotypes that exist in some localities. Specific agglutinins clump the spirochetes in successively larger clumps during the terminal stages of the disease. Agglutination-lysis then begins to disintegrate these clumps, and spirochetal degradation products are liberated, which may result in pyrexia. Death occurs most often 1-3 days after *Borrelia* disappear from the bloodstream. Spirochetal antibodies are readily detected in yolks of eggs laid by infected hens.

Treatment and Control: Several antibacterial agents are effective. The most widely used are penicillin derivatives, but the streptomycins, tetracyclines, and tylosin are also effective. The antibiotics can be completely efficacious if begun when the number of spirochetes per oil-immersion field is low or moderate; however, if large numbers of spirochetes are present in the bloodstream, the sudden liberation of large quantities of spirochetal degradation products can result in higher mortality than no treatment.

Control must be directed against the biologic vector. *Argas* ticks are notable for their long lifespan, ability to survive for extended periods without a blood meal, efficiency in transmitting the spirochete, and ability to remain securely hidden in cracks and crevices often beyond the effective reach of pesticides. Accordingly, control is difficult. A combination of tick eradication and immunization is the most effective means of control.

Immunization can be highly successful and, next to eradication of the biologic vector, is the preferred method of control. Bacterins prepared from local strains of *Borrelia* have been used with success. Vaccines may be prepared from formalin- or phenol-inactivated material from lysates of blood, tissues, embryos, or eggs infected with *B anserina*, and may be lyophilized or liquid. Whole-egg propagated bacterins are usually given in 1 or 2 IM injections. Little if any cross-protection is afforded to different serotypes. Birds normally have protective immunity after recovering from natural infection.

COLIBACILLOSIS

(Colisepticemia, *Escherichia coli* infection)

Colibacillosis occurs as an acute fatal septicemia or subacute pericarditis and airsacculitis. It is a common systemic disease of economic importance in poultry and is seen worldwide.

Etiology and Pathogenesis: *Escherichia coli* is a gram-negative, rod-shaped bacterium normally found in the intestines of poultry and most other animals; although most are nonpathogenic, a limited number produce extraintestinal infections. Pathogenic strains are commonly of the O1, O2, and O78 serotypes, but serotypes O11, O15, O18, O51, O115, and O132 have also been reported for *E coli* isolates associated with cellulitis and colibacillosis. There is considerable diversity of serogroups among clinical isolates, and only a small percentage of these isolates belong to serotypes O1, O2, or O78. In fact, 18-29% of avian *E coli* isolates cannot be typed. Therefore, no single *E coli* serotype used as a bacterin can provide full protection against all of the serotypes that cause *E coli* infections. Virulence factors include the ability to resist phagocytosis, utilization of highly efficient iron acquisition systems, resistance to killing by serum, production of colicins, and adherence to respiratory epithelium. Virulent *E coli* are generally nontoxigenic, poorly invasive, and do not possess common adhesins.

Large numbers of *E coli* are maintained in the poultry house environment through fecal contamination. Initial exposure to pathogenic *E coli* may occur in the hatchery from infected or contaminated eggs, but systemic infection usually requires predisposing environmental factors or infectious causes. Mycoplasmosis, infectious bronchitis, Newcastle disease, hemorrhagic enteritis, and turkey bordetellosis precede colibacillosis. Poor air quality and other environmental stresses may also predispose to *E coli* infections.

Systemic infection occurs when large numbers of pathogenic *E coli* gain access to the bloodstream from the respiratory tract or intestine. Bacteremia progresses to septicemia and death, or the infection extends to serosal surfaces, pericardium, joints, and other organs.

Clinical Findings and Lesions: Signs are nonspecific and vary with age, organs involved, and concurrent disease. Young birds dying of acute septicemia have few lesions except for enlarged, hyperemic liver and spleen with increased fluid in body cavities. Birds that survive septicemia develop subacute fibrinopurulent airsacculitis, pericarditis, perihepatitis, and lymphocytic depletion of the bursa and thymus. (Unusually pathogenic salmonellae produce similar lesions in chicks.) Although airsacculitis is a classic lesion of colibacillosis, whether it results from primary respiratory exposure or from extension of serositis is unclear. Sporadic lesions include pneumonia, arthritis, osteomyelitis, and salpingitis.

Diagnosis: Unlike pathogenic *E coli* associated with illnesses in other animal species, avian isolates are generally nonhemolytic on sheep (5%) blood agar. Isolation of a pure culture of *E coli* from heart blood, liver, or typical visceral lesions in a fresh carcass indicates primary or secondary colibacillosis. Consideration should be given to predisposing infections and environmental factors. Pathogenicity of isolates is established when parenteral inoculation of young chicks or poults results in fatal septicemia or typical lesions within 3 days. Pathogenicity can also be detected by inoculation of the allantoic sac of 12-day-old chick embryos. Resulting gross lesions include cranial and skin hemorrhages in addition to encephalomalacia in embryos inoculated with virulent isolates.

Treatment and Control: Treatment strategies include attempts to control predisposing infections or environmental factors and early use of antibacterials indicated by susceptibility tests. Most isolates are resistant to tetracyclines, streptomycin, and sulfa drugs, although therapeutic success can sometimes be achieved with tetracycline. In fact, 90% of clinical isolates are resistant to tetracycline, with 60% of isolates resistant to 5 or more antibiotics. Fluoroquinolone use is controversial because the use of these drugs in commercial broilers is believed to select for resistant *Campylobacter* spp associated with human foodborne infections. Commercial bacterins, administered to breeder hens or chicks, have provided some protection against homologous *E coli* serotypes.

DUCK VIRAL HEPATITIS

Duck viral hepatitis is an acute, highly contagious, viral disease of young ducklings characterized by a short incubation period, sudden onset, high mortality, and characteristic liver lesions. The disease is of economic importance in all duck-raising areas of the world. Three distinct types of duck hepatitis virus (DHV) have been isolated from diseased ducklings. A natural outbreak of DHV Type I has been reported in mallard ducklings; experimental DHV Type I infections have been produced in goslings, turkey poults, young pheasants, quail, and guinea fowl. The viruses that cause hepatitis in ducklings should not be confused with duck hepatitis B virus, a hepadnavirus infection of older ducks.

Etiology: The originally described, most widespread, and most virulent DHV Type I is an enterovirus in the family Picornaviridae and is readily propagated in chick and duck embryos. It does not produce hemagglutinins. Field experience with DHV Type I indicates that egg transmission does not occur. The disease can be transmitted experimentally by parenteral or oral administration of infected tissues.

Viruses differing from classic DHV Type I have been recognized as causes of hepatitis in ducklings. DHV Type II is considered to be an astrovirus and is difficult to propagate under laboratory conditions; DHV Type III is a member of the Picornaviridae, is antigenically distinct from Type I virus, and can be propagated in duck (but not chick) embryos. A distinct serologic variant of DHV Type I, named DHV Type Ia, has also been described.

Clinical Findings: The incubation period for Type I virus is 18-48 hr. Affected ducklings become lethargic, lose balance, paddle spasmodically, and die within minutes, typically with opisthotonos. Although adults may become infected, clinical signs have not been seen in ducks >7 wk old. Mortality may be as high as 95% in ducklings. Practically all deaths occur within 1 wk after onset of signs.

The clinical course of DHV Type II infection is similar to that of Type I and can occur in ducklings immune to Type I infection. DHV Type III infections occur in ducklings despite immunity to Type I virus. The clinical course of Type III infection is less severe, and mortality is rarely >30%.

Lesions: The lesions caused by all 3 types of DHV are similar. The liver is enlarged and covered with hemorrhagic foci up to 1 cm in diameter. The spleen may be enlarged and mottled. Kidneys may be swollen, and renal blood vessels congested.

Diagnosis: A presumptive diagnosis can be based on the history and lesions. Sudden onset, rapid spread, and short course, together with characteristic liver lesions, are highly suggestive of duck viral hepatitis. Type I virus may be isolated in duck embryos, day-old ducklings, and duck-embryo liver cell cultures, or less easily in chicken embryos. The virus can be identified by neutralization with specific antisera or by inoculation into both susceptible and immune ducklings. Type II and III viruses are not neutralized by classic Type I antiserum.

Prevention and Treatment: Prevention is by strict isolation, particularly during the first 5 wk of age. Contact with wild waterfowl should be avoided. Rats have been reported as a reservoir host of the virus; therefore, pest control is indicated.

Immunization of breeder ducks with modified live virus vaccines, using Type I, II, and III viruses, provides parenteral immunity that effectively prevents high losses in young ducklings. The Type I virus vaccine is administered SC in the neck to breeder ducks at 16, 20, and 24 wk of age and every 12 wk thereafter throughout the laying period. Three immunizations are advisable for passive protection of ducklings.

An inactivated DHV Type I vaccine for use in breeder ducks that have been previously primed with live DHV Type I virus has been described. A single dose of the inactivated vaccine, given IM before the birds come into lay, provides passive immunity for a complete laying cycle to progeny ducklings.

The chick-embryo origin, modified live Type I virus vaccine also can be used for early vaccination of ducklings susceptible to Type I (progeny of nonimmune breeders). This vaccine is administered SC or by foot web stab in a single dose to day-old ducklings. Vaccinated ducklings rapidly develop an active immunity over 3-4 days.

Antibody against Type I virus, prepared from the eggs of hyperimmunized chickens, administered SC in the neck at the time of initial loss, is an effective flock treatment.

ENTEROCOCCOSIS

The application of new bacteriologic techniques, especially DNA-DNA and DNA-rRNA hybridization has led to the reclassification of Lancefield group D streptococci as *Enterococcus* spp. (For a discussion of diseases caused by the Lancefield antigenic serogroup C and other *Streptococci* spp, *see* STREPTOCOCCOSIS, p 2266.)

Enterococcus spp in avian species are worldwide in distribution. Enterococci are ubiquitous in nature and commonly found in various poultry environments. *Enterococcus* spp are considered normal microflora of the intestinal tract of poultry and other birds. A high percentage of ready-to-eat poultry products are contaminated with *Enterococcus* spp; however, no resultant food poisoning in humans has been reported.

Etiology and Epidemiology: The genus *Enterococcus* is composed of gram-positive, spherical bacteria occurring singly, in pairs, or in short chains, which are nonmotile, nonsporeforming, facultative anaerobes. They are catalase-negative and ferment sugars, usually to lactic acid. Common avian isolates can be differentiated by their ability to ferment mannitol, sorbitol, and L-arabinose and by their growth on MacConkey agar without crystal violet or salt. (Other types of MacConkey agar inhibit *Enterococcus* and may provide false-negative results.) *Enterococcus* spp isolated from avian species and associated with disease include *E faecalis, E faecium, E durans, E avium,* and *E hirae. E faecalis* affects birds of all ages; it is a serious disease occurring in embryos and young chicks from fecal-contaminated eggs. *E faecium* is a cause of mortality in ducklings.

Enterococci are transmitted most commonly via oral and aerosol routes. However, transmission can occur through skin injuries, especially in caged layers. Aerosol transmission of *E faecalis* results in acute septicemia in chickens. Concurrent enteric infections or any condition compromising the intestinal villous epithelium, allowing penetration of resident enterococci, can result in septicemia, bacterial endocarditis, or both. Incubation periods range from 1 day to several weeks, with 5-21 days most common. Endocarditis can occur when a septicemic enterococcal infection progresses to a subacute or chronic stage. *Enterococcus* spp have been associated with brain necrosis and encephalomalacia in young chickens. Some enterococci, however, have been demonstrated to have a beneficial effect on growth and feed efficiency and are being studied as potential probiotics.

Clinical Findings: *Enterococcus* spp in poultry can result in 2 distinct clinical forms of disease, acute and subacute/chronic. In the acute form, clinical signs are related to septicemia and include depression, lethargy, lassitude, pale combs and wattles, ruffled feathers, diarrhea, fine head tremors, and decrease or cessation of egg production. Often, only dead birds are found. In the subacute/chronic form, depression, loss of body weight, lameness, and head tremors may be observed. Body temperature is elevated in birds with persistent bacteremia. Clinically affected birds eventually die if not treated. Egg transmission or fecal contamination of hatching eggs results in late embryo mortality and an increased number of chicks or poults unable to "pip" or penetrate through the shell at hatch.

Lesions: Gross lesions of enterococci infection in acute disease include splenomegaly, hepatomegaly (with or without foci), enlarged kidneys, and congestion of subcutaneous tissue. Omphalitis or enlarged yolk sacs may be seen in chicks or poults infected at hatching. Hepatomegaly, splenic necrosis, fibrinous pericarditis, perihepatitis, and airsacculitis are observed in ducks infected with *E faecium*. Lesions of chronic enterococcal infections include fibrinous arthritis and/or tenosynovitis, osteomyelitis, fibrinous pericarditis and perihepatitis, necrotic myocarditis, and valvular vegetative endocarditis similar to that observed with *Streptococcus zooepidemicus* infection (*see* STREPTOCOCCOSIS, p 2266). Additional gross lesions associated with valvular endocarditis include an enlarged, pale, flaccid heart; pale to hemorrhagic areas in the myocardium; infarcts in the liver, spleen, or heart; and, less commonly, infarcts in the lung, kidney, and brain.

On microscopic examination, the liver has dilated sinusoids congested with RBC and increased heterophils. Splenomegaly is characterized by congestion and hyperplasia of cells in the mononuclear phagocytic system. Valvular lesions consist primarily of fibrin with bacteria, heterophils, macrophages, and fibroblasts. Other microscopic lesions related to endocarditis include cerebral vasculitis and infarcts, leptomeningitis, glomerulonephritis, and thrombosed pulmonary vessels. Focal granulomas can be found in virtually any tissue as a result of septic emboli. Aggregates of bacteria are present throughout necrotic areas with a zone of heterophils just within the necrotic border, a characteristic feature of the lesion. Gram-positive bacterial colonies are readily observed in thrombosed vessels and within necrotic foci.

Diagnosis: Demonstration of bacteria typical of enterococci in blood or impression smears of affected heart valves or lesions from birds with typical clinical signs will provide a presumptive diagnosis of enterococcosis. Isolation of *Enterococcus* spp (without fecal contamination) from typical lesions will confirm the diagnosis. Enterococci are easily isolated on blood agar or more specific differential media, which should help differentiate species. Fermentation of mannitol, sorbitol, and arabinose, and growth on MacConkey agar (without crystal violet or salt) can also aid in differentiating enterococci from *Streptococcus* spp. Preferred tissues for culture include liver, spleen, blood, yolk, embryo fluids, or any suspected lesion. Diagnosis of bacterial endocarditis is based on valvular vegetations with secondary infarcts of myocardium, liver, or spleen. In suspected cases, it is important to culture lesions to establish a definitive diagnosis and rule out other bacteria.

Differential diagnosis includes other bacterial septicemic diseases, eg, staphylococcosis, streptococcosis, colibacillosis, pasteurellosis, and erysipelas.

Treatment and Prevention: Treatment includes use of antibiotics such as penicillin, erythromycin, novobiocin, oxytetracycline, chlortetracycline, or tetracycline in acute and subacute infections. Clinically affected birds respond well early in the course of the disease. As the disease progresses within a flock, treatment efficacy decreases. Antibacterial sensitivity should be performed on bacterial isolates in any clinical cases of enterococcosis before treatment begins. There is no treatment for poultry with bacterial endocarditis.

Prevention and control requires reducing stress and preventing immunosuppressive diseases and conditions. Proper cleaning and disinfection can reduce environmental enterococcal resident flora to minimize external exposure.

ERYSIPELAS

Erysipelas in poultry is seen worldwide, mainly as an acute septicemia. Outbreaks usually occur suddenly, with a few birds being found dead followed by increasing mortality on subsequent days. Mortality may range from <1% to 50%. From an economic standpoint, turkeys are the most important poultry species affected, but serious outbreaks have occurred in chickens, ducks, and geese. Mammals are also affected, with swine being the most economically important species. Infection in reptiles and amphibians has also been reported. The organism has been isolated from the surface slime on fish, which may serve as a source of infection for other species. People usually become infected when the organism enters through cuts in the skin. There have been no reports of people becoming infected by the oral route. The disease in humans (**erysipeloid**) is most common in people who handle infected tissues such as veterinarians, butchers, and fish handlers. Erysipeloid in people may be a localized or a septicemic and occasionally fatal infection. (*See also* ERYSIPELAS IN MAMMALS, p 505.)

Etiology: The causative agent is *Erysipelothrix rhusiopathiae*, a facultatively anaerobic, intracellular bacterium. A second genomic species, *E tonsillarum*, has been described but is not considered pathogenic for poultry. Morphologically, *E tonsillarum* cannot be distinguished from *E rhusiopathiae*. *E rhusiopathiae* stains gram-positive but tends to decolorize, particularly in older cultures. The organism is nonmotile, does not form spores, and produces no known toxins. There is no flagellum but a capsule has been demonstrated. The cellular morphology of *E rhusiopathiae* is variable. Cells freshly isolated from tissues during acute infection or from smooth colonies are straight or slightly curved small rods that may occur in short chains. Cells from older cultures or rough colonies tend to become filamentous and may be confused with mycelia. The filamentous form occurs more frequently after repeated passages on artificial media.

E rhusiopathiae grows readily on ordinary culture media containing the blood or sera of various animals. Growth is enhanced by reducing the oxygen content or increasing the carbon dioxide level to 5-10%. Optimal incubation temperature is 35-37°C, and the optimal pH range is 7.4-7.8.

The organism is not readily destroyed by the usual laboratory disinfectants, and it may survive in litter or soil for various lengths of time; therefore, disinfection of premises is difficult. *E rhusiopathiae* may also survive smoking and pickling processes. It is inactivated by a 1:1,000 concentration of bichloride of mercury, 0.5% sodium hydroxide solution, 3.5% liquid cresol, 5% solution of phenol, or 0.5% formalin.

Though different serotypes of *E rhusiopathiae* exist, no correlation has been shown to exist between the serotype, chemical structure, or biochemical pattern, and the manifestation of the septicemic, urticarial, or endocardial forms of erysipelas.

Epidemiology: Erysipelas occurs sporadically in poultry of all ages. Turkeys are susceptible regardless of sex or age. Recent evidence indicates that there may be a genetically related resistance in turkeys. The incidence in males is reported to be higher, but this is not supported by experimental data. Erysipelas may affect the fertility of males and may contribute to downgrading and processing losses. Infection results from entrance of the organisms through breaks in the skin, through the mucous membranes such as during artificial insemination, by ingestion of contaminated foodstuffs (particularly cannibalism of infected carcasses), and possibly by mechanical transmission via biting insects. Fighting and cannibalism increase losses.

The organism is shed in feces from infected animals and contaminates the soil, in which it may survive for long periods depending on temperature and pH. Seasonal changes in climate such as the onset of cold, rainy weather have been associated with disease occurence. Poultry, as well as other animals, may be carriers and shed the organism without showing clinical signs of disease.

In nonvaccinated flocks, morbidity and mortality may reach 40-50%, but mortality is usually limited to <15%. In vaccinated flocks, some birds may be depressed for a short period and recover. Mortality in vaccinated and nonvaccinated poultry is influenced by the virulence of the organism.

Clinical Findings: Erysipelas is primarily an acute infection that results in sudden death. In an affected flock, a few birds may be depressed but easily aroused; within 24 hr, a few birds will be dead. Just before death, some birds may be very droopy, with an unsteady gait. Chronic clinical disease in a flock is not usual but does occur; birds may have cutaneous lesions and swollen hocks. Turkeys with vegetative endocarditis usually do not have clinical signs and may die suddenly. Erysipelas should be suspected in flocks that have been artificially inseminated 4-5 days before an episode of death without clinical signs. Clinical signs in chickens include general weakness, depression, diarrhea, and sudden death. In laying hens, egg production may drop markedly.

Lesions: At necropsy, a generalized darkening of the skin or various sized areas of diffuse darkening is common. The liver and spleen are usually enlarged and friable and may be mottled. There may be other gross lesions such as peritonitis, pericarditis, catarrhal exudate in the GI tract, and degeneration of fat associated with the thigh and heart.

Diagnosis: Infections with *E coli* or *Pasteurella multocida*, as well as salmonellosis and peracute Newcastle disease may be confused with the septicemic form of erysipelas. Urticaria and endocarditis may be caused by other miscellaneous bacterial or fungal pathogens. Noninfectious differential diagnoses include poisoning, stampede injuries, or predators. A presumptive diagnosis can be based on an impression smear of the liver or spleen or on a smear of cardiac blood or bone marrow that shows gram-positive, slender, pleomorphic rods. Bone marrow is the tissue of choice in partially decomposed specimens. Isolation and identification of *E rhusiopathiae* is necessary for definitive diagnosis. Identification can be made by fluorescent antibody staining, PCR, or a mouse protection test; however, the isolate must be pathogenic for mice. A mouse ear scarification model has been described and is particularly helpful for mixed cultures. Caution must be used in attempting reisolation, because the organism produces pinpoint colonies that may be easily overlooked or masked by faster-growing bacteria. Highly selective media are available for reisolation.

Treatment and Control: Antibiotic resistance of *E rhusiopathiae* has not been reported. The antibiotic of choice is a rapid-acting penicillin such as potassium or sodium penicillin. As soon as a presumptive diagnosis is made, penicillin should be administered IM at 10,000 u/lb body wt, simultaneously with a full dose of erysipelas bacterin. In situations in which it is impractical to handle every bird, administration of penicillin in the drinking water at 10,000,000 u/gal. for 4-5 days greatly reduces losses. Sulfonamides and oral oxytetracyline are not effective; broad-spectrum antibiotics, eg, erythromycin, are effective. Antibiotic in feed or water treats only those in the flock that are still eating and drinking normally and may not have dramatic results. Vaccination with a bacterin helps protect those birds in the flock not yet infected. Antibiotic therapy or vaccination does not eliminate the carrier state.

Vaccination will control erysipelas. Both inactivated and live vaccines are available for use in turkeys; only vaccines approved for use in turkeys should be used. The use of bacterins in flocks used for meat is useful but labor intensive. For breeders, the bacterin should be given every 2-4 mo. The use of live vaccines administered in the drinking water does not require handling each bird and, therefore, is less stressful.

There are no specific husbandry recommendations other than sound management practices for the control of erysipelas in poultry, particularly in endemic areas.

FATTY LIVER SYNDROME

Fatty liver syndrome was first described in the 1950s as excessive fat in the liver associated with varying degress of hemorrhage. The condition is almost universally confined to caged birds fed high-energy diets, and is most often seen in summer months. The liver is usually enlarged, yellow or putty colored, and very friable. The abdominal cavity contains large amounts of fat. Fatty liver syndrome without excessive body fat is thought to be associated with mycotoxins (eg, aflatoxins) in feed. *See* MYCOTOXICOSES, p 2246. The affected birds may also have pale combs. The ovary is usually active and the metabolic and physical stress associated with oviposition may be factors that induce the fatal hemorrhage, although mortality generally is <5%.

Because fatty liver syndrome seems to occur only when birds are in a positive energy balance, the monitoring of body weight is a good diagnostic tool. Through force-feeding techniques, it has been shown that fatty liver syndrome is caused by an oversupply of energy rather than by an excess of any specific nutrient, such as fat or carbohydrate. The condition can be induced experimentally in layers and even male birds by the administration of estrogen, reinforcing the concept that it occurs more frequently in high-producing birds that presumably are producing estrogen from very active ovaries.

The condition is easy to recognize at necropsy due to the liver hemorrhage and also the fact that the liver is often enlarged and engorged with fat. This makes the liver friable, and it is difficult to remove each lobe in one piece. The pale yellow color of the liver, while characteristic, is not always specific to this condition. Normal layers fed appreciable quantities of yellow corn will also have a yellow liver. Also, liver color may be indicative of dietary xanthophylls rather than fatty liver syndrome, because the condition can be induced by force-feeding semi-purified diets devoid of pigment; these birds lack the characteristic yellow liver. Birds with fatty liver syndrome have 40-70% fat in the liver dry matter. In many studies, the degree of fatty liver syndrome is described via a liver hemorrhage score, which is usually based on a scale from 1-5, in which 1 = no hemorrhage, 2 = 1-5 hemorrhages, 3 = 6-15 hemorrhages, 4 = 16-25 hemorrhages, and 5 = >25 hemorrhages, including a massive, usually fatal, hemorrhage.

Attempts have been made to prevent or treat the condition through diet modification. Substituting carbohydrate with supplemental fat, while not increasing the energy content of the dietary, seems to be beneficial. Presumably such modification means that the liver needs to synthesize less fat for yolk. Replacement of corn with other cereals, such as wheat and barley, is often beneficial. However, this substitution may involve a reduction in dietary energy level or may necessitate the use of additional fat to maintain isoenergetic conditions, and these 2 factors are known to influence fatty liver syndrome. The syndrome has reportedly been reduced through the use of various byproduct feeds such as distiller's grains and solubles, fish meal, and alfalfa meal. Although the mode of action is unclear, unintentional supplementation of selenium may be involved. Addition of 6% oat hulls to the feed has been successful at times. Fatty liver syndrome is best prevented by not allowing an excessive positive energy balance in older birds. Body weight can be monitored and when potential problems are seen, remedial action taken to limit energy intake through the use of lower energy diets and/or change in feed management. A wide energy:protein ratio in the diet will aggravate fatty liver syndrome. On farms with history of fatty liver syndrome, the diet should be supplemented with 0.3 ppm selenium, up to 100 IU vitamin E/kg diet, and appropriate levels of an antioxidant such as ethoxyquin.

FLIP-OVER DISEASE

(Sudden death syndrome, Heart attack, Acute death syndrome, Fatal syncope, Lung edema, Lung congestion, Dead in good condition)

Flip-over disease has been reported in most areas of the world that intensively raise broilers. Young, healthy, fast-growing broiler chickens die suddenly with a short, terminal, wing-beating convulsion. Many affected broilers just "flip over" and die on their backs; 60-80% are males. The condition is uncommon or unrecognized when low-density feed is used and the ratio of feed intake to weight gain is >2.5 at 6 wk, or when broilers take 8 wk to reach 2 kg.

Etiology and Epidemiology: The cause is unknown but probably is a metabolic disease related to carbohydrate metabolism, cell membrane integrity, and intracellular electrolyte balance. Death may result from ventricular fibrillation. The modern broiler tends to overeat and continues to grow rapidly while maintaining a low feed-to-gain ratio. Flip-over appears to be related to high carbohydrate intake. It is not known whether a genetic predisposition exists.

Incidence in a rapidly growing healthy broiler flock is typically 1-4%.

Clinical Findings: Broilers show no premonitory signs. They appear healthy and may be feeding, sparring, walking, or resting, but suddenly extend their necks, gasp or squawk, and die rapidly with a short period of wing beating and leg movement, during which they frequently flip onto their backs. They also may be found dead on their sides or breasts.

Flip-over may occur as early as day 3 and may continue until 10-12 wk in roaster flocks. Peak mortality varies but usually is between days 12 and 28, although it can be as early as day 9. It may occur after day 28, particularly if growth is restricted in young broilers. Mortality of 0.25-0.5% per day can occur for 1-3 days.

Lesions: Confirmation is difficult because no specific gross or histologic lesions are present. Dead birds are well fleshed, have an empty or partially filled crop containing normal ingesta, and feed in the gizzard. The abdomen is distended because the bird is fat and because the intestines are dilated and filled with semisolid digesta and mucus (as in any broiler that dies with the intestine full of feed). There is no evidence of stasis. The muscles are mottled red and white with congestion of the dependent muscles. Organs are moderately to severely congested. There may be small hemorrhages in the liver and kidney. The ventricles of the heart are contracted (but not hypertrophied), and the atria are dilated and blood filled. (If autolysis is advanced, the ventricles may be dilated.) The lungs are congested and frequently edematous; however, pulmonary edema increases with time after death and is not prominent in broilers that are examined within a few minutes after death. The gallbladder may be small or empty (as it is in many broilers on full feed).

Diagnosis: Good broilers found dead on their backs may be assumed to have died of flip-over because that position is rare in death from other causes except cardiac tamponade, asphyxia, and ascites syndrome (p 2269). Birds in good condition on their sides or breasts, scattered in a random fashion in the pen also usually are considered to be dead from flip-over. Diagnosis is supported by the full GI tract (particularly the full intestine); large, pale liver; large, normal bursa; contracted ventricles and dilated, blood-filled atria; lung congestion and edema; and the lack of pathologic lesions.

The condition called sudden death syndrome in Australia in broiler breeders coming into production is a different disease; it is reported to be caused by potassium deficiency. Similar mortality caused by a combination of high environmental temperature and hypophosphatemia or by acute hypocalcemia has been reported in North America.

Sudden death in turkeys may be caused by choke, aortic rupture (p 2197), focal (obstructive) granulomatous pneumonia, or by hypertrophic cardiomyopathy (p 2200) with lung congestion and edema, splenomegaly, and perirenal hemorrhage (p 2199).

Prevention and Control: The incidence of flip-over disease can be minimized by slowing the growth rate of broilers, particularly during the first 3 wk of life. Growth rate can be moderated by controlling nutrient intake. This can be accomplished by reducing day length (number of hours of light per day), providing a ration low in energy and protein, or limiting the amount of feed provided to broilers.

FOWL CHOLERA

Fowl cholera is a contagious, widely distributed disease that affects domestic and wild birds. It usually occurs as a septicemia of sudden onset with high morbidity and mortality, but chronic and asymptomatic infections also occur.

Etiology and Transmission: *Pasteurella multocida*, the causal agent, is a small, gram-negative, nonmotile rod that may exhibit pleomorphism after repeated subculture. In freshly isolated cultures or in tissues, the bacteria have a bipolar appearance when stained with Wright's stain. Although *P multocida* may infect a wide variety of animals, strains isolated from nonavian hosts generally do not produce fowl cholera. Strains that cause fowl cholera represent a number of immunotypes, which complicates widespread prevention by using bacterins. The organism is susceptible to ordinary disinfectants, sunlight, drying, and heat. Turkeys are more susceptible than chickens, older chickens are more susceptible than young ones, and some breeds of chickens are more susceptible than others.

Chronically infected birds are considered to be a major source of infection. Dissemination of *P multocida* within a flock is primarily by excretions from mouth, nose, and conjunctiva of diseased birds that contaminate their environment.

Clinical Findings: These vary greatly depending on the course of disease. In acute fowl cholera, dead birds are usually the first indication of disease. Fever, depression, anorexia, mucoid discharge from the mouth, ruffled feathers, diarrhea, and increased respiratory rate are usually seen. Pneumonia is particularly common in turkeys.

In chronic fowl cholera, signs and lesions are generally related to localized infections. Sternal bursae, wattles, joints, tendon sheaths, and footpads are often swollen because of accumulated fibrinosuppurative exudate. There may be exudative conjunctivitis and pharyngitis. Torticollis may result when the meninges, middle ear, or cranial bones are infected.

Lesions: Many of the lesions are related to vascular disturbances. Hyperemia is especially evident in the vessels of the abdominal viscera. Petechial and ecchymotic hemorrhages are common, particularly in subepicardial and subserosal locations. Increased amounts of peritoneal and pericardial fluids are frequently seen. The liver may be swollen and often develops multiple, small, necrotic foci.

Diagnosis: A presumptive diagnosis may be based on the characteristic signs and lesions and demonstration of gram-negative, bipolar organisms in blood and other tissues. A more conclusive diagnosis requires isolation and identification of *P multocida*.

Prevention: Good management practices are essential to prevention. Rodents, which are often carriers of *P multocida*, must be excluded from poultry houses. Adjuvant bacterins are widely used and generally effective; autogenous bacterins are recommended when polyvalent bacterins are found to be ineffective. Attenuated vaccines are available for administration in drinking water to turkeys and by wing-web inoculation to chickens. These live vaccines can effectively induce immunity against different serotypes of *P multocida*. They are recommended for use in healthy flocks only.

Treatment: Sulfonamides and antibiotics are commonly used; early treatment and adequate dosages are important. Sensitivity testing often aids in drug selection. Sulfaquinoxaline sodium in feed or water usually controls mortality, as do sulfamethazine and sulfadimethoxine. Sulfas should be used with caution in breeders because of potential toxicity. High levels of tetracycline antibiotics in the feed (0.04%), drinking water, or administered parenterally may be useful. Penicillin is often effective for sulfa-resistant infections.

GOOSE PARVOVIRUS INFECTION

(Derzsy's disease, Goose viral hepatitis)

Goose parvovirus infection is a highly contagious and fatal disease of goslings and Muscovy ducklings. Goose parvovirus has been reported from all the major goose-farming countries of Europe and the Far East where the disease is of serious economic significance. Muscovy ducks and several hybrid duck breeds are also susceptible to another parvovirus that has been shown to be antigenically related to goose parvovirus. The former has been isolated from an outbreak among Muscovy ducks in California, but goose parvovirus has not been detected in the USA.

Etiology: Goose parvovirus is a member of the family Parvoviridae and has recently been shown to be related to the human dependovirus genus. Apart from the Muscovy duck parvovirus, to which it is closely related, goose parvovirus shows no similarity to the other avian or mammalian parvoviruses. Following primary infection, the virus replicates in the intestinal wall and after a short viremic phase reaches the heart, liver, and other organs.

Transmission and Epidemiology: The virus is excreted in large amounts in the feces of infected birds, resulting in rapid spread by direct and indirect means. Outbreaks are often initiated in susceptible goslings following transmission of the virus via eggs laid by infected breeder geese. Evidence suggests that older subclinically infected geese may act as carriers. Infected eggs are often the source of the virus when outbreaks of goose parvovirus occur in countries or geographic locations formerly free of the disease. No other avian or biologic vectors have been identified.

Clinical Findings: In susceptible goslings and ducklings, clinical signs vary according to the age of the birds. The course of the disease in birds <1 wk old is rapid with anorexia and death occurring within 2-5 days. Mortality can reach 100% in birds that are infected in the hatchery. In older birds, the disease follows a more protracted course characterized by ocular and nasal discharge, a profuse white diarrhea, and weakness. The eyelids and uropygial glands are red and swollen. Birds surviving the acute stage show profound growth retardation with loss of feathers and reddening of the skin, particularly on the back. Birds may stand in a "penguin-like" posture due to accumulation of ascitic fluid in the abdomen. In 2- to 4-wk-old birds, mortality can reach 10%, but morbidity levels may be much higher. No clinical signs are seen in older birds, although adults will respond immunologically.

Lesions: Gross lesions include the presence of a fibrinous pseudomembrane covering the tongue and oral cavity, perihepatitis, pericarditis, pulmonary edema, liver dystrophy, and catarrhal enteritis. In acute cases, the heart is characteristically rounded at the apex with a pale myocardium. The main microscopic lesions are pronounced degenerative changes in the myocardial cells and the presence of Cowdry type-A intranuclear inclusion bodies.

Diagnosis: A presumptive diagnosis is based on the characteristic clinical course, age incidence, and gross and histologic lesions. Confirmation can be obtained following isolation of the parvovirus in cell cultures or embryonated eggs derived from susceptible geese and Muscovy ducks. Presence of the virus can be confirmed by electron microscopic examination of infected cultures and neutralization with specific goose parvovirus antiserum. Diagnosis can also be confirmed by direct detection of antigen or virus in tissues from infected birds, by immunofluorescence, or by the use of PCR. Serologic tests for goose parvovirus include virus neutralization, agar gel precipitation, and ELISA.

Although goose parvovirus causes disease in both geese and Muscovy ducks, recent studies have shown that Muscovy ducks are also infected with another antigenically related parvovirus. This virus causes serious disease in Muscovy ducklings but not in goslings and can be detected and differentiated using molecular methods. Differential diagnoses should also include duck viral enteritis (duck plague, *see* p 2208), which affects all types of waterfowl. Duck viral hepatitis (*see* p 2222) causes a fatal disease in ducklings but is not pathogenic for goslings or Muscovy ducklings. *Riemerella anatipestifer* and *P multocida* bacteria may also cause high mortality in goslings and Muscovy ducklings but can be differentiated by bacterial isolation and identification.

Prevention and Treatment: Goslings should be hatched together only from flocks that are known to be free of goose parvovirus, as many outbreaks are attributed to the practice of custom hatching eggs from various sources. Eggs should be imported only from countries that can guarantee freedom from goose parvovirus. Geese that have survived an outbreak should not be used for breeding purposes. Both live and inactivated oil emulsion vaccines are available and are widely used in countries where the disease is endemic. Vaccination of breeding flocks induces high levels of maternal antibody in the progeny.

HELMINTHIASIS

(Nematode and cestode infections)

About 100 worm species have been recognized in wild and domestic birds in the USA. Nematodes (roundworms) are the most significant in number of species and in economic impact. Of species found in commercial poultry, the common roundworm (*Ascaridia galli*) is by far the most common. Many field studies show that poultry maintained under free-range conditions may be heavily parasitized; therefore, control measures such as preventing infections or chemotherapy are likely to improve weight gain and egg production. In surveys of poultry raised under nonconfinement conditions throughout the world, an incidence of infection >80% is not uncommon.

Generally, nematodes have separate sexes that have morphologic differences; eg, males of *Tetrameres* spp are elongate and slender, while gravid females are globe-shaped. The size and shape of nematode species vary widely; ascarids are sturdy and long (up to 4.5 in. [116 mm]); capillarids are more delicate, slender, and long (2.3 in. [60 mm]); and other nematodes are much shorter (0.08-0.48 in. [2-12 mm]).

Cestodes (tapeworms) also vary in size. *Raillietina* spp may be >12 in. (30 cm), while *Davainea proglottina* often is <0.16 in. (4 mm). The proglottids of individual tapeworms are hermaphroditic. Tapeworms have been recovered in the thousands from individual chickens and turkeys.

See TABLE 5 for information on common nematodes and cestodes of poultry.

Transmission: Modern confinement rearing of poultry has significantly reduced the frequency and variety of these endoparasite infections, which were common earlier in range birds and in backyard flocks. However, severe parasitism still may occur in floor-reared layers, breeders, turkeys, or pen-reared game birds. Contributing factors may be the use of built-up litter (which fosters the propagation of intermediate hosts and the accumulation of infective eggs), and the resistance of the parasites to therapeutic drugs. Range infections of nematodes such as *Heterakis gallinarum* and *Syngamus trachea* may increase due to seasonal or climatic abundance of specific invertebrate hosts, eg, large numbers of earthworms brought to the surface by spring rains. Other species have been associated with large numbers of darkling beetles, which may act as mechanical vectors of infective eggs.

Nematodes have either a species-specific, direct life cycle with bird-to-bird transmission by ingestion of infective eggs or larvae, or an indirect cycle that requires an intermediate host (eg, insects, snails, or slugs). Eggs of many nematode species are resistant to low temperatures and disinfectants, but may be more susceptible to heat and desiccation.

The life cycle of *A galli* is simple and direct. Eggs in the droppings become infective in 10-12 days under optimal conditions. The infective eggs are ingested and hatch in the proventriculus, and the larvae live free in the lumen of the duodenum for the first 9 days. They then penetrate the mucosa, causing hemorrhages, return to the lumen by 17-18 days, and reach maturity at 28-30 days. Levels of infection are often underestimated, as early larval stages are barely visible and can remain for long periods within intestinal tissues, while adult stages in the lumen are generally fewer in number. Maturation of larval stages can be hampered by adult worm numbers, thereby increasing the time larval stages remain in intestinal tissues and continue to cause damage.

The life cycle of *H gallinarum* is similar to that of *A galli*. The greatest production of eggs for each egg ingested occurs in the ring-necked pheasant, followed by the guinea fowl and chicken. The larvae are closely associated with the cecal tissue, but a true tissue phase rarely occurs. Most of the adult worms are found at the blind end of the ceca.

TABLE 5. Common Helminths of Poultry ▶

Parasite	Host	Intermediate Host or Life Cycle	Organ Infected	Pathogenicity
Nematodes				
Amidostomum anseris	Duck, goose, pigeon	Direct	Gizzard	Severe
Ascaridia dissimilis	Turkey	Direct	Small intestine	Moderate
Ascaridia galli	Chicken, turkey, duck, quail	Direct	Small intestine	Moderate
Capillaria caudinflata (columbae)	Chicken, turkey, duck, game birds, pigeon	Earthworms	Small intestine	Moderate to severe
Capillaria contorta (annulata)	Chicken, turkey, duck, game birds	None or earthworms	Mouth, esophagus, crop	Severe
Capillaria obsignata	Chicken, turkey, goose, pigeon, quail	Direct	Small intestine, ceca	Severe
Cheilospirura hamulosa	Chicken, turkey, game birds	Grasshoppers, beetles	Gizzard	Moderate
Cyathostoma bronchialis	Turkey, duck	Direct or earthworm	Trachea	Severe
Cyrnea colini	Turkey, game birds	Cockroaches	Proventriculus	Mild
Dispharynx nasuta	Chicken, turkey, game birds, pigeon	Sowbugs	Proventriculus	Moderate to severe
Gongylonema ingluvicola	Chicken, game birds	Beetles, cockroaches	Crop, esophagus, proventriculus	Mild
Heterakis gallinarum	Chicken, turkey, duck, game birds	Direct	Ceca	Mild, but transmits agent of histomoniasis
Heterakis isolonche	Quail, duck, pheasant	Direct	Ceca	Severe

Earthworms may ingest the eggs of the cecal worm and serve as a source of infection when ingested by poultry.

The life cycle of *Capillaria* may be direct (*C obsignata*), require an intermediate host such as earthworms (*C caudinflata*), or be either direct or use earthworms (*C contorta*). Larval development in the egg takes 8-15 days depending on temperature. Worms reach maturity in 20-26 days after ingestion by the final host.

The gapeworm *Syngamus trachea* inhabits the trachea and lungs of many domestic and various wild birds. Infection may occur directly by ingestion of infective eggs or larvae; however, severe field infection is associated with ingestion of transport hosts

◀ **TABLE 5.** *(continued)*

Parasite	Host	Intermediate Host or Life Cycle	Organ Infected	Pathogenicity
Ornitho-strongylus quadriradiatus	Pigeon, dove	Direct	Small intestine	Severe
Oxyspirura mansoni	Chicken, turkey, guinea fowl, quail	Cockroaches	Eye	Moderate
Strongyloides avium	Chicken, turkey, quail, goose	Direct	Ceca	Moderate
Subulura brumpti	Chicken, turkey, duck, game birds	Earwigs, grasshoppers, beetles, cockroaches	Ceca	Mild
Syngamus trachea	Chicken, turkey, pheasant, quail	None or earthworm	Trachea	Severe
Tetrameres americana	Chicken, turkey, duck, game birds, pigeon	Grasshoppers, cockroaches	Proventriculus	Moderate to severe
Tricho-strongylus tenuis	Chicken, turkey, duck, game birds, pigeon	Direct	Ceca	Severe
Cestodes				
Choanotaenia infundibulum	Chicken	House flies	Upper intestine	Moderate
Davainea proglottina	Chicken	Slugs, snails	Duodenum	Severe
Metroliasthes lucida	Turkey	Grasshoppers	Intestine	Unknown
Raillietina cesticillus	Chicken	Beetles	Duodenum, jejunum	Mild
Raillietina echinobothrida	Chicken	Ants	Lower intestine	Severe, nodules
Raillietina tetragona	Chicken	Ants	Lower intestine	Severe

such as earthworms, snails, slugs, and arthropods (eg, flies). Many gapeworm larvae may encyst and survive within a single invertebrate for years. Although gapeworms are not a problem in confinement-reared poultry, they cause serious economic losses in game-farm pens and in range-reared chickens, pheasants, turkeys, and peacocks. *Cyatho-stoma bronchialis* is the gapeworm of geese and ducks.

Eggs of *Oxyspirura mansoni*, Manson's eyeworm, are deposited in the eye, reach the pharynx via the nasolacrimal duct, are swallowed, passed in the feces, and ingested by the Surinam cockroach, *Pycnoscelus surinamensis*. Larvae reach the infective stage in the roach.

When infected intermediate hosts are eaten, liberated larvae migrate up the esophagus to the mouth and then through the nasolacrimal duct to the eye, where the cycle is completed.

Cestodes require an intermediate host (eg, insects, crustaceans, earthworms, or snails). Floor layers, breeders, and broilers are infected with *Raillietina cesticillus* by ingestion of the intermediate host, small beetles that breed in contaminated litter. Cage layers in unscreened houses may become infected with *Choanotaenia infundibulum* by eating its intermediate host, the house fly.

Over 3,000 of the microscopic tapeworm *D proglottina* have been recovered from a single bird. Several species of slugs and snails serve as intermediate hosts, and >1,500 infective parasites have been recovered from a single slug.

Pathogenesis and Clinical Findings: *Ascaridia, Heterakis*, and *Capillaria* spp are widely distributed and cause such nonspecific signs as general unthriftiness, inactivity, depressed appetite, and retarded growth; death may result. A mere few ascarids may depress weight, and larger numbers may block the intestinal tract. Ascarids may migrate up the oviduct (via the cloaca) to become enshelled later within the egg (an aesthetic, but not a public health problem, avoidable by careful egg-candling before the release of eggs to market). *A dissimilis* (turkey roundworm) may also migrate out of the intestine, through the portal system, and into the liver causing hepatic granulomas.

H gallinarum, a mild pathogen, in large numbers may cause thickening, inflammation, or nodulation in the cecal walls. Infection with *H gallinarum* has been associated with cecal and hepatic granulomas. *Heterakis isolonche*, highly pathogenic in pheasants, may cause 50% mortality. *H gallinarum* carries *Histomonas meleagridis*, the protozoa that causes blackhead (p 2238).

C contorta in the mucosae of the crop and esophagus, and *C obsignata* in the wall of the small intestine, cause marked thickening and inflammation of the organs. Birds harboring large numbers of these threadlike worms become weak and emaciated and may die.

Young birds are the most severely affected by gapeworms. Sudden death and verminous pneumonia characterize early outbreaks. Signs of gasping, choking, shaking of the head, inanition, emaciation, and suffocation may follow. Necropsy reveals adult gapeworms obstructing the lumina of the trachea, bronchi, and lungs. Respiratory inflammation may be present. The blood-red, female gapeworm is usually found in copulation with a much smaller, paler male with its head embedded deep in the host tissue. The joined pair have a "Y"-shaped or forked appearance.

O mansoni is a slender nematode, 12-18 mm, found beneath the nictitating membrane of chickens and other fowl in tropical and subtropical regions. The parasite causes various degrees of inflammation, lacrimation, corneal opacity, and disturbed vision.

Among other nematodes, *Amidostomum anseris* attacks the gizzard lining of ducks and geese and causes dark discoloration, necrosis, and sloughing at the parasitic loci. *Dispharynx nasuta* causes ulceration, thickening, and maceration of the proventriculus; heavily infected birds may die. *Tetrameres americana*, a bright red worm discernible through the proventricular wall, causes diarrhea, emaciation, and with heavy infection, death. *Trichostrongylus tenuis* causes inflamed ceca, weight loss, anemia, and death, especially in young birds. *Ornithostrongylus quadriradiatus*, a blood-sucking parasite, causes pigeons to regurgitate bile-stained fluid mixed with food; greenish mucoid diarrhea from hemorrhagic intestines, emaciation, and death follow.

Most pathogenic tapeworms are found in the small intestine; the scolex, usually buried in the mucosa, generally causes mild lesions. *Davainea proglottina* may cause weight loss. *Raillietina tetragona* causes weight loss and decreased egg production; *R echinobothrida* produces granulomas at its attachment sites ("nodular disease").

Diagnosis: A reliable diagnosis can be made only by accurate identification of the individually recovered parasites; careful and complete necropsy techniques are essential. Only by specific recognition of the parasite can meaningful recommendations be made on flock therapy and management.

Treatment and Control: Improvement of sanitary practices and application of approved insecticides to soil and litter when premises are unoccupied may interrupt the life cycle of the parasite by destroying its intermediate host. When the premises are re-stocked, groups of birds of different species or ages should be widely separated to avoid spread of parasites. Approved compounds are very limited in the USA. Because of frequently changing regulations, the status of any medication should be checked prior to its administration. Approved drugs for the USA are listed in the FDA's Green Book and in the commercially available Feed Compendium. The Green Book and current updates are available online at http://www.fda.gov/cvm/greenbook/greenbook.html.

Only approved drugs may be used in birds producing eggs or meat for the commercial market. Label directions and recommended doses should be followed precisely, with scrupulous adherence to withdrawal times.

Piperazine compounds are relatively nontoxic and widely used against ascariasis. Several piperazine salts are available internationally. Because only the piperazine moiety is efficacious, doses should be calculated based on mg of active piperazine/bird. Pipera-zine should be completely consumed by birds within a few hours because only relatively high concentrations of the drug eliminate worms. It may be given to chickens as a single dose, 50-100 mg/bird, or at 0.2-0.4% in the feed or at 0.1-0.2% in the drinking water; it may be administered to turkeys at 100 mg/bird <12 wk old, 100-400 mg/bird ≥12 wk old, or in feed or water concentrations as for chickens. Some practitioners recommend the addi-tion of molasses to unmedicated water after piperazine administration, so as to induce an osmotic flushing, theoretically removing any of the remaining worms from the intesti-nal tract. The medications must also be withdrawn in turkeys 14 days prior to slaughter. There is increasing evidence of significant piperazine resistance in the USA.

Fenbendazole is approved in the USA for use in growing turkeys at the rate of 14.5 g/ton of feed (16 ppm), fed continuously as the sole ration for 6 days for the removal of *A dissimilis* and *Heterakis gallinarum.*

Phenothiazine controls cecal worms in chickens at 0.5 g/bird, in turkeys at 1 g/bird, given in 1 day. Combined in drinking water, as a 1-day treatment, phenothiazine (0.5-0.56%) and piperazine (0.11%) treat heterakids and ascarids.

Thiabendazole at 0.05% in the feed continuously for 2 wk can eliminate gapeworms from pheasants, and when given continuously for ≥4 days is said to help prevent and control infections.

Hygromycin B, 0.00088-0.00132% in feed is used to control ascarids, cecal worms, and capillarids. Coumaphos, 0.004% in feed for 10-14 days for replacements, or 0.003% in feed for 14 days for layers, has been commonly used against capillarids.

As a treatment for Manson's eyeworm, a local anesthetic can be applied to the eye, and the worms in the lacrimal sac exposed by lifting the nictitating membrane. A 5% cresol solution (1-2 drops) placed in the lacrimal sac kills the worms immediately. The eye should be irrigated with sterile water immediately to wash out the debris and excess solution. The eyes improve within 48-72 hr and gradually become clear if the destructive process caused by the parasite is not too far advanced.

Several compounds are reported to be effective against nematode infections but are not currently approved for use in the USA. In chickens, *A galli, H gallinarum,* and *C obsignata* were removed by tetramisole at 40 mg/kg. Pyrantel tartrate was highly effec-tive against *A galli* and somewhat effective against *Capillaria.* Levamisole at a level of 25-30 mg/kg appears to be effective against *A dissimilis, H gallinarum,* and *C obsig-nata;* it can also be given in the drinking water at 30-60 ppm. Injection SC of 1 mL of 10% methyridine in the pectoral region or leg of pigeons removed *Capillaria,* but the drug must be handled with care as contact with skin may produce lesions. Coumaphos re-moves *Capillaria* in quail. Haloxon at 25 and 50 mg/kg, or at 750 ppm in the feed for 5-7 days, has good activity against *Capillaria* in chickens and quail.

Fenbendazole at 20 mg/kg for 3-4 days is effective for removing gapeworms in pheas-ants. Tetramisole at 3.6 mg/kg for 3 consecutive days in the drinking water removes gapeworms. Poultry treated while larvae are migrating in the body develop immunity to gapeworms, even though therapy may abort larval migration. Levamisole fed at a level of 40 ppm for 2 days or at 2 g/gal. drinking water for 1 day each month has proved to be an effective control in game birds. Mebendazole fed prophylactically at 64 ppm or curatively at 125 ppm is effective in turkey poults. Cambendazole provided control when given in 3 treatments of 50 mg/kg for chickens and 20 mg/kg for turkeys.

There have been some reports of experimental drug treatment for other nematodes. Cambendazole (60 mg/kg), pyrantel (100 mg/kg), citrin (40 mg/kg), mebendazole (10 mg/kg for 3 days), and fenbendazole have been reported to be effective against *Amidostomum anseris*. *Trichostrongylus tenuis* is controlled by cambendazole (30 mg/kg), pyrantel (50 mg/kg), thiabendazole (75 mg/kg), mebendazole (10 mg/kg for 3 days), and citrin (40 mg/kg). At recommended levels for chickens, mebendazole has some reported effect against *Dispharynx nasuta*, tetramisole against *Subulura brumpti* and *Strongyloides avium*, and piperazine against *Tetrameres*.

Poultry producers wanting to treat for tapeworms should be aware that expulsion of the parasite will be a short-term remedy if the scolex is not removed or if the intermediate host is not eliminated as a source of reinfection. Butynorate in combination with piperazine and phenothiazine as a feed additive or individual tablets has shown some efficacy. Other promising experimental drugs include chlorophene and niclosamide. None is approved in the USA.

HEMORRHAGIC ENTERITIS OF TURKEYS AND MARBLE SPLEEN DISEASE OF PHEASANTS

Hemorrhagic enteritis is an acute GI disorder affecting young turkeys. In its most severe form, it is characterized by depression, bloody droppings, and substantial mortality. Marble spleen disease is an acute respiratory disease of pheasants characterized by depression, enlarged mottled spleens, pulmonary congestion, and death. Both diseases are caused by similar viruses. Species-specific differences in clinical response are thought to be related to differences in the target organs for anaphylaxis and variation in viral pathotype. Infection with less virulent pathotypes in either host may often go undetected until secondary bacterial infections begin to develop as a result of viral-induced immunosuppression.

Etiology and Epidemiology: The etiologic agent is a nonenveloped, icosahedral DNA virus, 70-90 nm in diameter. It is a member of the family Adenoviridae and has recently been assigned to the new genus *Siadenovirus*. Based on differences in clinical presentation within host species, numerous viral pathotypes appear to exist. These differ slightly at the DNA level but are indistinguishable serologically.

Both hemorrhagic enteritis and marble spleen disease are geographically widespread and considered endemic in areas where turkeys and pheasants are raised commercially. The usual route of infection is oral, and virus is often introduced onto previously uninfected premises via personnel or equipment contaminated with infectious feces. Turkey poults and pheasants <4 wk of age are resistant to infection due to age-related resistance or, more commonly, the presence of maternal antibody. The virus may survive under moist conditions (ie, in litter) well beyond the refractory period. As infection begins to cycle through a flock, large quantities of virus are shed in the feces, which facilitates rapid spread through susceptible birds. Morbidity usually approaches 100% for both hemorrhagic enteritis and marble spleen disease.

Clinical Findings: In commercial operations, hemorrhagic enteritis typically affects turkeys 6-12 wk of age. In outbreaks involving highly virulent pathotypes, clinical signs can include depression, pallor, and bloody droppings. Acute mortality ranges from <1% to 60% with an average of 10-15% over a 2-wk period. Birds that survive the acute phase experience a transient immunosuppression related to the lymphotrophic, lymphocytopathic nature of the virus. This often manifests itself in the form of secondary bacterial infections, eg, colibacillosis, p 600) ~10-14 days after initial exposure to the virus. Thus, a second peak in mortality, potentially overlapping the first, may be seen and, in less virulent outbreaks, may actually dominate the clinical picture. The second wave of mortality often lasts 2-4 wk and is characterized by lesions commonly associated with bacterial respiratory disease or septicemia, eg, fibrinopurulent pneumonia, airsacculitis, pericarditis, peritonitis, perihepatitis, hepatomegaly, and splenomegaly. Concomitant or prior exposure to Newcastle disease virus (p 2255), *Bordetella avium* (p 2300), or *Mycoplasma* spp (p 2242) is known to exacerbate the problem. Similar multiple agent interactions have been implicated in mortality associated with the use of vaccines for hemorrhagic enteritis.

Marble spleen disease typically affects pheasants 3-8 mo of age. Onset is acute, with dyspnea, asphyxiation, and sudden death occurring as a result of pulmonary congestion and edema. Mortality is commonly 2-3% but can reach 15%. Secondary bacterial infections as a result of immunosuppression have also been noted.

Lesions: Necropsy of moribund or dead birds infected with hemorrhagic enteritis virus reveals gross congestion and intraluminal hemorrhage in the proximal small intestine. The spleen is usually enlarged, friable, and mottled, except in birds that have hemorrhaged extensively. Histopathologic changes in the duodenum include congestion, hemorrhage, and necrosis of the intestinal epithelium. This lesion in particular is thought to be the result of a virally induced, cytokine-mediated anaphylactic reaction, with the GI tract being considered the target shock organ in the turkey. Basophilic intranuclear inclusions can be found in lymphocytes and macrophages in a variety of tissues but predominantly in the spleen where lymphoreticular hyperplasia and lymphoid necrosis are noted.

On histopathologic evaluation of pheasants with marble spleen disease, flooding of the atria and tertiary bronchi with fibrin and RBC, as well as generalized vascular congestion and focal necrosis, are often seen in the lung. As with hemorrhagic enteritis, this response may be anaphylactic in nature, with the lung being considered the target shock organ in the pheasant. Splenomegaly with lymphoreticular hyperplasia and lymphoid necrosis also occur and are the characteristic lesions for which marble spleen disease is named. Basophilic intranuclear inclusions may be found in a variety of tissues excluding the GI tract with the highest concentration of virus again being found in the spleen.

Diagnosis: Diagnosis of virulent outbreaks of hemorrhagic enteritis or marble spleen disease can often be made based on clinical signs and gross lesions. Confirmation is by histopathology and the presence of seroprecipitating virus in the spleen as determined by agar gel immunodiffusion. PCR techniques to detect hemorrhagic enteritis viral DNA in tissue have also been described and are in regular use in select laboratories. To determine whether hemorrhagic enteritis or marble spleen disease is a predisposing factor in cases of bacterial respiratory disease or septicemia, or to verify a primary diagnosis, acute and convalescent sera (3 wk apart) can be tested using either agar gel immunodiffusion or ELISA. In turkeys, differential diagnoses include colibacillosis, pasteurellosis, paratyphoid, and erysipelas. Reticuloendotheliosis or lymphoproliferative disease should be considered when lymphoreticular hyperplasia is the predominant lesion. GI lesions without splenic involvement should evoke consideration of other viral, bacterial, parasitic, and toxic enteritides of turkeys. In pheasants with acute respiratory disease, differential diagnoses include Newcastle disease, avian influenza, and in the case of birds reared in confinement, gaseous toxins.

Treatment, Control, and Prevention: Virulent outbreaks of hemorrhagic enteritis have been successfully treated and controlled by SC injection of exposed birds with 0.5-1.0 mL of antiserum obtained from recovered flocks. It is presumed that a similar approach may be effective for pheasants. In anticipation of secondary bacterial complications, antibiotics may be used, but if possible, an informed choice should be made based on current antibiotic susceptibility profiles for locally obtained *Escherichia coli* isolates. In addition to good biosecurity, prevention hinges on the use of vaccines administered in the water at ~4-5 wk of age. Commercially available tissue culture products and crude splenic preparations containing avirulent isolates produce lifelong protection. Vaccines intended for use in turkeys should not be used in pheasants, and vice versa, because the avirulent isolates used for vaccinating one species are typically virulent in the other. Due to potential for interaction with other agents, including live vaccines, regular disease monitoring and careful integration of hemorrhagic enteritis and marble spleen disease vaccines into flock vaccination protocols is encouraged. Intuitively, vaccines should not be administered to birds exhibiting signs of illness or within 2 wk of any other vaccination.

HISTOMONIASIS

(Blackhead, Infectious enterohepatitis)

Histomoniasis is caused by a protozoan that infects the ceca, and later the liver, of turkeys, chickens, and occasionally other galliform birds. In turkeys, most infections are fatal; in other birds, mortality is less common.

Etiology: The protozoan parasite *Histomonas meleagridis* is transmitted most often in embryonated eggs of the cecal nematode *Heterakis gallinarum*, and sometimes directly by contact with infected birds. Outbreaks spread quickly through flocks by direct contact. A large percentage of chickens harbor this worm, and histomonads have been located in adult worms of both sexes. Three species of earthworms can harbor *H gallinarum* larvae containing *H meleagridis*, which are infective to both chickens and turkeys. *H meleagridis* survives for long periods within *Heterakis* eggs, which are resistant and may remain viable in the soil for years. Histomonads are released from *Heterakis* larvae in the ceca a few days after entry of the nematode and replicate rapidly in cecal tissues. The parasites migrate into the submucosa and muscularis mucosae and cause extensive and severe necrosis. Histomonads reach the liver either by the vascular system or via the peritoneal cavity, and rounded necrotic lesions quickly appear on the liver surface. Histomonads interact with other gut organisms, such as bacteria and coccidia, and depend on these for full virulence.

Traditionally, histomoniasis has been thought of as affecting turkeys, while doing little damage to chickens. However, outbreaks in chickens may cause high morbidity, moderate mortality, and extensive culling. Liver lesions tend to be less severe in chickens, but morbidity can be especially high in young layer or breeder pullets. Tissue responses to infection may resolve in 4 wk, but birds may be carriers for another 6 wk.

Clinical Findings: Signs are apparent 7-12 days after infection and include listlessness, drooping wings, unkempt feathers, and yellow droppings. The origin of the name "blackhead" is obscure. Young birds have a more acute disease and die within a few days after signs appear. Older birds may be sick for some time and become emaciated before death.

Lesions: The primary lesions are in the ceca, which exhibit marked inflammatory changes and ulcerations, causing a thickening of the cecal wall. Occasionally these ulcers erode the cecal wall, leading to peritonitis and involvement of other organs. The ceca contain a yellowish green, caseous exudate or, in later stages, a dry, cheesy core. Liver lesions are highly variable in appearance; in turkeys, they may be up to 4 cm in diameter and involve the entire organ. The liver and cecal lesions together are pathognomonic. However, the liver lesions must be differentiated from those of tuberculosis, leukosis, avian trichomoniasis, and mycosis. In some cases, especially in chickens, histopathologic examination is helpful. Histomonads are intercellular, although they may be so closely packed as to appear intracellular. The nuclei are much smaller than those of the host cells, and the cytoplasm less vacuolated. Scrapings from the liver lesions or ceca may be placed in isotonic saline solution for direct microscopic examination; *Histomonas* spp must be differentiated from other cecal flagellates.

Prevention and Treatment: Because healthy chickens often carry infected cecal worms, any contact between chickens and turkeys should be avoided. Grouse and quail also may carry the infection to turkey yards. Because *H gallinarum* ova can survive in soil for many months or years, turkeys should not be put on ground contaminated by chickens. Once established in a flock, infection spreads rapidly without the use of a carrier.

The only drug used for the control (prophylaxis) of histomoniasis in the USA is nitarsone at 0.01875% of feed until 5 days before marketing. There is no effective treatment available commercially. Nitroimidazoles such as ronidazole, ipronidazole, and dimetridazole are effective for treatment or prevention but are not available in the USA. Frequent worming of flocks with benzimidazole anthelminthics helps reduce exposure to heterakid worms that carry the infection.

INFECTIOUS BURSAL DISEASE

(Gumboro disease)

Etiology and Transmission: Infectious bursal disease is caused by a birnavirus (IBDV) that is most readily isolated from the bursa of Fabricius but may be isolated from other organs. It is shed in the feces and transferred from house to house by fomites. It is very stable and difficult to eradicate from premises.

IBDV may be isolated in 8- to 11-day-old, antibody-free chicken embryos with inocula from birds in the early stages of disease. The chorioallantoic membrane is more sensitive to inoculation than is the allantoic sac. IBDV also may be isolated in cell cultures derived from the cloacal bursa and established cell lines, and some strains may be isolated in chicken-embryo fibroblasts. Cell-culture-adapted strains of IBDV produce a cytopathic effect and may be used for quantitative serologic tests. Two serotypes of IBDV have been identified; within them, antigenic variation between strains is considerable. Serotype 2 infects chickens and turkeys but does not cause clinical disease or immunosuppression.

"Variant" strains of IBDV, which have major antigenic differences from the "standard" strains, cause immunosuppression but not clinical disease in older chickens.

Clinical Findings: Infectious bursal disease is highly contagious; results of infection depend on age and breed of chicken and virulence of the virus. Infections may be subclinical or clinical. Infections before 3 wk of age are usually subclinical. Chickens are most susceptible to clinical disease at 3-6 wk, but severe infections have occurred in Leghorn chickens up to 18 wk old.

Early **subclinical infections** are the most important form of the disease because of economic losses. They cause severe, long-lasting immunosuppression due to destruction of immature lymphocytes in the bursa of Fabricius, thymus, and spleen. The humoral (B cell) immune response is most severely affected; the cell-mediated (T cell) immune response is affected to a lesser extent. Chickens immunosuppressed by early IBDV infections do not respond well to vaccination and are predisposed to infections with normally nonpathogenic viruses and bacteria. Common diseases are usually exacerbated by IBDV infections. Subclinical infections by the "variant" strains occur in immature birds, and severe longterm immunosuppression and bursal atrophy result from early infections.

In **clinical infections**, onset of the disease is sudden after an incubation of 3-4 days. Chickens exhibit severe prostration, incoordination, watery diarrhea, soiled vent feathers, vent picking, and inflammation of the cloaca. Losses range to >20%. Recovery occurs in <1 wk, and broiler weight gain is delayed by 3-5 days. The presence of maternal antibody will modify the clinical course of the disease. Virulence of field strains of the virus varies considerably. Very virulent (vv) strains of the virus that cause high mortality and morbidity were detected first in Europe. These spread throughout the Old World in the last decade and in 1999 were in South America. The vv strains have not been detected in the USA.

Lesions: At necropsy, the cloacal bursa is swollen, edematous, yellowish, and occasionally hemorrhagic, especially in birds that have died of the disease. Congestion and hemorrhage of the pectoral, thigh, and leg muscles is common. Chickens recovered from IBDV infections have small, atrophied, cloacal bursas due to the destruction and lack of regeneration of the bursal follicles.

Control: There is no treatment. Depopulation and rigorous disinfection of contaminated farms have achieved limited success. Live vaccines of chick-embryo or cell-culture origin and of varying virulence can be administered by eye drop, drinking water, or SC routes at 1-21 days of age. The immune response can be altered by maternal antibody, and the more virulent vaccine strains can override higher levels of antibody.

High levels of maternal antibody during early brooding of chicks in broiler flocks (and in some commercial layer operations) can minimize early infection, subsequent immunosuppression, or both. Breeder flocks should be vaccinated one or more times during the growing period, first with a live vaccine and again just before egg production with an oil-adjuvanted, inactivated vaccine. Inactivated vaccines of chick-embryo, bursa, or cell-culture origin are available. The latter vaccines induce higher, more uniform, and more persistent levels of antibody than do live vaccines. The immune status of breeder flocks should be monitored periodically with a quantitative serologic test such as virus neutralization or ELISA. If antibody levels fall, hens should be revaccinated to maintain adequate immunity in the progeny.

LISTERIOSIS

Listeriosis is quite rare in birds and usually occurs as a septicemia or sometimes as a localized encephalitis. Encephalitis combined with septicemia has been seen in young geese. Chickens, turkeys, geese, ducks, canaries, and parrots appear to be the most commonly affected avian species.

In workers at poultry-processing plants, conjunctivitis due to *Listeria monocytogenes* has been linked to handling of apparently normal but infected chickens. Human infections have also resulted from consumption of contaminated poultry or poultry products. Abortions and congenitally infected babies have been associated with handling of *L monocytogenes*-positive birds or those that have died with the disease, but these cases were not confirmed.

Etiology and Epidemiology: *L monocytogenes* is a gram-positive, coccoid to bacillus-shaped, nonsporeforming bacteria that tends to form long filaments, particularly in older cultures. Based on somatic and flagellar antigens, several serotypes have been described. *L monocytogenes* can be cultured on blood and tryptose agar or brain-heart infusion. It is widely distributed among avian species. The organism is common in feces and soil, with numbers increasing in late winter and early spring. It has been isolated from apparently normal birds and from birds dying of causes other than uncomplicated listeriosis; therefore, it is possible that carrier birds play an important role in the perpetuation of the disease in birds and mammals. It is commonly associated with concurrent diseases such as coccidiosis, infectious coryza, salmonellosis, and parasitic infections demonstrating the largely opportunistic character of the organism.

Clinical Findings: Young birds appear to be more susceptible than mature ones. Transmission and subsequent infections occur by ingestion of contaminated nasal secretions, feces, and soil. Infection can also occur via inhalation and wound contamination. In most avian species, the incubation period has not been documented; in turkeys, it is 16 hr to 52 days. Frequently, *L monocytogenes* infections are subclinical. Chickens and turkeys are relatively resistant to natural infection. However, signs of infection are suggestive of a septicemia and include depression, listlessness, and peracute death. In this form, it is common to find only dead birds. In the subacute and chronic forms, signs are related to encephalitis and include torticollis, stupor, paresis, and paralysis. Adult birds may die suddenly with septicemia, while young birds tend to have chronic infections. Emaciation and diarrhea are seen in some affected birds.

Lesions: In uncomplicated listeriosis, lesions include multiple areas of degeneration and necrosis of the myocardium with congestion, increased pericardial fluid, and pericarditis. Petechial hemorrhages can be seen in the proventriculus and heart. Splenomegaly and hepatomegaly with bile retention and focal areas of necrosis are common. In the encephalitic form, no gross brain lesions are seen; microscopically, however, gliosis in the cerebellum with microabscesses containing gram-positive bacteria are present in the midbrain and medulla.

Diagnosis: Listeriosis can be suspected based on the history, clinical signs, necropsy lesions, and microscopic observation of the bacteria in the myocardial fibrils, hepatocytes, or both. The diagnosis can be confirmed by isolation from the blood, liver, heart, spleen, or brain of a gram-positive, nonacid-fast, nonsporeforming bacillus that is catalase-positive, motile, aerobic, and that ferments sugars. Isolation by direct culture of the affected tissues may not be successful because of low concentration of organisms in the tissues; however, recovery increases significantly if a portion of the specimen is refrigerated for 4-8 wk and subcultured weekly. Chick embryos are readily infected and can be used for organism identification.

Differential diagnoses include colibacillosis, pasteurellosis, erysipelas, velogenic viscerotropic Newcastle disease, and many other acute and chronic bacterial diseases.

Treatment and Control: The organism is often resistant to many of the commonly used antibiotics. However, the tetracyclines have been efficacious in both the acute and subacute forms when given at 25 mg/kg, PO, SID for 1 wk. Treatment of the chronic form is usually unsuccessful. Widespread use of antimicrobials in the feed for growth promotion may have prophylactic value. Rigid sanitation and disinfection procedures with culling and isolation of affected birds may be helpful. Prevention should focus on identifying and eliminating the source of infection.

MALABSORPTION SYNDROME

(Runting-stunting syndrome, Pale bird syndrome)

Malabsorption syndrome is characterized by stunted growth and a lack of skin pigmentation in growing chickens, most commonly meat type or broilers. It has been identified in virtually all countries in which intensive poultry production occurs.

Etiology and Transmission: Mycotoxins and several viruses, including enteroviruses, parvoviruses, astroviruses, caliciviruses, arenaviruses, and reoviruses have been implicated. Although the etiology is believed to be complex, only mycotoxins, enteroviruses, and reoviruses have thus far been identified as potential etiologic factors. The specific feedborne mycotoxins involved and concentration needed to induce the syndrome are not well understood. Numerous enteric viruses are prevalent worldwide in commercially produced poultry. Transmission of viruses occurs via fecal-oral routes.

Clinical Findings: The disease is typically recognized in broiler chicks 1-3 wk old. It is characterized by stunted growth; lack of pigmentation in the skin, feet, or beak; slow feathering; broken or twisted feathers; undigested feed in the feces; and/or poor feed conversion ratios. Diarrhea is common during the initial phases. Severely affected birds do not respond immediately to changes in feed or management practices and are usually culled from flocks before processing.

Lesions: The severity and type of lesions resulting from both field and laboratory infections vary with the particular agents or combinations of agents involved. Lesions often include enlarged proventriculi, small gizzards, and orange mucus in the small-intestinal lumen. No consistent microscopic lesions are found. Encephalomalacia or rickets may be seen occasionally, presumably as a result of malabsorption or malassimilation of nutrients.

Diagnosis: Clinical signs and lesions permit a presumptive diagnosis, although a similar gross appearance can be caused by a retrovirus (*see* RETICULOENDOTHELIOSIS, p 2253). More conclusive diagnostic evidence includes finding either viruses in the lesions or dietary toxins.

Prevention and Control: There is no effective treatment for severely affected birds. Sanitation and disinfection will reduce the burden of challenge caused by multiple infectious organisms. There are no vaccines that will prevent malabsorption syndrome. Reovirus vaccines can prevent the stunting and poor feed conversions that occur with pathogenic reovirus infections. Feeds should be analyzed for dietary toxins, and high levels of toxins should not knowingly be fed to commercial poultry.

MYCOPLASMOSIS

Several *Mycoplasma* spp have been isolated from avian hosts; *M gallisepticum*, *M iowae*, *M meleagridis*, and *M synoviae* are the most important. Mycoplasmas are fastidious bacteria, 0.3-0.8 μm in diameter; they lack a cell wall and require a rich growth medium containing serum. They do not survive for more than a few days outside the host and are vulnerable to common disinfectants. Each has distinctive epidemiologic and pathologic characteristics.

MYCOPLASMA GALLISEPTICUM INFECTION
(PPLO infection, Chronic respiratory disease, Infectious sinusitis)

M gallisepticum infection is commonly designated as chronic respiratory disease in chickens and as infectious sinusitis in turkeys. Infection may also be seen in pheasants, chukar partridges, and peafowl. Infection in pigeons, quail, ducks, geese, and psittacine birds should be considered. Passerine-type birds are quite resistant, although *M gallisepticum* is the major cause of natural outbreaks of conjunctivitis in wild house finches (*Carpodacus mexicanus*) in the eastern USA. The disease is worldwide. Its effects are most severe in large commercial operations during winter.

M gallisepticum is the most pathogenic avian mycoplasma; however, strains may differ markedly in virulence. Primary isolation is made in enriched broth medium containing 10-15% serum, then plated on agar. Typical colonies are identified by immunofluorescence.

Transmission, Epidemiology, and Pathogenesis: In the USA, most breeder flocks are free of *M gallisepticum*, and outbreaks are due to lateral transmission from infected chickens; however, in some parts of the world, egg transmission is a major source of infection. The incidence of egg transmission is highly variable, ranging up to 30-40% during the first 2 mo after infection of susceptible birds in production. The transmission rate then lessens and is inconsistent (0-5%) until the end of production. Birds infected before the onset of production transmit through the egg at a much lower rate, if at all. The infection may be dormant in the infected chick for days to months, but when the flock is stressed, aerosol transmission occurs rapidly and infection spreads through the flock. Live virus vaccination, natural virus infection, cold weather, or crowding may initiate the spread. In addition, the infection may be carried by personnel (especially from an infected to a clean flock), fomites, or introduction of infected birds. In many flocks, the source of infection cannot be determined.

The epithelium of the upper air passages is most susceptible to infection; however, in severe, acute disease the infection is also found in the lower respiratory tract. There is a marked interaction between respiratory viruses, *Escherichia coli*, and *M gallisepticum* in the pathogenesis of chronic respiratory disease. Once infected, birds remain carriers for life.

Clinical Findings: In chickens, infection may be inapparent or result in varying degrees of respiratory distress, with slight to marked rales, difficulty breathing, coughing, and/or sneezing. Morbidity is high and mortality low in uncomplicated cases. Nasal discharge and frothiness about the eyes may be present. In turkeys, the disease is generally more severe than in chickens, and swelling of the paranasal sinus is common. Feed efficiency and weight gains are reduced. Broilers and market turkeys may suffer high condemnations at processing due to airsacculitis. In laying flocks, birds may fail to reach peak egg production, and the overall production rate is lower than normal.

Lesions: Uncomplicated *M gallisepticum* infections in chickens result in relatively mild sinusitis, tracheitis, and airsacculitis. *E coli* infections are often concurrent and result in severe air sac thickening and turbidity, with exudative accumulations, fibrinopurulent pericarditis, and perihepatitis, particularly in broilers. Turkeys develop severe mucopurulent sinusitis and varying degrees of tracheitis and airsacculitis. The mucous membranes are thickened, hyperplastic, necrotic, and infiltrated with inflammatory cells. Lymphofollicular areas are found in the submucosa.

Diagnosis: Agglutination reactions and ELISA are commonly used for diagnosis. *M gallisepticum* should be confirmed by isolation and identification, PCR, or hemagglutination-inhibition because nonspecific false agglutination reactions are common, especially after the inoculation of inactivated, oil-emulsion vaccines or *M synoviae* infection. Isolates must be identified, because birds may also be infected with nonpathogenic *Mycoplasma* spp. PCR is commonly used to rapidly detect the organism in upper respiratory tissues. Newcastle disease, infectious bronchitis, influenza, and other respiratory pathogens should be considered in the differential diagnosis.

Treatment and Control: In the field, many cases of *M gallisepticum* infection are complicated by other pathogenic bacteria; thus, effective treatment must also attack the secondary invader. Most strains of *M gallisepticum* are sensitive to a number of antibiotics, such as chlortetracycline, erythromycin, oxytetracycline, spectinomycin, tiamulin, tylosin, or a fluoroquinolone such as enrofloxacin. Antibiotic is usually given in the feed or water for 5-7 days; however, in turkeys, antibiotic may be given initially by injection, followed by feed or water medication. Antibiotics may alleviate the clinical signs and lesions but do not eliminate infection.

Eradication of *M gallisepticum* from chicken and turkey breeding stock is well advanced in the USA and several other countries. The most effective control program is to identify breeders without serum agglutination or ELISA titers and to maintain seronegative stock. In valuable breeding stock, treatment of eggs, usually with tylosin or heat, may be used to eliminate egg transmission to progeny. Medication is not a good long-term control method but is of value in treating individual infected flocks.

The use of birds free of *M gallisepticum* is desirable, but infection in multiple-age commercial egg farms where depopulation is not feasible is a problem. An inactivated, oil-emulsion bacterin is available in most countries; it prevents egg production losses but not infection. A live vaccine has been licensed in the USA for use in infected, multiple-age layer flocks but may be used only with permission of the state veterinarian. The vaccine consists of a mild strain of *M gallisepticum* (F-strain) and is usually given at ~10-14 wk of age. F-strain is of low pathogenicity for chickens but is fully virulent for turkeys. Vaccinated birds remain carriers, and immunity lasts through the laying season. Recently, 2 nonpathogenic live vaccine strains (6/85 and ts-11) have been introduced; these strains offer the advantage of improved safety and are in widespread use in commercial layers.

MYCOPLASMA IOWAE INFECTION

M iowae was originally thought to be of low pathogenicity in producing air sac lesions in chickens and turkeys, but it is a potentially important cause of reduced hatchability in turkeys. Antigenicity and pathogenicity vary considerably among *M iowae* strains. *M iowae* is resistant to 1% bile salts, and an enriched medium similar to those used for other avian mycoplasmas is suitable.

Infection was common in turkey flocks in Europe and North America, but the infection rate has now been reduced by intensive eradication efforts in breeding stocks. It is a relatively uncommon infection of chickens. *M iowae* is egg transmitted, but little is known of other aspects of its epidemiology.

Many strains of *M iowae* are lethal to turkey embryos. After experimental inoculation of young poults, stunting, poor feathering, and various skeletal deformities such as tenosynovitis and chondrodystrophy develop, but the mechanism is unknown. These effects have not been recognized in the field, probably because most infected birds die before hatching. Older birds appear to be quite resistant.

Clinical Findings, Lesions, and Diagnosis: Affected turkey breeder flocks show no clinical signs other than reduced hatchability (usually 2-5%). In many flocks, the hatchability returns to normal after 1-2 mo.

Most embryos die during the mid to late stages of incubation. Dead turkey embryos are edematous, congested, and stunted; they may have clubbed down. Poults challenged in ovo or at 1 day of age may develop various skeletal deformities such as rotated tibia, deviated toes, chondrodystrophy, or erosion of the articular cartilage of the hock joint. Feathers may also be poorly developed. Chicks challenged at 1 day of age may develop tenosynovitis and ruptured tendons.

Turkeys apparently have a poor antibody response, and no reliable serologic test is available. Diagnosis relies on isolation and identification of the causative agent.

Treatment and Control: The best method of control is to maintain flocks free of *M iowae*; however, because serology is unreliable, this may be difficult. Dipping hatching eggs in solutions of enrofloxacin has significantly reduced losses in hatchability.

MYCOPLASMA MELEAGRIDIS INFECTION

M meleagridis infection is a widespread, egg-transmitted disease of turkeys found worldwide. The primary lesion in the progeny is airsacculitis. *M meleagridis* is thought to be a specific pathogen for turkeys, and the organism is commonly found in the respiratory and reproductive tracts. It has been eradicated in most basic breeder and many commercial flocks.

M meleagridis was recognized as a pathogen of turkeys after widespread elimination of the bacteria from breeding stock.

Transmission and Pathogenesis: Infection is established primarily through egg transmission, which can be as high as 30-50% or higher early in the production cycle. However, transmission of *M meleagridis* is also related to genital contact. Early infections usually become quiescent at sexual maturity. In the tom, the phallus and adjacent tissues are infected and contaminate semen, thus infecting the vagina of the hen. Hens may retain infection in the bursa of Fabricius, which serves as a source of infection of the reproductive tract after rupture of the cloacal-vaginal occluding membrane at puberty. Infection ascends the reproductive system and may reach the surface of the ovary. The high rate of egg transmission of *M meleagridis* is from infection of the reproductive tract being incorporated into the egg after ovulation. Infection of the respiratory tract leads to transmission among birds in young flocks and may be a factor in the spread to flocks previously free of infection. Hatchery transmission is also possible.

The marked difference in the pathogenicity of various strains of *M meleagridis* results in variable clinical manifestations. The high incidence of air sac infection in poults suggests a symbiotic host-parasite relationship. *M meleagridis* may be involved in crooked necks and leg deformities, but the pathogenesis of this syndrome is not clear. The vaginas of naturally infected hens are free of infection 1-3 mo after the source of infection is removed. Immunity is not permanent, and hens can be reinfected with contaminated semen.

Clinical Findings: Embryo infection appears to reduce hatchability, poult quality, and growth rate. Superimposed stress may cause considerable mortality in poults during the first few weeks. Infection during early rapid growth of hock joints, periarticular tissues, cervical vertebrae, and adjacent bone may produce major bone deformities such as crooked necks and hocks. Rales may develop in poults 3-8 wk old and persist for several weeks without significant mortality or serious interference with growth.

Lesions: Day-old poults have thoracic airsacculitis with thickening, turbidity, and marked caseous exudate. In 1-3 wk, the lesions may extend to the abdominal air sacs. These lesions recede with age. The air sac lesions of roaster and mature birds are probably related to other factors. Tracheitis may be present, but sinusitis does not occur.

Microscopic lesions in hens consist of lymphocytic foci in the fimbria, uterus, and vagina. In young poults, inflammatory lesions are seen in the air sacs and lungs.

Diagnosis: A high incidence of air sac lesions in day-old poults suggests *M meleagridis* infection. The serum plate agglutination or ELISA test may be used. Confirmation is generally by hemagglutination-inhibition, isolation and identification of the organism, or both. *M gallisepticum*, chlamydiae, bacteria, and respiratory viruses such as influenza must be eliminated as causes of air sac infection.

Treatment and Control: The commercial use of flocks free of *M meleagridis* should be monitored by serology and/or by examining pipped embryos or cull poults for airsacculitis. Semen used for insemination must be free of *M meleagridis*. Dipping eggs in tylosin or another suitable antibiotic reduces the incidence of transmission in infected flocks and may improve weight gains and feed conversion ratios. Inoculation SC of a suitable antibiotic at 1 day of age or water medication for the first 5-10 days appears to reduce airsacculitis caused by *M meleagridis* and may improve weight gain.

MYCOPLASMA SYNOVIAE INFECTION
(Infectious synovitis)

M synoviae was first recognized as an acute to chronic infection of chickens and turkeys that produced an exudative tendinitis and bursitis; it now occurs most frequently as a subclinical infection of the upper respiratory tract. *M synoviae* infection is also a complication of airsacculitis in association with Newcastle disease or infectious bronchitis. It is seen primarily in chickens and turkeys, but ducks, geese, guinea fowl, parrots, pheasants, and quail may also be susceptible. Serum (preferably swine serum) and nicotinamide adenine dinucleotide are required for growth on artificial media.

Transmission, Epidemiology, and Pathogenesis: *M synoviae* is egg-transmitted, but the rate is low (probably <5%), and some hatches of progeny may be free of infection. Egg transmission is greatest during the first 1-2 mo after infection of susceptible breeders. Lateral transmission is similar to that of *M gallisepticum*, but the rate of spread is generally more rapid.

M synoviae isolates vary widely in pathogenicity. Isolates from cases of airsacculitis are more apt to produce air sac lesions than isolates from synovial fluid or membranes. Some strains produce the typical clinical disease of synovitis. The paucity of natural outbreaks of clinical synovitis in chickens in recent years may be related to the adaptation of *M synoviae* to the respiratory tract; however, clinical synovitis in turkeys is relatively common.

Clinical Findings: Although slight rales may be present in birds with respiratory infection, usually no signs are noticed. Younger birds, especially those under stress or suffering concurrent infections, are more likely to be affected. Outbreaks of infectious synovitis occur most commonly in chickens at 4-6 wk and in turkeys at 10-12 wk. Lame birds tend to sit. The more severely affected birds are depressed and are found around the feeders and waterers. Swellings of the hocks and footpads are seen. Morbidity is 2-15%, and mortality 1-10%. The effect on egg production is minimal, but instances of egg production losses have occurred.

Lesions: In the respiratory syndrome, airsacculitis occurs when the bird is stressed from Newcastle disease, infectious bronchitis, or improper ventilation. In many cases, air sac lesions resolve after 1-2 wk. Early in synovitis, the liver is enlarged and sometimes green. The spleen is enlarged, and the kidneys are enlarged and pale. A yellow to gray, viscid exudate is present in almost all synovial structures; it is most commonly seen in the keel bursa, hock, and wing joints. In chronic cases, this exudate may become inspissated and orange.

Diagnosis: A presumptive diagnosis can be based on the lesions and clinical signs, but laboratory confirmation is necessary. Skeletal abnormalities must be eliminated as the cause of lameness. The disease must be differentiated from viral tenosynovitis and from staphylococcal and other bacterial infections.

The serum plate agglutination or ELISA test is used to detect infected flocks, but cross-reactions with *M gallisepticum* and other nonspecific reactions may occur. Reactors are confirmed as positive by hemagglutination-inhibition or by isolation and identification of the organism. PCR may be used to rapidly detect the organism in infected tissues. In turkeys, the agglutination test for *M synoviae* may not be reliable.

Treatment and Control: Serologic testing and isolation similar to those for *M gallisepticum* have resulted in eradication of the infection in most primary breeder flocks of chickens and turkeys. Administration of a tetracycline antibiotic in the feed may be beneficial in treatment or prevention of synovitis. When airsacculitis is a problem, preventive antibiotic therapy during the time of respiratory reaction to Newcastle disease and infectious bronchitis vaccine may be helpful. Medication of breeder flocks is of little value in preventing egg transmission.

MYCOTOXICOSES

A mycotoxicosis is a disease caused by a toxin produced by a fungus. In poultry, this usually results when fungi grow in grains and feeds. Hundreds of mycotoxins have been identified and many are pathogenic. Mycotoxins may have additive or even synergistic effects with other mycotoxins, infectious agents, and nutritional deficiencies. Many are chemically stable and maintain toxicity over time. (*See also* MYCOTOXICOSES, p 2408.)

The significance of mycotoxin problems in poultry is probably considerable but yet insidious. The impact on poultry production may be best measured indirectly by the improvements in weight gain, feed efficiency, pigmentation, egg production, and reproductive performance that accompany effective control programs for mycotoxins.

Aflatoxicosis: The aflatoxins are toxic and carcinogenic metabolites of *Aspergillus flavus, A parasiticus,* and others. Aflatoxicosis in poultry primarily affects the liver, but can involve immunologic, digestive, and hematopoietic functions. It affects weight gain, feed intake, feed conversion efficiency, pigmentation, processing yield, egg production, male and female fertility, and hatchability. Some effects are directly attributable to toxins, while others are indirect, such as reduced feed intake. Susceptibility to aflatoxins varies, but in general, ducklings, turkeys, and pheasants are susceptible, while chickens, Japanese quail, and guinea fowl are relatively resistant.

Clinical signs vary from general unthriftiness to high morbidity and mortality. At necropsy, the lesions are found mainly in the liver, which can be reddened due to necrosis and congestion or yellow due to lipid accumulation. Hemorrhages may also occur. In chronic aflatoxicosis, the liver becomes yellow to gray and atrophied. The aflatoxins are carcinogenic, but tumor formation is rare with the natural disease, probably because the animals do not live long enough for this to occur.

Fusariotoxicosis: The genus *Fusarium* produces many mycotoxins injurious to poultry. The trichothecene mycotoxins produce caustic and radiomimetic patterns of disease exemplified by T-2 toxin and diacetoxyscirpenol (DAS). Deoxynivalenol (vomitoxin, DON) and zearalenone are common trichothecene mycotoxins that are relatively nontoxic for poultry, but may cause disease in pigs.

Fusariotoxicosis in poultry caused by the trichothecenes results in feed refusal, caustic injury to the oral mucosa and areas of the skin in contact with the mold, acute digestive disease, and injury to the bone marrow and immune system. Lesions include necrosis and ulceration of the oral mucosa, reddening of the GI mucosa, mottling of the liver, atrophy of the spleen and other lymphoid organs, and visceral hemorrhages. In laying hens, egg production decreases, accompanied by depression, recumbency, feed refusal, and cyanosis of the comb and wattles. Ducks and geese develop necrosis and pseudomembranous inflammation of the esophagus, proventriculus, and gizzard.

Other *Fusarium* mycotoxins cause defective growth of long bones. The fumonisin mycotoxins produced by *F moniliforme* impair feed conversion without causing specific lesions. Moniliformin is also produced by *F moniliforme* and is cardiotoxic and nephrotoxic in poultry. *F moniliforme* causes ear rot, kernel rot, and stalk rot of unharvested corn and is found in stored high-moisture shelled corn, and on other grains that appear sound.

Ochratoxicosis: Ochratoxins are among the mycotoxins most toxic to poultry. These nephrotoxic metabolites are produced chiefly by *Penicillium viridicatum* and *Aspergillus ochraceus* in grains and feed. Ochratoxicosis causes primarily renal disease but also affects the liver, immune system, and bone marrow. Severe intoxication causes reduced spontaneous activity, huddling, hypothermia, diarrhea, rapid weight loss, and death. Moderate intoxication impairs weight gain, feed conversion, pigmentation, carcass yield, egg production, fertility, and hatchability.

Ergotism: Toxic ergot alkaloids are produced by *Claviceps* spp, which are fungi that attack cereal grains. Rye is especially affected, but also wheat and other leading cereal grains. The mycotoxins form in the sclerotium, a visible, hard, dark mass of mycelium that displaces the grain tissue. Within the sclerotium are the ergot alkaloids, which affect the nervous system, causing convulsive and sensory neurologic disorders; the vascular system, causing vasoconstriction and gangrene of the extremities; and the endocrine system, influencing the neuroendocrine control of the anterior pituitary.

In chicks, the toes become discolored due to vasoconstriction and ischemia. In older birds, vasoconstriction affects the comb, wattles, face, and eyelids, which become atrophied and disfigured. Vesicles and ulcers develop on the shanks of the legs and on the tops and sides of the toes. In laying hens, feed consumption and egg production are reduced.

Citrinin Mycotoxicosis: Citrinin is produced by *Penicillium* and *Aspergillus* and is a natural contaminant of corn, rice, and other cereal grains. Citrinin causes a diuresis that results in watery fecal droppings and reductions in weight gain. At necropsy, lesions involve chiefly the kidney. Citrinin acts directly on the kidney to transiently alter tubular transport processes.

Oosporein Mycotoxicosis: Oosporein is a mycotoxin produced by *Chaetomium* spp that causes gout and high mortality in poultry. *Chaetomium* spp are found on feeds and grains, including peanuts, rice, and corn. Oosporein mycotoxicosis is seen as visceral and articular gout related to impaired renal function and elevated plasma concentrations of uric acid. Chickens are more sensitive to oosporein than turkeys. Water consumption increases during intoxication, and fecal droppings become unformed and fluid.

Cyclopiazonic Acid: This is a metabolite of *Aspergillus flavus*, which is the predominant producer of aflatoxin in feeds and grains. In chickens, cyclopiazonic acid causes impaired feed conversion, decreased weight gain, and mortality. Lesions develop in the proventriculus, gizzard, liver, and spleen. The proventriculus is dilated and the mucosa is thickened and sometimes ulcerated.

Sterigmatocystin: This biogenic precursor to aflatoxin is hepatotoxic and hepatocarcinogenic but is less common than aflatoxin.

Diagnosis: Mycotoxicosis should be suspected when the history, signs, and lesions are suggestive of feed intoxication. Toxin exposure associated with consumption of a new batch of feed may result in subclinical or transient disease. Chronic or intermittent exposure can occur in regions where grain and feed ingredients are of poor quality, and feed storage is substandard or prolonged. Impaired production can be an important clue to a mycotoxin problem, as can improvement due to correction of feed management deficiencies.

Definitive diagnosis involves detection and quantitation of the specific toxin(s). This can be difficult because of the rapid and voluminous use of feed and ingredients in poultry operations. Diagnostic laboratories differ in the capability to conduct screening and confirmation tests for the different mycotoxins and should be contacted before sending samples. Feed and also birds that are sick or recently dead should be submitted. A complete diagnostic evaluation including necropsy, histopathology, bacterial and viral cultures, and serology should accompany feed analysis if mycotoxicosis is suspected. Other diseases that occur concurrently with mycotoxins can adversely affect production and should be considered. A flock rarely has a single disease. Sometimes, a mycotoxicosis is suspected but not confirmed by feed analysis. In these situations, a complete laboratory evaluation can exclude other significant diseases.

Feed and ingredient samples should be properly collected and promptly submitted for analysis. Mycotoxin formation can be localized in a batch of feed or grain. Multiple samples taken from different sites increase the likelihood of confirming a mycotoxin formation zone (hot spot).

Samples should be collected at sites of ingredient storage, feed manufacture and transport, feed bins, and feeders. Fungal activity increases as feed is moved from the feed mill to the feeder pans. Samples of 500 g (1 lb) should be collected and submitted in separate containers. Clean paper bags, properly labeled, are adequate. Sealed plastic or glass containers are appropriate only for short-term storage and transport, because feed and grain rapidly deteriorate in airtight containers.

Treatment: The toxic feed should be removed and replaced with unadulterated feed. Concurrent diseases should be treated to alleviate disease interactions, and substandard management practices must be corrected. Some mycotoxins increase requirements for vitamins, trace minerals (especially selenium), protein, and lipids, and can be compensated for by feed supplementation and water-based treatment. Nonspecific toxicologic therapies using activated charcoal (digestive tract adsorption) in the feed have a sparing effect but are not practical for larger production units.

Prevention: The focus should be on using feed and ingredients free of mycotoxins and on management practices that prevent mold growth and mycotoxin formation during feed transport and storage. Regular inspection of feed mills and feeding systems can identify flow problems, which allow residual feed and enhance fungal activity and mycotoxin formation. Mycotoxins can form in decayed, crusted feed in feeders, feed mills, and storage bins; appropriate cleaning can be immediately beneficial. Temperature extremes cause moisture condensation and migration in bins and promote mycotoxin formation.

Ventilation of poultry houses to avoid high relative humidity also decreases the moisture available for fungal growth and toxin formation in the feed. Pelleting of feed also reduces moisture. Antifungal agents added to feeds to prevent fungal growth have no effect on toxin already formed but may be cost-effective in conjunction with other feed management practices. Organic acids (propionic acid, 500-1,500 ppm [0.5-1.5 g/kg]) are effective inhibitors, but the effectiveness may be reduced by the particle size of feed ingredients and the buffering effect of certain ingredients. Sorbent compounds such as hydrated sodium calcium aluminosilicate (HSCAS) are effective in binding and preventing absorption of aflatoxin. Esterified-glucomannan, a cell wall derivative of *Saccharomyces cerevisiae*, is protective against aflatoxin B_1 and ochratoxin and has moderate binding activity for fumonisins, zearalenone, and T-2 toxin.

NEOPLASMS

Depending on whether the etiologic agent is known, neoplasms of poultry are divided into 2 categories: virus-induced neoplasms and neoplasms of unknown etiology. There are 3 economically important virus-induced neoplastic diseases of poultry: Marek's disease, caused by a herpesvirus, and avian leukosis/sarcoma and reticuloendotheliosis, caused by retroviruses.

A rare neoplastic disease of turkeys known as lymphoproliferative disease that has been reported in Europe and Israel is induced by yet another retrovirus distinct from both the leukosis/sarcoma and reticuloendotheliosis viruses. The incidence of lymphoproliferative disease of turkeys has always been sporadic and is not discussed in this chapter.

Neoplasms of unknown etiology are classified according to their morphologic characteristics; they include a wide variety of benign and malignant neoplasms. Of these tumors, dermal squamous cell carcinoma, multicentric histiocytosis, and adenocarcinoma are the most commonly seen in the field.

MAREK'S DISEASE

Chickens are the most important natural host for Marek's disease virus, a highly cell-associated but readily transmitted alphaherpesvirus with lymphotropic properties of gammaherpesviruses. Quail can be naturally infected and turkeys can be infected experimentally. However, severe clinical outbreaks of Marek's disease in commercial turkey flocks, with mortality from tumors reaching 40-80% between 8-17 wk of age, were reported recently in France, Israel, and Germany. In some of these cases, the affected turkey flocks were raised in proximity to broilers. Turkeys are also commonly infected with turkey herpesvirus, an avirulent strain related to Marek's disease virus. Other birds and mammals appear to be refractory to the disease or infection.

Marek's disease is one of the most ubiquitous avian infections; it is identified in chicken flocks worldwide. Every flock, except for those maintained under strict pathogen-free conditions, may be presumed to be infected. Although clinical disease is not always apparent in infected flocks, a subclinical decrease in growth rate and egg production may be economically important.

Etiology: Three serotypes of the cell-associated herpesvirus are recognized. Serotypes 1 and 2 designate virulent and avirulent chicken isolates, respectively; serotype 3 designates the related avirulent turkey herpesvirus. Serotypes 2 and 3, as well as attenuated serotype 1 viruses, have been used as vaccines. Serotypes are identified by reaction with type-specific monoclonal antibodies or by biological characteristics such as host range, pathogenicity, growth rate, and plaque morphology. Currently, virulent serotype 1 strains are further divided into pathotypes, which are often referred to as mild (m), virulent (v), very virulent (vv), and very virulent plus (vv+) Marek's disease virus strains.

Transmission and Epidemiology: The disease is highly contagious and readily transmitted among chickens. The virus matures into a fully infective, enveloped form in the epithelium of the feather follicle, from which it is released into the environment. It may survive for months in poultry house litter or dust. Dust or dander from infected chickens is particularly effective in transmission. Once the virus is introduced into a chicken flock, regardless of vaccination status, infection spreads quickly from bird to bird. Infected chickens continue to be carriers for long periods and act as sources of infectious virus. Shedding of infectious virus can be reduced, but not prevented, by prior vaccination. Unlike serotypes 1 and 2, which are highly contagious, turkey herpesvirus is not readily transmissible among chickens (although it is easily transmitted among turkeys, its natural host). Attenuated serotype 1 strains vary greatly in their transmissibility among chickens; the most highly attenuated are not transmitted. Marek's disease virus is not vertically transmitted. The incidence of Marek's disease is quite variable in commercial flocks and depends on strain and dose of virus, age at exposure, maternal antibody, host gender and genetics, other concurrent diseases, and several environmental factors including stress.

Pathogenesis: Currently, 4 arbitrary phases of infection in vivo are recognized: 1) early productive-restrictive virus infection causing primarily degenerative changes, 2) latent infection, 3) a second phase of cytolytic, productive-restrictive infection coincident with permanent immunosuppression, and 4) a proliferative phase involving nonproductively infected lymphoid cells that may or may not progress to the point of lymphoma formation. Productive infection may occur transiently in B lymphocytes within a few days after infection with virulent serotype 1 strains and is characterized by antigen production, which leads to cell death. Productive infection also occurs in the feather follicle epithelium, in which enveloped virions are produced. Latent infection of activated T cells is responsible for the longterm carrier state. No antigens are expressed, but virus can be recovered from lymphocytes by co-cultivation with susceptible cells in tissue cultures. Some T cells, latently infected with oncogenic serotype 1 strains, undergo neoplastic transformation. These transformed cells, provided they escape the immune system of the host, may multiply to form characteristic lymphoid neoplasms. Cell-mediated and humoral immune responses are both directed against viral antigens, with cell-mediated immunity probably being the most important.

Clinical Findings and Lesions: Typically, affected birds show only depression before death, although emaciation may be noted. A transient paralysis syndrome (unilateral leg paresis) has been associated with Marek's disease, causing a characteristic posture of one leg held forward and the other held backward as lesions progress. Chickens become ataxic for periods of several days and then recover. This syndrome is rare in immunized birds.

Enlarged nerves are one of the most consistent gross lesions in affected birds. Various peripheral nerves, but particularly the vagus, brachial, and sciatic, become enlarged and lose their striations. Diffuse or nodular lymphoid tumors may be seen in various organs, particularly the liver, spleen, gonads, heart, lung, kidney, muscle, and proventriculus. Lymphoid infiltrates may expand the iris muscle and distort the shape of the pupil. Enlarged feather follicles (commonly termed skin leukosis) may be noted in broilers after defeathering during processing and are a cause for condemnation. The bursa is only rarely tumorous and more frequently is atrophic. Histologically, the lesions consist of a mixed population of small, medium, and large lymphoid cells plus plasma cells and large anaplastic lymphoblasts. These cell populations undoubtedly include both tumor cells and reactive inflammatory cells. When the bursa is involved, the tumor cells typically appear in interfollicular areas.

Diagnosis: Usually, diagnosis is based on enlarged nerves and lymphoid tumors in various viscera. The rareness of bursal tumors helps distinguish this disease from lymphoid leukosis (*see* p 2251); also, Marek's disease can develop in chickens as young as 3 wk of age, whereas lymphoid leukosis typically is seen in chickens >14 wk of age. Reticuloendotheliosis, although rare, can easily be confused with Marek's disease because both diseases feature enlarged nerves and T-cell lymphomas in visceral organs. A diagnosis based on typical gross lesions may be confirmed histologically, or better, by demonstration of predominant T-cell populations and Marek's viral DNA in lymphomas by histochemistry and PCR, respectively. Furthermore, Marek's disease lymphomas will usually lack evidence of clonally integrated avian retroviruses or alteration of the cellular oncogene *c-myc*.

Control: Vaccination is the central strategy for the prevention and control of Marek's disease. The efficacy of vaccines can be improved, however, by strict sanitation to reduce or delay exposure and by breeding for genetic resistance. Probably the most widely used vaccine consists of turkey herpesvirus. Bivalent vaccines consisting of turkey herpesvirus and either the SB-1 or 301B/1 strains of serotype 2 Marek's disease virus have been used to provide additional protection against challenge with virulent serotype 1 isolates. Several attenuated serotype 1 Marek's disease vaccines are also available; of these, the CV1988/Rispens strains appears particularly effective. A synergistic effect on protection, noted mainly between serotype 2 and 3 strains, has prompted the empirical use of other virus mixtures. Because vaccines are administered at hatching and require 1-2 wk to produce an effective immunity, exposure of chickens to virus should be minimized during the first few days after hatching. Vaccines are also effective when administered to embryos at the 18th day of incubation. In ovo vaccination is now performed by automated technology and is widely used for vaccination of commercial broiler chickens, mainly because of reduced labor costs and greater precision of vaccine administration. Proper handling of vaccine during thawing and reconstitution is crucial to ensure that adequate doses are administered. Cell-associated vaccines are generally more effective than cell-free vaccines because they are neutralized less by maternal antibodies. Under typical conditions, vaccine efficacy is usually >90%. Since the advent of vaccination, losses from Marek's disease have been reduced dramatically in broiler and layer flocks. However, disease may become a serious problem in individual flocks or in selected geographic areas (eg, the Delmarva broiler industry). Of the many causes proposed for these excessive losses, early exposure to very virulent virus strains appears to be among the most important. Using fowlpox virus and herpesvirus of turkeys as vectors, experimental recombinant vaccines have been shown to be effective against challenge with virulent Marek's disease virus.

LEUKOSIS/SARCOMA GROUP

Under natural conditions, lymphoid leukosis has been the most common form of the leukosis/sarcoma group of diseases seen in chicken flocks, although recently myeloid leukosis has become prevalent. Members of the leukosis/sarcoma group of avian retroviruses, including avian leukosis viruses, that were formerly placed in a subgenus termed avian type C oncornaviruses have recently been termed alpharetroviruses. Members of this group of viruses have similar physical and molecular characteristics and share a common group-specific antigen.

Avian leukosis occurs naturally only in chickens. Experimentally, some of the viruses of the leukosis/sarcoma group can infect and produce tumors in other species of birds or even mammals. The infection is known to exist in virtually all chicken flocks except for some SPF flocks from which it has been eradicated. The frequency of infection has been reduced substantially in the primary breeding stocks of several commercial poultry breeding companies. In recent years this control program has expanded, and infection has become infrequent or absent in certain commercial flocks. The frequency of avian leukosis tumors even in heavily infected flocks is typically low (<4%), and disease is often inapparent. Up to 1.5% excess mortality per wk has been reported in commercial broiler-breeder flocks naturally infected with subgroup J avian leukosis virus.

Etiology: Avian leukosis is caused by certain members of the leukosis/sarcoma group of avian retroviruses. These viruses are commonly called avian leukosis viruses and belong to subgroups A, B, C, D, E, and J. Subgroups A and B have been most prevalent in western countries, until the emergence of subgroup J. Since the initial isolation of subgroup J virus in England, the virus has been isolated from broiler-breeder stocks experiencing myeloid neoplasms (myelocytoma) in many other countries. Subgroup E avian leukosis viruses are endogenous viruses produced by viral genes integrated into the host cell DNA and are only rarely oncogenic. The subgroups have distinct antigenicities and cellular host ranges that are determined by viral envelope glycoproteins. Some antigenic variation, demonstrated by cross-neutralization, also occurs within subgroups. All field strains of avian leukosis virus are oncogenic, although some differences in oncogenicity and replicative ability have been recognized.

Transmission and Epidemiology: Chickens are the natural hosts for all viruses of the leukosis/sarcoma group; these viruses have not been isolated from other avian species except pheasants, partridges, and quail. Avian leukosis virus is shed by the hen into the albumen or yolk, or both; infection probably occurs after the onset of incubation. Congenitally infected chickens fail to produce neutralizing antibodies and usually remain viremic for life. Horizontal infection after hatching is also important, especially when chicks are exposed immediately after hatching to high doses of virus, eg, in feces of congenitally infected chicks or in contaminated vaccines. Horizontally infected chickens have a transient viremia followed by antibody production. The earlier the infection, the more likely it is to lead to tolerance, persistent viremia, and tumors. Other factors known to increase the susceptibility of chickens to horizontal infection include the absence of maternal antibodies and the presence of endogenous retroviruses, especially those associated with the late feathering (K) gene. Tumors are more frequent in congenital than in horizontal infections, but many more chickens are exposed horizontally than congenitally. Rates of embryo transmission typically are 1-10%; virtually all chicks in an infected flock are exposed by contact. Congenital and, in some cases, early horizontal infection can induce permanent carrier states characterized by shedding of virus or antigen into the environment and into eggs. Late infection (ie, inoculation at 12-20 wk of age) is unlikely to lead to virus shedding. The virus is not highly contagious compared with other viral agents and is readily inactivated by disinfectants. Transmission can be reduced or eliminated by strict sanitation. After the infection is eradicated, standard disease control and sanitation practices can keep chicken flocks free of the disease. The role of males in transmission of avian leukosis virus is uncertain. Infected cocks apparently do not influence the rate of congenital infection of progeny. Cocks may act only as virus carriers and sources of contact or venereal infection to other birds.

Pathogenesis: Lymphoid leukosis is a clonal malignancy of the bursal-dependent lymphoid system. Transformation invariably occurs in the intact bursa, often as early as 4-8 wk after infection. These tumors require 14-16 wk to develop. Death rarely occurs before 14 wk of age and is more frequent around the time of sexual maturity. The disease can be prevented, even up to 5 mo of age, by treatments that destroy the bursa. The tumors are composed almost entirely of B lymphocytes that, in many instances, have IgM on their surfaces. No antitumor immune response has been recognized. Antibodies are readily induced after infection, except when tolerance occurs.

The induction of lymphoid leukosis tumors can be enhanced in chickens coinfected with serotype 2 Marek's disease virus, a common vaccine virus. This enhancement requires a genetically susceptible chicken and early infection with lymphoid leukosis virus in addition to serotype 2 Marek's disease vaccination. Because most commercial chicken strains are resistant, and lymphoid leukosis virus infection has been largely eradicated from susceptible stocks, enhancement is not currently recognized as a field problem.

A subclinical disease syndrome characterized by depressed egg production in the absence of tumor formation is more important economically than mortality from lymphoid leukosis. Chickens with subclinical disease usually shed virus or viral antigen into the albumen of eggs. The pathogenic mechanisms are poorly understood.

Myeloid leukosis is a malignancy of myeloid precursors arising from the bone marrow. Its pathogenesis is not well understood.

Clinical Findings and Lesions: Chickens with lymphoid leukosis show nonspecific clinical signs including inappetence, weakness, diarrhea, dehydration, and emaciation. Infected chickens become depressed before death. Palpation often reveals an enlarged bursa and sometimes an enlarged liver. Infected birds may not necessarily develop tumors, but they may lay fewer eggs.

Diffuse or nodular lymphoid tumors are common in the liver, spleen, and bursa, and are found occasionally in the kidneys, gonads, and mesentery. Involvement of the bursa has been considered virtually pathognomonic, although bursal lymphomas are now known to also be induced by reticuloendotheliosis virus. Sometimes the bursal tumors are small and observed only after careful examination of the mucosal surface of the organ. Usually, no enlargement of peripheral nerves is apparent, although such lesions have been noted after experimental inoculation of subgroup J virus. Microscopically, the tumor cells are uniform, large lymphocytes. Mitotic figures are frequent.

Outbreaks of neoplasms other than lymphoid leukosis such as myelocytomas, hemangiomas, and renal tumors have also been noted in meat-type chickens infected with subgroup J avian leukosis virus. Myelocytomatosis and skeletal myelocytomas may cause protuberances on the head, thorax, and shanks. Myelocytomas may develop in the orbit of the eye, causing hemorrhage and blindness. Hemangiomas may be seen in the skin, appearing as "blood blisters," which may rupture causing hemorrhage. Renal tumors may cause paralysis due to pressure on the sciatic nerve. Microscopically, especially in cases of myelocytomas induced by subgroup J avian leukosis virus, the liver shows a massive intravascular and extravascular accumulation of myelocytes characterized by the presence of cytoplasmic eosinophilic granules.

Most strains of leukosis/sarcoma viruses also induce nonlymphoid tumors (including sarcomas), erythroblastosis, myeloblastosis, myelocytomas, hemangiomas, nephroblastomas, osteopetrosis, and related neoplasms. The nature of the tumors and their frequency depend on virus and chicken strain, age, dose, and route of infection. Occasional outbreaks of predominantly one type of tumor are seen in the field. The Rous sarcoma virus, a member of this group, has been widely studied in the laboratory. Each strain usually causes a predominantly neoplastic disease and can be distinguished on the basis of pathogenicity. Some viruses (eg, Rous sarcoma and erythroblastosis viruses) contain a viral oncogene that leads to neoplasm induction within a short incubation period, but such viruses are rare in the field. Viruses with a viral oncogene are often defective for replication and require the presence of a nondefective helper virus to replicate.

Diagnosis: Because avian leukosis virus is widespread among chickens, virus isolation and the demonstration of antigen or antibody have limited or no value in diagnosing field cases of lymphomas. Gross characteristics of diagnostic significance include the tumorous involvement of the liver, spleen, or bursa in the absence of peripheral nerve lesions. Tumors occur in birds >14 wk old. In lymphoid leukosis, the lymphoid cells are histologically uniform in character, large, and contain IgM and B-cell markers on their surface. Tumors can be differentiated from those of Marek's disease by gross and microscopic pathology (although this can be difficult in practice) and by molecular techniques that demonstrate the characteristic clonal integration of proviral DNA into the tumor cell genome with the associated disruption of the *c-myc* oncogene. Lymphoid leukosis cannot easily be differentiated from B-cell lymphomas caused by reticuloendotheliosis virus except by virologic assays; however, such tumors probably are extremely rare. ELISA kits for detection of antibodies to avian leukosis virus subgroups A, B, and J are available commercially.

Control: Lymphoid leukosis appears to be controlled best by reduction and eventual eradication of the causative virus. Breeder flocks are evaluated for viral shedding by testing for viral antigens in the albumen of eggs with enzyme immunoassays or by biologic assays for infectious virus. Eggs from shedder hens are discarded, so that progeny flocks typically have reduced levels of infection. If raised in small groups, infection-free flocks can be derived with relative ease. These control measures are applied only to primary breeder flocks. Voluntary programs to reduce viral infection have already reduced mortality from lymphoid leukosis and improved egg production in most layer strains; similar programs are underway in certain meat strains. Some breeders favor, and have virtually achieved, total eradication, while others favor a reduced level of viral infection. Some chickens have specific genetic resistance to infection with certain subgroups of virus. Although genetic cellular resistance will unlikely replace the need for reduction or eradication of the virus, the cellular receptor gene has been cloned, and quick molecular assays for viral susceptibility could be developed. Thus far, vaccination for tumor prevention has not been promising. However, recombinant vaccines lacking infectious avian leukosis virus can induce antibodies in breeders to ensure protective maternal antibodies in progeny chicks and may be an attractive adjunct to eradication programs.

RETICULOENDOTHELIOSIS

Reticuloendotheliosis designates a group of pathologic syndromes in several avian species caused by reticuloendotheliosis virus, a member of the avian retrovirus group. Chickens, turkeys, ducks, geese, and quail, and rarely guinea fowl, peafowl, and prairie chickens have experienced natural infection and disease; probably many species of birds can be infected. Mammals appear refractory, although certain mammalian cell cultures are susceptible.

Reticuloendotheliosis virus is not as ubiquitous as Marek's disease and avian leukosis viruses, but is more widely distributed than once believed. Serologic surveys suggest that the virus is prevalent in both chicken and turkey flocks in many countries, including the USA.

Etiology: Reticuloendotheliosis virus is a retrovirus that is immunologically, morphologically, and structurally distinct from the leukosis/sarcoma group of avian retroviruses. Because of the phylogenetic relationship between reticuloendotheliosis virus and mammalian C-type retroviruses, reticuloendotheliosis virus has recently been placed in the genus mammalian C-type. Although all isolates belong to a single serotype, 3 subtypes of reticuloendotheliosis virus have been identified on the basis of neutralization tests and differential reactivity with monoclonal antibodies. Isolates can be classified as either nondefective or defective. Most field isolates appear to be nondefective for replication in cell cultures and contain no viral oncogene. One unique laboratory strain (strain T) is defective for replication in cell cultures and contains a viral oncogene, *v-rel*, that is responsible for an acute reticulum cell neoplasia in experimentally inoculated chicks; this neoplasm prompted the name reticuloendotheliosis but does not occur commonly in the field.

Transmission and Epidemiology: Horizontal transmission is probably more important than vertical, although both have been documented in chickens and turkeys. Transmission by mosquitos and other blood-sucking insects is suspected. The virus has been isolated from litter. A high rate of congenital infection has been demonstrated in naturally infected turkeys, but such flocks are probably rare. The virus has been transmitted accidentally through use of contaminated vaccines. Most commonly, however, flocks seroconvert after 10 wk of age without clinical disease or virus shedding to progeny. Experimentally, contact transmission occurs, but the virus is neither highly contagious nor highly stable in the environment. Partial or complete genomic insertion of reticuloendotheliosis virus in the genome of other avian viruses, namely fowlpox and Marek's disease viruses, has recently been described. However, the significance of such insertion in transmission of reticuloendotheliosis virus is not known.

Pathogenesis: The nondefective subgroups in strains of reticuloendotheliosis virus produce 3 distinct syndromes: non-neoplastic runting, acute neoplastic disease, and chronic neoplastic disease resulting in B and T lymphomas. Typically, the runting syndrome is seen 4-10 wk after administration of contaminated vaccines to day-old chicks. Chronic neoplastic disease has been induced experimentally in chickens, turkeys, and ducks; one type occurs in chickens after latent periods of >4 mo and appears identical to lymphoid leukosis—the tumors are composed of B cells, are bursal-dependent, and have IgM on their surface. Acute neoplasia, which develops after a latent period of 6-8 wk, also has been seen in chickens, turkeys, ducks, and quail. This tumor in chickens involves T cells and may be confused with Marek's disease.

Clinical Findings and Lesions: The runting syndrome is characterized by weight loss, paleness, occasional paralysis, and abnormal feathering (Nakanuke disease). Death from neoplasia is preceded by depression and occasionally by some of the same clinical changes described for the runting syndrome.

Lesions include bursal and thymic atrophy, enlarged nerves, anemia, and abnormal feathering. Of these, the abnormal feathering, in which the barbules are compressed to the shaft over a small part of its length, may be of diagnostic value. Neoplasms typically involve the liver, spleen, intestine, and heart. The bursa is involved in the chronic B-cell lymphomas of chickens in a manner similar to that of lymphoid leukosis. Nonbursal (T-cell) lymphomas with shorter latent periods and lesions superficially resembling those of Marek's disease also are recognized in chickens. In turkeys, prominent lesions include enlarged livers and nodular lesions on the intestines; the bursa is only rarely tumorous. The tumors, regardless of type or host species, are usually composed of uniform, large, lymphoreticular cells.

Diagnosis: The lesions induced by reticuloendotheliosis virus are so diverse and resemble so closely those of other tumors that diagnosis at necropsy is difficult; virus or antibody detection tests are useful in confirmation. The nerve lesions are usually less extensive and may contain more plasma cells than in Marek's disease, but in other cases are difficult to differentiate by histology. The runting syndrome is easily confused with immunosuppressive syndromes caused by other viral agents. The chronic B-cell lymphomas induced experimentally in chickens cannot easily be distinguished from those of lymphoid leukosis except by virus studies, including PCR. Similarly, the T-cell lymphomas of chickens cannot easily be distinguished from Marek's disease except by virus studies. However, both B- and T-cell lymphomas induced by reticuloendotheliosis virus contain a clonally integrated DNA provirus usually associated with the *c-myc* oncogene, which can be demonstrated by appropriate molecular methods. The chronic lymphomas that are seen in turkeys must be differentiated from lymphoproliferative disease of turkeys based on histology, virus isolation, and characterization of the virus-associated reverse transcriptase for activity in the presence of manganese or magnesium ions. Techniques based on immunocytochemistry with monoclonal antibodies to cellular, tumor, and viral antigens, or molecular hybridization can be used in the differential diagnosis of avian viral lymphomas, including reticuloendotheliosis.

Control: No control measures are currently practiced. An experimental recombinant fowlpox virus vaccine has been developed. Some breeder companies wish to avoid sero-conversion of their primary breeder stocks to obviate restrictions on export of progeny to certain countries, but reliable techniques to prevent horizontal transmission have not been developed.

NEOPLASMS OF UNKNOWN ETIOLOGY

Of the numerous tumors of unknown etiology in poultry, dermal squamous cell carcinoma, multicentric histiocytosis, and adenocarcinomas are the most common, but appear to be of limited economic importance.

Dermal Squamous Cell Carcinoma: These neoplasms occur at relatively high frequencies in some broiler flocks and are a cause of condemnations. Typically, the lesions are seen during processing as crater-like eruptions on the defeathered skin. An etiologic agent has not been identified, and the true neoplastic nature of the lesion has not been confirmed. Transmissibility of this tumor has neither been demonstrated nor ruled out.

Multicentric Histiocytosis: This condition of young broiler chickens is characterized by both splenomegaly and hepatomegaly. Miliary 0.5-5 mm, white to yellow nodules can be seen in the spleen, liver, and kidneys. Microscopically, nodules of spindle-shaped cells diffusely expand periarteriolar lymphoid sheaths. These histiocytic cells contain elongated oval, fusiform, or more bizarrely configured nuclei. No definitive etiologic agent has been identified. In some cases, the DNA that was extracted from lesions of naturally diseased broiler chickens did not contain sequences specific for exogenous avian leukosis/sarcoma viruses, reticuloendotheliosis viruses, or Marek's disease virus. A somewhat similar condition with lesions, termed "histiocytic sarcomatosis," has been described in meat-type chickens experimentally infected with subgroup J avian leukosis virus.

Adenocarcinomas: Adenocarcinomas of the ovary or oviduct are relatively common incidental tumors in mature chickens. These neoplasms often are characterized by multiple miliary implant tumors on the mesentery and other visceral surfaces, frequently accompanied by ascites. These tumors are not known to be virus-induced or to be transmissible.

NEWCASTLE DISEASE AND OTHER PARAMYXOVIRUS INFECTIONS

NEWCASTLE DISEASE
(Avian pneumoencephalitis)

Newcastle disease is an acute viral disease of domestic poultry and many other bird species. It is a worldwide problem that presents primarily as a respiratory disease, but depression, nervous manifestations, or diarrhea may be the predominant clinical form. Mortality is variable. Occurrence of a virulent form of the disease is reportable and may result in trade restrictions.

Etiology and Pathogenesis: Newcastle disease is caused by an RNA virus, Newcastle disease virus (NDV), synonymous with avian paramyxovirus-1 which is in the genus Avulavirus, family Paramyxoviridae. Isolates are classified into 1 of 3 virulence groups by chicken embryo and chicken inoculation as virulent (velogenic), moderately virulent (mesogenic), or of low virulence (lentogenic). Lentogenic strains are used widely as live vaccines in healthy chickens. Clinical manifestations vary from high morbidity and mortality to asymptomatic infections. The severity of an infection is dependent on virus virulence and the age, immune status, and susceptibility of the host species. Chickens are the most and waterfowl the least susceptible of domestic poultry.

Epidemiology and Transmission: Virulent NDV strains are endemic in poultry in most of Asia, Africa, and some countries of North, Central, and South America. Other countries, including the USA and Canada, are free of those strains and maintain that status with import restrictions and eradication by destroying diseased poultry. Cormorants, pigeons, and imported psittacine species have also been sources of virulent NDV infections of poultry. Low virulence NDV is prevalent in poultry and wild birds, especially waterfowl. Infection of domestic poultry with low virulence NDV contributes to lower productivity.

Infected birds shed virus in exhaled air, respiratory discharges, and feces. Virus is shed during incubation, during the clinical stage, and for a varying but limited period during convalescence. Virus may also be present in eggs laid during clinical disease and in all parts of the carcass during acute virulent infections. Chickens are readily infected by aerosols and by ingesting contaminated water or food. Infected chickens are the primary source of virus, but other domestic and wild birds may be sources of NDV. Transfer of virus, especially in infective feces, by the movement of people and contaminated equipment is the main method of spread between poultry flocks.

Clinical Findings: Onset is rapid, and signs appear throughout the flock within 2-12 days (average 5) after aerosol exposure. Spread is slower if the fecal-oral route is the primary means of transmission, particularly for caged birds. Young birds are the most susceptible. Observed signs depend on whether the infecting virus has a predilection for respiratory, digestive, or nervous systems. Respiratory signs of gasping, coughing, sneezing, and rales predominate in low virulence infections. Nervous signs of tremors, paralyzed wings and legs, twisted necks, circling, clonic spasms, and complete paralysis may accompany, but usually follow, the respiratory signs in neurotropic velogenic disease. Nervous signs with diarrhea are typical in pigeons, and nervous signs are frequently seen in cormorants and exotic bird species. Respiratory signs with depression, watery-greenish diarrhea, and swelling of the tissues of the head and neck are typical of the most virulent form of the disease, viscerotropic velogenic Newcastle disease (VVND, also called exotic Newcastle disease), although nervous signs may also be seen. Varying degrees of depression and inappetence are observed. A partial or complete cessation of egg production may occur. Eggs may be abnormal in color, shape, or surface, and have watery albumen. Mortality is variable but can be as high as 100%.

Lesions: Remarkable gross lesions are usually observed only with VVND. Petechiae may be seen on the serous membranes; hemorrhages of the proventricular mucosa and intestinal serosa are accompanied by multifocal, necrotic hemorrhagic areas on the mucosal surface of the intestine, especially at lymphoid foci such as cecal tonsils. Splenic necrosis and hemorrhage and edema around the thymus may also be observed. In contrast, the lesions in birds infected with lower virulence NDV strains may be limited to congestion and mucoid exudates seen in the respiratory tract with opacity and thickening of the air sacs. Secondary bacterial infections will increase the severity of the respiratory lesions.

Diagnosis: Diagnosis may be confirmed by isolation of a hemagglutinating virus identified by inhibition with Newcastle disease antiserum. A rise in hemagglutination-inhibition antibodies in paired serum samples also confirms the disease. The acute form should be differentiated from highly pathogenic avian influenza (p 2297). Virulence of an isolate is established by the rapidity of killing day-old chicks inoculated by the intracerebral route, the intracerebral pathogenicity index, or by the presence of a specified amino acid motif at the cleavage site of the fusion protein (F) precursor (FO). Reference laboratories use monoclonal antibodies to detect antigenic differences and nucleotide sequence analysis to detect genetic differences for comparison of isolates from different outbreaks and to identify the source of those infections.

Prevention: Live lentogenic vaccines, chiefly B1 and LaSota strains, are widely used and typically administered to poultry by mass application in drinking water or by spray. Alternatively, individual administration is via the nares or conjunctival sac. Healthy chicks are vaccinated as early as day 1-4 of life. However, delaying vaccination until the second or third week avoids maternal antibody interference with an active immune response. *Mycoplasma*, some other bacteria, and other viruses affecting the respiratory tract, if present, may act synergistically with some vaccines to aggravate the vaccine reaction after spray administration.

Oil-adjuvanted inactivated vaccines are also used following live vaccine in breeders and layers and may be used alone in situations where use of live virus may be contraindicated. In countries where virulent NDV is endemic, a combination of live virus and inactivated vaccine can be used; or alternatively, if permitted by law, a live mesogenic strain vaccine may be used in older birds. The frequency of revaccination to protect chickens throughout life largely depends on the risk of exposure and virulence of the field virus challenge.

Zoonotic Risk: Newcastle disease viruses, whether virulent field viruses or live vaccine, can produce a transitory conjunctivitis in humans, but the condition has been limited primarily to laboratory workers and vaccination teams exposed to large quantities of virus. Before poultry vaccination was widely practiced, conjunctivitis from NDV infection occurred in crews eviscerating poultry in processing plants. The disease has not been reported in people who rear poultry or consume poultry products.

OTHER AVIAN PARAMYXOVIRUS INFECTIONS

Avian paramyxovirus infections have been reported in chickens and turkeys in association with respiratory disease or decreases in egg production.

Etiology and Epidemiology: There are 9 recognized serotypes of avian paramyxoviruses (PMV-1 to PMV-9). Newcastle disease virus (PMV-1, *see* above) is the most important pathogen of this group for poultry, but PMV-2, -3, -6, and -7 are occasionally associated with disease in chickens and turkeys.

PMV-2 has been isolated from wild birds, mainly passerines, and caged psittacine species. Primary infections in poultry are believed to be the result of contact with wild birds. The method of transmission to chickens or turkeys is unclear. PMV-3 has been isolated from imported exotic and other bird species held in captivity. Psittacines appear to be the primary host, although PMV-3 will spread among passerines in captivity. There are no reports of isolation of PMV-3 from wild birds. The method of transmission among turkeys is unclear, and spread within a flock is usually slow.

Clinical Findings: Infections by PMV-2, -3, -6, and -7 in turkeys have produced mild to severe respiratory disease, drops in egg production, reduced hatchability and infertility of eggs, and increased numbers of white-shelled eggs. Infection with PMV-2 has produced mild respiratory disease in chickens, but PMV-2 infection is usually most severe in turkeys, especially breeders. Infection is more severe when accompanied by secondary pathogens.

Diagnosis: Most diagnoses are made by clinical signs and confirmed by serology. PMV-2, -3, -6, and -7 can be isolated from tracheal or cloacal swabs or tissue samples from infected birds by inoculating the allantoic cavity of 8- to 10-day-old embryonating chicken eggs. Confirmation of the virus as PMV can be done by hemagglutination inhibition tests with specific antiserum to individual serotypes. However, PMV-1 (Newcastle disease virus) and PMV-3 may cross-react in hemagglutination inhibition tests (and in other serologic tests such as ELISA), which causes interpretation problems in vaccinated birds. Birds vaccinated against Newcastle disease show a rise in hemagglutination inhibition titers to both viruses if subsequently infected with PMV-3.

Prevention and Control: No vaccines are available for PMV-2, -6, and -7. Inactivated oil emulsion vaccines have been used in turkey breeder flocks against PMV-3. These are injected twice, 4 wk apart, before the birds begin to lay (usually when 20-24 wk old). The risk of introducing PMV-2 and other paramyxoviruses may be minimized by bird-proofing poultry houses and using good hygiene and biosecurity practices. Treatment of secondary bacterial infections with antibiotics has had some success. PMV-3 appears to spread slowly.

OMPHALITIS

(Navel ill, "Mushy chick" disease, Yolk sac infection)

Omphalitis is a condition characterized by infected yolk sacs, often accompanied by unhealed navels in young fowl. It is infectious but noncontagious and associated with excessive humidity and marked contamination of the hatching eggs or incubator.

The affected chicks or poults usually appear normal until a few hours before death. Depression, drooping of the head, and huddling near the heat source usually are the only signs. The navel may be inflamed and fail to close, producing a wet spot on the abdomen; a scab may be present. Opportunistic bacteria (coliforms, staphylococci, *Pseudomonas* spp, and *Proteus* spp) are often involved, and mixed infections are common. Proteolytic bacteria are prevalent in outbreaks. The yolk sac is not absorbed and often is highly congested or may contain solidified pieces of yolk material; peritonitis may be extensive. Edema of the sternal subcutis may be seen. Mortality often begins at hatching and continues to 10-14 days of age, with losses up to 15% in chickens and 50% in turkeys. Chilling or overheating during shipment may increase losses. Persistent, unabsorbed, infected yolks often produce chicks or poults with reduced weight gain.

There is no specific treatment; antibiotic use is based on the prevalent bacterial type involved, but is probably of little value. The disease is prevented by careful control of temperature, humidity, and sanitation in the incubator. Only clean, uncracked eggs should be set. If it is necessary to set dirty eggs, they should be segregated from clean eggs. Sanitizing detergents must be used according to directions if eggs are washed. Time, temperature, and frequent changes of water are as critical as the concentration of sanitizer in both wash and rinse water. The rinse should be warmer than the wash water (which should be warmer than the internal temperature of the egg), but should not be >60°C.

The incubator should be cleaned and disinfected thoroughly between hatches. If fumigation is to be done with formaldehyde, vents should be closed. Thirty mL of 40% formaldehyde per 0.6 m^3, or paraformaldehyde (in the strength recommended by the manufacturer), should be allowed to evaporate in the closed incubator or hatcher. The machines are readily contaminated after fumigation unless the exterior of the machines and the rooms in which they are located are cleaned and disinfected.

POISONINGS

Generally, birds are less susceptible to poisoning than are mammals, and instances of toxicosis usually indicate departure from feed additive or drug label recommendations. However, the possibility of residues of toxic substances in eggs or poultry meat is of concern. Label recommendations regarding withdrawal times for all potentially toxic substances should be followed scrupulously.

See also the TOXICOLOGY section, p 2337 et seq.

INORGANIC SOURCES

Calcium: Excessive calcium intake in broiler chicks results in urolithiasis with urate deposits on the abdominal viscera and in the joints. Tetanic convulsions can also be seen in chicks consuming excess calcium. Calcium levels >2% will induce these lesions in broilers. Feeding calcium in excess of 3% before the onset of egg production will induce the same lesions in egg-type or meat-type pullets.

Carbon Monoxide: This poisoning commonly arises from exhaust fumes when chicks are being transported by truck or from improper ventilation in hatchers. Mortality may be high unless fresh air is provided immediately. At necropsy, the beak is cyanotic, and a characteristic bright pink color is noted throughout the viscera, particularly the lungs. Diagnosis can be confirmed by a spectroscopic analysis of the blood.

Copper: Copper sulfate in a single dose of >1 g is fatal. The signs are watery diarrhea and listlessness. A catarrhal gastroenteritis and burns or erosions in the lining of the gizzard, accompanied by a greenish, seromucous exudate throughout the intestinal tract, are found at necropsy.

Diazinon: Diazinon is an organic phosphate that is commonly used for the control of a variety of insects around poultry houses. It should not be used inside poultry houses. Some producers have used diazinon in poultry houses for the control of fire ants. Chickens will consume the diazinon crystals, which results in lacrimation, diarrhea, dyspnea, and death. Necropsy lesions include lung edema, fatty livers, and severe enteritis. The diazinon crystals can be seen in the crop and gizzard contents.

Lead: Lead poisoning usually is caused by paint or orchard-spray material. Metallic lead in amounts of 7.2 mg/kg body wt is lethal. Signs are depression, inappetence, emaciation, thirst, and weakness. Greenish droppings are commonly seen within 36 hr. As poisoning progresses, the wings may be extended downward. Young birds may die within 36 hr after ingestion. Acute lead poisoning may be diagnosed from the history and necropsy findings of a greenish brown gizzard mucosa, enteritis, and degeneration of the liver and kidney. Chronic poisoning results in emaciation and in atrophy of the liver and heart. The pericardium is distended with fluid, the gallbladder is thickened and enlarged, and urate deposits are usually found in the kidneys. Ingestion of lead shot often occurs in wild waterfowl on heavily gunned feeding grounds. Retention of only a few lead pellets in the gizzard can kill a duck.

Mercury: Poisoning occurs from mercurial disinfectants and fungicides, including mercurous chloride (calomel) and bichloride of mercury (corrosive sublimate). Clinical findings are progressive weakness and incoordination. Diarrhea may occur, depending on the amount ingested. The caustic action of the chemical may produce gray areas in the mouth and esophagus, which usually ulcerate if the bird lives >24 hr. Catarrhal inflammation of the proventriculus and intestines may occur; if a large amount of mercury is ingested, extensive hemorrhage may occur in those organs. The kidneys are pale and studded with small, white foci. The liver shows fatty degeneration.

Salt: The addition of 0.5% salt (NaCl) to the ration of chickens and turkeys is recommended, but amounts >2% are usually considered dangerous. Rations for chicks have contained as much as 8% without injurious effect, but in poults, rations containing 4% were harmful and levels of 6-8% have resulted in mortality. The addition of 2% NaCl to the feed, or 4,000 ppm in the water, depresses growth in young ducks and lowers the fertility and hatchability of the eggs in breeding stock.

Salt levels high enough to produce poisoning may be reached when salty protein concentrates (eg, fish meal) are added to rations already fortified with salt or when the salt is poorly incorporated in the feed. Sporadic poisoning also has been reported from accidental ingestion of rock salt or salt provided for other livestock. Necropsy findings are not diagnostic; enteritis and ascites are common. Watery droppings and wet litter often are suggestive of a high salt intake. Edema of the testicle is pathognomonic of salt toxicity in young birds.

Selenium: Ingestion of feeds containing >5 ppm of selenium decreases the hatchability of eggs due to deformities of the embryos, which are unable to emerge from the shell because of beak anomalies. Eyes may be unilaterally hypoplastic or aplastic, and feet and wings may be deformed or underdeveloped. Selenium at 10 ppm, as in seleniferous grains in the laying ration, usually reduces hatchability to zero. Young laying hens entering egg production are more susceptible than older hens.

Mature birds seem to tolerate more selenium in their feed than do pigs, cattle, or horses and do not exhibit signs of poisoning other than poor hatchability of their eggs. Starting rations containing 8 ppm selenium have reduced the growth rate of chicks, but 4 ppm had no noticeable effect. Rations containing as little as 2.5 ppm have resulted in meat and eggs with concentrations of selenium in excess of the suggested tolerance limit in foods. Sodium arsenite and some of the organic arsenicals, when administered to laying hens with selenium, have increased hatchability.

Sulfur: Sulfur is often used in broiler houses in an attempt to improve growth rate and feed conversion and to minimize bacterial disease. The compound is applied to the floor after the litter has been removed. If the amount of new litter placed in the house is inadequate, young chicks will come in contact with the sulfur, resulting in conjunctivitis and cutaneous burns, especially under the wings and on the legs. Clinically, the birds appear cold and tend to huddle; in many instances, death will occur due to the birds piling-up, causing overheating and suffocation. When sulfur comes into contact with moisture, sulfuric acid is produced, which results in the burns.

ORGANIC SOURCES

Various organic chemicals are dangerous, especially those used to treat seed grain.

Coffee Weed Seed: *Cassia obtusifolia* seeds are frequently found in corn and soybeans. When present at ≥2%, they reduce feed intake and lower body weights, increase feed conversion in broilers, and significantly depress egg production in laying birds. Necropsy lesions are absent.

Crotalaria: Seeds of many species are toxic to chickens. Concentrations >0.05% in the feed produce signs of toxicosis. At 0.2%, weight gain is reduced markedly; 0.3% causes death in 18 days. Lesions consist of ascites, swelling or cirrhosis of the liver, and hemorrhages. Resistance to the toxin increases with age.

Gossypol: Cottonseed meal contains appreciable amounts of gossypol, which produces severe cardiac edema that results in dyspnea, weakness, and anorexia. When fed to laying hens, gossypol also causes egg-yolk discoloration.

Lasalocid: Lasalocid is an anticoccidial compound that has been used in hot summer months because it increases water consumption. When used at other times of the year, the level of salt in the ration is reduced to prevent excessive water elimination and wet litter problems. If the salt level is reduced too much, it will result in stunting, increased lameness, and a characteristic clinical picture in broilers manifested by the bird walking on its toes. This clinical syndrome has been called lasolocid toxicity when, in reality, it is due to low levels of salt in the feed.

Monensin: This ionophore coccidiostat is widely used in the broiler industry. At levels >120 ppm, it reduces feed intake and weight gain; in layers, egg production is reduced. Signs of toxicity include a characteristic paralysis in which the legs are extended backward. Mortality occurs in naive turkeys if they are switched to a feed that contains monensin. They become paralyzed with the legs extended backward; no lesions are seen at necropsy.

Nicarbazin: This coccidiostat is used in broilers. It should not be fed to layers, as it can cause discoloration and reduced hatchability of eggs (although the effect is reversible once the nicarbazin is withdrawn). It also may result in reduced heat tolerance in birds exposed to high temperature and humidity.

Nitrofurazone: This has been used to treat several bacterial diseases in poultry, but is no longer approved for use in the USA. When fed at 0.022%, it causes hyperexcitability manifest by rapid movements, loud squawking, and frequent falling forward. In turkeys, which are more sensitive to nitrofurazone than are chickens, it produces cardiac dilatation, ascites, and when fed at 0.033%, death.

3-Nitro-4-hydroxyphenylarsonic Acid: When this compound, widely used in feed to improve weight gain and feed efficiency, is improperly mixed or fed at a level 2-3 times higher than normal, it induces a high-pitched chirp and a "duck-walking" stance. Cervical paralysis is frequently seen in chickens that consume excessive amounts. Clinical signs are usually reversible in a few minutes. Chronic exposure may produce intrahepatic cholangitis.

Polychlorinated Biphenyls (PCB): Residues have been reported in the fatty tissue of chickens and turkeys in excess of the 5 ppm permitted in edible tissue, and in egg products in excess of the permitted 0.5 ppm. PCB depress egg production and hatchability, and levels of 50 ppm result in cirrhosis of the liver and ascites in broilers and a drop in egg production and hatchability in hens. (*See also* HALOGENATED CYCLIC HYDROCARBON POISONING, p 2367.)

Quaternary Ammonia: Quaternary-ammonia-based compounds are widely used as disinfectants. (*See also* ANTISEPTICS AND DISINFECTANTS, p 2153.) Turkeys are very sensitive; levels of 150 ppm result in substantial mortality. Clinical signs include reduced water intake, nasal and ocular discharge, facial swelling, and gasping. Necropsy lesions include caseous ulcers at the base of the tongue and commissures of the mouth.

Salinomycin: Salinomycin is commonly used as an anticoccidial compound in the broiler industry. When used at 60 g/ton of feed, the compound is safe. Toxicities occur when broiler feed containing salinomycin is accidentally fed to naive breeder hens. Clinical signs in these hen flocks include paralysis with the legs extended backward and decreased feed consumption, egg production, and hatchability. Levels of salinomycin >10 g/ton in breeder-hen feed are sufficient to produce these clinical signs. Necropsy lesions are absent in birds with this clinical picture.

Sulfaquinoxaline: Sulfonamides are widely used for treatment of several bacterial and protozoal infections in poultry. Sulfaquinoxaline, when fed at 0.25%, results in severe pancytopenia. Hemorrhages are common on the legs, breast muscle, and in virtually all abdominal organs. The bone marrow is pale, and the blood is slow to clot. Toxicity is frequently seen in hot weather when sulfaquinoxaline is provided in drinking water. Water consumption increases rapidly as the temperature increases, which leads to increased drug intake. This toxicity usually is responsive to vitamin K therapy.

Thiram: Thiram is used to treat seed corn. It is toxic to chicks at 40 ppm and to goslings at 150 ppm; it causes leg deformities and weight loss. At 10 ppm, it causes soft-shelled eggs, and at 40 ppm, egg production and hatchability are reduced. Turkey poults tolerate up to 200 ppm.

Toxic Fat: A crystalline halogen has been identified as the "toxic fat" factor in some feeds. In young pullets, it reduces growth, retards sexual development, and increases mortality. Hatchability is decreased. Turkeys and ducks are less susceptible than chickens. Signs of intoxication include ruffled feathers, droopiness, and dyspnea. Lesions include ascites and hydropericardium, liver necrosis, subepicardial hemorrhage, and bile duct hyperplasia. Although the amount of toxin varies in feeds from different sources, 0.25-0.5% fed for 35-150 days produces typical lesions.

RIEMERELLA ANATIPESTIFER INFECTION

(New duck disease, Infectious serositis, *Pasteurella anatipestifer* infection)

Infection with *Riemerella (Pasteurella) anatipestifer* is a contagious, widely distributed disease that primarily affects young ducks and turkeys. Other waterfowl, chickens, and pheasants also may be affected. The epidemiology and pathogenesis are not understood. Ducks are believed to be infected by the respiratory route or when *R anatipestifer* is introduced into toenail scratches of the webbed foot. Turkeys may be infected by injuries or by the respiratory route when another pathogen disrupts the respiratory epithelium.

Affected ducks, usually 2-7 wk old, often have ocular and nasal discharges, mild coughing and sneezing, tremors of the head and neck, and incoordination. Stunting may occur. Fibrinous exudate in the pericardial cavity and over the surface of the liver is the most characteristic lesion. Fibrinous airsacculitis is common, and infection of the CNS can result in fibrinous meningitis. The spleen and liver may be swollen. Pneumonia may be seen. Mortality is usually 2-30%.

Affected turkeys, usually 5-15 wk old, often exhibit dyspnea, droopiness, hunched back, lameness, and a twisted neck. Fibrinous pericarditis and epicarditis are the most pronounced lesions. There may also be fibrinous perihepatitis, airsacculitis, and purulent synovitis. Osteomyelitis, meningitis, and focal pneumonia are seen occasionally. Mortality is 5-60%, and condemnations are 3-13%.

Diagnosis is based on signs, lesions, and isolation and identification of the causative organism, because other diseases, particularly colibacillosis (p 600) and chlamydiosis (p 2216), may produce similar lesions. Chocolate agar medium is recommended for isolation, although blood agar is also used, with incubation at 37°C in a candle jar or under

5% carbon dioxide. The isolate should be serotyped because the information may be needed for vaccine selection and epidemiology. Biochemical characteristics can be used to differentiate this organism from other bacteria that cause important diseases of ducks and turkeys, particularly *Escherichia coli* and *Pasteurella multocida*. Impression smears help to determine whether chlamydia is involved.

Careful management practices are important for prevention of infection. Rigid sanitation and depopulation are necessary for elimination of the disease. A bacterin and, more recently, a live vaccine, which include the 3 most common immunotypes of *R anatipestifer*, are available for use in turkeys. An autogenous oil-emulsion bacterin can be used in ducks. A combination of penicillin and streptomycin, or sulfaquinoxaline can be used for initial treatment, but an antibiotic sensitivity test should be performed.

SALMONELLOSES

Historically, the 3 salmonellae infections in poultry causing severe economic losses are *Salmonella pullorum*, *S gallinarum*, and *S arizonae*. Through the institution of control programs, the incidence of infections with these salmonellae has decreased dramatically. In addition to the above salmonellae, *S paratyphoid* infections in poultry are relatively common and have public health significance because of the consumption of contaminated poultry products.

S pullorum and *S gallinarum* are highly host-adapted to chickens and turkeys. *S arizonae* is most important in turkeys, with chickens occasionally affected. There are ~2,000 nonhost-adapted species (paratyphoid) that may be transmitted to almost all animals (*see also* SALMONELLOSIS, p 156).

PULLORUM DISEASE

Etiology and Transmission: Infections with *Salmonella pullorum* usually cause very high mortality (potentially approaching 100%) in young chickens and turkeys. In adult chickens mortality may be high, but frequently there are no clinical signs. Pullorum disease was once common but has been eradicated from most commercial chicken stock, although it may occur in other avian species (eg, guinea fowl, quail, pheasants, sparrows, parrots, canaries, and bullfinches). Infection in mammals is rare.

Transmission is primarily through the egg but also occurs via direct or indirect contact with infected birds. Infection transmitted via egg or hatchery contamination usually results in death during the first few days of life up to 2-3 wk of age.

Clinical Findings and Lesions: Affected birds huddle near a heat source, are anorectic, appear weak, and have whitish fecal pasting around the vent (diarrhea). Survivors frequently become asymptomatic carriers with localized infection of the ovary. Some of the eggs laid by such hens hatch and produce infected progeny.

Lesions in young birds usually include unabsorbed yolk sacs and classic gray nodules in the liver, spleen, lungs, heart, gizzard, and intestine. Firm, cheesy material in the ceca (cecal cores) and raised plaques in the mucosa of the lower intestine are sometimes seen. Occasionally, synovitis is prominent. Adult carriers usually have no gross lesions but may have nodular pericarditis, fibrinous peritonitis, or hemorrhagic, atrophic regressing ovarian follicles with caseous contents. In mature chickens, chronic infections produce lesions that are indistinguishable from those of fowl typhoid (*see* below).

Diagnosis: Lesions may be highly suggestive, but diagnosis should be confirmed by isolation, identification, and serotyping of *S pullorum*. Infections in mature birds can be identified by serologic tests, followed by necropsy evaluation complemented by microbiologic culture and typing for confirmation. Official testing recommendations are outlined in the USA National Poultry Improvement Program (NPIP).

Treatment and Control: Treatment of infected flocks to alleviate the perpetuation of the carrier state is not recommended. Control is based on routine serologic testing of breeding stock to assure freedom from infection.

FOWL TYPHOID

Etiology and Epidemiology: The causal agent is *Salmonella gallinarum*. The incidence of fowl typhoid is low in the USA and Canada, but much higher in other countries. Although *S gallinarum* is egg-transmitted and produces lesions in chicks and poults similar to those produced by *S pullorum*, there is a much greater tendency to spread among growing or mature flocks. Mortality in young birds is similar to *S pullorum* infection but may be higher in older birds.

Clinical Findings and Lesions: Clinical signs and lesions in young birds are similar to those of infection with *S pullorum*. The older bird may be pale, dehydrated, and have diarrhea. Lesions in the older bird may include a swollen, friable, and often bile-stained liver, with or without necrotic foci, enlarged spleen and kidneys, anemia, and enteritis.

Diagnosis: Diagnosis should be confirmed by isolation and identification and serotyping of *S gallinarum* (NPIP testing procedure).

Treatment and Control: Treatment and control are as for pullorum disease (*see* above). There are no federally licensed vaccines in the USA. In other countries, vaccines (killed or modified live) made from a rough strain of *S gallinarum* (9R) have been useful in controlling mortality. More recently, vaccines derived from outer membrane proteins, mutant strains, and a virulence-plasmid-cured derivative of *S gallinarum* have shown promise in protecting birds against challenge. The standard serologic tests for pullorum disease are equally effective in detecting fowl typhoid.

ARIZONA INFECTION
(Paracolon infection)

Arizona infection is an acute or chronic egg-transmitted infection, primarily of turkeys, caused by *Salmonella arizonae*.

Etiology, Clinical Findings, and Lesions: Many serotypes have been identified from various birds, mammals, and reptiles. Foodborne infections occasionally occur in humans. Reptiles, wild birds, rats, and mice are frequently infected and are thought to act as a reservoir of infection for poultry.

Clinical signs and lesions are not distinctive. Mortality is usually limited to the first 3-4 wk of age, and adult carriers may not develop appreciable clinical signs. Infection tends to persist in a flock. Poults are diarrheic, listless, and unthrifty; in some flocks, birds may develop eye opacity and blindness. Neurologic signs occur due to infection of the brain.

Lesions include unabsorbed yolk sacs, enlarged and mottled livers, congestion in the duodenum, and caseous cecal cores. Some birds develop peritonitis, salpingitis, local ovarian infections, or ophthalmitis. Purulent material may be seen in the meninges.

Diagnosis: Diagnosis is based on isolation and identification of the organism. Affected eyes and brain are excellent sites for isolation. Environmental samples also may be used for detecting the microbe. Egg transmission levels are often high; therefore, culture of dead embryos, eggshells, and cull poults may identify infected breeding stock. Effective serologic tests have not been developed.

Treatment and Control: Killed vaccines (bacterins) have been used in infected breeder flocks to reduce egg transmission and to develop breeding flocks free of *S arizonae*. Early fumigation of hatching eggs and rigorous hatchery sanitation also aid in reducing transmission. Antibiotics are given by injection to day-old poults to minimize mortality. Birds may still carry and shed the organism even after treatment.

PARATYPHOID INFECTIONS

Etiology, Clinical Findings, and Lesions: Paratyphoid infections can be caused by any one of the many nonhost-adapted salmonellae. These *Salmonella* may infect many types of birds, mammals, reptiles, and insects. Paratyphoid infections are of public health significance via contamination and mishandling of poultry products. *Salmonella typhimurium*, *S enteritidis*, and *S heidelberg* are among the most common salmonella infections in poultry, although infections may be produced by 10-20 different serotypes in the USA. Some species or strains are more pathogenic than others. The prevalence of other species varies widely by geographic location and season.

Transmission usually occurs horizontally from infected birds, contaminated environments, or infected rodents. With the exception of *S enteritidis*, transmission of most serotypes to progeny from infected breeders is mainly through fecal contamination of the eggshell. Infected birds remain carriers.

Clinical Findings and Lesions: Although not common, clinical signs are sometimes seen in young birds. Mortality is most often limited to the first few weeks of age. Depression, poor growth, weakness, diarrhea, and dehydration are hallmarks of the disease, although these clinical signs are not distinctive.

Lesions may include an enlarged liver with focal necrosis, unabsorbed yolk sac, enteritis with necrotic lesions in the mucosa, and cecal cores. Infections occasionally localize in the eye or synovial tissues. Conversely, there may be no lesions due to acute death caused by septicemia. Isolation, identification, and serotyping of the causal agent are essential for diagnosis. Serology is not highly reliable.

Treatment and Control: General control measures for the paratyphoid *Salmonella* include strict sanitation in the hatchery, fumigation of hatching eggs, pelleting of feed to destroy salmonellae, cleaning and disinfection of poultry houses, rodent control, and use of competitive exclusion products. Several antibacterial agents help prevent mortality but cannot eliminate flock infection. Maintenance of poultry in confinement and exclusion of all pets, wild birds, and rodents help prevent introduction of infection.

Salmonella enteritidis (a paratyphoid *Salmonella* serotype) is a major food safety concern, primarily for the egg-laying industry. Possible sources in commercial layers include transmission from breeders, contaminated environments, infected rodents, and contaminated feed. Transmission to progeny from breeders is mainly through eggshell contamination, although, unlike other paratyphoid *Salmonella*, transovarial transmission may also occur. The NPIP now includes *S enteritidis* control measures in breeders, including depopulation of infected flocks, cleaning and disinfection of pullet and layer houses, extensive and improved rodent control programs, use of competitive exclusion products, vaccination, and proper handling and refrigeration of eggs.

STAPHYLOCOCCOSIS

All avian species appear to be susceptible to staphylococcosis, which is common worldwide wherever poultry are reared. *Staphylococcus aureus* is usually the causative agent, but there is increasing evidence that other *Staphylococcus* species may also be involved. The disease condition can vary depending on where and how the bacteria enter the host; infections have been reported in the bones, joints, tendon sheaths, skin, sternal bursa, navel, yolk sac, liver, lungs, and eyelids. Septicemic infection has also been seen in laying chickens, with death occurring very quickly.

Etiology: *S aureus* is a gram-positive coccus that appears in grape-like clusters on a stained smear. It is usually isolated on blood agar, on which it produces circular, smooth, white to orange colonies, 1-3 mm in diameter, within 24 hr. *S aureus* is facultatively anaerobic, β hemolytic, catalase positive, fermentative for glucose and mannitol, and coagulase positive. For many years, only coagulase-positive strains were considered to be of any clinical significance; however, in recent years, *S hyicus*, *S epidermidis*, and *S gallinarum* have been isolated from clinical materials.

Transmission, Epidemiology, and Pathogenesis: *S aureus* and other *Staphylococcus* species are part of the normal flora on the skin and mucous membranes and are not thought to produce disease unless there is some breakdown in an environmental or immune system barrier. Most infections occur because of a wound, damage to the mucous membranes, or both. Infection can also occur in the hatchery as a result of contamination of an open navel. Birds that are immunosuppressed are also subject to staphylococcal infections. Staphylococcal septicemia is usually seen in laying chickens only in very hot weather. Once in the host, *S aureus* usually travels to the metaphyseal area of a nearby joint and causes osteomyelitis with subsequent spread to the joint. *S aureus* can produce disease locally at the site of entry, but the tendency to spread to the bones and joints is probably the most important feature of this disease.

Clinical Findings: Infection most often manifests as a synovitis, with lameness being the most common clinical presentation. The bones and associated joints most frequently affected are the proximal tibiotarsus and proximal femur; the proximal tarsometatarsus, distal femur, and tibiotarsus are also involved when infection is extensive. Other common lesions include navel and yolk sac infections. Lesions that have been reported include green liver in turkeys, and liver spots and granulomas. In acute infections, mortality may be the only clinical observation.

   Lesions: Lesions in the bone are focal yellow areas of necrosis, while lesions in joints consist of purulent exudate. Chicks with navel infection have navel areas that are dark and wet. Infected yolk sacs are retained longer than normal and are abnormal in color, consistency, and odor. Gangrenous dermatitis is seen in chickens that are immunosuppressed and is a combination of *S aureus* and *Clostridium septicum*. Affected areas are usually dark (hemorrhagic) and crepitant. Green liver has been a problem in turkeys and has been associated with osteomyelitis and synovitis at the processing plant. Liver spots and granulomas have been a cause of liver condemnation. In acute infections, necrosis and vascular congestion is observed in the liver, spleen, and/or kidneys.

Diagnosis: *S aureus* is easily isolated from stab swabs of affected material on sheep or bovine blood agar. Most strains of *S aureus* are β hemolytic, while most other strains of *Staphylococcus* are not. Swabs can be streaked onto selective media such as mannitol-salt agar or phenylethyl alcohol agar. These media inhibit the growth of gram-negative bacteria. The coagulase test is used to establish the significance of an isolate; only coagulase-positive isolates are considered to be pathogenic. Differential diagnosis includes *Escherichia coli* and *Pasteurella multocida*.

Treatment and Prevention: Staphylococcosis can be successfully treated with antibiotics, but a sensitivity test should be performed because antibiotic resistance is common. Antibiotics used to treat *Staphylococcus* infections include penicillin, erythromycin, lincomycin, and spectinomycin. Because wounds are a major cause of infection, it is important to reduce all potential sources of injury (eg, sharp objects) to the bird. Splinters in litter, sharp rocks, wire from cages, sharp edges or nails on floor slats, and fighting have been associated with the disease, as well as beak and toe trimming procedures in young chickens and turkeys. Good litter management is important in controlling footpad erosions to prevent infection. Hatchery sanitation is also important to reduce the numbers of bacteria, including *S aureus*, which is a hearty bacterium that can be difficult to kill using normal sanitation procedures. Bacterins have not been effective against *S aureus*, but there have been reports that competitive exclusion using a strain of *S epidermidis* has been effective in young, growing turkeys.

Zoonotic Risk: *S aureus* can cause food poisoning. Enterotoxin-producing strains are found on poultry, and proper precautions should be taken during handling and cooking.

STREPTOCOCCOSIS

Streptococcosis in avian species is worldwide in distribution, occurring as both acute septicemic and chronic infections with mortality ranging from 0.5% to 50%. Infection is considered secondary, because streptococci may form part of the normal intestinal and mucosal flora of most avian species, including wild birds, and are commonly found in various poultry environments.

Streptococci were previously classified in both Lancefield antigenic serogroups C and D. Lancefield group D *Streptococcus* spp are commonly referred to as "fecal streps." The application of new bacteriologic techniques, especially DNA-DNA and DNA-rRNA hybridization has led to the reclassification of the Lancefield group D streptococci to the *Enterococcus* spp. Bacteria identified by genus only in earlier reports could have been classified as *Enterococcus* spp in current nomenclature instead of *Streptococcus* spp. For diseases caused by the Lancefield antigenic serogroup D, *see* ENTEROCOCCOSIS, p 2223.

Etiology and Epidemiology: The genus *Streptococcus* is composed of gram-positive, spherical bacteria occurring singly, in pairs, or in short chains, which are nonmotile, nonsporeforming, facultative anaerobes. They are catalase-negative and ferment sugars, usually to lactic acid. *Streptococcus* spp isolated from avian species and associated with disease include *S zooepidemicus* (occasionally referred to as *S gallinarum*), *S bovis*, and *S dysgalactiae*. *S mutans*, a common bacterium in the human oral cavity, has been associated with septicemia and mortality in geese; contaminated drinking water and poor quality litter were possible predisposing factors. Naturally occurring infections of *S bovis* causing acute septicemia and joint infections have been found in racing pigeons. *S dysgalactiae* has been cultured from broiler chickens with cellulitis, a condition observed on the skin and subcutaneous tissue at processing. *Streptococcus* spp have been isolated from lesions of osteomyelitis in turkeys. Naturally occurring and experimental poultry infections resulting in bacterial endocarditis are commonly associated with streptococci and other bacteria. Transmission occurs most commonly via oral and aerosol routes. However, transmission can occur through skin injuries, especially in caged layers. Aerosol transmission of *S zooepidemicus* can result in acute septicemia in chickens.

Clinical Findings: *S zooepidemicus* is found almost exclusively in mature chickens but has been documented as a cause of mortality in wild birds. Incubation periods range from 1 day to several weeks, with 5-21 days most common. Endocarditis occurs when septicemic streptococcal infection progresses to a subacute or chronic stage. Lameness may also be observed in subacute or chronic infections. In *S zooepidemicus* infections, clinical signs are typical of an acute septicemic infection and include lassitude, blood-stained tissue and feathers around the head, yellow droppings, emaciation, and pale combs and wattles. Cyanosis in the terminal stages has been described. Mortality varies, but may reach 50%. In layers, egg production may drop as much as 15%. *Streptococcus* spp have also been isolated in cases of acute fibrinopurulent conjunctivitis. In pigeons, *S bovis* infection produces acute onset of mortality with occasional lameness, inappetence, diarrhea, and the inability to fly.

Lesions: Gross lesions of *S zooepidemicus* in acute disease include splenomegaly, hepatomegaly (with or without miliary to 1-cm foci that are red, tan, or white), enlarged kidneys, congestion of subcutaneous tissue, and peritonitis. Subcutaneous and pericardial fluid may appear serosanguineous. Bloodstained feathers around the mouth and head with blood coming from the mouth may occur. In broilers, cellulitis involving the skin and subcutaneous tissues can be observed at processing and has been associated with both *Escherichia coli* and *S dysgalactiae*. Lesions of chronic streptococcal infections include fibrinous arthritis and/or tenosynovitis, osteomyelitis, salpingitis, fibrinous pericarditis, necrotic myocarditis, and valvular endocarditis. Vegetative valvular lesions are usually yellow, white, or tan small, raised rough areas on the valvular surface. Valve lesions are most consistently found on the mitral valve but may be found on other valves. Microscopically, valvular lesions consist primarily of fibrin with bacteria, heterophils, macrophages, and fibroblasts. Focal granulomas can be found in virtually any tissue as a result of septic emboli. Gram-positive bacterial colonies are readily observed in thrombosed vessels and within necrotic foci with tissue Gram stains.

Diagnosis: Demonstration of bacteria typical of streptococci in blood films or impression smears of affected heart valves or lesions from birds with typical signs and lesions allows a presumptive diagnosis of streptococcosis. Isolation of *Streptococcus* spp from typical lesions in poultry with appropriate clinical signs confirms the diagnosis. Streptococci are easily isolated in blood agar. Fermentation of mannitol, sorbitol, arabinose, and growth on MacConkey agar can also aid in differentiation of streptococci in Lancefield serogroup D from *S zooepidemicus* and other Lancefield serogroup C streptococci. Preferred tissues for culture include liver, spleen, blood, yolk, embryo fluids, or any tissue with lesions. Bacterial endocarditis can be diagnosed based on valvular vegetations with secondary infarcts of myocardium, liver, and/or spleen. In suspected cases, it is important to culture lesions to establish a definitive diagnosis and rule out other bacteria. A rapid detection test by latex agglutination has been described for identification of antigenic serogroup C streptococci in animals.

Differential diagnosis includes other bacterial septicemic diseases, eg, staphylococcosis, enterococcosis, colibacillosis, pasteurellosis, and erysipelas.

Treatment and Control: Treatment includes use of antibiotics such as penicillin, erythromycin, novobiocin, oxytetracycline, chlortetracycline, and tetracycline in acute and subacute infections. Clinically affected birds respond well early in the course of the disease. As the disease progresses within a flock, treatment efficacy decreases. Antibacterial sensitivity should be performed on bacterial isolates. There is no treatment for poultry with bacterial endocarditis. In vitro sensitivity to *S bovis* in pigeons has been demonstrated with penicillins, macrolides, lincomycin, tetracyclines, chloramphenicol, and nitrofurans.

Prevention requires reducing stress and preventing immunosuppressive diseases and conditions. Proper cleaning and disinfection can reduce environmental streptococcal resident flora to minimize external exposure. The use of formaldehyde reduces the total count of *Streptococcus* spp in hatchers by as much as 86%.

TUBERCULOSIS

Tuberculosis is a slowly spreading, chronic, granulomatous bacterial infection, characterized by gradual weight loss. All birds appear to be susceptible, although to variable degrees; pheasants seem to be highly susceptible, while the disease is uncommon in turkeys. Tuberculosis is more prevalent in captive than in wild birds. Tuberculosis is unlikely to occur in commercial poultry due to the short life span and husbandry practices used. (*See also* TUBERCULOSIS in mammals, p 549).

Etiology and Epidemiology: *Mycobacterium avium* var *avium* is the cause. Serologic identification of isolates is essential to differentiate strains of *M avium* that cause disease in chickens and birds (serovars 1, 2, and 3) from other serovars that fail to produce disease in these species. *M tuberculosis* has infrequently been isolated from parrots and canaries. *M avium* is very resistant; it can survive in soil for up to 4 yr, in 3% hydrochloric acid for ≥2 hr, and in 4% sodium hydroxide for ≥30 min. Tuberculosis is found worldwide, most commonly in small, barnyard flocks and in zoo aviaries; it is rarely found in young flocks. Wild birds, such as cranes, sparrows, starlings, and raptors, have been found to be infected. Tuberculosis has been found in emus and other ratites.

Infected birds with advanced lesions excrete the organism in their feces. Cadavers and offal may infect predators and cannibalistic flockmates. Rabbits, pigs, and mink are readily infected. Cattle exposed to contaminated feces may respond to mammalian tuberculin and to johnin. *M avium* may cause disease in humans; serovar 1, often isolated from tuberculous chickens, has been isolated from people with acquired immunodeficiency syndrome.

Clinical Findings and Diagnosis: Signs usually do not develop until late in the infection when birds become thin and sluggish, and lameness may be seen. In chickens, granulomatous nodules of varying size are usually found in the liver, spleen, bone marrow, and intestine. Some exotic species may have lesions in the liver and spleen without intestinal involvement, but bone marrow and small mesenteric nodules may be found. Lesions are not calcified.

Live birds may be tested with avian tuberculins, although these are of little value in birds that do not have wattles. Large numbers of acid-fast bacteria in smears from lesions provide a tentative diagnosis.

Control: Chemotherapy is ineffective. In commercial poultry flocks, relatively rapid turnover of populations, together with improved general sanitation, has largely eliminated this once common infection. Infected poultry should be destroyed, and housing facilities thoroughly cleaned and disinfected using cresylic compounds. Dirt-floored houses should have several inches of the floor removed and replaced with dirt from a place where poultry have not been maintained. All openings should be screened against wild birds. Avian tuberculosis in zoos is difficult to eradicate. New additions to the aviary should be quarantined for 2-3 mo. The movement of ratites through sales and the long life of these animals have made tuberculosis a major concern for ratite producers. Isolation of ratites purchased at sales is essential to prevent the introduction of tuberculosis into established flocks.

VIRAL HEPATITIS OF TURKEYS

Turkey viral hepatitis is an acute, highly contagious, frequently subclinical disease of turkey poults 5 wk of age. The disease is widespread and common in some areas with morbidity rates of up to 100%. Mortality has been reported only in poults, is confined to a 4- to 8-day period, and may reach 25%.

Etiology: A picorna-like virus from poults with typical lesions has been reported, but its etiologic role has not been conclusively established. The causal virus has not been fully classified. It is isolated without difficulty from the liver and a variety of other tissues, including the pancreas, spleen, and kidney, as well as feces. The virus is isolated less consistently from older birds. It grows readily in the yolk sac of 5- to 7-day-old chick or turkey embryos. It is thermostabile; resistant to ether, phenol, and creolin but not formalin; and susceptible to high, but not low pH.

Clinical Findings: Disease is usually subclinical and becomes apparent only when the birds are stressed. Affected birds are stunted and unthrifty. Morbidity and mortality vary according to the severity of stress. In poults <5 wk old, morbidity may reach 100% and mortality 10-25%. Breeder flocks may suffer from decreased production, fertility, and hatchability.

Lesions: Gross lesions are confined to the liver and pancreas. In the liver, foci of necrosis are 1-3 mm in diameter and may be confluent. Areas of hemorrhage or congestion are also present and frequently obscure the degenerative changes. Occasionally, the liver is diffusely bile-stained. Liver lesions may resemble those of bacterial infections, particularly from *Salmonella* spp, *Pasteurella multocida*, or *Escherichia coli* and infections caused by Group 1 and Group 2 avian adenovirus and reovirus. The liver lesions may resemble those of blackhead (histomoniasis, p 2238), but the absence of cecal lesions in turkey viral hepatitis helps to differentiate the 2 diseases. The pancreas frequently exhibits relatively large, circular, gray areas of degeneration. In the subclinical form, lesions are less extensive, and hepatic hemorrhage or congestion is seldom prominent. Affected tissues return to normal in 3-4 wk.

Diagnosis: Paratyphoid and paracolon infections (p 2264) produce necrotic areas in the liver that can be confused with those of viral hepatitis. These and other bacterial and mycotic infections must be differentiated by appropriate culturing techniques. Histomoniasis usually produces concurrent cecal lesions unless modified by medication. In the latter case, histologic examination or demonstration of the respective etiologic agents is necessary.

Control: There is no known treatment. Secondary bacterial invasion does not appear to be important, but if it occurs, it should be treated on the basis of specific etiology. Although recovered birds demonstrate resistance to infection, neutralizing antibodies have not been detected. Improved sanitation may be of value in preventing dissemination of the agent.

MISCELLANEOUS CONDITIONS OF POULTRY

ASCITES SYNDROME
(Waterbelly, Right ventricular failure, Pulmonary hypertension syndrome)

Ascites is an accumulation of noninflammatory transudate in one or more of the peritoneal cavities or potential spaces. The fluid, which accumulates most frequently in the 2 ventral hepatic, peritoneal, or pericardial spaces, may contain yellow protein clots. Ascites may result from increased vascular hydraulic pressure, vascular damage, increased tissue oncotic pressure, decreased vascular oncotic (usually colloidal) pressure, or blockage of lymph drainage.

The most common cause of ascites is increased vascular hydraulic pressure in the venous system, which is most commonly caused by right ventricular failure (RVF) or hepatic fibrosis.

In poultry, RVF is usually secondary to valvular insufficiency and may result from inflammatory (myocarditis, valvular endocarditis) or degenerative disease of the myocardium or valves or from congenital heart disease. In turkeys, spontaneous cardiomyopathy (p 2200) is a common cause of ascites. However, the most common cause of ascites in meat-type chickens is RVF in response to increased pulmonary arterial resistance. Pulmonary hypertension occurs frequently in chickens secondary to the hypoxia of altitude with resultant polycythemia and increased blood viscosity. It also occurs frequently secondary to the red blood cell rigidity of sodium toxicity and less frequently from lung pathology. When ascites occurs at low altitudes in meat-type chickens, which have a high metabolic oxygen requirement, it is usually caused by primary or spontaneous pulmonary hypertension because of insufficient capacity of the pulmonary capillaries.

In poultry, liver damage may be caused by aflatoxin or by toxins from plants such as *Crotalaria*. In broiler chickens, obstructive cholangiohepatitis (caused by *Clostridium perfringens* infection) is the most common cause of the liver damage, which results in ascites. In both meat-type ducks and breeders, amyloidosis of the liver frequently causes ascites.

Pathogenesis and Epidemiology: Pulmonary hypertension syndrome (PHS) is caused by increased pressure in the pulmonary arteries when the heart tries to pump more blood through the lungs to meet the body's oxygen requirement. The resultant volume and pressure overload on the right ventricle cause dilatation and hypertrophy of the right ventricular wall, valvular insufficiency, RVF, and ascites.

Bird lungs are rigid and fixed in the thoracic cavity. The capillaries can expand very little to accommodate increased blood flow. Lung size in proportion to body weight, and particularly to muscle mass, decreases as meat-type chickens grow. Increased blood flow results in primary pulmonary hypertension and cor pulmonale with sporadic cases of RVF and ascites in fast-growing broilers. Predisposing factors that increase oxygen demand (eg, cold), reduce oxygen-carrying capacity of the blood (eg, acidosis, carbon monoxide), increase blood volume (eg, sodium), or interfere with blood flow through the lung (eg, lung pathology that narrows or occludes capillaries, increased RBC rigidity, or polycythemia with increased blood viscosity) may result in flock outbreaks of PHS with or without ascites.

The incidence of PHS is >2% in some broiler and many roaster flocks and is occasionally 15-20% in other roaster flocks. Right ventricular hypertrophy is the response to an increased workload and eventually leads to RVF if the volume or pressure load persists. Hypertrophy of the right ventricular wall is directly related to pulmonary hypertension, and the ratio of the right ventricle to the total ventricular mass can be used as a measure of the increased pressure load on the right ventricle.

Clinical Findings: Occasionally, young broilers develop PHS, particularly if increased sodium or lung pathology (eg, aspergillosis) is involved, but in primary pulmonary hypertension, mortality is greatest after 5 wk of age. Clinical signs are not seen until RVF occurs and ascites develops. Clinically affected broilers are cyanotic, the abdominal skin may be red, and peripheral vessels congested. Because growth stops as RVF develops, affected broilers may be smaller than their pen mates. However, rapid growth rate is a known predisposing factor, and sometimes the largest broilers are affected, with occurrence in males more frequent than in females. The ascites increases the respiratory rate and reduces exercise tolerance. Affected broilers frequently die on their backs, and differential diagnosis includes flip-over disease (p 2227). Not all broilers that die from PHS have ascites. Death may occur suddenly before clinical signs are seen.

Lesions: Most lesions are the result of increased venous hydraulic pressure secondary to RVF. There is a variable amount of clear yellow fluid and clots of fibrin in the hepatoperitoneal spaces. The liver may be swollen and congested, or firm and irregular with edema, and have clotted protein adherent to the surface. It may be nodular or shrunken; it may be white with subcapsular edema and a thickened capsule, or have large or small blebs of fluid between the capsule and the visceral peritoneum. Hydropericardium is mild to marked, and occasionally there is pericarditis with adhesions. Right ventricular dilatation and mild to marked hypertrophy of the right ventricular wall may be noted. The right atrium and vena cava are very dilated. Occasionally, there is thinning of the left ventricle. The lungs are extremely congested and edematous. The intestine may or may not be empty.

Diagnosis: Broilers that die from ascites or suddenly as the result of RVF or pulmonary hypertension can be identified by the enlarged heart; enlarged, thickened right ventricle; or fluid in the body cavities and heart sac. If the wall of the right ventricle is enlarged or thickened, the broiler has probably died from PHS, even if there is no fluid in the body or heart sac.

Control: Reducing the birds' metabolic oxygen requirement by slowing growth or reducing feed can prevent ascites caused by PHS. Environmental temperature, humidity, and air movement should be controlled to prevent excessive loss of body heat, particularly in the early neonatal period. Ascites caused by other factors (eg, sodium, lung damage, liver damage, etc) can be prevented by avoiding the etiologic agents involved. Altitudes >3,000 ft (900 m) are unsatisfactory for meat-type chickens, and growth must be slowed to prevent mortality. More care to prevent chilling is also necessary at higher altitudes.

BREAST BLISTERS

In chickens and turkeys, a bursa lined with synovial membrane normally exists over the anterior projection of the keel bone. When this bursa becomes inflamed by trauma or infection, fluid or exudate accumulates and appears as a fluid-filled blister 1-3 cm in diameter. Causes of trauma to this bursa include poor feathering, hard flooring, and leg weakness, which is associated with increased recumbency. Some young turkeys have pointed keels, which can lead to increased bursal trauma, but as the size of their breast muscle increases and trauma decreases, lesions may regress. Infectious causes of sternal bursitis include *Mycoplasma synoviae*, *Staphylococcus*, and *Pasteurella* spp.

BREAST BUTTONS

These are lesions found in a similar location to breast blisters. They have a hard crust on the surface and a core of dead skin and granulomatous reaction extending into the subadjacent subcutis. Their etiology is not well defined but they are not due to the causes listed above for breast blisters. Rather they may be chemical burns due to prolonged contact of poorly feathered skin with wet litter containing ammonia or toxins.

CANNIBALISM

Cannibalism is an abnormal behavior of chickens and turkeys most often manifested as vent-picking or picking at unfeathered skin on the head, comb, wattles, or toes. No single cause has been identified, but overcrowding, excessive light intensity, and nutritional imbalances are directly correlated with its occurrence. Additionally, in overly fat pullets entering egg production or hens in production, mucosa will protrude from the vent during and after egg laying, and this red tissue will attract pecking. Other factors that predispose to cannibalism are insufficient feeder space, mineral and vitamin deficiencies, skin injuries, and failure to remove dead birds daily. Other than the loss of birds due to pecking trauma, cannibalism often leads to transmission of infectious diseases (eg, erysipelas) and botulism.

Control depends on correcting or reducing the above risk factors and trimming the sharp distal end of the upper beak to prevent pecking. Trimming of the tip of the beak distal to the nostrils is often done at 1 day of age and repeated between 6 and 12 wk of age in maturing pullets or turkeys. Cautery often is required to provide hemostasis.

FLUKE INFECTIONS

Modern poultry production methods have diminished the incidence of fluke infections, although the parasites persist in poultry allowed contact with snails or other hosts and in some wild birds.

Prosthogonimus macrorchis, the oviduct fluke of poultry, infects birds after they consume infective metacercariae in larval or mature dragonflies, the secondary host. The fluke matures in ~2 wk in the bursa of Fabricius or, in gallinaceous birds without a functional bursa (eg, chickens, turkeys, pheasants), in the oviduct.

Light infections without clinical signs appear in ducks and other birds with a functional bursa. In gallinaceous birds, heavy infections in the oviduct cause inappetence, droopiness, weight loss, calcareous cloacal discharge, depressed egg production, and an increase in soft-shelled eggs. Lesions range from mild inflammation to distention or rupture of the oviduct; death may result. Diagnosis by fecal examination is unreliable because fluke eggs are not consistently present. Adult flukes may appear in the bird's eggs or be found in the oviduct on necropsy.

To prevent fluke transmission, birds must be kept from feeding on dragonflies. There is no effective treatment approved for use in poultry. Carbon tetrachloride, a common remedy, is highly toxic to chickens and other birds.

Collyriclum faba, another common fluke in birds, appear as subcutaneous cysts 4-6 mm in diameter (usually containing 2 adults) anywhere on the body but more frequently near the vent in turkeys, chickens, and other birds. The cysts ooze an exudate, which attracts flies and predisposes to bacterial infection. Signs in young birds include locomotor difficulty and inappetence; death may result in heavy infections. The parasites can be removed surgically. The life cycle is unknown but probably involves snails and insects such as dragonflies or mayflies. Prevention of infection requires restricting birds from areas frequented by aquatic insects.

GOUT

Avian species excrete nitrogenous wastes as urates bound in colloidal form with mucus in their urine. Renal disease decreases the clearance of uric acid from the blood, which results in acute or chronic hyperuricemia, and the excess uric acid precipitates on either visceral or articular surfaces (gout). Urate deposits are white and semisolid and must be differentiated from yellow fibrinous or purulent inflammatory exudates that are secondary to infectious causes such as synovitis, peritonitis, perihepatitis, and pericarditis.

Acute urate deposition occurs after rapidly progressing renal failure, or as a terminal event with acute decompensation of chronic renal disease. Deposits develop most commonly on the pericardium, peritoneum, and liver capsule, and rarely on synovial surfaces of joints and tendons. They are usually present for too short a time to induce significant inflammation. Most clinical cases of acute renal failure and urate deposition in commercial poultry are due to dehydration, ingestion of feed containing >3% calcium by nonlaying chickens, renal infection by nephrotropic strains of infectious bronchitis virus, or infection with avian nephritis virus. Other avian species commonly develop visceral deposits secondary to nephrotoxin exposure, most commonly aminoglycoside antibiotics or heavy metals.

Chronic urate deposition is less common and occurs after longterm increases in serum levels of uric acid. Deposits develop on synovial membranes in the toes and wing joints and incite a chronic granulomatous reaction to urate crystals (tophi). Chronic urate deposition may be seen in chickens that have hereditary defects in uric acid metabolism or that are fed excessive protein.

Urolithiasis is common in older laying chickens. Brittle, white, staghorn calcium urate calculi form in one or both ureters. Most cases are due to feeding high-calcium laying feed to hens not in egg production, infection with infectious bronchitis virus, or severe vitamin A deficiency. If blockage is complete, acute postrenal failure develops, and birds die with acute urate deposition on visceral surfaces or less commonly in joint spaces. If blockage is incomplete or unilateral, chickens survive in compensated renal failure, and chronic urate deposits form in joint spaces.

PENDULOUS CROP

Incidence of pendulous crop is low in flocks of chickens and turkeys. The crop is visibly distended and contains foul-smelling fluid, feed, and litter. Digestion is impaired, and affected birds become thin or emaciated. If these birds survive, they often are condemned or trimmed at processing to reduce contamination by ingesta.

The etiology is not known, but a hereditary predisposition has been suggested in turkeys. Incidence may increase with erratic feed or water consumption. Experimentally feeding rations containing cerelose as a substitute for starch can cause pendulous crops. Vagus nerve damage has also been postulated as a cause. There is no known efficacious treatment.

ECTOPARASITES

BEDBUGS

Cimex lectularius is a common bloodsucking parasite in temperate and subtropical climates that attacks poultry, humans, and most other mammals. It is rare in modern laying operations, but breeding houses and pigeon lofts may become heavily infested. The life cycle may be completed in 4-6 wk or extend much longer because nymphs can withstand fasting for ~70 days, and adults for up to 12 mo. Feeding usually occurs at night. Bedbugs become engorged within 10 min, then hide in cracks and crevices. If attacked by large numbers of bedbugs, birds may become anemic. Bites are usually followed by swelling and itching due to the injection of saliva into the wound.

Control is best accomplished by thoroughly cleaning the houses, reducing hiding places for the bedbugs, and high-pressure spraying of the houses as for control of fowl ticks (*see* below).

FLEAS

The **sticktight flea**, *Echidnophaga gallinacea*, is unique among poultry fleas in that the adults become sessile parasites and usually remain attached to the skin of the head for days or weeks. The adult females forcibly eject their eggs so that they reach surrounding litter. The larvae develop best in sandy, well-drained litter. Hosts of the adult flea include chickens, turkeys, pigeons, pheasants, quail, humans, and many other mammals. Irritation and blood loss may cause anemia and death, particularly in young birds. The **Western hen flea**, *Ceratophyllus niger*, seems to be confined to the Pacific coast area of the USA. This flea actually breeds in droppings and feeds on birds only occasionally. The **European chick flea**, *C gallinae*, is widespread in the USA. It breeds in nests and litter and is on the birds only to feed. It attacks many other birds besides chickens.

The most important control measures are removing infested litter and dusting the litter surface with carbaryl, coumaphos, or malathion to kill immature fleas. Insect growth regulators such as methoprene are also effective. Sticktight fleas can be controlled by topical application of pyrethrin.

FLIES AND GNATS

Biting Midge

Culicoides spp (Ceratopogonidae) transmit a malaria-like organism, *Haemoproteus nettionis*, to wild and domestic ducks. They also transmit the skin mite *Myialges anchora* (Epidermoptidae).

Black Fly

Simulium spp (Simuliidae), also known as buffalo gnats and turkey gnats, are bloodsuckers and transmit leucocytozoonosis (p 2193) to ducks, turkeys, and other birds. They are most abundant in the north temperate and subarctic zones, but many species are found in tropical areas. They often attack in swarms and cause anemia and death of birds either directly or through disease transmission. Control is extremely difficult because immature stages are restricted to running water, which is often some distance from the poultry farm. Larval control can be achieved with applications of temephos, chlorphoxim, or *Bacillus thuringiensis israelensis* during early spring before adults emerge. Screens of 24 mesh per in. (2.54 cm) or smaller are required for adult control. Measures recommended for mosquito control in houses are applicable to black fly control.

Pigeon Fly

Pseudolynchia canariensis (Hippoboscidae) is an important parasite of pigeons in warm or tropical areas. It may transmit *Haemoproteus columbae*, which causes pigeon malaria. It may also cause heavy losses in squabs. The pigeon loft should be cleaned every 20 days, and squabs can be dusted with pyrethrum powder.

FOWL TICKS

Argas persicus is found worldwide in tropical and subtropical countries and is the vector of *Borrelia anserina* (spirochetosis, p 2219). In the USA, the *A persicus* complex has been divided to include *A sanchezi* and *A radiatus* in addition to *A persicus*. These ticks are particularly active in poultry houses during warm, dry weather. All stages may be found hiding in cracks and crevices during the day. Larvae can be found on the birds because they remain attached and feed for 2-7 days. Nymphs and adults feed at night in ~15-30 min. Nymphs feed and molt several times before reaching the adult stage. Adults feed repeatedly, and the females lay 50-100 eggs after each feeding. Adult females may live ≥4 yr without a blood meal.

In addition to being vectors of some poultry diseases (eg, spirochetosis, aegyptianellosis), fowl ticks produce anemia (most important), weight loss, depression, toxemia, and paralysis. Egg production decreases. Red spots can be seen on the skin where the ticks have fed. Because the ticks are nocturnal, the birds may show some uneasiness when roosting. Death is rare, but production may be severely depressed.

After houses are cleaned, walls, ceilings, cracks, and crevices should be treated thoroughly (using a high-pressure sprayer) with carbaryl, coumaphos, malathion, stirofos, or a mixture of stirofos and dichlorvos. Cracks and crevices should be filled in.

LICE

Avian lice, which belong to the order Mallophaga, have a life cycle of ~3 wk and normally feed on bits of skin or feather products. Lice may live for several months on the host but remain alive only for ~1 wk off the host. Humans and other mammals may harbor avian lice, but only temporarily.

In intensive poultry systems, the most common and economically important louse to both chickens and turkeys is *Menacanthus stramineus*, the chicken body louse. It punctures soft quills near their base or gnaws the skin at the base of the feathers and feeds on the blood. Chickens are less commonly infested with *Menopon gallinae* (on feather shafts), *Lipeurus caponis* (mainly on the wing feathers), *Cuclotogaster heterographus* (mainly on the head and neck), *Goniocotes gallinae* (very small, in the fluff), *Goniodes gigas* (the large chicken louse), *Goniodes dissimilis* (the brown chicken louse), *Menacanthus cornutus* (the body louse), *Uchida pallidula* (the small body louse), or *Oxylipeurus dentatus*. Turkeys may also be infested with *Chelopistes meleagridis* (the large turkey louse), *Oxylipeurus polytrapezius* (the slender turkey louse), or *Menacanthus stramineus* (the chicken body louse).

Because lice transfer from one bird species to another when the hosts are in close contact, other domestic and caged birds may be infested with species of Mallophaga that are usually host-specific.

Heavy populations of the chicken body louse decrease reproductive potential in males, egg production in females, and weight gain in growing chickens. The skin irritations are also sites for secondary bacterial infections. Other species of lice are not highly pathogenic to mature birds but may be fatal to chicks. Examination of birds, particularly around the vent and under the wings, reveals eggs or moving lice on the skin or feathers.

Lice are usually introduced to a farm through infested equipment (eg, crates or egg flats) or by galliform birds. Lice are best controlled on caged chickens or turkeys by spraying with pyrethroids, carbaryl, coumaphos, malathion, or stirofos. Birds on the floor are more easily treated by scattering carbaryl, coumaphos, malathion, or stirofos dust on the litter.

MITES

The most economically important of the many external parasites of poultry are mites of the families Dermanyssidae (chicken mite, northern fowl mite, and tropical fowl mite) and Trombiculidae (turkey chigger).

Chicken Mite
(Red mite, Roost mite, Poultry mite)

Dermanyssus gallinae infests chickens, turkeys, pigeons, canaries, and various wild birds. While rare in modern commercial cage-layer operations, it is found in breeder and small farm flocks. Chicken mites are nocturnal feeders that hide during the day under manure, on roosts, and in cracks and crevices of the chicken house, where they deposit eggs. Populations develop rapidly during the warmer months and more slowly in cold weather; the life cycle may be completed in only 1 wk. A house may remain infested for 6 mo after birds are removed.

Transmission of the chicken mite, as well as the northern fowl mite and the tropical fowl mite (*see* below), is by mite dispersion or by contact with infested birds, animals, or inanimate objects. In the integrated poultry industry, mites are dispersed most frequently on inanimate objects such as egg flats, crates, or coops, or by personnel going from house to house or farm to farm.

Heavy infestations of either chicken mites or northern fowl mites decrease reproductive potential in males, egg production in females, and weight gain in young birds. Chicken mites may be found in the chicken houses during the day, particularly in cracks or where roost poles touch supports, or on birds at night. Northern fowl mites are found on eggs or by parting feathers in the vent area.

Obtaining mite-free birds and using good sanitation practices are important to prevent a buildup of mite populations. Once poultry have been infested with northern fowl mites, control may be achieved by spraying or dusting the birds and litter with carbaryl, coumaphos, malathion, stirofos, or a pyrethroid compound in areas where the parasites have not developed resistance to these chemicals. Miticide spray treatments must be applied with sufficient force to penetrate the feathers in the vent area. Nicotine sulfate is an effective fumigant for mites but is particularly hazardous. Pyrethrins and piperonyl butoxide are initially active but have poor residual killing power. For control of chicken mites, in addition to treating the birds, the inside of the house and all hiding places for the mite (such as roosts, behind nest boxes, and cracks and crevices) must be treated thoroughly using a high-pressure sprayer. Dimethoate and fenthion may be used as residual house sprays when poultry are not present. Systemic control with ivermectin (1.8-5.4 mg/kg) or moxidectin (8 mg/kg) is effective for short periods, but the high dosages are expensive, close to toxic levels, and require repeated use.

Common Chigger

Trombicula alfreddugesi and other chigger species (harvest mites, red bugs) infest birds as well as humans and other mammals. Heavily parasitized birds become droopy, refuse to eat, and may die from starvation and exhaustion. Larvae may be found either singly or in clusters on the ventral portion of the birds. Control on the range is aided by keeping the grass cut short and dusting with sulfur or malathion.

Depluming Mite

Neocnemidocoptes gallinae burrow into the epidermis at the base of feather shafts and cause intense irritation and feather pulling in chickens, pheasants, pigeons, and geese in spring and summer. Affected birds should be isolated and treated with ivermectin.

Feather Mite

Most feather mites belong to the families Analgidae (Analgesidae), Pterolichidae, and Proctophyllodidae and are rare on modern poultry ranches. They do little economic damage but may reduce egg production via malnutrition, feather loss, and dermatitis. Affected birds should be dusted with pyrethrin or carbaryl powder.

Northern Fowl Mite

Ornithonyssus sylviarum is the most important parasite of caged layers and breeding chickens in the USA and is a serious pest of chickens throughout the temperate zone of other countries. On turkeys, it is second in importance only to the turkey chigger in areas where the turkey chigger is found. It has been reported from many species of birds and from rats, mice, and humans; however, fertile populations are reported only on birds. Northern fowl mites are obligate bloodsucking parasites that normally spend their entire life cycle (~1 wk) on the host. Off the host, mites may live up to 2 mo, depending on temperature and relative humidity. In heavy infestations, the feathers, particularly in the vent area, are blackened. The mites, their eggs, cast skins, and excrement can be seen on the feathers and skin of the bird when the feathers are parted, and the skin may be scabbed and cracked. Mites are often seen on the eggs.

For clinical findings and control, *see* CHICKEN MITE, above.

Scaly Leg Mite

Knemidocoptes mutans is a small, spherical, sarcoptic mite that usually tunnels into the tissue under the scales of the legs. It is rare in modern poultry facilities, but when found, it is usually on older birds on which the irritation and exudation cause the legs to become thickened, encrusted, and unsightly. This mite may occasionally attack the comb and wattles. The entire life cycle is in the skin; transmission is by contact.

For control, affected birds should be culled or isolated, and houses cleaned and sprayed frequently as recommended for the chicken mite (*see* above). Individual birds should be treated with oral or topical ivermectin.

Subcutaneous Mite

Laminosioptes cysticola is a small parasite that is most often diagnosed by observing white to yellowish caseocalcareous nodules ~1-3 mm in diameter in the subcutis. Careful examination of the skin and subcutis of birds under a dissecting microscope frequently reveals the mites. Destroying the bird has been the best control for this parasite, but ivermectin may be effective.

Tropical Fowl Mite

Ornithonyssus bursa is distributed throughout the warmer regions of the world and has been reported in Texas, Florida, Illinois, Indiana, Maryland, and New York. It closely resembles the northern fowl mite (*see* above) in its biology and habits but lays a greater proportion of its eggs in the nest. Hosts include chickens, turkeys, ducks, pigeons, sparrows, starlings, mynah birds, and humans. Western equine encephalomyelitis virus has been recovered from this mite.

For clinical findings and control, *see* CHICKEN MITE, above.

Turkey Chigger

The larvae of *Neoschongastia americana* are parasitic on numerous birds. Across the southern USA, they are the major pest of turkeys ranged on heavy clay soils in the summer. The chiggers feed in groups of up to 100 mites/lesion for 8-15 days. Turkeys may have 25-30 lesions each. One lesion, 3 mm in diameter, may cause significant downgrading at market time. To prevent downgrading, turkeys must be protected for ≥4 wk before marketing.

Sprays or dusts of malathion or chlorpyrifos on turkey ranges control chiggers. A preventive measure now used in many turkey-growing areas includes a shift from range to confinement rearing, or use of sheds to provide shade.

MOSQUITOS

Mosquitos that feed on poultry usually belong to the genera *Culex*, *Aedes*, or *Psorophora*. Mosquitos may transmit several diseases, and large numbers decrease egg production or cause death. Virus is transmitted from infected birds to other birds primarily by mosquitos, although it has been transmitted directly from bird to bird in the laboratory. It has been found in >110 species of birds in America, including chickens, turkeys, pigeons, budgerigars, cockatiels, ducks, finches, and birds of prey. (*See* WEST NILE VIRUS, p 2289.)

Removal of mosquito-breeding habitats by emptying water-filled containers, clearing pool and pond edges of emergent vegetation, draining swampy areas, and filling low areas that collect water are the best physical control measures. Insecticidal control involves chemicals such as malathion, propoxur, permethrin, chlorpyrifos, or temephos. Insect growth regulators such as methoprene and diflubenzuron are also effective. Microbial control uses *Bacillus thuringiensis israelensis*. Screening to prevent mosquito entry, residual wall sprays, or fogging within poultry houses also aids in control.

FOWLPOX

FOWLPOX IN CHICKENS AND TURKEYS

Fowlpox is a slow-spreading viral infection of chickens and turkeys characterized by proliferative lesions in the skin (cutaneous form) that progress to thick scabs and by lesions in the upper GI and respiratory tracts (diphtheritic form). It is seen worldwide.

Etiology and Epidemiology: The large DNA virus (an avipoxvirus, family Poxviridae) is highly resistant and may survive for several years in dried scabs. Field and vaccine strains have only minor differences in their genomic profiles, although the strains can be differentiated to some extent by restriction endonuclease analysis, and immunoblotting.

Recently, molecular analyses of vaccine and field strains of fowlpox viruses have shown some significant differences. The virus is present in large numbers in the lesions and is usually transmitted by contact through abrasions of the skin. Skin lesions (scabs) shed from the recovering birds in poultry houses can become a source of aerosol infection. Mosquitos and other biting insects may serve as mechanical vectors. Transmission within flocks is rapid when mosquitos are plentiful. Some affected birds may become carriers, and the disease may be reactivated by stress (eg, moulting) or by immunosuppression due to other infections. The disease tends to persist for extended periods in multiple-age poultry complexes.

Clinical Findings: Only a few birds develop lesions at one time. Lesions are prominent in some birds and may significantly decrease flock performance. The cutaneous form is characterized by nodular lesions on various parts of the unfeathered skin of chickens and on the head and upper neck of turkeys. Generalized lesions of feathered skin may also be seen. In some cases, lesions are limited chiefly to the feet and legs. The lesion is initially a raised, blanched, nodular area that enlarges, becomes yellowish, and progresses to a thick, dark scab. Multiple lesions usually develop and often coalesce. Lesions in various stages of development may be found on the same bird. Localization around the nostrils may cause nasal discharge. Cutaneous lesions on the eyelids may cause complete closure of one or both eyes.

In the diphtheritic form, lesions develop on the mucous membranes of the mouth, esophagus, pharynx, larynx, and trachea (wetpox or fowl diphtheria). Occasionally, lesions are seen almost exclusively in one or more of these sites. Caseous patches firmly adherent to the mucosa of the larynx and mouth or proliferative masses may develop. Mouth lesions interfere with feeding. Tracheal lesions cause difficulty in respiration and may simulate infectious laryngotracheitis (p 2305) in chickens. Laryngeal and tracheal lesions in chickens must be differentiated from those of laryngotracheitis.

Often, the course of the disease in a flock is protracted. Extensive infection in a layer flock results in decreased egg production. Cutaneous infections alone ordinarily cause low or moderate mortality, and these flocks generally return to normal production after recovery. Mortality is usually high in the generalized or diphtheritic form.

Diagnosis: Cutaneous infections usually produce characteristic gross and microscopic lesions. When only small lesions are present, it is often difficult to distinguish them from abrasions caused by fighting. Microscopic examination of affected tissues stained with H&E reveals eosinophilic cytoplasmic inclusion bodies. Cytoplasmic inclusions are also detectable by fluorescent antibody and immunohistochemical methods. The elementary bodies in the inclusion bodies can be detected in smears from lesions stained by the Gimenez method. Viral particles with typical poxvirus morphology can be demonstrated by negative-staining electron microscopy as well as in ultrathin sections of the lesions. The virus can be isolated by inoculating chorioallantoic membrane of developing chicken embryos, susceptible birds, or cell cultures of avian origin. Chicken embryos (9-12 days old) are the preferred and most convenient host for virus isolation.

Field isolates and vaccine strains of fowlpox virus can be compared by restriction endonuclease analysis of viral genomes. This method is useful for comparing closely related DNA genomes. However, because of the large size of the genome, minor differences are difficult to detect by this method. Detailed genetic analysis reveals differences between vaccine strains and field strains responsible for outbreaks of fowlpox in previously vaccinated chicken flocks. While vaccine strains of fowlpox virus contain remnants of long terminal repeats of reticuloendotheliosis virus (REV), most field strains contain full-length REV in their genome.

Nucleic acid probes derived from cloned genomic fragments of fowlpox virus can also be used for diagnosis. This procedure is especially useful for differentiation of the diphtheritic form of fowlpox (involving the trachea) from infectious laryngotracheitis.

PCR can be used to amplify genomic DNA sequences of various sizes using specific primers. This procedure is useful when an extremely small amount of viral DNA is present in the sample. PCR has been used effectively to differentiate field and vaccine strains of fowlpox virus.

Recently, 2 monoclonal antibodies that recognize different fowlpox virus antigens have been developed. These monoclonal antibodies can be used for strain differentiation by immunoblotting.

The complete sequence of the fowlpox virus genome has been identified recently and is useful in comparing the sequences of selected genes of other avian poxviruses.

Prevention and Treatment: Where pox is prevalent, chickens and turkeys should be vaccinated with live-embryo or cell-culture-propagated virus. The most widely used vaccines are attenuated fowlpox virus and pigeonpox virus isolates of high immunogenicity and low pathogenicity. A turkeypox vaccine has been developed to control pox in turkey flocks in which fowlpox vaccine has been ineffective. This virus appears to be immunologically different from fowlpox virus. In high-risk areas, vaccination with an attenuated vaccine of cell-culture origin in the first few weeks of life and revaccination at 12-16 wk is often sufficient. Health of birds, extent of exposure, and type of operation determine the timings of vaccinations. Because the infection spreads slowly, vaccination is often useful in limiting spread in affected flocks if administered when <20% of the birds have lesions. Because passive immunity may interfere with multiplication of vaccine virus, progeny from recently vaccinated or recently infected flocks should be vaccinated only after passive immunity has declined. Vaccinated birds should be examined 1 wk later for swelling and scab formation ("take") at the site of vaccination. Absence of "take" indicates lack of potency of vaccine, passive or acquired immunity, or improper vaccination. Revaccination with another serial lot of vaccine may be indicated.

Naturally infected or vaccinated birds develop humoral as well as cell-mediated immune responses. Humoral immune responses can be measured by ELISA or virus neutralization tests.

POX IN OTHER AVIAN SPECIES

Infections with avian poxvirus have been seen in a variety of wild and pet birds. Some isolates are primarily infectious for only the homologous host, whereas others are infectious for one or more additional species. Classification has usually been based on host pathogenicity or cross-protection studies. Canarypox infection is usually severe, and mortality sometimes approaches 100%. Cutaneous lesions may develop, as may systemic infection with cytoplasmic inclusion bodies detected in lesions on histologic examination. A commercial canarypox virus vaccine for canaries is available in the USA. Poxvirus infection in psittacines may also be severe, especially in blue-fronted Amazon parrots. Poxviruses isolated from psittacines appear to be antigenically different from poxviruses of other avian species.

Genomic profiles of canarypox, mynahpox, and quailpox viruses show marked differences from fowlpox virus when their DNA is compared after restriction endonuclease digestion. Quailpox virus shows marked antigenic differences from fowlpox virus and, although some cross-reacting antigens are present, provides limited or no cross-protection against fowlpox virus. A quailpox virus vaccine is available commercially. Avianpox virus infection has been considered as a population-limiting factor in endangered Hawaiian forest birds. Avianpox viruses isolated from Hawaiian crows (*Corvus hawaiiansis*), Hawaiian geese (*Branta sandvicensis*), Palila (*Loxiodes bailleui*), and Apapane species (*Himatione sanguinea*) are different from each other as well as from fowlpox virus. Similarly, a poxvirus isolated from an Andean condor (*Vultur gryphus*) at the San Diego Zoo is antigenically, genetically, and biologically different from fowlpox virus.

GANGRENOUS DERMATITIS

(Necrotic dermatitis, Gangrenous cellulitis, Clostridial dermatomyositis)

Gangrenous dermatitis is characterized by a sudden onset, sharp increase in mortality, and gangrenous necrosis of the skin over the wings, thighs, breast, and head. It occurs sporadically in chickens 4-16 wk old, affects broiler and layer replacement stocks, and occasionally causes outbreaks in turkeys.

Etiology, Transmission, and Epidemiology: Gangrenous skin necrosis may be associated with various aerobic and anaerobic bacteria; however, *Clostridium septicum*, *Clostridium perfringens* type A, and *Staphylococcus aureus*, either singly or in combination are most often involved. Combined infections are often more severe. Young chicks immunosuppressed by infectious bursal disease (p 2239) or chick anemia virus are predisposed. The disease may occur secondary to avian adenovirus or reticuloendothelial virus infections as well. Skin lesions due to trauma, wet litter, picking, or treading wounds may provide entry sites for causative bacteria. The disease has been reproduced by SC or IM inoculation of *S aureus*, *C septicum*, or *C perfringens* type A. Inoculated chickens develop gangrenous necrosis of the skin and underlying musculature and can die within 12-72 hr. Systemic effects arise from invading bacteria and their elaborated exotoxins.

Clinical Findings and Lesions: The first sign is usually a sudden dramatic increase in mortality in the affected flock. Overall mortality is 10-60%. Affected chickens are extremely depressed, lethargic, and prostrate, and die within 8-24 hr. Red to black patches of moist, gangrenous skin are seen over the breast, abdomen, wing tips, or thighs. Feather loss or sloughing of the epidermis is common. When clostridial infection occurs, palpation of the affected areas often reveals crepitation due to gas bubbles in the subcutis and musculature. At necropsy, there is an accumulation of gaseous, serosanguineous fluid in the subcutis, and the musculature has a pale cooked appearance. The liver and spleen are enlarged and may contain infarcts or pale focal areas of necrosis. The kidneys are usually swollen, and the lungs may be congested and edematous or necrotic. Atrophy of the bursa of Fabricius may be found in birds that were exposed to infectious bursal disease virus in the first few weeks after hatching.

Diagnosis: Histopathologic demonstration of gangrenous necrosis with numerous coccoid bacteria or large, gram-positive rods with or without spores in affected tissues is sufficient to confirm a clinical diagnosis. Isolation of the etiologic agent (*C septicum*, *C perfringens*, or *S aureus*), together with the history and clinical findings, differentiate gangrenous dermatitis from exudative diathesis and other diseases involving the skin.

Treatment and Control: Maintaining proper litter conditions, minimizing traumatic injury, and controlling cannibalism can help prevent the disease. A program to vaccinate breeders against infectious bursal disease to establish healthy, immunocompetent, replacement stock has also been useful. Administration of oxytetracycline in the feed at 0.02% rapidly reduces mortality in field outbreaks of clostridial infections. Chlortetracycline, oxytetracycline, erythromycin, or penicillin in the water have proved beneficial for staphylococcal infections, depending on the results of antibiotic sensitivity testing.

DISORDERS OF THE SKELETAL SYSTEM

Skeletal disorders cause lameness from biomechanical dysfunction and result in poor growth, culled birds, increased mortality (caused by starvation and dehydration), and carcass condemnation and downgrading. Production characteristics of modern poultry lines (eg, body weight in broiler chickens, egg production in laying hens) place high demands on the skeletal system, and inadequacies in nutrition or husbandry will often result in skeletal diseases. Skeletal disorders may be primarily infectious or noninfectious; both may be seen concurrently within a flock. Before postmortem examination, flocks should be assessed; live, lame birds should be examined, and an opinion as to general flock health, litter quality, and management should be formed. Serum samples may be collected for viral and mycoplasmal serology.

Noninfectious Skeletal Disorders

Rotational (Torsional) and Angular (Valgus/Varus) Deformity: These deformities often are seen as distinct flock problems. Bones all exhibit some degree or combination of lateral, medial, anterior, or posterior bend. They also show some torsion (rotation) about their long axis. The most common abnormalities are valgus deformity of the intertarsal joint and excessive external rotation of the tibiotarsus. Valgus/varus deformity is associated with rapid growth and little exercise. The incidence can be reduced by slowing growth rate at an early age by feed restriction or lighting programs. It may also be due to chondrodystrophy due to B vitamin or trace mineral deficiencies. Rotated tibia has been a major problem in turkeys and a minor problem in Leghorns and guinea fowl. The cause is poorly understood but has been associated with early rickets. Poor mineralization of the bone, as in rickets, increases the ease of deformation of the bone and therefore the incidence and severity of deformities. Rickets may be associated with nutritional deficiencies, enteric disease, or malabsorption.

Spondylopathies: Vertebral deformities and/or displacements (spondylopathies) are common in thoracic vertabrae, particularly the fifth or free thoracic vertabrae. Spondylolisthesis is the most common deformity, but incidence is low in most flocks of broiler chickens. It causes posterior paralysis due to spinal cord compression.

Dyschondroplasia: Dyschondroplastic lesions are masses of avascular cartilage extending from the growth plate into the metaphysis and are attributed to the failure of chondrocytes to differentiate. This results in a focal thickening of the growth plate in the proximal tibiotarsus (tibial dyschondroplasia) or sometimes the proximal tarsometatarsus. The lesion in the proximal tibiotarsus is often associated with anterior bowing of the tibiotarsus and sometimes fractures below the plug of cartilage. Factors shown to influence the incidence and severity of dyschondroplasia include genetic selection, calcium:phosphorus ratios in feed, metabolic acidosis through excess chloride in feed, acid/base balance, and mycotoxins. In a flock of modern broilers, the cause may be marginal inadequacies in dietary calcium or a calcium:phosphorus imbalance.

Rickets: Rickets develops in growing birds due to deficiency of calcium or phosphorus (p 2320) or insufficient vitamin D (p 2330). Malabsorption can also cause a mineral deficiency. In rickets, a failure of bone mineralization leads to flexibility of long bones. Bone ashing and estimates of calcium and phosphorus content combined with bone pathology are useful diagnostic tools. Bacterial infections are common in bones with rickets.

Plantar Pododermatitis: Ulceration of the metatarsal and digital footpads is a common cause of lameness in meat-type poultry. Wet or poor quality litter is the common cause, although a biotin deficiency will cause plantar pododermatitis even when litter quality is good. Ulcerated footpads may become secondarily infected and caked with litter.

Osteopenia (Osteoporosis and Osteomalacia): Osteopenia is a consequence of osteoporosis, a deficiency in the quantity of fully mineralized, structural bone. Cage layer fatigue describes a syndrome in which laying hens become paralyzed in their cages. The bones of the birds are osteopenic. The sternum is often deformed, and fractures causes infolding of the ribs at the junctions of the sternal and vertebral portions. Fractures can also occur in the long bones and vertebrae. The medullary bone is osteomalacic. The syndrome is due in part to a lack of exercise and high egg production, but severe problems are associated with inadequate calcium, phosphorus, or vitamin D. Calcium requirements during growth and before and during lay vary markedly. Sources of calcium that enable the slow release of mineral, such as oyster shell, appear to give the best results.

Amyloidosis: Extensive amyloid arthropathy is primarily caused by *Enterococcus faecalis*, but not by all isolates. Clinical cases are seen only occasionally and are most frequently seen in the hock joint of a few replacement pullets or broiler breeders. Cases may be attributed to the contamination of a previously sterile vaccine diluent with *E faecalis* during administration (eg, Marek's vaccine in day-old chicks).

Infectious Skeletal Disorders

Coagulase-positive staphylococci (*see also* STAPHYLOCOCCOSIS, p 2264) are frequently responsible for bacterial infections in the bones and joints of broiler chickens. *Mycoplasma synoviae* (p 2245) may also play a role in infectious bone disorders and can be monitored serologically.

In broilers, bacterial infections are most common in the proximal femur and proximal tibiotarsus when the birds are >22 days of age. In the proximal femur, the condition is also referred to as femoral head necrosis. Recent reports indicate this is the most common cause of lameness in broilers. The etiology appears dependent on vertically transmitted staphylococci in combination with a challenge by immunosuppressive viruses (eg, INFECTIOUS BURSAL DISEASE, p 2239). Floor eggs have been shown to be common carriers of staphylococci, so their use should be minimal. A high standard of hatchery hygiene can reduce this risk. Formaldehyde fumigation within the hatchers is also likely to help. In addition, hatchery fluff samples can be examined to monitor for contamination with staphylococci.

Staphylococcal infections in joints and tendons are also seen in breeders. Outbreaks are likely to be due to management practices or other diseases causing stress and/or joint and tendon trauma (eg, competition over feed space, heavy coccidiosis challenge). Insufficient lighting in the rear of cages appears to predispose to an increase in bacterial tenosynovitis.

Escherichia coli is often responsible for flock outbreaks of arthritis and osteomyelitis in broiler chickens and turkeys. These outbreaks may be associated with respiratory disease. *Pasteurella multocida* has been isolated from arthritic joints in broiler breeders following use of live vaccines. Other sporadic causes of arthritis in poultry include *Salmonella* spp and *Streptobacillus moniliformis*. Viral arthritis due to a reovirus has been reported as a significant cause of lameness in some parts of the world (*see* VIRAL ARTHRITIS, p 2284). The virus is egg transmitted. Vaccines against the condition have been developed.

Control: Bacterial bone and joint infections often show a poor response to antibiotic treatment. Antibiotics may be used to control the bacteremia contributing to new cases and to modify the bacterial flora within a flock. When individual birds are of high value, injections of long-acting antibiotics may improve some less severe cases. Control requires minimizing sources of infection and stock susceptibility.

MYOPATHIES

Minimal Myopathy

A minimal myopathy is seen in otherwise normal meat-type poultry. Affected individuals show no clinical signs and their muscles are grossly normal, but microscopically there is mild myofiber degeneration and fat accumulation between myofibers. Focal or multifocal scattered myofibers are hyalinized and mineralized. More severe examples of this lesion contain individual myofiber necrosis, increased fat, and fibroplasia between fibers. No specific cause has been determined for these minimal changes.

Deep Pectoral Myopathy
(Degenerative myopathy, Green muscle disease)

In this myopathy, there is degeneration, necrosis, and fibrosis of the deep pectoral (supracoracoideus) muscle in heavy meat birds (chickens, turkeys), most often turkey breeder hens. Flock incidence as high as 25% has been reported with few birds developing the disease before 24 wk of age. The major loss is from downgrading or condemnation at processing.

The myopathy may be unilateral or bilateral with the central one-third to two-thirds of the muscle affected. Early, the involved muscle is pale, swollen, and edematous. Later, affected tissue is sharply demarcated from adjacent, viable muscle; eventually, it is encapsulated, resulting in dry, green, necrotic muscle enclosed in a thick fibrous capsule.

The defect can be identified by a depression of the breast over affected muscles or by transillumination of carcasses at slaughter.

The deep pectoral muscle functions to elevate the wing. Although well-developed in modern meat birds, it is little used. After episodes of prolonged wing flapping (such as occurs during handling), when lame birds use their wings to assist ambulation, or when the bird is placed on its back, the muscle swells within the dense fascial covering normally surrounding it. This swelling collapses vessels supplying the muscle, leading to ischemia, tissue hypoxia, and muscle necrosis. The lesion can be produced artificially by stimulating the deep pectoral muscle to contract and can be prevented by surgically opening the fascial sheath covering the muscle.

Incidence can be decreased by careful handling of susceptible birds to prevent excessive wing flapping and, as a longterm method, by selective breeding because the condition is heritable. Supplementing rations with selenium, vitamin E, or methionine has not influenced incidence.

Nutritional Myopathy

Nutritional myopathy in poultry, waterfowl, and ostriches is selenium-responsive. Cysteine also may have a beneficial effect in chicks. Lesions have been reported in skeletal, heart, and smooth muscle (gizzard and intestine) of ducks, turkeys, and chickens. Arsenic, zinc, copper, and other metals are antagonistic to selenium, and exposure to these other metals may precipitate outbreaks. Gross lesions, with pale foci or streaking, are similar to those of nutritional myopathies in mammals. Microscopic changes include focal or widespread myofiber swelling, edema, hyalinization, mineralization, degeneration, and lysis with infiltration of macrophages and heterophils. Hypercellularity from proliferation of sarcolemmal nuclei may be prominent if regeneration is occurring. Poultry feeds in many parts of the world contain added selenium at 0.1-0.4 ppm to prevent this myopathy.

Toxic Myopathy

Ionophore toxicity causes muscle damage with incoordination, leg weakness, diarrhea, dyspnea, and reduced feed intake and weight. Stunting may also occur. Type I (red or fat-metabolizing) fibers are most susceptible. Lesions may also be found in heart and gizzard muscle. Adult birds (chickens, turkeys, ratites) and birds with no previous exposure are more sensitive to ionophore coccidiostats. Gross and histologic changes are similar to those of nutritional myopathy (see p 948). Toxicity of ionophores is increased if they are used in conjunction with tiamulin, erythromycin, or chloramphenicol.

Cassia (coffee weed) toxicity can produce clinical signs and gross and histologic changes in muscle similar to those seen in ionophore toxicity.

Exertional Myopathy

Myopathy induced by muscle activity develops when local muscle hypoxia or metabolic byproducts of muscle metabolism (lactic acid), or both, exceed the capacity of the vascular system to remove them. These substances accumulate locally, causing muscle and vascular damage. Mediators of inflammation are activated, resulting in edema and hyperemia.

Exertional myopathy can be caused by isometric muscle activity (eg, transport, capture, or restraint myopathy as with turkey leg edema syndrome) or kinetic muscle activity (eg, subgastrocnemial ischemic myopathy of male broiler breeders, polymyopathy of male turkeys). Early gross lesions include pallor with edema or bloodstained transudate. There is swelling, degeneration, necrosis, and mineralization of muscle fibers, with edema, hemorrhage, and infiltration of heterophils and macrophages.

Mechanically Induced Myopathy

Avascular necrosis caused by pressure in heavy birds that are down because of lameness or leg deformity is seen occasionally and occurs most frequently in the breast muscle. On gross examination, the tissue is firm and pale. Histologic examination reveals swelling, hyalinization, and necrosis of fibers with edema, heterophils, and macrophages at the periphery.

Rupture of the gastrocnemius tendon is common in meat-type chickens, particularly roasters and breeders, and rare in turkeys. The rupture is due to application of excess weight to tendons that have been previously damaged (most frequently by reoviral, staphylococcal, or toxic tendonitis) with subsequent intra- and peritendonal fibroplasia. This fibroplasia makes the tendon larger but weaker due to replacement of normal strong, dense tendon connective tissue with weak, dense, irregular tissue. Synechial connections between the tendon and its sheath may also be produced, limiting the tendon's range of motion. Application of normal or excess weight to these previously damaged tendons results in partial or complete tearing or rupture. Rupture of the tendon of one leg puts stress on the other tendon, and bilateral rupture is frequent. Affected birds are lame or "down on their hocks" (creepers). Hemorrhage from the injury is visible as red, blue, or green discoloration in the tissue above the hock on the back of the leg and results in condemnation of the affected part at processing (red-leg, green-leg). The ruptured tendon can be palpated as a hard mass on the back of the leg above the hock.

Transport Myopathy of Turkeys
(Leg edema syndrome)

Heavy toms are primarily affected, although transport myopathy also develops in hens, especially in flocks in the upper midwest of the USA. About 5% of all flocks are affected, and morbidity within the flock is 2-70%. Transport myopathy occurs sporadically but is most common during fall and early winter. A high incidence has occurred in sequential flocks from the same farm. Incidence is likely to be higher in flocks raised in confinement than in range flocks.

The cause is unknown, but transport myopathy is associated with increased body size and weight, increased transport time to processing plant, cool ambient temperatures, and valgus leg deformities. The pathogenesis is presumed to be due to impaired circulation; the resulting muscle ischemia and acute necrosis lead to edema that tends to be manifested in the large potential space in the subcutis of the medial thigh. Signs are rarely seen on the farm.

Often, only 1 leg is affected. No evidence of external trauma is seen. Skin over edematous subcutaneous tissue is pale, feather follicles are less visible, and the skin slips easily over underlying muscle when moved. Occasionally, there is crepitation. Affected areas are dark when the edematous areas contain blood. Typically, when lesions are cut, the edematous subcutis is a few to several millimeters thick and is amber, occasionally green, or rarely red. Purulent exudate is absent, which distinguishes transport myopathy from cellulitis. If hemorrhage is present, the adductor muscle usually is torn. Removal of affected legs at processing results in carcass downgrading. Microscopically, acute multifocal muscle necrosis is found, primarily in the adductor muscles. Sometimes, subacute or chronic lesions also are seen, which suggest earlier episodes of myopathy. Serum CK increases sharply between farm and processing.

Programs designed to improve leg strength and conformation and to reduce trauma during transportation help reduce the incidence. Supplemental vitamin E also may be useful. If possible, flocks with a high incidence of valgus leg deformities should be marketed early at a processing plant nearby.

Rupture of the Peroneus (Fibularis) Longus Muscle

The origin of the peroneus muscle is on the proximal end of the tibiotarsus and patellar tissue, with attachments to other muscles in that area. In turkeys, the insertion appears to be in 3 places. A small band of tissue from the medial side of the muscle runs to the lateral tibial condyle. The main muscle tendon crosses the lateral side of the hock and joins other tendons that extend the hock and may affect foot and toe movement. The muscle is thin and wide, covering the anterior and lateral surface of the leg. It has a heavy aponeurosis in which the tendon is embedded. Rupture of the aponeurosis and muscle occurs as a 1-2 cm horizontal wound on the anterior surface of the muscle. It occurs above the middle of the tibiotarsus at the top of the ossifying tendon where the tendon attaches to the muscle. Rupture occurs at 10-14 wk, the age at which turkey leg tendons become ossified, reducing the elasticity of the tissue in that location.

Incidence appears to be increasing. It is most frequent in females and may affect up to 5% of the flock. The separation of the muscle likely occurs slowly, caused by activity such as repeated springing, in turkeys that are becoming heavier and maturing earlier each year. The attachments of this muscle suggest that antagonistic activity is possible. Affected birds are not lame, but the resulting hemorrhage causes a red, blue, or green discoloration under the skin on the anterior of the drumstick ventral to the rupture. The affected portion is trimmed at processing.

VIRAL ARTHRITIS

(Reoviral infection, Tenosynovitis)

Reoviruses are ubiquitous in chickens and turkeys; some strains become viremic and localize in the large joints, resulting in arthritis, tendinitis, and synovitis. Most birds are thought to be susceptible to respiratory-intestinal strains of reoviruses. Chickens and, to a lesser degree, turkeys are susceptible to viral arthritis, which is seen worldwide. Reoviruses also have been associated with pericarditis and myocarditis, hydropericardium, pasting, malabsorption, and femoral head necrosis, although further study is needed to define their role. (*See also* MALABSORPTION SYNDROME, p 339.)

Transmission and Pathogenesis: The disease is egg-transmitted and is of short duration except when lateral transmission in a flock is prolonged. Respiratory and digestive infections may occur but are of short duration; however, the virus survives in tendon sheaths for extended periods. The virus is spread via aerosols, fomites, and mechanical means, and is resistant to heat and chemical inactivation.

Several antigenic subtypes of avian reoviruses have been identified; however, there appears to be significant cross-protection among most of the isolates or subtypes. Pathogenicity of the isolates varies widely. Serious outbreaks of viral arthritis are followed by a decreased incidence in later hatch groups of birds from the same parent flock. This may be related to decreased egg transmission and development of parental immunity. Day-old chicks are more susceptible than older birds when exposed by natural means. The earlier in life the chick is infected, the longer the virus persists in the tissues.

Clinical Findings: The arthritic form (tenosynovitis) usually is seen in broilers 4-8 wk old as unilateral or bilateral swellings of the tendons of the shank and above the hock; it can also be found in much older chickens. The birds walk with a stilted gait. In severely affected flocks, rupture of the gastrocnemius tendon is frequent, and many cull birds are seen around the feeders and waterers. Mortality is 2-10% and morbidity 5-50%. Severely affected birds rarely recover; less severely affected birds recover in 4-6 wk. The infection is inapparent in many birds. Feed efficiency and rate of gain are decreased.

Lesions: An acute, fulminating infection is occasionally seen in young chicks and embryos with cardiomegaly, hepatomegaly, and splenomegaly with necrotic foci. Edema of the tendons of the leg is marked, petechial hemorrhages develop in the synovial membranes above the hock, and fusion and calcification of the tendon bundles are common. Blood clots and hemorrhages are seen with rupture of the gastrocnemius tendon. Pitted erosions of the cartilage of the distal tibiotarsus are seen with flattening of the condyles. Histologically, the synovial cells are hypertrophied, hyperplastic, and infiltrated by lymphocytes and macrophages. The synovia contain heterophils and macrophages. Infiltration of heterophils or lymphocytes, or both, between myocardial fibers is a constant finding. However, the infiltrating heterophils are difficult to distinguish from the clusters of young, proliferating heterophils (ectopic myelopoiesis) that are present in the heart muscle of all young, rapidly growing broiler chickens.

Diagnosis: A presumptive diagnosis can be based on unilateral or bilateral swelling of the tendons of the shank and tendon bundle above the hock and on the inflammatory changes in the tendons and synovia described above. Virus from affected tissues can be isolated in primary kidney, liver, or lung cells, or in the yolk sac or chorioallantoic membrane of embryonating chicken eggs. The agar-gel-precipitin test is usually positive, and most birds are positive early in the infection. Virus neutralization tests and challenge of immunized chickens are used to detect the specific serotype. Culture procedures should be used to differentiate mycoplasmal and other bacterial infections. Other causes of lameness should be considered.

Treatment and Control: There is no treatment. Maternal antibody prevents early infection in chicks and should reduce or prevent egg transmission. Because egg transmission is the principal means of spread, it is desirable to have the breeder flock immune. Such a program should be directed to the serotypes present in the flock. Adult birds are less susceptible to clinical disease if exposed by natural routes.

AVIAN ENCEPHALOMYELITIS

(Epidemic tremor)

Avian encephalomyelitis is a worldwide viral disease of Japanese quail, turkeys, chickens, and pheasants, characterized by ataxia and tremor of the head, neck, and limbs. Ducklings, pigeons, and guinea fowl are susceptible to experimental infection. The causative picornavirus can be grown in chicken embryos from nonimmune hens. It is transmitted for ~1 wk through a portion of eggs laid by infected hens, and then spreads laterally in the hatcher or brooder to susceptible hatchmates.

Clinical Findings: Signs commonly appear at 7-10 days of age, although they may be present at hatching or delayed for several weeks. The main signs are unsteadiness, sitting on hocks, paresis, and even complete inability to move. Muscular tremors are best seen after exercising the bird; holding the bird on its back in the cupped hand helps in detection. Typically, about 5% of the flock is affected, although morbidity and mortality may be much higher. The disease in adult birds is inapparent except for a transient drop in egg production. The disease in turkeys is often milder than in chickens.

Lesions: No gross lesions of the nervous system are seen. Lymphocytic accumulations in the gizzard muscle may be visible as grayish areas. Lens opacities may develop weeks after infection. Microscopic lesions in the CNS consist of neuronal axon-type degeneration ("ghost" cells) in the brain, particularly in the brain stem and in the anterior horn cells of the spinal cord. Gliosis and lymphocytic perivascular cuffing can also be seen. Visceral microscopic lesions consist of lymphoid follicles in the muscular tissue of the gizzard, proventriculus, and myocardium, while numerous lymphoid follicles can be found in the pancreas.

Diagnosis: Avian encephalomyelitis must be differentiated from avian encephalomalacia (vitamin E deficiency), rickets, vitamin B_1 or B_2 deficiency, Newcastle disease, eastern encephalitis, Marek's disease, and encephalitis caused by bacteria, fungi (eg, aspergillosis), or mycoplasmas. Diagnosis is based on history, signs, and histologic study of brain, spinal cord, proventriculus, gizzard, and pancreas. Virus isolation in eggs free of avian encephalomyelitis antibody is sometimes necessary for confirmation. Serologic testing of paired samples is helpful, using virus neutralization or ELISA tests. Microscopic lesions are sparse and may not be found in infected adults.

Prevention and Treatment: Immunization of breeder pullets 10-15 wk old with a commercial live vaccine is advised to prevent vertical transmission of the virus to progeny and to provide them with maternal immunity against the disease. Vaccination of table-egg flocks is also advisable to prevent a temporary drop in egg production. Affected chicks and poults are ordinarily destroyed because few recover. A combination vaccine for fowlpox and avian encephalomyelitis for wing-web administration is widely used. The disease does not affect humans or other mammals.

BOTULISM

(Limberneck, Western duck sickness)

Botulism is an intoxication caused by ingesting *Clostridium botulinum* exotoxin or by absorbing toxin produced in the alimentary tract (toxico-infection). (*See also* BOTULISM, p 490.)

Etiology: *C botulinum* is a gram-positive, sporeforming, anaerobic bacterium that inhabits soils and marine and freshwater sediments. It is commonly found in the gut of poultry and wild birds and in litter, feed, and water in broiler chicken houses. Intoxications are sporadic in poultry, but massive mortality has occurred in waterfowl in western North America. Outbreaks in poultry and waterfowl are predominately caused by type C toxin, and types A and E are less frequently incriminated.

Type C intoxications are found in chickens, turkeys, ducks, and pheasants. However, the disease has been identified in 117 species of feral birds representing 22 families. Mammalian species affected by type C toxin include mink, ferrets, cattle, pigs, dogs, horses, laboratory rodents, and various zoo animals. Botulism was reported in ruminants fed poultry manure contaminated with *C botulinum* type C spores. The zoonotic potential of type C botulism is minimal. Only 4 poorly documented type C botulism intoxications have been reported in people, but cases have occurred in nonhuman primates.

Transmission, Epidemiology, and Pathogenesis: Ingested preformed toxin, absorbed into the blood, binds to nerve terminals and blocks release of acetylcholine. The result is flaccid muscle paralysis. Death is due to cardiac and respiratory arrest.

Toxin is elaborated in dead carcasses after postmortem release of the organism from the gut. Maggots acquire toxin from carcass tissues and, when eaten by scavenging poultry, serve as a source of neurotoxin. Alternatively, if toxin levels are sufficiently high in carcass tissues, cannibalism can initiate disease. Other feed sources have been implicated in outbreaks in backyard poultry flocks. Botulism in water fowl may result after ingesting dead invertebrates found in water that contains decaying vegetation.

Toxico-infectious botulism is reported to occur in intensively reared broiler flocks housed on litter. Mortality may range from a few birds to 40% of a flock. The conditions that allow toxin elaboration in the alimentary tract are not clearly understood because *C botulinum* can be recovered from normal chickens on farms without histories of outbreaks. However, two outbreaks of type *C botulinum* in commercial broiler flocks were associated with elevated iron content from feed and water sources. Iron promotes the proliferation of enteric bacteria, including *C botulinum*.

Clinical Findings: Clinical signs in poultry and wild birds are similar. Flaccid paralysis of the legs, wings, neck, and eyelids is seen. Paralytic signs progress cranially from the legs to include the wings, neck, and eyelids. "Limberneck," the common name of botulism, describes neck paralysis. In affected waterfowl, neck paralysis can lead to drowning. Affected chickens have ruffled feathers. Signs in broiler chickens may also include diarrhea with excess urates in the loose droppings.

Lesions: No characteristic gross lesions develop.

Diagnosis: Definitive diagnosis requires demonstration of the toxin in serum, liver homogenates, or crop or GI washings from morbid birds. Mice injected with samples of such material become paralyzed and die unless protected with specific typing serum.

Leg paralysis is the only sign in mild intoxications, which must be differentiated from Marek's disease, drug and chemical toxicities, or appendicular skeletal problems. In waterfowl, botulism must be differentiated from fowl cholera and chemical toxicities, especially lead poisoning.

Treatment and Prevention: Affected birds may recover without treatment. Numerous treatments have been reported, including use of bacitracin (100 g/ton in feed) or streptomycin (1 g/L in water), but none have been uniformly successful.

Collection and disposal of dead birds is important in preventing and limiting outbreaks, especially in pheasant and broiler chicken flocks. Fly control may reduce risk of toxic maggots in the environment. Some, but not all, recurrent outbreaks in broiler flocks may be prevented by cleaning and disinfecting with products effective against spore-forming bacteria. Disinfection around poultry houses is suggested because spores are found outside the houses and can be reintroduced into housing. Litter treatments, although not always effective, have included sodium bisulfate at 1 lb/1,000 sq ft (1 kg/200 sq m). In waterfowl outbreaks, ducks should be dispersed from affected areas and water levels stabilized. Elimination of large shallow areas may prevent conditions favorable for decay of vegetation and die-off of invertebrates.

Active immunization with inactivated type C bacterin-toxoids has been successful in pheasant operations but is not cost effective in commercial chickens and wild ducks. Treatment with type-specific antitoxin is effective but not practical.

VIRAL ENCEPHALITIDES

Encephalitis in poultry and farm-reared gamebirds may be caused by several different arboviruses. These include eastern equine encephalitis (EEE) virus, western equine encephalitis (WEE) virus, Highlands J (HJ) virus, Israel turkey meningoencephalitis virus, and West Nile Virus (p 2289). The term "arbovirus," an abbreviation of arthropod-borne virus, is used to describe a virus that replicates in a hematophagous (bloodsucking) arthropod and is transmitted by bite to a vertebrate host.

Eastern Equine Encephalitis: Eastern equine encephalitis (EEE) is most commonly seen as a disease of horses (see EQUINE ENCEPHALOMYELITIS, p 1027); however, many outbreaks of EEE in farm-raised ring-necked pheasants and Chukar partridges have been identified. EEE occurs only sporadically in other species of poultry (turkeys, ducks) and game birds (ratites). EEE virus exists primarily in the eastern and central parts of North America, throughout Central America and the Caribbean, and in eastern parts of South America. In the USA, EEE has been identified in most states east of the Mississippi River, as well as Louisiana and Texas; it is seen most often in Atlantic seaboard and Gulf Coast states. Reports of EEE virus in Europe and Asia have not been confirmed.

EEE outbreaks generally occur in late summer and fall as a consequence of increasing numbers of mosquito vectors. *Culiseta melanura*, an ornithophilic mosquito, is the principal vector; however, the virus also has been identified in a variety of other mosquitos. *C melanura* is the likely vector responsible for transmission to poultry and game birds. Wild birds, primarily the smaller species of Passeriformes, are the principal vertebrate hosts of EEE virus. These birds rarely become ill but serve as maintenance and amplifying hosts for the virus in the transmission cycle.

Epornitics of EEE virus infection in pheasants are believed to be initiated by mosquito-borne infection of 1 or more birds in a flock, with subsequent spread within the flock occurring as a result of feather picking and cannibalism. In ratites, the virus may be transmitted by the fecal-oral route.

Clinical disease produced by EEE virus in poultry and game birds usually is attributed to CNS infection with or without involvement of viscera. However, EEE also may produce visceral infections with little or no involvement of CNS tissues, especially in ratites.

Pheasants develop incoordination, depression, leg paralysis, torticollis, and tremors. Mortality may be as high as 80%. Gross lesions are not observed; however, microscopic changes in the CNS may include lymphocytic encephalitis, vasculitis, patchy necrosis, neuronal degeneration, and meningeal inflammation.

Chukar partridges exhibit clinical signs of depression, somnolence, and high mortality (30-80%). Pale, focal areas generally are present on hearts of affected birds, and spleens are mottled and enlarged. Microscopic lesions in the brain consist of gliosis, satellitosis, and perivascular lymphocytic infiltration. Myocardial lesions include multifocal necrosis and lymphocytic infiltration.

EEE virus infection in turkeys is characterized by drowsiness, incoordination, progressive weakness, paralysis of legs and wings, and low mortality (<5%). In turkeys, EEE virus also has been identified as a cause of decreased egg production.

Ducklings infected with EEE virus develop a paralytic disease characterized by sudden onset, posterior paresis, and paralysis; mortality rates in affected flocks range from 2-60%. Microscopic lesions consist of edema of spinal cord white matter, lymphocytic meningitis, and microgliosis.

Ratites exhibit depression, hemorrhagic diarrhea, emesis of blood-stained ingesta, and high mortality (up to 80%). Hemorrhagic enteritis is the principal lesion observed at postmortem examination. Microscopic lesions include necrosis of hepatocytes and intestinal mucosa.

Western Equine Encephalitis (WEE): This virus has many characteristics in common with EEE virus; however, it is rarely associated with diseases in avian species. WEE virus has been reported to cause encephalitis and high mortality in turkeys; affected turkeys exhibited somnolence, tremors, and leg paralysis. WEE virus may also cause decreased egg production in turkeys.

WEE is identified mainly in western parts of the USA and Canada, Central America, and South America. In the USA and Canada it is transmitted principally by *Culiseta tarsalis*, a mosquito vector that is relatively common west of the Mississippi River.

Highlands J Virus: Highlands J (HJ) virus is a cause of encephalitis in Chukar partridges. Chukars exhibit somnolence, ruffled feathers, and recumbency prior to death. HJ virus infection in this species is associated with high mortality. Microscopic lesions primarily consist of lymphocytic meningoencephalitis and focal myocardial necrosis. HJ virus has been shown to cause decreased egg production in turkeys. The virus has been identified only in eastern parts of the USA.

Israel Turkey Meningoencephalitis: This disease has been reported only in turkeys and generally is seen only in birds >10 wk of age. It has been reported in Israel and South Africa. While the specific vector has not been identified, the seasonal incidence and sporadic occurrence in flocks on the same farms strongly suggest that it is transmitted by insect vectors, most likely mosquitos and *Culicoides* spp flies. Turkeys exhibit neurologic dysfunction characterized by progressive paresis and paralysis, with variable mortality. Morbidity and mortality rates generally average 15-30% but may be as high as 80%. Turkey breeder hens exhibit a severe drop in egg production. Gross lesions in affected turkeys include splenomegaly or atrophy of the spleen, catarrhal enteritis, and myocarditis. The principal microscopic lesions are meningoencephalitis characterized by submeningeal and perivascular lymphocytic infiltration and focal myocardial necrosis.

Diagnosis: Diagnosis of EEE, WEE, and HJ virus or Israel turkey meningoencephalitis infection may be confirmed by isolation and identification of the virus, detection of viral antigens in tissues by immunohistochemistry, detection of viral RNA in tissues using reverse transcriptase PCR, and serologic testing. Virus can be isolated by inoculation of newborn mice, day-old chickens, embryonated chicken eggs, or a variety of cell cultures. Brain, spleen, liver, and serum are the preferred materials for diagnostic analyses.

Arbovirus infections must be distinguished from other causes of neurologic disease in poultry and game birds such as Newcastle disease virus, avian encephalomyelitis virus, botulism, and listeriosis.

Prevention and Control: EEE, WEE, and HJ virus infection and Israel turkey meningoencephalitis are best prevented by measures aimed at reducing vector populations. Such measures include reduction of vector habitats by modifying the environment or by chemical spraying. If feasible, farms that raise susceptible avian species should be located away from swamps and other areas that provide habitat for vectors.

Formalin-inactivated EEE virus vaccines, prepared for use in horses, have been used to protect pheasants against EEE, although their efficacy has been questioned. One-tenth the equine dose of either an eastern or bivalent eastern and western vaccine is injected into the pectoral muscle, preferably at 5-6 wk of age or when birds are released from the brooder house.

Israel turkey meningoencephalitis also can be controlled by vaccination. A live attenuated vaccine has been prepared by serial passage of virus in Japanese quail kidney cells; this vaccine has been shown to be highly efficacious and is commercially available.

Zoonotic Risk: EEE and WEE viruses are zoonotic agents and potential causes of significant human disease. These viruses result in neurologic disease that may progress to paralysis, convulsions, coma, and death. The case fatality rate for EEE virus in humans is 50-75%, and survivors often have permanent neurologic sequelae. WEE virus is less severe, with a case-fatality rate of ~3-7%. Most infections are subclinical. Human infection usually is acquired by mosquito bite; laboratory and clinically acquired infections are rare. However, care should be taken to avoid contact or droplet exposure when handling suspect infected birds or performing necropsies.

WEST NILE VIRUS INFECTION IN POULTRY

See also WEST NILE ENCEPHALOMYELITIS, p 1077.

West Nile virus (WNV), a flavivirus related to the St. Louis encephalitis/Japanese encephalitis complex, was first isolated from the blood of a febrile Ugandan woman in 1937. The virus was first described as the cause of a West Nile fever epidemic in humans in Israel in 1951; in a later outbreak, severe meningoencephalitis was seen in elderly patients. The role of mosquitos in viral transmission was clearly delineated in a series of field studies in Egypt in the 1950s. Wild birds were identified as the reservoir of the virus around the same time. Cases of West Nile fever in horses were reported several years later. WNV was first associated with disease in domestic avian species in 1997, when flocks of young geese in Israel were affected with a neuroparalytic disease. In August 1999, the disease appeared for the first time in the Western Hemisphere when wild and zoo birds, horses, and humans died in the northeast USA, notably in the New York City area.

Etiology and Epidemiology: WNV is considered to be endemic in many countries of Africa, Asia, southern Europe, and North America. Epidemics appear in the human population at infrequent intervals in some of these countries, and there is evidence for viral transmission between Africa and Europe by migrating birds. Most outbreaks have occurred from mid-July through October when cold nights reduce mosquito vector activity, notably *Culex* spp.

Geese are the only known natural hosts of WNV among domestic avian species. Most of the flocks affected in the Israel outbreaks were 5-9 wk old, but goslings as young as 3 wk and as old as 11 wk were also affected. Adult breeding flocks were clinically unaffected but virus neutralizing antibodies were found. Mortality of young Muscovy ducks but not young chickens or turkey poults was induced experimentally with a WNV isolate.

Transmission: The principal route of viral transmission is by the bite of a mosquito (primarily *Culex* spp). In the USA during 1999 and 2000, most of the viral isolates were made from *C pipiens* and *C restvans*. In Africa and the Middle East, the usual vector is *C univittatus*, and in Europe, *C pipiens* and *C modestus*. WNV has also been isolated from at least 10 tick species.

Clinical Findings: Affected geese show various degrees of neurologic involvement ranging from recumbency to leg and wing paralysis. Affected birds are either reluctant or unable to move when disturbed. Signs of incoordination are pronounced and some birds flip over while attempting to stand. Naturally affected geese show torticollis and opisthotonos. Mortality rates of 20-60% have been reported, probably due to horizontal spread of the virus.

Lesions: Pathologic changes include pallor of the myocardium and occasionally of the kidneys, splenomegaly, and hepatomegaly. The meningeal blood vessels are injected. Microscopic brain lesions consist of lymphocytic perivascular infiltration and neuronal degeneration. Small necrotic foci are present in the myocardium but lymphocytic infiltration is minimal.

Diagnosis: The tissues of choice for isolating virus from paralytic or dead birds are the brain, spleen, and kidneys. Homogenates are inoculated into the brain of newborn mice, embryonated eggs by the yolk sac route, or Vero and mosquito cell line cultures. Reverse transcriptase PCR with RNA extracted from either brain material or cell culture supernatant can also be performed. TakMan technology for rapid molecular diagnosis of field-collected mosquitos and avian tissues has been introduced recently. Immunohistochemistry can be used on formalin-fixed paraffin-embedded tissues, in particular brain and kidney, to visualize viral antigens in infected birds. Several forms of ELISA have also been developed for flaviviruses.

Neurologic signs in young geese must be distinguished from those caused by *Riemerella* (*Pasteurella*) infections, especially *R anatipestifer*. Other bacteria include *Streptococcus gallolyticus*, and *Erysipelothrix*, *Listeria*, and *Salmonella* spp. Neurotropic viruses include Newcastle disease, which is rare in geese, and avian influenza. Ionophore intoxication can induce paralytic signs. *Aspergillus* also causes brain lesions and caseous nodules in the lungs.

Prevention and Control: Mosquito control is a mandatory component of any arboviral disease control program. Unfortunately, this is difficult to implement in a rural environment because of the distances that mosquitos can fly or be carried by prevailing winds. Standing water and similar insect breeding sites in the vicinity of densely populated avian farms should be treated with larvicides. Poultry houses should be constructed to be insect free. Because many arboviral diseases are zoonoses, much can be achieved by cooperation with human disease surveillance agencies.

Control of WNV in geese is confined to vaccinating young flocks at risk, especially those raised during July through November when *Culex* spp are most numerous. Because of confounding factors such as possible horizontal transmission of virus, all birds in the flock should be vaccinated. Due to the age-related susceptibility to the virus, goslings should be immunized as young as possible, preferably at 3 wk old. Currently, WNV vaccines are not available commercially, although several types have been developed. Laboratory trials have been performed with a formaldehyde-inactivated suckling mouse brain-derived product. Over 75% of geese vaccinated with a single dose of vaccine at 3 wk of age were protected, and 94% protection was achieved with 2 doses spaced 2 wk apart. The duration of immunity was estimated to last until 12 wk of age. Inactivated vaccines prepared from chick embryos or Vero cells are not protective because of their low antigenic mass. A single dose of a live attenuated vaccine derived from high mosquito cell passage induced immunity to intracerebral challenge in young geese. Mosquito feeding experiments and back passage reversions to virulence studies have yet to be completed.

ARTIFICIAL INSEMINATION

Low fertility in turkeys, resulting from unsuccessful mating as a consequence of large, heavily muscled birds or of reduced libido, is a serious and costly problem in the production of hatching eggs. Artificial insemination (AI) is widely used to overcome this problem. AI has not found wide application in chickens but is routinely used in special breeding work.

Collecting semen from a chicken or turkey is done by stimulating the copulatory organ to protrude by massaging the abdomen and the back over the testes. This is followed quickly by pushing the tail forward with one hand and, at the same time, using the thumb and forefinger of the same hand to "milk" semen from the ducts of this organ. Semen flow response is quicker and easier to stimulate in chickens than in turkeys. The semen may be collected with an aspirator or in a small tube or any cup-like container. In turkeys, the volume averages ~0.35-0.5 mL, with a spermatozoon concentration of 6 to >8 billion/mL.

In chickens, volume is 2-3 times that of turkeys, but the concentration is about one-half. Collected semen is usually pooled.

Chicken and turkey semen begin to lose fertilizing ability when stored >1 hr. Liquid cold (4°C) storage of turkey and chicken semen can be used to transport semen and maintain spermatozoal viability for ~6-12 hr. When using liquid cold storage for >1 hr, turkey semen must be diluted with a semen extender at least 1:1 and then agitated slowly (150 rpm) to facilitate oxygenation; chicken semen should be diluted and then cooled—agitation is not necessary. Several commercial semen extenders are available and are routinely used, particularly for turkeys. Extenders enable more precise control over inseminating dose and facilitate filling of tubes. Results may be comparable to those using undiluted semen when product directions are followed. Dilution should result in an insemination dose containing ~300 million viable spermatozoa.

For insemination, pressure is applied to the left side of the abdomen around the vent. This causes the cloaca to evert and the oviduct to protrude so that a syringe or plastic straw can be inserted ~1 in. (2.5 cm) into the oviduct and the appropriate amount of semen delivered. As the semen is expelled by the inseminator, pressure around the vent is released, which assists the hen in retaining sperm in the vagina or the oviduct. Due to the high sperm concentration of turkey semen, 0.025 mL (~2 billion spermatozoa) of undiluted pooled semen, inseminated at regular intervals of 10-14 days, yields optimal fertility. In chickens, due to the lower spermatozoon concentration and shorter duration of fertility, 0.05 mL of undiluted pooled semen, at intervals of 7 days, is required. The hen's squatting behavior indicates receptivity and the time for the first insemination. For maximal fertility, inseminations may be started before the initial oviposition. Fertility tends to decrease later in the season; therefore, it may be justified to inseminate more frequently or use more cells per insemination dose.

Chicken and turkey semen may be frozen, but reduced fertility limits usage to special breeding projects. Under experimental conditions, fertility levels of 90% have been obtained in hens inseminated at 3-day intervals with 400-500 million frozen-thawed chicken spermatozoa.

DISORDERS OF THE REPRODUCTIVE SYSTEM

Cystic Right Oviduct

Fluid accumulation in the vestigial right oviduct is a common finding in hens. The abdominal cyst is filled with clear fluid and is attached to the right side of the cloacal wall. The cyst may vary in size from barely perceptible to 15-20 cm in diameter. An increased incidence has been observed in flocks after infectious bronchitis virus outbreaks. Oviductal cysts are a necropsy finding that rarely, if ever, affect flock performance.

Defective or Abnormal Eggs

Most "ridged," "sunburst," "slab-sided," soft-shelled, or double-shelled eggs are the result of eggs colliding in the shell gland when an ovum (yolk) is released too soon after the previous one. Necropsy examinations have demonstrated that 2 full-sized eggs can be found in the shell gland pouch. As the second egg comes in contact with the first, pressure is exerted, disrupting the pattern of mineralization. The first egg acquires a white band and chalky appearance, while the second egg is flattened on its contiguous surface (ie, slab-sided). Pimpled or rough eggs may have been retained too long in the shell gland. Blood spots result when a follicle vessel along the stigma ruptures as the ovum is being released. Meat spots occur when a piece of follicle membrane or residual albumen from the previous day is incorporated into the developing egg.

Many abnormalities occur as "accidents" (no specific cause), but the incidence is much higher in hens subjected to stressful management conditions, rough handling, or vaccination during production. A significant increase in the number of soft-shelled eggs is also common as a result of viral disease such as infectious bronchitis, egg drop syndrome, and exotic Newcastle disease.

Small eggs with no yolk form around a nidus of material (residual albumen) in the magnum of the oviduct. Small eggs with reduced albumen and eggs with defective shells may be the result of damage to the epithelium of the magnum or shell gland.

Very rarely, foreign material that enters the oviduct through the vagina (eg, a roundworm) may be incorporated into an egg.

Egg-bound or Impacted Oviducts

A fully formed egg may lodge in the shell gland or vagina because the egg is too big (eg, double-yolked) or because of hypocalcemia, calcium tetany, or previous trauma (pecking) to the vent and/or vagina. This condition may be more prevalent in pullets that are brought into production before body development is adequate or in hens that are extremely obese. It occurs more often during spring and summer months due to over-stimulation of birds by increasing light intensity and day length. This is a medical emergency in pet birds but is usually recognized only at necropsy in poultry. When impaction occurs, eggs that continue to form create layers of albumen and yolk material, and the oviduct becomes very large. Some eggs are refluxed to the abdominal cavity, and affected hens assume a penguin-like posture.

Egg Peritonitis
(Egg yolk peritonitis)

Egg peritonitis is characterized by fibrin or albumen-like material with a cooked appearance among the abdominal viscera. It is a common cause of sporadic death in layers, but in some flocks may become the major cause of death and give the appearance of a contagious disease. It is diagnosed at necropsy. Peritonitis follows reverse movement of albumen and *Escherichia coli* bacteria from the oviduct into the abdomen. If the incidence is high, culture should be done to differentiate between *Pasteurella* (fowl cholera) or *Salmonella* infection.

When hens have too many large ovarian follicles, a problem described as erratic oviposition and defective egg syndrome (EODES) is seen in broiler breeders. This condition is accompanied by a high incidence of double-yolked eggs, prolapses of the oviduct, internal ovulation, and/or internal laying that often results in egg peritonitis and mortality. EODES is prevented by avoiding light stimulation of underweight pullets too early and following body weight and lighting recommendations for each breeder strain. Overweight hens may also have a higher incidence of erratic ovulations and mortality associated with egg peritonitis.

False Layer

These hens ovulate normally, but the yolk is dropped into the abdominal cavity rather than being collected by the oviduct because of obstruction of the oviduct after infection with *E coli* or *Mycoplasma gallisepticum*. The yolk is absorbed from the abdominal cavity. The hen looks like a normal layer but does not produce eggs. Hypoplasia of the ovary and oviduct has been associated with infectious bronchitis virus infections (*see* p 2302) at an early age (1-2 wk). Atresia or even atrophy of the ovary are caused by severe stress, chronic infections, and feed refusal due to mycotoxins in the feed.

Hypocalcemia, Sudden Death, Osteoporosis, or Cage Layer Fatigue

Pullets or hens with insufficient dietary calcium, phosphorus, or vitamin D_3 may die suddenly or be found paralyzed from hypocalcemia while shelling an egg. This may be associated with high production and withdrawal of calcium from bones for egg shell production, in which case the main lesion may be osteoporosis. At necropsy, there is an egg in the shell gland and the ova are not regressed. There are no other lesions, although medullary bone may be lacking. Paralyzed hens respond to calcium IV, and this response may be useful in diagnosis.

Hens with osteoporosis may show similar signs at necropsy, or the ova may be regressing with no egg in the oviduct. The femur is always fragile, and medullary bone is always absent in osteoporosis. These hens may also respond to calcium IV if there are no fractures of the legs or vertebrae. Osteoporosis is a major cause of death in high-production flocks. The use of large particle size calcium (limestone, oyster shell) in the diet may be beneficial. High rates of mortality due to fractures are common in birds affected with osteoporosis. This situation is more common in birds in wood-slatted houses due to the trauma caused by jumping on and off the slats. Ruptured egg follicles indicating trauma can be found during necropsy examination of these birds.

In recent years, a condition known as hypocalcemia or calcium tetany (paralysis) has been seen in high-yielding broiler breeders. Careful postmortem examination reveals a fully active ovary and the presence of a partially or fully formed egg in the shell gland in the absence of other lesions. This indicates that the hen used all available calcium from the bloodstream in an effort to complete the egg shell. The condition is common in flocks with poor body weight uniformity that are fed high-calcium diets in the weeks prior to the onset of lay and brought into production by drastic increases in day length and feed allocation. Hypocalcemia can be prevented by management practices that promote body weight uniformity and avoid excessive/premature allocation of high-calcium diets and light stimulation. Mortality can be reduced by the administration ("topping of the feed") of 5 g of oyster shell per hen for 3 consecutive days, and addition of vitamin D_3 to the drinking water. This treatment should be suspended for 3 days and then repeated. Severe cases will require continual treatment for 2-3 wk (3 days of treatment, followed by 3 days without).

Mortality and the presence of an egg in the shell gland also can be caused by a condition referred as to sudden death syndrome, first reported in Australia. This is believed to be caused by marginal levels of potassium and phosphorus in the diet, resulting in cardiomyopathy.

Internal Layer

In these hens, partially or fully formed eggs are found in the abdominal cavity. Such eggs reach the cavity by reverse peristalsis of the oviduct. If they have no shell, they are often misshapen due to partial or complete absorption of the contents. Frequently, only empty shell membranes are present. No control or treatment is known. This condition is related to erratic ovulation and defective eggs (*see* above).

Infertility

Because males may have a harem of females that they defend from other males, infertility is more important in the male than in females. However, obese females may be less efficient in transporting sperm to the infundibulum resulting in reduced fertilization of the ovum as it is released from the ovary. The male must be dominant to the females or mating will not occur. Commercial turkey hens are inseminated artificially with semen collected from the stags and used the same day. (*See* ARTIFICIAL INSEMINATION, p 2290). Parthenogenesis is responsible for some infertility in turkeys. There are host sperm glands in the oviduct of females, and live sperm can be retained for 3-4 wk. Waterfowl have a rudimentary penis, and prolapse of the penis is occasionally reported in drakes. There is no treatment.

Neoplasia

The most frequent tumor of the reproductive system is carcinoma of the oviduct. Neoplastic cells are shed from tumors in the oviduct into the abdominal cavity. They implant on the ovary, pancreas, and other viscera and produce multiple, hard, yellow nodules. They may block lymph return and result in ascites. The incidence increases with age, and this tumor may be a frequent cause of death after 2 yr. Affected hens are condemned at processing.

Leiomyoma of the broad ligament is an estrogen-induced hypertrophy of the smooth muscle of the broad ligament. It is benign and is an incidental finding at necropsy or processing.

A variety of ovarian and testicular tumors has been described. Marek's disease (p 2248) is also found frequently in the ovary.

Oophoritis and Ovary Regression

Regression of the ovary may result in leakage of free yolk into the abdomen (yolk peritonitis); this rarely causes death except when yolk material migrates through the air sacs to the lung and causes foreign body pneumonia. Free yolk occurs in many cases of acute illness, injury, or forced molt. Regression of the ovary is frequently caused by low body weight, deliberate reduction of feed, overcrowding, or lack of feeder space. Infectious diseases such as exotic Newcastle disease, fowl cholera, pullorum disease, and avian influenza are known to cause this condition. It can also result from severe stress, which is often accompanied by feather molt, emaciation, and dehydration.

Prolapse of the Oviduct

When an egg is laid, the vagina everts through the cloaca to deliver the egg. If there has been injury to the vagina, such as from a large egg, or if the hen is fat, the vagina may not retract immediately. This may result in cannibalism (p 2271). When the protruding organ is pecked by others in the flock, the complete oviduct and parts of the adjacent intestinal tract may be pulled from the abdominal cavity ("peckout"). Alternatively, the vagina swells, cannot retract, and remains prolapsed ("blowout"). The hen dies from shock. A high incidence has been associated with excessive/premature photostimulation, early laying (inadequate body size), large eggs, double-yolked eggs, and obesity. Cannibalism may be prevented by beak trimming, maintaining appropriate stocking density, and avoiding nutritional deficiencies.

Salpingitis

Salpingitis is an inflammation of the oviduct, which may contain liquid or caseous exudate. In young pullets, it is often due to *Mycoplasma gallisepticum*, *E coli*, *Salmonella* spp, or *Pasteurella multocida* (fowl cholera) infection and can result in reduced egg production. It is a frequent lesion in female broilers and ducks at processing. On gross examination, salpingitis may be difficult to differentiate from impacted oviduct in adults. As the oviduct becomes nonfunctional, the ovaries are usually atrophied. Unless associated with an infectious problem, this condition tends to be found sporadically during necropsy of cull hens.

Sex Reversal

If the normal left ovary of a hen is destroyed by infection, the vestigial right organ may develop as a testicle and the hen may develop male characteristics. Neoplasia in the adrenal glands or ovary that result in the production of testosterone could also cause the development of male secondary sexual characteristics (comb and wattles) in affected females.

EGG DROP SYNDROME

Egg drop syndrome (EDS) is characterized by production of soft-shelled and shell-less eggs in apparently healthy birds. It has been recognized worldwide, except in the USA.

Etiology: The causal adenovirus is widely distributed in both wild and domestic ducks, geese, coots, and grebes. Antibody has also been detected in herring gulls, owls, storks, and swans. The adenovirus group antigen cannot be demonstrated by conventional means, and EDS virus also differs from other avian adenoviruses by strongly agglutinating avian RBC. The virus achieves high titers in embryonating eggs or in cell cultures of duck or goose origin. It replicates well in chick kidney or chick-embryo liver cells and to a lesser degree in chick-embryo fibroblasts. It does not grow in embryonating chick eggs or in mammalian cells.

The resistant virus has 1 serotype but at least 3 genotypes: 1 associated with classical EDS, 1 with ducks in the UK, and 1 with EDS in Australia.

Epidemiology: The natural hosts for EDS virus are ducks and geese, and the disease has been described in Japanese quail (*Coturnix coturnix japonica*). Three types of disease are recognized in chickens. Classical EDS probably was due to contamination of a vaccine for Marek's disease grown in duck-embryo fibroblasts and subsequent adaptation of the virus to chickens. Basic breeding stock was infected, and the virus was transmitted vertically through the egg. The virus often remained latent until the chick reached sexual maturity, when it was excreted in the eggs and droppings to infect susceptible contacts. Because the virus is vertically transmitted and is reactivated around peak egg production, there was an apparent breed and age susceptibility. However, all ages and breeds of chickens are susceptible, although the disease tends to be most severe in heavy broiler-breeders or brown egg producers.

Arising from the classical form, endemic EDS has been reported in many areas and is usually seen in commercial egg producers. Flocks become infected at any stage in lay. Contaminated egg collection trays are one of the main forms of horizontal transmission, and outbreaks are often associated with a common egg-packing station.

Rare, sporadic EDS has been recognized in isolated flocks. It appears to be due either to contact with domestic ducks or geese or, more often, to water contaminated with wildfowl droppings. The risk is that these introductions could become endemic.

The main method of horizontal spread is through contaminated eggs; droppings also are infective. Humans and contaminated fomites such as crates or trucks can spread virus, which also can be transmitted by needles when vaccinating and drawing blood. Insect transmission is possible but not proved.

Pathogenesis: After horizontal or experimental infection, the virus grows to low titers in the nasal mucosa. This is followed by viremia, virus replication in lymphoid tissue, and then massive replication for ~8 days in the oviduct, especially in the pouch shell gland region. Changes in the eggshell occur coincidentally. Both the exterior and interior of eggs produced between 8 and ~18 days after infection contain virus. A copious exudate in the lumen of the oviduct is rich in virus, and this contaminates the droppings. Unlike other fowl adenoviruses, there is little, if any, growth in the epithelial cells of the intestine.

Chicks hatched from infected eggs may excrete virus and develop antibody. More often, the virus remains latent, and antibody does not develop until the bird starts to lay, at which time the virus reactivates and grows in the oviduct, repeating the cycle.

Clinical Findings: In flocks without antibody, the first sign is loss of color in pigmented eggs, quickly followed by soft-shelled and shell-less eggs. Diarrhea and a transient dullness may be seen before the eggshell changes. Birds tend to eat the shell-less eggs, which therefore may be missed unless a search is made for the membranes. Egg production falls 10-40% mainly because of the shell-less eggs. In flocks in which there has been some spread of virus and some of the birds have antibody (usually 10-20%), the condition is seen as a failure to achieve predicted production targets; careful examination shows that these flocks are experiencing a series of small EDS episodes. Birds with antibody slow the spread of virus.

There is no effect on fertility or hatchability of those eggs suitable for setting.

Lesions: The major pathologic changes are seen in the pouch shell gland. Surface epithelial cells develop intranuclear inclusion bodies and degenerate; they are replaced by squamous, cuboidal, or undifferentiated columnar cells. There is moderate to severe inflammatory infiltration of the mucosa.

Diagnosis: In classical EDS, the combination of poor eggshell quality at peak production in healthy birds is almost diagnostic. With endemic or sporadic EDS, disease can be seen in laying birds of any age. In cage units, spread can be slow, and the clinical signs, may be overlooked or perceived as a small depression (2-4%) of egg yield.

EDS can be distinguished from Newcastle disease (p 2255) and influenza virus infections (p 2297) by the absence of illness, and from infectious bronchitis (p 2302) by the eggshell changes that occur at or just before the drop in egg production and by the absence of ridges and malformed eggs sometimes seen in infectious bronchitis.

EDS should be suspected whenever peak egg production parameters are not met; however, the observation of clinical signs alone does not provide enough reliable information for diagnosis. The virus can be isolated by inoculating embryonating duck eggs or duck- or chick-embryo liver cell cultures. It is important to select birds producing abnormal eggs, but this can be difficult, especially if the birds are on litter. An easier method is to feed affected eggs to antibody-free hens. Virus isolation from the pouch shell gland of these hens can be attempted when the first abnormal eggs are produced.

The hemagglutination inhibition test (high levels of hemagglutinins are produced) using fowl RBC or the ELISA test are the serologic and diagnostic tests of choice. In addition, the serum neutralization test can be used for confirmation. The double immunodiffusion test also has been used. If one adenovirus has been isolated, restriction endonuclease analysis can be used to classify the virus as EDS. When selecting birds for diagnosis, especially in cage units, it is important to bleed only birds that have produced affected eggs.

Control: There is no treatment. The classical form has been eradicated from primary breeders. Washing and disinfecting plastic egg trays before use can control the endemic form. The sporadic form can be prevented by separating chickens from other birds, especially waterfowl. General sanitary precautions are indicated, and potentially contaminated water should be chlorinated before use.

Inactivated vaccines with oil adjuvant are available and, if properly made, control the disease. They reduce but do not prevent virus shedding. These vaccines are given during the growing phase, usually at 14-18 wk, and can be combined with other vaccines such as for Newcastle disease. Sentinel birds are frequently placed along with vaccinated chickens to detect the presence of virus in the flock. Sentinel chickens will become serologically positive on hemagglutination inhibition test.

AIR SAC MITE

Cytodites nudus is a small cosmopolitan mite occasionally noticed as white spots on the bronchi, lungs, air sacs, and abdominal organs of chickens, turkeys, pheasants, pigeons, and mallards. (*See also* p 1465.) These mites are readily transmissible between birds, but the method of transfer is unknown. They are rarely found in commercial industries. The life cycle involves a larval and 2 nymphal stages. Infestation densities vary, and clinical signs range from none to weakness, weight loss, pneumonia, peritonitis, obstruction of respiratory passages, and death. Recommended treatments include ivermectin, a nearby dichlorvos pest strip (placed out of reach of the birds), or a pyrethrin/piperonyl butoxide spray.

ASPERGILLOSIS

(Brooder pneumonia, Mycotic pneumonia, Pneumomycosis)

Aspergillosis is a disease, usually of the respiratory system, of chickens, turkeys, and less frequently ducklings, pigeons, canaries, geese, and many other wild and pet birds. In chickens and turkeys, the disease may be endemic on some farms; in wild birds, it appears to be sporadic, frequently affecting only an individual bird. It is usually seen in birds 7-40 days old. (*See also* ASPERGILLOSIS in mammals, p 511, and CAGED BIRDS, p 1451.)

Etiology and Epidemiology: *Aspergillus fumigatus* is a common cause of the disease. However, several other *Aspergillus* spp may be incriminated.

Chicks and poults may become infected during hatching as a result of inhaling large numbers of spores in heavily contaminated hatching machines or from contaminated litter. In older birds, infection is caused primarily by inhalation of spore-laden dust from contaminated litter or feed or dusty range areas.

Clinical Findings and Lesions: Dyspnea, hyperpnea, somnolence, and other signs of nervous system involvement, inappetence, emaciation, and increased thirst may be seen. The encephalitic form is most common in turkeys. In chicks or poults up to 6 wk, the lungs are most frequently involved. Pulmonary lesions are characterized by cream-colored plaques a few mm to several cm in diameter; occasionally, mycelial masses may be seen within the air passages on gross examination. The plaques also may be found in the syrinx, air sacs, liver, intestines, and occasionally the brain. An ocular form, in which large plaques may be expressed from the medial canthus, has been seen in chickens and turkeys.

Diagnosis: The fungus can be demonstrated by culture or by microscopic examination of fresh preparations. One of the plaques is teased apart and placed on a suitable medium, usually resulting in a pure culture of the organism. Histopathologic examination using a special fungus stain reveals granulomas containing mycelia. Pathogenicity of the isolate is confirmed by injecting it into the air sacs of susceptible 3-wk-old chicks.

Differential diagnoses include infectious bronchitis, Newcastle disease, infectious laryngotracheitis, *Dactylaria* infection, and nutritional encephalomalacia.

Treatment and Control: Treatment of affected birds is considered useless. Strict adherence to sanitation procedures in the hatchery minimizes early outbreaks. Grossly contaminated eggs should not be set for incubation because they may explode and disseminate spores throughout the hatching machine. Contaminated hatchers should be fumigated with formaldehyde or thiabendazole (120-360 g/m^3). Avoiding moldy litter or ranges serves to prevent outbreaks in older birds. Pens should be sprayed with nystatin, and all equipment cleaned and disinfected.

AVIAN INFLUENZA

(Fowl plague)

Avian influenza (AI) viruses infect domestic poultry and wild birds. In domestic poultry, AI viruses are typically of low pathogenicity (LP), causing subclinical infections, respiratory disease, or drops in egg production. However, a few AI viruses cause severe systemic infections with high mortality. This highly pathogenic (HP) form of the disease has historically been called fowl plague. In most wild birds, AI viral infections are subclinical.

Etiology: Avian influenza viruses are type A orthomyxoviruses characterized by antigenically homologous nucleoprotein and matrix internal proteins, which are identified by serology in agar gel immunodiffusion (AGID) tests. AI viruses are further divided into 15 hemagglutinin (H1-15) and 9 neuraminidase (N1-9) subtypes based on hemagglutinin inhibition and neuraminidase inhibition tests, respectively. Most AI viruses (H1-15 subtypes) are of LP, but some of the H5 and H7 AI viruses are HP for chickens, turkeys, and related gallinaceous domestic poultry.

Epidemiology and Transmission: LP viruses are distributed worldwide and are recovered frequently from clinically normal shorebirds and migrating waterfowl. Occasionally, LP viruses are recovered from imported pet birds and ratites. The viruses may be present in backyard flocks and other birds sold through live-poultry markets, but most commercially raised poultry in developed countries are free of AI viruses. The HP viruses arise from mutation of some H5 and H7 LP viruses and cause devastating epizootics. Depopulation and quarantine programs are used to quickly eliminate the HP viruses.

The incubation period is highly variable and ranges from a few days to 1 wk. Transmission between individual birds is by ingestion or inhalation. Experimentally, cats have been infected with 1 strain of H5N1 Asian HP AI following respiratory exposure, ingestion of infected chickens, or contact with infected cats. Potentially, domestic house cats could serve as a transmission vector between farms, but the ability of other AI viruses, including other H5N1 strains, to infect cats is unknown. Transmission between farms is the result of breaches in biosecurity practices, principally by movement of infected birds or contaminated feces and respiratory secretions on fomites such as equipment or clothing. Airborne dissemination may be important over limited distances.

Clinical Findings and Lesions: Clinical signs, severity of disease, and mortality rates vary depending on AI virus strain and host species.

Low Pathogenicity AI Viruses: These AI viruses typically produce respiratory signs such as ocular and nasal discharge and swollen infraorbital sinuses. Sinusitis is common in domestic ducks, quail, and turkeys. Lesions in the respiratory tract typically include congestion and inflammation of the trachea and lungs. In layers and breeders, there may be decreased egg production or fertility, ova rupture (evident as yolk in the abdominal cavity) or involution, or mucosal edema and inflammatory exudates in the lumen of the oviduct. Some layer and breeder chickens may have acute renal failure and visceral urate deposition (visceral gout). The morbidity and mortality is usually low unless accompanied by secondary bacterial or viral infections or aggravated by environmental stress factors.

High Pathogenicity AI Viruses: Even in the absence of secondary pathogens, HP viruses cause severe, systemic disease with high mortality in chickens, turkeys, and other gallinaceous birds. In peracute cases, clinical signs or gross lesions may be lacking before death. However, in acute cases, lesions may include cyanosis and edema of the head, comb, and wattle; edema and discoloration of the shanks and feet due to subcutaneous ecchymotic hemorrhages; petechial hemorrhages on visceral organs and in muscles; and blood-tinged oral and nasal discharges. In severely affected birds, greenish diarrhea is common. Birds that survive the fulminating infection may develop CNS involvement evident as torticollis, opisthotonos, or incoordination. The location and severity of microscopic lesions are highly variable and may consist of edema, hemorrhage, and necrosis in parenchymal cells of multiple visceral organs, skin, and CNS.

Diagnosis: AI viruses can be readily isolated from tracheal and cloacal swabs. They grow well in the allantoic sac of embryonating chicken eggs and agglutinate RBC. The hemagglutination is not inhibited by Newcastle disease or other paramyxoviral antiserum. AI viruses are identified by demonstrating the presence of 1) influenza A matrix or nucleoprotein antigens using AGID or other suitable immunoassays, or 2) viral RNA using an influenza A specific RT-PCR tests.

Differential Diagnosis: LP AI must be differentiated from other respiratory diseases or causes of decreased egg production including: 1) acute to subacute viral diseases such as infectious bronchitis, infectious laryngotracheitis, lentogenic Newcastle disease, and infections by other paramyxoviruses; 2) bacterial diseases such as mycoplasmosis, infectious coryza, ornithobacteriosis, turkey coryza, and the respiratory form of fowl cholera; and 3) fungal diseases such as aspergillosis. HP AI must be differentiated from other causes of high mortality such as velogenic Newcastle disease, peracute septicemic fowl cholera, heat exhaustion, and severe water deprivation.

Prevention and Treatment: Vaccines can prevent clinical signs and death. Furthermore, viral replication and shedding from the respiratory and GI tracts may be reduced in vaccinated birds. Specific protection is achieved through autogenous virus vaccines or from vaccines prepared from AI virus of the same hemagglutinin subtype. Antibodies to the viral neuraminidase antigens may provide some protection. Currently, only inactivated whole AI virus and recombinant fowlpox-AI-H5 vaccines are licensed in the USA. The use of AI vaccine requires approval of the state veterinarian. In addition, use of H5 and H7 AI vaccines in the USA requires USDA approval. Treating LP-affected flocks with broad-spectrum antibiotics to control secondary pathogens and increasing house temperatures may reduce morbidity and mortality. Treatment with antiviral compounds is not approved or recommended. Suspected outbreaks should be reported to appropriate regulatory authorities.

Zoonotic Risk: Avian influenza viruses exhibit host adaptation and rarely infect humans, usually as isolated individual cases without human-to-human transmission. In the 1997 Hong Kong outbreak, the risk factor for human infection was direct contact with infected poultry, but not the handling, cooking, or consumption of poultry meat. In 2004, HP AI of strain H5N1 infected poultry and wild birds in 9 Asian countries. In Thailand and Vietnam, 37 human cases were confirmed, with a case fatality rate of 68%.

AVIAN PNEUMOVIRUS

(Turkey rhinotracheitis, Avian rhinotracheitis, Swollen head syndrome)

Avian pneumoviruses have been implicated in the upper respiratory tract disease of turkeys and chickens known as turkey rhinotracheitis. The virus has also been associated with swollen head syndrome of chickens. First described in south Africa in the late 1970s, avian pneumovirus soon appeared in Europe and the Middle East. The disease has now been reported from all the major poultry-producing areas in the world except for Australasia. The virus has also been detected in pheasants and guinea fowl, and serologic evidence suggests other avian species are susceptible. Recent studies have indicated an antigenic relationship with a newly discovered human pneumovirus isolated from children with respiratory tract disease.

Etiology: Avian pneumoviruses are members of the subfamily Pneumovirinae, belonging to the family Paramyxoviridae. The subfamily consists of 2 genera: Pneumovirus, consisting of mammalian respiratory syncytial viruses and mouse pneumovirus, and Metapneumovirus, in which avian pneumoviruses are placed. Based on observed differences following sequence analysis of the viral genes, at least 3 subtypes of the virus have been described (A, B, C). Subtype C viruses appear to be the only subtype found in North America and have not been reported in other parts of the world.

Transmission and Epidemiology: Following infection, the virus is shed from the nares and trachea but not in the feces. After initial introduction of the virus, the disease spreads rapidly within a geographic area or country. The methods by which the virus is spread are unclear and often unpredictable. Direct contact attributed to movement of infected birds, personnel, equipment, and vehicles have all been implicated, while airborne transmission has also been reported to occur. There is no published evidence of vertical transmission via the egg, even though the virus has, on occasion, been detected in the reproductive tract of laying birds. Persistence of the virus in turkeys and chickens has not been demonstrated and, following experimental infection, virus was detected for 6-7 days only after inoculation.

Wild birds have been implicated in the spread of avian pneumovirus, particularly waterfowl and gulls.

Clinical Findings: Clinical signs in turkey poults include snicking, rales, sneezing, nasal discharge, foamy conjunctivitis, swollen infraorbital sinuses, and submandibular edema. Coughing and head shaking are frequently observed in older poults. In laying birds, egg production may drop up to 70% with an increased incidence of poor shell quality and peritonitis. Coughing associated with lower respiratory tract involvement may lead to prolapses of the uterus in laying turkeys.

Morbidity in birds of all ages is usually described as up to 100% with mortality ranging from 0.4% to as high as 50%, particularly in fully susceptible young poults. Secondary pathogens and management factors significantly influence the levels of morbidity and mortality.

Infection in chickens and pheasants is less clearly defined and may not always be associated with clinical signs. Avian pneumovirus is associated with swollen head syndrome in chickens. This condition is characterized by swelling of the peri- and infraorbital sinuses, torticollis, cerebral disorientation, and opisthotonos. Typically, <4% of the flock is affected, although respiratory signs may be widespread. Mortality is rarely >2%. In broiler breeders and commercial layers, egg production and quality are frequently affected. Evidence suggests that infectious bronchitis virus (p 2302) and *Escherichia coli* may also be associated with swollen head syndrome.

Lesions: In turkeys, excess mucus found in the nares, sinuses, and trachea is clear at first but rapidly becomes mucopurulent. When bacteria are involved, typical lesions of colisepticemia are frequently seen in various organs. The oviducts of affected breeders may contain inspissated albumen and solid yolk. Egg peritonitis may be associated with oviduct regression. Microscopic examination of the upper respiratory tract 1-2 days after infection reveals localized lesions, including loss of cilia, increased glandular activity, congestion, and mild mononuclear infiltration of the submucosa. Inflammatory infiltration of the submucosa can be observed with some mild lesions in the trachea between days 3 and 5. Similar but milder lesions can be observed in affected chickens.

Diagnosis: Taking samples from the upper respiratory tract of birds in the very early stages of the disease is extremely important when attempting virus isolation. Early investigators found that tracheal organ cultures prepared from turkey or chicken embryos, or 1- to 2-day-old chicks, were the most sensitive for primary isolation of avian pneumoviruses. Ciliostasis may occur within 7 days of inoculation or on passage. The virus has also been isolated following the inoculation of 6- to 8-day-old embryonated chicken or turkey eggs via the yolk sac route and identified by electron microscopy, virus neutralization, and molecular techniques. Cell cultures have not proved successful for the primary isolation of the virus. However, once the virus has been isolated and adapted in the systems above, it will grow in a variety of avian and mammalian cultures.

PCR tests have been developed and are widely used to detect the virus in clinical material, particularly respiratory swabs. Some PCR tests have been constructed so that the subtype as well as the identity of virus can be determined from the clinical sample. Antigen detection tests have also been developed, including immunofluorescence and immunoperoxidase assays on both fixed and unfixed tissues.

Due to difficulties in isolating and identifying pneumoviruses, serologic assays have been developed to confirm infection in commercial chickens and turkeys. A number of commercially prepared ELISA kits are available and are used most commonly, but other techniques including virus neutralization and indirect immunofluorescence have also been used. As with all serologic tests, both acute and convalescent samples should be submitted for analysis. The sera should be heated to 56°C for 30 min and stored at -20°C if delays in testing are unavoidable. While ELISA that use either subgroup A or B strains as antigens detect antibodies to both of these subgroups, the homologous antigen should be used for the efficient detection of subgroup C.

Differential Diagnosis: Paramyxoviruses (particularly Newcastle disease and paramyxovirus 3), infectious bronchitis virus, and influenza viruses may cause respiratory disease and egg production problems in chickens and turkeys that closely resemble pneumovirus infection. These viruses can be differentiated on the basis of morphology, hemagglutinating and neuraminidase activity, and molecular characteristics. A wide range of bacteria and *Mycoplasma* spp can cause clinical signs very similar to those of avian pneumovirus. These agents are frequently present as secondary opportunistic pathogens and may mask the presence of the pneumovirus.

Prevention and Treatment: Good management practices can significantly reduce the severity of infection, especially in turkeys; in particular, optimal ventilation, stocking densities, temperature control, litter quality, and biosecurity all have a positive influence on the disease. Some success in reducing disease severity by controlling secondary adventitious bacteria with antibiotics has also been reported.

Both live and inactivated vaccines are available for immunization of chickens and turkeys and are widely used in countries where the disease is endemic. Live vaccines stimulate both local and systemic immunity in the respiratory tract, and cross-protection between subtypes can occur. To produce complete protection in adult birds, oil-adjuvanted inactivated vaccines are administered to birds previously primed with live vaccines.

BORDETELLOSIS

(Turkey coryza, *Bordetella avium* rhinotracheitis)

Avian bordetellosis is a highly infectious, acute upper respiratory tract disease of turkeys characterized by high morbidity and usually low mortality. Other synonyms previously used for the disease include, *Alcaligenes* rhinotracheitis, adenovirus-associated respiratory disease, acute respiratory disease syndrome, and turkey rhinotracheitis.

Although the disease primarily affects turkeys, quail are also susceptible, and it is an opportunistic infection in chickens. Damage to the upper respiratory tract, from prior exposure to an upper respiratory disease vaccine such as infectious bronchitis or Newcastle disease virus, or an environmental irritant such as ammonia, is necessary to induce clinical signs in Leghorn chickens.

Bordetellosis has been identified in almost every area of the world where turkeys are intensively reared. Historically, it has been severe in focal areas and rare or non-apparent in other locations. The reasons for these epidemiologic differences are not known.

Etiology and Pathogenesis: The causative agent is a gram-negative, nonfermentative, motile, aerobic bacillus. When the bacillus is grown in broth media high in nutrients, filamentous forms can be observed. *Bordetella avium* grows on many different media, including MacConkey agar, Bordet-Gengou agar, veal infusion broth, trypticase soy broth, blood agar, and brain-heart infusion broth. Strains of *B avium* typically produce small (0.2-1 mm diameter after 24 hr incubation), compact, translucent, glistening pearl-like colonies with smooth edges. Following serial passage in the laboratory, a rough colony type with a dry appearance and a serrated, irregular edge can be observed for some isolates. Rough colonies represent a global suppression of virulence factors in *B avium* termed antigenic variation and are nonpathogenic.

The mechanism of pathogenesis involves ability of *B avium* to deciliate the tracheal epithelium. Certain strains of the bacteria adhere to the ciliated pseudostratified columnar epithelium and produce toxins, some of which appear to be similar to those from other *Bordetella* spp. Toxins and virulence factors associated with pathogenic strains of *B avium* include a heat-labile toxin, tracheal cytotoxin, dermonecrotic toxin, osteotoxin, and adherence factors associated with the hemagglutinin. Damage to the tracheal cartilage with distortion and discoloration of the tracheal rings is often observed and thought to be caused by the osteotoxin. Some mortality is due to suffocation from a combination of increased mucus production in the trachea and tracheal collapse.

Damage to the upper respiratory tract can lead to secondary infections with *Escherichia coli* or other agents, which can significantly increase the severity of the disease. In many cases, turkeys infected solely with *B avium* recover within 4-6 wk without serious consequences.

Epidemiology and Transmission: Morbidity is usually 80-100% in young turkeys. Mortality can range from 0% in the uncomplicated disease to >40% if secondary invaders are present. Mortality can increase and clinical signs can become severe if young turkeys infected with *B avium* also become infected with other agents (eg, *E coli*, Newcastle disease virus) or when environmental conditions in turkey barns are less than optimal. Bordetellosis is a major initiator of colibacillosis in turkeys. There is an age-related resistance to the disease. Turkeys >4-5 wk old are largely refractory to the disease, but not infection.

B avium is highly contagious and easily transmitted from infected turkeys to susceptible birds by direct contact. It can also be transmitted through contaminated drinking water, feed, and litter, which can remain infectious for 1-6 mo.

Clinical Findings: Clinical signs of the disease usually occur 7-10 days after infection and include sinusitis with a clear nasal discharge that can be observed when pressure is applied to the nares. Foamy-watery eyes, a snick or cough, mouth breathing, dyspnea, tracheal rales, and altered vocalization are also characteristic. Complicated disease can result in more exaggerated signs including airsacculitis.

Lesions: Lesions are primarily found in the upper respiratory tract and consist of nasal and tracheal exudates, collapse of cartilaginous rings, and progressive loss of ciliated epithelium. In the uncomplicated disease, the tracheal epithelium can return to normal 4-6 wk after the onset of clinical signs.

At necropsy, turkeys with characteristic bordetellosis have watery eyes and extensive mucus in the sinuses and trachea, which rarely extends below the tracheal bifurcation. The lining of the trachea may have extremely mild hemorrhage in some cases and softening of the tracheal rings is usually felt. In addition, a dorsal/ventral flattening of the trachea can sometimes be observed. Pneumonia and airsacculitis are observed only when the disease is complicated by another disease agent.

Diagnosis: Diagnosis of infection is confirmed by isolation of *B avium* on MacConkey agar and identification using standard biochemical assays. Nonfermenting, small, slow-growing colonies from specimens from the anterior trachea are typical. The bacterium is best isolated from the anterior trachea; cultures taken from the sinuses frequently become overgrown with other faster-replicating bacteria such as *Proteus* spp.

Serology is also important, and both microagglutination (detects IgM) and ELISA (detects IgG) tests are available. The microagglutination test can detect specific antibodies ~1 wk after infection. The ELISA test generally detects specific antibodies >2 wk after infection and has the added benefit of detecting maternal antibody. Monoclonal antibody-based agglutination and indirect immunofluorescent tests as well as PCR tests have also been used to identify *B avium*.

Other nonfermenters, *B bronchiseptica* and *B hinzii*, can sometimes be isolated from the trachea and must be differentiated from *B avium*. Pathogenic *B avium* can be differentiated by growth and colony morphology on MacConkey agar, no growth on minimal essential medium, a negative urease reaction, and hemagglutination of guinea pig erythrocytes.

Treatment: Treatment with antimicrobial agents has not been effective, even though *B avium* may be highly sensitive. The tracheal epithelium of the turkey is a difficult location to medicate even though blood levels of the antimicrobial appear to be adequate. Resistance to streptomycin, sulfonamides, and tetracycline has been observed for some strains of *B avium*. Antimicrobial therapy may be helpful for secondary colibacillosis.

Control and Prevention: Vaccination with bacterins and a live temperature-sensitive mutant vaccine have given mixed results depending on the age of the turkey and the method of administration. Typically, turkeys >3 wk old respond positively to vaccination with the live temperature-sensitive vaccine. Vaccination is not widely practiced by turkey breeders, and the immunity that is passed to progeny generally comes from natural infections.

B avium is easily tracked between farms. Thus, prevention should include a good biosecurity program with rigorous cleanup and disinfection after field outbreaks. Most of the commonly used disinfectants are effective.

Zoonotic Risk: *B avium* does not cause disease in humans, but a closely related organism, *B hinzii*, also isolated from poultry, has been associated with septicemia and bacteremia in older or immunocompromised people.

INFECTIOUS BRONCHITIS

Infectious bronchitis is an acute, rapidly spreading, viral disease of chickens characterized by respiratory signs, decreased egg production, and poor egg quality. Some strains of the causative virus, infectious bronchitis virus (IBV), are nephropathogenic. The latter strains produce interstitial nephritis resulting in significant mortality. Infectious bronchitis is of major economic importance to commercial chicken producers worldwide.

Etiology and Epidemiology: IBV, a coronavirus, is worldwide in distribution and has numerous serotypes. Two or more serotypes may be seen simultaneously in one geographic region. IBV is shed by infected chickens in respiratory discharges and feces. The highly contagious virus is spread by airborne droplets, ingestion of contaminated feed and water, and contaminated equipment and clothng of caretakers. Naturally infected chickens and those vaccinated with live IBV may intermittently shed virus for many weeks or even months. Virus infection in layers and breeders occurs cyclically as immunity declines or on exposure to different serotypes.

Clinical Findings: Signs occur after an incubation period of 18-48 hr. Spread to other birds is rapid, and morbidity may be nearly 100%. The nature and severity of the disease are influenced by the age and immune status of the flock and virulence of the causal strain. Young chickens cough, sneeze, and have tracheal rales for 10-14 days. Wet eyes and dyspnea may be seen, and facial swelling may also occur ccasionally, particularly with concurrent bacterial infection of the sinuses. In broiler chickens, IBV infection is a major cause of poor feed conversion, reduced growth rate, and condemnation of meat at processing. Nephropathogenic strains can produce interstitial nephritis with high mortality (up to 60%) in young chickens. In most outbreaks, however, mortality is 5%, although secondary bacterial infections may cause higher losses.

In layers, egg production may drop 5-50%, and eggs are often misshapen, thin-shelled, and contain watery albumen. Egg production and egg quality generally return to near normal levels in most birds on recovery.

Lesions: Respiratory tract lesions include mucoid exudate in the trachea and bronchi, generally without hemorrhage. Caseous plugs may be found in the trachea of young birds. Air sacs are thickened and opaque. Secondary bacterial infections in meat-type birds, especially with coliform bacteria, produce caseous airsacculitis, perihepatitis, and pericarditis. Nephropathogenic strains produce swollen, pale kidneys, with tubules and ureters distended with urates. In layers, urolithiasis is associated with virus infection and certain dietary factors.

Diagnosis: Diagnosis cannot be based solely on clinical signs because of similarities to mild respiratory forms of Newcastle disease, laryngotracheitis, and infectious coryza. Seroconversion or a rise in IBV antibody titer shown by ELISA, hemagglutination inhibition, or virus neutralization tests can be used for diagnosis given a history of respiratory disease or reduced egg production. A definitive diagnosis is generally based on virus isolation and identification. Virus can be isolated by inoculation of bacteria-free tissue homogenates of trachea, cecal tonsils, and kidneys into 9- to 11-day-old chicken embryos. Several blind passages of the virus may be necessary for isolation of some field strains. The virus produces embryo stunting, curling, and urate deposits in the mesonephros, with variable mortality. Because the virus exhibits great antigenic variation, the serotype should be identified if possible. Serotypes are conventionally identified with the aid of known serotype-specific chicken antisera in the virus neutralization test. However, the virus neutralization test is expensive, time consuming, and not readily available; therefore, it is not commonly used. A limited number of serotype-specific monoclonal antibodies (MAb) have been developed for serotyping purposes. However, direct application of MAb-based immunohistochemical procedures for detection of viral antigen in infected chicken tissues is not considered dependable because of the low concentration of the antigen in the tissues. The MAb have been best used after the virus is propagated by passage in chicken embryos, in which case the virus can be detected in the cells associated with the chorioallantoic membranes by immunofluorescence or immunoperoxidase staining, or in the allantoic fluid by ELISA.

Analyses of the viral genome for the purpose of identifying the virus serotype are now commonly used. These methods are based on the application of reverse transcriptase PCR (RT-PCR), using-specific oligonucleotide primers, to produce DNA copies of IBV genes, usually of the S1 part of the spike glycoprotein gene. Subsequently, the RT-PCR product is subjected to restriction fragment length polymorphism (RFLP) or analyzed by nucleotide sequencing. For RFLP, the RT-PCR product is digested with a set of specific restriction endonucleases, and the digested nucleic acid fragments are separated by gel electrophoresis. The specific pattern of their separation in the gel is compared with those of the standard strains for identification.

Control: No available medication alters the course of the disease, although antibiotic therapy may reduce mortality due to secondary infections. Increasing the temperature in the poultry house and under the hover by 5-10°F (3-5°C) may lower mortality.

Attenuated vaccines used for immunization may produce mild respiratory signs. Live vaccines are initially given to chicks 1-14 days old by spray, drinking water, or eyedrop. Revaccination is common. Live or adjuvanted killed vaccines are sometimes used in breeders and layers to prevent egg production losses.

Many serotypes are recognized, and a number of new or variant serotypes have been reported, which pose problems in immunization and diagnosis. If possible, selection of vaccine should be based on knowledge of the prevalent serotype(s) on the premises. The most commonly used live vaccines in the USA contain strains of IBV serotypes Massachusetts, Connecticut, and Arkansas. Vaccination with selected variant serotypes is practiced in some areas. Outbreaks with mortality due to nephritis have been associated with several variant strains in Australia and the USA. Infection with standard as well as variant serotypes have been associated with egg production losses in vaccinated layer flocks.

INFECTIOUS CORYZA

Infectious coryza is an acute respiratory disease of chickens characterized by nasal discharge, sneezing, and swelling of the face under the eyes. It is distributed worldwide. The disease is seen only in chickens; reports of the disease in quail and pheasants probably describe a similar disease that is caused by a different etiologic agent.

In developed countries such as the USA, the disease is seen primarily in pullets and layers and occasionally in broilers. In the USA, it is most prevalent in commercial flocks in California and the southeast, although northeastern USA has recently experienced significant outbreaks. In developing countries, the disease often is seen in very young chicks, even as young as 3 wk of age. Poor biosecurity, poor environment, and the stress of other diseases are probably the main reasons why infectious coryza is more of a problem in developing countries. The disease has no public health significance.

Etiology: The causative bacterium, *Haemophilus paragallinarum (gallinarum)* is a gram-negative, pleomorphic, nonmotile, catalase-negative, microaerophilic rod that requires nicotinamide adenine dinucleotide (V-factor) for in vitro growth. When grown on blood agar with a staphylococcal nurse colony that excretes the V-factor, the satellite colonies appear as dewdrops, growing adjacent to the nurse colony. V-factor-independent *H paragallinarum* have been recovered in South Africa and Mexico. The most commonly used serotyping scheme is the Page scheme, which groups *H paragallinarum* isolates into 3 serovars (A, B, and C) that correlate with immunotype specificity.

Epidemiology and Transmission: Chronically ill or healthy carrier birds are the reservoir of infection. Chickens of all ages are susceptible, but susceptibility increases with age. The incubation period is 1-3 days, and the disease duration is usually 2-3 wk. Under field conditions, the duration may be longer in the presence of concurrent diseases, eg, mycoplasmosis.

Infected flocks are a constant threat to uninfected flocks. Transmission is by direct contact, airborne droplets, and contamination of drinking water. "All-in/all-out" management has essentially eradicated infectious coryza from many commercial poultry establishments in the USA. Commercial farms that have multiple-age flocks tend to perpetuate the disease. Egg transmission does not occur. Molecular techniques such as restriction endonuclease analysis and ribotyping have been used to trace outbreaks of infectious coryza.

Clinical Findings: In the mildest form of the disease, the only signs may be depression, a serous nasal discharge, and occasionally slight facial swelling. In the more severe form, there is severe swelling of one or both infraorbital sinuses with edema of the surrounding tissue, which may close one or both eyes. In adult birds, especially males, the edema may extend to the intermandibular space and wattles. The swelling usually abates in 10-14 days; however, if secondary infection occurs, swelling can persist for months. There may be varying degrees of rales depending on the extent of infection. In Argentina, a septicemic form of the disease has been reported, probably due to concurrent infections. Egg production may be delayed in young pullets and severely reduced in producing hens. Birds may have diarrhea, and feed and water consumption usually is decreased during acute stages of the disease.

Lesions: In acute cases, lesions may be limited to the infraorbital sinuses. There is a copious, tenacious, grayish, semifluid exudate. As the disease becomes chronic or other pathogens become involved, the sinus exudate may become consolidated and turn yellowish. Other lesions may include conjunctivitis, tracheitis, bronchitis, and airsacculitis, particularly if other pathogens are involved. The histopathologic response of respiratory organs consists of disintegration and hyperplasia of mucosal and glandular epithelia and edema with infiltration of heterophils, macrophages, and mast cells.

Diagnosis: Isolation of a gram-negative, satellitic, catalase-negative organism from chickens in a flock with a history of a rapidly spreading coryza is diagnostic. The catalase test is essential, as nonpathogenic *Haemophilus* organisms, which are catalase-positive, are present in both healthy and diseased chickens. A PCR test that can be used on the live chicken and that has proved superior to culture, even in developing countries, has been developed. Production of typical signs after inoculation with nasal exudate from infected into susceptible chickens is also reliable diagnostically. No suitable serologic test exists; a hemagglutination-inhibition test is the best of the available tests. Swelling of the face and wattles must be differentiated from that seen in fowl cholera (p 2228). Other diseases that must be considered are mycoplasmosis, laryngotracheitis, Newcastle disease, infectious bronchitis, avian influenza, swollen head syndrome (ornithobacterosis), and vitamin A deficiency.

While currently found only in South Africa and Mexico, the presence of a V-factor-independent *H paragallinarum* must also be considered. The *H paragallinarum* PCR is an ideal diagnostic tool in this situation.

Control and Treatment: Prevention is the only sound method of control. "All-in/all-out" farm programs with sound management and isolation methods are the best way to avoid the disease. Replacements should be raised on the same farm or obtained from clean flocks. If replacement pullets are to be placed on a farm that has a history of infectious coryza, bacterins are available to help prevent and control the disease. USDA-licensed bacterins are available, and bacterins also are produced within states for intrastate use. Bacterins also are produced in many other countries. Because serovars A, B, and C are not cross-protective, it is essential that bacterins contain the serovars present in the target population. Vaccination should be completed ~4 wk before infectious coryza usually breaks out on the individual farm. Antibodies detected by the hemagglutination-inhibition test after bacterin administration correlate with protective immunity. Controlled exposure to live organisms also has been used to immunize layers in endemic areas.

Because early treatment is important, water medication is recommended immediately until medicated feed is available. Erythromycin and oxytetracycline are usually beneficial. Several new-generation antibiotics (eg, fluoroquinolones, macrolides) are active against infectious coryza. Various sulfonamides, sulfonamide-trimethoprim, and other combinations have been successful but must not be used in layers. In more severe outbreaks, although treatment may result in improvement, the disease may recur when medication is discontinued.

Preventive medication may be combined with a vaccination program, if started pullets are to be reared or housed on infected premises.

INFECTIOUS LARYNGOTRACHEITIS

Infectious laryngotracheitis (ILT) is an acute, highly contagious, herpesvirus infection of chickens and pheasants characterized by severe dyspnea, coughing, and rales. It can also be a subacute disease with lacrimation, tracheitis, conjunctivitis, and mild rales. It has been reported from most areas of the USA in which poultry are intensively reared, as well as from many other countries.

Clinical Findings: In the acute form, gasping, coughing, rattling, and extension of the neck during inspiration are seen 5-12 days after natural exposure. Reduced productivity is a varying factor in laying flocks. Affected birds are anorectic and inactive. The mouth and beak may be bloodstained from the tracheal exudate. Mortality varies, but may reach 50% in adults, and is usually due to occlusion of the trachea by hemorrhage or exudate. Signs usually subside after ~2 wk, although birds may cough for 1 mo. Strains of low virulence produce little or no mortality with slight respiratory signs and lesions and a slight decrease in egg production.

After recovery, some birds remain carriers for extended periods and become a source of infection for susceptible birds. The latent virus can be reactivated under stressful conditions. Infection also may be spread mechanically. Several epidemics have been traced to the transport of birds in contaminated crates.

Diagnosis: The acute disease is characterized by the clinical signs and by finding blood, mucus, and yellow caseous exudate or a hollow caseous cast in the trachea. Microscopically, a desquamative, necrotizing tracheitis is characteristic. In the subacute form, punctiform hemorrhagic areas in the trachea and larynx, and conjunctivitis with lacrimation permit a presumptive diagnosis. In uncomplicated cases, the air sacs usually are not involved. The diagnosis may be confirmed by demonstrating intranuclear inclusion bodies in the tracheal epithelium early in the course of the disease; by isolating and identifying the specific virus in chick embryos, tissue culture, or chickens; or by inoculating the infraorbital sinus or vent of known immune and susceptible birds. Chicken embryos (9-12 days old) are preferred for virus isolation. Chorioallantoic membrane of developing chicken embryos is inoculated with the specimen. Microscopic examination of the chorioallantoic membrane lesion shows intranuclear inclusions. ILT must be differentiated from the diphtheritic form of fowlpox (p 2276), especially with tracheal lesions. Fowlpox virus produces intracytoplasmic inclusions.

Field isolates and vaccine strains of ILT virus can be compared by restriction endonuclease analysis of viral genomes. This method is useful for comparing closely related DNA genomes and in the epidemiology of the disease. However, significant differences may not be apparent between field and vaccine strains of ILT virus.

Nucleic acid probes prepared from cloned genomic fragments of ILT virus can also be used for diagnosis. This procedure is especially useful for differentiation of ILT from the diphtheritic form of fowlpox with tracheal lesions.

PCR, which can amplify ILT virus genomic DNA sequences of various sizes using specific primers, is useful when an extremely small amount of viral DNA is present in the sample. Restriction fragment length polymorphism of PCR products with restriction enzymes can be used to differentiate strains.

Prevention and Treatment: Some relief from signs is obtained by keeping the birds quiet, lowering the dust level, and using mild expectorants, being careful that they do not contaminate feed or water. Vaccination should be practiced in endemic areas and on farms where a specific diagnosis is made. Immediate vaccination of adults in the face of an outbreak shortens the course of the disease. Vaccination is best done with modified strains of low virulence applied to the conjunctiva (eye drop). Results are less consistent with mass methods of vaccination such as spray or drinking water administration. Broiler flocks in some areas where the disease is endemic must be vaccinated when young, but this is unlikely to be effective if done at <4 wk of age. Some vaccine producers recommend revaccination when birds are to be held to maturity. Recently, a recombinant fowlpox virus-vectored vaccine expressing genes from ILT virus has become available commercially.

QUAIL BRONCHITIS

Quail bronchitis is a naturally occurring, highly contagious, often fatal respiratory disease of bobwhite quail, seen both in the wild and in captivity. The disease is of major economic significance to gamebird breeders and has a worldwide distribution. It is a serious disease on certain farms where quail are pen-raised, and particularly when quail of different ages are maintained on the same premises.

The causative agent is a Group I serotype 1 adenovirus that can be readily isolated from the respiratory tract of acutely affected birds. The virus is also easily isolated from fecal samples, intestine, liver, and occasionally the bursa of Fabricius. It is highly contagious and spreads rapidly through multiple-age units. Other avian species, particularly chickens, may be carriers.

Clinical signs include respiratory distress, coughing, sneezing, rales, and lacrimation. Loose, watery droppings are common in some acutely affected older birds. Conjunctivitis, mild to severe tracheitis (the trachea may be completely filled with mucus), airsacculitis, hepatitis, and gaseous distention of the intestines may be seen. Multiple pale, pinpoint (3 mm) foci of necrosis in the liver and mottling and enlargement of the spleen are common lesions in infected birds. Mortality may reach 100% in birds <2 wk old but is usually <25% in birds >4 wk old.

The disease is often self-limiting. Experimental vaccines have proven ineffective in preventing quail bronchitis. There is no specific treatment, but increasing the brooder temperature by 3-5°F (1.5-3°C), preventing "piling up," and avoiding contact between older and younger birds and other avian species are of value, as are strict isolation and sanitation. Immunity is long lasting, possibly for life, and recovered birds can be retained for breeders. New birds should not be introduced to premises without a 30-day quarantine.

NUTRITION AND MANAGEMENT: POULTRY

NUTRITIONAL REQUIREMENTS

Poultry continue to rank high in their ability to convert feed into food products. Such high efficiency has increased progressively in recent decades. The nutrient requirement figures published in *Nutrient Requirements of Poultry* (National Academy of Sciences, 1994) are the most recent available and should be viewed as minimal nutrient needs for poultry. They are derived from experimentally determined levels after an extensive review of the published data. Criteria used to determine the adequacy of a given nutrient include growth, feed efficiency, health, productivity, and quality of poultry product. These requirements do not, however, include a margin of safety. Consequently, under practical conditions in which there may be different strains, energy content of the diets, environmental temperatures, type of floor, availability of nutrients from various feedstuffs, destruction or loss of nutrients in the gut, pro-oxidants, intestinal parasites, mycotoxins, diseases, and many other stresses, nutritionists should make the proper adjustment by adding a margin of safety to the nutrient requirements.

Water: Many factors influence water intake, including environmental temperature, relative humidity, composition of the diet, birds' productivity (rate of growth or egg production), and the individual bird's ability to resorb water in the kidney. As a result, precise water requirements cannot be determined. However, water is of vital importance and is considered an essential nutrient. Water deprivation for ≥12 hr has an adverse effect on growth of young poultry and egg production of layers; water deprivation for ≥36 hr results in a marked increase in mortality of both young and mature poultry. Cool, clean water must be available at all times.

Energy, Protein, and Amino Acids: The apparent metabolizable energy (AME_n) and the true metabolizable energy (TME_n) values are used for numerous feedstuffs in poultry rations. AME_n is the gross energy of the feed minus the gross energy of the excreta after a correction for the nitrogen retained in the body. Similarly, TME_n is the gross energy of the feed consumed minus the gross energy of the excreta of food origin after a correction for the nitrogen retained in the body. AME_n and TME_n are similar for many ingredients. However, the 2 values could differ substantially for some ingredients such as feather meal, rice bran, wheat middlings, and corn distiller's grains with solubles. AME_n is the energy value used by most poultry nutritionists in feed formulation.

Because chickens and other fowl can adjust their feed intake over a considerable range of feed energy levels to meet their daily energy needs, dietary energy levels are used to set the levels of other nutrients, including protein and amino acids. As a result, the concept of the calorie to protein and amino acids ratio has been used extensively in poultry feed formulation. However, recent research indicated that changes in feed intake of both broilers and layers were not inversely proportional to changes in dietary energy levels. This is particularly true when birds were fed high-energy diets (layers) or moderate-to high-energy diets (broilers). Consequently, the use of these specific ratios must be carefully evaluated. Because factors other than dietary energy could also affect feed intake, including ambient temperature (which can have a considerable impact on feed consumption), nutrient density in the ration should be adjusted to provide appropriate nutrient intake based on requirements and the actual feed intake.

The energy values listed in the nutrient requirement tables in this chapter (TABLE 6, TABLE 7, TABLE 8, TABLE 9, TABLE 10, TABLE 11, TABLE 12, TABLE 13, TABLE 14, and TABLE 15) should be regarded as guidelines rather than absolute requirements. Also, some of the amino acid values were established by direct experimentation, while other values were calculated, assuming the amino acid requirements to be proportional to protein requirements. The amino acids shown in these tables are considered essential for poultry.

TABLE 6. Nutrient Requirements of Growing Pullets[*]

Age (wk)	0-6	6-12	12-18	18 to 1st Egg
White-egg Layers				
Body weight (g)[†]	**450**	**980**	**1,375**	**1,475**
Protein	18	16	15	17
Arginine	1.0	0.83	0.67	0.75
Lysine	0.85	0.60	0.45	0.52
Methionine	0.30	0.25	0.20	0.22
Methionine + cystine	0.62	0.52	0.42	0.47
Threonine	0.68	0.57	0.37	0.47
Tryptophan	0.17	0.17	0.11	0.12
Calcium	0.90	0.80	0.80	2.00
Phosphorus, available	0.40	0.35	0.30	0.32
Brown-egg Layers				
Body weight (g)[†]	**500**	**1,100**	**1,500**	**1,600**
Protein	17	15	14	16
Arginine	0.94	0.78	0.62	0.72
Lysine	0.80	0.56	0.42	0.49
Methionine	0.28	0.23	0.19	0.21
Methionine + cystine	0.59	0.49	0.39	0.44
Threonine	0.64	0.53	0.35	0.44
Tryptophan	0.16	0.13	0.10	0.11
Calcium	0.90	0.80	0.80	2.0
Phosphorus, available	0.40	0.35	0.30	0.35

[*]Requirements are listed as percentages of diet. Nutrient levels should be adjusted to meet specific strain requirements, level of feed intake, and body weight and skeletal development.
[†]Average body weight at end of each period

TABLE 7. Nutrient Requirements of Laying Hens at Different Feed Intakes*

Pounds (approx.)/100 birds/day	18	20	22	24	26
Grams of feed/bird/day	80	90	100	110	120
White-egg Layers					
Protein	18.8	16.7	15.0	13.6	12.5
Arginine	0.88	0.78	0.70	0.64	0.58
Lysine	0.86	0.77	0.69	0.63	0.58
Methionine	0.38	0.33	0.30	0.27	0.25
Methionine + cystine	0.73	0.64	0.58	0.53	0.48
Threonine	0.59	0.52	0.47	0.43	0.39
Tryptophan	0.20	0.18	0.16	0.15	0.13
Calcium	4.12	3.67	3.30	3.00	2.75
Phosphorus, available	0.31	0.28	0.25	0.23	0.21
Brown-egg Layers					
Protein	22.5	20.0	18.0	16.4	15.0
Arginine	1.06	0.94	0.85	0.77	0.71
Lysine	1.05	0.93	0.84	0.76	0.70
Methionine	0.45	0.40	0.36	0.33	0.30
Methionine + cystine	0.89	0.79	0.71	0.65	0.59
Threonine	0.71	0.63	0.57	0.52	0.48
Tryptophan	0.24	0.21	0.19	0.17	0.16
Calcium	5.00	4.44	4.00	3.64	3.33
Phosphorus, available	0.38	0.33	0.30	0.27	0.25

*Requirements are listed as percentages of diet.

Poultry can synthesize glycine but often not in sufficient amounts. Cystine and tyrosine are considered essential even though they can be synthesized from methionine and phenylalanine, respectively.

In practical feed formulation, methionine can spare choline as a methyl donor, and tryptophan can be used to synthesize niacin. These relationships are important because the 2 vitamins can be supplied in diets more economically than the 2 amino acids.

Body weight and composition are important factors in rearing pullets of any strain for maximum egg production. Most strains of White Leghorn chickens have relatively low body weights and do not tend, under normal feeding, to become obese. Feed should be unrestricted to enable these birds to reach adequate body weights at onset of lay. There may be times when, for various reasons, pullets are to be delayed in coming into production. Under such circumstances, feed restriction is necessary to restrict body weight gain of the pullets. For brown-egg strains of chickens, some degree of restriction is often practiced (~90% of ad lib feeding). Some type of feed restriction program is particularly important for broiler-strain pullets, which tend to become obese if fed ad lib. Feed inake of the broiler breeder is also restricted during the laying period.

Pullets now come into production and reach peak production weeks earlier than they did several years ago. This is true both for commercial layers and broiler breeders. Thus, it is of utmost importance that the starting, growing, and developer feeds are fully adequate for development of strong pullets of normal body weight at onset of lay.

TABLE 8. Nutrient Requirements of Broilers[*]

Age[†] kcal AME$_n$/kg diet[‡]	0-3 wk 3,200	3-6 wk 3,200	6-8 wk 3,200
Crude protein[§]	23.00	20.00	18.00
Arginine	1.25	1.10	1.00
Glycine + serine	1.25	1.14	0.97
Histidine	0.35	0.32	0.27
Isoleucine	0.80	0.73	0.62
Leucine	1.20	1.09	0.93
Lysine	1.10	1.00	0.85
Methionine	0.50	0.38	0.32
Methionine + cystine	0.90	0.72	0.60
Phenylalanine	0.72	0.65	0.56
Phenylalanine + tyrosine	1.34	1.22	1.04
Proline	0.60	0.55	0.46
Threonine	0.80	0.74	0.68
Tryptophan	0.20	0.18	0.16
Valine	0.90	0.82	0.70

[*]Requirements are listed as percentages of diet.

[†]The 0- to 3-, 3- to 6-, and 6- to 8-wk intervals for nutrient requirements are based on chronology for which research data were available; however, these nutrient requirements are often implemented at younger age intervals or on a weight-of-feed consumed basis.

[‡]These are typical dietary energy concentrations. Different energy values may be appropriate depending on local ingredient prices and availability.

[§]Broiler chickens do not have a requirement for crude protein per se. However, there should be sufficient crude protein to ensure an adequate nitrogen supply for synthesis of nonessential amino acids. Suggested requirements for crude protein are typical of those derived with corn-soybean meal diets, and levels can be reduced when synthetic amino acids are used.

Vitamins: One IU of **vitamin A** activity is equivalent to 1.3 μg of pure retinol (or 0.344 μg of retinyl acetate). In chickens, 0.6 μg of β-carotene is considered equivalent to 1 IU of vitamin A. However, young chicks are not efficient in using β-carotene. The vitamin A requirements currently recommended are based on use of stabilized vitamin A preparations and thus are somewhat lower than previously recommended levels.

Requirements for **vitamin D** are expressed in IU. Birds use vitamin D_3 from fish oils and irradiated animal sterols quite effectively but cannot use vitamin D_2. Metabolic forms of vitamin D have been isolated and synthesized; these are 25-hydroxy vitamin D_3, which is synthesized in the liver, and 1,25-dihydroxy vitamin D_3, which is synthesized in the kidneys. One IU of vitamin D represents the vitamin D activity of 0.025 μg of pure vitamin D_3.

One IU of **vitamin E** is equivalent to 1 mg of synthetic dl-α-tocopherol acetate. Vitamin E requirements vary with the type and level of fat in the diet, the levels of selenium and trace minerals, and the presence or absence of other antioxidants.

Choline is required as an integral part of the body phospholipid, as a part of acetyl-choline, and as a source of methyl groups. Growing chickens can use betaine as a methylating agent, but betaine cannot replace choline in preventing perosis. Betaine is widely distributed in practical feedstuffs and may be important in sparing choline. Adequate dietary vitamin B_{12} helps pullets develop the ability to biosynthesize choline. The choline requirement values apply to diets containing the specified levels of vitamin B_{12}.

Minerals: The calcium requirement of laying hens is difficult to define. Too much dietary calcium interferes with the use of several other minerals, as well as fat, and tends to reduce palatability. For laying, the recommended level of 3.6-5.0% is adequate in most cases, depending on strain, level of egg production, body weight, and egg mass. Older hens, and especially those subjected to high environmental temperature, may require levels up to and perhaps >3.75%.

Unidentified Nutrients: The chick has requirements for 40 nutrients, together with an adequate level of metabolizable energy. Some unidentified growth and hatchability factors may improve performance under certain stress conditions. However, with the identification of vitamins and the significant role of many trace elements, many poultry nutritionists disregard the importance of such factors.

ANTIBIOTICS

Antibiotics at low levels (5-25 mg/kg of feed, depending on the antibiotic) are used in poultry feeds to improve growth rate and feed efficiency. However, in some countries, regulations restrict this usage for certain antibiotics.

FEEDING AND MANAGEMENT PRACTICES

Success of the feeding program should be measured by how it achieves the breeder's goals for proper weight and development specific to each strain. Feed and the length of time required for attaining certain weights in pullets and turkeys are presented in the growth and feed tables. *See* TABLE 6, TABLE 7, TABLE 8, TABLE 9, TABLE 10, TABLE 11, TABLE 12, TABLE 13, TABLE 14, and TABLE 15, which can be used as a guide in estimating the amount of feed required. These figures may vary considerably due to differences in the nutrient density of feed, strain or breed of bird, amount of feed wasted, and environmental temperature.

Most diets used in feeding poultry are nutritionally "complete" diets that are commercially mixed, ie, prepared by feed manufacturing companies, most of which employ trained nutritionists. The formulation and mixing of poultry feeds requires knowledge and experience in purchasing ingredients, experimental testing of formulas, laboratory control of ingredient quality, and computer applications. Improper mixing can result in vitamin and mineral deficiencies, lack of protection against disease, or drug toxicity.

The physical form of the feed influences the expected results. Most feeds for starting and growing birds are produced as pellets or crumbles. In the pelleting process, the mash is treated with steam and then passed through a suitably sized die under pressure. The pellets are then cooled quickly and dried by means of a forced air draft. The conditions under which pelleting occurs (eg, use of an expander rather than an extruder, exposure to high temperature, use of soft pellets) have an important effect on the nutritional quality of the pellets, or of the crumbles that are produced by crushing the pellets.

FEEDING METHODS

For newly hatched birds of any species, a "complete" feed in crumble form is the program of choice, regardless of other considerations. A "complete" feed program for growing stock, particularly for laying and breeding stock, is also highly recommended. Advantages of the "complete" feed program over the "mash and grain" system include the simplicity of feeding, accuracy of medication, improved balance of dietary nutrients, and superior feed conversion efficiency.

Regardless of the system of feeding, recommendations of the feed manufacturer or the strain's breeder company should be followed with regard to the feeding of extra calcium, grit, or whole grain. Fresh, clean water should be readily available.

VACCINATION PROGRAMS

See TABLE 16, TABLE 17, TABLE 18, TABLE 19, TABLE 20, and TABLE 21.

TABLE 9. Protein and Amino Acid Requirements of Turkeys[*]

Energy base kcal ME/kg diet[†]	Age (wk)			
	Male: 0-4 Female: 0-4 2,800	4-8 4-8 2,900	8-12 8-11 3,000	12-16 11-14 3,100
Protein	28.0	26	22	19
Arginine	1.6	1.4	1.1	0.9
Glycine + serine	1.0	0.9	0.8	0.7
Histidine	0.58	0.5	0.4	0.3
Isoleucine	1.1	1.0	0.8	0.6
Leucine	1.9	1.75	1.5	1.25
Lysine	1.6	1.5	1.3	1.0
Methionine	0.55	0.45	0.4	0.35
Methionine + cystine	1.05	0.95	0.8	0.65
Phenylalanine	1.0	0.9	0.8	0.7
Phenylalanine + tyrosine	1.8	1.6	1.2	1.0
Threonine	1.0	0.95	0.8	0.75
Tryptophan	0.26	0.24	0.2	0.18
Valine	1.2	1.2	0.9	0.8

[*]Requirements are listed as percentages of diet.
[†]These are typical ME concentrations for corn-soya diets. Different ME values may be appropriate if other ingredients predominate.

MANAGEMENT OF GROWING CHICKENS

Heated brooders for chicks are surrounded by a chick guard to keep the birds near the heat source. At placement the brooder floor temperature should be between 85-90°F (29.4-32.2°C). As the birds become older, the brooder temperature is lowered 5°F (2.8°C) each week until the temperature is 70°F (21.1°C). The chick guard is typically removed at 1 wk of age, and the birds then have the run of the whole pen. Ample space should be provided for feeders and waterers, which should be well distributed in the pen.

At least 3 in. (7.5 cm) of suitable litter, clean for each brood and spread to an even depth, should be provided at the start. Litter must be free of mold; it should absorb moisture without caking, be nontoxic, and of large enough particle size to discourage consumption. Chicks are started with 24 hr of light for several days; thereafter, light is reduced. Both length of day and intensity of light are important. Lighting programs vary widely, depending on whether housing is windowless or open-sided, and should comply with recommendations of major breeders in similar situations.

Feeding systems are often combined with day-length control during rearing to influence the rate at which birds mature. Under certain conditions, pullets may be debeaked at 4-7 days of age. In controlled environment housing, day lengths are controlled more precisely; with dim lights, debeaking may be delayed until later in the growing period.

Pullets should be treated for external and internal parasites as required. Vaccination should be used to control problem diseases of the area (see p 2311).

Many pullets are reared in cages. The cage manufacturer usually supplies specific instructions regarding heating, bird density, and feeding space. Most commercial rations are fortified with sufficient nutrients to meet the requirements of cage-reared birds.

MANAGEMENT OF LAYING CHICKENS

Most laying pullets are housed in cages and should be moved to these facilities at least 1 wk before egg production begins. Breeders moved from a growing house to an

◀ **TABLE 9.** *(Continued)*

	Age (wk)		
16-20 14-17 3,200	20-24 17-20 3,300	Holding 2,900	Breeding Hens 2,900
16.5	14	12	14
0.75	0.6	0.5	0.6
0.6	0.5	0.4	0.5
0.25	0.2	0.2	0.3
0.5	0.45	0.4	0.5
1.0	0.8	0.5	0.5
0.8	0.65	0.5	0.6
0.25	0.25	0.2	0.2
0.55	0.45	0.4	0.4
0.6	0.5	0.4	0.55
0.9	0.9	0.8	1.0
0.6	0.5	0.4	0.45
0.15	0.13	0.1	0.13
0.7	0.6	0.5	0.58

Adapted, with permission, from *Nutrient Requirements of Poultry*, 1994, National Academy of Sciences, National Academy Press, Washington, DC.

TABLE 10. Nutrient Requirements of Pheasants[*]

Energy base kcal ME/kg diet[†]	0-4 wk 2,800	4-8 wk 2,800	9-17 wk 2,700	Breeding 2,800
Protein (%)	28	24	18	15
Glycine + serine (%)	1.8	1.55	1	0.5
Lysine (%)	1.5	1.40	0.8	0.68
Methionine + cystine (%)	1.0	0.93	0.6	0.6
Linoleic acid (%)	1	1	1	1
Calcium (%)	1.0	0.85	0.53	2.5
Phosphorus, available (%)	0.55	0.5	0.45	0.40
Sodium (%)	0.15	0.15	0.15	0.15
Chlorine (%)	0.11	0.11	0.11	0.11
Iodine (mg)	0.3	0.3	0.3	0.3
Riboflavin (mg)	3.4	3.4	3.0	4.0
Pantothenic acid (mg)	10	10	10	16
Niacin (mg)	70	70	40	30
Choline (mg)	1,430	1,300	1,000	1,000

[*]Requirements are listed as percentages or as mg/kg of diet. For values not listed, *see* REQUIRE-MENTS OF TURKEYS (TABLE 9 and TABLE 15) as a guide.

[†]These are typical dietary energy concentrations

Adapted, with permission, from *Nutrient Requirements of Poultry*, 1994, National Academy of Sciences, National Academy Press, Washington, DC.

TABLE 11. Nutrient Requirements of Bobwhite Quail[*]

Energy base kcal ME/kg diet[†]	Starting 2,800	Growing 2,800	Breeding 2,800
Protein (%)	26	20	24
Glycine + serine (%)	—	—	—
Lysine (%)	—	—	—
Methionine + cystine (%)	1.0	0.75	0.90
Linoleic acid (%)	1	1	1
Calcium (%)	0.65	0.65	2.4
Phosphorus, available (%)	0.45	0.30	0.7
Sodium (%)	0.15	0.15	0.15
Chlorine (%)	0.11	0.11	0.11
Iodine (mg)	0.3	0.3	0.3
Riboflavin (mg)	3.8	3.0	4.0
Pantothenic acid (mg)	12	9	15
Niacin (mg)	30	30	20
Choline (mg)	1,500	1,500	1,000

[*]Requirements are listed as percentages or as mg/kg of diet. For values not listed, *see* REQUIRE-MENTS OF LAYING HENS AND LEGHORN-TYPE CHICKENS (TABLE 7 and TABLE 14) as a guide.
[†]These are typical dietary energy concentrations.

Adapted, with permission, from *Nutrient Requirements of Poultry*, 1994, National Academy of Sciences, National Academy Press, Washington, DC.

adult house should also be given at least 1 wk to adjust to their new environment before the stress of egg production begins. Beaks should be retrimmed as necessary, and cull birds removed at the time of rehousing.

Feeders and waterers should be of the proper type, size, and height for the stock and management system. Feeders that are too shallow, too narrow, or lacking a lip or flange on the upper edge may permit excess feed waste. Uneven distribution of waterers or lack of water space results in reduced intake and thus reduced performance.

Artificial Lights: Day length should be increased gradually as the pullets come into egg production and should reach a 14- to 16-hr light period/day at peak production for both market-egg and hatching-egg layers. An intensity of at least one foot-candle of light (10 lux) at the feed trough should be provided; this is about equal to one 60-watt light bulb to each 100 sq ft (~9 sq m), hanging 7 ft (2.1 m) above the birds. Production may decrease if day length or light intensity is reduced during the laying period. With cage systems of all types, illumination is more even if smaller wattage bulbs placed closer together are used, rather than large bulbs suspended over the center of each aisle. With tiered cages, the bulbs are suspended 6-7 in. (15-18 cm) above the level of the top cage.

Record Keeping: Successful intensive poultry keeping requires good records of all flock activities, including hatch date, regular body weights (to ensure that the pullets will have reached optimal body weight when they are brought into egg production), lighting program, house temperatures, disease history, medication and vaccination dates, quantity and type of feed given (important in calculating efficiency of feed utilization), and mortality.

Floor Space, Feeding, and Watering Requirements: Egg-production birds usually spend their entire lives in cages. While some broiler breeders are similarly housed, most are reared on litter floors or in pens in which up to two-thirds of the floor is slatted. For

TABLE 12. Nutrient Requirements of Pekin Ducks*

Energy base kcal ME/kg diet[†]	Starting (0-2 wk) 2,900	Growing (2-7 wk) 2,900	Breeding 2,900
Protein (%)	22	16	15
Arginine (%)	1.1	1.0	—
Lysine (%)	0.9	0.65	0.6
Methionine + cystine (%)	0.7	0.55	0.5
Calcium (%)	0.65	0.6	2.75
Phosphorus, available (%)	0.40	0.30	0.30
Sodium (%)	0.15	0.15	0.15
Chlorine (%)	0.12	0.12	0.12
Magnesium (mg)	500	500	500
Manganese (mg)	50	?	?
Zinc (mg)	60	?	?
Selenium (mg)	0.2	?	?
Vitamin A (IU)	2,500	2,500	4,000
Vitamin D (IU)	400	400	900
Vitamin K (mg)	0.5	0.5	0.5
Riboflavin (mg)	4	4	4
Pantothenic acid (mg)	11	11	11
Niacin (mg)	55	55	55
Pyridoxine (mg)	2.5	2.5	3.0

*Requirements are listed as percentages or as units or mg/kg of diet. For nutrients not listed, *see* NUTRIENT REQUIREMENTS OF BROILERS (TABLE 8) as a guide.
[†]These are typical dietary energy concentrations.

Adapted, with permission, from *Nutrient Requirements of Poultry*, 1994, National Academy of Sciences, National Academy Press, Washington, DC.

TABLE 13. Nutrient Requirements of Geese*

Energy base kcal ME/kg diet[†]	Starting (0-4 wk) 2,900	Growing (after 4 wk) 2,900	Breeding 2,900
Protein (%)		15	15
Lysine (%)	1.0	0.85	0.6
Methionine + cystine (%)	0.6	0.5	0.5
Calcium (%)	0.65	0.6	2.25
Phosphorus, available (%)	0.3	0.3	0.3
Vitamin A (IU)	1,500	1,500	4,000
Vitamin D (IU)	200	200	200
Riboflavin (mg)	3.8	2.5	4.0
Pantothenic acid (mg)	15	10	10
Niacin (mg)	65	35	20

*Requirements are listed as percentages or as units or mg/kg of diet. For nutrients not listed, *see* REQUIREMENTS OF BROILERS (TABLE 8) as a guide.
[†]These are typical dietary energy concentrations.

Adapted, with permission, from *Nutrient Requirements of Poultry*, 1994, National Academy of Sciences, National Academy Press, Washington, DC.

TABLE 14. Linoleic Acid, Mineral, and Vitamin Requirements of Leghorn-type Chickens[*]

Age	0-6 wk	6-18 wk	18 wk to 1st egg	Layers	Breeders
Linoleic acid (%)	1.00	1.00	1.00	1.00	1.00
Potassium (%)	0.25	0.25	0.25	0.15	0.15
Sodium (%)	0.15	0.15	0.15	0.15	0.15
Chlorine (%)	0.15	0.15	0.15	0.13	0.13
Magnesium (mg)	600	500/400	400	500	500
Manganese (mg)	60	30	30	20	20
Zinc (mg)	40	35	35	35	45
Iron (mg)	80	60	60	45	60
Copper (mg)	5	4	4	?	?
Iodine (mg)	0.35	0.35	0.35	0.035	0.01
Selenium (mg)	0.15	0.1	0.1	0.06	0.06
Vitamin A (IU)	1,500	1,500	1,500	3,000	3,000
Vitamin D_3 (IU)	200	200	300	300	300
Vitamin E (IU)	10	5	5	5	10
Vitamin K (mg)	0.5	0.5	0.5	0.5	1.0
Riboflavin (mg)	3.6	1.8	2.2	2.5	3.6
Pantothenic acid (mg)	10	10	10	2	7
Niacin (mg)	27	10	10	10	10
Vitamin B_{12} (mg)	0.009	0.003	0.004	0.004	0.08
Choline (mg)	1,300	900/500	500	1,050	1,050
Biotin (mg)	0.15	0.1	0.1	0.1	0.1
Folacin (mg)	0.55	0.25	0.25	0.25	0.35
Thiamine (mg)	1.0	1.0/0.8	0.8	0.7	0.7
Pyridoxine (mg)	3	3	3	2.5	4.5

[*]Requirements are listed as percentages or as units or mg/kg of diet. Assumes an average daily intake of 110 g of feed/hen/day.

Adapted, with permission, from *Nutrient Requirements of Poultry*, 1994, National Academy of Sciences, National Academy Press, Washington, DC.

egg-strain pullets that are reared in cages, there is little chance of altering the feeding and watering space available, but periodic checks are necessary to ensure that feed and water are being continuously supplied. With the success of nipple- and cup-waterers and the various types of automatic feeding systems, it becomes more difficult to give specific recommendations for feeding and watering space. Decisions must be made about optimal floor space and feeding and watering requirements based on advice from equipment manufacturers, primary breeders, careful observation, and past experience as to productivity. *See* TABLE 22 and TABLE 23 for space requirements for egg-strain and meat-strain birds. Environmental housing and various types of ventilation may alter these specifications.

Layers per Cage: Within the guidelines indicated in TABLE 22 and TABLE 23, most colony cages house 5-10 layers. The ideal flock size depends on several factors, including labor and cost, and is best determined only by the individual poultry manager or producer.

ORGANIC PRODUCTION PRACTICES

Organic Poultry: According to livestock standards, birds for slaughter designated as organic must be raised under organic management starting no later than the second day of life. Preventive management practices, including the use of vaccines to keep animals healthy are used, but no hormones can be given to promote growth, nor can antibiotics be used for any reason. Organic management standards prohibit producers from withholding treatment from a sick or injured animal; however, animals treated with a prohibited medication may not be sold as organic. All organically raised animals must have access to the outdoors; they may be temporarily confined only for reasons of health, safety, or to protect soil or water quality. Producers and handlers of any agricultural commodity or product, whether raw or processed, including any commodity or product derived from livestock that is marketed in the USA for human or livestock consumption may seek certification under the National Organic Program (NOP) as an organic producer or handler. (The term "consumption" is not limited to products that are used for food.) To qualify for certification, the producer or handler must comply with all applicable production, handling, and labeling regulations under the NOP, including the requirements concerning the use of natural and synthetic substances.

To label a product as "100% organic," an accredited certifying agent must certify "organic," or "made with organic (specified ingredients) by the producer or handler." USDA's Agricultural Marketing Service (AMS) is developing regulations for the use of the term "organic" on the labeling of food products. A proposed rule discussing this issue published in the *Federal Register* in 1997 resulted in ~280,000 public comments. AMS is planning to reissue a proposed rule that will address these issues and seek further comments.

The National Organic Standards Board (NOSB), formed because of the Organic Food Production Act (OFPA), continues to advise AMS on promulgating OFPA regulations. Because USDA has not yet defined the term organic, it may not be used by itself as a claim on the labeling of meat and poultry products, except as part of the signature line on labels (ie, if "organic" is part of the company's incorporated name and it is deemed not to be misleading). The AMS, supported by the activities of the NOP and NOSB, continues to be the focal point for the USDA's efforts to define organic and establish the circumstances under which it applies to agricultural products, including meat and poultry products. Therefore, any labeling statement that uses the term organic would have to be in accordance with the promulgated final rules. These rules will also address accreditation of certifying entities.

Animal Production Claims and "Natural" Claims: The USDA Food Safety and Inspection Service (FSIS) permits the claim "certified organic by (a certifying entity)" along with the use of animal production claims and the term "natural." FSIS permits the application of "animal production claims," ie, truthful statements about how the animals from which meat and poultry products are derived or raised, on the labeling of meat and poultry products. For many years, animal production claims have served as an alternative to the use of the term organic on the labeling of meat and poultry products in the absence of a uniformly accepted definition. Thus, producers may wish to continue the use of animal production claims (eg, "Raised Without Added Hormones," "Free Range") on meat and poultry labeling. The system FSIS has in place for evaluating the necessary supporting documentation to ensure the accuracy of animal production claims, such as producer affidavits and raising protocols, will continue to be used whenever these types of claims are made.

The term "natural" may be used when products contain no artificial ingredients and are no more than minimally processed in accordance with FSIS Policy Memo 055. This term may be used in combination with the claim "certified organic by (a certifying entity)" when the conditions of the policy are met.

NUTRITIONAL DEFICIENCIES

A nutritional deficiency can arise simply due to a nutrient being omitted from the diet, or due to interaction between nutrients or between nutrients and antinutritional

TABLE 15. Linoleic Acid, Mineral, and Vitamin Requirements of Turkeys*

Energy base kcal ME/kg diet[†]	Male: 0-4 Female: 0-4 2,800	4-8 4-8 2,900	8-12 8-11 3,000	12-16 11-14 3,100
		Age (wk)		
Linoleic acid (%)	1.0	1.0	0.8	0.8
Calcium (%)	1.2	1.0	0.85	0.75
Phosphorus, available (%)	0.6	0.5	0.42	0.38
Potassium (%)	0.7	0.6	0.5	0.5
Sodium (%)	0.17	0.15	0.12	0.12
Chlorine (%)	0.15	0.14	0.14	0.12
Magnesium (mg)	500	500	500	500
Manganese (mg)	60	60	60	60
Zinc (mg)	70	65	50	40
Iron (mg)	80	60	60	60
Copper (mg)	8	8	6	6
Iodine (mg)	0.4	0.4	0.4	0.4
Selenium (mg)	0.2	0.2	0.2	0.2
Vitamin A (IU)	5,000	5,000	5,000	5,000
Vitamin D[‡] (IU)	1,100	1,100	1,100	1,100
Vitamin E (IU)	12	12	10	10
Vitamin K (mg)	1.75	1.5	1.0	0.75
Riboflavin (mg)	4.0	3.6	3.0	3.0
Pantothenic acid (mg)	10	9	9	9
Niacin (mg)	60	60	50	50
Vitamin B_{12} (mg)	0.003	0.003	0.003	0.003
Choline (mg)	1,600	1,400	1,100	1,100
Biotin (mg)	0.2	0.2	0.125	0.125
Folacin (mg)	1.0	1.0	0.8	0.8
Thiamine (mg)	2	2	2	2
Pyridoxine (mg)	4.5	4.5	3.5	3.5

*Requirements are listed as percentages or as units or mg/kg of diet.
[†]These are typical ME concentrations for corn-soya diets. Different ME values may be appropriate if other ingredients predominate.
[‡]These concentrations of vitamin D are satisfactory when the dietary concentrations of calcium and available phosphorus conform with those in this table.

factors. The latter situations are difficult to diagnose because, on analysis, the diet is found to contain a normal level of the suspect nutrient. Micronutrients are often packaged into premixes, so it is rare to see classic individual deficiency signs—rather the effect is a compilation of many individual metabolic conditions. In many instances, a correct diagnosis can be made only by obtaining complete information about diet and management, clinical signs in the affected living birds, and results of necropsies and tissue analyses.

The composition of individual ingredients in a diet is variable; some nutrients are comparatively unstable, while others are unavailable in their natural form. A diet that, by

TABLE 15. (continued)

Age (wk)			
16-20 14-17 3,200	20-24 17-20 3,300	Holding 2,900	Breeding Hens 2,900
0.8	0.8	0.8	1.0
0.65	0.55	0.5	2.25
0.32	0.28	0.25	0.35
0.4	0.4	0.4	0.6
0.12	0.12	0.12	0.15
0.12	0.12	0.12	0.12
500	500	500	500
60	60	60	60
40	40	40	65
50	50	50	60
6	6	6	8
0.4	0.4	0.4	0.4
0.2	0.2	0.2	0.2
5,000	5,000	5,000	5,000
1,100	1,100	1,100	1,100
10	10	10	25
0.75	0.5	0.5	1.0
2.5	2.5	2.5	4.0
9	9	9	16
40	40	40	40
0.003	0.003	0.003	0.003
950	800	800	1,000
0.100	0.100	0.100	0.2
0.7	0.7	0.7	1.0
2	2	2	2
3.0	3.0	3.0	4.0

Adapted, with permission, from *Nutrient Requirements of Poultry*, 1994, National Academy of Sciences, National Academy Press, Washington, DC.

analysis, appears to contain just enough of one or more nutrients may actually be deficient to some degree. Stress due to bacterial, parasitic, or viral infections; high or low temperatures; low humidity; or drugs may either interfere with absorption of a nutrient or increase the quantity required. Thus, a toxin, microorganism, or other stressor may destroy or render unavailable a particular nutrient that is present in the diet at normally adequate levels.

Only deficiencies occurring in practical diets in the field are discussed below.

PROTEIN AND AMINO ACID DEFICIENCIES

The optimal level of balanced protein intake changes according to age; for growing chicks it is ~18-23% of the diet; for growing poults and gallinaceous upland game birds,

TABLE 16. Vaccination Program for Broilers*

Age	Vaccine	Route	Type
1 day	Marek's disease[†]	SC	Turkey herpesvirus and SB-1
1 day or	Newcastle disease	Coarse spray	B1
14-21 days	Newcastle disease	Water or coarse spray	B1 or LaSota
1 day or	Infectious bronchitis	Coarse spray	Massachusetts
14-21 days	Infectious bronchitis	Water or coarse spray	Massachusetts
14-21 days	Infectious bursal disease	Water	Intermediate

*This is an example of a typical vaccination program. Individual programs are highly variable and reflect local conditions, disease prevalence, severity of challenge, and individual preferences.
[†]Most USA commercial broiler hatcheries use an in ovo vaccination system for Marek's disease at 17-19 days of embryonation.

Infectious bursal disease vaccine (mild strain) may be combined with Marek's disease vaccines.

Connecticut strain often combined with Massachusetts. Bronchitis vaccine is usually combined with Newcastle.

Other bronchitis strains such as Arkansas 99 and Florida 88 are included in some areas.

Vaccinations at 14-21 days are optional. A single drinking water application for Newcastle disease/bronchitis is common also.

~26-30%; and for growing ducklings and goslings, ~20-22%. If the protein and component amino acid content of the diet is below these levels, birds tend to grow more slowly. Even when a diet contains the recommended quantities of protein, satisfactory growth also requires sufficient quantities and proper balance of all the essential amino acids.

Few specific signs are associated with a deficiency of the various amino acids, except for a peculiar cup-shaped appearance of the feathers in chickens with arginine deficiency and loss of pigment in some of the wing feathers in bronze turkeys with lysine deficiency. All deficiencies of essential amino acids result in retarded growth or reduced egg size or egg production. Some deficiencies or even imbalances of amino acids may be related to management problems such as hysteria, "pickouts" and "blowouts," and fatty liver syndrome.

MINERAL DEFICIENCIES

Calcium and Phosphorus Imbalances

A deficiency of either calcium or phosphorus in the diet of young growing birds results in abnormal bone development even when the diet contains adequate vitamin D_3. This condition, rickets, can also be caused by a dietary deficiency of vitamin D_3 (p 2329), which is necessary for absorption of calcium. A deficiency of either calcium or phosphorus results in lack of normal skeletal calcification. Rickets is seen mainly in growing birds. Calcium deficiency in adult laying hens usually results in reduced shell quality and osteoporosis. This depletion of bone structure causes a disorder commonly referred to as "cage layer fatigue." When calcium is mobilized from bone to overcome a dietary deficiency, the cortical bone erodes and is unable to support the weight of the hen.

Rickets: Rickets most commonly occurs in young meat birds. The primary pathologic change is inadequate bone mineralization. Calcium deficiency at the cellular level is the main problem, which may result from feeding a diet deficient or imbalanced in calcium, phosphorus, or vitamin D_3. Young broilers and poults exhibit lameness, usually around 10-14 days of age. Their bones are rubbery, and the rib cage is flattened and beaded at the attachment of the vertebrae. Rachitic birds exhibit a very disorganized cartilage matrix, with an irregular penetration of vascular canals. Rickets is not caused by a failure in the initiation of bone mineralization, but rather by the early maturation of this process. There is often an enlargement of the ends of the long bones, with a widening of the

TABLE 17. Vaccination Program for Broiler Breeders*

Age	Vaccine	Route	Type
1 day	Marek's disease	SC	Turkey herpesvirus
6-7 days	Tenosynovitis	SC	Live (Mild)
14-21 days	Newcastle/infectious bronchitis	Water	B1/Mass
14-28 days	Infectious bursal disease	Water	Intermediate
4 wk	Newcastle/infectious bronchitis	Water or coarse spray	B1/Mass
6-8 wk	Tenosynovitis	SC	Live (Mild)
8-10 wk	Infectious bursal disease	Water or coarse spray	Live
8-10 wk	Newcastle/infectious bronchitis	Water or coarse spray	B1 or LaSota/Mass
10-12 wk	Encephalomyelitis	Wing web	Live, chick-embryo origin
10-12 wk	Fowlpox	Wing web	Modified live
10-12 wk	Chicken infectious anemia	Wing web	Modified live
10-12 wk	Laryngotracheitis	Intraocular	Modified live
10-12 wk	Tenosynovitis	Parenteral	Inactivated
10-12 wk or	Fowl cholera	Parenteral	Inactivated
	Fowl cholera	Wing web	Live CU, PM-1, or M9
12-14 wk	Newcastle/infectious bronchitis	Water or aerosol	B1 or LaSota/Mass
14-18 wk or	Fowl cholera	Parenteral	Inactivated
	Fowl cholera	Wing web	Live CU, PM-1, or M9
16-18 wk	Infectious bursal disease	Parenteral	Inactivated
16-18 wk	Tenosynovitis	Parenteral	Inactivated
16-18 wk and every	Newcastle/infectious bronchitis	Water or aerosol	B1 or LaSota/Mass
60-90 days or 18 wk	Newcastle/infectious bronchitis	Parenteral	Inactivated

*This is an example of a vaccination program. Individual programs are highly variable and reflect local conditions, disease prevalence, severity of challenge, and individual preferences.

SB-1 or MDV301 may be combined with turkey herpesvirus in some areas.

Vaccination for fowlpox and laryngotracheitis depends on local requirements.

Other strains of infectious bronchitis (Connecticut, Arkansas 99, Florida 88, etc) are included in some areas.

epiphyseal plate. A determination of whether rickets is due to deficiencies of calcium, phosphorus, or vitamin D_3, or to an excess of calcium (which induces a phosphorus deficiency) may require analysis of blood phosphorus levels and parathyroid activity.

In most field cases of rickets, a deficiency of vitamin D_3 is suspected, due to simple dietary deficiency, inadequate potency of the D_3 supplement, or other factors that reduce the absorption of vitamin D_3. Rickets can best be prevented by providing adequate levels and potency of vitamin D_3 supplements, and by ensuring that the diet is formulated to

TABLE 18. Vaccination Program for Commercial Layers[*]

Age	Vaccine	Route	Type
1 day	Marek's disease	SC	Turkey herpesvirus and SB-1
14-21 days	Newcastle/infectious bronchitis	Water	B1/Mass
14-21 days	Infectious bursal disease	Water	Intermediate
5 wk	Newcastle/infectious bronchitis	Water or coarse spray	B1/Mass
8-10 wk	Newcastle/infectious bronchitis	Water or coarse spray	B1 or LaSota/Mass
10-12 wk	Encephalomyelitis	Wing web	Live, chick-embryo origin
10-12 wk	Fowlpox	Wing web	Modified live
10-12 wk	Laryngotracheitis	Intraocular	Modified live
10-14 wk	*Mycoplasma gallisepticum*[†]	Intraocular or spray	Mild live strain
or 18 wk	*M gallisepticum*	Parenteral	Inactivated
12-14 wk	Newcastle/infectious bronchitis	Water or aerosol	B1 or LaSota/Mass
16-18 wk and every	Newcastle/infectious bronchitis	Water or aerosol	B1 or LaSota/Mass
60-90 days or 18 wk	Newcastle/infectious bronchitis	Parenteral	Inactivated

[*]This is an example of a vaccination program. Individual programs are highly variable and reflect local conditions, disease prevalence, severity of challenge, and individual preferences.[†]

[†]The use of *M gallisepticum* vaccine is regulated or prohibited in some states. SB-1 or MDV301 may be combined with turkey herpesvirus in some areas. Vaccination for infectious bursal disease, laryngotracheitis, and fowlpox depends on local requirements. Other strains of infectious bronchitis (Connecticut, Arkansas 99, Florida 88, etc) are included in some areas. *M gallisepticum* and *Haemophilus gallinarum* (coryza) are used only on infected, multiage premises in some areas.

provide optimal utilization of fat-soluble compounds. Diets must also provide a correct calcium:phosphorus ratio. For this reason, ingredients that are notoriously variable in their content of these minerals should be used with caution.

Tibial Dyschondroplasia (Osteochondrosis): Tibial dyschondroplasia is characterized by an abnormal cartilage mass in the proximal head of the tibiotarsus. It is seen in all fast-growing meat birds but is most common in broiler chickens. Signs can occur early, but more usually are seen at 21-35 days of age. Birds are reluctant to move, and when forced to walk, do so with a swaying motion or stiff gait. Tibial dyschondroplasia results from disruption of the normal metaphyseal blood supply in the proximal tibiotarsal growth plate, where the disruption in nutrient supply means that the normal process of ossification does not occur. The abnormal cartilage is composed of severely degenerated cells, with cytoplasm and nuclei appearing shrunken.

The exact cause of tibial dyschondroplasia is unknown, although a genetic component is likely in some cases. Dietary electrolyte imbalances, and particularly high levels of chloride, seem to be a major contributor in many field outbreaks. More tibial dyschondroplasia is also seen when the level of dietary calcium is low relative to that of available phosphorus. Treatment involves dietary adjustment of the calcium:phosphorus ratio, consideration of dietary electrolyte balance, and higher levels of (or more potent)

TABLE 19. Vaccination Program for Turkeys[*]

Age (wk)[†]	Market Turkeys	Breeder Hens	Breeder Toms
2-3	ND[‡] B1-B1[§] or LaSota, DW[¶] or spray	ND, B1-B1 or LaSota, DW or spray	ND, B1-B1 or LaSota, DW or spray
4	Hemorrhagic enteritis, DW	Hemorrhagic enteritis, DW	Hemorrhagic enteritis, DW
6	Fowl cholera,[#] DW (live) or SC (inactivated)	Fowl cholera, DW (live) or SC (inactivated)	Fowl cholera, DW (live) or SC (inactivated)
9-10	ND, LaSota, DW or spray	ND, LaSota, DW or spray	ND, LaSota, DW or spray
12	Fowl cholera, DW (live) or SC (inactivated)	Fowl cholera, DW (live) or SC (inactivated)	Fowl cholera, DW (live) or SC (inactivated)
15	ND, LaSota, DW or spray	ND, LaSota, DW or spray	ND, LaSota, DW or spray
18	—	Fowl cholera, DW (live) or SC (inactivated)	Fowl cholera, DW (live) or SC (inactivated)
21	—	ND, LaSota, DW or spray	ND, LaSota, DW or spray
24	—	Fowl cholera, DW (live) or SC (inactivated)	Fowl cholera, DW (live) or SC (inactivated)
26	—	Erysipelas, DW (live) or SC (inactivated) Pox, WW[¶]	Erysipelas, DW (live) or SC (inactivated) Pox, WW
28	—	ND, SC (inactivated) Fowl cholera, DW (live) or SC (inactivated) Encephalomyelitis, DW	ND, SC (inactivated) Fowl cholera, DW (live) or SC (inactivated) Encephalomyelitis, DW

[*]Recommendations are for production areas where the diseases listed are common. In addition, other vaccinations may be advisable if previous experience indicates prevalence of certain diseases in the area. These may include turkey bordetellosis eye drop vaccine at 1 day old and in water or spray at 14 days old, or bacterin; paramyxovirus 3 and influenza A (prevalent hemagglutinin) at 26-28 and 40 wk old; erysipelas—live or killed products might be required for market turkeys, and repeated vaccinations might be required for breeders; and salmonellosis bacterins at 24 and 28 wk old.
[†]Recommended age at vaccination is an approximation.
[‡]ND = Newcastle disease
[§]Spray ND vaccines should not be used for birds suffering from respiratory disease; in such cases and at that age, the mild B1-B1 strain vaccine could be used in water. Timing of vaccination depends on maternal antibody levels.
[¶]DW = drinking water; WW = wing web stab
[#]Live fowl cholera vaccines should be used only in healthy flocks.

vitamin D_3 supplementation. Diet changes rarely result in complete recovery. Tibial dyschondroplasia can be prevented by reducing growth rate; however, programs of feed restriction must be considered in relation to economic consequences.

Cage Layer Fatigue: High-producing laying hens maintained in cages sometimes show paralysis around the time of peak egg production due to a fracture of the vertebrae

TABLE 20. Vaccination Program for Duck Breeders

Age	Vaccine	Route	Type
1 day old	*Riemerella anatipestifer*	Aerosol	Live vaccine[*]
10-14 days	*R anatipestifer*	Drinking Water	Live vaccine[*]
3 wk	*R anatipestifer*	SC	Bacterin[†]
4 wk	Duck viral hepatitis	SC	Live vaccine[‡] (Type 1)
4 wk	Duck viral enteritis	SC	Live vaccine[‡]
10 and 20 wk[§]	*R anatipestifer*	SC	Bacterin[†]
10 and 20 wk	Duck viral hepatitis	SC	Killed virus vaccine (Type 1)

[*]A live, avirulent vaccine consisting of the 3 major serotypes (1, 2 and 5) of *R anatipestifer*.
[†]A formalin-inactivated cell suspension of the 3 major serotypes (1, 2, and 5) of *R anatipestifer*. Bacterins and killed virus vaccines are administered SC in the neck.
[‡]A modified live virus vaccine of chick embryo origin.
[§]White Pekin breeder ducks normally start egg production at 24 wk of age. Egg production can be accelerated or delayed and breeder vaccination should be completed before the onset of egg production to optimize the passage of parental immunity to the progeny.

TABLE 21. Vaccination Program for Commercial Ducklings

Age	Vaccine	Route	Type
1 day old	*Riemerella anatipestifer*	Aerosol	Live vaccine[*]
10-14 days	*R anatipestifer*	Drinking Water	Live vaccine[*]
3 wk	*R anatipestifer*	SC	Bacterin[†]

[*]A live, avirulent vaccine consisting of the 3 major serotypes (1, 2, and 5) of *R anatipestifer*.
[†]A formalin-inactivated cell suspension of the 3 major serotypes (1, 2, and 5) of *R anatipestifer* is recommended for preventive immunization on farms where the disease is endemic or epidemic. An *E coli* bacterin can also be used where field challenge warrants. Ducklings should not be vaccinated within 21 days of slaughter.

that subsequently affects the spinal cord. The fracture is caused by an impaired calcium flux related to the high output of calcium in the eggshell. Because medullary bone reserves become depleted, the bird uses cortical bone as a source of calcium for the eggshell. The condition is rarely seen in floor-housed birds, suggesting that reduced activity or exercise is a predisposing factor. Affected birds are invariably found on their sides in the back of the cage. At the time of initial paralysis, birds appear healthy and often have a shelled egg in the oviduct and an active ovary. Death occurs from starvation or dehydration because the birds cannot reach feed or water.

Affected birds will recover if moved to the floor. A high incidence of cage layer fatigue can be prevented by ensuring the normal weight-for-age of pullets at sexual maturity and by giving pullets a high-calcium diet (minimum 3.5% calcium) for at least 14 days prior to first oviposition.

Diets must provide adequate quantities of calcium and phosphorus to prevent deficiencies. However, feeding diets that contain >2.5% calcium during the growing period produces a high incidence of nephrosis, visceral gout, calcium urate deposits in the ureters, and sometimes high mortality. Feeding high levels of calcium to pullets 2 wk before the onset of egg production is not harmful and may improve productivity.

Eggshell strength can be improved by feeding ~50% of the dietary calcium supplement in the form of oyster-shell flakes or coarse limestone, with the remaining half as

TABLE 22. Minimum Space Requirements for White Leghorn Egg-strain Birds[*]

	Age (wk)		
	0-6	7-17	18 onward
Cages			
Floor area per bird (sq in.)	25	45	60
Straight trough feeder space per bird, not less than (in.)	2	2.5	3
Waterers			
Birds per nipple	15	10	8
Birds per cup	25	15	12
Trough space per bird (in.)	1	1	2
Litter and Slats			
Floor area—litter only or combined with slats (sq ft/bird)	0.5	1	1-1.5
Straight trough feeder space per bird (in.)	1	2	3.5
Pans (15 in. [38 cm] diameter) per 100 birds			
Full fed	3	4	5
Restricted	—	5	
Waterers			
Birds per fount	100	50	25
Trough space per bird (in.)	1	1	2

[*]Requirements for White Leghorns and brown-egg layers are different.

TABLE 23. Space Requirements for Meat-strain Birds

Age	Floor Space	Feeder Space[*]	Cups or Founts[*] (per 1,000 birds)
From day 1	Heated area 5 sq ft brooder/100 chicks	10 trays/1,000 (feed little and often)	8
From wk 1	1 sq ft/bird	2 in./bird	20
From wk 8	2 sq ft/bird	4 in./bird	30
Mated adults	All litter: 3 sq ft/bird ½ to ⅔ slats: 2¼ sq ft/bird	4 in./bird	30 (60 in hot weather)

[*]For feeder and drinking trough space, both sides of the trough should be counted. Drinking trough space (all ages) is 1 in. (2.5 cm) per bird but doubled for adults in hot weather.

ground limestone. Oyster shell or any other form of calcium supplement should never be added without an equivalent reduction in the amount of limestone; feeding too much calcium reduces feed consumption and egg production. Offering the coarse supplement permits the birds to satisfy their requirements when they need it most, or allows the coarse material to be retained in the gizzard where the calcium can be absorbed continuously. A readily assimilable calcium and/or calcium phosphate supplement is effective if started very soon after paralysis due to calcium deficiency develops.

Manganese Deficiency

A deficiency of manganese in the diet of young growing chickens is one of the causes of perosis and of thin-shelled eggs and poor hatchability (*see also* CALCIUM AND PHOSPHORUS IMBALANCES, p 2320, and VITAMIN D DEFICIENCY, p 2330). It may also cause chondrodystrophy.

Perosis, which occurs in young chicks, is characterized by enlargement and malformation of the tibiometatarsal joint, twisting and bending of the distal end of the tibia and the proximal end of the tarsometatarsus, thickening and shortening of the leg bones, and slippage of the gastrocnemius or Achilles tendon from its condyles. Higher intakes of calcium or phosphorus will aggravate the condition due to reduced absorption of magnesium by precipitated calcium phosphate in the intestinal tract. In laying hens, reduced egg production, markedly reduced hatchability, and eggshell thinning are often noted.

A manganese-deficient breeder diet can result in chondrodystrophy in chick embryos. This condition is characterized by shortened and thickened legs, shortened wings, a "parrot beak" brought about by a disproportionate shortening of the lower mandible, globular contour of the head due to anterior bulging of the skull, edema usually occurring just above the atlas joint of the neck and extending posteriorly, protruding abdomen (apparently due to a relatively large amount of unassimilated yolk), and retarded growth of down and feathers. In the young chick, nervous signs may also be noted, which are characterized by a "star-gazing" posture similar to that observed in cases of thiamine deficiency. This posture is a result of defective or absent otoliths in the inner ear.

Prevention of perosis requires a diet adequate in all necessary nutrients, especially manganese, choline, niacin, biotin, and folic acid. Deformities cannot be corrected by feeding more manganese. Effects of manganese deficiency on egg production are fully corrected by a diet that contains manganese at 30-40 mg/kg, provided that the diet does not contain excess calcium and phosphorus. Calcium intake may be excessive if calcium supplements are provided free-choice. When meat meal is used as the principal source of protein, the feed may contain excess phosphorus.

Iron and Copper Deficiencies

Deficiencies of both iron and copper can lead to anemia. Iron deficiency causes a severe anemia with a reduction in PCV. In color-feathered strains, there is also loss of pigmentation in the feathers. The birds' requirements for RBC synthesis take precedence over metabolism of feather pigments, although if a fortified diet is introduced, all subsequent feather growth is normal. Iron may be needed not only for the red feather pigments, which are known to contain iron, but also to function in an enzyme system involved in feather pigmentation. Ochratoxin at 4-8 µg/g diet also causes an iron deficiency characterized by hypochromic microcytic anemia. Aflatoxin also reduces iron absorption. High levels of iron salts can lead to formation of insoluble phosphates in the digesta, with reduced phosphorus absorption and subsequent incidence of rickets. Insoluble iron phosphates produce a colloidal suspension that may also adsorb vitamins and other trace minerals. Such problems will not occur unless supplements exceed normal levels by at least 10-fold.

Young chicks become lame in 2-4 wk when fed a copper-deficient diet. Bones are fragile and easily broken, epiphyseal cartilage becomes thickened, and vascular penetration of the thickened cartilage is markedly reduced. These bone lesions in chickens are quite different from those seen in other farm animals and resemble the bone changes noted in birds with vitamin A deficiency. Copper-deficient chickens also show ataxia and spastic paralysis.

Copper deficiency in birds, and especially in turkeys, can lead to rupture of the aorta. The biochemical lesion in the copper-deficient aorta is likely related to failure to synthesize desmosine, the cross-link precursor of elastin. The lysine content of copper-deficient elastin is 3 times that seen in control birds, suggesting failure to incorporate lysine into the desmosine molecule. In field cases of naturally occurring aortic rupture, many birds have <10 ppm copper in the liver, compared with 15-30 ppm normally seen in birds of comparable age. High levels of sulfate, molybdenum, and ascorbic acid can reduce liver copper levels. A high incidence of aortic rupture has been seen in turkeys fed

4-nitrophenylarsonic acid. The problem can be resolved by feeding higher levels of copper, suggesting that products such as 4-nitro may complex with copper.

Most practical diets for poultry contain adequate iron and copper. Nevertheless, feed manufacturers often add small amounts as an insurance measure.

Iodine Deficiency

Iodine deficiency results in a decreased output of thyroxine from the thyroid gland, which in turn stimulates the anterior pituitary to produce and release increased amounts of thyroid stimulating hormone (TSH). This increased production of TSH results in stimulation, with subsequent enlargement of the thyroid gland, termed a goiter. This enlarged gland is an attempt by the thyroid to increase the secretory surface of the thyroid follicles by hypertrophy and hyperplasia of these follicles.

Lack of thyroid activity or inhibition of the thyroid by administration of thiouracil or thiourea causes hens to cease laying and become obese, and also results in the growth of abnormally long, lacy feathers. Administration of thyroxine or iodinated casein reverses the effects on egg production, with eggshell quality returning to normal. The iodine content of an egg is markedly influenced by the hen's intake of iodine. Eggs from a breeder fed an iodine-deficient diet will exhibit reduced hatchability and delayed yolk sac absorption. Rapeseed meal and, to a lesser extent, canola meal contain goitrogens that cause thyroid enlargement in young birds. Iodine deficiency in poultry is easily prevented by supplementing the feed with as little as 0.35 mg of iodine/kg.

Magnesium Deficiency

Natural feed ingredients are rich in magnesium, thus deficiency is rare. Magnesium is rarely added to diets in the mineral premix. Newly hatched chicks fed a diet devoid of magnesium live only a few days. They grow slowly when fed diets low in magnesium, are lethargic, and often pant and gasp. When disturbed, they exhibit brief convulsions and go into a comatose state, which is sometimes temporary but more often fatal. Mortality is quite high on diets only marginally deficient in magnesium, even though growth of survivors may approach that of control birds.

A magnesium deficiency in the diet of laying hens results in a rapid decline in egg production, blood hypomagnesemia, and a marked withdrawal of magnesium from bones. Egg size, shell weight, and the magnesium content of yolk and shell are decreased. Increasing the dietary calcium of laying hens accentuates these effects. Magnesium seems to play a central role in eggshell formation, although it is not clear whether there is a structural need or whether magnesium simply gets deposited as a cofactor along with calcium.

Requirements for most breeds of chicken appear to be ~500-600 ppm magnesium, a level that is usually achieved with contributions by natural feed ingredients.

Potassium, Sodium, and Chloride Deficiency

While requirements for potassium, sodium, and chloride have been clearly defined, it is also important to maintain a balance of electrolytes in the body. Often termed dietary electrolyte balance or acid-base balance, the effects of deficiency of any one element are often the consequence of alteration to this important balance as it affects osmoregulation.

Simple Deficiency: A deficiency of chloride causes ataxia with classic signs of nervousness, often induced by sudden noise or fright. The main sign of hypokalemia is an overall muscle weakness characterized by weak extremities, poor intestinal tone with intestinal distention, cardiac weakness, and weakness and ultimately failure of the respiratory muscles. Hypokalemia is apt to occur during severe stress. Plasma protein is elevated, causing the kidney, under the influence of adrenocortical hormone, to discharge potassium into the urine. During adaptation to the stress, blood flow to the muscle gradually improves, and the muscle begins to retrieve lost potassium. As liver glycogen is restored, potassium returns to the liver. This may result in temporary prolongation of the hypokalemia. Effects of administering potassium salts to chickens during and following severe stress periods have not been adequately investigated.

When fed a diet low in protein and potassium or when starving, animals grow slowly but do not show a potassium deficiency. Potassium derived from metabolized tissue protein replaces that lost in the urine and lacking in the diet. Under such conditions, less potassium is needed. The ratio of potassium to nitrogen in urine is relatively constant and is the same as that found in fresh muscle. Thus, tissue nitrogen and potassium are released together from metabolized tissue.

A deficiency of sodium leads to a lowering of osmotic pressure and a change in acid-base balance in the body. Cardiac output and blood pressure fall, hematocrit increases, elasticity of subcutaneous tissues decreases, and adrenal function is impaired. This leads to an increase in blood uric acid levels, which can result in shock and death. A less severe sodium deficiency in chicks can result in retarded growth, soft bones, corneal keratinization, impaired food utilization, and a decrease in plasma volume. In layers, reduced egg production, poor growth, and cannibalism may be noted. A number of diseases can result in sodium depletion from the body (eg, GI losses from diarrhea or urinary losses from renal or adrenal damage).

Electrolyte Imbalance: Most commonly, electrolyte balance is described by the simple formula of $Na^+ + K^+ - Cl^-$ expressed as mEq/kg (or mEq/g) of diet. Generally, an overall diet balance of 250 mEq/kg is optimal for normal physiologic function. The primary role of electrolytes is to maintain body water and ionic balance. Thus, requirements for elements such as sodium, potassium, and chlorine cannot be considered individually, as it is the overall balance that is important. Electrolyte balance is affected by 3 factors, namely the balance and proportion of these electrolytes in the diet, endogenous acid production, and the rate of renal clearance.

In most situations, the body attempts to maintain the balance between cations and anions in the body such that physiologic pH is maintained. If conditions in the body result in a shift toward acid or base conditions, physiologic defense mechanisms alter metabolism to maintain normal pH. Actual electrolyte imbalances rarely occur because these regulatory mechanisms must ensure optimal cellular pH and osmolarity. Electrolyte balance can therefore more correctly be described as the mechanisms that must occur in the body to achieve normal physiologic pH.

Electrolyte imbalance causes a number of metabolic disorders in birds, most notably tibial dyschondroplasia and respiratory alkalosis in layers. Tibial dyschondroplasia in young broiler chickens can be effected by the electrolyte balance of the diet. The unusual development of the cartilage plug at the growth plate of the tibia can be induced by a number of factors, although its incidence can be greatly increased by metabolic acidosis induced by feeding products such as NH_4Cl. Tibial dyschondroplasia occurs more frequently when the diet contains an excess of sodium relative to potassium and a very high level of chloride.

Overall electrolyte balance is always important, but is most critical when chloride or sulfur levels are high. With low dietary chloride levels, there is often little response to the manipulation of electrolyte balance; however, when dietary chloride levels are high, making adjustments to the dietary cations is critical to maintain overall balance. Alternatively, chloride levels can be reduced, although chickens have requirements ~0.12-0.15% of the diet, and deficiency signs will develop with dietary levels <0.12%. Therefore, care must be taken to meet the minimum chloride requirements when, for example, $NaHCO_3$ replaces NaCl in a diet.

Selenium Deficiency

A deficiency of selenium in growing chickens causes exudative diathesis. The early signs (unthriftiness, ruffled feathers) usually occur at 5-11 wk of age. The edema results in weeping of the skin, which is often seen on the inner surface of the thighs and wings. The birds bruise easily; large scabs often form on old bruises. In laying hens, the tissue damage is unusual, but egg production, hatchability, and feed conversion are adversely affected.

The metabolism of selenium is closely linked to that of vitamin E, and signs of deficiency can sometimes be treated with either the mineral or the vitamin. Vitamin E can spare selenium in its role as an antioxidant, and so some selenium-responsive conditions can also be treated by supplemental vitamin E. In most countries, there are limits to the quantity of selenium that can be added to a diet; the upper limit is usually 0.3 ppm.

The commonly used forms are sodium selenate and sodium selenite and, more recently, organic selenium chelates. Feeds grown on high-selenium soils may be used in poultry rations and are good sources of selenium. Fish meal and dried brewer's yeast are also good sources.

Zinc Deficiency

Zinc requirements and signs of deficiency are influenced by dietary ingredients. In semipurified diets, it is difficult to show a response to levels much above 25-30 mg/kg diet, whereas in practical corn-soy diets, requirement values are increased to 60-80 mg/kg. Such variable needs likely relate to phytic acid content of the diet, because this ligand is a potent zinc chelator. If phytase enzyme is used in diets, presumably the need for supplemental zinc will be reduced.

In young chicks, signs of zinc deficiency include retarded growth, shortening and thickening of leg bones and enlargement of the hock joint, scaling of the skin (especially on the feet), very poor feathering, reduced feed utilization, loss of appetite, and in severe cases, mortality. While zinc deficiency can reduce egg production in aging hens, the most striking effects are seen in developing embryos. Chicks hatched from zinc-deficient hens are weak and cannot stand, eat, or drink. They have accelerated respiratory rates and labored breathing. If the chicks are disturbed, the signs are aggravated and the chicks often die. Retarded feathering and frizzled feathers are also found. However, the major defect is grossly impaired skeletal development. Zinc-deficient embryos show micromelia, curvature of the spine, and shortened, fused thoracic and lumbar vertebrae. Toes often are missing and, in extreme cases, the embryos have no lower skeleton or limbs. Some embryos are rumpless, and occasionally the eyes are absent or not developed.

VITAMIN DEFICIENCIES

Vitamin deficiencies are most commonly due to inadvertent omission of a vitamin premix from the birds' diet. Multiple signs are therefore seen, although in general, problems with deficiencies of the B vitamins appear first. Because there are some stores of the fat-soluble vitamins in the body, it often takes longer for these deficiencies to affect the bird.

Treatment and prevention rely on an adequate dietary supply, usually protected by gelatin microencapsulation, that also contains an antioxidant. Vitamin destruction in feeds is a factor of time, temperature, and humidity. For most feeds, vitamin efficiency is little affected over 2-mo storage within mixed feed.

Vitamin A Deficiency

Adult birds, depending on liver storage, could be fed a vitamin A-deficient diet for 2-5 mo before signs of deficiency develop. As the deficiency progresses, birds become emaciated and weak with ruffled feathers. Egg production drops markedly, hatchability decreases, and embryonic mortality with incubated eggs increases. As egg production declines, there will likely be atretic follicles in the ovary, some of which show signs of hemorrhage. A watery discharge from the eyes may also be noted. As the deficiency continues, milky white, cheesy material accumulates in the eyes, making it impossible for the birds to see (xerophthalmia). The eye, in many cases, may be destroyed.

The first lesion usually noted in adult birds is in the mucous glands of the alimentary tract. The normal epithelium of the glands is replaced by a stratified squamous, keratinized layer, which blocks the ducts of the mucous glands, resulting in distention and necrosis. Small, white pustules may be found in the nasal passages, mouth, esophagus, and pharynx, and may extend into the crop. Breakdown of the mucous membrane may allow pathogenic microorganisms to invade these tissues and cause secondary infections.

Depending on the quantity of vitamin A passed on from the breeder hen, day-old chicks reared on a vitamin A-deficient diet may show signs within a week. However, chicks with a good reserve of vitamin A may not exhibit signs of deficiency for up to 7 wk. Gross signs in chicks include anorexia, growth retardation, drowsiness, weakness, incoordination, emaciation, and ruffled feathers. If the deficiency is severe, the chicks may exhibit an ataxia similar to that noted with a vitamin E deficiency (*see* below). The yellow pigment in the shanks and beaks is usually lost, and the comb and wattles are pale. A cheesy material may be noted in the eyes, but xerophthalmia is seldom seen because chicks usually die before the eyes become affected. Infection may play a role in many of the deaths noted with acute vitamin A deficiency.

Young chicks with a chronic vitamin A deficiency may also show pustules in the mucous membrane of the esophagus that can extend down the respiratory tract. Kidneys may be pale and the tubules distended due to the uric acid deposits. In extreme cases, the ureters may be filled with urates. Blood levels of uric acid can rise from a normal of ~5 mg to as high as 40 mg/100 mL of blood. Vitamin A deficiency does not interfere with uric acid metabolism but does prevent normal excretion of uric acid from the kidney. Histologic findings include atrophy of the cytoplasm and a loss of the cilia in the columnar, ciliated epithelium.

While vitamin A-deficient chicks can show ataxia, similar to that noted with vitamin E deficiency, no gross lesions are found in the brain of vitamin A-deficient chicks as compared with degeneration of the Purkinje cells in the cerebellum of vitamin E-deficient chicks (*see* below). Also, the livers of ataxic vitamin A-deficient chicks contain little or no vitamin A.

Vitamin D₃ Deficiency

Abnormal development of the bones is discussed under calcium and phosphorus deficiencies (p 2320) and manganese deficiency (p 2326). Vitamin D_3 is required for the normal absorption and metabolism of calcium and phosphorus. A deficiency can result in rickets in young growing chickens or in osteoporosis and poor eggshell quality in laying hens, even though the diet may be well supplied with calcium and phosphorus.

Laying hens fed a vitamin D_3-deficient diet exhibit loss of egg production within 2-3 wk, and depending on the degree of deficiency, shell quality deteriorates almost instantaneously. Using a corn-soybean meal diet with no supplemental vitamin D_3, shell weight decreases dramatically by about 150 mg/day within 7 days. The less obvious decline in shell quality with suboptimal supplements is more difficult to diagnose than that seen with absolute deficiency, as it is very difficult to assay vitamin D_3 in complete feeds.

There is a significant increase in plasma $1,25(OH)_2D_3$ of birds producing good vs poor eggshells. Feeding purified $1,25(OH)_2D_3$ improves the shell quality of these inferior layers, suggesting a potential inherent problem with metabolism of cholecalciferol.

Retarded growth and severe leg weakness are the first signs noted when chicks are deficient in vitamin D_3. Also, beaks and claws become soft and pliable. Chicks may have trouble walking and will take a few steps before squatting on their hocks. They often sway from side to side while resting, suggesting loss of equilibrium. Feathering is usually poor, and an abnormal banding of feathers is seen in colored breeds. With chronic vitamin D_3 deficiency, marked skeletal disorders are noted. The spinal column may bend downward, and the sternum may deviate to one side. These structural changes reduce the size of the thorax with subsequent crowding of the internal organs. A characteristic finding in chicks is a beading of the ribs at the junction of the spinal column along with downward, and posterior bending. Poor calcification can be seen at the epiphysis of the tibia and femur. By dipping the split bone in a silver nitrate solution and allowing it to stand under an incandescent light for a few minutes, the calcified areas are easily distinguished from the areas of uncalcified cartilage.

In the laying hen, signs of gross pathology are usually confined to the bones and parathyroid glands. Bones are soft and easily broken, and the ribs may become beaded. The ribs may also show spontaneous fractures in the sternovertebral region. Histologic examination shows deficiency of calcification in the long bones, with excess of osteoid tissue and parathyroid enlargement.

Adding synthetic $1,25(OH)_2D_3$ to the diet of susceptible chicks does reduce the incidence of this condition. Although the response is not dramatic and is quite variable, results suggest that some leg abnormalities may be a consequence of inefficient metabolism of cholecalciferol.

Vitamin E Deficiency

The 3 main disorders seen in chicks deficient in vitamin E are encephalomalacia, exudative diathesis, and muscular dystrophy. The occurrence of these conditions depends on various dietary and environmental factors.

Encephalomalacia is seen in commercial flocks if diets are low in vitamin E, an antioxidant is either omitted or not present in sufficient quantities, or the diet contains a reasonably high level of an unstable, unsaturated fat. For exudative diathesis to occur, the diet must be deficient in both vitamin E and selenium. Signs of muscular dystrophy are rare in chicks, as the diet must be deficient in both sulfur amino acids and vitamin E. Because the sulfur amino acids are necessary for growth, a deficiency severe enough to induce muscular dystrophy is unlikely to occur under commercial conditions. Signs of exudative diathesis and muscular dystrophy can be reversed in chicks by supplementing the diet with liberal amounts of vitamin E, assuming the deficiency is not too advanced. Encephalomalacia may or may not respond to vitamin E supplementation, depending on the extent of the damage to the cerebellum.

The classical sign of encephalomalacia is ataxia, which results from hemorrhage and edema within the molecular and granular layers of the cerebellum, with pyknosis and eventual disappearance of the Purkinje cells and separation of the molecular and granular layers of the cerebellar folia. Due to its inherently low level of vitamin E, the cerebellum is particularly susceptible to lipid peroxidation. In prevention of encephalomalacia, vitamin E functions as a biologic antioxidant. The quantitative need for vitamin E for this function depends on the amount of linoleic acid and polyunsaturated fatty acids in the diet. Over prolonged periods, antioxidants will prevent encephalomalacia in chicks when added to diets with very low levels of vitamin E, or in chicks fed vitamin E-depleted purified diets. Chicks hatched from breeders that are given additional dietary vitamin E are also less susceptible to lipid peroxidation in the brain. The fact that antioxidants can help prevent encephalomalacia but fail to prevent exudative diathesis or muscular dystrophy in chicks, strongly suggests that vitamin E is acting as an antioxidant. Exudative diathesis results in a severe edema caused by a marked increase in capillary permeability. Electrophoretic patterns of the blood show a decrease in albumin levels, whereas exudative fluids contained a protein pattern similar to that of normal blood plasma.

A vitamin E deficiency accompanied by a sulfur amino acid deficiency results in a severe muscular dystrophy in chicks by ~4 wk of age. This condition is characterized by degeneration of the muscle fibers, usually in the breast but sometimes also in the leg muscles. Histologic examination shows Zenker's degeneration, with perivascular infiltration and marked accumulation of infiltrated eosinophils, lymphocytes, and histocytes. Accumulation of these cells in dystrophic tissue results in an increase in lysosomal enzymes, the function of which appears to be the breakdown and removal of the products of dystrophic degeneration. Initial studies involving the effects of dietary vitamin E on muscular dystrophy showed that the addition of selenium at 1-5 mg/kg diet reduced the incidence of muscular dystrophy in chicks receiving a vitamin E-deficient diet that was low in methionine and cysteine, but did not completely prevent the disease. However, selenium was completely effective in preventing muscular dystrophy in chicks when the diet contained a low level of vitamin E, which by itself had no effect on the disease.

Studies on the interrelationships between antioxidants, linoleic acid, selenium, and sulfur amino acids have brought some order to the previous confusion about the role of vitamin E in chick nutrition. It is now apparent that selenium and vitamin E play supportive roles in several processes, one of which involves cysteine metabolism and its role in the prevention of muscular dystrophy in the chicken. Glutathione peroxidase is soluble and is therefore located in the aqueous portions of the cell, while vitamin E is located mainly in the hydrophobic environments of membranes and in lipid storage cells. The overlapping manner in which vitamin E and selenium function in the cellular antioxidant system suggest that they spare one another in the prevention of deficiency signs.

Vitamin K Deficiency

Impairment of blood coagulation is the major clinical sign of vitamin K deficiency. With a severe deficiency, subcutaneous and internal hemorrhages can prove fatal. Vitamin K deficiency results in a reduction in prothrombin content of the blood; in the young chick, plasma levels are as low as 2% of what is considered normal. Because the prothrombin content of newly hatched chicks is only about 40% that of adult birds, the young chick is readily affected by a vitamin K-deficient diet. A carryover of vitamin K from the dam to eggs, and subsequently hatched chicks, has been demonstrated, so breeder diets should be well fortified. Hemorrhagic syndrome in day-old chicks has been attributed to a deficiency of vitamin K in the diet of the breeder hens. Gross deficiency of vitamin K results in such a prolonged blood clotting time that severely deficient chicks may bleed to death from a slight bruise or other injury. Borderline deficiencies often cause small hemorrhagic blemishes. Hemorrhages may appear on the breast, legs, wings, in the abdominal cavity, and on the surface of the intestine. Chicks are anemic, which may be due in part to loss of blood but also to the development of hypoplastic bone marrow. Although blood-clotting time is a fairly good measure of vitamin K deficiency, a more accurate measure is obtained by determining the prothrombin time. Prothrombin times in severely deficient chicks may be extended from a normal of 17-20 sec to 5-6 min or longer. No major heart lesions are seen in vitamin K-deficient chicks such as those that occur in pigs.

A vitamin K deficiency in poultry may be related to low dietary levels of the vitamin, low levels in the maternal diet, degree of intestinal synthesis, extent of coprophagy, presence of sulfur drugs and other feed additives in the diet, and the presence of disease. Chicks with coccidiosis may have severe damage to their intestinal wall, leading to excessive bleeding in addition to depressed vitamin K absorption. Antimicrobial agents can suppress intestinal synthesis of vitamin K, leaving the bird completely dependent on the diet for its supply of the vitamin.

Vitamin B$_{12}$ Deficiency

Vitamin B$_{12}$ is an essential part of several enzyme systems, with most reactions involving the transfer or synthesis of one-carbon units (eg, methyl groups). While the most important function of vitamin B$_{12}$ is in the metabolism of nucleic acids and proteins, it also functions in carbohydrate and fat metabolism.

In growing chickens, a deficiency of B$_{12}$ results in reduced weight gain and feed intake, along with poor feathering and nervous disorders. While deficiency may lead to perosis, this is probably a secondary effect due to a dietary deficiency of methionine, choline, or betaine as sources of methyl groups. Vitamin B$_{12}$ may alleviate perosis due to its effect on the synthesis of methyl groups. Further clinical signs reported in poultry are anemia, gizzard erosion, and fatty infiltration of heart, liver, and kidneys. Laying hens appear to be able to maintain body weight and egg production in spite of a dietary deficiency of vitamin B$_{12}$, although egg size may be reduced. Hatchability can be markedly reduced in breeders, but several months may be needed for signs to appear. Changes noted in embryos from B$_{12}$-deficient breeders include a general hemorrhagic condition, fatty liver, fewer myelinated fibers in the spinal cord, and high incidence of embryo deaths at 17 days incubation.

Choline Deficiency

In addition to poor growth, the outstanding sign of choline deficiency in chicks and poults is perosis. Perosis is first characterized by pinpoint hemorrhages and a slight puffiness about the hock joint, followed by an apparent flattening of the tibiometatarsal joint caused by a rotation of the metatarsus. The metatarsus continues to twist and may become bent or bowed so that it is out of alignment with the tibia. When this condition exists, the leg cannot adequately support the weight of the bird. The articular cartilage is displaced, and the Achilles tendon slips from its condyles. Perosis is not a specific deficiency sign; it appears with several nutrient deficiencies.

Although choline deficiency readily develops in chicks fed diets low in choline, a deficiency in laying hens is not easily produced. Eggs contain approximately 12-13 mg of choline/g of dried whole egg. A large egg contains about 170 mg of choline, found almost entirely in the phospholipids. Thus, there appears to be a considerable need for choline to produce an egg. In spite of this, producing a marked choline deficiency in laying hens has been difficult even when highly purified diets essentially devoid of choline were provided for a prolonged period of time. The choline content of eggs was not lowered, suggesting synthesis by the bird.

Niacin (Nicotinic Acid) Deficiency

There is good evidence that poultry—even chick and turkey embryos—can synthesize niacin, but at a rate that is too slow for optimal growth. It has been claimed that a marked deficiency of niacin cannot occur in chickens unless there is a deficiency of tryptophan, an amino acid and a niacin precursor.

A niacin deficiency is characterized by severe metabolic disorders in the skin and digestive organs. The first signs are usually loss of appetite, retarded growth, general weakness, and diarrhea. There is conflicting evidence as to whether broilers respond, in terms of growth and feed utilization, to niacin supplementation. However, it has been clearly established that chicks do have a requirement for niacin. Deficiency produces an enlargement of the tibiotarsal joint, bowing of the legs, poor feathering, and dermatitis on the head and feet.

Niacin deficiency in chicks can also result in "black tongue," in which the tongue, oral cavity, and esophagus become inflamed at ~2 wk of age. In the niacin-deficient hen, weight loss, reduced egg production, and a marked decrease in hatchability can result. Turkeys, ducks, pheasants, and goslings are much more severely affected by niacin deficiency than are chickens. Their apparently higher requirements are likely related to their less efficient conversion of tryptophan to niacin. Ducks and turkeys with a niacin deficiency show a severe bowing of the legs and an enlargement of the hock joint. The main difference between the leg seen in niacin deficiency and perosis seen in manganese and choline deficiency is that with niacin deficiency the Achilles tendon seldom slips from its condyles.

Pantothenic Acid Deficiency

Pantothenic acid is the prosthetic group of coenzyme A, an important coenzyme involved in many reversible acetylation reactions in carbohydrate, fat, and amino acid metabolism. Signs of deficiency relate to general avian metabolism.

The major lesions of pantothenic acid deficiency involve the nervous system, the adrenal cortex, and the skin. Deficiency may result in reduced egg production; however, a marked drop in hatchability is usually noted prior to this event. Embryos from hens with pantothenic acid deficiency may have subcutaneous hemorrhages and severe edema, with most other mortality showing up during the later part of the incubation period. In chicks, the first signs are reduced growth and feed consumption; poor feather growth, with feathers becoming ruffled and brittle; and a rapidly developing dermatitis. Corners of the beak and the area below the beak are usually the worst affected, but the condition is also noted on the feet. In severe cases, the skin of the feet may cornify, and wart-like lumps may be seen on the balls of the feet. The foot problem often leads to bacterial infection.

Liver concentration of pantothenic acid is reduced during a deficiency, with the liver becoming atrophied. A faint to dirty yellow color may be noted. Nerve fibers of the spinal cord may show myelin degeneration. Panthothenic acid-deficient chicks show lymphoid cell necrosis in the bursa of Fabricius and thymus, together with lymphocytic paucity in the spleen. The foot condition in chicks and the poor feathering are difficult to differentiate from signs of a biotin deficiency. In a pantothenic acid deficiency, dermatitis of the feet is usually noted first on the toes; in contrast, in a biotin deficiency dermatitis primarily affects the footpads and is usually more severe than that in a pantothenic acid deficiency. Ducks do not show the usual signs noted for chickens and turkeys, except for in retarded growth, but mortality can be quite high.

Riboflavin Deficiency

Many tissues may be affected by riboflavin deficiency, although the epithelium and the myelin sheaths of some of the main nerves are major targets. Changes in the sciatic nerves produce "curled-toe" paralysis in growing chickens. Egg production is affected, and riboflavin-deficient eggs do not hatch. When chicks are fed a diet deficient in riboflavin, their appetite is fairly good but they grow slowly, become weak and emaciated, and develop diarrhea between the first and second weeks. Deficient chicks are reluctant to move unless forced and then frequently walk on their hocks with the aid of their wings. The leg muscles are atrophied and flabby, and the skin is dry and harsh. In advanced stages of deficiency, the chicks lie prostrate with their legs extended, sometimes in opposite directions. The characteristic sign of riboflavin deficiency is a marked enlargement of the sciatic and brachial nerve sheaths, with sciatic nerves usually showing the most pronounced effects. Histologic examination of the affected nerves shows degenerative changes in the myelin sheaths that, when severe, pinch the nerve, producing a permanent stimulus that results in curled-toe paralysis.

Signs of riboflavin deficiency in the hen are decreased egg production, increased embryonic mortality, and an increase in size and fat content of the liver. Hatchability decreases within 2 wk when hens are fed a riboflavin-deficient diet but returns to near normal when riboflavin is restored. Embryos from the eggs of hens receiving riboflavin-deficient diets are dwarfed and show characteristically defective down ("clubbed" down). The nervous system of these embryos shows degenerative changes much like those described in riboflavin-deficient chicks.

Signs of riboflavin deficiency first appear at 10 days of incubation, when embryos become hypoglycemic and accumulate intermediates of fatty acid oxidation. Although flavin-dependent enzymes are depressed with riboflavin deficiency, the main effect seems to be impaired fatty acid oxidation, which is a critical function in the developing embryo. An autosomal recessive trait blocks the formation of riboflavin-binding protein, which is needed for transport of riboflavin to the egg. While the adults appear normal, their eggs fail to hatch regardless of dietary riboflavin content. As eggs become deficient in riboflavin, the egg albumen loses its characteristic yellow tinge. In fact, albumen color score has been used to assess riboflavin status of birds.

Chicks receiving diets only partially deficient in riboflavin may recover spontaneously, indicating that the requirement rapidly decreases with age. A 100-μg dose should be sufficient for treatment of riboflavin-deficient chicks, followed by incorporation of an adequate level in the diet. However, when the curled-toe deformity is longstanding, irreparable damage has occurred in the sciatic nerve, and the administration of riboflavin is no longer curative.

Folic Acid (Folacin) Deficiency

A folacin deficiency results in a macrocytic (megaloblastic) anemia and leukopenia. Tissues with a rapid turnover, such as epithelial linings, GI tract, epidermis, and bone marrow, as well as cell growth and tissue regeneration, are principally affected. Poultry seem more susceptible than other farm animals to a folacin deficiency.

Deficiency results in poor feathering, slow growth, an anemic appearance, and perosis. As anemia develops, the comb becomes waxy white, and pale mucous membranes in the mouth are noted. Elevated erythrocyte phosphoribosylpyrophosphate concentration can be used as a diagnostic tool in folate-deficient chicks. There may also be damage to liver parenchyma and depleted glycogen reserves. While turkey poults show some of the same signs as chickens, mortality is usually higher and the birds develop a spastic type of cervical paralysis that results in the neck becoming stiff and extended.

The abnormal feather condition in chickens leads to weak and brittle shafts. Depigmentation develops in colored feathers due to a deficiency of the vitamin. While a folacin deficiency can result in reduced egg production, the main sign noted with breeders is a marked decrease in hatchability associated with an increase in embryonic mortality, usually during the last few days of incubation. Embryos have deformed beaks and often a bending of the tibiotarsus. While birds may exhibit perosis, the lesions seen differ histologically from those seen as a consequence of choline or manganese deficiency. Abnormal structure of the hyaline cartilage and retardation of ossification are noted with folacin deficiency. Increasing protein content of the diet increases the severity of perosis in chicks receiving diets low in folic acid, as there is an increased folacin demand for uric acid synthesis.

Biotin Deficiency

Biotin deficiency results in dermatitis of the feet and the skin around the beak and eyes similar to that described for pantothenic acid (*see* above). Perosis and footpad dermatitis are also characteristic signs. While signs of classical biotin deficiency are rare, occurrence of fatty liver and kidney syndrome (FLKS) is important to commercial poultry producers. FLKS was first described in Denmark in 1958, but was not a major concern until the late 1960s, especially in Europe and Australia. Chicks ~3 wk of age become lethargic and unable to stand, then die within hours. Mortality is usually quite low at 1-2% but can reach 20-30%. Postmortem examination reveals pale liver and kidney with accumulation of fat.

The condition was usually confined to wheat-fed birds and was most problematic in low-fat, high-energy diets. High vitamin supplementation in general corrected the problem, and biotin was isolated as the causative agent. It is now known that biotin in wheat has exceptionally low availability. The trigger of high-energy diets led to investigation of biotin in carbohydrate metabolism. Chicks suffering from FLKS are invariably hypoglycemic, highlighting the importance of biotin in 2 key enzymes: pyruvate carboxylase and acetyl Co-A carboxylase. Acetyl Co-A carboxylase appears to preferentially sequester biotin, such that with low biotin availability and need for high de novo fat synthesis (high energy, low-fat diet), pyruvate carboxylase activity is severely compromised. Even with this imbalance, birds are able to grow. However, with a concurrent deprivation in feed intake or increased demand for glucose, hypoglycemia develops, leading to adipose catabolism and the characteristic accumulation of fat in both liver and kidney. Birds with FLKS rarely show signs of classic biotin deficiency.

Plasma biotin levels <100 ng/100 mL may indicate a deficiency. However, recent evidence suggests that plasma biotin levels are quite insensitive to the birds' biotin status, and that biotin levels in the liver or kidney are more useful indicators. Plasma pyruvic carboxylase is positively correlated with dietary biotin concentration, and levels plateau much later than does the growth response to biotin.

Embryos are also sensitive to biotin status. Congenital perosis, ataxia, and characteristic skeletal deformities may be seen in embryos and newly hatched chicks when the dams are fed a low-biotin diet. Deformities can be prevented by adding biotin to the diet. Embryonic deformities include a shortened tibiotarsus that is bent posteriorly, a much shortened tarsometatarsus, shortening of the bones of the wing and skull, and shortening and bending of the anterior end of the scapula. Syndactyly—an extensive webbing between the third and fourth toes—in biotin-deficient embryos has been noted. Such embryos are chondrodystrophic and characterized by reduced size, parrot beak, crooked tibia, and shortened or twisted tarsometatarsus.

Pyridoxine (Vitamin B$_6$) Deficiency

A vitamin B$_6$ deficiency causes retarded growth, dermatitis, and anemia. Because a major role of the vitamin is in protein metabolism, deficiency can result in reduced nitrogen retention. A deficiency can result in a marked increase in iron and a decrease in copper levels of the serum; iron utilization appears to be markedly decreased. The resulting anemia is believed to be the result of a disturbance in the synthesis of the protoporphyrins. Anemia is often noted in ducks, but seldom seen in chickens and turkeys. Young chicks may show nervous movements of the legs when walking and often undergo spasmodic convulsions, leading to death. During convulsions, chicks may run about aimlessly, flapping their wings and falling with jerking motions. The greater intensity of activity, resulting from pyridine deficiency, distinguishes these signs from those of encephalomalacia. A marked gizzard erosion has been noted in vitamin B$_6$-deficient chicks. It can be prevented by inclusion of 1% taurocholic acid in the diet, leading to the speculation that pyridoxine is involved in taurine synthesis and is important for gizzard integrity. In pyridoxine deficiency, collagen maturation is incomplete, suggesting that this vitamin is essential for integrity of the connective tissue matrix. A chronic or borderline deficiency can result in perosis, with one leg usually being crippled and one or both middle toes bent inward at the first joint.

In adult birds, pyridoxine deficiency results in reduced appetite, leading to reduced egg production and a decline in hatchability. Severe deficiency can cause a rapid involution of the ovary, oviduct, comb, and wattles, and of the testis in cockerels. Feed consumption in B_6-deficient hens and cockerels declines sharply, but inanition is not responsible for the marked effects of vitamin B_6 deficiency on sexual development. Although a partial molt is observed in some hens, the molt is not serious, and hens return to normal egg production within 2 wk following provision of a normal dietary level of pyridoxine.

Thiamine Deficiency

Polyneuritis in birds represents the later stages of a thiamine deficiency, probably caused by buildup of the intermediates of carbohydrate metabolism. In the initial stages of deficiency, lethargy and head tremors may be noted. A marked decrease in appetite is also seen in birds fed a thiamine-deficient diet. Poultry are also susceptible to neuromuscular problems, resulting in impaired digestion, general weakness, star-gazing, and frequent convulsions.

Polyneuritis may be seen in mature birds ~3 wk after they are fed a thiamine-deficient diet. As the deficiency progresses to the legs, wings, and neck, birds may sit on flexed legs and draw back their heads in a star-gazing position. Retraction of the head is due to paralysis of the anterior neck muscles. Soon after this stage, chickens lose the ability to stand or sit upright and topple to the floor, where they may lie with heads still retracted. Thiamine deficiency may also lead to a decrease in body temperature and respiratory rate. Testicular degeneration may be noted, and the heart may show slight atrophy. Birds consuming a thiamine-deficient diet soon show severe anorexia. They lose all interest in feed and will not resume eating unless given thiamine. If a severe deficiency has developed, thiamine must be force-fed or injected to induce eating.

TOXICOLOGY
INTRODUCTION

Toxicology is the study of the harmful effects of chemical compounds on biologic systems, including their properties, actions, and effects. The toxic agent is referred to as a toxicant or poison. The term **toxin** refers to poisons produced by a biologic source (eg, venoms, plant toxins); the redundant term biotoxin is occasionally used. **Toxicosis, poisoning,** and **intoxication** are synonymous terms for the disease produced by a toxicant. **Toxicity** (sometimes incorrectly used instead of poisoning) refers to the amount of a toxicant necessary to produce a detrimental effect. **Hazard** describes the likelihood of poisoning under conditions of use.

If 2 poisons act via similar mechanisms on the same organs, their combined effects may be additive. Synergism is the amplification of the combined actions of 2 or more agents having the same biologic effects. Antagonism is the inhibition or elimination of the effect of one agent by another; it may be chemical or functional.

Toxicant accumulation and biomagnification occurs when absorption exceeds the capacity of the body to destroy or excrete a xenobiotic (foreign) compound. Likewise, the terms are applied to the environment, an ecosystem, species, etc, when a compound increases because of increased application or decreased destruction or disappearance. These elements are used with ecotoxicology, the study of the relation of potentially toxic chemicals in living organisms and their environment. When residual compounds are introduced into plant or animal species early in the ecosystem food chain, the levels tend to be successively higher in the next species that feeds on the contaminated plant or animal; eg, predatory birds, which are at the "end" of the food chain, often have the highest levels of certain residual chemicals.

Tolerance is the ability of an organism to show less response to a specific dose of a chemical than it demonstrated on a prior occasion; it refers to acquired, not innate, resistance.

Dose Expressions: All toxic effects are dose dependent. (By usual standards, allergens or inducers of idiosyncratic reactions may appear to be exceptions, although even with these, presumably some dose is too small to cause detectable effects.) A dose may cause undetectable, therapeutic, toxic, or lethal effects. Further, the effective dose may differ from molecule to cell to organ or to body level (or fetus vs mother). Usually, a dose is expressed as the amount of compound per unit of body wt and the toxicant concentration as ppm or ppb. These quantitative expressions also are used for feedstuffs, water, air, tissue levels, etc.

The LD_{50} is the dose that is lethal to 50% of a test sample. It is an estimator of lethality and the most common expression used to rate the potency of toxicants. Other terms used for prediction of illness or lethality include: no observed effect level (NOEL), maximum nontoxic dose (MNTD), and maximum tolerated dose or minimum toxic dose (MTD).

Elimination Expressions: The elimination or disappearance (by metabolic change) of a chemical from an organ or the body is expressed in terms of **half-life** ($t_{1/2}$). This is the amount of time required for the disappearance of half the compound. The rate of elimination is usually dependent on the concentration of the compound: a constant fraction (eg, $1/2$) is eliminated per unit of time (referred to as first-order kinetics); or a metabolic reaction may dictate the rate of elimination, and a constant amount is eliminated per unit of time (zero-order kinetics). Different body compartments will likely have different elimination rates. A 2-compartment system is used to describe the situation in which elimination is initially rapid, eg, from the central or plasma component, and subsequently slower from the peripheral component, eg, liver, kidney, or fat.

Acute toxicosis refers to effects during the first 24-hr period. Effects produced by prolonged exposure ($\geq$3 mo) are referred to as **chronic toxicosis**. Terms such as subacute and subchronic are used to cover the large gap between acute and chronic. Regardless of terms, the duration of exposure can alter the toxicity of an agent; this is reflected by the chronicity factor (CF), the ratio of the acute to chronic LD_{50} dose. The biologic system may develop tolerance so that after prolonged exposure, a higher dose may be tolerated (eg, potassium cyanide, CF = 0.04). Other compounds are metabolized and eliminated in much the same manner regardless of the duration of exposure, and the lethal dose does not change appreciably (eg, caffeine, CF = 1.3). However, due to increased sensitization or cumulative effects, prolonged exposure to a toxicant may cause the chronic lethal dose to be much lower than the acute lethal dose (eg, warfarin, CF = 20).

METABOLISM OF POISONS

Absorption occurs by way of the alimentary tract, skin, lungs, or via the eye, mammary gland, or uterus, as well as from sites of injection. Toxic effects may be local, but the poison must be dissolved and absorbed to some extent to affect the cell. The primary factor affecting absorption is solubility. Insoluble salts and ionized compounds are poorly absorbed, while lipid-soluble substances are generally readily absorbed, even through intact skin. For example, barium is toxic, but barium sulfate can be used for intestinal contrast radiography because of low absorption.

Distribution or translocation of the toxicant follows via the bloodstream to reactive sites, including storage depots. The liver receives the portal circulation and is the organ most commonly involved with intoxication (and detoxification). The selective deposit of foreign chemicals in various tissues depends on receptor sites. The ease of chemical distribution depends largely on its water solubility. Polar- or aqueous-soluble agents tend to be excreted by the kidneys; lipid-soluble chemicals are more likely to be excreted via the bile and accumulate in fat depots. The highest concentration of a poison within an animal is not necessarily found in the organ or tissue on which it exerts its maximal effect (the target organ), eg, lead may be found in highest concentrations in bone, which is neither a site for toxic effects nor a reliable tissue for toxicologic interpretation. Knowledge of the translocation characteristics of poisons is necessary for proper selection of organs for analysis.

Metabolism or biotransformation of toxicants occurs in most cases and is an "attempt to detoxify." In some cases, the metabolized xenobiotic agent is more toxic than the original compound; this may be referred to as lethal synthesis. Metabolism of many organophosphorous insecticides produces metabolites more toxic than the initial (or parent) compounds (eg, parathion to paraxon).

There are 2 phases of metabolism. Phase I includes oxidation, reduction, and hydrolysis mechanisms. These reactions, catalyzed by hepatic enzymes, generally convert foreign compounds to derivatives for Phase II reactions, although the products of Phase I may be excreted as such if polar solubility permits translocation. Phase II principally involves conjugation or synthesis reactions. Common conjugates include glucuronides, acetylation products, and combinations with glycine. Metabolism of xenobiotic agents seldom follows a single pathway. Usually, a fraction is excreted unchanged, and the rest is excreted or stored as metabolites. Significant differences in metabolic mechanisms exist between species. For example, because cats lack forms of glucuronyl transferase, their ability to conjugate compounds such as morphine and phenols is compromised. In some cases, the increased tolerance to subsequent exposures of a toxicant is due to enzyme induction initiated by the previous exposure.

Excretion of most toxicants and their metabolites is by way of the kidneys. Many polar and high-molecular-weight compounds are excreted by way of the bile. An enterohepatic cycle occurs when these products are excreted from the liver via bile, reabsorbed from the intestine, and returned to the liver. Milk is also an excretion pathway for some toxicants. The excretion rate may be of primary concern because some toxicants can cause violative residues in food-producing animals. The route of administration, dose, and condition of the animal—to name a few factors—can have a profound effect on excretion rates.

FACTORS AFFECTING THE ACTIVITY OF POISONS

Poisoning potential is usually determined more by the multitude of related factors than by the actual toxicity of the poison. Exposure-related, biologic, or chemical factors regulate absorption, metabolism, and elimination, and thus, influence the clinical consequences (if any).

Factors Related to Exposure: The dose is a primary concern; however, the exact intake of poison is seldom known. Duration and frequency of exposure are important. The route of exposure affects absorption, translocation, and perhaps metabolic pathways. The time of administration relative to periods of stress, food intake, etc, may also be a factor, eg, following ingestion of some toxicants, emesis may occur if the stomach is empty, but if partly filled, the toxicant is retained and poisoning can occur. Environmental factors, such as temperature, humidity, and barometric pressure, affect rates of consumption and even the occurrence of some toxic agents. Many mycotoxins and poisonous plants are correlated with seasonal or climatic changes, eg, the ischemic effects of ergot poisoning are more often observed during the winter cold, and plant nitrate levels are affected by rainfall amounts.

Biologic Factors: Various species and strains within species react differently to a particular poison because of variations in absorption, metabolism, or elimination. Functional differences in species may also affect the likelihood of poisoning (eg, species unable to vomit can be intoxicated with a lower dose of some agents).

The age and size of the animal are primary factors in poisoning. Metabolism and translocation of xenobiotic agents are compromised by the underdeveloped microsomal enzyme system in young animals; membrane permeability and hepatic and renal clearance capabilities vary with age, species, and health. Generally, the amount of toxicant required to cause poisoning is correlated to body weight, but with greater body weight, a disproportionate increase in toxicity (per unit body weight) of a compound often occurs.

Body surface area may correlate more closely with the toxic dose; no measurement parameter is consistent for every situation.

Nutritional and dietary factors, hormonal and health status, organ pathology, stress, and sex all affect poisoning. Nutritional factors may directly affect the toxin (ie, by altering absorption) or indirectly affect the metabolic processes or availability of receptor sites. (The copper-molybdenum-sulfate interaction is an example of both.)

Chemical Factors: The chemical nature of a toxicant determines solubility, which in turn influences absorption. Nonpolar or lipid-soluble substances tend to be more readily absorbed than polar or ionized substances. The vehicle or carrier of the toxic compound also affects its availability for absorption. Isomers, including optical isomers, vary in toxicity (eg, the γ isomer of hexachlorocyclohexane [Lindane] is more toxic than other isomers).

Adjuvants are formulation factors used to alter the toxicologic effect of the active ingredient (eg, piperonyl butoxide enhances the insecticidal activity of pyrethrins). Binding agents, enteric coating, and sustained-release preparations influence absorption of the active ingredient. Generally, as absorption is delayed, toxicity decreases. Flavoring agents affect palatability, and thus the amount ingested.

Droplet size is an important consideration in sprays and dips because the dose increases with larger droplet size. This is one of many reasons to adhere closely to label instructions and recommended applications. Only formulations intended for animals should be used.

Contaminants and impurities may affect poisoning or be the primary toxicant (eg, dioxins, p 2367).

DIAGNOSIS

As with any disease, diagnosis is based on history, clinical signs, lesions, laboratory examinations, and in some cases, bioassay procedures. Circumstantial evidence is valuable and should be noted, but does not replace a thorough clinical and postmortem examination. Histories from animal owners may stress obvious factors and omit subtle, important details. "Sudden death" is often actually "tardy observation."

Pertinent data and samples should be submitted to the diagnostic laboratory. A complete history is necessary for developing the scheme of laboratory investigation and may be valuable in case of litigation. Information should be detailed. For example, a notation of CNS signs is insufficient; most animals exhibit some type of CNS signs prior to death. Exact actions and signs should be described. Examples of pertinent information include the following: 1) number of animals exposed/sick/dead, age, weight, and a chronology of morbidity and mortality; 2) clinical signs and course of the disease; 3) any prior disease conditions; 4) lesions observed at necropsy, with careful examination of ingesta; 5) response to treatment (medication should be listed to avoid analytic confusion); 6) related events, eg, feed change, water source, other medications, feed additives, pesticide applications; 7) description of facilities (a drawing may be helpful), access to refuse, machinery, etc; and 8) recent past locations and when moved. The diagnostic laboratory should be contacted if there are questions regarding the appropriate sample, amount, or container. (*See also* COLLECTION AND SUBMISSION OF LABORATORY SAMPLES, p 1333, and TABLE 1. Guidelines for Submitting Samples for Toxicologic Examination, p 1336.)

PRINCIPLES OF THERAPY

At initial examination, certain immediate, life-saving measures may be needed. Beyond this, treatment for poisoning includes 3 basic principles: 1) prevention of further absorption, 2) supportive/symptomatic treatment, and 3) specific antidotes.

Prevention of Further Absorption: Topically applied toxicants usually can be removed by thorough washing with soap and water; clipping of the hair or wool may be necessary. However, emesis is of value in dogs, cats, and pigs if done within a few hours of ingestion. Emesis is contraindicated when the swallowing reflex is absent; the animal is convulsing; corrosive agents, volatile hydrocarbons, or petroleum distillates are involved; or risk of aspiration pneumonia is imminent. Oral emetics include syrup of ipecac (10-20 mL, PO in dogs), and hydrogen peroxide (2 mL/kg, PO). Apomorphine can be used in dogs parenterally at a dose of 0.05-0.1 mg/kg.

Gastric lavage, using an endotracheal tube and the largest bore stomach tube possible, is done on the unconscious or anesthetized animal. The head is lowered to a 30° angle, and 10 mL of lavage fluid (water or saline) per kg of body wt is gently flushed into the stomach, then removed. This process is repeated until returned fluid is clear. Cathartics and laxatives may be indicated in some instances for more rapid elimination of the toxicant from the GI tract. A gastrotomy or rumenotomy may be necessary when lavage techniques are insufficient (or too slow in ruminants).

When the poison cannot be physically removed, certain agents administered orally can adsorb it and prevent its absorption from the alimentary tract. Activated charcoal (1-2 g/kg) is effective in adsorbing a wide variety of compounds and usually is the adsorbant and detoxicant of choice when poisoning is suspected.

Supportive Therapy: This often is necessary until the toxicant can be metabolized and eliminated. The type of support required depends on the animal's clinical condition and may include control of convulsive seizures, maintenance of respiration, treatment for shock, correction of electrolyte and fluid loss, control of cardiac dysfunction, and alleviation of pain.

Specific Antidotes: Antidotes (when known) are listed for each toxicant. Some form complexes with the toxicant (eg, the oximes bind with organophosphorous insecticides, EDTA chelates lead); others block or compete for receptor sites (eg, vitamin K competes with the receptor for coumarin anticoagulants), and a few affect metabolism of the toxicant (eg, nitrite and thiosulfate ions release and bind cyanide).

ALGAL POISONING

Algal poisoning is often an acute, fatal condition caused by high concentrations of toxic blue-green algae (more commonly known as cyanobacteria—literally blue-green bacteria) in the drinking water. Fatalities and severe illness of livestock, pets, wildlife, birds, and fish from heavy growths of waterblooms of blue-green algae occur in almost all countries of the world. Poisoning usually occurs during warm seasons when the waterblooms are more intense and of longer duration. Most poisonings occur among animals drinking algal-infested freshwater, but marine animals, especially maricultured fish and shrimp, are also affected. The toxins of cyanobacteria comprise 5 distinct chemical classes collectively called cyanotoxins.

Etiology, Epidemiology, and Pathogenesis: Although toxic strains within species of *Anabaena, Aphanizomenon, Cylindrospermopsis, Microcystis, Nodularia, Nostoc,* and *Planktothrix (Oscillatoria)* are responsible for most cases of toxicity, there are >30 species of cyanobacteria that can be associated with toxic waterblooms. Neurotoxic alkaloids (called anatoxins) can be produced by *Anabaena, Aphanizomenon,* and *Planktothrix,* while saxitoxins can be produced by *Anabaena, Aphanizomenon,* and *Lyngbya.* Hepatotoxic peptides (called microcystins and nodularins) can be produced by *Anabaena, Microcystis, Nodularia, Nostoc,* and *Planktothrix. Cylindrospermopsis* can produce a potent hepatotoxic alkaloid called cylindrospermopsin. Some genera, especially *Anabaena,* can produce both neuro- and hepatotoxins. If a toxic waterbloom contains both types of toxins, the neurotoxin signs are usually observed first because their effects occur much sooner (minutes) than the hepatotoxins (1 to a few hours).

Poisoning usually does not occur unless there is a heavy waterbloom that forms a dense surface scum. Factors that contribute to heavy waterblooms are nutrient-rich eutrophic to hypereutrophic water and warm, sunny weather. Agriculture practices (eg, runoff of fertilizers and animal wastes) that lead to nutrient enrichment often contribute to waterbloom formation. The problem is augmented by light winds or wind conditions that lead to leeward shore concentrations of cyanobacteria in areas where livestock drink. Experiments with both toxin groups have revealed a steep dose-response curve, with up to 90% of the lethal dose being ingested without measurable effect. Animal size and species sensitivity influence the degree of intoxication. Monogastric animals are less sensitive than ruminants and birds. Depending on bloom densities and toxin content, animals may need to ingest only a few ounces or up to several gallons to experience acute or lethal toxicity.

While the species sensitivity and signs of poisoning can vary depending on the type of exposure, the gross and histopathologic lesions are quite similar among species poisoned by the hepatopeptides and neurotoxic alkaloids. Death from hepatotoxicosis induced by cyclic peptides is generally accepted as being the result of intrahepatic hemorrhage and hypovolemic shock. This conclusion is based on large increases in liver weight as well as in hepatic hemoglobin and iron content that account for blood loss sufficient to induce irreversible shock. In animals that live more than a few hours, hyperkalemia or hypoglycemia, or both, may lead to death from liver failure within a few days.

Neurotoxicosis, with death occurring in minutes to a few hours from respiratory arrest, may result from ingestion of the cyanobacteria that produce neurotoxic alkaloids. Species and strains of *Anabaena, Aphanizomenon*, and *Planktothrix* can produce a potent, postsynaptic cholinergic (nicotinic) agonist called anatoxin-a that causes a depolarizing neuromuscular blockade. Strains of *Anabaena* can produce an irreversible organophosphate anticholinesterase called anatoxin-a(s). *Anabaena, Aphanizomenon*, and *Lyngbya* can produce the potent, presynaptic sodium channel blockers called saxitoxins.

Clinical Findings and Lesions: One of the earliest effects (15-30 min) of microcystin poisoning is increased serum concentrations of bile acids, alkaline phosphatase, γ-glutamyltransferase, and AST. The WBC count and clotting times increase. Death may occur within a few hours (usually within 4-24 hr), up to a few days. Death may be preceded by coma, muscle tremors, paddling, and dyspnea. Watery or bloody diarrhea may also be seen. Gross lesions include hepatomegaly due mostly to intrahepatic hemorrhage. Intact clumps of greenish algae can be found in the stomach and GI tract, and there is a greenish algal stain on the mouth, nose, legs, and feet. Hepatic necrosis begins centrilobularly and proceeds to the periportal regions. Hepatocytes are disassociated and rounded. After death, debris from disassociated hepatocytes can be found in the pulmonary vessels and kidneys. Clinical signs of neurotoxicosis progress from muscle fasciculations to decreased movement, abdominal breathing, cyanosis, convulsions, and death. Signs in birds are similar but include opisthotonos. In smaller animals, death is often preceded by leaping movements. Cattle and horses that survive acute poisoning may experience photosensitization in areas exposed to light (nose, ears, and back), followed by hair loss and sloughing of the skin.

Diagnosis: Diagnosis is based primarily on history (recent contact with an algal bloom), signs of poisoning, and necropsy findings. Samples of the waterbloom should be taken as soon as possible for microscopic examination to confirm the presence of the toxigenic cyanobacteria and for toxin analysis. Although there are nontoxic and toxic strains of all the known toxic species, it is not possible to identify a toxic strain by visual examination. Cyanobacteria are detected by light microscopy, identified using morphologic characteristics, and counted per standard volume of water. Standard protocols for sampling and monitoring cyanobacteria as well as practical keys for the identification of toxic species are available.

Some laboratories can analyze for the toxins either by chemical or biologic assay. Animal bioassays (mouse tests) have traditionally been used for detecting the presence of the entire range of cyanotoxins based on survival times and signs of poisoning. These tests provide a definitive indication of toxicity, although they cannot be used for precise quantification of compounds in water or for determining compliance with standards for environmental levels. A number of analytic techniques are available for determining microcystins in water. Analytic techniques must provide for quantitative comparison to the guideline value in terms of toxicity equivalents. The technique most suitable in this regard is high-performance liquid chromatography, although it may still involve estimation of the concentration, and therefore only an estimate of toxicity. Commercial standards for some microcystins, nodularin, and saxitoxins are available, while those for anatoxins and cylindrospermopsin should be available shortly. Newer methods of immunoassay are also available, including commercial ELISA kits in both laboratory and field formats.

Treatment: After removal from the contaminated water supply, affected animals should be placed in a protected area out of direct sunlight. Ample quantities of water and good quality feed should be made available. Because the toxins have a steep dose-response curve, surviving animals have a good chance for recovery. While therapies for cyanobacterial poisonings have not been investigated in detail, activated charcoal slurry is likely to be of benefit. In laboratory studies, an ion-exchange resin such as cholestyramine has proved useful to absorb the toxins from the GI tract, and certain bile acid transport blockers such as cyclosporin A, rifampin, and silymarin injected before dosing of microcystin have been effective in preventing hepatotoxicity. No therapeutic antagonist has been found effective against anatoxin-a, cylindrospermopsin, or the saxitoxins, but atropine and activated charcoal reduce the muscarinic effects of the anticholinesterase anatoxin-a(s).

Prevention: Removal of animals from the affected water supply is essential. If no other water supply is available, animals should be allowed to drink only from shore areas kept free (by prevailing winds) of dense surface scums of algae. Some efforts have been made to erect surface barriers (logs or floating plastic booms) to keep shore areas free of surface scum, but these are not very successful. Cyanobacteria can be controlled by adding copper sulfate ($CuSO_4$) or other algicidal treatments to the water. The usual treatment is 0.2-0.4 ppm, equivalent to 0.65-1.3 oz/10,000 gal. of water or 1.4-2.8 lb/acre-foot of water. Livestock (especially sheep) should not be watered for at least 5 days after the last visible evidence of the algal bloom. $CuSO_4$ is best used to prevent bloom formation, and care should be taken to avoid water that has dead algae cells, either from treatment with algicide or natural aging of the bloom, because most toxin is freed in the water only after breakdown of the intact algae cells.

Source water management techniques for control of cyanobacterial growth include flow maintenance in regulated rivers, water mixing techniques for both the elimination of stratification and the reduction of nutrient release from sediments in reservoirs, and the use of algicides in dedicated water supply storages. Algicides will disrupt cells and liberate intracellular toxins. Algicide use should be in accordance with local environment and chemical registration regulations. In situations where multiple offtakes are available, the selective withdrawal of water from different depths can minimize the intake of high surface accumulations of cyanobacterial cells.

Water treatment techniques can be highly effective for removal of both cyanobacterial cells and microcystins with the appropriate technology. As with other cyanotoxins, a high proportion of microcystins remain intracellular unless cells are lysed or damaged, and can therefore be removed by coagulation and filtration in a conventional treatment plant. Treatment of water containing cyanobacterial cells with oxidants such as chlorine or ozone, while killing cells, will result in the release of free toxin. Therefore, the practice of prechlorination or preozonation is not recommended without a subsequent step to remove dissolved toxins.

Microcystins are readily oxidized by a range of oxidants, including ozone and chlorine. Adequate contact time and pH control are needed to achieve optimal removal of these compounds, which will be more difficult in the presence of whole cells. Microcystins, anatoxin-a, cylindrospermopsin and some saxitoxins are also adsorbed from solution by both granular activated carbon and, less efficiently, by powdered activated carbon. The effectiveness of the process should be determined by monitoring toxin in the product water.

ARSENIC POISONING

Arsenic poisoning in animals is caused by several different types of inorganic and organic arsenical compounds. Toxicity varies with factors such as oxidation state of the arsenic, solubility, species of animal involved, and duration of exposure. Therefore, the toxic effects produced by phenylarsonic feed additives and other inorganic and organic compounds must be distinguished. (*See also* p 2369.)

INORGANIC ARSENICALS

These include arsenic trioxide, arsenic pentoxide, sodium and potassium arsenate, sodium and potassium arsenite, and lead or calcium arsenate. Trivalent arsenicals, also known as arsenites, are more soluble and therefore more toxic than the pentavalents or arsenate compounds. The lethal oral dose of sodium arsenite in most species is from 1-25 mg/kg. Cats may be more sensitive. Arsenates (pentavalents) are 5-10 times less toxic than arsenites. Poisoning is now relatively infrequent due to decreased use of these compounds as pesticides, ant baits, and wood preservatives. Arsenites are used to some extent as dips for tick control. Lead arsenate is sometimes used as a taeniacide in sheep.

Toxicokinetics and Mechanism of Action: Soluble forms of arsenic compounds are well absorbed orally. Following absorption, most of the arsenic is bound to RBC; it distributes to several tissues, with the highest levels found in liver, kidneys, heart, and lungs. In subchronic or chronic exposures, arsenic accumulates in skin, nails, hooves, sweat glands, and hair. The majority of the absorbed arsenic is excreted in the urine as inorganic arsenic or in methylated form.

The mechanism of action of arsenic toxicosis varies with the type of arsenical compound. Generally, tissues that are rich in oxidative enzymes such as the GI tract, liver, kidneys, lungs, endothelium, and epidermis are considered more vulnerable to arsenic damage. Trivalent inorganic and aliphatic organic arsenic compounds exert their toxicity by interacting with sulfhydryl enzymes, resulting in disruption of cellular metabolism. Arsenate can uncouple oxidation and phosphorylation.

Clinical Findings: Poisoning is usually acute with major effects on the GI tract and cardiovascular system. Arsenic has a direct effect on the capillaries, causing damage to microvascular integrity, transudation of plasma, loss of blood, and hypovolemic shock. Profuse watery diarrhea, sometimes tinged with blood, is characteristic, as are severe colic, dehydration, weakness, depression, weak pulse, and cardiovascular collapse. The onset is rapid, and signs are usually seen within a few hours (or up to 24 hr). The course may run from hours to several weeks depending on the quantity ingested. In peracute poisoning, animals may simply be found dead.

Lesions: In peracute toxicosis, no significant lesions may be seen. Inflammation and reddening of GI mucosa (local or diffuse) may be seen followed by edema, rupture of blood vessels, and necrosis of epithelial and subepithelial tissue. Necrosis may progress to perforation of the gastric or intestinal wall. GI contents are often fluid, foul smelling, and blood tinged; they may contain shreds of epithelial tissue. There is diffuse inflammation of the liver, kidneys, and other visceral organs. The liver may have fatty degeneration and necrosis, and the kidneys have tubular damage. In cases of cutaneous exposure, the skin may exhibit necrosis and be dry or leathery.

Diagnosis: Chemical determination of arsenic in tissues (liver or kidney) or stomach contents provides confirmation. Liver and kidneys of normal animals rarely contain >1 ppm arsenic (wet wt); toxicity is associated with a concentration >3 ppm. The determination of arsenic in stomach contents is of value usually within the first 24-48 hr after ingestion. The concentration of arsenic in urine can be high for several days after ingestion. Drinking water containing >0.25% arsenic is considered potentially toxic, especially for large animals.

Treatment: In animals with recent exposure and no clinical signs, emesis should be induced (in capable species), followed by activated charcoal with a cathartic (efficacy of charcoal in arsenic toxicosis remains to be determined) and then oral administration of GI protectants (small animals, 1-2 hr after charcoal) such as kaolin-pectin, and fluid therapy as needed. In animals already showing clinical signs, aggressive fluid therapy, blood transfusion (if needed), and administration of dimercaprol (British antilewisite, 4-7 mg/kg, IM, TID for 2-3 days or until recovery). In large animals, thioctic acid (lipoic acid or α-lipoic acid) may be used alone (50 mg/kg, IM, TID, as a 20% solution) or in combination with dimercaprol (3 mg/kg, IM, every 4 hr for the first 2 days, QID for the third day, and BID for the next 10 days or until recovery). In large animals, the efficacy of dimercaprol alone is questionable. Sodium thiosulfate has also been used, PO, at 20-30 g in 300 mL of water in horses and cattle, one-fourth this dose in sheep and goats, and 0.5-3 g in small animals or as a 20% solution, IV, at 30-40 mg/kg, 2-3 times/day for 3-4 days or until recovery. The water-soluble analogs of dimercaprol, 2,3-dimercaptopropane-1-sulfonate (DMPS) and dimercaptosuc-cinic acid (DMSA), are considered to be less toxic and more effective and could be given orally. D-Penicillamine has been reported to be an effective arsenic chelator in humans. It has a wide margin of safety and could be used in animals at 10-50 mg/kg, PO, 3-4 times/day for 3-4 days. Supportive therapy may be of even greater value, particularly when cardiovascular collapse is imminent, and should involve IV fluids to restore blood volume and correct dehydration. Kidney and liver function should be monitored during treatment.

ORGANIC ARSENICALS

Phenylarsonic organic arsenicals are relatively less toxic than inorganic compounds or aliphatic and other aromatic organic compounds.

Aliphatic organic arsenicals include cacodylic acid and acetarsonic acid. These are generally used as stimulants in large animals, but their use is no longer common. Some aliphatic arsenicals such as monosodium methanearsonate (MSMA) and disodium methanearsonate (DSMA) are occasionally used as cotton defoliants or crabgrass killers. Persistence of MSMA or DSMA in the soil and their tendency to accumulate in plants creates a potential for arsenic poisoning, especially in grazing animals. Clinical signs, lesions, and treatment of aliphatic organic arsenicals are similar to those of inorganic arsenicals.

Aromatic organic arsenicals include trivalent phenylorganicals such as thiacetarsamide and arsphenamine for the treatment of adult heartworms in dogs and pentavalent compounds such as phenylarsonic acids and their salts. Thiacetarsamide and arsphenamine are no longer used commonly, especially since the recent introduction of melarsomine dihydrochloride (*see also* HEARTWORM DISEASE, p 100).

Phenylarsonic compounds are used as feed additives to improve production in swine and poultry rations and also to treat dysentery in pigs. The 3 major compounds in this class are arsanilic acid, roxarsone (4-hydroxy-3-nitrophenylarsonic acid), and nitarsone (4-nitro-phenylarsonic acid).

Etiology: Toxicosis results from an excess of arsenic-containing additives in pig or poultry diets. Severity and rapidity of onset are dose-dependent. Signs may be delayed for weeks after incorporation of 2-3 times the recommended (100 ppm) levels or may occur within days when the excess is >10 times the recommended levels. Chickens are tolerant of arsanilic acid; however, roxarsone can produce toxicosis in turkeys at only twice the recommended dose (50 ppm). Roxarsone also has a higher toxicity in pigs as compared with other phenylarsonics.

Clinical Findings and Diagnosis: The earliest sign in pigs may be a reduction in weight gain, followed by incoordination, posterior paralysis, and eventually quadriplegia. Animals remain alert and maintain good appetite. Blindness is characteristic of arsanilic acid intoxication but not of other organic arsenicals. In ruminants, phenylarsonic toxicosis is similar to inorganic arsenic poisoning. There are usually no specific lesions present in phenylarsonic poisoning. Demyelination and gliosis of peripheral nerves, the optic tract, and optic nerves are usually seen on histopathology. Analyses of feed for the presence of high levels of phenylarsonics confirm the diagnosis.

Phenylarsonic poisoning in pigs should be differentiated from salt poisoning, insecticide poisoning, and pseudorabies. In cattle, arsenic poisoning should be differentiated from other heavy metal (lead) poisoning, insecticide poisoning, and infectious diseases such as bovine viral diarrhea.

Treatment and Prognosis: There is no specific treatment, but the neurotoxic effects are usually reversible if the offending feed is withdrawn within 2-3 days of onset of ataxia. Once paralysis occurs, the nerve damage is irreversible. Blindness is also usually irreversible, but animals retain their appetite, and weight gain is good if competition for food is eliminated. Recovery may be doubtful when the exposure is long and the onset of intoxication slow.

BRACKEN FERN POISONING

Bracken fern (*Pteridium aquilinum* [*Pteris aquilina*]) is widely distributed in upland and marginal areas throughout North and South America, Europe, Australia, and Asia. Ingestion of significant quantities produces signs of acute poisoning related to thiamine deficiency in monogastric animals and bone marrow depletion (aplastic anemia) in ruminants. The toxic effects appear to be cumulative and may require 1-3 mo to develop, depending on the species of animal, quantity consumed, time of year, and other factors. Both leaves and rhizomes contain the toxic principles, which vary in concentration with the season. Most acute poisonings are seen after periods of drought when grazing is scarce; however, the plant is toxic even when present as a contaminant in hay, and cases have occurred in stabled animals.

Longterm, low-level consumption has been associated with other clinical syndromes. **Enzootic hematuria** with hemorrhages or tumors in the bladder is seen in cattle in many areas of the world, and similar tumors have been seen in sheep. **Bright blindness** with retinal degeneration and hyperreflectivity of the tapetum is found in hill sheep in parts of England, and a similar condition has been recognized in cattle grazing bracken in Wales. Ingestion of bracken fern has been implicated in the occurrence of tumors in the upper GI tract of cattle in areas of Brazil and Scotland.

Some epidemiologic evidence suggests that regular consumption of milk from cattle with access to bracken may be associated with an increased risk of human esophageal or gastric cancer, but this is still under investigation. A greater risk to humans is direct consumption of the fern itself, a practice that continues in various countries throughout the world and is indeed promoted in some North American publications.

Etiology: Bracken fern contains a number of toxic factors, some of which are not yet fully characterized. Poisoning in nonruminants is due to a thiaminase; the effects are essentially those of vitamin B_1 deficiency, with myelin degeneration of the peripheral nerves. Horses seem to be particularly susceptible, while disease in pigs is rare. Thiamine deficiency is generally not a problem in ruminants because the vitamin is synthesized in the rumen, but polioencephalomalacia (p 1061) associated with impaired thiamine metabolism in sheep has been attributed to consumption of bracken fern and rock or mulga fern (*Cheilanthes sieberi*) in Australia.

The nature of the bone marrow toxin (aplastic anemia factor) to which cattle are particularly susceptible has not been defined, although the compound ptaquiloside has been suggested. The toxin causes death of precursor cells in the marrow so that cells with a shorter life span (the platelets) are affected first. An initial leukocytosis is followed by granulocytopenia and thrombocytopenia with resultant increased susceptibility to infection and tendency to spontaneous hemorrhage.

Bladder tumors, carcinoma of the urothelium, and hemangioendotheliomas in naturally occurring enzootic hematuria suggest that bracken fern may act as a carcinogen. This has been confirmed experimentally—inclusion of bracken fern in the diet of rats, mice, guinea pigs, quail, and Egyptian toads has resulted in tumors at various sites depending on the species and duration of feeding. Identical tumors can be produced by feeding ptaquiloside. Studies suggest that upper GI tract tumors in cattle may be due to the combined action of bracken fern and bovine papilloma virus (BPV). Bracken fern in combination with either BPV types 2 or 4 is believed to cause tumors in cattle. A flavonoid isolated from bracken fern, quercetin, is essential to fully transform bovine cells exposed to BPV type 4 in vitro.

Clinical Findings: In horses, signs of bracken-induced thiamine deficiency (bracken staggers) include anorexia, weight loss, incoordination, and a crouching stance with back and neck arched and feet placed wide apart. When forced to move, trembling muscles are noted. In severe cases, tachycardia and arrhythmias are present; death (usually 2-10 days after onset) is preceded by convulsions, clonic spasms, and opisthotonos. The rectal temperature is usually normal but may reach 104°F (40°C).

In pigs, signs of thiamine deficiency are less distinct and may resemble heart failure. Affected pigs show anorexia and weight loss. Death can occur suddenly after recumbency and dyspnea.

In cattle, acute bracken poisoning causes an acute hemorrhagic syndrome or, in some cases, sudden death. Affected cattle are weak, rapidly lose weight, and are pyrexic (106-110°F [41-43°C]); many have difficulty breathing and have icteric or pale mucosae with petechiae. Clots of blood may be passed in the feces, and there is often bleeding from body orifices. The blood frequently fails to clot normally; where tabanid flies are abundant, the skin of affected cattle is marked by streaks of blood where the insects have fed. The disease is almost always fatal; necropsy reveals multiple hemorrhages throughout the carcass. Necrotic ulcers may be present in the GI tract and bruising in the muscles. Swelling of the larynx and difficulty breathing has been reported in young cattle.

Chronic enzootic hematuria in cattle is characterized by intermittent hematuria and, ultimately, death due to anemia. The bladder contains small hemorrhages, dilated vessels, or tumors, which can be vascular, fibrous, or epithelial. In many cases, a mixture of lesions is found.

Bright blindness in sheep is a progressive retinal atrophy that derives its name from the hyperreflectivity of the tapetum. Affected sheep are permanently blind and adopt a characteristic alert attitude. The pupils respond poorly to light, and ophthalmoscopic examination of sheep with advanced disease reveals narrowing of arteries and veins and a pale tapetum nigrum with fine cracks and spots of gray.

Diagnosis: Other plants, such as horsetail (*Equisetum arvense*) and turnip (*Beta vulgaris*), can induce thiamine deficiency. In horses, the condition must be distinguished from other neurologic disorders, including rabies or poisoning due to *Crotalaria* sp or ragwort (*Senecio jacobea*). Blood thiamine levels decrease from an average normal of 80-100 µg/L to 25-30 µg/L, while blood pyruvate levels increase from a normal of ~20-30 µg/L to 60-80 µg/L; comparison with a sample from an unexposed animal of similar age and type will mitigate problems associated with correlating data from different analytic protocols. In pigs, the signs and lesions may indicate heart failure. Definitive diagnosis is established by demonstrating decreased blood thiamine levels or an increase in blood pyruvate with a decrease in RBC transketolase activity.

The acute hemorrhagic syndrome in cattle is distinctive, but signs may be confused with those of any acute septicemia (including anthrax) or other forms of poisoning such as mycotoxicosis, or poisoning by sweet clover or trichloroethylene-extracted soybean meal. Hematologic examination shows a loss of platelets from the blood, normally accompanied by loss of WBC, and pancytopenia in advanced stages.

Chronic enzootic hematuria must be distinguished from other causes of "red water," eg, the hemoglobinemia of babesiosis (p 20). Occasionally, cases are complicated by co-existing chronic pyelonephritis.

The retinal changes of bright blindness in sheep are characteristic but subtle, so diagnosis requires the exclusion of other causes of blindness, including pregnancy toxemia, infectious keratoconjunctivitis, and cataracts.

Treatment: Treatment of thiamine deficiency in horses is highly effective if diagnosis is made early. Injection of a thiamine solution at 5 mg/kg is suggested, given initially IV every 3 hr, then IM for several days. Oral supplementation may be required for an additional 1-2 wk, although SC injection of 100-200 mg daily for 6 days has been successful in some cases. Thiamine treatment should also include animals similarly exposed but not yet showing signs, as they can develop days or weeks after removal from the source of bracken.

In acutely affected cattle, mortality is usually >90%, and the platelet count is the best prognostic indicator. Animals should be removed from contaminated pasture, but it is often difficult to convince farmers that the plant is poisonous because the disease can appear up to 2 wk after livestock are removed from the fern-infested area. Treatment with DL-batyl alcohol to stimulate the bone marrow is of doubtful value. Antibiotics may be useful to prevent secondary infections. Blood or even platelet transfusions from a donor not grazing bracken may be appropriate, but large volumes are required (minimum of 2-4 L blood). Granulocyte-macrophage colony-stimulating factor has been used to treat aplastic anemia in humans.

The other syndromes are essentially untreatable and must be controlled by preventing access to the fern.

Prevention: Bracken is usually grazed for want of more suitable food, although individual animals may develop a taste for the plant, particularly the young tender shoots and leaves. Early spring (tender bracken shoots) or late summer (poor pasture conditions) are the times when the problem is most often manifest. The disease has been prevented in ruminants and horses by improved pasture management and fertilization or by alternating bracken-contaminated and noncontaminated pasture at 3-wk intervals.

Fern growth can be retarded by close grazing or trampling in alternate grazing pasture systems. In time, a pasture can be freed of bracken using this approach or by regular cutting of the mature plant or, if the land is suitable, by deep plowing. Herbicide treatment using asulam or glyphosate can be an effective method of control, especially if combined with cutting before treatment. Biologic control by the use of microorganisms or insects has been considered, but the longterm implications are not clear.

CANTHARIDIN POISONING

(Blister beetle poisoning)

In nature, cantharidin is found in beetles belonging to the Meloidae family. Over 200 species of these beetles occur throughout the continental USA, but members of the genus *Epicauta* are most frequently associated with toxicosis in horses. The striped blister beetles (*E occidentalis*, *E temexia*, and *E vittata*) are particularly troublesome in the southwestern USA. The black blister beetle, *E pennsylvanica*, has caused toxicosis in horses in Illinois. Cantharidin is the sole toxin, but its concentration in beetles varies widely.

Blister beetles usually feed on various weeds and occasionally move into alfalfa fields in large swarms. These insects are gregarious and may be found in hay in large numbers when it is baled. One flake of alfalfa may contain several hundred beetles, but a flake from the other end of the same bale may have none. Animals are usually exposed by eating alfalfa hay or alfalfa products that have been contaminated with blister beetles.

Pathogenesis: Cantharidin is an odorless, colorless compound that is soluble in various organic solvents but only slightly soluble in water. It is highly irritating and causes acantholysis and vesicle formation when in contact with skin or mucous membranes. After ingestion, it is absorbed from the GI tract and rapidly excreted by the kidneys. The minimum lethal oral dose in horses has not been established, but it appears to be <1 mg/kg body wt. As little as 4-6 g of dried beetles may be fatal to a horse. The toxicity of cantharidin does not decrease in stored hay, and cantharidin is also toxic to people, cattle, sheep, goats, dogs, cats, rabbits, and rats.

Clinical Findings: The severity of clinical signs associated with cantharidin toxicosis vary according to dose. Signs may range from mild depression or discomfort to severe pain, shock, and death. Typical signs are related to GI and urinary tract irritation, endotoxemia and shock, hypocalcemia, and myocardial dysfunction. The onset and duration of signs can vary from hours to days. The signs seen most frequently include varying degrees of abdominal pain, depression, anorexia, and frequent attempts to drink small amounts of water or submerge the muzzle in water. Some horses show only signs of depression or make frequent attempts to urinate. Urine may be blood-tinged or contain blood clots but frequently appears normal. A striking clinical feature is that affected horses invariably have dark, congested mucous membranes, even if other systemic signs of toxicosis are minimal. Sweating, delayed capillary refill time, increased heart and respiratory rates, and increased rectal temperature are other common signs. Less frequent signs include oral erosions; salivation; synchronous diaphragmatic flutter; a stiff, short-strided gait; and diarrhea that may contain blood. Horses that ingest a massive amount of toxin may show signs of severe shock and die within hours.

Diagnosis: Both high-performance liquid chromatography and gas chromatography or mass spectrometry analyses are sensitive, reliable methods of detecting cantharidin in gastric contents or in urine. The concentration of cantharidin in urine becomes negligible in 3-4 days, so urine should be collected early in the course of disease if it is to be analyzed. Microscopic evaluation of stomach contents (and often cecal contents) of fatally poisoned horses may reveal fragments of the insect, which can be positively identified if from one of the 3-striped species.

Certain laboratory findings are particularly helpful in differentiating cantharidin toxicosis from other causes of acute abdominal crisis. Serum calcium concentration is usually markedly decreased and may remain low for a prolonged time. Serum magnesium concentration is also typically low, and concentration of serum creatine kinase usually increases markedly within 24 hr of onset. In acutely affected horses, urinalysis typically reveals markedly decreased specific gravity (usually <1.010) and varying degrees of hematuria. Peritoneal fluid usually contains increased protein (>4 g/dL) but normal numbers of WBC and normal fibrinogen concentration. Other laboratory abnormalities may include mild increases of serum urea nitrogen and creatinine and development of hypoproteinemia. Acutely affected horses are almost always hyperglycemic.

Treatment: There is no specific antidote for cantharidin, but prompt, vigorous symptomatic therapy is necessary for successful treatment. Oral administration of mineral oil aids in evacuation of the GI tract, and repeated dosing may be indicated. Activated charcoal PO may be helpful if given early. Calcium and magnesium supplementation for prolonged periods is almost always indicated. Other symptomatic therapy includes administration of fluids, analgesics, and diuretics and maintenance of normal blood pH and serum electrolyte concentrations. The prognosis for affected horses improves daily if no complications occur.

Prevention: Prevention is aimed at feeding beetle-free hay. The hay field must be scouted before it is cut and during baling, because the insects can be crushed in the cutting and crimping process as well as during baling. Areas of the field that contain swarms of beetles must be avoided for a few days because most of the insects will leave. Once the beetles have left, these areas can be harvested.

First-cutting hay is almost always free of blister beetles, because the insects overwinter as subadults and usually do not emerge until late May or June in the southwestern USA. Likewise, the last cutting of hay is often safe, because it is usually harvested after the adult insects are no longer active.

COAL-TAR POISONING

A variety of coal-tar derivatives induce acute to chronic disease in animals. Clinical effects are acute to chronic hepatic damage with signs of icterus, ascites, anemia, and death. Coal-tar pitch poisoning has been reported from Canada, Germany, Ireland, Poland, and the USA. Toxicosis in domestic food animals and pets has been reported.

Etiology: The distillation of coal tar yields a variety of compounds, 3 of which are notably toxic: cresols (phenolic compounds), crude creosote (composed of cresols, heavy oils, and anthracene), and pitch. Tars are also produced from crude petroleum or wood. Creosote contains less volatile liquid and solid aromatic hydrocarbons of coal tar and some phenols. Cresols, composed mainly of hydroxytoluenes, are used as disinfectants. Coal-tar and pine-tar pitch are the brown to black, amorphous, polynuclear hydrocarbon residues left after coal tar is redistilled. Access of animals to coal tars is often by direct chewing on or consumption of product, rather than inclusion in feed or water. Clay pigeons, tar paper, creosote-treated wood, and bitumen-based flooring are typical sources.

Phenol is the most important toxicant in coal-tar products. The approximate oral acute LD_{50} of phenol for most species is 0.5 g/kg, except for cats, which are more susceptible due to their limited ability to conjugate and excrete phenols.

Cresols, which are mixtures of methylphenols, are used as disinfectants and are readily absorbed through the skin. The lethal dose is 100-200 mg/kg, except in cats, which are especially sensitive. Because creosote derived from coal tar is toxic to wood-destroying fungi and insects, it is used as a wood preserver. Sows confined to wooden farrowing crates treated with 3 brush applications of creosote were reported to have stillborn pigs, and the surviving pigs grew slowly. Some sources suggest that coal tars reduce absorption of vitamin A by sows. Other species are less susceptible (eg, the lethal dose of creosote in calves is 4 g/kg). Pitch is used as a binder in clay pigeons, road asphalt, insulation, and tar paper and roofing compounds, and to cover iron pipes and line wooden water tanks. Pigs that consume 15 g of clay pigeons over a 5-day period will die. Floor slabs with one-third lignite pitch reduced growth rate in pigs ~25%.

Clinical Findings: The cresols are locally corrosive; they stimulate the CNS and depress the heart, which results in vascular collapse. Capillary damage and hepatic or renal damage can occur. Death can occur from 15 min to several days after exposure. The first sign of pitch poisoning often is several dead pigs. Other pigs are depressed, and signs may progress to weakness, ataxia, sternal recumbency, icterus, coma, and death. Secondary anemia may develop. Associated problems have included stillbirths in pigs and hyperkeratosis in calves. Blood glucose is reduced terminally, while thymol turbidity and serum chloride and phosphorus are increased.

  Lesions: Cresols and creosote produce contact irritation and nonspecific liver and kidney lesions. In pitch poisoning, the liver is markedly swollen with a diffuse, mottled appearance. The lobules are clearly outlined by a light-colored zone, and their centers contain deep-red dots the size of a pinhead. There is centrilobular liver necrosis, with blood replacing the lost cells and filling the center of the lobule. Renal tubular degeneration and necrosis also can be present. The blood clots slowly or not at all. The carcass is icteric. Excessive fluid is found in the peritoneal cavity.

Diagnosis: Differential diagnoses include toxic plant poisonings (*Crotalaria, Senecio,* cocklebur), aflatoxicosis, fumonisin toxicosis, gossypol toxicosis, yellow phosphorus poisoning, and vitamin E or selenium deficiency. Fragments of clay pigeons, tar paper, or other sources of coal tars found in the GI tract, or chemical detection of coal-tar products in liver, kidney, serum, or urine, aid in confirming the diagnosis. A rapid presumptive test is to mix 1 mL of urine with 0.1 mL of 20% ferric chloride; purple color is indicative of phenol, but results should be confirmed by a laboratory.

Treatment: There is no specific antidote for animals with frank signs. For recent oral exposure, activated charcoal and saline cathartics may reduce absorption. Supportive therapy to combat shock, respiratory failure, and acidosis could be useful for valuable individual animals. Demulcents or egg whites orally may help to reduce local corrosive effects in the stomach and intestines. Oral antibiotics and high-quality-protein diets may aid recovery.

COPPER POISONING

  Acute or chronic copper poisoning is encountered in most parts of the world. Sheep are affected most often, although other species are also susceptible. In various breeds of dogs, especially Bedlington Terriers, an inherited sensitivity to copper toxicosis similar to Wilson's disease in humans has been identified. Acute poisoning is usually seen after accidental administration of excessive amounts of soluble copper salts, which may be present in anthelmintic drenches, mineral mixes, or improperly formulated rations. Many factors that alter copper metabolism influence chronic copper poisoning by enhancing the absorption or retention of copper. Low levels of molybdenum or sulfate in the diet are important examples. Primary chronic poisoning is seen most commonly in sheep when excessive amounts of copper are ingested over a prolonged period. The toxicosis remains subclinical until the copper that is stored in the liver is released in massive amounts. Blood copper concentrations increase suddenly, causing lipid peroxidation and intravascular hemolysis. The hemolytic crisis may be precipitated by many factors, including transportation, pregnancy, lactation, strenuous exercise, or a deteriorating plane of nutrition.

  Phytogenous and hepatogenous factors influence secondary chronic copper poisoning. Phytogenous chronic poisoning is seen after ingestion of plants, such as subterranean clover (*Trifolium subterraneum*), that produce a mineral imbalance and result in excessive copper retention. The plants that are not hepatotoxic contain normal amounts of copper and low levels of molybdenum. The ingestion of plants such as *Heliotropium europaeum* or *Senecio* spp (p 2506) for several months may cause hepatogenous chronic copper poisoning. These plants contain hepatotoxic alkaloids, which result in retention of excessive copper in the liver.

Acute poisoning may follow intakes of 20-100 mg of copper/kg in sheep and young calves and of 200-800 mg/kg in mature cattle. Chronic poisoning of sheep may occur with daily intakes of 3.5 mg of copper/kg when grazing pastures that contain 15-20 ppm (dry matter) of copper and low levels of molybdenum. Clinical disease may occur in sheep that ingest cattle rations, which normally contain higher levels of copper, or when their water is supplied via copper plumbing; cattle are more resistant to copper poisoning than sheep, and thus are not affected in these instances. Young calves or sheep injected with soluble forms of copper may develop acute clinical signs of toxicity. Copper is used as a feed additive for pigs at 125-250 ppm; levels >250 ppm are dangerous—although as for sheep, other factors may be protective, eg, high levels of protein, zinc, or iron. Chronic copper toxicosis is more apt to occur with low dietary intake of molybdenum and sulfur. Reduced formation of copper molybdate or copper sulfide complexes in tissues impairs the excretion of copper in urine or feces.

Clinical Findings: Acute copper poisoning causes severe gastroenteritis characterized by abdominal pain, diarrhea, anorexia, dehydration, and shock. Hemolysis and hemoglobinuria may develop after 3 days if the animal survives the GI disturbances. The sudden onset of clinical signs in chronic copper poisoning is associated with the hemolytic crisis. Affected animals exhibit depression, weakness, recumbency, rumen stasis, anorexia, thirst, dyspnea, pale mucous membranes, hemoglobinuria, and jaundice. Several days or weeks before the hemolytic crisis, liver enzymes, including ALT and AST, are usually increased. During the hemolytic crisis, methemoglobinemia, hemoglobinemia, and decreases in PCV and blood glutathione are usually seen. In camelid species such as alpacas or llamas, no hemolytic crisis is observed, although extensive liver necrosis remains a predominant sign. Morbid animals often die within 1-2 days. Herd morbidity is often <5%, although usually >75% of affected animals die. Losses may continue for several months after the dietary problem has been rectified. Severe hepatic insufficiency is responsible for early deaths. Animals that survive the acute episode may die of subsequent renal failure.

Lesions: Acute copper poisoning produces severe gastroenteritis with erosions and ulcerations in the abomasum of ruminants. Icterus develops in animals that survive >24 hr. Tissues discolored by icterus and methemoglobin are characteristic of chronic poisoning. Swollen, gunmetal-colored kidneys, port-wine-colored urine, and an enlarged spleen with dark brown-black parenchyma are manifestations of the hemolytic crisis. The liver is enlarged and friable. Histologically, there is centrilobular hepatic and renal tubular necrosis.

Diagnosis: Evidence of blue-green ingesta and increased fecal (8,000-10,000 ppm) and kidney (>15 ppm, wet wt) copper levels are considered significant in acute copper poisoning. In chronic poisoning, blood and liver copper concentrations are increased during the hemolytic period. Blood levels often rise to 5-20 μg/mL, as compared with normal levels of ~1 μg/mL. Liver concentrations >150 ppm (wet wt) are significant in sheep. The concentration of copper in the tissue must be determined to eliminate other causes of hemolytic disease.

Treatment and Control: Often, treatment is not successful. GI sedatives and symptomatic treatment for shock may be useful in acute toxicity. Penicillamine (50 mg/kg, PO, SID, for 6 days) or calcium versenate may be useful if administered in the early stages of disease. Experimentally, ammonium tetrathiomolybdate (15 mg/kg, IV, on alternate days) is effective for the treatment and prevention of copper poisoning. Daily administration of ammonium molybdate (100 mg) and sodium sulfate (1 g) reduces losses in affected lambs. Dietary supplementation with zinc acetate (250 ppm) may be useful to reduce the absorption of copper. Plant eradication or reducing access to plants that cause phytogenous or hepatogenous copper poisoning is desirable. Primary chronic or phytogenous poisoning may be prevented by top-dressing pastures with 1 oz of molybdenum per acre (70 g/hectare) in the form of molybdenized superphosphate or by molybdenum supplementation or restriction of copper intake.

CYANIDE POISONING

Cyanide inhibits cytochrome oxidase and causes death from histotoxic anoxia. (*See also* SORGHUM POISONING, p 2520.)

Etiology: Cyanides are found in plants, fumigants, soil sterilizers, fertilizers, and rodenticides (eg, calcium cyanomide). Toxicity can result from improper or malicious use, but in the case of livestock, the most frequent cause is ingestion of plants that contain cyanogenic glycosides. These include *Triglochin maritima* (arrow grass), *Hoecus lunatus* (velvet grass), *Sorghum* spp (Johnson grass, Sudan grass, common sorghum), *Prunus* spp (apricot, peach, chokecherry, pincherry, wild black cherry), *Sambucus canadensis* (elderberry), *Pyrus malus* (apple), *Zea mays* (corn), and *Linum* spp (flax). The seeds (pits) of several plants such as the peach have been the source of cyanogenic glycosides in many cases. *Eucalyptus* spp, kept as ornamental houseplants, have been implicated in deaths of small animals. The cyanogenic glycosides in plants yield free hydrocyanic acid (HCN), otherwise known as prussic acid, when hydrolyzed by β-glycosidase or when other plant cell structure is disrupted or damaged, eg, by freezing, chopping, or chewing. Microbial action in the rumen can further release free cyanide.

Apple and other fruit trees contain prussic acid glycosides in leaves and seeds but little or none in the fleshy part of the fruits. In *Sorghum* spp forage grasses, leaves usually produce 2-25 times more HCN than do stems; seeds contain none. New shoots from young, rapidly growing plants often contain high concentrations of prussic acid glycosides. The cyanogenic glycoside potential of plants can be increased by heavy nitrate fertilization, especially in phosphorus-deficient soils. Spraying of cyanogenic forage plants with foliar herbicides such as 2,4-D can increase their prussic acid concentrations for several weeks after application.

The cyanogenic glycoside potential is slow to decrease in drought-stricken plants containing mostly leaves. Grazing stunted plants during drought is the most common cause of poisoning of livestock by plants that produce prussic acid.

Frozen plants may release high concentrations of prussic acid for several days. After wilting, release of prussic acid from plant tissues declines. Dead plants have less free prussic acid. When plant tops have been frosted, new shoots may regrow at the base; these can be dangerous because of glycoside content and because livestock selectively graze them.

Ruminants are more susceptible than monogastric animals, and cattle slightly more so than sheep. Hereford cattle have been reported to be less susceptible than other breeds.

Clinical Findings: Signs can occur within 15-20 min to a few hours after animals consume toxic forage. Excitement can be displayed initially, accompanied by rapid respiration rate. Dyspnea follows shortly, with tachycardia. Salivation, excess lacrimation, and voiding of urine and feces may occur. Vomiting may occur, especially in pigs. Muscle fasciculation is common and progresses to generalized spasms before death. Animals stagger and struggle before collapse. Mucous membranes are bright red but may become cyanotic terminally. Death occurs during severe asphyxial convulsions. The heart may continue to beat for several minutes after struggling and breathing stops. The whole syndrome usually does not exceed 30-45 min. Most animals that live ≥2 hr after onset of clinical signs recover, unless continuous absorption of cyanide from the GI tract occurs.

Lesions: In acute or peracute cyanide toxicoses, blood may be bright cherry red initially but can be dark red if necropsy is delayed; it may clot slowly or not at all. Mucous membranes may also be pink initially, then become cyanotic after respiration ceases. The rumen may be distended with gas, and the odor of "bitter almonds" may be detected after opening. Agonal hemorrhages of the heart may be seen. Liver, serosal surfaces, tracheal mucosa, and lungs may be congested or hemorrhagic; some froth may be seen in respiratory passages. Neither gross nor histologic lesions are consistently seen.

Multiple foci of degeneration or necrosis may be seen in the CNS of dogs chronically exposed to sublethal amounts of cyanide. These lesions have not been reported in livestock.

Diagnosis: Appropriate history, clinical signs, postmortem findings, and demonstration of HCN in rumen (stomach) contents or other diagnostic specimens support a diagnosis of cyanide poisoning. Specimens recommended for cyanide analyses include the suspected source (plant or otherwise), rumen or stomach contents, heparinized whole blood, liver, and muscle. Antemortem whole blood is preferred; other specimens should be collected as soon as possible after death, preferably within 4 hr. Specimens should be sealed in an airtight container, refrigerated or frozen, and submitted to the laboratory without delay. When cold storage is unavailable, immersion of specimens in 1-3% mercuric chloride has been satisfactory.

Hay, green chop, silage, or growing plants containing >220 ppm cyanide as HCN on a wet-weight (as is) basis are very dangerous as animal feed. Forage containing <100 ppm HCN, wet weight, is usually safe to pasture. Analyses performed on a dry-weight basis have the following criteria: >750 ppm HCN is hazardous, 500-750 ppm HCN is doubtful, and <500 ppm HCN is considered safe.

Normally expected cyanide concentrations in blood of most animal species are usually <0.5 µg/mL. Minimal lethal blood concentrations are ~3.0 µg/mL or less. Cyanide concentrations in muscle are similar to those in blood, but concentrations in liver are generally lower than those in blood.

Differential diagnoses include poisonings by nitrate or nitrite, urea, organophosphate, carbamate, chlorinated hydrocarbon pesticides, and toxic gases (carbon monoxide and hydrogen sulfide), as well as infectious or noninfectious diseases that cause sudden death.

Treatment, Control, and Prevention: Immediate treatment is necessary. Sodium nitrite (10 g/100 mL of distilled water or isotonic saline) should be given IV at 20 mg/kg body wt, followed by sodium thiosulfate (20%), IV, at ≥500 mg/kg; the latter may be repeated as needed with little hazard. Sodium nitrite therapy may be carefully repeated at 10 mg/kg, every 2-4 hr or as needed. In one study investigating cyanide poisoning treatment in dogs, either dimethylaminophenol (DMAP) IM at 5 mg/kg or hydroxylamine hydrochlorine IM at 50 mg/kg were as effective as nitrite and thiosulfate.

Sodium thiosulfate alone is also an effective antidotal therapy at ≥500 mg/kg, IV, plus 30 g/cow, PO, to detoxify any remaining HCN in the rumen. Oxygen may be helpful in supplementing nitrite or thiosulfate therapy, especially in small animals. Hyperbaric oxygen therapy (100% oxygen breathed intermittently at a pressure >1 atmosphere absolute) causes an above normal partial pressure of oxygen (PO_2) in arterial blood and markedly increases the amount of oxygen dissolved in plasma. Oxygen-dependent cellular metabolic processes benefit from heightened oxygen tension in capillaries and enhanced oxygen diffusion from capillaries to critical tissues. Activated charcoal is not efficacious in absorbing cyanide and thus is not recommended PO for antidotal therapy.

Caution is indicated in treatment. Many clinical signs of nitrate and prussic acid poisoning are similar, and injecting sodium nitrite induces methemoglobinemia identical to that produced by nitrate poisoning. If in doubt of the diagnosis, methylene blue, IV, at 4-22 mg/kg, may be used to induce methemoglobin. Because methylene blue can serve as both a donor and acceptor of electrons, it can reduce methemoglobin in the presence of excess methemoglobin or induce methemoglobin when only hemoglobin is present (but sodium nitrite is the more effective treatment for cyanide poisoning if the diagnosis is certain).

Pasture grasses (eg, Sudan grass and sorghum-Sudan grass hybrids) should not be grazed until they are 15-18 in. tall to reduce danger from prussic acid poisoning. Forage sorghums should be several feet tall. Animals should be fed before first turning out to pasture; hungry animals may consume forage too rapidly to detoxify HCN released in the rumen. Animals should be turned out to new pasture later in the day; prussic acid release potential is reported to be highest during early morning hours. Free-choice salt and mineral with added sulfur may help protect against prussic acid toxicity. Grazing should be monitored closely during periods of environmental stress, eg, drought or frost. Abundant regrowth of sorghum can be dangerous; these shoots should be frozen and wilted before grazing.

Green chop forces livestock to eat both stems and leaves, thereby reducing problems caused by selective grazing. Cutting height can be raised to minimize inclusion of regrowth.

Sorghum hay and silage usually lose ≥50% of prussic acid content during curing and ensiling processes. Free cyanide is released by enzyme activity and escapes as a gas. Although a rare occurrence, hazardous concentrations of prussic acid may still remain in the final product, especially if the forage had an extremely high cyanide content before cutting. Hay has been dried at oven temperatures for up to 4 days with no significant loss of cyanide potential. These feeds should be analyzed before use whenever high prussic acid concentrations are suspected. Potentially toxic feed should be diluted or mixed with grain or forage that is low in prussic acid content to achieve safe concentrations in the final product.

ETHYLENE GLYCOL TOXICITY

All animals are susceptible to ethylene glycol (EG) toxicity, but it is most common in dogs and cats. Most intoxications are associated with ingestion of radiator antifreeze, which is usually 95% EG. The widespread availability of antifreeze, its sweet taste and small minimum lethal dose, and the lack of public awareness of the toxicity (ie, improper storage and disposal) contribute to the frequency of this intoxication. In addition, antifreeze may be ingested because it is the only available liquid in cold weather or by way of intentional poisoning. Other sources of EG include some heat-exchange fluids used in solar collectors and ice-rink freezing equipment and some brake and transmission fluids. Cutaneous absorption from topical products that contain EG has been reported to cause toxicity in cats.

EG intoxication occurs most commonly in temperate and cold climates because antifreeze is used both to decrease the freezing point and to increase the boiling point of radiator fluid. In colder climates, the incidence of EG intoxications is seasonal with most cases occurring in the fall, winter, and early spring.

The minimum lethal dose of undiluted EG is 1.4 mL/kg body wt in cats, 4.4 mL/kg in dogs, 7-8 mL/kg in poultry, and 2-10 mL/kg in cattle (younger animals may be more susceptible).

Pathogenesis: EG is rapidly absorbed from the GI tract; in dogs, peak blood concentrations of EG occur within 3 hr of ingestion. About 50% of ingested EG is excreted unchanged by the kidneys; however, a series of oxidation reactions in the liver and kidneys metabolize the remaining EG. Toxic metabolites of EG cause severe metabolic acidosis and renal tubular epithelial damage.

The first of 2 rate-limiting biotransformation steps is the production of glycoaldehyde from EG by the enzyme alcohol dehydrogenase. Glycoaldehyde is then rapidly metabolized to glycolic acid. The oxidation of glycolic acid to glyoxylic acid is the second rate-limiting step, which allows glycolic acid to accumulate, resulting in acidosis and nephrosis. Glyoxylic acid is rapidly metabolized to formic acid, carbon dioxide, glycine, serine, and oxalate. Oxalate is not further metabolized and is cytotoxic to the renal tubular epithelium and exacerbates the metabolic acidosis. Glycolic acid and oxalate are the metabolites thought to be most responsible for acute tubular necrosis associated with EG ingestion. Oxalate also combines with calcium to form a soluble complex that is excreted via glomerular filtration. Calcium oxalate crystals form within the lumina of tubules as the concentration of the glomerular filtrate increases and the pH decreases (smaller numbers of calcium oxalate crystals may also be observed in the adventitia of blood vessel walls throughout the body).

Clinical Findings: Clinical signs are dose- and time-dependent and can be divided into those caused by unmetabolized EG and those caused by its toxic metabolites. The onset of clinical signs is almost immediate and resembles alcohol (ethanol) intoxication. Dogs and cats exhibit vomiting due to GI irritation, polydipsia and polyuria, and neurologic signs (CNS depression, stupor, ataxia, knuckling, decreased withdrawal and righting reflexes). Polydipsia occurs due to osmotic stimulation of the thirst center, and polyuria occurs due to an osmotic diuresis. As CNS depression increases in severity, dogs and cats drink less; however, the osmotic diuresis continues and results in dehydration. Dogs may appear to transiently recover from these CNS signs ~12 hr after ingestion.

Oliguric acute renal failure usually develops between 12 and 24 hr in cats and between 36 and 72 hr in dogs. Signs include lethargy, anorexia, dehydration, vomiting, diarrhea, oral ulcers, salivation, tachypnea, and possibly seizures or coma. The kidneys are often swollen and painful on abdominal palpation.

Pigs ingesting EG are usually depressed, weak, and reluctant to move; knuckling, posterior ataxia, trembling, collapse, abdominal distention, pulmonary edema, and muffled heart sounds are common sequelae. Poultry may become drowsy, ataxic, dyspneic, and recumbent; torticollis, ruffled feathers, and watery droppings are also seen. Cattle may become depressed, tachypneic, and ataxic, and develop paraparesis or recumbency. Epistaxis and hemoglobinuria have also been seen in cattle that have ingested large doses of EG.

Lesions: Renal tubular epithelial necrosis with calcium oxalate crystals in the tubular lumina is the characteristic finding of EG intoxication. Calcium oxalate crystals appear birefringent when viewed with polarized light. Pulmonary edema and hemorrhagic gastroenteritis are common secondary findings in dogs and cats. Pigs and cattle often develop renal and perirenal edema. Pigs may also have pulmonary edema with tan fluid in the pleural and peritoneal cavities. Poultry usually do not develop gross lesions.

Diagnosis: Diagnosis is often difficult due to nonspecific multisystemic signs that may appear similar to other types of CNS disease or trauma, gastroenteritis, pancreatitis, ketoacidotic diabetes mellitus, and acute renal failure due to renal ischemia or other nephrotoxicants. If ingestion of EG is not witnessed, diagnosis is usually based on a combination of history, physical examination, and laboratory data.

Within 3 hr of ingestion of toxic doses of EG, dogs and cats develop normochloremic metabolic acidosis with an increased anion gap, minimally concentrated or isosthenuric urine with an acidic pH, and marked serum hyperosmolality with an increased osmolal gap. Serum osmolality can be increased as much as 100 mOsm/kg above normal (280-310 mOsm/kg) within 3 hr of EG ingestion. The difference between measured and calculated $(1.86 [Na^+ + K^+] + glucose/18 + BUN/2.8 + 9)$ osmolality is referred to as the osmolal gap. The gap is caused by the presence of unmeasured osmotically active particles (eg, ethylene glycol) in the serum. Calcium oxalate crystalluria is commonly seen as early as 3 and 6 hr after ingestion in cats and dogs, respectively. Monohydrate calcium oxalate crystals (clear, 6-sided prisms) are more common than dihydrate calcium oxalate crystals (maltese cross or envelope-shaped). EG concentrations in serum and urine are detectable by 1-2 hr after ingestion. Commercial test kits can detect serum EG concentrations of ≥50 mg/dL. Some antifreeze preparations contain fluorescein, which appears bright yellow-green when viewed under a Wood's lamp. Urine fluorescence has been used as a qualitative adjunctive test in suspected EG ingestions in humans and may be of value in veterinary medicine. Hyperphosphatemia has been seen in dogs within 3 hr of ingestion of commercial antifreeze solutions that contain phosphate rust inhibitors. This hyperphosphatemia resolves before the onset of EG-induced acute renal failure and azotemia, then recurs when the animal becomes azotemic.

Treatment: The prognosis varies inversely with the amount of time that elapses between ingestion and initiation of treatment. Treatment is aimed at decreasing absorption of ingested EG, increasing excretion of unmetabolized EG, preventing metabolism of EG, and correcting the metabolic acidosis that occurs with EG metabolism. Further absorption of EG is prevented by induction of emesis or gastric lavage (or both) followed by administration of activated charcoal and sodium sulfate within 1-2 hr of ingestion. Once absorption has occurred, excretion of EG is increased by fluid therapy designed to correct dehydration and increase urine production. To prevent metabolism of EG, the activity of alcohol dehydrogenase is decreased by direct inactivation or by competitive inhibition. 4-Methylpyrazole (4-MP, fomepizole) effectively inactivates alcohol dehydrogenase in dogs without the side effects of ethanol and is the treatment of choice. The dose of 4-MP (5% solution [50 mg/mL]) is 20 mg/kg body wt, IV, initially, followed by 15 mg/kg, IV, at 12 and 24 hr, and 5 mg/kg, IV, at 36 hr. Commercial formulations of 4-MP are available.

In cats, 4-MP is ineffective at the canine dosage, and ethanol, a competitive inhibitor of alcohol dehydrogenase, is the treatment of choice. The recommended dose is 5 mL of 20% ethanol/kg body wt diluted in IV fluids and given as a drip over 6 hr for 5 treatments, and then over 8 hr for 4 more treatments.

The metabolic acidosis associated with metabolism of EG is corrected by administration of sodium bicarbonate. The formula $0.3 - (0.5 \times \text{kg body wt}) \times (24 - \text{plasma bicarbonate})$ is used to determine the dose, in mEq of bicarbonate. One-half of this dose should be given IV slowly to prevent overdose, and plasma bicarbonate concentrations should be monitored every 4-6 hr. Additional doses of bicarbonate based on the above formula are frequently necessary. Monitoring urine pH may also be helpful with a goal of maintaining the urine pH between 7.0 and 7.5.

In dogs and cats with azotemia or in oliguric acute renal failure, inhibition of alcohol dehydrogenase is of little benefit because almost all of the EG has already been metabolized. The prognosis for these animals is guarded to poor. Treatment should include correction of fluid, electrolyte, and acid-base disorders and, if possible, establishment of diuresis.

Propylene Glycol Toxicosis

Although less toxic than EG, ingestion of propylene glycol (PG) may be associated with a toxic syndrome similar to the acute phase of EG toxicosis. The oral LD_{50} of PG in dogs is ~9 mL/kg. In cats, ingestion of a diet containing 6-12% PG can result in Heinz body formation and decreased RBC survival. Treatment of PG toxicosis is largely supportive— the use of alcohol dehydrogenase inhibitors is not indicated. Ingestion of PG may result in false positive EG test kit results.

FLUORIDE POISONING

(Fluorosis)

Fluorides are widely distributed in the environment and originate naturally from rocks and soil or from industrial processes. Water supplies for human consumption have been adjusted to contain 1 ppm to prevent dental caries. Fluorine at 1-2 mg/kg in animal rations is considered adequate. The maximal tolerable level varies by species, eg, 40-50 ppm for cattle and horses, and 200 mg/kg for chickens. (The terms "fluorine" and "fluoride" are used interchangeably.)

Etiology: Toxic quantities of fluorides occur naturally, eg, certain rock phosphates and the superphosphates produced from them, partially defluorinated phosphates, and the phosphatic limestones. In certain areas, drinking water from deep wells may contain high levels of fluorides. Volcanic ash may be high in fluoride. Wastes from industrial processes, fertilizers, and mineral supplements are the most common causes of chronic fluorosis. The fluorine-containing gases and dusts from manufacturing of fertilizers, mineral supplements, metal ores (steel and aluminum), and certain enamelling processes may contaminate forage crops. Contamination of the surrounding area, particularly in the direction of the prevailing wind, may extend 5-6 miles. Forage crops grown on high-fluorine soils have increased levels due to mechanical contamination with soil particles. Feed-grade phosphates must contain no more than 1 part of fluorine to 100 parts phosphorus. A 100-g tube of fluoride toothpaste may contain 75-500 mg of sodium fluoride, depending on the brand.

There is a general correlation between solubility of a fluoride and its toxicity. Of the common fluorides, sodium fluoride is the most toxic, and calcium fluoride the least toxic. The fluorides of rock phosphates and most cryolites are of intermediate toxicity. Soluble fluorides originating from industrial fumes or dusts are more toxic than fluoride in rock phosphate.

Fluoride binds to Ca^{2+}, Mg^{2+}, and Mn^{2+}, acting as a direct cellular poison (including bacterial cells, hence its use in dental hygiene). At high levels most fluorides are corrosive to tissue. In bone, fluoride binds calcium and replaces the hydroxyl groups in the mineral

part of bone, which is mostly hydroxyapatite. In teeth developed during fluoride ingestion, the enamel is less soluble (protective) and more dense (brittle, if excessive). In addition, faulty mineralization of teeth and bones occurs when excessive fluoride interferes
with intracellular calcium metabolism and damages ameloblasts and odontoblasts.

Clinical Findings: Acute poisoning from inhalation of fluorine-containing gases or
from ingestion of rodenticides or ascaricides containing fluoride is rare. Oral cleaning
products present a danger to pets, especially dogs. The fatal dose of sodium fluoride is
5-10 mg/kg and toxic effects occur below 1 mg/kg. Fluoride (75-90% absorbed by 90 min)
lowers serum calcium and magnesium. Clinically, gastroenteritis and cardiac (ventricular tachycardia and ECG abnormalities) and nervous signs may be followed within a few
hours by collapse and death.

The signs of fluorosis from chronic ingestion are the same regardless of the source of
fluoride. Levels too low to produce skeletal signs can cause changes in the enamel of
developing teeth, leading to chalkiness or mottling, staining, and rapid and irregular
wear. When exposure occurs after dental development, the teeth remain normal even if
severe skeletal fluorosis develops. Clinical signs, apart from mild tooth lesions, occur in
many animals when bone fluoride reaches 4,000 ppm. Skeletal fluorosis results in accelerated bone resorption and remodeling with production of exostoses and sclerosis. Metabolically active bones (ribs, mandible, and long bones) and growing bones in the
young are most affected. Affected animals are lame, and feed and water intake and
weight gain are decreased. Severely diseased cattle may move around on their knees
due to spurring and bridging of the joints in the late stages. When the skeleton becomes
saturated (30-40 times normal bone content), "flooding" of the soft tissue occurs, which
causes a rise in plasma fluorides and metabolic breakdown evidenced by a loss of appetite and listlessness.

Lesions: Acute ingestion of high levels of fluoride causes inflammation of the gut
and degenerative changes in the lungs, liver, and kidneys. In chronic cases, mottling,
staining, and excessive wearing occur in teeth that develop during the time of excessive
fluoride ingestion. A more advanced stage of fluorosis is marked by skeletal abnormalities; the bones become chalky white, soft, thickened, and in the extreme, develop exostoses that may be palpated, especially along the long bones and on the mandible in animals exposed at any age.

Diagnosis: Urine fluoride levels are time dependent due to rapid elimination. In cases of
known ingestion, serum calcium and magnesium levels are beneficial. Casual observation
of affected animals may suggest chronic debilitating arthritis; osteoporosis; or deficiency
of calcium, phosphorus, or vitamin D. Lameness in advanced cases may be wrongly attributed to an accident. Nonspecific staining seen in cattle teeth may be confused with incipient fluorosis. A developing fluoride toxicosis can be recognized by the following criteria
(from most to least reliable): 1) chemical analyses to determine the amount of fluorine in
the diet, urine, bones, and teeth; 2) tooth effects, in animals exposed at time of permanent
teeth development; 3) lameness, as the result of fluoride accumulation in bone; and 4) systemic evidence as reflected by anorexia, inanition, and cachexia.

The normal levels of fluorine in livestock are considered to be <0.2 ppm in plasma,
1-8 in urine, 200-600 in bones, and 200-500 in teeth. Normal bovine urine contains <5 ppm
fluorine; in borderline toxicity, urine contains 20-30 ppm, and in cattle with systemic
signs, >35 ppm. In pigs, bones appear normal with 3,000-4,000 ppm fluorine, and levels of
<4,500 ppm in compact bones from cattle are considered innocuous. In cattle, toxicosis
is associated with levels of >5,500 ppm in compact bone and >7,000 ppm in cancellous
bone; in sheep, levels are believed to be lower (2,000-3,000 ppm in compact bone and
4,000-6,000 ppm in cancellous bone).

Treatment and Control: Acutely exposed animals require calcium gluconate (IV)
and oral magnesium hydroxide or milk to bind fluoride before absorption. In chronic
exposure, control is difficult unless animals are removed from affected areas. It has been
suggested that affected areas may be used for animals with a relatively short production
life, eg, pigs, poultry, or finishing cattle and sheep. Feeding calcium carbonate, aluminum

oxide, aluminum sulfate, magnesium metasilicate, or boron has either decreased absorption or increased excretion of fluoride, and thus could offer some control of chronic fluorosis under some conditions. However, no treatment has been shown to cure the chronic effects of fluorine toxicity.

FOOD HAZARDS

AVOCADO

Ingestion of avocado (*Persea americana*) has been associated with myocardial necrosis in mammals and birds and with sterile mastitis in lactating mammals. Cattle, goats, horses, mice, rabbits, guinea pigs, rats, sheep, budgerigars, canaries, cockatiels, ostriches, chickens, turkeys, and fish are susceptible. Caged birds appear more sensitive to the effects of avocado, while chickens and turkeys appear more resistant. A single case report exists of 2 dogs developing myocardial damage secondary to avocado ingestion.

Etiology: Ingestion of fruit, leaves, stems, and seeds of avocado has been associated with toxicosis in animals; leaves are the most toxic part. The Guatemalan varieties of avocado have been most commonly associated with toxicosis.

Purified persin at 60-100 mg/kg causes mastitis in lactating mice and doses >100 mg/kg result in myocardial necrosis. Goats develop severe mastitis when ingesting 20 g of leaves/kg, whereas 30 g of leaves/kg results in cardiac injury. Acute cardiac failure developed in sheep fed avocado leaves at 25 g/kg for 5 days; 5.5 g/kg of leaves fed for 21 days or 2.5 g/kg for 32 days caused chronic cardiac insufficiency. Budgerigars fed 1 g of avocado fruit developed agitation and feather pulling, while 8.7 g of mashed avocado fruit resulted in death within 48 hr.

Pathogenesis: Avocado causes necrosis and hemorrhage of mammary gland epithelium of lactating mammals and myocardial necrosis in birds and mammals. The toxic principle, persin, extracted from avocado leaves has caused lesions similar to those reported in natural cases.

Clinical Findings: In lactating animals, mastitis occurs within 24 hr of exposure to avocado, accompanied by a 75% decrease in milk production. Affected mammary glands are firm, swollen, and produce watery, curdled milk. Lactation may provide a degree of protection against myocardial injury at lower doses. In nonlactating mammals, or at higher doses, myocardial insufficiency may develop within 24-48 hr of ingestion and is characterized by lethargy, respiratory distress, subcutaneous edema, cyanosis, cough, exercise intolerance, and death. Horses may develop edema of the head, tongue, and brisket. Birds develop lethargy, dyspnea, anorexia, subcutaneous edema of neck and pectoral regions, and death.

Lesions: Mammary glands are edematous and reddened, with watery, curdled milk. In animals with cardiac insufficiency, there is congestion of lungs and liver, often with dependent subcutaneous edema. There may be free fluid within the abdominal cavity, pericardial sac, and thoracic cavity; pulmonary edema may be present. The heart may contain pale streaks. Histopathologic lesions in the mammary gland include degeneration and necrosis of secretory epithelium, with interstitial edema and hemorrhage. Myocardial lesions include degeneration and necrosis of myocardial fibers, which are most pronounced in ventricular walls and septum; interstitial hemorrhage and/or edema may be present. In horses, symmetric ischemic myopathy of head muscles and tongue, as well as ischemic myelomalacia of the lumbar spinal cord, have been described.

Diagnosis: Diagnosis of avocado toxicosis relies on history of exposure and clinical signs. There are no readily available specific tests that will confirm diagnosis. Differential diagnoses include other causes of mastitis (eg, infectious) and other myocardial disorders, including ionophore toxicosis, yew toxicosis, vitamin E/selenium deficiency, gossypol, cardiac glycoside toxicosis (eg, oleander), cardiomyopathy, and infectious myocarditis.

Treatment: NSAID and analgesics may benefit animals with mastitis. Treatment for congestive heart failure (eg, diuretics, antiarrhythmic drugs) may be of benefit, but may not be economically feasible in livestock.

BREAD DOUGH

Raw bread dough made with yeast poses mechanical and biochemical hazards when ingested, including gastric distention, metabolic acidosis, and CNS depression. Although any species is susceptible, dogs are most commonly involved due to their indiscriminate eating habits.

Pathogenesis: The warm, moist environment of the stomach serves as an efficient incubator for the replication of yeast within the dough. The expanding dough mass causes distention of the stomach, resulting in vascular compromise to the gastric wall similar to that seen in gastric dilatation/volvulus. With sufficient gastric distention, respiratory compromise occurs. Yeast fermentation products include ethanol, which is absorbed into the bloodstream, resulting in inebriation and metabolic acidosis.

Clinical Findings: Early clinical signs may include unproductive attempts at emesis, abdominal distention, and depression. As ethanol intoxication develops, the animal becomes ataxic and disoriented. Eventually, profound CNS depression, weakness, recumbency, coma, hypothermia, or seizures may be seen. Death is usually due to the effects of the alcohol, rather than from gastric distention; however, the potential for dough to trigger gastric dilatation/volvulus in susceptible dog breeds should not be overlooked.

Diagnosis: A presumptive diagnosis can be based on history of exposure and clinical signs. Blood ethanol levels are consistently elevated in cases of bread dough toxicosis. Differential diagnoses include gastric dilatation/volvulus, foreign body obstruction, ethylene glycol toxicosis, and ingestion of other CNS depressants (eg, benzodiazepines).

Treatment: With recent ingestions in asymptomatic animals, emesis may be attempted, although the glutinous nature of bread dough may make removal via emesis difficult. In animals where emesis (whether induced or spontaneous) has been unsuccessful, gastric lavage may be attempted. Cold water introduced into the stomach may slow the rate of yeast fermentation and aid in removal of dough. In some cases, surgical removal of the dough mass may be required. Animals presenting with signs of alcohol toxicosis should be stabilized and any life-threatening conditions corrected before attempts to remove the dough are made. Alcohol toxicosis is managed by correcting acid/base abnormalities, managing cardiac arrhythmias as needed, and maintaining normal body temperature. Providing fluid diuresis to enhance alcohol elimination may be helpful in some cases. Anecdotally, yohimbine (0.1 mg/kg, IV) has been used to stimulate severely comatose dogs with alcohol toxicosis.

CHOCOLATE

Chocolate toxicosis may result in potentially life-threatening cardiac arrhythmias and CNS dysfunction. Chocolate poisoning occurs most commonly in dogs, although many species are susceptible. Contributing factors include indiscriminate eating habits and readily available sources of chocolate. Deaths have also been reported in livestock fed cocoa byproducts and in animals consuming mulch from cocoa-bean hulls.

Etiology: Chocolate is derived from the roasted seeds of *Theobroma cacao*. The toxic principles in chocolate are the methylxanthines theobromine (3,7-dimethylxanthine) and caffeine (1,3,7-trimethylxanthine). Although the concentration of theobromine in chocolate is 3-10 times that of caffeine, both constituents contribute to the clinical syndrome seen in chocolate toxicosis. The exact amount of methylxanthines in chocolate varies due to natural variation of cocoa beans and variation within brands of chocolate products. However, in general, the total methylxanthine concentration of dry cocoa powder is ~800 mg/oz (28.5 mg/g), unsweetened (baker's) chocolate is ~450 mg/oz (16 mg/g), semisweet chocolate and sweet dark chocolate is ~150-160 mg/oz (5.4-5.7 mg/g), and milk chocolate is ~64 mg/oz (2.3 mg/g). White chocolate is an insignificant source of methylxanthines. Cocoa bean hulls contain ~255 mg/oz (9.1 mg/g) methylxanthines.

The LD_{50} of caffeine and theobromine are reportedly 100-200 mg/kg, but severe signs and deaths may occur at much lower doses and individual sensitivity to methylxanthines varies. In general, mild signs (vomiting, diarrhea, polydipsia) may be seen in dogs ingesting 20 mg/kg, cardiotoxic effects may be seen at 40-50 mg/kg, and seizures may occur at doses ≥60 mg/kg. One ounce of milk chocolate per pound of body weight is a potentially lethal dose in dogs.

Pathogenesis: Theobromine and caffeine are readily absorbed from the GI tract and are widely distributed throughout the body. They are metabolized in the liver and undergo enterohepatic recycling. Methylxanthines are excreted in the urine as both metabolites and unchanged parent compounds. The half-lives of theobromine and caffeine in dogs are 17.5 hr and 4.5 hr, respectively.

Theobromine and caffeine competitively inhibit cellular adenosine receptors, resulting in CNS stimulation, diuresis, and tachycardia. Methylxanthines also increase intracellular calcium levels by increasing cellular calcium entry and inhibiting intracellular sequestration of calcium by the sarcoplasmic reticulum of striated muscle. The net effect is increased strength and contractility of skeletal and cardiac muscle. Methylxanthines may also compete for benzodiazepine receptors within the CNS and inhibit phosphodiesterase, resulting in increased cyclic AMP levels. Methylxanthines may also increase circulating levels of epinephrine and norepinephrine.

Clinical Findings: Clinical signs of chocolate toxicosis usually occur within 6-12 hr of ingestion. Initial signs may include polydipsia, vomiting, diarrhea, abdominal distention, and restlessness. Signs may progress to hyperactivity, polyuria, ataxia, tremors, and seizures. Tachycardia, premature ventricular contractions, tachypnea, cyanosis, hypertension, hyperthermia, bradycardia, hypotension, or coma may occur. Hypokalemia may occur late in the course of the toxicosis, contributing to cardiac dysfunction. Death is generally due to cardiac arrhythmias, hyperthermia, or respiratory failure. The high fat content of chocolate products may trigger pancreatitis in susceptible animals.

Lesions: No specific lesions may be found in animals succumbing to chocolate toxicosis. Hyperemia, hemorrhages, or congestion of multiple organs may occur as agonal changes. Severe arrhythmias may result in pulmonary edema or congestion. Chocolate or cocoa bean hulls may be present in the alimentary tract at necropsy.

Diagnosis: Diagnosis is based on history of exposure, along with clinical signs. Amphetamine toxicosis, ma huang/guarana (ephedra/caffeine) toxicosis, pseudoephedrine toxicosis, cocaine toxicosis, and ingestion of antihistamines or other CNS stimulants should be considered in the differential diagnosis.

Treatment: Stabilization of symptomatic animals is a priority in treating chocolate toxicosis. Methocarbamol (50-220 mg/kg, slow IV; no more than 330 mg/kg/24 hr) or diazepam (0.5-2.0 mg/kg, slow IV) may be used for tremors and/or mild seizures; barbiturates may be required for severe seizures. Arrhythmias should be treated as needed: propranolol (0.02-0.06 mg/kg, slow IV) or metoprolol (0.2-0.4 mg/kg, slow IV) for tachyarrhythmias, atropine (0.01-0.02 mg/kg) for bradyarrhythmias, and lidocaine (1-2 mg/kg, IV, followed by 25-80 µg/kg/min infusion) for refractory ventricular tachyarrhythmias. Fluid diuresis may assist in stabilizing cardiovascular function and hasten urinary excretion of methylxanthines.

Once animals have stabilized, or in animals presenting before clinical signs have developed (eg, within 1 hr of ingestion), decontamination should be performed. Induction of emesis using apomorphine or hydrogen peroxide should be initiated; in animals that have been sedated due to seizures, gastric lavage may be considered. Activated charcoal (1-4 g/kg, PO) should be administered; because of the enterohepatic recirculation of methylxanthines, repeated doses should be administered every 8 hr in symptomatic animals (control vomiting with metoclopramide, 0.2-0.4 mg/kg, SC or IM, QID as needed).

Other treatment for symptomatic animals includes thermoregulation, correcting acid/base and electrolyte abnormalities, monitoring cardiac status via electrocardiography, and urinary catheter placement (methylxanthines and their metabolites can be reabsorbed across the bladder wall). Clinical signs may persist up to 72 hr in severe cases.

MACADAMIA NUTS

Ingestion of macadamia nuts by dogs has been associated with a nonfatal syndrome characterized by vomiting, ataxia, weakness, hyperthermia, and depression. Dogs are the only species in which signs have been reported.

Etiology: Macadamia nuts are cultivated from *Macadamia integrifolia* in the continental USA and *Macadamia tetraphylla* in Hawaii and Australia. The mechanism of toxicity is not known. Dogs have shown signs after ingesting 2.4 g of nuts/kg body weight. Dogs experimentally dosed at 20 g/kg of commercially prepared macadamia nuts developed clinical signs within 12 hr and were clinically normal without treatment within 48 hr.

Clinical Findings: Within 12 hr of ingestion, dogs develop weakness, depression, vomiting, ataxia, tremors, and/or hyperthermia. Tremors may be secondary to muscle weakness. Macadamia nuts may be identified in vomitus or feces. Mild transient elevations in serum triglycerides, lipases, and alkaline phosphatase were reported in some dogs experimentally dosed with macadamia nuts; these values quickly returned to baseline. Signs generally resolve within 12-48 hr.

Diagnosis: Diagnosis is based on history of exposure, along with clinical signs. Differential diagnoses include ethylene glycol toxicosis, ingestion of hypotensive agents, and infectious diseases (eg, viral enteritis).

Treatment: For asymptomatic dogs with recent ingestion of more than 1-2 g/kg, emesis should be induced; activated charcoal may be of benefit with large ingestions. Fortunately, most symptomatic dogs will recover without any specific treatment. Severely affected animals may be given supportive treatment such as fluids, analgesics, or antipyretics.

RAISINS/GRAPES

Ingestion of grapes or raisins has resulted in development of anuric renal failure in some dogs. Cases reported to date have been in dogs; an anecdotal report exists of a cat developing renal failure following ingestion of 1 cup of organic raisins. It is not known why many dogs can ingest grapes or raisins with impunity while others develop renal failure following ingestion. The condition has not been reproduced experimentally.

Pathogenesis: The mechanism of toxicity is unknown. Affected dogs develop anuric renal failure within 72 hr of ingestion of grapes or raisins. Estimated amounts of grapes associated with renal injury in dogs are ~32 g/kg; amounts of raisins associated with signs range from 11-30 g/kg.

Clinical Findings: Most affected dogs develop vomiting and/or diarrhea within 6-12 hr of ingestion of grapes or raisins. Other signs include lethargy, anorexia, abdominal pain, weakness, dehydration, polydipsia, and tremors (shivering). Oliguric or anuric renal failure develops within 24-72 hr of exposure; once anuric renal failure develops, most dogs die or are euthanized. Transient elevations in serum glucose, liver enzymes, pancreatic enzymes, serum calcium, or serum phosphorus develop in some dogs.

Diagnosis: Diagnosis is based on history of exposure, along with clinical signs. Other causes of renal failure (eg, ethylene glycol, cholecalciferol) should be considered in the differential diagnosis.

Treatment: Prompt decontamination of significant ingestion of raisins or grapes is recommended. Emesis can be induced with 3% hydrogen peroxide (2 mL/kg; no more than 45 mL), followed by activated charcoal. With large ingestions or in cases where vomiting and/or diarrhea has spontaneously developed within 12 hr of ingestion of grapes or raisins, aggressive fluid diuresis for 48 hr is recommended. Renal function and fluid balance should be monitored during fluid administration. For oliguric dogs, urine production may be stimulated by using dopamine (0.5-3 µg/kg/min, IV) and/or furosemide (2 mg/kg, IV). Anuric dogs are unlikely to survive unless peritoneal dialysis or hemodialysis is performed, and even then the prognosis is guarded.

GOSSYPOL POISONING

Gossypol poisoning, which is usually subacute to chronic, cumulative, and sometimes insidious, follows consumption of cottonseed or cottonseed products that contain excess free gossypol. It is of most concern in domestic livestock, especially immature ruminants and pigs. However, gossypol toxicosis can also affect high-producing dairy cows with high feed intake and other mature ruminants fed excess gossypol for long periods of time. It has also been reported in dogs fed cottonseed meal in diets.

Etiology: Gossypol, the predominant pigment and probably the major toxic ingredient in the cotton plant (*Gossypium* spp), and other polyphenolic pigments are contained within small discrete structures called pigment glands found in various parts of the cotton plant. Gossypol occurs in cottonseed as both protein-bound and free forms; only the free form is toxic. Gossypol content of cottonseeds varies from a trace to >6% and is affected by plant species and variety and by environmental factors such as climate, soil type, and fertilization. Gossypol is a natural component of all but the rarely produced "glandless" variety of cotton.

Cottonseed is processed into edible oil, meal, linters (short fibers), and hulls. Cottonseed meal is marketed with 50-90% protein, depending on intended use. Cottonseed and cottonseed meal are widely used as protein supplements in animal feed. Cottonseed oil soapstock (foots) is the principal byproduct of cottonseed oil refining. Cottonseed soapstocks are being increasingly used as animal feed additives; cottonseed hulls are used as a source of additional fiber in animal feeds and usually contain much lower gossypol concentrations than do whole cottonseeds.

Lipid-soluble gossypol is readily absorbed from the GI tract. It is highly protein-bound to amino acids, especially lysine, and to dietary iron. Conjugation, metabolism, and urinary excretion of gossypol is limited; most is eliminated in the feces.

All animals are susceptible, but monogastrics, immature ruminants, and poultry appear to be affected most frequently. Pigs, guinea pigs, and rabbits are reported to be sensitive. Dogs and cats appear to have intermediate sensitivity. Holstein calves seem to be the most sensitive of cattle breeds. Horses appear relatively unaffected. Toxic effects usually only occur after longterm exposure to gossypol, often after weeks to months.

Clinical Findings: Signs may relate to effects on the cardiac, hepatic, renal, reproductive, or other systems. Prolonged exposure can cause acute heart failure resulting from cardiac necrosis. Also, a form of cardiac conduction failure similar to hyperkalemic heart failure can result in sudden death with no visible cardiac lesions. Pulmonary effects and chronic dyspnea are most likely secondary to cardiotoxicity from congestive heart failure.

Hepatotoxicity can be a primary effect from direct damage to hepatocytes or metabolism of phenolic compounds to reactive intermediates, or liver necrosis may be secondary to congestive heart failure. Gossypol inhibits glutathione-S-transferase, impairing the liver's ability to metabolize xenobiotic compounds. Hematologic effects include anemia with reduced numbers of RBC and increased RBC fragility, decreased oxygen release from oxyhemoglobin, and reduced oxygen-carrying capacity of blood with lowered Hgb and PCV values due to complexing of iron by gossypol.

Reproductive effects include reduced libido with decreased spermatogenesis and sperm motility, as well as sperm abnormalities (which may be reversible) resulting from enzyme inhibition of steroid synthesis in testicular Leydig cells in males. Effects in females may include irregular cycling, luteolytic disruption of pregnancy, and direct embryotoxicity. Green discoloration of egg yolks and decreased egg hatchability have been reported in poultry.

Signs of prolonged excess gossypol exposure in many animals are weight loss, weakness, anorexia, and increased susceptibility to stress. Young lambs, goats, and calves may suffer cardiomyopathy and sudden death; if the course is more chronic, they may be depressed, anorectic, and have pronounced dyspnea. Adult dairy cattle may show weakness, depression, anorexia, edema of the brisket, and dyspnea, and also have gastroenteritis, hemoglobinuria, and reproductive problems. In monogastric animals, acute exposure may result in sudden circulatory failure, while subacute exposure may result in pulmonary edema secondary to congestive heart failure; anemia may be another common sequela. Violent dyspnea ("thumping") is the outstanding clinical sign in pigs. In dogs, gossypol poisoning is primarily reflected by cardiotoxic effects; condition deteriorates progressively, and ascites may be marked. Affected dogs may show polydipsia and have serum electrolyte imbalances, most notably hyperkalemia, with pronounced ECG abnormalities.

Lesions: Some animals have no obvious gross postmortem lesions, but copious amounts of tan to red-tinged fluid with fibrin clumps are frequently found in abdominal, thoracic, and pericardial cavities. An enlarged, flabby, pale, streaked, and mottled heart with pale myocardial streaking, enlarged and dilated ventricles, and valvular edema may be evident. Skeletal muscles may also be pale. A froth-filled trachea and edematous, congested lungs are common, with interstitial pulmonary edema and markedly edematous interlobular septa. Generalized icterus and an enlarged, congested, mottled or golden, friable liver with distinct lobular patterns can be seen. The kidneys, spleen, and other splanchnic organs may be congested, possibly with petechiae; mild renal tubular nephrosis may be present. Hemoglobinuria and edema and hyperemia of the visceral mucosa may occur. Cardiomyopathy in affected dogs has been characterized as focal or general, granular myocardial degeneration with edema between and within myofibers; severe abnormalities in contractility have resulted in right-sided congestive heart failure without pronounced dilatation, and pulmonary or hepatic changes can be minimal.

Diagnosis: Diagnosis is based on the following: 1) a history of dietary exposure to cottonseed meal or cottonseed products over a relatively long period; 2) signs, especially sudden death or chronic dyspnea, affecting multiple animals within a group; 3) lesions consistent with the reported syndrome and associated cardiomyopathy and hepatopathy, with increased amounts of fluids in various body cavities; 4) no response to antibiotic therapy; and 5) the presence of significant concentrations of free gossypol in the diet. Analyses of dietary components for free gossypol must be correlated with history, clinical signs, and postmortem findings. However, as with many feed-induced toxicoses, the responsible feed may be already completely consumed and not available for analysis. Free gossypol at >100 mg/kg (100 ppm) of feed in the diet of pigs or young ruminants <4 mo old supports a presumptive diagnosis. Adult ruminants can detoxify higher concentrations of gossypol, but intake should still be <1,000 ppm in the diet. However, dietary gossypol concentrations of 400-600 ppm in mature ruminants have caused toxicity after longterm exposure; rumen function is a variable, as is binding of gossypol to available proteins. Adverse effects on semen quality (decreased sperm motility and morphologic abnormalities) occurred in young bulls fed a concentrate containing 1,500 ppm free gossypol (providing 8.2 g free gossypol/head/day). Cottonseed meal containing 26.6% (266,000 ppm) total gossypol and 0.175% (1,750 ppm) free gossypol was toxic when fed to adult dogs for an unspecified length of time; however, the equivalent oral dosage of free gossypol fed was <6 mg/kg/day. Gossypol can accumulate in liver and kidney, which are additional specimens for postmortem analyses. In sheep, gossypol concentrations (free or bound) >10 ppm in the kidneys and >20 ppm in the liver suggest excess gossypol exposure. However, background and significantly increased tissue gossypol concentrations have not been determined in all animal species, so tissue analyses may be of limited diagnostic value.

Differential diagnoses include poisonings by cardiotoxic ionophoric antibiotics (eg, monensin, lasalocid, salinomycin, narasin) and ammonia, nutritional or metabolic disorders (eg, selenium, vitamin E, or copper deficiency), infectious diseases, noninfectious diseases (eg, pulmonary adenomatosis, emphysema), mycotoxicoses caused by *Fusarium*-contaminated grain, and toxicoses caused by plants with cardiotoxic and other effects.

Cardiotoxic plants, which may cause confusing or similar clinical signs and postmortem lesions, include English yew (*Taxus baccata*), Japanese yew (*T cuspidata*), laurel (*Kalmia* spp), azalea (*Rhododendron* spp), oleander (*Nerium oleander*), yellow oleander or yellow-be-still tree (*Thevetia peruviana*), purple foxglove (*Digitalis purpurea*), lily-of-the-valley (*Convallaria majalis*), dogbane (*Apocynum* spp), coffee senna (*Cassia occidentalis*), bracken fern (*Pteridium aquilinum*), white snakeroot (*Eupatorium rugosum*), death camas (*Zygadenus* spp), lantana (*Lantana camara*), monkshood (*Aconitum napellum*), and milkweed (*Asclepias* spp).

Prevention, Treatment, and Control: There is no effective treatment. Adsorbents such as activated charcoal and saline cathartics are of little value due to the chronic exposure and cumulative nature of gossypol. If gossypol toxicity is suspected, all cottonseed products should be removed from the diet immediately. However, severely affected animals may still die up to 2 wk later. Recovery depends primarily on the extent of toxic cardiopathy. Because exposure is usually chronic and life-threatening lesions may be advanced before a diagnosis is made, a favorable prognosis for complete recovery may be unrealistic. Mild to moderate myocardial lesions may be reversible with time if stress is minimized and animals are carefully handled. However, poor weight gains in affected livestock and increased susceptibility to stress may persist for several weeks after cottonseed products are removed from the diet. A high-quality diet supplemented with lysine, methionine, and fat-soluble vitamins should be included in supportive therapy.

A high intake of protein, calcium hydroxide, or iron salts appears to be protective in cattle. Cattle should also be given ≥40% of dry-matter intake from a forage source. Added iron of up to 400 ppm in swine diets and up to 600 ppm in poultry diets was reported to be effective in preventing signs and tissue residues of dietary gossypol exposure when used in ratios of 1:1 to 4:1 of iron to free gossypol. The best preventative approach is analysis of all dietary components containing cottonseed products prior to incorporating into animal diets as part of a managed feeding program. Potentially toxic dietary components should be mixed or diluted with cottonseed (gossypol)-free feedstuffs to achieve a safe and acceptable gossypol content in the final ration.

Prevention of tissue residues in animal organ meats consumed by humans is an important public health consideration for those individuals already consuming cottonseed oil and cottonseed flour products in their daily diets. Until pharmacokinetic parameters of gossypol are more completely characterized in all food animal species, immediate salvage and consumption of animals surviving excess gossypol exposure is not recommended. Only those animals living for ≥1 mo after exposure should be considered safe for human food sources.

HALOGENATED AROMATIC POISONING

(PCB, PBB, Dioxins, and others)

Common persistent halogenated aromatics (PHA) include polychlorinated and polybrominated biphenyls (PCB, PBB), naphthalenes, benzenes, and diphenyl ethers (PCDE, PBDE), as well as a number of pesticides such as DDT (p 2395). Unwanted byproducts formed during manufacture and heating or burning of chlorophenoxy herbicides (p 2369), chlorophenols (p 2429), or PCB include polychlorinated dibenzofurans (PCDF) and dibenzo-*p*-dioxins (PCDD). Triclosan is a hydroxylated PCDE commonly used in household products as a bacteriostat. PBDE are increasingly common in the environment due to their wide use as flame retardants in plastics and electronic components. PCB, marketed in the USA as Aroclors, are the most environmentally abundant of the halogenated aromatics and are still found in products from North America, Western Europe, or Japan produced before 1979. PCB manufacture and use continued in other areas up to the 1990s. The most common PCB-containing products still in use include electrical transformers and capacitors and fluorescent light ballasts. These should be considered to contain PCB if manufactured before 1980 unless they are labeled to the contrary. Other uses resulting in persistent contamination around farms and small animal facilities include hydraulic and heat transfer fluids, epoxy paints, and construction adhesives.

Polyhalogenated aromatics are chemically stable, lipid soluble, and bioaccumulative. They are rapidly absorbed by all routes of exposure and accumulate in adipose tissue, from where they are gradually eliminated during fat mobilization. Persistence, bioaccumulation, types of toxic effects, and potencies vary considerably among the many different compounds. PCB, PCDF, PCDD, and naphthalenes are always present as mixtures. Typically, representatives from all 4 classes as well as halogenated aromatic pesticides are present.

Livestock feed and pet food contamination as well as fish and fish meal were previously considered the major sources of exposure. It is now known that airborne (vapor phase) and forage exposures are nearly universal, although at considerably lower levels.

Most toxic effects of halogenated aromatics are subtle and delayed, but may be additive. Effects may include: 1) wasting (weight loss not necessarily accompanied by decreased food consumption; however, complex environmental mixtures with net antiestrogenic activity may increase food consumption, body weight and body fat), 2) skin disorders (chloracne, edema, alopecia, hyperkeratosis), 3) immune suppression, 4) enlarged liver with fatty change and enzyme induction, 5) endocrine disruption (antiestrogenicity; hypothyroxinemia, often without an increase in TSH), 6) reproductive disorders (abnormal cycling, reduced conception, fetotoxicity and fetal resorption, teratogenesis), and 7) carcinogenesis. Birds and guinea pigs are particularly susceptible to effects mediated by the Aryl hydrocarbon receptor (AhR), while hamsters and voles are more resistant. The most prevalent halogenated aromatics are noncoplanar, have little affinity for the AhR, and cause health effects by multiple mechanisms. They induce a different profile of xenobiotic metabolizing enzymes than do AhR agonists and tend to be weakly estrogenic rather than antiestrogenic. Noncoplanar PCB also inhibit gonadal and (probably) adrenal gland steroidogenesis. Fertility can be decreased by both coplanar and noncoplanar compounds. The less chlorinated and *ortho*-rich PCB stimulate ryanodine-sensitive intracellular calcium channels (*see also* MALIGNANT HYPERTHERMIA, p 832) and have a number of subtle effects on learning, memory, and behavior. These PCB are at higher proportions in the vapor phase, forages, and in many fish.

A unique hyperplastic gastritis has been observed in monkeys, swine, and rats exposed to PCB. Erosions in the mucosa are accompanied by autophagous parietal cells with mucus-secreting cells becoming dominant. These changes appear to be of systemic origin rather than from direct gastric irritation. Cattle with a high PCB burden (PCB-containing oil in back rubbers) became ill and suffered mortality when shipped; there were severe intestinal hemorrhages which may be a later stage of the stomach inflammation in monogastric species. Although weight gain may appear normal, decrements in feed efficiency have been demonstrated in swine.

Many effects are subtle and may not become apparent until the animal is stressed or, in the case of prepubertal exposure, reaches adulthood. There are no diagnostic signs specific to these broad-acting and subtle poisons; diagnostic confirmation relies on chemical analysis suggested by the clinical history. Initial diagnosis is based on a complete history, visual inspection of the premises for potential exposures, and elimination of more common etiologies. These compounds are readily detected in serum or whole blood as well as body fat, milk fat, liver, feed, and other suspected sources. Fluid samples for residue analysis should be collected in clean, acetone-rinsed glass or stainless steel containers with caps lined with acetone-rinsed teflon or aluminum foil. Solid samples may be wrapped in aluminum foil and frozen. The dull side of the foil should be in contact with the sample; the shiny side is coated with waxes that interfere with the analysis. Plastics should be avoided.

Treatment is most likely to be beneficial when instituted as soon as possible following acute exposure. It is based on discovering and eliminating the source of exposure, bathing animals with detergent and cool water after dermal exposure (do not scrub vigorously). Repeated large oral doses of activated charcoal (1-4 g/kg small animals; 1-2 g/kg large animals) or gastric lavage may be of benefit after oral exposure. The charcoal will trap some PHA in the intestine preventing absorption into the body and reducing fatty tissue concentrations. Also, oral activated charcoal can trap some PHA mobilized from the fat and excreted in bile into the intestines, thus preventing re-uptake and reducing the body burden. It is important to minimize stress and optimize environmental conditions following severe exposures. Residue levels above the MRL make these livestock unsaleable. For breeding stock and pets, elimination is hastened by weight loss, parturition, or lactation. Offspring, which are usually exposed in utero if the mother encounters PHA while pregnant, should not be suckled from contaminated mothers. Studies in humans suggest physical, reproductive, cognitive, concentration, and social deficits in offspring of mothers, long after exposure. This suggests that animals may be of doubtful value as breeding stock. Males, if suitably fertile, should remain useful.

HERBICIDE POISONING

Herbicides are used routinely to control noxious plants. Most of these chemicals, particularly the more recently developed synthetic organic herbicides, are quite selective for specific plants and have low toxicity for mammals; other less selective compounds (eg, arsenicals, chlorates, dinitrophenols) are more toxic to animals. Most toxicity problems in animals result from exposure to excessive quantities of herbicides because of improper or careless use or disposal of containers. When used properly, problems are rare.

Vegetation treated with herbicides at proper rates normally will not be hazardous to animals, including humans. Particularly after the herbicides have dried on the vegetation, only small amounts can be dislodged. When herbicide applications have been excessive, damage to lawns, crops, or other foliage is often evident.

The residue potential for most of these agents is low. However, the possibility of residues should be explored if significant exposure of food-producing animals occurs. The time recommended before treated vegetation is grazed or used as animal feed is available for a number of products.

Some of the more commonly used herbicides are discussed below. More specific information is available on the label and from the manufacturer, cooperative extension service, or poison control center. In addition, selected information on herbicides available for use on common field, vegetable, and fruit crops in the USA and Canada is included (see TABLE 1) as a guideline for common toxicologic concerns. These include the toxicity of a chemical relative to other herbicides (acute toxicity, LD_{50}), the amount an animal can be exposed to without being affected (no effect level, NOEL), and the likelihood of problems caused by dermal contact (dermal LD_{50}, eye and skin irritation). These chemicals are used widely in food crop production and are an important source of environmental exposure to avian and aquatic species, both wild and domesticated. The species data in TABLE 1 cover the most common animal toxicology models and data on animals with important economic or sociologic relevance.

Herbicide poisoning is a rare finding in veterinary practice. With few exceptions, it is only when animals gain direct access to the product that acute poisoning occurs. Acute signs usually will not lead to a diagnosis, although acute GI signs are frequent. All common differential diagnoses should be excluded in animals showing signs of a sudden onset of disease or sudden death. The case history is critical. Sickness following feeding, spraying of pastures or crops adjacent to pastures, a change in housing, or direct exposure may lead to a tentative diagnosis of herbicide poisoning. Frequently, the nature of exposure is hard to identify because of storage of herbicides in mis- or unlabeled containers. Unidentified spillage of liquid from containers or powder from broken bags near a feed source, or visual confusion with a dietary ingredient or supplement, may cause the exposure. Once a putative chemical source has been identified, an animal poison control center should be contacted for information on treatments, laboratory tests, and likely outcome.

Chronic disease caused by herbicides is even more difficult to diagnose. It may include a history of herbicide use in proximity to the animals or animal feed or water source, or a gradual change in the animals' performance or behavior over a period of weeks, months, or even years. Occasionally, it involves manufacture or storage of herbicides nearby. Samples of possible sources (ie, contaminated feed and water) for residue analysis, as well as tissues from exposed animals taken at necropsy, are essential. Months or even years may be required to successfully identify a problem of chronic exposure.

If poisoning is suspected, the first step in management is to halt further exposure. Animals should be separated from any possible source before attempting to stabilize and support them. If there are life-threatening signs, efforts to stabilize animals by general mitigation methods should be started. Any treatments undertaken should make a clear improvement in the most affected animals, as the physical act of handling and treatment, although logical, may make their condition worse. Specific antidotal treatments, when available, may help to confirm the diagnosis. As time permits, a more detailed history and investigation should be completed. The owner should be made aware of the need for full disclosure of facts in order to successfully determine the source of poisoning, eg, unapproved use or failure to properly store a chemical.

Inorganic Herbicides

These older herbicides are generally cheaper, more toxic, and more likely to cause problems than newer compounds. Their use has been mostly curtailed in developed countries.

Arsenicals: The use of **inorganic arsenicals** (sodium arsenite and arsenic trioxide) as herbicides has been reduced greatly because of livestock losses, environmental persistence, and their association with carcinogenesis. Sodium arsenate and chromic copper arsenate do not have active EPA registration. Arsenic derivatives continue to be available in other parts of the world in wood preservatives and insecticide formulations. These compounds can be hazardous to animals when used as recommended. Ruminants (even deer) are apparently attracted to and lick plants poisoned with arsenite.

The highly soluble **organic arsenicals** (methane arsonate, methyl arsonic acid) can concentrate in pools in toxic quantities after a rain has washed them from recently treated plants. Arsenicals are used as desiccants or defoliants on cotton, and residues of cotton harvest fed to cattle may contain toxic amounts of arsenic. Signs and lesions caused by organic arsenical herbicides resemble those of inorganic arsenical poisoning. Single toxic oral doses for cattle and sheep are 22-55 mg/kg body wt. Poisoning may be expected from smaller doses if consumed on successive days. Dimercaprol (3 mg/kg for large animals, and 2.5-5 mg/kg for small animals, IM, every 4-6 hr) is the recommended therapy. Sodium thiosulfate also has been used (20-30 g, PO in ~300 mL of water for cattle; one-fourth this dose for sheep); however, a rationale for its use is not established, and it may be unrewarding. (*See also* ARSENIC POISONING, p 2346.)

Ammonium Sulfamate: Ammonium sulfamate currently has no active EPA registration in the USA. It is used to kill brush and poison ivy. Ruminants apparently can metabolize this chemical to some extent and, in some studies, exposed animals made better gains than did controls. However, sudden deaths have occurred in cattle and deer that consumed treated plants. Large doses (>1.5 g/kg body wt) induce ammonia poisoning in ruminants. Treatment is designed to lower rumen pH by dilution with copious amounts of water to which weak acetic acid (vinegar) has been added.

Borax: Borax has been used as a herbicide, an insecticide, and a soil sterilant. It is toxic to animals if consumed in moderate to large doses (>0.5 g/kg). Poisoning has not been reported when borax was used properly but has occurred when it was accidentally added to livestock feed and when borax powder was scattered in the open for cockroach control. Principal signs of acute poisoning are diarrhea, rapid prostration, and perhaps convulsions. An effective antidote is not known. Balanced electrolyte fluid therapy with supportive care is indicated.

Sodium Chlorate: This is now seldom used as a herbicide but remains registered. Treated plants and contaminated clothing are highly combustible and constitute fire hazards. In addition, many cases of chlorate poisoning of livestock have occurred both from ingestion of treated plants and from accidental consumption of feed to which it was mistakenly added as salt. Cattle sometimes are attracted to foliage treated with sodium chlorate. Considerable quantities must be consumed before signs of toxicity appear. The minimum lethal dose is 1.1 g/kg body wt for cattle, 1.54-2.86 g/kg for sheep, and 5.06 g/kg for poultry. Ingestion results in hemolysis of RBC and conversion of Hgb to methemoglobin. Treatment with methylene blue (10 mg/kg) must be repeated frequently because, unlike the nitrites, the chlorate ion is not inactivated during the conversion of Hgb to methemoglobin and is capable of producing an unlimited quantity of methemoglobin as long as it is present in the body. Blood transfusions may reduce some of the tissue anoxia caused by methemoglobin; IV isotonic saline can hasten elimination of the chlorate ion. Mineral oil containing 1% sodium thiosulfate will inhibit further absorption of chlorate in monogastric animals.

Organic Herbicides

Anilide or Amide Compounds (propanil, cypromid, clomiprop): These herbicides are plant growth regulators, and some members of this group are more toxic than others. Hemolysis, methemoglobinemia, and immunotoxicity have occurred after experimental exposure to propanil. The half-life in catfish is >15 days. See ORGANOPHOSPHATE COMPOUNDS, below, for discussion of bensulide.

Bipyridyl Compounds or Quaternary Ammonium Herbicides (diquat, paraquat): The bipyridyl compounds are nonvolatile desiccant herbicides used at rather low rates of 2 oz/acre (150 mL/hectare). These compounds act rapidly, are inactivated on soil contact, and rapidly decompose in light. They produce toxic effects in the tissues of exposed animals by development of free radicals. Tissues can be irritated after contact (eg, mouth lesions after recent spraying of pastures). Skin irritation and corneal opacity occur on external exposure to these chemicals, and inhalation is dangerous. Animals, including humans, have died as a result of drinking from contaminated containers.

Paraquat and diquat have somewhat different mechanisms of action. Diquat exerts most of its harmful effects in the GI tract. Animals drinking from an old diquat container showed anorexia, gastritis, GI distension, and severe loss of water into the lumen of the GI tract. Signs of renal impairment, CNS excitement, and convulsions occur in severely affected individuals. Lung lesions are uncommon.

Paraquat has a biphasic toxic action after ingestion. Immediate effects include excitement, convulsions or depression and incoordination, gastroenteritis with anorexia, and possibly renal involvement and respiratory difficulty. Eye, nasal, and skin irritation can be caused by direct contact, followed within days to 2 wk by pulmonary lesions as a result of lipid-membrane peroxidation and thus destruction of the type I alveolar pneumocytes. This is reflected in progressive respiratory distress and is evident on necropsy as pulmonary edema, hyaline membrane deposition, and alveolar fibrosis. Toxicity of paraquat is enhanced by deficiency of vitamin E or selenium, oxygen, and low tissue activity of glutathione peroxidase.

Due to slow absorption of these chemicals, intensive oral administration of adsorbants in large quantities and cathartics is advised. Bentonite or Fuller's earth is preferred, but activated charcoal will suffice. In conjunction with supportive therapy, eg, vitamin E and selenium, excretion is accelerated by forced diuresis induced by mannitol and furosemide. Oxygen therapy should not be used, and some suggest only 15% oxygen in inspired air.

Carbamate and Thiocarbamate Compounds (terbucarb, asulam, carboxazole, EPTC, pebulate, triallate, vernolate, butylate, thiobencarb): These herbicides are moderately toxic; however, they are used at low concentrations, and poisoning problems would not be expected from normal use. Massive overdosage, as seen with accidental exposure, produces symptoms similar to the insecticide carbamates, with lack of appetite, depression, respiratory difficulty, mouth watering, diarrhea, weakness, and seizures. Thiobencarb has induced toxic neuropathies in neonatal and adult laboratory rats. It appears to increase permeability of the blood-brain barrier.

TABLE I. Herbicide Poisoning ▶

Compound	Acute Oral LD$_{50}$—Rat	NOEL* (oral)	Acute Dermal LD$_{50}$
Acetochlor	2,148 mg/kg	Dog, 1 yr 12 mg/kg/day	Rabbit 4,166 mg/kg
Acifluorfen	1,300 mg/kg (F)	Rat, 2 yr 180 ppm	Rabbit >2,000 mg/kg
Acrolein[†]	29 mg/kg	Rat, 13 wk 150 mg/L in drinking water	Rabbit 231 mg/kg
Alachlor	930-1,200 mg/kg	Dog, 90 day <200 mg/kg/day	Rabbit 13,300 mg/kg
α-Metolachlor	2,675-2,952 mg/kg		Rat 2,020 mg/kg
Atrazine	3,080 mg/kg	Dog, 1 yr 150 ppm; Rat, 2 yr 10 ppm	Rabbit 7,500 mg/kg
Amitrole	4,080 mg/kg (M)	Rat, 13 wk 2 mg/kg/day	Rat >5,000 mg/kg
Ammonium sulfamate[†]	3,900 mg/kg	Rat, 105 days 10,000 mg/kg/day	
Bensulfron methyl	>5,000 mg/kg	Rat, dog 2 yr 750 ppm in diet	Rat >2,000 mg/kg
Bensulide	271-770 mg/kg	Dog, 90 days 12.5 mg/kg/day	Rabbit 3,950 mg/kg
Bentazon	1,100 mg/kg (cat 500 mg/kg)	Rat, 90 days 3.5 mg/kg/day; Dog, 90 days 7.5 mg/kg/day	Rat >2,500 mg/kg
Bispyribac sodium		Rat, 2 yr 1.1 mg/kg/day (M) 1.4 mg/kg/day (F)	
Borax	2,000-6,000 mg/kg		
Bromacil	5,200 mg/kg	Rat, dog, 2 yr 250 mg/kg/day	Rabbit >5,000 mg/kg
Bromoxynil	779 mg/kg	Rat, 90 days 50 mg/kg/day	Rabbit >2,000 mg/kg
Butylate[†]	5,431 mg/kg (M) 4,659 mg/kg (F)	Rat, 2 yr 20 mg/kg/day Dog, 1 yr 25 mg/kg/day	Rabbit >4,640 mg/kg
Carfentrazone ethyl	>5,000 mg/kg	Rat, 2 yr 9 mg/kg/day (M) 3 mg/kg/day (F)	Rat >5,000 mg/kg
Chloramben[†]	5,620 mg/kg		Rabbit >3,160 mg/kg

TABLE I. (continued)

Avian Toxicity	Toxicity to Fish in Water	Skin and Eye Irritation
LC$_{50}$ 5 day Bobwhite quail and Mallard duck 5,620 mg/kg	LC$_{50}$ 96 hr Rainbow trout 0.45 mg/L	Skin–mild Eye–mild
LC$_{50}$ 8 day Mallard duck >10,000 mg/kg	LC$_{50}$ 96 hr Rainbow trout 31 mg/L	Skin–moderate Eye–severe
LD$_{50}$ (oral) Bobwhite quail 19.0 mg/kg Mallard duck 9.1 mg/kg	LC$_{50}$ 24 hr Bluegill and Rainbow trout 0.024 mg/L	Skin–severe Eye–severe
LC$_{50}$ 8 day Bobwhite quail and Mallard duck >5,000 mg/kg	LC$_{50}$ 96 hr Bluegill 2.8 mg/L Rainbow trout 5.3 mg/L	Skin–mild
		Skin–slight Eye–mild
LC$_{50}$ 8 day Mallard duck >10,000 ppm in diet	LC$_{50}$ 96 hr Rainbow trout 8.8 mg/L	Skin–slight
LD$_{50}$ Mallard duck 2,000 mg/kg		Skin–mild Eye–mild
LD$_{50}$ Bobwhite quail 3,000 mg/kg	LC$_{50}$ 48 hr Carp 1,000-2,000 mg/L	Skin–none
	LC$_{50}$ 96 hr Bluegill and Rainbow trout >150 ppm	Skin–none Eye–serious
LD$_{50}$ Bobwhite quail, 3 wk 50 mg/kg poor hatchability	LC$_{50}$ 96 hr Bluegill 1.4 mg/L Rainbow trout 0.7 mg/L	Eye–none
LD$_{50}$ Japanese quail 720 mg/kg Mallard duck 2,000 mg/kg	LC$_{50}$ 96 hr Bluegill 616 mg/L Rainbow trout 1,060 mg/L	Slight irritant
LC$_{50}$ Bobwhite quail and Mallard duck >5,620 ppm	LC$_{50}$ 96 hr Bluegill and Rainbow trout >100 ppm	Skin–minor Eye–minor
LC$_{50}$ 8 day Bobwhite quail and Mallard duck >10,000 mg/kg	LC$_{50}$ 48 hr Bluegill 71 mg/L Rainbow trout 56 mg/L	Skin–irritating Eye–irritating
Acute LD$_{50}$ Bobwhite quail 100 mg/kg Mallard duck 200 mg/kg	LC$_{50}$ 96 hr Rainbow trout 0.05 mg/L	Skin–none Eye–none
LC$_{50}$ 8 day Bobwhite quail 40,000 mg/kg Mallard duck 46,400 ppm in diet	LC$_{50}$ 96 hr Bluegill 6.9 mg/L Rainbow trout 4.2 mg/L	Skin–moderate Eye–mild
LC$_{50}$ Bobwhite quail and Mallard duck >5,620 ppm	LC$_{50}$ 96 hr Bluegill 2.0 ppm and Rainbow trout 16 ppm	Skin–none-slight Eye–minimum
LC$_{50}$ 8 day Mallard duck >4,640 mg/kg/day	Not toxic to fish	Skin–mild Eye–mild

(continued)

TABLE I. Herbicide Poisoning (*continued*) ▶

Compound	Acute Oral LD$_{50}$—Rat	NOEL* (oral)	Acute Dermal LD$_{50}$
Chlor-propham	4,100-7,000 mg/kg	Rat, dog, 2 yr 100-350 mg/kg/day	
Chlorsulfu-ron	5,545 mg/kg (M) 6,293 mg/kg (F)	Rat, 2 yr 100 ppm in diet	Rabbit >3,400 mg/kg
Chlorthal dimethyl	3,000-12,000 mg/kg	Rat, 2 yr <50 mg/kg/day	Rabbit >2,000 mg/kg
Clethodim	1,630 mg/kg (M) 1,360 mg/kg (F)	Dog, 1 yr >1 mg/kg/day	Rabbit >5,000 mg/kg
Clodinafop propargyl	1,392 mg/kg (M) 2,271 mg/kg (F)	Dog, 90 days 0.346 mg/kg/day (M), 1.89 mg/kg/day (F)	Rabbit >2,000 mg/kg
Clomazone	2,077 mg/kg (M) 1,369 mg/kg (F)	Dog, 1 yr <2.5 mg/kg/day	Rabbit >2,000 mg/kg
Clopyralid	>4,300 mg/kg	Rat, 2 yr 50 mg/kg/day	Rabbit >2,000 mg/kg
Cloransulam-methyl	>5,000 mg/kg	Dog, 1 yr 10 mg/kg/day	Rabbit >2,000 mg/kg
Copper chelate†	498 mg/kg		Rabbit >2,000 mg/kg
Copper sulfate	470 mg/kg		Rabbit >8,000 mg/kg
Cyanazine†	182-334 mg/kg	Dog, 2 yr <225 mg/kg/day	Rabbit >2,000 mg/kg
Cycloate	2,000-3,190 mg/kg	Dog 240 mg/kg/day	Rabbit >4,640 mg/kg
Cyhalofop-butyl	>5,000 mg/kg	Dog 46.7 mg/kg/day (M) 45.9 mg/kg/day (F)	Rat >5,000 mg/kg
2,4-D	370-700 mg/kg	Rat, 2 yr 50 mg/kg/day	Rabbit >2,000 mg/kg
2,4-D dimethy-lamine	949-4,650 mg/kg	Dog, 1 yr 1 mg/kg/day	Rabbit >2,000 mg/kg
2,4-D isooc-tyl ester	500-700 mg/kg	Dog, 1 yr 1 mg/kg/day	Rabbit >2,000 mg/kg

◀ TABLE I. *(continued)*

Avian Toxicity	Toxicity to Fish in Water	Skin and Eye Irritation
LD_{50} 8 day Mallard duck >2,000 mg/kg	LC_{50} 48 hr Bluegill 6.3-6.8 mg/L Rainbow trout 3-6 mg/L	Skin–moderate Eye–moderate
LC_{50} 8 day Mallard duck >5,000 mg/kg	LC_{50} 96 hr Rainbow trout >250 mg/L	Skin–none Eye–mild
LD_{50} young Bobwhite quail 5,500 mg/kg	Not toxic to fish	Skin–none Eye–mild
LC_{50} 8 day Bobwhite quail 4,270 ppm Mallard duck 3,978 ppm in diet	LC_{50} Bluegill 13 ppm Rainbow trout 18 ppm	Skin–none Eye–moderate
LC_{50} Birds >5,000 ppm	LC_{50} Freshwater fish 0.30 ppm	Skin–none Eye–slight‡ to severe§
LD_{50} 8 day Bobwhite quail and Mallard duck 5,620 ppm in diet	LC_{50} 96 hr Bluegill 34 mg/L Rainbow trout 19 mg/L	Skin–mild Eye–moderate
LC_{50}, Bobwhite quail and Mallard duck >4,640 ppm in diet	LC_{50} 96 hr Bluegill 125 mg/L Rainbow trout 103.5 mg/L	Skin–mild Eye–severe
LC_{50} 5 day Bobwhite quail and Mallard duck >5,620 ppm	LC_{50} 96 hr Bluegill >154 ppm Rainbow trout >86 ppm	Skin–none Eye–slight
LC_{50} 8 day Mallard duck >1,000 ppm in diet	LC_{50} 96 hr Bluegill 1.2-7.5 mg/L Rainbow trout <0.2-4 mg/L	Skin–slight Eye–moderate
$LD_{50 \text{ (oral)}}$ Pheasant 1,000 ppm in diet (estimated)	LC_{50} 96 hr Bluegill 4.4-7.3 mg/L Rainbow trout 0.135 mg/L	Skin–moderate Eye–severe
LD_{50} Bobwhite quail 400 mg/kg Mallard duck >2,000 mg/kg	LC_{50} 96 hr Bluegill 23 mg/L Rainbow trout 9 mg/L	Skin–none Eye–mild
LC_{50} 7 day Bobwhite quail >56,000 mg/kg	LC_{50} 96 hr Rainbow trout 5.6 mg/L	Skin–none Eye–none
	LC_{50} 96 hr Bluegill >99.2 mg/L Rainbow trout >1.65 mg/L	Skin–none Eye–minimal
LC_{50} 8 day Mallard duck >4,640 mg/kg	LC_{50} 96 hr Bluegill >300 mg/L Rainbow trout 800 mg/L‡	Skin–none Eye–moderate
LC_{50} 8 day Mallard duck, >5,600 ppm	LC_{50} 96 hr Bluegill 524 mg/L Rainbow trout 250 mg/L	Skin–minimal Eye–severe
As for 2,4-D (above)		Skin–none Eye–severe

(continued)

TABLE I.   Herbicide Poisoning (continued)

Compound	Acute Oral LD$_{50}$—Rat	NOEL* (oral)	Acute Dermal LD$_{50}$
Dazomet	551-646 mg/kg (M); 335-562 mg/kg (F)	Rat, 2 yr 1.6 mg/kg/day	Rabbit >2,000 mg/kg
Dicamba	1,700 mg/kg	Rat, 2 yr 125 mg/kg/day Dog, 2 yr 50 mg/kg day	Rabbit >2,000 mg/kg
Dichlobenil	>3,160-4,250 mg/kg	Rat, 2 yr >20 ppm in diet Pig, 6 mo >50 ppm in diet	Rabbit >1,350 mg/kg
Dichlorprop	700 mg/kg (M) 500 mg/kg (F)	Rat, 4 mg/kg	Mouse 1,400 mg/kg
Diclosulam	>5,000 mg/kg	0.05 mg/kg	Rabbit >2,000 mg/kg
Difenzoquat (methylsulfate)	617 mg/kg (M) 373 mg/kg (F)	Dog, 1 yr 20 mg/kg/day	Rabbit >2,000 mg/kg
Diflufen-zopyr	1,600 to >5,000 mg/kg	Dog, 1 yr 28 mg/kg/day (M) 26 mg/kg/day (F)	Rabbit >5,000 mg/kg
Dimethena-mid	1,293 mg/kg	Dog, 1 yr 50-250 ppm in diet	Rabbit >2,000 mg/kg
Dithiopyr	>5,000 mg/kg	Dog, 1 yr <0.5 mg/kg/day	Rabbit >5,000 mg/kg
Diuron	3,400 mg/kg	Dog, 2 yr 25 mg/kg	Rat >2,000 mg/kg
EPTC	1,630 mg/kg	Dog, 90 day 20 mg/kg	Rabbit 5,000 mg/kg
Ethalfluralin	Rat, >5,000 mg/kg (dog, cat >200 mg/kg)	Rat, mouse, 90 day 68 mg/kg	Rabbit >2,000 mg/kg
Ethephon	1,600-4,229 mg/kg	Rat, 2 yr 375 mg/kg/day Mouse, 78 wk 4.5 mg/kg/day; (lowers cholinesterase)	Rabbit >5,000 mg/kg
Fenoxaprop	2,357 mg/kg (M) 2,500 mg/kg (F)	Dog 2 yr 0.375 mg/kg/day	Rabbit >1,000 mg/kg
Fenoxaprop-p-ethyl	4,430 mg/kg	Dog, 2 yr 0.9 mg/kg/day	Rat >5,000 mg/kg

TABLE I. (continued)		
Avian Toxicity	**Toxicity to Fish in Water**	**Skin and Eye Irritation**
LD_{50} Bobwhite quail 415 ppm in diet	LC_{50} Rainbow trout 0.16; 2.4-16.2 mg/L	Skin–mild Eye–severe
LC_{50} 8 day Bobwhite quail and Mallard duck >4,600 mg/kg	LC_{50} 96 hr Bluegill and Rainbow trout >1,000 mg/L	Skin–moderate Eye–extreme
LC_{50} 8 day Mallard duck >5,200 ppm in diet	LC_{50} 96 hr Bluegill and Rainbow trout 7 mg/L	Skin–none Eye–mild to moderate
LC_{50} Upland birds, waterfowl >10,000 ppm in diet	LC_{50} Bluegill 1.1 mg/L Rainbow trout 100-200 mg/L	Skin–none Eye–none
	LC_{50} Most sensitive aquatic species 10-100 mg/L	Skin–moderate Eye–moderate
LC_{50} 8 day Bobwhite quail and Mallard duck 4,640 ppm in diet	LC_{50} 96 hr Bluegill 696 mg/L Rainbow trout 711 mg/L	Skin–mild Eye–mild
LC_{50} Avian, Mallard >5,620 ppm	LC_{50} Bluegill 135 ppm Rainbow trout 106 ppm	Skin–very slight Eye–mild to slight
LC_{50} Bobwhite quail and Mallard duck >5,620 ppm in diet	LC_{50} Bluegill 6.4 mg/L Rainbow trout 2.6 mg/L	Skin–mild Eye–moderate
LC_{50} Bobwhite quail and Mallard duck >5,260 ppm in diet	LC_{50} Bluegill 0.7 mg/L Rainbow trout 0.5 mg/L	Skin–slight Eye–moderate
LC_{50} Bobwhite quail 1,730 ppm Mallard duck >5,000 ppm in diet	LC_{50} Bluegill 7.4 mg/L Rainbow trout 4.3 mg/L	Skin–none Eye–mild
LC_{50} 7 day Bobwhite quail 20,000 ppm in diet	LC_{50} Bluegill 27 mg/L Rainbow trout 19 mg/L	Skin–mild Eye–mild
LC_{50} 8 day Bobwhite quail and Mallard duck >5,000 ppm	LC_{50} Bluegill 0.03-0.1 mg/L Rainbow trout 0.037-0.136 mg/L	Skin–slight to moderate Eye–slight
LC_{50} 8 day Mallard duck >10,000 ppm	LC_{50} 96 hr Bluegill 222-300 mg/L Rainbow trout 254-350 mg/L	Skin–corrosive Eye–corrosive
LD_{50} Japanese quail >5,000 mg/kg	LC_{50} Bluegill 3.3 mg/L Rainbow trout 3.4 mg/L	Skin–slight Eye–serious nonreversible corneal opacity
LC_{50} 8 day Bobwhite quail and Mallard duck 5,620 ppm	LC_{50} Bluegill 0.31 mg/L Rainbow trout 0.46 mg/L[‡]	Skin–slight Eye–moderate

(continued)

TABLE 1. Herbicide Poisoning (continued)

Compound	Acute Oral LD$_{50}$—Rat	NOEL* (oral)	Acute Dermal LD$_{50}$
Flamprop-methyl†	1,210 mg/kg	Dog, 2 yr 10 mg/kg/day	Rat >294 mg/kg
Fluazifop-p-butyl	3,680-4,096 mg/kg (M) 2,451-2,721 mg/kg (F)‡	Rat, 90 day >10 mg/kg/day	Rabbit >2,400 mg/kg
Flucarba-zone-sodium	>5,000 mg/kg	Dog, 1 yr 35.9 mg/kg/day	Rat >5,000 mg/kg
Flufenacet	1,617 mg/kg (M) 589 mg/kg (F)	Dog, 1 yr 1.29 mg/kg/day	Rat >2,000 mg/kg
Flumesulam	3,245 to >5,000 mg/kg		Rat >2,000 mg/kg
Flumiclorac	3,200 to >5,000 mg/kg	Dog, 1 yr 100 mg/kg/day	Rat >2,000 mg/kg
Fluroxypyr	>5,000 mg/kg	Dog, 1 yr 150 mg/kg/day	Rat >2,000 mg/kg
Fluthiacet	>5,000 mg/kg	Dog, 1 yr 57.6 mg/kg/day (M) 30.3 mg/kg/day (F)	Rat >2,000 mg/kg
Foramsulfu-ron	>3,881 mg/kg	Rat, 2 yr 849 mg/kg/day (M) 1,135 mg/kg/day (F)	Rat >5,000 mg/kg
Fosamine ammonium†	24,000 mg/kg	Rat, 90 day 1,000 mg/kg	Rabbit >1,683 mg/kg
Glufosinate (ammonium salt)	1,510-2,030 mg/kg	Dog, 1 yr 5 mg/kg/day	Rat >1,390 mg/kg
Glyphosate	5,600 mg/kg	Dog, 2 yr >500 mg/kg/day	Rabbit >5,000 mg/kg
Halosulfuron	1,287 mg/kg	Dog, 13 wk 10 mg/kg/day	Rat >5,000 mg/kg
Hexazinone	1,690 mg/kg	Rat, 2 yr 250 mg/kg in diet	Rabbit >5,278 mg/kg
Imazamox	>5,000 mg/kg		Rat >4,000 mg/kg

TABLE I. (continued)

Avian Toxicity	Toxicity to Fish in Water	Skin and Eye Irritation
LD_{50} Bobwhite quail 4,640 mg/kg Mallard duck >1,000 mg/kg	LC_{50} 96 hr Rainbow trout 4.7 mg/L	Skin–none Eye–none
LD_{50} 5 day Bobwhite quail >4,659 ppm Mallard duck >4,321 ppm	LC_{50} 96 hr Bluegill 0.5 mg/L Rainbow trout 1.4 mg/L	Skin–slight Eye–mild
$NOEC^{¶}$ (reproduction) Mallard duck 233 mg/kg/day	NOEL (chronic) Rainbow trout 2.75 mg/L$^{#}$	Skin–none Eye–minimal
LC_{50} 5 day Bobwhite quail >5,317 ppm Mallard duck >4,970 ppm	LC_{50} Bluegill 2.26-2.4 ppm Rainbow trout 3.49-5.84 ppm	Skin–none Eye–minimal
LC_{50} Mallard duck >5,620 ppm	LC_{50} Bluegill >300 ppm Rainbow trout >293 ppm	Skin–moderate Eye–severe
LC_{50} Mallard duck >5,620 ppm	LC_{50} 96 hr Bluegill 17.4 mg/L Rainbow trout 1.1 mg/L	Skin–severe Eye–moderate
LC_{50} 5 day Mallard duck >5,000 ppm	LC_{50} 96 hr Bluegill 14.3 mg/L Rainbow trout 13.4-100 mg/L	Skin–none Eye–slight
LC_{50} 5 day Bobwhite quail and Mallard duck >5,620 ppm	LC_{50} 96 hr Bluegill 140 μg/L Rainbow trout 43 μg/L	Skin–none Eye–minimal
LC_{50} Bobwhite quail and Mallard duck >5,000 ppm		Skin–moderate Eye–mild
LD_{50} Mallard duck >10,000 ppm in diet	LC_{50} Bluegill 670 mg/L Rainbow trout 1,000 mg/L	Skin–none Eye–moderate to severe
LC_{50} 5 day Japanese quail >5,000 mg/kg	LC_{50} 96 hr Bluegill 56-75 mg/L Rainbow trout >26.7 mg/L	Skin–slight Eye–moderate to severe
LC_{50} 8 day Bobwhite quail and Mallard duck 4,500 ppm in diet	LC_{50} 96 hr Bluegill 120 mg/L Rainbow trout 86 mg/L	Skin–none Eye–slight to moderate
LC_{50} 5 day Bobwhite quail and Mallard duck >5,620 ppm	LC_{50} 96 hr Bluegill >118 mg/L Rainbow trout >131 mg/L	Skin–slight Eye–slight
LC_{50} 5-8 day Bobwhite quail and Mallard duck >10,000 ppm in diet	LC_{50} 96 hr Bluegill 370-420 mg/L Rainbow trout 320-420 mg/L	Skin–none Eye–severe but reversible
LC_{50} Mallard duck >5,672 ppm	LC_{50} 96 hr Bluegill >119 ppm Rainbow trout >122 ppm	Skin–none Eye–none

(continued)

TABLE I.	Herbicide Poisoning (*continued*)		▶
Compound	Acute Oral LD$_{50}$—Rat	NOEL[*] (oral)	Acute Dermal LD$_{50}$
Imazapyr	>5,000 mg/kg	Rat, 300 mg/kg/day (teratology)	Rabbit >2,000 mg/kg
Imazethapyr	>5,000 mg/kg	Dog, 1 yr 25 mg/kg/day	Rabbit >2,000 mg/kg
Isoxaflutole	>5,000 mg/kg	Dog, 1 yr 1,200 ppm	Rat >2,000 mg/kg
Linuron	1,200-1,500 mg/kg	Dog, 2 yr 6.25 mg/kg/day (observed anemia)	Rabbit >5,000 mg/kg
Maleic hydrazide	>5,000 mg/kg (acid) >6,950 mg/kg (Na$^+$salt) >3,900 mg/kg (K$^+$salt)	Dog, 1 yr 25 mg/kg	Rabbit >20,000 mg/kg
MCPA	700-1,160 mg/kg	Rat, 7 mo 100 mg/kg/day (lowers wt gain)	Rabbits 3,400-4,800 mg/kg
MCPB	4,700 mg/kg	Rat, 6 mo 1.6 mg/kg/day	Rat >2,000 mg/kg
Mecoprop	930-1,210 mg/kg	Rat, 90 day 3.8 mg/kg/day Dog, 90 day 15 mg/kg/day	Rabbit 900 mg/kg
Mesotrione	>5,050 mg/kg		Rat >5,050 mg/kg
Metam (sodium and isothiocyanate)	1,800 mg/kg (M) 1,700 mg/kg (F) 97 mg/kg (isothiocyanate)	Rat, 65 day (inhalation, in inspired air) 6 hr/day for 5 day/wk at 0.045 mg/L	Rabbit 10,000 ppm mg/kg [‡]
Methyl bromide	Acute LC$_{50}$ (inhalation) 4.5 mg/L air	Safe threshold for humans 0.065 mg/L air	
Methyl isothiocyanate[†]	82 mg/kg (M)	Dog, 2 yr 10 mg/L in drinking water	Rabbit 202 mg/kg (F) 145 mg/kg (M)
Metobromuron	2,450-2,500 mg/kg	Rat, 2 yr 250 mg/kg/day Dog 100 mg/kg/day	Rabbit >2,000 mg/kg
Metolachlor	800-2,500 mg/kg	Rat, 90 day 1,000 mg/kg Dog, 90 day 500 mg/kg	Rabbit >5,000 mg/kg
Metribuzin	1,090-2,300 mg/kg (cat >500 mg/kg)	Rat, 2 yr 5 mg/kg Dog, 2 yr 2.5 mg/kg	Rat, rabbit >20,000 mg/kg

TABLE I. (continued)		
Avian Toxicity	**Toxicity to Fish in Water**	**Skin and Eye Irritation**
LC$_{50}$ 8 day Bobwhite quail and Mallard duck >5,000 ppm in diet	LC$_{50}$ 96 hr Bluegill and Rainbow trout >100 mg/L	Skin–mild Eye–more severe
LD$_{50}$ Bobwhite quail and Mallard duck >2,150 ppm in diet	LC$_{50}$ 96 hr Bluegill 420 mg/L Rainbow trout 340 mg/L	Skin–mild Eye–irritation reversible
LC$_{50}$ 5 day Bobwhite quail and Mallard duck >4,255 ppm	LC$_{50}$ 96 hr mg/L Bluegill >4.5 mg/L Rainbow trout >1.7 mg/L	Skin–minimal Eye–minimal
LC$_{50}$ 5-8 day Japanese quail >5,000 ppm Mallard duck 3,083 ppm in diet	LC$_{50}$ 96 hr Bluegill and Rainbow trout 16 mg/L	Skin–mild Eye–moderate
LD$_{50}$ Bobwhite quail and Mallard duck >10,000 mg/kg	LC$_{50}$ 96 hr Bluegill 1,608 mg/L Rainbow trout 1,435 mg/L	Skin–slight Eye–severe
LD$_{50}$ Bobwhite quail 377 mg/kg	LC$_{50}$ 96 hr Bluegill and Rainbow trout 90 mg/L	Skin–slight Eye–moderate
LC$_{50}$ 8 day Bobwhite quail and Mallard duck >5,000 ppm in diet	LC$_{50}$ 96 hr Bluegill 14 mg/L Rainbow trout 4.3 mg/L	Skin–moderate Eye–moderate
LC$_{50}$ Bobwhite quail and Mallard duck 5,000-5,500 ppm in diet	LC$_{50}$ 96 hr Bluegill >100 mg/L Rainbow trout 124-mg/L	Skin–slight Eye–intense
LD$_{50}$ Bobwhite quail, >2,000 mg/kg Mallard duck >5,200 mg/kg	LC$_{50}$ 96 hr Bluegill and Rainbow trout >120 mg/L	Skin–slight Eye–moderate
LC$_{50}$ Bobwhite quail, >10,000 Mallard duck >5,000 ppm in diet	LC$_{50}$ 96 hr Bluegill 0.047 mg/L Rainbow trout 0.029 mg/L	Skin–corrosive Eye–corrosive
	Acute toxicity Bluegill 11 mg/L	Skin–severe Eye–severe
LC$_{50}$ 5 day Mallard duck 10,936 mg/kg	LC$_{50}$ 96 hr Bluegill 0.13 mg/L Rainbow trout 0.37 mg/L	Skin–corrosive Eye–severe
LC$_{50}$ 8 day Bobwhite quail >20,000 ppm Mallard duck >4,640 ppm in diet	LC$_{50}$ 96 hr Bluegill 4 mg/L Rainbow trout 3 mg/L	Skin–moderate Eye–moderate
LC$_{50}$ 5 day Bobwhite quail and Mallard duck >10,000 ppm in diet	LC$_{50}$ 96 hr Bluegill 15 mg/L Rainbow trout 3 mg/L	Skin–slight Eye–mild
LC$_{50}$ Bobwhite quail and Mallard duck >4,000 ppm in diet	LC$_{50}$ 96 hr Bluegill 80 mg/L Rainbow trout 64-76 mg/L	Skin–none Eye–none

(continued)

TABLE I.   Herbicide Poisoning (continued)

Compound	Acute Oral LD$_{50}$—Rat	NOEL (oral)[*]	Acute Dermal LD$_{50}$
Napropamide	>5,000-4,680 mg/kg (M-F)[‡]	Dog, 13 wk <100 mg/kg	Rabbit >4,640 mg/kg
Naptalam[†]	>5,000 mg/kg 1,770 mg/kg (Na$^+$ salt)	Rat, dog, 90 day 1,000 mg/kg (Na$^+$ salt)	Rabbit >20,000 mg/kg
Nicosulfuron	Mouse >5,000 mg/kg	Dog 1 yr >5,000 ppm in diet (M)	Rat, Rabbit >2,000 mg/kg
Oxadiazon	>5,000 mg/kg	Rat, dog, 2 yr 100 mg/kg	Rabbit >2,000 mg/kg
Oxyfluorfen	Rat, dog >5,000 mg/kg	Rat 2 yr 2.0 mg/kg Dog 2.5 mg/kg	Rabbit >5,000 mg/kg
Paraquat (dichloride)	283 mg/kg (finished product)	Rat 2 yr 1.25 mg/kg Dog 1 yr 0.45 mg/kg	Rat >2,000 mg/kg (finished product)
Pebulate[†]	1,120 mg/kg	Rat 2 yr 15 ppm in diet (eye lesions)	Rabbit 4,640 mg/kg
Pendimethalin	1,050 to >5,000 mg/kg	Dog 2 yr 12.5 mg/kg/day	Rabbit >5,000 mg/kg
Phenmedipham	8,000 mg/kg (dog >4,000 mg/kg, chicken >3,000 mg/kg)	Dog 2 yr >1,000 ppm in diet	Rat >2,000 mg/kg Rabbit[#] >10,000 mg/kg[§]
Picloram	5,000-8,200 mg/kg (sheep >1,000 mg/kg, cattle >750 mg/kg)	Rat, 2 yr 150 mg/kg/day	Rabbit >4,000 mg/kg
Prometryn	3,750-5,235 mg/kg	Dog, 90 day <200 ppm in diet	Rabbit >2,000 to >3,100 mg/kg
Propanil	1,080 to >2,500 mg/kg Dog 1,217 mg/kg[‡]	Dog, 2 yr <85 ppm in diet	Rabbit >5,000 mg/kg
Propoxycarbazone	>5,000 mg/kg	Dog, 1 yr 258 mg/kg (M) 55.7 mg/kg (F)	Rat >5,000 mg/kg
Propyzamide[†]	8,350-5,620 mg/kg (M-F) Dog >10,000 mg/kg	Dog, 2 yr >7.5 ppm in diet	Rabbit 3,160 mg/kg
Pyrazon	3,030-3,600 mg/kg	Dog, 2 yr 1,500 ppm in diet	Rat >2,000 mg/kg

TABLE I. (continued)

Avian Toxicity	Toxicity to Fish in Water	Skin and Eye Irritation
LC$_{50}$ 5 day Bobwhite quail >5,600 ppm Mallard duck 7,200 ppm in diet	LC$_{50}$ 96 hr Bluegill 20-30 mg/L Rainbow trout 9-16 mg/L	Skin–none Eye–none
LC$_{50}$ 8 day Bobwhite quail 5,600 ppm Mallard duck >10,000 ppm in diet	LC$_{50}$ 96 hr Bluegill 354 mg/L Rainbow trout 76 mg/L	Skin–mild Eye–moderate
LC$_{50}$ Bobwhite quail and Mallard duck >5,620 ppm in diet	LC$_{50}$ 96 hr Bluegill and Rainbow trout >1,000 mg/L	Skin–none Eye–moderate
LC$_{50}$ Bobwhite quail and Mallard duck >5,620 ppm in diet	LC$_{50}$ 96 hr Bluegill 12.5 mg/L Rainbow trout 2 mg/L	Skin–moderate Eye–mild
LC$_{50}$ Bobwhite quail >5,000 Mallard duck >4,000 ppm in diet	LC$_{50}$ 96 hr Bluegill 0.2 mg/L Rainbow trout 0.41 mg/L	Skin–none Eye–moderate
LC$_{50}$ 5 day Bobwhite quail 981 ppm Mallard duck 4,048 ppm in diet	LC$_{50}$ 96 hr Rainbow trout 26 mg/L	Skin–slight Eye–moderate
LC$_{50}$ Bobwhite quail and Mallard duck >2,400 ppm in diet	LC$_{50}$ 96 hr Bluegill and Rainbow trout 7.4 mg/L	Skin–slight Eye–mild
LC$_{50}$ 8 day Bobwhite quail 3,149 ppm Mallard duck 10,900 ppm in diet	LC$_{50}$ 96 hr Bluegill 0.199 mg/L Rainbow trout 0.138 mg/L	Skin–none Eye–mild
LC$_{50}$ 4 day Bobwhite quail >2,480 ppm in diet	LC$_{50}$ 96 hr Bluegill 760 mg/L LC$_{50}$ 21 day Rainbow trout >210 mg/L	Skin–moderate Eye–severe[§]
LD$_{50}$ 8 day Bobwhite quail >2,500 Mallard duck >5,000 mg/kg	LC$_{50}$ 96 hr Bluegill 14.5 mg/L Rainbow trout 19.3 mg/L	Skin–mild Eye–moderate
LC$_{50}$ 5-7 day Bobwhite quail and Mallard duck >10,000 ppm in diet	LC$_{50}$ 96 hr Bluegill 10 mg/kg Rainbow trout 2.5-2.9 mg/L	Skin–none Eye–slight
LC$_{50}$ 8 day Bobwhite quail 2,861 ppm Mallard duck 5,627 ppm in diet	LC$_{50}$ 96 hr Bluegill 2.3 mg/L Rainbow trout 4.6 mg/L	Skin–moderate Eye–serious
		Skin–slight Eye–minimal
LC$_{50}$ 8 day Bobwhite quail and Mallard duck >10,000 ppm in diet	LC$_{50}$ 96 hr Bluegill 100 mg/L Rainbow trout 72 mg/L	Skin–slight Eye–moderate
	LC$_{50}$ Bluegill 40 mg/L	Skin–slight Eye–slight

(continued)

Compound	Acute Oral LD$_{50}$—Rat	NOEL* (oral)	Acute Dermal LD$_{50}$
Pyridate	1,285-1,412 mg/kg‡	Dog 1 yr 30 mg/kg/day	Rabbit >2,000 mg/kg
Pyrithiobac-sodium	4,000 mg/kg	Rat (longterm) 59 mg/kg	Rat >2,000 mg/kg
Quinclorac	3,060 mg/kg (M) 2,190 mg/kg (F)	Dog, 1 yr 142 mg/kg/day (M) 140 mg/kg/day (F)	Rat >2,000 mg/kg
Quizalofop-p-ethyl	1,210-1,670 mg/kg (M) 1,182-1,480 mg/kg (F)	Dog, 1 yr <10 mg/kg/day	Rat, mouse, rabbit >10,000 mg/kg
Rimsulfuron	>5,000 mg/kg	Dog 1 yr 50 ppm in diet	Rabbit >2,000 mg/kg
Sethoxydim	3,200 mg/kg (M) 2,676 mg/kg (F)	Dog, 1 yr >8.86-9.41 mg/kg (M-F)	Rat, mouse >5,000 mg/kg
Siduron	>7,500 mg/kg	Rat, 2 yr 500 ppm in diet	Rabbit >5,500 mg/kg
Simazine	>5,000 mg/kg	Rat 2 yr >5 mg/kg/day	Rabbit >10,200 mg/kg
Sodium chlorate	1,200-7,000 mg/kg		Rabbit 500 mg/kg
Sulfentra-zone	2,416-3,297 mg/kg	Rat 10 mg/kg/day oral development studies	Rat >5,000 mg/kg
Sulfosulfur-on	>5,000 mg/kg	Mouse 90 days 7,000 mg/kg of diet	Rat >5,000 mg/kg
Tebuthiuron	644 mg/kg (Dog >500 mg/kg, Cat >200 mg/kg)	Dog 1 yr >25 mg/kg/day	Rabbits >200 mg/kg
Thiazopyr	>5,000 mg/kg	Dog, 1 yr 0.8 mg/kg/day#	Rat >5,000 mg/kg
Thifensulfur-on-methyl	>5,000 mg/kg	Rat, 2 yr 25 ppm in diet	Rabbit >2,000 mg/kg
Tralkoxydim	1,258 mg/kg (M) 934 mg/kg (F)	Rat (teratogen) 30 mg/kg	Rat >2,000 mg/kg
Triallate†	800-2,165 mg/kg‡	Dog, 2 yr 15 mg/kg/day (highest tested)	Rabbit 8,200 mg/kg

◀ **TABLE I.** (continued)

Avian Toxicity	Toxicity to Fish in Water	Skin and Eye Irritation
LC_{50} 8 day Bobwhite quail >5,000 ppm in diet	LC_{50} 96 hr Rainbow trout >1.2 mg/L	Skin–none Eye–slight
LC_{50} Bobwhite quail and Mallard duck >6,300 ppm	LC_{50} 96 hr Bluegill 5.8 mg/L Rainbow trout 8.2 mg/L	Skin–mild[§] Eye–moderate[§]
LD_{50} Bobwhite quail and Mallard duck >5,000 mg/kg	LC_{50} 96 hr Bluegill and Rainbow trout >100 mg/L	Skin–irritating Eye–moderate
LC_{50} 8 day Bobwhite quail and Mallard duck >5,000 ppm in diet	LC_{50} 96 hr Bluegill 0.46-2.8 mg/L Rainbow trout 10.7 mg/L	Skin–none Eye–slight
LC_{50} 8 day Bobwhite quail and Mallard duck >5,600 ppm in diet	LC_{50} 96 hr Bluegill and Rainbow trout >1,000 mg/L	Skin–none Eye–moderate
LC_{50} 8 day Bobwhite quail >5,620 ppm Mallard duck >2,510 ppm in diet	LC_{50} 96 hr Bluegill 100 mg/L Rainbow trout 32 mg/L	Skin–mild Eye–mild
LC_{50} Bobwhite quail and Mallard duck >10,000 mg/kg	LC_{50} 48 hr Carp 18 mg/L	Skin–slight Eye–slight
LC_{50} 8 day Bobwhite quail >5,260 ppm Mallard duck 10,000 ppm in diet	LC_{50} 96 hr Bluegill and Rainbow trout >100 mg/L	Skin–none Eye–none
	LC_{50} 48 hr Various fish 10,000 mg/L	Skin–moderate Eye–moderate
LD_{50} Bobwhite quail and Mallard duck >5,620 ppm	LC_{50} 96 hr Bluegill 93.8 mg/L Rainbow trout >130 mg/L	Skin–mild Eye–moderate
LD_{50} Bobwhite quail and Mallard duck 5,620 ppm	LC_{50} 96 hr Rainbow trout >97 mg/L	Skin–slight Eye–slight
LD_{50} Bobwhite quail and Mallard duck >2,500 mg/kg	LC_{50} 96 hr Bluegill 112 mg/L Rainbow trout 144 mg/L	Skin–slight Eye–slight
LD_{50} Bobwhite quail and Mallard duck 5,328 mg/kg	LC_{50} Bluegill and Rainbow trout 3.5 mg/L	Skin–slight Eye–slight
LC_{50} 8 day Bobwhite quail and Mallard duck >5,620 mg/kg	LC_{50} 96 hr Bluegill and Rainbow trout 100 mg/L	Skin–none Eye–moderate
LD_{50} Mallard duck >3,020 mg/kg	LC_{50} 96 hr Bluegill >6.1 mg/L Rainbow trout >7.2 mg/L	Skin–mild Eye–mild
LC_{50} 8 day Bobwhite quail and Mallard duck >5,000 mg/kg	LC_{50} 96 hr Bluegill 1.3 mg/L Rainbow trout 1.2 mg/L	Skin–moderate Eye–slight

(continued)

TABLE I.   Herbicide Poisoning (continued)

Compound	Acute Oral LD$_{50}$—Rat	NOEL* (oral)	Acute Dermal LD$_{50}$
Triasulfuron	>5,000 mg/kg	Dog, 1 yr 129 mg/kg/day	Rat >2,000 mg/kg
Tribenuron-methyl	>5,000 mg/kg	Dog, 1 yr 875 ppm in diet	Rabbit >2,000 mg/kg
Trichloracetic acid	3,200-5,000 mg/kg		Rat >2,000 mg/kg
Triclopyr	630-729 mg/kg	Rat, 2 yr 3.0 mg/kg/day	Rabbit >2,000 mg/kg
Trifluralin	>5,000 mg/kg (dog >2,000 mg/kg)	Dog, 2 yr 18.75 mg/kg/day	Rabbit >2,000 mg/kg
Vernolate†	1,200-1,900 mg/kg‡	Dog, 90 day >38 mg/kg/day	Rabbit >1,955 mg/kg

*NOEL = No effect level; daily dose or ppm concentration in diet
† No active EPA registration
‡ Technical grade chemical

Aromatic/Benzoic Acid Compounds (chloramben, dicamba): The herbicides in this group have a low order of toxicity to domestic animals, and poisoning after normal use has not been reported. Environmental persistence and toxicity to wildlife is also low for this group. The signs and lesions are similar to those described for the phenoxyacetic compounds (*see* below).

Phenoxyacetic and Phenoxybutyric Compounds (2,4-D [2-4-dichlorophenoxyacetic acid], 2,4,5-T [2,4,5-trichlorophenoxyacetic acid], 2,4-DB, MCPA): These acids and their salts and esters are commonly used to control undesirable plants. As a group, they are essentially nontoxic to animals exposed to properly treated forage. When large doses are fed experimentally, general depression, anorexia, weight loss, tenseness, and muscular weakness (particularly of the hindquarters) are noted. Large doses in cattle may interfere with rumen function. Dogs may develop myotonia, ataxia, posterior weakness, vomiting, diarrhea, and metabolic acidosis. (The oral LD$_{50}$ for 2,4-D and 2,4,5-T in dogs is ~100 mg/kg body wt.) Even large doses, up to 2 g/kg, have not been shown to leave residues in the fat of animals. These compounds are plant growth regulators, and treatment may result in increased palatability of some poisonous plants as well as increased nitrate and cyanide content.

The use of 2,4,5-T was curtailed because extremely toxic contaminants, collectively called dioxins (TCDD and HCDD), were found in technical grade material (*see also* p 2367). The 2,3,7,8-TCDD is considered carcinogenic, mutagenic, teratogenic, fetotoxic, and able to cause reproductive damage and other toxic effects. Although manufacturing methods have reduced the level of the contaminants, use of this herbicide is very limited worldwide. Its EPA registration was canceled and it is no longer manufactured in the USA.

Dinitrophenolic Compounds (dinoseb, binapacryl, DNOC): The old 2-4 dinitrophenol and dinitrocresol compounds were highly toxic to all classes of animals (eg, LD$_{50}$ of 20-56 mg/kg body wt). Poisoning can occur if animals are sprayed accidentally or have immediate access to forage that has been sprayed, because these compounds are readily absorbed through skin or lungs. Dinitrophenolic herbicides markedly increase oxygen

TABLE I. *(continued)*

Avian Toxicity	Toxicity to Fish in Water	Skin and Eye Irritation
LC_{50} 8 day Bobwhite quail and Mallard duck >5,000 ppm	LC_{50} 96 hr Bluegill and Rainbow trout >100 ppm	Skin–none Eye–none
LC_{50} Bobwhite quail and Mallard duck >5,620 ppm	LC_{50} 96 hr Bluegill 760 mg/L Rainbow trout 730 mg/L	Skin–none Eye–mild/moderate
LD_{50} Chicken 4,280 mg/kg	Not toxic to fish	Skin–severe Eye–severe
LC_{50} 8 day Bobwhite quail 2,935 ppm Mallard duck >5,401 ppm in diet	LC_{50} 96 hr Bluegill 148 mg/L Rainbow trout 117 mg/L	Skin–none Eye–slight[‡]
LC_{50} 8 day Bobwhite quail and Mallard duck >5,000 ppm in diet	LC_{50} 96 hr Bluegill 0.05-0.07 mg/L Rainbow trout 0.02-0.06 mg/L	Skin–none Eye–moderate
LC_{50} 7 day Bobwhite quail 12,000 ppm in diet[‡]	LC_{50} 96 hr Bluegill 8.4 mg/L Rainbow trout 9.6 mg/L[‡]	Skin–none Eye–none

[§]Commercial formulation
[¶]NOEC = No effect concentration
[#]Active ingredient

consumption and deplete glycogen reserves. Clinical signs include fever, dyspnea, acidosis, tachycardia, and convulsions, followed by coma and death with a rapid onset of rigor mortis. Cataracts can occur in animals with chronic dinitrophenol intoxication. Exposure to dinitro compounds may cause yellow staining of the skin, conjunctiva, or hair. An effective antidote is not known. Affected animals should be cooled and sedated to help control hyperthermia. Phenothiazine tranquilizers are contraindicated; however, diazepam can be used to calm the animal. Atropine sulfate, aspirin, and antipyretics should not be used. Administration (IV) of large doses of carbohydrate solutions and parenteral vitamin A may be useful. If toxic amounts of one of these is ingested and the animal is alert, emetics should be administered in animals that readily vomit (eg, not horses); if the animal is depressed, gastric lavage should be performed. Treatment with activated charcoal should follow.

Organophosphate Compounds (glyphosate, bensulide): These are widely used herbicides with low toxicity, although fish and pond life have been killed experimentally. Sprayed forage appears to be preferred by cattle for 5-7 days after application and causes little or no problem. Acute LD_{50} in rats is >5.6 g/kg.

A few dogs and cats show eye, skin, and upper respiratory tract signs when exposed during or subsequent to an application to weeds or grass. Nausea, vomiting, staggering, and hind-leg weakness have been seen in dogs and cats that were exposed to fresh chemical on treated foliage. The signs usually disappear when exposure ceases, and minimal symptomatic treatment is needed. Washing the chemical off the skin, evacuating the stomach, and tranquilizing the animal are usually sufficient. Massive exposure with acute signs due to accidental contact should be handled as an organophosphate poisoning (p 2398).

Bensulide, listed as a plant growth regulator, has an oral LD_{50} in rats of 271-770 mg/kg, in dogs the lethal dose is ~200 g/kg. The most prominent clinical sign is anorexia, but other signs are similar to 2,4-D poisoning.

Triazolopyrimidine Compounds (bromacil, terbacil): These compounds can cause mild toxic signs at levels of 50 mg/kg body wt in sheep, 250 mg/kg in cattle, and 500 mg/kg in poultry when given daily for 8-10 doses. Signs include bloat, incoordination, depression, and anorexia. Application rates of ~5 lb/acre (5.6 kg/hectare) can be hazardous, especially for sheep, but no field cases of toxicity have been reported.

Phenyl or Substituted Urea Compounds (diuron, fenuron, linuron, monolinuron): Exposure to toxic amounts of these herbicides is unlikely with recommended application and handling of containers. Signs and lesions are similar to those described for the phenoxyacetic herbicides (*see* above). The substituted urea herbicides induce hepatic microsomal enzymes and may alter metabolism of other xenobiotic agents. Altered calcium metabolism and bone morphology have been seen in laboratory animals.

Polycyclic Alkanoic Acids or Aryloxyphenoxypropionic Compounds (diclofop, fenoxaprop, fenthiaprop, fluazifop, haloxyfop): Members of this group that are approved as herbicides are of moderately low toxicity with acute oral LD_{50} doses from 950 mg/kg to >4,000 mg/kg. (Haloxyfop-methyl is an exception and has an LD_{50} in male rats of ~400 mg/kg.) They tend to be more toxic if exposure is dermal. The dermal LD_{50} of diclofop in rabbits is only 180 mg/kg.

Triazinylsulfonylurea or Sulfonylurea Compounds (chlorsulfuron, sulfometuron, ethametsulfuron, chloremuron): Toxicity in this group appears to be quite low. The oral acute LD_{50} in rats is in the range of 4,000-5,000 mg/kg. The dermal acute LD_{50} in rabbits is ~2,000 mg/kg.

Triazine, Methylthiotriazine, Triazinone Compounds (atrazine, cyanazine, prometryn, metribuzin, simazine): Although these herbicides are widely used, incidents of poisoning are uncommon. Occasionally, accidental exposure of animals to large dosages (eg, open containers, spills) can cause toxic effects and even death. (Doses of 500 mg of simazine/kg or 30 mg of atrazine/kg for 36-60 days were lethal to sheep.) Generally, single doses >100-200 mg/kg body wt can be detrimental; repeat administration may reduce the toxic dose to <100 mg/kg body wt. Deaths have been reported in sheep and horses grazing triazine-treated pastures 1-7 days after spraying. Cumulative effects are not evident. The signs and lesions are similar to those described for the phenoxyacetic compounds (*see* above).

The oral LD_{50} of metribuzin is 2,200 mg/kg in rats and 500-1,000 mg/kg in birds. No harmful effects were apparent when it was fed to dogs at 100 ppm in the diet.

HOUSEHOLD HAZARDS

See also RODENTICIDE POISONING, p 2508; TOXICITIES FROM HUMAN DRUGS, p 2525; PLANTS POISONOUS TO ANIMALS, p 2432; and FOOD HAZARDS, p 2361.

Hazardous chemicals (eg, products containing alcohols,, bleaches, or corrosives) found in the home represent a significant risk of toxicosis in companion animals. It can often be difficult to determine the toxicant(s) consumed and amount ingested. Often a diagnosis must be based on owner report of possible exposure and the development of appropriate clinical signs.

ALCOHOLS

Alcohol toxicosis results in metabolic acidosis, hypothermia, and CNS depression. All species are susceptible.

Etiology: Ethanol, methanol, and isopropanol are the alcohols most frequently encountered in veterinary medicine. Ethanol is present in a variety of alcoholic beverages, some rubbing alcohols, drug elixirs, and fermenting bread dough (p 2362). Methanol is most commonly found in windshield washer fluids (windshield "antifreeze"). The lethal oral dose of methanol in dogs is 4-8 mL/kg, although significant clinical signs may be seen at lower doses. Isopropanol is twice as toxic as ethanol and is found in rubbing alcohols and in alcohol-based flea sprays for pets. Oral doses of isopropanol ≥0.5 mL/kg may result in significant clinical signs in dogs.

Pathogenesis: All alcohols are rapidly absorbed via the GI tract and most are well absorbed dermally; toxicosis from overspraying pets with alcohol-based flea sprays is not uncommon. Alcohols reach peak plasma levels within 1.5-2 hr and are widely distributed throughout the body. They are metabolized in the liver to acetaldehyde (ethanol), formaldehyde (methanol), and acetone (isopropanol); these intermediate metabolites are then further converted to acetic acid, formic acid, and/or carbon dioxide. (In humans and some other primates, accumulation of formic acid results in retinal and neuronal damage; nonprimates are efficient at eliminating formic acid and therefore do not develop the blindness and cerebral necrosis seen in primates). Alcohols are eliminated via the urine as parent compound as well as metabolites. In dogs, up to 50% of a dose of methanol may be eliminated unchanged via the lungs.

Alcohols are GI irritants, and ingestion may result in vomiting and hypersalivation. Alcohols and their metabolites are potent CNS depressants, affecting a variety of neurotransmitters within the nervous system. Metabolites such as acetaldehyde may stimulate the release of catecholamines, which can affect myocardial function. Metabolic acidosis results from the formation of acidic intermediates, and both parent compounds and metabolites contribute to increases in osmolal gap. Hypothermia may develop due to peripheral vasodilation, CNS depression, and interference with thermoregulatory mechanisms. Hypoglycemia develops secondary to alcohol-induced depletion of pyruvate, resulting in inhibition of gluconeogenesis.

Clinical Findings and Diagnosis: Signs generally begin within 30-60 min of ingestion and include vomiting, diarrhea, ataxia, disorientation (inebriation), depression, tremors, and dyspnea. Severe cases may progress to coma, hypothermia, seizures, bradycardia, and respiratory depression. Death is generally due to respiratory failure, hypothermia, hypoglycemia and/or metabolic acidosis. Pneumonia secondary to aspiration of vomitus is possible.

The determination of blood alcohol levels may help to confirm the diagnosis of alcohol intoxication.

Treatment: Stabilization of severely symptomatic animals is a priority. Adequate ventilation should be maintained, and cardiovascular and acid/base abnormalities should be corrected. Seizures can be controlled with diazepam (0.5-2 mg/kg, IV) as needed. For asymptomatic animals, induction of emesis may be of benefit in the first 20-40 min following ingestion. Activated charcoal is not thought to appreciably bind small chain alcohols and is not often recommended. Bathing with mild shampoo is recommended for significant dermal exposures. Supportive care, including thermoregulation and fluid diuresis to enhance alcohol elimination, should be administered. Anecdotally, yohimbine (0.1 mg/kg, IV) has been used to stimulate respiration in severely comatose dogs with alcohol toxicosis.

CHLORINE BLEACHES

Exposure to undiluted chlorine bleaches may result in alimentary, dermal, and ocular irritation or ulceration as well as significant respiratory irritation. All species are susceptible. Due to the countercurrent anatomy and physiology of the avian lung, caged birds are at increased risk of succumbing to fumes from bleaches and other cleaning agents.

Etiology: Chlorine bleaches are primarily used as household cleaners and pool sanitizers. Household bleaches tend to contain sodium hypochlorite at 3-10%, and pH of these products may range from 9.0 (mildly irritating) to >11 (corrosive). Pool treatments may contain lithium, calcium, or sodium hypochlorites at concentrations up to 70-80%, with pH that may range from acidic to alkaline. Pets may be exposed by chewing on containers of undiluted product, drinking from buckets containing product diluted in water, or swimming in recently treated pools.

Pathogenesis: The relative hazard of a particular bleach product depends on the concentration of hypochlorite, pH, and dilution of the product. In general, levels of hypochlorite <10% tend to be mild irritants; however, if the product has a pH >11 or <3.5, alkaline or acid corrosive injury may occur. Dilution of bleaches with water per label directions will often reduce the corrosive potential of these products and make them little more than mild GI or ocular irritants. Mixing of hypochlorite and ammonia produces highly toxic chloramine gas that can cause acute respiratory distress or delayed onset of pulmonary edema within 12-24 hr of exposure.

Clinical Findings and Lesions: Ingestion of dilute or moderate pH household bleach products rarely causes more than mild vomiting, hypersalivation, depression, anorexia, and/or diarrhea. Concentrated (>10%) bleach products or products with pH >11 may cause significant GI corrosive injury. Ingestion or inhalation of significant amounts of chlorine bleach occasionally results in hypernatremia, hyperchloremia, and/or metabolic acidosis. Acute inhalation may result in immediate coughing, gagging, sneezing, or retching. In addition to the immediate respiratory signs, animals exposed to concentrated chlorine fumes may develop pulmonary edema 12-24 hr after exposure. Ocular exposures may result in epiphora, blepharospasm, eyelid edema, and/or corneal ulceration. Dermal exposure may result in mild dermal irritation and bleaching of the hair coat. Oral, dermal, and ocular irritation or ulceration are possible. Respiratory lesions may include tracheitis, bronchitis, alveolitis, and pulmonary edema.

Treatment: For oral exposures, emesis and activated charcoal are contraindicated; instead, dilution with milk or water is recommended. Any spontaneous vomiting should be managed, and animals should be monitored for development of GI irritation/ulceration (*see* CORROSIVES, below). In cases where protracted vomiting causes electrolyte or hydration abnormalities, fluid therapy may be of benefit. For respiratory exposures, the animal should be moved to an area with fresh air and monitored for dyspnea. Stabilization of severely dyspneic animals is a must; pulmonary edema should be treated as needed. Bathing with mild shampoo and thorough rinsing is recommended for significant dermal exposures. Ocular exposures should be treated with 10-20 min of ocular irrigation with physiologic saline followed by fluorescein staining of the cornea to detect corneal injury.

CORROSIVES

Acid or alkaline corrosives produce significant local tissue injury that can result in full thickness burns of skin, cornea, and the mucosa of the oral cavity, esophagus, and stomach. All species are susceptible. Heavy coats may provide some protection from dermal exposure.

Etiology: Corrosives are divided into acid and alkaline corrosives. Acidic household products include anti-rust compounds, toilet bowl cleaners, gun-cleaning fluids, automotive batteries, swimming pool cleaning agents, and etching compounds. Alkaline corrosive agents include drain openers, automatic dishwasher detergents, toilet bowl cleaners, radiator cleaning agents, and swimming pool algaecides and "shock" agents. In general, alkaline products with pH >11 pose risk of significant corrosive injury.

Pathogenesis: Acids produce immediate coagulative necrosis of tissue and impart significant pain on contact, which may limit exposure. Alkaline agents produce immediate, penetrating liquefactive necrosis of tissue; the lack of significant discomfort on contact with alkaline products may result in prolonged exposure. For these reasons, burns from alkaline products tend to be deeper and more extensive than burns from acidic agents. Burns from alkaline agents may take up to 12 hr following exposure to become fully apparent, whereas the extent of acid burns is usually evident shortly after contact. Esophageal burns are more common with alkaline agents, and the absence of significant oral burns does not necessarily indicate that no esophageal damage has developed. Full thickness ulceration of the esophagus may result in pleuritis or peritonitis due to leakage of ingesta into body cavities. Esophageal burns may result in stricture formation during healing, resulting in dysphagia, megaesophagus, and aspiration pneumonia. Additionally, although the contents of the stomach may serve to buffer and dilute corrosive agents, gastric ulceration and possibly perforation may occur with significant exposures. Respiratory exposure to corrosives (especially acids) may result in respiratory distress, tracheobronchitis, or pneumonitis. Dermal or ocular exposures may result in severe ulceration of dermis or cornea.

Clinical Findings and Lesions: Clinical signs that may occur following ingestion of corrosive agents include vocalization, lethargy, polydipsia, vomiting (with or without blood), abdominal pain, dysphagia, pharyngeal edema, dyspnea, and oral, esophageal, and/or gastric ulceration. In severe cases, shock may develop rapidly following exposure. Lesions are initially milky white to gray but gradually will turn black as eschar formation occurs. Sloughing of necrotic tissue may occur within days of exposure. Dyspnea, cyanosis, and pulmonary edema may occur secondary to inhaled corrosive agents. Dermal exposure may result in significant burns, with local pain, erythema, and tissue sloughing. Ocular exposure may cause blepharospasm, epiphora, eyelid edema, conjunctivitis, or corneal ulceration. Burns of skins, corneas, and alimentary mucosa range from mild ulceration to full thickness necrosis with extensive tissue sloughing. Peritonitis or pleuritis may develop secondary to perforating ulcers of esophagus or stomach. Respiratory lesions may include tracheitis, bronchitis, pneumonitis, pulmonary edema, or aspiration pneumonia.

Treatment: Because of the rapid action of corrosive agents, much of the damage from exposure occurs before treatment can be initiated. Stabilization of animals presenting as dyspneic, in shock, or with severe electrolyte abnormalities is always a priority. For recent oral exposures, immediate dilution with water or milk should be done. Under no circumstances should emesis be attempted due to the risk of further mucosal exposure to corrosive material. Likewise, gastric lavage is contraindicated due to risk of perforation of weakened esophageal/gastric walls and risk of further exposure of mucosa to the corrosive material as it is removed. Attempts to chemically neutralize an acid with weak alkali (or alkali with weak acid) are also contraindicated due to the production of exothermic reactions that can result in thermal burns. Activated charcoal is ineffective in cases involving ingestion of corrosives, and the presence of charcoal on damaged mucosa may impede wound healing. Following dilution, general supportive care should be instituted, including monitoring for respiratory difficulty, pain management, antibiotics (if ulcers are present), and anti-inflammatories as needed. Endoscopic evaluation of the esophagus and stomach for ulceration should be performed ~12 hr after exposure; this time frame will allow the full extent of tissue injury to become apparent. The use of corticosteroids in cases with significant esophageal mucosal injury is controversial. Corticosteroids decrease inflammation and may aid in minimizing stricture formation, but they also suppress the immune system and may enhance susceptibility to secondary infection. In animals with significant oral and/or esophageal burns, gastrostomy tubes may be necessary to provide nutrition while affected tissues heal. Dermal or ocular exposures should be managed by flushing with copious amounts of water or physiologic saline; eyes should be flushed for a minimum of 20 min, followed by fluorescein staining. Standard topical treatments for dermal or ocular burns should be instituted as needed.

Alkaline Batteries

Ingestion of alkaline batteries poses a risk of both alimentary tract corrosive injury and foreign body obstruction. Dogs are most commonly involved.

Etiology: Alkaline batteries are present in many household electronic products, including remote controls, hearing aids, toys, watches, computers, and calculators. Most alkaline dry cell batteries use potassium hydroxide or sodium hydroxide to generate currents. Nickel-cadmium and lithium batteries also tend to contain alkaline material.

Pathogenesis: The alkaline gel in batteries causes liquefactive necrosis of tissues upon contact, resulting in burns that can penetrate deeply into tissue. Lithium disc or "button" batteries may lodge in the esophagus and generate a current against the esophageal walls, resulting in circular ulcers that have the potential to be perforating. Some battery casings may contain metals such as zinc or mercury, posing hazards of foreign body obstruction and metal toxicosis if they remain in the stomach for prolonged periods. Additionally, small batteries (especially disc batteries) may be inhaled and pose a choking hazard.

Clinical Findings and Lesions: *See* CORROSIVES (above) for discussion of alkaline burns. Foreign body obstruction may present as vomiting, anorexia, abdominal discomfort, or tenesmus. Respiratory obstruction due to battery inhalation may present with acute onset of dyspnea and cyanosis. Mucosal burns may occur within the oral cavity, esophagus, and, less commonly, stomach. Perforation of the esophagus may lead to secondary pyothorax, while gastric perforation may result in acute blood loss and/or peritonitis.

Diagnosis: Radiographs can help to confirm the diagnosis as well as the location of the battery. Differential diagnoses include GI or respiratory foreign bodies and other oral, dermal, or ocular corrosive agents.

Treatment: For batteries swallowed intact without any chewing, induction of emesis may result in expulsion. Due to the risk of leakage of alkaline gel onto oral and esophageal mucosa during vomiting, emesis should not be induced if there is any possibility that the battery casing has been punctured. When disc batteries have been ingested, 20 mL boluses of tap water every 15 min will decrease the severity and delay the development of current-induced esophageal ulceration. The decision on whether to remove a battery from the stomach depends on the size of the animal, battery size, and evidence of battery puncture. Radiography may be performed to determine the location of the battery casing; generally, batteries that have passed through the pylorus will pass through the intestinal tract uneventfully (adding bulk to the diet and judicious use of cathartics may facilitate passage). Serial radiography to verify battery location is recommended until the battery is expelled. Batteries that do not pass through the pylorus within 48 hr of ingestion are unlikely to pass on their own and may require surgical or endoscopic removal. Batteries that have obviously been punctured should be removed surgically to prevent gastric or intestinal ulceration due to leakage of alkaline gel. Endoscopic removal is not recommended in cases in which it is suspected that the casing has been punctured. Treatment of cases with suspected oral, esophageal, or gastric ulceration is the same as other alkaline corrosive injuries (*see* CORROSIVES, above). Dermal or ocular exposures to alkaline gels should be managed by copious rinsing of the area with tap water (skin) or physiologic saline solution (eyes). The affected areas should be monitored for development of ulcers and topical therapy administered as needed.

Cationic Detergents

Exposure to cationic detergents may result in local corrosive tissue injury as well as severe systemic effects. All species are susceptible. Cats are at increased risk of oral exposure due to grooming habits.

Etiology: Cationic detergents are present in a variety of algaecides, germicides (including quaternary ammonium compounds), sanitizers, fabric softeners (including dryer softener sheets), and liquid potpourris. Concentrations of cationic detergents ≤2% have been associated with oral mucosal ulcers in cats.

Pathogenesis: Cationic detergents are locally corrosive agents, causing dermal, ocular, and mucosal injury similar to that of alkaline corrosive agents. Additionally, exposure to cationic detergents may result in systemic effects ranging from CNS depression to pulmonary edema. The mechanism for these systemic effects is not known.

Clinical Findings and Lesions: Signs of oral exposure include oral ulceration, stomatitis, pharyngitis, hypersalivation, swollen tongue, depression, vomiting, abdominal discomfort, and increased upper respiratory noises within 6-12 hr of ingestion. Affected animals frequently have significant fever and elevations in WBC counts. Systemic effects include metabolic acidosis, CNS depression, hypotension, coma, seizures, muscular weakness and fasciculation, collapse, and pulmonary edema. Dermal irritation, erythema, ulceration, and pain are possible with dermal contact. Conjunctivitis, blepharospasm, eyelid edema, lacrimation, and corneal ulceration may be seen secondary to ocular exposure. Lesions can include GI, ocular, or dermal irritation or ulceration.

Treatment: Systemic signs should be treated symptomatically, eg, diazepam (0.5-2.0 mg/kg, slow IV) for seizures, fluid therapy for hypotension, etc. Due to the potential for corrosive mucosal injury, induction of emesis and administration of activated charcoal are contraindicated with cationic detergents. For recent oral exposures, milk or water can be given for dilution and the animal monitored for development of oral or esophageal burns. Oral burns should be treated the same as other corrosive injuries (*see* above). Dermal and ocular exposures should be managed by thorough flushing of the affected area with tepid water or physiologic saline, followed by monitoring for development of dermal or ocular irritation or ulceration. Topical treatment for dermal or ocular burns should be instituted as needed; in severe cases analgesics may be indicated.

DETERGENTS, SOAPS, AND SHAMPOOS

Exposures to products containing anionic and nonionic detergents generally cause mild GI irritation that responds well to symptomatic care. All animals are susceptible.

Etiology: Mild detergents, soaps, and shampoos contain anionic and nonionic detergents; products included in this group include human and pet shampoos, liquid hand dishwashing soaps, bar bath soaps (except homemade soaps, which may contain lye), many laundry detergents, and many household all-purpose cleaners. Most are of moderate pH, but agents with pH >11 (eg, electric dishwasher detergents) are alkaline corrosives and should be treated as such (*see* above).

Pathogenesis: Anionic and nonionic detergents are mild irritants; many have been pH adjusted to have minimal dermal irritation, although ocular and mucosal irritation is possible. There is no appreciable systemic absorption of these agents, and toxicity is limited to ocular, oral, or GI irritation, which is usually mild and self-limiting.

Clinical Findings: Nausea, vomiting, and diarrhea are the most common signs. Secondary dehydration and electrolyte imbalance may develop in rare instances secondary to protracted vomiting or diarrhea. Mild ocular irritation is possible, with lacrimation and blepharospasm. No significant lesions beyond mild local irritation are seen.

Treatment: Dilution with milk or water may reduce the risk of spontaneous vomiting. Vomiting is usually self-limiting and responds to short periods of food and water restriction. In severe cases or in animals with sensitive stomachs, antiemetics may be required (eg, metoclopramide, 0.2-0.4 mg/kg, PO, SC, or IM, QID). Rarely, parenteral fluid therapy is required to correct electrolyte or hydration abnormalities due to protracted vomiting or diarrhea. For ocular exposures, irrigation of eyes using tepid water or physiologic saline for 5 min will usually suffice.

INSECTICIDE AND ACARICIDE (ORGANIC) TOXICITY

Pesticide labels must carry warnings against use on unapproved species or under untested circumstances. These warnings may pertain to acute or chronic toxicity, or to residues in meat, milk, or other animal products. Because labels change to meet current government regulations, it is important that label directions accompanying the product *always* be read and followed.

Each exposure, no matter how brief or small, results in some of the compound being absorbed and perhaps stored. Repeated short exposures may eventually result in intoxication. Every precaution should be taken to minimize human exposure. This may include frequent changes of clothing with bathing at each change, or if necessary, the use of respirators, rain gear, and gloves impervious to pesticides. Respirators must have filters approved for the type of insecticide being used (eg, ordinary dust filters will not protect the operator from phosphorous fumes). Such measures are generally sufficient to guard against intoxication. Overexposure to chlorinated hydrocarbon insecticides is difficult to measure except by the occurrence of signs of poisoning.

The cholinesterase-inhibiting property of organophosphates may be used to indicate degree of exposure if the activity of the blood enzyme is determined frequently. In humans, serum esterase is usually inhibited first and, in the absence of declining RBC activity, indicates a recent exposure of only moderate degree. Depression of the RBC-enzyme activity indicates a more severe acute exposure or chronic exposure. (Normal cholinesterase activity values vary a great deal in unexposed individuals, and a determination of activity has significance only when compared with the normal value for that individual.)

In addition to their effects on humans, organic pesticides may have deleterious effects on fish and wildlife as well as on domestic species. In no event should amounts greater than those specifically recommended be used, and maximum precautions should be taken to prevent drift or drainage to adjoining fields, pastures, ponds, streams, or other premises outside the treatment area.

The safety and exposure level of these compounds in target species has been carefully established, and application recommendations and regulations must be followed. Individuals, including veterinarians, have been prosecuted for failure to follow label directions or to heed label warnings and for failure to warn animal owners of the necessary precautions.

An ideal insecticide or acaricide should be efficacious without risk to livestock or persons making the application and without leaving residues in tissues, eggs, or milk. Few compounds satisfy all these requirements.

Poisoning by organic insecticides and acaricides may be caused by direct application, by ingestion of contaminated feed or forage treated for controlling of plant parasites, or by accidental exposure. This discussion is limited to only those insecticides or acaricides most frequently hazardous to livestock or likely to leave residues in animal products.

Chemical synthesis rarely yields 100% of the product of interest, and normally there are, in variable proportions, structurally related compounds that have biologic effects different from the compound sought. A prime example is tetrachlorodiphenylethane (TDE or "Rhothane," also called DDD): the p,p'-isomer is an effective insecticide of low toxicity for most mammals; the o,p'-isomer causes necrosis of the adrenal glands of humans and dogs and is used to treat certain adrenal malfunctions.

Products stored under temperature extremes or held in partially emptied containers for long periods may deteriorate. Storing a chemical in anything but the original container is hazardous as in time its identity may be forgotten. Accidental contact with animals or humans may then have disastrous consequences. Consumer-mixed and unapproved combinations can be very dangerous and should never be used.

A number of carbamate and organophosphate insecticides that bind serine esterases (eg, carbaryl, dichlorvos, methiocarb, carbofuran, paraoxon, mevinophos, aldicarb, and monocrotophos) are also immunotoxic. Impaired macrophage signalling through interleukin I and II appears to be involved, and the insecticide levels that cause this effect are very low. This can lead to subtle but damaging influences on the health of exposed animals.

CARBAMATE INSECTICIDES

Carbaryl: The oral LD_{50} in rats is 307 mg/kg body wt and >500 mg/kg, dermally. A 2% spray is nontoxic to calves; 4% is nontoxic to mature cattle when applied dermally.

Carbofuran: The oral LD_{50} is 8 mg/kg body wt in rats and 19 mg/kg in dogs. The minimum toxic dose in cattle and sheep is 4.5 mg/kg, becoming lethal at 18 and 9 mg/kg, respectively. Pigs have been poisoned after drinking water contaminated by this compound.

Methomyl: The oral LD_{50} in rats is 17 mg/kg body wt. Cattle have been reported to be poisoned after consumption of forage inadvertently sprayed with this compound.

Propoxur: The oral LD_{50} is 95 mg/kg body wt in rats and >800 mg/kg in goats.

Clinical Findings: The carbamate insecticides act similarly to the organophosphates (p 2398) in that they inhibit cholinesterase at nerve junctions. However, the inhibiting bond is much less durable, and frequently the inhibition of blood esterase is not evident at the laboratory because of this reversibility. Signs include hypersalivation, GI hypermotility, abdominal cramping, vomiting, diarrhea, sweating, dyspnea, cyanosis, miosis, muscle fasciculations (in extreme cases, tetany followed by weakness and paralysis), and convulsions. Death usually results from hypoxia due to bronchoconstriction and pulmonary edema.

Diagnosis: This usually depends on history of exposure to a particular carbamate and response to atropine therapy. However, when a history of carbamate poisoning is not provided, but cholinergic signs and a clear positive response to atropine suggest carbamate or organophosphate poisoning, cholinesterase levels should be determined in serum, RBC, or brain tissue and, if lowered, will be confirmatory. Screening GI contents for carbamate insecticides may be helpful.

Treatment: Treatment of carbamate poisoning is similar to that of organophosphate poisoning in that atropine sulfate injections readily reverse the effects. Recommended dosages for atropine are as follows: dogs and cats—dosed to effect (repeated as needed), usually 0.2-2 mg/kg, parenterally, one-fourth of the dose given IV and the remainder given SC (cats should be dosed at the lower end of the range); cattle and sheep—0.6-1 mg/kg, one-fourth of the dose IV and the remainder SC, repeated as needed; horses and pigs—0.1-0.2 mg/kg, IV, repeated as needed.

Pralidoxime (2-PAM) has been used to treat carbamate poisoning but its value is controversial. Poisoning may be caused by a mixture of organophosphates and carbamate, and 2-PAM may be beneficial. Signs of excessive cholinergic activity may warrant its use, in case the cause is organophosphate exposure. 2-PAM administration can be fatal if given too rapidly; it must be given slowly (ie, in 5% saline over a 10-min period). *See also* ORGANOPHOSPHATES, p 2398.

CHLORINATED HYDROCARBON COMPOUNDS

Due to tissue residues and chronic toxicity, use of these agents is drastically curtailed. Only lindane and methoxychlor are approved for use on or around livestock. Nevertheless, in a recent surveillance study, 51% of the cattle (mainly originating from Colorado) had detectable residues of chlorinated hydrocarbon insecticides including heptachlor, heptachlor epoxide, lindane, and oxychlordane.

Aldrin is a potent insecticide similar to dieldrin with the same order of toxicity (*see* below). It is no longer registered in the USA but was used for termite control.

Benzene hexachloride (BHC, hexachlorocyclohexane) was a useful insecticide for large animals and dogs but is highly toxic to cats in the concentrations necessary for parasite control. Only the γ isomer (lindane) is a useful insecticidal agent; the other isomers are stored for excessively long periods in body tissues. Lindane, which contains >99% of the γ isomer, should be used in preference to the technical grade of BHC, which contains several isomers.

Cattle in good condition have tolerated 0.2% lindane applications, but stressed, emaciated cattle have been poisoned from spraying or dipping in 0.075% lindane. Horses and pigs appear to tolerate 0.2-0.5%, and sheep and goats ordinarily tolerate 0.5% applications. Emaciation and lactation increase the susceptibility of animals to poisoning by lindane; such animals should be treated with extreme caution. Young calves are very susceptible to lindane and are poisoned by a single oral dose of 4.4 mg/kg body wt. Mild signs appear in sheep given 22 mg/kg, and death occurs at 100 mg/kg. Adult cattle have tolerated 13 mg/kg without signs. BHC is stored in body fat and excreted in milk.

Chlordane is no longer registered as an insecticide in the USA. Exposure occurs when livestock consume treated plants or when they come in direct contact through carelessness and accidents. Very young calves have been killed by doses of 44 mg/kg, and the minimum toxic dose for cattle is ~88 mg/kg. Cattle fed chlordane at 25 ppm of their diet for 56 days showed 19 ppm in their fat at the end of the feeding. Topical emulsions and suspensions have been used safely on dogs at concentrations up to 0.25%, provided freshly diluted materials were used; dry powders up to 5% have been safe. The no effect level in dogs in a 2-yr feeding study was 3 mg/kg. Pigeons and Leghorn cockerels and pullets suffered no effects after 1-2 mo exposure to vapors emanating from chlordane-treated surfaces.

Dieldrin is not a registered pesticide in the USA. Residues limit its application, and it is one of the most toxic chlorinated hydrocarbon insecticides. Young dairy calves are poisoned by 8.8 mg/kg body wt, PO, but tolerate 4.4 mg/kg, while adult cattle tolerate 8.8 mg/kg and are poisoned by 22 mg/kg. Pigs tolerate 22 mg/kg and are poisoned by 44 mg/kg. Horses are poisoned by 22 mg/kg. Because of its effectiveness against insect pests on crops and pasture and the low dosage per acre, dieldrin is not likely to poison livestock grazing the treated areas. Diets containing 25 ppm of dieldrin have been fed to cattle and sheep for 16 wk without harmful effects other than residues in fat, which are slow to disappear. Great care must be exercised in marketing animals that have grazed treated areas or consumed products from previously treated areas. There is a zero tolerance level for residues in edible tissues.

Statements pertaining to dieldrin also apply, in general, to **endrin**, the most toxic of the 3 chlorinated cyclodiene insecticides.

Heptachlor is not currently registered in the USA and is not recommended for use on livestock in the USA. Because it is very effective against certain plant-feeding insects, it is encountered from time to time in some geographic areas grazed by livestock. Young dairy calves tolerate dosages as high as 13 mg/kg body wt but are poisoned by 22 mg/kg. Sheep tolerate 22 mg/kg but are poisoned by 40 mg/kg. Diets containing 60 ppm of heptachlor have been fed to cattle for 16 wk without harmful effects other than residues in fat. Heptachlor is converted to heptachlor epoxide by animals and stored in body fat. For this reason, a specific analysis performed for heptachlor usually yields negative results, while that for epoxide is positive.

Methoxychlor is one of the safest chlorinated hydrocarbon insecticides and one of the few with active registration in the USA. Young dairy calves tolerate 265 mg/kg body wt; 500 mg/kg is mildly toxic. While 1 g/kg produces rather severe poisoning in young calves, sheep are not affected. One dog was given 990 mg/kg daily for 30 days without showing signs. Six applications to cattle of a 0.5% spray at 3-wk intervals produces fat residues of 2.4 ppm; ~0.4 ppm of methoxychlor is found in milk 1 day after spraying a cow with a 0.5% concentration. Methoxychlor sprays are not approved for use on animals producing milk for human consumption. Cattle and sheep store essentially no methoxychlor when fed 25 ppm in the total diet for 112 days. If methoxychlor is used as recommended, the established tolerance in fat will not be exceeded. Commercial products are available for garden, orchard, and field crops and for horses and ponies.

Numerous reports suggest that methoxychlor has negative reproductive effects in laboratory animal experiments, but this has not been seen in the field.

Toxaphene is no longer under active registration in the USA. It has been used with reasonable safety if recommendations were followed, but it can cause poisoning when applied or ingested in excessive quantities. Dogs and cats are particularly susceptible. Young calves have been poisoned by 1% toxaphene sprays, while all other farm animals except poultry can withstand 1% or more as sprays or dips. Chickens have been poisoned by dipping in 0.1% emulsions, and turkeys have been poisoned by spraying with 0.5% material. Toxaphene is primarily an acute toxicant and does not persist long in the tissues. Adult cattle have been mildly intoxicated by 4% sprays and severely affected by 8%. Adult cattle have been poisoned from being dipped in emulsions that contained only 0.5% toxaphene (an amount ordinarily safe) because the emulsions had begun to break down, allowing the fine droplets to coalesce into larger droplets that readily adhere to the hair of cattle. The resultant dosage becomes equivalent to that obtained by spray treatments of much higher concentrations. Toxaphene is lethal to young calves at 8.8 mg/kg body wt but not at 4.4 mg/kg. The minimum toxic dose for cattle is ~33 mg/kg, and for sheep between 22 and 33 mg/kg. Spraying Hereford cattle 12 times at 2-wk intervals with 0.5% toxaphene produced a maximum residue of 8 ppm in fat. Cattle fed 10 ppm of toxaphene in the diet for 30 days had no detectable toxaphene tissue residues, while steers fed 100 ppm for 112 days stored only 40 ppm in their fat (this amount was eliminated 2 mo after the toxaphene was discontinued).

Clinical Findings: The chlorinated hydrocarbon insecticides are general CNS stimulants. They produce a great variety of signs—the most obvious are neuromuscular tremors and convulsions—and there may be obvious behavioral changes common to other poisonings and CNS infections. Body temperature may be very high. Affected animals are generally first noted to be more alert or apprehensive. Muscle fasciculation occurs, becoming visible in the facial region and extending backward until the whole body is involved. Large doses of DDT, DDD, and methoxychlor cause progressive involvement leading to trembling or shivering, followed by convulsions and death. With the other chlorinated hydrocarbons, the muscular twitchings are followed by convulsions, usually without the intermediate trembling. Convulsions may be continuous, clonic, or tonic lasting from a few seconds to several hours, or intermittent and leading to the animal becoming comatose. High fever may accompany convulsions, particularly in warm environments. Behavioral changes such as abnormal postures (eg, resting the sternum on the ground while remaining upright in the rear, keeping the head down between the forelegs, "head pressing" against a wall or fence, or continual chewing movements) may be seen. Occasionally, an affected animal becomes belligerent and attacks other animals, people, or moving objects. Vocalization is common. Some animals are depressed, almost oblivious to their surroundings, and do not eat or drink; they may last longer than those showing more violent symptoms. Usually, there is a copious flow of thick saliva and urinary incontinence. In certain cases, the clinical signs alternate, with the animal first being extremely excited, then severely depressed. The severity of the signs seen at a given time is not a sure prognostic index. Some animals have only a single convulsion and die, while others suffer innumerable convulsions but subsequently recover. Animals showing acute excitability often have a fever >106°F (41°C). The signs of poisoning by these insecticides are highly suggestive but not diagnostic; other poisons and encephalitis or meningitis must be considered.

Signs of acute intoxication by chlordane in birds are nervous chirping, excitability, collapse on hocks or side, and mucous exudates in the nasal passages. Signs of subacute and chronic intoxication are molting, dehydration and cyanosis of the comb, weight loss, and cessation of egg production.

Lesions: If death has occurred suddenly, there may be nothing more than cyanosis. More definite lesions occur as the duration of intoxication increases. Usually, there is congestion of various organs (particularly the lungs, liver, and kidneys) and a blanched appearance of all organs if the body temperature was high before death. The heart generally stops in systole, and there may be many hemorrhages of varying size on the epicardium. The appearance of the heart and lungs may suggest a peracute pneumonia and, if the animal was affected for more than a few hours, there may be pulmonary edema. The trachea and bronchi may contain a blood-tinged froth. In many cases, the CSF volume is excessive, and the brain and spinal cord frequently are congested and edematous.

Diagnosis: Chemical analysis of brain, liver, kidney, fat, and stomach or rumen contents is necessary to confirm the poisoning. The suspected source, if identified, should also be analyzed. Brain levels of the insecticide are the most useful. Whole blood, serum, and urine from live animals may be analyzed to evaluate exposure in the rest of the herd or flock. In food animal poisoning, if exposure is more than just the animals visibly affected, fat biopsies from survivors may be necessary to estimate the potential residue.

Treatment: There are no known specific antidotes. When exposure is by spraying, dipping, or dusting, a thorough bathing without irritating the skin (no brushes), using detergents and copious quantities of cool water is recommended. If exposure is by ingestion, gastric lavage and saline purgatives are indicated. The use of digestible oils such as corn oil is contraindicated; however, heavy-grade mineral oil plus a purgative hastens the removal of the chemical from the intestine. Activated charcoal appears to be useful in preventing absorption from the GI tract. When signs are excitatory, a sedative anticonvulsant such as a barbiturate or diazepam is indicated. Anything in the environment that stresses the animal—noise, handling etc—should be reduced or removed if possible. If the animal shows marked depression, anorexia, and dehydration, therapy should be directed toward rehydration and nourishment either IV or by stomach tube. Residues in exposed animals may be reduced by giving a slurry of activated charcoal or providing charcoal in feed. Feeding phenobarbital, 5 g/day, may hasten residue removal.

INSECTICIDES DERIVED FROM PLANTS

Most insecticides derived from plants (eg, derris [rotenone] and pyrethrum) have traditionally been considered safe for use on animals. **Nicotine** in the form of nicotine sulfate is an exception. Unless it is carefully used, poisoning may result. Affected animals show tremors, incoordination, nausea, and disturbed respiration, and finally coma and death. Necropsy lesions include pale mucous membranes, dark blood, hemorrhages on the heart and in the lungs, and congestion of the brain. Treatment consists of removing the material by washing or by gastric lavage with tannic acid, administering activated charcoal, providing artificial respiration, and treating for cardiac arrest and shock. Mildly affected animals recover rapidly and spontaneously.

Pyrethrins: This is a closely related group of naturally occurring compounds that are the active insecticidal ingredients of pyrethrum. Pyrethrum is extracted from the flowers of *Chrysanthemum cinerariaefolium* and has been an effective insecticide for many years. Synergists, such as piperonyl butoxide, sesamex, piperonyl cyclonene, etc, are added to increase stability and effectiveness. This is accomplished by inhibiting mixed function oxidases, enzymes that destroy pyrethrum; unfortunately, this also potentiates mammalian toxicity.

Pyrethroids: These are synthetic derivatives of natural pyrethrins and include allethrin, cypermethrin, decamethrin, fenvalerate, fluvalinate, permethrin, and tetramethrin. Generally, these compounds are more effective and less toxic to mammals than natural pyrethrins; they appear to be not well absorbed from the skin (however, allergic manifestations through skin contact and inhalation are common in humans). Mildly affected animals as well as those in early stages of toxicosis often show hypersalivation, vomiting, diarrhea, mild tremors, hyperexcitability, or depression. This syndrome may be confused with organophosphate or carbamate toxicosis. More severely affected animals can have hyperthermia, hypothermia, dyspnea, severe tremors, disorientation, and seizures. Death is due to respiratory failure. Clinical signs usually begin within a few hours of exposure, but the onset may be altered by the rate of dermal absorption or the timing of grooming behavior.

Generally, treatment is not required after ingestion of a dilute pyrethrin or pyrethroid preparations. Because the chief hazard may be the solvent, induction of emesis may be contraindicated. A slurry of activated charcoal at 2-8 g/kg may be administered, followed by a saline cathartic (magnesium or sodium sulfate [10% solution] at 0.5 mg/kg). Vegetable oils and fats, which promote the intestinal absorption of pyrethrum, should be avoided. If dermal exposure occurs, the animal should be bathed with a mild detergent and cool water. The area should be washed very gently so as not to stimulate the circulation and enhance skin absorption. Initial assessment of the animal's respiratory and cardiovascular integrity is important. Further treatment involves symptomatic and supportive care. Seizures should be controlled with either diazepam (administered to effect at 0.2-2 mg/kg, IV) or methocarbamol (55-220 mg/kg, IV, not exceeding 200 mg/min). Phenobarbital or pentobarbital (IV), to effect, can be used if diazepam or methocarbamol are too short acting.

d-Limonene: This is used for the control of fleas on cats and for other insect pests. Adult fleas and eggs appear to be most sensitive to d-limonene, which is more effective if combined with piperonyl butoxide. At recommended dosages, the solution containing d-limonene appears to be safe, but increasing the concentration 5-10 fold in sprays or dips increases the severity of toxic signs, which include salivation, muscle tremors, ataxia, and hypothermia. The inclusion of piperonyl butoxide in the formulation potentiates the toxicity in cats. Allergies have also been reported in people in contact with d-limonene, and it appears to increase dermal absorption of some chemicals. When orally administered to dogs, d-limonene causes vomiting (median effective dose 1.6 mL/kg).

ORGANOPHOSPHATES

Organophosphates (OP) have replaced the banned organochlorine compounds and are a major cause of animal poisoning. They vary greatly in toxicity, residue levels, and excretion. Many OP have been developed for plant and animal protection, and in general, they offer a distinct advantage by producing little tissue and environmental residue.

Many of the OP now used as pesticides are not potent inhibitors of esterases until activated in the liver by microsomal oxidation enzymes; they are generally less toxic, and intoxication occurs more slowly. Certain OP preparations are microencapsulated, and the active compound is released slowly; this increases the duration of activity and reduces their toxicity, but the toxic properties are still present. (*See also* p 2393.)

Organophosphate Insecticides with Active EPA Registration (as of 2002)

Azinphos-methyl (or -ethyl): The maximum nontoxic oral dose is 0.44 mg/kg body wt for calves, 2.2 mg/kg for cattle and goats, and 4.8 mg/kg for sheep.

Chlorpyrifos: The oral LD_{50} is 500 mg/kg body wt in goats and 97 mg/kg in rats. In comparison with calves, steers, and cows, bulls (particularly of the exotic breeds) are highly susceptible to a single dose of chlorpyrifos.

Coumaphos: Coumaphos is used against cattle grubs and a number of other ectoparasites and for treatment of premises. The maximum concentration that may be safely used on adult cattle, horses, and pigs is 0.5%. Young calves and all ages of sheep and goats must not be sprayed with concentrations >0.25%; 0.5% concentrations may be lethal. Adult cattle may show mild toxicity at 1% concentrations.

Diazinon: Young calves appear to tolerate 0.05% spray but are poisoned by 0.1% concentrations. Adult cattle may be sprayed at weekly intervals with 0.1% concentrations without inducing poisoning. Young calves tolerate 0.44 mg/kg body wt, PO, but are poisoned by 0.88 mg/kg. Cattle tolerate 8.8 mg/kg, PO, but are poisoned by 22 mg/kg. Sheep tolerate 17.6 mg/kg but are poisoned by 26 mg/kg.

Dichlorvos: Dichlorvos has many uses on both plants and animals. It is rapidly metabolized and excreted, and residues in meat and milk are not a problem if label directions are followed. It is of moderate toxicity, with a minimum toxic dose of 10 mg/kg body wt in young calves and 25 mg/kg in horses and sheep. The LD_{50} in rats is 25-80 mg/kg, PO. A 1% dust was not toxic to cattle. Flea collars containing dichlorvos may cause skin reactions in some pets.

Dimethoate: When administered PO, the minimum toxic dose for young dairy calves was ~48 mg/kg body wt, while 22 mg/kg was lethal for cattle 1 yr old. Daily doses of 10 mg/kg for 5 days in adult cattle lowered blood cholinesterase activity to 20% of normal but did not produce poisoning. Horses have been poisoned by doses of 60-80 mg/kg, PO. When applied topically, 1% sprays have been tolerated by calves, cattle, and adult sheep.

Disulfoton: The maximum nontoxic oral dose is 0.88 mg/kg body wt for young calves, 2.2 mg/kg for cattle and goats, and 4.8 mg/kg for sheep. Poisoning has occurred in cattle after consuming harvested forages previously sprayed with this insecticide.

Fenthion: Minimum toxic dose, PO, is 25 mg/kg body wt for cattle; 50 mg/kg is lethal to sheep.

Malathion: Malathion is one of the safest organophosphates. Young calves tolerate 0.5% but not 1% sprays; adult cattle tolerate 2% sprays. Given PO, it is toxic at 100 mg/kg but not 55 mg/kg body wt; young calves tolerate 11 mg/kg but are poisoned by 22 mg/kg. Malathion is excreted in cow's milk.

Methyl Parathion: The LD_{50} in rats from a single oral dose is 9-25 mg/kg body wt compared with 3-13 mg/kg for ethyl parathion. Microencapsulation of this compound decreases its toxicity, and the lethal dose in cattle has been increased from a 0.5% to a 2% spray.

Naled: The oral LD_{50} in rats is 430 mg/kg body wt.

Oxydemeton-methyl: The maximum nontoxic oral dose is 0.88 mg/kg body wt for young calves, 2.2 mg/kg for cattle, and 4.8 mg/kg for sheep and goats.

Parathion: Parathion (diethyl parathion) is widely used for control of plant pests and is approximately one-half as toxic as TEPP (*see* below). It is used as a dip and spray for cattle in some countries (not in the USA). Most cases of occupational insecticide poisonings in humans have been attributed to parathion or its degradation products. As a 0.02% spray, it produces signs of poisoning in young calves and occasional transitory signs at 0.01%. Parathion is lethal to sheep at 22 mg/kg body wt, PO, but not at 11 mg/kg. Young dairy calves are poisoned by 0.44 mg/kg, while 44 mg/kg is required to poison older cattle. Parathion is used extensively to control mosquitos and insects in orchards and on market garden crops. Normally, because so little is used per acre, it presents no hazard to livestock. However, because of its potency, care should be taken to prevent accidental exposure. Parathion does not produce significant residues in animal tissues.

Phorate: The minimum toxic dose PO is 0.25 mg/kg body wt in calves, 0.75 mg/kg in sheep, and 1 mg/kg in cattle.

Phosmet: The minimum oral toxic dose PO is 25 mg/kg body wt in cattle and calves and 50 mg/kg in sheep.

Temephos: The oral LD_{50} for rats is 1 g (or more)/kg body wt, while the dermal LD_{50} is >4 g/kg.

Tetrachlorvinphos: Tetrachlorvinphos has low toxicity in dogs; chronic feeding studies indicate the lowest effect level (LEL) was 50 mg/kg/day and the no observed effect level (NOEL) 3.13 mg/kg/day. The minimum toxic dose in pigs is 100 mg/kg.

Trichlorfon: As a spray, trichlorfon at a 1% concentration is tolerated by adult cattle; given PO, it is tolerated by young dairy calves at 4.4 mg/kg body wt but produces poisoning at 8.8 mg/kg. Adult cattle, sheep, and horses appear to tolerate 44 mg/kg, while 88 mg/kg produces poisoning. Dogs were unaffected when fed 1,000 ppm of trichlorfon for 4 mo. Trichlorfon is metabolized rapidly.

Organophosphate Insecticides with No Active EPA Registration (as of 2002)

Carbophenothion: Dairy calves <2 wk of age sprayed with water-based formulations showed poisoning at 0.05% or higher concentrations, and adult cattle were poisoned by spraying with 1%. Sheep and goats have been poisoned by 22 mg/kg body wt, PO, but not by 8 mg/kg. The LD_{50} for rats is ~31 mg/kg; a daily dosage of 2.2 mg/kg for 90 days produced poisoning. Dogs tolerated a diet containing 32 ppm for 90 days.

Chlorfenvinphos: Adult cattle were poisoned by 5% or higher sprays, while young calves were poisoned only when the concentration was raised to 2%. The minimum oral toxic dose appears to be ~22 mg/kg for cattle of all ages. The acute oral LD_{50} for rats is 10-39 mg/kg.

Crotoxyphos: Crotoxyphos is of rather low toxicity; however, Brahman cattle are markedly more susceptible than European breeds. Cattle (except as above), sheep, goats, and pigs all tolerate sprays containing crotoxyphos at 0.5% levels or higher. Toxic doses appears to be in the 2% range, except for in Brahman cattle, in which 0.144%-0.3% may be toxic.

Demeton: The oral LD_{50} is 8 mg/kg body wt in goats and 2 mg/kg in rats; the dermal LD_{50} in rats is 8 mg/kg.

Dioxathion: Dioxathion is a mixture of cis- and trans-isomers (70%) and reaction products (30%). Used on both plants and animals, it is rapidly metabolized and not likely to produce residues in meat greater than the 1 ppm official tolerance. Concentrations of 0.15% or greater are generally used on animals. The minimum toxic dose in calves is 5 mg/kg body wt. Sprays of 0.5% in cattle and sheep or 0.25% in goats and pigs are nontoxic. Dioxathion at 8.8 mg/kg, PO, has killed young calves, and it produced intoxication at 4.4 mg/kg.

EPN: EPN is related to parathion (*see* above) and is about one-half as toxic when applied externally; when given PO, it is about equally toxic. Dogs were not poisoned at doses >100 mg/kg.

Famphur: The maximum nontoxic dose is 10 mg/kg body wt in calves and 50 mg/kg in cattle, sheep, and horses. This compound is effective against warbles in cattle, but (as for all grubicides) directions must be followed as to time of application; larvae killed while migrating and the resultant local reaction can cause serious problems.

Mevinphos: The LD_{50} in rats is 3 mg/kg body wt, PO or topically.

Ronnel (Fenchlorphos): Ronnel produces mild signs of poisoning in cattle at 132 mg/kg body wt, but severe signs do not appear until the dosage is >400 mg/kg. The minimum toxic dose in sheep is 400 mg/kg. Concentrations as high as 2.5% in sprays have failed to produce poisoning of cattle, young dairy calves, or sheep. Poisoning usually occurs in 2 stages. The animal first becomes weak and, although able to move about normally, may be placid. Diarrhea, often flecked with blood, may also be seen. Salivation and dyspnea then appear if the dose was high enough. Blood cholinesterase activity declines slowly over 5-7 days. Ronnel produces residues in meat and milk; strict adherence to label restrictions is essential. The residues may be removed by giving the animal activated charcoal for several days.

Ruelene: Ruelene is active both as a systemic and contact insecticide in livestock, has some anthelmintic activity, and has rather low toxicity. Dairy calves have been poisoned by 44 mg/kg body wt, PO, while adult cattle require 88 mg/kg for the same effect. Sheep are moderately intoxicated by 176 mg/kg; Angora goats are about twice as sensitive. Pigs have been poisoned by 11 mg/kg and horses by 44 mg/kg. Most livestock tolerate a 2% topical spray.

Terbufos: This soil insecticide is used to control corn rootworms. The minimum oral toxic dose is ~1.5 mg/kg body wt for sheep and cattle. Cases of intoxication in cattle have occurred. Ingestion of 7.5 mg/kg was lethal to heifers.

Tetraethyl Pyrophosphate (TEPP): TEPP is one of the most acutely toxic insecticides. Although not used on animals, accidental exposure occurs occasionally. One herd of 29 cattle (including calves and adults) was accidentally sprayed with 0.33% TEPP emulsion; all died within 40 min.

Clinical Findings: In general, OP pesticides have a narrow margin of safety, and the dose-response curve is quite steep. Signs of OP poisoning are those of cholinergic overstimulation, which can be grouped under 3 categories: muscarinic, nicotinic, and central. Muscarinic signs, which are usually first to appear, include hypersalivation, miosis, frequent urination, diarrhea, vomiting, colic, and dyspnea due to increased bronchial secretions and bronchoconstriction. Nicotinic effects include muscle fasciculations and weakness. The central effects include nervousness, ataxia, apprehension, and seizures. Cattle and sheep commonly show severe depression. CNS stimulation in dogs and cats usually progresses to convulsions. Some OP (eg, amidothioates) do not enter the brain easily, so that CNS signs are mild. Onset of signs after exposure is usually within hours but may be delayed for >2 days. Severity and course of intoxication are influenced principally by the dosage and route of exposure. In acute poisoning, the primary clinical signs may be respiratory distress and collapse followed by death due to respiratory muscle paralysis.

Diagnosis: An important diagnostic aid is the cholinesterase activity in blood and brain. Unfortunately, the depression of blood cholinesterase does not necessarily correlate with the severity of poisoning; signs are seen when nerve cholinesterase is inhibited, and the enzyme in blood reflects, only in a general way, the levels in nervous tissue. The key factor appears to be the rate at which the enzyme activity is reduced. Analyses performed after exposure may be negative because OP do not remain long in tissues as the parent compound. Chlorinated OP compounds have greater potential for tissue residue. Frozen stomach and rumen samples should be analyzed for the pesticide because OP are generally more stable in acids.

Lesions: Animals with acute OP poisoning have nonspecific or no lesions. Pulmonary edema and congestion, hemorrhages, and edema of the bowel and other organs may be found. Animals surviving >1 day may become emaciated and dehydrated.

Treatment: Three categories of drugs are used to treat OP poisoning: 1) muscarinic blocking agents, 2) cholinesterase reactivators, and 3) emetics, cathartics, and adsorbants to decrease further absorption. Atropine sulfate blocks the central and peripheral muscarinic effects of OP; it is administered to effect in dogs and cats, usually at a dosage of 0.2-2 mg/kg body wt (cats are dosed at the lower end of the range), every 3-6 hr or as often as clinical signs indicate. For horses and pigs, the dosage is 0.1-0.2 mg/kg, IV, repeated every 10 min as needed; for cattle and sheep, the dosage is 0.6-1 mg/kg, one-third given IV, the remainder IM or SC, and repeated as needed. Atropinization is adequate when the pupils are dilated, salivation ceases, and the animal appears more alert. Animals initially respond well to atropine sulfate; however, the response diminishes after repeated treatments. Overtreatment with atropine should be avoided. Atropine does not alleviate the nicotinic cholinergic effects, such as muscle fasciculations and muscle paralysis, so that death from massive overdoses of OP can still occur. Including diazepam in the treatment reduced the incidence of seizures and increased survival of nonhuman primates experimentally.

Using barbiturates to treat the convulsions must be done very carefully, as they seem to be potentiated by anticholinesterases.

An improved treatment combines atropine with the cholinesterase-reactivating oxime, 2-pyridine aldoxime methchloride (2-PAM, pralidoxime chloride). The dosage of 2-PAM is 20-50 mg/kg body wt, given as a 5% solution IM or by slow IV (over 5-10 min), repeated as needed. IV 2-PAM must be given very slowly to avoid musculoskeletal paralysis and respiratory arrest. Response to cholinesterase reactivators decreases with time after exposure; therefore, treatment with oximes must be instituted as soon as possible (within 24-48 hr). The rate at which the enzyme/organophosphate complex becomes unresponsive to activators varies with the particular pesticide.

Removal of the poison from the animal also should be attempted. If exposure was dermal, the animal should be washed with detergent and water (about room temperature) but without scrubbing and irritating the skin. Emesis should be induced if oral exposure occurred <2 hr previously; emesis is contraindicated if the animal is depressed. Oral administration of mineral oil decreases absorption of pesticide from the GI tract. Activated charcoal (3-6 g/kg as a water slurry) adsorbs OP and helps elimination in the feces. This is particularly recommended in cattle. Continued absorption of OP from the large amount of ingesta in the rumen has caused prolonged toxicosis in cattle. Artificial respiration or administration of oxygen may be required. Phenothiazine tranquilizers should be avoided, as well as the xanthine stimulants theophylline and aminophylline. Succinylcholine should not be used for at least 10 days after OP exposure.

Delayed Neurotoxicity from Triaryl Phosphates

For some time, compounds known as triaryl phosphates (eg, triosthocresyl phosphate) have been used as flame retardants, plasticizers, lubricating oils, and hydraulic fluids. They are weak cholinesterase inhibitors, but do inhibit "neurotoxic esterase," located in the brain and spinal cord. A form of delayed neurotoxicity results from the inhibition of neurotoxic esterase. Triaryl phosphates have caused accidental poisonings in humans and other species (mostly cattle). Some OP insecticides (eg, PEN, leptophos) can also cause delayed neurotoxicity; however, field cases have been rare. The lesions associated with delayed neurotoxicity include demyelination of peripheral and spinal motor tracts due to loss of neurotoxic esterase function. Clinical signs associated with delayed neurotoxicity include muscle weakness and ataxia that progresses to flaccid paralysis of the hindlimbs. Signs are usually not manifest until 8-21 days after exposure to a neurotoxic triaryl phosphate. There are no specific antidotes.

PESTICIDE POTENTIATING AGENTS

Piperonyl butoxide is used as a potentiator in many pesticide formulations including pyrethrins, pyrethroids, and d-limonene. It decreases breakdown of the chemical in the animal or insect's body by inhibiting mixed function oxidase enzymes and makes the pesticide more toxic to the insect—and the host. Animals that are debilitated or have decreased drug metabolizing capability become more susceptible to the pesticide. However, toxins that must be activated in the body to a toxic form are frequently less toxic when piperonyl butoxide exposure occurs at the same time. This effect has been seen in many species, including cats, dogs, rats, humans, etc. Cimetidine, a drug that reduces stomach acid secretion by blocking gastric H_2 receptors, and the antibiotic chloramphenicol have the same effect.

SOLVENTS AND EMULSIFIERS

Solvents and emulsifiers are required in most liquid insecticide preparations. Usually they have low toxicity, but like the petroleum products (which many are), they must be considered as possible causes of poisoning. In direct treatment with pesticides, emulsification must be thorough with an average droplet size of 5 microns (preferably smaller), or excessive amounts may stick to treated animals. Treatment should be as for petroleum product poisoning (p 2430).

Acetone: GI irritation, narcosis, and kidney and liver damage are the main signs. Treatment consists of gastric lavage, oxygen, and a low-fat diet. Additional supportive treatment to alleviate clinical signs may be given.

Isopropyl Alcohol: The signs are GI pain, cramps, vomiting, diarrhea, and CNS depression (dizziness, stupor, coma, death from respiratory paralysis). The liver and kidneys are reversibly affected. Dehydration and pneumonia may occur. Treatment consists of emetics, gastric lavage, milk PO, oxygen, and artificial respiration.

Methanol: Nausea, vomiting, gastric pain, reflex hyperexcitability, opisthotonos, convulsions, fixed pupils, and acute peripheral neuritis are typical. Large overdoses can lead to blindness. Toxic effects are due in part to the alcohol itself, and in part to formic acid produced by its oxidation. Treatment should include emetics (apomorphine) followed by gastric lavage with 4% sodium bicarbonate, saline laxative, oxygen therapy, sodium bicarbonate solution IV, and analgesics; however, the prognosis is poor. Intensive and prolonged alkalinization is the mainstay of treatment. Ethanol retards the oxidation of methanol and may be given as an adjunct therapy.

SULFUR AND LIME-SULFUR

Sulfur and lime-sulfur are 2 of the oldest insecticides. Elemental sulfur is practically devoid of toxicity, although poisoning has occurred occasionally when large amounts were mixed in cattle feed. Specific toxic dosages are not known but probably exceed 4 g/kg body wt. Lime-sulfur, which is a complex of sulfides, may cause irritation, discomfort, or blistering but rarely causes death. Treatment consists of removing residual material and applying bland protective ointments plus any supportive measures that may be indicated.

IRON TOXICITY IN NEWBORN PIGS

Reports of toxicity after SC or IM injection of iron preparations in newborn piglets are sporadic, and the risk is not high; however, toxicity does occur occasionally. In some litters, death occurs quickly from 30 min to 6 hr after injection; in others, death is delayed for 2-4 days. (*See also* NONREGENERATIVE ANEMIAS, p 13.)

Three forms of toxicity may be seen. In the first form, damage to the muscles around the injection site causes potassium, among other substances, to be released; the blood potassium level rises and interferes with the heart's action. Usually, the whole litter is affected. Piglets may appear anemic, become weak, cannot stand, and have muscle tremors followed by convulsions. Respiratory distress may be seen. There is swelling at the injection site. On necropsy, skin and muscles may appear pale, and there is edema and a brownish black discoloration at the injection site. Waxy degeneration of skeletal and heart muscle may be seen; there may be hemorrhages in the heart and necrosis of the liver and kidneys.

In the second, less acute form of toxicity, the excess iron appears to block the body's defense mechanisms by overwhelming the phagocytic cells, which increases the likelihood of infection. Death occurs in ~2-4 days. In young piglets, the most likely infection is an *Escherichia coli* enteritis and, although some of the changes seen in the first form may be seen at necropsy, they are less obvious, and the enteritis contributes markedly to death.

The most important precipitating factor of iron toxicosis in pigs is a low vitamin E or selenium status of the sow. If either nutrient is low in the sow, pigs will either be born deficient in vitamin E or selenium or the colostrum will not be able to provide adequate amounts of these nutrients to nursing pigs to meet their antioxidant needs. Supplementing the sow's diet with 50 IU of vitamin E/kg and 0.15 mg of selenium/kg will improve the status of the sow and prevent iron toxicity in the piglets. Injections of vitamin E/selenium during late gestation may also help prevent iron toxicity in piglets.

A third, more rare form of toxicity is associated with **calciphylaxis**, the massive mobilization of calcium after injection of iron preparations, both in the presence and absence of supplementary vitamin D. It occurs within several days of iron injection and is associated with development of hard swellings at injection sites. Death may occur, and calcification in other parts of the body may be seen at necropsy.

LEAD POISONING

In veterinary medicine, lead poisoning is most common in dogs and cattle. Lead poisoning in other species is limited by reduced accessibility, more selective eating habits, or lower susceptibility. In cattle, many cases are associated with seeding and harvesting activities when used oil and battery disposal from machinery is handled improperly. Other sources of lead include paint, linoleum, grease, lead weights, lead shot, and contaminated foliage growing near smelters or along roadsides. Lead poisoning is also encountered in urban environments, and renovation of old houses that have been painted with lead-based paint has been associated with lead poisoning in small animals and children.

Pathogenesis: Absorbed lead enters the blood and soft tissues and eventually redistributes to the bone. The degree of absorption and retention is influenced by dietary factors such as calcium or iron levels. In ruminants, particulate lead lodged in the reticulum slowly dissolves and releases significant quantities of lead. Lead has a profound effect on sulfhydryl-containing enzymes, the thiol content of erythrocytes, antioxidant defenses, and tissues rich in mitochondria, which is reflected in the clinical syndrome. In addition to the cerebellar hemorrhage and edema associated with capillary damage, lead is also irritating, immunosuppressive, gametotoxic, teratogenic, nephrotoxic, and toxic to the hematopoietic system.

Clinical Findings: Acute lead poisoning is more common in young animals. The prominent clinical signs are associated with the GI and nervous systems. In cattle, signs that appear within 24-48 hr of exposure include ataxia, blindness, salivation, spastic twitching of eyelids, jaw champing, bruxism, muscle tremors, and convulsions.

Subacute lead poisoning, usually seen in sheep or older cattle, is characterized by anorexia, rumen stasis, colic, dullness, and transient constipation, frequently followed by diarrhea, blindness, head pressing, bruxism, hyperesthesia, and incoordination. Chronic lead poisoning, which is occasionally seen in cattle, may produce a syndrome that has many features in common with acute or subacute lead poisoning.

GI abnormalities, including anorexia, colic, emesis, and diarrhea or constipation, may be seen in dogs. Anxiety, hysterical barking, jaw champing, salivation, blindness, ataxia, muscle spasms, opisthotonos, and convulsions may develop. CNS depression rather than CNS excitation may be evident in some dogs.

In horses, lead poisoning usually produces a chronic syndrome characterized by weight loss, depression, weakness, colic, diarrhea, laryngeal or pharyngeal paralysis (roaring), and dysphagia that frequently results in aspiration pneumonia.

In avian species, anorexia, ataxia, loss of condition, wing and leg weakness, and anemia are the most notable signs.

Lesions: Animals that die from acute lead poisoning may have few observable gross lesions. Oil or flakes of paint or battery may be evident in the GI tract. The caustic action of lead salts causes gastroenteritis. In the nervous system, edema, congestion of the cerebral cortex, and flattening of the cortical gyri are present. Histologically, endothelial swelling, laminar cortical necrosis, and edema of the white matter may be evident. Tubular necrosis and degeneration and intranuclear acid-fast inclusion bodies may be seen in the kidneys. Osteoporosis has been described in lambs. Placentitis and accumulation of lead in the fetus may result in abortion.

Diagnosis: Lead levels in various tissues may be useful to evaluate excessive accumulation and to reflect the level or duration of exposure, severity, and prognosis and the success of treatment. Concentrations of lead in the blood at 0.35 ppm, liver at 10 ppm, or kidney cortex at 10 ppm are consistent with a diagnosis of lead poisoning in most species.

Hematologic abnormalities, which may be indicative but not confirmatory of lead poisoning, include anemia, anisocytosis, poikilocytosis, polychromasia, basophilic stippling, metarubricytosis, and hypochromia. Blood or urinary δ-aminolevulinic acid and free erythrocyte protoporphyrin levels are sensitive indicators of lead exposure but may not be reliable indicators of clinical disease. Radiologic examination may be useful to determine the magnitude of lead exposure.

Lead poisoning may be confused with other diseases that cause nervous or GI abnormalities. In cattle, such diseases may include polioencephalomalacia, nervous coccidiosis, tetanus, hypovitaminosis A, hypomagnesemic tetany, nervous acetonemia, arsenic or mercury poisoning, brain abscess or neoplasia, rabies, listeriosis, and *Haemophilus* infections.

In dogs, rabies, distemper, and hepatitis may appear similar to lead poisoning.

Treatment: If tissue damage is extensive, particularly to the nervous system, treatment may not be successful. In livestock, calcium disodium edetate (Ca-EDTA) is given IV or SC (110 mg/kg/day) divided into 2 treatments daily for 3 days; this treatment should be repeated 2 days later. In dogs, a similar dose divided into 4 treatments/day is administered SC in 5% dextrose for 2-5 days. After a 1-wk rest period, an additional 5-day treatment may be required if clinical signs persist. No approved veterinary product containing Ca-EDTA is commercially available at present.

Thiamine (2-4 mg/kg/day SC) alleviates clinical manifestations and reduces tissue deposition of lead. Combined Ca-EDTA and thiamine treatment appears to produce the most beneficial response.

D-Penicillamine can be administered PO to dogs (110 mg/kg/day) for 2 wk. However, undesirable side effects such as emesis and anorexia have been associated with this treatment. D-Penicillamine is not recommended for livestock. Succimer (meso 2,3-dimercaptosuccinic acid, DMSA) is a chelating agent that has proven to be effective in dogs (10 mg/kg, PO, TID for 10 days) and is also useful in birds. Fewer side effects have been associated with DMSA as compared with Ca-EDTA.

Cathartics such as magnesium sulfate (400 mg/kg, PO) or a rumenotomy may be useful to remove lead from the GI tract. Barbiturates or tranquilizers may be indicated to control convulsions. Chelation therapy, in combination with antioxidant treatment, may limit oxidative damage associated with acute lead poisoning. Antioxidants such as n-acetylcysteine (50 mg/kg, PO, SID) have been used in combination with DMSA.

Mobilization of lead at parturition, excretion of lead into milk, and lengthy withdrawal times in food-producing animals raise considerable controversy regarding the rationale for treatment from both public health and animal management perspectives.

MERCURY POISONING

Mercury exists in a variety of organic and inorganic forms. The replacement of commercial mercurial compounds, including antiseptics (eg, mercurochrome), diuretics, and fungicides by other agents has decreased the likelihood of mercurial toxicosis; however, the possibility of exposure to environmental sources of organic methylmercury exists.

Inorganic Mercurials: These include the volatile elemental form of mercury (used in thermometers) and the salted forms (mercuric chloride [sublimate] and mercurous chloride [calomel]). Ingested inorganic mercury is poorly absorbed and low in toxicity. Large amounts of these mercurials are corrosive and may produce vomiting, diarrhea, and colic. Renal damage also occurs, with polydipsia and anuria in severe cases. In rare cases of chronic inorganic mercurial poisoning, the CNS effects resemble those of organic mercury poisoning. Mercury vapor from elemental mercury produces corrosive bronchitis and interstitial pneumonia and, if not fatal, may lead to neurologic signs as do organic forms.

Emesis followed by initiation of chelation therapy (*see* below) is recommended after acute oral ingestion. Oral administration of sodium thiosulfate to bind mercury still in the gut may be beneficial.

Organic Mercury: Inorganic mercury is converted to the organic alkyl forms, methylmercury and ethylmercury, by microorganisms in the sediment of rivers, lakes, and seas. Marine life accumulate the most toxic form, methylmercury, and fish must be monitored for contamination. There are reports of commercial cat food causing severe neurologic disturbances in cats fed an exclusive tuna diet for 7-11 mo.

The organic mercurials are absorbed via all routes and bioaccumulate in the brain and to some extent in the kidneys and muscle. Aryl mercurials (eg, phenylmercury fungicide) are slightly less toxic and less prone to bioaccumulation. Animals poisoned by organic mercury exhibit CNS stimulation and locomotor abnormalities after a lengthy latent period (weeks). Signs may include blindness, excitation, abnormal behavior and chewing, incoordination, and convulsions. Cats show hindleg rigidity, hypermetria, cerebellar ataxia, and tremors. Mercury is also a mutagen, teratogen, and a carcinogen, and is embryocidal. Differential diagnoses include conditions with tremors and ataxia as predominant signs, such as ingestion of other metals and insecticides and cerebellar lesions due to trauma or feline parvovirus.

Histologic lesions include degeneration of neurons and perivascular cuffing in the cerebrocortical gray matter, cerebellar atrophy of the granular layer, and damage to Purkinje cells. Laboratory diagnosis must differentiate between normal concentrations of mercury in tissue (especially whole blood, kidney, and brain) and feed (<1 ppm) and concentrations associated with poisoning.

Neurologic signs may be irreversible once they develop. Chelation therapy with dimercaprol (3 mg/kg body wt, IM, every 4 hr for the first 2 days, QID on the third day, and BID for the next 10 days or until recovery is complete) has been beneficial. When available, the water soluble, less toxic analog of dimercaprol, 2,3-dimercaptosuccinic acid, is the chelator of choice for organic mercury poisoning. Penicillamine (15-50 mg/kg, PO) may be used only after the gut is free of ingested mercury and renal function has been established.

METALDEHYDE POISONING

Metaldehyde is the active ingredient in molluscicides used especially during the wet season for slug and snail control in domestic gardens. In certain locations, it is also used for rat control. (*See also* p 2508.) Metaldehyde comes as a liquid or bait (3.5%) combined with bran, either as flakes or pellets, and is palatable to pets and farm animals. Some products also contain arsenic or a cholinesterase-inhibiting insecticide, which is usually less toxic at the dosage used than the metaldehyde. All species are susceptible to metaldehyde poisoning (lethal dose 100-300 mg/kg); dogs are the species most frequently poisoned (3 oz of bait is toxic to a 30-lb dog). When ingested, a portion of the metaldehyde is partially hydrolyzed in stomach acid to acetaldehyde and absorbed, while the remaining metaldehyde is well absorbed from the intestines. The great variability in onset of clinical signs of metaldehyde poisoning appears to be dependent on gastric contents and the rate of stomach emptying. Metaldehyde and acetaldehyde contribute to a decrease in brain serotonin, noradrenaline, and γ-aminobutyric acid (GABA), which is proportional to the increase in muscle activity and CNS excitatory signs.

Clinical signs of toxicosis are similar in all mammals. Nervous signs are prominent. Initial signs may include severe muscle tremors, ataxia, hyperesthesia, tachycardia, hyperthermia, and hyperpnea, followed by nystagmus, opisthotonos, and continuous tonic convulsions. Nystagmus is most severe in cats. Nervous signs are more continuous and less exaggerated by stimulation than in strychnine poisoning (p 2521), which may appear clinically similar. Emesis, diarrhea, hypersalivation, and dyspnea, in all species, and profuse sweating in horses, are also seen.

Severe acidosis develops due to acid metabolites and high muscle activity in all species. Cholinergic signs (especially pupillary constriction) and a drop in blood cholinesterase may occur if the product contains a carbamate or organophosphate. In high-level exposure, death (4-24 hr) is from respiratory failure, while survivors may develop liver failure (3-4 days). Necropsy lesions are nonspecific and include congestion and edema of the liver, kidneys, and lungs, and intestinal hemorrhage. A mild formaldehyde-like odor may be present on opening the stomach or rumen. Stomach content, rapidly frozen, is the preferred sample for analysis due to the low levels and rapid loss of acetaldehyde from tissue (liver and urine).

An emetic (eg, apomorphine) in acute exposure may not be necessary because metaldehyde is a gastric irritant. However, gastric lavage with sodium bicarbonate is recommended. Diazepam (2-5 mg/kg, IV) to effect is preferred to reduce excitement and convulsions; acepromazine has been used successfully. Barbiturates (which compete with acetaldehyde degradation) are indicated only if the animal does not respond, and gas anesthesia is suggested to maintain severely affected animals. Horses benefit from xylazine plus acepromazine. In large animals, activated carbon (1-3 g/kg, repeated every 4-8 hr at half the original dose if necessary) reduces further absorption (metaldehyde is fat soluble). Aggressive fluid therapy with sodium lactate to reduce acidosis is essential, and dextrose or calcium borogluconate is used to prevent possible liver damage. Muscle relaxants, eg, methocarbamol, assist in reducing muscle activity and pain. Cold water rinses are recommended when fever is severe. Prognosis is good if hyperthermia and seizures are not severe and prolonged, but longterm aggressive therapy is required (≥4 days).

MOLYBDENUM POISONING

Molybdenum is an essential micronutrient that forms molybdenoenzymes, which are necessary for the health of all animals. In ruminants, the dietary intake of excessive molybdenum causes, in part, a secondary hypocuprosis. Toxicosis due to massive doses of molybdenum is rare. Domestic ruminants are much more susceptible to molybdenum toxicity than nonruminants. The resistance of other species is at least 10 times that of cattle and sheep.

Etiology: The metabolism of copper, molybdenum, and inorganic sulfate is a complex and incompletely understood interrelationship. It appears that the ruminal interaction of molybdates and sulfides gives rise to thiomolybdates (mono-, di-, tri-, and tetrathiomolybdates). Copper reacts with thiomolybdates (primarily tri-and tetrathiomolybdates) in the rumen to form an insoluble complex that is poorly absorbed. On this basis, tetrathiomolybdate is used in treating and preventing copper toxicity (p 2353) in sheep. Some thiomolybdates are absorbed and decrease blood copper availability and also appear to directly inhibit copper-dependent enzymes. Therefore, the susceptibility of ruminants to molybdenum toxicity depends on a number of factors: 1) copper content of the diet and intake of the animal—tolerance to molybdenum toxicity decreases as the content and intake of copper decrease; 2) the inorganic sulfate content of the diet—high dietary sulfate with low copper exacerbates the condition, while low dietary sulfate causes high blood molybdenum levels due to decreased excretion; 3) chemical form of the molybdenum—water-soluble molybdenum in growing herbage is most toxic, while curing decreases toxicity; 4) presence of certain sulfur-containing amino acids; 5) species of animal—cattle are less tolerant than sheep; 6) age—young animals are more susceptible; 7) season of year—plants concentrate molybdenum beginning in spring (maximum level reached in fall); and 8) botanic composition of the pasture—legumes take up more of the element than other plant species.

Molybdenum toxicity associated with copper deficiency has been seen in areas with peat or muck soils, where plants grow in alkaline sloughs (eg, western USA), as a result of industrial contamination (mining and metal alloy production), where excess molybdenum-containing fertilizer has been applied, and where applications of lime appeared to increase plant molybdenum uptake.

In the diet of cattle, copper:molybdenum ratios of 6:1 are considered ideal; 2:1-3:1, borderline; and <2:1, toxic. Dietary molybdenum of >10 ppm can cause toxicity regardless of copper intake; as little as 1 ppm may be hazardous if copper content is <5 ppm (dry-weight basis). Mixing errors may occur; concentrations above 1,000 mg/kg (as sodium molybdate) cause growth retardation while concentrations of 2,000-4,000 mg/kg cause death within 40 days.

Clinical Findings and Diagnosis: Most of the clinical signs attributed to molybdenum toxicity arise from impaired copper metabolism and are the same as those produced by simple copper deficiency. Molybdenum toxicity in cattle is characterized by persistent, severe scouring with passage of liquid feces full of gas bubbles (**peat scours** or **teart**). Depigmentation, resulting in fading of the hair coat, is most noticeable in black animals and especially around the eyes, which gives a spectacled appearance. Other signs include unthriftiness, anemia, emaciation, joint pain (lameness), osteoporosis, and decreased fertility. Effects on reproduction, particularly in heifers, include delayed puberty, decreased weight at puberty, and reduced conception rates. It appears that fertility is uniquely vulnerable to the effects of molybdenum or thiomolybdates and alone responds indirectly to copper acting as an antidote. Some studies have suggested that relatively low levels of molybdenum may exert these direct effects on certain metabolic processes, particularly reproduction, independent of alterations in copper metabolism. Sheep, and young animals in particular, show stiffness of the back and legs with a reluctance to rise (called enzootic ataxia in Australia). Joint and skeletal lesions appear to be due to defects in development of connective tissue and growth plates. Clinical signs appear within 1-2 wk of grazing affected pasture.

In molybdenum toxicity, low copper levels in blood and tissue and the occurrence of clinical signs of copper deficiency in cattle are poorly correlated. A provisional diagnosis can be made if the diarrhea stops within a few days of oral dosing with copper sulfate; the diagnosis is further supported if other causes of diarrhea and unthriftiness (including GI parasites) are ruled out. Diagnosis is confirmed by demonstrating abnormal concentrations of molybdenum and copper in blood or liver and by a high dietary intake of molybdenum relative to copper.

The disease may be confused with many other enteritides and is commonly mistaken for internal parasitism, especially in young cattle. In pastured animals, it is not uncommon for the diseases to occur simultaneously.

Effects in cattle and sheep poisoned with massive concentrations of molybdenum are unlike the chronic induced copper deficiency described above. Cattle lose appetite within 3 days and deaths begin to occur within 1 wk and continue for months after exposure ends. Animals appear lethargic, display hind limb ataxia that progresses to involve the front limbs, salivate profusely, and produce scant, mucoid feces. The molybdenum is toxic to hepatocytes and renal tubular epithelial cells, producing periacinar to massive hepatic necrosis and nephrosis.

Prevention and Treatment: Signs of severe acute toxicosis are reversed by providing copper sulfate in the diet. In areas where the molybdenum content of the forage is <5 ppm, the use of 1% copper sulfate ($CuSO_4 \cdot 5H_2O$) in salt has provided satisfactory control of molybdenosis. With higher levels of molybdenum, 2% copper sulfate has been successful; up to 5% has been used in a few regions where the molybdenum levels are very high. In areas where, for various reasons, cattle do not consume mineral supplements, the required copper may be supplied as a drench given weekly, as parenterally administered repository copper preparations, or as a top-dressing to the pasture. Copper glycinate injectable has been used successfully as an adjunct to therapy.

MYCOTOXICOSES

For discussion of POULTRY MYCOTOXICOSES, *see* p 2246.

Acute or chronic toxicoses can result from exposure to feed or bedding contaminated with toxins that may be produced during growth of various saprophytic or phytopathogenic fungi or molds on cereals, hay, straw, pastures, or any other fodder. A few principles characterize mycotoxic diseases: 1) the cause may not be immediately identified; 2) they are not transmissible from one animal to another; 3) treatment with drugs or antibiotics has little effect on the course of the disease; 4) outbreaks are usually seasonal because particular climatic sequences may favor fungal growth and toxin production; 5) study indicates specific association with a particular feed; and 6) although large numbers of fungi found on examination of feedstuff does not necessarily indicate that toxin production has occurred.

Confirmation of diagnosis of mycotoxic disease requires a combination of information. Detection of fungal spores alone, even at high concentrations, is not sufficient for diagnosis; fungal spores or even mold growth may be present without formation of mycotoxins. Especially important in diagnosis is the presence of a disease documented to be caused by a known mycotoxin, combined with detection of the mycotoxin in either feedstuffs or animal tissues.

Sometimes more than one mycotoxin may be present in feedstuffs, and their different toxicologic properties may cause clinical signs and lesions that are not consistent with those seen when animals are dosed experimentally with pure, single mycotoxins. Several mycotoxins are immunosuppressive, which may allow viruses, bacteria, or parasites to create a secondary disease that is more obvious than the primary.

In reaching a diagnosis of mycotoxicosis characterized by reduced feed intake, reproductive failure, or increased infectious disease due to immunosuppression, differential diagnoses must be carefully established and eliminated by a combination of thorough clinical and historical evaluation, examination of production records, and close attention to appropriate diagnostic testing.

There are no specific antidotes for mycotoxins; removal of the source of the toxin (ie, the moldy feedstuff) eliminates further exposure. The absorption of some mycotoxins (eg, aflatoxin) has been effectively prevented by aluminosilicate. If financial circumstances do not allow for disposal of the moldy feed, it can be blended with unspoiled feed just before feeding to reduce the toxin concentration or fed to less susceptible species. When contaminated feed is blended with good feed, care must be taken to prevent further mold growth by the toxigenic contaminants. This may be accomplished by thorough drying or by addition of organic acids (eg, propionic acid) to prevent mold growth.

Important mycotoxic diseases occur in domestic animals worldwide (TABLE 2).

Sampling and Submitting Feeds for Laboratory Analysis: Much of the error in detecting mycotoxins in feed results from sampling (or subsampling) rather than from analytical methodology. Samples can be taken at various stages—from growing crops or during transport or storage. Whenever possible, samples should be taken after particulate size has been reduced (eg, by shelling or grinding) and soon after blending has occurred (as in harvesting, loading, or grinding). Sampling is most effective if small samples are taken at periodic, predetermined intervals from a moving stream of grain or feed. These individual stream samples should be combined and mixed thoroughly, after which a subsample of 10 lb (4.5 kg) should be taken.

Probe sampling is acceptable when grain has been recently blended but is less reliable because different microenvironments within the storage facility may cause areas of mold or mycotoxin concentration. A suggested method of probe sampling is to sample at 5 locations, each 1 ft (30 cm) from the periphery of a bin, plus once in the center. This should be done for each 6 ft (2 m) of bin depth. Thus, taller bins would require more samples, and the total weight should be >10 lb.

Dry samples are preferable for transport and storage. Samples should be dried at 176-194°F (80-90°C) for ~3 hr to reduce moisture to 12-13%. If mold studies are to be done, drying at 140°F (60°C) for 6-12 hr should preserve fungal activity.

Containers should be appropriate for the nature of the sample. For dried samples, paper or cloth bags are recommended. Plastic bags should be avoided unless grain is dried thoroughly. Plastic bags are useful for high-moisture samples only if refrigeration, freezing, or chemicals are used to retard mold growth during transport and storage. Once a sample has been cooled or frozen, warming may induce condensation and allow mold growth.

TABLE 2.   Mycotoxicoses in Domestic Animals

Disease	Toxins (when known)	Fungi or Molds	Regions Where Reported
Aflatoxicosis	Aflatoxins	*Aspergillus flavus, A parasiticus*	Widespread (warmer climatic zones)
Diplodiosis	Unknown	*Diplodia zeae*	South Africa
Ergotism	Ergot alkaloids	*Claviceps purpurea*	Widespread
	Paspalinine and paspalitrems, tremorgens	*C paspali, C cinerea*	Widespread
Estrogenism and vulvo-vaginitis	Zearalenone	*Fusarium graminearum* Perfect state: *Gibberella zeae*	Widespread
Facial eczema (Pithomycotoxicosis)	Sporidesmins	*Pithomyces chartarum*	Widespread
Fescue foot	Ergovaline	*Acremonium coenophialum*	USA, Australia, New Zealand, Italy
Leukoencephalomalacia	Fumonisin B_1	*Fusarium moniliforme*	Egypt, USA, South Africa, Greece
Mold nephrosis	*See* ochratoxicosis (below)		
Mycotoxic lupinosis (as distinct from alkaloid poisoning)	Phomopsins	*Phomopsis leptostromiformis*	Widespread
Ochratoxicosis	Ochratoxin, also citrinin	*Aspergillus ochraceus* and others, *Penicillium viridicatum, P citrinum*	Widespread
Perennial ryegrass staggers	Lolitrems	*Acremonium loliae,* an endophyte fungus confined to *Lolium perenne*	Australia, New Zealand, Europe, USA
Poultry hemorrhagic syndrome	Probably aflatoxins and rubratoxins	Probably *Aspergillus flavus, A clavatus, Penicillium purpurogenum, Alternaria* sp	USA

◀ **TABLE 2.** (continued)

Contaminated Toxic Foodstuff	Animals Affected	Signs and Lesions
Moldy peanuts, soybeans, cottonseeds, rice, sorghum, corn (maize), other cereals	All poultry, pigs, cattle, sheep, dogs	Major effects in all species are slow growth and hepatotoxicosis. See also p 2412, and POULTRY MYCOTOXICOSES, p 2246.
Moldy corn (maize)	Cattle, sheep	Nervous system disorders, cold and insensitive limbs. Recovery usual on removal of source.
Seedheads of many grasses, grains	Cattle, horses, pigs, poultry	Peripheral gangrene, late gestation suppression of lactation initiation. See p 2414.
Seedheads of paspalum grasses	Cattle, horses, sheep	Acute tremors and ataxia. See PASPALUM STAGGERS, p 2421.
Moldy corn (maize) and pelleted cereal feeds, standing corn, corn silage, other grains	Pigs, cattle, sheep, poultry	Vulvovaginitis in pigs, anestrus or pseudopregnancy in mature sows, early embryonic death of swine embryos, estrogenism in cattle and sheep, reduced egg production in poultry. See also p 2415.
Toxic spores on pasture litter	Sheep, cattle, farmed deer	See also p 2417.
Tall fescue grass (Festuca arundinacea)	Cattle, horses	Lameness, weight loss, hyperthermia, dry gangrene of extremities, agalactia, thickened fetal membranes. See also p 2418.
Moldy corn (maize)	Horses, other Equidae, pigs	Depends on degree and specific site of brain lesion. See also p 2419.
Moldy seed, pods, stubble, and haulm of several Lupinus spp affected by Phomopsis stem blight	Sheep, occasionally cattle, horses, pigs	Lassitude, inappetence, stupor, icterus, marked liver injury. Usually fatal. See also p 2420.
Moldy barley, corn (maize), wheat	Pigs, poultry	Perirenal edema, enlarged pale kidneys with cortical cysts, and tubular degeneration and fibrosis; immunosuppression, polyuria and polydipsia.
Endophyte-infected ryegrass pastures	Sheep, cattle, horses, deer	Tremors, incoordination, collapse, convulsive spasms. See RYEGRASS STAGGERS, p 2512.
Moldy grain and meal	Growing chickens	Depression, anorexia, no weight gain, widespread internal hemorrhages, sometimes aplastic anemia, death. See MYCOTOXICOSES, p 2246.

(continued)

TABLE 2. Mycotoxicoses in Domestic Animals (continued) ▶

Disease	Toxins (when known)	Fungi or Molds	Regions Where Reported
Pulmonary edema, emphysema	4-Ipomeanol	*Fusarium solani*	USA
Porcine pulmonary edema	Fumonisin B_1 and Fumonisin B_2	*Fusarium moniliforme* and *F proliferatum*	USA, South Africa
Slobbers	Slaframine (and swainsonine)	*Rhizoctonia leguminicola*	USA
Sweet clover poisoning	Dicumarol	*Penicillium* spp, *Mucor* spp, *Aspergillus* spp	North America
Tremorgen ataxia syndrome	Penitrems, verruculogen, paxilline, fumitremorgens, aflatrems, roquefortine	*Penicillium crustosum, P puberulum, P verruculosum, P roqueforti, Aspergillus flavus, A fumigatus, A clavatus*, and others	USA, South Africa, probably worldwide
Trichothecene toxicosis			
Fusariotoxicosis, vomiting and feed refusal in pigs	Nonmacrocyclic trichothecenes (deoxynivalenol, T-2 toxin, diacetoxyscirpenol, many other trichothecenes)	*Fusarium sporotrichioides, F culmorum, F graminearum, F nivale*; other fungal species	Widespread (except for deoxynivalenol, more likely in temperate to colder climates)
Stachybotryotoxicosis	Macrocyclic trichothecenes (satratoxin, roridin, verrucarin)	*Stachybotrys atra (alternans)*	Former USSR, southeast Europe
Myrotheciotoxicosis, Dendrodochiotoxicosis	Macrocyclic trichothecenes (verrucarins, roridins, etc)	*Myrothecium verrucaria, M roridum*	Southeast Europe, former USSR
	Macrocyclic trichothecenes (baccharinoids)	*Myrothecium verrucaria*	Brazil

AFLATOXICOSIS

Aflatoxins are produced by toxigenic strains of *Aspergillus flavus* and *A parasiticus* on peanuts, soybeans, corn (maize), and other cereals either in the field or during storage when moisture content and temperatures are sufficiently high for mold growth. Usually, this means consistent day and night temperatures >70°F. The toxic response and disease in mammals and poultry varies in relation to species, sex, age, nutritional status,

TABLE 2. (continued)

Contaminated Toxic Foodstuff	Animals Affected	Signs and Lesions
Moldy sweet potatoes	Cattle	Pulmonary edema, leading to interstitial pneumonia and emphysema.
Corn	Swine	Acute interlobular pulmonary edema and hydrothorax cause anoxia and cyanosis. Survivors may develop icterus and chronic hepatotoxicosis.
Blackpatch-diseased legumes (notably red clover) eaten as forage or hay	Sheep, cattle	Salivation, bloat, diarrhea, sometimes death. Recovery usual when removed from clover. *See also* p 173 and p 2421.
Sweet clover (*Melilotus* spp)	Cattle, horses, sheep	*See also* p 2523.
Moldy feed	All species	Tremors, polypnea, ataxia, collapse, convulsive spasms.
Cereal crops, moldy roughage	Pigs, cattle, horses, poultry	Vomiting, feed refusal, loss of appetite and milk production, diarrhea, staggers, skin irritation, immunosuppression; recovery on removal of contaminated feed. *See also* p 2421.
Moldy roughage, other contaminated feed	Horses, cattle, sheep, pigs	Stomatitis and ulceration, anorexia, leukopenia, extensive hemorrhages in many organs, inflammation and necrosis in the gut, immunosuppression.
Moldy rye stubble, straw	Sheep, cattle, horses	Acute—diarrhea, respiratory distress, hemorrhagic gastroenteritis, immunosuppression, death. Chronic—ulceration of GI tract, unthriftiness, gradual recovery.
Plants of *Baccharis* spp that contain the toxins	Cattle, other herbivores	Epithelial necrosis of GI tract.

and the duration of intake and level of aflatoxins in the ration. Earlier recognized disease outbreaks called "moldy corn toxicosis," "poultry hemorrhagic syndrome," and "*Aspergillus* toxicosis" may have been caused by aflatoxins.

Aflatoxicosis occurs in many parts of the world and affects growing poultry (especially ducklings and turkey poults), young pigs, pregnant sows, calves, and dogs. Adult cattle, sheep, and goats are relatively resistant to the acute form of the disease but are susceptible if toxic diets are fed over long periods. Experimentally, all species of animals tested have shown some degree of susceptibility. Dietary levels of aflatoxin (in ppb) generally tolerated are ≤50 in young poultry, ≤100 in adult poultry, ≤50 in weaner pigs, ≤200 in finishing pigs, <100 in calves, and <300 in cattle. Dietary levels as low as 10-20 ppb may result in measurable metabolites of aflatoxin (aflatoxin M_1 and M_2) being excreted in milk; feedstuffs that contain aflatoxins should not be fed to dairy cows.

Aflatoxins bind to macromolecules, especially nucleic acids and nucleoproteins. Their toxic effects include mutagenesis due to alkylation of nuclear DNA, carcinogenesis, teratogenesis, reduced protein synthesis, and immunosuppression. Reduced protein synthesis results in reduced production of essential metabolic enzymes and structural proteins for growth. The liver is the principal organ affected. High doses of aflatoxins result in severe hepatocellular necrosis; prolonged low dosages result in reduced growth rate and liver enlargement.

Clinical Findings: In acute outbreaks, deaths occur after a short period of inappetence. Subacute outbreaks are more usual, and unthriftiness, weakness, anorexia, and sudden deaths can occur. Generally, aflatoxin concentrations in feed >1,000 ppb are associated with acute aflatoxicosis. Frequently, there is a high incidence of concurrent infectious disease, often respiratory, that responds poorly to the usual chemotherapy.

Lesions: In acute cases, there are widespread hemorrhages and icterus. The liver is the major target organ. Microscopically, the liver shows marked fatty accumulations and massive centrilobular necrosis and hemorrhage. In subacute cases, the hepatic changes are not so pronounced, but the liver is somewhat enlarged and firmer than usual. There may be edema of the gallbladder. Microscopically, the liver shows proliferation and fibrosis of the bile ductules; the hepatocytes and their nuclei (megalocytosis) are enlarged. The GI mucosa may show glandular atrophy and associated inflammation. In the kidneys, there may be tubular degeneration and regeneration. Prolonged feeding of low concentrations of aflatoxins may result in diffuse liver fibrosis (cirrhosis) and carcinoma of the bile ducts or liver.

Diagnosis: Disease history, necropsy findings, and microscopic examination of the liver should indicate the nature of the hepatotoxin, but hepatic changes are somewhat similar in *Senecio* poisoning (p 2506). The presence and levels of aflatoxins in the feed should be determined. Aflatoxin M_1 can be detected in urine or kidney or in milk of lactating animals if toxin intakes are high.

Control: Contaminated feeds can be avoided by monitoring batches for aflatoxin content. Young, newly weaned, pregnant, and lactating animals require special protection from suspected toxic feeds. Dilution with noncontaminated feedstuff is one possibility. Ammoniation of grain reduces contamination but is not currently approved for use in food animals.

Hydrated sodium calcium aluminosilicates (HSCAS) have shown promise in reducing the effects of aflatoxin when fed to pigs or poultry; at 10 lb/ton (5 kg/tonne), they provided substantial protection against dietary aflatoxin. HSCAS reduced, but did not eliminate, residues of aflatoxin M_1 in milk from dairy cows fed aflatoxin B_1.

ERGOTISM

This worldwide disease of farm animals results from continued ingestion of sclerotia of the parasitic fungus *Claviceps purpurea*, which replaces the grain or seed of rye and other small grains or forage plants, such as the bromes, bluegrasses, and ryegrasses. The hard, black, elongated sclerotia may contain varying quantities of ergot alkaloids, of which ergotamine and ergonovine (ergometrine) are pharmacologically most important. Cattle, pigs, sheep, and poultry are involved in sporadic outbreaks, and most species are susceptible.

Etiology: Ergot causes vasoconstriction by direct action on the muscles of the arterioles, and repeated dosages injure the vascular endothelium. These actions initially reduce blood flow and eventually lead to complete stasis with terminal necrosis of the extremities due to thrombosis. A cold environment predisposes the extremities to gangrene. In addition, ergot has a potent oxytocic action and also causes stimulation of the CNS, followed by depression. Ergot alkaloids inhibit pituitary release of prolactin in many mammalian species, with failure of both mammary development in late gestation and delayed initiation of milk secretion, resulting in agalactia at parturition.

Clinical Findings and Lesions: Cattle may be affected by eating ergotized hay or grain or occasionally by grazing seeded pastures that are infested with ergot. Lameness, the first sign, may appear 2-6 wk or more after initial ingestion, depending on the concentration of alkaloids in the ergot and the quantity of ergot in the feed. Hindlimbs are affected before forelimbs, but the extent of involvement of a limb and the number of limbs affected depends on the daily intake of ergot. Body temperature and pulse and respiration rates are increased. **Epidemic hyperthermia** and hypersalivation may also occur in cattle poisoned with *C purpurea* (*see also* FESCUE POISONING, p 2418).

Associated with the lameness are swelling and tenderness of the fetlock joint and pastern. Within ~1 wk, sensation is lost in the affected part, an indented line appears at the limit of normal tissue, and dry gangrene affects the distal part. Eventually, one or both claws or any part of the limbs up to the hock or knee may be sloughed. In a similar way, the tip of the tail or ears may become necrotic and slough. Exposed skin areas, such as teats and udder, appear unusually pale or anemic. Abortion is not seen.

The most consistent lesions at necropsy are in the skin and subcutaneous parts of the extremities. The skin is normal to the indented line, but beyond, it is cyanotic and hardened in advanced cases. Subcutaneous hemorrhage and some edema occur proximal to the necrotic area.

In pigs, ingestion of ergot-infested grains may result in reduced feed intake and reduced weight gain. If fed to pregnant sows, ergotized grains result in lack of udder development with agalactia at parturition, and the piglets born may be smaller than normal. Most of the litter die within a few days due to starvation. No other clinical signs or lesions are seen.

Clinical signs in sheep are similar to those in cattle. Additionally, the mouth may be ulcerated, and marked intestinal inflammation may be seen at necropsy. A convulsive syndrome has been associated with ergotism in sheep.

Diagnosis: Diagnosis is based on finding the causative fungus (ergot sclerotia) in grains, hay, or pastures provided to livestock showing signs of ergotism. Ergot alkaloids may be extracted and detected in suspect ground grain meals.

Identical signs and lesions of lameness, and sloughing of the hooves and tips of ears and tail, are seen in fescue foot in cattle grazing in winter on tall fescue grass infected with an endophyte fungus, in which the ergot alkaloid ergovaline is considered a major toxic principle. In gilts and sows, lactation failure not associated with ergot alkaloids is prevalent and must be differentiated from prolactin inhibition due to ergot.

Control: Ergotism can be controlled by an immediate change to an ergot-free diet. Under pasture feeding conditions, frequent grazing or topping of pastures prone to ergot infestation during the summer months reduces flower-head production and helps control the disease. Grain that contains even small amounts of ergot should not be fed to pregnant or lactating sows.

ESTROGENISM AND VULVOVAGINITIS

(*Fusarium* estrogenism)

Fusarium spp molds are extremely common and often contaminate growing plants and stored feeds. Corn (maize), wheat, and barley are commonly contaminated. In moderate climates under humid weather conditions, *F graminearum* may produce zearalenone, one of the resorcyclic acid lactones (RAL). Zearalenone (formerly called F_2 toxin) is a potent nonsteroidal estrogen and is the only known mycotoxin with primarily estrogenic effects. Often, zearalenone is produced concurrently with deoxynivalenol. Depending on the ratio of these 2 mycotoxins, signs of reduced feed intake or reproductive dysfunction may predominate, but presence of deoxynivalenol may limit exposure to zearalenone, thus reducing its practical effect.

Zearalenone binds to receptors for estradiol-17-β, and this complex binds to estradiol sites on DNA. Specific RNA synthesis leads to signs of estrogenism. Zearalenone is a weak estrogen with potency 2-4 times less than estradiol. Under controlled administration, zearalanol, a closely related RAL, is widely used in cattle as an anabolic agent.

Estrogenism due to zearalenone was first clinically recognized as vulvovaginitis in prepubertal gilts fed moldy corn (maize), but zearalenone is occasionally reported as a disease-causing agent in sporadic outbreaks in dairy cattle, sheep, chickens, and turkeys. High dietary concentrations are required to produce disease in cattle and sheep, and extremely high dosages are required to affect poultry.

Etiology: Zearalenone has been detected in corn, oats, barley, wheat, and sorghum (both fresh and stored); in rations compounded for cattle and pigs; in corn ensiled at the green stage; and rarely in hay. It has been detected occasionally in samples from pastures in temperate climates at levels thought to be sufficient to cause reproductive failure of grazing herbivores.

Clinical Findings: The condition cannot be distinguished from excessive estrogen administration. Physical and behavioral signs of estrus are induced in young gilts by as little as 1 ppm dietary zearalenone. In pigs, zearalenone primarily affects weaned and prepubertal gilts, causing hyperemia and enlargement of the vulva. There is hypertrophy of the mammary glands and uterus, with occasional prolapse of the uterus in severe cases. In multiparous sows, signs include diminished fertility, anestrus, reduced litter size, smaller offspring, and probably fetal resorption. Constant estrus or pseudopregnancy may be seen.

Zearalenone causes reproductive toxicosis in sexually mature sows by inhibiting secretion and release of follicle-stimulating hormone (FSH) resulting in arrest of preovulatory ovarian follicle maturation. Reproductive effects in sexually mature sows depend on time of consumption. Zearalenone fed at 3-10 ppm on days 12-14 of the estrous cycle in open gilts results in retention of the corpora lutea and prolonged anestrus (pseudopregnancy) for up to 40-60 days. Zearalenone fed at ≥30 ppm in early gestation (7-10 days post-mating) may prevent implantation and cause early embryonic death.

In cattle, dietary concentrations >10 ppm may cause reproductive dysfunction in dairy heifers, while mature cows may tolerate up to 20 ppm. Clinical signs include weight loss, vaginal discharge, nymphomania, uterine hypertrophy, and in pregnant heifers, abortion 1-3 mo after conception—usually followed by multiple returns to service.

Young males, both swine and cattle, may become infertile, with atrophy of the testes.

Ewes may show reduced reproductive performance (reduced ovulation rates and numbers of fertilized ova, and markedly increased duration of estrus) and abortion or premature live births.

Lesions: Lesions in pigs include ovarian atrophy and follicular atresia, uterine edema, cellular hypertrophy in all layers of the uterus, and a cystic appearance in degenerative endometrial glands. The mammary glands show ductal hyperplasia and epithelial proliferation. Squamous metaplasia is seen in the cervix and vagina.

Diagnosis: This is based on reproductive performance in the herd or flock, clinical signs, and history of diet-related occurrence. Chemical analysis of suspect feed for zearalenone and careful examination of reproductive organs at necropsy are required. As a bioassay, virgin prepubertal mice fed diets or extracts of zearalenone-contaminated feed demonstrate enlarged uteri and vaginal cornification typical of estrogens.

Differential diagnoses include reproductive tract infections and other causes of impaired fertility such as diethylstilbestrol in the diet of housed stock. In grazing herbivores, especially sheep, the plant estrogens (eg, isoflavones associated with some varieties of subterranean and red clovers, and coumestans in certain fodders [eg, alfalfa]) should be considered.

Control: Unless stock are severely or chronically affected, usually reproductive functions recover and signs regress 1-4 wk after intake of zearalenone stops. However, multiparous sows may remain anestrous up to 8-10 wk.

Management of swine with hyperestrogenism should include changing the grain immediately. Signs should stop within 1 wk. Animals should be treated symptomatically for vaginal or rectal prolapse and physical damage to external genitalia. For sexually mature sows with anestrus, one 10-mg dose of prostaglandin $F_{2\alpha}$, or two 5-mg doses on successive days, has corrected anestrus caused by retained corpora. Alfalfa and alfalfa meal fed to swine at 25% of the ration may reduce absorption and increase fecal excretion of zearalenone, but this is often not considered practical. Bentonite added to contaminated diets has been generally ineffective against zearalenone.

FACIAL ECZEMA
(Pithomycotoxicosis)

In this mycotoxic disease of grazing livestock, the toxic liver injury commonly results in photodynamic dermatitis. In sheep, the face is the only site of the body that is readily exposed to ultraviolet light, hence the common name. The disease is most common in New Zealand but also occurs in Australia, France, South Africa, several South American countries, and probably North America. Sheep, cattle, and farmed deer of all ages can contract the disease, but it is most severe in young animals.

Etiology and Pathogenesis: Sporidesmins are secondary metabolites of the saprophytic fungus *Pithomyces chartarum*, which grows on dead pasture litter. The warm ground temperatures and high humidity required for rapid growth of this fungus restrict disease occurrence to hot summer and autumn periods shortly after warm rains. By observing weather conditions and estimating toxic spore numbers on pastures, danger periods can be predicted and farmers alerted.

The sporidesmins are excreted via the biliary system, in which they produce severe cholangitis and pericholangitis as a result of tissue necrosis. Biliary obstruction may be seen, which restricts excretion of bile pigments and results in jaundice. Similarly, failure to excrete phylloerythrin in bile leads to photosensitization.

Previous ingestion of toxic spores causes potentiation, thus a succession of small intakes of the spores can lead to subsequent severe outbreaks.

Clinical Findings, Lesions, and Diagnosis: Few signs are apparent until photosensitization and jaundice appear ~10-14 days after intake of the toxins. Animals frantically seek shade. Even short exposure to the sun rapidly produces the typical erythema and edema of photodermatitis in unpigmented skin. The animals suffer considerably, and deaths occur from one to several weeks after photodermatitis appears.

Characteristic liver and bile duct lesions are seen in all affected animals whether photosensitized or not. In acute cases showing photodermatitis, livers are initially enlarged, icteric, and have a marked lobular pattern. Later, there is atrophy and marked fibrosis. The shape is distorted, and large nodules of regenerated tissue appear on the surface. In subclinical cases, livers often develop extensive areas in which the tissue is depressed and shrunken below the normal contour, which distorts and roughens the capsule. Generally, these areas are associated with fibrosis and thickening of corresponding bile ducts. The bladder mucosa commonly shows hemorrhagic or bile-pigment-stained ulcerative erosions with circumscribed edema.

The clinical signs together with characteristic liver lesions are pathognomonic. In live animals, high levels of hepatic enzymes may reflect the extensive injury to the liver.

Control: To minimize intake of pasture litter and toxic spores, short grazing should be avoided. Other feedstuffs should be fed during danger periods; encouraging clover dominance in pastures helps to provide a milieu unsuited to growth and sporulation of *P chartarum* on litter.

The application of benzimidazole fungicides to pastures considerably restricts the buildup of *P chartarum* spores and reduces pasture toxicity. A pasture area calculated at 1 acre (0.45 hectare)/15 cows or 100 sheep should be sprayed in midsummer with a suspension of thiabendazole. When danger periods of fungal activity are predicted, animals should be allowed only on the sprayed areas. The fungicide is effective within 4 days after spraying, provided that no more than 1 in. (2.5 cm) of rain falls within 24 hr during the 4-day period. After this time, heavy rainfall does little to reduce the effectiveness of spraying because the thiabendazole becomes incorporated within the plants. Pastures will then remain safe for ~6 wk, after which spraying should be repeated to ensure protection over the entire dangerous season.

Sheep and cattle can be protected from the effects of sporidesmin if given adequate amounts of zinc. Zinc may be administered by drenching with zinc oxide slurry, by spraying pastures with zinc oxide, or by adding zinc sulfate to drinking water.

Sheep may be selectively bred for natural resistance to the toxic effects of sporidesmin. The heritable trait for resistance is high. Ram sires are now being selected in stud and commercial flocks for resistance either by natural field challenge or by low-level, controlled dosage of ram lambs with sporidesmin.

FESCUE POISONING

Fescue Lameness
(Fescue foot)

Fescue lameness, which resembles ergot poisoning, is believed to be caused by ergot alkaloids, especially ergovaline, in tall fescue (*Festuca arundinacea*). It begins with lameness in one or both hindfeet and may progress to necrosis of the distal part of the affected limb(s). The tail and ears also may be affected independently of the lameness. In addition to gangrene of these extremities, animals may show loss of body mass, an arched back, and a rough coat. Outbreaks have been confirmed in cattle and similar lesions have been reported in sheep.

Tall fescue is a cool-season perennial grass adapted to a wide range of soil and climatic conditions; it is used in Australia and New Zealand for stabilizing the banks of watercourses. It is the predominant pasture grass in the transition zone in the eastern and central USA. Fescue lameness has been reported in Kentucky, Tennessee, Florida, California, Colorado, and Missouri, as well as in New Zealand, Australia, and Italy.

The causative toxic substance has actions similar to those produced by sclerotia of *Claviceps purpurea*. However, ergot poisoning (*see* p 2414) is not the cause of fescue lameness. Ergotism is most prevalent in late summer when the seed heads of grass mature. Fescue lameness is most common in late fall and winter and has been reproduced in cattle by feeding dried fescue free of seed heads and ergot.

Two fungi from toxic pastures have been implicated in fescue lameness. The clavicipitaceous endophyte fungus *Acremonium coenophialum* can synthesize ergot alkaloids in culture. The ergot alkaloid ergovaline has been detected in toxic fescue and is strongly implicated in some of the fescue toxicosis syndromes. However, the complete etiology of fescue foot remains unresolved.

Some reports indicate an increased incidence of fescue lameness as plants age and after severe droughts. Strains of tall fescue vary in their toxicity (eg, Kentucky-31 is more toxic than Fawn) due to variation in infection level with the fungus and to high variability within a strain. In some Kentucky-31 fescues, infection levels cannot be detected. High nitrogen applications appear to enhance the toxicity. Susceptibility of cattle is subject to individual variation.

Low environmental temperature is thought to exacerbate the lesions of fescue lameness; however, high temperatures increase the severity of a toxic problem known as **epidemic hyperthermia** or "summer syndrome," in which a high proportion of a herd of cattle exhibits hypersalivation and hyperthermia. It appears that the toxin is a vasoconstrictor that induces hyperthermia in hot weather and results in cold extremities during cold weather. Another cause of this is poisoning with *C purpurea* (ergot alkaloids).

Erythema and swelling of the coronary region occur, and cattle are alert but lose weight and may be seen "paddling" or weight-shifting. The back is slightly arched, and knuckling of a hind pastern may be an initial sign. There is progressive lameness, anorexia, depression, and later, dry gangrene of the distal limbs (hindlimbs first). Signs usually develop within 10-21 days after turnout into a fescue-contaminated pasture in fall. A period of frost tends to increase the incidence.

For control, all infected forage should be removed.

Summer Fescue Toxicosis

This warm season condition is characterized by reduced feed intake and weight gains or milk production. The toxin(s) affects cattle, sheep, and horses during the summer when they are grazing or being fed tall fescue forage or seed contaminated with the endophytic fungus *Acremonium coenophialum*. The severity of the condition varies from field to field and year to year.

Signs other than reduced performance, which may appear within 1-2 wk after fescue feeding is started, include fever, tachypnea, rough coat, lower serum prolactin levels, and excessive salivation. The animals seek wet spots or shade. Lowered reproductive performance also has been reported. Agalactia has been reported for both horses and cattle. Thickened placentas, delayed parturition, birth of weak foals, and agalactia have been reported in horses. The severity increases when environmental temperatures are >75-80°F (24-27°C) and if high nitrogen fertilizer has been applied to the grass.

For control, toxic tall fescue pastures must be destroyed and reseeded with seed that does not contain endophytic fungus because transfer of the fungus from plant to plant is primarily, if not solely, through infected seed. Not using pastures during hot weather, diluting tall fescue pastures with interseeded legumes, clipping pastures to reduce seed formation, or offering other feedstuffs helps reduce severity. (*See also* ABDOMINAL FAT NECROSIS, p 306.)

FUMONISIN TOXICOSIS

Equine leukoencephalomalacia is a mycotoxic disease of the CNS that affects horses, mules, and donkeys. It occurs sporadically in North and South America, South Africa, Europe, and China. It is associated with the feeding of moldy corn (maize), usually over a period of several weeks. Fumonisins are produced worldwide primarily by *Fusarium moniliforme* Sheldon and *F proliferatum*. Conditions favoring fumonisin production appear to include a period of drought during the growing season with subsequent cool, moist conditions during pollination and kernel formation. Three toxins produced by the fungi have been classified as fumonisin B_1 (FB$_1$), B_2 (FB$_2$), and B_3 (FB$_3$). Current evidence suggests that FB$_1$ and FB$_2$ are of similar toxicity, whereas FB$_3$ is relatively nontoxic. Major health effects are observed in Equidae and swine.

Signs in Equidae include apathy, drowsiness, pharyngeal paralysis, blindness, circling, staggering, and recumbency. The clinical course is usually 1-2 days but may be as short as several hours or as long as several weeks. Icterus may be present if the liver is involved. The characteristic lesion is liquefactive necrosis of the white matter of the cerebrum. The necrosis is usually unilateral but may be asymmetrically bilateral. Some horses may have hepatic necrosis similar to that seen in aflatoxicosis. Horses may develop leukoencephalomalacia from prolonged exposure to as little as 8-10 ppm fumonisins in the diet.

Fumonisins have also been reported to cause acute epidemics of disease in weanling or adult pigs, characterized by pulmonary edema and hydrothorax. **Porcine pulmonary edema** (PPE) is usually an acute, fatal disease and appears to be caused by pulmonary hypertension with transudation of fluids in the thorax resulting in interstitial pulmonary edema and hydrothorax. Acute PPE results after consumption of fumonisins for 3-6 days at dietary concentrations >100 ppm. Morbidity within a herd may be >50%, and mortality among affected pigs ranges from 50 to 100%. Signs include acute onset of dyspnea, cyanosis of mucous membranes, weakness, recumbency, and death, often within 24 hr after the first clinical signs. Affected sows in late gestation that survive acute PPE may abort within 2-3 days, presumably as a result of fetal anoxia. Prolonged exposure of pigs to sublethal concentrations of fumonisins results in hepatotoxicosis characterized by reduced growth; icterus; and increased serum levels of cholesterol, bilirubin, AST, lactate dehydrogenase, and γ-glutamyltransferase.

The biochemical mechanism of action for PPE or liver toxicosis is believed to be due to the ability of fumonisins to interrupt sphingolipid synthesis in many animal species.

Cattle, sheep, and poultry are considerably less susceptible to fumonisins than are horses or swine. Cattle and sheep tolerate fumonisin concentrations of 100 ppm with little effect. Dietary concentrations of 200 ppm cause inappetence, weight loss, and mild liver damage. Poultry are affected by concentrations >200-400 ppm and may develop inappetence, weight loss, and skeletal abnormalities.

No treatment is available. Avoidance of moldy corn is the only prevention, although this is difficult because it may not be grossly moldy or it may be contained in a mixed feed. However, most of the toxin is present in broken kernels or small, poorly formed kernels. Therefore, cleaning grain to remove the screenings markedly reduces fumonisin concentration. Corn suspected of containing fumonisins should not be given to horses.

MYCOTOXIC LUPINOSIS

Lupines (*Lupinus* spp) cause 2 distinct forms of poisoning in livestock—lupine poisoning and lupinosis. The former is a nervous syndrome caused by alkaloids present in bitter lupines; the latter is a mycotoxic disease characterized by liver injury and jaundice, which results mainly from the feeding of sweet lupines. Lupinosis is important in Australia and South Africa and also has been reported from New Zealand and Europe. There is increasing use of sweet lupines, either as forage crops or through feeding of their residues after grain harvest, as strategic feed for sheep in Mediterranean climate zones. Sheep, and occasionally cattle and horses, are affected, and pigs are also susceptible.

Etiology and Pathogenesis: The causal fungus is *Phomopsis leptostromiformis*, which causes *Phomopsis* stem-blight, especially in white and yellow lupines; blue varieties are resistant. It produces sunken, linear stem lesions that contain black, stromatic masses, and it also affects the pods and seeds. The fungus is also a saprophyte and grows well on dead lupine material (eg, haulm, pods, stubble) under favorable conditions. It produces phomopsins as secondary metabolites on infected lupine material, especially after rain.

Clinical changes are mainly attributable to toxic hepatocyte injury, which causes mitotic arrest in metaphase, isolated cell necrosis, and hepatic enzyme leakage, with loss of metabolic and excretory function.

Clinical Findings, Lesions, and Diagnosis: Early signs in sheep and cattle are inappetence and listlessness. Complete anorexia and jaundice follow, and ketosis is common. Cattle may show lacrimation and salivation. Sheep may become photosensitive. In acute outbreaks, deaths occur in 2-14 days.

In acute disease, icterus is marked. Livers are enlarged, orange-yellow, and fatty. More chronic cases show bronze- or tan-colored livers that are firm, contracted in size, and fibrotic. Copious amounts of transudates may be found in the abdominal and thoracic cavities and in the pericardial sac.

Feeding of moldy lupine material, together with clinical signs and increased levels of serum liver enzymes, strongly indicate lupinosis.

Control: Frequent surveillance of sheep and of lupine fodder material for characteristic black spot fungal infestation, especially after rains, is advised. The utilization of lupine cultivars, bred and developed for resistance to *P leptostromiformis* is advocated. Oral doses of zinc (≥0.5 g/day) have protected sheep against liver injury induced by phomopsins.

PASPALUM STAGGERS

This incoordination results from eating paspalum grasses infested by *Claviceps paspali*. The life cycle of this fungus is similar to that of *C purpurea* (*see* ERGOTISM, p 2414). The yellow-gray sclerotia, which mature in the seed heads in autumn, are round, roughened, and 2-4 mm in diameter. Ingestion of sclerotia causes nervous signs in cattle most commonly, but horses and sheep also are susceptible. Guinea pigs can be affected experimentally. The toxicity is not ascribed to ergot alkaloids; the toxic principles are thought to be paspalinine and paspalitrem A and B, tremorgenic compounds from the sclerotia.

A sufficiently large single dose causes signs that persist for several days. Animals display continuous trembling of the large muscle groups; movements are jerky and incoordinated. If they attempt to run, the animals fall over in awkward positions. Affected animals may be belligerent and dangerous to approach or handle. After prolonged exposure, condition is lost and complete paralysis can occur. The time of onset of signs depends on the degree of the infestation of seed heads and the grazing habits of the animals. Experimentally, early signs appear in cattle after ~100 g/day of sclerotia has been administered for >2 days. Although the mature ergots are toxic, they are most dangerous just when they are maturing to the hard, black (sclerotic) stage.

Recovery follows removal of the animals to feed not contaminated with sclerotia of *C paspali*. Animals are less affected if left alone and provided readily available nutritious forages. Care should be taken to prevent accidental access to ponds or rough terrain where accidental trauma or drowning could occur. Topping of the pasture to remove affected seed heads has been effective in control.

SLAFRAMINE TOXICOSIS

Trifolium pratense (red clover) may become infected with the fungus *Rhizoctonia leguminocola* (black patch disease), especially in wet, cool years. Rarely, other legumes (white clover, alsike, alfalfa) may be infected. Slaframine is an indolizidine alkaloid recognized as the toxic principle, and it is stable in dried hay and probably in silage. Horses are highly sensitive to slaframine, but clinical cases occur in cattle as well. Profuse salivation (salivary syndrome) develops within hours after first consumption of contaminated hay; signs also include mild lacrimation, diarrhea, mild bloat, and frequent urination. Morbidity can be high, but death is not expected, and removal of contaminated hay allows recovery and return of appetite within 24-48 hr. A related alkaloid, swainsonine, produced by *R leguminicola*, has caused a lysosomal storage disease from prolonged exposure, but its importance in the salivary syndrome is not confirmed. Diagnosis is tentatively based on recognition of the characteristic clinical signs and the presence of "black patch" on the forages. Chemical detection of slaframine or swainsonine in forages helps to confirm the diagnosis. There is no specific antidote to slaframine toxicosis, although atropine may control at least some of the prominent salivary and GI signs. Removal of animals from the contaminated hay is essential. Prevention of *Rhizoctonia* infection of clovers has been difficult. Some clover varieties may be relatively resistant to black patch disease. Reduced usage of red clover for forages or dilution with other feeds is helpful.

TRICHOTHECENE TOXICOSIS

The trichothecene mycotoxins are a group of closely related secondary metabolic products of several families of imperfect, saprophytic, or plant pathogenic fungi such as *Fusarium, Trichothecium, Myrothecium, Cephalosporium, Stachybotrys, Trichodesma, Cylindrocarpon,* and *Verticimonosporium* spp. On the basis of molecular structure, the trichothecenes are classed as nonmacrocyclic (eg, deoxynivalenol [DON] or vomitoxin, T-2 toxin, diacetoxyscirpenol, and others) or macrocyclic (satratoxin, roridin, verrucarin).

The trichothecene mycotoxins are highly toxic at the subcellular, cellular, and organic system level. They swiftly penetrate cell lipid bilayers, thus allowing access to DNA, RNA, and cellular organelles. Trichothecenes inhibit protein synthesis by affecting polyribosomes to interfere with the initiation phase of protein synthesis. At the subcellular level, these toxins inhibit protein synthesis and covalently bond to sulfhydryl groups.

Trichothecene mycotoxins are generally cytotoxic to most cells, including neoplastic cells; they are not mutagenic. Toxicity of the trichothecenes is based on direct cytotoxicity and is often referred to as a radiomimetic effect (eg, bone marrow hypoplasia, gastroenteritis, diarrhea, hemorrhages). The cutaneous cytotoxicity that follows administration of these compounds is a nonspecific, acute, necrotizing process with minimal inflammation of both the epidermis and dermis. Stomatitis, hyperkeratosis with ulceration of the esophageal portion of the gastric mucosa, and necrosis of the GI tract have been seen after ingestion of trichothecenes.

Given in sublethal toxic doses via any route, the trichothecenes are highly immunosuppressive in mammals; however, longterm feeding of high levels of T-2 toxin does not seem to activate latent viral or bacterial infections. The main immunosuppressive effect of the trichothecenes is at the level of the T-suppressor cell, but the toxins may affect function of helper T cells, B cells, or macrophages, or the interaction among these cells.

Hemorrhagic diathesis may occur after thrombocytopenia or defective intrinsic or extrinsic coagulation pathways. It appears that hemorrhage results from depression of clotting factors, thrombocytopenia, inhibition of platelet function, or possibly a combination of these.

Refusal to consume contaminated feedstuff is the typical sign, which limits development of other signs. If no other food is offered, animals may eat reluctantly, but in some instances, excessive salivation and vomiting may occur. In the past, the ability to cause vomiting had been ascribed to DON only, hence the common name, **vomitoxin**. However, other members of the trichothecene family also can induce vomiting.

Feed refusal caused by DON is a learned response known as taste aversion. It may be related to neurochemical changes in serotonin, dopamine, and 5-hydroxyindoleacetic acid. Feed refusal response to vomitoxin varies widely among species. DON in swine causes conditioned taste aversion, and swine would be expected to recognize new flavors (eg, flavoring agents) added to DON-containing feed and thus develop aversion to the new taste as well. Provision of uncontaminated feed usually leads to resumption of eating within 1-2 days.

In swine, reduced feed intake may occur at dietary concentrations as low as 1 ppm, and refusal may be complete at 10 ppm. Ruminants generally will readily consume up to 10 ppm dietary vomitoxin, and poultry may tolerate as much as 100 ppm. Horses may accept as much as 35-45 ppm dietary DON without feed refusal or adverse clinical effects. Related effects of weight loss, hypoproteinemia, and weakness may follow prolonged feed refusal. There is little credible evidence that vomitoxin causes reproductive dysfunction in domestic animals.

Irritation of the skin and mucous membranes and gastroenteritis are another set of signs typical of trichothecene toxicosis. Hemorrhagic diathesis can occur, and the radiomimetic injury (damage to dividing cells) is expressed as lymphopenia or pancytopenia. Paresis, seizures, and paralysis occur in almost all species. Eventually, hypotension may lead to death. Many of the severe effects described for experimental trichothecene toxicosis are due to dosing by gavage. From a practical perspective, high concentrations of trichothecenes often cause feed refusal and therefore are self-limiting as a toxic problem.

Due to the immunosuppressive action of trichothecenes, secondary bacterial, viral, or parasitic infections may mask the primary injury. The lymphatic organs are smaller than normal and may be difficult to find on necropsy.

Although no specific name has been given to most nonmacrocyclic trichothecene-related diseases, the term **fusariotoxicosis** is often used. Some other names used are moldy corn poisoning in cattle, bean hull poisoning of horses, and feed refusal and emetic syndrome in pigs. A condition in chickens, referred to as "rickets in broilers," is also thought to be caused by trichothecenes.

Macrocyclic trichothecene-related diseases have received a number of specific names. The best known is **stachybotryotoxicosis** of horses, cattle, sheep, pigs, and poultry, first diagnosed in the former USSR but occurring also in Europe and South Africa. Cutaneous and mucocutaneous lesions, panleukopenia, nervous signs, and abortions have been seen. Death may occur in 2-12 days.

Myrotheciotoxicosis and **dendrodochiotoxicosis** have been reported from the former USSR and New Zealand. The signs resemble those of stachybotryotoxicosis, but death may occur in 1-5 days.

Diagnosis: Because the clinical signs are nonspecific, or masked by secondary infections and disease, diagnosis is difficult. Analysis of feed is often costly and time consuming but ideally should be attempted. Interim measures are carefully examining feedstuff for signs of mold growth or caking of feed particles and switching to an alternative feed supply. Change of feed supply often results in immediate improvement and thus may provide one more clue that the original feed was contaminated.

Control: Symptomatic treatment and feeding of uncontaminated feed are recommended. Steroidal anti-shock and anti-inflammatory agents, such as methylprednisolone, prednisolone, and dexamethasone, have been used successfully in experimental trials. Poultry and cattle are more tolerant of trichothecenes than are pigs.

NITRATE AND NITRITE POISONING

Many species are susceptible to nitrate and nitrite poisoning, but cattle are affected most frequently. Ruminants are especially vulnerable because the ruminal flora reduces nitrate to ammonia, with nitrite (~10 times more toxic than nitrate) as an intermediate product. Nitrate reduction (and nitrite production) occurs in the cecum of equids but not to the same extent as in ruminants. Young pigs also have GI microflora capable of reducing nitrate to nitrite, but mature monogastric animals (except equids) are more resistant to nitrate toxicosis because this pathway is age-limited.

Acute intoxication is manifested primarily by methemoglobin formation (nitrite ion in contact with RBC oxidizes ferrous iron in Hgb to the ferric state, forming stable methemoglobin incapable of oxygen transport) and resultant anoxia. Secondary effects due to vasodilatory action of the nitrite ion on vascular smooth muscle may occur. The nitrite ion may also alter metabolic protein enzymes. Ingested nitrates may directly irritate the GI mucosa and produce abdominal pain and diarrhea.

Although usually acute, the effects of nitrite or nitrate toxicity may be subacute or chronic and are reported to include retarded growth, lowered milk production, vitamin A deficiency, minor transitory goitrogenic effects, abortions and fetotoxicity, and increased susceptibility to infection. Chronic nitrate toxicosis remains a controversial issue and is not as yet well characterized, but most current evidence does not support allegations of lowered milk production in dairy cows due to excessive dietary nitrate exposure alone.

Etiology: Nitrates and nitrites are used in pickling and curing brines for preserving meats, certain machine oils and antirust tablets, gunpowder and explosives, and fertilizers. They may also serve as therapeutic agents for certain noninfectious diseases, eg, cyanide poisoning. Toxicoses occur in unacclimated domestic animals most commonly from ingestion of plants that contain excess nitrate, especially by hungry animals engorging themselves and taking in an enormous body burden of nitrate. Nitrate toxicosis can also result from accidental ingestion of fertilizer or other chemicals. Nitrate concentrations may be hazardous in ponds that receive extensive feedlot or fertilizer runoff; these types of nitrate sources may also contaminate shallow, poorly cased wells. Although nitrate concentrations are increasing in groundwater in the USA, well water is rarely the sole cause of excess nitrate exposure.

Water with both high nitrate content and significant coliform contamination has greater potential to affect health adversely and lower productivity than do either nitrate or bacteria alone. Livestock losses have occurred during cold weather due to the concentrating effect of freezing, which increases nitrate content of remaining water in stock tanks.

Crops that readily concentrate nitrate include cereal grasses (especially oats, millet, and rye), corn (maize), sunflower, and sorghums. Weeds that commonly have high nitrate concentrations are pigweed, lamb's quarter, thistle, Jimson weed, fireweed (*Kochia*), smartweed, dock, and Johnson grass. Anhydrous ammonia and nitrate fertilizers and soils naturally high in nitrogen tend to increase nitrate content in forage.

Excess nitrate in plants is generally associated with damp weather conditions and cool temperatures (55°F [13°C]), although high concentrations are also likely to develop when growth is rapid during hot, humid weather. Drought conditions, particularly if occurring when plants are immature, may leave the vegetation with high nitrate content. Decreased light, cloudy weather, and shading associated with crowding conditions can also cause increased concentrations of nitrates within plants. Well-aerated soil with a low pH, and low or deficient amounts of molybdenum, sulfur, or phosphorus in soil tend to enhance nitrate uptake, whereas soil deficiencies of copper, cobalt, or manganese tend to have opposing effects. Anything that stunts growth increases nitrate accumulation in the lower part of the plant. Phenoxy acid derivative herbicides, eg, 2,4-D and 2,4,5-T, applied to nitrate-accumulating plants during early stages, cause increased growth and a high nitrate residual (10-30%) in surviving plants, which are lush and eaten with apparent relish even though previously avoided.

Nitrate, which does not selectively accumulate in fruits or grain, is found chiefly in the lower stalk with lesser amounts in the upper stalk and leaves. Nitrate in plants can be converted to nitrite under the proper conditions of moisture, heat, and microbial activity after harvesting.

Clinical Findings: Signs of nitrite poisoning usually appear suddenly due to tissue hypoxia and low blood pressure as a consequence of vasodilation. Rapid, weak heartbeat with subnormal body temperature, muscular tremors, weakness, and ataxia are early signs of toxicosis when methemoglobinemia reaches 30-40%. Brown, cyanotic mucous membranes develop rapidly as methemoglobinemia exceeds 50%. Dyspnea, tachypnea, anxiety, and frequent urination are common. Some monogastric animals, usually because of excess nitrate exposure from nonplant sources, exhibit salivation, vomiting, diarrhea, abdominal pain, and gastric hemorrhage. Affected animals may die suddenly without appearing ill, in terminal anoxic convulsions within 1 hr, or after a clinical course of 12-24 hr or longer. Acute lethal toxicoses almost always are due to development of ≥80% methemoglobinemia. Under certain conditions, adverse effects may not be apparent until animals have been eating nitrate-containing forages for days to weeks. Some animals that develop marked dyspnea recover but then develop interstitial pulmonary emphysema and continue to suffer respiratory distress; most of these recover fully within 10-14 days. Abortion and stillbirths may be seen in some cattle 5-14 days after excessive nitrate/nitrite exposure, but likely only in cows that have survived a ≥50% methemoglobinemia for 6-12 hr or longer. Prolonged exposure to excess nitrate coupled with cold stress and inadequate nutrition may lead to the alert downer cow syndrome (p 957) in pregnant beef cattle; sudden collapse and death can result.

Lesions: Blood that contains methemoglobin usually has a chocolate-brown color, although dark red hues may also be seen. There may be pinpoint or larger hemorrhages on serosal surfaces. Dark brown discoloration evident in moribund or recently dead animals is not pathognomonic, however, and other methemoglobin inducers must be considered. If necropsy is postponed too long, the brown discoloration may disappear with conversion of methemoglobin back to Hgb.

Diagnosis: Excess nitrate exposure can be assessed by laboratory analysis for nitrate in both pre- and postmortem specimens. High nitrate and nitrite values in postmortem specimens may be an incidental finding, indicative only of exposure and not toxicity. Plasma is the preferred premortem specimen, because some plasma-protein-bound nitrate could be lost in the clot if serum was collected. Nitrite present in whole blood also continues to react with Hgb in vitro, so these specimens must be centrifuged immediately and plasma separated to prevent erroneous values of both. Additional postmortem specimens from either toxicoses or abortions include ocular fluids, fetal pleural or thoracic fluids, fetal stomach contents, and maternal uterine fluid. All specimens should be frozen in clean plastic or glass containers before submission, except when whole blood is collected for methemoglobin analysis. Because the amount of nitrate in rumen contents is not representative of concentrations in the diet, evaluation of rumen contents is not indicated.

Bacterial contamination of postmortem specimens, especially ocular fluid, is likely to cause conversion of nitrate to nitrite at room temperature or higher; such specimens may have abnormally high nitrite concentrations with reduced to absent nitrate concentrations. Endogenous biosynthesis of nitrate and nitrite by macrophages stimulated by lipopolysaccharide or other bacterial products may also complicate interpretation of analytical findings; this should be considered as a possible maternal or fetal response to an infectious process.

Methemoglobin analysis alone is not a reliable indicator of excess nitrate or nitrite exposure except in acute toxicosis, because 50% of methemoglobin present will be converted back to Hgb in ~2 hr, and alternate forms of nonoxygenated Hgb that may be formed by reaction with nitrite are not detected by methemoglobin analysis. Nitrate and nitrite concentrations >20 μg NO_3/mL and >0.5 μg NO_2/mL, respectively, in maternal and perinatal serum, plasma, ocular fluid, and other similar biologic fluids are usually indicative of excessive nitrate or nitrite exposure in most domestic animal species; nitrate concentrations of up to 40 μg NO_3/mL have been present in the plasma of healthy calves at birth, but are reduced rapidly as normal neonatal renal function eliminates nitrate in the urine. Normally expected nitrate and nitrite concentrations in similar diagnostic specimens are usually <10 μg NO_3/mL and <0.2 μg NO_2/mL, respectively. Nitrate and nitrite concentrations >10 but <20 μg NO_3/mL and >0.2 but <0.5 μg NO_2/mL, respectively, are suspect and indicate nitrate or nitrite exposure of unknown duration, extent, or origin. The possible contribution of endogenous nitrate or nitrite synthesis by activated macrophages must also be considered. The biologic half-life of nitrate in beef cattle, sheep, and ponies was determined to be 7.7, 4.2, and 4.8 hr, respectively, so it will be at least 5 biologic half-lives (24-36 hr) before elevated nitrate concentrations from excessive nitrate exposure diminish to normally expected values, allowing additional time for valid premortem specimen collection.

A latent period may exist between excessive maternal dietary nitrate exposure and equilibrium in perinatal ocular fluids. Aqueous humor is actively secreted into the anterior chamber at a rate of ~0.1/mL/hr, and nitrate and nitrite are thought to enter the globe of the eye by this mechanism. Equilibrium between aqueous and vitreous humor is by passive diffusion rather than by active secretion, so nitrate or nitrite may be present in comparatively lesser concentrations in vitreous humor after acute exposure.

Field tests for nitrate are presumptive and should be confirmed by standard analytical methods at a qualified laboratory. The diphenylamine blue test (1% in concentrated sulfuric acid) is more suitable to determine the presence or absence of nitrate in suspected forages. Nitrate test strips (dipsticks) are effective in determining nitrate values in water supplies and can be used to evaluate nitrate and nitrite content in serum, plasma, ocular fluid, and urine.

Differential diagnoses include poisonings by cyanide, urea, pesticides, toxic gases (eg, carbon monoxide, hydrogen sulfide), chlorates, aniline dyes, aminophenols, or drugs (eg, sulfonamides, phenacetin, and acetaminophen), as well as infectious or noninfectious diseases (eg, grain overload, hypocalcemia, hypomagnesemia, pulmonary adenomatosis, or emphysema) and any sudden unexplained deaths.

Treatment: Slow IV injection of 1% methylene blue in distilled water or isotonic saline should be given at 4-22 mg/kg body wt, or more, depending on severity of exposure. Lower dosages may be repeated in 20-30 min if the initial response is not satisfactory. Lower dosages of methylene blue can be used in all species, but only ruminants can safely tolerate higher dosages. If additional exposure or absorption occurs during therapy, retreating with methylene blue every 6-8 hr should be considered. Rumen lavage with cold water and antibiotics may stop the continuing microbial production of nitrite.

Control: Animals may adapt to higher nitrate content in feeds, especially when grazing summer annuals such as sorghum-Sudan hybrids. Multiple, small feedings help animals adapt. Trace mineral supplements and a balanced diet may help prevent nutritional or metabolic disorders associated with longterm excess dietary nitrate consumption. Feeding grain with high-nitrate forages may reduce nitrite production. Forage nitrate concentrations >1% nitrate dry-weight basis (10,000 ppm NO_3) may cause acute toxicoses in unacclimated animals, and forage nitrate concentrations ≤5,000 ppm NO_3 (dry-weight basis) are recommended for pregnant beef cows. However, even forage concentrations of 1,000 ppm NO_3 dry-weight basis have been lethal to hungry cows engorging themselves in a single feeding within an hour, so the total dose of nitrate ingested is a deciding factor.

High-nitrate forages may also be harvested and stored as ensilage rather than dried hay or green chop; this may reduce the nitrate content in forages by up to 50%. Raising cutter heads of machinery during harvesting operations selectively leaves the more hazardous stalk bases in the field.

Hay appears to be more hazardous than fresh green chop or pasture with similar nitrate content. Heating may assist bacterial conversion of nitrate to nitrite; feeding high-nitrate hay, straw, or fodder that has been damp or wet for several days, or stockpiled, green-chopped forage should be avoided. Large round bales with excess nitrate are especially dangerous if stored uncovered outside; rain or snow can leach and subsequently concentrate most of the total nitrate present into the lower third of these bales.

Water transported in improperly cleaned liquid fertilizer tanks may be extremely high in nitrate. Young unweaned livestock, especially neonatal pigs, can be more sensitive to nitrate in water.

NONPROTEIN NITROGEN POISONING

(Ammonia toxicosis)

Poisoning by ingestion of excess urea or other sources of nonprotein nitrogen (NPN) is usually acute, rapidly progressive, and highly fatal. Sources of NPN have different toxicities in various species, but mature ruminants are affected most commonly. After ingestion, NPN undergoes hydrolysis and releases excess ammonia (NH_3) into the GI tract, which is absorbed and leads to hyperammonemia.

Etiology: The most common sources of NPN in feeds are urea, urea phosphate, ammonia (anhydrous), and salts such as monoammonium and diammonium phosphate. Because feed-grade urea is unstable, it is formulated (usually pelleted) to prevent degradation to NH_3. Biuret, a less toxic source of NPN, is used less frequently than in the past. Natural protein sources such as rice hulls, cottonseed meal, and straw or other low-quality forages may be treated with anhydrous ammonia to increase available nitrogen in supplemented livestock diets. Most sources of NPN are provided to ruminants by direct addition of dry supplement to a complete mixed or blended diet, by free-choice access to NPN-containing range blocks or cubes, or by lick tank systems combined with molasses as a supplement. Ammonia or NPN poisoning is a common sequela of abrupt change to urea or other NPN in the diet when only natural protein was previously fed; animals have to be gradually acclimated to NPN so that rumen microflora can increase in numbers to use the NH_3 produced. Also, farm animals sometimes drink liquid fertilizers or ingest dry granular fertilizers that contain ammonium salts or urea.

Ruminants are most sensitive because urease is normally present in the functional rumen after 50 days of age. Dietary exposure of unacclimated ruminants to 0.3-0.5 g of urea/kg body wt may cause adverse effects; doses of 1-1.5 g/kg are usually lethal. Urease activity in the equine cecum is ~25% that of the rumen, and horses may receive NPN as a feed additive; however, horses are more sensitive to urea than other monogastrics, and doses ≥4 g/kg can be lethal. Ammonium salts at 0.3-0.5 g/kg may be toxic in all species and ages of farm animals; doses ≥1.5 g/kg usually are fatal. Pigs and neonatal calves are generally unaffected by ingestion of urea except for a transient diuresis.

Livestock may require days or weeks for total adaptation before rumen microflora can utilize the gradually increasing amounts of urea or other NPN in the diets; however, adaptation is lost relatively quickly (1-3 days) once NPN is removed from the diet.

Diets low in energy and high in fiber are more commonly associated with NPN toxicosis, even in acclimated animals. Highly palatable supplements (such as liquid molasses or large protein blocks crumbled by precipitation) or improperly maintained lick tanks may lead to consumption of lethal amounts of NPN.

A related CNS disorder in cattle fed ammoniated high-quality hay, silage, molasses, and protein blocks is thought to be caused by the formation of 4-methylimidazole (4-MI) through the action of NH_3 on soluble carbohydrates (reducing sugars) in these feedstuffs. Cattle fed dietary components containing 4-MI develop a syndrome known as the "bovine bonkers syndrome," named for the wildly aberrant behavior exhibited. Signs relate to CNS effects, with stampeding, ear twitching, trembling, champing, salivating, and convulsions. Because nursing calves are affected, the toxic principle apparently is excreted in milk. Ammoniated low-quality forages do not have sufficient concentrations of reducing sugars to form 4-MI, and thus serve as a relatively safe nitrogen source to acclimated animals.

A related disorder involves accidental excessive exposure of ruminants (cattle and sheep) to raw soybeans. Soybeans have high concentrations of both carbohydrates and proteins, as well as urease. Overconsumption can cause acute carbohydrate fermentation and excessive ammonia release, resulting in ammonia toxicosis and lactic acidosis. Affected animals have engorged rumens with a gray, lava-like, amorphous mass inside.

Clinical Findings: The period from urea ingestion to onset of clinical signs is 20-60 min in cattle, 30-90 min in sheep, and longer in horses. Early signs include muscle tremors (especially of face and ears), exophthalmia, abdominal pain, frothy salivation, polyuria, and bruxism. Tremors progress to incoordination and weakness. Pulmonary edema leads to marked salivation, dyspnea, and gasping.

Horses may exhibit head pressing; cattle are often agitated, hyperirritable, violent, and belligerent as toxicosis progresses; sheep usually appear depressed. An early sign in cattle is ruminal atony; as toxicosis progresses, ruminal tympany is usually evident, and violent struggling and bellowing, a marked jugular pulse, severe twitching, tetanic spasms, and convulsions may be seen. Affected cattle with violent or belligerent aberrant behavior may have produced some 4-MI in vivo through reaction of excessive NH_3, released from NPN, with carbohydrates and reducing sugars in the rumen. The PCV and serum concentrations of NH_3, glucose, lactate, potassium, phosphorus, AST, ALT, and BUN usually are significantly increased.

As death nears, animals become cyanotic, dyspneic, anuric, and hyperthermic, and blood pH decreases from 7.4 to 7.0. Regurgitation may occur, especially in sheep. Death related to excess NPN usually occurs within 2 hr in cattle, 4 hr in sheep, and 3-12 hr in horses. Survivors recover in 12-24 hr with no sequelae.

Lesions: Carcasses of animals dying of NPN poisoning appear to bloat and decompose rapidly, with no specific characteristic lesions. Frequently, pulmonary edema, congestion, and petechial hemorrhages may be seen. Mild bronchitis and catarrhal gastroenteritis are often reported. Regurgitated and inhaled rumen contents are commonly found in the trachea and bronchi, especially in sheep. The odor of NH_3 may or may not be apparent in ingesta from a freshly opened rumen or cecum. A ruminal or cecal pH ≥ 7.5 from a recently dead animal is highly suggestive of NPN poisoning. The ruminal pH remains stable for several hours after death under most circumstances but continues to rise in NPN toxicosis.

Diagnosis: Ammonia or NPN poisoning is suggested by signs, lesions, history of acute illness, and dietary exposure. Exposure to excess NPN may be evaluated through laboratory analysis for the ammonia nitrogen (NH_3-N) in both antemortem and postmortem specimens and for urea or other NPN in suspected feeds and other dietary sources. Specimens for NH_3-N analysis include ruminal-reticular fluid, serum, whole blood, and urine. All specimens should be frozen immediately after collection and thawed only for analysis; alternatively, ruminal-reticular fluid may be preserved with a few drops of saturated mercuric chloride solution added to each 100 mL of specimen.

Animals dead more than a few hours in hot ambient temperatures or 12 hr in moderate climates probably have undergone too much autolysis to be of diagnostic value.

The amount of urea or the equivalent NPN in biologic specimens is meaningless; however, urea and NPN should be determined in representative feeds and other dietary sources. Values for urea and NPN in feed permit calculation of the protein equivalent (1 part protein = 0.34 parts urea; 1 part urea = 2.92 parts protein) in feed as well as the total estimated dose of NPN ingested.

Concentrations of ≥ 2 mg/100 mL NH_3-N in blood or serum indicate excess NPN exposure. The concentration of NH_3-N in ruminal-reticular fluid is >80 mg/100 mL in most cases of NPN poisoning and may be >200 mg/100 mL. Acclimated ruminants fed diets high in legume hay, soybean meal, cottonseed meal, linseed meal, fish meal, or milk byproducts may have NH_3-N concentrations in rumen fluid approaching 60 mg/100 mL with no apparent toxicity. The pH of ruminal-reticular fluid should also be determined; a pH of 7.5-8 (at time of death) is indicative of NPN toxicity.

Differential diagnoses include poisonings by nitrate/nitrite, cyanide, organophosphate/carbamate pesticides, raw soybean overload, 4-methylimidazole, lead, chlorinated hydrocarbon pesticides, and toxic gases (carbon monoxide, hydrogen sulfide, nitrogen dioxide); acute infectious diseases; and noninfectious diseases such as encephalopathies (eg, leukoencephalomalacia, hepatic encephalopathy, polioencephalomalacia), enterotoxemia or rumen autointoxication, protein engorgement, grain engorgement, ruminal tympany, and pulmonary adenomatosis. Nutritional and metabolic disorders related to hypocalcemia, hypomagnesemia, and other elemental aberrations should also be considered.

Treatment: Examination and treatment may be difficult because of violent behavior. Animals that are recumbent and moribund usually do not respond favorably to treatment.

If possible, affected animals should be treated by ruminal infusion of 5% acetic acid (0.5-2 L in sheep and goats and 2-8 L in cattle). Ruminal-reticular fluid specimens for analysis should be taken before acetic acid therapy. Concomitant infusion of iced (0-4°C) water (up to 40 L in adult cattle, proportionally less in sheep and goats) is also recommended. Acetic acid lowers rumen pH and prevents further absorption of NH_3; administration may have to be repeated if affected animals again show clinical signs. Acetic acid also inactivates existing NH_3 in the GI tract and rapidly forms ammonium acetate, which can be used by rumen microflora but does not release NH_3. Cold water lowers the rumen temperature and dilutes the reacting media, which slows urease activity. In valuable animals, removed rumen contents should be replaced with a hay slurry, and a transfer of some rumen contents from a healthy animal may serve as an inoculum to restore normal function. Ruminal tympany should be corrected if indicated, and a trocar may be installed to prevent recurrence.

Pulmonary edema is difficult to treat, although lowering blood pressure with α-adrenergic blocking agents such as ergotamine may help.

Supportive therapy is also indicated; isotonic saline solutions IV correct dehydration, and calcium gluconate and magnesium solutions IV relieve tetanic seizures.

Prevention and Control: Urea should not be fed at a rate exceeding 2-3% of the concentrate or grain portion of ruminant diets and should be limited to ≤1% of the total diet. Additionally, NPN should constitute no more than one-third of the total nitrogen in the ruminant diet. Once the decision is made to feed NPN, animals must be slowly adapted to, and maintained on, a consistent dietary NPN content with no significant deviation. Temporary absences of NPN from the diet should be avoided at all costs. While properly adapted adult cattle can tolerate up to 1 g urea/kg body wt/day, a safer feeding rate is no more than half that amount.

PENTACHLOROPHENOL POISONING

(Penta poisoning)

Penta has been used as a fungicide, molluscicide, insecticide, and as a wood preservative, but registration for its use in lumber in the USA was canceled in 1986. Gradually, other registrations for this agent have been canceled and it is now only registered for industrial purposes; agricultural and domestic uses are prohibited. It is rated by the World Health Organization as highly hazardous.

It can be absorbed through intact skin and lungs and is an intense irritant to the skin and mucous membranes. When absorbed, it increases metabolism by uncoupling cellular phosphorylation. Animals fed in troughs made of lumber treated with penta may salivate and have irritated oral mucosa. Vaporization or leaching of penta in pens, enclosures, homes, and barns has caused illness and death. Signs of poisoning include nervousness, rapid pulse and respiratory rate, weakness, muscle tremors, fever, and convulsions, followed by death. Chronic poisoning results in fatty liver, nephrosis, and weight loss. Additional problems reported when penta-contaminated shavings are used as bedding include "off flavors" in broilers, impaired immune response in chickens, and possibly decreased fertility in boars.

Commercial lots of technical-grade penta contain small but biologically significant amounts of highly toxic impurities (dioxins and furans), and material available today is manufactured so that these toxic ingredients are kept at as low a concentration as possible. Penta can cause residues in animal tissues. Also, a significant amount of hexachlorobenzene is metabolized in animal tissues to penta. Pentachlorophenol is considered to be a carcinogen and a tumor promoter, although studies have shown that the pure material does not increase the incidence of tumors in rats and mice; the technical-grade material has also been shown to be immunotoxic in laboratory studies. Penta must be handled very carefully and kept away from animal contact.

Whole blood analysis for penta may aid in the diagnosis of poisoning; diagnosis is usually made on the basis of the signs and the proximity of treated lumber in the animal's environment.

Acute toxic doses of penta range from 27-350 mg/kg and the fetotoxic NOEL is 10 mg/kg in rats.

There is no known antidote. Termination of exposure, bathing dermally exposed animals, oral administration of activated charcoal, and supportive therapy may be indicated. Bathing should be done gently with cold water and detergent so as not to cause vasodilation and increased absorption. Cattle, pigs, and chickens exposed to wood treated with commercial grade penta that contained these contaminants had increased mortality, decreased productivity, and other less specific herd health problems. (*See* HALOGENATED AROMATIC POISONING, p 2367.) Antipyretics, eg, aspirin and acetaminophen, should not be used. Treatment involves cooling the animal and removing it from the source of poison and administering fluids, electrolytes, and anticonvulsants.

PETROLEUM PRODUCT POISONING

Ingestion or inhalation of—or skin contact with—petroleum, petroleum condensate, gasoline, diesel fuel, kerosene, crude oil, or other hydrocarbon mixtures may cause illness and occasionally death in domestic and wild animals. Both dogs and cats may ingest petroleum products during grooming if their fur becomes contaminated. Dogs may ingest these products directly when they are left in open containers. Inhalation may occur when animals are confined in poorly ventilated areas where these chemicals have been used or stored. Cattle, and less frequently sheep or goats, may ingest such products because they are curious or seeking salt or other nutrients, water is not available, or food or water is contaminated. A cow may consume several gallons at one time.

Petroleum fractions have been used as insecticides and acaricides for many years, either alone or as part of formulations. Small quantities of these may be applied to the skin with few or no harmful effects, but large quantities and prolonged exposure can induce severe reactions. Pipeline breaks, accidental release from storage tanks, and tank car accidents may contaminate land and water supplies. Animals may have access to open or leaky containers of fuel or other hydrocarbon materials. The lower the molecular weight and the higher the degree of unsaturation or aromaticity, the greater the volatility. More volatile hydrocarbons are more lipid soluble and therefore more readily absorbed by inhalation or ingestion. Crude petroleum that has lost much of its lighter, more volatile components through weathering may still be hazardous.

Crude oil and gasoline contain varying amounts of aromatic hydrocarbons including benzene, toluene, ethyl-benzene, and xylene. For example, gasoline in the USA typically contains up to 2% benzene. Gasoline in some other countries may contain up to 5% benzene. These compounds, if ingested or inhaled in sufficient amounts, can have acute and chronic effects different from the other hydrocarbons that make up the majority of oil and gas products. Benzene, for example, is a known carcinogen at high levels of exposure and has a variety of hemotoxic properties. Toluene can cause profound neurologic signs and damage at sufficient doses.

Variation in composition of petroleum and petroleum-derived hydrocarbon mixtures explains some of the differences in toxic effects. Mixtures of low viscosity (eg, gasoline, naphtha, kerosene) have a high aspiration hazard and irritant activity on pulmonary tissues. Gasoline and naphtha fractions may induce vomiting, which contributes to aspiration hazard. Fractions more viscous than kerosene are less likely to be inhaled and, even if aspirated, are somewhat less damaging to lung tissue. Older formulations of lubricating oils and greases can be particularly hazardous because of toxic additives or contaminants (eg, lead).

Clinical Findings: Petroleum hydrocarbon toxicity may involve the respiratory, GI, or integumentary systems or the CNS. In most cases of ingestion, no clinical signs are observed. Pneumonia due to aspiration of hydrocarbons into the lungs is usually the most serious consequence of ingestion of these materials. Aspiration can occur during vomition or eructation of rumen contents. Acute bloat is not a consistent finding but has been reported to cause death very shortly after consumption of highly volatile hydrocarbons such as gasoline or naphtha. CNS effects are usually associated with aspiration. CNS signs may be a result of the anesthetic-like action of low-molecular-weight aliphatic hydrocarbons and/or cerebral anoxia that can result from lung damage or displacement of oxygen by the more volatile hydrocarbons. Some compounds when absorbed in high doses may sensitize the myocardium to endogenous catecholamines. Anorexia, decreased rumen motility, and mild depression may begin in ~24 hr and last 3-14 days depending on dose and content. Hypoglycemia may be seen several days after ingestion. These signs and weight loss may be the only responses seen in animals that do not bloat or aspirate oil. Some animals fail to reestablish normal rumen function after ingestion and can develop a chronic wasting condition.

After ingestion of oil, the feces may not be affected until several days later, at which time they become dry and formed in the case of kerosene or lighter hydrocarbon fractions; in contrast, heavier hydrocarbon mixtures tend to be cathartic. Oil may be found in feces and rumen contents up to 2 wk following ingestion. Regurgitated or vomited oil may be seen on the muzzle and lips. Signs attributable to pulmonary adsorption of hydrocarbons or cerebral anoxia include excitability (associated with aromatic fractions—benzene, toluene, etc), depression (aliphatic or saturated low-molecular-weight hydrocarbons), shivering, head tremors, visual dysfunction (sometimes associated with lead contamination), and incoordination. Acute pneumonia and possibly pleuritis (coughing, tachypnea, shallow respiration, reluctance to move, head held low, weakness, oily nasal discharge, dehydrated appearance) are seen in some animals that aspirate highly volatile mixtures; death usually are seen within days. Respiratory signs may be limited to dyspnea shortly before death in animals that aspirate heavier hydrocarbons. Increased PCV, Hgb, and BUN, indicating mild to moderate hemoconcentration, are associated with development of pneumonia. Neutropenia, lymphopenia, and eosinopenia occur initially and are followed by a relative increase in neutrophils.

There are a few anecdotal reports of abortion following exposure. Laboratory data in rodents support the occurrence of increased fetal loss and decreased fetal growth. However, the doses necessary to affect the fetus were also sufficient to profoundly affect maternal health and weight.

Lesions: Aspiration pneumonia is the most consistent postmortem finding in animals that did not die of bloat. This may be accompanied by tracheitis, pleuritis, and hydrothorax if highly volatile fractions such as gasoline or naphtha are involved. Lung lesions are usually bilateral and found in the caudoventral apical, cardiac, cranioventral diaphragmatic, and intermediate lobes. Affected portions are dark red and consolidated and may contain multiple abscesses. Encapsulated pulmonary abscesses may be found in cattle surviving up to several months after aspiration. Skin lesions may be obvious after repeated topical application or severe exposure and include drying, cracking, or blistering.

Diagnosis: A hydrocarbon odor may be detected in lungs, ruminal contents, and feces. Even if ingested in large doses, hydrocarbons may not be visible in ruminal contents after ~4 days. Adding warm water to the GI contents may cause any oily contents to collect at the surface, but finding oil in the GI tract does not in itself justify a diagnosis of poisoning; most oils have low toxicity if not aspirated. Samples of GI contents, lung, liver, kidney, and the suspected source should be collected for chemical analysis to demonstrate presence of hydrocarbons in tissue (particularly lung) and GI contents and to match those found in tissues and ingesta with the suspected source. Samples must be carefully protected from cross-contamination during necropsy and transportation to the laboratory. Check with the diagnostic laboratory to ensure collection equipment and transport containers are appropriate to prevent evaporative loss of important components and contamination. Positive chemical findings together with appropriate clinical and pathologic findings are confirmatory. Diagnosis in oil-field situations has historically been complicated by involvement of other toxicants, eg, explosives, lead from grease and "pipe dope," arsenicals, organophosphate esters, caustics (acids or alkalis), and saltwater.

Treatment: Bloat pressure should be released by passing a stomach tube if absolutely necessary to save the life of the animal; using a trocar risks forcing oil into the peritoneal cavity, which results in peritonitis. Passing a stomach tube dramatically increases the risk of aspiration and extreme caution is necessary. In the absence of bloat, the prime objectives are to prevent aspiration and to mitigate GI dysfunction. Rumenotomy to remove ruminal contents and replace them with healthy ruminal material is safer. More chronic cases involving primarily hypofunction of the rumen may also respond to this procedure. Cathartics, if used, should be of the saline type; however, there is no evidence that they improve prognosis. Activated charcoal has occasionally been suggested for use in small animals. Although it does not effectively adsorb petroleum distillates, it may be given if necessary to adsorb additives and other contaminants. Care should be taken to avoid inducing vomiting and aspiration.

Animals with evidence of respiratory involvement may require broad-spectrum antibiotic treatment. Pathogens can be introduced into the lungs from aspirated rumen contents mixed with the hydrocarbons. The use of steroids in hydrocarbon aspiration may further reduce the chance for recovery. Treatment of aspiration pneumonia (p 1176) is rarely effective, and the prognosis is poor. However, because signs of aspiration may not appear for several days, prognosis based on initial clinical findings may be misleading.

Most high-molecular-weight compounds pass through the digestive tract unchanged. Most of the petroleum hydrocarbons are highly lipophilic and will be stored for varying times in tissues with high lipid content including fat, nervous tissue, and the liver. Some of the absorbed compounds are metabolized into more toxic byproducts (eg, benzene, toluene, n-hexane). Although most of these compounds do not remain in the body for prolonged periods, little is known about exactly how long tissue levels persist in highly exposed animals. The potential for tissue residues must be considered prior to the slaughter of animals intended for human consumption.

In poisoning or damage due to cutaneous exposure, the material should be removed from the skin with the aid of soap or mild detergents and copious amounts of cool water. The skin should not be brushed or abraded. Further treatment depends on the clinical signs and is largely restricted to supportive therapy.

Petroleum hydrocarbon poisoning can be avoided only by preventing access to these materials through proper storage of home and farm chemicals and well maintained fencing around high-risk petroleum facilities.

Effects of Oil and Gas Fields on Cattle Health and Production: Anecdotal reports in the literature have documented producer concerns about the effect of oil fields on cattle health and production. Some recent observational studies have suggested that exposure to emissions from sour gas processing plants and sour gas flares (natural gas containing hydrogen sulfide) may be associated with an increased risk of certain reproductive losses in cattle. Current research is re-examining these findings and exploring the impact of oil and gas field emissions on the immune system.

PLANTS POISONOUS TO ANIMALS

HOUSEPLANTS AND ORNAMENTALS

Plants are an important part of the decor of homes; pets often chew on or ingest these plants, which can result in toxicoses (see TABLE 3). Inquiries to poison control centers on plants ingested by children <5 yr old are estimated at 5-10% of all inquiries. Similar estimates (though not documented) could be made for pets.

Little research has been done on the toxicity of houseplants. Most are hybrids, and selecting for growth outside their natural environment could affect their degree of toxicity. Age of the pet, boredom, and changes in the surroundings are factors that may affect the incidence of poisoning. Puppies and kittens are very inquisitive, and mouth or chew almost everything. Pets (especially single household pets) of all ages may become bored or restless if left alone or confined for too long at any one time, and chewing on objects for relief is common. Pets of all ages also explore changes in their environment; for example, pets commonly chew the leaves or ripe berries of potentially poisonous plants that are placed in the home during holidays.

RANGE PLANTS OF TEMPERATE NORTH AMERICA

Poisonous plants are among the important causes of economic loss to the livestock industry and should be considered when evaluating illness and decreased productivity in livestock (*see* TABLE 4). Poisonous plants can affect animals in many ways, including death, chronic illness and debilitation, decreased weight gain, abortion, birth defects, increased parturition interval, and photosensitization. In addition to these more obvious losses, other considerations include loss of forage, additional fencing, increased labor and management costs, and frequently interference with proper harvesting of forage.

Most poisonous range plants fall into 2 general categories: those that are indigenous to a range and increase with heavy grazing, and those that invade after overgrazing or disturbance of the land. Among those not in these categories are certain locoweeds and larkspurs, both of which form part of the normal range plant community. Poisonous plants can be found in most plant communities and should be considered in most grazing situations.

Livestock poisoning by plants often can be traced to problems of management or range condition, rather than simply to the presence of poisonous plants. Usually, animals are poisoned because hunger or other conditions cause them to graze abnormally. Overgrazing, trucking, trailing, corralling, or introducing animals onto a new range tend to induce hunger or change behavior, and poisoning may occur.

Not all poisonous plants are unpalatable, and they are not restricted to overgrazed ranges and pastures. Furthermore, poisonous plants do not always kill or otherwise harm animals when consumed. Many plants can be either useful forage or toxic. For example, plants such as lupine and greasewood may be part of an animal's diet, and the animal is poisoned only when it consumes too much of the plant too fast. To prevent poisoning, it is important to understand the factors involved when a useful forage becomes a poisonous plant.

Definitive diagnosis of suspect plant poisonings is difficult. It is important to be familiar with the poisonous plants growing in the specific area and to be acutely aware of those plants and the conditions under which livestock may be poisoned. A tentative diagnosis is possible if the following information is available: 1) any local soil deficiencies or excesses (which may complicate plant toxicities or simply confuse as to cause of a syndrome), 2) the syndromes associated with each of the poisonous plants in the area, 3) the time of year during which each is most likely to cause problems, 4) the detailed history of the animal(s) over the last 6-8 mo, and 5) any change of management or environmental condition that may cause an animal to change its diet or grazing habits (in some cases, eg, locoism, this may be all that is required in addition to identification of the plant involved). Identification of the plant is important, whatever its stage of growth, and is especially useful if it can be identified in the stomach contents of the poisoned animal. Chemical analysis of toxicants often is not useful. Metabolic profiles are useful for some toxicities, and in some, the necropsy lesions are distinctive.

IMPORTANT POISONOUS PLANTS OF AUSTRALIA

Plants recorded as definitely or probably toxic to animals in Australia total >1,000. This chapter includes only those plants with a significant impact (TABLE 5). The most comprehensive reference text on poisonous plants in Australia remains Everist SL (1981) *Poisonous Plants of Australia*. The general points made above on poisoning by range plants in North America apply broadly to Australian conditions as well. It is essential in many cases to confirm the identity of suspected poisonous plants by having a representative specimen carrying flowers, fruit, or both (or spores in the case of ferns) examined by a professional botanist, who may be consulted at state herbariums in Australian state capital cities. Several of the non-native plants (eg, foxglove, oleander) that are listed in TABLE 4 also occur in Australia.

TABLE 3. Poisonous Houseplants and Ornamentals ▶

Scientific Name (Family)	Common Name	Important Characteristics
Agave americana (Agavaceae)	Century plant, American aloe	Clumps of thick, long strap-shaped blue/green leaves with hook (margin) and pointed spines (tip). Central flower stalk with small tubular flowers in clusters.
Aglaonema modestum (Araceae)	Chinese evergreen, Painted drop tongue	Central stem with solid medium green or splotched gray/green leaves; small greenish flowers.
Aloe Barbadensis (vera) (Liliaceae)	Barbados aloe, Curacao aloe	Succulent herb with cluster of narrow fleshy, spinous or coarsely serrated margin leaves, with hook spines on leaf margin. Dense spiked tubular yellow flowers at end of single stalk.
Brunfelsia pauciflora varfloribunda (Solanaceae)	Yesterday-today-and-tomorrow, Lady-of-the-night	Evergreen shrubs to small trees with alternate, undivided, toothless, thick, rather leathery, lustrous leaves. Winter-blooming; large showy sometimes fragrant flowers, clustered or solitary at the branch ends, with 5-lobed tubular calyx, 5 petals, and funnel-shaped corolla. Fruits berry-like capsules.
Caladium spp (Araceae)	Caladium, Fancy leaf caladium, Angel wings	Perennial herbs with simple, heart-shaped, thin, highlighted veins, variegated leaves; yellow-green spathe; grown from rhizomes.
Cannabis sativa (Cannabaceae)	Mary Jane, Marijuana, Grass, Pot, Hashish, Indian hemp, Reefer, Weed	Annual herb, grown from seeds, ≥6 ft tall; Leaves opposite or alternate, palmately compound with 5-7 linear, coarsely dentate leaflets; small green flowers at tip (male) or along entire length (female) of branch; fruits achenes. Grown for its fiber; legally cultivated under federal license only.
Capsicum annuum (Solanaceae)	Cherry pepper, Chili pepper, Ornamental pepper, Capsicum	Annual shrub; branched, erect stem; dark, glossy, ovate, entire margin leaves; white flowers. Fruits—shiny berries of various colors, shapes, sizes.
Chlorophytum spp (Liliaceae)	Spider plant, St. Bernard's lily, Airplane plant	Rhizomatous herbs with leaves slightly glossy, succulent, narrow, strap-like, green—some with a broad, yellow or white band down the middle; long, cream, hanging stems with small, white flowers developing into plantlets. Often grown in hanging baskets.

Comments and Toxic Principles and Effects	**Treatment**
Sap contains calcium oxalate crystals; saponins and acrid volatile oil in leaves and seeds. On ingestion, causes dermal and oral mucosal irritation and edema.	Symptomatic
The entire plant contains calcium oxalate crystals. On ingestion, causes oral mucosal irritation and edema.	Symptomatic
Contains anthraquinone glycosides (barbaloin, emodin) and chrysophanic acid in the latex of the leaves; higher concentrations in younger leaves. On ingestion, causes abrupt, severe diarrhea and/or hypoglycemia, with vomiting in some cases.	Symptomatic—control diarrhea and fluid loss.
Alkaloid components (atropine, scopolamine, hyoscyamine) found in the flowers, leaves, bark, and roots. On ingestion, animals show tachycardia, dry mouth, dilated pupils, ataxia, tremors, depression, urinary retention, and sometimes coma (deep sedation). Not reported to cause death.	In severely depressed animals, stimulants (respiratory and cardiac), along with supportive therapy recommended.
Calcium oxalate crystals and unknowns found in all parts, especially rhizomes. Ingestion causes immediate intense pain, local irritation to mucous membranes, excess salivation, swollen tongue and pharynx, diarrhea, and dyspnea. Pets' access to plant associated with rhizomes brought indoors for winter storage.	Symptomatic
Leaves, stems, and flower buds of mature plants contain tetrahydrocannabinol (THC) and related compounds. THC concentrations vary with plant variety (1-6%), parts (female flowers have highest concentrations), processing (extracts have as much as 28%), sex, and growing conditions. Lethal dose for dogs >3.0 g/kg body wt. Pets' exposure usually from accidental access to this plant being used for in-home treatment of cancer patient or for illegal recreational uses by owner. Pets (dogs primarily) show ataxia, vomiting, mydriasis, prolonged depression, tachycardia or bradycardia, salivation, hyperexcitability, tremors, and hypothermia. Death results when vital CNS regulatory centers are severely depressed.	Remove animal from source. Effectiveness of emetics limited by antiemetic effect of THC. Oral tannic acid, activated charcoal followed by saline cathartics have been recommended. Stimulants (cardiac and respiratory) along with supportive therapy essential in severely depressed animals. Recovery slow at best. *See also* p 2540.
Capsaicinoids (capsaicin) in the mature fruits, solanine and scopoletin in foliage; irritating to the GI tract, with vomiting and diarrhea. Not likely to be lethal.	Symptomatic; irritation relief—cool water irrigation, topical or oral mineral or vegetable oil. Rarely topical anesthetics.
More commonly grown today for its filtering ability. Pet animals (especially cats) reach these plants either by climbing or when plantlets fall from mature stems. Unknown toxin(s) found in leaves and plantlets. Vomiting, salivation, retching, and transient anorexia seen in cats within hours of ingestion. Deaths and diarrhea not reported.	Symptomatic

(continued)

TABLE 3. Poisonous Houseplants and Ornamentals (*continued*) ▶

Scientific Name (Family)	Common Name	Important Characteristics
Colchicum autumnale (Liliaceae, Colchicaceae)	Autumn crocus, Crocus, Fall crocus, Meadow saffron, Wonder bulb	Popular house or yard plant, perennial herb, ovoid underground corm covered with brown membrane or scales. Leaves large, lanceolate, basal, ovate, smooth, ribbed, appear in spring and die back before flowering. Flowers tubular, solitary, pale purple or white appearing in fall; fruit a 3-celled ovoid capsule with numerous seeds.
Convallaria majalis (Liliaceae)	Lily-of-the-valley, Conval lily, May-flower	Herbaceous perennial from slender running rhizome; stem leafless, bearing a 1-sided raceme of nodding white, aromatic, bell-shaped flowers; leaves 2 or 3, basal to 1 ft long. Fruit a red berry but seldom formed.
Cyclamen spp (Primulaceae)	Cyclamen, Snow-bread, Shooting star	Herbaceous plants, grown from rhizomes or tubers. Petioled, heart-shaped, deep green intermixed with lighter green coloration (same leaf), serrated leaves; stems upright, with a terminal pink or white butterfly-like flower.
Dieffenbachia spp (Araceae)	Dumbcane	Fairly tall, erect, unbranched, fleshy plant; stem girdled with leaf scars; leaves large, thickly veined, sheath-like petioles, white or yellow spots on blade.
Digitalis purpurea (Scrophulariacae)	Foxglove	Erect biennial with simple, petioled (long on lower, short or sessile on upper), alternate, toothed, hairy, ovate to lanceolate leaves. Purple, pink, red, white, or yellow tubular flowers (with spots) in terminal racemes; fruit is a capsule with many seeds.
Dracaena spp (Agavaceae)	Dragon tree	Robust palm-like house plant with lance-shaped, thin, variegated, alternate, nonpetioled leaves. Yellow, red, or green stripes along leaf margins in some species. Lower leaves are lost, leaf scars remain and clearly demarcated, terminal leaves retained as plant matures.

TABLE 3.   (continued)

Comments and Toxic Principles and Effects	Treatment
Colchicine and related alkaloids found throughout plant. These alkaloids are heat stable and not affected by drying. Colchicine is used experimentally in genetic investigations, and medically in the treatment of gout in humans. It is cumulative and slowly excreted. Milk of lactating animals is a major excretory pathway. Observed clinical signs are thirst, difficult swallowing, abdominal pain, profuse vomiting and diarrhea, weakness, and shock within hours of ingestion. Death from respiratory failure.	Prolonged course due to slow excretion of colchicine. Gastric lavage; supportive care for dehydration and electrolyte losses (fluid therapy); CNS, circulatory, and respiratory disturbances. Analgesics and atropine recommended for abdominal pain and diarrhea.
Cardiac glycosides (convallarin, convallamarin, convallatoxin), irritant saponins found in leaves, flowers, rhizome, and water in which flowers have been kept. Variable latent period depending on dose. GI signs (vomiting, trembling, abdominal pain, diarrhea), progressive cardiac irregularities (irregular heart beats, A-V block), and death. Hyperkalemia in acute cases. Gastroenteritis, petechial hemorrhages throughout.	Aimed at gut decontamination (gastric lavage) and at correcting bradycardia (atropine), conduction defects (phenytoin), and electrolyte imbalance such as hyperkalemia (IV electrolytes). Electrocardiographic and serum potassium monitoring necessary.
Triterpinoid saponins found in tuberous rhizomes cause GI irritation, thereby increasing systemic absorption and severe toxicity. Anorexia, diarrhea, convulsions, and paralysis are observed clinical signs. Pets have greater access to these plants over winter months (both pets and plants are indoors).	Symptomatic
Calcium oxalate crystals and unknown toxic proteins (possibly asparagine or protoanemonin) in all parts, including sap. On ingestion, immediate intense pain, burning, and inflammation of mouth and throat, anorexia, vomiting, and possibly diarrhea, with tongue extended, head shaking, excessive salivation, and dyspnea. Immediate pain limits amount consumed. Death infrequent.	Symptomatic
Cardiac glycosides (digitoxin, digitalin, digoxin, and others), saponins, and alkaloids found throughout plant. Potency not affected by drying. Generally, acute abdominal pain, vomiting, bloody diarrhea, frequent urination, irregular slow pulse, tremors, convulsions, and rarely death.	Symptomatic
Alkaloids, saponins, and resin found in leaves. Vomiting and severe diarrhea indicative of GI irritation expected. Clinical cases have not been reported.	Symptomatic, to correct fluid and electrolyte imbalance.

(continued)

TABLE 3.   Poisonous Houseplants and Ornamentals (continued) ▶

Scientific Name (Family)	Common Name	Important Characteristics
Euphorbia pulcherrima (Euphorbiaceae)	Poinsettia, Christmas flower, Christmas star	Perennial shrub with milky, white sap throughout. Leaves alternate, petioled, distinctly veined, entire or lobed, and conspicuously bright red, pink, or white (terminal leaves), lower leaves remain green. Flowers small and inconspicuous.
Hyacinthus spp (Liliaceae)	Hyacinths	Garden ornamentals that grow from bulbs (close resemblance to onion bulbs) and flower in early spring. Bulbs harvested and stored in fall for replanting in spring.
Ilex aquifolium (Aquifoliaceae)	English holly, European holly	Evergreen shrub with leaves leathery, glossy upper surface, spiny toothed, alternate, and petioled; fruits red to yellow berries with many seeds and aromatic taste.
Kalanchoe spp (Crassulaceae)	Kalanchoe, Air-plant, Cathedral-bells	Winter flowering, herbaceous, succulent, nonhardy annuals or perennials. Fleshy, serrate or crenate, opposite, petioled leaves. Bright red, orange, or pink flowers in umbel. Stems become woody and untidy with age.
Lilium longiflorum; L tigrinum (Liliaceae)	Easter lily, Trumpet lily	Plants grown from bulbs; leaves alternate or whorled, sessile, linear or lanceolate blades; large showy funnelform flowers; Fruits capsules with numerous, flat seeds.
Narcissus spp (Amaryllidaceae)	Daffodils	Same as for *Hyacinthus*, above
Persea americana (Lauraceae)	Avocado pear, Alligator pear	Trees or shrubs with long branches arising from terminal buds, widely cultivated for its fruits. Three commonly cultivated races (Mexican, Guatemalan, and West Indies). Leaves ovate-elliptical, entire, alternate, veined, dark-green above and paler below, papery to the feel. Flowers inconspicuous, yellow-green in axillary or terminal panicles; fruit berry, ovoid to pyriform in shape with thick, leathery, glossy dark green skin over lime-green to yellow flesh and a smooth, ovoid, solitary seed.
Philodendron spp (Araceae)	Philodendron	Climbing vines with aerial roots; leaves (major attraction as a houseplant) are large, unlobed or pinnately lobed and heart-shaped; rarely flowering.

◀ **TABLE 3.** *(continued)*

Comments and Toxic Principles and Effects	Treatment
Milky sap contains unknown toxic principle(s); irritates mucous membranes and causes excessive salivation and vomiting but not death. Toxicity (hybrid species) not supported experimentally. Toxic diterpenes (ingenol derivatives) found in other *Euphorbia* spp have not been found in this species.	Symptomatic; gastric lavage, activated charcoal, and saline cathartics should be considered.
Calcium oxalate crystals and alkaloids (their toxic potential yet to be defined) found in bulbs. After ingestion of toxic dose (bulbs), vomiting, diarrhea, and rare deaths reported. Bulbs in storage may be accessible to pets.	Symptomatic
Saponins; an alkaloid (theobromine), triterpene compounds, and unknown compounds with digitalis-like cardiotonic activity have been found in leaves, fruits, and seeds. Abdominal pain, vomiting, and diarrhea seen after ingestion of ≥2 berries. Death rare.	Symptomatic (at best)
Cardiac glycosides found in leaves. Within hours of ingesting toxic dose, depression, rapid breathing, teeth grinding, ataxia, paralysis, opisthotonos (rabbit), and death (rat).	Symptomatic; atropine has been effective in rabbits.
Unknown toxin found throughout plants. Renal failure in cats 2-4 days post-ingestion. Not reported toxic to other species. Vomiting, depression, loss of appetite within 12 hr post-ingestion. Elevated creatinine, BUN, phosphorus, and potassium indicate toxicity.	Emetics, activated charcoal, saline cathartic, and nursing care—as for renal failure— within hours of ingestion. Delayed treatment is associated with poor prognosis.
All above-ground parts (leaves in particular) reported toxic to cattle, horses, goats, rabbits, canaries, ostriches, and fish. Responsible toxin a monoglyceride. Oil found in fruits used for cosmetic purposes. Toxicity associated with noninfectious agalactia (cattle, rabbits, goats), pulmonary congestion, cardiac arrhythmia, submandibular edema, acute death (rabbits, cage birds, goats), respiratory distress, generalized congestion, subcutaneous edema, and hydropericardium (suggestive of cardiac failure [caged birds]). In caged birds, clinical signs may be seen within 24 hr (usually after ≥12 hr), with death 1-2 days after exposure.	Primarily symptomatic and supportive. *See also* p 2361.
Calcium oxalate crystals and unidentified proteins throughout entire plant. On ingestion, immediate pain, local irritation to mucous membranes, excessive salivation, edematous tongue and pharynx, dyspnea, and renal failure. Excitability, nervous spasms, convulsions, and occasional encephalitis reported in cats.	Symptomatic

(continued)

TABLE 3. Poisonous Houseplants and Ornamentals (continued) ▶

Scientific Name (Family)	Common Name	Important Characteristics
Phoradendron flavescens (Viscaceae)	Mistletoe	Perennial parasitic shrub that grows on deciduous trees. Evergreen, ovoid, opposite leaves on round, highly branched, green stem. White berries with single seed. Brought into homes during Christmas season.
Rhododendron spp (Ericaceae)	Azalea, Rhododendron	Evergreen or deciduous shrub with simple, alternate, entire leaves; funnel-shaped flowers in terminal umbel-like clusters or solitary and of various colors; fruits are capsules with many seeds.
Sansevieria spp (Agavaceae)	Sansevieria, Snake plant, Mother-in-law's tongue	Hardy, succulent houseplant. Leaves erect, elongate, lanceolate, and flat or cylindrical, dark green with or without a yellow stripe along the margins, and horizontal gray bands throughout; many yellow star-like flowers on tall central raceme or spike.
Schefflera spp (Araliaceae)	Schefflera, Umbrella tree	Fast-growing evergreen with glossy, palmately compound leaves that hang and spread, appearing like an umbrella. Depending on the species, leaflets increase with plant maturity and become more compact; veins pronounced; margins entire to slightly crenate.
Solanum pseudocapsicum (Solanaceae)	Jerusalem cherry	Shrub with simple, lanceolate, entire or slightly serrated leaves. Small star-shaped white flowers. Ripe fruits are red, shiny berries with many white seeds.
Taxus spp (Taxaceae)	Yew	Evergreen tree or small erect shrub with alternate, needle-like, glossy (upper surface), dull (lower surface) leaves. Seeds (generally 1 per fruit), black-brown or green, nearly enclosed in a cup-shaped, fleshy, red covering (aril).
Zamia pumila (Zamiaceae)	Coontie, Florida arrowroot, Seminole bread, Cycad	Palm-like plant with thick underground fleshy, tuberous stem from which grow few pinnately compound, palm-like leaves ~2 ft long; cones containing inch-long, shiny, orange-red seeds.

TABLE 3. *(continued)*

Comments and Toxic Principles and Effects	Treatment
Amines (β-phenylethylamine, acetylcholine, choline, and tyramine), toxic proteins (viscotoxins), and unknowns in all parts. Vomiting, profuse diarrhea, dilated pupils, rapid labored breathing, shock, and death from cardiovascular collapse within hours of ingesting toxic dose.	Symptomatic
Andromedotoxins (grayanotoxins) found in all parts, including pollen and nectar. Within hours of ingestion of toxic dose (1 g/kg), salivation, lacrimation, vomiting, diarrhea, dyspnea, muscle weakness, convulsions, coma, and death. Signs may last several days, but toxin is not cumulative.	Symptomatic; gastric lavage, activated charcoal, saline cathartics, calcium injection, and antibiotics to control possible pneumonia suggested.
Hemolytic saponin and organic acids found in leaves and flowers. Vomiting, salivation, diarrhea, and hemolysis related to GI activity of these compounds.	Symptomatic; fluids and electrolytes may be necessary.
Oxalate found in the leaves. Mucous membrane irritation, salivation, anorexia, vomiting, and if severe enough, diarrhea.	Symptomatic
Solanocapsine and related alkaloids found in leaves and fruits. Anorexia, abdominal pain, vomiting, hemorrhagic diarrhea, salivation, progressive weakness or paralysis, dyspnea, bradycardia, circulatory collapse, dilated pupils, and convulsions reported.	Symptomatic; gastric lavage, activated charcoal, electrolytes and fluids, and anticonvulsants suggested.
The alkaloids (taxines and ephedrine), cyanide, and volatile oils found throughout plant except the fleshy aril. Nervousness, trembling, ataxia, dyspnea, collapse; bradycardia progressing to cardiac standstill and death without struggle. Empty right side of heart; dark, tarry blood in left side of heart; limited nonspecific postmortem lesions.	Symptomatic at best; usually futile once clinical signs appear. Atropine may be helpful.
The glucoside cycasin and its aglycone methylazoxymethanol (a colon-specific carcinogen in mice) found in leaves, seeds, and stem. Ingestion associated with hepatic and GI disturbances and ataxia. Clinical signs are persistent vomiting, diarrhea, abdominal pain, depression, and muscular paralysis. A neurologic condition characterized by hindleg paralysis (hyperextension followed by incomplete extension) has been reported in cattle.	No specific therapy; IV fluids and symptomatic care recommended.

TABLE 4. Poisonous Range Plants of Temperate North America ▶

Scientific and Common Names	Habitat and Distribution	Affected Animals
Dangerous Season: SPRING and FALL		
Cicuta spp Water hemlock	Open, moist to wet environments; throughout North America	All
Hymenoxys odorata Bitterweed	Roadways, lakebeds, flooded areas, overgrazed range; southwest	Sheep, rarely cattle
Hymenoxys richardsonii Pingue, Colorado rubber weed	Arid foothills (6,000-8,000 ft [1,800-2,400 m]); western	Sheep, cattle, goats
Dangerous Season: SPRING		
Nolina texana Sacahuista, Beargrass	Open areas on rolling hills and slopes; southwest	Sheep, cattle, goats
Peganum harmala African rue	Arid to semiarid ranges; southwest	Cattle, sheep, probably horses
Phytolacca americana Pokeweed, Poke	Disturbed rich soils such as recent clearings, pastures, waste areas; eastern	Pigs, cattle, sheep, horses, humans

TABLE 4. (continued)

Important Characteristics	Toxic Principle and Effects	Comments and Treatment
Dangerous Season: SPRING and FALL		
White flower, umbels. Veins of leaflets ending at notches. Stems hollow except at nodes. Tuberous roots from chambered rootstock.	Resinoids (cicutoxin, cicutol) in roots, stem base, young leaves. Toxicity retained when dry, except in hay. Rapid onset of clinical signs, with death in 15-30 min. Salivation, muscular twitching, dilated pupils. Violent convulsions, coma, death. Poisoning in humans common.	Sedatives to control spasm and heart action. Prognosis good if alive 2 hr after ingestion.
Multibranched annual or perennial up to 2 ft high. Yellow flower head. Leaves divided into narrow glandular segments.	Sesquiterpene lactone (hymenovin) in fresh or dry plant. Salivation, vomiting, green nasal discharge, depression, anorexia, abdominal pain. Lesions include inflammation of GI tract, foreign body pneumonia, renal degeneration.	Toxin cumulative. Avoid overgrazing. Remove from pasture.
Perennial herb. Leaves bright green, divided into narrow glandular segments.	Same as for *H odorata* (above).	Same as for *H odorata.*
Dangerous Season: SPRING		
Perennial with many clustered, long narrow leaves. Stem mostly underground. Several flower stems with many small, white flowers in clusters.	Unidentified hepatotoxin (buds, flowers, fruit). Photosensitization, anorexia, icterus, prostration. Dark urine, yellowish discharge from eyes, nostrils. Lesions include hepatic and renal degeneration, GI inflammation.	Remove animals from area where plant grows during blooming season. *See* PHOTOSENSITIZATION, p 794.
Multibranched, leafy, perennial, bright green, succulent herb. Leaves divided. Flowers white, single.	Alkaloids (seeds, leaves, stems; seeds more toxic). Anorexia, hindleg weakness, knuckling of fetlock, listlessness, excess salivation, subnormal temperature, pollakiuria. Lesions include gastroenteritis, with hemorrhages on heart and under liver capsule.	Unpalatable. Eaten only under drought conditions.
Tall (to 9 ft), glabrous, green, red-purple, perennial herbs. Berries black-purple, staining, in drooping racemes.	Oxalic acid, a saponin (phytolaccotoxin), and an alkaloid (phytolaccin) in all parts; roots most toxic. Vomiting, abdominal pain, bloody diarrhea, hemolytic anemia, drop in production (dairy cattle). Terminal convulsions, death from respiratory failure. Lesions include ulcerative gastritis, mucosal hemorrhage, dark liver.	Oils and protectants (GI tract). Dilute acetic acid PO, stimulants. Blood transfusion (hemolytic anemia).

(continued)

TABLE 4. Poisonous Range Plants (*continued*) ▶

Scientific and Common Names	Habitat and Distribution	Affected Animals
	Dangerous Season: SPRING (*continued*)	
Quercus spp Oaks	Most deciduous woods; throughout North America	All grazing animals, mostly cattle
Sarcobatus vermiculatus Greasewood	Alkaline or saline bottom soils, not in higher mountains; arid west. Dangerous season spring; may be year-round.	Sheep, cattle
Xanthium spp Cocklebur	Fields, waste places, exposed shores of ponds or rivers; throughout North America. Dangerous season spring and occasionally fall.	All animals, more common in pigs
Zygadenus spp Death camas	Foothill grazing lands, occasionally boggy grasslands, low open woods; throughout North America	Sheep, cattle, horses
	Dangerous Season: SPRING and SUMMER	
Aesculus spp Buckeye	Woods and thickets; eastern USA and California	All grazing animals
Amianthium muscaetoxicum Fly poison, Staggergrass, Crow poison	Open woods, fields, and acid bogs; eastern	All grazing animals

◀ **TABLE 4.** (continued)

Important Characteristics	Toxic Principle and Effects	Comments and Treatment
Dangerous Season: SPRING (continued)		
Mostly deciduous trees, rarely shrubs, with 2-4 leaves clustered at tips of all twigs.	Gallotannin thought to be the toxin (young leaves and swollen or sprouting acorn). Anorexia, rumen stasis, constipation, followed by dark tarry diarrhea, dry muzzle, frequent urination, rapid weak pulse, death. Lesions include perirenal edema, nephrosis, gastroenteritis.	Diet must consist of >50% oak buds and young leaves for a period of time. Increased BUN with diet history diagnostic. Treatment symptomatic. Oral ruminatorics helpful. *See also* p 2507.
Large deciduous shrub with spiny stems. Fleshy, alternate, round in cross-section. Flowers inconspicuous.	Oxalates (sodium and potassium). Dyspnea, weakness, depression, some salivation, atony of GI tract, coma, death. Hyperkalemia, hypocalcemia, increased BUN. Lesions include hemorrhage and edema of rumen wall, ascites, swollen kidneys (renal tubular necrosis and dilation).	Toxic when large quantity consumed in short time. Do not allow hungry animals to graze plant.
Coarse annual herb. Fruit covered with spines, 2-beaked, with 2 compartments.	Carboxyatractyloside (seeds and young seedlings). Anorexia, depression, nausea, vomiting, weakness, rapid weak pulse, dyspnea, muscle spasms, convulsions. Lesions include GI inflammation, acute hepatitis, nephritis.	Seedlings or grain contaminated with seeds. Oils and fats PO may be beneficial; warmth, stimulants IM.
Perennial, bulbous, unbranched herbs with basal, flat, grass-like leaves. Flowers greenish, yellow, or pink; in racemes or panicles. No onion odor.	Steroidal alkaloids, glycoalkaloids, and ester alkaloids (all parts). Salivation, vomiting, muscle weakness, ataxia or prostration, fast weak pulse, coma, death. No distinctive lesions.	Seeds most toxic. Leaves and stems lose toxicity as plant matures. Atropine sulfate and picrotoxin SC.
Dangerous Season: SPRING and SUMMER		
Trees or shrubs. Leaves opposite and palmately compound. Seeds large, glossy brown, with large white scar.	Glycoside, aesculin; also alkaloids and saponins in all parts, especially seeds and leaves. Depression, incoordination, twitching, paralysis, inflammation of mucous membranes.	Young shoots and seeds especially poisonous. Stimulants and purgatives.
Bulbous perennial herb. Leaves basal, linear. White flowers in a compact raceme, the pedicels subtended by short, brownish bracts.	Unidentified alkaloid, similar to those with *Zygadenus* (all parts). Salivation, vomiting, rapid and irregular respiration, weakness, death from respiratory failure.	No practical treatment. Especially dangerous for animals new to pasture. Keep animals well fed.

(continued)

TABLE 4. Poisonous Range Plants (continued) ▶

Scientific and Common Names	Habitat and Distribution	Affected Animals
Dangerous Season: SPRING and SUMMER (continued)		
Cassia obtusifolia Coffeepod, Sicklepod	Found in cultivated (corn, soybean, or sorghum) and abandoned fields, along fences, roadsides; naturalized in eastern USA	All grazing animals, mostly cattle, and poultry p 2260
Cassia occidentalis Coffee senna, Coffee weed, Styptic weed, Wild coffee	Common along roadsides, waste areas and pastures; naturalized in eastern USA	Cattle, horses, chickens, goats, sheep, rabbits
Delphinium spp Larkspurs	Either cultivated or wild, usually in open foothills or meadows and among aspen; mostly western. Dangerous season spring and summer, also seeds in fall.	All grazing animals, mostly cattle
Descurainia pinnata Tansy mustard	Dense stands especially in wet years; arid southwest	Cattle

(Continued)

Important Characteristics	Toxic Principle and Effects	Comments and Treatment
TABLE 4. *(continued)*		
Dangerous Season: SPRING and SUMMER *(continued)*		
Annual shrub frequently found in same fields as *C occidentalis*. Distinguishing features include leaflets fewer in number and more rounded. Seed pods long, round to 4-sided and more curved. Seeds shiny, brown, and rhomboid.	Toxic principles thought to be same as in *C occidentalis*. Clinical signs, although similar, less severe with *C obtusifolia*.	Treatment ineffective in down animals; salvaging most economic. Heat labile toxins not known to persist as residue. Meat from affected animals should be safe for human consumption.
Annual herb >3 ft tall, with glandular, alternate pinnately compound leaves (8-12 ovate to lanceolate leaflets, terminal pair largest). Flowers yellow, axillary, solitary, or in short racemes. Long, flat, straight to slightly curved pods with clearly outlined seed contents. Of the pods, seeds, and wilted foliage, seeds are most toxic.	Anthraquinones (emodinglycosides and oxymethylanthraquinone), chrysarobin and lectin (toxalbumins), and alkaloids are associated with GI dysfunction and myodegeneration. Afebrile, ataxic, with diarrhea and coffee-color urine, recumbent but eat and are alert shortly before death. Increased serum CPK and isocitric dehydrogenase activities; hyperkalemia and myoglobinuria frequent. Lesions include cardiac and skeletal muscle degeneration. Congestion, fatty degeneration and centrilobular necrosis (liver) in addition to tubular degeneration (kidneys) also reported. Death probably due to hyperkalemic heart failure.	No specific treatment known. Symptomatic and supportive care essential. Although gross lesions similar to those of vitamin E/selenium deficiency, this therapy is contraindicated. Mineralocorticoid therapy may facilitate potassium excretion. Remove animals from source. Salvaging for economic reasons (*see Cassia obtusifolia* above).
Annual or perennial erect herbs. Flowers each with 1 spur, in racemes. Perennial with tuberous roots. Leaves palmately lobed or divided.	Polycyclic diterpenoid alkaloids (eg, delphinine) in all parts, fresh or dry. Straddled stance, arched back, repeated falling, forelegs first. Constipation, bloat, salivation, vomiting. Death (respiratory and cardiac failure). Most often no lesions.	Young plants and seeds more toxic. Toxicity decreases with maturity.
Annual to 2 ft tall, stem and leaves covered with fine pubescence. Leaves alternate, deeply pinnately dissected. Inflorescence on elongated raceme. Flower small with 4 spreading yellow to yellow-green petals. Fruit-copula with 2 carpels and long waxy seeds in 2 rows.	Toxic principle unknown; must be grazed over relatively long period. Partial or complete blindness, inability to use tongue or swallow, "paralyzed tongue," "blind staggers," wandering, head pressing, emaciation, death if not treated.	Administer 2-3 gal. (8-12 L) water BID with stomach tube. Include nourishment if animal weak. Prognosis good if treatment started early. Possibly mustards cause same condition.

(continued)

TABLE 4. Poisonous Range Plants (continued) ▶

Scientific and Common Names	Habitat and Distribution	Affected Animals
Dangerous Season: SPRING and SUMMER (continued)		
Lantana spp Lantana	Ornamentals and wild; in lower coastal plain of southeast USA, and southern California	All grazing animals except horses
Tetradymia spp Horsebrush	Arid foothills and higher desert and sagebrush ranges, dense stands along trails; western	Sheep
Veratrum spp False hellebore, Skunk cabbage	Low, moist woods and pastures, and high mountain valleys; throughout North America	Sheep, cattle
Dangerous Season: SUMMER and FALL		
Acer rubrum Red maple	Moist land and swamps; eastern	Horses
Apocynum spp Dogbanes	Open woods, roadsides, fields; throughout North America	All

◄ **TABLE 4.** *(continued)*

Important Characteristics	Toxic Principle and Effects	Comments and Treatment
Dangerous Season: SPRING and SUMMER (continued)		
Shrubs. Young stems 4-angled. Leaves opposite. Flowers in flat-topped clusters, yellow, pink, orange, or red. Berries black.	Triterpenes (lantadene A and B) and unknowns in all parts, especially leaves and green berries. Anorexia, jaundice, watery feces, photosensitization. Lesions include degenerative changes in liver and kidneys. Death due to liver insufficiency, renal failure, myocardial damage.	Remove plants from pasture. Keep animals out of light sources after eating plant.
Shrubs with yellow flowers in spring, not later. Leaves spiny, silvery white. Early deciduous.	Furanoeremophilanes (tetradymol and others). Photosensitization, "bighead," loss of hair and wool, skin ulcerations, blindness, secondary infections. Lesions include dermal necrosis and edema, hepatic and renal degeneration. Abortions may occur.	Photosensitization seen when animals ingest other green forages together with this plant. Remove animals from plant source and sunlight. Antihistamines, topical antibiotics, and parenteral corticosteroids beneficial. Recovery slow and possibly incomplete.
Erect herbs. Leafy throughout, leaves large and plaited. Flowers small and white or greenish.	Steroidal alkaloids. Vomiting, excess salivation, cardiac arrhythmia, bradycardia, dyspnea, muscle weakness and paralysis, coma, congenital cyclops in lambs from ewes exposed to *V californicum*.	Respiratory and heart stimulants.
Dangerous Season: SUMMER and FALL		
A large tree at maturity. Leaves opposite, 2-6 in. across, palmately 3- or 5-lobed each, roughly triangular, and coarsely toothed. Red to yellow polygamous flowers. Fruit, a pair of 1-seeded winged units connected at base.	Unknown toxic principle(s) in wilted leaves. Methemoglobinemia, Heinz body anemia, and intravascular hemolysis; weakness, polypnea, tachycardia, depression, icterus, cyanosis, brownish discoloration of blood and urine.	Not common. Methemoglobinemia a prognostic indicator. Isotonic fluids, oxygen, and blood transfusion can be helpful. Methylene blue therapy not rewarding.
Erect, branching, perennial herb with milky sap arising from creeping underground root stock. Leaves opposite. Flowers white to greenish white in terminal clusters. Fruit long, slender, paired, with silky-haired seeds.	A resinoid and glucoside with some cardioactivity found in leaves and stems of green or dry plants. Increased temperature and pulse, dilated pupils, anorexia, discolored mucous membranes, cold extremities, death.	IV fluids and gastric protectants suggested.

(continued)

TABLE 4. Poisonous Range Plants (continued) ▶

Scientific and Common Names	Habitat and Distribution	Affected Animals
Dangerous Season: SUMMER and FALL (continued)		
Centaurea repens Russian knapweed	Waste areas, roadsides, railroads, and overgrazed rangeland; not common in cultivated or irrigated pastures; mostly western and upper midwestern USA	Horses
Centaurea solstitialis Yellow star thistle, Yellow knapweed	Waste areas, roadsides, pastures; mostly western	Horses
Eupatorium rugosum White snakeroot	Woods, cleared areas, waste places, usually the moister and richer soils; eastern	Sheep, cattle, horses
Hypochaeris radicata Flatweed, Cat's-ear, Gosmore	Native to the Mediterranean and South America; widely distributed in the USA—Pacific states, eastern/southeastern USA	Horses
Oxytenia acerosa Copperweed	Arid, alkaline soils in foothills, sagebrush plains; southwest	Cattle, sheep

Important Characteristics	Toxic Principle and Effects	Comments and Treatment
Dangerous Season: SUMMER and FALL *(continued)*		
Perennial weed with slender rhizomes. Stems erect and well branched. Leaves pinnately lobed to entire, not spiny, narrowed basally but not petioled and of decreasing length up the plant. Thinly pubescent or glabrous. Blue, pink, or white flowers. One-seeded fruit with whitish, slightly ridged attachment scar.	Unidentified alkaloid in fresh or dried plant. Chronic exposure, acute onset of signs. Inability to eat or drink, facial dystonia, chewing, yawning, standing with head down, severe facial edema, gait normal, head pressing, aimless walking or excitement most severe the first 2 days, become static thereafter. Death from starvation, dehydration, aspiration pneumonia.	More toxic than *C solstitialis* (*see* below) but with similar pathology and prognosis. Some relief with massive doses of atropine but not an effective treatment. Euthanasia recommended.
Annual weed. Leaves densely covered with cottony hair. Terminal spreading cluster of bright yellow flowers with spines below. Branches winged.	Unidentified alkaloid. Involuntary chewing movements, twitching of lips, flicking of tongue. Mouth commonly held open. Unable to eat; death from dehydration, starvation, aspiration pneumonia.	Horses graze because of lack of other forage. Extended period of consumption essential for toxicity. Liquefactive necrosis of substantia nigra and globus pallidus (brain) pathognomonic. No treatment. Euthanasia recommended.
Erect perennial herb. Tremetol leaves, opposite, simple, serrated. Flowers small, white, and many. Often grows in large patches.	Complex benzyl alcohol (tremetol in leaves and stems). Excreted via milk; cumulative. Weight loss, weakness, trembling (muzzle and legs) prominent after exercise, constipation, acetone odor, fatty degeneration of liver, partial paralysis of throat, death in 1-3 days.	"Milk sickness" or "trembles." Treatment symptomatic. Heart and respiratory stimulants and laxative may be necessary. Remove animal from access to plant, discard milk (hazardous to humans).
Perennial herb with viscid sap, stemless. Simple, serrated to lobed, basal, alternate leaves. One to several bright yellow flowers per plant.	Unknown; associated with but not proven cause of a neurologic condition in horses—stringhalt (hypermetria/hyperflexion of pelvic limb) in dry years. Sudden onset of abnormal gait; flexion/delayed extension of hocks, knuckling of carpal joints, laryngeal hemiplasia; spontaneous recovery possible, but condition could be permanent.	Tranquilizers, sedatives, mephenesin, and thiamine (questionable effectiveness); longterm phenytoin therapy seems helpful. Treatment with baclofen also reported helpful. Surgery (pelvic tenotomy of the lateral digital extensors) reported helpful.
Tall, perennial herb with narrow leaflets. Flowers in many heads resembling goldenrod.	Unknown; all above-ground parts, green or dry. Anorexia, marked depression, weakness, coma; death without struggle within 1-3 days.	Supplement diet or change pasture.

(continued)

TABLE 4. Poisonous Range Plants (continued) ▶

Scientific and Common Names	Habitat and Distribution	Affected Animals
Dangerous Season: SUMMER and FALL (continued)		
Perilla frutescens Perilla mint, Beefsteak plant	Ornamental originally from India, escaped to moist pastures, fields, roadsides, and waste places; eastern	Cattle primarily, horses and other livestock susceptible
Prosopis glandulosa Mesquite	Dry ranges, washes, draws; southwest	Primarily cattle, also goats; sheep resistant
Robinia pseudoacacia Black locust, False acacia, Locust tree	Open woods, roadsides, pinelands, on clay soils preferably; eastern USA	All grazing animals, mostly horses
Rumex crispus Curly dock, Dock, Sorrel	Commonly found on acid or sterile, graveled, seasonally moist soils of waste places, pastures, and fields throughout USA.	Cattle, sheep

◀ **TABLE 4.** *(continued)*

Important Characteristics	Toxic Principle and Effects	Comments and Treatment
Dangerous Season: SUMMER and FALL (continued)		
Annual, freely branched, squared stems. Opposite, purple or green, coarsely serrated leaves. White to purple flowers. Strong pungent odor when crushed.	Green or dry, 3-substituted furans (perilla ketone, egomaketone, isoegomaketone). Signs 2-10 days after exposure include dyspnea (especially on exhaling), open-mouth breathing, lowered head, reluctance to move, death on exertion. Lesions include pulmonary emphysema and edema.	Treatment ineffective once clinical signs severe. Parenteral steroids, antihistamines, and antibiotics may help. Handle gently (prevents exertion and death).
Deciduous shrub or small tree with smooth or furrowed gray bark, paired spines. Leaves divided. Legume pod long, constricted between seeds.	Unknown principle in the beans. Chronic wasting with rumen atony, excess salivation, continuous chewing. Partial paralysis of tongue, facial muscle tremor, submandibular edema, anemia. Lesions include emaciation, small firm kidneys and liver, gastroenteritis, filled rumen.	High sucrose content of beans alters rumen microflora, inhibiting cellulose digestion and B vitamin synthesis if grazed for extended period.
Tree or shrub. Deciduous, alternate, pinnately compound (>10 elliptic to ovate leaflets) leaves. Pair of spines at base of each leaf. Flowers in loose, fragrant, white to cream, drooping racemes. Flattened, brown pods containing 4-8 seeds.	The glycoside robitin, a lectin (hemagglutinin), and the phytotoxins robin and phasin found throughout plant, although flowers have been suggested as the toxic principles. Diarrhea, anorexia, weakness, posterior paralysis, depression, mydriasis, cold extremities; frequently laminitis and weak pulse. Death infrequent; recovery period extensive. Postmortem lesions restricted to GI tract.	Laxatives and stimulants suggested. Treatment symptomatic.
Perennial herb with erect stems, 3-4 ft tall. Leaves alternate, lanceolate to elliptic, finely crisped margins, base obtuse to cuneate, petioles form sheath around stem. Flowers small, numerous, greenish, in long terminal panicles; fruit an achene, papery 3-winged, with lustrous brown seeds.	Oxalic acid and soluble oxalate in leaves, stem, and seeds. Acute course (hypocalcemia, labored breathing, anorexia, depression, muscle fasciculation, tremor, weakness, teeth grinding, pulmonary edema, tetany, seizure, recumbency, and prostration), subacute course (hypocalcemia, altered kidney functions), or chronic course (renal fibrosis, renal insufficiency, and urolithiasis). Hemorrhage, edema (rumen and abomasal walls), and ascites (intestinal mucosa) seen in toxic cases. Death resulting from shock and hemorrhagic ruminitis.	In acute cases, death is too rapid for any treatment. Symptomatic and supportive care can be helpful. Remove animals from source. Calcium IV to correct hypocalcemia is ineffective. Give lime water to precipitate oxalate and prevent absorption. Allow animals to develop tolerance to oxalate by exposure to small amounts over time. Do not allow animals to graze pasture or offer hay highly contaminated with oxalate-producing plants.

(continued)

TABLE 4. Poisonous Range Plants *(continued)* ▶

Scientific and Common Names	Habitat and Distribution	Affected Animals
Dangerous Season: SUMMER and FALL (continued)		
Solanum spp Nightshades, Jerusalem cherry, Potato, Horse nettle, Buffalo bur	Fence rows, waste areas, grain and hay fields; throughout North America	All
Dangerous Season: FALL and WINTER		
Allium cepa, A canadense Onions (cultivated and wild)	Cultivated and grown on rich soils throughout USA.	Cattle, horses, sheep, dogs
Daubentonia (Sesbania) punicea Rattlebox, Purple sesbane	Cultivated and escaped, in waste places; southeastern USA coastal plain	All
Halogeton glomeratus Halogeton	Deserts, overgrazed areas, winter ranges, alkaline soils; western	Sheep, cattle
Haplopappus heterophyllus Rayless goldenrod, Burroweed	Dry plains, grasslands, open woodlands, and along irrigation canals; southwest	Cattle, sheep, horses

◀ **TABLE 4.** *(continued)*

Important Characteristics	Toxic Principle and Effects	Comments and Treatment
Dangerous Season: SUMMER and FALL (continued)		
Fruits small; yellow, red, or black when ripe; structurally like tomatoes; clustered on stalk arising from stem between leaves	Glycoalkaloid solanine (leaves, shoots, unripe berries). Acute hemorrhagic gastroenteritis, weakness, excess salivation, dyspnea, trembling, progressive paralysis, prostration, death.	Pilocarpine, physostigmine, GI protectants. Seeds may contaminate grain.
Dangerous Season: FALL and WINTER		
Biennials and perennials, bulb plants, onion odor. Leaves basal, green, hollow, cylindrical (*A cepa*), lustrous green, flat (*A canadense*); flowers on hollow flowering stalks, terminal umbels of many small blooms; fruits 3-celled capsules with many seeds.	N-propyl disulfide, an oxidant, in all parts. Livestock readily consume onions; anemia develops within days of exposure. Toxicosis in cattle associated with prolonged ingestion of large amounts of onions. N-propyl disulfide inhibits RBC glucose-6-phosphate dehydrogenase, leading to hemolysis and formation of Heinz bodies. Clinical signs are hemoglobinuria, diarrhea, loss of appetite, jaundice, ataxia, collapse, and possible death if untreated. Hemolytic anemia reported in livestock ingesting wild onions. Heinz body anemia; swollen, pale, necrotic liver; hemosiderin in liver, kidneys, and spleen are reported pathologic lesions.	Clinical signs similar to toxicity induced by S-methylcysteine sulfoxide (a rare toxic amino acid in *Brassica* spp) in livestock. Susceptibility to onion poisoning varies across animal species: cattle more susceptible than horses and dogs, which are more susceptible than sheep and goats. Remove animals from source and prevent future access to cull onions. Symptomatic and supportive care essential.
Shrub. Flowers orange. Legume pods longitudinally 4-winged.	Rapid pulse, weak respiration, diarrhea, death.	Seeds poisonous. Remove animal from source. Saline purgatives.
Annual herb. Leaves fleshy, round in cross-section, tip with stiff hair. Axillary flowers inconspicuous. Fruits bracted and conspicuous.	Oxalic acid, oxalate. Acute course. Rapid labored respiration, depression, weakness, coma, death. Lesions include hemorrhages and edema of rumen wall, swollen kidneys, oxalate crystals in kidneys and rumen wall.	Toxic dose consumed over short period. Increase water consumption.
Bushy perennial 2-4 ft tall, with many yellow flowerheads. Leaves alternate, linear, sticky.	Complex benzyl alcohol (tremetol); resin acid; primarily nursing young and nonlactating animals. Reluctance to move, trembling, weakness, vomiting, dyspnea, constipation, prostration, coma, death.	"Milk sickness." Remove young and discard milk (hazardous to humans).

(continued)

TABLE 4. Poisonous Range Plants (continued) ▶

Scientific and Common Names	Habitat and Distribution	Affected Animals
Dangerous Season: FALL and WINTER (continued)		
Juglans nigra Black walnut	Native to eastern USA; now from eastern seacoast, west to Michigan and most of the Midwest, south to Georgia and Texas	Horses
Melilotus officinalis and *M alba* Sweet clover, White sweet clover	Commonly found on alkaline soils, fields, roadsides, and waste places; forage crop in southern and northern USA	Most commonly cattle, also horses and sheep
Notholaena sinuata cochisensis Jimmy fern, Cloak fern	Dry rocky slopes and crevices, chiefly limestone areas; southwest	Sheep, goats, cattle
Sesbania vesicaria Bladderpod, Rattlebox, Sesbane, Coffeebean	Mostly open, low ground, abandoned cultivated fields; southeastern USA coastal plain	All
Sophora secundiflora Mescal bean, Frijolito, Mountain laurel	Hills and canyons, limestone soils; southwestern Texas into Mexico	Cattle, sheep, goats

(continued)

◀ **TABLE 4.** (continued)

Important Characteristics	Toxic Principle and Effects	Comments and Treatment
Dangerous Season: FALL and WINTER (continued)		
Tree with deciduous, alternate, pinnately compound leaves (numerous lanceolate leaflets with serrated margins); leaflets in middle are largest. Male and female flowers on same tree but different inflorescences. Thick husked nut does not open when ripe. Twigs have chambered pith.	Juglone, phenolic derivative of naphthoquinone. Shavings with as little as 20% black walnut toxic within 24 hr of exposure. Reluctance to move; depression; increased temperature, pulse, respiration rate, abdominal sounds, digital pulse, hoof temperature; distal limb edema; lameness. Severe laminitis with continued exposure.	Nonfatal; laminitis and edema of lower limbs. Remove shavings promptly. Treat for limb edema and laminitis. Improvement in 24-48 hr with no sequelae.
Annual or biennial herb 3-6 ft tall. Leaves alternate, pinnately compound with 3 obovate leaflets, serrated margins. Yellow or white flowers on racemes. Small 1-seeded pods.	*See* SWEET CLOVER POISONING, p 2523.	*See* p 2523.
Evergreen, perennial, erect fern with divided leaves, folding when dry. Leaflets about as wide as long, scaly on back.	Unknown (excreted in milk). Nervous syndrome, incoordination, arched back, trembling, increased respiratory rate and pulse. Death when not allowed to rest.	Avoid driving during danger period. Provide ample watering, placed to avoid long walks. Allow rest if signs occur.
Tall annual. Legume pods flat, tapered at both ends, 2-seeded. Leaves pinnate, divided. Flowers yellow.	Unknown (green plant and seeds). In ruminants, hemorrhagic diarrhea, shallow rapid respiration, fast irregular pulse, coma, death. Lesions include hemorrhages in abomasum and intestines, dark tarry blood.	Green seeds are more toxic. Remove animal from source immediately. General supportive treatment—saline purgatives, rumen stimulants, IV fluids.
Evergreen shrub or small tree. Leaves alternate, divided, and leathery. Flowers violet-blue, fragrant. Seeds large and bright red with hard seed coat, in legume pod.	Quinolizidine alkaloid (seeds and probably leaves). Violent trembling, stiff gait, falling on exercise, recumbent for a few minutes, becoming alert and eating.	Toxic effect not cumulative, consume large amounts quickly. Seeds more dangerous when crushed.

(continued)

TABLE 4. Poisonous Range Plants (continued) ▶

Scientific and Common Names	Habitat and Distribution	Affected Animals
Dangerous Season: FALL, WINTER, and SPRING		
Melia azedarach Chinaberry	Fence rows, brush, waste places; southeast	Pigs and sheep, others less susceptible
Dangerous Season: ALL SEASONS		
Acacia berlandieri Guajillo	Semiarid rangelands; southwestern Texas into Mexico	Sheep, goats
Agave lechuguilla Lechuguilla	Low limestone hills, dry valleys, and canyons; southwest. Dangerous all seasons, especially spring.	Sheep, goats, cattle, usually during drought
Agrostemma githago Corn cockle	Weed, grainfields, and waste areas; throughout North America	All
Asclepias spp Milkweeds	Dry areas, usually waste places, roadsides, streambeds	All
Astragalus spp, *Oxytropis* spp (certain species only) Locoweed	Mostly western	All grazing animals
Astragalus spp (certain species only) Milk vetch, etc (many common names)	Nearly all	All grazing animals

◀ **TABLE 4.** *(continued)*

Important Characteristics	Toxic Principle and Effects	Comments and Treatment
Dangerous Season: FALL, WINTER, and SPRING		
Small to medium deciduous tree. Fruit cream or yellow with a furrowed globose stone, persisting on tree through winter. Large amount required for intoxication.	Several alkaloids and a saponin (all parts), fruit most toxic. Restlessness, vomiting, constipation, cyanosis, rapid pulse, dyspnea, death within 24 hr.	Gastroenteritis usual. Recovery may be spontaneous. Laxatives and GI protectants suggested.
Dangerous Season: ALL SEASONS		
Deciduous shrub or small tree. Leaf divided. Flowers white to yellowish in dense heads. Fruit a legume with margins thickened.	Amine, N-methyl-β-phenylethylamine. Chronic course. Ataxia of hindquarters (limberleg), marked excitation, prostration, remain alert, death from starvation.	Dominates vegetation in some areas. Valuable to sheep industry due to high nutritive value and dominance. Supplement during drought to reduce possibility of poisoning.
Perennial, stemless, with thick, fleshy, tapered leaves having sharply serrated margins. Flowers infrequently with tall terminal panicle.	Unidentified hepatotoxin (causing photosensitivity) and a toxic saponin (abortifacient action). Subacute course. Listlessness, anorexia, icterus, yellow discharge from eyes and nostrils, photosensitization, coma, death.	Remove animals from range and provide shade. *See* PHOTOSENSITIZATION, p 794.
Green winter annual with silky-white hairs, opposite leaves, purple flowers, black seeds.	Saponin (githagenin) in seeds. Acute course. Profuse watery diarrhea, vomiting, dullness, general weakness, tachypnea, hemoglobinuria, death.	Oils and GI protectants. Neutralize toxin (dilute acetic acid PO). Blood transfusions may be necessary.
Perennial erect herbs with milky sap. Seeds silky-hairy from elongated pods.	Steroid glycosides and toxic resinous substances (all parts), green or dry. Staggering, tetanic convulsions, bloating, dyspnea, dilated pupils, rapid and weak pulse, coma, death.	Sedatives, laxatives, and IV fluids suggested.
Stemmed or stemless perennial herbs. Leaves alternate and pinnately compound. Flowers leguminous. Chronic intoxication.	Swainsonine. Depression, emaciation, incoordination, dry lusterless hair. Abortions. Neurovisceral cytoplasmic vacuolation, congestive right heart failure in cattle grazing at high altitudes.	Avoid grazing of source. Both green and dry plants toxic.
As above.	Miserotoxin, other aliphatic nitro compounds. Posterior paralysis, goose-stepping, depression, rough coat, pulmonary emphysema, acute death, cord demyelination.	Avoid grazing of preflower stage.

(continued)

TABLE 4. Poisonous Range Plants (continued) ▶

Scientific and Common Names	Habitat and Distribution	Affected Animals
Dangerous Season: ALL SEASONS (continued)		
Astragalus spp (certain species only—selenium accumulators) Many common names	Seleniferous areas, mostly western and midwestern	All grazing animals
Baccharis spp Silverling, Bacharis, Yerba-de-pasmo	Open areas, often moist; eastern and southwestern	Cattle
Brassica, Raphanus, Descurainia spp Mustards, Crucifers, Cress	Fields, roadsides; throughout North America	Cattle, horses, pigs
Cestrum diurnum, C nocturnum Day-blooming jessamine and night-blooming jessamine, respectively	Open woods and fields; Gulf Coast states (Florida, Texas) and California	Cattle, horses, and dogs (ingesting cholecalciferol-based rodenticides)
Conium maculatum Poison hemlock	Roadside ditches, damp waste areas; throughout North America	All

TABLE 4. (continued)		
Important Characteristics	Toxic Principle and Effects	Comments and Treatment
Dangerous Season: ALL SEASONS (continued)		
As above.	Selenium (chronic). Slow growth, reproductive failure, loss of hair, sore feet, acute death.	Avoid grazing seleniferous plants for extended periods. *See* SELENIUM POISONING, p 2516.
Shrubs. Numerous small, whitish flowers. Leaves resin-dotted, and persistent southward.	Unidentified. Acute course. Bloat, staggering, trembling, restlessness, polypnea, tachycardia, death.	Most dangerous in early growing stage. Toxin concentrated in leaves and flowers. No specific treatment.
Annual herbaceous weeds with terminal clusters of yellowish flowers and slender, elongated seed pods.	Glucosinolates (isothiocyanate, thiocyanates, nitrites) in seeds and vegetative parts, fresh or dry. Acute/chronic course. Anorexia, severe gastroenteritis, salivation, diarrhea, paralysis, photosensitization, hemoglobinuria.	Remove from source. Administer GI protectants (mineral oil).
Evergreen shrubs or tall bush; leaves alternate, ovate smooth-edged; flowers white, tubular, small clusters, fragrant by day; fruit, a greenish-white to lavender (immature), becoming dark purple to black (mature), fleshy berry, with several small, black, oblong seeds, dispersed by birds in droppings. Leaves longer, night fragrant flowers, white fruits at maturity (*C nocturnum*).	Atropine-like alkaloids (fruit), saponins (fruit and sap), and glycosides of 1,25-dihydroxycholecalciferol (leaves primarily, stem, fruits, and roots) are found. Gastroenteritis develops on ingestion of fruits. Vomiting, depression, anorexia, chronic weight loss with normal appetite, choppy stiff gait, increased pulse, persistent hypercalcemia and hyperphosphatemia, calcinosis (aorta, carotid and pulmonary arteries, tendons, ligaments, and kidneys), parathyroid atrophy, thyroid (C-cell) hypertrophy, and osteopetrosis reported with chronic ingestion of leaves.	Prevent further access of animals to plants. In early stages, treatment might be effective and cost effective. Correct fluid and electrolyte imbalances in cases with persistent vomiting or diarrhea. Reduce or prevent hypercalcemia (calciuresis, diuretics, steroids, calcitonin). Maintenance therapy of diuretics and steroids may be necessary.
Purple-spotted hollow stem. Leaves resemble parsley, parsnip odor when crushed. Taproot. Flowers white, in umbels.	Piperidine alkaloids (coniine and others) in vegetative parts. Acute course. Dilated pupils; weakness; staggering gait; slow pulse, progressing to rapid and thready. Slow, irregular breathing; death from respiratory failure. Teratogenic in cattle.	Coniine excreted via lungs and kidneys, mousy odor of breath and urine diagnostic. Administer saline cathartics; neutralize alkaloids with tannic acid, together with stimulants.

(continued)

TABLE 4. Poisonous Range Plants (continued) ▶

Scientific and Common Names	Habitat and Distribution	Affected Animals
Dangerous Season: ALL SEASONS (continued)		
Crotalaria spp Crotalaria, Rattlebox	Fields and roadsides; eastern and central USA	All
Cynoglossum officinale Hound's tongue	Common in waste places, roadsides, and pastured areas throughout USA.	Cattle, sheep, horses
Datura stramonium Jimson weed, Thorn apple	Fields, barn lots, trampled pastures, and waste places on rich bottom soils; throughout North America	All
Drymaria pachyphylla Inkweed, Drymary	Heavy alkaline clay soil in low areas or dry, over-grazed pastures; southwest.	Cattle, sheep, goats

◀ TABLE 4. *(continued)*

Important Characteristics	Toxic Principle and Effects	Comments and Treatment
Dangerous Season: ALL SEASONS *(continued)*		
Annual or perennial legume. Yellow flowers in racemes, pods inflated. Bracts at base of pedicels of flowers and fruits persistent. Leaves simple or divided. Seeds in harvested grain.	Pyrrolizidine alkaloid (monocrotaline) and other unidentified alkaloids (all parts, especially seeds). Chronic course. Chickens— diarrhea, pale comb, ruffled feathers; horses—unthriftiness, ataxic, walking in circles, icterus; cattle— bloody diarrhea, icterus, rough coat, edema, weakness. Death may occur from a few weeks to months after ingestion.	Cumulative, fresh or dry. No treatment.
Annual or biennial herbaceous plant, rough hairy stem and foliage, 3-4 ft tall. Leaves alternate, oblanceolate, narrowed to petiole (lower), lanceolate, sessile, clasping (upper). Flowers numerous in coiled racemes, without bracts, blue, purple, or white blooms. Fruit, bur-like from 4 nutlets, thickly covered with hooked prickles.	Pyrrolizidine alkaloids (0.6-2.1% of dry matter) including heliosupine and echinatine in the foliage. Unpleasant odor discourages consumption when fresh, becomes palatable in hay and is readily consumed. Toxic insult primarily hepatic and chronic in nature. Pyrrolizidine alkaloids (inactive) undergo hepatic metabolization to active intermediates—pyrroles (alkylating agent), which are toxic. Clinical signs are anorexia, depression, rough hair coat, hemorrhage, tenesmus, bloody feces, ataxia, jaundice, death. Hepatic lesions of necrosis, edema, megalocytosis, bile duct hyperplasia, and cytoplasmic vacuolation reported.	Know source and quality of hay. Treatment symptomatic and supportive at best. Affected animals seldom recover.
Leaves wavy. Flower large (4 in.), white, tubular. Fruit a spiny pod, 2 in. (5 cm) long.	Tropane alkaloids (atropine, scopolamine, hyoscyamine) in all parts, seeds in particular. Acute course. Weak rapid pulse and heartbeat, dilated pupils, dry mouth, incoordination, convulsions, coma.	All parts, mainly in hay or silage. Urine from animal dilates pupils of laboratory animals (diagnostic). Treatment nonspecific; cardiac and respiratory stimulants (physostigmine, pilocarpine, arecoline).
Multibranched, succulent, prostrate annual. Opposite leaves. Small white flowers.	Unknown toxin. Diarrhea, restlessness, depression, coma, death. Lesions include gastroenteritis with congestion of liver, kidneys, spleen. Petechial hemorrhages on heart.	Dangerous during drought, after rain, or at night. Avoid overstocking to improve range.

(continued)

TABLE 4.   Poisonous Range Plants (continued) ▶

Scientific and Common Names	Habitat and Distribution	Affected Animals
Dangerous Season: ALL SEASONS (continued)		
Festuca arundinacea Tall fescue	A coarse, hardy, drought-resistant grass; Pacific Northwest, Missouri, Oklahoma, and Kentucky; major pasture grass in southeastern USA	Mostly cattle and horses
Gelsemium sempervirens Yellow jessamine, Evening trumpet flower, Carolina jessamine	Open woods, thickets; southeast	All
Gutierrezia microcephala Broomweed, Snakeweed, Slinkweed, Turpentine weed	Widespread over dry range and desert; primarily south-west	Cattle, sheep, goats, pigs
Helenium hoopesii Orange sneezeweed	Moist slopes and well-drained mountain mead-ows; western	Sheep, rarely cattle
Helenium microcephalum Small head sneezeweed	Moist ground; southern	Cattle, sheep, goats
Hypericum perforatum St. John's-wort, Goatweed, Klamath weed	Dry soil, roadsides, pas-tures, ranges; throughout North America	Sheep, cattle, horses, goats
Kalmia spp Laurel, Ivybush, Lambkill	Rich moist woods, mead-ows, or acid bogs; eastern and northwestern. Danger-ous all seasons, especially winter and spring.	All, often sheep

◀ **TABLE 4.** *(continued)*

Important Characteristics	Toxic Principle and Effects	Comments and Treatment
Dangerous Season: ALL SEASONS *(continued)*		
Coarse, deeply rooted perennial grass. Broad, dark-green, ribbed, rough upper surface, and smooth sheathed leaves. Grows in clumps.	*See* FESCUE POISONING, p 2418.	*See* p 2418.
Climbing or trailing vines. Evergreen, entire, opposite leaves. Yellow tubular flowers, very fragrant.	Alkaloids (gelsemine and others, related to strychnine) in all parts. Acute course. Weakness, incoordination, dilated pupils, convulsions, coma, death within 48 hr. Limberneck in fowl.	No specific treatment. Relaxants and sedatives suggested.
Multibranched, perennial, resinous shrub. Yellow-flowered heads.	Unknown. Acute poisoning, anorexia, listlessness, hematuria, diarrhea followed by constipation. In cattle, abortions with retained placenta, stillbirths, or premature and weak calves.	Supplementing diet will help but not entirely prevent abortion in cattle.
Perennial herb. Orange sunflower-like heads or yellow flowers. Leaves alternate.	Sesquiterpene lactones (helenalin, hymenoxin). Subacute course (spewing sickness). Depression, weakness, restlessness, stiff gait, salivation, pronounced vomiting, emaciation, eventual death.	Cumulative. Aspiration pneumonia frequent. Remove from access to plant. Graze sneezeweed areas for only short periods of time. Can graze intermittently with some success.
Annual, erect herb, simple-stemmed below, bushy above. Stem winged. Narrow leaves throughout. Flowers in small heads; disk pale red-brown, rays yellow.	Sesquiterpene lactone (helenalin) in flowering stage. Depression, weakness, restlessness, stiff gait, salivation, vomiting.	Cumulative. Remove from pasture. Cathartics may help.
Perennial herb or woody below. Leaves opposite, dotted. Flowers many, yellow, with many stamens.	Photodynamic pigment (hypericin). Subacute course. Photosensitization, pruritus and erythema, blindness, convulsions, diarrhea, hypersensitivity to cold water contact, death.	Remove animals from source and sunlight. Corticosteroids parenterally, topical broad-spectrum antibiotics.
Woody shrub. Evergreen, glossy leaves. Flowers pink to rose, showy.	Resinoid (andromedotoxin) and a glucoside (arbutin) in vegetative parts. Acute course. Incoordination, excess salivation, vomiting, bloat, weakness, muscular spasms, coma, death.	Undigested rumen contents and ingesta in lungs at necropsy. Laxatives, demulcents, nerve stimulants, atropine.

(continued)

TABLE 4. Poisonous Range Plants (continued) ▶

Scientific and Common Names	Habitat and Distribution	Affected Animals
Dangerous Season: ALL SEASONS (continued)		
Kochia scoparia Kochia	Throughout North America	Cattle
Ligustrum spp Privet, Ligustrum, Hedge plant	An ornamental; common as hedge; found at abandoned farm home sites, along fences, and in bottomlands.	All livestock
Lupinus spp Lupines, Bluebonnet	Dry to moist soils, road-sides, fields, and mountains; throughout, but poisoning mostly western	Sheep, cattle, goats, horses, pigs
Nandina domestica Nandina, Heavenly bamboo, Chinese sacred bamboo	Common ornamental in southern USA	All grazing animals, especially ruminants
Nerium oleander Oleander	Common ornamental in southern regions	All

TABLE 4. (continued)		
Important Characteristics	Toxic Principle and Effects	Comments and Treatment
Dangerous Season: ALL SEASONS (continued)		
Annual to 5 ft tall. Many branched stems give bushy appearance. Leaves petiolate, lanceolate, thin, and flat. Fruit has 5 wedge-shaped wings.	An alkaloid has been suggested. This plant may also accumulate nitrate and oxalate. Photosensitization, polioencephalomalacia, which seems intensified by slow growth and sulfates.	Harvested foliage is source of toxin. Protect from sun in case of photosensitization; treat polioencephalomalacia with vitamin B.
Shrubs up to 15 ft tall. Simple, opposite, short-petioled, evergreen or deciduous leaves. Numerous small, white flowers in panicles. Fruit is 1- to 2-seeded, black or dark blue berry that persists throughout winter.	Ligustrin, ligustron, syringin, syringopictrin, and other unknown compounds in leaves and fruit. Primarily GI irritants. Diarrhea, abdominal pain, incoordination, paresis, weak pulse, hypothermia, convulsions, sometimes death.	Treatment symptomatic and supportive; correct dehydration.
Perennials. Leaves simple or palmately divided. Flowers blue, white, red, or yellow in terminal raceme.	Quinolizidine alkaloids (20 known) concentrated in seeds (fresh and dry); some piperidine alkaloids. Acute course. Inappetence, dyspnea, struggle, convulsions, death from respiratory paralysis. Some species teratogenic in cattle.	Do not disturb sick animals; remove from source as they begin to recover. No effective treatment, but survivors recover completely. *See also* p 2420.
Upright, unbranched, and multistemmed, evergreen shrub, 3-7 ft tall. Alternate, bi- to tripinnately compound leaves; leaflets subsessile, elliptic-lanceolate, half as wide as long, entire, leathery, metallic bluish-green becoming purple in fall. Small, white flowers; 2-seeded, bright red berries in large panicles persist throughout fall and winter.	Cyanogenic glycosides in foliage and fruits, hydrolyzed in GI tract to free cyanide, thereby affecting cellular respiration. *See* CYANIDE POISONING, p 2355. Prognosis good if animal survives for 1 hr after signs begin.	Acute outcome precludes effective treatment for most; IV sodium nitrite/sodium thiosulfate treatment of choice. Picrate test indicates toxic potential of the plant. *See* CYANIDE POISONING, p 2355.
Evergreen shrub or tree. Leaves whorled and prominently, finely, pinnately veined beneath. Flowers showy, white to deep pink.	Digitoxin-type glycosides (oleandroside, nerioside, and others) in all parts, fresh or dry. Acute course. Severe gastroenteritis, vomiting, diarrhea, increased pulse rate, weakness, death.	No specific treatment. Atropine in conjunction with propranolol reported helpful.

(continued)

TABLE 4. Poisonous Range Plants *(continued)* ▶

Scientific and Common Names	Habitat and Distribution	Affected Animals
Dangerous Season: ALL SEASONS (continued)		
Photinia fraseri, *P serrulata, P glabra* Fraser's photinia, Chinese photinia, Red leaf photinia, Red tip photinia	Common ornamental (hedge or screen) in southern USA	All grazing animals, mostly ruminants
Pinus ponderosa Western yellow pine	Coniferous forests of Rocky Mountains at moderate elevations; western. Dangerous all seasons, especially winter.	Cattle
Prunus caroliniana Laurel cherry, Cherry laurel	Woods, fence rows, and often escaped from cultivation; southern regions. Dangerous all seasons, especially winter and spring.	All grazing animals
Prunus spp Chokecherries, Wild cherries, Peaches	Waste areas, fence rows, woods, orchards, prairies, dry slopes	All grazing animals, mostly cattle and sheep
Psilostrophe spp Paperflowers	Open range lands and pastures; southwest	Sheep
Pteridium aquilinum Bracken fern	Dry poor soil, open woods, sandy ridges	All grazing animals
Ricinus communis Castor bean	Cultivated in southern regions	All

TABLE 4.	(continued)	
Important Characteristics	**Toxic Principle and Effects**	**Comments and Treatment**
Dangerous Season: ALL SEASONS (continued)		
Evergreen shrubs, 10-15 ft tall. Alternate, oblong-ovate serrated leaves, copper-red (when young) turning dark green in 2-4 wk. Prominent, whitish flowers in spring; showy, red berries in fall.	Same as for *N domestica* (above).	Same as for *N domestica.*
Tree, 150-180 ft. Leaves in groups of 3, yellowish green, 7-11 in. long. Bark platy, reddish orange.	Unknown toxin. Chronic course. Abortions in late gestation, still-births or weak calves, depressed, edema of vulva and udder, retained placenta.	Pine-needle ingestion during last half of gestation—may abort after single exposure. Keep pregnant cows away from source.
Leaves evergreen, shiny, leathery. Broken twigs with strong cherry bark odor. Fruit black.	Hydrocyanic acid (wilted leaves, bark, and twigs). Peracute course. Difficult breathing, bloat, staggering, convulsions, followed by prostration and death. Mucous membranes and blood bright red.	*See* CYANIDE POISONING, p 2355.
Large shrubs or trees. Flowers white or pink. Cherries or peaches. Crushed twigs with strong odor.	Glycoside-yielding cyanide (rumen hydrolysis). Excitement leading to depression, dyspnea, incoordination, convulsions, prostration. Death may occur in 15 min from asphyxiation.	Mucous membranes, bright pink color; blood, bright red color. *See* CYANIDE POISONING, p 2355.
Perennial composite. Erect, woolly stems branching from base. Many small heads of yellow flowers.	Sesquiterpene lactone. Depression, incoordination, anorexia, weakness, trembling, rapid irregular pulse and respiration, coughing, vomiting, aspiration pneumonia, death.	Antimicrobial actions of sesquiterpene lactone in rumen affect metabolism. Supplement diet with sodium sulfate and high protein.
Leaves firm, leathery, 3-pinnate.	*See* BRACKEN FERN POISONING, p 2349.	*See* p 2349.
Large, palmately lobed leaves. Seeds resembling engorged ticks, usually 3 in somewhat spiny pod.	Phytotoxin—ricin in all parts (seeds especially toxic). Acute to chronic course (death or recovery). Violent purgation, straining with bloody diarrhea, weakness, salivation, trembling, incoordination.	Diagnosis based on presence of seeds, RBC agglutination, precipitin test. Specific antiserum, ideal antidote; sedatives, arecoline hydrobromide, followed by saline cathartics suggested.

(continued)

TABLE 4. Poisonous Range Plants (*continued*) ▶

Scientific and Common Names	Habitat and Distribution	Affected Animals
Dangerous Season: ALL SEASONS (continued)		
Senecio spp Groundsel, Senecio	Grassland areas; mostly western	Cattle, horses, sheep to a limited extent in USA
Sorghum halepense Johnson grass	Weed of open fields and waste places; southern and scattered north to New York and Iowa	All grazing animals
Sorghum vulgare Sorghum, Sudan grass, Kafir, Durra, Milo, Broom-corn, Schrock, etc	Forage crops and escapes; throughout North America	All
Taxus spp Yew	Most of North America; Japanese and English yew common ornamentals	All
Triglochin spp Arrowgrass	Salt marshes, wet alkaline soils, lake shores. Dangerous all seasons, especially dry season.	Sheep, cattle

TABLE 4. (continued)		
Important Characteristics	**Toxic Principle and Effects**	**Comments and Treatment**
Dangerous Season: ALL SEASONS (continued)		
Perennial or annual herbs. Heads of yellow flowers with whorl of bracts below.	Pyrrolizidine alkaloids, volatile oils, and nitrogen oxides (fresh or dry). Acute poisoning not common. Dullness, aimless walking, increased pulse, rapid respiration, weakness, colic, delayed death (days to months). In cattle, prolapsed rectum from persistent straining. In horses, nervous signs evident in later stages.	Liver biopsy diagnostic in early stages. Liver function test of value for subclinical condition in cattle. No general treatment. *See also* p 2506.
Coarse grass with large rhizomes and white midvein on leaf. Topped by large, open panicle.	Same as for *S vulgare* (below).	Same as for *S vulgare*.
Coarse grasses with terminal flower cluster. Some to 8 ft tall.	Hydrocyanic acid (drought, trampling, frost, second growth) and nitrate (heavy in vegetative parts). Acute course. Difficult breathing, bloat, staggering, convulsions, death. Blood bright red (cyanide) or chocolate brown (nitrate).	Hay safe for cyanide (volatile), not safe for nitrate (analyze). *See* CYANIDE POISONING, p 2355, and NITRATE AND NITRITE POISONING, p 2423.
Evergreen perennial tree or shrub. Bark reddish brown then flaking in scales. Leaves linear, 0.5-1 in. (1.5-2.5 cm) long, 2-ranked on twig, upper surface dark green, lower yellow-green, midribs prominent. Flowers unisexual, inconspicuous. Fruit single stony seed. Bright scarlet color.	Toxic alkaloids in bark, leaves, seeds. Gaseous distress, diarrhea, vomiting, tremors, dyspnea, dilated pupils, respiratory difficulty, weakness, fatigue, collapse, coma, convulsions, bradycardia, circulatory failure, death. Death may be rapid.	Poisoning usually results when branches and trimmings fed to livestock.
Grasslike, except leaves are thick. Heads of fruits globular on erect raceme. Flowers inconspicuous.	Hydrocyanic acid in leaves. Salivation, dyspnea, excitement followed by depression, incoordination, prostration, convulsions followed by death from anoxia.	Often, animals found dead. *See* CYANIDE POISONING, p 2355.

TABLE 5.   Important Poisonous Vascular Plants of Australia ▶

Scientific and Common Names*	Plant Characteristics	Habitat and Distribution†
Abrus precatorius Gidee-gidee, Rosary pea, Precatory bean, Jequirity bean, Crab's eye	Vine with compound leaves and sprays of pink pea-type flowers followed by curled pods containing red and black seeds	Widespread in tropical Australia
Acacia georginae Georgina gidyea	Small tree with dark gray fissured flaky bark, "leaves" (phyllodes) gray-green tapered at both ends with parallel veins and clusters of yellow fluffy globular flowers in the "leaf" forks followed by flat curved and coiled seed pods	Arid zone; eastern central Australia
Adonis microcarpa Pheasant's eye	Annual herb with highly divided (ferny) leaves and glossy scarlet 5- to 8-petalled flowers	Weed of cultivation in temperate regions
Ageratina (Eupatorium) adenophora Crofton weed	Shrub with numerous upright stems 1-2 m high; leaves opposite and trowel-shaped; white flowers in dense clusters at ends of stems	Naturalized weed of pastures in eastern coastal regions
Agrostis avenacea Blown grass, Blow-away grass	Grass, tufted with spreading seedhead	Coastal and inland areas of subtropical and temperature regions
Alstonia constricta Bitter bark, Quinine tree	Tree up to 12 m, frequently suckering to form thickets; corky bark; leaves opposite; milky sap; cream, star-shaped flowers in clusters at ends of branches; long narrow pods with seeds bearing silky hair tufts	Widespread in coastal and inland southern Queensland and northeastern New South Wales
Ammi majus Bishop's weed	Annual herb with upright stems, ferny leaves and small white flowers in flat-topped clusters	Weed of cultivation in temperate regions
Anthoxanthum odoratum Sweet vernal grass	Grass, tufted upright with tapered cylindrical seedhead	Coastal and subcoastal in temperate regions. A weed of pasture.

TABLE 5. (continued)		
Affected Animals	**Toxic Principle and Effects**	**Comments and Treatment‡**
Ruminants, horses, humans	Abrin (toxalbumin) causing severe gastroenteritis	Seeds are the toxic part of the plant. No effective treatment is known.
Cattle, horses, dogs (secondary poisoning)	Fluoroacetate—sudden death. Dogs scavenging carcasses of poisoned livestock can be poisoned.	Pods and young foliage are most toxic. No effective treatment is known.
Ruminants, horses, pigs	Cardiac glycosides—cardiac arrhythmias, diarrhea with blood, dyspnea, sudden death	Both seeds and whole plants have caused toxicity. Cardiac glycosides—oral activated charcoal, 5 g/kg with electrolyte replacement solution; treat arrhythmias with atropine and propranolol; horses should receive analgesics/antispasmodics.
Horses	Unidentified toxin causes coughing and decreased exercise tolerance progressing to dyspnea from chronic pulmonary inflammation and fibrosis. Heart failure occurs in some cases.	Flowering plants are the most toxic. No effective treatment is known.
Ruminants, horses	Corynetoxins (tunicaminylu-racils produced by *Rathayi-bacter toxicus* bacteria in seedhead nematode galls) cause "floodplain staggers" with convulsions and death in most cases. *See* p 2512.	Corynetoxins—a cyclodextrin toxin binding agent is under development as an antidote. Immunization is being developed for prevention.
Ruminants; dogs may be poisoned by meat from poisoned ruminants.	Indole alkaloids (alstonine, alstonidine)—tetanic spasms of skeletal muscles	Leaves and fruit are toxic. Deny further access to plants. Serious cases may benefit from heavy sedation.
Ruminants, horses	Furanocoumarins—primary photosensitization, including corneal edema	Supportive therapy for photosensitization (shade, anti-inflammatory, rehydration). No specific therapy available. Deny further access to plants.
Cattle	Dihydroxycoumarin produced in moldy hay or silage causes coagulation defects and extensive hemorrhage in affected animals.	Toxin will be transported across the placenta and through milk. Treat with vitamin K_1 injections.

(continued)

TABLE 5. Important Poisonous Vascular Plants (continued) ▶

Scientific and Common Names*	Plant Characteristics	Habitat and Distribution†
Arctotheca calendula Cape weed	Annual herb with leaves in rosette; hairy on lower surfaces; bright yellow daisy-type flowers with dark centers	Weed of cultivation in southern regions
Argemone spp Mexican poppies	Upright thistle-like herbs with variegated gray-green deeply divided spiny leaves, large pale or deep yellow 4- to 6-petalled flowers followed by seed capsules with small dark seeds; cut stems exude bright yellow sap.	Widespread weeds of cultivation
Asclepias curassavica Red-head cotton-bush, Red cotton	Shrub with upright stems, milky sap, simple tapered leaves, red and yellow flowers and tapered seed pods with tufted seeds	Weed of pasture and cultivation in northern regions
Atalaya hemiglauca Whitewood	Small tree <6 m high with pale gray flaky bark with compound leaves consisting of 1-3 pairs of narrow leaflets and cream flowers in bunches at the end of branches, followed by winged fruit	Inland regions of mainland states
Avena sativa Oats	Grass, upright	Crop in temperate and subtropical areas
Bowenia spp Byfield "fern", Zamia "fern" There are 2 species, both endemic to Australia.	Fern-like plants with groups of leathery highly-divided leaves arising from underground trunks. Sexes are separate, bearing cones at the apex of the plant.	Open forests and rainforests of northeastern Australia; cultivated in gardens
Brachiaria spp Signal grass, Para grass	Grasses, tufted or sprawling	Cultivated tropical pasture grasses

◀ **TABLE 5.** *(continued)*

Affected Animals	Toxic Principle and Effects	Comments and Treatment[‡]
Ruminants	Nitrates—methemoglobinemia	Toxicity is most likely from rapid large plant intakes. Nitrates—IV methylene blue.
Poultry, ruminants	Isoquinoline alkaloids cause heart failure with cardiomyopathy, pulmonary and subcutaneous edema.	Seeds are the most toxic part, but dry plants in hay may be toxic. No effective treatment is known. Seeds crushed and exposed to sunlight are detoxified.
Cattle	Cardiac glycosides—cardiac arrhythmias, diarrhea with blood, dyspnea, sudden death	Cardiac glycosides—oral activated charcoal, 5 g/kg with electrolyte replacement solution; treat arrhythmias with atropine and propranolol; horses should receive analgesics/antispasmodics.
Horses	Unidentified toxin. A syndrome of cardiac failure is reported with severe edematous swelling of the head, muscle weakness, and myoglobinuria.	Young shoots and fruit are regarded as the toxic parts. Poisoning occurs when the plant forms a large proportion of the diet. No effective treatment is known.
Ruminants	Nitrates—methemoglobinemia. Unknown toxin in "rusty" or "red-tipped" fodder oats causes transient hyperesthesia and diarrhea in cattle. Unknown photosensitizing toxin	Nitrate toxicity is most likely from rapid large plant intakes. Nitrates—IV methylene blue. Supportive therapy for photosensitization (shade, anti-inflammatory, rehydration). No specific therapy available.
Cattle	Unidentified neurotoxin—permanent spinal cord degeneration with posterior ataxia in cattle ("zamia staggers"). Methylazoxymethanol—liver necrosis	Seeds and young leaves are the most toxic parts. No effective treatment is known.
Ruminants, horses	Steroidal saponins—hepatogenous photosensitization in ruminants. Calcium oxalate crystals deny calcium to horses producing nutritional secondary hyperparathyroidism (lameness, weight loss, jaw swelling).	Supportive therapy for photosensitization (shade, anti-inflammatory, rehydration). No specific therapy available. Calcium oxalate (horses)—remove from the pasture and remineralize bones by feeding a mineral supplement with a Ca:P ratio of 2:1, 2 kg/horse/wk for 6 mo.

(continued)

TABLE 5. Important Poisonous Vascular Plants (continued) ▶

Scientific and Common Names*	Plant Characteristics	Habitat and Distribution†
Brachyachne spp Native couches	Grasses, sprawling or erect with digitate seed heads	Native pasture grasses of northern inland regions
Brunfelsia spp Francisia, Yesterday-today-and-tomorrow	Shrub with dense foliage and conspicuous broad flowers opening purple and fading to white and followed by brown to black berries	Cultivated garden plant
Bryophyllum (Kalanchoe) spp Mother-of-millions	Erect succulent herbs with fleshy leaves (pencil-shaped to broad and lobed depending on species) and clusters of hanging tubular flowers with red petals at the top of stems	Naturalized weedy garden escape of north-eastern regions; prefers shaded habitat on leaf litter
Cascabela thevetia (Thevetia peruviana) Yellow oleander	Shrub or small tree; tapered leaves; bright yellow trumpet-shaped flowers; fleshy fruit turning black when ripe	Cultivated garden plant; naturalized in some areas
Castanospermum australe Black bean	Tree, usually up to 20 m high with compound leaves and clusters of red and yellow pea-type flowers on branches, followed by large seed pods containing large fleshy brown seeds	Riverine forest of eastern Australia; sparingly cultivated
Cenchrus ciliaris Buffel grass	Grass, tufted forming tussocks with crowded seedheads containing numerous bristly spikelets	Naturalized tropical pasture grass; weedy in arid zone
Cestrum parqui Green cestrum	Multistemmed erect shrub with leaves tapered at both ends and clusters of tubular yellow flowers at the end of stems, followed by black berries	Cultivated garden plant; naturalized in eastern Australia

TABLE 5. (continued)

Affected Animals	Toxic Principle and Effects	Comments and Treatment[‡]
Ruminants	Cyanogenic glycosides—sudden death	Toxicity is most likely from rapid large plant intakes. Cyanogenic glycosides—IV sodium thiosulfate, 660 mg/kg plus an oral dose (30 g cattle, 5 g sheep). Repeat treatment may be needed for relapse.
Dogs	Unidentified toxin causing vomiting, diarrhea, muscle tremors, and clonic/tonic convulsions	Fruits are toxic. Dogs attracted to ripe fruits will eat large amounts. Treat with an emetic followed by oral activated charcoal, 1-3 g/kg plus a saline cathartic, with an anticonvulsant or anesthetic to treat seizures.
Cattle	Cardiac glycosides—cardiac arrhythmias, diarrhea with blood, dyspnea, sudden death	Flowering plants are most toxic and poisoning cases are confined to winter when the plants flower. Cardiac glycosides—oral activated charcoal, 5 g/kg with electrolyte replacement solution; treat arrhythmias with atropine and propranolol.
Cattle, horses	Cardiac glycosides—cardiac arrhythmias, diarrhea with blood, dyspnea, sudden death	Cardiac glycosides—oral activated charcoal, 5 g/kg with electrolyte replacement solution; treat arrhythmias with atropine and propranolol; horses should receive analgesics/antispasmodics.
Cattle, horses	Unidentified toxin causing GI tract irritation; castanospermine (polyhydroxy alkaloid), a glucosidase inhibitor, is not responsible for poisoning.	Toxicity only occurs with persistent consumption of large numbers of ripe seeds, most likely under drought conditions. No effective treatment is known.
Ruminants, horses	Soluble oxalates—hypocalcemia, nephrosis in ruminants but not horses. Calcium oxalate crystals deny calcium to horses, producing nutritional secondary hyperparathyroidism (lameness, weight loss, jaw swelling).	Ruminants are susceptible only if very hungry and have access to very lush grass. Soluble oxalates—calcium borogluconate injection (prognosis guarded). Calcium oxalate (horses)—remove from the pasture and remineralize bones by feeding a mineral supplement with a Ca:P ratio of 2:1, 2 kg/horse/wk for 6 mo.
Ruminants	Diterpenoid (kaurene) glycosides parquin and carboxyparquin cause acute coagulation necrosis of periacinar hepatocytes with rapid death after hepatoencephalopathy in some cases	No effective treatment is known.

(continued)

TABLE 5. Important Poisonous Vascular Plants (continued) ▶

Scientific and Common Names*	Plant Characteristics	Habitat and Distribution†
Cheilanthes sieberi Mulga fern	Small upright fern with dark stems and small leaves. A xerophytic (drought-resistant) fern, often the first green plant available in pasture after drought-breaking rains	Widespread in woodlands of inland and coastal parts of subtropical and temperate regions
Citrullus spp Colocynth, Pie melons *Cucumis* spp Paddy melons	Vines with yellow flowers and melon-like fruit	Widespread weeds of inland arid regions
Corchorus olitorius Jute	Erect annual herb with alternate leaves, each bearing 2 elongated basal stipules, yellow 5-petalled flowers, dark cylindrical seed pods	Weed of cultivation and pasture in northern Australia
Crotalaria spp Rattlepods	Herbs to shrubs with either simple or trifoliate leaves and bright yellow pea-type flowers on spikes, followed by inflated seedpods	Native and naturalized in subtropical and tropical areas; some species are weeds of cultivation and pasture.
Cryptostegia grandiflora Rubber vine	Vine, multistemmed with oval leaves, pink trumpet-shaped flowers and rigid paired pods	Weed of pasture in northeastern regions

TABLE 5. (continued)		
Affected Animals	**Toxic Principle and Effects**	**Comments and Treatment‡**
Cattle, sheep	Ptaquiloside (*see Pteridium* above). Thiaminase (*see Marsilea* below).	Ptaquiloside—no effective treatment is known. Thiaminase—IV thiamine (vitamin B$_1$) is effective.
Cattle	Cucurbitacins—irritation of the upper GI tract and increased permeability of blood vessels producing sudden death with diarrhea	Ripe fruits are the most toxic part of the plants. Poisoning occurs when cattle have access to large quantities. No effective treatment is known. Rumenotomy to remove fruits could be considered.
Cattle, horses, pigs	Cardiac glycosides—cardiac arrhythmias, diarrhea with blood, dyspnea, sudden death	Seeds are toxic as contaminants of fed grains. Cardiac glycosides—oral activated charcoal, 5 g/kg with electrolyte replacement solution; treat arrhythmias with atropine and propranolol; horses should receive analgesics/antispasmodics.
Ruminants, horses, pigs	Pyrrolizidine alkaloids—chronic hepatopathy causing weight loss, irritability and compulsive walking (horses) or weight loss and persistent diarrhea with tenesmus (cattle). Rarely, horses may develop pulmonary adenomatosis and severe dyspnea after eating certain species that contain monocrotaline and similar pneumotoxic alkaloids. Pigs develop nephrosis rather than hepatopathy. Unknown toxin(s) in *C aridicola* and *C medicaginea* causes severe esophageal ulceration in horses.	15 species have been associated with toxicity of animals in Australia. Pigs have been poisoned by *C retusa* seeds contaminating feed grain. No effective treatment for hepatotoxicity. If a stomach tube can be passed in cases of esophageal ulceration, affected horses should recover with symptomatic treatment. *See* p 2506.
Cattle, horses	Cardiac glycosides—cardiac arrhythmias, diarrhea with blood, dyspnea, sudden death	Cardiac glycosides—oral activated charcoal, 5 g/kg with electrolyte replacement solution; treat arrhythmias with atropine and propranolol; horses should receive analgesics/antispasmodics.

(continued)

TABLE 5. Important Poisonous Vascular Plants (*continued*) ▶

Scientific and Common Names*	Plant Characteristics	Habitat and Distribution†
Cupressus macrocarpa Monterey cypress	Tree, densely branched with dark green foliage to 20 m high	Cultivated in temperate areas, often as wind-break trees
Cycas spp Zamias, zamia "palm" 27 species endemic to Australia. *C revoluta* Sago "palm" from the Japanese islands is cultivated in gardens.	Tree-like plants with trunks surmounted by rosettes of leathery leaves with numerous leaflets. Sexes are separate. Male cones produced at the apex; female cones divided into separate leaf-like structures bearing naked seeds on their margins.	Open forest and wood-lands of northern Australia, mostly coastal to subcoastal; some cultivated in gardens
Dactyloctenium radulans Button grass	Grass, spreading from central tuft with spikelets in star-like clusters	Widespread native pasture grass in all mainland states
Dendrocnide spp Stinging trees	Shrubs to trees with broad heart-shaped leaves bearing numerous stinging hairs with small flowers in bunches, followed by fleshy fruits	Rainforests of northeastern regions
Duboisia hopwoodii Pituri	Shrub, up to 3 m high with long narrow leaves and groups of white bell-shaped, purple-striped flowers at ends of branches, followed by black berries	Arid regions from central Australia to the western coast
Duboisia myoporoides and D leichhardtii Corkwoods	Small trees with corky bark with simple leaves and white tubular flowers in bunches at branch ends, followed by black berries	Coastal and inland eastern Australia
Echium plantagineum Patterson's curse, Salvation Jane	Annual herb with rosette of broad hairy leaves and erect flowering stalk with blue flowers crowded along one side of the curled spikes at the end of the branches	Weed of cultivation and pasture in southern regions

TABLE 5. (continued)

Affected Animals	Toxic Principle and Effects	Comments and Treatment[‡]
Cattle	Isocupressic acid and/or vasoactive lipids—abortion/premature birth	No effective treatment is known. Separating livestock from windbreaks by fencing provides effective prevention.
Cattle, dogs	Unidentified neurotoxin causing permanent spinal cord degeneration with posterior ataxia in cattle ("zamia staggers"). Methylazoxymethanol—liver necrosis. Dogs eating seeds of cultivated specimens of C revoluta have been affected.	Seeds and young leaves are the most toxic parts. No effective treatment is known.
Cattle, sheep	Nitrates—methemoglobinemia	Dangerous only when growing in heavily fertilized soils such as in stockyards and available to hungry animals. Nitrates—IV methylene blue
Horses, humans	Moroidin (a bicyclic octapeptide) is thought at least partly responsible for intense and persistent local pain caused by contact with stinging hairs on the leaf surfaces. Horses can be driven to frenzy by contact. Pain in humans can persist for several weeks after contact.	No effective treatment is known. Prompt euthanasia should be considered in affected horses.
Ruminants	Nicotine causing incoordination, muscle tremors, dilated pupils (impaired vision), recumbency, clonic seizures, diarrhea.	No effective treatment is known. Affected animals left undisturbed often recover.
Ruminants, horses	Tropane alkaloids causing dilated pupils (impaired vision), tachycardia, convulsions; paralytic ileus or impaction colic, gastric rupture, and hemorrhagic gastroenteritis are reported in horses.	Physostigmine
Cattle, horses, sheep	Pyrrolizidine alkaloids—chronic hepatopathy causing mostly weight loss, irritability and compulsive waling (horses) or weight loss and persistent diarrhea with tenesmus (cattle)	No effective treatment is known.

(continued)

TABLE 5. Important Poisonous Vascular Plants *(continued)* ▶

Scientific and Common Names*	Plant Characteristics	Habitat and Distribution†
Eremophila maculata Spotted emu bush	Densely branched shrub, 1-2 m high with dark green tapered leaves and red tubular flowers with spotted throats carried on S-shaped stalks, followed by round hard fruits with papery skin	Inland regions of mainland states
Eremophila (Myoporum) deserti Ellangowan poison bush, Turkey bush and *M accuminatum* Boobialla	Shrubs or small trees with leaves tapered at both ends and small white bell-shaped flowers, hairy inside, followed by purple, black, or yellow berries	Inland regions of mainland states
Erythrophleum chlorostachys Cooktown ironwood, Camel poison	Tree, up to 15 m with compound leaves consisting of leaflets with unequal amounts of blade on either side of the midvein, flower spikes with yellow-green flowers, followed by dry brown flat seed pods	Open woodland in northern Australia
Eucalyptus cladocalyx Sugar gum	Tree, up to 30 m with white or yellow-brown smooth bark, adult leaves strongly different shade of green on upper and lower surfaces (discolorous), rubbed buds, white flowers and barrel-shaped fruit	Southeastern states; commonly grown as windbreaks
Euphorbia spp Spurges	Prostrate to erect succulent herbs with milky sap and unusual inflorescences (cyathiums)	Toxic species occur in inland areas
Gastrolobium spp Poison bushes	Shrubs, most with opposite leaves or leaves in rosettes around stems, terminal racemes of pea-type flowers with red and yellow or all-red petals, followed by small hairy seed pods	Most species are concentrated in shrublands or southwestern Australia with one species in central and northeastern Australia

◀ **TABLE 5.** *(continued)*

Affected Animals	Toxic Principle and Effects	Comments and Treatment[‡]
Ruminants	Cyanogenic glycosides—sudden death	Young leaves are the most toxic part of the plant. Toxicity is most likely from rapid large plant intakes. Cyanogenic glycosides—IV sodium thiosulfate, 660 mg/kg, plus an oral dose (30 g cattle, 5 g sheep). Repeat for relapses.
Ruminants	Furanosesquiterpenes cause acute coagulation necrosis of hepatocytes with rapid death after hepatoencephalopathy in some cases.	Some individual plants are nontoxic. No effective treatment is known.
Ruminants, horses	Diterpenoid alkaloids and cinnamic acid derivatives; produce sudden death with effects similar to those of cardiac glycosides.	All parts can be fatally toxic in small doses. Suckers accessible to grazing animals. No effective treatment is known, but the regimen for cardiac glycosides could be applied, eg, oral activated charcoal, 5 g/kg with electrolyte replacement solution; treat arrhythmias with atropine and propranolol; horses should receive analgesics/antispasmodics.
Ruminants	Cyanogenic glycosides—sudden death	Young leaves are the most toxic part of the plant. Toxicity is most likely from rapid large plant intakes. Cyanogenic glycosides—IV sodium thiosulfate, 660 mg/kg plus an oral dose (30 g cattle, 5 g sheep). Repeat for relapses.
Ruminants	Irritant toxins of uncertain identity—alimentary tract irritation, diarrhea. Cyanogenic glycosides suspected in some species—sudden death	Toxicity is most likely from rapid large plant intakes. Irritant toxins—no effective treatment is known. Cyanogenic glycosides—IV sodium thiosulfate, 660 mg/kg plus an oral dose (30 g cattle, 5 g sheep). Repeat for relapses.
Ruminants, horses, dogs (secondary poisoning)	Fluoroacetate—sudden death. Dogs scavenging carcasses of poisoned livestock can be poisoned.	34 species are toxic and 8 more are suspected as toxic. No effective treatment is known.

(continued)

TABLE 5. Important Poisonous Vascular Plants (continued)

Scientific and Common Names[*]	Plant Characteristics	Habitat and Distribution[†]
[*]*Glyceria maxima* Reed sweet grass	Grass, erect 90-250 cm high, with an open branched seedhead	Temperate regions in semiaquatic habitats such as on the margins of water storage dams
[*]*Gomphocarpus* spp Balloon cotton	Shrub with upright stems, milky sap, simple tapered leaves, white flowers, and inflated seed pods with tufted seeds	Weed of pasture and cultivation in northern regions
[*]*Heliotropium europaeum* Common heliotrope *H amplexicaule* Blue heliotrope	Annual herbs with branched stems bearing green to gray-green simple leaves and flowering stems with white (*H europaeum*) or blue (*H amplexicaule*) flowers crowded on one side of the curled spikes at the ends of branches	Weeds of cultivation and pasture in southern regions
Heterodendron oleifolium Boonaree, Rosewood, Bullock bush	Tree, up to 7 m high with dark gray furrowed and flaky bark, pale green inconspicuous flowers, followed by rounded fruits	Inland regions of mainland states
[*]*Homeria flaccida* One-leaf cape tulip; [*]*H miniata* Two-leaf cape tulip	Herbs growing from underground corms, forming a leaf or leaves and branched flowering stems with 6-petalled, salmon-pink flowers	Naturalized in temperate regions of southern Australia
Hoya australis Wax flower	Vine with fleshy round leaves, milky sap, and bunches of waxy white flowers	Rocky areas and vine forests ("dry" rainforests) in coastal and subcoastal Queensland and New South Wales

TABLE 5.	(continued)	
Affected Animals	**Toxic Principle and Effects**	**Comments and Treatment**[‡]
Ruminants	Cyanogenic glycosides—sudden death.	Cyanide toxicity is most likely from rapid large plant intakes, eg, by hungry animals. cyanogenic glycosides—IV sodium thiosulfate, 660 mg/kg plus an oral dose (30 g cattle, 5 g sheep). Repeat treatment may be needed for relapses.
Cattle	Cardiac glycosides—cardiac arrhythmias, diarrhea with blood, dyspnea, sudden death.	Cardiac glycosides—oral activated charcoal, 5 g/kg with electrolyte replacement solution; treat arrhythmias with atropine and propranolol; horses should receive analgesics/antispasmodics
Cattle, horses, pigs, sheep, poultry	Pyrrolizidine alkaloids—chronic hepatopathy causing mostly weight loss, irritability and compulsive walking (horses) or weight loss and persistent diarrhea with tenesmus (cattle).	Seeds of *H europaeum* contaminating feed wheat have poisoned pigs and poultry. No effective treatment is known.
Ruminants	Cyanogenic glycosides—sudden death.	The plant is regarded as safe fodder unless fed in large amounts during droughts. Toxicity is most likely from rapid large plant intakes. Cyanogenic glycosides—IV sodium thiosulfate, 660 mg/kg plus an oral dose (30 g cattle, 5 g sheep). Repeat for relapses.
Ruminants, horses	Cardiac glycosides—cardiac arrhythmias, diarrhea with blood, dyspnea, sudden death.	Toxicity has occurred from access in pasture or in hay. Cardiac glycosides—oral activated charcoal, 5 g/kg with electrolyte replacement solution; treat arrhythmias with atropine and propranolol; horses should receive analgesics/antispasmodics.
Cattle, sheep	Unidentified neurotoxin—muscle tremors, ataxia, collapse, clonic/tetanic convulsions	No effective treatment is known.

(continued)

TABLE 5. Important Poisonous Vascular Plants (*continued*) ▶

Scientific and Common Names*	Plant Characteristics	Habitat and Distribution†
Indigofera linnaei Birdsville indigo, 9-leaved indigo	Prostrate herb with compound leaves and tight clusters of scarlet, pea-type flowers followed by hairy seed pods	Widespread in tropical Queensland, Northern Territory and Western Australia
Ipomoea batatus Sweet potato	Vine with arrowhead-shaped leaves and trumpet-shaped pink flowers	Cultivated crop
Ipomoea muelleri Poison morning glory	Vine with arrowhead-shaped leaves and trumpet-shaped pink flowers	Central and northwestern regions
Ipomea calobra Weir vine	Vine with arrowhead-shaped leaves and trumpet-shaped pink flowers	Localized to clay soils of Maranoa district, Queensland
Isotropis spp Lamb poisons, Granny bonnets, Poison sage	Shrubs or herbs with pea-type flowers with conspicuous radiating branched lines on the back of the large erect standard petal; flowers are purple, yellow, or orange	Most species confined to southwestern Australia with one in central Australia
Jatropha spp	Shrubs and small trees with inconspicuous or bright red flowers and seed pods	Cultivated garden plants, some species are naturalized and weedy in northern Australia
Lamium amplexicaule Dead nettle	Erect herb up to 30 cm high with opposite, rounded, lobed leaves on square stems and tubular pinkish flowers subtended by cup-shaped leaves around the stem	Widespread weed of cultivation
Leiocarpa (Ixiolaena) brevicompta Flat billy buttons, Plains plover daisy	Low-growing shrub up to ~30 cm tall with numerous flat-topped, dense yellow flower heads	Heavy clay soils of the floodplains of the Darling river system in Queensland and New South Wales

TABLE 5. *(continued)*

Affected Animals	Toxic Principle and Effects	Comments and Treatment‡
Horses, dogs (secondary poisoning)	Probable nitrotoxin causing lethargy, spinal cord damage and posterior ataxia in horses. Indospicine residues in horse meat has caused severe hepatopathy in dogs.	Horses are poisoned when the plant forms a dominant part of pastures in inland areas and is grazed for several weeks. No specific effective treatment is known, but horses drenched with gelatine in warm water, 450 g/kg for 3 days improved. Fencing off the plant, heavy grazing by small ruminants or feeding horses good quality lucerne hay, peanut meal, or cotton seed meal can prevent cases.
Ruminants	Pneumotoxic furanoterpenes (3-substituted furans)—severe dyspnea from interstitial pneumonia and edema	Only moldy tubers are toxic. Removal of moldy tubers from the feed results in recovery in most affected animals.
Ruminants, horses	Unknown toxin, probably calystegines—incoordination, nervous derangement	No effective treatment is known.
Ruminants, horses	Calystegines, swainsonine—acquired lysosomal storage of mannose leading to incoordination, nervous derangement, weight loss, polyuria.	Animals are reputed to develop a craving for the plants. Toxicity requires access for 4 wk or more. No effective treatment is known. Less severely-affected animals recover if access is prevented.
Ruminants	Iforrestine (heterocyclic alkaloid)—nephrosis.	No effective treatment is known.
Ruminants, horses	Irritant toxins of uncertain identity—alimentary tract irritation, diarrhea.	No effective treatment is known.
Ruminants, horses	Unidentified toxin causing incoordination.	Removal from access to plants will result in recovery in most cases.
Sheep	Crepenynic acid and other fatty acids cause striated muscle degeneration manifest as sudden death, severely reduced exercise tolerance, muscle weakness and recumbency.	Toxicity is from eating mature seedheads in quantity. No effective treatment is known. Affected sheep will recover in some cases.

(continued)

TABLE 5. Important Poisonous Vascular Plants (continued) ▶

Scientific and Common Names[*]	Plant Characteristics	Habitat and Distribution[†]
Lepidozamia spp Zamias There are 2 species, both endemic to Australia, 1 commonly cultivated in gardens.	Tree-like plants with trunks surmounted by rosettes of leaves with numerous leaflets. Sexes are separate, bearing cones at the apex of the plant.	Open forests and rain-forests of northeastern Australia; cultivated in gardens
*Leucaena leucocephala	Shrub to small tree with bipinnate (fern-like) leaves, pale yellow globular flowers, followed by long flat brown seed pods	Cultivated and naturalized browse shrub in tropical regions; weedy in some situations
*Lolium perenne Perennial ryegrass	Grass, tufted with flattened, flowering spike with spikelets arranged in a zig-zag pattern	Cultivated temperate pasture grass
*Lolium rigidum Annual ryegrass	Grass, tufted with flattened, flowering spike with spikelets arranged in a zig-zag pattern	Cultivated temperate pasture grass; naturalized weed in southern Australia
Lotus spp Birdsfoot trefoils	Herbs with compound leaves consisting of 5 leaflets, 3 at the tip and 2 at the base and pea-type flowers with red, yellow, pale pink, or white petals	Subtropical and temperate regions in all states

◀ **TABLE 5.** *(continued)*

Affected Animals	Toxic Principle and Effects	Comments and Treatment‡
Cattle	Unidentified neurotoxin—permanent spinal cord degeneration with posterior ataxia in cattle (zamia staggers). Methylazoxymethanol—liver necrosis	Seeds and young leaves are the most toxic parts. No effective treatment is known.
Ruminants, horses	Mimosine and derivatives—hair loss (ruminants, horses); goiter, cataracts and buccal erosions (ruminants)	No effective treatment is known. Ruminal bacterium (*Synergistes jonesii*) detoxifies mimosine and derivatives. Detoxification capacity is retained as long as mimosine is in the diet, the bacteria surviving up to 9 mo after access stops. Ferrous sulfate supplementation may help monogastric animals.
Ruminants	Lolitrems (tremorgenic mycotoxins from the endophytic fungus *Neotyphodium lolii* cause perennial ryegrass staggers (muscle tremor, head bobbing/weaving, stiff high-stepping gait, collapse, recovery if undisturbed). Nitrates—methemoglobinemia.	Lolitrems are concentrated in leaf sheaths, making toxicity most likely on well-cropped pasture. No effective therapy available. Nitrates—IV methylene blue. *See* p 2512.
Ruminants, horses	Corynetoxins (tunicaminyluracils produced by *Rathayibacter toxicus* bacteria in seedhead nematode galls) cause annual ryegrass toxicity with convulsions and death in most cases. Ergot alkaloids when seeds infested by *Claviceps purpurea* (rye ergot) cause agalactia and hyperthermia in pigs and cattle fed grain contaminated with ergot bodies.	Corynetoxins—a cyclodextrin toxin binding agent is under development as an antidote. Immunization is being developed for prevention. Ergot alkaloids—dopamine antagonists may be helpful, domperidone, metaclopromide, reserpine. *See* p 2512.
Ruminants	Cyanogenic glycoside—sudden death	Toxicity is most likely from rapid large plant intakes. Cyanogenic glycosides—IV sodium thiosulfate, 660 mg/kg plus an oral dose (30 g cattle, 5 g sheep). Repeat for relapses.

(continued)

TABLE 5. Important Poisonous Vascular Plants (continued) ▶

Scientific and Common Names*	Plant Characteristics	Habitat and Distribution†
Lupinus spp Lupines	Robust herbs with compound leaves with radiating leaflets and flower spikes crowded with pea-type yellow, white, or blue flowers, followed by hairy seed pods	Cultivated grain crops in southern regions
Lythrum hyssopifolia Lesser loosestrife	Herb with ribbed stems and simple small leaves with single pink to purple tubular flowers in leaf axils	Weed of pasture in temperate areas
Macadamia spp	Trees with oblong leaves carrying a few marginal spines, and hanging sprays of cream flowers, followed by a globular fruit containing a hard brown nut	Cultivated tree; nuts harvested as food
Macrozamia spp Zamias, Burrawang, Zamia "palm" There are ~40 species, all endemic to Australia.	Tree-like plants with trunks surmounted by rosettes of leathery leaves with numerous leaflets. Small species have no trunks. Sexes are separate, bearing cones at the apex of the plant.	Open forests and woodlands of southern and central Australia; some cultivated in gardens
Malva parviflora Marsh or small flowered mallow	Herb with rounded 7-lobed pleated leaves on stalks and with white to very pale pink or lavender flowers in clusters in the leaf forks, followed by button-shaped fruit	Widespread weed of cultivation
Marsilea drummondii Common nardoo	Aquatic fern; fronds with 4 leaflets; spores in hairy capsules at ground level	Widespread on floodplains in inland regions of eastern states and in coastal subtropical western Australia
Medicago spp Medics, Lucerne	Herbs with trifoliate leaves and small yellow or bluish pea-type flowers, followed by twisted seed pods	Subtropical and temperate regions in all states
Melia azedarach australasica White cedar	Deciduous tree with compound leaves, sprays of lilac flowers, followed by clusters of oval yellow fruits	Native to tropical and subtropical rainforest; cultivated garden plant, street and shade tree

(continued)

◀ **TABLE 5.** *(continued)*

Affected Animals	Toxic Principle and Effects	Comments and Treatment‡
Ruminants	Phomopsins produced by the fungus *Diaporthe toxica* growing in dead plants—chronic hepatopathy causing weight loss and jaundice with photosensitization in some cases and myopathy in others.	Most toxicity occurs if dry lupine stubble is grazed after grain harvest. No effective treatment is known. Selenium/vitamin E may help myopathy cases. Immunization against phomopsins is being developed as a control measure.
Sheep	Unidentified toxin causing renal tubular and hepatocyte necrosis	Poisoning commonly occurs when sheep are grazed on crop stubbles in which the plant is dominant. No effective treatment is known.
Dogs	Unidentified toxin; produce muscular weakness and joint pain	Both fresh and roasted kernels are potentially toxic. Clinical signs are transient with recovery occurring within 24 hr, with or without symptomatic treatment. *See* p 2364.
Cattle, sheep (rare), dogs	Unidentified neurotoxin—permanent spinal cord degeneration with posterior ataxia in cattle (zamia staggers). Methylazoxymethanol—animals eating seeds of cultivated specimens of *M riedlei* have been affected.	Seeds and young leaves are the most toxic parts. No effective treatment is known.
Ruminants, poultry	Unidentified toxin causing skeletal muscle necrosis. Nitrates—methemoglobinemia. Malvic acid causes pink discoloration of egg whites and pasty yolks from hens eating seeds (or leaves)	Toxicity is most likely from rapid large plant intakes. Nitrates—IV methylene blue.
Sheep, horses	Thiaminase—polioencephalomalacia in sheep; "bracken staggers" in horses	The plant contains 100 times more thiaminase than bracken. Poisoning occurs when stock graze dried floodplains dominated by nardoo. IV thiamine (vitamin B_1) is effective in many cases.
Ruminants	Unidentified photosensitizing toxin. Phytoestrogens—infertility (rare)	No effective treatment is known.
Pigs	Tetranortriterpenes cause severe gastroenteritis	Fruits are the toxic part of the plant. Some individual trees are nontoxic. No effective treatment is known.

(continued)

TABLE 5. Important Poisonous Vascular Plants (continued) ▶

Scientific and Common Names[*]	Plant Characteristics	Habitat and Distribution[†]
[*]*Mesembryanthemum* spp Ice plants	Succulent prostrate herbs	Cultivated in gardens; naturalized in south-western Australia
Morinda reticulata Mapoon, Adaa	Shrub with stems either self-supporting or scrambling over adjacent plants with leathery, opposite-paired leaves and groups of small flowers with a prominent large white leaf-like bract immediately below	Open woodland of Cape York peninsula
Neobassia proceriflora Soda bush	Annual upright many branched small shrub with red striped stems and short blue-green succulent leaves	Inland areas of eastern and central states
Neptunia amplexicaulis Selenium weed	Prostrate herb with compound leaves with a leaf-like, heart-shaped stipule at the junction of leaf stalk and stem and with small yellow globular flowers on stiff stalks, followed by clusters of dark brown seed pods	Native to Richmond-Hughenden area of northern Queensland
Nicotiana spp Native tobaccos	Erect herbs with soft dull green leaves and tall flower spikes with tubular white flowers, followed by thin-walled pods	Mostly inland regions of all mainland states
[*]*Oxalis pes-caprae* Soursob	Perennial prostrate herb with trifoliate spotted leaves and clusters of bright yellow, tubular, 5-petalled flowers on stalks	Widespread weed of pasture and cultivation in temperate areas
Panicum spp There are ~30 native and ~10 introduced species in Australia.	Grasses, tufted with open seed heads with spikelets attached on individual stalks	Native and naturalized pasture grasses, tropical to temperate regions

◀ **TABLE 5.** *(continued)*

Affected Animals	Toxic Principle and Effects	Comments and Treatment[‡]
Ruminants	Soluble oxalates— hypocalcemia, nephrosis	Toxicity is most likely from rapid large plant intakes, eg, by hungry animals. Soluble oxalates—calcium borogluconate injection (prognosis guarded).
Horses	Selenium as selenoamino acids—hair loss from mane and tail, lameness with cracking and shedding of hooves in severe cases	No effective treatment is known.
Ruminants	Soluble oxalates— hypocalcemia, nephrosis	Toxicity is most likely from rapid large plant intakes. Soluble oxalates—calcium borogluconate injection (prognosis guarded).
Horses, ruminants (rare)	Selenium as selenoamino acids—hair loss from mane and tail; lameness with cracking and shedding of hooves in severe cases	No effective treatment is known.
Ruminants	Nicotine causing incoordination, muscle tremors, dilated pupils (impaired vision), recumbency, clonic seizures, diarrhea.	No effective treatment is known. Affected animals left undisturbed often recover.
Ruminants	Soluble oxalates—hypocalcemia, nephrosis. Chronic intake causes chronic nephrosis and kidney failure.	Toxicity is most likely from rapid large plant intakes. Soluble oxalates—calcium borogluconate injection (prognosis guarded). No effective treatment is known for chronic toxicity.
Ruminants, horses	Steroidal saponins cause hepatogenous photosensitization in ruminants. Calcium oxalate crystals deny calcium to horses, producing nutritional secondary hyperparathyroidism (lameness, weight loss, jaw swelling).	Supportive therapy for photosensitization (shade, anti-inflammatory, rehydration). No specific therapy available. Calcium oxalate (horses)—remove from the pasture and remineralize bones by feeding a mineral supplement with a Ca:P ratio of 2:1, 2 kg/horse/wk for 6 mo.

(continued)

TABLE 5. Important Poisonous Vascular Plants (continued) ▶

Scientific and Common Names[*]	Plant Characteristics	Habitat and Distribution[†]
Paspalum spp	Grasses, tufted with erect branched seedhead	Cultivated tropical to subtropical pasture grass
Pennisetum clandestinum Kikuyu grass	Grass, creeping forming a dense sward and with very inconspicuous flowers/seeds	Cultivated tropical to subtropical pasture grass
Persicaria spp Smart weeds	Herbs with soft leaves and tubular stipules clasping the stem where leaves join; spikes or pink flowers	Weeds of waterway and reservoir margins in eastern states
Phalaris aquatica Australian phalaris, Toowoomba canary grass	Grass, clumped with a compact cylindrical seedhead	Cultivated temperate pasture grass
Pimelea trichostachya, P simplex, P elongata Flaxweeds	Upright annual herbs with opposite leaves on multiple branches, each ending in a flower spike carrying numerous flask-shaped green or yellow-green flowers; hairy to different degrees depending on species	In dense populations in disturbed habitats in inland northeastern regions
Polypogon monspeliensis Annual beard grass	Grass, tufted with compact cylindrical seedheads	Coastal and inland areas of subtropical and temperate regions; seasonally flooded areas

◀ **TABLE 5.** *(continued)*

Affected Animals	Toxic Principle and Effects	Comments and Treatment[‡]
Ruminants, horses	Paspalitrems from *Claviceps paspali* ergots in seedheads—muscular tremors and incoordination	The clinical syndrome is reversible if affected animals are removed from ergotized pasture.
Ruminants, horses	Unidentified toxin causes upper alimentary tract distension and irritation and nephrosis ("kikuyu poisoning") in ruminants. Calcium oxalate crystals deny calcium to horses, producing nutritional secondary hyperparathyroidism (lameness, weight loss, jaw swelling).	"Kikuyu poisoning" predisposing factors are poorly understood, but believed to be stressors such as drought and insect attack. No effective treatment is known. There is a high case fatality rate. Calcium oxalate (horses)—remove from the pasture and remineralize bones by feeding a mineral supplement with a Ca:P ratio of 2:1, 2 kg/horse/wk for 6 mo.
Ruminants	Unidentified toxin causing photosensitization	Supportive therapy for photosensitization (shade, anti-inflammatory, rehydration). No specific therapy available. Deny further access to plants.
Ruminants	Indole alkaloids causing "phalaris staggers" with hyperexcitability, muscle tremors and paresis	No specific effective therapy is available. Prevent by dosing with slow-release cobalt preparations (cobalt bullets) before grazing.
Cattle	Simplexin (irritant diterpenoid) causes a unique syndrome in cattle only consisting of chronic right-sided heart failure, anemia, and persistent diarrhea. If other animal species are forced to eat the plants (a very rare occurrence), only diarrhea occurs.	Plants are very unpalatable. Ingestion normally occurs after the plants die and their fragments contaminate other pasture components. Poisoning cases are most likely after more-than-normal winter rains promote dense growth of the plants and then less-than-normal rains in the following summer allow dry plant fragments to remain on pasture. No effective treatment is known.
Ruminants, horses	Corynetoxins (tunicaminyluracils produced by *Rathayibacter toxicus* bacteria in seedhead nematode galls) cause "Stewart range syndrome" with convulsions and death in most cases	Corynetoxins—a cyclodextrin toxin binding agent is under development as an antidote. Immunization is being developed for prevention.

(continued)

TABLE 5. Important Poisonous Vascular Plants (continued) ▶

Scientific and Common Names[*]	Plant Characteristics	Habitat and Distribution[†]
Portulaca oleracea Pigweed, Inland pigweed, Munyeroo	Prostrate succulent herb with thick branched brown or red stems and wedge-shaped leaves and yellow flowers	Widespread native weed of cultivation and disturbed habitats including stockyards
Pteridium esculentum Austral bracken	Robust large fern; simple fronds with recurved margins	Coastal and subcoastal regions; native to open forests; weed of pasture
Raphanus raphanistrum Wild radish	Herb with coarse rosette of leaves at ground level and branched flowering stems with 4-petalled white, yellow or pink flowers	Widespread weed of cultivation in temperate areas
Rapistrum rugosum Turnip weed	Herb with coarse rosette of leaves at ground level and branched flowering stems with 4-petalled yellow flowers	Widespread weed of cultivation
Rhodomyrtus macrocarpa Finger cherry, Native loquat, Wannakai	Shrub or small tree with opposite broad leaves carrying oil glands, white 5-petalled flowers, followed by fleshy cylindrical globular to oblong red fruit	Rainforests of north-eastern Queensland
Rumex spp Docks; *Acetosella vulgaris* Sheep sorrel	Herbs with rosettes of broad leaves and tall branched flowering stems carrying green to red flowers and seed pods	Weeds of temperate pasture mostly in south-eastern states
Salsola kali Soft roly-poly	Annual upright herb with gray-green succulent leaves and dry fruits with a circular, papery wing	Widespread weed of all mainland states
Salvia reflexa Mint weed	Erect herb with square stems and blue-green leaves with felty hairs and pale blue tubular flowers in opposite pairs along stems	Widespread weed in inland Queensland and New South Wales

TABLE 5. (continued)

Affected Animals	Toxic Principle and Effects	Comments and Treatment[‡]
Ruminants	Soluble oxalates—hypocalcemia, nephrosis. Nitrates—methemoglobinemia	Most poisonings are of hungry animals with access to lush plants in stockyards. Soluble oxalates—calcium borogluconate injection (prognosis guarded). Nitrates—IV methylene blue.
Cattle, horses	Ptaquiloside—thrombocytopenia and neutropenia resulting in widespread hemorrhage and terminal septicemia; chronic intake (>2 yr) is associated with urinary bladder neoplasia and chronic hematuria in cattle (rarely in sheep). Thiaminase—"bracken staggers" (ataxia and cardiac dysfunction) in horses (rare)	Young fronds are the most toxic part of the plant. Ptaquiloside—no effective treatment is known. "Bracken staggers" of horses—IV thiamine (vitamin B_1).
Ruminants	S-methylcysteine sulfoxide (SMCO)—hemolysis	SMCO—No effective treatment is known.
Ruminants	SMCO—hemolysis. Probably sulfur—polioencephalomalacia	SMCO—No effective treatment is known. Polioencephalomalacia—thiamine may not be effective.
Ruminants, humans	Unidentified toxin causes permanent blindness from optic nerve degeneration	Leaves and fruits have poisoned ruminants; fruits poison humans. No effective treatment is known.
Ruminants	Soluble oxalates—hypocalcemia, nephrosis	Toxicity is most likely from rapid large plant intakes. Soluble oxalates—calcium borogluconate injection (prognosis guarded).
Ruminants	Soluble oxalates—hypocalcemia, nephrosis	Toxicity is most likely from rapid large plant intakes. Soluble oxalates—calcium borogluconate injection (prognosis guarded).
Ruminants	Nitrates—methemoglobinemia	Toxicity is most likely from rapid large plant intakes. Plants contaminating hay can cause poisoning. Nitrates—IV methylene blue.

(continued)

TABLE 5.   Important Poisonous Vascular Plants *(continued)* ▶

Scientific and Common Names[*]	Plant Characteristics	Habitat and Distribution[†]
Sarcostemma brevipedicellatum Caustic vine, Caustic bush, Pencil caustic	Leafless gray-green succulent shrub or scrambling vine with small bunches of waxy white flowers and long pods with milky sap	Widespread in northern areas, both coastal and inland
Schoenus asperocarpus Poison sedge	Grass-like tussock of thin leaves with flower spikes extending above the leaves and bearing flowers (spikelets) in a zig-zag arrangement surrounded by broad brown square-tipped bracts	Southwestern Australia
[*]*Senecio jacobaea* Ragwort	Erect herb with finely-divided leaves and bright yellow daisy-type flowers in clusters at the top of the plant	Weed of pasture and cultivation in southern regions
Senecio linearifolius Fireweed	Erect shrub with long pointed leaves and flower heads in bunches resembling those of ragwort	Coastal and subcoastal New South Wales, Victoria, and Tasmania
Senecio lautus Fireweed, Variable groundsel	Erect herb with leaves either simple or with dissected edges and clusters of yellow daisy-type flowers	Widespread south of 20°S latitude on heavy clay soils
[*]*Senecio madagascariensis* Fireweed	Very similar to *S lautus* and distinguished by 20-21 bracts under the flower head compared with 11-14 in *S lautus*	Naturalized in eastern coastal subtropical and temperate regions
Senecio quadridentatus Cotton fireweed	Erect herb with narrow leaves covered in cottony hair and with bunches of small slender flower heads at the top of the stems	Weed of pasture and cultivation in southeastern regions
[*]*Senna occidentalis* Coffee senna [*]*S obtusifolia* Sickle pod	Small shrubs with compound leaves and clusters of open yellow flowers and flat long or curved seed pods	Naturalized in northern coastal and subcoastal Australia

◀ **TABLE 5.** *(continued)*

Affected Animals	Toxic Principle and Effects	Comments and Treatment[‡]
Cattle, sheep	Unidentified neurotoxin, suspected to be similar to cynanchoside—collapse, clonic convulsions	No effective treatment is known.
Ruminants	Galegine—acute pulmonary edema	No effective treatment is known.
Cattle, horses	Pyrrolizidine alkaloids—chronic hepatopathy causing mostly weight loss, irritability and compulsive walking (horses) or weight loss and persistent diarrhea with tenesmus (cattle)	No effective treatment is known. *See* p 2506.
Cattle, horses	Pyrrolizidine alkaloids—chronic hepatopathy causing mostly weight loss, irritability (horses) or weight loss and persistent diarrhea with tenesmus (cattle)	No effective treatment is known. *See* p 2506.
Cattle, horses	Pyrrolizidine alkaloids—chronic hepatopathy causing mostly weight loss, irritability and compulsive walking (horses) or weight loss and persistent diarrhea with tenesmus (cattle)	No effective treatment is known. *See* p 2506.
Cattle, horses	Pyrrolizidine alkaloids—chronic hepatopathy causing mostly weight loss, irritability and compulsive walking (horses) or weight loss and persistent diarrhea with tenesmus (cattle)	No effective treatment is known. *See* p 2506.
Cattle, horses	Pyrrolizidine alkaloids—chronic hepatopathy causing mostly weight loss, irritability and compulsive walking (horses) or weight loss and persistent diarrhea with tenesmus (cattle)	No effective treatment is known. *See* p 2506.
Ruminants	Unidentified toxin causing striated muscle degeneration and necrosis with myoglobinuria	Seeds and seed pods are the most toxic. No effective treatment is known.

(continued)

TABLE 5. Important Poisonous Vascular Plants (continued) ▶

Scientific and Common Names*	Plant Characteristics	Habitat and Distribution†
Setaria sphacelata	Grass, tall, tufted with a long compact cylindrical seedhead	Cultivated tropical pasture grass
Silybum marianum Variegated thistle	Herb with broad green and white leaves edged with small yellow spines, pink thistle-type flower heads	Weed of cultivation in southern and eastern regions
Solanum spp Nightshades, Potato weeds	Herbs to large soft-wood shrubs with star-shaped, 5-petalled white or purple flowers with prominent erect yellow staminodes centrally, followed by fleshy green, black, yellow, or red fruit	Widespread throughout all states; some as weeds of pasture or cultivation
Stachys arvensis Stagger weed	Erect herb up to 30 cm high with opposite round-lobed leaves on square stems and tubular pinkish flowers	Widespread weed of cultivation
Stemodia kingii	Erect herb with pale blue tubular flowers	Inland regions of Western Australia
Stypandra glauca Blind grass	Erect perennial herb with grass-like green leaves and terminal flower heads with pendulous, 6-petalled blue flowers with 6 prominent yellow anthers	Mostly in southwestern Australia with populations in New South Wales
Swainsona spp Darling or Swainson peas	Herbs with compound leaves with many leaflets and usually large, showy pea-type flowers with blue, pink, purple, or red petals, followed by inflated seed pods	Subtropical and temperate regions in all states
Terminalia oblongata oblongata Yellow wood	Deciduous tree up to 8-12 m tall with dark gray, furrowed bark, leaves simple in clusters on branches, small white flowers and fruits with a central oval seed enclosed in 2 papery wings	Confined to the McKenzie River basin of northeastern Queensland

Affected Animals	Toxic Principle and Effects	Comments and Treatment[‡]
Ruminants, horses	Soluble oxalates—hypocalcemia, nephrosis in ruminants, very rarely horses. Calcium oxalates crystals deny calcium to horses, producing nutritional secondary hyperparathyroidism (lameness, weight loss, jaw swelling).	Toxicity from soluble oxalates is most likely from rapid large plant intakes. Soluble oxalates—calcium borogluconate injection (prognosis guarded). Calcium oxalate (horses)—remove from the pasture and remineralize bones by feeding a mineral supplement with a Ca:P ratio of 2:1, 2 kg/horses/wk for 6 mo.
Ruminants	Nitrates—methemoglobinemia	Toxicity is most likely from rapid large plant intakes. Nitrates—IV methylene blue.
Ruminants	Glycosidic steroidal alkaloids cause gastroenteritis with diarrhea. They are poorly absorbed, but if absorption occurs, hemolysis (hemoglobinuria), depression, and stupor may occur.	No specific effective treatment is known. Dosing with activated charcoal and rehydration appear to be rational responses.
Ruminants, horses	Unidentified toxin causing incoordination	Removal from access to plants will result in recovery in most cases.
Ruminants	Cucurbitacins—irritation of the upper GI tract and increased permeability of blood vessels producing sudden death with diarrhea	No effective treatment is known.
Ruminants, horses	Stypandrol—degeneration of retina and optic nerves and tracts causing permanent blindness	No effective treatment is known.
Ruminants, horses	Swainsonine (an indolizidine alkaloid) produces acquired lysosomal storage of mannose leading to incoordination, nervous derangement, weight loss, infertility, abortion	Animals are reputed to develop a craving for the plants. Toxicity requires access for at least 2 wk (horses) or 4 wk (ruminants). No effective treatment is known. Less severely-affected animals will recover if access is prevented.
Cattle, sheep	Hydrolyzable tannins; cattle—hepatogenous photosensitization and/or nephrosis; sheep—convulsions	Toxicity is most likely from large plant intakes. No effective treatment is known.

(continued)

TABLE 5.   Important Poisonous Vascular Plants (continued) ▶

Scientific and Common Names*	Plant Characteristics	Habitat and Distribution†
Trachyandra divaricata Branched onion weed	Herb with rosette of fleshy green linear leaves and an erect dichotomously-branched flower spike with numerous darkly-striped white flowers	Naturalized in coastal southwestern Australia; small populations also in New South Wales and South Australia
Trachymene glaucifolia, T ochracea, T cyanantha Wild parsnips	Annual herbs with rosettes of divided leaves at ground level and upright flowering stems bearing clusters of small flowers in flat-topped bunches	Subtropical inland areas of eastern states, in grasslands or woodlands
Trema tomentosa Poison peach	Small tree with alternate leaves tapered at each end with toothed margins and rough texture, very small white flowers in clusters in the leaf angles, followed by small black fruits	Coastal and inland northern and eastern Australia
Trianthema spp Red spinach, Hogweed, Black or Giant pigweed	Succulent prostrate herbs	Widespread in semiarid and arid regions of northern Australia
Tribulus terrestris Caltrop, Puncture vine	Prostrate herb with branching stems and compound leaves with yellow 5-petalled flowers and spiny burrs	Widespread in all mainland states; weed of pasture
Trifolium spp Clovers	Herbs with trifoliate leaves and tight clusters of pea-type flowers with white, yellow, or pink petals	Cultivated pasture legumes in temperate regions
Urochloa panicoides Liverseed grass	Grass, prostrate or erect with hairy leaves and branched seedheads	Naturalized in Queensland and New South Wales
Verbesina encelioides Crownbeard	Erect herb with stem-clasping leaves and bright yellow daisy-type flower heads	Weed of pasture in eastern regions; prefers sandy soils
Vicia spp Woolly-pod vetch, Popany vetch	Herbs with compound leaves ending in tendrils and pink or purple pea-type flowers	Pasture legume in subtropical and temperate regions in all states

TABLE 5. *(continued)*

Affected Animals	Toxic Principle and Effects	Comments and Treatment‡
Horses, sheep	Unknown toxin causing ataxia and recumbency with degeneration of CNS tissues and intense lipofuscinosis of neurons.	No effective treatment is known.
Sheep	Unidentified teratogenic toxin causing limb deviations through interference with normal development of long bone growth plates—"bent-leg" of lambs. Some association with infertility (low lambing percentages). Unidentified (cardiac?) toxin causing sudden death in sheep under stress of mustering. Unidentified toxin causing diarrhea in young sheep.	No effective treatment is known. Many lambs affected at birth will recover.
Ruminants, horses	Unidentified hepatotoxin causes acute coagulation necrosis of periacinar hepatocytes with rapid death after hepatoencephalopathy in some cases.	No effective treatment is known.
Ruminants	Soluble oxalates—hypocalcemia, nephrosis. Nitrates—methemoglobinemia	Toxicity is most likely from rapid large plant intakes. Soluble oxalates—calcium borogluconate injection (prognosis guarded). Nitrates—IV methylene blue.
Sheep	Steroidal saponins cause hepatogenous photosensitization. β-carboline alkaloids cause progressive irreversible posterior ataxia.	Toxicity is most likely when the plant dominates available feed. Wilting is thought to enhance toxicity by steroidal saponins. No effective treatment is known.
Sheep	Unidentified photosensitizing toxin. Phytoestrogens—infertility	No effective treatment is known.
Ruminants	Nitrates—methemoglobinemia	Toxicity is most likely from rapid large plant intakes. Nitrates—IV methylene blue.
Ruminants, pigs	Galegine—acute pulmonary edema	Toxicity is most likely from rapid large plant intakes. No effective treatment is known.
Cattle (usually Aberdeen Angus, Friesian, and their cross-breeds), horses (rare).	Unidentified toxin can produce systemic eosinophilic granulomas in multiple organs.	Toxicity occurs when grazing dense swards of the plants. Skin lesions must be differentiated from photosensitization. No effective treatment is known.

(continued)

TABLE 5. Important Poisonous Vascular Plants *(continued)* ▶

Scientific and Common Names[*]	Plant Characteristics	Habitat and Distribution[†]
Wedelia asperrima Yellow daisy, Sunflower daisy	Erect herb with branched stems, leaves rough to the touch, yellow daisy-type flower heads	Grasslands of northern Australia
Wikstroemia indica Tie bush	Shrub up to 1-2 m high with red-brown bark, opposite leaves tapered at each end, greenish-yellow tubular flowers followed by red or orange fleshy fruits	Woodlands and forests of coastal eastern Australia
Xanthium occidentale Noogoora burr	Upright herb with branches carrying broad-lobed rough leaves on stalks, clusters of oblong brown burrs covered with hooked spines	Widespread weed of cultivation and pasture
Xanthorrhoea johnsonii, X fulva Grass trees	Rosette of numerous grass-like leaves arising from a trunk (caudex) constructed of leaf bases of fallen leaves, with a tall flower spike with a long cylindrical compact mass of flowers and bracts. *X fulva* does not develop a caudex.	Coastal and subcoastal regions of eastern Australia
Zantedeschia aethiopica Calla lily, Arum lily	Herb with dark green fleshy leaves with upright white tubular flower (spathe) with yellow stalk (spadix) in its center.	Cultivated garden plant, naturalized in coastal southern (particularly southwestern) Australia
Zea may Maize	Grass, erect, robust	Cultivated grain crop
Zieria arborescens Stinkwood	Shrub to tree with trifoliate leaves and bunches of small white flowers	Forests of southeastern mainland and Tasmania

[*]Plants introduced to Australia (not indigenous) are indicated by an asterisk (*) in front of the scientific name.

[†]For detailed information on plant distribution, consult Australia's Virtual Herbarium website (http://www.chah.gov.au/avh.html).

TABLE 5. (continued)

Affected Animals	Toxic Principle and Effects	Comments and Treatment[‡]
Ruminants	Diterpenoid (kaurene) glyco-side—wedeloside—causes acute coagulation necrosis of periacinar hepatocytes with rapid death after hepatoen-cephalopathy in some cases.	Toxicity is most likely from rapid large plant intakes. No effective treatment is known.
Cattle, deer	Irritant diterpenoid—alimentary tract irritation, diarrhea. Dicoumarin derivative—anti-coagulant effect seen only in deer	No effective treatment is known.
Ruminants, pigs	Diterpenoid (kaurene) glyco-side—carboxyatractyloside—causes acute coagulation necrosis of periacinar hepatocytes with rapid death after hepa-toencephalopathy in some cases	Only the cotyledonary (seed) leaves or burrs are toxic. Toxicity occurs commonly on river flats after rain or flooding. No effective treatment is known.
Cattle	Unidentified toxin—transient spinal cord dysfunction causing posterior ataxia and urinary incontinence	Flower spikes are the most toxic part of the plants. There may be a delay of several days between last access to the plants and onset of the syndrome. Supportive care is required. Most affected animals recover completely with symptomatic treatment.
Ruminants, horses, dogs, cats	Raphide calcium oxalate crystals—buccal irritation	Effects are likely to be transient and not require therapy unless laryngeal edema occurs.
Ruminants	Nitrates—methemoglobine-mia. Cyanogenic glycosides—sudden death	Nitrates—IV methylene blue. Cyanogenic glycosides—IV sodium thiosulfate, 660 mg/kg plus an oral dose (30 g cattle, 5 g sheep). Repeat treatment may be needed for relapses.
Cattle	Unidentified pneumotoxin causing severe pulmonary edema and emphysema	No effective treatment is known.

[‡]Effective therapeutic regimens are not known for many acute poisonings. The use of activated charcoal as an adsorbent for organic toxins should be considered for these.

PYRROLIZIDINE ALKALOIDOSIS

(Seneciosis, *Senecio* poisoning, Ragwort toxicity)

Typically, pyrrolizidine alkaloidosis is a chronic poisoning that results in hepatic failure. It is caused by many toxic plants, most commonly of the genera *Senecio, Crotalaria, Heliotropium, Amsinckia, Echium, Cynoglossum,* and *Trichodesma.* These plants grow mainly in temperate climates, but some (eg, *Crotalaria* spp) require tropical or subtropical climates. The plants most often implicated are ragwort (*S jacobea*), woolly groundsel (*S redellii, S longilobus*), rattleweed (*Crotalaria retusa*), and seeds of yellow tarweed (*A intermedia*).

Cattle, horses, farmed deer, and pigs are most susceptible; sheep and goats require ~20 times more plant material than cattle. Individual susceptibility varies greatly within species; young growing animals are most susceptible.

Etiology and Pathogenesis: More than 30 toxic factors (alkaloids with a pyrrolizidine base) have been found in the plants. It is likely that their toxic effects are unique. *Senecio jacobea* contains jacobine; retrorsine, seneciphylline, and monocrotaline are other pyrrolizidine alkaloids frequently incriminated in toxicities.

These plants, which under normal conditions are avoided by grazing animals, may be eaten during drought conditions. Some animals may eat these plants preferentially as roughage when they are available on extremely lush pasture. Animals are also poisoned by eating the plant material in hay, silage, or pellets. Seeds from *Crotalaria, Amsinckia,* and *Heliotropium* spp, which have been harvested with grain, have caused the disease in horses, cattle, pigs, and poultry.

The toxic alkaloids are metabolized to highly reactive pyrroles, which produce cytotoxic effects on target sites, most commonly the nuclei of hepatocytes. Other target sites may include the epithelial and vascular tissues of the kidneys and lungs. The pyrroles cross-link DNA strands and also unite DNA with nucleoproteins such as actin. These molecular alterations are presumed to create the antimitotic and megalocytic effects characteristic of pyrrolizidine alkalosis.

Clinical Findings: The clinical signs and hepatic pathology are similar in all animal species regardless of the species of plant involved or the toxic pyrrolizidine alkaloids it contains. Acute intoxication is characterized by sudden death from hemorrhagic liver necrosis and visceral hemorrhages. This is a rare event, as the poor palatability of these plants makes rapid ingestion of large quantities of the toxins uncommon. More chronic exposure is typical, and the liver reflects the cumulative and progressive effects of repeated ingestion of small doses of toxin. Clinical signs may not be seen for several weeks or months after initial exposure. Consumption of the offending plant may even have ceased months earlier. The ongoing hepatic damage in these instances is suspected to be due to the recycling of toxic pyrroles as they are released from one dying cell and taken up by another. Clinical progression may also be altered by concurrent hepatic pathology; a hemolytic crisis may be precipitated in sheep with excessive hepatic copper stores (*see* COPPER POISONING, p 2353).

In horses and cattle, signs include loss of condition, anorexia, dullness, and constipation or diarrhea. Tenesmus and passing of bloodstained feces may be followed by rectal prolapse, especially in cattle. Ascites and icterus may be present, and cattle and sheep sometimes show intermittent photosensitization. Some animals become progressively weaker and reluctant to move. Others exhibit signs of hepatic encephalopathy such as head-pressing, aimless wandering, ataxia, or even frenzied and aggressive behavior. Pica may be seen. Death may occur suddenly or after prolonged recumbency with hepatic coma and high levels of ammonia in the blood.

Lesions: In acute cases, the liver may be enlarged, hemorrhagic, and icteric. In chronic cases, it is atrophied, fibrous, finely nodular, and usually pale with a glistening surface due to fibrous thickening of the capsule. Other livers are markedly icteric. The gallbladder is often edematous and grossly distended with thick, mucoid bile. Edema of the abomasum and segments of the bowel, mesentery, and associated lymph nodes is common, and there may be ascites. In some cases, numerous small hemorrhages are present in the abdominal serous membranes.

Characteristic histologic changes occur in the liver. Irreversible enlargement of individual hepatocytes (megalocytosis) is often seen; it is conspicuous in horses and sheep but less pronounced in cattle. In cattle, marked perivenous fibrosis of sublobular veins is usually present, but this is not a consistent finding in horses and sheep. In all species, increases in connective tissue, both within and around the lobules, are marked. Bile duct hyperplasia is variable but may be the most striking microscopic change seen in some livers. Pigs may show pulmonary congestion, hemorrhage, septal fibrosis, alveolar epithelialization, and emphysema. Renal tubular lining cells and glomerular epithelial cells also may be individually enlarged.

Diagnosis: A diagnosis based on history, clinical signs, and gross necropsy findings can usually be confirmed by histologic examination of liver and renal tissue. Chemical analyses of the liver for toxic metabolites are available for confirmation of exposure but are seldom necessary. When hepatic cirrhosis is extensive, hypoalbuminemia and hyperglobulinemia develop. Serum levels of fibrinogen, bilirubin, γ-glutamyltransferase, and glutamate dehydrogenase may be increased, but it should be recognized that the insidious nature of this disease can result in surprisingly mild serum biochemical changes. Other hepatotoxins, such as copper or aflatoxin, as well as infections such as chronic fascioliasis, must be considered before making the diagnosis.

Treatment and Control: Further intake of toxic plant material must be prevented. Animals showing signs rarely recover, and lesions present in asymptomatic animals may progress and result in further losses over several months. Because high protein intake may prove harmful, rations high in carbohydrates are indicated. Methionine in 10% dextrose solution, IV, may be of value in treating horses.

The diminished ability of the liver to regenerate after pyrrolizidine alkaloid poisoning suggests a guarded prognosis. Preventing further outbreaks by reducing or eliminating contributory factors should be stressed.

Sheep are commonly used for grazing control of these plants, but this practice carries risks unless sheep destined for early slaughter are used. Biologic control of plants with predator moths, flea beetles, and seed flies has met with variable success. *Senecio* and related toxic species in pastures have been controlled satisfactorily by annual herbicide applications, preferably in spring before hay or silage conservation. Measures that enhance destruction of the alkaloids in the rumen of sheep also have shown some promise.

QUERCUS POISONING

(Oak bud poisoning, Acorn poisoning)

Most animals are susceptible to *Quercus* poisoning, although cattle and sheep are affected most often. Most species of oak (*Quercus* spp) found in Europe and North America are considered toxic. Clinical signs occur several days after consumption of large quantities of young oak leaves in the spring or green acorns in the fall. High mortality is often observed. Malformed calves and abortions have been reported in dams consuming acorns during the second trimester of pregnancy. The toxic principle, which appears to be gallotannins, polyhydroxyphenolic compounds, or their metabolites, causes GI and renal dysfunction. Signs include anorexia, depression, emaciation, dehydration, rumen stasis, tenesmus, smell of ammonia on the breath, serous ocular or nasal discharge, polydipsia, polyuria, hematuria, icterus, and constipation followed by mucoid to hemorrhagic diarrhea. Renal insufficiency may be evidenced by increased BUN and creatinine, proteinuria, hyperphosphatemia, hypocalcemia, and urine with a low specific gravity. Pale swollen kidneys, perirenal edema, subcutaneous edema, ascites, and hydrothorax are common necropsy findings. Edema and subserosal petechial or ecchymotic hemorrhage of intestinal mucosa and ulceration of the esophagus and rumen may be seen. Diagnosis is based on clinical findings, necropsy, history, and histopathologic examination of the kidney (ie, nephrosis). Other common diseases that resemble oak poisoning include pigweed (*Amaranthus* spp) poisoning and aminoglycoside antibiotic poisoning.

Consumption of a pelleted ration supplement (1 kg/head/day) containing 10-15% calcium hydroxide plus access to more palatable feeds may be used as a preventive measure if exposure to acorns or oak leaves cannot be avoided. Calcium hydroxide, ruminatorics, and purgatives (such as mineral oil [1 L/500 kg], sodium sulfate [1 kg/400 kg], or magnesium sulfate [450 g/400 kg]) may be effective antidotes if administered early in the course of disease. Fluid therapy to correct dehydration and acidosis and transplantation of ruminal microflora may be beneficial. Clinical recovery usually occurs within 60 days but is rare if renal dysfunction is severe.

RODENTICIDE POISONING

Many poisons have been used against rodent pests. Farm animals, pets, and wildlife often gain access to these poisons via the baits or the poisoned rodents or by malicious intent. This discussion covers the most commonly used rodenticides. Strychnine poisoning (p 2521) is discussed separately.

Anticoagulant Rodenticides (Warfarin and Congeners): Potentially dangerous to all mammals and birds, anticoagulant rodenticides are the most frequent cause of poisoning in pets. Pets and wildlife may be poisoned directly from baits or indirectly by consumption of poisoned rodents. Intoxications in domestic animals have resulted from contamination of feed with anticoagulant concentrate, malicious use of these chemicals, and feed mixed in equipment used to prepare rodent bait.

All anticoagulants have the basic coumarin or indanedione nucleus. The "first-generation" anticoagulants (warfarin, pindone, coumafuryl, coumachlor, isovaleryl indanedione, and others less frequently used) require multiple feedings to result in toxicity. The "intermediate" anticoagulants (chlorophacinone and in particular diphacinone) require fewer feedings than "first-generation" chemicals, and thus are more toxic to nontarget species. The "second-generation" anticoagulants (brodifacoum and bromadiolone) are highly toxic to nontarget species (dogs, cats, and potentially livestock) after a single feeding.

The anticoagulants antagonize vitamin K, which interferes with the normal synthesis of coagulation proteins (factors I, II, VII, IX, and X) in the liver; thus, adequate amounts are not available to convert prothrombin into thrombin. A latent period, dependent on species, dose, and activity, is required, during which clotting factors already present are used up. New products have a longer biologic half-life and therefore prolonged effects (which require prolonged treatment). For example, the half-life in canine plasma of warfarin is 15 hr, diphacinone is 5 days, and bromadiolone is 6 days, with maximum effects estimated at 12-15 days. Brodifacoum may continue to be detectable in serum for up to 24 days.

Clinical signs generally reflect some manifestation of hemorrhage, including anemia, hematomas, melena, hemothorax, hyphema, epistaxis, hemoptysis, and hematuria. Signs dependent on hemorrhage, such as weakness, ataxia, colic, and polypnea, may be seen. Depression and anorexia occur in all species even before bleeding occurs.

Anticoagulant rodenticide toxicosis is usually diagnosed based on history of ingestion of the substance. Differential diagnoses when massive hemorrhage is encountered include disseminated intravascular coagulation, congenital factor deficiencies, von Willebrand's disease, platelet deficiencies, and canine ehrlichiosis. A prolonged prothrombin, partial thromboplastin, or thrombin time in the presence of normal fibrinogen, fibrin degradation products, and platelet counts is strongly suggestive of anticoagulant rodenticide toxicosis, as is a positive therapeutic response to vitamin K_1.

Vitamin K_1 is antidotal. Recommended dosages vary from 0.25-2.5 mg/kg in warfarin (coumarin) exposure, to 2.5-5 mg/kg in the case of long-acting rodenticide intoxication (diphacinone, brodifacoum, bromadiolone). Vitamin K_1 is administered SC (with the smallest possible needle to minimize hemorrhage) in several locations to speed absorption. IV administration of vitamin K_1 is contraindicated, as anaphylaxis may occasionally result. The oral form of K_1 may be used daily after the first day, commonly at the same level as the loading dose (divided BID). Fresh or frozen plasma (9 mL/kg) or whole blood (20 mL/kg) IV is required to replace needed clotting factors and RBC if bleeding is severe. One week of vitamin K_1 treatment is usually sufficient for first-generation anticoagulants. For intermediate and second-generation anticoagulants or if anticoagulant type is unknown, treatment should continue for 2-4 wk to control longterm effects. Administration of oral vitamin K_1 with a fat-containing ration, such as canned dog food, increases its bioavailability 4-5 times as compared with vitamin K_1 given PO alone.

Coagulation should be monitored weekly until values remain normal for 5-6 days after cessation of therapy. Vitamin K_3 given as a feed supplement is ineffective in the treatment of anticoagulant rodenticide toxicosis. Additional supportive therapy may be indicated, including thoracocentesis (to relieve dyspnea due to hemothorax) and supplemental oxygen if needed.

ANTU (α-Naphthylthiourea): ANTU causes local gastric irritation; when absorbed, it increases permeability of the lung capillaries in all animals, although species variability in dose response is marked. Properties of ANTU, when compared with those of warfarin, have led to near abandonment of its use. Dogs and pigs are occasionally poisoned; ruminants are resistant. Animals with an empty stomach readily vomit after ingestion of ANTU; however, food in the stomach decreases the stimulation to vomit, and fatal quantities may be absorbed. Signs include vomiting, hypersalivation, coughing, and dyspnea. Animals prefer to sit. Severe pulmonary edema, moist rales, and cyanosis are present. Dependent signs include weakness; ataxia; rapid, weak pulse; and subnormal temperature. Death from hypoxia may occur within 2-4 hr of ingestion, while animals that survive 12 hr may recover.

The lesions are suggestive. The most striking findings are pulmonary edema and hydrothorax. Hyperemia of the tracheal mucosa; mild to moderate gastroenteritis; marked hyperemia of the kidneys; and a pale, mottled liver are found in most cases. Tissue for chemical analysis must be obtained within 24 hr.

Emetics should be used only if respiratory distress is not evident. Prognosis is grave when severe respiratory signs occur. Agents providing sulfhydryl groups, eg, n-amyl mercaptan, sodium thiosulfate (10% solution), or n-acetylcysteine are beneficial. Positive-pressure oxygen therapy, an osmotic diuretic (eg, mannitol), and atropine (0.02-0.25 mg/kg) may relieve the pulmonary edema.

Bromethalin: This nonanticoagulant, single-dose rodenticide is a neurotoxin that appears to uncouple oxidative phosphorylation in the CNS. CSF pressure increases, which places pressure on nerve axons and results in decreased conduction of nerve impulses, paralysis, and death. In dogs, a dose of 1.67 mg/kg is toxic, and 2.5 mg/kg (25 g of bait/kg body wt) is lethal.

Bromethalin can cause either an acute or a chronic syndrome. The acute effects follow consumption of ≥5 mg/kg bromethalin. Signs, which include hyperexcitability, muscle tremors, grand mal seizures, hindlimb hyperreflexia, CNS depression, and death, may appear ~10 hr after ingestion. Chronic effects are seen with lower dosages and may appear 24-86 hr after ingestion. This syndrome is characterized by vomiting, depression, ataxia, tremors, and lateral recumbency. The effects may be reversible if exposure to bromethalin is discontinued. Bromethalin toxicosis should be considered when cerebral edema or posterior paralysis is present.

Treatment should be directed at blocking absorption from the gut and reducing cerebral edema. Use of mannitol as an osmotic diuretic and corticosteroids have been suggested but have shown little effect in dogs poisoned by bromethalin. Use of activated charcoal for several days may improve the recovery rate.

Cholecalciferol: Although this rodenticide was introduced with claims that it was less toxic to nontarget species than to rodents, clinical experience has shown that rodenticides containing cholecalciferol are a significant health threat to dogs and cats.

Cholecalciferol produces hypercalcemia, which results in systemic calcification of soft tissue, leading to renal failure, cardiac abnormalities, hypertension, CNS depression, and GI upset.

Signs generally develop within 18-36 hr of ingestion and can include depression, anorexia, polyuria, and polydipsia. As serum calcium concentrations increase, clinical signs become more severe. Serum calcium concentrations >16 mg/dL are not uncommon. GI smooth muscle excitability decreases and is manifest by anorexia, vomiting, and constipation. Hematemesis and hemorrhagic diarrhea may develop as a result of dystrophic calcification of the GI tract and should not lead to a misdiagnosis of anticoagulant rodenticide toxicosis. Loss of renal concentrating ability is a direct result of hypercalcemia. As hypercalcemia persists, mineralization of the kidneys results in progressive renal insufficiency.

Diagnosis is based on history of ingestion, clinical signs, and hypercalcemia (see also p 444). Other causes of hypercalcemia, such as hyperparathyroidism, normal juvenile hypercalcemia, paraneoplastic hypercalcemia, hemoconcentration (hyperproteinemia), and diffuse osteoporosis should be ruled out. Gross lesions associated with hypercalcemia include pitted, mottled kidneys; diffuse hemorrhage of the GI mucosa; and roughened, raised plaques on the great vessels and on the surface of the lungs and abdominal viscera.

Recommended therapy includes gastric evacuation, generally followed by administration of activated charcoal at 2-8 g/kg body wt in a water slurry. Calciuresis is accomplished with 0.9% sodium chloride solution and administration of furosemide (initial bolus of 5 mg/kg, IV, followed by a constant rate IV infusion of 5 mg/kg/hr) and corticosteroids (prednisolone, 1-2 mg/kg, BID). Furosemide and prednisolone should be continued for 2-4 wk, and the serum calcium concentration monitored at 24 hr, 48 hr, and 2 wk after cessation of treatment. Additionally, calcitonin may be used at 4-6 IU/kg, SC, every 2-3 hr, until the serum calcium stabilizes at <12 mg/dL. The IV use of calcium chelators such as Na-EDTA has been used in severe cases, but this use is experimental and requires close monitoring of blood calcium to prevent hypocalcemia. The dose of prednisolone should be tapered if it is administered for >2 wk to prevent acute adrenocortical insufficiency. Continuous peritoneal dialysis may be considered if the animal is in renal failure. A low-calcium diet should be provided in all cases of significant exposure to cholecalciferol rodenticides.

Recently, pamidronate disodium, a specific inhibitor of bone resorption used for the treatment of hypercalcemia of malignancy and Paget's disease in humans, has shown promise in the treatment of cholecalciferol toxicosis in dogs. It is given slowly IV at 1.3-2.0 mg/kg in saline solution over 2-4 hr. Two infusions are given 4 days apart. Pamidronate disodium has a long-lasting inhibitory action on bone resorption, thus requiring only limited infusions. Total serum calcium and BUN should be monitored 2 and 4 days after the last infusion.

Metaldehyde: This polymer of acetaldehyde is used as a snail or slug bait, to which dogs and livestock may be exposed. (See also METALDEHYDE POISONING, p 2406.) Toxic effects are due to absorption of limited acetaldehyde from metaldehyde hydrolysis in the stomach, but primarily to the metaldehyde itself. Signs range from salivation and vomiting to anxiety and incoordination with muscle tremors, fasciculations, and hyperesthesia leading to continuous muscle spasms, prostration, and death. Generally, the muscle spasms are not initiated by external stimuli, but excessive muscular activity is common, often producing high body temperatures. Differential diagnoses include strychnine poisoning and anticholinesterase insecticide toxicity. The finding of metaldehyde bait or pellets in the vomitus and the possible odor of acetaldehyde from stomach contents or on the animal's breath may assist in diagnosis.

Treatment is most effective if initiated early. Further toxicant absorption should be prevented by induced emesis, gastric lavage, and oral dosing with activated charcoal. Hyperesthesia and muscle activity may be controlled with diazepam at 2-5 mg, IV, or light barbiturate anesthesia and muscle relaxants as needed. IV fluid therapy with lactated Ringer's solution or 5% glucose should be aggressive to promote toxin excretion and to combat dehydration and the acidosis induced by the excessive muscle activity. Continuous supportive care is important. Prognosis is heavily determined by the exposure dose, but if death does not occur earlier, animals poisoned by metaldehyde may show clinical improvement 24-36 hr after initial onset of signs.

Phosphorus: In its white (or yellow) form, phosphorus is hazardous to all domestic animals and is locally corrosive and hepatotoxic when absorbed. Phosphorus is infrequently used as a rodenticide today, but dogs occasionally become exposed through ingestion of fireworks that contain white phosphorus. The onset of signs of poisoning is sudden. Early signs include vomiting, severe diarrhea (often hemorrhagic), colic, and a garlic-like odor to the breath. Apparent recovery can occur up to 4 days after ingestion, but additional signs of acute liver damage may develop, including hemorrhages, abdominal pain, and icterus. Hepatic encephalopathy is followed by convulsions and death. Lesions include severe gastroenteritis; fatty liver; multiple hemorrhages; and black, tarry blood that fails to clot. Body tissues and fluids may be phosphorescent, and the gastric contents have a garlic odor. Death is due to hepatic and renal failure.

Prognosis is grave unless treatment is instituted early. A 1% solution of copper sulfate is an effective emetic and also forms a nonabsorbable copper phosphide complex. Gastric lavage with a 0.01-0.1% potassium permanganate solution or a 0.2-0.4% copper sulfate solution should be followed by activated charcoal adsorbent and 30 min later by a saline cathartic. Any fat in the diet must be avoided for 3-4 days or longer because fats favor additional absorption of phosphorus. Mineral oil orally has been recommended because it dissolves phosphorus and prevents absorption.

Red Squill: This rodenticide is a cardiac glycoside derived from the plant *Urginea maritima*. It is of limited current use. Because rats are incapable of vomiting, red squill is more toxic to that species. It is unpalatable to domestic animals but, when eaten, usually induces vomiting in dogs and cats. Large quantities are required for toxicity in farm animals. It is considered relatively safe, but dogs, cats, and pigs have been poisoned. Signs are vomiting, ataxia, and hyperesthesia followed by paralysis, depression, or convulsions. Bradycardia and cardiac arrhythmias may end in cardiac arrest. The clinical course seldom is longer than 24-36 hr.

Treatment consists of supportive therapy and evacuation of the GI tract using gastric lavage and saline cathartics. Atropine sulfate SC at 6- to 8-hr intervals may prevent cardiac arrest. Phenytoin at 35 mg/kg, TID, should be given to dogs to suppress arrhythmias.

Sodium Monofluoroacetate (1080): 1080 is a colorless, odorless, tasteless, water-soluble chemical that is highly toxic (0.1-8 mg/kg) to all animals, including humans. Its use is restricted to certain commercial applications. Fluoroacetate is metabolized to fluorocitrate, which blocks the tricarboxylic acid cycle—a mechanism necessary for cellular energy production. It causes toxic effects by overstimulating the CNS, resulting in death by convulsions, and by causing alteration of cardiac function that results in myocardial depression, cardiac arrhythmias, ventricular fibrillation, and circulatory collapse. CNS stimulation is the main effect in dogs, while the cardiac effects predominate in horses, sheep, goats, and chickens. Pigs and cats appear about equally affected by both.

A characteristic lag phase of ≥30 min after ingestion occurs before the onset of nervousness and restlessness. Marked depression and weakness follow in all species except dogs and pigs. Affected animals rapidly become prostrate, and the pulse is weak and 2-3 times normal rate. Death is due to cardiac failure. Usually, dogs and pigs rapidly develop tetanic convulsions similar to those of strychnine poisoning. Many exhibit severe pain. Vomiting is prominent in pigs. Dogs usually have urinary and fecal incontinence and exhibit frenzied running. The course is rapid; affected animals die within hours after signs appear. Few animals that develop marked signs recover. Congestion of organs, cyanosis, subepicardial hemorrhages, and a heart stopped in diastole are common necropsy findings.

Emetics are contraindicated if clinical signs are present. Gastric lavage and adsorbents (activated charcoal, 0.5 g/kg) are recommended. Prognosis is grave if clinical signs are severe. Barbiturates are preferred for controlling seizures. Glyceryl monoacetate (monacetin) has been used with inconsistent results as a competitive antagonist of fluoroacetate. The recommended dose is 0.55 mL/kg, IM, or IV in 5 parts of sterile saline solution, every 30 min for several hours.

The danger of secondary poisoning due to ingestion of rodents killed with 1080 is high and has led to restrictions in its use (and use of fluoroacetamide) in the USA. Only certified, insured exterminators can purchase 1080, and a black dye must be mixed with it for identification.

Sodium Fluoroacetamide (1081): 1081 causes signs similar to those of 1080 (*see* above) and requires the same treatment.

Thallium Sulfate: This general cellular poison can affect all species of animals. It has been banned for use as a rodenticide. Onset of clinical signs may be delayed 1-3 days and, although all body systems are affected, the most prominent signs are of the GI, respiratory, integumentary, and nervous systems. Signs include gastroenteritis (occasionally hemorrhagic), abdominal pain, dyspnea, blindness, fever, conjunctivitis, gingivitis, and tremors or seizures. After 4-5 days and an apparent recovery, or after repeated small doses, a chronic dermatitis characterized by alopecia, erythema, and hyperkeratosis occurs. Necrosis of many tissues is a common necropsy finding.

Treatment of the acute phase of thallium poisoning includes emetics, gastric lavage with a 1% sodium iodide solution, and IV administration of 10% sodium iodide. Diphenylthiocarbazone (dithizone, 70 mg/kg, PO, TID) is antidotal but must be given within 24 hr of exposure. At the same time and for 14 days thereafter, Prussian blue 100 mg/kg should be given BID in oral aqueous suspension to stop enterohepatic recirculation of the thallium and to enhance its excretion in the feces. Symptomatic treatment of the diarrhea and convulsions is needed with particular attention to fluid and electrolyte balance, nutrient needs, prevention of secondary infection, and good nursing care.

Zinc Phosphide and Aluminum Phosphide: Zinc phosphide has been used extensively around farms and barns because affected rats tend to die in the open. Toxicity is due to liberation of phosphine gas at the acid pH in the stomach. The gas results in direct GI tract irritation along with cardiovascular collapse. The toxic dose is ~40 mg/kg, and onset is rapid in animals with a full stomach. Clinical signs include vomiting, abdominal pain, and aimless running and howling, followed by depression, dyspnea, and convulsions (which may resemble those seen in strychnine or fluoroacetate poisoning). Death is due to respiratory arrest. The odor of acetylene is present in vomitus or stomach contents. Less frequent lesions include visceral congestion and pulmonary edema. Diagnosis is based on history of exposure to zinc phosphide, suggestive clinical signs, and detection of zinc phosphide in stomach contents. Zinc levels in the blood, liver, and kidneys may be increased. Treatment must include supportive therapy, calcium gluconate, and appropriate fluids to reduce acidosis. Sodium bicarbonate (in cattle, 2-4 L of 5%), PO, to neutralize stomach acidity is recommended.

RYEGRASS TOXICITY

ANNUAL RYEGRASS STAGGERS

This often fatal neurotoxic disease occurs in livestock of any age that graze pastures in which annual ryegrass (*Lolium rigidum*) is present and in the seedhead stage of growth. It occurs in western and southern Australia and in South Africa from November to March. Hay of *Festuca rubra commutata* (Chewing's fescue) with *Rathayibacter (Clavibacter) toxicus*-infected seedhead galls has caused a similar disease in cattle and horses in Oregon. Outbreaks of ergot alkaloid toxicity in cattle on *Lolium rigidum* have been reported in South Africa and should not be confused with annual ryegrass staggers.

In Australia, the responsible corynetoxins (members of the tunicaminyluracil group) are produced in seedhead galls induced by the nematode *Anguina funesta* and colonized by *Rathayibacter toxicus*. These bacteria-infected galls are present in infected annual ryegrass pastures from early spring onward, but they are most toxic when the plants senesce. Hence, animals show no sign of toxicity until late spring and summer. Spread of bacteria-infested nematodes to adjacent healthy annual ryegrass pastures is slow.

The corynetoxins are highly toxic glycolipids that inhibit specific glycosylation enzymes and therefore deplete or reduce activity of essential glycoproteins. Experimentally, the corynetoxins deplete fibronectins and cause failure of the hepatic reticuloendothelial system. Cardiovascular function and vascular integrity are consequently impaired, and peripheral circulation and oxygen distribution compromised. Tunicamycin irreversibly downregulates the expression of γ-aminobutyric acid$_A$ receptors and causes cell death in cultured brain neurons. Hence, the clinical expression of the disorder is nervous.

Outbreaks occur 2-6 days after animals graze a pasture that contains annual ryegrass infected at a toxic level. Deaths occur within hours, or up to 1 wk after onset of signs. Characteristic neurologic signs are similar to those of perennial ryegrass staggers (see below). However, mortality from annual ryegrass toxicity is commonly 40-50%, occasionally greater. The lesions include congestion, edema, hemorrhage of the brain and lungs, and degeneration of the liver and kidneys.

Diagnosis is based on the characteristic neurologic signs of tremors, incoordination, rigidity, and collapse when stressed, with animals often becoming apparently normal again when left undisturbed. When animals are severely affected, nervous spasms supervene, and convulsions could be precipitated by either forced exercise or high ambient temperatures. A thorough history and evaluation of the pastures will assist in differentiation of staggers caused by other grasses such as perennial ryegrass, phalaris, and the ergots of paspalum and other grasses. Polioencephalomalacia and enterotoxemia are other differential diagnoses.

Clinical signs identical to those of annual ryegrass toxicity have recently been described in Australia in animals grazing Agrostis avenacea (annual blown grass), Polypogon monspeliensis (annual beard grass), or Ehrharta longiflora (annual veldtgrass) infected with nematode galls containing R toxicus. These diseases have been called flood plain staggers, Stewart range syndrome, and veldtgrass staggers, respectively. Although the same bacterium is responsible for all the diseases, the Anguina nematode vectors of R toxicus for these 3 grasses are different species than the A funesta associated with annual ryegrass toxicity. Whereas the inflorescences of annual ryegrass infected with A funesta usually appear normal, nematode-infested inflorescences of these other grasses show distinctive signs.

A significant increase in survival of sheep experimentally poisoned with tunicamycin was observed following treatment with derivatives of β-cyclodextrin. The promising result with this toxin-binding agent offers hope for treatment of animals once they have become affected with annual ryegrass staggers. Losses from the disorder can be minimized by early recognition of signs and removal to safe grazing or by reducing grazing pressure. Gall identification is difficult in annual ryegrass pastures, and in south Australia the bacterium in emerging seedheads is detected and quantified by ELISA. Early detection of toxic fields enables farmers to mow the heads off grass or to allow grazing before the grass becomes too toxic. Grazing of hay aftermath from toxic pastures should be avoided. Burning annual ryegrass pastures in the fall destroys most of the galls colonized by bacteria and minimizes the risk of toxicity in the following season.

PERENNIAL RYEGRASS STAGGERS

This neurotoxic condition of grazing livestock of all ages occurs only in late spring, summer, and fall and only in pastures in which perennial ryegrass (Lolium perenne) or hybrid ryegrass are the major components. Sheep, cattle, horses, farmed deer, and llamas are susceptible. In New Zealand, a high incidence most years causes considerable loss and seriously disrupts management procedures and stock movement. Perennial ryegrass staggers occurs sporadically in parts of North and South America, Europe, and Australia.

The tremorgenic neurotoxins responsible are lolitrems, mainly lolitrem B. These indole diterpene alkaloids are produced in perennial and hybrid ryegrasses infected with the endophytic fungus Neotyphodium (Acremonium) lolii. The amounts of fungal hyphae and lolitrem B in infected plants increase to toxic levels as the temperature rises in late spring and decrease again to safe levels in the cooler seasons. Mycelia of the fungus are present in all above-ground parts of infected plants but are especially concentrated in leaf sheaths, flower stalks, and seed. Infected plants exhibit no signs, and the fungus is spread only through infected seed. Viability of the endophyte gradually declines when infected seed is stored at ambient temperatures and moderate to high humidity, so that few seeds contain viable endophyte after 2 yr. Neurotoxic tremorgens are believed to cause incoordination by interference with neuronal transmission in the cerebral cortex through production of a reversible biochemical lesion; no specific histologic lesion is recognized. *N lolii* also produces the ergopeptine alkaloid ergovaline, which is the alkaloid responsible for fescue toxicosis. Ergovaline raises the temperature of animals in the warmer months of the year, inducing heat stress. It also depresses prolactin levels, and reduced milk yield in cows has been recorded in New Zealand and Australia.

Signs develop gradually over a few days. Fine tremors of the head and nodding movements are the first signs noted in animals approached quietly and watched carefully. Noise, sudden exercise, or fright elicits more severe signs of head nodding with jerky movements and incoordination when first moved. Running movements are stiff and bounding with marked incoordination and often result in collapse in lateral recumbency with opisthotonos, nystagmus, and flailing of stiffly extended limbs. In less severe cases, the attack soon subsides and within minutes the animal regains its feet. If again forced to run, the episode is repeated. Signs are most severe when the animal is heat stressed.

Within flocks and herds, individual susceptibility varies greatly, and this trait is heritable. In outbreaks, morbidity may reach 80-90%, but mortality is low (0-5%). Deaths are usually accidental, often by drowning when drinking from ponds or streams, or due to the inability to forage for food and water.

The strict seasonal occurrence of characteristic tremors, incoordination, and collapse in several or many animals grazing predominantly perennial ryegrass pastures strongly implicates this disease. Reference to the botanical composition of the pastures will exclude annual ryegrass toxicity (*see* above) and paspalum staggers (p 2421), which have similar clinical signs and seasonality. Microscopic examination of the leaf sheaths of the ryegrass sward will reveal the extent of endophyte infection.

Because movement and handling of animals exacerbates signs, individual treatment is generally impractical. Recovery is spontaneous in 1-2 wk if animals are moved to nontoxic pastures or crops.

Because the endophyte and the lolitrems and ergovaline are not uniformly distributed within ryegrass plants, control by grazing management can help reduce or prevent the disease. Lolitrems and ergovaline are concentrated in the leaf sheath and inflorescences. If pastures are not overgrazed down into the leaf sheath zone or grazed when the plants are flowering, then animals should be relatively safe even when a high proportion of the ryegrass plants are infected with endophytes. Encouragement of growth of other grass species and legumes in established swards also reduces the intake of toxic grass.

Safe new pastures can be established using ryegrass seed with little or no endophyte infection. Alternatively, seed that has been stored at ambient temperatures for 18-24 mo probably contains few viable endophytes and would produce nontoxic pastures. However, the presence of endophyte in grasses makes the plants resistant to attack from many insects and so these pastures are more persistent than endophyte-free pastures. Cultivars of ryegrass artificially infected with a strain of endophyte that does not produce lolitrem B or ergovaline are now available in New Zealand. Signs of ryegrass staggers have not been seen in animals grazing these grasses.

SALT TOXICITY

Salt toxicity (sodium chloride, NaCl), which is more appropriately called "water deprivation sodium ion toxicosis" can result when excessive quantities of salt are ingested and intake of potable water is limited. Salt toxicity is unlikely to occur as long as salt-regulating mechanisms are intact and fresh drinking water is available. It has been reported in virtually all species of animals all over the world. In the USA, it is more common in swine (the most sensitive species), cattle, and poultry. Sheep are relatively resistant. The acute oral lethal dose of salt is 2.2 g/kg in swine and 6.0 g/kg in sheep.

Etiology: Salt toxicity is directly related to water consumption. Water intake in animals can be reduced significantly or abolished completely due to factors such as mechanical failure of waterers, overcrowding, unpalatable medicated water, new surroundings, or frozen water. With water deprivation, sodium propionate, acetate, or carbonate can produce the same toxicosis as sodium chloride.

Feeder pigs on feed containing only 0.25% salt have had salt poisoning when water intake was limited, yet even 13% salt in feed may not produce poisoning when adequate fresh water is consumed. Swine feed should contain 0.5-1% salt, and fresh drinking water should always be available. Feeding whey or brine containing 3-4% salt can result in toxicosis in most livestock and poultry species. Similarly, ingestion of 1-3 kg of salt in deprived animals can result in salt toxicosis even when water is available, especially in cattle.

Chickens can tolerate up to 0.25% salt in drinking water but are susceptible to sodium ion toxicosis when water intake is restricted. Wet mash containing 2% salt caused poisoning in ducklings. High salt content in wet mash is more likely to cause poisoning than in dry feed, probably because birds eat more wet mash.

Cattle and sheep on range can develop salt poisoning when a high percentage of mineral supplement is provided, and the water supply is limited or saline. Sheep can tolerate 1% salt in drinking water; however, 1.5% may be toxic. It is generally recommended that drinking water should contain <0.5% total salt for any species of livestock. Chronic salt poisoning in cattle can cause gastroenteritis, depressed appetite, weight loss, and dehydration.

Clinical Findings: In pigs, early signs (rarely seen) may be increased thirst, pruritus, and constipation. Affected pigs may be blind, deaf, and oblivious to their surroundings; they will not eat, drink, or respond to external stimuli. They may wander aimlessly, bump into objects, circle, or pivot around a single limb. After 1-5 days of limited water intake, intermittent seizures occur with the pig sitting on its haunches, jerking its head backward and upward, and finally falling on its side in clonic-tonic seizures and opisthotonos. Terminally, pigs may lie on their sides, paddling in a coma, and die within a few to 48 hr.

In cattle, signs of acute salt poisoning involve the GI tract and CNS. Salivation, increased thirst, vomiting (regurgitation), abdominal pain, and diarrhea are followed by ataxia, circling, blindness, seizures, and partial paralysis. Cattle sometimes manifest belligerent and aggressive behavior. A sequela of salt poisoning in cattle is dragging of hindfeet while walking or, in more severe cases, knuckling of the fetlock joint.

In poultry, increased thirst, dyspnea, fluid discharge from the beak, weakness, diarrhea, and leg paralysis are some of the common signs of salt poisoning.

Lesions: During the first 48 hr, swine develop eosinopenia, eosinophilic cuffs around vessels in the cerebral cortex and adjacent meninges, and cerebral edema or necrosis. After 3-4 days, eosinophilic cuffs are usually no longer present. The GI mucosa may be inflamed and congested and may have pinpoint, blood-filled ulcers. Cattle do not have eosinophilic cuffs; they have gastric inflammation or ulceration (or both), edema of skeletal muscles, and hydropericardium. Chickens have hydropericardium.

In acute cases, no gross lesions may be present in any species.

Diagnosis: Serum and CSF concentrations of sodium >160 mEq/L, especially when CSF has a greater sodium concentration than serum, are indicative of salt poisoning. In brain (cerebrum), >1,800 ppm of sodium (wet wt) is compatible with toxicosis. Characteristic brain lesions and analyses of feed or water for sodium content are useful for establishing a diagnosis.

In swine, differential diagnoses include insecticide poisoning (organochlorine, organophosphorous, and carbamate), phenylarsonic poisoning, and pseudorabies. In cattle, differential diagnoses include insecticide and lead poisoning, polioencephalomalacia, hypomagnesemic tetany, and the nervous form of ketosis.

Treatment: There is no specific treatment. Immediate removal of offending feed or water is imperative. Fresh water must be provided to all animals, initially in small amounts at frequent intervals. Ingestion of large amounts of water may exacerbate neurologic signs due to brain edema. Severely affected animals should be given water via stomach tube. The mortality rate may be >50% in affected animals regardless of treatment. In small animals, slow administration of hypertonic dextrose or isotonic saline may be useful.

SELENIUM TOXICOSIS

Selenium is an essential element that has a narrow margin of safety. Feed supplements containing 0.1-0.3 ppm selenium are added to the diet to prevent deficiency diseases such as white muscle disease in cattle and sheep, hepatosis dietetica in pigs, and exudative diathesis in chickens. The maximum tolerable level for selenium in most livestock feed is considered to be 2 ppm or as high as 5 ppm, although some believe that levels as high as 4-5 ppm can inhibit growth.

Selenium is a component of the glutathione peroxidase enzyme that acts as an antioxidant during release of energy. In excess, selenium has 2 general effects: the direct inhibition of cellular oxidation/reduction reactions, and the replacement of sulfur in the body. The inhibition of numerous cellular functions by high levels of selenium results in acute generalized cytotoxicity. The replacement of sulfur by chronic intake of selenium leads to altered structure and function of cellular components. Altered sulfur-containing amino acids (methionine, cystine) affects cell division and growth. Especially susceptible are the cells that form keratin (keratinocytes) and the sulfur-containing keratin molecule. Selenium therefore weakens the hooves and hair, which tend to fracture when subjected to mechanical stress.

Etiology: All animal species are susceptible to selenium toxicosis. However, poisoning is more common in forage-eating animals such as cattle, sheep, and horses that may graze selenium-containing plants. Plants may accumulate selenium when the element is found at high levels—generally in alkaline soil with little rainfall (<50 cm). Selenium accumulating plants have been categorized. Obligate indicator plants require large amounts of selenium for growth and contain high concentrations (often >1,000 ppm). Facultative indicator plants absorb and tolerate high levels of soil selenium accumulating up to 100 ppm under these conditions, but they do not require selenium. Nonaccumulator plants passively absorb low levels of selenium (1-25 ppm) from the soil. Poisoning may also occur in swine and poultry consuming grain raised on seleniferous soils or, more commonly, due to error in feed formulation. Selenium toxicosis after ingestion of selenium-containing shampoos or excess selenium tablets is rare in pets. Several factors are known to alter selenium toxicity; however, in general, a single acute oral dose of selenium in the range of 1-5 mg/kg is lethal in most animals. Parenteral selenium products are also quite toxic, especially to young animals, and have caused deaths in baby pigs, calves, and dogs at doses as low as 1.0 mg/kg.

Diagnosis: Severity of selenium toxicosis depends on the quantity ingested and duration of exposure. Poisoning in animals is characterized as acute, subchronic, or chronic. Diagnosis is based on clinical signs; necropsy findings; and laboratory confirmation of presence of high selenium levels in an animal's diet (feed, forage, grains), blood, or tissues (kidney, liver). Selenium levels in the diet >5 ppm may produce signs after prolonged exposure. Levels of 10-25 ppm could produce severe signs. In acute toxicosis, the blood selenium concentration may reach 25 ppm, and in chronic toxicosis, it may be 1-4 ppm. Kidney or liver may contain 4-25 ppm in both acute and chronic poisoning.

CHRONIC SELENIUM TOXICOSIS
(Alkali disease)

Chronic selenium poisoning usually develops when livestock consume seleniferous forages and grains containing 5-50 ppm of selenium for many weeks or months. Naturally occurring seleno-amino acids in plants are readily absorbed. Until recently, 2 types of chronic selenium poisoning were recognized—alkali disease and blind staggers. Blind staggers is no longer believed to be caused by selenium but by sulfate toxicity due to consumption of high-sulfate alkali water. Excess sulfate (>2% of diet) leads to polioencephalomacia and the classical signs of blind staggers. Animals consuming milk vetch (*Astragalus bisulcatus*) have demonstrated clinical signs similar to blind staggers. Although milk vetch contains high levels of selenium, evidence now indicates that the alkaloid swainsonine in milk vetch, responsible for locoism, produces the signs.

Clinical Findings: Alkali disease has been reported in cattle, sheep, and horses. Affected animals are dull, emaciated, and lack vitality. The most distinctive lesions are those involving the keratin of the hair and hooves. The animal has a rough hair coat and the long hairs of the mane and tail break off at the same level giving a "bob" tail and "roached" mane appearance. Abnormal growth and structure of horns and hooves results in circular ridges and cracking of the hoof wall at the coronary band. Extremely long, deformed hooves that turn upwards at the ends may be seen. Subsequent lameness is compounded by degeneration of joint cartilage and bone. Reduced fertility and reproductive performance occurs especially in sheep. Reproductive performance may be depressed with a dietary level of selenium lower than that required to produce typical signs of alkali disease. Other lesions may include anemia, liver cirrhosis and ascites, and atrophy of the heart.

Birds also may be affected with chronic selenium toxicosis. Eggs with >2.5 ppm selenium from birds in high selenium areas have low hatchability, and the embryos are usually deformed. Teratologic effects include underdeveloped feet and legs, malformed eyes, crooked beaks, and ropy feathers. This has been a problem with waterfowl in southern California, where selenium was leached by agricultural water and concentrated in lakes by runoff.

Blood levels of selenium in chronic cases are usually 1-4 ppm. Other changes in blood include decreased fibrinogen level and prothrombin activity; increased serum alkaline phosphatase, ALT, AST, and succinic dehydrogenase; and reduced glutathione. Hair may have >5 ppm selenium in chronic poisoning. A "garlicky" odor on the animal's breath may be noted.

Treatment and Control: There is no specific treatment for selenium toxicosis. Eliminating the source and exposure and symptomatic and supportive care of the animal should be started as soon as possible. Addition of substances that antagonize or inhibit the toxic effects of selenium in the diet may help reduce the risk of selenium toxicosis. A high protein diet, linseed oil meal, sulfur, arsenic, silver, copper, cadmium, and mercury have reduced selenium toxicity in laboratory animals, but their use under field conditions is limited. Addition of arsenic salt at 0.00375% to enhance biliary excretion of selenium or use of a high-protein diet to bind free selenium may help reduce incidence of selenium poisoning in cattle.

Soil and forages should be tested regularly in high-selenium areas.

SUBCHRONIC SELENIUM TOXICOSIS

Pigs fed a diet supplemented with selenium >20-50 ppm for >3 days develop a subchronic selenium toxicosis characterized by neurologic abnormalities. Animals are initially ataxic and uncoordinated followed by anterior paresis, then quadriplegia. Pigs continue to eat. The hooves show breaks and impaired growth similar to those seen in cattle; alopecia is observed. In sows, conception rate decreases and number of pigs born dead increases. Lesions of subchronic toxicosis include focal symmetric poliomyelomalacia, which is most prominent in the cervical and thoracic spinal cord. Death may result from complications of permanent paralysis. Hoof and hair damage is similar to but in most cases less severe than that observed in chronic selenium toxicosis. Treatment is similar to that for chronic toxicosis, but spinal lesions are usually permanent.

ACUTE SELENIUM TOXICOSIS

Acute selenium poisoning due to consumption of plants with levels >50 ppm (dosages 3-20 mg/kg) is rare but has caused large losses in cattle, sheep, and pigs. Animals usually avoid these plants because of their offensive odor; however, when pasture is limited, accumulator plants may be the only food available. Young animals are most susceptible to acute parenteral selenium toxicosis with dosages of 0.2-0.5 mg/kg. Clinical signs are different from those of chronic selenosis and are characterized by abnormal behavior, respiratory difficulty, gastrointestinal upset, and sudden death. Abnormal posture and depression, anorexia, unsteady gait, diarrhea, colic, increased pulse and respiration rates, frothy nasal discharge, moist rales, and cyanosis may be noted.

Death usually follows within a few hours of consumption or injection. The major lesions are lung edema and congestion, and necrosis of multiple organs, including lung, liver, and kidney. Sheep usually do not show these signs, but instead become depressed and die suddenly.

Blood selenium concentration in acute poisoning is much higher than in chronic poisoning. In acute cases, blood selenium may reach 25 ppm. Treatment consists of symptomatic and supportive care. Acetylcysteine to boost glutathione levels is beneficial.

SNAKEBITE

Venomous snakes fall into 2 classes: 1) the elapines, which include the cobra, mamba, and coral snakes; and 2) the 2 families of viperines, the true vipers (eg, puff adder, Russell's viper, and common European adder) and the pit vipers (eg, rattlesnakes, cottonmouth moccasin, copperhead, and fer-de-lance). Poisonous North American snakes include pit vipers and coral snakes.

Elapine snakes have short fangs and tend to hang on and "chew" venom into their victims. Their venom is neurotoxic and paralyzes the respiratory center. Animals that survive these bites seldom have any sequelae. Viperine snakes have long, hinged, hollow fangs; they strike, inject venom (a voluntary action), and withdraw. Many bites by vipers reportedly do not result in injection of substantial quantities of venom. Viperine venom is typically hemotoxic, necrotizing, and anticoagulant, although a neurotoxic component is present in the venom of some species, eg, the Mojave rattlesnake (*Crotalus scutulatus scutulatus*).

Fatal snakebites are more common in dogs than in any other domestic animal. Due to the relatively small size of some dogs in proportion to the amount of venom injected, the bite of even a small snake may be fatal. Because of their size, horses and cattle seldom die as a direct result of snakebite, but deaths may follow bites on the muzzle, head, or neck when dyspnea results from excessive swelling. Serious secondary damage sometimes occurs; livestock bitten near the coronary band may slough a hoof.

Snakebite, with envenomation, is a true emergency. Rapid examination and appropriate treatment are paramount. Owners should not spend time on first aid other than to keep the animal quiet and limit its activity.

Diagnosis: In many instances, the bite has been witnessed, and diagnosis is not a problem. However, many conditions thought by the owner to be snakebites are actually fractures, abscesses, spider envenomations, or allergic reactions to insect bites or stings. When possible, owners should be instructed to bring the *dead* snake along with the bitten animal; they should be warned not to mutilate the snake's head because identification may depend on the morphology of the head. Many bites do not result in envenomation, or are made by nonpoisonous snakes.

Typical pit viper bites are characterized by severe local tissue damage that spreads from the bite site. The tissue becomes markedly discolored within a few minutes, and dark, bloody fluid may ooze from the fang wounds if not prevented by swelling. Frequently, the epidermis sloughs when the overlying hair is clipped or merely parted. Hair may hide the typical fang marks. Sometimes, only one fang mark or multiple punctures are present. In elapine snakebites, pain and swelling are minimal; systemic neurologic signs predominate.

Treatment: Intensive therapy should be instituted as soon as possible because irreversible effects of venom begin immediately after envenomation.

Animals bitten by an elapine may be treated with antivenin (which may be available on an as-needed basis through larger human hospital emergency rooms) and supportive care, including anticonvulsants if necessary. A polyvalent antivenin (horse-serum origin) against North American pit vipers is readily available and should be used in all cases of substantial pit viper envenomation.

The progression of events after pit viper envenomation can be divided into 3 phases: the first 2 hr, the ensuing 24 hr, and a variable period (usually ~10 days) afterward. The first 2 hr is the acute stage in which untreated, severely envenomized animals usually die. If death does not occur during this period, and the untreated animal is not in shock or depressed, the prognosis usually is favorable. The acute phase can be prolonged for several hours by use of corticosteroids and, if they are administered, prognostication should be withheld. If the animal is active and alert after 24 hr, death due to the direct effects of the venom is unlikely. The third phase is a convalescent period in which infection (possibly anaerobic) may be of concern. If necrosis has been extensive, sloughing occurs and may be so severe as to involve an entire limb.

An attempt to estimate the severity of envenomation should be made. Although not infallible, it is prudent to consider the size of the snake both as an indicator of the quantity of venom injected, and as it relates to the size of the victim. In dogs and cats, mortality is generally higher from bites to the thorax or abdomen than from bites to the head or extremities. However, this may relate to the size and vulnerability of the victim because smaller animals are more likely to be bitten on the body. Sensitivity to the venom of pit vipers varies among domestic animals. In decreasing order, sensitivity is reportedly horse, sheep, goat, dog, rabbit, pig, and cat. If there has been a previous bite, the victim may have developed some degree of active humoral immunity and be less vulnerable to the toxic effects of the venom.

Treatment for pit viper envenomation should be directed toward preventing or controlling shock, neutralizing venom, preventing or controlling disseminated intravascular coagulation, minimizing necrosis, and preventing secondary infection. Any dog or cat presented within 24 hr of a snakebite showing signs of pit viper envenomation requires intensive treatment, starting with IV fluids to combat hypotension. The use of corticosteroids has been questioned, principally because they alone do not alter the ultimate outcome. They do, however, prolong the clinical course and therefore allow more time in which to institute curative measures. Rapid-acting corticosteroids may help to control shock, protect against tissue damage, and minimize the likelihood of allergic reactions to antivenin. Antivenin is highly beneficial because its action is the only direct and specific mechanism for neutralizing snake venom. Smaller animals probably receive a larger dose (per unit body wt) of venom than more massive animals and, accordingly, require proportionally larger doses of antivenin. Up to 100 mL of antivenin may be necessary for small dogs bitten by a large snake; 5-10 mL may be injected into the tissues around the bite, and the remainder given IV. The efficacy of antivenin is diminished if the bite occurred >24 hr previously. In the event of an anaphylactoid reaction to the heterologous (horse) serum components in antivenin, 0.5-1 mL of 1:1,000 epinephrine should be administered SC. If disseminated intravascular coagulation occurs, appropriate treatment, including blood products and heparin sodium (in mini dose at 5-10 U/kg/hr or low dose at 50-100 U/kg, TID), should be administered SC.

Broad-spectrum antibiotics should be given to prevent wound infection and other secondary infections. Several potential pathogens, including *Pseudomonas aeruginosa*, *Clostridium* spp, *Corynebacterium* spp, and staphylococci have been isolated from rattlesnakes' mouths. Antibiotics should be continued until all superficial lesions have healed.

Tetanus antitoxin also should be administered; other supportive treatment (eg, blood transfusion in the case of hemolytic or anticoagulant venoms) is administered as needed. In most cases, surgical excision is impractical or unwarranted. Antihistamines have been reported to be contraindicated, but diphenhydramine hydrochloride is frequently given along with antivenin to treat snakebite in humans.

Other procedures to neutralize venom (high-voltage, low-amperage electric shock and trypsin) have not proved effective in controlled studies.

SORGHUM POISONING

(Sudan grass poisoning)

Sorghum poisoning has been seen primarily in the southwestern USA and reported almost exclusively in horses, although a similar syndrome has been reported in sheep and cattle. Lathyrogenic nitriles such as β-cyanoalanine, cyanogenic glycosides, and nitrates have been suggested as causative agents. The syndrome develops in horses after they have grazed hybrid Sudan pastures for weeks to months and produces axonal degeneration and myelomalacia in the spinal cord and cerebellum. (*See also* CYANIDE POISONING, p 2355.) Consumption of the seed will not produce the syndrome.

Sorghum poisoning is characterized by posterior incoordination, cystitis, urinary incontinence (which predisposes both male and female horses to cystitis), and alopecia on the hindlegs due to urine scald. The incoordination may progress to flaccid paralysis. Deformities of the fetal musculoskeletal system (arthrogryposis) and abortion during late pregnancy may occur. Consumption of sorghum hybrids with low cyanogenic potential or restriction of access to sorghum grasses may limit the incidence. Affected horses often die from pyelonephritis. Treatment with antibiotics may be helpful, but a full recovery is rare.

SPIDER BITES

Envenomation of animals by spiders is relatively uncommon and difficult to recognize. It may be suspected on clinical signs, but confirmatory evidence is rare. Spiders of medical importance in the USA do not inflict particularly painful bites, so it is unusual for a spider bite to be suspected until clinical signs appear. It is also unlikely that the offending spider will remain in close proximity to the victim for the time (30 min to 6 hr) required for signs to develop. Almost all spiders are venomous, but few possess the attributes necessary to cause clinical envenomation in mammals—mouth parts of sufficient size to allow penetration of the skin and toxin of sufficient quantity or potency to result in morbidity.

The spiders in the USA that are capable of causing clinical envenomation belong to 2 groups—widow spiders (*Latrodectus* spp) and brown spiders (mostly *Loxosceles* spp).

Widow Spiders: Widow spiders usually bite only when accidental skin contact occurs. The most common species is the black widow, *Latrodectus mactans*, characterized by a red hourglass shape on the ventral abdomen. In the western states, the western black widow, *L hesperus*, predominates, while the brown widow, *L bishopi*, is found in the south, and the red widow, *L geometricus*, is found in Florida.

Latrodectus venom is one of the most potent biologic toxins. The most important of its 5 or 6 components is a neurotoxin that causes release of the neurotransmitters norepinephrine and acetylcholine at synaptic junctions, which continues until the neurotransmitters are depleted. The resulting severe, painful cramping of all large muscle groups accounts for most of the clinical signs.

Unless there is a history of a widow spider bite, diagnosis must be based on clinical signs, which include restlessness with apparent anxiety or apprehension; rapid, shallow, irregular respiration; shock; abdominal rigidity or tenderness; and painful muscle rigidity, sometimes accompanied by intermittent relaxation (which may progress to clonus and eventually to respiratory paralysis). Partial paresis also has been described.

An antivenin (equine origin) is commercially available but is usually reserved for confirmed bites of high-risk individuals (very young or very old). Symptomatic treatment is usually sufficient but may require a combination of therapeutic agents. Calcium gluconate IV (10 mL of a 10% solution is the usual human dose) is reportedly helpful. Meperidine hydrochloride or morphine, also given IV, provides relief from pain and produces muscle relaxation. Muscle relaxants and diazepam are also beneficial. Tetanus antitoxin also should be administered. Recovery may be prolonged; weakness and even partial paralysis may persist for several days.

Brown Spiders: There are at least 10 species of *Loxosceles* spiders in the USA, but the brown recluse spider, *L reclusa*, is the most common, and envenomation by it is typical. These spiders have a violin-shaped marking on the cephalothorax, although it may be indistinct or absent in some species. In the northwestern USA, the unrelated spider *Tegenaria agrestis* reportedly causes a clinically indistinguishable dermonecrosis in humans and presumably in other animals. Brown recluse spider venom has vasoconstrictive, thrombotic, hemolytic, and necrotizing properties. It contains several enzymes, including a phospholipase (sphingomyelinase D) that attacks cell membranes. Pathogenetic mechanisms of the characteristic dermal necrosis are poorly understood, but activation of complement, chemotaxis, and accumulations of neutrophils affect (or amplify) the process.

A history of a bite by a "fiddleback" brown spider is useful but rare. A presumptive diagnosis may be based on the presence of a discrete, erythematous, intensely pruritic skin lesion that may have irregular ecchymoses. Within 4-8 hr, a vesicle develops at the bite wound, and sometimes a blanched zone circumscribes the erythematous area, imparting a "bull's-eye" appearance to the lesion. The central area sometimes appears pale or cyanotic. The vesicle may degenerate to an ulcer that, unless treated in a timely manner, may enlarge and extend to underlying tissues, including muscle. Sometimes, a pustule follows the vesicle and, on its breakdown, a black eschar remains. The final tissue defect may be extensive and indolent and require months to heal. However, medical authorities claim that not all brown recluse spider bites result in severe, localized dermal necrosis.

Systemic signs sometimes accompany brown recluse spider envenomation and may not appear for 3-4 days after the bite. Hemolysis, thrombocytopenia, and disseminated intravascular coagulation are more likely to occur in cases with severe dermal necrosis. Fever, vomiting, edema, hemoglobinuria, hemolytic anemia, renal failure, and shock may result from systemic loxoscelism.

In known bites, early treatment can be successful, but unfortunately, many cases are not recognized until cutaneous necrosis has become extensive; treatment at that stage is less rewarding but is still of value. Immediate application of cold packs is beneficial, and if administered early, corticosteroids protect against cutaneous necrosis by stabilizing cell membranes and suppressing chemotaxis. Corticosteroids also tend to protect against systemic involvement. Radical excision has been advocated, but its value is questionable. Dapsone, an inhibitor of leukocyte function, which is frequently used in the treatment of leprosy, is currently considered the drug of choice for brown recluse spider bites. In humans, it is administered at 100 mg, BID for 14-25 days. Broad-spectrum antibiotics are useful in preventing secondary infection, and tetanus immunoprophylaxis should be considered.

STRYCHNINE POISONING

Strychnine is an indole alkaloid obtained from the seeds of the Indian tree *Strychnos nux-vomica*. It is mainly used as a pesticide to control rats, moles, gophers, and coyotes. Commercial baits (usually <0.5%) are pelleted and often dyed red or green. Strychnine is highly toxic to most domestic animals. Its oral LD_{50} in dogs, cattle, horses, and pigs is between 0.5-1 mg/kg, and in cats is 2 mg/kg. Malicious or accidental strychnine poisoning, although not very common in the USA, occurs mainly in small animals, especially dogs and occasionally cats, and rarely in livestock.

Pathogenesis: Strychnine is ionized in an acidic pH and then rapidly and completely absorbed in the small intestine. It is metabolized in the liver by microsomal enzymes. The highest concentrations of strychnine are found in the blood, liver, and kidneys. Strychnine and its metabolites are excreted in the urine. Depending on the quantity ingested and treatment measures taken, most of the toxic dose is eliminated within 24-48 hr.

Strychnine inhibits competitively and reversibly the inhibitory neurotransmitter glycine at postsynaptic neuronal sites in the spinal cord and medulla. This results in unchecked reflex stimulation of motor neurons affecting all the striated muscles. Because the extensor muscles are relatively more powerful than the flexor muscles, they predominate to produce generalized rigidity and tonic-clonic seizures. Death results from anoxia and exhaustion.

Clinical Findings: The onset of strychnine poisoning is fast. After oral exposure, clinical signs may appear within 30-60 min. Presence of food in the stomach can delay onset. Early signs, which may often be overlooked, consist of apprehension, nervousness, tenseness, and stiffness. Vomiting usually does not occur. Severe tetanic seizures may appear spontaneously or may be initiated by stimuli such as touch, sound, or a sudden bright light. An extreme and overpowering extensor rigidity causes the animal to assume a "sawhorse" stance. Hyperthermia (104-106°F [40-41°C]) due to stiffness and seizures is often present in dogs. The tetanic convulsions may last from a few seconds to ~1 min. Respiration may stop momentarily. Intermittent periods of relaxation are seen during convulsions but become less frequent as the clinical course progresses. The mucous membranes become cyanotic, and the pupils dilated. Frequency of the seizures increases, and death eventually occurs from exhaustion or asphyxiation during seizures. If untreated, the entire syndrome may last only 1-2 hr. There are no characteristic necropsy lesions. Sometimes, due to prolonged convulsions before death, agonal hemorrhages of heart and lungs and cyanotic congestion from anoxia may be seen. Animals dying from strychnine poisoning have rapid rigor mortis.

Diagnosis: Tentative diagnosis of strychnine poisoning is usually based on history of exposure and clinical signs. Recovery of strychnine alkaloid from the stomach contents, vomitus, liver, kidneys, or urine should be considered diagnostic. Sometimes, urine may not have a detectable amount of strychnine present; therefore, multiple samples should be collected and analyzed.

Strychnine poisoning can be confused with poisonings by several other substances such as metaldehyde; organochlorine, organophosphate, or carbamate insecticides; fluoroacetate (1080); zinc phosphide; nicotine; 4-aminopyridine; or human medications (tricyclic antidepressants, 5-fluorouracil, metronidazole, isoniazid). Acute, massive hepatic necrosis (hepatic encephalopathy) can also produce clinical signs that resemble those of strychnine poisoning.

Treatment: Strychnine poisoning is an emergency, and treatment should be instituted quickly. Treatment should be aimed at decontamination, control of seizures, prevention of asphyxiation, and supportive care.

Decontamination consists of removal of gastric contents by inducing emesis or gastric lavage, and binding of remaining bait in the GI tract with activated charcoal. Due to the rapid onset of clinical signs, emesis may be of limited value in most cases. If exposure is recent and no clinical signs are present, emesis should be induced with 3% hydrogen peroxide (small animals and pigs) at 1-2 mL/kg, PO, maximum 3 tbsp, repeated once after 30 min if vomiting has not occurred; or apomorphine (dogs only) at 0.03 mg/kg, IV, or 0.04 mg/kg, IM; or xylazine (dogs or cats) at 0.5-1 mg/kg, IV or IM. If emesis cannot be induced, gastric lavage should be performed with tepid water. Animals that are already seizuring should be anesthetized first (with pentobarbital) and an endotracheal tube passed before gastric lavage. After emesis or gastric lavage, activated charcoal should be administered at 2-3 g/kg in small animals and 0.5-1 g/kg in large animals with magnesium sulfate at 250 mg/kg, PO.

Seizures should be controlled in small animals with pentobarbital, IV to effect, repeated as necessary. Muscle relaxants such as methocarbamol at 100-200 mg/kg, IV, also work well; they should be repeated as needed with a maximum dose of 330 mg/kg/day. In large animals, chloral hydrate or xylazine can be used to control seizures. Other medications such as glyceryl guaiacolate (5%, 110 mg/kg), diazepam, and xylazine have been used in dogs to control seizures with variable success.

Severely affected dogs should be intubated and artificial respiration provided. Acidification of urine with ammonium chloride (100 mg/kg, BID, PO) may be useful for iontrapping and urinary excretion of the alkaloid. Intravenous fluids should be administered to force diuresis and maintain normal kidney function. Hyperthermia treatment (fans, cool bath) should be given if necessary. Acid-base balance should be monitored and corrected as needed.

SWEET CLOVER POISONING

Sweet clover poisoning, an insidious hemorrhagic disease, is seen in animals that consume toxic quantities of spoiled sweet clover (*Melilotus officinalis* and *M alba*) hay or silage.

Etiology: During the process of spoiling, the harmless natural coumarins in sweet clover are converted to toxic dicumarol. Any method of hay storage that allows molding of sweet clover promotes the likelihood of formation of dicumarol in the hay. Weathered, large round bales, particularly the outer portions, usually contain the highest levels of dicumarol. When toxic hay or silage is consumed, hypoprothrombinemia results, presumably because dicumarol combines with the proenzyme required for synthesis of prothrombin (by preventing formation of the active enzyme). It probably also interferes with synthesis of factor VII and other coagulation factors. (*See* HEMOSTATIC DISORDERS, p 37.) Dicumarol levels of 20-30 mg/kg of hay are usually required to cause poisoning in cattle. The toxic agent crosses the placenta in pregnant animals, and newborn animals may be affected at birth. All species of animals studied are susceptible, but instances of poisoning have involved mainly cattle and, to a limited extent, sheep, pigs, and horses.

Clinical Findings and Lesions: Clinical signs are referable to hemorrhages that result from faulty blood coagulation. The time between consumption of toxic sweet clover and appearance of clinical disease varies greatly and depends on the dicumarol content of the particular sweet clover variety being fed, age of the animals, and the amount of feed consumed. If the dicumarol content of the ration is low or variable, animals may consume it for months before signs of disease appear.

The first indication of dicumarol poisoning may be the death of one or more animals. In affected animals, the first signs may be stiffness and lameness, due to bleeding into the muscles and joints. Hematomas, epistaxis, or GI bleeding may be seen. Death may occur suddenly with little preliminary evidence of disease and is caused by massive hemorrhage or bleeding after injury, surgery, or parturition. Neonatal deaths rarely occur without signs in the dam.

Hemorrhage is the characteristic necropsy finding; large extravasations of blood are common in subcutaneous and connective tissues.

Diagnosis: This is based on a history of continuous consumption of sweet clover hay or silage over relatively long periods, compatible signs and lesions, and markedly prolonged blood clotting time or demonstration of reduced prothrombin content of the plasma. The nature of the coagulopathy can be confirmed in the laboratory when the prothrombin time (PT) is prolonged. Sweet clover poisoning is normally a herd problem; signs of hemorrhage or slow blood clotting in only one animal from a group makes this diagnosis unlikely. Most diseases with hemorrhagic manifestations, such as blackleg, pasteurellosis, bracken fern poisoning, and aplastic anemia, can be readily differentiated based on clinical, pathologic, and hematologic findings. This is the only commonly acquired disease, except purpura hemorrhagica (common only in horses) and rodenticide poisoning (p 2508), in which such large hemorrhages occur.

Congenital or inherited diseases affecting coagulation factors or blood platelets (eg, hemophilia A) also may be characterized by large hemorrhages.

Treatment: The hypoprothrombinemia, hemorrhages, and anemia can be immediately corrected, to a degree, by IV administration of whole blood. Recommended dosages range from 2-10 L of fresh blood per 1,000 lb (450 kg) body wt. Animals used as a source of blood must not be receiving sweet clover feed. All animals with marked signs should receive a transfusion, which can be repeated if necessary. In addition, all severely affected animals should receive parenteral administration of synthetic vitamin K_1 (phytonadione). SC or IM injection is recommended to avoid the substantial risk of anaphylaxis; SC vitamin K_1 may not be as effective as IM treatment. There appears to be little advantage in outcome from IV administration. The usual dose recommended for cattle is 1 mg/kg, BID-TID for 2 days. Although it is more costly, vitamin K_1 is more effective than K_3 (menadione) in experimental studies and is the preferred treatment. Because reversal of the dicumarol by vitamin K_1 requires synthesis of coagulation proteins, significant improvement in homeostasis requires several hours, and >24 hr is required to completely restore coagulation. Either vitamin K_1 or a blood transfusion is sufficient to correct mild cases of intoxication if feeding toxic hay is stopped.

Prevention: Cultivars of sweet clover, low in coumarin and safe to feed (eg, Polara), have been developed. If one of these is not available, the only certain method of prevention is to avoid feeding sweet clover hay or silage. Although well-cured sweet clover is not dangerous, the absence of visible spoilage is insufficient evidence of safety. There is no quick chemical test for dicumarol, but suspect feed can be fed to rabbits, which develop fatal hemorrhages more rapidly than cattle. This can be combined with periodic determination of PT in the rabbits to speed up the test results. Unfortunately, some rabbits are refractory to dicumarol, which complicates negative test results.

A simple management technique involves alternating sweet clover hay suspected of containing dicumarol with other roughage such as alfalfa or a grass-legume hay mixture. A 7- to 10-day period on the sweet clover hay is followed by an equal time on the alternate hay. Alternating the forage can successfully prevent poisoning but does not completely prevent prolonged bleeding times. Some animals are at greater risk of serious hemorrhaging at calving (or lambing). They should not receive sweet clover hay for a minimum of 2-3 wk, and preferably 4 wk, prior to parturition. The goal is to allow the animal's clotting system to fully reestablish competency before a hemorrhagic stress. Dehorning and castration should also be avoided in animals consuming sweet clover hay at least until a full withdrawal period has been achieved.

TOAD POISONING

Dogs and, less frequently, cats may be poisoned by oral exposure to many types of toads. Severity varies greatly, depending on extent of contact and type of toad. Venom is produced by all toads, but its potency varies with species and apparently between geographic locations within individual species. Toad venom, a defensive mechanism, is secreted by glands located dorsal and posterior to the eyes and by other dermal structures, including warts. The venom, a thick, creamy white, highly irritating substance, can be expelled quickly by the contraction of periglandular muscles in the skin. Its many components include bufagins, which have digitalis-like effects, catecholamines, and serotonin. The most toxic species in the USA appears to be the giant or marine toad, *Bufo marinus*, an introduced species that is established in Florida, Hawaii, and Texas. Mortality is 20-100% in untreated cases, depending on venom potency.

Diagnosis: Encounters with toads are most common in warm or mild weather. Signs of poisoning are variable and range from local effects to convulsions and death. Severity depends on host factors, extent of exposure, length of time since exposure, and species of toad. Local effects (profuse, sometimes frothy salivation, accompanied by vigorous head shaking, pawing at the mouth, and retching) are immediate, probably because the venom is extremely irritating. Vomiting is not unusual, especially in severe cases, and although it may persist for several hours, no further signs may develop in poisoning by common indigenous toads. With more severe intoxication, as from *B marinus*, cardiac arrhythmias, dyspnea, cyanosis, and seizures are characteristic. Both cardiac and CNS involvement are life-threatening.

Treatment: A specific antidote for the toxins in toad venom is not available. Therapy is directed at minimizing absorption of the venom and controlling the associated clinical signs. Minimal treatment may be required after exposure to venom in areas where less toxic toads are found. The mouth should be immediately and thoroughly flushed with copious amounts of water. The victim should be prevented from inhaling aerosols of saliva or water that contain toad venom. Atropine may reduce the volume of saliva and the risk of aspiration. More severely affected animals require more extensive therapy. Cardiac arrhythmias should be identified and controlled using standard treatment protocols (*see also* ARRHYTHMIAS, p 78). If bradyarrhythmias exist, atropine or dopamine should be considered; tachyarrhythmias should be treated with lidocaine, phenytoin, propranolol, or procainamide hydrochloride. CNS excitation, if present, should be controlled by pentobarbital anesthesia, diazepam, or a combination of the two. Thiamylal, halothane, and other forms of anesthesia may be contraindicated because they may predispose to ventricular fibrillation. Supplemental oxygen and mechanical ventilation may also be needed if cyanosis and dyspnea are prominent.

TOXICITIES FROM HUMAN DRUGS

TOXICITIES FROM OVER-THE-COUNTER DRUGS

Human drugs or nutritional supplements available without a prescription are known as over-the-counter (OTC) medications. Exposures to OTC drugs in pets can be accidental or intentional. A valid client-patient-veterinarian relationship must exist for veterinarians to recommend extra-label use of these drugs to their clients. Safety of most OTC drugs has not been determined in animals, as most are not approved for veterinary use by the FDA. Veterinarians should understand the potential risks of using OTC medications and communicate them to their clients.

COLD AND COUGH MEDICATIONS

Antihistamines

Antihistamines are H_1-receptor antagonists that provide symptomatic relief of allergic signs caused by histamine release, including pruritus and anaphylactic reactions. They are also used as sedatives and antiemetics. Antihistamines belong to different classes and are categorized as first- or second-generation (also called nonsedating) antihistamines. First-generation antihistamines may cause adverse effects because of their cholinergic activity and ability to cross the blood-brain barrier. Second-generation antihistamines are more lipophilic than first-generation antihistamines and are thought to lack CNS and cholinergic effects at therapeutic doses. Antihistamines are often found in combination with other ingredients in many OTC cold, sinus, and allergy medications.

Chlorpheniramine is a first-generation propylamine-derivative antihistamine. Oral absorption of chlorpheniramine in dogs is rapid and complete, reaching peak plasma concentrations in 30-60 min. Chlorpheniramine maleate undergoes substantial first-pass effect. Chlorpheniramine and its metabolites are primarily excreted in urine. The recommended dose in cats and dogs is 1-2 mg and 2-8 mg respectively, PO, BID-TID. Mild clinical signs such as depression and GI upset have been reported for dosages <1 mg/kg. Significant clinical signs such as ataxia, tremors, depression or hyperactivity, hyperthermia, and seizures may be seen within 6 hr of ingestion of large amounts.

Dimenhydrinate and **diphenhydramine** are first-generation ethanolamine-derivative antihistamines. Diphenhydramine is well absorbed orally in people, but undergoes first-pass metabolism in the liver with only 40-60% of the drug reaching the systemic circulation. Peak plasma concentrations of ethanolamine-derivative antihistamines occur within 1-5 hr; elimination half-lives vary from 2.4-10 hr. A recommended dose for dimenhydrinate and diphenhydramine in cats and dogs is 4-8 mg/kg and 2-4 mg/kg, respectively. Hyperactivity or depression, hypersalivation, tachypnea, and tachycardia are the most common adverse signs reported with these antihistamines, generally within 1 hr of exposure.

Promethazine hydrochloride is an ethylamino derivative of phenothiazine and first-generation antihistamine used for the management of motion sickness. Promethazine is widely distributed in body tissues and readily crosses the placenta. Overdoses may result in CNS depression or excitation. CNS depression was reported in a dog 30 min after ingesting 1 mg/kg of promethazine.

Meclizine is a first-generation piperazine-derivative antihistamine commonly used as an antiemetic. Peak plasma concentrations occur within 2-3 hr of oral administration. Meclizine is primarily excreted as metabolites in urine, with a reported serum half-life of 6 hr. In cases involving <33 mg/kg of meclizine in dogs, only mild hyperactivity or depression has been reported.

Loratadine is a tricyclic long-acting antihistamine with selective peripheral histamine H_1-receptor antagonist activity. In humans, loratadine is well absorbed orally and extensively metabolized to an active metabolite. Most of the parent drug is excreted unchanged in the urine. The mean elimination half-life in humans is 8.4 hr. Loratadine appears to have a large margin of safety in laboratory animals. No deaths were reported at oral doses up to 5 g/kg in rats and mice. In rats, mice, and monkeys, no clinical signs were observed at 10 times the maximum recommended human daily oral dose.

Treatment: Treatment of antihistamine toxicosis is primarily symptomatic and supportive. Emesis should only be considered in asymptomatic patients. Activated charcoal may be useful for recent ingestion. Cardiovascular function and body temperature should be closely monitored. Diazepam can be used to control seizures or seizure-type activity. Physostigmine is recommended to counteract the CNS anticholinergic effects of antihistamine overdoses in people, although the risk of seizures associated with this drug may limit its use. IV fluids should be given as needed.

DECONGESTANTS

Imidazoline Decongestants

The imidazoline derivatives, **oxymetazoline**, **xylometazoline**, **tetrahydrozoline**, and **naphazoline** are found in topical ophthalmic and nasal decongestants available OTC. They are generally used as topical vasoconstrictors in the nose and eyes for temporary relief of nasal congestion due to colds, hay fever or other upper respiratory allergies, or sinusitis.

Imidazolines are sympathomimetic agents, with primary effects on α-adrenergic receptors and little if any effect on β-adrenergic receptors. Oxymetazoline is readily absorbed orally. Effects on α-receptors from systemically absorbed oxymetazoline hydrochloride may persist for up to 7 hr after a single dose. The elimination half-life in humans is 5-8 hr. It is excreted unchanged both by the kidneys (30%) and in feces (10%).

Clinical Findings: In dogs, signs of intoxication may include vomiting, bradycardia, cardiac arrhythmias, poor capillary refill time, hypotension or hypertension, panting, increased upper respiratory sounds, depression, weakness, nervousness, hyperactivity, or shaking. These signs appear within 30 min to 4 hr postexposure. In general, imidazoline decongestant exposure may affect the GI, cardiopulmonary, and nervous systems.

Treatment: Decontamination may not be practical due to the rapid absorption and onset of clinical signs. Heart rate and rhythm and blood pressure should be assessed, and an ECG obtained if needed. IV fluids should be given, along with atropine at 0.02 mg/kg, IV, if bradycardia is present. Diazepam (0.25-0.5 mg/kg, IV) can be given if CNS signs (eg, apprehension, shaking) are present. Serum electrolytes (ie, potassium, sodium, chloride) should be assessed and corrected as needed. Yohimbine, which is a specific α_2-adrenergic antagonist, can also be used at 0.1 mg/kg, IV, and repeated in 2-3 hr if needed.

Pseudoephedrine and Ephedrine

Pseudoephedrine is a sympathomimetic drug, which occurs naturally in plants of the genus *Ephedra*. Pseudoephedrine is a stereoisomer of ephedrine and is available as the hydrochloride or sulfate salt. Ephedrine and pseudoephedrine are common OTC medications used as nasal decongestants; these drugs are not currently affected by the FDA ban on products containing ephedra. Both ephedrine and pseudoephedrine have α- and β-adrenergic agonist effects. The pharmacologic effects of the drugs are due to direct stimulation of adrenergic receptors and the release of norepinephrine.

In humans, pseudoephedrine is rapidly absorbed orally. The onset of action is 15-30 min, with peak effects within 30-60 min. It is incompletely metabolized in the liver. Approximately 90% of the drug is eliminated through the kidneys. Renal excretion is accelerated in acidic urine. Elimination half-life varies between 2-21 hr, depending on urinary pH.

Clinical Findings: Pseudoephedrine and ephedrine overdose can result in mydriasis, tachycardia, hypertension, sinus arrhythmias, agitation, anxiety, hyperactivity, tremors, head bobbing, hiding, and vomiting. Clinical signs can be seen at 5-6 mg/kg and death may occur at 10-12 mg/kg.

Treatment: Treatment of pseudoephedrine toxicosis consists of decontamination, controlling the CNS and cardiovascular effects, and supportive care. Vomiting should be induced, followed by administration of activated charcoal with a cathartic. If the animal's condition contraindicates induction of emesis, a gastric lavage with a cuffed endotracheal tube should be performed. Hyperactivity, nervousness, or seizures can be controlled with acepromazine (0.05-1.0 mg/kg, IM, IV, or SC), chlorpromazine (0.5-1.0 mg/kg, IV), phenobarbital (3-4 mg/kg, IV), or pentobarbital to effect. Diazepam should be avoided as it can exaggerate hyperactivity. Phenothiazines should be used with caution as they can lower the seizure threshold, lower blood pressure, and cause bizarre behavioral changes. Tachycardia can be controlled with propranolol at 0.02-0.04 mg/kg, IV, repeated if needed. IV fluids should be given. Acidifying the urine with ammonium chloride (50 mg/kg, PO, QID) or ascorbic acid (20-30 mg/kg, IM or IV, TID) may enhance urinary excretion of pseudoephedrine. Acid-base status should be monitored if ammonium chloride or ascorbic acid is given. Electrolytes, heart rate and rhythm, and blood pressure should be monitored. Excessive trembling or shaking can cause myoglobinuria; if this occurs, kidney function should be monitored. Clinical signs of toxicosis can last 1-4 days. The presence of pseudoephedrine in urine can support the diagnosis.

ANALGESICS

Nonsteroidal Anti-inflammatory Drugs (NSAID)

NSAID are the most commonly used class of human medications in the world. Due to their widespread availability and use, acute accidental ingestion of human NSAID in dogs and cats is quite common. Ibuprofen, aspirin, and naproxen are some of the most commonly encountered NSAID in pet animals.

NSAID inhibit the enzyme cyclooxygenase (COX; also referred to as prostaglandin synthetase), blocking the production of prostaglandins (PG). It is believed that most NSAID act through COX inhibition, although they may also have other mechanisms of action. (See also NONSTEROIDAL ANTI-INFLAMMATORY DRUGS, p 2131.)

Ibuprofen, 2-(4-isobutylphenyl) propionic acid, is used for its anti-inflammatory, antipyretic, and analgesic properties in animals and humans. It is rapidly absorbed orally in dogs with peak plasma concentrations seen in 30 min to 3 hr. Presence of food can delay absorption and the time to reach peak plasma concentration. The mean elimination half-life is ~4.6 hr. Ibuprofen is metabolized in the liver to several metabolites, which are mainly excreted in the urine within 24 hr. The major metabolic pathway is via conjugation with glucuronic acid, sometimes preceded by oxidation and hydroxylation.

Ibuprofen has been recommended in dogs at 5 mg/kg. However, prolonged use at this dosage may cause gastric ulcers and perforations. GI irritation or ulceration, GI hemorrhage, and renal damage are the most commonly reported toxic effects of ibuprofen ingestion in dogs. In addition, CNS depression, hypotension, ataxia, cardiac effects, and seizures can be seen. Ibuprofen has a narrow margin of safety in dogs. Dogs dosed with ibuprofen at 8-16 mg/kg/day, PO for 30 days showed gastric ulceration or erosions, along with other clinical signs of GI disturbances. An acute single ingestion of 100-125 mg/kg can lead to vomiting, diarrhea, nausea, abdominal pain, and anorexia. Renal failure may follow dosages of 175-300 mg/kg. CNS effects (ie, seizures, ataxia, depression, coma) in addition to renal and GI signs can be seen at dosages >400 mg/kg. Dosages >600 mg/kg are potentially lethal in dogs.

Cats are susceptible to ibuprofen toxicosis at approximately half the dosage required to cause toxicosis in dogs. Cats are especially sensitive because they have a limited glucuronyl-conjugating capacity. Ibuprofen toxicity is more severe in ferrets than in dogs that consume similar dosages. Typical toxic effects of ibuprofen in ferrets involve the CNS, GI, and renal systems.

Aspirin (acetylsalicylic acid), the salicylate ester of acetic acid, is the prototype of salicylate drugs. It is a weak acid derived from phenol. The oral bioavailability of aspirin may vary due to differences in drug formulation. Aspirin reduces prostaglandin and thromboxane synthesis by COX inhibition. Salicylates also uncouple mitochondrial oxidative phosphorylation and inhibit specific dehydrogenases. Platelets are incapable of synthesizing new cyclooxygenase, leading to an effect on platelet aggregation.

Aspirin is rapidly absorbed from the stomach and proximal small intestine in monogastric animals. The rate of absorption depends on gastric emptying, tablet disintegration rates, and gastric pH. Peak salicylate levels are reached 0.5-3 hr after ingestion. Topically applied salicylic acid can be absorbed systemically.

Aspirin is hydrolyzed to salicylic acid by esterases in the liver and, to a lesser extent, in the GI mucosa, plasma, RBC, and synovial fluid. Salicylic acid is 50-70% protein bound, especially to albumin. Salicylic acid readily distributes to extracellular fluids and to the kidneys, liver, lungs, and heart. Salicylic acid is eliminated by hepatic conjugation with glucuronide and glycine. Renal clearance is enhanced by an alkaline urinary pH. There are significant differences in the elimination and biotransformation of salicylates among different species. Plasma half-lives vary from 1-37.6 hr in animals.

Aspirin toxicosis is usually characterized by depression, fever, hyperpnea, seizures, respiratory alkalosis, metabolic acidosis, coma, gastric irritation or ulceration, liver necrosis, or increased bleeding time. Seizures may occur as a consequence of severe intoxication, although the exact etiology is unknown.

Cats are deficient in glucuronyl transferase and have a prolonged excretion of aspirin (the half-life in cats is 37.5 hr). No clinical signs of toxicosis occurred when cats were given 25 mg/kg of aspirin every 48 hr for up to 4 wk. Dosages of 5 grains (325 mg), BID, can be lethal to cats.

Dogs tolerate aspirin better than cats; however, prolonged use can lead to the development of gastric ulcers. Dosages of 25 mg/kg, TID, of regular aspirin have caused mucosal erosions in 50% of dogs after 2 days. Gastric ulcers were seen by day 30 in 66% of dogs given aspirin at 35 mg/kg, PO, TID. Similarly, 43% of dogs given aspirin at 50 mg/kg, PO, BID, showed gastric ulcers after 5-6 wk of dosing. Acute ingestion of 450-500 mg/kg can cause GI disturbances, hyperthermia, panting, seizures, or coma. Alkalosis due to stimulation of the respiratory center can occur early in the course of intoxication. Metabolic acidosis with an elevated anion gap usually develops later.

Naproxen, a propionic acid-derivative NSAID is available OTC as an acid or the sodium salt. It is available as 200-550 mg tablets or gelcaps or as a suspension (125 mg/5 mL). Structurally and pharmacologically, naproxen is similar to carprofen and ibuprofen. In humans and dogs, it is used for its anti-inflammatory, analgesic, and antipyretic properties.

Oral absorption of naproxen in dogs is rapid, with peak plasma concentration reached in 0.5-3 hr. The reported elimination half-life in dogs is 34-72 hr. Naproxen is highly protein bound (>99.0%). In dogs, naproxen is primarily eliminated through the bile, whereas in other species, the primary route of elimination is through the kidneys. The long half-life of naproxen in dogs appears to be due to its extensive enterohepatic recirculation.

Several cases of naproxen toxicosis in dogs have been described. Dosages of 5.6-11.1 mg/kg, PO, for 3-7 days have caused melena, frequent vomiting, abdominal pain, perforating duodenal ulcer, weakness, stumbling, pale mucous membranes, regenerative anemia, neutrophilia with a left shift, increased BUN and creatinine, and decreased total protein. Acute toxicity from a single oral dose has been described at 35 mg/kg. Cats may be more sensitive to naproxen toxicity than dogs due to their limited glucuronyl-conjugating capacity.

Acetaminophen is a synthetic nonopiate derivative of p-aminophenol widely used in humans for its antipyretic and analgesic properties. Its use has largely replaced salicylates due to the reduced risk of gastric ulceration.

Acetaminophen is rapidly absorbed from the GI tract. Peak plasma concentrations are usually seen within an hour, but can be delayed with extended-release formulations. It is uniformly distributed into most body tissues. Protein binding varies from 5-20%. The metabolism of acetaminophen involves 2 major conjugation pathways in most species. Both involve cytochrome P-450 metabolism, followed by glucuronidation or sulfation.

Cats are more sensitive to acetaminophen toxicosis because they are deficient in glucuronyl transferase and therefore have limited capacity to glucuronidate this drug. In cats, acetaminophen is primarily metabolized via sulfation; when this pathway is saturated, toxic metabolites are produced. In dogs, signs of acute toxicity are usually not observed unless the dosage of acetaminophen exceeds 100 mg/kg. Clinical signs of methemoglobinemia have been reported in 3 out of 4 dogs at 200 mg/kg. Toxicity can be seen at lower dosages with repeated exposures. In cats, toxicity can occur with 10-40 mg/kg.

Methemoglobinemia and hepatotoxicity characterize acetaminophen toxicosis. Renal injury is also possible. Cats primarily develop methemoglobinemia within a few hours, followed by Heinz body formation. Methemoglobinemia makes mucous membranes brown or muddy in color, and is usually accompanied by tachycardia, hyperpnea, weakness, and lethargy. Other clinical signs of acetaminophen toxicity include depression, weakness, hyperventilation, icterus, vomiting, hypothermia, facial or paw edema, cyanosis, dyspnea, hepatic necrosis, and death. Liver necrosis is more common in dogs than in cats. Liver damage in dogs is usually seen 24-36 hr after ingestion. Centrilobular necrosis is the most common form of hepatic necrosis seen with acetaminophen toxicity.

Treatment: Treatment of NSAID toxicosis consists of early decontamination, protection of the GI tract and kidneys, and supportive care. Vomiting should be induced in recent exposures, followed by administration of activated charcoal with a cathartic. Activated charcoal can be repeated in 6-8 hr to prevent NSAID reabsorption from enterohepatic recirculation. Use of H_2-receptor antagonists (ranitidine, famotidine, cimetidine) may not prevent GI ulcers but can be useful in treating them. Omeprazole, which is a proton pump inhibitor used for inhibiting gastric acid secretions, can be used instead of an H_2-blocker at 0.5-1.0 mg/kg, PO, SID, in dogs. Sucralfate (dog: 0.5-1 g, PO, BID-TID; cat: 0.25-0.5 tablet, PO, BID-TID) reacts with hydrochloric acid in the stomach and forms a paste-like complex that binds to the proteins in ulcers and protects them from further damage. Because sucralfate requires an acidic environment, it should be given ≥30 min before administering H_2 antagonists. Misoprostol (dog: 1-3 µg/kg, PO, TID) has recently been shown to prevent GI ulceration when used concomitantly with aspirin and other NSAID.

IV fluids should be given at a diuretic rate if the potential for renal damage exists. Alkalinization of the urine with sodium bicarbonate results in ion trapping of salicylates in kidney tubules and can increase their excretion. However, ion trapping should be used judiciously and only in cases where the acid-base balance can be monitored closely. Baseline renal function should be monitored and rechecked at 48 and 72 hr. Prognosis depends on the dose ingested and how soon the animal receives treatment following exposure.

Treatment of Acetaminophen Toxicity: The objectives of treating acetaminophen toxicosis are early decontamination, prevention or treatment of methemoglobinemia and hepatic damage, and provision of supportive care. Induction of emesis is useful when performed early. This should be followed by administration of activated charcoal with a cathartic. Activated charcoal may be repeated because acetaminophen undergoes some enterohepatic recirculation. Administration of N-acetylcysteine (NAC), a sulfur-containing amino acid, can reduce the extent of liver injury or methemoglobinemia. NAC provides sulfhydryl groups, directly binds with acetaminophen metabolites to enhance their elimination, and serves as a glutathione precursor. It is available as a 10% or 20%

2530 ■ TOXICITIES FROM HUMAN DRUGS

solution. The loading dose is 140 mg/kg of a 5% solution IV or PO (diluted in 5% dextrose or sterile water), followed by 70 mg/kg, PO, QID for generally 7 more treatments. Vomiting can occur with oral NAC. NAC is not labeled for IV use; however, it can be administered as a slow IV (over 15-20 min) with a 0.2 micron bacteriostatic filter. Activated charcoal and oral NAC should be administered 2 hr apart as activated charcoal could adsorb NAC. Liver enzymes should be monitored and rechecked at 24 and 48 hr. The animal should also be monitored for methemoglobinemia, Heinz body anemia, and hemolysis. Fluids and blood transfusions should be given as needed. Ascorbic acid (30 mg/kg, PO or injectable, BID-QID) may further reduce methemoglobin levels. Cimetidine (5-10 mg/kg, PO, IM, or IV), a cytochrome P-450 inhibitor, may help reduce formation of toxic metabolites and prevent liver damage.

GASTROINTESTINAL DRUGS

H₂-Receptor Antagonists

H_2-receptor antagonists are structural analogs of histamine, commonly used to treat GI ulcers, erosive gastritis, esophagitis, and gastric reflux. They act at the H_2 receptors of parietal cells to competitively inhibit histamine, reducing gastric acid secretions during basal conditions and when stimulated by food, amino acids, pentagastrin, histamine, or insulin. Cimetidine, famotidine, and ranitidine are examples of this group, also commonly referred to as H_2 blockers. These drugs are rapidly absorbed, reaching peak plasma concentrations within 1-3 hr. Ranitidine is widely distributed throughout the body. H_2 blockers are primarily metabolized in the liver. Famotidine and ranitidine are excreted in the urine as metabolites and unchanged drug, while cimetidine is eliminated in feces. The elimination half-life for all 3 drugs is ~2.2 hr in dogs. Because cimetidine may inhibit the hepatic microsomal enzyme system, ingestion of an H_2 blocker may result in reduced metabolism of certain drugs, including β blockers, calcium channel blockers, diazepam, metronidazole, and theophylline.

H_2 blockers have a wide margin of safety, with acute oral overdoses typically resulting in minor effects such as vomiting, diarrhea, anorexia, and dry mouth. Serious adverse effects, such as tremors, hypotension, and bradycardia, are more likely to occur with IV H_2-blocker overdoses. The minimum lethal dose of famotidine in dogs is >2 g/kg, PO, and 300 mg/kg, IV. Most exposures require only monitoring and supportive care, although massive overdoses may also warrant decontamination.

Antacids

Antacids come in pill and liquid forms, and are frequently used to treat GI upset. Common antacids include calcium carbonate, aluminum hydroxide, and magnesium hydroxide (milk of magnesia). These agents are poorly absorbed orally. Calcium- and aluminum-containing antacids generally cause constipation, while magnesium-containing antacids tend to cause diarrhea. Some products contain both aluminum and magnesium salts in an attempt to balance their constipating and laxative effects. Acute single ingestion of calcium salts may cause transient hypercalcemia, but is unlikely to be associated with significant systemic effects. Induction of emesis within 2-3 hr of exposure may be helpful in preventing severe GI upset.

Multivitamins and Iron

The common ingredients in multivitamins include: ascorbic acid (vitamin C), cyanocobalamin (vitamin B_{12}), folic acid, thiamine (vitamin B_1), riboflavin (vitamin B_2), niacin (vitamin B_3), biotin, pantothenic acid, pyridoxine (vitamin B_6), calcium, phosphorus, iodine, iron, magnesium, copper, zinc, and vitamins A, D, and E. Among these ingredients, iron and vitamins A and D may cause significant systemic signs. Acute ingestion of other listed ingredients in companion animals can result in self-limiting GI upset (eg, vomiting, diarrhea, anorexia, lethargy). However, toxicity is typically rare in pets.

Multivitamin preparations contain varying amounts of **iron**. Unless otherwise listed, iron should be assumed to be elemental iron. Various iron salts may contain 12-48% elemental iron. Iron has direct caustic or irritant effects on the GI mucosa. It can also be a direct mitochondrial poison. Once the iron-carrying capacity of serum has been exceeded, free iron is deposited in the liver where it damages mitochondria, leading to necrosis of periportal hepatocytes. Signs of iron toxicosis usually develop within 6 hr. Initial vomiting and diarrhea, with or without blood, may be followed by hypovolemic shock, depression, fever, acidosis, and liver failure 12-24 hr later, often with a period of apparent recovery in between. Oliguria and anuria secondary to shock-induced renal failure may also occur. Ingestion of >20 mg/kg of elemental iron generally warrants decontamination and administration of GI protectants. Additional treatment and monitoring will be necessary for patients that have ingested >60 mg/kg of elemental iron. Milk of magnesia can complex with iron to decrease its absorption from the GI tract. Serum iron levels and the total iron binding capacity should be checked at 3 hr and again at 8-10 hr post-exposure. If serum iron is >300 µg/dL, or greater than the total iron binding capacity, chelation therapy may be needed. Desferoxamine (40 mg/kg, IM, every 4-8 hr) is a specific iron chelator and is most effective within the first 24 hr post-ingestion, before iron has been distributed from blood to tissues. Other signs should be treated symptomatically.

Even though **vitamin A** toxicity following consumption of large amounts of fish oil or bear's liver has been well documented, it is less likely to occur following acute ingestion of multivitamins. The amount of vitamin A needed to cause toxic effects is 10-1,000 times the dietary requirements for most species. The vitamin A requirement for cats is 10,000 IU/kg of diet fed, with levels up to 100,000 IU/kg of diet considered to be safe. For dogs, the requirement is 3,333 IU/kg of diet fed, with up to 333,300 IU/kg of diet considered to be safe. Signs associated with acute vitamin A toxicity include general malaise, anorexia, nausea, peeling skin, weakness, tremors, convulsions, paralysis, and death.

Vitamin D is included in many calcium supplements to aid the absorption of the calcium. Most vitamins contain cholecalciferol (vitamin D_3). After consumption, cholecalciferol is converted into 25-hydroxycholecalciferol (calcifediol) in the liver, which is subsequently converted to the active metabolite 1,25-dihydroxycholecalciferol (calcitriol) in the kidneys. One IU of vitamin D_3 is equivalent to 0.025 µg of cholecalciferol. Even though the oral LD_{50} of cholecalciferol in dogs has been reported as 88 mg/kg, signs have been seen at dosages as low as 0.5 mg/kg. Vomiting, depression, polyuria, polydipsia, and hyperphosphatemia may be seen within 12 hr of a significant vitamin D exposure, followed by hypercalcemia and acute renal failure 24-48 hr post-exposure. In addition to renal failure, the kidneys, heart, and GI tract may show signs of necrosis and mineralization. Initial treatment should include decontamination and assessment of baseline calcium, phosphorus, BUN, and creatinine. Multiple doses of activated charcoal with a cathartic should be administered. If clinical signs of toxicosis develop, treatment consists of saline diuresis and the use of furosemide, corticosteroids, and phosphate binders. Specific agents such as (salmon) calcitonin or pamidronate may be needed for patients that remain hypercalcemic despite symptomatic treatment. Stabilization of serum calcium may require days of treatment due to the long half-life of calcifediol (16-30 days).

TOPICAL PREPARATIONS

Zinc Oxide

Zinc oxide ointments or creams are commonly used as topical skin protectants, astringents, and bactericidal agents. Most ointments contain 10-40% zinc oxide. Ingestion of zinc oxide-containing products usually results in gastric irritation (vomiting) and diarrhea, without the intravascular hemolysis, and liver and renal damage associated with elemental zinc ingestion. Signs are usually seen within 2-4 hr of a significant exposure. Vomiting animals should be managed symptomatically and supportively.

NUTRITIONAL SUPPLEMENTS

Ma Huang (Ephedrine) and Guarana (Caffeine)

Several herbal supplements, sold with the claim of providing weight loss and energy, contain guarana (*Paullinia cupana*), a natural source of caffeine, and ma huang (*Ephedra sinica*), a natural source of ephedrine. In humans, use of herbal supplements containing guarana and ma huang have been linked to acute hepatitis, nephrolithiasis, hypersensitivity myocarditis, and sudden death. In dogs, accidental ingestion of herbal supplements containing ma huang and guarana can have synergistic effects when ingested together and can lead to severe hyperactivity, tremors, seizures, vomiting, tachycardia, hyperthermia, and death within a few hours of exposure. The use of ephedra-containing supplements has recently been banned by the FDA. For treatment, *see* PSEUDOEPHEDRINE AND EPHEDRINE, p 2526.

5-Hydroxytryptophan

Several OTC herbal supplements containing 5-hydroxytryptophan (5-HTP) or *Griffonia* seed extracts claim to treat depression, headaches, insomnia, and obesity. Orally, 5-HTP is rapidly absorbed and constitutively converted to serotonin (5-hydroxytryptamine). In cases of 5-HTP overdose, excessive concentrations of serotonin at target cells (GI, CNS, cardiovascular, and respiratory systems) can lead to a serotonin-like syndrome in dogs (eg, seizures, depression, tremors, ataxia, vomiting, diarrhea, hyperthermia, transient blindness, and death). Clinical signs can develop within 4 hr after ingestion and last up to 36 hr. Treatment consists of early decontamination, control of CNS signs (diazepam, barbiturates), thermoregulation (cool water bath, fans), fluid therapy, and administration of a serotonin antagonist such as cyproheptadine (1.1 mg/kg, PO or rectally).

TOXICITIES FROM PRESCRIPTION DRUGS

Pets commonly ingest prescription medications, from countertops, pill minders, mail-order packages, or other sources. Veterinarians can prescribe certain human drugs in animals. Safety data for human prescription drugs in certain animals species may not be available, as most are not approved for veterinary use by the FDA. A valid client-patient-veterinarian relationship must exist for veterinarians to recommend extra-label use of human prescription medications to their clients.

CARDIOVASCULAR MEDICATIONS

See also SYSTEMIC PHARMACOTHERAPEUTICS OF THE CARDIOVASCULAR SYSTEM, p 1966.

Angiotensin-converting Enzyme (ACE) Inhibitors

Several ACE inhibitors (eg, enalapril, captopril, lisinopril) are used therapeutically in dogs and cats. The primary concern in cases of acute ACE inhibitor overdose is usually marked hypotension. If hypotension is severe, secondary renal damage may result. Onset occurs within a few hours of exposure, depending on the agent (extended-release formulations may have a delayed onset of action). Other clinical signs of overdose may include vomiting, poor mucous membrane color, weakness, and tachycardia or bradycardia. Activated charcoal is effective in binding the drug from the GI tract if administered within 1-2 hr of ingestion. Blood pressure should be monitored and IV fluids given at twice the maintenance rate if hypotension develops. Renal function should be monitored if severe or persistent hypotension develops.

Calcium Channel Blockers

Calcium channel blockers (eg, diltiazem, amlodipine, verapamil) inhibit movement of calcium from extracellular sites through cell membrane-based calcium channels. The most common signs seen with overdoses of calcium channel blockers are hypotension, bradycardia, GI upset, and heart block. Reflex tachycardia may develop in response to the drop in blood pressure.

Management of an acute overdose includes correcting hypotension and rhythm disturbances. In general, emesis is not recommended unless induced within minutes of witnessed ingestion—the increased vagal tone can worsen the bradycardia. Activated charcoal binds unabsorbed drug in the GI tract and is most useful in the first 1-2 hr after ingestion; if a sustained-release product was ingested, repeat doses of activated charcoal every 4-6 hr for a total of 2-4 doses can provide additional benefit. Specific therapies should be instituted based on blood pressure, heart rate, ECG, and blood chemistry profiles. IV fluids are recommended; calcium gluconate should be added if chemistries reveal hypocalcemia. Atropine (0.02-0.04 mg/kg) can be given for bradycardia; isoproterenol can be used if the ECG indicates atrioventricular block. For persistent hypotension not corrected by administration of IV fluids, dopamine (1-20 μg/kg/min) or dobutamine (2-20 μg/kg/min) can be given via continuous IV infusion. Calcium channel blockers may interact with almost any other cardioactive medication, resulting in more profound bradycardia, hypotension, and depression of cardiac contractility.

β Blockers

Drugs in this class (eg, propanolol, atenolol, timolol) act by competitively inhibiting catecholamine binding to β-adrenergic receptor sites. The most common signs of overdose are bradycardia and hypotension; respiratory depression, coma, seizures, hyperkalemia, and hypoglycemia may occur. It is also possible to precipitate congestive heart failure. Significant clinical signs may arise even at therapeutic (published) doses—no approved veterinary products are on the market.

Because of rapid absorption, emesis should only be induced within minutes of ingestion. Administration of activated charcoal should be considered if either multiple tablets or capsules or sustained-release formulation tablets are ingested. Heart rate and clinical condition should be monitored for at least 2-4 hr for the development of signs. If clinical signs do develop, blood chemistries should also be measured. Hypotension should be treated with IV fluids; atropine can be used for bradycardia. If hyperkalemia is confirmed, administration of insulin, followed by IV glucose, may drive the excess potassium back into the cells.

Diuretics

Oral diuretic agents include thiazides (eg, chlorothiazide, hydrochlorothiazide), loop diuretics such as furosemide, and potassium-sparing agents such as spironolactone (an aldosterone antagonist) and triamterene. Osmotic diuretics, administered by injection, include mannitol and urea. The most common signs of diuretic overdose include vomiting, depression, polyuria, polydipsia, and electrolyte changes. Electrolytes, especially potassium, may shift subsequent to a very large ingestion of a diuretic. Management should include monitoring hydration and electrolytes, with correction as needed.

TRANQUILIZERS, ANTIDEPRESSANTS, SLEEP AIDS, AND ANTICONVULSANTS

See also SYSTEMIC PHARMACOTHERAPEUTICS OF THE NERVOUS SYSTEM, p 2019.

Benzodiazepines

These drugs bind γ-aminobutyric acid (inhibitory neurotransmitter) receptors and are used for seizure control and as anxiolytics. While diazepam is probably best known in the veterinary field, alprazolam, chlordiazepoxide, clonazepam, lorazepam, oxazepam, and triazolam are all commonly prescribed medications. In general, all are rapidly and fairly completely absorbed, lipophilic, and highly protein bound. Metabolism is mostly by glucuronidation, so cats may be more sensitive to adverse effects. Several have active metabolites (eg, diazepam, clorazepate) and consequently have much longer duration of signs. The most common signs seen, at a wide range of dosages, are CNS depression, respiratory depression, ataxia, weakness, disorientation, nausea, and vomiting. Some animals, especially at high doses, may show CNS excitation instead of depression (paradoxical reaction), which may be followed by CNS depression. Other common signs are hypothermia, hypotension, tachycardia, muscle hypotonia, and meiosis.

Emesis can be induced if ingestion is recent and no clinical signs are present. Gastric lavage, followed by administration of activated charcoal can be performed if the ingested amount is very high. The patient should be kept warm and quiet and closely monitored for responsiveness to stimuli and adequate breathing. IV fluids will help support blood pressure. If severe respiratory depression develops, the reversal agent flumazenil can be given at a dose of 0.01 mg/kg, slow IV, in both cats and dogs. Flumazenil has a short half-life, so it may need to be repeated. Benzodiazepines should not be used to control CNS excitation due to a paradoxical reaction. In such situations, low doses of barbiturates may be useful to control initial CNS excitation.

Antidepressants

Antidepressants fall into several classes. An overdose of almost any of them can result in development of serotonin syndrome (*see* below).

Selective Serotonin Reuptake Inhibitors: This group of antidepressant agents include sertraline, fluoxetine, paroxetine, and fluvoxamine. They block the activity of serotonin receptors at presynaptic membranes and have little effect on other neurotransmitters.

Tricyclic Antidepressants: These antidepressants (eg, amitriptyline, clomipramine, nortriptyline) are commonly used psychoactive agents. They are structurally similar to the phenothiazines, with a similar anticholinergic, adrenergic, and α-blocking properties. Following absorption, these agents are extensively bound to plasma proteins and also bind to tissue and cellular sites, including the mitochondria. Cyclic antidepressants block the amine pump and stop neuronal reuptake of norepinephrine, serotonin, and dopamine. These agents also appear to have a slight α-adrenergic blocking effect. Tricyclics may exert their major toxicity via a nonspecific membrane-stabilizing effect, similar to chlorpromazine and the β-blockers. Tricyclics also have central and peripheral anticholinergic activity, along with antihistaminic effects. Clinical signs of toxicosis include CNS stimulation (agitation, confusion, pyrexia), cardiac arrythmias, hypertension, myoclonus, nystagmus, seizures, metabolic acidosis, urinary retention, dry mouth, mydriasis, and constipation. This may be followed by CNS depression (lethargy), ataxia, hypothermia, respiratory depression, cyanosis, hypotension, and coma.

Treatment: Emesis should be induced in cases of recent exposure if the animal is asymptomatic. This can be followed by activated charcoal (even several hours after ingestion) plus a cathartic such as sorbital or sodium sulfate (magnesium sulfate is contraindicated, as it can add to CNS depression). Diazepam can be given to control seizures. Serotonin syndrome signs should be managed as needed. Heart rate and rhythm should be monitored and cardiac arrythmias treated. Atropine should not be used to control bradycardia as it can aggravate anticholinergic effects of tricyclic antidepressants.

Serotonin Syndrome: This group of clinical signs usually includes 3 of the following features: altered mental status, agitation, myoclonus, hyperreflexia, tremors, diarrhea, incoordination, and fever. It often occurs after overdose or ingestion of substances that result in elevated free levels of serotonin, such as antidepressants or profound stimulants (eg, amphetamines, cocaine, pseudoephedrine, and ephedra). Cyproheptadine is a serotonin antagonist often used for treatment. It is available only as a tablet, but can be dissolved in a small amount of saline and administered per rectum at 1.1 mg/kg in dogs or 2 mg/dose in cats. If there is a good response to the initial dose, it can be repeated if signs recur.

Barbiturates

Both long-acting and short-acting barbiturates may be encountered. The long-acting group includes phenobarbital, mephobarbital, and primadone—all commonly used as anticonvulsants or sedatives. The short-acting (butabarbital, pentobarbital, secobarbital) and ultra short-acting (thiamylal and thiopental) barbiturates are used mainly for induction of anesthesia and seizure control. All are readily absorbed from the gut and have extensive liver metabolism; metabolites are primarily excreted via the kidneys. The onset of clinical signs varies from 15 min to several hours, and duration can be up to several days for the long-acting class. The most common signs are sedation, ataxia, respiratory depression, coma, loss of reflexes, hypotension, and hypothermia.

Management is aimed at life support while attempting to remove unmetabolized drug from the system. Emesis should be induced if the exposure is very recent and the animal is asymptomatic. Gastric lavage while protecting the airway can remove much of the drug still in the stomach. Activated charcoal readily adsorbs barbiturates; small doses repeated every 4-6 hr can further decrease the body burden, even if overdose has resulted from use of an injectable product. IV fluids can be given to support blood pressure. Respiratory effort and effectiveness needs to be closely monitored; treatment may require a respirator. Support for maintaining body temperature may be necessary.

Sleep Aids

Zolpidem and zaleplon are the newest drugs used as sleep aids and have a mechanism of action similar to the benzodiazepines. These agents have a very rapid onset (usually <30 min) and a similarly short half-life. While the expected result from ingestion would be marked sedation, they have been associated with paradoxical excitement. Dosages as low as 0.22 mg/kg have resulted in sedation and ataxia, and dogs have developed tremors, vocalizing, and pacing at dosages as low as 0.6 mg/kg.

GI decontamination can be performed if the ingestion was recent and no signs are seen. For mild signs, keeping the pet quiet and in a safe place may suffice. If paradoxical excitement develops, symptomatic treatment should be given and will vary with the signs and their intensity. Hyperexcitation may be controlled with acepromazine or other phenothiazines. Use of valium may aggravate signs of CNS depression. Flumazenil (0.01 mg/kg, IV) can be used if clinical signs of toxicosis are severe.

Phenothiazine Tranquilizers

The most commonly used phenothiazines in veterinary medicine are acepromazine, chlorpromazine, and promazine. In domestic animals, they are used as tranquilizers, preanesthetic agents, antiemetics, and for the treatment of CNS agitation following specific drug overdoses (amphetamines, cocaine). The most common signs of overdose are sedation, weakness, ataxia, collapse, behavioral changes, hypothermia, hypotension, tachycardia, and bradycardia.

Treatment consists of symptomatic and supportive care. Due to rapid onset of CNS signs, emesis should only be attempted in a recent exposure and should be followed by administration of activated charcoal and a cathartic. Repeated doses of activated charcoal may be helpful, especially for large ingestions. Hypotension should be treated with IV fluids. Dopamine may be used if fluid administration does not correct hypotension. Body temperature, heart rate, and blood pressure should be monitored and treated symptomatically.

MUSCLE RELAXANTS

The most commonly encountered centrally acting muscle relaxants include baclofen and cyclobenzaprine. Baclofen is rapidly absorbed orally. The onset of clinical signs of toxicosis may be <30 min to 2 hr following ingestion. The most common signs of toxicosis are vocalization, salivation, vomiting, ataxia, weakness, tremors, shaking, coma, seizures, bradycardia, hypothermia, and blood pressure abnormalities. Cyclobenzaprine, often used in management of acute muscle spasms, is almost completely absorbed after an oral dose, with peak plasma levels in 3-8 hr. It has extensive liver metabolism and undergoes enterohepatic recirculation. The most common signs seen in both dogs and cats include depression and ataxia.

Treatment of muscle relaxant overdose consists of symptomatic and supportive care. Vomiting should be induced if the exposure is recent and no clinical signs are present, followed by administration of activated charcoal. Respiratory support (ie, ventilator) should be provided if needed. Recumbent or comatose animals should be monitored for hypothemia and aspiration. IV fluids should be given as needed.

TOPICAL AGENTS

There are many topical preparations that pets ingest, often resulting in only mild gastroenteritis. For example, ingestion of most corticosteroid-containing creams or ointments usually results in only mild to moderate stomach upset, polydipsia, and polyphagia. However, ingestion of certain topical agents in pet animals, such as 5-fluorouracil and calcipotriene, can be deadly even at low doses.

5-Fluorouracil

5-Fluorouracil (5-FU) is available as an ointment (1% or 5%) or topical solution (1%, 2%, or 5%). It is used in the treatment of skin cancers and solar keratoses in humans. Most exposures result from accidental ingestion, although occasionally 5-FU is used extra-label in pets. Ingestion in dogs and cats leads to the onset of signs within a few hours. In dogs, signs have been seen at dosages as low as 8.6 mg/kg, with the minimum lethal dose reported as 20 mg/kg. Initial signs include severe vomiting, which may progress to bloody vomiting and diarrhea. Signs often progress to severe tremors, ataxia, and seizures. In cats and dogs, 5-FU may be converted to fluorocitrate and interfere with the Kreb's cycle, which may be one cause of seizures and ataxia. Generally, 5-FU destroys rapidly dividing cells, affecting the GI tract, liver, kidneys, CNS, and bone marrow. The mortality rate among dogs ingesting 5-FU is high.

All 5-FU exposures in pets should be treated aggressively. Treatment consists primarily of symptomatic and supportive care. Emesis should be induced and the animal given activated charcoal and a cathartic if it is asymptomatic and the ingestion has occurred within 1 hr. If the animal is symptomatic (eg, vomiting or seizuring) it should be stabilized first. The GI tract should be protected with sucralfate (1 g in large dogs, 0.5 g in small dogs, PO, TID) and inhibitors of gastric acid secretion such as cimetidine. Diazepam may be used initially to control seizures and tremors, but in severe cases it is usually not effective and other antiseizure medications such as pentobarbital (3-15 mg/kg, IV slowly to effect) or phenobarbital (3-30 mg/kg, slowly IV to effect) can be used. Constant rate infusion using diazepam or barbiturates has been recently shown to be successful in controlling severe seizures. If this also fails to control CNS signs, gas anesthetics (eg, isoflurane) and propofol (4-6 mg/kg, IV or as a continuous drip 0.6 mg/kg/min) can be tried. IV fluids should be given and body temperature monitored. Monitoring electrolytes, serum chemistries (liver-specific enzymes and renal function), and CBC is usually required for ~2 wk. Surviving dogs may show evidence of bone marrow suppression later. For severe neutropenia in dogs, administration of filgrastim or granulocyte colony stimulating factor at 4-6 µg/kg, SC may be useful.

Calcipotriene

Calcipotriene, used to treat psoriasis in humans, is available as an ointment or cream (0.005% or 50 µg/g). Calcipotriene is a novel structural analog of calcitriol (1,25-dihydroxycholecalciferol), the most active metabolite of cholecalciferol (vitamin D_3). Accidental ingestion of 40-60 µg/kg of calcipotriene in dogs has been associated with life-threatening hypercalcemia. Clinical signs usually occur within 24-72 hr of ingestion and include anorexia, vomiting, diarrhea, polyuria, polydipsia, depression, and weakness. Serum calcium is usually elevated within 12-24 hr and may remain above normal for weeks. This is usually accompanied by an increase in serum phosphorous concentration and calcium phosphorous product (Ca × P) and soft tissue mineralization. Acute renal failure as evidenced by elevated BUN and creatinine levels, coma, and death occur in severe or untreated cases.

Treatment of calcipotriene toxicosis involves standard decontamination (emesis induction, administration of activated charcoal and a cathartic) and reduction of serum calcium concentrations by saline diuresis, furosemide, and corticosteroids, with or without salmon calcitonin treatment (see PRINCIPLES OF TREATMENT OF HYPERCALCEMIA, p 448). Recent reports indicate that concurrent use of pamidronate (1.3-2 mg/kg diluted in saline and given IV over 2 hr) in dogs may be a useful adjunctive therapy. Calcipotriene toxicosis cases usually require monitoring of serum calcium, phosphorous, BUN, and creatinine for several days or even weeks. Signs of renal failure are managed with ongoing supportive fluids.

PRESCRIPTION NONSTEROIDAL ANTI-INFLAMMATORY DRUGS

For a general discussion of commonly seen adverse effects and treatment of NSAID toxicosis, *see* NONSTEROIDAL ANTI-INFLAMMATORY DRUGS, p 2527.

Carprofen

Carprofen is a proprionic acid-derived NSAID of the carbazole class approved for the relief of pain and inflammation associated with osteoarthritis and surgery in dogs. Carprofen is well absorbed orally with peak serum levels occurring in 1-3 hr. It is metabolized in the liver primarily via glucuronidation and oxidation. Because cats are deficient in glucuronyl transferase, they are particularly sensitive to toxicosis. Most of the drug is eliminated in the feces, with some enterohepatic recirculation; 10-20% is eliminated in urine. The mean half-life in dogs is ~8 hr after oral dosing. Carprofen seems to be well tolerated by dogs. Like most other NSAID, it has the potential to adversely affect the GI, renal, and hepatic systems. Idiosyncratic hepatocellular toxicosis characterized by hepatocellular necrosis, cholestasis, anorexia, lethargy, icterus, vomiting, increased hepatic enzymes, and hyperbilirubinemia has been reported in dogs following administration of therapeutic (approved) dosages.

Etodolac

Etodolac is an indole acetic acid-derivative NSAID labeled for use in dogs to treat pain and inflammation associated with osteoarthritis. It is rapidly absorbed orally, with peak serum concentrations seen 2 hr after dosing. It is primarily eliminated through the bile. The elimination half-life is 8-12 hr. Etodolac appears to be well tolerated by dogs when used at the labeled dosage (10-15 mg/kg, PO, SID) for 1 yr. With multiple doses, clinical signs of toxicity such as GI ulcers, vomiting, diarrhea, and weight loss can be seen at 40 mg/kg. Six of 8 dogs died or became moribund due to GI ulceration at 80 mg/kg.

Deracoxib

Deracoxib has been recently approved for control of inflammation and pain associated with osteoarthritis and postoperative pain and inflammation associated with orthopedic surgery in dogs. The approved oral dose of deracoxib for the control of pain and inflammation is 1-2 mg/kg/day; the dose for postoperative orthopedic pain is 3-4 mg/kg/day, not to exceed 7 days of administration. Deracoxib is well absorbed orally. It is extensively metabolized in the liver. The majority of the parent drug and its metabolites are eliminated through the bile, with a plasma elimination half-life of ~3 hr. Deracoxib administration to healthy young dogs at 10 mg/kg for 14 days resulted in erosions and ulcers in the jejunum. At 25, 50, and 100 mg/kg for 14 days, weight loss, vomiting, and melena occurred. In a 6-mo study, dose-dependent focal renal tubular degeneration and regeneration was seen in some dogs at 6, 8, and 10 mg/kg.

TOXICITIES FROM ILLICIT AND ABUSED DRUGS

Exposures to illicit or abused drugs in pet animals can be accidental, intentional, or malicious. Occasionally, drug-sniffing dogs also ingest these substances. Due to the illegal nature of illicit or abused drugs, owners may provide inaccurate, incomplete, or misleading exposure histories. Illicit drugs are often adulterated with other pharmacologically active substances, making the diagnosis even more difficult.

In suspected cases of illicit or abused drug exposure, an attempt should be made to gather information about the animal's environment; amount of exposure; and the onset time of clinical signs and their type, severity, and duration. These questions will help include or exclude possible exposure to an illicit or abused drug. Illicit and abused drugs are often known by street names that vary from area to area. A call to a local police station, or animal or human poison control center, can be extremely helpful in identifying the illicit substance. Most human hospitals, emergency clinics, or veterinary diagnostic laboratories have illicit drug screens available and can check for the presence of illicit drugs or their metabolites in different body fluids. The presence of a parent drug or its metabolites in blood or urine may help confirm the exposure in suspect cases. Veterinarians should contact these laboratories for the types of samples needed and time required for completion.

Commonly available over-the-counter drug test kits may be helpful in ruling out a suspected case of illicit drug toxicosis. These test kits are inexpensive, efficient, and easy to use. They are designed to detect drug metabolites in the urine and can detect most commonly available illicit or recreational drugs such as amphetamines, cocaine, marijuana, opiates, and barbiturates. The sensitivities and specificities of these test kits may vary. The instructions provided with each kit should be followed carefully for best results.

Cocaine

Cocaine (benzoyl-methylecgonine) alkaloid is obtained from the leaves of the coca plant, *Erythroxylon coca* and *E monogymnum*. Some common street names for cocaine are coke, gold dust, stardust, snow, "C", white girl, white lady, baseball, and speedball (cocaine and heroin). Cocaine alkaloid from coca leaves is processed into cocaine hydrochloride salt. The salt is not suitable for smoking because heat decomposes it. The salt is then reprocessed to form cocaine alkaloid or free base (a process called freebasing or base balling), which is colorless, odorless, transparent, and more heat stable. Free base cocaine is also called crack, rock, or flake. Cocaine is cut (diluted) several times before it reaches the user. Xanthine alkaloids, local anesthetics, and decongestants are some of the most common adulterants.

Cocaine is a schedule II drug approved for human use. Its medical uses are restricted to topical administration as a local anesthetic on mucous membranes of the oral, laryngeal, and nasal cavities. Mostly, it is used as a recreational drug.

Pharmacokinetics and Toxicity: Cocaine is absorbed from most routes. Orally, it is better absorbed in an alkaline medium (ie, intestine). In humans, ~20% of an oral dose is absorbed. The reported plasma half-life is 0.9-2.8 hr. Cocaine is extensively metabolized by liver and plasma cholinesterases to several inactive metabolites that are primarily excreted in the urine. The acute LD_{50} of IV-administered cocaine hydrochloride in dogs is 13 mg/kg; the LD_{100} in dogs and cats is 12 mg/kg and 15 mg/kg, respectively. The oral LD_{50} in dogs is believed to be 2-4 times more than the IV dose.

Pathogenesis: Cocaine acts on the sympathetic division of the autonomic nervous system. It blocks the reuptake of dopamine and norepinephrine in the CNS leading to feelings of euphoria, restlessness, and increased motor activity. Cocaine can also decrease concentrations of serotonin or its metabolites. Topical use of cocaine causes vasoconstriction of small vessels. Hyperthermia in cocaine toxicosis may develop either due to increased heat production from muscular activity or due to decreased heat loss from vasoconstriction.

Clinical Findings and Diagnosis: Hyperactivity, shaking, ataxia, panting, agitation, nervousness, seizures, tachycardia, acidosis, or hyperthermia characterize cocaine toxicosis. CNS depression and coma may follow CNS excitation. Death may be due to hyperthermia, cardiac arrest, or respiratory arrest.

Diagnosis is based on a history of exposure and the presence of characteristic clinical signs. Identification of cocaine in plasma, stomach contents, or urine can confirm exposure. Differential diagnoses include amphetamines, pseudoephedrine, ephedrine, caffeine, chocolate, metaldehyde, strychnine, tremorgenic mycotoxins, lead, nicotine, permethrin (cats) and other pesticides, and encephalitis.

Treatment: The objectives of treatment are GI decontamination, stabilization of CNS and cardiovascular effects, thermoregulation, and supportive care. Animals with clinical signs should be stabilized first before attempting decontamination. Emesis can be induced in a recent exposure if the animal is asymptomatic and has the ability to guard its airway via a gag reflex. This should be followed by administration of activated charcoal with a cathartic. If the animal's condition contraindicates induction of emesis (eg, presence of CNS signs or extreme tachycardia) a gastric lavage with a cuffed endotracheal tube to reduce the risk of aspiration should be performed. A dose of activated charcoal with a cathartic should be left in the stomach after the lavage.

Controlling the CNS signs may require use of more than one anticonvulsant. Clinical signs of CNS excitation can be controlled with diazepam. However, the effects of diazepam are short-lived and repeated administration may be needed to control signs of CNS excitation. Phenothiazine tranquilizers such as acepromazine (0.05-1.0 mg/kg, IV, IM, or SC) or chlorpromazine (0.5-1.0 mg/kg, IV or IM) usually work well to control the CNS effects. Phenothiazines should be used cautiously as they may lower the seizure threshold. If phenothiazines are ineffective, phenobarbital at 3-4 mg/kg, IV, or pentobarbital, IV to effect, could be used. If CNS signs are uncontrolled from the preceding measures, a gas anesthetic such as isoflurane may be useful.

Blood pressure, heart rate and rhythm, ECG, and body temperature should be monitored frequently and treated as needed. Propranolol at 0.02-0.06 mg/kg, IV, TID-QID or other β-blocking agents can be used to control tachycardia. After stabilization of CNS and cardiovascular effects, IV fluids should be administered and electrolyte changes monitored and corrected as needed. Treatment and monitoring should continue until all clinical signs have resolved.

Amphetamines and Related Drugs

Amphetamines and their derivatives are CNS and cardiovascular system stimulants commonly used in humans for depression of appetite, narcolepsy, attention deficit disorder, Parkinsonism, and some behavior disorders. Some commonly encountered amphetamines or related drugs are benzphetamine, dextroamphetamine, pemoline, methylphenidate, phentermine, diethylpropion, phendimetrazine, methamphetamine, and phenmetrazine. Amphetamines are sold on the street with common names such as speed, bennies, or uppers. Commonly used adulterants are caffeine, ephedrine, or phenylpropanolamine.

Pharmacokinetics and Toxicity: Amphetamines are rapidly absorbed in the GI tract, reaching a peak plasma concentration in 1-2 hr. Sustained-release formulations have a delayed absorption. The plasma half-life of amphetamines depends on the urinary pH. With an alkaline pH, the half-life is 15-30 hr; with an acidic urinary pH the half-life is 8-10 hr. The acute oral LD_{50} of amphetamine in rats and mice is 10-30 mg/kg. In humans, deaths from metamphetamine have been reported at 1.3 mg/kg following ingestion.

Pathogenesis: Amphetamine stimulates the release of norepinephrine, affecting both α- and β-adrenergic receptor sites. Amphetamine also stimulates catecholamine release centrally in the cerebral cortex, medullary respiratory center, and reticular activating system. It increases the amount of catecholamine at nerve endings by increasing release and inhibiting reuptake and metabolism. The neurotransmitters that are affected in the CNS are norepinephrine, dopamine, and serotonin.

Clinical Findings and Diagnosis: Clinical signs of amphetamine and cocaine toxicosis are similar and difficult to differentiate clinically. The only difference may be the longer duration of clinical signs of amphetamine toxicosis due to a longer half-life compared to cocaine. The most commonly reported signs are hyperactivity, aggression, hyperthermia, tremors, ataxia, tachycardia, hypertension, mydriasis, circling, and death.

Diagnosis is as for cocaine (*see* above) and relies mostly on owner knowledge of exposure. Most amphetamines and related drugs or their metabolites are detectable in the stomach contents and urine. They are difficult to detect in plasma unless large amounts have been ingested.

Treatment: Phenothiazines are preferred for controlling CNS signs in amphetamine toxicosis (*see* treatment of cocaine toxicosis, above). Other anticonvulsants, such as diazepam, barbiturates, or isoflurane, may be used if needed. Acidifying the urine with ammonium chloride (25-50 mg/kg/day, PO, QID) or ascorbic acid (20-30 mg/kg, PO, SC, IM, or IV) may enhance amphetamine elimination in the urine. However, this should be done only if acid-base status can be monitored. Heart rate and rhythm, body temperature, and electrolytes should be monitored and treated as needed.

Marijuana (Cannabis)

Marijuana refers to a mixture of cut, dried, and ground flowers, leaves, and stems of the leafy green hemp plant *Cannabis sativa*. The plant grows in most tropical and temperate regions of the world. Marijuana is the principal drug produced from the hemp plant. There are several cannabinoids present in the plant resin but delta-9-tetrahydrocannabinol (THC) is considered the most active and main psychoactive agent. The concentration of THC in marijuana varies between 1-8%. Hashish is the resin extracted from the top of the flowering plant and is higher in THC concentration than marijuana. Street names for marijuana include pot, Mary Jane, hashish, weed, grass, THC, ganja, bhang, and charas. Pure THC is available by prescription under the generic name dronabinol. A synthetic cannabinoid, nabilone, is also available. Marijuana or hashish sold on the streets may be contaminated with phencyclidine, LSD, or other drugs.

Marijuana is a schedule I controlled substance mostly used by people as a recreational drug. It is also used as an antiemetic for chemotherapy patients and to decrease intraocular pressure in glaucoma patients. Some clinicians advocate the use of dronabinol as an appetite stimulant, but the dysphoric effects of this drug outweigh any benefit of appetite stimulation.

Pharmacokinetics and Toxicity: The most common route of exposure is oral. After ingestion, THC goes through a substantial first pass effect. It is metabolized by liver microsomal hydroxylation and nonmicrosomal oxidation. In dogs, the onset of clinical signs occurs within 30-90 min and can last up to 72 hr. THC is highly lipophilic and readily distributes to the brain and other fatty tissues following absorption. The oral LD_{50} of pure THC in rats and mice is 666 mg/kg and 482 mg/kg, respectively. However, clinical effects of marijuana are seen at much lower doses than this.

Pathogenesis: THC is believed to act on a unique receptor in the brain that is selective for cannabinoids and is responsible for the CNS effects. Cannabinoids can enhance the formation of norepinephrine, dopamine, and serotonin. They can also stimulate release of dopamine and enhance γ-aminobutyric acid turnover.

Clinical Findings and Diagnosis: The most common signs of marijuana toxicosis are depression, ataxia, bradycardia, hypothermia, vocalization, hypersalivation, vomiting, diarrhea, urinary incontinence, seizures, and coma.

Diagnosis is based on a history of exposure and typical clinical signs. THC is difficult to detect in body fluids because of the low levels found in the plasma. Urine testing in the early course of exposure may help confirm the diagnosis. Marijuana toxicosis can be confused with ethylene glycol (antifreeze, p 2357) or ivermectin toxicosis; hypoglycemia; or benzodiazepine, barbiturate, or opioid overdose.

Treatment: Treatment consists of supportive care. The animal should be decontaminated if the exposure is recent and there are no contraindications. Comatose animals should be given IV fluids, treated for hypothermia, and rotated frequently to prevent dependent edema or decubital ulceration. Diazepam can be given for sedation or to control seizures. Treatment and monitoring should be maintained until all clinical signs have resolved (up to 72 hr in dogs).

Opiates

The term opiate initially referred to all naturally occurring alkaloids obtained from the sap of the opium poppy (*Papaver somniferum*). Opium sap contains morphine, codeine, and several other alkaloids. Currently, opioid refers to all drugs, natural or synthetic, that have morphine-like actions or actions that are mediated through opioid receptors. Structurally, opioids can be divided into 5 classes. Some of the common agents within each class are: 1) phenanthrenes—morphine, heroin, hydromorphone, oxymorphone, hydrocodone, codeine, and oxycodone; 2) morphinan—butorphanol; 3) diphenylheptanes—methadone and propoxyphene; 4) phenylpiperidines—meperidine, diphenoxylate, fentanyl, loperamide, and profadol; and 5) benzomorphans—pentazocine and buprenorphine. A new synthetic opiate, tramadol, is a derivative of codeine and has become a widely used veterinary analgesic.

Opioids are used primarily for analgesia. In addition, they are also used as cough suppressants and for the treatment of diarrhea. Occasionally, opioids are also used for sedation before surgery and as a supplement to anesthesia.

Pharmacokinetics and Toxicity: Opioids are generally well absorbed following oral, rectal, or parenteral administration. Some more lipophilic opioids are also absorbed through nasal, buccal, respiratory (heroin, fentanyl, buprenorphine), or transdermal (fentanyl) routes. For some opioids, there is variable reduction in bioavailability due to a first pass effect when given orally. Opioids generally undergo hepatic metabolism with some form of conjugation, hydrolysis, oxidation, dealkylation, or glucuronidation. Because cats are deficient in glucuronidation, the half-life of some opioids in cats may be prolonged. Following absorption, opioids are rapidly cleared from blood and stored in kidney, liver, brain, lung, spleen, skeletal muscle, and placental tissue. Most of the opioid metabolites are excreted through the kidneys.

Toxicity of opioids in animals is highly variable. In dogs, 100-200 mg/kg of morphine administered SC or IV is considered lethal. The estimated lethal dose of codeine in adult humans is 7-14 mg/kg. In infants, 2.5 mg of hydrocodone has been lethal.

Pathogenesis: The effects of opioids are due to their interaction with opiate receptors (μ, κ, δ, σ, and ε) that are found in the limbic system, spinal cord, thalamus, hypothalamus, striatum, and midbrain. Opioids may be agonists, mixed agonist-antagonists, or antagonists at these receptors. Agonists bind and activate a receptor, whereas antagonists bind without causing activation.

Clinical Findings: The primary effects of opioids are on the CNS, respiratory, cardiovascular, and GI systems. Commonly reported clinical signs of toxicosis include CNS depression, drowsiness, ataxia, vomiting, seizures, miosis, coma, respiratory depression, hypotension, constipation/defecation, and death. Some animals—especially cats, horses, cattle, or swine—can show CNS excitation instead of CNS depression.

Diagnosis: Diagnosis of opioid toxicosis is based on history of exposure and the types of clinical signs (CNS and respiratory depression) present. Plasma opioid levels are usually not clinically useful. Urine may be used to determine exposure to opioids using some of the over-the-counter illicit drug kits (manufacturer's instructions should be followed). Opioid toxicosis should be differentiated from antifreeze toxicosis, ivermectin, benzodiazepines, barbiturates, marijuana, and hypoglycemia-inducing conditions.

Treatment: Clinical signs can be reversed with the opiate antagonist naloxone. The dosages in different animals are: dog and cat, 0.002-0.04 mg/kg, IV, IM or SC; rabbit and rodent, 0.01-0.1 mg/kg, SC or IP; horse, 0.01-0.02 mg/kg, IV. Administration of naloxone should be repeated as needed because its duration of action may be shorter than the opioid being treated. Animals should be closely monitored for respiratory depression and ventilatory support provided if needed. Other signs should be treated symptomatically.

ZINC TOXICOSIS

Zinc is an essential trace metal that plays an important role in many biologic processes. It is ubiquitous in nature and exists in many forms. The ingestion of some forms leads to creation of toxic zinc salts in the acidic gastric environment. Zinc toxicity has been documented in humans as well as in a wide range of large, small, exotic, and wild animals. It is seen commonly in pet dogs, possibly because of a higher degree of dietary indiscretion and greater levels of exposure to zinc-containing substances. Common sources of zinc include batteries, automotive parts, paints, zinc-oxide creams, herbal supplements, zippers, board-game pieces, screws and nuts on pet carriers, and the coating on galvanized metals such as pipes and cookware. One of the most well known sources of zinc that causes toxicity following ingestion is the USA Lincoln penny. Some pennies minted during 1983, and all pennies minted since, are 97.5% zinc by weight.

Pathogenesis: The low pH in the stomach causes the formation of soluble zinc salts. These are absorbed from the duodenum and rapidly distributed to the liver, kidneys, prostate, muscles, bones, and pancreas. Zinc salts have direct irritant and corrosive effects on tissue, interfere with the metabolism of other ions such as copper, calcium, and iron, and inhibit erythrocyte production and function. The mechanisms by which zinc exerts these toxic effects are not completely understood. The median lethal dose (LD_{50}) of zinc salts in cases of acute toxicity has been reported to be ~100 mg/kg. Also, diets containing high levels of zinc (>2,000 ppm) have been reported to cause chronic zinc toxicosis in large animals.

Clinical Signs and Lesions: Clinical signs vary based on the duration and degree of exposure. Signs progress from anorexia and vomiting to more advanced symptoms such as diarrhea, lethargy, icterus, shock, intravascular hemolysis, hemoglobinuria, cardiac arrhythmias, and seizures. Large animals often show decreases in weight gain and milk production, and lameness has been reported in foals secondary to epiphyseal swelling.

Major histopathologic findings include hepatocellular centrolobular necrosis with hemosiderosis and vacuolar degeneration, renal tubular necrosis with hemoglobin casts, and pancreatic duct necrosis with fibrosis of the interlobular fat.

Diagnosis: Radiodense material is easily seen on radiographs of the GI tract in animals with zinc-containing foreign bodies. Changes in the CBC, chemistry profile, urinalysis, and coagulation profile reflect the degree of toxicity to various organ systems. The hemogram typically reveals a regenerative hemolytic anemia characterized by changes in erythrocyte morphology. The leukogram often shows a neutrophilic leukocytosis secondary to stress, pancreatitis, and a regenerative bone marrow. Serum chemistry changes that are seen secondary to hepatic damage include elevations in bilirubin, the transaminases, and alkaline phosphatase. As zinc accumulates in the pancreas, increases in amylase and lipase can be seen following pancreatitis and pancreatic necrosis. Glomerular damage and renal tubular epithelial necrosis result in elevations in BUN, creatinine, amylase, and urine protein. Hemoglobinuria can be differentiated from hematuria during urinalysis; the urine color will not clear after centrifugation in the presence of hemoglobinuria. Prolongation of prothrombin time and activated partial thromboplastin time can result from toxic effects on the synthesis or function of coagulation factors.

The hematologic and clinical findings in animals with zinc toxicosis are similar to the changes in animals with immune-mediated hemolytic anemia (IMHA). Misdiagnosis of a primary autoimmune disorder can lead to the inappropriate use of immunosuppressive drugs. Zinc toxicosis can cause the direct antiglobulin test (direct Coombs' test) to be positive in the absence of a primary autoimmune disorder. The direct Coombs' test is therefore not reliable when differentiating between zinc intoxication and IMHA.

Definitive diagnosis of zinc poisoning is achieved by measuring zinc levels in blood or other tissue. In dogs and cats, the normal serum zinc level is 0.7-2 µg/mL. Serum samples can be submitted in green-top heparinized tubes or in royal blue-top trace element tubes. Methods for quantifying zinc levels from saliva and hair have not been validated in domestic animals, and measuring zinc in urine is unreliable because elimination of zinc through the kidneys is variable.

Differential diagnoses should include any infectious, toxic, immune-mediated, neoplastic, genetic, or other medical disorder characterized by clinical signs and laboratory test results similar to those seen in cases of zinc toxicity. These include IMHA, hypophosphatemia, splenic torsion, babesiosis, ehrlichiosis, heartworm disease, leptospirosis, hemobartonellosis, feline leukemia infection, hemangiosarcoma, lymphosarcoma, phosphofructokinase or pyruvate-kinase deficiency, and toxicity from acetaminophen, naphthalene, paradichlorobenzene, *Allium*, lead, or copper.

Treatment and Prevention: After stabilizing the animal with fluids, oxygen, and blood products as necessary, removal of the source of zinc as early as possible is paramount. This often requires surgery or endoscopy. Inducing emesis to remove chronic gastric zinc foreign bodies is typically not rewarding because zinc objects often adhere to the gastric mucosa.

Diuresis with a balanced crystalloid solution is indicated to promote renal excretion of zinc and prevent hemoglobinuric nephrosis.

There is debate regarding the necessity of chelation therapy in cases of zinc toxicosis. Animals can recover from zinc intoxication following only supportive care and removal of the source. However, chelation therapy enhances elimination of zinc and thus may accelerate recovery. Calcium disodium ethylenediaminetetraacetate (Ca-EDTA) successfully chelates zinc when given at 100 mg/kg/day IV or SC for 3 days (diluted and divided into 4 doses), but may exacerbate zinc-induced nephrotoxicity. Although they have been used to treat animals with zinc toxicity, D-penicillamine and dimercaprol (British antilewisite) have not been specifically validated for this purpose. Reported doses are 110 mg/kg/day for 7-14 days for D-penicillamine, and 3-6 mg/kg TID for 3-5 days for dimercaprol. Chelation therapy with any of these agents should be monitored with serial serum zinc levels to help determine the appropriate duration of treatment.

If diagnosed early and treated aggressively, the outcome is often favorable for animals with zinc toxicosis. Eliminating sources of zinc from the environment is essential in preventing recurrence.

■ ■ ■

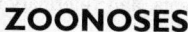

ZOONOSES

The emergence and reemergence of zoonotic diseases present challenges not only to veterinarians, but also to all professions concerned with public health. Since the 19th century, the veterinary profession in the USA has been at the forefront of control and eradication of animal diseases, including bovine pleuropneumonia, foot-and-mouth disease, Texas fever, bovine tuberculosis, brucellosis, vesicular exanthema, and classical swine fever (see TABLE 1). The early cooperation of veterinarians and public health physicians gave impetus to the eradication of bovine tuberculosis first in Denmark, Sweden, Finland, and Norway and then in the USA and Canada. Unfortunately, bovine tuberculosis has emerged in Mexico along the border with the USA and has caused human disease and dairy cow infections from California to Texas. Bovine tuberculosis and brucellosis remain major problems in the developing world.

People with acquired immune deficiency syndrome (AIDS) are much more susceptible, in general, to zoonotic diseases, including tuberculosis and other related mycobacterial infections; toxoplasmosis; cryptosporidial enteritis, foodborne *Salmonella* infections, and other enteric organisms; *Campylobacter*; *Listeria*; and *Yersinia*. It is possible that other zoonotic diseases that are dormant or infrequent (eg, leptospirosis, plague, glanders, melioidosis, and pseudoglanders) may emerge in individuals with AIDS or other immunocompromising conditions. Many of these are latent or nonpathogenic serovars. AIDS-like infections have been described in lions and the tropical cats of Africa as well as in domesticated cats. None have caused human disease.

In Australia and Malaysia, new diseases have been reported in horses and swine that also affect humans. They are caused by a morbillivirus—a measles-like virus related to canine distemper and rinderpest viruses. Another virus killed many wild felids in a zoo in Egypt. Many emerging viral diseases that have a rodent or unknown animal host have caused devastating fatal diseases in humans in Africa and South America, eg, Lassa fever, an arenavirus serologically related to lymphocytic choriomeningitis, and South American hemorrhagic diseases of Argentina and Bolivia. In Africa, Ebola fever and Marburg disease, the latter a dormant monkey disease, have caused death in medical personnel and in patients. Crimean-Congo hemorrhagic fever has caused death in African travelers and in the Middle East in abattoir workers.

The death of veterinarians in the western USA from plague, and reports of serious illness in veterinary technicians and cat owners, has focused attention on both domestic and feral cats and the larger mountain lion or bobcats as carriers of this ancient disease. Dogs and wild canids are likewise involved in plague regions of the USA. The involvement of cats since the 1970s is evidence of the dynamics of zoonotic diseases in a changing environment. Human populations may be pressuring old habitats, or there may be more subtle changes. The plague bacterium (*Yersinia pestis*) may be more adept at finding new hosts or new foci, as seen in other emerging diseases.

Although Lyme borreliosis has been recognized as an important zoonotic disease in North America, other forms of borreliosis have appeared in the USA and abroad for decades.

The Hantaan virus complex was first noted in 1951 in Korea, where it caused a hemorrhagic disease with renal syndrome. Various forms of the disease exist worldwide, and it is a major public health problem in China. In the USA, 2 fatal forms of the disease have been reported, namely, nephritic and pneumonic (in addition to latent infections).

Hantaan virus has caused infections in laboratory rodents, and veterinary technicians have been infected in Asia and Europe.

The naturally occurring oral bacterium of the dog and cat *Capnocytophaga canimorsus* can cause disease and even death in persons with other debilitating illness, eg, alcoholism. *Yersinia enterocolitica* in an infected dog can be a hazard to humans, as can *Bartonella* in infected cats.

Prion diseases have been described in North America, Europe, and Asia and are known to affect sheep, cattle, elk, and deer as well as wild and domestic felids. The bovine prion disease is reported to have caused >140 human cases with 100% mortality in the UK. Although the incidence is <1/1,000,000, the threat of prion diseases to human and animal health is of major concern.

Exposure to animals kept as pets is steadily increasing as the number of pets increases in the USA and other affluent countries. The types of animals kept as pets are also increasing. Examples of these are the "exotic pets" that have become popular in many parts of the world, eg, prairie dogs, that have brought plague, tularemia, and even monkeypox out of the wild into people's homes. The desire of humans to touch wild animals or have contact with farm animals has resulted in the establishment of "petting zoos." Contact with farm or wild animals may expose children or other visitors to organisms such as *Escherichia coli* O157:H4 or even rabies. Public health officials in the USA, Canada, and Britain are trying to control these "zoos" through inspections and rules, including microbicidal handwashing following exposures.

TABLE I. Global Zoonoses*

Disease	Causative Organism	Principal Animals Involved
BACTERIAL DISEASES		
Anthrax	*Bacillus anthracis*	Cattle, sheep, goats, horses, wild herbivorous animals
Bordetellosis	*Bordetella bronchiseptica*	Dogs, rabbits, guinea pigs
Borreliosis	*Borrelia spp*	Rodents
Lyme disease	*B burgdorferi*	Deer, wild rodents
Relapsing fever	*B recurrentis* (Louseborne or epidemic)	No animal reservoir for the transmitting lice
	(Tickborne or endemic)	Wild rodents
Southern tick-associated rash illness	*B lonestari*	Uncertain
Brucellosis	*Brucella abortus*	Cattle, bison, elk, caribou
	B melitensis	Goats, sheep, camels
	B suis	Swine and wild pigs
	B canis	Dogs, coyotes

Another source of infection is exemplified by the severe acute respiratory syndrome epidemic caused by a novel coronavirus that appeared in southern China in 2003, first among food preparation workers exposed to civet cats and other "exotic animals" during their preparation as special foods.

The 21st century holds the threat of even more emerging diseases, nurtured by an ever-increasing human population. Control of zoonotic diseases and protection of the public health will become even more challenging as world population increases. When overpopulation and crowding occur, water shortages occur, hygiene often cannot be maintained, and malnutrition develops, leading to disease and epidemics. Surveillance and reporting of disease is the first line of defense. Knowledge of the epidemiology of the disease organisms is the first step in initiating a control program. The ultimate objective is to protect and preserve both human and animal health.

Zoonoses are generally defined as animal diseases that are transmissible to humans. However, there are several diseases listed below that occur primarily in humans and that may also be transmitted between humans and animals, with some animals serving as reservoirs for human infection (eg, *Trichuris trichiura*). The following common bacterial and viral diseases of humans are not found as naturally occurring diseases in animals (ie, animals are not a reservoir): diphtheria (*Corynebacterium diphtheriae*), Legionnaires' disease (*Legionella pneumoniae, L pneumophila*, and related organisms), syphilis (*Treponema pallidum*), trachoma (*Chlamydia trachomatis*), typhoid fever (*Salmonella typhi*), poliomyelitis, hepatitis B, mumps, chickenpox, smallpox, and measles.

◄ TABLE I. (continued)

Known Distribution	Probable Means of Spread to Humans	Clinical Manifestations in Humans
BACTERIAL DISEASES		
Worldwide; common in Africa, Asia, South America, eastern Europe	Occupational exposure; foodborne in Africa, Russia, and Asia; occasionally wounds or insect bites; rarely airborne	Ulcerative skin lesions, pneumonia, sepsis
Worldwide	Exposure to saliva or sputum	Pertussis-like pneumonia, usually in immunocompromised
Worldwide	*Ornithodoros* spp	Fever to sepsis
Worldwide	*Ixodes* spp	Target lesions, arthritis, sepsis
Epidemic	Crushing infected lice	Relapsing fever (every 3-5 days; up to 10 episodes), sepsis
Epidemic	Tick bites	
Southern USA	*Amblyomma americanum*	Similar to Lyme disease
Worldwide, except North America	Occupational and recreational exposure	Fever, often subacute and undulant to sepsis
Worldwide	Milk, cheese, contact	As above plus arthritis
Northern hemisphere	Rarely airborne	As above plus endocarditis
Rare		

(continued)

TABLE I.   Global Zoonoses* (continued) ▶

Disease	Causative Organism	Principal Animals Involved
BACTERIAL DISEASES (*continued*)		
Campylobacter enteritis	*Campylobacter jejuni*	Cattle, swine, poultry, dogs, cats, wild birds
	C coli, C fetus, C laridis	Nonhuman primates, laboratory animals, domestic pigs
Capnocytophaga infection	*Capnocytophaga canimorsus, C cynodegmi*	Dogs, cats
Cat scratch disease	*Bartonella henselae, B quintana*	Cats
Clostridial diseases (*See also* TETANUS, below.)	*Clostridium perfringens*, type A	Domestic animals
	C septicum C novyi	Domestic and wild animals
Enterohemorrhagic *Escherichia coli* infections (Enterotoxigenic, enteroinvasive, enteropathogenic, and enteroaggressive strains are not considered zoonotic.)	*E coli* O157:H7; also implicated are types O26:H11, O111:H8, O104:H21, and O48:H21	Cattle, humans
Erysipeloid	*Erysipelothrix rhusiopathiae*	Swine, turkeys, pigeons, marine mammals, fish
Glanders	*Burkholderia mallei*	Equids
Leprosy	*Mycobacterium leprae*	Armadillos
Leptospirosis	*Leptospira interrogans* (200 serovars) in 23 serogroups	Domestic and wild animals, common in rodents, dogs
Listeriosis	*Listeria monocytogenes* types 1/2a, 1/2b, 4b	Numerous mammals, birds
Melioidosis (Pseudoglanders)	*Pseudomonas pseudomallei*	Rodents, sheep, goats, horses, swine, nonhuman primates, kangaroos, zoo animals

TABLE I. (continued)		
Known Distribution	**Probable Means of Spread to Humans**	**Clinical Manifestations in Humans**
	BACTERIAL DISEASES (continued)	
Worldwide	Mainly foodborne, milk, waterborne, or occupational	Enteritis, arthritis, sepsis
Less frequent		Enteritis, sepsis
USA	Bites or scratches	Fever to sepsis
Worldwide	Scratches, bites, "licks"	Lymphadenopathy to sepsis; skin lesions in AIDS
Worldwide	Foodborne; occasionally wound contaminant	Enteritis, gas gangrene, sepsis
Worldwide	Wound infection	
North and South America, Europe, South Africa, Japan, Australia	Ingestion of undercooked ground beef, or food or water contaminated with bovine feces	Enteritis, hemolytic uremic syndrome
Worldwide	Occupational, recreational exposure	Cellulitis, sepsis
Rare except for some regions in Asia	Occupational exposure	Mucous membrane or skin lesions, pneumonia, fever to sepsis
Southern Texas and Louisiana	Transmission of animal leprosy to humans suspected—never confirmed	Various skin lesions, sensory nerve lesions and deficits, nasal mucosal lesions
Worldwide	Occupational and recreational exposure; water- and foodborne	Fever, rash, pneumonia, meningitis, hepatic and renal failure
Worldwide in cool environments	Foodborne among domestic animals by ensilage and hay; raw contaminated milk, cheese, mud, water, and vegetables are infectious; nosocomial infection in hospitals and institutions	Enteritis, meningitis, sepsis, fetal infection
Asia, Africa, Australia, South America and USA; rare	Wound infection and ingestion; organisms live in soil and surface water	Skin and pulmonary lesions, hepatitis, organ abscesses

(continued)

TABLE I.   Global Zoonoses* (continued) ▶

Disease	Causative Organism	Principal Animals Involved
BACTERIAL DISEASES (continued)		
Mycobacteriosis	Mycobacterium avium-intracellulare complex	Many species of mammals, some birds
	M paratuberculosis	Cattle, occasionally sheep and other ruminants
	Mycobacteria other than tuberculosis (includes M simiae)	Cattle, other ruminants
Pasteurellosis	Pasteurella multocida and other species	Many species of animals, especially dogs and cats
Plague	Yersinia pestis	Rodents, cats, rabbits, squirrels, related animals
Psittacosis and ornithosis	Chlamydophila psittaci	Parakeets, pigeons, parrots, turkeys, ducks, geese, etc; other isolates in cattle, sheep, goats, opossums, etc, rarely cause disease in humans
Rat bite fever	Streptobacillus moniliformis	Rodents
	Spirillum minus	Rodents
Salmonellosis	Salmonella enterica (2,000 serovars, 200 seen in the USA)	Poultry, swine, cattle, horses, dogs, cats, wild mammals and birds, reptiles, amphibians, crustaceans
Streptococcal infections	Streptococcus pyogenes, other group A streptococci, uncommonly groups B-G	Cattle (S agalactiae), swine (S suis), horses (S equi); occasionally other animals including dogs, cats
Tetanus	Clostridium tetani	Principally herbivores, but all animals may be intestinal carriers
Tuberculosis (See also MYCOBACTERIOSIS, above.)	Mycobacterium bovis	Cattle, swine, monkeys, and other animals
	M tuberculosis	Monkeys, other nonhuman primates, rarely dogs, cats, and other domestic animals, Asian elephants

◄ TABLE I.	(continued)	
Known Distribution	Probable Means of Spread to Humans	Clinical Manifestations in Humans
BACTERIAL DISEASES (continued)		
Worldwide	Primarily waterborne	Pulmonary disease in elderly; disseminated in immunocompromised, especially AIDS patients
Worldwide		Chronic, intermittent diarrhea
Worldwide	Water and/or soil	Skin and pulmonary lesions
Worldwide	Wounds, scratches, bites	Wound infections, cellulitis, sepsis, meningitis
Foci in Western USA, South America, Asia and Africa; rare	Fleas, aerosols, handling infected animals	Ulcerative skin lesions, lymphadenopathy (buboes), pneumonia, sepsis
Worldwide; common	Exposure to aerosols	Pneumonia, sepsis
Worldwide; rare	Bites of rodents; can be water- or foodborne	Fever, peripheral rash, arthritis, sepsis
Asia		Fever, rash with plaques, wound reactivates, sepsis
Worldwide; very common	Foodborne infection, especially in the elderly, infants, or immunosuppressed; occupational and recreational exposure	Enteritis to sepsis
Worldwide	Ingestion especially of raw milk; direct contact	Pharyngitis, cellulitis, pneumonia, meningitis, arthritis, sepsis
Worldwide	Wound infection and injections	Muscle spasms and contractions (especially facial), seizures, high mortality
Worldwide; rare in USA, Canada, Europe	Ingestion, inhalation, occupational exposure	Skin lesions, adenitis, enteritis
Worldwide	Exposure to animals infected with human type tuberculosis	Pulmonary disease, adenitis, meningitis, disseminated organ abscesses

(continued)

TABLE I. Global Zoonoses* (continued) ▶

Disease	Causative Organism	Principal Animals Involved
BACTERIAL DISEASES (continued)		
Tularemia	*Francisella tularensis* Type A virulent, type B less virulent	Wild animals, rabbits, rodents, cats, sheep
Vibriosis	*Vibrio parahaemolyticus* (Kanagawa phenomenon) *V vulnificus* Other noncholera vibrios	Marine shellfish
	V cholerae Non O1/O139, mostly halophilic	Crabs, shrimp, mussels
Yersiniosis	*Yersinia pseudotuberculosis* (6 serotypes)	Mammals, birds, puppies, kittens
	Y enterocolitica (50 serotypes)	Domestic animals especially pigs, dogs, cats
RICKETTSIAL DISEASES		
Boutonneuse fever, tick bite fever	*Rickettsia conorii*, related *Rickettsia*	Dogs, rodents, other animals
Ehrlichiosis	*Ehrlichia chaffeensis*	Deer, rodents, horses, dogs
	Anaplasma (Ehrlichia) phagocytophilum	As above
	E sennetsu	Uncertain
	E ewingi	Uncertain
Eperythrozoonosis	*Mycoplasma (Eperythrozoon)* spp	Livestock
Murine typhus	*Rickettsia typhi (R mooseri)* and related species	Rats, cats, opossums, skunks, raccoons
North Asian tick-borne rickettsiosis	*Rickettsia siberica*	Wild rodents
Q fever (Query fever)	*Coxiella burnetii*	Sheep, cattle, goats, cats, dogs, rodents, other mammals, birds, ticks
Queensland tick typhus	*Rickettsia australis*	Bandicoots, rodents
Rickettsial pox	*Rickettsia akari*	Mice

◀ **TABLE I.** *(continued)*

Known Distribution	Probable Means of Spread to Humans	Clinical Manifestations in Humans
BACTERIAL DISEASES *(continued)*		
Circumpolar in America, Europe, Asia	Occupational and recreational exposure; insect bites; ingestion; inhalation	Ulcerative skin lesions, pharyngitis, adenitis, enteritis, pneumonia, sepsis
Pacific basin, warm shores of Asia	Ingestion	Enteritis
Australia, North America; probably worldwide	Ingestion; wound infection	Ulcerating, bullous skin lesions to necrotizing fasciitis, enteritis; sepsis especially severe in immunocompromised host (mortality ≤50%)
Worldwide except Europe; epidemic in some developing countries	Ingestion; wound infection	Severe, voluminous diarrhea, dehydration; deadly if untreated
Temperate zones	Ingestion; recreational exposure	Mesenteric adenitis, enteritis
		Enteritis ± bloody stools or erythema nodosum, arthritis, sepsis
RICKETTSIAL DISEASES		
Europe, Asia, Africa	Bite of infected ticks	Eschar, adenitis, rash, fever
USA Japan	Ticks	Human monocytic ehrlichiosis
Worldwide	Ticks	Human granulocytic ehrlichiosis (HGE)
Japan		Fever, adenopathy, sepsis, fever
Missouri	Dogs	HGE
Worldwide (animals); reports of human infection in China, Yugoslavia	Direct contact; transplacental, vectorborne	Anemia, hemolytic jaundice, fever, lymphadenopathy, hemoglobinuria; many cases asymptomatic
Worldwide	Infected rodent fleas, possibly cat fleas	Fever, central rash, relatively mild
Siberia, Mongolia, China	Bite of infected ticks	Similar to Boutonneuse fever
Worldwide; common	Mainly airborne; exposure to placenta, birth tissues, animal excreta; occasionally ticks and milk	Fever, pneumonia, hepatitis, endocarditis
Australia	Bite of infected *Ixodes* tick	Similar to Boutonneuse fever
Eastern USA, Africa, Russia; rare	Bite of infected rodent mites, *Liponyssoides* spp	Eschar, rash, fever, mild

(continued)

TABLE I. Global Zoonoses* (continued) ▶

Disease	Causative Organism	Principal Animals Involved
RICKETTSIAL DISEASES (continued)		
Rocky Mountain spotted fever	*Rickettsia rickettsii*	Rabbits, field mice, dogs
Spotted fever group	*R parkeri*	Dogs and possibly cats
Scrub typhus	*Orientia tsutsugamushi* and related species	Rodents
Typhus	*Rickettsia prowazekii*	Flying squirrels
FUNGAL DISEASES		
Actinomycosis	*Actinomyces israelii*, rarely other *Actinomyces* spp	Mammals
Aspergillosis Allergic broncho-pulmonary aspergillosis	*Aspergillus* spp	Birds and mammals; principally environmental in decaying vegetation or grains
Blastomycosis	*Blastomyces dermatitidis*	Dogs, cats, horses, sea mammals; principally environmental in moist soil
Candidiasis (Moniliasis)	*Candida* spp	Principally human reservoirs, occasionally birds and mammals
Coccidioidomycosis	*Coccidioides immitis*	Cattle, sheep, horses, dogs, wild cats, desert rodents, other animals; principally environmental in specific arid foci
Cryptococcosis	*Cryptococcus neoformans*	Pigeons, cockatoos, cats, other mammals; principally environmental
Dermatophilosis	*Dermatophilus congolensis*	Cattle, horses, deer, sheep, other mammals
Histoplasmosis	*Histoplasma capsulatum*	Dogs; principally environmental in river valleys
Nocardiosis	*Nocardia asteroides* *N brasiliensis* *N caviae*	Cattle, dogs, other mammals, fish; principally environmental in decomposing organic matter

(continued)

◀ **TABLE I.** (continued)

Known Distribution	Probable Means of Spread to Humans	Clinical Manifestations in Humans
RICKETTSIAL DISEASES (*continued*)		
Western hemisphere	Bite of infected ticks, especially *Dermacentor variabilis, D andersoni;* also from crushing tick	Fever, rash ± petechiae, sepsis
Western hemisphere	Likely Gulf Coast tick *Amblyomma maculatum* and other *Amblyomma* spp	Fever, mild headache, diffuse myalgia and arthralgia, rash
"Typhus islands" in Asia, Australia, East Indies	Bite of infected larval trombiculid mites	Eschar, rash, fever, ± pneumonia
Eastern USA	Squirrel fleas or ticks suspected	Fever, rash, sepsis
FUNGAL DISEASES		
Worldwide	Contact; rare	Fever, sepsis
Worldwide; sporadic	Environmental exposure	Pneumonia with dissemination in immunocompromised; chronic pulmonary disease ± fungus ball
Worldwide	Environmental exposure; also reported by animal exposure	Pneumonia, skin or bone lesions
Worldwide	Direct contact; often endogenous in humans	Skin and mucous membrane lesions; sepsis and dissemination to organs in immunocompromised
Southwestern USA, Mexico, Central and South America	Environmental exposure	Self-limited febrile illness; persistent meningitis or osteomyelitis in immunocompromised
Worldwide	Environmental exposure, especially pigeon nests	Self-limiting pulmonary granulomas; meningitis and dissemination in immunocompromised
Worldwide	Contact; arthropod vectors	Pustular desquamative dermatitis
Worldwide	Environmental exposure; grows abundantly in feces of chickens, blackbirds, bats	Flu-like, pneumonia, dissemination in immunocompromised
Worldwide	Environmental exposure	Pneumonia, dissemination in immunocompromised

(continued)

TABLE I. Global Zoonoses* (continued)

Disease	Causative Organism	Principal Animals Involved
FUNGAL DISEASES (continued)		
Pneumocystis pneumonia	*Pneumocystis carinii* (human strain); recent evidence places this as a fungus rather than protozoa	Rodents, dogs, cats, cattle (animal strains)
Rhinosporidiosis	*Rhinosporidium seeberi*	Horses, cattle, mules, dogs, and birds; unidentified environmental reservoirs
Ringworm (Dermatophytosis)	*Microsporum, Trichophyton,* and *Epidermophyton* spp	Dogs, cats, cattle, rodents, other animals
Sporotrichosis	*Sporothrix schenckii*	Horses, other domestic and laboratory animals, birds; primarily environmental in vegetation (moss) and wood
PARASITIC DISEASES		
Protozoans		
Babesiosis	*Babesia microti* *B bovis*	Wild rodents, cattle
	B divergens	Cattle, other mammals
Balantidiasis	*Balantidium coli*	Swine, rats, nonhuman primates
Chagas' disease (American trypanosomiasis)	*Trypanosoma cruzi*	Opossums, rodents, armadillos, dogs, cats, other wild and domestic animals
Cryptosporidiosis	*Cryptosporidium parvum*	Cattle, other animals
Giardiasis	*Giardia lamblia*	Beavers, porcupines, dogs, other animals
Leishmaniasis Kalaazar (visceral)	*Leishmania donovani* and other species	Wild canids and dogs

◀ **TABLE I.** (continued)

Known Distribution	Probable Means of Spread to Humans	Clinical Manifestations in Humans
FUNGAL DISEASES (continued)		
Worldwide; common in AIDS patients	Environmental exposure; person to person; source yet to be determined, nor have animal strains been verified as human pathogens	Pneumonia, fever, nonproductive cough
Worldwide, endemic in South Asia	Environmental exposure	Nasal and other mucous membrane masses and polyps; may cause obstruction
Worldwide	Direct contact with infected animals, fomites	Skin and hair lesions; rare skin dissemination in immunocompromised
Worldwide	Occupational contact, including with animals	Ulcerative skin lesions may follow course of draining lymphatics of arms and legs; may disseminate in immunocompromised
PARASITIC DISEASES		
Protozoans		
Worldwide; rare	Bite of infected *Ixodes* ticks	Fever and hemolytic anemia, especially severe in immunocompromised (asplenic and elderly); recurrent or chronic infection may develop; dual infection with *B burgdorferi* may worsen both diseases
Europe		
Worldwide; low incidence	Ingestion, especially of water	Enteritis or gastroenteritis
Western hemisphere—Southern USA, Mexico, Central and South America	Fecal material of triatoma bug, including Reduviidae (also called cone-nosed, kissing, or assassin bug); contaminates bite wounds, abrasions, or mucous membranes; blood transfusion; congenitally; tissue transplantation (infrequent)	Acute—erratic fever, adenopathy, hepatosplenomegaly, skin lesions, myocarditis, or encephalitis; worse in immunocompromised Chronic—cardiomyopathy, megaesophagus, megacolon
Worldwide	Occupational contact and ingestion; waterborne	Enteritis, cholera-like and persistent in immunocompromised; cholecystitis
Worldwide; common	Water and less often food; person to person	Enteritis; may be persistent
Southern Asia, South America, Africa	Bite of infected phlebotomine sand flies	Fever, hepatosplenomegaly, pancytopenia

(continued)

TABLE I. Global Zoonoses* (continued) ▶

Disease	Causative Organism	Principal Animals Involved
PARASITIC DISEASES		
Protozoans (continued)		
Cutaneous and mucosal	L tropica L braziliensis complex	Canids, marsupials, sloths, wild mammals, rodents
Malaria of nonhuman primates	At least 20 species of Plasmodium	Monkeys, chimpanzees
Microsporidiosis	Microsporidia Enterocytozoon bieneusis Encephalitozoon cuniculi; E intestinalis; E hellem	Various wild and domestic animals, primates, rodents, psittacine birds
Sarcocystosis (Sarcosporidiosis)	Sarcocystis suihominis	Swine
	S hominis	Cattle
Toxoplasmosis	Toxoplasma gondii	Mammals, especially cats, food animals, birds
Trypanosomiasis (African sleeping sickness)	Trypanosoma brucei T brucei rhodesiense T brucei gambiense	Wild and domestic dogs, ruminants, hyenas, carnivores
Trematodes (Flukes)		
Clonorchiasis	Clonorchis sinensis (Chinese liver fluke)	Dogs, cats, swine, rats, wild animals
Dicrocoeliasis	Dicrocoelium dendriticum (Lancet fluke)	Ruminants
	D hospes (Lancet fluke)	Ruminants
Echinostomiasis	Echinostoma ilocanum and other Echinostoma spp	Cats, dogs, rodents, fish
Fascioliasis	Fasciola hepatica	Cattle, sheep, other large ruminants (eg, water buffalo)
	F gigantica	

◀ **TABLE I.** *(continued)*

Known Distribution	Probable Means of Spread to Humans	Clinical Manifestations in Humans
PARASITIC DISEASES		
Protozoans (continued)		
		Papules to ulcers; may spread to oral mucous membranes and persist or recur
Tropical Americas, Asia, Africa	Anopheline mosquitos	Fever; human infection rare
Worldwide	Zoonotic transmission: fecal-oral; direct contact; waterborne possible; person to person common	Keratitis (pain, redness, and visual blurring); acute diarrhea (traveler's diarrhea); chronic diarrhea (immunocompromised)
Worldwide	Ingestion of raw pork or beef; ingestion of feces	Meat yields intestinal form, usually mild; feces yield muscular form, usually asymptomatic; muscular pain and eosinophilia reported
	Ingestion of raw beef; ingestion of feces	Meat yields intestinal form, usually mild; feces yield muscular form, usually asymptomatic; muscular pain and eosinophilia reported
Worldwide; common	Ingestion of oocysts shed in feces of infected cats or found in meat or raw milk	Fever and adenopathy; disseminated, multiorgan disease in immunocompromised, including brain abscess; infection of fetus may result in severe damage to CNS
Africa; common below the Sahara desert	Bite of infected tsetse fly (*Glossina* spp)	Painful chancre at bite site, fever, headache, adenopathy, rash, somnolence; gambiense disease may last years; rhodesiense disease may last weeks; both usually fatal without treatment
Trematodes (Flukes)		
Asia	Ingestion of raw or partially cooked infected freshwater fish	Cholecystitis symptoms; chronic infections associated with cirrhosis or cholangiocarcinoma
Worldwide	Ingestion of infected ants	Abdominal discomfort
Africa		
Asia	Ingestion of uncooked fish, shellfish, or contaminated water	Abdominal discomfort, diarrhea
Worldwide	Ingestion of contaminated greens, eg, watercress	Biliary colic and obstructive jaundice
Africa and western Pacific		Biliary colic and obstructive jaundice; migrating inflammatory skin lesions

(continued)

TABLE I. Global Zoonoses* (continued) ▶

Disease	Causative Organism	Principal Animals Involved
	Trematodes *(continued)*	
Fasciolopsiasis	*Fasciolopsis buski*	Swine, dogs
Gastrodiscoidiasis	*Gastrodiscoides hominis*	Swine, rats
Heterophyiasis	*Heterophyes* and other heterophids	Cats, dogs, foxes, fish-eating birds
Metagonimiasis	*Metagonimus yokogawai*	Cats, dogs, other fish-eating mammals, fish
Opisthorchiasis	*Opisthorchis felineus* (cat liver fluke)	Cats, dogs, foxes, swine
	O viverrini (small liver fluke)	Dogs, cats, fish-eating mammals
	Amphimerus pseudofelineus	Dogs, cats, coyotes, opossums
Paragonimiasis (Lung fluke disease)	*Paragonimus westermani, P africanus, P mexicanus,* and other species	Dogs, cats, swine, wild carnivores
Schistosomiasis (Bilharziasis)	*Schistosoma japonicum*	Cattle, buffalo, swine, dogs, cats, rodents
	S hematobium	Humans are the only reservoir
	S mansoni	Baboons, rodents, cattle, dogs
	S mattbeei	Cattle
	S mekongi	Dogs, monkeys
	S intercalatum	Cattle, sheep, antelope, goats
Swimmer's itch	Schistosome cercariae	Birds, mammals

◀ **TABLE I.** (continued)

Known Distribution	Probable Means of Spread to Humans	Clinical Manifestations in Humans
Trematodes (continued)		
Asian pig-raising regions	Ingestion of raw tubers and nuts of aquatic plants	Enteritis with diarrhea, constipation, vomiting, anorexia; facial, abdominal, extremity edema may occur
Asia	Snails (metacercariae encyst on plants)	Mild diarrhea
Nile delta, Turkey, Asia	Ingestion of undercooked fish	Diarrhea with mucus; rarely heart or CNS involvement
Asia, Europe, Siberia	Ingestion of undercooked fish	Diarrhea with mucus
Eastern Europe, Asia, Siberia	Ingestion of uncooked fish containing encysted larvae	All may produce fever, biliary colic, enlarged liver due to cholangitis, abscess, or cholangiocarcinoma
Thailand, Laos	Ingestion of undercooked fish containing encysted larvae	
USA, Central and South America	Undetermined	
China, India, Myanmar, Africa, tropical America	Ingestion of raw or partially cooked, infected freshwater crustaceans	Pulmonary disease resembling tuberculosis; less often meningoencephalitis and skin nodules with dissemination
Southeast Asia, China, Philippines	Penetration of unbroken skin by cercariae larva from infected snails in water	Acute (especially *S japonicum, S mansoni*)—Katayama's fever with fever, chills, cough, diarrhea, hepatosplenomegaly Chronic—colonic polyposis with bloody diarrhea; portal hypertension with hematemesis and splenomegaly, hemorrhagic cystitis, and ureteritis, which can progress to bladder cancer; pulmonary hypertension; glomerulonephritis; and CNS manifestations
Africa, the Middle East		
Africa, Arabia, tropical America		
Southern Africa		
Southeast Asia		
Central Africa		
Worldwide	Penetration of unbroken skin by cercariae from infected snails in fresh- and saltwater	Self-limiting urticaria

(continued)

TABLE I. Global Zoonoses* (continued) ▶

Disease	Causative Organism	Principal Animals Involved
	Cestodes (Tapeworms)	
Asian taeniasis	Taenia asiatica	Domestic and wild pigs, cattle, monkeys
Bertielliasis	Bertiella studeri B mucronata	Primates, oribatid mites
Coenuriasis	Taenia multiceps	Definitive hosts of all species are other canids, sheep, other herbivores
	T serialis	Lagomorphs
	T brauni	Wild rodents
Diphyllobothriasis (Fish tapeworm infection)	Diphyllobothrium latum (Dibothriocephalus latus), D pacificum	Humans, dogs, bears, fish-eating animals, freshwater fish
Dipylidiasis (Dog tapeworm infection)	Dipylidium caninum	Dogs, cats, fleas
Echinococcosis	Echinococcus granulosus	Dogs, sheep, cattle, swine, rodents, deer, moose
	E multilocularis	Foxes, microtine rodents, coyotes, dogs, wolves, cats, voles, lemmings, shrews
	E vogeli	Bush and hunting dogs, agouti, pacas, spiny rats
Hymenolepiasis (Dwarf tapeworm infection)	Hymenolepis nana	Humans, rodents
Inermicapsifer infection	Inermicapsifer madagascariensis	Rodents
Mouse or rat tapeworm	Hymenolepis nana H diminuta	Rats, mice
Raillietina infection	Raillietina spp	Birds, mammals
Sparganosis	Spirometra spp (pseudophyllidean tapeworms, second larval stage)	Monkeys, cats, pigs, dogs, weasels, rats, chickens, snakes, frogs, mice

◀ **TABLE 1.** *(continued)*

Known Distribution	Probable Means of Spread to Humans	Clinical Manifestations in Humans
	Cestodes (Tapeworms)	
East and southeast Asia	Ingestion of undercooked meat	Vague abdominal complaints; dissemination
Asia, South America, Africa	Ingestion of infected arthropods	Abdominal pain, vomiting, diarrhea, constipation
Worldwide in scattered foci	Ingestion of tapeworm eggs in canine feces	Painless skin swelling; rarely neurologic involvement, including eye
Africa, Europe, USA; rare		
Africa		
Worldwide	Ingestion of raw or partially cooked infected fish	Usually asymptomatic; may cause mild abdominal distress; rare megaloblastic anemia
Worldwide	Ingestion of dog or cat fleas	Usually in children, asymptomatic or mild abdominal distress; proglottids in stool resemble cucumber seeds
Worldwide but mostly in Mediterranean region and southern South America	Ingestion of tapeworm eggs	Cause space-occupying lesions of organs, eg, lung, liver, kidney, etc; rarely CNS
Alaska, Canada, Asia, Central Europe	Ingestion of tapeworm eggs	Usually involves liver with mass lesions, occasionally lung or CNS
Central and South America	Ingestion of tapeworm eggs	Usually involves liver, may invade adjacent tissues
Worldwide	Accidental ingestion of tapeworm eggs or infected insects	Mild abdominal distress, may be accompanied by nausea or vomiting
Africa, southeast Asia, tropical America	Ingestion of infected arthropods	Mild abdominal symptoms, if any
Worldwide	Ingestion of cysticercoids in fleas, mealworms, etc, in food	Mild abdominal symptoms of short duration
Tropical America, east Asia, Australia, Africa	Ingestion of infected arthropods	Vague discomfort
Worldwide; uncommon	Ingestion of infected cyclops or raw infected animal flesh or application of animal flesh to human	Nodular, itchy skin lesions that can migrate; conjunctival and eyelid lesions; other organ involvement including CNS

(continued)

TABLE I. Global Zoonoses* (continued) ▶

Disease	Causative Organism	Principal Animals Involved
Cestodes (continued)		
Taeniasis		
Beef tapeworm disease	*Taenia saginata*	Cattle, water buffalo, reindeer, camels
Pork tapeworm disease Cysticercosis and neurocysticercosis	*T solium*	Swine, humans
Nematodes (Roundworms)		
Angiostrongyliasis	*Parastrongylus (Angiostrongylus) costaricensis*	Cotton rats, slugs
	A cantonensis	Rats, snails, slugs, prawns, fish, land crabs, *Bandicota* spp
Anisakiasis	Larvae of *Anisakis* and *Pseudoterranova* spp	Marine invertebrates, fish, mammals
Capillariasis		
Hepatic capillariasis	*Capillaria hepatica*	Rodents, other wild and domestic animals
Intestinal capillariasis	*C philippinensis*	Aquatic birds, freshwater fish
Pulmonary capillariasis	*C aerophila*	Dogs, cats, other carnivores
Dioctophymosis (Giant kidney worm infection)	*Dioctophyma renale*	Dogs, mink, other carnivores, frogs, fish
Dracunculiasis (Guinea worm infection)	*Dracunculus medinensis*	Humans
	D insignis	Raccoons, mink, dogs

◀ **TABLE I.** (continued)

Known Distribution	Probable Means of Spread to Humans	Clinical Manifestations in Humans
	Cestodes (continued)	
Worldwide	Ingestion of undercooked meat containing larvae of *T saginata*	Bowel infection from larvae causes mild abdominal discomfort and proglottid passage; eggs do not cause disseminated disease
Worldwide where swine are reared (rare in USA, Canada, UK, Scandinavia)	Ingestion of undercooked pork containing *C cellulosae*; direct or autogenous transmission of *T solium* ova in humans may lead to cysticercosis	Usually asymptomatic for years until cysticerci result in inflammation in CNS (seizures) or less often in eye or heart; autoinfection with eggs may occur as well as infection of other humans; adult stage infection (taeniasis) mild or asymptomatic
	Nematodes (Roundworms)	
Central and South America, USA	Accidental ingestion of slugs or plants contaminated by their secretions	*P costaricensis* may cause a syndrome resembling appendicitis, especially in children, called abdominal or intestinal angiostrongyliasis
Japan, east and southeast Asia to Australia, Pacific Islands, Africa		Eosinophilic meningitis, ocular involvement occurs with decreased vision, eye muscle paralysis
Japan, Holland, Scandinavia, western South America, western Europe, USA	Ingestion of undercooked marine fish, squid, octopus	Gastroenteritis with upper quadrant pain may be accompanied by hematemesis; cough if oropharynx is involved
Worldwide in scattered foci	Ingestion of embryonated eggs in soil	Acute or subacute hepatitis with marked eosinophilia
Northern Philippines, Thailand, east Asia, and Egypt	Ingestion of infected fish	Enteropathy with protein loss and malabsorption, vomiting
Worldwide	Accidental ingestion of infective eggs in soil or contaminated food	Fever, cough, bronchospasm
Europe, Asia, North and South America; rare	Ingestion of infected fish or frog's liver and mesentery	Flank pain, renal colic, hematuria, ureteral obstruction
Asia and Africa; common	Ingestion of infected cyclops in water	Vesicular skin lesion that opens to reveal worm; allergic reaction and secondary infection may occur
North America	Ingestion of frogs and other paratenic hosts	

(continued)

TABLE I. Global Zoonoses[*] (continued) ▶

Disease	Causative Organism	Principal Animals Involved
	Nematodes (continued)	
Filariasis		
Dirofilariasis	Dirofilaria immitis	Dogs, cats, raccoons, bears, mosquitos
Malayan filariasis	Brugia malayi	Cats, other carnivores, monkeys, mosquitos
Tropical eosinophilia	B pahangi	
Gnathostomiasis	Gnathostoma spinigerum	Dogs, cats, wild carnivores, copepods, freshwater fish
Gongylonemiasis	Gongylonema pulchrum	Ruminants, domestic and wild swine, other mammals; beetles
Larva migrans, cutaneous (See also GNATHOSTOMIASIS, above.)	Ancylostoma braziliense, A caninum, Uncinaria stenocephala	Cats, dogs, wild carnivores
	Strongyloides stercoralis	Cats, dogs, sheep, swine, etc
Larva migrans, visceral (See also ANGIOSTRONGYLIASIS and ANISAKIASIS, above.)	Toxocara canis, T cati	Dogs, cats
	Baylisascaris procyonis	Raccoons
Oesophagostomiasis Ternidensiasis	Oesophagostomum spp, Ternidens diminutus	Primates
Strongyloidiasis	Strongyloides stercoralis S fuelleborni	Dogs, cats, foxes, primates

◀ **TABLE I.** *(continued)*

Known Distribution	Probable Means of Spread to Humans	Clinical Manifestations in Humans
Nematodes (continued)		
Worldwide	Bite of infected mosquitos	Fever, cough acutely, resulting in infarct or coin lesion in the lungs; often asymptomatic; rarely involves eye
Asia; common	Bite of infected mosquitos	Cutaneous lesion may include lymph nodes
		Cutaneous lesion may include lymph nodes
East Asia, India, Australia	Ingestion of infected fish or poultry	Migratory skin lesions; may involve viscera or CNS
Worldwide; rare	Ingestion of infected arthropods	Intestinal discomfort
Worldwide in tropics and subtropics; common	Contact with infective larvae that penetrate skin	Itchy, serpiginous, migrating skin lesions, usually of extremities; wheezing, cough, and urticaria may occur
Worldwide in tropics and subtropics; rare to common	Contact with infective larvae that penetrate skin	Itchy, urticarial lesions, usually on buttocks, groin, or trunk (autoinfection), along with GI symptoms; dissemination with pulmonary or CNS disease may occur in immunocompromised
Worldwide	Ingestion of embryonated eggs shed in feces of dogs and cats	Fever, wheezing cough; nodular rash on trunk and extremities; may wax and wane for months; eye involvement (ocular migrans) may resemble retinoblastoma
North America, Europe	Accidental ingestion of embryonated eggs in soil or fecal contaminated material	Can cause fatal meningoencephalitis in infants (neural larval migrans); increased frequency of ocular disease in children but can occur in adults
Asia, Africa, South America	Ingestion of infective larvae in soil	Abdominal pain (may be right lower quadrant) and masses; may have mild fever
Worldwide; rare to common	Contact with infective larvae that penetrate skin	Frequently asymptomatic; clinical features include abdominal pain, diarrhea, urticarial rash (waist, buttocks); disseminated strongyloidiasis with abdominal pain and distention, shock, pulmonary and neurologic complications, septicemia, and death may occur in immunocompromised

(continued)

TABLE I. Global Zoonoses* (continued) ▶

Disease	Causative Organism	Principal Animals Involved
Nematodes (continued)		
Thelaziasis	*Thelazia* spp	Dogs, cats, other domestic and wild animals, flies
Trichinosis (Trichinellosis)	*Trichinella spiralis* and subspecies, *T nativa, T britovi, T nelsoni, T pseudospiralis*	Swine, rodents, bears, horses, wild carnivores, marine mammals; both in the neoarctic and the tropics
Trichostrongyliasis	*Trichostrongylus* spp	Cattle, sheep, wild ruminants
Trichuriasis (Whipworm infection)	*Trichuris trichiura* and other *Trichuris* spp	Humans, other primates
Acanthocephalans		
Macracanthorhynchosis	*Macracanthorhynchus hirudinaceus* and other species	Domestic and wild pigs, beetles, squirrels, muskrats, arctic foxes, dogs, sea otters, crustaceans, fish
Annelids (Leeches)		
Hirudiniasis	*Limnatis nilotica* and other leeches	Cattle, buffalo, horses, sheep, dogs, pigs
ARTHROPOD DISEASES		
Acariasis (Mange)	Mites of *Sarcoptes, Cheyletiella, Dermanyssus,* and *Ornithonyssus* spp	Domestic animals
Myiasis	*Cochliomyia hominivorax* (screwworm)	Mammals
	Chrysomya bezziana	Mammals
	Cordylobia anthropophaga (Tumbu fly)	Mammals
	Cuterebra spp	Mammals
	Dermatobia hominis (human bot fly)	Mammals
	Gasterophilus spp (equine bot fly)	Mammals
	Hypoderma lineatum	Mammals
	Hypoderma bovis (warbles)	Mammals
	Oestrus ovis Rhinoestrus purpurensis	Bovidea
	Wohlfahrtia spp	Bovidea

TABLE I. (continued)

Known Distribution	Probable Means of Spread to Humans	Clinical Manifestations in Humans
Nematodes (continued)		
East and south Asia; rare	Infected insects	Conjunctivitis
Worldwide, especially subarctic region	Ingestion of pork and flesh of wild animals containing viable cysts	Gastroenteritis followed by fever, severe myalgia, facial swelling; CNS or myocardial involvement may follow
Worldwide	Ingestion of infective larvae on plant foods or in soil	Asymptomatic or mild enteritis
Worldwide; common	Ingestion of embryonated eggs on plant foods or in soil	Asymptomatic or mild enteritis
Acanthocephalans		
Worldwide; uncommon	Ingestion of infected beetles	Enteritis, may lead to gut perforation
Annelids (Leeches)		
Africa, Asia, Europe, Chile	Direct contact with leeches	Attaches to skin to suck blood; secondary infection may occur
ARTHROPOD DISEASES		
Worldwide	Contact with infected individuals or animals; contaminated clothing	Itchy skin lesions
Tropical America	Can invade living tissue; necrotic tissue ingested	Dermal and subdermal wounds; nasal myiasis; intestinal myiasis; usually mild; some may be migratory and destructive causing burrows and boils
Asia, Africa		
Africa		
North America		
South America, Mexico		
Worldwide		
North America, Europe		
Asia, north Africa		
Worldwide	Eggs and their larva	
North America, Europe, north Africa, Asia		

(continued)

TABLE I. Global Zoonoses* (continued) ▶

Disease	Causative Organism	Principal Animals Involved
ARTHROPOD DISEASES (*continued*)		
Nanophyetiasis	*Troglotrema salmincola*	Raccoons, skunks, snails
Pentastomid infections	*Linguatula serrata* *Armillifer* spp (tongue worms)	Dogs, snakes, other vertebrates
Tick paralysis	Envenomization of ticks *Dermacentor andersoni, D variabilis*, and sometimes *Ixodes, Haemaphysalis, Rhinocephalus*, and *Argas* spp	Various animals
Tunga infections	*Tunga penetrans* (sand fleas, jiggers)	Humans, dogs, pigs, other mammals
VIRAL DISEASES		
California group infections	Bunyavirus spp	Ground squirrels, other rodents
LaCrosse encephalitis		
Tahyna fever		Hares, rodents, other mammals
Central European tickborne encephalitis	Central European encephalitis virus (flavivirus)	Rodents, hedgehogs, birds, goats, sheep
Colorado tick fever	Colorado tick fever virus	Ground squirrels, chipmunks, porcupines, small rodents
Contagious ecthyma (Orf)	Orf virus (parapox)	Sheep, goats, wild ungulates
Cowpox	Cowpox virus	Cattle, rodents, cats, zoo cats
Eastern equine encephalomyelitis	Eastern equine encephalomyelitis virus (alphavirus)	Wild birds, domestic fowl, horses, mules, donkeys
Encephalomyocarditis	Encephalomyocarditis virus (picornavirus)	Rats, mice, squirrels, swine, nonhuman primates, elephants

◀ **TABLE I.** (*continued*)

Known Distribution	Probable Means of Spread to Humans	Clinical Manifestations in Humans
ARTHROPOD DISEASES (*continued*)		
North America, Russia	Ingestion of fish or roe	Mild enteritis
Northern hemisphere Worldwide	Ingestion of infected animal tissues, water, or vegetation	Usually asymptomatic; pressure from larvae may cause symptoms in lung or other organs, including CNS and eye
North America, Australia, South Africa, Ethiopia	Direct contact (attachment) with tick	Gastroenteritis followed by ascending lower neuron paralysis; paresthesia may be noted
Subtropical Africa, Americas, south Asia	Contact with contaminated soil	Penetration of skin and burrowing result in pain and itching; may be secondarily infected
VIRAL DISEASES		
USA, Canada	Mosquito (*Aedes* spp) bites	Fever, encephalitis with seizures, paralysis, and other focal neurologic signs
Europe, Africa		
Europe	*Ixodes* tick bites; may be milkborne	Biphasic illness with encephalitis occurring in second febrile phase; paralysis or neuropsychiatric symptoms may develop
Western USA; common	Tick (*Dermacentor andersoni*) bites	2- to 3-phase illness with meningoencephalitis occurring in late phases; abdominal pain and vomiting may occur
Worldwide; common	Occupational exposure	Papule(s) that umbilicate and ulcerate, usually on hands; dissemination rare
Worldwide; rare	Contact exposure	Vesicles that become pustular, usually on hands; regional adenopathy
Western hemisphere	Mosquito (*Culiseta melanura* and *Aedes* spp) bites	Nonspecific febrile illness to encephalitis which may be severe and accompanied by seizures; neurologic sequelae occur in 30-50% of encephalitis cases
Worldwide	Environmental contamination	Rare, acute myocarditis

(*continued*)

TABLE I. Global Zoonoses* (continued) ▶

Disease	Causative Organism	Principal Animals Involved
VIRAL DISEASES (continued)		
Far eastern tick-borne encephalitis (Russian spring-summer encephalitis)	Far eastern (Russian spring-summer encephalitis) virus (flavivirus)	Birds, small mammals, sheep
Foot-and-mouth disease	Foot-and-mouth disease virus (aphthovirus types A, O, C, SAT, and Asia)	Cattle, swine, related cloven-hoofed animals
Hendra virus infection	Hendra virus	Horses, fruit bats (reservoir)
Hepatitis E	Hepatitis E virus	Swine, deer, others
Herpes B virus disease	Cercopithecine herpesvirus 1 (Herpesvirus simiae, B virus)	Old World monkeys; cell cultures
Influenza type A (synonyms: swine flu, avian flu, Hong Kong flu)	Influenza virus (myxovirus)	Birds, swine, other wild and domestic mammals; migratory waterfowl serve as reservoirs and carriers for highly pathogenic avian influenza
Japanese B encephalitis	Japanese encephalitis virus (flavivirus)	Swine, wild birds, horses
Louping ill	Louping ill virus (flavivirus)	Sheep, goats, grouse, small rodents
Lymphocytic choriomeningitis	Lymphocytic choriomeningitis virus (arenavirus)	House mice, dogs, monkeys, guinea pigs, hamsters
Menangle virus infection	Menangle virus	Fruit bats, pigs

◀ **TABLE I.** (continued)

Known Distribution	Probable Means of Spread to Humans	Clinical Manifestations in Humans
VIRAL DISEASES (continued)		
Asia, Europe; rare	Tick (*Ixodes persulcatus* and *I ricinus*) bites	Similar to central European tickborne encephalitis; flaccid paralysis of shoulders and arms may be seen; fatality rate 20-25%; neurologic sequelae in 30-60% of survivors
Europe, Asia, Africa, South America	Contact exposure	Humans can become carriers but not ill
Australia (Queensland)	Direct contact with infected animals or contaminated tissue	Respiratory infection, encephalitis
Worldwide	Fecal, oral spread; consumption of raw or undercooked liver	Fever, GI symptoms, jaundice; may be prolonged; worse in pregnancy
Worldwide; rare	Monkey bites and scratches, occupational exposure	Vesicular skin lesions followed by severe encephalitis with seizures, paralysis, coma; 70% mortality
Worldwide; common	Contact exposure; animals rarely a source	Upper and lower respiratory symptoms; may progress to influenza, pneumonia, or secondary bacterial pneumonia; seasonally endemic or epidemic
Asia, Pacific islands from Japan to the Philippines	Mosquito (*Culex tritaeniorhynchus*, other *Culex* spp) bites	Fever, GI symptoms to severe encephalitis with seizures, paralysis; neurologic sequelae in up to 80% of survivors
Great Britain, Northern Ireland; rare	Tick (*Ixodes ricinus*) bites	Biphasic illness with meningoencephalitis in second phase; relatively mild compared with central European tickborne encephalitis, which it resembles
Worldwide	Host excretions and secretions	Ranges from mild flu-like illness to biphasic with severe meningitis in second phase; arthritis, parotitis, and orchitis may occur; may be teratogenic or cause abortion
Australia	Respiratory secretions, feces	Fever

(continued)

TABLE I. Global Zoonoses* (continued)

Disease	Causative Organism	Principal Animals Involved
VIRAL DISEASES (continued)		
Milker's nodules (Pseudocowpox)	Pseudocowpox virus (parapoxvirus)	Cattle
Monkeypox	Monkeypox virus	Nonhuman primates, Gambian rats, other African rodents; prairie dogs, other pet rodents in USA
Murray Valley encephalitis	Murray Valley encephalitis virus (flavivirus)	Wild birds
Newcastle disease	Newcastle disease virus (paramyxovirus)	Fowl, wild birds
Nipah virus infection	Nipah virus	Swine, dogs, fruit bats, other animals
Rabies and rabies-related infections	Lyssaviruses Rabies virus Duvenhage virus Mokola virus Ibadan shrew virus	Wild and domestic canids, mustelidae, viverridae, vampire and insectivorous bats
	Obodhiang virus	Fruit bats
Ross River fever	Ross River virus (alphavirus)	Undetermined
St. Louis encephalitis	St. Louis encephalitis virus (flavivirus)	Wild birds, domestic fowl
Severe acute respiratory syndrome (SARS)	Coronavirus	Civet cats most likely
Sindbis virus disease	Sindbis virus (alphavirus)	Birds
Tanapox	Tanapox virus	Asian and African monkeys
Venezuelan equine encephalomyelitis	Venezuelan equine encephalitis virus (alphavirus)	Rodents, equids

◀ **TABLE I.** *(continued)*

Known Distribution	Probable Means of Spread to Humans	Clinical Manifestations in Humans
	VIRAL DISEASES *(continued)*	
Worldwide; common	Occupational exposure	Papular to nodular red skin lesions; painless and self-limiting
West and central Africa; rare	Contact; aerosols	Usually mild, smallpox-like disease; even milder in those vaccinated for smallpox; lymphadenopathy prominent
Australia, New Guinea; rare	Mosquito (*Culex annulirostris*) bites	Asymptomatic infection in 99%; when disease occurs it can be severe encephalitis with neurologic sequelae
Worldwide; common	Occupational exposure	Can cause self-limiting conjunctivitis
Malaysia	Direct contact with infected animals or contaminated tissue	Fever, headache, vomiting, encephalitis; 30% mortality
Worldwide except Australia, New Zealand, UK, Ireland, Scandinavia, Japan, Taiwan; many smaller islands, including Hawaii, are free of infection	Bites of diseased animals; aerosols in closed environments	Paresthesias or pain at bite site, fever, myalgia, mood changes progress to hyperventilation, general paresthesias, paresis, seizures, hydrophobia; mortality >99% in symptomatic infection; other strains of virus very rare, but deadly
Australia, South Pacific Islands	Mosquito (*Culex annulirostris* and *Aedes* spp) bites	Fever, arthralgia, rash, may persist for months; purpura on lower extremities
Western hemisphere	Mosquito (*Culex tarsalis*, *C pipiens-quinquefasciatus* complex, *C nigripalpus*) bites	Encephalitis with cerebellar signs, hepatitis, dysuria; more severe in elderly
China, southeast Asia	Direct contact suspected, person to person	Fever, myalgia, headache, diarrhea, pneumonia; case fatality rate 10%
Eastern hemisphere; rare	Mosquito (*Culex* spp) bites	Fever, arthritis, rash that may become hemorrhagic, prominent myalgia
Asia, Africa, and in monkey colonies	Contact; aerosols	Fever, 1 or 2 papulovesicular lesions, often on extremities
Western hemisphere; common	Mosquito (*Monsonia*, *Aedes*, *Culex* spp) bites	Most have nonspecific febrile illness; <5% progress to encephalitis with mortality rate of 20%

(continued)

TABLE I. Global Zoonoses* (continued) ▶

Disease	Causative Organism	Principal Animals Involved
VIRAL DISEASES (continued)		
Vesicular stomatitis	Vesicular stomatitis virus (Indiana and New Jersey strains)	Swine, cattle, horses, bats, rodents, other wild mammals
Viral hemorrhagic fevers (HF)		
Arenaviridae		
Lassa fever	Lassa virus (arenavirus)	Wild rodents
New World HF	Arenavirus	Rodents
Argentinean HF	Junin virus	
Bolivian HF	Machupo virus	
Brazilian HF	Sabia virus	
Venezuelan HF	Guanarito virus	
Bunyaviridae		
Crimean-Congo HF	Nairovirus	Cattle, rodents, sheep, goats, hares, birds
Hantaviral diseases		Rodents
Hantaviral pulmonary syndrome	Sin Nombre virus, Black Creek Canal virus	*Peromyscus* spp *Sigmodon hispidus*
Hemorrhagic fever with renal syndrome	Hantaan virus, Dobrava virus, Puumala virus, Seoul virus	*Apodemus, Clethrionomys, Rattus* spp
Rift Valley fever	Phlebovirus	Sheep, goats, cattle, camels

◄ **TABLE I.** (*continued*)

Known Distribution	Probable Means of Spread to Humans	Clinical Manifestations in Humans
VIRAL DISEASES (*continued*)		
North and South America	Contact exposure and insect bites, including mosquitos and biting flies (*Phlebotomus* spp)	Fever (± biphasic), myalgia, pharyngitis, cervical adenopathy, oral or rectal vesicles
Africa	Rodent excretions, secretions or tissues; person to person	Gradual onset of myalgia and fever; may develop severe swelling of head and neck; pleural/pericardial effusions; hemorrhagic syndrome less common
Americas	Rodent excretions, secretions, or tissues; person to person	Gradual onset of myalgia and fever; may develop petechial hemorrhage, bleeding, CNS symptoms
Africa, Middle East, central Asia, eastern Europe	Tick (*Hyalomma* and *Boophilus* spp) bites; occupational risk among animal workers	Fever, headache, pharyngitis, abdominal symptoms, petechial rash, hemorrhage; very severe in pregnant women
Worldwide	Aerosols from rodent excretions and secretions	
USA, may be more widespread throughout Americas		Fever, myalgia, respiratory failure, thrombocytopenia; mortality 40-50%
China, Siberia, Korea, Manchuria, Japan, Balkan countries, Europe		Abrupt onset of fever, back pain, petechiae, hemorrhage, renal failure with oliguria; mortality 5-15%
Africa; common to rare	Mosquitos (*Aedes* spp); contact on autopsy or handling fresh meat	May show biphasic illness, bradycardia, petechiae, hemorrhage

(*continued*)

TABLE I. Global Zoonoses* (continued) ▶

Disease	Causative Organism	Principal Animals Involved
	VIRAL DISEASES (*continued*)	
Filoviridae		
Ebola HF Marburg HF	Marburg and Ebola viruses	Primates suspected
Flaviviridae		
Kyasanur forest disease	Kyasanur forest virus	Rodents, monkeys
Omsk hemorrhagic fever	Omsk hemorrhagic fever virus	Rodents, muskrats
Yellow fever	Yellow fever virus	Monkeys, baboons
Wesselsbron fever	Wesselsbron virus (flavivirus)	Sheep
West Nile fever	West Nile virus (flavivirus)	Wild birds, horses, other mammals
Western equine encephalomyelitis	Western equine encephalomyelitis virus (alphavirus)	Wild birds, domestic fowl, horses, mules, donkeys, bats, reptiles, amphibians
Yabapox	Yabapox virus	African monkeys
	PRION DISEASES	
Variant Creutzfeldt-Jakob disease	Prion protein—likely from bovine spongiform encephalopathy	Cattle

◀ **TABLE I.** (continued)

Known Distribution	Probable Means of Spread to Humans	Clinical Manifestations in Humans
	VIRAL DISEASES (continued)	
Central and southern Africa	Contact with infected tissues	Abrupt onset of fever; joint and muscle pain, headache, gastro-enteritis with vomiting; maculo-papular rash with desquamation; hepatitis and widespread hemorrhages 3-4 days after onset; mortality 50-90% for Ebola, 20-30% for Marburg
India	Tick (*Haemaphysalis spinigera*) bites	Fever, rash, bradycardia; course may be biphasic with remission followed by menin-goencephalitis
Omsk, Siberia; rare	Tick (*Dermacentor* spp) bites; direct contact with *D marginatus*	Biphasic illness with encephali-tis occurring in second phase; sequelae, including deafness, relatively common
Tropical America, Africa	Mosquito (*Aedes aegypti* in urban cycles, *Haemagogus* spp in jungle cycles in South America, *Aedes* spp in jungle cycles in Africa) bites	Fever, myalgia, prostration, progressing to jaundice, brady-cardia; liver and renal failure in 20-50%; often fatal with hemor-rhagic manifestations
Southern Africa, south-east Asia	Mosquito (*Aedes, Manso-nia, Culex* spp) bites	Fever, myalgia, and hyperesthe-sia of skin ± maculopapular rash; self-limiting
Eastern and Western hemisphere; common	Mosquito (primarily *Culex* spp) bites; blood transfu-sion, tissue transplant rarely; may be milkborne	Fever, rash, worse in elderly; encephaliçtis may be accompa-nied by flaccid paresis and res-piratory failure
Western and Central USA, Canada, South America	Mosquito (*Culex tarsalis* in USA, other *Culex* and *Aedes* spp outside USA)	Febrile illness to encephalitis; worse in infants and children in whom neurologic sequelae are more likely
Africa; rare	Contact; aerosols	Indurated, painful skin lesion
	PRION DISEASES	
Primarily in England, sporadic cases in France, Ireland, Italy, Canada	Ingestion of beef	Rapidly fatal neurodegenera-tive disorder similar to sporadic Cruetzfeldt-Jakob disease

*Many proven zoonoses, including some relatively rare arthropodborne viral infections and helminth infections have been omitted, as well as those diseases caused by fish and reptile toxins.

■ ■ ■

REFERENCE GUIDES

TABLE 1. Rectal Temperatures[*]

Species	°F ± 1°	°C ± 0.5°
Cattle		
Beef cow	101	38.3
Dairy cow	101.5	38.6
Cat	101.5	38.6
Dog	102	38.9
Goat	102.3	39.1
Horse		
Mare	100	37.8
Stallion	99.7	37.6
Pig	102.5	39.2
Rabbit	103.1	39.5
Sheep	102.3	39.1

[*]Adapted from Andersson B.E. and Jónasson H., Temperature Regulation and Environmental Physiology, in *Dukes' Physiology of Domestic Animals*, 11th ed., Swenson M.J. and Reece W.O., Eds. Copyright©1993 by Cornell University.

TABLE 2. Heart Rates[*]

Species	bpm (range)
Cat	120-140
Chick	350-450
Chicken (adult)	250-300
Dairy cow	48-84
Dog	70-120
Elephant	25-40
Goat	70-80
Guinea Pig	200-300
Hamster	300-600
Horse	28-40
Mouse	450-750
Ox	36-60
Pig	70-120
Rabbit	180-350
Rat	250-400
Rhesus monkey	80-300
Sheep	70-80

[*]Adapted in part from Detweiler D.K., Regulation of the Heart, in *Dukes' Physiology of Domestic Animals*, 11th ed., Swenson M.J. and Reece W.O. Eds. Copyright©1993 by Cornell University.

TABLE 3. Resting Respiratory Rates*

Species	Breaths/min (range)
Cat	16-40
Dairy cow	26-50
Dog	18-34
Horse	10-14
Pig	32-58
Sheep	16-34

*Adapted from Reece W.O., Respiration in Mammals, in *Dukes' Physiology of Domestic Animals,* 11th ed., Swenson M.J. and Reece W.O. Eds. Copyright©1993 by Cornell University.

TABLE 4. Urine Volume and Specific Gravity*

Species	Volume (mL/kg body wt/day)	Specific Gravity (range)
Cat	10-20	1.020-1.040
Cow	17-45	1.030-1.045
Dog	20-100	1.016-1.060
Goat	10-40	1.015-1.045
Horse	3-18	1.025-1.060
Pig	5-30	1.010-1.050
Sheep	10-40	1.015-1.045

*Adapted from Reece W.O., Water Balance and Excretion, in *Dukes' Physiology of Domestic Animals,* 11th ed., Swenson M.J. and Reece W.O. Eds. Copyright©1993 by Cornell University.

TABLE 5. Temperature Equivalents and Conversions

Celsius (°C)	$°C = (°F - 32) \times 5/9$ $°F = (°C \times 9/5) + 32$	Fahrenheit (°F)
0	Freezing	32
36.0		96.8
36.5		97.7
37.0		98.6
37.5		99.5
38.0		100.4
38.5		101.3
39.0		102.2
39.5		103.1
40.0		104.0
40.5		104.9
41.0		105.8
41.5		106.7
42.0		107.6
100	Boiling	212

TABLE 6. Hematologic Reference Ranges[*] ▶

	Conventional (USA) Units	SI Units	Dog	Cat	Cow
PCV (hematocrit)	%	$\times 10^{-2}$ L/L	37-55 (25-34)[†]	30-45 (24-34)[†]	24-46
Hemoglobin (Hgb)	g/dL	$\times 10$ g/L	12-18	8-15	8-15
Red blood cells	$\times 10^6/\mu L$	$\times 10^{12}$ g/L	5.5-8.5	5-10	5-10
Reticulocytes	%	%	0-1.5	0-1	0
Mean corpuscular volume	fL	fL	60-77	39-55	40-60
Mean corpuscular Hgb	pg	pg	19.5-24.5	13-17	11-17
Mean corpuscular Hgb concentration	g/dL	$\times 10$ g/L	32-36	30-36	30-36
Platelets	$\times 10^5/\mu L$	$\times 10^{11}$/L	2-9	3-7	1-8
White blood cells	$\times 10^3/\mu L$	$\times 10^9$/L	6-17	5.5-19.5	4-12
Neutrophils (segmented)	% $\times 10^3/\mu L$	% $\times 10^9$/L	60-70 3-11.4	35-75 2.5-12.5	15-45 0.6-4
Neutrophils (band)	% $\times 10^3/\mu L$	% $\times 10^9$/L	0-3 0-0.3	0-3 0-0.3	0-2 0-0.12
Lymphocytes	% $\times 10^3/\mu L$	% $\times 10^9$/L	12-30 1-4.8	20-55 1.5-7	45-75 2.5-7.5
Monocytes	% $\times 10^3/\mu L$	% $\times 10^9$/L	3-10 0.15-1.35	1-4 0-0.85	2-7 0.025-0.85
Eosinophils	% $\times 10^3/\mu L$	% $\times 10^9$/L	2-10 0.1-0.75	2-12 0-0.75	2-20 0-2.4
Basophils	% $\times 10^3/\mu L$	% $\times 10^9$/L	rare	rare	0-2 0-0.2
Myeloid/erythroid ratio			0.75-2.4:1	0.6-3.9:1	0.3-1.8:1
Plasma proteins[#]	g/dL	$\times 10$ g/L	6-7.5	6-7.5	6-8
Plasma fibrinogen	g/dL	$\times 10$ g/L	0.15-0.3	0.15-0.3	0.1-0.6

[*]Adapted, with permission, in part from Duncan J.R. and Prasse K.W., *Veterinary Laboratory Medicine*, 2nd ed., Iowa State University Press, 1986.
[†]5- to 6-wk-old pups, kittens; 3- to 45-day-old pigs
[‡]Lower in foals and cold-blooded horses
[§]Heterophil
[#]Lower in young animals

◀ **TABLE 6.** *(continued)*

Horse	Pig	Sheep	Goat	Rabbit	Llama	Vietnamese Potbellied Pig	Ostrich
32-48‡	36-43 (26-35)†	27-45	22-38	33-50	29-39	37-51	32
10-18	9-13	9-15	8-12	10-17	13-18	11-15	12
6-12	5-7	9-15	8-18	5-8	11-18	6-8	1.7
0	0-12	0	0				
34-58	52-62	28-40	16-25	58-67	21-28	47-68	174
13-19	17-24	8-12	5.2-8	17-24	43-47	14-22	61
31-37	29-34	31-34	30-36	29-37		28-33	33
1-6	2-5	2.5-7.5	3-6	2.5-6.5			
6-12	11-22	4-12	4-13	5-12.5	7.5-21.5	19-38	5.5
30-75	20-70	10-50	30-48	20-75	60-74	18-63	63§
3-6	2-15	0.7-6.0	1.2-7.2	1-9.4	4.6-16	3.3-24	3.4
0-1	0-4	0	rare		0-1	0-1	
0-0.1	0-0.8				0-0.35	0-0.4	
25-60	35-75	40-75	50-70	30-85	13-35	24-70	34
1.5-5	3.8-16.5	2-9	2-9	1.6-10.6	1-7.5	4.5-27	188
1-8	0-10	0-6	0-4	1-4	1-4	3-13	2.8
0-0.6	0-1	0-0.75	0-0.55	0.05-0.5	0.05-0.8	0.6-5.0	0.15
1-10	0-15	0-10	1-8	1-4	0-15	1-12	0.3
0-0.8	0-1.5	0-1	0.05-0.65	0.05-0.5	0-3.3	0.2-4.6	0.02
0-3	0-3	0-3	0-1	1-7	0-2	0	0.2
0-0.3	0-0.5	0-0.3	0-0.12	0.05-0.9	0-0.4	0-0.4	
0.9-3.8:1	1.2-2.2:1	0.8-1.7:1	0.7-1.0:1				
6-8.5	6-8	6-7.5	6-7.5	5.4-8.3		5.4-8.5	
0.1-0.4	0.2-0.4	0.1-0.5	0.1-0.4	0.2-0.4	0.1-0.4	0.1-0.4	

TABLE 7. Serum Biochemical Reference Ranges[*]

In Conventional (USA) Units	Units	Dog	Cat	Cow	Horse
ALT	u/L	8.2-57	8.3-53	6.9-35	2.7-21
Amylase	u/L	270-1,462	371-1,193	41-98	47-188
Alk phos[†]	u/L	10.6-101	12-65	18-153	70-227
AST	u/L	8.9-49	9.2-40	45-110	116-287
Creatine kinase	u/L	14-120	17-150	14-107	34-166
GGT[†]	u/L	1.0-9.7	1.8-12	4.9-26	2.7-22
LDH[†]	u/L	24-219	35-225	309-938	102-341
SDH[†]	u/L	3.1-7.6	2.4-6.1	6.1-18	1.2-8.5
Bicarbonate	mEq/L	18-25	16-22	21-29	22-29
Bilirubin	mg/dL	0.1-0.6	0.1-0.5	0.0-0.8	0.3-3.0
Calcium	mg/dL	8.7-11.8	7.9-10.9	8.4-11.0	10.4-13.4
Chloride	mEq/L	102-117	108-130	96-109	97-110
Cholesterol	mg/dL	116-254	71-161	62-193	71-142
Creatinine	mg/dL	0.5-1.6	0.5-1.9	0.6-1.8	0.9-2.0
Glucose	mg/dL	62-108	61-124	42-75	62-114
Magnesium	mg/dL	1.7-2.7	1.9-2.8	1.7-3.0	1.8-2.7
Phosphorus	mg/dL	2.9-6.2	4.0-7.3	4.3-7.8	2.3-5.4
Potassium	mEq/L	3.8-5.6	3.8-5.3	4.0-5.8	2.8-4.7
Protein	g/dL	5.5-7.5	5.7-8.0	6.2-8.2	5.7-7.9
Albumin	g/dL	2.6-4.0	2.4-3.8	2.8-3.9	2.5-3.8
Globulin	g/dL	2.1-3.7	2.4-4.7	2.9-4.9	2.4-4.6
Sodium	mEq/L	140-154	146-159	135-148	133-147
Urea nitrogen	mg/dL	8.8-26	15-31	7.8-25	10.4-25
In SI Units					
Bicarbonate	mmol/L	18-25	16-22	21-29	22-29
Bilirubin	μmol/L	0.9-10.6	1.2-7.9	0.7-14	5.4-51
Calcium	mmol/L	2.2-3.0	2.0-2.7	2.1-2.8	2.6-3.3
Chloride	mmol/L	102-117	108-130	96-109	97-110
Cholesterol	mmol/L	3.0-6.6	1.8-4.2	1.6-5.0	1.8-3.7
Creatinine	μmol/L	44-138	49-165	56-162	77-175
Glucose	mmol/L	3.4-6.0	3.4-6.9	2.3-4.1	3.5-6.3
Magnesium	mmol/L	0.7-1.1	0.8-1.2	0.7-1.2	0.7-1.1
Phosphorus	mmol/L	1.0-2.0	1.3-2.4	1.4-2.5	0.7-1.7
Potassium	mmol/L	3.8-5.6	3.8-5.3	4.0-5.8	2.8-4.7
Protein	g/L	55-75	57-80	62-82	57-79
Albumin	g/L	26-40	24-38	28-39	25-38
Globulin	g/L	21-37	24-47	29-49	24-46
Sodium	mmol/L	140-154	146-159	135-148	133-147
Urea nitrogen	mmol/L	3.1-9.2	5.5-11.1	2.8-8.8	3.7-8.8

[*]Adapted, with permission, primarily from Boyd J.W., The interpretation of serum biochemistry test results in domestic animals, in *Veterinary Clinical Pathology*, Veterinary Practice Publishing Co., 13(2), 1984.

[†]Alk phos = alkaline phosphatase; GGT = gamma glutamyltransferase; LDH = lactate dehydrogenase; SDH = sorbitol dehydrogenase

◀ **TABLE 7.** *(continued)*

Pig	Sheep	Goat	Rabbit	Llama	Vietnamese Potbellied Pig	Ostrich
22-47	15-44	15-52	48-80		23-83	20
44-88	140-270		167-315			
41-176	27-156	61-283	4-16	30-780	35-563	32-98
15-55	49-123	66-230	14-113	110-250	<109	131-486
66-489	7.7-101	16-48	218-2,705	30-400		294
31-52	20-44	20-50	0-14	5-29	21-57	2.1
160-425	83-476	79-265	34-129			
0.5-4.9	3.5-21	9.3-21		85-740		
18-27	20-27		16-38			
0.0-0.5	0.0-0.5	0.1-0.2	0-0.7	0-0.1	<0.3	
9.3-11.5	9.3-11.7	9.0-11.6	5.6-12.5	7.7-9.4	10.2-12.2	10.7-14
97-106	101-113	100-112	92-112	106-118	91-103	100
81-134	44-90	65-136	10-80			
0.8-2.3	0.9-2.0	0.7-1.5	0.5-2.5	1.5-2.9	0.4-1.1	0.1-0.4
66-116	44-81	48-76	75-155	90-140	68-155	245
2.3-3.5	2.0-2.7	2.1-2.9			1.5-3.8	
5.5-9.3	4.0-7.3	3.7-9.7	4.0-6.9	4.6-9.8	5.0-10.7	4.0-9.9
4.4-6.5	4.3-6.3	3.8-5.7	3.6-6.9	4.3-5.6	3.9-5.9	3.0
5.8-8.3	5.9-7.8	6.1-7.5	5.4-8.3	5.5-7.0	4.6-7.8	3.8
2.3-4.0	2.7-3.7	2.3-3.6	2.4-4.6	3.5-4.4	3.1-4.3	1.8
3.9-6.0	3.2-5.0	2.7-4.4	1.5-2.8	1.7-3.5	1.5-3.5	2.0
139-153	142-160	137-152	131-155	147-158	134-150	147
8.2-25	10-26	13-26	13-29	13-32	10.8-47	1.1
In SI Units						
18-27	20-27		16-38			
0.3-8.2	0.7-8.6	1.7-4.3	0-12	1.7	5.0	
2.3-2.9	2.3-2.9	2.3-2.9	1.4-3.1	2-2.4	2.5-3.1	2.7-3.5
97-106	101-113	100-112	92-112	106-118	91-103	100
2.1-3.5	1.1-2.3	1.7-3.5	0.3-2.1			
70-208	76-174	60-135	44-221	133-256	35-97	8.8-35
3.7-6.4	2.4-4.5	2.7-4.2	4.1-8.5	5.0-7.7	3.8-8.5	14
0.9-1.4	0.8-1.1	0.9-1.2			0.7-1.9	
1.8-3.0	1.3-2.4	1.2-3.1	1.3-2.2	1.5-3.2	1.6-3.4	1.3-3.2
4.4-6.5	4.3-6.3	3.8-5.7	3.6-6.9	4.3-5.6	3.9-5.9	3.0
58-83	59-78	61-75	54-83	55-70	46-78	38
23-40	27-37	23-36	24-46	35-44	31-43	18
39-60	32-50	27-44	15-28	17-35	15-35	20
139-153	142-160	137-152	131-155	147-158	134-150	147
2.9-8.8	3.7-9.3	4.5-9.2	4.6-10.4	4.6-11.4	3.9-17	0.4

TABLE 8. Clinical Chemistry SI Conversion Factors*

	Conventional (USA) Units	Conversion Factor (×)	SI Units
Alkaline phosphatase	IU/L	1.0	U/L
ALT	U/L	1.0	U/L
Albumin	g/dL	10.0	g/L
Ammonia (NH_4)	µg/dL	0.5872	µmol/L
Amylase	Somogyi units	1.85	U/L
AST	U/L	1.0	U/L
Bilirubin	mg/dL	17.10	µmol/L
Calcium	mg/dL	0.25	mmol/L
Carbon dioxide	mEq/L	1.0	mmol/L
Chloride	mEq/L	1.0	mmol/L
Cholesterol	mg/dL	0.026	mmol/L
Copper	µg/dL	0.16	µmol/L
Cortisol	µg/dL	0.0276	µmol/L
Creatine kinase	IU/L	1.0	U/L
Creatinine	mg/dL	88.40	µmol/L
Fibrinogen	mg/dL	0.01	g/L
Glucose	mg/dL	0.055	mmol/L
Iron, binding	µg/dL	0.179	µmol/L
Iron, total	µg/dL	0.179	µmol/L
Lipase	IU/L	1	U/L
	Cherry-Crandall U	278	U/L
Magnesium	mEq/L	0.5	mmol/L
Osmolality	Osm/kg	1.0	mmol/L
Phosphorus	mg/dL	0.323	mmol/L
Potassium	mEq/L	1.0	mmol/L
Protein, total	g/dL	10.0	g/L
Sodium	mEq/L	1.0	mmol/L
Triglycerides	mg/dL	0.011	mmol/L
Tri-iodothyronine (T_3)	µg/dL	15.6	nmol/L
Thyroxine (T_4)	µg/dL	12.87	nmol/L
Urea nitrogen	mg/dL	0.357	mmol/L
Uric acid	mg/dL	0.059	mmol/L
Urine protein/creatinine ratio	g/g	0.113	g/mmol
Xylose absorption	mg/dL	0.067	mmol/L

*Adapted from *Veterinary Laboratory Medicine: Interpretation and Diagnosis*, Meyer D.H., Coles E.H., Rich L.J., 2nd ed., Copyright, 1998, with permission from Elsevier.

TABLE 9. Weight to Body Surface Area Conversion[*]

Body surface area (BSA) in square meters = $K \times$ (body wt in grams$^{2/3}$) $\times 10^{-4}$
K = constant (10.1 for dogs and 10.0 for cats)

Dogs				Cats	
Body wt (kg)	BSA (m^2)	Body wt (kg)	BSA (m^2)	Body wt (kg)	BSA (m^2)
0.5	0.06	26	0.88	0.5	0.06
1	0.10	27	0.90	1	0.10
2	0.15	28	0.92	1.5	0.12
3	0.20	29	0.94	2	0.15
4	0.25	30	0.96	2.5	0.17
5	0.29	31	0.99	3	0.20
6	0.33	32	1.01	3.5	0.22
7	0.36	33	1.03	4	0.24
8	0.40	34	1.05	4.5	0.26
9	0.43	35	1.07	5	0.28
10	0.46	36	1.09	5.5	0.29
11	0.49	37	1.11	6	0.31
12	0.52	38	1.13	6.5	0.33
13	0.55	39	1.15	7	0.34
14	0.58	40	1.17	7.5	0.36
15	0.60	41	1.19	8	0.38
16	0.63	42	1.21	8.5	0.39
17	0.66	43	1.23	9	0.41
18	0.69	44	1.25	9.5	0.42
19	0.71	45	1.26	10	0.44
20	0.74	46	1.28		
21	0.76	47	1.30		
22	0.78	48	1.32		
23	0.81	49	1.34		
24	0.83	50	1.36		
25	0.85				

[*]Adapted from Rosenthal R.C., Chemotherapy, in *Textbook of Veterinary Internal Medicine: Diseases of the Dog and Cat*, 4th ed., Ettinger S.J. and Feldman E.C., Eds. Copyright, 1995, with permission from Elsevier.

TABLE 10.   Metric System Prefixes and Symbols

Factor	Prefix	Symbol	Factor	Prefix	Symbol
10^{18}	exa	E	10^{-1}	deci	d
10^{15}	peta	P	10^{-2}	centi	c
10^{12}	tera	T	10^{-3}	milli	m
10^{9}	giga	G	10^{-6}	micro	μ
10^{6}	mega	M	10^{-9}	nano	n
10^{3}	kilo	k	10^{-12}	pico	p
10^{2}	hecto	h	10^{-15}	femto	f
10	deka	da	10^{-18}	atto	a

TABLE 11.   Weights and Measures Equivalents and Conversions

Length	1 m = 39.37 in.	
	1 yd = 91.44 cm	
	1 ft = 30.48 cm	
	1 in. = 2.54 cm	
Weight*	1 kg = 2.205 lb	1 lb = 0.454 kg
	1 g = 0.035 oz	1 oz = 28.35 g
	1 mg = 0.015 grain	1 grain = 64.8 mg
	1 ton = 2,000 lb	
	1 metric ton = 1,000 kg = 2,205 lb	
Capacity		*Imperial system:*
	1 gal. = 3.785 L	1 gal. = 4.55 L
	1 quart = 0.946 L	1 quart = 1.136 L
	1 pint = 473.2 mL	1 pint = 568.26 mL
	1 oz = 29.57 mL	
	1 tablespoon = 15 mL	
	1 teaspoon = 5 mL	

*Avoirdupois (used in the USA as the common system of measuring weight) unless otherwise specified

TABLE 12. Percentage, ppm, and ppb Conversions

ppm	ppb	Percentage
0.001	1	0.0000001
0.01	10	0.000001
0.1	100	0.00001
1	1,000	0.0001
10		0.001
100		0.01
1,000		0.1
10,000		1

Other useful conversions: 1 mg/kg = 1 ppm
1 g/ton = 1.1 ppm
100 g/ton = 110 ppm

TABLE 13. Milligram-milliequivalent Conversions and Atomic Weights

The milliequivalent (mEq) is the unit of measure often used for electrolytes. It indicates the chemical activity, or combining power, of an element relative to the activity of 1 mg of hydrogen. Thus, 1 mEq is represented by 1 mg of hydrogen (1 mole) or 23 mg of Na^+, 39 mg of K^+, etc.

$$mEq/L = \frac{(mg/L) \times valence}{molecular\ weight}$$

$$mg/L = \frac{(mEq/L) \times molecular\ weight}{valence}$$

Ion	Atomic Weight	Valence
Hydrogen (H)	1	1
Carbon (C)	12	4
Nitrogen (N)	14	3
Oxygen (O)	16	2
Sodium (Na)	23	1
Magnesium (Mg)	24	2
Phosphate (P)*	31	3, 5
Chlorine (Cl)	35.5	1
Potassium (K)	39	1
Calcium (Ca)	40	2

*As phorphorus, inorganic

TABLE 16. Percentage, ppm, and ppb Conversions

Percentage	ppb	ppm
0.0000001	1	0.001
0.000001	10	0.01
0.00001	100	0.1
0.0001	1,000	1
0.001		10
0.01		100
0.1		1,000
1		10,000

Other useful conversions: 1 mg/L = 1 ppm.
1 atm = 1.1 ppm
110 g/m = 110 ppm

TABLE 17. Milligram Equivalent Conversions and Atomic Weights

The milliequivalent (meq/L) is the unit of measure often used for electrolytes. It indicates the chemical activity of combining power of an element relative to the activity of 1 meq of hydrogen. Thus, 1 meq is represented by 1 mg of hydrogen, 1 mg/L or 23 mg of Na^+, 39 mg of K^+, etc.

$$meq/L = \frac{(mg/L) \times valence}{molecular\ weight}$$

$$mg/L = \frac{(meq/L) \times molecular\ weight}{valence}$$

Ion	Atomic Weight	Valence
Hydrogen (H)	1	1
Carbon (C)	12	4
Nitrogen (N)	14	3,5
Oxygen (O)	16	2
Sodium (Na)	23	1
Magnesium (Mg)	24	2
Phosphate (P)	31	3,5
Chlorine (Cl)	35.5	1
Potassium (K)	39	1
Calcium (Ca)	40	2

As phosphate, inorganic

INDEX

Page numbers in **bold type** indicate principal references.

1080 poisoning 2511
1081 poisoning 2512

A

Aardvarks, nutrition 1855
Abamectin 2113, 2121
Abattoir sanitation 1385
Abdominal
  counterpressure 1402
  distention 125
    large animals 201
  fat necrosis **306**
  pain 126
  ping 125
  trauma 1400
Abdominocentesis 89
  horses 1427
Abducent nerve 985
Aberrant
  leucocytozoonosis, birds 2193
  parasites 1035
Abnormal
  beak growth, turtles and tortoises 1614
  behavior 1292
    ingestive, dogs and cats 1320
  fetal development, calves 1752
  teeth
    eruption, large animals 141
    number 132
    position and direction 133
Abomasum
  diseases 177
  disorders **193**
  displaced, 193, 1842
  impaction, dietary 198
  right torsion of 193
  ulcers 196
  volvulus 193
Abortion
  cattle 1098, 1752
    contagious 1110
    mycotic 1100
  chinchillas 1622
  enzootic
    ewes 1102
    goats 1103
  epizootic bovine 1101
  foothill 1101

goats 1103
  chlamydophilial 1103
  horses 1106, 1766
    bacterial 1108
  large animals **1097**
  pigs 1104
  sheep 1101
  small animals 1793
  virus, equine 1203
Abscesses
  chinchillas 1620
  foot, sheep 943
  hamsters 1637
  liver 287, 288
    cattle 299
  rabbits 1577
  reptiles 1605
  spinal, pigs 940
  subsolar, horses 910
  toe
    cattle 879
    sheep 947
  udder 1147
Absidia sp 1100
Absolute polycythemia 57
Absorption of drugs 1941
Abuse, animal 1330
Acacia berlandieri 2458
Acanthamoeba castellani 1045
Acanthocephala
  fish 1504
  marine mammals 1538
  small animals 359
Acanthocephaliasis 2568, 2569
Acantholysis 653
  familial 683
Acanthoma
  infundibular keratinizing
    767
  papillary 418
Acanthomatous epulis 313
Acanthosis nigricans **789**
Acariasis 2568
  cutaneous 742
  gerbils 1627
  hamsters 1638
  marine mammals 1538
  mice and rats 1650
  pulmonary, primates 1552

W